Williams
GYNECOLOGY

NOTICE

Medicine is an ever-changing science. As new research and clinical experience broaden our knowledge, changes in treatment and drug therapy are required. The authors and the publisher of this work have checked with sources believed to be reliable in their efforts to provide information that is complete and generally in accord with the standards accepted at the time of publication. However, in view of the possibility of human error or changes in medical sciences, neither the authors nor the publisher nor any other party who has been involved in the preparation or publication of this work warrants that the information contained herein is in every respect accurate or complete, and they disclaim all responsibility for any errors or omissions or for the results obtained from use of the information contained in this work. Readers are encouraged to confirm the information contained herein with other sources. For example and in particular, readers are advised to check the product information sheet included in the package of each drug they plan to administer to be certain that the information contained in this work is accurate and that changes have not been made in the recommended dose or in the contraindications for administration. This recommendation is of particular importance in connection with new or infrequently used drugs.

Williams GYNECOLOGY

FOURTH EDITION

Barbara L. Hoffman, MD
John O. Schorge, MD
Lisa M. Halvorson, MD
Cherine A. Hamid, MD
Marlene M. Corton, MD
Joseph I. Schaffer, MD

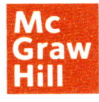

New York   Chicago   San Francisco   Lisbon   London   Madrid   Mexico City
Milan   New Delhi   San Juan   Seoul   Singapore   Sydney   Toronto

Williams Gynecology, Fourth Edition

3 4 5 6 7 8 9 LWI 25 24 23

ISBN 978-1-260-45686-8
MHID 1-260-45686-2

This book was set in Adobe Garamond by Aptara, Inc.
The editors were Jason Malley and Christie Naglieri.
The production supervisor was Richard Ruzycka.
Project management was provided by Indu Jawwad, Aptara, Inc.
The designer was Alan Barnett.
The cover designer was W2 Design.

Library of Congress Cataloging-in-Publication Data

Library of Congress Control Number: 2019949852
Cataloging in Publication data available on request from publisher.

IN MEMORIAM
Kristin Paulson Landon

Early in production of this edition, our *Williams* family lost a dedicated member of the team in Ms. Kristin Landon. We knew her as our valued copyeditor for many editions of both *William Obstetrics* and *Williams Gynecology*. However, Kristin's life was multifaceted, with talents that included analytic chemist, musician, cooking enthusiast, and writer. Indeed, her published science fiction novels include the *Hidden Worlds* trilogy and *Windhome*. We knew Kristin as an integral member of our textbook team. Her precision added clarity to our efforts and made our textbooks better.

DEDICATION

This edition of Williams Gynecology is dedicated to Dr. Karen Bradshaw, who has served as an Editor of Williams Gynecology since its inaugural edition. We are especially grateful for her tenacity during the formative years of our project and her academic support to bring our first edition to print. Our text's content has benefited greatly from her clinical acumen coupled with a mastery of the evidence-based literature. Her clear, concise chapters distilled challenging reproductive endocrinology tenets into easily understood concepts that translate to the bedside. Indeed, her many teaching awards throughout her career attest to this gift.

Dr. Bradshaw's roots at the University of Texas Southwestern run deep and include her medical school years, residency training, and fellowship study in Reproductive Endocrinology and Infertility. Early in her career as a faculty member at UTSW, she became Director of the Assisted Reproductive Technologies Program. Subsequently, she helped develop the Pediatric Gynecology Service at Children's Hospital, which was a first for Dallas and continues to this day. This was the first of many collaborative and multidisciplinary projects that typify her career. As another example, she was instrumental in expanding the field of minimally invasive surgery (MIS) at our institution and initiated the Laparoscopy Teaching Service. She partnered with the Department of Surgery and was provided a joint appointment to foster MIS development. She served on the Southwestern Minimally Invasive Surgery Executive Committee from its inception in 1997 until her retirement in 2019.

In addition to academics, Dr. Bradshaw was clinically and administratively active in our expanding private practice on campus. As an advocate of health for women as they entered and advanced through menopause, she was the first holder of the Helen J. and Robert S. Strauss and Diana L. and Richard C. Strauss Distinguished Professorship in Women's Health. Her vision led to development of a single, multidisciplinary site to care for the various health aspects of mature women. This was subsequently endowed and became the Lowe Foundation Center for Women's Preventative Health Care.

During her academic career, Dr. Bradshaw promoted academic excellence at UTSW. She served administratively on numerous academic committees involved with medical school, residency, and specialty training. Moreover, Karen was a passionate advocate for the advancement of women in academia at our institution. She was also a voice on the national academic stage. Karen served on the Board of the American Society of Reproductive Endocrinology and Infertility and extensively participated in their postgraduate training efforts. She filled prominent leadership roles in the Society for Reproductive Endocrinology and Infertility, including president. In both organizations, she actively advanced both residency and fellowship training in the specialty.

For us in the Department of Obstetrics and Gynecology, Dr. Bradshaw has played an important role as mentor and colleague. Her experience and clinical expertise have been invaluable, and she has provided guidance for challenging gynecology cases. On so many levels, we have benefitted greatly from her academic and clinical contributions.

CONTENTS

SECTION 1

GENERAL GYNECOLOGY

SECTION 2

REPRODUCTIVE ENDOCRINOLOGY, INFERTILITY, AND THE MENOPAUSE

SECTION 3

FEMALE PELVIC MEDICINE AND RECONSTRUCTIVE SURGERY

SECTION 4

GYNECOLOGIC ONCOLOGY

SECTION 5

ASPECTS OF GYNECOLOGIC SURGERY

SECTION 6

ATLAS OF GYNECOLOGIC SURGERY

EDITORS

Barbara L. Hoffman, MD
Distinguished Professor in Obstetrics and Gynecology,
    in Honor of F. Gary Cunningham, M.D.
Professor, Department of Obstetrics and Gynecology
University of Texas Southwestern Medical Center

John O. Schorge, MD, FACOG, FACS
Chief, Division of Gynecologic Oncology
Professor, Department of Obstetrics and Gynecology
Tufts University School of Medicine

Lisa M. Halvorson, MD
Rockville, Maryland

Cherine A. Hamid, MD
Associate Professor, Department of Obstetrics and Gynecology
University of Texas Southwestern Medical Center
Medical Director–Gynecology Clinics
Parkland Health and Hospital Systems, Dallas, Texas

Marlene M. Corton, MD, MSCS
Director, Anatomical Education and Research
Professor, Department of Obstetrics and Gynecology
University of Texas Southwestern Medical Center

Joseph I. Schaffer, MD, MBA
Holder, Frank C. Erwin, Jr. Professorship in Obstetrics and Gynecology
Director, Division of Gynecology
Director, Division of Female Pelvic Medicine and Reconstructive
    Surgery
Professor, Department of Obstetrics and Gynecology
University of Texas Southwestern Medical Center
Chief of Gynecology
Parkland Health and Hospital Systems, Dallas, Texas

Atlas Art Director

Lewis E. Calver, MS, CMI, FAMI

CONTRIBUTORS

Emily H. Adhikari, MD
Assistant Professor, Division of Maternal–Fetal Medicine
Department of Obstetrics and Gynecology
University of Texas Southwestern Medical Center
Medical Director of Perinatal Infectious Disease
Parkland Health and Hospital Systems, Dallas, Texas
Chapter 3: Gynecologic Infection

Sunil Balgobin, MD
Assistant Professor, Department of Obstetrics and Gynecology
University of Texas Southwestern Medical Center
Chapter 12: Pelvic Pain
Chapter 40: Intraoperative Considerations

Rachel A. Bonnema, MD, MS, FACP
Associate Chief, Division of General Internal Medicine
Associate Professor, Department of Internal Medicine
University of Texas Southwestern Medical Center
Chapter 1: Well Woman Care

Anna R. Brandon, PhD, MCS, ABPP
Department of Psychiatry, Division of Clinical Psychology
University of Texas Southwestern Medical Center
Chapter 14: Psychosocial Issues and Female Sexuality

Alison Brooks Heinzman, MD, FACOG
Director, Medical Student Clerkship
Assistant Professor, Department of Women's Health
The University of Texas at Austin Dell Medical School
Chapter 39: Preoperative Considerations

Matthew J. Carlson, MD
Associate Director, Residency Obstetrics and Gynecology
Assistant Professor, Department of Obstetrics and Gynecology
University of Texas Southwestern Medical Center
Chapter 34: Uterine Sarcoma

Kelley S. Carrick, MD
Professor, Department of Pathology
University of Texas Southwestern Medical Center
Director of Surgical Pathology Images for Williams Gynecology

Stephanie Y. Chang, MD
Associate Director, Residency Obstetrics and Gynecology
Associate Director, Fellowship Minimally Invasive Gynecologic Surgery
Assistant Professor, Department of Obstetrics and Gynecology
University of Texas Southwestern Medical Center
Chapter 8: Abnormal Uterine Bleeding

Marlene M. Corton, MD, MSCS
Director, Anatomical Education and Research
Professor, Department of Obstetrics and Gynecology
University of Texas Southwestern Medical Center
*Chapter 25: Anal Incontinence, Anorectal Disorders,
   and Rectovaginal Fistula*
Chapter 38: Anatomy
Chapter 43: Surgeries for Benign Gynecologic Disorders
Chapter 45: Surgeries for Pelvic Floor Disorders

F. Gary Cunningham, MD
Beatrice & Miguel Elias Distinguished Chair in
   Obstetrics and Gynecology
Professor, Department of Obstetrics and Gynecology
University of Texas Southwestern Medical Center
Chapter 6: First-Trimester Abortion

Kevin J. Doody, MD
Director, Center for Assisted Reproduction, Bedford, TX
Clinical Professor, Department of Obstetrics and Gynecology
University of Texas Southwestern Medical Center
Chapter 21: Treatment of the Infertile Couple

David M. Euhus, MD
Professor, Department of Surgery
Johns Hopkins Hospital/University
Chapter 13: Breast Disease

Veronica Gomez-Lobo, MD
Director of Pediatric and Adolescent Gynecology
Eunice Kennedy Shriver National Institute of Child Health
   and Human Development
Professor of Obstetrics and Gynecology
Georgetown University
Chapter 19: Anatomic Disorders

William F. Griffith, MD
Professor, Department of Obstetrics and Gynecology
University of Texas Southwestern Medical Center
Medical Director, OB/GYN Emergency Services
Director, Vulvology Clinic
Co-Director, Dysplasia Services
Parkland Health and Hospital System, Dallas, Texas
Chapter 4: Benign Disorders of the Lower Reproductive Tract
Chapter 29: Preinvasive Lesions of the Lower Anogenital Tract

Lisa M. Halvorson, MD
Rockville, Maryland
Chapter 6: First-Trimester Abortion
Chapter 16: Reproductive Endocrinology
Chapter 17: Amenorrhea
Chapter 20: Evaluation of the Infertile Couple

Cherine A. Hamid, MD
Associate Professor, Department of Obstetrics and Gynecology
University of Texas Southwestern Medical Center
Medical Director–Gynecology Clinics
Parkland Health and Hospital Systems, Dallas, Texas
Chapter 10: Benign Adnexal Mass
Chapter 39: Preoperative Considerations
Chapter 40: Intraoperative Considerations
Chapter 42: Postoperative Considerations
Chapter 43: Surgeries for Benign Gynecologic Disorders

Barbara L. Hoffman, MD
Distinguished Professor in Obstetrics and Gynecology,
    in Honor of F. Gary Cunningham, M.D.
Professor, Department of Obstetrics and Gynecology
University of Texas Southwestern Medical Center
Chapter 1: Well Woman Care
Chapter 3: Gynecologic Infection
Chapter 5: Contraception and Sterilization
Chapter 7: Ectopic Pregnancy
Chapter 8: Abnormal Uterine Bleeding
Chapter 9: Benign Uterine Pathology
Chapter 10: Benign Adnexal Mass
Chapter 11: Pelvic Pain
Chapter 40: Intraoperative Considerations
Chapter 43: Surgeries for Benign Gynecologic Disorders

Jason Jarin, MD
Assistant Professor, Department of Obstetrics and Gynecology
Division of Pediatric and Adolescent Gynecology
University of Texas Southwestern Medical Center
Children's Health
Chapter 1: Well Woman Care

Andrew M. Kaunitz, MD, FACOG, NCMP
University of Florida Term Professor and Associate Chairman
Department of Obstetrics and Gynecology
University of Florida College of Medicine–*Jacksonville*
Medical Director and Director of Menopause and Gynecologic
    Ultrasound Services
UF Women's Health Specialists–Emerson
Chapter 22: Menopause

Erika L. Kelley, PhD
Assistant Professor, Department of Reproductive Biology
Case Western Reserve University School of Medicine
Clinical Psychologist, Division of Behavioral Medicine, Department
    of Obstetrics & Gynecology
MacDonald Women's Hospital, University Hospitals Cleveland
    Medical Center
Chapter 14: Psychosocial Issues and Female Sexuality

Kimberly A. Kho, MD, MPH, MSCS, FACOG
Helen J. and Robert S. Strauss and Diana K. and Richard C. Strauss
    Chair in Women's Health
Associate Professor, Department of Obstetrics and Gynecology
Director, Fellowship in Minimally Invasive Gynecologic Surgery
University of Texas Southwestern Medical Center
Chapter 41: Minimally Invasive Surgery Fundamentals
Chapter 44: Minimally Invasive Surgery

Young B. Kim, MD
Associate Professor, Department of Obstetrics and Gynecology
Tufts University School of Medicine
Chapter 33: Endometrial Cancer

Sheryl A. Kingsberg, PhD
Professor, Departments of Reproductive Biology and Psychiatry
Case Western Reserve University School of Medicine
Chief, Division of Behavioral Medicine, Department of Obstetrics &
    Gynecology
MacDonald Women's Hospital, University Hospitals Cleveland
    Medical Center
Chapter 14: Psychosocial Issues and Female Sexuality

Alexander Kotlyar, MD
Instructor, Department of Obstetrics, Gynecology, and Reproductive
    Sciences
Yale School of Medicine, Yale University

Jayanthi S. Lea, MD
Patricia Duniven Fletcher Distinguished Professor in Gynecologic
    Oncology
Director, Gynecologic Oncology Fellowship Program
Associate Professor, Department of Obstetrics and Gynecology
University of Texas Southwestern Medical Center
Chapter 31: Vulvar Cancer
Chapter 46: Surgeries for Gynecologic Malignancies

Melissa M. Mauskar, MD
Assistant Professor, Departments of Dermatology and Obstetrics and
    Gynecology
University of Texas Southwestern Medical Center
Chapter 4: Benign Disorders of the Lower Reproductive Tract

John E. Mignano, MD, PhD
Associate Professor, Department of Radiation Oncology
Tufts University School of Medicine
Chapter 28: Principles of Radiation Therapy

David Scott Miller, MD, FACOG, FACS
Dallas Foundation Chair in Gynecologic Oncology
Director, Gynecologic Oncology Fellowship Program
Director of Gynecologic Oncology
Professor, Department of Obstetrics and Gynecology
University of Texas Southwestern Medical Center
Medical Director of Gynecology Oncology
Parkland Health and Hospital System, Dallas, Texas
Chapter 34: Uterine Sarcoma

Wilmer Moreno, MD
Assistant Professor, Department of Obstetrics and Gynecology
University of Texas Southwestern Medical Center
Chapter 7: Ectopic Pregnancy

Elysia Moschos, MD
Professor, Department of Obstetrics and Gynecology
University of Texas Southwestern Medical Center
Administrative Director of Gynecologic Ultrasound
Parkland Health and Hospital System
Chapter 2: Techniques Used for Imaging in Gynecology

David M. Owens, MD
Assistant Professor, Department of Obstetrics and Gynecology
University of Texas Southwestern Medical Center
Chapter 12: Pelvic Pain

JoAnn V. Pinkerton, MD, FACOG, NCMP
Professor of Obstetrics and Gynecology
Division Director of Midlife Health
The University of Virginia Health System
Charlottesville, Virginia
Emeritus Executive Director, The North American Menopause Society
Chapter 22: Menopause

David D. Rahn, MD
Associate Professor, Department of Obstetrics and Gynecology
University of Texas Southwestern Medical Center
Chapter 23: Urinary Incontinence

Debra L. Richardson, MD, FACOG, FACS

Associate Professor, Department of Obstetrics and Gynecology

Stephenson Cancer Center, University of Oklahoma Health Sciences Center

Chapter 30: Cervical Cancer
Chapter 32: Vaginal Cancer

David E. Rogers, MD, MBA

Associate Professor, Department of Obstetrics and Gynecology

University of Texas Southwestern Medical Center

Chapter 41: Minimally Invasive Surgery Fundamentals
Chapter 44: Minimally Invasive Surgery

John O. Schorge, MD, FACOG, FACS

Chief, Division of Gynecologic Oncology

Professor, Department of Obstetrics and Gynecology

Tufts University School of Medicine

Chapter 27: Principles of Chemotherapy
Chapter 34: Uterine Sarcoma
Chapter 35: Epithelial Ovarian Cancer
Chapter 36: Ovarian Germ Cell and Sex Cord–Stromal Tumors
Chapter 37: Gestational Trophoblastic Disease
Chapter 46: Surgeries for Gynecologic Malignancies

Joseph I. Schaffer, MD, MBA

Holder, Frank C. Erwin, Jr. Professorship in Obstetrics and Gynecology

Director, Division of Gynecology

Director, Division of Female Pelvic Medicine and Reconstructive Surgery

Professor, Department of Obstetrics and Gynecology

University of Texas Southwestern Medical Center

Chief of Gynecology

Parkland Health and Hospital System, Dallas, Texas

Chapter 24: Pelvic Organ Prolapse
Chapter 45: Surgeries for Pelvic Floor Disorders

Geetha Shivakumar, MD, MSCS

Mental Health Trauma Services, Dallas VA Medical Center

Associate Professor, Department of Psychiatry

University of Texas Southwestern Medical Center

Chapter 14: Psychosocial Issues and Female Sexuality

Gretchen S. Stuart, MD, MPHTM, FACOG

Director, Family Planning Program

Director, Fellowship in Family Planning

Professor, Department of Obstetrics and Gynecology

University of North Carolina at Chapel Hill

Chapter 5: Contraception and Sterilization
Chapter 6: First-Trimester Abortion

Hugh S. Taylor, MD

Professor and Chair, Department of Obstetrics, Gynecology and Reproductive Sciences

Yale School of Medicine, Yale University

Chapter 11: Endometriosis

Mayra J. Thompson, MD, FACOG

Professor, Department of Obstetrics and Gynecology

University of Texas Southwestern Medical Center

Chapter 41: Minimally Invasive Surgery Fundamentals

Diane M. Twickler, MD, FACR

Dr. Fred Bonte Professorship in Radiology

Distinguished Teaching Professor

Department of Radiology Vice Chairman for Academic Affairs

Professor, Departments of Radiology and Obstetrics and Gynecology

University of Texas Southwestern Medical Center

Clifford Y. Wai, MD

Director, Fellowship Program in Female Pelvic Medicine and Reconstructive Surgery

Professor, Department of Obstetrics and Gynecology

University of Texas Southwestern Medical Center

Chapter 23: Urinary Incontinence
Chapter 26: Genitourinary Fistula and Urethral Diverticulum

Claudia L. Werner, MD

Professor, Department of Obstetrics and Gynecology

University of Texas Southwestern Medical Center

Medical Director of Dysplasia Services

Co-Director Vulvology Clinic

Parkland Health and Hospital System, Dallas, Texas

Chapter 29: Preinvasive Lesions of the Lower Anogenital Tract

Ellen E. Wilson, MD

Professor, Department of Obstetrics and Gynecology

University of Texas Southwestern Medical Center

Director of Pediatric and Adolescent Gynecology Program

Children's Medical Center, Dallas, Texas

Chapter 15: Pediatric and Adolescent Gynecology
Chapter 18: Polycystic Ovarian Syndrome and Hyperandrogenism

ARTISTS

Primary Atlas Artist

Lewis E. Calver, MS, CMI, FAMI

Contributing Atlas Artists

Katherine Brown
Graduate, Biomedical Communications Graduate Program
University of Texas Southwestern Medical Center at Dallas

SangEun Cha
Graduate, Biomedical Communications Graduate Program
University of Texas Southwestern Medical Center at Dallas

T. J. Fels
Graduate, Biomedical Communications Graduate Program
University of Texas Southwestern Medical Center at Dallas

Erin Frederikson
Graduate, Biomedical Communications Graduate Program
University of Texas Southwestern Medical Center at Dallas

Alexandra Gordon
Graduate, Biomedical Communications Graduate Program
University of Texas Southwestern Medical Center at Dallas

Kimberly Hoggatt Krumwiede, MA, PhD
Associate Dean for Academic Affairs
Distinguished Teaching Professor
University of Texas Southwestern School of Health Professions

Richard P. Howdy, Jr.
Former Instructor, Biomedical Communications Graduate Program
University of Texas Southwestern Medical Center at Dallas

Belinda Klein
Graduate, Biomedical Communications Graduate Program
University of Texas Southwestern Medical Center at Dallas

Anne Matuskowitz
Graduate, Biomedical Communications Graduate Program
University of Texas Southwestern Medical Center at Dallas

Lindsay Oksenberg
Graduate, Biomedical Communications Graduate Program
University of Texas Southwestern Medical Center at Dallas

Jordan Pietz
Graduate, Biomedical Communications Graduate Program
University of Texas Southwestern Medical Center at Dallas

Marie Sena
Graduate, Biomedical Communications Graduate Program
University of Texas Southwestern Medical Center at Dallas

Maya Shoemaker
Graduate, Biomedical Communications Graduate Program
University of Texas Southwestern Medical Center at Dallas

Jennie Swensen
Graduate, Biomedical Communications Graduate Program
University of Texas Southwestern Medical Center at Dallas

Amanda Tomasikiewicz
Graduate, Biomedical Communications Graduate Program
University of Texas Southwestern Medical Center at Dallas

Kimberly VanExel
Graduate, Biomedical Communications Graduate Program
University of Texas Southwestern Medical Center at Dallas

Kristin Yang
Graduate, Biomedical Communications Graduate Program
University of Texas Southwestern Medical Center at Dallas

PREFACE

Williams Gynecology provides a thorough, evidence-based presentation of gynecology's depth and breadth. In Section 1, general gynecology topics are covered. Section 2 provides chapters covering reproductive endocrinology and infertility. The developing field of female pelvic medicine and reconstructive surgery is presented in Section 3. In Section 4, gynecologic oncology is discussed.

Traditionally, gynecologic information has been offered either as a didactic text or a surgical atlas. Instead, because the day-to-day activity of a gynecologist blends these two, we did the same with our text. The initial four sections of our book describe the evaluation and medical treatment of gynecologic problems. The remaining two sections focus on the surgical patient. Section 5 offers detailed anatomy and a discussion of perioperative considerations. Our final section presents an illustrated atlas for the surgical correction of conditions described in Sections 1 through 4. In addition, chapters are extensively complemented by illustrations, photographs, diagnostic algorithms, and treatment tables. To interconnect this content, readers will find page references within one chapter that will direct them to complementary content in another.

ACKNOWLEDGMENTS

During the creation and production of our textbook, we were lucky to have the assistance and support of countless talented professionals both within and outside our department. First, a task of this size could not be completed without the unwavering support provided by our Department Chairman, Dr. Steven Bloom, and Vice-Chairpersons, Drs. Barry Schwarz and Catherine Spong. Their financial and academic endorsement of our efforts has been essential. Without their academic vision, this undertaking could not have flourished. In addition, Dr. F. Gary Cunningham provided the academic vision that led to the creation of this text. Dr. Cunningham has been the senior author for eight editions of Williams Obstetrics. His dedication to evidence-based medicine set the bar on which our textbook was built. We feel privileged to have learned the craft of clear, concise academic summary from a consummate master.

In constructing a compilation of this breadth, physicians from several departments and their expertise were needed to add vital, contemporaneous information. From the Department of Pathology, Dr. Kelley Carrick shared her expertise and generously shared from her cadre of outstanding images. She translated her extensive knowledge of gynecologic pathology into concepts relevant for the general gynecologist. We appreciate the contributions of Dr. Agnieszka Dombrowska of Johns Hopkins University. She added her great expertise to our chapter on breast disease. Dr. Kevin Doody lent his considerable clinical and academic prowess in the treatment of infertility. He was also a kind benefactor of many spectacular clinical photographs and contributed these generously to numerous chapters. This is also true of Dr. David Rogers, Ellen Wilson, and William Griffith, who have been champions in expanding our academic image library. Sonographer Jason McWhirt at Parkland Hospital has similarly been a tremendous advocate in securing images of common and unique gynecologic pathology. In sum, their stunning images add to the academic richness of this edition.

New beautiful and detailed artwork in our atlas this edition was drawn by Mr. Lewis Calver. Again for this edition, he paired his academic talents with Dr. Marlene Corton to create urogynecologic images. Lew also partnered with Drs. Cherine Hamid, Patrick Weix, and Kimberly Kho to create academically new presentations for other sections of our surgical atlas. These renderings were crafted and tailored with the gynecologic surgeon in mind to depict important techniques and anatomy for these surgeries. We also acknowledge our atlas artists from the first three editions, who are listed in subsequent pages.

We are truly indebted to our administrative staff. For this project, we were lucky to have Ms. Toshia Lee serve as our primary administrative assistant. We greatly appreciated her cheery professionalism, relentless commitment to our project, and efficiency. Our words fall well short in expressing our gratitude to her for her heroic efforts. She was assisted by Ms. Regina Williams and Ms. Tabitha Brumfield. Their dedicated work ethic, eagerness to assist, attention to detail, and pleasant professionalism made our chapters crisp and accurate. None of our image and text production would have been possible without brilliant information technology support. Knowledgeable and responsive, Mr. Charles Richards has assisted our project since the first edition. We could not do our job without his expertise.

Williams Gynecology was sculpted into its final form by the talented and dedicated group at McGraw-Hill Education. Senior Project Development Editor Ms. Christie Naglieri has brought her considerable publishing knowledge, energetic work ethic, and creativity to our project. Her attention to detail and organizational talents have kept our project on track with efficiency and style. Ms. Leah Carton served as editorial coordinator, and we extend warm thanks for her tremendous support. Her efficiency, professionalism, hard work, accuracy, and positive attitude made coordination of this project a dream. Mr. Rick Ruzycka served as production supervisor and has been a long-time advocate of our books. We are so appreciative of his expertise and knowledge. Executive Editor Mr. Jason Malley has taken our project under his care and has adeptly shepherded it to completion. We happily look forward to many future collaborative editions together.

Without the thoughtful, creative efforts of many, our textbook would be a barren wasteland of words. Integral to this process is Jason M. McAlexander, Biomedical Media Manager at MPS North America, LLC. His artistic team assisted us in creating and revising many of our text images. Their attention to detail and accurate renderings added important academic support to our words.

Our text took its final shape under the watchful care of our compositors at Aptara, Inc. Specifically, we thank Ms. Indu Jawwad for her talents in skillfully and expediently coordinating and overseeing composition. Her dedicated attention to detail and organization were vital to completion of our project. Her pleasant professionalism was appreciated daily. Also at Aptara, Mr. Mahender Singh served a crucial task of quality control and assisted in creating beautiful chapter layouts to highlight our content aesthetically and informatively. We thank the entire Aptara team for their dedication to our books. Special thanks go to Mr. Greg Feldman. As copyeditor for our project, Greg has added precision and clarity to our efforts. His pleasant professionalism and expertise has made our text better.

We offer a sincere "thank you" to our residents in training. Their curiosity keeps us energized to find new and effective ways to convey age-old as well as cutting-edge concepts. Their logical questions lead us to holes in our text, and thereby, always help us to improve our work. Moreover, many of the photographs in this textbook were gathered with the help of our many residents.

Furthermore, the contributors to this text owe a significant debt to the women who have allowed us to participate in their care. The images and clinical expertise presented in this text would not have been possible without their collaborative spirit to help us move medical knowledge forward.

Lastly, we offer an enthusiastic and heartfelt "thank you" to our families and friends. Without their patience, generosity, and encouragement, this task would have been impossible. For them, too many hours with "the book" left them with new responsibilities. And importantly, time away from home left precious family memories and laughs unrealized. We sincerely thank you for your love and support.

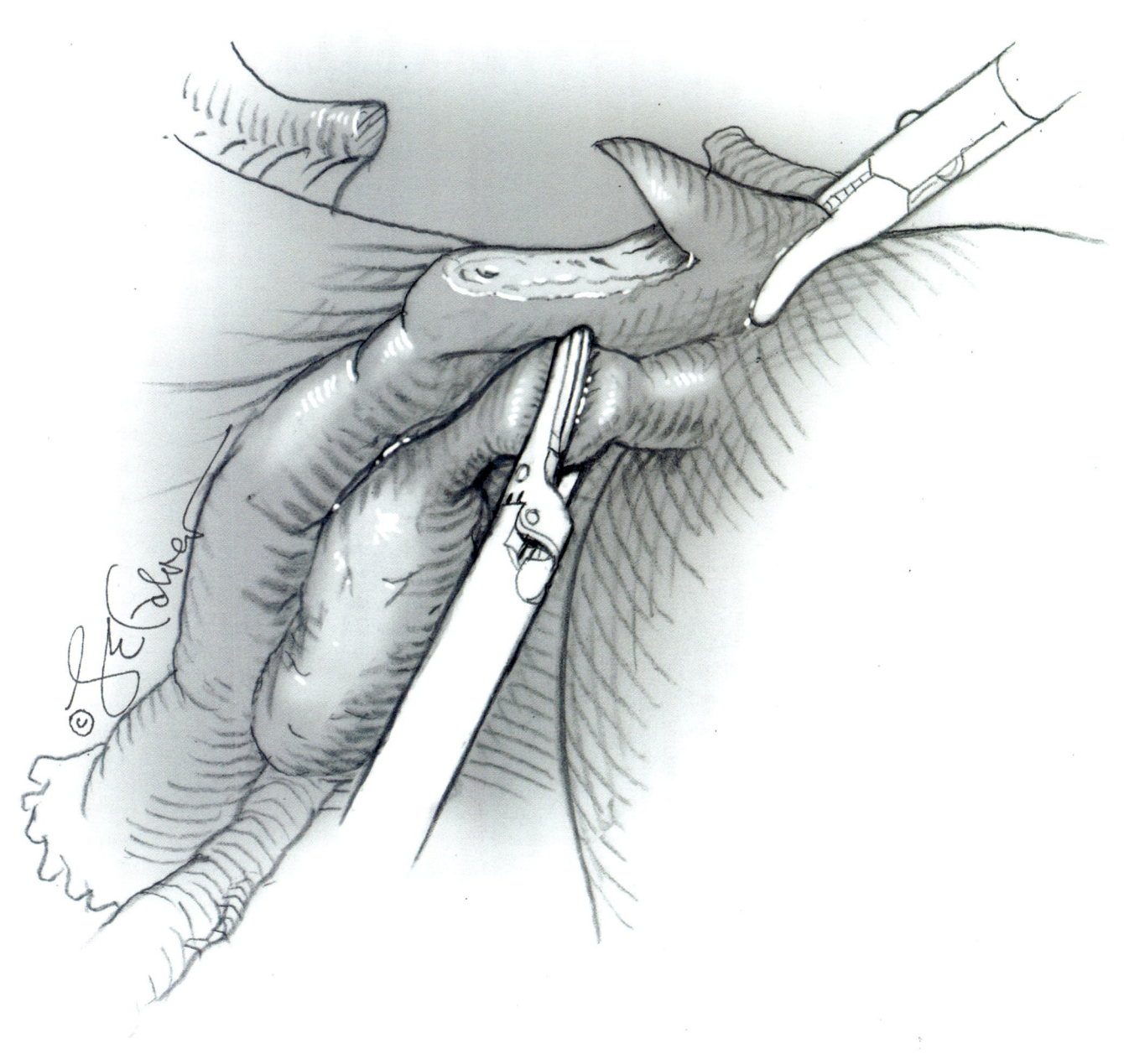

CHAPTER 1

Well Woman Care

Serving as both specialist and primary care provider, gynecologists provide patient screening, emphasize ideal health behaviors, and coordinate appropriate consultation for care beyond their scope of practice. Various organizations provide regularly updated preventive care recommendations. Guidelines commonly accessed are those from the American College of Obstetricians and Gynecologists (ACOG), Centers for Disease Control and Prevention (CDC), U.S. Preventive Services Task Force (USPSTF), and American Cancer Society.

MEDICAL HISTORY

During a comprehensive well woman visit, patients are first queried regarding new or ongoing illness. To assist with evaluation, complete medical, social, surgical, and family histories are obtained. Specific gynecologic topics usually cover current and prior contraceptives; results from prior sexually transmitted disease (STD) testing, cervical cancer screening, or other gynecologic tests; sexual history, described in Chapter 3 (p. 63); and menstrual history, outlined in Chapter 8 (p. 182). Obstetric questions chronicle circumstances around deliveries, losses, or complications. Screening for intimate partner violence (p. 24)

or depression is also completed (p. 19). Discussion might also assess the patient's support system and any cultural or spiritual beliefs that might affect her general health care. Last, a review of systems, whether performed by the clinician or office staff, can add clarity to new patient problems.

PHYSICAL EXAMINATION

■ Breast Examination

Many women present to their gynecologist with complaints specific to the breast or pelvis. Accordingly, these are often areas of increased focus, and their evaluation is described here.

Self breast examination (SBE) is an examination performed by the patient herself to detect abnormalities. In contrast, clinical breast examination (CBE) is completed by a health care professional and may identify a small portion of breast malignancies not detected with mammography. In addition, CBE may identify cancer in young women, who are not typical candidates for mammography (McDonald, 2004). Overall, however, studies show that SBE and CBE raise diagnostic testing rates for ultimately benign breast disease and are ineffective in lowering breast cancer mortality rates (Kösters, 2008; Thomas, 2002). Accordingly, several organizations have removed SBE and CBE from their recommended screening practices (Oeffinger, 2015; Siu, 2016). However, the American College of Obstetricians and Gynecologists (2017b) encourages breast self-awareness, which focuses on breast appearance and architecture and may include SBE. It also recommends that women receive a CBE every 1 to 3 years between ages 20 and 39. At age 40, CBE is completed annually. Specific mammography guidelines are listed in Chapter 13 (p. 293).

During CBE, the breasts are initially viewed as a woman sits on the table's edge with hands placed at her hips and with pectoralis muscles flexed. Alone, this position enhances asymmetry. Additional arm positions, such as placing arms above the head, do not add vital information. Breast skin is inspected for breast erythema; retraction; scaling, especially over the nipple; and edema, which is termed peau d'orange change. The breast and axilla are also observed for contour symmetry.

Following inspection, axillary, supraclavicular, and infraclavicular lymph nodes are palpated most easily with a woman seated and her arm supported by the examiner (Fig. 1-1). The axilla is bounded by the pectoralis major muscle ventrally and the latissimus dorsi muscle dorsally. Lymph nodes are detected as the examiner's hand glides from high to low in the axilla and momentarily compresses nodes against the lateral chest wall. In a thin patient, one or more normal, mobile lymph nodes less

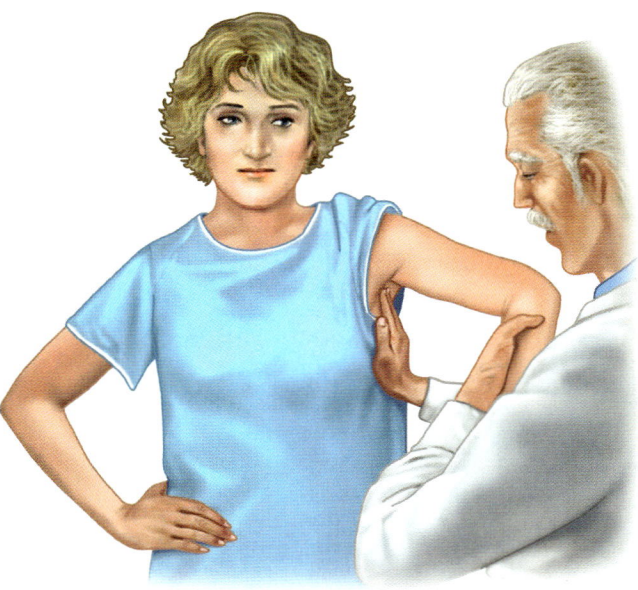

FIGURE 1-1 One method of axillary lymph node palpation. Finger tips extend to the axillary apex and compress tissue against the chest wall in the rolling fashion shown in Figure 1-2. The patient's arm is supported by the examiner.

than 1 cm in diameter may commonly be appreciated. The first lymph node to become involved with breast cancer metastasis (the sentinel node) is nearly always located just behind the midportion of the pectoralis major muscle belly.

Breast palpation is completed with a woman supine and with one hand above her head to stretch breast tissue across the chest wall. Examination includes breast tissue bounded by the clavicle, sternal border, inframammary crease, and midaxillary line. Breast palpation within this pentagonal area is approached in a linear fashion. Technique uses the finger pads in a continuous rolling, gliding, circular motion (Fig. 1-2). At each palpation point, tissue is assessed both superficially and deeply.

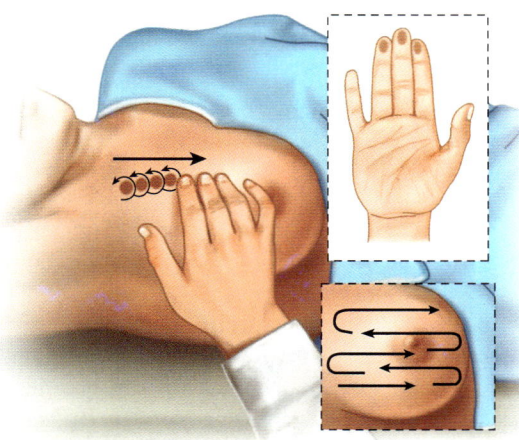

FIGURE 1-2 Recommended patient positioning and palpation technique. One inset shows the path of palpation. The other illustrates use of finger pads and a circular rolling motion to palpate the entire breast.

During CBE, intentional attempts at nipple discharge expression are not required unless a *spontaneous* discharge has been described by the patient.

If abnormal breast findings are noted, they are described by their location in the right or left breast, clock position, distance from the areola, and size. Evaluation and treatment of breast and nipple diseases are described in Chapter 13 (p. 280).

During examination, patients are educated that new axillary or breast masses, noncyclic breast pain, spontaneous nipple discharge, new nipple inversion, and breast skin changes such as dimpling, scaling, ulceration, edema, or erythema should prompt evaluation. This constitutes breast self-awareness. Patients who desire to perform SBE are counseled on its benefits, limitations, and potential harms and instructed to complete SBE the week after menses.

■ Pelvic Examination

Pelvic examination is typically performed with a patient supine, legs in dorsal lithotomy position, and feet resting in stirrups. The head of the bed is elevated 30 degrees to relax abdominal wall muscles for bimanual examination. A woman is assured that she may stop or pause the examination at any time. Moreover, each part of the evaluation is announced or described before its performance. Recommended STD screening is discussed prior to examination, and necessary samplers are assembled (Table 1-1).

Inguinal Lymph Nodes and Perineal Inspection

Pelvic cancers and infections may drain to the inguinal lymph nodes, and these are palpated during examination. Following this, a methodical inspection of the perineum extends from the mons pubis ventrally, to the labiocrural folds laterally, and to the anus. Notably, infections and neoplasms that involve the vulva can also involve perianal skin. Some clinicians additionally palpate for Bartholin and paraurethral gland pathology. However, in most cases, patient symptoms and asymmetry in these areas will dictate the need for this specific evaluation.

Speculum Examination

Both metal and plastic specula are available for this examination, each in various sizes to accommodate vaginal length and laxity. The plastic speculum may be equipped with a small light that provides illumination, whereas metal specula require an external light source. Preference between these two types is provider dependent.

The vagina and cervix are typically viewed after placement of either a Graves or Pederson speculum (Fig. 1-3). Prior to insertion, a speculum may be warmed with running water or by warming lights built into some examination tables. In addition, lubrication may add comfort to insertion. Gel lubricants do not raise unsatisfactory Pap smear cytology rates or decrease *Chlamydia trachomatis* detection rates compared with water (Griffith, 2005). If gel lubrication is used, a dime-sized aliquot is applied sparingly to the outer surface of the speculum blades.

Immediately before insertion, the labia minora are gently separated, and the urethra is identified. Because of urethral sensitivity, the speculum is inserted well below the meatus. Alternatively, prior to speculum placement, an index finger may be placed in the vagina, and pressure exerted against the

TABLE 1-1. Sexually Transmitted Disease Screening Guidelines for Nonpregnant, Sexually Active Asymptomatic Women

Infectious Agent	Screening Recommendations	Risk Factors
C trachomatis + N gonorrhoeae	All ≤24 yr; those older with risks Timing: annually or if new or persistent factors since last negative result	New or multiple partners; partner with STD or multiple partners; inconsistent condom use; sex work; current or prior STD
T pallidum	Those with risks	Sex work; incarceration; HIV; high local prevalence
HIV virus	All aged 13–64 yrs: one time[a] Those with risks: periodically	Multiple partners; injection drug use; sex work; concurrent STD; MSM; at-risk partners; initial TB diagnosis
HCV	All aged 18–79 yrs: one time Those with risk factors: periodical y	Injection/intranasal drug use; dialysis; infected mother; blood products before 1992; unregulated tattoo; high-risk sexual behavior
HBV	Those with risk factors	HIV; injection drug use; affected family or partner; multiple partners; high-prevalence country of origin[b]
HSV	No routine screening	

[a]Centers for Disease Control and Prevention (2015) and American College of Obstetricians and Gynecologists (2017d) recommend one-time screening between ages 13 and 64 years. The U.S. Preventive Services Task Force uses a 15–65 yr age range.
[b]Regions of the world with high or intermediate prevalence of include much of Eastern Europe, Asia, Africa, the Middle East, and the Pacific Islands.
C trachomatis = Chlamydia trachomatis; HBV = hepatitis B virus; HCV = hepatitis C virus; HIV = human immunodeficiency virus; HSV = herpes simplex virus; MSM = men having sex with men; N gonorrhoeae = Neisseria gonorrhoeae; STD = sexually transmitted disease; TB = tuberculosis; T pallidum = Treponema pallidum.
Compiled from those above and Centers for Disease Control and Prevention, 2015; LeFevre, 2014a,b; Moyer, 2013a,b; U.S. Preventive Services Task Force, 2016c,d, 2019.

posterior wall. A woman is then encouraged to relax this wall to improve comfort with speculum insertion. This practice may prove especially helpful for women undergoing their first examination and for those with infrequent coitus, dyspareunia, or heightened anxiety.

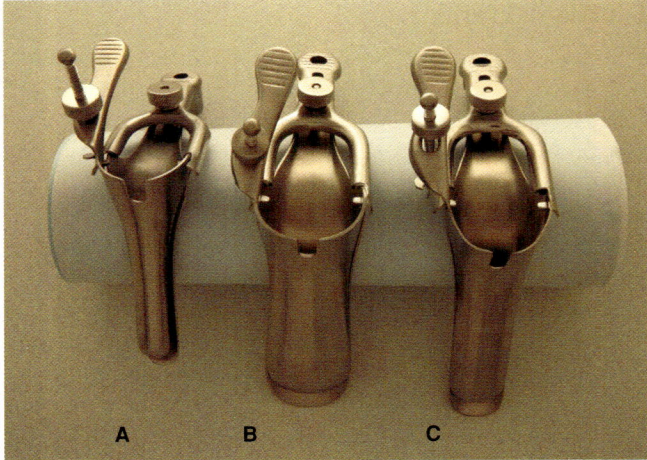

FIGURE 1-3 Vaginal specula. **A.** Pediatric Pederson speculum. This may be selected for child, adolescent, or virginal adult examination. **B.** Graves speculum. This may be selected for examination of parous women with relaxed or collapsing vaginal walls. **C.** Pederson speculum. This may be selected for sexually active women with adequate vaginal wall tone. (Reproduced with permission from US Surgitech, Inc.)

With speculum insertion, the vagina commonly contracts, and a woman may note pressure or discomfort. A pause at this point typically is followed by vaginal muscle relaxation. As the speculum bill is completely inserted, it is angled approximately 30 degrees downward to reach the cervix. Commonly, the uterus is anteverted, and the ectocervix lies against the posterior vaginal wall.

As the speculum is opened, the ectocervix can be identified. Vaginal walls and cervix are inspected for masses, ulceration, or unusual discharge. As outlined in Chapter 29 (p. 630), cervical cancer screening is often completed. Additional swabs for STD screening, culture, or microscopic evaluation can be collected as needed.

Bimanual Examination

Most often, the bimanual examination is performed after the speculum evaluation. Some clinicians prefer to complete the bimanual portion first to better identify cervical location prior to speculum insertion. Either process is appropriate. Uterine and adnexal size, mobility, and tenderness can be assessed during this examination. For women with prior hysterectomy and adnexectomy, bimanual examination is still valuable and can be used to exclude other pelvic pathology.

To begin, a gloved index and middle finger are inserted together into the vagina until the cervix is reached. To ease insertion, a water-based lubricant can be initially applied to these gloved fingers. Once the cervix is reached, uterine orientation can be quickly assessed by sweeping the index finger inward along the

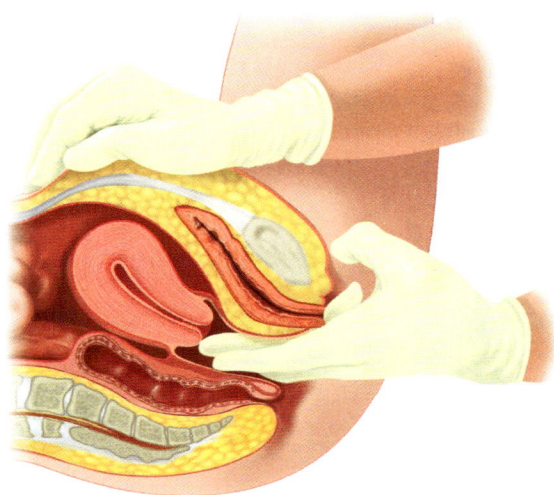

FIGURE 1-4 Bimanual examination. Fingers beneath the cervix lift the uterus toward the anterior abdominal wall. A hand placed on the abdomen detects upward pressure from the uterine fundus. Examination allows assessment of uterine size, mobility, and tenderness.

anterior surface of the cervix. In those with an anteverted position, the uterine isthmus is noted to sweep upward, whereas in those with a retroverted position, a soft bladder is palpated. However, in those with a retroverted uterus, if a finger is swept along the cervix's posterior aspect, the isthmus is felt to sweep downward. With a retroverted uterus, this same finger is continued posteriorly to the fundus and then side-to-side to assess uterine size and tenderness.

To determine the size of an anteverted uterus, fingers are placed beneath the cervix, and upward pressure tilts the fundus toward the anterior abdominal wall. A clinician's opposite hand is placed against the abdominal wall to locate the upward fundal pressure (Fig. 1-4).

To assess adnexa, the clinician uses two vaginal fingers to lift the adnexa from the posterior cul-de-sac or from the

ovarian fossa toward the anterior abdominal wall. The adnexum is trapped between these vaginal fingers and the clinician's other hand, which is exerting downward pressure against the lower abdomen. For those with a normal-sized uterus, this abdominal hand is typically best placed just above the inguinal ligament.

Rectovaginal Examination

The decision to perform rectovaginal evaluation varies among providers. Some prefer to complete this evaluation on all adults, whereas others elect to perform rectovaginal examination for those with specific indications. These may include pelvic pain, an identified pelvic mass, rectal symptoms, or risks for colon cancer.

Gloves are changed between bimanual and rectovaginal examinations to avoid contamination of the rectum with potential vaginal pathogens. Initially, an index finger is placed into the vagina and a middle finger into the rectum (Fig. 1-5). These fingers are swept against one another in a scissoring fashion to assess the rectovaginal septum for scarring or peritoneal studding. The index finger is removed, and the middle finger completes a circular sweep of the rectal vault to exclude masses. If immediate diagnostic fecal occult blood testing is indicated, it may be performed with a sample from this portion of the examination. As noted later, this single fecal occult blood testing does not constitute adequate colorectal cancer screening.

■ Examination Interval

An initial reproductive health visit is recommended between ages 13 and 15 years (American College of Obstetricians and Gynecologists, 2016b). This visit initiates discussion between an adolescent and health care provider on issues of puberty, menstruation, contraception, and STD protection. Although not mandated, a pelvic examination may be necessary if gynecologic symptoms are described.

For women older than 21, the American College of Obstetricians and Gynecologists (2016c) recommends annual well woman visits for examination, screening, counseling, and immunizations based on age and risk factors. In many cases, physical examination includes a pelvic examination to assess specific symptoms or to complete cervical cancer or STD screening. However, outside these indications, the American College of Physicians, the American Academy of Family Physicians (2017), and USPSTF (2017) recommend against screening pelvic examination for asymptomatic, nonpregnant, adult women. They cite potential harms that include discomfort, anxiety, and overtreatment (Qaseem, 2014). In contrast, potential benefits are early detection of dermatologic changes or of vulvar or vaginal cancer. Thus, the American College of Obstetricians and Gynecologists (2018b) recommends a patient-provider discussion of the benefits and risks of pelvic examination in the asymptomatic, nonpregnant, adult woman who does not require genital screening.

■ Care of the Transgender Patient

"Transgender" refers to individuals whose gender identity, expression, and behavior differ from those typically associated with their gender assigned at birth (World Professional

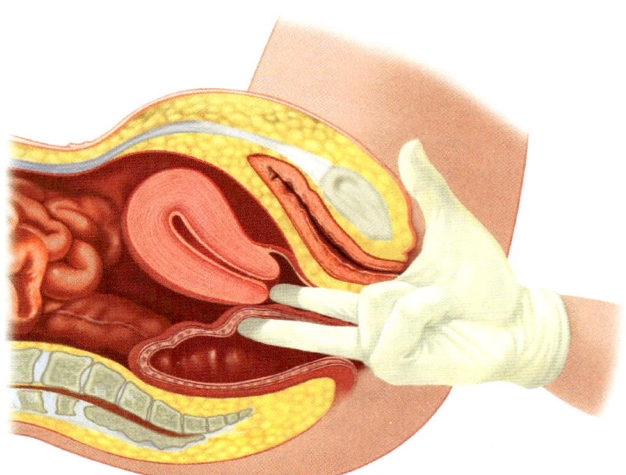

FIGURE 1-5 Rectovaginal examination.

TABLE 1-2. Gender Terminology

Transgender: Individuals whose gender identity, expression and behavior differ to varying degrees from those typically ascribed to their sex at birth

Cisgender: Individuals whose gender identity aligns with their sex at birth

Gender dysphoria: Distress that is caused by a discrepancy between a person's assigned gender at birth and the person's gender identity

Gender identity: An individual's intrinsic sense of being male, female, or an alternative gender (gender variant) that is independent of the gender assigned at birth

Sexual orientation: An individual's attraction to members of the same sex and/or a different sex (i.e., lesbian, gay, bisexual, heterosexual, or asexual)

Gender expression: The manner used by individuals to present themselves socially that may or may not be congruent with their gender identity

Gender variance/gender nonconformity: Expression of gender identity that that does not fully adhere to either male or female gender norms

Female-to-male (trans men): Individuals assigned female gender at birth who are changing to a more masculine body/gender role

Male-to-female (trans women): Individuals assigned male gender at birth who are changing to a more feminine body/gender role

Data from World Professional Association for Transgender Health, 2012.

Association for Transgender Health, 2012). Also, an individual's gender identity is independent of their sexual orientation or gender expression (Table 1-2). Despite agreement on these concepts, no definition of "transgender" is universally accepted.

In 2016 in the United States, an estimated 0.6 percent of adults, which approximates 1.4 million, identified as transgender (Flores, 2016). However, global prevalence rates of transgender populations have not been established. In part, differing behavioral expression of gender likely affects rates across cultures.

Despite growing awareness of transgender issues within the medical community, individuals continue to face significant barriers to both medical and mental health care (American College of Obstetricians and Gynecologists, 2011). For example, transgender adolescents compose up to 40 percent of homeless youth, and this can limit health care access (Ray, 2006). Further, medical schools teach little about sexuality in general and even less about the unique aspects of transgender health. This knowledge gap prepares few providers to address specific transgender needs (Mayer, 2008).

In 2017, the Endocrine Society updated clinical practice guidelines to provide an evidence-based standard for the care of transgender persons (Hembree, 2017). The American College of Obstetricians and Gynecologists (2011) urges obstetrician-gynecologists to be willing and able either to provide care for these individuals or to refer them for routine care or gender-affirming treatment. Thus, an understanding of current practices and long-term health risks is essential.

One first step in eliminating barriers is creation of a welcoming and inclusive clinical environment for transgender persons. Intake forms ideally incorporate sexual minorities in the gender field and use terms such as "relationship status" instead of "marital status." Providers begin the visit with an open dialogue that asks for a preferred name and pronoun.

A history of their gender experience ideally uses open-ended questions to ascertain the age at their initial transition, prior supplement or hormone use, and its duration. Importantly, not all transgender patients have undergone surgical transition, and many opt for medical therapy alone. Clarifying prior gender-affirming and sexual practices allows adequate assessment of an individual's medical risks and reproductive needs. Assumptions regarding a patient's sexual orientation or practices are best avoided (Gay and Lesbian Medical Association, 2006).

Prior to physical examination, each patient's individual comfort level with being examined is assessed. A problem-oriented examination usually suffices, and a genital examination is not indicated unless needed for a specific complaint or routine screening.

Medical Management of Gender Dysphoria

Gender dysphoria is the condition commonly ascribed to transgender individuals seeking medical care (see Table 1-2). The *Diagnostic and Statistical Manual of Mental Disorders, Fifth Edition* (DSM-5) defines it as the distress experienced by persons whose gender identity is incongruent to the gender they were assigned at birth (American Psychiatric Association, 2013). This diagnosis is best made by a qualified mental health provider. Following diagnosis, initiation of proper gender-affirming hormone therapy improves health outcomes and quality of life in these individuals (Gorin-Lazard, 2012). Those with gender dysphoria often have concurrent psychosocial or psychiatric issues. Thus, patients receiving hormone therapy are recommended to receive continuing psychotherapy (Spack, 2013).

In female-to-male transgender persons, the primary goals of testosterone therapy are cessation of menses and virilization. An increase in muscle mass and decline in fat mass are other effects. Testosterone is typically administered intramuscularly (IM) or subcutaneously every 1 to 2 weeks. To induce puberty in adolescents, initial testosterone doses may begin at 25 mg weekly. Doses increase incrementally every 3 to 6 months to reach the typical adult maintenance dose, which is 50 to 100 mg weekly (Hembree, 2017). Creams and patches are not

TABLE 1-3. Medical Management of Gender Dysphoria

	Puberty Suppression	FTM	MTF
Medications	Provide GnRH analogues: Implant (histrelin) Intramuscular (leuprolide)	Testosterone Parenteral (IM or SC) Oral Transdermal	Estrogen Oral Transdermal Parenteral Antiandrogens Spironolactone
Anticipated effects	Prevent secondary sexual characteristics of the assigned gender	Deepened voice Facial/body hair growth ↑ libido Amenorrhea Clitoral enlargement ↑ percentage muscle mass compared to body fat	Breast growth ↓ testicle size ↓ percentage muscle mass compared to body fat Antiandrogens may reduce effects of endogenous testosterone
Anticipated risks	May decrease BMD (may theoretically be reversed with sex hormone therapy)	Polycythemia Weight gain Acne Androgenic hair loss Sleep apnea	VTE Gallstones ↑ liver enzyme levels Weight gain Hypertriglyceridemia
No risk increase/ data inconclusive		BMD loss Breast cancer Cervical cancer Ovarian cancer Uterine cancer	Breast cancer

BMD = bone mineral density; FTM = female to male; GnRH = gonadotropin-releasing hormone; IM = intramuscular; MTF = male to female; SC = subcutaneous; VTE = venous thromboembolism.

as widely prescribed as data are limited regarding their use for puberty induction.

Serum testosterone levels are measured every 2 to 3 months to ensure that levels are in the normal physiologic range for males (320 to 1000 ng/dL). Importantly, the most common adverse effects of exogenous testosterone are erythrocytosis and more atherogenic lipid levels (Bhasin, 2006). Accordingly, patients undergo periodic laboratory testing while receiving treatment. Panels include a complete blood count (CBC), liver function tests (LFTs), and lipid and hemoglobin A_{1c} levels (Spack, 2013).

In male-to-female transgender individuals, feminizing therapy is often begun to promote breast growth, redistribute body fat, and reduce body hair growth. Estrogen, either conjugated equine estrogens or 17β-estradiol, is typically administered orally, transdermally, or parenterally (estrogen esters). Puberty induction with 17β-estradiol may begin with a 1-mg oral daily dose that is incrementally increased every 3 to 6 months to reach the typical adult maintenance doses of 4 to 6 mg daily. Similarly, transdermal estrogen may begin with a patch that delivers 0.1 mg/d estradiol daily and is changed once or twice weekly depending on brand. Dosing can then be incrementally raised to a daily 0.4 mg/d dose, which is achieved by wearing multiple 0.1 mg/d patches (Deutsch, 2018). As with any patient undergoing chronic estrogen replacement therapy, transgender women are screened and counseled regarding the higher risk

for thromboembolic disease, liver dysfunction, and hypertension (Spack, 2013). Effects of hormone therapy and different methods of administration are summarized in Table 1-3.

Concurrently, testosterone is ideally lowered to premenopausal levels (<50 ng/dL). For this degree of suppression, treatment with estrogen alone is insufficient. Thus, adjuncts, such as progestins with antiandrogen activity or GnRH agonists, are options. Another is spironolactone, which directly blocks androgen receptor binding.

With therapy, serum testosterone and estradiol levels are measured every 3 months to ensure that serum estradiol levels do not exceed the peak physiologic range for premenopausal females. The preferred range is 100 to 200 pg/mL (Spack, 2013). Estrogen therapy can promote pituitary lactotroph cell growth. And, several reports describe prolactinomas occurring after long-term, high-dose estrogen therapy. Accordingly, periodic serum prolactin level testing is recommended (Hembree, 2017).

Surgical Management of Gender Dysphoria

Most, but not all, transgender individuals consider gender-affirming surgeries necessary to complete their transition. These procedures are classified as those that directly impair fertility and those that do not. The former include hysterectomy and gonadectomy, and in minors, performance of these is typically controlled by governing laws (Hembree, 2017). However, less-legislated procedures may be considered in both minors and adults who have been living in their new gender role and have been receiving hormonal therapy for approximately 12 months. Such surgeries include mastectomy and breast reconstruction and other procedures meant to feminize or masculinize the face and body. Consensus among the patient, physician, and the mental health provider is advisable.

Female-to-male transgender individuals commonly choose total hysterectomy, and both vaginal and laparoscopic approaches are options. Of these, the vaginal approach appears to be more cost-effective and amenable to subsequent phalloplasty, which is creation of a phallus, if elected (O'Hanlan, 2007). The gynecologist also provides essential counseling regarding retention or removal of ovaries. This decision is made with utmost respect for the patient's autonomy and is directed by their desire for removal of their female gonads and their plans for future fertility. Gynecologic considerations also include comorbid pathology, such as endometriosis or positive *BRCA* gene mutation status, which may favor oophorectomy. As another counseling point, future disruption of their testosterone therapy due to financial constraints could pose osteoporosis risks from lack of exogenous steroid hormones. Primary ovarian retention may mitigate this risk.

During female-to-male transition, mastectomy is also often undertaken, as testosterone therapy has little effect on breast regression. In adults, discussion regarding mastectomy usually takes place after androgen therapy has begun. Other procedures available to transgender males have been less satisfactory and not as widely sought. Surgical creation of a neopenis is still cost-prohibitive and typically requires multiple stages. That said, newer surgical techniques are yielding improved cosmetic results (Monstrey, 2007).

Male-to-female transgender surgery can involve penile and testicular excision and creation of a neovagina. Postoperatively, significant risks for vaginal and urethral stenosis persist, and lifelong vaginal dilation is required to maintain neovagina patency. Other cosmetic procedures include breast augmentation and facial feminizing surgery. These reconstructive procedures are best performed by urologists, gynecologists, or plastic surgeons with experience and specialized training in this field.

Adolescent Care

The effects of gender dysphoria in adolescents are potentiated by the unwanted physical changes that accompany puberty. Medical treatment of gender dysphoria during puberty improves psychological functioning in this group (de Vries, 2011). The Endocrine Society suggests suppression of pubertal development in adolescents who meet criteria for gender dysphoria (Hembree, 2017).

Puberty suppression is commonly accomplished with gonadotropin-releasing hormone (GnRH) analogues in the form of the histrelin implant (Supprelin LA) or depot leuprolide acetate (Lupron). Histrelin is a single subcutaneous implant that delivers the GnRH agonist over 12 months. Depot leuprolide acetate is administered IM in distinct doses that supply activity for 1 month or for 3 months. With these agents, gonadotropin suppression is profound (Chap. 9, p. 208).

Suppression is considered once Tanner stage 2 development is reached (Fig. 15-3, p. 322), that is, before the physical signs of puberty have significantly progressed. GnRH agonists offer the advantage of complete reversibility. However, their overall effect on bone density is not well studied. Accordingly, the Endocrine Society recommends that bone mineral density testing be completed annually (Hembree, 2017). They also support initiation of gender-affirming hormones in adolescents by age 16, although use in 14-year-old adolescents has been described (de Vries, 2014).

Long-Term Considerations

Transgender aging is an underexplored field (Fredriksen-Goldsen, 2014). The American College of Obstetricians and Gynecologists (2018a) advocates against routine discontinuation of systemic hormone therapy in postmenopausal women if used for the management of persistent vasomotor symptoms. However, no such recommendations exist for gender-affirming hormones in transgender persons receiving long-term therapy.

Both testosterone and estrogen therapy pose many of the same medical risks in both trans- and cisgender populations. However, their use in transgender persons is complicated by prolonged exposure to exogenous high-dose hormones and the potential negative secondary effects of early gonadectomy. In addition to monitoring weight and blood pressure and directed physical examination, routine health evaluation should seek lifestyle risk factors (such as smoking) and concurrent use of medications that can heighten the risks of long-term gender-affirming hormone therapy. Laboratory testing described earlier is standard for transgender adults (p. 7).

For transgender males, age-appropriate screening for breast cancer is continued as recommended by the American Cancer Society (Smith, 2018a). Long-term estrogen use does not raise the breast cancer risk in this group. But, breast cancer has been reported in transgender males even following mastectomy and highlights the need for continued screening (Shao, 2011). No cases of endometrial cancer have been reported in transgender males following long-term testosterone treatment. That said, individuals who maintain their uterus and ovaries are counseled regarding the potential risk of endometrial hyperplasia resulting from the aromatization of testosterone to estradiol (Futterweit, 1998; Moore, 2003). Thus, transgender males who present with abnormal uterine bleeding (AUB) following prolonged amenorrhea may benefit from evaluation similar to that in cisgender women with AUB. Evaluation for AUB may be considered if bleeding persists despite 6 to 12 months of suppressed luteinizing hormone and follicle-stimulating hormone levels and a testosterone level in the male range. If cervical tissue is still present, cervical cancer screening is performed as recommended by the American College of Obstetricians and Gynecologists (Chap. 29, p. 630).

Transgender women should continue routine screening for prostate and breast cancer. Breast cancer has been reported in transgender females undergoing long-term estrogen therapy. That said, no long-term studies have determined the actual risk of breast cancer in this population (Ganly, 1995). Although the overall benefit of screening mammography for transgender females has not been established, breast cancer screening as in the general population is reasonable (Hembree, 2017).

Prolonged use of gender-affirming hormones has potentially negative effects on ovarian and testicular function. Thus, a discussion regarding plans for future childbearing is essential (Mayer, 2008). These discussions ideally take place prior to initiation of hormone therapy. Fertility preservation options offered to transgender individuals mirror those suitable to their cisgender counterparts (Chap. 21, p. 466). Conversely, unintended pregnancies have occurred in transgender men receiving testosterone. Thus, contraceptive needs are addressed in patients who have maintained their uterus (Light, 2014). Contraceptive options for transgender men do not differ from those for cisgender women (Chap. 5, p. 111). Testosterone is not a form of contraception, and this should be emphasized during patient discussion.

PREVENTIVE CARE

Gynecologists have an opportunity to evaluate their patients for leading causes of female morbidity and mortality and intervene accordingly. In 2016, screening recommendations by the American College of Obstetricians and Gynecologists (2016c) were updated. The USPSTF regularly revises its screening guidelines, which can be accessed at www.USPreventiveServicesTaskForce.org. Many of these topics are covered in other text chapters. Some remaining important subjects are presented in the following sections.

■ Immunization

The need for new or repeat administration of vaccines is best reviewed periodically. Table 1-4 summarizes recommended schedules, precautions, and contraindications for these adult vaccines, and as of 2019, a link is provided to the full schedules at: http://www.cdc.gov/vaccines/schedules. In general, any vaccine may be coadministered with another type at the same visit.

■ Cancer Screening

Colon Cancer

In the United States, colon cancer is the third leading cause of cancer death in women, behind lung and breast cancer (Siegel, 2019). Incidence and mortality rates from this cancer have declined during the past two decades, largely due to improved screening tools. No trials have directly compared any of the screening tools. Instead, identifying an acceptable screening strategy for an individual patient may improve overall compliance and screening completion rates (U.S. Preventive Services Task Force, 2016a).

Guidelines recommend screening average-risk patients for colorectal cancer from age 50 to 75 with any of the methods shown in Table 1-5 (Smith, 2018a). Black women in the United States have a higher incidence of colorectal cancer, and the U.S. Multi-Society Task Force on Colorectal Cancer recommends discussing initial screening at age 45 (Rex, 2017). Health care disparities related to race and colon cancer are complex, and patient-oriented outcome studies are lacking to strongly support this earlier screening. Other organization guidelines, including those of the USPSTF (2016a), have not yet supported this earlier screening age.

Direct visualization methods can detect cancer *and* precancerous lesions. Of these, colonoscopy visualizes the entire colon, and biopsy can be performed simultaneously if needed. Stool-based tests include fecal occult blood test, fecal immunochemical test, and stool DNA tests.

Because colonoscopy allows for both screening and simultaneous diagnostic evaluation, it is often the preferred colorectal cancer screening test. For the patient with average risk and normal findings, testing is repeated every 10 years. In the United States, the direct visualization method offered may depend on a patient's insurance plan coverage.

Fecal occult blood testing (gFOBT) is an adequate *annual* screening method when two or three stool samples are

TABLE 1-4. Summary of Recommendations for Adult Immunization

Vaccine and Route	Reason to Vaccinate	Vaccine Administration	Contraindications and Precautions[a,b]
Influenza[c] **IIV** *or* **RIV** *Give SC*	• All adults	• Yearly • October is ideal, or as long as virus is circulating	**Precaution** • GBS within 6 wk of prior vaccine • IIV: egg allergy
Pneumococcal PCV13 *Give IM* **PPSV23** *Give IM or SC*	• All ≥65 yr • Chronic illness[d]; asplenia; immunocompromise; smokers	• Age ≥65 yr without health issues: PCV13, then PPSV23 after 1 yr ***or*** PPSV23, then PCV13 after 1 yr • Variant regimens for other indications[d]	
Hepatitis A *Give IM*	• Desires immunity • Contact or travel risk[e]; other health indications[d]	• Two doses: 0 and 6 months	
Hepatitis B *Give IM*	• Desires immunity • Contact or travel risks[e]; other health indications[d]	• Three doses: 0, 1, and 6 months	

(Continued)

TABLE 1-4. Summary of Recommendations for Adult Immunization *(Continued)*

Vaccine and Route	Reason to Vaccinate	Vaccine Administration	Contraindications and Precautions[a,b]
Combined Hepatitis A + B *Give IM*	• Indications for hepatitis A or B	• Three doses: 0, 1, and 6 months	
Tdap Td *Give IM*	• All adults • Pregnancy	• No prior vaccine: 1 dose Tdap • Td booster every 10 yr • At-risk wounds: booster Td dose if ≥5 yr since prior dose • Pregnancy: Tdap dose at 27–36 wk regardless of prior dosing	**Contraindication** • Tdap: encephalopathy after prior vaccine **Precaution** • GBS within 6 wk of prior vaccine • Tdap: unstable neurologic condition
Varicella *Give SC*	• Lacks immunity	• Two doses: 0 and 1 month • Nonimmune gravida: give series postpartum	**Contraindications** • Pregnancy • Immunocompromise **Precaution** • Recent antibody-containing blood products • Hold "-cyclovir" antivirals[f] 14 days after vaccine
Zoster RZV *Give IM* **ZVL** *Give SC*	• RZV: ≥50 yr *or* • ZVL: ≥60 yr	• Two doses: 0, 2–6 months • One dose	**ZVL Contraindications** • Immunocompromise • Pregnancy **Precaution** • Hold "-cyclovir" antivirals[f] 14 days after vaccine
MMR *Give SC*	• Lacks immunity	• One dose • Nonimmune gravida: give postpartum	**Contraindications** • Immunocompromise • Pregnancy **Precaution** • Prior thrombocytopenia • Recent antibody-containing blood products
HPV *Give IM*	• Desires immunity • Ages 9 to 45 yr	• Three doses: 0, 1, and 6 months	**Precaution** • Pregnancy

[a]Previous anaphylactic reaction to any of a vaccine's components serves as a contraindication for any vaccine.
[b]Moderate to severe illness is a precaution to vaccination. Mild illness is not a contraindication.
[c]Several influenza vaccines are available and listed at: https://www.cdc.gov/flu/protect/vaccine/vaccines.htm.
[d]Full guidelines found at http://www.cdc.gov/vaccines/schedules/downloads/adult/adult-combined-schedule.pdf.
[e]A list is found at https://wwwnc.cdc.gov/travel/page/yellowbook-home.
[f]These include acyclovir, famciclovir, valacyclovir.
GBS = Guillain-Barré syndrome; HPV = human papillomavirus; IIV = inactivated influenza vaccine; IM = intramuscular; MMR = measles, mumps, rubella; PCV = pneumococcal conjugate vaccine; PPSV = pneumococcal polysaccharide vaccine; RIV = recombinant influenza vaccine; RZV = recombinant zoster vaccine; SC = subcutaneous; Td = tetanus, diphtheria; Tdap = tetanus, diphtheria, activated pertussis; ZV_ = zoster vaccine live.
From Dooling, 2018; Food and Drug Administration, 2018; Kim, 2019.

TABLE 1-5. Screening Guidelines for the Early Detection of Colorectal Cancer and Adenomas for Average-Risk Women Aged 50 to 75 years[a]

Direct Visualization Tests		
Test	**Interval**	**Key Issues for Informed Decisions**
Colonoscopy	10 years	Bowel prep required; conscious sedation provided
FSIG	5 years	Bowel prep required, sedation usually not provided Positive findings usually merit colonoscopy
CT Colonography	5 years	Bowel prep required, polyps ≥6 mm merit colonoscopy; incidental extracolonic findings are common and can result in unnecessary diagnostic testing
Stool-based Tests		
Test	**Interval**	**Key Issues for Informed Decisions**
gFOBT	Annually	Two to three stool samples *collected at home* (a single sample gathered during an office examination is insufficient); positive results merit colonoscopy
FIT	Annually	Single specimen *collected at home*; positive results merit colonoscopy
FIT-DNA	3 years	Lower specificity/higher sensitivity than FIT; positive results merit colonoscopy

[a]One method is selected.
FIT = fecal immunochemical test; FSIG = flexible sigmoidoscopy; gFOBT = guaiac-based fecal occult blood test.
Adapted from Rex, 2017; Smith, 2018a; U.S. Preventive Services Task Force, 2016a.

self-collected by the patient and the cards are returned for analysis. This method relies on a chemical oxidation reaction between the heme moiety of blood and alpha guaiaconic acid, a component of guaiac paper. However, gFOBT is not specific for human blood, and some factors can yield false-positive results. Ingestion of red meat or iron is an example. In contrast, vitamin C may preemptively react with the reagents and lead to false-negative results (Park, 2010). All of these must be eliminated for 3 days before testing. In addition, women should avoid nonsteroidal antiinflammatory drugs (NSAIDs) 7 days prior to testing to limit risks of gastric irritation and bleeding. These restrictions are cumbersome for some patients and lead to noncompliance.

Alternatively, the fecal immunochemical test (FIT) relies on an immune reaction to human hemoglobin. Similar to gFOBT, the FIT test is performed for annual screening on patient-collected stool samples but does not require pretesting dietary limitations. Advantages to FIT include greater specificity for human blood, and thus fewer false-positive results and improved accuracy for detecting colorectal cancer (U.S. Preventive Services Task Force, 2016a). An emerging screening strategy combines FIT with testing for altered DNA biomarkers in cells shed into the stool (FIT-DNA). One Food and Drug Administration (FDA)-approved test, Cologuard, screens stool for both DNA and hemoglobin biomarkers that are associated with colorectal cancer (Imperiale, 2014). Positive test results from any of these three stool tests warrant further evaluation by colonoscopy.

During patient evaluation of pelvic complaints such as pain, a gynecologist not uncommonly performs gFOBT testing for diagnostic purposes on a single stool sample obtained during digital rectal examination. As noted, this single stool sample is not adequate colorectal cancer screening.

These guidelines are appropriate for those with average risk. High-risk factors include a personal history of colorectal cancer or adenomatous polyps, a first-degree relative with colon cancer or adenomas, chronic inflammatory bowel disease, prior cancer-related abdominopelvic radiation, or known or suspected hereditary syndrome such as hereditary nonpolyposis colon cancer (Lynch syndrome) or familial adenomatous polyposis (Smith, 2018a).

Lung Cancer

In the United States, this cancer is estimated to account for 13 percent of all new cancers diagnosed in women in 2019 (Siegel, 2019). It is now the leading cause of cancer-related death in both men and women. Cumulative exposure to tobacco smoke is an important risk factor for lung cancer; thus all smokers should be advised of tobacco-use risks and encouraged to stop. A list of potential aids is found on page 13.

Lung cancer screening with low-dose computed tomography (CT) scanning is recommended for individuals aged 55 to 74, who have a 30-pack-year or longer history, who actively smoke or quit within the past 15 years, and who lack life-limiting comorbidities (Tanoue, 2015). One remembers that pack-year determination is calculated by multiplying the number of packs smoked per day by the number of years the person has smoked. By convention, one pack contains 20 cigarettes. Although a common diagnostic test, chest radiography is not recommended as a lung cancer screening tool.

Skin Cancer

The incidence of skin cancers (melanoma and non-melanomas) has risen in the United States during the past three decades. In 2019, melanoma was expected to account for 1 percent of all cancer deaths in women (Siegel, 2019). Skin cancer risks include fair complexion, use of indoor tanning beds, history of sunburns, family or personal history of skin cancer, and personal history of numerous moles (>100). The USPSTF (2016b) notes insufficient evidence to recommend whole body screening by physician or patient for skin cancer in the general adult population. It does advise clinicians to use the "ABCDE" system—asymmetry, border irregularity, color, diameter (>6 mm), and evolving over time—to evaluate skin lesions of concern and refer appropriately.

Lifestyle Changes

Smoking

Tobacco use is the leading preventable cause of disease, disability, and death in the United States and has been linked with certain cancers, cardiovascular disease, chronic lung diseases, and stroke (Barboza, 2016). Moreover, specific to women's health, smoking is linked to diminished fertility, pregnancy complications, and postoperative complications.

Almost 70 percent of adults who smoke daily are interested in quitting, and approximately half attempted to quit in the previous year. Guidelines from the USPSTF recommend that clinicians ask all patients about tobacco use, advise them to stop, and provide brief behavioral interventions (Siu, 2015a).

Behavioral interventions can be effective for any health-related lifestyle change. The five A's framework is a useful strategy for engaging patients and is tailored for smoking cessation in this example.

- Ask: every patient about tobacco use
- Advise: all users to quit
- Assess: her willingness to quit and decide if she is in a (1) precontemplation, (2) contemplation, (3) preparation, or (4) action phase. Her stage of readiness guides further discussion
- Assist: her attempts to quit (develop plan together)
- Arrange: for follow-up

Many behavioral interventions are available including local or community group programs, brief in-person behavioral counseling sessions, or even telephone counseling interventions. Patients can be referred to the National Cancer Institute's smoking cessation website: www.smokefree.gov or toll-free quit line: 1-800-QUIT-NOW. These supports provide free, evidence-based information, professional assistance, and in some cases free or discounted cessation medications.

Pharmacotherapy interventions approved by the FDA are bupropion SR, varenicline, and nicotine replacement therapy. These can be used in combination with behavioral interventions, and their use together can improve cessation rates. If appropriate, pharmacologic treatments to aid smoking cessation can be offered to all interested women and are listed in Table 1-6. Gynecologists who are proficient in the use of these therapies may prescribe. Referral is also appropriate (American College of Obstetricians and Gynecologists, 2014).

Exercise

Exercise is known to help prevent coronary artery disease, diabetes, osteoporosis, obesity, depression, insomnia, and multiple types of cancer (Piercy, 2018). Many of these associations result from the effects of exercise to help lower blood pressure, improve blood sugar control, reduce weight, and decrease low-density lipoprotein (LDL) cholesterol levels (Eckel, 2014).

In 2018, an estimated 10 percent of the premature mortality rate was associated with inadequate physical activity (Piercy, 2018). Recommendations from the U.S. Department of Health and Human Services (2018) include moderate-intensity activity for at least 150 minutes each week *or* vigorous-intensity activities for 75 minutes each week. When counseling patients on physical activity, the "talk test" is helpful to determine activity intensity. Generally, a woman doing moderate-intensity aerobic exercise can talk, but not sing, during the activity. A person doing vigorous-intensity activity generally cannot say more than a few words without pausing for a breath. Current evidence also supports raising routine daily physical activity levels, such as taking the stairs rather than the elevator (Piercy, 2018).

Research supports biweekly muscle-strengthening exercise that involves all the major muscle groups. Sedentary behavior, specifically time spent sitting, has also become of interest. Guidelines are beginning to address risks, but no recommendations are currently available.

Obesity

Associated Risks and Diagnosis

In 2016, 40 percent of women in the United States were obese, and this reflects a steady rise over the previous decade (Hales, 2018). Possible consequences include diabetes mellitus, nonalcoholic fatty liver disease, hypertension, hyperlipidemia, heart disease, osteoarthritis, and obstructive sleep apnea. Gynecologic issues related to obesity include abnormal menstruation, risks for endometrial neoplasia, and worsening polycystic ovary syndrome. Some hormonal contraceptives and emergency contraceptives may have lower efficacy in obese women. And, during pregnancy, obese women suffer higher rates of cesarean delivery, gestational diabetes, preeclampsia, and postpartum hemorrhage, among others (Hawkins, 2018). Even if not trained as weight management specialists, clinicians ideally screen for obesity, provide initial obesity evaluation and management, and refer as needed.

Screening is accomplished with calculation of body mass index (BMI). BMI, although not a direct measure of body fat content, is valuable in assessing the risk for weight-related complications. Several online calculators can be found. For adolescents (and children), BMI is adjusted for age and gender and calculated as a percentile. A BMI calculator for adolescents can be found at http://apps.nccd.cdc.gov/dnpabmi/.calculator.aspx. Table 1-7 reflects the definitions for underweight, overweight, and obesity for adolescents and adults. Adult obesity is further divided. Class 1 is a BMI 30 to 34.9 kg/m^2, class 2 is 35 to 39.9 kg/m^2, and class 3 is ≥40 kg/m^2. Class 3 obesity is often referred to as extreme obesity.

No standard single or panel laboratory test is indicated for an obese woman. Evaluation for comorbidities is tailored and factors her family and social histories. Blood pressure measurement, fasting lipid and glucose level screening, and thyroid function testing can all be considered for these patients during initial evaluation.

TABLE 1-6. Drugs Used for Smoking Cessation

Agent	Brand Name	Initial Dosing	Maintenance	Therapy Duration	Additional Considerations
Nicotine Replacement					
Patch[d]	Habitrol Nicoderm CQ	If >10 CPD: a 21-mg patch is reapplied daily wk 1–6 If <10 CPD: 14-mg patch for wk 1–6	14-mg patch is used wk 7–8	8–12 wk	
Gum[d]	Nicorette 2 mg 4 mg (if ≥25 CPD)	1 piece every 1–2 hr for wk 1–6 (maximum 24 pieces/d)	1 piece every 2–4 hr for wk 7–9	12 wk	Not chewed like regular gum, "chew and park" Not for those with extensive dental work
Lozenge[b]	Commit 2 mg 4 mg (if smokes <30 min after waking)	1 piece every 1–2 hr for wk 1–6 (maximum 20 pieces/d)	1 piece every 2–4 hr for wk 7–9	12 wk	Do not eat 15 min prior
Inhaler[d]	Nicotrol		6 (average use) to 16 cartridges puffed qd for 12 wk	12–24 wk	More expensive
Nasal spray[d]	Nicotrol		1 dose = 1 spray to each nostril per hr (maximum 5 doses/hr & 40/d)	12–24 wk	More expensive
Nicotine Agonists					
Varenicline[c]	Chantix	0.5 mg PO qd for 3 d, then 0.5 mg PO bid for next 4 d	1 mg PO bid	12 wk	Start 1 wk before quit date Avoid if history of suicide ideation or attempt; nausea is common
CNS Agents					
Bupropion[c]	Wellbutrin SR Zyban	1–2 wk prior to cessation: 150 mg PO qd for 3 d	150 mg PO bid	7–12 wk; may use for 6 mo.	Start 1 wk before quit date Avoid in patients with disordered eating, seizures, insomnia
Nortriptyline[a,d]		25 mg PO qd with gradual increase	75–100 mg PO qd	12 wk; may use for 6 mo.	Start at least 10 d before quit date
Clonidine[a,c]	Catapres-TTS	0.1-mg transdermal patch is changed weekly	0.1- to 0.2-mg transdermal patch weekly		Use limited by: dry mouth, sedation, postural hypotension

[a]Recommended as second-line agents by U.S. Department of Health and Human Services (Fiori, 2008).
[b]Has not been evaluated by the Food and Drug Administration (FDA) for pregnancy.
[c]Considered an FDA pregnancy category C drug.
[d]Considered an FDA pregnancy category D drug.
bid = twice daily; CNS = central nervous system; CPD = cigarettes per day; PO = orally; qd = daily.

TABLE 1-7. Definitions of Abnormal Weight for Adults and Adolescents Using Body Mass Index

Age Group	Underweight	Overweight	Obese	Extreme Obesity
Adolescent	<5th percentile for age	85th to 95th percentile for age	>95th percentile for age	
Adult	<18.5	25–29.9	Class I: 30–34.9 Class 2: 35–39.9	Class 3: ≥40

For a woman with an elevated BMI, a clinician assesses her readiness for change and thereby, provides appropriate guidance, support, or referral. In addition, questions regarding previous attempts at weight loss, social hurdles that impede diet and exercise change, and detrimental eating habits are discussed.

Treatment

Effective weight loss is best achieved by assisting patients in making healthier dietary, physical activity, and behavioral choices that will lead to a net negative caloric balance. The initial goal is to achieve a 5 to 10 percent weight loss over the initial 6 months of treatment (Jensen, 2014; National Heart, Lung, and Blood Institute, 2013). Caloric reduction is the most important component, whereas increased and sustained physical activity is particularly important in maintenance. Table 1-8 illustrates recommended guidelines to direct therapy for overweight or obese women. Several clinician and patient aids can be found in *Managing Overweight or Obesity in Adults*, available at: www.nhlbi.nih.gov/health-topics/managing-overweight-obesity-in-adults.

One of the most effective strategies encourages self-monitoring with a diet/activity calorie tracker. Many free versions are accessible either online or through smartphone applications. One sponsored by the U.S. Department of Agriculture is available at: www.choosemyplate.gov. Women are encouraged to follow a low-calorie diet that yields a 500 kcal/d deficit. This is an intake of 1200 to 1500 kcal/d (Jensen, 2014; National Heart, Lung, and Blood Institute, 2013). Specific daily calorie requirements by gender and age from the Institute of Medicine (2002) are listed at: www.health.gov/dietaryguidelines/2015/guidelines/appendix-2/.

In addition to diet and exercise, pharmacologic or surgical options may be advised for selected obese patients. Table 1-9 outlines specifics of weight loss medications. Orlistat (Xenical) is a reversible inhibitor of gastric and pancreatic lipases and blocks the digestion and absorption of approximately 30 percent of dietary fat (Kushner, 2018). This drug is approved for over-the-counter use at half the prescription strength (Allī). Because of its action, fatty stools and increased defecation are common side effects. Severe liver injury has been reported rarely, and labeling reflects this risk (Food and Drug Administration, 2010). Orlistat can reduce the absorption of fat-soluble vitamins, and patients are advised to take a daily oral multivitamin (Bray, 2013). Combination oral contraceptive action is not reduced by orlistat (Hartmann, 1996). This agent is not recommended during pregnancy but does not appear teratogenic (Källén, 2014). Orlistat is poorly absorbed, and thus theoretically is unlikely to reach significant breast milk levels (Briggs, 2017).

Four medications have been approved by the FDA since 2012: lorcaserin, phentermine-topiramate, naltrexone-bupropion, and liraglutide. Each suppresses appetite, and all are approved in conjunction with a reduced-calorie diet. These medications have met stringent FDA requirements, which included predetermined measures of effectiveness (5 percent mean weight loss after 1 year) and postmarketing long-term cardiovascular disease outcome trials (Kushner, 2018). The FDA recommends evaluation of weight loss after 3 to 4 months. This is based on observations that those who fail to lose weight early are less successful at 1 year. Choice of a specific agent is individualized and may be driven by comorbidities. For example, liraglutide might be more appropriate for a woman with diabetes (Khera, 2016). None of these are recommended during pregnancy or lactation.

Lorcaserin is a serotonin-receptor agonist used to suppress appetite. Naltrexone SR-bupropion SR (Contrave) is a combination of naltrexone, which is FDA approved for the treatment of alcohol dependence and opioid blockade, and bupropion, an antidepressant and smoking cessation aid.

Phentermine-topiramate (Qsymia) is a combination medication and is gradually titrated upward as needed. This drug has fetotoxicity potential and prescribing providers must participate in a Risk Evaluation and Mitigation Strategy (REMS) program. REMS are safety strategies mandated by the FDA to help manage known risks associated with a medicine yet still allow patients to have access to the benefits of a given drug.

Liraglutide is a glucagon-like peptide-1 receptor agonist delivered by self-administered subcutaneous injection. In studies, mean

TABLE 1-8. Treatment Recommendations According to BMI

Treatment	BMI 25–26.9	BMI 27–29.9	BMI 30–34.9	BMI 35–39.9	BMI ≥ 40
Diet, activity, behavioral therapy	WCM	WCM	+	+	+
Pharmacotherapy	—	WCM	+	+	+
Surgery	—	—	—	WCM	+

+ represents the use of indicated treatment regardless of comorbidities; BMI = body mass index; WCM = with comorbidities (type 2 DM, hypertension, obstructive sleep apnea, heart disease).

TABLE 1-9. Drugs Used for Weight Loss

Agent (Brand Name)	Oral[a] Daily Dosing	Mechanism	Placebo-subtracted Wt. Loss at 1 Year (%)	Adverse Effects
Gastrointestinal Fat Blocker				
Orlistat (Xenical, Alli)	120 mg three times	Blocks digestion and absorption of fat	n/a (6.2 kg avg. wt. loss)	Oily stools, fecal urgency or fecal incontinence
Appetite Suppressant				
Lorcaserin (Belviq)	10 mg twice	Serotonin receptor agonist	3.2	Headache, dizziness, increased heart rate or blood pressure
Phentermine/ topiramate (Qsymia)	3.75 mg/23 mg once for 2 wks, then 7.5 mg/46 mg once for 12 wks	Similar to amphetamines, appetite suppressed and satiety enhanced	8.4	Paraesthesia, dizziness, dysgeusia, insomnia, constipation, dry mouth
Naltrexone/bupropion (Contrave)	8 mg/90 mg (1 tab); titrate up by 1 tab each wk to reach 2 tabs twice daily	Opioid antagonist, antidepressant	4.0	Headache, GI side effects, insomnia, dry mouth
Liraglutide (Saxenda)	0.6 mg SC; titrate up by 0.6 mg SC each wk to reach 3 mg SC once daily	GLP-1 agonist, slows gastric emptying, decreases food intake	5.0	GI side effects

[a]Except for liraglutide.
GI = gastrointestinal; GLP-1 = glucagon-like peptide-1 receptor agonist; n/a = not available; SC = subcutaneously; Wt. = weight.

weight loss averages 6 to 8 percent (Davies, 2015; Pi-Sunyer, 2015). Liraglutide has an associated risk for pancreatitis. Because of this and an unclear risk of medullary thyroid carcinoma, the FDA requires participation in a REMS program. This drug is contraindicated for women with a family or personal history of medullary thyroid carcinoma or multiple endocrine neoplasia (Novo Nordisk, 2017).

Bariatric surgery is an important consideration for women with BMIs ≥40 or with BMIs ≥35 if other comorbid conditions are present (Garber, 2018). Of available laparoscopic procedures, three are more commonly performed and fall into two categories: restrictive (gastric banding, gastric sleeve) or malabsorptive (gastric bypass). Gastric banding places an adjustable plastic ring around the stomach to limit food intake. Sleeve gastrectomy removes 80 percent of the body of the stomach, creating a tubular sleeve appearance. Restrictive procedures produce modest weight loss and carry low surgical complication rates (Wolfe, 2016).

The Roux-en-Y gastric bypass creates a small stomach pouch that is connected directly to the jejunum to bypass the duodenum. This reduces calorie and nutrient absorption and can lead to substantial weight loss in individuals with morbid obesity. Gastric bypass has been linked with improvement in comorbid risk factors and decreased mortality rates. However, common long-term problems can include malabsorption of micronutrients such as iron, folate, calcium/vitamin D, and vitamin B_{12} (Abdeen, 2016).

Following bariatric surgery, patients are advised to delay pregnancy for 12 to 24 months (American College of Obstetricians and Gynecologists, 2017a). Rapid weight loss during this time poses theoretical risks for intrauterine fetal-growth restriction and nutritional deprivation. However, as weight is lost, fertility rates overall appear to improve, and risks for pregnancy rise (Merhi, 2009). Thus, effective contraception is needed. Most contraceptive methods appear to be as effective in women with elevated BMIs compared with normal-weight controls. However, the contraceptive patch (OrthoEvra) is less effective in those weighing more than 90 kg (Zieman, 2002). Specific to those with malabsorptive bariatric surgery types, oral contraception efficacy may be lower due to poor absorption (Curtis, 2016). Last, due to its risk for associated weight gain, depot medroxyprogesterone acetate (Depo-Provera) may be an unpopular choice in women trying to lose weight.

■ Cardiovascular Disease

This is the leading cause of death in the United States. In 2011 to 2014, 36 percent of women were affected by cardiovascular disease (CVD), and more than 410,000 women died from its complications (Benjamin, 2018). Stratification of CVD predispositions can identify vulnerable patients for management or referral (Table 1-10). Ideal goals for exercise, glucose and lipid levels, blood pressure, and smoking cessation are discussed in other sections of this chapter.

TABLE 1-10. Classification of Cardiovascular Disease (CVD) in Women

≥1 assigns high-risk status	Known CHD or CVD Peripheral arterial disease Abdominal aortic aneurysm End-stage renal disease Diabetes mellitus
≥1 assigns at-risk status	Smoking SBP ≥120 or DBP ≥80 mm Hg, or treated hypertension Total cholesterol ≥200 mg/dL, HDL <50 mg/dL, or treated dyslipidemia Obesity Poor diet Physical inactivity Family history of premature CVD Metabolic syndrome Autoimmune collagen-vascular disease Prior PIH or gestational DM

CHD = coronary heart disease; CVD = cardiovascular disease; DBP = diastolic blood pressure; DM = diabetes mellitus; HDL = high-density lipoprotein; PIH = pregnancy-induced hypertension; SBP = systolic blood pressure.
Abbreviated from Mosca, 2011.

■ Chronic Hypertension

Nearly 45 million American women are hypertensive, and this accounted for 33 percent of U.S. women from 2011 to 2014. The risk of hypertension rises with age and is higher for black women compared with those of other races (Benjamin, 2018). Chronic hypertension raises the risks for myocardial infarction, stroke, congestive heart failure, renal disease, and peripheral vascular disease. Moreover, chronic hypertension and its potential therapies may limit contraception choices for some women. Thus, gynecologists ideally are familiar with criteria used to diagnose hypertension. Although many may choose to refer patients for hypertension treatment, gynecologists should be aware of target goals and long-term risks associated with this disease.

For adult screening, the American Heart Association (2017) recommends blood pressure assessment starting at age 20 and repeated evaluation every 2 years if initially normal (Table 1-11). For patients with elevated pressures, assessment is at least annually.

With screening, blood pressures are best taken with a woman seated in a chair with the tested arm resting on a table, at the level of the heart. Ideally, the patient has been able to rest quietly for a few minutes prior to measurement and to have refrained from tobacco and caffeine use immediately prior to testing. An appropriately sized cuff is selected, and the cuff bladder should encircle at least 80 percent of the arm. Hypertension is diagnosed if readings are elevated on at least two separate office visits over one or more weeks.

With the diagnosis of chronic hypertension, assessment then follows for both modifiable and nonmodifiable CVD risk

TABLE 1-11. Blood Pressure Categories in Women

BP Category	SBP (mm Hg)		DBP (mm Hg)
Normal	<120	and	<80
Elevated	120–129	and	<80
Stage 1 HTN	130–139	or	80–89
Stage 2 HTN	>140	or	>90

DBP = diastolic blood pressure; HTN = hypertension; SBP = systolic blood pressure.
Adapted from Whelton, 2018, with permission.

factors. Thus, routine laboratory tests recommended before initiating therapy include an electrocardiogram, urinalysis, blood glucose level, complete blood count, lipid profile, thyroid testing, and serum potassium and creatinine level measurement. A more extensive search for identifiable underlying causes is not generally indicated unless hypertension is not controlled with initial treatment (Table 1-12) (Whelton, 2018).

For treatment, lifestyle changes that mirror those for CVD are encouraged. However, if blood pressure is significantly elevated or resistant to lifestyle modification alone, then pharmacologic treatment may be needed to decrease long-term complications. Recommendations are shown in Table 1-13, and the target blood pressure with treatment is <130/80 mm Hg.

■ Stroke

This is the fifth leading cause of death in the United States, and in 2014, approximately 425,000 American women suffered a new or recurrent stroke (Benjamin, 2018). Gender-specific risk

TABLE 1-12. Identifiable Causes of Hypertension

Common	Renal parenchymal disease
	Renovascular disease
	Primary aldosteronism
	Obstructive sleep apnea
	Drug/alcohol
	  Caffeine
	  Smoking
	  Alcohol
	  NSAIDs
	  Oral contraceptives
	  Cyclosporine
	  Decongestant/anorectics
	  Herbal medicines (ephedra, ma huang)
	  Cocaine and amphetamines
	Adrenal steroids

Uncommon	Pheochromocytoma Thyroid or parathyroid disease Cushing syndrome Coarctation of the aorta Congenital adrenal hyperplasia

NSAIDs = nonsteroidal antiinflammatory drugs.

TABLE 1-13. Initial Drug Therapy for Adults with Hypertension

Health Status	Treatment
General	Nonblack: thiazide-type diuretic, ACEI, ARB, or CCB
	Black: thiazide-type diuretic or CCB
Renal disease	ACEI or ARB

ACEI = angiotensin-converting enzyme inhibitor; ARB = angiotensin-receptor blocker; BP = blood pressure; CCB = calcium-channel blocker.

factors for stroke in women include hypertension, atrial fibrillation, migraines with aura, and combination oral contraceptives. Low-dose aspirin use for the primary prevention of CVD is recommended only in women aged 50 to 59 years who have a ≥10 percent CVD risk (using the risk calculator outlined next) and are not at increased risk for bleeding (Bibbins-Domingo, 2016). No consensus describes the optimal dose or frequency of aspirin for stroke prevention. For women aged ≥60, the conversation balances risks of bleeding complications from aspirin against the benefits of stroke prevention for a given patient.

■ Dyslipidemia

Hypercholesterolemia

Serum cholesterol is known to be related to atherosclerotic CVD (ASCVD). The lipoprotein carriers are LDL, high-density lipoprotein (HDL), and very low-density lipoprotein (VLDL), and LDL is the dominant atherogenic form (Grundy, 2019). Other ASCVD risk factors include smoking, hypertension, dysglycemia, and advancing age. Using these, prediction models can estimate the risk of developing ASCVD. One tool is available through a smartphone application or accessible online at www.tools.acc.org/ASCVD-Risk-Estimator-Plus.

Preventively, adults aged ≥20 years ideally have lipids measured (either fasting or nonfasting) every 5 years. This profile includes measurement of total, LDL, and HDL cholesterol levels and triglyceride concentrations. If the initial nonfasting lipid profile reveals a triglycerides level ≥400 mg/dL, a fasting lipid is then performed (Grundy, 2019).

Lowering LDL levels is associated with reduced rates of ASCVD. Initial management usually begins with lifestyle and dietary changes. Lipid-lowering treatment for primary prevention is added for: (1) those with persisting LDL levels ≥190 mg/dL, (2) those aged 40 to 75 years with diabetes and LDL levels ≥70 mg/dL, and (3) those aged 40 to 75 years with an estimated 10-year risk of a cardiovascular event that is at least 7.5 percent (Stone, 2014). The risk estimator referenced above can help guide providers through recommendations and offer therapeutic advice.

Hypertriglyceridemia

Triglycerides are not directly atherogenic. Instead, they represent an important biomarker of CVD risk because of their association with proinflammatory, proatherogenic proteins found on all classes of the plasma lipoproteins. Because hypertriglyceridemia is associated with many other unique CVD risk factors, the benefit of lowering triglycerides directly remains uncertain (Jellinger, 2017). Triglycerides are particularly responsive to dietary adjustments, specifically restricting fat and carbohydrates. Omega-3 supplementation can also help lower levels. Medication therapy is reserved for those with triglyceride levels ≥500 mg/dL and is implemented to lower these levels to prevent pancreatitis.

■ Diabetes Mellitus

Diabetes is common, and approximately 14.9 million adult women in the United States are diabetic (Centers for Disease Control and Prevention, 2017a). The long-term consequences of this endocrine disorder are serious and include coronary heart disease, stroke, peripheral vascular disease, nephropathy, neuropathy, and retinopathy.

The USPSTF recommends screening of all adults aged 40 to 70 who are overweight or obese (Siu, 2015b). However, the American Diabetes Association (2019) recommends that screening be considered at 3-year intervals in those aged ≥45 or in those with a BMI ≥25 and one other risk factor (Table 1-14).

Diabetes and prediabetes may be diagnosed by various laboratory tests listed in Table 1-15. Measurement of plasma glucose concentration is performed on venous samples, and the aforementioned values are based on the use of such methods. Capillary blood glucose testing using a blood glucometer is an effective monitoring tool but is not recommended for diagnostic use.

For those diagnosed with diabetes, referral to an internist is usually indicated. Control of blood glucose levels reduces microvascular complications such as CVD, neuropathy, and nephropathy. Lifestyle optimization is essential for all patients with diabetes, and weight loss is recommended for overweight or obese patients with prediabetes or diabetes mellitus type 2. If lifestyle modification is insufficient for glucose control, many therapeutic options are available for patients in lieu of insulin. To lower diabetic morbidity, therapy goals for otherwise normal patients include hemoglobin A_{1c} levels below

TABLE 1-14. Adult Risk Factors for Diabetes

Age ≥45 years
Body mass index ≥25
Affected first-degree relative
Physical inactivity
Ethnicity: African-, Hispanic-, Native-, and Asian-Americans; Pacific Islanders
Prior prediabetes-range test values
Prior gestational diabetes mellitus
Hypertension (≥140/90 mm Hg or on therapy)
HDL cholesterol <35 mg/dL and/or triglyceride level >250 mg/dL
Polycystic ovary syndrome
Acanthosis nigricans
Cardiovascular disease

HDL = high-density lipoprotein.

TABLE 1-15. Diagnostic Criteria for Diabetes Mellitus

HbA$_{1C}$ ≥6.5%

or

Fasting plasma glucose ≥126 mg/dL. Fasting is no caloric intake for at least 8 hr

or

2-hr plasma glucose ≥200 mg/dL during an OGTT

or

Symptoms of diabetes plus random plasma glucose concentration ≥200 mg/dL. Classic symptoms of diabetes include polyuria, polydipsia, and unexplained weight loss

Criteria for Increased Diabetes Risk (prediabetes)

Fasting plasma glucose: 100–125 mg/dL

or

2-hr plasma glucose during 75-g OGTT: 140–199 mg/dL

or

HbA$_{1C}$: 5.7–6.4%

FPG = fasting plasma glucose; HbA$_{1c}$ = hemoglobin A$_{1c}$; OGTT = oral glucose tolerance test.

6.5 percent, blood pressure readings <130/80 mm Hg, LDL levels <100 mg/dL, triglyceride levels <150 mg/dL, weight control, and smoking cessation (Garber, 2018).

Patients with prediabetes, that is, impaired fasting glucose or impaired glucose tolerance, have an elevated risk for developing diabetes. To avert or delay this, management includes greater physical activity and weight loss, drugs such as metformin, nutritional counseling, and yearly diabetes screening. Medications, including weight loss medications discussed earlier, can be considered for those meeting criteria (p. 14).

■ Metabolic Syndrome

The metabolic syndrome refers to a clustering of specific CVD risk factors with the underlying pathophysiology thought to be related to insulin resistance (Grundy, 2005; Kahn, 2005). The components include insulin resistance, visceral obesity, hypertension, and low HDL but high triglyceride levels.

When the metabolic syndrome was initially identified, it served as a useful paradigm to draw attention to the fact that CVD risk factors often clustered in patients. Over time, as risk assessments and screening guidelines have advanced, the clinical usefulness of the metabolic syndrome has waned. If identified, management of the syndrome does not differ from management of individual risk factors and focuses on lifestyle modification discussed in earlier sections.

■ Thyroid Disease

The risk of thyroid disease accrues with age, and dysfunction is more common in women. Expert panels disagree regarding thyroid screening of the general population. Only the American Thyroid Association recommends that adults, especially women, be screened for thyroid dysfunction by measurement of a serum thyroid-stimulating hormone (TSH) concentration, beginning at age 35 and then again every 5 years. Other organizations' guidelines recommend screening in older women or those with risk factors for thyroid disease (LeFevre, 2015). People at higher risk include the elderly and those with prior head or neck radiation, thyroid surgery, autoimmune disease, type 1 diabetes mellitus, affected first-degree relative, pituitary disease, or lithium use.

■ Geriatric Screening

Women are now living longer, and the current life expectancy for women in the United States is 81 years (Arias, 2017). As a woman moves past menopause, many of her health care needs may not be gynecologic.

Of these, functional status is a patient's ability to perform both basic and complex activities for independent living. Basic activities are grooming and toileting, whereas bill paying and housekeeping are more complex instrumental activities of daily living (Katz, 1963; Lawton, 1969). Declines in functional status are linked to higher risks of hospitalization, institutionalization, and death. Identifying this status loss may permit early intervention.

Loss of cognitive function may present as short- and long-term memory loss, difficulty with problem solving, or inattention to personal hygiene. Although not expert in the diagnosis of cognitive problems, a gynecologist can perform initial screening that either reassures or prompts more formal evaluation by a geriatrician or neurologist. During Medicare Annual Wellness Visits (AWV), cognitive evaluation is a mandatory component.

For screening purposes, the test choice ideally matches the level of concern. For patients in whom cognitive impairment is thought unlikely, the clock-drawing test can provide reassurance. For this test, a person is asked to draw a clock with "the hands set to 10 past 11." A correct clock has numbers 1 through 12 labeled correctly in a clockwise fashion, with two arms (of any length) pointing at the correct numbers for the time requested. Any error or refusal to complete the clock is considered abnormal.

The Mini-Cog Test can also screen for mild cognitive impairment in the primary care setting (Janssen, 2017). The Mini-Cog test requires approximately 3 minutes to administer and begins by giving the patient three items to remember early in the interview. Later in discussion, she is asked to recall those three items. For a Mini-Cog Test result suggestive of dementia, referral to an internist, geriatrician, or neurologist is indicated.

Last, in those for whom impairment is a possibility, the Montreal cognitive assessment (MOCA) can be used to screen (Nasreddine, 2005). This tool assesses different cognitive domains and may characterize a cognitive impairment more precisely than the clock or Mini-Cog tests.

■ Mental Health
Depression

For women of all ages, mood disorders are pervasive and account for significant morbidity and mortality. These are discussed in detail in Chapter 14 (p. 302) and should be screened for

TABLE 1-16. Insomnia Medications Approved by the U.S. Food and Drug Administration

Medication: Brand	Dose
Benzodiazepines	
Temazepam: Restoril	7.5–30 mg
Estazolam: ProSom	0.5–2 mg
Triazolam: Halcion	0.125–0.25 mg
Flurazepam: Dalmane	15–30 mg
Quazepam: Doral	7.5–15 mg
Benzodiazepine-receptor Agonists	
Eszopiclone: Lunesta	1–3 mg
Zolpidem: Ambien,	5–10 mg
Ambien CR[a]	6.25–12.5 mg
Intermezzo[b]	1.75 mg
Zaleplon: Sonata	5–20 mg
Melatonin-receptor Agonist	
Ramelteon: Rozerem	8 mg
Melatonin-receptor Agonist	
Doxepin: Silenor	3–6 mg
Dual Orexin-receptor Antagonist	
Suvorexant: Belsomra	5–20 mg

[a]Extended release form.
[b]Indicated for middle-of-night awakening.

during routine health visits. For depression, the Personal Health Questionnaire-2 (PHQ2) is a simple, two-question screening tool (Kroenke, 2003). Questions are: "During the past 2 weeks, have you felt down, depressed, or hopeless?" and "Have you felt little interest or pleasure in doing things?" A positive screening result should prompt evaluation for depression (Chap. 14, p. 303).

Insomnia

Insomnia is common. It is defined as trouble initiating or maintaining sleep, despite adequate opportunity and circumstances for sleep, and is associated with daytime consequences (Sateia, 2017). Insomnia may be primary or may be secondary to other conditions such as depression, restless leg syndrome, stimulant use, menopause symptoms, and sleep apnea (Baker, 2018).

Insomnia is typically treated first with cognitive-behavioral therapy (CBT) (Sateia, 2017). Cognitive therapy is aimed at changing patients' beliefs and attitudes regarding sleep. Components include control of sleep timing and duration, attempts to improve the bedroom environment, or relaxation or biofeedback techniques. Medications may be added to aid sleep, and many work via benzodiazepine receptors. Table 1-16 lists medications FDA-approved for insomnia. Although lacking an FDA indication for insomnia, commonly prescribed agents are benzodiazepines, sedating antidepressants, sedating antipsychotics, and anticonvulsants (Buysse, 2013). Shared decision-making is ideally used for insomnia pharmacotherapy as evidence is insufficient to support use of medications, both FDA-approved and off label, for chronic insomnia.

■ Preconceptional Counseling

Value lies in counseling women before conception so that each pregnancy is planned with the goal to achieve the best maternal and fetal outcomes. With this in mind, topics found in Table 1-17 are ideally addressed.

TABLE 1-17. Preconceptional Counseling Topics

Topic	Recommendations
Abnormal weight	Calculate BMI yearly. $BMI \geq 25 \ kg/m^2$: Counsel on diet. Test for DM and metabolic syndrome if indicated $BMI \leq 18.5 \ kg/m^2$: Assess for eating disorder
Exercise	Uncomplicated pregnancy, engage in exercise before, during, and after
Substance abuse	Discuss perinatal effects of opioids, cocaine, methamphetamine, alcohol, smoking. Offer cessation options
Heart disease	Optimize function. Discuss warfarin, ACE inhibitor, and ARB teratogenicity, and if possible, switch agents prior to conception. Offer genetic counseling to women with congenital cardiac anomalies.
Hypertension	*Long-standing HTN*: assess ventricular hypertrophy, retinopathy, and renal disease. Discuss ACE inhibitor and ARB teratogenicity, and switch agents prior to conception
Asthma	Optimize function. Provide appropriate influenza and pneumococcal vaccines
Thrombophilia	Question for personal or family history of thrombotic events or recurrent poor pregnancy outcomes. If found, screen those contemplating pregnancy. Offer genetic counseling to those with known thrombophilia. Discuss warfarin teratogenicity, and switch agent, if possible, prior to conception
Renal disease	Optimize HTN. Discuss ACE inhibitor and ARB teratogenicity, and switch agents prior to conception
GI disease	*Inflammatory bowel disease*: Counsel on subfertility and risks of adverse pregnancy outcomes. Discuss MTX and mycophenolate mofetil, and switch agents, if possible, prior to conception

(Continued)

TABLE 1-17. Preconceptional Counseling Topics *(Continued)*

Topic	Recommendations
Liver disease	*Hepatitis B*: Vaccinate all high-risk women prior to conception (Table 1-1, p. 4). Counsel chronic carriers on transmission prevention to partners and fetus *Hepatitis C*: Screen as indicated in Table 1-1, p. 4. Counsel affected women on risks of perinatal transmission. Refer for antiviral treatment, discuss risks of treatment during pregnancy
Blood disorders	*Iron-deficiency anemia:* Offer iron supplementation *Sickle-cell disease:* Screen all black women. Test partner as indicated *Thalassemias:* Screen all women *von Willebrand disease:* Counsel regarding postpartum hemorrhage risk
Diabetes	Optimize glucose control, especially periconceptionally due to known teratogenicity. Evaluate for retinopathy, nephropathy, HTN
Thyroid disease	Screen those with thyroid disease symptoms. Ensure iodine-sufficient diet. Treat overt hyper- or hypothyroidism prior to conception
CT disease	*RA and other inflammatory arthritides*: Counsel on flare risk after pregnancy. Discuss MTX and leflunomide teratogenicity, and switch agents prior to conception *SLE*: Optimize disease. Discuss mycophenolate mofetil and cyclophosphamide teratogenicity, and switch agents, if possible, prior to conception
Neurologic disorder	*Seizure disorder:* Optimize control using monotherapy, if possible
Psychiatric disorder	*Depression:* Screen for symptoms. If affected, counsel on risks of treatment and of untreated illness and high risk of peripartum exacerbation
Skin disease	Discuss isotretinoin and etretinate teratogenicity, and switch agents prior to conception
Cancer	*Current:* Counsel on fertility preservation options prior to cancer therapy and on decreased fertility following certain agents. Offer genetic counseling to those with mutation-linked cancers. Evaluate cardiac function in those given cardiotoxic agents. Discuss SERM teratogenicity, and switch agents prior to conception. Discuss possible teratogenic effects of chemotherapy if continued during pregnancy *Prior:* Update mammography for those given childhood chest radiotherapy. Discuss pregnancy risks of childhood abdominopelvic radiation (Chap. 28, p. 616)
Infectious diseases	*Influenza:* Vaccinate all women prior to flu season *Malaria:* Avoid travel to endemic areas; chemoprophylaxis during conception *Rubella* or *Varicella:* Assess immunity, vaccinate as needed, and offer effective BCM during next 3 mos. *Tuberculosis:* Screen high-risk women and treat *Tetanus:* Update vaccination, as needed *Zika:* Abstain or use condoms after possible exposure for males (3 mos.) or females (2 mos.)
STDs	*Gonorrhea, syphilis, chlamydial infection:* Screen per Table 1-1 (p. 4) and treat as indicated *HIV:* For infection, treat prior to conception to decrease perinatal transmission. For discordant couple prevention, discuss PrEP if male partner viral load is not suppressed or is unknown (Chap. 3, p. 87). *HPV:* Screen per guidelines (Chap. 29, p. 630). Vaccinate as indicated *HSV:* Provide serological screening to asymptomatic women with affected partners. Counsel affected women on perinatal transmission risks and prophylaxis during the third trimester and labor

ACE = angiotensin-converting enzyme; ARB = angiotensin-receptor blocker; BMI = body mass index; CT = connective tissue; DM = diabetes mellitus; GI = gastrointestinal; HIV = human immunodeficiency virus; HPV = human papillomavirus; HSV = herpes simplex virus; HTN = hypertension; MTX = methotrexate; PrEP = preexposure prophylaxis; RA = rheumatoid arthritis; SERM = selective estrogen-receptor modulator; SLE = systemic lupus erythematosus; STD = sexually transmitted disease.

Compiled from American College of Obstetricians and Gynecologist, 2017c,e, 2019; Centers for Disease Control and Prevention, 2017b, 2018b; Jack, 2008; Kim, 2018.

VIOLENCE AGAINST WOMEN

■ Sexual Violence

Sexual violence is a broad term that includes rape, unwanted genital touching, intimidation to acquiesce to sex, and forced viewing of or involvement in pornography (Basile, 2014). *Rape* is a legal term and in the United States refers to penetration or attempted penetration of a body orifice without consent and with force or the threat of force or incapacity (Federal Bureau of Investigation, 2013). A few states mandate clinicians to report rape of a competent adult to a law enforcement agency, and one list is provided by the National District Attorney Association (2016). In other states, law enforcement is involved at the patient's request. For the elderly and children, reporting is mandatory.

Large population-based surveys indicate a lifetime prevalence for sexual violence of 19 percent among women (Smith, 2017). Certain populations are at greater risk and include the disabled; lesbian, bisexual, or transgender individuals; college students; and persons younger than 24 years (Basile, 2016; Fedina, 2018; Taylor, 2016; Walters, 2013).

Examination and Documentation

Initial evaluation of a sexual violence victim concentrates on identifying serious injuries that may be genital or often nongenital (Riggs, 2000; Zilkens, 2017a). Once life-threatening injuries are excluded, a systematic, thorough, and compassionate approach to obtaining a history and collecting evidence is essential for appropriate treatment of the victim and for future prosecution of her assailant (American College of Obstetricians and Gynecologists, 2016a).

Valid evidence may be collected from 3 to 7 days after sexual assault, and timing varies by jurisdiction. Immediate examination enhances the opportunity to obtain valuable physical evidence. Consent is obtained prior to examination and evidence collection and is essential for entry of evidence in a court. Most states have standardized kits for collection, and completed kits are stored in a locked site to ensure that legal evidence procedures are maintained. Evidence collection does not commit a victim to pressing criminal charges. A patient is also counseled that she may terminate an examination if it is too emotionally or physically painful.

Evidence gathering follows the steps outlined in Table 1-18 (Department of Justice, 2013). In approximately 25 percent of female rape victims, evidence of anogenital injury is detected (Larsen, 2015; Zilkens, 2017b). Frequent injury types include tears, ecchymosis, abrasions, redness, and swelling (TEARS) (Slaughter, 1997). Common sites include the posterior fourchette, inner labial minora, and hymen. Colposcopy is used if available, and this technique raises detection rates of more subtle injuries (Astrup, 2012; Lenahan, 1998).

Treatment

Pregnancy Prevention. Medication prophylaxis to prevent pregnancy following sexual assault can be provided to at-risk women with reproductive organs. Among reproductive-aged victims, the risk of rape-related pregnancy approximates 5 percent per rape (Holmes, 1996). Emergency contraception can be administered for up to 120 hours after rape but is most effective in the first 24 hours (Table 5-10, p. 131).

A negative pregnancy test to exclude a preexisting pregnancy is confirmed before administering emergency contraception. This is especially true for ulipristal (Ella), a progesterone antagonist,

---

TABLE 1-18. Important Elements of Examination and Evidence Collection Following Sexual Assault

Physical Examination
Perform full body examination; record injuries on body diagram
Inspect vulva, inner thighs, anus, and buttock; add colposcopic inspection if available; record injuries on anogenital diagram
Inspect vagina and cervix; add colposcopic inspection if available

Evidence Collection
Collect clothing and associated debris as a patient disrobes onto cloth sheet
Comb head hair; trim any matted hair that contains secretions. Cut head hairs from patient for comparison[a]
Comb pubic hair; trim any matted hair that contains secretions. Cut pubic hair from patient for comparison[a]
Scrape debris from beneath fingernails if the victim scratched assailant's skin or clothing
Collect swabs from vagina, mouth, and anus if penetrated during assault
Wipe sites of possible secretion exposure with saline moistened swab; save and label swab. Common examples include inner labia minora, perineum, breasts, or neck
Smear each swab onto individual microscope slide; save and label slide[a]

Laboratory Testing
Obtain toxicology testing if examination suggests or if patient states drugging
Collect patient's blood or saliva to serve as DNA reference
Obtain swabs and blood for STD testing and prophylaxis as detailed in Table 1-19.

[a]Collection practices varies by jurisdiction.
STD = sexually transmitted disease.
From Department of Justice, 2013.

TABLE 1-19. Pregnancy and Sexually Transmitted Disease Prophylaxis Following Sexual Assault

Testing

Pregnancy test (urine or serum); repeat at 4–6 wks
Serum testing for hepatitis B surface antigen, surface antibody, and core antibody
Serum testing for HIV and syphilis; repeat at 4–6 wks and 3 mos.
NAAT for *Neisseria gonorrhoeae* and *Chlamydia trachomatis* from each penetrated site
NAAT for *Trichomonas vaginalis* from vagina
Microscopic evaluation of saline wet mount of vaginal discharge
If HIV PEP[a] is planned, add HCV antibody. Draw serum LFTs and serum creatinine level[b] and repeat both at 4–6 wks

Treatment

Levonorgestrel, ulipristal, or Yuzpe method for candidates: all dosages in Table 5-10 (p. 131)
Ceftriaxone 250 mg intramuscularly, single dose[c]
Azithromycin 1 g orally, single dose[c]
Metronidazole 2 g orally, single dose[c]
Hepatitis B vaccination if not previously vaccinated (Table 1-1, p. 4)
HPV vaccination if not previously vaccinated (Table 1-1, p. 4)
If exposure ≤72 hrs ago, HIV PEP offered to suitable candidates (see text). Regimen given daily for 28 days:
    Tenofovir disoproxil fumarate/emtricitabine (Truvada[d]) once daily **plus** raltegravir 400 mg (Isentress) twice daily

[a]Questions regarding PEP can be directed to the Clinician Consultation Center at 1-888-448-4911.
[b]With renal dysfunction and creatinine clearance <60 mL/min, tenofovir disoproxil fumarate/emtricitabine is not recommended, and consultation for other regimens is suggested.
[c]Antibiotic alternatives for exposure to *N gonorrhoeae*, *C trachomatis*, and *T vaginalis* are found in Chapter 3 (p. 56).
[d]Caution in those with chronic hepatitis B.
CBC = complete blood count; HCV = hepatitis C virus; HIV = human immunodeficiency virus; HPV = human papillomavirus; LFTs = liver function tests; NAAT = nucleic acid amplification test; PEP = postexposure prophylaxis.
Compiled from Centers for Disease Control and Prevention, 2015, 2016, 2018a; Seña, 2015.

because of fetal loss risks if used in the first trimester. With estrogen/progestin combinations, nausea and vomiting is a potential side effect, and an antiemetic can be prescribed 30 minutes prior to hormone administration (Table 42-9, p. 916).

Patients are informed that their next menses may be delayed following this prophylaxis. Although current regimens are 74 to 89 percent effective, pregnancy testing is repeated at the follow-up visit at 4 to 6 weeks (Task Force on Postovulatory Methods of Fertility Regulation, 1998; Trussell, 1996; Yuzpe, 1982).

Sexually Transmitted Disease Prevention. The risk of acquiring an STD after rape has been estimated but varies by circumstances. The risk for trichomoniasis approximates 12 percent; gonorrhea, 4 percent to 12 percent; chlamydial infection, 2 to 14 percent; and syphilis, 5 percent (Jenny, 1990; Schwarcz, 1990). General recommendations for STD screening and for prophylaxis are listed in Table 1-19.

Of these, postexposure prophylaxis (PEP) for human immunodeficiency virus (HIV) is recommended in selected cases following sexual assault. These include rape by an assailant known to be HIV infected or by a person of unknown HIV status if exposure represents a substantial risk for acquisition (Seña, 2015). With known HIV infection, the estimated acquisition risk is 1 per 10,000 receptive penile-vaginal exposures and 138 per 10,000 receptive penile-anal exposures (Patel, 2014). HIV transmission associated with receptive oral intercourse is rare.

For potential HIV PEP candidates, the risks and side effects of the medications and need for close monitoring are discussed. Nausea is a common side effect. Thus, a prescription for an antiemetic such as promethazine, to be used as needed, is commonly provided. Importantly, if an initial HIV test result in the victim is positive, PEP is stopped and replaced with appropriate long-term antiretroviral therapy.

Because of the emotional intensity of the experience, a woman may not recall all the information provided, and thus written instructions are helpful. Survivors are referred to local rape crisis centers and encouraged to visit within 1 to 2 days. Sexual assault victims receive subsequent medical reevaluation 1 to 2 weeks later. After 4 to 6 weeks, if initial test results were negative for pregnancy, HIV, or syphilis, these are repeated (see Table 1-19). These later tests capture conditions that may have been undetectable during initial screening. HIV is again screened for at 3 months (Centers for Disease Control and Prevention, 2016). Additional hepatitis B and HPV vaccines are provided as dictated by vaccination schedule (p. 9).

Psychological Response to Sexual Assault. Survivors of sexual assault may display an array of reactions that frequently include anxiety, agitation, crying, or a quiet, removed affect. Burgess and Holmstrom (1974) first characterized the "rape trauma syndrome" and its two response phases. The first acute disorganization phase lasts several weeks and is followed by a reorganization phase, lasting several weeks to years. Acutely, shock and disbelief, fear, shame, self-blame, humiliation, anger, isolation, grief, somatic manifestations, and loss of control are common. During the reorganization phase, feelings of vulnerability, despair, guilt, and shame may continue. Longitudinal data indicate that sexual assault survivors are at increased lifetime risk for posttraumatic stress disorder (PTSD), mood disorders, somatic symptoms, and suicide contemplation or attempt (Linden, 2011; Smith, 2017). Health care providers ideally enlist the input of social workers or rape crisis counselors to help evaluate the patient's immediate and future emotional and safety needs.

■ Child Sexual Abuse

Definitions of sexual abuse in the child mirror those in the adult (Basile, 2014; Federal Bureau of Investigation, 2013). From one large U.S. survey, the estimated overall prevalence of youth sexual violence for females is 8 percent (Merrick, 2018). Thus, indicators that should prompt evaluation include: (1) statements by the minor or family of abuse, (2) genital or anal injury without concordant history of unintentional trauma, (3) identification of semen or pregnancy, or (4) STD diagnosis beyond the incubation period of vertical (natal mother-to-child) transmission. Health care providers in the United States are mandated to report suspected child maltreatment to an appropriate agency, such as child protective services or a law enforcement agency (Child Welfare Information Gateway, 2016).

Determining whether anogenital findings in children are normal variants or indicative of assault can be difficult, and these have been categorized according to the likelihood of associated sexual abuse. An exhaustive list of normal and indeterminate signs has been compiled by Adams and associates (2018), and those considered diagnostic are listed in Table 1-20. A provider completing the examination should have formal training in the evaluation of suspected child sexual abuse. Importantly, acute injuries associated with child sexual abuse heal and resolve

rapidly. Thus, examination is completed as soon as assault is suspected (Smith, 2018b). As signs may be subtle, a careful history and full examination are carried out with the aid of photodocumentation, preferably using a colposcope.

The prevalence of STDs in child victims of sexual abuse is low (Girardet, 2009a). Thus, the decision to obtain specimens from a child is individualized. Situations that typically prompt child testing include: (1) signs or complaints of genital penetration or of an STD, (2) one STD already diagnosed, (3) suspected assailant with a high risk for STDs, (4) another household member with an STD, (5) abuse by a stranger, or (6) community with a high STD rate (Centers for Disease Control and Prevention, 2015).

Recommended testing includes a nucleic acid amplification test (NAAT) for *Neisseria gonorrhoeae* and *C trachomatis* from urine or vagina. Culture and wet mount evaluation of a vaginal swab specimen are preferred for *Trichomonas vaginalis* infection (Adams, 2018). Decisions regarding serologic testing for *Treponema pallidum*, HIV, and hepatitis B virus are individualized.

Although STDs found beyond the neonatal period raise suspicious for sexual abuse, this has exceptions. Perinatal transmission of *N gonorrhoeae*, *C trachomatis,* HIV, *T pallidum*, and *T vaginalis* is possible. Outside this circumstance, these infections suggest sexual contact. In contrast, herpes simplex virus, human papillomavirus, and *Molluscum contagiosum* infections can be transmitted nonsexually (Adams, 2018). Most hepatitis B virus infections in children result from household exposure to those chronically infected with the virus.

Routine STD prophylaxis for children who have been sexually abused is generally not recommended due to lower rates of infection and a greater guarantee of scheduled follow-up for test results. However, if the clinical setting dictates or if test results are found to be positive for infection, antibiotics are provided. Rates of HIV transmission following sexual abuse are also very low in children (Girardet, 2009b). However, HIV PEP is well tolerated by children and can be offered based on

---

TABLE 1-20. Findings of Sexual Contact in Suspected Child Sexual Abuse

Acute genital laceration or extensive bruising[a]
Acute perianal laceration
Hymeneal petechiae or abrasions
Perianal or fourchette scarring[a]
Healed hymeneal cleft(s) below 3 or 9 o'clock locations that extends to hymeneal base.
Signs of female genital mutilation (see Table 1-21)
Bite marks
Torn oral frenulum
Positive testing for *Neisseria gonorrhoeae, Chlamydia trachomatis, HIV, Treponema pallidum*[b]
Pregnancy
Sperm identified in specimens taken directly from a child's body

[a]If other medical conditions such as Crohn disease, coagulopathy, accident, or labial adhesion not explanatory for findings.
[b]If perinatal transmission, transmission from blood products, and needle contamination have been excluded.
HIV = human immunodeficiency virus.
Compiled from Adams, 2007, 2018; Chiesa, 2017.

the clinical setting and within the first 72 hours. The CDC (2015) recommends consulting professionals who specialize in care of HIV-infected children.

■ Elder Abuse

This is an intentional act or failure to act by a trusted individual that causes or creates a risk of harm to an older adult. Elder abuse may include neglect or physical, psychologic, sexual, or financial abuse (Hall, 2016). Approximately 10 percent of the elderly are mistreated each year (Acierno, 2010). Identified risk factors are caregiver stress, patient cognitive impairment, need for assistance with daily life activities, conflicted family relationships, and poor social support (Hoover, 2014). Similar to other forms of violence, elderly victims can suffer subsequent depression, anxiety, PTSD, and poor self-reported health (Acierno, 2017; Wong, 2017).

Signs that can be associated with abuse are decubitus ulcers, poor hygiene, poor adherence to medication regimens, or signs of trauma, sexual assault, dehydration, or malnutrition. Psychologic clues include depression, anxiety, cowering, vague somatic complaints, and social withdrawal (Lachs, 2015). Physicians are mandated in most states to report suspicion of elder abuse, and each state's "mandatory reporting" requirements are posted by the Department of Justice (2016). Sexual and physical assault will involve local law enforcement. Reports of other abuse forms are typically filed with the Adult Protective Services agency of the given state (National Adult Protective Services, 2018).

■ Intimate Partner Violence

Intimate-partner violence (IPV) refers to harm inflicted by one intimate partner on the other, with the intent of causing pain or controlling the other's behavior. *Domestic violence, violence against women,* and *gender-based violence* are older synonyms. *Honor-based violence (HBV)* is a subcategory in which male family members act against female members to maintain family honor in the community.

IPV takes various forms and includes sexual violence, physical violence, stalking, and psychological aggression or coercion (Breiding, 2015). Most victims have been assaulted more than once and often over the course of years. In the United States, nearly one third of women experienced physical violence by an intimate partner in their lifetime, one quarter suffered severe violence, and 16 percent have described contact sexual violence (Smith, 2017). Rates of IPV are higher in adolescents and those who witnessed violence as a child (Jung, 2019; Kann, 2018; Smith, 2017). Pregnant women may also be victims, and homicide is the leading cause of death during pregnancy (Palladino, 2011; Shadigian, 2005).

Diagnosis

Numerous health complications follow IPV. Short-term sequelae include acute injuries, pregnancy, and STD acquisition (Smith, 2017). Gravely, in the United States in 2015, 45 percent of female homicides were IPV-related (Jack, 2018). Long term, mental health consequences such as PTSD, anxiety, depression, suicide attempt, and substance abuse are prominent (Iverson, 2013). Chronic somatic complaints often focus on gastrointestinal dysfunction,

genitourinary pain, and other chronic pain (Campbell, 2002; Centers for Disease Control and Prevention, 2008). Effects on sexual function are discussed in Chapter 14 (p. 313).

Women who have been assaulted are far more likely to seek help from their medical provider. Although some clinicians may feel awkward asking patients, researchers agree that the single most important thing a physician can do for a battered woman is to ask about violence (American College of Obstetricians and Gynecologists, 2012). Additionally, symptoms or behaviors that may be associated with victimization are investigated. Numerous formal assessment tools are available from the CDC (Basile, 2007).

Management

If a patient discloses IPV, a clinician should validate and normalize a patient's perspective. Patients are counseled that many women have assault experiences, that most are afraid to confide these, that memories of the experience can be painful, and that a fear of future assaults is a reasonable fear. Following a patient's disclosure, a provider expresses concern for the woman's health and safety and conveys a willingness to discuss relationship issues at any time. Moreover, information describing community resources is offered. The National Domestic Violence Hotline (1-800-799-SAFE (7233)) is a nonprofit telephone referral service with access to more than 5000 shelters nationally.

Battery is a crime, yet few states specifically require mandatory reporting of IPV. Accordingly, each clinician should know their state laws, and one list has been compiled by Durborow and associates (2013). In addition, providers ideally thoroughly document physical findings of violence. Such data may be required if criminal charges are pursued.

■ Female Genital Mutilation

This practice refers to medically unnecessary vulvar modification. In the United States, it is a federal crime to perform unnecessary genital surgery on a girl younger than 18 years or to send or attempt to send her outside the country so it can be performed. That said, female genital mutilation (FGM) is practiced in countries within Africa, the Middle East, and Asia. As many as 200 million women worldwide have undergone one of these procedures, and approximately 513,000 girls in the United States were at risk for this practice in 2012 (Goldberg, 2016; UNICEF, 2016). Cultural sensitivity is imperative, because many women may be offended by the suggestion that they have been assaulted or mutilated (American College of Obstetricians and Gynecologists, 2014). The World Health Organization (2008) classifies genital mutilations into four types (Table 1-21).

Long-term complications from surgery and its associated scarring include infertility, chronic vulvar pain, diminished sexual quality of life, propensity for urogenital infection, difficulty passing menstrual blood, and formation of a vulvar neuroma, epidermoid cyst, or keloid (Almroth, 2005; Andersson, 2012; World Health Organization, 2018). Moreover, cervical cancer screening may not be possible.

In general, women with significant symptoms following type III procedures are candidates for *defibulation*. This procedure sharply divides scar tissue at the midline to reopen the

TABLE 1-21. World Health Organization Classification of Female Genital Mutilation

Type Ia	Prepuce (clitoral hood) removal
Ib	Prepuce, clitoris removal
Type IIa	Labia minora removal
IIb	Labia minora, clitoris removal
IIc	Labia majora and minora, clitoris removal
Type IIIa	Removal and surgical apposition of labia minora ± clitoris removal
IIIb	Removal and surgical apposition of labia majora ± clitoris removal
Type IV	Pricking, piercing, incising, scraping, cautery, or other genital injury

vulva (Chap. 43, p. 992). Following surgery, sexual functioning is typically improved (Krause, 2011; Nour, 2006). Also, gravidas with type III FGM may benefit from lower rates of both cesarean delivery and higher-order perineal laceration following defibulation (Berg, 2018).

In contrast, results of clitoral reconstruction are mixed, and outcome data are limited. Surgery provides a visible clitoris in approximately 75 percent of cases. Average improvement scores for desire, dyspareunia, pleasure, and sexual frequency range from 40 to 60 percent. However, worsening of these last four parameters is seen in 2 to 20 percent of women (Berg, 2018). During presurgical evaluation for clitoral reconstruction, patients may be best served by a team that includes gynecologic, psychological, and sexual counseling to discuss treatment options (De Schrijver, 2016).

REFERENCES

Abdeen G, le Roux CW: Mechanism underlying the weight loss and complications of Roux-en-Y gastric bypass. Obes Surg 26(2):410, 2016

Acierno R, Hernandez MA, Amstadter AB, et al: Prevalence and correlates of emotional, physical, sexual, and financial abuse and potential neglect in the United States: the National Elder Mistreatment Study. Am J Public Health 100(2):292, 2010

Acierno R, Hernandez-Tejada MA, Anetzberger GJ, et al: The National Elder Mistreatment Study: an 8-year longitudinal study of outcomes. J Elder Abuse Negl 29(4):254, 2017

Adams JA, Farst KJ, Kellogg ND: Interpretation of medical findings in suspected child sexual abuse: an update for 2018. J Pediatr Adolesc Gynecol 31(3):225, 2018

Adams JA, Kaplan RA, Starling SP, et al: Guidelines for medical care of children who may have been sexually abused. J Pediatr Adolesc Gynecol 20:163, 2007

Almroth L, Elmusharaf S, El Hadi N, et al: Primary infertility after genital mutilation in girlhood in Sudan: a case-control study. Lancet 366:385, 2005

American Academy of Family Physicians: Screening pelvic exam. 2017. Available at: https://www.aafp.org/patient-care/clinical-recommendations/all/screening-pelvic-exam.html. Accessed November 19, 2018

American College of Obstetricians and Gynecologists: Health care for transgender individuals. Committee Opinion No. 512, December 2011

American College of Obstetricians and Gynecologists: Intimate partner violence. Committee Opinion No. 518, February 2012

American College of Obstetricians and Gynecologists: Guidelines for Women's Health Care, 4th ed. Washington, ACOG, 2014

American College of Obstetricians and Gynecologists: Sexual assault. Committee Opinion No. 592, April 2014, Reaffirmed 2016a

American College of Obstetricians and Gynecologists: The initial reproductive health visit. Committee Opinion No. 598, May 2014, Reaffirmed 2016b

American College of Obstetricians and Gynecologists: Well-woman visit. Committee Opinion No. 534, August 2012, Reaffirmed 2016c

American College of Obstetricians and Gynecologists: Bariatric surgery and pregnancy. Practice Bulletin No. 105, June 2009, Reaffirmed 2017a

American College of Obstetricians and Gynecologists: Breast cancer risk assessment and screening in average-risk women. Practice Bulletin No. 179, July 2017b

American College of Obstetricians and Gynecologists: Physical activity and exercise during pregnancy and the postpartum period. Committee Opinion No. 650, December 2015, Reaffirmed 2017c

American College of Obstetricians and Gynecologists: Routine human immunodeficiency virus screening. Committee Opinion No. 596, May 2014, Reaffirmed 2017d

American College of Obstetricians and Gynecologists: Carrier screening in the age of genomic medicine. Committee Opinion No. 690, March 2017e

American College of Obstetricians and Gynecologists: Hormone therapy and heart disease. Committee Opinion No. 565, June 2013, Reaffirmed 2018a

American College of Obstetricians and Gynecologists: The utility of and indications for routine pelvic examination. Committee Opinion No. 754, October 2018b

American College of Obstetricians and Gynecologists, American Society for Reproductive Medicine: Prepregnancy Counseling. Committee Opinion No. 762, January 2019

American Diabetes Association: 2. Classification and diagnosis of diabetes: standards of medical care in diabetes—2019. Diabetes Care 42(Suppl 1):S13, 2019

American Heart Association: Understanding blood pressure readings. 2017. Available at: https://www.heart.org/en/health-topics/consumer-healthcare/what-is-cardiovascular-disease/heart-health-screenings. Accessed January 19, 2019

American Psychiatric Association: Diagnostic and Statistical Manual of Mental Disorders, 5th ed. Arlington, APA, 2013

Andersson SH, Rymer J, Joyce DW, et al: Sexual quality of life in women who have undergone female genital mutilation: a case-control study. BJOG 119(13):1606, 2012

Arias E, Heron M, Xu J: United States life tables, 2014. Natl Vital Stat Rep 66(4):1, 2017

Astrup BS, Ravn P, Lauritsen J, et al: Nature, frequency and duration of genital lesions after consensual sexual intercourse: implications for legal proceedings. Forensic Sci Int 219:50, 2012

Baker FC, de Zambotti M, Colrain IM, et al: Sleep problems during the menopausal transition: prevalence, impact, and management challenges. Nat Sci Sleep 10:73, 2018

Barboza JL, Patel R, Patel P, et al: An update on the pharmacotherapeutic interventions for smoking cessation. Expert Opin Pharmacother 17(11):1483, 2016

Basile KC, Breiding MJ, Smith SG: Disability and risk of recent sexual violence in the United States. Am J Public Health 106(5):928, 2016

Basile KC, Hertz MF, Back SE: Intimate partner violence and sexual violence victimization assessment instruments for use in healthcare settings: version 1. Atlanta, Centers for Disease Control and Prevention, 2007

Basile KC, Smith SG, Breiding MJ, et al: Sexual violence surveillance: uniform definitions and recommended data elements, version 2.0. Atlanta, National Center for Injury Prevention and Control, 2014

Benjamin EJ, Virani SS, Callaway CW, et al: Heart disease and stroke statistics—2018 update: a report from the American Heart Association. Circulation 137(12):e67, 2018

Berg RC, Taraldsen S, Said MA, et al: The effectiveness of surgical interventions for women with FGM/C: a systematic review. BJOG 125(3):278, 2018

Bhasin S, Cunningham GR, Hayes FJ, et al: Testosterone therapy in adult men with androgen deficiency syndromes: an Endocrine Society clinical practice guideline. J Clin Endocrinol Metab 91(6): 1995, 2006

Bibbins-Domingo K, U.S. Preventive Services Task Force: Aspirin use for the primary prevention of cardiovascular disease and colorectal cancer: U.S. Preventive Services Task Force recommendation statement. Ann Intern Med 164:836, 2016

Borson S, Scanlan J, Brush M, et al: The Mini-Cog: a cognitive "vital signs" measure for dementia screening in multi-lingual elderly. Int J Geriatr Psychiatry 15:1021, 2000

Bray G, Look M, Ryan D: Treatment of the obese patient in primary care: targeting and meeting goals and expectations. Postgrad Med 125(5):67, 2013

Breiding MJ, Basile KC, Smith SG, et al: Intimate partner violence surveillance: uniform definitions and recommended data elements, version 2.0. Atlanta, National Center for Injury Prevention and Control, 2015

Briggs GG, Freeman RK, Tower CV, et al: Drugs in Pregnancy and Lactation, 11th ed. Philadelphia, Wolters Kluwer, 2017, p 1079

Burgess AW, Holmstrom LL: Rape trauma syndrome. Am J Psychiatry 131(9):981, 1974

Buysse DJ: Insomnia. JAMA 309(7):706, 2013

Campbell JC: Health consequences of intimate partner violence. Lancet 359(9314):1331, 2002

Centers for Disease Control and Prevention: Adverse health conditions and health risk behaviors associated with intimate partner violence—United States, 2005. MMWR 57(5):113, 2008

Centers for Disease Control and Prevention: Interim statement regarding potential fetal harm from exposure to dolutegravir—implications for HIV post—exposure prophylaxis (PEP). 2018a. Available at: https://www.cdc.gov/hiv/pdf/basics/cdc-hiv-dolutegravir-alert.pdf. Accessed November 11, 2018

Centers for Disease Control and Prevention: National diabetes statistics report, 2017a. Atlanta, U.S. Department of Health and Human Services, 2017

Centers for Disease Control and Prevention: Sexually transmitted diseases treatment guidelines, 2015. MMWR 64(3):1, 2015

Centers for Disease Control and Prevention: Updated guidelines for antiretroviral postexposure prophylaxis after sexual, injection drug use, or other non-occupational exposure to HIV—United States, 2016. 2016. Available at: https://www.cdc.gov/hiv/pdf/programresources/cdc-hiv-npep-guidelines.pdf. Accessed November 11, 2018

Centers for Disease Control and Prevention: US Public Health Service: pre-exposure prophylaxis for the prevention of HIV infection in the United States—2017 update: a clinical practice guideline. 2017b. Available at: https://www.cdc.gov/hiv/pdf/risk/prep/cdc-hiv-prep-guidelines-2017.pdf. Accessed November 20, 2018

Centers for Disease Control and Prevention: Women and their partners trying to become pregnant. 2018b. Available at: https://www.cdc.gov/pregnancy/zika/women-and-their-partners.html. Accessed November 20, 2018

Chiesa A, Goldson E: Child sexual abuse. Pediatr Rev 38(3):105, 2017

Child Welfare Information Gateway: Mandatory reporters of child abuse and neglect. Washington, Department of Health and Human Services, 2016

Curtis KM, Jatlaoui TC, Tepper NK, et al: U.S. Selected practice recommendations for contraceptive use, 2016. MMWR 65(4):1, 2016

Davies MJ, Bergenstal R, Bode B, et al: Efficacy of liraglutide for weight loss among patients with type 2 diabetes: the SCALE diabetes randomized clinical trial. JAMA 314:687, 2015

De Schrijver L, Leye E, Merckx M: A multidisciplinary approach to clitoral reconstruction after female genital mutilation: the crucial role of counselling. Eur J Contracept Reprod Health Care 21(4):269, 2016

de Vries AL, McGuire JK, Steensma TD, et al: Young adult psychological outcome after puberty suppression and gender reassignment. Pediatrics 134(4):696, 2014

de Vries AL, Steensma TD, Doreleijers TA, et al: Puberty suppression in adolescents with gender identity disorder: a prospective follow-up study. J Sex Med 8(8):2276, 2011

Department of Justice: A national protocol for sexual assault medical forensic examinations: adults/adolescents, second edition. Washington, Office on Violence Against Women, 2013

Department of Justice: State elder abuse statutes. 2016. Available at: https://www.justice.gov/elderjustice/elder-justice-statutes-0. Accessed November 18, 2018

Deutsch MB: Overview of feminizing hormone therapy. 2018. Available at: http://transhealth.ucsf.edu/trans?page=guidelines-feminizing-therapy. Accessed November 27, 2018

Dooling KL, Guo A, Patel M, et al: Recommendations of the Advisory Committee on Immunization Practices for use of herpes zoster vaccines. MMWR 67:103, 2018

Durborow N, Lizdas KC, O'Flaherty A, et al: Compendium of state and U.S. territory statutes and policies on domestic violence and health care. San Francisco, Futures Without Violence, 2013

Eckel RH, Jakicic JM, Ard JD, et al: 2013 AHA/ACC guideline on life-style management to reduce cardiovascular risk: a report of the American College of Cardiology/American Heart Association Task Force on Practice Guidelines. Circulation 129(25 Suppl 2):S76, 2014

Federal Bureau of Investigation: Summary reporting system (SRS) user manual version 1.0. 2013. Available at: https://ucr.fbi.gov/nibrs/summary-reporting-system-srs-user-manual. Accessed November 11, 2018

Fedina L, Holmes JL, Backes BL: Campus sexual assault: a systematic review of prevalence research from 2000 to 2015. Trauma Violence Abuse 19(1):76, 2018

Fiore MC, Jaen CR, Baker TB: Treating tobacco use and dependence: 2008 update. Rockville, U.S. Department of Health and Human Services, 2008

Flores AR, Herman JL, Gates GJ, et al: How many adults identify as transgender in the United States? Los Angeles, The Williams Institute, 2016

Food and Drug Administration: Completed safety review of Xenical/Alli (orlistat) and severe liver injury. 2010. http://www.fda.gov/Drugs/DrugSafety/PostmarketDrugSafetyInformationforPatientsandProviders/ucm213038.htm. Accessed February 13, 2015

Food and Drug Administration: FDA approves expanded use of Gardasil 9 to include individuals 27 through 45 years old. 2018. Available at: https://www.fda.gov/NewsEvents/Newsroom/PressAnnouncements/ucm622715.htm. Accessed November 3, 2018

Fredriksen-Goldsen KI, Cook-Daniels L, Kim HJ, et al: Physical and mental health of transgender older adults: an at-risk and underserved population. Gerontologist 54(3):488, 2014

Futterweit W: Endocrine therapy of transsexualism and potential complications of long-term treatment. Arch Sex Behav 27(2):209, 1998

Ganly I, Taylor EW: Breast cancer in a trans-sexual man receiving hormone replacement therapy. Br J Surg 82:341, 1995

Garber AJ, Abrahamson MJ, Barzilay JI, et al: Consensus statement by the AACE and ACE on the comprehensive type 2 diabetes management algorithm—2018 executive summary. Endocr Pract 24(1):91, 2018

Gay and Lesbian Medical Association: Guidelines for care of lesbian, gay, bisexual and transgender patients. Washington, GLMA, 2006

Girardet RG, Lahoti S, Howard LA, et al: Epidemiology of sexually transmitted infections in suspected child victims of sexual assault. Pediatrics 124(1):79, 2009a

Girardet RG, Lemme S, Biason TA, et al: HIV post-exposure prophylaxis in children and adolescents presenting for reported sexual assault. Child Abuse Negl 33:173, 2009b

Goldberg H, Stupp P, Okoroh E, et al: Female genital mutilation/cutting in the United States: updated estimates of women and girls at risk, 2012. Public Health Rep 131(2):340, 2016

Gorin-Lazard A, Baumstarck K, Boyer L: Is hormonal therapy associated with better quality of life in transsexuals? A cross sectional study. J Sex Med 9(2):531, 2012

Griffith WF, Stuart GS, Gluck KL, et al: Vaginal speculum lubrication and its effects on cervical cytology and microbiology. Contraception 72(1):60, 2005

Grundy SM, Cleeman JI, Daniels SR, et al: Diagnosis and management of the metabolic syndrome: an American Heart Association/National Heart, Lung, and Blood Institute scientific statement. Circulation 112(17):2735, 2005

Grundy SM, Stone NJ, Bailey AL, et al: 2018 AHA/ACC/AACVPR/AAPA/ABC/ACPM/ADA/AGS/APhA/ASPC/NLA/PCNA Guideline on the Management of Blood Cholesterol. Circulation 139(25):e1082, 2019

Hales CM, Fryar CD, Carroll MD, et al: Trends in obesity and severe obesity prevalence in US youth and adults by sex and age, 2007–2008 to 2015–2016. JAMA 319(16):1723, 2018

Hall JE, Karch DL, Crosby AE: Elder abuse surveillance: uniform definitions and recommended core data elements for use in elder abuse surveillance, version 1.0. Atlanta, National Center for Injury Prevention and Control, 2016

Hartmann D, Güzelhan C, Zuiderwijk PB, et al: Lack of interaction between orlistat and oral contraceptives. Eur J Clin Pharmacol 50(5):421, 1996

Hawkins JS, Casey BM: Obesity. In Cunningham FG, Leveno KL, Bloom SL, et al: Williams Obstetrics, 25th ed. New York, McGraw-Hill, 2018

Hembree WC, Cohen-Kettenis PT, Gooren L, et al: Endocrine treatment of gender-dysphoric/gender-incongruent persons: an Endocrine Society clinical practice guideline. J Clin Endocrinol Metab 102(11):3869, 2017

Holmes MM, Resnick HS, Kilpatrick DG, et al: Rape-related pregnancy: estimates and descriptive characteristics from a national sample of women. Am J Obstet Gynecol 175(2):320, 1996

Hoover RM, Polson M: Detecting elder abuse and neglect assessment and intervention. Am Fam Physician 89(6):453, 2014

Imperiale TF, Ransohoff DF, Itzkowitz SH, et al: Multitarget stool DNA testing for colorectal-cancer screening. N Engl J Med 370(14):1287, 2014

Institute of Medicine: Dietary reference intakes for energy, carbohydrate, fiber, fat, fatty acids, cholesterol, protein, and amino acids. Washington, The National Academies Press, 2002

Iverson KM, McLaughlin KA, Gerber MR, et al: Exposure to interpersonal violence and its associations with psychiatric morbidity in a U.S. national sample: a gender comparison. Psychol Violence 3(3):273, 2013

Jack BW, Atrash H, Coonrod DV, et al: The clinical content of preconception care: an overview and preparation of this supplement. Am J Obstet Gynecol 199(6 Suppl 2):S266, 2008

Jack SP, Petrosky E, Lyons BH, et al: Surveillance for violent deaths—National Violent Death Reporting System, 27 states, 2015. MMWR 67(11):1, 2018

Janssen J, Koekkoek PS, Moll van Charante EP, et al: How to choose the most appropriate cognitive test to evaluate cognitive complaints in primary care. BMC Fam Pract 18(1):101, 2017

Jellinger PS, Handelsman Y, Rosenblit PD, et al: American Association of Clinical Endocrinologists and American College of Endocrinology guidelines for management of dyslipidemia and prevention of cardiovascular disease—executive summary. Endocr Pract 23(4):479, 2017

Jenny C, Hooton TM, Bowers A, et al: Sexually transmitted diseases in victims of rape. N Engl J Med 322(11):713, 1990

Jensen MD, Ryan DH, Apovian CM, et al: 2013 AHA/ACC/TOS guideline for the management of overweight and obesity in adults: a report of the American College of Cardiology/American Heart Association Task Force on Practice Guidelines and The Obesity Society. Circulation 129(25 Suppl 2): S102, 2014

Jung H, Herrenkohl TI, Skinner ML, et al: Gender differences in intimate partner violence: a predictive analysis of IPV by child abuse and domestic violence exposure during early childhood. Violence Against Women. 25(8):903, 2019

Kahn R, Buse J, Ferrannini E, et al: The metabolic syndrome: time for a critical appraisal: joint statement from the American Diabetes Association and the European Association for the Study of Diabetes. Diabetes Care 28(9): 2289, 2005

Källén BA: Antiobesity drugs in early pregnancy and congenital malformations in the offspring. Obes Res Clin Pract 8(6):e571, 2014

Kann L, McManus T, Harris WA, et al: Youth risk behavior surveillance—United States, 2017. MMWR 67(8):1, 2018

Katz S, Ford, AB, Moskowitz RW, et al: Studies of illness in the aged. The index of ADL: a standardized measure of biological and psychosocial function. JAMA 185:914, 1963

Khera R, Murad MH, Chandar AK, et al: Association of pharmacological treatments for obesity with weight loss and adverse events: a systematic review and meta-analysis. JAMA 315(22):2424, 2016

Kim DK, Hunter P: Advisory Committee on Immunization Practices recommended immunization schedule for adults aged 19 years or older—United States, 2019. MMWR 68(5):115, 2019

Kösters JP, Gøtzsche PC: Regular self-examination or clinical examination for early detection of breast cancer. Cochrane Database Syst Rev 3:CD003373, 2008

Krause E, Brandner S, Mueller MD, et al: Out of Eastern Africa: defibulation and sexual function in woman with female genital mutilation. J Sex Med 8(5):1420, 2011

Kroenke K, Spitzer RL, Williams JB: The Patient Health Questionnaire—2: validity of a two-item depression screener. Med Care 41(11):1284, 2003

Kushner RF: Weight loss strategies for treatment of obesity: lifestyle management and pharmacotherapy. Prog Cardiovasc Dis 61(2):246, 2018

Lachs MS, Pillemer KA: Elder abuse. N Engl J Med 373(20):1947, 2015

Larsen ML, Hilden M, Lidegaard Ø: Sexual assault: a descriptive study of 2500 female victims over a 10-year period. BJOG 122(4):577, 2015

Lawton MP, Brody EM: Assessment of older people: self-monitoring and instrumental activities of daily living. Gerontologist 9:179, 1969

LeFevre ML, U.S. Preventive Services Task Force: Screening for chlamydia and gonorrhea: U.S. Preventive Services Task Force recommendation statement. Ann Intern Med 161(12):902, 2014a

LeFevre ML, U.S. Preventive Services Task Force: Screening for hepatitis B virus infection in nonpregnant adolescents and adults: U.S. Preventive Services Task Force recommendation statement. Ann Intern Med 161(1):58, 2014b

LeFevre ML, U.S. Preventive Services Task Force: Screening for thyroid dysfunction: U.S. Preventive Services Task Force recommendation statement. Ann Intern Med 162(9):641, 2015

Lenahan LC, Ernst A, Johnson B: Colposcopy in evaluation of the adult sexual assault victim. Am J Emerg Med 16(2):183, 1998

Light AD, Obedin-Maliver J, Sevelius JM, et al: Transgender men who experienced pregnancy after female-to-male gender transitioning. Obstet Gynecol 124(6):1120, 2014

Linden JA: Care of the adult patient after sexual assault. N Engl J Med 365:834, 2011

Mayer K, Bradford J, Makadon H, et al: Sexual and gender minority health: what we know and what needs to be done. Am J Public Health 98(6):989, 2008

McDonald S, Saslow D, Alciati MH: Performance and reporting of clinical breast examination: a review of the literature. CA Cancer J Clin 54:345, 2004

Merhi ZO: Impact of bariatric surgery on female reproduction. Fertil Steril 92(5):1501, 2009

Merrick MT, Basile KC, Zhang X, et al: Characterizing sexual violence victimization in youth: 2012 National Intimate Partner and Sexual Violence Survey. Am J Prev Med 54(4):596, 2018

Monstrey S, De Cuypere G, Ettner R: Surgery: female-to-male patient. In Ettner SR, Monstrey S, Eyler AE (eds): Principles of Transgender Medicine and Surgery. New York, Haworth Press, 2007, p 135

Moore E, Wisniewski A, Dobs A: Endocrine treatment of transsexual people: a review of treatment regimens, outcomes, and adverse effects. J Clin Endocrinol Metab 88:3467, 2003

Mosca L, Benjamin EJ, Berra K, et al: Effectiveness-based guidelines for prevention of cardiovascular disease in women—2011 update. Circulation 123:1243, 2011

Moyer VA, U.S. Preventive Services Task Force: Screening for hepatitis C virus infection in adults: U.S. Preventive Services Task Force recommendation statement. Ann Intern Med 159(5):349, 2013a

Moyer VA, U.S. Preventive Services Task Force: Screening for HIV: U.S. Preventive Services Task Force recommendation statement. Ann Intern Med 159(1):51, 2013b

Nasreddine ZS, Phillips NA, Bedirian V, et al: The Montreal Cognitive Assessment, MoCA: a brief screening tool for mild cognitive impairment. J Am Geriatr Soc 53(4):695, 2005

National Adult Protective Services: Get help. 2018. Available at: http://www.napsa-now.org/get-help/help-in-your-area/. Accessed November 18, 2018

National District Attorney Association: Reporting requirements related to rape of competent adult victims. Arlington, National District Attorney Association, 2016

National Heart, Lung, and Blood Institute: Managing overweight and obesity in adults: systematic evidence review from the obesity expert panel, 2013. Available at: https://www.nhlbi.nih.gov/health-topics/managing-overweight-obesity-in-adults. Accessed December 9, 2018

Nour NM, Michels KB, Bryant AE: Defibulation to treat female genital cutting: effect on symptoms and sexual function. Obstet Gynecol 108(1):55, 2006

Novo Nordisk: Saxenda REMS program. 2017. Available at: https://www.saxendarems.com/. Accessed December 9, 2018

Oeffinger KC, Fontham ET, Etzioni R, et al: Breast cancer screening for women at average risk: 2015 Guideline Update from the American Cancer Society. JAMA 314(15):1599, 2015

O'Hanlan KA, Dibble SL, Young-Spint M: Total laparoscopic hysterectomy for female-to-male transsexuals. Obstet Gynecol 110(5):1096, 2007

Palladino CL, Singh V, Campbell J, et al: Homicide and suicide during the perinatal period: findings from the National Violent Death Reporting System. Obstet Gynecol 118(5):1056, 2011

Park DI, Ryu S, Kim YH, et al: Comparison of guaiac-based and quantitative immunochemical fecal occult blood testing in a population at average risk undergoing colorectal cancer screening. Am J Gastroenterol 105(9):2017, 2010

Patel P, Borkowf CB, Brooks JT, et al: Estimating per-act HIV transmission risk: a systematic review. AIDS 28(10):1509, 2014

Pi-Sunyer X, Astrup A, Fujioka K, et al: A randomized, controlled trial of 3.0 mg of liraglutide in weight management. N Engl J Med 373(1):11, 2015

Piercy KL, Troiano RP, Ballard RM, et al: The physical activity guidelines for Americans. JAMA 320(19):2020, 2018

Qaseem A, Humphrey LL, Harris R, et al: Screening pelvic examination in adult women: a clinical practice guideline from the American College of Physicians. Ann Intern Med 161:67, 2014

Ray N: Lesbian, gay, bisexual and transgender youth: an epidemic of homelessness. New York, National Gay and Lesbian Task Force Policy Institute, 2006

Rex DK, Boland CR, Dominitz JA, et al: Colorectal cancer screening: recommendations for physicians and patients from the U.S. Multi-Society Task Force on colorectal cancer. Gastroenterology 153(1):307, 2017

Riggs N, Houry D, Long G, et al: Analysis of 1,076 cases of sexual assault. Ann Emerg Med 35(4):358, 2000

Sateia MJ, Buysse DJ, Krystal AD, et al: Clinical practice guideline for the pharmacologic treatment of chronic insomnia in adults: an American Academy of Sleep Medicine clinical practice guideline. J Clin Sleep Med 13(2):307, 2017

Schwarcz SK, Whittington WL: Sexual assault and sexually transmitted diseases: detection and management in adults and children. Rev Infect Dis 12 (S6):682, 1990

Seña AC, Hsu KK, Kellogg N, et al: Sexual assault and sexually transmitted infections in adults, adolescents, and children. Clin Infect Dis 61(8 suppl):S856, 2015

Shadigian E, Bauer ST: Pregnancy-associated death: a qualitative systematic review of homicide and suicide. Obstet Gynecol Surv 60(3):183, 2005

Shao T, Grossbard ML, Klein P: Breast cancer in female-to-male transsexuals: two cases with a review of physiology and management. Clin Breast Cancer 11(6):417, 2011

Siegel RL, Miller KD, Jemal A: Cancer statistics, 2019. CA Cancer J Clin 69(1):7, 2019

Siu AL, U.S. Preventive Services Task Force: Behavioral and pharmacotherapy interventions for tobacco smoking cessation in adults, including pregnant women: U.S. Preventive Services Task Force recommendation statement. Ann Intern Med 163(8):622, 2015a

Siu AL, U.S. Preventive Services Task Force: Screening for abnormal blood glucose and type 2 diabetes mellitus: U.S. Preventive Services Task Force recommendation statement. Ann Intern Med. 163(11):861, 2015b

Siu AL, U.S. Preventive Services Task Force: Screening for breast cancer: U.S. Preventive Services Task Force recommendation statement. Ann Intern Med 164(4):279, 2016

Slaughter L, Brown CR, Crowley S, et al: Patterns of genital injury in female sexual assault victims. Am J Obstet Gynecol 176(3):609, 1997

Smith RA, Andrews KS, Brooks D, et al: Cancer screening in the United States, 2018: a review of current American Cancer Society guidelines and current issues in cancer screening. CA Cancer J Clin 68(4):297, 2018a

Smith SG, Chen J, Basile KC, et al: The National Intimate Partner and Sexual Violence Survey (NISVS): 2010–2012 state report. Atlanta, National Center for Injury Prevention and Control, 2017

Smith TD, Raman SR, Madigan S, et al: Anogenital findings in 3569 pediatric examinations for sexual abuse/assault. J Pediatr Adolesc Gynecol 31(2):79, 2018b

Spack NP: Management of transgenderism. JAMA 309(5):478, 2013

Stone NJ, Robinson JG, Lichtenstein AH, et al: 2013 ACC/AHA guideline on the treatment of blood cholesterol to reduce atherosclerotic cardiovascular risk in adults: a report of the American College of Cardiology/American Heart Association Task Force on Practice Guidelines. Circulation 29(25 Suppl 2): S1, 2014

Tanoue LT, Tanner NT, Gould MK, et al: Lung cancer screening. Am J Respir Crit Care Med 191(1):19, 2015

Task Force on Postovulatory Methods of Fertility Regulation: Randomized controlled trial of levonorgestrel versus the Yuzpe regimen of combined oral contraceptives for emergency contraception. Lancet 352(9126):428, 1998

Taylor BG, Mumford EA: A national descriptive portrait of adolescent relationship abuse: results from the national survey on teen relationships and intimate violence. J Interpers Violence 31(6):963, 2016

Thomas DB, Gao DL, Ray RM: Randomized trial of breast self-examination in Shanghai: final results. J Natl Cancer Inst 94(19):1445, 2002

Trussell J, Ellertson C, Stewart F: The effectiveness of the Yuzpe regimen of emergency contraception. Fam Plann Perspect 28 (2):58, 1996

UNICEF: Female genital mutilation/cutting: a global concern. 2016. Available at: https://data.unicef.org/resources/female-genital-mutilationcutting-global-concern/. Accessed November 15, 2018

U.S. Department of Health and Human Services: Physical Activity Guidelines for Americans, 2nd ed. Washington, U.S. Department of Health and Human Services, 2018

U.S. Preventive Services Task Force: Colon cancer: screening. 2016a. Available at: https://www.uspreventiveservicestaskforce.org/Page/Document/Update SummaryFinal/colorectal-cancer-screening2?ds=1&s=colon%20cancer. Accessed January 8, 2019

U.S. Preventive Services Task Force: Draft recommendation statement hepatitis C virus infection in adolescents and adults: screening. Available at: https://www.uspreventiveservicestaskforce.org/Page/Document/draft-recommendation-statement/hepatitis-c-screening1. Accessed September 8, 2019

U.S. Preventive Services Task Force, Bibbins-Domingo K, Grossman DC: Screening for gynecologic conditions with pelvic examination: US Preventive Services Task Force recommendation statement. JAMA 317(9):947, 2017

U.S. Preventive Services Task Force, Bibbins-Domingo K, Grossman DC, et al: Screening for skin cancer: US Preventive Services Task Force recommendation statement. JAMA 316(4):429, 2016b

U.S. Preventive Services Task Force, Bibbins-Domingo K, Grossman DC, et al: Screening for syphilis infection in nonpregnant adults and adolescents: US Preventive Services Task Force recommendation statement. JAMA 315(21):2321, 2016c

U.S. Preventive Services Task Force, Bibbins-Domingo K, Grossman DC, et al: Serologic screening for genital herpes infection: US Preventive Services Task Force recommendation statement. JAMA 316(23):2525, 2016d

Walters ML, Chen J, Breiding MJ: The National Intimate Partner and Sexual Violence Survey (NISVS): 2010 findings on victimization by sexual orientation. Atlanta, National Center for Injury Prevention and Control, 2013

Whelton PK, Carey RM, Aronow WS, et al: 2017 ACC/AHA/AAPA/ABC/ACPM/AGS/APhA/ASH/ASPC/NMA/PCNA guideline for the prevention, detection, evaluation, and management of high blood pressure in adults: executive summary: a report of the American College of Cardiology/American Heart Association Task Force on Clinical Practice Guidelines. Hypertension 71(6):1269, 2018

Wolfe BM, Kvach E, Eckel RH: Treatment of obesity: weight loss and bariatric surgery. Circ Res 118(11):1844, 2016

Wong JS, Waite LJ: Elder mistreatment predicts later physical and psychological health: results from a national longitudinal study. J Elder Abuse Negl 29(1):15, 2017

World Health Organization: Care of Women and Girls Living with Female Genital Mutilation: a Clinical Handbook. Geneva, World Health Organization, 2018

World Health Organization: Eliminating female genital mutilation. Geneva, World Health Organization, 2008

World Professional Association for Transgender Health: Standards of Care for the Health of Transsexual, Transgender, and Gender Nonconforming People, 7th ed. 7th Version. Illinois, WPATH, 2012

Yuzpe AA, Smith RP, Rademaker AW: A multicenter clinical investigation employing ethinyl estradiol combined with DL-norgestrel as postcoital contraceptive agent. Fertil Steril 37(4):508, 1982

Zieman M, Guillebaud J, Weisberg E, et al: Contraceptive efficacy and cycle control with the Ortho Evra/Evra transdermal system: the analysis of pooled data. Fertil Steril 77:S13, 2002

Zilkens RR, Smith DA, Kelly MC, et al: Sexual assault and general body injuries: a detailed cross-sectional Australian study of 1163 women. Forensic Sci Int 279:112, 2017a

Zilkens RR, Smith DA, Phillips MA, et al: Genital and anal injuries: a cross-sectional Australian study of 1266 women alleging recent sexual assault. Forensic Sci Int 275:195, 2017b

CHAPTER 2

Techniques Used for Imaging in Gynecology

Several technical advances in recent decades currently allow superb imaging of female pelvic structures. As a result, use of sonography in gynecology now equals that in obstetrics. Enhancements to traditional sonography continue to fill important clinical gaps. For example, technical refinements now allow three-dimensional (3-D) imaging to rival the roles of computed tomography (CT) and magnetic resonance (MR) imaging for many conditions. In addition, application of MR imaging now includes MR-guided high-intensity focused-ultrasound therapy, used for uterine leiomyomas.

SONOGRAPHY

■ Physics

In sonography, the picture displayed on a screen is produced by sound waves reflected back from an imaged structure. To begin, alternating current is applied to a transducer containing piezoelectric crystals, which convert electric energy to high-frequency sound waves. A water-soluble gel applied to the skin acts as a coupling agent. Sound waves then pass through tissue layers, encounter an interface between tissues of different densities, and are reflected back to the transducer. Converted back into electric energy, they are displayed on a screen.

Dense material, such as bone, or a synthetic material, such as an intrauterine device (IUD), produces high-velocity reflected waves, also termed *echoes*, which are displayed on a screen as white. These are described as *echogenic*. Conversely, fluid is *anechoic*, generates few reflected waves, and appears black on

a screen. Middle-density tissues variably reflect waves to create various shades of gray, and images are described as *hypoechoic* or *hyperechoic* relative to tissues immediately adjacent to them. Images are generated so quickly—50 to 100 frames per second—that the picture on the screen appears to move in real time.

Sound reflection is greatest when the difference between the acoustic impedance of two structures is large. This explains why cysts are so well demonstrated with sonography. Strong echoes are produced from the cyst walls, but no echoes arise from the cyst fluid. As more sound traverses the cyst, more echoes are received from the area behind the cyst, a feature known as *through transmission* or *acoustic enhancement* (Fig. 2-1). In contrast, with a dense structure, the sound passing through it is diminished, which creates a band of reduced echoes beyond it, known as *acoustic shadowing* (Fig. 2-2).

The frequency of emitted ultrasound waves is expressed in megahertz (MHz), which means million vibrations per second. The frequency is inversely related to its wavelength. Thus, transducers emitting pulses of high frequency generate waves of shorter length, which result in higher spatial resolution or sharpness between interfaces but achieve less penetration. Curved transducers provide a wider field of view but often generate lower-frequency waves than linear transducers. Higher-frequency probes (10 to 15 MHz) are used to image superficial structures, such as breast masses or lost etonogestrel implants in the upper arm. Lower frequencies are required to image deeper structures. As such, transabdominal transducers are typically in the

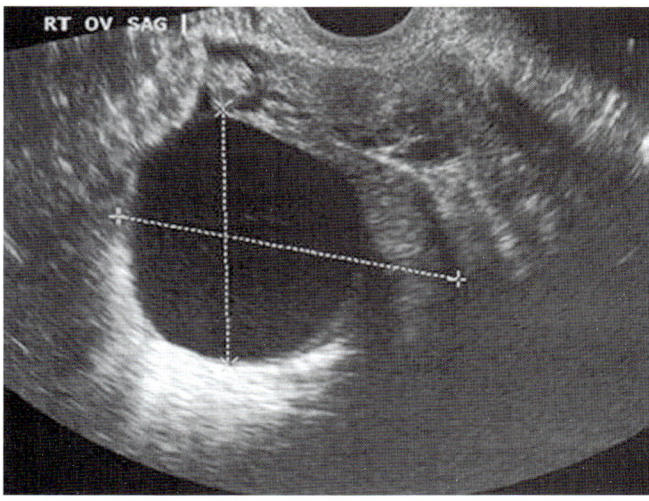

FIGURE 2-1 Transvaginal sonogram of a premenopausal ovary containing a follicular cyst. The cyst fluid appears black or anechoic. Note the white or hyperechoic area under the cyst, a sonographic feature called *posterior acoustic enhancement* or *through transmission*.

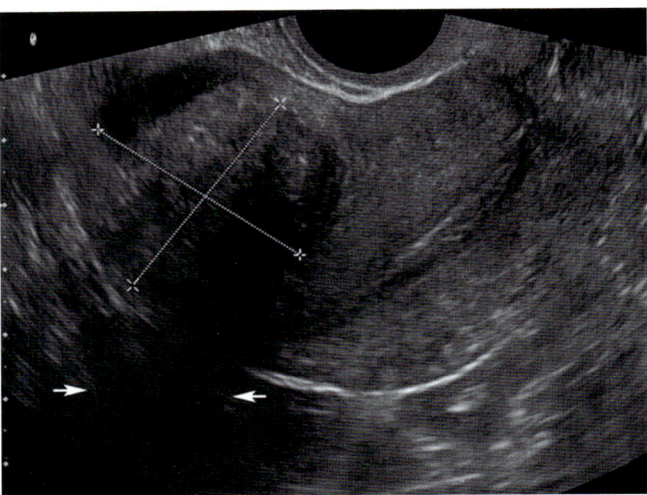

FIGURE 2-2 Transvaginal sonogram shows a leiomyoma marked by calipers and demonstrates *posterior acoustic shadowing* (*arrows*).

3 to 5 MHz range, whereas transvaginal transducers are generally 5 to 10 MHz.

■ Examination Techniques

Guidelines for sonographic examination of the female pelvis have been established by The American Institute of Ultrasound in Medicine (2014). These serve as quality assurance standards for patient care and provide assistance to practitioners performing sonography. Guidelines describe equipment and documentation and may be accessed at: http://www.aium.org/resources/guidelines/femalePelvis.pdf.

All probes are cleaned after each examination, and vaginal probes are covered by a protective sheath prior to insertion. A female staff member should always chaperone transvaginal sonography. Guidelines describe the examination steps for each organ and anatomic region in the female pelvis. For the uterus, uterine size, shape, orientation, and description of the endometrium, myometrium, and cervix are documented. The examination and its interpretation are permanently recorded, appropriately labeled, and placed in the medical record. A copy is also kept by the facility performing the study.

Grayscale Imaging

Various examination techniques can be used for sonographic study of the female pelvis. Of these, transabdominal evaluation, using a curved-array 3- to 5-MHz transducer, is the first component of general gynecologic examinations. It provides global identification of all pelvic organs and their spatial relationships. In a nonpregnant patient, a full bladder is preferred for adequate viewing, as it pushes the uterus upward from behind the pubic symphysis and displaces small bowel from the field of view. Moreover, the bladder acts as an *acoustic window*, to improve ultrasound wave transmission. In patients with large lesions or masses located superior to the bladder dome, transabdominal sonography provides a panoramic view for greater disease evaluation. Still, endometrial cavity assessment is limited with a transabdominal approach and often requires the transvaginal technique.

Transvaginal sonography (TVS) uses higher-frequency (5- to 10-MHz) transducers and is the second component of general gynecologic examinations. Because of its greater sensitivity and spatial image resolution, TVS is ideal for interrogating pelvic anatomy within the confines of the true pelvis. With larger masses, imaging may be incomplete and is complemented by transabdominal sonography.

For TVS, the probe is positioned in the vaginal fornices to place the transducer close to the region of interest and thereby lessen beam attenuation by superficial soft tissues. In contrast to transabdominal imaging, the bladder is emptied prior to a transvaginal study. TVS has few limitations. The only two absolute contraindications are imperforate hymen and patient refusal. A relative contraindication is a patient with a virginal or strictured introitus. These women, however, can usually undergo comfortable examination with proper counseling.

Transrectal and *transperineal techniques* employ transrectal probes and conventional transducers placed over the perineal region, respectively, for image acquisition. Much less commonly used, they are selected for indications such as pelvic floor imaging (p. 38).

Harmonic Imaging

This recent modification of sonography improves image quality by using several frequencies at once from the transmitted ultrasound beam instead of just a single frequency. Newer probes and postprocessing features enhance image resolution, particularly at surface interfaces. Visual artifacts that arise from superficial structures such as adipose are reduced. As such, tissue harmonic imaging is routinely used in our institution's ultrasound examinations.

Doppler Technology

This ultrasound technique can be performed with either transabdominal or transvaginal sonography to determine blood flow through pelvic organs, based on the red blood cell (RBC) velocity within vessels, especially arteries. *Color Doppler* captures and characterizes the spectral waveform of flow through certain vessels seen during real-time imaging. Ratios are often used to compare these different waveform components. The simplest is the systolic-diastolic ratio (S/D ratio), which compares the maximal (or peak) systolic flow and end-diastolic flow to evaluate downstream impedance to flow (Fig. 2-3). Of arterial Doppler spectral waveform parameters, the *resistance index* and *pulsatility index* also are commonly calculated. These quantitative indices estimate the impedance to RBC velocity within the artery by expressing the differences between the peak systolic and end-diastolic velocities.

A second application is *color Doppler mapping*, in which the color-coded pulsed-Doppler velocity information is superimposed on the real-time grayscale image. The color is scaled such that the color brightness is proportional to the flow velocity. Additionally, color Doppler also provides information regarding blood flow direction, and color is assigned to this. Flow approaching the transducer is customarily displayed in red, and flow away from it is shown in blue.

Color Doppler is not applied during every general gynecologic examination. One frequent indication is adnexal mass

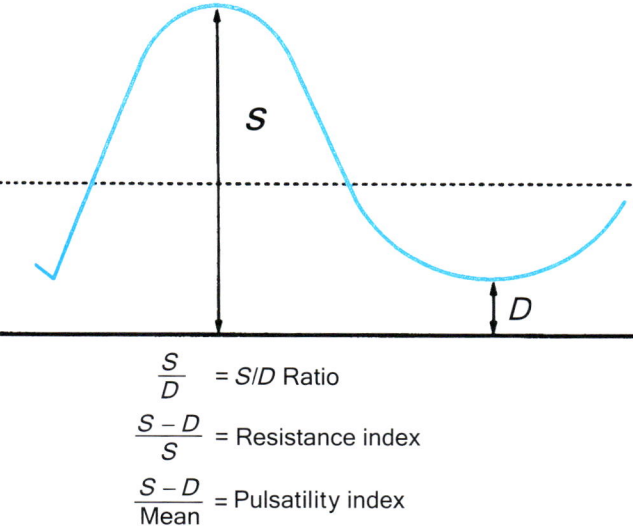

$$\frac{S}{D} = S/D \text{ Ratio}$$

$$\frac{S-D}{S} = \text{Resistance index}$$

$$\frac{S-D}{\text{Mean}} = \text{Pulsatility index}$$

FIGURE 2-3 Doppler systolic–diastolic waveform indices of blood flow velocity. *S* represents the peak systolic flow or velocity, and *D* indicates the end-diastolic flow or velocity. The mean, which is the time-average mean velocity, is calculated from computer-digitized waveforms. (Reproduced with permission from Dashe, 2018.)

interrogation. Neovascularity within cancer is composed of abnormal vessels that lack smooth muscle and contain multiple arteriovenous shunts. Consequently, low-impedance flow is expected with such masses (Fig. 2-4) (Timmerman, 2016; Weiner, 1992). Other indications include evaluation of ovarian masses for torsion, detection of extrauterine vascularity associated with ectopic pregnancy, and assessment of uterine perfusion in patients with leiomyomas and endometrial disorders (Navve, 2013; Wang, 2016a). Because of safety concerns regarding the higher intensities generated by color and spectral Doppler, use of Doppler imaging in the first trimester is discouraged, unless clear indications are present.

Power Doppler imaging also maps RBC motion. It detects the energy of Doppler signals generated from moving RBCs using

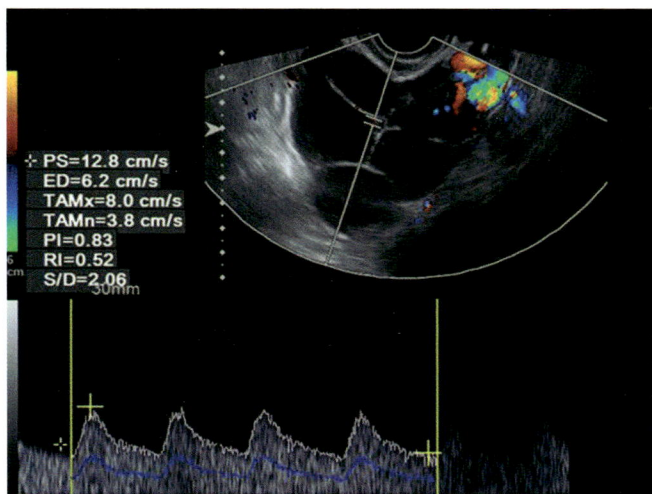

FIGURE 2-4 Complex ovarian mass with irregular cystic areas demonstrating low-impedance (pulsatility index = 0.83) flow in a septation.

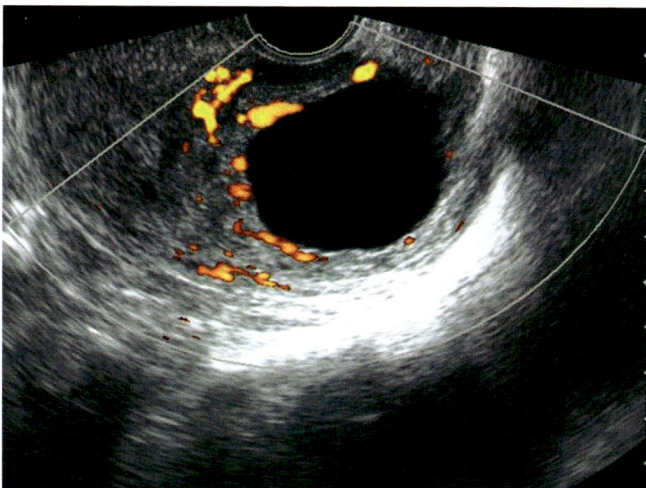

FIGURE 2-5 Power Doppler evaluation of a gestational sac in the lower uterine segment. Circular flow is depicted, consistent with the peritrophoblastic flow of an implanted pregnancy.

signal-to-noise characteristics of the vessels compared with surrounding tissues. This modality gives no information regarding blood flow direction, and thus data are displayed as a single color, usually yellow or orange. However, power Doppler is more sensitive to low-flow velocities, such as in veins and small arteries. Although employed less often than color Doppler mapping, power Doppler can gather additional information regarding endometrial and ovarian abnormalities (Fig. 2-5).

Saline-Infusion Sonography

Also called *sonohysterography*, saline-infusion sonography (SIS) displays detailed endometrial cavity anatomy by distending the cavity with sterile saline (American College of Obstetricians and Gynecologists, 2016). It is commonly selected after an endometrial mass is identified or suspected during general TVS. SIS can also assist in some infertility investigations and aid viewing of the central endometrial echo if it is poorly imaged because of uterine position or pathology.

After voiding, a woman first undergoes a comprehensive TVS evaluation. A vaginal speculum is then inserted, and the vagina and cervix are swabbed with an antiseptic solution. A catheter primed with sterile saline is advanced into the cervical canal and past the internal os. We do not routinely use a tenaculum for this. Contact with the uterine fundus is ideally avoided when advancing the catheter to avert pain or vasovagal response. It can also shear away endometrium, causing false-positive results. Once in the lower uterine segment, the catheter balloon is inflated. The speculum is carefully removed, the transvaginal probe is reinserted, and sterile saline is injected through the catheter at a rate based on the patient's tolerance. Usually not more than 5 to 40 mL is required to distend the endometrial cavity, depending on the patient's hormonal status and intracavitary pathology (Fig. 2-6). During this time, the cavity is observed with TVS. The sonographer scans in the longitudinal plane, imaging from one cornu to the other, and in the transverse plane, from the top of the fundus to the cervix. Endometrial surface irregularities are well delineated by the anechoic contrast of saline. At the procedure's conclusion,

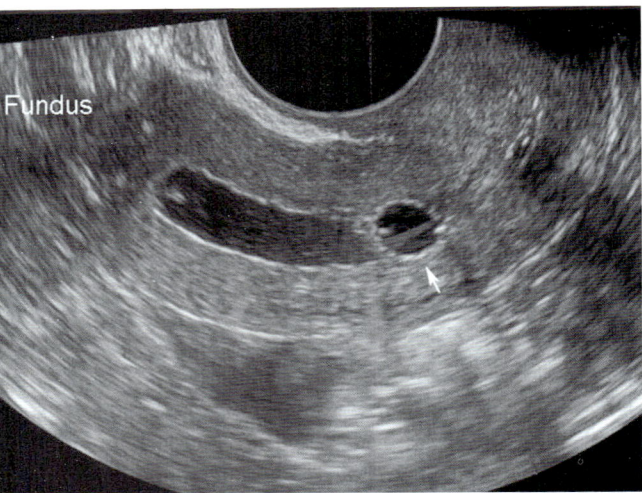

FIGURE 2-6 Saline-infusion sonography of a normal endometrial cavity. The infusion catheter balloon (*arrow*) is seen in the uterine isthmus.

the catheter is withdrawn under sonographic visualization. The uterine isthmus, endocervical canal, and upper vagina and vaginal fornices also may be evaluated, and this technique is referred to as *sonovaginography*. On average, the entire procedure lasts 5 to 10 minutes.

Many different catheter systems are available, including rigid systems and flexible catheters with and without attached balloons. We use a 7F SIS balloon catheter set, which tamponades the internal cervical os. This blockade prevents backflow of the distending medium and provides stable filling and adequate distention. We have found it easy to place and well tolerated (Fig. 2-7). Several distending solutions have been described, including saline, lactated Ringer solution, and 1.5-percent glycine. Sterile saline is inexpensive and provides optimal imaging. Alternatively, gel and foam substances have been developed to avoid backflow problems. However, these alternative products have not been extensively investigated and are not used widely in clinical practice.

In the premenopausal woman, SIS is best performed within the first 10 days of the menstrual cycle, and optimally on cycle days 4, 5, or 6 when the lining is thinnest. This timing is recommended to avoid misinterpreting menstrual blood clots as intrauterine pathology or missing pathology obscured by thick endometrial growth. In addition, such timing usually precludes disturbing a potential pregnancy. For the postmenopausal woman, timing of the procedure is not cycle-dependent.

Complications of SIS are minimal, and the risk of infection is <1 percent (Bonnamy, 2002). The American College of Obstetricians and Gynecologists (2018) recommends prophylactic antibiotics for women with prior pelvic inflammatory disease (PID) or identified hydrosalpinges, in which cases doxycycline 100 mg orally twice daily is prescribed for 5 days. Although not evidence based, we also routinely give a single dose of doxycycline, 200 mg orally, following SIS in women with diabetes and to infertile patients because of the risk for significant tubal damage associated with pelvic infection. Pain is usually minimal. In our experience, women with prior tubal ligation have greater discomfort, likely because fluid is unable to efflux through the fallopian tubes. A nonsteroidal antiinflammatory drug (NSAID) given 30 minutes prior to the procedure will typically minimize discomfort.

Contraindications to SIS include hematometra, pregnancy, active pelvic infection, or obstruction such as with an atrophic or stenotic cervix or vagina. In postmenopausal women with cervical stenosis, we have found the following steps to be helpful. First, a 200-μg misoprostol tablet is taken orally the evening before and the morning of the procedure. During SIS, a paracervical block with 1-percent lidocaine without epinephrine is provided; a tenaculum is placed on the cervix for traction; and the cervix undergoes sonographically guided sequential cervical dilation with lacrimal duct dilators. To overcome severe cervical stenosis, Pisal and colleagues (2005) inserted a 20-gauge spinal needle directly into the uterine cavity under sonographic guidance to deliver the saline.

Hysterosalpingo-Contrast Sonography

In the past, a fallopian tube could be detected with sonography only when distended by fluid, such as with obstruction. Injection of echogenic contrast during real-time sonography,

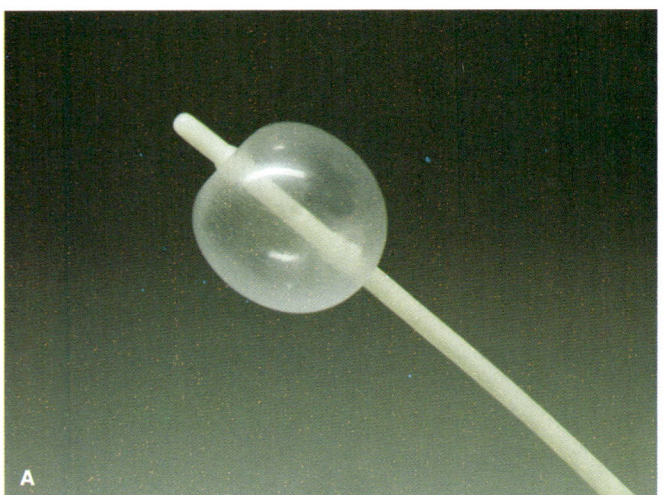

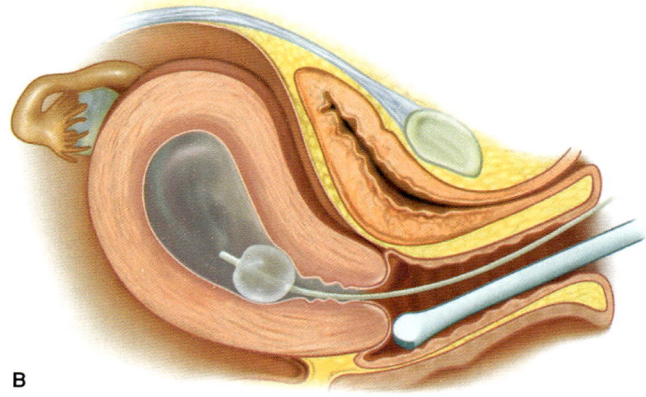

FIGURE 2-7 A. Saline-infusion sonography catheter. **B.** Saline-infusion sonography technique.

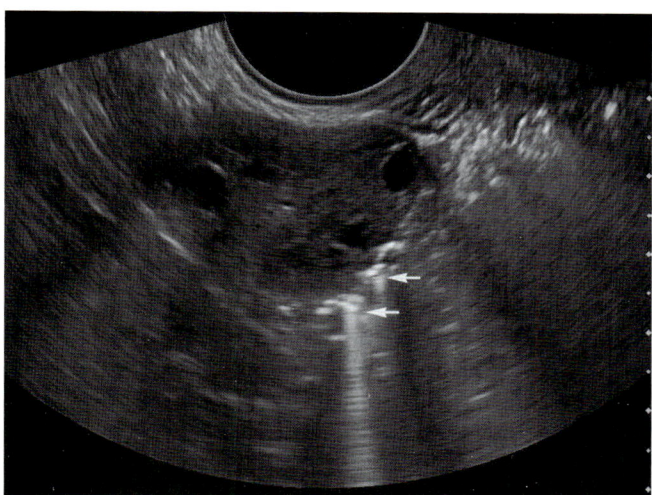

FIGURE 2-8 Transvaginal image of an ovary with echogenic bubbles adjacent to it (*arrows*) as seen during hysterosalpingo-contrast sonography (HyCoSy). The air in the saline contrast produces the bright echo and ring-down artifacts. Visualization of these echoes adjacent to the ovary represents contrast exiting the tube, consistent with tubal patency.

called *sonosalpingography, sonohysterosalpingography,* or *hystero-salpingo-contrast sonography (HyCoSy),* is now an accurate first-line procedure to assess tubal patency (Lo Monte, 2015).

HyCoSy is done in a manner similar to SIS. Fluid egress from the uterine cavity is blocked by a balloon catheter within the cervical canal. Using transvaginal sonography, the fallopian tubes are identified at the point where they join the uterine cornua. A hyperechoic sonographic contrast medium (Echovist, Albunex, or Infoson) is injected through the catheter to fill the cavity and then the fallopian tubes (Fig. 2-8). Air coupled with sterile saline solution is another contrast option. With either medium choice, patent tubes appear hyperechoic as they fill with contrast. Color or pulsed Doppler techniques raise the diagnostic accuracy of HyCoSy by showing flow velocity within the tubes (Kupesic, 2007). We use the FemVue Sono Tubal Evaluation System, which simultaneously introduces air and sterile saline in a controlled fashion. The positive pressure flow of the echogenic mixture creates "scintillations" that are visually followed using real-time ultrasound. In patent tubes, flow proceeds from the uterotubal junction, through the length of the tube, and out the fimbriated end. Bubbles then surround the ovary or fill the posterior cul-de-sac. At present no large studies quantitate a risk for post-HyCoSy pelvic infection, and our periprocedural antibiotic prophylaxis mirrors that for SIS.

HyCoSy performed in conjunction with SIS provides a comprehensive "one-stop" outpatient assessment of tubal patency, adnexal architecture, and uterine cavity and myometrial anatomy. Comparable to hysterosalpingography (HSG) in detecting tubal pathology and anatomy, HyCoSy is well tolerated and avoids x-ray exposure or iodine-related allergic reaction (Lo Monte, 2015; Luciano, 2014).

However, HyCoSy does have limitations. First, similar to HSG, tubal spasm can provide false-positive occlusion results with HyCoSy. In addition, a patent tube does not always correlate with normal tubal function. Second, the entire fallopian tube often cannot be visualized due to normal tubal tortuosity. To that end, recent studies have evaluated the combination of 3-D sonography with HyCoSy for more accurate delineation of tubal anatomy (Alcázar, 2016; Exacoustos, 2017; Wang, 2016b).

Three-Dimensional Sonography

Technical Aspects. The ability to obtain certain views of pelvic organs in two dimensions is inherently limited. Transabdominally, the bony pelvis prevents scanning from the pelvic sidewall. Transvaginally, the views obtainable are restricted by the range of vaginal probe mobility. Sonography scanners now can collect 3-D data and represent it on a two-dimensional (2-D) screen. With 3-D imaging, any desired plane through a pelvic organ can be obtained, regardless of the sound beam orientation during acquisition. For example, the "face-on" or coronal plane through the uterus is routinely seen in 3-D imaging but is rarely viewed during 2-D scanning. This view of the uterus is essential for assessing the external contour, particularly of the fundus, for congenital uterine anomaly diagnosis.

With 3-D sonography, a volume, rather than a slice, of sonographic data is acquired and stored. The stored data can be reformatted and analyzed in numerous ways, and navigation through the saved volume can show countless planes. At any time, the volume can be retrieved, studied, reconstructed, and reinterpreted as needed. In addition, the level of energy with 3-D sonography is no higher than with 2-D, and manipulations of the obtained volumes are performed "off-line" to avoid additional ultrasound scanning time.

The three main components of 3-D sonography are volume acquisition, processing, and display. First, the preferred method to acquire volumes is automated and uses a dedicated 3-D probe that contains a mechanized drive. When these probes are activated, the transducer elements automatically sweep through the operator-selected region of interest, called a *volume box,* while the probe is held stationary.

After the appropriate volume is acquired, the user can begin to process the volume using the modes available in the ultrasound machine. The acquired volume can be displayed multiple ways. The most common is multiplanar reconstruction, in which three perpendicular planes, sagittal (the longitudinal plane that divides the body into right and left sections), axial (the transverse plane that divides the body into top and bottom sections), and coronal (the frontal plane that divides the body into front and back sections), are displayed simultaneously. Correlation between the three planes in the multiplanar display is accomplished by placing the planar center dot at the point of interest in one plane and observing the location of the corresponding center dots in the other two planes (Fig. 2-9A–C).

Abuhamad and associates (2006) have described a straightforward postprocessing technique that aids in the manipulation of 3-D volumes of the uterus, called the *Z technique.* The anatomic basis of the Z technique is such that, in aligning the midsagittal and midtransverse planes of the uterus parallel to the horizontal axis, the midcoronal plane of the uterus will easily and consistently be displayed. In addition, all or part of the saved volume can be processed into a rendered image that can

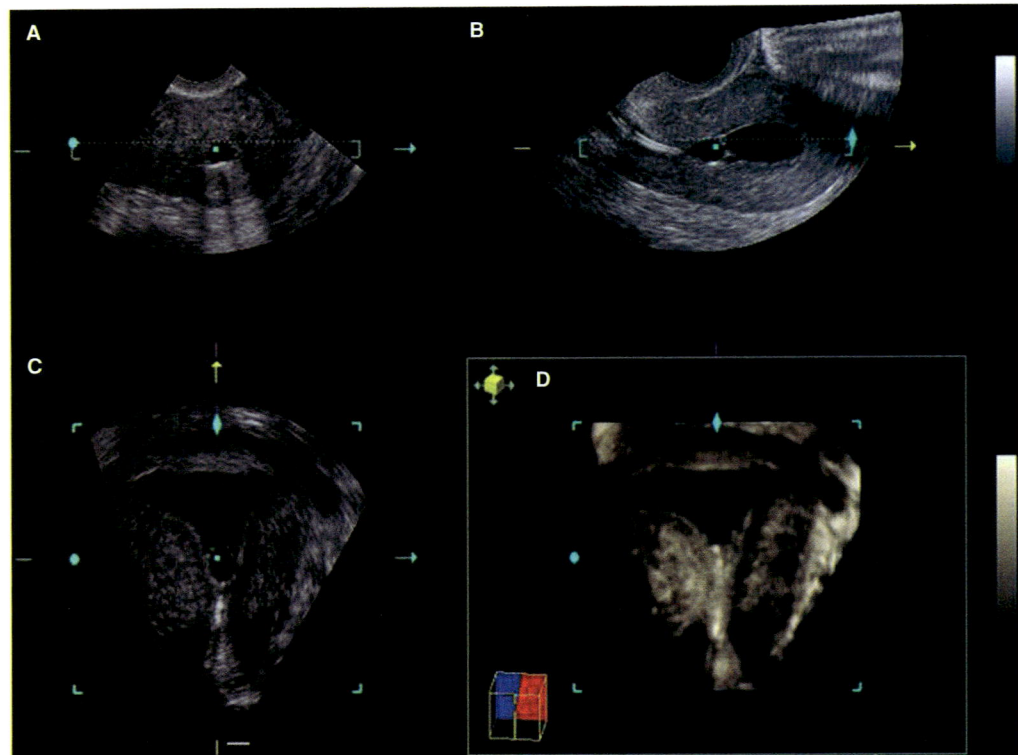

FIGURE 2-9 Multiplanar display of a 3-dimensional volume of a uterus and normal endometrial cavity during saline-infusion sonography. The views were obtained from a midsagittal reference plane using the Z technique. The planes are as follows: **A.** transverse, **B.** sagittal, **C.** coronal, **D.** rendered image.

be shown alone or in correlation with the multiplanar display. A rendered image is a "sum" of all the coronal planar images (see Fig. 2-9D). This is the display method that has been publicized in obstetrics, when showing the image of a fetal face in utero.

The inverse mode is a rendering technique of the entire volume in which all cystic areas within the volume become digitally opaque and all solid areas become transparent. This technique is useful when trying to see cystic areas that might be hidden in a volume, such as within an ovarian mass. Last, the volume can be displayed in parallel tomographic slices, similar to the displays used by CT and MR imaging.

3-D imaging is not without shortcomings. With 3-D sonography, the same type of acoustic artifacts that occur with 2-D imaging are encountered, such as acoustic shadowing and enhancement, refraction and reverberation, and motion artifacts from bowel peristalsis and vascular pulsation. Another potential pitfall in 3-D imaging of the pelvis involves spatial orientation within the saved volume data. Uterine flexion or version or left versus right may not be readily apparent on review of saved volumes. As such, during the preliminary real-time scanning, the operator must determine the orientation of the area of interest and notate it accordingly.

Another problem is related to the limited size of the volume box. Because of this, the entire uterus is often not acquired in a single volume. In some cases, it may be necessary to acquire two volumes, one for the cervix and a second for the uterine body. Likewise, a very large adnexal mass may not be imaged completely in any single volume of data obtained transvaginally.

The size of the volume box provided by the abdominal probe is greater. Thus with 3-D sonography, a large mass may need to be imaged transabdominally instead of transvaginally.

Clinical Use. Because it can study organs in numerous scanning planes, 3-D imaging has become invaluable in gynecology to assess the uterine cavity, complex ovarian masses, ovarian fertility reserve, uterine anomalies, and interstitial pregnancies. It simultaneously provides anatomic and dynamic information from pelvic floor structures and also from mesh implants.

Of these, mapping leiomyoma location relative to the endometrial cavity and surrounding structures is an essential step in triaging patients for treatment (Chap, 9, p. 206). For such mapping, 3-D sonography, in particular 3-D SIS, has been used in place of convention SIS or MR imaging (Keizer, 2018; Mavrelos, 2011). In patients receiving gonadotropin-releasing hormone (GnRH) agonists or following uterine artery embolization (UAE), 3-D sonography can also monitor leiomyoma volume reductions. However, following UAE, MR imaging is more often used.

Abnormalities of the endometrium and adjacent myometrium, especially focal endometrial thickenings such as polyps and cancer, may be better defined with 3-D technology (Fig. 2-10) (Benacerraf, 2008). In a recent Cochrane database review, 3-D SIS offered uterine cavity and endometrial thickness visualization rates comparable to hysteroscopy (Nieuwenhuis, 2017). We now routinely implement 3-D imaging for evaluation of abnormal endometrium during our TVS studies and with all SIS procedures.

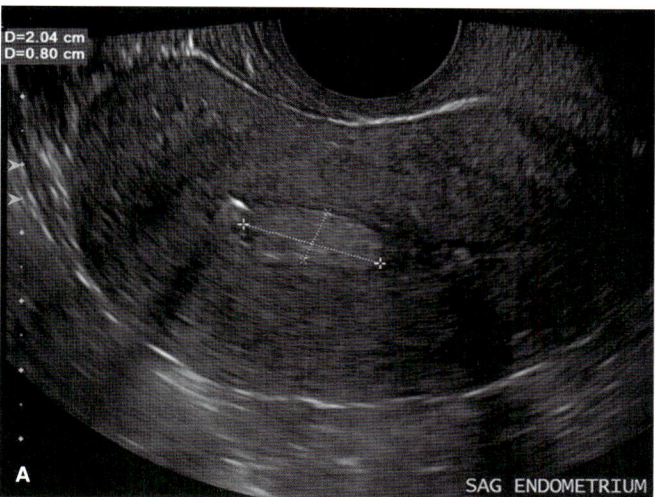
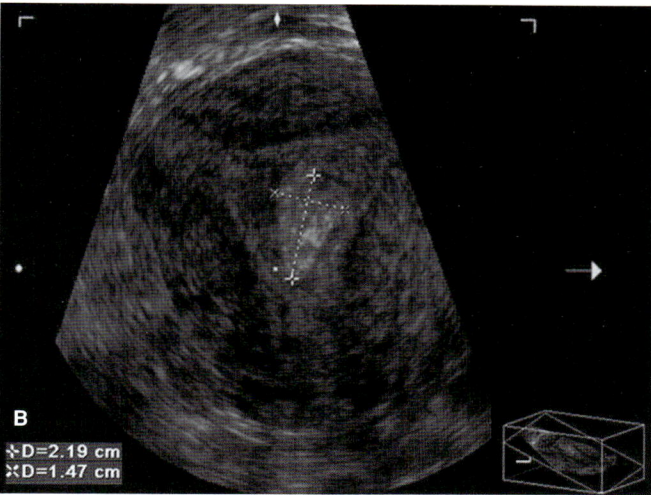

FIGURE 2-10 A. Transvaginal sonogram displays endometrial polyp measured by calipers. **B.** Three-dimensional image in the coronal plane of a polyp (*calipers*).

Although investigational, 3-D sonography with power Doppler angiography (3D-PDA) can help discriminate benign from malignant endometrial disease in women with postmenopausal bleeding and a thickened endometrium (Makled, 2013). Endometrial lesions in infertile women are another potential indication (Ni, 2019). 3D-PDA can assess endometrial volume, which may more accurately reflect true tissue volume than a 2-D endometrial thickness measurement. Another tool, 3-D power Doppler imaging enhanced by intravenous (IV) contrast, also is being studied to distinguish benign endometrial polyps from endometrial cancer (Lieng, 2008; Song, 2009).

IUD positioning within the endometrial cavity can be documented adequately in most cases with traditional 2-D TVS. That said, 3-D sonography offers improved visualization, especially with the levonorgestrel-containing IUDs (Moschos, 2011). The coronal plane images, which are not possible with 2-D imaging, provide views of the arms and shaft of the device and their

relation to the endometrial cavity (Benacerraf, 2009). At our institution, patients undergoing gynecologic sonography with an IUD in situ, regardless of the study indication, have both a standard 2-D evaluation and a 3-D volume acquisition of the uterus. The coronal view of the endometrial cavity is reconstructed to establish IUD type, location, and positioning (Fig. 2-11). TVS also is an acceptable method to confirm proper Essure coil positioning (Fig. 2-12) (Carretti, 2019; Legendre, 2010).

For adnexal mass interrogation, most agree that 3-D sonography provides detailed internal anatomy (Alcázar, 2003). Moreover, 3D-PDA displays the internal architecture and also the neovascularization characteristic of malignant neoplasms. However, 3D-PDA does not significantly improved diagnostic accuracy compared with that of grayscale and 2-D power Doppler imaging (Jokubkiene, 2007; Ohel, 2010).

In reproductive medicine, 3-D imaging acquires more precise ovarian volumes and follicle counts than measurements

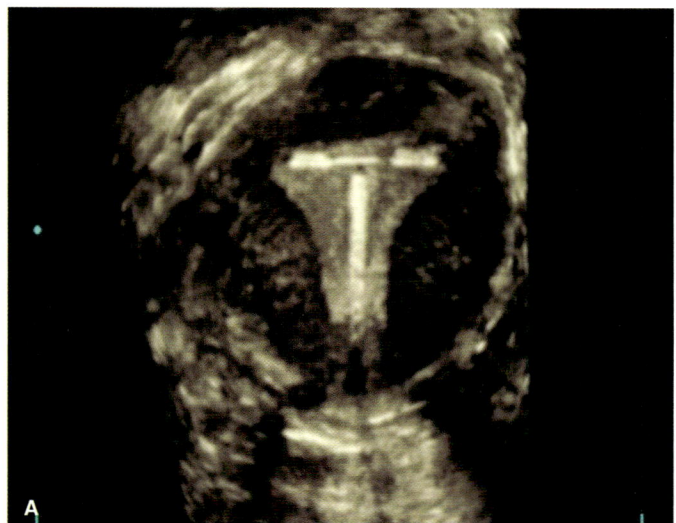
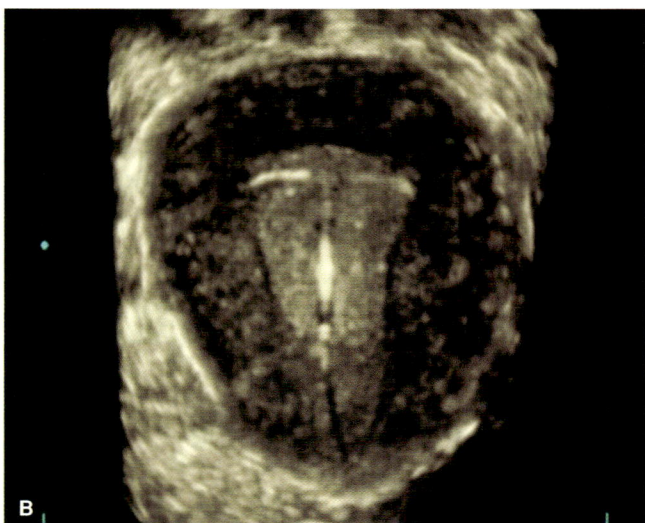

FIGURE 2-11 Intrauterine devices (IUDs). The coronal planes of 3-dimensional sonography best depict the type and positioning of the Copper T 380A IUD (ParaGard) **(A)** and levonorgestrel-containing IUD (Mirena) **(B)** within the endometrial cavity.

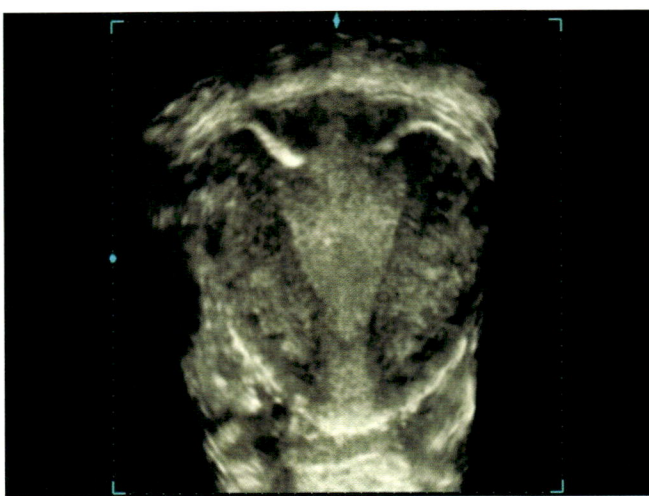

FIGURE 2-12 Essure contraception. Three-dimensional image in the coronal plane demonstrates the microinsert coils in the bilateral cornua of the uterus, corresponding to proper placement of the devices.

estimated from 2-D imaging. It is becoming the preferred ultrasound technique for infertility ovarian evaluation (Nylander, 2017; Peres Fagundes, 2017). Moreover, 3-D sonography can also examine endometrial vascularity and volume to help predict endometrial receptivity prior to ovarian stimulation (Wu, 2003; Zollner, 2012).

For congenital müllerian uterine anomalies, 3-D ultrasound is as sensitive as hysteroscopy and as accurate as MR imaging. It provides detailed images of both endometrial cavity shape and external fundal contour (Bermejo, 2010; Ghi, 2009). Because the uterine horns and fundal contour are displayed clearly in the same plane, müllerian anomalies can be differentiated (p. 41) (Troiano, 2004). This can help preoperative planning.

For pelvic reconstructive surgery indications, 3-D ultrasound can evaluate pelvic floor anatomy and pelvic support. In addition, polypropylene mesh implants appear as echogenic interwoven interfaces with ultrasound. In contrast, these are poorly depicted with radiography or MR imaging. As a result, 3-D vaginal and perineal sonography is now selected for this evaluation (Dietz, 2012, 2017; Fleischer, 2012). However, cranial aspects of mesh or retropubic mesh may be poorly imaged with 3-D ultrasound. For these patients, MR imaging may be helpful.

As a second indication, postprocessing reconstruction in a coronal plane improves views of the urethra and the periurethral tissue, which are inaccessible with 2-D ultrasound techniques. 3-D images are obtained with abdominal transducers using a translabial-transperineal approach or with transvaginal probes using specialized rotational transducers (Dietz, 2007, 2012; Santoro, 2011).

In women with pelvic floor dysfunction, the reconstructed ultrasound images afforded by 3-D ultrasound are particularly useful to quantify the degree of levator ani muscle defects (Dietz, 2017; Hedge, 2017). Perhaps most importantly, 3-D imaging can provide not only anatomic but also dynamic information about the pelvic floor structures, as imaging can

be executed with the patient performing the Valsalva maneuver or actively contracting the pelvic floor musculature (Fleischer, 2012).

Contrast-Enhanced Sonography

This newer technique couples IV contrast with traditional sonography. With contrast-enhanced sonography, the density (or signal intensity) of a focal lesion and its density compared with the surrounding normal organ tissue can be enhanced.

Ultrasound contrast agents used intravenously are small, stabilized microbubbles, usually 1 to 10 μm in diameter, and composed of perfluorocarbon or nitrogen gas encapsulated in albumin, phospholipid, or polymer shells. The gas-liquid interface contributes to the echogenicity of the microbubbles. Also, a high impedance mismatch between the microbubbles and adjacent RBCs in the blood vessels causes greater scatter and reflection of the ultrasound sound beam. This heightens the ultrasound signal and thereby increases brightness or echogenicity (Hwang, 2010). The degree of echo enhancement depends on many factors, including microbubble size, contrast agent density, bubble compressibility, and the interrogating ultrasound frequency. The greater the size, density, and compressibility of the agent, the more reflection and echogenicity are elicited (Eckersley, 2002).

For ovarian cancer, contrast-enhanced sonography may highlight tumor neovascularization in developing microscopic tumors (Wu, 2015). In addition, because vascular channels associated with malignancy are often incompetent, the resultant extravasation of RBCs and contrast agent may be detected (Fleischer, 2008). Accordingly, its preoperative interrogation of cervical and endometrial carcinomas can help determine the extent of invasion (Song, 2009; Zheng, 2018).

Other promising clinical applications of contrast-enhanced sonography include monitoring tumor and therapeutic angiogenesis, inflammation assessment, evaluation of ischemia and reperfusion injury, early detection of transplant rejection, and targeted drug delivery (Hwang, 2010; Peng 2016).

Sonoelastography

Elastography is an ultrasound imaging technique that measures tissue stiffness in both physiologic and pathologic states. With this modality, a source of "stress" promotes tissue deformation to assess stiffness (Stoelinga, 2014). For gynecologic imaging, vibration sonoelastography employs low-amplitude, low-frequency shear waves that propagate through the organ of interest. Simultaneously, real-time color Doppler techniques generate an image of tissue movement in response to the external vibrations (Taylor, 2000). For example, if a hard inhomogeneous mass, such as a tumor, lies within a region of soft tissue, the vibration amplitude is decreased at the tumor site.

Potential areas of investigation include distinguishing endometrial polyps from submucous pedunculated myomas, endometrial cancer from benign endometrial thickening, cervical cancer from normal cervical stroma, and leiomyomas from adenomyosis (Stoelinga, 2014, 2018). Moreover, uterine and cervical stiffness during pregnancy may help predict or manage preterm or postterm complications (Xie, 2018).

Focused-Ultrasound Therapy

Ultrasound energy during conventional imaging propagates harmlessly through tissue with little energy being absorbed. This energy is deposited as heat but dissipates by the cooling effects of perfusion and conduction. No harmful effects have been recorded at the intensities used for diagnostic purposes (American Institute of Ultrasound in Medicine, 2009).

If, however, the ultrasound beam carries high energy and is brought into tight focus, this energy is rapidly converted into heat. When target spot temperatures rise above 55°C, proteins are denatured, cells die, and coagulative necrosis follows. In contrast, surrounding tissues are warmed but not to lethal temperatures. In gynecology, this tool offers an option for leiomyoma ablation (Chap. 9, p. 210).

■ Normal Sonographic Findings

Reproductive Tract Organs

In the reproductive years, a normal uterus measures approximately 7.5 × 5.0 × 2.5 cm but is smaller in prepubertal, postmenopausal, or hypoestrogenized women. Normal uterine stroma returns low-level, uniform echoes, and the endometrial and endocervical canals are indicated by linear echogenic stripes that represent the interfaces between mucus and mucosa (Fig. 2-13). The cervix is best visualized transvaginally with the tip of the probe placed 2 to 3 cm from it. The endocervical canal is a continuation of the endometrial cavity and appears as a thin echogenic line (Fig. 2-14). The vagina is seen as a hypoechoic tubular structure with an echogenic lumen that curves inferiorly over the muscular perineal body at the introitus.

The ovaries are ellipsoid and normally lie in the ovarian fossa with their long axes parallel to the internal iliac vessels (Fig. 2-15). Ovarian volume ranges from 4 to 10 cubic centimeters depending on hormonal status (Cohen, 1990). Ovarian volume is calculated using the formula for an ellipse: $\pi/6 \times (A \times B \times C)$. In this formula, A, B, and C are the ovarian diameters in centimeters, measured in the three different planes.

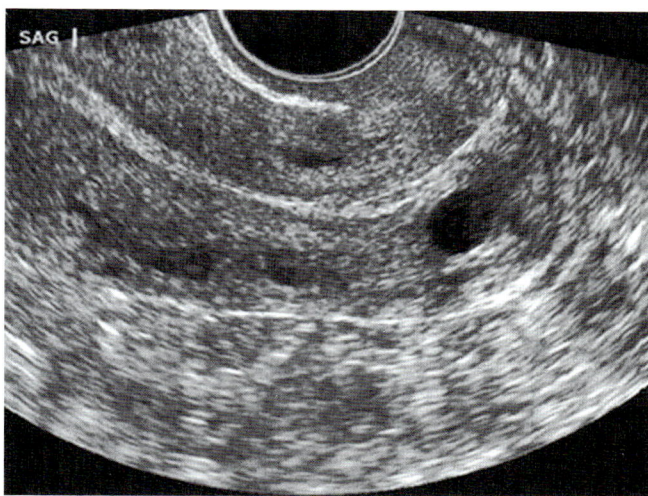

FIGURE 2-14 Transvaginal sonogram in the sagittal plane of a uterine cervix. An endocervical cyst is seen posterior to the thin, echogenic endocervical canal.

Ovarian follicles appear as spherical anechoic structures within the ovary and may reach a normal size of 3 cm. Normal fallopian tubes are not visible.

Endometrium

Functionally, the endometrium has two main layers: the *stratum basale*, which comprises the densely cellular supporting stroma and varies little with menstrual cycle phase, and the *stratum functionale*, which proliferates during each cycle and partially desquamates at menses. These layers cover the entire cavity.

Sonographically, the endometrium's appearance during the menstrual cycle correlates with the phasic changes in its histologic anatomy. During the follicular phase, when the endometrium is provided estrogen from ovarian folliculogenesis, the stratum basale appears echogenic due to spectral reflections from the mucus-laden glands. In contrast, the stratum functionale is relatively hypoechoic because of its orderly arrangement

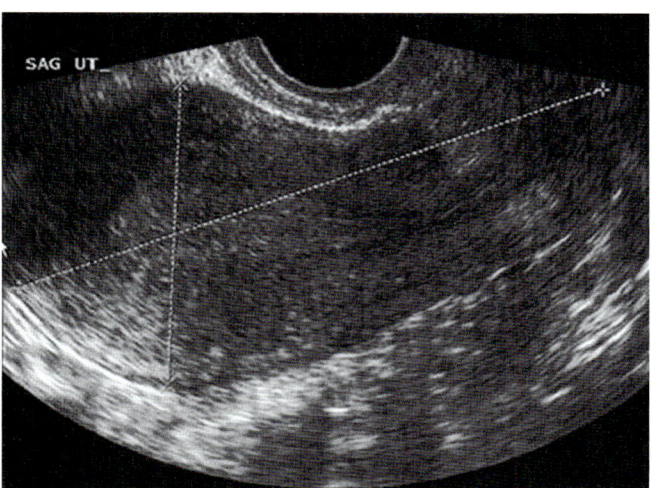

FIGURE 2-13 Transvaginal sonogram in the sagittal plane of an anteverted anteflexed uterus. Calipers demonstrate measurements of the uterine length (+) and the anterior-posterior dimension (×).

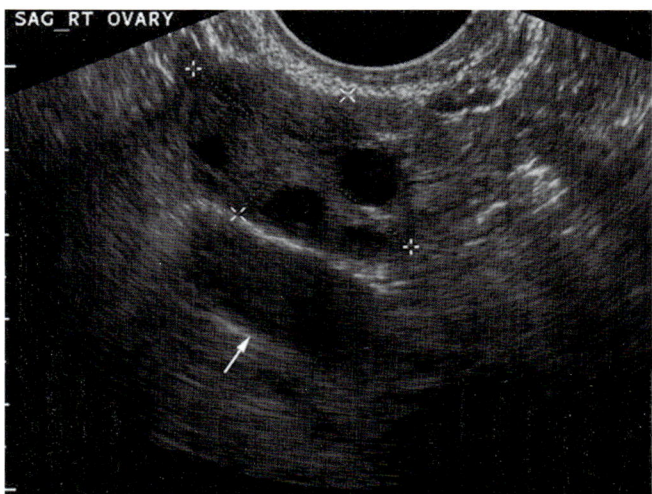

FIGURE 2-15 Transvaginal sonogram in the sagittal plane of an ovary (*calipers*) in a premenopausal woman. The ovary normally lies in the ovarian fossa, anterior to the internal iliac vessel (*arrow*).

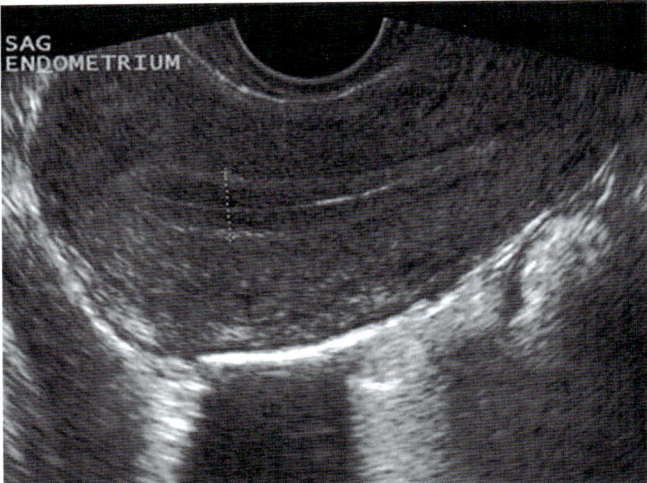

FIGURE 2-16 Transvaginal sonogram in the sagittal plane of a characteristic trilaminar proliferative endometrium. Calipers demonstrate proper measurement of the "double-layer" thickness made of the alternating hyper-hypo-hyperechogenic lines.

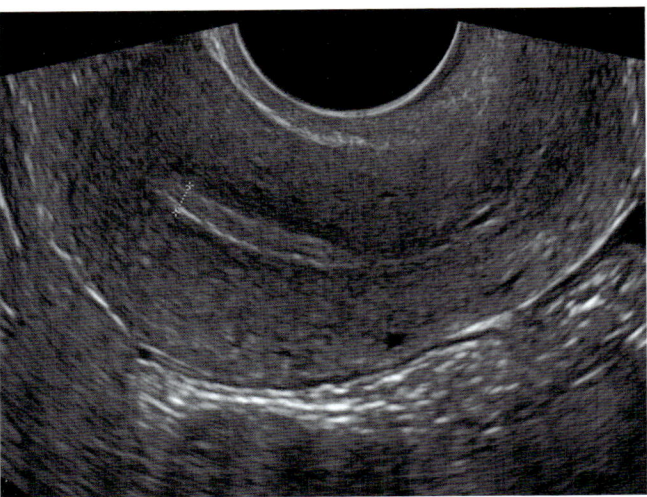

FIGURE 2-18 Transvaginal sonogram in the sagittal plane of a menstrual-phase endometrium, which is marked by calipers.

of glands that lack secretions. The central opposing surfaces of these two endometrial layers manifest as a highly reflective, thin midline strip. Together, the three echogenic lines create the characteristic trilaminar appearance of the proliferative endometrium (Fig. 2-16).

To measure the *endometrial thickness*, one caliper is placed at the echogenic interface of the anterior basale layer and myometrium. The other is positioned at the similar echogenic interface of the posterior basale layer. It thus represents a "double thickness." The hypoechoic halo outside of and adjacent to the endometrium is not included in the measurement, as this is actually the inner compact layer of myometrium. Sonographically, the endometrium is measured from a sagittal or long-axis image of the uterus in the plane where the central endometrial echo is contiguous with the endocervical canal and is distinct from the myometrium. Endometrial thickness correlates approximately with the day of the menstrual cycle up to day 7 or 8.

With ovulation and progesterone production from the corpus luteum, glandular enlargement and secretory vacuoles are seen histologically. During this secretory phase, the endometrium achieves its maximum thickness as the stroma becomes more vascular and edematous. Sonographically, these changes cause the endometrium to appear echogenic (Fig. 2-17).

With menstruation, the endometrium displays as a slightly irregular echogenic interface, which derives from sloughed tissue and blood. The thinnest endometrial measurements are found at the conclusion of menses (Fig. 2-18).

With cessation of estrogen stimulation, the endometrium atrophies, and cyclic sloughing ceases. The postmenopausal endometrium appears thin and uniform (Fig. 2-19).

Pelvic Floor

Sonography is widely used to evaluate pelvic floor anatomy and function (Dietz, 2017). First, various 2-D techniques,

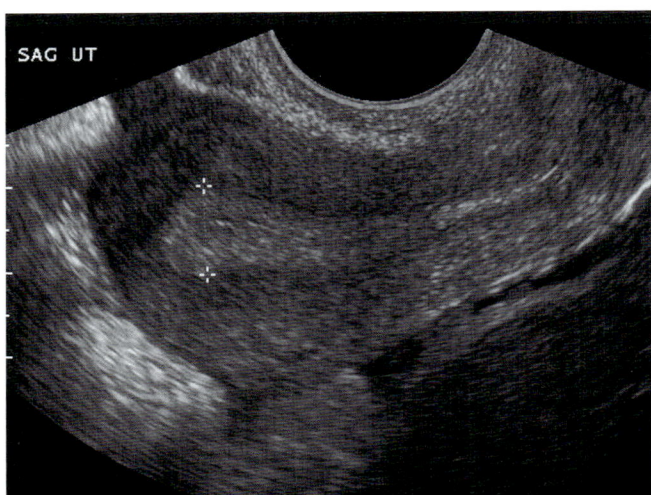

FIGURE 2-17 Transvaginal sonogram in the sagittal plane of a secretory endometrium. The endometrium, which is marked by calipers, has become uniformly echogenic.

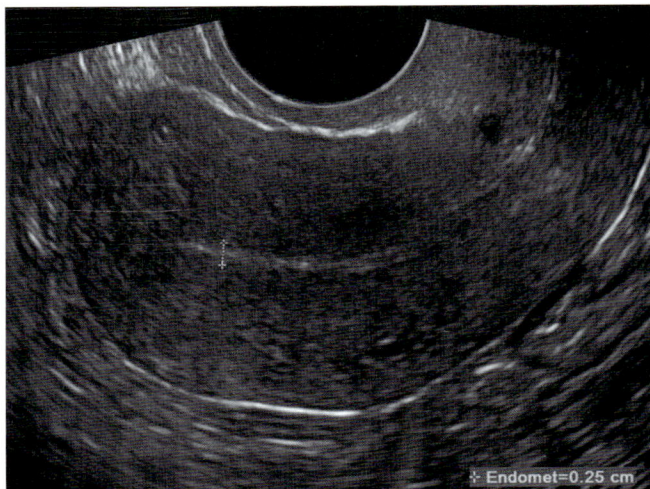

FIGURE 2-19 Transvaginal sonogram in the sagittal plane of an atrophic postmenopausal endometrium, which is marked by calipers.

including transvaginal, transrectal, transperineal, and intra-urethral sonography, can display urethral anatomy. In addition, anorectal morphology and the pelvic floor both can be assessed with vaginal sonography using a rotating endorectal probe or standard transvaginal probe (Chap. 25, p. 564). Less commonly, transrectal sonography can assess anal sphincter morphology after childbirth. This method requires special equipment and distention of the anal canal. The technique has limited value in the immediate puerperium and only provides information regarding the anal sphincter. Thus, without levator ani muscle assessment, the posterior compartment is incompletely evaluated.

Perineal sonography requires filling the bladder with approximately 300 mL of saline. With the woman either supine or erect, a 3.5- to 6-MHz curved-array transducer is placed in sagittal orientation to the perineum. This allows real-time imaging of the pubic symphysis, levator ani muscles, urethra, bladder neck, bladder, vagina, rectal ampulla, and anal canal simultaneously and with little transducer manipulation (Dietz, 2017; Schaer, 1995; Vellucci, 2018). Last, 3-D ultrasound is increasingly selected, and evaluation of pelvic anatomy, support, and mesh implants are some indications.

CLINICAL APPLICATIONS OF SONOGRAPHY

Transvaginal sonography is often preferred for early evaluation of pelvic pain, abnormal uterine bleeding, pelvic mass, early pregnancy complications, and infertility practices. Many of these topics and their radiologic characteristics are covered in other chapters. Some remaining important subjects are presented in the following sections.

■ Intraabdominal Fluid

During general sonographic evaluation of the pelvis, a small amount of free fluid, as little as 10 mL, is commonly present in the posterior cul-de-sac (Khalife, 1998). If free fluid is seen

extending to the fundus of the uterus, it is considered moderate in amount. Once identified, moderate free fluid should prompt further evaluation of the paracolic gutters and Morison pouch in the right upper quadrant to assess the fluid's extent (Fig. 2-20). If it fills these areas, then the minimum volume of intraperitoneal fluid approximates 500 mL (Abrams, 1999; Branney, 1995). Large amounts of anechoic free peritoneal fluid generically described as *ascites* suggest a volume status abnormality or an infectious or inflammatory etiology. Free fluid that contains low-level echoes or echogenic debris is consistent with hemoperitoneum with clot, such as with a ruptured hemorrhagic ovarian cyst or ectopic pregnancy.

Focused assessment with sonography for trauma (FAST) is a limited sonographic examination directed solely to help diagnosis intraperitoneal bleeding. With FAST, four specific areas are imaged: perihepatic (right upper quadrant), perisplenic (left upper quadrant), pelvis, and pericardium. For intraperitoneal free fluid identification, FAST is a rapid, noninvasive, bedside test and has significant advantages compared with diagnostic peritoneal lavage or with CT. However, FAST has a significant false-negative rate (Scalea, 1999). This stems in part from examination being carried out early when only a small amount of free fluid may have collected in dependent portions of the peritoneal cavity.

■ Malignant Ovarian Characteristics

Sonography is commonly the initial and often the only imaging procedure performed during pelvic and ovarian mass evaluation, as most can be correctly categorized based on grayscale and Doppler ultrasound characteristics. Found in Table 10-2 (p. 221), recommendations from a Society of Radiologists in Ultrasound consensus conference summarize a reasonable management approach to asymptomatic ovarian and other adnexal cysts imaged sonographically (Levine, 2010).

Sonography is the best preoperative diagnostic technique to determine the malignant potential of an ovarian mass

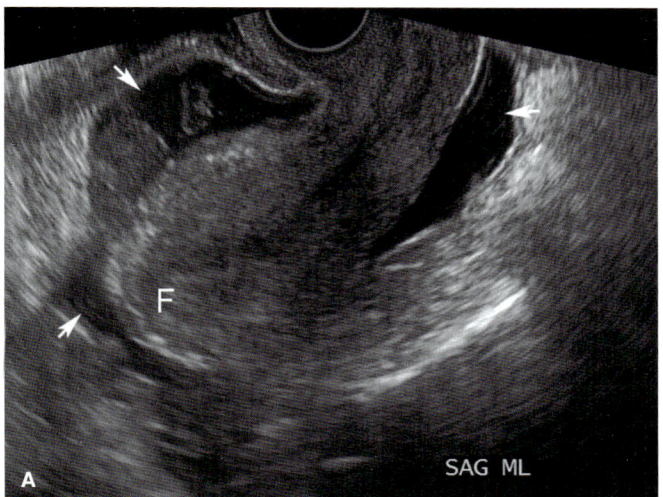

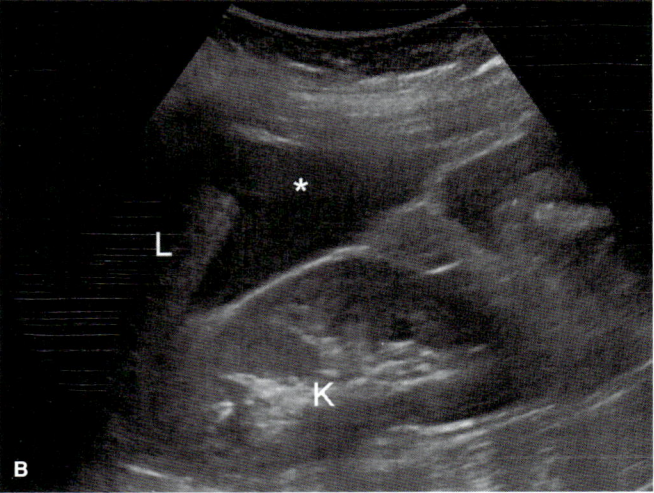

FIGURE 2-20 Hemoperitoneum. **A.** In this transvaginal image, a large amount of free fluid (*arrows*) is seen in the posterior cul-de-sac, above the fundus of the uterus, and in the anterior cul-de-sac. Floating clot is also seen in the anterior cul-de-sac. **B.** Transabdominal image of Morison pouch in the right upper quadrant. Free fluid, corresponding to the dark anechoic area (*asterisk*), is visualized between the liver edge (*L*) and the kidney (*K*), which suggests a large-volume hemoperitoneum.

(Twickler, 2010). To this end, morphologic scoring systems based on number and thickness of septa, presence and number of papillations, and proportion of solid tissue within the mass have been proposed to standardize findings (DePriest, 1993; Sassone, 1991). When size, morphology, and structure of adnexal masses are combined with color Doppler and spectral analysis of flow signals, the specificity and positive predictive value of sonographic diagnosis are increased (Buy, 1996; Fleischer, 1993; Jain, 1994; Kinkel, 2000). The International Ovarian Tumor Analysis (IOTA) Group has developed the most accurate mathematic model to date to calculate the malignancy risk of an adnexal mass based on sonographic features (Timmerman, 2005, 2016). We use the Ovarian Tumor Index developed by Twickler and colleagues (1999) at our institution.

Neovascularity secondary to angiogenesis within a malignant neoplasm increases color Doppler flow signals. These new vessels are abnormal, lack smooth muscle, and contain multiple arteriovenous shunts. Consequently, low-impedance flow is expected with such masses (see Fig. 2-4) (Kurjak, 1992; Weiner, 1992). Moreover, most malignant lesions appear well-vascularized and display flow signals in both peripheral and central regions—including within septations and solid tumor areas. In contrast, most benign tumors appear poorly vascularized. Of Doppler parameters, the color content of a tumor probably reflects tumor vascularity better than any other. The overall impression of this vascularity reflects both the number and size of vessels and their functional capacity. The IOTA group scoring system uses this subjective semiquantitative assessment of flow to describe the vascular features of ovarian masses (Ameye, 2009; Timmerman, 2005). A four-point color score is used to describe tumor blood flow only within septa and solid portions of the mass (Timmerman, 2000). However, because of overlap of vascular parameters between malignant and benign neoplasms, a firm differential diagnosis based on spectral Doppler evaluation alone is not possible (Valentin, 1997).

■ Pelvic Inflammatory Disease

With acute salpingitis, pelvic sonography is commonly performed as part of an acute pain assessment. However, large studies evaluating its sensitivity, specificity, or overall usefulness for PID diagnosis are lacking (Romosan, 2014). Sonographic findings vary according to disease severity, and in early infection, anatomy may appear normal. With progression, early nonspecific findings include free pelvic fluid, endometrial thickening, endometrial cavity distention by fluid or gas, and indistinct borders of the uterus and ovaries. Enlarged ovaries with increased numbers of small cysts—a "polycystic ovary appearance"—can correlate with PID. With treatment, this ovarian enlargement resolves (Cacciatore, 1992).

Sonographic findings of the fallopian tubes are the most striking and specific landmarks of PID (Fig. 2-21). Although normal tubes are rarely seen unless surrounded by ascites, tubal wall inflammation allows visualization with sonography. As the lumen occludes distally, the tube distends and fills with pus. Various appearances result. The tube may become ovoid or pear shaped, filling with fluid that may be anechoic or echoic. The tubal wall becomes thickened, measuring ≥5 mm, and

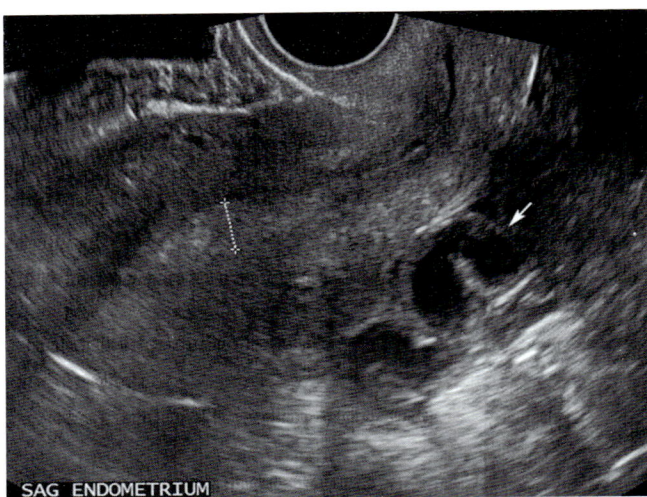

FIGURE 2-21 Transvaginal sonogram of an inflamed, dilated fallopian tube (*arrow*) demonstrating thickened tubal walls, incomplete septa, and intratubal fluid.

incomplete septa are common as the tube folds back on itself. If the distended tube is viewed in cross section it may demonstrate the cogwheel sign, due to thickened endosalpingeal folds (Timor-Tritsch, 1998). Typically, the swollen fallopian tubes extend posteriorly into the cul-de-sac, rather than extending cephalad and anterior to the uterus as large ovarian tumors tend to do. Fluid-debris levels are often visualized in the dilated tubes, and rarely, gas-fluid levels or echogenic bubbles of gas are seen. Color and power Doppler show increased flow from hyperemia in the walls and in incomplete septa of the inflamed tubes (Tinkanen, 1993).

As the disease progresses, the ovary can become involved. When an ovary adheres to the fallopian tube, but is still visualized, it is called a *tuboovarian complex*. In contrast, a *tuboovarian abscess (TOA)* results from a complete breakdown of ovarian and tubal architecture such that the separate structures are no longer identified (Fig. 2-22). If the contralateral side was

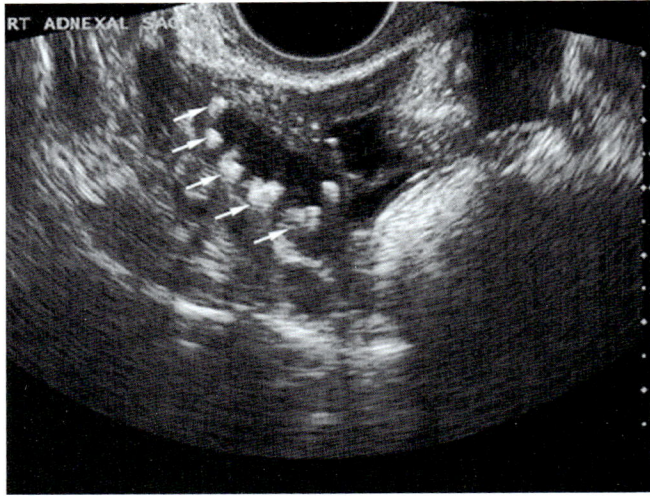

FIGURE 2-22 "Beads on a string" sign. The echogenic mural nodules shown here (*arrows*) within this tuboovarian abscess are thought to represent flattened and fibrotic endosalpingeal folds of the inflamed fallopian tube.

not affected initially, it may become so. When both tubes are inflamed and occluded, the entire complex typically acquires a U-shape as it fills the cul-de-sac, extending from one adnexal region to the other. The lateral and posterior uterine borders become obscure, and individual tubes and ovaries cannot be distinguished. In women not responding to medical therapy, sonography or CT can be used to guide percutaneous or transvaginal drainage of TOAs.

Findings of chronic PID include hydrosalpinx. As discussed in Chapter 10 (p. 229), several sonographic findings such as its tubular shape, incomplete septa, and hyperechoic mural nodules can help to distinguish a hydrosalpinx from other cystic adnexal lesions. If color flow is detected in a hydrosalpinx, it tends to be less exuberant than flow seen in acute PID. Molander and colleagues (2002) found a higher pulsatility index in patients with a chronic hydrosalpinx (1.5 ± 0.1) than with acute PID (0.84 ± 0.04).

A small number of women with prior PID may have a peritoneal inclusion cyst. These form when ruptured ovarian cyst fluid is trapped around the ovary by adhesions. This diagnosis is suspected if the ovary is surrounded by fluid loculations created by thin septations.

■ Infertility

For female infertility evaluation, sonography can help identify abnormal pelvic anatomy, detect contributory pathology, and evaluate cyclic physiologic uterine and ovarian changes. During treatment, sonography aids ovarian surveillance to guide management.

Sonography easily demonstrates many uterine defects that may affect both gamete passage and ovum implantation. TVS can display submucous leiomyomas and polyps, but their relationships with the endometrial surface are better seen with SIS. As a screening tool for cavity evaluation in this setting, SIS appears to be twice as accurate as HSG or TVS (Seshadri, 2015). Many infertility specialists now incorporate SIS as a first-line screening tool for uterine evaluation before embryo transfer in women undergoing IVF, ovum donation, or IVF-surrogacy. Intrauterine adhesions, also termed *synechiae*, are displayed as hypoechoic lines disrupting the echogenic endometrium. These are more definitively seen during SIS as echogenic bands extending from one endometrial surface to the other (Fig. 2-23).

TVS also can help detect congenital uterine anomalies related to infertility or early spontaneous abortion. The addition of 3-D techniques raises sonographic test performance to a level similar to that of HSG, laparoscopy, and MR imaging. Thereafter, MR imaging is used to characterize and evaluate complicated or equivocal cases, especially preoperatively (p. 49).

Of abnormalities, a fusion anomaly, such as uterus didelphys, can be accurately diagnosed by sonography. In this setting, two divergent uterine horns are separated by a deep fundal cleft, and a wide angle separates the two endometrial cavities (Fig. 2-24). In contrast, bicornuate and septate uterine anomalies are less confidently differentiated by traditional 2-D TVS techniques. Ideally, the angle between the two endometrial cavities is ≥105° for bicornuate uterus, but ≤75° for septate uterus. The fundal shape shows a >1-cm notch for bicornuate uterus, but a <1-cm notch for septate uterus (Reuter, 1989).

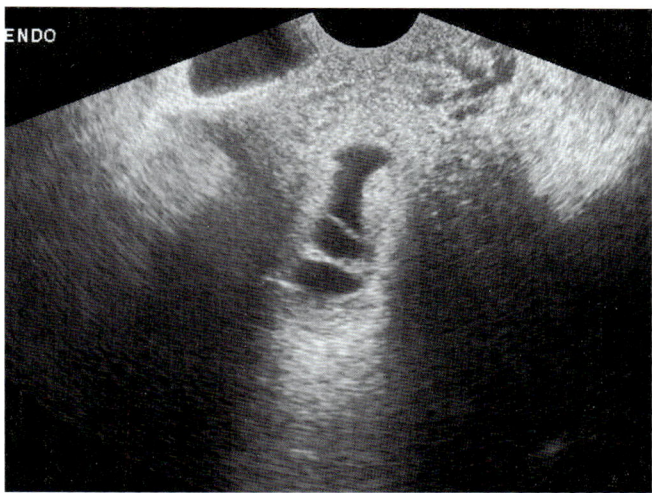

FIGURE 2-23 Asherman syndrome. Transvaginal saline-infusion sonography demonstrates echogenic intrauterine synechiae.

However, in many cases, the distinctions between bicornuate and septate uteri are subtle. In a 3-D coronal plane, relationship between the uterine fundus and the *intercornual line*—the line joining both horns of the uterine cavity—can be measured to aid diagnosis (Fig. 2-25). Similarly, arcuate versus partial septate uteri can be correctly differentiated using quantitative measurements of the endometrial cavity fundal indentation depth in the coronal plane. Combining 3-D TVS findings with SIS provides accuracy up to 90 percent to distinguish the two anomalies. Although MR imaging is frequently employed, 3-D sonography is considered by many to be the best noninvasive method for distinguishing between these uterine anomalies (Bermejo, 2010).

A unicornuate uterus without a rudimentary horn is seen as a small, well-formed elliptical uterus that deviates to one side. The fundus is concave. With 3-D imaging, the unicornuate uterus has a classic "banana" configuration (Fig. 2-26). In 65 percent of cases, however, the unicornuate uterus is associated with a

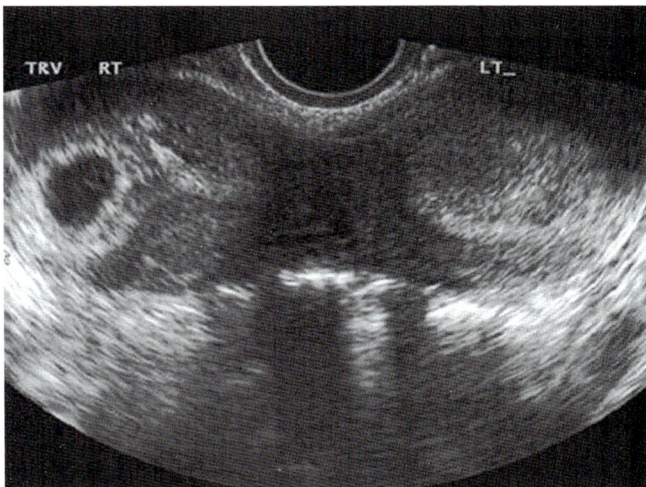

FIGURE 2-24 Uterus didelphys. Transvaginal sonogram in the transverse plane best depicts the two completely separate uterine horns. A gestational sac is evident in the right uterus.

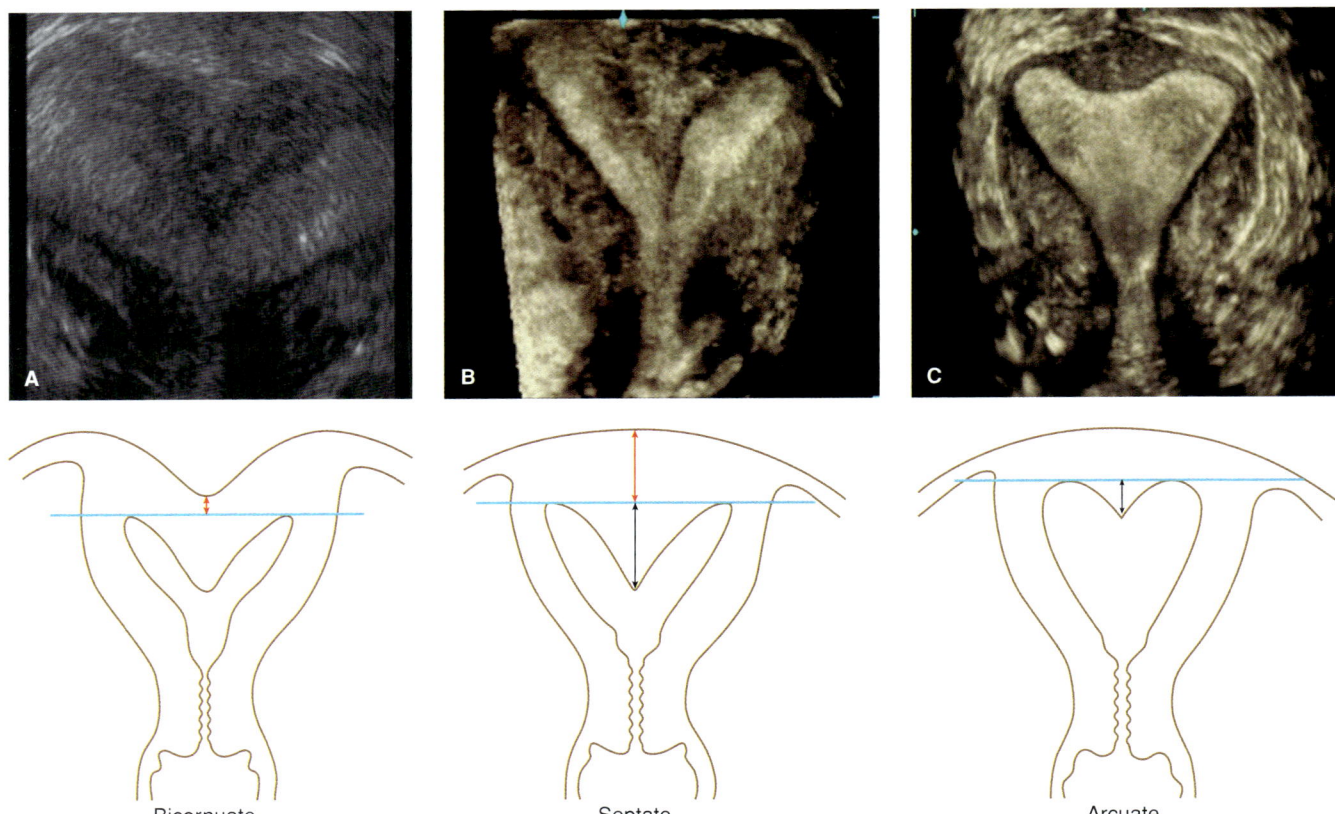

FIGURE 2-25 Three-dimensional (3-D) images of müllerian uterine anomalies in the coronal plane and corresponding diagrammatic uteri. **A.** Bicornuate uterus. This 3-D rendered image demonstrates a concave external fundal contour that dips to a point near the intercornual line. This point lies no further than 5 mm from the intercornual line (*red line*), which characterizes a bicornuate uterus. The 5-mm defining distance, either above or below the intercornual line, is used to differentiate bicornuate and septate uteri. **B.** Septate uterus. This image depicts the narrow angle between the two small endometrial cavities, which is characteristic of a septate uterus, and shows a normal uterine serosal contour. This contour extends >5 mm (*red line*) above the intercornual line, which is characteristic of a septate uterus. The septum ends at the uterine isthmus and does not extend into the cervix. Thus, this anomaly is properly termed *subseptate*. **C.** Arcuate uterus. This image illustrates the normal uterine contour and obtuse angle of the endometrial cleft that is characteristic of an arcuate uterus. The cleft extends <15 mm (*black line*) below the intercornual line, which is characteristic of arcuate uterus. In diagram B, the distance (*black line*) between the cleft and intercornual line is >15 mm, which reflects a septate uterus. This 15-mm defining distance is used to differentiate arcuate and septate uteri.

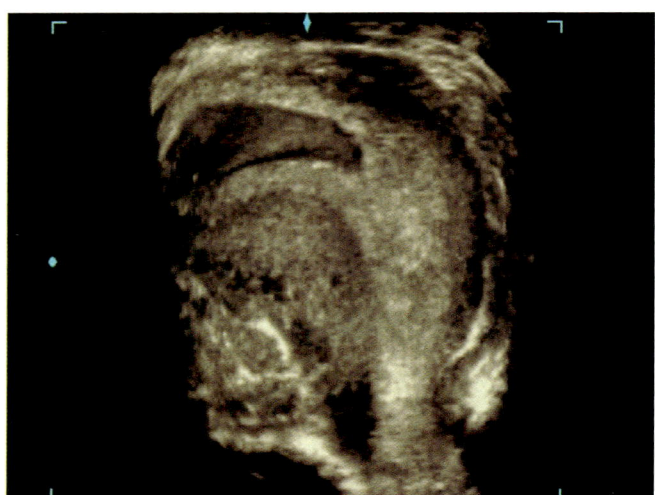

FIGURE 2-26 Unicornuate uterus. The coronal plane of 3-dimensional sonography illustrates the classic "banana" configuration. A gestational sac is seen within the endometrial cavity.

rudimentary horn, which is difficult to recognize sonographically (Fig. 19-11, p. 420) (Jayasinghe, 2005). A rudimentary horn is often misdiagnosed as a uterine or adnexal mass. Complete evaluation of these cases often requires MR imaging. With most uterine anomalies, especially if unilateral, proper positioning of the kidneys should be documented with transabdominal imaging. This is because of the close link between reproductive and urinary anomalies. Last, in women with complex anomalies associated with vaginal agenesis or imperforate hymen, hematocolpos is often seen and frequently is associated with hematometra or hematosalpinx.

Pelvic endometriosis is a prominent cause of infertility, and sonography is the most common imaging procedure in suspected cases. It is most effective to evaluate endometriotic ovarian cysts, and its capability to detect small implants and adhesions is limited. Endometriomas exhibit various sonographic appearances, the most frequent being a pelvic mass with a thick wall and diffuse low-level echoes within the cyst (Fig. 11-4, p. 239). Magnetic resonance imaging is more specific than sonography for identifying endometriomas, and thus, it is indicated in cases with unclear anatomy sonographically (Fig. 11-5, p. 240).

Sonography is invaluable for infertility treatment surveillance. First, folliculogenesis both in normal and stimulated cycles can be monitored. Observation of a developing follicle and ovulation prediction allow optimal timing for postcoital testing, human chorionic gonadotropin (hCG) administration, intercourse, insemination, and ovum collection. At ovulation, the dominant follicle usually disappears, and fluid is observed in the cul-de-sac. At the follicular site, the corpus luteum appears as an irregular oval containing a small quantity of fluid, internal echoes, and a thick wall. In general, blood flow in the ovulating ovary diminishes throughout the menstrual cycle. At ovulation, blood flow velocities dramatically rise in vessels surrounding the corpus luteum because of neovascularization and are seen as low-impedance waveforms. In women undergoing in vitro fertilization (IVF), low ovarian vessel impedance may correlate directly with pregnancy rates (Majeed, 2018).

Sonography can be used to guide interventional maneuvers such as oocyte retrieval and transfer of embryos into the endometrial cavity (Figs. 21-10 and 21-12, p. 465). In stimulated cycles, sonographic detection of too many follicles allows withholding of hCG induction to prevent ovarian hyperstimulation syndrome (Fig. 21-4, p. 457). If this develops, sonography is used to grade disease severity through measurements of ovarian size, detection of ascites, and analysis of renal flow resistances.

■ Ultrasound Beyond the Pelvis

Ultrasound is used throughout the body. It is often the initial tool in radiologic evaluation, given its lack of ionizing radiation, low cost, and availability. In the abdomen, common indications for solid organ evaluation include abdominal and flank pain, jaundice, hematuria, organomegaly, or palpable mass. Abnormal blood tests, including elevated liver function tests and creatinine, also may be indications for an abdominal ultrasound. Typically, a limited or right upper quadrant ultrasound includes the liver, gallbladder, common bile duct, pancreas, and right kidney. A complete abdominal ultrasound adds the spleen, left kidney, and images of the aorta and inferior vena cava in the upper abdomen. Ideally, a patient has fasted prior to sonographic evaluation of the abdomen. This minimizes bowel gas and permits adequate gallbladder distention. A renal ultrasound focuses on the kidneys, proximal collecting systems, and urinary bladder. Outside of the abdomen and pelvis, a gynecologist may select ultrasound to evaluate superficial structures, like the thyroid gland and breasts. Breast imaging is discussed fully in Chapter 13 (p. 279).

Compression Sonography

Compression sonography, often combined with color Doppler sonography, is the initial test currently used to detect deep-vein thrombosis (DVT) (Hanley, 2018; Needleman, 2018). Leg vein interrogation is divided into two components. First, the groin and thigh are examined with the patient supine. Then, the popliteal region is evaluated with the patient sitting or lying on her side with the thigh abducted and externally rotated. Some institutions also evaluate the calf veins. Impaired visibility, noncompressibility, and the typical echo pattern of a thrombosed vein confirm the diagnosis (Fig. 2-27).

Examination of the femoral, popliteal, and calf trifurcation veins in symptomatic patients is more than 90-percent sensitive and greater than 99-percent specific for proximal DVT (Davis, 2001). Moreover, in 220 patients with suspected DVT, Lensing and coworkers (1989) compared compression sonography with contrast venography, which is the gold standard for DVT detection. Both the common femoral and popliteal veins were fully compressible—no thrombosis—in 142 of 143 patients who had a normal venogram (99-percent specific). All 66 patients with proximal vein thrombosis had noncompressible femoral or popliteal veins or both (100-percent sensitive).

For detecting calf vein thrombosis, compression sonography is significantly less reliable. Eventually, isolated calf thromboses extend into the proximal veins in up to a fourth of cases. They do so within 1 to 2 weeks of presentation and thus are usually detected by serial sonographic compression examinations (Bates, 2004). The safety of withholding anticoagulation for those symptomatic patients who have a normal compression examination has been established (Birdwell, 1998; Friera, 2002). Importantly, normal venous sonographic findings do not necessarily exclude pulmonary embolism (PE) because the thrombosis may have already embolized or because it arose from deep pelvic veins, which are inaccessible to sonographic evaluation (Goldhaber, 2004).

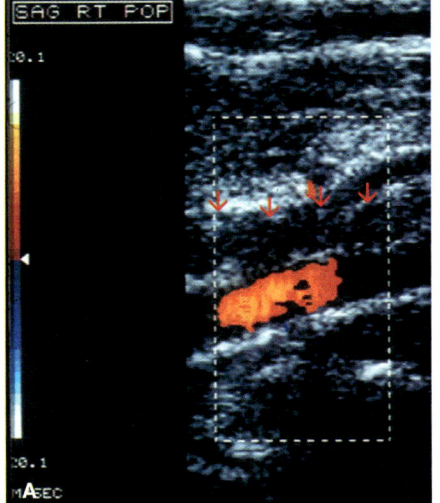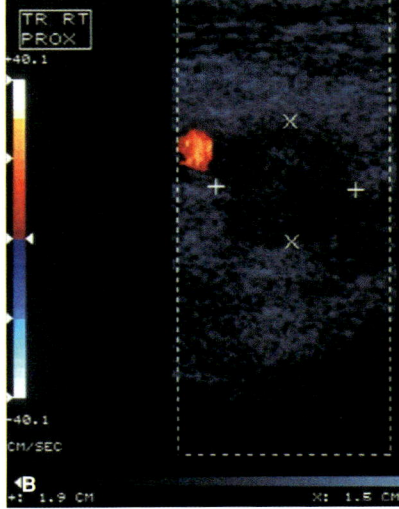

FIGURE 2-27 Sagittal **(A)** and transverse **(B)** images from a lower extremity. Color Doppler ultrasound study in a woman with popliteal vein thrombosis. **A.** Red arrows demarcate the popliteal vein with no flow suggesting clot in the lumen, which sits above the artery demonstrating normal flow as evidenced by the red color map. **B.** The transverse image shows the large size of the vein due to the thrombus (*cursors*), as well as normal flow in the artery, evidenced by the red color map.

RADIOGRAPHY

Radiographs are used in gynecologic practice in a manner similar to other medical specialties. Of frequently used studies, the *acute abdominal series* includes an upright radiograph of the chest to exclude free air under the diaphragm, an upright film of the abdomen to exclude air-fluid levels within bowel loops, and a supine image to measure bowel loop widths. It is commonly selected as an initial modality if bowel obstruction or perforation is a concern. Importantly, images from those with recent laparotomy or laparoscopy often show expected subdiaphragmatic air. In contrast, a single supine radiograph of the abdomen is called a KUB (kidneys, ureters, and bladder). It may help identify an extrauterine location of a missing IUD or a collecting-system stone.

In women with gynecologic malignancies, radiographs also may be informative. Examples are chest radiographs to screen for pulmonary metastases during cancer staging and during surveillance after initial treatment. As discussed in the next sections, several specialized radiographic procedures are especially useful or specific for gynecology.

■ Intravenous Pyelography

Excretory urography, also called *intravenous pyelography (IVP)*, provides serial images of the urinary tract. The initial radiograph, termed a *scout film*, helps identify radiopaque urinary calculi. IV contrast is then administered, and the concentrating function of the proximal tubules renders renal parenchyma radiodense within 1 to 3 minutes. This *nephrogram phase* displays renal size, contour, and axis. Next, a radiograph obtained 5 minutes after agent injection depicts contrast excreted into the collecting system. During this *pyelogram phase,* the calyces and proximal ureters are evaluated for symmetry and excretion promptness. Serial imaging is obtained as the more distal collecting system and bladder are opacified by contrast, and a final postvoid radiograph completes the series.

Up to 5 to 10 percent of women have an allergic reaction to iodide during IVP, and 1 to 2 percent of reactions are life threatening. In addition, hyperosmolar ionic contrast can be nephrotoxic because of direct tubular insult and ischemic injury. Notably, women with diabetes, renal impairment, and congestive heart failure are at high risk for this contrast nephrotoxicity. As alternatives, nonionic low and isoosmolar iodinated contrast media carry a five- to 30-fold lower incidence of allergic reactions and are less nephrotoxic (Mishell, 1997). Because of this improved safety profile, most centers no longer use intravascular hyperosmolar ionic contrast.

Preoperatively, IVP may be selected to identify urinary anomalies coexistent with congenital reproductive tract defects or confirm lower urinary tract compression by an adjacent pelvic mass. However, many preoperative IVPs have been replaced with multiphasic CT urography protocols performed on multislice CT scanners (Beyersdorff, 2008). For example, as it now is a suitable element of cervical cancer staging, many clinicians substitute CT imaging for IVP in initial cervical cancer evaluation. Of value, CT allows the cervix, parametria, uterus, adnexa, retroperitoneal lymph nodes, liver, and ureters to be imaged concurrently.

For suspected nephrolithiasis, the American College of Radiology recommends primary evaluation using noncontrast CT given its superior sensitivity for these stones (Moreno, 2015). To evaluate hematuria, noncontrast combined with contrast-enhanced CT images (CT urography) is most appropriate because of its improved sensitivity for renal and urothelial masses. Although IVP has higher in-plane spatial resolution, the current recommendations are to move immediately to initial one-step CT evaluation as CT is frequently needed regardless of IVP results to delineate abnormalities (Cowan, 2007, 2012). That said, IVP may still play a role, especially in resource-poor areas, in postoperative patients, and in those for whom radiation exposure is ideally minimized. Specifically, IVP delivers an average adult effective dose of 1 to 10 mSv, whereas CT urography carries an average adult effective dose of 10 to 30 mSv (Moreno, 2015).

■ Voiding Cystourethrography and Positive Pressure Urethrography

These radiographic procedures are used to evaluate the female urethra. Voiding cystourethrography (VCUG) is performed by placing a small catheter into the urinary bladder to instill contrast media. If present, diverticula that open into the urethra will fill with contrast. In cases of suspected vesicovaginal or urethrovaginal fistula, the contrast trail connecting the two involved structures is seen.

In comparison, MR imaging permits superior visualization of urethral abnormalities and is more sensitive than VCUG or positive pressure urethrography (PPUG) for delineating diverticula with complex structure (Chou, 2008; Neitlich, 1998). For this reason, VCUG is currently more often used to evaluate lower urinary tract injury, such as fistulas, and patients with prolonged urinary retention, incontinence, or suspected vesicoureteral reflux.

Described in more detail in Chapter 26 (p. 583), PPUG use has declined. This stems mainly from fewer technicians trained to complete the study, difficulty finding appropriate equipment, and the higher sensitivity of MR imaging.

■ Hysterosalpingography

This radiographic imaging technique is typically used during infertility evaluations to assess the endocervical canal, the endometrial cavity, and the fallopian tube lumina by injecting radiopaque contrast material through the cervical canal (Chap. 20, p. 438). An average HSG study is performed in 10 minutes, involves approximately 90 seconds of fluoroscopic time, and has an average radiation exposure to the ovaries of 0.01 to 0.02 Gy. As discussed previously (p. 32), hysterosalpingo-contrast sonography is used by some initially in place of HSG to assess tubal patency.

Hysterosalpingography is performed between cycle days 5 and 10. During this time, cessation of menstrual flow minimizes infection and the risk of flushing an ovum from the fallopian tube following ovulation. The test causes cramping, and an NSAID taken 30 minutes prior to the procedure may limit discomfort. To begin, a designated balloon-tipped injection catheter or acorn cannula is introduced just beyond the internal os in the lower endometrial cavity, as this location is more comfortable for the patient. However, the catheter may also be positioned just beyond the external os within the endocervical canal if necessary. A paracervical block may be indicated in selected patients, such as those with cervical stenosis. Because rapid injection may cause tubal spasm, slow contrast injection of usually no more than 3 to 4 mL of contrast medium allows a clear outline of the uterine cavity. Generally, few radiographic views are needed: a preliminary view before injecting contrast, a view showing uterine cavity filling, and the third demonstrating spill of contrast from the tubes into the peritoneal cavity. An additional image with the catheter deflated and pulled back into the endocervical canal will typically be obtained at the conclusion of the examination to evaluate the lower uterine cavity and internal os.

A normal endometrial cavity is usually triangular or sometimes T-shaped in the anteroposterior (AP) projection (Fig. 20-6, p. 439). In a lateral view, it is oblong. The contour of the endometrium is usually smooth. It occasionally has polypoid filling defects that can be isolated or diffuse and can be difficult to distinguish from endometrial polyps or hyperplasia. Inadvertent injection of air bubbles introduces artifact. In these instances, SIS is often later obtained to further interrogate the endometrial cavity.

Contraindications to HSG include acute pelvic infection, active uterine bleeding, pregnancy, and iodine allergy. HSG complications are rare but can be serious. Of these, the overall risk of acute pelvic infection serious enough to require hospitalization is <1 percent but can reach 3 percent in women with prior pelvic infection (Stumpf, 1980). In patients with no history of pelvic infection, HSG is performed without prophylactic antibiotics. If HSG demonstrates dilated fallopian tubes, doxycycline, 100 mg orally twice daily for 5 days, is given to reduce the incidence of post-HSG PID. In patients with a history of pelvic infection, doxycycline can be administered before the procedure and continued if dilated fallopian tubes are found (American College of Obstetricians and Gynecologists, 2018). Pelvic pain, uterine perforation, and vasovagal reactions also may occur. From the contrast, allergic reaction and entry into the vascular system from high injection pressure are potential risks.

■ Selective Salpingography

In some cases, it is not possible to distinguish whether tubal blockage seen by HSG is caused by anatomic occlusion or tubal spasm. Described in Chapter 44 (p. 1067), hysteroscopic tubal cannulation can further clarify and treat many cases of proximal tubal occlusion. Alternatively, transcervical selective salpingography and tubal catheterization (SS-TC) under fluoroscopic guidance is another suitable procedure. Similar to HSG, it is performed during the follicular phase. The tubal catheter is forwarded through the cervix and advanced by tactile sensation to the tubal ostium. The position of the catheter is checked fluoroscopically, and water- or oil-soluble contrast is injected. If the obstruction is overcome, the tubal contour is outlined with contrast agent. If the proximal tubal obstruction persists, a guide wire is threaded through the inner cannula of the catheter, advanced toward the obstruction, and gently manipulated to overcome the blockage. The guide wire is then withdrawn, and contrast medium is injected through the catheter to confirm patency. This fluoroscopic tool is effective at diagnosing and treating proximal tubal blockage, as discussed in Chapter 21 (p. 459) (Capitanio, 1991; Thurmond, 1991).

■ Bone Densitometry

Depending on its mineral density, bone absorbs x-rays to different degrees. Because of this, bone density can be determined, and most measurements provide site-specific information. However, these studies do not assess current or past bone remodeling rates. Thus, sequential density measurements are necessary to monitor rates of bone loss over time (Kaplan, 1995).

Dual-energy x-ray absorptiometry (DEXA) measures integral bone (cortical and trabecular bone) mineral density and is the preferred method to diagnose osteoporosis and monitor treatment (Fig. 22-9, p. 488). DEXA employs two x-ray beams of differing energy levels and accurately measures bone density in the hip and spine. The spine is commonly scanned between the first and fourth lumbar vertebrae. DEXA measurements are accurate; radiation dose is low (<5 mrem); and patient acceptability is high because the procedure time is usually only 5 to 15 minutes (Jergas, 1993). Of disadvantages, DEXA is a 2-D technique that cannot distinguish between cortical and trabecular bone. In addition, bone spurs, aortic calcifications, and arthritis may falsely elevate reported bone density.

Quantitative computed tomography (QCT) evaluates bone mineral in high-turnover trabecular bone. QCT uses multiple x-rays to provide a cross-sectional view of the vertebral body. As the rate of turnover in trabecular bone is nearly eight times that in cortical bone, this technique can detect early metabolic changes in this highly vulnerable tissue. It provides a volumetric density, which is an advantage in situations in which DEXA may underestimate bone mineral density (Damilakis, 2007). Although its precision is excellent, it has never been validated for World Health Organization (WHO) criteria and is not routinely used as a screening modality.

COMPUTED TOMOGRAPHY

This procedure involves multiple exposures of thin x-ray beams that are translated to 2-D axial images, termed a *slice*, of the particular area of interest. Multiple slices of the targeted body part are obtained along its length. Multiple-channel helical CT, also called *spiral CT*, allows for continuous acquisition of images in a spiral and the potential for image reformatting in multiple planes. This technique is much faster and permits images to be manipulated for analysis after they have been acquired. Many variables affect radiation dose, especially slice thickness and number of cuts obtained. If a study is performed with multiple phases of contrast, each added phase or acquisition multiplies the total patient dose of radiation.

IV contrast enables superior evaluation of solid organ parenchyma and vasculature. By adding IV contrast, masses become more obvious due to density differences. Dedicated thin-slice evaluation of vasculature, termed CT angiography (CTA) can be done throughout the body. Traditional (fluoroscopic) angiography is still performed, but cross-sectional CT imaging provides accurate information and is technically easier. As discussed earlier, IV nonionic low and isoosmolar iodinated contrast media can induce nephrotoxicity and are used with caution in patients with or with risks for renal insufficiency. IV hydration before and after an examination can help reduce contrast-induced nephrotoxicity. One option is 0.9-percent saline at 100 mL/hr beginning 6 to 12 hours before imaging and continuing 4 to 12 hours after the examination (American College of Radiology, 2018).

Oral contrast may enhance CT images if gastrointestinal disease is sought or if bowel must be differentiated from adjacent structures. Positive oral contrast is most frequently used and is dense (white) on scan images. Patients with documented allergies to IV contrast are rarely allergic to oral contrast. Intraluminal contrast in the rectum or urinary bladder also is dense (white) and can be used to address a specific concern, such as rectovaginal fistula or bladder injury, respectively.

■ Normal Pelvic Anatomy

The uterus appears as a homogenous, soft tissue oval or triangle situated posterior to the bladder (Fig. 2-28). The uterine walls enhance after IV contrast. However, unlike sonography and MR imaging, the endometrium is poorly delineated by CT imaging. The cervix also may not enhance like the remainder of the uterus, and the inner stromal layer typically enhances less than the outer stromal layer (Yitta, 2011). The endocervical canal, which can be identified by MR imaging, is indistinct using CT imaging. The lateral margins of the cervix can typically be differentiated from parametrial fat because of differences in density. However, CT is not sensitive for parametrial involvement in the setting of cervical cancer (Hricak, 2005). Imaging of the vagina and vulva is very limited with CT. Typically, the ovaries are relatively hypodense, vary in appearance and position, and are usually situated lateral to the uterus.

■ Imaging Following Gynecologic Surgery

CT is well suited to diagnose potential complications of gynecologic procedures. For ureteral injuries, CT with IV contrast

or CT urography is useful. To detect obstruction or injury, CT images are obtained after the kidneys have excreted the contrast and have opacified the collecting systems. High-density (white) contrast that abruptly stops within the ureter suggests obstruction. With ureteral disruption, contrast may flow freely from the injury site or may form an encapsulated collection, a *urinoma* (Titton, 2003).

For bladder injury, CT cystography may be informative. For this, the bladder is retrograde filled with 300 to 400 mL of dilute iodinated contrast by gravity drip. This is followed by helical CT of the bladder with multiplanar reformations (Chan, 2006). The technique is sensitive and specific for diagnosis of extraperitoneal and intraperitoneal bladder rupture and can also demonstrate fistulas connecting to the bladder (Jankowski, 2006; Yu, 2004).

CT also outperforms conventional radiography and barium studies for diagnosing bowel complications, such as small bowel obstruction (Maglinte, 1993). For characterizing an abdominal-pelvic fluid collection such as abscess or hematoma, CT with intravenous and oral contrast may be more helpful than other imaging tools (Fig. 3-8, p. 71) (Gjelsteen, 2008).

■ Gynecologic Malignancy

In most instances, sonography is the preferred initial method of evaluating the female pelvis. For additional information, MR imaging is now often preferable to CT imaging because it avoids radiation exposure and iodinated IV contrast, provides excellent soft-tissue contrast, and displays pelvic structures in multiple planes. However, in many settings, the greater availability of CT is another advantage compared with MR imaging. In addition, to evaluate and monitor gynecologic malignancies, CT imaging is probably the most frequently used imaging technique. Although its sensitivity for intraperitoneal metastases is limited, CT can estimate bulky metastases, such as in women with advanced ovarian cancer.

MAGNETIC RESONANCE IMAGING

With this technology, images are constructed based on the radiofrequency signal emitted by hydrogen nuclei after they have been "excited" by radiofrequency pulses in the presence of a strong magnetic field. The radiofrequency signal emitted has characteristics called *relaxation times*. These include the T1 relaxation time and the T2 relaxation time. The signal intensity of one tissue compared with another, that is, the contrast, can be manipulated by adjusting parameters of the acquisition. Examples are varying the elapsed time between applications of radiofrequency pulses, which is called *repetition time,* and the time between a radiofrequency pulse and sampling the emitted signal, called the *echo delay time.*

Sequences with a short repetition time and short echo delay time are called *T1-weighted*. Sequences with a long repetition time and long echo delay time are regarded as *T2-weighted*. As examples, the hydrogen molecules in a water-containing area have longer relaxation times than those in a solid tissue. Thus, on T1-weighted images, urine in the bladder will appear dark or have low signal intensity. On T2-weighted images, the same urine

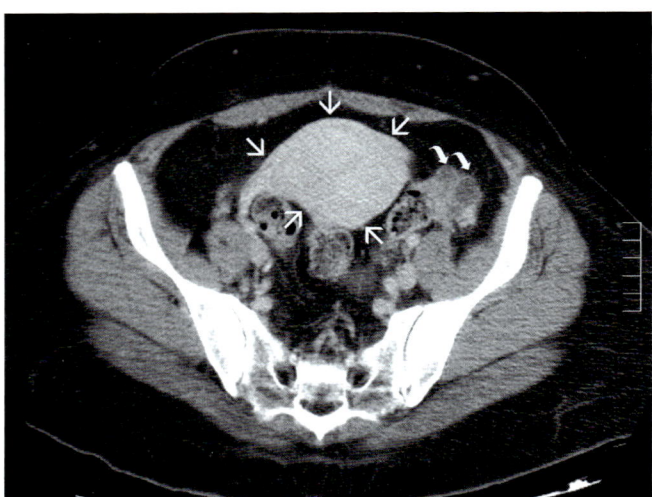

FIGURE 2-28 Computed tomography (CT) of the female pelvis in the axial plane demonstrates the normal uterus (*arrows*) as well as cysts in the left ovary (*curved arrows*).

will appear bright or have high signal intensity. By manipulating multiple parameters and imaging planes, MR imaging can achieve superior soft-tissue contrast. The strength of the magnetic field within the bore of the magnet is measured in tesla (T) (1 tesla = 10,000 gauss). For reference, the earth's magnetic field is approximately 0.5 gauss. Most clinical magnets used for MR imaging are 1.5 to 3 T or 15,000 to 30,000 gauss.

■ Technique

The standard imaging technique for the pelvis includes both T1- and T2-weighted sequences that are acquired in at least two planes, usually axial and sagittal. The T2-weighted sequence provides detailed definition of internal organ architecture, such as the uterus, vagina, and ovaries. The T1-weighted sequence clearly delineates organ boundaries and surrounding fat, allows optimal visualization of lymph nodes, and is necessary for tissue and fluid content characterization.

To aid accurate diagnosis, highly paramagnetic gadolinium-based contrast agents (GBCA) are often administered prior to imaging. The most frequently used GBCA types are extracellular agents administered intravenously. Gadolinium shortens the T1 relaxation time of adjacent protons. This increases signal intensity on T1-weighted images to enhance information regarding tissue vascularity (Gandhi, 2006). Side effects are rare, and MR contrast can be used even in those with prior reactions to other contrast agents (American College of Radiology, 2018). MR contrast is given in concentrations and doses significantly lower than that used in CT imaging, undergoes renal excretion within 24 hours, and is safe for patients with mildly compromised renal function. Of note, the Food and Drug Administration recommends caution in administering IV GBCA to patients with moderate to end-stage renal disease due to the rare but serious risk of developing nephrogenic systemic fibrosis (NSF). The risks and benefits of using GBCA are discussed by the requesting physician and radiologist. Written informed consent from the patient is obtained if GBCA use is required for those with a severely diminished glomerular filtration rate. Providing hemodialysis immediately after administration of GBCA for patients in this renal category for NSF prevention has not been proven.

In addition to intravascular GBCA, water-soluble ultrasound gel can be placed endoluminally in the vagina or the rectum to better delineate anatomy. This technique can also aid detection of fistulas or congenital vaginal septa (Gupta, 2016).

Additional imaging parameters include fat saturation to detect bulk fat and opposed-phase imaging to highlight microscopic fat. Diffusion-weighted imaging (DWI) with quantitative measurement of apparent diffusion coefficient (ADC) characterizes proton movement in tissues. Highly cellular tissues restrict random Brownian motion and yield a high DWI signal and low ADC value. This cellularity information can help identify tumor, abscess, and lymph nodes (Moore, 2014).

■ Safety

To date, harmful or mutagenic effects have not been reported from MR imaging at field strengths used clinically, that is, 3 T or lower. Additionally, the American College of Radiology

TABLE 2-1. Safety of MR Imaging with Some Implanted Devices

Device	Safe (S), Conditional (C), or Unsafe (U)	
	1.5 T	3 T
Intrauterine Devices		
Paragard	S	C
Mirena	S	S
Skyla	—	C
Tubal Occlusion Devices		
Essure	S	C
Adiana (Silicone)	S	S
Adiana (Radiopaque)	S	C
Filshie Clips	S	C
Hulka (Clemens) Clip	S	C
Implants		
Implanon/Nexplanon	S	S
Saline or silicone breast	S	S
Tissue expander with non-magnetic injection site	S	—
Tissue expander with magnetically localizable injection site	U	U
Biopsy Needles/Markers		
Localization wires	U	U
Biopsy needles	U	U
Coaxial needles	U	U
Breast biopsy markers (e.g., HydroMARK)	S	C

considers MR imaging in pregnancy to be risk free, regardless of trimester. Using the ALARA (as low as reasonably achievable) principle, imaging during pregnancy is typically limited to 1.5 T. Moreover, GBCA is not used routinely in pregnancy due to the theoretic risk of toxic gadolinium ion dissociation into the amnionic fluid (American College of Radiology, 2017).

Some, but not all, devices preclude MR imaging. For example, many implanted devices unique to women can be safely imaged (Table 2-1). Contraindications to entering the MR environment include mechanically, electrically, or magnetically activated implanted devices such as internal cardiac pacemakers, neurostimulators, cardiac defibrillators, electronic infusion pumps, and cochlear implants. Certain intracranial aneurysm clips and any metallic foreign body in the globe of the eye contraindicate scanning. Before the patient enters the MR environment, radiology personnel should obtain documentation of the type of patient implant (manufacturer, model and type) and verify its MR safety rating.

■ Use in Gynecology

Although sonography is widely used for suspected gynecologic disease, MR imaging may add information when sonographic

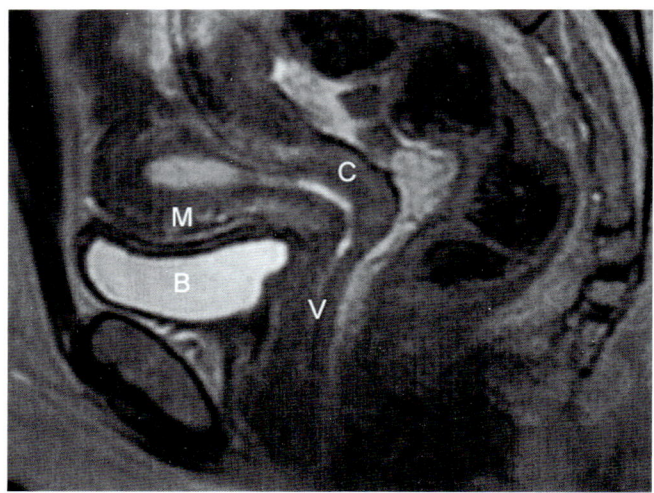

FIGURE 2-29 Sagittal T2-weighted magnetic resonance (MR) image of a normal uterus and cervix (C). B = bladder; M = myometrium; V = vagina.

findings are equivocal. Specifically, its multiplanar imaging, superior soft-tissue contrast, and large field of view are distinct MR imaging advantages. Accordingly, common indications for MR imaging include distorted pelvic anatomy, large masses that are poorly delineated with sonography, indeterminate cases of adenomyosis, and endometrial disorders in poor surgical candidates. In some instances, pelvic MR imaging may help tailor management. Also, MR imaging can be selected for primary evaluation and subsequent surveillance of pelvic malignancies.

■ Normal Findings

The pelvic organs show generally moderate to low signal intensity on T1-weighted images. T2-weighted images of the menstrual uterus depict a high-signal-intensity endometrium; contiguous low-signal-intensity inner myometrium, which is the junctional zone; and a moderate-signal-intensity outer myometrium (Fig. 2-29) (McCarthy, 1986).

The cervix can be distinguished from the uterine body by its prominent fibrous stroma, which has an overall lower signal intensity. The internal architecture of the cervix is seen on T2-weighted images as central high signal intensity (endocervical glands and mucus) surrounded by low signal intensity (fibrous stroma) and peripheral moderate signal intensity (smooth muscle intermixed with fibrous stroma) (Lee, 1985). Similarly, T2-weighted images of the vagina display central high-signal-intensity mucosa and mucus, which is surrounded by a low-signal-intensity muscular wall (Hricak, 1988). Ovaries are normally seen on the T2-weighted sequence as stroma with moderately high signal intensity that contains very high-signal-intensity follicles (Dooms, 1986). The fallopian tubes are not typically visualized. Hormonal status influences the MR appearance of all structures and reflects associated physiologic changes.

■ Benign Disease

Leiomyomas

For suspected leiomyomas, the initial imaging technique is sonography. However, its limited field of view, image resolution that declines with increasing patient body fat, and distorted anatomy from large or multiple myomas are potential hindrances (Wolfman, 2006). False-negative rates may reach 20 percent with TVS, and tumors measuring <2 cm are routinely missed (Gross, 1983). Thus, MR imaging is used when TVS findings are equivocal or nondiagnostic (Ascher, 2003). For conservative myoma treatment, the effects of GnRH agonist therapy to shrink tumor volume can be quantified with MR imaging (Lubich, 1991). Moreover, MR imaging is warranted before UAE or focused-ultrasound myoma treatments and often selected prior to hysteroscopic myoma resection. In these cases, imaging verifies leiomyoma location, seeks tumor qualities that portend outcome success or failure, and excludes other causes of patient symptoms such as unsuspected malignancy or indeterminate intracavitary masses (Cura, 2006; Rajan, 2011).

Shown in Figure 2-30, leiomyomas have a variable but characteristic MR appearance and thus can be differentiated from

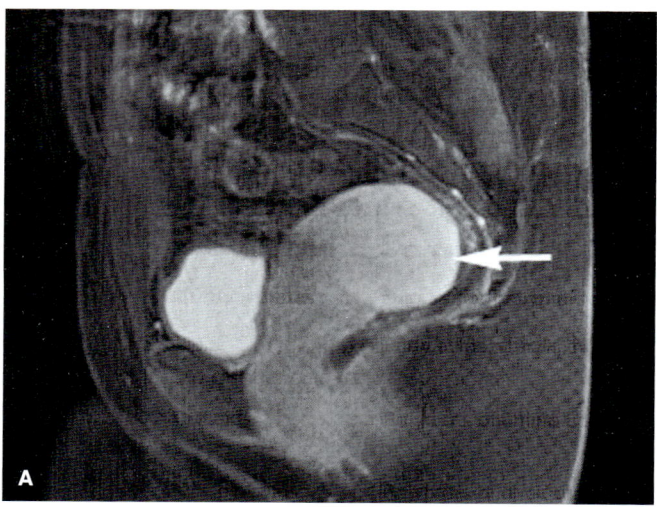

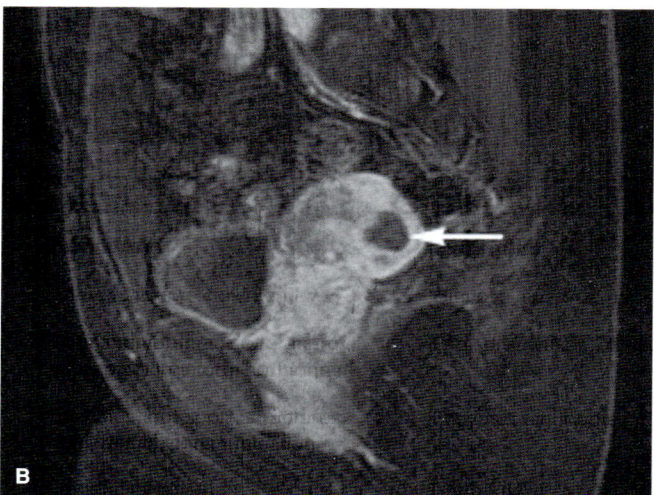

FIGURE 2-30 A. Sagittal T1-weighted post-contrast image demonstrates a 5.6-cm enhancing leiomyoma at the uterine fundus (*arrow*). **B.** Sagittal T1-weighted post-contrast image of the same patient 2 months after uterine artery embolization demonstrates lack of enhancement in the fibroid and significant interval decrease in size (now measuring 2 cm).

adenomyosis or adenomyoma with 90-percent accuracy (Mark, 1987; Togashi, 1989). This is important when myomectomy is considered. Leiomyomas, even those as small as 0.5 cm, are best seen on T2-weighted images and appear as round, sharply marginated masses with low signal intensity relative to the myometrium. Tumors >3 cm often are heterogeneous because of varying degrees and types of degeneration (Hricak, 1986; Yamashita, 1993). With MR imaging, multiplanar views allow for accurate tumor localization as subserosal, intramural, or submucosal. Moreover, pedunculated myomas and their bridging stalk can be defined. Of myoma types, intramural or subserosal leiomyomas are frequently circumscribed by a high-signal-intensity rim that represents edema from dilated lymphatics and veins.

Of treatment options, magnetic resonance–guided focused ultrasound (MRgFUS), also called *magnetic resonance high-intensity focused ultrasound (MR-HIFU)*, directs high-power ultrasound pulses—*sonications*—into the myoma. Without MR guidance, focused-ultrasound therapy is hampered by imprecise beam targeting. Fortunately, excellent soft-tissue resolution with MR imaging enables precise tissue targeting. Moreover, MR imaging can measure accurate, near real-time thermometry. This permits power adjustments to reach adequate treatment temperatures yet minimize thermal injury. Pulse duration lasts generally 15 seconds, and a cooling interval is inserted between pulses. The average procedure duration approximates 3.5 hours (Hindley, 2004). This has improved with updated devices. Outcomes, candidate selection, and comparisons with UAE are described in Chapter 9 (p. 209).

Congenital Anomalies

Discussed in Chapter 19 (p. 419), müllerian duct anomalies comprise a spectrum of developmental malformations. In the past, full evaluation required laparoscopy, laparotomy, HSG, and hysteroscopy. These invasive techniques were largely replaced by MR imaging, which has an accuracy of up to 100 percent (Carrington, 1990; Fielding, 1996).

MR imaging is particularly adept at differentiating septate and bicornuate uteri, which is imperative as these two have differing clinical implications and surgical management. IV contrast is not routinely needed. If a vaginal septum is suspected clinically, ultrasound gel placed within the vagina prior to imaging may be helpful (Gupta, 2016). T2-weighted images and coronal planes are typically the most informative. With these, the septate uterus generally displays a convex fundal contour. The bicornuate uterus typically has a significant fundal notch >1 cm. However, any notch depth within 5 mm of the intercornual line qualifies for bicornuate (Behr, 2012). The endometrial cavities of a bicornuate uterus have a normal width and communicate. Although a less-reliable marker, an intercornual distance typically measures >4 cm with a bicornuate uterus (Carrington, 1990; Fedele, 1989).

With a septate uterus, a fibrous septum divides the two uterine horns. Collagen has low signal intensity on both T1- and T2-weighted images, whereas the intervening myometrium of a bicornuate uterus has high signal intensity on T2-weighted images. The fundal contour of the septate uterus can be convex, flattened, or mildly concave, but if present, the fundal

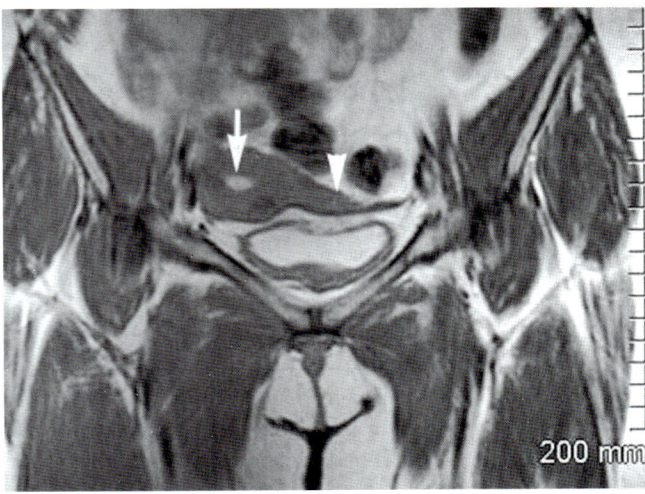

FIGURE 2-31 Unicornuate uterus. This coronal T2-weighted image demonstrates a protrusion of myometrial tissue from the left lateral uterine body (*arrowhead*). It is isointense to myometrium but does not demonstrate normal uterine zonal anatomy. Specifically, endometrium (*arrow*) is noted in the developed right uterine horn but not in the left rudimentary horn.

notch lies >5 mm above the intercornual line (Behr, 2012). Also in contrast to the bicornuate uterus, the intercornual distance of a septate uterus is not increased, and thus each uterine cavity is smaller than usual (Carrington, 1990; Forstner, 1994).

MR imaging also offers detailed evaluation of a unicornuate uterus, especially in evaluation for a rudimentary horn (Fig. 2-31). On MR imaging, if endometrial tissue is present within a rudimentary horn, zonal anatomy will be preserved. Moreover, communication of an endometrium-containing rudimentary horn is of considerable clinical importance (Chap. 19, p. 422). In a menstruating woman, a noncommunicating horn containing endometrium will often be evident as a hematometra when the cavity becomes distended with blood. MR imaging can also identify uterine didelphys, agenesis, or hypoplasia.

Other Gynecologic Indications

MR imaging is equivalent or superior to sonography to diagnose adenomyosis and has a sensitivity of 88 to 93 percent and a specificity of 66 to 99 percent (Ascher, 1994; Dueholm, 2001; Reinhold, 1996). Compared with sonography, MR imaging reliably diagnoses adenomyosis, particularly focal adenomyomas, in the setting of concomitant pathology such as leiomyomas. In addition, MR imaging reproducibility allows accurate treatment monitoring (Reinhold, 1995).

With adenomyosis, the low-signal-intensity junctional zone (inner myometrium) on T2-weighted images measures >12 mm (Fig. 2-32). A normal junctional zone can be up to 8 mm, and measurements from 8 to 12 mm are considered indeterminate (Novellas, 2011). Low-signal-intensity areas of adenomyosis often contain internal ovoid or punctate foci of increased signal on both T1- and T2-weighted images. These foci are nests of ectopic endometrium with dilated endometrial glands, with or without hemorrhage (Reinhold, 1995, 1996). Contrast

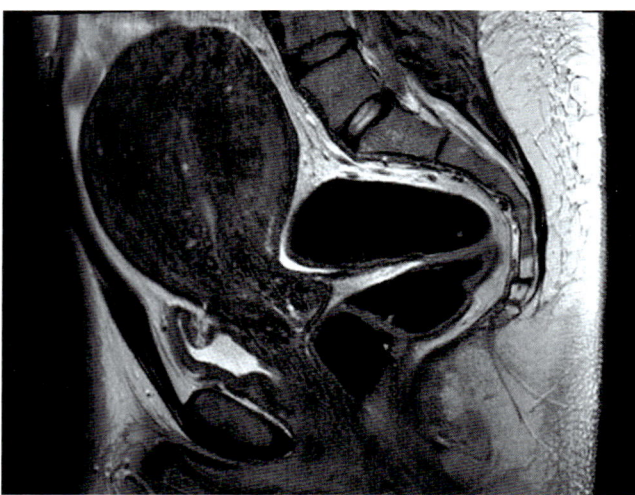

FIGURE 2-32 Sagittal T2-weighted magnetic resonance image of a uterus with diffuse adenomyosis. Adenomyosis is shown as circumferential thickening of the junctional zone.

administration does not increase the diagnostic accuracy for adenomyosis (Outwater, 1998).

For polyps and endometrial hyperplasia, TVS and SIS are common diagnostic tools. MR imaging may be helpful if these modalities are nondiagnostic in a patient who is a poor surgical candidate for direct endometrial sampling. However, distinguishing intracavitary myomas and endometrial polyps can be problematic with MR imaging if necrosis and inflammation are present.

For diagnosing ovarian endometriomas, MR imaging offers 98-percent specificity, which is similar to TVS. These cysts show imaging characteristics of old blood products that include "shading" signal loss on T2-weighted images and a hyperintense signal on T1-weighted images (Chamie, 2011). However, MR imaging differs from TVS in that it can provide evaluation for endometriosis in locations that are not easy to access sonographically or laparoscopically, especially in the setting of advanced disease. For diagnosing pelvic deep infiltrating endometriosis, MR imaging has a sensitivity of 90 percent, specificity of 91 percent, and accuracy of 91 percent (Bazot, 2004). Additional endometriosis features include the stellate margins of fibrotic plaques, tethering, and obliteration of normal pelvic spaces. On T1-weighted images, foci with hyperintense signals aids diagnosis of multifocal lesions involving the bladder, rectum, or ureters.

For other adnexal masses, MR imaging can further characterize anatomy if sonography is nondiagnostic or inconclusive. MR imaging frequently provides added information regarding soft-tissue composition and the origin and extent of pelvic pathology that may be nongynecologic. Although both sonography and MR imaging are highly sensitive for the detection of adnexal malignancy, MR imaging is slightly more specific (Adusumilli, 2006; Jeong, 2000; Yamashita, 1995).

■ Gynecologic Malignancies

For cervical cancer, imaging can be a component of strict clinical staging (Chap. 30, p. 661). Also, MR imaging is an excellent adjunct for preoperative assessment of gynecologic neoplasms.

Its superior soft-tissue contrast and ability to image directly in multiple planes allow evaluation for local tumor extension and lymphadenopathy.

Although CT imaging is typically used for assessment of nodal disease and distant metastases, MR imaging consistently outperforms clinical and CT evaluation of cervical cancer in the assessment of local tumor extension (Choi, 2004; Hricak, 1996, 2007). Current recommendations for MR imaging of cervical cancer include tumors with a transverse diameter >2 cm based on physical examination, endocervical or predominately infiltrative tumors that cannot be accurately assessed clinically, and women who are pregnant or have concomitant uterine lesions that make evaluation difficult (Ascher, 2001; Hricak, 2007). When the extent of parametrial and sidewall invasion is unclear clinically, MR imaging can play an important role as it has a 95- to 98-percent negative predictive value for parametrial invasion (Hricak, 2007; Subak, 1995).

For endometrial carcinoma, surgery is currently the most accurate preoperative staging method. MR imaging may assess the degree of myometrial and cervical extension, which can affect the planned hysterectomy type, extent of lymph node dissection, and decision to provide neoadjuvant intracavitary radiation (Boronow, 1984; Frei, 2000). MR imaging has 92-percent accuracy in staging endometrial cancer, and 82-percent accuracy in assessing myometrial invasion depth (Hricak, 1987). Thus, MR imaging is often considered if lymph node metastases are likely, such as from a high-grade tumor; with papillary or clear cell histology; with cervical invasion; or if multifactorial assessment of myometrial, cervical, and lymph node involvement is required (Ascher, 2001).

For ovarian neoplasms, MR imaging is reserved for evaluation when TVS or CT scanning is indeterminate or nondiagnostic, or in cases with a desire to minimize ionizing radiation (Kang, 2018). However, in a Society of Radiologists in Ultrasound consensus statement, MR imaging was recommended to assess simple ovarian cysts >7 cm. This factored sonography's limitations in detecting mural nodules in larger ovarian masses (Ekerhovd, 2001; Levine, 2010). MR imaging also can better determine adnexal mass origin as uterine, ovarian, or nongynecologic. For those of the ovary, MR imaging helps clarify whether the mass is neoplastic or functional and is malignant or benign. MR imaging of an adnexal mass ideally includes gadolinium-enhanced images to assess tumor vascularity and incorporates fat-saturation techniques to differentiate blood from fat (Ascher, 2001). Although histology cannot be diagnosed, imaging findings that are suspicious for malignancy include enhancing solid components, thick septations, nodules, or papillary projections.

Sensitivity of MR imaging for detecting adnexal pathology ranges from 87 to 100 percent, which is comparable to sonography and CT scanning (Siegelman, 1999). The advantages of MR imaging compared with CT scanning in the evaluation of suspected ovarian cancer include its superior contrast resolution and greater sensitivity for detecting uterine invasion, extrapelvic peritoneal and lymph node metastases, and tumor extension to omentum, bowel, bone, and vessels (Low, 1995; Tempany, 2000). However, MR imaging has a lower sensitivity for implants <1 cm compared with CT (Sala, 2013).

◼ Urogynecology

Pelvic floor evaluations previously performed fluoroscopically are now more often performed with MR imaging. MR imaging provides detailed soft-tissue evaluation of the female urethra, levator ani muscles, and adjacent pelvic structures (Pannu, 2002). Contrast agents placed in the vagina, rectum, and/or bladder can enhance imaging.

Functional data also can be obtained. For example, dynamic MR imaging is completed as the patient performs the Valsalva maneuver. With MR defecography, the patient both performs Valsalva maneuver and defecates rectal contrast (ultrasound gel) during rapid cine acquisitions. Protocols vary significantly from center to center, and upright open MR units are not universally available. We employ supine MR defecography at our institution (Khatri, 2015; Kumar, 2014). MR defecography can evaluate patients with pelvic organ descent, incontinence, constipation, and defecatory dysfunction. It may add information prior to complex pelvic floor reconstruction or after failed previous repairs (Macura, 2006).

NUCLEAR MEDICINE

Nuclear medicine examinations are used similarly in the gynecologic patient as in other medical specialties. Small amounts of radioactive material are ingested or injected to diagnose, and at times treat, various diseases. Thyroid studies use radioactive iodine to assess or ablate function. Bone scans may be elected to seek metastatic disease. Various renal scans can offer information regarding renal function, perfusion, and possible obstruction. Ventilation-perfusion (V/Q) scans can help identify pulmonary emboli. Controversy remains regarding whether pulmonary artery CTA or V/Q scan is most appropriate in pulmonary emboli evaluation. The V/Q scan does not use nephrotoxic agents and is often preferred in those with renal insufficiency. However, radiopharmaceuticals are not always readily available, and thus pulmonary artery CTA is frequently employed.

Positron emission tomography (PET) uses short-lived radiochemical compounds to serve as tracers for measuring specific metabolic processes suggestive of malignancy or infection (Juweid, 2006). This enables detection of early cancer biochemical anomalies that precede structural changes. With FDG-PET, a radiolabeled analogue of glucose, 2-[^{18}F]fluoro-2-deoxy-D-glucose (FDG), is injected intravenously and is taken up by metabolically active cells such as tumor cells. PET provides a poor depiction of detailed anatomy, thus scans are frequently read side-by-side or fused with CT scans. The combination allows correlation of metabolic and anatomic data. As a result, current PET scanners are now commonly integrated with CT scanners, and the two scans can be performed during the same session.

PET/CT has become a vital clinical tool, particularly for cancer diagnosis and management. The most common PET radiochemical tracer used clinically is FDG. This tracer highlights areas of accelerated glycolysis, which is common in neoplastic cells (Goh, 2003).

Several studies have demonstrated high sensitivity and specificity of FDG-PET for the initial staging of cervical cancer. This may be most valuable in patients with no evidence of extrapelvic metastatic disease by MR or CT imaging (Gjelsteen, 2008; Park, 2005). The ability of FDG-PET imaging to assess nodal status in cervical cancer has both prognostic and therapeutic implications (Fig. 2-33). Prior to lymph node radiation treatment planning, the added anatomic data obtained with PET/CT can be used to guide intensity-modulated radiotherapy

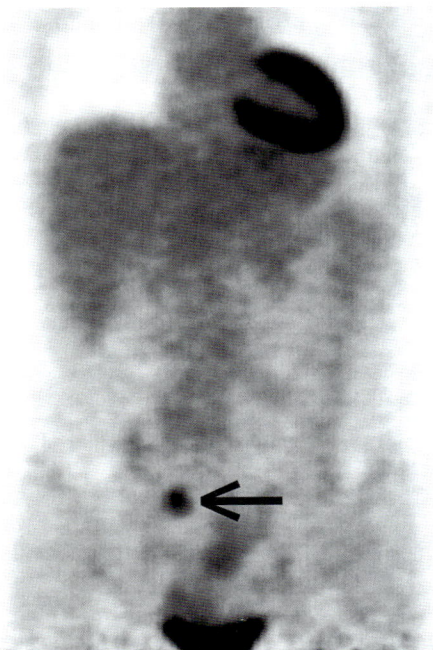
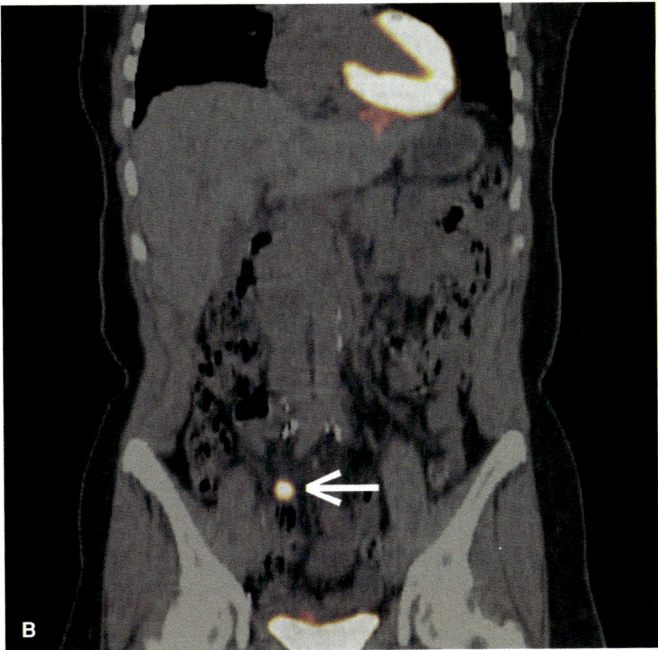

FIGURE 2-33 Positron emission tomography (PET) **(A)** and PET-computed tomography (PET-CT) fusion **(B)** images of a woman with recurrence of ovarian cancer. Arrows demarcate abnormal uptake of tracer in the pelvis that represented a 1-cm lymph node. The biopsy of this lymph node revealed recurrent ovarian cancer. (Reproduced with permission from Dr. Dana Mathews.)

(Chap. 28, p. 612). This significantly reduces the amount of radiation delivered to surrounding normal structures (Havrilesky, 2003; Wong, 2004).

INTERVENTIONAL RADIOLOGY

In gynecology, procedures often provided by interventional radiologists include image-guided biopsy or drainage. In those with advanced cervical cancer, percutaneous nephrostomy may be needed to preserve renal function or to decompress an infected collecting system. UAE is a vascular intervention that employs angiography to delineate the uterine arteries. Once catheterized, each artery is injected with embolic particles to occlude uterine vasculature. Discussed in Chapter 9 (p. 209), UAE can provide definitive independent treatment of uterine leiomyomas. Although adenomyosis was initially thought to be a contraindication for UAE success, studies are now showing durable treatment efficacy (Kim, 2007). Given the frequent concomitant presence of adenomyosis and uterine leiomyomata, treatment success and improvement in symptoms also have been reported in populations with both diseases after UAE (Froeling, 2012). Rarely, UAE may be selected to control severe uterine bleeding in women who are not considered surgical candidates.

REFERENCES

Abrams BJ, Sukmvanich P, Seibel R, et al: Ultrasound for the detection of intraperitoneal fluid: the role of Trendelenburg position. Am J Emerg Med 17:117, 1999

Abuhamad AZ, Singleton S, Zhao Y, et al: The Z technique: an easy approach to the display of the mid-coronal plane of the uterus in volume sonography. J Ultrasound Med 25:607, 2006

Adusumilli S, Hussain HK, Caoili EM, et al: MR imaging of sonographically indeterminate adnexal masses. AJR 187:732, 2006

Alcázar JL, Galan MJ, Garcia-Manero M, et al: Three-dimensional sonographic morphologic assessment in complex adnexal masses: preliminary experience. J Ultrasound Med 22:249, 2003

Alcázar JL, Martinez-Astorquiza Corral T, Orozco R, et al: Three-dimensional hysterosalpingo-contrast-sonography for the assessment of tubal patency in women with infertility: a systematic review with meta-analysis. Gynecol Obstet Invest 81(4):289, 2016

American College of Obstetricians and Gynecologists: Sonohysterography. Technology Assessment No. 12, August 2016

American College of Obstetricians and Gynecologists: Prevention of infection after gynecologic procedures. Practice Bulletin No. 195, June 2018

American College of Radiology: ACR Manual on Contrast Media, Version 10.3, Reston, American College of Radiology, 2018

American College of Radiology: ACR practice parameter for performing and interpreting magnetic resonance imaging (MRI). Reston, American College of Radiology, 2017

American Institute of Ultrasound in Medicine: Guidelines for performance of the ultrasound examination of the female pelvis. 2014. Available at: https://www.aium.org/resources/guidelines/femalepelvis.pdf. Accessed April 22, 2019

American Institute of Ultrasound in Medicine: Official statement on heat. AIUM Bioeffects Committee, 2009

Ameye L, Valentin L, Testa AC, et al: A scoring system to differentiate malignant from benign masses in specific ultrasound-based subgroups of adnexal tumors. Ultrasound Obstet Gynecol 33:92, 2009

Ascher SM, Arnold LL, Patt RH, et al: Adenomyosis: prospective comparison of MR imaging and transvaginal sonography. Radiology 190:803, 1994

Ascher SM, Jha RC, Reinhold C: Benign myometrial conditions: leiomyomas and adenomyosis. Top Magn Reson Imaging 14:281, 2003

Ascher SM, Takahama J, Jha RC: Staging of gynecologic malignancies. Top Magn Reson Imaging 12:105, 2001

Bates SM, Ginsberg JS: Treatment of deep-vein thrombosis. N Engl J Med 351:268, 2004

Bazot M, Darai E, Hourani R, et al: Deep pelvic endometriosis: MR imaging for diagnosis and prediction of extension of disease. Radiology 232:379, 2004

Behr S, Courtier J, Qayyum A: Imaging of müllerian duct anomalies. Radiographics 32:E233, 2012

Benacerraf BR, Shipp TD, Bromley B: Three-dimensional ultrasound detection of abnormally located intrauterine contraceptive devices which are a source of pelvic pain and abnormal bleeding. Ultrasound Obstet Gynecol 34:110, 2009

Benacerraf BR, Shipp TD, Bromley B: Which patients benefit from a 3D reconstructed coronal view of the uterus added to standard routine 2D pelvic sonography? AJR 190:626, 2008

Bermejo C, Martinez Ten P, Cantarero R, et al: Three-dimensional ultrasound in the diagnosis of müllerian duct anomalies and concordance with magnetic resonance imaging. Ultrasound Obstet Gynecol 35:593, 2010

Beyersdorff D, Zhang J, Schoder H, et al: Bladder cancer: can imaging change patient management? Curr Opin Urol 18:98, 2008

Birdwell BG, Raskob GE, Whitsett TL, et al: The clinical validity of normal compression ultrasonography in outpatients suspected of having deep venous thrombosis. Ann Intern Med 128:1, 1998

Bonnamy L, Marret H, Perrotin F, et al: Sonohysterography: a prospective survey of results and complications in 81 patients. Eur J Obstet Gynecol Reprod Biol 102:42, 2002

Boronow RC, Morrow CP, Creasman WT, et al: Surgical staging in endometrial cancer: clinical-pathologic findings of a prospective study. Obstet Gynecol 63:825, 1984

Branney SW, Wolfe RE, Moore EE, et al: Quantitative sensitivity of ultrasound in detecting free intraperitoneal fluid. J Trauma 39:375, 1995

Buy JN, Ghossain MA, Hugol D, et al: Characterization of adnexal masses: combination of color Doppler and conventional sonography compared with spectral Doppler analysis alone and conventional sonography alone. AJR 166:385, 1996

Cacciatore B, Leminen A, Ingman-Friberg S, et al: Transvaginal sonographic findings in ambulatory patients with suspected pelvic inflammatory disease. Obstet Gyncol 80:912, 1992

Capitanio GL, Ferraiolo A, Croce S, et al: Transcervical selective salpingography: a diagnostic and therapeutic approach to cases of proximal tubal injection failure. Fertil Steril 55:1045, 1991

Carretti M, Dos Santos Simões R, Bernardo WM, et al: Accuracy of ultrasonography in the evaluation of tubal sterilization microinsert positioning: systematic review and meta-analysis. J Ultrasound Med 38:289, 2019

Carrington BM, Hricak H, Nuruddin RN, et al: Müllerian duct anomalies: MR imaging evaluation. Radiology 176:715, 1990

Chamie L, Blasalg R, Pereira R, et al: Findings of pelvic endometriosis at transvaginal US, MR imaging, and laparoscopy. Radiographics 31:E77, 2011

Chan DP, Abujudeh HH, Cushing GL Jr, et al: CT cystography with multiplanar reformation for suspected bladder rupture: experience in 234 cases. AJR 187:1296, 2006

Choi SH, Kim SH, Choi HJ, et al: Preoperative magnetic resonance imaging staging of uterine cervical carcinoma: results of prospective study. J Comput Assist Tomogr 28:620, 2004

Chou CP, Levenson RB, Elsayes KM, et al: Imaging of female urethral diverticulum: an update. Radiographics 28(7):1917, 2008

Cohen HL, Tice HM, Mandel FS: Ovarian volumes measured by US: bigger than we think. Radiology 177:189, 1990

Cowan NC: CT urography for hematuria. Nat Rev Urol 9:218, 2012

Cowan NC, Turney BW, Taylor NJ, et al: Multidetector computed tomography urography for diagnosing upper urinary tract urothelial tumour. BJU Int 99:1363, 2007

Cura M, Cura A, Bugnone A: Role of magnetic resonance imaging in patient selection for uterine artery embolization. Acta Radiol 47:1105, 2006

Damilakis J, Maris T, Karantanas A: An update on the assessment of osteoporosis using radiologic techniques. Eur Radiol 17:1591, 2007

Dashe JS, Twickler DM: Fetal imaging. In Cunningham FG, Leveno KJ, Bloom SL, et al (eds): Williams Obstetrics, 25th ed. New York, McGraw-Hill Education, 2018, p 213

Davis JD: Prevention, diagnosis, and treatment of venous thromboembolic complications of gynecologic surgery. Am J Obstet Gynecol 184:759, 2001

DePriest PD, Shenson D, Fried A, et al: A morphology index based on sonographic findings in ovarian cancer. Gynecol Oncol 51:7, 1993

Dietz HP: Mesh in prolapse surgery: an imaging perspective. Ultrasound Obstet Gynecol 40:495, 2012

Dietz HP: Quantification of major morphological abnormalities of the levator ani. Ultrasound Obstet Gynecol 29:329, 2007

Dietz HP: Pelvic floor ultrasound: a review. Clin Obstet Gynecol 60:58, 2017

Dooms GC, Hricak H, Tscholakoff D: Adnexal structures: MR imaging. Radiology 158:639, 1986

Dueholm M, Lundorf E, Hansen E, et al: Magnetic resonance imaging and transvaginal ultrasonography for the diagnosis of adenomyosis. Fertil Steril 76:588, 2001

Eckersley RJ, Sedelaar JP, Blomley MJ, et al: Quantitative microbubble enhanced transrectal ultrasound as a tool for monitoring hormonal treatment of prostate carcinoma. Prostate 51:256, 2002

Ekerhovd E, Wienerroith H, Staudach A, et al: Preoperative assessment of unilocular adnexal cysts by transvaginal ultrasonography: a comparison between ultrasonographic morphologic imaging and histopathologic diagnosis. Am J Obstet Gynecol 184:48, 2001

Exacoustos C, Pizzo A, Lazzeri L, et al: Three-dimensional hysterosalpingo contrast sonography with gel foam: methodology and feasibility to obtain 3-dimensional volumes of tubal shape. J Minim Invasive Gynecol 24:827, 2017

Fedele L, Dorta M, Brioschi D, et al: Magnetic resonance evaluation of double uteri. Obstet Gynecol 74:844, 1989

Fielding JR: MR imaging of müllerian anomalies: impact on therapy. AJR 167:1491, 1996

Fleischer AC, Harvey SM, Kurita SC, et al: Two-/three-dimensional transperineal sonography of complicated tape and mesh implants. Ultrasound Q 28:243, 2012

Fleischer AC, Lyshchik A, Jones HW Jr, et al: Contrast-enhanced transvaginal sonography of benign versus malignant ovarian masses: preliminary findings. J Ultrasound Med 27:1011, 2008

Fleischer AC, Rodgers WH, Kepple DM, et al: Color Doppler sonography of ovarian masses: a multiparameter analysis. J Ultrasound Med 12:41, 1993

Forstner R, Hricak H: Congenital malformations of uterus and vagina. Radiology 34:397, 1994

Frei KA, Kinkel K, Bonel HM, et al: Prediction of deep myometrial invasion in patients with endometrial cancer: clinical utility of contrast-enhanced MR imaging—a meta-analysis and Bayesian analysis. Radiology 216:444, 2000

Friera A, Gimenez NR, Caballero P, et al: Deep vein thrombosis: can a second sonographic examination be avoided? AJR 178:1001, 2002

Froeling V, Scheurig-Muenkler C, Hamm B, et al: Uterine artery embolization to treat uterine adenomyosis with or without uterine leiomyomata results of symptom control and health-related quality of life 40 months after treatment. Cardiovasc Intervent Radiol 25:523, 2012

Gandhi S, Brown M, Wong J, et al: MR contrast agents for liver imaging: what, when, how. Radiographics 26:1621, 2006

Ghi T, Casadio P, Kuleva M, et al: Accuracy of three-dimensional ultrasound in diagnosis and classification of congenital uterine anomalies. Fertil Steril 92:808, 2009

Gjelsteen A, Ching BH, Meyermann MW, et al: CT, MRI, PET, PET/CT, and ultrasound in the evaluation of obstetric and gynecologic patients. Surg Clin North Am 88:361, 2008

Goh AS, Ng DC: Clinical positron emission tomography imaging—current applications. Ann Acad Med Singapore 32:507, 2003

Goldhaber SZ: Pulmonary embolism. Lancet 363:1295, 2004

Gross BH, Silver TM, Jaffe MH: Sonographic features of uterine leiomyomas: analysis of 41 proven cases. J Ultrasound Med 2:401, 1983

Gupta MK, Khatri G, Bailey A, et al: Endoluminal contrast for the abdominal and pelvic magnetic resonance imaging. Abdom Radiol (NY) 41(7):1378, 2016

Hanley M, Steigner ML, Ahmed O, et al: ACR Appropriateness Criteria®: suspected lower-extremity deep vein thrombosis. J Am Coll Radiol 15(11S): S413, 2018

Havrilesky LJ, Wong TZ, Secord AA, et al: The role of PET scanning in the detection of recurrent cervical cancer. Gynecol Oncol 90:186, 2003

Hegde A, Aguilar VC, Davila G: Levator ani defects in patients with stress urinary incontinence: three-dimensional endovaginal ultrasound assessment. Int Urogynecol J 28:85, 2017

Hindley J, Gedroyc WM, Regan L, et al: MRI guidance of focused ultrasound therapy of uterine fibroids: early results. AJR 183:1713, 2004

Hricak H, Chang YCF, Thurnher S: Vagina: evaluation with MR imaging. I. Normal anatomy and congenital anomalies. Radiology 169:169, 1988

Hricak H, Gatsonis C, Chi D, et al: Role of imaging in pretreatment evaluation of early invasive cervical cancer: results of the intergroup study American College of Radiology Imaging Network 6651–Gynecologic Oncology Group 183. J Clin Oncol 23(36):9329, 2005

Hricak H, Gatsonis C, Conkley F, et al: Early invasive cervical cancer: CT and MRI imaging in preoperative evaluation-ACRIN/GOG comparative study of diagnostic performance and interobserver variability. Radiology 245:491, 2007

Hricak H, Powell CB, Yu KK, et al: Invasive cervical carcinoma: role of MR imaging in pretreatment work-up—cost minimization and diagnostic efficacy analysis. Radiology 198:403, 1996

Hricak H, Stern JL, Fisher MR, et al: Endometrial carcinoma staging by MR imaging. Radiology 162:297, 1987

Hricak H, Tscholakoff D, Heinrichs L, et al: Uterine leiomyomas: correlation of MR histopathologic findings, and symptoms. Radiology 158:385, 1986

Hwang M, Lyshchik A, Fleischer A: Molecular sonography with targeted microbubbles: current investigations and potential applications. Ultrasound Q 26:75, 2010

Jain KA: Prospective evaluation of adnexal masses with endovaginal gray-scale and duplex and color Doppler US: correlation with pathologic findings. Radiology 191:63, 1994

Jankowski JT, Spirnak JP: Current recommendations for imaging in the management of urologic traumas. Urol Clin North Am 33:365, 2006

Jayasinghe Y, Rane A, Stalewski H, et al: The presentation and early diagnosis of the rudimentary uterine horn. Obstet Gynecol 105:1456, 2005

Jeong Y, Outwater EK, Kang HK: Imaging evaluation of ovarian masses. Radiographics 20:144, 2000

Jergas M, Genant HK: Current methods and recent advances in the diagnosis of osteoporosis. Arthritis Rheum 36:1649, 1993

Jokubkiene L, Sladkevicius P, Valentin L: Does three-dimensional power Doppler ultrasound help in discrimination between benign and malignant ovarian masses? Ultrasound Obstet Gynecol 29:215, 2007

Juweid ME, Cheson BD: Positron-emission tomography and assessment of cancer therapy. N Engl J Med 354:496, 2006

Kang SK, Reinhold C, Atri M, et al: ACR appropriateness criteria® staging and follow-up of ovarian cancer. J Am Coll Radiol 15(5S):S198, 2018

Kaplan FS: Prevention and management of osteoporosis. Clin Symp 1995, p 47

Keizer AL, Nieuwenhuis LL, Twisk JW, et al: Role of 3-dimensional sonography in the assessment of submucous fibroids: a pilot study. J Ultrasound Med 37:191, 2018

Khalife S, Falcone T, Hemmings R, et al: Diagnostic accuracy of transvaginal ultrasound in detecting free pelvic fluid. J Reprod Med 43:795, 1998

Khatri G, Bailey AA, Bacsu C, et al: Influence of rectal gel volume on defecation during dynamic pelvic floor magnetic resonance imaging. Clin Imaging 39(6):1027, 2015

Kim M, Kim S, Kim N, et al: Long-term results of uterine artery embolization for symptomatic adenomyosis. AJR 188:176, 2007

Kinkel K, Hricak H, Lu Y, et al: US characterization of ovarian masses: a metaanalysis. Radiology 217:803, 2000

Kumar N, Khatri G, Xi Y, et al: Valsalva maneuvers versus defecation for MRI assessment of multi-compartment pelvic organ prolapse. American Roentgen Ray Society Annual Meeting, San Diego, May 4–9, 2014

Kupesic A, Plavsic BM: 2D and 3D hysterosalpingo-contrast-sonography in the assessment of uterine cavity and tubal patency. Eur J Obstet Gynecol Reprod Biol 113:64, 2007

Kurjak A, Schulman H, Sosic A, et al: Transvaginal ultrasound, color flow, and Doppler waveform of the postmenopausal adnexal mass. Obstet Gynecol 80:917, 1992

Lee JKT, Gersell DJ, Balfe DM, et al: The uterus: in vitro MR anatomic correlation of normal and abnormal specimens. Radiology 157:175, 1985

Legendre G, Gervaise A, Levaillant JM, et al: Assessment of three-dimensional ultrasound examination classification to check the position of the tubal sterilization microinsert. Fertil Steril 94:2732, 2010

Lensing AW, Prandoni P, Brandjes D, et al: Detection of deep-vein thrombosis by real-time B-mode ultrasonography. N Engl J Med 320:342, 1989

Levine D, Brown DL, Andreotti RF, et al: Management of asymptomatic ovarian and other adnexal cysts imaged at ultrasound: Society of Radiologists in Ultrasound consensus conference statement. Ultrasound Q 26:121, 2010

Lieng M, Qvigstad E, Dahl GF, et al: Flow differences between endometrial polyps and cancer: a prospective study using intravenous contrast-enhanced transvaginal color flow Doppler and three-dimensional power Doppler ultrasound. Ultrasound Obstet Gynecol 32:935, 2008

Lo Monte G, Capobianco G, Piva I, et al: Hysterosalpingo contrast sonography (HyCoSy): let's make the point! Arch Gynecol Obstet 291:19, 2015

Low RN, Carter WD, Saleh F, et al: Ovarian cancer: comparison of findings with perfluorocarbon-exchanged MR imaging, In-111-CYT-103 immunoscintigraphy, and CT. Radiology 195:391, 1995

Lubich LM, Alderman MG, Ros PR: Magnetic resonance imaging of leiomyomata uteri: assessing therapy with the gonadotropin-releasing hormone agonist leuprolide. Magn Reson Imaging 9:331, 1991

Luciano DE, Exacoustos C, Luciano AA: Contrast ultrasonography for tubal patency. J Minim Invasive Gynecol 21:994, 2014

Macura KJ: Magnetic resonance imaging of pelvic floor defects in women. Top Magn Reson Imaging 17:417, 2006

Maglinte DD, Gage SN, Harmon BH, et al: Obstruction of the small intestine: accuracy and role of CT in diagnosis. Radiology 188:61, 1993

Majeed A, Divyashree PS, Rao KA: Perifollicular vascularity in poor ovarian responders in In-vitro fertilization cycles. J Hum Reprod Sci 11:242, 2018

Makled AK, Elmekkawi SF, El-Refaie TA, et al: Three-dimensional power Doppler and endometrial volume as predictors of malignancy in patients with postmenopausal bleeding. J Obstet Gynaecol Res 39:1045, 2013

Mark AS, Hricak H, Heinrichs LW: Adenomyosis and leiomyoma: differential diagnosis by means of magnetic resonance imaging. Radiology 163:527, 1987

Mavrelos D, Naftalin J, Hoo W, et al: Preoperative assessment of submucous fibroids by three-dimensional saline contrast sonohysterography. Ultrasound Obstet Gynecol 38:350, 2011

McCarthy S, Tauber C, Gore J: Female pelvic anatomy: MR assessment of variations during the menstrual cycle and with use of oral contraceptives. Radiology 160:119, 1986

Mishell DR Jr, Stenchever MA, Droegemueller W, et al (eds): Comprehensive Gynecology, 3rd ed. St. Louis, Mosby, 1997, p 691

Molander P, Sjoberg J, Paavonen J, et al: Transvaginal power Doppler findings in laparoscopically proven acute pelvic inflammatory disease. Ultrasound Obstet Gynecol 17:233, 2002

Moore W, Khatri G, Madhuranthakam A, et al: Added value of diffusion-weighted acquisitions in MRI of the abdomen and pelvis. AJR 202:995, 2014

Moreno CC, Beland MD, Goldfarb S, et al: ACR Appropriateness Criteria®: acute onset flank pain—suspicion of stone disease. Reston, American College of Radiology, 2015

Moschos E, Twickler DM: Does the type of intrauterine device affect conspicuity and position evaluation with 2D and 3D ultrasound imaging? AJR 196:1439, 2011

Navve D, Hershkovitz R, Zetounie E, et al: Medial or lateral location of the whirlpool sign in adnexal torsion: clinical importance. J Ultrasound Med 32:1631, 2013

Needleman L, Cronan JJ, Lilly MP, et al: Ultrasound for lower extremity deep venous thrombosis: multidisciplinary recommendations from the Society of Radiologists in Ultrasound consensus conference. Circulation 137(14):1505, 2018

Neitlich JD, Foster HE, Glickman MG, et al: Detection of urethral diverticula in women: comparison of a high resolution fast spin echo technique with double balloon urethrography. J Urol 159:408, 1998

Ni J, Han B, Liang J, et al: Three-dimensional 3D ultrasound combined with power Doppler for the differential diagnosis of endometrial lesions among infertile women. Int J Gynaecol Obstet 145:212, 2019

Nieuwenhuis LL, Hermans FJ, Bij de Vaate AJ, et al: Three-dimensional saline infusion sonography compared to two-dimensional saline infusion sonography for the diagnosis of focal intracavitary lesions. Cochrane Database Syst Rev 5:CD011126, 2017

Novellas S, Chassang M, Delotte J, et al: MRI characteristics of the uterine junctional zone: from normal to the diagnosis of adenomyosis. AJR 196:1206, 2011

Nylander M, Frøssing S, Bjerre AH, et al: Ovarian morphology in polycystic ovary syndrome: estimates from 2D and 3D ultrasound and magnetic resonance imaging and their correlation to anti-Müllerian hormone. Acta Radiol 58:997, 2017

Ohel I, Sheiner E, Aricha-Tamir B, et al: Three-dimensional power Doppler ultrasound in ovarian cancer and its correlation with histology. Arch Gynecol Obstet 281:919, 2010

Outwater EK, Siegelman ES, Van Deerlin V: Adenomyosis: current concepts and imaging considerations. AJR 170:437, 1998

Pannu HK: Magnetic resonance imaging of pelvic organ prolapse. Abdom Imaging 27:660, 2002

Park W, Park YJ, Huh SJ, et al: The usefulness of MRI and PET imaging for the detection of parametrial involvement and lymph node metastasis in patients with cervical cancer. Jpn J Clin Oncol 35:260, 2005

Peng C, Liu LZ, Zheng W, et al: Can quantitative contrast-enhanced ultrasonography predict cervical tumor response to neoadjuvant chemotherapy? Eur J Radiol 85:2111, 2016

Peres Fagundes PA, Chapon R, Olsen PR, et al: Evaluation of three-dimensional SonoAVC ultrasound for antral follicle count in infertile women: its agreement with conventional two-dimensional ultrasound and serum levels of anti-Müllerian hormone. Reprod Biol Endocrinol 15:96, 2017

Pisal N, Sindos M, O'Riordian J, et al: The use of spinal needle for transcervical saline infusion sonohysterography in presence of cervical stenosis. Acta Obstet Gynecol Scand 84:1019, 2005

Rajan D, Margau R, Kroll R, et al: Clinical utility of ultrasound versus magnetic resonance imaging for deciding to proceed with uterine artery embolization for presumed symptomatic fibroids. Clin Radiol 66:57, 2011

Reinhold C, Atri M, Mehio AR, et al: Diffuse uterine adenomyosis: morphologic criteria and diagnostic accuracy of endovaginal sonography. Radiology 197:609, 1995

Reinhold C, McCarthy S, Bret PM, et al: Diffuse adenomyosis: comparison of endovaginal US and MR imaging with histopathologic correlation. Radiology 199:151, 1996

Reuter KL, Daly DC, Cohen SM: Septate versus bicornuate uteri: errors in imaging diagnosis. Radiology 172:749, 1989

Romosan G, Valentin L: The sensitivity and specificity of transvaginal ultrasound with regard to acute pelvic inflammatory disease: a review of the literature. Arch Gynecol Obstet 289:705, 2014

Sala E, Rockall A, Freeman S, et al: The added role of MR imaging in treatment stratification of patients with gynecologic malignancies: what the radiologist needs to know. Radiology 266:718, 2013

Santoro GA, Wieczorek AP, Dietz HP, et al: State of the art: an integrated approach to pelvic floor ultrasonography. Ultrasound Obstet Gynecol 37:381, 2011

Sassone AM, Timor-Tritsch IE, Artner A, et al: Transvaginal sonographic characterization of ovarian disease: evaluation of a new scoring system to predict ovarian malignancy. Obstet Gynecol 78:70, 1991

Scalea TM, Rodriquez A, Chiu WC, et al: Focused assessment with sonography for trauma (FAST): results from an international consensus conference. J Trauma 46:466, 1999

Schaer GN, Koechli OR, Schuessler B, et al: Perineal ultrasound for evaluating the bladder neck in urinary stress incontinence. Obstet Gynecol 85:220, 1995

Seshadri S, Khalil M, Osman A, et al: The evolving role of saline infusion sonography (SIS) in infertility. Eur J Obstet Gynecol Reprod Biol 185:66, 2015

Siegelman ES, Outwater EK: Tissue characterization in the female pelvis by means of MR imaging. Radiology 212:5, 1999

Song Y, Yang J, Liu Z, et al: Preoperative evaluation of endometrial carcinoma by contrast-enhanced ultrasonography. BJOG 116:294, 2009

Stoelinga B, Hehenkamp WJK, Brolmann HAM et al: Real-time elastography for assessment of uterine disorders. Ultrasound Obstet Gynecol 43:218, 2014

Stoelinga B, Hehenkamp WJK, Nieuwenhuis LL, et al: Accuracy and reproducibility of sonoelastography for the assessment of fibroids and adenomyosis, with magnetic resonance imaging as reference standard. Ultrasound Med Biol 44:1654, 2018

Stumpf PG, March CM: Febrile morbidity following hysterosalpingography: identification of risk factors and recommendations for prophylaxis. Fertil Steril 33:487, 1980

Subak LL, Hricak H, Powell CB, et al: Cervical carcinoma: computed tomography and magnetic resonance imaging for preoperative staging. Obstet Gynecol 86:43, 1995

Taylor LS, Porter BC, Rubens DJ, et al: Three-dimensional sonoelastography: principles and practices. Phys Med Biol 45:1477, 2000

Tempany C, Dou K, Silverman S, et al: Staging of advanced ovarian cancer: comparison of imaging modalities report from the Radiological Diagnostic Oncology Group. Radiology 215:761, 2000

Thurmond AS: Selective salpingography and fallopian tube recanalization. AJR 156:33, 1991

Timmerman D, Testa AC, Bourne T, et al: Logistic regression model to distinguish between the benign and malignant adnexal mass before surgery: a multicenter study by the International Ovarian Tumor Analysis Group. J Clin Oncol 23:8794, 2005

Timmerman D, Valentin L, Bourne T, et al: Terms, definitions and measurements to describe the sonographic features of adnexal tumors: a consensus opinion from the International Ovarian Tumor Analysis (IOTA) group. Ultrasound Obstet Gynecol 16:500, 2000

Timmerman D, Van Calster B, Testa A, et al: Predicting the risk of malignancy in adnexal masses based on the simple rules from the International Ovarian Tumor Analysis group. Am J Obstet Gynecol 214:424, 2016

Timor-Tritsch IE, Lerner JP, Monteagudo A, et al: Transvaginal sonographic markers of tubal inflammatory disease. Ultrasound Obstet Gynecol 12:56, 1998

Tinkanen H, Kujansuu E: Doppler ultrasound findings in tubo-ovarian infectious complex. J Clin Ultrasound 21:175, 1993

Titton RL, Gervais DA, Hahn PF, et al: Urine leaks and urinomas: diagnosis and imaging guided intervention. Radiographics 23:1133, 2003

Togashi K, Ozasa H, Konishi I: Enlarged uterus: differentiation between adenomyosis and leiomyoma with MRI. Radiology 171:531, 1989

Troiano R, McCarthy S: Müllerian duct anomalies: imaging and clinical issues. Radiology 233:19, 2004

Twickler DM, Forte TB, Santos-Ramos R, et al: The Ovarian Tumor Index predicts risk for malignancy. Cancer 86:2280, 1999

Twickler DM, Moschos E: Ultrasound and assessment of ovarian cancer risk. AJR 194:322, 2010

Valentin L: Gray scale sonography, subjective evaluation of the color Doppler image and measurement of blood flow velocity for distinguishing benign and malignant tumor of suspected adnexal origin. Eur J Obstet Gynecol Reprod Biol 72:63, 1997

Vellucci F, Regini C, Barbanti C, et al: Pelvic floor evaluation with transperineal ultrasound: a new approach. Minerva Ginecol 70:58, 2018

Wang XW, Tian JW, Wang HK: Diagnostic value of transvaginal color Doppler ultrasound on endometrial lesions. Eur J Gynaecol Oncol 37:842, 2016a

Wang Y, Qian L: Three- or four-dimensional hysterosalpingo contrast sonography for diagnosing tubal patency in infertile females: a systematic review with meta-analysis. Br J Radiol 89(1063):20151013, 2016b

Weiner Z, Thaler I, Beck D, et al: Differentiating malignant from benign ovarian tumors with transvaginal color flow imaging. Obstet Gynecol 79:159, 1992

Wolfman DJ, Ascher SM: Magnetic resonance imaging of benign uterine pathology. Top Magn Reson Imaging 17:399, 2006

Wong TZ, Jones EL, Coleman RE: Positron emission tomography with 2-deoxy-2-[^{18}F]fluoro-d-glucose for evaluating local and distant disease in patients with cervical cancer. Mol Imaging Biol 6:55, 2004

Wu HM, Chiang CH, Huang HY, et al: Detection of the subendometrial vascularization flow index by three-dimensional ultrasound may be useful for predicting the pregnancy rate for patients undergoing *in vitro* fertilization-embryo transfer. Fertil Steril 79:507, 2003

Wu Y, Peng H, Zhao X: Diagnostic performance of contrast-enhanced ultrasound for ovarian cancer: a meta-analysis. Ultrasound Med Biol 41:967, 2015

Xie M, Zhang X, Yu M, et al: Evaluation of the cervix after cervical conization by transvaginal elastography. J Ultrasound Med 37:1109, 2018

Yamashita Y, Torashima M, Hatanaka Y, et al: Adnexal masses: accuracy of characterization with transvaginal US and precontrast and postcontrast MR imaging. Radiology 194:557, 1995

Yamashita Y, Torashima M, Takahashi M: Hyperintense uterine leiomyoma at T2-weighted MR imaging: differentiation with dynamic enhanced MR imaging and clinical implications Radiology 189:721, 1993

Yitta S, Hecht E, Mausner E, et al: Normal or abnormal? Demystifying uterine and cervical contrast enhancement at multidetector CT. Radiographics 31:647, 2011

Yu NC, Raman SS, Patel M, et al: Fistulas of the genitourinary tract: a radiologic review. Radiographics 24:1331, 2004

Zheng W, Chen K, Peng C, et al: Contrast-enhanced ultrasonography vs MRI for evaluation of local invasion by cervical cancer. Br J Radiol 91:20170858, 2018

Zollner U, Specketer MT, Dietl J, et al: 3D-Endometrial volume and outcome of cryopreserved embryo replacement cycles. Arch Gynecol Obstet 286:517, 2012

Gynecologic Infection

NORMAL VAGINAL FLORA

The vaginal flora of a normal, asymptomatic, reproductive-aged woman includes multiple aerobic, facultative anaerobic, and obligate anaerobic species. Of these, anaerobes predominate and outnumber aerobic species approximately 10 to 1 (Bartlett, 1977). These bacteria exist with the host in a symbiotic relationship, which is alterable depending on the microenvironment.

Certain bacterial species normally found in vaginal flora have access to the upper reproductive tract. The female upper reproductive tract is not sterile, and the presence of these bacteria does not indicate active infection (Hemsell, 1989; Spence, 1982). Together, these findings illustrate the potential for infection following gynecologic surgery and the need for antimicrobial prophylaxis.

■ Vaginal pH

Typically, the vaginal pH ranges between 4 and 4.5. This is due in part to gram-positive aerobic *Lactobacillus* species producing lactic acid, fatty acids, and other organic acids. Other bacteria also can add organic acids from protein catabolism, and anaerobic bacteria donate by amino acid fermentation.

Glycogen, which is present in healthy vaginal mucosa, provides nutrients for many vaginal ecosystem species and is metabolized to lactic acid (Boskey, 2001). Glycogen content within vaginal epithelial cells normally diminishes after menopause and is low in childhood. As a result, postmenopausal women not receiving estrogen replacement and young girls have a lower prevalence of *Lactobacillus* species and less acid production compared with that of reproductive-aged women. This leads to a rise in vaginal pH. For menopausal women, hormone replacement therapy restores vaginal lactobacilli populations, which protect against vaginal pathogens (Dahn, 2008).

■ Altered Flora

Changing other elements of the vaginal ecology may alter the prevalence of various species and may lead to infection. With the menstrual cycle, transient changes in flora are observed. These are predominantly during the first days of the cycle and are presumed to be associated with hormonal changes (Keane, 1997). Menstrual fluid can serve as a nutrient source for several bacterial species, resulting in their overgrowth. The role of this in the development of upper reproductive tract infection following menstruation is unclear, but an association may be present. For example, women symptomatic with acute gonococcal upper reproductive tract infection classically are menstruating or have just completed their menses. Last, treatment with broad-spectrum antibiotics may result in symptoms attributed to inflammation from *Candida albicans* or other *Candida* species by eradicating other balancing species in the flora.

■ Bacterial Vaginosis (BV)

This common, complex, and poorly understood clinical syndrome reflects vaginal flora in which anaerobic species are overrepresented. These include *Gardnerella*, *Prevotella*, *Mobiluncus*, and *Bacteroides* species; *Atopobium vaginae*; and BV-associated bacteria, provisionally named BVAB1, BVAB2, and BVAB3. These latter three are newly recognized bacteria found in women with BV (Fredricks, 2005). BV is also associated with a significant reduction of normal *Lactobacillus* species.

Molecular ribosomal RNA gene sequencing techniques have greatly aided classification of specific bacteria within vaginal flora ecosystems, which are also called *vaginal microbiota* or *vaginal biomes*. There are five types of vaginal microbiota, referred to as *community state types (CSTs)*. CSTs are defined by their specific clustering of specific species. And, a woman can be categorized to one of these five CSTs based on her vaginal microbiota composition (Ravel, 2011). Researchers have begun to quantify the risk of BV by these CST groups. Specifically, CSTs I, II, III, and V are lactobacilli rich. In contrast, CST IV is a heterogeneous microbiota of strict anaerobes and is associated with BV. CSTs vary racially, and CST IV is also the most common in asymptomatic, healthy black women (Fettweis, 2014).

In evaluating risks for BV, this condition is not considered by the Centers for Disease Control and Prevention (CDC) (2015) to be a sexually transmitted disease (STD). However, a greater risk of BV is associated with multiple or new sexual partners, female partners, and oral sex, whereas condom use lowers the risk (Fethers, 2008). Moreover, rates of STD acquisition are increased in affected women, and a possible role of sexual transmission in the pathogenesis of recurrent BV has been proposed (Atashili, 2008; Bradshaw, 2006; Wiesenfeld, 2003). Other potential risks are douching, black race, smoking, and intrauterine device (IUD) use.

BV is the most common cause of vaginal discharge among reproductive-aged women. Of symptoms, a nonirritating, malodorous vaginal discharge is characteristic but may not always be present. The vagina is usually not erythematous, and cervical examination reveals no abnormalities.

For diagnosis, clinical criteria first proposed by Amsel and associates (1983) include: (1) microscopic evaluation of a vaginal-secretion saline preparation, (2) release of volatile amines produced by anaerobic metabolism, and (3) determination of the vaginal pH. A saline preparation, also known as a "wet prep," contains a swab-collected sample of discharge mixed with drops of saline on a microscope slide. Clue cells are the most reliable indicators of BV and were originally described by Gardner and Dukes (1955) (Fig. 3-1). These vaginal epithelial cells contain many attached bacteria, which create a poorly defined stippled cellular border. At least 20 percent of the epithelial cells should be clue cells. The positive predictive value of this test for BV is 95 percent.

Adding 10-percent potassium hydroxide (KOH) to a fresh sample of vaginal secretions releases volatile amines that have a

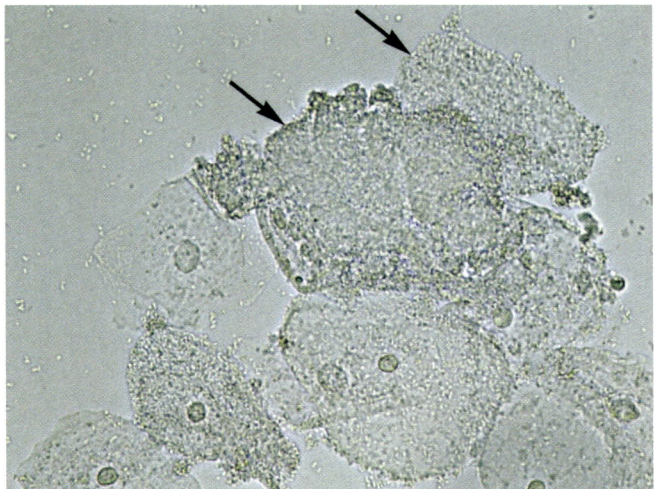

FIGURE 3-1 Photomicrograph of saline wet preparation reveals clue cells. Several of these squamous cells are heavily studded with bacteria. Clue cells are covered to the extent that cell borders are blurred and nuclei are not visible (*arrows*). (Reproduced with permission from Dr. Lauri Campagna and Mercedes Pineda, WHNP.)

fishy odor. This is often colloquially referred to as a "whiff test." The odor is frequently evident even without KOH. Similarly, alkalinity of seminal fluid and blood are responsible for foulodor complaints after intercourse and with menses. The finding of both clue cells and a positive whiff test result is pathognomonic, even in asymptomatic patients.

Characteristically with BV, the vaginal pH is >4.5, and this stems from diminished acid production by bacteria. Similarly, *Trichomonas vaginalis* infection also is associated with anaerobic overgrowth and elaboration of amines. Thus, women diagnosed with BV should have no microscopic evidence of trichomoniasis.

Used primarily in research studies rather than clinical practice, the Nugent Score is a system employed for diagnosing BV. During microscopic examination of a gram-stained vaginal discharge smear, scores are calculated by assessing bacteria staining and morphology.

Last, molecular DNA assays against the more frequent organisms found in women with BV have suitable accuracy (Coleman, 2018). However, these tests assess for bacteria that may also be part of normal flora in asymptomatic women. Moreover, compared with traditional methods, molecular tests have yet to show superior health outcomes but do add substantial cost.

Several gynecologic adverse health outcomes have been observed in women with BV. These include vaginitis, endometritis, postabortal endometritis, pelvic inflammatory disease (PID) unassociated with *Neisseria gonorrhoeae* or *Chlamydia trachomatis*, susceptibility to human immunodeficiency virus (HIV) acquisition, and acute pelvic infections following pelvic surgery, especially hysterectomy (Atashili, 2008; Larsson, 1989, 1991, 1992; Soper, 1990). Pregnant patients with BV have an elevated risk of preterm delivery and postpartum endometritis (Hillier, 1995; Watts, 1990).

Several regimens are available for nonpregnant women (Table 3-1). The newest of these is secnidazole, a 5-nitroimidazole in granule form taken once orally (Schwebke, 2017). Cure rates with regimens in Table 3-1 range from 80 to 90 percent at 1 week, but within 3 months, 30 percent of women have experienced a recurrence. Many of these are correlated with heterosexual contact (Amsel, 1983; Gardner, 1955; Wilson, 2004). However, treatment of male sexual partners does not benefit women with this recurring condition and is not recommended. Moreover, other forms of therapy such as introduction of lactobacilli, acidifying vaginal gels, and use of probiotics have shown inconsistent efficacy (Senok, 2009).

Limited evidence supports specific ways to prevent BV. Alteration of previously mentioned risk factor behaviors can be considered. Of these, some data suggest elimination or diminished use of vaginal douches may have benefits (Brotman, 2008; Klebanoff, 2010).

GENITAL ULCER INFECTIONS

Ulceration defines complete loss of the epidermal covering with invasion into the underlying dermis. In contrast, *erosion* describes partial loss of the epidermis without dermal penetration. These are distinguished by clinical examination. Biopsies are generally not helpful. But if taken, samples obtained from the edge of new lesions are the most likely to be informative.

TABLE 3-1. Single-Agent Bacterial Vaginosis Treatment

Recommended regimens	
Metronidazole (Flagyl)	500 mg orally twice daily for 7 days
Metronidazole gel 0.75% (Metrogel vaginal)	5 g (1 full applicator) intravaginally once daily for 5 days
Clindamycin cream[a] 2% (Cleocin, Clindesse)	5 g (1 full applicator) intravaginally at bedtime for 7 days
Alternative regimens	
Secnidazole (Solosec)	2 g orally once[b]
Tinidazole (Tindamax)	2 g orally once daily for 2 days
	1 g orally once daily for 5 days
Clindamycin	300 mg orally twice daily for 7 days
Clindamycin ovules[a] (Cleocin)	100 mg intravaginally at bedtime for 3 days

[a]Clindamycin cream and ovules are oil-based and might weaken latex condoms and diaphragms for 5 days after use.
[b]These granules are mixed with applesauce, yogurt, or pudding and are not chewed.
From the Centers for Disease Control and Prevention, 2015; Schwebke, 2017.

Importantly, biopsy is mandatory if carcinoma is suspected, and Figure 4-2 (p. 94) illustrates technique.

Most young sexually active women in the United States who have genital ulcers will have herpes simplex virus (HSV) infection or syphilis. Rarely, some will have chancroid, lymphogranuloma venereum, or granuloma inguinale. Essentially all are sexually transmitted and are associated with higher risk for HIV transmission.

As a general rule, females diagnosed with one STD are offered testing for others. This typically includes testing for syphilis, gonorrhea, and HIV, chlamydial, and hepatitis B infections. Sexual contacts require evaluation, and both require reassessment following treatment.

■ Herpes Simplex Virus Infection

Genital herpes is the most prevalent genital ulcer disease and is a chronic viral infection. After crossing an epithelial barrier, the virus enters sensory nerve endings and undergoes retrograde axonal transport to the dorsal root ganglion. Here, the virus develops lifelong latency. Spontaneous reactivation by various events results in anterograde transport of virus to the surface. The virus is shed, with or without lesion formation. It is postulated that immune mechanisms control latency and reactivation.

There are two types of herpes simplex virus, HSV-1 and HSV-2. HSV-1 is the predominant cause of oral lesions and often is acquired in childhood. Additionally, HSV-1 is now the most frequent agent of genital lesions in Hispanic and white women (Bernstein, 2013). This rise in the prevalence of HSV-1 genital disease may stem from an increase in oral–genital sexual practices. Another explanation is that HSV-1 acquisition has declined in childhood as a result of improved living conditions and hygiene. Without prior exposure, this renders people without HSV-1 antibodies susceptible to genital acquisition of HSV-1 or -2. HSV-2 causes primarily genital lesions and is the most common source of genital disease in black women (Fanfair, 2013). Of all females aged 14 to 49 years in the United States, 16 percent have suffered a genital HSV-2 infection, and nearly 55 percent are seropositive to HSV-1 (Bradley, 2014).

Most women who have been infected with either HSV-1 or HSV-2 lack a formal diagnosis because of mild or unrecognized infections. Infected patients can shed infectious virus while asymptomatic, and most infections are transmitted sexually by patients who are unaware of their infection. Compared with men, women have more severe symptoms with primary and recurrent infection.

Symptoms

Patient symptoms at initial presentation will depend primarily on whether a patient during the current episode has antibody from previous exposure. If a patient has no antibody, the attack rate in an exposed person approaches 70 percent. The mean incubation period is approximately 1 week. Up to 90 percent of those who are symptomatic with their initial infection will have another episode within a year.

The virus infects viable epidermal cells, the response to which is erythema and papule formation. With cell death and cell wall lysis, blisters form (Fig. 3-2). The covering then disrupts, leaving a usually painful ulcer. These lesions develop crusting and heal but may become secondarily infected. The three stages of lesions are: (1) vesicle with or without pustule formation, which lasts approximately a week; (2) ulceration; and (3) crusting. Virus is predictably shed during the first two phases.

Burning and severe pain accompany initial vesicular lesions. With ulcers, urinary frequency and/or dysuria from direct contact of urine with ulcers may be complaints. Rarely, local swelling can result from vulvar lesions and cause urethral obstruction. Alternatively or additionally, herpetic lesions can involve the vagina, cervix, bladder, anus, and rectum. Commonly, low-grade fever, headache, and myalgias are noted.

Viral load undoubtedly contributes to the number, size, and distribution of lesions. Normal host defense mechanisms inhibit viral growth, and healing starts within 1 to 2 days. Early treatment with an antiviral medication decreases the viral load. Immune-deficient patients have greater susceptibility and display diminished immune response and delayed healing.

For a previously uninfected patient, the period of new lesion formation and time to healing are both longer. Pain persists for

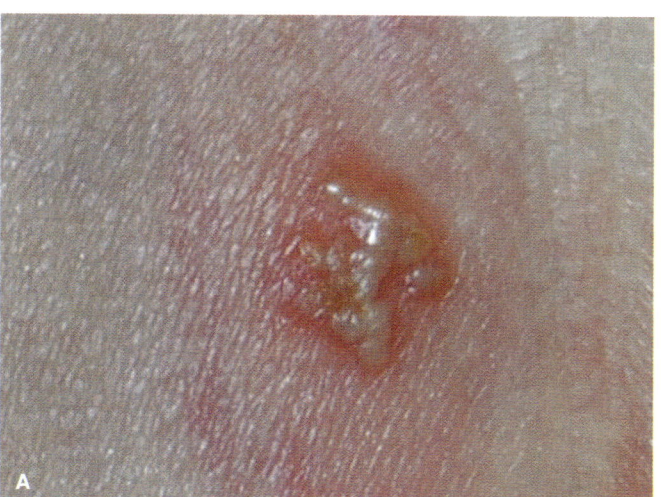 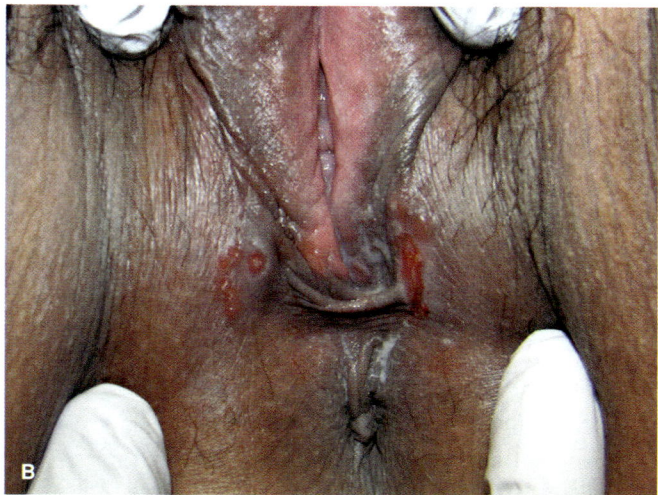

FIGURE 3-2 Genital herpetic ulcers. **A.** Vesicles prior to ulceration. **B.** Punctate (*left*) or "knife-cut" (*right*) ulcers are common lesions. (Reproduced with permission from Dr. William Griffith.)

the first 7 to 10 days, and lesions heal by 2 to 3 weeks. If a patient has had prior exposure to HSV-2, their initial episode is significantly less severe, and time to healing approximates 2 weeks.

Recurrence following HSV-2 infection is common, and almost two thirds of patients have a prodrome prior to lesion onset. Heralding paresthesias are frequently described as pruritus or tingling in the area prior to vesicle formation. However, prodromal symptoms may develop without actual lesion formation. Clinical manifestations for women with recurrences are more limited, with only approximately 1 week of symptoms.

Diagnosis

The gold standard for diagnosing genital herpes was previously cell culture. Specificity is high, but sensitivity is low and declines as lesions heal. Nucleic acid amplification test (NAAT) testing is many times more sensitive than culture and can detect HSV DNA shed from epithelia without vesicular lesions (LeFoff, 2014). Moreover, results generally are available in 1 to 2 days. Importantly, a negative culture or polymerase chain reaction (PCR) result does not mean that there is no herpetic infection. In contrast, false-positive results are rare.

HSV is surrounded by envelope glycoproteins, and glycoprotein G is the antigen of interest. Serologic assays are available to detect antibodies formed against the HSV type-specific glycoproteins, namely glycoprotein G2 (HSV-2) or glycoprotein G1 (HSV-1). Assay specificity is ≥96 percent, and the sensitivity of HSV-2 antibody testing ranges from 80 to 98 percent. Importantly, with serologic screening, only immunoglobulin G (IgG) antibody assays are ordered. Although these tests may be used to confirm herpes simplex infection, seroconversion following initial infection takes approximately 3 weeks (Ashley-Morrow, 2003). Immunoglobulin M (IgM) testing is not recommended. This can lead to ambiguous results as the IgM assays are not type-specific and also may be positive during a recurrent outbreak. Thus, in clinically obvious cases, immediate treatment and additional STD screening can be initiated following physical examination alone.

Serologic screening for HSV in the asymptomatic general population is not recommended. However, HSV serologic testing can be considered for HIV-infected individuals or for women presenting for an STD evaluation, especially for those with multiple partners and for those in demographics with high prevalence (Fanfair, 2013). It can also add management information for couples thought but not confirmed to be discordant for infection (Centers for Disease Control and Prevention, 2015).

Treatment

The CDC provides and regularly updates guidelines for the treatment of all STDs. These are found on the CDC website at: www.cdc.gov/std/tg2015/default.htm. For HSV, currently available antiviral therapy is listed in Table 3-2. Although these agents may hasten healing and improve symptoms, therapy does not eradicate latent virus or affect future rates of recurrent infection. Analgesia with nonsteroidal antiinflammatory drugs or, if severe, a mild narcotic such as acetaminophen with codeine may be prescribed. In addition, topical anesthetics such as lidocaine ointment may provide relief. Local hygiene to prevent secondary bacterial infection is important.

For women with established HSV-2 infection, therapy may not be necessary if symptoms are mild and tolerable. Episodic therapy for recurrent disease is ideally initiated at least within 1 day of lesion outbreak or during the prodrome. Patients may be given a prescription ahead of time so that medication is available to begin therapy with prodrome onset.

If episodes recur at frequent intervals, a woman may elect daily suppressive therapy, which reduces recurrences by 70 to 80 percent (Centers for Disease Control and Prevention, 2015). Suppressive therapy may eliminate recurrences and decreases sexual transmission. Once-daily dosing may result in enhanced compliance and lower cost.

Patient education is mandatory, and specific topics include prodrome recognition, recurrence triggers, methods to reduce sexual transmission, and obstetric consequences. Acquisition of this infection may have significant psychological impact, and several websites provide patient information and support. A useful CDC website is www.cdc.gov/std/Herpes/STDFact-Herpes.htm.

TABLE 3-2. Oral Agents for Genital Herpes Simplex Infection

First clinical episode
Acyclovir 400 mg three times daily for 7–10 days
or
Acyclovir 200 mg five times daily for 7–10 days
or
Famciclovir (Famvir) 250 mg three times daily for 7–10 days
or
Valacyclovir (Valtrex) 1 g twice daily for 7–10 days

Episodic therapy for recurrent disease
Acyclovir 400 mg three times daily for 5 days
or
Acyclovir 800 mg twice daily for 5 days
or
Acyclovir 800 mg three times daily for 2 days
or
Famciclovir 125 mg twice daily for 5 days
or
Famciclovir 1 g twice daily for 1 day
or
Famciclovir 500 mg once, then 250 mg twice daily for 2 days
or
Valacyclovir 500 mg twice daily for 3 days
or
Valacyclovir 1 g once daily for 5 days

Suppressive therapy
Acyclovir 400 mg twice daily
or
Famciclovir 250 mg twice daily
or
Valacyclovir 0.5 or 1 g once daily

From the Centers for Disease Control and Prevention, 2015.

Prevention

Women with genital herpes should refrain from sexual activity with uninfected partners when prodrome symptoms or lesions are present. Latex condom use potentially lowers the risk for herpetic transmission (Martin, 2009). Suppressive therapy with oral valacyclovir 0.5 g daily reduces sexual transmission by almost 50 percent among couples discordant for HSV-2 (Corey, 2004). Unfortunately, preventive herpes vaccine trials have failed to demonstrate protective immunity in the genital tract (Belshe, 2012; Shin, 2013).

■ Syphilis

Pathophysiology

Syphilis is an STD caused by the spirochete *Treponema pallidum*, which is a slender, spiral-shaped organism with tapered ends. Women at highest risk are those from lower socioeconomic groups, adolescents, those with early onset of sexual activity, and those with many sexual partners. The number of

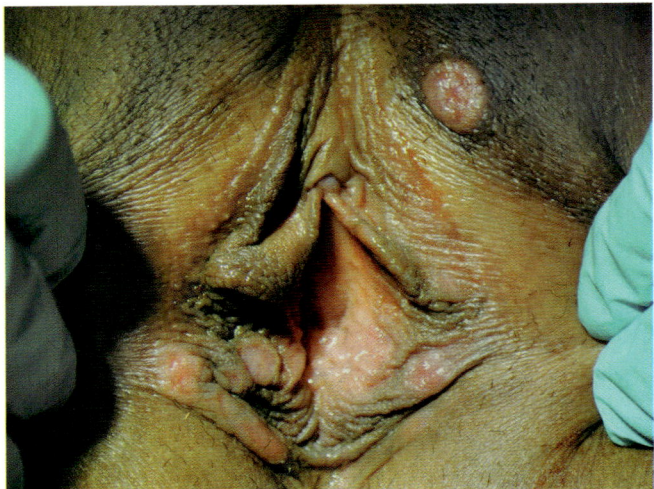

FIGURE 3-3 Several vulvar syphilitic chancres. Lesions that lie directly across the vulvar midline from each other are sometimes referred to as "kissing" lesions.

syphilis cases has risen almost every year in the United States since 2001. In 2017, more than 100,000 cases of syphilis, which included all stages, were reported to the CDC (2018a).

The natural history of syphilis in untreated patients can be divided into four stages. Of these, primary and secondary syphilis represent incident infection. With primary syphilis, the hallmark lesion is the *chancre*, in which spirochetes are abundant. Classically, it is an isolated, nontender ulcer with raised, rounded borders and an uninfected base (Fig. 3-3). However, it may become secondarily infected and painful. Chancres are often found on the cervix, vagina, or vulva but may also form in the mouth or around the anus. The mean incubation period is 3 weeks, but lesions can develop 10 days to 3 months after exposure. Without treatment, lesions spontaneously heal within 6 weeks.

With *secondary syphilis,* bacteremia develops 6 weeks to 6 months after a chancre appears. Its hallmark is a maculopapular rash that may involve the entire body and includes the palms, soles, and mucous membranes (Fig. 3-4). Mucosal lesions, called *mucous patches,* actively shed spirochetes. In warm, moist body areas, this rash may produce broad, pink or gray-white, highly infectious plaques called *condylomata lata*. Because syphilis is a systemic infection, other manifestations may include fever and malaise. Less commonly, cranial nerve dysfunction, meningitis, hepatitis, nephrotic syndrome, and arthritis develop.

Untreated, the manifestations of secondary syphilis resolve, and latent syphilis is diagnosed using serologic tests. During *early latent syphilis*, which is diagnosed within 1 year of infection, secondary signs and symptoms may recur. *Late latent syphilis* is defined as a period greater than 1 year after the initial infection.

Tertiary syphilis is the phase of untreated syphilis that may appear up to 20 years after latency. During this phase, cardiovascular, central nervous system, and musculoskeletal involvement become apparent. However, cardiovascular and neurosyphilis are half as common in females as in males.

Diagnosis

A definitive diagnosis requires direct detection of spirochetes within a lesion sample. However, most cases are diagnosed presumptively

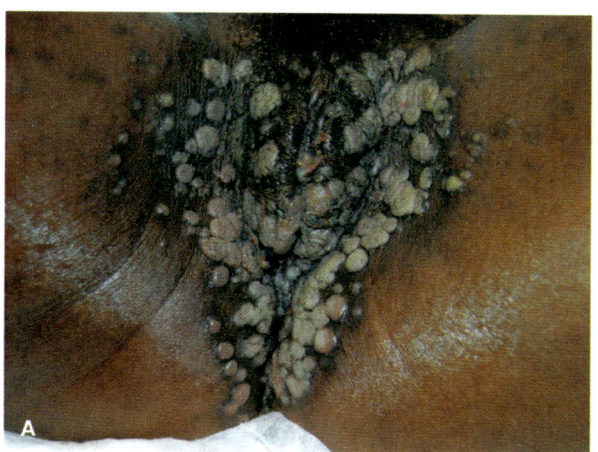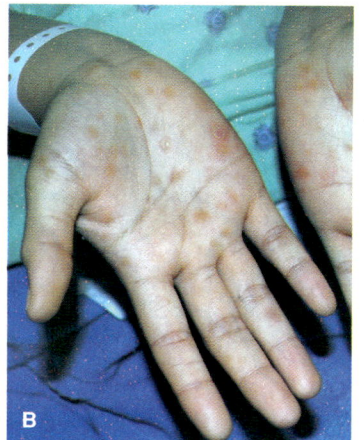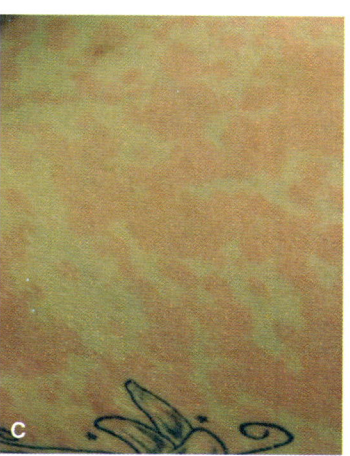

FIGURE 3-4 Secondary syphilis. **A.** Woman with multiple condyloma lata on her labia. Soft, flat, moist, pink-tan papules and nodules on the perineum and perianal area are typical. (Reproduced with permission from Dr. George Wendel.) **B.** Woman with multiple keratotic papules on her palms. With secondary syphilis, disseminated papulosquamous eruptions may be seen on the palms, soles, or trunk. (Reproduced with permission from Dr. Devin Macias.) **C.** Characteristic rash on this woman's torso. (Reproduced with permission from Dr. Eddie McCord.)

using clinical assessment plus serologic testing. Serologic testing includes both nontreponemal and treponemal-specific tests. The two nontreponemal tests are the Venereal Disease Research Laboratory (VDRL) and the rapid plasma reagin (RPR) tests. Both tests measure patient IgM and IgG antibodies formed against cardiolipin that is released from damaged host cells and possibly also from treponemes. Notably, these same antibodies can also be produced in response to recent vaccination, febrile illness, pregnancy, or chronic conditions such as intravenous (IV) drug abuse, systemic lupus erythematosus, aging, or cancer. These all serve as potential sources of false-positive results (Larsen, 1995). With true infection, seroconversion occurs at approximately 3 weeks but can take up to 6 weeks (Peeling, 2004). Thus, women with very early primary syphilis can have initially false-negative serologic test results.

With positive nontreponemal test results, findings are quantified and expressed as titers. In the traditional screening

algorithm, a positive nontreponemal test result in a woman who has not been treated previously for syphilis will prompt clinical assessment and confirmation with a treponemal-specific test. These are either the fluorescent treponemal antibody-absorption (FTA-ABS) or *Treponema pallidum* particle agglutination (TP-PA). These species-specific tests remain positive for life following infection. If the treponemal-specific test results also are positive, treatment is then provided. In a woman previously treated for syphilis, a fourfold (two dilution) rise in nontreponemal titer suggests reinfection, and retreatment is provided.

In an alternative "reverse" screening algorithm, a treponemal-specific enzyme or chemiluminescence immunoassay (EIA or CIA) is used first. If positive results are found, RPR or VDRL testing is then performed along with clinical assessment to determine timing of infection (Table 3-3). In this scenario, a positive screening EIA or CIA result reflects either *current* or

TABLE 3-3. Interpretation of Serologic Tests Using Reverse Sequence Syphilis Screening

Treponemal Test	VDRL or RPR	TP-PA	Possible Interpretations
Nonreactive	Nonreactive[a]		1. Absence of syphilis 2. Very early syphilis before seroconversion
Reactive[b]	Nonreactive	Reactive Reactive Nonreactive	1. Prior treated syphilis 2. Untreated syphilis 3. False-positive treponemal test[c]
Reactive	Reactive		1. Active syphilis 2. Recently treated syphilis with nontreponemal titers that have not yet become nonreactive 3. Treated syphilis with persistent titers[d]
Nonreactive	Reactive[a]		1. False-positive nontreponemal test

[a]Usually not performed if the initial treponemal test is negative.
[b]By 2 different methods if the nontreponemal test is nonreactive.
[c]May be seen in pregnancy or among immigrants with previous exposure to endemic treponematoses.
[d]Successful treatment is usually considered with a fourfold decline in titers (e.g., from 1:32 to 1:8).
RPR = rapid plasma reagin; TP-PA = *Treponema pallidum* particle agglutination; VDRL = Venereal Disease Research Laboratory.
Derived from Centers for Disease Control and Prevention, 2011.

past infection because treponemal-specific antibodies typically remain positive for life. For patients with discordant screening results (EIA/CIA+ and RPR/VDRL-), TP-PA is performed. If the TP-PA result is positive and documentation of prior syphilis treatment is lacking, antibiotics are then administered. Management of patients using the reverse algorithm relies heavily on disease history and physical findings.

Following treatment of patients diagnosed using either the traditional or reverse algorithm, sequential nontreponemal tests are performed. During this surveillance, the same type of test—either RPR or VDRL-is ideally used for consistency. A fourfold titer decline is expected by 6 to 12 months after therapy for primary or secondary syphilis. Patients with latent syphilis or initially low nontreponemal antibody titers are less likely to achieve a fourfold drop. Although nontreponemal tests usually become nonreactive after treatment, some women may have persistently low titer results. These patients are described as *serofast*.

Treatment

Penicillin is the first-line therapeutic agent for this infection, and benzathine penicillin is primarily chosen. Specific recommendations for therapy by the CDC (2015) are listed in Table 3-4. Within the first 24 hours after treatment of early disease, an acute, self-limited febrile response, termed a *Jarisch-Herxheimer reaction*, may develop and is associated with headache and myalgia.

Up to 10 percent of the general population may manifest an allergic reaction to penicillins. The lowest risk is associated with oral preparations, whereas the highest follows those combined with procaine and given intramuscularly (IM). For patients with penicillin allergy who cannot be surveilled posttherapy or whose compliance is questioned, skin testing, desensitization, and treatment with IM benzathine penicillin is recommended (Wendel, 1985). Desensitization can be performed relatively safely and outlined at the CDC website: www.cdc.gov/std/tg2015/pen-allergy.htm.

After initial treatment, women are seen at 6-month intervals for clinical evaluation and serologic retesting. If the expected

TABLE 3-4. Treatment of Syphilis

Primary, secondary, early latent (<1 year) syphilis
Recommended regimen:
   Benzathine penicillin G, 2.4 million units IM once
   Alternative oral regimens (penicillin-allergic, nonpregnant women): Doxycycline 100 mg orally twice daily for 2 weeks

Late latent, tertiary, and cardiovascular syphilis
Recommended regimen:
   Benzathine penicillin G, 2.4 million units IM weekly times 3 doses
   Alternative oral regimen (penicillin-allergic, nonpregnant women): Doxycycline 100 mg orally twice daily for 4 weeks

From the Centers for Disease Control and Prevention, 2015.

fourfold titer decline does not occur, possible reinfection or treatment failure is considered. Retreatment recommendation is benzathine penicillin G, 2.4 million units IM weekly for 3 weeks.

■ Chancroid

Chancroid, granuloma inguinale, and lymphogranuloma venereum are each rare STDs in the United States. Thus, any evaluation of genital ulcer disease first includes testing to exclude syphilis and HSV infection, which are much more common.

Chancroid is caused by *Haemophilus ducreyi*, and following exposure, incubation usually spans 3 to 10 days. One or more erythematous papules then become pustular and ulcerate. These painful genital ulcers classically have soft irregular margins and friable bases. In addition, many patients develop tender inguinal lymphadenopathy. If large and fluctuant, these *buboes* may suppurate and form fistulas.

Previously, definitive diagnosis required growth of *H ducreyi* in cell culture, but now the accepted standard for diagnosis is a NAAT (Romero, 2017). No *H ducreyi* PCR is Food and Drug Administration (FDA)-cleared in the United States (Copeland, 2016). A presumptive diagnosis can be made from a Gram stain of lesion contents that show small gram-negative rods in a chain. Superficial debris is ideally first removed.

For treatment, the CDC's (2015) recommended regimens include either a single dose of oral azithromycin (1 g) or of IM ceftriaxone (250 mg). Second-line, multidose options are ciprofloxacin or erythromycin base.

■ Granuloma Inguinale

Also known as donovanosis, granuloma inguinale is caused by the gram-negative bacterium *Klebsiella granulomatis*. Incubation may last from days to weeks, and infection presents with painless inflammatory nodules that progress to highly vascular, nontender ulcers. These ulcers heal by fibrosis, which can result in scarring resembling keloids. Lymph nodes are usually uninvolved.

Culturing this organism is difficult, and FDA-approved PCR tests for *K granulomatis* are lacking (Copeland, 2016). Instead, diagnosis is confirmed by identification of Donovan bodies, which appear as a "closed safety pin" during microscopic cytologic evaluation following Wright-Giemsa staining.

Treatment recommended by the CDC (2015) is azithromycin 1 g once weekly for at least 3 weeks and until lesions are completely healed. Alternative regimens include doxycycline, ciprofloxacin, trimethoprim-sulfamethoxazole, or erythromycin base. Improvement will be evident within the first few treatment days, but resolution may be lengthy and relapses have been reported.

■ Lymphogranuloma Venereum

This ulcerative genital disease is caused by *C trachomatis* serotypes L1, L2, and L3. Although uncommon in the United States, rates have risen in men having sex with men (Stoner, 2015). Incubation ranges from 3 days to 2 weeks, and lymphogranuloma venereum (LGV) is divided into three stages: (1) small painless papule, (2) regional lymphadenopathy, and (3) anogenitorectal fibrosis (Ceovic, 2015). In the primary stage, initial papules heal quickly and without scarring. During the second stage, inguinal and femoral lymph nodes progressively enlarge. Painful nodes can mat together on either side of the inguinal ligament to create a "groove sign." Nodes may then rupture and lead to chronically draining sinuses. Malaise, fever, and arthralgias also can be comorbid. In the third stage, tissue destruction and scarring are prominent, and sequela of lymphatic obstruction can develop.

LGV may be diagnosed by positive chlamydial testing. Specifically, culture or immunofluorescence or NAAT testing of samples from genital lesions, affected lymph nodes, or rectum are suitable. Moreover, a chlamydial serologic titer that is >1:64 can support the diagnosis. For treatment, the CDC (2015) recommends doxycycline, 100 mg orally twice daily for 21 days. An alternative is erythromycin base.

INFECTIOUS VAGINITIS

Symptomatic vaginal discharge most often reflects BV, candidiasis, or trichomoniasis. *Aerobic vaginitis* is a newly described disturbance of vaginal microbiota that leads to inflammation and discharge. Microscopic discharge evaluation shows increased white blood cell (WBC) counts, a greater number or aerobic species, but diminished lactobacilli counts (Sherrard, 2018). This is described further in Chapter 4 (p. 107).

BV typically evokes complaints of foul discharge odor without irritation. In contrast, if abnormal discharge is associated with vulvar burning, irritation, or itching, then *vaginitis* is diagnosed. Between 7 and 70 percent of women who have vaginal discharge complaints will have no definitive diagnosis (Anderson, 2004). For those in whom identifiable infection is absent, an inflammatory diagnosis and treatment for infection should not be given. In such instances, a woman may seek reassurance, having concern about a recent sexual exposure, and STD screening may alleviate this.

■ Initial Evaluation

During initial steps, a provider obtains information regarding prior vaginal infections and their treatment, symptom duration, specifics of self-treatment with over-the-counter (OTC) preparations, and a complete menstrual and sexual history. The salient features of a menstrual history are outlined in Chapter 8 (p. 182). A sexual history typically includes questions regarding age at coitarche, date of most recent sexual activity, number of recent partners, gender of those partners, use of condom protection, method of birth control, prior STD history, and type of sexual practices—anal, oral, or vaginal.

A thorough physical examination of the vulva, vagina, and cervix also is performed. Several etiologies may be identified in the office by microscopic examination of the discharge (Table 3-5). First, a saline preparation, described earlier, can be inspected (p. 57). A "KOH-prep" contains a swab-collected sample of discharge mixed with several drops of 10-percent potassium hydroxide. KOH leads to osmotic swelling and then lysis of squamous cell membranes. This visually clears the microscopic view and aids identification of fungal buds or hyphae, whose cell walls remain intact. Finally, vaginal pH analysis may add supportive information. Vaginal pH can be estimated using chemical testing paper strips. Appropriate readings are obtained by pressing a test strip directly to the upper vaginal wall and resting it there for a few seconds to absorb vaginal fluid. Once the strip is removed, its color is matched to the color indicator chart on the test strip dispenser. Importantly, blood and semen are alkaline and often will artificially elevate pH. Unfortunately, inexpensive laboratory tests such as these are not as accurate as a clinician would hope (Landers, 2004; Lowe, 2009).

A laboratory PCR panel specific for candidal species, *T vaginalis*, and BV species is now available (Gaydos, 2017a). This FDA market-authorized panel shows greater sensitivity than the clinical tests described in the prior paragraphs (Schwebke, 2018). However, in addition to added cost, it is unclear which

TABLE 3-5. Characteristics of Some Vaginal Infections

Category	Complaint	Discharge	KOH "Whiff Test"	Vaginal pH	Microscopic Findings
Normal	None	White, clear	–	3.8–4.2	NA
BV	Odor, increased after intercourse and/or menses	Thin, gray or white, adherent, often increased	+	>4.5	Clue cells, bacteria clumps (saline wet prep)
Candidiasis	Itching, burning, discharge	White, curdy	–	<4.5	Hyphae and buds (10-percent KOH solution wet prep)
Trichomoniasis	Frothy discharge, odor, dysuria, pruritus, spotting	Green-yellow, frothy, adherent, increased	±	>4.5	Motile trichomonads (saline wet prep)
Aerobic vaginitis[a]	Thin, watery discharge, pruritus	Purulent	–	>4.5	Many WBCs

[a]*Escherichia coli* or streptococcal or staphylococcal species.
BV = bacterial vaginosis; KOH = potassium hydroxide; NA = not applicable; WBC = white blood cell.

women may benefit because many cases of vaginitis can be diagnosed solely by clinical means.

■ Fungal Infection

C albicans can be found in the vagina of asymptomatic patients and is a commensal of the mouth, rectum, and vagina. However, imbalance between this yeast and its host can develop and can lead to vulvovaginal candidiasis. Occasionally, other *Candida* species may be involved and include *C tropicalis* and *C glabrata,* among others. Candidiasis is seen more often in patients with immunosuppression, diabetes mellitus, pregnancy, and recent broad-spectrum antibiotic use (Nyirjesy, 2013). Sexual transmission is uncommon, and treatment of sexual partners is unnecessary.

With candidiasis, vulvar pruritus, burning, erythema, and edema with excoriations are common (Fig. 3-5). The typical vaginal discharge is described as curdy or cottage cheese–like. Microscopic examination of vaginal discharge with saline and with 10-percent KOH preparations allows yeast identification. *C albicans* is dimorphic, with both yeast buds and hyphal forms. It may be present in the vagina as a filamentous fungus (pseudohyphae) or as germinated yeast with mycelia. Vaginal candidal culture is not routinely recommended. However, it may be indicated for those who fail empiric treatment and for women with evidence of infection yet absence of microscopic yeast.

The CDC classifies vulvovaginal candidiasis (2015) into "uncomplicated" and "complicated." Uncomplicated cases are sporadic or infrequent, are mild to moderate in symptom severity, are likely caused by *C albicans*, and involve immunocompetent women. For both uncomplicated and complicated infection, effective treatment formulations are listed in Table 3-6. Conceptually, the vagina can be considered a reservoir for which treatment lowers the infectious load, whereas the vulva is more often the site of symptoms (Donders, 2017). Thus, several of the listed products are combination packs that contain separate treatments for both vagina and vulva. For uncomplicated infection, azoles are extremely effective, and women require specific follow-up only if therapy is unsuccessful.

However, 10 to 20 percent of women have complicated candidiasis. This term encompasses infections with frequent recurrence or greater symptom severity, those from non-*albicans* species, or those in immunosuppressed patients. For women with complicated infection, cultures are obtained to direct care, and longer therapy may be needed to achieve clinical cure. Examples include local intravaginal therapy for 7 to 14 days.

By definition, *recurrent disease* reflects four or more candidal infections during a year. For recurrent *C albicans* disease, local intravaginal therapy for 7 to 14 days is an option. Alternatively, oral fluconazole (Diflucan) in 100-mg, 150-mg, or 200-mg strengths once every third day for a total of three doses (day 1, 4, and 7) may be chosen. Suppressive maintenance for recurrence prevention is with oral fluconazole, 100 to 200 mg weekly for 6 months. Non-*albicans* candidal species are less responsive to topical azole therapy. For non-*albicans* recurrent infection, a 600-mg boric acid gelatin capsule intravaginally at bedtime for 2 weeks may be successful. Prefilled capsules can be purchased OTC or can be assembled personally by filling a 0-size gelatin capsule with boric acid powder.

Oral azole therapy has been associated with serum liver enzyme elevation. Additionally, interactions with multiple medications that include certain antacid, antihypertensive, antiseizure, antiretroviral, immunosuppressive, and antilipidemic drugs have been reported (Brüggemann, 2009). In cases in which prolonged oral therapy is not feasible due to potential interactions, local intravaginal therapy once or twice weekly may give a similar clinical response.

Last, probiotics have been suggested as treatment or adjuncts to traditional therapy. However, evidence to support either role is not robust (Xie, 2017). Moreover, agreement on the preferred bacterial species is lacking.

■ Trichomoniasis

This infection is the most prevalent nonviral STD worldwide (Newman, 2015). And, in one large U.S. national survey, the prevalence was 1.8 percent in women aged 18 to 59 (Patel, 2018).

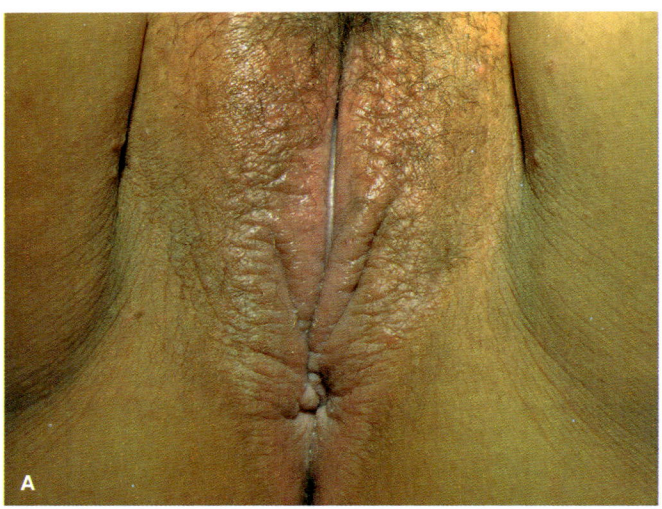
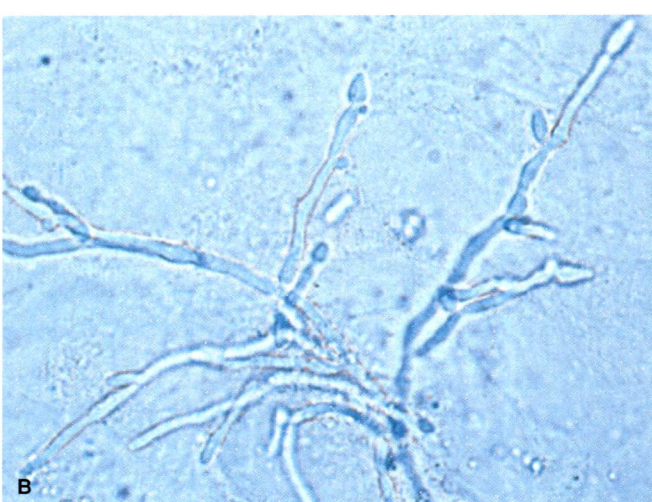

FIGURE 3-5 Candidal infection. **A.** Mild erythema and edema of the affected vulva creates a slightly leathery skin texture. (Reproduced with permission from Dr. Savita Joglekar.) **B.** *Candida albicans* in a potassium hydroxide preparation. Serpentine pseudohyphae are seen. (From Hansfield, 2001, with permission.)

TABLE 3-6. Topical Agents for the Treatment of Candidiasis[a]

Drug	Brand Name	Formulation	Dosage
Butoconazole	Gynazole-1[b]	2% vaginal cream	1 app vaginally, once
Clotrimazole	–	1% vaginal cream	1 app vaginally for 7 d
	Trivagizole	2% vaginal cream	1 app vaginally for 3 d
Clotrimazole + betamethasone	Lotrisone[a]	1% clotrimazole with 0.05% betamethasone vaginal cream	Apply cream topically twice daily[c]
Miconazole	–	100 mg vaginal supp	1 supp daily for 7 d
	Monistat 7, Miconazole 7	2% vaginal cream	1 app vaginally for 7 d
	Monistat 3 LESS MESS Ovule	200 mg vaginal ovule	1 ovule vaginally for 3 d
	Monistat 3 Suppositories	200 mg vaginal supp	1 supp vaginally for 3 d
	Monistat 3, Miconazole 3	4% vaginal cream	1 app vaginally for 3 d
	Monistat 1 LESS MESS Ovule	1200 mg ovule	1 ovule vaginally, once
Terconazole[b]		80 mg vaginal supp	1 supp daily for 3 d
		0.4% vaginal cream	1 app vaginally 7 d
		0.8% vaginal cream	1 app vaginally 3 d
Tioconazole	Monistat 1 Prefilled Ointment, Vagistat-1	6.5% vaginal ointment	1 app vaginally, once

[a]Some products offer suppository/cream combination products for intravaginal and introital use.
[b]Prescription required.
[c]Maximum use recommended is 2 weeks.
app = applicatorful; supp = suppository.

Unlike other STDs, its incidence appears to increase with patient age (Stemmer, 2018). Most men are asymptomatic, but up to 70 percent of male partners of women with vaginal trichomoniasis will have trichomonads in their urinary tract (Seña, 2007).

Diagnosis

Incubation with *T vaginalis* requires 3 days to 4 weeks, and the vagina, urethra, endocervix, and bladder can be infected. No symptoms are noted in up to one half of women with trichomoniasis, and such colonization can persist for months or years. Notably, trichomoniasis is associated with a nearly twofold greater risk for HIV acquisition (McClelland, 2007; Laga, 1993). In those with complaints, vaginal discharge is typically described as foul, thin, and yellow or green. Dysuria, dyspareunia, vulvar pruritus, vaginal spotting, and lower abdominal pain also may be noted.

Of clinical findings, the vagina contains the discharge just described, and subepithelial hemorrhages or "strawberry spots" dot the vagina and cervix. Vaginal pH is often elevated. Microscopically, WBC numbers are increased in saline preparations of the discharge. Trichomonads are oval anaerobic protozoa that are slightly larger than a WBC and have anterior flagella (Fig. 3-6). Microscopic identification of these motile parasites is diagnostic. However, trichomonads are less motile with cooling, and slides ideally are examined within 10 to 30 minutes (Kingston, 2003; Stoner, 2013). Inspection of a saline preparation is highly specific, yet its sensitivity ranges from 40 to 70 percent (Nathan, 2015; Nye, 2009; Schwebke, 2018).

Laboratory-based NAATs for trichomonal DNA are the most sensitive and specific tests (Meites, 2015). Suitable specimens include endocervical swab, vaginal swab, or urine. However, NAAT testing adds cost, and results are not immediately available. Alternatively, point-of-care in-clinic testing is possible but again adds cost and is not recommended for asymptomatic patients. Of these, the OSOM Trichomonas Rapid Test is an immunochromatographic assay that provides results in 10 minutes. It offers 88-percent sensitivity and 99-percent specificity (Huppert, 2005, 2007). With similar accuracy, the Solana Trichomonas Assay uses a DNA hybridization probe and yields results within 1 hour (Gaydos, 2017b). Although these molecular tests may add accuracy compared with microscopy, diagnostic test selection ideally factors patient risks and symptoms, laboratory capabilities, and cost.

Culture and antimicrobial susceptibility analysis play a lesser diagnostic role and are elected mainly in cases of persistent infection or suspected treatment failure. For culture, the commercially available InPouch system provides suitable sensitivity, 100-percent specificity, and results within 3 days (Hobbs, 2013). Diamond's media for culture is less widely available and requires 7 days. Last, trichomonads can also be noted on Pap screening slides and diagnostic sensitivity approximates 60 percent (Wiese, 2000). If trichomonads are reported from a Pap test, confirmation by microscopic evaluation of a saline preparation is encouraged prior to treatment (American College of Obstetricians and Gynecologists, 2017b).

Treatment

Oral regimens recommended by the CDC (2015) are either metronidazole 2 g once or tinidazole (Tindamax) 2 g once.

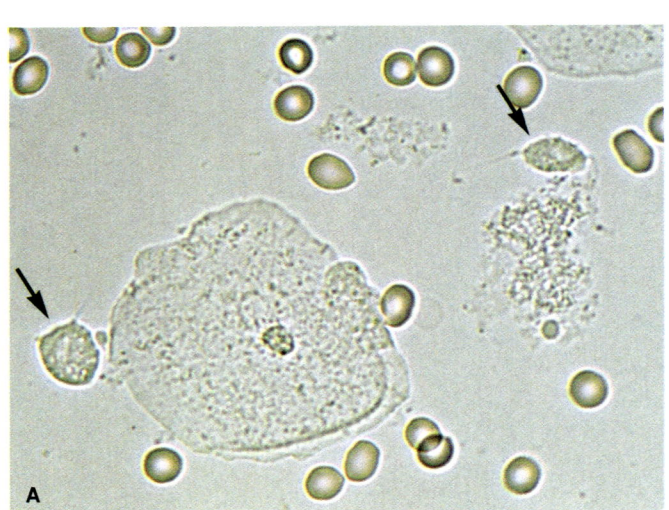
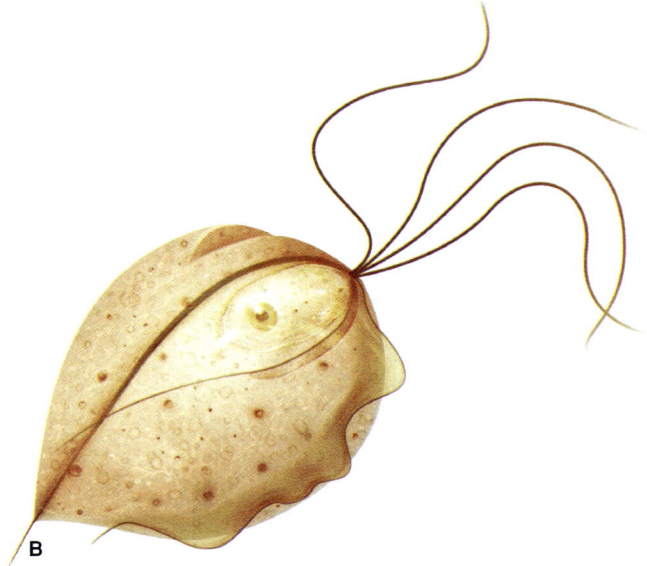

FIGURE 3-6 Trichomonads. **A.** Photomicrograph of a vaginal smear saline preparation containing trichomonads (*arrows*). (Reproduced with permission from Dr. Lauri Campagna and Rebecca Winn, WHNP.) **B.** Drawing depicts anatomic features of trichomonads. Flagella allow this parasite to be motile.

Although each is effective, some report that an oral 7-day treatment regimen with metronidazole 500 mg twice daily is more effective in compliant patients and produces fewer side effects (Howe, 2017). However, compliance may be poor because of longer treatment length. Up to 12 percent of patients taking oral metronidazole may have nausea or an unpleasant metallic taste. Because of drug disulfiram-like effects, patients should abstain from alcohol during use and for 24 hours following metronidazole therapy and for 72 hours after tinidazole.

Affected women who become asymptomatic or who are initially asymptomatic do not require routine reevaluation. However, recurrences occur in approximately 30 percent of patients. Importantly, NAATs cannot distinguish live from dead (adequately treated) trichomonads. Thus, repeat NAAT testing is ideally delayed for 3 weeks following treatment (Williams, 2014). Sex partners are encouraged to seek treatment, and patients are reminded to abstain from sex until they and their partners are cured. Condom use may be protective.

Infrequently, patients may have strains that are highly resistant to metronidazole, but these organisms are usually sensitive to tinidazole. If cure is not achieved by a single dose or then by a subsequent 7-day course of metronidazole, oral tinidazole 2 g daily for 7 days is considered. If treatment fails following adherence to multiple 1-week regimens and reinfection is excluded, culture and susceptibility testing is considered with the assistance of CDC (404-718-4141). Cases of allergy to these two nitroimidazoles require desensitization by a specialist (Helms, 2008).

SUPPURATIVE CERVICITIS

◼ *Neisseria Gonorrhoeae*

N gonorrhoeae is a gram-negative coccobacillus that invades columnar and transitional epithelial cells of the cervix while sparing the vaginal squamous epithelium. Many women with cervical *N gonorrhoeae* are asymptomatic. For this reason, women at risk are screened periodically. Risk factors for gonococcal carriage and potential upper reproductive tract infection that merit screening are: age ≤24 years, prior or current STDs, new or multiple sexual partners, a partner with other concurrent partners, a partner with an STD, lack of barrier protection in those without a monogamous relationship, and commercial sex work (U.S. Preventive Services Task Force, 2014). Screening for women at low risk is not recommended.

Diagnosis

Symptomatic lower female reproductive tract gonorrhea can present as vaginitis or cervicitis. Those with cervicitis commonly describe a profuse, odorless, nonirritating, and white-to-yellow vaginal discharge. Microscopic inspection of secretions in a saline preparation typically reveals ≥20 WBCs per high-power field. Patients may report intermenstrual or postcoital vaginal bleeding. Gentle passage of a cotton swab into the cervical os often produces endocervical bleeding. Gonococcus can also infect the Bartholin and Skene glands, as well as the urethra, and ascend into the endometrium and fallopian tube to cause upper reproductive tract infection.

For gonococcal identification, NAATs are available and have replaced culture in most laboratories. Previously, acceptable specimens were recovered only from the endocervix or urethra. However, NAAT collection kits are now available for collection from the vagina, endocervix, or urine. For women without a cervix following hysterectomy, first-void urine samples are collected. For those with a cervix, vaginal-swab specimens are as sensitive and specific as cervical-swab specimens. Urine samples, although acceptable, are least preferred for those with a cervix (Centers for Disease Control and Prevention, 2014a). However, if selected, the initial urine stream, not the midstream, is collected. Of note, these NAAT tests are not FDA-cleared for diagnostic identification of rectal or pharyngeal disease, and laboratories must establish performance specifications to meet standards for NAAT testing of these extragenital specimens. If NAAT is not available for these specimen types, cultures are obtained for rectal and pharyngeal specimens. In women with vaginal symptoms and who practice anal intercourse, consideration is given to rectal screening. One study of urban STD clinics found that approximately 20 percent of rectal chlamydia and gonorrhea infections would be missed if only cervical, vaginal, or urine samples were obtained (Llata, 2018).

Treatment

CDC recommendations for dual therapy of uncomplicated cervical, urethral, or rectal infection are outlined in Table 3-7. Importantly, widespread quinolone-resistant gonococci in the United States prompted removal of this antibiotic class from the CDC STD guidelines, and declining effectiveness of cefixime has shifted its role to an alternative agent (Centers for Disease Control and Prevention, 2015). Uncomplicated gonococcal pharyngeal infection treatment mirrors the recommended regimen in Table 3-7. Test-of-cure cultures are not usually necessary unless an alternative to ceftriaxone is used to treat pharyngeal gonorrhea infection.

In cases of cephalosporin allergy, one potential option is single oral doses of gemifloxacin 320 mg plus azithromycin 2 g. Another is single doses of gentamicin 240 mg IM plus oral azithromycin 2 g. For azithromycin allergy, ceftriaxone alone suffices. However, if the alternative regimen with cefixime is used, then doxycycline, 100 mg orally twice daily for 7 days, replaces the azithromycin (Centers for Disease Control

---

TABLE 3-7. Single-Dose Treatment of Uncomplicated Gonococcal Infection of the Cervix, Urethra, or Rectum[a]

Recommended regimen
Ceftriaxone (Rocephin) 250 mg IM[b]
PLUS
Azithromycin (Zithromax) 1 g orally once

Alternative regimen
Cefixime (Suprax) 400 mg orally once
PLUS
Azithromycin 1 g orally once

---

[a]Test of cure is not required. Persons with persistent symptoms of gonococcal infection or whose symptoms recur shortly after treatment are reevaluated by culture for *N gonorrhoeae*. If positive, isolates are submitted for resistance testing. Suspected treatment failures are reported to the CDC within 24 hours.
[b]Other cephalosporin options include: (1) ceftizoxime (Cefizox) 500 mg IM, (2) cefoxitin (Mefoxin) 2 g IM given with probenecid 1 g orally, or (3) cefotaxime (Claforan) 500 mg IM. From the Centers for Disease Control and Prevention, 2015.

and Prevention, 2015). Abstinence is practiced until therapy is completed and until women and their treated sexual partners have symptom resolution. Screening for reinfection is now recommended 3 months after treatment or at the next opportunity within 12 months following treatment. Earlier test-of-cure-sampling is not recommended and risks identifying dead, treated gonococci.

To prevent and control STDs, guidelines for expedited partner therapy (EPT) have been created by the CDC. EPT is the delivery of a prescription by persons infected with an STD to their sexual partners without clinical assessment of the partners. EPT ideally does not replace traditional strategies, such as standard patient referral, when these are available. Although acceptable for treatment of heterosexual contacts with gonorrhea or chlamydial infection, data do not support EPT for trichomoniasis or syphilis. Although sanctioned by the CDC, EPT is not legal in some states within the United States. Moreover, the risk of litigation in the event of adverse outcomes may be elevated when a practice has uncertain legal status or is outside formally accepted community practice standards (Centers for Disease Control and Prevention, 2006). The legal status of EPT in each of the 50 states can be found at: www.cdc.gov/std/ept/legal/default.htm.

Chlamydia Trachomatis

This organism is among the most prevalent of the STD species recovered in the United States. Its prevalence is highest in individuals <25 years, and this was 4.3 percent in national survey estimates from 2013 to 2017 (Centers for Disease Control and Prevention, 2018a). Since many with this organism are asymptomatic, women with the same risks that prompt gonococcal screening, listed in the last section, are screening candidates.

This obligate intracellular parasite is dependent on host cells for survival. It infects columnar epithelial cells, and endocervical glandular infection leads to mucopurulent discharge or endocervical secretions. If infected, the endocervical tissue is commonly edematous and hyperemic. Urethritis also can develop, and dysuria is prominent.

Microscopic inspection of secretions in a saline preparation typically reveals ≥20 WBCs per high-power field. Also, NAAT, culture, and enzyme-linked immunosorbent assay (ELISA) are available for endocervical specimens. Of these, NAAT is recommended for its high sensitivity and specificity and technical feasibility. Also, combined gonococcal and chlamydial tests are widely used. As with gonorrhea testing, newer NAAT collection kits permit specific collection from the vagina, the endocervix, or urine (p. 66). Vaginal-swab specimens are as sensitive and specific as cervical-swab specimens. Urine samples, although acceptable, are least preferred for women with a cervix. However, for women following hysterectomy, first-void urine samples are preferred. Again, these molecular tests are not FDA-cleared for diagnostic identification of rectal or pharyngeal disease, but some laboratories have established specifications for performance of the test in extragenital specimens. As noted earlier, rectal screening is considered for women with vaginal symptoms and who practice anal intercourse.

TABLE 3-8. Oral Treatments of Chlamydial Infection

Recommended regimen
Azithromycin 1 g once
or
Doxycycline 100 mg twice daily for 7 days

Alternative regimens
Erythromycin base 500 mg four times daily for 7 days
or
Erythromycin ethyl succinate 800 mg four times daily for 7 days
or
Levofloxacin (Levaquin) 500 mg once daily for 7 days
or
Ofloxacin (Floxin) 300 mg twice daily for 7 days

From Centers for Disease Control and Prevention, 2015.

Recommended therapy for *C trachomatis* infection is described in Table 3-8. Azithromycin has the obvious therapeutic compliance advantage. Azithromycin is a broad-spectrum macrolide antibiotic with activity against many gram-positive and gram-negative bacteria. Mean concentrations in tissue are manyfold higher than those reached in serum and persist for several days (Parnham, 2014).

After therapy, women treated for chlamydial infection are retested 3 months after treatment or at the next opportunity up to 12 months following treatment. Abstinence is recommended until a woman and her partner(s) are treated and are asymptomatic. As with gonorrhea in heterosexual partners, EPT is sanctioned by the CDC for selected patients (p. 67).

■ *Mycoplasma Genitalium*

This bacterium has only recently been considered significant as a potential public health risk for its role in female reproductive tract pathology (Weisenfeld, 2017). Most female carriers are asymptomatic, but it has been linked in some but not all studies to urethritis, cervicitis, PID, and tubal-factor infertility (Lis, 2015). Thus, in women with persistent or recurrent urethritis, cervicitis, or PID, *M genitalium* is considered. It has a much more established role in male urethritis (Daley, 2014). As such, gynecologists may more frequently encounter the exposed female partner of an infected male.

In prevalence studies, *M genitalium* is common in groups at risk for STDs (Getman, 2016; Trent, 2018). However, a consensus on screening criteria is hindered by lack of a NAAT that is FDA-approved and available outside a research setting. Currently, the CDC (2015) comments that NAAT testing for women exposed to *M genitalium* and treatment of subsequently identified infections can be considered. In Europe, NAATs for this organism are more widely available. Guidelines there for testing include women with STD exposure or symptoms of infection (Jensen, 2016). In these cases, samples from voided urine, the vagina, or the endocervix are appropriate (Lillis, 2011).

Without specific diagnostic testing, women are often empirically treated for persistent urethritis or cervicitis or for *M genitalium* exposure. Azithromycin 1 g orally once is recommended and is more effective than doxycycline. Antibiotic-resistant strains are not uncommon, and for treatment failure, moxifloxacin 400 mg orally once daily for 7 to 14 days may be used. This same moxifloxacin regimen for 14 days may be considered for women with PID who fail to respond after 7 to 10 days of standard regimens and in whom *M genitalium* is detected (Centers for Disease Control and Prevention, 2015; Manhart, 2015).

PELVIC INFLAMMATORY DISEASE

With this infection of the upper female reproductive tract, all reproductive tract organs may be involved. However, the organ of importance, with or without abscess formation, is the fallopian tube. Because tubal-factor infertility, ectopic pregnancy, and chronic pelvic pain are known sequelae of clinical and subclinical infection, clinicians ideally carry a low threshold for diagnosing and treating PID. The true prevalence of PID is unknown, due to difficulty in accurately diagnosing pelvic infection. Among females aged 15 to 44 years, the self-reported prevalence rate in 2013 was 4 percent, which was lower than the rate in 1995 (8.6 percent) (Kreisel, 2017; Leichliter, 2013). Greater STD screening is one suggested cause for this decline (Nelson, 2001; Owusu Edusei, 2010).

PID may be classified as acute, subclinical, or chronic. Acute PID, which is defined as lasting <30 days, represents most cases. Chronic PID is generally associated with *Mycobacterium tuberculosis* or *Actinomyces* species and is described later (p. 72).

■ Microbiology and Pathogenesis

Classic acute PID is associated with and secondary to *N gonorrhoeae* infection, and *C trachomatis* also can be recovered. The gonococcus incites a direct inflammatory response in the human endocervix, endometrium, and fallopian tube and is one of the true pathogens of human fallopian tube epithelial cells. In contrast, intracellular *C trachomatis* does not cause an acute inflammatory response, and little *direct* permanent damage results from chlamydial tubal involvement (Patton, 1983). However, cell-mediated immune mechanisms may be responsible for later tissue injury (Tiitinen, 2006). Specifically, persistent chlamydial antigens can trigger a delayed hypersensitivity reaction with continued tubal scarring and destruction (Toth, 2000). Another species frequently found is *T vaginalis*. The presence of *M genitalium* in women with PID has been described, but its pathogenesis is less well understood (Baczynska, 2007; Short, 2009). In sum, risks for PID mirror those for STDs. Also, the lower reproductive tract flora in women with PID and in those with BV includes predominately anaerobic species. PID shares an association with BV, but causation is unclear (Ness, 2004, 2005).

Despite the association between PID and chlamydial infection or gonorrhea, many cases of PID are culture-negative for an STD (Burnett, 2012; Goller, 2017). In these cases, upper tract infection is believed to be caused by bacteria that ascend from the lower reproductive tract. Ascension is enhanced by loss of endocervical barriers that can accompany menstruation, BV, and gonococcal or chlamydial infection. Last, direct extension from inflammatory GI disease, especially a ruptured appendiceal or diverticular abscess, for example, also can lead to salpingitis and PID.

Diagnosis

Subclinical Pelvic Inflammatory Disease

Subclinical PID is an upper genital tract infection without symptoms. It is an ultimate diagnosis given to women with tubal-factor infertility who lack a history compatible with acute PID (Wiesenfeld, 2005, 2012). Many of these patients have antibodies to *C trachomatis* and/or *N gonorrhoeae* (Sellors, 1988; Tjiam, 1985). At laparoscopy or laparotomy, affected women may have evidence of prior tubal infection such as adhesions or hydrosalpinges, but for the most part, the fallopian tubes are grossly normal. Internally, however, tubes show flattened mucosal folds, extensive deciliation of the epithelium, and secretory epithelial cell degeneration (Patton, 1989).

Acute Pelvic Inflammatory Disease

Symptoms and Physical Findings. Acute PID is diagnosed if uterine tenderness, adnexal tenderness, *or* cervical motion tenderness is present and other etiologies are excluded or unlikely. One or more of the following enhances diagnostic specificity: (1) oral temperature >38.3°C (101.6°F), (2) mucopurulent cervical discharge or cervical friability, (3) abundant WBCs on saline microscopy of cervical secretions, (4) elevated erythrocyte sedimentation rate (ESR) or C-reactive protein (CRP), and (5) presence of cervical *N gonorrhoeae* or *C trachomatis* (Centers for Disease Control and Prevention, 2015). Thus, a diagnosis of PID is typically based on clinical findings.

Symptoms of acute PID characteristically develop during or following menstruation. These can include lower abdominal and/or pelvic pain, yellow or green vaginal discharge, heavy menstrual bleeding, fever, nausea, vomiting, diarrhea, dysmenorrhea, and dyspareunia. Patients also may have complaints suggesting urinary tract infection (UTI). Unfortunately, no single symptom is associated with a physical finding that is specific for this diagnosis. Accordingly, other possible sources of acute pelvic pain are considered and listed in Table 12-1 (p. 255).

Of findings, mucopurulent endocervicitis is common and is diagnosed visually and microscopically. During bimanual pelvic examination, affected women will usually have pelvic organ tenderness. Cervical motion tenderness (CMT) is typically elicited by quickly moving the cervix with examining vaginal fingers. This reflects pelvic peritonitis and can be considered a vaginal "rebound" test. If a woman has pelvic peritonitis secondary to bacteria and pus that has exuded from the fimbriated end of the fallopian tube into the pelvis, this rapid peritoneal movement usually causes a marked pain response. Tapping the posterior cul-de-sac with an examining finger will give the examiner similar information. This latter maneuver usually causes a patient significantly less pain because less inflamed peritoneum is stretched.

Abdominal peritonitis may be identified by deep palpation and quick release of a hand placed on the abdomen—a test for rebound. Alternatively, an examining hand may be positioned with a palm against a woman's midabdomen and gently and quickly moved back and forth (shake). This can identify abdominal peritonitis, often with less patient discomfort.

In women with PID and peritonitis, usually only the lower abdomen is involved. However, inflammation of the liver capsule, which can accompany PID, may lead to right upper quadrant pain, a condition known as *Fitz-Hugh-Curtis syndrome*. Classically, symptoms of this perihepatitis include sharp, pleuritic right upper quadrant pain that accompanies pelvic pain. The upper abdominal pain may refer to the shoulder or upper arm. Importantly, during examination, if all abdominal quadrants are involved, suspicion for a ruptured tuboovarian abscess (TOA) is heightened.

Testing. For reproductive-aged women, pregnancy complications can be identified by serum or urine beta–human chorionic gonadotropin testing. A complete blood count (CBC) is selected as a baseline test to help exclude hemoperitoneum and identify WBC elevation. In those with significant nausea and vomiting or Fitz-Hugh-Curtis syndrome, liver enzyme values can be normal or mildly elevated. If properly collected, urinalysis findings for infection will be absent. Saline preparation of cervical or vaginal discharge typically shows sheets of WBCs. In women with suspected acute PID, endocervical testing for both *N gonorrhoeae* and *C trachomatis* is performed as described earlier (p. 66). Screening for other STDs also is completed. Although an endometrial biopsy that reveals acute endometritis is a specific criterion, this is mainly used in research settings. In general, the delay between collection and reporting precludes its clinical utility.

Sonography. In women with marked abdominal pain and tenderness, appreciation of upper reproductive tract organs during bimanual examination may be limited, and sonography is a primary imaging tool. Normal fallopian tubes are rarely imaged. However, with acute tubal inflammation, the tube swells, its lumen occludes distally, it distends, and its walls and endosalpingeal folds thicken. Characteristic acute findings include: (1) distended, ovoid-shaped tube filled with anechoic or echogenic fluid, (2) fallopian tube wall thickening, (3) incomplete internal septa, and (4) a "cogwheel" appearance when inflamed tubes are imaged in cross section (Timor-Tritsch, 1998) (Fig. 3-7). If color or power Doppler is applied, marked vascularity with low-impedance blood flow, which reflects hyperemia, is seen within thickened fallopian tube walls and septa (Molander, 2001; Romosan, 2013). Sonography also may be used to identify a TOA or exclude other pathology as the pain source. If sonography does not lead to a clear diagnosis, computed tomography (CT) scanning may be useful and especially with right upper quadrant pain suggestive of perihepatitis (Kim, 2009). Classic findings of acute PID on CT imaging include fallopian tube thickening and pelvic fat stranding (Jung, 2011). Magnetic resonance (MR) imaging is a suitable, although infrequently used, alternative.

Laparoscopy. Historically, in Scandinavian countries, women with suspected PID underwent laparoscopy for diagnosis. Tubal serosal hyperemia, tubal wall edema, and purulent exudate issuing

Treatment of Acute Pelvic Inflammatory Disease

The most successful patient outcomes follow early diagnosis and prompt, appropriate therapy. The primary therapy goal is to eradicate bacteria, relieve symptoms, and prevent sequelae.

Failed outpatient therapy
Noncompliant with medications
White blood cell count >15,000/mm³
Nausea/vomiting precluding oral therapy

PID = pelvic inflammatory disease.

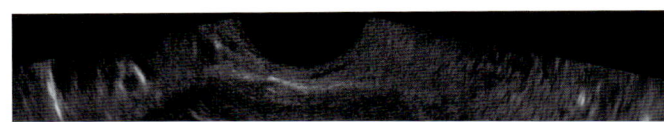

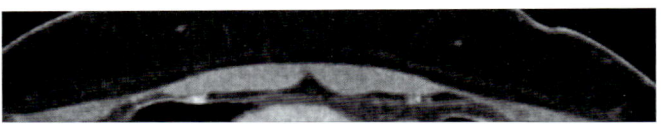

Oral Treatment

In women with a mild to moderate clinical presentation, outpatient treatment and inpatient therapy yield comparable results. Clinical treatment with oral therapy is also appropriate for women with HIV infection and PID. This group has the same species recovered compared with non-HIV-infected patients, and their response to therapy is similar.

If women have more than moderate disease, they require hospitalization. For women with outpatient treatment, one study showed that women treated as outpatients took 70 percent of prescribed doses, and for less than 50 percent of their outpatient treatment days (Dunbar-Jacob, 2004). Thus, if patients are treated as outpatients, an initial parenteral dose may be beneficial. Women treated as outpatients are reevaluated in approximately 72 hours by phone or in person. If women do not respond to oral therapy within 72 hours, parenteral therapy is initiated either as an inpatient or as an outpatient if home nursing care is available. This assumes that the diagnosis is confirmed at reevaluation.

Specific oral treatment recommendations from the CDC are found in Table 3-11. Anaerobes are believed by some to play an important role in upper tract infection and are treated. Hence, metronidazole may be added to improve anaerobic coverage. If patients have BV or trichomoniasis, then metronidazole addition is required, although perhaps not for 14 days.

Parenteral Treatment

Any woman who has criteria as outlined in Table 3-10 is hospitalized for parenteral treatment for at least 24 hours. Following this, if home parenteral treatment is available, this is a reasonable option. Alternatively, a woman who responds clinically to initial parenteral antibiotics may be discharged on one of the oral regimens in Table 3-11.

Recommendations for parenteral antibiotic treatment of PID are found in Table 3-9. Of these antibiotics, oral and parenteral routes of doxycycline have almost identical bioavailability, but parenteral doxycycline is caustic to veins. Many prospective clinical trials have shown that either of the listed cephalosporins alone, without doxycycline, will result in a clinical cure. For that reason, doxycycline administration could be reserved until the patient can take oral medication. Parenteral

TABLE 3-11. Outpatient Treatment of PID

Ceftriaxone (Rocephin) 250 mg IM once[a,b]
PLUS
Doxycycline 100 mg orally twice daily for 14 days
with or without
Metronidazole (Flagyl) 500 mg orally twice daily for 14 days

[a]Cefoxitin (Mefoxin) 2 g IM with 1 g oral probenecid once may replace ceftriaxone.
[b]Other parenteral third-generation cephalosporin IM given in a single dose such as ceftizoxime or cefotaxime may replace ceftriaxone.
IM = intramuscular; PID = pelvic inflammatory disease.
From Centers for Disease Control and Prevention, 2015.

therapy is continued for 24 hours after the patient clinically improves. The oral doxycycline 100 mg twice daily is continued to complete 14 days of therapy. Alternatively, if the IV gentamycin/clindamycin regimen is used, transition to a 14-day oral agent may involve clindamycin orally four times daily or doxycycline 100 mg twice daily.

Chronic Pelvic Inflammatory Disease

This is defined as PID lasting longer than 30 days, and one cause is *Actinomyces israelii*. This is a gram-positive, slow-growing, anaerobic bacterium found to be part of the indigenous genital flora of healthy women (Persson, 1984). Pelvic infection and abscess are rare, even in those identified to harbor the bacteria.

With infection, findings include fever, weight loss, abdominal pain, and abnormal vaginal bleeding or discharge. Actinomyces is sensitive to penicillins. Prolonged parenteral antibiotic administration is required for 4 to 6 weeks followed by oral antibiotics for 6 to 12 months.

Some have found *Actinomyces* species more frequently in the vaginal flora of IUD users, and rates of colonization rise with duration of IUD use (Curtis, 1981). *Actinomyces* is also identified in Pap smears, and Fiorino (1996) cited a 7-percent incidence in IUD users compared with <1 percent in nonusers. In the absence of symptoms, the incidental finding of *Actinomyces* in a Pap sample may be managed conservatively. Other suitable options include extended oral antibiotic treatment with the IUD in place, IUD removal, or IUD removal followed by antibiotic treatment (American College of Obstetricians and Gynecologists, 2017a). Reviews by Lippes (1999) and Westhoff (2007) support IUD retention and observation. If signs or symptoms of infection do develop in a woman who harbors *Actinomyces*, the device is removed and antimicrobial therapy is instituted.

Although rare in the United States, salpingitis and endometritis can originate from pulmonary tuberculosis. *Mycobacterium tuberculosis* is thought to be blood-borne, but ascension may still be a possible route. Importantly, with infection, an associated pelvic mass, ascites, omental inflammation, and peritoneal studding or thickening may mimic peritoneal spread of malignancy. Once diagnosed, treatment is best coordinated with an infectious disease specialist.

INFECTIOUS WARTS AND PAPULES

External Genital Warts

These lesions originate from human papillomavirus (HPV) infection, and 86 percent of genital wart cases stem from HPV 6 or 11 (Garland, 2009). From one large insurance database, the incidence ranged from 0.1 to 0.3 percent in reproductive-aged women (Flagg, 2018). Logically, genital wart incidence is lowest in those previously vaccinated against HPV. Genital wart prevention is one indication for the nonavalent vaccine (Gardasil), which protects against 9 HPV serotypes, including 6 and 11 (Table 1-4, p. 9).

Genital warts appear as flat papules or classic verrucous, exophytic lesions, termed *condyloma acuminata* (Fig. 3-9)

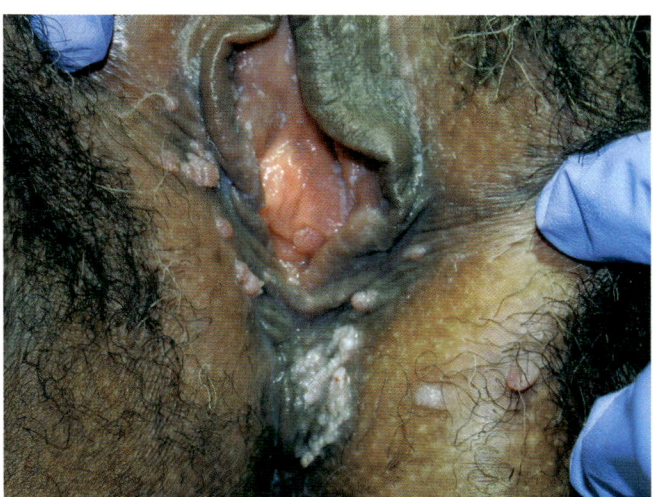

FIGURE 3-9 Condyloma acuminata. Multiple exophytic verrucous warts are seen on the labia and perineum.

(Beutner, 1998). External genital warts can develop at sites in the lower reproductive tract, urethra, anus, or mouth. They are usually asymptomatic but can be pruritic or painful depending on their size and location. Warts are typically diagnosed by clinical inspection. Biopsy is not required unless coexisting neoplasia is suspected, the diagnosis is unclear, or the patient is immunosuppressed (Park, 2015). Similarly, HPV serotyping is not required for routine diagnosis.

Condyloma acuminata may remain unchanged or spontaneously resolve, and the effect of treatment on future viral transmission is unclear. However, many women prefer removal, and lesions can be removed or destroyed with sharp excision,

electrosurgical needle-tip excision, cryotherapy, or laser ablation. Alternatively, topical agents can be applied to resolve lesions (Table 3-12). One of these, 5-percent imiquimod cream (Aldara), is an immunomodulatory topical treatment for genital warts (Yan, 2006). Also, a 3.75-percent imiquimod cream (Zyclara) is effective (Baker, 2011). Imiquimod enhances local production of immune-stimulating cytokines to promote a response against HPV (Miller, 1999). Another topical immune-modulating agent is a 15-percent sinecatechins ointment (Veregen) derived from green tea leaf extracts (Meltzer, 2009; Tatti, 2008). Podofilox, also termed podophyllotoxin, is an antimitotic agent that disrupts viral activity by inducting local tissue necrosis. Available in a 0.5-percent solution or gel (Condylox), it can be self-applied by the patient (Komericki, 2011; Yan, 2006). The more concentrated 10 to 25-percent podophyllin resin is no longer a recommended regimen due to risks of systemic toxicity. Of other agents, trichloroacetic acid and bichloroacetic acid are proteolytic and are applied serially to warts. Intralesional interferon, photodynamic therapy, or topical cidofovir are second-tier alternative regimens listed by the CDC (2015). All topical treatments in this section can result in skin irritation, which at times may require treatment breaks.

Of therapy choices, no data suggest the superiority of one treatment. Thus, in general, treatment is selected based on clinical circumstances and patient and provider preferences (Werner, 2017). Importantly, no treatment option, even surgical excision, boasts 100-percent clearance rates. Indeed, clearance rates range from 30 to 80 percent. Accordingly, recurrences are common following treatment, particularly in women with HIV. Biopsy is considered for atypical or recalcitrant lesions, which may harbor concomitant intraepithelial neoplasia (Massad, 2011).

TABLE 3-12. Recommended Treatment of External Genital Warts

Patient-applied
Imiquimod 5% cream (Aldara). Apply a thin layer and rub until absorbed once daily at bedtime, three times a week, up to 16 wks. After 6 to 10 hr, the area is washed with soap and water.
or
Imiquimod 3.75% cream (Zyclara). Apply a thin layer once daily at bedtime, up to 8 wks. After 8 hr, the area is washed with soap and water.
or
Podofilox 0.5% solution or gel (Condylox). Apply the solution with a cotton swab or the gel with a finger to genital warts twice daily for 3 d, followed by 4 d of no therapy. This cycle is repeated up to four cycles. The area treated does not exceed 10 cm², and the total volume of podofilox is limited to 0.5 mL/d.
or
Sinecatechins 15% ointment (Veregen). Apply a 0.5-cm strand to each wart with a finger three times daily, up to 16 wks. It is not washed off, and sexual contact is avoided when ointment is present.

Provider-administered
Cryotherapy with liquid nitrogen or cryoprobe. Repeat applications every 1 to 2 wks.
or
Trichloroacetic acid (TCA) or **bichloroacetic acid** (BCA) 80 to 90 percent. Apply a small amount only to the warts and allowed to dry, which creates a white "frosting." This is repeated weekly if necessary. If an excess amount is applied, the treated area is powdered with talc, baking soda, or liquid soap to remove unreacted acid.
or
Surgical removal by scissor, shave excision, curettage, or electrosurgery needle.

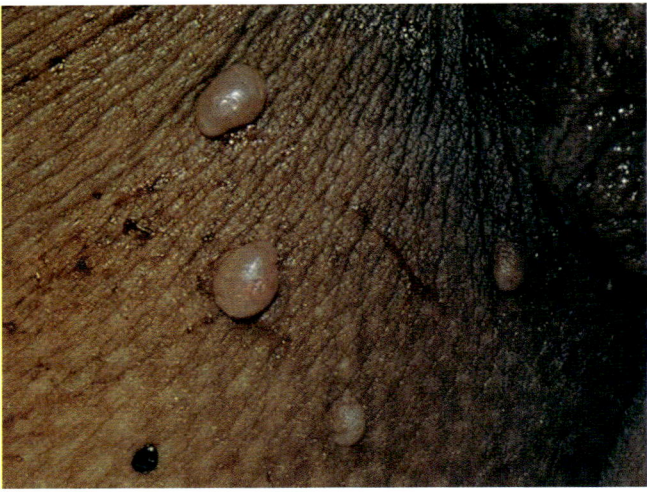

FIGURE 3-10 Molluscum contagiosum. Labial lesions are flesh-colored, dome-shaped papules with central umbilication.

Molluscum Contagiosum

This skin infection is caused by the molluscum contagiosum virus, which is transmitted by direct human-to-human contact or by infected fomites. Molluscum contagiosum is contagious until lesions resolve, and an incubation period of 2 to 7 weeks is typical. Infection gives rise to multiple, 2- to 5-mm, flesh-colored papules with central umbilication (Fig. 3-10). These are commonly found on the vulva, thighs, or buttocks.

These papules are typically diagnosed by visual inspection alone. With an unclear diagnosis, biopsy is considered. Histologically, the classic cup-shaped lesion has normal basal layers but surface keratinocytes acquire eosinophilic *molluscum bodies* that contain virus particles. Alternatively, material from a lesion can be collected on a swab, applied to a slide, and submitted for diagnostic staining. With this, molluscum bodies are diagnostic.

Most lesions spontaneously regress within 6 to 12 months. If removal is preferred, lesions may be treated by cryotherapy, electrosurgical needle coagulation, or sharp needle-tip curettage of a lesion's umbilicated center. These methods have not demonstrated superior results compared with spontaneous healing. Some topical agents used for genital warts may be considered (Tyring, 2003). However, no single treatment is superior. Of these, topical imiquimod is ineffective and may cause severe application-site reactions (van der Wouden, 2017).

PRURITIC INFESTATIONS

Scabies

Sarcoptes scabiei infects skin and result in an intensely pruritic rash. This mite is crab-shaped, and the female digs into the skin and remains there for approximately 30 days, elongating her burrow. Several eggs are laid daily and begin hatching after 3 to 4 days. The baby mites furrow their own burrows, becoming reproductive adults in approximately 10 days. The number of adult mites present on an affected patient averages a dozen. Sexual transmission is the most likely cause of initial infection, but household contacts can become infected. Shared or crowded housing is another risk.

Burrows are thin elevated skin tracks measuring 5 to 10 mm in length. A delayed hypersensitivity reaction (type 4) to the mites, eggs, and feces develops and results in erythematous papules, vesicles, or nodules in association with skin burrows. Secondary infection, however, may develop and hide these tracks. Most common infestation sites include the hands, wrist, elbows, groin, and ankles. Itching and dermatologic changes in these areas are the predominant symptoms.

Definitive testing requires scraping across the burrow with a scalpel blade and mixing these fragments in immersion oil on a microscope slide. Identification of mites, eggs, egg fragments, or fecal pellets is diagnostic (Fig. 3-11). For treatment, 5-percent permethrin cream (Elimite) is a recommended agent. A thin layer is applied from the neck downward with special attention to pruritic areas and the hands, feet, and genital regions. Ideally, all family members are treated with the exception of infants younger than 2 years. Eight to 14 hours after application, a shower or bath is taken to remove the medication. Only one application is necessary. Another option is a 200-µg/kg single oral dose of ivermectin (Stromectol) given initially and then repeated 2 weeks later. Bed linens and recently worn clothing

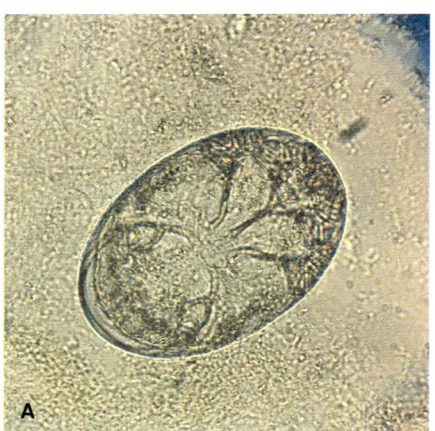
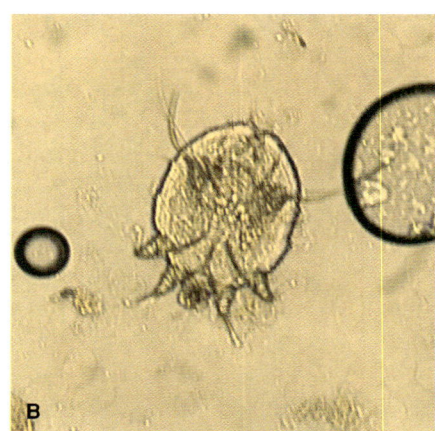
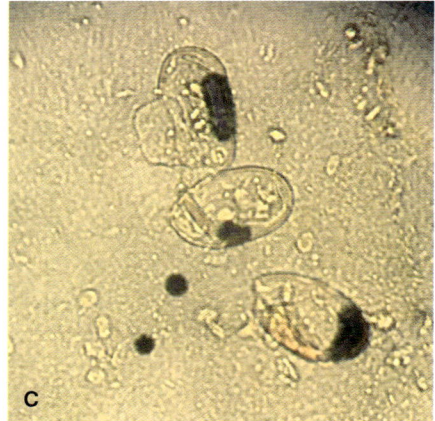

FIGURE 3-11 Microscopic images of *Sarcoptes scabiei*. **A.** A mite is seen prior to hatching. **B.** Hatched mite. **C.** Remnant egg casings following hatching and smaller fecal particles.

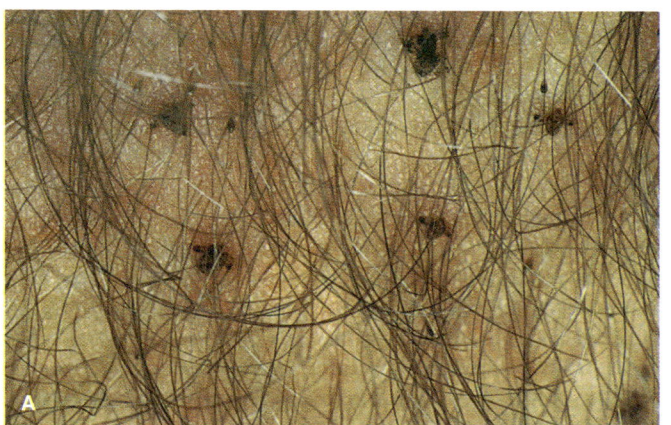 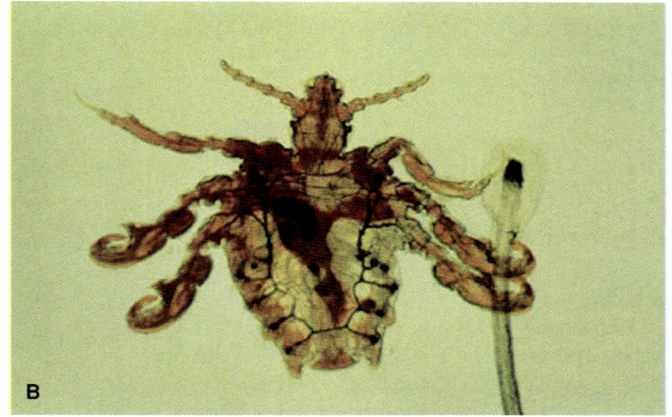

FIGURE 3-12 *Phthirus pubis.* **A.** Pubic lice are seen attached to hair. In addition, nits are seen as dark dots adhered to pubic hair. (From Morse, 2003, with permission.) **B.** Photomicrograph of *Phthirus pubis.* Claw-like legs are ideally suited for clinging to hair shafts. (From Birnbaum, 2010, with permission.)

are washed to prevent reinfection. A 1-percent lindane lotion is less-preferred due to associated risk of seizures. An antihistamine can help reduce pruritus, which may also be treated with a hydrocortisone-containing cream in adults or with emollients in infants. If these lesions become infected, antibiotics directed against skin flora may be necessary.

Pediculosis

Lice are small ectoparasites that measure approximately 1 mm (Fig. 3-12). Three species infest humans and include the body louse (*Pediculus humanus*), the crab louse (*Phthirus pubis*), and the head louse (*Pediculus humanus capitis*). Lice attach to the base of human hair with claws that vary in diameter between species. This claw diameter determines the infestation site. For this reason, the crab louse is found on pubic hair and other hair of similar diameter, such as axillary and facial hair, including eyelashes and eyebrows. Pubic lice are usually sexually transmitted, whereas head and body lice may be transmitted by sharing personal objects such as combs, brushes, and clothing.

Each female adult pubic louse lays approximately four eggs a day, which are glued to the base of hairs. Incubation approximates 1 month. Their attached eggs, termed *nits*, can be seen attached to the hair shaft away from the skin line as hair growth progresses. These nits usually require a magnifying glass for identification. Moreover, suspicious flecks on pubic hair or in clothing can be examined microscopically to see the characteristic louse. Lice depend on frequent human blood meals, and pubic lice must travel for new attachment sites. The main symptom from louse attachment and biting is pruritus.

Some pediculicides kill only adult lice, whereas others are ovicidal as well. A single application is usually effective, but a second dose is recommended within 7 to 10 days to kill new hatches. OTC cream rinses or shampoos contain 1-percent permethrin (Nix) or pyrethrins with piperonyl butoxide (Rid, Pronto, R & C). These remain on affected areas for 10 minutes. CDC (2015) alternative regimens include 0.5-percent malathion lotion (Ovide) applied for 8 to 12 hours. Also, ivermectin, 250 μg/kg orally once, can be taken and then repeated in 2 weeks.

In selected cases, 1-percent lindane shampoo can be used, but again, this is less favored due to potential neurotoxicity. Last, eyelash and eyebrow treatment is problematic. These areas are best treated by applying petrolatum (Vaseline) with a cotton swab at night and washing it off in the morning. Bedding and infested clothing are washed and dried with a heat cycle.

In spite of treatment, pruritus may continue and can be relieved by oral antihistamines, topical antiinflammatory cream, or both. The patient is reevaluated after 1 week to document louse eradication. If lesions become secondarily infected, antibiotic therapy may be necessary. Patient screening for other STDs is encouraged. Other family members and sexual contacts require evaluation for infestation.

URINARY TRACT INFECTIONS

Acute cystitis accounts for most symptomatic bacterial lower UTIs. Women have many more UTIs than men because of their pelvic anatomy. Bacteria ascend from the short, colonized urethra and easily enter the bladder and perhaps then the kidneys. Sexual intercourse increases bladder inoculation. Also, contributing to contamination, the warm moist vulva and rectum are both in close proximity. Indeed, the bacterial species most frequently recovered from infected urine cultures is *E coli*. Other identified species are *Klebsiella pneumoniae*, *Proteus mirabilis*, and *Staphylococcus saprophyticus* (Echols, 1999; Czaja, 2007). Once in the bladder, bacteria may ascend within the ureters into the renal pelvis and cause upper tract infection. Less often, the renal parenchyma can be infected by blood-borne organisms, especially during staphylococcal bacteremia.

Acute Bacterial Cystitis

Diagnosis

With acute bacterial cystitis, frequent complaints in otherwise healthy, immunocompetent nonpregnant women are dysuria, frequency, urgency, hematuria, and incontinence. With one or more of these symptoms, the probability of infection is 50 percent. This rises to 90 percent when symptoms of vaginitis are

TABLE 3-13. Exclusions from "Uncomplicated" Cystitis

Diabetes
Pregnancy
Immunosuppression
Symptoms >7 days
Postmenopausal hematuria
Recent UTI or urologic surgery
Documented urologic abnormalities
Recent hospital or nursing home discharge
Documented temperature above 38°C (100.4°F)
Abdominal and/or pelvic pain, nausea, vomiting
Symptoms of vaginitis (vaginal discharge/vulvar irritation)
Persisting symptoms despite >3 days of treatment of
 urinary tract infection

UTI = urinary tract infection.

absent (Bent, 2002). If the patient prefers, most women can be treated based solely on symptoms for an isolated episode of acute uncomplicated bacterial cystitis. However, patients are instructed that fever >38°C (100.4°F) and persistence or recurrence of hematuria, dysuria, and frequency, despite treatment, merit further attention.

In women with complicated or recurrent infections or with persistent or new symptoms during treatment, physical examination can be informative (Table 3-13). For example, hematuria in a postmenopausal woman may reflect cervical, uterine, or colonic bleeding that is most evident to them at the time of urination. Similarly, burning with urination may indicate vulvitis. Coupled with examination, urinalysis and urine culture are obtained for suspected complicated infection.

For a culture specimen to be informative, it must be accurately collected. A "clean catch" midstream voided urine specimen is usually sufficient. A patient is counseled on the steps of urine specimen collection, which are designed to prevent contamination by other bacteria from the vulva, vagina, and rectum. More than one bacterial species identified in a urine culture usually indicates specimen collection contamination. Initially, a patient spreads her labia and wipes the periurethral area from front to back with an antiseptic tissue. With labia spread, she begins urinating but does not collect the initial stream. A "midstream" sample is then collected into a sterile cup. After collection, the specimen is delivered promptly to the laboratory and is plated for culture within 2 hours of collection unless it is refrigerated.

Culture. Urine culture allows accurate identification of an inciting pathogen and susceptibility testing of that pathogen to various antibiotics. Classically, significant bacteriuria is defined as $\geq 10^5$ bacteria (colony-forming units [cfu]) per milliliter of urine. If urine is collected by either suprapubic aspirate or catheterization, colony counts $\geq 10^2$ cfu/mL are diagnostic. As an exception, Hooton and coworkers (2013) demonstrated that *E coli* in midstream urine is highly predictive of bladder bacteriuria even at very low counts of 10^2 cfu/mL.

Although anaerobic bacteria are part of the vaginal, colonic, and skin flora, they rarely cause UTIs. Hence, urine culture reports do not note anaerobes unless laboratory staff

is specifically instructed to look for these species. Fungi are reported but are rare causes of acute cystitis.

Culture is the gold standard, and bacterial species may be identified preliminarily, but a final urine culture report usually is not available for 48 hours. However, rapid test surrogates for culture can support a UTI diagnosis and include microscopy, nitrite testing, and leukocyte esterase testing. Empiric treatment is initially begun but is modified, as needed, after culture results are available.

Culture Surrogates. *Gram staining* is a simple, rapid, and sensitive method for detecting a concentration $\geq 10^5$ cfu/mL of a bacterial species. Rapid identification allows appropriate selection of empiric antimicrobial therapy. However, realistically, such testing is typically limited to patients with complicated UTIs or acute pyelonephritis. Instead, *simple microscopic examination* of a centrifuged urine specimen allows identification of both pyuria and bacteriuria in the sediment. A specimen is examined expeditiously because WBCs deteriorate quickly in urine that has not been appropriately preserved. Standards to define pyuria are inadequate, other than gross counts. Accordingly, the rapid test for leukocyte esterase has become a surrogate for the microscopic WBC count.

Leukocyte esterase testing measures esterase enzyme found in urinary WBCs. If used alone diagnostically, this test has poor sensitivity (Devillé, 2004). Specifically, if specimens are contaminated with vaginal or colonic bacteria or with trichomonads, test results can be falsely positive for uropathogens. Conversely, very concentrated urine or urine with significant proteinuria, ketonuria, or glucosuria will risk false-negative results (Susianti, 2015). The test is most beneficial for its high negative predictive value, which approximates 95 percent (Sawyer, 1984).

Nitrites are produced from nitrates metabolized by bacteria, especially the gram-negative uropathogen family. However, this marker does not identify *Pseudomonas* species or gram-positive pathogens such as staphylococci, streptococci, and enterococci. First morning urine specimens are ideally tested, because more than 4 hours are required for bacteria to convert nitrates to nitrites at levels that are detectable. As a single test, the sensitivity of a positive nitrite test is poor. However, its negative predictive value approximates 90 (Deville, 2004; Marques, 2017).

Together, combined nitrite and leukocyte esterase negative results from a clean-catch, uncontaminated, voided specimen offer a sensitivity of 80 to 90 percent and negative predictive value of 96 percent (Deville, 2004; Marques, 2017; Patel, 2005). Notably, substances that turn the urine red, such as the bladder analgesic phenazopyridine (Pyridium) or ingestion of beets, can lead to false-positive nitrite or leukocyte esterase test results. Vitamin C can cause false-negative readings (Lee, 2017).

Treatment

Treatment options for uncomplicated UTIs are found in (Table 3-14). Notably, during the past two decades, the frequency of infections caused by group B *Streptococcus* and *Klebsiella* species has risen, whereas *E coli* infection rates have diminished. Also, in many locations, sensitivity patterns in *E coli* may warrant avoidance of trimethoprim-sulfamethoxazole as initial empiric treatment. Importantly, for a given patient, FDA

TABLE 3-14. Treatment of Urinary Tract Infection

Infection Category	Antimicrobial Regimen
Uncomplicated cystitis	
Recommended regimens	Nitrofurantoin macrocrystals/monohydrate (Macrobid) 100 mg twice daily for 5–7 days
	or
	Nitrofurantoin macrocrystals (Macrodantin) 100 mg four times daily for 7 days
	or
	Fosfomycin tromethamine (Monurol) single 3-g dose once
	or
	Trimethoprim-sulfamethoxazole DS 160/800 mg (Bactrim DS, Septra DS) twice daily for 3 days[a]
	or
	Trimethoprim-sulfamethoxazole (Bactrim, Septra) 100 mg twice daily for 3 days[a]
Alternative regimens	Specific β-lactams in 3- to 7-day regimens[b]
	or
	Ciprofloxacin (Cipro) 250 mg twice daily for 3 days
	or
	Norfloxacin (Noroxin) 400 mg twice daily for 3 days
	or
	Levofloxacin (Levaquin) 250 mg daily for 3 days
Outpatient pyelonephritis	
Recommended regimens	Ciprofloxacin 500 mg twice daily for 7 days[c]
	or
	Ciprofloxacin 1000 mg daily for 7 days[c]
	or
	Levofloxacin 750 mg daily for 5 days[c]
	or
	Trimethoprim-sulfamethoxazole DS 160/800 mg twice daily for 14 days[c]
Alternative regimens	Specific β-lactams for 10–14 days[b,c]

[a]Not recommended as first line where local resistance rates of *E coli* exceed 20%.
[b]Suitable agents include amoxicillin-clavulanate, cefdinir, cefaclor, cefpodoxime-proxetil.
[c]If the prevalence of fluoroquinolone resistance is thought to exceed 10%, then an initial, single intravenous dose of a long-acting parenteral antimicrobial, such as 1 g of ceftriaxone or a consolidated 24-hr dose of an aminoglycoside, is recommended.
DS = double strength.
From American College of Obstetricians and Gynecologists, 2016; Gupta, 2011, 2017.

(2018) warnings regarding fluoroquinolone-associated peripheral neuropathy, tendonitis, hypoglycemia, and mental confusion should be weighed against clinical drug benefits.

For significant dysuria, up to 2 days of a bladder analgesic such as phenazopyridine (Pyridium), 200 mg orally up to three times daily, may give significant relief. However, gastrointestinal (GI) upset, yellow-orange stained urine and clothing, and hemolysis in patients with glucose-6-phosphate dehydrogenase (G6PD) deficiency are potential side effects.

Following treatment, recurrences may develop. In healthy women, recurrent UTI is defined as two or more episodes of symptomatic cystitis within 6 months or three infections within 1 year. Greater oral fluid intake may lower recurrences (Hooton, 2018). For reinfection linked to intercourse, low-dose postcoital antimicrobial therapy with an appropriate agent found in Table 3-14 is usually effective at preventing UTI recurrence. Otherwise, low-dose antimicrobial prophylaxis for 6 to 12 months may be effective but is associated with more side effects. Importantly, evidence of superiority of any particular regimen is lacking (Albert, 2004). In postmenopausal women, vaginal estrogen may be particularly helpful to reduce recurrent UTI (Mody, 2014). Nonantimicrobial prophylactic strategies lack strong evidence but may be considered (Beerepoot, 2016; Jepson, 2012). Of these, proanthocyanidins are considered the important component in cranberry-containing products and inhibit *E coli* adherence to uroepithelium (Gupta, 2007). Last, urologic evaluation of the urinary tract is considered for women with recurrent UTI following modification of known risk factors.

■ Asymptomatic Bacteriuria

This is defined as isolation of a specified quantitative count of bacteria in an appropriately collected urine specimen obtained from a person without symptoms or signs referable to UTI (Rubin, 1992). In healthy nonpregnant women, the prevalence of this condition rises with age. It is associated with sexual activity and is more common in diabetics. Moreover, one fourth to one half of elderly women in long-term care facilities have bacteriuria, which is seen primarily in those with chronic neurologic illness and functional impairment.

The Infectious Disease Society of America recommends that nonpregnant premenopausal women not be screened or treated for asymptomatic bacteriuria (Nicolle, 2019). The same is true for diabetic women and for older persons living in the community.

■ Acute Pyelonephritis

This is defined as infection of the renal parenchyma and pelvicalyceal system. Acute pyelonephritis is typically accompanied by fever and flank or back pain, in addition to symptoms of lower urinary tract infection.

Studies in young healthy women with normal urinary tracts indicate that 7 to 14 days of oral therapy are sufficient for compliant women with mild infection (Gupta, 2011). In one study of more than 50 college women with acute uncomplicated pyelonephritis, resistance to trimethoprim-sulfamethoxazole was seen in 30 percent (Hooton, 1997). Accordingly, for outpatient therapy, an oral fluoroquinolone is recommended treatment unless a pathogen is susceptible to trimethoprim-sulfamethoxazole. Oral fluoroquinolones have excellent bioavailability, tissue penetration, broad-spectrum antibacterial activity, and long half-lives. At initial diagnosis, clinicians may also administer a parenteral dose prior to starting oral therapy (see Table 3-14). This is especially true if the prevalence of fluoroquinolone resistance is thought to exceed 10 percent. Alternatively, if a causative organism is gram-positive, then amoxicillin-clavulanate, cefdinir, cefaclor, or cefpodoxime-proxetil are recommended options (Gupta, 2011).

Hospitalization with intravenous hydration and antibiotic therapy is indicated for women who display significant clinical findings at initial evaluation or who fail to improve with outpatient therapy. Clinical factors that favor admission include vomiting, elevated serum creatinine level, high fever, marked leukocytosis, or other signs of sepsis. Patient factors are advanced age, nursing home residency, abnormal urinary tract anatomy, and severe comorbid health conditions (Kang, 2013; Stalenhoef, 2017). Appropriate initial IV regimens include a fluoroquinolone; an aminoglycoside with or without ampicillin; an extended-spectrum cephalosporin or extended-spectrum penicillin with or without an aminoglycoside; or a carbapenem. The choice among these agents is based on local resistance data and is then tailored based on culture-derived susceptibility.

POSTOPERATIVE INFECTION

Development of a postoperative infection can create significant patient morbidity, most seriously sepsis. Risks for postoperative infection are varied and include both patient- and procedure-related factors. Of these, the degree of wound contamination at the time of surgery plays an important role. Because most gynecologic surgeries are elective, a gynecologist has time and opportunity to decrease microbial inoculum. Thus, BV, trichomoniasis, cervicitis, and urinary tract or respiratory infections ideally are treated and eradicated prior to surgery.

■ Wound Classification

Surgical wounds are classified according to the degree of bacterial contamination of the operative site at the time of surgery (Mangram, 1999). In general, as the number of operative site bacteria (inoculum) rises, so too does the postoperative infection rate.

Clean wounds are most commonly found in procedures performed for nontraumatic indications, that are without operative site inflammation, and that avoid the respiratory, GI, and genitourinary tracts. No breaks occur in surgical technique. Thus, most laparoscopic and adnexal surgeries are in this category. Postoperative infection rates range from 1 to 5 percent. Prophylactic antibiotics do not lower these rates and are not required.

Clean contaminated wounds are those in which the respiratory, GI, genital, or urinary tract is entered under controlled conditions and without unusual bacterial contamination. Criteria further define that there is no break in surgical technique. Infection rates range from 5 to 15 percent. This group encompasses many gynecologic procedures including total hysterectomy, cervical conization, and dilation and curettage (D & C). Of these, hysterectomy is the gynecologic procedure most frequently followed by surgical site infection. These procedures are usually elective, and only hysterectomy and obstetric D & C require antimicrobial prophylaxis to reduce postoperative infection rates (American College of Obstetricians and Gynecologists, 2018).

Contaminated wounds reflect operations with major breaks in sterile technique or gross GI spillage or incisions in which acute, nonpurulent inflammation is encountered. Infection rates approximate 10 to 25 percent. For this reason, a minimum of 24 hours of perioperative antimicrobial administration is required, and delayed wound closure may be selected. Laparoscopy or laparotomy for acute salpingitis is included in this category.

Dirty or infected wounds are typically old traumatic wounds or those that involve existing clinical infection or perforated viscera. If an abscess is present, wounds are considered dirty. These operative sites are clinically infected at the time of surgery, and subsequent postsurgical infection rates range from 30 to 100 percent. Accordingly, therapeutic antimicrobial therapy is required, and these wounds typically close by secondary intention.

■ Surgical Site Infection Classification

Criteria for classifying postoperative surgical site infections (SSIs) are provided by the CDC (2019) (Table 3-15). The incisional group is further subdivided into superficial and deep classes (Fig. 3-13). Organ/space infections may develop in spaces or organs other than that opened by the original incision or manipulated during the surgical procedure. Specific sites include the vaginal cuff, urinary tract, and intraabdominal sites. Of note, vaginal cuff infections are generally considered in the organ/space class, presuming they meet at least one of these criteria: purulent drainage from the cuff, abscess at the cuff, or pathogens cultured from fluid or tissue obtained from the cuff. Pelvic infections such as adnexal infection, pelvic abscess, or infected pelvic hematoma also fall into the category of organ/space infection.

TABLE 3-15. Criteria for Defining Surgical Site Infections (SSIs)

Superficial incisional
Involves only skin and subcutaneous tissue of the incision
Develops within 30 days of surgical procedure
Features at least one of the following:
    Purulent drainage from the superficial incision
    Bacteria in culture obtained aseptically from fluid or tissue from the superficial incision
    Incision deliberately opened by surgeon and is culture positive (or not cultured) *and* patient has at least one of the
        following incisional signs or symptoms:
        Tenderness or pain
        Heat or redness
        Localized swelling
    SSI diagnosis made by surgeon or attending physician
Stitch abscesses are not included in this category
Diagnosis of "cellulitis," by itself, does not meet criterion for SSI

Deep incisional
Involves the deep soft tissues (muscle and fascia) of the incision
Develops within 30 days of surgical procedure
Features at least one of the following:
    Purulent drainage from deep incision of surgical site (but not organ or space component)
    Deep incision that spontaneously dehisces or is deliberately opened by a surgeon and is culture-positive (or not cultured)
        and patient has at least one of the following signs or symptoms:
        Temperature ≥38°C (100.4°F)
        Localized pain or tenderness
    Abscess or other infection found by reoperation, histopathology, or radiology

Organ/space
Involves any body part that was opened or manipulated during the operative procedure, excluding the skin incision, fascia,
    or muscle layers
Develops within 30 days of the surgical procedure
Features at least one of the following:
    Purulent drainage from a drain placed through a stab wound into the organ/space
    Bacteria obtained aseptically from tissue or fluid in that organ/space
    Abscess found by reoperation, histopathology, or radiology
Vaginal cuff infection with purulence, abscess, and/or positive tissue or fluid culture is included in this category

From Centers for Disease Control and Prevention, 2019.

■ Diagnosis

Physical Findings

Postoperative febrile morbidity is defined as an oral temperature of ≥38°C (≥100.4°F) on two or more occasions, 4 or more hours apart, and 24 or more hours following surgery. Importantly, postoperative febrile morbidity usually is *not* associated with other symptoms or signs of infection and does *not* require antimicrobial therapy. It resolves without antibiotic treatment in the absence of other signs of infection, but detailed evaluation is required to exclude infectious sources.

Evaluation of a patient with postoperative fever requires a thorough history and a careful physical examination to seek surgical and nonsurgical sources. This search is often complemented by laboratory testing and imaging. Nonsurgical causes of fever may include pulmonary complications, IV site phlebitis, and UTI. Investigation of these is found in Chapter 42 (p. 921).

Operative site pain (incisional, lower abdominal, pelvic, and/or lower back) following surgery is normal. However, patients with an operative site infection report worsening pain at the surgery site, and increasing tenderness is present during physical examination. With superficial SSI, pain is superficial and localized to the incision. With pelvic infection, there is deep lower abdominal and/or pelvic pain, and the most common infection sites are the parametria and the vaginal cuff. Pelvic abscess or infected pelvic hematoma is less common, and pain is central.

Abdominal palpation is an integral part of SSI diagnosis. Avoiding the abdominal incision if present, a surgeon slowly, gently, and deeply palpates the lower abdomen over the surgical site following hysterectomy and normally elicits patient discomfort. Tenderness does not mean an acute surgical abdomen or infection. In the immediate postoperative period, this tenderness is expected and resolves quickly within days. Women

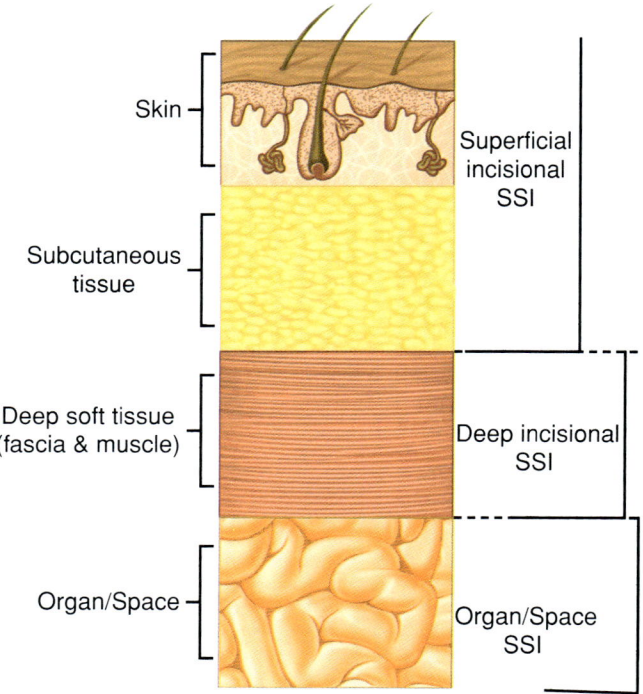

FIGURE 3-13 Anatomy and classification of surgical site infections (SSI).

Labels in figure: Skin, Subcutaneous tissue, Deep soft tissue (fascia & muscle), Organ/Space, Superficial incisional SSI, Deep incisional SSI, Organ/Space SSI

who develop pelvic cellulitis or cuff cellulitis will have increasing tenderness at gentle depression of the lower abdominal wall over the infected area. Tenderness may be bilateral, but more commonly is more marked on one side. Peritoneal signs are not present. Cellulitis, whether it involves the parametria, adnexa, or vaginal cuff, is not associated with a mass.

In those without worsening lower abdominal pain and tenderness, a bimanual examination is not necessary for asymptomatic temperature elevation. However, with a combination of fever, increasing tenderness, and new-onset pain, a gentle bimanual examination is required to accurately identify the infection site and to exclude or diagnose a mass. Speculum examination usually is not required, and findings from this inspection are similar with or without an existing infection. As is true for routine pelvic examination, most information at bimanual examination is obtained from the vaginal fingers. Bowel function is usually not altered by soft-tissue cellulitis but can be by pelvic abscess or infected pelvic hematoma.

Testing

Pelvic infections following hysterectomy are polymicrobial, and thus, it is difficult to identify true pathogens. Namely, bacteria recovered transvaginally from the pelves of infected and clinically uninfected women are similar. Accordingly, routine transvaginal culturing of women with cuff or pelvic cellulitis does not add useful information. Moreover, a surgeon should not wait for culture results before starting empiric broad-spectrum antibiotic therapy. However, if initial therapy is partially effective or unsuccessful, a culture will more predictably identify pathogen(s) since therapy will have eradicated other species. The antibiotic regimen is then modified, and culture results may direct this change. In contrast, abscess or infected hematoma

fluid are cultured since those species are less likely to be vaginal contaminants. The same is true for any fluid or purulent material present in an abdominal incision.

For many postoperative SSIs, imaging is not mandatory. However, if additional anatomic information is needed, transvaginal sonography or CT scanning is most often used, and selection depends on clinical circumstances and suspected etiology. If a mass is appreciated clinically, transvaginal sonography can identify a vaginal cuff abscess or infected cuff hematoma. In those with less specific findings, CT scanning with IV and oral contrast is more likely to aid diagnosis of a broader list of etiologies. Serum creatinine levels are obtained prior to IV contrast, which can be nephrotoxic.

■ Specific Infections

Vaginal Cuff Cellulitis

Essentially all women develop this infection at the vaginal surgical margin after hysterectomy. Normal healing is characterized by small-vessel engorgement, which results in erythema and heat. Vascular stasis with endothelial leakage follows and results in interstitial edema, which causes induration. This area is tender, microscopic evaluation of a wet prep reveals numerous WBCs, and discharge is seen in the vagina. This process usually subsides, does not require treatment, and does not require reporting as a SSI.

The few women who do require treatment are usually those who present after hospital discharge with mild, but increasing, new-onset lower abdominal pain and have a yellow vaginal discharge (Fig. 3-14). Findings are as above, but the vaginal cuff is tenderer than anticipated at this interval from the initial surgical procedure. Oral antimicrobial therapy with a single broad-spectrum agent is appropriate (Table 3-16). The combination of amoxicillin and clavulanic acid (Augmentin) provides excellent oral broad-spectrum antibiotic coverage. Dual-agent regimens are another option (Lachiewicz, 2015). A patient is then reevaluated in several days to assess therapeutic efficacy. This may be completed by phone or with an examination if necessary.

Pelvic Cellulitis

Commonly following hysterectomy, pelvic cellulitis develops when host humoral and cellular defense mechanisms, combined with preoperative antibiotic prophylaxis, cannot overcome the bacterial inoculum and inflammatory process at the vaginal cuff. This process spreads into the parametria resulting in lower abdominal pain, regional tenderness, and fever, usually during the late second or third postoperative day. Peritoneal signs are absent, bowel and urinary functions are normal, but the patient may note anorexia.

With pelvic cellulitis, hospitalization and treatment with an IV broad-spectrum antibiotic regimen found in Table 3-16 are indicated until a patient is afebrile for 24 to 48 hours. She then may be discharged home. Single-agent therapeutic regimens are as effective as combination-agent regimens. These infections are polymicrobial, and the regimen selected must have coverage for gram-positive and gram-negative aerobic and anaerobic bacteria. Most patients requiring hospitalization for IV antibiotic therapy are discharged with a 5- to 7-day oral antimicrobial prescription.

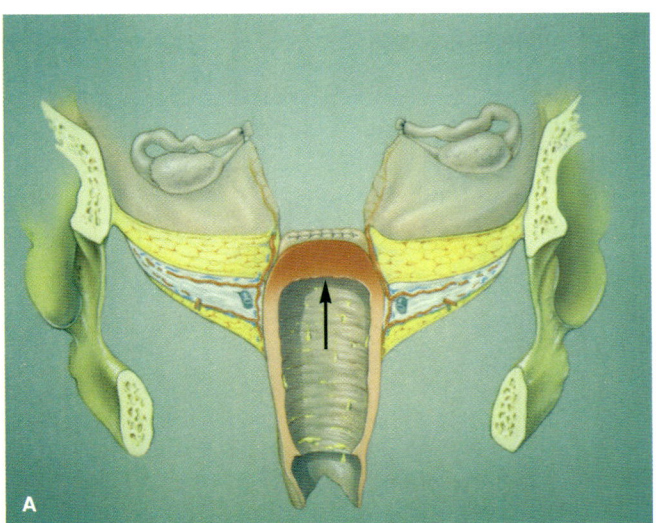

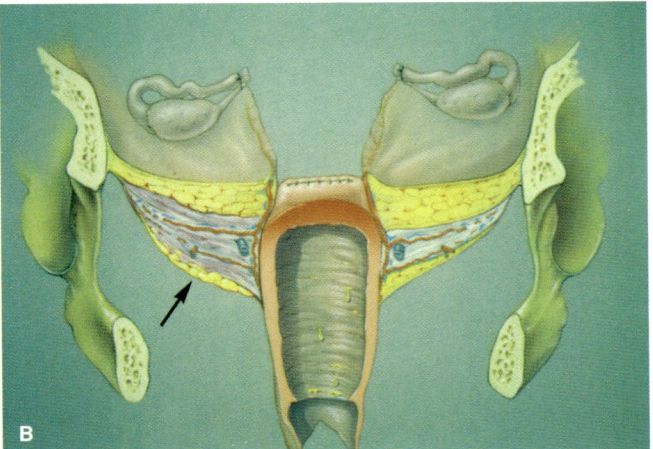

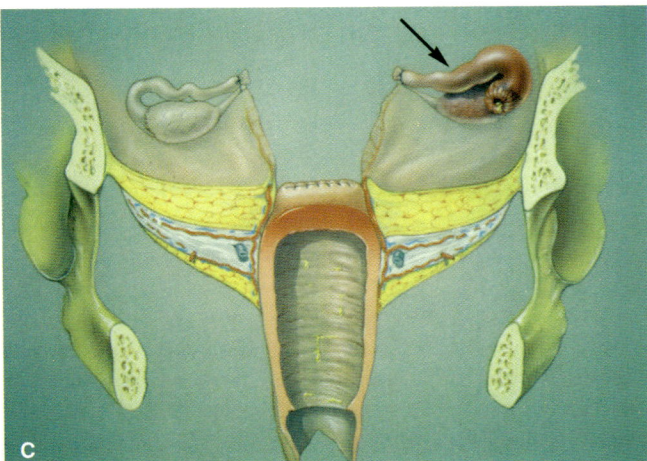

FIGURE 3-14 Organ/space infections. **A.** Vaginal cuff cellulitis. The vaginal surgical margin is edematous, hyperemic, and tender, and there are purulent secretions in the vagina. Parametria and adnexa are normal during gentle bimanual examination. **B.** Pelvic cellulitis in the right parametrium. It is indurated and tender to palpation; no mass is present. **C.** Adnexal infection after hysterectomy. The parametria are normal. Tenderness without a mass is appreciated in the adnexal area.

Of potential IV or oral agents shown in Table 3-16, second-generation cephalosporins have activity against aerobic gram-positive cocci and some gram-negative aerobic and anaerobic bacteria. Third-generation cephalosporins provide gram-positive activity, even greater gram-negative coverage, and some anaerobic effects. With penicillins, the β-lactam ring provides antibacterial activity, which is directed primarily against gram-positive aerobic bacteria. However, pharmacologic manipulation has also created penicillins with added antibacterial spectra that are suitable for pelvic infection. Some bacteria produce an enzyme (β-lactamase) that opens the β-lactam ring and inactivates the drug. Inhibitors of β-lactamase are clavulanic acid, sulbactam, and tazobactam, and these have been combined with several penicillins to enhance their antibacterial spectrum. Additionally, oral probenecid can be administered separately with penicillins. This drug lowers the renal-tubular secretion rate of these antibiotics and is used to raise penicillin or cephalosporin plasma levels.

For gram-negative pathogens, the aminoglycoside gentamicin is primarily selected because of its low cost and clinical efficacy. However, this drug has the potential for nephrotoxicity, and risk factors include older age, renal insufficiency, hypotension, volume depletion, frequent dosing intervals, longer treatment, multiple co-antibiotics, or multisystem disease. For serious pelvic infection, gentamycin is often combined with clindamycin to achieve adequate pathogen coverage. Clindamycin is primarily active against aerobic gram-positive bacteria and most anaerobic bacteria. Its added activity against methicillin-resistant *Staphylococcus aureus* (MRSA) has increased its use in these cases. Metronidazole may be used instead of clindamycin for women with serious postoperative pelvic infections, including pelvic abscess. It is active only against obligate anaerobes and must be combined with agents effective against gram-positive and gram-negative aerobic bacterial species, such as ampicillin and gentamicin.

Adnexal Infection

This infection is uncommon and presents identically to that of pelvic cellulitis. The difference is in the location of tenderness during bimanual pelvic examination. The cuff and parametrial areas are not usually tender, but the adnexa are. This infection may also develop after tubal ligation, surgical therapy for ectopic pregnancy, or other adnexal surgery. Empiric antibiotic regimens are identical to those for pelvic cellulitis (see Table 3-16).

Ovarian Abscess

A rare but life-threatening complication following primarily vaginal hysterectomy is ovarian abscess. Presumably with this infection, surgery is performed in the late proliferative phase of an ovulatory menstrual cycle, and ovaries are in close proximity to the vaginal cuff. As expected, physiologic cuff cellulitis develops normally, but when ovulation occurs, local bacteria gain access to the ovulation site and the corpus luteum. The corpus luteum often is hemorrhagic, and the blood in this functional cyst provides a perfect medium for bacterial growth.

Affected women have an essentially normal postoperative course until approximately 10 days following surgery. At this time, they experience acute unilateral lower abdominal pain, which then involves multiple quadrants. These symptoms reflect rupture of their abscess and abdominal peritonitis. Sepsis commonly follows,

TABLE 3-16. Empiric Antimicrobial Regiments for Postgynecologic Surgery Infections

Regimen	Dose
Single-agent intravenous	
Cephalosporin	
Cefoxitin (Mefoxin)	2 g every 6 hr
Cefotetan (Cefotan)	2 g every 12 hr
Cefotaxime (Claforan)	1–2 g every 8 hr
Penicillin with or without β-lactamase inhibitor	
Piperacillin	4 g every 6 hr
Piperacillin/tazobactam (Zosyn)	3.375 g every 6 hr
Ampicillin/sulbactam (Unasyn)	3 g every 6 hr
Ticarcillin/clavulanate (Timentin)	3.1 g every 4–6 hr
Carbapenems	
Imipenem/cilastatin (Primaxin)	500 mg every 8 hr
Meropenem (Merrem)	500 mg every 8 hr
Ertapenem (Invanz)	1 g once daily
Combination agent intravenous	
Metronidazole (Flagyl)	Loading dose 15 mg/kg; maintenance 7.5 mg/kg every 6 hr
Ampicillin	2 g every 6 hr
Gentamicin	3–5 mg/kg once daily
OR	
Clindamycin	900 mg every 8 hr
Gentamicin	3–5 mg/kg once daily
with or without ampicillin	2 g every 6 hr
Oral agents	
Amoxicillin/clavulanate (Augmentin) alone	875 mg/125 mg twice daily
Metronidazole	500 mg every 12 hr
PLUS	
Trimethoprim-sulfamethoxazole DS 160/800 mg	160/800 every 12hr
Metronidazole	500 mg every 12 hr
PLUS	
Ciprofloxacin (Cipro)	500 mg every 12 hr

and this is a true gynecologic emergency. Immediate exploratory laparotomy is necessary, with IV administration of perioperative broad-spectrum antimicrobials, abscess evacuation, and adnexectomy if easily accessible. At a minimum, necrotic tissues are debrided, which may require oophorectomy. After hospital discharge, oral antibiotics are typically continued for an additional 5 to 7 days, and this is variable depending on the clinical course.

Similarly, women rarely may develop a TOA identical to that seen as an end result of acute PID. This process can be managed medically with IV antimicrobials, and surgery is usually not required unless rupture follows. Depending on size and location, percutaneous drainage may be considered. Broad-spectrum antibiotics are continued until a woman has been afebrile for 48 to 72 hours. Then, IV antibiotics may be replaced by oral agents, which are continued outpatient to complete a 2-week course.

Pelvic Abscess/Infected Pelvic Hematoma

Pelvic abscess not involving an adnexal structure may also uncommonly complicate hysterectomy (Fig. 3-15). This develops from blood, serum, and/or lymph collections following hysterectomy that provide an excellent milieu for the overgrowth of bacteria inoculated into the adjacent tissues during surgery.

An infected surgical pelvic hematoma may present similarly. A classic history in this case is a postoperative hemoglobin level that is significantly lower than predicted by measured intraoperative blood loss, and this reflects postsurgical bleeding. Unlike women who develop tissue cellulitis following surgery and whose early symptom of infection is pain, women with an infected hematoma will have low-grade temperature elevation (>37.8°C) as their early finding. Pain is a late symptom for these women. As prevention, women with an unexplained postoperative hemoglobin drop but no fever are discharged with instructions to monitor their temperature twice daily for approximately 1 week. Temperatures ≥37.8°C typically prompt evaluation.

Signs and symptoms of pelvic abscess or infected hematoma are midline, and a mass is typically discernible centrally. Pelvic abscesses often remain confined to the extraperitoneal space, and a patient does not usually develop peritonitis. Some may develop diarrhea due to the proximity of the rectum, which is usually adjacent to the infected space. Transvaginal sonography

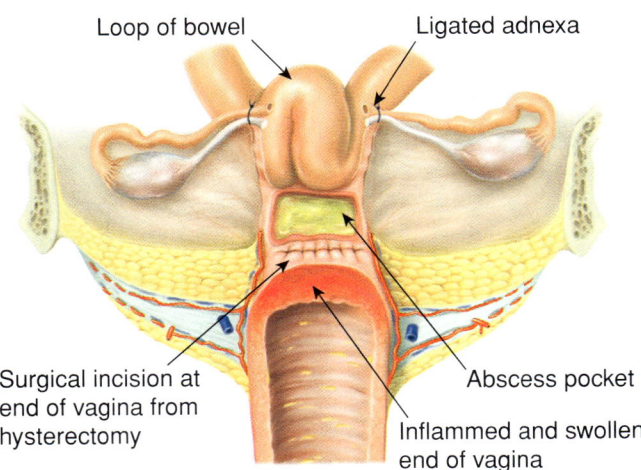

Loop of bowel   Ligated adnexa

Surgical incision at end of vagina from hysterectomy

Abscess pocket

Inflamed and swollen end of vagina

FIGURE 3-15 Pelvic abscess or infected hematoma that is extraperitoneal and cephalad to the vaginal margins.

can accurately characterize the dimensions (Fig. 3-16). In those with a less clear clinical picture, CT scanning may be more effective to exclude other fever etiologies. For both, hospital readmission for broad-spectrum IV antibiotics is usually necessary (see Table 3-16). Additionally, opening the vaginal surgical margin, if possible, to allow drainage will aid treatment. Both these can be drained with sonographic transvaginal guidance or in the operating room.

Combination IV antibiotics are administered until a woman has been afebrile 48 to 72 hours. IV antibiotics may then be replaced by oral agents, which are continued outpatient to complete a 2-week course of therapy, if the abscess or hematoma is not drained. If drained, then oral agents continued for 5 to 7 days following IV agents typically is sufficient.

Abdominal Incision Infection

The superficial and easily accessible location of this infection aids its diagnosis. Abdominal incisions are usually the most

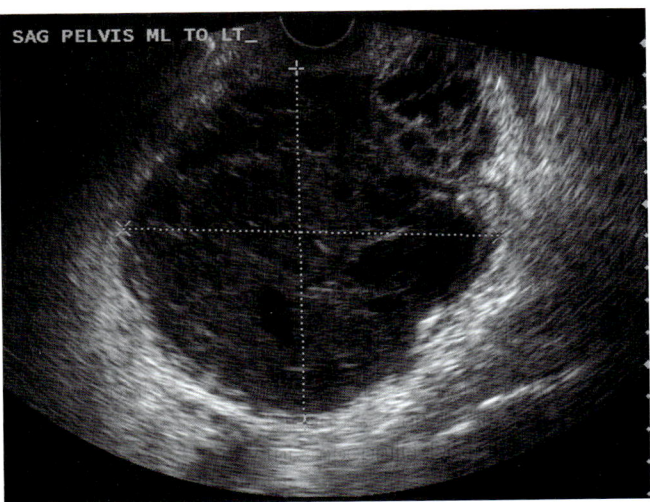

SAG PELVIS ML TO LT_

FIGURE 3-16 Transvaginal sonogram of an infected pelvic hematoma following hysterectomy. This 11 × 12 cm collection of blood and clot was drained vaginally in the operative room. (Reproduced with permission from Dr. Elysia Moschos.)

uncomfortable following gynecologic surgery, but pain diminishes daily. Erythema and heat are the first physical signs of this infection, which is usually diagnosed on the fourth or fifth postoperative day. A hematoma or seroma may develop in the abdominal wall incision without infection.

Drainage and documentation of an intact fascial incision are basics of abdominal incision infection, hematoma, or seroma treatment. These steps may be performed at the bedside with locally injected lidocaine or in the operative room depending on extent, risk of comorbid fascial dehiscence, and patient tolerance.

If soft-tissue cellulitis is adjacent to the incision, antimicrobial therapy is required. If the initial surgery was a clean procedure, then *Staphylococcus* species predominate. Instead, following clean-contaminated or dirty procedures, isolated organisms commonly include gram-negative bacteria such as *E coli*, *Pseudomonas aeruginosa*, and *Enterobacter* species and gram-positive bacteria, namely, *Staphylococcus* and *Enterococcus* species (Kirby, 2009). Anaerobes are typically not prominent pathogens in these infections but may be present, especially following hysterectomy. Thus, these infections are usually polymicrobial, and antibiotics found in Table 3-16 are suitable.

Subsequent local care with wet-to-dry dressings stimulates fibroblastic proliferation and development of healthy granulation tissue. Moistening the dry dressing prior to its removal will ease removal and decrease patient discomfort. In most cases, wounds are irrigated with normal saline. For some complicated wounds, early wound irrigation with hypochlorous acid (Vashe Wound Solution) is chosen for its antimicrobial properties and skin-neutral pH. Povidone-iodine, iodophor gauze, hydrogen peroxide, and sodium hypochlorite (Dakin solution) are typically avoided once infection has resolved, as they are caustic to healing tissues. Some recommend their use early but follow with normal saline irrigation.

Once uninfected granulation tissue is established, healing may continue by secondary intention. For larger wounds, secondary surgical closure can be considered. Negative-pressure wound therapy provided by vacuum-assisted wound closure devices is available for more serious or larger wounds.

Toxic Shock Syndrome

This condition, caused by an exotoxin (TSS toxin-1) produced by *S aureus*, appears approximately 2 days following surgery or menstruation onset. Menstrual-associated toxic shock syndrome (TSS) rates have diminished following changes in tampon composition and use. For TSS, the vagina or wound must be colonized by a toxigenic staphylococcal strain, and the patient must lack the specific antibody that can block the superantigen.

The classic TSS symptoms include fever, malaise, and diarrhea. If postoperative, signs of wound infection are minimal. A patient has conjunctival and pharyngeal hyperemia without purulence. The tongue is usually reddened, and the skin on the trunk is erythematous but not painful or pruritic. Temperatures are usually above 38.8°C, and orthostatic hypotension or shock may be present. This syndrome results from host cytokines released in response to superantigenic properties of the toxin. The criteria for this diagnosis are presented in Table 3-17.

The wound, if present, is treated like any other wound. It is cultured to confirm presence of *S aureus*. However, results from

TABLE 3-17. Criteria for Diagnosis of Toxic Shock Syndrome

Major criteria

Hypotension
  Orthostatic syncope
  Systolic BP <90 mm Hg for adults
Diffuse macular erythroderma
Temperature ≥38.9°C
Late skin desquamation, particularly on hands, palms, and soles (1–2 weeks after rash onset)

Minor criteria (organ system involvement)

Gastrointestinal: diarrhea or vomiting
Mucous membranes: oral, pharyngeal, conjunctival, and/or vaginal erythema
Muscular: myalgia or creatinine level greater than twice normal
Renal: BUN and creatinine greater than twice normal or >5 WBCs/hpf in urine, without concurrent UTI
Hematologic: platelet count <100,000 per mm³
Hepatic: ALT, AST, and/or bilirubin levels greater than twice normal
Central nervous system: altered consciousness without focal localizing signs

ALT = alanine aminotransferase; AST = aspartate aminotransferase; BP = blood pressure; BUN = blood urea nitrogen; hpf = high-power field; UTI = urinary tract infection; WBC = white blood cell.

other cultures (e.g., blood, throat, and cerebrospinal fluid) will be negative. To meet the strict criteria, a woman must have all major and at least three minor criteria. If this is suspected early and therapy is initiated, the complete syndrome may not develop. If obtained, serologies for Rocky Mountain spotted fever, measles, and leptospirosis are negative. Viral infection and group A streptococci also can cause a similar presentation.

While awaiting culture results for selection of specific anti-staphylococcal antibiotics, empiric therapy covers both methicillin-susceptible and methicillin-resistant *S aureus*. Vancomycin (15 to 20 mg/kg/dose) can be given every 8 to 12 hours, not exceeding 2 g per dose. Regardless, the hallmark of therapy is entire system support with large volumes of IV fluids and electrolytes to replace massive body fluid losses from diarrhea, capillary leakage, and insensible loss. These patients may develop signifi-

cant edema and are best managed in an intensive care unit. Even with appropriate management, the death rate can be as high as 5 percent because of subsequent acute respiratory distress syndrome (ARDS), disseminated intravascular coagulopathy (DIC), or hypotension unresponsive to therapy. This syndrome may also follow gynecologic surgical procedures such as D & C, hysterectomy, urethral suspension, and tubal ligation.

Necrotizing Fasciitis

Risk factors for this postoperative incision infection are age older than 50 years, arteriosclerotic heart disease, diabetes mellitus, obesity, debilitating disease, smoking, and previous radiation therapy, all of which are associated with decreased tissue perfusion. In our clinical service, vulvar infection in obese diabetic women is a prominent risk (Fig. 3-17). Only approximately 20 percent

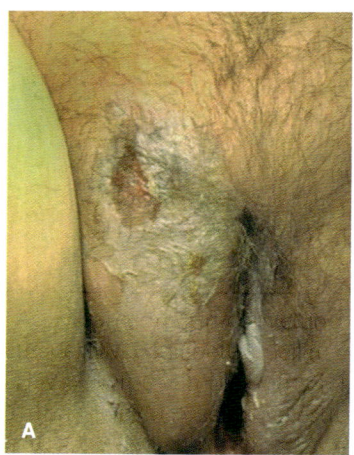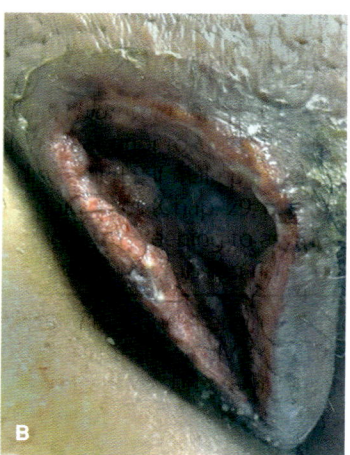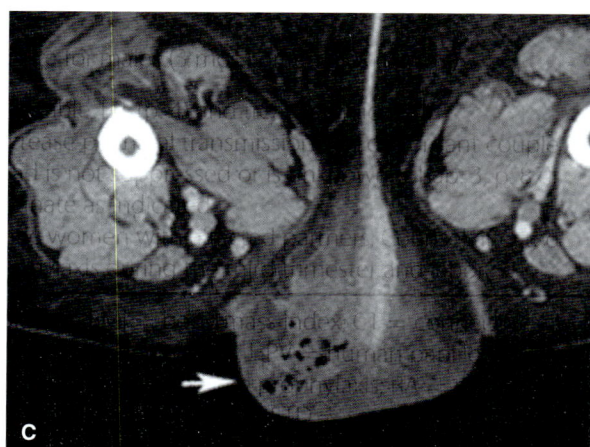

FIGURE 3-17 Vulvar necrotizing fasciitis in an obese, diabetic patient. **A.** Preoperative image of the right labium majus shows mild erythema and moderate edema. A discrete erosion is seen within an area of peeling skin. **B.** After debridement, the extent of tissue destruction is evident. **C.** A diagnostic computed tomography image of this patient shows subcutaneous gas, which is seen as multiple dark round areas within the labium majus (*arrow*).

of cases follow surgery. Bacteria recovered from women with this infection are similar to those recovered from any postoperative gynecologic infection site, namely predominantly *E coli*, *Escherichia faecalis*, *Bacteroides* species, *Peptostreptococcus* species, *S aureus*, and groups A and B hemolytic streptococci.

Although this postoperative superficial incisional infection begins like any other postoperative infection with pain and erythema, its hallmark is subcutaneous and superficial fascial necrosis, manifested by excessive tissue edema in adjacent areas. Blisters or bullae form in tissue that has become avascular and is discolored. Crepitus or induration and edema beyond the region of visible erythema may be present. Tissue destruction is far more extensive than is evident by surface examination, and myonecrosis may be present. The skin will slip over underlying tissue, and if incised, due to the lack of vascularity, there is no bleeding but instead usually a thin, gray transudate. Severe systemic toxicity and fever may develop. In obvious cases, no imaging is needed, and patients are prepared for surgical debridement. In less-clear cases, radiographs or CT scans, if these can be quickly obtained, may add information by revealing gas in affected tissues produced by clostridial species such as *Clostridium perfringens* (see Fig. 3-17) (Ballard, 2018).

Although broad-spectrum antibiotic administration is required, the cornerstone of treatment is prompt recognition and immediate surgical removal of necrotic tissue to a level at which viable bleeding tissue is reached. To achieve this, excision of large tissue volumes is often needed. Although this is potentially disfiguring, postponing surgery while waiting for antimicrobial activity only raises the volume of tissue death. Gynecologists may enlist assistance from a general surgeon or gynecologic oncologist if extensive debridement into the abdominal wall, posterior perineal triangle, buttock, or inner thigh is anticipated. Early fatality rates for patients with this infection approximated 20 percent in the systematic review of 1463 patients by Goh and associates (2014).

Wounds are left open and treated as described earlier (p. 83). Assistance from a general or plastic surgeon for potential grafting is often necessary.

Methicillin-Resistant *Staphylococcus Aureus*

Any of the polymicrobial infections discussed in this section may be complicated by MRSA. To cover MRSA, suitable outpatient oral antibiotics for uncomplicated infection include trimethoprim-sulfamethoxazole DS (160 mg/800 mg) twice daily, clindamycin 300 or 450 mg three times daily, doxycycline or minocycline 100 mg twice daily, or linezolid (Zyvox) 600 mg twice daily. For complicated infections, the Infectious Disease Society of America recommends MRSA coverage with IV vancomycin, IV or oral clindamycin, IV or oral linezolid 600 mg twice daily, IV daptomycin (Cubicin) 4 mg/kg once daily, or IV telavancin (Vibativ) 10 mg/kg once daily (Liu, 2011).

Of these agents, vancomycin is active only against aerobic gram-positive bacteria. It is primarily used by the gynecologist to treat patients with severe allergic reaction to other antibiotics or for MRSA infections. The most significant of vancomycin's side effects is its potential nephrotoxicity, which is enhanced with aminoglycoside therapy. However, the most remarkable is the "red man" syndrome, which is a dermal response to histamine release that creates an erythematous pruritic rash and potentially

TABLE 3-18. Risk Factors for Postoperative Surgical Site Infection

Preoperative
Smoking
Obesity
Poor nutrition
Diabetes mellitus
ASA category ≥3
Immunosuppression
Prior adjacent surgery
Skin shaving at surgical site
Recent skin or soft tissue infection

Perioperative
Emergent procedure
Excessive blood loss
Non–β-lactam prophylaxis
Intraoperative hypothermia
Perioperative hyperglycemia
Laparotomy for abdominal entry
Inadequate antibiotic prophylaxis
Failure to close wound dead space
Higher category wound classification
Prolonged surgical procedure (>3.5 hr)
Non–chlorhexidine-alcohol skin preparation
Foreign body placement (catheter, drain, etc.)
Inadequate irrigation and removal of wound contaminants
Extensive electrosurgical coagulation use or tissue dissection

ASA = American Society of Anesthesiologists.
From Ban, 2017; Lake, 2013; Mahdi, 2014; Steiner, 2017; Uppal, 2016.

hypotension. Intravenous administration over 1 hour or administration of an antihistamine may be protective.

Prevention

Because of its greater bacterial exposure, hysterectomy raises the risk of the just described surgical site infections. Other risk factors are listed in Table 3-18.

As prevention, obvious skin or reproductive tract infections are cleared prior to elective surgery. Also, antibiotic prophylaxis immediately before surgery reduces the risk of SSI following abdominal hysterectomy (Ayeleke, 2017). Specifically, SSIs develop in 20 to 30 percent of women after vaginal or abdominal hysterectomy. This rate drops to 15 to 25 percent with preoperative antibiotic prophylaxis. Suitable antibiotics for prophylaxis are listed in Table 39-8 (p. 832). Other preventions are discussed in Chapter 42 (p. 922).

OTHER GYNECOLOGIC INFECTIONS

■ Vulvar Abscess

These infections develop similarly to other superficial abscesses but have the potential for significant expansion due to the loose areolar subcutaneous tissue in this area. Risk factors include diabetes, obesity, perineal shaving, and immuno-suppression. Common isolates include *Staphylococcus*, group B *Streptococcus*, *Enterococcus* species, *E coli*, and *P mirabilis*. Importantly, Thurman (2008) and Kilpatrick (2010) and their coworkers found MRSA in 40 to 60 percent of cultured vulvar abscesses.

In early stages, surrounding cellulitis may be the most prominent finding and only a small or no abscess is identified. In these cases, sitz baths and oral antibiotics are reasonable. Sizes large than this may be treated with incision and drainage, abscess packing if indicated, and oral antibiotics to treat surrounding cellulitis. For uncomplicated infection, suitable oral agents will be broad-spectrum and will cover MRSA. Trimethoprim-sulfamethoxazole, clindamycin, or doxycycline is a suitable choice, among others. However, for those with a large abscess, immunosuppression, or diabetes, hospitalization and IV antibiotic therapy is often preferred. Again, coverage for MRSA is included in acceptable IV regimens (see Table 3-16).

Large abscesses often require admission for drainage under anesthesia. This provides adequate pain control for abscess drainage and for abscess cavity exploration to disrupt loculated areas of pus. This is illustrated in Chapter 43 (p. 986).

■ Bartholin Gland Duct Abscess

This infection is managed primarily by drainage (Fig. 3-18). Drainage with either Word catheter placement or marsupialization can typically be completed in an outpatient setting and is described in Chapter 43 (p. 980). Neither technique is clearly superior and depends on clinical circumstance (Kroese, 2017). Antibiotics are often added to treat surrounding tissue cellulitis. The most common bacteria isolated from these abscesses include anaerobic *Bacteroides* and *Peptostreptococcus* species and aerobic *E coli*, *S aureus*, *Streptococcus* species, and *E faecalis* (Kessous, 2013; Krissi, 2016). Also, *N gonorrhoeae* and *C trachomatis* may be identified (Bleker, 1990). Thus, polymicrobial coverage is selected, and suitable single-agent oral outpatient therapy includes, among others, trimethoprim-sulfamethoxazole, amoxicillin-clavulanate, or second-generation cephalosporins. In most cases, abscess aerobic

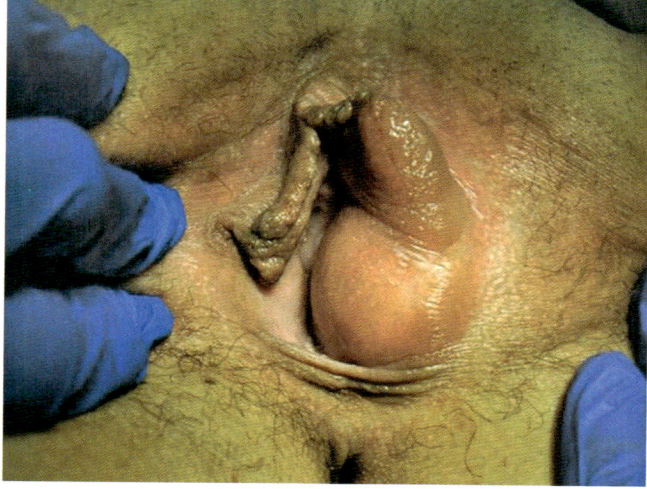

FIGURE 3-18 Left Bartholin gland duct abscess and associated edema of the labium minus.

cultures are obtained. Depending on patient risks, NAATs for *N gonorrhoeae* and *C trachomatis* and screening for other STDs may be included.

HUMAN IMMUNODEFICIENCY VIRUS

■ Pathogenesis

This single-stranded RNA virus causes chronic infection and progressive depletion of specific T lymphocytes known as *CD4 cells*. HIV-1 and HIV-2 are the two distinct viral types. HIV-1 is the most widespread, whereas HIV-2 is found mainly in Africa. The HIV virus is transmitted by either direct inoculation with infected blood or by transepithelial migration across a mucosal barrier. Subsequently, the virus targets CD4 cells by fusing their viral envelope glycoproteins to target cell surface receptors. The viral RNA genome is reverse transcribed into viral DNA, which then integrates into the host genome, leading to further virus replication and transcription. During approximately 10 years without treatment, cycles of CD4 cell infection and depletion coupled with chronic T cell activation and apoptosis eventually lead to late-stage infection (Hazenberg, 2000). Acquired immunodeficiency syndrome (AIDS), also known as stage 3 infection, is the most advanced stage of HIV infection and is diagnosed in those meeting specific criteria. These are a CD4 count <200 cell/μL and AIDS-defining criteria that include *Pneumocystis jirovecii* pneumonia, Kaposi sarcoma, invasive cervical cancer, and others (Selik, 2014).

■ Screening and Diagnosis

Screening for HIV is recommended at least one time for all women aged 13 to 64 years. Screening is also offered to women seeking evaluation and treatment of STDs or those with other identified risk factors (Centers for Disease Control and Prevention, 2015; American College of Obstetricians and Gynecologists, 2019). STD screening guidelines for nonpregnant, sexually active, asymptomatic women are listed in Table 1-1 (p. 4).

HIV infection may be characterized as acute or chronic, and current diagnostic tests help distinguish the two (Table 3-19). The recommended initial screening test is an FDA-approved, fourth-generation antigen/antibody combination immunoassay that detects both HIV-1 and HIV-2 antibodies and HIV-1 p24 antigen. This antigen is produced before antibody formation in HIV-1 infection (Centers for Disease Control and Prevention, 2014b). No further testing is indicated if the initial screen is nonreactive.

If reactive ("positive"), specimens are tested with an FDA-approved antibody immunoassay that differentiates between HIV-1 and HIV-2 antibodies ("differentiation assay"). In chronic infection, both the initial combination immunoassay and the antibody differentiation assay for the specific HIV type are reactive. In acute infection, specimens may be reactive by fourth-generation combination assay but nonreactive or indeterminate on the differentiation assay. In this case, an FDA-approved HIV-1 NAAT is performed, which identifies early HIV RNA production prior to antibody formation. If the NAAT result is nonreactive ("negative"), the possibility of a false-positive combination immunoassay is considered.

TABLE 3-19. Laboratory Results for Diagnosis of HIV Infection

HIV 1/2 Ag/Ab Combination Immunoassay	HIV 1/2 Differentiation Assay	HIV-1 NAAT	Interpretation
Nonreactive	n/a	n/a	HIV negative
Reactive	HIV-1 positive	n/a	HIV-1 positive
Reactive	HIV positive nontypeable (undifferentiated)	n/a	HIV positive
Reactive	HIV indeterminate	Detected Not detected	Acute HIV-1 positive HIV negative
Reactive	HIV antibody negative	Detected Not detected	Acute HIV-1 positive HIV negative
Reactive	HIV antibody negative or indeterminate	Invalid or not performed	Inconclusive

Ab = antibody; Ag = antigen; HIV = human immunodeficiency virus; n/a = not applicable; NAAT = nucleic acid amplification test.
From Centers for Disease Control and Prevention, 2014c.

If an initial laboratory-based screening antigen/antibody combination assay is not available, an FDA-approved point-of-care or "rapid" test such as Alere Determine HIV 1/2 Ag/Ab Combo test may be used (Centers for Disease Control and Prevention, 2017). However, this single-use test is less sensitive for acute infection than laboratory-based screening tests.

■ **Prevention**

Prophylaxis to prevent HIV infection may be provided either post- or preexposure. First, occupational or nonoccupational exposure may warrant postexposure prophylaxis (PEP). The initial evaluation determines the timing of exposure, the HIV status of the source (when possible), the type of infectious fluid(s), and exposure site. Additionally, rapid HIV screening of the exposed person is completed at this first visit. If results are positive, initiation of lifelong antiretroviral therapy (ART), rather than short-term prophylaxis, is warranted. Prompt initiation of PEP should not be delayed in a high-risk exposure and may be continued or stopped after the initial evaluation is complete.

If PEP is elected following a high-risk sexual encounter, prophylaxis with a 28-day course of an approved antiretroviral regimen is initiated within 72 hours (Centers for Disease Control and Prevention, 2016). Guidelines and PEP regimens are discussed in Chapter 1 (p. 22).

Following a high-risk occupational exposure from an HIV-positive individual, an identical 28-day regimen is offered. When the HIV status of the source is unknown, use of PEP is decided on a case-by-case basis with expert consultation (Kuhar, 2013). Exposures across broken skin or mucosal membranes or needle-stick injuries are considered significant. Infectious fluids include blood, semen, vaginal secretions, and cerebrospinal, synovial, pleural, peritoneal, pericardial, and amnionic fluids.

For women with ongoing risk factors for HIV acquisition, ongoing preventive measures are necessary. Risk factors may include: ongoing sexual relationship with an HIV-positive (serodifferent) partner, infrequent condom use with one or more partners who are bisexual males or who inject drugs, and a recent (with the past 6 months) syphilis or gonorrhea diagnosis. If risks are identified, behavioral interventions are initially recommended. Consistent condom use is associated with an 80-percent reduction in transmission among heterosexual couples (Weller, 2002). Additionally, for a woman with a known serodifferent sexual partner, treatment of the partner with ART reduces the transmission risk by more than 90 percent. Achieving viral suppression in the affected partner provides effective prevention (Cohen, 2016).

Daily pharmacologic preexposure prophylaxis (PrEP) with antiretroviral agents is considered in combination with safer sex practices for adults at highest risk and is now a Grade A recommendation for men and women with certain risk factors. Women at highest risk include those with serodifferent partner(s) living with HIV, inconsistent condom use with a partner whose HIV status is unknown and is at high risk (injects drugs or has sex with men and women), and those with a diagnosis of syphilis or gonorrhea within the past 6 months (U.S. Preventive Services Task Force, 2019). Adherence to the medication is essential. The extent to which PrEP contributes to prevention among individuals with a serodifferent partner who is already taking suppressive ART is not known. The CDC offers guidelines for PrEP risk assessment, initial laboratory studies, and ongoing STD screening and monitoring for side effects (Centers for Disease Control and Prevention, 2018b). Additionally, the National Clinicians Consultation Center PrEPline is available at 1-855-448-7737.

■ **Treatment**

If HIV infection is diagnosed, referral to an infectious disease specialist for prompt initiation of ART is recommended. Primary therapeutic targets for antiretroviral drugs include the viral reverse transcriptase enzyme, which converts HIV RNA into DNA inside the host cell; the integrase enzyme, which aids incorporation of HIV DNA into the host genome; and the viral protease enzyme responsible for creating mature viral particles. The initial regimen for a newly diagnosed patient includes two nucleoside reverse transcriptase inhibitors (NRTIs) in combination with a third agent from the integrase inhibitor (INSTI) class, protease inhibitor (PI) class, or non-nucleoside reverse transcriptase inhibitor (NNRTI) class (Panel on Antiretroviral Guidelines for Adults and Adolescents, 2018). When selecting initial ART, medical comorbidities, fertility desires, convenience, and patient motivation are considered. If a patient taking PrEP is diagnosed with HIV infection, PrEP is stopped until a full-dose ART regimen can be initiated (Centers for Disease Control and Prevention, 2018b). All partners with unknown HIV status are referred for testing.

REFERENCES

Albert X, Huertas I, Pereiró II, et al: Antibiotics for preventing recurrent urinary tract infection in non-pregnant women. Cochrane Database Syst Rev 3:CD001209, 2004

American College of Obstetricians and Gynecologists: Treatment of urinary tract infections in nonpregnant women. Practice Bulletin No. 91, March 2008, Reaffirmed 2016

American College of Obstetricians and Gynecologists: Long-acting reversible contraception: implants and intrauterine devices. Practice Bulletin No. 186, November 2017a

American College of Obstetricians and Gynecologists: Vaginitis. Practice Bulletin No. 72 May 2006, Reaffirmed 2017b

American College of Obstetricians and Gynecologists: Prevention of infection after gynecologic procedures. Practice Bulletin No. 195, June 2014, Reaffirmed 2018

American College of Obstetricians and Gynecologists: Routine human immunodeficiency virus screening. Committee Opinion No. 596, May 2014, Reaffirmed 2019

American College of Radiology: ACR–SIR–SPR practice parameter for specifications and performance of image-guided percutaneous drainage/aspiration of abscesses and fluid collections. Resolution No. 13, 2018

Amsel R, Totten PA, Spiegel CA, et al: Nonspecific vaginitis. Diagnostic criteria and microbial and epidemiologic associations. Am J Med 74:14, 1983

Anderson MR, Klink K, Kohrssen A: Evaluation of vaginal complaints. JAMA 291:1368, 2004

Ashley-Morrow R, Krantz E, Wald A: Time course of seroconversion by HerpeSelect ELISA after acquisition of genital herpes simplex virus type 1 (HSV-1) or HSV-2. Sex Transm Dis 30(4):310, 2003

Atashili J, Poole C, Ndumbe PM, et al: Bacterial vaginosis and HIV acquisition: a meta-analysis of published studies. AIDS 22(12):1493, 2008

Ayeleke RO, Mourad S, Marjoribanks J, et al: Antibiotic prophylaxis for elective hysterectomy. Cochrane Database Syst Rev 6:CD004637, 2017

Baczynska A, Funch P, Fedder J, et al: Morphology of human Fallopian tubes after infection with Mycoplasma genitalium and Mycoplasma hominis—in vitro organ culture study. Hum Reprod 22(4):968, 2007

Ballard DH, Raptis CA, Guerra J, et al: Preoperative CT findings and interobserver reliability of Fournier gangrene. AJR Am J Roentgenol 211(5):1051, 2018

Baker DA, Ferris DG, Martens MG, et al: Imiquimod 3.75% cream applied daily to treat anogenital warts: combined results from women in two randomized, placebo-controlled studies. Infect Dis Obstet Gynecol 2011:806105, 2011

Ban KA, Minei JP, Laronga C, et al: American College of Surgeons and Surgical Infection Society: surgical site infection guidelines, 2016 update. J Am Coll Surg 224(1):59, 2017

Bartlett JG, Onderdonk AB, Drude E, et al: Quantitative bacteriology of the vaginal flora. J Infect Dis 136(2):271, 1977

Beerepoot M, Geerlings S: Non-antibiotic prophylaxis for urinary tract infections. Pathogens 5(2):E36, 2016

Belshe RB, Leone PA, Bernstein DI, et al: Efficacy results of a trial of a herpes simplex vaccine. N Engl J Med 366(1):34, 2012

Bent S, Nallamothu BK, Simel DL, et al: Does this woman have an acute uncomplicated urinary tract infection? JAMA 287(20):2701, 2002

Bernstein DI, Bellamy AR, Hook EW 3rd, et al: Epidemiology, clinical presentation, and antibody response to primary infection with herpes simplex virus type 1 and type 2 in young women. Clin Infect Dis 56(3):344, 2013

Beutner KR, Reitano MV, Richwald GA, et al: External genital warts: report of the American Medical Association Consensus Conference. AMA Expert Panel on External Genital Warts. Clin Infect Dis 27:796, 1998

Birnbaum DM: Microscopic findings. In Knoop KJ, Stack LB, Storrow AB (eds): Atlas of Emergency Medicine, 3rd ed. New York, McGraw-Hill, 2010

Bleker OP, Smalbraak DJ, Schutte MF: Bartholin's abscess: the role of Chlamydia trachomatis. Genitourin Med 66:24, 1990

Boskey ER, Cone RA, Whaley KJ, et al: Origins of vaginal acidity: high D/L lactate ratio is consistent with bacteria being the primary source. Hum Reprod 16(9):1809, 2001

Bradley H, Markowitz LE, Gibson T, et al: Seroprevalence of herpes simplex virus types 1 and 2—United States, 1999–2010. J Infect Dis 209(3):325, 2014

Bradshaw CS, Morton AN, Garland SM, et al: Higher-risk behavioral practices associated with bacterial vaginosis compared with vaginal candidiasis. Obstet Gynecol 106:105, 2005

Bradshaw CS, Morton AN, Hocking J, et al: High recurrence rates of bacterial vaginosis over the course of 12 months after oral metronidazole therapy and factors associated with recurrence. J Infect Dis 193:1478, 2006

Brotman RM, Klebanoff MA, Nansel TR, et al: A longitudinal study of vaginal douching and bacterial vaginosis—a marginal structural modeling analysis. Am J Epidemiol 168(2):188, 2008

Brüggemann R, Alffenaar J, Blijlevens N, et al: Clinical relevance of the pharmacokinetic interactions of azole antifungal drugs with other coadministered agents. Clin Inf Dis 48(10):1441, 2009

Burnett AM, Anderson CP, Zwank MD: Laboratory-confirmed gonorrhea and/or chlamydia rates in clinically diagnosed pelvic inflammatory disease and cervicitis. Am J Emerg Med 30(7):1114, 2012

Centers for Disease Control and Prevention: Expedited partner therapy in the management of sexually transmitted diseases. Atlanta, U.S. Department of Health and Human Services, 2006

Centers for Disease Control and Prevention: Discordant results from reverse sequence syphilis screening–five laboratories, United States, 2006–2010. MMWR 60(5):133, 2011

Centers for Disease Control and Prevention: Procedure-associated module: surgical site infection (SSI) event. 2014a. Available at: http://www.cdc.gov/nhsn/PDFs/pscManual/9pscSSIcurrent.pdf. Accessed March 10, 2019

Centers for Disease Control and Prevention: Recommendations for the laboratory-based detection of Chlamydia trachomatis and Neisseria gonorrhoeae–2014. MMWR 63(2):1, 2014b

Centers for Disease Control and Prevention, Association of Public Health Laboratories: Laboratory testing for the diagnosis of HIV infection: updated recommendations. 2014c. Available at http://stacks.cdc.gov/view/cdc/23447. Accessed March 17, 2019

Centers for Disease Control and Prevention: Sexually transmitted diseases treatment guidelines, 2015. MMWR 59(12):1, 2015

Centers for Disease Control and Prevention: Updated guidelines for antiretroviral postexposure prophylaxis after sexual, injection drug use, or other nonoccupational exposure to HIV—United States, 2016. 2016. Available at: https://www.cdc.gov/hiv/pdf/programresources/cdc-hiv-npep-guidelines.pdf. Accessed November 11, 2018

Centers for Disease Control and Prevention: Technical update: use of the determine HIV 1/2 Ag/Ab combo test with serum or plasma in the laboratory algorithm for HIV diagnosis. 2017. Available at https://stacks.cdc.gov/view/cdc/48472. Accessed March 17, 2019

Centers for Disease Control and Prevention: Sexually transmitted disease surveillance, 2017. Atlanta, U.S. Department of Health and Human Services, 2018a

Centers for Disease Control and Prevention: US Public Health Service: Preexposure prophylaxis for the prevention of HIV infection in the United States—2017 update: a clinical practice guideline. 2018b. Available at: https://www.cdc.gov/hiv/pdf/risk/prep/cdc-hiv-prep-guidelines-2017.pdf. Accessed March 17, 2019

Centers for Disease Control and Prevention: Surgical site infection (SSI) event. 2019. Available at: https://www.cdc.gov/nhsn/pdfs/pscmanual/9pscssicurrent.pdf. Accessed March 16, 2019

Ceovic R, Gulin SJ: Lymphogranuloma venereum: diagnostic and treatment challenges. Infect Drug Resist 8:39, 2015

Cohen MS, Chen YQ, McCauley M, et al: Antiretroviral therapy for the prevention of HIV-1 transmission. N Engl J Med 375(9):830, 2016

Coleman JS, Gaydos CA: Molecular diagnosis of bacterial vaginosis: an update. J Clin Microbiol 56(9):e00342, 2018

Copeland NK, Decker CF: Other sexually transmitted diseases chancroid and donovanosis. Dis Mon 62(8):306, 2016

Corey L, Wald A, Patel R, et al: Once-daily valacyclovir to reduce the risk of transmission of genital herpes. N Engl J Med 350:11, 2004

Curtis EM, Pine L: Actinomyces in the vaginas of women with and without intrauterine contraceptive devices. Am J Obstet Gynecol 140:880, 1981

Czaja CA, Scholes D, Hooton TM, et al: Population-based epidemiologic analysis of acute pyelonephritis. Clin Infect Dis 45(3):273, 2007

Dahn A, Saunders S, Hammond JA, et al: Effect of bacterial vaginosis, Lactobacillus and Premarin estrogen replacement therapy on vaginal gene expression changes. Microbes Infect 10(6):620, 2008

Daley G, Russell D, Tabrizi S, et al: Mycoplasma genitalium: a review. Int J STD AIDS 25(7):475, 2014

Devillé WL, Yzermans JC, van Duijn NP, et al: The urine dipstick test useful to rule out infections. A meta-analysis of the accuracy. BMC Urol 4:4, 2004

Dewitt J, Reining A, Allsworth JE, et al: Tuboovarian abscesses: is size associated with duration of hospitalization & complications? Obstet Gynecol Int 2010:847041, 2010

Donders GG, Sobel JD: Candida vulvovaginitis: a store with a buttery and a show window. Mycoses 60(2):70, 2017

Dunbar-Jacob J, Sereika SM, Foley SM, et al: Adherence to oral therapies in pelvic inflammatory disease. J Womens Health 13:285, 2004

Echols RM, Tosiello RL, Haverstock DC, et al: Demographic, clinical, and treatment parameters influencing the outcome of acute cystitis. Clin Infect Dis 29(1):113, 1999

Fan H, Wang TT, Ren G, et al: Characterization of tubo-ovarian abscess mimicking adnexal masses: comparison between contrast-enhanced CT, (18)F-FDG PET/CT and MRI. Taiwan J Obstet Gynecol 57(1):40, 2018

Fanfair RN, Zaidi A, Taylor LD, et al: Trends in seroprevalence of herpes simplex virus type 2 among non-Hispanic blacks and non-Hispanic whites aged 14 to 49 years—United States, 1988 to 2010. Sex Transm Dis 40(11):860, 2013

Fethers KA, Fairley CK, Hocking JS, et al: Sexual risk factors and bacterial vaginosis: a systematic review and meta-analysis. Clin Infect Dis 47(11):1426, 2008

Fettweis JM, Brooks JP, Serrano MG, et al: Differences in vaginal microbiome in African American women versus women of European ancestry. Microbiology 160(Pt 10):2272, 2014

Fiorino AS: Intrauterine contraceptive device-associated actinomycotic abscess and Actinomyces detection on cervical smear. Obstet Gynecol 87:142, 1996

Flagg EW, Torrone EA: Declines in anogenital warts among age groups most likely to be impacted by human papillomavirus vaccination, United States, 2006–2014. Am J Public Health 108(1):112, 2018

Food and Drug Administration: FDA reinforces safety information about serious low blood sugar levels and mental health side effects with fluoroquinolone antibiotics; requires label changes. 2018. Available at: https://www.fda.gov/Drugs/DrugSafety/ucm611032.htm. Accessed March 10, 2019

Fredricks DN, Fiedler TL, Marrazzo JM: Molecular identification of bacteria associated with bacterial vaginosis. N Engl J Med 353:1899, 2005

Gardner HL, Dukes CD: Haemophilus vaginalis vaginitis: a newly defined specific infection previously classified non-specific vaginitis. Am J Obstet Gynecol 69:962, 1955

Garland SM, Steben M, Sings HL, et al: Natural history of genital warts: analysis of the placebo arm of 2 randomized phase III trials of quadrivalent human papillomavirus (types 6, 11, 16, and 18) vaccine. J Infect Dis 199(6):805, 2009

Gaydos CA, Beqaj S, Schwebke JR, et al: Clinical validation of a test for the diagnosis of vaginitis. Obstet Gynecol 130(1):181, 2017a

Gaydos CA, Schwebke J, Dombrowski J, et al: Clinical performance of the Solana® Point-of-Care Trichomonas Assay from clinician-collected vaginal swabs and urine specimens from symptomatic and asymptomatic women. Expert Rev Mol Diagn 17(3):303, 2017b

Getman D, Jiang A, O'Donnell M, et al: Mycoplasma genitalium prevalence, coinfection, and macrolide antibiotic resistance frequency in a multicenter clinical study cohort in the United States. J Clin Microbiol 54(9):2278, 2016

Gjelland K, Ekerhovd E, Granberg S: Transvaginal ultrasound-guided aspiration for treatment of tubo-ovarian abscess: a study of 302 cases. Am J Obstet Gynecol 193:1323, 2005

Goh T, Goh LG, Ang CH, et al: Early diagnosis of necrotizing fasciitis. Br J Surg 101(1):e119, 2014

Goller JL, De Livera AM, Fairley CK, et al: Characteristics of pelvic inflammatory disease where no sexually transmitted infection is identified: a cross-sectional analysis of routinely collected sexual health clinic data. Sex Transm Infect 93(1):68, 2017

Gupta K, Chou MY, Howell A, et al: Cranberry products inhibit adherence of p-fimbriated Escherichia coli to primary cultured bladder and vaginal epithelial cells. J Urol 177(6):2357, 2007

Gupta K, Grigoryan L, Trautner B: Urinary tract infection. Ann Intern Med 167(7):ITC49, 2017

Gupta K, Hooton TM, Naber KG, et al: International clinical practice guidelines for the treatment of acute uncomplicated cystitis and pyelonephritis in women: a 2010 update by the Infectious Diseases Society of America and the European Society for Microbiology and Infectious Diseases. Clin Infect Dis 52(5):e103, 2011

Hadgu A, Westrom L, Brooks CA, et al: Predicting acute pelvic inflammatory disease: a multivariate analysis. Am J Obstet Gynecol 155:954, 1986

Hansfield HH: Vaginal infections. In Color Atlas and Synopsis of Sexually Transmitted Diseases. New York, McGraw-Hill, 2001, p 169

Hazenberg MD, Hamann D, Schuitemaker H, et al: T cell depletion in HIV-1 infection: how CD4+ T cells go out of stock. Nat Immunol 1(4):285, 2000

Helms DJ, Mosure DJ, Secor WE, et al: Management of Trichomonas vaginalis in women with suspected metronidazole hypersensitivity. Am J Obstet Gynecol 198(4):370 e371, 2008

Hemsell DL, Obregon VL, Heard MC, et al: Endometrial bacteria in asymptomatic, nonpregnant women. J Reprod Med 34:872, 1989

Hiller N, Fux T, Finkelstein A, et al: CT differentiation between tubo-ovarian and appendiceal origin of right lower quadrant abscess: CT, clinical, and laboratory correlation. Emerg Radiol 23(2):133, 2016

Hillier SL, Nugent RP, Eschenbach DA, et al: Association between bacterial vaginosis and preterm delivery of a low-birth-weight infant. The Vaginal Infections and Prematurity Study Group. N Engl J Med 333:1737, 1995

Hobbs MM, Seña AC: Modern diagnosis of Trichomonas vaginalis infection. Sex Transm Infect 89(6):434, 2013

Holmes NE, Howden BP: What's new in the treatment of serious MRSA infection? Curr Opin Infect Dis 27(6):471, 2014

Hooton TM, Roberts PL, Cox ME, et al: Voided midstream urine culture and acute cystitis in premenopausal women. N Engl J Med 369(20):1883, 2013

Hooton TM, Stamm WE: Diagnosis and treatment of uncomplicated urinary tract infection. Infect Dis Clin North Am 11:551, 1997

Hooton TM, Vecchio M, Iroz A, et al: Effect of increased daily water intake in premenopausal women with recurrent urinary tract infections: a randomized clinical trial. JAMA Intern Med 178(11):1509, 2018

Howe K, Kissinger PJ: Single-dose compared with multidose metronidazole for the treatment of trichomoniasis in women: a meta-analysis. Sex Transm Dis 44(1):29, 2017

Huppert JS, Batteiger BE, Braslins P, et al: Use of an immunochromatographic assay for rapid detection of Trichomonas vaginalis in vaginal specimens. J Clin Microbiol 43:684, 2005

Huppert JS, Mortensen JE, Reed JL, et al: Rapid antigen testing compares favorably with transcription-mediated amplification assay for the detection of Trichomonas vaginalis in young women. Clin Infect Dis 45(2):194, 2007

Jensen JS, Cusini M, Gomberg M, et al: 2016 European guideline on Mycoplasma genitalium infections. J Eur Acad Dermatol Venereol 30(10):1650, 2016

Jepson RG, Williams G, Craig JC: Cranberries for preventing urinary tract infections. Cochrane Database Syst Rev 10: CD001321, 2012

Joesoef MR, Westrom L, Reynolds G, et al: Recurrence of ectopic pregnancy: the role of salpingitis. Am J Obstet Gynecol 165:46, 1991

Jung SI, Kim YJ, Park HS, et al: Acute pelvic inflammatory disease: diagnostic performance of CT. J Obstet Gynaecol Res 37(3):228, 2011

Kang C, Kim K, Lee SH, et al: A risk stratification model of acute pyelonephritis to indicate hospital admission from the ED. Am J Emerg Med 31(7):1067, 2013

Keane FE, Ison CA, Taylor-Robinson D: A longitudinal study of the vaginal flora over a menstrual cycle. Int J STD AIDS 8:489, 1997

Kessous R, Aricha-Tamir B, Sheizaf B, et al: Clinical and microbiological characteristics of Bartholin gland abscesses. Obstet Gynecol 122(4):794, 2013

Kilpatrick CC, Alagkiozidis I, Orejuela FJ, et al: Factors complicating surgical management of vulvar abscess. J Reprod Med 55(3-4):139, 2010

Kim JY, Kim Y, Jeong WK, et al: Perihepatitis with pelvic inflammatory disease (PID) on MDCT: characteristic findings and relevance to PID. Abdom Imaging 34(6):737, 2009

Kingston MA, Bansal D, Carlin EM: 'Shelf life' of Trichomonas vaginalis. Int J STD AIDS 14(1):28, 2003

Kirby JP, Mazuski JE: Prevention of surgical site infection. Surg Clin North Am 89(2):365, 2009

Klebanoff MA, Nansel TR, Brotman RM, et al: Personal hygienic behaviors and bacterial vaginosis. Sex Transm Dis 37(2):94, 2010

Komericki P, Akkilic-Materna M, Strimitzer T, et al: Efficacy and safety of imiquimod versus podophyllotoxin in the treatment of anogenital warts. Sex Transm Dis 38(3):216, 2011

Kreisel K, Torrone E, Bernstein K, et al: Prevalence of pelvic inflammatory disease in sexually experienced women of reproductive age—United States, 2013–2014. MMWR 66(3):80, 2017

Krissi H, Shmuely A, Aviram A, et al: Acute Bartholin's abscess: microbial spectrum, patient characteristics, clinical manifestation, and surgical outcomes. Eur J Clin Microbiol Infect Dis 35(3):443, 2016

Kroese JA, van der Velde M, Morssink LP, et al: Word catheter and marsupialisation in women with a cyst or abscess of the Bartholin gland (WoMan-trial): a randomised clinical trial. BJOG 124(2):243, 2017

Kuhar DT, Henderson DK, Struble KA, et al: Updated US Public Health Service guidelines for the management of occupational exposures to human immunodeficiency virus and recommendations for postexposure prophylaxis. Infect Control Hosp Epidemiol 34(9):875, 2013

Lachiewicz MP, Moulton LJ, Jaiyeoba O: Pelvic surgical site infections in gynecologic surgery. Infect Dis Obstet Gynecol 2015:614950, 2015

Laga M, Manoka A, Kivuvu M, et al: Non-ulcerative sexually transmitted diseases as risk factors for HIV-1 transmission in women: results from a cohort study. AIDS 7(1):95, 1993

Lake AG, McPencow AM, Dick-Biascoechea MA, et al: Surgical site infection after hysterectomy. Am J Obstet Gynecol 209(5):490.e1, 2013

Landers DV, Sweet RL: Tubo-ovarian abscess: contemporary approach to management. Rev Infect Dis 5(5):876, 1983

Landers DV, Wiesenfeld HC, Heine RP, et al: Predictive value of the clinical diagnosis of lower genital tract infection in women. Am J Obstet Gynecol 190:1004, 2004

Larsen SA, Steiner BM, Rudolph AH: Laboratory diagnosis and interpretation of tests for syphilis. Clin Microbiol Rev 8:1, 1995

Larsson PG, Bergman B, Försum U, et al: Mobiluncus and clue cells as predictors of pelvic inflammatory disease after first trimester abortion. Acta Obstet Gynecol Scand 68:217, 1989

Larsson PG, Platz-Christensen JJ, Försum U, et al: Clue cells in predicting infections after abdominal hysterectomy. Obstet Gynecol 77:450, 1991

Larsson PG, Platz-Christensen JJ, Thejls H, et al: Incidence of pelvic inflammatory disease after first-trimester legal abortion in women with bacterial vaginosis after treatment with metronidazole: a double-blind, randomized study. Am J Obstet Gynecol 166:100, 1992

Lee W, Kim Y, Chang S, et al: The influence of vitamin C on the urine dipstick tests in the clinical specimens: a multicenter study. J Clin Lab Anal 31(5), 2017

LeFoff J, Pere H, Belec L: Diagnosis of genital herpes simplex virus infection in the clinical laboratory. Virol J 11:83, 2014

Leichliter JS, Chandra A., Aral SO: Correlates of self-reported pelvic inflammatory disease treatment in sexually experienced reproductive aged women in the United States, 1995 and 2006–2010. Sex Transm Dis 40(5):413, 2013

Lillis RA, Nsuami MJ, Myers L, et al: Utility of urine, vaginal, cervical, and rectal specimens for detection of Mycoplasma genitalium in women. J Clin Microbiol 49(5):1990, 2011

Lippes J: Pelvic actinomycosis: a review and preliminary look at prevalence. Am J Obstet Gynecol 180:265, 1999

Liu C, Bayer A, Cosgrove SE, et al: Clinical practice guidelines by the Infectious Diseases Society of America for the treatment of methicillin-resistant Staphylococcus aureus infections in adults and children: executive summary. Clin Infect Dis 52(3):285, 2011

Lis R, Rowhani-Rahbar A, Manhart LE: Mycoplasma genitalium infection and female reproductive tract disease: a meta-analysis. Clin Inf Dis 61(3):418, 2015

Llata E, Braxton J, Asbel L, et al: Rectal Chlamydia trachomatis and Neisseria gonorrhoeae infections among women reporting anal intercourse. Obstet Gynecol 132(3):692, 2018

Lowe NK, Neal JL, Ryan-Wenger NA: Accuracy of the clinical diagnosis of vaginitis compared with a DNA probe laboratory standard. Obstet Gynecol 113(1):89, 2009

Mahdi H, Goodrich S, Lockhart D, et al: Predictors of surgical site infection in women undergoing hysterectomy for benign gynecologic disease: a multicenter analysis using the national surgical quality improvement program data. J Minim Invasive Gynecol 21(5):901, 2014

Mangram AJ, Horan TC, Pearson ML, et al: Guideline for prevention of surgical site infection, 1999. Hospital Infection Control Practices Advisory Committee. Infect Control Hosp Epidemiol 20(4):250, 1999

Manhart LE, Jensen JS, Bradshaw CS, et al: Efficacy of antimicrobial therapy for Mycoplasma genitalium infections. Clin Infect Dis 61(8 Suppl):S802, 2015

Marques AG, Doi AM, Pasternak J, et al: Performance of the dipstick screening test as a predictor of negative urine culture. Einstein (Sao Paulo) 15(1):34, 2017

Martin ET, Krantz E, Gottlieb SL, et al: A pooled analysis of the effect of condoms in preventing HSV-2 acquisition. Arch Intern Med 169(13):1233, 2009

Massad LS, Xie X, Darragh T, et al: Genital warts and vulvar intraepithelial neoplasia: natural history and effects of treatment and human immunodeficiency virus infection. Obstet Gynecol 118:831, 2011

McClelland RS, Sangare L, Hassan WM, et al: Infection with Trichomonas vaginalis increases the risk of HIV-1 acquisition. J Infect Dis 195(5):698, 2007

Meites E, Gaydos CA, Hobbs MM, et al: A review of evidence-based care of symptomatic trichomoniasis and asymptomatic Trichomonas vaginalis Infections. Clin Infect Dis 61(8 Suppl):S837, 2015

Meltzer SM, Monk BJ, Tewari KS: Green tea catechins for treatment of external genital warts. Am J Obstet Gynecol 200(3):233.e1, 2009

Miller RL, Gerster JF, Owens ML, et al: Imiquimod applied topically: a novel immune response modifier and new class of drug. Int J Immunopharmacol 21(1):1, 1999

Mody L, Juthani-Mehta M: Urinary tract infections in older women: a clinical review. JAMA 311(8):844, 2014

Molander P, Sjöberg J, Paavonen J: Transvaginal power Doppler findings in laparoscopically proven acute pelvic inflammatory disease. Ultrasound Obstet Gynecol 17:233, 2001

Morse S, Long J: Infestations. In Morse S, Ballard RC, Holmes KK, et al (eds): Atlas of Sexually Transmitted Diseases. 3rd ed. Edinburgh, Mosby, 2003

Nathan B, Appiah J, Saunders P, et al: Microscopy outperformed in a comparison of five methods for detecting Trichomonas vaginalis in symptomatic women. Int J STD AIDS 26(4):251, 2015

Nelson HD, Helfand M: Screening for chlamydial infection. Am J Prev Med 20(3 Suppl):95, 2001

Ness RB, Hillier SL, Kip KE, et al: Bacterial vaginosis and risk of pelvic inflammatory disease. Obstet Gynecol 104:761, 2004

Ness RB, Kip KE, Hillier SL, et al: A cluster analysis of bacterial vaginosis-associated microflora and pelvic inflammatory disease. Am J Epidemiol 162(6):585, 2005

Newman L, Rowley J, Vander Hoorn S, et al: Estimates of the prevalence and incidence of four curable sexually transmitted infections in 2012 based on systematic review and global reporting. PLoS One 10(12):e0143304, 2015

Nicolle LE, Gupta K, Bradley SF, et al: Clinical practice guideline for the management of asymptomatic bacteriuria: 2019 update by the Infectious Diseases Society of America. Clin Infect Dis 68(10):1611, 2019

Nye MB, Schwebke JR, Body BA: Comparison of APTIMA Trichomonas vaginalis transcription-mediated amplification to wet mount microscopy, culture, and polymerase chain reaction for diagnosis of trichomoniasis in men and women. Am J Obstet Gynecol 200(2):188.e1, 2009

Nyirjesy P, Sobel JD: Genital mycotic infections in patients with diabetes. Postgrad Med 125(3):33, 2013

Owusu Edusei K Jr, Bohm MK, Chesson HW, et al: Chlamydia screening and pelvic inflammatory disease: insights from exploratory time-series analyses. Am J Prev Med 38(6):652, 2010

Panel on Antiretroviral Guidelines for Adults and Adolescents: Guidelines for the use of antiretroviral agents in adults and adolescents living with HIV. 2018. Available at: http://aidsinfo.nih.gov/contentfiles/lvguidelines/AdultandAdolescentGL.pdf. Accessed March 17, 2019

Park IU, Introcaso C, Dunne EF: Human papillomavirus and genital warts: a review of the evidence for the 2015 Centers for Disease Control and Prevention sexually transmitted diseases treatment guidelines. Clin Infect Dis 61(8 Suppl):S849, 2015

Parnham MJ, Erakovic Haber V, et al: Azithromycin: mechanisms of action and their relevance for clinical applications. Pharmacol Ther 143:225, 2014

Patel EU, Gaydos CA, Packman ZR, et al: Prevalence and correlates of Trichomonas vaginalis infection among men and women in the United States. Clin Infect Dis 67(2):211, 2018

Patel HD, Livsey SA, Swann RA, et al: Can urine dipstick testing for urinary tract infection at point of care reduce laboratory workload? J Clin Pathol 58(9):951, 2005

Patton DL, Halbert SA, Kuo CC, et al: Host response to primary Chlamydia trachomatis infection of the fallopian tube in pig-tailed monkeys. Fertil Steril 40:829, 1983

Patton DL, Moore DE, Spadoni LR, et al: A comparison of the fallopian tube's response to overt and silent salpingitis. Obstet Gynecol 73:622, 1989

Peeling RW, Ye H: Diagnostic tools for preventing and managing maternal and congenital syphilis: an overview. Bull World Health Organ 82(6):439, 2004

Persson E, Holmberg K: A longitudinal study of Actinomyces israelii in the female genital tract. Acta Obstet Gynecol Scand 63:207, 1984

Ravel J, Gajer P, Abdo Z, et al: Vaginal microbiome of reproductive-age women. Proc Natl Acad Sci U S A 108 (1 Suppl):4680, 2011

Reed SD, Landers DV, Sweet RL: Antibiotic treatment of tuboovarian abscess: comparison of broad-spectrum beta-lactam agent agents versus clindamycin-containing regimens. Am J Obstet Gynecol 164(6 Pt 1):1556, 1991

Romero L, Huerfano C, Grillo-Ardila CF: Macrolides for treatment of Haemophilus ducreyi infection in sexually active adults. Cochrane Database Syst Rev 12:CD012492, 2017

Romosan G, Bjartling C, Skoog L, et al: Ultrasound for diagnosing acute salpingitis: a prospective observational diagnostic study. Hum Reprod 28(6):1569, 2014

Rubin RH, Shapiro ED, Andriole VT, et al: Evaluation of new anti-infective drugs for the treatment of urinary tract infection. Infectious Diseases Society of America and the Food and Drug Administration. Clin Infect Dis 15(1 Suppl):S216, 1992

Sawyer KP, Stone LL: Evaluation of a leukocyte dip-stick test used for screening urine cultures. J Clin Microbiol 20(4):820, 1984

Schwebke JR, Gaydos CA, Nyirjesy P, et al: Diagnostic performance of a molecular test versus clinician assessment of vaginitis. J Clin Microbiol 56(6):e00252, 2018

Schwebke JR, Morgan FG Jr, Koltun W, et al: A phase-3, double-blind, placebo-controlled study of the effectiveness and safety of single oral doses of secnidazole 2 g for the treatment of women with bacterial vaginosis. Am J Obstet Gynecol 217(6):678.e1, 2017

Selik RM, Mokotoff ED, Branson B, et al: Revised surveillance case definition for HIV infection—United States, 2014. MMWR 63(3):1, 2014

Sellors JW, Mahony JB, Chernesky MA, et al: Tubal factor infertility: an association with prior chlamydial infection and asymptomatic salpingitis. Fertil Steril 49(3):451, 1988

Seña AC, Miller WC, Hobbs MM, et al: Trichomonas vaginalis infection in male sexual partners: implications for diagnosis, treatment, and prevention. Clin Infect Dis 44(1):13, 2007

Senok AC, Verstraelen H, Temmerman M, et al: Probiotics for the treatment of bacterial vaginosis. Cochrane Database Syst Rev 4:CD006289, 2009

Sherrard J, Wilson J, Donders G, et al: 2018 European (IUSTI/WHO) International Union against sexually transmitted infections (IUSTI) World Health Organisation (WHO) guideline on the management of vaginal discharge. Int J STD AIDS 29(13):1258, 2018

Shin H, Iwasaki A: Generating protective immunity against genital herpes. Trends Immunol 34(10):487, 2013

Short VL, Totten PA, Ness RB, et al: Clinical presentation of Mycoplasma genitalium infection versus Neisseria gonorrhoeae infection among women with pelvic inflammatory disease. Clin Infect Dis 48(1):41, 2009

Soper DE, Bump RC, Hurt WG: Bacterial vaginosis and trichomoniasis vaginitis are risk factors for cuff cellulitis after abdominal hysterectomy. Am J Obstet Gynecol 163:1016, 1990

Spence MR, Blanco LJ, Patel J, et al: A comparative evaluation of vaginal, cervical and peritoneal flora in normal, healthy women: a preliminary report. Sex Transm Dis 9(1):37, 1982

Stalenhoef JE, van der Starre WE, Vollaard AM, et al: Hospitalization for community-acquired febrile urinary tract infection: validation and impact assessment of a clinical prediction rule. BMC Infect Dis 17(1):400, 2017

Steiner HL, Strand EA: Surgical-site infection in gynecologic surgery: pathophysiology and prevention. Am J Obstet Gynecol 217(2):121, 2017

Stemmer SM, Mordechai E, Adelson ME, et al: Trichomonas vaginalis is most frequently detected in women at the age of peri-/premenopause: an unusual pattern for a sexually transmitted pathogen. Am J Obstet Gynecol 218(3):328. e1, 2018

Stoner BP, Cohen SE: Lymphogranuloma venereum 2015: clinical presentation, diagnosis, and treatment. Clin Infect Dis 61 (8 Suppl):S865, 2015

Stoner KA, Rabe LK, Meyn LA, et: Survival of Trichomonas vaginalis in wet preparation and on wet mount. Sex Transm Infect 89(6):485, 2013

Susianti H, Lie S: Auto identify discrepancies between urine test strip and sediment results using cross check function on fully automated urine analyzer. Int Clin Pathol J 1(4):87, 2015

Tatti S, Swinehart JM, Thielert C, et al: Sinecatechins, a defined green tea extract, in the treatment of external anogenital warts: a randomized controlled trial. Obstet Gynecol 111(6):1371, 2008

Tepper NK, Steenland MW, Gaffield ME, et al: Retention of intrauterine devices in women who acquire pelvic inflammatory disease: a systematic review. Contraception 87(5):655, 2013

Thurman AR, Satterfield TM, Soper DE: Methicillin-resistant Staphylococcus aureus as a common cause of vulvar abscesses. Obstet Gynecol 112:538, 2008

Tiitinen A, Surcel HM, Halttunen M, et al: Chlamydia trachomatis and chlamydial heat shock protein 60-specific antibody and cell-mediated responses predict tubal factor infertility. Hum Reprod 21(6):1533, 2006

Timor-Tritsch IE, Lerner JP, Monteagudo A, et al: Transvaginal sonographic markers of tubal inflammatory disease. Ultrasound Obstet Gynecol 12(1):56, 1998

Tjiam KH, Zeilmaker GH, Alberda AT, et al: Prevalence of antibodies to Chlamydia trachomatis, Neisseria gonorrhoeae, and Mycoplasma hominis in infertile women. Genitourin Med 61(3):175, 1985

Toth M, Patton DL, Campbell LA, et al: Detection of chlamydial antigenic material in ovarian, prostatic, ectopic pregnancy and semen samples of culture-negative subjects. Am J Reprod Immunol 43(4):218, 2000

Trent M, Coleman JS, Hardick J, et al: Clinical and sexual risk correlates of Mycoplasma genitalium in urban pregnant and non-pregnant young women: cross-sectional outcomes using the baseline data from the Women's BioHealth Study. Sex Transm Infect 94(6):411, 2018

Tyring SK: Molluscum contagiosum: the importance of early diagnosis and treatment. Am J Obstet Gynecol 189(3 Suppl):S12, 2003

Uppal S, Harris J, Al-Niaimi A, et al: Prophylactic antibiotic choice and risk of surgical site infection after hysterectomy. Obstet Gynecol 127(2):321, 2016

U.S. Preventive Services Task Force: Clinical summary. Chlamydia and gonorrhea: screening. 2014. Available at: http://www.uspreventiveservicestaskforce.org/Page/Document/ClinicalSummaryFinal/chlamydia-and-gonorrhea-screening. Accessed April 13, 2019

U.S Preventive Services Task Force: Preexposure prophylaxis for the prevention of HIV infection: recommendation statement. JAMA 321:22, 2019

van der Wouden JC, van der Sande R, Kruithof EJ, et al: Interventions for cutaneous molluscum contagiosum. Cochrane Database Syst Rev 5:CD004767, 2017

Watts DH, Krohn MA, Hillier SL, et al: Bacterial vaginosis as a risk factor for postcesarean endometritis. Obstet Gynecol 75:52, 1990

Weisenfeld HC, Manhart LE: Mycoplasma genitalium in women: current knowledge and research priorities for this recently emerged pathogen. J Inf Dis 216(2 suppl):S389, 2017

Weller S, Davis K: Condom effectiveness in reducing heterosexual HIV transmission. Cochrane Database Syst Rev 1:CD003255, 2002

Wendel GD Jr, Stark BJ, Jamison RB, et al: Penicillin allergy and desensitization in serious infections during pregnancy. N Engl J Med 312:1229, 1985

Werner RN, Westfechtel L, Dressler C, et al: Self-administered interventions for anogenital warts in immunocompetent patients: a systematic review and meta-analysis. Sex Transm Infect 93(3):155, 2017

Westhoff C: IUDs and colonization or infection with Actinomyces. Contraception 75:S48, 2007

Westrom L, Joesoef R, Reynolds G, et al: Pelvic inflammatory disease and fertility. A cohort study of 1,844 women with laparoscopically verified disease and 657 control women with normal laparoscopic results. Sex Transm Dis 19:185, 1992

Wiese W, Patel SR, Patel SC, et al: A meta-analysis of the Papanicolaou smear and wet mount for the diagnosis of vaginal trichomoniasis. Am J Med 108(4):301, 2000

Wiesenfeld HC, Hillier SL, Krohn MA, et al: Bacterial vaginosis is a strong predictor of Neisseria gonorrhoeae and Chlamydia trachomatis infection. Clin Infect Dis 36(5):663, 2003

Wiesenfeld HC, Hillier SL, Meyn LA, et al: Subclinical pelvic inflammatory disease and infertility. Obstet Gynecol 120(1):37, 2012

Wiesenfeld HC, Sweet RL, Ness RB, et al: Comparison of acute and subclinical pelvic inflammatory disease. Sex Transm Dis 32(7):400, 2005

Williams JA, Ofner S, Batteiger BE, et al: Duration of polymerase chain reaction-detectable DNA after treatment of Chlamydia trachomatis, Neisseria gonorrhoeae, and Trichomonas vaginalis infections in women. Sex Transm Dis 41(3):215, 2014

Wilson J: Managing recurrent bacterial vaginosis. Sex Transm Infect 80:8, 2004

Xie HY, Feng D, Wei DM, et al: Probiotics for vulvovaginal candidiasis in non-pregnant women. Cochrane Database Syst Rev 11: CD010496, 2017

Yan J, Chen SL, Wang HN, et al: Meta-analysis of 5% imiquimod and 0.5% podophyllotoxin in the treatment of condylomata acuminata. Dermatology 213(3):218, 2006

CHAPTER 4

Benign Disorders of the Lower Reproductive Tract

The lower reproductive tract, comprising the vulva, vagina, and cervix, exhibits a wide spectrum of benign and neoplastic diseases. Disorder characteristics often overlap, and thus differentiating normal variants, benign disease, and potentially serious lesions can be challenging. Lower reproductive tract infection is a frequent cause and discussed in Chapter 3 (p. 56), whereas congenital anomalies and preinvasive neoplasia are infrequent and described in Chapters 19 (p. 406) and 29 (p. 620). The benign lesions highlighted in this chapter are common, and mastery of their identification and treatment is essential.

VULVAR LESIONS

Vulvar skin is more permeable than surrounding tissues because of differences in structure, hydration, occlusion, and susceptibility to friction (Farage, 2004). Accordingly, pathology can develop in this area, although frequency estimates are difficult because of patient underreporting and clinician misdiagnosis. Lesions may develop from allergen or irritant exposure, infection, trauma, autoimmunity, or neoplasia. As a result, symptoms may be acute or chronic and include pain, pruritus, dyspareunia, bleeding, and discharge, which all may affect a woman's sense of well-being. Effective therapies are available for most disorders, yet embarrassment and fear may be significant roadblocks for many women.

■ General Approach

The initial encounter includes reassurance that the patient's complaints will be investigated thoroughly. Women often minimize and may be uncomfortable with describing their symptoms. They may describe protracted histories of assorted diagnoses and treatments by numerous providers and may voice frustration and doubt that relief is possible. Patients are not promised a cure but rather that efforts will be made to control their symptoms. This can require multiple visits, tissue sampling, treatment attempts, and even a multidisciplinary plan. A patient-provider partnership approach to management enhances compliance and satisfaction with care. Patients are often relieved to learn that their complaints and conditions are not unique. Thus, referral to national websites and support groups is usually welcomed.

■ Diagnosis

History

Scheduling adequate time for the initial evaluation is a wise investment, and detailed patient questionnaires are invaluable. First, symptoms are clarified as to their onset, duration, precise location, and association with vaginal complaints. Vulvar pruritus is often referred to as "vaginal," thus symptom location is ideally clarified. A thorough medical history addresses systemic illnesses, medications, and known allergies. Obstetric, sexual, and psychosocial histories and any potentially provocative events around the time of symptom onset often suggest etiologies. Hygiene and sexual practices are investigated in detail.

Of symptoms, vulvar pruritus is frequent with many dermatoses. Patients may have been previously diagnosed with psoriasis, eczema, or dermatitis at other body sites. Isolated vulvar pruritus may be associated with a new medication. Most often, vulvar pruritus stems from an irritant or allergic contact dermatitis. Common offenders include urine, moist wipes, or washing with strongly scented body soaps or laundry products. Excessive washing and use of wash cloths can result in skin drying and mechanical trauma. Washing often becomes more aggressive with pruritus as patients assume their hygiene is lacking. Any of these practices can create an escalating itch-scratch cycle or exacerbate the symptoms of other preexisting dermatoses. Last, patients frequently use nonprescription remedies for relief of vulvovaginal itching or perceived odor. These products commonly contain multiple known contact allergens, and their use is discouraged (Table 4-1).

TABLE 4-1. Common Vulvar Irritants and Allergens[a]

General Categories	Examples
Antiseptics	Povidone iodine, hexachlorophene
Body fluids	Semen or saliva
Body soaps	Scented soaps, bath salts, shampoos, conditioners
Condoms	Lubricant or spermicide containing
Contraceptive creams, jellies, foams	Nonoxynol-9, lubricants
Dyes	
Emollients	Lanolin, jojoba oil, glycerin
Toilet paper	Colored or scented
Laundry products	Detergents, softeners, dryer sheets
Rubber products	Including latex
Menstrual products	Pad, tampons
Sanitary wipes	Adult or baby wipes
Tea tree oil	
Topical agents:	
Anesthetics	Benzocaine, lidocaine, dibucaine
Antibacterials	Neomycin, bacitracin, polymyxin
Antimycotics	Imidazoles, nystatin
Corticosteroids	
Medications	TCA, 5-FU, podofilox or podophyllin
Vaginal hygiene products	Perfumes, deodorants

5-FU = 5-fluorouracil; TCA = trichloroacetic acid.
[a]Categories arranged alphabetically.
Compiled from American College of Obstetricians and Gynecologists, 2016a; Marren, 1992; Margesson, 2004.

Physical Examination

Examination of the vulva and surrounding skin is completed using adequate lighting, optimal patient positioning, and a magnifying lens. Both focal and generalized skin changes are carefully noted, as neoplasia may arise within a field of generalized dermatosis. Abnormal pigmentation, skin texture, nodularity, or vascularity is evaluated. Touch with a small blunt probe such as a cotton swab defines the anatomic boundaries of generalized symptoms and precisely locates focal complaints (Fig. 4-1). Both photographs and diagrams noting vulvar findings and symptoms can be stored in the medical record to aid treatment assessment over time.

Vaginal complaints or vulvar conditions without obvious etiology typically prompt vaginal examination. Careful inspection may reveal generalized inflammation or atrophy, abnormal discharge, or focal mucosal lesions such as erosions. In these cases, saline preparation of secretions for microscopic evaluation ("wet prep"), vaginal pH testing, potassium hydroxide (KOH) testing, and a standard genital aerobic culture are collected to detect a possible etiology.

A general skin examination, including the oral mucosa and axillae, may suggest the cause of some vulvar conditions. A focused neurologic examination to evaluate lower extremity sensation and strength as well as perineal sensation and tone may help evaluate vulvar dysesthesias.

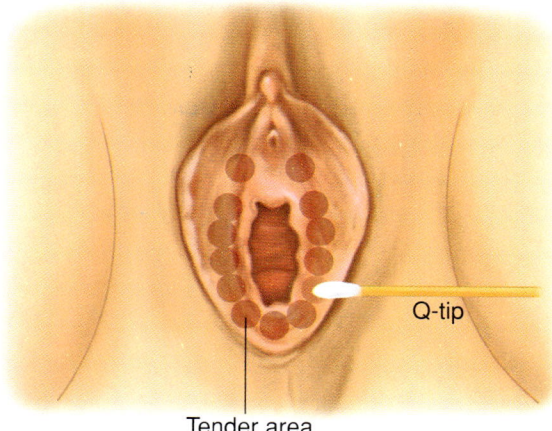

Tender area   Q-tip

FIGURE 4-1 Pain can be assessed and mapped by systematically touching a cotton-tip applicator to the vulva.

Vulvar Biopsy

Vulvar skin changes are frequently nonspecific and may require biopsy for accurate diagnosis. Biopsy is recommended if the cause of symptoms is not obvious; if focal, hyper-/hypopigmented, or exophytic lesions are present; or if initial empiric treatment fails. During biopsy, ulcerative and erosive lesions are sampled at their edges, whereas indurated areas are biopsied in their thickest region (Mirowski, 2004). Conditions with multiple morphologies may require more than one biopsy for diagnosis.

The steps for vulvar biopsy are shown in **Figure 4-2**. First, the biopsy site is cleaned with an antimicrobial agent and infiltrated with a 1- or 2-percent lidocaine solution. Biopsy is performed most easily with a Keyes skin punch. Its open, circular blade is designed to remove a shallow disc of tissue when gently pressed against the skin and rotated. Keyes punches are available in various diameters, which range from 2 to 6 mm. Size selection is based on lesion dimensions and on clinical goals of sampling versus excision. Vulvar skin and lesion thicknesses vary, and these are assessed prior to biopsy to avoid over-rotation of or undue pressure on the Keyes punch. Too deep a biopsy will leave a depressed scar. Rotation and pressure should ideally stop when decreased resistance is felt, signaling the dermis has been reached. The tissue disc core is then freed at its base with fine scissors. Larger punch biopsies (4- to 6-mm) may require closure with an absorbable suture or gelfoam.

For raised or pedunculated lesions, fine scissors may be used. Occasionally, a no. 15 blade scalpel is selected for larger focal lesions. Tissue is excised parallel to the natural skin folds, and if needed, the defect is sutured to aid healing and minimize scarring.

An alternative sampling technique is *modified snip excision*. With this, a stitch is begun on one side of the lesion and advanced beneath it to exit on the opposite side. The tissue is gently tented upward, and fine Gradle scissors are used to snip below the stitch to remove an ellipse of tissue. Larger lesions, for which simple closure would create significant incision tension, may be removed as in a wide local excision (Chap. 43, p. 1006).

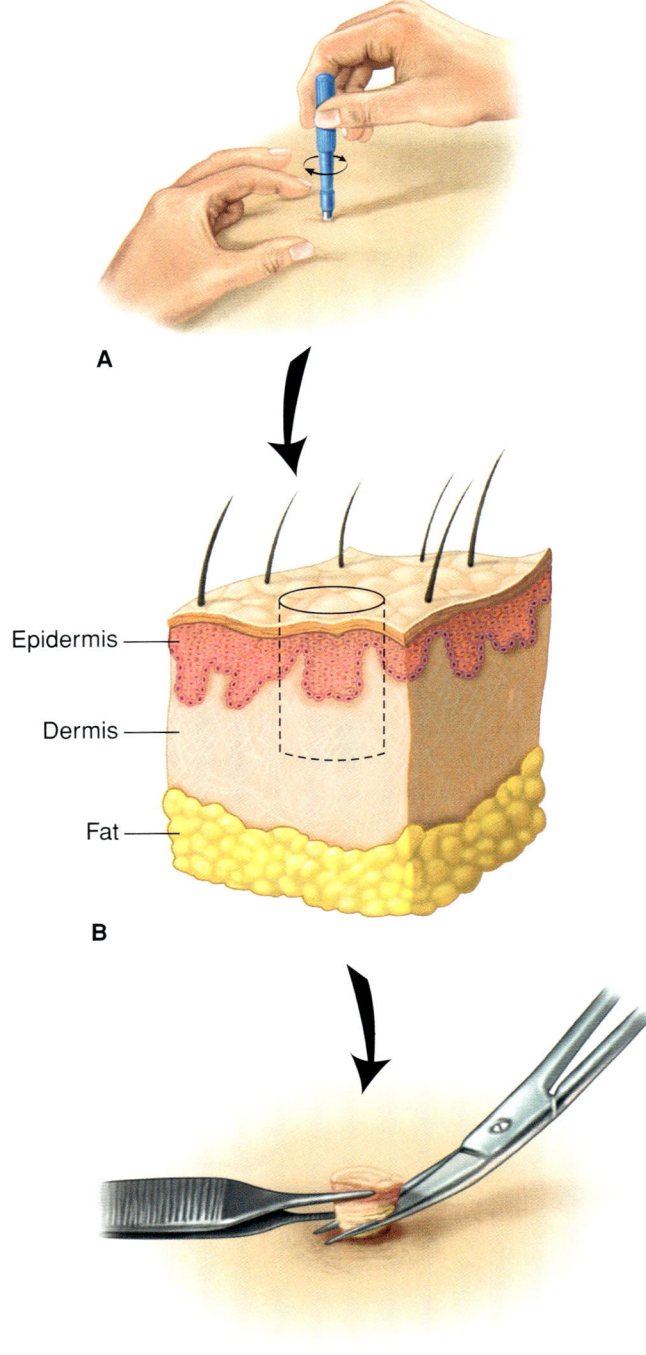

A

Epidermis

Dermis

Fat

B

C

FIGURE 4-2 Vulvar biopsy steps. **A.** A Keyes punch biopsy is placed against the biopsy site. Gentle downward pressure is exerted as the punch is rotated. **B.** A core biopsy is created that extends through the epidermis and into the dermis. **C.** The tip of a fine needle is used to elevate the core, while fine scissors incise its base.

Following biopsy, direct pressure with topical aluminum chloride, Monsel paste, or silver nitrate stick can control bleeding. The last two may permanently discolor the skin and confuse subsequent examinations. If needed, simple interrupted stitches using a fine, rapidly absorbable suture provide hemostasis and edge approximation. Nonnarcotic oral analgesics generally relieve postbiopsy discomfort, if present.

VULVAR DERMATOSES

■ Lichen Simplex Chronicus

The International Society for the Study of Vulvovaginal Disease (ISSVD) provides classification systems for vulvar abnormalities (Lynch, 2007, 2012). Of these, lichen simplex chronicus originates from an itch-scratch cycle that leads to chronic trauma from rubbing and scratching (Lynch, 2004). The skin responds by thickening with exaggerated gray, leathery-appearing skin markings termed *lichenification*. Skin changes are usually bilateral and symmetric and may extend beyond the labia majora. Intense vulvar pruritus causes functional and psychologic distress, and sleep is often disrupted. This is often the end stage of other dermatologic conditions that include lichen sclerosus, atopic dermatitis, or psoriasis. Other irritants such as tight clothing, heat, sweating, or products listed in Table 4-1 may cause this condition (Virgili, 2003). Finally, neurologic or psychiatric disorders may results in repetitive scratching and are ideally addressed (Guerrero, 2015). A detailed history typically leads to the diagnosis.

Treatment involves halting the itch-scratch cycle. First, provocative stimuli are eliminated, and topical corticosteroid ointments help reduce inflammation. In addition, lubricants, such as plain petrolatum or vegetable oil, and cool sitz baths help to restore the skin's barrier function. Oral antihistamine use, trimmed fingernails, and cotton gloves worn at night can help decrease scratching during sleep. Depending on the degree of inflammation, treatment from 4 to 12 weeks is needed to alleviate symptoms. Histology classically shows thickening of both the epidermis (acanthosis) and the stratum corneum (hyperkeratosis). This condition often reoccurs, thus education and maintenance therapy with bland emollients is important. In refractory cases, questions regarding new irritant exposures and a trial of higher potency corticosteroid are reasonable. If symptoms fail to resolve, biopsy is indicated to exclude other pathology.

■ Lichen Sclerosus

This classically presents in postmenopausal women and prepubertal girls, although cases are found less often in premenopausal women and men (Fig. 15-8, p. 325). In one referral dermatologic clinic, lichen sclerosus was found in 1:300 to 1:1000 patients with a tendency toward whites (Goldstein, 2005a). Others estimate an incidence of childhood lichen sclerosus to be 1 in 900 (Powell, 2001).

The cause of lichen sclerosus remains unknown, although infectious, hormonal, genetic, and autoimmune etiologies have been suggested. Approximately 20 to 30 percent of patients with lichen sclerosus have other autoimmune disorders, such as Graves disease, types 1 and 2 diabetes mellitus, systemic lupus erythematosus, and achlorhydria, with or without pernicious anemia (Bor, 1969; Kahana, 1985; Poskitt, 1993). Accordingly, concurrent testing for these is indicated if other suggestive findings are present.

Diagnosis

Although sometimes asymptomatic, most individuals with lichen sclerosus complain of anogenital symptoms that often

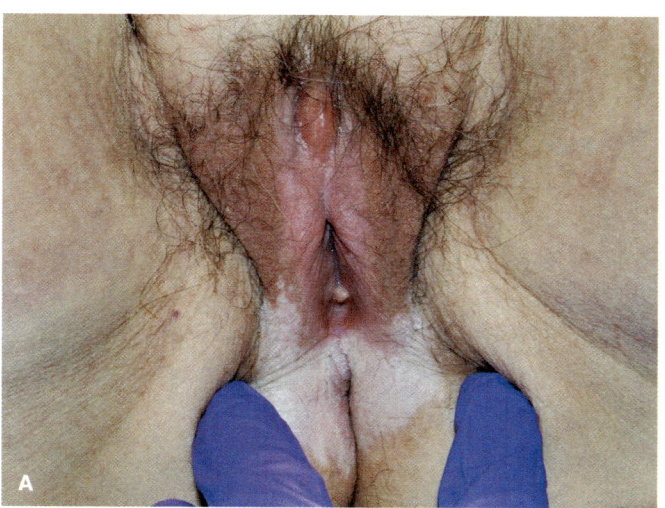
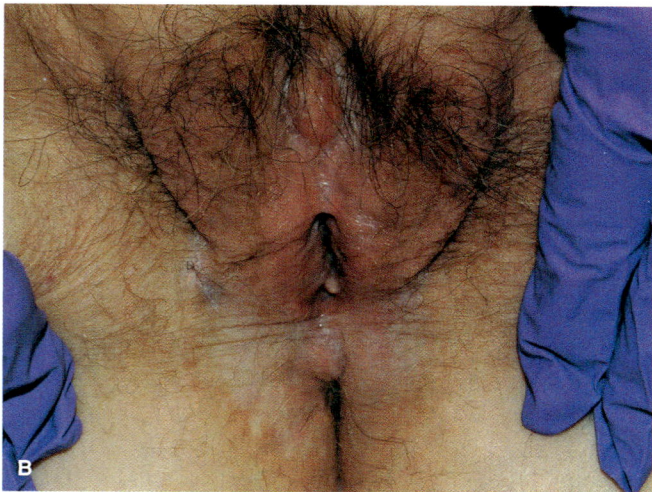

FIGURE 4-3 Vulvar lichen sclerosus. **A.** Note the thin and pale vulvar skin, loss of labia minora architecture, labia minora fusion beneath the clitoris, and hourglass distribution around vulva and anus. **B.** Skin fullness and texture improved following several weeks of topical corticosteroid ointment. (Reproduced with permission from Dr. David D. Rahn.)

worsen at night. Inflammation of local terminal nerve fibers is suspected. Pruritus-induced scratching creates a repetitive cycle that may lead to excoriations and vulvar skin thickening. Late symptoms can include burning and dyspareunia due to vulvar skin fragility and structural changes.

Perianal involvement is frequently seen. The typical white, atrophic papules may coalesce into porcelain-white plaques that distort normal vulvar anatomy. As a result, labia minora regression, clitoral concealment, urethral obstruction, and introital stenosis can develop. The skin generally appears thinned and crinkled. Over time, involvement may extend to the perineum and anus to form a "figure-eight" or "hourglass" shape (Fig. 4-3) (American College of Obstetricians and Gynecologists, 2016a). Thickened white plaques, areas of erythema, or nodularity should prompt biopsy to exclude preinvasive and malignant lesions. This characteristic clinical picture and histologic findings typically confirm the diagnosis. In long-standing cases, histologic findings may be nonspecific, and clinical suspicion will guide treatment.

Treatment and Surveillance

Curative therapies are not available for lichen sclerosus. Thus, treatment goals are symptom control and prevention of anatomic distortion. Despite its classification as a nonneoplastic dermatosis, patients with lichen sclerosus have a higher risk of vulvar malignancy. Malignant transformation within lichen sclerosus develops in 5 percent of patients in whom histologic cellular atypia may precede a diagnosis of invasive squamous cell carcinoma. Accordingly, lifetime surveillance of women with lichen sclerosus every 6 to 12 months is suggested (Lee, 2015). Persistently symptomatic, new, or changing lesions are biopsied (American College of Obstetricians and Gynecologists, 2016a).

As with all vulvar disorders, hygiene recommendations focus on minimizing chemical and mechanical skin irritation (Table 4-2). The chronicity of lichen sclerosus and lack of cure elicits an array of emotions. Support groups dedicated to this condition, such as that found at www.lichensclerosus.org, offer needed psychologic support.

Corticosteroids. First-line therapy is an ultrapotent topical corticosteroid preparation, which offers effective antiinflammatory, antipruritic, and vasoconstrictive properties. Examples are 0.05-percent clobetasol propionate, 0.05-percent halobetasol propionate, or 0.05-percent betamethasone dipropionate ointment. Ointment formulations are preferred to creams due to their protective and less irritating properties (Table 4-3). Common side effects such as striae and telangiectasias can develop if medication is used incorrectly. Theoretic adrenocorticosuppression and iatrogenic Cushing syndrome may be risks if topical corticosteroid preparations are used in large doses for extended periods.

Treatment initiation within 2 years of symptom onset usually prevents significant scarring, but no treatment scheme is universally accepted for topical corticosteroid use. Current recommendations are once- to twice-daily treatment for up

---

TABLE 4-2. Vulvar Hygiene Recommendations

Avoid using gels, scented bath products, moisturizing wipes, and soaps, as they may contain irritants

Avoid douching

Use aqueous creams to clean the vulva and thoroughly rinse with tepid water

Avoid using a harsh washcloth to clean the vulva

After bathing, sparingly apply an emollient, such as plain petrolatum, to moist vulva epithelium

Dab the vulva gently to dry

Avoid wearing tight-fitting pants

Select white cotton underwear

Avoid washing undergarments in commercial washing detergents. Wash and rinse these items separately. Consider using a multirinse process with cold water to remove any remaining detergent residue

Consider wearing skirts and no underwear at home and at night to avoid friction and aid drying

TABLE 4-3. Topical Medication Guide

Steroid Class Potency	Generic Name	Brand Names (available forms)
Ultrapotent	Betamethasone dipropionate augmented 0.05% Clobetasol propionate 0.05% Diflorasone 0.05% Halobetasol propionate 0.05%	Diprolene (oint., gel) Temovate (cream, gel, oint.) Psorcon (cream, oint.) Ultravate (cream, oint.)
High	Amcinonide 0.1% Betamethasone dipropionate 0.05% Desoximetasone 0.05%, 0.25% Diflorasone diacetate 0.05% Fluocinonide 0.05% Fluocinolone acetonide 0.2% Halcinonide 0.1% Triamcinolone 0.5%	Cyclocort (cream, oint., lotion) Diprolene, Diprosone (cream) Topicort (cream) Psorcon (cream, oint.) Lidex (cream, gel, oint.) Synalar-HP (cream) Halog (cream, oint., solution) Aristocort, Kenalog (cream, oint.)
Intermediate	Betamethasone valerate 0.1% Desonide 0.05% Fluocinolone acetonide 0.025% Flurandrenolide 0.025%, 0.05% Fluticasone 0.005%, 0.05% Hydrocortisone butyrate 0.1% Hydrocortisone valerate 0.2% Mometasone furoate 0.1% Prednicarbate 0.1% Triamcinolone 0.025%, 0.1%	Valisone (cream, lotion, oint.) DesOwen (cream, oint., lotion) Synalar (cream, oint.) Cordran (cream, oint.) Cutivate 0.005% (oint.), 0.05% (cream) Locoid (cream, oint., solution) Westcort (cream, oint.) Elocon (cream, oint., lotion) Dermatop (cream, oint.) Aristocort, Kenalog (cream, oint., lotion)
Low	Alclometasone dipropionate 0.05% Betamethasone valerate 0.01% Fluocinolone acetonide 0.01% Hydrocortisone 1%, 2.5%	Aclovate (cream, oint.) Valisone (cream, lotion) Synalar (solution) Generic OTC versions 1% or 2.5% (cream, oint., lotion)

Oint. = ointment; OTC = over the counter.

to three months depending on disease thickness. Studies now show that maintenance therapy of three times weekly, even in asymptomatic patients, significantly decreases the development of squamous cell carcinoma (Lee, 2015). During initial treatment, some patients may also require oral antihistamines, particularly at night, to control itching.

Corticosteroids can also be injected into affected areas, a treatment offered by specialty clinics familiar with techniques and potential complications. One study of eight patients evaluated the efficacy of once-monthly intralesional infiltration of 25 to 30 mg of triamcinolone hexacetonide for a total of 3 months. Severity scores declined in all categories including symptoms, gross appearance, and histopathologic findings (Mazdisnian, 1999).

Other Topical Treatments. *Estrogen cream* is not a primary therapy for lichen sclerosus. However, its addition is indicated for menopausal atrophy, labial fusion, and dyspareunia. Testosterone ointment has failed to show efficacy in trials and is no longer recommended (Bornstein, 1998; Sideri, 1994). *Retinoids* historically used in the past for lichen sclerosus have fallen out of favor given their epithelial irritation side effects. *Topical calcineurin inhibitors* such as tacrolimus (Protopic) and

pimecrolimus (Elidel) have antiinflammatory and immuno-modulating effects. These are indicated for moderate to severe eczema and have been evaluated for lichen sclerosus (Goldstein, 2011; Hengge, 2006). However, one double-blind, randomized study found topical clobetasol propionate to be more effective in treating vulvar lichen sclerosus than topical tacrolimus (Funaro, 2014). In the face of Food and Drug Administration (FDA) (2015) concerns regarding its link to various cancers, clinicians ideally exercise caution when prescribing tacrolimus for extended periods.

Last, *phototherapy* after pretreatment using 5-aminolevulinic acid was investigated in one small series of 12 postmenopausal women with advanced lichen sclerosus. Significant reductions in patient symptoms and short-term improvement for up to 9 months were noted (Hillemanns, 1999). Fractionated carbon dioxide (CO_2) laser has been combined with long-term topical corticosteroids for severe hypertrophic lichen sclerosus (Lee, 2016). However, it is not FDA approved for treatment of lichen sclerosus, and additional studies are needed.

Surgery. Surgical intervention is reserved for significant sequelae and not for primary treatment of uncomplicated lichen sclerosus. For introital stenosis, Rouzier and coworkers (2002)

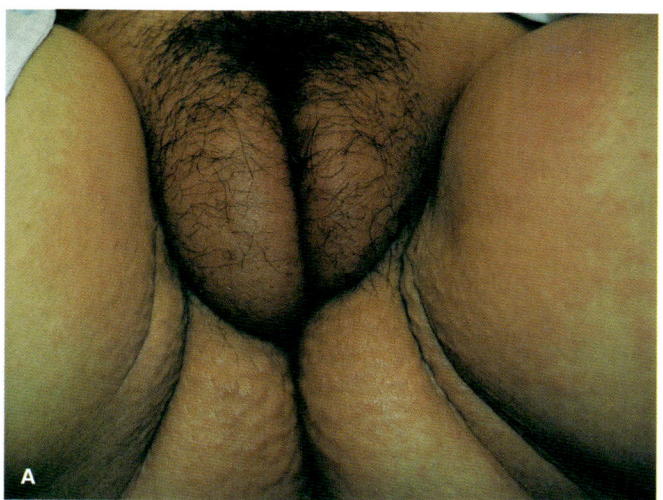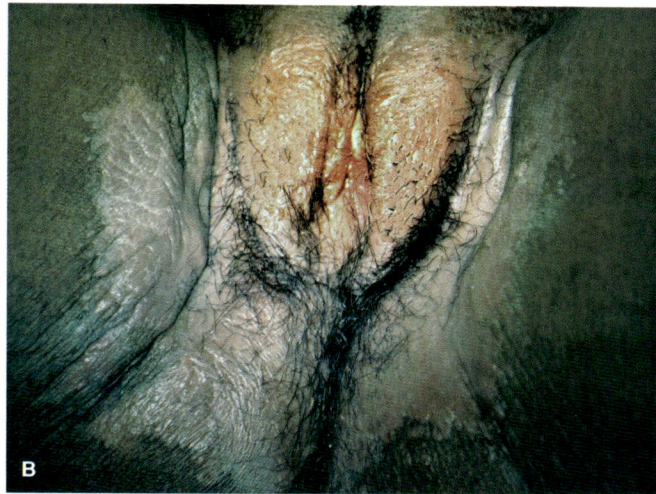

FIGURE 4-4 Vulvar contact dermatitis. **A.** Reaction to povidone-iodine solution. Contact sites show symmetric erythema and edema on the vulva, inner thighs, and buttocks. (Reproduced with permission from Dr. Alicia N. Kiszka.) **B.** Chronic dermatitis creates thick, leathery skin.

described marked improvements in dyspareunia and quality of sexual intercourse if perineoplasty was performed (Chap. 43, p. 988). Vaginal dilation and corticosteroids are recommended following most surgical corrections of introital stenosis. For symptomatic clitoral adhesions, surgical dissection can be used to free the hood from the glans. Reagglutination can be averted using nightly application of ultrapotent topical corticosteroid ointment. After the surgical site is healed, clobetasol application is decreased to twice weekly (Goldstein, 2007).

■ Inflammatory Dermatoses

Contact Dermatitis

A primary irritant or allergen creates vulvar skin inflammation, termed *contact dermatitis* (Fig. 4-4). This condition is common and affects all ages. In unexplained cases of vulvar pruritus and inflammation, irritant contact dermatitis is diagnosed in up to 54 percent of patients (Fischer, 1996).

Irritant contact dermatitis classically presents as immediate burning and stinging upon exposure to an offending agent. In contrast, patients with *allergic contact dermatitis* experience a delayed onset and an intermittent course of pruritus and localized erythema, edema, and vesicles or bullae (Margesson, 2004). A detailed history will help distinguish between the two and help identify the irritant (see Table 4-1).

With allergic contact dermatitis, patch testing may aid in identifying responsible allergen(s). Associated conditions, such as candidiasis, psoriasis, seborrheic dermatitis, and squamous cell carcinoma, can be excluded through appropriate use of cultures and biopsy. Classic histologic features are mild spongiosis, epidermal cell necrosis, and neutrophilic infiltrate of the epidermis.

Treatments for both entities involve elimination of the offending agent(s), restoration of the natural protective skin barrier, inflammation reduction, and scratch cessation (Table 4-4) (Farage, 2004; Margesson, 2004).

Intertrigo

Friction between moist skin surfaces produces this chronic condition. Found most often in labiocrural folds, intertrigo can also develop in the inguinal or intergluteal regions or below a lower abdominal panniculus. Superimposed bacterial and fungal infections may complicate the condition.

If untreated, the initial erythematous phase can progress to intense inflammation with erosions, exudate, fissuring, maceration, and crusting (Mistiaen, 2004). Symptoms typically include burning and itching. With long-standing intertrigo, hyperpigmentation and verrucous changes can develop.

Treatment entails the use of drying agents such as antifungal powders or zinc oxide paste and application of mild topical corticosteroids for inflammation. If skin changes do not respond, then seborrheic dermatitis, psoriasis, atopic dermatitis, pemphigus vegetans, or even scabies are considered. If the area is superinfected with bacteria or yeast, directed therapy is provided (Chap. 3, p. 65).

TABLE 4-4. Treatment of Vulvar Contact Dermatitis

1. Stop offending agents and/or practices
2. Correct vulvar skin barrier function
   a. Sitz bath twice daily with plain water
   b. Application of plain petrolatum
3. Treat any underlying infection
   a. Oral antifungal therapy
   b. Oral antibiotic administration
4. Reduce inflammation
   a. Topical corticosteroids twice daily for 1–3 weeks
      i. 0.05% clobetasol propionate ointment
      ii. 0.1% triamcinolone ointment
   b. Systemic corticosteroids for severe irritation
5. Break the itch-scratch cycle
   a. Cool packs (avoid ice packs, which may injure skin)
   b. Plain, cold yogurt on a sanitary napkin for 5–10 minutes
   c. Consider an SSRI (sertraline [Zoloft] 50–100 mg) or an antihistamine (hydroxyzine [Vistaril] 25–100 mg)

SSRI = selective serotonin-reuptake inhibitor.

To prevent recurrences, obese patients are encouraged to lose weight. Other preventions include light-weight, loose-fitting clothing made of natural fibers, improved skin ventilation, and thorough drying between skin folds after bathing (Janniger, 2005).

Atopic Dermatitis

This classically presents in the first 5 years of life as a severe pruritic eruption. Scaly patches with fissuring are evident. Atopic dermatitis follows a chronic, relapsing course, and affected individuals may later develop allergic rhinitis and asthma (Spergel, 2003).

Topical corticosteroids and immunomodulators, such as tacrolimus, can control flares (Leung, 2004). For dry skin, moisturizing with emollients can offer relief.

Psoriasis

Approximately 1 to 2 percent of the United States' population is affected by psoriasis (Gelfand, 2005). Psoriasis is a T-cell–mediated autoimmune process in which proinflammatory cytokines induce keratinocyte and endothelial cell proliferation. Typically, thick, red plaques covered with silvery scales are found on extensor limb surfaces. Occasionally, lesions involve the mons pubis or labia. Here, vulvar plaques are well defined and dull red and often lack the characteristic silver scale of psoriasis (Fig. 4-5). Psoriasis can be exacerbated by nervous stress and menses, with remissions experienced during summer months and pregnancy. Pruritus may be minimal or absent, and this condition is often diagnosed by skin findings alone.

For treatment, topical corticosteroids are widely used because of their rapid efficacy. High-potency corticosteroids are applied to affected areas twice daily for 2 to 4 weeks and then reduced to weekly applications. Diminishing response and skin atrophy are potential disadvantages of long-term corticosteroid use, and recalcitrant cases are best managed by a dermatologist. Vitamin D analogues, such as calcipotriene (Dovonex), are similar in efficacy to potent corticosteroids and avoid skin atrophy. However, these are frequently associated with local irritation (Smith, 2006). Phototherapy offers short-term relief, but long-term treatment plans require a multidisciplinary team (Griffiths, 2000). For moderate to severe psoriasis, several FDA-approved immunomodulating biologic agents are available such as infliximab, adalimumab, etanercept, and ustekinumab (Smith, 2009).

Lichen Planus

This uncommon disease involves both cutaneous and mucosal surfaces and affects genders equally between ages 30 and 60 years (Mann, 1991). Genital lichen planus affects 1 to 2 percent of the general United States' population (Zendels, 2015).

Although not completely understood, T-cell–mediated autoimmunity directed against basal keratinocytes is thought to underlie its pathogenesis (Goldstein, 2005b). Lichen planus may be drug-induced, and nonsteroidal antiinflammatory drugs, β-blocking agents, methyldopa, penicillamine, and quinine drugs have been implicated. Vulvar lichen planus can present as one of three variants: (1) erosive, (2) papulosquamous, or (3) hypertrophic. Of these, erosive lichen planus is the most common vulvovaginal form and the most difficult variant to treat.

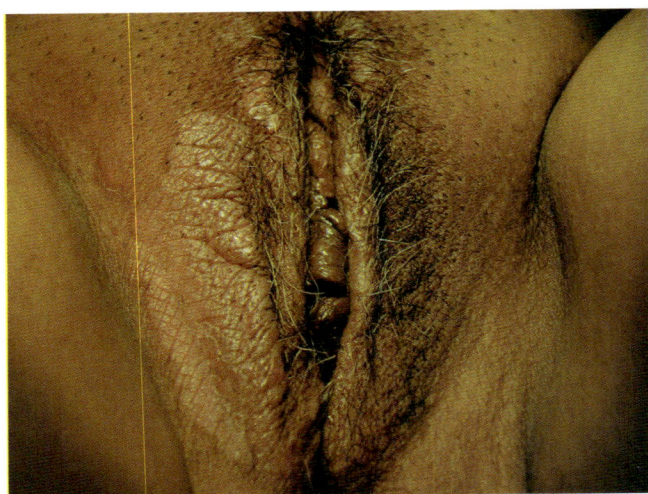

FIGURE 4-5 Psoriasis. Raised plaques are seen on the vulva. (Reproduced with permission from Dr. Saly Thomas.)

Diagnosis. Table 4-5 summarizes the most common imitations of lichen planus. Women typically complain of chronic vaginal discharge with intense vulvovaginal pruritus, burning pain, dyspareunia, and postcoital bleeding. On inspection, papules classically are brightly erythematous or violaceous, flat-topped, shiny polygons. These are most commonly found on the trunk, buccal mucosa, or extremity flexor surfaces (Goldstein, 2005b; Zellis, 1996). Lacy, white striations (Wickham striae) are frequently found in conjunction with the papules and may also be present on the buccal mucosa (Fig. 4-6). In the posterior vestibule, well-defined erosions can extend to the labia, resulting in agglutination. With speculum insertion, vulvar skin and vaginal mucosa may bleed easily, and a copious vaginal discharge may be present. Vaginal erosions can produce adhesions and synechiae, which may lead to vaginal obliteration.

TABLE 4-5. Differential Diagnosis of Lichen Planus

Class of Lichen Planus	Mimicking Condition
Erosive lichen planus	Lichen sclerosus
	Pemphigoid vulgaris
	Mucous membrane pemphigoid
	Behçet disease
	Plasma cell vulvitis
	Erythema multiforme major
	Stephen-Johnson syndrome
	Desquamative inflammatory vaginitis
Papulosquamous lichen planus	Molluscum contagiosum
	Genital warts
Hypertrophic lichen planus	Squamous cell carcinoma

Compiled from Goldstein, 2005b; Kaufman, 1974; Moyal-Barracco, 2004.

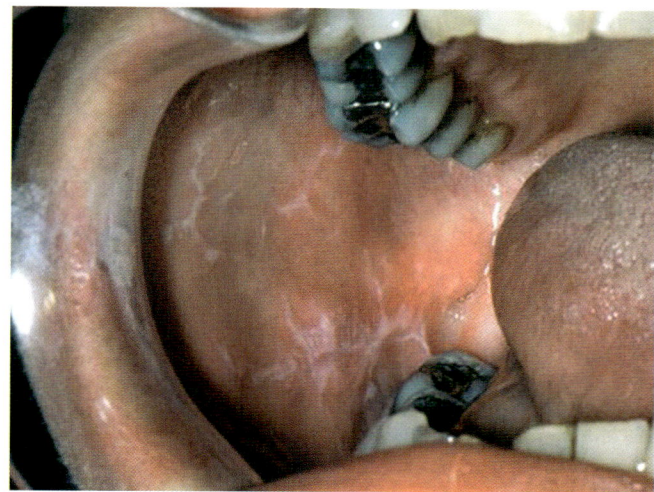

FIGURE 4-6 Oral lichen planus. Mucosal lesions manifest commonly as lacy, white striations (Wickham striae), although white papules or plaques, erosions, or blisters may also be seen. Oral lesions predominantly affect the buccal mucosa, tongue, and gingiva. (Reproduced with permission from Dr. Edward Ellis.)

Women with suspected lichen planus require a thorough dermatologic survey looking for extragenital lesions. Nearly one quarter of women with oral lesions will have vulvovaginal involvement, and most with erosive vulvovaginal lichen planus have oral involvement (Cooper, 2006). Diagnosis is confirmed by biopsy of the linear, white border at the junction of normal skin and erosive disease.

Vulvar Lichen Planus Treatment. Pharmacotherapy remains the first-line treatment for this condition. Additionally, vulvar hygiene, discontinuing any medications associated with lichenoid changes, and psychologic support are instituted.

Erosive vulvar lichen planus is treated initially with ultrapotent topical corticosteroid ointments. One regimen is 0.05-percent clobetasol propionate applied daily for up to 3 months and then slowly tapered. Refractory cases are common, and nearly

40 percent of patients will need more than one treatment to control disease progression (Bradford, 2013).

Vaginal Lichen Planus Treatment. Commonly prescribed to treat hemorrhoids, corticosteroid suppositories containing 25 mg of hydrocortisone and used vaginally can be helpful. In one regimen, these are inserted twice daily, and then the dosage is tapered for symptom remission maintenance (Anderson, 2002). For poorly responding patients, compounding pharmacies can provide a 100-mg hydrocortisone suppository. Potent corticosteroids are prescribed judiciously, as systemic absorption may lead to adrenocorticosuppression (Moyal-Barracco, 2004). Combining local corticosteroid therapy with vaginal dilator use may help restore coital function in patients with moderate vaginal synechiae.

If topical medications fail for either vulvar or vaginal lichen planus, systemic treatment with prednisone 40 to 60 mg daily for up to 4 weeks may modulate symptoms (Moyal-Barracco, 2004). Although no alternative systemic medications have been fully studied, methotrexate, hydroxychloroquine, and mycophenolate mofetil administered by providers familiar with their use are effective within a multidisciplinary approach (Eisen, 1993; Frieling, 2003; Lundqvist, 2002). Surgical adhesiolysis is a last resort. In general, vulvovaginal lichen planus is a chronic, recurrent disease for which symptomatic improvement is possible, but complete control is unlikely.

Hidradenitis Suppurativa

This chronic disease is manifested by recurrent papular inflammatory lesions that may lead to abscess, fistula formation, and scarring predominantly in apocrine gland–bearing skin (Fig. 4-7). In order of frequency, affected areas include the axillae; inguinal, perianal, and perineal skin; inframammary regions; and retroauricular skin. Chronic inflammation obstructs skin follicles, and subcutaneous abscess formation, skin thickening, and deformity follows. Abscesses typically form sinus tracts, and the resulting disfigurement and chronic purulent drainage can be devastating physically, emotionally, and sexually. Described

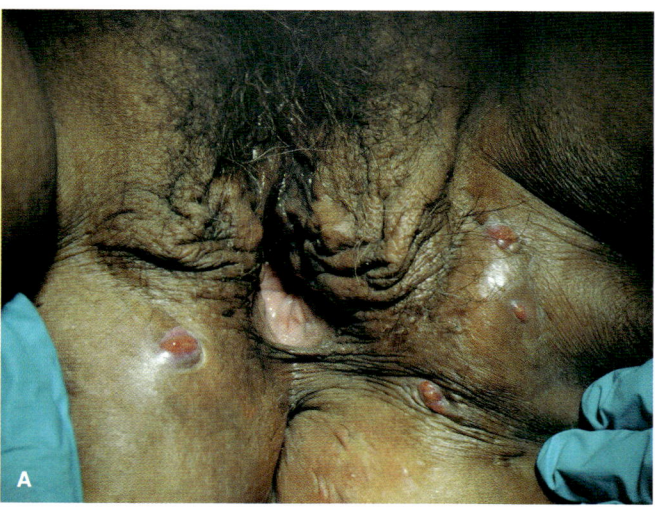

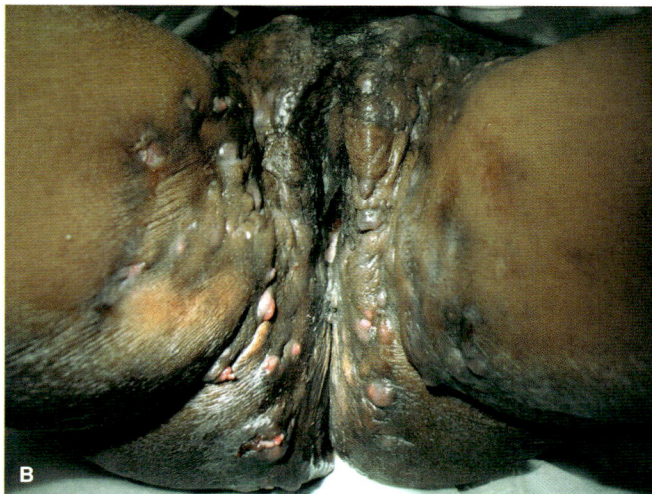

FIGURE 4-7 Hidradenitis suppurativa. **A.** This case of Hurley stage II shows several distinct fistulous tracts that end in raised nodules of granulation tissue (Reproduced with permission from Dr. David Rogers). **B.** In this Hurley stage III case, multiple and connecting tracts drain purulent fluid and create marked disfiguration.

by the Hurley classification, stage I has transient inflammatory lesions without scarring. Stage II shows single or widely spaced lesions with sinus tracts and scarring. Diffuse involvement and multiple connecting tracts between abscesses characterize stage III (Hurley, 1989).

The etiology of hidradenitis suppurativa is unknown. More than one quarter of patients will report a family history of disease, and an autosomal dominant inheritance pattern is hypothesized (der Werth, 2000). Although Mortimer and colleagues (1986) found higher plasma concentrations of androgens in women with hidradenitis suppurativa, others have not replicated this finding (Barth, 1996).

Treatment of early presenting cases includes local hygiene, weight reduction in obese patients, topical or oral antibiotics, and warm compresses. For mild episodic disease as needed, an initial treatment of topical 1-percent clindamycin solution applied twice daily plus benzoyl-peroxide wash three times weekly is often effective. Local cysts may be treated with injections of triamcinolone acetonide rather than incision and drainage (Riis, 2016). Used individually, appropriate long-term oral antibiotics with antiinflammatory effects include: tetracycline, 500 mg twice daily; erythromycin, 500 mg twice daily; doxycycline, 100 mg twice daily; or minocycline, 100 mg twice daily. A 10-week course of clindamycin, 300 mg twice daily, plus rifampicin, 600 mg twice daily, also has shown efficacy (Gener, 2009).

As reviewed by Rhode and associates (2008), other treatment modalities offer varying efficacies. These include systemic cyproterone acetate (an antiandrogen available in Europe), corticosteroids, isotretinoin, cyclosporine, and infliximab. In their evidence-based review, Alhusayen and Shear (2012) suggest antibiotics or agents targeting tumor necrosis factor alpha (TNF-α) are effective for hidradenitis. Nonmedical therapies include laser and phototherapy. Severe, refractory cases may require surgical excision that often involves extensive resection of the vulva and surrounding areas (Rhode, 2008). Hu and Haefner (2018) have published their successful treatment of severe disease after vulvectomy with skin grafting and vacuum-assisted closure. Unfortunately, postoperative local recurrences can develop.

Aphthous Ulcers

Nearly 25 percent of women in the second and third decade of life will experience these self-limited mucosal lesions. Classically found on nonkeratinized oral mucosa, aphthous ulcers may also develop on vulvovaginal surfaces. Lesions are painful and can recur every few months. Distinguishing an aphthous ulcer from genital herpes may require herpes simplex virus (HSV) polymerase chain reaction (PCR) testing and/or targeted biopsies. Histologically, aphthous ulcers show a mononuclear infiltrate with a fibrin coating. Although the etiology is unknown, immune-mediated epithelial cell damage is one theory (Rogers, 1997). Other described triggers include stress, trauma, infection, hormonal fluctuation, and nutritional deficiencies of vitamin B_{12}, folate, iron, or zinc (Torgerson, 2006). The ulcers are normally self-limited, but persistent lesions can lead to painful scarring (Rogers, 2003). If large mutilating aphthae develop in an adolescent

girl, nonsexual acute genital ulceration (NAGU) is suspected. Aphthae may also be the first cutaneous manifestation of systemic diseases, described next.

No cure is available, yet treatment goals include basic vulvar skin hygiene and pain management with topical analgesics such as 5-percent lidocaine ointment. High-potency topical corticosteroids can be applied at ulceration onset. In cases resistant to topical corticosteroids, oral corticosteroids can help decrease inflammation. Finally, colchicine, dapsone, and thalidomide can be effective for recalcitrant cases (Steward, 2017).

MANIFESTATIONS OF SYSTEMIC DISEASE

Systemic illnesses may initially manifest on the vulvar or vaginal mucosa as bullous, solid, or ulcerative lesions. Examples include systemic lupus erythematosus, human immunodeficiency virus infection, erythema multiforme, Stevens-Johnson syndrome, pemphigus, pemphigoid, sarcoidosis, and syphilis. A thorough history and physical examination usually suffice to link genital lesions with preexisting conditions. However, biopsy of vulvovaginal lesions may provide a new and unexpected diagnosis if the disorder has not yet manifest elsewhere.

■ Acanthosis Nigricans

This condition is characterized by velvety to warty, brown to black, poorly marginated plaques. These changes are typically found at skin flexures, especially on the neck, axillae, and labiocrural folds (Fig. 18-6, p. 395).

Acanthosis nigricans is commonly associated with obesity, diabetes mellitus, and polycystic ovarian syndrome. Thus, if signs or symptoms of these are present, appropriate evaluation is indicated. Common to these conditions, insulin resistance with compensatory hyperinsulinemia is thought to promote the skin thickening of acanthosis nigricans. Insulin binds to insulin-like growth factor receptors and leads to keratinocyte and dermal fibroblast proliferation (Hermanns-Le, 2004). Rarely, acanthosis nigricans is caused by other insulin-resistance or fibroblast growth-factor disorders (Saraiya, 2013).

Treatment of acanthosis nigricans has not been evaluated in randomized trials. However, weight loss can ameliorate insulin resistance, which may lead to plaque improvement. In those prescribed metformin for glucose control, improved acanthosis nigricans has been demonstrated (Romo, 2008). Topical retinoids may have benefit but are often irritating (Patel, 2018). Last, topical vitamin D analogs such as calcipotriene can promote plaque improvement (Bohm, 1998).

■ Crohn Disease

Up to one third of women with Crohn disease suffer from anogenital involvement, which may precede gastrointestinal (GI) symptoms and a formal Crohn disease diagnosis. Vulvar lesions are commonly "metastatic" in that they show typical Crohn disease granulomatous inflammation but are not contiguous

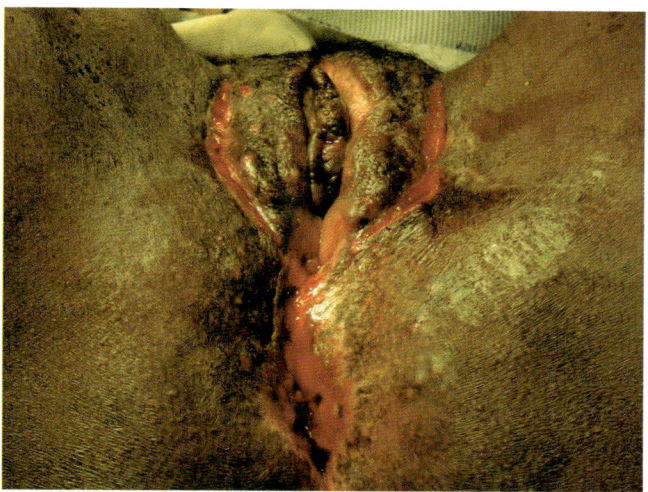

FIGURE 4-8 Vulvar Crohn disease. Knife-cut ulcers in the labiocrural folds and perineum are commonly seen with vulvar Crohn disease. (Reproduced with permission from Dr. F. Gary Cunningham.)

with the affected GI site (Sides, 2013). However, vulvar and perianal abscesses and fistulae can extend directly from GI tract lesions. The four manifestation types are vulvar edema (usually asymmetric), ulceration, hypertrophic lesions, and chronic abscesses (Barret, 2014). Linear "knife-cut" ulcerations and other lesions often affect inguinal, labiocrural, and interlabial folds (Fig. 4-8). All can be asymptomatic but may cause burning or pruritus.

Therapy for GI Crohn disease generally benefits external Crohn lesions. Vulvar lesions unrelated to GI disease activity often respond to prolonged courses of oral metronidazole alone or in conjunction with corticosteroids (Andreani, 2010). Anti-TNF-α agents (infliximab or adalimumab) show promising results (Laftah, 2015). Surgery often can be avoided or delayed with appropriate vulvar care, nutrition, and close collaboration with a gastroenterologist. As a last resort, excision of fistulous tracts and other refractory lesions or vulvectomy is an option. However, either can be complicated by poor healing and scarring (Sides, 2013). Regardless of management, recurrence is common.

■ Behçet Disease

This rare systemic vasculitis most commonly affects patients in their twenties and thirties and those of Asian or Middle Eastern descent. Behçet disease is characterized by mucocutaneous lesions (ocular, oral, and genital) and associated systemic vasculitis. Oral and genital ulcers appear similar to aphthous ulcers and generally heal within 7 to 10 days. Nevertheless, associated pain can be debilitating. Treatment for these lesions mirrors that for aphthous ulcers.

The exact etiology of Behçet disease remains unknown, although genetic and autoimmune etiologies are suspected. Vasculitis dominates the disease process, which may involve the brain, GI tract, joints, lungs, and great vessels. Accordingly, for those suspected of Behçet disease, referral to a rheumatologist for additional testing and treatment is recommended.

DISORDERS OF PIGMENTATION

Benign variations of vulvar, perineal, and perianal skin pigmentation are commonly encountered, especially in women with darker skin. Diffuse areas of increased pigmentation are usually encountered on the labia minora and fourchette. Areas tend to be bilateral and symmetric and have flat tone and normal texture. With gentle stretching, the color attenuates evenly. However, this may also be seen with pigment variation of chronic inflammatory dermatoses.

Some benign vulvar lesions may also be pigmented. These include benign melanosis, lentigines, cherry hemangiomas, angiokeratomas, and seborrheic keratosis (Heller, 2013). Focal dyspigmentation raises concern for premalignant or malignant conditions, and prompt biopsy avoids diagnostic delay. As discussed in Chapter 29 (p. 645), high-grade intraepithelial neoplasia or invasive cancer can appear white (hyperkeratotic) or hyperpigmented and can present with or without symptoms. Melanoma is discussed in Chapter 31 (p. 685).

■ Nevus

Discrete, rounded, pigmented lesions, known as nevi or moles, are easily overlooked on the vulva. These warrant close surveillance as more than half of all melanomas arise from preexisting nevi (Kaufman, 2005). Congenital and dysplastic nevi have the most malignant potential.

Common nevi are classified into three groups: junctional, compound, and dermal, depending on whether the melanotic nevus cells are located at the epidermis-dermis junction, extend into the dermis, or evolve over time to reside entirely within the dermis. Dermal nevi may appear bluish or have normal skin coloration depending on the depth of the nevus cells and may be raised, papillary, or pedunculated.

Recommendations vary regarding biopsy of pigmented vulvar lesions. The American College of Obstetricians and Gynecologists (2016a) recommends biopsy of all such lesions. Others suggest nevus-sampling criteria used elsewhere on the body. Namely, asymmetry, uneven pigmentation, irregular border, diameter >5 mm, or erosion or fissuring merits biopsy (Edwards, 2010). Burning or itching also raises concern. Histologic atypia requires full lesion excision with adequate margins. Atypia or anatomically challenging biopsies, such as those near the clitoris, may prompt referral to clinicians with specialized knowledge and experience with these lesions. Small, bland nevi that are not biopsied warrant a careful descriptive or photographic entry into the medical record and surveillance at least annually until the lesion is deemed stable. Self-examination is encouraged, and changes in lesion or symptoms are important.

■ Vitiligo

Loss of epidermal melanocytes can result in depigmented skin, termed vitiligo (Fig. 4-9). No race or ethnicity has greater risks for vitiligo, but the disease may be more disfiguring and distressing for darker-skinned individuals (Grimes, 2005).

Although the etiology remains unknown, genetic factors are most likely (Zhang, 2005). Approximately 20 percent of patients have at least one affected first-degree relative. Vitiligo

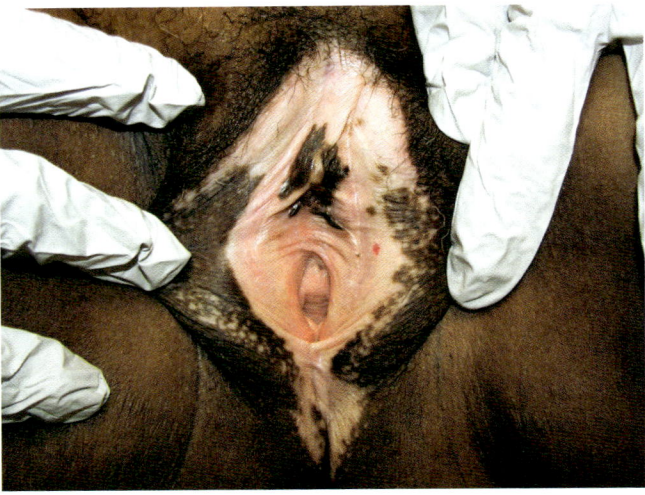

FIGURE 4-9 Vulvar vitiligo.

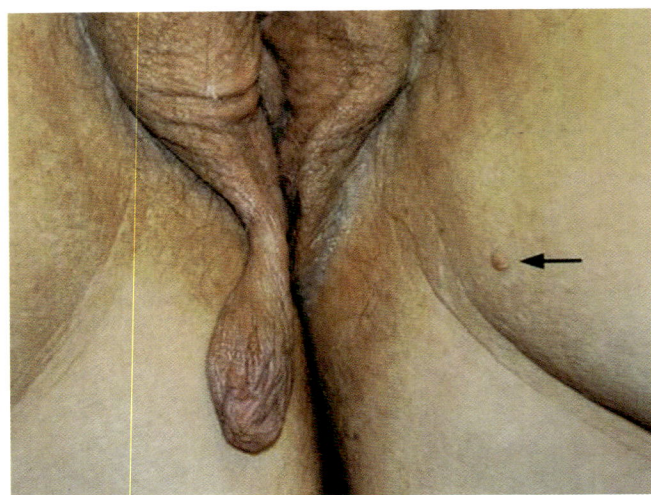

FIGURE 4-10 Vulvar acrochordons (skin tags). Lesions typically are small (*arrow*) and require no intervention. The larger vulvar acrochordon shown here was excised due to mechanical symptoms from its size.

may be mediated by an autoimmune process that destroys melanocytes. Autoimmune diseases such as Hashimoto thyroiditis, Graves disease, diabetes mellitus, rheumatoid arthritis, psoriasis, and vulvar lichen sclerosus are associated with vitiligo (Boissy, 1997; Vrijman, 2012).

Most commonly, depigmentation is symmetric and generalized, although distribution may be acral (limbs, ears) and localized. Sometimes confused with the epithelial changes seen with lichen sclerosus, vitiligo preserves normal skin texture and contour and is otherwise asymptomatic. No cure is presently available for vitiligo, and spontaneous repigmentation is rare. Several treatments for vitiligo include narrowband ultraviolet (UV) B phototherapy, excimer laser therapy, and topical immunomodulators (Baciqalupi, 2012). Most cases are self-limited, and explanation of the condition alone is sufficient.

SOLID VULVAR TUMORS

Most solid vulvar tumors are benign and arise from local tissue. Less commonly, malignant lesions arise on the vulva and are typically of squamous cell epithelial origin. Rarely, solid vulvar tumors develop as metastatic lesions. Accordingly, many growths warrant biopsy if not obviously diagnosed visually.

■ Epidermal and Dermal Lesions

Acrochordons, commonly known as skin tags, are benign, soft fibroepithelial lesions. Most often seen on the neck, axilla, or groin, these skin-colored polypoid masses are usually devoid of hair and generally measure 1 to 6 mm in diameter but can grow larger (Fig. 4-10). They are mistaken for vulvar condylomata, and therapeutic unresponsiveness by presumed genital warts should prompt removal for histologic analysis. Surgical removal is likewise recommended for chronic irritation or cosmetic concerns. Small lesions are easily removed under local anesthesia in an office setting. Acrochordons have been linked to diabetes mellitus, and insulin-mediated fibroblast proliferation may explain this relationship (Demir, 2002).

Seborrheic keratosis may be observed in women with concurrent lesions on the neck, face, or trunk. These lesions typically appear sharply circumscribed, slightly raised, and waxy or scaly. The malignant potential of these slow-growing lesions is minimal, therefore excision is offered only in cases of discomfort or disfigurement.

Keratoacanthoma is a rapidly growing keratinocyte proliferation originating in a pilosebaceous gland. Rarely developing on the vulva, lesions begin as firm, round papules that progress to a dome-shaped nodule with a central crater. Untreated, the lesion usually spontaneously regresses within 4 to 6 months and leaves only a slightly depressed scar. Controversy surrounds its malignant potential (Ko, 2010; Savage, 2014). Some consider keratoacanthoma benign, whereas others classify it as a well-differentiated squamous cell carcinoma. Nevertheless, its histologic resemblance to this cancer merits surgical excision in most cases with a 4- to 5-mm margin.

Syringoma is a benign eccrine (sweat gland) tumor found most frequently on the lower eyelid, neck, and face. Rarely, the vulva may be involved bilaterally with multiple 1- to 4-mm firm papules. The clinical appearance of vulvar syringoma is not pathognomonic, thus vulvar punch biopsy will establish the diagnosis and exclude malignancy. Treatment is not required. However, for those with pruritus, mild-potency topical corticosteroids and antihistamines may be helpful. In those with refractory pruritus, surgical excision or lesion ablation can be offered.

■ Subcutaneous Masses

Leiomyoma of the vulva is a rare tumor felt to arise either from smooth muscle within the vulva's erectile tissue or from transmigration through the round ligament. Surgical excision to exclude leiomyosarcoma is sound, and recurrence has been reported (Nielsen, 1996).

Fibroma is a benign tumor rarely arising from deep vulvar connective tissue by fibroblast proliferation. Lesions are primarily found on the labia majora and range from 0.6 to 8 cm in diameter. Larger lesions often become pedunculated with a long stalk and may cause pain or dyspareunia. Surgical excision is indicated for symptomatic lesions or if the diagnosis is unclear.

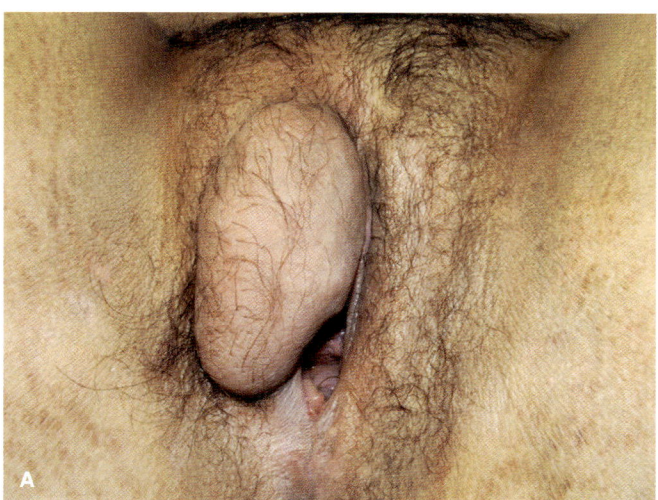
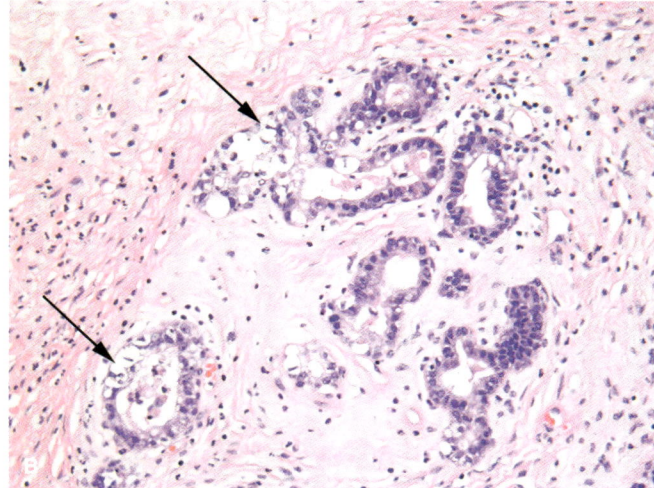

FIGURE 4-11 Ectopic breast tissue. **A.** This chronic vulvar mass grew slightly during pregnancy and then dramatically enlarged 3 days following an uncomplicated vaginal birth. This corresponded with lactation. **B.** Histologic evaluation following excision shows glands typical of breast tissue (*arrow*).

Lipoma is a soft sessile or pedunculated mass composed of mature adipose cells. Similar to fibromas, observation is reasonable in the absence of patient complaints, although symptoms may prompt surgical excision. These lesions lack a fibrous connective tissue capsule. Thus, complete dissection can require a larger incision and can be complicated by bleeding.

Ectopic breast tissue may develop along the theoretical milk lines, which extend bilaterally from the axilla through the breast to the mons pubis. Uncommonly found in the vulva, extramammary breast tissue is hormonally sensitive and may enlarge in response to pregnancy or exogenous hormones (Fig. 4-11). Importantly, these typically soft masses may also develop breast pathologies including fibroadenoma, phyllodes tumor, Paget disease, and invasive adenocarcinoma.

CYSTIC VULVAR TUMORS

■ Bartholin Gland Duct Cyst and Abscess

Mucus produced to lubricate the vulva originates in part from the Bartholin glands. Obstruction of this gland's duct is common and may follow infection, trauma, mucus changes, or congenitally narrowed ducts. However, the underlying cause is often unclear.

In some cases, cyst contents may become infected and lead to abscess formation. These tend to develop in populations with demographic profiles similar to those at high risk for sexually transmitted infections (Aghajanian, 1994). However, a wide spectrum of organisms has been cultured. *Escherichia coli* is the most common isolate, but other gram-positive and gram-negative aerobes and anaerobes are found (Kessous, 2013; Mattila 1994; Tanaka, 2005). Infrequently, *Neisseria gonorrhoeae* or *Chlamydia trachomatis* is identified.

Diagnosis and Treatment

Most Bartholin gland cysts are small and asymptomatic except for minor discomfort during sexual contact (Fig. 4-12). With larger or infected cysts, however, patients may complain of severe vulvar pain that precludes walking, sitting, or coitus (Fig. 3-18, p. 86).

On physical examination, cysts typically are unilateral, round or ovoid, and fluctuant or tense. If infected, they display surrounding erythema and are tender. The mass is usually located in the inferior labia majora or lower vestibule. Whereas most cysts and abscesses lead to labial asymmetry, smaller cysts may be detected only by palpation. Bartholin abscesses on the verge of spontaneous decompression will exhibit an area of softening, where rupture will most likely occur.

Small, asymptomatic Bartholin gland duct cysts require no intervention except exclusion of neoplasia in women older than 40 years. If symptomatic, a cyst may be managed with one of several techniques. These include incision and drainage (I & D), marsupialization, and Bartholin gland excision, which are described and illustrated in Chapter 43 (p. 980). Abscesses are treated with I & D or marsupialization.

Malignancy

After menopause, Bartholin gland duct cysts and abscesses are uncommon and should raise concern for possible neoplasia.

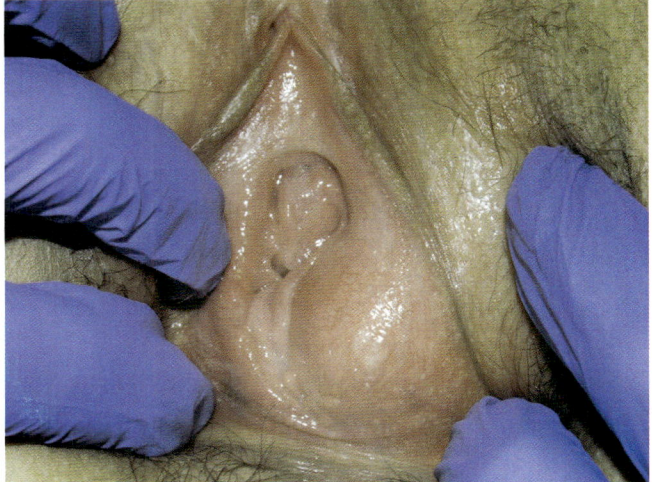

FIGURE 4-12 Bartholin gland duct cyst seen as an asymmetric bulge in the left lower vestibule.

However, carcinoma of the Bartholin gland is rare, and its incidence approximates 0.1 per 100,000 women (Visco, 1996). Most are squamous carcinomas or adenocarcinomas (Heller, 2014). Given the rarity of these cancers, Bartholin gland excision is typically not indicated. Alternatively, in women older than 40 years, drainage of the cyst and biopsy of cyst wall sites adequately excludes malignancy (Visco, 1996).

Urethral Diverticulum and Skene Gland

Ductal occlusion of the Skene gland or paraurethral glands may lead to paraurethral cystic enlargement and possible abscess formation. Their symptoms and treatment are described in Chapter 26 (p. 581).

Epidermal Inclusion Cysts

These cysts, also known as sebaceous cysts, are commonly found on the vulva, and less so in the vagina. Although histologically similar and lined by squamous epithelium, it is unclear if they represent separate entities. Vulvar epidermoid cysts typically form from plugged pilosebaceous units (Fig. 4-13). However, epidermoid cysts can also follow traumatic implantation of epidermal cells into deeper tissues and are filled with keratin.

Epidermal inclusion cysts are variably sized, are typically round or ovoid, and are skin colored, yellow, or white. Grossly, cysts are usually filled with viscous, gritty, or caseous foul-smelling material. Epidermoid cysts are generally asymptomatic and require no further evaluation. If symptomatic or secondarily infected, incision and drainage is recommended.

VULVODYNIA

Shown in Table 4-6, the ISSVD in 2015 defined *vulvodynia* as "vulvar pain of at least 3 months duration, without clear identifiable cause, which may have potential associated factors"

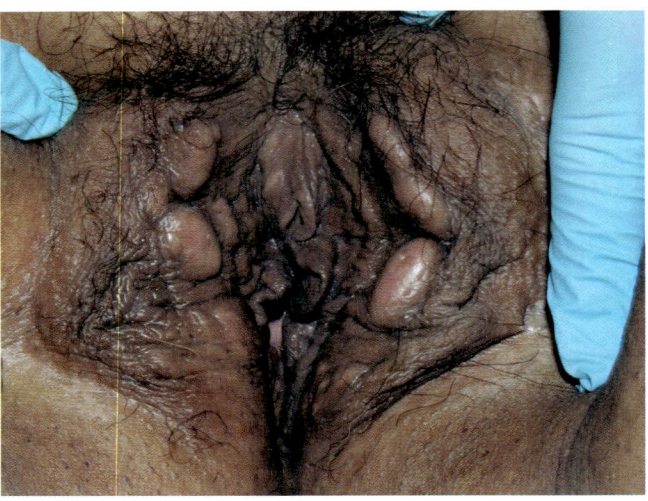

FIGURE 4-13 Multiple, mobile, knotty epidermal inclusion cysts line the inner labia majora.

(Bornstein, 2016). In distinction, *persistent vulvar pain* is attributable to a specific condition (see Table 4-6). The term *vestibulitis* was eliminated from ISSVD terminology because inflammatory changes are not consistently documented.

From limited studies, the prevalence of vulvodynia in the general population is 3 to 11 percent (Lavy, 2007; Reed, 2004, 2014). One study estimated that each year 1 in 50 women will develop vulvodynia (Reed, 2008). All ethnicities and a wide age range are affected.

The underlying cause of vulvodynia is multifactorial and varies among individuals (Stockdale, 2014). Potential factors associated with vulvodynia include other pain syndromes, genetic influences, hormonal factors, inflammation, musculoskeletal dysfunction, neurologic mechanisms, psychosocial elements, and structural defects (Bornstein, 2016). Ultimately, identification of these associated factors will guide individualized treatment planning.

TABLE 4-6. 2015 Consensus Terminology and Classification of Persistent Vulvar Pain and Vulvodynia

Vulvar pain caused by a specific disorder
 Infectious (e.g., recurrent candidiasis, herpes)
 Inflammatory (e.g., lichen sclerosus, lichen planus, immunobullous disorders)
 Neoplastic (e.g., Paget disease, squamous cell carcinoma)
 Neurologic (e.g., postherpetic neuralgia, nerve compression or injury, neuroma)
 Trauma (e.g., female genital cutting, obstetrical)
 Iatrogenic (e.g., postoperative, chemotherapy, radiation)
 Hormonal deficiencies (e.g., genitourinary syndrome of menopause [vulvovaginal atrophy], lactational amenorrhea)

Vulvodynia—vulvar pain of at least 3 months' duration, without clear identifiable cause, which may have potential associated factors
 The following are the descriptors:
 Localized (e.g., vestibulodynia, clitorodynia) or generalized or mixed (localized and generalized)
 Provoked (e.g., insertional, contact) or spontaneous or mixed (provoked and spontaneous)
 Onset (primary or secondary)
 Temporal pattern (intermittent, persistent, constant, immediate, delayed)

From Bornstein, 2016, with permission.

TABLE 4-7. Appropriate Vulvodynia Questions

Pain onset date? A precipitating event?
Pain onset gradual or sudden?
Is pain intermittent, constant, immediate, or delayed?
Describe the pain and its intensity.
Aggravating factors? Is pain provoked or spontaneous?
Relieving factors? Prior therapy?
Associated symptoms? Urinary? GI? Dermatologic?
Does pain lessen quality of life? Limit activities?
    Disturb sexual function?

GI = gastrointestinal

Diagnosis

Typically, evaluation and management are delayed for years due to patient embarrassment, attempts at self-treatment, and lack of knowledge that it is a medical condition. Diagnosis and treatment delays, often by multiple providers, are common (Harlow, 2003, 2014).

An evidence-based approach to diagnose vulvodynia and its associated factors is essential (Haefner, 2005; Stockdale, 2014). Given that vulvodynia is a diagnosis of exclusion, a thorough history that includes medical, sexual, and surgical inquiries aids diagnosis (Table 4-7) (American College of Obstetricians and Gynecologists, 2016b).

As noted, vulvodynia is categorized as spontaneous (unprovoked), triggered by physical pressure (provoked), or mixed. Pain is further categorized by its general or local anatomic distribution, its onset, and its temporal pattern. Sensations may be constant, intermittent, or episodic with exacerbations noted premenstrually (Arnold, 2006). Vulvodynia is described variably as burning, rawness, itching, or cutting pain within affected areas (Bergeron, 2001).

Questioning seeks to identify frequently associated pain syndromes or psychologic disorders. These may include irritable bowel syndrome, interstitial cystitis, painful bladder syndrome, fibromyalgia, and mood or posttraumatic stress disorders. A history of recurrent infectious diseases such as herpes simplex or zoster is sought. Past surgical or obstetric procedures may help identify pudendal nerve injury. A sexual history may reveal clues of past or current abuse, unfavorable coital patterns, female sexual dysfunction, relationship disharmony, and contraceptive modalities that could provoke vulvodynia (Chap. 14, p. 313). Additionally, clinicians inquire about recurrent candidiasis; prior genital trauma, including childbirth-related injuries; and current hygiene practices. Specifically, questions regarding genital shaving, type of undergarment fabric worn, and use of products in Table 4-1 can be helpful. Prior therapies are documented to avoid unnecessary treatment repetition.

Next, a thorough examination excludes other possible pathologies. Inspection of the external vulva for lesions or irritation is followed by examination of the vestibule looking for focal, usually mild, erythema at vestibular gland openings. Use of a magnifying lens is important, and directed biopsies of nonerythematous epithelial changes may be helpful. Of note, Bowen

and associates (2008) found clinically relevant dermatoses in 61 percent of refractory vulvodynia patients referred to their tertiary care vulvovaginal clinic.

Systematic pain mapping of the vestibule, perineum, and inner thigh is completed, and documentation serves as a reference to assess treatment success (see Fig. 4-1). A cotton swab is used to check for allodynia and hyperesthesia. The swab end can first be unwound to form a cotton-fiber wisp. Subsequently, the wooden stick is broken to form a sharp point to retest the same areas. Pain scale scores of mild, moderate, or severe are recorded and followed over time.

Last, a saline "wet prep" of vaginal secretions and vaginal pH testing assist in excluding hormonal or infectious causes. Testing as clinically indicated for yeast and HSV is similarly helpful (Chap. 3, pp. 58 and 64).

Treatment

Like other chronic pain conditions, vulvodynia is challenging to treat. Importantly, all vulvodynia treatment is individualized and may require a multidisciplinary approach that includes medical therapy, pelvic floor physical therapy, and psychotherapy. However, due to the lack of well-designed randomized trials, no specific therapy for vulvodynia demonstrates superiority. Often, a combination of several therapeutic options is required to relieve symptoms (Haefner, 2005; Landry, 2008). Approaches are described further by Stockdale (2014) and the American College of Obstetricians and Gynecologists (2016b). Encouragingly, from one 2-year study, the annual remission rate for women with vulvodynia was 11 percent (Reed, 2008). Without improvement, surgical excision is a final option.

Behavioral and Physical Therapy

The first step in managing all vulvar disorders includes vulvar care as summarized in Table 4-2. Also, provision of accurate medical information can help resolve some patient concerns and questions associated with vulvodynia. The National Vulvodynia Association offers patient information and support and can be accessed online at www.nva.org.

Compared with the general population, no differences in marital contentment or psychologic distress are found (Bornstein, 1999). That said, education regarding foreplay, sexual positions, lubrication, and alternatives to vaginal intercourse are offered if potentially helpful. Female sexual dysfunction and its treatment are further discussed in Chapter 14 (p. 312).

Back pain, pelvic floor muscle spasm, or vaginismus may be the underlying cause of vulvodynia, and pelvic floor muscle examination is described and illustrated in Chapter 12 (p. 260). A physical therapist familiar with treating these concerns may provide internal and external massage, myofascial release techniques, acupressure, joint manipulation, electrical stimulation, therapeutic ultrasonography, and pelvic floor muscle retraining to improve symptoms (Bergeron, 2002).

Dietary oxalates excreted into urine have been suggested to aggravate symptoms, but evidence is limited and shows contradictory results (Baggish, 1997; Harlow, 2008). Similarly, support for supplementing with calcium citrate to balance the urine oxalates is scarce (Solomons, 1991).

TABLE 4-8. Nonsurgical Vulvodynia Treatment

Vulvar care	See Table 4-2
Topical agents	2% lidocaine jelly or 5% lidocaine ointment, apply precoitally Gabapentin 2% to 6% ointment or cream, apply two or three times daily
Antidepressant	Amitriptyline, initially 5–25 mg orally daily, then increase daily dose by 10–25 mg each week. Maximum dose 150 mg daily Duloxetine (Cymbalta), 30 mg orally daily. May increase to 60 mg daily
Anticonvulsant	Gabapentin, 100 mg orally three times daily and gradually increase as needed over 6–8 weeks. Maximum dose 1200 mg three times daily.
Local injection	1 mL 1% lidocaine plus 1 mL betamethasone (6 mg/mL) or 10 mg lidocaine plus 40 mg methylprednisolone acetate in 10 mL normal saline
Biofeedback	
Sex counseling	

Data from Boardman, 2008; Murina, 2001; Reed, 2006; Segal, 2003; Stockdale, 2014.

Medications

Agents for vulvodynia treatment may be administered topically, orally, or intralesionally (Table 4-8). Of topical agents, 2-percent lidocaine mucosal jelly or 5-percent lidocaine ointment applied sparingly to the vestibule prior to coitus is often a first-line choice. However, randomized trials do not show a statistically significant difference between these and placebo. Other topical anesthetic preparations are reported to have variable success. However, caution is exercised with benzocaine, which is associated with higher rates of contact dermatitis.

Eva and coworkers (2003) found lower estrogen-receptor expression in women with vulvodynia. However, topical or intravaginal estrogen therapy has yielded mixed results.

As reported by Boardman and associates (2008), topical gabapentin cream is well tolerated, is effective, and avoids the potential side effects of systemic gabapentin therapy. In their study, 0.5 mL of a compounded 2-, 4-, or 6-percent gabapentin-containing cream was applied three times daily for at least 8 weeks to affected vulvar areas.

Of oral medications, antidepressants and anticonvulsants are reported to help vulvodynia. However, polypharmacy is ideally avoided, and clinicians prescribe one drug at a time. Additionally, contraception is required for reproductive-aged patients. Tricyclic antidepressants (TCAs) are widely used for vulvodynia, and reported response rates may reach nearly 60 percent in nonrandomized trials (Pagano, 1999; Reed, 2006). In our experience, amitriptyline started at doses of 5 to 25 mg orally nightly and increased as needed by 10 to 25 mg each week yields good results for some patients. Final daily doses do not exceed 150 mg. Importantly, compliance is encouraged during the nearly 4-week lag required to achieve significant pain relief. Alternatively, duloxetine (Cymbalta), which is a serotonin-norepinephrine-reuptake inhibitor, has fewer anticholinergic effects.

Cases resistant to antidepressants may be treated with the anticonvulsant gabapentin (Harris, 2007). Oral gabapentin is initiated at a dosage of 100 mg three times daily and gradually increased within 6 to 8 weeks to a maximal daily dose of 1200 mg three times daily. Once this dose is reached, pain is reassessed after 1 to 2 weeks (Haefner, 2005). Most support for gabapentin comes from case series. One recent randomized trial found no improvement in pain scores but did find improvement in sexual functioning scores (Brown, 2018; Bachmann, 2019).

Topical corticosteroids generally do not help patients with vulvodynia. However, injections using a combination of corticosteroids and local anesthetics have been used for localized vulvodynia in case reports (Murina, 2001; Segal, 2003). Alternatively, botulinum toxin A injection into the levator ani muscles has been reported effective for vulvodynia-related vaginismus (Bertolasi, 2009; Morrissey, 2015).

Surgery

Women with vulvodynia who fail to improve despite aggressive medical therapy are candidates for surgery. Options include local excision of a precise pain locus, complete resection of the vestibule (vestibulectomy), or resection of the vestibule and perineum (perineoplasty) (Chap. 43, p. 988). From a series of 155 treated women, Traas and colleagues (2006) reported high success rates with vestibulectomy among women younger than 30 years. Perineoplasty is the most extensive of the three procedures. Its incision extends from just below the urethra to the perineal body, usually terminating above the anal orifice. This procedure may be selected if significant perineal scarring is suspected to contribute to dyspareunia. Overall, improvement rates for appropriately selected patients are high following vulvar excision procedures. However, surgery is reserved for those with severe, localized, long-standing vestibular pain who have failed significant attempts at conservative, multidisciplinary management. It is best performed by gynecologists skilled in vulvar excisional surgery.

VULVOVAGINAL TRAUMA

■ Vulvar Hematoma

This may develop in the relatively vascular vulva following straddle injury, trauma from coitus or assault, or vulvovaginal

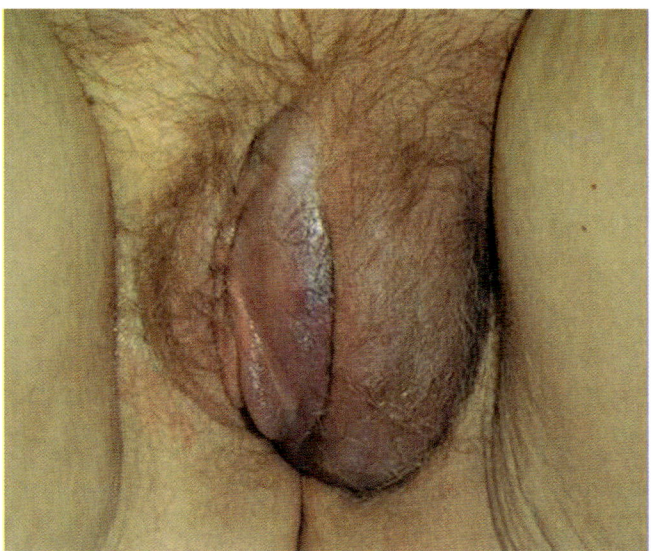

FIGURE 4-14 Vulvar hematoma.

procedures. Hematomas may develop within subcutaneous tissues or within the superficial perineal pouch of the anterior perineal triangle (Fig. 38-26, p. 815). Within the latter, laceration of the vestibular bulb, clitoral crus, or branches of the internal pudendal vessels may create a sizable mass (Fig. 4-14). Given the protected anatomic location and adipose padding of the labia majora, traumatic vulvar injuries are rare in adults. These are much more frequent in children who lack such padding. Differentiating straddle injury and sexual abuse in children is often challenging, as injury patterns are not reliably discriminating.

Often requiring a general anesthetic, thorough examination of the vulva and vagina will estimate hematoma stability and the integrity of the surrounding bowel, bladder, urethra, and rectum. If no associated organ injury is found, the venous origin of most vulvar hematomas makes them candidates for conservative management with cool packs, pain control, and Foley catheter bladder drainage as needed. In general, large or rapidly expanding hematomas are surgically explored to secure bleeding vessels. However, following incision and clot evacuation, a cavity is often seen without an identifiable bleeding vessel. To prevent reaccumulation, the cavity is closed in layers with absorbable or delayed-absorbable suture using a running or interrupted stitch closure.

■ Vaginal Laceration

Penetrating trauma accounts for most vaginal injuries. Common causes include pelvic fracture, forced inanimate objects, coitus, and hydraulic forces such as those experienced with water skiing. Atrophic vaginal changes can predispose to injury.

With extensive laceration, examination under anesthesia is usually necessary to perform a thorough assessment and to exclude intraperitoneal damage. Moreover, if the peritoneal cavity has been breached, abdominal cavity exploration by laparotomy or laparoscopy is often needed to exclude visceral injury and supralevator or retroperitoneal hematoma.

Treatment goals include hemostasis and restoration of normal anatomy. Irrigation, debridement, and primary repair are key steps during initial management. The vaginal mucosa is typically reapproximated with running or interrupted stitches with absorbable or delayed-absorbable suture. Uncommonly, infection dictates laceration healing by secondary intention. Nonexpanding hematomas may be managed conservatively, whereas expanding masses often require evacuation and isolation of bleeding vessels. Angiography coupled with embolization is another option. With laceration or hematoma, postoperatively, a vaginal pack can help tamponade any continued bleeding.

VAGINAL CONDITIONS

■ Foreign Body

Trauma or chronic irritation from a foreign body placed into the vagina can affect all ages. Objects vary by age group, and small objects may become lodged in a child's vagina during play (Fig. 15-11, p. 329). An adolescent may be unable to retrieve or may be unaware of a vaginal tampon or piece of broken condom. In adults, sexual misadventure or abuse can usually explain most objects found.

Three notable items include a retained tampon or contraceptive sponge and the vaginal pessary. Women with a retained tampon or sponge typically complain of foul-smelling vaginal discharge with some associated pruritus, discomfort, or unscheduled bleeding. A history of multiple unsuccessful retrieval attempts may be elicited. In the absence of leukocytosis, fever, or evidence of an endometritis or salpingitis, simple removal is sufficient treatment. Vaginal lavage to cleanse the vagina is not indicated and may actually increase the risk of ascending infection. Toxic shock syndrome has been described with both tampons and contraceptive sponges, and its management is outlined in Chapter 3 (p. 83). Vaginal pessaries are frequently selected to conservatively treat pelvic organ prolapse or incontinence. Associated complications with these devices and their management are described fully in Chapter 24 (p. 548).

■ Desquamative Inflammatory Vaginitis

Desquamative inflammatory vaginitis (DIV) is likely a severe form of aerobic vaginitis (AV) (Sherrard, 2018). This uncommon chronic inflammatory vaginitis develops primarily in perimenopausal women, and white women appear to be more often affected. Although the etiology of DIV is unknown, it may represent a variant of erosive vaginal lichen planus (Edwards, 1988). In contrast, AV may be secondary to an overgrowth of aerobic microbes such as *E coli*, group B streptococcus, and *Staphylococcus aureus* (Donders, 2002). Possible triggers include diarrhea or antibiotic use (Bradford, 2010).

Copious vaginal discharge, introital burning, dyspareunia, and vaginal irritation, all refractory to common therapies, is a typical presentation. On examination, a diffuse, exudative, purulent yellow or green discharge is seen on the vaginal walls. Varying degrees of vestibular-vaginal erythema or ulceration are noted. Microscopy reveals many polymorphonuclear and parabasal cells but a reduced lactobacilli population. Pathogens such as trichomonads or yeast forms are absent. The vaginal pH is elevated, and exclusionary test results for gonorrhea and Chlamydia infection are negative. The profuse leukorrhea may lead to an erroneous diagnosis of pelvic inflammatory disease or cervicitis, but pelvic tenderness is absent.

Although no randomized clinical trials are available, Sobel (2011) reports favorable outcomes with 2-percent intravaginal clindamycin cream or an intravaginal hydrocortisone cream or suppositories for 4 to 6 weeks. Whether the efficacy of clindamycin is due to its antibacterial or antiinflammatory properties is unknown (Bradford, 2010). This is a chronic condition, and prolonged treatment courses, relapses, and need for retreatment are common.

■ Diethylstilbestrol-induced Reproductive Tract Abnormalities

In the mid-1900s, diethylstilbestrol (DES), a synthetic nonsteroidal estrogen, was prescribed to women in the United States for several pregnancy-related problems. Daughters exposed in utero to DES had congenital reproductive tract anomalies and demonstrated higher rates of vaginal clear cell adenocarcinoma (Herbst, 1971). More commonly, *vaginal adenosis,* which is an area(s) of columnar epithelium within the vaginal squamous mucosa, is found in these women. Vaginal adenosis typically appears as red, granular patches. Symptoms include vaginal irritation, vaginal discharge, and intermenstrual or postcoital bleeding. A fuller discussion of DES-related defects is found in Chapter 19 (p. 424).

■ Gartner Duct Cyst

Most vaginal cysts are epidermoid cysts, urethral diverticula, or Gartner duct cysts. The last are uncommon vaginal cysts developing from mesonephric (Wolffian) duct remnants (Chap. 19, p. 406). They are typically asymptomatic and found within the lateral vaginal wall during routine examination. Symptoms, if present, include dyspareunia, vaginal pain, and difficulty inserting tampons. Examination reveals a tense cyst that is palpable or seen to bulge beneath the vaginal wall. Observation is reasonable in most cases. Marsupialization or excision may be appropriate for symptomatic Gartner duct cysts.

CERVICAL LESIONS

■ Eversion

The squamocolumnar junction (SCJ) borders between the columnar epithelium of the endocervix and the squamous epithelium of the ectocervix. As described in Chapter 29 (p. 621), endocervical tissue in some women may migrate outward from the endocervical canal in a process termed *eversion,* which is thought to be hormonally mediated. As a result, the SCJ lies further distally from the external cervical os. Eversion is a normal finding. However, asymmetry of the columnar epithelium surrounding the cervical os can mimic an erosive lesion, and cervical biopsy can aid clarity in this case.

■ Nabothian Cyst

Mucus-secreting columnar cells line the endocervical canal. During squamous metaplasia, squamous epithelium may cover functional

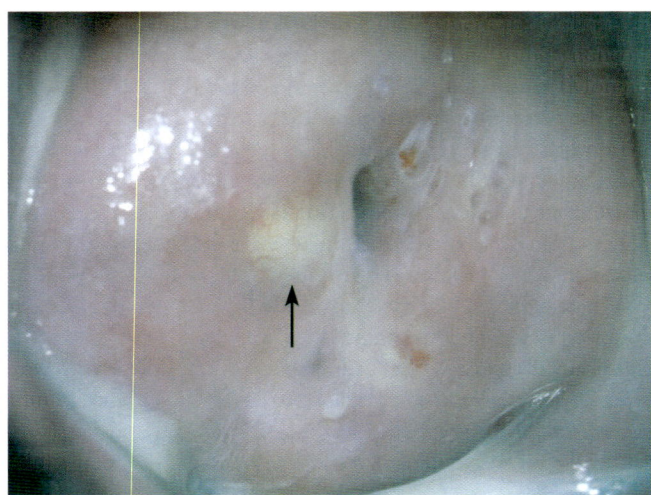

FIGURE 4-15 Cervical nabothian cyst (*arrow*) is seen as a raised, symmetric, smooth, yellow lesion on the ectocervix.

glandular cells, and secretions may accumulate. As this benign process continues, smooth, clear, pale white or yellow, rounded elevations can form and are visible during routine examination (Fig. 4-15). They are also frequently seen as well-defined anechoic sonolucency along the endocervical canal (Fig. 2-14, p. 37).

Nabothian cysts typically do not warrant therapy. However, if they grow large enough to make Pap testing or cervical examination difficult or cause symptoms, they can be opened with a biopsy forceps and drained. Moreover, if the diagnosis of a cervical mass is uncertain, biopsy for histologic confirmation is obtained.

■ Endocervical Polyp

One of the most common benign neoplasms of the cervix is a hyperplastic projection of endocervical tissue known as an *endocervical polyp* (Fig. 8-10, p. 190). These are usually found during routine pelvic examination and are generally asymptomatic. Polyps may be associated with leukorrhea or postcoital spotting, and additional discussion is found in Chapter 8.

■ Cervical Stenosis

This narrowing of the cervical canal or opening may be congenital or acquired. Congenital stenosis is rare and likely due to segmental müllerian hypoplasia (Chap. 19, p. 421). In contrast, acquired stenosis is usually iatrogenic due to scarring after cervical excisional procedures such as cold-knife conization and loop electrosurgical excision. This complication is estimated to follow 3 to 8 percent of such procedures (Brun, 2002). Infection, neoplasia, severe atrophy, and radiation changes are less frequent causes.

Diagnosis is based on symptoms and physical findings, as a precise and universally accepted definition is lacking. Symptoms of stenosis in menstruating women include dysmenorrhea, amenorrhea, and infertility. An inability to introduce a dilator into the endocervical canal is generally considered diagnostic. Postmenopausal women are usually asymptomatic until fluid, exudates, or blood accumulates behind the obstruction. These collections are discussed additionally in Chapter 9 (p. 212). If obstruction is complete, a soft, enlarged uterus from trapped intracavitary fluid is sometimes palpable.

Cervical stenosis is relieved by introduction of dilators, which may require anesthesia and treatment may be followed by recurrences. Preprocedural misoprostol may aid by softening the cervix (Chap. 41, p. 899). In postmenopausal women, pretreatment for several weeks with vaginal estrogen cream may also assist dilation. Surgical techniques to overcome stenosis are described fully in Chapter 41 (p. 903).

REFERENCES

Aghajanian A, Bernstein L, Grimes DA: Bartholin's duct abscess and cyst: a case-control study. South Med J 87(1):26, 1994

Alhusayen R, Shear NH: Pharmacologic interventions for hidradenitis suppurativa: what does the evidence say? Am J Clin Dermatol 13(5):283, 2012

American College of Obstetricians and Gynecologists: Diagnosis and management of vulvar skin disorders. Practice Bulletin No. 93, May 2008, Reaffirmed 2016a

American College of Obstetricians and Gynecologists: Persistent vulvar pain. Committee Opinion No. 673, September 2016b

Anderson M, Kutzner S, Kaufman RH: Treatment of vulvovaginal lichen planus with vaginal hydrocortisone suppositories. Obstet Gynecol 100(2):359, 2002

Andreani SM, Ratnasingham K, Dang HH, et al: Crohn's disease of the vulva. Int J Surg 8(1):2, 2010

Arnold LD, Bachmann GA, Rosen R, et al: Vulvodynia: characteristics and associations with comorbidities and quality of life. Obstet Gynecol 107(3):617, 2006

Bachmann GA, Brown CS, Phillips NA, et al: Gabapentin Study Group. Effect of gabapentin on sexual function in vulvodynia: a randomized, placebo-controlled trial. Am J Obstet Gynecol 220(1):89.e1, 2019

Bacigalupi RM, Postolova A, Davis RS: Evidence-based, non-surgical treatments for vitiligo: a review. Am J Clin Dermatol 13(4):217, 2012

Baggish MS, Sze EH, Johnson R: Urinary oxalate excretion and its role in vulvar pain syndrome. Am J Obstet Gynecol 177(3):507, 1997

Barret M, de Parades V, Battistella M, et al: Crohn's disease of the vulva. J Crohns Colitis 8(7):563, 2014

Barth JH, Layton AM, Cunliffe WJ: Endocrine factors in pre- and postmenopausal women with hidradenitis suppurativa. Br J Dermatol 134(6):1057, 1996

Bergeron S, Binik YM, Khalife S, et al: Vulvar vestibulitis syndrome: reliability of diagnosis and evaluation of current diagnostic criteria. Obstet Gynecol 98(1):45, 2001

Bergeron S, Brown C, Lord MJ, et al: Physical therapy for vulvar vestibulitis syndrome: a retrospective study. J Sex Marital Ther 28(3):183, 2002

Bertolasi L, Frasson E, Cappelletti JY, et al: Botulinum neurotoxin type A injections for vaginismus secondary to vulvar vestibulitis syndrome. Obstet Gynecol 114(5):1008, 2009

Boardman LA, Cooper AS, Blais LR, et al: Topical gabapentin in the treatment of localized and generalized vulvodynia. Obstet Gynecol 112(3):579, 2008

Böhm M, Luger T, Metie D: Treatment of mixed-type acanthosis nigricans with topical calcipotriol. Br J Derm 139(5):932, 1998

Boissy RE, Nordlund JJ: Molecular basis of congenital hypopigmentary disorders in humans: a review. Pigment Cell Res 10(1-2):12, 1997

Bor S, Feiwel M, Chanarin I: Vitiligo and its aetiological relationship to organ-specific autoimmune disease. Br J Dermatol 81(2):83, 1969

Bornstein J, Goldstein AT, Stockdale CK, et al: 2015 ISSVD, ISSWSH, and IPPS consensus terminology and classification of persistent vulvar pain and vulvodynia. Obstet Gynecol 127(4):745, 2016

Bornstein J, Heifetz S, Kellner Y, et al: Clobetasol dipropionate 0.05% versus testosterone propionate 2% topical application for severe vulvar lichen sclerosus. Am J Obstet Gynecol 178(1 Pt 1):80, 1998

Bornstein J, Zarfati D, Goldik Z, et al: Vulvar vestibulitis: physical or psychosexual problem? Obstet Gynecol 93(5 Pt 2):876, 1999

Bowen AR, Vester A, Marsden L, et al: The role of vulvar skin biopsy in the evaluation of chronic vulvar pain. Am J Obstet Gynecol 199(5):467.e1, 2008

Bradford J, Fischer G: Desquamative inflammatory vaginitis: differential diagnosis and alternate diagnostic criteria. J Low Genit Tract Dis 14(4):306, 2010

Bradford J, Fischer G: Management of vulvovaginal lichen planus: a new approach. J Low Genit Tract Dis 17(1):28, 2013

Brown CS, Bachmann GA, Wan J, et al: Gabapentin for the treatment of vulvodynia: a randomized controlled trial. Obstet Gynecol 131(6):1000, 2018

Brun J, Youbi A, Hocke C: Complications, sequelae and outcome of cervical conizations: evaluation of three surgical technics. J Gynecol Obstet Bio Reprod 31(6):558, 2002

Cooper SM, Wojnarowska F: Influence of treatment of erosive lichen planus of the vulva on its prognosis. Arch Dermatol 142(3):289, 2006

Demir S, Demir Y: Acrochordon and impaired carbohydrate metabolism. Acta Diabetol 39(2):57, 2002

der Werth JM, Williams HC: The natural history of hidradenitis suppurativa. J Eur Acad Dermatol Venereol 14(5):389, 2000

Donder G: Definition of a type of abnormal vaginal flora that is distinct from bacterial vaginosis: aerobic vaginitis. BJOG 109:1, 2002

Edwards L: Pigmented vulvar lesions. Dermatol Ther 23(5):449, 2010

Edwards L, Friedrich EG Jr: Desquamative vaginitis: lichen planus in disguise. Obstet Gynecol 71(6 Pt 1):832, 1988

Eisen D: The therapy of oral lichen planus. Crit Rev Oral Biol Med 4(2):141, 1993

Eva LJ, MacLean AB, Reid WM, et al: Estrogen receptor expression in vulvar vestibulitis syndrome. Am J Obstet Gynecol 189(2):458, 2003

Farage M, Maibach HI: The vulvar epithelium differs from the skin: implications for cutaneous testing to address topical vulvar exposures. Contact Dermatitis 51(4):201, 2004

Fischer GO: The commonest causes of symptomatic vulvar disease: a dermatologist's perspective. Australas J Dermatol 37(1):12, 1996

Food and Drug Administration: Tacrolimus (marketed as Protopic Ointment) Information, 2015. Available at: http://www.fda.gov/Drugs/DrugSafety/PostmarketDrugSafetyInformationforPatientsandProviders/ucm107845.htm. Accessed February 12, 2019

Frieling U, Bonsmann G, Schwarz T, et al: Treatment of severe lichen planus with mycophenolate mofetil. J Am Acad Dermatol 49:1063, 2003

Funaro D: A double-blind, randomized prospective study evaluating topical clobetasol propionate 0.05% versus topical tacrolimus 0.1% in patients with vulvar lichen sclerosus. J Am Acad Dermatol 71(1):84, 2014

Gelfand JM Stern RS, Nijsten T: The prevalence of psoriasis in African Americans: results from a population-based study. J Am Acad Dermatol 52(1):23, 2005

Gener G, Canoui-Poitrine F, Revuz JE, et al: Combination therapy with clindamycin and rifampicin for hidradenitis suppurativa: a series of 116 consecutive patients. Dermatology 219(2):148, 2009

Goldstein AT, Burrows LJ: Surgical treatment of clitoral phimosis caused by lichen sclerosus. Am J Obstet Gynecol 196(2):126.e1, 2007

Goldstein AT, Creasey A, Pfau R, et al: A double-blind, randomized controlled trial of clobetasol versus pimecrolimus in patients with vulvar lichen sclerosus. J Am Acad Dermatol 64(6):e99, 2011

Goldstein AT, Marinoff SC, Christopher K, et al: Prevalence of vulvar lichen sclerosus in a general gynecology practice. J Reprod Med 50:477, 2005a

Goldstein AT, Metz A: Vulvar lichen planus. Clin Obstet Gynecol 48(4):818, 2005b

Griffiths CE, Clark CM, Chalmers RJ, et al: A systematic review of treatments for severe psoriasis. Health Technol Assess 4(40):1, 2000

Grimes PE: New insights and new therapies in vitiligo. JAMA 293(6):730, 2005

Guerrero A, Vankatesan A: Inflammatory vulvar dermatoses. Clin Obstet Gynecol 58:464, 2015

Haefner HK, Collins ME, Davis GD, et al: The vulvodynia guideline. J Low Genit Tract Dis 9(1):40, 2005

Harlow BL, Abenhaim HA, Vitonis AF, et al: Influence of dietary oxalates on the risk of adult-onset vulvodynia. J Reprod Med 53(3):171, 2008

Harlow BL, Kunitz CG, Nguyen RH, et al: Prevalence of symptoms consistent with a diagnosis of vulvodynia: population-based estimates from 2 geographic regions. Am J Obstet Gynecol 210(1):40.e1, 2014

Harlow BL, Stewart EG: A population-based assessment of chronic unexplained vulvar pain: have we underestimated the prevalence of vulvodynia? J Am Med Womens Assoc 58(2):82, 2003

Harris G, Horowitz B, Borgida A: Evaluation of gabapentin in the treatment of generalized vulvodynia, unprovoked. J Reprod Med 52(2):103, 2007

Heller D: Pigmented vulvar lesions—a pathology review of lesions that are not melanoma. J Low Genit Tract Dis 17(3):320, 2013

Heller DS, Bean S: Lesions of the Bartholin gland: a review. J Low Genit Tract Dis 18(4):351, 2014

Hengge UR, Krause W, Hofmann H, et al: Multicentre, phase II trial on the safety and efficacy of topical tacrolimus ointment for the treatment of lichen sclerosus. Br J Dermatol 155(5):1021, 2006

Herbst AL, Ulfelder H, Poskanzer DC: Adenocarcinoma of the vagina. Association of maternal stilbestrol therapy with tumor appearance in young women. N Engl J Med 284(15):878, 1971

Hermanns-Le T, Scheen A, Pierard GE: Acanthosis nigricans associated with insulin resistance: pathophysiology and management. Am J Clin Dermatol 5(3):199, 2004

Hillemanns P, Untch M, Prove F, et al: Photodynamic therapy of vulvar lichen sclerosus with 5-aminolevulinic acid. Obstet Gynecol 93(1):71, 1999

Hu J, Haefner HK: The management of vacuum-assisted closure following vulvectomy with skin grafting. Plast Reconstr Surg Glob Open 6(4):e1726, 2018

Hurley HJ: Axillary hyperhidrosis, apocrine bromhidrosis, hidradenitis suppurativa and familial benign pemphigus: surgical approach. In Roenigk RK, Roenigk HH (eds): Dermatologic Surgery. New York, Marcel Dekker, 1989, p 729

Janniger CK, Schwartz RA, Szepietowski JC, et al: Intertrigo and common secondary skin infections. Am Fam Physician 72(5):833, 2005

Kahana M, Levy A, Schewach-Millet M, et al: Appearance of lupus erythematosus in a patient with lichen sclerosus et atrophicus of the elbows. J Am Acad Dermatol 12(1 Pt 1):127, 1985

Kaufman RH, Faro S, Brown D: Benign Diseases of the Vulva and Vagina, 5th ed. Philadelphia, Mosby, 2005

Kaufman RH, Gardner HL, Brown D Jr, et al: Vulvar dystrophies: an evaluation. Am J Obstet Gynecol 120(3):363, 1974

Kessous R, Aricha-Tamir B, Sheizaf B, et al: Clinical and microbiological characteristics of Bartholin gland abscesses. Obstet Gynecol 122(4):794, 2013

Ko CJ: Keratoacanthoma: facts and controversies. Clin Dermatol 28(3):254, 2010

Laftah Z, Bailey C, Zaheri S, et al: Vulval Crohn's disease: a clinical study of 22 patients. J Crohns Colitis 9(4):318, 2015

Landry T, Bergeron S, Dupuis MJ, et al: The treatment of provoked vestibulodynia. Clin J Pain 24:155, 2008

Lavy RJ, Hynan LS, Haley RW: Prevalence of vulvar pain in an urban, minority population. J Reprod Med 52:59, 2007

Lee A, Bradford J, Fischer G: Long-term management of adult vulvar lichen sclerosus: a prospective cohort study of 507 women. JAMA Dermatol 151:1061, 2015

Lee A, Lim A, Fischer G: Fractional carbon dioxide laser in recalcitrant vulval lichen sclerosus. Australas J Dermatol 57(1):39, 2016

Leung DY, Boguniewicz M, Howell MD, et al: New insights into atopic dermatitis. J Clin Invest 113(5):651, 2004

Lundqvist EN, Wahlin YB, Hofer PA: Methotrexate supplemented with steroid ointments for the treatment of severe erosive lichen ruber. Acta Derm Venereol 82:63, 2002

Lynch PJ: Lichen simplex chronicus (atopic/neurodermatitis) of the anogenital region. Dermatol Ther 17(1):8, 2004

Lynch PJ, Moyal-Barracco M, Bogliatto F, et al: 2006 ISSVD classification of vulvar dermatoses: pathological subsets and their clinical correlates. J Reprod Med 52(1):3, 2007

Lynch PJ, Moyal-Barracco M, Scurry J et al: 2011 ISSVD terminology and classification of vulvar dermatological disorders: an approach to clinical diagnosis. J Reprod Med 16(4):339, 2012

Mann MS, Kaufman RH: Erosive lichen planus of the vulva. Clin Obstet Gynecol 34(3):605, 1991

Margesson LJ: Contact dermatitis of the vulva. Dermatol Ther 17(1):20, 2004

Marren P, Wojnarowska F, Powell S: Allergic contact dermatitis and vulvar dermatoses. Br J Dermatol 126(1):52, 1992

Mattila A, Miettinen A, Heinonen PK: Microbiology of Bartholin's duct abscess. Infect Dis Obstet Gynecol 1(6):265, 1994

Mazdisnian F, Degregorio F, Mazdisnian F, et al: Intralesional injection of triamcinolone in the treatment of lichen sclerosus. J Reprod Med 44(4):332, 1999

Mirowski GW, Edwards L: Diagnostic and therapeutic procedures. In Edwards L (ed): Genital Dermatology Atlas. Philadelphia, Lippincott Williams & Wilkins, 2004, p 9

Mistiaen P, Poot E, Hickox S, et al: Preventing and treating intertrigo in the large skin folds of adults: a literature overview. Dermatol Nurs 16(1):43, 2004

Morrissey D, El-Khawand D, Ginzburg N, et al: Botulinum toxin a injections into pelvic floor muscles under electromyographic guidance for women with refractory high-tone pelvic floor dysfunction: a 6-month prospective pilot study. Female Pelvic Med Reconstr Surg 21(5):277, 2015

Mortimer PS, Dawber RP, Gales MA, et al: Mediation of hidradenitis suppurativa by androgens. Br Med J (Clin Res Ed) 292(6515):245, 1986

Moyal-Barracco M, Edwards L: Diagnosis and therapy of anogenital lichen planus. Dermatol Ther 17(1):38, 2004

Murina F, Tassan P, Roberti P, et al: Treatment of vulvar vestibulitis with submucous infiltrations of methylprednisolone and lidocaine. An alternative approach. J Reprod Med 46(8):713, 2001

Nielsen GP, Rosenberg AE, Koerner FC, et al: Smooth-muscle tumors of the vulva. A clinicopathological study of 25 cases and review of the literature. Am J Surg Pathol 20(7):779, 1996

Pagano R: Vulvar vestibulitis syndrome: an often unrecognized cause of dyspareunia. Aust N Z J Obstet Gynaecol 39(1):79, 1999

Patel NU, Roach C, Alinia H, et al: Current treatment options for acanthosis nigricans. Clin Cosmet Investig Dermatol 11:407, 2018

Poskitt L, Wojnarowska F: Lichen sclerosus as a cutaneous manifestation of thyroid disease. J Am Acad Dermatol 28(4):665, 1993

Powell J, Wojnarowska F: Childhood vulvar lichen sclerosus: an increasingly common problem. J Am Acad Dermatol 44(5):803, 2001

Reed BD, Caron AM, Gorenflo DW, et al: Treatment of vulvodynia with tricyclic antidepressants: efficacy and associated factors. J Low Genit Tract Dis 10(4):245, 2006

Reed BD, Crawford S, Couper M, et al: Pain at the vulvar vestibule: a web-based survey. J Low Genit Tract Dis 8:48, 2004

Reed BD, Haefner HK, Sen A, et al: Vulvodynia incidence and remission rates among adult women. Obstet Gynecol 112:231, 2008

Reed BD, Legocki LJ, Plegue MA, et al: Factors associated with vulvodynia incidence. Obstet Gynecol 123(2 Pt 1):225, 2014

Rhode JM, Burke WM, Cederna PS, et al: Outcomes of surgical management of stage III vulvar hidradenitis suppurativa. J Reprod Med 53:420, 2008

Riis PT, Boer J, Prens E, et al: Intralesional triamcinolone for flares of hidradenitis suppurativa: a case series. J Am Acad Dermatol 75(6):1151, 2016

Rogers RS III: Complex aphthosis. Adv Exp Med Biol 528:311, 2003

Rogers RS III: Recurrent aphthous stomatitis: clinical characteristics and associated systemic disorders. Semin Cutan Med Surg 16(4):278, 1997

Romo A, Benavides S: Treatment options in insulin resistance obesity-related acanthosis nigricans. Ann Pharmacother 42(7):1090, 2008

Rouzier R, Haddad B, Deyrolle C, et al: Perineoplasty for the treatment of introital stenosis related to vulvar lichen sclerosus. Am J Obstet Gynecol 186(1):49, 2002

Saraiya A, Al-Shoha A, Brodell RT: Hyperinsulinemia associated with acanthosis nigricans, finger pebbles, acrochordons, and the sign of Leser-Trélat. Endocr Pract 19(3):522, 2013

Savage JA, Maize JC Sr: Keratoacanthoma clinical behavior: a systematic review. Am J Dermatopathol 36(5):422, 2014

Segal D, Tifheret H, Lazer S: Submucous infiltration of betamethasone and lidocaine in the treatment of vulvar vestibulitis. Eur J Obstet Gynecol Reprod Biol 107(1):105, 2003

Sherrard J, Wilson J, Donders G, et al: 2018 European (IUSTI/WHO) International Union Against Sexually Transmitted Infections (IUSTI) World Health Organization (WHO) guideline on the management of vaginal discharge. Int J STD AIDS 29(13):1258, 2018

Sideri M, Origoni M, Spinaci L, et al: Topical testosterone in the treatment of vulvar lichen sclerosus. Int J Gynaecol Obstet 46(1):53, 1994

Sides C, Trinidad MC, Heitlinger L, et al: Crohn disease and the gynecologic patient. Obstet Gynecol Surv 68(1):51, 2013

Smith CH, Anstey AV, Barker JN, et al: British Association of Dermatologists' guideline for biologic interventions for psoriasis 2009. Br J Dermatol 161(5):987, 2009

Smith CH, Barker JN: Psoriasis and its management. BMJ 333(7564):380, 2006

Sobel JD, Reichman O: Diagnosis and treatment of desquamative inflammatory vaginitis. Am J Obstet Gynecol 117(4):850, 2011

Solomons CC, Melmed MH, Heitler SM: Calcium citrate for vulvar vestibulitis. A case report. J Reprod Med 36(12):879, 1991

Spergel JM, Paller AS: Atopic dermatitis and the atopic march. J Allergy Clin Immunol 112(Suppl 6):S118, 2003

Steward KM: Challenging ulcerative vulvar conditions: hidradenitis suppurativa, Crohn disease, and aphthous ulcers. Obstet Gynecol Clin North Am 44(3):453, 2017

Stockdale CK, Lawson HW: 2013 Vulvodynia Guideline update. J Low Genit Tract Dis 18(2):93, 2014

Tanaka K, Mikamo H, Ninomiya M, et al: Microbiology of Bartholin's gland abscess in Japan. J Clin Microbiol 43(8):4258, 2005

Torgerson RR, Marnach ML, Bruce AJ, et al: Oral and vulvar changes in pregnancy. Clin Dermatol 24(2):122, 2006

Traas MA, Bekkers RL, Dony JM, et al: Surgical treatment for the vulvar vestibulitis syndrome. Obstet Gynecol 107(2 Pt 1):256, 2006

Virgili A, Bacilieri S, Corazza M: Evaluation of contact sensitization in vulvar lichen simplex chronicus. A proposal for a battery of selected allergens. J Reprod Med 48(1):33, 2003

Visco AG, Del Priore G: Postmenopausal Bartholin gland enlargement: a hospital-based cancer risk assessment. Obstet Gynecol 87(2):286, 1996

Vrijman C, Kroon MW, Limpens J, et al: The prevalence of thyroid disease in patients with vitiligo: a systematic review. Br J Dermatol 167(6):1224, 2012

Zellis S, Pincus SH: Treatment of vulvar dermatoses. Semin Dermatol 15(1):71, 1996

Zendels K: Genital lichen planus: update on diagnosis and treatment. Seminar Cutan Med Surg 34:182, 2015

Zhang XJ, Chen JJ, Liu JB: The genetic concept of vitiligo. J Dermatol Sci 39(3):137, 2005

CHAPTER 5

Contraception and Sterilization

Today, the variety of effective fertility regulation methods continues to grow. Contraceptive availability is paramount for the care of women, as approximately half of pregnancies in the United States are unintended (Finer, 2016). And related, in 2014, nearly 11 percent of sexually active fertile women in the United States not pursuing pregnancy did not use any birth control method (Kavanaugh, 2018). These statistics have prompted a reexamination of contraceptive counseling to prevent unplanned pregnancy.

Contraceptive methods are grouped according to their effectiveness. *Top-tier* or *first-tier methods* are those that are most effective and are characterized by their ease of use (Fig. 5-1). These methods require minimal user motivation or intervention and have a typical-use pregnancy rate <1 per 100 women during the first year of use (Table 5-1) (Guttmacher Institute, 2018; Trussell, 2018). As expected, these first-tier methods provide the longest duration of contraception after initiation and require the fewest number of return visits. Top-tier methods include various methods of male and female sterilization, intrauterine contraceptive devices, and contraceptive implants. The last two are considered *long-acting reversible contraceptives (LARCs)*. Although counseling is provided for all contraceptive methods, a reduction in the unintended pregnancy rate may be better achieved by increasing top-tier method use.

Second-tier methods include systemic hormonal contraceptives that are available as oral tablets, intramuscular injections, transdermal patches, or transvaginal rings. In sum, their typical-use pregnancy rate is 4 to 7 per 100 users during the first year (see Table 5-1). Perfect-use rates reflect the pregnancy rate if a method is used flawlessly. With second-tier methods, the greater difference between perfect- and typical-use rates most likely stems from a failure to redose at the appropriate interval. Automated reminder systems for these second-tier methods have shown limited efficacy (Halpern, 2013).

Third-tier methods include condoms for men and women, withdrawal, and fertility awareness methods such as cycle beads.

The typical-use pregnancy rate is 13 to 24 pregnancies per 100 users in the first year (Guttmacher Institute, 2018). However, efficacy rises with consistent and correct use.

Fourth-tier methods include spermicidal preparations, which have a typical-use failure rate of 28 percent per 100 first-year users (Guttmacher Institute, 2018).

MEDICAL ELIGIBILITY CRITERIA

In 2016, the Centers for Disease Control and Prevention published updated *United States Medical Eligibility Criteria (US MEC)* for contraceptive use in the United States (Curtis, 2016).

TABLE 5-1. Contraceptive Failure Rates During the First Year of Method Use in Women in the United States

Method[a]	Perfect Use	Typical Use
Top tier: most effective		
Intrauterine devices:		
52-mg LNG-IUS	0.1	0.1
T 380A copper	0.6	0.8
Etonogestrel implant	0.1	0.1
Female sterilization	0.5	0.5
Male sterilization	0.1	0.15
Second tier: very effective		
Combination pill	0.3	7
Vaginal ring	0.3	7
Patch	0.3	7
DMPA	0.2	4
Progestin-only pill	0.3	7
Third tier: effective		
Condom		
Male	2	13
Female	5	21
Diaphragm with spermicides	16	24
Fourth tier: least effective		
Spermicides	18	28
Sponge		
Multiparas	20	27
Nulliparas	9	14

[a]Methods organized according to tiers of efficacy.
DMPA = depot medroxyprogesterone acetate;
LNG-IUS = levonorgestrel-releasing intrauterine system.

Description	Method examples	Pregnancy per 100 woman years

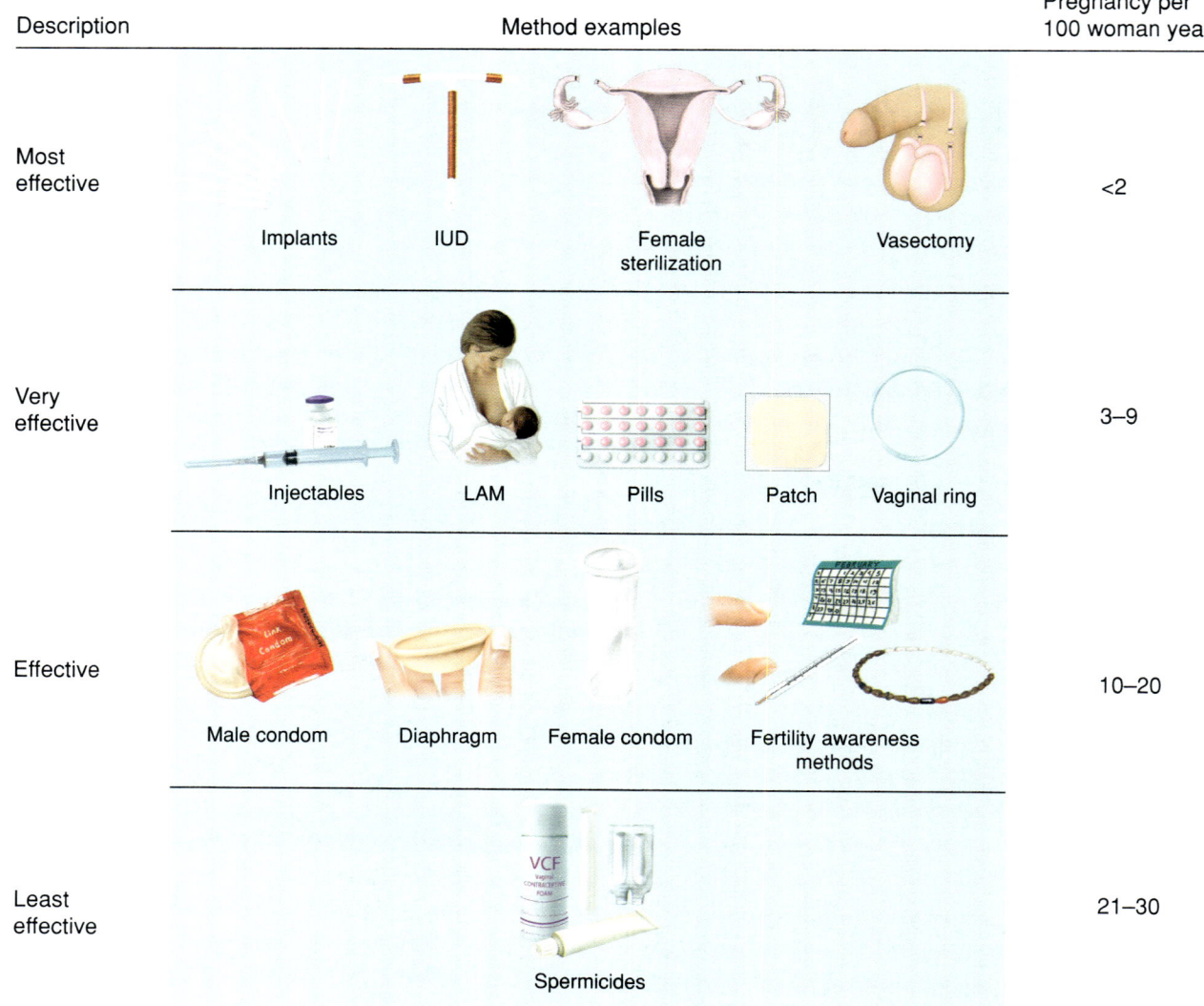

Most effective	Implants IUD Female sterilization Vasectomy	<2
Very effective	Injectables LAM Pills Patch Vaginal ring	3–9
Effective	Male condom Diaphragm Female condom Fertility awareness methods	10–20
Least effective	Spermicides	21–30

FIGURE 5-1 Contraceptive methods arranged by effectiveness.

These US MEC guidelines are available and updated regularly at the CDC website: www.cdc.gov/reproductivehealth/contraception/mmwr/mec/summary.html. In the US MEC, many contraceptive methods are classified into six groups by their similarity: combination hormonal contraceptive (CHC), progestin-only pill (POP), depot medroxyprogesterone acetate (DMPA), implants, levonorgestrel-releasing intrauterine system (LNG-IUS), and copper intrauterine device (Cu-IUD). For a given health condition, each method is categorized 1 through 4. The score describes a method's safety profile for a typical woman with that condition: (1) no restriction of method use, (2) method advantages outweigh risks, (3) method risks outweigh advantages, or (4) method poses unacceptably high health risk.

■ Lactation

Lactation is one factor addressed in the US MEC guidelines. Approximately 20 percent of breast-feeding women will ovulate by 3 months postpartum. Ovulation often precedes menstruation, and these women are at risk for unplanned pregnancy. For women who breastfeed intermittently, effective contraception should begin as if they were not breastfeeding. Moreover, contraception is essential after the first menses unless pregnancy is planned.

Of available methods, the Cu-IUD does not affect lactation because it lacks hormones. The category 2 status in Table 5-2 reflects a higher rate of expulsion if placed place in the puerperium but later than 10 minutes after delivery.

Starting hormonal contraceptives during the puerperium is ideally a shared decision-making process between provider and new mother (Bryant, 2019). Theoretically, systemic progestins may interfere with initial breast milk production. This is reflected in their peripartum US MEC category 2 status during the first 4 weeks postpartum. In reviews, authors describe the lack of evidence to support a negative effect of progestin contraception on lactation (Gurtcheff, 2011; Lopez, 2015c; Phillips, 2016; Tepper, 2016b). However, because progestins are metabolized variably among individuals, alteration in breastfeeding due to individual differences is possible. CHCs are category 2 status or higher because the estradiol component may raise the risk of venous thromboembolism (VTE), especially during the puerperium.

TABLE 5-2. U.S. Medical Eligibility Criteria for Use of Various Contraceptive Methods While Breastfeeding

Method[a]	Category
CHCs[b]	
Breastfeeding	
<21 d	4
21 d–<30 d	3
30–42 d[c]	2
>42 d	2
Non-breastfeeding	
<21 d	4
21–42 d[c]	2
>42 days	1
DMPA, POPs, Implants	
Breastfeeding	
<1 month	2
≥1 month	1
Non-breastfeeding	1
LNG-IUS	
Breastfeeding or not	
<10 min	2
10 min to ≤4 weeks	2
≥4 weeks	1
Puerperal sepsis	4
Cu-IUD	
Breastfeeding or not	
<10 min	1
10 min to ≤4 weeks	2
≥4 weeks	1
Puerperal sepsis	4

[a]Time reflects time from delivery.
[b]Combined hormonal contraceptive (CHC) group includes pills, vaginal ring, and patch.
[c]Associated risks that increase puerperal category score include: age ≥35, transfusion at delivery, BMI ≥30, PPH, cesarean delivery, smoking, preeclampsia.
Cu-IUD = copper-bearing intrauterine device; DMPA = depot medroxyprogesterone acetate; LNG-IUS = levonorgestrel-releasing intrauterine system; POPs = progestin-only pills.
Summarized from Curtis, 2016.

Adolescents

The adolescent birth rate in the United States reached an all-time low in 2017 (Martin, 2018). Despite this, adolescent pregnancy rate in this country is the highest among industrialized countries and is 22 births per 1000 women aged 15 to 19 years. IUDs and implants are safe for adolescents and thus are recommended by national bodies such as the American College of Obstetricians and Gynecologists (2018a) and the American Academy of Pediatrics (2014). Importantly, in 2011, 75 percent of adolescent pregnancies were unintended (Finer, 2016). Thus, effective contraception

counseling ideally is provided *before* the onset of sexual activity. In most states, minors have explicit legal authority to consent to contraceptive services, and in many areas, publicly funded clinics provide free contraception to adolescents (Guttmacher Institute, 2014). Moreover, contraception can be provided without a pelvic examination or cervical cancer screening.

■ Perimenopause

In the perimenopause, ovulation becomes irregular and fertility wanes. However, pregnancies do occur, and in women aged >40 years, nearly half of all pregnancies are unintended (Finer, 2011). Importantly, pregnancy with advanced maternal age carries greater risk for pregnancy-related morbidity and mortality. Women in this group may also have coexistent medical problems that may preclude certain contraceptive methods. Last, perimenopausal symptoms may be improved with hormonal contraceptive methods. Women are encouraged to continue contraceptive use until they have achieved a full year of amenorrhea.

TOP-TIER CONTRACEPTIVE METHODS

■ Intrauterine Contraception

Intrauterine contraception (IUC) is now used by almost 12 percent of all contraceptive users in the United States (Fig. 5-2) (Guttmacher Institute, 2018). This is a sixfold rise since 2002. Still, this rate is much lower compared with the worldwide IUC use rate of 14 percent and the rate in China (40 percent) (United Nations, 2013).

Some barriers to IUC use in the United States include cost, politics, and provider failure to offer or encourage this method. Despite higher up-front costs, the extended span of effective IUC use results in competitive cost effectiveness compared with other contraceptive forms.

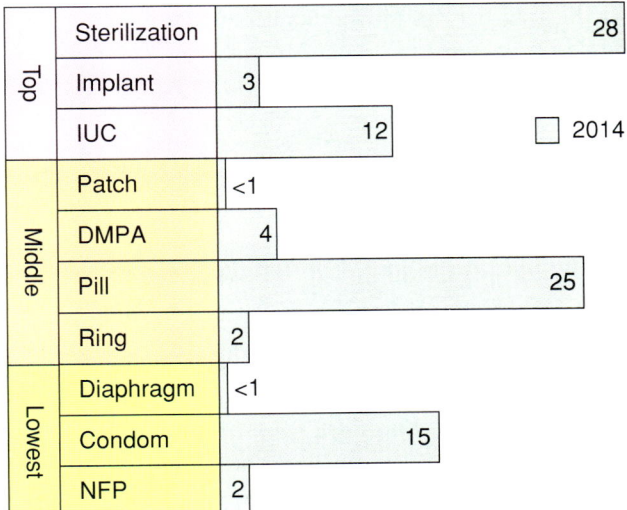

FIGURE 5-2 Rates of contraceptive methods used in the last month by women in the United States, 2014. These do not sum to 100 percent, as withdrawal method and emergency contraception values were not included. DMPA = depot medroxyprogesterone acetate. IUC = intrauterine contraception; NFP = natural family planning.

TABLE 5-3. Properties of Intrauterine Devices

Active Agent	Quantity of Active Agent	Width × Height (mm)	Inserter Tube Diameter (mm)	FDA-Approved Duration of Use (years)	String Color	Silver Ring	Brand Name
LNG	52 mg	32 × 32	4.4	5	Tan	No	Mirena
LNG	52 mg	32 × 32	4.8	5	Blue	No	Liletta
LNG	19.5 mg	28 × 30	3.8	5	Blue	Yes	Kyleena
LNG	13.5 mg	28 × 30	3.8	3	Tan	Yes	Skyla, Jaydess
Copper	380 mm^2	32 × 36	—	10	White	No	ParaGard

LNG = levonorgestrel.

Levonorgestrel-Releasing Intrauterine System

These contraceptives have become more popular in the United States, and currently four types of levonorgestrel-releasing intrauterine systems are approved by the Food and Drug Administration (FDA) (Table 5-3). These contraceptive systems are T-shaped polyethylene structures with the stem encased by a cylinder containing polydimethylsiloxane and levonorgestrel (Fig. 5-3). The cylinder has a permeable membrane that regulates continuous daily hormone release. Although similarly shaped, each device type can be distinguished by its size, string color, and presence or absence of a silver band at the junction of the stem and arms.

Several progestin-mediated mechanisms may explain the contraceptive action of the LNG-IUS. The progestin renders the endometrium atrophic; it stimulates thick cervical mucus that blocks sperm penetration into the uterus; and it may decrease tubal motility, thereby preventing ovum and sperm union. The progestin may also inhibit ovulation, but this is inconsistent (Nilsson, 1984).

Shown in Table 5-4 are the contraindications to use of LNG-IUS. Women who have had a prior ectopic pregnancy may be at higher risk for another because of diminished tubal motility from progestin action. In women with uterine leiomyomas, placement of the LNG-IUS may be problematic if the uterine cavity is distorted. Although not a strict limit, many studies have included only uteri measuring ≤12-week size.

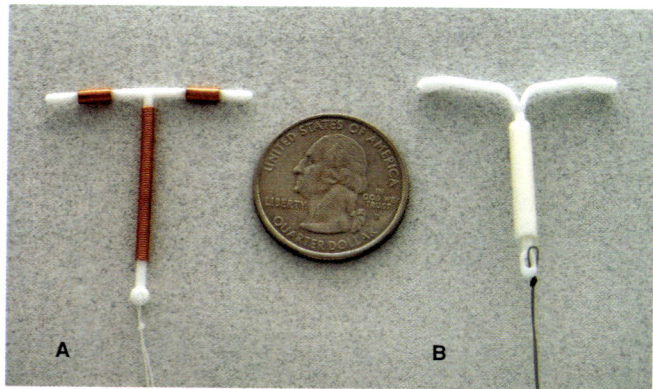

FIGURE 5-3 Intrauterine contraceptive devices. **A.** Copper-containing device. **B.** Levonorgestrel-releasing device.

Copper-T 380A Intrauterine Device

Marketed as ParaGard, this device is composed of a stem wrapped with 314 mm^2 of fine copper wire, and each arm has a 33-mm^2 copper bracelet. The sum of these is 380 mm^2 of copper. As shown in Figure 5-3, two strings extend from the base of the stem. The Cu-T 380A is approved for 10 years of continuous use, although it has been shown to prevent pregnancy with continuous use for up to 20 years (Bahamondes, 2005).

The intense local inflammatory response induced in the uterus by copper-containing devices leads to lysosomal activation and other inflammatory actions that are spermicidal (Alvarez, 1988; Ortiz, 1987). In the unlikely event that fertilization does occur, the same inflammatory actions are directed against the blastocyst. And finally, the endometrium becomes hostile for implantation.

Counseling for Intrauterine Contraception

Infection. Several improvements have created safer and more effective models. That said, some unwanted side effects and misconceptions persist surrounding their use.

First, fear of IUD-associated infections precluded use in the past. Improved device design has mitigated these concerns appreciably. In addition, several well-designed studies have shown that sexual behavior and sexually transmitted disease (STD) are important risk factors.

With current devices, prophylactic antibiotics are unnecessary with insertion for women at low risk for STDs (American College of Obstetricians and Gynecologists, 2018c). Of the <1 in 100 women who develop an infection within 20 days of IUD insertion, most have a concomitant unrecognized cervical infection. Accordingly, women at higher risk for lower genital tract STDs are screened either before or at the time of IUD insertion (Centers for Disease Control and Prevention, 2015; Turok, 2016). If this STD test result is positive and the patient is asymptomatic, the IUD may remain and targeted antibiotics are provided. Alternatively, a small number of pelvic infections are presumed to be caused by intrauterine contamination with normal flora at the time of insertion. Thus, antibiotics selected for treatment of symptomatic pelvic infection within the early weeks following IUD insertion should be broad-spectrum to adequately cover all these organisms.

Long-term IUC use is not associated with a greater pelvic infection rate in women at low risk for STDs. Indeed, these long-term users have a pelvic infection rate comparable with

TABLE 5-4. Contraindications to IUD Use

Copper-containing
Pregnancy or suspicion of pregnancy
Uterine abnormality with distorted uterine cavity
Acute PID, or current behavior suggesting a high risk for PID
Postpartum endometritis or postabortal endometritis in the past 3 months
Known or suspected uterine or cervical malignancy
Genital bleeding of unknown etiology
Mucopurulent cervicitis
Wilson disease
Allergy to any component of ParaGard
A previously placed IUD that has not been removed

Levonorgestrel-releasing
Pregnancy or suspicion of pregnancy
Uterine abnormality with distorted uterine cavity
Acute PID or history of unless there has been a subsequent intrauterine pregnancy
Postpartum endometritis or infected abortion in the past 3 months
Known or suspected uterine or cervical neoplasia
Uterine bleeding of unknown etiology
Untreated acute cervicitis or vaginitis or other lower genital tract infections
Acute liver disease or liver tumor (benign or malignant)
Increased susceptibility to pelvic infection
A previously placed IUD that has not been removed
Hypersensitivity to any component of Mirena
Known or suspected breast cancer or other progestin-sensitive cancer

IUD = intrauterine device; PID = pelvic inflammatory disease.

that of combination oral contraceptive users. Any pelvic infection after 45 to 60 days is considered sexually transmitted and appropriately treated as described in Chapter 3 (p. 115). Unless a tuboovarian abscess has formed, women who develop a genital tract infection with an IUD in place do not need to have the IUD removed. Close clinical reevaluation, which would be warranted for outpatient management of any patient with pelvic inflammatory disease, is warranted (Centers for Disease Control and Prevention, 2015).

Special concerns have arisen for women in whom *Actinomyces* species are identified in the lower genital tract, most commonly during Pap test reporting. Fiorino (1996) noted a 7-percent incidence in the Pap smears of IUD users compared with a 1-percent incidence in nonusers. Currently, in the absence of symptoms, incidental identification of *Actinomyces* species in cytologic specimens has uncertain significance. For an asymptomatic woman, the American College of Obstetricians and Gynecologists (2017) favors expectant management. Other treatment options include oral antibiotics, IUD removal, or antibiotics plus IUD removal. Symptomatic pelvic actinomycosis is rare but tends to be indolent and severe. Treatment is described in Chapter 3 (p. 72).

Young Nulliparas. Young nulliparas, including adolescents, can safely use IUC (American College of Obstetricians and Gynecologists, 2018a; Lohr, 2017). Revised labeling now places no restrictions on IUC use based on parity. A 1-percent lidocaine paracervical block placed immediately before IUD insertion can significantly lower pain scores for nulliparas aged 14 to 22 years (Akers, 2017). However, for all women, misoprostol administration prior to IUD insertion does not enhance insertion success and may increase associated insertional pain (Matthews, 2016; Lathrop, 2013).

Human Immunodeficiency Virus-Infected Women. Intrauterine contraception is appropriate for women with human immunodeficiency virus (HIV) infection who meet other usual criteria for IUD insertion. Neither device type is associated with higher IUD complication rates if used in this population. Moreover, IUDs do not appear to adversely affect viral shedding or antiretroviral therapy efficacy (Tepper, 2016a).

Postabortion or Postpartum Placement. An ideal time to improve successful provision of contraception is immediately following abortion or delivery. For women with an induced or spontaneous first- or second-trimester abortion, IUC can be placed immediately after uterine evacuation. Insertion techniques depend upon uterine size. After first-trimester evacuation, the uterine cavity length seldom exceeds 12 cm. In these instances, the IUD can be placed using the inserter provided in the package. If the uterine cavity is larger, the IUD can be placed using ring forceps with sonographic guidance.

In women for whom an IUD is placed immediately after induced abortion, the repeat induced abortion rate is only one third of the rate of women not choosing immediate IUD placement (Goodman, 2008; Heikinheimo, 2008). As perhaps expected, the risk of IUD expulsion is slightly higher when placed immediately after abortion or miscarriage, but the advantages of preventing unplanned pregnancies seem to outweigh this (Bednarek, 2011; Fox, 2011; Okusanya, 2014).

Insertion of an IUD immediately following vaginal or cesarean delivery at or near term also has been studied. Moreover, for puerpera at highest risk for future pregnancy complications, the Society for Maternal Fetal Medicine (2019) encourages immediate postpartum LARC insertion for candidates. Placement by hand or by using an instrument has a similar expulsion rate (Xu, 1996).

As with postabortion insertion, expulsion rates by 6 months are higher than those in women whose IUD is placed after complete uterine involution (Lopez, 2015a). In one study, the expulsion rate in the former group was nearly 25 percent (Chen, 2010). Even in these circumstances, however, immediate placement may be beneficial because in some populations up to 40 percent of women do not return for a postpartum clinic visit (Ogburn, 2005). Finally, postpartum placement is category 1 or 2 by the US MEC, that is, its advantages consistently outweigh the risks if puerperal infection is absent (see Table 5-2).

Despite these findings, many choose to delay insertion for several weeks postpartum. Insertion at 2 weeks is quite satisfactory, and in the Parkland System Family Planning Clinics, insertion is scheduled at 6 weeks postpartum to ensure complete uterine involution.

Menstrual Changes. Commonly, IUC may be associated with changes in menstrual patterns. Women who choose the Cu-T 380A are informed that dysmenorrhea and heavier bleeding with menses may develop. Objectively, no clinically significant hemoglobin changes are generally expected (Tepper, 2013). Treatment with a nonsteroidal anti-inflammatory drug (NSAID) will usually diminish the amount of bleeding—even normal amounts—and also relieve dysmenorrhea (Grimes, 2006). Intermenstrual bleeding, however, is typically not improved with these agents (Godfrey, 2013).

With the LNG-IUS, women are counseled to expect irregular spotting for up to 6 months after insertion and thereafter to expect monthly menses to be lighter or even absent. The LNG-IUS device reduces menstrual blood loss and is an effective treatment for some women with heavy menstrual bleeding. This is often associated with improved dysmenorrhea.

Expulsion or Perforation. Approximately 5 percent of women will spontaneously expel their IUD during the first year of use. This is most likely during the first month. Accordingly, a woman is instructed to periodically palpate the marker strings protruding from the cervical os. This can be accomplished by either sitting on the edge of a chair or squatting down and then advancing the middle finger into the vagina until the cervix is reached. Following IUD insertion, women are reappointed for a visit within several weeks, usually after completion of menses. At this meeting, any side effects are addressed, and IUD placement is confirmed by visualizing the marker strings. Some recommend barrier contraception to ensure contraception during this first month. This may be especially desirable if a device has been expelled previously.

The uterus may be perforated either with a uterine sound or with an IUD. Perforations may be clinically apparent or silent.

Their frequency depends on operator skill and is estimated to be 1 to 2 per 1000 insertions (Barnett, 2017). In some cases, a partial perforation during insertion results in the IUD later migrating through the uterine wall.

Marker Strings. In some cases, the IUD marker strings may not be palpated or seen during speculum examination. During the investigation, a nonpregnant patient should use alternative contraception. Possibilities are that the device was expelled silently, the device has partially or completely perforated the uterus, the woman is pregnant and the enlarging uterus has drawn the device upward, or the marker strings are temporarily hidden within the endocervical canal. An IUD should not be considered expelled unless it was seen by the patient.

Initially, an endocervical brush or similar instrument can be used to gently draw the string out of the cervical canal. If this is unsuccessful, at least two options are available. After pregnancy has been excluded, the uterine cavity is gently probed using an instrument such as Randall stone forceps or a rod with a hooked end. The strings or device will often be found with this method. If not successful, at this juncture, or possibly as a first choice, transvaginal sonography (TVS) is performed. As described in Chapter 2 (p. 35), 3-dimensional TVS better defines device positioning (Moschos, 2011). If the device is not seen within the uterine cavity or uterine walls, an abdominal radiograph, with or without a uterine sound in place, may localize it. Another option includes office hysteroscopy.

Management decisions depend upon device location and presence of an intrauterine pregnancy. First, a device may penetrate the uterine wall in varying degrees and should be removed. Devices with a predominantly intrauterine location are typically managed by hysteroscopic removal. In contrast, devices that have nearly completely perforated through the uterine wall are more easily removed laparoscopically.

For women with an intraabdominal IUD, an inert-material device located outside the uterus may cause harm, but not universally. Bowel perforations of both large and small bowel as well as bowel fistulas have been reported. In more typical situations, once identified laparoscopically, inert devices can easily be retrieved via laparoscopy. Conversely, an extrauterine copper-bearing device induces intense inflammation with adhesions. Thus, they are more firmly adhered, and laparotomy may become necessary (Balci, 2010). IUDs adhered to the omentum or small bowel may move with these organs from their preoperative radiographic location. Rarely, intraoperative radiography or fluoroscopy may be needed to localize such devices.

In those with pregnancy and an IUD, early pregnancy identification is important. Up to approximately 14 weeks' gestation, the IUD strings may be visible within the cervix, and if seen, they are grasped to remove the entire IUD. This action reduces subsequent complications such as spontaneous abortion, sepsis, and preterm birth (Brahmi, 2012). Tatum and colleagues (1976) reported an abortion rate of 54 percent with the device left in place compared with a rate of 25 percent if it was promptly removed. In another study of Cu-IUDs, outcomes were compared in the two groups of women with and without IUD removal as well as with the general obstetric population. In general, the group of women with an IUD left in place had the worst outcomes.

If pregnancy continuation is desired, IUD removal is recommended. However, if the strings are not visible, attempts to locate and remove the device may result in pregnancy loss. This risk must be weighed against the risk of leaving the device in place. If removal is attempted, TVS can be used. If attempts at removal are followed by evidence for uterine infection, then antibiotics are begun and followed by prompt uterine evacuation.

Ectopic Pregnancy. IUC is effective in preventing all pregnancies. However, the IUC mechanisms of action are more effective in preventing intrauterine implantation. Thus, if IUC fails, a higher proportion of pregnancies are likely to be ectopic (Furlong, 2002).

Insertion Procedures

Before IUD insertion, the FDA requires that a woman be given a brochure detailing the side effects and apparent risks from its use. Timing of insertion influences the ease of placement as well as pregnancy and expulsion rates. When done toward the end of normal menstruation, when the cervix is usually softer and somewhat more dilated, insertion may be easier, and early pregnancy can be excluded. However, insertion is not limited to this time. For a woman who is sure she is not pregnant and does not want to be pregnant, insertion may be carried out any time during the menstrual cycle. Insertion immediately postpartum or postabortion is also feasible and discussed earlier (p. 115).

Prior to insertion, a pelvic examination is completed to identify uterine position and size. Abnormalities are evaluated as they may contraindicate the device. Evidence for infection such as a mucopurulent discharge or significant vaginitis is appropriately treated and resolved before insertion.

For pain management, the most effective method of analgesia has not been established, and patient and provider preference direct selection. Applying lidocaine-prilocaine cream locally or placing paracervical blockade prior to insertion is helpful (Samy, 2019). As noted on page 115, young nulliparas may suffer less pain if a paracervical block with 1-percent lidocaine is given immediately before IUD insertion (Akers, 2017).

Ketorolac or naproxen also has some evidence-based support. But most other NSAIDs, topical lidocaine gel, or misoprostol do not reduce insertion pain (Lopez, 2015b; Samy, 2019).

Immediately prior to initiating the insertion procedure a bimanual examination is performed to assess the size, shape, and position of the uterus. After speculum placement, the cervical surface is cleaned with an antiseptic solution, and a tenaculum is placed on the cervical lip. The uterus is sounded to guide correct depth placement. Specific insertional steps for a given IUD are outlined and illustrated in the prescribing information document accompanying each IUD. If, during insertion, correct IUD positioning is uncertain, then placement may be checked by inspection with sonography. If not positioned completely within the uterus, the device is removed and replaced with a new one. An expelled or partially expelled device should not be reinserted.

■ Progestin Implants

Contraception can be provided by a progestin-containing device that is implanted subdermally and releases hormone over many years. The devices are coated with a polymer to prevent fibrosis. Several systems have been developed, but only one is available in the United States. The initial implant, the Norplant System, released levonorgestrel from six Silastic rods but was withdrawn from the U.S. market. Supposedly, the silicone-based rods caused ill-defined symptoms that were reversed with removal. A newer two-rod levonorgestrel system, Jadelle, has received FDA approval but is not marketed or distributed in the United States (Sivin, 2002). Sino-implant II is a structurally and pharmacologically similar system to Jadelle. It provides contraception for 5 years and is approved for use by several countries in Asia and Africa (Steiner, 2010).

The implant Nexplanon is currently the only subdermal contraceptive implant marketed in the United States. This single-rod subdermal implant contains 68 mg of the progestin etonogestrel covered by an ethylene vinyl acetate copolymer. Nexplanon has replaced the earlier etonogestrel implant, Implanon.

For Nexplanon, contraception is provided by progestin released continuously to suppress ovulation, thicken cervical mucus, and induce endometrial atrophy. The etonogestrel implant will provide contraception for up to 3 years. At this time, the device is removed, and another rod may be placed within the same incision site. Contraindications for this device are similar to those cited for other progestin-containing methods. Specifically, these include pregnancy, thrombosis or thromboembolic disorders, benign or malignant hepatic tumors, active liver disease, undiagnosed abnormal genital bleeding, or breast cancer (Merck, 2018). Importantly, patients are counseled that Nexplanon causes *irregular bleeding* that does not normalize over time. Thus, women who cannot tolerate unpredictable and irregular spotting or bleeding should select an alternative method.

Nexplanon is inserted subdermally. In 2018, Merck released new recommendations for the location of the Nexplanon insertion. The Nexplanon should be placed overlying the triceps muscle 8 to 10 cm from the medial epicondyle of the humerus and 3 to 5 cm medial to the sulcus (groove) that lies between the biceps and triceps muscles (Merck, 2018). This location is intended to avoid the large blood vessels and nerves lying within and surrounding the sulcus. Subdermal placement is essential, and deeper insertion can risk nerve injury and intravascular migration (Odom, 2017; Rowlands, 2017). Immediately following insertion, the provider and patient should document that the device is palpable beneath the skin.

When Nexplanon is removed, this superficial location allows in-office extraction of the implant. Prior to removal, pressure on the proximal end of the device should elevate its distal tip. An inability to appreciate the distal tip may indicate a deep device. In this instance, removal by a provider with experience and an understanding of upper arm anatomy is preferred (American College of Obstetrics and Gynecology, 2019b; Laumonerie, 2018). For routine cases, following surgical cleansing of the site, a small incision is made large enough to admit hemostat tips. The implant is grasped and removed. If desired, a new rod can be placed at the same time. With the newer recommendations for the location of insertion, the replacement rod may need to be placed in a different location.

If Nexplanon is not palpable, it can be imaged by radiography. Norplant and Jadelle also are radiopaque. This is an advantage compared with Implanon, which was not radiopaque and required sonography with a 10- to 15-MHz sonographic transducer or MR imaging for identification (Shulman, 2006). In the rare event that an etonogestrel implant cannot be palpated or identified radiologically, the manufacturer can be contacted (1-877-888-4231) and arrangements made for etonogestrel level measurement (Merck, 2018).

■ Permanent Contraception—Sterilization

In 2014, surgical sterilization was one of the most commonly reported forms of contraception in childbearing-aged women in the United States (Guttmacher Institute, 2018). These procedures cannot be tracked accurately because most interval tubal sterilizations and vasectomies are performed in ambulatory surgical centers. However, according to the National Survey of Family Growth, approximately 643,000 female tubal sterilizations are performed annually in the United States (Chan, 2010).

Female Tubal Sterilization

This is usually accomplished by occlusion or division of the fallopian tubes to prevent ovum passage and fertilization. According to the National Health Statistics Report, 25 percent of contracepting women in the United States use this method (Daniels, 2015). Tubal sterilization procedures are performed in conjunction with approximately 7 percent of deliveries (Moniz, 2017). Procedures with this timing are termed *puerperal sterilization*. A tubal sterilization procedure done at a time unrelated to recent pregnancy is called *nonpuerperal tubal sterilization* or *interval sterilization*. Currently, nonpuerperal tubal sterilization is mainly accomplished via laparoscopy.

Tubal Interruption Methods. Three methods, along with their modifications, are used for tubal interruption. These include application of various permanent rings or clips to the fallopian tubes; electrocoagulation of a tubal segment; or ligation with suture material, with or without removal of a tubal segment. In a Cochrane review, Lawrie and colleagues (2016) concluded that all of these are effective in preventing pregnancy.

Electrocoagulation is used for destruction of a segment of tube and can be accomplished with either unipolar or bipolar current. Although unipolar coagulation has the lowest long-term failure rate, it also has the highest serious complication rate. For this reason, of the two, bipolar coagulation is favored by most (American College of Obstetricians and Gynecologists, 2019a).

Mechanical methods of tubal occlusion can be accomplished with: (1) a silicone rubber band such as the Falope Ring or the Tubal Ring, (2) the spring-loaded Hulka-Clemens clip—also known as the Wolf clip, or (3) the silicone-lined titanium Filshie clip. The steps to these procedures are described in Chapter 44 (p. 1019). In a randomized trial of 2746 women, Sokal and associates (2000) compared the Tubal Ring and Filshie clip and reported similar rates of safety and 1-year pregnancy rates of 1.7 per 1000 women. All of these mechanical occlusion methods have favorable long-term success rates.

Suture ligation with tubal segment excision is more often used for puerperal sterilization. Methods include Parkland, Pomeroy, and modified Pomeroy, which are illustrated in Chapter 43 (p. 943).

The type of abdominal entry for sterilization is variable. Laparoscopic tubal ligation is the leading method used in this country for nonpuerperal female sterilization. This is frequently done in an ambulatory surgical setting under general anesthesia, and the woman can be discharged several hours later. Alternatively, some choose minilaparotomy using a 3-cm suprapubic incision. This is especially popular in resource-poor countries. With either laparoscopy or minilaparotomy, major morbidity is rare. Minor morbidity, however, was twice as common with minilaparotomy in a review by Kulier and associates (2004). Finally, the peritoneal cavity can also be entered by colpotomy through the posterior vaginal fornix, although this approach is infrequently used.

Counseling. Indications for this elective procedure for sterilization include a request for sterilization with clear understanding that this is permanent and irreversible. Each woman is counseled regarding all alternative contraceptive options and their efficacy. Many women may also have questions or misunderstanding regarding possible long-term outcomes after female sterilization. As with any operation, surgical risks are assessed, and occasionally the procedure may be contraindicated.

Risk-Reducing Salpingectomy. The Society of Gynecologic Oncology currently recommends consideration of opportunistic bilateral salpingectomy as a preventive measure against serous ovarian and peritoneal cancers among women who are at average risk of ovarian cancer and are undergoing other pelvic surgery or sterilization at the completion of childbearing (Walker, 2015). Most pelvic serous cancers are thought to originate in the distal fallopian tube (Erickson, 2013). And, although currently theoretical, bilateral salpingectomy may lower ovarian cancer rates (Falconer, 2015; Lessard-Anderson, 2014). As discussed in Chapter 35 (p. 736), this may be especially relevant for women at greatest risk for these cancers, namely, women with *BRCA1* or *BRCA2* mutation. If risk-reducing salpingectomy is elected in women with *BRCA* mutations, the pathology requisition form should state this genetic information. This prompts more thorough tubal specimen sectioning and evaluation.

In low-risk women, because the ovarian cancer risk is less than 2 percent, risk-reducing salpingectomy as a sole procedure is likely unwarranted. However, if tubal sterilization is planned, women are counseled regarding risks and benefits of salpingectomy compared with tubal interruption. Data from epidemiologic studies find that tubal interruption offers an approximate 30-percent decline in ovarian cancer rates (Rice, 2012; Sieh, 2013). From similar studies, salpingectomy may reduce the risk by 42 to 78 percent (Gockley, 2018). As another advantage, subsequent tubal surgery may be avoided following total salpingectomy. Retrospective studies have reported that laparoscopic salpingectomy has similar blood loss and complication rate compared with tubal interruption (Kim, 2019; Powell, 2017; Westberg, 2017). However, no prospective studies of sufficient size or duration have yet been done to demonstrate the true risk and benefit ratio for women. Salpingectomy slightly lengthens operating time and may require additional laparoscopic ports. Lastly, with total salpingectomy for sterilization, few data describe the potential effects on ovarian reserve from blood supply disruption. In one small study comparing the two surgeries, no differences in the antimüllerian hormone level, which is a measure of ovarian reserve, were found (Ganer Herman, 2017; Findley 2013). Thus, women who are at average risk and who are requesting permanent contraception should be fully counselled on the risks and benefits of bilateral salpingectomy versus tubal interruption.

Regret. Invariably, some women will later express regrets regarding sterilization. From a CREST study, Jamieson and coworkers (2002) reported that by 5 years, 7 percent of women undergoing tubal ligation had regrets. This is not limited to female sterilization, as 6 percent of women whose husbands had undergone vasectomy had similar remorse. The cumulative probability of regret within 14 years of sterilization was 20 percent for women aged 30 or younger at sterilization compared with only 6 percent for those older than 30 years (Hillis, 1999).

No woman should undergo tubal sterilization believing that subsequent fertility is guaranteed either by surgical reanastomosis or by assisted reproductive techniques. These are technically difficult, expensive, and not always successful. Pregnancy rates vary greatly depending upon age, the amount of tube remaining, and the technology used. Pregnancy rates range from 50 to 90 percent with surgical reversal (Deffieux, 2011). Of note, pregnancies that result after tubal sterilization reanastomosis are at risk to be ectopic.

Method Failure. Reasons for interval tubal sterilization failure are not always apparent, but some have been identified. First, surgical error may occur and likely accounts for 30 to 50 percent of cases. Second, tubal fistula may complicate occlusion methods. Although usually encountered with electrocoagulation procedures, fistulas from inadequate or defective electric current delivery are now less likely because an amp meter is used routinely. In some cases, sterilization failure may follow spontaneous reanastomosis of the tubal segments. With faulty clips, occlusion is incomplete. Last, luteal phase pregnancy may occur and describes the situation in which a woman is already pregnant when the procedure is performed. This can often be avoided by scheduling surgery during the menstrual cycle's follicular phase and by preoperative human chorionic gonadotropin (hCG) testing.

The best estimated overall failure rate with laparoscopic tubal sterilization is from the CREST studies reported by Peterson and coworkers (1999). The reported failure rate was 1.3 percent of 10,685 tubal sterilization surgeries. Shown in Figure 5-4, rates vary for different procedures. And even with the same operation, failure rates vary. For example, with electrocoagulation, if fewer than three tubal sites are coagulated, the 5-year cumulative pregnancy rate approximates 12 per 1000 procedures. However, it is only 3 per 1000 if three or more sites are coagulated. The lifetime increased cumulative failure rates over time are supportive that failures after 1 year are not likely due to technical errors.

With method failure, pregnancies following tubal sterilization have a high incidence of being ectopically implanted compared with the rate in a general gynecologic population.

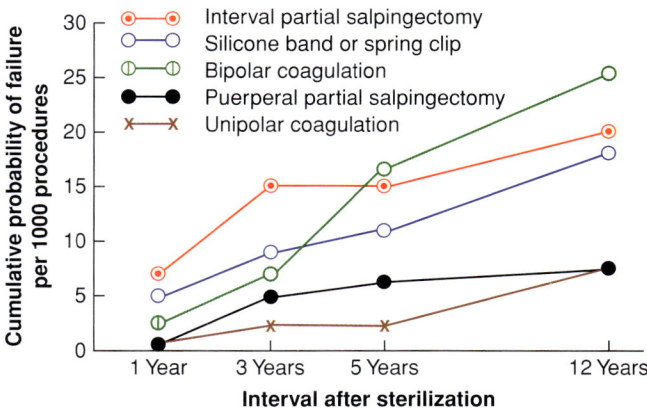

FIGURE 5-4 Data from the U.S. Collaborative Review of Sterilization (CREST) shows the cumulative probability of pregnancy per 1000 procedures by five methods of tubal sterilization.

These rates are especially high following electrocoagulation procedures, in which up to 65 percent of pregnancies are ectopic. With failures following other methods—ring, clip, tubal resection—this percentage is only 10 percent (Peterson, 1999). Importantly, ectopic pregnancy must be excluded when any symptoms of pregnancy develop in a woman who has undergone tubal sterilization.

Other Effects. Several studies have evaluated the risk of heavy menstrual bleeding and intermenstrual bleeding following tubal sterilization, and many report no link (DeStefano, 1985; Shy, 1992). In addition, Peterson and coworkers (2000) compared long-term outcomes of 9514 women who had undergone tubal sterilization with a cohort of 573 women whose partners had undergone vasectomy. Risks for heavy menstrual bleeding, intermenstrual bleeding, and dysmenorrhea were similar in each group. Perhaps unexpectedly, women who had undergone sterilization had *decreased* duration and volume of menstrual flow, they reported *less* dysmenorrhea, but they had an *increased* incidence of cycle irregularity.

Other long-term effects have also been studied. It is controversial whether risks for subsequent hysterectomy are elevated (Pati, 2000). In a CREST surveillance study, Hillis and associates (1997) reported that 17 percent of women undergoing tubal sterilization subsequently had undergone hysterectomy by 14 years. Although they did not compare this incidence with a control cohort, the indications for hysterectomy were similar to those for nonsterilized women who had undergone a hysterectomy. Women are highly unlikely to develop salpingitis following sterilization (Levgur, 2000).

Some psychological sequelae of sterilization were evaluated in a CREST study by Costello and associates (2002). Tubal ligation did not change sexual interest or pleasure in 80 percent of women. In the remaining 20 percent who reported a change, 80 percent described the changes to be positive.

Transcervical Sterilization

Sterilization may theoretically be completed using a transcervical approach to reach the tubal ostia. However, no methods using this approach are currently approved in the United States.

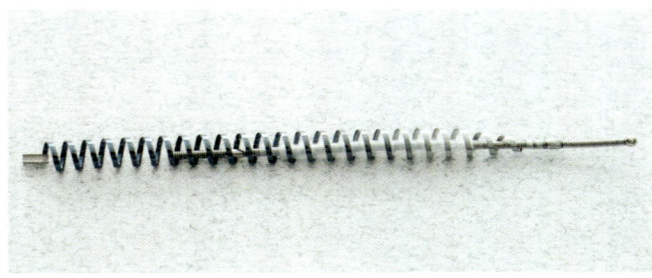

FIGURE 5-5 Microinsert used in the Essure Permanent Birth Control System.

Mechanical methods employ insertion of a device into the proximal fallopian tubes via hysteroscopy. Both the Essure system and the Adiana Permanent Contraception system have been removed from the U.S. market.

The Essure Permanent Birth Control System consists of a microinsert made of a stainless steel inner coil that is enclosed in polyester fibers. These fibers are surrounded by an expandable outer coil made of *nitinol*—a nickel and titanium alloy used in coronary artery stents (Fig. 5-5). Fibroblastic proliferation within the fibers causes tubal occlusion. Essure contraceptive failure rates range from <1 percent to 5 percent (Gariepy, 2014; Munro, 2014).

Chronic pelvic pain after hysteroscopic sterilization may develop in 2 to 6 percent of those with inserts (Chudnoff, 2015; Kamencic, 2016; Yunker, 2015). Pain may stem from tubal perforation, device migration, or the device itself (Adelman, 2014). For those desiring removal, one method is described in Chapter 44 (p. 1024). Importantly, device removal is not curative in all symptomatic patients (Clark, 2017; Maassen, 2019).

As with all sterilization procedures, Essure placement should be considered permanent. The success rate of subsequent spontaneous pregnancy after microsurgery tubal reversal ranges between 0 and 36 percent (Fernandez, 2014; Monteith, 2014).

Chemical agents may also be placed into the uterine cavity or tubal ostia to incite an inflammatory response to cause tubal occlusion. A method that has been used worldwide in more than 100,000 women consists of using an IUD-type inserter to place quinacrine pellets. It is effective, especially considering its simplicity. Pregnancy rates reported by Sokal and colleagues (2008) were 1 and 12 percent at 1 and 10 years, respectively. The World Health Organization (WHO) (2009) recommended against its use because of carcinogenesis concerns. Evidence is contradictory, and some consider it a potential option for resource-poor countries (Lippes, 2015).

Hysterectomy

For a woman with uterine or other pelvic disease for which hysterectomy may be indicated, this may be the ideal form of sterilization.

Male Sterilization

Vasectomy is performed for approximately one-half million men each year in the United States (Ostrowski, 2018). The office procedure is done with local analgesia and usually takes ≤20 minutes to complete. As illustrated in Figure 5-6, a small

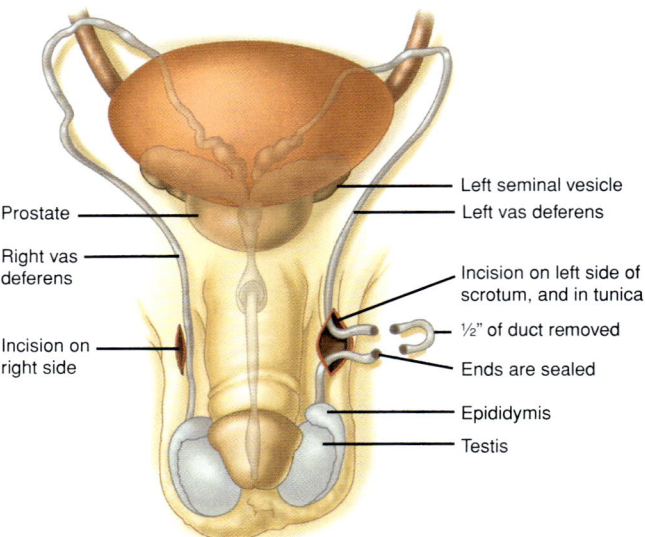

FIGURE 5-6 Vasectomy. On the left, the incision site is shown. On the right, a portion of the vas deferens has been excised.

incision is made in the scrotum, and the lumen of the vas deferens is disrupted to block sperm traveling from the testes. Vasectomy is highly effective and has a failure rate <1 percent (Michielsen, 2010). Causes include failure from unprotected intercourse too soon after vasectomy, incomplete vas deferens occlusion, or recanalization following suitable separation.

Sterility following vasectomy is not immediate nor is its onset reliably predictable. The time until complete expulsion of sperm stored distal to the vas deferens interruption is variable and requires approximately 3 months or 20 ejaculations. Thus, another form of contraception is used until azoospermia is documented. Although most recommend that semen be analyzed until two consecutive sperm counts are zero, Bradshaw and coworkers (2001) reported that a single azoospermic semen analysis is sufficient.

Fertility Restoration. After vasectomy, fertility may be restored either by surgical reanastomosis techniques or by sperm retrieval from the testis. Surgical reversal techniques and perioperative evaluation have been reviewed by the American Society for Reproductive Medicine (2008). Sperm retrieval combined with in vitro fertilization techniques avoids such reversal surgeries and is described in Chapter 21 (p. 464). From their review, Shridharani and Sandlow (2010) concluded that microsurgical reversal is cost effective, but comparative trials with sperm retrieval methods are needed.

Long-Term Effects. Regret of sterilization was discussed on page 119. Other than this, long-term consequences are rare (Amundsen, 2004). However, because antibodies directed at spermatozoa frequently develop in these men, there were initial concerns that these might cause systemic disease. Putative risks were analyzed by Köhler and coworkers (2009) and include cardiovascular disease, immune-complex disorders, psychological changes, male genital cancers, and frontotemporal dementia. Their findings and those of others are not convincing for a greater risk of cardiovascular disease or accelerated atherogenesis from vasectomy (Schwingl, 2000). Moreover, rates of testicular or prostate cancers do not appear increased with this procedure (Holt, 2008; Köhler, 2009).

SECOND-TIER CONTRACEPTIVE METHODS

Contraceptives considered to be *very effective* are the hormone-containing preparations that include combination oral contraceptives (COCs), progestin-only contraceptive pills, and contraceptives with estrogens and/or progestins that are made systemically available by injection, transdermal patch, or intravaginal ring. When used as intended, these methods are effective, however, their efficacy is user dependent. Thus, *typical use* considers each woman's compliance with taking a daily pill, changing transdermal patches or rings, or presenting for an injection (see Table 5-1). Such "real world" use significantly diminishes their efficacy, and for women in the United States, these contraceptives have a first-year pregnancy rate of 4 to 7 per 100 users (Trussell, 2018).

■ Combined Hormonal Contraceptives

These are contraceptives that contain an estrogen and a progestin. As such, several underlying conditions are considered contraindications (Table 5-5). CHCs are available in the United States in three formats—combination oral contraceptive pills, the transdermal patch, and the intravaginal contraceptive ring. Because of limited data for the transdermal and transvaginal methods relative to that for COCs, their use is usually considered along with the combined oral form.

Pharmacology

CHCs provide multiple contraceptive actions. The most important is ovulation inhibition by suppression of hypothalamic gonadotropin-releasing hormone, which prevents pituitary secretion of follicle-stimulating hormone (FSH) and luteinizing hormone (LH). Estrogens suppress FSH release and stabilize the endometrium to prevent intermenstrual bleeding—referred to as *breakthrough bleeding* in this setting. Progestins inhibit ovulation by suppressing LH, they thicken cervical mucus to restrict sperm passage, and they render the endometrium unfavorable for implantation. Thus, CHCs have contraceptive effects from both hormones and, when taken daily for 3 out of every 4 weeks, provide virtually absolute protection against conception.

Until recently, only two estrogens were available for use in oral contraceptives in the United States. These were *ethinyl estradiol* and its less commonly used 3-methyl ether, *mestranol* (Table 5-6). In 2010, a third estrogen compound—*estradiol valerate*—was approved by the FDA. Most currently available progestins are *19-nortestosterone* derivatives. However, drospirenone is a spironolactone analogue, and the dose of drospirenone in COCs currently marketed has properties similar to 25 mg of this diuretic (Seeger, 2007). It displays antiandrogenic activity, and its antimineralocorticoid properties may, in theory, cause potassium retention, leading to hyperkalemia. Thus, drospirenone is not prescribed for those with renal or adrenal insufficiency or with hepatic dysfunction. Moreover, monitoring of serum potassium levels is recommended in the first month for patients chronically treated concomitantly with any drug associated with potassium retention (Bayer HealthCare Pharmaceuticals, 2012). Several studies have shown improvement in symptoms for women with premenstrual dysphoric disorder (PMDD) who use a drospirenone-containing COC, Yaz (Lopez, 2012; Yonkers, 2005). For this pill, the FDA has approved its indications to include treatment of PMDD and moderate acne vulgaris for women requesting oral contraception.

TABLE 5-5. Contraindications to the Use of Combination Oral Contraceptives

Pregnancy
Uncontrolled hypertension
Smokers older than 35 years
Diabetes with vascular involvement
Cerebrovascular or coronary artery disease
Migraines with associated focal neurologic deficits
Thrombophlebitis or thromboembolic disorders
History of deep-vein thrombophlebitis or thrombotic disorders
Thrombogenic heart arrhythmias or thrombogenic cardiac valvulopathies
Undiagnosed abnormal genital bleeding
Known or suspected breast carcinoma
Cholestatic jaundice of pregnancy or jaundice with pill use
Hepatic adenomas or carcinomas or active liver disease with abnormal liver function
Endometrial cancer or other known or suspected estrogen-dependent neoplasia

TABLE 5-6. Estrogen and Progestins Used in FDA-Approved Oral Contraceptive Pills

Combination Pills	
Estrogen Type (pill dose)	**Paired Progestin[a]**
Ethinyl estradiol 10 μg	Norethindrone acetate
Ethinyl estradiol 20 μg	Desogestrel
	Drospirenone
	Levonorgestrel
	Norethindrone acetate
Ethinyl estradiol 25 μg	Desogestrel
	Norgestimate
Ethinyl estradiol 30–35 μg	Desogestrel
	Drospirenone
	Ethynodiol diacetate
	Levonorgestrel
	Norethindrone
	Norethindrone acetate
	Norgestimate
	Norgestrel
Ethinyl estradiol 50 μg	Ethynodiol diacetate
	Norgestrel
Estradiol valerate 2 mg	Dienogest
Mestranol 50 μg	Norethindrone

[a]Progestins are listed alphabetically.
FDA = Food and Drug Administration.

Progestins were initially selected for their progestational potency. However, they are often compared, marketed, and prescribed based on their presumed estrogenic, antiestrogenic, and androgenic effects. However, the doses of progestins used in combined contraceptive formulations are so low that none of these purported negative side effects are actually manifested clinically. In fact, an important effect of CHCs is enhanced production of sex hormone–binding globulin (SHBG) by the liver and production is promoted mostly by the estrogen component of CHCs. Elevated SHBG levels lower serum free testosterone levels and thereby limit 5α-reductase, the enzyme necessary to convert testosterone to its active form, dihydrotestosterone. For this reason, progestins can be expected to have salutary effects on androgen-related conditions such as acne (Rosen, 2003; Thorneycroft, 1999).

Combined Oral Contraceptive Pills

Formulations. COCs are marketed in a bewildering variety. Currently, the daily estrogen content in most COCs varies from 20 to 50 μg of ethinyl estradiol, and most pills contain 35 μg or less (see Table 5-6). Of note, in 2011, the FDA approved the first pill containing only 10 μg of ethinyl *estradiol—Lo Loestrin Fe*. For current formulations, the lowest acceptable dose is governed by the ability to prevent unacceptable breakthrough bleeding.

With COCs, the progestin dose can be constant throughout the cycle—*monophasic pills*—but the dose frequently is varied—*biphasic* and *triphasic pills* (Fig. 5-7). In some of these, the estrogen dose is also varied during the cycle. Such *multiphasic pills* were developed to reduce the amount of total progestin per cycle without sacrificing contraceptive efficacy or cycle control. The reduction is achieved by beginning with a low dose of progestin and raising it later in the cycle. Theoretically, the lower total dose minimizes the intensity of progestin-induced metabolic changes and adverse side effects. Disadvantages of multiphasic formulations include confusion caused by the multicolored pills, and some brands contain five colors. Also, breakthrough bleeding or spotting rates are likely higher compared with monophasic pills (Woods, 1992).

In a few COCs, inert placebo pills have been replaced by tablets containing iron. These have the suffix Fe added to their name. In addition, Beyaz has a form of folate—levomefolate calcium—within both its active and placebo pills.

Administration. Women may begin COCs on a *quick start* method. With this, pills are started on any day of the cycle, commonly the day prescribed. This approach improves short-term compliance (Westhoff, 2002, 2007a). A more traditional schedule—the *Sunday start*—requires pill initiation on the first Sunday following the onset of menses. If menses begin on a Sunday, pills are started that day. Last, both Sunday start and quick start methods require use of an additional method for 1 week to protect against conception, unless the pill is started on the first day of a menstrual cycle, in which case an additional contraceptive method is unnecessary.

To obtain maximum efficacy and promote regular use, most manufacturers offer dispensers that provide 21 sequential color-coded tablets containing hormones, followed by seven inert tablets of another color (see Fig. 5-7B). Some newer, lower-dose pill regimens continue active hormones for 24 days, followed by 4 days of inert pills (see Fig. 5-7C). The goal of these 24/4 regimens is to improve the efficacy of very low-dose COCs. Importantly, for maximum contraceptive efficiency, each woman should adopt an effective scheme for ensuring consistent daily or nightly self-administration.

During COC use, if one dose is missed, conception is unlikely with higher-dose monophasic COCs. When this is recognized, taking that day's pill plus the missed pill will minimize breakthrough bleeding. The remainder of the pill pack is then completed with one pill taken daily.

If several doses are missed, or if a dose is missed with the lower-dose pills, then two pills are taken but an effective barrier technique is added for the subsequent 7 days. The remainder of the pack is completed with one pill taken daily. Alternatively, a new pack can be started and a barrier method added as additional contraception for a week. With any scenario of missed pills, if withdrawal bleeding does not occur during the placebo pills, the pills are continued, but the woman should seek medical attention to exclude pregnancy. Fortunately, CHCs are not teratogenic if taken accidentally during early pregnancy (Charlton, 2016).

Transdermal System

One transdermal system is available in the United States—*Ortho Evra patch*. The patch has an inner layer with an adhesive and hormone matrix and an outer water-resistant layer. The patch is applied to the buttocks, upper outer arm, lower abdomen, or upper torso but avoids the breasts. It delivers daily a dose of 150 μg of the progestin norelgestromin and 20 μg of ethinyl estradiol. A new patch is applied each week for 3 weeks, followed by a patch-free week to allow withdrawal bleeding.

Initial concerns questioned the patch efficacy in obese women. However, evidence informing use of the transdermal patch among

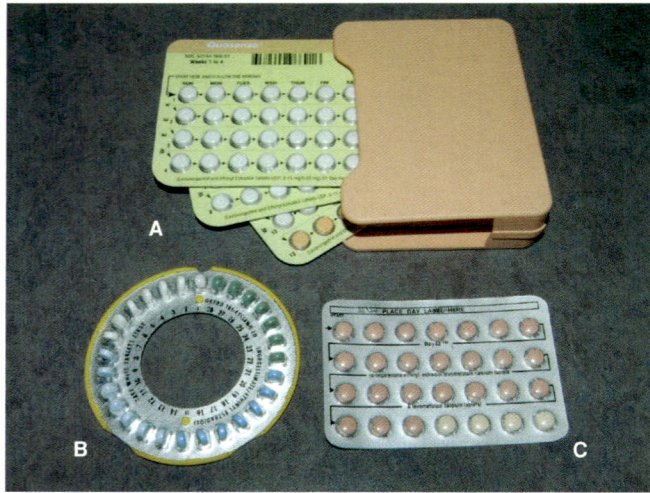

FIGURE 5-7 Various combined oral contraceptive (COC) pills. **A.** Extended-use COCs. Each of the three sequential cards of pills is taken. Placebo pills (*peach*) are found in the bottom card. **B.** 21/7 triphasic COCs. Active pills are taken for 3 weeks and are followed by seven placebo pills (*green*). With triphasic pills, the combination of estrogen and progestin varies with color changes, in this case, from white to blue to dark blue. **C.** 24/4 monophasic COCs. Monophasic pills contain a constant dose of estrogen and progestin throughout the pill pack. With 24/4 dosing regimens, the number of placebo pills is decreased to four.

women with a body mass index (BMI) ≥25 is low quality and limited (Lopez, 2016). Currently, no recommendations suggest a transdermal patch dosing change for women with a BMI >30 (Curtis, 2016). The patch's other metabolic and physiologic effects mirror those seen with low-dose COCs, with the caveat that accumulated experience is limited. The patch is suitable for women who prefer weekly applications to daily dosing and who meet the other criteria for CHC administration.

Another concern was that CHC delivered by the patch may be associated with a higher risk for VTE and other vascular complications. This followed reports that patch use was associated with greater hepatic synthesis of procoagulants compared with COC or vaginal ring use (Jensen, 2008; White, 2006). Although peak serum estrogen levels were lower with patch versus COC use, total exposure was greater—a relatively greater net estrogen effect (Kluft, 2008; van den Heuvel, 2005). Despite lack of a convincing clinical association, the FDA in 2008 ordered patch labeling to state that users *may* be at higher risk for developing VTE. To date, conclusive evidence for greater morbidity with the patch compared with other CHC forms is lacking (Jick, 2010; Tepper, 2017).

Transvaginal Ring

One intravaginal hormonal contraceptive is available in the United States—*NuvaRing*. It is a flexible polymer ring with a 54-mm outer diameter and a 50-mm inner diameter (Fig. 5-8). Its core releases a daily dose of 15 µg ethinyl estradiol and 120 µg of the progestin etonogestrel. These doses effectively inhibit ovulation, and the failure rate is reported to be 0.65 pregnancies per 100 woman-years (Mulders, 2001; Roumen, 2001).

Prior to dispensing, the pharmacy must keep rings refrigerated. Once dispensed, their shelf life is 4 months. The ring is initially inserted within 5 days after the onset of menses. After 3 weeks, it is removed for 1 week to allow withdrawal bleeding. Then, a new ring is inserted. Breakthrough bleeding is uncommon. Up to 20 percent of women and 35 percent of men reported being able to feel the ring during intercourse. If bothersome, the ring may be removed for coitus, but it should be replaced within 3 hours.

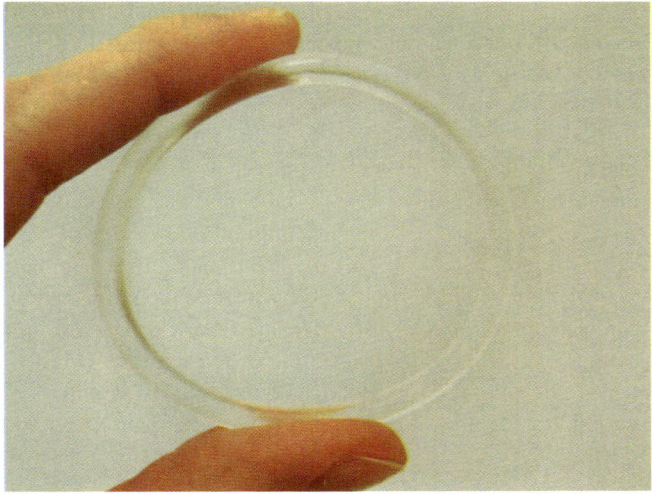

FIGURE 5-8 Estrogen- and progestin-releasing vaginal contraceptive ring.

Extended-Cycle Contraception

The use of CHCs continuously for more than 28 days has become increasingly popular. Benefits include fewer episodes of cyclic bleeding, diminished menstrual symptoms, and lower costs. Several prepackaged formulations are available, but extended-cycle contraception can also be achieved in other ways. Namely, the standard 21- or 28-day COC packs, with the placebo pills discarded, can be used continuously. Also, either the transdermal patch or the vaginal ring can be used without the 1-week hormone-free interval.

Several factors unique to extended-cycle CHCs are important. Some of these are shared with continuous progestin contraceptive methods such as implants or injections. The principal change is loss of menstrual normalcy that manifests as less frequent, lighter, and generally unpredictable bleeding episodes. For example, amenorrhea of 6 months or more is reported to affect 8 to 63 percent of extended-cycle users. Although considered a benefit by most women, it is far from a guaranteed one. More often, women have fewer bleeding episodes per month. This allows repair of associated anemia in those who had heavy menstrual bleeding prior to extended-cycle use.

However, these characteristics also render some women reluctant to use this method, as it may be considered "unnatural" to miss monthly menses. Some are concerned that amenorrhea may be a sign of pregnancy, may diminish future fertility, or may increase endometrial neoplasia risk. Rather, findings support a *lower* risk for endometrial malignancy with cyclic CHC use. Thus on a biological basis, it seems reasonable to conclude that this protective effect would also apply to continuous CHC use. Moreover, hypothalamic-pituitary-ovarian suppression is greater with continuous use and reduces the possibility of escape ovulation caused by delayed start of a new contraceptive cycle.

Drug Interactions

Interactions between CHCs and various other medications take two forms. First, hormonal contraceptives may interfere with the actions of some drugs shown in Table 5-7. As an example, levels of the anticonvulsant lamotrigine are typically lowered by CHCs (p. 126).

In contrast, some drugs shown in Table 5-8 may diminish the effectiveness of CHCs. In many cases, genes coding for cytochrome oxidase system enzymes are either stimulated or suppressed. Notably, antibiotics other than rifampin do not lower clinical efficacy of COCs (Simmons, 2018). Also, most antiretroviral regimens for treatment of human immunodeficiency infection (HIV) are compatible with CHCs. Of exceptions, efavirenz may lower CHC efficacy, whereas CHCs may diminish fosamprenavir effectiveness (Curtis, 2016; Nanda, 2017). For other HIV agents, similar potential interactions can be researched at the University of California, San Francisco HIV InSite website: http://hivinsite.ucsf.edu/insite?page=ar-00-02.

These interactions often require that the dose of contraceptive or that of the other drug be adjusted to ensure efficacy. Alternatively, choosing another contraceptive method may be preferable.

Use with Medical Disorders

A summary of health benefits associated with combination hormonal contraceptives is found in Table 5-9. Despite this,

TABLE 5-7. Drugs Affected by Combination Oral Contraceptives (COCs)

Interacting Drug	Documentation	Management
Analgesics		
Acetaminophen	Adequate	Possible dose increase needed
Aspirin	Probable	Possible dose increase needed
Meperidine	Suspected	Possible dose decrease needed
Morphine	Probable	Possible dose increase needed
Anticoagulants		
Dicumarol, warfarin	Controversial	
Antidepressants		
Imipramine	Suspected	Reduce dosage about a third
Tranquilizers		
Diazepam, alprazolam	Suspected	Reduce dose
Temazepam	Possible	Possible dose increase needed
Other benzodiazepines	Suspected	Observe for increased effect
Antiinflammatories		
Corticosteroids	Adequate	Watch for increased effect, decrease dose accordingly
Bronchodilators		
Aminophylline, theophylline	Adequate	Reduce starting dose by a third
Antihypertensives		
Cyclopenthiazide	Adequate	Increase dose
Metoprolol	Suspected	Possible dose decrease needed
Other		
Troleandomycin	Suspected liver damage	Avoid
Cyclosporine	Possible	May use smaller dose
Antiretrovirals	Variable	See manufacturer or other[a]
Lamotrigine	Adequate	With monotherapy or when given with drugs that are not known to alter lamotrigine levels, then avoid COCs

[a]University of California at San Francisco (UCSF): HIV Insite, 2014.
From Gaffield, 2011; Nanda, 2017; Wallach, 2000.

TABLE 5-8. Drugs That May Reduce COC Efficacy

Antitubercular drug
Rifampin

Antifungal drug
Griseofulvin

Anticonvulsants and sedatives
Phenytoin, barbiturates, primidone, carbamazepine, oxcarbazepine, topiramate, rufinamide, felbamate

Antiretroviral drug
Efavirenz

Herbal medicine
St. John's Wort

COC = combination oral contraceptives; EE = ethinyl estradiol.
Summarized from Back, 1980; Berry-Bibee, 2016; Curtis, 2016; Gaffield, 2011; Nanda, 2017; Reimers, 2015; Van Dijke, 1984.

interactions of CHCs with some chronic medical disorders may constitute relative or absolute contraindication to CHC use. These are described in the following sections.

Obese and Overweight Women. In general, CHCs are highly effective in obese women (Lopez, 2016). However,

TABLE 5-9. Some Benefits of Combination Estrogen Plus Progestin Oral Contraceptives

Acne improvement
Increased bone density
Prevention of atherogenesis
Fewer premenstrual complaints
Inhibition of hirsutism progression
Decreased risk of ectopic pregnancy
Decreased activity of rheumatoid arthritis
Reduced menstrual blood loss and anemia
Reduction in various benign breast diseases
Improved dysmenorrhea from endometriosis
Decreased risk of endometrial and ovarian cancer
Decreased incidence and severity of acute salpingitis

obesity may result in altered pharmacokinetics of some CHC methods. That said, data regarding overweight women are conflicting regarding greater pregnancy risk due to decreased CHC efficacy from lowered bioavailability (Brunner, 2005; Edelman, 2009; Holt, 2005; Westhoff, 2010). Importantly, in some women, obesity may be synergistic with other conditions, described next, that may render CHCs a less optimal contraceptive method.

Excessive weight gain is a concern with use of any hormonal contraceptive. Gallo and associates (2014) again concluded in their review that available evidence was insufficient to determine the influence of CHCs on weight gain, although no large effect was obvious.

Diabetes Mellitus. Higher-dose COCs were associated with insulin antagonistic properties, particularly those mediated by progestins. However, with current low-dose CHCs, these concerns have been mitigated. In healthy women, large, long-term prospective studies have found that COCs do not increase the risk for diabetes (Rimm, 1992). Moreover, these agents do not appear to raise the risk for overt diabetes in women with prior gestational diabetes (Kjos, 1998). Last, use of these contraceptives is approved for nonsmoking diabetic women who are younger than 35 years and who have no associated vascular disease (American College of Obstetricians and Gynecologists, 2019d).

Cardiovascular Disease. In general, severe cardiovascular disorders limit the use of CHCs. For less severe disorders, however, current formulations do not raise associated risks.

First, low-dose CHCs do not appreciably raise the absolute risk of clinically significant hypertension (Chasan-Taber, 1996). However, it is common practice for patients to return 8 to 12 weeks following CHC initiation for evaluation of blood pressure and other symptoms. For those with already established chronic hypertension, CHC use is permissible in those with well-controlled, otherwise uncomplicated hypertension (American College of Obstetricians and Gynecologists, 2019d). Severe forms of hypertension, especially those with end-organ involvement, usually preclude CHC use.

Women who have had a documented *myocardial infarction* should not be given CHCs. That said, these contraceptives do not elevate the de novo risk for myocardial ischemia in nonsmoking women younger than 35 years (Margolis, 2007; Mishell, 2000; World Health Organization, 1997). Smoking by itself, however, is a potent risk factor for ischemic heart disease, and CHCs used after age 35 years act synergistically to enhance this risk.

Cerebrovascular Disorders. Women who have had either an *ischemic* or *hemorrhagic stroke* should not use CHCs. But the incidence in nonsmoking young women is low, and use of CHCs does not raise the risk for either type of stroke in these women (World Health Organization, 1996). Stroke is more commonly encountered in those who smoke, have hypertension, or have migraine headaches with visual aura *and* who use CHCs (MacClellan, 2007).

Migraine headaches may be a risk factor for strokes in some young women. One systematic review reported that women using COCs who had migraine headaches had a two- to fourfold greater risk for stroke compared with nonusers (Tepper, 2016c).

The American College of Obstetricians and Gynecologists (2019d), because the absolute risk is low, has concluded that CHCs may be considered for young nonsmoking women who have migraine headaches without focal neurologic changes. For many of these women, an intrauterine contraceptive method or a progestin-only pill may be more appropriate.

Venous Thromboembolism. Early in CHC history, it was apparent that *deep-vein thrombosis* and *pulmonary embolism* risks were significantly elevated in women who used these contraceptives (Realini, 1985). These risks were found to be estrogen-dose related and have been appreciably lowered with evolution of low-dose formulations that contain only 20 to 35 μg of ethinyl estradiol (Westhoff, 1998). Of note, a possible increased VTE risk with drospirenone-containing COCs has been shown in two studies. The FDA has encouraged an assessment of benefits and of VTE risks in users of these pills (Food and Drug Administration, 2012; Jick, 2011; Parkin, 2011).

Mishell and coworkers (2000) concluded that VTE risk is three- to fourfold higher in current COC users compared with nonusers. However, the risk without contraception is low—approximately 1 per 10,000 woman years—and thus the incidence with CHCs is only 3 to 4 per 10,000 woman years. Importantly, these CHC-enhanced risks appear to dissipate rapidly once contraceptive treatment is discontinued. And, of equal importance, these VTE risks are still lower than those estimated during pregnancy, which has an incidence of 5 to 6 per 10,000 woman years.

Several cofactors raise the incidence of VTE in women using estrogen-containing contraceptives or those who are pregnant or postpartum. These include one or more of the many *thrombophilias,* which include *protein C or S deficiency* or *factor V Leiden mutation* (Chap. 39, p. 834) (Mohllajee, 2006). Other factors that raise VTE risks are hypertension, obesity, diabetes, smoking, and a sedentary lifestyle (Pomp, 2007, 2008).

Older studies indicated a twofold higher risk for *perioperative VTE* in CHC users (Robinson, 1991). Data are lacking with the low-dose formulations currently used, and thus the American College of Obstetricians and Gynecologists (2019d) recommends balancing VTE risks against those of unintended pregnancy during the 4 to 6 weeks required preoperatively for thrombogenic effects of CHCs to dissipate. For women undergoing major surgery with prolonged immobility, CHCs are halted perioperatively.

Systemic Lupus Erythematosus. The use of CHCs in women with otherwise uncomplicated systemic lupus erythematosus (SLE) has been the "poster child" for evidence-based clinical research. In the past, and with good reason, CHCs were contraindicated in women with SLE. This was because of their underlying high risk to develop venous and arterial thrombosis along with the thrombogenic effects of older high-dose COC pills. The safety of the low-dose modern COCs in many women with SLE was shown in two randomized trials (Petri, 2005; Sánchez-Guerrero, 2005). Importantly, CHCs are not appropriate in women with SLE who have positive testing for antiphospholipid antibodies or have other known contraindications to CHC use. Affected women with these antibodies have elevated clotting risks.

Seizure Disorders. Approximately 1 million women of reproductive age in the United States are diagnosed with some form of epilepsy. As shown in Tables 5-7 and 5-8, metabolism and clearance of some CHCs are appreciably altered by some, but not all, of the commonly used anticonvulsants. One mechanism with several antiepileptic drugs is potent induction of cytochrome P450 system enzymes. In turn, this boosts contraceptive steroid metabolism, and serum levels of these decrease by as much as half (American College of Obstetricians and Gynecologists, 2019d; Zupanc, 2006).

These metabolic interactions usually do not result in increased seizure activity. One possible exception is combined use of CHCs and monotherapy with the anticonvulsant lamotrigine. Serum anticonvulsant levels decline by up to 50 percent, which may raise seizure risks (Gaffield, 2011).

Evidence-based guidelines for use of contraceptives by women with epilepsy are listed in the US MEC. Use of CHCs in epileptic women is rated as category 1. However, CHCs used concurrently with some anticonvulsants may reduce contraceptive or anticonvulsant effectiveness. Thus, epileptic women using cytochrome P450 enhancing anticonvulsants are counseled regarding alternate contraceptive methods if feasible. If not, a COC containing at least 30 μg of ethinyl estradiol should be used. For those using lamotrigine monotherapy, CHCs are not recommended.

Although they are not CHCs, progestin-only containing preparations also are affected by use of anticonvulsants that induce the cytochrome P450 enzyme system. These result in decreased serum progestin levels and lower rates of effective ovulation suppression and pose an unacceptable risk of unplanned pregnancy.

Liver Disease. Both estrogens and progestins have known effects on hepatic function. Cholestasis and cholestatic jaundice, which develop more commonly in pregnancy, also are infrequently induced by CHC use. Because susceptibility is likely due to an inherited gene mutation of bilirubin transport, cholestasis with CHCs is more likely in women also affected during a pregnancy. Discontinuing CHCs typically resolves symptoms. Whether these cholestatic effects of CHCs also raise risks for subsequent cholelithiasis and cholecystectomy is unclear. Any elevated risk is likely to be small, and the known effects of increasing parity on gallbladder disease must also be considered.

Regarding women with viral hepatitis or cirrhosis, the WHO has provided recommendations (Kapp, 2009b). For women who have active hepatitis, CHCs should not be initiated, but these may be continued in women who experience a flare of their liver disease while already taking CHCs. Use of progestin-only contraception in these women is not restricted. With cirrhosis, mild compensated disease does not limit the use of CHCs or progestin-only methods. However, in those with severe decompensated disease, all hormonal types are avoided.

Neoplastic Diseases. Stimulatory effects of sex steroids on some cancers are a concern. It would appear, however, that overall these hormones do not *cause* cancer (Hannaford, 2007). A report from the Collaborative Group on Epidemiological Studies of Ovarian Cancer (2008) verified earlier studies that showed a protective effect against endometrial and ovarian cancers

(Cancer and Steroid Hormone Study, 1987a,b). However, this protection wanes as duration from pill discontinuance lengthens (Tworoger, 2007). Reports concerning possible increased risks for premalignant and malignant changes of the liver, cervix, and breast are conflicting and are presented next.

First, *hepatic focal nodular hyperplasia* and *benign hepatic adenomas* were previously linked with older higher-dose estrogen-containing COCs. However, studies that evaluated women taking contemporary low-dose COCs reported no such association (Hannaford, 1997; Heinemann, 1998). Similarly, earlier correlations between CHCs and hepatocellular carcinoma have been refuted (Maheshwari, 2007; World Health Organization, 1989). For women with known tumors, COCs may be used in those with focal nodular hyperplasia, but avoided in those with benign hepatic adenoma and hepatocellular carcinoma (Kapp, 2009a).

Second, *cervical dysplasia* and *cervical cancer* rates are higher in COC users. These risks increase with duration of use. But, according to the International Collaboration of Epidemiological Studies of Cervical Cancer (2007), if COC use is discontinued, by 10 years the risk becomes comparable with that of never-users. The reasons for this neoplasia risk are speculative and may be related to more frequent human papillomavirus (HPV) exposure because of decreased use of barrier methods. It may also be related to the more frequent cytologic screening that COC users may have. Moreover, COCs may favor persistence of HPV infection and HPV oncogene expression (de Villiers, 2003). Importantly, if cervical dysplasia is treated, the recurrence rate is not higher in CHC users.

Last, *breast cancer* is stimulated by female sex steroid hormones, but it is still unclear whether CHCs have an adverse effect on tumor growth or development. The Collaborative Group on Hormonal Factors in Breast Cancer (1996) analyzed data from studies that included more than 53,000 women with breast cancer and 100,000 nonaffected women. They found a significant 1.24-fold higher risk for current COC users. This risk declined to 1.16 for those 1 to 4 years after discontinuing COCs and 1.07 for those at 5 to 9 years. The risks were not influenced by age at first use, duration of use, family history of breast cancer, first use prior to pregnancy, or the dose or type of hormone used. This lack of correlation serves to question any causal role of COCs in breast tumorigenesis.

The Collaborative Group investigators also found that COC-associated tumors tended to be to be less aggressive and that cancers were detected at earlier stages. They suggested that the increased cancer diagnosis may have been because of more intensive surveillance among users. In a case-control study—4575 cases and 4682 controls—no relationship was found with either current or past COC use and breast cancer (Marchbanks, 2002). Finally, women heterozygous for *BRCA1* or *BRCA2* gene mutations do not have a higher incidence of breast or ovarian cancer with COC use (Brohet, 2007). With regard to benign breast disease, Vessey and Yeates (2007) reported that COC use apparently *lowered* the relative risk.

■ Progestin-Only Contraceptives

Contraceptives that contain only a progestin were developed to obviate the unwanted side effects of estrogens. Progestins can be delivered by several routes that include tablets, injections, intrauterine devices, and subdermal implants.

Progestin-Only Pills

Also called *mini-pills*, POPs are taken daily. They do not reliably inhibit ovulation, but instead thicken cervical mucus and decidualize and atrophy the endometrium. Because mucus changes do not persist beyond 24 hours, to be maximally effective, a pill is ideally taken at the same time daily. Their use has not achieved widespread popularity because of a much higher incidence of irregular bleeding and a slightly higher pregnancy rate than that seen with CHCs (see Table 5-1).

POPs have minimal if any effect on carbohydrate metabolism and coagulation factors. They do not cause or exacerbate hypertension and thus may be ideal for some women at higher risk for other cardiovascular complications. Because they do not impair milk production, POPs are suitable for lactating women. When used in combination with breastfeeding, POPs are virtually 100-percent effective for up to 6 months (Betrabet, 1987; Shikary, 1987). POPs should not be taken by women with unexplained uterine bleeding, breast cancer, hepatic neoplasms, pregnancy, or active severe liver disease (Janssen Pharmaceuticals, 2017).

Compliance is essential to POP use. If a pill is taken even 4 hours late, an additional form of contraception must be used for the next 48 hours. This may contribute to another major drawback, which is a higher risk for contraceptive failure compared with CHCs. Moreover, with failure, the proportion of pregnancies that are ectopic is increased (Sivin, 1991).

Another disadvantage is irregular uterine bleeding. This may be characterized by amenorrhea, intermenstrual bleeding, or prolonged heavy menstrual bleeding. As with other progestin-containing contraceptive methods, functional ovarian cysts develop with a greater frequency, although they usually do not require intervention (Hidalgo, 2006; Inki, 2002).

Injectable Progestins

Formulations. Three injectable depot progesterone preparations are used worldwide. This method is popular in the United States and is used by approximately 5 percent of women choosing a contraceptive (Daniels, 2015). Injectable progestins have mechanisms of action similar to those for oral progestins and include greater cervical mucus viscosity, creation of an endometrium unfavorable for implantation, and unpredictable ovulation suppression.

Injectable preparations include depot medroxyprogesterone acetate—marketed as *Depo-Provera*. A 150-mg dose is given by intramuscular injection every 90 days. A derivative of DMPA is marketed as *depo-subQ provera 104*, and a 104-mg dose is given subcutaneously every 90 days. Because absorption is slower with subcutaneous injections, the 104-mg dose is equivalent to the 150-mg intramuscular preparation (Jain, 2004). With either method, if the initial dose is given within the first 5 days following menses onset, no back-up contraception is necessary (Haider, 2007). A third injectable depot progestin that is not currently available in the United States is norethindrone enanthate, which is marketed as *Norgest*, and a 200-mg dose is injected intramuscularly every 2 months.

Injectable progestins have contraceptive efficacy equivalent or better than that of COCs. With perfect use, DMPA has a pregnancy rate of 0.2 percent, but typical-use failure rates are as high as 7 percent at 12 months (Trussell, 2018). Depot progesterone does not suppress lactation, and iron-deficiency anemia is less likely in long-term users because of less menstrual bleeding. Progestin injectables should not be taken by women with pregnancy, unexplained uterine bleeding, breast cancer, active or history of thromboembolic disease, cerebrovascular disease, or significant liver disease (Pfizer, 2017).

As with most progestin-only contraceptive methods, DMPA does not significantly affect lipid metabolism, glucose levels, hemostatic factors, liver function, thyroid function, and blood pressure (Dorflinger, 2002). Moreover, these have not been shown to elevate the risk for VTE, stroke, or cardiovascular disease (Mantha, 2012; World Health Organization, 1998). Despite this, manufacturer prescribing information often lists thrombosis or thromboembolic conditions as contraindications. However, for individuals with these disorders, US MEC considers progestin-containing methods category 2.

Notable Effects. Patients interested in DMPA should be familiar with its potential effects and side effects. First, as is typical of progestin-only contraception, DMPA usually causes irregular menstrual-type bleeding. Cromer and coworkers (1994) reported that one fourth of women discontinued its use in the first year because of irregular bleeding. Amenorrhea may develop after extended use, and women are counseled about this benign effect.

Prolonged ovulation suppression may also persist after DMPA injections are stopped. In an earlier study by Gardner and Mishell (1970), one fourth of women did not resume regular menses for up to a year. Accordingly, DMPA may not be the best choice for women who plan to use contraception only briefly before attempting conception.

Bone mineral density can also be significantly diminished because of lowered estrogen levels and is most worrisome in long-term users. This loss is particularly relevant for adolescents because bone density accrues most rapidly from ages 10 to 30 years (Sulak, 1999). Additionally, decreased bone mineral density may be a concern for perimenopausal women, who will shortly be entering the menopause, a time of known accelerated bone loss. These concerns prompted the FDA in 2004 to require a black-box warning that DMPA "should be used as a long-term birth control method—longer than 2 years—only if other birth-control methods are inadequate." There are some mitigating factors that balance this concern. First, although bone loss is greatest during the first 2 years, it subsequently slows appreciably. Second, most bone lost during contraceptive use is restored within 5 years after its discontinuance (Clark, 2006; Harel, 2010). In sum, the American College of Obstetricians and Gynecologists (2019c) has concluded that concerns of bone density loss should not prevent or limit use of this contraceptive method.

Of potential cancer risks, cervical carcinoma in-situ rates are possibly raised with DMPA use. However, risks for cervical cancer or for hepatic neoplasms are not higher with this method (Thomas, 1995). Advantageously, ovarian and endometrial cancer rates are *decreased* (Kaunitz, 1996; World Health Organization, 1991). In addition, Skegg and colleagues (1995) pooled the results of the New Zealand and WHO case-control studies that included almost 1800 women with breast cancer. Compared with 14,000 controls, DMPA contraceptive use was associated with a twofold cancer risk in the first 5 years of use. However, the overall risk was not increased.

Of other effects, some women report breast tenderness with DMPA use. Depression also has been noted, but a causal link is unproven. Finally, although weight gain is often attributed to depot progestins, not all studies have shown this (Bahamondes, 2001; Mainwaring, 1995; Moore, 1995; Taneepanichskul, 1998). Beksinska and coworkers (2010) reported that adolescents who used intramuscular DMPA gained 2.3 kg more weight during a 4- to 5-year interval compared with weight gained by adolescents who used COCs. Subcutaneous DMPA also may cause modest weight gain in most women (Westhoff, 2007b). Because women who gain weight in the first 6 months of use are more likely to have long-term progressive weight gain, Le and coworkers (2009) suggest that these women may benefit from early counseling.

THIRD-TIER CONTRACEPTIVE METHODS

Contraceptive methods in this group are considered moderately effective. One type includes barrier methods, which are designed to prevent functional sperm from reaching and fertilizing the ovum. The other category consists of fertility awareness methods. Perhaps more so than with other contraceptive methods, moderately effective methods have the highest success rates when used by couples who are dedicated to their use.

■ Barrier Methods

These methods include vaginal diaphragms and male and female condoms. As shown in Table 5-1, the reported pregnancy rate for these methods with perfect use varies from 2 to 16 percent in the first year of use and is highly dependent on correct and consistent use.

Male Condom

Most condoms are made from latex rubber, and various sizes are manufactured to accommodate anatomy. Less commonly, polyurethane or lamb cecum is used.

The efficacy of condoms is enhanced appreciably with a reservoir tip. Lubricants should be water based because oil-based products destroy latex condoms and diaphragms (Waldron, 1989). Key steps to ensure maximal condom effectiveness include: (1) used with every coitus, (2) placed before penis and vagina contact, (3) withdrawn while penis still erect, (4) its base held during withdrawal, and (5) used with spermicide.

A distinct advantage of condoms is that, when used properly, they provide considerable—not absolute—protection against many STDs. Condoms also help prevent premalignant cervical changes, probably by blocking HPV transmission (Winer, 2006).

For latex-sensitive individuals, alternative condoms are available. Condoms made from lamb intestines—*natural skin* or *lambskin condoms*—are effective, but they do not provide

protection against STDs. Nonallergenic condoms are made with a synthetic thermoplastic elastomer, such as polyurethane, which is also used in some surgical gloves. These are effective against STDs but have significantly higher breakage and slippage rates compared with those of latex condoms (Gallo, 2006). In a randomized trial of 901 couples, Steiner and associates (2003) documented breakage and slippage with 8.4 percent of polyurethane condoms compared with only 3.2 percent of latex condoms. They also reported that 6-month typical pregnancy probabilities were 9.0 percent with polyurethane condoms but only 5.4 percent with latex ones.

Female Condom

Manufactured by many companies under different names, female condoms prevent pregnancy and STDs. One brand available in the United States is the *FC2 Female Condom*—a polyurethane cylindrical sheath with a flexible polyurethane ring at each end (Fig. 5-9). The open ring remains outside the vagina, and the closed internal ring is fitted behind the symphysis and beneath the cervix like a diaphragm (Fig. 5-10). It should not be used with a male condom because together they may slip, tear, or become displaced. In vitro tests show the female condom to be impermeable to HIV, cytomegalovirus, and hepatitis B virus. As shown in Table 5-1, the pregnancy rate is higher than with the male condom.

Diaphragm Plus Spermicide

The diaphragm consists of a circular rubber dome of various diameters supported by a circumferential metal spring (Fig. 5-11). When used in combination with spermicidal jelly or cream, it can be very effective. The spermicide is applied to the cervical surface centrally in the cup and along the rim. The device is then placed in the vagina so that the cervix, vaginal fornices, and anterior vaginal wall are partitioned effectively from the remainder of the vagina and the penis. At the same time, the centrally placed spermicidal agent is held against the cervix by the diaphragm. When appropriately positioned, the rim is lodged deep into the posterior vaginal fornix. Superiorly,

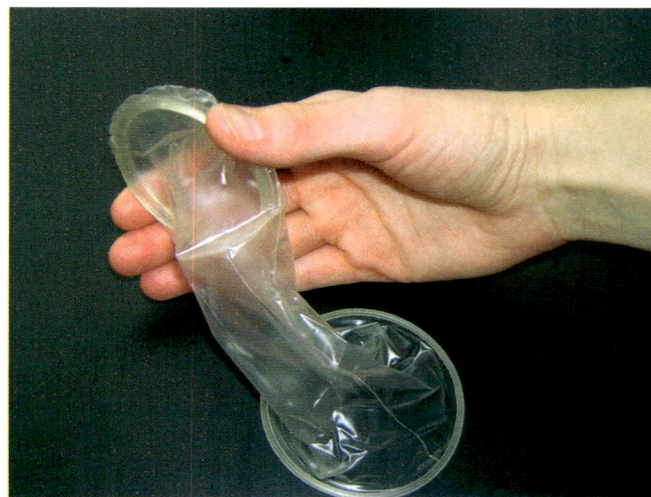

FIGURE 5-9 Female condom. (Reproduced with permission of The Cervical Barrier Advancement Society and Ibis Reproductive Health.)

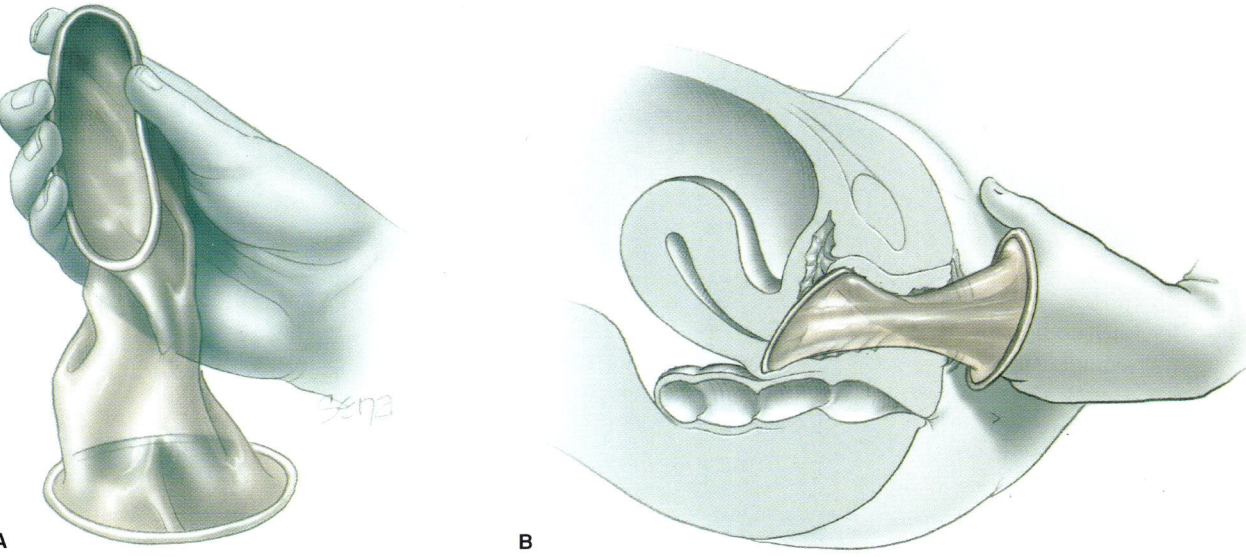

FIGURE 5-10 Female condom insertion and positioning. **A.** The inner ring is squeezed for insertion and is placed similarly to a diaphragm. **B.** The inner ring is pushed inward with an index finger.

the rim lies in close proximity to the inner surface of the symphysis immediately below the urethra (Fig. 5-12). If the diaphragm is too small, it will not remain in place. If too large, it will be uncomfortable when positioned. Because the variables of size and spring flexibility must be specified, the diaphragm is available only by prescription. Because of the requirement for proper placement, the diaphragm may not be an effective choice for women with significant pelvic organ prolapse. The malpositioned uterus can cause unstable diaphragm positioning that results in expulsion.

For use, the diaphragm and spermicidal agent can be inserted well before intercourse, but if more than 2 hours elapse, additional spermicide is placed in the upper vagina for maximum protection. Spermicide is similarly placed before each episode of coitus. The diaphragm is not removed for at least 6 hours after intercourse. Because toxic shock syndrome has been described following its use, the diaphragm is not left in place for longer than 24 hours.

Proper diaphragm use requires a high level of motivation. Vessey and coworkers (1982) reported a pregnancy rate of only 1.9 to 2.4 per 100 woman-years for compliant users. In a small study, Bounds and associates (1995) reported a much higher failure rate of 12.3 per 100 woman years. The unintended pregnancy rate is lower in women older than 35 years compared with younger women.

Cervical Cap

This reusable, washable, silicone barrier device surrounds the cervix to block sperm passage and is combined with a spermicide. Marketed in the United States, FemCap is currently

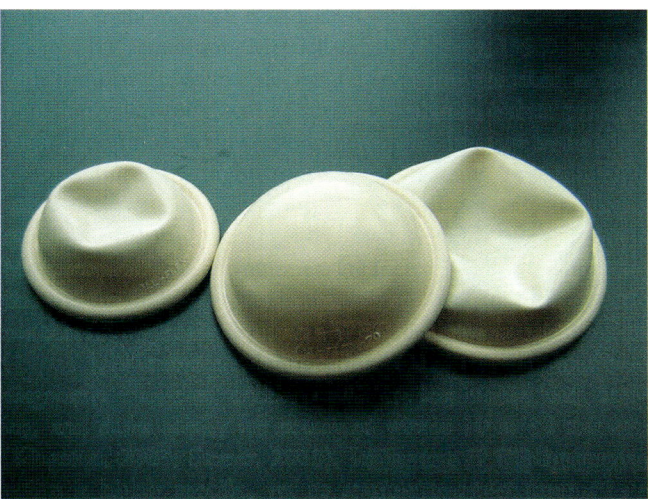

FIGURE 5-11 Group of three diaphragms. (Reproduced with permission from The Cervical Barrier Advancement Society and Ibis Reproductive Health.)

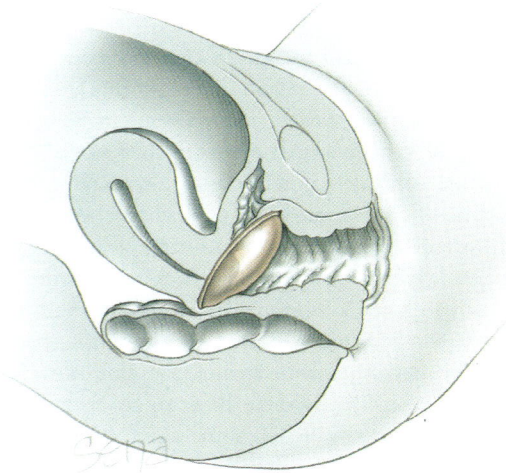

FIGURE 5-12 A diaphragm in place creates a physical barrier between the vagina and cervix.

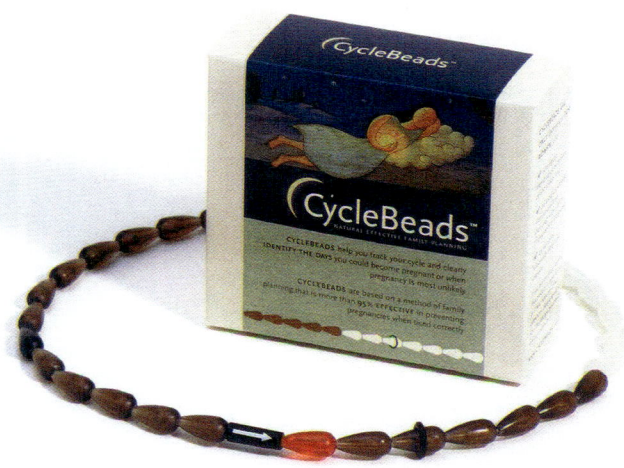

FIGURE 5-13 CycleBeads. During use, the red bead denotes menses onset, and the small black band is advanced for each day of the menstrual cycle. When the white beads are reached, abstinence is observed until brown beads begin again. (Reproduced with permission from Cycle Technologies.)

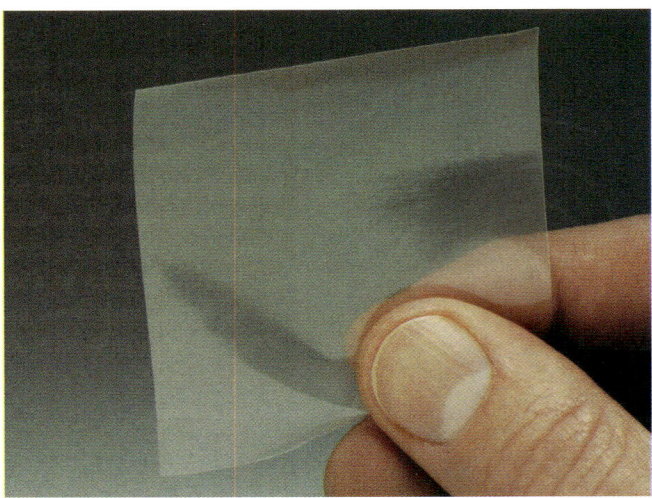

FIGURE 5-14 Vaginal contraceptive film. The film is first folded in half and then folded up and over the tip of the inserting finger. Once inserted near the cervix, the film will dissolve to provide spermicide.

available in 22-, 26-, and 30-mm diameters to accommodate cervical size. It may be inserted any time prior to intercourse and must be left in place for at least 8 hours thereafter. Spermicide dosing and redosing mirrors that with a diaphragm.

■ Fertility Awareness–Based Methods

This form of contraception involves identification of the fertile days of the menstrual cycle (Fig. 5-13). The couple may then avoid intercourse or use a barrier method during those days. The comparative efficacy of fertility awareness–based methods remains unknown (Peragallo Urrutia, 2018). Clearly, proper instruction is critical, and complex charting is involved. These charts, as well as detailed advice, are available from the FertilityUK for the United Kingdom at: www.fertilityuk.org.

FOURTH-TIER CONTRACEPTIVE METHODS

■ Spermicides

These contraceptives are marketed variously as creams, jellies, suppositories, aerosol foams, and film (Fig. 5-14). They are used widely in the United States, and most are available without a prescription. Probable users include women who find other methods unacceptable. They are useful especially for women who need temporary protection, for example, during the first week after starting CHC or while nursing.

Spermicidal agents provide a physical barrier to sperm penetration and a chemical spermicidal action. The active ingredient is nonoxynol-9 or octoxynol-9. Importantly, spermicides must be deposited high in the vagina in contact with the cervix shortly before intercourse. Their duration of maximal effectiveness is usually no more than 1 hour. Thereafter, they must be reinserted before repeat intercourse. Douching, if practiced, is avoided for at least 6 hours after intercourse.

High pregnancy rates are primarily attributable to inconsistent use rather than to method failure. Even if inserted regularly

and correctly, however, spermicides are reported to have a failure rate of up to 28 pregnancies per 100 woman-years with perfect use (see Table 5-1). If pregnancy does occur with use, spermicides are not teratogenic (Briggs, 2017).

Spermicides that primarily contain nonoxynol-9 do not provide protection against STDs. Also, long-term use of nonoxynol-9 was reported to have minimal effects on vaginal flora (Schreiber, 2006).

■ Contraceptive Sponge

The contraceptive sponge *Today* was reintroduced into the United States in 2005. Sold over the counter, it consists of a nonoxynol-9–impregnated polyurethane disc that can be inserted for up to 24 hours prior to intercourse (Fig. 5-15). The

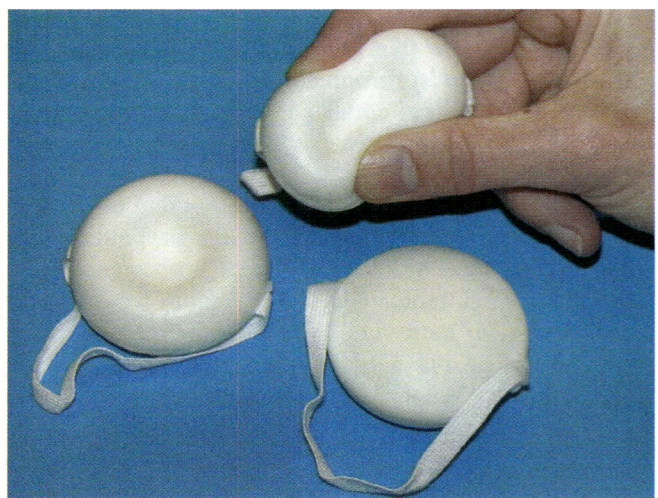

FIGURE 5-15 Vaginal sponge. When in position, the sponge dimple apposes the cervix surface, and the ribbon loop faces outward to allow easy hooking with a finger for removal.

disc is moistened and placed directly against the cervix. While in place, the sponge provides contraception regardless of the number of coital episodes. For efficacy, it remains in place for 6 hours after intercourse, and to lower irritation and infection risks, it remains no longer than 30 hours (Mayer Laboratories, 2011). Although perhaps more convenient, the sponge is less effective than the diaphragm or condom.

EMERGENCY CONTRACEPTION

Emergency contraception (EC) is appropriate for women presenting for contraceptive care following consensual but unprotected sexual intercourse or following sexual assault. If used correctly, several methods will substantially lower the likelihood of an unwanted pregnancy in these women. Methods currently available include sex steroid–containing compounds, antiprogesterone compounds, and the Cu-IUD (Table 5-10). Because duration of use is short, women with conditions that might normally contraindicate hormonal forms may be given these for EC.

Information regarding EC is made available to health care providers or patients by several 24-hour sources:

- American Congress of Obstetricians and Gynecologists: www.acog.org
- Emergency Contraception Hotline and website: 1-888-NOT-2-LATE (888-668-2528) and www.not-2-late.com
- Reproductive Health Technologies Project: rhtp.org/work/contraception/emergency-contraception/.

■ Hormone-Based Options
Mechanisms of Action

Hormonal contraceptives have different mechanisms of action depending on which day of the menstrual cycle intercourse occurs and which day the tablets are given (Croxatto, 2003). One major mode is inhibition or delay of ovulation (Marions, 2004). Other suggested mechanisms include endometrial changes that prevent implantation, interference with sperm transport or penetration, and impaired corpus luteum function (American College of Obstetricians and Gynecologists, 2018b). Despite these effects, every method used for postcoital contraception will have failures. Pregnancies that develop despite emergency hormonal contraception appear unaffected by this prophylaxis. Moreover, emergency hormonal contraception is not a form of medical abortion. Rather, this method prevents ovulation or implantation.

Except perhaps the copper IUD, other EC methods generally will not prevent pregnancy resulting from subsequent episodes of intercourse during the same cycle. Accordingly, use of a barrier technique is recommended until the next menses. When menstruation is delayed 3 weeks past its expected onset, the likelihood of pregnancy is increased and appropriate testing is instituted.

Estrogen-Progestin Combinations

Also known as the *Yuzpe method*, these COC-containing regimens shown in Table 5-10 have been approved by the FDA for use as EC (Yuzpe, 1974). Pills should be taken within 72 hours

TABLE 5-10. Methods Available for Use as Emergency Contraception

Method	Formulation	Pills per Dose
Progestin-only pill		
Plan B[a]	0.75 mg levonorgestrel	1
Plan B One-Step[b]	150 mg levonorgestrel	1
SPRM pill		
Ella[b]	30 mg ulipristal acetate	1
COC pills[a,c,d]		
Ogestrel	0.05 mg ethinyl estradiol + 0.5 mg norgestrel[e]	2
Lo/Ovral	0.03 mg ethinyl estradiol + 0.3 mg norgestrel[e]	4
Trivora (pink)	0.03 mg ethinyl estradiol + 0.125 mg levonorgestrel	4
Aviane	0.02 mg ethinyl estradiol + 0.1 mg levonorgestrel	5
Copper-containing IUD		
ParaGard T 380A		

[a]Treatment consists of doses taken 12 hours apart.
[b]Treatment consists of a single dose taken once.
[c]Use of an antiemetic agent before taking the medication will lessen the risk of nausea, which is a common side effect.
[d]A listing of other suitable COCs and dosing is found at https://ec.princeton.edu/questions/dose.html#dose.
[e]Norgestrel contains two isomers, and only one of these isomers is bioactive, namely levonorgestrel. Thus, the amount of norgestrel needed for efficacy is twice that of the levonorgestrel-based regimens.
COC = combination oral contraceptive; IUD = intrauterine device; SPRM = selective progesterone-receptor modulator.

of intercourse, are more effective the sooner they are taken, but may be given up to 120 hours. Initial dosing is followed 12 hours later by a second dose.

Efficacy is defined by the number of pregnancies observed after treatment divided by the estimated number that would have occurred with no treatment. This *prevented fraction* ranges widely between reports and averages 75 percent with COC regimens (American College of Obstetricians and Gynecologists, 2018b).

Nausea and vomiting are common with COC regimens because of their high estrogen doses. An oral antiemetic taken at least 1 hour before each dose may reduce symptoms. In randomized trials, a 1-hour pretreatment dose of either 50-mg meclizine or 10-mg metoclopramide was effective (Ragan, 2003; Raymond, 2000). If vomiting occurs within 2 hours of a dose, a replacement dose is given.

Progestin-Only Regimens

A progestin-only method of EC is marketed as *Plan B* and *Plan B One-Step*. Plan B consists of two tablets, each containing 0.75 mg of levonorgestrel. The first dose is taken within 72 hours of unprotected coitus but may be given as late as 120 hours, and the second dose is taken 12 hours later (see Table 5-10). Ngai and associates (2005) also showed that a 24-hour interval between dosing is effective. Plan B One-Step is a single, 1.5-mg levonorgestrel dose, which is taken ideally with 72 hours or up to 120 hours following intercourse.

Most studies, including a multicenter WHO trial, indicate that the progestin-only regimens are more effective than COC regimens to prevent pregnancy (von Hertzen, 2002). The American College of Obstetricians and Gynecologists (2018b) cites an approximately 50-percent lower pregnancy rate with levonorgestrel compared with COCs. Ellertson and colleagues (2003) reported a 55-percent pregnancy prevention rate even if Plan B was taken as late as 4 to 5 days after unprotected intercourse. From small studies, newer pharmacokinetic data suggest lower bioavailability of a 1.5-mg dose in obese women compared with normal-weight patients (Natavio, 2019; Praditpan, 2017). Still, the pregnancy rate in obese women prescribed this EC type was only 2 percent in one pooled analysis (Festin, 2017).

Selective Progestin-Receptor Modulators

In 2010, ulipristal acetate—*Ella*—was FDA approved for post-coital contraception. It is taken as a single 30-mg tablet up to 120 hours after unprotected intercourse (Brache, 2010). This agent, described in Chapter 9 (p. 208), provides contraceptive activity by delaying ovulation. Compared with levonorgestrel in randomized trials, ulipristal acetate proved slightly more effective (Crenin, 2006; Glasier, 2010). Side effects include nausea and delay of subsequent menses.

■ Copper-Containing Intrauterine Devices

Insertion of a Cu-IUD is an effective postcoital contraceptive method and can be inserted up to 5 days following unprotected intercourse in IUC candidates. It is the most effective method of EC, and one systematic review of 42 studies calculated a pregnancy rate of 0.1 percent (Cleland, 2012). A secondary advantage is that this method also puts in place an effective 10-year method of contraception.

REFERENCES

Adelman MR, Dassel MW, Sharp HT: Management of complications encountered with Essure hysteroscopic sterilization: a systematic review. J Minim Invasive Gynecol 21(5):733, 2014

Akers AY, Steinway C, Sonalkar S, et al: Reducing pain during intrauterine device insertion: a randomized controlled trial in adolescents and young women. Obstet Gynecol 130(4):795, 2017

Alvarez F, Brache V, Fernandez E, et al: New insights on the mode of action of intrauterine contraceptive devices in women. Fertil Steril 49(5):768, 1988

American Academy of Pediatrics: Contraception for adolescents. Pediatrics 134(4):e1244, 2014

American College of Obstetricians and Gynecologists: Long-acting reversible contraception: implants and intrauterine devices. Practice Bulletin No. 186, November 2017

American College of Obstetricians and Gynecologists: Adolescents and long-acting reversible contraception: implants and intrauterine devices. Committee Opinion No. 735, May 2018a

American College of Obstetricians and Gynecologists: Emergency contraception. Practice Bulletin No. 152, September 2015, Reaffirmed 2018b

American College of Obstetricians and Gynecologists: Prevention of infection after gynecologic procedures. Practice Bulletin No. 195, June 2018c

American College of Obstetricians and Gynecologists: Benefits and risks of sterilization. Practice Bulletin No. 208, March 2019a

American College of Obstetricians and Gynecologists: Clinical challenges of long-acting reversible contraceptive methods. Committee Opinion No. 672, September 2016, Reaffirmed 2019b

American College of Obstetricians and Gynecologists: Depot medroxyprogesterone acetate and bone effects. Committee Opinion No. 602, June 2014, Reaffirmed 2019c

American College of Obstetricians and Gynecologists: Use of hormonal contraception in women with coexisting medical conditions. Practice Bulletin No. 206, February 2019d

American Society for Reproductive Medicine: Vasectomy reversal. Fertil Steril 90(5 Suppl):S78, 2008

Amundsen GA, Ramakrishnan K: Vasectomy: a "seminal" analysis. South Med J 97:54, 2004

Back DJ, Breckenridge AM, Crawford FE, et al: The effect of rifampicin on the pharmacokinetics of ethynyl estradiol in women. Contraception 21(2):135, 1980

Bahamondes L, Del Castillo S, Tabares G, et al: Comparison of weight increase in users of depot medroxyprogesterone acetate and copper IUD up to 5 years. Contraception 64(4):223, 2001

Bahamondes L, Faundes A, Sobreira-Lima B, et al: TCu 380A IUD: a reversible permanent contraceptive method in women over 35 years of age. Contraception 72(5):337, 2005

Balci O, Mahmoud AS, Capar M, et al: Diagnosis and management of intra-abdominal, mislocated intrauterine devices. Arch Gynecol Obstet 281(6):1019, 2010

Barnett C, Moehner S, Do Minh T, et al: Perforation risk and intra-uterine devices: results of the EURAS-IUD 5-year extension study. Eur J Contracept Reprod Health Care 22(6):424, 2017

Bayer HealthCare Pharmaceuticals: Yasmin, drospirenone and ethinyl estradiol tablets: prescribing information. Wayne, Bayer HealthCare Pharmaceuticals, 2018. Available at: https://resources.bayer.com.au/resources/uploads/PI/file9448.pdf. Accessed March 11, 2019

Bednarek PH, Creinin MD, Reeves MF, et al: Immediate versus delayed IUD insertion after uterine aspiration. N Engl J Med 364(23):2208, 2011

Beksinska ME, Smit JA, Kleinschmidt I, et al: Prospective study of weight change in new adolescent users of DMPA, NET-EN, COCs, nonusers and discontinuers of hormonal contraception. Contraception 81(1):30, 2010

Berry-Bibee EN, Kim MJ, Tepper NK, et al: Co-administration of St. John's wort and hormonal contraceptives: a systematic review. Contraception 94(6):668, 2016

Betrabet SS, Shikary ZK, Toddywalla VS, et al: ICMR Task Force Study on hormonal contraception. Transfer of norethindrone (NET) and levonorgestrel (LNG) from a single tablet into the infant's circulation through the mother's milk. Contraception 35:517, 1987

Bounds W, Guillebaud J, Dominik R, et al: The diaphragm with and without spermicide. A randomized, comparative efficacy trial. J Reprod Med 40:764, 1995

Brache V, Cochon L, Jesam C, et al: Immediate pre-ovulatory administration of 30 mg ulipristal acetate significantly delays follicular rupture. Hum Reprod 25(9):2256, 2010

Bradshaw HD, Rosario DJ, James MJ, et al: Review of current practice to establish success after vasectomy. Br J Surg 88:290, 2001

Brahmi D, Steenland MW, Renner RM, et al: Pregnancy outcomes with an IUD in situ: a systematic review. Contraception 85(2):131, 2012

Briggs GG, Freeman RK, et al (eds): Drugs in Pregnancy and Lactation, 11th ed. Philadelphia, Wolters Kluwer, 2017, p 1025

Brohet RM, Goldgar DE, Easton DF, et al: Oral contraceptives and breast cancer risk in the international BRCA 1/2 carrier cohort study: a report from EMBRACE, GENEPSO, GEO-HEBON, and the IBCCS Collaborating Group. J Clin Oncol 25:5327, 2007

Brunner LR, Hogue CJ: The role of body weight in oral contraceptive failure: results from the 1995 national survey of family growth. Ann Epidemiol 15:492, 2005

Bryant AG, Lyerly AD, DeVane-Johnson S, et al: Hormonal contraception, breastfeeding and bedside advocacy: the case for patient-centered care. Contraception 99(2):73, 2019

Cancer and Steroid Hormone Study of the Centers for Disease Control and the National Institute of Child Health and Development: Combination oral contraceptive use and the risk of endometrial cancer. JAMA 257:796, 1987a

Cancer and Steroid Hormone Study of the Centers for Disease Control and the National Institute of Child Health and Development: The reduction in risk of ovarian cancer associated with oral-contraceptive use. N Engl J Med 316:650, 1987b

Centers for Disease Control and Prevention: Sexually transmitted diseases treatment guidelines, 2015. MMWR 64(3):1, 2015

Chan LM, Westhoff CL: Tubal sterilization trends in the United States. Fertil Steril 94(1):1, 2010

Charlton BM, Mølgaard-Nielsen D, Svanström H, et al: Maternal use of oral contraceptives and risk of birth defects in Denmark: prospective, nationwide cohort study. BMJ 352:h6712, 2016

Chasan-Taber L, Willett WC, Manson JE, et al: Prospective study of oral contraceptives and hypertension among women in the United States. Circulation 94:483, 1996

Chen BA, Reeves MF, Hayes JL, et al: Postplacental or delayed insertion of the levonorgestrel intrauterine device after vaginal delivery: a randomized controlled trial. Obstet Gynecol 116(5):1079, 2010

Chudnoff SG, Nichols JE Jr, Levie M: Hysteroscopic Essure inserts for permanent contraception: extended follow-up results of a phase III multicenter international study. J Minim Invasive Gynecol 22(6):951, 2015

Clark MK, Sowers M, Levy B, et al: Bone mineral density loss and recovery during 48 months in first-time users of depot medroxyprogesterone acetate. Fertil Steril 86(5):1466, 2006

Clark NV, Rademaker D, Mushinski AA, et al: Essure removal for the treatment of device-attributed symptoms: an expanded case series and follow-up survey. J Minim Invasive Gynecol 24(6):971, 2017

Cleland K, Zhu H, Goldstuck N, et al: The efficacy of intrauterine devices for emergency contraception: a systematic review of 35 years of experience. Hum Reprod 27(7):1994, 2012

Collaborative Group on Epidemiological Studies of Ovarian Cancer: Ovarian cancer and oral contraceptives: collaborative reanalysis of data of 45 epidemiological studies including 23,257 women with ovarian cancer and 87,303 controls. Lancet 371:303, 2008

Collaborative Group on Hormonal Factors in Breast Cancer: Breast cancer and hormonal contraceptives: collaborative reanalysis of individual data on 53,297 women with breast cancer and 100,239 women without breast cancer from 54 epidemiological studies. Lancet 347:1713, 1996

Costello C, Hillis S, Marchbanks P, et al: The effect of interval tubal sterilization on sexual interest and pleasure. Obstet Gynecol 100:3, 2002

Creinin MD, Schlaff W, Archer DF, et al: Progesterone receptor modulator for emergency contraception: a randomized controlled trial. Obstet Gynecol 108(5):1089, 2006

Cromer BA, Smith RD, Blair JM, et al: A prospective study of adolescents who choose among levonorgestrel implant (Norplant), medroxyprogesterone acetate (Depo-Provera), or the combined oral contraceptive pill as contraception. Pediatrics 94:687, 1994

Croxatto HB, Ortiz ME, Muller AL: Mechanisms of action of emergency contraception. Steroids 68:1095, 2003

Curtis KM, Tepper NK, Jatlaoui TC, et al: U.S. medical eligibility criteria for contraceptive use, 2016. MMWR 65(3):1, 2016

Daniels K, Daugherty J, Jones J, et al: Current contraceptive use and variation by selected characteristics among women aged 15–44: United States, 2011–2013. Natl Health Stat Report 86:1, 2015

de Villiers EM: Relationship between steroid hormone contraceptives and HPV, cervical intraepithelial neoplasia and cervical carcinoma. Int J Cancer 103(6):705, 2003

Deffieux X, Morin Surroca M, Faivre E, et al: Tubal anastomosis after tubal sterilization: a review. Arch Gynecol Obstet 283(5):1149, 2011

DeStefano F, Perlman JA, Peterson HB, et al: Long term risk of menstrual disturbances after tubal sterilization. Am J Obstet Gynecol 152:835, 1985

Dorflinger LJ: Metabolic effects of implantable steroid contraceptives for women. Contraception 65(1):47, 2002

Edelman AB, Carlson NE, Cherala G, et al: Impact of obesity on oral contraceptive pharmacokinetics and hypothalamic-pituitary-ovarian activity. Contraception, 80(2):119, 2009

Ellertson C, Evans M, Ferden S, et al: Extending the time limit for starting the Yuzpe regimen of emergency contraception to 120 hours. Obstet Gynecol 101:1168, 2003

Erickson BK, Conner MG, Landen CN Jr: The role of the fallopian tube in the origin of ovarian cancer. Am J Obstet Gynecol 209(5):409, 2013

Falconer H, Yin L, Grönberg H, et al: Ovarian cancer risk after salpingectomy: a nationwide population-based study. J Natl Cancer Inst 107(2), 2015

Fernandez H, Legendre G, Blein C, et al: Tubal sterilization: pregnancy rates after hysteroscopic versus laparoscopic sterilization in France, 2006–2010. Eur J Obstet Gynecol Reprod Biol 180:133, 2014

Festin MPR, Peregoudov A, Seuc A, et al: Effect of BMI and body weight on pregnancy rates with LNG as emergency contraception: analysis of four WHO HRP studies. Contraception 95(1):50, 2017

Findley AD, Siedhoff MT, Hobbs KA, et al: Short-term effects of salpingectomy during laparoscopic hysterectomy on ovarian reserve: a pilot randomized controlled trial. Fertil Steril 100(6):1704, 2013

Finer LB, Zolna MR: Declines in unintended pregnancy in the United States, 2008–2011. N Engl J Med 374(9):843, 2016

Finer LB, Zolna MR: Unintended pregnancy in the United States: incidence and disparities, 2006. Contraception 84(5):478, 2011

Fiorino AS: Intrauterine contraceptive device–associated actinomycotic abscess and *Actinomyces* detection on cervical smear. Obstet Gynecol 87:142, 1996

Food and Drug Administration: Drug safety communication: updated information about the risk of blood clots in women taking birth control pills containing drospirenone. Rockville, Food and Drug Administration, 2012

Fox MC, Oat-Judge J, Severson K, et al: Immediate placement of intrauterine devices after first and second trimester pregnancy termination. Contraception 83(1):34, 2011

Furlong LA: Ectopic pregnancy risk when contraception fails. J Reprod Med 47:881, 2002

Gaffield ME, Culwell KR, Lee CR: The use of hormonal contraception among women taking anticonvulsant therapy. Contraception 83(1):16, 2011

Gallo MF, Grimes DA, Lopez LM, et al: Non-latex versus latex male condoms for contraception. Cochrane Database Syst Rev 1:CD003550, 2006

Gallo MF, Lopez LM, Grimes DA, et al: Combination contraceptives: effects on weight. Cochrane Database Syst Rev 1:CD003987, 2014

Ganer Herman H, Gluck O, Keidar R, et al: Ovarian reserve following cesarean section with salpingectomy vs tubal ligation: a randomized trial. Am J Obstet Gynecol 217(4):472, 2017

Gardner JM, Mishell DR Jr: Analysis of bleeding patterns and resumption of fertility following discontinuation of a long-acting injectable contraceptive. Fertil Steril 21:286, 1970

Gariepy AM, Creinin MD, Smith KJ, et al: Probability of pregnancy after sterilization: a comparison of hysteroscopic versus laparoscopic sterilization. Contraception 90(2):174, 2014

Glasier AF, Cameron ST, Fine PM, et al: Ulipristal acetate versus levonorgestrel for emergency contraception: a randomised non-inferiority trial and meta-analysis. Lancet 375(9714):555, 2010

Gockley AA, Elias KM: Fallopian tube tumorigenesis and clinical implications for ovarian cancer risk-reduction. Cancer Treat Rev 69:66, 2018

Godfrey EM, Folger SG, Jeng G, et al: Treatment of bleeding irregularities in women with copper-containing IUDs: a systematic review. Contraception 87(5):549, 2013

Goodman S, Henlish SK, Reeves MF, et al: Impact of immediate postabortal insertion of intrauterine contraception on repeat abortion. Contraception 78:143, 2008

Grimes DA, Hubacher D, Lopez LM, et al: Non-steroidal anti-inflammatory drugs for heavy bleeding or pain associated with intrauterine-device use. Cochrane Database Syst Rev 4:CD006034, 2006

Gurtcheff SE, Turok DK, Stoddard G, et al: Lactogenesis after early postpartum use of the contraceptive implant: a randomized controlled trial. Obstet Gynecol 117(5):1114, 2011

Guttmacher Institute: Contraceptive use in the United States. 2018. Available at: https://www.guttmacher.org/fact-sheet/contraceptive-use-united-states. Accessed February 27, 2019

Guttmacher Institute: An overview of consent to reproductive health services by young people. 2014. Available at: https://www.guttmacher.org/state-policy/explore/overview-minors-consent-law. Accessed February 19, 2019

Haider S, Darney PD: Injectable contraception. Clin Obstet Gynecol 50(4):898, 2007

Halpern V, Grimes DA, Lopez L, et al: Strategies to improve adherence and acceptability of hormonal methods of contraception. Cochrane Database Syst Rev 10:CD004317, 2013

Hannaford PC, Kay CR, Vessey MP, et al: Combined oral contraceptives and liver disease. Contraception 55:145, 1997

Hannaford PC, Selvaraj S, Elliott AM, et al: Cancer risk among users of oral contraceptives: cohort data from the Royal College of General Practitioners oral contraception study. BMJ 335(7621):651, 2007

Harel Z, Johnson CC, Gold MA, et al: Recovery of bone mineral density in adolescents following the use of depot medroxyprogesterone acetate contraceptive injections. Contraception 81(4):281, 2010

Heikinheimo O, Gissler M, Suhonen S: Age, parity history of abortion and contraceptive choices affect the risk of repeat abortion. Contraception 78:149, 2008

Heinemann LA, Weimann A, Gerken G, et al: Modern oral contraceptive use and benign liver tumors: the German Benign Liver Tumor Case-Control study. Eur J Contracept Reprod Health Care 3(4):194, 1998

Hidalgo MM, Lisondo C, Juliato CT, et al: Ovarian cysts in users of Implanon and Jadelle subdermal contraceptive implants. Contraception 73(5):532, 2006

Hillis SD, Marchbanks PA, Tylor LR, et al: Poststerilization regret: findings from the United States Collaborative Review of Sterilization. Obstet Gynecol 93:889, 1999

Hillis SD, Marchbanks PA, Tylor LR, et al: Tubal sterilization and long-term risk of hysterectomy: findings from the United States Collaborative Review of Sterilization. Obstet Gynecol 89(4):609, 1997

Holt SK, Salinas CA, Stanford JL: Vasectomy and the risk of prostate cancer. J Urol 180(6):2565, 2008

Holt VL, Scholes D, Wicklund KG, et al: Body mass index, weight, and oral contraceptive failure risk. Obstet Gynecol 105:46, 2005

Inki P, Hurskainen R, Palo P, et al: Comparison of ovarian cyst formation in women using the levonorgestrel-releasing intrauterine system vs. hysterectomy. Ultrasound Obstet Gynecol 20(4):381, 2002

International Collaboration of Epidemiological Studies of Cervical Cancer: Cervical cancer and hormonal contraceptives: collaborative reanalysis of individual data for 16,573 women with cervical cancer and 35,509 women without cervical cancer from 24 epidemiological studies. Lancet 370: 1609, 2007

Jain J, Dutton C, Nicosia A, et al: Pharmacokinetics, ovulation suppression and return to ovulation following a lower dose subcutaneous formulation of Depo-Provera. Contraception 70(1):11, 2004

Jamieson DJ, Kaufman SC, Costello C, et al: A comparison of women's regret after vasectomy versus tubal sterilization. Obstet Gynecol 99:1073, 2002

Janssen-Ortho: Micronor: prescribing information. Titusville, Janssen Ortho, 2017

Jensen JT, Burke AE, Barnhart KT, et al: Effects of switching from oral to transdermal or transvaginal contraception on markers of thrombosis. Contraception 78(6):451, 2008

Jick SS, Hagberg KW, Kaye JA: ORTHO EVRA and venous thromboembolism: an update. Contraception 81(5):452, 2010

Jick SS, Hernandez RK: Risk of non-fatal venous thromboembolism in women using oral contraceptives containing drospirenone compared with women using oral contraceptives containing levonorgestrel: case-control study using United States claims data. BMJ 342:d2151, 2011

Kamencic H, Thiel K, Karreman E, et al: Does Essure cause significant de novo pain? A retrospective review of indications for second surgeries after Essure placement. J Minim Invasive Gynecol 23(7):1158, 2016

Kapp N, Curtis KM: Hormonal contraceptive use among women with liver tumors: a systematic review. Contraception 80(4):387, 2009a

Kapp N, Tilley IB, Curtis KM: The effects of hormonal contraceptive use among women with viral hepatitis or cirrhosis of the liver: a systematic review. Contraception 80(4):381, 2009b

Kaunitz AM: Depot medroxyprogesterone acetate contraception and the risk of breast and gynecologic cancer. J Reprod Med 45:419, 1996

Kavanaugh ML, Jerman J: Contraceptive method use in the United States: trends and characteristics between 2008, 2012 and 2014. Contraception 97(1):14, 2018

Kim AJ, Barberio A, Berens P, et al: The trend, feasibility, and safety of salpingectomy as a form of permanent sterilization. J Minim Invasive Gynecol 26(7):1363, 2019

Kjos SL, Peters RK, Xiang A, et al: Contraception and the risk of type 2 diabetes mellitus in Latina women with prior gestational diabetes mellitus. JAMA 280:533, 1998

Kluft C, Meijer P, LaGuardia KD, et al: Comparison of a transdermal contraceptive patch vs. oral contraceptives on hemostasis variables. Contraception 77(2):77, 2008

Köhler TS, Fazili AA, Brannigan RE: Putative health risks associated with vasectomy. Urol Clin North Am 36(3):337, 2009

Kulier R, Boulvain M, Walker D, et al: Minilaparotomy and endoscopic techniques for tubal sterilization. Cochrane Database Syst Rev 3:CD001328, 2004

Laumonerie P, Blasco L, Tibbo ME, et al: Peripheral nerve injury associated with a subdermal contraceptive implant: illustrative cases and systematic review of literature. World Neurosurg 111:317, 2018

Lathrop E, Haddad L, McWhorter CP: Self-administration of misoprostol prior to intrauterine device insertion among nulliparous women: a randomized controlled trial. Contraception 88(6): 725, 2013

Lawrie TA, Kulier R, Nardin JM: Techniques for the interruption of tubal patency for female sterilization. Cochrane Database Syst Rev 8:CD003034, 2016

Le YC, Rahman M, Berenson AB: Early weight gain predicting later weight gain among depot medroxyprogesterone acetate users. Obstet Gynecol 114(2 Pt 1):279, 2009

Lessard-Anderson CR, Handlogten KS, Molitor RJ, et al: Effect of tubal sterilization technique on risk of serous epithelial ovarian and primary peritoneal carcinoma. Gynecol Oncol 135(3): 423, 2014

Levgur M, Duvivier R: Pelvic inflammatory disease after tubal sterilization: a review. Obstet Gynecol Surv 55:41, 2000

Lippes J: Quinacrine sterilization: the imperative need for clinical trials. Fertil Steril 77:1106, 2002

Lippes J: Quinacrine sterilization (QS): time for reconsideration. Contraception 92(2):91, 2015

Lohr PA, Lyus R, Prager S: Use of intrauterine devices in nulliparous women. Contraception 95(6), 2017

Lopez LM, Bernholc A, Chen M, et al: Hormonal contraceptives for contraception in overweight or obese women. Cochrane Database Syst Rev 8:CD008542, 2016

Lopez LM, Bernholc A, Hubacher D, et al: Immediate postpartum insertion of intrauterine device for contraception. Cochrane Database Syst Rev 6:CD003036, 2015a

Lopez LM, Bernholc A, Zeng Y, et al: Interventions for pain with intrauterine device insertion. Cochrane Database Syst Rev 7:CD007373, 2015b

Lopez LM, Grey TW, Stuebe AM, et al: Combined hormonal versus nonhormonal versus progestin-only contraception in lactation. Cochrane Database Syst Rev 3:CD003988, 2015c

Lopez LM, Kaptein AA, Helmerhorst FM: Oral contraceptives containing drospirenone for premenstrual syndrome. Cochrane Database Syst Rev 2:CD006586, 2012

Maassen LW, van Gastel DM, Haveman I, et al: Removal of Essure sterilization devices: a retrospective cohort study in the Netherlands. J Minim Invasive Gynecol 26(6):1056, 2019

MacClellan LR, Giles W, Cole J, et al: Probable migraine with visual aura and risk of ischemic stroke: the stroke prevention in young women study. Stroke 38(9):2438, 2007

Maheshwari S, Sarraj A, Kramer J, et al: Oral contraception and the risk of hepatocellular carcinoma. J Hepatol 47:506, 2007

Mainwaring R, Hales HA, Stevenson K, et al: Metabolic parameters, bleeding, and weight changes in U.S. women using progestin only contraceptives. Contraception 51:149, 1995

Mantha S, Karp R, Raghavan V, et al: Assessing the risk of venous thromboembolic events in women taking progestin-only contraception: a meta-analysis. BMJ 345:e4944, 2012

Marchbanks PA, McDonald JA, Wilson HG, et al: Oral contraceptives and the risk of breast cancer. N Engl J Med 346:2025, 2002

Margolis KL, Adami HO, Luo J, et al: A prospective study of oral contraceptive use and risk of myocardial infarction among Swedish women. Fertil Steril 88(2):310, 2007

Marions L, Cekan SZ, Bygdeman M, et al: Effect of emergency contraception with levonorgestrel or mifepristone on ovarian function. Contraception 69:373, 2004

Martin JA, Hamilton BE, Osterman MJ, et al: Births: final data for 2017. Natl Vital Stat Rep 67(8):1, 2018

Matthews LR, O'Dwyer L, O'Neill E: Intrauterine device insertion failure after misoprostol administration: a systematic review. Obstet Gynecol 128(5):1084, 2016

Mayer Laboratories: Today sponge. Consumer information leaflet. 2011. Available at: http://www.todaysponge.com/pdf/todaysponge-pi2.pdf. Accessed March 11, 2019

Merck: Nexplanon: prescribing information. 2018. Available at: https://www.merck.com/product/usa/pi_circulars/n/nexplanon/nexplanon_pi.pdf. Accessed March 11, 2019

Michielsen D, Beerthuizen R: State-of-the art of non-hormonal methods of contraception: VI. Male sterilization. Eur J Contracept Reprod Health Care 15(2):136, 2010

Mishell DR Jr: Oral contraceptives and cardiovascular events: summary and application of data. Int J Fertil 45:121, 2000

Mohllajee AP, Curtis KM, Martins SL, et al: Does use of hormonal contraceptives among women with thrombogenic mutations increase their risk of venous thromboembolism? A systemic review. Contraception 73:166, 2006

Moniz MH, Chang T, Heisler M, et al: Inpatient postpartum long-acting reversible contraception and sterilization in the United States, 2008–2013. Obstet Gynecol 129(6):1078, 2017

Monteith CW, Berger GS, Zerden ML: Pregnancy success after hysteroscopic sterilization reversal. Obstet Gynecol 124(6):1183, 2014

Moore LL, Valuck R, McDougall C, et al: A comparative study of one-year weight gain among users of medroxyprogesterone acetate, levonorgestrel implants, and oral contraceptives. Contraception 52:215, 1995

Moschos E, Twickler DM: Does the type of intrauterine device affect conspicuity on 2D and 3D ultrasound? AJR Am J Roentgenol 196(6):1439, 2011

Mulders TM, Dieben T: Use of the novel combined contraceptive vaginal ring NuvaRing for ovulation inhibition. Fertil Steril 75:865, 2001

Munro MG, Nichols JE, Levy B, et al: Hysteroscopic sterilization: 10-year retrospective analysis of worldwide pregnancy reports. J Minim Invasive Gynecol 21(2):245, 2014

Nanda K, Stuart GS, Robinson J, et al: Drug interactions between hormonal contraceptives and antiretrovirals. AIDS 31(7):917, 2017

Natavio M, Stanczyk FZ, Molins EA, et al: Pharmacokinetics of the 1.5 mg levonorgestrel emergency contraceptive in women with normal, obese and extremely obese body mass index. Contraception 99(5):306, 2019

Ngai SW, Fan S, Li S, et al: A randomized trial to compare 24 h versus 12 h double dose regimen of levonorgestrel for emergency contraception. Hum Reprod 20:307, 2005

Nilsson CG, Lahteenmaki P, Luukkainen T: Ovarian function in amenorrheic and menstruating users of a levonorgestrel-releasing intrauterine device. Fertil Steril 41:52, 1984

Odom EB, Eisenberg DL, Fox IK: Difficult removal of subdermal contraceptive implants: a multidisciplinary approach involving a peripheral nerve expert. Contraception 96(2):89, 2017

Ogburn JA, Espey E, Stonehocker J: Barriers to intrauterine device insertion in postpartum women. Contraception 72(6):426, 2005

Okusanya BO, Oduwole O, Effa EE: Immediate postabortal insertion of intrauterine devices. Cochrane Database Syst Rev 6:CD001777, 2014

Ortiz ME, Croxatto HB: The mode of action of IUDs. Contraception 36:37, 1987

Ostrowski KA, Holt SK, Haynes R, et al: Evaluation of vasectomy trends in the United States. Urology 118:76, 2018

Parkin L, Sharples K, Hernandez RK, et al: Risk of venous thromboembolism in users of oral contraceptives containing drospirenone or levonorgestrel: nested case-control study based on UK General Practice Research Database. BMJ 342:d2139, 2011

Pati S, Cullins V: Female sterilization: evidence. Obstet Gynecol Clin North Am 27:859, 2000

Peragallo Urrutia R, Polis CB, Jensen ET, et al: Effectiveness of fertility awareness-based methods for pregnancy prevention: a systematic review. Obstet Gynecol 132(3):591, 2018

Peterson HB, Jeng G, Folger SG, et al: The risk of menstrual abnormalities after tubal sterilization. N Engl J Med 343:1681, 2000

Peterson HB, Xia Z, Wilcox LS, et al: Pregnancy after tubal sterilization with bipolar electrocoagulation. U.S. Collaborative Review of Sterilization Working Group. Obstet Gynecol 94:163, 1999

Petri M, Kim MY, Kalunian KC, et al: Combined oral contraceptives in women with systemic lupus erythematosus. N Engl J Med 353:2550, 2005

Pfizer: Depo-Provera: prescribing information. 2017. Available at: http://labeling.pfizer.com/showlabeling.aspx?id=522. Accessed March 11, 2019

Phillips SJ, Tepper NK, Kapp N, et al: Progestogen-only contraceptive use among breastfeeding women: a systematic review. Contraception 94(3):226, 2016

Pomp ER, le Cessie S, Rosendaal FR, et al: Risk of venous thrombosis: obesity and its joint effect with oral contraceptive use and prothrombotic mutations. Br J Haematol 139(2):289, 2007

Pomp ER, Rosendaal FR, Doggen CJ: Smoking increases the risk of venous thrombosis and acts synergistically with oral contraceptive use. Am J Hematol 83:97, 2008

Powell CB, Alabaster A, Simmons S, et al: Salpingectomy for sterilization: change in practice in a large integrated health care system, 2011–2016. Obstet Gynecol 130(5):961, 2017

Praditpan P, Hamouie A, Basaraba CN, et al: Pharmacokinetics of levonorgestrel and ulipristal acetate emergency contraception in women with normal and obese body mass index. Contraception 95(5):464, 2017

Ragan RE, Rock RW, Buck HW: Metoclopramide pretreatment attenuates emergency contraceptive-associated nausea. Am J Obstet Gynecol 188:330, 2003

Raymond EG, Creinin MD, Barnhart KT, et al: Meclizine for prevention of nausea associated with use of emergency contraceptive pills: a randomized trial. Obstet Gynecol 95:271, 2000

Realini JP, Goldzieher JW: Oral contraceptives and cardiovascular disease: a critique of the epidemiologic studies. Am J Obstet Gynecol 152:729, 1985

Reimers A, Brodtkorb E, Sabers A: Interactions between hormonal contraception and antiepileptic drugs: clinical and mechanistic considerations. Seizure 28:66, 2015

Rice MS, Murphy MA, Tworoger SS: Tubal ligation, hysterectomy and ovarian cancer: a meta-analysis. J Ovarian Res 5(1):13, 2012

Rimm EB, Manson JE, Stampfer MJ, et al: Oral contraceptive use and the risk of type 2 (non-insulin-dependent) diabetes mellitus in a large prospective study of women. Diabetologia 35:967, 1992

Robinson GE, Burren T, Mackie IJ, et al: Changes in haemostasis after stopping the combined contraceptive pill: implications for major surgery. BMJ 302:269, 1991

Rosen MP, Breitkopf DM, Nagamani M: A randomized controlled trial of second-versus third-generation oral contraceptives in the treatment of acne vulgaris. Am J Obstet Gynecol 188:1158, 2003

Roumen F, Apter D, Mulders TM, et al: Efficacy, tolerability and acceptability of a novel contraceptive vaginal ring releasing etonogestrel and ethinyl estradiol. Hum Reprod 16:469, 2001

Rowlands S, Mansour D, Walling M: Intravascular migration of contraceptive implants: two more cases. Contraception 95(2):211, 2017

Samy A, Abbas AM, Mahmoud M, et al: Evaluating different pain lowering medications during intrauterine device insertion: a systematic review and network meta-analysis. Fertil Steril 111(3):553, 2019

Sánchez-Guerrero J, Uribe AG, Jiménez-Santana L, et al: A trial of contraceptive methods in women with systemic lupus erythematosus. N Engl J Med 353:2539, 2005

Schreiber CA, Meyn LA, Creinin MD, et al: Effects of long-term use of nonoxynol-9 on vaginal flora. Obstet Gynecol 107:136, 2006

Schwingl PJ, Guess HA: Safety and effectiveness of vasectomy. Fertil Steril 73:923, 2000

Seeger JD, Loughlin J, Eng PM, et al: Risk of thromboembolism in women taking ethinyl estradiol/drospirenone and other oral contraceptives. Obstet Gynecol 110:587, 2007

Shikary ZK, Betrabet SS, Patel ZM, et al: ICMR Task Force Study on hormonal contraception. Transfer of levonorgestrel (LNG) administered through different drug delivery systems from the maternal circulation via breast milk. Contraception 35:477, 1987

Shridharani A, Sandlow JL: Vasectomy reversal versus IVF with sperm retrieval: which is better? Curr Opin Urol 20(6):503, 2010

Shulman LP, Gabriel H: Management and localization strategies for the nonpalpable Implanon rod. Contraception 73(4):325, 2006

Shy KK, Stergachis A, Grothaus LG, et al: Tubal sterilization and risk of subsequent hospital admission for menstrual disorders. Am J Obstet Gynecol 166:1698, 1992

Sieh W, Salvador S, McGuire V, et al: Tubal ligation and risk of ovarian cancer subtypes: a pooled analysis of case-control studies. Int J Epidemiol 42(2):579, 2013

Simmons KB, Haddad LB, Nanda K, et al: Drug interactions between nonrifamycin antibiotics and hormonal contraception: a systemic review. Am J Obstet Gynecol 218(1):88, 2018

Sivin I: Alternative estimates of ectopic pregnancy risks during contraception. Am J Obstet Gynecol 165:1900, 1991

Sivin I, Nash H, Waldman S: Jadelle levonorgestrel rod implants: a summary of scientific data and lessons learned from programmatic experience. New York, Population Council, 2002

Skegg DC, Noonan EA, Paul C, et al: Depot medroxyprogesterone acetate and breast cancer. JAMA 273:799, 1995

Society for Maternal-Fetal Medicine, Vricella LK, Gawron LM, et al: Society for Maternal-Fetal Medicine (SMFM) Consult Series #48: Immediate postpartum long-acting reversible contraception for women at high-risk for medical complications. Am J Obstet Gynecol 220(5):B2, 2019

Sokal D, Gates D, Amatya R, et al: Two randomized controlled trials comparing the Tubal Ring and Filshie Clip for tubal sterilization. Fertil Steril 74:3, 2000

Sokal DC, Hieu do T, Loan ND, et al: Contraceptive effectiveness of two insertions of quinacrine: results from 10-year follow-up in Vietnam. Contraception 78(1):61, 2008

Steiner M, Lopez M, Grimes D, et al: Sino-implant (II)—a levonorgestrel-releasing two-rod implant: systematic review of the randomized controlled trials. Contraception 81(3)197, 2010

Steiner MJ, Dominik R, Rountree W, et al: Contraceptive effectiveness of a polyurethane condom and a latex condom: a randomized controlled trial. Obstet Gynecol 101:539, 2003

Sulak PJ, Haney AF: Unwanted pregnancies: understanding contraceptive use and benefits in adolescents and older women. Am J Obstet Gynecol 168:2042, 1993

Sulak PJ, Kaunitz AM: Hormonal contraception and bone mineral density. Dialogues Contraception 6:1, 1999

Taneepanichskul S, Reinprayoon D, Khaosaad P: Comparative study of weight change between long-term DMPA and IUD acceptors. Contraception 58:149, 1998

Tatum HJ, Schmidt FH, Jain AK: Management and outcome of pregnancies associated with Copper-T intrauterine contraceptive device. Am J Obstet Gynecol 126:869, 1976

Tepper NK, Curtis KM, Nanda K, et al: Safety of intrauterine devices among women with HIV: a systematic review. Contraception 94(6):713, 2016a

Tepper NK, Dragoman MV, Gaffield ME, et al: Nonoral combined hormonal contraceptives and thromboembolism: a systematic review. Contraception 95(2):130, 2017

Tepper NK, Phillips SJ, Kapp N, et al: Combined hormonal contraceptive use among breastfeeding women: an updated systematic review. Contraception 94(3):262, 2016b

Tepper NK, Steenland MW, Marchbanks PA, et al: Hemoglobin measurement prior to initiating copper intrauterine devices: a systematic review. Contraception 87(5):639, 2013

Tepper NK, Whiteman MK, Zapata LB, et al: Safety of hormonal contraceptives among women with migraine: a systematic review. Contraception 94(6):630, 2016c

Thomas DB, Ye Z, Ray RM, et al: Cervical carcinoma in situ and use of depo-medroxyprogesterone acetate (DMPA). Contraception 51:25, 1995

Thorneycroft IH, Stanczyk FZ, Bradshaw KD, et al: Effect of low-dose oral contraceptives on androgenic markers and acne. Contraception 60:255, 1999

Trussell J: Estimates of contraceptive failure from the 2002 National Survey of Family Growth. Contraception 78(1):85, 2008

Trussell J, Aikens AR, Micks E, et al: Efficacy, safety, and personal considerations. In Hatcher RA, Nelson AL, Trussell J, et al (eds): Contraceptive Technology, 21st ed. New York, Ayer Company, 2018, p 100

Turok DK, Eisenberg DL, Teal SB, et al: A prospective assessment of pelvic infection risk following a same-day sexually transmitted infection testing and levonorgestrel intrauterine system placement. Am J Obstet Gynecol 215(5):599, 2016

Tworoger SS, Fairfield KM, Colditz GA, et al: Association of oral contraceptive use, other contraceptive methods, and infertility with ovarian cancer risk. Am J Epidemiol 166(8):894, 2007

United Nations, Department of Economic and Social Affairs Population Division: World contraceptive patterns, 2013. New York, United Nations, 2013

University of California at San Francisco: HIV Insite: database of antiretroviral drug interactions. 2014. Available at: http://hivinsite.ucsf.edu/InSite. Accessed March 11, 2019

van den Heuvel MW, van Bragt A, Alnabawy AK, et al: Comparison of ethinylestradiol pharmacokinetics in three hormonal contraceptive formulations: the vaginal ring, the transdermal patch and an oral contraceptive. Contraception 72(3):168, 2005

van Dijke CP, Weber JC: Interaction between oral contraceptives and griseofulvin. BMJ 288(6424):1125, 1984

Vessey M, Yeates D: Oral contraceptives and benign breast disease: an update of findings in a large cohort study. Contraception 76(6):418, 2007

Vessey MP, Lawless M, Yeates D: Efficacy of different contraceptive methods. Lancet 1:841, 1982

von Hertzen H, Piaggio G, Ding J, et al: Low dose mifepristone and two regimens of levonorgestrel for emergency contraception: a WHO multicentre randomized trial. Lancet 360:1803, 2002

Waldron T: Tests show commonly used substances harm latex condoms. Contracept Tech Update 10:20, 1989

Wallach M, Grimes DA (eds): Modern Oral Contraception. Updates from The Contraception Report. Totowa, Emron, 2000, pp 26, 90, 194

Walker JL, Powell CB, Chen LM, et al: Society of Gynecologic Oncology recommendations for the prevention of ovarian cancer. Cancer 121(13):2108, 2015

Westberg J, Scott F, Creinin MD: Safety outcomes of female sterilization by salpingectomy and tubal occlusion. Contraception 95(5):505, 2017

Westhoff C, Heartwell S, Edwards S, et al: Initiation of oral contraceptive using a quick start compared with a conventional start: a randomized controlled trial. Obstet Gynecol 109:1270, 2007a

Westhoff C, Jain JK, Milsom I, et al: Changes in weight with depot medroxyprogesterone acetate subcutaneous injection 104 mg/0.65 mL. Contraception 75(4):261, 2007b

Westhoff C, Kerns J, Morroni C, et al: Quick start: novel oral contraceptive initiation method. Contraception 66:141, 2002

Westhoff CL: Oral contraceptives and thrombosis: an overview of study methods and recent results. Am J Obstet Gynecol 179:S38, 1998

Westhoff CL, Torgal AH, Mayeda ER, et al: Pharmacokinetics of a combined oral contraceptive in obese and normal-weight women. Contraception, 81(6):474, 2010

White T, Ozel B, Jain JK, et al: Effects of transdermal and oral contraceptives on estrogen-sensitive hepatic proteins. Contraception 74(4):293, 2006

Winer RL, Hughes JP, Feng Q, et al: Condom use and the risk of genital human papillomavirus infection in young women. N Engl J Med 354:2645, 2006

Woods ER, Grace E, Havens KK, et al: Contraceptive compliance with a levonorgestrel triphasic and a norethindrone monophasic oral contraceptive in adolescent patients. Am J Obstet Gynecol 166:901, 1992

World Health Organization: Acute myocardial infarction and combined oral contraceptives: results of an international multi-center case-control study. Lancet 349:1202, 1997

World Health Organization: Cardiovascular disease and use of oral and injectable progestogen-only contraceptives and combined injectable contraceptives. Results of an international, multicenter, case-control study. Contraception 57:315, 1998

World Health Organization: Combined oral contraceptives and liver cancer. Int J Cancer 43:254, 1989

World Health Organization: Depot-medroxyprogesterone acetate (DMPA) and risk of endometrial cancer. Int J Cancer 49:186, 1991

World Health Organization: Ischaemic stroke and combined oral contraceptives: results of an international, multi-center case-control study. Lancet 348:498, 1996

World Health Organization: The safety of quinacrine when used as a method of non-surgical sterilization in women. Interim statement. Geneva, WHO, 2009

Xu JX, Rivera R, Dunson TR, et al: A comparative study of two techniques used in immediate postplacental insertion (IPPI) of the Copper T-380A IUD in Shanghai, People's Republic of China. Contraception 54(1):33, 1996

Yonkers KA, Brown C, Pearlstein TB, et al: Efficacy of a new low-dose oral contraceptive with drospirenone in premenstrual dysphoric disorder. Obstet Gynecol 106:492, 2005

Yunker AC, Ritch JM, Robinson EF, et al: Incidence and risk factors for chronic pelvic pain after hysteroscopic sterilization. J Minim Invasive Gynecol 22(3):390, 2015

Yuzpe AA, Thurlow HJ, Ramzy I, et al: Post coital contraception—a pilot study. J Reprod Med 13:53, 1974

Zapata LB, Whiteman MK, Tepper NK, et al: Intrauterine device use among women with uterine fibroids: a systematic review. Contraception 82(1):41, 2010

Zupanc M: Antiepileptic drugs and hormonal contraceptives in adolescent women with epilepsy. Neurology 66(Suppl 3):S37, 2006

CHAPTER 6

First-Trimester Abortion

TERMINOLOGY

Abortion is the spontaneous or induced termination of pregnancy before fetal viability. Thus, miscarriage and abortion appropriately are terms used interchangeably in a medical context. But, because popular use of abortion by laypersons implies a deliberate intact pregnancy termination, many prefer miscarriage for spontaneous fetal loss. Both terms will be used throughout this chapter.

For statistical and legal purposes, viability is usually defined by pregnancy duration and fetal birthweight. The Centers for Disease Control and Prevention (CDC) and the World Health Organization (WHO) define abortion as any pregnancy termination—spontaneous or induced—before 20 weeks' gestation or with a fetus born weighing <500 g. Confusion may be introduced by individual states whose laws define abortion more widely.

Technologic developments have revolutionized current abortion terminology. Transvaginal sonography (TVS) and precise measurement of serum beta human chorionic gonadotropin (β-hCG) concentrations help to identify extremely early pregnancies and to clarify intrauterine versus ectopic location. The term *pregnancy of unknown location (PUL)* aids timely identification and management of ectopic pregnancy. In the context of early pregnancies, five categories have been proposed: definite ectopic pregnancy, probable ectopic, PUL, probable intrauterine pregnancy (IUP), and definite IUP (Barnhart, 2011). Management options for ectopic pregnancies are described in Chapter 7 (p. 168). Of IUPs, those that spontaneously abort during the first trimester, that is, within the first $12^{6/7}$ weeks of gestation, are also defined as *early pregnancy loss* by the American College of Obstetricians and Gynecologists (2018a). *Recurrent pregnancy loss* is variably defined but is meant to identify women with repetitive miscarriage.

If studies are confined to first-trimester abortions, up to 70 percent are *anembryonic*, that is, with no identifiable embryonic elements (Du, 2018; Soler, 2017). The previous term *blighted ovum* is no longer preferred. The remaining pregnancies are *embryonic* miscarriages, which may be further grouped as either those with chromosomal anomalies—*aneuploid abortions*, or those with a normal chromosomal complement—*euploid abortions*.

SPONTANEOUS ABORTION

■ Incidence

More than 80 percent of spontaneous abortions occur during the first 12 weeks of gestation (American College of Obstetricians and Gynecologists, 2018a). Their rate increases significantly with advancing maternal age. For example, the clinical miscarriage rate nearly doubles with maternal or paternal age older than 40 (Gracia, 2005; Kleinhaus, 2006).

The reported incidence of spontaneous abortion varies with the sensitivity of methods used to identify them. Wilcox and colleagues (1988) studied 221 healthy women through 707 menstrual cycles. They used highly specific assays sensitive to minute concentrations of maternal serum β-hCG and found that 31 percent of pregnancies were lost after implantation. Importantly, two thirds of these very early losses were *clinically silent*.

TABLE 6-1. Chromosomal Findings in Early Abortuses

Chromosomal Studies	Reported Incidence Range (Percent)
Normal (euploid)	
46,XY and 46,XX	45–55
Abnormal (aneuploid)	
Autosomal trisomy	22–32
Monosomy X (45,X)	5–20
Triploidy	6–8
Tetraploidy	2–4
Structural anomaly	2
Double or triple trisomy	0.7–2

Data from Eiben, 1990; Kajii, 1980; Simpson, 1980, 2007.

Fetal Factors

Approximately half of embryonic first-trimester miscarriages are aneuploid. This incidence declines markedly with advancing gestation at the time of pregnancy loss. In general, aneuploid fetuses abort earlier than those with a normal chromosomal complement. Kajii (1980) reported that 75 percent of aneuploid fetuses aborted before 8 weeks, whereas the rate of euploid abortions peaks at approximately 13 weeks. Almost 95 percent of chromosomal abnormalities in aneuploid fetuses are caused by maternal gametogenesis errors (Jacobs, 1980). Importantly, the American College of Obstetricians and Gynecologists (2018a) does not recommend routine use of chromosomal microarray analysis of first-trimester fetal tissues.

Aneuploid Abortion

Trisomy describes the condition in which three copies of a given chromosome are present. Shown in Table 6-1, *autosomal trisomy* is the most frequently identified chromosomal anomaly in early miscarriages. Although most trisomies result from *isolated nondisjunction*, balanced structural chromosomal rearrangements are present in one partner in approximately 2 percent of couples with recurrent pregnancy loss (Barber, 2010).

Monosomy X (45,X) is the single most common specific chromosomal abnormality, also known as *Turner syndrome*. Most affected fetuses spontaneously abort, but some are liveborn females (Chap. 19, p. 412). Conversely, *autosomal monosomy* is rare and incompatible with life.

Ploidy describes the number of complete chromosome sets. *Triploidy* is often associated with hydropic or molar placental degeneration (Chap. 37, p. 777). Of hydatidiform moles, partial moles are characteristically triploid. The associated triploid fetuses frequently abort early, and those born later are all nonviable and grossly malformed. Advanced maternal and paternal ages do not increase the incidence of triploidy. *Tetraploid* fetuses most often abort early in gestation and are rarely liveborn.

Chromosomal structural abnormalities infrequently cause abortion. Neonates with a balanced translocation who are liveborn usually appear normal, but as adults they may experience recurrent pregnancy loss (p. 145).

Euploid Abortion

The causes of euploid abortions are poorly understood, but various maternal medical disorders, uterine defects, and environmental and lifestyle conditions have been implicated. The subsequent etiologies are most logically discussed with sporadic spontaneous abortion. Those most strongly linked to recurrent loss are described later (p. 144).

Maternal Factors

Medical Disorders

Pregnancy loss is clearly associated with diabetes mellitus and thyroid disorders, as discussed on page 149. Inflammatory bowel disease and systemic lupus erythematosus—especially antiphospholipid syndrome—may independently also raise the risk (Khashan, 2012; Ling, 2018; Wu, 2018). Beyond these, few acute or chronic diseases convey early pregnancy risk.

Infection

Only a few organisms are proven to cause abortion. In general, systemic infections likely infect the fetoplacental unit by a blood-borne route. Others may infect locally via maternal genitourinary infection or colonization. Importantly, some infections truly cause miscarriage, whereas others may serve as only an associated marker.

Chlamydia trachomatis is suspected to cause abortion. The mechanism is unclear, but this infection may adversely affect outcome by infecting the fetus, by stimulating a fetal inflammatory response, or by promoting an excessive maternal immunologic reaction (Baud, 2011; Prasad, 2017). An association between *bacterial vaginosis* and first-trimester miscarriage is controversial (Haahr, 2019; Kuon, 2017). Of others, one metaanalysis showed that Ebola virus and *Mycoplasma genitalium* infection were significantly associated with spontaneous abortion (Lis, 2015; Lyman, 2018). Data concerning the abortifacient effects of some other infections are conflicting. Namely, roles for *Mycoplasma hominis* and *Ureaplasma urealyticum* are unclear (Quinn 1983a,b; Temmerman, 1992). Human immunodeficiency virus infection is not associated with excessive abortion risks (Haddad, 2017). Of other viruses, human papilloma virus (HPV) infects trophoblasts, but it does not appear to play a role in miscarriage (Ambühl, 2017). Infections caused by parvovirus, cytomegalovirus, herpes simplex virus, or *Listeria monocytogenes* likely have no abortifacient effects (Brown, 1997; Feldman, 2010; Yan, 2015). Last, several infections cause abortion in livestock, but data remain inconclusive in humans. These include *Brucella abortus*, *Campylobacter fetus*, and *Toxoplasma gondii* (Feldman, 2010; Hide, 2009).

Imaging and Surgery

With low-dose radiation from diagnostic imaging, embryofetal risks appear to be minimal. Current evidence suggests that malformation, growth restriction, or miscarriage rates are not increased from a radiation dose less than 0.05 Gy (5 rad). Indeed, Brent (2009) concluded that gross congenital malformation rates would not be higher with exposure to less than 0.2 Gy (20 rad). Because diagnostic x-rays seldom exceed 0.1 Gy (10 rad),

Strzelczyk and associates (2007) concluded that these procedures are unlikely to cause disordered embryogenesis. With computed tomography, radiation doses can be higher. Thus, modified protocols or substitution with magnetic resonance (MR) imaging is preferred. Importantly, with MR imaging, use of gadolinium is not recommended unless benefits outweigh risks (American College of Radiology, 2018).

For surgery during pregnancy, the risk of miscarriage is not well studied. No currently used anesthetic agents have teratogenic effects when used at any gestational age. *Uncomplicated* surgical procedures—including abdominal or pelvic surgery—do not appear to increase the miscarriage risk (Mazze, 1989). The American College of Obstetricians and Gynecologists (2019c) recommends that elective surgery be postponed until delivery and nonurgent surgery be performed in the second trimester. This practice lowers the theoretical risk for miscarriage or preterm contractions. Laparoscopy also is suitable, and adaptations for pregnancy are described in Chapter 41 (p. 875) (Pearl, 2017).

Ovarian tumors or cysts can be safely resected without causing pregnancy loss. An important exception involves early removal of the corpus luteum or the ovary in which it resides. If performed prior to 10 weeks' gestation, supplemental progesterone is given. Between 8 and 10 weeks, a single 150-mg injection of intramuscular 17-hydroxyprogesterone caproate is given at the time of surgery. If the corpus luteum is excised between 6 to 8 weeks, two additional 150-mg injections are given 1 and 2 weeks after the first. Other suitable progesterone replacement regimens include: (1) micronized vaginal progesterone (Prometrium) 200 mg twice or three times daily; (2) 8-percent progesterone vaginal gel (Crinone) 90 mg once or twice daily; (3) progesterone vaginal insert (Endometrin) 100 mg twice or three times daily; (4) micronized oral progesterone (Prometrium) 200 mg orally twice or three times daily; or (5) progesterone in oil (compounded in a specialty pharmacy) 50 to 100 mg daily intramuscular injection. Any of these regimens is continued until 10 weeks' gestation.

Trauma seldom causes first-trimester miscarriage, and although Parkland Hospital is a busy trauma center, this is an infrequent association. Major trauma—especially abdominal—can cause fetal loss but is more likely as pregnancy advances.

Radiotherapy and Chemotherapy

In utero exposure to radiation may be abortifacient, teratogenic, or carcinogenic depending on the level of exposure and stage of fetal development. Threshold doses that cause abortion are not precisely known but definitely lie within the therapeutic doses used for maternal disease treatment (Williams, 2010). Methotrexate is a known teratogen, and its effects on early pregnancy are described later (p. 153).

Female cancer survivors who were treated in the past with abdominopelvic radiotherapy may be at higher risk for miscarriage. Wo and Viswanathan (2009) reported a two- to eight-fold greater risk for miscarriage, perinatal mortality, preterm delivery, and low-birthweight and growth-restricted neonates in women with prior radiotherapy. Hudson (2010) found a higher miscarriage risk in those given radiotherapy and chemotherapy in the past for a childhood cancer.

Medications and Vaccines

Certain medications are known abortifacients and include progesterone antagonists, prostaglandin E_1 (misoprostol), and methotrexate. A complete listing of medications associated with miscarriage lies outside this chapter's scope. The prescribing information document for each drug is best consulted prior to use.

Many routine immunizations can be given safely during pregnancy. Most studies have demonstrated safety of both the HPV and influenza vaccines if given in early pregnancy (Donahue, 2017; McMillan, 2015; Scheller, 2017). However, most live-virus vaccines are proscribed during pregnancy (Table 1-4, p. 11). That said, robust evidence to link live-virus vaccines with miscarriage is lacking.

Nutritional Factors and Weight

Dietary deficiency of any one nutrient or moderate deficiency of all nutrients does not appear to be an important cause of abortion. Even in extreme cases—for example, hyperemesis gravidarum—abortion is rare. Dietary quality may be important, and miscarriage risk is reportedly reduced in women who consume fruit, vegetables, whole grains, and fish (Gaskins, 2015).

Data also suggest that extremes in weight can be deleterious. Obesity is associated with subfertility, raises the risk of miscarriage, and results in a host of other adverse pregnancy outcomes (Boots, 2014). In one study of 6500 women with in vitro fertilization (IVF)-conceived pregnancies, the pregnancy and live birth rates were reduced progressively for each incremental rise in body mass index (BMI) units (Bellver, 2010a). Although the risks for many adverse late-pregnancy outcomes decline after bariatric surgery, its salutary effect on the miscarriage rate is unclear (Guelinckx, 2009).

Low BMI in some but not all studies has been associated with greater miscarriage risk (Balsells, 2016; Metwally, 2010). A cohort of more than 90,000 women demonstrated that the primary modifiable prepregnant risk factors for miscarriage are being underweight, obese, or aged 30 years or older at conception (Feodor Nilsson, 2014).

Behavior

Of lifestyle choices, alcohol use has been best studied in pregnancy. Earlier observations were that both miscarriage and fetal anomaly rates rose with alcohol abuse rates during the first 8 weeks of gestation (Floyd, 1999). Such outcomes likely are dose related, although safe levels have not been identified. Maconochie (2007) observed a significantly greater risk only with regular or heavy alcohol use. In some studies, low-level alcohol consumption apparently did not significantly raise the abortion risk (Avalos, 2014; Feodor Nilsson, 2014). In contrast, Danish National Birth Cohort data suggest an adjusted hazard ratio for first-trimester fetal death of 1.66 with as few as two drinks per week (Andersen, 2012).

In the United States, 7 percent of women who delivered in 2016 were cigarette smokers (Drake, 2018). Cigarettes may cause early pregnancy loss by several mechanisms that also cause adverse late-pregnancy outcomes (Pineles, 2014). Some but not all studies link smoking with abortion risk and find a dose-response effect (Nielsen, 2006; Westreich, 2017).

"Heavy" caffeine consumption has been associated with greater abortion risk, and this association is enhanced in smokers (Morales–Suárez–Valera, 2018). Studies of "moderate" intake—less than 200 mg daily—do not demonstrate a higher risk (Savitz, 2008; Weng, 2008). Currently, the American College of Obstetricians and Gynecologists (2018d) concludes that moderate consumption likely is not a major abortion risk and that any associated risk with higher intake is unsettled.

The adverse effects of illicit drugs on early pregnancy loss also are unclear. Although cocaine was linked to an increased miscarriage rate in one study, reanalysis refuted this conclusion (Mills, 1999; Ness, 1999).

Occupation and Environment

Some environmental toxins such as benzene are implicated in fetal malformations, but data regarding miscarriage risk are less clear (Lupo, 2011). Earlier reports implicated arsenic, lead, formaldehyde, benzene, and ethylene oxide (Barlow, 1982). More recently, evidence suggests that bisphenol A, polychlorinated biphenyls, and DDT (dichlorodiphenyltrichloroethane) may raise miscarriage rates (Krieg, 2016). Nevertheless, DDT-containing insecticides are endorsed by the WHO (2011) for mosquito control to prevent malaria.

Few studies have assessed occupational exposure and abortion risks. An elevated risk has been described for dental assistants exposed to 3 or more hours of *nitrous oxide* per day in offices without gas-scavenging equipment (Rowland, 1995). In their metaanalysis, Dranitsaris and colleagues (2005) found a small incremental risk for spontaneous abortion in women who worked with cytotoxic antineoplastic chemotherapeutic agents.

■ Clinical Classification

As a group, abortion can be divided clinically several ways. Commonly used categories include threatened, inevitable, incomplete, complete, and missed abortion. When the products of conception and uterus become infected, the term *septic abortion* is used.

Threatened Abortion

The diagnosis of *threatened abortion* is presumed when bloody vaginal discharge or blood exits through a closed internal cervical os during the first 20 weeks of gestation. In early pregnancy, bleeding is common and includes that with blastocyst implantation at the time of expected menses. Approximately one fourth of pregnant women experiences first-trimester spotting or bleeding. Of these, 43 percent will subsequently miscarry. Bleeding is by far the most predictive risk factor for pregnancy loss, but this risk is substantially less if fetal cardiac activity is seen sonographically (Tongsong, 1995). However, the combination of bleeding and uterine cramping predicts a poor prognosis for pregnancy continuation. Even if miscarriage does not follow early bleeding, the risks for later adverse pregnancy outcomes are elevated (Table 6-2). In a study of almost 1.8 million pregnancies, the risk for many of these pregnancy complications rose threefold (Lykke, 2010).

TABLE 6-2. Increased Incidence of Some Adverse Outcomes in Women with Threatened Abortion

Maternal	Perinatal
Placenta previa	Preterm ruptured
Placental abruption	membranes
Manual removal of placenta	Preterm birth
Cesarean delivery	Low-birthweight infant
	Fetal-growth restriction
	Perinatal death

From Johns, 2006; Lykke, 2010; Saraswat, 2010; Wijesiriwardana, 2006.

Diagnosis. In a woman with an early pregnancy, vaginal bleeding will prompt evaluation. The primary goal is to diagnose abnormal pregnancies that include spontaneous abortion, ectopic pregnancy, or molar pregnancy. With initial physical evaluation, abdominal tenderness and its location are sought. During speculum examination, blood flow from the cervix is assessed, and a swab or ring forceps gently probes for internal cervical os integrity. The external os is less informative and is often slightly dilated in parous women. Of laboratory tests, hematocrit, blood type, and a quantitative serum β-hCG level are determined. Last, TVS can help ascertain if the fetus is alive and if it is within the uterus. Repeat evaluations are often necessary as neither β-hCG nor TVS has 100-percent accuracy for the diagnosis of pregnancy location or fetal viability. Several predictive models based on serum β-hCG levels done 48 hours apart have been described (Barnhart, 2010; Condous, 2007). Of these, serum β-hCG levels with a robust uterine pregnancy should increase at least 33 to 49 percent every 48 hours depending on the baseline level (American College of Obstetricians and Gynecologists, 2018f). In contrast, Table 7-2 (p. 165) depicts serum β-hCG level disappearance in women with a PUL and bleeding who ultimately went on to have an early miscarriage.

A serum progesterone level can be added to provide information, although its sensitivity is poor. Levels <5 ng/mL suggest a dying pregnancy. Values >20 ng/mL support the diagnosis of a healthy pregnancy. However, progesterone levels often lie between these thresholds, are then considered indeterminate, and thus are less informative.

TVS can document the location and viability of a gestation. If this cannot be done, then a PUL is diagnosed. Notably, a consensus conference in 2012 concluded that prior sonographic criteria for fetal viability yielded unacceptably high rates of viable IUPs being falsely diagnosed as nonviable or as PULs (American College of Obstetricians and Gynecologists, 2018a; Doubilet, 2014). Such errors can lead to unnecessary surgical or medical treatment, interruption of a viable IUP, or incorrect assumption that a woman is at recurrent risk for an ectopic pregnancy. Because of this, as shown in Table 6-3, more stringent guidelines were proposed to diagnose pregnancy failure (Doubilet, 2014).

TABLE 6-3. Society of Radiologists in Ultrasound Guidelines for Early Pregnancy Loss Diagnosis

Diagnostic Sonographic Findings
CRL ≥7 mm and no heartbeat
MSD ≥25 mm and no embryo
Absence of embryo with heartbeat ≥2 weeks after a scan showed a gestational sac without a yolk sac
Absence of embryo with heartbeat ≥11 days after a scan showed a gestational sac with a yolk sac

CRL = crown-rump length; MSD = mean sac diameter.

One early TVS sign of an IUP is the gestational sac. This anechoic fluid collection represents the exocoelomic cavity. It may be encircled by two echogenic external layers, the *double-decidual sign*, which represent the decidua parietalis and decidua capsularis (Fig. 6-1). The gestational sac can usually be seen by 4.5 weeks with maternal β-hCG levels between 1500 and 2000 mIU/mL (Barnhart, 1994). More recently, Connolly and colleagues (2013) reported that a threshold value of 3500 mIU/mL may be required to detect a gestational sac in 99 percent of cases. This level is now recommended by the American College of Obstetricians and Gynecologists (2018f). Importantly, a gestational sac may appear similar to other intrauterine fluid accumulations such as the *pseudogestational sac (pseudosac)* present with ectopic pregnancy (Fig. 7-4, p. 165). A pseudosac may be excluded once a definite yolk sac or embryo is seen inside the sac. The diagnosis of an IUP should be made cautiously if the yolk sac is not yet seen (American College of Obstetricians and Gynecologists, 2018g).

The yolk sac is a circular, 3- to 5-mm-diameter anechoic structure. It is typically seen within the gestational sac at approximately 5.5 weeks' gestation and with a mean sac diameter (MSD) ≥10 mm. At approximately 6 weeks' gestation, a 1- to 2-mm embryo adjacent to the yolk sac can be found (see Fig. 6-1). Absence of an embryo in a sac with a MSD of 16 to 24 mm is suspicious for pregnancy failure (Doubilet, 2014). Cardiac motion can be detected at 6 to 6.5 weeks' gestation, at an embryonic length of 1 to 5 mm. Shown in Table 6-3, absent cardiac activity at certain stages can be used to diagnose pregnancy failure.

Management. With threatened abortion, bed rest is often recommended but does not improve outcomes. Neither has treatment with a host of medications and hormones that include progesterone and chorionic gonadotropin (Devaseelan, 2010). Acetaminophen-based analgesia will help relieve cramping discomfort. If anemia or hypovolemia is significant from active bleeding, pregnancy evacuation is generally indicated. In cases in which there is a live fetus, less often, some instead may choose transfusion and further observation.

Inevitable Abortion

Amnionic fluid leaking through a dilated cervix portends almost certain abortion. Sonography will usually show markedly diminished fluid volume. Following such membrane rupture,

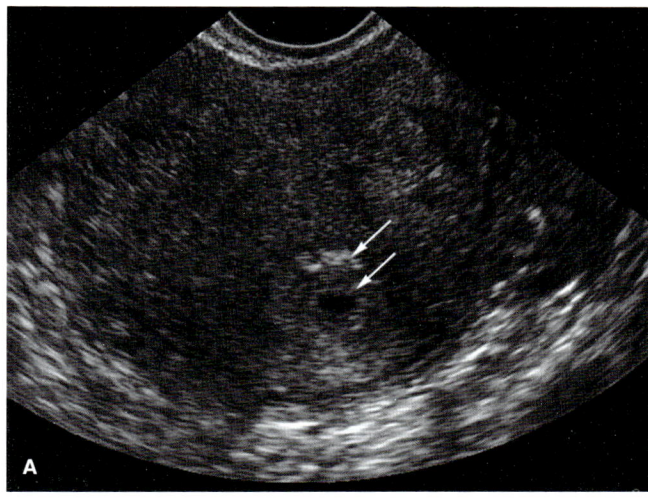

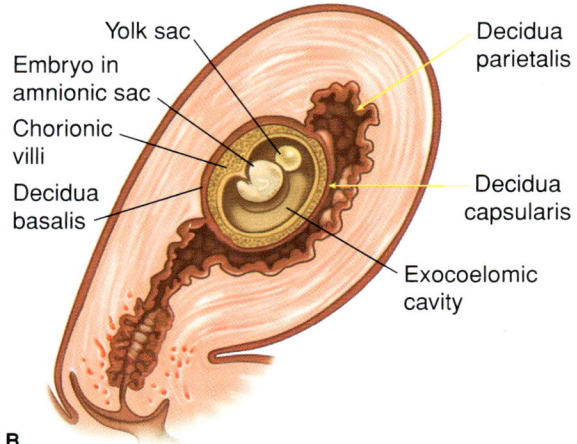

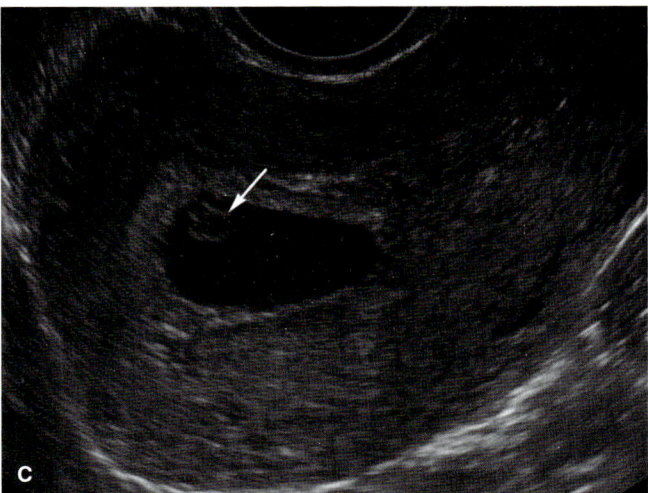

FIGURE 6-1 Early intrauterine pregnancy. **A.** Sonogram shows the anechoic gestational sac surrounded by two concentric echogenic layers, which are the inner decidua capsularis (*arrow*) and the peripheral decidua parietalis (*arrow*). **B.** The drawing shows the anatomy of an early pregnancy. **C.** The yolk sac (*arrow*) is circular and anechoic, and in this image, it lies to the right of its adjacent embryo.

TABLE 6-4. Randomized Controlled Studies for Management of Early Pregnancy Loss

Study	Inclusion Criteria	No.	Treatment Arms	Outcomes
Nguyen (2005)	Incomplete SAB	149	(1) PGE_1, 600 µg orally (2) PGE_1, 600 µg orally initially and at 4 hour	60% completed at 3 d 95% at 7 d; 3% curettage
Zhang (2005)	Pregnancy failure[a]	652	(1) PGE_1, 800 µg vaginally (2) Vacuum aspiration	71% completed at 3 d; 16% failure 97% successful
Trinder (2006) (MIST Trial)	Incomplete SAB; missed AB	1200	(1) Expectant (2) PGE_1, 800 µg vaginally ± 200 mg mifepristone (3) Suction curettage	50% curettage 38% curettage 5% repeat curettage
Dao (2007)	Incomplete SAB	447	(1) PGE_1, 600 µg orally (2) Vacuum aspiration	95% completed 100% completed
Torre (2012)	First-trimester miscarriage[b]	174	(1) Immediate—PGE_1, 200 µg orally Day 2—400 µg vaginally (2) Delayed—no treatment; TVS days 7 and 14	81% completed 19% curettage 57% completed 43% curettage

[a]Includes anembryonic gestation, embryonic or fetal death, without signs of incomplete SAB.
[b]Includes anembryonic gestation, embryonic or fetal death, or incomplete or inevitable SAB.
SAB = spontaneous abortion; PGE_1 = prostaglandin E_1; TVS = transvaginal sonography.

either uterine contractions begin promptly or infection develops. Rarely is a gush of vaginal fluid during the first half of pregnancy without serious consequence.

In the rare case, fluid may have collected previously between the amnion and chorion and may not be associated with pain, fever, or bleeding. TVS will typically show normal fluid volume. If a live fetus and normal fluid volume is documented, diminished activity with observation is reasonable. After 48 hours, if no additional amnionic fluid has escaped and no bleeding, cramping, or fever is noted, a woman may resume ambulation. Initial abstinence from intercourse and exercise also is recommended. Instead, with bleeding, cramping, or fever, abortion is considered inevitable, and the uterus is evacuated.

Incomplete Abortion

With first-trimester losses, death of the embryo or fetus nearly always precedes spontaneous expulsion. Death of the conceptus is usually accompanied by hemorrhage into the decidua basalis. This is followed by adjacent tissue necrosis that stimulates uterine contractions and expulsion. An intact gestational sac is generally filled with fluid and may or may not contain an embryo or fetus. With miscarriage, bleeding usually begins first, and abdominal cramping follows hours to days later. Low-midline rhythmic cramps; persistent low backache with pelvic pressure; or dull and midline suprapubic discomfort are common symptoms.

Partial or complete placental separation and dilation of the cervical os is termed *incomplete abortion*. The fetus and the placenta may remain entirely within the uterus or partially extrude through the dilated os. Before 10 weeks, they are frequently expelled together, but later in pregnancy, they deliver separately. Management options of incomplete abortion include curettage,

medical abortion, or expectant management in clinically stable women (Table 6-4) (Kim, 2017). With surgical therapy, additional cervical dilation may be necessary before suction curettage is performed (p. 152). In others, retained placental tissue simply lies loosely within the cervical canal and allows easy extraction with ring forceps. The removed products of conception are sent to pathology for standard histologic analysis. By this, products of conception are confirmed, and gestational trophoblastic disease is excluded.

Complete Abortion

In some cases, expulsion of the entire pregnancy is completed before a patient presents for care. In such cases, a history of heavy bleeding, cramping, and tissue passage at home is common. On pelvic examination, the cervical os is closed. Patients are encouraged to bring in passed tissue, which may be a complete gestation, blood clots, or a decidual cast. The last is a layer of endometrium in the shape of the uterine cavity that when sloughed can appear as a collapsed sac (Fig. 7-7, p. 167).

If a gestational sac is not identified grossly in the expelled specimen, sonography is performed to differentiate a complete abortion from threatened abortion or ectopic pregnancy. With TVS, characteristic intrauterine findings of a complete abortion include a thickened endometrium without a gestational sac. However, this does not guarantee a recent IUP. Condous and associates (2005) described 152 women with heavy bleeding, an empty uterus with endometrial thickness <15 mm, and a diagnosis of completed miscarriage. Of these, 6 percent were subsequently found to have an ectopic pregnancy. Thus, a diagnosis of complete abortion should not be made unless an intrauterine pregnancy was previously diagnosed sonographically or passage of a gestational sac has been confirmed.

In unclear settings, serial serum β-hCG measurements aid clarification. With complete abortion, these levels drop quickly. Pocius and coworkers (2017) found a mean serum decline of 70 percent after 2 days and a minimum decline of 36 percent. After 4 days, these values were 91 percent and 64 percent, respectively.

Missed Abortion—Early Pregnancy Loss

The term *missed abortion* requires clarification. Historically, the term was used to describe dead products of conception that were retained for weeks or months in a uterus with a closed cervical os. Despite this, concurrent early pregnancy findings of amenorrhea, nausea and vomiting, breast changes, and uterine growth appeared normal. To elucidate these disparities, Streeter (1930) studied aborted fetuses and observed that the mean interval from death to abortion was approximately 6 weeks.

This historical description of missed abortion is in contrast to that defined currently based on results of serial serum β-hCG assays and TVS (Fig. 6-2 and Table 6-3). With these tools, fetal or embryonic death is confirmed relatively rapidly—even in early pregnancies. Although many classify this as a missed abortion, the term is used interchangeably with *early pregnancy loss* (Silver, 2011). Management options include dilation and curettage, medical abortion, or expectant management (see Table 6-4).

Septic Abortion

Horrific infections and maternal deaths associated with septic abortions have become rare with legalized abortion. With current abortion practices, rates are <1 percent (Achilles, 2011; Upadhyay, 2015). That said, elective abortion, either surgical or medical, is occasionally complicated by severe and even fatal infections. Bacteria gain uterine entry and colonize dead conception products. Organisms may invade myometrial tissues and extend to cause parametritis, peritonitis, septicemia, and rarely, endocarditis (Vartian, 1991).

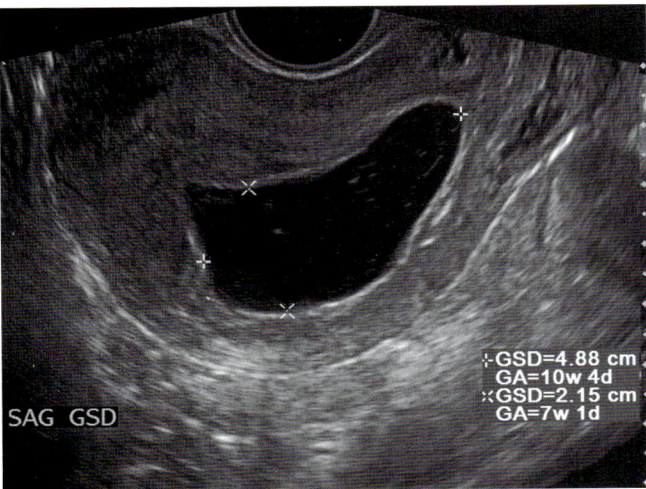

FIGURE 6-2 Transvaginal sonogram in the sagittal plane showing a gravid uterus. Calipers mark the sac borders of this anembryonic gestation.

Infections are usually polymicrobial. But, significant necrotizing infections and toxic shock syndrome can be caused by group A streptococcus—*S pyogenes* (Daif, 2009). In addition, rare but severe infections with otherwise low-virulence organisms have complicated medical abortions. These include deaths from toxic shock syndrome due to *Clostridium perfringens* (Centers for Disease Control and Prevention, 2005). Similar infections caused by *Clostridium sordellii* and *novyi* have clinical manifestations that begin within a few days after an abortion. Women may be afebrile when first seen with prominent endothelial injury, capillary leakage, hemoconcentration, hypotension, and a profound leukocytosis (Fischer, 2005; Herrera, 2016; Ho, 2009). Maternal deaths from these clostridial species approximate 0.58 per 100,000 medical abortions (Meites, 2010).

Treatment of infected abortion or postabortal sepsis includes prompt administration of broad-spectrum antibiotics. Suitable regimens are found in Table 3-16 (p. 82). For women with septic incomplete abortion or for those with retained fragments, intravenous antimicrobial therapy is promptly followed by uterine evacuation. Most women respond to this treatment within 1 to 2 days and are discharged when afebrile. Continued outpatient oral antibiotic treatment is likely unnecessary (Savaris, 2011). Rarely, sepsis causes acute respiratory distress syndrome, acute kidney injury, or disseminated intravascular coagulopathy. In these cases, intensive supportive care is essential.

To prevent postabortal sepsis, prophylactic antibiotics are given at the time of surgical evacuation of incomplete or induced abortion. Guidelines recommend doxycycline as a sole 200-mg oral preoperative dose (American College of Obstetricians and Gynecologists (2018a,e)).

■ Management

Unless there is serious bleeding or infection, management of spontaneous abortion can be individualized. Any of three management options is reasonable—expectant, medical, or surgical (see Table 6-4). Each has its own risks and benefits. For example, the first two are associated with unpredictable bleeding, and some women will require unscheduled curettage. Nevertheless, expectant management for suspected first-trimester miscarriage results in spontaneous resolution of pregnancy in more than 80 percent of women (Luise, 2002). Whereas surgical treatment is definitive and predictable, it is invasive and not necessary for all women. If anemia or hypovolemia is significant, pregnancy evacuation is generally indicated.

Several randomized studies that compared these management schemes have been reviewed (Kim, 2017; Neilson, 2013; Wu, 2017). A major drawback cited for between-study comparisons was varied inclusion criteria and techniques. For example, studies that included women with vaginal bleeding enhanced the success of medical therapy compared with studies that excluded such women (Creinin, 2006).

The selected studies in Table 6-4 permit some generalizations. First, success is dependent on the type of early pregnancy loss, that is, incomplete versus missed abortion. Second, expectant management of spontaneous incomplete abortion has failure rates as high as 50 percent. Curettage results in a quick resolution that is 95- to 100-percent successful. Last, medical therapy failure rates with prostaglandin E_1 (PGE_1) may be related to dose, route, and form—tablet, gel, dissolved—and rates vary from 5 to 40 percent. The addition of mifepristone and laminaria appear to improve efficacy of PGE_1 (Dunford, 2018; Khooshideh, 2017; Schreiber, 2018). Importantly, subsequent pregnancy rates do not differ among these management methods (Smith, 2009).

As a single agent for medical management, a common standard is misoprostol, given 800 µg vaginally as a single dose (American College of Obstetricians and Gynecologists, 2016b). The dose may be repeated in 1 to 2 days. If mifepristone is selected for pretreatment to misoprostol, an oral dose of 200 mg is given prior to the misoprostol 800-µg vaginal dose (Schreiber, 2018).

During spontaneous miscarriage, 2 percent of D-negative women will become isoimmunized if not provided passive isoimmunization. With an induced abortion, this rate may reach 5 percent. The American College of Obstetricians and Gynecologists (2017a) recommends anti-Rh_0(D)immunoglobulin given as 300 µg intramuscularly (IM) for all gestational ages. Alternatively, some give 50 µg IM for pregnancies ≤12 weeks and 300 µg for ≥13 weeks.

With a threatened abortion, immunoglobulin prophylaxis is controversial, and recommendations are limited by scarce evidence-based data (Hannafin, 2006; Weiss, 2002). Up to 12 weeks' gestation, prophylaxis is optional for women with threatened abortion and a live fetus. At Parkland Hospital, we administer a 50-µg dose to all D-negative women with first-trimester bleeding.

RECURRENT MISCARRIAGE

Terms used to describe repetitive early spontaneous pregnancy losses include *recurrent miscarriage, recurrent spontaneous abortion,* and *recurrent pregnancy loss (RPL)* with the last term gaining popularity. The term *habitual abortion* was used in the past and currently is not preferred. Approximately 1 to 2 percent of fertile couples experience RPL. Most women with recurrent miscarriage have embryonic or early fetal loss. Recurrent anembryonic miscarriage or those with consecutive losses after 14 weeks are much less common.

The definition of RPL varies across professional societies, and revisions stem from new information regarding etiology. It was previously defined as three or more consecutive losses. Now, the American Society for Reproductive Medicine (ASRM) (2012, 2013) and the European Society of Human Reproduction and Embryology (2017) define RPL as the loss of two or more pregnancies (Khalife, 2019; Youssef, 2019). ASRM requires pregnancies to be confirmed by β-hCG levels and either sonographic or histopathologic findings. Losses need not be consecutive. Moreover, the classic definition of pregnancy loss at gestational age <20 weeks or with a fetal weight <500 g is less strictly adhered to. These changes are supported by a study of more than 1000 women in which those with two pregnancy losses had a prevalence of abnormal test findings similar to that of women with three or more losses (Jaslow, 2010). Other evaluation considerations include maternal age

TABLE 6-5. Predicted Success Rate of Subsequent Pregnancy According to Age and Number of Previous Miscarriages

| Age (years) | No. of Previous Miscarriages | | | |
| | 2 | 3 | 4 | 5 |
	Predicted Success of Subsequent Pregnancy (%)			
20	92	90	88	85
25	89	86	82	79
30	84	80	76	71
35	77	73	68	62
40+	69	64	58	52

and the interval between pregnancies. Evaluation and treatment are considered earlier in couples with concordant subfertility.

Shown in Table 6-5, the success rate of a subsequent viable pregnancy declines as age increases and as the number of consecutive losses rises. Remarkably, the chances for a successful pregnancy are >50 percent even after five losses in women aged <45 years (Brigham, 1999). Following more than 150,000 miscarriages, Bhattacharya and coworkers (2010) reported miscarriage rate as it related to the number of prior losses (Table 6-6). In both studies, the risk for subsequent miscarriage was similar following either two or three losses.

◼ Etiology

Of the many putative causes of early RPL, only three are widely accepted: parental chromosomal abnormalities, antiphospholipid antibody syndrome, and acquired or congenital uterine abnormalities. Other suspected but not proven causes are alloimmunity, endocrinopathies, and environmental toxins. Discussed earlier, very few infections are firmly associated with early pregnancy loss (p. 138). It is even less likely that infections would cause recurrent miscarriage because most are isolated events or stimulate protective maternal antibodies.

The timing of the recurrent losses may provide a clue to their etiology. For a given individual with RPL, each miscarriage tends to occur near the same gestational age (Heuser, 2010). Genetic factors most frequently result in early embryonic losses, whereas autoimmune or anatomic abnormalities more likely

TABLE 6-6. Predicted Miscarriage Rate with Subsequent Pregnancy Based on Number of Prior Miscarriages[a]

| | Previous Pregnancy Losses | | | |
	0	1	2	3
Pregnancies (n)	143,595	6577	700	115
Subsequent risk for miscarriage	7.0%	13.9%	26.1%	27.8%

[a]Nonconsecutive miscarriages showed the same pattern of risk as consecutive miscarriages.

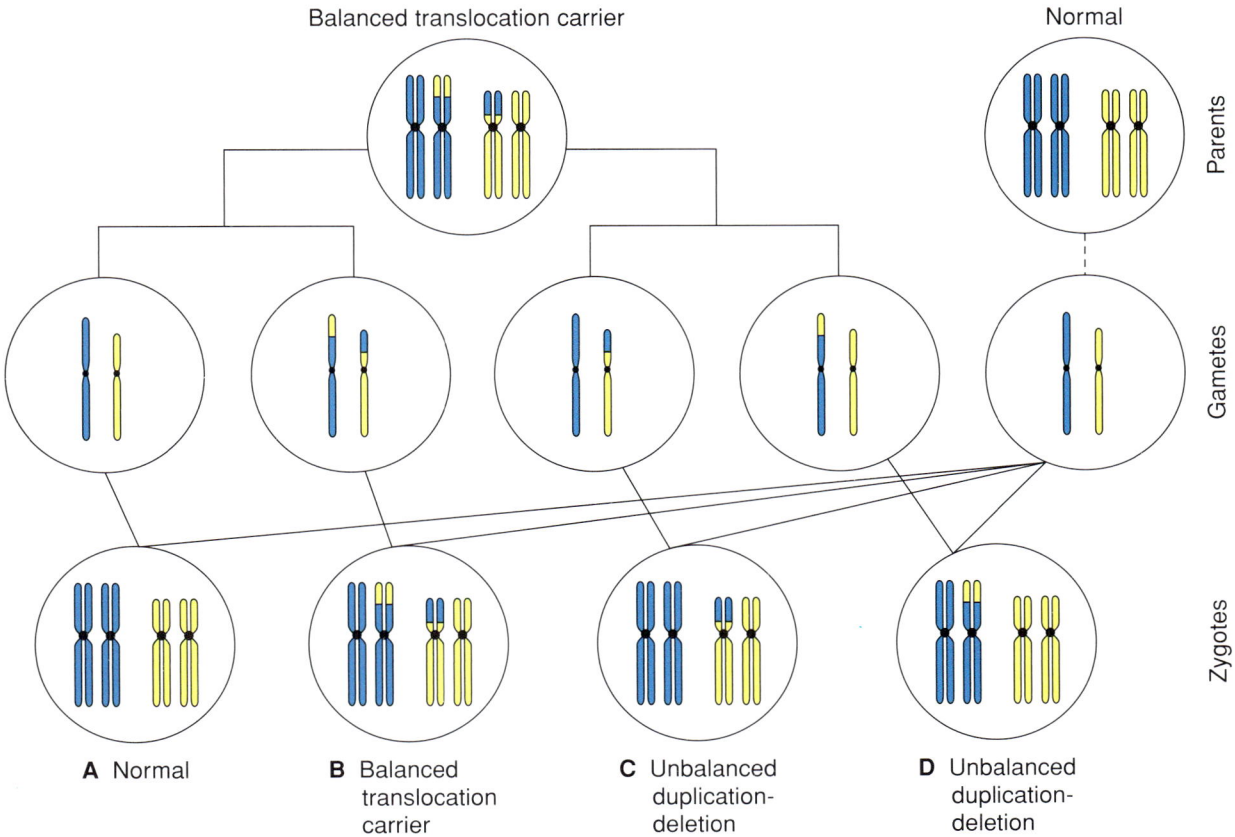

Balanced translocation carrier   Normal

Parents

Gametes

Zygotes

A Normal   **B** Balanced translocation carrier   **C** Unbalanced duplication-deletion   **D** Unbalanced duplication-deletion

FIGURE 6-3 Gametes produced by a balanced translocation carrier. (Reproduced with permission from Dashe, 2018.)

lead to second-trimester losses. Although many causes of RPL parallel those of sporadic miscarriage, the relative incidence differs between the two categories. For example, recurrent first-trimester losses have a significantly lower incidence of genetic abnormalities than observed in sporadic losses. In one series, the products of conception had a normal karyotype in half of recurrent miscarriages but in only a fourth of sporadic losses (Sullivan, 2004).

■ Parental Chromosomal Abnormalities
Parental Karyotype

An abnormal parental karyotype is estimated to account for 2 to 5 percent of RPL cases, and karyotype evaluation of both parents is recommended by the American Society for Reproductive Medicine (2012). Data from 8000 couples with two or more miscarriages demonstrated structural chromosomal anomalies in 3 percent—a fivefold greater incidence than observed for the general population. In the parents, balanced reciprocal translocations accounted for 50 percent of identified abnormalities; robertsonian translocations for 24 percent; and X chromosome mosaicism such as 47,XXY—*Klinefelter syndrome*—for 12 percent. Inversions and various other anomalies made up the remainder. The women were twice as likely as the men to harbor the cytogenetic abnormality (Tharapel, 1985). The likelihood of a karyotypic abnormality does not differ between consecutive or nonconsecutive pregnancy losses (van den Boogaard, 2010).

As noted, balanced translocations are the most common structural chromosomal abnormality and result in several possible genetic outcomes in the conceptus: normal, the same balanced translocation, or an unbalanced translocation (Fig. 6-3). Offspring who inherit the balanced translocation also are likely to experience recurrent miscarriage. With an unbalanced translocation, the conceptus will either spontaneously abort or produce an anomalous, frequently stillborn fetus. Thus, a history of second-trimester loss or fetal anomaly raises suspicion that one parent may have an abnormal chromosome pattern.

Sperm DNA Testing

The male genetic contribution to recurrent pregnancy loss has gained greater attention. In couples with RPL, some but not all studies report higher rates of aneuploidy and DNA fragmentation in sperm from a male partner (Bellver, 2010b; Ramasamy, 2015; Robinson, 2012). Additional areas of study include Y chromosome microdeletion, structural chromosomal abnormalities, and shortened telomere length (Ibrahim, 2018).

Although unlikely to be as critical as maternal age, increasing paternal age was significantly associated with a higher abortion risk in one study of more than 92,000 births (Kleinhaus, 2006). This risk was lowest before age 25 years, after which it progressively rose at 5-year intervals. A detrimental effect of paternal age on pregnancy outcomes following intrauterine insemination and IVF also is reported (Belloc, 2008; Robertshaw, 2014). At this time, semen analysis and assays for DNA integrity or other genetic abnormalities are not recommended as part of RPL evaluation (American Society for Reproductive Medicine, 2012).

Screening Products of Conception

Some recommend that fetal tissue be routinely analyzed for chromosomal abnormalities following a second consecutive miscarriage (Stephenson, 2006). One reason cited is that an abnormal karyotype suggests a sporadic loss and therefore does not predict a greater risk for loss with a subsequent pregnancy. Conversely, an abortus with a normal karyotype might suggest an alternative cause and imply a need for earlier evaluation.

Opponents of such routine karyotyping cite its high cost and possibility of misleading results. This applies particularly if the abnormal cells are derived from a pregnancy with placental mosaicism. Moreover, detection of a 46,XX karyotype may simply reflect contamination with maternal tissues. In sum, karyotyping of products of conception may not accurately reflect fetal karyotype. Because of the expense and limited information provided, we do not recommend this as a routine part of the evaluation at present.

Some are promoting the use of even more complex and expensive genetic techniques. Testing options include comparative genomic hybridization, chromosomal microarray, and copy number sequence technologies. These approaches can detect chromosomal changes below the threshold of sensitivity for conventional cytogenetic analysis (Gao, 2012; Lui, 2015). Some current practicality concerns are being mitigated by the advent of highly accurate 24-chromosome microarray technology and decreasing expense (Popescu, 2018). Thus, future recommendations may change.

Currently, we recommend that RPL evaluation should include a standard karyotype of both parents. More detailed chromosomal evaluation should remain investigational.

Whole Genome Sequencing

Specific genes responsible for human disorders now can be identified through DNA sequencing of the whole genome (whole genome sequencing) or the coding part of the genome (exome). Originally cost prohibitive, associated expense is now at levels in line with routine clinical practice. Thus, this approach has been used successfully in several specialties, but less so in the reproductive field. One hurdle is the ability to distinguish benign from causative variants in the DNA nucleotide sequence. Despite this, important information is expected from this work in the near future (Rajcan-Separovic, 2019).

Treatment

Individualized treatment is indicated in couples with a structural genetic abnormality. Approaches include IVF with preimplantation genetic testing (PGT) or the use of donor gametes. These techniques are described in Chapter 21 (p. 466). Depending on the timing of prior losses, chorionic villus sampling or amniocentesis also may be considered. In one retrospective study of couples with known translocations, PGT was found to increase the successful pregnancy rate and decrease the length of time to conception (Fischer, 2010). Even so, the prognosis is generally good without intervention for couples with a balanced translocation. Franssen and colleagues (2006)

compared couples with a balanced translocation and noncarrier couples. In both groups, 85 percent of couples had a healthy child, although the miscarriage rate was higher for the carrier couples.

Some have recommended PGT even in couples with normal karyotypes who have idiopathic RPL (Vitez, 2019). However, results from a large prospective cohort trial found no support for this practice (Platteau, 2005). Currently, the American Society for Reproductive Medicine (2012) does not recommend PGT in couples who are chromosomally normal.

■ Anatomic Factors

Several uterine abnormalities have been implicated in RPL and other adverse pregnancy outcomes but not in infertility (Reichman, 2010). According to Devi Wold and associates (2006), 15 percent of women with three or more consecutive miscarriages will be found to have an acquired or congenital uterine anomaly. The likelihood of identifying an abnormality is similar whether a patient has experienced two, three, or four consecutive miscarriages. This suggests that cavity evaluation after two miscarriages is reasonable (Seckin, 2012).

Acquired Uterine Defects

Acquired uterine abnormalities associated with pregnancy loss include intrauterine synechiae, leiomyoma, and endometrial polyps. Of these, intrauterine synechiae—also known as *intrauterine adhesions* or as *Asherman syndrome*—usually result from destruction of large areas of endometrium by curettage or ablative procedures. Characteristic multiple filling defects are seen during hysterosalpingography (HSG) or saline-infusion sonography (Fig. 2-23, p. 41 and Fig. 20-6, p. 439). As treatment, directed hysteroscopic lysis of adhesions is preferable to curettage, as discussed and illustrated in Section 44-18 (p. 1069). In one study, adhesiolysis lowered the miscarriage rate from 79 to 22 percent and raised the successful term pregnancy rate from 18 to 69 percent (Katz, 1996). Other studies report similar outcomes with prognosis correlating with disease severity (Al-Inany, 2001; Goldenberg, 1995).

Uterine leiomyomas are found in a large proportion of adult women and can cause miscarriage, especially if located near the placental implantation site. Common sense suggests that detrimental effects should be greater for submucous compared with intramural leiomyomas, and for large versus small tumors. However, uterine cavity distortion is apparently not requisite for bad outcomes, although conclusive data are lacking (Saravelos, 2011). In support, in women undergoing IVF, pregnancy outcomes were adversely affected by submucous but not subserosal or intramural leiomyomas (Jun, 2001; Ramzy, 1998). In contrast, a metaanalysis reported higher rates of adverse pregnancy outcomes—including miscarriage—following IVF in women with intramural myomas (Sunkara, 2010).

Currently, although based on poor-quality data, most agree that consideration be given to excision of submucosal and intracavitary leiomyomas in women with recurrent miscarriage (American Society for Reproductive Medicine, 2017). Uterine artery embolization to treat myomas may increase the risk for subsequent miscarriage and may not be advisable (Homer,

2010). For endometrial polyps, hysteroscopic removal is generally recommended. However, data are limited, particularly for single or small polyps. In all these cases, reproductive benefits are weighed against surgical risks, which include de novo synechiae formation.

Cervical insufficiency, also known as *incompetent cervix*, may develop following surgical or birth trauma. It may also be associated with a molecular defect in collagen synthesis (Dukhovny, 2009). Cervical insufficiency does not cause first-trimester miscarriage but is associated with a greater risk for second-trimester loss. The classic presentation is painless cervical dilation after 16 to 18 weeks' gestation. Cervical insufficiency is often treated surgically with cerclage placement. Interested readers are referred to Chapter 18 of *Williams Obstetrics*, 25th edition (Hoffman, 2018).

Developmental Anomalies

Congenital malformations of the müllerian duct also may have adverse pregnancy effects. Anomalies include unicornuate, bicornuate, septate, arcuate, and didelphic uteri. Cited prevalence rates for müllerian anomalies vary widely. This likely reflects differences in criteria to define normalcy and in the diagnostic modality employed. Anomalies are often first detected by HSG or routine TVS. Further characterization by 3-dimensional TVS (3-D TVS) and MR imaging may be helpful (Fig. 2-25, p. 42).

In one study of more than 573,000 women, the observed incidence was 1 anomaly in 600 fertile women and 1 in 30 infertile women. The overall incidence was 1 in 200 (Nahum, 1998). Much higher rates are reported using 3-D TVS, perhaps due to its greater sensitivity. Salim and associates (2003) described nearly 2500 women using 3-D TVS. Anomalies were identified in 24 percent of women with RPL, but in only 5 percent of controls. Authors of one metaanalysis concluded that uterine anomalies are present in approximately 17 percent of patients with RPL, 7.3 percent of infertile women, and 6.7 percent of women in the general population (Saravelos, 2008).

The distribution of anomalies and associated loss rates are shown in Table 6-7. Unicornuate, bicornuate, and septate uteri

---

TABLE 6-7. Estimated Prevalence of Some Congenital Uterine Malformations and Their Associated Pregnancy Loss Rate

Uterine Anomaly[a]	Proportion (%)	SAB Rate (%)[b]
Bicornuate	39	40–70
Septate or unicornuate	14–24	34–88
Didelphys	11	40
Arcuate	7	—
Hypo- or aplastic	4	—

[a]Estimated overall prevalence 1:200 women (Nahum, 1998).
[b]Includes first- and second-trimester spontaneous abortions (SABs).
Data from Buttram, 1979; Nahum, 1998; Reddy, 2007; Valli, 2001.

---

are all associated with increased early miscarriage and second-trimester loss, fetal malpresentation, and preterm labor rates (Reichman, 2010).

Improving early pregnancy outcome by uterine anomaly correction has proved difficult. Nevertheless, in one observational study, pregnancy outcomes were reviewed following hysteroscopic removal of a septum in women with more than two prior miscarriages (Saygili-Yilmaz, 2003). The miscarriage rate declined from 96 to 10 percent following surgery, and the term pregnancy rate rose from 0 to 70 percent. Another metaanalysis reported that hysteroscopic septum resection was associated with a markedly reduced probability of spontaneous abortion compared with untreated women (Venetis, 2014). Based on these reports and the relative safety of surgical correction, most experts recommend hysteroscopic resection of a uterine septum in women with RPL (American Society for Reproductive Medicine, 2012). The procedure is described in Section 44-16 (p. 1065).

In contrast, surgical repair of a bicornuate uterus requires laparotomy and full-thickness incision of the uterine wall (Fig. 19-12, p. 423). Disadvantages to uterine metroplasty include the requirement of cesarean delivery to prevent uterine rupture in subsequent pregnancy. This surgery also is linked to a high rate of postoperative pelvic adhesion formation and subsequent infertility. Thus, uterine metroplasty is generally not recommended except for women who have had a very high number of pregnancy losses. Additional discussion regarding the incidence, clinical impact, and treatment of congenital anatomic abnormalities can be found in Chapter 19 (p. 419). The use of a gestational carrier may be an option in women who are not surgical candidates or for whom surgery is unsuccessful.

▪ Immunologic Factors

The immune system also plays an important role in RPL. Yetman and Kutteh (1996) estimated that 15 percent of more than 1000 women with recurrent miscarriages had recognized immunologic factors. Two primary pathophysiologic models are the *autoimmune theory*—immunity against "self," and the *alloimmune theory*—immunity against antigens from another person.

Autoimmune Factors

RPL has a long-recognized association with systemic lupus erythematosus (Clowse, 2008). Subsequently, many women with lupus were identified to have antiphospholipid antibodies—a family of autoantibodies directed against phospholipid-binding plasma proteins (Erkan, 2011). Between 5 and 15 percent of women with RPL have clinically significant antiphospholipid antibodies compared with only 2 to 5 percent of controls (Branch, 2010).

These antiphospholipid antibodies in conjunction with specific clinical findings are termed the *antiphospholipid antibody syndrome—APS* (American College of Obstetrics and Gynecology, 2017c). Criteria for its diagnosis are shown in Table 6-8. Positive tests are repeated at a minimum of 12 weeks with strict requirements for acceptable laboratory methods and interpretation (Miyakis, 2006). This is the only autoimmune disorder that is clearly linked to pregnancy loss. Miscarriage

TABLE 6-8. Clinical and Laboratory Criteria for Diagnosis of Antiphospholipid Antibody Syndrome[a]

Clinical Criteria

Obstetric:

One or more unexplained deaths of a morphologically normal fetus at or beyond 10 weeks,

or

Severe preeclampsia or placental insufficiency necessitating delivery before 34 weeks,

or

Three or more unexplained consecutive spontaneous abortions before 10 weeks

Vascular: One or more episodes of arterial, venous, or small vessel thrombosis in any tissue or organ

Laboratory Criteria[b]

Presence of lupus anticoagulant according to guidelines of the International Society on Thrombosis and Hemostasis,

or

Medium or high serum levels of IgG or IgM anticardiolipin antibodies,

or

Anti-β2 glycoprotein-I IgG or IgM antibody

[a]At least one clinical and one laboratory criteria must be present for diagnosis.
[b]These tests must be positive on two or more occasions at least 12 weeks apart.
IgG = immunoglobulin G; IgM = immunoglobulin M.
Modified from Branch, 2010; Erkan, 2011; Miyakis, 2006.

due to APS most often occurs after 10 weeks. APS is more commonly associated with fetal death, preterm delivery, early-onset preeclampsia, and fetal-growth restriction stemming from placental insufficiency and placental thromboses (Clark, 2007a,b).

The mechanisms by which antiphospholipid antibodies result in miscarriage are unclear but can be divided into three general categories—thrombosis, inflammation, and abnormal placentation (Meroni, 2010). With *thrombosis,* it has been proposed that antiphospholipid antibodies act on trophoblast and endothelial surfaces to inhibit annexin A5 function. Annexin A5 is a natural anticoagulant that prevents the activation of factor X and prothrombin (Rand, 2010). Antiphospholipid antibodies may also activate complement to intensify hypercoagulability, which leads to recurrent placental thromboses. *Acute local inflammatory responses* at the placental–maternal interface also may be induced by antiphospholipid antibodies. Last, *placentation* may be affected directly by these antibodies through impaired decidual expression of integrins and cadherins. This can inhibit placental proliferation and syncytial development. Notably, defective decidual trophoblast invasion—not placental thrombosis—is the most common histologic abnormality identified in APS-related early pregnancy loss (Di Simone, 2007).

Several other *antilipid antibody idiotypes* have been described (Bick, 2006). Their measurement is expensive and frequently poorly controlled, and the relevance of results in the evaluation of RPL is uncertain. Results are likewise inconclusive regarding testing for other antibodies including rheumatoid factor, antinuclear antibodies, and those for celiac disease. Currently, testing for these additional antibodies is not recommended during RPL evaluation.

Antiphospholipid Antibody Syndrome Treatment.
Various treatments have been proposed for women with APS and RPL (Kutteh, 2014). Studies have compared single-agent or combination therapies using unfractionated heparin, low-molecular-weight heparin (LMWH), low-dose aspirin, glucocorticoids, or intravenous immunoglobulin (IVIG). Concomitant use of glucocorticoids and heparin generally is not recommended. Compared with single-treatment regimens, this combination may increase the maternal fracture risk without improving outcome. In addition, IVIG is not endorsed for RPL.

For women with APS, one reviewer group concluded that the combination of unfractionated heparin and low-dose aspirin significantly benefitted pregnancy outcome in those with prior first-trimester pregnancy losses (Ziakas, 2010). They found no improvement with LMWH and aspirin combinations. Similar conclusions were reached in a Cochrane Database Review (Empson, 2012).

Guidelines from the American College of Obstetricians and Gynecologists (2018b) suggest that women with RPL and APS who have not had a thrombotic event receive prophylactic low-dose aspirin—81 mg orally per day—and heparin when pregnancy is diagnosed. This is continued until delivery and 6 weeks postpartum. Heparin regimens vary, but unfractionated heparin—5000 to 10,000 units subcutaneously daily—is common. Some experts suggest initiating low-dose aspirin prior to conception (Kutteh, 2014). At a minimum, careful clinical surveillance to ensure early pregnancy identification seems prudent.

Alloimmune Factors

The immune tolerance of the mother to a semiallogeneic fetus remains incompletely understood (Williams, 2012). An attractive theory suggests that normal pregnancy requires the expression of blocking factors that prevent maternal rejection of paternally derived foreign fetal antigens. The pregnant woman ostensibly will not produce these blocking factors if she shares human leukocyte antigens (HLAs) with the father.

Other alloimmune disorders that have been posited to cause recurrent miscarriage include altered natural killer cell activity and increased levels of lymphocytotoxic antibodies.

Various tests and treatment options have been developed to address this issue. None has withstood rigorous scrutiny. In an attempt to correct the dysregulated response to fetal antigens, proposed therapies include paternal or third-party leukocyte immunization and IVIG. Three randomized clinical trials failed to demonstrate any benefit of IVIG or placebo in patients with idiopathic miscarriage (Stephenson, 2010). A 2014 Cochrane Review concluded that none of the studied immunotherapies provided a significant benefit over placebo in improving live birth rate or lowering the future miscarriage risk of women with RPL (Wong, 2014). Consequently, immunotherapy is not recommended for RPL.

■ Endocrinologic Factors
Luteal Phase Defect

Arredondo and Noble (2006) estimated that 8 to 12 percent of recurrent miscarriages are the result of endocrine factors. The greater incidence of miscarriage in these disorders is most frequently attributed to abnormal folliculogenesis with subsequent abnormal luteal function. This so-called *luteal phase defect (LPD)* is postulated to be associated with inadequate endometrial development at implantation. Treatment for presumed LPD has included progesterone supplementation, hCG administration to enhance corpus luteum function, or ovulation induction with agents such as clomiphene citrate to generate additional corpora lutea. A recent metaanalysis concluded that progestogen treatment may lead to a slight reduction in the number of miscarriages but was based on relatively poor-quality data and mixed study designs (Haas, 2018). At this time, progesterone treatment is not recommended despite its minimal risks and expense. Although controversial for LPD, progesterone supplementation is clearly indicated until 8 to 10 weeks in women who have had a corpus luteum removed surgically (p. 139).

Thyroid Disease

Although the mechanisms by which they may adversely affect early pregnancy remain unclear, thyroid disorders, hyperprolactinemia, diabetes mellitus, and polycystic ovarian syndrome (PCOS) merit discussion. Of these, thyroid disorders have long been suspected to cause early pregnancy loss and other adverse pregnancy outcomes. First, severe iodine deficiency—infrequent in developed countries—is associated with excessive miscarriage rates (Castañeda, 2002). In addition, women with hyperthyroidism have greater risks for both spontaneous abortion and stillbirth (Andersen, 2014).

Thyroid hormone insufficiency is common, but the degree of insufficiency varies. In pregnancy, overt hypothyroidism is rare, but the incidence of subclinical hypothyroidism approximates 2 percent (Casey, 2005). Autoimmune *Hashimoto thyroiditis* is a usual cause, and its incidence and severity accrue with age. Despite this common prevalence, any effects of hypothyroidism on early pregnancy loss remain unclear (Krassas, 2010). That said, De Vivo (2010) reported that subclinical thyroid hormone deficiency may be associated with very early pregnancy loss.

The prevalence of abnormally high serum levels of antibodies to thyroid peroxidase or thyroglobulin is nearly 15 percent in pregnant women (Abbassi-Ghanavati, 2010; Haddow, 2011). Most of these women are euthyroid, but those with clinical hypothyroidism tend to have higher concentrations of antibodies. Even in euthyroid women, however, antibodies are a marker for increased miscarriage risk (Chen, 2011; Thangaratinam, 2011).

In sum, current recommendations suggest that all women with RPL undergo thyroid function testing. This includes antibody testing for anti–thyroid peroxidase antibodies (Amrane, 2019). Overt hypo- or hyperthyroidism should be treated to prevent pregnancy complications. It remains unclear whether patients with subclinical hypothyroidism or thyroid autoimmunity should receive treatment (Vissenberg, 2012). Treatment may be considered in patients with both a TSH level above 2.5 mIU/L and positive antibody testing (American Society for Reproductive Medicine, 2015).

Hyperprolactinemia

Cyclic ovulation may become dysfunctional in response to elevated serum prolactin levels such as occurs with prolactinoma. Prolactin also may have direct effects on the endometrium. Hirahara (1998) reported an increase in the successful pregnancy rate for patients with hyperprolactinemia treated with the dopamine agonist bromocriptine. Although data are few, many experts still suggest measuring prolactin levels in patients with RPL.

Diabetes Mellitus

Type 1 diabetes substantively raises risks for spontaneous abortion and major congenital malformations (Greene, 1999). This directly relates to the degree of periconceptional glycemic and metabolic control. Importantly, this risk is greatly mitigated with optimal metabolic control. The miscarriage rate in women with excellent control rivals that of nondiabetic women (Mills, 1988).

In addition, diabetic women with RPL may also have greater degrees of insulin resistance than diabetic women without miscarriages (Craig, 2002). This suggests that ovarian insulin resistance may be contributory, as discussed next.

Polycystic Ovarian Syndrome

Women with PCOS generally have been considered to carry an elevated miscarriage risk. However, this association has been questioned (Cocksedge, 2009). For example, inhibition of serum luteinizing hormone (LH) during a gonadotropin ovulation-induction cycle failed to improve pregnancy outcomes in a controlled trial. This argues against a role for the elevated LH levels seen in PCOS (Clifford, 1996).

Data implicating hyperinsulinemia in pregnancy loss are somewhat stronger. Insulin modulates insulin-like growth factor actions in the ovary, thereby affecting folliculogenesis and steroid production. Retrospective and case-control studies concluded that metformin (Glucophage) lowered miscarriage rates in women with PCOS (Glueck, 2002; Nawaz, 2010). Metformin lowers hepatic glucose production and enhances insulin sensitivity and thereby lowers insulin levels. However, a systematic review of randomized trials found no improvement in abortion risk with metformin treatment (Palomba, 2009). At this time, routine metformin treatment for women with PCOS solely to treat pregnancy loss is not recommended.

Thrombophilias

The coagulation cascade can be altered by several single-gene mutations that affect pro- or anticoagulant proteins. Mutations predisposing to thrombosis—collectively termed *thrombophilias*—are caused by mutations of the genes for factor V Leiden, prothrombin, antithrombin, and protein C and protein S. These are described further in Chapter 39 (p. 834). In the past, several of these thrombophilias were suspected to cause RPL. However, large prospective cohort studies have refuted these associations, and testing for these abnormalities for RPL is no longer recommended (American College of Obstetricians and Gynecologists, 2018b; American Society of Reproductive Medicine, 2012).

Evaluation and Treatment

Some considerations for evaluation and management of women with RPL are outlined in Table 6-9. Timing and extent of evaluation is based on maternal age, coexistent infertility,

symptoms, and level of patient anxiety. In our view, after a thorough history and clinical examination, a modicum of testing is done that is directed to likely causes. General testing may include parental karyotyping, uterine cavity evaluation, and testing for APS. Screening for inherited thrombophilias, endocrine disorders, or LPD has progressively less support. Evaluation also assesses the potential need for psychologic support (Koert, 2019).

Unfortunately, a putative cause will be identified in only about half of couples with RPL. Empiric treatment for unexplained pregnancy loss is discouraged. Even for those with no explanatory findings, couples are cautiously assured that the chances of successfully achieving a live birth are reasonably good (Branch, 2010). Reassuringly, a large cohort study did not detect higher rates of adverse pregnancy outcomes in patients with a history of RPL. Specific assessed outcomes included congenital anomalies, aneuploidy, neonatal asphyxia, or small-for-gestational-age neonates (Sugiura-Ogasawara, 2019).

Although age dependent, the results shown in Tables 6-5 and 6-6 forecast a reasonable prognosis for a successful subsequent pregnancy even after five recurrent losses. Couples may be anxious to try any treatment. However, the lack of definitive benefits for many of these is carefully considered and appropriate counseling offered.

TABLE 6-9. Tests Used for Evaluation of Couples with Recurrent Pregnancy Loss

Etiology	Diagnostic Evaluation	Possible Therapies
Genetic[a]	Karyotype partners	Genetic counseling, donor gametes
Anatomic[a]	Sonohysterography Hysterosalpingogram MR imaging	Septum transection, myomectomy, or adhesiolysis
Immunologic[a]	Lupus anticoagulant Anticardiolipin antibodies Anti-β2 glycoprotein-I antibody	Heparin + aspirin
Endocrinologic[b]	TSH ± TPOAb Prolactin Fasting glucose, Hgb A_{1c} Day 3 FSH, estradiol Midluteal progesterone	Levothyroxine Dopamine agonist Metformin Counseling Progesterone
Thrombophilic[c]	Antithrombin deficiency Protein C or S deficiency Factor V Leiden mutation Prothrombin mutation } No proven treatment Hyperhomocysteinemia	Folic acid
Toxic	Tobacco, alcohol use Exposure to toxins, chemicals Obesity	Eliminate consumption Behavior modification Weight loss

[a]Testing for these disorders is generally supported by the literature and expert opinion. One or a combination of these tests may be indicated.
[b]Ongoing controversy regarding testing. Strongest support for thyroid function testing.
[c]Current recommendations against testing. Included for historic reference.
FSH = follicle-stimulating hormone; MR = magnetic resonance; TSH = thyroid-stimulating hormone; TPOAb = thyroid peroxidase antibody.
Modified from Brezina, 2013; Fritz, 2011; Reddy, 2007.

INDUCED ABORTION

■ Rates

The term *induced abortion* defines the medical or surgical termination of pregnancy before the time of fetal viability. Definitions to describe its incidence include the *abortion ratio*, which is the number of abortions per 1000 live births, and the *abortion rate*, which is the number of abortions per 1000 reproductive-aged women per year.

The Guttmacher Institute reported that 926,200 abortions were performed in the United States in 2014 (Guttmacher, 2019). The Centers for Disease Control and Prevention (CDC) reported an abortion ratio of 188 in 2015 (Jatlaoui, 2018). Most women selecting induced abortion are in their twenties, and 91 percent of abortions in 2015 were performed at a gestational age ≤13 weeks. Only 1.3 percent was performed at a gestational age ≥21 weeks. Notably, 25 percent of all abortions were early medication abortions. This reflects a 114 percent rise compared with the number of medication abortions reported in 2006 (Jatlaoui, 2018).

Worldwide, an estimated 56 million induced abortions occur each year. Women in developing regions have a higher likelihood to select abortion than those in developed regions. Yet, abortion tends to be safer in countries with higher gross national incomes. An estimated 25 million abortions annually are considered unsafe, and Africa and Latin America carry the highest rates (World Health Organization, 2018). In 2012, unsafe abortion was linked to complications in an estimated 6.9 million women worldwide and to 8 percent of maternal deaths.

■ Indications

Induced abortions are performed for social, economic, or maternal health indications. Medical and surgical conditions include persistent cardiac decompensation, pulmonary arterial hypertension, advanced hypertensive vascular disease, diabetes with end-stage organ failure, and malignancy.

■ Abortion in the United States

Legality

The legality of abortion was established by the United States Supreme Court in the case of *Roe v. Wade* in 1973. The Court defined the extent to which states might regulate abortion and ruled that first-trimester procedures must be left to the medical judgment of the physician. After this, the state could regulate abortion procedures in ways reasonably related to maternal health. Subsequent to viability, the state could promote its interest in the potential of human life and regulate and even proscribe abortion, except for the preservation of the life or health of the mother. The legal definition of abortion itself is removal of or termination of a pregnancy prior to viability.

Other legislation soon followed. The 1976 Hyde Amendment forbids use of federal funds to provide abortion services except in cases of rape, incest, or life-threatening circumstances. The effect is that most states do not provide public funds for abortion

expenses. However, 16 states fund all or most abortions. At least 13 states restrict abortion coverage by private insurance carriers (Guttmacher, 2019).

The Supreme Court in 1992 reviewed *Planned Parenthood v. Casey* and upheld the fundamental right to abortion but established that regulations before viability are constitutional as long as they do not impose an "undue burden" on the woman. Subsequently, many states have passed legislation that imposes counseling requirements, waiting periods, parental consent or notification for minors, facility requirements, and funding restrictions. One major abortion restriction decision was the 2007 Supreme Court decision that reviewed *Gonzales v. Carhart* and upheld the 2003 Partial-Birth Abortion Ban Act. This was problematic because no medically approved definition describes partial-birth abortion.

The Supreme Court decision of *Whole Woman's Health v. Hellerstedt* decided that two provisions in a Texas law created an undue burden and thus violated the Constitution. The first required a physician who performed abortions to have hospital admitting privileges. The second required clinics that provided abortions to have facilities comparable to an ambulatory surgical center.

More than 400 laws restricting access to abortion have been passed in the United States since 2011 (Inman, 2018). In the first 5 months of 2019, seven states have passed legislation to ban first-trimester abortion. These bans currently are, or are expected to be, held up in court.

Access

A woman's chance of receiving the abortion services that best meet her needs varies considerably by locale (National Academies of Sciences, Engineering, and Medicine, 2018). For example, in a survey of Texas women after drastic family planning funding cuts were instituted, 7 percent of women reported an attempt to self-induce abortion. This is significantly higher than the 2 percent rate reported in a U.S. national survey in 2008 (Grossman, 2014). As a correlate, access to safe, legal abortion is the most effective prevention to maternal morbidity.

The American College of Obstetricians and Gynecologists (2019a,b) calls for increased advocacy to overturn restrictions, improve access, and codify abortion as a fundamental component of women's health care. The College (2014, 2016b) supports the legal right of women to obtain an abortion and considers this a medical matter between a woman and her physician.

Training

Because of abortion controversy, training for residents and postgraduate fellows has been both championed and assailed. The Accreditation Council for Graduate Medical Education mandates that obstetrics and gynecology residency programs must provide abortion training or access to training, and this must be part of the planned curriculum (Accreditation Council for Graduate Medical Education, 2017).

The American College of Obstetricians and Gynecologists (2019b) outlines legislative, institutional, and social barriers to abortion training and supports the use of "opt-out" programs. In these, abortion training is integrated as a standard part of the residency schedule, but residents with religious or moral objections can decline to participate. The Kenneth J. Ryan Residency Training Program was established in 1999 to improve residency training in abortion and family planning. By 2019, more than 70 Ryan programs have been started in the United States and in Canada. However, one survey of U.S. residency program directors found that abortion training was not available in 5 percent of programs and was optional in 31 percent (Steinauer, 2018). In Canada, up to 15 percent of residents report having limited access to abortion training within their residency (Liauw, 2016).

Other programs teach residents technical aspects through management of early incomplete and missed abortions and through uterine evacuation for fetal death, severe fetal anomalies, and life-threatening maternal medical or surgical disorders (Steinauer, 2005). Freedman and coworkers (2010) rightly emphasize that abortion training should include discussion of the social, moral, and ethical aspects of the procedure.

Formal fellowships in Family Planning are 2-year postgraduate programs. By 2019, these are located in 26 departments of obstetrics and gynecology and in two departments of family medicine. Training includes experience with high-level research and uterine evacuation for induced and spontaneous abortion.

Abortion Providers

The American College of Obstetricians and Gynecologists (2016a) respects the need and responsibility of health-care providers to determine their individual positions on induced abortion. The College also emphasizes the need to provide standard-of-care counseling and timely referral if providers have individual beliefs that preclude pregnancy termination. Up to 97 percent of obstetrician-gynecologists may encounter women seeking an abortion, but only 24 percent reported having performed one in the year from 2016 to 2017 (Grossman, 2019; Stulberg, 2011). Most practitioners help women find an abortion provider (Harris, 2011). In any event, physicians who care for women must be familiar with abortion techniques so that referrals for care and management of complications are appropriate.

■ Counseling before Abortion

Three basic choices are available to a woman considering an abortion. Women may continue pregnancy with its risks and parental responsibilities, may continue pregnancy with arranged adoption, or may elect pregnancy termination with its risks. Knowledgeable and compassionate counselors should objectively describe and provide information regarding these choices for informed decision making (Templeton, 2011).

ABORTION TECHNIQUES

In the absence of serious maternal medical disorders, abortion procedures can be done in an outpatient setting (Levy, 2019). First-trimester abortion can be performed with either medication or surgery. With medication abortion, surgery and the need for sedation are usually avoided. Medication terminations have lower average costs and may allow for more privacy during the termination.

■ Surgical Abortion

Surgical abortion methods are predominantly completed transvaginally through an appropriately dilated cervix. Rarely, pregnancies are evacuated transabdominally either by hysterotomy or hysterectomy. Electric vacuum aspiration (EVA) of the uterus is the most commonly used form and is illustrated in Chapter 43 (p. 972). Instead, manual vacuum aspiration (MVA) is done with a cannula that attaches to a handheld syringe for its vacuum source.

Cervical Preparation

Unless a woman presents with an incomplete or inevitable abortion, preoperative cervical softening and dilation is common prior uterine evacuation. Cervical preparation softens and slowly dilates the cervix. Medical or mechanical approaches are available, and both aim to minimize the degree of mechanical dilation and thereby lower cervix or uterine trauma risk. Cervical preparation is also associated with less pain, a technically easier procedure, and shorter operating times (Kapp, 2010).

For pregnancies ≤8 weeks, preprocedural cervical ripening is usually unnecessary. After this time, some recommend that osmotic dilators be placed the day prior or misoprostol given 2 to 4 hours before the procedure (Table 6-10). Adolescents, nulliparas, or women with gestations ≥12 weeks may especially benefit from preoperative cervical preparation (Allen, 2016). For gestational age ≥12 weeks, the type and length of time of cervical preparation varies by clinician, patient, and clinical setting. The Society of Family Planning offers excellent clinical guidelines at www.societyfp.org/home (Fox, 2014; Newmann, 2008).

Of medical options for cervical preparation, many clinicians provide a 400-μg buccal misoprostol dose at least 3 hours before uterine vacuum aspiration (Allen, 2016). For gestational ages >20 weeks, mifepristone, a progesterone antagonist, can be given as a 200-mg oral dose (Fox, 2014; Goldberg, 2015).

Of mechanical options, hygroscopic dilators draw water from cervical tissues and expand to gradually dilate the cervix. One type is derived from various species of *Laminaria* algae that are harvested from the ocean floor (Chap. 43, p. 972). Another is Dilapan-S, which is composed of an acrylic-based gel. Each is available in varying diameters.

Electric Vacuum Aspiration

In this method, also known as *dilation and curettage (D & C)*, a cannula is attached to tubing and an electric-powered vacuum source empties the uterus. Suction aspiration is highly effective and obviates the need for sharp curettage, which carries attendant risks for traumatic injury. To begin, the surgeon first dilates the cervix. The pregnancy is then evacuated by suctioning out the contents. Suction is recommended for gestational ages ≤15 weeks.

Manual Vacuum Aspiration

MVA is accomplished with a suction cannula attached to a self-locking syringe for the suction source. Advantages of MVA are that it is portable, is quieter than EVA, and does not require electricity. However, MVA may be limited by the volume that the aspirator can hold. Thus, at gestational

TABLE 6-10. Suggested Cervical Preparation Regimens for Aspiration and D & E Procedures

EGA	Cervical Preparation
<12 weeks	Consider misoprostol 400 μg buccally 3 hours before procedure if: Age <20 years Nulliparous No prior vaginal delivery
≥12 to <15 weeks	Misoprostol 400 μg buccally 3 hours before procedure if: Age <20 years Nulliparous No prior vaginal delivery
≥15 to <17 weeks	Dilapan-S (quantity: 1–4 for ≥4 hours) Laminaria (quantity: 1–7 for ≥4 hours) *or* Misoprostol 400 μg buccally ≥3 hours before procedure
≥17 to <20 weeks	Dilapan-S (quantity: 2–5 for ≥4 hours) *plus* Laminaria (quantity 1 to aid dilator removal) *or* Laminaria (quantity: 6–10 usually overnight) *or* Misoprostol 400 μg buccally for ≥3 hours; may require repeated doses; generally reserved for highly experienced surgeons
≥20 weeks	May require multiple sets of dilators ± mifepristone or misoprostol

D & E = dilation and evacuation; EGA = estimated gestational age.

ages >9 weeks, MVA procedures are lengthier than EVA ones, because the syringe requires repeated emptying. Time can be shortened by using multiple aspirators, which can be changed out.

The technique employs a hand-operated 60-mL syringe and cannula. A vacuum is created in the syringe attached to the cannula, which is inserted transcervically into the uterus. The vacuum produces suction pressures up to 60 mm Hg. MVA complications are similar to EVA (Goldberg, 2004).

Dilation and Evacuation

Dilation and evacuation (D & E) involves cervical dilation followed by evacuation of the fetus and placenta via a combination of tissue forceps and suction cannula. Unless the cervix is already dilated, preoperative cervical preparation is essential to provide an adequate diameter to evacuate the larger tissue volume. For this, ripening options discussed earlier may require up to 48 hours for sufficient effect (see Table 6-10).

D & E is the most frequently used method for second-trimester uterine evacuation in the United States. For these pregnancies, it is generally safer and faster than labor induction (American College of Obstetricians and Gynecologists, 2017b). In addition, risks for a second procedure to remove retained products are lower with D & E than with labor induction (Bryant, 2011).

Many clinicians routinely perform D & E with sonographic guidance. This guides tissue extraction, directs instrument insertion, and confirms complete tissue evacuation. Bierer or Sopher forceps for tissue extraction are valuable adjuncts and are designed to cause minimal trauma to the surrounding endometrium. D & E completion is confirmed with identification of all fetal parts (four extremities, spine, and calvarium). For missing parts, the uterus can be gently explored with these forceps under sonographic guidance.

■ Medication Abortion

Throughout history, many natural substances have been given for alleged abortifacient effects. Currently, mifepristone is the most widely used medication for induced abortion (Table 6-11). Two other studied agents are misoprostol and methotrexate. The American College of Obstetricians and Gynecologists and the Society of Family Planning regularly update clinical guidelines for management of medication abortion (American College of Obstetricians and Gynecologists, 2016b).

As noted earlier, mifepristone is a progesterone-receptor antagonist. It primes the myometrium and cervix for prostaglandin activity. Clark and associates (2006) reported that mifepristone causes cervical collagen degradation, possibly from greater matrix metalloproteinase expression. Misoprostol is a PGE_1 analogue that directly stimulates the myometrium. Methotrexate is an antimetabolite that stops cell division. It halts fetal growth and placental implantation. These last two are teratogens, and a commitment to complete the abortion is required once these drugs are given. Methotrexate can lead to pulmonary atresia, craniosynostosis, and limb deficiencies (Hyoun, 2012; Nurmohamed, 2011). With misoprostol, the central nervous system, limbs, genitalia, eye, and palate may be affected (Gonzalez, 1998; Vargas, 2000).

Medication abortion is suitable for women who desire privacy or wish to avoid a procedure, if possible. This approach can be performed safely at home and is well tolerated and

TABLE 6-11. Common Medication Regimens for Early Pregnancy Termination

Mifepristone/Misoprostol
[a]Mifepristone, 200 mg orally followed 24–48 hours later by:
[b]Misoprostol, 400 µg vaginally, buccally, or sublingually

Misoprostol Alone
[c]800 µg vaginally or sublingually, repeated for up to three doses

Methotrexate/Misoprostol
[d]Methotrexate, 50 mg/m² intramuscularly or orally followed by:
[e]Misoprostol, 800 µg vaginally in 3–7 days. Repeat if needed 1 week after methotrexate initially given

[a]Doses of 200 versus 600 mg are similarly effective.
[b]Oral route may be less effective; possibly more side effects, namely, nausea and diarrhea. Sublingual route has more side effects than vaginal route. Shorter intervals (6 hours) with PGE₁ given after mifepristone may be less effective than when given >36 hours.
[c]Intervals 3–12 hours given vaginally; 3–4 hours given sublingually.
[d]Efficacy similar for routes of administration.
[e]Similar efficacy when given on day 3 versus day 5.
Data from Borgatta, 2001; Coyaji, 2007; Creinin, 2001, 2007; Fekih, 2010; Guest, 2007; Hamoda, 2005; Honkanen, 2004; Jain, 2002; Kulier, 2011; Pymar, 2001; Raghavan, 2009; Schaff, 2000; Shannon, 2006; von Hertzen, 2003, 2007, 2009, 2010; Winikoff, 2008.

effective through 70 days' gestation. The failure rate quoted in most studies is 3 percent (American College of Obstetricians and Gynecologists, 2016b). Contraindications to medication abortion broadly are a patient's unwillingness to have a procedure in the event of heavy bleeding or ongoing pregnancy; an in situ intrauterine device; a confirmed or suspected ectopic pregnancy; and severe anemia, coagulopathy, or anticoagulant use. Additionally, patients who undergo medication abortion should be committed to returning for a follow-up visit.

Contraindications to mifepristone are current long-term systemic corticosteroid therapy, chronic adrenal failure, or allergy to mifepristone. A known allergy to misoprostol is its main limitation to use. Contraindications to methotrexate are listed in Table 7-3 (p. 168).

Provision of mifepristone requires completion of a manufacturer's patient agreement form (Danco Laboratories, 2016). For providers who want to dispense mifepristone in their practice, the drug is available through a *risk evaluation and mitigation strategy (REMS)* program. REMS are U.S. Food and Drug Administration (FDA)-mandated safety strategies to help manage known medicine risks yet still allow access to the drug's benefits (Danco Laboratories, 2019).

Thorough counseling should include a description of cramping and bleeding during conceptus passage. Bleeding that soaks two or more pads per hour for more than 2 consecutive hours warrants a provider discussion or evaluation. Women without bleeding within 24 hours of taking misoprostol should contact their clinician because they may be at risk of ectopic pregnancy or abortion failure.

Updated labeling by the FDA (2016) now matches evidence-based regimens. For gestations up to 70 days' gestation, labeling recommends that a single 200-mg oral dose of mifepristone be administered in the provider's office. After 24 to 48 hours, an 800-µg buccal dose of misoprostol is taken at home. For most women, the pregnancy is expelled after 2 to 24 hours. A woman

is reassessed after 7 to 14 days with TVS or serum β-hCG level to confirm no ongoing pregnancy and medication abortion completion. One study reported that a multilayered sonographic pattern indicated a successful abortion (Tzeng, 2013).

Unnecessary surgical intervention in women undergoing medication abortion can be avoided by the proper interpretation of postabortal sonogram findings. Specifically, if no gestational sac is seen and bleeding is not heavy, intervention is unnecessary. This is true even when, as is common, the uterus contains sonographically evident debris. Assessment of the clinical course along with bimanual pelvic examination is generally adequate.

ABORTION CONSEQUENCES

Morbidity and mortality associated with abortion is very low. Potential short-term morbidity of induced abortion includes retained tissue, hemorrhage, and infection, each in approximately equal frequency (Niinimäki, 2009; von Hertzen, 2010). In a review of more than 233,000 medication abortions, 0.65 percent was complicated by significant adverse events. Most of these were an ongoing pregnancy (Cleland, 2013). From one systematic review of first-trimester aspiration, the overall major complications rate was ≤1.0 percent (White, 2015). The rate of any complication leading to an emergency department visit was 2 percent in one California study (Upadhyay, 2015).

Complication rates rise with increasing gestational age in both spontaneous and induced abortions. For example, retained tissue occurs more frequently following second-trimester loss (40 percent) compared with earlier losses (17 percent) (van den Bosch, 2008).

Mortality rates from induced abortion performed by trained clinicians, especially during the first 2 months of pregnancy, are less than 1 death per 100,000 procedures (Grimes, 2006; Jatlaoui, 2018). Moreover, pregnancy-associated mortality is 14-fold greater than abortion-related mortality (8 versus

0.6 deaths per 100,000) (Raymond, 2012). Early abortions are even safer, and the relative mortality risk of abortion approximately doubles for each 2 weeks after 8 weeks' gestation. The CDC identified six abortion-related deaths in the United States in 2014 (Jatlaoui, 2018).

Most modern studies and systematic reviews conclude that first-trimester medication and vacuum aspiration abortion do not raise rates of preterm birth in subsequent pregnancies (Kc, 2017; Moreau, 2005; Shah, 2009). Rates of infertility or ectopic pregnancy also are not significantly higher after induced abortion (Atrash, 1997; Shannon, 2004; Stubblefield, 1984). Exceptions may stem from postabortal infections, especially those caused by chlamydial species. It may be most reasonable to compare women undergoing a pregnancy termination with those having a first-trimester miscarriage. In this later group, the 5-year live-birth rate approximates 80 percent (Smith, 2009).

Schneider and associates (1991) described 21 cases in which women who had a hygroscopic dilator placed changed their minds. Of 17 women who chose to continue their pregnancy, 14 carried to term, two delivered preterm, and one miscarried 2 weeks later. None suffered infection-related morbidity, including three untreated women with cervical cultures positive for *Chlamydia trachomatis*. In spite of this generally reassuring report, it seems prudent to presume irrevocability with regard to dilator placement and abortion.

Induced abortion does not negatively affect a woman's mental health. The Turnaway Study is a prospective longitudinal study that followed more than 500 women for 5 years after having obtained or been denied an abortion. Findings showed that induced abortion does not increase a woman's risk of posttraumatic stress, depression, anxiety, low self-esteem, or poor life satisfaction (Biggs, 2017). Effects of being denied an abortion may be more detrimental to psychologic well-being than obtaining a wanted procedure. Modern prospective studies report no association between breast cancer and induced abortion (American College of Obstetricians and Gynecologists, 2018b).

POSTABORTAL CONTRACEPTION

Ovulation may resume as early as 2 weeks after an early pregnancy loss, whether spontaneous or induced. Accordingly, effective contraception should be initiated soon after abortion unless another pregnancy is desired immediately. An intrauterine device can be inserted after the procedure is completed (Bednarek, 2011; Shimoni, 2011). Alternatively, any of the hormonal contraceptive methods discussed in Chapter 5 can be initiated at this time (Madden, 2009; Reeves, 2007).

REFERENCES

Abbassi-Ghanavati M, Casey BM, Spong CY, et al: Pregnancy outcomes in women with thyroid peroxidase antibodies. Obstet Gynecol 116:381, 2010
Accreditation Council for Graduate Medical Education: Clarification on requirements regarding family planning and contraception. Review Committee for Obstetrics and Gynecology. 2017. Available at: http://www.acgme.org/portals/0/pfassets/programresources/220_obgyn_abortion_training_clarification.pdf. Accessed on June 2, 2019
Achilles SL, Reeves MF, Society of Family Planning: Prevention of infection after induced abortion: release date October 2010: SFP guideline 20102. Contraception 83(4):295, 2011
Al-Inany H: Intrauterine adhesions. An update. Acta Obstet Gynecol Scand 80:986, 2001
Allen RH, Goldberg AB: Cervical dilation before first-trimester surgical abortion (<14 weeks' gestation). Contraception 93(4):277, 2016
Ambühl LMM, Leonhard AK, Widen Zakhary C, et al: Human papillomavirus infects placental trophoblast and Hofbauer cells, but appears not to play a causal role in miscarriage and preterm labor. Acta Obstet Gynecol Scand 96(10):1188, 2017
American College of Obstetricians and Gynecologists: College statement of policy: abortion policy. 2014. Available at: https://www.acog.org/-/media/Statements-of-policy/Public/sop069.pdf?dmc = 1&ts = 20190602T1940544584. Accessed on June 2, 2019
American College of Obstetricians and Gynecologists: The limits of conscientious refusal in reproductive medicine. Committee Opinion No. 385, November 2007, Reaffirmed 2016a
American College of Obstetricians and Gynecologists, Society of Family Planning: Medical management of first-trimester abortion. Practice Bulletin No. 143, March 2014, Reaffirmed 2016b
American College of Obstetricians and Gynecologists: Prevention of Rh D alloimmunization. Practice Bulletin No. 181, August 2017a
American College of Obstetricians and Gynecologists: Second-trimester abortion. Practice Bulletin No. 135, June 2013, Reaffirmed 2017b
American College of Obstetricians and Gynecologists: Antiphospholipid syndrome. Practice Bulletin No. 132, December 2012, Reaffirmed 2017c
American College of Obstetricians and Gynecologists: Early pregnancy loss. Practice Bulletin No. 200, August 2019b/2018a
American College of Obstetricians and Gynecologists: Induced abortion and breast cancer risk. Committee Opinion No. 434, June 2009, Reaffirmed 2018b
American College of Obstetricians and Gynecologists: Inherited thrombophilias in pregnancy. Practice Bulletin No. 197, July 2018c
American College of Obstetricians and Gynecologists: Moderate caffeine consumption during pregnancy. Committee Opinion No. 462, August 2010, Reaffirmed 2018d
American College of Obstetricians and Gynecologists: Prevention of infection after gynecologic procedures. Practice Bulletin No. 195, June 2018e
American College of Obstetricians and Gynecologists: Tubal ectopic pregnancy. Practice Bulletin No. 193, March 2018f
American College of Obstetricians and Gynecologists: Ultrasound in pregnancy. Practice Bulletin No. 175, December 2016, Reaffirmed 2018g
American College of Obstetricians and Gynecologists: Abortion training and education. Committee Opinion No. 612, November 2014, Reaffirmed 2019a
American College of Obstetricians and Gynecologists: Increasing access to abortion. Committee Opinion No. 613, November 2014, Reaffirmed 2019b
American College of Obstetricians and Gynecologists, American Society of Anesthesiologists: Nonobstetric surgery during pregnancy. Committee Opinion No. 775, April 2019c
American College of Radiology: ACR Manual on Contrast Media, Version 10.3, Reston, American College of Radiology, 2018
American Society for Reproductive Medicine: Definitions of infertility and recurrent pregnancy loss. Fertil Steril 99(1):63, 2013
American Society for Reproductive Medicine: Evaluation and treatment of recurrent pregnancy loss: a committee opinion. Fertil Steril 98 (5):1103, 2012
American Society for Reproductive Medicine: Removal of myomas in asymptomatic patients to improve fertility and/or reduce miscarriage rate: a guideline. Fertil Steril 108(3):416, 2017
American Society for Reproductive Medicine: Subclinical hypothyroidism in the infertile female population: a guideline. Fertil Steril 104(3):545, 2015
Amrane S, McConnell R: Endocrine causes of recurrent pregnancy loss. Semin Perinatol 43(2):80, 2019
Andersen AM, Andersen PK, Olsen J, et al: Moderate alcohol intake during pregnancy and risk of fetal death. Int J Epidemiol 41(2):405, 2012
Andersen SL, Olsen J, Wu CS, et al: Spontaneous abortion, stillbirth and hyperthyroidism: a Danish population-based study. Eur Thyroid J 3(3):164, 2014
Arredondo F, Noble LS: Endocrinology of recurrent pregnancy loss. Semin Reprod Med 1:33, 2006
Atrash HK, Strauss LT, Kendrick JS, et al: The relation between induced abortion and ectopic pregnancy. Obstet Gynecol 89(4):512, 1997
Avalos LA, Roberts SC, Kaskutas LA, et al: Volume and type of alcohol during early pregnancy and the risk of miscarriage. Subst Use Misuse 49:1437, 2014
Balsells M, García-Patterson A, Corcoy R: Systematic review and meta-analysis on the association of prepregnancy underweight and miscarriage. Eur J Obstet Gynecol Reprod Biol 207:73, 2016
Barber JC, Cockwell AE, Grant E: Is karyotyping couples experiencing recurrent miscarriage worth the cost? BJOG 117:885, 2010

Barlow S, Sullivan FM: Reproductive Hazards of Industrial Chemicals: an Evaluation of Animal and Human Data. New York, Academic Press, 1982

Barnhart K, Mennuti MT, Benjamin I, et al: Prompt diagnosis of ectopic pregnancy in an emergency department setting. Obstet Gynecol 84(6):1010, 1994

Barnhart K, van Mello NM, Bourne T, et al: Pregnancy of unknown location: a consensus statement of nomenclature, definitions, and outcome. Fertil Steril 95(3):857, 2011

Barnhart KT, Sammel MD, Appleby D, et al: Does a prediction model for pregnancy of unknown location developed in the UK validate on a US population? Hum Reprod 25(10):2434, 2010

Baud D, Goy G, Jaton K, et al: Role of *Chlamydia trachomatis* in miscarriage. Emerg Infect Dis 17(9):1630, 2011

Bednarek PH, Creinin MD, Reeves MF, et al: Immediate versus delayed IUD insertion after uterine aspiration. N Engl J Med 364(21):2208, 2011

Belloc S, Cohen-Bacrie P, Benkhalifa M, et al: Effect of maternal and paternal age on pregnancy and miscarriage rates after intrauterine insemination. Reprod Biomed Online 17(3):392, 2008

Bellver J, Ayllón Y, Ferrando M, et al: Female obesity impairs in vitro fertilization outcome without affecting embryo quality. Fertil Steril 93(2):447, 2010a

Bellver J, Meseguer M, Muriel L, et al: Y chromosome microdeletions, sperm DNA fragmentation and sperm oxidative stress as causes of recurrent spontaneous abortion of unknown etiology. Hum Reprod 25(7):1713, 2010b

Bhattacharya S, Townend J, Bhattacharya S: Recurrent miscarriage: are three miscarriages one too many? Analysis of a Scottish population-based database of 151,021 pregnancies. Eur J Obstet Gynecol Reprod Biol 150:24, 2010

Bick RL, Baker WF Jr: Hereditary and acquired thrombophilia in pregnancy. In Bick RL (ed): Hematological Complications in Obstetrics, Pregnancy, and Gynecology. Cambridge, Cambridge University Press, 2006, p 122

Biggs MA, Upadhyay UD, McCulloch CE, et al: Women's mental health and well-being 5 years after receiving or being denied an abortion: a prospective, longitudinal cohort Study. JAMA Psychiatry 74(2): 169, 2017

Boots CE, Bernardi LA, Stephenson MD: Frequency of euploid miscarriage is increased in obese women with recurrent early pregnancy loss. Fertil Steril 102(2):455, 2014

Borgatta L, Burnhill MS, Tyson J, et al: Early medical abortion with methotrexate and misoprostol. Obstet Gynecol 97:11, 2001

Branch DW, Gibson M, Silver RM: Recurrent miscarriage. N Engl J Med 363: 18, 2010

Brent RL: Saving lives and changing family histories: appropriate counseling of pregnant women and men and women of reproductive age, concerning the risk of diagnostic radiation exposures during and before pregnancy. Am J Obstet Gynecol 200(1):4, 2009

Brezina PR, Kutteh WH: Classic and cutting-edge strategies for the management of early pregnancy loss. Obstet Gynecol Clin North Am 41(1):1, 2014

Brigham SA, Conlon C, Farquharson RG: A longitudinal study of pregnancy outcome following idiopathic recurrent miscarriage. Hum Reprod 14(11):2868, 1999

Brown ZA, Selke S, Zeh J, et al: The acquisition of herpes simplex virus during pregnancy. N Engl J Med 337:509, 1997

Bryant AG, Grimes DA, Garrett JM, et al: Second-trimester abortion for fetal anomalies or fetal death: labor induction compared with dilation and evacuation. Obstet Gynecol 117(4):788, 2011

Casey BM, Dashe JS, Wells CE, et al: Subclinical hypothyroidism and pregnancy outcomes. Obstet Gynecol 105(2):239, 2005

Castañeda R, Lechuga D, Ramos RI, et al: Endemic goiter in pregnant women: utility of the simplified classification of thyroid size by palpation and urinary iodine as screening tests. BJOG 109:1366, 2002

Centers for Disease Control and Prevention: *Clostridium sordellii* toxic shock syndrome after medical abortion with mifepristone and intravaginal misoprostol—United States and Canada, 2001–2005. MMWR 54(29):724, 2005

Chen L, Hu R: Thyroid autoimmunity and miscarriage: a meta-analysis. Clin Endocrinol 74(4):513, 2011

Clark CA, Spitzer KA, Crowther MA, et al: Incidence of postpartum thrombosis and preterm delivery in women with antiphospholipid antibodies and recurrent pregnancy loss. J Rheumatol 34(5):992, 2007a

Clark EA, Silver RM, Branch DW: Do antiphospholipid antibodies cause preeclampsia and HELLP syndrome? Curr Rheumatol Rep 9:219, 2007b

Clark K, Ji H, Feltovich H et al: Mifepristone-induced cervical ripening: structural, biomechanical, and molecular events. Am J Obstet Gynecol 194:1391, 2006

Cleland K, Creinin M, Nucatola D, et al: Significant adverse events and outcomes after medical abortion. Obstet Gynecol 121(1):166, 2013

Clifford K, Rai R, Watson H, et al: Does suppressing luteinizing hormone secretion reduce the miscarriage rate? Results of a randomized controlled trial. BMJ 312:1508, 1996

Clowse ME, Jamison M, Myers E, et al: A national study of the complications of lupus in pregnancy. Am J Obstet Gynecol 199:127.e1, 2008

Cocksedge KA, Saravelos SH, Metwally M, et al: How common is polycystic ovary syndrome in recurrent miscarriage? Reprod Biomed Online 19(4):572, 2009

Condous G, Okaro E, Khalid A, Bourne T: Do we need to follow up complete miscarriages with serum human chorionic gonadotrophin levels? BJOG 112:827, 2005

Condous G, Van Calster B, Kirk E, et al: Clinical information does not improve the performance of mathematical models in predicting the outcome of pregnancies of unknown location. Fertil Steril 88(3):572, 2007

Connolly A, Ryan DH, Stuebe AM, et al: Reevaluation of discriminatory and threshold levels for serum β-hCG in early pregnancy. Obstet Gynecol 121(1):65, 2013

Coyaji K, Krishna U, Ambardekar S, et al: Are two doses of misoprostol after mifepristone for early abortion better than one? BJOG 114(3):271, 2007

Craig TB, Ke RW, Kutteh WH: Increase prevalence of insulin resistance in women with a history of recurrent pregnancy loss. Fertil Steril 78:487, 2002

Creinin MD, Huang X, Westhoff C, et al: Factors related to successful misoprostol treatment for early pregnancy failure. Obstet Gynecol 107:901, 2006

Creinin MD, Pymar HC, Schwartz JL: Mifepristone 100 mg in abortion regimens. Obstet Gynecol 98:434, 2001

Creinin MD, Schreiber CA, Bednarek P, et al: Mifepristone and misoprostol administered simultaneously versus 24 hours apart for abortion: a randomized controlled trial. Obstet Gynecol 109(4):885, 2007

Daif JL, Levie M, Chudnoff S, et al: Group A *Streptococcus* causing necrotizing fasciitis and toxic shock syndrome after medical termination of pregnancy. Obstet Gynecol 113(2 Pt 2):504, 2009

Danco Laboratories: Ordering mifeprex. 2019. Available at: https://www.earlyoptionpill.com/for-health-professionals/ordering-mifeprex/. Accessed June 5, 2019

Danco Laboratories: Patient agreement form. 2016. Available at: https://www.earlyoptionpill.com/wp-content/uploads/2016/03/Patient-Agreement-Form-March2016-1.pdf. Accessed June 4, 2019

Dao B, Blum J, Thieba B, et al: Is misoprostol a safe, effective and acceptable alternative to manual vacuum aspiration for postabortion care? Results from a randomized trial in Burkina Faso, West Africa. BJOG 114(11):1368, 2007

Dashe JS, Cunningham FG: Genetics. In Cunningham FG, Leveno KJ, Bloom SL, et al (eds): Williams Obstetrics, 25th ed. New York, McGraw-Hill, 2018, p 262

De Vivo A, Mancuso A, Giacobbe A, et al: Thyroid function in women found to have early pregnancy loss. Thyroid 20(6):633, 2010

Devaseelan P, Fogarty PP, Regan L: Human chorionic gonadotropin for threatened abortion. Cochrane Database Syst Rev 5:DC007422, 2010

Devi Wold AS, Pham N, Arici A: Anatomic factors in recurrent pregnancy loss. Semin Reprod Med 1:25, 2006

Di Simone N, Meroni PL, D'Asta M, et al: Pathogenic role of anti-beta2-glycoprotein I antibodies on human placenta: functional effects related to implantation and roles of heparin. Hum Reprod Update 13(2):189, 2007

Donahue JG, Kieke BA, King JP, et al: Association of spontaneous abortion with receipt of inactivated influenza vaccine containing H1N1pdm09 in 2010–11 and 2011–12. Vaccine 35(40):5314, 2017

Doubilet PM, Benson CB, Bourne T, et al: Diagnostic criteria for nonviable pregnancy early in the first trimester. N Engl J Med 369(15):1443, 2014

Drake P, Driscoll AK, Mathews TJ: Cigarette smoking during pregnancy: United States, 2016. NCHS Data Brief 305:1, 2018

Dranitsaris G, Johnston M, Poirier S, et al: Are health care providers who work with cancer drugs at an increased risk for toxic events? A systematic review and meta-analysis of the literature. J Oncol Pharm Pract 2:69, 2005

Du Y, Chen L, Lin J, et al: Chromosomal karyotype in chorionic villi of recurrent spontaneous abortion patients. Biosci Trends 12(1):32, 2018

Dukhovny S, Zutshi P, Abbott JF: Recurrent second trimester pregnancy loss: evaluation and management. Curr Opin Endocrinol Diabetes Obes 16:451, 2009

Dunford A, Fyfe R: Combination therapy with mifepristone and misoprostol for the management of first trimester miscarriage: Improved success. Aust N Z Obstet Gynaecol 58(4):438, 2018

Eiben B, Bartels I, Bahr-Prosch S, et al: Cytogenetic analysis of 750 spontaneous abortions with the direct-preparation method of chorionic villi and its implications for studying genetic causes of pregnancy wastage. Am J Hum Genet 47:656, 1990

Empson M, Lassere M, Craig J, et al: Prevention of recurrent miscarriage for women with antiphospholipid antibody or lupus anticoagulant. Cochrane Database Syst Rev 2:CD002859, 2012

Erkan D, Kozora E, Lockshin MD: Cognitive dysfunction and white matter abnormalities in antiphospholipid syndrome. Pathophysiology 18(1):93, 2011

European Society of Human Reproduction and Embryology: ESHRE information for couples with recurrent pregnancy loss. 2017. Available at: https://www.eshre.eu/Guidelines-and-Legal/Guidelines/Recurrent-pregnancy-loss.aspx Accessed July 3, 2019

Fekih M, Fathallah K, Ben Regaya L, et al: Sublingual misoprostol for first trimester termination of pregnancy. Int J Gynaecol Obstet 109(1):67, 2010

Feldman DM, Timms D, Borgida AF: Toxoplasmosis, parvovirus, and cytomegalovirus in pregnancy. Clin Lab Med 30(3):709, 2010

Feodor Nilsson S, Andersen PK, Strandberg-Larsen K, et al: Risk factors for miscarriage from a prevention perspective: a nationwide follow-up study. BJOG 121(11):1375, 2014

Fischer J, Colls P, Esudero T, et al: Preimplantation genetic diagnosis (PGD) improves pregnancy outcome for translocation carriers with a history of recurrent losses. Fertil Steril 94(1):283, 2010

Fischer M, Bhatnagar J, Guarner J, et al: Fatal toxic shock syndrome associated with *Clostridium sordellii* after medical abortion. N Engl J Med 353:2352, 2005

Floyd RL, Decoufle P, Hungerford DW: Alcohol use prior to pregnancy recognition. Am J Prev Med 17:101, 1999

Food and Drug Administration: Labeling for mifepristone (Mifeprex). 2016. Available at: https://www.accessdata.fda.gov/drugsatfda_docs/label/2016/020687s020lbl.pdf. Accessed June 3, 2019

Fox MC, Krajewski CM: Cervical preparation for second-trimester surgical abortion prior to 20 weeks' gestation: SFP Guideline #2013-4. Contraception 89(2):75, 2014

Franssen MTM, Korevaar JC, van der Veen F, et al: Reproductive outcome after chromosome analysis in couples with two or more miscarriages: case-control study. BMJ 332:750, 2006

Freedman L, Landy U, Steinauer J: Obstetrician-gynecologist experiences with abortion training: physician insights from a qualitative study. Contraception 81(6):525, 2010

Fritz MA, Speroff L, (eds): Recurrent early pregnancy loss. In Clinical Gynecologic Endocrinology and Infertility, 8th ed. Philadelphia, Lippincott Williams & Wilkins, 2011, p 1220

Gao J, Liu C, Yao F, et al: Array-based comparative genomic hybridization is more informative than conventional karyotyping and fluorescence in situ hybridization in the analysis of first-trimester spontaneous abortion. Mol Cytogenet 5(1):33, 2012

Gaskins AJ, Toth TL, Chavarro JE: Prepregnancy nutrition and early pregnancy outcomes. Curr Nutr Rep 4(3):265, 2015

Glueck CJ, Want P, Goldenberg N, et al: Pregnancy outcomes among women with polycystic ovary syndrome treated with metformin. Hum Reprod 17:2858, 2002

Goldberg AB, Dean G, Kang MS, et al: Manual versus electric vacuum aspiration for early first-trimester abortion: a controlled study of complication rates. Obstet Gynecol 103:101, 2004

Goldberg AB, Fortin JA, Drey EA, et al: Cervical preparation before dilation and evacuation using adjunctive misoprostol or mifepristone compared with overnight osmotic dilators alone: a randomized controlled trial. Obstet Gynecol 126(3):599, 2015

Goldenberg M, Sivan E, Sharabi Z, et al: Reproductive outcome following hysteroscopic management of intrauterine septum and adhesions. Hum Reprod 10:2663, 1995

Gonzalez CH, Marques-Dias MJ, Kim CA, et al: Congenital abnormalities in Brazilian children associated with misoprostol misuse in first trimester of pregnancy. Lancet 351(9116):1624, 1998

Gracia CR, Sammel MD, Chittams J, et al: Risk factors for spontaneous abortion in early symptomatic first-trimester pregnancies. Obstet Gynecol 106:993, 2005

Greene MF: Spontaneous abortions and major malformations in women with diabetes mellitus. Semin Reprod Endocrinol 17:127, 1999

Grimes DA: Estimation of pregnancy-related mortality risk by pregnancy outcome, United States, 1991 to 1999. Am J Obstet Gynecol 194:92, 2006

Grossman D, Grindlay K, Altshuler AL, et al: Induced abortion provision among a national sample of obstetrician-gynecologists. Obstet Gynecol 133:477, 2019

Grossman D, White K, Hopkins K, et al: The public health threat of anti-abortion legislation. Contraception 89:73, 2014

Guelinckx I, Devlieger R, Vansant G: Reproductive outcome after bariatric surgery: a critical review. Hum Reprod Update 15(2):189, 2009

Guest J, Chien PF, Thomson MA, et al: Randomised controlled trial comparing the efficacy of same-day administration of mifepristone and misoprostol for termination of pregnancy with the standard 36 to 48 hour protocol. BJOG 114(2):207, 2007

Guttmacher Institute: An overview of abortion laws. 2019. Available at: https://www.guttmacher.org/state-policy/explore/overview-abortion-laws. Accessed June 2, 2019

Haahr T, Zacho J, Bräuner M, et al: Reproductive outcome of patients undergoing in vitro fertilisation treatment and diagnosed with bacterial vaginosis or abnormal vaginal microbiota: a systematic PRISMA review and meta-analysis. BJOG 126(2):200, 2019

Haas DM, Hathaway TJ, Ramsey PS: Progestogen for preventing miscarriage in women with recurrent miscarriage of unclear etiology. Cochrane Database Syst Rev 10:CD003511, 2018

Haddad LB, Wall KM, Mehta CC, et al: Trends of and factors associated with live-birth and abortion rates among HIV-negative women. Am J Obstet Gynecol 216(1):71, 2017

Haddow JE, McClain MR, Palomaki GE, et al: Thyroperoxidase and thyroglobulin antibodies in early pregnancy and placental abruption. Obstet Gynecol 117:287, 2011

Hamoda H, Ashok PW, Flett GM, et al: A randomised controlled trial of mifepristone in combination with misoprostol administered sublingually or vaginally for medical abortion up to 13 weeks of gestation. BJOG 112:1102, 2005

Hannafin B, Lovecchio F, Blackburn P: Do Rh-negative women with first trimester spontaneous abortions need Rh immune globulin? Am J Obstet Gynecol 24:487, 2006

Harris LH, Cooper A, Rasinski KA, et al: Obstetrician-gynecologists' objections and willingness to help patients obtain an abortion. Obstet Gynecol 118(4):905, 2011

Herrera C, Meehan R, Podduturi V, et al: Maternal death due to *Clostridium novyi* in an injection drug user. Obstet Gynecol 128(4):876, 2016

Heuser C, Dalton J, Macpherson C, et al: Idiopathic recurrent pregnancy loss recurs at similar gestational ages. Am J Obstet Gynecol 203(4):343.e1, 2010

Hide G, Morley EK, Hughes JM, et al: Evidence for high levels of vertical transmission in Toxoplasma gondii. Parasitology 136(14):1877, 2009

Hirahara F, Andoh N, Sawai K, et al: Hyperprolactinemic recurrent miscarriage and results of randomized bromocriptine treatment trials. Fertil Steril 70(2):246, 1998

Ho CS, Bhatnagar J, Cohen AL, et al: Undiagnosed cases of fatal Clostridium-associated toxic shock in Californian women of childbearing age. Am J Obstet Gynecol 201:459.e1, 2009

Hoffman BL, Cunningham FG: First-trimester loss. In Cunningham FG, Leveno KL, Bloom SL, et al (eds): Williams Obstetrics, 25th ed. New York, McGraw-Hill, 2018, p 354

Homer H, Saridogan E: Uterine artery embolization for fibroids is associated with an increased risk of miscarriage. Fertil Steril 94(1):324, 2010

Honkanen H, Piaggio G, Hertzen H, et al: WHO multinational study of three misoprostol regimens after mifepristone for early medical abortion. BJOG 111(7):715, 2004

Hudson MM: Reproductive outcomes for survivors of childhood cancer. Obstet Gynecol 116:1171, 2010

Hyoun SC, Običan SG, Scialli AR: Teratogen update: methotrexate. Birth Defects Res A Clin Mol Teratol 94(4):187, 2012

Ibrahim Y, Johnstone E: The male contribution to recurrent pregnancy loss. Transl Androl Urol 7(3 suppl):S317, 2018

Inman S: More than 400 abortion restrictions passed since 2011—states working overtime to cut access. 2018. Available at: https://thehill.com/opinion/healthcare/386976-more-than-400-abortion-restrictions-passed-since-2011-states-working. Accessed June 2, 2019

Jacobs PA, Hassold TJ: The origin of chromosomal abnormalities in spontaneous abortion. In Porter IH, Hook EB (eds): Human Embryonic and Fetal Death. New York, Academic Press, 1980, p 289

Jain JK, Harwood B, Meckstroth KR, et al: A prospective randomized, double-blinded, placebo-controlled trial comparing mifepristone and vaginal misoprostol to vaginal misoprostol alone for elective termination of early pregnancy. Hum Reprod 17:1477, 2002

Jaslow CR, Carney JL, Kutteh WH: Diagnostic factors identified in 1020 women with two versus three or more recurrent pregnancy losses. Fertil Steril 93(4):1234, 2010

Jatlaoui TC, Mandel MG, et al: Abortion Surveillance—United States, 2018. MMWR 67(13):1, 2018

Johns J, Jauniaux E: Threatened miscarriage as a predictor of obstetric outcome. Obstet Gynecol 107:845, 2006

Jun SH, Ginsburg ES, Racowsky C, et al: Uterine leiomyomas and their effect on in vitro fertilization outcome: a retrospective study. J Assist Reprod Genet 18:139, 2001

Kajii T, Ferrier A, Niikawa N, et al: Anatomic and chromosomal anomalies in 639 spontaneous abortions. Hum Genet 55:87, 1980

Kapp N, Lohr PA, Ngo TD, et al: Cervical preparation for first trimester surgical abortion. Cochrane Database Syst Rev 2:CD007207, 2010

Katz A, Ben-Arie A, Lurie S, et al: Reproductive outcome following hysteroscopic adhesiolysis in Asherman's syndrome. Int J Fertil Menopausal Stud 41:462, 1996

Kc S, Hemminki E, Gissler M, et al: Perinatal outcomes after induced termination of pregnancy by methods: a nationwide register-based study of first births in Finland 1996–2013. PLoS One 12(9):e0184078, 2017

Khalife D, Ghazeeri G, Kutteh W: Review of current guidelines for recurrent pregnancy loss: new strategies for optimal evaluation of women who may be superfertile. Semin Perinatol 43(2):105, 2019

Khashan AS, Quigley EM, McNamee R, et al: Increased risk of miscarriage and ectopic pregnancy among women with irritable bowel syndrome. Clin Gastroenterol Hepatol 10(8):902, 2012

Khooshideh M, Yarmohammadi N, Shahriari A, et al: Sublingual misoprostol plus laminaria for cervical preparation before surgical management of late first trimester missed abortions, a randomized controlled trial. J Matern Fetal Neonatal Med 30(3):317, 2017

Kim C, Barnard S, Neilson JP, et al: Medical treatments for incomplete miscarriage. Cochrane Database Syst Rev 1:CD007223, 2017

Kleinhaus K, Perrin M, Friedlander Y, et al: Paternal age and spontaneous abortion. Obstet Gynecol 108:369, 2006

Koert E, Malling GM, Sylvest R, et al: Recurrent pregnancy loss: couples' perspectives on their need for treatment, support and follow up. Hum Reprod 34(2):291, 2019

Krassas GE, Poppe K, Glinoer D: Thyroid function and human reproductive health. Endo Rev 31:702, 2010

Krieg SA, Shahine LK, Lathi RB: Environmental exposure to endocrine-disrupting chemicals and miscarriage. Fertil Steril 106(4):941, 2016

Kulier R, Kapp N, Gülmezoglu AM, et al: Medical methods for first trimester abortion. Cochrane Database Syst Rev 11:CD002855, 2011

Kuon RJ, Togawa R, Vomstein K, et al: Higher prevalence of colonization with *Gardnerella vaginalis* and gram-negative anaerobes in patients with recurrent miscarriage and elevated peripheral natural killer cells. J Reprod Immunol 120:15, 2017

Kutteh WH, Hinote CD: Antiphospholipid antibody syndrome. Obstet Gynecol Clin North Am 41(1):113, 2014

Levy BS, Ness DL, Weinberger SE: Consensus guidelines for facilities performing outpatient procedures: evidence over ideology. Obstet Gynecol 133(2):255, 2019

Liauw J, Dineley B, Gerster K, et al: Abortion training in Canadian obstetrics and gynecology residency programs. Contraception 94:478, 2016

Ling N, Lawson E, von Scheven E: Adverse pregnancy outcomes in adolescents and young women with systemic lupus erythematosus: a national estimate. Pediatr Rheumatol Online J 16(1):26, 2018

Lis R, Rowhani-Rahbar A, Manhart LE: *Mycoplasma genitalium* infection and female reproductive tract disease: a meta-analysis. Clin Infect Dis 61(3):418, 2015

Lui S, Song L, Cram DS, et al: Traditional karyotyping versus copy number variation sequencing for detection of chromosomal abnormalities associated with spontaneous miscarriage. Ultrasound Obstet Gynecol 46:472, 2015

Luise C, Jermy K, May C, et al: Outcome of expectant management of spontaneous first trimester miscarriage: observational study. BMJ 324:873, 2002

Lupo PJ, Symanski E, Waller DK, et al: Maternal exposure to ambient levels of benzene and neural tube defects among offspring, Texas, 1999–2004. Environ Health Perspect 119:397, 2011

Lykke JA, Dideriksen KL, Lidegaard Ø, et al: First-trimester vaginal bleeding and complications later in pregnancy. Obstet Gynecol 115:935, 2010

Lyman M, Mpofu JJ, Soud F: Maternal and perinatal outcomes in pregnant women with suspected Ebola virus disease in Sierra Leone, 2014. Int J Gynaecol Obstet 142(1):71, 2018

Maconochie N, Doyle P, Prior S, et al: Risk factors for first trimester miscarriage—results from a UK-population-based case-control study. BJOG 114:170, 2007

Madden T, Westhoff C: Rates of follow-up and repeat pregnancy in the 12 months after first-trimester induced abortion. Obstet Gynecol 113:663, 2009

Mazze RI, Källén B: Reproductive outcome after anesthesia and operation during pregnancy: a registry study of 5405 cases. Am J Obstet Gynecol 161:1178, 1989

McMillan M, Porritt K, Kralik D, et al: Influenza vaccination during pregnancy: a systematic review of fetal death, spontaneous abortion, and congenital malformation safety outcomes. Vaccine 33(18):2108, 2015

Meites E, Zane S, Gould C: Fatal *Clostridium sordellii* infections after medical abortions. N Engl J Med 363(14):1382, 2010

Meroni PL, Tedesco F, Locati M, et al: Anti-phospholipid antibody mediated fetal loss: still an open question from a pathogenic point of view. Lupus 19:453, 2010

Metwally M, Saravelos SH, Ledger WL, et al: Body mass index and risk of miscarriage in women with recurrent miscarriage. Fertil Steril 94(1):290, 2010

Mills JL: Cocaine, smoking, and spontaneous abortion. N Engl J Med 340(5):380, 1999

Mills JL, Simpson JL, Driscoll SG, et al: Incidence of spontaneous abortion among normal women and insulin-dependent diabetic women whose pregnancies were identified within 21 days of conception. N Engl J Med 319:1618, 1988

Miyakis S, Lockshin MD, Atsumi T, et al: International consensus statement on an update of the classification criteria for definite antiphospholipid syndrome (APS). J Thromb Haemost 4:295, 2006

Morales-Suárez-Varela M, Nohr EA, Olsen J, et al: Potential combined effects of maternal smoking and coffee intake on foetal death within the Danish National Cohort. Eur J Public Health 28(2):315, 2018

Moreau C, Kaminski M, Ancel PY, et al: Previous induced abortions and the risk of very preterm delivery: results of the EPIPAGE study. BJOG 112:430, 2005

Nahum GG: Uterine anomalies. How common are they, and what is their distribution among subtypes? J Reprod Med 43(10):877, 1998

National Academies of Science Engineering and Medicine: The safety and quality of abortion care in the United States. 2018. Available at: http://www.nationalacademies.org/hmd/Reports/2018/the-safety-and-quality-of-abortion-care-in-the-united-states.aspx. Accessed on June 2, 2019

Nawaz FH, Rizvi J: Continuation of metformin reduces early pregnancy loss in obese Pakistani women with polycystic ovarian syndrome. Gynecol Obstet Invest 69(3):184, 2010

Neilson JP, Gyte GM, Hickey M, et al: Medical treatments for incomplete miscarriage (less than 24 weeks). Cochrane Database Syst Rev 3:CD007223, 2013

Ness RB, Grisso JA, Hirschinger N, et al: Cocaine and tobacco use and the risk of spontaneous abortion. N Engl J Med 340(5):333, 1999

Newmann S, Dalve-Endres A, Drey EA: Society of Family Planning clinical guidelines. Cervical preparation for surgical abortion from 20 to 24 weeks' gestation. Contraception 77(4):308, 2008

Nguyen NT, Blum J, Durocher J, et al: A randomized controlled study comparing 600 versus 1200 μg oral misoprostol for medical management of incomplete abortion. Contraception 72:438, 2005

Nielsen A, Hannibal CG, Lindekilde BE, et al: Maternal smoking predicts the risk of spontaneous abortion. Acta Obstet Gynecol Scand 85(9):1057, 2006

Niinimäki M, Pouta A, Bloigu A, et al: Immediate complications after medical compared with surgical termination of pregnancy. Obstet Gynecol 114:795, 2009

Nurmohamed L, Moretti ME, Schechter T, et al: Outcome following high-dose methotrexate in pregnancies misdiagnosed as ectopic. Am J Obstet Gynecol 205:533.e1, 2011

Oakeshott P, Hay P, Hay S, et al: Association between bacterial vaginosis or chlamydial infection and miscarriage before 16 weeks' gestation: prospective, community based cohort study. BMJ 325:1334, 2002

Palomba S, Falbo A, Orio F Jr, et al: Effect of preconceptional metformin on abortion risk in polycystic ovary syndrome: a systematic review and meta-analysis of randomized controlled trials. Fertil Steril 92(5):1646, 2009

Pearl JP, Price RR, Tonkin AE, et al: SAGES guidelines for the use of laparoscopy during pregnancy. Surg Endosc 31(10):3767, 2017

Pineles BL, Park E, Samet JM: Systematic review and meta-analysis of miscarriage and maternal exposure to tobacco smoke during pregnancy. Am J Epidemiol 179(7):807, 2014

Platteau P, Staessen C, Michiels A, et al: Preimplantation genetic diagnosis for aneuploidy screening in patients with unexplained recurrent miscarriages. Fertil Steril 83(2):393, 2005

Pocius KD, Bartz D, Maurer R, et al: Serum human chorionic gonadotropin (hCG) trend within the first few days after medical abortion: a prospective study. Contraception 95(3):263, 2017

Popescu F, Jaslow CR, Kutteh WH: Recurrent pregnancy loss evaluation combined with 24-chromosome microarray of miscarriage tissue provides a probable or definite cause of pregnancy loss in over 90% of patients. Hum Reprod 33(4):579, 2018

Prasad P, Singh N, Das B, et al: Differential expression of circulating Th1/Th2/Th17 cytokines in serum of *Chlamydia trachomatis*-infected women undergoing incomplete spontaneous abortion. Microb Pathog 110:152, 2017

Pymar HC, Creinin MD, Schwartz JL: Mifepristone followed on the same day by vaginal misoprostol for early abortion. Contraception 64:87, 2001

Quinn PA, Shewchuck AB, Shuber J, et al: Efficacy of antibiotic therapy in preventing spontaneous pregnancy loss among couples colonized with genital mycoplasmas. Am J Obstet Gynecol 145:239, 1983a

Quinn PA, Shewchuck AB, Shuber J, et al: Serologic evidence of *Ureaplasma urealyticum* infection in women with spontaneous pregnancy loss. Am J Obstet Gynecol 145:245, 1983b

Raghavan S, Comendant R, Digol I, et al: Two-pill regimens of misoprostol after mifepristone medical abortion through 63 days' gestational age: a randomized controlled trial of sublingual and oral misoprostol. Contraception 79(2):84, 2009

Rajcan-Separovic E: Next generation sequencing in recurrent pregnancy loss-approaches and outcomes. Eur J Med Genet Apr 13, 2019 [Epub ahead of print]

Ramasamy R, Scovell JM, Kovac JR, et al: Fluorescence in situ hybridization detects increased sperm aneuploidy in men with recurrent pregnancy loss. Fertil Steril 103(4):906, 2015

Ramzy AM, Sattar M, Amin Y, et al: Uterine myomata and outcome of assisted reproduction. Hum Reprod 13:198, 1998

Rand JH, Wu XX, Quinn AS, et al: The annexin A5-mediated pathogenic mechanism in the antiphospholipid syndrome: role in pregnancy losses and thrombosis. Lupus 19(4):460, 2010

Raymond E, Grimes D: The comparative safety of legal induced abortion and childbirth in the United States. Obstet Gynecol 119(2, Part 1):215, 2012

Reddy UM: Recurrent pregnancy loss: nongenetic causes. Contemp OB/GYN 52:63, 2007

Reeves MF, Smith KJ, Creinin MD: Contraceptive effectiveness of immediate compared with delayed insertion of intrauterine devices after abortion. Obstet Gynecol 109:1286, 2007

Reichman DE, Laufer MR: Congenital uterine anomalies affecting reproduction. Best Pract Res Clin Obstet Gynecol 24(2):193, 2010

Robertshaw I, Khoury J, Abdallah ME, et al: The effect of paternal age on outcome in assisted reproductive technology using the ovum donation model. Reprod Sci 21(5):590, 2014

Robinson L, Gallos ID, Conner SJ, et al: The effect of sperm DNA fragmentation on miscarriage rates: a systematic review and meta-analysis. Hum Reprod 27(10):2908, 2012

Rowland AS, Baird DD, Shore DL, et al: Nitrous oxide and spontaneous abortion in female dental assistants. Am J Epidemiol 141:531, 1995

Salim R, Regan L, Woelfer B, et al: A comparative study of the morphology of congenital uterine anomalies in women with and without a history of recurrent first trimester miscarriage. Hum Reprod 18:162, 2003

Saraswat L, Bhattacharya S, Maheshwari A, et al: Maternal and perinatal outcome in women with threatened miscarriage in the first trimester: a systematic review. BJOG 117:245, 2010

Saravelos SH, Cocksedge KA, Li TC: Prevalence and diagnosis of congenital uterine anomalies in women with reproductive failure: a critical appraisal. Hum Reprod Update 14(5):415, 2008

Saravelos SH, Yan J, Rehmani H, et al: The prevalence and impact of fibroids and their treatment on the outcome of pregnancy in women with recurrent miscarriage. Hum Reprod 26:3274, 2011

Savaris RF, Silva de Moraes G, Cristovam RA, et al: Are antibiotics necessary after 48 hours of improvement in infected/septic abortions? A randomized controlled trial followed by a cohort study. Am J Obstet Gynecol 204:301. e1, 2011

Savitz DA, Chan RL, Herring AH, et al: Caffeine and miscarriage risk. Epidemiology 19:55, 2008

Saygili-Yilmaz E, Yildiz S, Erman-Akar M, et al: Reproductive outcome of septate uterus after hysteroscopic metroplasty. Arch Gynecol Obstet 4:289, 2003

Schaff EA, Fielding SL, Westhoff C, et al: Vaginal misoprostol administered 1, 2, or 3 days after mifepristone for early medical abortion. A randomized trial. JAMA 284:1948, 2000

Scheller NM, Pasternak B, Mølgaard-Neilsen D, et al: Quadrivalent HPV vaccination and the risk of adverse pregnancy outcomes. N Engl J Med 376(13): 1223, 2017

Schneider D, Golan A, Langer R, et al: Outcome of continued pregnancies after first and second trimester cervical dilatation by laminaria tents. Obstet Gynecol 78:1121, 1991

Schreiber CA, Creinin MD, Atrio J, el at: Mifepristone pretreatment for the medical management of early pregnancy loss. N Engl Med 378: 2161, 2018

Seckin B, Sarikaya E, Oruc AS, et al: Office hysteroscopic findings in patients with two, three, and four or more, consecutive miscarriages. Eur J Contracept Reprod Health Care 17(5):393, 2012

Shah PS, Zao J, Knowledge synthesis group of determinants of preterm/LBW births: induced termination of pregnancy and low birthweight and preterm birth: a systematic review and meta-analyses. BJOG 116(11):1425, 2009

Shannon C, Brothers LP, Philip NM, et al: Ectopic pregnancy and medical abortion. Obstet Gynecol 104(1):161, 2004

Shannon C, Wiebe E, Jacot F: Regimens of misoprostol with mifepristone for early medical abortion: a randomized trial. BJOG 113:621, 2006

Shimoni N, Davis A, Ramos M, et al: Timing of copper intrauterine device insertion after medical abortion. Obstet Gynecol 118(3):623, 2011

Silver RM, Branch DW, Goldenberg R, et al: Nomenclature for pregnancy outcomes. Obstet Gynecol 118(6):1402, 2011

Simpson JL: Causes of fetal wastage. Clin Obstet Gynecol 50(1):10, 2007

Simpson JL: Genes, chromosomes, and reproductive failure. Fertil Steril 33(2): 107, 1980

Smith LF, Ewings PD, Guinlan C: Incidence of pregnancy after expectant, medical, or surgical management of spontaneous first trimester miscarriage: long term follow-up of miscarriage treatment (MIST) randomized controlled trial. BMJ 339:b3827, 2009

Soler A, Morales C, Mademont-Soler I, et al: Overview of chromosome abnormalities in first trimester miscarriages: A series of 1,011 consecutive chorionic villi sample karyotypes. Cytogenet Genome Res 152(2):81, 2017

Steinauer J, Drey EA, Lewis R, et al: Obstetrics and gynecology resident satisfaction with an integrated, comprehensive abortion rotation. Obstet Gynecol 105:1335, 2005

Steinauer JE, Turk JK, Pomerantz T, et al: Abortion training in US obstetrics and gynecology residency programs. Am J Obstet Gynecol 219:86.e1, 2018

Stephenson MD: Management of recurrent early pregnancy loss. J Reprod Med 51:303, 2006

Stephenson MD, Kutteh WH, Purkiss S, et al: Intravenous immunoglobulin and idiopathic secondary recurrent miscarriage: a multicentered randomized placebo-controlled trial. Hum Reprod 25(9):2203, 2010

Streeter GL: Focal deficiencies in fetal tissues and their relation to intra-uterine amputation. Carnegie Institute of Washington 1930, Publication No. 414, p 5

Strzelczk JJ, Damilakis J, Marx MV, et al: Facts and controversies about radiation exposure, part 2: low-level exposures and cancer risk. J Am Coll Radiol 4(1):32, 2007

Stubblefield PG, Monson RR, Schoenbaum SC, et al: Fertility after induced abortion: a prospective follow-up study. Obstet Gynecol 63(2):186, 1984

Stulberg DB, Dude AM, Dahlguist I, et al: Abortion provision among practicing obstetrician-gynecologists. Obstet Gynecol 118(3):609, 2011

Sugiura-Ogasawara M, Ebara T, Yamada Y, et al: Adverse pregnancy and perinatal outcome in patients with recurrent pregnancy loss: Multiple imputation analyses with propensity score adjustment applied to a large-scale birth cohort of the Japan Environment and Children's Study. Am J Reprod Immunol 81(1):e13072, 2019

Sullivan AE, Silver RM, LaCoursiere DY, et al: Recurrent fetal aneuploidy and recurrent miscarriage. Obstet Gynecol 104:784, 2004

Sunkara SK, Khairy M, El-Toukhy T, et al: The effect of intramural fibroids without uterine cavity involvement on the outcome of IVF treatment: a systematic review and meta-analysis. Hum Reprod 25(2):418, 2010

Temmerman M, Lopita MI, Sanghvi HC, et al: The role of maternal syphilis, gonorrhoea and HIV-1 infections in spontaneous abortion. Int J STD AIDS 3:418, 1992

Templeton A, Grimes D: A request for abortion. N Engl J Med 365(23):2198, 2011

Thangaratinam S, Tan A, Knox E, et al: Association between thyroid autoantibodies and miscarriage and preterm birth: meta-analysis of evidence. BMJ 342:d2616, 2011

Tharapel AT, Tharapel SA, Bannerman RM: Recurrent pregnancy losses and parental chromosome abnormalities: a review. BJOG 92:899, 1985

Tongsong T, Srisomboon J, Wanapirak C, et al: Pregnancy outcome of threatened abortion with demonstrable fetal cardiac activity: a cohort study. J Obstet Gynaecol 21:331, 1995

Torre A, Huchon C, Bussieres L, et al: Immediate versus delayed medical treatment for first-trimester miscarriage: a randomized trial. Am J Obstet Gynecol 206:215.e1, 2012

Trinder J, Brocklehurst P, Porter R, et al: Management of miscarriage: expectant, medical, or surgical? Results of randomized controlled trial (miscarriage treatment (MIST) trial). BMJ 332(7552):1235, 2006

Tzeng CR, Hwang JL, Au HK, et al: Sonographic patterns of the endometrium in assessment of medical abortion outcomes. Contraception 88(1):153, 2013

Upadhyay UD, Desai S, Zlidar V, et al: Incidence of emergency department visits and complications after abortion. Obstet Gynecol 125(1):175, 2015

Valli E, Zupi E, Marconi D, et al: Hysteroscopic findings in 344 women with recurrent spontaneous abortion. J Am Assoc Gynecol Laparosc 8(3):398, 2001

van den Boogaard E, Kaandorp SP, Franssen MT, et al: Consecutive or nonconsecutive recurrent miscarriage: is there any difference in carrier status? Hum Reprod 25(6):1411, 2010

van den Bosch T, Daemen A, Van Schoubroeck D, et al: Occurrence and outcome of residual trophoblastic tissue: a prospective study. J Ultrasound Med 27(3):357, 2008

Vargas FR, Schuler-Faccini L, Brunoni D, et al: Prenatal exposure to misoprostol and vascular disruption defects: a case-control study. Am J Med Genet 95(4):302, 2000

Vartian CV, Septimus EJ: Tricuspid valve group B streptococcal endocarditis following elective abortion. Review Infect Dis 13:997, 1991

Venetis CA, Papadopoulos SP, Campo R, et al: Clinical implications of congenital uterine anomalies: a meta-analysis of comparative studies. Reprod Biomed Online 29(6):665, 2014

Vissenberg R, van den Boogaard E, van Wely M, et al: Treatment of thyroid disorders before conception and in early pregnancy: a systematic review. Hum Reprod Update 18(4):360, 2012

Vitez SF, Forman EJ, Williams Z: Preimplantation genetic diagnosis in early pregnancy loss. Semin Perinatol 43:116, 2019

von Hertzen H, Honkanen H, Piaggio G, et al: WHO multinational study of three misoprostol regimens after mifepristone for early medical abortion. I: Efficacy. BJOG 110:808, 2003

von Hertzen H, Huong NTM, Piaggio G, et al: Misoprostol dose and route after mifepristone for early medical abortion: a randomized controlled non-inferiority trial. BJOG 117(10):1186, 2010

von Hertzen H, Piaggio G, Huong NT, et al: Efficacy of two intervals and two routes of administration of misoprostol for termination of early pregnancy: a randomised controlled equivalence trial. Lancet 369(9577):1938, 2007

von Hertzen H, Piaggio G, Wojdyla D, et al: Two mifepristone doses and two intervals of misoprostol administration for termination of early pregnancy: a randomized factorial controlled equivalence trial. BJOG 116(3):381, 2009

Weiss J, Malone F, Vidaver J, et al: Threatened abortion: a risk factor for poor pregnancy outcome—a population based screening study (the FASTER Trial). Am J Obstet Gynecol 187:S70, 2002

Weng X, Odouki R, Li DK: Maternal caffeine consumption during pregnancy and the risk of miscarriage: a prospective cohort study. Am J Obstet Gynecol 198:279.e1, 2008

Westreich D, Cates J, Cohen M, et al: Smoking, HIV, and risk of pregnancy loss. AIDS 31(4):553, 2017

White KE, Carroll E, Grossman D: Complications from first-trimester aspiration abortion: a systematic review of the literature. Contraception 92(5):422, 2015

Wijesiriwardana A, Bhattacharya S, Shetty A, et al: Obstetric outcome in women with threatened miscarriage in the first trimester. Obstet Gynecol 107:557, 2006

Wilcox AF, Weinberg CR, O'Connor JF, et al: Incidence of early loss of pregnancy. N Engl J Med 319:189, 1988

Williams PM, Fletcher S. Health effects of prenatal radiation exposure. Am Fam Physician 82(5):488, 2010

Williams Z: Inducing tolerance to pregnancy. N Engl J Med 367(12):1159, 2012

Winikoff B, Dzuba IG, Creinin MD, et al: Two distinct oral routes of misoprostol in mifepristone medical abortion: a randomized controlled trial. Obstet Gynecol 112(6):1303, 2008

Wo JY, Viswanathan AN: Impact of radiotherapy on fertility, pregnancy, and neonatal outcomes in female cancer patients. Int J Radiat Oncol Biol Phys 73(5):1304, 2009

Wong LF, Porter TF, Scott JR: Immunotherapy for recurrent miscarriage. Cochrane Database Syst Rev 10:CD000112, 2014

World Health Organization: Preventing unsafe abortion. 2018. Available at: https://www.who.int/en/news-room/fact-sheets/detail/preventing-unsafe-abortion. Accessed June 4, 2019

World Health Organization: The use of DDT in malaria vector control: WHO position statement Geneva, World Health Organization, 2011

Wu HL, Marwah S, Wang P, et al: Misoprostol for medical treatment of missed abortion: a systematic review and network meta-analysis. Sci Rep 7(1):1664, 2017

Wu J, Ma J, Bao C: Pregnancy outcomes among Chinese women with and without systemic lupus erythematosus: a retrospective cohort study. BMJ Open 8(4):e020909, 2018

Yan XC, Wang JH, Wang B, et al: Study of human cytomegalovirus replication in body fluids, placental infection, and miscarriage during the first trimester of pregnancy. J Med Virol 87(6):1046, 2015

Yetman DL, Kutteh WH: Antiphospholipid antibody panels and recurrent pregnancy loss: prevalence of anticardiolipin antibodies compared with other antiphospholipid antibodies. Fertil Steril 66:540, 1996

Youssef A, Vermeulen N, Lashley EE, et al: Comparison and appraisal of (inter)national recurrent pregnancy loss guidelines. Reprod Biomed Online 39(3):497, 2019

Zhang J, Gilles JM, Barnhart K, et al: A comparison of medical management with misoprostol and surgical management for early pregnancy failure. N Engl J Med 353:761, 2005

Ziakas PD, Pavlou M, Voulgarelis M: Heparin treatment in antiphospholipid syndrome with recurrent pregnancy loss: a systematic review and meta-analysis. Obstet Gynecol 115(6):1256, 2010

CHAPTER 7

Ectopic Pregnancy

EPIDEMIOLOGY

An ectopic or extrauterine pregnancy is one in which the blastocyst implants anywhere other than the endometrial lining of the uterine cavity. Nearly 95 percent of ectopic pregnancies implant in the fallopian tube. Other sites are shown in Figure 7-1, which reflects data from 1800 surgically treated ectopic pregnancies (Bouyer, 2002). Rare, bilateral ectopic pregnancies have been described (al-Awwad, 1999).

The reported incidence of ectopic pregnancy is usually calculated as the number of treated cases divided by the total of all pregnancies. Nationally, the rates in 2013 from one large private insurance database and from Medicaid claims were 1.54 percent and 1.38 percent, respectively (Tao, 2017). Stulberg and coworkers (2014) reviewed Medicaid data from 2004 to 2008 from 14 states and found a similar national rate.

Although ectopic pregnancy accounts for a small proportion of all pregnancies, it disparately accounts for 3 percent of all pregnancy-related deaths (Creanga, 2017). Still, current diagnostic and treatment protocols have substantially lowered fatality rates. One analysis showed a 56-percent decline in the ectopic pregnancy mortality ratio between the 1980 to 1984 epoch and the 2003 to 2007 epoch (Creanga, 2011). From the same Medicaid database noted earlier, Stulberg and coworkers

(2016) noted that 53 percent of ectopic-related deaths occurred in black women. Inadequate access to gynecologic and prenatal care may partially explain this trend.

RISK FACTORS

Several risks have been linked with ectopic pregnancy. As shown in Table 7-1, abnormal fallopian tube anatomy that alters normal embryo transport underlies most cases. For example, prior tubal pregnancy raises risks. In one study of more than 1000 treated ectopic pregnancies, the recurrence rate was 10 percent (de Bennetot, 2012). Surgeries for fertility restoration, for ectopic pregnancy, or for sterilization also confer a higher risk.

Pelvic inflammatory disease (PID) originating from *Neisseria gonorrhoeae* or *Chlamydia trachomatis* is a potent risk factor for tubal injury and ectopic pregnancy. Recurrent chlamydial infection causes intraluminal inflammation, subsequent fibrin deposition, and tubal scarring (Hillis, 1997). Moreover, persistent chlamydial antigens can trigger a delayed hypersensitivity reaction with continued injury despite negative culture results (Toth, 2000). *N gonorrhoeae* induces a potent acute inflammatory neutrophil influx, which raises levels of destructive matrix metalloproteinases (Stevens, 2018). These lytic enzymes damage and scar fallopian tubal epithelium.

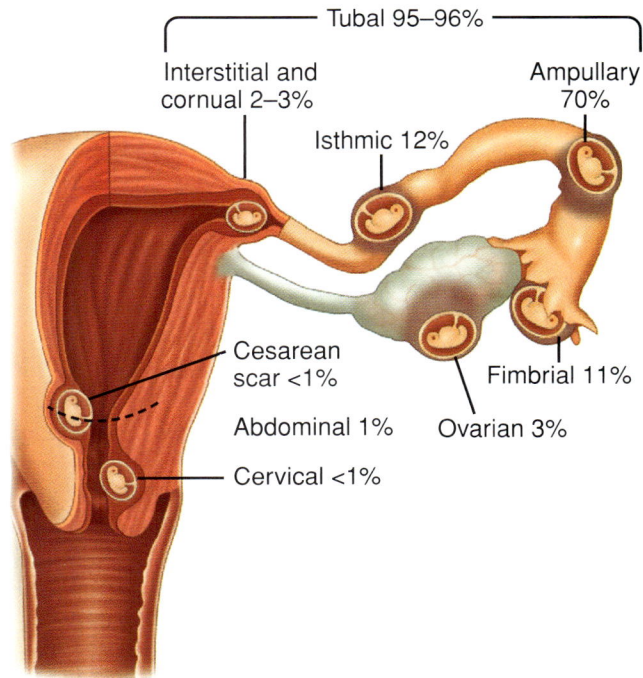

FIGURE 7-1 Various sites and frequency of ectopic pregnancies.

TABLE 7-1. Risk Factors for Ectopic Pregnancy

Factor	Odds Ratio (95% CI)
Prior ectopic pregnancy	12.5 (7.5, 20.9)
Prior tubal surgery	4.0 (2.6, 6.1)
Smoking >20 cigarettes per day	3.5 (1.4, 8.6)
PID confirmed by laparoscopy or positive test for *Chlamydia trachomatis*	3.4 (2.4, 5.0)
≥3 prior miscarriages	3.0 (1.3, 6.9)
Age ≥40 years	2.9 (1.4, 6.1)
Prior medical or surgical abortion	2.8 (1.1, 7.2)
Infertility >1 year	2.6 (1.6, 4.2)
Lifelong sexual partners >5	1.6 (1.2, 2.1)
Prior IUD use	1.3 (1.0, 1.8)

IUD = intrauterine device; PID = pelvic inflammatory disease; STD = sexually transmitted disease.
Data from Bouyer, 2003; Buster, 1999.

Smoking elevates the ectopic pregnancy risk more than threefold in women who smoke more than one pack of cigarettes daily (Saraiya, 1998). Among smokers undergoing assisted reproductive technology, the risk of ectopic pregnancy was 15 times higher in one metaanalysis (Waylen, 2009). The mechanism of this association is unclear, but smoking alters fallopian tube physiology and may affect embryo transport (Shaw, 2010).

Assisted reproductive technology (ART) confers an increased risk for ectopic pregnancy. In women undergoing in vitro fertilization (IVF), the main risk factor for ectopic pregnancy is tubal factor infertility (Li, 2015a). Perkins and associates (2015) reviewed nearly 600,000 pregnancies from 2001 to 2011 conceived by IVF and found a 1.7-percent rate of ectopic pregnancy. Some newer practices are associated with slightly fewer extrauterine implantations. For example, with fresh, nondonor transfers, the ectopic rate drops as the number of embryos transferred is reduced. Also, the transfer of day-5 or day-6 embryos compared with day-3 embryos lowers ectopic pregnancy risk (Du, 2017; Fang, 2015). Last, transfer of frozen-thawed embryos rather than fresh embryos leads to decreased rates (Londra, 2015). Importantly, "atypical" implantation—that is, interstitial, abdominal, cervical, ovarian, or heterotopic—is more common following ART procedures.

Increasing maternal age raises risks of ectopic pregnancy, and patients older than 40 carry the highest risk (Tao, 2017). This has been attributed to age-related hormonal changes that alter tubal function (Coste, 2000).

Contraception lowers overall pregnancy rates and thereby lowers the risk of ectopic pregnancy. However, if pregnancy does occur, some methods increase the relative incidence of ectopic pregnancy (Li, 2014a). Examples include the levonorgestrel-releasing intrauterine system (LNG-IUS) and copper intrauterine device (IUD). In one study of 61,448 IUD users, only 118 contraceptive failures were reported, but 21 of these (18 percent) were ectopic pregnancies (Heinemann, 2015).

Progestin-only contraceptive pills also pose a slightly greater risk because of their effects to diminish tubal motility.

If pregnancy occurs after tubal sterilization, the ectopic risk accrues as the time from primary surgery increases. This risk is also greater if electrosurgery methods were used (Malacova, 2014; Peterson, 1997). Although the Essure device for transcervical sterilization has been withdrawn from the U.S. market, many women still rely on this method. In one study, only nine of 722 contraceptive failures (1.25 percent) were ectopic pregnancies (Perkins, 2016).

Altered tubal anatomy can stem from peritubal adhesions subsequent to salpingitis, appendicitis, endometriosis, or other intraabdominal inflammatory processes. Anatomy is also altered with salpingitis isthmica nodosa. In this condition, epithelium-lined diverticula extend into a hypertrophied muscularis layer (Bolaji, 2015; Kutluay, 1994). Finally, congenital fallopian tube anomalies, especially those secondary to in utero diethylstilbestrol exposure, can predispose (Hoover, 2011).

PATHOPHYSIOLOGY

Once normal tubal transport has been disrupted, outcomes of ectopic pregnancy include *tubal rupture*, *tubal abortion*, or *pregnancy failure* with resolution. With tubal rupture, the invading trophoblast and associated hemorrhage tear rents in the fallopian tube. In this genesis, fallopian tube anatomy plays an important role. Specifically, the fallopian tube lacks a submucosal layer beneath its epithelium (Senterman, 1988). Therefore, a fertilized ovum can easily burrow through the epithelium and implant within the tube's muscularis layer (Fig. 7-2). As rapidly proliferating trophoblasts erode the muscularis layer, maternal blood pours into the spaces within the trophoblastic or the adjacent tissue. Rupture is usually spontaneous but can also follow trauma such as that associated with bimanual pelvic examination or coitus.

With tubal abortion, the pregnancy instead may pass out the distal fallopian tube. This outcome depends in part on the initial implantation site, and distal implantations are favored. Subsequently, hemorrhage may cease and symptoms eventually disappear. However, bleeding can persist as long as some products remain in the tube.

With spontaneous failure, the pregnancy dies and is reabsorbed. Of ectopic pregnancies that fail, β-human chorionic gonadotropin (hCG) levels typically are low and likely reflect dying trophoblast.

After tubal implantation, ectopic pregnancy development may follow an acute or chronic course. *Acute ectopic pregnancy* is more common and follows the pathogenesis described in the prior paragraphs. Compared with chronic ectopic pregnancy, acute ectopic pregnancy has higher serum β-hCG levels at initial presentation. The absolute depth of trophoblast invasion into the tubal wall and tubal wall rupture correlates with these high serum levels (Erol, 2015). Also with the acute form, their rapid growth leads to an immediate diagnosis from painful tubal distention or from rupture. Indeed, compared with chronic ectopic pregnancy, acute ectopic pregnancy carries a higher risk of tubal rupture (Barnhart, 2003c).

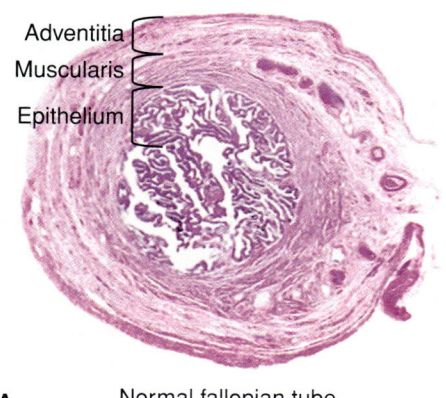

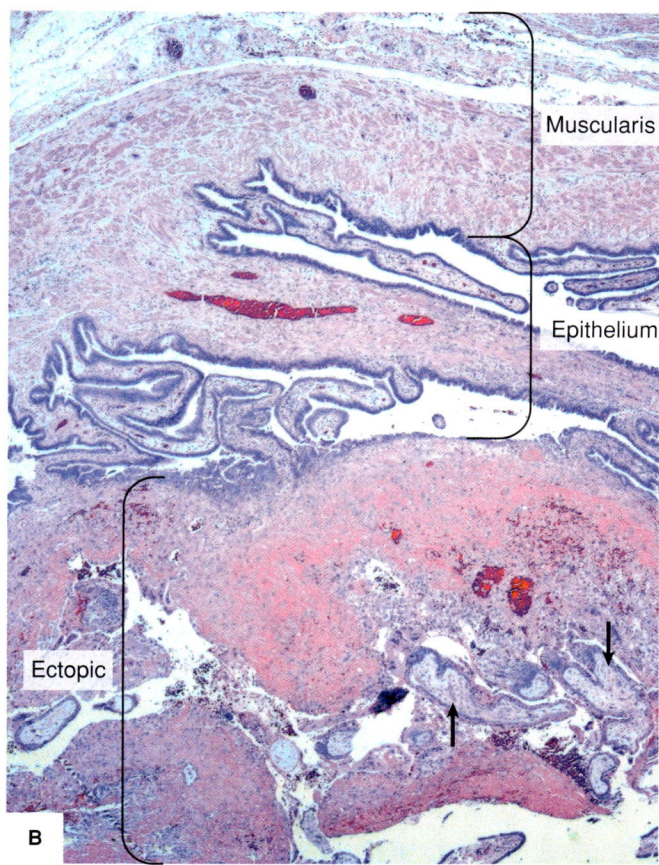

FIGURE 7-2 Photomicrograph of fallopian tubes. **A.** Normal ampullary portion of a fallopian tube. (Reproduced with permission from Dr. Kelley Carrick.) **B.** Ectopic tubal pregnancy. Chorionic villi (*arrows*) can be seen within the tubal lumen. (Reproduced with permission from Dr. Raheela Ashfaq.)

Chronic ectopic pregnancy is much less common. Minor repeated ruptures or tubal abortion incites an inflammatory response that leads to formation of a pelvic mass. This mass contains old blood and gestational tissue surrounded by adhesions. Trophoblastic tissue dies early, and β-hCG testing may be negative or may show very low, static levels. Chronic ectopic pregnancies typically rupture late, if at all, but commonly form a complex pelvic mass. This often is the indication that prompts diagnostic surgery (Cole, 1982; Uğur, 1996).

CLINICAL MANIFESTATIONS

The classic symptom triad of ectopic pregnancy is amenorrhea followed by vaginal bleeding and ipsilateral abdominal pain. However, as women seek care earlier, the ability to diagnose ectopic pregnancy before rupture—even before the onset of symptoms—is not unusual. Of other symptoms, banal pregnancy discomforts such as breast tenderness and nausea may accompany more ominous findings. These include shoulder pain worsened by inspiration, which is caused by phrenic nerve irritation from subdiaphragmatic blood. Vasomotor disturbances such as vertigo and syncope may reflect hemorrhage-related hypovolemia.

Of physical findings, some hypovolemic women show orthostatic changes, and the shock index is one evaluation tool. This index is calculated as the heart rate divided by systolic blood pressure and can assess trauma patients for hypovolemic or septic shock. The normal range lies between 0.5 and 0.7 for nonpregnant patients. A shock index >0.85 and a systolic blood pressure <110 mmHg are highly suggestive of a potentially life-threatening gynecologic emergency, such as a ruptured ectopic pregnancy (Birkhahn, 2003; Polena, 2015). Despite these findings of advanced hypovolemia, normal vital signs are unreliable to exclude earlier stages of tubal rupture and blood loss.

Abdominal and pelvic findings may also be notoriously few in women before tubal rupture. With rupture, however, many will have marked tenderness on both abdominal and pelvic examination, and pain is aggravated with cervical manipulation. A pelvic mass, including fullness posterolateral to the uterus, can be gently palpated in some affected women. Initially, an ectopic pregnancy may feel soft and elastic, whereas extensive intraluminal hemorrhage produces a firmer consistency. Many times, discomfort precludes palpation of the mass, and limiting examinations may help avert iatrogenic rupture.

DIAGNOSIS

Ectopic pregnancy is considered in any reproductive-aged woman with pain, uterine bleeding, and/or anemia. Symptoms of ectopic pregnancy can mimic multiple entities (Table 12-1, p. 255). Broadly, these can first be divided into complications of early pregnancy or not. Thus, in those without prior hysterectomy, urine pregnancy testing is indicated. If testing is positive, transvaginal sonography and serial serum β-hCG measurements are the most valuable diagnostic aids. Additionally, because ectopic pregnancy can lead to significant bleeding, a hemogram is an additional fast and effective initial screen.

■ Laboratory Findings

Serum β-hCG Measurements

Human chorionic gonadotropin is a glycoprotein produced by syncytiotrophoblast of the placenta and can be detected in serum as early as 8 days after the luteinizing hormone (LH) surge. Current pregnancy tests have lower limits of detection that are 20 to 25 mIU/mL for urine and ≤5 mIU/mL for serum (Greene, 2015). Importantly, given an interassay variability of 5 to 10 percent, interpretation of serial values is more reliable when performed by the same laboratory (Desai, 2014).

With a robust intrauterine pregnancy (IUP), early studies suggest that serum β-hCG levels should rise at least 53 to 66 percent every 48 hours (Barnhart, 2004; Kadar, 1982). A more conservative rise of 35 percent in 48 hours is now often used, and this lowers the potential disruption of normal IUPs (Seeber, 2006). With multifetal gestation, this same anticipated rate of rise is expected (Chung, 2006).

Importantly, a similar 53-percent or greater rise at 48 hours can be seen with ectopic pregnancy cases (Silva, 2006). Moreover, inadequately rising serum β-hCG levels indicate only a dying pregnancy, not its location. Thus, β-hCG levels are coupled with sonography and other clinical findings.

Past this 48 hours, adding a third serum β-hCG level on day 4 or 7 may better determine the location and viability of the pregnancy (Morse, 2012; Zee, 2014). This is weighed against an increased chance of ectopic pregnancy rupture during these extra diagnostic days.

Serum Progesterone Levels

Serum progesterone concentration is used by some to aid ectopic pregnancy diagnosis when serum β-hCG levels and sonographic findings are inconclusive (Stovall, 1992). Serum progesterone concentration varies minimally between 5 and 10 weeks' gestation, thus a single value is sufficient. From studies, a single serum progesterone level <6 ng/mL (<20 nmol/L) has a specificity of 99 percent to predict a nonviable pregnancy in women without clear sonographic evidence of pregnancy location (Van Calster, 2016; Verhaegen, 2012). Ultimately, serum progesterone levels can be used to buttress a clinical impression, but again they cannot reliably differentiate between ectopic and intrauterine pregnancies (Guha, 2014).

■ Sonography

High-resolution sonography has revolutionized the management of women with a suspected ectopic pregnancy. With transvaginal sonography (TVS), an intrauterine gestational sac is usually visible between 4½ and 5 weeks, the yolk sac appears between 5 and 6 weeks, and a fetal pole with cardiac activity is first detected at 5½ to 6 weeks. With transabdominal sonography, these structures are visualized slightly later. The sonographic diagnosis of ectopic pregnancy rests on visualization of an adnexal mass separate from the ovary (Fig. 7-3). Definitive criteria include either an extrauterine yolk sac or embryo.

When ectopic pregnancy is part of a differential diagnosis, serum β-hCG testing is used to define expected sonographic findings. Each institution must define a β-hCG discriminatory value for TVS, that is, the lower limit at which an examiner can

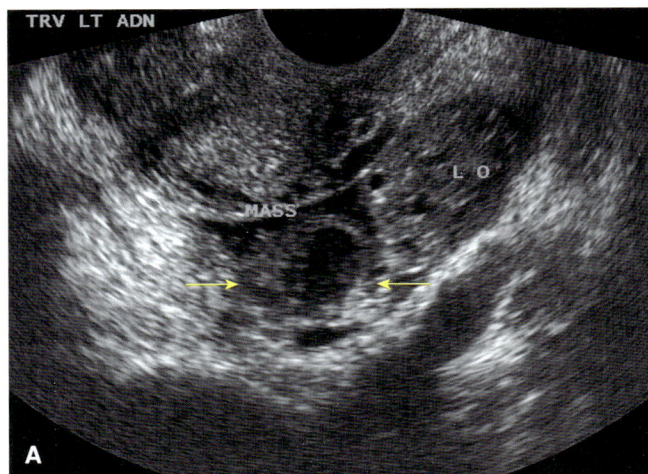

Inhomogeneous mass

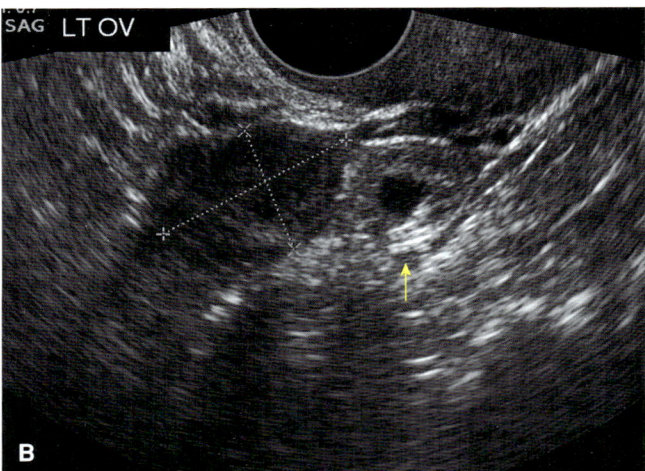

Mass with empty extrauterine sac

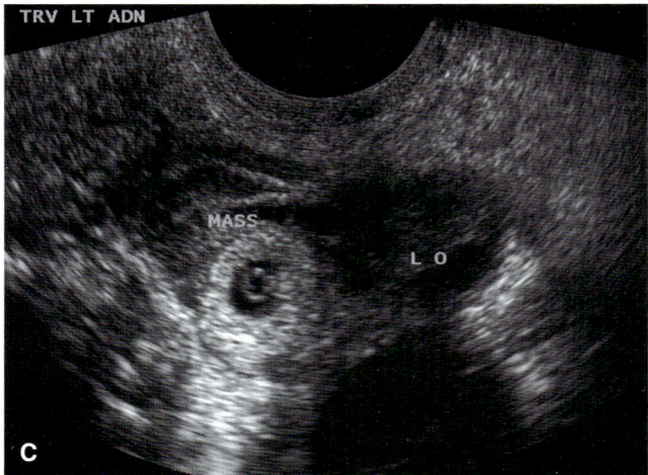

Mass with yolk sac

FIGURE 7-3 Transvaginal sonographic findings with various ectopic pregnancies. For sonographic diagnosis, an ectopic mass should be seen in the adnexa separate from the ovary and may be seen: **(A)** as an inhomogeneous adnexal mass (*yellow arrows*), **(B)** as an empty extrauterine sac with a hyperechoic ring (*arrow*), or **(C)** as a yolk sac and/or fetal pole with or without cardiac activity within an extrauterine sac. LO = left ovary. (Reproduced with permission from Dr. Elysia Moschos.)

reliably visualize an IUP. Early threshold values were ≥1500 or ≥2000 mIU/mL, but others subsequently have suggested an even higher threshold (Barnhart, 1994; Mehta, 1997). Specifically, Connolly and associates (2013) noted that with live IUPs, a gestational sac was seen 99 percent of the time with a discriminatory level of >3510 mIU/mL. The American College of Obstetricians and Gynecologists (2018) recognizes this more conservative threshold. Even with β-hCG levels above the chosen discriminatory value, technical challenges such as leiomyomas, adenomyosis, multifetal gestation, or IUD can hinder the ability to accurately diagnose an intrauterine gestation (Gurel, 2007; Ko, 2014).

When β-hCG levels are above the set discriminatory value, absence of an IUP may suggest an abnormal pregnancy. These include an ectopic pregnancy, an incomplete abortion, or a resolving completed abortion. For example, despite total passage of products of conception with complete abortion, β-hCG testing may still be positive while original β-hCG is metabolized and cleared. Early multifetal gestation also remains a possibility (Ko, 2014). Without clear evidence for ectopic pregnancy, serial β-hCG level assessment is reasonable in a hemodynamically stable patient. This averts unnecessary MTX administration to a failing IUP and avoids harming an early normal multifetal intrauterine pregnancy.

Conversely, when β-hCG values lie below the discriminatory value, sonographic findings are typically nondiagnostic. With this *pregnancy of unknown location (PUL)*, serial β-hCG level assays are done to identify patterns that indicate either a growing or failing IUP. As noted, thriving IUPs show a minimum 35-percent rise in β-hCG levels after 2 days. Conversely, PULs that ultimately are found to be failing IUPs show a characteristic decline (Table 7-2). Levels that rise or fall outside these expected parameters raise the concern for ectopic pregnancy.

In an attempt to unify the language used with sonographic evaluation of early pregnancies, a consensus statement was drafted with five categories: (1) definitive ectopic pregnancy (extrauterine gestational sac with yolk sac and/or embryo), (2) probable ectopic pregnancy (inhomogeneous adnexal mass or extrauterine halo-like structure), (3) probable IUP (intrauterine echogenic sac), (4) definite IUP (intrauterine gestational sac with yolk sac and/or embryo), and (5) PUL (lacking signs of either ectopic pregnancy or IUP) (Barnhart, 2011).

Systematic sonographic evaluation is critical to establish the correct diagnosis. Most begin with the endometrial cavity. In pregnancies conceived spontaneously, identification of an IUP effectively excludes the possibility of ectopic implantation. When ART is employed, however, careful examination of the tube and ovary is performed even with an IUP because heterotopic pregnancy rates may be as high as 1 per 1000 (Perkins, 2015). An intracavitary fluid collection caused by sloughing of the decidua can create a *pseudogestational sac*, or *pseudosac*. As shown in Figure 7-4, this one-layer collection typically lies in the midline of the uterine cavity. In contrast, a normal gestational sac is eccentrically located, that is, lying within one side of the endometrial stripe more than the other (Dashefsky, 1988). Another intracavitary finding of ectopic pregnancy is a trilaminar endometrial pattern, which represents two adjacent edematous proliferative-phase endometrial layers (Fig. 2-16, p. 38) (Lavie, 1996). For the diagnosis of ectopic pregnancy, this finding's specificity is 93 percent but sensitivity is only 21 percent (Col-Madendag, 2010). Endometrial stripe thickness has not been well correlated with ectopic pregnancy. However, Moschos and Twickler (2008b) determined that in PULs, none that ultimately proved to be normal IUPs had a stripe thickness <8 mm.

The fallopian tubes and ovaries are also inspected. Seeing an extrauterine yolk sac or embryo clearly confirms an ectopic pregnancy, although such findings are less common (Paul, 2000). In some cases, a *halo* or tubal ring can be seen. This ring surrounds an anechoic center and is covered by a thin hypoechoic

TABLE 7-2. Percentage Decline of Initial Serum β-hCG Levels in Those with PUL and Ultimately Diagnosed with Spontaneous Abortion

| Initial hCG (mIU/mL) | Percentage Decline[a] | | |
	By Day 2 Expected % (Minimum %)	By Day 4 Expected % (Minimum %)	By Day 7 Expected % (Minimum %)
50	68 (12)	78 (26)	88 (34)
100	68 (16)	80 (35)	90 (47)
300	70 (22)	83 (45)	93 (62)
500	71 (24)	84 (50)	94 (68)
1000	72 (28)	86 (55)	95 (74)
2000	74 (31)	88 (60)	96 (79)
3000	74 (33)	88 (63)	96 (81)
4000	75 (34)	89 (64)	97 (83)
5000	75 (35)	89 (66)	97 (84)

[a]The percentage decline is given as the expected decline. The minimum expected decline in parentheses is the 95th percentile value. Declines less than this minimum may reflect retained either intrauterine or extrauterine trophoblast.
Data from Barnhart, 2004; Chung, 2006.

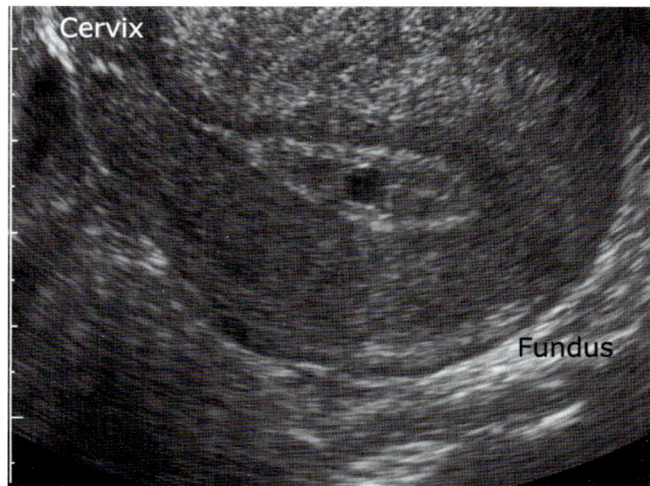

FIGURE 7-4 Transvaginal sonography of a pseudogestational sac within the endometrial cavity. Note its circular shape and central location, which are characteristic of these fluid collections. (Reproduced with permission from Dr. Elysia Moschos.)

area caused by subserosal tubal edema. According to Burry and associates (1993), this has a positive predictive value of 92 percent and a specificity of 95 percent. Alternatively, a more solid, inhomogeneous complex adnexal mass is usually caused by hemorrhage within the ectopic sac or by an ectopic pregnancy that has ruptured into the tube. Overall, approximately 60 percent of ectopic pregnancies are seen as an inhomogeneous mass adjacent to the ovary; 30 percent appear as a hyperechoic ring; and 8 percent have an obvious gestational sac with a fetal pole (Nadim, 2018). In women undergoing sonography for ectopic pregnancy concerns, specificity is 95 to 99 percent and positive predictive value is 96 percent for ectopic pregnancy when an extraovarian adnexal mass is found (Brown, 1994; Nadim, 2018). However, not all extraovarian adnexal masses represent an ectopic pregnancy, and integration of sonographic findings with other clinical information is necessary.

With transvaginal color Doppler imaging, placental blood flow within the periphery of an ectopic pregnancy—the *ring of fire*—can be seen (Fig. 7-5). However, this ring can also be noted with a corpus luteum of pregnancy. Another technique to help characterize a suspicious mass involves an examiner gently palpating an adnexum that is placed between the vaginal probe and the examiner's abdominal hand during real-time scanning. A mass that moves separately from the ovary suggests a tubal pregnancy, whereas a mass that moves synchronously more likely represents an intraovarian structure (Levine, 2007).

Also during sonographic evaluation of the pelvis, TVS can detect as little as 50 mL of free peritoneal fluid in the posterior cul-de-sac (Fig. 7-6). This may be intraabdominal bleeding or physiologic peritoneal fluid. A large volume of fluid or fluid that is echogenic is more worrisome for hemoperitoneum. In addition, transabdominal right upper quadrant sonographic imaging helps assess the extent of hemoperitoneum. Blood in the paracolic gutters and Morison pouch indicates significant hemorrhage. Specifically, free fluid in Morison pouch typically is not seen until a hemoperitoneum reaches 400 to 700 mL (Branney, 1995; Rodgerson, 2001). Detection of peritoneal fluid in conjunction with an adnexal mass and positive pregnancy testing is

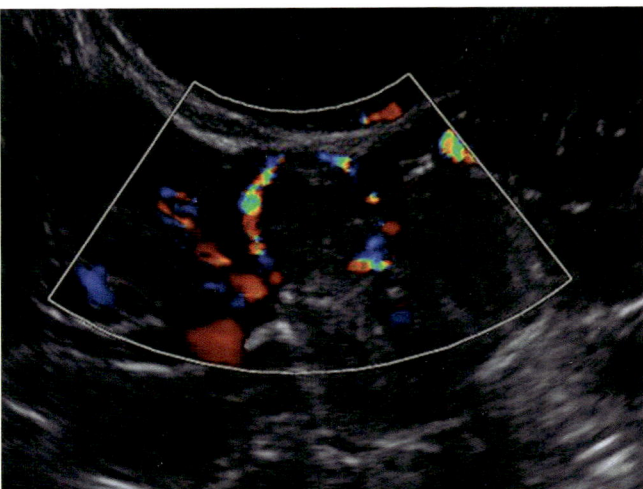

FIGURE 7-5 Color Doppler transvaginal sonography of an ectopic pregnancy. The "ring of fire" reflects placental blood flow around the periphery of the pregnancy. This finding, however, may also be seen with corpus luteum cysts.

highly predictive of ectopic pregnancy (Nyberg, 1991). That said, despite technologic advances, the absence of suggestive findings does not exclude ectopic pregnancy. Moreover, in rare instances, an hCG-secreting tumor can produce the triad of adnexal pathology, ascites, and positive hCG testing (Chap. 16, p. 338). Thus, in all circumstances, clinical integration is essential.

■ Culdocentesis

With a 16- to 18-gauge spinal needle, the posterior cul-de-sac can be entered through the posterior vaginal fornix. The aspirate characteristics, in conjunction with clinical findings, may help clarify the diagnosis. Colorless or yellow clear peritoneal fluid is designated as a negative test. If fragments of an old clot or nonclotting blood are found in the aspirate when placed into a dry, clean test tube, then hemoperitoneum is diagnosed. If the aspirated blood clots after it is withdrawn, this may signify

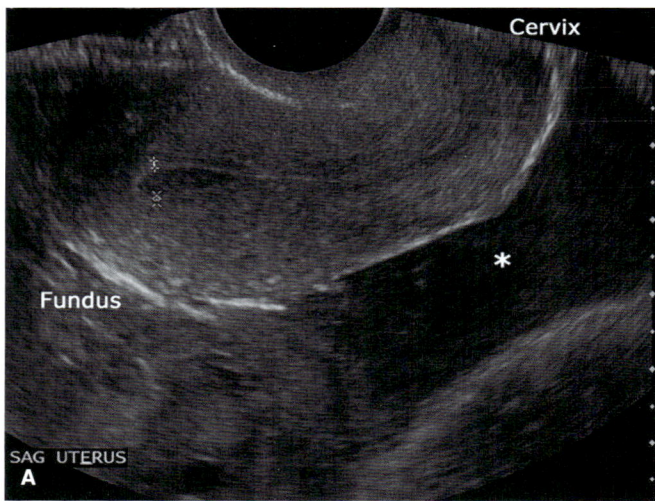

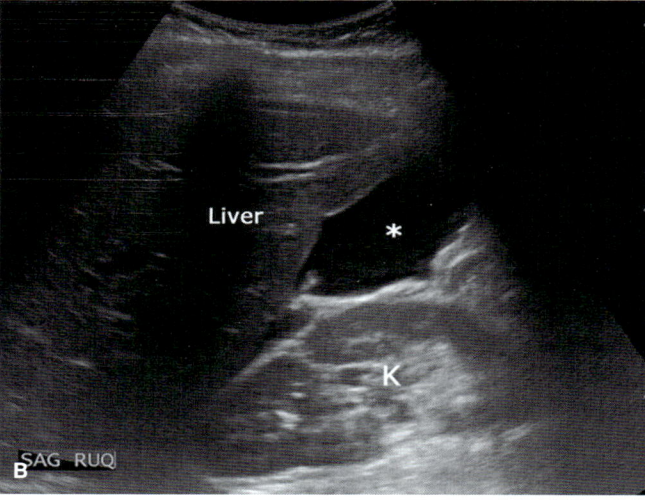

FIGURE 7-6 A. Transvaginal sonography displays hypoechoic fluid (*asterisk*) in the posterior cul-de-sac. **B.** Right upper quadrant sonogram shows anechoic fluid (*asterisk*) in Morison pouch between the liver and kidney (*K*).

active intraperitoneal bleeding or puncture of an adjacent vessel. If fluid cannot be aspirated, the test can only be interpreted as unsatisfactory. Purulent fluid suggests an infection-related etiology such as salpingitis or appendicitis. Feculent material may originate from a perforated colon or an inadvertent puncture of the rectum during culdocentesis.

Several studies have challenged the usefulness of this bedside test, and culdocentesis mostly has been replaced by TVS (Glezerman, 1992; Vermesh, 1990). Sonography with findings of echogenic fluid to establish hemoperitoneum is more sensitive and specific than culdocentesis—100 and 100 percent versus 66 and 80 percent, respectively. Also, for most women, sonography is better tolerated.

■ Endometrial Evidence

Several endometrial changes are associated with ectopic pregnancy. These include decidua found in 42 percent of samples, secretory endometrium in 22 percent, and proliferative endometrium in 12 percent, all with an absence of trophoblast (Lopez, 1994). Decidua is endometrium that is hormonally prepared for pregnancy, and the degree to which the endometrium is converted with ectopic pregnancy is variable. Thus, in addition to bleeding, women with ectopic tubal pregnancy may pass a *decidual cast*, which is the entire sloughed endometrium that takes the form of the endometrial cavity (Fig. 7-7). Decidual sloughing may also occur with an IUP abortion. Thus, tissue is carefully evaluated visually and then histologically for evidence of a conceptus. If no clear gestational sac is visually seen or if no villi are identified histologically within the cast, then the possibility of ectopic pregnancy must still be entertained.

Dilation and curettage (D & C) can help clarify the diagnosis in persistent or unclear PUL cases. Villi in the surgical sample support an intrauterine location. This strives to avoid treating the mother and exposing a potential IUP to methotrexate, a known teratogen (p. 169). Less often, in cases of diagnosed ectopic pregnancy, some also recommend curettage prior to methotrexate treatment to confirm the absence of intrauterine villi (Barnhart,

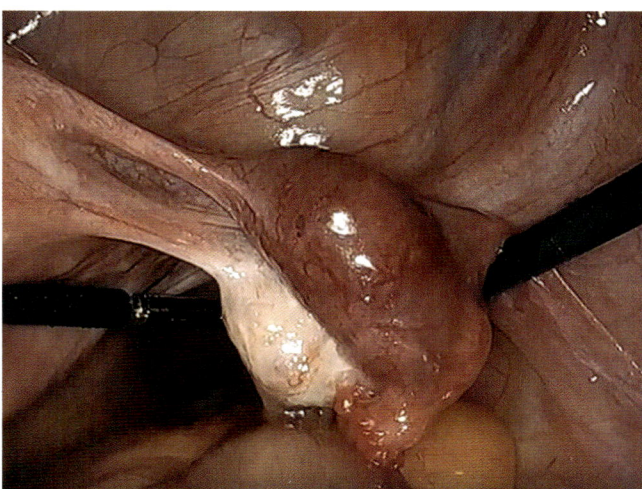

FIGURE 7-8 Laparoscopic photograph of a right-sided ectopic pregnancy shows a distended tubal ampulla. (Reproduced with permission from Dr. Lisa Chao.)

2002; Chung, 2011; Shaunik, 2011). This averts maternal, and possible IUP, exposure to potential drug side effects. Nevertheless, the need, method, and risks of surgical endometrial sampling must carefully be weighed against the evidence supporting the diagnosis of ectopic pregnancy and drug risks in a given patient.

Endometrial biopsy with a Pipelle catheter or endometrial aspiration was studied as an alternative to surgical curettage and found inferior (Barnhart, 2003b; Insogna, 2017). By comparison, frozen section of surgical curettage fragments to identify products of conception is accurate in more than 90 percent of cases (Barak, 2005; Li, 2014b; Spandorfer, 1996).

■ Summary of Diagnostic Evaluation

Confirmation by diagnostic laparoscopy remains the gold standard for ectopic pregnancy diagnosis (Fig. 7-8). That said, with sensitive diagnostic modalities available, ectopic pregnancy can typically be diagnosed prior to surgery, and use of an evidence-based approach can assist. First, after appropriate clinical evaluation, all reproductive-aged women with any suspicion of pregnancy are tested using a sensitive urine β-hCG assay. Following positive testing, TVS is completed for all women with first-trimester pain or bleeding. If sonographic findings are not diagnostic and concerns for ectopic pregnancy complications are not urgent, serial serum β-hCG levels are measured until discriminatory zone levels are reached. TVS is then repeated. The interval between serum testing after the first 48 hours, however, is currently not well defined. The American College of Obstetricians and Gynecologists (2018) recommends serum β-hCG level testing every 2 to 7 days depending on the level of change. Those with a higher ectopic pregnancy risk are typically tested more frequently. D & C or diagnostic laparoscopy or both can be considered to help clarify cases concerning for, but not clearly diagnostic of, ectopic pregnancy.

Because ectopic pregnancies can rupture even at low β-hCG levels, serum β-hCG values are usually followed until they lie below the "negative" result threshold for the given assay. Rupture at low values likely reflects partial disruption of the

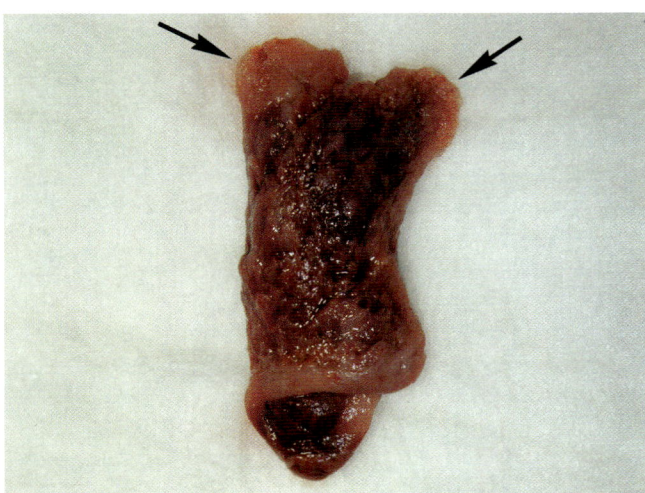

FIGURE 7-7 In this decidual cast, arrows mark the area that conformed to the cornua. (From Hoffman, 2018, with permission.)

vascular connection between trophoblast and maternal vessels. That said, one recent study of more than 1500 PULs showed that a β-hCG value drop of 85 percent between the initial draw and day-4 values or 95-percent decline by day 7 excluded 100 percent of ectopic pregnancies (Cameron, 2016).

To better define PULs and their ectopic risk, several protocols and risk calculators have been evaluated. These ideally limit overtesting of pregnancies yet still identify high-risk pregnancies for close surveillance (Van Calster, 2013, 2016). These have not been sufficiently validated in United States populations (Barnhart, 2010).

MANAGEMENT

Once diagnosed, ectopic pregnancies can be managed surgically, medically with methotrexate (MTX), or expectantly. Because of the potential for life-threatening bleeding, careful patient selection is essential.

With the ending of any early pregnancy, Rh status is assessed. Alloimmunization is a possibility in D-negative women. Therefore, 300 μg of anti-D immune globulin is given to these women if the father of the baby has the D antigen or if his status is unknown (Krause, 1996).

■ Medical Management

For most ectopic pregnancies, medical therapy is preferred, if feasible, to avoid surgical risks. However, before consideration of this option, important criteria must be met. Namely, evidence for tubal rupture and hemodynamic instability are absent, and the patient must lack MTX contraindications (Table 7-3). Other considerations include reasonably close access to an emergency department and a commitment to be compliant with surveillance laboratory testing.

Some classic predictors of success with MTX use are the initial serum β-hCG level, ectopic pregnancy size, and fetal cardiac activity. Of these, the β-hCG level is the single best prognostic indicator of treatment success. In their classic study, Lipscomb and colleagues (1999) found that an initial serum value <5000 mIU/mL was associated with a success rate of 92 percent, whereas an initial concentration >15,000 mIU/mL had a success rate of only 68 percent. This trend has been confirmed by many. In a more recent study, the failure rate associated with β-hCG levels >4500 mIU/mL was 65 percent (Cohen, 2014). Although not exclusionary, rapidly rising β-hCG levels in the 48 hours before MTX therapy may also portend a higher failure rate (Cohen, 2017; Dudley, 2004). Specifically, a rise >50 percent is cited by the American Society for Reproductive Medicine (2013) as a predictor.

The effect of size on success rates with medical therapy has fewer supporting data, although many early trials used "large size" as an exclusion criterion. In one study, the success rate with single-dose methotrexate was 93 percent in cases with ectopic masses ≤3.5 cm, whereas success rates were between 87 and 90 percent when the mass was >3.5 cm (Lipscomb, 1998). These authors also found ectopic pregnancies measuring ≤4 cm and lacking cardiac activity to be suitable candidates.

Cardiac activity seen sonographically is also a relative contraindication to medical therapy. Most studies report a greater failure rate if cardiac activity is noted. Still, a success rate of 87 percent has been reported (Lipscomb, 1998).

Methotrexate

This medication stalls cell growth and protein production by competitively inhibiting the enzyme dihydrofolate reductase (Berlin, 1963). Possible MTX side effects include stomatitis, conjunctivitis, transient liver dysfunction, myelosuppression,

TABLE 7-3. Medical Treatment Protocols for Ectopic Pregnancy

	Single Dose	Multidose
Dosing	One dose; repeat if necessary	Up to four doses of both drugs until serum β-hCG declines by 15%
Medication dosage		
Methotrexate	50 mg/m² BSA (day 1)	1 mg/kg, days 1, 3, 5, and 7
Leucovorin	NA	0.1 mg/kg days 2, 4, 6, and 8
Serum β-hCG level	Days 1, 4, and 7	Days 1, 3, 5, and 7
Indication for additional dose	• If serum β-hCG level does not decline by 15% from day 4 to day 7 • <15% decline during weekly surveillance	If serum β-hCG declines <15% between days 1 & 3, give additional dose; repeat serum β-hCG in 48 hours and compare with previous value; maximum four doses
Surveillance	Once 15% decline achieved, draw weekly serum β-hCG level until undetectable	

Methotrexate Contraindications		
Sensitivity to MTX	Intrauterine pregnancy	Peptic ulcer disease
Tubal rupture	Hepatic, renal, or hematologic dysfunction	Immunodeficiency
Breastfeeding	Active pulmonary disease	

BSA = body surface area; β-hCG = β-human chorionic gonadotropin; MTX = methotrexate; NA = not applicable.

mucositis, pulmonary damage, and anaphylactoid reactions (Conway, 2015; Salliot, 2009; Shao, 2018; Soysal, 2016; Troeltzsch, 2013). In some cases, leucovorin (folinic acid) is given following treatment to blunt or reverse MTX side effects. Such therapy is termed *leucovorin rescue* and discussed in Chapter 27 (p. 592).

To help select suitable MTX candidates, several laboratory tests are obtained. First, MTX is renally cleared, and significant renal dysfunction precludes its use (Rheumatoid Arthritis Clinical Trial Archive Group, 1995). Thus, a serum creatinine level is reviewed. Second, MTX can be hepato- and myelotoxic, and complete blood count (CBC) and liver function tests (LFTs) establish a baseline. Last, blood type and Rh status are determined. All except blood typing are considered surveillance laboratory tests and are repeated prior to additional MTX doses (Lipscomb, 2007).

With administration, women are counseled to avoid several aggravating agents until treatment is completed. These are: (1) folic acid–containing supplements, which can competitively reduce methotrexate binding to dihydrofolate reductase; (2) nonsteroidal antiinflammatory drugs, which reduce renal blood flow and delay drug excretion; (3) alcohol, which can predispose to concurrent hepatic enzyme elevation; (4) sunlight, which can provoke MTX-related dermatitis; and (5) sexual activity, which can rupture the ectopic pregnancy (American College of Obstetricians and Gynecologists, 2018).

Importantly, MTX is a teratogen that can lead to severe embryopathy including pulmonary atresia, craniosynostosis, and limb deficiencies (Hyoun, 2012; Nurmohamed, 2011). Thus, to avoid inadvertent fetal exposure, MTX is ideally used when a confident diagnosis of ectopic pregnancy is made. PUL is a transition diagnosis and is not suitable for MTX administration.

During the first few days following MTX administration, some abdominal pain is common, and patients are so counseled. This separation pain presumably results from tubal distention caused by tubal abortion or hematoma formation or both (Stovall, 1993). Mild analgesics are typically sufficient. In few cases, inpatient observation with serial hematocrit determinations and gentle abdominal examinations help assess the need for surgical intervention.

Dosing Options

The two most common regimens are listed in Table 7-3, and doses are given IM. With single-dose therapy, the dose is 50 mg/m^2 body surface area (BSA), and BSA can be derived using various Internet-based BSA calculators. At our institution, patients are observed for 30 minutes following MTX injections to exclude adverse reaction.

During single-dose therapy, a serum β-hCG level is measured on the day of MTX administration, and this is repeated on days 4 and 7 following injection. Day-4 levels may rise or fall. Although both trends are acceptable, falling levels are linked to higher resolution rates (Agostini, 2007; Nguyen, 2010; Skubisz, 2013). Next, a comparison is made between day 4 and 7 serum values. If the value declines by ≥15 percent, weekly serum β-hCG levels are then drawn until they measure <2 mIU/mL. A decline <15 percent is seen in approximately 20 percent of treated women. In such cases, a CBC, creatinine

level, and LFTs are rechecked. If these surveillance tests are normal, a second IM 50-mg/m^2 dose based on BSA is given. The date of this second injection will become the new day 1, and the protocol is restarted. Others have tried, without success, to develop more convenient, yet reliable, serum β-hCG monitoring protocols (Dai, 2017; Kirk, 2007; Thurman, 2010). In the end, the original day-4-to-7 guidelines have been validated.

Shown in Table 7-3, multidose therapy provides MTX (1 mg/kg) treatment with leucovorin (0.1 mg/kg) therapy on alternating days. A maximum of four doses of MTX can be given, and each is followed by the adjunctive doses of leucovorin 24 hours later. After the first dyad of injections, a serum β-hCG concentration is measured. Values between days 1 and 3 are anticipated to drop by ≥15 percent. If not and if surveillance tests are normal, an additional MTX/leucovorin alternating dyad is given. A serum β-hCG level is repeated 2 days later. Once a decline >15 percent is achieved, weekly serum β-hCG level testing then begins until values are undetectable.

Comparing the efficacy of single- versus multidose MTX, Lipscomb and colleagues (2005) studied 643 consecutively treated patients. They found no significant differences in treatment duration, serum β-hCG levels, or success rates between the multi- and single-dose protocols—95 and 90 percent, respectively. Barnhart and coworkers (2003a) performed a metaanalysis of 26 studies that included 1327 women treated with MTX for ectopic pregnancy. The success rates were 88 percent with single-dose and 92 percent for multidose treatment. Last, in a randomized trial with 70 patients, Tabatabaii and associates (2012) found resolution rates of 83 percent with single-dose and 87 percent with multidose regimens, respectively. At our institution, we use single-dose IM MTX.

A hybrid "two dose" MTX protocol strives to balance the efficacy and convenience of the two most commonly used protocols (Barnhart, 2007). However, comparisons of the single-dose and two-dose MTX protocols found equivalent success rates (Mergenthal, 2016; Song, 2016).

Surveillance

Posttherapy monitoring assesses treatment success and screens for signs of persistent ectopic pregnancy. In the absence of symptoms, bimanual examinations are limited to avoid the theoretical risk of manual tubal rupture. Importantly, sonographic monitoring of ectopic mass dimensions can be misleading after serum β-hCG levels have declined to <15 mIU/mL. Brown and colleagues (1991) described persistent masses to be resolving hematomas rather than persistent trophoblastic tissue. For this reason, posttherapy sonography is reserved for suspected complications such as tubal rupture. Approximate time to resolution for all women averages 36 days, but in some, treatment requires as long as 109 days (Lipscomb, 1998).

After successful medical therapy with MTX, pregnancy is delayed for at least 3 months, as this drug may persist in human tissues for months after a single dose (Hackmon, 2011). Although data are very limited, conception before this waiting period appears reassuring. In one study, 45 women who conceived <6 months after MTX had similar pregnancy outcomes compared with 80 women who conceived >6 months after MTX (Svirsky, 2009). In the long term, ovarian reserve does not appear diminished with MTX use for this indication (Hill, 2014; Ohannessian, 2014).

Surgical Management

For surgical removal of an ectopic pregnancy, two procedures—salpingectomy or salpingostomy—are options. With salpingectomy, the entire fallopian tube is removed, and this is suitable for ruptured or unruptured tubes. With rare exception, the entire conceptus is removed with the fallopian tube. Thus, cases of persistent trophoblastic tissue with salpingectomy are uncommon.

In contrast, salpingostomy is typically used to remove a small, unruptured pregnancy yet preserve the fallopian tube. For this, a 15-mm linear incision is made on the antimesenteric border of the fallopian tube over the pregnancy. The products usually will extrude from the incision and can be carefully removed (Chap. 44, p. 1028). Main risks include postoperative bleeding from the tubal incision or trophoblast left within the tube that later causes tubal rupture.

For salpingostomy, a suitable candidate is one who is hemodynamically stable and desires fertility preservation. This applies especially if the other fallopian tube is absent or damaged. In addition to tubal attributes, serum β-hCG levels may influence patient selection. One retrospective study found that ectopic resolution rates were lower following salpingostomy in women in whom the initial serum β-hCG level was >8000 mIU/mL (Milad, 1998). Supportive evidence for this comes from Natale and coworkers (2003), who reported that serum β-hCG levels >6000 mIU/mL have a high risk of implantation into the tubal muscularis. Such implantation would hinder complete trophoblast removal during surgery.

Although salpingectomy achieves a higher initial surgical resolution rate, one concern was that later fertility rates would be lower than those following salpingostomy. In response, two randomized trials have compared laparoscopic outcomes between these two procedures in women with a normal contralateral fallopian tube. The European Surgery in Ectopic Pregnancy (ESEP) study randomized 231 women to salpingectomy and 215 to salpingostomy. After surgery and in subsequent pregnancies, the cumulative rates of ongoing pregnancy by natural conception did not differ significantly between groups–56 versus 61 percent, respectively (Mol, 2014). Again, in the DEMETER trial, the subsequent 2-year rate for achieving an IUP did not significantly differ between groups–64 versus 70 percent, respectively (Fernandez, 2013). One large cohort study had similar findings (Li, 2015b). Thus, if the contralateral fallopian tube appears normal, salpingectomy is a reasonable treatment option that avoids the 5- to 8-percent complication rate caused by persistent or recurrent ectopic pregnancy in the same tube (Rulin, 1995). For women with an abnormal-appearing contralateral tube, salpingostomy is a conservative option for fertility preservation.

Regarding abdominal entry for ectopic surgery, several studies have compared laparotomy with laparoscopy for completion of either salpingectomy or salpingostomy (Murphy, 1992; Lundorff, 1991; Vermesh, 1989). For either tubal surgery, both entry options yielded equivalent ectopic resolution rates and subsequent IUP rates. Moreover, in studies of salpingostomy specifically, tubal patency rates were similar, but fewer adnexal adhesions formed following laparoscopy. However, in one

systematic review, laparoscopic salpingostomy had a 13-percent rate of persistent trophoblastic disease compared with a rate of 3 percent with laparotomic salpingostomy (Mol, 2008).

In sum, laparoscopy is the preferred surgical treatment for ectopic pregnancy unless a woman is hemodynamically unstable. As experience has accrued, cases previously managed by laparotomy—for example, ruptured tubal pregnancies with hemoperitoneum—can safely be managed laparoscopically by those with suitable expertise (Cohen, 2013; Sagiv, 2001). That said, the lowered venous return and cardiac output associated with the pneumoperitoneum of laparoscopy must be factored into the decision to select minimally invasive surgery for a hypovolemic woman.

Before surgery, future fertility desires are discussed. In women desiring permanent sterilization, the unaffected tube can be removed concurrently with salpingectomy for the affected fallopian tube.

Medical versus Surgical Therapy

Multidose MTX treatment and laparoscopic salpingostomy have been compared in one randomized trial of 100 patients. The authors found no differences for rates of tubal preservation, primary treatment success, and subsequent fertility (Dias Pereira, 1999; Hajenius, 1997).

For single-dose MTX, its efficacy compared with laparoscopic salpingostomy shows conflicting results. In one randomized trial, single-dose MTX was less successful in pregnancy resolution, whereas in the other, single-dose MTX was equally effective (Saraj, 1998; Sowter, 2001). Krag Moeller and associates (2009) reported during a median surveillance period of 8.6 years that ectopic-resolution success rates and cumulative spontaneous IUP rates were not significantly different between those managed by laparoscopic salpingostomy and those treated with single-dose MTX.

Salpingectomy effectively removes the entire conceptus and yields high resolution rates. It thus outperforms MTX in this regard. Yet, when future fertility and ectopic pregnancy recurrence rates are analyzed, both salpingectomy and MTX therapy show comparable results (de Bennetot, 2012; Irani, 2017). In another study, surgery, MTX, or expectant management all yielded statistically similar subsequent spontaneous IUP rates (Demirdag, 2017).

In sum, medical or surgical management offer similar outcomes in women who are hemodynamically stable, have serum β-hCG concentrations <5000 mIU/mL, and have a small pregnancy with no fetal cardiac activity. Despite lower success rates with medical therapy for women with larger tubal size, higher serum β-hCG levels, and fetal cardiac activity, medical management can be offered to the motivated woman who understands the risks of emergency surgery in the event of treatment failure.

Expectant Management

In anticipation that a tubal ectopic pregnancy will spontaneously resolve, close observation is reasonable in select women without pain or significant bleeding. A commitment to surveillance visits and relative proximity to an emergency department are other safeguards. Importantly, this differs from expectant management of a PUL during its evaluation.

Consensus guidelines are difficult to formulate from available small studies, which have markedly disparate inclusion criteria. Despite this, predictive factors for success include a low initial serum β-hCG concentration, a significant drop in levels over 48 hours, and a sonographic inhomogeneous mass rather than a tubal halo or other gestational structure. For example, initial values <175 mIU/mL predict spontaneous resolution in 88 to 96 percent of attempts (Elson, 2004; Kirk, 2011). Initial values <1000 mIU/mL have success rates ranging from 71 to 92 percent (Jurkovic, 2017; Mavrelos, 2013; Silva, 2015).

Regarding subsequent fertility, Shalev and associates (1995) found no difference in rates of ipsilateral tubal patency, recurrent ectopic pregnancy, or 1-year fertility with either success or failed expectant management. In another study, expectant management and salpingectomy had similar rates of recurrent ectopic or of subsequent spontaneous IUP (Helmy, 2007).

Resolution time with expectant management approximates 3 weeks, and β-hCG concentrations are followed to undetectable levels (Mavrelos, 2015). Close monitoring is warranted during this time because the risk of tubal rupture persists despite low or declining serum β-hCG levels (Fu, 2007). Moreover, an argument could be made that the minimal side effects of MTX may make it preferable to expectant-care disadvantages. These include a potentially prolonged surveillance, patient anxiety, and tubal rupture risk.

■ Persistent Ectopic Pregnancy

Incomplete eradication of trophoblastic tissue and its continued growth causes tubal rupture in 3 to 20 percent of women following conservative surgical or medical treatment of ectopic pregnancy (Graczykowski, 1999). Rarely, surgically dislodged trophoblast can also secondarily implant on abdominal surfaces and bleed. Thus, abdominal pain following ectopic pregnancy treatment prompts immediate suspicion for persistent trophoblast proliferation.

Following salpingostomy, persistent ectopic pregnancy can complicate very early pregnancies (Nathorst-Böös, 2004). And,

as discussed earlier, higher initial β-hCG levels that may reflect greater tubal muscularis invasion are another predictor (Lund, 2002). To obviate persistent trophoblast, Graczykowski and associates (1997) administered a prophylactic MTX dose of 1 mg/m² BSA postoperatively. This reduced the incidence of persistent ectopic pregnancy and shortened the length of surveillance. But again, this is balanced against MTX side effects. Our practice is to watch hormone levels rather than to use prophylactic MTX.

The optimal monitoring schedule to identify persistent ectopic pregnancy after surgical therapy has not been determined. Protocols describe serum β-hCG level monitoring from every 3 days to every 2 weeks. Spandorfer and associates (1997) estimated the risk of persistent ectopic pregnancy based on serum β-hCG levels done on the first postoperative day after salpingostomy. They observed that if serum β-hCG levels fell by >50 percent compared with presurgical values, there were no treatment failures within the first 9 days, and thus repeat serum β-hCG determinations 1 week after surgery were appropriate. Conversely, if serum levels fell by <50 percent, there was a 3.5-fold greater risk of failure within the first week, thus necessitating earlier postoperative evaluation. Currently, standard therapy for persistent ectopic pregnancy in clinically stable women is single-dose MTX with 50 mg/m² BSA.

CESAREAN SCAR PREGNANCY

Among women with a prior cesarean delivery, implantation within a prior cesarean hysterotomy scar develops in approximately 1 in 2000 pregnancies (Seow, 2004). Similar to patients with ectopic pregnancy in other locations, affected women may have vaginal bleeding or abdominal pain, but up to 33 percent are asymptomatic (Rotas, 2006).

Cesarean scar pregnancies (CSPs) are usually diagnosed in the first trimester, and transvaginal sonography is essential (Fig. 7-9). Diagnostic criteria include: (1) an empty uterine

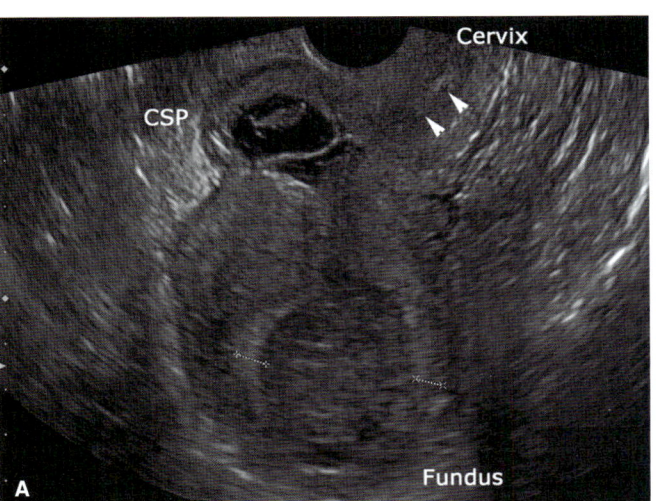
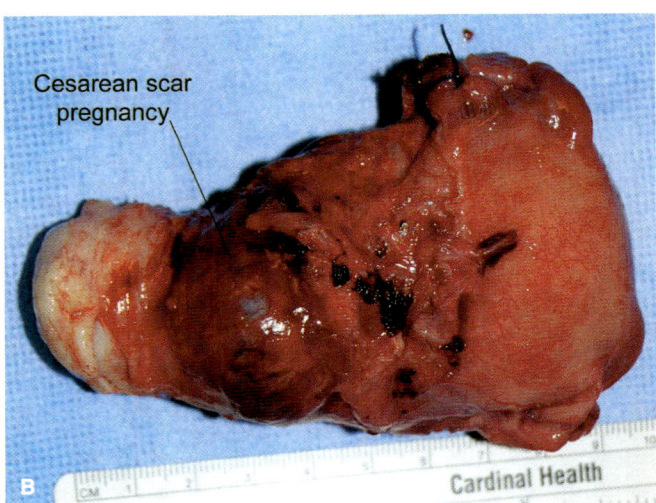

FIGURE 7-9 Cesarean scar pregnancy. **A.** Transvaginal sonogram of a uterus with a cesarean scar pregnancy (*CSP*) in a sagittal plane. The diagnosis is suggested by sonographic criteria indicative of CSP. First, the uterine cavity contains only heterogeneous echoes suggestive of clot. The endometrium is measured by calipers here. An empty cervical canal is identified by a bright hyperechoic endocervical stripe (*white arrowheads*). Last, an intrauterine mass is seen in the anterior part of the uterine isthmus. **B.** Hysterectomy specimen containing a cesarean scar pregnancy. The fundus lies to the right. (Reproduced with permission from Dr. Sunil Balgobin.)

cavity and empty endocervical canal, (2) placenta or gestational sac embedded in the hysterotomy scar niche, (3) a thin myometrial mantle between the gestational sac and bladder, and (4) a prominent vascular pattern at the scar (Timor-Tritsch, 2012). Mimics include a spontaneous expelling abortus or a cervicoisthmic implantation. To help differentiate these, inability to displace or propel the gestational sac from its position using gentle pressure applied by the endovaginal probe suggests implantation (Jurkovic, 2003; Moschos, 2008a).

For management, insights into the pathogenesis of CSPs are providing new options. Namely, growing evidence suggests that some of these pregnancies will not behave as a typical ectopic pregnancy, and thus rates of rupture and bleeding are lower. Instead, CSPs are thought by some to be a precursor of morbidly adherent placenta (Rac, 2016; Timor-Tritsch, 2014). As such, a significant percentage of affected pregnancies will progress to a viable-aged neonate, albeit with the complications associated with placenta accreta (Cali, 2018; Timor-Tritsch, 2015). These include preterm delivery, hemorrhage, and hysterectomy.

With expectant care of CSPs, one systematic review of 69 patients found that uterine rupture or dehiscence complicated 10 percent of all cases (Cali, 2018). During the first or second trimester, hysterectomy was performed in 15 percent. For the 40 patients progressing to the third trimester, 17 had placenta percreta, 23 patients underwent hysterectomy, and two patients had uterine rupture or dehiscence. For all trimesters, 60 percent of cases ultimately underwent hysterectomy. More reassuringly, in early pregnancies without cardiac activity, 70 percent had uncomplicated miscarriage, whereas 30 percent required surgical or medical intervention. None required hysterectomy. Thus, women accepting expectant care are ideally well counseled on these potential obstetric complications.

Patients may prefer to avoid these risks and seek pregnancy termination. From one literature review, the most successful interventions include: (1) laparoscopic uterine isthmic resection; (2) transvaginal resection of the isthmus through an anterior colpotomy, created similarly to anterior entry during vaginal hysterectomy; (3) uterine artery embolization (UAE) followed by D & C with or without hysteroscopy; and (4) hysteroscopic resection (Birch Petersen, 2016; Wang, 2014). In some instances, hysterectomy is required or may be elected in those not desiring future fertility (Hudeck, 2014; Sadeghi, 2010).

Medical management is an option for those hoping to avoid surgery. However, compared with surgery, pregnancy resolution rates are more varied. In one systematic review, local MTX injection alone provided a success rate of approximately 60 percent, and systemic plus local MTX injection raised the rate to nearly 80 percent (Maheaux-Lacroix, 2017). More recently, a novel double-balloon catheter, in which the balloons lie in tandem, has been used in a few case series (Monteagudo, 2018; Timor-Tritsch, 2016). The cephalad balloon tightly fills the endometrial cavity to prevent device expulsion, whereas the lower balloon interrupts the CSP via mechanical pressure and tamponades any potential bleeding.

Subsequent normal pregnancies can follow CSP, but recurrence rates are high. In one recent series of ten subsequent pregnancies in women with a prior CSP, four were recurrent CSPs (Grechukhina, 2018).

INTERSTITIAL PREGNANCY

This ectopic pregnancy implants within the proximal tubal segment that lies within the muscular uterine wall. Swelling lateral to the insertion of the round ligament is the characteristic anatomic finding (Fig. 7-10). Incorrectly, these are sometimes called *cornual pregnancies*, but this term correctly describes conceptions that develop in the horns of uteri with müllerian anomalies (Moawad, 2010). Cornual pregnancies are described in Chapter 19 (p. 422). In the past, interstitial conceptions classically ruptured later than pregnancies found in other tubal portions. This is attributed to the greater distensibility of the myometrium covering the fallopian tube's interstitial segment. Risk factors are similar to those for other ectopic locations, although prior ipsilateral salpingectomy is a specific risk factor for interstitial pregnancy (Lau, 1999).

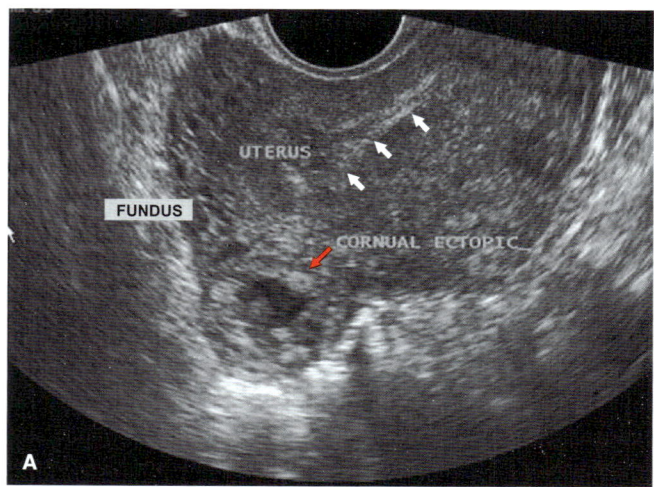
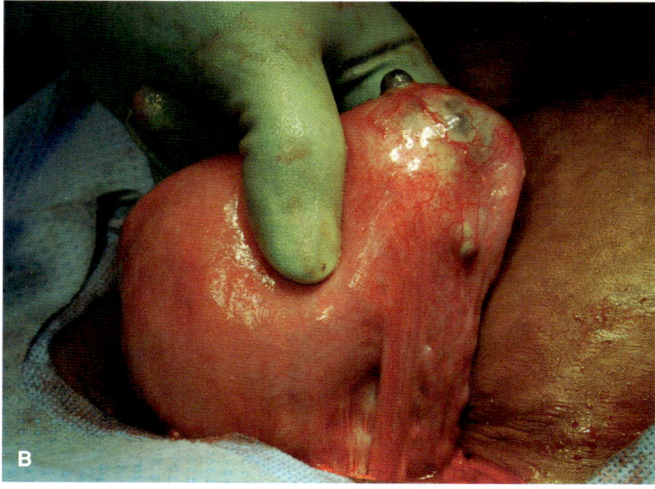

FIGURE 7-10 Interstitial pregnancy. **A.** Transvaginal sonogram, parasagittal view showing an empty uterine cavity (*white arrows*) and a mass lateral to the uterine fundus (*red arrow*). (Reproduced with permission from Dr. Elysia Moschos.) **B.** Interstitial pregnancy prior to resection. (Reproduced with permission from Dr. Mario Castellanos.)

Distinct from interstitial pregnancy, the term *angular pregnancy* describes intrauterine implantation in one of the lateral angles of the uterus and medial to the uterotubal junction and round ligament. This distinction is important because angular pregnancies can sometimes be carried to term but have a greater risk of abnormal placentation or uterine rupture late in pregnancy (Arleo, 2014; Jansen, 1981).

Diagnostically, symptoms of interstitial pregnancy mirror those of pregnancies at other tubal sites. Sonographically, criteria include a gestational sac that lies outside the endometrial cavity and >1 cm away from the endometrium. The sac is intramyometrial but is covered only by a <5-mm muscular mantle. Last, an echogenic line, known as the *interstitial line sign*, may be seen extending between the gestational sac and endometrial cavity and most likely represents the interstitial portion of the fallopian tube (Ackerman, 1993; Timor-Tritsch, 1992). Improved imaging from 3-dimensional sonography may help differentiate angular and interstitial gestations (Tanaka, 2014).

For interstitial pregnancies, surgical management involves cornual resection or evacuation by laparotomy or laparoscopy (Chap. 43, p. 947). Rather than conservative management with MTX, surgery is often preferred because of the proximity of these pregnancies to both the uterine and ovarian arteries. Hemorrhage with rupture can be severe and is associated with mortality rates as high as 2.5 percent (Tulandi, 2004). Also, although the risk of recurrence in a subsequent pregnancy is rare, cornuectomy has the lowest associated rates (Egger, 2017).

If elected, MTX can be administered in several routes. Jermy and colleagues (2004) reported a 94-percent success with systemic IM MTX using a dose of 50 mg/m^2 BSA (see Table 7-3). Others employ a traditional multidose MTX regimen (Hiersch, 2014). Direct MTX injection into the gestational sac also offers comparable success (Framarino-dei-Malatesta, 2014).

Last, uterine artery MTX infusion and then embolization—"chemoembolization"—combined with systemic methotrexate has shown promise (Krissi, 2014).

Following either medical or conservative surgical management, the risk of uterine rupture with subsequent pregnancies is unclear. Several small case series describe no uterine rupture in women delivering vaginally (Hoyos, 2019; Ng, 2009; Tulandi, 2004). In our and others' experiences, rupture rates are higher (Liao, 2017; Kim, 2017; Svenningsen, 2019). Thus, careful observation of these women during pregnancy, along with consideration of elective cesarean delivery, is reasonable.

CERVICAL PREGNANCY

This ectopic pregnancy location is rare, and risk factors are ART and prior D & C (Ginsburg, 1994; Hung, 1996). For cervical pregnancy confirmation, cervical glands must be found opposite the placental attachment site. Also, at least a portion of the placenta is located below the entrance of the uterine vessels or below the peritoneal reflection on the anterior and posterior uterine surface (Rubin, 1911). Sonographic criteria are shown in Figure 7-11.

For most hemodynamically stable women with a first-trimester cervical pregnancy, nonsurgical management with either single- or multidose systemic MTX can be administered (see Table 7-3) (Murji, 2015). Alternatively, 50 mg of MTX can be injected directly into the gestational sac (Jeng, 2007; Yamaguchi, 2017). Others describe MTX chemoembolization, as just described for interstitial pregnancy (Xiaolin, 2010). Higher risk of systemic MTX treatment failure is noted in those with a gestational age >9 weeks, β-hCG levels >10,000 IU/L, and fetal cardiac activity (Hung, 1996). For this reason, many induce fetal death with injection of potassium chloride (KCL)

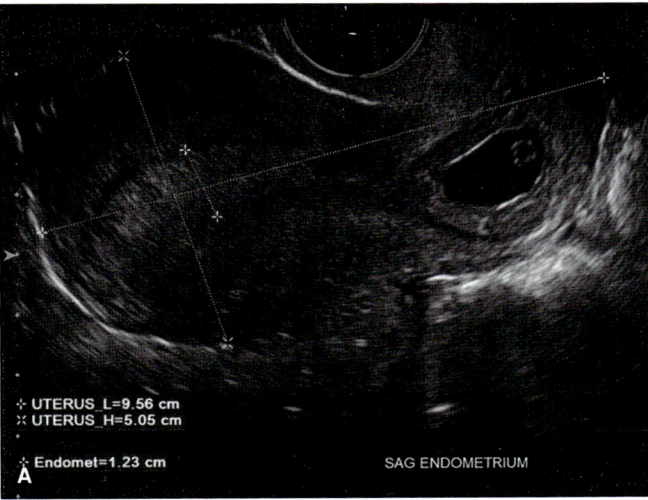 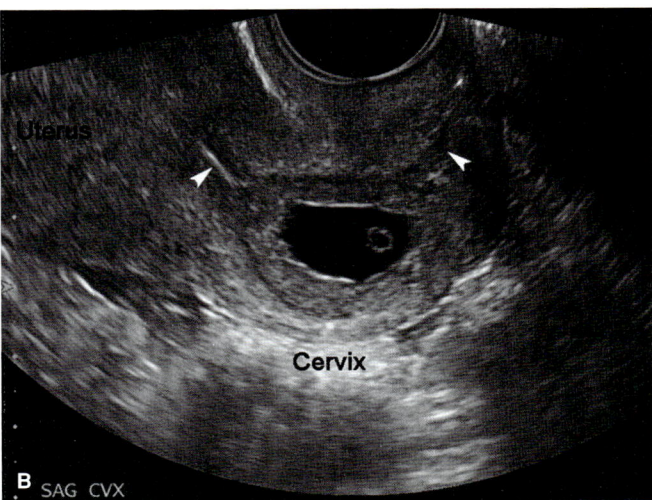

FIGURE 7-11 Cervical pregnancy. **A.** Transvaginal sonography, sagittal view of a uterus containing a cervical pregnancy. Calipers mark the uterine length and depth and endometrial thickness. Sonographic findings with cervical pregnancy may include: (1) an hourglass uterine shape and ballooned cervical canal; (2) gestational tissue at the level of the cervix; (3) absent intrauterine gestational tissue (*inner calipers*); and (4) a portion of the endocervical canal seen interposed between the gestation and the endometrial canal. An absent "sliding sign" helps differentiate a cervical pregnancy from the transcervical passage of a miscarriage. With the maneuver, gentle pressure is applied to the cervix by the vaginal probe, and the gestation sac of an abortus will move or slide against the endocervical canal. This will not be seen in an implanted cervical pregnancy. **B.** In this sonogram of the same cervix, a portion of the endocervical canal (*white arrowheads*) is seen on either side of the gestational sac. (Reproduced with permission from Dr. Angela R. Seasley.)

into the fetus or gestational sac (Jeng, 2007; Verma, 2009). One option is 1 mL of 2 mEq/mL KCL. UAE may be valuable to treat bleeding complications.

Although conservative management is feasible for many women with cervical pregnancies, surgical intervention also may be selected. Procedures include suction evacuation or hysterectomy. Moreover, in those with advanced gestations or with bleeding uncontrolled by conservative methods, hysterectomy is typically required. Prior to either procedure, UAE may be considered to limit intra- and postoperative bleeding (Hu, 2016; Trambert, 2005).

If suction evacuation is selected, dilatation is not required and incites brisk bleeding, as does sharp curettage. Aside from UAE, intraoperative hemorrhage can also be lessened by intracervical vasopressin injection or by a cerclage placed at the internal cervical os to compress feeding vessels (Ishikawa, 2016; Trojano, 2009). Also, cervical branches of the uterine artery can effectively be ligated with vaginal placement of hemostatic cervical sutures on the lateral aspects of the cervix at 3 and 9 o'clock (Bianchi, 2011). Following suctioning, in the event of hemorrhage, a 26F Foley catheter with a 30-mL balloon or the double-balloon catheter described earlier can be inflated to effect hemostasis and to monitor bloody drainage (p. 172) (Fylstra, 2014). The balloon remains inflated for 24 hours and is gradually deflated. In addition, UAE may be considered.

OVARIAN PREGNANCY

Ectopic implantation of the fertilized egg in the ovary is rare and is diagnosed if four clinical criteria are met. These include: (1) the ipsilateral tube is intact and distinct from the ovary; (2) the ectopic pregnancy occupies the ovary; (3) the ectopic pregnancy is connected by the ovarian ligament to the uterus; and (4) ovarian tissue can be demonstrated histologically in the placental tissue (Spiegelberg, 1878). Of risk factors, IVF and IUD use are prominent (Zhu, 2014).

In one review of 100 cases, nearly a third of women presented with hemodynamic instability because of rupture (Ko, 2012). In unruptured cases, the classic sonographic description is that of a cyst with a wide echogenic outer ring on or within the ovary. This may mimic a corpus luteum cyst (Comstock, 2005).

These pregnancies are managed surgically. With smaller ectopic pregnancies, ovarian wedging can be considered (Raziel, 2004). For larger or significantly ruptured lesions, oophorectomy is often required.

HETEROTOPIC PREGNANCY

A uterine pregnancy in conjunction with an extrauterine pregnancy is termed a *heterotopic pregnancy*. The natural incidence of these heterotopic pregnancies approximates 1 per 30,000 pregnancies (Reece, 1983). ART is one risk factor, and the heterotopic pregnancy rate approximates 9 per 10,000 in ART-treated women (Perkins, 2015). MTX is contraindicated due to the detrimental effects on the normal pregnancy (p. 169). Thus, most tubal pregnancies are excised surgically.

OTHER ECTOPIC PREGNANCY SITES

Abdominal pregnancy forms from implantation in the peritoneal cavity. This may result from primary implantation or may develop following tubal abortion and subsequent peritoneal implantation. Other less expected sites have been described in case reports and include the omentum, liver, and retroperitoneum, among others (Brouard, 2015; Liang, 2014; Watrowski, 2015).

A tubal pregnancy implanted toward the mesosalpinx may rupture into a space formed between the leaves of the broad ligament to become an *intraligamentous* or *broad ligament pregnancy*. Rents in prior cesarean scars serve as another conduit into this space (Rudra, 2013).

Intramural uterine pregnancies form at sites other than a cesarean scar, and risk factors are prior uterine surgeries, ART, or adenomyosis (Kirk, 2013; Memtsa, 2013). Clinically, these pregnancies can mimic invasive gestational trophoblastic tissue.

Rarely, ectopic pregnancies have been reported in women with prior hysterectomy (Fylstra, 2010). Presumably, a vaginal cuff fistula, a prolapsed fallopian tube, or a cervical stump allows sperm to access an ovulated ovum. For all these unique locations, surgical excision is generally required.

REFERENCES

Ackerman TE, Levi CS, Dashefsky SM, et al: Interstitial line: sonographic finding in interstitial (cornual) ectopic pregnancy. Radiology 189(1):83, 1993

Agostini A, Blanc K, Ronda I, et al: Prognostic value of human chorionic gonadotropin changes after methotrexate injection for ectopic pregnancy. Fertil Steril 88(2):504, 2007

al-Awwad MM, al Daham N, Eseet JS: Spontaneous unruptured bilateral ectopic pregnancy: conservative tubal surgery. Obstet Gynecol Surv 54:543, 1999

American College of Obstetricians and Gynecologists: Tubal ectopic pregnancy. Practice Bulletin No. 193, March 2018

American Society for Reproductive Medicine: Medical treatment of ectopic pregnancy: a committee opinion. Fertil Steril 100(3):638, 2013

Arleo EK, DeFilippis EM: Cornual, interstitial, and angular pregnancies: clarifying the terms and a review of the literature. Clin Imaging 38(6):763, 2014

Barak S, Oettinger M, Perri A, et al: Frozen section examination of endometrial curettings in the diagnosis of ectopic pregnancy. Acta Obstet Gynecol Scand 84:43, 2005

Barnhart K, Hummel AC, Sammel MD, et al: Use of "2-dose" regimen of methotrexate to treat ectopic pregnancy. Fertil Steril 87(2):250, 2007

Barnhart K, Mennuti MT, Benjamin I, et al: Prompt diagnosis of ectopic pregnancy in an emergency department setting. Obstet Gynecol 84:1010, 1994

Barnhart K, Sammel MD, Chung K, et al: Decline of serum human chorionic gonadotropin and spontaneous complete abortion: defining the normal curve. Obstet Gynecol 104:975, 2004

Barnhart K, van Mello NM, Bourne T, et al: Pregnancy of unknown location: a consensus statement of nomenclature, definitions, and outcome. Fertil Steril 95(3):857, 2011

Barnhart KT, Gosman G, Ashby R, et al: The medical management of ectopic pregnancy: a meta-analysis comparing "single dose" and "multidose" regimens. Obstet Gynecol 101:778, 2003a

Barnhart KT, Gracia CR, Reindl B, et al: Usefulness of Pipelle endometrial biopsy in the diagnosis of women at risk for ectopic pregnancy. Am J Obstet Gynecol 188:906, 2003b

Barnhart KT, Katz I, Hummel A, et al: Presumed diagnosis of ectopic pregnancy. Obstet Gynecol 100:505, 2002

Barnhart KT, Rinaudo P, Hummel A, et al: Acute and chronic presentation of ectopic pregnancy may be two clinical entities. Fertil Steril 80:1345, 2003c

Barnhart KT, Sammel MD, Appleby D, et al: Does a prediction model for pregnancy of unknown location developed in the UK validate on a US population? Hum Reprod 25(10):2434, 2010

Berlin NI, Rall D, Mead JA, et al: Folic acid antagonists: effects on the cell and the patient: combined clinical staff conference at the National Institutes of Health. Ann Intern Med 59:931, 1963

Bianchi P, Salvatori MM, Torcia F, et al: Cervical pregnancy. Fertil Steril 95(6):2123, 2011

Birch Petersen K, Hoffmann E, Rifbjerg Larsen C, et al: Cesarean scar pregnancy: a systematic review of treatment studies. Fertil Steril 105:958, 2016

Birkhahn RH, Gaeta TJ, Van Deusen SK, et al: The ability of traditional vital signs and shock index to identify ruptured ectopic pregnancy. Am J Obstet Gynecol 189:1293, 2003

Bolaji II, Oktaba M, Mohee K, et al: An odyssey through salpingitis isthmica nodosa. Eur J Obstet Gynecol Reprod Biol 184:73, 2015

Bouyer J, Coste J, Fernandez H, et al: Sites of ectopic pregnancy: a 10 year population-based study of 1800 cases. Hum Reprod 17:3224, 2002

Bouyer J, Coste J, Shojaei T, et al: Risk factors for ectopic pregnancy: a comprehensive analysis based on a large case-control, population-based study in France. Am J Epidemiol 157:185, 2003

Branney SW, Wolfe RE, Moore EE, et al: Quantitative sensitivity of ultrasound in detecting free intraperitoneal fluid. J Trauma 40(6):1052, 1995

Brouard KJ, Howard BR, Dyer RA: Hepatic pregnancy suspected at term and successful delivery of a live neonate with placental attachment to the right lobe of the liver. Obstet Gynecol 126(1):207, 2015

Brown DL, Doubilet PM: Transvaginal sonography for diagnosing ectopic pregnancy: positivity criteria and performance characteristics. J Ultrasound Med 13:259, 1994

Brown DL, Felker RE, Stovall TG, et al: Serial endovaginal sonography of ectopic pregnancies treated with methotrexate. Obstet Gynecol 77:406, 1991

Burry KA, Thurmond AS, Suby-Long TD, et al: Transvaginal ultrasonographic findings in surgically verified ectopic pregnancy. Am J Obstet Gynecol 168:1796, 1993

Buster JE, Pisarska MD: Medical management of ectopic pregnancy. Clin Obstet Gynecol 42:23, 1999

Calì G, Timor-Tritsch IE, Palacios-Jaraquemada J, et al: Outcome of cesarean scar pregnancy managed expectantly: systematic review and meta-analysis. Ultrasound Obstet Gynecol 51(2):169, 2018

Cameron KE, Senapati S, Sammel MD, et al: Following declining human chorionic gonadotropin values in pregnancies of unknown location: when is it safe to stop? Fertil Steril 105(4):953, 2016

Chung K, Chandavarkar U, Opper N, et al: Reevaluating the role of dilation and curettage in the diagnosis of pregnancy of unknown location. Fertil Steril 96(3):659, 2011

Chung K, Sammel MD, Coutifaris C, et al: Defining the rise of serum HCG in viable pregnancies achieved through use of IVF. Hum Reprod 21(3):823, 2006

Cohen A, Almog B, Cohen Y, et al: The role of HCG increment in the 48h prior to methotrexate treatment as a predictor for treatment success. Eur J Obstet Gynecol Reprod Biol 211:103, 2017

Cohen A, Almog B, Satel A, et al: Laparoscopy versus laparotomy in the management of ectopic pregnancy with massive hemoperitoneum. Int J Gynaecol Obstet 123(2):139, 2013

Cohen A, Zakar L, Gil Y, et al: Methotrexate success rates in progressing ectopic pregnancies: a reappraisal. Am J Obstet Gynecol 211(2):128, 2014

Cole T, Corlett RC Jr: Chronic ectopic pregnancy. Obstet Gynecol 59(1):63, 1982

Col-Madendag I, Madendag Y, Kanat-Pektas M, et al: Can sonographic endometrial pattern be an early indicator for tubal ectopic pregnancy and related tubal rupture? Arch Gynecol Obstet 281(2):189, 2010

Comstock C, Huston K, Lee W: The ultrasonographic appearance of ovarian ectopic pregnancies. Obstet Gynecol 105:42, 2005

Connolly A, Ryan DH, Stuebe AM, et al: Reevaluation of discriminatory and threshold levels for serum β-hCG in early pregnancy. Obstet Gynecol 121(1):65, 2013

Conway R, Low C, Coughlan RJ, et al: Risk of liver injury among methotrexate users: a meta-analysis of randomised controlled trials. Semin Arthritis Rheum 45(2):156, 2015

Coste J, Fernandez H, Joye N, et al: Role of chromosome abnormalities in ectopic pregnancy. Fertil Steril 74:1259, 2000

Creanga AA, Shapiro-Mendoza CK, Bish CL, et al: Trends in ectopic pregnancy mortality in the United States: 1980–2007. Obstet Gynecol 117(4):837, 2011

Creanga AA, Syverson C, Seed K, et al: Pregnancy-related mortality in the United States, 2011–2013. Obstet Gynecol 130(2):366, 2017

Dai Y, Zhang G, Zhu L, et al: Routine β-human chorionic gonadotropin monitoring for single-dose methotrexate treatment in ectopic pregnancy. J Minim Invasive Gynecol 24(7):1195, 2017

Dashefsky SM, Lyons EA, Levi CS, et al: Suspected ectopic pregnancy: endovaginal and transvesical US. Radiology 169:181, 1988

de Bennetot M, Rabischong B, Aublet-Cuvelier B, et al: Fertility after tubal ectopic pregnancy: results of a population-based study. Fertil Steril 98(5):1271, 2012

Demirdag E, Guler I, Abay S, et al: The impact of expectant management, systemic methotrexate and surgery on subsequent pregnancy outcomes in tubal ectopic pregnancy. Ir J Med Sci 186(2):387, 2017

Desai D, Lu J, Wyness SP, et al: Human chorionic gonadotropin discriminatory zone in ectopic pregnancy: does assay harmonization matter? Fertil Steril 101(6):1671, 2014

Dias Pereira G, Hajenius PJ, Mol BW, et al: Fertility outcome after systemic methotrexate and laparoscopic salpingostomy for tubal pregnancy. Lancet 353(9154):724, 1999

Du T, Chen H, Fu R, et al: Comparison of ectopic pregnancy risk among transfers of embryos vitrified on day 3, day 5, and day 6. Fertil Steril 108(1):108, 2017

Dudley PS, Heard MJ, Sangi-Haghpeykar H, et al: Characterizing ectopic pregnancies that rupture despite treatment with methotrexate. Fertil Steril 82(5):1374, 2004

Egger E: Recurrent interstitial pregnancy: a review of the literature. Geburtshilfe Frauenheilkd 77(4):335, 2017

Elson J, Tailor A, Banerjee S, et al: Expectant management of tubal ectopic pregnancy: prediction of successful outcome using decision tree analysis. Ultrasound Obstet Gynecol 23:552, 2004

Erol O, Suren D, Unal B, et al: Significance of trophoblastic infiltration into the tubal wall in ampullary pregnancy. Int J Surg Pathol 23(4):271, 2015

Fang C, Huang R, Wei LN, et al: Frozen-thawed day 5 blastocyst transfer is associated with a lower risk of ectopic pregnancy than day 3 transfer and fresh transfer. Fertil Steril 103(3):655, 2015

Fernandez H, Capmas P, Lucot JP, et al: Fertility after ectopic pregnancy: the DEMETER randomized trial. Human Reprod 28(5):1247, 2013

Framarino-dei-Malatesta M, Piccioni MG, Derme M, et al: Transabdominal ultrasound-guided injection of methotrexate in the treatment of ectopic interstitial pregnancies. J Clin Ultrasound 42(9):522, 2014

Fu J, Henne MB, Blumstein S, et al: Rupture of ectopic pregnancy with minimally detectable beta-human chorionic gonadotropin levels: a report of 2 cases. J Reprod Med 52(6):541, 2007

Fylstra DL: Cervical pregnancy: 13 cases treated with suction curettage and balloon tamponade. Am J Obstet Gynecol 210(6):581.e1, 2014

Fylstra DL: Ectopic pregnancy after hysterectomy: a review and insight into etiology and prevention. Fertil Steril 94(2):431, 2010

Ginsburg ES, Frates MC, Rein MS, et al: Early diagnosis and treatment of cervical pregnancy in an in vitro fertilization program. Fertil Steril 61(5):966, 1994

Glezerman M, Press F, Carpman M: Culdocentesis is an obsolete diagnostic tool in suspected ectopic pregnancy. Arch Gynecol Obstet 252(1):5, 1992

Graczykowski JW, Mishell DR Jr.: Methotrexate prophylaxis for persistent ectopic pregnancy after conservative treatment by salpingostomy. Obstet Gynecol 89(1):118, 1997

Graczykowski JW, Seifer DB: Diagnosis of acute and persistent ectopic pregnancy. Clin Obstet Gynecol 42(1):9, 1999

Grechukhina O, Deshmukh U, Fan L, et al: Cesarean scar pregnancy, incidence, and recurrence: five-year experience at a single tertiary care referral center. Obstet Gynecol 132(5):1285, 2018

Greene DN, Grenache DG, Education Committee of the Academy of Clinical Laboratory Physicians and Scientist: Pathology consultation on human chorionic gonadotropin testing for pregnancy assessment. Am J Clin Pathol 144(5):830, 2015

Guha S, Ayim F, Ludlow J, et al: Triaging pregnancies of unknown location: the performance of protocols based on single serum progesterone or repeated serum hCG levels. Human Reprod 29(5):938, 2014

Gurel S, Sarikaya B, Gurel K, et al: Role of sonography in the diagnosis of ectopic pregnancy. J Clin Ultrasound 35(9):509, 2007

Hajenius PJ, Engelsbel S, Mol BW, et al: Randomised trial of systemic methotrexate versus laparoscopic salpingostomy in tubal pregnancy. Lancet 350:774, 1997

Hackmon R, Sakaguchi S, Koren G: Effect of methotrexate treatment of ectopic pregnancy on subsequent pregnancy. Can Fam Physician 57(1):37, 2011

Heinemann K, Reed S, Moehner S, et al: Comparative contraceptive effectiveness of levonorgestrel-releasing and copper intrauterine devices: the European Active Surveillance Study for Intrauterine Devices. Contraception 91(4):280, 2015

Helmy S, Sawyer E, Ofili-Yebovi D, et al: Fertility outcomes following expectant management of tubal ectopic pregnancy. Ultrasound Obstet Gynecol 30(7):988, 2007

Hiersch L, Krissi H, Ashwal E, et al: Effectiveness of medical treatment with methotrexate for interstitial pregnancy. Aust N Z J Obstet Gynaecol 54(6):576, 2014

Hill MJ, Cooper JC, Levy G, et al: Ovarian reserve and subsequent assisted reproduction outcomes after methotrexate therapy for ectopic pregnancy or pregnancy of unknown location. Fertil Steril 101(2):413, 2014

Hillis SD, Owens LM, Marchbanks PA, et al: Recurrent chlamydial infections increase the risks of hospitalization for ectopic pregnancy and pelvic inflammatory disease. Am J Obstet Gynecol 176(1 pt 1):103, 1997

Hoffman BL: Ectopic pregnancy. In Cunningham FG, Leveno KJ, Bloom SL (eds): Williams Obstetrics, 25th ed. New York, McGraw-Hill Education, 2018, p 373

Hoover RN, Hyer M, Pfeiffer RM, et al: Adverse health outcomes in women exposed in utero to diethylstilbestrol. N Engl J Med 365(14):1304, 2011

Hoyos LR, Vilchez G, Allsworth JE, et al: Outcomes in subsequent pregnancies after wedge resection for interstitial ectopic pregnancy: a retrospective cohort study. J Matern Fetal Neonatal Med 32(14):2354, 2019

Hu J, Tao X, Yin L, et al: Successful conservative treatment of cervical pregnancy with uterine artery embolization followed by curettage: a report of 19 cases. BJOG 123(3 suppl):97, 2016

Hudecek R, Felsingerova Z, Felsinger M, et al: Laparoscopic treatment of cesarean scar ectopic pregnancy. J Gynecol Surg 30(5):309, 2014

Hung TH, Jeng CJ, Yang YC, et al: Treatment of cervical pregnancy with methotrexate. Int J Gynaecol Obstet 53:243, 1996

Hyoun SC, Običan SG, Scialli AR: Teratogen update: methotrexate. Birth Defects Res A Clin Mol Teratol 94(4):187, 2012

Insogna IG, Farland LV, Missmer SA, et al: Outpatient endometrial aspiration: an alternative to methotrexate for pregnancy of unknown location. Am J Obstet Gynecol 217(2):185.e1, 2017

Irani M, Robles A, Gunnala V, et al: Unilateral salpingectomy and methotrexate are associated with a similar recurrence rate of ectopic pregnancy in patients undergoing in vitro fertilization. J Minim Invasive Gynecol 24(5):777, 2017

Ishikawa H, Unno Y, Omoto A, et al: Local injection of diluted vasopressin followed by suction curettage for cervical ectopic pregnancy. Eur J Obstet Gynecol Reprod Biol 207:173, 2016

Jansen RP, Elliott PM: Angular intrauterine pregnancy. Obstet Gynecol 58(2):167, 1981

Jeng CJ, Ko ML, Shen J: Transvaginal ultrasound-guided treatment of cervical pregnancy. Obstet Gynecol 109(5):1076, 2007

Jermy K, Thomas J, Doo A, et al: The conservative management of interstitial pregnancy. BJOG 111:1283, 2004

Jurkovic D, Hillaby K, Woelfer B, et al: First-trimester diagnosis and management of pregnancies implanted into the lower uterine segment cesarean section scar. Ultrasound Obstet Gynecol 21(3):220, 2003

Jurkovic D, Memtsa M, Sawyer E, et al: Single-dose systemic methotrexate vs expectant management for treatment of tubal ectopic pregnancy: a placebo-controlled randomized trial. Ultrasound Obstet Gynecol 49(2):171, 2017

Kadar N, DeCherney AH, Romero R: Receiver operating characteristic (ROC) curve analysis of the relative efficacy of single and serial chorionic gonadotropin determinations in the early diagnosis of ectopic pregnancy. Fertil Steril 37:542, 1982

Kim MJ, Cha JH, Bae HS, et al: Therapeutic outcomes of methotrexate injection in unruptured interstitial pregnancy. Obstet Gynecol Sci 60(6):571, 2017

Kirk E, Condous G, Van Calster B, et al: A validation of the most commonly used protocol to predict the success of single-dose methotrexate in the treatment of ectopic pregnancy. Hum Reprod 22(3):858, 2007

Kirk E, McDonald K, Rees J, et al: Intramural ectopic pregnancy: a case and review of the literature. Eur J Obstet Gynecol Reprod Biol 168(2):129, 2013

Kirk E, Van Calster B, Condous G, et al: Ectopic pregnancy: using the hCG ratio to select women for expectant or medical management. Acta Obstet Gynecol Scand 90(3):264, 2011

Ko JK, Cheung VY: Time to revisit the human chorionic gonadotropin discriminatory level in the management of pregnancy of unknown location. J Ultrasound Med 33(3):465, 2014

Ko PC, Lo LM, Hsieh TT, et al: Twenty-one years of experience with ovarian ectopic pregnancy at one institution in Taiwan. Int J Gynaecol Obstet 119(2):154, 2012

Krag Moeller LB, Moeller C, Thomsen SG, et al: Success and spontaneous pregnancy rates following systemic methotrexate versus laparoscopic surgery for tubal pregnancies: a randomized trial. Acta Obstet Gynecol Scand 88(12):1331, 2009

Krause HG, Goh JT: Positive Kleihauer result following an ectopic pregnancy. Aust N Z J Obstet Gynaecol 36(3):324, 1996

Krissi H, Hiersch L, Stolovitch N, et al: Outcome, complications and future fertility in women treated with uterine artery embolization and methotrexate for non-tubal ectopic pregnancy. Eur J Obstet Gynecol Reprod Biol 182:172, 2014

Kutluay L, Vicdan K, Turan C, et al: Tubal histopathology in ectopic pregnancies. Eur J Obstet Gynecol Reprod Biol 57:91, 1994

Lau S, Tulandi T: Conservative medical and surgical management of interstitial ectopic pregnancy. Fertil Steril 72:207, 1999

Lavie O, Boldes R, Neuman M, et al: Ultrasonographic "endometrial three-layer" pattern: a unique finding in ectopic pregnancy. J Clin Ultrasound 24(4):179, 1996

Levine D: Ectopic pregnancy. Radiology 245(2):385, 2007

Li C, Zhao WH, Meng CX, et al: Contraceptive use and the risk of ectopic pregnancy: a multi-center case-control study. PLoS One 9(12):e115031, 2014a

Li C, Zhao WH, Zhu Q, et al: Risk factors for ectopic pregnancy: a multi-center case-control study. BMC Pregnancy Childbirth 15:187, 2015a

Li J, Jiang K, Zhao F: Fertility outcome analysis after surgical management of tubal ectopic pregnancy: a retrospective cohort study. BMJ Open 5(9):e007339, 2015b

Li Y, Yang Y, He QZ, et al: Frozen section of uterine curetting in excluding the possibility of ectopic pregnancy—a clinicopathologic study of 715 cases. Clin Exp Obstet Gynecol 41(4):419, 2014b

Liang C, Li X, Zhao B, et al: Demonstration of the route of embryo migration in retroperitoneal ectopic pregnancy using contrast-enhanced computed tomography. J Obstet Gynaecol Res 40(3):849, 2014

Liao CY, Tse J, Sung SY, et al: Cornual wedge resection for interstitial pregnancy and postoperative outcome. Aust N Z J Obstet Gynaecol 57(3):342, 2017

Lipscomb GH: Medical therapy for ectopic pregnancy. Semin Reprod Med 25(2):93, 2007

Lipscomb GH, Bran D, McCord ML, et al: Analysis of three hundred fifteen ectopic pregnancies treated with single-dose methotrexate. Am J Obstet Gynecol 178:1354, 1998

Lipscomb GH, Givens VM, Meyer NL, et al: Comparison of multidose and single-dose methotrexate protocols for the treatment of ectopic pregnancy. Am J Obstet Gynecol 192:1844, 2005

Lipscomb GH, McCord ML, Stovall TG, et al: Predictors of success of methotrexate treatment in women with tubal ectopic pregnancies. N Engl J Med 341:1974, 1999

Londra L, Moreau C, Strobino D, et al: Ectopic pregnancy after in vitro fertilization: differences between fresh and frozen-thawed cycles. Fertil Steril 104(1):110, 2015

Lopez HB, Micheelsen U, Berendtsen H, et al: Ectopic pregnancy and its associated endometrial changes. Gynecol Obstet Invest 38:104, 1994

Lund CO, Nilas L, Bangsgaard N, et al: Persistent ectopic pregnancy after linear salpingotomy: a non-predictable complication to conservative surgery for tubal gestation. Acta Obstet Gynecol Scand 81(11):1053, 2002

Lundorff P, Thorburn J, Hahlin M, et al: Laparoscopic surgery in ectopic pregnancy. A randomized trial versus laparotomy. Acta Obstet Gynecol Scand 70:343, 1991

Maheux-Lacroix S, Li F, Bujold E, et al: Cesarean scar pregnancies: a systematic review of treatment options. J Minim Invasive Gynecol 24(6):915, 2017

Malacova E, Kemp A, Hart R, et al: Long-term risk of ectopic pregnancy varies by method of tubal sterilization: a whole-population study. Fertil Steril 101(3):728, 2014

Mavrelos D, Memtsa M, Helmy S, et al: β-hCG resolution times during expectant management of tubal ectopic pregnancies. BMC Womens Health 15:43, 2015

Mavrelos D, Nicks H, Jamil A, et al: Efficacy and safety of a clinical protocol for expectant management of selected women diagnosed with a tubal ectopic pregnancy. Ultrasound Obstet Gynecol 42(1):102, 2013

Mehta TS, Levine D, Beckwith B: Treatment of ectopic pregnancy: is a human chorionic gonadotropin level of 2000 mIU/mL a reasonable threshold? Radiology 205:569, 1997

Memtsa M, Jamil A, Sebire N, et al: Rarity revisited: diagnosis and management of intramural ectopic pregnancy. Ultrasound Obstet Gynecol 42(3):359, 2013

Mergenthal MC, Senapati S, Zee J, et al: Medical management of ectopic pregnancy with single-dose and 2-dose methotrexate protocols: human chorionic gonadotropin trends and patient outcomes. Am J Obstet Gynecol 215(5):590.e1, 2016

Milad MP, Klein E, Kazer RR: Preoperative serum hCG level and intraoperative failure of laparoscopic linear salpingostomy for ectopic pregnancy. Obstet Gynecol 92:373, 1998

Moawad NS, Mahajan ST, Moniz MH, et al: Current diagnosis and treatment of interstitial pregnancy. Am J Obstet Gynecol 202(1):15, 2010

Mol F, Mol BW, Ankum WM, et al: Current evidence on surgery, systemic methotrexate and expectant management in the treatment of tubal ectopic pregnancy: a systematic review and meta-analysis. Hum Reprod Update 14(4):309, 2008

Mol F, van Mello NM, Strandell A, et al: Salpingotomy versus salpingectomy in women with tubal pregnancy (ESEP study): an open-label, multicentre, randomised controlled trial. Lancet 383(9927):1483, 2014

Monteagudo A, Calì G, Rebarber A, et al: Minimally invasive treatment of cesarean scar and cervical pregnancies using a cervical ripening double balloon catheter: expanding the clinical series. J Ultrasound Med 38(3):785, 2018

Morse CB, Sammel MD, Shaunik A, et al: Performance of human chorionic gonadotropin curves in women at risk for ectopic pregnancy: exceptions to the rules. Fertil Steril 97(1):101, 2012

Moschos E, Sreenarasimhaiah S, Twickler DM: First-trimester diagnosis of cesarean scar ectopic pregnancy. J Clin Ultrasound 36(8):504, 2008a

Moschos E, Twickler DM: Endometrial thickness predicts intrauterine pregnancy in patients with pregnancy of unknown location. Ultrasound Obstet Gynecol 32(7):929, 2008b

Murji A, Garbedian K, Thomas J, et al: Conservative management of cervical ectopic pregnancy. J Obstet Gynaecol Can 37(11):1016, 2015

Murphy AA, Nager CW, Wujek JJ, et al: Operative laparoscopy versus laparotomy for the management of ectopic pregnancy: a prospective trial. Fertil Steril 57:1180, 1992

Nadim B, Infante F, Lu C, et al: The morphological ultrasound types known as "blob" and "bagel" signs should be reclassified from probable to definite ectopic pregnancy. Ultrasound Obstet Gynecol 51:543, 2018

Natale A, Candiani M, Merlo D, et al: Human chorionic gonadotropin level as a predictor of trophoblastic infiltration into the tubal wall in ectopic pregnancy: a blinded study. Fertil Steril 79:981, 2003

Nathorst-Böös J, Rafik Hamad R: Risk factors for persistent trophoblastic activity after surgery for ectopic pregnancy. Acta Obstet Gynecol Scand 83(5):471 2004

Ng S, Hamontri S, Chua I, et al: Laparoscopic management of 53 cases of cornual ectopic pregnancy. Fertil Steril 92:448, 2009

Nguyen Q, Kapitz M, Downes K, et al: Are early human chorionic gonadotropin levels after methotrexate therapy a predictor of response in ectopic pregnancy? Am J Obstet Gynecol 202(6):630.e1, 2010

Nurmohamed L, Moretti ME, Schechter T, et al: Outcome following high-dose methotrexate in pregnancies misdiagnosed as ectopic. Am J Obstet Gynecol 205(6):533.e1, 2011

Nyberg DA, Hughes MP, Mack LA, et al: Extrauterine findings of ectopic pregnancy of transvaginal US: importance of echogenic fluid. Radiology 178:823, 1991

Ohannessian A, Loundou A, Courbière B, et al: Ovarian responsiveness in women receiving fertility treatment after methotrexate for ectopic pregnancy: a systematic review and meta-analysis. Hum Reprod 29(9):1949, 2014

Paul M, Schaff E, Nichols M: The roles of clinical assessment, human chorionic gonadotropin assays, and ultrasonography in medical abortion practice. Am J Obstet Gynecol 183:S34, 2000

Perkins KM, Boulet SL, Kissin DM, et al: Risk of ectopic pregnancy associated with assisted reproductive technology in the United States, 2001–2011. Obstet Gynecol 125(1):70, 2015

Perkins RB, Morgan JR, Awosogba TP, et al: Gynecologic outcomes after hysteroscopic and laparoscopic sterilization procedures. Obstet Gynecol 128(4):843, 2016

Peterson HB, Xia Z, Hughes JM, et al: The risk of ectopic pregnancy after tubal sterilization. U.S. Collaborative Review of Sterilization Working Group. N Engl J Med 336(11):762, 1997

Polena V, Huchon C, Varas Ramos C, et al: Non-invasive tools for the diagnosis of potentially life-threatening gynaecological emergencies: a systematic review. PLoS One 10(2):e0114189, 2015

Rac MW, Moschos E, Wells CE, et al: Sonographic findings of morbidly adherent placenta in the first trimester. J Ultrasound Med 35(2):263, 2016

Raziel A, Schachter M, Mordechai E, et al: Ovarian pregnancy-a 12-year experience of 19 cases in one institution. Eur J Obstet Gynecol Reprod Biol 114(1):92, 2004

Reece EA, Petrie RH, Sirmans MF, et al: Combined intrauterine and extrauterine gestations: a review. Am J Obstet Gynecol 146:323, 1983

Rheumatoid Arthritis Clinical Trial Archive Group: The effect of age and renal function on the efficacy and toxicity of methotrexate in rheumatoid arthritis. J Rheumatol 22(2):218, 1995

Rodgerson JD, Heegaard WG, Plummer D, et al: Emergency department right upper quadrant ultrasound is associated with a reduced time to diagnosis and treatment of ruptured ectopic pregnancies. Acad Emerg Med 8(4):331, 2001

Rotas MA, Haberman S, Levgur M: Cesarean scar ectopic pregnancies: etiology, diagnosis, and management. Obstet Gynecol 107(6):1373, 2006

Rubin IC: Cervical pregnancy. Surg Gynecol Obstet 13:625, 1911

Rudra S, Gupta S, Taneja BK, et al: Full term broad ligament pregnancy through a cesarean scar. Obstet Gynecol Sci 56(6):404, 2013

Rulin MC: Is salpingostomy the surgical treatment of choice for unruptured tubal pregnancy? Obstet Gynecol 86:1010, 1995

Sadeghi H, Rutherford T, Rackow BW: Cesarean scar ectopic pregnancy: case series and review of the literature. Am J Perinatol 27(2):111, 2010

Sagiv R, Debby A, Sadan O, et al: Laparoscopic surgery for extrauterine pregnancy in hemodynamically unstable patients. J Am Assoc Gynecol Laparosc 8:529, 2001

Salliot C, van der Heijde D: Long-term safety of methotrexate monotherapy in patients with rheumatoid arthritis: a systematic literature research. Ann Rheum Dis 68:1100, 2009

Saraiya M, Berg CJ, Kendrick JS, et al: Cigarette smoking as a risk factor for ectopic pregnancy. Am J Obstet Gynecol 178:493, 1998

Saraj AJ, Wilcox JG, Najmabadi S, et al: Resolution of hormonal markers of ectopic gestation: a randomized trial comparing single-dose intramuscular methotrexate with salpingostomy. Obstet Gynecol 92:989, 1998

Seeber BE, Sammel MD, Guo W, et al: Application of redefined human chorionic gonadotropin curves for the diagnosis of women at risk for ectopic pregnancy. Fertil Steril 86(2):454, 2006

Senterman M, Jibodh R, Tulandi T: Histopathologic study of ampullary and isthmic tubal ectopic pregnancy. Am J Obstet Gynecol 159:939, 1988

Seow KM, Huang LW, Lin YH, et al: Cesarean scar pregnancy: issues in management. Ultrasound Obstet Gynecol 23:247, 2004

Shalev E, Peleg D, Tsabari A, et al: Spontaneous resolution of ectopic tubal pregnancy: natural history. Fertil Steril 63:15, 1995

Shaunik A, Kulp J, Appleby DH, et al: Utility of dilation and curettage in the diagnosis of pregnancy of unknown location. Am J Obstet Gynecol 204(2): 130.e1, 2011

Shaw JL, Dey SK, Critchley HO, et al: Current knowledge of the aetiology of human tubal ectopic pregnancy. Hum Reprod Update 16(4):432, 2010

Shao SC, Yang YH, Chien PS, et al: Methotrexate-induced pancytopenia in a patient with ectopic pregnancy. Arch Med Sci 14(2):475, 2018

Silva C, Sammel MD, Zhou L, et al: Human chorionic gonadotropin profile for women with ectopic pregnancy. Obstet Gynecol 107:605, 2006

Silva PM, Araujo Júnior E, Cecchino GN, et al: Effectiveness of expectant management versus methotrexate in tubal ectopic pregnancy: a double-blind randomized trial. Arch Gynecol Obstet 291(4):939, 2015

Skubisz M, Dutton P, Duncan WC, et al: Using a decline in serum hCG between days 0–4 to predict ectopic pregnancy treatment success after single-dose methotrexate: a retrospective cohort study. BMC Pregnancy Childbirth 13:30, 2013

Song T, Kim MK, Kim ML, et al: Single-dose versus two-dose administration of methotrexate for the treatment of ectopic pregnancy: a randomized controlled trial. Hum Reprod 31(2):332, 2016

Sowter MC, Farquhar CM, Petrie KJ, et al: A randomized trial comparing single dose systemic methotrexate and laparoscopic surgery for the treatment of unruptured ectopic pregnancy. BJOG 108(2):192, 2001

Soysal S, Anık İlhan G, Vural M, et al: Severe methotrexate toxicity after treatment for ectopic pregnancy: a case report. Turk J Obstet Gynecol 13(4): 221, 2016

Spandorfer SD, Menzin AW, Barnhart KT, et al: Efficacy of frozen-section evaluation of uterine curettings in the diagnosis of ectopic pregnancy. Am J Obstet Gynecol 175(3 Pt 1):603, 1996

Spandorfer SD, Sawin SW, Benjamin I, et al: Postoperative day 1 serum human chorionic gonadotropin level as a predictor of persistent ectopic pregnancy after conservative surgical management. Fertil Steril 68:430, 1997

Spiegelberg O: Zur Casuistic der Ovarialschwangerschaft. Arch Gynaekol 13: 73, 1878

Stevens JS, Criss AK: Pathogenesis of Neisseria gonorrhoeae in the female reproductive tract: neutrophilic host response, sustained infection, and clinical sequelae. Curr Opin Hematol 25(1):13, 2018

Stovall TG, Ling FW: Single-dose methotrexate: an expanded clinical trial. Am J Obstet Gynecol 168:1759, 1993

Stovall TG, Ling FW, Andersen RN, et al: Improved sensitivity and specificity of a single measurement of serum progesterone over serial quantitative beta-human chorionic gonadotrophin in screening for ectopic pregnancy. Hum Reprod 7:723, 1992

Stulberg DB, Cain LR, Dahlquist I, et al: Ectopic pregnancy rates and racial disparities in the Medicaid population, 2004–2008. Fertil Steril 102(6):1671, 2014

Stulberg DB, Cain L, Dahlquist IH, et al: Ectopic pregnancy morbidity and mortality in low-income women, 2004–2008. Hum Reprod 31:666, 2016

Svenningsen R, Staff AC, Langebrekke A, et al: Fertility Outcome after cornual resection for interstitial pregnancies. J Minim Invasive Gynecol 26(5):865, 2019

Svirsky R, Rozovski U, Vaknin Z, et al: The safety of conception occurring shortly after methotrexate treatment of an ectopic pregnancy. Reprod Toxicol 27(1):85, 2009

Tabatabaii Bafghi A, Zaretezerjani F, Sekhavat L, et al: Fertility outcome after treatment of unruptured ectopic pregnancy with two different methotrexate protocols. Int J Fertil Steril 6:189, 2012

Tanaka Y, Mimura K, Kanagawa T, et al: Three-dimensional sonography in the differential diagnosis of interstitial, angular, and intrauterine pregnancies in a septate uterus. J Ultrasound Med 33(11):2031, 2014

Tao G, Patel C, Hoover KW: Updated estimates of ectopic pregnancy among commercially and Medicaid-insured women in the United States, 2002–2013. South Med J 110(1):18, 2017

Thurman AR, Cornelius M, Korte JE, et al: An alternative monitoring protocol for single-dose methotrexate therapy in ectopic pregnancy. Am J Obstet Gynecol 202(2):139.e1, 2010

Timor-Tritsch IE, Khatib N, Monteagudo A, et al: Cesarean scar pregnancies: experience of 60 cases. J Ultrasound Med 34(4):601, 2015

Timor-Tritsch IE, Monteagudo A, Bennett TA, et al: A new minimally invasive treatment for cesarean scar pregnancy and cervical pregnancy. Am J Obstet Gynecol 215(3):351.e1, 2016

Timor-Tritsch IE, Monteagudo A, Cali G, et al: Cesarean scar pregnancy is a precursor of morbidly adherent placenta. Ultrasound Obstet Gynecol 44(3): 346, 2014

Timor-Tritsch IE, Monteagudo A, Matera C, et al: Sonographic evolution of cornual pregnancies treated without surgery. Obstet Gynecol 79(6):1044, 1992

Timor-Tritsch IE, Monteagudo A, Santos R, et al: The diagnosis, treatment, and follow-up of cesarean scar pregnancy. Am J Obstet Gynecol 207(1): 44.e1, 2012

Toth M, Patton DL, Campbell LA, et al: Detection of chlamydial antigenic material in ovarian, prostatic, ectopic pregnancy and semen samples of culture-negative subjects. Am J Reprod Immunol 43:218, 2000

Trambert JJ, Einstein MH, Banks E, et al: Uterine artery embolization in the management of vaginal bleeding from cervical pregnancy: a case series. J Reprod Med 50:844, 2005

Troeltzsch M, von Blohn G, Kriegelstein S, et al: Oral mucositis in patients receiving low-dose methotrexate therapy for rheumatoid arthritis: report of 2 cases and literature review. Oral Surg Oral Med Oral Pathol Oral Radiol 115(5):e28, 2013

Trojano G, Colafiglio G, Saliani N, et al: Successful management of a cervical twin pregnancy: neoadjuvant systemic methotrexate and prophylactic high cervical cerclage before curettage. Fertil Steril 91(3):935.e17, 2009

Tulandi T, Al Jaroudi D: Interstitial pregnancy: results generated from the Society of Reproductive Surgeons Registry. Obstet Gynecol 103:47, 2004

Uğur M, Turan C, Vicdan K, et al: Chronic ectopic pregnancy: a clinical analysis of 62 cases. Aust N Z J Obstet Gynaecol 36(2):186, 1996

Van Calster B, Abdallah Y, Guha S, et al: Rationalizing the management of pregnancies of unknown location: temporal and external validation of a risk prediction model on 1962 pregnancies. Hum Reprod 28(3):609, 2013

Van Calster B, Bobdiwala S, Guha S, et al: Managing pregnancy of unknown location based on initial serum progesterone and serial serum hCG levels: development and validation of a two-step triage protocol. Ultrasound Obstet Gynecol 48(5):642, 2016

Verhaegen J, Gallos ID, van Mello NM, et al: Accuracy of single progesterone test to predict early pregnancy outcome in women with pain or bleeding: meta-analysis of cohort studies. BMJ 345:e6077, 2012

Verma U, Goharkhay N: Conservative management of cervical ectopic pregnancy. Fertil Steril 91(3):671, 2009

Vermesh M, Graczykowski JW, Sauer MV: Reevaluation of the role of culdocentesis in the management of ectopic pregnancy. Am J Obstet Gynecol 162:411, 1990

Vermesh M, Silva PD, Rosen GF, et al: Management of unruptured ectopic gestation by linear salpingostomy: a prospective, randomized clinical trial of laparoscopy versus laparotomy. Obstet Gynecol 73:400, 1989

Wang DB, Chen YH, Zhang ZF, et al: Evaluation of the transvaginal resection of low-segment cesarean scar ectopic pregnancies. Fertil Steril 101(2):602, 2014

Watrowski R, Lange A, Möckel J: Primary omental pregnancy with secondary implantation into posterior cul-de-sac: laparoscopic treatment using hemostatic matrix. J Minim Invasive Gynecol 22(3):501, 2015

Waylen AL, Metwally M, Jones GL, et al: Effects of cigarette smoking upon clinical outcomes of assisted reproduction: a meta-analysis. Human Reprod Update 15(1):31, 2009

Xiaolin Z, Ling L, Chengxin Y, et al: Transcatheter intraarterial methotrexate infusion combined with selective uterine artery embolization as a treatment option for cervical pregnancy. J Vasc Interv Radiol 21(6):836, 2010

Yamaguchi M, Honda R, Erdenebaatar C, et al: Treatment of cervical pregnancy with ultrasound-guided local methotrexate injection. Ultrasound Obstet Gynecol 50(6):781, 2017

Zee J, Sammel MD, Chung K, et al: Ectopic pregnancy prediction in women with a pregnancy of unknown location: data beyond 48 h are necessary. Human Reprod 29(3):441, 2014

Zhu Q, Li C, Zhao WH, et al: Risk factors and clinical features of ovarian pregnancy: a case-control study. BMJ Open 4(12):e006447, 2014

CHAPTER 8

Abnormal Uterine Bleeding

PATHOPHYSIOLOGY

The endometrium is the source of most abnormal reproductive tract bleeding. It consists of two distinct zones, the functionalis layer and the basalis layer (Fig. 8-1). The basalis layer lies in direct contact with the myometrium and beneath the functionalis layer. The basalis serves as a reservoir for regeneration of the functionalis layer following menses. In contrast, the functionalis layer lines the uterine cavity and undergoes dramatic change throughout the menstrual cycle. It ultimately sloughs during menstruation. Histologically, the functionalis has a surface epithelium and underlying subepithelial capillary plexus. Beneath these are stroma, glands, and interspersed leukocytes (Fig. 33-1, p. 701).

Blood reaches the uterus via the uterine and ovarian arteries (see Fig. 8-1). From these, the arcuate arteries arise to supply the myometrium. These in turn branch into the radial arteries, which extend toward the endometrium at right angles from the arcuate arteries. At the endometrium-myometrium junction, the radial arteries bifurcate to create the basal and spiral arteries. The basal arteries serve the basalis layer of the endometrium and are relatively insensitive to hormonal changes. The spiral arteries stretch to supply the functionalis layer and end in a subepithelial capillary plexus.

In human menstruation, progesterone plays a critical role. Two progesterone receptors (PR) are found in the endometrium, PRA and PRB. In the secretory phase, PRB levels decline in the stromal and glandular epithelial cells of the functionalis layer. However, PRA expression in this layer persists in the stromal cells, which thus remain responsive to progesterone and to its withdrawal (Maybin, 2015).

In the absence of pregnancy, the corpus luteum regresses and curtails progesterone production. Progesterone acts as an antiinflammatory agent, and thus its withdrawal raises cytokine levels in the endometrium. Elevated concentrations of cytokines prompt an influx of leukocytes, which release lytic enzymes. These matrix metalloproteinases break down the stroma and vascular architecture of the functionalis layer (Critchley, 2011). Subsequent bleeding and sloughing of this layer constitute menstruation (Jabbour, 2006). Concurrently, endometrial levels of tissue factor and plasminogen activator inhibitor-1 drop with progesterone withdrawal. These two proteins foster hemostasis during the luteal phase, but their decline promotes an environment conducive to bleeding and fibrinolysis (Lockwood, 2011). Last, progesterone withdrawal raises concentrations of cyclooxygenase-2, a necessary enzyme in prostaglandin PG synthesis. As a result, levels of prostaglandin $F_{2\alpha}$ ($PGF_{2\alpha}$) rise and cause intense spiral arteriole constriction. Explanations differ as to whether this vasoconstriction produces a hypoxia needed to prompt endometrial sloughing or whether it serves to minimizes menstrual blood loss (Maybin, 2015; Schatz, 2016).

Hemostasis and cessation of menstruation are dependent on the endometrial coagulation system. Initially, platelets aggregate and are activated in response to endothelial injury. This occurs by either platelet glycoprotein interaction with von Willebrand factor or tissue factor generation of thrombin. Subsequently, fibrin is formed through the coagulation cascade to help form a stable clot to seal bleeding vessels. In addition, the remaining endometrial arterioles constrict to limit further bleeding (Ferenczy, 2003). During menses, augmented endometrial glucocorticoid production also helps to control blood loss by dampening the inflammatory response.

Dysregulation in any of the above events can lead to abnormal menstruation and greater blood loss.

DEFINITIONS

Women normally menstruate every 28 ± 7 days. The average duration is 5 days, and menstrual blood loss volume does not normally exceed 80 mL. Variations in any of these norms constitute *abnormal uterine bleeding (AUB)*, which may be acute or chronic. Acute AUB is defined as bleeding sufficiently heavy to require immediate intervention to prevent ongoing losses. Chronic AUB is defined as bleeding that has been present

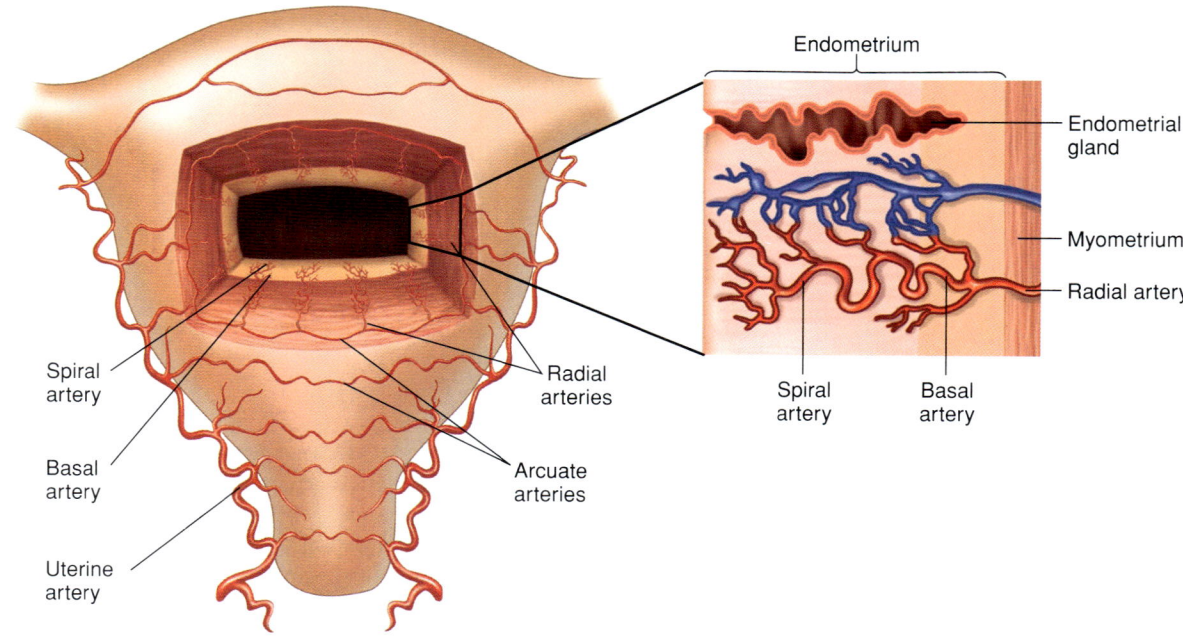

FIGURE 8-1 Drawing of uterine blood supply and endometrial anatomy.

during most of the prior 6 months. Because AUB can display several patterns, the descriptive terms listed next help standardize nomenclature (Munro, 2018).

Menses are ideally categorized by four qualities—volume, duration, frequency, and regularity (Table 8-1). *Heavy menstrual bleeding (HMB)*, which was formerly called menorrhagia, describes menstruation with excessive flow. Objectively, this has been defined as >80 mL of blood loss per menstrual period. Second, the duration of menses may vary, with *prolonged bleeding* lasting >8 days per menstrual period. In some cases, women may complain of both, which is described as *heavy, prolonged menstrual bleeding*. A third quality is frequency, which reflects the number of days between menses. *Frequent bleeding* describes menses with <24 days intervening. *Infrequent bleeding*, previously called oligomenorrhea, is defined by menses with >38 days intervening. Absence of menstrual bleeding in a 90-day period is defined as *amenorrhea*. Last, regularity describes the variability of cycle lengths. If cycle lengths vary from cycle to cycle by ≥10 days, they are considered irregular. As an example, one cycle length is 28 days, but the next is 60 days.

Previously, "dysfunctional uterine bleeding (DUB)" was often used to describe abnormal uterine bleeding without a clear underlying pathology. This term has now been abandoned in favor of describing the specific disorders (Fraser, 2011a).

Specific terms also describe nonmenstrual bleeding. *Intermenstrual bleeding* defines bleeding, usually brief, that occurs between fairly normal menses. This term replaces metrorrhagia. Intermenstrual bleeding may be further defined by clinical context. For example, intermenstrual bleeding prompted by vaginal intercourse is called *postcoital bleeding*. The terms *pre-* and *postmenstrual spotting* are self-explained. *Breakthrough bleeding* and *unscheduled bleeding* are terms associated with hormone administration. Another term, *withdrawal bleeding*, refers to the predictable bleeding that results from an abrupt decline in progesterone levels. Last, women may experience bleeding outside the reproductive years. *Precocious menstruation* is initiation of menses in childhood and described in Chapter 15 (p. 329). *Postmenopausal bleeding* is included in this chapter.

Although HMB is defined as menstrual blood loss >80 mL, evaluation can proceed based solely on a patient's description of

TABLE 8-1. Recommended Terminology for Normal and Abnormal Menses

Quality	Normal	Abnormal		Prior Terms
Volume	5–80 mL	Light (<5 mL)	Heavy (>80 mL)	hypomenorrhea, menorrhagia
Duration	≤8 d	Prolonged (>8 d)		hypomenorrhea, menorrhagia
Frequency: days between menses				
	24–38 d	Frequent (<24 d)	Infrequent (>38 d) Amenorrhea (>90 d)	polymenorrhea, oligomenorrhea
Regularity: numbers of days by which cycle lengths vary				
	≤7–9 d	Irregular ≥10 d		

flow that suggests HMB. Of objective methods, Hallberg and associates (1966) first described a technique to extract hemoglobin from sanitary napkins using sodium hydroxide. Hemoglobin is then converted to hematin and measured spectrophotometrically. This alkaline hematin technique has since been modified and revalidated for use with modern sanitary napkins that contain superabsorbent polymer granules (Magnay, 2010). Although used in research, this precise approach has obvious constraints in a routine clinical setting.

Other tools used to estimate menstrual blood loss include hemoglobin and hematocrit evaluation. Hemoglobin concentrations below 12 g/dL raise the chance of identifying HMB. A normal level, however, does not exclude HMB, as many women with clinically significant bleeding have normal values.

Another method involves estimating the number and type of pads or tampons used by a woman during menses. Warner and colleagues (2004) found positive correlations between objective HMB and passing clots more than 1 inch in diameter and changing pads more frequently than every 3 hours. Attempts to standardize this type of evaluation have led to the pictorial blood assessment chart (PBAC) (Fig. 8-2). Using a scoring sheet, patients are asked to record daily the number of sanitary products that are lightly, moderately, or completely saturated. Scores are assigned as follows: 1 point for each lightly stained tampon, 5 if moderately saturated, and 10 if completely soaked. Pads are similarly given ascending scores of 1, 5, and 20, respectively. Presence of small, 2-mm-diameter clots score 1 point, whereas 3-mm clots score 5. Points are then tallied for each day. Totals >100 points per menstrual cycle correlate with >80 mL objective blood loss (Higham, 1990).

As another option, a menstrual cup may offer a more direct method of measure. Seated in the vagina similar to a diaphragm, these cups allow trapping and collection of menstrual blood. Several times during the day, a woman can remove, empty, wash, and replace. Differing sizes and stiffness accommodate parous or nulliparous anatomy. Disposable brands are also available.

Menstrual calendars are another option to evaluate AUB and its patterns. With this, patients are asked to record dates and blood flow quantity throughout the month. These calendars can be used to aid diagnosis and to document improvement during medical treatment. Smartphone applications, or "apps," are similarly available to chart menstrual timing and flow (Moglia, 2016). Clue and iPeriod apps allow daily menstrual flow charting and comments. The Me-Period Flow Assessment specifically collects PBAC data.

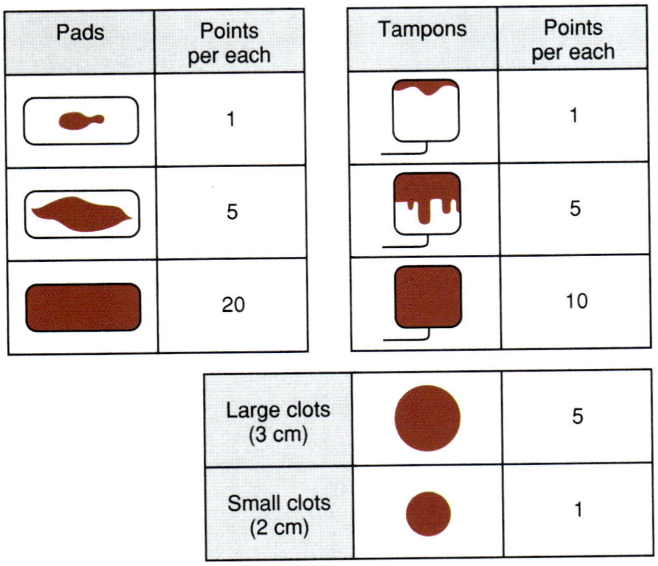

ETIOLOGY

Depending on whether subjective self-reporting or objective blood loss measurement is used, the true population rates of AUB can vary. Data may also differ depending on the definitions used for AUB. Commonly cited rates range from 10 to 30 percent (Liu, 2007; Matteson, 2013).

Age and reproductive status most greatly influence AUB incidence, and these factors can help prioritize potential etiologies. Prior to menarche, bleeding is investigated as an abnormal finding. In children, the vagina, rather than the uterus, is more frequently involved. True uterine bleeding usually results from increased exposure to endogenous or exogenous estrogen. Bleeding in this age group is discussed in Chapter 15 (p. 329).

In adolescence, AUB results from anovulation and coagulation defects at disproportionately higher rates compared with older reproductive-aged women (Ahuja, 2010). In contrast, benign or malignant neoplastic growths are less frequent. Pregnancy, sexually transmitted diseases (STDs), and sexual abuse are also possibilities in this population.

Following adolescence, the hypothalamic-pituitary-ovarian (HPO) axis matures, and anovulatory uterine bleeding is encountered less often. With greater sexual activity, rates of bleeding related to pregnancy and STDs rise. The incidences of bleeding from leiomyomas, adenomyosis, and endometrial polyps also increase with age.

During the perimenopause, as with perimenarchal girls, anovulatory uterine bleeding from HPO axis dysfunction is a more frequent finding (Chap. 22, p. 476). In contrast, the incidences of bleeding related to pregnancy and STDs decline. With aging, risks of benign and malignant neoplastic growth rise.

After menopause, bleeding typically can be traced to a benign origin such as endometrial or vaginal atrophy or polyps. Even so, malignant neoplasms, especially endometrial carcinoma, are found more often in this age group. Less commonly, estrogen-producing ovarian carcinoma may cause endometrial hyperplasia and uterine bleeding. Similarly, ulcerative vulvar, vaginal, or cervical neoplasms can be sources. Rarely, serosanguinous discharge from a fallopian tube cancer may appear as uterine bleeding. Thus, bleeding in this demographic usually prompts evaluation to exclude these cancers.

The causes of reproductive tract bleeding are numerous (Table 8-2). To organize the main causes of AUB, the International Federation of Gynecology and Obstetrics (FIGO) created a classification system using the acronym

Pads	Points per each		Tampons	Points per each
	1			1
	5			5
	20			10

Large clots (3 cm)		5
Small clots (2 cm)		1

FIGURE 8-2 Scoring for the pictorial bleeding assessment chart. Patients are counseled to evaluate the degree of saturation for each sanitary product used during menstruation. Total points are tallied for each menses. Point totals >100 per menses indicate heavy menstrual bleeding.

TABLE 8-2. Reproductive Tract Bleeding

Uterine Bleeding

PREGNANCY: Normal implantation, abortion, ectopic, mole

STRUCTURAL

Polyps: endometrial, endocervical

Adenomyosis

Leiomyomas

Malignancy:
Preinvasive: CIN, EIN
Cancer: cervical, endometrial, sarcoma

NONSTRUCTURAL

Coagulopathy: inherited, liver failure, immunologic

Ovulatory
Adolescent HPO immaturity
Perimenopausal follicle aging
Premature ovarian failure
Androgen excess: PCOS, CAH, Cushing syndrome/disease
Hypothyroidism
Obesity
Hyperprolactinemia: pituitary or hypothalamic disorder
HPO dysregulation: stress, anorexia, extreme exercise

Endometrial: Atrophy, intrinsic abnormality, endometrial hyperplasia, chronic endometritis

Iatrogenic:
Intrauterine device
Medications: sex steroid agent or SERM, anticoagulants, valproate, hyperprolactinemia-inducing agent

Not otherwise specified:
Infection: PID, cervicitis, TB, postabortal/postpartum
Arteriovenous malformation
Partial sequestration of menses: isthmocele, Asherman syndrome

Other Lower Genital Tract Bleeding

Malignancy: vaginal, vulvar, fallopian tube, ovarian hormone-producing

Traumatic: vulvar or vaginal trauma, foreign body

Partial outlet obstruction: transverse or longitudinal septum

Other: postsurgical granulation tissue, prolapsed fallopian tube, vaginal adenosis

CAH = congenital adrenal hyperplasia; CIN = cervical intraepithelial neoplasia; EIN = endometrial intraepithelial neoplasia; HPO = hypothalamic-pituitary-ovarian axis; PID = pelvic inflammatory disease; PCOS = polycystic ovarian syndrome; SERM = selective estrogen-receptor modulator; TB = tuberculosis.

PALM-COEIN (Munro, 2011, 2018). Letters are grouped by structural and nonstructural causes of AUB, respectively, and reflect the following categories: polyp, adenomyosis, leiomyoma, malignancy and hyperplasia, coagulopathy, ovulatory disorders, endometrial dysfunction, iatrogenic, and those not otherwise classified. Causes not otherwise classified can include conditions defined only by biochemical assays or those whose association with AUB is still poorly defined. Examples are isthmocele, arteriovenous malformations, and myometrial hypertrophy. Pregnancy is not considered in this system, but AUB is encountered in 15 to 20 percent of pregnancies (Everett, 1997; Weiss, 2004). Although frequently no reason is found in these cases, bleeding may reflect early abortion, ectopic pregnancy, cervical infection, gestational trophoblastic disease, cervical eversion, or polyp. Detailed discussions of bleeding associated with these are found in Chapters 6, 7, and 37.

DIAGNOSIS

■ History and Physical Examination

With AUB, the diagnostic goal is exclusion of pregnancy or cancer and identification of the underlying pathology to allow optimal treatment. During initial evaluation, a thorough patient history is collected. The menstrual history includes age at menarche, date of last menstrual period, birth control method, and the timing and amount of bleeding. A review of associated symptoms such as fever, fatigue, bulk symptoms, tissue passage, or pain can also direct evaluation. A family history inquires about members with AUB or other bleeding problems, and coagulopathy screening is described on page 193. Importantly, medications are reviewed, as abnormal bleeding can accompany the use of nonsteroidal antiinflammatory drugs (NSAIDs), anticoagulants, and agents with hyperprolactinemia as a potential side effect (Table 13-2, p. 285). Less robust evidence implicates herbal supplements that may affect coagulation, such as ginseng, garlic, ginkgo, dong quai, and St. John wort (Cordier, 2012).

Notably, most gynecologic disorders do not consistently display a specific bleeding pattern, and patients may complain of HMB or intermenstrual bleeding or both. Pain symptoms may be complex and include both cyclic and noncyclic patterns. Thus, the pattern for a particular woman may be of limited value in diagnosing the underlying cause of bleeding but can be used to assess improvement with treatment.

Of pain symptoms, dysmenorrhea often accompanies abnormal bleeding caused by structural abnormalities, infections, and pregnancy complications. This seems intuitive considering the role of prostaglandins in both HMB and dysmenorrhea. Painful intercourse and noncyclic pain are less frequent in women with AUB and usually suggest a structural or infectious source.

Gynecologic examination can also suggest an etiology. Moreover, it confirms the bleeding site as uterine, because vaginal, rectal, or urethral bleeding can present similarly. This is more difficult if there is no active bleeding, and urinalysis or stool guaiac evaluation can be helpful adjuncts.

In addition, blood tests, cervical cytology, sonography (with or without saline infusion), endometrial biopsy (EMB), and hysteroscopy are used primarily. In many cases, not all of these tools are required and instead can be individually selected based on patient variables, suspected diagnosis, available resources, and provider training.

Laboratory Evaluation

β-Human Chorionic Gonadotropin and Hematologic Testing

Miscarriage, ectopic pregnancies, and gestational trophoblastic disease can present with AUB and may cause life-threatening hemorrhage. Pregnancy complications are quickly excluded with determination of urine or serum β-human chorionic gonadotropin (hCG) levels. This test is typically obtained on all reproductive-aged women with a uterus.

In women with AUB, a complete blood count (CBC) will identify anemia, the degree of blood loss, and platelet count extremes. With chronic loss, erythrocyte indices will reflect a microcytic, hypochromic anemia and show declines in mean corpuscular volume (MCV), mean corpuscular hemoglobin (MCH), and mean corpuscular hemoglobin concentration (MCHC). Moreover, in women with classic iron-deficiency anemia from chronic blood loss, an elevated platelet count can be seen. In those for whom the cause of anemia is unclear, those with profound anemia, or those who fail to improve with oral iron therapy, iron studies are often indicated. Specifically, iron-deficiency anemia produces low serum ferritin and low serum iron levels but an elevated total iron-binding capacity. Laboratory testing for disordered hemostasis is considered for those taking anticoagulant agents or in women and adolescents with HMB and no other obvious cause.

Cervicitis Evaluation

Cervicitis often causes intermenstrual or postcoital spotting. Accordingly, microscopic examination of a saline preparation of cervical secretions, or "wet prep," can be informative. With mucopurulent discharge, sheets of neutrophils (>30 per high-power field) and red blood cells are typical. With trichomoniasis, motile trichomonads are found. Cervicitis-related bleeding is frequently reproduced during sampling from an inflamed cervix with a friable epithelium.

The association between mucopurulent cervicitis and cervical infection with *Chlamydia trachomatis* and *Neisseria gonorrhoeae* is well established (Brunham, 1984). Thus, the Centers for Disease Control and Prevention (CDC) (2015) recommend testing for both when mucopurulent cervicitis is found (Chap. 3, p. 66). Moreover, even without frank discharge, these organisms can cause endometritis (Wiesenfeld, 2002). Thus, bleeding or spotting alone may merit screening for these two infections in at-risk populations (Table 1-1, p. 4). Last, herpes simplex virus (HSV) may manifest as diffuse erosive and hemorrhagic ectocervical lesions. In patients with such findings who lack a known HSV history, swab of the lesion for polymerase chain reaction (PCR) or serologic testing can be obtained.

Cervical Cytology or Biopsy

Both cervical and endometrial cancers can bleed, and evidence for these tumors may be detected during diagnostic Pap testing. The most frequent abnormal cytologic results involve squamous cell pathology and may reflect cervicitis, intraepithelial neoplasia, or cancer. Less commonly, atypical glandular or endometrial cells are found. Thus, depending on the cytologic results and patient age, colposcopy with ectocervical biopsy, endocervical curettage, and/or EMB may be indicated as discussed in Chapter 29 (p. 633). Moreover, at times, a visibly suspicious vaginal or cervical lesion may bleed and warrant direct biopsy with Tischler forceps.

Endometrial Biopsy

Indications. In many women, endometrial pathology underlies their AUB. These endometrial entities can be divided theoretically into focal lesions (leiomyoma, polyp) or more global conditions (hyperplasia, cancer, endometritis). This artificial division can aid diagnostic tool selection. Namely, some modalities have greater sensitivity for focal disease detection, whereas others are more sensitive for global pathology. That said, no tool, including transvaginal sonography, is recommended for routine endometrial cancer screening in asymptomatic low-risk women (Smith, 2018).

With endometrial cancer, AUB is noted in most affected women. The incidence and risk of this cancer rises with age, and most affected women are postmenopausal (Siegel, 2019). Thus, in postmenopausal women with AUB, the need to exclude cancer intensifies, and EMB is typically indicated. Of premenopausal women with endometrial neoplasia, most are obese or have chronic anovulation or both. Specifically, the American College of Obstetricians and Gynecologists (2016a) recommends endometrial assessment in any woman older than 45 years with AUB. Endometrial sampling is also reasonable in those younger than 45 with failed initial medical management, persistent AUB, or a history of unopposed estrogen exposure such as seen in obesity or polycystic ovarian syndrome (PCOS). Other risk factors include diabetes, tamoxifen use, and genetic predisposition to uterine cancer (American College of Obstetricians and Gynecologists, 2015). Genetic syndromes and their corresponding genes include hereditary non-polypoid cancer of the colon or Lynch syndrome (*MLH1, MSH2, MSH6, PMS2*); Peutz-Jeghers (*STK11*); Cowden (*PTEN*); Li-Fraumeni (*TP53*); and polymerase proofreading-associated polyposis (*POLD1*) (Ring, 2017).

Sampling Methods. With endometrial sampling, diagnostic accuracy correlates positively with the amount of endometrial tissue collected (Reijnen, 2017). Thus, a preferred screening tool collects as much tissue as possible for evaluation. Also, both focal and global lesions ideally would be identified. Last, patient comfort, cost, inability to enter the cavity, and rates of insufficient tissue are factored.

For years, dilation and curettage (D & C) has been used for endometrial sampling. It offers a high rate of access to the endometrial cavity, and in one study, the inability to biopsy was only 0.5 percent (Hefler, 2008). Its sensitivity for endometrial hyperplasia or cancer exceeds 90 percent (Sany, 2012; Yarandi, 2010). That said, blind sampling can be incomplete and can miss pathology (Stock, 1975). This is especially true for focal lesions (Bettocchi, 2001). D & C also has associated surgical risks, expense, postoperative pain, and need for operative anesthesia. For these reasons, other suitable in-office substitutes have been evaluated.

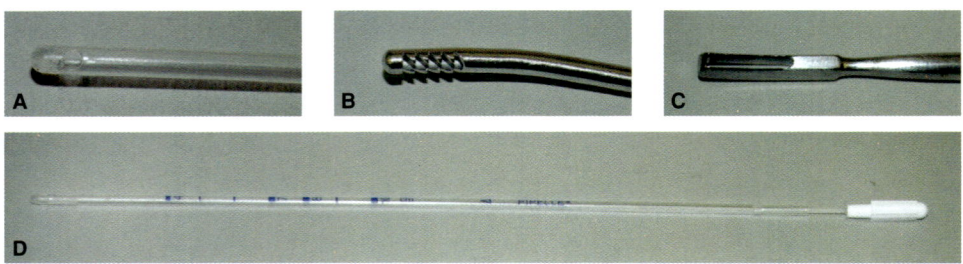

FIGURE 8-3 Endometrial sampling devices. **A.** Pipelle fluted tip. **B.** Novak curette tip. **C.** Kevorkian curette tip. **D.** Pipelle suction device.

Early office techniques used metal curettes, and Novak and Kevorkian curettes are examples (Fig. 8-3). Endometrial samples that are removed with these devices show significant positive correlation with histologic results obtained from hysterectomy specimens (Stovall, 1989). Thus, they are deemed adequate biopsy methods (Ferenczy, 1979). Disadvantages include patient discomfort and rare procedural complications such as uterine perforation and infection.

To minimize these, flexible plastic samplers have been evaluated for EMB. Advantageously, samples from these catheters have histologic findings for global pathology that are comparable with tissues obtained by D & C, hysterectomy, or stiff metal curette (Dijkhuizen, 2000; Stovall, 1991). Moreover, they afford greater patient comfort compared with D & C or in-office metal curettage. Of these disposable samplers, the Pipelle device is widely used (see Fig. 8-3).

Prior to performing EMB, pregnancy is excluded in women of reproductive age. With device insertion, patients frequently note cramping, which can be allayed by an oral preprocedural NSAID. For some, slow transcervical intrauterine instillation of 5 mL of 2-percent lidocaine solution using an 18-gauge angiocatheter can lower perceived pain scores (Dogan, 2004; Güler, 2010). Alternatively, 2-percent lidocaine gel can be applied, 1 mL at the tenaculum site and 2 mL into the endocervical canal (Karaca, 2016).

To begin, a speculum is placed, and the cervix is cleansed with an antibacterial solution, such as povidone-iodine solution. In many cases, a single-tooth tenaculum is needed to stabilize the cervix and permit passage of the Pipelle through the cervical os and into the endometrial cavity. When placing the tenaculum on the anterior cervical lip, closing the clamp slowly can decrease patient discomfort.

With sampling, the Pipelle is directed toward the fundus until resistance is met. Markings on the Pipelle allow measurement of uterine depth, and this value is recorded in the procedure note. The inner Pipelle stilette is then retracted to create suction within the cylinder. Several times, the Pipelle is withdrawn to the level of the internal cervical os and advanced back to the fundus. The device is gently turned during its advancement and retraction to allow thorough sampling of all endometrial surfaces. Once filled, the Pipelle is removed and its contents are emptied into a formalin-filled collection jar. The Pipelle tip should not be dipped into the formalin prior to reinsertion. Two to three insertions are performed to aid adequate sampling. Rarely, a vagal response can follow device insertion. In this instance, the procedure is terminated, and patient support is provided.

Despite its advantages, the Pipelle device does have limitations. First, a tissue sample may be *insufficient* or *scant* for histologic evaluation, and these are considered inadequate. In postmenopausal women, a significant percentage is subsequently found to have endometrial cancer or hyperplasia (Goebel, 2019; Kandil, 2014). For these inadequate samples in a postmenopausal patient with a low cancer risk, TVS is reasonable. A thin endometrial stripe typically reflects atrophy, and no further sampling is usually required if bleeding resolves. In these low-risk women, if a focal lesion is identified sonographically, hysteroscopy may be preferred. For an inadequate sample in those who carry a higher cancer risk and thus are better served by tissue biopsy, D & C offers higher rates of sufficient sampling (Arafah, 2014). Concurrent hysteroscopy during D & C can screen for focal lesions.

Premenopausal women with an inadequate sample are best served by D & C with hysteroscopy. Remember that patients in this group were initially sampled because of their inherent risks for endometrial cancer. That said, preoperative TVS can be added to help identify other possible AUB etiologies in this demographic.

A second limitation of Pipelle sampling is an inability to access the cavity. For example, cervical stenosis may obstruct sampling and techniques to overcome this are found in Chapter 41 (p. 903). A submucous leiomyoma near the isthmus is another frequent obstruction. Risks for stenosis include postmenopausal status, nulliparity, and prior cervical surgeries (Williams, 2008; Xie, 2018). With cervical stenosis, a second attempt following cervical ripening is common. A second failed EMB attempt or uterine myoma merits further investigation by D & C plus diagnostic hysteroscopy.

A third concern is the imperfect negative predictive value of Pipelle EMB. In one metaanalysis, the cancer-detection failure rate was 0.7 percent for all women biopsied (Clark, 2002a). Thus, a positive histologic result is accurate to diagnose cancer, but a negative result does not definitively exclude it. Therefore, if an EMB with normal tissue is obtained, but abnormal bleeding continues despite conservative treatment, or if the suspicion of endometrial cancer is high, then further sampling efforts are warranted.

Finally, endometrial sampling is associated with a greater percentage of false-negative results with focal pathology such as endometrial polyps (Demirkiran, 2012; Svirsky, 2008; Xie, 2018). Because of all these limitations with endometrial sampling, investigators have evaluated sonography, hysteroscopy, or both to replace or complement it.

In addition to the Pipelle device, the Tao Brush is another sampler. Once intracavitary, its long, bristled brush is rotated for sampling. Whereas the Pipelle obtains tissue for histologic examination, the Tao brush provides a specimen for cytologic evaluation. Although sensitivity values appear comparable to other techniques, this sampling method has not been widely adopted (Abdelazim, 2015; Del Priore, 2001).

■ Sonography

Transvaginal Sonography

Transvaginal sonography (TVS) is a widely available, cost-effective tool that is commonly used to evaluate AUB. TVS can be an adjunct to both EMB and hysteroscopy when evaluating the endometrium. However, because of greater patient comfort and improvements in imaging resolution, TVS is also frequently used as a primary diagnostic modality. Another advantage of TVS is its ability to assess the myometrium, uterine surfaces, and adnexa. As such, it offers anatomic information not afforded by hysteroscopy or EMB. Namely, pathology such as leiomyomas, adenomyosis, or estrogen-producing stromal ovarian tumors can be identified.

For *endometrial lesions*, TVS is most helpful and sensitive to define endometrial thickness. Imaged in a sagittal view, this thickness represents the opposed endometrial surfaces and appears as a hyperechoic endometrial stripe down the center of the uterine body (Fig. 8-4 and Fig. 2-16, p. 38). Intracavity fluid, if present, is not included in the calculation. Instead, the endometrial thickness on each side of the fluid is measured and then summed. Factors that can limit visualization and accuracy of endometrial measurement include patient obesity and other uterine pathology such as myomas and adenomyosis. In both premenopausal and postmenopausal women, a thick endometrium may reflect global pathology, or it may signal a focal lesion. However, the sensitivity of TVS to differentiate the two is poor. In such cases, saline-infusion sonography (SIS) or hysteroscopy, which are more effective for identifying focal lesions, can be informative.

In *postmenopausal women with AUB*, endometrial thickness has been correlated with endometrial cancer risk. Thickness measurements of 3.4 ± 1.2 mm typically reflect an atrophic endometrium, whereas much greater thicknesses correlate with endometrial hyperplasia, intraepithelial neoplasia, and endometrial cancer (Granberg, 1991). For endometrial cancer, negative predictive values >99 percent have been reported using a measurement ≤4 mm (Karlsson, 1995; Tsuda, 1997). This threshold does not appear to be affected by hormone replacement therapy (HRT) use (Smith-Bindman, 1998). In those using cyclic HRT, TVS is best performed 4 or 5 days following cycle bleeding cessation (Goldstein, 2001). For postmenopausal women with AUB, an endometrial thickness >4 mm typically requires additional evaluation with SIS, hysteroscopy, or EMB.

Although these criteria can safely reduce EMB rates for many patients, others consider false-negative rates too high with this strategy. In one retrospective cohort of 4000 postmenopausal women with bleeding, the sensitivity to diagnose endometrial cancer was 97 percent for a thickness ≤3 mm but 94 percent for a threshold of ≤4 mm (Wong, 2016). This was similar to a metaanalysis by Timmermans and associates (2010). In addition, in diabetic or obese women, the 4-mm guideline may be less predictive (van Doorn, 2004). Because of these concerns, some advocate hysteroscopy with direct biopsy or endometrial sampling to evaluate all postmenopausal bleeding (Litta, 2005; Tabor, 2002).

For low-cancer-risk postmenopausal women *without bleeding*, the risk of cancer or hyperplasia is low. This includes those found to have an endometrial thickness above accepted thresholds (Fleischer, 2001; Jokubkiene, 2016). The American College of Obstetricians and Gynecologists (2018c) notes that an endometrial thickness >4 mm in this population need not routinely prompt evaluation. Instead, further testing is directed by coexistent patient risks. According to the decision analysis by Smith-Bindman and colleagues (2004), however, endometrial sampling is suitable for a threshold thickness value >11 mm in asymptomatic postmenopausal women. Focal lesions are common in this subgroup and can contribute to the endometrial thickness measurement. Thus, SIS or hysteroscopy may be favored if additional evaluation is indicated (Schmidt, 2009; Wong, 2016).

For *premenopausal women with AUB*, researchers have also attempted to create endometrial thickness guidelines. Merz and colleagues (1996) found that the normal endometrial thickness in premenopausal women did not exceed 4 mm on day 4 of the menstrual cycle, nor did it measure more than 8 mm by day 8. However, endometrial thicknesses can vary considerably among premenopausal women, and evidence-based abnormal thresholds that have been proposed range from ≥4 mm to >16 mm (Breitkopf, 2004; Goldstein, 1997; Shi, 2008). Thus, a consensus for endometrial thickness guidelines has not been established for this group.

In addition to thickness, other sonographic qualities of the endometrium are also considered when evaluating AUB. Standardization of terms and definitions for these have been proposed but have not been robustly validated (Leone, 2010; Sladkevicius, 2018). Of findings, punctate cystic areas within the endometrium may indicate a polyp. Hypoechoic masses that distort the endometrium and originate from the inner layer of myometrium most likely are submucous leiomyomas. In postmenopausal women, endometrial cavity fluid is common and typically benign (Bar-Hava, 1998; Vuento, 1996). No sonographic findings are specific to endometrial cancer, but some findings have been linked with greater frequency (Fig. 33-3, p. 702). For example, intermingled hypo- and hyperechoic areas within the endometrium and an irregular endometrial-myometrial junction may indicate malignancy. Thus, with these

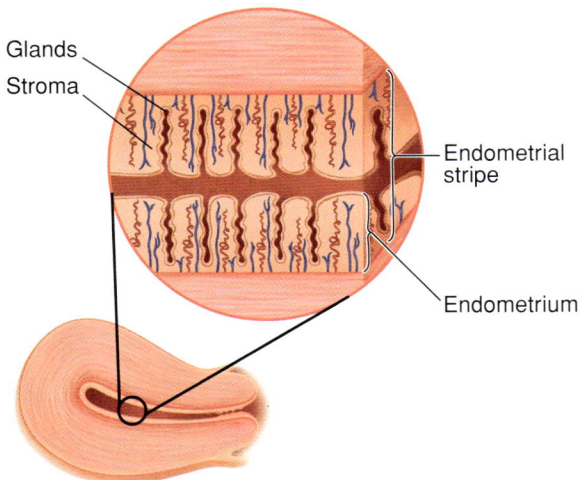

Glands
Stroma
Endometrial stripe
Endometrium

FIGURE 8-4 The sonographic endometrial stripe in a sagittal plane represents the thickness created by the apposed anterior and posterior endometrium. In premenopausal women, stripe thickness will vary during the menstrual cycle as the endometrium gradually thickens and then is sloughed.

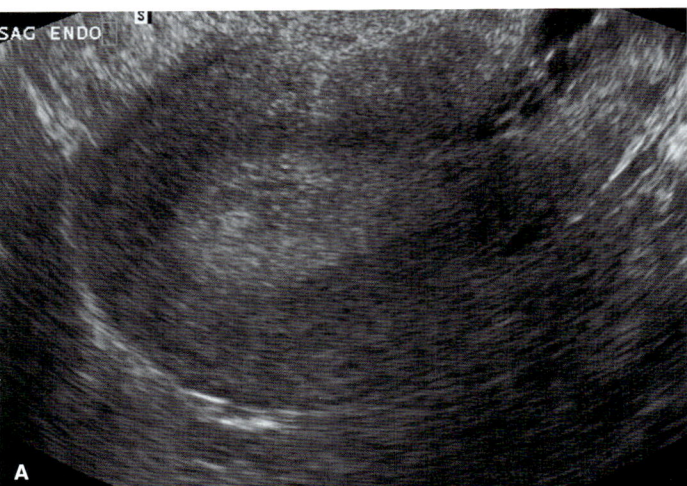
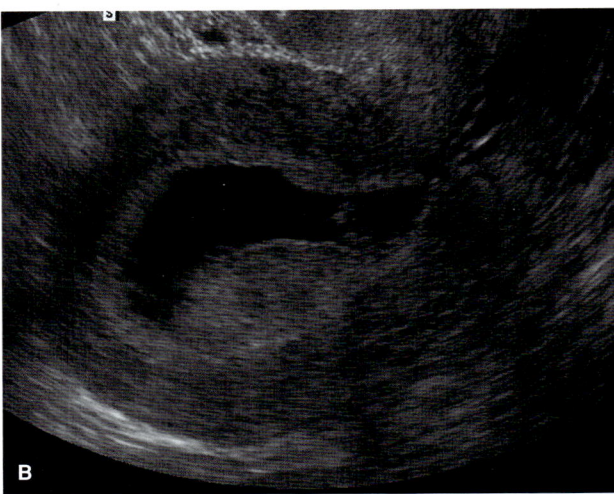

FIGURE 8-5 Transvaginal sonography of the uterus in the sagittal plane. **A.** The endometrium is thickened in this postmenopausal patient. **B.** Saline-infusion sonography reveals a posterior endometrial mass and further delineates its size and qualities. (Reproduced with permission from Dr. Elysia Moschos.)

findings, even with a normal endometrial thickness in post-menopausal patients, EMB or hysteroscopy with biopsy is considered to exclude malignancy (Sheikh, 2000).

Saline-Infusion Sonography

Also known as *sonohysterography* or *hysterosonography*, saline-infusion sonography (SIS) usually provides a detailed evaluation of the endometrial cavity (Chap. 2, p. 32). By distending the cavity with fluid, SIS allows identification of common endometrial masses associated with AUB. These lesions include endometrial polyps, submucous leiomyomas, and intracavitary blood clots, which all frequently create only a nondescript distortion or endometrial thickening when imaged with TVS (Fig. 8-5). Because SIS also images the myometrium, this modality can help differentiate lesions as being endometrial, submucous, or intramural.

To detect uterine cavitary focal lesions, SIS is often compared against hysteroscopy and provides similar diagnostic accuracy (Maheux-Lacroix, 2016; Seshadri, 2015). Importantly, neither can reliably discriminate between benign and malignant. Thus, because of the malignant potential of many focal lesions, biopsy or excision of most structural lesions, when identified, is recommended for those with risk factors. For this, operative hysteroscopy is typically used.

Although accurate for identifying focal lesions, SIS may not add to the value of TVS for evaluation of global lesions such as hyperplasia and cancer. Thus, in women with AUB for whom the exclusion of cancer is more relevant, SIS alone as an initial diagnostic tool may not have advantages over TVS.

SIS has other limitations. Contraindications include pregnancy, active pelvic infection, or stenosis (Chap. 2, p. 31). Additionally, SIS is cycle dependent and best performed in the proliferative phase of the menstrual cycle (American College of Obstetricians and Gynecologists, 2016b). By performing SIS prior to ovulation, interruption of an early pregnancy is avoided. Additionally, timing in the proliferative phase can minimize false-negative and false-positive results. Namely, a thick secretory endometrium may conceal or be mistaken for focal lesions such as small polyps or focal hyperplasia. In addition, SIS usually has

more patient discomfort than TVS, and approximately 5 percent of examinations cannot be completed because of cervical stenosis or patient discomfort. As expected, stenosis is more prevalent in postmenopausal women, and the incompletion rate mirrors that of diagnostic hysteroscopy.

Other Sonographic Techniques

In selected instances, other imaging modalities can provide information beyond that obtained from TVS and SIS, and these are described in Chapter 2. Doppler technology can be applied to ultrasound to assess vascularity. For example, a feeding vessel supplying a focal endometrial mass supports the diagnosis of endometrial polyp. Similarly, 3-dimensional (3-D) sonography and 3-D SIS are most helpful to clarify focal endometrial lesions (Benacerraf, 2008; Makris, 2007). However, even with enhanced sonographic visualization, 3-D SIS does not appear superior to two-dimensional SIS for this indication (Nieuwenhuis, 2017). With power Doppler, findings of multiple irregularly branching vessels can suggest malignancy (Dueholm, 2014). 3-D power Doppler has been employed to differentiate malignant and benign endometrium, but its value is still undefined (Dueholm, 2015; Opolskiene, 2010). Last, although preferred to computed tomography (CT), magnetic resonance (MR) imaging is rarely needed for AUB evaluation. However, MR imaging can display the endometrium in cases in which sonographic views are obstructed and in which SIS or hysteroscopy is not possible (Bennett, 2011).

◼ Hysteroscopy

With this procedure, a small-diameter endoscope is inserted into the endometrial cavity as explained in Chapter 41 (p. 899). The uterine cavity is then distended with saline or another medium for visualization. In addition, targeted hysteroscopic biopsy permits a histologic diagnosis of any abnormal areas (Ceci, 2002; Tinelli, 2008). Another main use of hysteroscopy is detection of focal intracavitary lesions, such as leiomyomas and polyps, which might be missed by EMB or TVS (Maheux-Lacroix,

2016; Tahir, 1999). When identified during hysteroscopy, these lesions can be simultaneously removed in the same session.

Because of these advantages, some advocate hysteroscopy as the primary tool for AUB diagnosis. However, the invasiveness and cost of hysteroscopy are balanced against improved diagnostic efficiency. Moreover, although accurate for identifying endometrial cancer, hysteroscopy is less accurate for endometrial hyperplasia or intraepithelial neoplasia (Gkrozou, 2015; Lasmar, 2006). Accordingly, some recommend EMB or endometrial curettage in conjunction with hysteroscopy (Ben-Yehuda, 1998; Clark, 2002b).

Hysteroscopy has other limitations. Cervical stenosis will sometimes block successful introduction of the endoscope. Alternatively, overdilation of the cervix may result in excessive backflow of the distention media and prohibit adequate distention of the cavity for viewing. Additionally, heavy bleeding may obscure and hinder an adequate examination. Hysteroscopy is also more expensive and technically challenging compared with TVS or SIS. Costs can be lowered if performed in the office rather than in an operative suite. However, patient discomfort may limit complete examination during some office procedures. Procedural pain may be diminished with use of a smaller diameter or flexible hysteroscope (Cicinelli, 2003; Paulo, 2015).

Another concern with hysteroscopy is the potential to seed the peritoneal cavity with malignant cells via retrograde flow of distention media through the fallopian tubes (Bradley, 2004; Zerbe, 2000). However, despite this, overall patient prognosis does not appear to be worsened in such cases (Chang, 2011; Soucie, 2012). The American College of Obstetricians and Gynecologists (2018a) considers hysteroscopy acceptable for AUB evaluation in those without advanced-stage uterine or advanced-stage cervical cancer.

■ Summary of Diagnostic Procedures

No one clear sequence of EMB, TVS, SIS, and hysteroscopy is superior during AUB evaluation. That said, TVS for several reasons is a logical first step. It is well tolerated, cost-effective, and requires relatively minimal technical skill (Figs. 8-6 and 8-7). In addition, it can reliably determine endometrial stripe thickness and whether a lesion is myometrial or endometrial. Once potential anatomic lesions have been identified, subsequent evaluation requires individualization. If endometrial hyperplasia or cancer is suspected, EMB offers advantages. Alternatively, possible focal lesions may be best investigated with hysteroscopy or SIS. Ultimately, the diagnostic goal is to identify and treat pathology and exclude endometrial neoplasia. Thus, test selection is guided by its accuracy in characterizing the most likely anatomic lesions, which are described in subsequent sections.

ENDOMETRIAL ABNORMALITIES

■ Hyperplasia and Intraepithelial Neoplasia

Several endometrial conditions linked with a relative estrogen excess can cause AUB. Estrogen promotes endometrial proliferation and growth, whereas progesterone limits this growth. With unbalanced estrogen stimulation, endometrial proliferation continues unchecked, leading to a spectrum of architectural and cytologic changes. These global conditions include disordered proliferative endometrium (DPE), endometrial hyperplasia without atypia, endometrial intraepithelial neoplasia (EIN), and endometrial cancer.

Remember that normal proliferative-phase endometrium contains regularly spaced glands that lie within stroma at a glands-to-stroma ratio of 1:1 (Fig. 33-1, p. 701). With DPE, the proliferative endometrium maintains this normal ratio overall but shows focal and mild gland dilation and crowding.

In contrast, *hyperplasia without atypia* shows more widespread gland crowding. Gland cytology is normal, and only occasional mitotic figures are seen. Hyperplasia without atypia is the term now recognized by the World Health Organization (WHO) and encompasses the former terms *simple hyperplasia without atypia* and *complex hyperplasia without atypia* (Zaino, 2014). Hyperplasia without atypia will typically regress after the unopposed estrogen environment is corrected. That said, 1 to 3 percent of untreated cases may progress to endometrioid adenocarcinoma.

EIN reflects a transition to a true premalignant lesion. It displays both gland crowding and abnormal gland nuclei. EIN comprises the former *simple hyperplasia with atypia* and *complex hyperplasia with atypia* (American College of Obstetricians and Gynecologists, 2017a). EIN significantly raises the risk of developing endometrial cancer, and its treatment is discussed in Chapter 33 (p. 703).

DPE and hyperplasia without atypia are best treated with progesterone. Common forms include oral medroxyprogesterone acetate (MPA), 10 to 20 mg daily; intramuscular DMPA, 150 mg every 3 months; or the levonorgestrel-releasing intrauterine system (LNG-IUS). Megestrol acetate, 40 to 200 mg orally daily, is also effective but used less frequently and mainly in those with EIN (Trimble, 2012). Consensus is lacking on optimal treatment length and route. That said, one randomized study showed the LNG-IUS or a continuous daily oral 10-mg dose of MPA was more effective in reestablishing a normal endometrium than was cyclic oral MPA (Ørbo, 2014).

To document resolution of hyperplasia without atypia, rebiopsy is recommended following progestin treatment and a subsequent withdrawal bleeding. However, consensus as to rebiopsy timing is lacking, and retesting after 3 to 6 months of treatment is used at our institution. Once normal endometrium is reestablished, no additional sampling is required unless new bleeding develops. Importantly, unless the underlying cause of unopposed estrogen is corrected, long-term progestin therapy is considered. Relapse rates following progestin discontinuation are high (Ørbo, 2016).

■ Metaplasia

Tissues derived from the müllerian ducts have remarkable capacity to undergo transformation into various epithelial types. This transformation is termed *metaplasia*. Endometrial metaplasia involving architecturally normal, or simple, glands usually reflects a benign reactive or hormonally driven process within the endometrium. However, endometrial metaplasia can also arise in association with EIN and endometrial adenocarcinoma (Carlson, 2008; Nicolae, 2011). Thus, if metaplastic change is associated with architectural abnormalities diagnostic of, or suspicious for, EIN or endometrial adenocarcinoma, further endometrial evaluation is warranted.

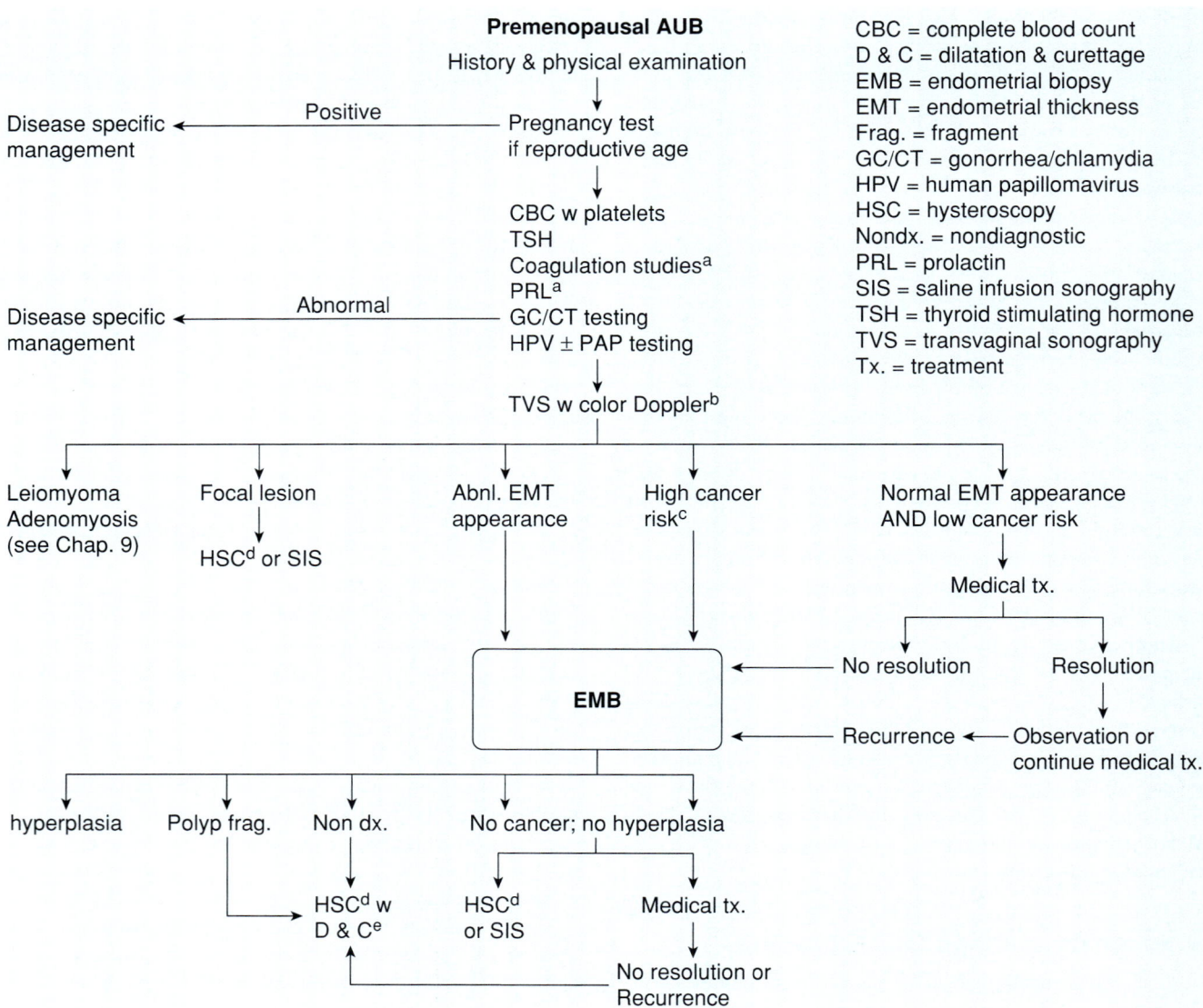

FIGURE 8-6 Diagnostic algorithm to identify endometrial pathology in premenopausal patients with abnormal uterine bleeding.
[a]Study obtained as indicated by patient history.
[b]When indicated, EMB as a primary step is suitable in settings without readily available TVS.
[c]Patients with chronic anovulation, obesity, ≥45 years of age, PCOS, tamoxifen use, diabetes, nulliparity, late menopause, unopposed estrogen use, and predisposing genetic syndromes.
[d]Other endoscopic devices to visualize the endometrial cavity are suitable.
[e]Depending on clinical setting, direct hysteroscopic sampling may suitably replace D & C.

Endometrial reactive changes comprise a heterogeneous group of endometrial morphology that can be associated with hormonal imbalance or recent inciting events such as infection, stromal breakdown, pregnancy, or instrumentation (Quick, 2018). Reactive changes are uncommonly linked to malignancy unless architectural abnormalities characterizing EIN or endometrial adenocarcinoma are also present (Nicolae, 2011).

■ Endometritis

In addition to cervicitis (p. 183), chronic endometritis has been linked to AUB in some but not all studies (Greenwood, 1981; Pitsos, 2009). Underlying infection is often implicated, and agents of bacterial vaginosis, *Mycoplasma* species (spp.),

Streptococcus spp., certain coliforms, *N gonorrhoeae*, and *C trachomatis* have each been identified (Cicinelli, 2008; Wiesenfeld, 2002). Thus, gonorrhea and chlamydial infection screening is reasonable in many sexually active patients with AUB, and positive results prompt treatment per CDC guidelines (2015) (Tables 3-9 and 3-11, p. 70). In other cases, chronic endometritis is linked to a structural cause such as endometrial polyp, intrauterine device (IUD), or submucous leiomyoma. It may also follow abortion or pregnancy.

Chronic endometritis is traditionally diagnosed histologically by plasma cell infiltration. In women undergoing diagnostic hysteroscopy, endometrial hyperemia, edema, and "micropolyps" measuring <1 mm can also suggest the diagnosis (Cicinelli, 2005).

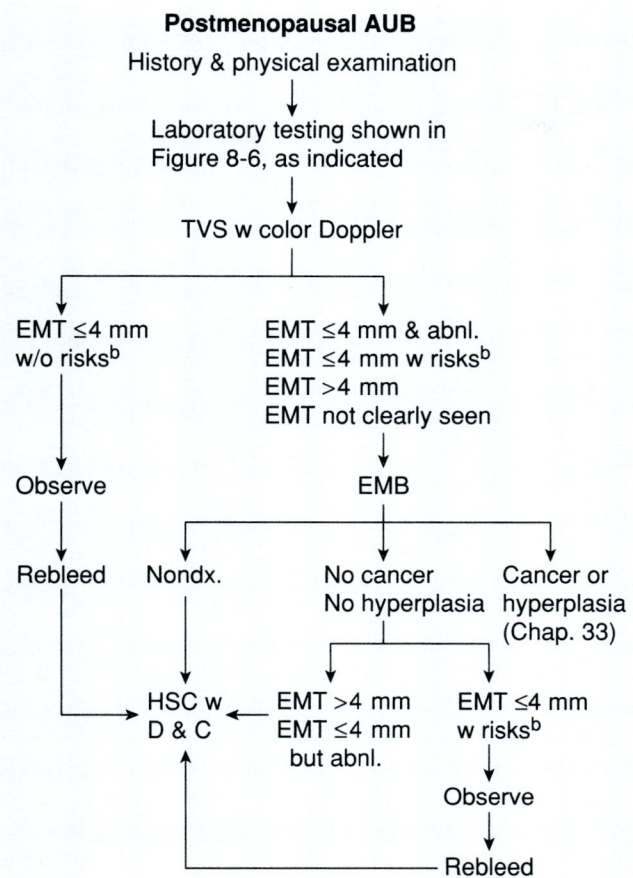

Postmenopausal AUB

History & physical examination

↓

Laboratory testing shown in
Figure 8-6, as indicated

↓

TVS w color Doppler

FIGURE 8-7 Diagnostic algorithm to identify endometrial pathology in postmenopausal patients with abnormal uterine bleeding.
[a]Study obtained as indicated by patient history.
[b]Chronic anovulation, obesity, ≥45 years of age, polycystic ovarian syndrome, tamoxifen use, diabetes, nulliparity, late menopause, unopposed estrogen use, and predisposing genetic syndromes.

Because infection may or may not underlie all cases of chronic endometritis, the decision to prescribe antibiotics can be challenging. And, few studies have evaluated the efficacy of antibiotics to resolve bleeding symptoms. At our institution, patients with documented histologic findings of endometritis are typically given a course of doxycycline, 100 mg orally twice daily for 10 days.

STRUCTURAL ABNORMALITIES

■ Uterine Enlargement

Structural abnormalities are frequent causes of AUB, and leiomyomas are by far the most common. Myomas, adenomyosis, and isthmoceles are presented in Chapter 9. Uterine and cervical neoplasms are discussed in Chapters 30, 33, and 34. As described in Chapter 19, partially obstructive congenital reproductive tract anomalies may at times cause chronic intermenstrual bleeding superimposed on normal menstrual cycling. Endometrial and endocervical structural abnormalities such as polyps and arteriovenous malformations are described here.

■ Endometrial Polyp

These soft, fleshy intrauterine growths are composed of endometrial glands, fibrous stroma, and surface epithelium. Intact polyps may be single or multiple, measure from a few millimeters to several centimeters, and be sessile or pedunculated (Fig. 8-8). Estrogen and progesterone are implicated in their growth, as higher receptor levels are noted within polyps compared with adjacent normal endometrium (Peres, 2018).

Polyps are common, and their prevalence in the general population approximates 9 percent (Dreisler, 2009a). In those with AUB, rates range from 10 to 30 percent (Bakour, 2000; Goldstein, 1997). Risk factors for developing endometrial polyps include increasing age, obesity, and tamoxifen use (Reslova, 1999). Although some studies suggest an association between HRT and polyp formation, others do not (Bakour, 2002; Dreisler, 2009a; Maia, 2004; Oguz, 2005). However, use of oral contraceptive pills appears to be protective (Dreisler, 2009b). For women taking tamoxifen, the LNG-IUS lowers endometrial polyp and endometrial hyperplasia rates. With LNG-IUS use, breast cancer recurrence rates are not higher in the short term, however long-term data are lacking regarding recurrence (Dominick, 2015).

Women with endometrial polyps may have no complaints, and polyps are identified during imaging for other indications (Goldstein, 2002). When symptomatic, polyps are frequently associated with HMB, prolonged bleeding, or intermenstrual bleeding. Infertility has also been linked indirectly with endometrial polyps. For example, small studies have shown higher pregnancy rates and fewer early pregnancy losses in infertile

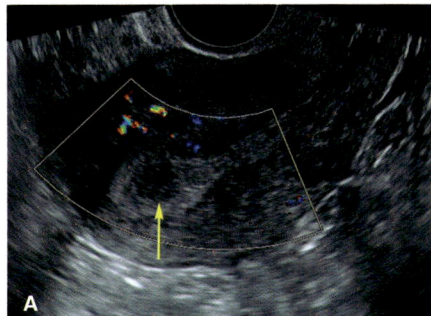
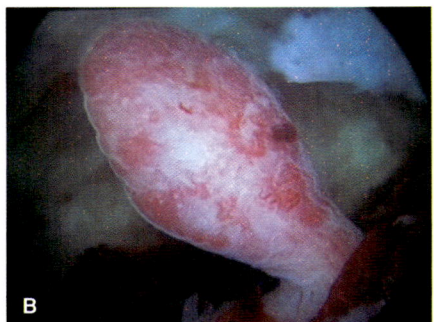
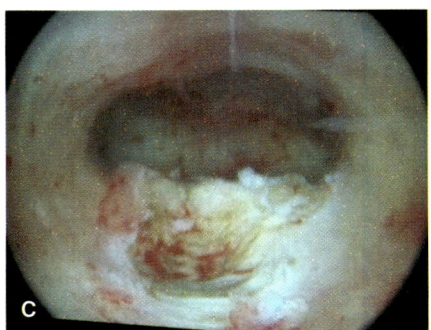

FIGURE 8-8 Endometrial polyp. **A.** Sagittal image of a uterus using transvaginal sonography with color Doppler. The yellow arrow points to the polyp, which is hypoechoic compared with the surrounding endometrium. **B.** Hysteroscopic image of same polyp. **C.** Endometrial cavity following polyp resection. (Reproduced with permission from Drs. David Rogers and Hillary Myears.)

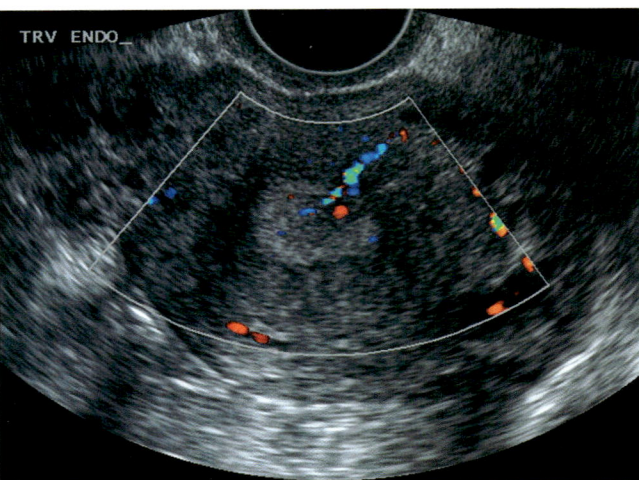

FIGURE 8-9 Transvaginal color Doppler sonography (TV-CDS) of an endometrial polyp. Color flow feature identifies a single feeder vessel, which is characteristic of a polyp. (Reproduced with permission from Dr. Elysia Moschos.)

women following hysteroscopic polyp excision (Pérez-Medina, 2005; Preutthipan, 2005; Stamatellos, 2008).

The main diagnostic tools include TVS with applied color Doppler, SIS, and hysteroscopy. In premenopausal women, TVS is best performed prior to day 10 of the cycle to lower the risk of false-positive findings from a normally thick secretory endometrium. With TVS, an endometrial polyp may appear as a nonspecific endometrial thickening or as a rounded hyperechoic mass within the cavity. Sonolucent cystic spaces corresponding to dilated endometrial glands are seen within some polyps. Importantly, polyps may appear similar to intracavity myomas. To help differentiate the two, TVS can be augmented with color or power Doppler. Endometrial polyps typically have only one arterial feeding vessel, whereas submucous leiomyomas generally received blood flow from several vessels arising from the inner myometrium (Fig. 8-9) (Cil, 2010; Fleischer, 2003).

SIS and hysteroscopy are both accurate in identifying endometrial polyps (Bittencourt, 2017; Soares, 2000). With SIS, polyps appear as echogenic, smooth, intracavitary masses with either broad bases or thin stalks (see Fig. 8-5B). With hysteroscopy, nearly all cases are identified with the added ability to remove the polyp concurrently.

The Pap test is an ineffective tool to identify polyps. However, 5 percent of postmenopausal women with benign endometrial cells detected on Pap testing are found to have endometrial polyps (Karim, 2002). Moreover, in postmenopausal women with atypical glandular cells of undetermined significance (AGUS), endometrial polyps were the most frequent underlying pathology found (Obenson, 2000).

EMB or D & C may also identify polyps. However, as previously discussed, blind sampling may completely miss or incompletely sample focal lesions.

Management of endometrial polyps is directed by symptoms and malignancy risk. Most polyps are benign, and premalignant or malignant transformation develops in only approximately 5 percent (Baiocchi, 2009; Ricciardi, 2014). The most consistent risks for transformation are postmenopausal status, age older than 60, and

abnormal bleeding. Some supporting data suggest that larger polyp size (>1.5 cm), tamoxifen use, diabetes, and obesity also confer a higher risk (Ferrazzi, 2009; Sasaki, 2018). Thus, operative hysteroscopic polypectomy may be most effective for symptomatic women or those with risk factors for malignant transformation. Procedural steps are described in Chapter 44 (p. 1056). During polypectomy, targeted sampling of the remaining endometrium is considered in those with endometrial cancer risk factors or with risks for malignant transformation within the polyp (Rahimi, 2009). Endometrial sampling during all polypectomy procedures also is reasonable, as previously undiagnosed endometrial cancer was found in 0.5 percent of more than 6000 women younger than 45 undergoing endometrial polypectomy (Yuk, 2018). Following polypectomy, subsequent polyp recurrence rates vary widely and can reach 45 percent (Gu, 2018; Yang, 2015).

Findings within a polyp are treated similarly to results found in nonpolypoid endometrium. For example, with polyps containing atypical hyperplasia, comorbid atypical hyperplasia or cancer in the remaining endometrium is found in one half to two thirds of hysterectomy specimens (Mittal, 2008; Naaman, 2015).

For asymptomatic women with small polyps and no malignant transformation risk factors, management can be more conservative (American Association of Gynecologic Laparoscopists, 2012). Some advocate removal of all endometrial polyps because premalignant and malignant transformation has been identified in even asymptomatic premenopausal women (Golan, 2010). However, the transformation risk in these patients with lesions measuring <15 mm is low (Ben-Arie, 2004). In addition, many polyps ≤10 mm will spontaneously resolve or slough (DeWaay, 2002; Wong, 2017). If conservative observation is elected, the optimum surveillance regimen for these women remains undefined.

■ Endocervical Polyp

These lesions represent overgrowths of benign endocervical stroma covered by mucinous columnar epithelium. They typically appear as single, red, smooth, elongated masses extending from the endocervical canal (Fig. 8-10). Polyps vary in size and

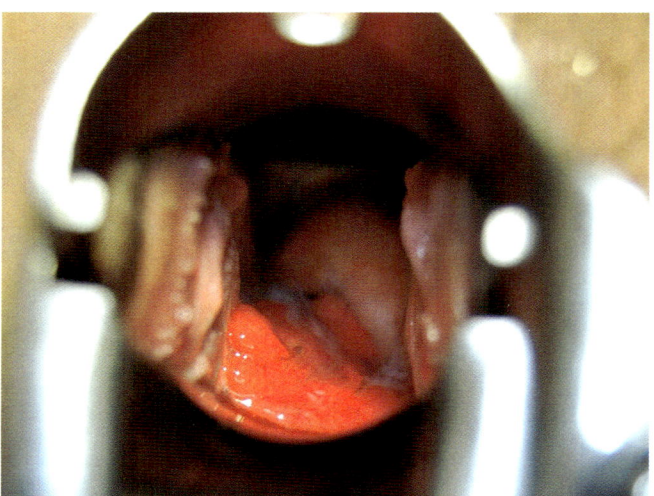

FIGURE 8-10 This endocervical polyp has a typical color and texture but is longer than most of these polyps.

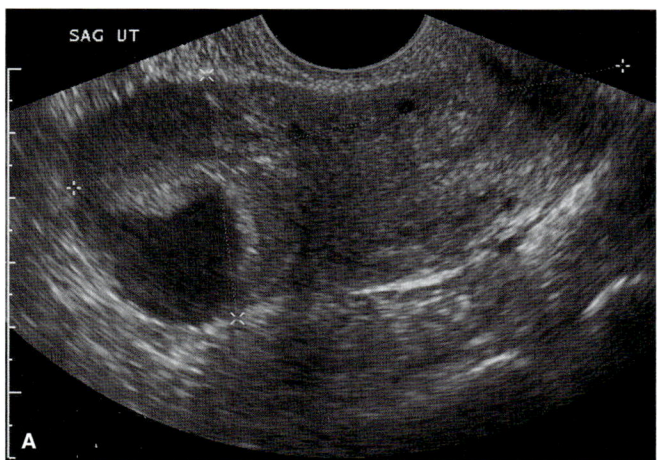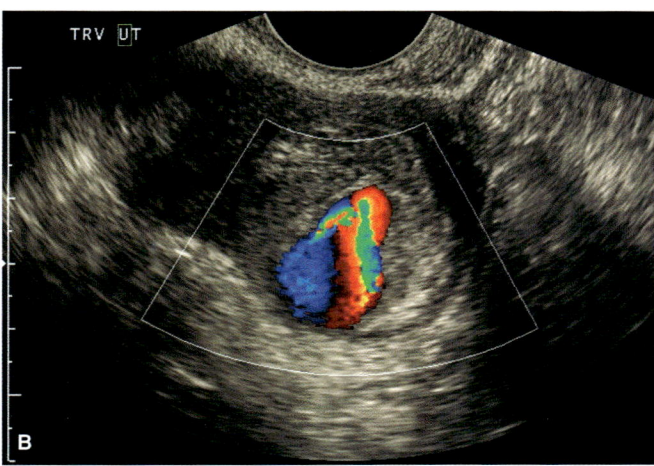

FIGURE 8-11 Transvaginal sonography of an arteriovenous malformation (AVM). **A.** Sagittal image of the uterus (*calipers*) with an irregular-shape anechoic space within the posterior fundal myometrium. **B.** Color Doppler evaluation of this area in the transverse plane demonstrates the classic mosaic color pattern of an AVM. (Reproduced with permission from Dr. Elysia Moschos.)

range from several millimeters to 2 or 3 cm. These common growths are found more frequently in multiparas and rarely in prepubertal females. Endocervical polyps are usually asymptomatic, but they can cause intermenstrual or postcoital bleeding or symptomatic vaginal discharge. Many endocervical polyps are identified by visual inspection during pelvic examination. In other instances, AGUS Pap smear findings may prompt investigation and lead to identification of endocervical polyps higher in the endocervical canal (Burja, 1999).

Endocervical polyps are typically benign, and premalignant or malignant transformation develops in less than 1 percent (Chin, 2008; Schnatz, 2009). However, cervical cancer can present as polypoid masses and can mimic these benign lesions. Others in the differential diagnosis include condyloma acuminata, leiomyoma, decidua, granulation tissue, or fibroadenoma. Most recommend removal and histologic evaluation of all polypoid lesions. However, studies have stratified affected patients by symptoms and cytology and found no preinvasive disease or cancer in endocervical polyps of asymptomatic women with normal cervical cytology (Long, 2013; MacKenzie, 2009).

For removal, if the stalk is slender, endocervical polyps are grasped by ring forceps. The polyp is twisted repeatedly about the base of its stalk. With repeated twisting, feeding vessels are strangulated, and its base will narrow and avulse. Monsel paste (ferric subsulfate) can be applied with direct pressure as needed to the resulting stalk stub to complete hemostasis. A thick pedicle may warrant surgical ligation and excision if heavier bleeding is anticipated. Patients are counseled that endocervical polyp recurrence rates range from 6 to 15 percent (Berzolla, 2007; Younis, 2010).

Arteriovenous Malformation

These rare structures contain a mixture of arterial, venous, and small capillary-like channels with fistulous connections. Uterine arteriovenous malformations (AVMs) may be congenital or acquired, and vessel sizes can vary considerably. Acquired AVMs are usually large vessels that develop after myometrial or intracavitary uterine surgery. Concurrent cervical or endometrial cancer, gestational trophoblastic disease, or IUD use are other associations (Ghosh, 1986). Uterine AVMs more frequently involve the corpus, but they may also be found in the cervix (Lowenstein, 2004). Affected patients often note HMB and perhaps intermenstrual bleeding that is unprovoked or that is triggered by a spontaneous miscarriage, curettage, or other intracavitary uterine surgery. Symptoms can appear slowly or suddenly with life-threatening hemorrhage (Timmerman, 2003).

In some cases, AVMs are first visualized with TVS because of its ready availability and widespread use. Sonographic characteristics are nonspecific and may include anechoic tubular structures within the myometrium (Fig. 8-11). Color Doppler or power Doppler ultrasound may provide a more specific image with bright, large-caliber vessels and multidirectional flow (Tullius, 2015). Angiography aids confirmation and can be used concurrently to perform vessel embolization (Cura, 2009). CT scanning with contrast, MR imaging, SIS, and hysteroscopy have also been used to image these.

AVMs are effectively treated by hysterectomy. Arterial embolization is another potential option (Barral, 2017). In one systematic review, the success rate with embolization was a 91 percent. A second embolization was required in some cases (Yoon, 2016).

EXTERNAL SOURCES

■ Intrauterine Device

The copper-containing IUD (ParaGard) alone can cause HMB or intermenstrual bleeding, but concurrent pregnancy, infection, or malpositioned device is first sought. Their management is discussed in Chapter 5 (p. 114). Once these are excluded, other AUB sources are investigated. With TVS, endometrial stripe evaluation may be limited by IUD shadowing. If needed, EMB with small catheters can be performed without device removal (Dean, 2018).

HMB attributed solely to a copper IUD can be treated or prevented with an empiric trial of NSAIDs taken during menses (Grimes, 2006). Intermenstrual bleeding, however, is typically not improved with these agents (Godfrey, 2013). For HMB treatment or prevention, limited evidence also supports tranexamic acid (Alanwar, 2018; Ylikorkala, 1983).

With the LNG-IUS, unscheduled spotting or light bleeding is expected during the first several months and decreases with continued use (Curtis, 2016b). Over time, the endometrium atrophies and leads to progestin-induced amenorrhea (McGavigan, 2003). However, if needed, treatment options mirror those for the copper IUD.

■ Hormonal Therapy

Other hormonal birth control methods typically lighten menstrual flow. However, breakthrough bleeding can be a common cause of early discontinuation.

With combination oral contraceptive (COCs), intermenstrual bleeding typically occurs early during use, and reassurance alone is suitable. Also, a medication inventory can identify new medications that might lower COC efficacy to incite such bleeding (Table 5-8, p. 124). If persistent, intermenstrual bleeding can typically be corrected by changing to a formulation with a higher estrogen dose (Table 5-6, p. 121).

In contrast, users of progestin-only contraceptive methods can experience breakthrough bleeding throughout the duration of use. Although this often improves with time, chronic breakthrough bleeding with these methods can be lessened by an estrogen supplement such as an oral daily 2-mg estradiol dose or 1.25-mg conjugated equine estrogen dose for 1 to 2 weeks. Alternatively, a COC can be added for 1 to 3 cycles (Zigler, 2017).

With *hormone replacement therapy*, irregular spotting or bleeding is also a well-known early side effect. With continuous therapy, lower initial doses may cause less estrogen stimulation of the endometrium and thus result in less bleeding (Archer, 2011). Importantly, compared with women on HRT who have attained amenorrhea, intrauterine pathology is four times more frequent in patients with continued abnormal bleeding past the first 6 months of HRT use and in those who have abnormal bleeding after achieving initial amenorrhea (Leung, 2003). Thus, further evaluation of AUB in these postmenopausal women should be considered.

Of the *selective estrogen-receptor modulators (SERMs)*, raloxifene, ospemifene, and bazedoxifene can each result in postmenopausal bleeding. However, this is much less frequent than with HRT (Christodoulakos, 2006; Kagan, 2018; Simon, 2013). These agents are discussed in Chapter 22.

Another SERM, tamoxifen, is used as an adjunct for treatment of estrogen-receptor-positive breast cancer. Although it diminishes estrogen action in breast tissue, tamoxifen stimulates endometrial proliferation. This SERM has been linked to hyperplasia, polyps, and adenocarcinoma of the endometrium and to uterine sarcomas (Cohen, 2004). Thus, in women with tamoxifen-associated AUB, evaluation is prudent. In contrast, for women who use tamoxifen but who do not have AUB, *screening* with TVS or EMB provides no endometrial cancer-lowering advantage and is not recommended (American College of Obstetricians and Gynecologists, 2017c).

■ Anticoagulants

The use of anticoagulants confers a risk of HMB or intermenstrual bleeding. The vitamin K antagonists are warfarin and heparin, and the direct oral anticoagulants (DOACs) include apixaban, rivaroxaban, dabigatran, and edoxaban. During AUB evaluation, patients are queried regarding recent dosing changes or antagonist medications. In addition, a prothrombin time (PT), partial thromboplastin time (PTT), and platelet count are usually obtained as bleeding may be related to excess anticoagulant activity.

Management of *chronic* anticoagulant-related AUB can be challenging. If anticoagulant levels lie in therapeutic range, an LNG-IUS, DMPA, or an oral daily progestin is an appropriate option for this indication (Culwell, 2009). Tranexamic acid is contraindicated due to theoretic risks of venous thromboembolism in this population (p. 195). Similarly, the US Medical Eligibility Criteria consider COCs to have risks that outweigh benefits in this setting (Curtis, 2016a). However, a few, including the International Society on Thrombosis and Haemostasis, consider COC use suitable for well-selected and compliant anticoagulated women with AUB (Baglin, 2012; Martinelli, 2016). If a surgical approach is ultimately desired, endometrial ablation or hysterectomy can be considered. Anticoagulation reversal for surgery differs depending on whether surgery is urgent or elective, and both instances are described in Chapter 39 (p. 828).

For acute severe HMB, anticoagulation is reversed. As a temporizing step, a Foley balloon can be inserted into the intrauterine cavity and inflated to tamponade bleeding. Foley balloon sizes range from the traditional 30 mL up to 80 mL, and selection can be tailored to endometrial cavity volume. For a typical uterus, intrauterine tamponade with a 30-mL balloon filled with saline is suitable. Also, the progestins in the table on page 195 can be used. No data describe the safety or risk of short-term, high-dose estrogens or of tranexamic acid in these cases. Surgery or uterine artery embolization (UAE) is associated with higher rates of intra- and postoperative bleeding or thromboembolic complications.

SYSTEMIC CAUSES

■ Kidney, Liver, and Thyroid Disease

Severe *renal dysfunction* often is accompanied by endocrine disturbances that can lead to AUB. This results from either hypoestrogenism or normal estrogen levels but anovulation (Cochrane, 1997; Matuszkiewicz-Rowińska, 2004). Of additional concern, bleeding may worsen the chronic anemia already associated with renal failure.

For AUB from anovulation, renal patients are treated with traditional methods outlined on page 196 (Guglielmi, 2013). Of specific options, COCs may be contraindicated with severe hypertension or with some systemic lupus erythematosus cases, both of which can complicate renal disease. Moreover, in those with renal disease, NSAIDs are avoided because they cause renal artery vasoconstriction to diminish glomerular function. If women with renal failure and HMB cannot take or do not respond to medical therapy, surgical treatments are considered. Of these, Jeong and coworkers (2004) noted decreased bleeding in 87 percent of 62 patients following endometrial ablation.

For women with renal disease and with bleeding attributed to estrogen-deficient atrophy, short-term estrogen use is suitable. However, guidelines and robust support for long-term estrogen replacement therapy (ERT) in this population are lacking. If considered, nonoral routes bypass the liver and theoretically may minimize blood pressure elevation. Thrombogenic effects and specifically dialysis-access thrombosis are also a concern (Ahmed, 2017). Last, significantly higher serum estrogen levels with ERT are found in women with advanced renal disease compared with healthy women. Thus, lowest doses and monitoring estrogen levels are reasonable (Mattix, 2000).

Liver dysfunction, depending on its severity, can lead to menstrual abnormalities (Stellon, 1986). The underlying mechanism for bleeding is not clear, but as in renal failure, HPO axis dysfunction is suggested. Additionally, hyperestrogenism from disrupted metabolism can lead to a disordered proliferative or hyperplastic endometrium (de Costa, 1992). Hemostatic dysfunction from poor coagulation factor synthesis may also contribute. Moreover, thrombocytopenia is common in women with portal hypertension and splenomegaly.

Evidence directing HMB treatment in women with liver disease is limited, and hormonal therapy may be inappropriate for some. In those with chronic viral hepatitis and normal transaminase levels or with mild compensated cirrhosis, hormonal contraceptive use is not restricted. In those with active hepatitis or a flare of their chronic viral disease, progestin-only contraception is acceptable. Estrogen-containing products, if already in use, may be continued, whereas initiation of these is avoided. In those with severe, decompensated cirrhosis, all hormonal contraception is avoided (Kapp, 2009). As one surgical option, endometrial ablation was effective and well tolerated in one small study of cirrhotic women (Liu, 2016).

Following liver or renal transplant, women may still be at risk for abnormal bleeding, and a few case series have shown higher rates of endometrial hyperplasia without atypia in transplant recipients with AUB (Bobrowska, 2006; Tohma, 2018).

Both *hyperthyroidism* and *hypothyroidism* can cause menstrual disturbances ranging from amenorrhea to HMB. In many women, these menstrual abnormalities antedate other clinical findings of thyroid disease (Joshi, 1993). Thus, in most women with chronic AUB, serum thyroid-stimulating hormone (TSH) level measurement is recommended. With hyperthyroidism, light or infrequent menses are more typical complaints (Krassas, 2010). With severe overt hypothyroidism, women commonly present with amenorrhea or anovulatory AUB (p. 194). These women can also display defects in hemostasis. This may be due to decreased coagulation factor levels, which have been identified in some hypothyroid patients. With either hypo- or hyperthyroidism, treatment of the underlying thyroid disorder usually corrects AUB (Krassas, 1999; Wilansky, 1989).

■ **Coagulopathy**

Normally, a clot forms from an aggregation of platelets, which is then stabilized by a fibrin net. Thus, many coagulation defects leading to HMB can be broadly categorized as either: (1) dysfunction of platelet adherence or (2) defects in platelet plug stabilization. First, during initial stages of hemostasis, platelets adhere to vessel wall breaks through binding of their receptors to exposed collagen. This bridging is dependent on von Willebrand factor, a plasma protein. Once bound, platelets are activated and release a potent agonist of their aggregation, thromboxane. Thus, low platelet number, defects in von Willebrand factor quality or quantity, platelet receptor defects, or thromboxane inhibitors may all lead to poor platelet adherence and HMB. Second, the coagulation cascade leads to fibrin, which stabilizes aggregated platelets. Thus, defects in the clotting factors that comprise this cascade may also predispose to AUB.

In general, coagulopathies are infrequent causes of gynecologic bleeding. However, in the subset of women with HMB and normal anatomy, the incidence is significantly higher (Eising, 2018; Philipp, 2005). This is especially true with adolescents presenting with AUB (Seravalli, 2013). In women with known inherited bleeding disorders, HMB is the most common complaint (Ragni, 2016).

For diagnosis, a history of easy bruising, bleeding complications with surgery or obstetric delivery, recurrent hemorrhagic ovarian cysts, epistaxis, and gastrointestinal bleeding or a family history of bleeding disorders raises concern for coagulopathy. Laboratory screening includes a CBC with platelets, PT, PTT, and fibrinogen level (American College of Obstetricians and Gynecologists, 2017d). More frequently identified coagulopathy disorders are von Willebrand disease, thrombocytopenia, and platelet dysfunction. Specific screening for each is discussed in subsequent sections.

Uncommon reasons include deficiencies of factor VIII and IX (hemophilia A and B) and other factor deficiencies. Acute treatment of these rare disorders is by factor replacement, and long-term management is similar to von Willebrand disease (vWD) (Mannucci, 2004).

Von Willebrand Disease

Von Willebrand factor (vWF) is a glycoprotein synthesized in endothelial cells and in megakaryocytes, which produce platelets. For coagulation, it is integral to platelet adherence at sites of endothelial injury and also prevents clearance of factor VIII. VWD is an inherited bleeding disorder that has several variants, which are characterized by either diminished amount or decreased function of vWF (Table 8-3). In general, type 3 vWD displays autosomal recessive transmission, whereas type 1 and most subtypes of type 2 show an autosomal dominant pattern.

The disorder is most common in Caucasians, and the prevalence of vWD approximates 1 percent in the general population (Rodeghiero, 2001). In screening for coagulopathy, women with vWD may display a prolonged PTT or may have normal results. If vWD is suspected clinically, specific tests include measurement of von Willebrand-ristocetin cofactor activity, vWF antigen concentration, and factor VIII activity (James, 2009b). Of note, factor VIII and vWF levels reach a nadir during menses and are relatively increased in women using COCs. However, testing need not be rescheduled nor COCs halted to complete patient evaluation (James, 2009a). Consultation with a hematologist is often recommended because the diagnosis of vWD, especially in its mild form, can be difficult.

TABLE 8-3. vWD Classification and Laboratory Values

Condition	Description of vWF Deficiency	Bleeding Propensity	vWf:RCo (IU/dL)	vWf:Ag (IU/dL)	FVIII Activity
Type 1	Quantitative: partial	Mild to Moderate	<30	<30	↓ or Normal
Type 2	Qualitative	Moderate	<30	<30–200	↓ or Normal
Type 3	Quantitative: virtually complete	High	<3	<3	↓↓↓(<10 IU/dL)
Normal			50–200	50–200	Normal

FVIII = coagulation factor VIII; vWD = von Willebrand disease; vWF = von Willebrand factor; vWF:Ag = von Willebrand factor antigen; vWF:RCo = von Willebrand factor: risocetin cofactor activity.
From Nichols, 2008, 2009.

Treatments for women with vWD and chronic HMB mirror that for primary endometrial dysfunction (p. 196) (Adeyemi-Fowode, 2017; Foster, 1995; Kingman, 2004). Importantly, agents that prevent platelet adhesion, such as aspirin or NSAIDs, are avoided (American College of Obstetricians and Gynecologists, 2017d).

For women with chronic HMB who do not respond to conventional treatment, a hematologist may be consulted for desmopressin or vWF concentrate use (Nichols, 2008). Desmopressin is a vasopressin analogue that promotes release of vWF from endothelial cells. In those with chronic HMB in whom desmopressin is ineffective or contraindicated, a vWF concentrate can be chosen (Holm, 2015).

In those with vWD-related chronic HMB and no longer desiring fertility, surgical intervention may be considered. Endometrial ablation offers preliminary improvement for affected women. However, it provides less long-term success than for those without a bleeding disorder (Rubin, 2004). Hysterectomy is curative, although rates of bleeding complications from hysterectomy in women with vWD are higher than those of unaffected women (James, 2009c). In preparation for surgical procedures, a hematologist can assist with desmopressin or vWF concentrate dosing.

For severe emergent bleeding, hormonal and antifibrinolytic options shown on page 195 are implemented while clotting factor deficiencies are corrected. In addition, desmopressin can be administered (Edlund, 2002). However, desmopressin is a potent antidiuretic agent. Thus, if multiple doses or shorter dosing intervals are used, then concurrent fluid restriction and monitoring for hyponatremia is advised (Rodeghiero, 2008). Additionally, if aggressive fluid resuscitation is needed, desmopressin may not be appropriate. In this case, vWF concentrates are used instead to quickly raise factor levels (James, 2011). Comprehensive management guidelines for vWD are also available from The National Heart, Lung, and Blood Institute at: http://www.nhlbi.nih.gov/files/docs/guidelines/vwd.pdf.

Platelets

Thrombocytopenia may be broadly categorized as resulting from: (1) increased platelet destruction, as with idiopathic thrombocytopenic purpura (ITP), (2) decreased platelet production, as with hematopoietic malignancy, or (3) increased platelet sequestration, as with splenomegaly.

Alternatively, normal platelet counts may be found, but *platelet dysfunction* leads to poor aggregation. One example is prolonged use of thromboxane inhibitors such as NSAIDs and aspirin. These drugs are often taken by women with AUB due to its close association with dysmenorrhea. Much less often, primary genetic defects in platelet receptors, such Bernard-Soulier syndrome and Glanzmann thrombasthenia, lead to platelet dysfunction and abnormal bleeding.

As a group, evidenced-based data directing the treatment of platelet-associated HMB are limited. For acute, severe HMB, platelet transfusion is considered for counts <20,000/μL or <50,000/μL with brisk bleeding. For those undergoing procedures, a transfusion threshold of ≤50,000/μL is often used, and for major surgery, ≤100,000/μL (James, 2011). Concurrently, treatment is tailored to the underlying cause of thrombocytopenia. Long-term, with the exception of NSAIDs, treatment options include those described later for AUB due to primary endometrial dysfunction (p. 196).

OVULATORY DISORDERS

A large percentage of women with AUB have anovulation as the underlying etiology, and the term AUB-O denotes the ovulatory dysfunction. The underlying causes of anovulation are varied and fully described in Chapter 17 (p. 371). Regardless of the reason, if ovulation does not occur, no progesterone is produced, and a proliferative endometrium persists. For this reason, women with AUB-O are at risk for developing endometrial hyperplasia, EIN, or endometrial cancer.

With AUB-O, bleeding episodes are variable, and classically, several months of amenorrhea are followed by HMB. Management of acute severe bleeding is described in the next section. For chronic management, correction of the underlying cause of anovulation is primary. If this is not possible, chronic progestin therapy replaces the physiologic progesterone that is absent. For women requiring contraception, COCs, progestin-only contraceptive pills, DMPA, LNG-IUS, and etonogestrel subdermal implant are options. In those not desiring contraception, cyclic monthly progesterone followed by withdrawal will typically regulate menses. Suitable oral daily doses given for 10 days each month include: (1) MPA [Provera], 5 or 10 mg; (2) norethindrone acetate (NETA [Aygestin]), 5 or 10 mg; or

(3) micronized progesterone, 300 mg (de Lignières, 1999; Munro, 2000). Another less frequently used choice is a gonad-otropin-releasing hormone (GnRH) agonist, which creates profound hypogonadism (Chap. 9, p. 207). The induced amenorrhea can be advantageous to permit severely anemic women with HMB to rebuild their red cell volume.

Surgery is rarely indicated for AUB-O, unless medical therapy fails, is contraindicated, or is not tolerated by the patient. Surgery may also be indicated if the patient has significant concomitant intracavitary lesions. In general, surgical options mirror those for abnormal bleeding associated with primary endometrial dysfunction (p. 197). However, special consideration is given to whether endometrial ablation should be used as first-line therapy for AUB-O. Namely, endometrial ablation is an effective treatment for AUB, but may cause broad intracavitary scar bands, termed synechiae. Acting as an obstruction, these may hinder subsequent satisfactory evaluation of the endometrium in those with AUB-O, who carry higher risks for endometrial hyperplasia, EIN, and cancer (American College of Obstetricians and Gynecologists, 2018b).

PRIMARY ENDOMETRIAL DYSFUNCTION

Unlike the clear mechanism underlying AUB-O, abnormal uterine bleeding from primary endometrial dysfunction (AUB-E) has no clear diagnostic features, and currently this is a diagnosis of exclusion. Suggested mechanisms include dysregulation of local endometrial hemostasis or deficiencies in endometrial repair. The resultant bleeding patterns may be HMB, intermenstrual bleeding, or prolonged bleeding.

■ Acute Hemorrhage Management

At times, women with AUB may have brisk bleeding that requires acute intervention. Fluid resuscitation is instituted as described in Chapter 40 (p. 862). Medical treatment is simultaneously administered to slow bleeding (Table 8-4). With any of these medication regimens, an intrauterine Foley balloon can be inflated concurrently to control brisk bleeding (p. 192).

As primary choices, equine estrogens can be given intravenously in 25-mg doses every 4 hours for up to three doses (DeVore, 1982). Once bleeding has slowed, patients can be transitioned to an oral taper using Premarin pills or more commonly COCs. These pill forms can also be selected primarily for less severe bleeding. With any of these high-dose choices, an antiemetic may be needed to control estrogen-related nausea. For COC administration, formulations containing at least 30 μg of ethinyl estradiol are selected (Table 5-6, p. 121). If bleeding is significant, the regimen begins with one pill every 6 hours until the bleeding has markedly diminished. For most women, bleeding will slow within 24 to 48 hours. After bleeding has ebbed, the COC dosage is decreased to one pill every 8 hours for the next 2 to 7 days and then to one pill every 12 hours for 2 to 7 days (James, 2011). Subsequently, once-daily dosing is continued for several weeks and then stopped to allow withdrawal menses. This type of dose-diminishing regimen is colloquially known as a "COC taper." This regimen is often individualized to the degree of patient bleeding and may include less frequent dosing

TABLE 8-4. Medical Treatment of Acute Severe AUB[a,b]

CEE[c,d]	25 mg IV every 4 hr, up to 3 doses
CEE[d,e]	2.5 mg every 6 hr
COCs[d,e] 30–50 μg	1 pill every 6 or 8 hr, up to 7 d
MPA[e]	10 mg every 4 hr
NETA[e]	5–10 mg every 4 hr
TXA[c]	10 mg/kg IV every 8 hr
TXA	1.3 g every 8 hr for 5 d

[a]Agents given orally except where noted as IV.
[b]For anemic patients, initiate oral iron supplements.
[c]If IV forms required, transition patients to oral agents once bleeding controlled.
[d]Antiemetics may aid nausea.
[e]Oral hormonal agent dosages are tapered by extending dosing from every 6 hr, to every 8 hr, to every 12 hr, and finally to daily. Each new dosing lasts 2 to 7 days depending on the level of concern for rebleeding.
AUB = abnormal uterine bleeding; CEE = conjugated equine estrogen (Premarin); COCs = combination oral contraceptive pills; d = day; hr = hour; IV = intravenous; MPA = medroxyprogesterone acetate; NETA = norethindrone acetate; TXA = tranexamic acid.
From DeVore, 1982; Munro, 2006; James, 2011.

or smaller doses. Following this taper, COCs may be discontinued or prescribed long-term for cycle control (Munro, 2006).

As an alternative to high-dose estrogen therapy for acute HMB, high-dose MPA (10 mg) or NETA (5 to 10 mg) can be used and administered orally every 4 hours. As with oral COCs, dosing is then tapered once bleeding has waned. One proposed taper stretches dosing to every 6 hours for 4 days, then every 8 hours for 3 days, then every 12 hours for 2 to 14 days. The progestin is then continued daily (James, 2011). Another primary regimen uses DMPA 150 mg intramuscularly and combines it with MPA 20 mg orally three times daily for 3 days. Here, the single depot injection serves as the taper (Ammerman, 2013).

Tranexamic acid (TXA) is also an option for acute HMB. This antifibrinolytic drug reversibly blocks lysine binding sites on plasminogen, thus allowing blood clots to persist to slow bleeding (Fig. 8-12). The usual IV dose is 10 mg/kg (maximum 600 mg/dose) every 8 hours. As bleeding declines or for less severe acute bleeding, oral TXA can be given in a dosage of 1.3 g (two tablets) three times daily (James, 2011). The drug has no effect on other blood coagulation parameters such as platelet count, PTT, and PT (Wellington, 2003). Contraindications are concurrent COC use, active thromboembolism, or history of or an intrinsic risk for thromboembolism.

■ Levonorgestrel-Releasing Intrauterine System

Chronic medical options for AUB-E include LNG-IUS, COCs, sustained progestins, TXA, NSAIDs, androgens, and GnRH agonists (Table 8-5). Of these, the LNG-IUS provides sustained progestin levels within the uterine cavity to atrophy the endometrium. It reduces menstrual loss by 74 to 97 percent

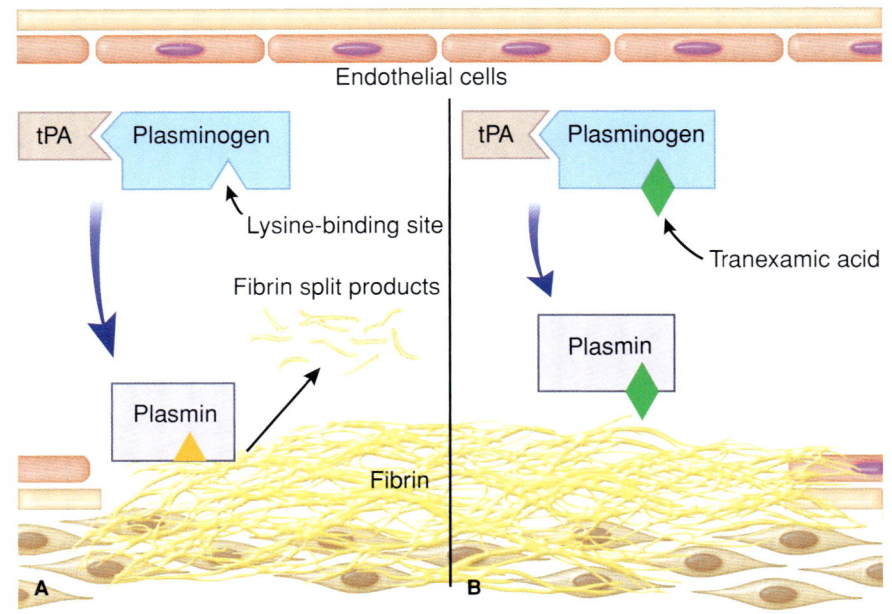

FIGURE 8-12 Tranexamic acid (TXA) mechanism of action. **A.** Normally, plasminogen binds with tissue plasminogen activator (tPA) to form plasmin. This binding degrades fibrin into fibrin degradation products and leads to clot lysis. **B.** TXA binds to the lysine-binding site on plasminogen. This new conformation blocks plasmin binding to fibrin. Fibrin strands are not broken, and a clot persists to slow bleeding.

In randomized trials of AUB-E, the LNG-IUS proved more effective in decreasing menstrual blood loss than NSAIDs given during menses; than oral progesterone given 21 days each cycle; or than COCs (Irvine, 1998; Reid, 2005; Shaaban, 2011). Other clinical trials have evaluated HMB more generally, bundling several AUB etiologies, including AUB-E. Gupta and coworkers (2013) noted higher associated quality-of-life scores with LNG-IUS compared with several traditional oral medical options. If compared with endometrial ablation, the LNG-IUS appears to have similar therapeutic effects for HMB in women followed 2 years after treatment (Kaunitz, 2009). One randomized trial compared LNG-IUS or hysterectomy for HMB and reported equal improvements in health status and quality of life at 1 year and again after 5 years (Hurskainen, 2001, 2004). However, by 5 years, 42 percent of those assigned to the LNG-IUS eventually underwent hysterectomy, and by 10 years, 46 percent (Heliövaara-Peippo, 2013).

after 3 months' use (Singh, 2005; Stewart, 2001). The LNG-IUS can be used in most women, including adolescents, as a first-line treatment for HMB. It is particularly useful for reproductive-aged women with AUB who wish to retain fertility. Contraindications are listed in Table 5-4 (p. 115).

■ Combination Oral Contraceptive Pills

These hormonal agents effectively treat AUB-E, and when used long term, menstrual blood loss is reduced by 40 to 70 percent (Jensen, 2011; Fraser, 1991, 2011b). Advantages to COCs include the additional benefits of reducing dysmenorrhea and

TABLE 8-5. Chronic Medical Treatment of AUB due to Primary Endometrial Dysfunction[a,b]

Agent	Brand	Dosage
LNG-IUS	Mirena	5-yr intrauterine use
COCs	Table 5-6[c]	One pill daily
DMPA	Depo-Provera	150 mg IM every 3 mo
NETA	Aygestin	5 mg, 3 times daily, days 5–26 of cycle
TXA[d]	Lysteda	1.3 g, 3 times daily × 5 d
NSAID[d]		
Mefenamic acid	Ponstel	500 mg, 3 times daily × 5 d
Naproxen	Naprosyn	550 mg on first day, then 275 mg daily
Ibuprofen	Motrin	600 mg, daily throughout menses
Flurbiprofen	Ansaid	100 mg, 2 times daily × 5 d
GnRH agonists	Lupron	3.75 mg, IM each month (up to 6 mo)

[a]All agents are administered orally except high-dose GnRH agonists, DMPA, and LNG-IUS.
[b]For anemic patients, also initiate oral iron supplementation.
[c]See Table 5-6, p. 121.
[d]Begin treatment with menses onset.
AUB = abnormal uterine bleeding; COCs = combination oral contraceptive pills; DMPA = depot medroxyprogesterone acetate; GnRH = gonadotropin-releasing hormone; IM = intramuscularly; LNG-IUS = levonorgestrel-releasing intrauterine system; NETA = norethindrone acetate; NSAID = nonsteroidal antiinflammatory drug; TXA = tranexamic acid.

providing contraception. Their presumed method of action is endometrial atrophy, although diminished prostaglandin synthesis and decreased endometrial fibrinolysis are other suggested actions (Irvine, 1999).

Tranexamic Acid

In women with AUB-E, fibrinolytic activity within the endometrium is increased compared with that of women with normal menses (Gleeson, 1994). Clinically, the antifibrinolytic effect of TXA reduces chronic bleeding in women with AUB-E by 40 to 50 percent (Bonnar, 1996; Lukes, 2010). In addition, it requires administration only during menstruation and has few minor reported side effects. The recommended dose is two 650-mg tablets orally taken three times daily for a maximum of 5 days during menses. Although used in other parts of the world for many years, oral TXA (Lysteda) was approved by the U.S. Food and Drug Administration (FDA) to treat HMB in 2009.

Nonsteroidal Antiinflammatory Drugs

These well-tolerated oral agents are commonly used to treat AUB-E, and rationale for their use stems from prostaglandin's suspected role in the pathogenesis of this endometrial dysfunction. Because women lose 90 percent of menstrual blood volume during the first 3 days of menses, NSAIDs are most effective if initiated just prior to or with menses onset and continued throughout its duration (Haynes, 1977). Thus, one advantage is that they are taken only during menstruation. Another advantage is that frequently associated dysmenorrhea also improves with NSAIDs.

So-called conventional NSAIDs nonspecifically inhibit both cyclooxygenase-1 (COX-1), an enzyme critical to normal platelet function, and cyclooxygenase-1 (COX-2), which mediates inflammatory response mechanisms. Thus, conventional NSAIDs such as ibuprofen and naproxen may not be ideal considering their inhibitory effects on platelet function. However, no data show an advantage with specific COX-2 inhibitors for HMB compared with conventional NSAIDs. Moreover, among conventional NSAIDS, one is not clinically superior to another, but responses to a particular agent may vary among individuals.

Although NSAIDs require only temporal dosing, are cost-effective, and are well tolerated, they often are only moderately effective for AUB-E and reduce menstrual bleeding by approximately 25 percent (Lethaby, 2013a). Thus, if greater reductions in blood loss are needed, other agents in this section may be more beneficial.

Other Agents

In contrast to AUB-O, AUB-E is relatively unresponsive to cyclic administration of oral progestins (Kaunitz, 2010; Preston, 1995). However, women with AUB-E may respond to longer treatment schedules. NETA, 5 mg, or MPA, 10 mg, each given orally three times daily for days 5 to 26 of each menstrual cycle have proved effective (Fraser, 1990; Irvine, 1998). Unfortunately, prolonged use of high-dose progestins is often associated with side effects such as mood changes, weight gain, bloating, headaches, and atherogenic lipid profile changes (Lethaby, 2008). Moreover, patients may find the dosing schedule challenging.

With GnRH agonists, the profound hypoestrogenic state created induces endometrial atrophy and amenorrhea in most women. Side effects include those typical for menopause, and thus associated bone loss precludes long-term use. This family of drugs, however, may be helpful for short-term use by inducing amenorrhea and allowing women to correct their anemia.

Of androgens, danazol creates a hypoestrogenic and hyperandrogenic environment to induce endometrial atrophy. For HMB, suggested dosing is 100 to 200 mg orally daily (Chimbira, 1980). Although effective, this agent has side effects that include weight gain, oily skin, and acne. Thus, some reserve danazol as a second-line drug for short-term use prior to surgery (Bongers, 2004). Another androgen, gestrinone, has mechanisms of action, side effects, and indications for HMB treatment similar to danazol. The recommended treatment dose is 2.5 mg orally twice weekly (Turnbull, 1990). The drug is used in other countries but is not approved for use in the United States.

Last, women with AUB may become anemic, and care typically is directed toward bleeding abatement and oral iron replacement. Anemia is effectively corrected with 150 to 200 mg of elemental iron daily. One common replacement regimen is ferrous sulfate, 325 mg tablet (contains 65 mg elemental iron) three times daily.

Uterine Procedures

For many women, conservative medical management may be unsuccessful or associated with significant side effects. Surgical management of HMB may include procedures to destroy the endometrium or hysterectomy.

Of these, *dilation and curettage* is rarely used for long-term treatment of AUB because its effects are temporary. Occasionally, D & C is performed to quickly remove endometrium and arrest acute, severe HMB refractory to high-dose estrogen administration (American College of Obstetricians and Gynecologists, 2017b). Notably, preprocedural TVS may be prudent as D & C may be ineffective or disadvantageous for women with an already thinned endometrium.

Endometrial resection or ablation attempts to permanently remove and destroy the uterine lining, using laser, radiofrequency, electrical, or thermal energies. Methods are considered first- or second-generation techniques according to when they were introduced into use and their need for concurrent hysteroscopic guidance (Chap. 44, p. 1061).

Several studies that compared first- and second-generation techniques have shown them equally effective to reduce HMB (Lethaby, 2013b). Similarly equivalent efficacy is seen among the various second-generation options (Daniels, 2012). After ablation, 70 to 80 percent of women experience significantly decreased flow, and 15 to 35 percent of these develop amenorrhea (Sharp, 2006). Increasing treatment failures due to endometrial regeneration accrue with time, and by 5 years following ablation, approximately 25 percent required additional surgery, in most cases hysterectomy (Cooper, 2011). However, the risk of reoperation following resection and ablation procedures is balanced by their significantly lower complication rates compared with hysterectomy.

TABLE 8-6. Endometrial Ablation

Contraindications

Pregnancy
Acute pelvic infection
Endometrial hyperplasia, EIN, or genital tract cancer
Desire to preserve fertility
Postmenopausal women
Expectation of amenorrhea
Large or distorted endometrial cavity[b]
Intrauterine device in place
Prior uterine surgery—classical cesarean delivery,
    transmural myomectomy

Caution

Those at risk for endometrial cancer[a]

---

[a]Risks include obesity, chronic anovulation, tamoxifen use, unopposed estrogen use, and diabetes mellitus.
[b]Each device has specific cavity-size limitations.
EIN = endometrial intraepithelial neoplasia.

After ablation, uterine cavity anatomy is often distorted by uterine wall agglutination and intracavitary synechiae. This may pose several long-term problems. First, focal hematometra from menstrual blood trapped behind synechiae can cause severe distention and cyclic pain (Chap. 44, p. 1061). Specifically, postablation tubal sterilization syndrome (PATSS) develops from menstrual blood sequestered between synechiae and previously occluded fallopian tubes. Second, because of distorted anatomy, 33 percent of endometrial sampling attempts may be inadequate, and endometrial stripe evaluation by TVS or hysteroscopic examination may be limited (Ahonkallio, 2009). As noted, endometrial ablation is not routinely recommended for patients at high risk for endometrial cancer. Other contraindications are listed in Table 8-6.

UAE is more commonly used to treat chronic HMB from uterine myomas and is described in Chapter 9 (p. 209). Rarely, this intervention may be considered emergently in women with excessive acute, severe HMB who fail conservation measures, especially those who refuse blood products or who have a coagulopathy. However, the latter may preclude femoral or radial artery cannulation, which is requisite for UAE.

Hysterectomy, despite the above measures, ultimately is chosen by more than half of women with HMB within 5 years of their referral to a gynecologist. In at least a third of these, an anatomically normal uterus is removed (Coulter, 1991). Removal of the uterus is the most effective treatment for bleeding, and overall patient satisfaction rates are high. Disadvantages to hysterectomy include more frequent and severe intraoperative and postoperative complications compared with either conservative medical or ablative surgical procedures. The procedure and its complications are discussed in detail in Chapter 43 (p. 956).

REFERENCES

Abdelazim IA, Abdelrazak KM, Elbiaa AA, et al: Accuracy of endometrial sampling compared to conventional dilatation and curettage in women with abnormal uterine bleeding. Arch Gynecol Obstet 291(5):1121, 2015

Adeyemi-Fowode OA, Santos XM, Dietrich JE, et al: Levonorgestrel-releasing intrauterine device use in female adolescents with heavy menstrual bleeding and bleeding disorders: single institution review. J Pediatr Adolesc Gynecol 30(4):479, 2017

Ahmed SB: Menopause and chronic kidney disease. Semin Nephrol 37(4):404, 2017

Ahonkallio SJ, Liakka AK, Martikainen HK, et al: Feasibility of endometrial assessment after thermal ablation. Eur J Obstet Gynecol Reprod Biol 147(1):69, 2009

Ahuja SP, Hertweck SP: Overview of bleeding disorders in adolescent females with menorrhagia. J Pediatr Adolesc Gynecol 23(6 Suppl):S15, 2010

Alanwar A, Abbas AM, Hussain SH, et al: Oral micronised flavonoids versus tranexamic acid for treatment of heavy menstrual bleeding secondary to copper IUD use: a randomised double-blind clinical trial. Eur J Contracept Reprod Health Care 23(5):365, 2018

American Association of Gynecologic Laparoscopists: AAGL practice report: practice guidelines for the diagnosis and management of endometrial polyps. J Minim Invasive Gynecol 19(1):3, 2012

American College of Obstetricians and Gynecologists: Endometrial cancer. Practice Bulletin No. 149, April 2015

American College of Obstetricians and Gynecologists: Diagnosis of abnormal uterine bleeding in reproductive-aged women. Practice Bulletin No. 128, July 2012, Reaffirmed 2016a

American College of Obstetricians and Gynecologists: Sonohysterography. Technology Assessment No. 12, August 2016b

American College of Obstetricians and Gynecologists: Endometrial intraepithelial neoplasia. Committee Opinion No. 631, May 2015, Reaffirmed 2017a

American College of Obstetricians and Gynecologists: Management of acute abnormal uterine bleeding in nonpregnant reproductive-aged women. Committee Opinion No. 557, April 2013, Reaffirmed 2017b

American College of Obstetricians and Gynecologists: Tamoxifen and uterine cancer. Committee Opinion No. 601, June 2014, Reaffirmed 2017c

American College of Obstetricians and Gynecologists: Von Willebrand disease in women. Committee Opinion No. 580, December 2013, Reaffirmed 2017d

American College of Obstetricians and Gynecologists: Hysteroscopy. Technology Assessment No. 13, May 2018a

American College of Obstetricians and Gynecologists: Management of abnormal uterine bleeding associated with ovulatory dysfunction. Practice Bulletin No. 136, July 2013, Reaffirmed 2018b

American College of Obstetricians and Gynecologists: The role of transvaginal ultrasonography in evaluating the endometrium of women with postmenopausal bleeding. Committee Opinion No. 734, May 2018c

Ammerman SR, Nelson AL: A new progestogen-only medical therapy for outpatient management of acute, abnormal uterine bleeding: a pilot study. Am J Obstet Gynecol 208(6):499.e1, 2013

Arafah MA, Cherkess Al-Rikabi A, et al: Adequacy of the endometrial samples obtained by the uterine Explora device and conventional dilatation and curettage: a comparative study. Int J Reprod Med. 2014:578193, 2014

Archer DF: Endometrial bleeding in postmenopausal women: with and without hormone therapy. Menopause 18(4):416, 2011

Baglin T, Bauer K, Douketis J, et al: Duration of anticoagulant therapy after a first episode of an unprovoked pulmonary embolus or deep vein thrombosis: guidance from the SSC of the ISTH. J Thromb Haemost 10(4):698, 2012

Baiocchi G, Manci N, Pazzaglia M, et al: Malignancy in endometrial polyps: a 12-year experience. Am J Obstet Gynecol 201(5):462.e1, 2009

Bakour SH, Gupta JK, Khan KS: Risk factors associated with endometrial polyps in abnormal uterine bleeding. Int J Gynecol Obstet 76(2):165, 2002

Bakour SH, Khan KS, Gupta JK: The risk of premalignant and malignant pathology in endometrial polyps. Acta Obstet Gynecol Scand 79:317, 2000

Bar-Hava I, Orvieto R, Ferber A, et al: Asymptomatic postmenopausal intrauterine fluid accumulation: characterization and significance. Climacteric 1(4):279, 1998

Barral PA, Saeed-Kilani M, Tradi F, et al: Transcatheter arterial embolization with ethylene vinyl alcohol copolymer (Onyx) for the treatment of hemorrhage due to uterine arteriovenous malformations. Diagn Interv Imaging 98(5):415, 2017

Benacerraf BR, Shipp TD, Bromley B: Which patients benefit from a 3D reconstructed coronal view of the uterus added to standard routine 2D pelvic sonography? AJR Am J Roentgenol 190(3):626, 2008

Ben-Arie A, Goldchmit C, Laviv Y, et al: The malignant potential of endometrial polyps. Eur J Obstet Gynecol Reprod Biol 115:206, 2004

Bennett GL, Andreotti RF, Lee SI, et al: ACR Appropriateness Criteria on abnormal vaginal bleeding. J Am Coll Radiol 8(7):460, 2011

Ben-Yehuda OM, Kim YB, Leuchter RS: Does hysteroscopy improve upon the sensitivity of dilatation and curettage in the diagnosis of endometrial hyperplasia or carcinoma? Gynecol Oncol 68:4, 1998

Berzolla CE, Schnatz PF, O'Sullivan DM, et al: Dysplasia and malignancy in endocervical polyps. J Womens Health 16(9):1317, 2007

Bettocchi S, Ceci O, Vicino M, et al: Diagnostic inadequacy of dilatation and curettage. Fertil Steril 75(4):803, 2001

Bittencourt CA, Dos Santos Simões R, et al: Accuracy of saline contrast sonohysterography in detection of endometrial polyps and submucosal leiomyomas in women of reproductive age with abnormal uterine bleeding: systematic review and meta-analysis. Ultrasound Obstet Gynecol 50(1):32, 2017

Bobrowska K, Kaminski P, Cyganek A, et al: High rate of endometrial hyperplasia in renal transplanted women. Transplant Proc 38(1):177, 2006

Bongers MY, Mol BW, Brolmann HA: Current treatment of dysfunctional uterine bleeding. Maturitas 47:159, 2004

Bonnar J, Sheppard BL: Treatment of menorrhagia during menstruation: randomised controlled trial of ethamsylate, mefenamic acid, and tranexamic acid. BMJ 313:579, 1996

Bradley WH, Boente MP, Brooker D, et al: Hysteroscopy and cytology in endometrial cancer. Obstet Gynecol 104(5 Pt 1):1030, 2004

Breitkopf DM, Frederickson RA, Snyder RR: Detection of benign endometrial masses by endometrial stripe measurement in premenopausal women. Obstet Gynecol 104(1):2004

Brunham RC, Paavonen J, Stevens CE, et al: Mucopurulent cervicitis—the ignored counterpart in women of urethritis in men. N Engl J Med 311(1):1, 1984

Burja IT, Thompson SK, Sawyer WL Jr, et al: Atypical glandular cells of undetermined significance on cervical smears. A study with cytohistologic correlation. Acta Cytol 43:351, 1999

Carlson JW, Mutter GL: Endometrial intraepithelial neoplasia is associated with polyps and frequently has metaplastic change. Histopathology 53(3):325, 2008

Ceci O, Bettocchi S, Pellegrino A, et al: Comparison of hysteroscopic and hysterectomy findings for assessing the diagnostic accuracy of office hysteroscopy. Fertil Steril 78(3):628, 2002

Centers for Disease Control and Prevention: Sexually transmitted diseases treatment guidelines, 2015. MMWR 64(3):1, 2015

Chang YN, Zhang Y, Wang YJ, et al: Effect of hysteroscopy on the peritoneal dissemination of endometrial cancer cells: a meta-analysis. Fertil Steril 96(4):957, 2011

Chimbira TH, Anderson AB, Naish C, et al: Reduction of menstrual blood loss by danazol in unexplained menorrhagia: lack of effect of placebo. BJOG 87:1152, 1980

Chin N, Platt AB, Nuovo GJ: Squamous intraepithelial lesions arising in benign endocervical polyps: a report of 9 cases with correlation to the Pap smears, HPV analysis, and immunoprofile. Int J Gynecol Pathol 27(4):582, 2008

Christodoulakos GE, Botsis DS, Lambrinoudaki IV, et al: A 5-year study on the effect of hormone therapy, tibolone and raloxifene on vaginal bleeding and endometrial thickness. Maturitas 53(4):413, 2006

Cicinelli E, De Ziegler D, Nicoletti R, et al: Chronic endometritis: correlation among hysteroscopic, histologic, and bacteriologic findings in a prospective trial with 2190 consecutive office hysteroscopies. Fertil Steril 89(3):677, 2008

Cicinelli E, Parisi C, Galantino P, et al: Reliability, feasibility, and safety of minihysteroscopy with a vaginoscopic approach: experience with 6,000 cases. Fertil Steril 80(1):199, 2003

Cicinelli E, Resta L, Nicoletti R, et al: Endometrial micropolyps at fluid hysteroscopy suggest the existence of chronic endometritis. Hum Reprod 20(5):1386, 2005

Cil AP, Tulunay G, Kose MF, et al: Power Doppler properties of endometrial polyps and submucosal fibroids: a preliminary observational study in women with known intracavitary lesions. Ultrasound Obstet Gynecol 35(2):233, 2010

Clark TJ, Mann CH, Shah N, et al: Accuracy of outpatient endometrial biopsy in the diagnosis of endometrial cancer: a systematic quantitative review. BJOG 109(3):313, 2002a

Clark TJ, Voit D, Gupta JK, et al: Accuracy of hysteroscopy in the diagnosis of endometrial cancer and hyperplasia: a systematic quantitative review. JAMA 288:1610, 2002b

Cochrane R, Regan L: Undetected gynaecological disorders in women with renal disease. Hum Reprod 12:667, 1997

Cohen I: Endometrial pathologies associated with postmenopausal tamoxifen treatment. Gynecol Oncol 94:256, 2004

Cooper K, Lee A, Chien P, et al: Outcomes following hysterectomy or endometrial ablation for heavy menstrual bleeding: retrospective analysis of hospital episode statistics in Scotland. BJOG 118(10):1171, 2011

Cordier W, Steenkamp V: Herbal remedies affecting coagulation: a review. Pharm Biol 50(4):443, 2012

Coulter A, Bradlow J, Agass M, et al: Outcomes of referrals to gynaecology outpatient clinics for menstrual problems: an audit of general practice records. BJOG 98:789, 1991

Critchley HO, Maybin JA: Molecular and cellular causes of abnormal uterine bleeding of endometrial origin. Semin Reprod Med 29(5):400, 2011

Culwell KR, Curtis KM: Use of contraceptive methods by women with current venous thrombosis on anticoagulant therapy: a systematic review. Contraception 80(4):337, 2009

Cura M, Martinez N, Cura A, et al: Arteriovenous malformations of the uterus. Acta Radiol 50(7):823, 2009

Curtis KM, Jatlaoui TC, Tepper NK, et al: U.S. selected practice recommendations for contraceptive use, 2016. MMWR 65(4):1, 2016a

Curtis KM, Tepper NK, Jatlaoui TC, et al: U.S. medical eligibility criteria for contraceptive use, 2016. MMWR 65(3):1, 2016b

Daniels JP, Middleton LJ, Champaneria R, et al: Second generation endometrial ablation techniques for heavy menstrual bleeding: network meta-analysis. BMJ 344:e2564, 2012

de Costa C, Jeremy R, Russell P: Alcoholic liver disease with subsequent hyperoestrogenism. Aust N Z J Obstet Gynaecol 32(2):179, 1992

de Lignières B: Oral micronized progesterone. Clin Ther 21(1):41, 1999

Dean G, Schwartz EB: Intrauterine devices (IUDs). In Hatcher RA, Nelson AL, Trussell J, et al (eds): Contraceptive Technology, 21th ed. New York, Ayer Company Publishers, 2018, p 178

Del Priore G, Williams R, Harbatkin CB, et al: Endometrial brush biopsy for the diagnosis of endometrial cancer. J Reprod Med 46(5):439, 2001

Demirkiran F, Yavuz E, Erenel H, et al: Which is the best technique for endometrial sampling? Aspiration (Pipelle) versus dilatation and curettage (D & C). Arch Gynecol Obstet 286(5):1277, 2012

DeVore GR, Owens O, Kase N: Use of intravenous Premarin in the treatment of dysfunctional uterine bleeding—a double-blind randomized control study. Obstet Gynecol 59:285, 1982

DeWaay DJ, Syrop CH, Nygaard IE, et al: Natural history of uterine polyps and leiomyomata. Obstet Gynecol 100:3, 2002

Dijkhuizen FP, Mol BW, Brölmann HA, et al: The accuracy of endometrial sampling in the diagnosis of patients with endometrial carcinoma and hyperplasia: a meta-analysis. Cancer 89(8):1765, 2000

Dogan E, Celiloglu M, Sarihan E, et al: Anesthetic effect of intrauterine lidocaine plus naproxen sodium in endometrial biopsy. Obstet Gynecol 103(2):347, 2004

Dominick S, Hickey M, Chin J, et al: Levonorgestrel intrauterine system for endometrial protection in women with breast cancer on adjuvant tamoxifen. Cochrane Database Syst Rev 12:CD007245, 2015

Dreisler E, Sorensen SS, Ibsen PH, et al: Prevalence of endometrial polyps and abnormal uterine bleeding in a Danish population aged 20–74 years. Ultrasound Obstet Gynecol 33(1):102, 2009a

Dreisler E, Sorensen SS, Lose G: Endometrial polyps and associated factors in Danish women aged 36–74 years. Am J Obstet Gynecol 200(2):147.e1, 2009b

Dueholm M, Christensen JW, Rydbjerg S, et al: Two- and three-dimensional transvaginal ultrasound with power Doppler angiography and gel infusion sonography for diagnosis of endometrial malignancy. Ultrasound Obstet Gynecol 45(6):734, 2015

Dueholm M, Møller C, Rydbjerg S, et al: An ultrasound algorithm for identification of endometrial cancer. Ultrasound Obstet Gynecol 43(5):557, 2014

Edlund M, Blombäck M, Fried G: Desmopressin in the treatment of menorrhagia in women with no common coagulation factor deficiency but with prolonged bleeding time. Blood Coagul Fibrinolysis 13(3):225, 2002

Eising HP, Roest M, de Groot PG, et al: High prevalence of reduced thrombin generation and/or decreased platelet response in women with unexplained heavy menstrual bleeding. Int J Lab Hematol 40(3):268, 2018

Everett C: Incidence and outcome of bleeding before the 20th week of pregnancy: prospective study from general practice. BMJ 315:32, 1997

Ferenczy A: Pathophysiology of endometrial bleeding. Maturitas 45(1):1, 2003

Ferenczy A, Shore M, Guralnick M, et al: The Kevorkian curette. An appraisal of its effectiveness in endometrial evaluation. Obstet Gynecol 54(2):262, 1979

Ferrazzi E, Zupi E, Leone FP, et al: How often are endometrial polyps malignant in asymptomatic postmenopausal women? A multicenter study. Am J Obstet Gynecol 200(3):235.e1, 2009

Fleischer AC, Shappell HW: Color Doppler sonohysterography of endometrial polyps and submucosal fibroids. J Ultrasound Med 22:601, 2003

Fleischer AC, Wheeler JE, Lindsay I, et al: An assessment of the value of ultrasonographic screening for endometrial disease in postmenopausal women without symptoms. Am J Obstet Gynecol 184(2):70, 2001

Foster PA: The reproductive health of women with von Willebrand disease unresponsive to DDAVP: results of an international survey. On behalf of the Subcommittee on von Willebrand Factor of the Scientific and Standardization Committee of the ISTH. Thromb Haemost 74(2):784, 1995

Fraser IS: Treatment of ovulatory and anovulatory dysfunctional uterine bleeding with oral progestogens. Aust N Z J Obstet Gynaecol 30(4):353, 1990

Fraser IS, Critchley HO, Broder M, et al: The FIGO recommendations on terminologies and definitions for normal and abnormal uterine bleeding. Semin Reprod Med 29(5):383, 2011a

Fraser IS, McCarron G: Randomized trial of 2 hormonal and 2 prostaglandin-inhibiting agents in women with a complaint of menorrhagia. Aust N Z J Obstet Gynaecol 31:66, 1991

Fraser IS, Römer T, Parke S, et al: Effective treatment of heavy and/or prolonged menstrual bleeding with an oral contraceptive containing estradiol valerate and dienogest: a randomized, double-blind Phase III trial. Hum Reprod 26:2698, 2011b

Ghosh TK: Arteriovenous malformation of the uterus and pelvis. Obstet Gynecol 68:40S, 1986

Gkrozou F, Dimakopoulos G, Vrekoussis T, et al: Hysteroscopy in women with abnormal uterine bleeding: a meta-analysis on four major endometrial pathologies. Arch Gynecol Obstet 291(6):1347, 2015

Gleeson NC: Cyclic changes in endometrial tissue plasminogen activator and plasminogen activator inhibitor type 1 in women with normal menstruation and essential menorrhagia. Am J Obstet Gynecol 171:178, 1994

Godfrey EM, Folger SG, Jeng G, et al: Treatment of bleeding irregularities in women with copper-containing IUDs: a systematic review. Contraception 87(5):549, 2013

Goebel EA, McLachlin CM, Ettler HC, et al: Insufficient and scant endometrial samples: determining clinicopathologic outcomes and consistency in reporting. Int J Gynecol Pathol 38(3):216, 2019

Golan A, Cohen-Sahar B, Keidar R, et al: Endometrial polyps: symptomatology, menopausal status and malignancy. Gynecol Obstet Invest 70(2):107, 2010

Goldstein RB, Bree RL, Benson CB, et al: Evaluation of the woman with postmenopausal bleeding: Society of Radiologists in Ultrasound—Sponsored Consensus Conference statement. J Ultrasound Med 20(10):1025, 2001

Goldstein SR, Monteagudo A, Popiolek D, et al: Evaluation of endometrial polyps. Am J Obstet Gynecol 186:669, 2002

Goldstein SR, Zeltser I, Horan CK, et al: Ultrasonography-based triage for perimenopausal patients with abnormal uterine bleeding. Am J Obstet Gynecol 177(1):102, 1997

Granberg S, Wikland M, Karlsson B, et al: Endometrial thickness as measured by endovaginal ultrasonography for identifying endometrial abnormality. Am J Obstet Gynecol 164:47, 1991

Greenwood SM, Moran JJ: Chronic endometritis: morphologic and clinical observations. Obstet Gynecol 58:176, 1981

Grimes DA, Hubacher D, Lopez LM, et al: Non-steroidal anti-inflammatory drugs for heavy bleeding or pain associated with intrauterine-device use. Cochrane Database Syst Rev 4:CD006034, 2006

Gu F, Zhang H, Ruan S, et al: High number of endometrial polyps is a strong predictor of recurrence: findings of a prospective cohort study in reproductive-age women. Fertil Steril 109(3):493, 2018

Guglielmi KE: Women and ESRD: modalities, survival, unique considerations. Adv Chronic Kidney Dis 20(5):411, 2013

Güler A, Sahin HG, Küçükaydın Z, et al: Comparison of the efficacy of intrauterine lidocaine, paracervical block and oral etodolac for decreasing pain in endometrial biopsy. J Turk Ger Gynecol Assoc 11(4):178, 2010

Gupta J, Kai J, Middleton L, et al: Levonorgestrel intrauterine system versus medical therapy for menorrhagia. N Engl J Med 368(2):128, 2013

Hallberg L, Hogdahl AM, Nilsson L, et al: Menstrual blood loss—a population study. Variation at different ages and attempts to define normality. Acta Obstet Gynecol Scand 45:320, 1966

Haynes PJ, Hodgson H, Anderson AB, et al: Measurement of menstrual blood loss in patients complaining of menorrhagia. BJOG 84:763, 1977

Hefler L, Leipold H, Hinterberger S, et al: Influence of the time interval between hysteroscopy, dilation and curettage, and hysterectomy on survival in patients with endometrial cancer. Obstet Gynecol 112(5):1098, 2008

Heliövaara-Peippo S, Hurskainen R, Teperi J, et al: Quality of life and costs of levonorgestrel-releasing intrauterine system or hysterectomy in the treatment of menorrhagia: a 10-year randomized controlled trial. Am J Obstet Gynecol 209(6):535.e1, 2013

Higham JM, O'Brien PM, Shaw RW: Assessment of menstrual blood loss using a pictorial chart. BJOG 97:734, 1990

Holm E, Abshire TC, Bowen J, et al: Changes in bleeding patterns in von Willebrand disease after institution of long-term replacement therapy: results from the von Willebrand Disease Prophylaxis Network. Blood Coagul Fibrinolysis 26(4):383, 2015

Hurskainen R, Teperi J, Rissanen P, et al: Clinical outcomes and costs with the levonorgestrel-releasing intrauterine system or hysterectomy for treatment of menorrhagia: randomized trial 5-year follow-up. JAMA 291:1456, 2004

Hurskainen R, Teperi J, Rissanen P, et al: Quality of life and cost-effectiveness of levonorgestrel-releasing intrauterine system versus hysterectomy for treatment of menorrhagia: a randomized trial. Lancet 357(9252):273, 2001

Irvine GA, Cameron IT: Medical management of dysfunctional uterine bleeding. Best Pract Res Clin Obstet Gynaecol 13:189, 1999

Irvine GA, Campbell-Brown MB, Lumsden MA, et al: Randomised comparative trial of the levonorgestrel intrauterine system and norethisterone for treatment of idiopathic menorrhagia. BJOG 105:592, 1998

Jabbour HN, Kelly RW, Fraser HM, et al: Endocrine regulation of menstruation. Endocr Rev 27(1):17, 2006

James AH, Kouides PA, Abdul-Kadir R, et al: Evaluation and management of acute menorrhagia in women with and without underlying bleeding disorders: consensus from an international expert panel. Eur J Obstet Gynecol Reprod Biol 158(2):124, 2011

James AH, Kouides PA, Abdul-Kadir R, et al: Von Willebrand disease and other bleeding disorders in women: consensus on diagnosis and management from an international expert panel. Am J Obstet Gynecol 201(1):12.e1, 2009a

James AH, Manco-Johnson MJ, Yawn BP, et al: Von Willebrand disease: key points from the 2008 National Heart, Lung, and Blood Institute guidelines. Obstet Gynecol 114(3):674, 2009b

James AH, Myers ER, Cook C, et al: Complications of hysterectomy in women with von Willebrand disease. Haemophilia 15(4):926, 2009c

Jensen JT, Parke S, Mellinger U, et al: Effective treatment of heavy menstrual bleeding with estradiol valerate and dienogest: a randomized controlled trial. Obstet Gynecol 117:777, 2011

Jeong KA, Park KH, Chung DJ, et al: Hysteroscopic endometrial ablation as a treatment for abnormal uterine bleeding in patients with renal transplants. J Am Assoc Gynecol Laparosc 11(2):252, 2004

Jokubkiene L, Sladkevicius P, Valentin L: Transvaginal ultrasound examination of the endometrium in postmenopausal women without vaginal bleeding. Ultrasound Obstet Gynecol 48(3):390, 2016

Joshi JV, Bhandarkar SD, Chadha M, et al: Menstrual irregularities and lactation failure may precede thyroid dysfunction or goitre. J Postgrad Med 39:137, 1993

Kagan R, Abreu P, Andrews E: Vaginal bleeding/spotting with conjugated estrogens/bazedoxifene, conjugated estrogens/medroxyprogesterone acetate, and placebo. Postgrad Med 130(8):687, 2018

Kandil D1, Yang X, Stockl T, et al: Clinical outcomes of patients with insufficient sample from endometrial biopsy or curettage. Int J Gynecol Pathol 33(5):500, 2014

Kapp N: WHO provider brief on hormonal contraception and liver disease. Contraception 80(4):325, 2009

Karaca I, Yapca OE, Adiyeke M, et al: Effect of cervical lidocaine gel for pain relief in Pipelle endometrial sampling. Eurasian J Med 48(3):189, 2016

Karim BO, Burroughs FH, Rosenthal DL, et al: Endometrial-type cells in cervico-vaginal smears: clinical significance and cytopathologic correlates. Diagn Cytopathol 26:123, 2002

Karlsson B, Granberg S, Wikland M, et al: Transvaginal ultrasonography of the endometrium in women with postmenopausal bleeding—a Nordic multicenter study. Am J Obstet Gynecol 172:1488, 1995

Kaunitz AM, Bissonnette F, Monteiro I, et al: Levonorgestrel-releasing intrauterine system or medroxyprogesterone for heavy menstrual bleeding: a randomized controlled trial. Obstet Gynecol 116(3):625, 2010

Kaunitz AM, Meredith S, Inki P, et al: Levonorgestrel-releasing intrauterine system and endometrial ablation in heavy menstrual bleeding: a systematic review and meta-analysis. Obstet Gynecol 113:1104, 2009

Kingman CE, Kadir RA, Lee CA, et al: The use of levonorgestrel-releasing intrauterine system for treatment of menorrhagia in women with inherited bleeding disorders. BJOG 111(12):1425, 2004

Krassas GE, Pontikides N, Kaltsas T, et al: Disturbances of menstruation in hypothyroidism. Clin Endocrinol 50:655, 1999

Krassas GE, Poppe K, Glinoer D: Thyroid function and human reproductive health. Endocr Rev 31(5):702, 2010

Lasmar RB, Barrozo PR, de Oliveira MA, et al: Validation of hysteroscopic view in cases of endometrial hyperplasia and cancer in patients with abnormal uterine bleeding. J Minim Invasive Gynecol 13(5):409, 2006

Leone FP, Timmerman D, Bourne T, et al: Terms, definitions and measurements to describe the sonographic features of the endometrium and intrauterine lesions: a consensus opinion from the International Endometrial Tumor Analysis (IETA) group. Ultrasound Obstet Gynecol 35(1):103, 2010

Lethaby A, Duckitt K, Farquhar C: Non-steroidal anti-inflammatory drugs for heavy menstrual bleeding. Cochrane Database Syst Rev 1:CD000400, 2013a

Lethaby A, Irvine G, Cameron I: Cyclical progestogens for heavy menstrual bleeding. Cochrane Database Syst Rev 1:CD001016, 2008

Lethaby A, Penninx J, Hickey M, et al: Endometrial resection and ablation techniques for heavy menstrual bleeding. Cochrane Database Syst Rev 8: CD001501, 2013b

Leung PL, Tam WH, Kong WS, et al: Intrauterine pathology in women with abnormal uterine bleeding taking hormone replacement therapy. J Am Assoc Gynecol Laparosc 10(2):260, 2003

Litta P, Merlin F, Saccardi C, et al: Role of hysteroscopy with endometrial biopsy to rule out endometrial cancer in postmenopausal women with abnormal uterine bleeding. Maturitas 50:117, 2005

Liu Q, Li XL, Liu JJ, et al: Efficacy and safety of endometrial ablation for treating abnormal uterine bleeding in pre- and postmenopausal women with liver cirrhosis. J Obstet Gynaecol Res 42(12):1753, 2016

Liu Z, Doan QV, Blumenthal P, et al: A systematic review evaluating health-related quality of life, work impairment, and health-care costs and utilization in abnormal uterine bleeding. Value Health 10(3):183, 2007

Lockwood CJ: Mechanisms of normal and abnormal endometrial bleeding. Menopause 18(4):408, 2011

Long ME, Dwarica DS, Kastner TM, et al: Comparison of dysplastic and benign endocervical polyps. J Low Genit Tract Dis 17(2):142, 2013

Lowenstein L, Solt I, Deutsch M, et al: A life-threatening event: uterine cervical arteriovenous malformation. Obstet Gynecol 103:1073, 2004

Lukes AS, Moore KA, Muse KN, et al: Tranexamic acid treatment for heavy menstrual bleeding: a randomized controlled trial. Obstet Gynecol 116(4): 865, 2010

MacKenzie IZ, Naish C, Rees CM, et al: Why remove all cervical polyps and examine them histologically? BJOG 116(8):1127, 2009

Magnay JL, Nevatte TM, Dhingra V, et al: Menstrual blood loss measurement: validation of the alkaline hematin technique for feminine hygiene products containing superabsorbent polymers. Fertil Steril 94(7):2742, 2010

Maheux-Lacroix S, Li F, Laberge PY, et al: Imaging for polyps and leiomyomas in women with abnormal uterine bleeding: a systematic review. Obstet Gynecol 128(6):1425, 2016

Maia H Jr, Maltez A, Studard E, et al: Effect of previous hormone replacement therapy on endometrial polyps during menopause. Gynecol Endocrinol 18: 299, 2004

Makris N, Kalmantis K, Skartados N, et al: Three-dimensional hysterosonography versus hysteroscopy for the detection of intracavitary uterine abnormalities. Int J Gynaecol Obstet 97(1):6, 2007

Mannucci PM, Duga S, Peyvandi F: Recessively inherited coagulation disorders. Blood 104:1243, 2004

Martinelli I, Lensing AW, Middeldorp S, et al: Recurrent venous thromboembolism and abnormal uterine bleeding with anticoagulant and hormone therapy use. Blood 127(11):1417, 2016

Matteson KA, Raker CA, Clark MA, et al: Abnormal uterine bleeding, health status, and usual source of medical care: analyses using the Medical Expenditures Panel Survey. J Womens Health 22(11):959, 2013

Mattix H, Singh AK: Estrogen replacement therapy: implications for post-menopausal women with end-stage renal disease. Curr Opin Nephrol Hypertens 9(3):207, 2000

Matuszkiewicz-Rowinska J, Skorzewska K, Radowicki S, et al: Endometrial morphology and pituitary-gonadal axis dysfunction in women of reproductive age undergoing chronic haemodialysis—a multicentre study. Nephrol Dial Transplant 19:2074, 2004

Maybin JA, Critchley HO: Menstrual physiology: implications for endometrial pathology and beyond. Hum Reprod Update 21(6):748, 2015

McGavigan CJ, Dockery P, Metaxa-Mariatou V, et al: Hormonally mediated disturbance of angiogenesis in the human endometrium after exposure to intrauterine levonorgestrel. Hum Reprod 18:77, 2003

Merz E, Miric-Tesanic D, Bahlmann F, et al: Sonographic size of uterus and ovaries in pre- and postmenopausal women. Ultrasound Obstet Gynecol 7(1):38, 1996

Mittal K, Da Costa D: Endometrial hyperplasia and carcinoma in endometrial polyps: clinicopathologic and follow-up findings. Int J Gynecol Pathol 21(1):45, 2008

Moglia ML, Nguyen HV, Chyjek K, et al: Evaluation of smartphone menstrual cycle tracking applications using an adapted APPLICATIONS scoring system. Obstet Gynecol 127(6):1153, 2016

Munro MG: Medical management of abnormal uterine bleeding. Obstet Gynecol Clin North Am 27(2):287, 2000

Munro MG, Critchley HO, Fraser IS: The FIGO classification of causes of abnormal uterine bleeding in the reproductive years. Fertil Steril 95(7):2204, 2011

Munro MG, Critchley HO, Fraser IS, et al: The two FIGO systems for normal and abnormal uterine bleeding symptoms and classification of causes of abnormal uterine bleeding in the reproductive years: 2018 revisions. Int J Gynaecol Obstet 143(3):393, 2018

Munro MG, Mainor N, Basu R, et al: Oral medroxyprogesterone acetate and combination oral contraceptives for acute uterine bleeding: a randomized controlled trial. Obstet Gynecol 108(4):924, 2006

Naaman Y, Diment J, Perlman S, et al: Can malignant potential of endometrial polyps be determined by incorporating the endometrial intraepithelial neoplasia (EIN) classification? Gynecol Oncol 136(2):254, 2015

Nichols WL, Hultin MB, James AH, et al: Von Willebrand disease (VWD): evidence-based diagnosis and management guidelines, the National Heart, Lung, and Blood Institute (NHLBI) Expert Panel report (USA). Haemophilia 14(2):171, 2008

Nichols WL, Rick ME, Ortel TL, et al: Clinical and laboratory diagnosis of von Willebrand disease: a synopsis of the 2008 NHLBI/NIH guidelines. Am J Hematol 84(6):366, 2009

Nicolae A, Preda O, Nogales FF: Endometrial metaplasias and reactive changes: a spectrum of altered differentiation. J Clin Pathol 64(2):97, 2011

Nieuwenhuis LL, Hermans FJ, Bij de Vaate AJ, et al: Three-dimensional saline infusion sonography compared to two-dimensional saline infusion sonography for the diagnosis of focal intracavitary lesions. Cochrane Database Syst Rev 5:CD011126, 2017

Obenson K, Abreo F, Grafton WD: Cytohistologic correlation between AGUS and biopsy-detected lesions in postmenopausal women. Acta Cytolog 44:41, 2000

Oguz S, Sargin A, Kelekci S, et al: The role of hormone replacement therapy in endometrial polyp formation. Maturitas 50(3):231, 2005

Opolskiene G, Sladkevicius P, Jokubkiene L, et al: Three-dimensional ultrasound imaging for discrimination between benign and malignant endometrium in women with postmenopausal bleeding and sonographic endometrial thickness of at least 4.5 mm. Ultrasound Obstet Gynecol 35(1):94, 2010

Ørbo A, Arnes M, Vereide AB, et al: Relapse risk of endometrial hyperplasia after treatment with the levonorgestrel-impregnated intrauterine system or oral progestogens. BJOG 123(9):1512, 2016

Ørbo A, Vereide A, Arnes M, et al: Levonorgestrel-impregnated intrauterine device as treatment for endometrial hyperplasia: a national multicenter randomized trial. BJOG 121(4):477, 2014

Paulo AA, Solheiro MH, Paulo CO: Is pain better tolerated with mini-hysteroscopy than with conventional device? A systematic review and meta-analysis: hysteroscopy scope size and pain. Arch Gynecol Obstet 282(5):987, 2015

Peres GF, Spadoto-Dias D, Bueloni-Dias FN, et al: Immunohistochemical expression of hormone receptors, Ki-67, endoglin (CD105), claudins 3 and 4, MMP-2 and -9 in endometrial polyps and endometrial cancer type I. OncoTargets Ther 11:3949, 2018

Pérez-Medina T, Bajo-Arenas J, Salazar F, et al: Endometrial polyps and their implication in the pregnancy rates of patients undergoing intrauterine insemination: a prospective randomised study. Hum Reprod 20:1632, 2005

Philipp CS, Faiz A, Dowling N, et al: Age and the prevalence of bleeding disorders in women with menorrhagia. Obstet Gynecol 105:61, 2005

Pitsos M, Skurnick J, Heller D: Association of pathologic diagnoses with clinical findings in chronic endometritis. J Reprod Med 54(6):373, 2009

Preston JT, Cameron IT, Adams EJ, et al: Comparative study of tranexamic acid and norethisterone in the treatment of ovulatory menorrhagia. BJOG 102:401, 1995

Preutthipan S, Herabutya Y: Hysteroscopic polypectomy in 240 premenopausal and postmenopausal women. Fertil Steril 83:705, 2005

Quick CM, Nucci MR, Crum CP, et al: Altered endometrial differentiation (metaplasia). In Crum CP, Nucci MR, Howitt BE, et al: Diagnostic Gynecologic and Obstetric Pathology, 3rd ed. Philadelphia, Elsevier, 2018, p 556

Ragni MV, Machin N, Malec LM, et al: Von Willebrand factor for menorrhagia: a survey and literature review. Haemophilia 22(3):397, 2016

Rahimi S, Marani C, Renzi C, et al: Endometrial polyps and the risk of atypical hyperplasia on biopsies of unremarkable endometrium: a study on 694 patients with benign endometrial polyps. Int J Gynecol Pathol 28(6):522, 2009

Reid PC, Virtanen-Kari S: Randomised comparative trial of the levonorgestrel intrauterine system and mefenamic acid for the treatment of idiopathic menorrhagia: a multiple analysis using total menstrual fluid loss, menstrual blood loss and pictorial blood loss measurements. BJOG 112:1121, 2005

Reijnen C, Visser NC, Bulten J, et al: Diagnostic accuracy of endometrial biopsy in relation to the amount of tissue. J Clin Pathol 70(11):941, 2017

Reslova T, Tosner J, Resl M, et al: Endometrial polyps. A clinical study of 245 cases. Arch Gynecol Obstet 262:133, 1999

Ricciardi E, Vecchione A, Marci R, et al: Clinical factors and malignancy in endometrial polyps. Analysis of 1027 cases. Eur J Obstet Gynecol Reprod Biol 183:121, 2014

Ring KL, Garcia C, Thomas MH, et al: Current and future role of genetic screening in gynecologic malignancies. Am J Obstet Gynecol 217(5):512, 2017

Rodeghiero F: Management of menorrhagia in women with inherited bleeding disorders: general principles and use of desmopressin. Haemophilia 14 (Suppl 1):21, 2008

Rodeghiero F, Castaman G: Congenital von Willebrand disease type I: definition, phenotypes, clinical and laboratory assessment. Best Pract Res Clin Haematol 14(2):321, 2001

Rubin G, Wortman M, Kouides PA: Endometrial ablation for von Willebrand disease-related menorrhagia—experience with seven cases. Haemophilia 10: 477, 2004

Sany O, Singh K, Jha S: Correlation between preoperative endometrial sampling and final endometrial cancer histology. Eur J Gynaecol Oncol 33(2):142, 2012

Sasaki LM, Andrade KR, Figueiredo AC, et al: Factors associated with malignancy in hysteroscopically resected endometrial polyps: a systematic review and meta-analysis. J Minim Invasive Gynecol 25(5):777, 2018

Schatz F, Guzeloglu-Kayisli O, Arlier S, et al: The role of decidual cells in uterine hemostasis, menstruation, inflammation, adverse pregnancy outcomes and abnormal uterine bleeding. Hum Reprod Update 22(4):497, 2016

Schmidt T, Breidenbach M, Nawroth F, et al: Hysteroscopy for asymptomatic postmenopausal women with sonographically thickened endometrium. Maturitas 62(2):176, 2009

Schnatz PF, Ricci S, O'Sullivan DM: Cervical polyps in postmenopausal women: is there a difference in risk? Menopause 16(3):524, 2009

Seravalli V, Linari S, Peruzzi E, et al: Prevalence of hemostatic disorders in adolescents with abnormal uterine bleeding. J Pediatr Adolesc Gynecol 26(5):285, 2013

Seshadri S, El-Toukhy T, Douiri A, et al: Diagnostic accuracy of saline infusion sonography in the evaluation of uterine cavity abnormalities prior to assisted reproductive techniques: a systematic review and meta-analyses. Hum Reprod Update 21(2):262, 2015

Shaaban MM, Zakherah MS, El-Nashar SA, et al: Levonorgestrel-releasing intrauterine system compared to low dose combined oral contraceptive pills for idiopathic menorrhagia: a randomized clinical trial. Contraception 83(1):48, 2011

Sharp HT: Assessment of new technology in the treatment of idiopathic menorrhagia and uterine leiomyomata. Obstet Gynecol 108(4):990, 2006

Sheikh M, Sawhney S, Khurana A, et al: Alteration of sonographic texture of the endometrium in post-menopausal bleeding. A guide to further management. Acta Obstet Gynecol Scand 79:1006, 2000

Shi AA, Lee SI: Radiological reasoning: algorithmic workup of abnormal vaginal bleeding with endovaginal sonography and sonohysterography. AJR Am J Roentgenol 191(6 Suppl):S68, 2008

Siegel RL, Miller KD, Jemal A: Cancer statistics, 2019. CA Cancer J Clin 69(1):7, 2019

Simon JA, Lin VH, Radovich C, et al: One-year long-term safety extension study of ospemifene for the treatment of vulvar and vaginal atrophy in postmenopausal women with a uterus. Menopause 20(4):418, 2013

Singh RH, Blumenthal P: Hormonal management of abnormal uterine bleeding. Clin Obstet Gynecol 48:337, 2005

Sladkevicius P, Installé A, Van Den Bosch T, et al: International Endometrial Tumor Analysis (IETA) terminology in women with postmenopausal bleeding and sonographic endometrial thickness ≥4.5 mm: agreement and reliability study. Ultrasound Obstet Gynecol 51(2):259, 2018

Smith RA, Andrews KS, Brooks D, et al: Cancer screening in the United States, 2018: a review of current American Cancer Society guidelines and current issues in cancer screening. CA Cancer J Clin 68(4):297, 2018

Smith-Bindman R, Kerlikowske K, Feldstein VA, et al: Endovaginal ultrasound to exclude endometrial cancer and other endometrial abnormalities. JAMA 280:1510, 1998

Smith-Bindman R, Weiss E, Feldstein V: How thick is too thick? When endometrial thickness should prompt biopsy in postmenopausal women without vaginal bleeding. Ultrasound Obstet Gynecol 24(5):558, 2004

Soares SR, Barbosa dos Reis MM, Camargos AF: Diagnostic accuracy of sonohysterography, transvaginal sonography, and hysterosalpingography in patients with uterine cavity diseases. Fertil Steril 73:406, 2000

Soucie JE, Chu PA, Ross S, et al: The risk of diagnostic hysteroscopy in women with endometrial cancer. Am J Obstet Gynecol 207(1):71.e1, 2012

Stamatellos I, Apostolides A, Stamatopoulos P, et al: Pregnancy rates after hysteroscopic polypectomy depending on the size or number of the polyps. Arch Gynecol Obstet 277(5):395, 2008

Stellon AJ, Williams R: Increased incidence of menstrual abnormalities and hysterectomy preceding primary biliary cirrhosis. Br Med J (Clin Res Ed) 293:297, 1986

Stewart A, Cummins C, Gold L, et al: The effectiveness of the levonorgestrel-releasing intrauterine system in menorrhagia: a systematic review. BJOG 108:74, 2001

Stock RJ, Kanbour A: Prehysterectomy curettage. Obstet Gynecol 45:537, 1975

Stovall TG, Ling FW, Morgan PL: A prospective, randomized comparison of the Pipelle endometrial sampling device with the Novak curette. Am J Obstet Gynecol 165:1287, 1991

Stovall TG, Solomon SK, Ling FW: Endometrial sampling prior to hysterectomy. Obstet Gynecol 73:405, 1989

Svirsky R, Smorgick N, Rozowski U, et al: Can we rely on blind endometrial biopsy for detection of focal intrauterine pathology? Am J Obstet Gynecol 199(2):115.e1, 2008

Tabor A, Watt HC, Wald NJ: Endometrial thickness as a test for endometrial cancer in women with postmenopausal vaginal bleeding. Obstet Gynecol 99:663, 2002

Tahir MM, Bigrigg MA, Browning JJ, et al: A randomised controlled trial comparing transvaginal ultrasound, outpatient hysteroscopy and endometrial biopsy with inpatient hysteroscopy and curettage. BJOG 106:1259, 1999

Timmerman D, Wauters J, Van Calenbergh S, et al: Color Doppler imaging is a valuable tool for the diagnosis and management of uterine vascular malformations. Ultrasound Obstet Gynecol 21:570, 2003

Timmermans A, Opmeer BC, Khan KS, et al: Endometrial thickness measurement for detecting endometrial cancer in women with postmenopausal bleeding: a systematic review and meta-analysis. Obstet Gynecol 116(1):160, 2010

Tinelli R, Tinelli FG, Cicinelli E, et al: The role of hysteroscopy with eye-directed biopsy in postmenopausal women with uterine bleeding and endometrial atrophy. Menopause 15(4 Pt 1):737, 2008

Tohma YA, Akilli H, Kirnap M, et al: Possible impact of immunosuppressive therapy regimens on histopathologic outcomes of abnormal uterine bleeding in solid-organ transplant recipients. Clin Transplant 32(8):e13305, 2018

Trimble CL, Method M, Leitao M, et al: Management of endometrial precancers. Obstet Gynecol 120(5):1160, 2012

Tsuda H, Kawabata M, Kawabata K, et al: Improvement of diagnostic accuracy of transvaginal ultrasound for identification of endometrial malignancies by using cutoff level of endometrial thickness based on length of time since menopause. Gynecol Oncol 64:35, 1997

Tullius TG Jr, Ross JR, Flores M, et al: Use of three-dimensional power Doppler sonography in the diagnosis of uterine arteriovenous malformation and follow-up after uterine artery embolization: case report and brief review of literature. J Clin Ultrasound 43(5):327, 2015

Turnbull AC, Rees MC: Gestrinone in the treatment of menorrhagia. BJOG 97(8):713, 1990

van Doorn LC, Dijkhuizen FP, Kruitwagen RF, et al: Accuracy of transvaginal ultrasonography in diabetic or obese women with postmenopausal bleeding. Obstet Gynecol 104:571, 2004

Vuento MH, Pirhonen JP, Mäkinen JI, et al: Endometrial fluid accumulation in asymptomatic postmenopausal women. Ultrasound Obstet Gynecol 8(1):37, 1996

Warner PE, Critchley HO, Lumsden MA, et al: Menorrhagia I: measured blood loss, clinical features, and outcome in women with heavy periods: a survey with follow-up data. Am J Obstet Gynecol 190:1216, 2004

Weiss JL, Malone FD, Vidaver J, et al: Threatened abortion: a risk factor for poor pregnancy outcome, a population-based screening study. Am J Obstet Gynecol 190:745, 2004

Wellington K, Wagstaff AJ: Tranexamic acid: a review of its use in the management of menorrhagia. Drugs 63:1417, 2003

Wiesenfeld HC, Hillier SL, Krohn MA, et al: Lower genital tract infection and endometritis: insight into subclinical pelvic inflammatory disease. Obstet Gynecol 100(3):456, 2002

Wilansky DL, Greisman B: Early hypothyroidism in patients with menorrhagia. Am J Obstet Gynecol 160:673, 1989

Williams AR, Brechin S, Porter AJ, et al: Factors affecting adequacy of Pipelle and Tao Brush endometrial sampling. BJOG 115(8):1028, 2008

Wong AS, Lao TT, Cheung CW, et al: Reappraisal of endometrial thickness for the detection of endometrial cancer in postmenopausal bleeding: a retrospective cohort study. BJOG 123(3):439, 2016

Wong M, Crnobrnja B, Liberale V, et al: The natural history of endometrial polyps. Hum Reprod 32(2):340, 2017

Xie B, Qian C, Yang B, et al: Risk factors for unsuccessful office-based endometrial biopsy: a comparative study of office-based endometrial biopsy (Pipelle) and diagnostic dilation and curettage. J Minim Invasive Gynecol 25(4):724, 2018

Yang JH, Chen CD, Chen SU, et al: Factors influencing the recurrence potential of benign endometrial polyps after hysteroscopic polypectomy. PLoS One 10(12):e0144857, 2015

Yarandi F, Izadi-Mood N, Eftekhar Z, et al: Diagnostic accuracy of dilatation and curettage for abnormal uterine bleeding. J Obstet Gynaecol Res 36(5):1049, 2010

Ylikorkala O, Viinikka L: Comparison between antifibrinolytic and antiprostaglandin treatment in the reduction of increased menstrual blood loss in women with intrauterine contraceptive devices. BJOG 90(1):78, 1983

Yoon DJ, Jones M, Taani JA, et al: A systematic review of acquired uterine arteriovenous malformations: pathophysiology, diagnosis, and transcatheter treatment. AJP Rep 6(1):e6, 2016

Younis MTS, Iram S, Anwar B, et al: Women with asymptomatic cervical polyps may not need to see a gynaecologist or have them removed: an observational retrospective study of 1126 cases. Eur J Obstet Gynecol Reprod Biol 150(2):190, 2010

Yuk JS, Shin JY, Moon HS, et al: The incidence of unexpected uterine malignancy in women undergoing hysteroscopic myomectomy or polypectomy: a national population-based study. Eur J Obstet Gynecol Reprod Biol 224:12, 2018

Zaino R, Carinelli SG, Ellenson LH, et al: Tumours of the uterine corpus: epithelial tumours and precursors. In: Kurman RJ, Carcanglu ML, Herrington CS, et al (eds): WHO Classification of Tumours of Female Reproductive Organs. 4th ed., Lyon, World Health Organization, 2014, p 125

Zerbe MJ, Zhang J, Bristow RE, et al: Retrograde seeding of malignant cells during hysteroscopy in presumed early endometrial cancer. Gynecol Oncol 79(1):55, 2000

Zigler RE, McNicholas C: Unscheduled vaginal bleeding with progestin-only contraceptive use. Am J Obstet Gynecol 216(5):443, 2017

CHAPTER 9

Benign Uterine Pathology

LEIOMYOMAS

■ Pathogenesis

Often simply called myomas, uterine leiomyomas are benign smooth-muscle neoplasms that typically originate from the myometrium. Their prevalence among women is generally cited as 10 to 20 percent, but is as high as 70 to 80 percent in sonographic studies (Baird, 2003; Marshall, 1997).

Grossly, a typical off-white, whorled leiomyoma is autonomous from its surrounding myometrium because of a thin, outer connective tissue layer (Fig. 9-1). This clinically important cleavage plane allows leiomyomas to be easily "shelled" from the uterus during surgery. The blood supply within these tumors is tenuous, and thus ischemia and necrosis develop frequently in myomas. Following necrosis, their smooth muscle is replaced with various degenerative substances. Forms include hyaline, calcific, cystic, myxoid, red, and fatty, and these gross changes should be recognized as normal variants.

Each leiomyoma is derived from a single progenitor myocyte. Following their genesis, uterine leiomyomas are estrogen- and progesterone-sensitive tumors. And, these tumors carry higher densities of both progesterone and estrogen receptors compared with their surrounding myometrium. Progesterone is considered the critical mitogen for uterine leiomyoma growth and development. In turn, estrogen functions to upregulate and maintain progesterone receptors (Ishikawa, 2010).

To help maintain and promote growth, leiomyomas themselves create a local hyperestrogenic environment (Bulun, 1994; Englund, 1998). Also, some conditions provide sustained estrogen exposure that encourages leiomyoma growth. Examples include early menarche, obesity, and polycystic ovarian syndrome (Wise, 2005,2007). Despite this hormonal responsiveness, myoma formation is not induced by combination oral contraceptive (COC) pills (Qin, 2013). And, depot medroxyprogesterone acetate (DMPA) use in young

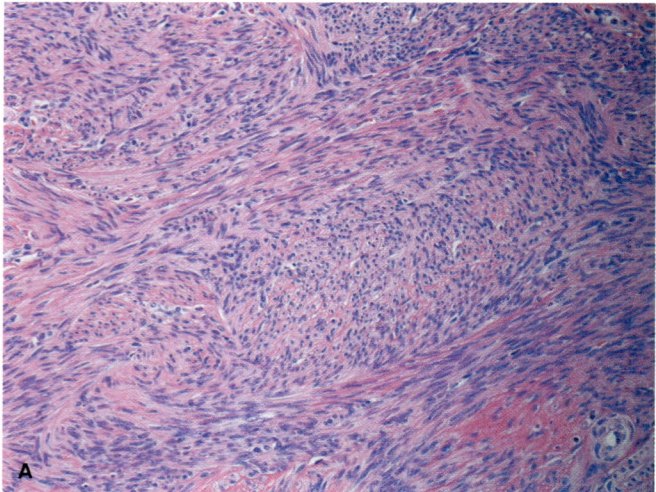
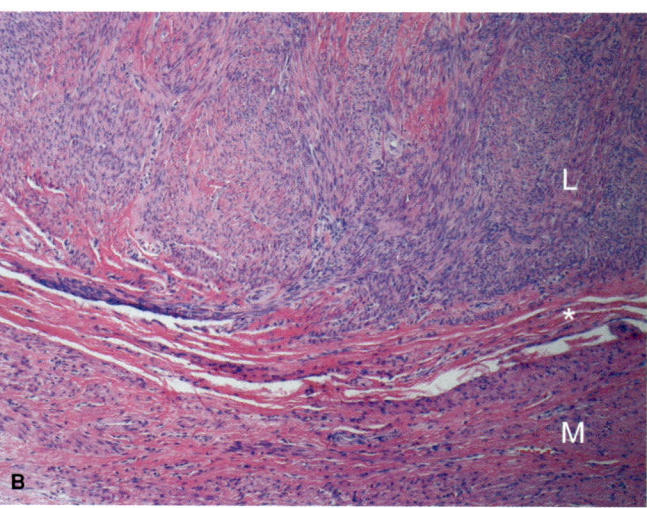

FIGURE 9-1 A. Microscopically, leiomyomas are composed of bland, spindled smooth-muscle cells characterized by elongate, blunt-ended nuclei and tapered eosinophilic cytoplasm. The cells are arranged in interlacing fascicles that intersect at right angles. **B.** The interface (*asterisk*) between the leiomyoma (*L*) and adjacent myometrium (*M*) can be seen grossly and microscopically. These tumors are usually more cellular than the surrounding myometrium. (Reproduced with permission from Dr. Kelley Carrick.)

African-American women is associated with lower myoma risk (Harmon, 2015).

For myoma development, race and age are notable factors. Myomas are rare in adolescence, but rates rise with age during the reproductive years. In one study, the cumulative incidence by age 50 years was nearly 70 percent in whites and more than 80 percent in African-American women (Baird, 2003). However, once in the menopause, accruing age lowers the incidence (Sommer, 2015). Leiomyomas are more common in African-American women compared with white, Asian, or Hispanic women (Marshall, 1997). Thus, as noted earlier, heredity and gene mutations play a seminal role in myoma development.

■ Classification

These tumors are classified numerically based on their location (Fig. 9-2) (Munro, 2018). *Subserosal leiomyomas* originate from myocytes adjacent to the uterine serosa. As variants, *parasitic leiomyomas* attach themselves to nearby pelvic structures from which they derive vascular support. These myomas then may or may not detach from the parent myometrium. *Intramural leiomyomas* are those with growth centered within the uterine walls. *Submucous leiomyomas* are proximate to the endometrium and grow toward and bulge into the endometrial cavity. Last, *pedunculated leiomyomas* attach only by a stalk to their progenitor myometrium. Type 0 and type 7 myomas are examples.

Submucous		4 Intramural
0 Pedunculated intracavity		5 Subserous ≥50% intramural
1 <50% intramural		6 Subserous <50% intramural
2 ≥50% intramural		7 Subserous pedunculated
3 100% intramural but contacts endometrium		8 Other (e.g., cervical, parasitic)

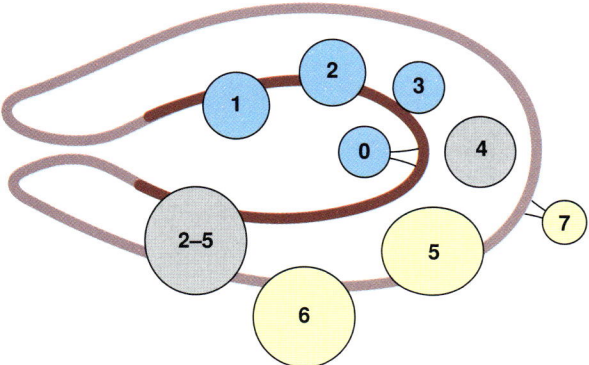

FIGURE 9-2 Leiomyomas categorized by the International Federation of Gynecology and Obstetrics (FIGO) system. Type 3, although completely intramural, is now considered to overlap with the submucous group because of its contact with the endometrium. Not shown, type 8 defines myomas that do not relate to the myometrium and include cervical, broad ligament, or parasitic myomas. Transmural lesions, an example labeled in here as "2-5," are categorized by both their endometrial and serosal components. In these cases, the endometrial surface is described first.

Infrequently, leiomyomas develop in the cervix or broad ligament and rarely in the ovary, fallopian tube, vagina, or vulva.

■ Symptoms

Bleeding

Most women with leiomyomas are asymptomatic. However, affected women may complain of bleeding, pain, pressure, or infertility. Of these, bleeding is common, especially heavy menstrual bleeding (HMB). Despite this, the underlying pathophysiology is unclear, and vasodilation of endometrial vessels and altered hemostasis are suspected mechanisms (Ikhena, 2018). In general, symptom risk rises with myoma size and number (Baird, 2015).

Pressure and Pain

A sufficiently large uterus can cause chronic pressure, urinary frequency, incontinence, or constipation. Aside from pressure, patients may also note chronic dysmenorrhea, dyspareunia, or noncyclical pelvic pain.

Acute pelvic pain is a less frequent complaint but is most often seen with a degenerating, a prolapsing, or a twisting leiomyoma. With leiomyoma degeneration, tissue necrosis classically causes acute pain, fever, and leukocytosis. This constellation mimics other acute pelvic pain sources. Thus, sonography is typically performed to help identify a cause, and usually a nondescript leiomyoma is found. Computed tomography (CT) may help exclude other etiologies or clarify pelvic anatomy obscured by multiple large leiomyomas. Treatment of myoma degeneration is nonsurgical and includes nonsteroidal antiinflammatory drugs (NSAIDs) and additional analgesics and antipyretics as needed. If differentiation between myoma degeneration and acute endomyometritis is unclear, broad-spectrum antibiotics may be administered. In most cases, symptoms improve within 24 to 48 hours. Also, the stalks of large pedunculated myomas can acutely twist to cause similar ischemia and pain. In this case, surgical severing of the stalk and myoma excision is curative.

Prolapse of a pedunculated tumor from the endometrial cavity can cause marked cramping or pain as the tumor stretches the endocervical canal to pass through it. Associated bleeding or serosanguinous discharge is common. Rarely, cervical stretching may prompt a vagal response or prolapse can lead to uterine inversion. With myoma prolapse, visual inspection is usually diagnostic. However, sonography is often performed to evaluate the size and number of other uterine leiomyomas and exclude other sources of pain. Surgical treatment involves severing the leiomyoma from its stalk as described in Chapter 43 (p. 954).

Fertility Issues

Leiomyomas can diminish fertility, but only 1 to 3 percent of infertility cases are due solely to leiomyomas (Buttram, 1981; Donnez, 2002). Instead, subfertility is more closely associated with submucous leiomyomas than with tumors located elsewhere (American Society for Reproductive Medicine, 2017). Improved pregnancy rates following hysteroscopic resection have provided most of the indirect evidence for this link (Casini,

2006; Surrey, 2005). In contrast, evidence does not implicate subserosal tumors. For intramural leiomyomas that do not distort the endometrial cavity, the relationship with subfertility is more tenuous, and evidence of benefits from myomectomy is conflicting (Christopoulos, 2017; Yan, 2014). Importantly, the strength of this evidence must be weighed against the morbidity associated with myomectomy. Namely, peritubal or intrauterine adhesions can threaten fertility, and myometrial defects lead to a risk of uterine rupture during subsequent pregnancies. If surgery is elected, conception attempts ideally follow complete surgical healing, if possible, to limit tumor recurrence risk.

Both uterine leiomyoma and spontaneous miscarriage are common, and an association between these has not been shown convincingly. Moreover, there is no conclusive evidence that surgical treatment reduces miscarriage rates (American Society for Reproductive Medicine, 2017; Pritts, 2009).

■ Diagnosis

Leiomyomas are often detected by pelvic examination with findings of uterine enlargement, irregular contour, or both. In reproductive-aged women, a urine or serum β-human chorionic gonadotropin (hCG) level excludes pregnancy, and sonography is done to define pelvic anatomy. Of modalities, transvaginal sonography (TVS) provides superior resolution, but some uteri are so large that transabdominal sonography is needed to image the entire corpus. Leiomyomas appear as focal masses with a heterogeneous texture. This varies from hypo- to hyperechoic depending on the ratio of smooth muscle to connective tissue and the presence of degenerative substances (Fig. 9-3). Calcifications appear hyperechoic and commonly rim the tumor or are randomly scattered throughout the mass. Cystic or myxoid degeneration typically dots the leiomyoma with multiple, smooth-walled, irregularly sized but generally small hypoechoic or anechoic areas.

The endometrial cavity is also inspected for submucous leiomyomas, endometrial polyps, or synechiae. With these focal

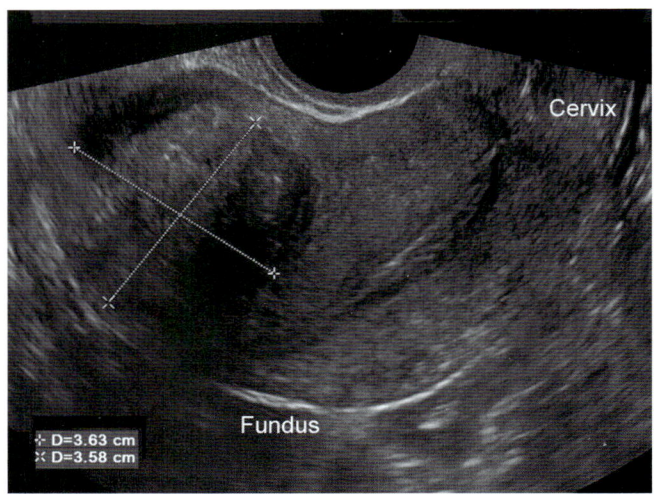

FIGURE 9-3 Transvaginal sonogram of a subserosal leiomyoma. Classically, sonography calipers are placed from outer border to outer border during myoma measurement.

lesions, the endometrium can appear thick or irregular during TVS, and adjunct imaging tools may help clarify anatomy. Of these, saline-infusion sonography (SIS) or hysteroscopy often best provide additional cavity information (Figs. 9-4 and 9-5). Also, three-dimensional (3-D) TVS and 3-D SIS can be valuable to define the cavity.

Leiomyomas have characteristic vascular patterns, and these can be identified by color Doppler and by power Doppler techniques. A peripheral circumferential rim of vascularity from which a few vessels arise to penetrate into the center of the tumor is a classic finding. Adenomyosis usually shows central rather than peripheral vascularity (Sharma, 2015). Polyps classically show one feeder vessel. As such, Doppler imaging can help differentiate these.

For the infertile woman, the endometrial cavity can be evaluated with hysterosalpingography (HSG), hysterosalpingocontrast sonography (HyCoSy), or hysteroscopy. The first two also offer the advantage of defining tubal patency.

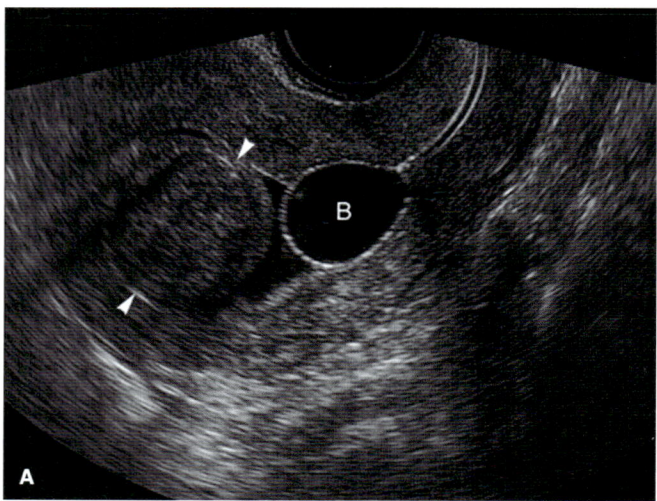
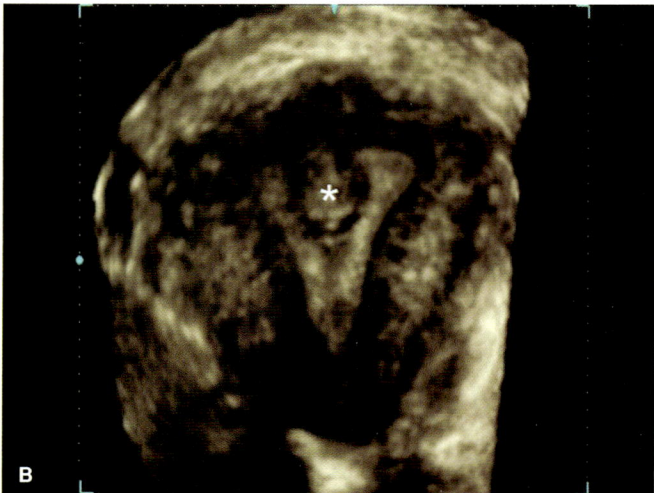

FIGURE 9-4 A. Submucous fibroid is clearly outlined during saline infusion sonography (SIS) (*arrowheads*). The SIS catheter balloon is seen in the lower uterine cavity (*B*). **B.** 3-D transvaginal sonogram of a submucous leiomyoma (*asterisk*). (Reproduced with permission from Dr. Elysia Moschos.)

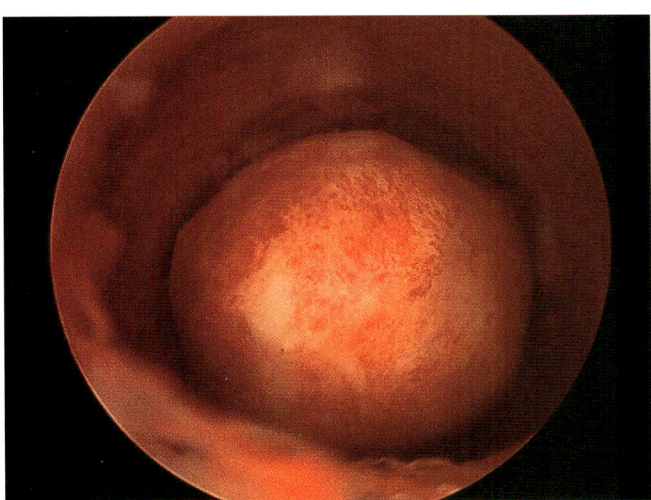

FIGURE 9-5 Hysteroscopic photograph of a submucous leiomyoma prior to resection. (Reproduced with permission from Dr. Karen Bradshaw.)

Magnetic resonance (MR) imaging may be required when imaging is limited by body habitus or distorted anatomy. On T2-weighted images, myomas usually are dark, homogeneous, and circumscribed. Notably, areas of degeneration create variations of this typical appearance. MR imaging allows more accurate assessment of the size, number, and location of leiomyomas. This can help identify appropriate candidates for hysterectomy alternatives such as uterine artery embolization (UAE) or myomectomy. Of note, for a dominant fundal uterine mass, MR imaging can also aid differentiation of a fundal leiomyoma, which is a suitable myomectomy indication, from a compact collection of adenomyosis, which is not. Another mimicker is leiomyosarcoma (LMS), which is often a single, large mass with cystic degeneration. MR imaging provides greater, but not perfect, accuracy for diagnosis of LMS (Bonneau, 2014).

CT is not widely used to further characterize myomas. However, as discussed earlier, it may aid initial diagnosis in patients with acute pain of unclear etiology.

■ Nonsurgical Management

Observation

Leiomyomas in general are slow-growing (DeWaay, 2002). Thus, regardless of their size, asymptomatic leiomyomas usually can be observed and surveilled with an annual pelvic examination (Parker, 1994). At times, adnexal assessment may be hindered by a large or irregular uterus or patient obesity. In these cases, some add annual sonographic surveillance (Cantuaria, 1998).

In contrast, symptomatic leiomyomas can be treated with long-term medical therapy discussed in the next sections (Table 9-1). In others, medical therapy is used only as a short-term preoperative adjunct. Also, because these tumors typically regress post-menopausally, some women choose medical treatment to relieve symptoms as a bridge to menopause.

Sex Steroid Hormones

Either COCs, continuous oral progestins, or DMPA can be used to induce endometrial atrophy and to decrease prostaglandin production. Despite this frequent practice, few studies have evaluated these specifically for leiomyoma-related bleeding (Kriplani, 2016; Sayed, 2011). Their use and expected effects are extrapolated from studies in women with nonmyomatous uteri.

Also in small studies, the levonorgestrel-releasing intrauterine system (LNG-IUS) significantly improved leiomyoma-related bleeding scores (Sayed, 2011; Socolov, 2011). However, for women with myomas, LNG-IUS expulsion rates are higher and range from 10 to 15 percent (Kriplani, 2012; Youm, 2014). Candidates should meet criteria listed in Table 5-4 (p. 115), and tumors that distort the endometrial cavity preclude LNG-IUS use (Bayer, 2017). Placement into the large cavities of enormous uteri is also avoided, as the device and its strings may migrate cephalad to make retrieval difficult. Although not a strict clinical limit, many studies have included only uteri measuring ≤12-week size.

Other sex steroid hormone options include the androgens danazol and gestrinone, which shrink leiomyoma volume and improve bleeding symptoms (Coutinho, 1989; De Leo, 1999). Unfortunately, their prominent side effects, which include acne and hirsutism, preclude their use as first-line agents.

GnRH Receptor Agents

Synthetic derivatives of gonadotropin-releasing hormone (GnRH) can function at the GnRH receptor as either agonists or antagonists. Despite their differing actions at the receptor, both groups ultimately incite profound systemic drops in estrogen and progesterone levels.

GnRH agonists are inactive if taken orally, but other preparations are available. Of these, leuprolide acetate (Lupron) is Food

TABLE 9-1. Indications for the Medical Treatment of Uterine Leiomyoma

Agent	NSAID	COC	DMPA	LNG-IUS	GnRH Agonist	Ulipristal[a]
Symptom						
Dysmenorrhea	+	+	+	+	+	+
Menorrhagia	–	+	+	+	+	+
Pelvic pressure	–	–	–	–	+	+
Infertility	–	–	–	–	+	–

[a]Available in Europe and Canada for preoperative use for this indication.
COC = combination oral contraceptive pills; DMPA = depot medroxyprogesterone acetate;
GnRH = gonadotropin-releasing hormone; LNG-IUS = levonorgestrel-releasing intrauterine system;
NSAID = nonsteroidal antiinflammatory drug.

and Drug Administration (FDA)-approved for leiomyoma treatment and is available in a 3.75-mg monthly dose or 11.25-mg 3-month intramuscular (IM) dose. Less frequently used GnRH agonists include goserelin (Zoladex), administered as a 3.6-mg monthly or 10.8-mg 3-month subcutaneous depot implant. Triptorelin (Trelstar) is given as a 3.75-mg monthly or 11.25-mg 3-month IM injection. Nafarelin (Synarel) is used in a 200-μg twice-daily nasal spray regimen. These latter three are not FDA-approved for leiomyoma treatment, but in off-label use they have proved effective (Donnez, 2003; Vercellini, 1998).

GnRH agonists shrink leiomyomas by targeting the growth effects of estrogen and progesterone. Initially, these agonists stimulate receptors on pituitary gonadotropes to cause a supraphysiological release of both luteinizing hormone (LH) and follicle-stimulating hormone (FSH). Also called a *flare*, this phase typically lasts 1 week. With their long-term action, however, agonists downregulate GnRH receptors in gonadotropes, thus desensitizing gonadotropes to further GnRH stimulation. Subsequently, lowered gonadotropin secretion leads to suppressed estrogen and progesterone levels 1 to 2 weeks after initial GnRH agonist administration (Broekmans, 1996).

Results with GnRH agonist treatment include dramatic decreases in uterine and leiomyoma volume. Most women experience a mean decline in uterine volume of 35 to 50 percent, and most of this occurs during the first 3 months of therapy (Donnez, 2012b; Friedman, 1991). As a result, smaller uterine size may allow a less complicated or extensive surgical procedure.

Clinical benefits of GnRH agonists include pain relief and diminished HMB, usually amenorrhea. For example, 90 to 97 percent of women achieve bleeding control by 3 months. The mean time to amenorrhea is 21 days (Donnez, 2012b; Friedman, 1991). Adjunctively, women can be given oral iron supplements to correct anemia.

Following their discontinuance, normal menses resume in 1 to 2 months (Letterie, 1989). Unfortunately, leiomyomas then regrow, and uterine volumes regain pretreatment sizes within 3 to 6 months (Friedman, 1991). Despite regrowth, symptom relief may persist for 6 to 12 months in many women given GnRH agonists (Scialli, 2000; Schlaff, 1989).

GnRH agonists have significant costs and side effects. Side effects mirror those of menopause and develop in up to 95 percent of treated women (Letterie, 1989). In addition, 6 months of agonist therapy can result in a 6-percent loss in trabecular bone, not all of which may be recouped following discontinuation (Scharla, 1990). As a result, these agents alone are not recommended for use longer than 6 months without add-back therapy.

To obviate side-effect severity, "add-back therapy" counters hypoestrogenic symptoms without negating the shrinking action (Friedman, 1994). This is made possible by the fact that the estrogen level required to improve vasomotor symptoms and minimize bone loss is below the estrogen threshold that would restimulate leiomyoma growth. Add-back therapy is typically begun 1 to 3 months following GnRH agonist initiation (Mizutani, 1998). Regimens include estrogen combined with a progestin, and those studied have generally been low-dose preparations equivalent to menopausal HRT. Of note, progestins,

such as norethindrone or medroxyprogesterone acetate, as a sole agent for add-back therapy have yielded contradictory results (Carr, 1993; Friedman, 1994). Last, although used less often, add-back therapy with selective estrogen-receptor modulators (SERMs), such as tibolone and raloxifene, also prevents bone loss (Palomba, 1998, 2004).

GnRH antagonists, elagolix and relugolix, are nonpeptide forms suitable for oral use, although not yet FDA-approved for this indication. As one advantage, the initial flare of gonadotropins is avoided. In randomized trials, both menstrual bleeding and myoma volumes declined (Archer, 2017; Carr, 2018; Osuga, 2019). As expected with GnRH suppression, hot flashes are a prominent side effect. However, add-back therapy attenuates both hot-flash severity and bone mineral density losses during 6 months of treatment. Yet, diminished menstrual blood loss is preserved.

Selective Progesterone-Receptor Modulators

As noted, progesterone is essential for myoma growth, and thus antagonists are another option. Agents are classified as *antiprogestins* if they universally prompt antagonist effects upon binding to the progesterone receptor. However, agents are termed *selective progesterone-receptor modulators (SPRMs)* if they exert antiprogestational effects in some tissues but progestational effects in others.

Ulipristal acetate (UPA) is an SPRM currently marketed in the United States as the emergency contraceptive Ella. For myoma treatment, UPA is available in Europe and Canada (Esmya, Fibristal) and prescribed in 5-mg oral daily doses for up to 12 weeks. UPA acts as a potent antiprogestin in myomas and shrinks their volume. UPA performs comparably with leuprolide acetate to shrink myoma volume and controlled heavy menstrual bleeding (Donnez, 2012b). But unlike GnRH-receptor agents, it avoids the gonadotropin flare and hypoestrogenic side effects. Estradiol levels lie in the midfollicular range (Donnez, 2016).

The effect of UPA on the endometrium is not that of a pure antagonist. Instead, a new category of endometrial changes are recognized with UPA use. These *progesterone-receptor-modulator–associated endometrial changes (PAECs)* reflect dyssynchronous growth between glands and stroma (Mutter, 2008). PAECs are not linked to short-term higher rates of endometrial hyperplasia or cancer. And, in the largest randomized studies of UPA, PAECs revert within 3 to 6 months following drug cessation (Donnez, 2012a,b). However, the long-term effects of PAECs are unclear, and this is the main reason that each treatment course is limited to 12 weeks. That said, repetitive courses of UPA have been evaluated (Donnez, 2016).

More recently, concerns have arisen regarding liver injury, and underlying liver disease is now a contraindication. The European Medicines Agency (2018) still permits one 12-week course preoperatively. Additional courses are allowed only to those who are not eligible for surgery. Serum liver-function testing is done pretreatment, then monthly during the first two 12-week courses, and finally 2 to 4 weeks posttreatment. Enzyme levels three or more times the upper normal limit should prompt treatment cessation.

Nonhormonal Options

Tranexamic acid (TXA) is an antifibrinolytic agent described fully in Chapter 8 (p. 196). Studies have not evaluated TXA specifically for myoma-related HMB. Subgroup analysis does provide some support for its use for this indication (Eder, 2013; Lukes, 2010).

The benefits of NSAIDs for leiomyoma-related bleeding are less clear, and studies have conflicting results (Anteby, 1985; Mäkäräinen, 1986). Thus, although NSAIDs are potentially helpful for myoma-related dysmenorrhea, available data do not robustly support their use as sole agents for leiomyoma-related HMB.

The enzyme aromatase converts androgens to estrogens and is active in the ovary, breast, endometrium, adipose, bone, and endothelium, among others. In myomas, aromatase contributes to the estrogen environment that propels and sustains myoma growth. In premenopausal women, inhibitors of aromatase appear to predominantly suppress estrogen production in myomas yet only partial suppress this activity in the ovary. Aromatase inhibitors (AIs) are not FDA-approved for leiomyoma treatment. But, in a few small studies, they decreased myoma volumes by approximately 50 percent and improved menstrual symptoms during 3-month therapies (Parsanezhad, 2010; Sayyah-Melli, 2017). AI side effects include hot flashes, nausea, and musculoskeletal pain. Moreover, AI use can augment FSH release, which can risk pregnancy or formation of multiple follicular cysts. Long-term effects on bone and cardiovascular health are also unclear. AIs are not widely used, and larger studies are needed.

Uterine Artery Embolization

Uterine artery embolization is an angiographic procedure that delivers synthetic particulate emboli into both uterine arteries. Uterine blood flow is thereby obstructed, producing ischemia and necrosis. Because vessels serving leiomyomas have a larger caliber, these microspheres are preferentially directed to the tumors, sparing the surrounding myometrium.

During UAE, an angiographic catheter is placed in one femoral artery and advanced under fluoroscopic guidance to sequentially catheterize both uterine arteries (Fig. 9-6). Failure to embolize both uterine arteries allows collateral circulation to sustain leiomyoma blood flow and is associated with a significantly lower success rate (Bratby, 2008).

UAE is a management option for women who might otherwise be considered candidates for hysterectomy or myomectomy. Based on current evidence, women who have not completed childbearing may be better served by myomectomy (Gupta, 2014). Other patient limitations are listed in Table 9-2, and many are associated with altered vascular anatomy. For example, GnRH agonists are thought to narrow vessels. Pedunculated submucous tumors are less suitable, as these tumors can infarct and slough. Pedunculated subserosal tumors were previously excluded, but the Society of Interventional Radiology has removed this caveat (Dariushnia, 2014).

Prior to UAE, a woman undergoes radiologic consultation and MR imaging to assess myoma qualities for success. The gynecologist screens for infection and for endometrial and cervical cancer. Before UAE, intrauterine devices are typically removed.

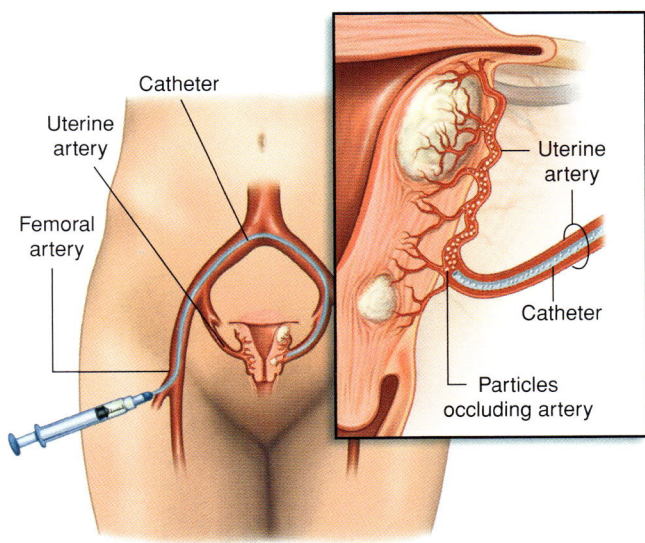

FIGURE 9-6 Diagram of uterine artery embolization (UAE).

Following UAE, pain management usually requires a 24- to 48-hour hospital admission. After discharge, most patients have pain controlled with NSAIDs and have a rapid return to daily activities. However, as a result of leiomyoma necrosis, patients can develop a *postembolization syndrome* that may require readmission. These symptoms are seen in 10 to 25 percent of cases, usually last 2 to 7 days, and are classically marked by pelvic pain, nausea, low-grade fever, and mild leukocytosis (Edwards, 2007; Hehenkamp, 2005,2006). Management includes supportive care and analgesia. Antibiotics are not typically required but may be administered if infectious endomyometritis is an alternative diagnosis.

TABLE 9-2. UAE Absolute and Relative Contraindications

Absolute
Pregnancy
Active uterine or adnexal infection
Suspected reproductive tract malignancy[a]

Relative	Reason
Coagulopathy	Bleeding complications
Renal impairment	Renal effects of contrast
Severe contrast allergy	Allergic reaction
Desire for future fertility	See text
Uterine size >20–24 weeks	Difficult to embolize
Prior salpingectomy or SO	Altered arterial anatomy
Prior pelvic radiation	Altered arterial anatomy
Large hydrosalpinx	Increased infection risk
GnRH agonist use	Narrows vascularity

[a]Unless performed as an adjunct to treatment.
GnRH = gonadotropin-releasing hormone; SO = salpingo-oophorectomy; UAE = uterine artery embolization.
Compiled from American College of Obstetricians and Gynecologists, 2016; Dariushnia, 2014; Stokes, 2010.

Bleeding and bulk relief is not immediate, but by 6 months clinical responses are significant (Moss, 2016). Several trials have shown high rates of patient satisfaction and symptom improvement (Edwards, 2007; Hehenkamp, 2008). Compared with hysterectomy, UAE is associated with shorter hospitalization, reduced 24-hour pain scores, and earlier return to daily activities. UAE also compares favorably with myomectomy for symptom relief (Goodwin, 2006; Manyonda, 2012). However, long-term surveillance reveals that 28 to 35 percent of UAE-treated patients will require a subsequent procedure, which in many cases is hysterectomy (Moss, 2011; de Bruijn, 2016).

Compared with surgery, UAE has comparable major complication rates but higher minor complication rates (Gupta, 2014). Leiomyoma tissue passage is common and seen in approximately 4 percent of cases (Toor, 2012). Necrotic leiomyomas that pass into the vagina usually can be removed in the office. Those retained in the uterine cavity or firmly attached to the uterine wall may require dilatation and evacuation (Spies, 2002). Groin hematoma and prolonged vaginal discharge are other frequent complications. Brief amenorrhea and associated transiently elevated FSH levels may last a few menstrual cycles after UAE. Permanent amenorrhea, however, develops occasionally, and more often in older reproductive-aged patients (Hehenkamp, 2007; Spies, 2005). This likely results from concurrent embolization of the ovaries. Pregnancy subsequent to UAE can pose complications. Although the number of evaluable pregnancies is small, consistent problems include higher rates of miscarriage, postpartum hemorrhage, and cesarean delivery (Homer, 2010).

In sum, UAE has typically low major complication rates and high symptom-relief scores. However, these are balanced against the need for ultimate reintervention in a significant number of women.

Magnetic Resonance–Guided Focused Ultrasound

With MR-guided focused ultrasound (MRgFUS), ultrasound energy is focused to heat and incite coagulative necrosis in selected myomas (Fig. 9-7). Concurrent MR imaging enables this energy to be precisely targeted and also provides real-time tissue temperature feedback to limit surrounding tissue injury. After treatment, gadolinium-enhanced MR images are obtained to measure the

nonperfused volume within the treated myomas. This correlates positively with tumor and symptom reduction (Park, 2014).

Also called MR-guided high-intensity focused ultrasound (MR-HIFU), this procedure requires only conscious sedation and is associated with rapid recovery. Sessions last 2 to 3 hours during which a patient lies prone within the MR imaging unit and the bladder is continuously drained.

For potential candidates, manufacturer contraindications are pregnancy, uterine malignancy, menopause, calcified myomas, general contraindications to MR imaging, and obstructions along the energy path. These latter include abdominal wall scars, bowel, or foreign bodies. In studies, other exclusion criteria have been current pelvic infection, uterine size >24 weeks, myoma size >10 cm, and myomas lying deeper than 12 cm from the skin surface (Kim, 2011; Pron, 2015). Also, failure or injury rates are greater with pedunculated serosal or submucous myomas, concurrent adenomyosis, tumors near vital structures, or more than four myomas (Mindjuk, 2015). Because of these limitations, many women are ineligible.

Early prospective studies show that MRgFUS improves quality-of-life scores and is well tolerated (Hindley, 2004). Potential minor complications include vaginal discharge, fever, hematuria, and abdominal wall edema. More serious conditions are venous thromboembolism, necrotic myoma tissue retained in the uterine cavity, heavy uterine bleeding, endometritis, and burns.

MRgFUS with the Exablate device is now permissible for women who desire fertility preservation. In one review of 102 pregnancies following MRgFUS, most of the 48 live births were full term and appropriately sized, 13 percent had antepartum spotting, 4 percent had placenta previa, and 4 percent required manual placenta removal (Keltz, 2017). Placenta accreta or uterine rupture was not noted.

Comparing UAE and MRgFUS, the FIRSTT randomized trial showed a 30-percent reintervention rate within 3 years after MRgFUS. The rate was only 13 percent for UAE (Laughlin-Tommaso, 2019). Other efficacy data are from nonrandomized cohorts that offer relatively short-term results. Improvement in symptoms scores ranges from 30 to 70 percent. But, similar to UAE, symptom relief wanes with time. At ≥12 months following MRgFUS, 13 to 24 percent sought alternative procedures for their symptoms, including hysterectomy (Kim, 2011; Machtinger, 2012; Mindjuk, 2015). Compared with UAE in one small study, MRgFUS was less successful in providing symptom improvement at 5 years, and 67 percent of women elected reintervention (Froeling, 2013).

As an alternative to MR guidance, a newer modality uses ultrasound imaging to focus ultrasound energy but is not yet FDA approved. Also, ultrasound-guided focused ultrasound (USgFUS) does not provide thermal feedback from the myoma. Limited data regarding its efficacy and safety concerns mirror those with MRgFUS (Chen, 2016; Parsons, 2017).

■ Surgery

Hysterectomy

For women with persistent symptoms despite conservative efforts, hysterectomy, myomectomy, endometrial ablation, and myolysis are options. Of these, hysterectomy is the definitive and

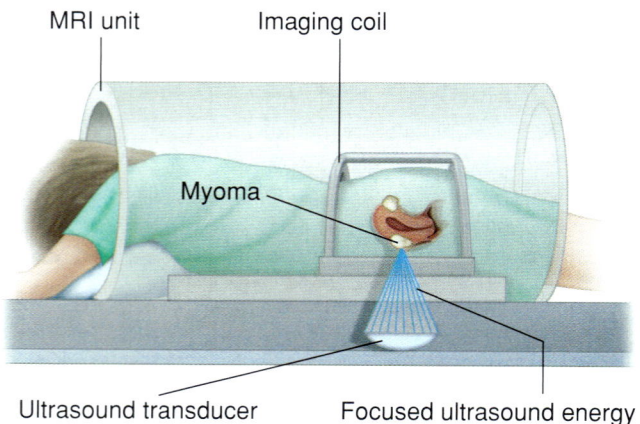

MRI unit   Imaging coil

Myoma

Ultrasound transducer   Focused ultrasound energy

FIGURE 9-7 Diagram of magnetic resonance-guided focused ultrasound.

most common surgery. It can be performed vaginally, abdominally, or laparoscopically depending on patient and uterine factors. Symptomatic cervical or broad ligament leiomyomas are best treated with hysterectomy.

Following hysterectomy, postoperative satisfaction rates are high, and data show superior rates compared with conservative options (Carlson, 1994; De Bruijn, 2016). However, benefits are balanced against the risks of major surgery.

Myomectomy

This uterus-preserving surgery excises myomas and is considered for women who desire fertility preservation or who decline hysterectomy. Contraindications are active infection, pregnancy, and suspected malignancy. Compared with hysterectomy, myomectomy poses a higher risk of myoma recurrence and incomplete symptom relief but has lower rates of injury to adjacent organs. Blood loss, surgery length, febrile morbidity, and hospital stays are comparable for surgery performed on uteri up to 16-week size (Iverson, 1996; Sawin, 2000).

Myomectomy can be performed hysteroscopically, laparoscopically, or via laparotomy, and these are illustrated in the atlas portion of this book. In general, predominantly intracavitary myomas are resected hysteroscopically, whereas subserosal or intramural myomas require laparotomy or laparoscopy for surgical excision.

For intracavitary myomas, hysteroscopic resection affords quicker recovery and less surgical morbidity than hysterectomy or laparoscopic myomectomy. The efficacy of hysteroscopic myomectomy positively correlates with percentage of excised volume, and the size, topography, extension, penetration, wall (STEPW) criteria can guide patient selection (Table 9-3) (Tsujioka, 2017). Resection is most effective with type 0 and type 1 tumors and with those measuring ≤3 cm (Mazzon, 2015). Although suitable for skilled surgeons, larger or type 2 myomas carry higher risks for incomplete resection, difficult visualization, uterine perforation, or reaching media volume limits (Arnold, 2016). For hysteroscopic myomectomy in general, 15 to 20 percent of treated women eventually require additional surgery (Emanuel, 1999; Hart, 1999).

In contrast, for women with subserosal or intramural myomas, surgeons must enucleate tumors buried in the muscular uterine walls and then reconstruct normal anatomy. As such, surgical complexity and subsequent risks are increased. This type of myomectomy usually improves pain and bleeding. For example, HMB improves in approximately 70 to 80 percent of patients (Buttram, 1981; Olufowobi, 2004). Reintervention rates are 10 to 15 percent (Hanafi, 2005; Yoo, 2007).

When selecting a surgical approach for subserosal or intramural myomas, several factors are weighed. Laparoscopic leiomyoma resection yields successful outcomes and recurrence rates that are comparable to those for laparotomy (Bhave Chittawar, 2014; Rossetti, 2001). Advantageously, shorter hospital stays and less febrile morbidity, blood loss, adhesion formation, and pain are found with laparoscopic resection (Jin, 2009; Takeuchi, 2002). However, uterine rupture in subsequent pregnancy, although rare, has higher rates following laparoscopic enucleation (Pop, 2018). Single-layer closures and thermal myometrial injury from greater electrosurgery use are proposed causes (Parker, 2010).

Patient selection criteria vary by surgeon, but for a laparoscopic approach limits can include large myoma size (≥6 to 10 cm), many tumors (≥3), and locations that require multiple incisions. In general, large intramural and multiple myomas require greater laparoscopic skill (Juhasz-Böss, 2017).

To overcome some of these limits, minilaparotomy techniques may be elected. However, similar to larger laparotomy incisions, minilaparotomy is faster but still underperforms laparoscopy with regard to patient pain scores, hospital stay, and blood loss (Alessandri, 2006; Palomba, 2007). Also, robot-assisted myomectomy has been described. Overall, this offers similar minimally invasive surgery (MIS) advantages but longer operating times and greater cost (Buckley, 2015). Moreover, due to poor tactile feedback from robotic instruments, myomas may be missed, leading to higher recurrence rates (Griffin, 2013).

In sum, for those considering myomectomy, hysteroscopic resection is preferred when possible. For remaining cases, selection varies depending on myoma characteristics and surgeon skill. MIS, when feasible, offers decreased postoperative pain and surgical complication rates comparable to laparotomy.

Endometrial Ablation

Several endometrium-destructive modalities are often elected for abnormal uterine bleeding due to endometrial dysfunction. These can be also used as a sole technique for myoma-related bleeding. However, data are conflicting as to whether the failure rate is higher in those with myomas (Klebanoff, 2017; Longinotti, 2008). Of note, most of these modalities have limitations regarding cavity length and degree of cavity distortion. That said, some data show efficacy if treating submucous myomas measuring ≤3 cm (Glasser, 2009). However, these specific tumors may be more suited to hysteroscopic resection. Instead, some have used ablation as an adjunct following hysteroscopic leiomyoma resection in women with HMB (Loffer, 2005).

Myolysis and Other Approaches

Myolysis describes procedures using tools that directly contact the myoma to incite myoma necrosis and subsequent shrinkage. With the various procedures, radiofrequency energy, laser vaporization, or cryotherapy ablates the myoma.

Of these, the Acessa system uses a monopolar radiofrequency needle that is inserted transabdominally into each tumor during

TABLE 9-3. STEPW Criteria for Hysteroscopic Myomectomy

Criteria	Points 0	1	2	Total
Size (cm)	≤2	>2–5	>5	
Topography	low	middle	upper	
Base width	≤⅓	>⅓–⅔	>⅔	
Penetration	0	≤50%	>50%	
Lateral wall	If along lateral wall, then +1			

Point totals from 0–4 = Group I; from 5–6 = Group II; from 7–9 = Group III. Surgical difficulty increases as point totals rise. Adapted from Wamsteker, 1993; Lasmar, 2005.

laparoscopy. Radiofrequency ablation (RFA) may be best suited for women with myomas <7 cm and uterine sizes <16 weeks. Exclusion criteria from studies have included myomas >10 cm, type 0 or type 1 myomas, pregnancy, infection, suspected malignancy, recent GnRH agonist use, suspected adenomyosis, and prior pelvic radiation. A desire for future fertility is not a contraindication. Data on pregnancy outcomes are few but encouraging (Keltz, 2017).

With this newer approach, early evidence shows a 50-percent improvement in symptom severity scores at 1 year (Chudnoff, 2013). In studies, reintervention rates were 11 percent at 3 years and 29 percent at 5 years (Berman, 2014; Iversen, 2017). Compared with laparoscopic myomectomy, RFA offers shorter operative and recovery times and less blood loss (Brucker, 2014). Short-term outcomes are comparable with those of laparoscopic myomectomy (Berman, 2014).

Different from myolysis, laparoscopic uterine artery occlusion (LUAO) attempts to achieve myoma necrosis by surgically sealing both the ovarian arteries and the uterine arteries near their origin from the internal iliac artery (Ambat, 2009). In studies, the reintervention rate at 16 months was 15 percent, but at 4 years it was 28 percent and similar to UAE (Hald, 2009; Mara, 2012). For now, the required advanced surgical skills and scarce long-term outcome data limit its use.

■ Rare Manifestations

Most myomas are treated as just described. However, uncommon tumor complications can also affected numerous other organ systems. First, deep-vein thromboembolism risks are increased in those with myomas weighing >1000 g (Shiota, 2011). Of uncommon urologic complications, acute urinary retention may stem from compression by a myoma or by an incarcerated myomatous uterus. As management, bladder drainage by Foley catheter or by intermittent self-catheterization is a temporizing option. In contrast, severe hydronephrosis originates from ureteral compression, usually at the pelvic brim (Alyeshmerni, 2011). Both retention and ureteral obstruction can be resolved with removal or shrinkage of myomas.

Also rarely, *myomatous erythrocytosis syndrome* can create an elevated red blood cell (RBC) count but not the pancytosis that characterizes polycythemia. This syndrome stems from excessive erythropoietin production, most likely by the myoma itself (Ono, 2014). Following hysterectomy, the RBC count returns to normal.

Leiomyomas infrequently may cause *pseudo-Meigs syndrome* (Yonehara, 2014). Traditionally, Meigs syndrome consists of ascites and pleural effusions that accompany a benign ovarian fibroma. However, any pelvic tumor can cause this. If due to a myoma, resolution of ascites and hydrothorax follows hysterectomy or myomectomy.

An autosomal dominant mutation in the *fumarate hydratase (FH)* gene underlies the rare *hereditary leiomyomatosis and renal cell cancer (HLRCC) syndrome*. Also called Reed syndrome, the classic triad is cutaneous and uterine leiomyomas and renal cell cancer (Miettinen, 2016).

Rarely, extrauterine smooth muscle tumors, which are benign yet infiltrative, may develop in women with concurrent or prior uterine leiomyomas, and this condition is termed leiomyomatosis. In such cases, malignant metastases from a leiomyosarcoma must be excluded.

Intravenous leiomyomatosis invades and extends serpiginously into the uterine veins, vena cava, and even cardiac chambers (Ma, 2016). With a multidisciplinary team, surgical resection, including hysterectomy and adnexectomy, is preferred treatment (Yang, 2018).

Benign metastasizing leiomyomas derive from morphologically benign uterine leiomyomas that disseminate hematogenously. The slow-growing lesions are found most often in the lungs (Barnaś, 2017). Once diagnosed, excision of symptomatic accessible lesions is reasonable. Multiple masses or pulmonary lesions can be surveilled if asymptomatic or can be treated with castrating surgery or drugs (Pacheco-Rodriguez, 2016).

Disseminated peritoneal leiomyomatosis (DPL) appears as numerous, small peritoneal nodules in the abdominal cavity and often mimics widespread peritoneal metastatic cancer. DPL is usually found in women of reproductive age and is often associated with pregnancy or COC use. Conservative surgery permits diagnosis. Then, treatment typically is cessation of exogenous hormones or antiestrogenic agents to prompt myoma regression (Bisceglia, 2014).

Last, with use of electromechanical morcellation during MIS, multiple small peritoneal leiomyomas may be found later after the primary surgery. Secondary implantation of myoma remnants is implicated, and these present similarly to parasitic leiomyomas or DPL (Tulandi, 2016).

HEMATOMETRA

In this condition, outflow obstruction traps blood and distends the uterus. Depending on the level of the genital tract blockage, blood can variably distend the vagina (hematocolpos), cervix (hematotrachelos), the uterus (hematometra), and fallopian tubes (hematosalpinx). Obstruction may be congenital, and these are described in Chapter 19. Acquired abnormalities such as scarring and neoplasms can also obstruct menstrual flow. As such, hematometra may follow radiation treatment, prolonged hypoestrogenism with atrophy, or surgeries of the endometrial cavity or endocervical canal, particularly cervical conization or endometrial ablation. With postablation tubal sterilization syndrome (PATSS), the occluded fallopian tube and postoperative obstructive synechiae serve as the outflow obstruction (Chap. 44, p. 1061) (McCausland, 2010). Other predisposing conditions are Asherman syndrome or malignancies of the uterus or cervix. Rarely, acute hematometra will follow suction aspiration of the gravid uterus and requires re-aspiration to alleviate (Chap. 43, p. 972) (Sherer, 2011).

Hematometra classically produces suprapubic or low back pain or pelvic fullness. With total obstruction, amenorrhea is noted. If significant, a large uterus can even compress the bladder or rectum to yield urinary retention or constipation. With partial obstruction, blood may erratically drain around the blockage and can be foul. Last, blood may become infected, and pyometra creates fever and leukocytosis.

Pelvic examination findings include an enlarged, soft, or even cystic midline uterine corpus that may be tender to palpation.

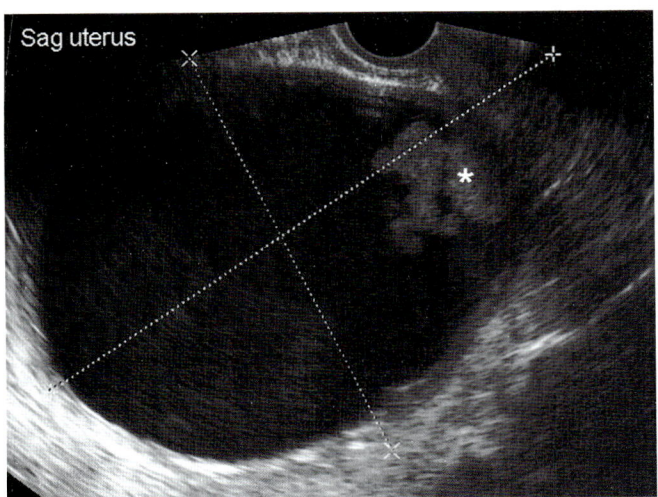

FIGURE 9-8 Sonographic transvaginal sagittal image of hematometra. The uterine walls and proximal cervix are dilated by retained blood, which appears hypoechoic. An obstructive cervical cancer is marked by an asterisk.

Urine or serum β-hCG assay is obtained to exclude pregnancy. Sonography is a principal diagnostic tool, and imaging shows a smooth, symmetric hypoechoic enlargement of the uterine cavity and low-level internal echoes (Fig. 9-8). A hematosalpinx is seen less commonly as a hypoechoic tubular structure lateral to the uterus. Although typically not required for the diagnosis, MR imaging can be used in some cases to help localize the obstruction and to provide additional anatomic information. Importantly, in cases in which the underlying cause is unclear, Pap testing and endocervical and endometrial biopsy are usually indicated to exclude malignancy.

For most cases of hematometra, relief of the obstruction and blood evacuation are goals. Cervical dilatation in the clinic or operating suite usually relieves the accumulation. Some have described hysteroscopy following dilatation to access blood pockets and to lyse adhesions in cases complicated by uterine synechiae (Cooper, 2000). Congenital abnormalities may require more extensive procedures to correct the obstruction.

ADENOMYOSIS

■ Pathophysiology

Adenomyosis is characterized by uterine enlargement caused by ectopic rests of endometrium—both glands and stroma—located deep within the myometrium (Fig. 9-9). These rests may be scattered throughout the myometrium—*diffuse adenomyosis*, or may form a localized nodular collection—*focal adenomyosis*. Incidences in hysterectomy specimens vary depending on the histologic criteria and on the degree of sectioning but range from 20 to 40 percent (Vercellini, 2006). In one clinic population undergoing TVS, adenomyosis was suspected in 21 percent (Naftalin, 2012).

On gross examination, the uterus is often globally enlarged, but this rarely exceeds 12-week size. The uterine surface is usually smooth, regular, reddish, and soft. The grossly cut myometrium typically appears spongy or trabeculated and shows focal areas of hemorrhage. An example is seen in the next section.

The most widely held theory regarding adenomyosis development describes the downward invagination of the endometrial basalis layer into the myometrium. Mechanisms are unknown, but prior uterine surgery and estrogen and progesterone likely play a role in its development and maintenance. Adenomyosis is also associated with aromatase expression and higher tissue estrogen levels (Yamamoto, 1993). This similar increase is also seen in leiomyomas, endometrial hyperplasia, and endometriosis, which are often coexistent with adenomyosis. However, endometriosis differs from adenomyosis in its pathogenesis and epidemiology. Adenomyosis derives from the basalis layer, but endometriosis stems from the functionalis.

Parity and age are significant risk factors for adenomyosis (Templeman, 2008). Specifically, nearly 90 percent of cases are in

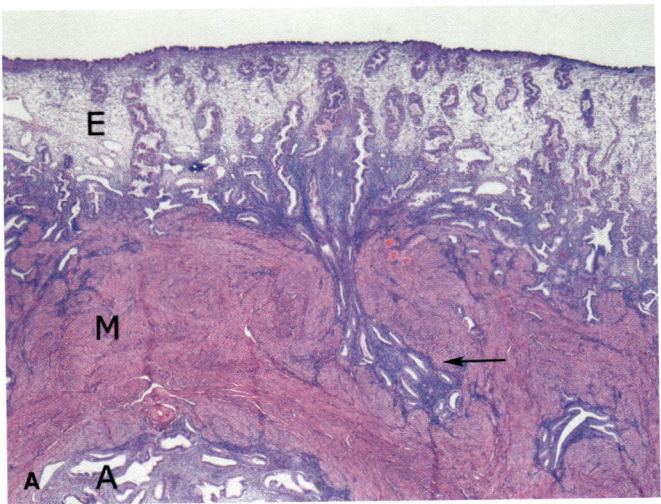

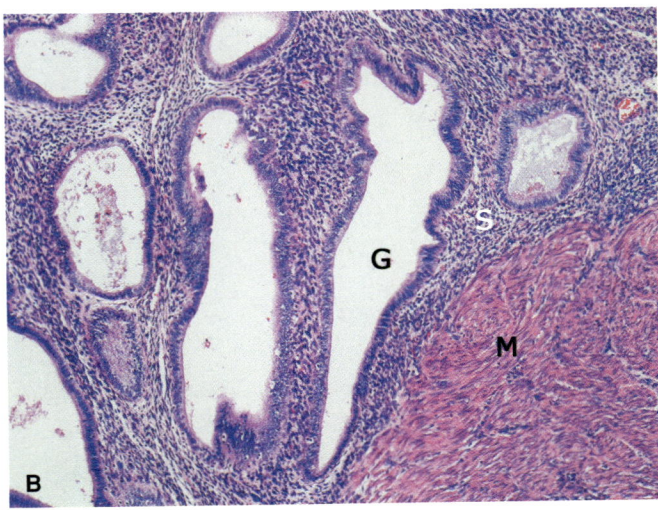

FIGURE 9-9 A. In adenomyosis, endometrial glands and their surrounding stroma dip irregularly into the myometrium (*arrow*). A = adenomyosis; E = endometrium; M = myometrium. **B.** Higher magnification view. Endometrial glands (*G*) and stroma (*S*) are seen adjacent to myometrium (*M*). (Reproduced with permission from Dr. Kelley Carrick.)

parous women, and nearly 80 percent develop in women in their 40s and 50s (Bird, 1972; Lee, 1984). It regresses after menopause.

Diagnosis

Approximately one third of women with adenomyosis have symptoms, and HMB and dysmenorrhea are common. Perhaps 10 percent complain of dyspareunia. Symptom severity correlates with increasing number of ectopic foci and extent of invasion (Levgur, 2000). Any link with subfertility is unclear, as data are scarce and poor quality (Maheshwari, 2012).

For diagnosis, transabdominal sonography inconsistently identifies the often subtle myometrial changes of adenomyosis, and imaging with TVS is preferred (Bazot, 2001). In comparison, MR imaging may be equal or slightly superior to TVS (Reinhold, 1996). Thus, MR imaging may be most appropriate when the diagnosis is inconclusive, when further delineation would affect patient management, or when coexisting uterine myomas distort anatomy (American College of Obstetricians and Gynecologists, 2016). With TVS, findings of diffuse adenomyosis may include: (1) anterior or posterior myometrial wall appearing thicker than its counterpart, (2) myometrial texture heterogeneity, (3) small myometrial hypoechoic cysts, which are cystic glands within ectopic endometrial foci, (4) striated projections extending from the endometrium into the myometrium, (5) ill-defined endometrial echo border, and (6) a globally enlarged uterus (Fig. 9-10). With application of color or power Doppler, diffuse vascularity may be seen in affected myometrium. Focal adenomyosis appears as a discrete hypoechoic nodule that may sometimes be differentiated from leiomyomas by its poorly defined margins, elliptical shape, minimal mass effect on surrounding tissues, and lack of calcifications, but presence of small anechoic myometrial cysts (Levy, 2013).

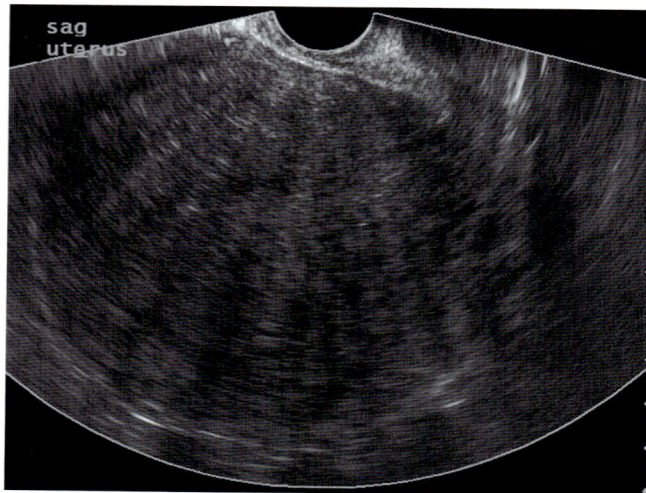

FIGURE 9-10 Transvaginal sagittal uterine image displaying globular uterine enlargement and heterogeneous myometrial texture. Uterine wall thickening can show anteroposterior asymmetry, and here the posterior wall is thicker. In this image, the endomyometrial junction is also poorly defined. Last, a "shutter blind" effect is thought to reflect endometrial gland invasion into the subendometrial tissue and appears as echogenic linear striations.

Management

Treatment goals are relief of pain and bleeding. Although supportive data specific to adenomyosis are limited, conservative therapy for symptomatic adenomyosis is similar to that for endometriosis. First, cyclic NSAIDs are often given with menses. In small studies, COCs and progestin-only regimens can be used to induce endometrial atrophy and lower endometrial prostaglandin production to improve dysmenorrhea and HMB (Muneyyirci-Delale, 2012; Osuga, 2017). Also, the LNG-IUS has proved effective for treatment of adenomyosis-related bleeding (Shaaban, 2015). Notably, expulsion rates may be higher in affected women (Youm, 2014). GnRH agonists are another effective choice, although their high cost and hypoestrogenic side effects typically limit long-term use. These agonists may be most helpful for women with adenomyosis-related subfertility or as relief prior to surgical treatment. Although danazol may be considered, it is often a less desirable option due to its androgenic side effects.

Hysterectomy is definitive treatment. As with other conditions, surgical route selection is influenced by uterine size and associated uterine or abdominopelvic pathology. Alternatively, global endometrial ablation or hysteroscopic endometrial resection has successfully treated dysmenorrhea and HMB caused by adenomyosis (Preutthipan, 2010). However, failure rates may be higher in women with adenomyosis (Wishall, 2014). By 3 years in one small study, 19 percent of ablation-treated women with adenomyosis ultimately underwent hysterectomy (Philip, 2018). Complete eradication of deep adenomyosis is problematic and is thought responsible for a significant number of treatment failures (Mengerink, 2015). Accordingly, some recommended imaging prior to ablation to identify these deep lesions and allow better patient selection (McCausland, 1996).

UAE can also relieve symptoms for some women with adenomyosis, although study sizes are small (Chen, 2006; Liang, 2018). One systematic review found that 90 percent of women with adenomyosis were improved short-term (de Bruijn, 2017). After 1 year, 74 percent still benefited. In another, investigators following women 1 to 5 years after UAE found 65 percent were still improved (Popovic, 2011). For focal adenomyomas, MRgFUS was effective in small case series (Yang, 2009; Zhang, 2014).

OTHER UTERINE ENTITIES

Myometrial hypertrophy is global uterine enlargement without identifiable pathology, especially in those with high parity (Traiman, 1996). Also known as gravid hypertrophy, one definition includes uterine weights >130 g for nulliparas and >210 g for multiparas (Zaloudek, 2011). Symptoms are infrequent, but HMB is a common complaint.

Uterine or cervical diverticula are sacculations that communicate with and extend out from the endometrial cavity or endocervical canal. Rarely, these are congenital anomalies developing from a localized duplication of the distal müllerian duct on one side (Engel, 1984). More often, defects are acquired, develop in the uterine isthmus, and follow cesarean delivery (Fig. 9-11). These *isthmoceles* may cause postmenstrual spotting or intermenstrual bleeding. Also termed *cesarean scar*

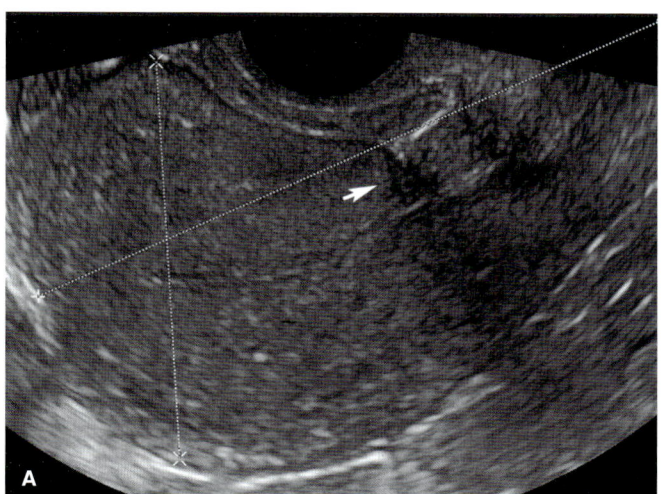 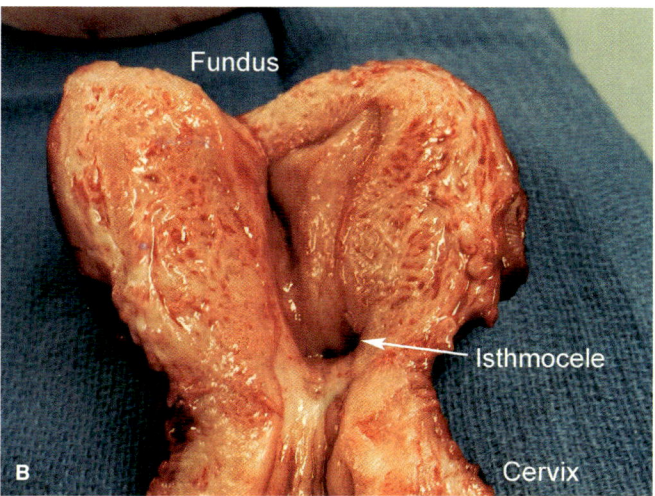

FIGURE 9-11 Isthmocele. **A.** In this sagittal sonogram, the cesarean scar niche is the hypoechoic triangle marked by the arrow. **B.** The same uterus is seen after hysterectomy. In this specimen, comorbid adenomyosis is identified by the highly trabeculated myometrium. (Reproduced with permission from Dr. David Rogers.)

defects, these niches can serve as a passive repository for menstrual blood and release it during postmenstrual days. Also, cesarean scar pregnancies may result from blastocyst implantation within the isthmocele (Chap. 7, p. 171).

Although niches can be seen during TVS, defects are best imaged by SIS and can be identified hysteroscopically (Antila-Långsjö, 2018; Bij de Vaate, 2011). MR imaging is also informative but less cost effective than SIS.

Endometrial suppression with COCs has been described (Tahara, 2006). Although data are lacking, progestins alone might also be helpful. The LNG-IUS appears less effective (Zhang, 2016a). Surgical options include hysterectomy or hysteroscopic shaving of niche edges plus ablation of the pouch base (Vervoort, 2018; Setubal, 2018). Another option is excision of the involved myometrium followed by reapproximation of muscle edges. This last method has been described laparoscopically and transvaginally (Zhang, 2016b). Data are limited regarding the superiority of one surgical approach compared with another for symptom relief or for future childbearing. However, in those with thinner myometrium (<3 mm) at the site, hysteroscopic resection may pose greater perforation risk (Sanders, 2018).

REFERENCES

Alessandri F, Lijoi D, Mistrangelo E, et al: Randomized study of laparoscopic versus minilaparotomic myomectomy for uterine myomas. J Minim Invasive Gynecol 13(2):92, 2006

Alyeshmerni D, Banovac F, Pehlivanova M, et al: Resolution of hydronephrosis after uterine artery embolization for fibroids. J Vasc Interv Radiol 22(6):865, 2011

Ambat S, Mittal S, Srivastava DN, et al: Uterine artery embolization versus laparoscopic occlusion of uterine vessels for management of symptomatic uterine fibroids. Int J Gynaecol Obstet 105(2):162, 2009

American College of Obstetricians and Gynecologists: Alternatives to hysterectomy in the management of leiomyomas. Practice Bulletin No. 96, August 2008, Reaffirmed 2016

American Society for Reproductive Medicine: Removal of myomas in asymptomatic patients to improve fertility and/or reduce miscarriage rate: a guideline. Fertil Steril 108(3):416, 2017

Anteby SO, Yarkoni S, Ever Hadani P: The effect of a prostaglandin synthetase inhibitor, indomethacin, on excessive uterine bleeding. Clin Exp Obstet Gynecol 12(3-4):60, 1985

Antila-Långsjö R, Mäenpää JU, Huhtala H, et al: Comparison of transvaginal ultrasound and saline contrast sonohysterography in evaluation of cesarean scar defect: a prospective cohort study. Acta Obstet Gynecol Scand 97(9):1130, 2018

Archer DF, Stewart EA, Jain RI, et al: Elagolix for the management of heavy menstrual bleeding associated with uterine fibroids: results from a phase 2a proof-of-concept study. Fertil Steril 108(1):152, 2017

Arnold A, Ketheeswaran A, Bhatti M, et al: A prospective analysis of hysteroscopic morcellation in the management of intrauterine pathologies. J Minim Invasive Gynecol 23(3):435, 2016

Baird DD, Dunson DB, Hill MC, et al: High cumulative incidence of uterine leiomyoma in black and white women: ultrasound evidence. Am J Obstet Gynecol 188(1):100, 2003

Baird DD, Saldana TM, Shore DL, et al: A single baseline ultrasound assessment of fibroid presence and size is strongly predictive of future uterine procedure: 8-year follow-up of randomly sampled premenopausal women aged 35–49 years. Hum Reprod 30(12):2936, 2015

Barnaś E, Książek M, Raś R, et al: Benign metastasizing leiomyoma: a review of current literature in respect to the time and type of previous gynecological surgery. PLoS One 12(4):e0175875, 2017

Bayer HealthCare Pharmaceuticals: Mirena (levonorgestrel-releasing intrauterine system). Highlights of prescribing information, 2017. Available at: https://labeling.bayerhealthcare.com/html/products/pi/Mirena_PI.pdf. Accessed September 9, 2018

Bazot M, Cortez A, Darai E, et al: Ultrasonography compared with magnetic resonance imaging for the diagnosis of adenomyosis: correlation with histopathology. Hum Reprod 16(11):2427, 2001

Berman JM, Guido RS, Garza Leal JG, et al: Three-year outcome of the Halt trial: a prospective analysis of radiofrequency volumetric thermal ablation of myomas. J Minim Invasive Gynecol 21(5):767, 2014

Bhave Chittawar P, Franik S, Pouwer AW, et al: Minimally invasive surgical techniques versus open myomectomy for uterine fibroids. Cochrane Database Syst Rev 10:CD004638, 2014

Bij de Vaate AJ, Brölmann HA, van der Voet LF, et al: Ultrasound evaluation of the cesarean scar: relation between a niche and postmenstrual spotting. Ultrasound Obstet Gynecol 37(1):93, 2011

Bird CC, McElin TW, Manalo-Estrella P: The elusive adenomyosis of the uterus—revisited. Am J Obstet Gynecol 112(5):583, 1972

Bisceglia M, Galliani CA, Pizzolitto S, et al: Leiomyomatosis peritonealis disseminata: report of 3 cases with extensive review of the literature. Adv Anat Pathol 21(3):201, 2014

Bonneau C, Thomassin-Naggara I, Dechoux S, et al: Value of ultrasonography and magnetic resonance imaging for the characterization of uterine mesenchymal tumors. Acta Obstet Gynecol Scand 93(3):261, 2014

Bratby MJ, Hussain FF, Walker WJ: Outcomes after unilateral uterine artery embolization: a retrospective review. Cardiovasc Intervent Radiol 31(2):254, 2008

Broekmans FJ: GnRH agonists and uterine leiomyomas. Human Reprod 11(Suppl 3):3, 1996

Brucker SY, Hahn M, Kraemer D, et al: Laparoscopic radiofrequency volumetric thermal ablation of fibroids versus laparoscopic myomectomy. Int J Gynaecol Obstet 125(3):261, 2014

Buckley VA, Nesbitt-Hawes EM, Atkinson P, et al: Laparoscopic myomectomy: clinical outcomes and comparative evidence. J Minim Invasive Gynecol 22(1):11, 2015

Bulun SE, Simpson ER, Word RA: Expression of the CYP19 gene and its product aromatase cytochrome P450 in human uterine leiomyoma tissues and cells in culture. J Clin Endocrinol Metab 78(3):736, 1994

Buttram VC Jr, Reiter RC: Uterine leiomyomata: etiology, symptomatology, and management. Fertil Steril 36(4):433, 1981

Cantuaria GH, Angioli R, Frost L, et al: Comparison of bimanual examination with ultrasound examination before hysterectomy for uterine leiomyoma. Obstet Gynecol 92(1):109, 1998

Carlson KJ, Miller BA, Fowler FJ Jr: The Maine Women's Health Study: II. Outcomes of nonsurgical management of leiomyomas, abnormal bleeding, and chronic pelvic pain. Obstet Gynecol 83(4):566, 1994

Carr BR, Marshburn PB, Weatherall PT, et al: An evaluation of the effect of gonadotropin-releasing hormone analogs and medroxyprogesterone acetate on uterine leiomyomata volume by magnetic resonance imaging: a prospective, randomized, double blind, placebo-controlled, crossover trial. J Clin Endocrinol Metab 76(5):1217, 1993

Carr BR, Stewart EA, Archer DF, et al: Elagolix alone or with add-back therapy in women with heavy menstrual bleeding and uterine leiomyomas: a randomized controlled trial. Obstet Gynecol 132(5):1252, 2018

Casini ML, Rossi F, Agostini R, et al: Effect of the position of fibroids on fertility. Gynecol Endocrinol 22:106, 2006

Chen CL, Liu P, Zeng BL, et al: Intermediate and long term clinical effects of uterine arterial embolization in treatment of adenomyosis. Zhonghua Fu Chan Ke Za Zhi 41(10):660, 2006

Chen R, Keserci B, Bi H, et al: The safety and effectiveness of volumetric magnetic resonance-guided high-intensity focused ultrasound treatment of symptomatic uterine fibroids: early clinical experience in China. J Ther Ultrasound 4(27):1, 2016

Christopoulos G, Vlismas A, Salim R, et al: Fibroids that do not distort the uterine cavity and IVF success rates: an observational study using extensive matching criteria. BJOG 124(4):615, 2017

Chudnoff SG, Berman JM, Levine DJ, et al: Outpatient procedure for the treatment and relief of symptomatic uterine myomas. Obstet Gynecol 121(5):1075, 2013

Cooper JM, Brady RM: Late complications of operative hysteroscopy. Obstet Gynecol Clin North Am 27(2):367, 2000

Coutinho EM, Gonçalves MT: Long-term treatment of leiomyomas with gestrinone. Fertil Steril 51(6):939, 1989

Dariushnia SR, Nikolic B, Stokes LS, et al: Quality improvement guidelines for uterine artery embolization for symptomatic leiomyomata. J Vasc Interv Radiol 25(11):1737, 2014

de Bruijn AM, Ankum WM, Reekers JA, et al: Uterine artery embolization vs hysterectomy in the treatment of symptomatic uterine fibroids: 10-year outcomes from the randomized EMMY trial. Am J Obstet Gynecol 215(6):745.e1, 2016

de Bruijn AM, Smink M, Lohle PN, et al: Uterine artery embolization for the treatment of adenomyosis: a systematic review and meta-analysis. J Vasc Interv Radiol 82(12):1629, 2017

De Leo V, la Marca A, Morgante G: Short-term treatment of uterine fibromyomas with danazol. Gynecol Obstet Invest 47(4):258, 1999

DeWaay DJ, Syrop CH, Nygaard IE, et al: Natural history of uterine polyps and leiomyomata. Obstet Gynecol 100(1):3, 2002

Donnez J, Donnez O, Matule D, et al: Long-term medical management of uterine fibroids with ulipristal acetate. Fertil Steril 105(1):165, 2016

Donnez J, Hervais Vivancos B, Kudela M, et al: A randomized, placebo-controlled, dose-ranging trial comparing fulvestrant with goserelin in premenopausal patients with uterine fibroids awaiting hysterectomy. Fertil Steril 79(6):1380, 2003

Donnez J, Jadoul P: What are the implications of myomas on fertility? A need for a debate? Human Reprod 17(6):1424, 2002

Donnez J, Tatarchuk TF, Bouchard P, et al: Ulipristal acetate versus placebo for fibroid treatment before surgery. N Engl J Med 366(5):409, 2012a

Donnez J, Tomaszewski J, Vázquez F, et al: Ulipristal acetate versus leuprolide acetate for uterine fibroids. N Engl J Med 366(5):421, 2012b

Eder S, Baker J, Gersten J, et al: Efficacy and safety of oral tranexamic acid in women with heavy menstrual bleeding and fibroids. Womens Health (Lond Engl) 9(4):397, 2013

Edwards RD, Moss JG, Lumsden MA, et al: Uterine-artery embolization versus surgery for symptomatic uterine fibroids. N Engl J Med 356(4):360, 2007

Emanuel MH, Wamsteker K, Hart AA, et al: Long-term results of hysteroscopic myomectomy for abnormal uterine bleeding. Obstet Gynecol 93(5 Pt 1):743, 1999

Engel G, Rushovich AM: True uterine diverticulum. A partial müllerian duct duplication? Arch Pathol Lab Med 108(9):734, 1984

Englund K, Blanck A, Gustavsson I, et al: Sex steroid receptors in human myometrium and fibroids: changes during the menstrual cycle and gonadotropin-releasing hormone treatment. J Clin Endocrinol Metab 83(11):4092, 1998

European Medicines Agency: Esmya. 2018. Available at: https://www.ema.europa.eu/en/medicines/human/referrals/esmya. Accessed November 10, 2018

Friedman AJ, Daly M, Juneau-Norcross M, et al: Long-term medical therapy for leiomyomata uteri: a prospective, randomized study of leuprolide acetate depot plus either oestrogen-progestin or progestin "add-back" for 2 years. Hum Reprod 9(9):1618, 1994

Friedman AJ, Hoffman DI, Comite F, et al: Treatment of leiomyomata uteri with leuprolide acetate depot: a double-blind, placebo-controlled, multicenter study. The Leuprolide Study Group. Obstet Gynecol 77(5):720, 1991

Froeling V, Meckelburg K, Schreiter NF, et al: Outcome of uterine artery embolization versus MR-guided high-intensity focused ultrasound treatment for uterine fibroids: long-term results. Eur J Radiol 82(12):2265, 2013

Glasser MH, Heinlein PK, Hung YY: Office endometrial ablation with local anesthesia using the HydroThermAblator system: comparison of outcomes in patients with submucous myomas with those with normal cavities in 246 cases performed over 5(1/2) years. J Minim Invasive Gynecol 16(6):700, 2009

Goodwin SC, Bradley LD, Lipman JC, et al: Uterine artery embolization versus myomectomy: a multicenter comparative study. Fertil Steril 85(1):14, 2006

Griffin L, Feinglass J, Garrett A, et al: Postoperative outcomes after robotic versus abdominal myomectomy. JSLS 17(3):407, 2013

Gupta JK, Sinha A, Lumsden MA, et al: Uterine artery embolization for symptomatic uterine fibroids. Cochrane Database Syst Rev 12:CD005073, 2014

Hald K, Noreng HJ, Istre O, et al: Uterine artery embolization versus laparoscopic occlusion of uterine arteries for leiomyomas: long-term results of a randomized comparative trial. J Vasc Interv Radiol 20(10):1303, 2009

Hanafi M: Predictors of leiomyoma recurrence after myomectomy. Obstet Gynecol 105(4):877, 2005

Harmon QE, Baird DD: Use of depot medroxyprogesterone acetate and prevalent leiomyoma in young African American women. Hum Reprod 30(6):1499, 2015

Hart R, Molnár BG, Magos A: Long term follow up of hysteroscopic myomectomy assessed by survival analysis. BJOG 106(7):700, 1999

Hehenkamp WJ, Volkers NA, Birnie E, et al: Pain and return to daily activities after uterine artery embolization and hysterectomy in the treatment of symptomatic uterine fibroids: results from the randomized EMMY trial. Cardiovasc Intervent Radiol 29(2):179, 2006

Hehenkamp WJ, Volkers NA, Birnie E, et al: Symptomatic uterine fibroids: treatment with uterine artery embolization or hysterectomy—results from the randomized clinical Embolisation versus Hysterectomy (EMMY) trial. Radiology 246(3):823, 2008

Hehenkamp WJ, Volkers NA, Broekmans FJ, et al: Loss of ovarian reserve after uterine artery embolization: a randomized comparison with hysterectomy. Hum Reprod 22(7):1996, 2007

Hehenkamp WJ, Volkers NA, Donderwinkel PF, et al: Uterine artery embolization versus hysterectomy in the treatment of symptomatic uterine fibroids (EMMY trial): peri- and postprocedural results from a randomized controlled trial. Am J Obstet Gynecol 193(5):1618, 2005

Hindley J, Gedroyc WM, Regan L, et al: MRI guidance of focused ultrasound therapy of uterine fibroids: early results. AJR Am J Roentgenol 183(6):1713, 2004

Homer J, Saridogan E: Uterine artery embolization for fibroids is associated with an increase risk of miscarriage. Fertil Steril 94(1):324, 2010

Ikhena DE, Bulun SE: Literature review on the role of uterine fibroids in endometrial function. Reprod Sci 25(5):635, 2018

Ishikawa H, Ishi K, Serna VA, et al: Progesterone is essential for maintenance and growth of uterine leiomyomata. Endocrinology 151(6):2433, 2010

Iversen H, Dueholm M: Radiofrequency thermal ablation for uterine myomas: long-term clinical outcomes and reinterventions. J Minim Invasive Gynecol 24(6):1020, 2017

Iverson RE Jr, Chelmow D, Strohbehn K, et al: Relative morbidity of abdominal hysterectomy and myomectomy for management of uterine leiomyomas. Obstet Gynecol 88(3):415, 1996

Jin C, Hu Y, Chen X, et al: Laparoscopic versus open myomectomy: a meta-analysis of randomized controlled trials. Eur J Obstet Gynecol Reprod Biol 145(1):14, 2009

Juhasz-Böss I, Jungmann P, Radosa J, et al: Two novel classification systems for uterine fibroids and subsequent uterine reconstruction after myomectomy. Arch Gynecol Obstet 295(3):675, 2017

Keltz J, Levie M, Chudnoff S: Pregnancy outcomes after direct uterine myoma thermal ablation: review of the literature. J Minim Invasive Gynecol 24(4):538, 2017

Kim HS, Baik JH, Pham LD, et al: MR-guided high-intensity focused ultrasound treatment for symptomatic uterine leiomyomata: long-term outcomes. Acad Radiol 18(8):970, 2011

Klebanoff J, Makai GE, Patel NR, et al: Incidence and predictors of failed second-generation endometrial ablation. Gynecol Surg 14(1):26, 2017

Kriplani A, Awasthi D, Kulshrestha V, et al: Efficacy of the levonorgestrel-releasing intrauterine system in uterine leiomyoma. Int J Gynaecol Obstet 116(1):35, 2012

Kriplani A, Srivastava A, Kulshrestha V, et al: Efficacy of ormeloxifene versus oral contraceptive in the management of abnormal uterine bleeding due to uterine leiomyoma. J Obstet Gynaecol Res 42(12):1744, 2016

Lasmar RB, Barrozo PR, Dias R, et al: Submucous fibroids: a new presurgical classification to evaluate the viability of hysteroscopic surgical treatment—preliminary report. J Minim Invasive Gynecol 12(4):308, 2005

Laughlin-Tommaso S, Barnard EP, AbdElmagied AM, et al: FIRSTT study: randomized controlled trial of uterine artery embolization vs focused ultrasound surgery. Am J Obstet Gynecol 220(2):174.e1, 2019

Lee NC, Dicker RC, Rubin GL, et al: Confirmation of the preoperative diagnoses for hysterectomy. Am J Obstet Gynecol 150(3):283, 1984

Letterie GS, Coddington CC, Winkel CA, et al: Efficacy of a gonadotropin-releasing hormone agonist in the treatment of uterine leiomyomata: long-term follow-up. Fertil Steril 51(6):951, 1989

Levgur M, Abadi MA, Tucker A: Adenomyosis: symptoms, histology, and pregnancy terminations. Obstet Gynecol 95(5):688, 2000

Levy G, Dehaene A, Laurent N, et al: An update on adenomyosis. Diagn Interv Imaging 94(1):3, 2013

Liang E, Brown B, Rachinsky M: A clinical audit on the efficacy and safety of uterine artery embolisation for symptomatic adenomyosis: results in 117 women. Aust N Z J Obstet Gynaecol 58(4):454, 2018

Loffer FD: Improving results of hysteroscopic submucosal myomectomy for menorrhagia by concomitant endometrial ablation. J Minim Invasive Gynecol 12(3):254, 2005

Longinotti MK, Jacobson GF, Hung YY, et al: Probability of hysterectomy after endometrial ablation. Obstet Gynecol 112(6):1214, 2008

Lukes AS, Moore KA, Muse KN, et al: Tranexamic acid treatment for heavy menstrual bleeding: a randomized controlled trial. Obstet Gynecol 116(4):865, 2010

Ma G, Miao Q, Liu X, et al: Different surgical strategies of patients with intravenous leiomyomatosis. Medicine (Baltimore) 95(37):e4902, 2016

Machtinger R, Inbar Y, Cohen-Eylon S, et al: MR-guided focus ultrasound (MRgFUS) for symptomatic uterine fibroids: predictors of treatment success. Hum Reprod 27(12):3425, 2012

Maheshwari A, Gurunath S, Fatima F, et al: Adenomyosis and subfertility: a systematic review of prevalence, diagnosis, treatment and fertility outcomes. Hum Reprod Update 18(4):374, 2012

Mäkäräinen L, Ylikorkala O: Primary and myoma-associated menorrhagia: role of prostaglandins and effects of ibuprofen. BJOG 93(9):974, 1986

Manyonda IT, Bratby M, Horst JS, et al: Uterine artery embolization versus myomectomy: impact on quality of life—results of the FUME (Fibroids of the Uterus: Myomectomy versus Embolization) Trial. Cardiovasc Intervent Radiol 35(3):530, 2012

Mara M, Kubinova K, Maskova J, et al: Uterine artery embolization versus laparoscopic uterine artery occlusion: the outcomes of a prospective, non-randomized clinical trial. Cardiovasc Intervent Radiol 35(5):1041, 2012

Marshall LM, Spiegelman D, Barbieri RL, et al: Variation in the incidence of uterine leiomyoma among premenopausal women by age and race. Obstet Gynecol 90(6):967, 1997

Mazzon I, Favilli A, Grasso M, et al: Predicting success of single step hysteroscopic myomectomy: a single centre large cohort study of single myomas. Int J Surg 22:10, 2015

McCausland AM, McCausland VM: Depth of endometrial penetration in adenomyosis helps determine outcome of rollerball ablation. Am J Obstet Gynecol 174(6):1786, 1996

McCausland AM, McCausland VM: Long-term complications of minimally invasive endometrial ablation devices. J Gynecol Surg 26(2):133, 2010

Mengerink BB, van der Wurff AA, ter Haar JF, et al: Effect of undiagnosed deep adenomyosis after failed NovaSure endometrial ablation. J Minim Invasive Gynecol 22(2):239, 2015

Miettinen M, Felisiak-Golabek A, Wasag B, et al: Fumarase-deficient uterine leiomyomas: an immunohistochemical, molecular genetic, and clinicopathologic study of 86 cases. Am J Surg Pathol 40(12):1661, 2016

Mindjuk I, Trumm CG, Herzog P, et al: MRI predictors of clinical success in MR-guided focused ultrasound (MRgFUS) treatments of uterine fibroids: results from a single centre. Eur Radiol 25(5):1317, 2015

Mizutani T, Sugihara A, Nakamuro K, et al: Suppression of cell proliferation and induction of apoptosis in uterine leiomyoma by gonadotropin-releasing hormone agonist (leuprolide acetate). J Clin Endocrinol Metab 83(4):1253, 1998

Moss J, Christie A: Uterine artery embolization for heavy menstrual bleeding. Womens Health (Lond) 12(1):71, 2016

Moss JG, Cooper KG, Khaund A, et al: Randomised comparison of uterine artery embolisation (UAE) with surgical treatment in patients with symptomatic uterine fibroids (REST trial): 5-year results. BJOG 118(8):936, 2011

Muneyyirci-Delale O, Chandrareddy A, Mankame S, et al: Norethindrone acetate in the medical management of adenomyosis. Pharmaceuticals 5(10):1120, 2012

Munro MG, Critchley HO, Fraser IS, et al: The two FIGO systems for normal and abnormal uterine bleeding symptoms and classification of causes of abnormal uterine bleeding in the reproductive years: 2018 revisions. Int J Gynaecol Obstet 143(3):393, 2018

Mutter GL, Bergeron C, Deligdisch L, et al: The spectrum of endometrial pathology induced by progesterone receptor modulators. Mod Pathol 21(5):591, 2008

Naftalin J, Hoo W, Pateman K, et al: How common is adenomyosis? A prospective study of prevalence using transvaginal ultrasound in a gynaecology clinic. Hum Reprod 27(12):343, 2012

Olufowobi O, Sharif K, Papaionnou S, et al: Are the anticipated benefits of myomectomy achieved in women of reproductive age? A 5-year review of the results at a UK tertiary hospital. J Obstet Gynaecol 24(4):434, 2004

Ono Y, Hidaka T, Fukuta K, et al: A case of myomatous erythrocytosis syndrome associated with a large uterine leiomyoma. Case Rep Obstet Gynecol 2014:602139, 2014

Osuga Y, Enya K, Kudou K, et al: Oral gonadotropin-releasing hormone antagonist relugolix compared with leuprorelin injections for uterine leiomyomas: a randomized controlled trial. Obstet Gynecol 133(3):423, 2019

Osuga Y, Fujimoto-Okabe H, Hagino A: Evaluation of the efficacy and safety of dienogest in the treatment of painful symptoms in patients with adenomyosis: a randomized, double-blind, multicenter, placebo-controlled study. Fertil Steril 108(4):673, 2017

Pacheco-Rodriguez G, Taveira-DaSilva AM, Moss J: Benign metastasizing leiomyoma. Clin Chest Med 37(3):589, 2016

Palomba S, Affinito P, Tommaselli GA, et al: A clinical trial of the effects of tibolone administered with gonadotropin-releasing hormone analogues for the treatment of uterine leiomyomata. Fertil Steril 70(1):111, 1998

Palomba S, Orio F Jr, Russo T, et al: Gonadotropin-releasing hormone agonist with or without raloxifene: effects on cognition, mood, and quality of life. Fertil Steril 82(2):480, 2004

Palomba S, Zupi E, Russo T, et al: A multicenter randomized, controlled study comparing laparoscopic versus minilaparotomic myomectomy: short-term outcomes. Fertil Steril 88(4):942, 2007

Park MJ, Kim YS, Rhim H, et al: Safety and therapeutic efficacy of complete or near-complete ablation of symptomatic uterine fibroid tumors by MR imaging-guided high-intensity focused US therapy. J Vasc Interv Radiol 25(2):231, 2014

Parker WH, Einarsson J, Istre O, et al: Risk factors for uterine rupture after laparoscopic myomectomy. J Minim Invasive Gynecol 17(5):551, 2010

Parker WH, Fu YS, Berek JS: Uterine sarcoma in patients operated on for presumed leiomyoma and rapidly growing leiomyoma. Obstet Gynecol 83(3):414, 1994

Parsanezhad ME, Azmoon M, Alborzi S, et al: A randomized, controlled clinical trial comparing the effects of aromatase inhibitor (letrozole) and gonadotropin-releasing hormone agonist (triptorelin) on uterine leiomyoma volume and hormonal status. Fertil Steril 93(1):192, 2010

Parsons JE, Lau MP, Martin PJ, et al: Pilot study of the Mirabilis System prototype for rapid noninvasive uterine myoma treatment using an ultrasound-guided volumetric shell ablation technique. J Minim Invasive Gynecol 24(4):579, 2017

Philip CA, Le Mitouard M, Maillet L, et al: Evaluation of NovaSure global endometrial ablation in symptomatic adenomyosis: a longitudinal study with a 36 month follow-up. Eur J Obstet Gynecol Reprod Biol 227:46, 2018

Pop L, Suciu ID, Oprescu D, et al: Patency of uterine wall in pregnancies following assisted and spontaneous conception with antecedent laparoscopic and abdominal myomectomies—a difficult case and systematic review. J Matern Fetal Neonatal Med 21:1, 2018

Popovic M, Puchner S, Berzaczy D, et al: Uterine artery embolization for the treatment of adenomyosis: a review. J Vasc Interv Radiol 22(7):901, 2011

Preutthipan S, Herabutya Y: Hysteroscopic rollerball endometrial ablation as an alternative treatment for adenomyosis with menorrhagia and/or dysmenorrhea. J Obstet Gynaecol Res 36(5):1031, 2010

Pritts EA, Parker WH, Olive DL: Fibroids and infertility: an updated systematic review of the evidence. Fertil Steril 91(4):1215, 2009

Pron G: Magnetic resonance-guided high-intensity focused ultrasound (MRgHIFU) treatment of symptomatic uterine fibroids: an evidence-based analysis. Ont Health Technol Assess Ser 15(4):1, 2015

Qin J, Yang T, Kong F, et al: Oral contraceptive use and uterine leiomyoma risk: a meta-analysis based on cohort and case-control studies. Arch Gynecol Obstet 288(1):139, 2013

Reinhold C, McCarthy S, Bret PM, et al: Diffuse adenomyosis: comparison of endovaginal US and MR imaging with histopathologic correlation. Radiology 199(1):151, 1996

Rossetti A, Sizzi O, Soranna L, et al: Long-term results of laparoscopic myomectomy: recurrence rate in comparison with abdominal myomectomy. Hum Reprod 16(4):770, 2001

Sanders AP, Murji A: Hysteroscopic repair of cesarean scar isthmocele. Fertil Steril 110(3):555, 2018

Sawin SW, Pilevsky ND, Berlin JA, et al: Comparability of perioperative morbidity between abdominal myomectomy and hysterectomy for women with uterine leiomyomas. Am J Obstet Gynecology 183(6):1448, 2000

Sayed GH, Zakherah MS, El-Nashar SA, et al: A randomized clinical trial of a levonorgestrel-releasing intrauterine system and a low-dose combined oral contraceptive for fibroid-related menorrhagia. Int J Gynaecol Obstet 112(2):126, 2011

Sayyah-Melli M, Mobasseri M, Gharabaghi PM, et al: Comparing the effect of aromatase inhibitor (letrozole) + cabergoline (Dostinex) and letrozole alone on uterine myoma regression, a randomized clinical trial. Eur J Obstet Gynecol Reprod Biol 210:257, 2017

Scharla SH, Minne HW, Waibel-Treber S, et al: Bone mass reduction after estrogen deprivation by long-acting gonadotropin-releasing hormone agonists and its relation to pretreatment serum concentrations of 1,25-dihydroxyvitamin D3. J Clin Endocrinol Metab 70(4):1055, 1990

Schlaff WD, Zerhouni EA, Huth JA, et al: A placebo-controlled trial of a depot gonadotropin-releasing hormone analogue (leuprolide) in the treatment of uterine leiomyomata. Obstet Gynecol 74(6):856, 1989

Scialli AR, Levi AJ: Intermittent leuprolide acetate for the nonsurgical management of women with leiomyomata uteri. Fertil Steril 74(3):540, 2000

Setubal A, Alves J, Osório F, et al: Treatment for uterine isthmocele, a pouch-like defect at the site of a cesarean section scar. J Minim Invasive Gynecol 25(1):38, 2018

Shaaban OM, Ali MK, Sabra AM, et al: Levonorgestrel-releasing intrauterine system versus a low-dose combined oral contraceptive for treatment of adenomyotic uteri: a randomized clinical trial. Contraception 92(4):301, 2015

Sharma K, Bora MK, Venkatesh BP, et al: Role of 3D ultrasound and Doppler in differentiating clinically suspected cases of leiomyoma and adenomyosis of uterus. J Clin Diagn Res 9(4):QC08, 2015

Sherer DM, Salame G, Shah T, et al: Transvaginal sonography of postabortal (Redo) syndrome. J Clin Ultrasound 39(3):155, 2011

Shiota M, Kotani Y, Umemoto M, et al: Deep-vein thrombosis is associated with large uterine fibroids. Tohoku J Exp Med 224(2):87, 2011

Socolov D, Blidaru I, Tamba B, et al: Levonorgestrel releasing-intrauterine system for the treatment of menorrhagia and/or frequent irregular uterine bleeding associated with uterine leiomyoma. Eur J Contracept Reprod Health Care 16(6):480, 2011

Sommer EM, Balkwill A, Reeves G, et al: Effects of obesity and hormone therapy on surgically-confirmed fibroids in postmenopausal women. Eur J Epidemiol 30(6):493, 2015

Spies JB, Myers ER, Worthington-Kirsch R, et al: The FIBROID Registry: symptom and quality-of-life status 1 year after therapy. Obstet Gynaecol 106(6):1309, 2005

Spies JB, Spector A, Roth AR, et al: Complications after uterine artery embolization for leiomyomas. Obstet Gynecol 100(5 Pt 1):873, 2002

Stokes LS, Wallace MJ, Godwin RB, et al: Quality improvement guidelines for uterine artery embolization for symptomatic leiomyomas. J Vasc Interv Radiol 21:1153, 2010

Surrey ES, Minjarez DA, Stevens JM, et al: Effect of myomectomy on the outcome of assisted reproductive technologies. Fertil Steril 83(5):1473, 2005

Tahara M, Shimizu T, Shimoura H: Preliminary report of treatment with oral contraceptive pills for intermenstrual vaginal bleeding secondary to a cesarean section scar. Fertil Steril 86(2):477, 2006

Takeuchi H, Kinoshita K: Evaluation of adhesion formation after laparoscopic myomectomy by systematic second-look microlaparoscopy. J Am Assoc Gynecol Laparosc 9(4):442, 2002

Templeman C, Marshall SF, Ursin G, et al: Adenomyosis and endometriosis in the California Teachers Study. Fertil Steril 90(2):415, 2008

Toor SS, Jaberi A, Macdonald DB, et al: Complication rates and effectiveness of uterine artery embolization in the treatment of symptomatic leiomyomas: a systematic review and meta-analysis. AJR Am J Roentgenol 199(5):1153, 2012

Traiman P, Saldiva P, Haiashi A, et al: Criteria for the diagnosis of diffuse uterine myohypertrophy. Int J Gynaecol Obstet 54(1):31, 1996

Tsujioka H, Matsuoka S, Sorano S, et al: Follow-up study of symptomatic submucous fibroids after hysteroscopic myomectomy. Clin Exp Obstet Gynecol 44(1):61, 2017

Tulandi T, Leung A, Jan N: Nonmalignant sequelae of unconfined morcellation at laparoscopic hysterectomy or myomectomy. J Minim Invasive Gynecol 23(3):331, 2016

Vercellini P, Crosignani PG, Mangioni C, et al: Treatment with a gonadotrophin releasing hormone agonist before hysterectomy for leiomyomas: results of a multicentre, randomised controlled trial. BJOG 105(11):1148, 1998

Vercellini P, Viganò P, Somigliana E, et al: Adenomyosis: epidemiological factors. Best Pract Res Clin Obstet Gynaecol 20(4):465, 2006

Vervoort A, van der Voet LF, Hehenkamp W, et al: Hysteroscopic resection of a uterine caesarean scar defect (niche) in women with postmenstrual spotting: a randomised controlled trial. BJOG 125(3):326, 2018

Wamsteker K, Emanuel MH, de Kruif JH: Transcervical hysteroscopic resection of submucous fibroids for abnormal uterine bleeding: results regarding the degree of intramural extension. Obstet Gynecol 82(5):736, 1993

Wise LA, Palmer JR, Spiegelman D, et al: Influence of body size and body fat distribution on risk of uterine leiomyomata in U.S. black women. Epidemiology 16(3):346, 2005

Wise LA, Palmer JR, Stewart EA, et al: Polycystic ovary syndrome and risk of uterine leiomyomata. Fertil Steril 87(5):1108, 2007

Wishall KM, Price J, Pereira N, et al: Postablation risk factors for pain and subsequent hysterectomy. Obstet Gynecol 124(5):904, 2014

Yamamoto T, Noguchi T, Tamura T, et al: Evidence for estrogen synthesis in adenomyotic tissues. Am J Obstet Gynecol 169(3):734, 1993

Yan L, Ding L, Li C, et al: Effect of fibroids not distorting the endometrial cavity on the outcome of in vitro fertilization treatment: a retrospective cohort study. Fertil Steril 101(3):716, 2014

Yang C, Fang H, Yang Y, et al: Diagnosis and surgical management of inferior vena cava leiomyomatosis. J Vasc Surg Venous Lymphat Disord 6(5):636, 2018

Yang Z, Cao YD, Hu LN, et al: Feasibility of laparoscopic high-intensity focused ultrasound treatment for patients with uterine localized adenomyosis. Fertil Steril 91:2338, 2009

Yonehara Y, Yanazume S, Kamio M, et al: Concentrated ascites re-infusion therapy for pseudo-Meigs' syndrome complicated by massive ascites in large pedunculated uterine leiomyoma. J Obstet Gynaecol Res 40(7):1944, 2014

Yoo EH, Lee PI, Huh CY, et al: Predictors of leiomyoma recurrence after laparoscopic myomectomy. J Minim Invasive Gynecol 14(6):690, 2007

Youm J, Lee HJ, Kim SK, et al: Factors affecting the spontaneous expulsion of the levonorgestrel-releasing intrauterine system. Int J Gynaecol Obstet 126(2):165, 2014

Zaloudek C, Hendrickson M, Soslow RA: Mesenchymal tumors of the uterus. In Kurman RJ, Ellenson LH, Ronnett BM (eds): Blaustein's Pathology of the Female Genital Tract, 6th ed. New York, Springer, 2011, p. 468

Zhang X, Li K, Xie B, et al: Effective ablation therapy of adenomyosis with ultrasound-guided high-intensity focused ultrasound. Int J Gynaecol Obstet 124(3):207, 2014

Zhang X, Yang M, Wang Q, et al: Prospective evaluation of five methods used to treat cesarean scar defects. Int J Gynaecol Obstet 134(3):336, 2016a

Zhang Y: A comparative study of transvaginal repair and laparoscopic repair in the management of patients with previous cesarean scar defect. J Minim Invasive Gynecol 23(4):535, 2016b

CHAPTER 10

Benign Adnexal Mass

OVARIAN CYSTS AS A GROUP

Ovarian masses are a frequent finding in general gynecology, and most are cystic (Fig. 10-1). Histologically, ovarian cysts are often divided into those derived from neoplastic growth, *ovarian cystic neoplasms*, and those created by disruption of normal ovulation, *functional ovarian cysts*. Differentiation of these is not always clinically apparent using either imaging or tumor markers. Thus, ovarian cysts are often managed as a single composite clinical entity, and the next sections describe this general approach. Later sections discuss discrete pathologies.

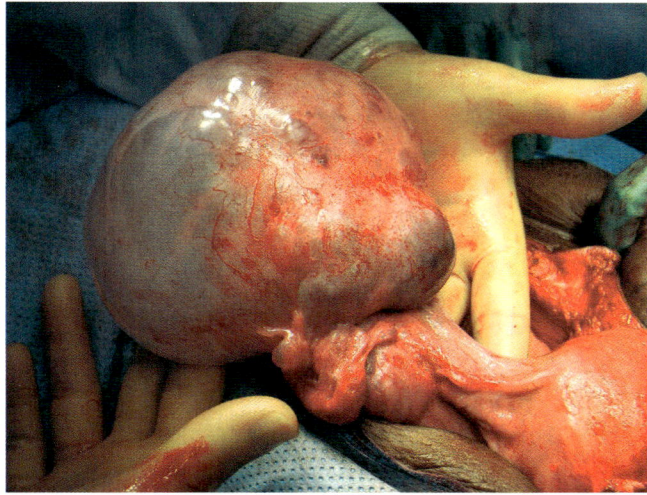

FIGURE 10-1 Intraoperative photograph of a large benign mucinous cystadenoma. The fimbriated end of the fallopian tube is seen below the ovary, and the uterus lies at the lower right. (Reproduced with permission from Dr. Eddie McCord.)

The exact mechanisms leading to cyst formation are unclear. Angiogenesis is an essential component of both the follicular and luteal phases of the ovarian cycle. It is also a component of various pathologic ovarian processes. Some include follicular cyst formation, polycystic ovarian syndrome (PCOS), ovarian hyperstimulation syndrome, and benign and malignant ovarian neoplasms.

The incidence of ovarian cysts varies only slightly with patient demographics and ranges from 5 to 15 percent (Dorum, 2005; Millar, 1993). Functional ovarian cysts make up a large portion. Neoplasms constitute most of the remainder, and these predominantly are benign. In their review of U.S. inpatient hospitalizations for 2010, Whiteman and colleagues (2010) reported that approximately 7 percent of gynecologic admissions were for benign ovarian cysts.

Management goals include identifying malignancy and treating symptoms while preserving ovarian function when possible and minimizing overtreatment. However, despite continuous improvement in diagnostic methods, it is often impossible to clinically differentiate between benign and malignant conditions. Thus, management must balance the surgical morbidity from excision of an innocent lesion with the risk of not removing an ovarian malignancy.

■ Symptoms

Most women with ovarian cysts are asymptomatic. If symptoms develop, pain is common. Dysmenorrhea may indicate endometriosis and an associated endometrioma. Intermittent or acute severe pain with vomiting often accompanies torsion. Other causes of acute pain include cyst rupture or tuboovarian abscess. In contrast, pressure or ache may be the sole symptom and can result from ovarian capsule stretching or cyst bulk. In ovarian malignancies, diagnosis depends on providers having a high index of suspicion in symptomatic women (Schorge, 2010). In some affected individuals, evidence of hormonal disruption is found. For example, excess estrogen production from granulosa cell stimulation may disrupt normal menstruation or initiate bleeding even in prepubertal or postmenopausal patients. Increased androgen levels produced by theca cell stimulation can virilize women.

■ Diagnosis

Tumor Markers

Many ovarian cysts are asymptomatic and found incidentally on routine pelvic examination or during imaging studies for another indication. Findings vary, but typically masses are mobile, cystic, nontender, and found lateral to the uterus.

Serum β-human chorionic gonadotropin (hCG) testing is invaluable for adnexal pathology evaluation. Detection of serum β-hCG may indicate ectopic pregnancy or a corpus luteum of pregnancy. Less commonly, β-hCG also can serve as a tumor marker in defining germ cell neoplasms.

Other tumor markers are typically proteins produced by cancer cells or by the body in response to tumor cells. Of markers used, cancer antigen 125 (CA125) is an antigenic determinant on a high-molecular-weight glycoprotein produced by mesothelial cells that line the peritoneal, pleural, and pericardial cavities. Serum CA125 levels are often elevated in women with epithelial ovarian cancer. Unfortunately, CA125 is not a tumor-specific antigen, and concentrations are elevated in up to 1 percent of healthy controls. Levels may also rise in women with nonmalignant disease such as leiomyomas, endometriosis, adenomyosis, and salpingitis. Despite these limitations, serum CA125 determinations may be helpful and are often obtained if ovarian cysts are large or have sonographically worrisome signs described in the next section. Cysts in patients who are postmenopausal or who carry a *BRCA* gene mutation also may warrant CA125 level evaluation (Chap. 35, p. 740).

Of other markers, elevated carcinoembryonic antigen (CEA) and cancer antigen 19-9 (CA19-9) levels arise from secretions of mucinous epithelial ovarian carcinomas. Serum alpha-fetoprotein (AFP) levels may be elevated in those patients with a rare endodermal sinus tumor or embryonal cell carcinoma. Increased serum levels of β-hCG may indicate an ovarian choriocarcinoma, a mixed germ cell tumor, or embryonal cell carcinoma. Inhibin A and B are markers for granulosa cell tumors. Last, lactate dehydrogenase (LDH) levels may be higher in those with dysgerminoma.

OVA1 is a biomarker blood test panel and considered a *multivariate index assay* that can be used in women with an identified ovarian mass warranting surgery (Ueland, 2011; Ware Miller, 2011). Scores ≥5.0 in premenopausal and scores ≥4.4 in postmenopausal women suggest a need for gynecologic oncologist consultation (Table 10-1).

Another marker, human epididymal protein 4 (HE4), is coupled with CA125 in the Risk of Ovarian Malignancy Algorithm (ROMA). This algorithm helps predict the likelihood of finding malignancy at surgery in women with known adnexal masses to aid presurgical triage. The ROMA score is derived from the results of both blood tests plus menopausal status (Moore, 2009, 2010).

Similarly, the risk of malignancy index (RMI) algorithm factors menopausal status, CA125 serum level, and sonographic score. This last element is derived from ovarian appearance, and presence of ascites or intraabdominal metastases (Jacobs, 1990; Karlsen, 2012).

None of these three tests is a screening tool, nor are their findings absolute. They are reserved for those with a known surgical mass to guide specialty referral.

Imaging

Sonography is a first-line tool to evaluate pelvic masses. Transabdominal scanning is performed first to avoid missing a large cyst that lies outside the pelvis. For lesions confined within the true pelvis, transvaginal sonography (TVS) has superior resolution. Characteristic findings for specific types of ovarian cysts have been defined to help discriminate malignant from benign lesions (Table 10-2). Specifically, thick septa with increased vascularity, papillary intracystic growths, and solid elements within the cyst raise concern.

Traditional grayscale sonography can be augmented with color Doppler. Described in Chapter 2 (p. 30), transvaginal color Doppler sonography depicts blood flow to and within a pelvic mass. This can add information regarding lesion structure, malignant potential, and possible torsion. However, for assessing simple ovarian cysts and the risk of malignancy, the application of color Doppler typically provides no significant advantage compared with conventional TVS (Vuento, 1995).

Sonographic color Doppler and spectral analysis of flow signals are combined with tumor size and morphology in several scoring systems to help differentiate malignant and benign masses (Chap. 2, p. 30). As an example, using these sonographic features, the International Ovarian Tumor Analysis (IOTA) Group developed accurate mathematic models to calculate malignancy risk (Timmerman, 2000, 2005, 2016). Several other sonographic scoring systems have been evaluated. At our institution, we use the Ovarian Tumor Index developed by Twickler and colleagues (1999).

TABLE 10-1. Indications for Referral of a Suspicious Ovarian Mass to a Gynecologic Oncologist

Clinical Indicator	Premenopausal Woman	Postmenopausal Woman
CA125	Very elevated	Elevated (>35 U/mL)
Sonography	Suggests malignancy	Suggests malignancy
Other imaging	Ascites	Ascites
	Abdominal or distant metastasis	Abdominal or distant metastasis
Physical finding	—	Nodular or fixed pelvic mass
Presurgical triage tool		
ROMA	Laboratory-dependent thresholds	
MIA (OVA1)	≥5.0	≥4.4
RMI	>200	>200

CA125 = cancer antigen 125; MIA = multivariate index assay; RMI = Risk of Malignancy Index; ROMA = Risk of Malignancy Algorithm.

TABLE 10-2. Recommended Management of Asymptomatic Ovarian Masses Found with Imaging

Type of Ovarian Mass	Recommendation
CYSTS WITH BENIGN QUALITIES	
Simple Cyst	Simple cysts, regardless of patient age, are typically benign
Premenopausal	
≤3 cm diameter	Normal anatomic finding
≤5 cm diameter	No additional treatment required
>5 but ≤7 cm diameter[a]	TVS repeated in 6–12 wks to document resolution; if persistent, then yearly TVS[b]
>7 cm diameter[a]	MRI or surgical evaluation
Postmenopausal	
≤1 cm diameter	Normal anatomic finding
≤5 cm diameter[a]	CA125 level; if normal level, then TVS repeated in 6–12 weeks; if persistent cyst, then yearly TVS[b]
>7 cm diameter[a]	MRI or surgical evaluation
Hemorrhagic Cyst[c]	
Premenopausal	
≤3 cm diameter CL	Normal anatomic finding
≤5 cm diameter	No additional treatment required
>5 but ≤7 cm diameter	TVS repeated in 6–12 weeks; if persistent, then consider MRI or surgical evaluation
Early postmenopausal[d] Any size	CA125 level; if normal, then TVS repeated in 6–12 weeks; if persistent cyst, then consider MRI or surgical evaluation
Late postmenopausal[d] Any size	Surgical evaluation
Endometrioma	TVS repeated in 6–12 weeks; if persistent, then yearly TVS[b]
Mature cystic teratoma	If not surgically removed[e], then yearly TVS[b]
Hydrosalpinx	May be observed as clinically indicated
Peritoneal inclusion cyst	May be observed as clinically indicated
CYSTS WITH INDETERMINATE, BUT PROBABLY BENIGN QUALITIES	
Indeterminate for: hemorrhagic cyst, mature cystic teratoma, endometrioma	
Premenopausal	TVS repeated in 6–12 weeks; if persistent cyst, then consider surgical evaluation or MRI
Postmenopausal	Consider surgical evaluation
Thin-walled cyst with single thin septation or focal cyst wall calcification	Same as for simple cyst
Multiple thin septations (<3 mm)	Consider surgical evaluation
Nodule (non-hyperechoic) without flow	Consider surgical evaluation or MRI
CYSTS WITH QUALITIES SUGGESTING MALIGNANCY	
Thick (>3 mm) irregular septations	Consider surgical evaluation
Nodule with blood flow	Consider surgical evaluation

[a]The American College of Obstetricians and Gynecologists (2016) recommends a threshold up to 10 cm for simple cysts in all age groups.
[b]Shorter time interval may be selected for surveillance as clinically indicated.
[c]Color Doppler as an adjunct is recommended to exclude solid components.
[d]All postmenopausal women with an adnexal mass also undergo breast and digital rectal examination and mammography, if not already performed in the last year due to the high rate of metastasis from other primary tumors to the ovary.
[e]Some studies have found that stable small mature cystic teratomas with a confident diagnosis may be observed in premenopausal women.
CA125 = cancer antigen 125; CL = corpus luteum; MRI = magnetic resonance imaging; TVS = transvaginal sonography.
From American College of Obstetricians and Gynecologists, 2016; Atri, 2019; Levine, 2010.

CHAPTER 10

Computed tomography (CT) or magnetic resonance (MR) imaging of an ovarian cyst may clarify situations in which anatomy or patient habitus complicates sonographic imaging. CT is best used when malignancy is suspected to evaluate for metastasis, ascites, or lymphadenopathy (American College of Obstetricians and Gynecologists, 2016). However, in most clinical settings, sonography alone is suitable (Atri, 2019; Outwater, 1996).

■ Management

Observation

In prepubertal and reproductive-aged women, most ovarian cysts are functional and spontaneously regress within 6 months of identification. For postmenopausal women with a simple ovarian cyst, expectant management also may be reasonable if several criteria are met. These are: (1) sonographic evidence of a thin-walled, unilocular cyst; (2) cyst diameter <5 cm; (3) no cyst enlargement during surveillance; and (4) normal serum CA125 level (Nardo, 2003). Moreover, the American College of Obstetricians and Gynecologists (2016) notes that simple cysts up to 10 cm in diameter by sonographic evaluation may safely be followed even in postmenopausal women. Consensus regarding an end point for observation is lacking. Some experts recommend 1 year of surveillance for patients with stable adnexal masses without solid components and 2 years for those with stable masses with solid components (Suh-Bergmann, 2014, 2015). With any surveillance plan, the risks of potentially serious pathology and patient anxiety are weighed against surgical morbidity.

Surgery

Both malignant and benign cysts show considerable morphologic similarity. For diagnosis, ovarian cyst aspiration usually is avoided because of possible intraperitoneal seeding by early-stage ovarian cancer. Moreover, false-positive and false-negative results are common (Martinez-Onsurbe, 2001; Moran, 1993). Accordingly, for many cases, cyst excision serves as the definitive diagnostic tool.

With suspected ovarian cancers, optimal surgical resection and proper staging by a gynecologic oncologist during the primary operation are major factors in long-term patient survival. Thus, women with pelvic masses and preoperative findings suspicious for malignancy are generally referred. The American College of Obstetricians and Gynecologists (2017) and Society of Gynecologic Oncologists have jointly presented guidelines regarding clinical criteria that should prompt preoperative referral to a gynecologic oncologist (see Table 10-2).

For the generalist, cysts presumed to be benign may be excised or the whole ovary may be removed. Of these, cystectomy offers the advantage of ovarian preservation but risks cyst rupture and content spill. With ovarian cancer, such spill and subsequent malignant seeding can worsen patient prognosis. Thus, the decision for one surgical technique in preference over the other is influenced by lesion size, patient age, and intraoperative findings. For example, in premenopausal women, smaller lesions generally require only cystectomy with preservation of reproductive function. Larger lesions may prompt oophorectomy because of their greater risk for rupture during enucleation, difficulty in reconstructing ovarian anatomy following large cyst removal, and the increased risk of malignancy in these bigger cysts. However, in postmenopausal women, oophorectomy is preferred because the risk for cancer is higher. The ovaries in these women are also no longer providing sufficient estrogen production or fertility potential (Okugawa, 2001).

The surgical route is also dictated by clinical factors. Laparoscopy and minilaparotomy are the more common approaches to a benign adnexal mass. Advantages of these minimally invasive techniques compared with laparotomy include reduced pain, length of stay, incidences of postoperative fever, and complication rates (Medeiros, 2009). However, during laparoscopic cystectomy or oophorectomy, cyst size must allow suitable optics. Moreover, laparoscopic instruments must have sufficient room to interact effectively and to create tissue tension. Contained cyst removal without morcellating the ovarian cortex also is desirable in cases with an intermediate risk of malignancy.

If these requisites cannot be achieved, minilaparotomy may be preferred. With smaller cysts, excision and removal can be completed through the incision. For larger cysts, primary decompression through the incision can then permit excision and extraction of the entire specimen.

Last, women with large cysts or other factors indicating a higher malignancy risk often are managed by laparotomy. With a greater potential for malignancy, a midline vertical incision provides a surgical field large enough for oophorectomy or cyst enucleation without tumor rupture and for surgical staging if malignancy is found.

Clinical findings of an unexpected malignancy at the time of surgery will dictate further actions. Multiple small lesions studding the peritoneal surface, ascites, and exophytic growths extending from the ovarian capsule should prompt collection of peritoneal fluid for cytologic study and intraoperative frozen section analysis. If cancer is found, a gynecologic oncologist is ideally consulted intraoperatively. At minimum, limited clinical staging, as discussed in Chapter 35 (p. 747), can be completed.

FUNCTIONAL OVARIAN CYSTS

These are common, originate from ovarian follicles, and are created during follicle maturation and ovulation. They are subcategorized as either *follicular cysts* or *corpus luteum cysts* based on both their pathogenesis and histologic qualities. They are not neoplasms and derive mass from accumulation of intrafollicular fluids rather than cellular proliferation. With follicular cyst formation, hormonal dysfunction prior to ovulation results in expansion of the follicular antrum with serous fluid. In contrast, excessive hemorrhage from the vascular corpus luteum following ovulation may fill its center to create a corpus luteum cyst. Thus, follicular and corpus luteum cysts differ in their genesis, but symptoms and management are similar.

■ Associated Factors

Of potential factors, high-dose combination oral contraceptives (COCs) suppress ovarian activity and protect against cyst development (Ory, 1974). However, in subsequent studies with low-dose pills, which contain 35 µg of ethinyl estradiol or less, COCs provided only modest protective effects (Holt, 2003; Lanes, 1992). By contrast, the incidence of follicular cysts is increased with many progestin-only contraceptives. Recall that continuous, low-dose progestins do not completely suppress ovarian function. As a result, dominant follicles may develop in response to gonadotropin secretion. Yet, the normal ovulatory process is frequently disrupted, and follicular cysts develop. Clinically, follicular cysts are found with greater frequency in those using the levonorgestrel-releasing intrauterine system (LNG-IUS) and progestin-releasing implants (Hidalgo, 2006; Nahum, 2015).

Both pre- and postmenopausal women treated with tamoxifen for breast cancer have a higher risk for benign ovarian cyst formation (Chalas, 2005; Simpkins 2005). Premenopausal women and women with greater body mass index are disparately affected. Most are functional cysts that resolve with time whether tamoxifen treatment is continued or discontinued (Cohen, 2003). If small simple cysts are found, sonographic surveillance is reasonable. If clinical signs of malignancy are present, surgical exploration is indicated, and tamoxifen is discontinued. Of other selective estrogen-receptor modulators, bazedoxifene, raloxifene, and ospemifene do not appear to raise ovarian cyst rates (Archer, 2015).

Several epidemiologic studies have linked smoking with functional cyst development (Holt, 2005; Wyshak, 1988). Although the exact mechanism(s) is unknown, changes in gonadotropin secretion and ovarian function are suspected (Michnovicz, 1986).

■ Diagnosis and Treatment

Functional cysts are managed similarly to other cystic ovarian lesions. Consequently, sonography is initially performed. Typical follicular cysts are completely rounded anechoic lesions with thin, regular walls (Fig. 10-2). Conversely, corpus luteum cysts are termed "great imitators" because of their varied and evolving sonographic characteristics (Fig. 10-3). With a corpus luteum, transvaginal sonography and applied color Doppler typically display a brightly colored ring because of enhanced vascularity surrounding the cyst. This *ring of fire* also is common to ectopic pregnancies (Fig. 7-5, p. 166).

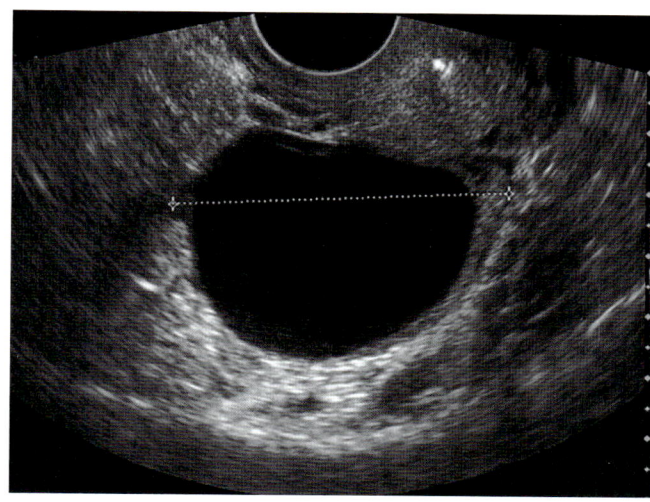

FIGURE 10-2 Sonographic transvaginal image of an ovary containing a follicular cyst. Note the smooth walls and lack of internal echoes. (Reproduced with permission from Dr. Elysia Moschos.)

If asymptomatic, women with findings of a functional ovarian cyst usually are observed. Spontaneous regression of these cysts is anticipated, and COC use does not hasten resolution (Grimes, 2014). Patients undergoing surveillance are advised of the symptoms of ovarian torsion. Surgical excision may be reasonable for large persistent cysts, usually those >10 cm, or for smaller ones producing persistently bothersome symptoms. Enlarging cysts are typically removed.

■ Theca Lutein Cysts

These are an uncommon type of follicular cyst, characterized by luteinization and hypertrophy of their theca interna layer. Bilateral, multiple smooth-walled cysts form and range in size from 1 to 4 cm in diameter. Termed *hyperreactio lutealis*, this condition is thought to be prompted by elevated luteinizing hormone or β-hCG levels. Commonly associated conditions include gestational trophoblastic disease, multifetal gestation, placentomegaly, and ovarian hyperstimulation during assisted reproductive techniques (Fig. 37-4, p. 776). These cysts typically resolve spontaneously following removal of the stimulating hormone source. However, prior to this, these bulky ovaries are at risk for torsion.

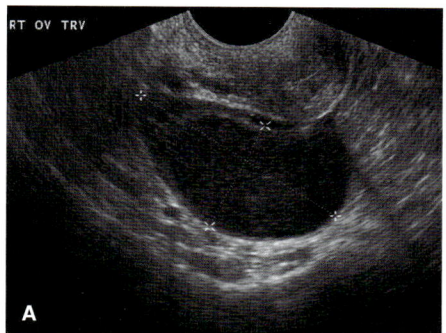
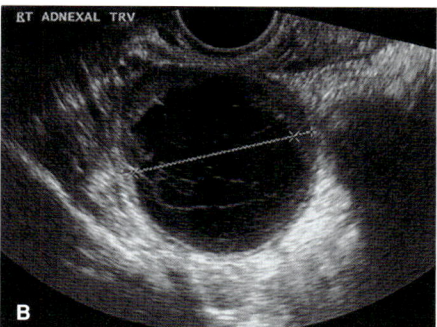
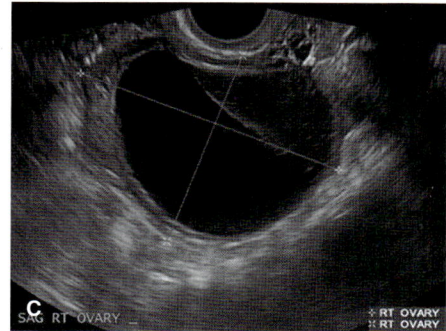

FIGURE 10-3 Sonographic transvaginal transverse images of hemorrhagic corpus luteum cysts. **A.** Diffuse low-level echoes, which are commonly associated with recent hemorrhage, are seen throughout this smooth-walled cyst. **B.** With evolution of the clot, a lacy reticular pattern develops. **C.** As the clot hemolyzes, a distinct line often forms between the serum and retracting clot. With further retraction, the clot may appear as an intramural nodule. (Reproduced with permission from Dr. Elysia Moschos.)

TABLE 10-3. WHO Histologic Classification of Predominant Ovarian Tumors

Epithelial
Serous
Mucinous
Endometrioid
Clear cell
Brenner
Seromucinous

Mesenchymal
Endometrioid stromal sarcoma

Mixed Epithelial/Mesenchymal
Adenosarcoma
Carcinosarcoma

Sex Cord–Stromal Tumors
   Pure stromal
   Fibroma
   Thecoma
   Leydig cell
   Steroid cell
   Pure sex cord
   Juvenile granulosa cell
   Adult granulosa cell
   Sertoli cell

Mixed Sex Cord–Stromal Tumors
   Sertoli–Leydig cell

Germ Cell Tumors
   Dysgerminoma
   Yolk sac
   Embryonal carcinoma
   Choriocarcinoma
   Mature teratoma
   Immature teratomas

Germ Cell/Sex Cord–Stromal Tumor
   Gonadoblastoma

WHO = World Health Organization.

BENIGN NEOPLASTIC OVARIAN CYSTS

These lesions, in combination with functional ovarian cysts, constitute most ovarian masses. Ovarian neoplasms can be distinguished histologically depending on their cell type of origin. These are grouped as epithelial tumors, germ cell tumors, sex cord–stromal tumors, and others shown in Table 10-3. Of benign ovarian neoplasms, serous and mucinous cystadenomas and mature cystic teratoma are the most common (Pantoja, 1975).

■ Benign Serous and Mucinous Tumors

These are members of the surface epithelial neoplasia group, and both are lined by cells similar to those lining the fallopian tube. *Benign serous tumors* are typically thin-walled, unilocular cysts filled with serous fluid (Fig. 10-4). They are bilateral in up to 20 percent of cases. *Benign mucinous tumors* are typically thicker-walled, mucoid-containing tumors that may be

small but can often attain large diameters. They may be uni- or multilocular.

In categorizing tumors within the epithelial family, benign tumors are designated as *adenomas*; malignant tumors, as *carcinomas*; and those with exuberant cellular proliferation without invasive behavior as *low malignant potential* (Chen, 2003). The prefix *cyst-* describes predominantly cystic neoplasms. In addition, in most of these tumors, the epithelial component dominates. In those in which ovarian stroma predominates, the suffix *–fibroma* is used. Thus, *serous cystadenofibroma* describes a benign, mainly cystic tumor of the ovarian epithelial tumor group in which stromal components predominate (Prat, 2009).

■ Ovarian Teratoma

These belong to the germ cell family of ovarian neoplasms. Teratomas arise from a single germ cell, and therefore may contain any of the three germ layers—ectoderm, mesoderm, or endoderm. These layers are typically disorganized.

Teratomas are classified as:

Immature teratoma—This neoplasm is malignant and described in Chapter 36 (p. 760). Immature tissues from one, two, or all three germ cell layers are found and often coexist with mature elements.

Mature teratoma—This benign tumor contains mature forms of the three germ cell layers:

1. Mature cystic teratoma develops into a cyst, is common, and may also be called *benign cystic teratoma* or *dermoid cyst.*
2. Mature solid teratoma has elements formed into a solid mass.
3. Fetiform teratoma or homunculus forms a doll-shape, as the germ cell layers display considerable normal spatial differentiation.

Monodermal teratoma—This benign tumor is composed either solely or predominantly of only one highly specialized tissue type. Of the monodermal teratomas, those composed dominantly of thyroid tissue are termed *struma ovarii.*

Of these teratoma types, mature cystic teratoma is by far the most common. These benign tumors constitute approximately 10 to 25 percent of all ovarian neoplasms and 60 percent of all benign ovarian neoplasms (Koonings, 1989; Peterson, 1955). These cystic tumors are typically slow growing, and most measure between 5 and 10 cm (Comerci, 1994). They are bilateral in approximately 10 percent of cases (Peterson, 1955). When sectioned, most cysts appear unilocular and typically contain one area of localized growth, which protrudes into the cystic cavity. Alternatively designated as *Rokitansky protuberance, dermoid plug, dermoid process, dermoid mamilla,* or *embryonal rudiment,* this protuberance can be absent or multiple.

Microscopically, endodermal or mesodermal derivatives may be found, but ectodermal elements usually predominate. The cyst is typically lined with keratinized squamous epithelium and contains abundant sebaceous and sweat glands. Hair and fatty secretions are often found within (Fig. 10-5). At times, bone and teeth are identified.

The Rokitansky protuberance is usually the site where the most varied tissue types are found and is a common location

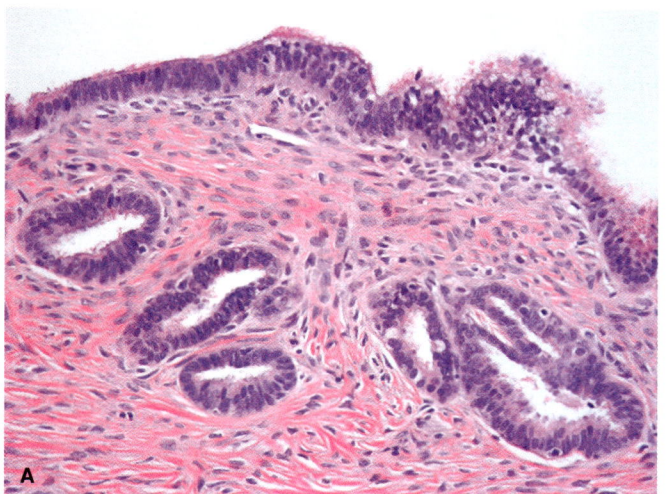

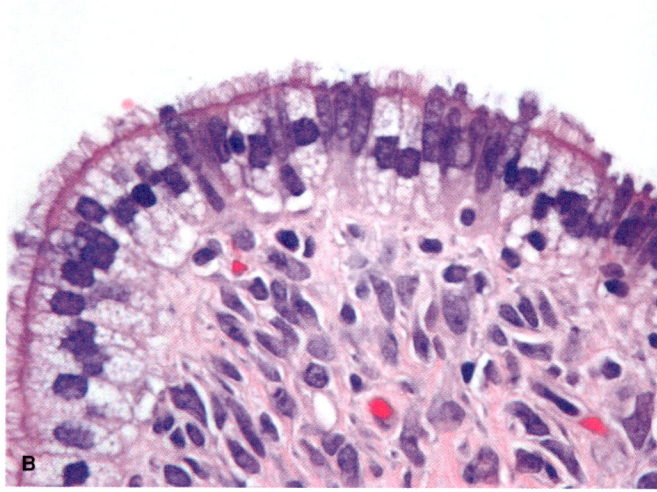

Serous cystadenoma

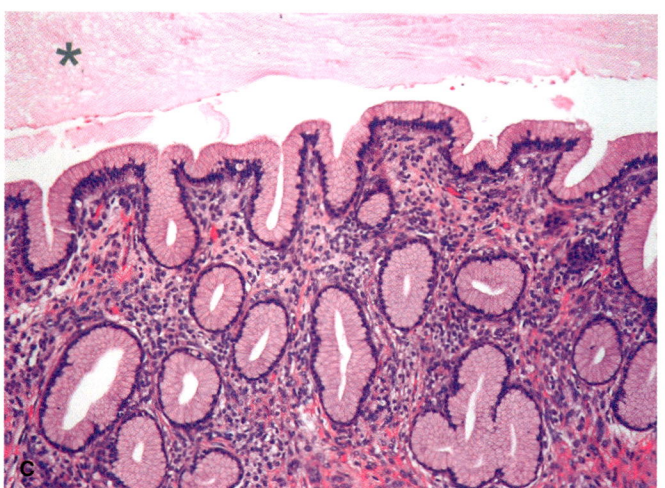

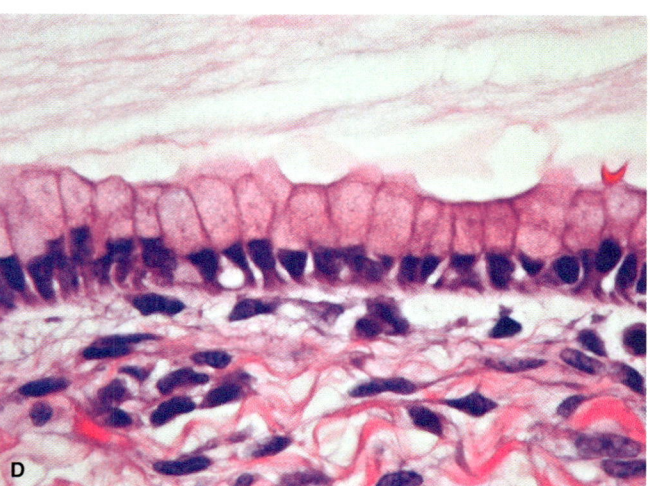

Mucinous cystadenoma

FIGURE 10-4 Serous **(A,B)** and mucinous **(C,D)** cystadenoma. **A.** This simple cyst has a fibrous wall and is lined by a single layer of benign, columnar tubal-type epithelium with cilia. **B.** High-power view of its ciliated, tubal-type lining. **C.** Mucinous cystadenomas are typically multiloculated cysts lined by a single layer of benign mucin-containing epithelium. Mucinous fluid is secreted by the epithelium and contained within the cystic mass. In this image, it is the amorphous material above the epithelium and is stained pink (*asterisk*). **D.** High-power view of simple columnar, mucin-containing epithelium. (Reproduced with permission from Dr. Kelley Carrick.)

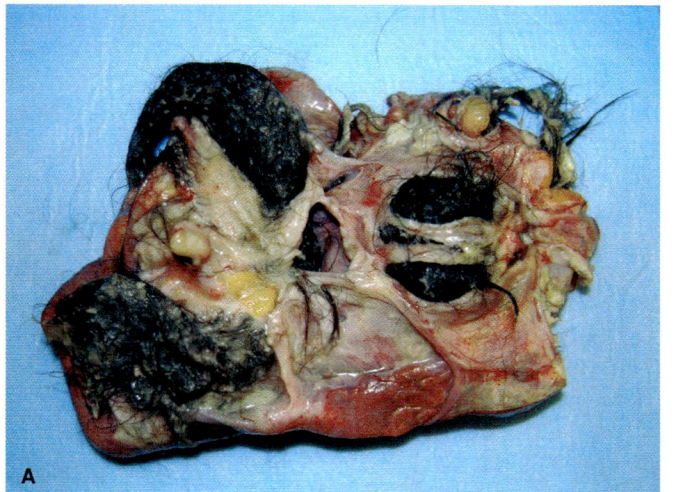

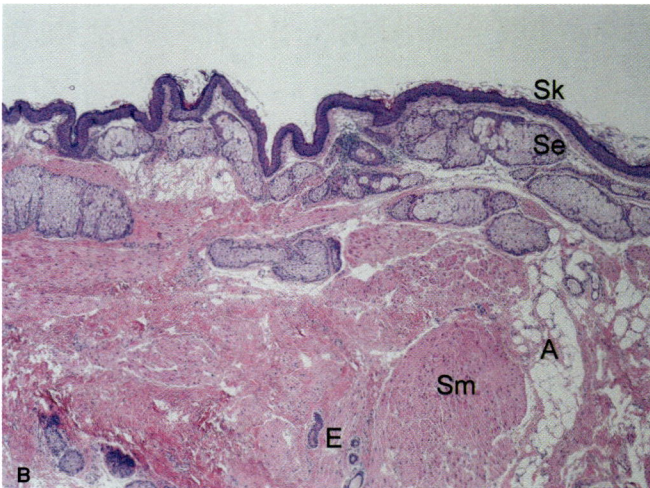

FIGURE 10-5 A. A sectioned mature cystic teratoma following cystectomy. Abundant hair, sebum, and teeth, which are all characteristic of these neoplasms, are evident. **B.** In this classic histologic example, ectodermal elements include skin (*Sk*), sebaceous (*Se*), and eccrine (*E*) glands, whereas mesodermal elements are smooth muscle (*Sm*) and adipose (*A*). (Reproduced with permission from Dr. Kelley Carrick.)

of malignant transformation. This transformation occurs in <2 percent of mature cystic teratomas (Black, 2015; Comerci, 1994). Patients older than 50 years or with masses >10 cm are at greater risk (Chiang, 2017; Park, 2008). Most malignant cases are squamous cell carcinoma.

The diverse tissues found within teratomas do not arise by fertilization of an ovum by sperm. Instead, they are thought to develop from genetic material contained within a single oocyte by asexual *parthenogenesis*. As a result, almost all mature cystic teratomas have a 46,XX karyotype (Linder, 1975).

Mature cystic teratomas often can undergo torsion, but cyst rupture is rare. Presumably, their thick cyst wall resists rupture compared with other ovarian neoplasms. If cysts do spill, acute peritonitis is common, and Fielder and associates (1996) attributed peritonitis to the sebum and hair contents. They showed the benefits of intraoperative lavage to prevent peritonitis and adhesion formation. Chronic leakage of teratoma contents is rare but can lead to granulomatous peritonitis.

Symptoms from these teratomas are similar to those of other ovarian cysts. However, ovarian teratomas can rarely cause immune-mediated encephalitis. Neurologic symptoms stem from antibodies to *N*-methyl-D-aspartate receptors (NMDARs), which have critical roles in synaptic transmission. The diagnosis is confirmed by detecting antibodies in the serum or cerebrospinal fluid. Teratomas are one of several potential causes of this anti-NMDAR encephalitis. The teratomas contain primitive neural tissue, which presumably provides the antigen that prompts NMDAR antibody formation. Teratoma resection is essential to encephalitis resolution, which can often be dramatic. Resection may be combined with immunotherapy (Yan, 2019). In one large series of 100 patients, 75 percent recovered, but 25 percent died or survived with severe deficits (Dalmau, 2008).

Sonography is the main imaging tool, and mature cystic teratomas display several characteristic features (Fig. 10-6). First, fat-fluid or hair-fluid levels are seen as a distinct linear demarcation. Here, intracystic serous fluid interfaces with sebum, which is liquid at body temperature. When floating, hair forms accentuated lines and dots that represent hair in longitudinal and transverse planes. The Rokitansky protuberance is a rounded mural nodule measuring 1 to 4 cm, is predominantly hyperechoic, and creates an acute angle with the cyst wall. Last, the "tip of the iceberg" sign is created by amorphous echogenic interfaces of fat, hair, and tissues in the foreground that shadow and thus obscure structures behind it (Guttman, 1977). Notably, these findings are not exclusive to mature cystic teratomas. For example, Patel and associates (1998) reported modest positive predictive values for these findings individually. However, they described values of 100 percent when two or more were found within a given lesion.

Of serum markers, increased CA19-9 and CA125 levels may be noted. Of the two, CA19-9 level elevations are seen more often and in approximately 30 percent of cases (Fan, 2016; Kim, 2011; Sagi-Dain, 2015). Thus, this marker occasionally may help differentiate cystic adnexal masses. That said, serum markers are not diagnostic and often unnecessary when the clinical picture is clear.

For most women with mature cystic teratoma, surgical excision provides a definitive diagnosis, affords relief of symptoms, and prevents torsion, rupture, and malignant transformation. Of surgical approaches, laparoscopy is appropriate, and route is selected as for other ovarian masses (p. 222). To prevent granulomatous peritonitis, the cyst can be enucleated over laparotomy sponges or an endoscopic bag to capture cyst spill (Kondo, 2010). Moreover, copious pelvic irrigation is a final surgical step if contents spill. In the past, the opposite ovary was explored because of the high frequency of bilateral lesions. However, given the accuracy of current sonographic imaging, this practice is no longer indicated for a normal-appearing contralateral ovary (Comerci, 1994).

Most of these masses are surgically removed, but a few studies support only surveillance. Especially those desiring future fertility, premenopausal women with cysts measuring <6 cm and with a confident diagnosis are reasonable potential candidates (Hoo, 2010; Pascual, 2017). These studies document slow tumor growth that averages <2 mm/year. If not removed, sonography is recommended every 6 to 12 months initially (Levine, 2010).

SOLID OVARIAN MASSES

Completely solid ovarian masses typically are benign. That said, these masses are still removed because of the inability to exclude malignancy in these tumors. Ovarian tumors that may present as a solid masses include: sex cord–stromal tumors, Krukenberg tumor, ovarian leiomyoma and leiomyosarcoma, carcinoid, primary lymphoma, and transitional cell tumors, also called Brenner tumors (Figs. 10-7 and 10-8). The most common solid tumors are fibromas or fibrothecomas, both typically benign stromal tumors and discussed in Chapter 36 (p. 767).

Solid adnexal masses may also represent nonneoplastic conditions. Ovarian remnant syndrome and ovarian retention syndrome stem from persistent functional ovarian tissue following surgery. These conditions most commonly cause pain and are discussed in Chapter 12 (p. 264). Rarely, congenital accessory ovaries may confuse sonographic findings and are discussed in Chapter 19 (p. 425).

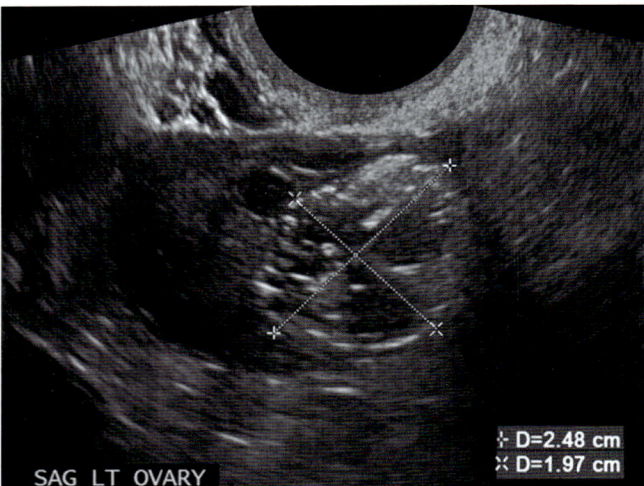

D=2.48 cm
D=1.97 cm
SAG LT OVARY

FIGURE 10-6 Sonogram revealing characteristics of mature cystic teratoma, which is measured by calipers. (Reproduced with permission from Dr. Elysia Moschos.)

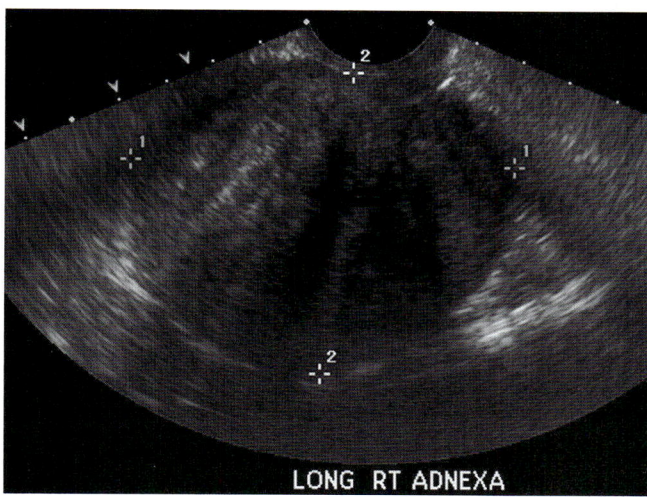

FIGURE 10-7 Transvaginal sonogram of a benign ovarian fibroma.

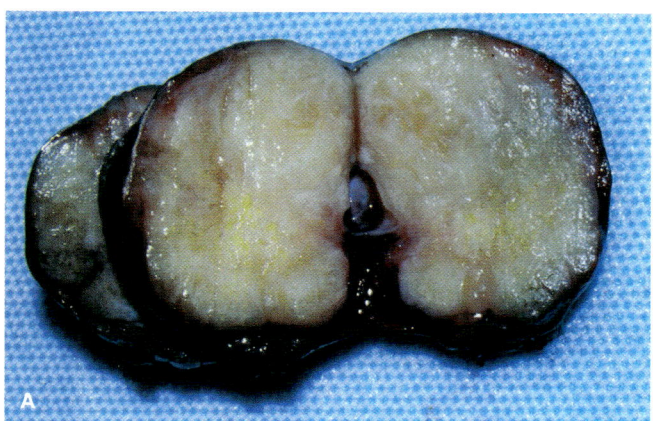

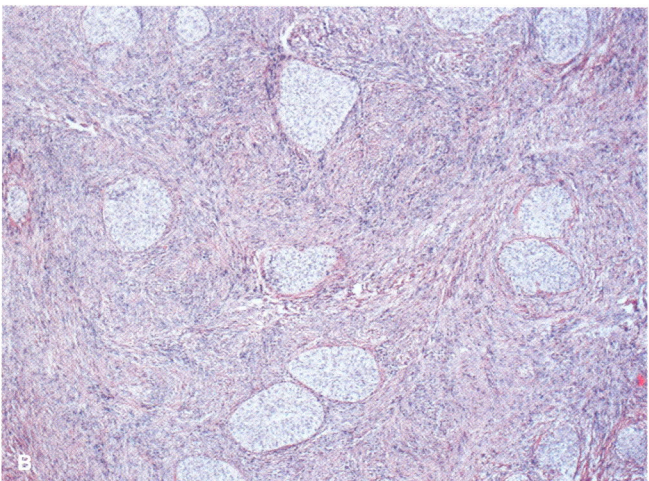

FIGURE 10-8 Photographs of a Brenner tumor following oophorectomy. **A.** A well-circumscribed, tan, rubbery mass with a smooth to slightly bosselated cut surface is characteristic. During preparation of this specimen for histologic assessment, black ink was applied to the external surface of the mass to allow identification of inner and outer surfaces during microscopic evaluation. **B.** Within densely fibrous stroma, sharply demarcated nests of transitional-type epithelial cells are found. These epithelial cells have prominent cell borders, lightly eosinophilic cytoplasm, and oval nuclei, without atypia or mitotic activity. (Reproduced with permission from Dr. Jason Mull.)

ADNEXAL TORSION

Torsion involves the twisting of adnexal components. Most often, the ovary and fallopian tube rotate as a single entity. Infrequently, an ovary may alone turn about its mesovarium, and rarely a fallopian tube twists alone about the mesosalpinx. Last, paraovarian mass may rotate independently and not involve the tube or ovary. Normal adnexa can twist, but in 50 to 80 percent of cases unilateral ovarian masses are identified (Nichols, 1985; Warner, 1985). Adnexal torsion accounts for 3 percent of gynecologic emergencies. Although this most commonly occurs during the reproductive years, postmenopausal women also can be affected. A disproportionate number of cases of adnexal torsion develop during pregnancy, and these compose 20 to 25 percent of all torsion cases.

Adnexal masses that possess greater mobility have greater torsion rates. Congenitally long uteroovarian ligaments create excessively mobile mesovaria and may raise the risk for even normal adnexa. Similarly, pathologically enlarged ovaries with a diameter >6 cm will typically rise from the true pelvis. Without these bony confines, mobility and torsion risk are increased. Accordingly, the highest rates of torsion are in adnexal masses measuring 6 to 10 cm (Houry, 2001). Torsion of the adnexa more commonly involves the right adnexa, likely because mobility of the left ovary is limited by the sigmoid colon (Hasiakos, 2008).

Two key points assist in initially maintaining blood flow to the involved adnexal structures despite twisting of their vascular pedicles. First, adnexa are supplied from the respective adnexal branches of both the uterine and ovarian vessels. During torsion, one of these, but not the other, may be involved. Second, although low-pressure veins draining the adnexa are compressed by the twisting pedicle, high-pressure arteries initially resist compression. As a result of this continued inflow but arrested egress of blood, the adnexa become congested and edematous but do not infarct. Consequently, torsion cases can often be conservatively managed at the time of surgery. With continued stromal swelling, however, arteries may become compressed, leading to infarction and necrosis that necessitate adnexectomy. Grossly, twisted adnexa are enlarged and often appear hemorrhagic (Fig. 10-9).

■ Diagnosis

Classically, the woman with adnexal torsion complains of sharp lower abdominal pain with sudden onset that worsens intermittently over several hours. The pain usually is localized to the involved side, with radiation to the flank, groin, or thigh. Low-grade fever suggests adnexal necrosis. Nausea and vomiting frequently accompany the pain.

Lack of clear physical findings can make diagnosis difficult. An adnexal mass may not be palpable, and during its early stages, significant discomfort may not be elicited during examination. Sonography plays an essential role. However, sonographic findings can vary widely depending on the degree of vascular compromise, the characteristics of any associated intraovarian or intratubal mass, and the presence or absence of adnexal hemorrhage. Sonographically, torsion may mimic

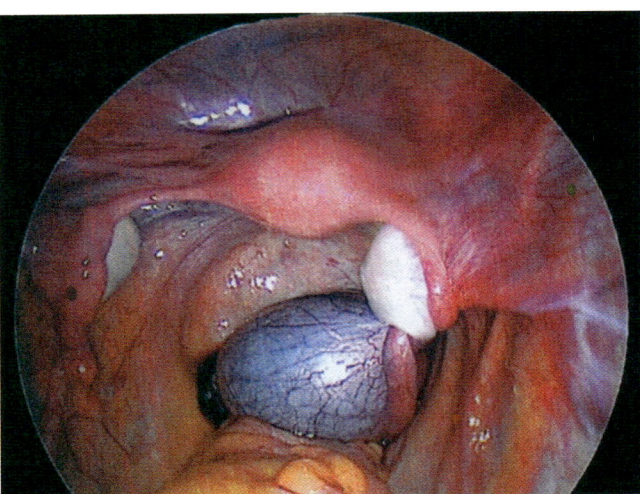

FIGURE 10-9 Laparoscopic photograph of adnexal torsion shows twisting of the fallopian tube and adjacent cyanotic paratubal cyst, which is distinct from the ovary. (Reproduced with permission from Dr. Ellen Wilson.)

ectopic pregnancy, tuboovarian abscess, hemorrhagic ovarian cyst, and endometrioma. Accordingly, rates of correct diagnosis range from 50 to 75 percent (Graif, 1984; Mashiach, 2011).

Despite these limitations, specific findings have been described. First, multiple follicles rimming an enlarged ovary reflect ovarian congestion and edema described earlier. The twisted pedicle may also appear as a bull's-eye target, whirlpool, or snail shell, that is, a rounded hyperechoic structure with multiple, inner, concentric hypoechoic rings. In affected women, application of color Doppler may show disruption of normal adnexal blood flow. However, in some cases, incomplete or intermittent torsion may variably display both venous and arterial flow. Thus, disruption of vascular flow is highly suggestive of torsion. However, torsion should not be discounted on the basis of a normal Doppler study alone, especially with clinically suggestive signs and symptoms.

Last, CT or MR imaging is usually not required. These may be helpful in complicated cases or in those with ambiguous clinical presentation such as seen with incomplete or chronic torsion (Rha, 2002).

■ Management

Salvage of the involved adnexa, resection of any associated cyst or tumor, and indicated oophoropexy are treatment goals. Importantly, rapid operative intervention is believed to improve the likelihood of ovarian conservation (Rossi, 2012; Rousseau, 2008). Findings of adnexal necrosis, rupture with significant hemorrhage, or suspicion of malignancy, however, may necessitate removal of adnexal structures. Salpingo-oophorectomy is reasonable in postmenopausal women with ovarian torsion.

Torsion may be evaluated by laparoscopy or laparotomy. Previously, adnexectomy was usually done to avoid possible thrombus release and subsequent embolism during untwisting. Evidence does not support this. McGovern and coworkers (1999) reviewed nearly 1000 cases of torsion and found the rare occurrence of pulmonary embolism in only 0.2 percent.

These cases of embolism were associated with adnexal excision, and none were linked to untwisting of the pedicle. In a study of 94 women with adnexal torsion, Zweizig and associates (1993) reported no increased morbidity in women undergoing untwisting of the adnexa compared with those undergoing adnexectomy.

For these reasons, detorsion of the adnexa is generally recommended. Within minutes following untwisting, congestion is relieved, and ovarian volume and cyanosis typically diminish. That said, a persistently black-bluish ovary is not pathognomonic for necrosis, and the ovary may still recover. Cohen and colleagues (1999) reviewed 54 cases in which adnexa were preserved regardless of their appearance following detorsion. They reported functional integrity and successful subsequent pregnancy in almost 95 percent. Bider and coworkers (1991) observed no increased postoperative infectious morbidity in cases similarly managed. Because adnexal necrosis may still occur, conservative management requires postoperative vigilance for fever, leukocytosis, and peritoneal signs.

Following detorsion, management of the adnexa is individualized. Specific ovarian lesions ideally are excised for pathologic diagnosis of the original mass and to prevent repeat torsion. However, cystectomy in a hemorrhagic, edematous ovary may be technically difficult. Therefore, some recommend cystectomy if the mass persists for 6 to 8 weeks after primary intervention (Adeyemi-Fowode, 2019; Rody, 2002).

The retorsion rate among fertile women was 28 percent in one review of 38 publications (Hyttel, 2015). To minimize these rates, unilateral or bilateral oophoropexy may be considered (Djavadian, 2004; Kives, 2017). Techniques to secure the ovary vary. These include shortening of the uteroovarian ligament with a running accordion stitch through the ligament. Instead, the ovary or the uteroovarian ligament can be sutured to the posterior aspect of the uterus, the lateral pelvic wall, or the round ligament (Fuchs, 2010; Weitzman, 2008). However, the effects of this positioning on ovum uptake and later fertility are unclear.

Management during pregnancy does not differ. However, if the corpus luteum is removed, progestational support is recommended until 10 weeks' gestation to maintain the pregnancy. Suitable progesterone replacement regimens include: (1) micronized vaginal progesterone (Prometrium) 200 mg twice or three times daily; (2) 8-percent progesterone vaginal gel (Crinone) 90 mg once or twice daily; (3) progesterone vaginal insert (Endometrin) 100 mg twice or three times daily; (4) micronized oral progesterone (Prometrium) 200 mg orally twice or three times daily; (5) progesterone in oil (compounded in a specialty pharmacy) 50 to 100 mg daily intramuscular injection; or (6) intramuscular 17-hydroxyprogesterone caproate 150-mg weekly injections.

PARAOVARIAN MASSES

Most paratubal/paraovarian cysts are not neoplastic and are either distended remnants of the paramesonephric duct or mesothelial inclusion cysts (**Fig. 10-10**). One autopsy series cited a rate of approximately 5 percent of adnexal cysts (Dorum, 2005). The most common paramesonephric cyst is the *hydatid*

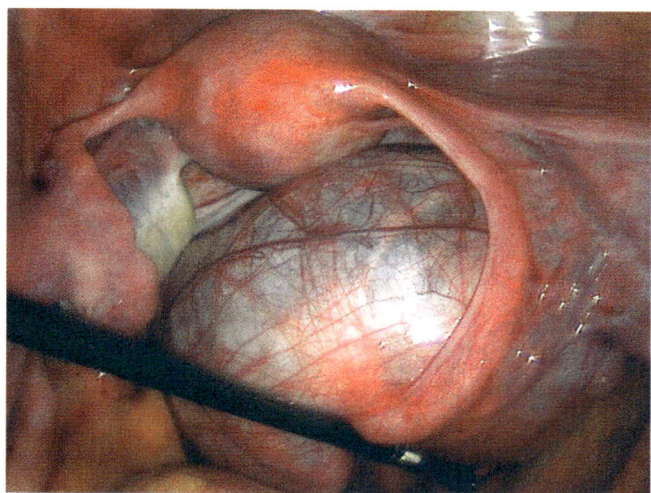

FIGURE 10-10 In this laparoscopic photograph, a large right paratubal cyst lies between its adjacent and outstretched fallopian tube and the uterus. (Reproduced with permission from Dr. Ellen Wilson.)

of Morgagni, which is pedunculated and typically dangles from one of the fimbria. Neoplastic paraovarian cysts are rare and histologically resemble tumors of ovarian origin. They are usually cystadenomas or cystadenofibromas and rarely malignant (Korbin, 1998).

Paratubal and paraovarian cysts are most commonly identified in asymptomatic women during surgery or sonography for other gynecologic problems. If symptoms develop, they mimic those of ovarian cysts. They are infrequently associated with complications such as hemorrhage, rupture, or torsion (Genadry, 1977).

Transvaginal sonography is often used as a primary evaluation tool for symptomatic women, and most of these cysts have thin, smooth walls and anechoic centers. However, sonography and MR imaging have limitations in differentiating between paraovarian and ovarian pathology (Ghossain, 2005). Thus, many women are managed as if diagnosed with a comparable ovarian cyst. When surgically managed, cystectomy or, less frequently, drainage and fulguration of the cyst wall are performed. When small and noted as an incidental intraoperative finding, these are generally excised, although this is not an evidence-based practice.

Of solid paraovarian tumors, leiomyomas are the most common and have pathophysiology identical to those within myometrium. Infrequently, congenital anomalies such as an accessory or supernumerary ovary, rudimentary uterine horn, or pelvic kidney may present as a pelvic mass with or without symptoms. One rare solid paraovarian tumor arises as a remnant of the wolffian duct and has been termed the *female adnexal tumor of probable wolffian origin* (Devouassoux-Shisheboran, 1999). Most reported cases are benign, but a few malignancies have been noted (Hong, 2018). These mirror the path of the embryologic wolffian duct and develop within the broad ligament or along the mesosalpinx (Kariminejad, 1973). Other rare paraovarian solid tumors include sarcomas, lymphoma, adenocarcinoma, pheochromocytoma, and choriocarcinoma.

Most paraovarian solid tumors are asymptomatic and identified on routine pelvic examination. Occasionally, there is unilateral pelvic and abdominal pain. Sonography and MR imaging are used to visualize these masses, although accurate differentiation between benign and malignant lesions is typically not possible. Thus, most solid masses are surgically removed.

FALLOPIAN TUBE PATHOLOGY

■ Hydrosalpinx

Fallopian tube neoplasms are rare, and most fallopian tube masses involve ectopic pregnancy or the sequelae of pelvic inflammatory disease (PID). Of these, hydrosalpinx is a chronic cystic swelling of the fallopian tube that forms following distal tubal obstruction. Causes include PID and endometriosis and rarely fallopian tube cancer. Grossly, the fine fimbria and tubal ostia are obliterated and replaced by a smooth, clubbed end (Fig. 10-11). The ballooned, thin walls of the elongated tube are translucent, and the tube is typically distended with a clear serous fluid. The ipsilateral ovary may be adhered to the hydrosalpinx.

Hydrosalpinx may be found in asymptomatic women during pelvic examination or imaging done for other indications. Some women note infertility or chronic pelvic pain. The differential diagnosis mimics that for other cystic pelvic lesions. In general, no laboratory test is helpful, and serum CA125 level testing results for presumed ovarian malignancy are typically normal.

Sonographic interrogation shows a thin-walled, cystic fusiform structure with incomplete septa and anechoic contents (Fig. 10-12A). In some, multiple hyperechoic mural nodules measuring 2 to 3 mm arch around the inner circumference of the tube to create the *beads on a string* sign. These nodules represent fibrotic endosalpingeal folds. Performed for fertility evaluation, hysterosalpingography shows ballooned, clubbed fallopian tubes filled with contrast (see Fig. 10-12).

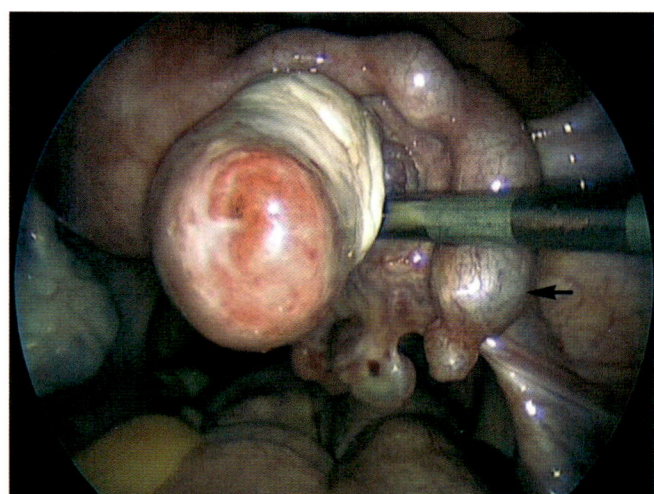

FIGURE 10-11 Laparoscopic photograph of a hydrosalpinx. Note the thin-walled ballooned fallopian tube and its clubbed end (*arrow*) draped around the blunt probe. A typical corpus luteum cyst is seen at the distal end of the ovary. (Reproduced with permission from Dr. Karen Bradshaw.)

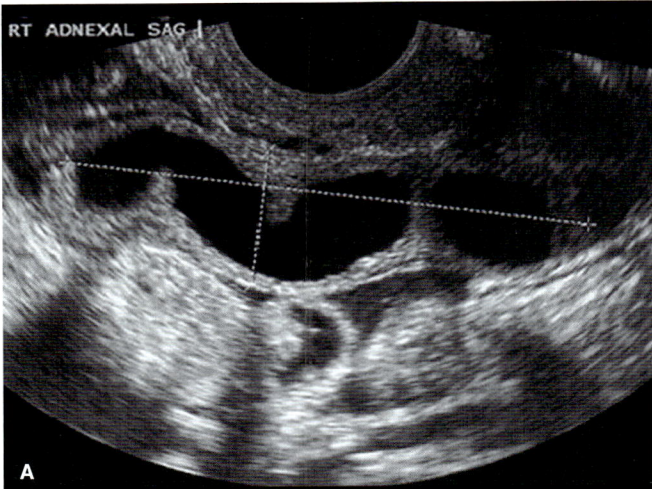
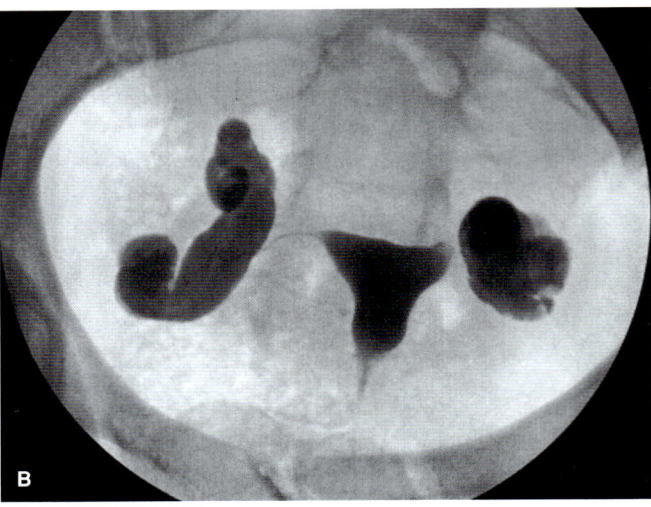

FIGURE 10-12 A. Transvaginal sonogram of a hydrosalpinx. Incomplete septa, which are folds of the dilated tube, are seen within this fusiform, fluid-filled structure. (Reproduced with permission from Dr. Elysia Moschos.) **B.** Hysterosalpingogram shows bilateral ballooned hydrosalpinges with clubbed ends. (Reproduced with permission from Dr. Kevin Doody.)

Management varies depending on the conviction of diagnosis, desire for future fertility, and associated symptoms. In asymptomatic women who have completed childbearing, and in whom the sonographic evidence supports the diagnosis of hydrosalpinx, expectant management is typical. In those with pelvic pain or infertility, or in whom the diagnosis is uncertain, diagnostic laparoscopy is often chosen.

For women not wishing to preserve fertility, laparoscopic treatment may include lysis of adhesions and salpingectomy. Conversely, in women who desire fertility, surgical intervention depends on the degree of tubal damage. As the degree of tubal distortion increases, fertility rates decline. In women with mild tubal disease, laparoscopic neosalpingostomy has resulted in 80-percent pregnancy rates and is a reasonable approach (Fig. 21-7, p. 460) (Milingos, 2000; Schlaff, 1990).

In those with severe tubal disease, in vitro fertilization (IVF) may offer a greater chance at conception. However, of infertile women undergoing IVF, women with hydrosalpinges have approximately half the pregnancy rate of those without dilated tubes (Camus, 1999; Zeyneloglu, 1998). The explanation is unclear, and theories include toxic hydrosalpinx fluid, lowered growth factor concentrations, and mechanical flushing of embryos by excess fluid (Loutradis, 2005; Lu, 2013; Strandell, 2002). If hydrosalpinges are resected prior to IVF, subsequent rates of pregnancy, implantation, and live births are improved (Johnson, 2010; Strandell, 1999). The American Society for Reproductive Medicine (2015) recommends such surgery prior to IVF.

Benign Neoplasms

These are rare in the fallopian tube. The most common benign tumor is mesothelioma, which is found in <1 percent of hysterectomy specimens (Pauerstein, 1968). Previously termed adenomatoid tumors, these 1- to 2-cm, well-circumscribed solid nodules arise in the tubal wall (Salazar, 1972). Tubal leiomyomas are uncommon and derive from the smooth muscle of

the tubal muscularis, from the broad ligament, or from vessels in either location.

The epithelium of the fallopian tube contains an intermixing of both ciliated and secretory cells. The secretory cell population increases with age, and cellular outgrowths can be seen histologically that contain only secretory cells (Li, 2013). These benign secretory cell outgrowths (SCOUTs) and their link to serous tubal intraepithelial carcinoma (STIC) and pelvic serous carcinoma are current research topics (Mehrad, 2010). These are described in Chapter 35 (p. 738).

Tuboovarian Abscess

This is an inflammatory mass involving the fallopian tube, ovary, and often surrounding structures. If an ovary adheres to the fallopian tube, but is still visually distinct, it is called a *tuboovarian complex*. In contrast, a *tuboovarian abscess* results from a complete breakdown of ovarian and tubal architecture such that the separate structures are no longer identified. Either is usually a consequence of PID, although occasionally endometritis and pelvic malignancy may be the generative source. Affected women usually have lower abdominal pain, fever, leukocytosis, and unilateral or bilateral adnexal masses. These abscesses and their management are more fully discussed in Chapter 3 (p. 70).

REFERENCES

Adeyemi-Fowode O, Lin EG, Syed F, et al: Adnexal torsion in children and adolescents: a retrospective review of 245 cases at a single institution. J Pediatr Adolesc Gynecol 32(1):64, 2019

American College of Obstetricians and Gynecologists: Evaluation and management of adnexal masses. Practice Bulletin No. 174, November 2016

American College of Obstetricians and Gynecologists: The role of the obstetrician-gynecologist in the early detection of epithelial ovarian cancer in women at average risk. Committee Opinion No. 716, September 2017

American Society for Reproductive Medicine: Role of tubal surgery in the era of assisted reproductive technology: a committee opinion. Fertil Steril 103(6):e37, 2015

Archer DF, Carr BR, Pinkerton JV, et al: Effects of ospemifene on the female reproductive and urinary tracts: translation from preclinical models into clinical evidence. Menopause 22(7):786, 2015

Atri M, Alabousi A, Reinhold C, et al: ACR Appropriateness Criteria® clinically suspected adnexal mass, no acute symptoms. J Am Coll Radiol 16(5S):S77, 2019

Bider D, Mashiach S, Dulitzky M, et al: Clinical, surgical and pathologic findings of adnexal torsion in pregnant and nonpregnant women. Surg Gynecol Obstet 173(5):363, 1991

Black JD, Roque DM, Pasternak MC, et al: A series of malignant ovarian cancers arising from within a mature cystic teratoma: a single institution experience. Int J Gynecol Cancer 25(5):792, 2015

Camus E, Poncelet C, Goffinet F, et al: Pregnancy rates after in-vitro fertilization in cases of tubal infertility with and without hydrosalpinx: a meta-analysis of published comparative studies. Hum Reprod 14(5):1243, 1999

Chalas E, Costantino JP, Wickerham DL, et al: Benign gynecologic conditions among participants in the Breast Cancer Prevention Trial. Am J Obstet Gynecol 192(4):1230, 2005

Chen VW, Ruiz B, Killeen JL, et al: Pathology and classification of ovarian tumors. Cancer 97(S10):2631, 2003

Chiang AJ, Chen MY, Weng CS, et al: Malignant transformation of ovarian mature cystic teratoma into squamous cell carcinoma: a Taiwanese Gynecologic Oncology Group (TGOG) study. J Gynecol Oncol 28(5):e69, 2017

Cohen I, Potlog-Nahari C, Shapira J, et al: Simple ovarian cysts in postmenopausal patients with breast carcinoma treated with tamoxifen: long-term follow-up. Radiology 227(3):844, 2003

Cohen SB, Oelsner G, Seidman DS, et al: Laparoscopic detorsion allows sparing of the twisted ischemic adnexa. J Am Assoc Gynecol Laparosc 6(2):139, 1999

Comerci JT Jr, Licciardi F, Bergh PA, et al: Mature cystic teratoma: a clinicopathologic evaluation of 517 cases and review of the literature. Obstet Gynecol 84(1):22, 1994

Dalmau J, Gleichman AJ, Hughes EG, et al: Anti-NMDA-receptor encephalitis: case series and analysis of the effects of antibodies. Lancet Neurol 7(12):1091, 2008

Devouassoux-Shisheboran M, Silver SA, Tavassoli FA: Wolffian adnexal tumor, so-called female adnexal tumor of probable Wolffian origin (FATWO): immunohistochemical evidence in support of a Wolffian origin. Hum Pathol 30(7):856, 1999

Djavadian D, Braendle W, Jaenicke F: Laparoscopic oophoropexy for the treatment of recurrent torsion of the adnexa in pregnancy: case report and review. Fertil Steril 82(4):933, 2004

Dorum A, Blom GP, Ekerhovd E, et al: Prevalence and histologic diagnosis of adnexal cysts in postmenopausal women: an autopsy study. Am J Obstet Gynecol 192(1):48, 2005

Fan JT, Yan HQ, Malla S, et al: The clinical significance of CA19-9 in ovarian mature cystic teratoma. Clin Exp Obstet Gynecol 43(4):522, 2016

Fielder EP, Guzick DS, Guido R, et al: Adhesion formation from release of dermoid contents in the peritoneal cavity and effect of copious lavage: a prospective, randomized, blinded, controlled study in a rabbit model. Fertil Steril 65(4):852, 1996

Fuchs N, Smorgick N, Tovbin Y, et al: Oophoropexy to prevent adnexal torsion: how, when, and for whom? J Minim Invasive Gynecol 17(2):205, 2010

Genadry R, Parmley T, Woodruff JD: The origin and clinical behavior of the parovarian tumor. Am J Obstet Gynecol 129(8):873, 1977

Ghossain MA, Braidy CG, Kanso HN, et al: Extraovarian cystadenomas: ultrasound and MR findings in 7 cases. J Comput Assist Tomogr 29(1):74, 2005

Goldberg J, Pereira L, Berghella V, et al: Pregnancy outcomes after treatment for fibromyomata: uterine artery embolization versus laparoscopic myomectomy. Am J Obstet Gynecol 191(1):18, 2004

Graif M, Shalev J, Strauss S, et al: Torsion of the ovary: sonographic features. AJR 143(6):1331, 1984

Grimes DA, Jones LB, Lopez LM, et al: Oral contraceptives for functional ovarian cysts. Cochrane Database Syst Rev 4:CD006134, 2014

Guttman PH Jr: In search of the elusive benign cystic ovarian teratoma: application of the ultrasound "tip of the iceberg" sign. J Clin Ultrasound 5(6):403, 1977

Hidalgo MM, Lisondo C, Juliato CT, et al: Ovarian cysts in users of Implanon and Jadelle subdermal contraceptive implants. Contraception 73(5):532, 2006

Holt VL, Cushing-Haugen KL, Daling JR: Oral contraceptives, tubal sterilization, and functional ovarian cyst risk. Obstet Gynecol 102(2):252, 2003

Holt VL, Cushing-Haugen KL, Daling JR: Risk of functional ovarian cyst: effects of smoking and marijuana use according to body mass index. Am J Epidemiol 161(6):520, 2005

Hong S, Cui J, Li L, et al: Malignant female adnexal tumor of probable wolffian origin: case report and literature review. Int J Gynecol Pathol 37(4):331, 2018

Hoo W, Yazebek J, Holland T, et al: Expectant management of ultrasonically diagnosed ovarian dermoid cysts: is it possible to predict the outcome? Ultrasound Obstet Gynecol 36(2):235, 2010

Houry D, Abbott JT: Ovarian torsion: a fifteen-year review. Ann Emerg Med 38(2):156, 2001

Hyttel TE, Bak GS, Larsen SB, et al: Re-torsion of the ovaries. Acta Obstet Gynecol Scand 94(3):236, 2015

Jacobs I, Oram D, Fairbanks J, et al: A risk of malignancy index incorporating CA 125, ultrasound and menopausal status for the accurate preoperative diagnosis of ovarian cancer. BJOG 97(10):922, 1990

Johnson NP, van Voorst S, Sowter MC: Surgical treatment for tubal disease in women due to undergo in vitro fertilisation. Cochrane Database Syst Rev 1:CD002125, 2010

Kariminejad MH, Scully RE: Female adnexal tumor of probable Wolffian origin. A distinctive pathologic entity. Cancer 31(3):671, 1973

Karlsen MA, Sandhu N, Høgdall C, et al: Evaluation of HE4, CA125, risk of ovarian malignancy algorithm (ROMA) and risk of malignancy index (RMI) as diagnostic tools of epithelial ovarian cancer in patients with a pelvic mass. Gynecol Oncol 127(2):379, 2012

Kim MJ, Kim NY, Lee DY, et al: Clinical characteristics of ovarian teratoma: age-focused retrospective analysis of 580 cases. Am J Obstet Gynecol 205(1):32.e1, 2011

Kives S, Gascon S, Dubuc E, et al: No. 341-diagnosis and management of adnexal torsion in children, adolescents, and adults. J Obstet Gynaecol Can 39:82, 2017

Kondo W, Bourdel N, Cotte B, et al: Does prevention of intraperitoneal spillage when removing a dermoid cyst prevent granulomatous peritonitis? BJOG 117(8):1027, 2010

Koonings PP, Campbell K, Mishell DR Jr, et al: Relative frequency of primary ovarian neoplasms: a 10-year review. Obstet Gynecol 74(6):921, 1989

Korbin CD, Brown DL, Welch WR: Paraovarian cystadenomas and cystadenofibromas: sonographic characteristics in 14 cases. Radiology 208(2):459, 1998

Kurman RJ, Carcangiu ML, Herrington CS, et al (eds): WHO Classification of Tumours of Female Reproductive Organs, 4th ed. Lyon, International Agency for Research on Cancer, 2014

Lanes SF, Birmann B, Walker AM, et al: Oral contraceptive type and functional ovarian cysts. Am J Obstet Gynecol 166(3):956, 1992

Levine D, Brown DL, Andreotti RF, et al: Management of asymptomatic ovarian and other adnexal cysts imaged at US: Society of Radiologists in Ultrasound Consensus Conference Statement. Radiology 256(3):943, 2010

Li J, Ning Y, Abushahin N, et al: Secretory cell expansion with aging: risk for pelvic serous carcinogenesis. Gynecol Oncol 131(3):555, 2013

Linder D, McCaw BK, Hecht F: Parthenogenic origin of benign ovarian teratomas. N Engl J Med 292(2):63, 1975

Loutradis D, Stefanidis K, Kousidis I, et al: Effect of human hydrosalpinx fluid on the development of mouse embryos and role of the concentration of growth factors in culture medium with and without hydrosalpinx fluid. Gynecol Endocrinol 20(1):26, 2005

Lu S, Peng H, Zhang H, et al: Excessive intrauterine fluid cause aberrant implantation and pregnancy outcome in mice. PLoS One 8(10):e7844, 2013

Martinez-Onsurbe P, Ruiz VA, Sanz Anquela JM, et al: Aspiration cytology of 147 adnexal cysts with histologic correlation. Acta Cytol 45(6):941, 2001

Mashiach R, Melamed N, Gilad N, et al: Sonographic diagnosis of ovarian torsion: accuracy and predictive factors. J Ultrasound Med 30(9):1205, 2011

McGovern PG, Noah R, Koenigsberg R, et al: Adnexal torsion and pulmonary embolism: case report and review of the literature. Obstet Gynecol Surv 54(9):601, 1999

Medeiros LR, Rosa DD, Bozzetti MC, et al: Laparoscopy versus laparotomy for benign ovarian tumour. Cochrane Database Syst Rev 2:CD004751, 2009

Mehrad M, Ning G, Chen EY, et al: A pathologist's road map to benign, precancerous, and malignant intraepithelial proliferations in the fallopian tube. Adv Anat Pathol 17(5):293, 2010

Michnovicz JJ, Hershcopf RJ, Naganuma H, et al: Increased 2-hydroxylation of estradiol as a possible mechanism for the anti-estrogenic effect of cigarette smoking. N Engl J Med 315(21):1305, 1986

Milingos SD, Kallipolitis GK, Loutradis DC, et al: Laparoscopic treatment of hydrosalpinx: factors affecting pregnancy rates. J Am Assoc Gynecol Laparosc 7:355, 2000

Millar DM, Blake JM, Stringer DA, et al: Prepubertal ovarian cyst formation: 5 years' experience. Obstet Gynecol 81(3):434, 1993

Moore RG, Jabre-Raughley M, Brown AK, et al: Comparison of a novel multiple marker assay vs the Risk of Malignancy Index for the prediction of epithelial ovarian cancer in patients with a pelvic mass. Am J Obstet Gynecol 203(3):228.e1, 2010

Moore RG, McMeekin DS, Brown AK, et al: A novel multiple marker bioassay utilizing HE4 and CA125 for the prediction of ovarian cancer in patients with a pelvic mass. Gynecol Oncol 112(1):40, 2009

Moran O, Menczer J, Ben Baruch G, et al: Cytologic examination of ovarian cyst fluid for the distinction between benign and malignant tumors. Obstet Gynecol 82(3):444, 1993

Nahum GG, Kaunitz AM, Rosen K, et al: Ovarian cysts: presence and persistence with use of a 13.5 mg levonorgestrel-releasing intrauterine system. Contraception 91(5):412, 2015

Nardo LG, Kroon ND, Reginald PW: Persistent unilocular ovarian cysts in a general population of postmenopausal women: is there a place for expectant management? Obstet Gynecol 102(3):589, 2003

Nichols DH, Julian PJ: Torsion of the adnexa. Clin Obstet Gynecol 28(2):375, 1985

Okugawa K, Hirakawa T, Fukushima K, et al: Relationship between age, histological type, and size of ovarian tumors. Int J Gynaecol Obstet 74(1):45, 2001

Ory H: Functional ovarian cysts and oral contraceptives. Negative association confirmed surgically. A cooperative study. JAMA 228(1):68, 1974

Outwater EK, Mitchell DG: Normal ovaries and functional cysts: MR appearance. Radiology 198(2):397, 1996

Pantoja E, Rodriguez-Ibanez I, Axtmayer RW, et al: Complications of dermoid tumors of the ovary. Obstet Gynecol 45(1):89, 1975

Park JY, Kim DY, Kim JH, et al: Malignant transformation of mature cystic teratoma of the ovary: experience at a single institution. Eur J Obstet Gynecol Reprod Biol 141(2):173, 2008

Pascual MA, Graupera B, Pedrero C, et al: Long-term results for expectant management of ultrasonographically diagnosed benign ovarian teratomas. Obstet Gynecol 130(6):1244, 2017

Patel MD, Feldstein VA, Lipson SD, et al: Cystic teratomas of the ovary: diagnostic value of sonography. AJR 171(4):1061, 1998

Pauerstein CJ, Woodruff JD, Quinton SW: Development patterns in "adenomatoid lesions" of the fallopian tube. Am J Obstet Gynecol 100(7):1000, 1968

Peterson WF, Prevost EC, Edmunds FT, et al: Benign cystic teratomas of the ovary: a clinico-statistical study of 1,007 cases with a review of the literature. Am J Obstet Gynecol 70(2):368, 1955

Prat J: Ovarian serous and mucinous epithelial-stromal tumors. In Robboy SJ, Mutter GL, Prat J, et al (eds): Robboy's Pathology of the Female Reproductive Tract, 2nd ed. Churchill Livingstone Elsevier, 2009, p 611

Rha SE, Byun JY, Jung SE, et al: CT and MR imaging features of adnexal torsion. Radiographics 22(2):283, 2002

Rody A, Jackisch C, Klockenbusch W, et al: The conservative management of adnexal torsion—a case-report and review of the literature. Eur J Obstet Gynecol Reprod Biol 101(1):83, 2002

Rossi BV, Ference EH, Zurakowski D, et al: The clinical presentation and surgical management of adnexal torsion in the pediatric and adolescent population. J Pediatr Adolesc Gynecol 25:109, 2012

Rousseau V, Massicot R, Darwish AA, et al: Emergency management and conservative surgery of ovarian torsion in children: a report of 40 cases. J Pediatr Adolesc Gynecol 21:201, 2008

Sagi-Dain L, Lavie O, Auslander R, et al: CA 19-9 in evaluation of adnexal mass: retrospective cohort analysis and review of the literature. Int J Biol Markers 30(3):e333, 2015

Salazar H, Kanbour A, Burgess F: Ultrastructure and observations on the histogenesis of mesotheliomas, "adenomatoid tumors," of the female genital tract. Cancer 29(1):141, 1972

Schlaff WD, Hassiakos DK, Damewood MD, et al: Neosalpingostomy for distal tubal obstruction: prognostic factors and impact of surgical technique. Fertil Steril 54(6):984, 1990

Schorge JO, Modesitt SC, Coleman RL, et al: SGO white paper on ovarian cancer: etiology, screening and surveillance. Gynecol Oncol 119(1): 7, 2010

Simpkins F, Zahurak M, Armstrong D, et al: Ovarian malignancy in breast cancer patients with an adnexal mass. Obstet Gynecol 105(3):507, 2005

Strandell A, Lindhard A: Why does hydrosalpinx reduce fertility? The importance of hydrosalpinx fluid. Hum Reprod 17(5):1141, 2002

Strandell A, Lindhard A, Waldenstrom U, et al: Hydrosalpinx and IVF outcome: a prospective, randomized multicentre trial in Scandinavia on salpingectomy prior to IVF. Hum Reprod 14(11):2762, 1999

Suh-Burgmann E, Hung YY, Kinney W: Outcomes from ultrasound follow-up of small complex adnexal masses in women over 50. Am J Obstet Gynecol 211(6):623.e1, 2014

Suh-Burgmann E, Kinney W: Potential harms outweigh benefits of indefinite monitoring of stable adnexal masses. Am J Obstet Gynecol 213(6):816.e1, 2015

Timmerman D, Testa AC, Bourne T, et al: Logistic regression model to distinguish between the benign and malignant adnexal mass before surgery: a multicenter study by the International Ovarian Tumor Analysis Group. J Clin Oncol 23:8794, 2005

Timmerman D, Valentin L, Bourne T, et al: Terms, definitions and measurements to describe the sonographic features of adnexal tumors: a consensus opinion from the International Ovarian Tumor Analysis (IOTA) group. Ultrasound Obstet Gynecol 16:500, 2000

Timmerman D, Van Calster B, Testa A, et al: Predicting the risk of malignancy in adnexal masses based on the simple rules from the International Ovarian Tumor Analysis group. Am J Obstet Gynecol 214:424, 2016

Twickler DM, Forte TB, Santos-Ramos R, et al: The Ovarian Tumor Index predicts risk for malignancy. Cancer 86:2280, 1999

Ueland FR, Desmone CP, Seamon LG, et al: Effectiveness of a multivariate index assay in the preoperative assessment of ovarian tumors. Obstet Gynecol 117(6):1289, 2011

Vuento MH, Pirhonen JP, Makinen JI, et al: Evaluation of ovarian findings in asymptomatic postmenopausal women with color Doppler ultrasound. Cancer 76(7):1214, 1995

Ware Miller R, Smith A, DeSimone CP, et al: Performance of the American College of Obstetricians and Gynecologists' ovarian tumor referral guidelines with a multivariate index assay. Obstet Gynecol 117(6):1298, 2011

Warner MA, Fleischer AC, Edell SL, et al: Uterine adnexal torsion: sonographic findings. Radiology 154(3):773, 1985

Weitzman VN, DiLuigi AJ, Maier DB, et al: Prevention of recurrent adnexal torsion. Fertil Steril 90(5):2018.e1, 2008

Whiteman MK, Kuklina E, Jamieson DJ, et al: Inpatient hospitalization for gynecologic disorders in the United States. Am J Obstet Gynecol 202(6):541.e1, 2010

Wyshak G, Frisch RE, Albright TE, et al: Smoking and cysts of the ovary. Int J Fertil 33(6):398, 1988

Yan B, Wang Y, Zhang Y, et al: Teratoma-associated anti-N-methyl-D-aspartate receptor encephalitis: a case report and literature review. Medicine (Baltimore) 98(21):e15765, 2019

Zeyneloglu HB, Arici A, Olive DL: Adverse effects of hydrosalpinx on pregnancy rates after in vitro fertilization-embryo transfer. Fertil Steril 70(3):492, 1998

Zweizig S, Perron J, Grubb D, et al: Conservative management of adnexal torsion. Am J Obstet Gynecol 168(6 Pt 1):1791, 1993

CHAPTER 11

Endometriosis

Endometriosis is a common gynecologic condition in which endometrial tissue is present outside the uterine cavity. Endometrial tissue located within the myometrium is termed *adenomyosis* and is discussed in Chapter 9 (p. 213). With its molecular basis further elucidated, endometriosis now is seen more as a systemic disease, with the implants of endometriosis leading to an inflammatory response. Although some women with endometriosis may be asymptomatic, many others present with subfertility or various forms of chronic pelvic pain (CPP). Endometriosis often strikes women during their early career or schooling, and the long-term harm to professional or social development can be profound (Lamvu, 2019). As endometriosis is an estrogen-dependent disease, hormone-based treatment is a mainstay of therapy. However, if disease is unresponsive to medical management, surgery may be required.

EPIDEMIOLOGY

Approximately 10 percent of all reproductive-aged women are affected by endometriosis (Rogers, 2009). Given that many women with endometriosis are asymptomatic, the true prevalence is difficult to quantify. Imaging modalities of any pelvic compartment generally have low specificities (Wall, 2015). Thus, the "gold standard" diagnostic method is laparoscopy, with or without biopsy for histologic diagnosis (Dunselman, 2014). With this, the annual incidence of surgically diagnosed endometriosis is 1.6 cases per 1000 reproductive-aged women (Houston, 1987). In asymptomatic women, the prevalence of endometriosis ranges from 6 to 11 percent, depending on the population studied and diagnostic mode (Buck Louis, 2011; Mahmood, 1991). Among patients with infertility, endometriosis is more common, and prevalence rates lie between 20 to 50 percent. In those with CPP, it ranges from 40 to 50 percent (Balasch, 1996; Eskenazi, 2001; Meuleman, 2009). Nearly two thirds of adolescents undergoing diagnostic laparoscopy for pelvic pain have evidence of endometriosis (Janssen, 2013).

Of potential risk factors, lower body mass appears to positively correlate with endometriosis risk (Peterson, 2013; Shah, 2013). Early menarche, especially before age 14, carries increased risk for endometriosis. Similarly, nulliparas have a higher risk that likely is secondary to a greater number of ovulatory cycles (Missmer, 2004; Treloar, 2010; Vercellini, 2010). Evidence for racial differences in prevalence is conflicting (Jacoby, 2010).

PATHOPHYSIOLOGY

Pathogenesis

The definitive cause of endometriosis remains unknown, but several theories are proposed. The most favored one describes retrograde menstruation through the fallopian tubes (Sampson 1927; Tal, 2019). The refluxed endometrial fragments invade the peritoneal mesothelium and develop a blood supply for implant survival and growth. In correlation, women with outflow tract obstruction also have a high incidence of endometriosis, which often resolves following obstruction relief (Sanfilippo, 1986; Williams, 2014). Interestingly, >90 percent of women experience retrograde menstruation, yet only a small fraction develop endometriosis (Halme, 1984). Thus, factors that enhance menstrual remnant implantation or defects in its clearance may contribute.

Retrograde menstruation does not account for endometriosis found outside the peritoneal cavity. To account for this, hematogenous or lymphatic spread is a suggested mode. For example, the eutopic endometrium of affected women has greater lymphatic vessel density, which likely promotes endometrial tissue entry into lymphatic circulation (Jerman, 2015). This may explain the spread of endometriosis into pelvic sentinel lymph nodes, groin, and retroperitoneum of affected women (Moore, 1988; Mourra, 2015; Tempfer, 2011).

Still, cases of endometriosis after hysterectomy or in men defy both of these theories. One explanation is the derivation of endometriosis from stem cells (Batt, 2013; Du, 2007; Sasson, 2008). Specifically, progenitor cells inside the endometrium and multipotent bone marrow cells both contribute to endometrial growth (Hufnagel, 2015; Schwab, 2005). Progenitor cells can slough and seed ectopic endometrial sites (Pluchino,

2016; Li, 2018). One immunohistochemical study found that affected patients shed more of their endometrial basalis layer, which is the site of many progenitor cells (Leyendecker, 2002). Mesenchymal cells, likely from the bone marrow, also can spread and differentiate into ectopic endometrial implants. These mesenchymal cells may underlie many of the extraperitoneal implants seen in endometriosis (Figueira, 2011; Kao, 2011).

Instead, the coelomic metaplasia theory describes pluripotent cells within the parietal peritoneum that transform to tissue histologically identical to normal endometrium. Since the ovary and the progenitor of the endometrium, the müllerian ducts, are both derived from coelomic epithelium, such metaplasia may help explain endometriosis involving the ovary. This process also may underlie cases of endometriosis in those without menstruation, such as premenarchal girls, males treated with estrogen and orchiectomy for prostate cancer, and patients with müllerian agenesis (Marsh, 2005; Taguchi, 2012; Troncon, 2014).

One final theory suggests that müllerian remnants left along their embryonic path undergo abnormal differentiation leading to endometriosis. This is based upon histologic studies in female fetuses showing ectopic endometrium (Batt, 2013; Signorile, 2012).

◼ Anatomic Sites

Endometriosis may develop anywhere within the pelvis and on other extrapelvic peritoneal surfaces. Most commonly, endometriosis is found in the dependent areas of the pelvis. The anterior and posterior cul-de-sacs, other pelvic peritoneum, the ovary, and uterosacral ligaments are frequently involved (Kennedy, 2005). Other sites are the rectovaginal septum, ureter, and bladder. Rarely, pericardium, surgical scars, and pleura may be affected. Implants may be superficial or they may be *deep infiltrating endometriosis (DIE)*, that is, infiltrative forms that involve vital structures such as bowel, bladder, and ureters. Some definitions of DIE also quantify invasion as >5 mm (Koninckx, 1994).

Ovarian endometriomas are frequent manifestations of endometriosis (Fig. 11-1). These smooth-walled, dark-brown ovarian cysts are filled with a chocolate-appearing fluid and may be uni- or multilocular. Their pathogenesis is unclear, yet three theories include invagination of ovarian cortex implants, coelomic metaplasia, and secondary involvement of functional ovarian cysts by endometrial implants located on the ovarian surface (Vignali, 2002). Continued menstruation into the cyst results in accumulation of old blood and cellular debris, forming the chocolate-appearing fluid.

◼ Molecular Mechanisms

Endometriosis is an estrogen-dependent chronic inflammatory disease with aberrant growth of ectopic endometrial tissue. These ectopic endometrial implants show molecular differences from the eutopic endometrium of unaffected women. *Eutopic endometrium* is that which lines the uterine cavity. The aberrant molecular mechanisms in endometriosis are yet to be fully defined. However, suspected underpinnings include an implant

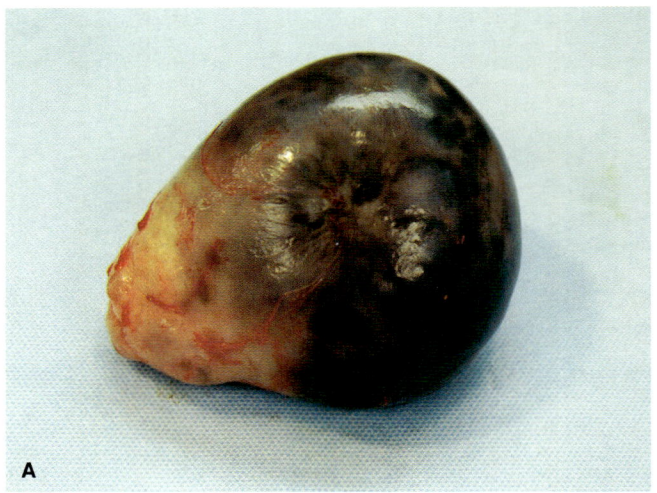

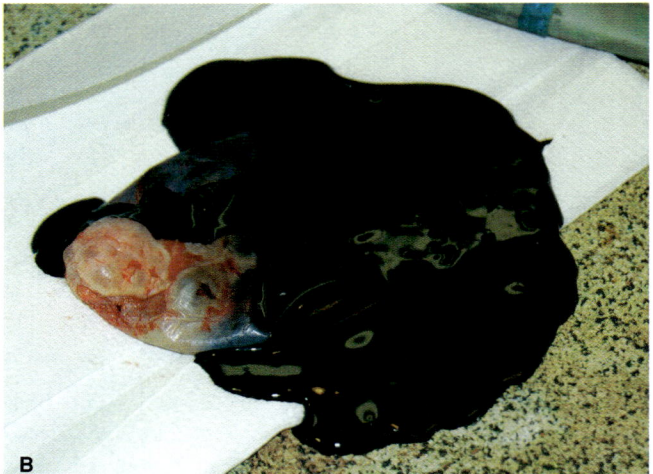

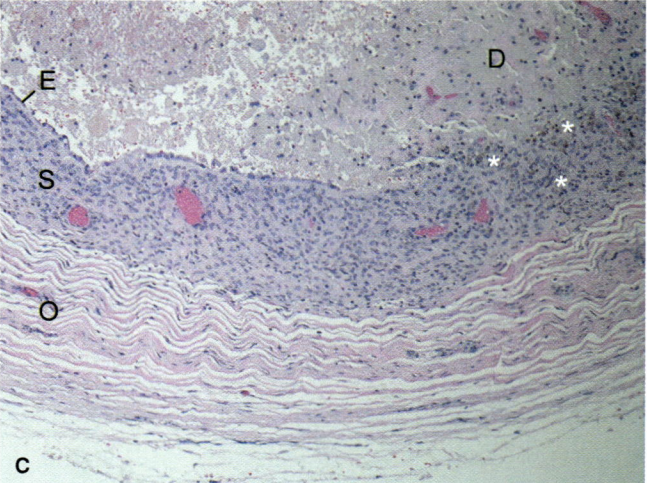

FIGURE 11-1 Endometrioma. **A.** Surgical specimen of an ovary containing an endometrioma. **B.** Dark, chocolate-like fluid had filled this cyst. (Photographs contributed by Dr. Roxanne Pero.) **C.** In ovarian endometriomas, endometrial-type epithelium (*E*) and subjacent stroma (*S*) line the cyst and are bordered peripherally by ovarian stroma (*O*). The golden brown pigment in the cyst wall (*asterisk*) is hemosiderin, indicating remote hemorrhage. Debris composed of necrotic and degenerating cells and remote hemorrhage occupies the interior of the cyst (*D*). It is the remote hemorrhage that confers the chocolate-like color to cyst fluid.

environment of estrogen dominance, estrogen dependence, and progesterone resistance; inflammation; escape from immune clearance; local invasion and neurovascularity development; and genetic predisposition.

Estrogen and Progesterone

Estrogen plays a causative role in endometriosis formation and is derived from multiple sources. First, most estrogen in women is produced directly by the ovaries. Second, peripheral tissues also produce estrogens through conversion of ovarian and adrenal androgens by the enzyme aromatase. Endometriotic implants express aromatase and 17β-hydroxysteroid dehydrogenase type 1, which are the enzymes responsible for conversion of androstenedione to estrone and of estrone to estradiol, respectively. Implants, however, are deficient in 17β-hydroxysteroid dehydrogenase type 2, which inactivates estrogen (Kitawaki, 1997; Zeitoun, 1998). Endometriotic stromal cells uniquely also express the full complement of genes in the steroidogenic cascade, which is sufficient to convert cholesterol to estradiol itself (Bulun, 2012). In sum, these enzymatic changes ensure that implants create an estrogenic environment. It also provides a rationale for aromatase inhibitor use in refractory clinical cases.

Normal progesterone effects are attenuated in endometriosis. This progesterone resistance is thought to stem from an overall low concentration of progesterone receptors within implants (Attia, 2000; Flores, 2018). Specifically, pathologic overexpression of estrogen receptor β in endometriosis suppresses estrogen receptor α expression. This diminishes estradiol-mediated induction of the progesterone receptor in endometriotic cells (Xue, 2007).

As one consequence of this resistance, survival of refluxed endometrium in affected women may be bolstered. Namely, normal endometrium has elevated levels of 17β-hydroxysteroid dehydrogenase type 2 in response to progesterone (Satyaswaroop, 1982). As a result, progesterone antagonizes the estrogen effects in normal endometrium during the luteal phase. Endometriosis, however, manifests a relative progesterone-resistant state, which prevents this antagonism in its implants (Patel, 2017).

Progesterone resistance may also enhance ectopic tissue implantation. First, mesothelium invasion can be aided by matrix metalloproteinases (MMPs). These are a group of collagenases implicated in endometrial turnover during normal menstruation. Progesterone represses MMP activity (Itoh, 2012). Thus, progesterone resistance within endometriotic implants may augment the MMP activity necessary for implant invasion.

Inflammation

Prostaglandin E_2 (PGE_2) is the most potent inducer of aromatase activity in endometrial stromal cells (Noble, 1997). Estradiol produced in response to the greater aromatase activity subsequently augments PGE_2 production (Gurates and Bulun 2003). This creates a positive feedback loop and potentiates the estrogenic effects. PGE_2 also augments MMP-2 activity, which can augment endometriosis angiogenesis (Jana, 2016).

In vitro inhibition of PGE_2 receptors, which are EP2 and EP4, decreases endometriotic lesion growth, angiogenesis, and innervation (Arosh, 2015). As a clinical correlate, nonsteroidal antiinflammatory drugs (NSAIDs) are used clinically to reduce prostaglandin formation and thereby decrease endometriosis-linked pain.

Immune System

With retrograde menstruation, refluxed menstrual tissue in most women is cleared by macrophages, natural killer (NK) cells, and lymphocytes. Accordingly, immune system dysfunction is one likely mechanism for endometriosis establishment (Seli, 2003). First, macrophages in greater numbers are found in the peritoneal cavity of affected women (Haney, 1981; Olive, 1985b). Although this increased population might logically act to suppress endometrial proliferation, macrophages in these affected women actually stimulate endometriotic tissue (Braun, 1994).

NK cells numbers are unaltered in the peritoneal fluid of affected women. However, their cytotoxicity against endometrium is diminished, especially in more advanced-stage endometriosis (Ho, 1995; Wilson, 1994). Several factors are suspected, but the exact reason for this decreased cytotoxicity is unclear.

Cellular immunity also is likely disordered in women with endometriosis. For example, the cytotoxic activity of T lymphocytes against autologous endometrium in affected women is impaired (Ulukus, 2005). Humoral immunity, which is B cell dependent, also is altered. IgG and IgA autoantibodies against endometrial and ovarian tissues are found in the sera and in cervical and vaginal secretions of affected women (Mathur, 1982; Odukoya, 1995). These results suggest that endometriosis has features similar to other autoimmune diseases.

Cytokines are involved in immune cell signaling. Numerous cytokines, especially interleukins, are identified in relevant tissues and are implicated in endometriosis pathogenesis (Arici, 1998; Mori, 1991; Tseng, 1996). Each of these cytokines produces or perpetuates a proinflammatory immune response.

Vascular endothelial growth factor (VEGF) is an angiogenic growth factor that is upregulated by estradiol in endometrial stromal cells and peritoneal fluid macrophages. Levels of this factor also are higher in the peritoneal fluid of affected women (McLaren, 1996).

Genetics

No mendelian genetic inheritance pattern has been identified for endometriosis. However, the greater incidence in first-degree relatives suggests a polygenic/multifactorial pattern. For example, in population studies, 4 to 8 percent of the female siblings or mothers of affected women had endometriosis (Dalsgaard, 2013). Studies also demonstrate concordance for endometriosis in monozygotic twin pairs (Saha, 2015; Treloar, 1999).

To assist with identifying candidate genes, researchers have used population-based genome-wide association study (GWAS). This method is founded on the principle that common diseases, such as endometriosis, are caused by genetic variants that are common themselves. From GWAS of endometriosis, several candidate genes and chromosomes have been identified for further investigation (Burney, 2013). In total, evidence from GWAS suggests that endometriosis inheritance is complex and likely polygenic.

Chronic Pain and Pain Sensitization

The exact mechanism for endometriosis-associated pain is not yet clear. Proinflammatory cytokines and prostaglandins released by endometriotic implants may be one source (Bulun, 2009). Nerve growth into endometriotic implants also has been implicated (Barcena de Arellano, 2011; McKinnon, 2012). Once an endometriotic lesion has been established, continued exposure of these sensory nerves to the implant's inflammatory environment can create central sensitization and CPP. The mechanism of central sensitization and its role in CPP is described fully in Chapter 12 (p. 254) (As-Sanie, 2013; Bajaj, 2003).

Moreover, in research studies, magnetic resonance (MR) imaging of brains of patients with CPP, either with and without endometriosis, shows consistent reduction in thalamic gray matter volume. However, no volume change is noted in the thalami of patients with endometriosis but no CPP (As-Sanie, 2012). Hypersensitization and expansion of pain sensory regions also is observed in patients with endometriosis and CPP (As-Sanie, 2013; Neziri, 2010). These findings suggest that the persistent pelvic pain of endometriosis may be inadequately treated by therapies that address the endometriotic implants alone.

CLASSIFICATION

The extent of endometriosis can vary widely between individuals. In an attempt to classify this, a scheme was developed by the American Society for Reproductive Medicine (1997) (Fig. 11-2). With this system, endometriosis on the peritoneum, ovaries, fallopian tubes, and cul-de-sac is scored during surgery. At these sites, points are assigned for disease surface area, degree of invasion, morphology, and extent of associated adhesions. Endometriotic lesions also are morphologically categorized as white, red, or black. In this system, endometriosis is classified as stage I (minimal), stage II (mild), stage III (moderate), and stage IV (severe).

Advantages of this scheme are its widespread implementation, its ease of use, and its four simple-to-comprehend stages. However, the system has limitations. It correlates poorly with infertility and pain symptoms (Guzick, 1997; Vercellini, 1996). This poor predictive ability stems in part from scores that are derived from subjective visual examination. Moreover, disease involving ureter, bowel, or other extrapelvic sites is not scored (Adamson, 2013). To address these shortcomings, other methods have been developed but are

yet to be widely used. These include the ENZIAN staging system to better represent DIE and the Endometrial Fertility Index (EFI) to predict fertility in endometriosis patients (Adamson, 2010; Haas, 2011). The World Endometriosis Society (WES) established consensus statements concerning the roles of these three assessment tools (Johnson, 2017).

SYMPTOMS

■ Pain

Women with endometriosis may be asymptomatic. However, compared with unaffected women, they are much more likely to have subfertility or CPP (Ballard, 2008). Dysmenorrhea,

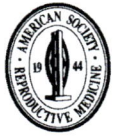

AMERICAN SOCIETY FOR REPRODUCTIVE MEDICINE REVISED CLASSIFICATION OF ENDOMETRIOSIS

Patient's Name _____ Date _____

Stage I   (Minimal) - 1-5
Stage II (Mild)   - 6-15   Laparoscopy_____ Laparotomy_____ Photography_____
Stage III (Moderate) - 16-40   Recommended Treatment_____
Stage IV (Severe)   - >40
Total_____   Prognosis_____

PERITONEUM	ENDOMETRIOSIS		<1cm	1-3cm	>3cm
	Superficial		1	2	4
	Deep		2	4	6
OVARY	R	Superficial	1	2	4
		Deep	4	16	20
	L	Superficial	1	2	4
		Deep	4	16	20

POSTERIOR CULDESAC OBLITERATION		Partial		Complete	
		4		40	

	ADHESIONS		<1/3 Enclosure	1/3-2/3 Enclosure	>2/3 Enclosure
OVARY	R	Filmy	1	2	4
		Dense	4	8	16
	L	Filmy	1	2	4
		Dense	4	8	16
TUBE	R	Filmy	1	2	4
		Dense	4*	8*	16
	L	Filmy	1	2	4
		Dense	4*	8*	16

*If the fimbriated end of the fallopian tube is completely enclosed, change the point assignment to 16.

Denote appearance of superficial implant types as red [(R), red, red-pink, flamelike, vesicular blobs, clear vesicles], white [(W), opacifications, peritoneal defects, yellow-brown], or black [(B) black, hemosiderin deposits, blue]. Denote percent of total described as R___%, W___% and B___%. Total should equal 100%.

Additional Endometriosis: _____   Associated Pathology: _____
_____   _____
_____   _____
_____   _____

To Be Used with Normal   To Be Used with Abnormal
Tubes and Ovaries   Tubes and/or Ovaries

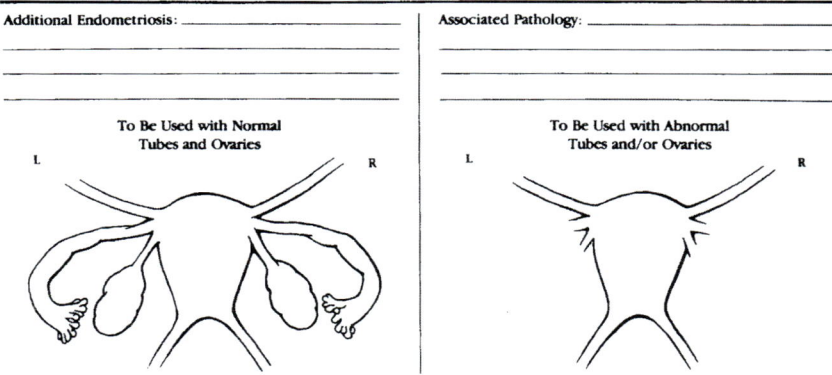

FIGURE 11-2 American Society for Reproductive Medicine Revised Classification of Endometriosis, 1997, with permission.

dyspareunia, and noncyclic pain are common pain manifestations. Less often, affected women may also note dyschezia (pain with defecation), dysuria, or abdominal wall pain (Schliep, 2015). The variability of implant location and inflammatory mediators help explain the differing pain manifestations.

To initially assess CPP, pain scoring tools such as the visual analogue scale (VAS) and the numerical rating scale (NRS) are options. These are shown in Figure 12-2 (p. 258) (Bourdel, 2015). Posttreatment scoring allows evaluation of treatment response.

Of pain types in endometriosis, dysmenorrhea typically precedes menses by 24 to 48 hours. Compared with primary dysmenorrhea, this pain is thought to be more severe, more progressive, and less responsive to NSAIDs and combination oral contraceptives (COCs) (Opoku-Anane, 2012). DIE also positively correlates with dysmenorrhea severity (Lafay Pillet, 2014). Although initially cyclic, pelvic pain may become constant because of ongoing fibrosis, scarring, and adhesion formation.

Endometriosis-associated dyspareunia often is related to rectovaginal septum, uterosacral ligament, or posterior cul-de-sac disease, although other involved sites can cause painful intercourse (Vercellini, 2007, 2012). Tension on diseased uterosacral ligaments during intercourse may trigger this pain (Fauconnier, 2002). Although some women with endometriosis describe a history of dyspareunia since coitarche, endometriosis-associated dyspareunia is suspected if pain develops after years of pain-free intercourse (Montagna, 2008).

Noncyclic CPP is another frequent symptom of endometriosis. Of women with CPP, approximately 33 percent are found to have endometriosis during laparoscopy (Howard, 2003). This percentage is even higher in adolescents with CPP (Janssen, 2013). As noted earlier, endometriosis stage often does not correlate with the pain severity (Fedele, 1992; Hsu, 2011; Vercellini, 1996). Greater positive correlation for pain is seen with DIE (Hsu, 2011; Porpora, 1999).

The site of chronic pain may vary according to the lesion location. With rectovaginal septum or uterosacral ligament involvement, pain may radiate to the rectum or lower back. Alternatively, pain radiating down the leg may reflect sciatic nerve involvement (Possover, 2011).

Women with endometriosis-related chronic pain may experience comorbid depression (Gambadauro, 2019). An initial depression screen described in Chapter 1 (p. 19) is suitable. Treatment options and indications for consultation are described in Chapter 14 (p. 302).

■ Infertility

The incidence of endometriosis in women with subfertility is 20 to 30 percent (Waller, 1993). Although wide variability is reported, patients with infertility appear to have a greater incidence of endometriosis than fertile controls (13 to 33 percent versus 4 to 8 percent) (D'Hooghe, 2003; Strathy, 1982). Furthermore, Matorras and colleagues (2001) noted an increased prevalence of more severe stages of endometriosis in women with infertility.

Adhesions are one intuitive explanation for endometriosis-related infertility. These may impair normal oocyte pick-up and transport by the fallopian tube. Beyond mechanical impairment, numerous subtle defects also appear to be involved. Such defects include perturbations in follicle development, ovulation, sperm function, embryo quality and development, and implantation (Macer, 2012; Stilley, 2012).

Concerning endometriosis stages, associations between infertility and milder forms of endometriosis are not robust (D'Hooghe, 1996; Schenken, 1980). However, an association is suggested by the differing prevalence of endometriosis between infertile and fertile women. For example, in one small study, women with minimal endometriosis had a 12-month cumulative pregnancy rate of 47 percent, which falls below that of normal fertile women (Rodriguez-Escudero, 1988). Additionally, a prospective cohort study demonstrated that women with minimal or mild endometriosis had a fecundity similar to that of those with unexplained infertility (Bérubé, 1998).

In moderate to severe endometriosis (stage III to IV), tubal and ovarian architecture are often distorted. As a result, impaired fertility would be expected. Few studies report fecundity rates in women with severe endometriosis. One investigation comparing mild, moderate, and severe endometriosis revealed a monthly fecundity rate of 8.7 percent in those with mild disease, 3.2 percent with moderate disease, and no pregnancies with severe disease (Olive, 1985a). In another, women with severe endometriosis undergoing in vitro fertilization (IVF) had poorer implantation and pregnancy rates compared with those with mild disease (Harb, 2013).

■ Symptoms from Specific Sites

Rectosigmoid Lesions

Defecatory pain develops much less often than other types of CPP in patients with endometriotic lesions on the rectosigmoid colon. Complaints may be chronic or cyclic, and they can be associated with constipation, diarrhea, or cyclic hematochezia (Roman, 2013). Thus, gastrointestinal causes of CPP also are entertained and excluded during evaluation (Chap. 12, p. 268). The origin of symptoms can be fixation of the rectum to adjacent anatomic structures or rectal wall inflammation.

Symptoms may also stem from DIE of the gastrointestinal tract, which complicates 5 to 12 percent of proven endometriosis cases. Bowel DIE predominantly involves rectosigmoid colon and much less so the small bowel, cecum, or appendix (Ruffo, 2014b). Lesions usually are confined to the subserosa and muscularis propria. Thus, colonoscopy offers poor diagnostic sensitivity (Milone, 2015). Rarely, more severe cases may involve the bowel wall transmurally and lead to intestinal obstruction or a clinical picture suggesting malignancy (Kaufman, 2011; Ruffo, 2014a).

For diagnosis, rectal DIE can be imaged by transvaginal sonography (TVS), and sensitivity approximates 73 to 80 percent. However, TVS techniques used for DIE have a learning curve, and these are predominantly performed at select tertiary care centers (Tammaa, 2014). MR imaging can clarify anatomy and degree of invasion, especially preoperatively (Bazot, 2009; Wall, 2015). For rectosigmoid DIE, MR imaging has a sensitivity and specificity of 92 and 96 percent, respectively (Bazot, 2017). However, most simple peritoneal lesions are not visualized, and laparoscopy typically provides definitive diagnosis.

Without obstructing symptoms, women may be considered for conservative management with hormonal therapy. However, treatment is often surgical, and cases often warrant a surgeon skilled in bowel surgery. Variables such as anatomic site, DIE depth, lesion size, and number of foci influence surgical planning. Colorectal segment resection is rarely necessary but should be an available option depending on the extent of lesion invasion. Less invasive techniques that shave down the lesion without opening the rectum or that excise discrete nodules also are described (Alabiso, 2015; Wolthuis, 2014).

Urinary Tract Lesions

Endometriosis should be considered if urinary tract symptoms persist despite negative urine culture results. Symptoms such as dysuria, suprapubic pain, urinary frequency, urgency, and hematuria are more common with bladder involvement by endometriosis (Gabriel, 2011; Seracchioli, 2010). Costovertebral angle pain may reflect ureteral endometriosis with obstruction and hydronephrosis that can progress eventually to loss of kidney function (Knabben, 2015).

In one large series, the prevalence of urinary tract DIE was 2.6 percent (Antonelli, 2006). Of the 31 patients, 12 had bladder endometriosis, 15 had ureteral endometriosis, and four had both ureteral and bladder involvement. TVS has suitable accuracy for bladder DIE but, as expected, is less sensitive for ureteral disease (Exacoustos, 2014a). In unclear cases, MR imaging can add additional anatomic information. Cystoscopy with biopsy also can help clarify the diagnosis.

Treatment is either medical or surgical. If elected, surgery for bladder invasion typically involves partial cystectomy. Surgeries for ureteral involvement vary by disease severity and involved segment. Operations may include: (1) freeing the tethered ureter by ureterolysis, (2) segmental resection and primary reanastomosis, or (3) ureter reimplantation into the bladder (Seracchioli, 2010).

Anterior Abdominal Wall

Some individuals with abdominal pain can have anterior abdominal wall endometriomas. Most of these lesions develop in an abdominal scar after uterine surgery or cesarean delivery, whereas others form unrelated to prior operations (Fig. 11-3) (Ding, 2013). Pfannenstiel incisions are disproportionately affected. Implants usually are found within the subcutaneous layer, are palpable, and can variably involve the adjacent fascia. Less often, the rectus abdominis muscle is infiltrated (Mostafa, 2013). Diagnostic tools are employed variably, and abdominal wall sonography, computed tomography (CT), MR imaging, and fine-needle aspiration are diagnostic options. The decision to perform concurrent TVS typically is guided by whether CPP symptoms coexist.

In most instances, implants are surgically excised for pain relief and diagnosis. For small implants, preoperative imaging may not be needed. But with larger implants and concerns for fascial or rectus abdominis muscle involvement, CT or MR imaging is helpful. Images can guide surgery planning and the possible need for abdominal wall mesh placement (Ecker, 2014).

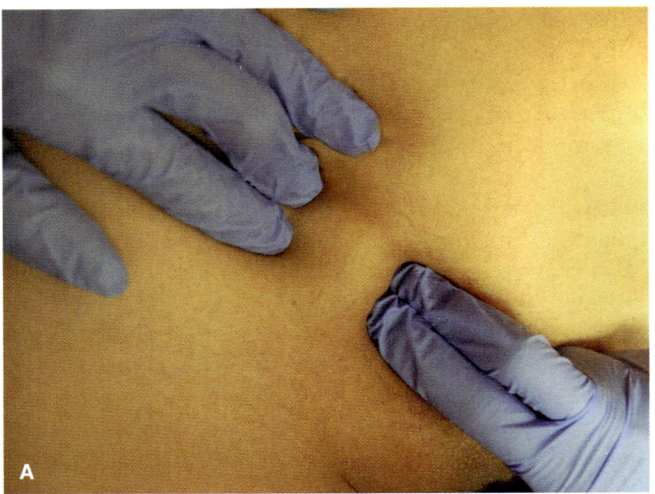

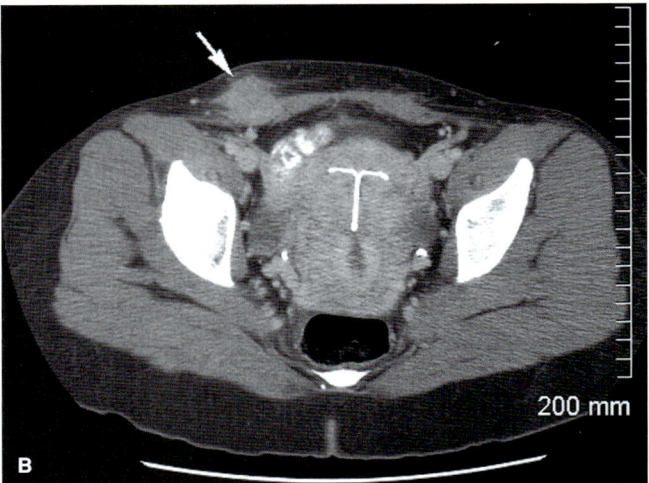

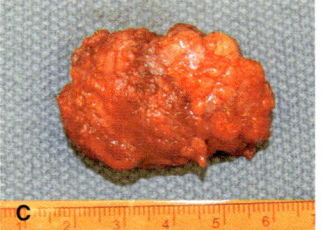
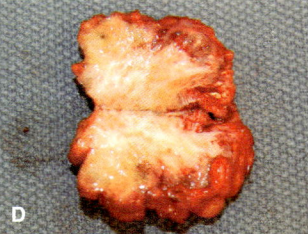

FIGURE 11-3 Endometriosis within a Pfannenstiel incision scar. **A.** Preoperative photograph delineates the borders of the mass. **B.** Computed tomography image shows a subcutaneous mass extending down to the anterior abdominal wall fascia on the left. **C.** Excised mass. **D.** Bivalved mass shows white fibrous scarring within yellow subcutaneous fat. Pathologic evaluation confirmed endometriosis. (Reproduced with permission from Dr. Christi Capet.)

Thoracic Lesions

Thoracic endometriosis defines implants inside the thoracic cavity that lead to symptoms described as menstrual or synonymously called *catamenial*. These include cyclic chest or shoulder pain, hemoptysis, or pneumothorax, which predominantly occurs on the right (Haga, 2014; Rousset-Jablonski, 2011; Tulandi, 2018). Chest CT is the preferred imaging modality (Rousset, 2014). For the case of catamenial pneumothorax, minimally invasive thoracoscopic surgery usually is indicated. This is often coupled with postoperative gonadotropin-releasing hormone (GnRH) or progestin therapy identical to that for pelvic endometriosis treatment (Alifano, 2010). Depending on findings, hemoptysis may be treated hormonally or surgically.

DIAGNOSTIC EVALUATION

■ Physical Examination

Endometriosis is confined predominantly to the pelvis, and visual cues often are lacking. Exceptions include endometriosis within an episiotomy or other surgical scar (Koger, 1993; Zhu, 2002). Rarely, endometriosis may develop spontaneously within the perineum or perianal region (Watanabe, 2003). Occasionally, blue or red powder-burn lesions are seen on the cervix or the posterior vaginal fornix. These lesions can be tender or bleed with contact. In one study, 14 percent of patients diagnosed with DIE had endometriotic findings seen by speculum evaluation (Chapron, 2002).

During bimanual examination, pelvic organ palpation often reveals suggestive anatomic abnormalities. Uterosacral ligament nodularity and tenderness may reflect active disease or scarring along the ligament. An enlarged, cystic adnexal mass may be an ovarian endometrioma, which can be mobile or adhered to other pelvic structures. A retroverted, fixed, tender uterus and a firm, fixed posterior cul-de-sac are other findings. However, examination is generally inaccurate in assessing the extent of endometriosis, especially if the lesions are extragenital (Bazot, 2009). Last, rectal examination may reveal rectovaginal septum nodularity or tenderness.

■ Laboratory Testing

Although not specific for endometriosis, various tests are used to diagnose other causes of pelvic pain. Initially, a complete blood count (CBC), human chorionic gonadotropin assay, urinalysis and urine cultures, vaginal cultures, and cervical swabs may be collected to exclude infections or pregnancy complications. If urinary tract endometriosis is suspected, creatinine levels can assess renal function.

Numerous serum markers have been studied as possible indicators of endometriosis. Cancer antigen 125 (CA125) is an antigenic determinant on a glycoprotein that is found in fallopian tube epithelium, endometrium, endocervix, pleura, and peritoneum. This marker is used in ovarian cancer evaluation and surveillance. With endometriosis, levels can be elevated and positively correlate with disease severity (Hornstein, 1995a). Unfortunately, the assay has poor sensitivity in detecting mild endometriosis and appears to be a better diagnostic test for stage III or IV endometriosis (Mol, 1998; Santulli, 2015). Other suspected biomarkers include VEGF, thyroid stimulating hormone (TSH), and cytokines such as interleukin 6 (IL-6) or IL-8. However, these and many others appear not to provide suitable clinical accuracy (May, 2010).

Recently, microRNAs have been assessed for this diagnostic role. MicroRNAs are RNA oligonucleotides, typically 18 to 22 nucleotides long, that are essential for modulating gene expression (Bartel, 2009). Several microRNAs are differentially

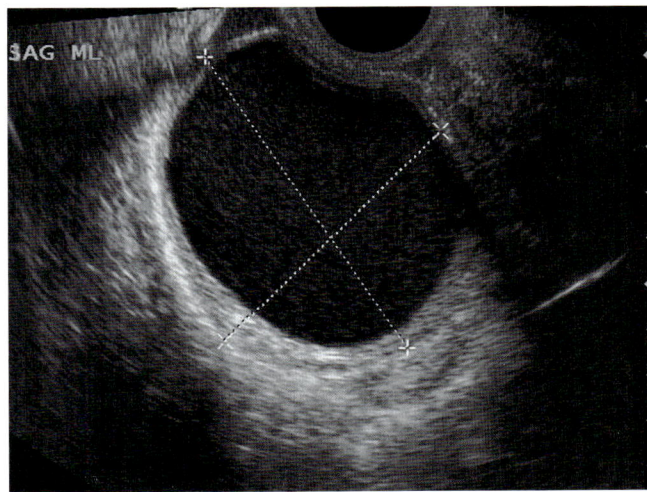

FIGURE 11-4 Transvaginal sonogram demonstrating ovarian endometrioma. A cyst with diffuse internal low-level echoes is seen.

expressed in endometriosis and include miR-125b-5p and the let-7 family of microRNAs. In the future, these may serve as a noninvasive diagnostic tool.

■ Diagnostic Imaging

Many women with endometriosis present with CPP, and thus TVS is an initial imaging tool. TVS has suitable accuracy for detecting endometriomas and aids exclusion of other pelvic pain sources. However, imaging of superficial endometriosis or associated adhesions is inadequate (Wall, 2015).

For endometriomas, TVS sensitivity and specificity range from 64 to 90 percent and from 22 to 100 percent, respectively (Moore, 2002). An endometrioma classically is cystic with homogeneous, low-level internal echoes, often described as having "ground glass" echogenicity. Surrounding ovarian tissue is normal (Fig. 11-4). As such, these may have an identical appearance to hemorrhagic corpus luteum cysts. Reimaging 6 to 8 weeks later can help differentiate these two. Corpora lutea typically will resolve but endometriomas persist. Most endometriomas are unilocular, but one to four thin septations can be found (Van Holsbeke, 2010). Less typically, these cysts can display thick septations or be thick-walled. Also less often, echogenic wall foci that lack flow when color Doppler is applied can be seen and typically are depositions of blood (Bhatt, 2006). Color Doppler TVS often demonstrates pericystic, but not intracystic, flow. Much less commonly, endometriomas can be found in postmenopausal women. These cysts often are multilocular, in contrast to those in reproductive-aged women.

As noted previously (p. 237), TVS for DIE involving the bowel and bladder has suitable accuracy (Exacoustos, 2014a; Hudelist, 2011). That said, for the diagnosis of rectal endometriosis, TVS is highly operator dependent, and experience is often lacking (Dunselman, 2014). Thus, MR imaging may clarify anatomy for equivocal sonographic findings and offers superior resolution at soft tissue interfaces (Fig. 11-5) (Bazot, 2017). In some DIE cases, MR imaging can assist preoperative planning.

CT scanning plays a limited role in the evaluation of endometriosis because of its poor sensitivity for small implants and

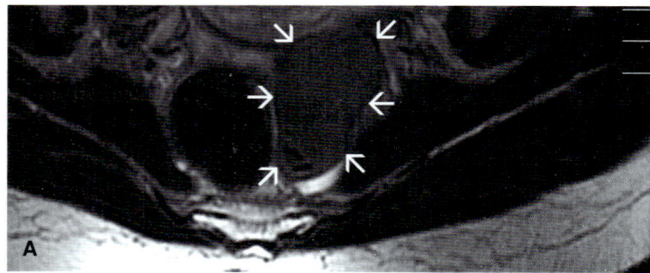

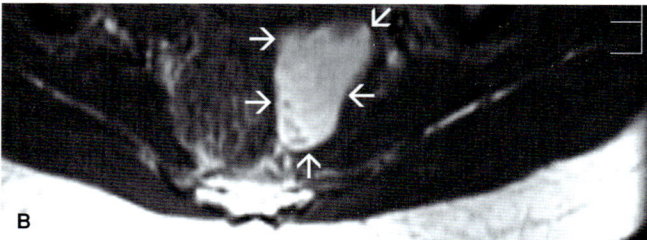

FIGURE 11-5 Magnetic resonance images of an endometrioma (*arrows*) just lateral to the rectum. **A.** Consistent with subacute blood, low-intensity signals are found on T2-weighted sequences. **B.** High-intensity signals are seen on T1-weighted sequences. (Reproduced with permission from Dr. Diane Twickler.)

plaques. Instead, CT is preferred for thoracic endometriosis and is suitable for abdominal wall endometrioma evaluation. In selected cases, CT may have a role in evaluating bowel or ureteral endometriosis (Exacoustos, 2014b).

Diagnostic Laparoscopy

Although imaging can add clinical information, laparoscopy is the primary method used for diagnosis (American College of Obstetricians and Gynecologists, 2018). Surgical findings are variable and may include discrete endometriotic lesions, endometrioma, or adhesions. Implants are typically found on pelvic organ serosa and pelvic peritoneum. Lesions are variably colored and can be red (red, red-pink, or clear), white (white or yellow-brown), and black (black or black-blue) (Fig. 11-6). White and red lesions most commonly correlate with the

characteristic histologic findings of endometriosis (Jansen, 1986). Dark lesions are pigmented by hemosiderin deposition from trapped menstrual debris. Endometriotic lesions also can differ morphologically. They may be smooth blebs on peritoneal surfaces, holes or defects within the peritoneum, or flat stellate lesions whose points are formed by surrounding scar. Endometriotic lesions can be superficial or can deeply invade the peritoneum or pelvic organs.

Laparoscopic visualization of ovarian endometriomas has a sensitivity and specificity of 97 percent and 95 percent, respectively (Vercellini, 1991). Thus, cyst biopsy rarely is required for diagnosis.

Pathologic Analysis

Current guidelines do not require biopsy and histologic evaluation for endometriosis diagnosis. However, some suggest that relying solely on laparoscopic findings in the absence of histologic confirmation results in overdiagnosis (Buck Louis, 2011; Wykes, 2004). Specifically, the greatest discordance between laparoscopic and histologic findings is noted in scarred lesions (Walter, 2001). Histologic diagnosis requires both endometrial glands and stroma found outside the uterine cavity (Fig. 11-7). Histologic hemosiderin deposition also is common. The gross appearance of endometriotic lesions often suggests microscopic findings. For example, histologically, red lesions are frequently vascularized, whereas white lesions more often display fibrosis and few vessels (Nisolle, 1997).

In general, endometriosis is characterized by long delays until diagnosis. We believe that clinical diagnosis can speed the time to recognition and treatment (Agarwal, 2019; Taylor, 2018). Cyclic and progressive pelvic pain without other clear etiologies most commonly reflects endometriosis. Clinical diagnosis with initiation of therapy is reasonable.

TREATMENT

Therapy for endometriosis depends on a woman's specific complaints, symptom severity, location of lesions, goals for

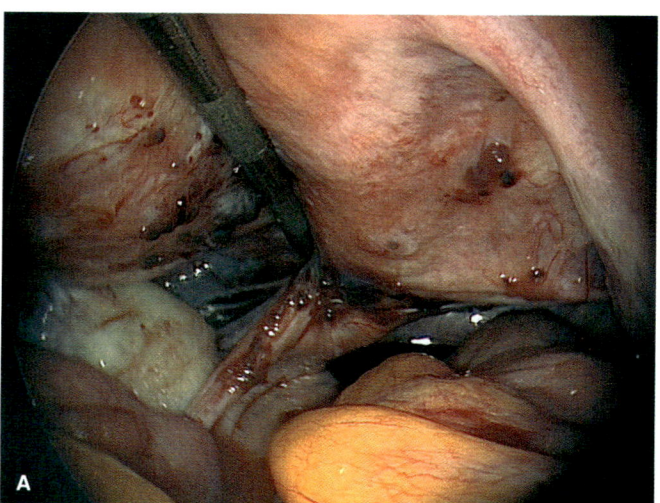

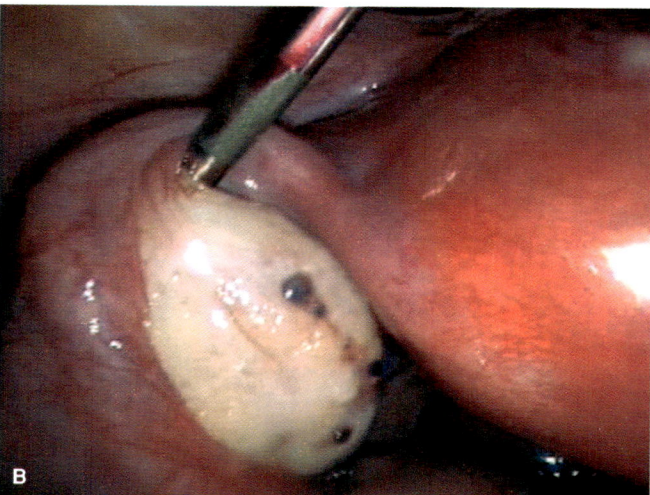

FIGURE 11-6 Endometriosis diagnosed during laparoscopy. **A.** Several red and clear endometriotic lesions seen on the pelvic peritoneum of the posterior cul-de-sac. **B.** Several brown-black lesions on the ovarian surface. (Reproduced with permission from Dr. David Rogers.)

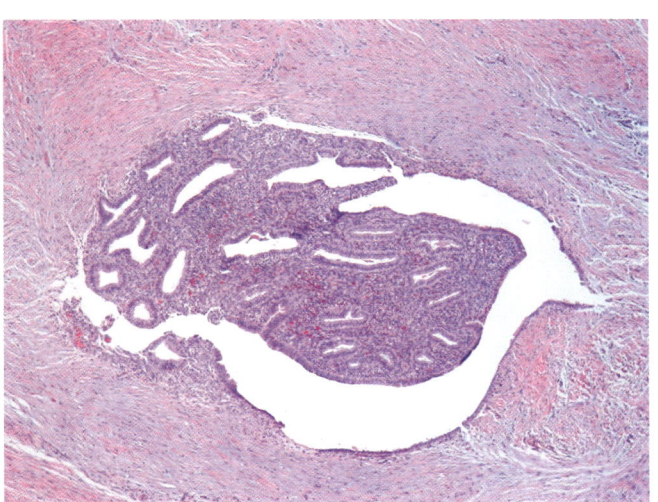

FIGURE 11-7 Endometriosis. This focus of endometrial glands and stroma was identified in the abdominal wall at the lateral aspect of a cesarean delivery scar. (Reproduced with permission from Dr. Kelley Carrick.)

treatment, and desire for future fertility (Fig. 11-8). If pain is prominent and conception is not currently desired, medical therapy usually is selected. Treatment strives to atrophy ectopic endometrium and lessen disease-associated inflammation. Agents include NSAIDs, COCs, oral progestins, androgens, GnRH agonists, GnRH antagonists, and aromatase inhibitors. For most, suitable initial regimens are NSAIDS combined with COCs or with a progestin. These agents may be initiated if endometriosis is suspected in a woman with CPP or may be started following diagnostic laparoscopy. Following laparoscopy, if initial therapy fails to control pain, switching to a different medication is suitable. With empiric therapy, if an initial agent(s) is ineffective, either diagnostic laparoscopy or medication change is indicated (American College of Obstetricians and Gynecologists, 2018). For those who fail to respond to progestin-containing options, a GnRH agent is reasonable. Although medical treatment improves pain, relapse rates are high with therapy discontinuation (Bozdag, 2015).

If infertility is the presenting symptom, fertility-preserving treatment without ovulation suppression will be required, as

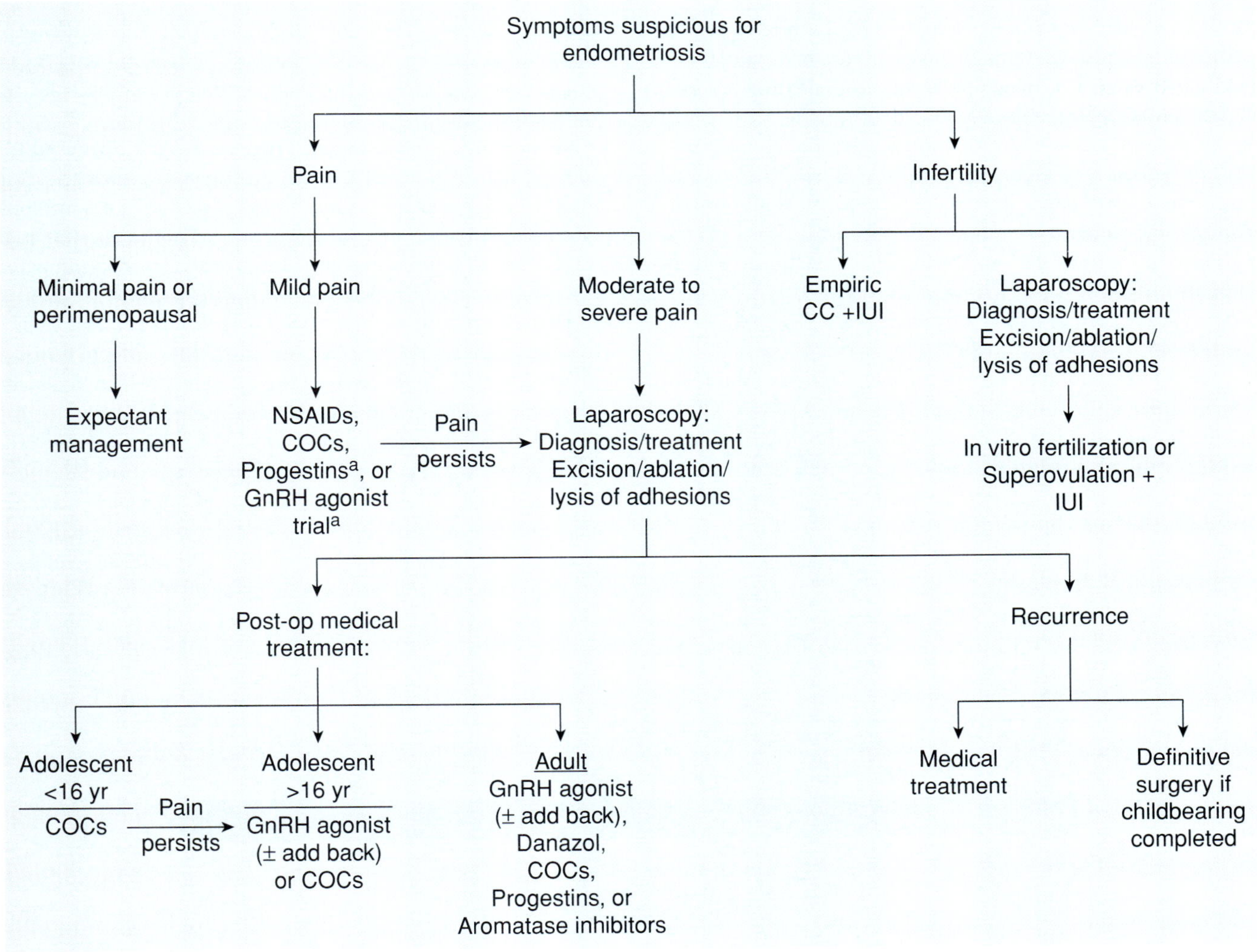

FIGURE 11-8 Diagnostic and treatment algorithm for women with presumptive or proven endometriosis. CC = clomiphene citrate; COCs = combination oral contraceptive pills; GnRH = gonadotropin-releasing hormone; IUI = intrauterine insemination; NSAIDs = nonsteroidal antiinflammatory drugs. [a]Agents not recommended for adolescents younger than 16 years.

outlined on page 274. In contrast, if the patient has severe, recalcitrant pain and has completed childbearing, definitive surgery may be indicated, as described on page 246.

Medical Treatment of Pain

Expectant Management

For many women, symptoms will preclude them from choosing expectant management. However, for those with mild symptoms or for asymptomatic women diagnosed incidentally, expectant management may be appropriate (Moen, 2002). Sutton and associates (1997) expectantly managed patients initially diagnosed by laparoscopy with minimal to moderate endometriosis. At second-look laparoscopy after 1 year, 29 percent of women had disease regression, 42 percent remained unchanged, and 29 percent had disease progression. Other investigators have shown similar rates of disease regression with expectant management (Thomas, 1987). These studies are confined to patients with minimal to moderate endometriosis. No well-designed trials have examined expectant management for severe disease.

Nonsteroidal Antiinflammatory Drugs

Both cyclooxygenase (COX)-1 and COX-2 enzymes promote synthesis of prostaglandins involved in the pain and inflammation associated with endometriosis. Specifically, endometriotic tissue expresses COX-2 at greater levels than eutopic endometrium (Cho, 2010). Accordingly, therapy aimed at lowering these prostaglandin levels helps alleviate endometriosis-associated pain. Indeed, NSAIDs often are first-line therapy in women with primary dysmenorrhea or CPP from suspected or known endometriosis. That said, study evidence supporting NSAIDs for this disease is scant and is extrapolated from efficacy data in primary dysmenorrhea (Kauppila, 1985; Marjoribanks, 2010).

The NSAIDs listed in Table 11-1 nonselectively inhibit both COX-1 and COX-2 enzymes. In contrast, selective COX-2 inhibitors specifically inhibit the COX-2 isoenzyme. Due to the cardiovascular risks with long-term use of selective COX-2 inhibitors, these medications are used at the lowest possible dose and for the shortest duration necessary (Jones, 2005). Thus, drugs in Table 11-1 are primarily selected.

Described earlier, central sensitization can lead to neuropathic pain in women with endometriosis. Multimodal approaches to chronic pain are discussed in Chapter 12 and listed in Table 12-5 (p. 263).

Combination Hormonal Contraceptives

These estrogen plus progestin-containing agents are a mainstay for the initial treatment of endometriosis-related pain. They inhibit gonadotropin release, decrease menstrual flow, and decidualize implants. As such, abundant study evidence supports use of COC pills or the contraceptive patch or ring to relieve endometriosis-related pain (Harada, 2008; Vercellini, 1993, 2010). These provide contraception and other noncontraceptive benefits, which are balanced against risks enumerated in Chapter 5 (p. 121).

COCs can be used conventionally in a cyclic regimen or may be used continuously without a break for withdrawal menses (American Society for Reproductive Medicine, 2014). The continuous regimen decreases the frequency of painful menses and improves CPP (Guzick, 2011). For endometriosis-related pain, monophasic COCs are preferred. Low-dose COCs (containing ≤20 μg ethinyl estradiol) are not superior to conventional-dose COCs for endometriosis treatment, but lower doses may lead to higher rates of breakthrough bleeding (Gallo, 2013).

Progestins

This family of hormones often is used for endometriosis therapy. Progestins antagonize the estrogenic effects on the endometrium. They cause initial decidualization and subsequent endometrial atrophy. For endometriosis treatment, oral progestins, depot progestins, or progestin-eluting intrauterine devices are options.

As supporting evidence, one randomized trial compared the effect of oral high-dose (100 mg) medroxyprogesterone acetate (MPA) daily given for 6 months and placebo. At second-look laparoscopy, partial or total resolution of peritoneal implants was noted in 60 percent of progestin-treated women compared with 18 percent of the placebo group. Furthermore, pelvic pain and defecatory pain were significantly reduced (Telimaa, 1987). In practice, MPA is prescribed in oral dosages ranging from 20 to 100 mg daily. Side effects of high-dose MPA included acne, edema, weight gain, and irregular menstrual bleeding.

Norethindrone acetate (NETA) is a 19-nortestosterone synthetic progestin. In one study, investigators administered an initial oral dosage of NETA, 5 mg daily, with increases of 2.5 mg daily until amenorrhea or a maximal dosage of 20 mg daily was reached. They found an approximately 90-percent reduction in dysmenorrhea and pelvic pain (Muneyyirci-Delale, 1998). Discussed later, NETA also is used as adjunct therapy with GnRH agents to blunt the bone loss linked with those drugs (DiVasta, 2015).

TABLE 11-1. Commonly Used Oral Nonsteroidal Antiinflammatory Drugs (NSAIDs) in the Treatment of Endometriosis-Associated Dysmenorrhea

Generic Name	Trade Name	Dosage
Ibuprofen	Motrin, Advil	400 mg every 4–6 h
Naproxen	Naprosyn, Aleve	500 mg initially, then 250 mg every 6–8 h
Naproxen sodium	Anaprox	550 mg initially, then 275 mg every 6–8 h
Mefenamic acid	Ponstel	500 mg initially, then 250 mg every 6 h
Ketoprofen	Orudis, Oruvail	50 mg every 6–8 h

Dienogest is another 19-nortestosterone synthetic progestin suitable for endometriosis. In one randomized study, it was significantly more effective than placebo for reducing endometriosis-associated pain when used orally at a dosage of 2 mg daily (Strowitzki, 2010a). Other trials show efficacy equivalent to that of GnRH agonists (Harada, 2009; Strowitzki, 2010b). Currently, this progestin alone is not available in the United States. It is, however, coupled with estradiol valerate in the Food and Drug Administration (FDA)-approved COC marketed as Natazia.

Alternatively, MPA may be given intramuscularly in depot form in a dosage of 150 mg every 3 months. In depot form, MPA may delay resumption of normal menses and ovulation and thus is less suitable for women contemplating imminent pregnancy. Subcutaneous formulation of MPA, marketed as Depo-SubQ Provera 104, also is effective (Schlaff, 2006).

Discussed in Chapter 5 (p. 127), the Depo-Provera package insert carries a "black box warning." This explains that prolonged DMPA use may result in bone mineral density (BMD) loss, that this loss is greater with increasing duration of use, and that the loss may not be completely reversible. Labeling recommends limiting use to 2 years unless other contraceptive methods are inadequate. Thus, the risks and benefits of treatment are weighed if contemplating long-term DMPA therapy. Bone density surveillance with dual energy x-ray absorptiometry (DEXA) scanning is not recommended (American College of Obstetricians and Gynecologists, 2019).

The levonorgestrel-releasing intrauterine system (LNG-IUS) (Mirena) delivers levonorgestrel directly to the endometrium and is approved for use up to 5 years. One small randomized trial that incorporated second-look laparoscopy showed improved endometriosis stage with both LNG-IUS and the comparator GnRH treatment. In other small randomized trials, the LNG-IUS provided improved symptoms compared against expectant management, DMPA, or GnRH agonists (Petta, 2005; Tanmahasamut, 2012; Vercellini, 2003b; Wong, 2010). The LNG-IUS also is effective for postoperative endometriosis suppression (Abou-Setta, 2013). However, in patients with bowel endometriosis, the LNG-IUS may be ineffective for symptoms (Hinterholzer, 2007). It likely also is less effective for other lesions types that are remote from the uterus. Contraindications to LNG-IUS use are listed in Chapter 5 (p. 115).

Intuitively, the Nexplanon implant that chronically releases the progestin etonogestrel might be considered for endometriosis. Data regarding its efficacy for this indication are limited. One small randomized study comparing this implant and DMPA reported comparable efficacy (Walch, 2009). A recent small prospective trial using a VAS score showed improved dysmenorrhea and dyspareunia at both 6 and 12 months compared with baseline scores (Sansone, 2018).

GnRH Agonists

Endogenous pulsatile release of GnRH prompts secretory activity of the gonadotropes within the anterior pituitary. Gonadotropin release from the pituitary then leads to ovarian steroidogenesis and ovulation. However, continuous, nonpulsatile GnRH administration results in pituitary desensitization and subsequent loss of ovarian sex steroid hormone production.

These features allow pharmacologic use of GnRH agonists for endometriosis treatment. With loss of ovarian estradiol production, the hypoestrogenic environment removes the stimulation normally provided to the endometriotic implants and creates a pseudomenopausal state during treatment. In addition to this direct effect, GnRH agonists also reduce COX-2 levels in patients with endometriosis (Kim, 2009).

GnRH agonists are inactive if taken orally, but intramuscular (IM), subcutaneous (SC), and intranasal preparations are available. Leuprolide acetate (Lupron Depot) is available in a 3.75-mg monthly dose or an 11.25-mg 3-month dose, both given IM. Less frequently used GnRH agonists include goserelin (Zoladex) administered as a 3.6-mg monthly or a 10.8-mg 3-month SC depot implant; triptorelin (Trelstar) given as a 3.75-mg monthly IM injection; and nafarelin (Synarel) used in a 200-mg twice-daily nasal spray regimen. All of these except triptorelin carry specific FDA approval for endometriosis treatment.

Pain Improvement. Empirically, GnRH agonists may be used *prior to laparoscopy* in women with CPP and clinical suspicion of endometriosis. In one study, pain scores after 3 months of GnRH agonist treatment significantly declined compared with those after placebo (Ling, 1999). Subsequent laparoscopy revealed that 93 percent of these women had surgically diagnosed endometriosis. In suspected cases, depot leuprolide acetate may be used empirically *in lieu of laparoscopy* for satisfactory symptom improvement. However, an empiric GnRH trial is not routinely offered to patients younger than 16 years. GnRH agonist effects on long-term BMD have not been adequately studied in this age group.

In those with *surgically confirmed* endometriosis, numerous studies demonstrate the effectiveness of GnRH agonist therapy to improve pain symptoms (Brown, 2010). The GnRH agonists provide greater relief when administered for 6 months compared with 3 months (Hornstein, 1995b). As noted in the prior sections, GnRH agonists compares favorably with other drugs used for endometriosis treatment. In one metaanalysis of postoperative GnRH therapy, GnRH treatment reduced the endometriosis recurrence risk compared with placebo or expectant management (Zheng, 2016). Although GnRH agonist treatment is highly effective, its cost and side effects often favor trials of COCs or progestins first.

Add-Back Therapy. Concerns regarding the effects of prolonged hypoestrogenism preclude extended treatment with GnRH agonists alone. Hypoestrogenic symptoms include hot flashes, insomnia, reduced libido, vaginal dryness, and headaches. Moreover, both spine and hip BMD decline at 3 and 6 months of GnRH agonist therapy, with only partial recovery at 12 to 15 months after treatment (Orwoll, 1994).

Because of the greater osteoporosis risk and vasomotor symptoms, hormone therapy usually is added. Daily progestins or a low-dose estrogen plus progestin regimen is suitable and is termed *add-back therapy*. With this therapy, a GnRH agonist may be used longer than 6 months (American College of Obstetricians and Gynecologists, 2018). The goal of add-back therapy is to supply sufficient estrogen to minimize GnRH agonist side effects yet still maintain a hypoestrogenic state to suppress endometriosis. Barbieri (1992) explained that tissues have varied sensitivity to estrogen, and a concentration of estrogen that will partially prevent bone loss may not stimulate endometrial growth. This "estrogen threshold" has not been established but is thought to approximate 30 to 40 pg/mL of estradiol.

Several regimens appear equally effective (Wu, 2014). In one 12-month study, NETA, 5 mg orally daily, with or without conjugated equine estrogen (Premarin) 0.625 mg orally daily, provided extended pain relief and preserved BMD (Hornstein, 1998). Another regimen of 25-μg transdermal estradiol plus daily 5 mg oral MPA showed that GnRH remained effective in reducing endometriosis pain (Edmonds, 1996). Traditional COCs also may be used effectively as add-back agents.

The extent of BMD decline has been evaluated with add-back therapy. Although bone loss was noted in all patients undergoing GnRH agonist treatment, the extent of loss was far lower or absent in the add-back group (Edmonds, 1994). Quality of life also is improved with add-back therapy (Zupi, 2004).

Ideally, this therapy is initiated simultaneously with the GnRH agonist. Little benefit is gained by deferring add-back therapy, and patients who receive add-back concurrently with agonist therapy have less bone loss (Al-Azemi, 2009; Kiesel, 1996). Pain relief is identical to those using GnRH agonist alone. Supplemental calcium as a 1000-mg total daily dose is recommended along with add-back regimens (American College of Obstetricians and Gynecologists, 2018).

GnRH Antagonists

GnRH antagonists are a newer category of GnRH analogues capable of suppressing gonadotropin production. Unlike GnRH agonists, GnRH antagonists do not produce an initial release or *flare* of gonadotropins. Thus, suppression of gonadotropins and of sex steroid hormones is immediate.

Elagolix is a nonapeptide, orally bioactive GnRH antagonist taken daily. One 24-week randomized trial showed similar efficacy between elagolix and DMPA for endometriosis-associated pain (Carr, 2014). Two phase III clinical trials assessed the clinical efficacy of a low-dose (150 mg daily) and a high-dose (200 mg twice daily) regimen provided for 6 months. Both regimens significantly reduced dysmenorrhea and nonmenstrual pelvic pain compared with placebo after 3 months. Compared with placebo, the high-dose regimen also led to lower levels of dyspareunia (Taylor, 2017). An extension of the above trials showed sustained improvements in dysmenorrhea, nonmenstrual pelvic pain, and dyspareunia at the 12-month mark. Greater effects were seen with the high-dose regimen (Surrey, 2018). Marketed in the United States as Orilissa, this agent appears best suited as second-line therapy after COCs.

Aromatase Inhibitors

In endometriotic tissue, estrogen may be produced locally through aromatization of circulating androgens. This may clarify the pathogenesis of postmenopausal endometriosis or may explain cases in which symptoms persist despite conventional treatment. Hormonal strategies described in prior sections target ovarian estrogen production but have little effect on estrogens produced from other sources. In contrast, aromatase inhibitors (AIs) block aromatase action and estradiol production in both the ovary and extraovarian sites. As a result, estrogen levels are dramatically suppressed, and AIs have hypoestrogenic side-effect profiles similar to those of GnRH agonists (Pavone, 2012). AIs used clinically include anastrozole (Arimidex) and letrozole (Femara).

A serious concern is ovarian cyst formation. Shown in Figure 21-3 (p. 456), by blocking the conversion of androgens to estrogens in ovarian granulosa cells, AIs reduce the negative feedback at the pituitary–hypothalamus level. This leads to increased GnRH secretion. Concomitant elevations in luteinizing hormone (LH) and follicle-stimulating hormone promote increased ovarian follicular development. Therefore, AIs always are combined with a progestins, COCs, or GnRH agonist to help blunt this significant side effect (Shippen, 2004).

Small studies that combined AIs with NETA or with COCs support this approach for pain relief (Amsterdam, 2005; Ferrero, 2009). However, due to side effects and limited data, such AI combinations are usually prescribed to women after other options for medical or surgical treatment have been exhausted (Dunselman, 2014).

Progesterone-Receptor Modulators

Progestins produce agonist effects upon binding to progesterone receptors. In contrast, progesterone antagonists and selective progesterone-receptor modulators (SPRMs) are agents that vary in their progesterone-receptor binding. Progesterone antagonists universally bind to and inactivate these receptors. SPRMS, depending on their individual pharmacologic profile, may activate or inactive progesterone receptors variably within different tissue types (Chap. 16, p. 366).

Of progesterone antagonists, mifepristone (Mifeprex) is currently FDA-approved solely for early pregnancy termination. When studied in patients with endometriosis, mifepristone reduced both pelvic pain and the extent of endometriosis (Kettel, 1996). Unfortunately, mifepristone's antiprogestational effects expose the endometrium to chronic unopposed estrogen. The resulting endometrial changes range from endometrial hyperplasia to a new category described as progesterone-receptor-modulator–associated endometrial changes (PAECs), described next (Mutter, 2008).

Of SPRMs, ulipristal acetate is available in the United States for emergency contraception as single-dose Ella. In Europe and Canada for presurgical treatment of leiomyomas, Esmya and Fibristal, respectively, are administered over several weeks. With long-term use, ulipristal acetate also is associated with endometrial PAECs, which carry unclear clinical significance for both eutopic and ectopic endometria. This limits its chronic use at this time. However, a recent systematic review of 10 studies and 1450 participants showed that ulipristal acetate–associated premalignant changes were rare (0.4 percent) and always reversible. PAEC developed in 40 to 80 percent of the participants that were treated with extended-use ulipristal acetate (De Milliano, 2017). Rare but serious liver injury also has been reported and is detailed in Chapter 9 (p. 208). Other SPRMs are still experimental at this time.

Selective Estrogen-Receptor Modulators

Bazedoxifene (BZA) is a third-generation selective estrogen-receptor modulator (SERM). Discussed in Chapter 22 (p. 482),

BZA is pharmacologically coupled with conjugated equine estrogen, and BZA/CEE (Duavee) is indicated for menopause symptom relief and osteoporosis prevention. BZA alone prompts lesion regression in an endometriosis rodent model (Lyu, 2015). Either alone or with a GnRH antagonist, BZA/CEE also was effective in a small case series for symptom suppression in patients with confirmed endometriosis (Hill, 2018).

Raloxifene is another SERM. Despite reassuring animal data showing implant regression, a subsequent trial using raloxifene in patients with endometriosis was stopped early due to early CPP relapse (Stratton, 2008; Yao, 2005).

Androgens

These agents are now used as second-line treatment for endometriosis due to their androgenic side effects. Danazol (Danocrine) is a synthetic 17α-ethinyl testosterone derivative. Its predominant action suppresses the midcycle LH surge to promote chronic anovulation (Floyd, 1980). It also occupies receptor sites on sex hormone–binding globulin to raise serum free testosterone levels and binds directly to androgen and progesterone receptors. In sum, danazol creates a hypoestrogenic, hyperandrogenic state that promotes endometriotic lesion atrophy (Godin, 2015).

Regarding efficacy, danazol given orally at dosages of 200 mg three times daily is superior to placebo to diminish endometriotic implant size and pelvic pain symptoms after 6 months of therapy (Telimaa, 1987). A metaanalysis of five clinical trials assessed danazol efficacy for endometriosis-associated symptoms, excluding infertility. Compared with placebo, danazol offered substantial pain relief (Selak, 2007).

The recommended dosage of danazol is 600 to 800 mg orally daily. Unfortunately, significant androgenic side effects develop and include acne, hot flashes, hirsutism, adverse serum lipid profiles, voice deepening (possibly irreversible), elevation of liver enzyme levels, and mood changes. Moreover, due to possible teratogenicity, this medication should be taken in conjunction with effective contraception. Because of its adverse side-effect profile, danazol is prescribed less frequently, and if administered, its duration is limited.

Gestrinone is an antiprogestational agent prescribed in Europe for endometriosis. It has antiprogestational, antiestrogenic, and androgenic effects. Gestrinone equals the effectiveness of danazol and of GnRH agonists for relief of endometriosis-related pain (Prentice, 2000). Furthermore, during 6 months of treatment, gestrinone was not associated with the BMD decline commonly seen with GnRH agonist use and was more effective in persistently decreasing moderate to severe pelvic pain (Gestrinone Italian Study Group, 1996). Unfortunately, one of the side effects of gestrinone appears to be lowering high-density lipoprotein (HDL) levels. Gestrinone can be administered as 2.5-mg oral twice weekly dose.

■ Surgical Treatment of Pain
Lesion Removal and Adhesiolysis

Because laparoscopy is the primary method for endometriosis diagnosis, concurrent surgical treatment is an attractive option. As evidence, diagnostic laparoscopy alone was compared with laparoscopic endometriotic lesion ablation plus uterine nerve ablation in one randomized trial. In the ablation group, 63 percent of women attained significant symptom relief compared with 23 percent in the expectant management group (Jones, 2001).

The optimal method to address endometriotic implants for maximal symptom relief is controversial. First, laser ablation does not appear to be more effective than conventional electrosurgical coagulation of endometriosis (Blackwell, 1991). Second, ablation and excision both appear to perform suitably. In one randomized trial, ablation was compared with excision of lesions in women with stage I or II endometriosis. At 6 months, similar reductions in pain scores were found (Wright, 2005). Another study showed no significant difference between ablation and excision at 12 months (Healey, 2010). However, at 5 years, the need for further hormonal or analgesic treatment was greater in the ablation group (Healey, 2014). For deeply infiltrative endometriosis, some authors have advocated radical surgical excision, although well-designed trials are lacking (Chapron, 2004).

Unfortunately, recurrence is common following surgical excision. Jones and associates (2001) demonstrated pain recurrence in 74 percent of patients at a mean time of 73 months postoperatively. The median time for recurrence was 20 months. After surgery for pain-related endometriosis, postoperative medical treatment may be elected to extend pain relief or treat residual pain. For this, the most rigorous evidence supports COCs or the LNG-IUS (Somigliana, 2014).

Adhesiolysis is postulated to effectively treat pain symptoms in women with endometriosis by restoring normal anatomy. However, most studies are poorly designed and retrospective. As a result, a definitive link between adhesions and pelvic pain is unclear (Hammoud, 2004). For example, one randomized trial demonstrated no overall pain relief from adhesiolysis compared with expectant management (Peters, 1992). However, within this study, one woman with severe, dense, vascularized bowel adhesions experienced pain relief following adhesiolysis.

Adhesion prevention during endometriosis surgery emphasizes sound surgical techniques described in Chapter 40 (p. 855). Of adhesion-prevention agents available in the United States, small studies show lower adhesions reformation rates with use of the cellulose barrier Interceed in endometriosis cases (Mais, 1995a; Sekiba, 1992). However, as noted by the American Society for Reproductive Medicine (2013), although peritoneal instillates and barriers may reduce postoperative adhesions, this has not translated clinically into improved pain, fertility, or bowel obstruction rates.

Endometrioma Resection

Endometriomas typically are treated surgically to exclude malignancy. To determine the best technique, both total ovarian cystectomy and aspiration coupled with cyst wall ablation have been compared. Of the two, cystectomy lowers endometrioma recurrence rates and pain symptoms and improves subsequent spontaneous pregnancy rates (Dan, 2013; Hart, 2008).

During surgery, steps are taken to preserve as much normal ovarian tissue as possible. To achieve this goal, electrosurgical coagulation of bleeding sites should be limited. As alternatives, some have described use of dilute vasopressin or ovarian suturing (Pergialiotis, 2015; Qiong-Zhen, 2014). Other technical steps are described in Chapters 43 (p. 939) and 44 (p. 1030). Despite cystectomy, endometriomas may recur. Liu and coworkers (2007) found an approximately 15 percent recurrence rate at 2 years following initial surgery.

Importantly, women who undergo endometrioma excision may subsequently have reduced *ovarian reserve*, that is, the capacity to provide ova capable of fertilization (Somigliana, 2012). Additionally, surgery also raises the risk for adhesion formation. Both effects may diminish future fertility. Accordingly, in a woman who is asymptomatic, has a small endometrioma that displays classic findings, has a known endometriosis diagnosis, and has normal or stable CA125 levels, surveillance is an option (American College of Obstetricians and Gynecologists, 2016, 2018). This approach may benefit asymptomatic women with recurrent endometriomas, as repeat surgery can again diminish reserve (Ferrero, 2015). Following initial diagnosis, repeat TVS is recommended 6 to 12 weeks later to exclude a hemorrhagic cyst. Endometriomas then may be sonographically surveilled in asymptomatic women yearly or sooner, at the clinician's discretion (Levine, 2010). The main disadvantage to observation is an inability to exclude ovarian malignancy, and thus patient counseling is essential.

Presacral Neurectomy

For some women, transection of the presacral nerves lying within the presacral space may provide relief of CPP (Fig. 38-23, p. 812). This surgery is most effective for midline pain.

For endometriosis, results from a randomized trial revealed significantly greater pain relief at 12 months postoperatively in women treated with presacral neurectomy (PSN) and endometriotic excision compared with that from endometriotic excision alone (86 percent versus 57 percent) (Zullo, 2003). However, all of these women had midline pain. One metaanalysis demonstrated a significant decline in CPP after PSN compared with more conservative procedures, but only in those with midline pain (Proctor, 2005). PSN may be performed laparoscopically, but it is technically challenging. Moreover, postoperative constipation and voiding dysfunction due to involved nerve disruption are common (Huber, 2015). For these reasons, PSN is used in a limited manner and not recommended routinely for endometriosis-related pain relief.

Laparoscopic uterosacral nerve ablation (LUNA) destroys nerve fibers that pass to the uterus through the uterosacral ligaments. No evidence supports LUNA for endometriosis-related pain (Vercellini, 2003a). In a randomized trial of 487 women with CPP and with or without minimal endometriosis, LUNA did not improve pain, dysmenorrhea, dyspareunia, or quality-of-life scores compared with laparoscopy without pelvic denervation (Daniels, 2009).

Abdominal versus Laparoscopic Approach

All of the surgical procedures listed above can be completed through open or laparoscopic approaches. First, for benign ovarian masses such as endometriomas, strong evidence supports laparoscopy (Mais, 1995b; Yuen, 1997). Laparoscopic treatment of endometrioma carries an associated 5-percent risk for

conversion to laparotomy. However, because of its efficacy and low rates of postoperative morbidity, laparoscopy is a preferred route when feasible (Canis, 2003).

For excision of endometriotic implants, laparoscopy is associated with demonstrated effectiveness and low morbidity rates. Moreover, adhesiolysis is preferred via laparoscopy when safe, and laparoscopy leads to less de novo adhesion formation than laparotomy (Gutt, 2004). Although requiring advanced skills, laparoscopic PSN appears to be as effective as laparotomy (Nezhat, 1992; Redwine, 1991).

Hysterectomy

This procedure is the definitive and most effective therapy for women with endometriosis who do not wish to retain fertility. It is appropriate for women with intractable pain, adnexal masses, or multiple previous conservative therapies or surgeries (American College of Obstetricians and Gynecologists, 2018). Hysterectomy for patients with endometriosis suitably may be completed laparoscopically, abdominally, or vaginally. However, adhesions and distorted anatomy secondary to endometriosis often makes a vaginal approach difficult, especially if adnexectomy is planned. Consequently, procedure route depends on equipment availability, operator experience, and disease extent.

Oophorectomy. Prior to hysterectomy for endometriosis, oophorectomy may be discussed. A general discussion of risks and benefits is found in Chapter 43 (p. 957). Specific to endometriosis, the benefits of pain relief and reoperation risks are measured against complications of hypoestrogenism.

In one study, of those with hysterectomy and bilateral salpingo-oophorectomy (BSO), 10 percent had recurrent CPP and 4 percent required reoperation. Compared with these women, those choosing ovarian conservation had a sixfold greater risk of recurrent pain and an eightfold greater risk of requiring additional surgery (Namnoum, 1995). In a second study, among all those choosing hysterectomy, ovarian conservation doubled the reoperation rate compared with those undergoing BSO (Shakiba, 2008). Moreover, in a subanalysis of those older than 40, ovary conservation lead to a sevenfold greater reoperation rate than BSO. However, in those younger than 40, reoperation rates did not differ whether ovaries were retained or removed. American College of Obstetricians and Gynecologists (2018) notes that ovarian conservation can be considered in patients undergoing hysterectomy if ovaries appear normal.

In epidemiologic studies, women with prior endometriosis have slightly greater ovarian cancer rates and higher proportions of clear cell and endometrioid subtypes (Kim, 2014; Pearce, 2012; Somigliana, 2006). That said, the risk is still small, and consensus guidelines do not recommend management changes based on this cancer potential (Dunselman, 2014).

Postoperative Hormone Replacement. Women with surgical menopause usually are younger and would likely benefit from estrogen replacement. Options are discussed in Chapter 22 (p. 479). Although evidence is lacking, some sources suggest that treatment in these women ideally continues until the time of expected natural menopause.

Unopposed estrogen is appropriate for hypoestrogenic women without a uterus. However, endometriosis recurrence has been reported with this therapy in women with severe endometriosis first treated with hysterectomy and BSO (Taylor, 1999). These symptoms required repeat surgery and did not recur with subsequent treatment with combined estrogen and progestin regimens. Additionally, cases of endometrial carcinoma have been reported in women with endometriosis treated with unopposed estrogen after hysterectomy and BSO (Reimnitz, 1988; Soliman, 2006). This is rare and may arise from incompletely resected pelvic endometriosis. Therefore, adding a progestin to estrogen replacement therapy can be considered in women with severe endometriosis that was treated surgically (Moen, 2010). However, the risks of malignancy are balanced against the adverse lipid changes and breast cancer risks associated with adding progesterone to estrogen replacement therapy.

The optimal timing for estrogen replacement initiation following hysterectomy with BSO is guided by limited data. One small study showed no significant differences in postoperative recurrent pain rates whether hormones were begun immediately after surgery or were delayed (Hickman, 1998).

Endometriosis-Related Infertility

For an asymptomatic woman with infertility, laparoscopy solely to exclude endometriosis is unwarranted (American Society for Reproductive Medicine, 2012). For those with endometriosis-related pain undergoing medical therapy, treatment does not raise fecundity (Hughes, 2007). An exception is the use of GnRH agonists for endometriosis treatment in patients who plan to undergo IVF or intracytoplasmic sperm injection (ICSI). Namely, a Cochrane review assessed three randomized trial of GnRH agonist treatment in patients with endometriosis planning IVF. Treatment significantly raised pregnancy rates (Sallam, 2006).

For women with infertility and minimal to mild endometriosis, surgical ablation may be beneficial, although the effect appears small (Marcoux, 1997). However, other researchers report a fertility benefit from surgical ablation for mild to moderate endometriosis (Parazzini, 1999). A metaanalysis of these two studies did demonstrate an advantage for laparoscopic surgery compared with diagnostic laparoscopy alone. Based on this study, nearly eight women would need to under laparoscopic surgery for one additional clinical pregnancy (Jacobson, 2002, 2010).

Moderate to severe endometriosis may be treated with surgery to restore normal anatomy and tubal function. However, for women with severe endometriosis, well-designed trials examining the role of surgery for subfertility are limited (Crosignani, 1996). In infertile women with stage III/IV endometriosis, clinicians can consider operative laparoscopy, instead of expectant management, to increase spontaneous pregnancy rates (Dunselman, 2014). However, after initial unsuccessful surgery for infertility, IVF is preferable to reoperation (Pagidas, 1996).

Alternatively, patients with endometriosis and infertility are candidates for fertility treatments such as controlled ovarian hyperstimulation, intrauterine insemination, and IVF (Chap. 21, p. 450). In particular, IVF is the most effective treatment for infertility in patients with endometriosis. Numerous studies show similar live-birth rates following IVF in patients with all stages of endometriosis (endometriomas excluded) and patients without this disease (Bukulmez, 2001; Opøien, 2012; Ozkan, 2008).

REFERENCES

Abou-Setta AM, Houston B, Al-Inany HG, et al: Levonorgestrel-releasing intrauterine device (LNG-IUD) for symptomatic endometriosis following surgery. Cochrane Database Syst Rev 1:CD005072, 2013

Adamson GD: Endometriosis fertility index: is it better than the present staging systems? Curr Opin Obstet Gynecol 25(3):186, 2013

Adamson GD, Pasta DJ: Endometriosis fertility index: the new, validated endometriosis staging system. Fertil Steril 94(5):1609, 2010

Agarwal SK, Chapron C, Giudice LC, et al: Clinical diagnosis of endometriosis: a call to action. Am J Obstet Gynecol 220(4): 354, 2019

Alabiso G, Alio L, Arena S, et al: How to manage bowel endometriosis: the ETIC approach. J Minim Invasive Gynecol 22(4):517, 2015

Al-Azemi M, Jones G, Sirkeci F, et al: Immediate and delayed add-back hormonal replacement therapy during ultra long GnRH agonist treatment of chronic cyclical pelvic pain. BJOG 116:1646, 2009

Alifano M: Catamenial pneumothorax. Curr Opin Pulm Med 16(4):381, 2010

Allen C, Hopewell S, Prentice A: Non-steroidal anti-inflammatory drugs for pain in women with endometriosis. Cochrane Database Syst Rev 4: CD004753, 2005

American College of Obstetricians and Gynecologists: Evaluation and management of adnexal masses. Practice Bulletin No. 174, November 2016

American College of Obstetricians and Gynecologists: Management of endometriosis. Practice Bulletin No. 114, July 2010, Reaffirmed 2018

American College of Obstetricians and Gynecologists: Depot medroxyprogesterone acetate and bone effects. Committee Opinion No. 602, June 2014, Reaffirmed 2019

American Society for Reproductive Medicine: Revised American Society for Reproductive Medicine classification of endometriosis: 1996. Fertil Steril 67:817, 1997

American Society for Reproductive Medicine: Endometriosis and infertility: a committee opinion. Fertil Steril 98(3):591, 2012

American Society for Reproductive Medicine, Society of Reproductive Surgeons: Pathogenesis, consequences, and control of peritoneal adhesions in gynecologic surgery: a committee opinion. Fertil Steril 99(6):1550, 2013

American Society for Reproductive Medicine: Treatment of pelvic pain associated with endometriosis: a committee opinion. Fertil Steril 101(4):927, 2014

Amsterdam LL, Gentry W, Jobanputra S, et al: Anastrazole and oral contraceptives: a novel treatment for endometriosis. Fertil Steril 84:300, 2005

Antonelli A, Simeone C, Zani D, et al: Clinical aspects and surgical treatment of urinary tract endometriosis: our experience with 31 cases. Eur Urol 49:1093, 2006

Arici A, Seli E, Zeyneloglu HB, et al: Interleukin-8 induces proliferation of endometrial stromal cells: a potential autocrine growth factor. J Clin Endocrinol Metab 83(4):1201, 1998

Arosh JA, Lee J, Balasubbramanian D, et al: Molecular and preclinical basis to inhibit PGE2 receptors EP2 and EP4 as a novel nonsteroidal therapy for endometriosis. Proc Natl Acad Sci U S A 112(31):9716, 2015

As-Sanie S, Harris RE, Harte SE, et al: Increased pressure pain sensitivity in women with chronic pelvic pain. Obstet Gynecol 122(5):1047, 2013

As-Sanie S, Harris RE, Napadow V, et al: Changes in regional gray matter volume in women with chronic pelvic pain: a voxel-based morphometry study. Pain 153(5):1006, 2012

Attia GR, Zeitoun K, Edwards D, et al: Progesterone receptor isoform A but not B is expressed in endometriosis. J Clin Endocrinol Metab 85:2897, 2000

Bajaj P, Bajaj P, Madsen H, et al: Endometriosis is associated with central sensitization: a psychophysical controlled study. J Pain 4(7):372, 2003

Balasch J, Creus M, Fabregues F, et al: Visible and non-visible endometriosis at laparoscopy in fertile and infertile women and in patients with chronic pelvic pain: a prospective study. Hum Reprod 11:387, 1996

Ballard KD, Seaman HE, de Vries CS, et al: Can symptomatology help in the diagnosis of endometriosis? Findings from a national case–control study—part 1. BJOG 115(11):1382, 2008

Barbieri RL: Hormone treatment of endometriosis: the estrogen threshold hypothesis. Am J Obstet Gynecol 166:740, 1992

Barcena de Arellano ML, Arnold J, Vercellino F, et al: Overexpression of nerve growth factor in peritoneal fluid from women with endometriosis may promote neurite outgrowth in endometriotic lesions. Fertil Steril 95(3):1123, 2011

Bartel DP: MicroRNAs: target recognition and regulatory functions. Cell 136(2):215, 2009

Batt RE, Yeh J: Müllerianosis: four developmental (embryonic) mullerian diseases. Reprod Sci 20(9):1030, 2013

Bazot M, Daraï E: Diagnosis of deep endometriosis: clinical examination, ultrasonography, magnetic resonance imaging, and other techniques. Fertil Steril 108(6):886, 2017

Bazot M, Lafont C, Rouzier R, et al: Diagnostic accuracy of physical examination, transvaginal sonography, rectal endoscopic sonography, and magnetic resonance imaging to diagnose deep infiltrating endometriosis. Fertil Steril 92(6):1825, 2009

Bérubé S, Marcoux S, Langevin M, et al: Fecundity of infertile women with minimal or mild endometriosis and women with unexplained infertility. The Canadian Collaborative Group on Endometriosis. Fertil Steril 69(6):1034, 1998

Bhatt S, Kocakoc E, Dogra VS: Endometriosis: sonographic spectrum. Ultrasound Q 22(4):273, 2006

Blackwell RE: Applications of laser surgery in gynecology. Hype or high tech? Surg Clin North Am 71:1005, 1991

Bourdel N, Alves J, Pickering G, et al: Systematic review of endometriosis pain assessment: how to choose a scale? Hum Reprod Update 21(1):136, 2015

Bozdag G: Recurrence of endometriosis: risk factors, mechanisms and biomarkers. Womens Health (Lond) 11(5):693, 2015

Braun DP, Muriana A, Gebel H, et al: Monocyte-mediated enhancement of endometrial cell proliferation in women with endometriosis. Fertil Steril 61:78, 1994

Brown J, Pan A, Hart RJ: Gonadotrophin-releasing hormone analogues for pain associated with endometriosis. Cochrane Database Syst Rev 12:CD008475, 2010

Buck Louis GM, Hediger ML, Peterson CM, et al: Incidence of endometriosis by study population and diagnostic method: the ENDO study. Fertil Steril 96(2):360, 2011

Bukulmez O, Yarali H, Gurgan T: The presence and extent of endometriosis do not effect clinical pregnancy and implantation rates in patients undergoing intracytoplasmic sperm injection. Eur J Obstet Gynecol Reprod Biol 96(1):102, 2001

Bulun SE: Endometriosis. N Engl J Med 360(3):268, 2009

Bulun SE, Monsavais D, Pavone ME, et al: Role of estrogen receptor-β in endometriosis. Semin Reprod Med 30(1):39, 2012

Burney RO: The genetics and biochemistry of endometriosis. Curr Opin Obstet Gynecol 25(4):280, 2013

Canis M, Mage G, Wattiez A, et al: The ovarian endometrioma: why is it so poorly managed? Laparoscopic treatment of large ovarian endometrioma: why such a long learning curve? Hum Reprod 18:5, 2003

Carr B, Dmowski WP, O'Brien C, et al: Elagolix, an oral GnRH antagonist, versus subcutaneous depot medroxyprogesterone acetate for the treatment of endometriosis: effects on bone mineral density. Reprod Sci 21(11):1341, 2014

Chapron C, Chopin N, Borghese B, et al: Surgical management of deeply infiltrating endometriosis: an update. Ann NY Acad Sci 1034:326, 2004

Chapron C, Dubuisson JB, Pansini V, et al: Routine clinical examination is not sufficient for diagnosing and locating deeply infiltrating endometriosis. J Am Assoc Gynecol Laparosc 9:115, 2002

Cho S, Park SH, Choi YS, et al: Expression of cyclooxygenase-2 in eutopic endometrium and ovarian endometriotic tissue in women with severe endometriosis. Gynecol Obstet Invest 69:93, 2010

Crosignani PG, Vercellini P, Biffignandi F, et al: Laparoscopy versus laparotomy in conservative surgical treatment for severe endometriosis. Fertil Steril 66(5):706, 1996

D'Hooghe TM, Bambra CS, Raeymaekers BM, et al: The cycle pregnancy rate is normal in baboons with stage I endometriosis but decreased in primates with stage II and stage III-IV disease. Fertil Steril 66:809, 1996

D'Hooghe TM, Debrock S, Hill JA, et al: Endometriosis and subfertility: is the relationship resolved? Semin Reprod Med 21:243, 2003

Dalsgaard T, Hjordt Hansen MV, Hartwell D, et al: Reproductive prognosis in daughters of women with and without endometriosis. Hum Reprod 28(8):2284, 2013

Dan H, Limin F: Laparoscopic ovarian cystectomy versus fenestration/coagulation or laser vaporization for the treatment of endometriomas: a meta-analysis of randomized controlled trials. Gynecol Obstet Invest 76(2):75, 2013

Daniels J, Gray R, Hills RK, et al: Laparoscopic uterosacral nerve ablation for alleviating chronic pelvic pain: a randomized controlled trial. JAMA 302:955, 2009

De Milliano I, Van Hattum D, Ket JC, et al: Endometrial changes during ulipristal acetate use: a systematic review. Eur J Obstet Gynecol Reprod Biol 214:56, 2017

Ding Y, Zhu J: A retrospective review of abdominal wall endometriosis in Shanghai, China. Int J Gynaecol Obstet 121(1):41, 2013

DiVasta AD, Feldman HA, Sadler Gallagher J, et al: Hormonal add-back therapy for females treated with gonadotropin-releasing hormone agonist for endometriosis: a randomized controlled trial. Obstet Gynecol 126(3):617, 2015

Du H, Taylor HS: Contribution of bone-marrow-derived stem cell to endometrium and endometriosis. Stem Cells 25(8):2082, 2007

Dunselman GA, Vermeulen N, Becker C, et al: ESHRE guideline: management of women with endometriosis. Hum Reprod 29(3):400, 2014

Ecker AM, Donnellan NM, Shepherd JP, et al: Abdominal wall endometriosis: 12 years of experience at a large academic institution. Am J Obstet Gynecol 211(4):363.e1, 2014

Edmonds DK: Add-back therapy in the treatment of endometriosis: the European experience. BJOG 103(14 suppl):10, 1996

Edmonds DK, Howell R: Can hormone replacement therapy be used during medical therapy of endometriosis? BJOG 101(10 suppl):24, 1994

Eskenazi B, Warner M, Bonsignore L, et al: Validation study of nonsurgical diagnosis of endometriosis. Fertil Steril 76:929, 2001

Exacoustos C, Malzoni M, Di Giovanni A, et al: Ultrasound mapping system for the surgical management of deep infiltrating endometriosis. Fertil Steril 102(1):143, 2014a

Exacoustos C, Manganaro L, Zupi E: Imaging for the evaluation of endometriosis and adenomyosis. Best Pract Res Clin Obstet Gynaecol 28(5):655, 2014b

Fauconnier A, Chapron C, Dubuisson JB, et al: Relation between pain symptoms and the anatomic location of deep infiltrating endometriosis. Fertil Steril 78:719, 2002

Fedele L, Bianchi S, Bocciolone L, et al: Pain symptoms associated with endometriosis. Obstet Gynecol 79:767, 1992

Ferrero S, Camerini G, Seracchioli R, et al: Letrozole combined with norethisterone acetate compared with norethisterone acetate alone in the treatment of pain symptoms caused by endometriosis. Hum Reprod 24(12):3033, 2009

Ferrero S, Scala C, Racca A, et al: Second surgery for recurrent unilateral endometriomas and impact on ovarian reserve: a case-control study. Fertil Steril 103(5):1236, 2015

Figueira PG, Abrão MS, Krikun G, et al: Stem cells in endometrium and their role in the pathogenesis of endometriosis. Ann N Y Acad Sci 1221:10, 2011

Flores VA, Vanhie A, Dang T, et al: Progesterone receptor status predicts response to progestin therapy in endometriosis. J Clin Endocrinol Metab 103(12):4561, 2018

Floyd WS: Danazol: endocrine and endometrial effects. Int J Fertil 25:75, 1980

Gabriel B, Nassif J, Trompoukis P, et al: Prevalence and management of urinary tract endometriosis: a clinical case series. Urology 78(6):1269, 2011

Gallo MF, Nanda K, Grimes DA, et al: 20 μg versus >20 μg estrogen combined oral contraceptives for contraception. Cochrane Database Syst Rev 8: CD003989, 2013

Gambadauro P, Carli V, Hadlaczky G: Depressive symptoms among women with endometriosis: a systematic review and meta-analysis. Am J Obstet Gynecol 220(3):230, 2019

Gestrinone Italian Study Group: Gestrinone versus a gonadotropin-releasing hormone agonist for the treatment of pelvic pain associated with endometriosis: a multicenter, randomized, double-blind study. Fertil Steril 66:911, 1996

Godin R, Marcoux V: Vaginally administered danazol: an overlooked option in the treatment of rectovaginal endometriosis? J Obstet Gynaecol Can 37(12):1098, 2015

Gurates B, Bulun SE: Endometriosis: the ultimate hormonal disease. Semin Reprod Med 21:125, 2003

Gutt CN, Oniu T, Schemmer P, et al: Fewer adhesions induced by laparoscopic surgery? Surg Endosc 18:898, 2004

Guzick DS, Huang LS, Broadman BA, et al: Randomized trial of leuprolide versus continuous oral contraceptives in the treatment of endometriosis-associated pelvic pain. Fertil Steril 95(5):1568, 2011

Guzick DS, Silliman NP, Adamson GD, et al: Prediction of pregnancy in infertile women based on the American Society for Reproductive Medicine's revised classification of endometriosis. Fertil Steril 67:822, 1997

Haas D, Chvatal R, Habelsberger A, et al: Comparison of revised American Fertility Society and ENZIAN staging: a critical evaluation of classifications of endometriosis on the basis of our patient population. Fertil Steril 95(5):1574, 2011

Haga T, Kataoka H, Ebana H, et al: Thoracic endometriosis-related pneumothorax distinguished from primary spontaneous pneumothorax in females. Lung 192(4):583, 2014

Halme J, Hammond MG, Hulka JF, et al: Retrograde menstruation in healthy women and in patients with endometriosis. Obstet Gynecol 64(2):151, 1984

Hammoud A, Gago LA, Diamond MP: Adhesions in patients with chronic pelvic pain: a role for adhesiolysis? Fertil Steril 82:1483, 2004

Haney AF, Muscato J, Weinberg JB: Peritoneal fluid cell populations in infertility patients. Fertil Steril 35:696, 1981

Harada T, Momoeda M, Taketani Y, et al: Dienogest is as effective as intranasal buserelin acetate for the relief of pain symptoms associated with endometriosis—a randomized, double blind, multicentre trial. Fertil Steril 91(3):675, 2009

Harada T, Momoeda M, Taketani Y, et al: Low-dose oral contraceptive pill for dysmenorrhea associated with endometriosis: a placebo-controlled, double-blind, randomized trial. Fertil Steril 90:1583, 2008

Harb H, Gallos I, Chu J, et al: The effect of endometriosis on in vitro fertilisation outcome: a systematic review and meta-analysis. BJOG 120(11):1308, 2013

Hart RJ, Hickey M, Maouris P, et al: Excisional surgery versus ablative surgery for ovarian endometriomata. Cochrane Database Syst Rev 2:CD004992, 2008

Healey M, Ang WC, Cheng C: Surgical treatment of endometriosis: a prospective randomized double-blinded trial comparing excision and ablation. Fertil Steril 94(7):2536, 2010

Healey M, Cheng C, Kaur H: To excise or ablate endometriosis? A prospective randomized double-blinded trial after 5-year follow-up. J Minim Invasive Gynecol 21(6):999, 2014

Hickman TN, Namnoum AB, Hinton EL, et al: Timing of estrogen replacement therapy following hysterectomy with oophorectomy for endometriosis. Obstet Gynecol 91(5 Pt 1):673, 1998

Hill AM, Lessey B, Flores VA, et al: Bazedoxifene/conjugated estrogens in combination with leuprolide for the treatment of endometriosis. Clin Case Rep 6(6):990, 2018

Hinterholzer S, Riss D, Brustmann H: Symptomatic large bowel endometriosis in a woman with a hormonal intrauterine device: a case report. J Reprod Med 52:1055, 2007

Ho HN, Chao KH, Chen HF, et al: Peritoneal natural killer cytotoxicity and CD25+ CD3+ lymphocyte subpopulation are decreased in women with stage III-IV endometriosis. Hum Reprod 10:2671, 1995

Hornstein MD, Harlow BL, Thomas PP, et al: Use of a new CA 125 assay in the diagnosis of endometriosis. Hum Reprod 10:932, 1995a

Hornstein MD, Surrey ES, Weisberg GW, et al: Leuprolide acetate depot and hormonal add-back in endometriosis: a 12-month study. Lupron Add-Back Study Group. Obstet Gynecol 91:16, 1998

Hornstein MD, Yuzpe AA, Burry KA, et al: Prospective randomized double-blind trial of 3 versus 6 months of nafarelin therapy for endometriosis associated pelvic pain. Fertil Steril 63:955, 1995b

Houston DE, Noller KL, Melton LJ III, et al: Incidence of pelvic endometriosis in Rochester, Minnesota, 1970–1979. Am J Epidemiol 125:959, 1987

Howard FM: The role of laparoscopy in the chronic pelvic pain patient. Clin Obstet Gynecol 46(4):749, 2003

Hsu AL, Sinaii N, Segars J, et al: Relating pelvic pain location to surgical findings of endometriosis. Obstet Gynecol 118(2 Pt 1):223, 2011

Huber SA, Northington GM, Karp DR: Bowel and bladder dysfunction following surgery within the presacral space: an overview of neuroanatomy, function, and dysfunction. Int Urogynecol J 26(7):941, 2015

Hudelist G, English J, Thomas AE, et al: Diagnostic accuracy of transvaginal ultrasound for non-invasive diagnosis of bowel endometriosis: systematic review and meta-analysis. Ultrasound Obstet Gynecol 37(3):257, 2011

Hufnagel D, Li F, Cosar E, et al: The role of stem cells in the etiology and pathophysiology of endometriosis. Semin Reprod Med 33(5):333, 2015

Hughes E, Brown J, Collins JJ, et al: Ovulation suppression for endometriosis. Cochrane Database Syst Rev 3:CD000155, 2007

Itoh H, Kishore AH, Lindqvist A, et al: Transforming growth factor β1 (TGFβ1) and progesterone regulate matrix metalloproteinases (MMP) in human endometrial stromal cells. J Clin Endocrinol Metab 97:888, 2012

Jacobson TZ, Barlow DH, Koninckx PR, et al: Laparoscopic surgery for subfertility associated with endometriosis. Cochrane Database Syst Rev 4:CD001398, 2002

Jacobson TZ, Duffy JM, Barlow D, et al: Laparoscopic surgery for subfertility associated with endometriosis. Cochrane Database Syst Rev 1:CD001398, 2010

Jacoby VL, Fujimoto VY, Giudice LC, et al: Racial and ethnic disparities in benign gynecologic conditions and associated surgeries. Am J Obstet Gynecol 202(6):514, 2010

Jana S, Chatterjee K, Ray AK, et al: Regulation of matrix metalloproteinase-2 activity by COX-2-PGE2-pAKT axis promotes angiogenesis in endometriosis. PLoS One 11(10):e0163540

Jansen RP, Russell P: Nonpigmented endometriosis: clinical, laparoscopic, and pathologic definition. Am J Obstet Gynecol 155:1154, 1986

Janssen EB, Rijkers AC, Hoppenbrouwers K, et al: Prevalence of endometriosis diagnosed by laparoscopy in adolescents with dysmenorrhea or chronic pelvic pain: a systematic review. Hum Reprod Update 19(5):570, 2013

Jerman LF, Hey-Cunningham AJ: The role of the lymphatic system in endometriosis: a comprehensive review of the literature. Biol Reprod 92(3):64, 2015

Johnson NP, Hummelshoj L, Adamson GD, et al: World Endometriosis Society consensus on the classification of endometriosis. Hum Reprod 32(2):315, 2017

Jones KD, Haines P, Sutton CJ: Long-term follow-up of a controlled trial of laser laparoscopy for pelvic pain. J Soc Laparoendosc Surg 5:111, 2001

Jones SC: Relative thromboembolic risks associated with COX-2 inhibitors. Ann Pharmacother 39:1249, 2005

Kao AP, Wang KH, Chang CC, et al: Comparative study of human eutopic and ectopic endometrial mesenchymal stem cells and the development of an in vivo endometriotic invasion model. Fertil Steril 95(4):1308, 2011

Kaufman LC, Smyrk TC, Levy MJ, et al: Symptomatic intestinal endometriosis requiring surgical resection: clinical presentation and preoperative diagnosis. Am J Gastroenterol 106(7):1325, 2011

Kauppila A, Rönnberg L: Naproxen sodium in dysmenorrhea secondary to endometriosis. Obstet Gynecol 65(3):379, 1985

Kennedy S, Bergqvist A, Chapron C, et al: ESHRE guideline for the diagnosis and treatment of endometriosis. Hum Reprod 20(10):2698, 2005

Kettel LM, Murphy AA, Morales AJ, et al: Treatment of endometriosis with the antiprogesterone mifepristone (RU486). Fertil Steril 65:23, 1996

Kiesel L, Schweppe KW, Sillem M, et al: Should add-back therapy for endometriosis be deferred for optimal results? BJOG 103(14 suppl):15, 1996

Kim HS, Kim TH, Chung HH, et al: Risk and prognosis of ovarian cancer in women with endometriosis: a meta-analysis. Br J Cancer 110:1878, 2014

Kim YA, Kim MR, Lee JH, et al: Gonadotropin-releasing hormone agonist reduces aromatase cytochrome P450 and cyclooxygenase-2 in ovarian endometrioma and eutopic endometrium of patients with endometriosis. Gynecol Obstet Invest 68:73, 2009

Kitawaki J, Noguchi T, Amatsu T, et al: Expression of aromatase cytochrome P450 protein and messenger ribonucleic acid in human endometriotic and adenomyotic tissues but not in normal endometrium. Biol Reprod 57:514, 1997

Knabben L, Imboden S, Fellmann B, et al: Urinary tract endometriosis in patients with deep infiltrating endometriosis: prevalence, symptoms, management, and proposal for a new clinical classification. Fertil Steril 103(1):147, 2015

Koger KE, Shatney CH, Hodge K, et al: Surgical scar endometrioma. Surg Gynecol Obstet 177:243, 1993

Koninckx PR, Oosterlynck D, D'Hooghe T, et al: Deeply infiltrating endometriosis is a disease whereas mild endometriosis could be considered a non-disease. Ann NY Acad Sci 734:333, 1994

Lafay Pillet MC, Huchon C, Santulli P, et al: A clinical score can predict associated deep infiltrating endometriosis before surgery for an endometrioma. Hum Reprod 29(8):1666, 2014

Lamvu G, Soliman AM, Manthena SR, et al: Patterns of prescription opioid use in women with endometriosis: evaluating prolonged use, daily dose, and concomitant use with benzodiazepines. Obstet Gynecol 133(6):1120, 2019

Levine D, Brown DL, Andreotti RF, et al: Management of asymptomatic ovarian and other adnexal cysts imaged at US: Society of Radiologists in Ultrasound Consensus Conference Statement. Radiology 256(3):943, 2010

Leyendecker G, Herbertz M, Kunz G, et al: Endometriosis results from the dislocation of basal endometrium. Hum Reprod 17(10):2725, 2002

Li F, Alderman MH III, Tal A, et al: Hematogenous dissemination of mesenchymal stem cells from endometriosis. Stem Cells 36(6):881, 2018

Ling FW: Randomized controlled trial of depot leuprolide in patients with chronic pelvic pain and clinically suspected endometriosis. Obstet Gynecol 93:51, 1999

Liu X, Yuan L, Shen F, et al: Patterns of and risk factors for recurrence in women with ovarian endometriomas. Obstet Gynecol 109(6):1411, 2007

Lyu H, Liu Y, Dang Q, et al: Effect of bazedoxifene on endometriosis in a rat model. Zhonghua Fu Chan Ke Za Zhi 50(4):291, 2015

Macer ML, Taylor HS: Endometriosis and infertility: a review of the pathogenesis and treatment of endometriosis-associated infertility. Obstet Gynecol Clin North Am 39(4):535, 2012

Mahmood TA, Templeton A: Prevalence and genesis of endometriosis. Hum Reprod 6(4):544, 1991

Mais V, Ajossa S, Marongiu D, et al: Reduction of adhesion reformation after laparoscopic endometriosis surgery: a randomized trial with an oxidized regenerated cellulose absorbable barrier. Obstet Gynecol 86(4 Pt 1):512, 1995a

Mais V, Ajossa S, Piras B, et al: Treatment of nonendometriotic benign adnexal cysts: a randomized comparison of laparoscopy and laparotomy. Obstet Gynecol 86:770, 1995b

Marcoux S, Maheux R, Berube S: Laparoscopic surgery in infertile women with minimal or mild endometriosis. Canadian Collaborative Group on Endometriosis. N Engl J Med 337:217, 1997

Marjoribanks J, Proctor M, Farquhar C, et al: Nonsteroidal anti-inflammatory drugs for dysmenorrhoea. Cochrane Database Syst Rev 1:CD001751, 2010

Marsh EE, Laufer MR: Endometriosis in premenarcheal girls who do not have an associated obstructive anomaly. Fertil Steril 83(3):758, 2005

Mathur S, Peress MR, Williamson HO, et al: Autoimmunity to endometrium and ovary in endometriosis. Clin Exp Immunol 50:259, 1982

Matorras R, Rodriguez F, Pijoan JI, et al: Women who are not exposed to spermatozoa and infertile women have similar rates of stage I endometriosis. Fertil Steril 76:923, 2001

May KE, Conduit-Hulbert SA, Villar J, et al: Peripheral biomarkers of endometriosis: a systematic review. Hum Reprod Update 16(6):651, 2010

McKinnon B, Bersinger NA, Wotzkow C, et al: Endometriosis-associated nerve fibers, peritoneal fluid cytokine concentrations, and pain in endometriotic lesions from different locations. Fertil Steril 97(2):373, 2012

McLaren J, Prentice A, Charnock-Jones DS, et al: Vascular endothelial growth factor is produced by peritoneal fluid macrophages in endometriosis and is regulated by ovarian steroids. J Clin Invest 98:482, 1996

Meuleman C, Vandenabeele B, Fieuws S, et al: High prevalence of endometriosis in infertile women with normal ovulation and normospermic partners. Fertil Steril 92:68, 2009

Milone M, Mollo A, Musella M, et al: Role of colonoscopy in the diagnostic work-up of bowel endometriosis. World J Gastroenterol 21(16):4997, 2015

Missmer SA, Hankinson SE, Spiegelman D, et al: Reproductive history and endometriosis among premenopausal women. Obstet Gynecol 104(5 Pt 1):965, 2004

Moen MH, Rees M, Brincat M, et al: EMAS position statement: managing the menopause in women with a past history of endometriosis. Maturitas 67(1):94, 2010

Moen MH, Stokstad T: A long-term follow-up study of women with asymptomatic endometriosis diagnosed incidentally at sterilization. Fertil Steril 78(4):773, 2002

Mol BW, Bayram N, Lijmer JG, et al: The performance of CA-125 measurement in the detection of endometriosis: a meta-analysis. Fertil Steril 70:1101, 1998

Montagna P, Capellino S, Villaggio B, et al: Peritoneal fluid macrophages in endometriosis: correlation between the expression of estrogen receptors and inflammation. Fertil Steril 90(1):156, 2008

Moore J, Copley S, Morris J, et al: A systematic review of the accuracy of ultrasound in the diagnosis of endometriosis. Ultrasound Obstet Gynecol 20:630, 2002

Moore JG, Binstock MA, Growdon WA: The clinical implications of retroperitoneal endometriosis. Am J Obstet Gynecol 158(6 Pt 1):1291, 1988

Mori H, Sawairi M, Nakagawa M, et al: Peritoneal fluid interleukin-1 beta and tumor necrosis factor in patients with benign gynecologic disease. Am J Reprod Immunol 26:62, 1991

Mostafa HA, Saad JH, Nadeem Z, et al: Rectus abdominis endometriosis. A descriptive analysis of 10 cases concerning this rare occurrence. Saudi Med J 34(10):1035, 2013

Mourra N, Cortez A, Bennis M, et al: The groin: an unusual location of endometriosis—a multi-institutional clinicopathological study. J Clin Pathol 68(7):579, 2016

Muneyyirci-Delale O, Karacan M: Effect of norethindrone acetate in the treatment of symptomatic endometriosis. Int J Fertil Womens Med 43:24, 1998

Mutter GL, Bergeron C, Deligdisch L, et al: The spectrum of endometrial pathology induced by progesterone receptor modulators. Mod Pathol 21(5):591, 2008

Namnoum AB, Hickman TN, Goodman SB, et al: Incidence of symptom recurrence after hysterectomy for endometriosis. Fertil Steril 64:898, 1995

Nezhat C, Nezhat F: A simplified method of laparoscopic presacral neurectomy for the treatment of central pelvic pain due to endometriosis. BJOG 99:659, 1992

Neziri AY, Haesler S, Petersen-Felix S, et al: Generalized expansion of nociceptive reflex receptive fields in chronic pain patients. Pain 151(3):798, 2010

Nisolle M, Donnez J: Peritoneal endometriosis, ovarian endometriosis, and adenomyotic nodules of the rectovaginal septum are three different entities. Fertil Steril 68:585, 1997

Noble LS, Takayama K, Zeitoun KM, et al: Prostaglandin E2 stimulates aromatase expression in endometriosis-derived stromal cells. J Clin Endocrinol Metab 82:600, 1997

Odukoya OA, Wheatcroft N, Weetman AP, et al: The prevalence of endometrial immunoglobulin G antibodies in patients with endometriosis. Hum Reprod 10:1214, 1995

Olive DL, Stohs GF, Metzger DA, et al: Expectant management and hydrotubations in the treatment of endometriosis-associated infertility. Fertil Steril 44:35, 1985a

Olive DL, Weinberg JB, Haney AF: Peritoneal macrophages and infertility: the association between cell number and pelvic pathology. Fertil Steril 44:772, 1985b

Opøien HK, Fedorcsak P, Omland AK, et al: In vitro fertilization is a successful treatment in endometriosis-associated infertility. Fertil Steril 97(4):912, 2012

Opoku-Anane J, Laufer MR: Prevalence of endometriosis in adolescent girls with chronic pelvic pain not responding to conventional therapy. Have we underestimated? J Pediatr Adolesc Gynecol 25(2):e50, 2012

Orwoll ES, Yuzpe AA, Burry KA, et al: Nafarelin therapy in endometriosis: long-term effects on bone mineral density. Am J Obstet Gynecol 171:1221, 1994

Ozkan S, Murk W, Arici A: Endometriosis and infertility: epidemiology and evidence-based treatments. Ann N Y Acad Sci 1127:92, 2008

Pagidas K, Falcone T, Hemmings R, et al: Comparison of reoperation for moderate (stage III) and severe (stage IV) endometriosis-related infertility with in vitro fertilization-embryo transfer. Fertil Steril 65:791, 1996

Parazzini F: Ablation of lesions or no treatment in minimal-mild endometriosis in infertile women: a randomized trial. Gruppo Italiano per lo Studio dell'Endometriosi. Hum Reprod 14:1332, 1999

Patel BG, Rudnicki M, Yu J, et al: Progesterone resistance in endometriosis: origins, consequences and interventions. Acta Obstet Gynecol Scand 96(6):623, 2017

Pavone ME, Bulun SE: Aromatase inhibitors for the treatment of endometriosis. Fertil Steril 98(6):1370, 2012

Pearce CL, Templeman C, Rossing MA, et al: Association between endometriosis and risk of histological subtypes of ovarian cancer: a pooled analysis of case-control studies. Lancet Oncol 13(4):385, 2012

Pergialiotis V, Prodromidou A, Frountzas M, et al: The effect of bipolar electrocoagulation during ovarian cystectomy on ovarian reserve: a systematic review. Am J Obstet Gynecol 213(5):620, 2015

Peters AA, Trimbos-Kemper GC, Admiraal C, et al: A randomized clinical trial on the benefit of adhesiolysis in patients with intraperitoneal adhesions and chronic pelvic pain. BJOG 99:59, 1992

Peterson CM, Johnstone EB, Hammoud AO, et al: Risk factors associated with endometriosis: importance of study population for characterizing disease in the ENDO Study. Am J Obstet Gynecol 208(6):451.e1, 2013

Petta CA, Ferriani RA, Abrao MS, et al: Randomized clinical trial of a levonorgestrel-releasing intrauterine system and a depot GnRH analogue for the treatment of chronic pelvic pain in women with endometriosis. Hum Reprod 20:1993, 2005

Pluchino N, Taylor HS: Endometriosis and stem cell trafficking. Reprod Sci 23(12):1616, 2016

Porpora MG, Koninckx PR, Piazze J, et al: Correlation between endometriosis and pelvic pain. J Am Assoc Gynecol Laparosc 6(4):429, 1999

Possover M, Schneider T, Henle KP: Laparoscopic therapy for endometriosis and vascular entrapment of sacral plexus. Fertil Steril 95(2):756, 2011

Prentice A, Deary AJ, Bland E: Progestagens and anti-progestagens for pain associated with endometriosis. Cochrane Database Syst Rev 2:CD002122, 2000

Proctor ML, Latthe PM, Farquhar CM, et al: Surgical interruption of pelvic nerve pathways for primary and secondary dysmenorrhoea. Cochrane Database Syst Rev 4:CD001896, 2005

Qiong-Zhen R, Ge Y, Deng Y, et al: Effect of vasopressin injection technique in laparoscopic excision of bilateral ovarian endometriomas on ovarian reserve: prospective randomized study. J Minim Invasive Gynecol 21(2):266, 2014

Redwine DB: Conservative laparoscopic excision of endometriosis by sharp dissection: life table analysis of reoperation and persistent or recurrent disease. Fertil Steril 56:628, 1991

Reimnitz C, Brand E, Nieberg RK, et al: Malignancy arising in endometriosis associated with unopposed estrogen replacement. Obstet Gynecol 71:444, 1988

Rodriguez-Escudero FJ, Neyro JL, Corcostegui B, et al: Does minimal endometriosis reduce fecundity? Fertil Steril 50:522, 1988

Rogers PA, D'Hooghe TM, Fazleabas A, et al: Priorities for endometriosis research: recommendations from an international consensus workshop. Reprod Sci 16(4):335, 2009

Roman H, Bridoux V, Tuech JJ, et al: Bowel dysfunction before and after surgery for endometriosis. Am J Obstet Gynecol 209(6):524, 2013

Rousset P, Rousset-Jablonski C, Alifano M, et al: Thoracic endometriosis syndrome: CT and MRI features. Clin Radiol 69(3):323, 2014

Rousset-Jablonski C, Alifano M, Plu-Bureau G, et al: Catamenial pneumothorax and endometriosis-related pneumothorax: clinical features and risk factors. Hum Reprod 26(9):2322, 2011

Ruffo G, Crippa S, Sartori A, et al: Management of rectosigmoid obstruction due to severe bowel endometriosis. Updates Surg 66(1):59, 2014a

Ruffo G, Scopelliti F, Manzoni A, et al: Long-term outcome after laparoscopic bowel resections for deep infiltrating endometriosis: a single-center experience after 900 cases. Biomed Res Int 2014:463058, 2014b

Saha R, Pettersson HJ, Svedberg P, et al: Heritability of endometriosis. Fertil Steril 104(4):947, 2015

Sallam HN, Garcia-Velasco JA, Dias S, et al: Long-term pituitary down-regulation before in vitro fertilization (IVF) for women with endometriosis. Cochrane Database Syst Rev 1:CD004635, 2006

Sampson JA: Peritoneal endometriosis due to menstrual dissemination of endometrial tissue into the peritoneal cavity. Am J Obstet Gynecol 14:442, 1927

Sanfilippo JS, Wakim NG, Schikler KN, et al: Endometriosis in association with uterine anomaly. Am J Obstet Gynecol 154:39, 1986

Sansone A, De Rosa N, Giampaolino P, et al: Effects of etonogestrel implant on quality of life, sexual function, and pelvic pain in women suffering from endometriosis: results from a multicenter, prospective, observational study. Arch Gynecol Obstet 298(4):731, 2018

Santulli P, Streuli I, Melonio I, et al: Increased serum cancer antigen-125 is a marker for severity of deep endometriosis. J Minim Invasive Gynecol 22(2):275, 2015

Sasson IE, Taylor HS: Stem cells and the pathogenesis of endometriosis. Ann N Y Acad Sci 1127:106, 2008

Satyaswaroop PG, Wartell DJ, Mortel R: Distribution of progesterone receptor, estradiol dehydrogenase, and 20 alpha-dihydroprogesterone dehydrogenase activities in human endometrial glands and stroma: progestin induction of steroid dehydrogenase activities in vitro is restricted to the glandular epithelium. Endocrinology 111:743, 1982

Schenken RS, Asch RH: Surgical induction of endometriosis in the rabbit: effects on fertility and concentrations of peritoneal fluid prostaglandins. Fertil Steril 34:581, 1980

Schlaff WD, Carson SA, Luciano A, et al: Subcutaneous injection of depot medroxyprogesterone acetate compared with leuprolide acetate in the treatment of endometriosis-associated pain. Fertil Steril 85(2):314, 2006

Schliep KC, Mumford SL, Peterson CM, et al: Pain typology and incident endometriosis. Hum Reprod 30(10):2427, 2015

Schwab KE, Chan RW, Gargett CE: Putative stem cell activity of human endometrial epithelial and stromal cells during the menstrual cycle. Fertil Steril 84(2 suppl):1124, 2005

Sekiba K: Use of Interceed(TC7) absorbable adhesion barrier to reduce postoperative adhesion reformation in infertility and endometriosis surgery. The Obstetrics and Gynecology Adhesion Prevention Committee. Obstet Gynecol 79(4):518, 1992

Selak V, Farquhar C, Prentice A, et al: Danazol for pelvic pain associated with endometriosis. Cochrane Database Syst Rev 4:CD000068, 2007

Seli E, Arici A: Endometriosis: interaction of immune and endocrine systems. Semin Reprod Med 21:135, 2003

Seracchioli R, Mabrouk M, Montanari G, et al: Conservative laparoscopic management of urinary tract endometriosis (UTE): surgical outcome and long-term follow-up. Fertil Steril 94(3):856, 2010

Shah DK, Correia KF, Vitonis AF, et al: Body size and endometriosis: results from 20 years of follow-up within the Nurses' Health Study II prospective cohort. Hum Reprod 28(7):1783, 2013

Shakiba K, Bena JF, McGill KM, et al: Surgical treatment of endometriosis: a 7-year follow-up on the requirement for further surgery. Obstet Gynecol 111(6):1285, 2008

Shippen ER, West WJ Jr: Successful treatment of severe endometriosis in two premenopausal women with an aromatase inhibitor. Fertil Steril 81(5):1395, 2004

Signorile PG, Baldi F, Bussani R, et al: Embryologic origin of endometriosis: analysis of 101 human female fetuses. J Cell Physiol 227(4):1653, 2012

Soliman NF, Hillard TC: Hormone replacement therapy in women with past history of endometriosis. Climacteric 9(5):325, 2006

Somigliana E, Berlanda N, Benaglia L, et al: Surgical excision of endometriomas and ovarian reserve: a systematic review on serum antimüllerian hormone level modifications. Fertil Steril 98(6):1531, 2012

Somigliana E, Vercellini P, Vigano P, et al: Postoperative medical therapy after surgical treatment of endometriosis: from adjuvant therapy to tertiary prevention. J Minim Invasive Gynecol 21(3):328, 2014

Somigliana E, Vigano P, Parazzini F, et al: Association between endometriosis and cancer: a comprehensive review and a critical analysis of clinical and epidemiological evidence. Gynecol Oncol 101:331, 2006

Stilley JA, Birt JA, Sharpe-Timms KL: Cellular and molecular basis for endometriosis-associated infertility. Cell Tissue Res 349(3):849, 2012

Strathy JH, Molgaard CA, Coulam CB, et al: Endometriosis and infertility: a laparoscopic study of endometriosis among fertile and infertile women. Fertil Steril 38:667, 1982

Stratton P, Sinaii N, Segars J, et al: Return of chronic pelvic pain from endometriosis after raloxifene treatment: a randomized controlled trial. Obstet Gynecol 111(1):88, 2008

Strowitzki T, Faustmann T, Gerlinger C, et al: Dienogest in the treatment of endometriosis-associated pelvic pain: a 12-week, randomized, double-blind, placebo-controlled study. Eur J Obstet Gynecol Reprod Biol 151(2):193, 2010a

Strowitzki T, Marr J, Gerlinger C, et al: Dienogest is as effective as leuprolide acetate in treating the painful symptoms of endometriosis: a 24-week, randomized, multicentre, open-label trial. Hum Reprod 25(3):633, 2010b

Surrey E, Taylor HS, Giudice L, et al: Long-term outcomes of elagolix in women with endometriosis: results from two extension studies. Obstet Gynecol 132(1):147, 2018

Sutton CJ, Pooley AS, Ewen SP, et al: Follow-up report on a randomized controlled trial of laser laparoscopy in the treatment of pelvic pain associated with minimal to moderate endometriosis. Fertil Steril 68:1070, 1997

Taguchi S, Enomoto Y, Homma Y: Bladder endometriosis developed after long-term estrogen therapy for prostate cancer. Int J Urol 19(10):964, 2012

Tal A, Tal R, Pluchino N, et al: Endometrial cells contribute to preexisting endometriosis lesions in a mouse model of retrograde menstruation. Biol Reprod 100(6):1453, 2019

Tammaa A, Fritzer N, Strunk G, et al: Learning curve for the detection of pouch of Douglas obliteration and deep infiltrating endometriosis of the rectum. Hum Reprod 29(6):1199, 2014

Tanmahasamut P, Rattanachaiyanont M, Angsuwathana S, et al: Postoperative levonorgestrel-releasing intrauterine system for pelvic endometriosis-related pain: a randomized controlled trial. Obstet Gynecol 119(3):519, 2012

Taylor HS, Adamson GD, Diamond MP, et: An evidence-based approach to assessing surgical versus clinical diagnosis of symptomatic endometriosis. Int J Gynaecol Obstet 142(2):131, 2018

Taylor HS, Giudice LC, Lessey BA, et al: Treatment of endometriosis-associated pain with elagolix, an oral GnRH antagonist. N Engl J Med 377(1):28, 2017

Taylor M, Bowen-Simpkins P, Barrington J: Complications of unopposed oestrogen following radical surgery for endometriosis. J Obstet Gynaecol 19:647, 1999

Telimaa S, Puolakka J, Ronnberg L, et al: Placebo-controlled comparison of danazol and high-dose medroxyprogesterone acetate in the treatment of endometriosis. Gynecol Endocrinol 1:13, 1987

Tempfer CB, Wenzl R, Horvat R, et al: Lymphatic spread of endometriosis to pelvic sentinel lymph nodes: a prospective clinical study. Fertil Steril 96(3):692, 2011

Thomas EJ, Cooke ID: Successful treatment of asymptomatic endometriosis: does it benefit infertile women? Br Med J (Clin Res Ed) 294:1117, 1987

Treloar SA, Bell TA, Nagle CM, et al: Early menstrual characteristics associated with subsequent diagnosis of endometriosis. Am J Obstet Gynecol 202(6):534.e1, 2010

Treloar SA, O'Connor DT, O'Connor VM, et al: Genetic influences on endometriosis in an Australian twin sample. Fertil Steril 71:701, 1999

Troncon JK, Zani AC, Vieira AD, et al: Endometriosis in a patient with mayer-rokitansky-küster-hauser syndrome. Case Rep Obstet Gynecol 2014:376231, 2014

Tseng JF, Ryan IP, Milam TD, et al: Interleukin-6 secretion in vitro is up-regulated in ectopic and eutopic endometrial stromal cells from women with endometriosis. J Clin Endocrinol Metab 81:1118, 1996

Tulandi T, Sirois C, Sabban H, et al: Relationship between catamenial pneumothorax or non-catamenial pneumothorax and endometriosis. J Minim Invasive Gynecol 25(3):480, 2018

Ulukus M, Arici A: Immunology of endometriosis. Minerva Ginecol 57(3):237, 2005

Van Holsbeke C, Van Calster B, Guerriero S, et al: Endometriomas: their ultrasound characteristics. Ultrasound Obstet Gynecol 35(6):730, 2010

Vercellini P, Aimi G, Busacca M, et al: Laparoscopic uterosacral ligament resection for dysmenorrhea associated with endometriosis: results of a randomized, controlled trial. Fertil Steril 80:310, 2003a

Vercellini P, Barbara G, Somigliana E, et al: Comparison of contraceptive ring and patch for the treatment of symptomatic endometriosis. Fertil Steril 93:2150, 2010

Vercellini P, Fedele L, Aimi G, et al: Association between endometriosis stage, lesion type, patient characteristics and severity of pelvic pain symptoms: a multivariate analysis on 1000 patients. Hum Reprod 22(1):266, 2007

Vercellini P, Frontino G, De Giorgi O, et al: Comparison of a levonorgestrel-releasing intrauterine device versus expectant management after conservative surgery for symptomatic endometriosis: a pilot study. Fertil Steril 80(2):305, 2003b

Vercellini P, Somigliana E, Buggio L, et al: "I can't get no satisfaction": deep dyspareunia and sexual functioning in women with rectovaginal endometriosis. Fertil Steril 98(6):1503, 2012

Vercellini P, Trespidi L, Colombo A, et al: A gonadotropin-releasing hormone agonist versus a low-dose oral contraceptive for pelvic pain associated with endometriosis. Fertil Steril 60:75, 1993

Vercellini P, Trespidi L, De Giorgi O, et al: Endometriosis and pelvic pain: relation to disease stage and localization. Fertil Steril 65:299, 1996

Vercellini P, Vendola N, Bocciolone L, et al: Reliability of the visual diagnosis of ovarian endometriosis. Fertil Steril 56:1198, 1991

Vignali M, Infantino M, Matrone R, et al: Endometriosis: novel etiopathogenetic concepts and clinical perspectives. Fertil Steril 78(4):665, 2002

Walch K, Unfried G, Huber J, et al: Implanon versus medroxyprogesterone acetate: effects on pain scores in patients with symptomatic endometriosis—a pilot study. Contraception 79(1):29, 2009

Wall DJ, Javitt MC, Glanc P, et al: ACR Appropriateness Criteria® infertility. Ultrasound Q 31(1):37, 2015

Waller KG, Lindsay P, Curtis P, et al: The prevalence of endometriosis in women with infertile partners. Eur J Obstet Gynecol Reprod Biol 48:135, 1993

Walter AJ, Hentz JG, Magtibay PM, et al: Endometriosis: correlation between histologic and visual findings at laparoscopy. Am J Obstet Gynecol 184:1407, 2001

Watanabe M, Kamiyama G, Yamazaki K, et al: Anal endosonography in the diagnosis and management of perianal endometriosis: report of a case. Surg Today 33:630, 2003

Williams CE, Nakhal RS, Hall-Craggs MA, et al: Transverse vaginal septae: management and long-term outcomes. BJOG 121(13):1653, 2014

Wilson TJ, Hertzog PJ, Angus D, et al: Decreased natural killer cell activity in endometriosis patients: relationship to disease pathogenesis. Fertil Steril 62:1086, 1994

Wolthuis AM, Meuleman C, Tomassetti C, et al: Bowel endometriosis: colorectal surgeon's perspective in a multidisciplinary surgical team. World J Gastroenterol 20(42):15616, 2014

Wong AY, Tang LC, Chin RK: Levonorgestrel-releasing intrauterine system (Mirena) and Depot medroxyprogesterone acetate (Depoprovera) as long-term maintenance therapy for patients with moderate and severe endometriosis: a randomised controlled trial. Aust N Z J Obstet Gynaecol 50(3):273, 2010

Wright J, Lotfallah H, Jones K, et al: A randomized trial of excision versus ablation for mild endometriosis. Fertil Steril 83:1830, 2005

Wu D, Hu M, Hong L, et al: Clinical efficacy of add-back therapy in treatment of endometriosis: a meta-analysis. Arch Gynecol Obstet 290(3):513, 2014

Wykes CB, Clark TJ, Khan KS: Accuracy of laparoscopy in the diagnosis of endometriosis: a systematic quantitative review. BJOG 111(11):1204, 2004

Xue Q, Lin Z, Cheng YH, et al: Promoter methylation regulates estrogen receptor 2 in human endometrium and endometriosis. Biol Reprod 77(4):681, 2007

Yao Z, Shen X, Capodanno I, et al: Validation of rat endometriosis model by using raloxifene as a positive control for the evaluation of novel SERM compounds. J Invest Surg 18(4):177, 2005

Yuen PM, Yu KM, Yip SK, et al: A randomized prospective study of laparoscopy and laparotomy in the management of benign ovarian masses. Am J Obstet Gynecol 177:109, 1997

Zeitoun K, Takayama K, Sasano H, et al: Deficient 17 beta-hydroxysteroid dehydrogenase type 2 expression in endometriosis: failure to metabolize 17 beta-estradiol. J Clin Endocrinol Metab 83:4474, 1998

Zheng Q, Mao H, Xu Y, et al: Can postoperative GnRH agonist treatment prevent endometriosis recurrence? A meta-analysis. Arch Gynecol Obstet 294(1):201, 2016

Zhu L, Wong F, Lang JH: Perineal endometriosis after vaginal delivery—clinical experience with 10 patients. Aust N Z J Obstet Gynaecol 42:565, 2002

Zullo F, Palomba S, Zupi E, et al: Effectiveness of presacral neurectomy in women with severe dysmenorrhea caused by endometriosis who were treated with laparoscopic conservative surgery: a 1-year prospective randomized double-blind controlled trial. Am J Obstet Gynecol 189:5, 2003

Zupi E, Marconi D, Sbracia M, et al: Add-back therapy in the treatment of endometriosis-associated pain. Fertil Steril 82:1303, 2004

CHAPTER 12

Pelvic Pain

PAIN PATHOPHYSIOLOGY

Pain in the lower abdomen and pelvis is a common complaint. Diagnosis can be challenging due to the wide differential diagnosis that spans multiple organ systems. Clinicians ideally should understand the mechanisms underlying human pain perception, which involves complex physical, biochemical, emotional, and social interactions.

Pain is a protective mechanism meant to warn of an immediate threat and to prompt withdrawal from noxious stimuli. Pain is usually followed by an emotional response and behavioral consequences. The mere threat of discomfort may elicit emotional responses even without actual injury.

When categorized, pain may be considered *somatic* or *visceral* depending on the type of afferent nerve fibers involved. Additionally, pain is described by the physiologic steps that produce it and can be defined as *inflammatory* or *neuropathic* (Kehlet, 2006). Both categories are helpful for diagnosis and treatment.

◼ Somatic or Visceral Pain

Somatic pain stems from nerve afferents of the somatic nervous system, which innervates the parietal peritoneum, skin, muscles, and subcutaneous tissues. Somatic pain is typically sharp and localized. It is found on either the right or left within dermatomes that correspond to the innervation of involved tissues (Fig. 12-1).

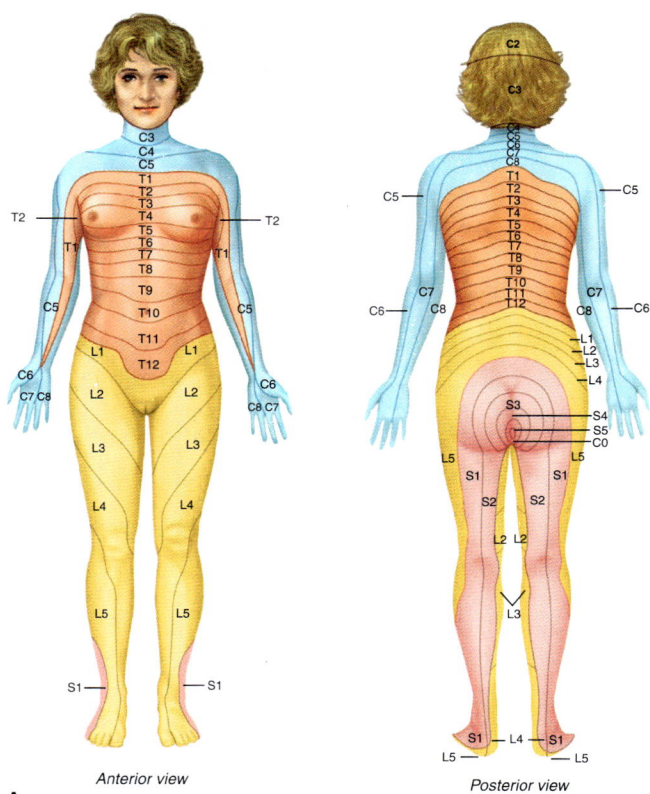

Anterior view   Posterior view

A

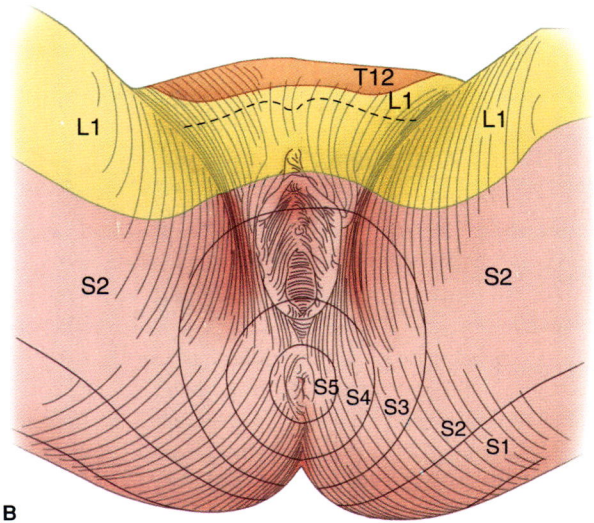

B

FIGURE 12-1 Dermatome maps. A dermatome is an area of skin supplied by a single spinal nerve. **A.** Body dermatomes. **B.** Perineal dermatomes.

In contrast, visceral pain stems from afferent fibers of the autonomic nervous system, which transmits information from the viscera and visceral peritoneum. Noxious stimuli typically include stretch, ischemia, or spasm of abdominal organs. The visceral afferent fibers that transfer these stimuli are sparse. Thus, the resulting diffuse sensory input leads to a generalized, dull ache.

Visceral pain often localizes to the midline because visceral innervation of abdominal organs is usually bilateral (Flasar, 2006). Also, visceral pain is typically localized by the brain's sensory cortex to an approximate spinal cord level that is determined by the embryologic origin of the involved organ. For example, pathology in midgut organs, such as the small bowel, appendix, and caecum, causes perceived periumbilical pain. In contrast, disease in hindgut organs, such as the colon and intraperitoneal portions of the genitourinary tract, causes midline suprapubic or hypogastric pain (Gallagher, 2004).

Visceral afferent fibers are poorly myelinated, and action potentials can easily spread from them to adjacent somatic nerves. As a result, visceral pain may at times be referred to dermatomes that correspond to these adjacent somatic nerve fibers (Giamberardino, 2003). In addition, both peripheral somatic and visceral nerves often synapse in the spinal cord at the same dorsal horn neurons. These neurons, in turn, relay sensory information to the brain. The cortex recognizes the signal as coming from the same dermatome regardless of its visceral or somatic nerve origin. This phenomenon is termed *viscerosomatic convergence* and makes it difficult for a patient to distinguish internal organ pain from abdominal wall or pelvic floor pain (Perry, 2003).

In contrast, *direct intraspinal neuronal reflexes* permit transmission of visceral nociceptive input to other pelvic viscera (viscerovisceral reflex), muscle (visceromuscular reflex), and skin (viscerocutaneous reflex). These intraspinal reflexes may explain why patients with endometriosis or interstitial cystitis/bladder pain syndrome (IC/BPS) manifest other pain syndromes such as vestibulitis, pelvic floor myalgia, or irritable bowel syndrome (IBS). Thus, unless the underlying chronic visceral pain source is identified and properly treated, referred pain and secondary pain syndromes may not be successfully eliminated (Perry, 2000).

Inflammatory Pain

With acute pain, noxious stimuli such as a knife cut, burn, or crush injury activate sensory pain receptors, more formally termed *nociceptors*. Action potentials travel from the periphery to dorsal horn neurons in the spinal cord. Here, reflex arcs may lead to immediate muscle contraction, which removes and protects the body from harm. Additionally, within the spinal cord, sensory information is augmented or dampened and may then be transmitted to the brain. In the cortex, it is recognized as pain (Janicki, 2003). After an acute stimulus is eliminated, nociceptor activity quickly diminishes.

If tissues are injured, inflammation usually follows. Chemical mediators of this process are prostaglandins, which are released from the damaged tissue, and cytokines, which are produced in white blood cells and endothelial cells. These sensitizing mediators lower the conduction threshold of nociceptors. This is termed *peripheral sensitization*. Similarly, neurons within the spinal cord and/or brain display enhanced excitability, termed *central sensitization*. As a result, within inflamed tissues, the perception of pain is increased relative to the strength of the external stimulus (Kehlet, 2006). Normally, as inflammation declines and healing ensues, the greater sensitivity to stimuli and thus the perception of pain subsides.

Neuropathic Pain

In some individuals, sustained noxious stimuli can lead to persistent central sensitization and permanent loss of neuronal inhibition. As a result, a lower threshold to painful stimuli remains despite resolution of the inciting stimuli (Butrick, 2003). This persistence characterizes *neuropathic pain*, which is felt to underlie many chronic pain syndromes. During central sensitization, neurons within spinal cord levels above or below those initially affected may eventually become involved, resulting in chronic pain that may be referred across several spinal cord levels. In addition, some evidence suggests that chronic pain states are also associated with regional brain morphology changes in regions known to regulate pain. This has been described as maladaptive central nervous system (CNS) plasticity (As-Sanie, 2012). The concept of neuropathic pain helps explain in part why many patients with chronic pain have discomfort disproportionately greater than the amount of coexistent disease.

Thus, in assessing patients with chronic pain, a clinician may find an ongoing inflammatory condition. In these cases, inflammatory pain dominates, and treatment is directed at resolving the underlying inflammatory condition. However, for many, evaluation may reveal no or minimal current pathology. In these cases, pain is neuropathic, and treatment thus focuses on management of pain symptoms themselves.

ACUTE PAIN

History

Acute pelvic pain is defined as pain in the lower abdomen or pelvis lasting <3 months. The range of causes is extensive, and a thorough history and physical examination can narrow the list (Table 12-1). Generally, potentially life-threatening or other urgent conditions are excluded first and include pregnancy complications, appendicitis, ovarian torsion, pelvic inflammatory disease (PID), and ruptured ovarian cyst or abscess.

During evaluation, a verbal description of the pain and its associated factors is essential. For example, duration can be informative, and pain with abrupt onset may be more often associated with organ torsion, rupture, or ischemia. Patients with acute pathology involving pelvic viscera may describe *visceral pain* that is midline, diffuse, dull, achy, or cramping. One example is the midline periumbilical pain of early appendicitis. Patients may repeatedly shift or roll to one side to find a comfortable position.

The underlying pelvic pathology may extend from the viscera to inflame the adjacent parietal peritoneum. In these cases, sharp *somatic pain* is described, which is localized, often unilateral,

TABLE 12-1. Etiologies of Acute Lower Abdominal and Pelvic Pain

Gynecologic

PID	Dysmenorrhea
Tuboovarian abscess	Mittelschmerz
Ectopic pregnancy	Ovarian mass
Incomplete abortion	Ovarian torsion
Prolapsing leiomyoma	Obstructed outflow tract

Gastrointestinal

Gastroenteritis	Inflammatory bowel disease
Colitis	Irritable bowel disease
Appendicitis	Obstructed small bowel
Diverticulitis	Mesenteric ischemia
Constipation	Malignancy

Urologic

Cystitis	Urinary tract stone
Pyelonephritis	Perinephric abscess

Musculoskeletal

Hernia	Abdominal wall trauma

Miscellaneous

Peritonitis	Sickle cell crisis
Diabetic ketoacidosis	Vasculitis
Herpes zoster	Abdominal aortic aneurysm rupture
Opiate withdrawal	

PID = pelvic inflammatory disease.

For example, vomiting has been found in approximately 75 percent of adnexal torsion cases (Descargues, 2001; Huchon, 2010). Conversely, if vomiting is noted prior to pain onset, a surgical abdomen is less likely (Miller, 2006).

■ Physical Examination

Examination begins with patient observation during initial questioning. Her general appearance, including facial expression, diaphoresis, pallor, and degree of agitation, often indicates the urgency of the clinical condition.

Elevated temperature, tachycardia, and hypotension will prompt an expedited evaluation, as the risk for intraabdominal pathology rises with their presence. Constant, low-grade fever is common in inflammatory conditions such as diverticulitis and appendicitis, and higher temperatures may be seen with PID, advanced peritonitis, or pyelonephritis.

Pulse and blood pressure evaluations ideally assess orthostatic changes if intravascular hypovolemia is suspected. A pulse rise of 30 beats per minute or a systolic blood pressure drop of 20 mm Hg or both, between lying and standing after 1 minute, is often reflective of hypovolemia. If noted, establishment of intravenous (IV) access and fluid resuscitation may be required prior to examination completion. Notably, certain neurologic disorders and medications, such as tricyclic antidepressants or antihypertensives, may produce similar orthostatic blood pressure changes.

Abdominal examination is essential. Visual inspection of the abdomen focuses on prior surgical scars, which raise the possibility of bowel obstruction from adhesions or incisional hernia. Additionally, abdominal distention may reflect bowel obstruction, perforation, ascites, or secondary intestinal dysmotility. After inspection, auscultation can identify hyperactive or high-pitched bowel sounds characteristic of bowel obstruction. Hypoactive sounds, however, are less informative.

Palpation of the abdomen systematically explores each quadrant and begins away from the area of indicated pain. Peritoneal irritation is suggested by rebound tenderness or by abdominal rigidity due to involuntary guarding or reflex spasm of the adjacent or involved abdominal muscles. A positive Carnett sign was found in one study to be 95-percent accurate at distinguishing between pain originating from abdominal wall pathology or from visceral sources (Thomson, 1977). Carnett sign is pain with elevation of the head and shoulders, and this lifting concurrently tenses the abdominal wall muscles. It is typical of anterior abdominal wall pathology.

Pelvic examination in general is performed in reproductive-aged women, as gynecologic pathology and pregnancy complications are a common pain source in this age group. The decision to pursue pelvic examination in geriatric and pediatric patients is based on clinical information.

Of findings, purulent vaginal discharge or cervicitis often accompanies reproductive tract infection. Vaginal bleeding can stem from pregnancy complications, reproductive tract neoplasia, or acute vaginal trauma. Leiomyomas, pregnancy, hematometra, and adenomyosis are frequent causes of uterine enlargement, and the last three may also create uterine softening. Cervical motion tenderness reflects peritoneal irritation from pus or blood. A tender adnexal or pelvic mass may reflect ectopic pregnancy;

and focused to a specific corresponding dermatome. Again using appendicitis as an example, the classic migration of pain to the site of peritoneal irritation in the right lower quadrant illustrates acute somatic pain. In other instances, sharp, localized pain may originate not from the parietal peritoneum, but from pathology in specific muscles or in isolated areas of skin or subcutaneous tissues. In these instances, with somatic pain, patients classically rest motionless to avoid movement of the affected peritoneum, muscle, or skin.

Colicky pain may reflect bowel obstructed by adhesion, neoplasia, stool, or hernia. It can also stem from greater bowel peristalsis in those with IBS, inflammatory bowel disease, or infectious gastroenteritis. Alternatively, colic may follow forceful uterine contractions with the passage of products of conception, pedunculated leiomyomas, or endometrial polyps. Last, stones in the lower urinary tract may cause spasms of pain as they are passed.

Associated symptoms may also direct diagnosis. For example, absence of dysuria, hematuria, frequency, or urgency will exclude urinary pathology in most instances. Gynecologic causes are often associated with vaginal bleeding, vaginal discharge, dyspareunia, or amenorrhea. Alternatively, exclusion of diarrhea, constipation, or gastrointestinal (GI) bleeding lowers the probability of GI disease.

Vomiting complaints, however, are less informative, although the temporal relationship of vomiting to the pain may be helpful. In the acute surgical abdomen, if vomiting occurs, it usually follows as a response to pain and results from vagal stimulation. This vomiting is typically severe and develops without nausea.

tuboovarian abscess; ovarian cyst with torsion, hemorrhage, or rupture; or nongynecologic pathology of the appendix or colon.

Rectal examination can add information regarding the source and size of pelvic masses and the possibility of colorectal disease. Stool guaiac testing for occult blood may add information in patients with rectal bleeding, painful defecation, or significant changes in bowel habits.

In emergency departments, women with acute pain may experience waits between their initial assessment and subsequent testing. For these patients, literature supports early administration of analgesia. Fears that analgesia will mask patient symptoms and hinder accurate diagnosis have not been supported (Manterola, 2011). Thus, barring significant hypotension or drug allergy, analgesia may be administered judiciously in these situations. In general, well-localized pain or tenderness, persisting longer than 6 hours and unrelieved by analgesics, has a greater likelihood of acute peritoneal pathology.

■ Laboratory Testing

Despite benefits from a thorough history and physical examination, the sensitivity of these two in diagnosing abdominal pain is low (Gerhardt, 2005). Thus, laboratory and diagnostic testing are typically required. First, either urine or serum β-human chorionic gonadotropin testing is recommended in those of reproductive age without prior hysterectomy. Complete blood count can identify hemorrhage, both uterine and intraabdominal, and can assess for infection. Urinalysis helps evaluate possible urolithiasis or cystitis. Microscopic evaluation and culture of vaginal discharge may add support to suspected cases of reproductive tract infection. Last, specific measures of GI dysfunction can be selected as indicated.

■ Radiologic Imaging

If an obstetric or gynecologic cause is suspected, transvaginal and transabdominal pelvic sonography are preferred modalities (Bhosale, 2016). Sonography is widely available, can usually be obtained quickly, requires little patient preparation, is relatively noninvasive, and avoids ionizing radiation. In most cases, transvaginal sonography (TVS) offers superior resolution of the reproductive organs (Chap. 2, p. 29). Transabdominal sonography may still be necessary if the uterus or adnexal structures are significantly large or lie beyond the transvaginal probe's field of view. In women with acute pain, the addition of Doppler studies is particularly useful if adnexal torsion or ectopic pregnancy is suspected (Twickler, 2010). Less common causes of acute pain amenable to sonographic diagnosis are perforation of the uterine wall by an intrauterine device or menstrual outflow obstruction from müllerian agenesis anomalies. For these, 3-dimensional (3-D) TVS has become invaluable (Bermejo, 2010; Moschos, 2011). Instead, computed tomography (CT) offers a more global examination that can identify numerous abdominal and pelvic conditions, often with a high level of confidence (Hsu, 2005). CT performs the best for identifying structural urinary tract and GI causes of acute pelvic pain (Bhosale, 2016).

The debate regarding CT safety and possible overuse is ongoing (Brenner, 2007). Of major concern is the potential higher cancer risk directly attributable to ionizing radiation

(Einstein, 2007). Investigators in a large multicenter analysis found the median effective radiation dose from a multiphase abdominopelvic CT scan was 31 mSv, and this correlates with a lifetime attributed risk of four cancers per 1000 patients (Smith-Bindman, 2009). However, in an acute setting, CT imaging benefits frequently outweigh this risk.

In some instances, plain film radiography is selected. Although its sensitivity is low for most gynecologic conditions, it still may be informative if bowel obstruction or perforation is suspected (Leschka, 2007). Dilated loops of small bowel, air-fluid levels, free air under the diaphragm, or the presence or absence of colonic gas are significant findings.

Magnetic resonance (MR) imaging may play a role if initial sonography is nondiagnostic. Common reasons include patient obesity and pelvic anatomy distortion secondary to large leiomyomas, müllerian anomalies, or exophytic tumor growth. As a first-line tool, MR imaging is often selected for pregnant patients, in whom ionizing radiation exposure is ideally limited. However, for most acute disorders, it provides little advantage over 3-D sonography or CT (Bermejo, 2010; Brown, 2005). Limited availability can be another disadvantage.

■ Laparoscopy

Operative laparoscopy is the primary treatment for suspected appendicitis, adnexal torsion, ruptured ectopic pregnancy, and ruptured ovarian cyst associated with ongoing hemorrhage. However, diagnostic laparoscopy may be indicated in patients with severe pain if no pathology can be identified after a conventional evaluation is completed (Sauerland, 2006).

The decision to perform a surgical procedure for acute pelvic pain can be challenging. In a patient with signs of peritoneal irritation, possible hemoperitoneum, shock, and/or impending sepsis, the decision to operate is made decisively unless contraindications to immediate surgery are present. Although patients with torsion are often stable, this condition is a surgical emergency due to the time urgency in relieving ischemia to preserve fertility and ovarian function (Sauerland 2006). Surgical intervention may also be expedited for conditions that are causing severe uncontrolled pain or are refractory to supportive or medical management.

CHRONIC PAIN

Persistent pain may be visceral, somatic, or mixed in origin. As a result, it may take several forms in women, and these include chronic pelvic pain (CPP), dysmenorrhea, dyspareunia, dysuria, musculoskeletal pain, intestinal cramping, or vulvodynia. Vulvodynia is discussed in Chapter 4 (p. 104). The list of possible underlying pathologies is extensive (Table 12-2). Moreover, pathology in one organ can commonly lead to dysfunction in adjacent systems and create overlapping symptoms (Maixner, 2016). A comprehensive evaluation of multiple organ systems and psychologic state is essential for complete treatment.

CHRONIC PELVIC PAIN

This common gynecologic problem has an estimated prevalence of 15 percent in reproductive-aged women (Mathias, 1996).

TABLE 12-2. Diseases That May Be Associated with Chronic Pelvic Pain in Women

Gynecologic

Endometriosis	Reproductive tract cancer	Chronic PID
Adenomyosis	Pelvic muscle trigger points	Chronic endometritis
Leiomyomas	Intrauterine contraceptive device	Vestibulitis
Abdominal adhesions	Outflow tract obstruction	Pelvic congestion syndrome
Endometrial/endocervical polyps	Ovarian retention syndrome	Broad ligament herniation
Ovarian mass	Ovarian remnant syndrome	Chronic ectopic pregnancy
Adnexal cysts		Postoperative peritoneal cysts
Pelvic organ prolapse		

Urologic

Chronic UTI	Urethral syndrome	Interstitial cystitis
Detrusor dyssynergia	Urethral diverticulum	Radiation cystitis
Urinary tract stone	Urinary tract cancer	

Gastrointestinal

Irritable bowel syndrome	Colitis	Celiac disease
Constipation	Inflammatory bowel disease	Chronic intermittent bowel obstruction
Diverticular disease	Gastrointestinal cancer	

Musculoskeletal

Hernias	Myofascial pain	Vertebral compression
Muscular strain	Levator ani syndrome	Disc disease
Faulty posture	Fibromyositis	Coccydynia
Degenerative joint disease	Spondylosis	Peripartum pelvic pain

Neurologic

Neurologic dysfunction	Neuralgia of iliohypogastric, ilioinguinal, lateral femoral cutaneous, or genitofemoral nerves	Spinal cord or sacral nerve tumor
Pudendal neuralgia		
Piriformis syndrome	Abdominal cutaneous nerve entrapment	

Miscellaneous

Psychiatric disorders
Physical or sexual abuse
Shingles

PID = pelvic inflammatory disease; UTI = urinary tract infection.

No definition is universally accepted. However, most include pain that: (1) is present for >6 months; (2) localizes to the pelvis, lower abdomen, lower back, medial thigh, or perineum; (3) has various pain manifestations; and (4) presents variably in duration and cyclicity (Doggweiler, 2017).

Causes of CPP are broad. Of gynecologic causes, endometriosis is the most prevalent and found in 70 to 90 percent of patients with pelvic pain (American Society for Reproductive Medicine, 2014). Dysmenorrhea is the most frequent endometriosis symptom, but intermittent or continuous nonmenstrual pain also may be present. Endometriosis is fully described in Chapter 11. Other etiologies are discussed subsequently.

■ History

A detailed history is integral to CPP diagnosis, and a pelvic pain questionnaire can be used initially. One example is available from the International Pelvic Pain Society at: https://www.pelvicpain.org/. Additionally, a body silhouette diagram can be provided to patients for them to mark specific sites of pain. The McGill Pain Questionnaire and Short Form combines a list of pain descriptors with a body map for patients to mark pain sites (Melzack, 1987). Pain scales also can quantify discomfort and include visual analogue scales (VAS) and verbal descriptor scales (VDS) (Fig. 12-2). At minimum, the series of questions found in Table 12-3 can provide valuable information.

First, of gynecologic factors, pregnancy and delivery can be traumatic to neuromuscular structures and is associated with pelvic organ prolapse, pelvic floor muscle myofascial pain syndromes, and symphyseal or sacroiliac joint pain. In addition, injury to the ilioinguinal or iliohypogastric nerves during Pfannenstiel incision for cesarean delivery may lead to lower abdominal wall pain even years after the initial injury (Whiteside, 2003). Following delivery, recurrent, cyclic pain and swelling in

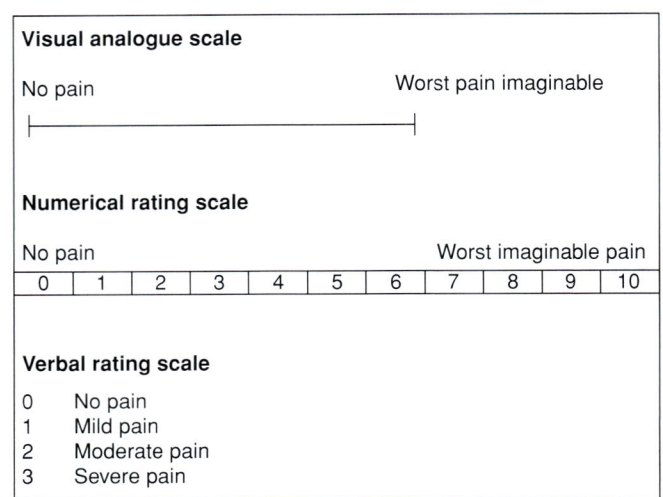

Visual analogue scale

No pain   Worst pain imaginable

|———————————————————————————|

Numerical rating scale

No pain   Worst imaginable pain

0	1	2	3	4	5	6	7	8	9	10

Verbal rating scale

0   No pain
1   Mild pain
2   Moderate pain
3   Severe pain

FIGURE 12-2 Rating scales for pain. The visual analogue, numeric, and verbal rating scales are shown.

the vicinity of a cesarean incision or within an episiotomy suggests endometriosis within the scar itself (Fig. 11-3, p. 238). In a nullipara with infertility, pain may stem more often from endometriosis, pelvic adhesions, or PID.

TABLE 12-3. Questions Relevant to Chronic Pelvic Pain

1. Describe the location, quality, severity, and timing of your pain.
2. When and how did your pain start and how has it changed?
3. What makes your pain better or worse?
4. What other symptoms or health problems do you have?
5. Do you have frequency, urgency, or bloody urine?
6. Do you have nausea or vomiting, diarrhea, constipation, or rectal bleeding?
7. Do you have pain with your periods?
8. Did your pain start initially as menstrual cramps?
9. Have you had surgery? What was the reason?
10. How many pregnancies have you had?
11. How did you deliver? Was there an episiotomy?
12. What form of birth control do you use and have you used in the past?
13. Have you ever been treated for a sexually transmitted disease or pelvic infection?
14. Do you have pain with deep penetration during intercourse?
15. Are you depressed or anxious?
16. Have you been treated for mental illness in the past?
17. Have you been or are you now being abused physically or sexually?
18. What prior evaluations or treatments have you had for your pain?
19. Have any of the previous treatments helped?
20. What medications are you taking now?
21. How has the pain affected your quality of life?
22. What do you believe or fear is causing your pain?

Second, prior abdominal surgery raises the risk for pelvic adhesions, especially if infection, bleeding, or large areas of denuded peritoneal surfaces were involved. Adhesions were found in 40 percent of patients who underwent laparoscopy for CPP suspected to be of gynecologic origin (Sharma, 2011). The incidence of adhesions increases with the number of prior surgeries (Dubuisson, 2010). Last, certain disorders persist or commonly recur, and thus information regarding prior surgeries for endometriosis, adhesive disease, or malignancy is sought.

Of psychologic risk factors, CPP and sexual abuse are significantly associated (Jamieson, 1997; Lampe, 2000). A metaanalysis found sexual abuse linked with a higher lifetime diagnosis rate of functional bowel disorders, fibromyalgia, psychogenic seizure disorder, and CPP (Paras, 2009). Additionally, for some women, CPP is an acceptable means to cope with social stresses. Thus, patients are questioned regarding intimate partner violence and satisfaction with family relationships. Furthermore, depression may cause or result from CPP, and Table 14-3 (p. 303) provides one assessment tool. Other conditions bearing similarities to CPP include fibromyalgia, chronic fatigue syndrome, temporomandibular disorder, and migraine. These are referred to as functional somatic syndromes, and CPP may be comorbid with each of these (Warren, 2011).

■ Physical Examination

In a woman with chronic pain, even routine examination may be extremely painful. Thus, examination proceeds slowly to allow relaxation between each step. Moreover, a patient is reassured that she may ask for the examination to stop at any time. Terms used to describe examination findings include *allodynia* and *hyperesthesia*, among others. Allodynia is a painful response to a normally innocuous stimulus, such as a cotton swab. Hyperalgesia is an extreme response to a painful stimulus.

Stance and Gait

Women with intraperitoneal pathology may compensate with changes in posture. Such adjustments can create secondary musculoskeletal sources of pain (p. 270). Alternatively, musculoskeletal structures may be the site of referred pain from these organs (Table 12-4). Initial studies estimated that 14 to 22 percent of women with CPP have pain arising primarily or secondarily from musculoskeletal sources (Reiter, 1991; Tu, 2006). In specialty clinics, in which a standard musculoskeletal examination is incorporated, the reported musculoskeletal dysfunction prevalence rises to 50 to 90 percent (Fitzgerald, 2011; Lamvu, 2015; Mieritz, 2016; Sedighimehr, 2018).

Initially, a woman is examined while standing. Posture is evaluated anteriorly, posteriorly, and laterally. Anteriorly, the umbilicus, symmetry of the anterior superior iliac spines (ASISs), and weight bearing is evaluated. If one leg bears most of the weight, the nonbearing leg is often externally rotated and slightly flexed at the knee. Next, the anterior abdominal wall and inguinal areas are inspected for hernias (p. 270). Inspection of the perineum and vulva with the patient standing may identify varicosities. These are often asymptomatic or may cause superficial discomfort. Such varicosities may coexist with internal pelvic varicosities, the underlying cause of pelvic congestion syndrome (p. 264).

TABLE 12-4. Musculoskeletal Origins of Chronic Pelvic Pain

Structure	Innervation	Referred Pain Site(s)
Hip	T12–S1	Lower abdomen; anterior medial thigh; knee
Lumbar ligaments, facets/disks	T12–S1	Low back; posterior thigh and calf; lower abdomen; lateral trunk; buttock
Sacroiliac joints	L4–S3	Posterior thigh; buttock; pelvic floor
Abdominal muscles	T5–L1	Abdomen; anteromedial thigh; sternum
Pelvic and back muscles		
Iliopsoas	L1–L4	Lateral trunk; lower abdomen; low back; anterior thigh
Piriformis	L5–S3	Low back, buttock; pelvic floor
Pubococcygeus	S1–L4	Pelvic floor; vagina; rectum; buttock
Obturator internal/external	L3–S2	Pelvic floor; buttock; anterior thigh
Quadratus lumborum	T12–L3	Anterior lateral trunk; anterior thigh; lower abdomen

Posteriorly, inspection for scoliosis and of horizontal stability of the shoulders, gluteal folds, and knee creases is completed. Asymmetry may reflect musculoskeletal disorders.

Lateral visual examination searches for lordosis and concomitant kyphosis. This combination has been noted in some women with CPP and termed *typical pelvic pain posture (TPPP)* (Fig. 12-3) (Baker, 1993). Also, abnormal tilt of the pelvic bones can be assessed by simultaneously placing an open palm on each side between the posterior superior iliac spine (PSIS) and the ASIS. Normally, the ASIS lies one quarter inch below the level of the PSIS, and greater distances may suggest abnormal tilt. Pelvic tilt may be associated with hip osteoarthritis and other orthopedic problems (Labelle, 2005; Yoshimoto, 2005).

To augment passive inspection, a woman is asked to perform a Valsalva maneuver. Diastasis of the rectus abdominis muscle or hernias may become evident. With diastasis, the borders of the rectus abdominis muscle can be palpated bilaterally along the entire length of the protrusion.

Mobility limitations also can be informative. Thus, a patient is asked to bend forward at the waist. Limitation in forward flexion may reflect primary orthopedic disease or adaptive shortening of back extensor muscles. This shortening is seen frequently in women with chronic pain and TPPP. In such cases, patients are unable to bend over at the waist to create the normal convex curve. Gait is evaluated by having the patient walk across the room. An antalgic gait, known as a limp, indicates a higher probability of musculoskeletal pain.

Muscle weakness may also indicate orthopedic disease. A Trendelenburg test, in which a patient is asked to balance on one foot, can indicate dysfunction of hip abductor muscles or hip joint. With a positive test, when a woman elevates a leg by flexing the hip, the ipsilateral iliac crest droops.

Sitting and Supine

A patient is next invited to sit on the examining table. Myofascial pain syndrome may involve pelvic floor muscles and often leads to a patient shifting weight to one buttock or sitting toward a chair's front edge.

Next, with the patient supine, the anterior abdominal wall is evaluated for abdominal scars. These may be sites of hernia or nerve entrapment or may indicate a risk for intraabdominal adhesive disease. Auscultation for bowel sounds and bruits follows. Increased bowel activity may reflect IBS or inflammatory bowel disease. Bruits prompt investigation for vascular pathology.

While supine, a woman is asked to demonstrate with one finger the point of maximal pain and then encircle the total surrounding area of involvement. Superficial palpation of the anterior abdominal wall by a clinician may reveal sites of tenderness or knotted muscle that may reflect nerve entrapment or myofascial pain syndrome (p. 270). Carnett sign, described on page 255, is typical of anterior abdominal wall pathology. Conversely, with pain originating from inside the abdominal cavity, discomfort usually decreases during this maneuver (Thomson, 1991). Last, deep palpation of the lower abdomen may identify pathology originating from pelvic viscera. Dullness to percussion or a shifting fluid wave can reflect ascites. Lower extremity mobility also is evaluated. In most cases, a woman can elevate her leg 80 degrees from the horizontal toward her head, termed a *straight leg test*. Pain with leg elevation may be seen with lumbar disc, hip joint, or myofascial pain syndromes.

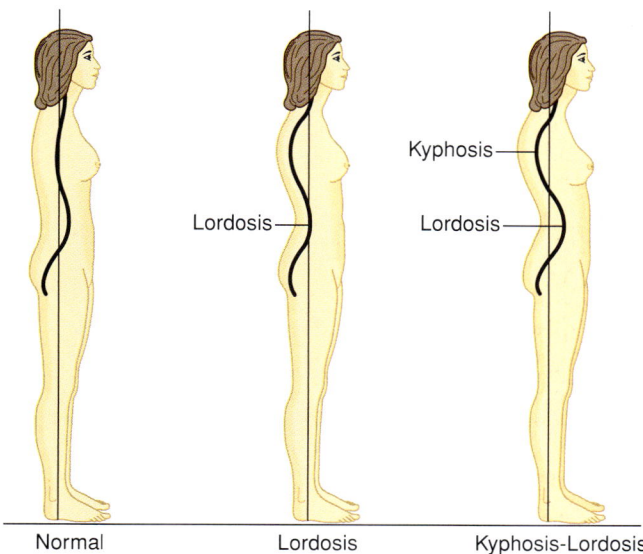

Normal   Lordosis   Kyphosis-Lordosis
(TPPP)

FIGURE 12-3 Concurrent lordosis and kyphosis are common postural changes associated with chronic pelvic pain. TPPP = typical pelvic pain posture.

Additionally, symphyseal pain with this test may indicate laxity in the symphysis pubis or pelvic girdle. Both the obturator and iliopsoas tests may indicate myofascial pain syndromes involving these muscles or disorders of the hip joint. With the obturator test, a supine patient brings one knee into 90 degrees of flexion while the same foot remains planted. The ankle is held stationary, but the knee is gently pulled laterally and then medially to assess for tenderness. With the iliopsoas test, a supine woman attempts to flex each hip separately against downward resistance from the examiner's hand placed on the ipsilateral anterior thigh. If pain is described with hip flexion, the test result is positive.

Pelvic Examination

Pelvic examination begins with inspection of the vulva for generalized changes and localized lesions. Vulvar erythema often reflects infectious vulvitis, described in Chapter 3 (p. 57), or vulvitis stemming from dermatoses (Chap. 4, p. 94). The vestibular area also is examined. Erythema of the vestibule, with or without punctate lesions, may indicate vestibulitis. Following this inspection, systematic pressure point palpation of the vestibule, shown in Figure 4-1 (p. 93), is completed using a small cotton swab to assess for pain. Last, the anocutaneous reflex, described in Chapter 24 (p. 544), may be performed to assess pudendal nerve integrity.

Prior to speculum examination, a single digit systematically evaluates the vagina. Pain elicited from pressure beneath the urethra may indicate urethral diverticulum. Pain with anterior vagina palpation under the trigone can reflect IC/BPS. Systematic sweeping pressure against the pelvic floor muscles along their length may identify isolated taut muscle knots from pelvic floor myofascial syndrome. Of these muscles, the pubococcygeus, iliococcygeus, and obturator internus muscles can usually be reached with a vaginal finger (Fig. 12-4). Next, insertion points

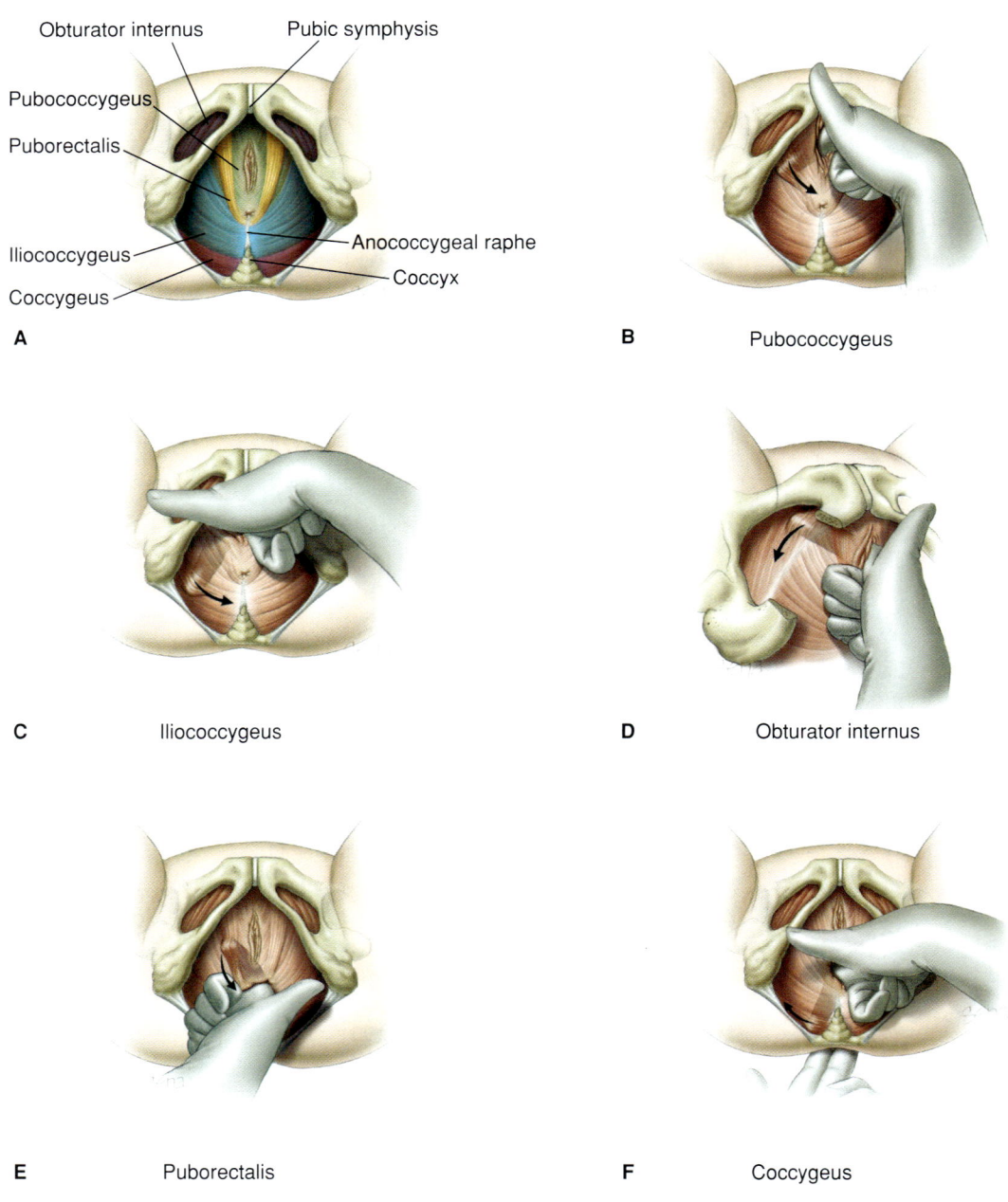

FIGURE 12-4 Pelvic floor muscle examination. (Reproduced with permission from Ms. Marie Sena.)

of the uterosacral ligaments are palpated. Tender nodularity has approximately 85-percent sensitivity and 5-percent specificity for the diagnosis of infiltrative endometriosis (Donnez, 1996). If pain follows gentle movement of the coccyx, then articular disease of the coccyx, termed *coccydynia*, is suspected. The importance of pelvic examination sequence cannot be overstated, as information from single-digit examination may be lost if preceded by bimanual examination.

Bimanual assessment of the uterus and adnexa investigates size, mobility, and tenderness. Specific benign pathologies of the uterus and adnexa are outlined in Chapters 9 and 10.

Rectal examination and rectovaginal palpation of the rectovaginal septum is included. Palpation of hard stool or hemorrhoids may indicate GI disorders, whereas nodularity of the rectovaginal septum may be found with endometriosis or neoplasia. Last, stool testing for occult blood may be performed during digital rectal examination at the initial visit.

■ Testing

For women with CPP, results from urinalysis and urine culture can indicate stones, malignancy, or recurrent urinary tract infection (UTI). Thyroid disease can affect physiologic functioning and may be found in those with bowel or bladder symptoms. Thus, serum thyroid-stimulating hormone (TSH) levels are commonly assayed. Diabetes can lead to neuropathy, and glucose levels can be assessed with urinalysis or serum screening.

Of radiologic imaging and endoscopy options, TVS is widely used by gynecologists to evaluate CPP for the same reasons described earlier (p. 256) (Hoyos, 2017). It is most effective for structural lesion identification. In those with suspected pelvic congestion syndrome, transvaginal color Doppler ultrasound is an adjunct to TVS (Phillips, 2014). Both TVS and MR imaging are recognized imaging modalities for diagnosing deep infiltrating pelvic endometriosis (Van den Bosch, 2018). In those with bowel symptoms, barium enema may indicate intraluminal or external obstructive lesions, malignancy, and diverticular or inflammatory bowel disease. However, flexible sigmoidoscopy and colonoscopy may offer more information because colonic mucosa can be directly inspected and biopsied.

Cystoscopy and laparoscopy can be employed, and patient symptoms will dictate their use. In those with symptoms of chronic pain and urinary symptoms, cystoscopy is often advised. For many women with no obvious cause of their CPP, laparoscopy can aid diagnosis (Cunanan, 1983; Kang, 2007). Laparoscopy allows direct identification and, in many cases, treatment of intraabdominal pathology. Therefore, laparoscopy is considered for CPP if initial evaluations are nondiagnostic.

■ Treatment

Nonpharmacologic Therapy

In many women with CPP, an identifying source is found and treatment is dictated by the diagnosis. However, in other cases, pathology may not be identified, and treatment is directed toward dominant symptoms.

Data addressing use of nonpharmacologic options for CPP are scarce, but benefits may be extrapolated from studies in other chronic pain syndromes. These therapies are typically low risk and may be advantageous in patients with multiple comorbidities, in those with drug intolerances or potential drug interactions, and for pain refractory to traditional therapies.

Of options, evidence supporting the role of dietary modification in CPP management is mainly limited to anecdotal reports or questionnaire-based surveys. Antiinflammatory, gluten-free, Paleo, and low fermentable oligosaccharides, disaccharides, monosaccharides, and polyols (low FODMAP) diets are the most commonly cited as potentially beneficial for chronic pain.

Pelvic Floor Physical Therapy

This specialized physical therapy focuses on pelvic floor, hips, back, and abdominal wall muscles. Interventions are customized and often include a combination of therapeutic exercises, manual manipulation, trigger point or myofascial release, acupressure, patient education, biofeedback, and muscle coordination training (Bradley, 2017; Vandyken, 2017). Clinical experience supports the role of pelvic floor physical therapy (PFPT) for pelvic pain conditions, but high-quality evidence is limited. One small study showed reduced pain for women with pelvic floor myalgia (Zoorob, 2015).

Patients likely to benefit from PFPT are those with pain reproducible during pelvic floor, abdominal wall, or back muscle palpation or contraction. Another is the group with significant deconditioning as a result of pain avoidance behaviors (Till, 2017). Patients with CPP are ideally referred to a physical therapist with specialized expertise in PFPT for this indication (Polackwich, 2015).

Psychotherapy

Psychotherapy, in the form of cognitive behavioral therapy, counseling, group therapy, biofeedback, and mindfulness-based strategies can be used for CPP. In a randomized trial of women with endometriosis-associated pelvic pain, psychotherapy combined with somatosensory stimulation improved pain, dyschezia, and quality of life (Meissner, 2016). Mindfulness-based strategies promote pain acceptance and nonreactive awareness rather than attempts to control or decrease pain itself (Sturgeon, 2014). In one metaanalysis, this intervention improved pain acceptance and reduce depression rates in patients with chronic pain conditions (Veehof, 2016). Patients with CPP and concurrent depression or anxiety may especially benefit from mindfulness-based interventions (Sephton, 2007).

Neuromodulation

Peripheral neuromodulation involves delivering electrical stimulation to a sensory nerve, which is thought to suppress nociceptive processing of pain signals (Ellrich, 2005). No consensus defines the optimal target or location for neuromodulation for CPP (Hunter, 2018). Modalities include transcutaneous electric nerve stimulation (TENS), intravaginal electrical stimulation (IVES), sacral neuromodulation, and percutaneous tibial nerve stimulation (PTNS).

Of these, TENS using skin electrodes placed at the T10 dermatome was compared with placebo for CPP treatment. After 2 weeks, VAS pain scores improved with TENS (Sharma, 2017).

IVES uses an intravaginal probe to emit electrical impulses to stimulate muscle contraction. Several Food and Drug

Administration (FDA)-approved devices are available for pelvic floor muscle re-education or rehabilitation to treat stress, urge, or mixed urinary incontinence. IVES has also been studied for CPP using frequencies below the threshold to induce muscle contraction. Despite its widespread therapeutic use for CPP indications, few rigorous studies have evaluated its efficacy for CPP. In one randomized trial comparing IVES and placebo for CPP, IVES significantly reduced pain intensity after 5 weeks of treatment (de Bernardes, 2010). However, no long-term follow-up was incorporated in this study.

Sacral neuromodulation is FDA approved only for treatment of overactive bladder, urinary retention, and chronic fecal incontinence. The only currently available method for transforaminal sacral nerve access is the InterStim Neurostimulator, which is fully described and illustrated in Chapter 45 (p. 1111). InterStim has been used off label to treat refractory CPP, IC/BPS, and pudendal neuralgia. Evidence shows symptom relief still at 12 months (Hunter, 2018).

PTNS delivers electrical pulses through a needle to stimulate the afferent fibers of the tibial nerve that runs posterior to the medial malleolus and extends to the sacral nerve plexus. Although currently approved by the FDA for treatment of overactive bladder, only a few small studies have assessed PTNS efficacy for CPP. In one small randomized trial that compared PTNS with usual care for CPP, pain and physical functioning were significantly improved. Moreover, benefits were sustained after 6 months (Istek, 2014).

Pharmacologic Options

Pharmacologic options for management for CPP include analgesics, opioids, hormones, antidepressants, and antiepileptic drugs. CPP often has a visceral and neuropathic pain component. Accordingly, effective drug combinations often work peripherally and in the CNS (Carey, 2016).

Nonopioid analgesics include nonsteroidal antiinflammatory drugs (NSAIDs) and acetaminophen. NSAIDs block inflammatory mediators through their inhibition of the cyclooxygenase enzyme, which reduces prostaglandin production. They are most useful if inflammatory states underlie the pain, and examples are found in Table 11-1 (p. 242). Acetaminophen has no antiinflammatory properties but may be useful as an analgesic, especially in patients with allergies or intolerances to NSAIDs.

Hormonal modulation may be most useful in patients with endometriosis-related CPP. However, pain from IC/BPS, IBS, inflammatory bowel disease, temporomandibular disorder, and migraine headaches may fluctuate with the menstrual cycle (Bharadwaj, 2015; LeResche, 2003; Powell-Boone, 2005). It follows that cycle suppression could improve symptoms. For this, off-label use of combination oral contraceptives (COCs) or progestin-only pills is a mainstay of hormonal modulation. Moreover, depot medroxyprogesterone acetate (DMPA), progestin implants, the levonorgestrel-releasing intrauterine system (LNG-IUS), and gonadotropin-releasing hormone (GnRH) agonists and antagonists are options. The oral GnRH antagonist elagolix is FDA-approved for the management of endometriosis-associated pain (Taylor, 2017).

Traditionally prescribed for neuropathic pain, gabapentin and pregabalin are anticonvulsants that act as calcium-channel blockers (Table 12-5). They have efficacy for nonspecific pain conditions and for fibromyalgia (Benzon, 2011). In gynecology, gabapentin has the most evidence of efficacy for women with CPP due to known gynecologic pathology (Lewis, 2016). Other anticonvulsants such as phenytoin, carbamazepine, and lamotrigine act by means of their sodium channel–blocking effects and are effective in many neuropathic pain conditions. However, studies evaluating their efficacy specifically for CPP are lacking.

Antidepressants can treat chronic pain syndromes, but limited evidence supports their usefulness for CPP. Of these, tricyclic antidepressants (TCAs) raise norepinephrine levels and are thought to modify descending pain pathways (Kremer, 2016). This makes them particularly effective for neuropathic pain, independent of their antidepressant effects. However, their use may be limited by significant anticholinergic side effects (Saarto, 2010). The serotonin- and norepinephrine-reuptake inhibitors (SNRIs) venlafaxine, duloxetine, and milnacipran have been studied in the management of chronic pain syndromes. Both TCAs and SNRIs at best modestly improve these pain syndromes, are often accompanied adverse effects that limit dosing and therapy, and have not been well studied for CPP. The benefits of selective serotonin-reuptake inhibitors (SSRIs) for anxiety and depression are well established. But, support of efficacy specifically for CPP is similarly lacking.

Opioid analgesia was reviewed in a 2018 metaanalysis of 96 randomized trials of patients with chronic noncancer pain. Opioid use was associated with significant but small improvements in pain and physical functioning compared with placebo. Comparisons of opioids with nonopioid alternatives (NSAIDs, TCAs, anticonvulsants) suggest that pain and physical functioning benefits may be similar, although the evidence was considered low to moderate quality (Busse, 2018).

In response to high rates of opioid use disorders in the United States, the Centers for Disease Control published guidelines in 2016 for the prescription of opioids for chronic nonmalignant pain (Nicol, 2017). These recommendations were based on three primary tenets. First, no evidence shows long-term improvement in function or pain between opioid and nonopioid alternatives. Second, opioid harms include overdose, opioid use disorder, and motor vehicle injuries. Last, nonpharmacologic and nonopioid pharmacologic treatments offer similar pain relief and less associated harm (Valentine, 2018).

Surgery

Hysterectomy and bilateral salpingo-oophorectomy (BSO) at times may serve as definitive management if thorough evaluation is complete and conservative therapies have failed. For many women with CPP, hysterectomy is effective in resolving pain and improving quality of life (Hartmann, 2004; Stovall, 1990). However, pain may not be resolved in a significant number. For example, one prospective study assessed 308 women for 1 year after hysterectomy performed for CPP. Of these, 75 percent had complete discomfort resolution, 21 percent had persistent but improved pain, and 5 had unchanged or worsening pain. Pain may persist despite hysterectomy more commonly in women who are <30 years, have mental illness, or have no identifiable pelvic pathology (Gunter, 2003). Almost

TABLE 12-5. Antidepressants and Antiseizure Drugs Used in Chronic Pain Syndromes

Drug (Brand name)	Dosage	Side Effects
ANTISEIZURE DRUGS		
Gabapentin (Neurontin)	100–300 mg at bedtime; increase by 100 mg every 3 days up to 1800 to 3600 mg per day taken in divided doses three times daily	Drowsiness, dizziness, fatigue, nausea, sedation, weight gain
Pregabalin (Lyrica)	150 mg at bedtime for diabetic neuropathy; 300 mg twice daily for postherpetic neuralgia	Drowsiness, dizziness, fatigue, nausea, sedation, weight gain
Lamotrigine (Lamictal)[a]	50 mg per day; increase by 50 mg every 2 weeks up to 400 mg per day	Dizziness, constipation, nausea; rarely, life-threatening rashes
Carbamazepine (Tegretol)	200 mg per day; increase by 200 mg per week up to 400 mg three times daily (1200 mg per day)	Dizziness, diplopia, nausea, aplastic anemia
Phenytoin (Dilantin)[a]	100 mg at bedtime; increase weekly up to 500 mg at bedtime	Blood dyscrasias, hepatotoxicity
ANTIDEPRESSANTS		
Tricyclic antidepressants		Dry mouth, constipation, urinary retention, sedation, weight gain
Amitriptyline (Elavil)[a] Imipramine (Tofranil)[a]	For both, 10–25 mg at bedtime; increase by 10–25 mg per week up to 75–150 mg at bedtime or a therapeutic drug level	Tertiary amines have greater anticholinergic side effects
Desipramine (Norpramin)[a] Nortriptyline (Pamelor)[a]	For both, 25 mg in the morning or at bedtime; increase by 25 mg per week up to 150 mg per day or a therapeutic drug level	Secondary amines have fewer anticholinergic side effects
SNRIs		
Venlafaxine (Effexor)[a]	37.5 mg per day; increase by 37.5 mg per week up to 225 mg per day	Nausea, sweating, sedation, dry mouth, anorexia, constipation, sweating
Duloxetine (Cymbalta)	60 mg once daily	
Milnacipran (Savella)	12.5 mg once daily and then escalate every few days through 12.5 mg and 25 mg twice daily to reach 50 mg twice daily	
SSRIs		
Fluoxetine (Prozac)[a]	For both, 10–20 mg per day; up to 80 mg per day for fibromyalgia	Nausea, sedation, decreased libido, sexual dysfunction, headache, weight gain
Paroxetine (Paxil)[a]		

[a]Not approved by the Food and Drug Administration for treatment of neuropathic pain.
SNRI = Serotonin- and norepinephrine-reuptake inhibitor; SSRI = Selective serotonin-reuptake inhibitor.

40 percent of women with no identified pelvic pathology will have persistent pain after hysterectomy (Hillis, 1995).

Failure of hysterectomy to relieve pain may be multifactorial. First, visceral reflexes may produce multiple pain syndromes within the same patient. Second, hysterectomy does not address nongynecologic etiologies for pelvic pain. Last, pain from IC/BPS, pelvic floor myofascial syndrome, or musculoskeletal disorders may worsen following surgery due to its potentially negative effects on innervation, musculature, or vasculature.

Accordingly, before hysterectomy is considered, efforts to accurately diagnose CPP causes and to conservatively manage pain are first exhausted. Women are given reasonable expectations for symptom relief from hysterectomy and informed of the potential for persistent or worsening pain. As with any operation, the anticipated benefits should outweigh potential risks.

■ Specific Causes of CPP
Pelvic Adhesions

Adhesions are fibrous connections that vary in vascularity and thickness between opposing organ surfaces or between an organ and abdominal wall. These develop secondarily and promoters include previous surgery, prior intraabdominal infection, and endometriosis. Less commonly, inflammation from radiation, chemical irritation, or foreign-body reaction may be causes. Pain is typically aggravated by sudden movement or intercourse. In those with pain, adhesions are believed to stretch the peritoneum or organ serosa as it moves (Demco, 2004; Suleiman, 2001).

These fibrous connections are common, and in laparoscopies performed for CPP, adhesions are found in approximately one quarter of cases (Howard, 1993). However, not all adhesive disease creates pain (Thornton, 1997).

To diagnose these, a history of prior surgeries and pain with abrupt movement are suggestive. Adhesions are poorly imaged. Although not used routinely, dynamic sonography techniques that push the transducer to incite movement or tethering between organs can be informative in some cases (Ayachi, 2018; Nezhat, 2014).

Surgical lysis is often used to treat affected women with associated pain (Fayez, 1994; Steege, 1991; Sutton, 1990). However, two randomized studies comparing adhesion lysis with expectant management found no difference in pain scores after 1 year (Peters, 1992; Swank, 2003). Others who support the continued judicious use of adhesiolysis in the treatment of pelvic pain question the statistical methods used in these studies (Roman, 2009). When performed, adhesiolysis is associated with a significant risk of adhesiogenesis, especially in cases involving endometriosis (Parker, 2005). Moreover, actual adhesive disease is often not reliably confirmed preoperative. Thus, the decision to pursue laparoscopic adhesiolysis is individualized. Pain-relief benefits are balanced against laparoscopy risks and the risk for new adhesion formation with surgery. Techniques to minimize adhesion formation are described in Chapter 40 (p. 855).

Ovarian Remnant Syndrome and Ovarian Retention Syndrome

After oophorectomy, remnants of an excised ovary may create symptoms that are termed *ovarian remnant syndrome*. Distinction is made between this syndrome and *ovarian retention syndrome*. Ovarian retention syndrome involves symptoms stemming from an ovary intentionally left at the time of previous gynecologic surgery (El Minawi, 1999). Although differentiated by the amount of ovarian tissue involved, both syndromes have nearly identical symptoms and are diagnosed and treated similarly.

Although an uncommon cause of CPP, women with symptomatic ovarian remnants most typically complain of chronic or cyclic pain or dyspareunia. Those with BSO performed for endometriosis may be at particular risk (Kho, 2012). The onset of symptoms is variable and may begin years following surgery (Nezhat, 2005). Women with these syndromes may have a pelvic mass palpable on bimanual examination. Sonography is often informative. In those with remnants, ovaries may be identified in some cases by a thin rim of ovarian cortex surrounding a coexistent ovarian cyst (Fleischer, 1998). Indeterminate cases may require CT or MR imaging. In cases in which ureteral compression is suspected, radiographic or CT pyelography or MR imaging may be indicated. Laboratory testing, specifically

follicle-stimulating hormone (FSH) levels, can aid diagnosis in reproductive-aged women with prior BSO. If these levels lie in the premenopausal range, then retained ovarian tissue is likely (Magtibay, 2005).

Although medical treatment has included hormonal manipulation to suppress functioning tissue, surgical excision is required in most symptomatic cases (Lafferty, 1996). Because the ureter or bladder is commonly intimately involved with adhesions encasing a remnant, laparotomy is reasonable in some cases. However, surgeons with advanced skills in minimally invasive surgery can achieve successful outcomes (Nezhat, 2005; Zapardiel, 2012).

Pelvic Congestion Syndrome

Retrograde blood flow through incompetent valves can often create tortuous, congested ovarian or pelvic veins. Chronic pelvic ache, pressure, and heaviness may result and is termed *pelvic congestion syndrome* (Beard, 1988). Currently, it is not clear whether congestion results from mechanical dilation, ovarian hormonal dysfunction, or both. Higher rates of ovarian varicosities and pelvic congestion syndrome are noted in parous women. A mechanical theory describes a dramatic increase in pelvic vein diameter during late pregnancy that leads to ovarian vein valve incompetence and pelvic varicosities. Estrogen is implicated in pelvic congestion syndrome in that it acts as a venous dilator. Moreover, pelvic congestion syndrome resolves following menopause, and antiestrogenic medical therapy can be effective (Farquhar, 1989; Gangar, 1993). Most likely, both factors play roles. The cause of pain with pelvic congestion also is unclear, but greater vessel dilation, concomitant stasis, and release of local nociceptive mediators are suggested mechanisms.

Affected women may describe pelvic ache or heaviness that may worsen premenstrually, after prolonged sitting or standing, or following intercourse. During physical examination, tenderness at the junction of the middle and lateral thirds of a line drawn between the symphysis and ASIS (the ovarian point) or direct ovarian tenderness may be found. In addition, varicosities in the thigh, buttocks, perineum, or vagina may be associated (Venbrux, 1999).

To initially investigate suspected cases, TVS or CT or MR venography is recommended. Sonographic findings with applied Doppler include a dilated tortuous ovarian vein with a diameter ≥6 mm, slow blood flow ≤3 cm/s, and a dilated arcuate vein in the myometrium that communicates to the pelvic varicosities (Fig. 12-5) (Park, 2004). With positive findings, retrograde ovarian and internal iliac venography is preferred if intervention is planned (Gloviczki, 2011). Diagnostic laparoscopy also can identify varicosities. However, because all these modalities are performed while a woman is supine or in Trendelenburg position, varicosities often decompress and may be missed. CO_2 insufflation pressure also contributes to the high false-negative rate of laparoscopy to diagnose pelvic varicosities.

Common treatments for pelvic congestion syndrome are hormonal suppression, ovarian vein embolization, or hysterectomy with BSO. First, medical treatment with medroxyprogesterone acetate, 30 mg orally daily, or with a GnRH agonist is effective for some women with pelvic congestion syndrome. Notably, symptoms typically recur after medication

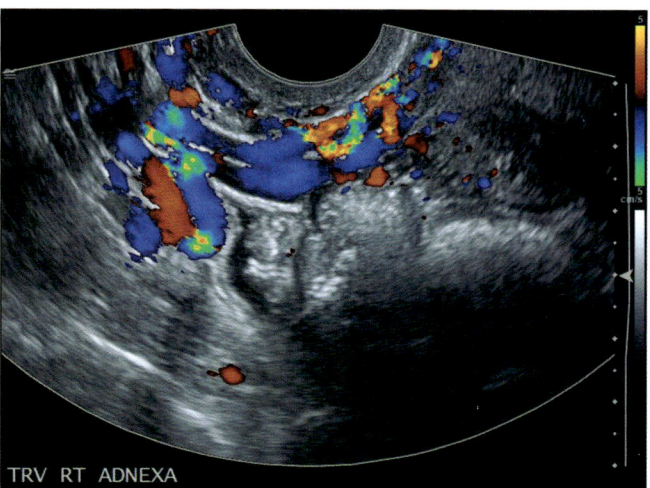

FIGURE 12-5 Color Doppler transvaginal image of tortuous and dilated pelvic vessels in the right adnexa in a patient with chronic pelvic pain. (Reproduced with permission from Dr. Elysia Moschos.)

is discontinued (Reginald, 1989; Soysal, 2001). Alternatively, vessel embolization can be effective, and pain improves in 70 to 80 percent of treated women (Hansrani, 2015). Last, in one study of 36 women who underwent hysterectomy and BSO for pelvic congestion syndrome with intractable pelvic pain, 12 of 36 had residual pain at 1 year (Beard, 1991). However, only one patient had pain that affected her daily life, and authors concluded that pain and quality-of-life scores were improved. Importantly, none of these options is definitive, and evidence-based studies supporting their efficacy are limited.

DYSMENORRHEA

Cyclic pain with menstruation is common and accompanies most menses (Weissman, 2004). This pain is classically described as cramping and is often accompanied by low backache, nausea and vomiting, headache, or diarrhea. The term *primary dysmenorrhea* describes cyclic menstrual pain without an identifiable associated pathology, whereas *secondary dysmenorrhea* frequently complicates endometriosis, leiomyomas, PID, adenomyosis, endometrial polyps, and menstrual outlet obstruction. For this reason, secondary dysmenorrhea may be associated with other gynecologic symptoms, such as dyspareunia, dysuria, abnormal bleeding, or infertility.

Compared with secondary dysmenorrhea, primary dysmenorrhea more commonly begins shortly after menarche. Pain characteristics, however, typically fail to differentiate between the two types, and primary dysmenorrhea is usually diagnosed following exclusion of known associated causes.

When other factors are removed, primary dysmenorrhea equally affects women regardless of race and socioeconomic status. However, increased pain duration or severity is positively associated with earlier age at menarche, long menstrual periods, smoking, and greater body mass index (BMI). In contrast, parity appears to improve symptoms (Harlow, 1996; Sundell, 1990).

Pathophysiologically, prostaglandins are implicated in dysmenorrhea. During endometrial sloughing, endometrial cells release prostaglandins as menstruation begins. Prostaglandins stimulate myometrial contractions and ischemia. Women with more severe dysmenorrhea have higher levels of prostaglandins in their menstrual fluid, and these levels are highest during the first 2 days of menstruation. Prostaglandins are also implicated in secondary dysmenorrhea. However, anatomic mechanisms also are suspected, depending on the type of accompanying pelvic disease.

■ Diagnosis

In women with menstrual cramps and no other associated findings or symptoms, no additional evaluation may be initially required, and empiric therapy can be prescribed (Proctor, 2006). If pelvic evaluation is incomplete due to body habitus, TVS may be informative to exclude structural pelvic pathology. If symptoms or physical examination suggest a specific source for secondary dysmenorrhea, evaluation is directed to confirm this suspicion.

■ Treatment

Of options, NSAIDs are often preferred. Because prostaglandins are suspected in the genesis of dysmenorrhea, NSAID administration is logical, and studies support their use (Marjoribanks, 2015). These drugs and their dosages are found in Table 11-1 (p. 242).

Steroid hormone contraception leads to endometrial atrophy and in turn to lower endometrial prostaglandin levels. Of choices, COCs are believed to improve dysmenorrhea by lowering prostaglandin production (Brill, 1991; Wong, 2009). In addition, extended or continuous administration of COCs, described in Chapter 5 (p. 122), may be helpful for women with pain not controlled by the traditional cyclic pill schedule (Sulak, 1997). Progestin-only contraceptives also are used for dysmenorrhea. Namely, the LNG-IUS, DMPA, or progestin-releasing implant is a reasonable choice (Lindh, 2013).

GnRH agonists, GnRH antagonists, and androgens are other options. The estrogen-lowering effects of these lead to endometrial atrophy and diminished prostaglandin production. Although GnRH agents and androgens such as danazol lessen dysmenorrhea, their substantial side effects preclude their routine and long-term use. A fuller discussion of these agents and their side effects is found in Chapter 11 (p. 243).

Cases of dysmenorrhea refractory to conservative management are unusual, and in such instances, surgery may be indicated. Hysterectomy is effective in treating dysmenorrhea, but those desiring future fertility may decline. For these women, presacral neurectomy (PSN) can be considered.

PSN involves interruption of somatic pain fibers from the uterus that course within the superior hypogastric plexus (Fig. 38-13, p. 802). This procedure is performed by incising the pelvic peritoneum over the sacrum and then identifying and transecting the sacral nerve plexus. PSN is technically challenging and requires familiarity with operating in the presacral space. PSN has central pelvic effects and is most effective for dysmenorrhea. Success rates range from 60 to 75 percent (Chen, 1997; Lee, 1986; Zullo, 2003). However, surgery can be associated with long-term postoperative constipation and urinary retention. Infrequently, intraoperative hemorrhage may be encountered from the middle sacral vessels, which run in the presacral space.

Laparoscopic uterosacral nerve ablation (LUNA) destroys nerve fibers that pass to the uterus through the uterosacral ligament. Current evidence does not support LUNA use for pelvic pain (Daniels, 2009, 2010; Proctor, 2005).

DYSPAREUNIA

Dyspareunia is defined as pain with intercourse. It is subclassified as *insertional*, that is, pain with vaginal entry, or *deep*, which is associated with deep penetration. Of insertional dyspareunia cases, most stem from vulvodynia, vulvitis, poor lubrication, or genitourinary symptoms of menopause (GSM), which is the new preferred term for vulvovaginal atrophy. Of deep dyspareunia cases, endometriosis, pelvic adhesions, and bulky leiomyomas are frequent causes. In many women, both insertional and deep dyspareunia may be present.

Additional terms include *primary dyspareunia*, which describes the onset of painful intercourse coincident with coitarche. *Secondary dyspareunia* is painful intercourse after a period of pain-free sexual activity. Sexual abuse, female genital mutilation, and congenital anomalies most frequently lead to primary dyspareunia, whereas sources of secondary dyspareunia are more varied. Last, dyspareunia is clarified as *generalized*, occurring in all episodes of intercourse, or as *situational*, associated with only specific partners or sexual positions. Changes in the Diagnostic and Statistical Manual of Mental Disorders (DSM-5) have merged dyspareunia and vaginismus into the term *genito-pelvic pain/penetration disorder* (American Psychiatric Association, 2013).

Dyspareunia is common, and in reproductive-aged women in the United States, the 12-month prevalence is 15 to 20 percent (Glatt, 1990; Laumann, 1999). Painful intercourse may be associated with vulvar, visceral, musculoskeletal, neurogenic, or psychosomatic disorders. Coexistent etiologies also may lead to similar symptoms. For example, women with vulvodynia in many cases have coexistent pelvic floor muscle spasm, both of which may cause dyspareunia (Reissing, 2005). Because of the frequent association between dyspareunia and CPP and frequent overlap of etiologies, physical examination and diagnostic testing often follow that for women with CPP (p. 258).

■ Diagnosis

During history taking, patients are questioned regarding associated symptoms such as vaginal discharge, vulvar pain, dysmenorrhea, CPP, dysuria, or scant lubrication. Onset of symptoms and their temporal association with obstetric delivery, pelvic surgery, sexual abuse, or menopause is often informative. In addition, dyspareunia may be found in those who breastfeed, presumably because of hypoestrogenism-derived vaginal atrophy seen with lactation (Buhling, 2006; Signorello, 2001). Psychosocial topics such as relationship satisfaction or depression also are covered. These elements and others related to female sexuality are fully discussed in Chapter 14.

Inspection of the vulva mirrors that for CPP. In particular, generalized erythema, episiotomy scars, or atrophy is sought. Erythema may indicate contact or allergic dermatitis or infection,

particularly fungal infection. Accordingly, a historical inventory of potential skin irritants, microscopy of a saline-mixed vaginal discharge, vaginal pH testing, and vaginal cultures are performed. Specifically, a vaginal fungal culture may be required in some cases as several noncandidal species may be poorly detected if microscopic analysis is solely used (Haefner, 2005).

Some studies, but not all, have found a positive correlation between the degree of pelvic organ prolapse and dyspareunia (Burrows, 2004; Ellerkmann, 2001). If noted, its degree is assessed as described in Chapter 24 (p. 537).

Physical examination evaluates the distal, mid-, and proximal vagina. Evaluation may first begin with palpation of the Bartholin and paraurethral glands. Additionally, cotton-swab testing is used to map painful areas (Fig. 4-1, p. 93). Next, insertion of a single digit into the distal vagina may elicit vaginismus, that is, reflex contraction of the muscles associated with distal vaginal penetration (Basson, 2010). This contraction response is normal, but prolonged spasm of the bulbospongiosus, pubococcygeus, piriformis, and obturator internus muscles may cause pain. Spasm is thought to be a conditioned response to current or former physical pain.

With deeper digital examination, midvaginal pain may be triggered. This can be seen with IC/BPS or urethral diverticula, with congenital anomalies, or after radiation therapy or pelvic reconstructive surgeries.

Deep dyspareunia is more commonly caused by disorders that also cause CPP. Focal points of this examination are discussed on page 260. Similarly, diagnostic testing for deep dyspareunia in large part mirrors that for CPP. Urine and vaginal cultures may indicate infection, and radiologic imaging may reveal structural visceral disease.

■ Treatment

Resolution of dyspareunia is highly dependent on the underlying cause. For those with vaginismus, structured desensitization is effective. Patients gradually gain control in comfortably inserting dilators of increasing size into the introitus. Concurrent psychological counseling in such cases is often indicated. Poor lubrication may be countered with education directed toward adequate arousal techniques and use of external lubricants. Discussed in Chapter 22 (p. 496), estrogen cream or the selective estrogen-receptor modulator ospemifene (Osphena) will usually resolve GSM. Elagolix is FDA approved for endometriosis-related dyspareunia at doses of 200 mg bid for 6 months.

Surgery may be indicated for structural pathologies and may include ablation of endometriosis, lysis of adhesions, and restoration of normal anatomy. For those with dyspareunia confidently attributed to a retroverted uterine position, uterine suspension was shown to be effective, although studies were small (Perry, 2005).

UROLOGIC ETIOLOGIES

■ Infection

Recurrent UTIs are defined as two or more symptomatic infections in 6 months or three episodes in 1 year (Smith, 2018). In addition to acute treatment, continuous or postcoital antibiotic prophylaxis or self-treatment for recurrences is an effective approach (Stamm, 1993). In postmenopausal women, topical vaginal estrogen alters the vaginal flora and significantly reduces the risk of UTI compared with placebo (Raz, 1993).

Dysuria and itching are prominent symptoms of infectious urethritis. This is commonly caused by *Neisseria gonorrhoeae*, *Chlamydia trachomatis*, and *Mycoplasma genitalium*, and less commonly by *Trichomonas vaginalis*, *Gardnerella vaginalis*, *Ureaplasma urealyticum*, herpes simplex virus, and some adenoviruses (Hakenberg, 2017). Thus, a sexual history is important, and testing for these infections may be indicated depending on history and physical examination findings. Suitable testing methods for these are found in Chapter 3 (p. 65).

■ Urethral Diverticulum

Classic symptoms associated with urethral diverticula are known as the "3D's" (dysuria, dyspareunia, postvoid dribbling). Women may also note recurrent UTI, vaginal wall tenderness, frequency, urgency, and chronic pelvic or urethral pain (Baradaran, 2016; El-Nasher, 2016; Foley, 2011; Romanzi, 2000). Clinical evaluation and treatment of urethral diverticula are discussed in Chapter 26 (p. 582).

■ Lower Urinary Tract Stones

Vesical calculi represent 5 percent of urinary tract stones and typically result from foreign bodies, obstruction, or infection (Philippou, 2012). Women with prolapse may develop bladder stones from urethral obstruction and urinary stasis. Vesical calculi may also form after antiincontinence procedures due to suture or mesh in the lower urinary tract (Philippou, 2012; Schwartz, 2000). The most common symptoms are terminal dysuria, pain, incontinence, urgency, and frequency (Stav, 2012). Bladder stones can be detected by radiography, sonography, CT, or cystoscopy (Stav, 2012). Referral to a urogynecologist or urologist for further management is appropriate.

■ Other Causes

As discussed in Chapter 11, symptoms of urinary tract endometriosis may include colicky flank pain, recurrent UTIs, frequency, urgency, and bladder pain during voiding (Berlanda, 2009). Leiomyomas, discussed in Chapter 9, and midurethral slings for stress urinary incontinence, detailed in Chapter 45, both may cause chronic pain and urinary tract symptoms (Abouassaly, 2004; Langer, 1990). Patients with neoplastic lesions such as bladder cancer may present with dysuria, hematuria, pain, and recurrent UTIs (Henning, 2013).

■ Interstitial Cystitis/Bladder Pain Syndrome

This condition describes a symptom complex that encompasses bladder, urethral, and pelvic pain, as well as lower urinary tract symptoms. The American Urological Association considers IC and BPS to be synonymous, and defines it as "an unpleasant sensation (pain, pressure, discomfort) perceived to be related to the urinary bladder, associated with lower urinary tract symptoms of more than six weeks duration, in the absence of infection or other identifiable causes" (Hanno, 2011). IC/BPS is estimated to affect 6.5 percent of women in the United States, and the condition is typically diagnosed after age 40 (Berry, 2011; Hanno, 2015).

The exact cause of IC/BPS is unknown. Two current theories focus on greater bladder mucosa permeability or mast cell activation. Glycosaminoglycans (GAG) are an important component of the mucin layer that covers and protects the bladder urothelium. One theory explains that IC/BPS symptoms originate from a defect in the protective bladder GAG component. This leads to increased permeability of the bladder mucosa to noxious agents (Parsons, 2007; Sant, 2007; Theoharides, 2001).

Diagnosis

IC/BPS is considered in women with unexplained CPP and voiding symptoms. By definition, it is a diagnosis of exclusion. Other conditions such as recurrent UTI, urethral diverticulum, bladder stone, endometriosis, leiomyomas, foreign bodies, and neoplasia can mimic IC/BPS. In one study, 45 percent of patients with an initial diagnosis of IC/BPS were found during further evaluation to have other common alternative diagnoses (Irwin, 2005).

Pain, including pelvic pressure and discomfort, is the hallmark symptom of IC/BPS. The pain is often related to bladder filling and associated with pain in the pelvis, lower abdomen, and back. Frequency and urgency also are typical complaints, but other symptoms include dyspareunia and postcoital ache. Symptoms may worsen premenstrually. Given the broad spectrum of triggers that include alcohol, caffeine, smoking, spicy foods, citrus fruits and juices, carbonated drinks, and potassium, patients may not relate exacerbation of their symptoms to these. Cranberry juice, frequently advised for UTI prevention, can acutely exacerbate pain from IC/BPS.

Single-digit vaginal examination in the patient with IC/BPS may demonstrate urethral or anterior vaginal/bladder base tenderness and pelvic floor hypertonus, tenderness, or trigger points. Laboratory examination classically includes urinalysis and culture, and unevaluated microhematuria typically prompts cytology, especially in smokers, to exclude urinary tract neoplasia. Cystoscopy and urodynamic studies may add clarity to complex presentations or exclude of other entities that mimic IC/BPS. However, consensus on cystoscopic or urodynamic criteria for IC/BPS is lacking (Hanno, 2011). Cystoscopically, *Hunner ulcers* are reddish-brown mucosal lesions with small vessels radiating toward a central scar. These ulcers are rare but considered diagnostic for IC. The more common finding is *glomerulations,* which are small petechiae or submucosal hemorrhages. However, these may be present in patients without IC/BPS symptoms and undergoing cystoscopy for other indications (Waxman, 1998). Urodynamic testing may reveal sensory urgency at low bladder volumes, decreased compliance, and diminished capacity. The potassium sensitivity test (PST) indicates greater urothelial permeability but is painful and may trigger a severe symptom flare. Moreover, a negative result does not eliminate suspicion for IC/BPS. In one study, 25 percent of patients meeting strict IC criteria had a negative PST result (Parsons, 1998).

Diagnosing IC/BPS can be challenging given its broad symptom spectrum, its frequent association with other pelvic pain syndromes, and its symptoms that overlap with other pain disorders. Moreover, uniform consensus on diagnostic criteria is lacking. Thus, the diagnosis of IC/BPS remains clinical. Not surprisingly, misdiagnosis, underdiagnosis, or delayed diagnosis of IC/BPS is common.

Treatment

A multidisciplinary approach to treatment should be emphasized (Nickel, 2011). The American Urological Association has provided evidence-based guidelines for IC/BPS management (Hanno, 2011, 2015). First-line treatment provides patient education and behavioral modification, especially avoidance of bladder irritants. In one prospective study, dietary manipulation improved symptoms and quality of life in patients with IC/BPS (Oh-Oka, 2017).

Second-tier options are pharmacologic agents or pelvic floor physical therapy to resolve trigger points or pelvic floor hypertonus. One small randomized trial showed reduced pain in affected women (FitzGerald, 2012). Suitable oral agents include amitriptyline, cimetidine, hydroxyzine, or pentosan polysulfate sodium (Elmiron). The choice is typically provider dependent and is influenced by patient characteristics, previous treatments, provider experience, and perhaps cost. Pentosan polysulfate sodium is a weak anticoagulant, but its mechanism of action for IC/BPS is unknown. Elmiron is FDA-approved for this indication, and the dosage is 100 mg three times daily. Doses ideally avoid meals. Also, intravesical therapy may consist of direct bladder instillation of heparin, lidocaine, or dimethyl sulfoxide (DMSO).

For patients who do not respond, third-line treatments include cystoscopy coupled with short-duration, low-pressure bladder distention and fulguration of Hunner ulcers. FDA approval is lacking for treatment with cyclosporin A, intradetrusor botulinum toxin A, sacral neuromodulation, and pudendal nerve stimulation. This last is similar to sacral neuromodulation, but instead the implanted electrode stimulates the pudendal nerve (Hunter, 2018). These third-tier methods may be considered in patients who fail to respond to other therapies. Last, major surgery such as cystoplasty or urinary diversion is performed rarely for carefully selected patients in whom all other therapies have failed to provide adequate symptom control.

Treatments that are not recommended due to poor efficacy or unacceptable adverse events include long-term antibiotic use, intravesical bacillus Calmette-Guérin or resiniferatoxin, high-pressure or long-term hydrodistension, and long-term oral corticosteroids (Hanno, 2011).

GASTROINTESTINAL DISEASE

GI disease is often found to underlie CPP and causes may be organic or functional (see Table 12-2). Thus, initial screening may follow that for CPP. However, symptoms such as fever, GI bleeding, weight loss, anemia, and abdominal mass will prompt a stronger search for organic pathology. Investigations may include sigmoidoscopy or colonoscopy to exclude inflammation, diverticula, or tumors. For those with diarrhea, stool examination for leukocytes or for ova and parasites may be indicated. Moreover, serologic testing for celiac disease can be

valuable. When indicated, TVS may aid in distinguishing GI from gynecologic pathology.

■ Colonic Diverticular Disease

Colon diverticula are small defects in the muscular layer of the colon through which colonic mucosa and submucosa herniate. Diverticular disease is common and typically affects the sigmoid or descending colon. Recurrent or chronic disease can lead to CPP (Morris, 2014). Chronic symptoms include abdominal pain that localizes to the left lower quadrant, obstipation, and rectal fullness. More seriously, diverticula may cause acute or chronic GI bleeding or may become infected. Clinically, infection can be difficult to distinguish from PID or tuboovarian abscess. In these cases, CT is the preferred imaging technique and has sensitivity for diagnosis of 94 percent and specificity of 99 percent (Lameris, 2008).

Chronic diverticular disease is usually treated with a high-fiber diet and long-term suppressive therapy with antibiotics. With acute severe infection, hospitalization, parenteral antibiotics, surgical or percutaneous abscess drainage, or partial colectomy may be required. Suspected rupture of a diverticular abscess with peritonitis is an indication for immediate surgical exploration (Morris, 2014).

■ Celiac Disease

This is an inherited autoimmune intolerance to gluten, which is a component of wheat, barley, or rye. In affected individuals, gluten ingestion creates an immune-mediated reaction that damages the small intestine mucosa and leads to varying degrees of malabsorption. Thus, treatment dictates a gluten-free diet for life (Rubio-Tapia, 2013). Celiac disease is common, and its incidence in the general population approaches 1 percent (Green, 2007).

The most common symptoms are abdominal pain and diarrhea. Other findings include weight loss, osteopenia, and fatigue from anemia, all of which stem from malabsorption. In addition, celiac disease has been associated with infertility, although the mechanism is not understood (Tersigni, 2014).

Celiac disease is suspected in those with characteristic findings and in those with a family history of the disorder. Diagnosis requires both duodenal biopsy and a positive response to a gluten-free diet. However, many physicians will screen with noninvasive serologic tests. Of these, testing for IgA antitissue transglutaminase antibodies is preferred. For this, patients maintain a gluten-containing diet during testing (Rubio-Tapia, 2013).

■ Functional Bowel Disorders

This group of functional disorders has symptoms attributable to the lower GI tract, and definitions are periodically updated. Those listed in Table 12-6 reflect Rome IV criteria (Drossman, 2016a,b). The diagnosis of these functional disorders always presumes the absence of a structural or biochemical explanation for symptoms.

Irritable Bowel Syndrome

This functional bowel disorder is defined as abdominal pain related to defecation and is associated with a change in bowel

TABLE 12-6. Functional Bowel Disorders and Definitions[a]

Irritable bowel syndrome (IBS)	Recurrent abdominal pain on average at least 1 day/week in the last 3 months associated with 2 or more of the following: (1) related to defecation; (2) associated with a change in stooling frequency; (3) associated with a change in form of stool
Functional abdominal bloating/distention	Must include *both* of the following: (1) recurrent bloating or distention on average at least 1 day/week; (2) insufficient criteria for a diagnosis of IBS or other functional GI disorder
Functional constipation	Must include *two or more* of the following: (1) straining during >25% of defecations; (2) lumpy or hard stools in >25% of defecations; (3) sensation of incomplete evacuation in >25% of defecations; (4) sensation of anorectal obstruction/blockage in >25% of defecations; (5) manual maneuvers to aid >25% of defecations; (6) fewer than three defecations per week Loose stools are rarely present without the use of laxatives Criteria insufficient for IBS
Functional diarrhea	Loose or watery stools without pain, occurring in >25% of stools
Unspecified functional bowel disorder	Bowel symptoms not attributable to an organic etiology that do not meet criteria for the previously defined categories
Opioid-induced constipation	New or worsening constipation related to opioid therapy with two of more of the same required criteria for functional constipation Loose stools are rarely present without the use of laxatives

[a]Criteria fulfilled for the last 3 months with symptom onset at least 6 months before diagnosis.
GI = gastrointestinal.
From Drossman, 2016b; Lacy, 2016.

habits. Criteria further mandate that symptoms are present for the last 3 months with symptom onset at least 6 months before diagnosis (Lacy, 2016). Subtypes are divided by the predominant stool pattern and include constipative, diarrheal, and mixed categories. Although defining criteria are listed in Table 12-6, other symptoms that support the diagnosis include straining, defecatory urgency, feeling of incomplete evacuation, passing mucus, and bloating.

IBS is common, and its general population prevalence approximates 10 percent (Canavan, 2014; Lovell, 2012). The prevalences of diarrhea-predominant and constipation-predominant IBS are equivalent, but constipation-predominant IBS may be more common in women (Saito, 2002, Lovell, 2012).

The pathophysiology of IBS is complex, and neural, hormonal, genetic, environmental, and psychosocial factors are variably involved (Drossman, 2002). The primary mechanism of IBS, however, is thought to stem from poorly regulated interactions between the CNS and the enteric nervous system (ENS). Such brain-gut dysfunction may eventually cause alterations of GI mucosal immune response, intestinal motility and permeability, and visceral sensitivity. In turn, these produce abdominal pain and altered bowel function (Mayer, 2008). Specifically, serotonin (5-hydroxytryptamine, 5-HT) is involved with regulating intestinal motility, visceral sensitivity, and gut secretion and is implicated in IBS (Atkinson, 2006; Gershon, 2005).

For young patients who have typical IBS symptoms and no organic disease symptoms, few tests are required. Testing is individualized, and factors that typically prompt greater evaluation include older patient age, longer duration and greater severity of symptoms, absent psychosocial factors, organic disease symptoms, and family history of GI disease.

Treatment. Nonpharmacologic approaches may improve symptoms. First, no specific diet suffices for all patients, but foods known to trigger symptoms are logically avoided. Combination probiotics in general improve global IBS symptoms, bloating, and flatulence, although data limit recommendation of preferred species (Ford, 2014a,c).

Drug therapy is directed toward dominant symptoms. For those with constipation-dominant IBS, commercial soluble fiber analogues or psyllium husk may help if increased dietary fiber is unsuccessful (Bijkerk, 2009). Of these, psyllium husk is gradually titrated to improve tolerability to a dosage of 3 to 5 g orally twice daily. Of note, dietary fiber is effective in treating constipation but is not effective for diarrhea-dominant IBS or for IBS-associated pain (Ruepert, 2011).

Of medical options, linaclotide (Linzess), a guanylate cyclase agonist, enhances fluid secretion and transit time (Chey, 2012b; Rao, 2012). It is taken orally as a 290-μg capsule once daily. Alternatively, lubiprostone (Amitiza) is a GI chloride-channel activator that is taken orally twice daily as an 8-μg capsule. It also enhances intestinal fluid secretion to improve intestinal motility (Chey, 2012a; Drossman, 2009).

For those with diarrhea-dominant symptoms, treatments often strive to slow bowel motility because as substances stay longer in the gut, more water is absorbed from fecal matter to bulk stools. Goals are improved abdominal pain and stool consistency. Indirect evidence supports loperamide (Imodium), 2 mg orally once or twice daily (Trinkley, 2014; Weinberg, 2014). Eluxadoline (Viberzi) acts peripherally on bowel opioid receptors to reduce visceral hypersensitivity without completely disrupting intestinal motility. It improves IBS symptoms when a 100-mg dose is taken twice daily (Lembo, 2016). Rifaximin (Xifaxan) is an oral, nonsystemic antibiotic that targets the gut microbiome to improve symptoms (Pimentel, 2011). Last, for those with severe diarrhea, alosetron (Lotronex), a selective serotonin 5-HT_3-receptor antagonist, interacts with ENS neuron receptors to aid IBS symptoms (Camilleri, 2000; Chey, 2004). However, due to cases of ischemic colitis associated with its use, alosetron is now available but providers are encouraged to participate in a modified risk evaluation and mitigation strategy (REMS) program that provides product updates when needed (Chang, 2006; Food and Drug Administration, 2016).

For patients with pain secondary to bowel spasm, antispasmodic agents decrease intestinal smooth muscle activity and are thought to improve abdominal discomfort. Agents available in the United States include dicyclomine (Bentyl) and hyoscyamine sulfate (Levsin). Dicyclomine is begun at 20 mg orally four times daily and increased after 1 week to 40 mg. Hyoscyamine sulfate is dosed at 0.25 to 0.5 mg orally daily and can be increased as needed up to four times daily. Although having benefits for IBS, the anticholinergic side effects of these agents often limit their long-term use (Ruepert, 2011; Schoenfeld, 2005). Peppermint oil, another effective antispasmodic, can be taken orally as over-the-counter capsules at dosages of 550 mg once daily or 187 mg three times daily (Khanna, 2014).

Tricyclic antidepressants may help patients with IBS both by an anticholinergic effect on the gut and by their mood-modifying action. TCAs may slow intestinal transit time and can be effective in treatment of diarrhea-dominant IBS (Hadley, 2005). Last, psychological or behavioral treatments may help some patients (Ford, 2014b).

■ Functional Anorectal Pain

Proctalgia fugax, levator ani syndrome, and unspecified functional anorectal pain are the three types of functional anorectal pain disorders described by Rome IV criteria (Rao, 2016). The term *chronic proctalgia* is excluded from the new classification.

Levator ani syndrome usually presents as a pressure or dull ache in the upper rectum that is often worse with sitting than with standing or lying. Four criteria are: (1) chronic or recurrent rectal pain or aching, (2) episodes lasting ≥30 minutes, (3) exclusion of organic rectal pain causes, and (4) tenderness during traction on the puborectalis muscle. These four must be present for the last 3 months and symptom onset should be at least 6 months before diagnosis. A diagnosis of *unspecified functional anorectal pain* can be made when the first three of these are present.

The levator ani muscles, including their supporting fascia, overlying parietal peritoneum, and intimately associated visceral peritoneum, are connected by common sensory nerves to the spinal cord. These are thought to provide the basis for viscerosomatic convergence (Spitznagle, 2014). Some suggest that pain stems from trigger points, described subsequently, in the levator ani muscles.

For levator ani syndrome treatment, biofeedback is preferred, but anal canal electrical stimulation or levator ani muscle massage is an option. Adjuvant treatments include warm sitz baths and medicines such as NSAIDs, other analgesics, muscle relaxants, and tranquilizers (Hull, 2009).

In contrast, *proctalgia fugax* presents as sudden, severe rectal pain, unrelated to defecation, that lasts for a few seconds to a few minutes and then completely disappears. Pain may disrupt normal activities and may awaken a patient from sleep. But, episodes rarely occur more than five times a year. Diagnosis is based on its characteristic symptoms and exclusion of organic anorectal or pelvic pathology (Rao, 2016). Proctalgia fugax is typically managed with explanation of the condition and reassurance.

MUSCULOSKELETAL ETIOLOGIES

Clinical syndromes involving the muscles, nerves, and skeletal system of the lower abdomen and pelvis are frequently encountered but often overlooked by gynecologists. Importantly, unrecognized musculoskeletal pain may lead to unnecessary surgery or promote development of pelvic pain syndromes.

■ Hernia

Defects in the anterior abdominal wall or femoral fascia can lead to herniation of bowel or other intraabdominal contents through these rents. Such herniation can create pain locally at the defect site or cause referred pain along the distribution of a compressed sensory nerve. Moreover, if blood supply to the contents is acutely compromised, then bowel obstruction or ischemia will require surgical intervention. Hernias that involve the anterior abdominal wall and pelvic floor are most commonly associated with CPP.

Hernias may develop at sites of inherent anatomic weakness, which may be congenital or acquired. Conditions that raise intraabdominal pressure such as pregnancy, ascites, peritoneal dialysis, and chronic cough are known risk factors. Of types, ventral hernias derive from fascial defects typically occurring in the midline and may develop at prior incision sites (Fig. 12-6). Umbilical hernias originate from umbilical ring weakness. Spigelian hernias are rare and develop along the lateral rectus abdominis muscle border, especially at this border's intersection with the arcuate line. Indirect inguinal hernias are those in which abdominal contents herniate through the internal inguinal ring and into the inguinal canal. Contents may then exit the external inguinal ring (Fig. 12-7). In contrast, contents of a direct inguinal hernia bulge directly through a fascial defect within the Hesselbach triangle.

For diagnosis, patients with CPP or abdominal pain ideally are examined while standing and also during Valsalva maneuver. Small ventral, umbilical, or incisional hernias may be repaired by gynecologic surgeons. In these cases, the hernia sac is excised and fascia reapproximated. Patients with larger hernias, which usually require mesh placement, or with hernias in the inguinal area are typically referred to a general surgeon.

■ Myofascial Pain Syndrome

Primary musculoskeletal conditions can lead to CPP (see Table 12-2). In other cases, secondary myofascial pain syndromes can originate from endometriosis, IC/BPS, or IBS. Such chronic visceral inflammatory conditions can create pathologic changes in nearby muscles and/or nerves to cause abdominal

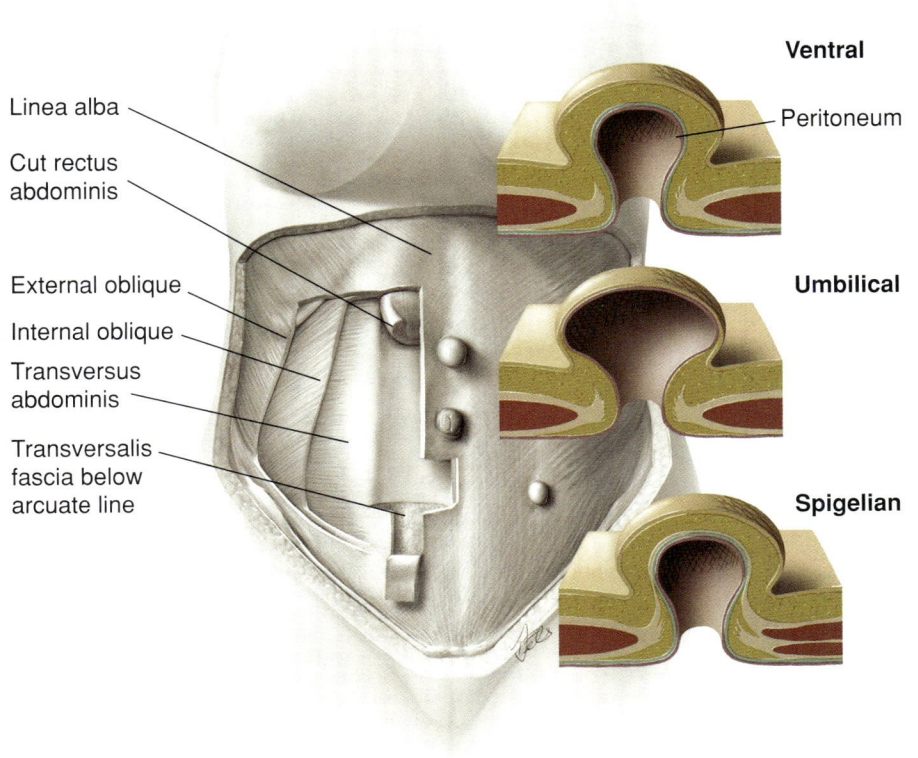

Linea alba

Cut rectus
abdominis

External oblique

Internal oblique

Transversus
abdominis

Transversalis
fascia below
arcuate line

Ventral

Peritoneum

Umbilical

Spigelian

FIGURE 12-6 Hernias that may involve the anterior abdominal wall. (Reproduced with permission from Mr. T. J. Fels.)

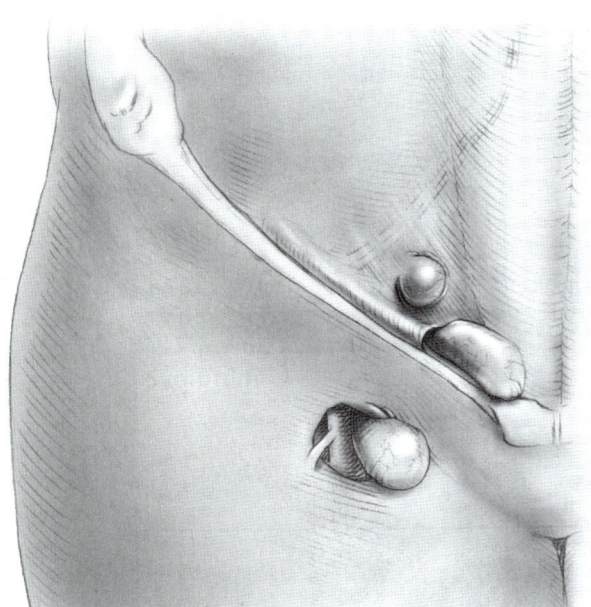

FIGURE 12-7 Indirect and direct inguinal hernias and femoral hernia. (Reproduced with permission from Mr. T. J. Fels.)

wall or pelvic floor pain. With myofascial pain, a hyperirritable area within a muscle promotes persistent fiber contraction (Simons, 1999). The primary reactive area within the muscle is termed a *trigger point (TrP)* and is identified as a palpable taut, ropy band.

TrPs are thought to form as the end point of a metabolic crisis within a muscle. Dysfunction of a neuromuscular endplate can lead to sustained acetylcholine release, persistent depolarization, sarcomere shortening, and creation of a taut muscle band. Affected fibers compress capillaries and decrease local blood flow. The resulting ischemia leads to release of substances that activate peripheral nerve nociceptors and in turn cause pain (McPartland, 2004). A persistent barrage of nociceptive signals from TrPs may eventually lead to central sensitization and the potential for neuropathic pain (p. 254). Signals may spread segmentally within the spinal cord to cause localized or referred pain (Gerwin, 2005). TrPs can also initiate viscerosomatic convergence that can generate autonomic responses such as vomiting, diarrhea, and bladder spasm.

TrPs can affect any muscle, and those involving muscles of the anterior abdominal wall, pelvic floor, and pelvic girdle can be sources of CPP. The incidence of myofascial disease is unknown, but in one study of more than 1100 women with CPP, 13 percent were diagnosed with myofascial pain syndrome (Bedaiwy, 2013). Prevalence appears to be greatest at ages between 30 and 50 years. Risk factors vary, although many TrPs can be traced to a prior specific trauma (Sharp, 2003). Accordingly, a detailed inventory of sports injuries, traumatic injuries, obstetric deliveries, surgeries, and work activities is essential.

Diagnosis

Having the patient mark painful sites on a body silhouette diagram can be an informative first step. Involvement of specific muscles will often give characteristic patterns. Patients typically describe the pain as aggravated by specific movement or activity and relieved by certain positions. Cold, damp exposure generally worsens pain. Pressure on a TrP causes discomfort and produces effects on a target area or *referral zone*. This specific and reproducible area of referral rarely coincides with dermatologic or neuronal distribution and is the feature that differentiates myofascial pain syndromes from fibromyalgia (Lavelle, 2007).

Muscle examination may be completed by flat palpation, pincer palpation, or deep palpation depending on muscle location. Flat palpation uses fingertips to roll over superficial

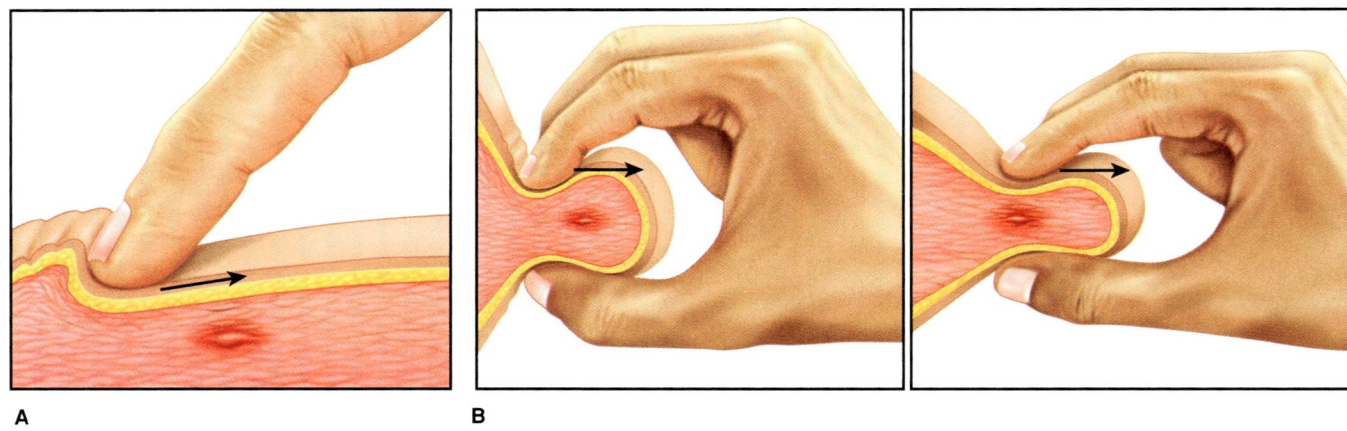

FIGURE 12-8 Techniques for trigger point palpation. **A.** With flat palpation, fingertips stroke across the muscle surface. **B.** With pincer palpation, the muscle is grasped and palpation for trigger points is completed as the muscle slips through the fingers.

muscles, which are accessible only at the surface (Fig. 12-8). This technique is commonly used to assess the anterior abdominal wall. In muscles with greater accessibility, pincer palpation grasps the muscle belly between the thumb and fingers. With any of the palpation techniques, spot tenderness and taut muscle bands are sought. Classically, the involved muscle displays weakness and restricted stretch. TrP pressure may also elicit a local muscle twitch response, reproduce a patient's referred pain, or both.

Specific Muscle Groups

Anterior abdominal wall muscles—that is, the rectus abdominis, the obliques, and transversus abdominis muscles—may all develop TrPs. Somatovisceral pelvic symptoms from these muscles can include diarrhea or urinary frequency, urgency, or retention. Rectus abdominis muscle TrPs are frequently found along the linea semilunaris, which is the term for this muscle's lateral margin (Suleiman, 2001). Additional rectus abdominis TrPs may develop at the muscle's insertion into the pubic bone and also below the umbilicus. Within the external oblique muscle, trigger points frequently involve its lateral attachment to the anterior iliac crest. Pain usually refers to the pubic bone.

After examination of the anterior abdominal wall, muscles of the pelvis are evaluated. Following careful inspection of the external genitalia, vaginal examination proceeds slowly and cautiously with the index finger only and initially without a palpating abdominal hand. Muscles within the pelvis include the levator ani, coccygeus, obturator internus, and deep transverse perineal and piriformis muscles, and these are assessed for painful TrPs (see Fig. 12-4) (Vercellini, 2009). TrPs involving these muscles and anal sphincter muscles are frequently associated with poorly localized pain that may be described as involving the coccyx, hip, or back (Fig. 12-9). Dyspareunia is common.

Treatment

Regardless of TrP location, the treatment goal is TrP inactivation, which then allows stretching and release of taut muscle bands. Of methods, TrP point massage or more aggressive ischemic compression massage are effective (Hull, 2009). Biofeedback, relaxation techniques, or psychotherapy may be helpful adjuncts. Analgesics, antiinflammatory drugs, muscle relaxants, or neuroleptics also may be prescribed. Finally, electrical stimulation, TrP dry needling, or TrP injection may be required. In those who are unresponsive to injection of local

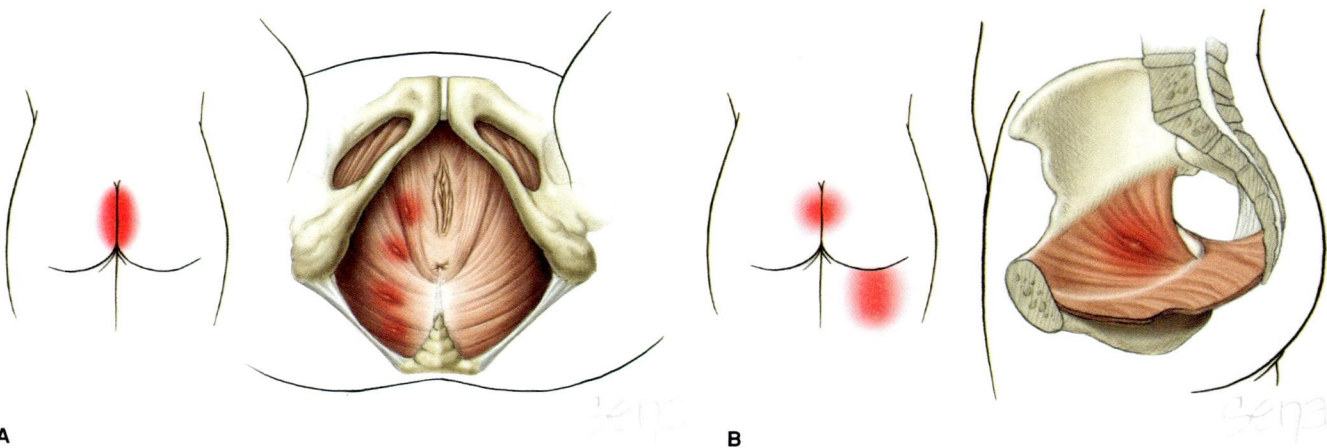

FIGURE 12-9 Trigger points and their extensive patterns of referred pain (*red shading*) **A.** Trigger points in the levator ani and coccygeus muscles. **B.** Trigger point in the obturator internus muscle. (Reproduced with permission from Ms. Marie Sena.)

anesthetic agents, botulinum toxin A injection may be considered (Gyang, 2013).

■ Peripartum Pelvic Pain Syndrome

Also known as *pelvic girdle pain*, this condition is characterized by persistent pain that begins during pregnancy or immediately postpartum. Pain is prominent around the sacroiliac joints and symphysis and is thought to originate from injury or inflammation of the pelvic and/or lower spine ligaments. Muscle weakness, postural adjustments of pregnancy, hormonal changes, and weight of the fetus and gravid uterus are all potential contributors (Mens, 1996). Pelvic girdle pain is common. Significant pain is estimated to afflict approximately 20 percent of gravidas and 7 percent of those during the 3 months following delivery (Albert, 2002; Wu, 2004). Diagnosis is usually clinical and based on findings during specific orthopedic joint manipulation tests. These are used to recreate or provoke the pain. Treatment includes physical therapy, exercise, and analgesics typically used for CPP, described on page 261 (Vermani, 2010; Vleeming, 2008).

NEUROLOGIC ETIOLOGIES

■ Anterior Abdominal Wall Nerve Entrapment Syndromes

With these, anterior cutaneous branches of the intercostal nerves or branches of the ilioinguinal, iliohypogastric, genitofemoral nerves, and lateral femoral cutaneous nerves are most commonly involved (Greenbaum, 1994). These peripheral nerves can be compressed within narrow anatomic canals or rings or beneath tight ligaments, fibrous bands, or sutures. For example, each anterior cutaneous branch of an intercostal nerve traverses anteriorly through the rectus abdominis muscle. Each branch and its corresponding vessels travels through a fibrous ring found within the lateral aspect of the rectus abdominis muscle (Fig. 12-10). These branches are often seen during Pfannenstiel incision creation as the anterior rectus sheath is dissected off each rectus belly (Fig. 43-2.3, p. 934). On crossing the anterior rectus sheath, each nerve branch divides and then courses within the subcutaneous layer. Within the fibrous ring, fat surrounding the neurovascular bundle appears to pad the enclosed structures (Srinivasan, 2002). However, if this bundle receives excessive intra- or extraabdominal pressure, compression of the bundle against the fibrous ring causes nerve ischemia and pain (Applegate, 1997).

Alternatively, nerve entrapment, injury, or neuroma formation may involve branches of the ilioinguinal, iliohypogastric, lateral femoral cutaneous, or genitofemoral nerves, as described in Chapter 40 (p. 842). Involvement may follow inguinal hernia repair, low transverse abdominal incisions, and lower abdominal laparoscopic trocar placement. Hypoesthesia is the more common finding with these injuries, but pain may variably develop within months of surgery or after several years.

Criteria for diagnosing nerve entrapment are clinical and include: (1) pain aggravated by patient movement or light skin pinching over the affected area and (2) pain improvement

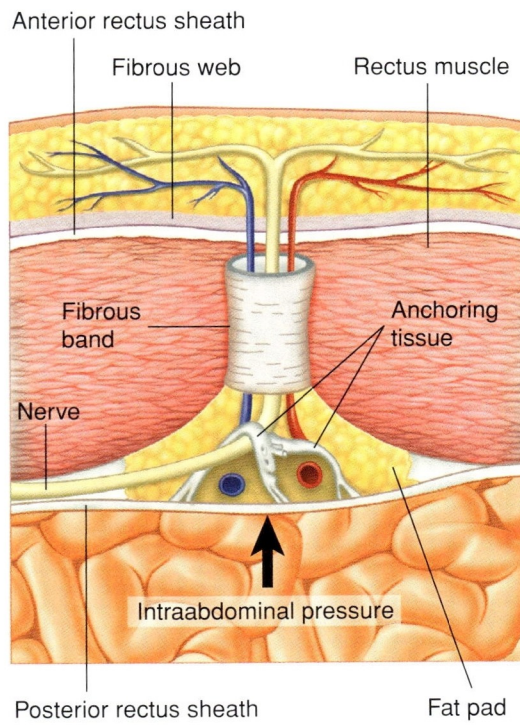

FIGURE 12-10 Nerve entrapment of the anterior cutaneous branches of one of the intercostal nerves. The nerve is compressed as it traverses the rectus abdominis muscle within a fibrous sheath.

following local anesthetic injection. In general, electromyography (EMG) is uninformative because it lacks adequate sensitivity (Knockaert, 1996). For local injection, 1- or 2-percent lidocaine and a 40-mg/mL concentration of triamcinolone can be combined in a 1:1 ratio. However, the corticosteroid may be omitted. Less than half a milliliter is injected at each pain site. Additional treatments can include oral analgesics, biofeedback, and gabapentin. If conservative options fail to bring sufficient relief, neurolysis with injection of 5- to 6-percent absolute alcohol or phenol, or surgical neurectomy may be required (Oor, 2016; Suleiman, 2001).

■ Pudendal Neuralgia

Neuralgia is sharp, severe, shooting pain that follows the distribution of the involved nerve. Pudendal nerve entrapment may create this type of pain on the perineum. The three branches of this nerve are the perineal nerve, the inferior rectal nerve, and the dorsal nerve to the clitoris (Fig. 25-1, p. 559). Thus, pain may involve, alone or in combination, the clitoris, vulva, or rectum. Pudendal neuralgia is rare, is usually unilateral, and typically develops after age 30. In affected individuals, allodynia and hyperesthesia may be extreme to the point of disability. The pain is aggravated by sitting, is relieved by sitting on a toilet seat or standing, and may progress during the day. Pudendal neuralgia has been associated with persistent genital arousal disorder (Pink, 2014).

The diagnosis of pudendal neuralgia is clinical, and *Nantes criteria* are used by many. As inclusion criteria, pain follows the pudendal nerve innervation path, is worse with sitting, has no associated sensory loss, does not awaken patients, and is relieved by nerve blockade (Labat, 2008). Clinical suspicion may be supported by objective testing. This may include neurophysiologic testing such as pudendal nerve motor latency and EMG, both described in Chapter 25 (p. 565). However, abnormal findings with these are not specific for pudendal neuralgia. Rarely, CT or MR imaging may be informative, although these may be performed to exclude other pathology (Khoder, 2014).

Treatment can involve physical therapy; behavioral modification; gabapentin or tricyclic antidepressants; pudendal nerve blockade, with or without corticosteroids; botulinum toxin A injection; and pudendal nerve stimulation. If these are unsuccessful, surgical nerve decompression may be elected.

■ Piriformis Syndrome

Compression of the sciatic nerve by the piriformis muscle may lead to buttock or low back pain in the distribution of the sciatic nerve (Broadhurst, 2004). This is termed the *piriformis syndrome.* Proposed mechanisms for compression include: contracture or spasm of the piriformis muscle from trauma, overuse and muscle hypertrophy, and congenital variations, in which the sciatic nerve or its divisions pass directly through this muscle (Hopayian, 2010).

Fishman and associates (2002) estimate the piriformis syndrome to be responsible for 6 to 8 percent of cases of low back pain and sciatica in the United States each year. Symptoms include pain and tenderness involving the buttocks, with or without radiation into the posterior thigh, and external tenderness near the greater sciatic notch. Pain is worse with activity, prolonged sitting, walking, and internal rotation of the hip (Hopayian, 2018; Kirschner, 2009). Dyspareunia has a common but variable association and has been demonstrated in 13 to 100 percent of cases (Hopayian, 2010).

Diagnosis of the syndrome is clinical and based on findings during specific orthopedic joint manipulation tests (Michel, 2013). Nerve conduction and EMG are typically nondiagnostic. MR imaging may be helpful by identifying a swollen or enlarged piriformis muscle or anatomic muscle variants (Vassalou, 2018). Treatment is conservative and includes physical therapy, NSAIDs, muscle relaxants, or neuropathic pain agents such as gabapentin, nortriptyline, or carbamazepine. Therapeutic injections of local anesthetics, with or without corticosteroids, or of botulinum toxin A may be used. Surgery is reserved for refractory cases.

REFERENCES

Abouassaly R, Steinberg JR, Lemieux M, et al: Complications of tension-free vaginal tape surgery: a multi-institutional review. BJU Int 94(1):110, 2004

Albert HB, Godskesen M, Westergaard JG: Incidence of four syndromes of pregnancy-related pelvic joint pain. Spine 27(24):2831, 2002

American Psychiatric Association: DSM-5: Diagnostic and Statistical Manual for Mental Disorders, 5th edition. Washington, American Psychiatric Press, 2013

American Society for Reproductive Medicine: Treatment of pelvic pain associated with endometriosis. Fertil Steril 101(4):927, 2014

Applegate WV, Buckwalter NR: Microanatomy of the structures contributing to abdominal cutaneous nerve entrapment syndrome. J Am Board Fam Pract 10:329, 1997

As-Sanie S, Harris RE, Napadow V, et al: Changes in regional gray matter volume in women with chronic pelvic pain: a voxel-based morphometry study. Pain 153(5):1006, 2012

Atkinson W, Lockhart S, Whorwell PJ, et al: Altered 5-hydroxytryptamine signaling in patients with constipation- and diarrhea-predominant irritable bowel syndrome. Gastroenterology 130(1):34, 2006

Ayachi A, Bouchahda R, Derouich S, et al: Accuracy of preoperative real-time dynamic transvaginal ultrasound sliding sign in prediction of pelvic adhesions in women with previous abdominopelvic surgery: prospective, multi-center, double-blind study. Ultrasound Obstet Gynecol 51(2):253, 2018

Baker PK: Musculoskeletal origins of chronic pelvic pain. Diagnosis and treatment. Obstet Gynecol Clin North Am 20:719, 1993

Baradaran N, Chiles LR, Freilich DA, et al: Female urethral diverticula in the contemporary era: is the classic triad of the "3Ds" still relevant? Urology 94:53, 2016

Basson R, Wierman ME, van Lankveld J, et al: Summary of the recommendations on sexual dysfunctions in women. J Sex Med 7(1 Pt 2):314, 2010

Beard RW, Kennedy RG, Gangar KF, et al: Bilateral oophorectomy and hysterectomy in the treatment of intractable pelvic pain associated with pelvic congestion. BJOG 98:988, 1991

Beard RW, Reginald PW, Wadsworth J: Clinical features of women with chronic lower abdominal pain and pelvic congestion. BJOG 95:153, 1988

Bedaiwy MA, Patterson B, Mahajan S: Prevalence of myofascial chronic pelvic pain and the effectiveness of pelvic floor physical therapy. J Reprod Med 58(11-12):504, 2013

Benzon H, Raja SN, Fishman SE, et al (eds): Essentials of Pain Medicine, 3rd ed. Philadelphia, Saunders, 2011, p 115

Berlanda N, Vercellini P, Carmignani L, et al: Ureteral and vesical endometriosis: two different entities sharing the same pathogenesis. Obstet Gynecol Surv 64(12):830, 2009

Bermejo C, Martínez Ten P, Cantarero R, et al: Three-dimensional ultrasound in the diagnosis of müllerian duct anomalies and concordance with magnetic resonance imaging. Ultrasound Obstet Gynecol 35(5):593, 2010

Berry SH, Elliott MN, Suttorp M, et al: Prevalence of symptoms of bladder pain syndrome/interstitial cystitis among adult females in the United States. J Urol 186:540, 2011

Bharadwaj S, Barber MD, Graff LA, et al: Symptomatology of irritable bowel syndrome and inflammatory bowel disease during the menstrual cycle. Gastroenterol Rep 3(3):185, 2015

Bhosale PR, Javitt MC, Atri M, et al: ACR Appropriateness Criteria® acute pelvic pain in the reproductive age group. Ultrasound Q 32(2):108, 2016

Bijkerk CJ, de Wit NJ, Muris JW, et al: Soluble or insoluble fibre in irritable bowel syndrome in primary care? Randomised placebo controlled trial. BMJ 339:b3154, 2009

Bradley MH, Rawlins A, Brinker CA: Physical therapy treatment of pelvic pain. Phys Med Rehabil Clin N Am 28(3):589, 2017

Brenner DJ, Hall EJ: Computed tomography—an increasing source of radiation exposure. N Engl J Med 357(22):2277, 2007

Brill K, Norpoth T, Schnitker J, et al: Clinical experience with a modern low-dose oral contraceptive in almost 100,000 users. Contraception 43:101, 1991

Broadhurst NA, Simmons DN, Bond MJ: Piriformis syndrome: correlation of muscle morphology with symptoms and signs. Arch Phys Med Rehabil 85(12):2036, 2004

Brown MA, Sirlin CB: Female pelvis. Magn Reson Imaging Clin North Am 13(2):381, 2005

Buhling KJ, Schmidt S, Robinson JN, et al: Rate of dyspareunia after delivery in primiparae according to mode of delivery. Eur J Obstet Gynecol Reprod Biol 124:42, 2006

Burrows LJ, Meyn LA, Walters MD, et al: Pelvic symptoms in women with pelvic organ prolapse. Obstet Gynecol 104(5 Pt 1):982, 2004

Busse JW, Wang L, Kamaleldin M, et al: Opioids for chronic noncancer pain: a systematic review and meta-analysis. JAMA 320(23):2448, 2018

Butrick CW: Interstitial cystitis and chronic pelvic pain: new insights in neuropathology, diagnosis, and treatment. Clin Obstet Gynecol 46:811, 2003

Butrick CW: Patients with chronic pelvic pain: endometriosis or interstitial cystitis/painful bladder syndrome? JSLS 11(2):182, 2007

Camilleri M, Northcutt AR, Kong S, et al: Efficacy and safety of alosetron in women with irritable bowel syndrome: a randomised, placebo-controlled trial. Lancet 355:1035, 2000

Canavan C, West J, Card T: The epidemiology of irritable bowel syndrome. Clin Epidemiol 6:71, 2014

Carey ET, As-Sanie S: New developments in the pharmacotherapy of neuropathic chronic pelvic pain. Future Sci OA 2(4): FSO148, 2016

Chang L, Chey WD, Harris L, et al: Incidence of ischemic colitis and serious complications of constipation among patients using alosetron: systematic review of clinical trials and post-marketing surveillance data. Am J Gastroenterol 101(5):1069, 2006

Chen FP, Soong YK: The efficacy and complications of laparoscopic presacral neurectomy in pelvic pain. Obstet Gynecol 90(6):974, 1997

Chey WD, Chey WY, Heath AT, et al: Long-term safety and efficacy of alosetron in women with severe diarrhea-predominant irritable bowel syndrome. Am J Gastroenterol 99:2195, 2004

Chey WD, Drossman DA, Johanson JF, et al: Safety and patient outcomes with lubiprostone for up to 52 weeks in patients with irritable bowel syndrome with constipation. Aliment Pharmacol Ther 35:587, 2012a

Chey WD, Lembo AJ, Lavins BJ, et al: Linaclotide for irritable bowel syndrome with constipation: a 26-week, randomized, double-blind, placebo-controlled trial to evaluate efficacy and safety. Am J Gastroenterol 107: 1702, 2012b

Cunanan RG Jr, Courey NG, Lippes J: Laparoscopic findings in patients with pelvic pain. Am J Obstet Gynecol 146:589, 1983

Daniels J, Gray R, Hills RK, et al: Laparoscopic uterosacral nerve ablation for alleviating chronic pelvic pain: a randomized controlled trial. JAMA 302(9):955, 2009

Daniels JP, Middleton L, Xiong T, et al: Individual patient data meta-analysis of randomized evidence to assess the effectiveness of laparoscopic uterosacral nerve ablation in chronic pelvic pain. Hum Reprod Update 16(6):568, 2010

de Bernardes NO, Marques A, Ganunny C, et al: Use of intravaginal electrical stimulation for the treatment of chronic pelvic pain: a randomized, double-blind, crossover clinical trial. J Reprod Med 55(1-2):19, 2010

Demco L: Pain mapping of adhesions. J Am Assoc Gynecol Laparosc 11:181, 2004

Descargues G, Tinlot-Mauger F, Gravier A, et al: Adnexal torsion: a report on forty-five cases. Eur J Obstet Gynecol Reprod Biol 98:91, 2001

Doggweiler R, Whitmore KE, Meijlink JM, et al: A standard for terminology in CPP syndromes: A report from the CPP working group of the international continence society. Neurourol Urodyn 36(4):984, 2017

Donnez J, Nisolle M, Smoes P, et al: Peritoneal endometriosis and "endometriotic" nodules of the rectovaginal septum are two different entities. Fertil Steril 66(3):362, 1996

Drossman DA, Camilleri M, Mayer EA, et al: AGA technical review on irritable bowel syndrome. Gastroenterology 123:2108, 2002

Drossman DA, Chang L, Chey WD, et al: Rome IV Functional Gastrointestinal Disorders: Disorders of Gut-Brain Interaction, Raleigh, Rome Foundation, Inc, 2016a

Drossman DA, Chey WD, Johanson JF, et al: Clinical trial: lubiprostone in patients with constipation-associated irritable bowel syndrome—results of two randomized, placebo-controlled studies. Aliment Pharmacol Ther 29:329, 2009

Drossman DA, Hasler WL: Rome IV-functional GI disorders: disorders of gut-brain interaction. Gastroenterology 150(6):1257, 2016b

Dubuisson J, Botchorishvili R, Perrette S, et al: Incidence of intraabdominal adhesions in a continuous series of 1000 laparoscopic procedures. Am J Obstet Gynecol 203(2):111.e1, 2010

Einstein AJ, Henzlova MJ, Rajagopalan S: Estimating risk of cancer associated with radiation exposure from 64-slice computed tomography coronary angiography. JAMA 298(3):317, 2007

El Minawi AM, Howard FM: Operative laparoscopic treatment of ovarian retention syndrome. J Am Assoc Gynecol Laparosc 6:297, 1999

El-Nashar SA, Singh R, Bacon MM, et al: Female urethral diverticulum: presentation, diagnosis, and predictors of outcomes after surgery. Female Pelvic Med Reconstr Surg 22(6):447, 2016

Ellerkmann RM, Cundiff GW, Melick CF, et al: Correlation of symptoms with location and severity of pelvic organ prolapse. Am J Obstet Gynecol 185:1332, 2001

Ellrich J, Lamp S: Peripheral nerve stimulation inhibits nociceptive processing: an electrophysiological study in healthy volunteers. Neuromodulation 8(4):225, 2005

Farquhar CM, Rogers V, Franks S, et al: A randomized controlled trial of medroxyprogesterone acetate and psychotherapy for the treatment of pelvic congestion. BJOG 96:1153, 1989

Fayez JA, Clark RR: Operative laparoscopy for the treatment of localized chronic pelvic-abdominal pain caused by postoperative adhesions. J Gynecol Surg 10:79, 1994

Fishman LM, Dombi GW, Michaelsen C, et al: Piriformis syndrome: diagnosis, treatment and outcome—a ten-year study. Arch Phys Med Rehabil 83:295, 2002

Fitzgerald CM, Neville CE, Mallinson T, et al: Pelvic floor muscle examination in female chronic pelvic pain. J Reprod Med 56(3-4):117, 2011

FitzGerald MP, Payne CK, Lukacz ES, et al: Randomized multicenter clinical trial of myofascial physical therapy in women with interstitial cystitis/painful bladder syndrome and pelvic floor tenderness. J Urol 187(6):2113, 2012

Flasar MH, Goldberg E: Acute abdominal pain. Med Clin North Am 90:481, 2006

Fleischer AC, Tait D, Mayo J, et al: Sonographic features of ovarian remnants. J Ultrasound Med 17:551, 1998

Foley CL, Greenwell TJ, Gardiner RA: Urethral diverticula in females. BJU Int 108(2 Suppl):20, 2011

Food and Drug Administration: Lotronex (alosetron hydrochloride) information. 2016. Available at: http://www.fda.gov/Drugs/DrugSafety/PostmarketDrugSafetyInformationforPatientsandProviders/ucm110450.htm. Accessed March 28, 2019

Ford AC, Moayyedi P, Lacy BE, et al: American College of Gastroenterology monograph on the management of irritable bowel syndrome and chronic idiopathic constipation. Am J Gastroenterol 109(1 Suppl):S2, 2014a

Ford AC, Quigley EM, Lacy BE, et al: Effect of antidepressants and psychological therapies, including hypnotherapy, in irritable bowel syndrome: systematic review and meta-analysis. Am J Gastroenterol 109(9):1350, 2014b

Ford AC, Quigley EM, Lacy BE, et al: Efficacy of prebiotics, probiotics, and synbiotics in irritable bowel syndrome and chronic idiopathic constipation: systematic review and meta-analysis. Am J Gastroenterol 109(10):1547, 2014c

Gallagher EJ: Acute abdominal pain. In Tintinalli JE, Kelen GD, Stapczynski JS, et al (eds): Tintinalli's Emergency Medicine: A Comprehensive Study Guide. New York, McGraw-Hill, 2004

Gangar KF, Stones RW, Saunders D, et al: An alternative to hysterectomy? GnRH analogue combined with hormone replacement therapy. BJOG 100:360, 1993

Gerhardt RT, Nelson BK, Keenan S, et al: Derivation of a clinical guideline for the assessment of nonspecific abdominal pain: the Guideline for Abdominal Pain in the ED Setting (GAPEDS) Phase 1 Study. Am J Emerg Med 23:709, 2005

Gershon MD: Nerves, reflexes, and the enteric nervous system: pathogenesis of the irritable bowel syndrome. J Clin Gastroenterol 39(4 Suppl 3):S184, 2005

Gerwin RD: A review of myofascial pain and fibromyalgia—factors that promote their persistence. Acupunct Med 23:121, 2005

Giambernardino MA: Referred muscle pain/hyperalgesia and central sensitisation. J Rehab Med (41 Suppl):85, 2003

Glatt AE, Zinner SH, McCormack WM: The prevalence of dyspareunia. Obstet Gynecol 75:433, 1990

Gloviczki P, Comerota AJ, Dalsing MC, et al: The care of patients with varicose veins and associated chronic venous diseases: clinical practice guidelines of the Society for Vascular Surgery and the American Venous Forum. J Vasc Surg 53(5 Suppl):2S, 2011

Green PH, Cellier C: Celiac disease. N Engl J Med 357(17):1731, 2007

Greenbaum DS, Greenbaum RB, Joseph JG, et al: Chronic abdominal wall pain. Diagnostic validity and costs. Dig Dis Sci 39:1935, 1994

Gunter J: Chronic pelvic pain: an integrated approach to diagnosis and treatment. Obstet Gynecol Surv 58:615, 2003

Gyang A, Hartman M, Lamvu G: Musculoskeletal causes of chronic pelvic pain: what a gynecologist should know. Obstet Gynecol 121(3):645, 2013

Hadley SK, Gaarder SM: Treatment of irritable bowel syndrome. Am Fam Physician 72:2501, 2005

Haefner HK, Collins ME, Davis GD, et al: The vulvodynia guideline. J Lower Gen Tract Dis 9:40, 2005

Hakenberg OW, Harke N, Wagenlehner F: Urethritis in men and women. Eur Urol 16(16 Suppl):144, 2017

Hanno PM, Burks DA, Clemens JQ, et al: AUA guideline for the diagnosis and treatment of interstitial cystitis/bladder pain syndrome. J Urol 185(6):2162, 2011

Hanno PM, Erickson D, Moldwin R, et al: Diagnosis and treatment of interstitial cystitis/bladder pain syndrome: AUA guideline amendment. J Urol 193(5):1545, 2015

Hansrani V, Abbas A, Bhandari S, et al: Trans-venous occlusion of incompetent pelvic veins for chronic pelvic pain in women: a systematic review. Eur J Obstet Gynecol Reprod Biol 185:156, 2015

Harlow SD, Park M: A longitudinal study of risk factors for the occurrence, duration and severity of menstrual cramps in a cohort of college women. BJOG 103:1134, 1996

Hartmann KE, Ma C, Lamvu GM, et al: Quality of life and sexual function after hysterectomy in women with preoperative pain and depression. Obstet Gynecol 104(4):701, 2004

Henning A, Wehrberger M, Madersbacher S, et al: Do differences in clinical symptoms and referral patterns contribute to the gender gap in bladder cancer? BJU Int 112(1):68, 2013

Hillis SD, Marchbanks PA, Peterson HB: The effectiveness of hysterectomy for chronic pelvic pain. Obstet Gynecol 86:941, 1995

Hopayian K, Danielyan A: Four symptoms define the piriformis syndrome: an updated systematic review of its clinical features. Eur J Orthop Surg Traumatol 28(2):155, 2018

Hopayian K, Song F, Riera R, et al: The clinical features of the piriformis syndrome: a systematic review. Eur Spine J 19(12):2095, 2010

Howard FM: Chronic pelvic pain. Obstet Gynecol 101:594, 2003

Howard FM: The role of laparoscopy in chronic pelvic pain: promise and pitfalls. Obstet Gynecol Surv 48:357, 1993

Hoyos LR, Benacerraf B, Puscheck EE: Imaging in endometriosis and adenomyosis. Clin Obstet Gynecol 60(1):27, 2017

Hsu CT, Rosioreanu A, Friedman RM, et al: Computed tomography imaging of the acute female pelvis. Contemporary Diagnostic Radiology 28(18):1, 2005

Huchon C, Fauconnier A: Adnexal torsion: a literature review. Eur J Obstet Gynecol 150(1):8, 2010

Hull M, Corton MM: Evaluation of the levator ani and pelvic wall muscles in levator ani syndrome. Urol Nurs 29(4):225, 2009

Hunter CW, Stovall B, Chen G, et al: Anatomy, pathophysiology and interventional therapies for chronic pelvic pain: a review. Pain Physician 21(2):147, 2018

Irwin P, Samsudin A: Reinvestigation of patients with a diagnosis of interstitial cystitis: common things are sometimes common. J Urol 174:584, 2005

Istek A, Gungor Ugurlucan F, Yasa C, et al. Randomized trial of long-term effects of percutaneous tibial nerve stimulation on chronic pelvic pain. Arch Gynecol Obstet 290(2): 291, 2014

Jamieson DJ, Steege JF: The association of sexual abuse with pelvic pain complaints in a primary care population. Am J Obstet Gynecol 177:1408, 1997

Janicki TI: Chronic pelvic pain as a form of complex regional pain syndrome. Clin Obstet Gynecol 46:797, 2003

Kang SB, Chung HH, Lee HP, et al: Impact of diagnostic laparoscopy on the management of chronic pelvic pain. Surg Endosc 21(6):916, 2007

Kehlet H, Jensen TS, Woolf CJ: Persistent postsurgical pain: risk factors and prevention. Lancet 367:1618, 2006

Khanna R, MacDonald JK, Levesque BG: Peppermint oil for the treatment of irritable bowel syndrome: a systematic review and meta-analysis. J Clin Gastroenterol 48(6):505, 2014

Kho RM, Abrao MS: Ovarian remnant syndrome: etiology, diagnosis, treatment and impact of endometriosis. Curr Opin Obstet Gynecol 24(4):210, 2012

Khoder W, Hale D: Pudendal neuralgia. Obstet Gynecol Clin North Am 41(3):443, 2014

Kirschner JS, Foye PM, Cole JL: Piriformis syndrome, diagnosis and treatment. Muscle Nerve 40(1):10, 2009

Knockaert DC, Boonen AL, Bruyninckx FL, et al: Electromyographic findings in ilioinguinal-iliohypogastric nerve entrapment syndrome. Acta Clin Belg 51:156, 1996

Kremer M, Salvat E, Muller A, et al: Antidepressants and gabapentinoids in neuropathic pain: mechanistic insights. Neuroscience 338:183, 2016

Labat JJ, Riant T, Robert R, et al: Diagnostic criteria for pudendal neuralgia by pudendal nerve entrapment (Nantes criteria). Neurourol Urodyn 27(4):306, 2008

Labelle H, Roussouly P, Berthonnaud E, et al: The importance of spino-pelvic balance in L5-S1 developmental spondylolisthesis: a review of pertinent radiologic measurements. Spine 30(6 Suppl):S27, 2005

Lacy BE, Mearin F, Chang L, et al: Bowel disorders. Gastroenterology 150(6):1393, 2016

Lafferty HW, Angioli R, Rudolph J, et al: Ovarian remnant syndrome: experience at Jackson Memorial Hospital, University of Miami, 1985 through 1993. Am J Obstet Gynecol 174:641, 1996

Laméris W, van Randen A, Bipat S, et al: Graded compression ultrasonography and computed tomography in acute colonic diverticulitis: meta-analysis of test accuracy. Eur Radiol 18(11):2498, 2008

Lampe A, Solder E, Ennemoser A, et al: Chronic pelvic pain and previous sexual abuse. Obstet Gynecol 96:929, 2000

Lamvu G, Nguyen RH, Burrows LJ, et al: The evidence-based vulvodynia assessment project. A national registry for the study of vulvodynia. J Reprod Med 60(5-6):223, 2015

Langer R, Golan A, Neuman M, et al: The effect of large uterine fibroids on urinary bladder function and symptoms. Am J Obstet Gynecol 163(4 Pt 1):1139, 1990

Laumann EO, Paik A, Rosen RC: Sexual dysfunction in the United States: prevalence and predictors. JAMA 281:537, 1999

Lavelle ED, Lavelle W, Smith HS: Myofascial trigger points. Med Clin North Am 91(2):229, 2007

Lee RB, Stone K, Magelssen D, et al: Presacral neurectomy for chronic pelvic pain. Obstet Gynecol 68(4):517, 1986

Lembo AJ, Lacy BE, Zuckerman MJ, et al: Eluxadoline for irritable bowel syndrome with diarrhea. N Engl J Med 374(3):242, 2016

LeResche L, Mancl L, Sherman JJ, et al: Changes in temporomandibular pain and other symptoms across the menstrual cycle. Pain 106(3):253, 2003

Leschka S, Alkadhi H, Wildermuth S, et al: Acute abdominal pain: diagnostic strategies. In Marincek B, Dondelinger RF (eds): Emergency Radiology. New York, Springer, 2007, p 411

Lewis SC, Bhattacharya S, Wu O, et al: Gabapentin for the management of chronic pelvic pain in women (GaPP1): a pilot randomised controlled trial. PloS One 11(4):e0153307, 2016

Lindh I, Milsom I: The influence of intrauterine contraception on the prevalence and severity of dysmenorrhea: a longitudinal population study. Hum Reprod 28(7):1953, 2013

Lovell RM, Ford AC: Global prevalence of, and risk factors for, irritable bowel syndrome: a meta-analysis. Clin Gastroenterol Hepatol 10:712, 2012

Magtibay PM, Nyholm JL, Hernandez JL, et al: Ovarian remnant syndrome. Am J Obstet Gynecol 193:2062, 2005

Maixner W, Fillingim RB, Williams DA, et al: Overlapping chronic pain conditions: implications for diagnosis and classification. J Pain 17(9 Suppl): T93, 2016

Manterola C, Vial M, Moraga J, et al: Analgesia in patients with acute abdominal pain. Cochrane Database Syst Rev 1:CD005660, 2011

Marjoribanks J, Ayeleke RO, Farquhar C, et al: Nonsteroidal anti-inflammatory drugs for dysmenorrhea. Cochrane Database Syst Rev 7:CD001751, 2015

Mathias SD, Kuppermann M, Liberman RF, et al: Chronic pelvic pain: prevalence, health-related quality of life, and economic correlates. Obstet Gynecol 87:321, 1996

Mayer E: Irritable bowel syndrome. N Engl J Med 358(16):1692, 2008

McPartland JM: Travell trigger points—molecular and osteopathic perspectives. J Am Osteopath Assoc 104:244, 2004

Meissner K, Schweizer-Arau A, Limmer A, et al: Psychotherapy with somatosensory stimulation for endometriosis-associated pain: a randomized controlled trial. Obstet Gynecol 128(5):1134, 2016

Melzack R: The short-form McGill Pain Questionnaire. Pain 30(2):191, 1987

Mens JM, Vleeming A, Stoeckart R, et al: Understanding peripartum pelvic pain: implications of a patient survey. Spine 21(11):1363, 1996

Michel F, Decavel P, Toussirot E, et al: The piriformis muscle syndrome: an exploration of anatomical context, pathophysiological hypotheses and diagnostic criteria. Ann Phys Rehabil Med 56(4):300, 2013

Mieritz RM, Thorhauge K, Forman A, et al: Musculoskeletal dysfunctions in patients with chronic pelvic pain: a preliminary descriptive survey. J Manipulative Physiol Ther 39(9):616, 2016

Miller SK, Alpert PT: Assessment and differential diagnosis of abdominal pain. Nurse Pract 31:38, 2006

Morris AM, Regenbogen SE, Hardiman KM, et al: Sigmoid diverticulitis: a systematic review. JAMA 311(3):287, 2014

Moschos E, Twickler DM: Does the type of intrauterine device affect conspicuity on 2D and 3D ultrasound? AJR Am J Roentgenol 196(6):1439, 2011

Nezhat C, Kearney S, Malik S, et al: Laparoscopic management of ovarian remnant. Fertil Steril 83:973, 2005

Nezhat CH, Dun EC, Katz A, et al: Office visceral slide test compared with two perioperative tests for predicting periumbilical adhesions. Obstet Gynecol 123(5):1049, 2014

Nickel JC, Tripp D, Gordon A, et al: Update on urologic pelvic pain syndromes: highlights from the 2010 international chronic pelvic pain symposium and workshop, August 29, 2010, Kingston, Ontario, Canada. Rev Urol 13(1):39, 2011

Nicol AL, Hurley RW, Benzon HT: Alternatives to opioids in the pharmacologic management of chronic pain syndromes: a narrative review of randomized, controlled, and blinded clinical trials. Anesth Analg 125(5):1682, 2017

Oh-Oka H: Clinical efficacy of 1-year intensive systematic dietary manipulation as complementary and alternative medicine therapies in female patients with interstitial cystitis/bladder pain syndrome. Urology 106(1):50, 2017

Oor JE, Ünlü Ç, Hazebroek EJ: A systematic review of the treatment for abdominal cutaneous nerve entrapment syndrome. Am J Surg 212(1):165, 2016

Paras ML, Murad MH, Chen LP, et al: Sexual abuse and lifetime diagnosis of somatic disorders: a systematic review and meta-analysis. JAMA 302(5):550, 2009

Park SJ, Lim JW, Ko YT, et al: Diagnosis of pelvic congestion syndrome using transabdominal and transvaginal sonography. AJR Am J Roentgenol 182:683, 2004

Parker JD, Sinaii N, Segars JH, et al: Adhesion formation after laparoscopic excision of endometriosis and lysis of adhesions. Fertil Steril 84:1457, 2005

Parsons CL: The role of the urinary epithelium in the pathogenesis of interstitial cystitis/prostatitis/ urethritis. Urology 69(4 Suppl):9, 2007

Parsons CL, Greenberger M, Gabal L, et al: The role of urinary potassium in the pathogenesis and diagnosis of interstitial cystitis. J Urol 159(6):1862, 1998

Perry CP: Peripheral neuropathies and pelvic pain: diagnosis and management. Clin Obstet Gynecol 46:789, 2003

Perry CP: Somatic referral. In Howard FM, Perry CP, Carter JE, et al (eds): Pelvic Pain: Diagnosis and Management. Philadelphia, Lippincott Williams & Wilkins, 2000, p 486

Perry CP, Presthus J, Nieves A: Laparoscopic uterine suspension for pain relief: a multicenter study. J Reprod Med 50:567, 2005

Peters AA, Trimbos-Kemper GC, Admiraal C, et al: A randomized clinical trial on the benefit of adhesiolysis in patients with intraperitoneal adhesions and chronic pelvic pain. BJOG 99:59, 1992

Philippou P, Moraitis K, Masood J, et al: The management of bladder lithiasis in the modern era of endourology. Urology 79(5):980, 2012

Phillips D, Deipolyi AR, Hesketh RL, et al: Pelvic congestion syndrome: etiology of pain, diagnosis, and clinical management. J Vasc Interv Radiol 25(5):725, 2014

Pimentel M, Lembo A, Chey WD, et al: Rifaximin therapy for patients with irritable bowel syndrome without constipation. N Engl J Med 364(1):22, 2011

Pink L, Rancourt V, Gordon A: Persistent genital arousal in women with pelvic and genital pain. J Obstet Gynaecol Can 36(4):324, 2014

Polackwich AS, Li J, Shoskes DA: Patients with pelvic floor muscle spasm have a superior response to pelvic floor physical therapy at specialized centers. J Urol 194: 1002 2015

Powell-Boone T, Ness TJ, Cannon R, et al: Menstrual cycle affects bladder pain sensation in subjects with interstitial cystitis. J Urol 174(5):1832, 2005

Proctor M, Farquhar C: Diagnosis and management of dysmenorrhoea. BMJ 332:1134, 2006

Proctor ML, Latthe PM, Farquhar CM, et al: Surgical interruption of pelvic nerve pathways for primary and secondary dysmenorrhoea. Cochrane Database Syst Rev 4:CD001896, 2005

Rao SS, Bharucha AE, Chiarioni G, et al: Functional anorectal disorders. Gastroenterology March 25, 2016 [Epub ahead of print]

Rao S, Lembo AJ, Shiff SJ, et al: A 12-week, randomized, controlled trial with a 4-week randomized withdrawal period to evaluate the efficacy and safety of linaclotide in irritable bowel syndrome with constipation. Am J Gastroenterol 107:1714, 2012

Raz R, Stamm WE: A controlled trial of intravaginal estriol in postmenopausal women with recurrent urinary tract infections. N Engl J Med 329(11):753, 1993

Reginald PW, Adams J, Franks S, et al: Medroxyprogesterone acetate in the treatment of pelvic pain due to venous congestion. BJOG 96:1148, 1989

Reissing ED, Brown C, Lord MJ, et al: Pelvic floor muscle functioning in women with vulvar vestibulitis syndrome. J Psychosom Obstet Gynecol 26:107, 2005

Reiter RC, Gambone JC: Nongynecologic somatic pathology in women with chronic pelvic pain and negative laparoscopy. J Reprod Med 36(4):253, 1991

Roman H, Hulsey TF, Marpeau L, et al: Why laparoscopic adhesiolysis should not be the victim of a single randomized clinical trial. Am J Obstet Gynecol 200(2):136.e1, 2009

Romanzi LJ, Groutz A, Blaivas JG: Urethral diverticulum in women: diverse presentations resulting in diagnostic delay and mismanagement. J Urol 164(2):428, 2000

Rubio-Tapia A, Hill ID, Kelly CP, et al: ACG clinical guidelines: diagnosis and management of celiac disease. Am J Gastroenterol 108(5):656, 2013

Ruepert L, Quartero AO, de Wit NJ, et al: Bulking agents, antispasmodics and antidepressants for the treatment of irritable bowel syndrome. Cochrane Database Syst Rev 8:CD003460, 2011

Saarto T, Wiffen PJ: Antidepressants for neuropathic pain: a Cochrane review. J Neurol Neurosurg Psychiatry 81(12):1372, 2010

Saito YA, Schoenfeld P, Locke GR III: The epidemiology of irritable bowel syndrome in North America: a systematic review. Am J Gastroenterol 97:1910, 2002

Sant GR, Kempuraj D, Marchand JE, et al: The mast cell in interstitial cystitis: role in pathophysiology and pathogenesis. Urology 69(4 Suppl):34, 2007

Sauerland S, Agresta F, Bergamaschi R, et al: Laparoscopy for abdominal emergencies: evidence-based guidelines of the European Association for Endoscopic Surgery. Surg Endosc 20:14, 2006

Schoenfeld P: Efficacy of current drug therapies in irritable bowel syndrome: what works and does not work. Gastroenterol Clin North Am 34:319, 2005

Schwartz BF, Stoller ML: The vesical calculus. Urol Clin N Am 27(2):333, 2000

Sedighimehr N, Manshadi FD, Shokouhi N, et al: Pelvic musculoskeletal dysfunctions in women with and without chronic pelvic pain. J Bodyw Mov Ther 22(1):92, 2018

Sephton SE, Salmon P, Weissbecker I, et al: Mindfulness meditation alleviates depressive symptoms in women with fibromyalgia: results of a randomized clinical trial. Arthritis Rheum 57(1):77, 2007

Sharma D, Dahiya K, Duhan N, et al: Diagnostic laparoscopy in chronic pelvic pain. Arch Gynecol Obstet 283(2):295, 2011

Sharma N, Rekha K, Srinivasan JK: Efficacy of transcutaneous electrical nerve stimulation in the treatment of chronic pelvic pain. J Midlife Health 8(1):36, 2017

Sharp HT: Myofascial pain syndrome of the abdominal wall for the busy clinician. Clin Obstet Gynecol 46:783, 2003

Signorello LB, Harlow BL, Chekos AK, et al: Postpartum sexual functioning and its relationship to perineal trauma: a retrospective cohort study of primiparous women. Am J Obstet Gynecol 184:881, 2001

Simons DG, Travell JG: Travell and Simons' Myofascial Pain and Dysfunction: the Trigger Point Manual, 2nd ed. Baltimore, Williams & Wilkins, 1999

Smith AL, Brown J, Wyman JF, et al: Treatment and prevention of recurrent lower urinary tract infections in women: a rapid review with practice recommendations. J Urol 200(6):1174, 2018

Smith-Bindman R, Lipson J, Marcus R, et al: Radiation dose associated with common computed tomography examinations and the associated lifetime attributable risk of cancer. Arch Intern Med 169(22):2078, 2009

Soysal ME, Soysal S, Vicdan K, et al: A randomized controlled trial of goserelin and medroxyprogesterone acetate in the treatment of pelvic congestion. Hum Reprod 16:931, 2001

Spitznagle TM, Robinson CM: Myofascial pelvic pain. Obstet Gynecol Clin North Am 41(3):409, 2014

Srinivasan R, Greenbaum DS: Chronic abdominal wall pain: a frequently overlooked problem. Practical approach to diagnosis and management. Am J Gastroenterol 97:824, 2002

Stamm WE, Hooton TM: Management of urinary tract infections in adults. N Engl J Med 329(18):1328, 1993

Stav K, Dwyer PL: Urinary bladder stones in women. Obstet Gynecol Surv 67(11):715, 2012

Steege JF, Stout AL: Resolution of chronic pelvic pain after laparoscopic lysis of adhesions. Am J Obstet Gynecol 165:278, 1991

Stovall TG, Ling FW, Crawford DA: Hysterectomy for chronic pelvic pain of presumed uterine etiology. Obstet Gynecol 75:676, 1990

Sturgeon JA: Psychological therapies for the management of chronic pain. Psychol Res Behav Manag 7:115, 2014

Sulak PJ, Cressman BE, Waldrop E, et al: Extending the duration of active oral contraceptive pills to manage hormone withdrawal symptoms. Obstet Gynecol 89:179, 1997

Suleiman S, Johnston DE: The abdominal wall: an overlooked source of pain. Am Fam Physician 64:431, 2001

Sundell G, Milsom I, Andersch B: Factors influencing the prevalence and severity of dysmenorrhoea in young women. BJOG 7:588, 1990

Sutton C, MacDonald R: Laser laparoscopic adhesiolysis. J Gynecol Surg 6:155, 1990

Swank DJ, Swank-Bordewijk SC, Hop WC, et al: Laparoscopic adhesiolysis in patients with chronic abdominal pain: a blinded randomised controlled multi-centre trial. Lancet 361:1247, 2003

Taylor HS, Giudice LC, Lessey BA, et al: Treatment of endometriosis-associated pain with elagolix, an oral GnRH antagonist. N Engl J Med 377(1):28, 2017

Tersigni C, Castellani R, de Waure C, et al: Celiac disease and reproductive disorders: meta-analysis of epidemiologic associations and potential pathogenic mechanisms. Hum Reprod Update 20(4):582, 2014

Theoharides TC, Kempuraj D, Sant GR: Mast cell involvement in interstitial cystitis: a review of human and experimental evidence. Urology 57(6 Suppl 1): 47, 2001

Thomson H, Francis DM: Abdominal-wall tenderness: a useful sign in the acute abdomen. Lancet 2(8047):1053, 1977

Thomson WH, Dawes RF, Carter SS: Abdominal wall tenderness: a useful sign in chronic abdominal pain. Br J Surg 78:223, 1991

Thornton JG, Morley S, Lilleyman J, et al: The relationship between laparoscopic disease, pelvic pain and infertility; an unbiased assessment. Eur J Obstet Gynaecol Reprod Biol 74:57, 1997

Till SR, Wahl H, As-Sanie S: The role of nonpharmacologic therapies in management of chronic pelvic pain: what to do when surgery fails. Curr Opin Obstet Gynecol 29(4):231, 2017

Trinkley KE, Nahata MC: Medication management of irritable bowel syndrome. Digestion 89(4):253, 2014

Tu FF, As-Sanie S, Steege JF: Prevalence of pelvic musculoskeletal disorders in a female chronic pelvic pain clinic. J Reprod Med 51(3):185, 2006

Valentine LN, Deimling TA: Opioids and alternatives in female chronic pelvic pain. Semin Reprod Med 36(2):164, 2018

Van den Bosch T, Van Schoubroeck D: Ultrasound diagnosis of endometriosis and adenomyosis: state of the art. Best Pract Res Clin Obstet Gynaecol 51:16, 2018

Vandyken C, Hilton S: Physical therapy in the treatment of central pain mechanisms for female sexual pain. Sex Med Rev 5(1):20, 2017

Vassalou EE, Katonis P, Karantanas AH: Piriformis muscle syndrome: a cross-sectional imaging study in 116 patients and evaluation of therapeutic outcome. Eur Radiol 28(2):447, 2018

Veehof MM, Trompetter HR, Bohlmeijer ET, et al: Acceptance- and mindfulness-based interventions for the treatment of chronic pain: a meta-analytic review. Cogn Behav Ther 45(1):5, 2016

Venbrux AC, Lambert DL: Embolization of the ovarian veins as a treatment for patients with chronic pelvic pain caused by pelvic venous incompetence (pelvic congestion syndrome). Curr Opin Obstet Gynecol 11:395, 1999

Vercellini P, Frontino G, Pisacreta A, et al: The pathogenesis of bladder detrusor endometriosis. Am J Obstet Gynecol 187(3):538, 2002

Vercellini P, Somigliana E, Viganò P, et al: Chronic pelvic pain in women: etiology, pathogenesis and diagnostic approach. Gynecol Endocrinol 25(3): 149, 2009

Vermani E, Mittal R, Weeks A: Pelvic girdle pain and low back pain in pregnancy: a review. Pain Pract 10(1):60, 2010

Vleeming A, Albert HB, Ostgaard HC, et al: European guidelines for the diagnosis and treatment of pelvic girdle pain. Eur Spine J 17(6):794, 2008

Warren JW, Morozov V, Howard FM: Could chronic pelvic pain be a functional somatic syndrome? Am J Obstet Gynecol 205(3):199.e1, 2011

Waxman JA, Sulak PJ, Kuehl TJ: Cystoscopic findings consistent with interstitial cystitis in normal women undergoing tubal ligation. J Urol 160:1663, 1998

Weinberg DS, Smalley W, Heidelbaugh JJ, et al: American Gastroenterological Association Institute Guideline on the pharmacological management of irritable bowel syndrome. Gastroenterology 147(5):1146, 2014

Weissman AM, Hartz AJ, Hansen MD, et al: The natural history of primary dysmenorrhoea: a longitudinal study. BJOG 111:345, 2004

Whiteside JL, Barber MD, Walters MD, et al: Anatomy of ilioinguinal and iliohypogastric nerves in relation to trocar placement and low transverse incisions. Am J Obstet Gynecol 189:1574, 2003

Wong CL, Farquhar C, Roberts H, et al: Oral contraceptive pill for primary dysmenorrhoea. Cochrane Database Syst Rev 4:CD002120, 2009

Wu WH, Meijer OG, Uegaki K, et al: Pregnancy-related pelvic girdle pain (PPP), I: terminology, clinical presentation, and prevalence. Eur Spine J 13(7):575, 2004

Yoshimoto H, Sato S, Masuda T, et al: Spinopelvic alignment in patients with osteoarthrosis of the hip: a radiographic comparison to patients with low back pain. Spine 30:1650, 2005

Zapardiel I, Zanagnolo V, Kho RM, et al: Ovarian remnant syndrome: comparison of laparotomy, laparoscopy and robotic surgery. Acta Obstet Gynecol Scand 91(8):965, 2012

Zoorob D, South M, Karram M, et al: A pilot randomized trial of levator injections versus physical therapy for treatment of pelvic floor myalgia and sexual pain. Int Urogynecol J 26(6):845, 2015

Zullo F, Palomba S, Zupi E, et al: Effectiveness of presacral neurectomy in women with severe dysmenorrhea caused by endometriosis who were treated with laparoscopic conservative surgery: a 1-year prospective randomized double-blind controlled trial. Am J Obstet Gynecol 189(1):5, 2003

Breast Disease

Breast disease in women encompasses a spectrum of benign and malignant disorders, which present most commonly as breast pain, nipple discharge, or palpable mass. The specific causes of these symptoms vary with patient age. Benign disorders predominate in young premenopausal women, whereas malignancy rates rise with advancing age. Evaluation of breast disorders usually requires the combination of a careful history, physical examination, imaging, and, when indicated, biopsy.

ANATOMY

■ Ductal System

The glandular portion of the breast is composed of 12 to 15 independent ductal systems that each drains approximately 40 lobules (Fig. 13-1). Each lobule consists of 10 to 100 milk-producing acini that empty into small terminal ducts (Fig. 13-2) (Parks, 1959). Histologically, acini and terminal ducts are lined by a cuboidal epithelium and an outer layer of myoepithelial cells. Terminal ducts drain into larger collecting ducts that merge into even larger ducts, which exhibit a saccular dilation just below the nipple called a *lactiferous sinus*.

In general, only six to eight openings are visible on the nipple surface. These drain the dominant ductal systems, which account for approximately 80 percent of the breast's glandular volume (Going, 2004). Minor ducts either terminate just below the nipple surface or open on the areola near the base of the nipple. The areola itself contains numerous lubricating sebaceous glands, called *Montgomery glands*, which are often visible as punctate prominences.

In addition to epithelial structures, the breast is composed of varying proportions of collagenous stroma and fat. The distribution and abundance of these stromal components accounts for a breast's consistency when palpated and for its imaging characteristics.

■ Lymphatic Drainage

Afferent lymphatic drainage of the breast is provided by dermal, subdermal, interlobar, and prepectoral systems (Fig. 13-3) (Grant, 1953). Each of these may be viewed as a lattice of valveless channels that interconnect with every other system and that ultimately drain into one or two axillary lymph nodes (the sentinel nodes). Because all of these systems are interconnected, the breast drains as a unit, and injection of colloidal dyes in any part of the breast at any level will result in accumulation of dye in the same one or two axillary sentinel lymph nodes. The axillary lymph nodes receive most of the lymphatic drainage of the breast and consequently are the nodes most frequently involved with breast cancer metastases (Hultborn, 1955). However, there are also alternate drainage pathways that do not appear to interconnect with other networks and that drain directly into internal mammary, supraclavicular, contralateral axillary, or abdominal lymph node basins.

DEVELOPMENT AND PHYSIOLOGY

During fetal development, the primordial breast arises from the basal layer of the epidermis. Before puberty, the breast is a rudimentary bud composed of a few branching ducts capped with alveolar buds, end buds, or small lobules (Osin, 1998). At puberty, usually between the ages of 10 and 13 years, ovarian estrogen and progesterone cooperate to direct organized communication between breast epithelial cells and mesenchymal cells, resulting in extensive branching of the ductal system and development of lobules (Ismail, 2003). Specific disorders of this

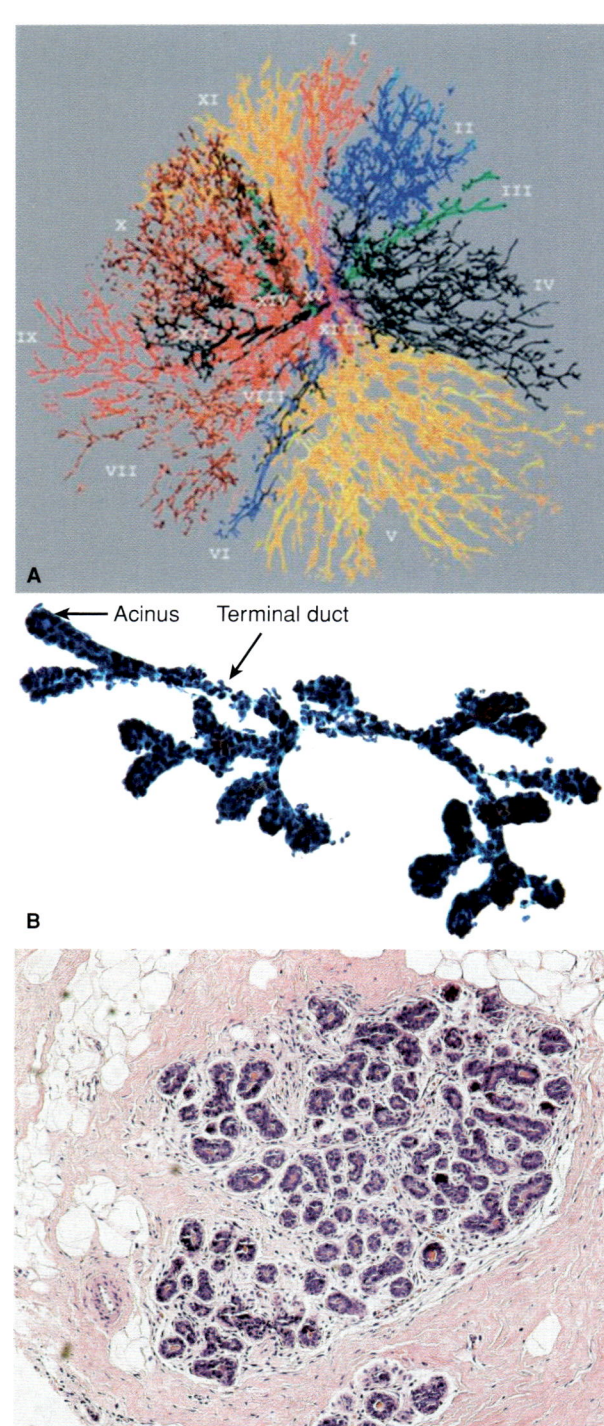

FIGURE 13-1 A. Ductal anatomy of the breast. (From Going, 2004, with permission.) **B.** Terminal duct—acinar structure from a fine-needle aspiration biopsy. **C.** Histology of a normal breast lobule. The terminal duct lobular units are surrounded by loosely cellular intralobular stroma, which consists of dense fibrous tissue admixed with adipocytes.

development are discussed in Chapter 15 (p. 328). Final differentiation of the breast is mediated by progesterone and prolactin and is not completed until the first full-term pregnancy (Grimm, 2002; Ismail, 2003).

During the reproductive years, terminal ducts near the acini and the acini themselves are most sensitive to ovarian hormones and prolactin. Most forms of benign and malignant breast disease arise in these terminal duct–acinar structures. Breast epithelial cells proliferate during the luteal phase of the menstrual cycle when estrogen and progesterone levels are elevated, and then undergo programmed cell death at the end of the luteal phase, when these hormone levels decline (Anderson, 1982; Soderqvist, 1997). This effect is mediated by paracrine signaling induced by estrogen receptor activation and is associated with greater water content in the extracellular matrix (Stoeckelhuber, 2002). This is often recognized as breast fullness and tenderness in the week preceding menses.

At menopause, when ovarian estrogen production ceases, breast lobules involute, and the collagenous stroma is replaced by fat. Estrogen receptor expression is negatively regulated by estrogen, and thus estrogen receptor expression rises after menopause (Khan, 1997). Despite a decline in ovarian estrogen production, postmenopausal women continue to produce estrogen through the action of the enzyme aromatase, which converts adrenal androgens to estrogen (Bulun, 1994). Aromatase is found in fat, muscle, and breast tissue.

EVALUATION OF A BREAST LUMP

It is not possible to distinguish benign from malignant or cystic from solid breast masses by clinical examination. However, findings from clinical examination, interpreted in conjunction with imaging and pathology (the triple test), contribute significantly to management decisions (Hermansen, 1987).

■ Physical Examination

The breast is comma shaped, and the comma's tail corresponds to the axillary tail of Spence. This extension can be large, especially during pregnancy and lactation, and is frequently mistaken for an axillary mass.

Clinical examination of the breast begins with inspection of the breast for dimpling, nipple retraction, or skin changes. This examination is fully described in Chapter 1 (p. 2). The presence and character of expressible nipple discharge is recorded. In addition, the location of a mass is specifically documented according to its clock position and then measured along its long axis using a ruler or caliper (Fig. 13-4). The distance from the center of the nipple to the center of the mass is specified. Since numerous health care providers are typically involved in the evaluation and management of the same breast mass, the most useful entry in the clinical record will define the location and size of the mass (e.g., right breast, 2-cm mass, 3:00, 4 cm from the nipple). Clinical examination alone can never exclude malignancy. However, noting that a mass has benign features such as smoothness, roundness, and mobility will factor into the ultimate decision to excise or observe a lesion. Evaluation also includes careful examination of the axillae, infraclavicular fossa, and supraclavicular fossa to identify lymphadenopathy.

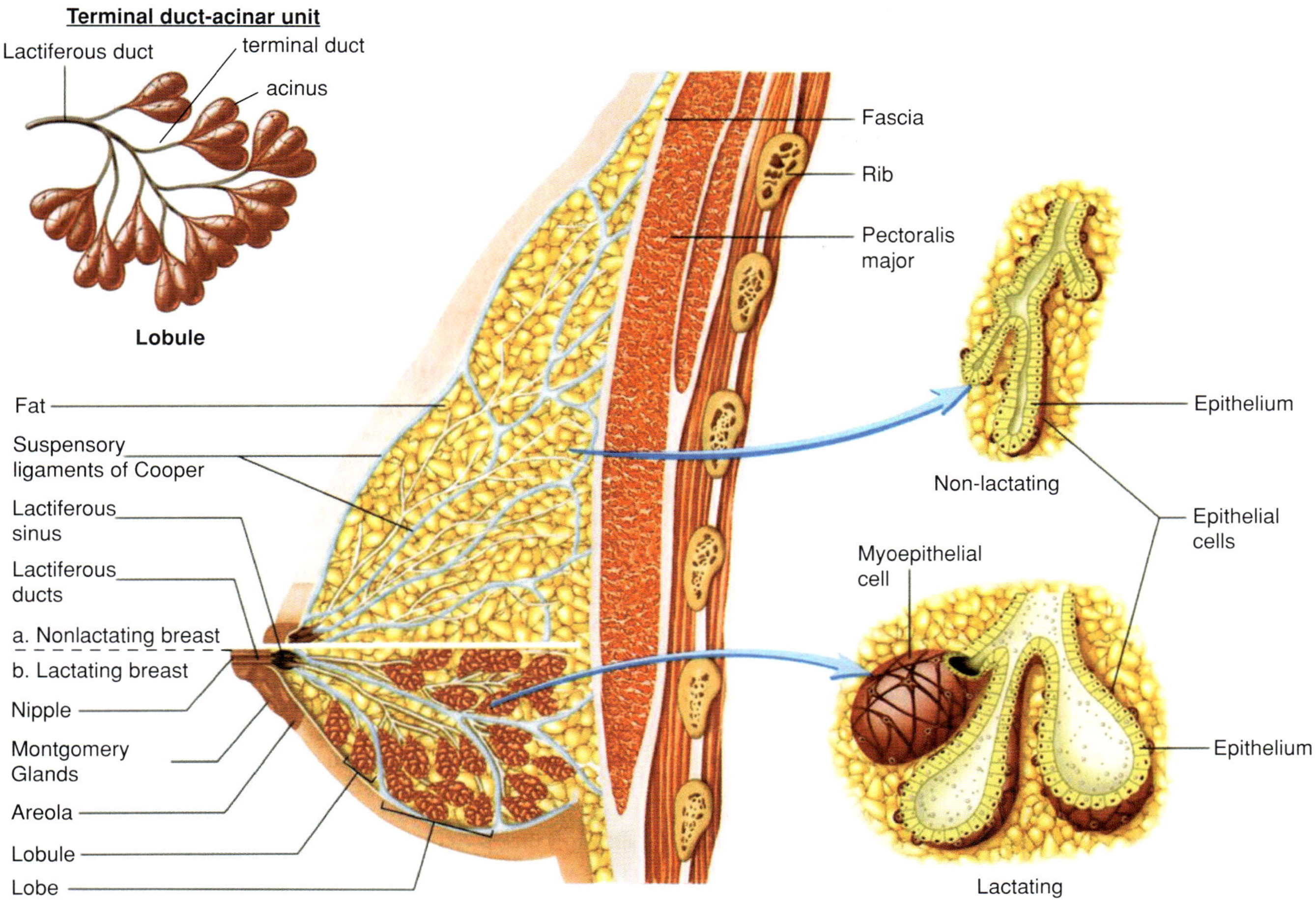

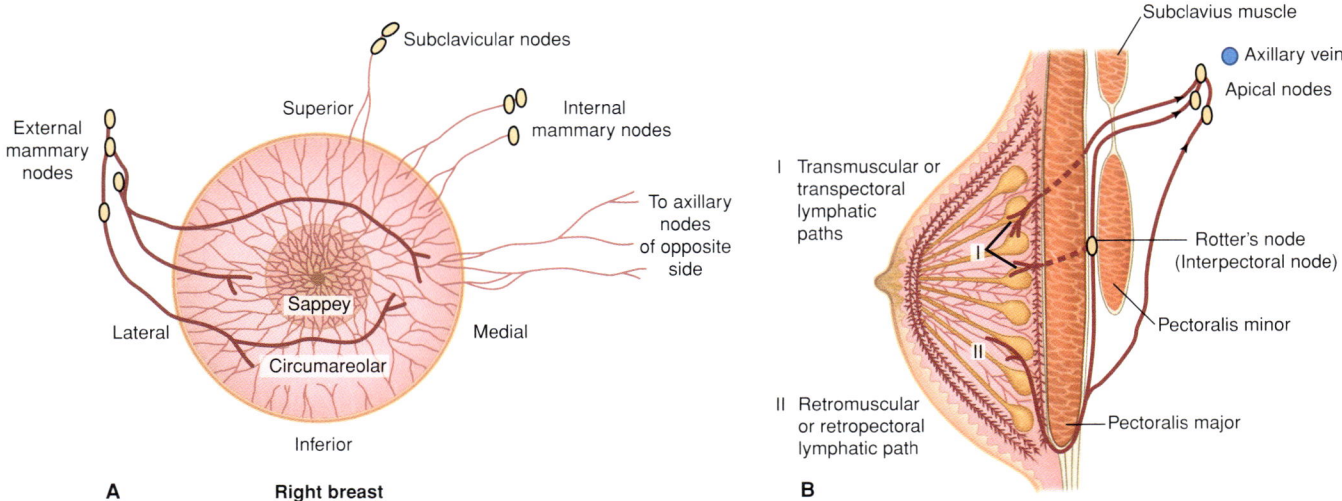

Terminal duct-acinar unit

Lactiferous duct

terminal duct

acinus

Lobule

Fat

Suspensory ligaments of Cooper

Lactiferous sinus

Lactiferous ducts

a. Nonlactating breast

b. Lactating breast

Nipple

Montgomery Glands

Areola

Lobule

Lobe

Fascia

Rib

Pectoralis major

Epithelium

Non-lactating

Epithelial cells

Myoepithelial cell

Epithelium

Lactating

FIGURE 13-2 Breast anatomy. (From Seeley, 2006, with permission.)

■ Diagnostic Imaging

Imaging of a suspected mass may begin with mammography that includes magnification, extra compression, or extra views beyond the usual medial lateral oblique and cranial caudal views that are typically used for screening. Unlike screening mammography, diagnostic mammography may be appropriate for women of any age. However, because of their radiosensitive breast tissue, mammography is generally avoided in women younger than 25 years, for whom magnetic resonance (MR) imaging is a suitable option. In addition, sonography is invaluable for determining whether a mass is cystic or solid and is a component of most diagnostic imaging algorithms. Certain features of solid masses, such

Subclavicular nodes

Superior

External mammary nodes

Internal mammary nodes

To axillary nodes of opposite side

Lateral

Sappey

Medial

Circumareolar

Inferior

A   **Right breast**

Subclavius muscle

Axillary vein

Apical nodes

I Transmuscular or transpectoral lymphatic paths

Rotter's node (Interpectoral node)

Pectoralis minor

II Retromuscular or retropectoral lymphatic path

Pectoralis major

B

FIGURE 13-3 Lymphatic drainage of the breast. **A.** Accessory drainage pathways. **B.** Classic axillary drainage pathways. (Redrawn from Grant, 1953, with permission.)

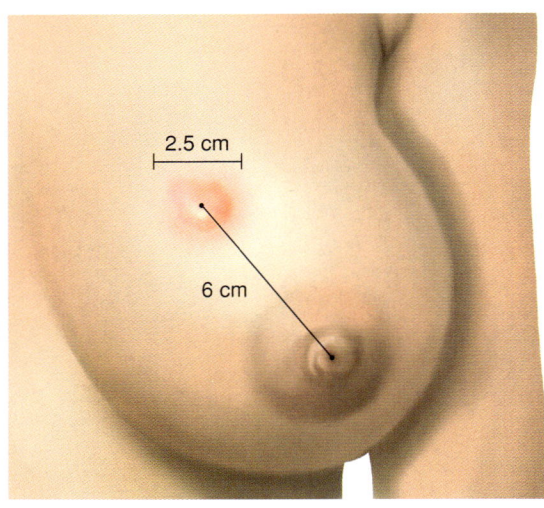

FIGURE 13-4 Recording the location of a breast mass as "Left breast, 2.5-cm mass, 10:00, 6 cm FN." FN = from the nipple.

as irregular margins, internal echoes, or a width-to-height ratio <1.7 may suggest malignancy (Stavros, 1995).

Diagnostic imaging results are summarized according to the Breast Imaging Reporting and Data System (BI-RADS) classification (Table 13-1) (D'Orsi, 2013). Lesions that are graded BI-RADS 5 are highly suggestive of malignancy, and ≥95 percent of these are ultimately proven to be cancerous. Decreasing numerical grades are associated with diminishing probability of malignancy.

■ Breast Biopsy

Evaluation of a solid breast mass is completed by needle biopsy. These biopsies should be performed after an imaging test or a minimum of 2 weeks prior to an imaging test. This is because resulting tissue trauma can produce image artifacts that simulate malignancy (Sickles, 1983). Options include fine-needle aspiration

(FNA) biopsy or core needle biopsy. The trend in recent years favors core needle biopsy (Tabbara, 2000). Although FNA takes less time to perform and is less expensive than core needle biopsy, it is less likely to provide a specific diagnosis and has a higher insufficient sample rate (Shannon, 2001). FNA retrieves clusters of epithelial cells that may be interpreted as benign or malignant, but it cannot reliably differentiate between benign proliferative lesions and fibroepithelial neoplasms or between ductal carcinoma in situ and invasive cancer (Boerner, 1999; Ringberg, 2001).

In contrast, core needle biopsy is performed using an automated device that takes one core at a time or is completed using a vacuum-assisted device that, once initially positioned, delivers multiple cores. Needle biopsy of solid masses should be done prior to excision, as the biopsy results contribute significantly to surgical planning (Cox, 1995).

■ Triple Test

The combination of clinical examination, imaging, and needle biopsy is called the *triple test* (Wai, 2013). When all three assessments suggest a benign lesion or all three suggest a breast cancer, the triple test is said to be concordant. A concordant benign triple test is >99-percent accurate, and breast lumps in this category can be followed by clinical examination alone at 6-month intervals. If any of the three assessments suggests malignancy, the lump should be excised regardless of results from the other two. It is always appropriate to offer excision of a fully evaluated breast lump, even after a benign concordant triple test result, as breast lumps can be a source of significant anxiety.

BENIGN LUMPS AND FIBROEPITHELIAL NEOPLASMS

■ Cysts

Most breast cysts arise from apocrine metaplasia of lobular acini. They are generally lined by a single layer of epithelium

TABLE 13-1. Breast Imaging Reporting and Data System (BI-RADS)

BI-RADS Category	Description	Examples
0	Additional views or sonography required	Focal asymmetry, microcalcifications, or a mass identified on a screening mammogram
1	No abnormalities identified	Normal fat and fibroglandular tissue
2	Not entirely normal, but definitely benign	Fat necrosis from a prior excision, stable biopsy-proven fibroadenoma, stable cyst
3	Probably benign	Circumscribed mass that has been followed for <2 years
4A	Low suspicion for malignancy, but intervention required	Probable fibroadenoma, complicated cyst
4B	Intermediate suspicion for malignancy, intervention required	Partially indistinctly marginated mass otherwise consistent with a fibroadenoma
4C	Moderate suspicion, but not classic for carcinoma	New cluster of fine pleomorphic calcifications, ill-defined irregular solid mass
5	Almost certainly malignant	Spiculated mass, fine linear and branching calcifications
6	Biopsy-proven carcinoma	Biopsy-proven carcinoma

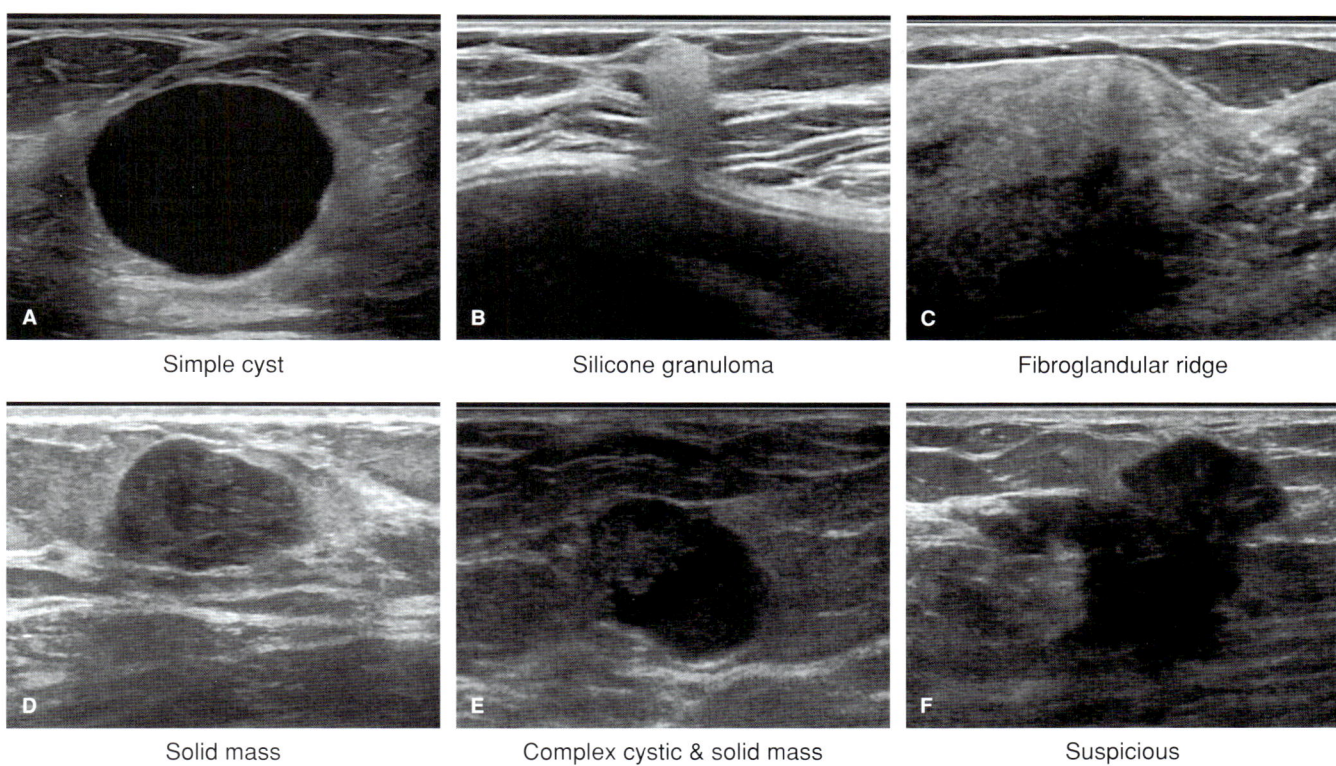

A	B	C
Simple cyst	Silicone granuloma	Fibroglandular ridge
D	E	F
Solid mass	Complex cystic & solid mass	Suspicious

FIGURE 13-5 Sonographic appearance of palpable breast masses. **A.** Simple cyst. **B.** Silicone granuloma. **C.** Fibroglandular ridge. **D.** Solid mass (benign phyllodes tumor). **E.** Complex cystic and solid mass (intracystic papillary carcinoma with low-grade ductal carcinoma in situ). **F.** Suspicious (invasive ductal carcinoma). (Reproduced with permission from Stephen J. Seiler, MD.)

that ranges from flattened to columnar. One autopsy series that included 725 women reported microcysts in 58 percent and cysts >1 cm in 21 percent (Davies, 1964). The incidence of breast cysts peaks between 40 and 50 years, and the lifetime incidence of palpable breast cysts is estimated to be 7 percent (Haagensen, 1986).

Breast cysts are diagnosed and classified by sonography. The three types of cysts are simple, complicated, and complex (Berg, 2003). Simple cysts are sonolucent, have a smooth margin, and show enhanced through-transmission (Fig. 13-5). These lesions do not require special management or monitoring, but they may be aspirated if painful. Recurrent cysts can be reimaged and reaspirated, but recurrent symptomatic cysts are best managed by excision.

Complicated cysts show internal echoes during sonography and can sometimes be indistinguishable from solid masses. Internal echoes are usually caused by proteinaceous debris. Consideration is given to aspirating complicated cysts. The aspirated material may be submitted for culture, if it is purulent, or for cytology, if worrisome clinical or imaging features are found. If the sonographic abnormality does not resolve completely with aspiration, a core-needle biopsy is usually performed.

Complex cysts show septa or intracystic masses during sonographic evaluation. An intracystic mass usually represents a papilloma, but medullary carcinoma, papillary carcinoma, and some infiltrating ductal carcinomas can present as complex cysts. Although some advocate core needle biopsy for the evaluation of complex cysts, this procedure can decompress a cyst, making it difficult to localize at the time of surgery. Additionally, papillary

lesions diagnosed by needle biopsy will require excision. Thus, it seems reasonable to recommend excision of all complex cysts.

■ Fibroadenoma

This is best considered a focal developmental abnormality of a terminal duct-lobular unit and not a true neoplasm. Histologically, fibroadenomas are composed of glandular and cystic epithelial structures surrounded by a cellular stroma. Fibroadenomas account for 7 to 13 percent of breast clinic visits and had a prevalence of 9 percent in one autopsy series (Dent, 1988; Franyz, 1951). They often present in adolescence, are recognized most frequently in premenopausal women, and usually spontaneously involute at menopause.

Fibroadenomas classified as benign concordant by the triple test can be safely followed without excision. Because some fibroadenomas may grow large, and because benign phyllodes tumors are often indistinguishable from fibroadenomas by imaging and needle biopsy, a fibroadenoma that is growing should be excised.

For most women with fibroadenomas, the risk of cancer is not increased. Exceptions are cases of complex fibroadenomas, fibroadenomas adjacent to another proliferative lesion, or those in women with a significant family breast cancer history (Greenberg, 1998).

■ Phyllodes Tumors

These are true biphasic neoplasms characterized by epithelial-lined spaces surrounded by cellular stroma. Both the epithelial and stromal components can be monoclonal and clonally related (Karim, 2013). Phyllodes tumors are classified as benign, borderline, or malignant, based on the degree of stromal cell atypia, number of mitoses, tumor margin characteristics, and abundance of stromal cells (Oberman, 1965). Phyllodes tumors account for less than 1 percent of breast neoplasms, and the median age at diagnosis is 40 years (Kim, 2013; Reinfuss, 1996). Malignant phyllodes tumors can metastasize to distant organs, with lung being the primary site. Chest radiographs or chest computed tomography (CT) scanning are appropriate staging tests for malignant cases. Phyllodes tumors rarely metastasize to lymph nodes, thus axillary staging is not required unless nodes clinically appear involved (Chaney, 2000).

Previously, treatment consisted of wide local excision with a minimum 1-cm margin, regardless of phyllodes grade. For benign phyllodes, data now show that excision with a negative or a 1-mm margin may be sufficient (Shaaban, 2017; Tremblay-LeMay, 2017). Positive margins warrant close observation but do not necessarily require reexcision (Moo, 2017). Wide excision with a 1-cm margin is still advised for borderline and malignant phyllodes.

Mastectomy may be required to achieve this margin, as the median tumor size at presentation is 5 cm. Local recurrence rates for completely excised tumors range from 8 percent for benign lesions to 36 percent for malignant ones. Distant metastases develop in <1 percent of benign phyllodes cases but in up to 17 percent of malignant ones (Tan 2016). Postoperative adjuvant radiation therapy may be indicated for high-risk cases (Barth, 2009).

NIPPLE DISCHARGE

Fluid can be expressed from the nipple ducts of at least 40 percent of premenopausal women, 55 percent of parous women, and 74 percent of women who have lactated within 2 years (Wrensch, 1990). The fluid generally issues from more than one duct and may range from milky white to dark green or brown. The green color is related to the content of cholesterol diepoxides and does not suggest underlying infection or malignancy (Petrakis, 1988).

Multiduct discharges that are elicited only following manual expression are considered physiologic and do not require additional evaluation. However, spontaneous discharges merit evaluation (Fig. 13-6). Spontaneous milky nipple discharge, also

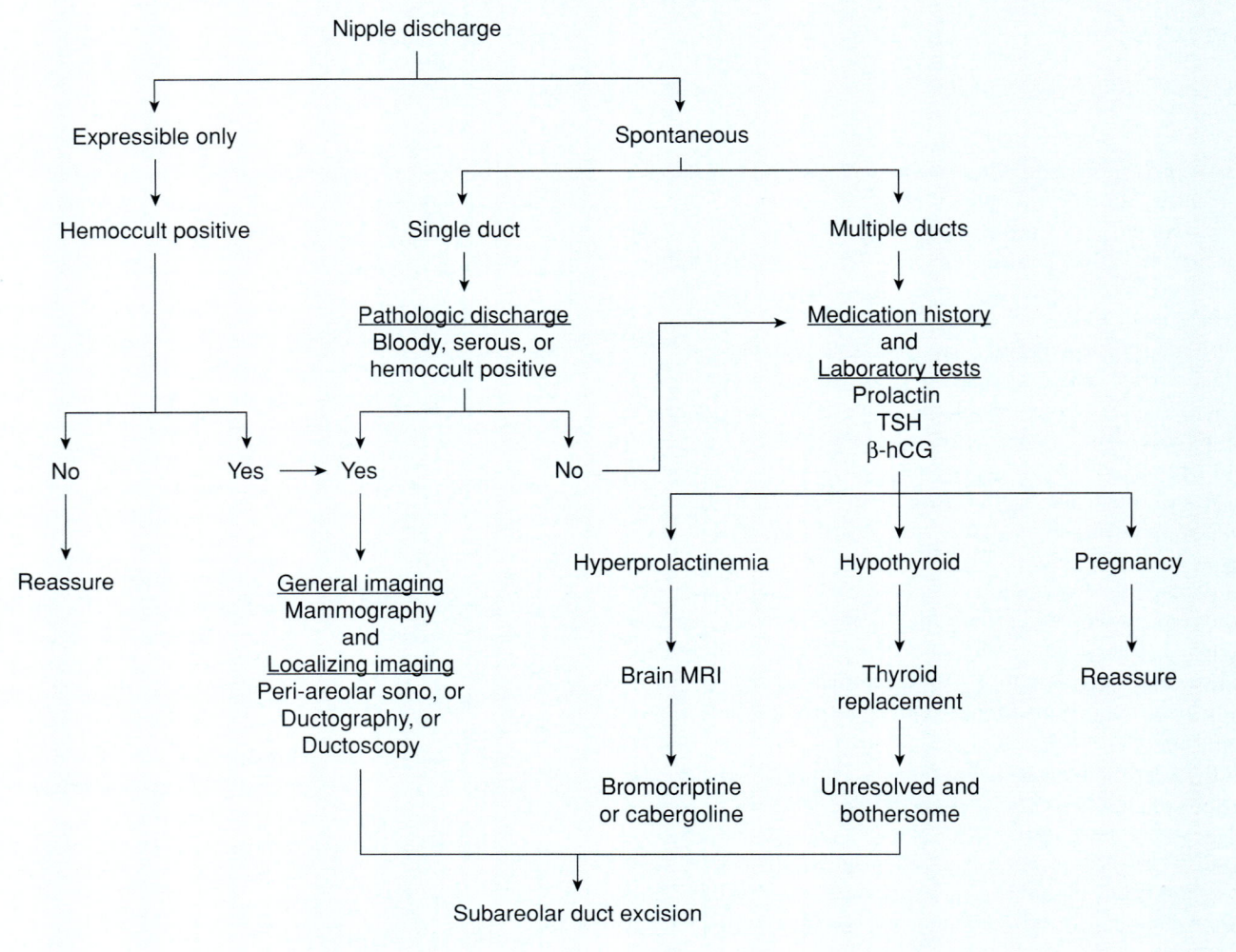

FIGURE 13-6 Diagnostic algorithm to evaluate nipple discharge. hCG = human chorionic gonadotropin; MRI = magnetic resonance imaging; TSH = thyroid-stimulating hormone.

TABLE 13-2. Causes of Galactorrhea

Idiopathic	**Systemic disorders**
Physiologic	Chronic renal failure
Lactation	Hypothyroidism
Breast stimulation	Cirrhosis
Stress	Pseudocyesis
	Seizures
Hypothalamic lesions	Ectopic tumor production
Tumors	**Pharmacologic**
Infiltrative disorders	Dopamine blocking agents
Irradiation	Phenothiazines: chlorpromazine, prochlorperazine
Trauma, surgery	Butyrophenones: haloperidol
Rathke cleft cyst	Thioxanthenes: thiothixene
Pituitary lesions	Benzamides: metoclopramide
Prolactinoma	Risperidone
Other tumors	Dopamine depletors: reserpine, opiates, α-methyldopa
Infiltrative disorders	H_2 antagonists: cimetidine, ranitidine
Lymphocytic hypophysitis	Serotonergic pathway stimulation: amphetamines
Empty sella	Calcium-channel blockers: verapamil
Intercostal nerve stimulation	Antidepressants: MAOI, TCA, SSRI
Chest wall lesions or surgery	Estrogen
Spinal cord injury	

H_2 = histamine 2; MAOI = monoamine oxidase inhibitor; TCA = tricyclic antidepressant; SSRI = selective serotonin-reuptake inhibitor.

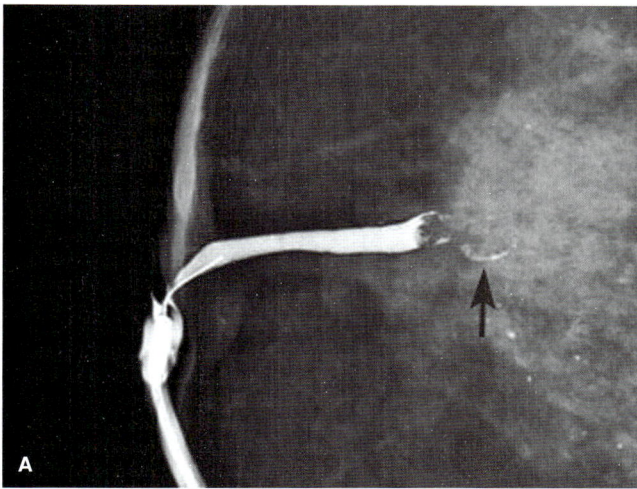
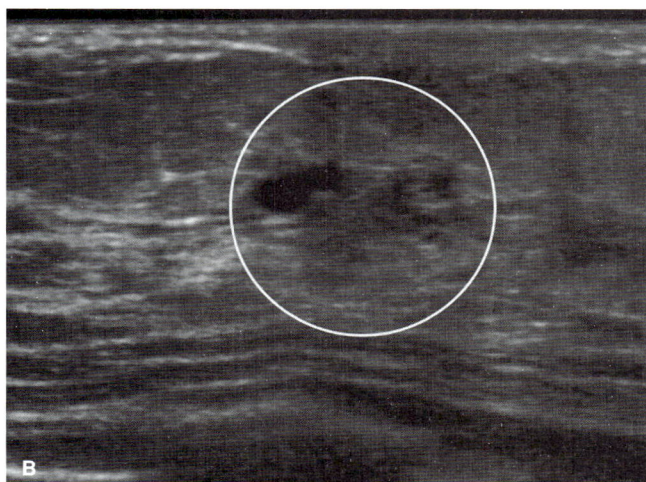

FIGURE 13-7 Imaging for a pathologic nipple discharge. **A.** Ductography shows a single dilated duct with an irregular filling defect (*arrow*). **B.** Periareolar sonogram demonstrates an irregular intraductal mass with microlobulated margins within the white circle. An excisional biopsy revealed a benign intraductal papilloma. (Reproduced with permission from Stephen J. Seiler, MD.)

called galactorrhea, results from various causes (Table 13-2) (Chap. 16, p. 360). Of these, pregnancy is a frequent cause of new-onset spontaneous discharge, and a bloody multiduct discharge during pregnancy is not uncommon.

Pathologic nipple discharge is defined as a spontaneous single-duct discharge that is serous or bloody. The rate of underlying malignancy ranges from approximately 2 percent for young women with no associated clinical or imaging findings to 20 percent for older women with associated findings (Cabioglu, 2003; Lau, 2005). Most pathologic nipple discharges are caused by benign intraductal papillomas, which are simple milk duct polyps (Urban, 1978). They arise in the major milk ducts, generally within 2 cm of the nipple, and contain a velvety papillary epithelium on a central fibrovascular stalk.

Evaluation of a pathologic nipple discharge begins with breast examination. Careful evaluation can frequently locate a trigger point on the areolar edge that elicits the discharge when pressed. Occult-blood testing and microscopic examination of the discharge can provide additional information. A glass slide that has been touched to the discharge and immediately fixed in 95-percent alcohol may be used for cytologic assessment. Nipple fluid samples are acellular in 25 percent of cases and thus cannot exclude an underlying malignancy (Papanicolaou,

1958). However, malignant cells, if found, are highly correlated with an underlying cancer (Gupta, 2004).

Following these examinations, diagnostic mammography and an assessment of the subareolar ducts by sonography or ductography are indicated. Diagnostic mammography is usually negative, but it may occasionally identify an underlying ductal carcinoma in situ. Mammary ductography, also known as *galactography*, requires cannulating the affected duct, injecting radiocontrast, and then performing mammography (Fig. 13-7).

An evaluation of the subareolar ducts, as described above, is required to localize an intraductal lesion for subsequent excision. However, pathologic nipple discharge is *definitively* diagnosed and treated by subareolar duct excision, which is also known as *microductectomy* (Locker, 1988). Subareolar duct excision can also be used to treat bothersome multiduct discharges not associated with prolactinoma.

BREAST INFECTIONS

■ Puerperal Infections

Breast infections are generally divided into puerperal, which develop during pregnancy and lactation, and nonpuerperal. Of these, pregnancy-related breast infection is characterized by warm, tender, diffuse breast erythema and is associated with systemic signs of infection such as fever, malaise, and leukocytosis. The most common organism is staphylococcal, and it is successfully treated with oral or intravenous antibiotics, depending on clinical severity. However, infection may also progress to form deep parenchymal abscesses (Branch-Elliman, 2012). Sonographic examination is highly sensitive for identifying underlying abscesses if mastitis does not improve rapidly with antibiotics or if an abscess is suggested clinically (Fig. 13-8). Women with puerperal mastitis ideally continue to breastfeed or breast pump during treatment to prevent milk stasis, which may contribute to infection progression (Thomsen, 1983). Cracked or excoriated nipples may provide entry for bacteria and are treated with lanolin-based lotions or ointments.

Appropriate antibiotics for puerperal mastitis include those covering staphylococcal species, although group A and B *Streptococcus*, *Corynebacterium*, and *Bacteroides* species and *Escherichia coli* are less frequently isolated. Commonly, cephalexin (Keflex) or dicloxacillin (Dynapen), each given at dosages of 500 mg orally four times daily, or the combination of amoxicillin and clavulanate (Augmentin), 500 mg orally three times daily, may be prescribed for 7 days. Erythromycin, 500 mg orally four times daily, will provide adequate coverage for those with a penicillin allergy. Methicillin-resistant *Staphylococcus aureus (MRSA)* is becoming a more prevalent community-acquired pathogen causing mastitis in pregnancy and the puerperium (Laibl, 2005; Stafford, 2008). If MRSA is suspected or if a patient fails to improve on an initial regimen, then trimethoprim-sulfamethoxazole double strength (Bactrim DS, Septra DS), one or two tablets orally twice daily, or clindamycin, 300 mg orally three times daily, is a suitable choice. In ill patients with extensive infection, hospitalization and intravenous antibiotics are typically required. In these complicated cases, MRSA coverage may be prudent, and clindamycin, 600 mg IV every 8 hours, or vancomycin, 1 g IV every 12 hours, can be administered. Intravenous antibiotics are typically given until the woman is afebrile for 24 to 48 hours. Oral antibiotics are then continued to complete a 7- to 10-day course.

An abscess that is initially present or that develops is drained. For smaller abscesses, sonographically guided needle aspiration using local analgesia has evidence-based support in small studies (Eryilmaz, 2005; Kang, 2016; Naeem, 2012). Incision and drainage may be needed for large abscesses or those failing to resolve with aspiration.

Focal mastitis may result from an infected galactocele. A tender mass will usually be palpable at the site of skin erythema. Needle aspiration of the galactocele and antibiotics are frequently all that is required, but recurrence or progression may mandate surgical drainage.

■ Nonpuerperal Infections

Uncomplicated cellulitis in a nonirradiated breast and in a nonpuerperal setting is uncommon. Accordingly, its presence prompts imaging and biopsies to exclude inflammatory breast cancer, described on page 296.

Nonpuerperal breast abscesses are generally classified as peripheral or subareolar. Peripheral abscesses usually are skin infections such as folliculitis or infection of epidermal inclusion cysts or Montgomery glands. These abscesses are all adequately treated by surgical drainage and then antibiotics discussed in the previous section. In contrast, subareolar abscesses arise from keratin-plugged milk ducts directly behind the nipple. The abscess itself usually presents under the areola, and fistulous communications between multiple abscesses are common (Kasales, 2014). Simple drainage is associated with a recurrence rate of nearly 40 percent, thus effective treatment requires subareolar duct excision and complete removal of sinus tracts. In general, surgical drainage of nonpuerperal breast abscesses is usually always accompanied by biopsy of the abscess wall, as breast cancer occasionally presents as an abscess (Benson, 1989; Watt-Boolsen, 1987).

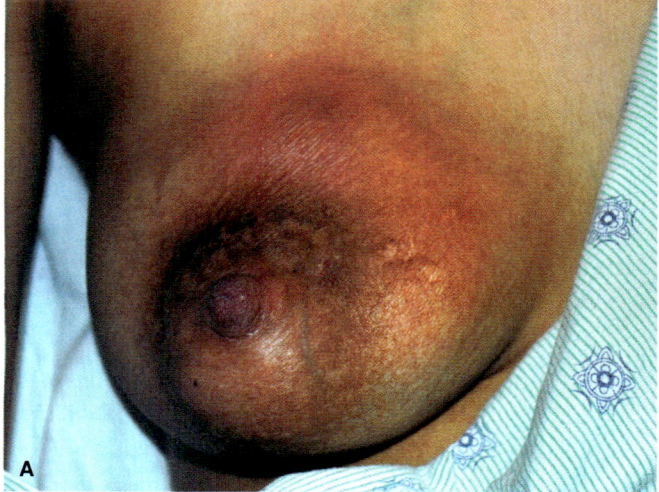
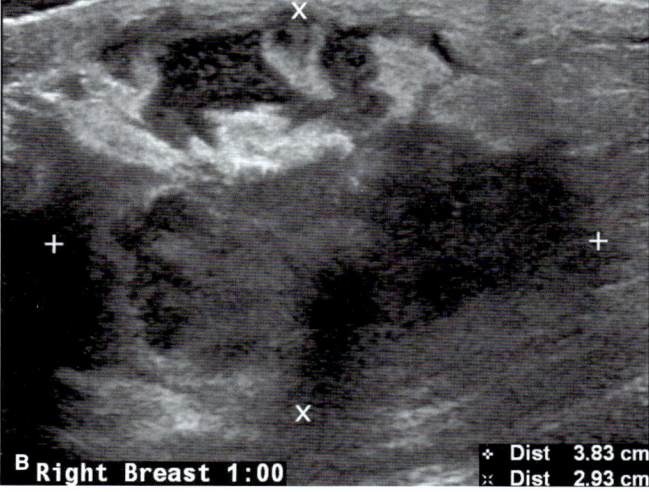

FIGURE 13-8 A. Puerperal right breast abscess. **B.** Breast sonogram displays the hypoechoic abscess contents, and calipers mark its borders. (Reproduced with permission from Dr. Agnieszka Dombrowska.)

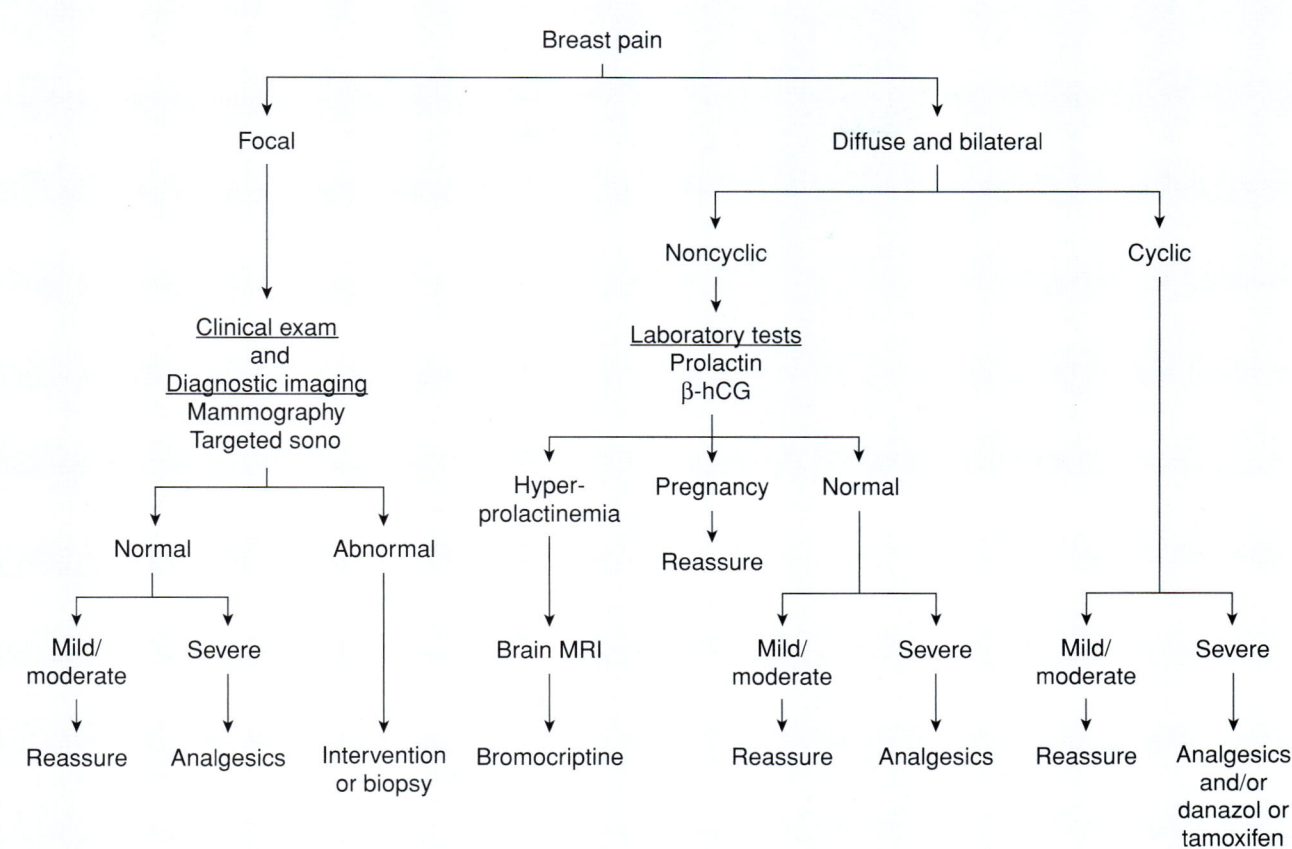

FIGURE 13-9 Diagnostic algorithm to evaluate mastalgia. Oil of evening primrose or vitamin E is frequently used for mild/moderate pain, but the effects are no better than placebo. hCG = human chorionic gonadotropin; MRI = magnetic resonance imaging.

Idiopathic granulomatous mastitis (IGM) is not a true infection. It is included in this section because the painful masses, fluid collections, skin erythema, ulceration, and draining sinus tracts are often confused with infection. Core needle biopsy will show noncaseating granulomas, and fluid aspirated from apparent "abscesses" is nearly always sterile. Tissue stains can be used to exclude tuberculosis or mycotic infection. Wegener granulomatosis and sarcoidosis are considered in the initial differential diagnosis. This is a self-limiting condition that may take years to resolve. Procedures should be minimized as they will often result in painful draining sinuses. High-dose corticosteroids or methotrexate have been used for treatment, but their efficacy is unclear (Mohammed, 2013; Pandey, 2014).

MASTALGIA

The prevalence of breast pain is 66 percent and is higher for women nearing menopause than for younger women (Euhus, 1997; Maddox, 1989). The precise etiology of mastalgia is unknown. Estrogen- and progesterone-mediated changes in interstitial water content and thus in interstitial pressure are implicated.

Mastalgia is generally classified as cyclic or noncyclic. Noncyclic mastalgia is often focal and shows no relationship to the menstrual cycle. Although focal mastalgia is frequently caused by a simple cyst, breast cancer occasionally presents as focal breast pain. Therefore, this complaint is evaluated

by careful clinical examination, targeted imaging, and needle biopsy of any palpable or imaging abnormalities.

In contrast, cyclic mastalgia is usually bilateral, diffuse, and most severe during the late luteal phase of the menstrual cycle (Gateley, 1990). It remits with the onset of menstruation. Cyclic mastalgia requires no specific evaluation and is generally managed symptomatically with nonsteroidal antiinflammatory agents (Fig. 13-9). Various other proposed treatments include bromocriptine, vitamin E, or oil of evening primrose. However, outcomes are no better than placebo in the best randomized clinical trials, except for bromocriptine in the subset of women with elevated prolactin levels (Kumar, 1989; Mansel, 1990). For the most severe cases, several agents are effective when administered during the last 2 weeks of the menstrual cycle. These include: (1) danazol, 200 mg orally daily; (2) the selective estrogen-receptor modifier toremifene (Fareston), 20 mg orally daily; or (3) tamoxifen (Nolvadex), 20 mg orally daily. Pregnancy must first be excluded and then avoided if these medications are used.

BENIGN BREAST DISEASE

■ Benign Breast Disease without Atypia

The primary tissue components of the breast are fat, fibrous stroma, and epithelial structures. The hormonally responsive

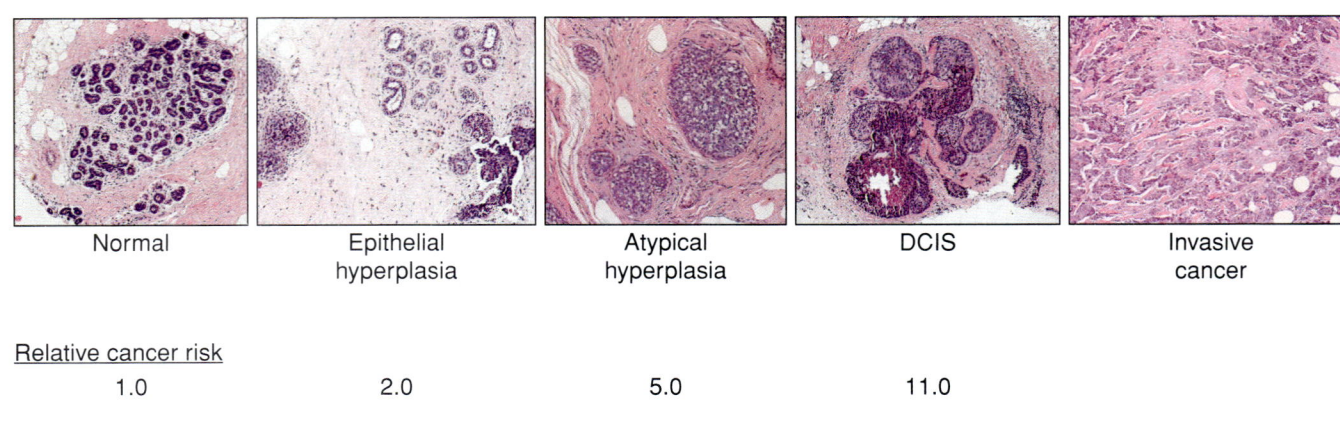

| Normal | Epithelial hyperplasia | Atypical hyperplasia | DCIS | Invasive cancer |

Relative cancer risk

| 1.0 | 2.0 | 5.0 | 11.0 | |

Tumor suppressor gene methylation

Allelic imbalances

Oncogene amplification

FIGURE 13-10 Histologic progression from normal breast tissue to cancer. DCIS = ductal carcinoma in situ.

component is the epithelium, but considerable paracrine communication exists between the epithelium and stroma. The natural hormonal changes of puberty, pregnancy, lactation, and menopause drive considerable physiologic remodeling of breast tissue during a woman's lifetime, but pathologic remodeling is observed in some. This is initially characterized by acinar dilation and fibrosis, termed *nonproliferative benign breast disease*. Depending on the extent and pattern of these changes, a breast may appear mammographically dense, feel nodular to palpation, or both. The term "fibrocystic change" is often used to refer to palpably nodular breast tissue or to the histologic pattern of dilated ducts and acini invested with dense collagenous stroma. This is not a significant breast cancer risk factor and does not require any special management.

When this change is accompanied by accumulation of luminal epithelial cells (e.g., epithelial hyperplasia), it is called *benign proliferative disease* (Fig. 13-10). This change has been linked to higher levels of estrogen, insulin, and certain inflammatory cytokines and to reduced levels of the beneficial adipokine adiponectin (Catsburg, 2014). Benign proliferative breast disease without atypia is a modest breast cancer risk factor, with a relative risk of 1.5 to 1.9 (Dupont, 1993; Hartmann, 2005; Sneige, 2002).

■ Benign Proliferative Disease with Atypia

Atypia refers to specific alterations in the size, shape, or nuclear features of individual epithelial cells in combination with the way groups of cells are organized. Atypical proliferation of ductal cells is termed atypical ductal hyperplasia (ADH), whereas similar changes in acinar cells are termed atypical lobular hyperplasia (ALH). As more and more terminal ducts or acini become involved, the condition is recognized as ductal carcinoma in situ (DCIS) or lobular carcinoma in situ (LCIS), respectively, which are discussed in later sections (Ringberg, 2001).

Benign proliferative disease with atypia historically accounts for 4 percent of benign breast lesions (Hartmann, 2005).

However, the incidence has declined coincident to reductions in hormone replacement therapy use (Menes, 2009).

Importantly, the difference between ADH and low-grade DCIS is based on the area occupied by the proliferative epithelial cells (Vandenbussche, 2013). Accordingly, surgical excision is usually recommended when ADH is diagnosed by core needle biopsy, as 4 to 38 percent of cases will be upgraded to in situ or invasive cancer. However, for ALH or LCIS diagnosed in core needle biopsy samples, excision is no longer recommended when imaging is not suspicious (Bevers, 2018).

Chemoprevention is an excellent option for high-risk women with atypical hyperplasia. These lesions are estrogen-driven, and tamoxifen reduces breast cancer risk by 52 to 86 percent for these women (Coopey, 2012; Fisher, 1999).

Benign proliferative disease with atypia is a marker of increased breast cancer risk. Relative risks are 4.5 to 5.0, and absolute risks approximate 1 percent per year for 20 to 30 years (Degnim, 2007; Dupont, 1993). This risk is higher for more extensive lesions. Risk does not appear to rise further with hormone replacement use.

LOBULAR CARCINOMA IN SITU

Similar to proliferative ductal lesion, LCIS differs from ALH by the greater extent of lobular cell proliferation with LCIS and increased acini distention. Two main types of LCIS are classic and pleomorphic. Classic LCIS is not associated with specific mammographic or palpable features and thus is only diagnosed incidentally. Classic LCIS has not traditionally been viewed as a direct precursor of breast cancer, but this view is changing. For example, although LCIS is associated with greater cancer risk for both breasts, women with LCIS most commonly develop carcinoma in the ipsilateral breast (Fisher, 2004b; Ottesen, 1993; Salvadori, 1991). Moreover, infiltrating lobular cancers frequently show associated LCIS, and a clonal relationship between LCIS and subsequent invasive cancer has been demonstrated (Abner, 2000; Andrade, 2012; Sasson, 2001).

With LCIS, the risk for developing breast cancer averages 1 percent per year. This can be modified upward by early age at diagnosis, family history of breast cancer, and extensive disease (Bodian, 1996). Classic LCIS is strongly estrogen receptor–positive, and tamoxifen reduces breast cancer risk by 56 percent in this setting (Fisher, 1999).

Pleomorphic lobular carcinoma in situ (P-LCIS) is thought to be more aggressive than classic LCIS. P-LCIS may be diagnosed as a palpable mass or on mammogram as fine pleomorphic calcifications or architectural distortion (Jorns, 2014; Savage, 2018). P-LCIS is a relatively new diagnosis, and there is no clear consensus on its treatment (Wazir, 2016).

When P-LCIS is diagnosed from a core needle biopsy sample, the final pathologic diagnosis will be upgraded to either DCIS or invasive cancer in 30 to 40 percent of cases (Fasola, 2018; Masannat, 2018). The more aggressive character of P-LCIS suggests that it may best be approached in a manner similar to DCIS (Masannat, 2018). Unlike the classic form of LCIS, P-LCIS should be considered for complete excision with negative margins (National Comprehensive Cancer Network, 2018). Occasionally P-LCIS is also treated with adjuvant radiotherapy. However, data are limited, and more evidence is needed.

The Ki67 index, a protein marker of cell proliferation, is often higher in pleomorphic LCIS than in classic LCIS. Similarly, Her-2/neu, a protein receptor associated with cancer proliferation, is more commonly amplified in P-LCIS. In contrast, estrogen and progesterone receptor expression is lower in P-LCIS than in classic LCIS (Chen, 2009). Although tamoxifen is an effective chemopreventive agent in classic LCIS, its efficacy for P-LCIS is unclear.

DUCTAL CARCINOMA IN SITU

DCIS can be understood as a condition in which cancer cells fill portions of a mammary ductal system without invading beyond the duct's basement membrane (Fig. 13-11) (Ringberg, 2001). Although DCIS cells have accumulated many of the DNA changes common to invasive breast cancer, they lack certain critical changes that would permit them to persist outside of the duct (Aubele, 2002). DCIS is currently classified as stage 0 breast cancer.

The U.S. incidence of DCIS has risen and plateaued in parallel with that of invasive breast cancer. DCIS currently accounts for 25 to 30 percent of all breast cancers in the United States. It is most commonly diagnosed by screening mammography as it is frequently associated with pleomorphic, linear, or branching calcifications (Fig. 13-12).

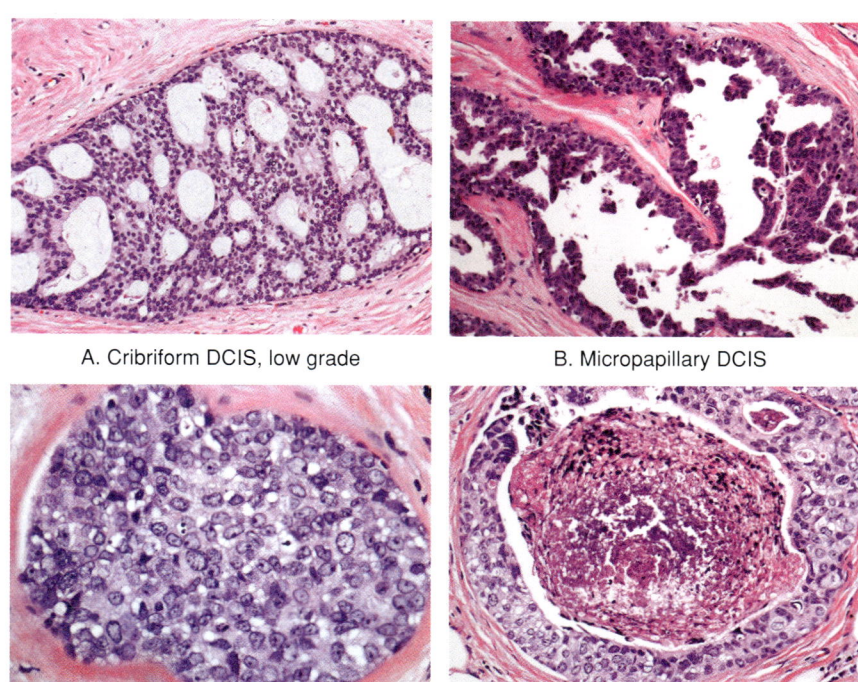

A. Cribriform DCIS, low grade   B. Micropapillary DCIS

C. Solid DCIS, high grade   D. DCIS with comedonecrosis

FIGURE 13-11 A–D. Morphologic types of ductal carcinoma in situ (DCIS). (Reproduced with permission from Dr. Sunati Sahoo, Pathology, UTSW Medical Center.)

Although considered stage 0 breast cancer, DCIS's classification as a carcinoma has spurred considerable debate. Namely, the chance of dying of breast cancer after a DCIS diagnosis is 3.3 percent at 20 years, and this is not reduced by mastectomy compared with breast-conserving therapy (Fig. 13-13) (Narod, 2015; Solin, 1996). The reason to treat DCIS is to reduce future invasive cancer risk. However, most DCIS lesions do not progress to invasive cancer, even if undertreated. Several clinical trials are currently evaluating observation with or without endocrine therapy as a management strategy.

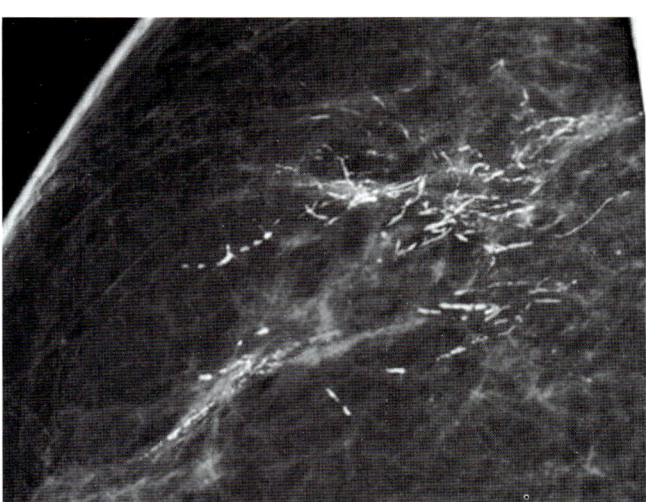

FIGURE 13-12 Fine linear-branching calcifications in a segmental distribution associated with ductal carcinoma in situ. (Reproduced with permission from Stephen J. Seiler, MD.)

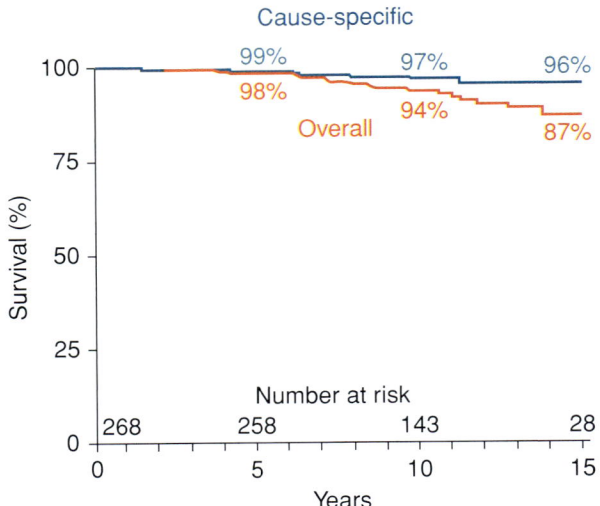

Cause-specific

99%   97%   96%

98%   94%   87%

Overall

Survival (%)

Number at risk

268   258   143   28

Years

FIGURE 13-13 Cause-specific and overall survival rates for ductal carcinoma in situ. (From Solin, 1996, with permission.)

Current guidelines recommend excision of DCIS with at least a 2-mm margin (Morrow, 2016). This may require mastectomy if DCIS is extensive or if there are other contraindications to breast conservation. When breast conservation is possible, postoperative breast irradiation will reduce the local recurrence rate by 50 percent (Fisher, 1993). Current interests are focused on recognizing which patients will or will not benefit from radiotherapy. Early age at diagnosis and palpable DCIS consistently predict greater recurrence risk and favor adjunctive radiation. Molecular assays for predicting this benefit are available commercially.

Axillary staging is generally not included in the management of DCIS. Some have advocated sentinel lymph node (SLN) biopsy for large, high-grade DCIS diagnosed by needle biopsy and treated by lumpectomy, as occult invasive cancer is diagnosed in 10 percent of these cases (Wilkie, 2005). SLN biopsy in conjunction with mastectomy is less controversial, as it is not possible to go back and perform SLN biopsy if an occult invasive cancer is diagnosed in this setting.

Adjuvant endocrine therapy (tamoxifen or aromatase inhibitor) is recommended for estrogen receptor–positive DCIS treated by breast conservation (Fisher, 1999). This is not associated with a statistically significant improvement in overall survival rates. However, it does significantly reduce the incidence of ipsilateral invasive cancer and also reduces the risk of contralateral breast cancer.

■ Paget Disease of the Nipple

This type of DCIS presents as a focal eczematous rash of the nipple (Fig. 13-14). Ductal carcinoma cells, responding to chemoattractants secreted by cells in the dermis, migrate to the surface of the nipple, inducing skin breakdown (Schelfhout, 2000). The condition is easily diagnosed histologically by punch biopsy or excision of the affected nipple tip after nipple-areolar blockade using local anesthetic. Evaluation also includes careful clinical examination, as an associated mass is identified in approximately 60 percent of cases (Ashikari, 1970). Among those with no palpable abnormalities, mammography will show suspicious densities or calcifications in 21 percent (Ikeda, 1993). An underlying DCIS is identified in about two thirds of cases, and an invasive cancer in approximately one third (Ashikari, 1970).

Treatment includes wide excision to achieve negative margins. Breast conservation requires central breast resection including the nipple-areolar complex and all identifiable underlying disease. Resection is followed by postoperative breast irradiation (Bijker, 2001). Axillary staging by SLN biopsy is not required unless an invasive component is identified or total mastectomy is performed.

BREAST CANCER RISK FACTORS

The most profound breast cancer risk factor is female gender. In addition, the incidence of breast cancer, as for most other cancers, increases with advancing age. Only 12 to 30 percent of breast cancer has a significant familial component, and apart from radiation exposure early in life, convincing environmental causes have not been elucidated (Baker, 2005; Locatelli, 2004). Breast cancer risk factors are listed in Table 13-3. In general, all of these risk factors are more prevalent in developed countries than in less-developed ones. Consequently, breast cancer is more common in industrialized cultures (Parkin, 2001).

■ Reproductive Factors
Ovulatory Cycles

Ovulatory menstrual cycles exert stress on the breast epithelium by inducing proliferation in the late luteal phase. If conception

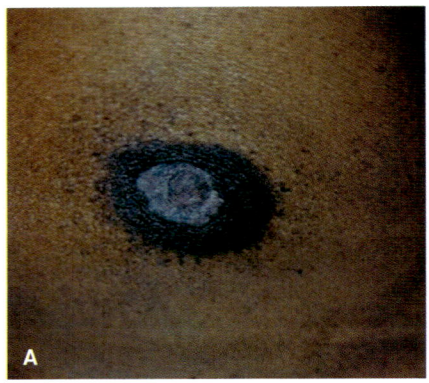
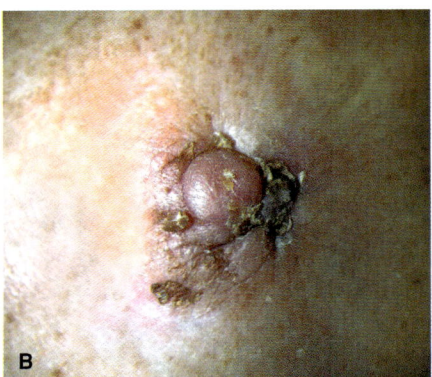
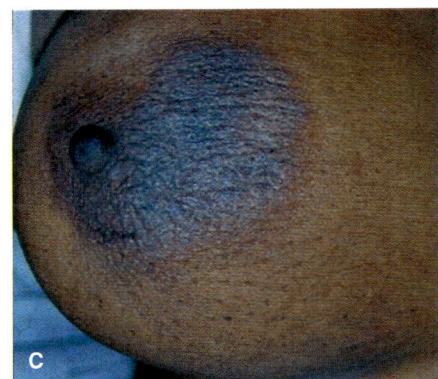

FIGURE 13-14 A and **B.** Paget disease of the nipple. **C.** Benign reactive dermatitis. (Reproduced with permission from Dr. Marilyn Leitch.)

TABLE 13-3. Common Risk Factors and Their Risk Ratios[a]

Genetic Risk Factors	Risk Ratio
Female gender	114
Age	4–158[b]
High-penetrance mutations: BRCA1, BRCA2, p53, STK11	26–36
Modest-penetrance mutations: PTEN, p16, PALB2, CDH1, NF1, CHEK2, ATM, BRIP1	2.0–2.7
Family: mother, daughter, sister	1.55–1.8
Family: aunt, niece, grandmother	1.15
Genetic polymorphisms: FGFR2, TNRC9, MAP3K1, LSP1, MRPS30	1.07–1.26
Other Factors	
Mantle radiation	5.6
Acini per lobule in benign breast tissue	
11–20	2.8
21–40	3.23
≥41	11.85
Mammographic density	
>25–50% (scattered)	2.4
>51–75% (heterogeneous)	3.4
>75% (dense)	5.3
Biopsy w LCIS	5.4
Biopsy w atypical hyperplasia	5
Increased BMD	2.0–2.5
Age at first birth >35	1.31–1.93
Obesity (BMI >30)	1.2–1.8
Any benign breast disease	1.47
Elevated circulating insulin	1.46
5 years of combined HRT	1.26–1.76
Elevated circulating estrogen	1.1–1.7
Nulliparity	1.26–1.55
Alcohol (>1 drink/day)	1.31
Age at menarche <12	1.21

[a]Risks listed by genetic or nongenetic and ordered by strength of association with breast cancer.
[b]Risk compared with women aged 20–29. The risk ratio increases approximately by 4 for every year older than 30.
BMD = bone mineral density; BMI = body mass index; HRT = hormone replacement therapy; LCIS = lobular carcinoma in situ.
Compiled from Beral, 2011; Bodian, 1996; Cauley, 1996; Claus, 1994; De Bruin, 2009; Easton, 2007; Freisinger, 2009; Fu, 2007; Gail, 1989; Gunter, 2009; Hankinson, 2005; Hulley, 2002; Kotsopoulos, 2010; Lalloo, 2006; Mavaddat, 2010; McKian, 2009; Phipps, 2010; Rossouw, 2002; Santen, 2005; Welsh, 2009; Zhou, 2011.

does not occur, proliferation is followed by programmed cell death (Anderson, 1982; Soderqvist, 1997). Early age at menarche is associated with earlier onset of ovulatory cycles and higher breast cancer risk (den Tonkelaar, 1996; Vihko, 1986). Conversely, early menopause, whether it is natural or surgical, is associated with a reduced breast cancer risk (Kvale, 1988). Pregnancy generates very high levels of circulating estradiol, which is associated with a transient rise in short-term risk. But pregnancy also induces terminal differentiation of breast epithelium and provides relief from ovarian cycling. Consequently, increasing parity is associated with reduced lifetime risk.

Pregnancy

The breast is unique among all human organs in that it exists as a primordium for a decade or more before entering a highly proliferative state at menarche, and then does not fully mature until the first live birth. Immature breast epithelium is more susceptible to carcinogens than postlactational epithelium (Russo, 1996). Thus, the longer a first live birth is delayed, the greater the breast cancer risk is. Specifically, a first live birth before the age of 28 years is associated with reduced breast cancer risk, whereas one occurring later is associated with elevated risk (Gail, 1989). Both early age at first live birth and greater numbers of live births are associated with a lower breast cancer risk (Layde, 1989; Pike, 1983).

■ Hormone Replacement Therapy

The postmenopausal use of combined estrogen and progestin hormone replacement therapy is a modest breast cancer risk factor, and relative risks range from 1.26 to 1.76 (Beral, 2011; Hulley, 2002; Rossouw, 2002). The risk is higher with longer durations of use and with a shorter interval between the onset of menopause and the start of the medication (Beral, 2011). Estrogen-only replacement is not convincingly associated with an increased breast cancer risk. However, a relationship between estrogen-only therapy and body mass index yields a lower risk for obese women and higher risk for thin women (Anderson, 2004).

BREAST CANCER RISK STRATIFICATION AND MANAGEMENT

Approaches for managing breast cancer risk include: (1) lifestyle modification to achieve and sustain ideal body weight, (2) enhanced surveillance that includes screening MR imaging, (3) chemoprevention with a selective estrogen-receptor modifier (SERM) or an aromatase inhibitor, and (4) prophylactic surgery that includes oophorectomy or mastectomy for those at highest risk (Cuzick, 2014; Domchek, 2010; Goss, 2011; Heemskerk-Gerritsen, 2007; Vogel, 2010). Beyond beneficial lifestyle modification, each intervention introduces new risks, and thus breast cancer risk quantification is essential for decision making.

The American Cancer Society has endorsed screening MR imaging for women with a lifetime breast cancer risk that exceeds 20 percent (Saslow, 2010). The Food and Drug Administration (FDA) has approved tamoxifen chemoprevention for women older than 35 years with >1.7 percent breast cancer risk over 5 years. Similarly, the SERM raloxifene (Evista) is approved for increased-risk postmenopausal women. To maximize benefit and minimize harm, breast cancer risk, age, race, and prior hysterectomy all factor into chemoprevention decisions (Freedman, 2011).

The foregoing highlights the importance of quantitative breast cancer risk stratification. Several computer models are available for this. The most widely used are the Gail model, available at www.cancer.gov/bcrisktool/ and the IBIS (Tyrer-Cuzick) model available at www.ems-trials.org/riskevaluator/ (Costantino, 1999; Gail, 1989; Rockhill, 2001; Tyrer, 2004). The Gail model is insufficient when there is a strong family history of breast cancer, male breast cancer, or ovarian cancer (Euhus, 2002). Genetic models such as BRCAPRO, Tyrer-Cuzick, or BOADICEA are more appropriate in these settings (Berry, 1997; Lee, 2014; Tyrer, 2004).

■ Breast Cancer Genetics

Twin studies suggest that only 12 to 30 percent of breast cancer is primarily genetic in origin, and modeling studies implicate autosomal dominant inheritance of single genes as the most important mechanism (Lichtenstein, 2000; Locatelli, 2004; Risch, 2001). Accordingly, genetic testing is one of the most powerful risk stratification tools available. It can identify women at very high risk for cancer who could reasonably consider risk-reducing surgery. In breast cancer patients, it can also contribute directly to decisions regarding surgery, radiation, and systemic therapies (Euhus, 2013). Mutations in *BRCA1*, *BRCA2*, *PALB2*, *CHEK2*, and *ATM* genes are the most frequently identified germline alterations in familial breast cancer, but the list of predisposition genes is growing (Table 13-4). Commercialized massive parallel sequencing, namely, next-generation sequencing, now allows testing for mutations in a few to dozens of genes simultaneously (Euhus, 2015).

Obtaining a reasonably detailed cancer family history is essential for identifying individuals who may benefit from genetic counseling and testing. At a minimum, the relationship and age at diagnosis is recorded for every cancer in the family. Family histories that may suggest inherited susceptibility include early-onset breast cancer (<50 years), bilateral breast cancer, male breast cancer, multiple affected relatives in one generation, breast cancer in multiple generations, development of cancers that are known to be associated with a particular syndrome, and two or more cancers in one relative, especially if they develop at an early age.

■ Hereditary Breast-Ovarian Cancer Syndrome

This syndrome accounts for 5 to 7 percent of breast cancers in the United States and is most frequently caused by *BRCA1* or *BRCA2* mutation (Malone, 2000). With *BRCA1* mutations, hallmarks include early age at breast cancer diagnosis (median 44 years); high-grade, estrogen-receptor– and progesterone-receptor–negative breast cancers; and associated ovarian cancer (Foulkes, 2004).

For *BRCA1* mutation carriers, the lifetime breast cancer risk ranges from 45 to 81 percent, and ovarian cancer risk from 16 to 54 percent (Antoniou, 2008; Brohet, 2014; Ford, 1998; King, 2003; Mavaddat, 2013). Individuals who have developed both breast and ovarian cancer have an 86-percent probability of carrying a *BRCA* mutation (Cvelbar, 2005).

Among *BRCA2* carriers, lifetime risk for breast cancer ranges from 27 to 85 percent, and ovarian cancer risk from 6 to 27 percent. Women with *BRCA2* mutations develop breast cancer later in life than *BRCA1* carriers, thus age at diagnosis is not usually a good criterion for recognizing this syndrome (Panchal, 2010). Similar to sporadic breast cancer, most *BRCA2*-associated breast cancers are hormone receptor–positive (Lakhani, 2002). Ovarian cancer is an associated cancer but develops less frequently than it does in *BRCA1*-affected families. Five to 13 percent of male breast cancers are associated with *BRCA2* mutations. For men, lifetime breast cancer risk is estimated at 1.8 percent with *BRCA1* mutations and 8.3 percent for *BRCA2* (Tai, 2007).

For affected women, early premenopausal bilateral oophorectomy reduces breast cancer risk by 37 to 72 percent and also lowers breast cancer–specific and all-cause mortality rates (Domchek, 2010; Finch, 2014; Kauff, 2008). This is discussed further in Chapter 35 (p. 736). Bilateral prophylactic mastectomy reduces breast cancer risk by more than 90 percent but does not appear to improve survival rates (Hartmann, 2001; Heemskerk-Gerritsen, 2007; Meijers-Heijboer, 2001).

With the introduction of next-generation sequencing panel tests, clinicians are increasingly confronted with rare syndromes for which data to guide management are limited (see Table 13-4) (Euhus, 2015). Involvement of professional genetic counselors and careful assessment of a three-generation family cancer history are essential for estimating and managing cancer risk.

Surgical options for breast cancers that arise in the context of an inherited predisposition syndrome are the same as for sporadic breast cancers (Pierce, 2010). However, patients are counseled that the lifetime risk for contralateral breast cancer risk may be as high as 83 percent for *BRCA1* mutation carriers and 62 percent for *BRCA2* carriers. Retrospective data suggest that bilateral mastectomy may improve survival rates for these women (Evans, 2013; Mavaddat, 2013; Metcalfe, 2014).

TABLE 13-4. Genetic Syndromes Associated with Increased Breast Cancer Risk

Syndrome Name	Genetic Mutation
Hereditary breast-ovarian cancer syndrome	BRCA1, BRCA2
Li-Fraumeni	p53
Cowden	PTEN
Peutz-Jegher	STK11
Hereditary diffuse gastric cancer	CDH1
PALB2	PALB2
ATM	ATM
CHEK2	CHEK2
RAD51C	RAD51C

BREAST CANCER SCREENING

In the United States, digital mammography has largely replaced film-screen mammography, and three-dimensional (3-D) tomosynthesis is gradually replacing two dimensional (2-D) mammography. This technique generates hundreds of images as the x-ray source arcs over the top of the breast. Digital reconstruction allows a radiologist to visually scroll through breast images and also significantly attenuates overlying breast densities at each level (Kopans, 2013). Compared with 2-D mammography, tomosynthesis reduces the false-positive rate (recall rate) by 15 to 30 percent and raises the cancer detection rate by 10 to 29 percent (Greenberg, 2014; Haas, 2013; Skaane, 2013). This is achieved with slightly higher radiation doses (Feng, 2012).

■ The Screening Mammography Controversy

In 2009, for women not at high risk for breast cancer, the U.S. Preventive Services Task Force recommended biennial screening mammography for women aged 50 to 74 years and individualized screening decisions for women aged 40 to 49. Nevertheless, several influential organizations including the American Cancer Society, the American College of Obstetricians and Gynecologists (2017), and the American College of Radiology have recommended that yearly screening mammography begin earlier (Monticciolo, 2017; Smith, 2018). The American College of Obstetricians and Gynecologists (2017) recommends offering annual or biennial screening beginning at age 40 years or at least by no later than age 50. The controversy centers on: (1) the true mortality rate benefit, (2) the harm from false-positive results, and (3) the harm from diagnosing clinically irrelevant breast cancers.

However, most data available for addressing these issues are derived from eight large, but older, randomized prospective trials. The most recent trial was completed in the 1980s. Recent technologic advances have significantly improved the sensitivity of mammography. However, breast cancer treatment has also advanced, reducing the mortality rate improvement from early detection. Based on 30-year-old data, it is generally agreed that screening mammography starting at age 50 reduces breast cancer mortality rates by approximately 27 percent, and one meta-analysis reported an 18-percent reduction for women aged 40 to 49 (Hendrick, 1997; Kerlikowske, 1997). However, screen-detected breast cancer is a heterogeneous disease. Some cancers will eventually develop clinical metastases no matter how small they are when first detected, and some will never become lethal no matter how long diagnosis is delayed. This latter form is the one most likely to be detected by periodic screening (length time bias).

The practice of screening mammography is based on the assumption that early intervention in some subgroup of tumors will interrupt progression and save lives. Since screening mammography inception, the detection of early-stage breast cancer has significantly risen, but the diagnosis of node-positive or metastatic disease has shown only a small decline (Bleyer, 2012). This suggests that many breast cancers will never progress (overdiagnosed) and that the fraction of breast cancers whose progression can be interrupted by surgery may be modest.

For now, annual mammography beginning at age 40, as recommended by several professional societies, is reasonable. But, women are counseled of the risks and benefits. Among 1000 U.S. women aged 50 years who are screened annually for a decade, 0.3 to 3.2 are estimated to avoid a breast cancer death, 490 to 670 will have at least 1 false alarm, and 3 to 14 will be overdiagnosed and treated needlessly (Welch, 2014). There is no arbitrary age above which screening should cease. Women should have at least 10 years of remaining life to realize a mortality benefit from screening mammography (Lee, 2013).

Women who are at high risk for breast cancer because of a breast cancer predisposition mutation, a strong family history of breast cancer, or a personal history of high-risk preneoplasia such as ADH, ALH, or LCIS often participate in enhanced surveillance. This consists of semiannual imaging that alternates mammography and breast MR imaging. MR imaging screening may start as early as age 25 for mutation carriers, but annual mammography is delayed until after age 30.

■ Breast Magnetic Resonance Imaging

Breast MR imaging is commonly used as an adjunct to screen high-risk women and to establish disease extent in certain breast cancer patients. It is more sensitive for breast cancer detection than is mammography, but it is expensive and has a high false-positive rate. In addition, some evidence links its use with higher mastectomy rates but without reducing reexcision rates or improving breast cancer outcome (Houssami, 2013, 2014; Pilewskie, 2014; Turnbull, 2010).

As noted, annual screening breast MR imaging is frequently selected for genetically high-risk women and in women with a lifetime breast cancer risk exceeding 20 percent (Saslow, 2010). This raises the diagnosis of smaller, lymph node–negative breast cancers but does not improve survival rates (Gareth, 2014; Moller, 2013).

Breast MR imaging should not be routinely performed in women with newly diagnosed breast cancer, but it is recommended for women with mammographically dense breasts. Its primary value is assessing response to neoadjuvant chemotherapy in women contemplating breast conservation and in evaluating women with breast cancer metastatic to axillary lymph nodes from an unknown primary (Morrow, 2011). Additionally, it can aid establishing the extent of disease prior to breast conservation for a subset of patients in whom uncertainty persists after careful clinical examination, mammography, and sonography.

■ Other Breast Imaging Modalities

Adding almost any imaging modality to screening mammography will incrementally raise the cancer detection rate but at the cost of a higher false-positive rate and more biopsies. Modalities that are occasionally useful, but not recommended for routine use, include screening sonography, breast-specific gamma imaging, and breast positron emission tomography (PET) (Kalinyak, 2014; Merry, 2014; Rechtman, 2014). These last two tests are associated with significantly higher radiation exposure. Evidence is accumulating that medical radiation exposure before age 30 can elevate breast cancer risk, and thus caution is advised (Berrington de Gonzalez, 2009; Pijpe, 2012).

Screening Physical Examination

The value of a screening clinical breast examination (CBE) performed by health care providers should not be neglected (Jatoi, 2003). Four of the large, randomized mammography trials mentioned earlier collected information on CBE and found that 44 to 74 percent of the breast cancers were detected by this approach. Among young women, sensitivity and specificity were higher for CBE than mammography.

In contrast, enthusiasm for patients to perform breast self-examination (BSE) has diminished after a large randomized trial from Shanghai found no improvement in mortality rates (Thomas, 2002). Although there is less interest in promoting regimented BSE, encouraging women to remain breast-aware is reasonable.

INVASIVE BREAST CANCER

In the United States, breast cancer is the most common cancer in women and the second most frequent cause of cancer-related mortality (second to lung) (Siegel, 2019). Although the incidence of breast cancer rose steadily in this country through the 1980s and 1990s, it has leveled at approximately 125 cases per year per 100,000 postmenopausal women and is declining for some ethnicities. Concurrently, survival rates steadily improve (Fig. 13-15).

Tumor Characteristics

Primary cancers of the breast constitute 97 percent of malignancies affecting the breast, whereas 3 percent represent metastases from other sites. The most common of these, in descending order, are the contralateral breast, sarcoma, melanoma, serous epithelial ovarian cancer, and lung cancer (DeLair, 2013). Cancers of mammary epithelial structures account for most of primary breast cancer. Infiltrating ductal carcinoma is the most common form of invasive breast cancer (~80 percent), and infiltrating lobular carcinoma is the second most frequent (~15 percent). Other malignancies such as phyllodes tumors, sarcoma, and lymphoma account for the remainder.

Apart from stage, the primary tumor characteristics that most influence prognosis and treatment decisions are hormone receptor status, nuclear grade, and Her-2/neu expression (Harris, 2007). Approximately two thirds of breast cancers are estrogen-receptor–positive and progesterone-receptor–positive. This feature is generally associated with a better prognosis and more treatment options.

Her-2/neu is a membrane tyrosine kinase that cooperates with other Her-family receptors to generate proliferation and survival signals in breast cancer cells. Approximately 20 percent of breast cancers have elevated expression of Her-2/neu (Masood, 2005). The list of medications that specifically target Her-2/neu overexpressing breast cancer is growing and includes trastuzumab (Herceptin), trastuzumab emtansine (Kadcyla), pertuzumab (Perjeta), neratinib (Nerlynx), and lapatinib (Tykerb) (Tolaney, 2014).

Gene expression profiling has identified several "intrinsic subtypes" of breast cancer with prognostic significance (Cadoo, 2013). Multigene assays are now available in the clinic for individualized prediction of prognosis and treatment response, especially for estrogen-receptor–positive tumors (Rouzier, 2013).

Breast Cancer Staging

Careful breast cancer staging is essential for predicting outcome, planning treatment, and comparing treatment effects in clinical trials. Each patient is assigned both a clinical and a pathologic stage. The clinical stage is based on examination and radiographic findings, whereas the pathologic stage is based on actual tumor measurements and histologic assessments of lymph nodes after primary surgery. Staging of breast cancer is based on anatomic features such as tumor size (T) and metastases to lymph nodes (N) or distant organs (M) and on the biologic features of the tumor. In 2018, the American Joint Committee on Cancer (AJCC) introduced this updated breast cancer staging system to better reflect true tumor behavior for treatment planning (Giuliano, 2017). The AJCC system incorporates additional prognostic factors to the TNM system. Biologic aspects are estrogen-receptor, progesterone-receptor, and HER-2/neu status; tumor grade; and sometimes the results of a molecular prognostic assay. The TNM information provides an anatomic stage, which may be adjusted to a higher or lower prognostic stage based on these biologic features.

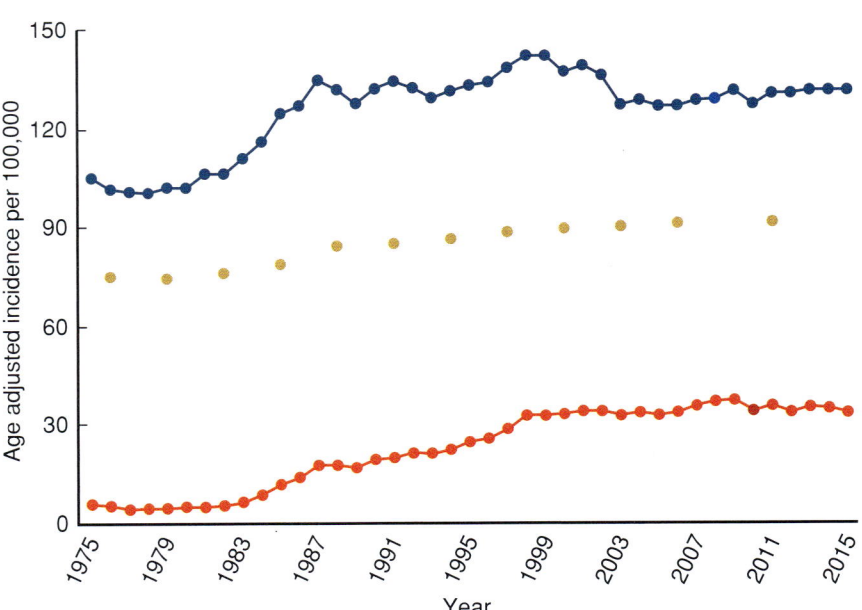

FIGURE 13-15 Trends in breast cancer incidence and survival in the United States. Curve of decreasing breast cancer rates in U.S. ● = incidence of invasive breast cancer; ● = incidence in situ; ● = 5-year survival.

The most common distant metastatic site in breast cancer is bone, followed by lung, liver, and brain. Thus, for newly diagnosed breast cancer patients, a complete blood count and liver function tests including alkaline phosphatase are recommended. Whole-body screening with CT of the chest, CT or MR imaging of the abdomen and pelvis, and bone scan or whole-body PET/CT are recommended only for clinical suspicion of metastases or for patients with clinical stage III disease (National Comprehensive Cancer Network, 2018).

■ Breast Cancer Treatment

Breast cancer is best managed by a multidisciplinary team of breast surgeons, medical oncologists, and radiation oncologists. Goals of surgery and radiation therapy are elimination of all local or regional tumor in a way that maximizes cosmesis and minimizes the risk of local or regional recurrence. Some evidence supports these local modalities to reduce the risk of subsequent metastases and therefore increase survival rates (Darby, 2011). However, a significant proportion of patients with apparently localized disease have tumor cells detectable in their blood or bone marrow at diagnosis (Braun, 2005; Giuliano, 2011a). Tumor size, nodal metastases, and biomarker profiles are used to recognize women at greater risk for disseminated disease. These women receive systemic treatment with chemotherapy, hormone manipulation, or targeted therapies to reduce the risk of metastasis and death (Dowsett, 2010; Peto, 2012).

Surgery

Halstead (1894) revolutionized breast cancer treatment by demonstrating improved outcome for patients treated with radical mastectomy. However, results from later randomized clinical trials have appropriately fostered a trend toward less aggressive surgery. Specifically, lumpectomy with postoperative radiation therapy results in the same breast cancer survival rate as total mastectomy (Fisher, 2002).

Axillary dissection—that is, near-complete axillary lymphadenectomy—also was once a standard in staging and treatment, but its role is diminishing (Rao, 2013). The procedure is still indicated for patients with clinically node-positive disease at diagnosis. However, it is frequently omitted in selected patients with clinically negative nodes but positive sentinel nodes, because radiation therapy and systemic adjuvant therapies achieve the same low axillary recurrence rate and the same survival rate (Galimberti, 2013; Giuliano, 2010,2011b). When required, axillary dissection results in lymphedema in 15 to 50 percent of women, depending on how it is measured (Morrell, 2005). Dissection is also associated with persistent shoulder or arm symptoms in up to 70 percent (Kuehn, 2000).

Radiation Therapy

After breast-conserving surgery, whole breast radiation reduces local recurrence from approximately 5 percent per year to 1 percent per year, although it may be omitted in elderly patients with favorable tumors (Fisher, 2002; Hughes, 2013). Shorter courses of partial breast irradiation may be appropriate in selected patients (Smith, 2009). Postmastectomy chest wall radiation improves survival in women with high-risk lymph node–positive breast cancer (Overgaard, 1999; Ragaz, 2005). Recent clinical trial data are driving a marked increase use of extended field radiation therapy (Early Breast Cancer Trialists' Collaborative Group, 2014).

Chemotherapy

In the past, adjuvant chemotherapy was reserved for patients with nodal metastases and was always given after definitive surgery. However, randomized prospective trials show that adjuvant chemotherapy also improves survival rates for high-risk node-negative patients (Fisher, 2004a). Increasingly, however, the decision for chemotherapy is influenced by specific measures of tumor biology including results from multigene assays (Rouzier, 2013; Sparano, 2008).

If used, adjuvant chemotherapy is usually administered after primary surgery but before radiation therapy. Neoadjuvant chemotherapy is given prior to definitive surgery and is gaining popularity. Neoadjuvant chemotherapy permits assessment of a given tumor's sensitivity to the selected agents, and tumor shrinkage permits less aggressive surgery (von Minckwitz, 2013).

Modern breast cancer chemotherapy often includes an anthracycline such as doxorubicin (Adriamycin) in conjunction with cyclophosphamide (Cytoxan) (Trudeau, 2005). The addition of a taxane has been shown to improve outcome (A'Hern, 2013). Platins such as cisplatin (Platinol) or carboplatin (Paraplatin) are increasingly used to replace doxorubicin when other cardiotoxic drugs such as trastuzumab are required. Platin may also be selected to treat certain tumor subtypes that have defects in homologous recombination, such as tumors associated with a *BRCA1* or *BRCA2* mutation. Chemotherapeutic agents are described more fully in Chapter 27 (p. 587).

Hormonal Therapy and Targeted Therapies

Adjuvant hormonal therapy is used for estrogen-receptor–positive tumors. In pre- or postmenopausal women, one option is the SERM tamoxifen (Jaiyesimi, 1995). As discussed in Chapter 27 (p. 598), important side effects of tamoxifen include menopausal symptoms, greater risk of thromboembolic events, and higher rates of endometrial polyps and endometrial cancer. Although this cancer risk is elevated, surveillance of the endometrium with routine transvaginal sonography or endometrial biopsy is not recommended. Endometrial evaluation is reserved for those with abnormal bleeding and follows that outlined in Chapter 8 (p. 182).

In postmenopausal women, aromatase inhibitors may be used. FDA-approved agents include anastrozole (Arimidex), letrozole (Femara), and exemestane (Aromasin) (Kudachadkar, 2005). In postmenopausal women, most circulating estradiol is derived from the peripheral conversion of androgens by the enzyme aromatase. Administration of aromatase inhibitors reduces circulating estradiol to nearly undetectable levels in these women. The addition of an aromatase inhibitor after tamoxifen is associated with a 23- to 39-percent improvement in the disease-free survival rate and a nearly 50-percent reduction in the contralateral breast cancer rate (Geisler, 2006). Although

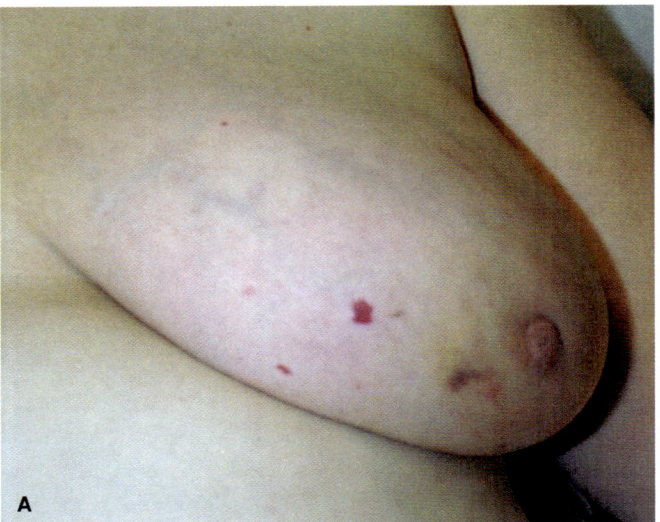
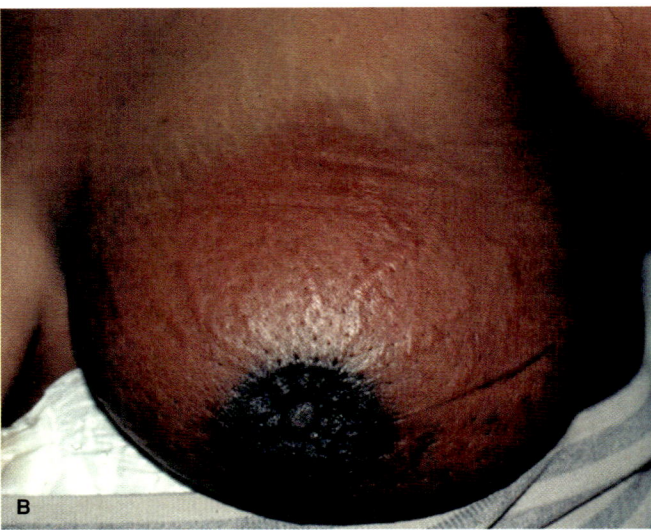

FIGURE 13-16 Photographs of inflammatory breast cancer. **A.** Subtle erythematous blush and edema in inflammatory breast cancer. **B.** Classic inflammatory breast cancer. (Reproduced with permission from Dr. Marilyn Leitch.)

tamoxifen is commonly used as an initial antihormonal therapy in postmenopausal women, transition to an aromatase inhibitor improves outcome (Johnston, 2014).

Unlike tamoxifen, aromatase inhibitors are associated with greater rates of bone loss and fractures. Accordingly, baseline bone mineral density testing and periodic monitoring is recommended. For women with mild or moderate bone loss, exercise and supplementation with vitamin D and calcium are encouraged. Various agents are available for managing severe loss, and a discussion of these drugs is found in Chapter 22 (p. 491).

Bisphosphonates such as zoledronic acid (Zometa) are often used to prevent cancer treatment–induced bone loss (Hadji, 2011). In addition, the combination of aromatase inhibitors and zoledronic acid appears to improve outcome in hormone receptor–positive breast cancer (Coleman, 2013).

Her-2/neu is currently the only target routinely exploited in the adjuvant therapy of early-stage breast cancer. However, other therapies that target specific biological pathways are improving outcomes, especially for metastatic breast cancer. Beyond tamoxifen and aromatase inhibition, advanced estrogen-receptor–positive breast cancer can be treated with the estrogen-receptor antagonist fulvestrant (Faslodex), by inciting cell cycle blockade with one of the several CDK4/6 inhibitors, or by inhibiting the mTOR pathway with everolimus (Afinitor) (Andre, 2014; Dhillon, 2013). Tumors that lack estrogen receptors, progesterone receptors, and Her-2/neu, so-called triple-negative breast cancers, have long been recognized as treatment resistant, but progress is being made. It is increasingly recognized that subsets of triple-negative breast cancer are sensitive to platinum-based chemotherapy, to poly ADP ribose polymerase (PARP) inhibition, and to immune checkpoint blockade. Comprehensive molecular profiling of tumors to identify targets for intervention is becoming more common but only rarely yields a clinically useful result (Frampton, 2013). These biologic agents for targeting cancer are described in Chapter 27 (p. 600).

■ Surveillance

Long-term surveillance of breast cancer patients after treatment includes periodic history and physical examination. Women who elect breast conservation are counseled that the remaining breast tissue requires surveillance indefinitely. Rates of ipsilateral or contralateral second primary breast cancers have been declining and now average 0.2 percent per year (Nichols, 2011). Rates are higher for younger patients and patients with estrogen receptor–negative disease. Laboratory and imaging tests are obtained to further evaluate specific signs or symptoms. Screening tests other than annual mammography to identify asymptomatic recurrences are not recommended (Khatcheressian, 2013).

■ Inflammatory Breast Cancer

Inflammatory breast cancer accounts for 1 to 5 percent of breast cancers (Chang, 1998; Dawood, 2010). This cancer presents with skin changes that can range from a faint red blush to a flaming-red rash associated with skin edema (peau d'orange change) (Fig. 13-16). It is distinguished from a neglected advanced primary breast cancer by its rapid onset and progression within just a few weeks. The cancer spreads rapidly throughout the entire breast and creates diffuse induration. As a result, the breast may enlarge to two to three times its original volume within weeks (Taylor, 1938).

Although mastitis or even congestive heart failure can produce a similar clinical appearance, inflammatory breast cancer must be definitively excluded. This always includes diagnostic mammography and punch biopsy of the skin. However, it also may require multiple biopsies and additional imaging such as MR imaging. Treatment begins with induction chemotherapy, followed by modified radical mastectomy (total mastectomy and axillary dissection). This is followed by postoperative chest wall irradiation with or without additional chemotherapy (Cariati, 2005). The 5-year survival rate is 30 to 55 percent, which is significantly worse than for neglected advanced primary breast cancer (Brenner, 2002; Harris, 2003).

REFERENCES

Abner AL, Connolly JL, Recht A, et al: The relation between the presence and extent of lobular carcinoma in situ and the risk of local recurrence for patients with infiltrating carcinoma of the breast treated with conservative surgery and radiation therapy. Cancer 88:1072, 2000

A'Hern RP, Jamal-Hanjani M, Szasz AM, et al: Taxane benefit in breast cancer—a role for grade and chromosomal stability. Nat Rev Clin Oncol 10(6):357, 2013

American College of Obstetricians and Gynecologists: Breast cancer risk assessment and screening in average-risk women. Practice Bulletin No. 179, July 2017

Anderson GL, Limacher M, Assaf AR, et al: Effects of conjugated equine estrogen in postmenopausal women with hysterectomy: the Women's Health Initiative randomized controlled trial. JAMA 291:1701, 2004

Anderson TJ, Ferguson DP, Raab G: Cell turnover within "resting" human breast: influence of parity, contraceptive pill, age and laterality. Br J Cancer 46(3):276, 1982

Andrade VP, Ostrovnaya I, Seshan VE, et al: Clonal relatedness between lobular carcinoma in situ and synchronous malignant lesions. Breast Cancer Res 14:R103, 2012

Andre F, O'Regan R, Ozguroglu M, et al: Everolimus for women with trastuzumab-resistant, HER2-positive, advanced breast cancer (BOLERO-3): a randomised, double-blind, placebo-controlled phase 3 trial. Lancet Oncol 15:580, 2014

Antoniou AC, Cunningham AP, Peto J, et al: The BOADICEA model of genetic susceptibility to breast and ovarian cancers: updates and extensions. Br J Cancer 98:1457, 2008

Ashikari R, Park K, Huvos AG, et al: Paget's disease of the breast. Cancer 26:680, 1970

Aubele M, Werner M, Hofler H: Genetic alterations in presumptive precursor lesions of breast carcinomas. Anal Cell Pathol 24:69, 2002

Baker SG, Lichtenstein P, Kaprio J, et al: Genetic susceptibility to prostate, breast, and colorectal cancer among Nordic twins. Biometrics 61(1):55, 2005

Barth RJ Jr, Wells WA, Mitchell SE, et al: A prospective, multi-institutional study of adjuvant radiotherapy after resection of malignant phyllodes tumors. Ann Surg Oncol 16:2288, 2009

Benson EA: Management of breast abscesses. World J Surg 13:753, 1989

Beral V, Reeves G, Bull D, et al: Breast cancer risk in relation to the interval between menopause and starting hormone therapy. J Natl Cancer Inst 103:296, 2011

Berg WA, Campassi CI, Loffe OB: Cystic Lesions of the breast: sonographic-pathologic correlation. Radiology 227:183, 2003

Berrington de Gonzalez A, Berg CD, Visvanathan K, et al: Estimated risk of radiation-induced breast cancer from mammographic screening for young BRCA mutation carriers. J Natl Cancer Inst 101:205, 2009

Berry DA, Parmigiani G, Sanchez S, et al: Probability of carrying a mutation of breast-ovarian cancer gene BRCA1 based on family history. J Natl Cancer Inst 89:227, 1997

Bevers TB, Helvie M, Bonaccio E, et al: Breast cancer screening and diagnosis, version 3.2018, NCCN clinical practice guidelines in oncology. J Natl Compr Canc Netw 16(11):1362, 2018

Bijker N, Rutgers EJ, Duchateau L, et al: Breast-conserving therapy for Paget disease of the nipple: a prospective European Organization for Research and Treatment of Cancer study of 61 patients. Cancer 91:472, 2001

Bleyer A, Welch HG: Effect of three decades of screening mammography on breast-cancer incidence. N Engl J Med 367:1998, 2012

Bodian CA, Perzin KH, Lattes R: Lobular neoplasia. Long-term risk of breast cancer and relation to other factors. Cancer 78:1024, 1996

Boerner S, Fornage BD, Singletary E, et al: Ultrasound-guided fine-needle aspiration (FNA) of nonpalpable breast lesions. Cancer 87(1):19, 1999

Branch-Elliman W, Golen TH, Gold HS, et al: Risk factors for *Staphylococcus aureus* postpartum breast abscess. Clin Infect Dis 54(1):71, 2012

Braun S, Vogl FD, Naume B, et al: A pooled analysis of bone marrow micrometastasis in breast cancer. N Engl J Med 353:793, 2005

Brenner B, Siris N, Rakowsky E, et al: Prediction of outcome in locally advanced breast cancer by post-chemotherapy nodal status and baseline serum tumour markers. Br J Cancer 87:1404, 2002

Brohet RM, Velthuizen ME, Hogervorst FB, et al: Breast and ovarian cancer risks in a large series of clinically ascertained families with a high proportion of BRCA1 and BRCA2 Dutch founder mutations. J Med Genet 51(2):98, 2014

Buckley ES, Webster F, Hiller JE, et al: A systematic review of surgical biopsy for LCIS found at core needle biopsy—do we have the answer yet? Eur J Surg Oncol 40:168, 2014

Bulun SE, Simpson ER: Competitive RT-PCR analysis indicates levels of aromatase cytochrome P450 transcripts in adipose tissue of buttocks, thighs, and abdomen of women increase with advancing age. J Clin Endocrinol Metab 78:428, 1994

Cabioglu N, Hunt KK, Singletary S, et al: Surgical decision making and factors determining a diagnosis of breast carcinoma in women presenting with nipple discharge. J Am Coll Surg 196:354, 2003

Cadoo KA, Traina TA, King TA: Advances in molecular and clinical subtyping of breast cancer and their implications for therapy. Surg Oncol Clin North Am 22:823, 2013

Cariati M, Bennett-Britton TM, Pinder SE, et al: "Inflammatory" breast cancer. Surg Oncol 14:133, 2005

Catsburg C, Gunter MJ, Chen C, et al: Insulin, estrogen, inflammatory markers, and risk of benign proliferative breast disease. Cancer Res 74:3248, 2014

Cauley JA, Lucas FL, Kuller LH, et al: Bone mineral density and risk of breast cancer in older women: the study of osteoporotic fractures. Study of Osteoporotic Fractures Research Group. JAMA 276:1404, 1996

Chaney AW, Pollack A, Mcneese MD, et al: Primary treatment of cystosarcoma phyllodes of the breast. Cancer 89:1502, 2000

Chang S, Parker SL, Pham T, et al: Inflammatory breast carcinoma incidence and survival. The surveillance, epidemiology, and end results program of the National Cancer Institute, 1975–1992. Cancer 82:2366, 1998

Chen YY, Hwang ES, Roy R, et al: Genetic and phenotypic characteristics of pleomorphic lobular carcinoma in situ of the breast. Am J Surg Pathol 33(11):1683, 2009

Claus EB, Risch N, Thompson WD: Autosomal dominant inheritance of early-onset breast cancer. Implications for risk prediction. Cancer 73(3):643, 1994

Coleman R, de Boer R, Eidtmann H, et al: Zoledronic acid (zoledronate) for postmenopausal women with early breast cancer receiving adjuvant letrozole (ZO-FAST study): final 60-month results. Ann Oncol 24:398, 2013

Coopey SB, Mazzola E, Buckley JM, et al: The role of chemoprevention in modifying the risk of breast cancer in women with atypical breast lesions. Breast Cancer Res Treat 136:627, 2012

Costantino JP, Gail MH, Pee D, et al: Validation studies for models projecting the risk of invasive and total breast cancer incidence. J Natl Cancer Inst 91:1541, 1999

Cox CE, Reintgen DS, Nicosia SV, et al: Analysis of residual cancer after diagnostic breast biopsy: an argument for fine-needle aspiration cytology. Ann Surg Oncol 2:201, 1995

Cuzick J, Sestak I, Forbes JF, et al: Anastrozole for prevention of breast cancer in high-risk postmenopausal women (IBIS-II): an international, double-blind, randomised placebo-controlled trial. Lancet 383:1041, 2014

Cvelbar M, Ursic-Vrscaj M, Rakar S: Risk factors and prognostic factors in patients with double primary cancer: epithelial ovarian cancer and breast cancer. Eur J Gynaecol Oncol 26:59, 2005

Darby S, McGale P, Correa C, et al: Effect of radiotherapy after breast-conserving surgery on 10-year recurrence and 15-year breast cancer death: meta-analysis of individual patient data for 10,801 women in 17 randomised trials. Lancet 378:1707, 2011

Davies HH, Simons M, Davis JB: Cystic disease of the breast. Relationship to carcinoma. Cancer 17:757, 1964

Dawood S: Biology and management of inflammatory breast cancer. Expert Rev Anticancer Ther 10:209, 2010

De Bruin ML, Sparidans J, van't Veer MB, et al: Breast cancer risk in female survivors of Hodgkin's lymphoma: lower risk after smaller radiation volumes. J Clin Oncol 27:4239, 2009

Degnim AC, Visscher DW, Berman HK, et al: Stratification of breast cancer risk in women with atypia: a Mayo cohort study. J Clin Oncol 25:2671, 2007

DeLair DF, Corben AD, Catalano JP, et al: Non-mammary metastases to the breast and axilla: a study of 85 cases. Mod Pathol 26:343, 2013

den Tonkelaar I, de Waard F: Regularity and length of menstrual cycles in women aged 41–46 in relation to breast cancer risk: results from the DOM-project. Breast Cancer Res Treat 38(3):253, 1996

Dent DM, Macking EA, Wilkie W: Benign breast disease clinical classification and disease distribution. Br J Clin Pract 42 (Suppl 56):69, 1988

Dhillon S: Everolimus in combination with exemestane: a review of its use in the treatment of patients with postmenopausal hormone receptor-positive, HER2-negative advanced breast cancer. Drugs 73:475, 2013

Domchek SM, Friebel TM, Singer CF, et al: Association of risk-reducing surgery in BRCA1 or BRCA2 mutation carriers with cancer risk and mortality. JAMA 304:967, 2010

D'Orsi CJ, Sickles EA, Mendelson EB, et al (eds): ACR BI-RADS Atlas, Breast Imaging Reporting and Data System. Reston, American College of Radiology, 2013

Dowsett M, Cuzick J, Ingle J, et al: Meta-analysis of breast cancer outcomes in adjuvant trials of aromatase inhibitors versus tamoxifen. J Clin Oncol 28:509, 2010

Dupont WD, Parl FF, Hartman WH, et al: Breast cancer risk associated with proliferative breast disease and atypical hyperplasia. Cancer 71:1258, 1993

Early Breast Cancer Trialists' Collaborative Group, McGale P, Taylor C, et al: Effect of radiotherapy after mastectomy and axillary surgery on 10-year recurrence and 20-year breast cancer mortality: meta-analysis of individual patient data for 8135 women in 22 randomised trials. Lancet 383(9935):2127, 2014

Easton DF, Pooley KA, Dunning AM, et al: Genome-wide association study identifies novel breast cancer susceptibility loci. Nature 447:1087, 2007

Eryilmaz R, Sahin M, Hakan Tekelioglu M, et al: Management of lactational breast abscesses. Breast 14(5):375, 2005

Euhus DM: Genetic testing today. Ann Surg Oncol 21(10):3209, 2015

Euhus DM, Leitch AM, Huth JF, et al: Limitations of the Gail model in the specialized breast cancer risk assessment clinic. Breast J 8:23, 2002

Euhus DM, Robinson L: Genetic predisposition syndromes and their management. Surg Clin North Am 93(2):341, 2013

Euhus DM, Uyehara C: Influence of parenteral progesterones on the prevalence and severity of mastalgia in premenopausal women. A multi-institutional cross-sectional study. J Am Coll Surg 184:596, 1997

Evans DG, Ingham SL, Baildam A, et al: Contralateral mastectomy improves survival in women with BRCA1/2-associated breast cancer. Breast Cancer Res Treat 140:135, 2013

Fasola CE, Chen JJ, Jensen KC, et al: Characteristics and clinical outcomes of pleomorphic lobular carcinoma in situ of the breast. Breast J 24(1):66, 2018

Feng SS, Sechopoulos I: Clinical digital breast tomosynthesis system: dosimetric characterization. Radiology 263:35, 2012

Finch AP, Lubinski J, Moller P, et al: Impact of oophorectomy on cancer incidence and mortality in women with a BRCA1 or BRCA2 mutation. J Clin Oncol 32:1547, 2014

Fisher B, Anderson S, Bryant J, et al: Twenty-year follow-up of a randomized trial comparing total mastectomy, lumpectomy, and lumpectomy plus irradiation for the treatment of invasive breast cancer. N Engl J Med 347:1233, 2002

Fisher B, Costantino J, Redmond C, et al: Lumpectomy compared with lumpectomy and radiation therapy for the treatment of intraductal breast cancer. N Engl J Med 328:1581, 1993

Fisher B, Dignam J, Wolmark N, et al: Tamoxifen in treatment of intraductal breast cancer: National Surgical Adjuvant Breast and Bowel Project B-24 randomised controlled trial. Lancet 353(9169):1993, 1999

Fisher B, Jeong JH, Anderson S, et al: Treatment of axillary lymph node-negative, estrogen receptor-negative breast cancer: updated findings from National Surgical Adjuvant Breast and Bowel Project clinical trials. J Natl Cancer Inst 96:1823, 2004a

Fisher ER, Land SR, Fisher B, et al: Pathologic findings from the National Surgical Adjuvant Breast and Bowel Project: twelve-year observations concerning lobular carcinoma in situ. Cancer 100:238, 2004b

Ford D, Easton DF, Stratton M, et al: Genetic heterogeneity and penetrance analysis of the BRCA1 and BRCA2 genes in breast cancer families. Am J Hum Genet 62:676, 1998

Foulkes WD, Metcalfe K, Sun P, et al: Estrogen receptor status in BRCA1- and BRCA2-related breast cancer: the influence of age, grade, and histological type. Clin Cancer Res 10:2029, 2004

Frampton GM, Fichtenholtz A, Otto GA, et al: Development and validation of a clinical cancer genomic profiling test based on massively parallel DNA sequencing. Nat Biotechnol 31:1023, 2013

Franyz VK, Pickern JW, Melcher GW, et al: Incidence of chronic cystic disease in so-called normal breast: a study based on 225 post-mortem examinations. Cancer 4:762, 1951

Freedman AN, Yu B, Gail MH, et al: Benefit/risk assessment for breast cancer chemoprevention with raloxifene or tamoxifen for women age 50 years or older. J Clin Oncol 29:2327, 2011

Freisinger F, Domchek SM: Clinical implications of low-penetrance breast cancer susceptibility alleles. Current oncology reports 11:8, 2009

Fu R, Harris EL, Helfand M, et al: Estimating risk of breast cancer in carriers of BRCA1 and BRCA2 mutations: a meta-analytic approach. Stat Med 26:1775, 2007

Gail MH, Brinton LA, Byar DP, et al: Projecting individualized probabilities of developing breast cancer for white females who are being examined annually. J Natl Cancer Inst 81:1879, 1989

Galimberti V, Cole BF: Axillary versus sentinel-lymph-node dissection for micrometastatic breast cancer—authors' reply. Lancet Oncol 14:e251, 2013

Gareth ED, Nisha K, Yit L, et al: MRI breast screening in high-risk women: cancer detection and survival analysis. Breast Cancer Res Treat 145:663, 2014

Gateley CA, Mansel RE: Management of cyclic breast pain. Br J Hosp Med 43:330, 1990

Geisler J, Lonning PE: Aromatase inhibitors as adjuvant treatment of breast cancer. Crit Rev Oncol Hematol 57:53, 2006

Giuliano AE, Connolly JL, Edge SB, et al: Breast cancer-major changes in the American Joint Committee on Cancer eighth edition cancer staging manual. CA Cancer J Clin 67(4):290, 2017

Giuliano AE, Hawes D, Ballman KV, et al: Association of occult metastases in sentinel lymph nodes and bone marrow with survival among women with early-stage invasive breast cancer. JAMA 306:385, 2011a

Giuliano AE, Hunt KK, Ballman KV, et al: Axillary dissection vs no axillary dissection in women with invasive breast cancer and sentinel node metastasis: a randomized clinical trial. JAMA 305:569, 2011b

Giuliano AE, McCall L, Beitsch P, et al: Locoregional recurrence after sentinel lymph node dissection with or without axillary dissection in patients with sentinel lymph node metastases: the American College of Surgeons Oncology Group Z0011 randomized trial. Ann Surg 252:426, 2010

Going JJ, Moffat DF: Escaping from Flatland: clinical and biological aspects of human mammary duct anatomy in three dimensions. J Pathology 203(1):538, 2004

Goss PE, Ingle JN, Ales-Martinez JE, et al: Exemestane for breast-cancer prevention in postmenopausal women. N Engl J Med 364:2381, 2011

Grant RN, Tabah EJ, Adair FE: The surgical significance of the subareolar lymph plexus in cancer of the breast. Surgery 33(1):71, 1953

Greenberg JS, Javitt MC, Katzen J, et al: Clinical Performance metrics of 3D Digital breast tomosynthesis compared with 2D digital mammography for breast cancer screening in community practice. AJR Am J Roentgenol 203(3):687, 2014

Greenberg R, Skornick Y, Kaplan O: Management of breast fibroadenomas. J Gen Intern Med 13(9):640, 1998

Grimm SL, Seagroves TN, Kabotyanski EB, et al: Disruption of steroid and prolactin receptor pattern in the mammary gland correlates with a block in lobuloalveolar development. Mol Endocrinol 16:2675, 2002

Gunter MJ, Hoover DR, Yu H, et al: Insulin, insulin-like growth factor-I, and risk of breast cancer in postmenopausal women. J Natl Cancer Inst 101:48, 2009

Gupta RK, Gaskell D, Dowle CS, et al: The role of nipple discharge cytology in the diagnosis of breast disease: a study of 1948 nipple discharge smears from 1530 patients. Cytopathology 15:326, 2004

Haagensen CD: Gross cystic disease. In Diseases of the Breast. Philadelphia, WB Saunders, 1986, p 250

Haas BM, Kalra V, Geisel J, et al: Comparison of tomosynthesis plus digital mammography and digital mammography alone for breast cancer screening. Radiology 269:694, 2013

Hadji P, Aapro MS, Body JJ, et al: Management of aromatase inhibitor-associated bone loss in postmenopausal women with breast cancer: practical guidance for prevention and treatment. Ann Oncol 22:2546, 2011

Haffty BG, Harrold E, Khan AJ, et al: Outcome of conservatively managed early-onset breast cancer by BRCA1/2 status. Lancet 359:1471, 2002

Halstead W: The results of operations for cure of cancer of the breast performed at Johns Hopkins Hospital. Johns Hopkins Hosp Bull 4:497, 1894

Hankinson SE: Endogenous hormones and risk of breast cancer in postmenopausal women. Breast Dis 24:3, 2005

Harris EE, Schultz D, Bertsch H, et al: Ten-year outcome after combined modality therapy for inflammatory breast cancer. Int J Radiat Oncol Biol Phys 55:1200, 2003

Harris L, Fritsche H, Mennel R, et al: American Society of Clinical Oncology 2007 update of recommendations for the use of tumor markers in breast cancer. J Clin Oncol 25:5287, 2007

Hartmann LC, Sellers TA, Frost MH, et al: Benign breast disease and the risk of breast cancer. N Engl J Med 353:229, 2005

Hartmann LC, Sellers TA, Schaid DJ, et al: Efficacy of bilateral prophylactic mastectomy in BRCA1 and BRCA2 gene mutation carriers. J Natl Cancer Inst 93:1633, 2001

Heemskerk-Gerritsen BA, Brekelmans CT, Menke-Pluymers MB, et al: Prophylactic mastectomy in BRCA1/2 mutation carriers and women at risk of hereditary breast cancer: long-term experiences at the Rotterdam Family Cancer Clinic. Ann Surg Oncol 14:3335, 2007

Hendrick RE, Smith RA, Rutledge JH 3rd, et al: Benefit of screening mammography in women aged 40–49: a new meta-analysis of randomized controlled trials. J Natl Cancer Inst Monogr 22:87, 1997

Hermansen C, Skovgaard Poulsen H, Jensen J, et al: Diagnostic reliability of combined physical examination, mammography, and fine-needle puncture ("triple-test") in breast tumors. A prospective study. Cancer 60:1866, 1987

Houssami N, Turner R, Macaskill P, et al: An individual person data meta-analysis of preoperative magnetic resonance imaging and breast cancer recurrence. J Clin Oncol 32:392, 2014

Houssami N, Turner R, Morrow M: Preoperative magnetic resonance imaging in breast cancer: meta-analysis of surgical outcomes. Ann Surg 257:249, 2013

Hughes KS, Schnaper LA, Bellon JR, et al: Lumpectomy plus tamoxifen with or without irradiation in women age 70 years or older with early breast cancer: long-term follow-up of CALGB 9343. J Clin Oncol 31:2382, 2013

Hulley S, Furberg C, Barrett-Connor E, et al: Noncardiovascular disease outcomes during 6.8 years of hormone therapy: Heart and Estrogen/progestin Replacement Study follow-up (HERS II). JAMA 288:58, 2002

Hultborn KA, Larsen LG, Raghnult I: The lymph drainage from the breast to the axillary and parasternal lymph nodes, studied with the aid of colloidal Au[198]. Acta Radiol 45:52, 1955

Ikeda DM, Helvie MA, Frank TS, et al: Paget's disease of the nipple: radiologic-pathologic correlation. Radiology 189:89, 1993

Ismail PM, Amato P, Soyal SM, et al: Progesterone involvement in breast development and tumorigenesis—as revealed by progesterone receptor "knockout" and "knockin" mouse models. Steroids 68:779, 2003

Jaiyesimi IA, Buzdar AU, Decker DA, et al: Use of tamoxifen for breast cancer: twenty-eight years later. J Clin Oncol 13:513, 1995

Jatoi I: Screening clinical breast exam. Surg Clin North Am 83:789, 2003

Johnston SR, Yeo B: The optimal duration of adjuvant endocrine therapy for early stage breast cancer—with what drugs and for how long? Curr Oncol Rep 16:358, 2014

Jorns J, Sabel MS, Pang JC: Lobular neoplasia: morphology and management. Arch Pathol Lab Med 138(10):1344, 2014

Kalinyak JE, Berg WA, Schilling K, et al: Breast cancer detection using high-resolution breast PET compared to whole-body PET or PET/CT. Eur J Nucl Med Mol Imaging 41:260, 2014

Kang YD, Kim YM: Comparison of needle aspiration and vacuum-assisted biopsy in the ultrasound-guided drainage of lactational breast abscesses. Ultrasonography 35(2):148, 2016

Karim RZ, O'Toole SA, Scolyer RA, et al: Recent insights into the molecular pathogenesis of mammary phyllodes tumours. J Clin Pathol 66:496, 2013

Kasales CJ, Han B, Smith JS Jr, et al: Nonpuerperal mastitis and subareolar abscess of the breast. AJR Am J Roentgenol 202(2):W133, 2014

Kauff ND, Domchek SM, Friebel TM, et al: Risk-reducing salpingo-oophorectomy for the prevention of BRCA1- and BRCA2-associated breast and gynecologic cancer: a multicenter, prospective study. J Clin Oncol 26:1331, 2008

Kerlikowske K: Efficacy of screening mammography among women aged 40 to 49 years and 50 to 69 years: comparison of relative and absolute benefit. J Natl Cancer Inst Monogr 22:79, 1997

Khan SA, Rogers MA, Khurana KK, et al: Estrogen receptor expression in benign breast epithelium and breast cancer risk. J Natl Cancer Inst 89:37, 1997

Khatcheressian JL, Hurley P, Bantug E, et al: Breast cancer follow-up and management after primary treatment: American Society of Clinical Oncology clinical practice guideline update. J Clin Oncol 31(7):961, 2013

Kim S, Kim JY, Kim do H, et al: Analysis of phyllodes tumor recurrence according to the histologic grade. Breast Cancer Res Treat 141:353, 2013

King MC, Marks JH, Mandell JB: Breast and ovarian cancer risks due to inherited mutations in BRCA1 and BRCA2. Science 302:643, 2003

Kopans DB: Digital breast tomosynthesis: a better mammogram. Radiology 267:968, 2013

Kotsopoulos J, Chen WY, Gates MA, et al: Risk factors for ductal and lobular breast cancer: results from the Nurses' Health Study. Breast Cancer Res 12:R106, 2010

Kudachadkar R, O'Regan RM: Aromatase inhibitors as adjuvant therapy for postmenopausal patients with early stage breast cancer. CA Cancer J Clin 55:145, 2005

Kuehn T, Klauss W, Darsow M, et al: Long-term morbidity following axillary dissection in breast cancer patients—clinical assessment, significance for life quality and the impact of demographic, oncologic and therapeutic factors. Breast Cancer Res Treat 64:275, 2000

Kumar S, Mansel RE, Scanlon F: Altered responses of prolactin, luteinizing hormone and follicle stimulating hormone secretion to thyrotrophin releasing hormone/gonadotrophin releasing hormone stimulation in cyclical mastalgia. Br J Surg 71:870, 1989

Kvale G, Heuch I: Menstrual factors and breast cancer risk. Cancer 62:1625, 1988

Laibl VR, Sheffield JS, Roberts S, et al: Clinical presentation of community-acquired methicillin-resistant *Staphylococcus aureus* in pregnancy. Obstet Gynecol 106:461, 2005

Lakhani SR, Van De Vijver MJ, Jacquemier J, et al: The pathology of familial breast cancer: predictive value of immunohistochemical markers estrogen receptor, progesterone receptor, HER-2, and p53 in patients with mutations in BRCA1 and BRCA2. J Clin Oncol 20:2310, 2002

Lalloo F, Varley J, Moran A, et al: BRCA1, BRCA2 and TP53 mutations in very early-onset breast cancer with associated risks to relatives. Eur J Cancer 42:1143, 2006

Lau S, Küchenmeister I, Stachs A, et al: Pathological nipple discharge: surgery is imperative in postmenopausal women. Ann Surg Oncol 12:246, 2005

Layde PM, Webster LA, Baughman LA, et al: The independent associations of parity, age at first full term pregnancy, and duration of breastfeeding with the risk of breast cancer. Cancer and Steroid Hormone Study Group. J Clin Epidemiol 42:963, 1989

Lee AJ, Cunningham AP, Kuchenbaecker KB, et al: BOADICEA breast cancer risk prediction model: updates to cancer incidences, tumour pathology and web interface. Br J Cancer 110:535, 2014

Lee CH, Dershaw DD, Kopans D, et al: Breast cancer screening with imaging: recommendations from the Society of Breast Imaging and the ACR on the use of mammography, breast MRI, breast ultrasound, and other technologies for the detection of clinically occult breast cancer. J Am Coll Radiol 7:18, 2010

Lee SJ, Boscardin WJ, Stijacic-Cenzer I, et al: Time lag to benefit after screening for breast and colorectal cancer: meta-analysis of survival data from the United States, Sweden, United Kingdom, and Denmark. BMJ 346:e8441, 2013

Lichtenstein P, Holm NV, Verkasalo PK, et al: Environmental and heritable factors in the causation of cancer—analyses of cohorts of twins from Sweden, Denmark, and Finland. N Engl J Med 343:78, 2000

Locatelli I, Lichtenstein P, Yashin AI: The heritability of breast cancer: a Bayesian correlated frailty model applied to Swedish twins data. Twin Res 7(2):182, 2004

Locker AP, Galea MH, Ellis IO, et al: Microdochectomy for single-duct discharge from the nipple. Br J Surg 75:700, 1988

Lyman GH, Temin S, Edge SB, et al: Sentinel lymph node biopsy for patients with early-stage breast cancer: American Society of Clinical Oncology clinical practice guideline update. J Clin Oncol 32:1365, 2014

Maddox PR, Mansel RE: Management of breast pain and nodularity. World J Surg 13:699, 1989

Malone KE, Daling JR, Neal C, et al: Frequency of BRCA1/BRCA2 mutations in a population-based sample of young breast carcinoma cases. Cancer 88:1393, 2000

Mansel RE, Dogliotti L: European multicenter trial of bromocriptine in cyclical mastalgia. Lancet 335:190, 1990

Masannat YA, Husain E, Roylance R, et al: Pleomorphic LCIS what do we know? A UK multicenter audit of pleomorphic lobular carcinoma in situ. Breast 38:120, 2018

Masood S: Prognostic/predictive factors in breast cancer. Clin Lab Med 25:809, 2005

Mavaddat N, Peock S, Frost D, et al: Cancer risks for BRCA1 and BRCA2 mutation carriers: results from prospective analysis of EMBRACE. J Natl Cancer Inst 105:812, 2013

Mavaddat N, Pharoah PD, Blows F, et al: Familial relative risks for breast cancer by pathological subtype: a population-based cohort study. Breast Cancer Res 12:R10, 2010

McKian KP, Reynolds CA, Visscher DW, et al: Novel breast tissue feature strongly associated with risk of breast cancer. J Clin Oncol 27:5893, 2009

Meijers-Heijboer H, van Geel B, van Putten WL, et al: Breast cancer after prophylactic bilateral mastectomy in women with a BRCA1 or BRCA2 mutation. N Engl J Med 345:159, 2001

Menes TS, Kerlikowske K, Jaffer S, et al: Rates of atypical ductal hyperplasia have declined with less use of postmenopausal hormone treatment: findings from the Breast Cancer Surveillance Consortium. Cancer Epidemiol Biomarkers Prev 18(11):2822, 2009

Merry GM, Mendelson EB: Update on screening breast ultrasonography. Radiol Clin North Am 52:527, 2014

Metcalfe K, Gershman S, Ghadirian P, et al: Contralateral mastectomy and survival after breast cancer in carriers of BRCA1 and BRCA2 mutations: retrospective analysis. BMJ 348:g226, 2014

Mohammed S, Statz A, Lacross JS, et al: Granulomatous mastitis: a 10 year experience from a large inner city county hospital. J Surg Res 184(1):299, 2013

Moller P, Stormorken A, Jonsrud C, et al: Survival of patients with BRCA1-associated breast cancer diagnosed in an MRI-based surveillance program. Breast Cancer Res Treat 139:155, 2013

Monticciolo DL, Newell MS, Hendrick RE, et al: Breast cancer screening for average-risk women: recommendations from the ACR Commission on Breast Imaging. J Am Coll Radiol 14(9):1137, 2017

Moo TA, Alabdulkareem H, Tam A, et al: Association between recurrence and re-excision for close and positive margins versus observation in patients with benign phyllodes tumors. Ann Surg Oncol 24(10):3088, 2017

Morrell RM, Halyard MY, Schild SE, et al: Breast cancer-related lymphedema. Mayo Clin Proc 80:1480, 2005

Morrow M, Van Zee KJ, Solin LJ, et al: Society of Surgical Oncology-American Society for Radiation Oncology-American Society of Clinical Oncology consensus guideline on margins for breast-conserving surgery with whole-breast irradiation in ductal carcinoma in situ. Ann Surg Oncol 23(12):3801, 2016

Morrow M, Waters J, Morris E: MRI for breast cancer screening, diagnosis, and treatment. Lancet 378:1804, 2011

Naeem M, Rahimnajjad MK, Rahimnajjad NA, et al: Comparison of incision and drainage against needle aspiration for the treatment of breast abscess. Am Surg 78(11):1224, 2012

Narod SA, Iqbal J, Giannakeas V, et al: Breast cancer mortality after a diagnosis of ductal carcinoma in situ. JAMA Oncol 1(7):888, 2015

National Comprehensive Cancer Network: Breast cancer, version 3.2018: lobular carcinoma in situ. 2018. Available at: https://www2.tri-kobe.org/nccn/guideline/breast/english/breast.pdf. Accessed February 10, 2019

Nichols HB, Berrington de González A, Lacey JV Jr, et al: Declining incidence of contralateral breast cancer in the United States from 1975 to 2006. J Clin Oncol 29(12):1564, 2011

Oberman HA: Cystosarcoma phyllodes: a clinicopathologic study of hypercellular periductal neoplasms of the breast. Cancer 28:697, 1965

Osin PP, Anbazhagan R, Bartkova J, et al: Breast development gives insights into breast disease. Histopathology 33:275, 1998

Ottesen GL, Graversen HP, Blichert-Toft M, et al: Lobular carcinoma in situ of the female breast. Short-term results of a prospective nationwide study. The Danish Breast Cancer Cooperative Group. Am J Surg Pathol 17:14, 1993

Overgaard M, Jensen MB, Overgaard J, et al: Postoperative radiotherapy in high-risk postmenopausal breast-cancer patients given adjuvant tamoxifen: Danish Breast Cancer Cooperative Group DBCG 82c randomised trial. Lancet 353:1641, 1999

Panchal S, Bordeleau L, Poll A, et al: Does family history predict the age at onset of new breast cancers in BRCA1 and BRCA2 mutation-positive families? Clin Genet 77:273, 2010

Pandey TS, Mackinnon JC, Bressler L, et al: Idiopathic granulomatous mastitis—a prospective study of 49 women and treatment outcomes with steroid therapy. Breast J 20:258, 2014

Papanicolaou GN, Holmquist DG, Bader GM, et al: Exfoliative cytology in the human mammary gland and its value in the diagnosis of breast cancer and other diseases of the breast. Cancer 11:377, 1958

Parkin DM: Global cancer statistics in the year 2000. Lancet Oncol 2:533, 2001

Parks AG: The micro-anatomy of the breast. Ann R Coll Surg Engl 25:235, 1959

Peto R, Davies C, Godwin J, et al: Comparisons between different polychemotherapy regimens for early breast cancer: meta-analyses of long-term outcome among 100,000 women in 123 randomised trials. Lancet 379:432, 2012

Petrakis NL, Miike R, King EB, et al: Association of breast fluid coloration with age, ethnicity and cigarette smoking. Br Cancer Res Treat 11:255, 1988

Phipps AI, Li CI, Kerlikowske K, et al: Risk factors for ductal, lobular, and mixed ductal-lobular breast cancer in a screening population. Cancer Epidemiol Biomarkers Prev 19:1643, 2010

Pierce LJ, Phillips KA, Griffith KA, et al: Local therapy in BRCA1 and BRCA2 mutation carriers with operable breast cancer: comparison of breast conservation and mastectomy. Breast Cancer Res Treat 121:389, 2010

Pijpe A, Andrieu N, Easton DF, et al: Exposure to diagnostic radiation and risk of breast cancer among carriers of BRCA1/2 mutations: retrospective cohort study (GENE-RAD-RISK). BMJ 345:2012

Pike MC, Krailo MD, Henderson BE, et al: Hormonal risk factors, breast tissue age and the age-incidence of breast cancer. Nature 303:767, 1983

Pilewskie M, Olcese C, Eaton A, et al: Perioperative breast MRI is not associated with lower locoregional recurrence rates in DCIS patients treated with or without radiation. Ann Surg Oncol 21:1552, 2014

Ragaz J, Olivotto IA, Spinelli JJ, et al: Locoregional radiation therapy in patients with high-risk breast cancer receiving adjuvant chemotherapy: 20-year results of the British Columbia randomized trial. J Natl Cancer Inst 97:116, 2005

Rao R, Euhus D, Mayo HG, et al: Axillary node interventions in breast cancer: a systematic review. JAMA 310:1385, 2013

Rechtman LR, Lenihan MJ, Lieberman JH, et al: Breast-specific gamma imaging for the detection of breast cancer in dense versus nondense breasts. AJR Am J Roentgenol 202:293, 2014

Reinfuss M, Mitus J, Duda K, et al: The treatment and prognosis of patients with phyllodes tumor of the breast: an analysis of 170 cases. Cancer 77:910, 1996

Ringberg A, Anagnostaki L, Anderson H, et al: Cell biological factors in ductal carcinoma in situ (DCIS) of the breast-relationship to ipsilateral local recurrence and histopathological characteristics. Eur J Cancer 37:1514, 2001

Risch N: The genetic epidemiology of cancer: interpreting family and twin studies and their implications for molecular genetic approaches. Cancer Epidemiol Biomarkers Prev 10:733, 2001

Rockhill B, Spiegelman D, Byrne C, et al: Validation of the Gail model of breast cancer risk prediction and implications for chemoprevention. J Natl Cancer Inst 93:358, 2001

Rossouw JE, Anderson GL, Prentice RL, et al: Risks and benefits of estrogen plus progestin in healthy postmenopausal women: principal results from the Women's Health Initiative randomized controlled trial. JAMA 288(3):321, 2002

Rouzier R, Pronzato P, Chereau E, et al: Multigene assays and molecular markers in breast cancer: systematic review of health economic analyses. Breast Cancer Res Treat 139:621, 2013

Russo IH, Russo J: Mammary gland neoplasia in long-term rodent studies. Environ Health Perspect 104:938, 1996

Sadek BT, Shenouda MN, Abi Raad RF, et al: Risk of local failure in breast cancer patients with lobular carcinoma in situ at the final surgical margins: is re-excision necessary? Int J Radiat Oncol Biol Phys 87:726, 2013

Salvadori B, Bartoli C, Zurrida S, et al: Risk of invasive cancer in women with lobular carcinoma in situ of the breast. Eur J Cancer 27:35, 1991

Santen RJ, Mansel R: Benign breast disorders. N Engl J Med 353:275, 2005

Saslow D, Boetes C, Burke W, et al: American Cancer Society guidelines for breast screening with MRI as an adjunct to mammography. CA Cancer J Clin 57:75, 2010

Sasson AR, Fowble B, Hanlon AL, et al: Lobular carcinoma in situ increases the risk of local recurrence in selected patients with stages I and II breast carcinoma treated with conservative surgery and radiation. Cancer 91:1862, 2001

Savage JL, Jeffries DO, Noroozian M, et al: Pleomorphic lobular carcinoma in situ: imaging features, upgrade rate, and clinical outcomes. AJR Am J Roentgenol 211(2):462, 2018

Schelfhout VR, Coene ED, Delaey B, et al: Pathogenesis of Paget's disease: epidermal heregulin-alpha, motility factor, and the HER receptor family. J Natl Cancer Inst 92(8):622, 2000

Seeley RR, Stephens TD, Tate P: Reproductive system. In Anatomy and Physiology, 7th ed. New York, McGraw-Hill, 2006, p 1058

Seynaevea C, Verhooga LC, van de Boscha LM, et al: Ipsilateral breast tumour recurrence in hereditary breast cancer following breast-conserving therapy. Eur J Cancer 40:1150, 2004

Shaaban M, Barthelmes L: Benign phyllodes tumours of the breast: (over) treatment of margins – a literature review. Eur J Surg Oncol 43(7):1186, 2017

Shannon J, Douglas-Jones AG, Dallimore NS: Conversion to core biopsy in preoperative diagnosis of breast lesions: is it justified by results? J Clin Pathol 54:762, 2001

Sickles EA, Klein DL, Goodson WH, et al: Mammography after needle aspiration of palpable breast masses. Am J Surg 145:395, 1983

Siegel RL, Miller KD, Jemal A: Cancer statistics, 2019. CA Cancer J Clin 69(1):7, 2019

Skaane P, Bandos AI, Gullien R, et al: Comparison of digital mammography alone and digital mammography plus tomosynthesis in a population-based screening program. Radiology 267:47, 2013

Smith BD, Arthur DW, Buchholz TA, et al: Accelerated partial breast irradiation consensus statement from the American Society for Radiation Oncology (ASTRO). Int J Radiat Oncol Biol Phys 74:987, 2009

Smith RA, Andrews KS, Brooks D, et al: Cancer screening in the United States, 2018: a review of current American Cancer Society guidelines and current issues in cancer screening. CA Cancer J Clin 68(4):297, 2018

Sneige N, Wang J, Baker BA, et al: Clinical, histopathologic, and biologic features of pleomorphic lobular (ductal-lobular) carcinoma in situ of the breast: a report of 24 cases. Mod Pathol 15:1044, 2002

Soderqvist G, Isaksson E, von Schoultz B, et al: Proliferation of breast epithelial cells in healthy women during the menstrual cycle. Am J Obstet Gynecol 176:123, 1997

Solin LJ, Kurtz J, Fourquet A, et al: Fifteen-year results of breast-conserving surgery and breast irradiation for the treatment of ductal carcinoma in situ of the breast. J Clin Oncol 14:754, 1996

Sparano JA, Paik S: Development of the 21-gene assay and its application in clinical practice and clinical trials. J Clin Oncol 26:721, 2008

Stafford I, Hernandez J, Laibl V, et al: Community-acquired methicillin-resistant *Staphylococcus aureus* among patients with puerperal mastitis requiring hospitalization. Obstet Gynecol 112:533, 2008

Stavros AT, Thickman D, Rapp CL, et al: Solid breast nodules: use of sonography to distinguish between benign and malignant lesions. Radiology 196:123, 1995

Stoeckelhuber M, Stumpf P, Hoefter EA, et al: Proteoglycan-collagen associations in the non-lactating human breast connective tissue during the menstrual cycle. Histochem Cell Biol 118(3):221, 2002

Tabbara SO, Frost AR, Stoler MH, et al: Changing trends in breast fine-needle aspiration: results of the Papanicolaou Society of Cytopathology Survey. Diagn Cytopathol 22:126, 2000

Tai YC, Domchek S, Parmigiani G, et al: Breast cancer risk among male BRCA1 and BRCA2 mutation carriers. J Natl Cancer Inst 99:1811, 2007

Tan BY, Acs G, Apple SK, et al: Phyllodes tumours of the breast: a consensus review. Histopathology 68(1):5, 2016

Taylor G, Meltzer A: Inflammatory carcinoma of the breast. Am J Cancer 33:33, 1938

Thomas DB, Gao DL, Ray RM, et al: Randomized trial of breast self-examination in Shanghai: final results. J Natl Cancer Inst 94:1445, 2002

Thomsen AC, Hansen KB, Moller B: Leukocyte counts and microbiological cultivation in the diagnosis of puerperal mastitis. Am J Obstet Gynecol 146:938, 1983

Tolaney S: New HER2-positive targeting agents in clinical practice. Curr Oncol Rep 16:359, 2014

Tremblay-LeMay R, Hogue JC, Provencher L, et al: How wide should margins be for phyllodes tumors of the breast? Breast J 23(3):315, 2017

Trudeau M, Charbonneau F, Gelmon K, et al: Selection of adjuvant chemotherapy for treatment of node-positive breast cancer. Lancet Oncol 6:886, 2005

Turnbull L, Brown S, Harvey I, et al: Comparative effectiveness of MRI in breast cancer (COMICE) trial: a randomised controlled trial. Lancet 375:563, 2010

Tyrer J, Duffy SW, Cuzick J: A breast cancer prediction model incorporating familial and personal risk factors. Stat Med 23(7):1111, 2004

Urban J, Egeli R: Non-lactational nipple discharge. CA Cancer Journal Clin 28:3, 1978

U.S. Preventive Services Task Force: Screening for breast cancer: U.S. Preventive Services Task Force recommendation statement. Ann Intern Med 151(10):716, 2009

Vandenbussche CJ, Khouri N, Sbaity E, et al: Borderline atypical ductal hyperplasia/low-grade ductal carcinoma in situ on breast needle core biopsy should be managed conservatively. Am J Surg Pathol 37:913, 2013

Vihko RK, Apter DL: The epidemiology and endocrinology of the menarche in relation to breast cancer. Cancer Surv 5:561, 1986

Virnig BA, Tuttle TM, Shamliyan T, et al: Ductal carcinoma in situ of the breast: a systematic review of incidence, treatment, and outcomes. J Natl Cancer Inst 102:170, 2010

Vogel VG, Costantino JP, Wickerham DL, et al: Update of the National Surgical Adjuvant Breast and Bowel Project Study of Tamoxifen and Raloxifene (STAR) P-2 Trial: preventing breast cancer. Cancer Prev Res (Phila) 3:696, 2010

von Minckwitz G: Neoadjuvant therapy: what are the lessons so far? Hematol Oncol Clin North Am 27:767, 2013

Wai CJ, Al-Mubarak G, Homer MJ, et al: A modified triple test for palpable breast masses: the value of ultrasound and core needle biopsy. Ann Surg Oncol 20:850, 2013

Watt-Boolsen S, Rasmussen NR, Blichert-Toft M: Primary periareolar abscess in the non-lactating breast: risk of recurrence. Am J Surg 155:571, 1987

Wazir U, Wazir A, Wells C, et al: Pleomorphic lobular carcinoma in situ: current evidence and a systemic review. Oncol Lett 12(6):4863, 2016

Welch HG, Passow HJ: Quantifying the benefits and harms of screening mammography. JAMA Intern Med 174:448, 2014

Welsh ML, Buist DS, Aiello Bowles EJ, et al: Population-based estimates of the relation between breast cancer risk, tumor subtype, and family history. Breast Cancer Res Treat 114:549, 2009

Wilkie C, White L, Dupont E, et al: An update of sentinel lymph node mapping in patients with ductal carcinoma in situ. Am J Surg 190:563, 2005

Wrensch WR, Petrakis NL, Gruenke LD, et al: Factors associated with obtaining nipple aspirate fluid: analysis of 1428 women and literature review. Br Cancer Res Treat 15:39, 1990

Zhou WB, Xue DQ, Liu XA, et al: The influence of family history and histological stratification on breast cancer risk in women with benign breast disease: a meta-analysis. J Cancer Res Clin Oncol 137:1053, 2011

Psychosocial Issues and Female Sexuality

Thirty years ago, psychiatrist George Engel coined a term to describe a developing paradigm for patient care, the "biopsychosocial model" (Engel, 1977). In the years since, this model has also incorporated cultural and spiritual factors. When conceptualizing a woman's understanding of her reproductive events, this model highlights the distinction between disease, a pathologic process, and illness, a patient's experience of that process. At times, psychologic health is linked directly with reproductive health. As an example, infertility can lead to mood and anxiety disorders. In contrast, preexisting psychologic distress might be an insidious cause of a health problem. For example, higher hysterectomy rates are noted in women with a low tolerance for the physical discomfort of menstruation.

Years before Engel's work, Erik Erikson (1963) created a model that describes psychologic maturation in stages across the life span. Specifically, adolescents are confronted with identity development; reproductive-aged women with intimacy concerns; peri- and early menopausal women with productivity issues; and older women with life review. Combining Erikson's developmental model with a biopsychosociocultural model provides a dimensional perspective to aid evaluation, diagnosis, and treatment of any patient.

Most patients with psychiatric illness are first seen in primary care settings, and gynecologists often are the first to evaluate a woman with psychiatric distress. The clinical interview in Table 14-1 provides an example of an assessment that includes all domains from the biopsychosociocultural model.

MOOD DISORDERS

Mood, anxiety, and alcohol or substance use disorders are three families of psychiatric disorders commonly seen and often comorbid with reproductive events. These three groups are defined by specific criteria described by the *Diagnostic and Statistical Manual of Mental Disorders, Fifth Edition* (DSM-5) (American Psychiatric Association, 2013). Each family of disorders is characterized by predominant features, and each disorder within those families is identified by specific symptoms of that feature.

Of these families, mood disorders are categorized as *depressive disorders* (major depressive disorder, persistent depressive

TABLE 14-1. Psychiatric Assessment of Women

Component	Consideration
Present or past psychiatric illness	Relation to reproductive triggers: pregnancy, menses, menopause, etc.
Medications	All medications and supplements; exogenous hormones
Diet	Abnormal eating patterns; diet pills, laxatives, diuretics
Substance use	Covert use, particularly prescription drugs
Family history	Including reproductive event–related symptoms/disorders
Medical history	Autoimmune disease, which can present with psychiatric symptoms
Reproductive history	Premenstrual, pregnancy, pregnancy loss, postpartum or perimenopausal context of symptoms
Social	Current or past sexual, physical, or emotional abuse. Note sexual preference and current relationship satisfaction
Cultural	Norms and beliefs of community/family
Spiritual	Rituals, guidelines, and attributes of a "good" life
Economic	Ability to meet ongoing financial needs

TABLE 14-2. Diagnostic Criteria for a Major Depressive Episode

A. **≥5 criteria present during the same 2-week period and represent change from previous functioning. At least one of these is:**
Depressed mood most of the day, nearly every day
Markedly diminished interest/pleasure in most activities, most of the day, most days

The balance of 5 from these:
Significant weight loss/gain, change in appetite, or failure to make expected gains
Insomnia or hypersomnia nearly every day
Psychomotor agitation or retardation nearly every day, *observable by others*
Fatigue or loss of energy nearly every day
Feelings of worthlessness or excessive or inappropriate guilt nearly every day
Diminished ability to think or concentrate or indecisiveness
Recurrent thoughts of death, recurrent suicidal ideation, plans, or attempt

B. Symptoms cause significant distress or impairment in functioning
C. Symptoms are not due to a substance or a general medical condition
D. Symptoms not accounted by other psychiatric disorder
E. No prior mania or hypomania

Data from American Psychiatric Association, 2013.

disorder, premenstrual dysphoric disorder, other specified depressive disorder, and unspecified depressive disorder) or as *bipolar and related disorders* (bipolar I, bipolar II, cyclothymic disorder, other specified bipolar disorder, and unspecified bipolar disorder). Bipolar disorders are first characterized by abnormally and persistently elevated, expansive, or irritable mood (sometimes described as "energy") alternating with depressed mood. Other characteristics are impulsiveness, high-risk behavior, and difficulty sleeping. As with all psychiatric disorders, these characteristics must represent a change in functioning and be severe enough to impair occupational or social relationships.

For depressive disorders, symptoms include those in Table 14-2. The lifetime prevalence in the general U.S. population approximates 20 percent (Kessler, 2005; National Institute of Mental Health, 2016). As such, depression is a major cause of disability, and females are 1.6 times more likely than males to suffer from a major depressive episode (Substance Abuse and Mental Health Services Administration, 2013). Women also may experience one or more comorbid psychiatric disorders, most often an anxiety disorder and/or substance use disorder.

Self-report questionnaires are generally used to identify individuals who require further psychiatric evaluation (screening measures) and may also assess the frequency and intensity of depressive symptoms (severity measures). The Quick Inventory of Depressive Symptomatology-Self Report (QIDS-SR) is one such tool easily implemented for clinical use (Tables 14-3 and 14-4)

TABLE 14-3. The Quick Inventory of Depressive Symptomatology (16-Item) (Self-Report) (QIDS-SR$_{16}$)

CHECK THE ONE RESPONSE TO EACH ITEM THAT BEST DESCRIBES YOU FOR THE PAST SEVEN DAYS.

During the past seven days...

1. Falling Asleep:
☐ 0 I never take longer than 30 minutes to fall asleep.
☐ 1 I take at least 30 minutes to fall asleep, less than half the time.
☐ 2 I take at least 30 minutes to fall asleep, more than half the time.
☐ 3 I take more than 60 minutes to fall asleep, more than half the time.

2. Sleep During the Night:
☐ 0 I do not wake up at night.
☐ 1 I have a restless, light sleep with a few brief awakenings each night.
☐ 2 I wake up at least once a night, but I go back to sleep easily.
☐ 3 I awaken more than once a night and stay awake for 20 minutes or more, more than half the time.

3. Waking Up Too Early:
☐ 0 Most of the time, I awaken no more than 30 minutes before I need to get up.
☐ 1 More than half the time, I awaken more than 30 minutes before I need to get up.
☐ 2 I almost always awaken at least one hour or so before I need to, but I go back to sleep eventually.
☐ 3 I awaken at least one hour before I need to, and can't go back to sleep.

4. Sleeping Too Much:
☐ 0 I sleep no longer than 7–8 hours/night, without napping during the day.
☐ 1 I sleep no longer than 10 hours in a 24-hour period including naps.
☐ 2 I sleep no longer than 12 hours in a 24-hour period including naps.
☐ 3 I sleep longer than 12 hours in a 24-hour period including naps.

(Continued)

TABLE 14-3. The Quick Inventory of Depressive Symptomatology (16-Item) (Self-Report) (QIDS-SR$_{16}$) *(Continued)*

During the past seven days...

5. Feeling Sad:
- ☐ 0 I do not feel sad.
- ☐ 1 I feel sad less than half the time.
- ☐ 2 I feel sad more than half the time.
- ☐ 3 I feel sad nearly all of the time.

Please complete either 6 or 7 (not both)

6. Decreased Appetite:
- ☐ 0 There is no change in my usual appetite.
- ☐ 1 I eat somewhat less often or lesser amounts of food than usual.
- ☐ 2 I eat much less than usual and only with personal effort.
- ☐ 3 I rarely eat within a 24-hour period, and only with extreme personal effort or when others persuade me to eat.

-OR-

7. Increased Appetite:
- ☐ 0 There is no change from my usual appetite.
- ☐ 1 I feel a need to eat more frequently than usual.
- ☐ 2 I regularly eat more often and/or greater amounts of food than usual.
- ☐ 3 I feel driven to overeat both at mealtime and between meals.

Please complete either 8 or 9 (not both)

8. Decreased Weight (Within the Last Two Weeks):
- ☐ 0 I have not had a change in my weight.
- ☐ 1 I feel as if I have had a slight weight loss.
- ☐ 2 I have lost 2 pounds or more.
- ☐ 3 I have lost 5 pounds or more.

-OR-

9. Increased Weight (Within the Last Two Weeks):
- ☐ 0 I have not had a change in my weight.
- ☐ 1 I feel as if I have had a slight weight gain.
- ☐ 2 I have gained 2 pounds or more.
- ☐ 3 I have gained 5 pounds or more.

During the past seven days...

10. Concentration/Decision-Making:
- ☐ 0 There is no change in my usual capacity to concentrate or make decisions.
- ☐ 1 I occasionally feel indecisive or find that my attention wanders.
- ☐ 2 Most of the time, I struggle to focus my attention or to make decisions.
- ☐ 3 I cannot concentrate well enough to read or cannot make even minor decisions.

11. View of Myself:
- ☐ 0 I see myself as equally worthwhile and deserving as other people.
- ☐ 1 I am more self-blaming than usual.
- ☐ 2 I largely believe that I cause problems for others.
- ☐ 3 I think almost constantly about major and minor defects in myself.

12. Thoughts of Death or Suicide:
- ☐ 0 I do not think of suicide or death.
- ☐ 1 I feel that life is empty or wonder if it's worth living.
- ☐ 2 I think of suicide or death several times a week for several minutes.
- ☐ 3 I think of suicide or death several times a day in some detail, or I have made specific plans for suicide or have actually tried to take my life.

13. General Interest:
- ☐ 0 There is no change from usual in how interested I am in other people or activities.
- ☐ 1 I notice that I am less interested in people or activities.
- ☐ 2 I find I have interest in only one or two of my formerly pursued activities.
- ☐ 3 I have virtually no interest in formerly pursued activities.

During the past seven days...

14. Energy Level:
- ☐ 0 There is no change in my usual level of energy.
- ☐ 1 I get tired more easily than usual.
- ☐ 2 I have to make a big effort to start or finish my usual daily activities (for example, shopping, homework, cooking, or going to work).
- ☐ 3 I really cannot carry out most of my usual daily activities because I just don't have the energy.

15. Feeling Slowed Down:
- ☐ 0 I think, speak, and move at my usual rate of speed.
- ☐ 1 I find that my thinking is slowed down or my voice sounds dull or flat.
- ☐ 2 It takes me several seconds to respond to most questions, and I'm sure my thinking is slowed.
- ☐ 3 I am often unable to respond to questions without extreme effort.

16. Feeling Restless:
- ☐ 0 I do not feel restless.
- ☐ 1 I'm often fidgety, wringing my hands, or need to shift how I am sitting.
- ☐ 2 I have impulses to move about and am quite restless.
- ☐ 3 At times, I am unable to stay seated and need to pace around.

From Rush, 2003, with permission.

TABLE 14-4. Quick Inventory of Depressive Symptomatology-Self Report (QIDS-SR$_{16}$) Scoring Instructions

1. Enter the highest score on any one of the four sleep items (items 1 to 4)
   Enter the highest score on any one of the four weight items (items 6 to 9)
   Enter the highest score on either of the two psychomotor items (items 15 and 16)
2. There will be one score for each of the nine Major Depressive Disorder symptom domains
3. Add the scores of the nine items (sleep, weight, psychomotor changes, depressed mood, decreased interest, fatigue, guilt, concentration, and suicidal ideation) to obtain the total score; total scores range from 0 to 27
4. 0–5: no depressive symptoms; 6–10: mild symptoms; 11–15: moderate symptoms; 16–20: severe symptoms; 21–27: very severe symptoms

From Rush, 2003.

(Rush, 2003). Further information regarding the instrument is available at www.ids-qids.org. By patient report, this questionnaire assesses symptom severity required by DSM-5 criteria to diagnosis major depressive disorder. Ultimately, diagnosing mood disorders requires assessment by a trained clinician.

ANXIETY DISORDERS

Anxiety disorders have the highest prevalence rates in the United States. Lifetime rates approximate 30 percent, and as with depression, women are 1.6 times more likely to be diagnosed than men (Kessler, 2005). Criteria established in the DSM-5 provide guidelines to help distinguish anxiety disorders from normally expected worries (Table 14-5).

SUBSTANCE USE DISORDERS

In the United States, the lifetime prevalence for alcohol and substance use disorders approximates 15 percent. This diagnosis is twice as likely in males, although rates in women are rising (Kessler, 2005). Indicators of substance misuse are found in Table 14-6. Often substance use disorders coexist with mood and anxiety disorders. Additional information regarding commonly abused substances is found at the National Institute on Drug Abuse website www.drugabuse.gov.

EATING DISORDERS

Specific feeding and eating disorders classified by the DSM-5 and relevant to women's health care are anorexia nervosa,

bulimia nervosa, binge-eating disorder, and unspecified feeding or eating disorder (Tables 14-7 and 14-8). The core symptoms of both anorexia and bulimia are preoccupation with weight gain and excessive self-evaluation of weight and body shape, accompanied by either restriction of food intake (anorexia) or the use of compensatory behaviors to prevent weight gain after binge eating (bulimia). Binge-eating disorder is differentiated by consuming larger amounts of food, lacking a sense of control over the eating, but not engaging in subsequent weight-loss behaviors. These disorders are 10 to 20 times more common in females than in males, particularly in those aged 15 to 24 years (Mitchell, 2006). In young females, an estimated 4 percent suffer from anorexia, 1 to 1.5 percent from bulimia, and 1.6 percent from binge-eating disorder. While anorexia usually begins early in adolescence and peaks around age 17, bulimia nervosa typically has a later onset than anorexia and is more prevalent over the life span (Hoek, 2006). Pathologic eating is also found in older women, particularly binge-eating disorder and unspecified eating disorder (Mangweth-Matzek, 2014).

The exact etiology of such abnormal consumption is unknown. However, evidence suggests a strong familial aggregation for eating disorders (Trace, 2013). Twin studies yield estimates of heritability ranging from 28 to 74 percent for anorexia nervosa, 55 to 65 percent for bulimia nervosa, and 33 to 45 percent for binge-eating disorder (Hübel, 2018). Biologic, environmental, and psychologic factors all interact with and influence the expression of genetic risk (Culbert, 2015). Factors may include abnormalities in neuropeptides and neurotransmitter levels, altered hypothalamic-pituitary-adrenal and hypothalamic-pituitary-gonadal axes, and family and sociocultural

TABLE 14-5. Diagnostic Criteria for Generalized Anxiety Disorder

A. Excessive anxiety and worry occurring more days than not for at least 6 months, about a number of events or activities
B. The person finds it difficult to control the worry
C. The anxiety and worry are associated with ≥3 of the following six symptoms:

Easily fatigued	Irritability
Muscle tension	Disturbed sleep
Difficulty concentrating	Restless or keyed up

D. The anxiety, worry, or physical symptoms cause clinically significant distress or impairment in social, occupational, or other important areas of functioning
E. The disturbance is not due to physiological effects of a substance or another medical condition
F. Symptoms not better explained by another mental disorder

Data from American Psychiatric Association, 2013.

TABLE 14-6. Diagnostic Criteria for Substance Use Disorder

A maladaptive pattern of substance use, leading to clinically significant impairment or distress, as manifested by two or more of the following, occurring at any time in the same 12-month period:

Consumption of larger amounts or over a longer period than was intended
Desire or unsuccessful efforts to cut down
Increased time spent in activities seeking the substance
Cravings or urges
Failure to fulfill major obligations
Continued use despite recurrent problems
Giving up important social, occupational, or recreational activities
Use in physically hazardous situations
Persistent use despite knowledge of problem
Tolerance develops to the substance
Substance cessation leads to withdrawal symptoms

Data from American Psychiatric Association, 2013.

influences (Stoving, 2001). Although previously thought to be culture-bound to the Western world, eating disorders appear to be distributed throughout the world (Kolar, 2016; Pike, 2015; Thomas, 2016).

■ Diagnosis

Anorexia nervosa is divided into two subtypes: (1) a restricting type and (2) a binge-eating/purging type, which is distinguished from bulimia by the patient weighing less than the minimum standard for normal. Symptoms begin as unique eating habits that become more and more restrictive. Advanced symptoms may include extreme food intake restriction and excessive exercise. Up to 50 percent of anorectics also show bulimic behavior, and these types may alternate during the course of anorexic illness. Bulimic-type anorectics have been found to engage in two distinct behavior patterns, those who binge and purge and those who solely purge.

Diagnosis of anorexia is initially challenging, as patients often defend their eating behaviors upon confrontation and rarely recognize their illness. They increasingly isolate themselves socially as their disorder progresses. Multiple somatic complaints such as gastrointestinal symptoms and cold intolerance are common. In the disorder's later stages, weight loss becomes more apparent, and medical complications may prompt patients to seek help. Findings often include dental problems, general nutritional

deficiency, electrolyte abnormalities (hypokalemia and alkalosis), and decreased thyroid function. Electrocardiogram changes such as QT prolongation (bradycardia) and inversion or flattened T-waves may be noted. Rare complications include gastric dilation, arrhythmias, seizure, and death.

Bulimia nervosa is identified by periods of uncontrolled eating of high-calorie foods (binges), followed by compensatory behaviors such as self-induced vomiting, fasting, excessive exercise, or misuse of laxatives, diuretics, or emetics. Unlike patients with anorexia, those with bulimia often recognize their maladaptive behaviors. Severity is based on the frequency of the inappropriate behaviors, clinical symptoms, and level of disability. Most bulimics have normal weights, although their weight may fluctuate. Physical changes may be subtle and include dental problems, swollen salivary glands, or knuckle calluses on the dominant hand. Termed *Russell sign*, calluses form in response to repetitive contact with stomach acid or teeth during purging (Strumia, 2005).

Binge-eating disorder is distinct from anorexia and bulimia. It is characterized by ingesting large amounts of food within a short time and is accompanied by feelings that one cannot control the amount of food eaten. Severity is assessed according to the number of gorging episodes per week. Binge-eating is associated with obesity. That said, most obese individuals do not necessarily engage in binge episodes and consume comparatively fewer calories than those with the syndrome. Prevalence in

TABLE 14-7. Diagnostic Criteria for Anorexia Nervosa

A. Refusal to maintain body weight at or above a minimal normal weight for age and height
B. Intense fear of gaining weight or becoming fat, even though underweight
C. Disturbance in the way in which one's body weight or shape is experienced, undue influence of body weight or shape on self-evaluation, or denial of the seriousness of the current low weight

Restricting Type: No binge-eating or purging behaviors

Binge-Eating/Purging Type: Binge-eating and self-induced vomiting, or the misuse of laxatives, diuretics, or enemas

Data from American Psychiatric Association, 2013.

TABLE 14-8. Diagnostic Criteria for Bulimia Nervosa

A. Recurrent episodes of binge eating
    Eating, in a discrete period of time, an amount of food definitely larger than most people would eat in a similar period of time under similar circumstances
    A sense of lack of control over eating during the episode
B. Recurrent inappropriate compensatory behavior to prevent weight gain, such as self-induced vomiting; misuse of laxatives, diuretics, enemas, or other medications; fasting; or excessive exercise
C. Binge eating and inappropriate compensatory behaviors both occur, on average, at least once a week for 3 months
D. Self-evaluation is unduly influenced by body shape and weight
E. The disturbance does not occur exclusively during episodes of anorexia nervosa

Data from American Psychiatric Association, 2013.

the United States approximates 1.6 percent for females and 0.8 percent for males. In middle-aged women, binge-eating is more common than anorexia or bulimia (Mangweth-Matzek, 2014).

All these are complex disorders that affect both psychologic and physical systems and are often comorbid with depression and anxiety. Rates of mood symptoms approximate 50 percent, and anxiety symptoms, 60 percent (Braun, 1994). Simple phobia and obsessive-compulsive behaviors may coexist. In many cases, patients with anorexia have rigid, perfectionistic personalities and low sexual interest. Patients with bulimia often display sexual conflicts, problems with intimacy, and impulsive suicidal tendencies.

■ Treatment

A multidisciplinary approach benefits the treatment of eating disorders. Practice approaches include: (1) nutritional rehabilitation, (2) psychosocial treatment that includes individual and family therapies, and (3) pharmacotherapeutic treatment of concurrent psychiatric symptoms. Online resources for information and support are provided by the National Eating Disorder Association, www.edap.org and Academy for Eating Disorders, www.aedweb.org.

Data concerning the long-term physical and psychologic prognosis of women with eating disorders are limited. Most may symptomatically improve with aging. However, complete recovery from anorexia nervosa is rare, and many continue to have distorted body perceptions and peculiar eating habits. Overall, the prognosis for bulimia is better than for anorexia.

MENSTRUATION-RELATED DISORDERS

Frequently, reproductive-aged women experience symptoms during the late luteal phase of their menstrual cycle. Collectively these complaints are termed *premenstrual syndrome (PMS)* or, when more severe and disabling, *premenstrual dysphoric disorder (PMDD)*. Nearly 300 different symptoms have been reported and typically include both psychiatric and physical complaints. For most women, these are self-limited. However, approximately 15 percent report moderate-to-severe complaints that cause some impairment or require special consideration (Wittchen, 2002). Current estimates are that 3 to 8 percent of menstruating women meet the strict criteria for PMDD (Halbreich, 2003b).

■ Pathophysiology

Still under investigation, PMDD is thought to spring from genetic factors, psychosocial factors (particularly stress), and an altered sensitivity to the normal hormonal fluctuations that influence CNS functioning (Hantsoo, 2015). Because of the timing of symptoms, current thinking is that hormonal fluctuation is the key trigger.

First, estrogen and progesterone are integral to the menstrual cycle. The cyclic complaints of PMS begin following ovulation and resolve with menses. PMS is less common in women with surgical oophorectomy or drug-induced ovarian hypofunction, such as with gonadotropin-releasing hormone (GnRH) agonists (Cronje, 2004; Wyatt, 2004). Moreover, women with anovulatory cycles appear protected. One potential effect stems from estrogen and progesterone's influence on CNS neurotransmitters: serotonin, noradrenaline, and gamma-aminobutyric acid (GABA). The predominant action of estrogen is neuronal excitability, whereas progestins are inhibitory (Halbreich, 2003a). Menstruation-related symptoms are believed to be associated with neuroactive progesterone metabolites. Of these, allopregnanolone is a potent modulator of GABA receptors, and its effects mirror those of low-dose benzodiazepines, barbiturates, and alcohol. These effects may include loss of impulse control, negative mood, and aggression or irritability (Bäckström, 2014). Wang and colleagues (1996) noted fluctuations in allopregnanolone across the various menstrual cycle phases. These changes were implicated with PMS symptom severity.

Second, evidence also supports a role for serotonergic system dysregulation in PMS pathophysiology. Decreased serotonergic activity has been noted in the luteal phase. Moreover, trials of serotonergic treatments show PMS symptom reduction (Marjoribanks, 2013).

Third, sex steroids also interact with the renin-angiotensin-aldosterone system (RAAS) to alter electrolyte and fluid balance. The antimineralocorticoid properties of progesterone and possible estrogen activation of the RAAS system may explain PMS symptoms of bloating and weight gain.

The most recent agent implicated in PMDD is brain-derived neurotrophic factor (BDNF). Neurotrophins are involved in neuronal survival, synaptic signaling, and synaptic integration, and BDNF is considered one the most important. BDNF is modified by estradiol and demonstrates cyclic fluctuation across the menstrual cycle. In women with PMDD, levels of BDNF are significantly higher during the luteal phase than in the follicular phase (Oral, 2015). Last, differences brain structure and function have been noted between women with and without PMDD in small imaging studies (Baller, 2013; Ossewaarde, 2013).

■ Diagnosis

PMDD is identified in the DSM-5 by the presence of at least five symptoms accompanied by significant psychosocial or functional impairment (Table 14-9). PMS refers to the presence of numerous symptoms that are not associated with significant impairment. During evaluation, the revised criteria in DSM-5 recommend that clinicians confirm symptoms by prospective patient mood charting for at least two menstrual cycles. In certain instances, complaints may be an exacerbation of an underlying primary psychiatric condition(s). Thus, other common psychiatric conditions such as depression and anxiety disorders are excluded. Additionally, other medical conditions that have a multisystem presentation are considered. These include hypothyroidism, systemic lupus erythematosus, endometriosis, anemia, fibromyalgia, chronic fatigue syndrome, fibrocystic breast disease, irritable bowel syndrome, and migraine.

■ Treatment

Therapy for PMDD and PMS includes psychotropic agents, ovulation suppression, and dietary modification. Generalists may consider treatment of cases with mild-to-moderate severity. However, if treatment fails or if symptoms are severe, then psychiatric referral may be indicated (Reid, 2018).

Selective serotonin-reuptake inhibitors (SSRIs) are considered primary therapy for psychologic symptoms of PMDD and PMS, and fluoxetine, sertraline, and paroxetine are Food and Drug Administration (FDA) approved for this indication (Table 14-10). Standard dosages are administered in either continuous or luteal-phase (14 days prior to expected menses) dosing regimens. Several well-controlled trials of SSRIs show these drugs to be efficacious and well tolerated (Shah, 2008). In addition, short-term use of anxiolytics such as alprazolam or buspirone offers added benefits to some women with prominent anxiety. However, in prescribing benzodiazepines, caution is taken in women with prior history of substance abuse (Nevatte, 2013).

Because gonadal hormonal dysregulation is implicated in the genesis of PMS symptoms, ovulation suppression is another option. Some data supports use of combination oral contraceptive (COC) pills in general for premenstrual mood symptoms. Moreover, in randomized trials, *Yasmin*, a COC containing the spironolactone-like progestin drospirenone, showed therapeutic benefits. It carries an FDA indication for PMDD treatment in women who desire contraception (Pearlstein, 2005; Yonkers, 2005). Alternatively, GnRH agonists are another means of ovulation suppression. These agents are infrequently selected due to their hypoestrogenic side effects and risks. If elected for PMDD and used longer than 6 months, add-back therapy, as discussed in Chapter 11 (p. 243), can potentially blunt these effects. Rarely, symptoms warrant bilateral oophorectomy, and a trial of GnRH agonists prior to surgery may be prudent to determine the potential efficacy of castration. Last, the synthetic androgen danazol also suppresses ovulation, but androgen-related acne and hair growth are usually poorly tolerated.

Of other possible agents, prostaglandin inhibitors such as ibuprofen and naproxen offer benefits through their anti-inflammatory effects and alleviate cramping and headaches associated with PMS (Table 11-1, p. 242). Diuretics such as combined hydrochlorothiazide and triamterene (Dyazide) and spironolactone (Aldactone) may be prescribed to alleviate fluid retention and leg edema. Monitoring for potential side effects such as orthostatic hypotension and hypokalemia is essential.

Diet, in particular foods and beverages high in sugar and caffeine, can aggravate premenstrual symptoms in some women. Calcium, 600 mg orally twice daily, has shown benefits. Theoretically, this corrects deficiency-related symptoms such as muscle cramps (Thys-Jacobs, 2000). Vitamins such as pyridoxine (vitamin B_6) and vitamin E may offer some relief. Pyridoxine is a cofactor to tryptophan hydroxylase, which is the key enzyme in serotonin synthesis (Wyatt, 1999). The recommended dose of pyridoxine

---

TABLE 14-9. Diagnostic Criteria for Premenstrual Dysphoric Disorder

A. ≥5 symptoms below: occur in most cycles during the week before menses onset, improve within a few days after menses onset, and diminish in the week post-menses

B. One (or more) of the following symptoms must be present:
Marked affective lability
Marked irritability or anger or increased interpersonal conflicts
Marked depressed moods, feelings of hopelessness, or self-deprecating thoughts
Marked anxiety, tension

C. One (or more) of the following symptoms must be also present:
Decreased interest
Difficulty concentrating
Easy fatigability, low energy
Increase or decrease in sleep
Feelings of being overwhelmed
Physical symptoms such as breast tenderness, muscle or joint aches, "bloating" or weight gain
Note: Criteria A–C must be present for most menstrual cycles in the preceding year.

D. Symptoms are associated with significant distress or interferences with work, school, relationships

E. The disturbance is not merely an exacerbation of another disorder such as major depression, panic disorder, persistent depressive disorder, or a personality disorder.

F. Criterion A should be confirmed by prospective daily ratings in at least two symptomatic cycles.

G. The symptoms are not due to physiological effects of a substance or another medical condition.

Data from American Psychiatric Association, 2013.

TABLE 14-10. List of Common Psychotropic Medications

Drug Class	Indication	Examples[a]	Brand Name	Commonly Reported Side Effects
Selective serotonin-reuptake inhibitors (SSRIs)	Depressive, anxiety, and premenstrual disorders	Fluoxetine Citalopram Escitalopram Sertraline Paroxetine Fluvoxamine	Prozac, Sarafem Celexa Lexapro Zoloft Paxil Luvox	Nausea, headache, insomnia, diarrhea, dry mouth, sexual dysfunction
Serotonin noradrenergic-reuptake inhibitors (SNRIs)	Depressive, anxiety, and premenstrual disorders	Venlafaxine XR Duloxetine Levomilnacipran Desvenlafaxine	Effexor Cymbalta Fetzima Pristiq	Dry mouth, anxiety, agitation, dizziness, somnolence, constipation
Tricyclic and tetracyclic antidepressants	Depressive and anxiety disorders	Desipramine Nortriptyline Amitriptyline Doxepin Maprotiline	Norpramin Pamelor, Aventyl Elavil Sinequan Ludiomil	Drowsiness, dry mouth, dizziness, blurred vision, confusion, constipation, urinary retention and frequency
Benzodiazepines	Anxiety disorders	Alprazolam Clonazepam Diazepam	Xanax Klonopin Valium	Drowsiness, ataxia, sleep changes, impaired memory, hypotension
Others	Depressive disorders	Nefazodone Trazodone Bupropion SR, XL	Serzone Desyrel Wellbutrin	Headache, dry mouth, orthostatic hypotension, somnolence
		Mirtazapine	Remeron	Dry mouth, increased appetite, somnolence, constipation
		Vilazodone	Viibryd	Diarrhea, nausea, dry mouth
		Aripiprazole[a]	Abilify	Weight gain, akathisia, extrapyramidal signs, somnolence
		Vortioxetine	Brintellix	Constipation, nausea, vomiting
	Anxiety disorders	Buspirone Hydroxyzine	Buspar Vistaril, Atarax	Dizziness, drowsiness, headache
	Sleep agents	Zaleplon Zolpidem Ramelteon Eszopiclone	Sonata Ambien, Intermezzo, Edluar, Zolpimist Rozerem Lunesta	Headache, somnolence, amnesia, fatigue

[a]Adjunctive treatment in patients receiving antidepressants.
SR = sustained release; XR/XL = extended release.

is 50 to 100 mg/d, but doses exceeding 100 mg/d are avoided to prevent pyridoxine toxicity. Magnesium in combination with vitamin B$_6$ appears to reduce anxiety-related premenstrual symptoms (De Souza, 2000). Of nonpharmacologic alternatives to treatment, acupuncture, bright-light therapy, exercise, and omega fatty acids have some evidence-based support (Brandon, 2014).

PERINATAL DISORDERS

In general, psychiatric disorders during pregnancy have a course and presentation similar to that in nonpregnant women. For this reason, there are no distinct diagnostic criteria for psychiatric disorders experienced in the context of pregnancy and the puerperium.

■ Perinatal Depression

In the revised DSM-5, a major depressive episode with onset during pregnancy or within 4 weeks following childbirth is categorized by a specifier term noting "with peripartum onset." Some women experience the first onset of depression during this time, whereas others are vulnerable for relapse (Cohen, 2006a). Etiologic studies have been inconclusive, but both hormonal changes and psychosocial stressors are implicated (Bloch, 2006; Boyce, 2005). Other risks include life stress, poor social support, and maternal anxiety (Lancaster, 2010).

Treatment is critical, as suicide is a leading cause of maternal death in developed countries (Centre for Maternal and Child Enquiries, 2011). Accordingly, health professionals are encouraged to thoroughly assess psychiatric and psychosocial history to enable early identification, prevention, and treatment of perinatal depression. The American College of Obstetricians and Gynecologists (2018) recently advised obstetric care providers to screen perinatal women at least once during the perinatal period for depression and anxiety using a standardized, validated tool. Even if screening occurs during pregnancy, providers are also urged to complete a full assessment of emotional well-being during the postpartum visit.

To screen for and assess severity of peripartum depressive symptoms, the Edinburgh Postnatal Depression Scale (EPDS) is one tool specifically developed for pregnancy (Cox, 1987). Unlike screening measures that score symptoms characteristic of pregnancy itself (appetite, weight change, sleep disturbance, and fatigue), the EPDS assesses neurovegetative symptoms that are more specific to depression. Available in numerous languages, the EPDS is an efficient way to identify patients at risk for perinatal depression. It is available through the American Academy of Pediatrics at: www2.aap.org/sections/scan/practicingsafety/toolkit_resources/module2/epds.pdf.

Antepartum

From a global perspective, the pooled prevalence of perinatal depression is estimated to be 12 percent (Woody, 2017). Specific to pregnancy, depression has been estimated to be highest (11 percent) in the first trimester and falls to 8.5 percent in the second and third trimesters (Gaynes, 2005). For treatment, the American Psychiatric Association and American College of Obstetricians and Gynecologists issued pregnancy guidelines for depression management that recommend careful risk and benefit analysis of existing treatment (especially medications) (Yonkers, 2009). For major depression, psychotropic medication and psychotherapy have the largest evidence-based support (Stuart, 2014). However, data also note efficacy for several complementary interventions (Deligiannidis, 2014). The FDA (2006, 2011b) recommends careful and transparent risk assessment during pregnancy before prescribing psychotropic medications. The FDA (2014) has also eliminated the letter risk categories (A, B, C, D and X). Currently, the Pregnancy and Lactation Labeling Rule (PLLR) specifically highlights risks and benefits of the medication to mother and fetus and its benefit for the underlying illness. Additional guidance is found in *Williams Obstetrics*, 25th edition (Dashe, 2018). Nonpharmacologic and complementary approaches are also potential options for depressive symptoms during pregnancy. These include acupuncture, bright light therapy, exercise, omega fatty acid supplementation, and yoga and massage therapies (Field, 2012; Manber, 2010; Shivakumar, 2011; Su, 2008; Wirz-Justice, 2011). Electroconvulsive therapy (ECT) is reserved for those unresponsive to pharmacotherapy. In one review, ECT was 78-percent effective, but maternal and fetal complication rates were 5 and 3 percent, respectively (Andersen, 2009).

Postpartum

Depression after childbirth is largely divided into three categories: "postpartum blues," postpartum depression, and postpartum psychosis. The strongest predictors of postpartum depression include prior history of depression or anxiety, family history of

psychiatric illness, poor marital relationship, limited social support, and stressful life events in the previous 12 months (Boyce, 2005; Sayil, 2007).

Postpartum blues describes a transient state of heightened emotional reactivity that can develop in up to 50 percent of women. The onset is 2 to 14 days after childbirth, and its duration is less than 2 weeks (Gaynes, 2005). Blues generally require no intervention. Rest and social support contribute significantly to remission. However, postpartum blues do constitute a significant risk factor for subsequent depression during the puerperium.

Postpartum depression, as noted, includes onset during pregnancy and within 4 weeks following delivery. However, in research and most clinical settings, any depression developing within 12 months following childbirth is considered to have postpartum onset (Sharma, 2014). With this definition, the prevalence of postpartum depression globally ranges from 12 to 26 percent (Gaynes, 2005; Shorey, 2018). Postpartum depression warrants careful assessment by a mental health professional, and treatment is initiated immediately to minimize impaired caregiving. Infants of depressed mothers exhibit cognitive, temperamental, and developmental differences compared with those of unaffected mothers (Kaplan, 2009; Newport, 2002). SSRIs are usually first-line agents, although fluoxetine use is discouraged due to relatively high concentrations in breast milk (Sie, 2012). Psychosocial interventions, especially interpersonal therapy and cognitive-behavioral therapy, are also effective in treating postpartum depression (Sockol, 2015, 2018). In refractory cases, two hospital-based treatments can be considered. ECT, mentioned earlier, may improve symptoms (Gressier, 2015; Rundgren, 2018). Brexanolone is an allopregnanolone analogue and administered by infusion over a 48-hour period. Plasma allopregnanolone levels rise in connection with progesterone throughout pregnancy, and after childbirth these concentrations decrease abruptly. In small randomized trials, the drug significantly reduced Hamilton Rating Scale for Depression scores compared with placebo (Kanes, 2017; Meltzer-Brody, 2018). It has been recently FDA-approved for treatment of postpartum depression and is undergoing further evaluation. Additionally, for both clinicians and patients, Postpartum Support International is an excellent resource and is found at www.postpartum.net.

Last, *postpartum psychosis* develops uncommonly in new mothers, and its onset is generally within 2 weeks of childbirth (Gaynes, 2005; VanderKruik, 2017). The risk for this severe form of depression is increased for women who have had prior mood disorders. Particularly, prior postpartum psychosis increases a woman's risk with subsequent deliveries by 30 to 50 percent (American Psychiatric Association, 2013). Evaluation and antipsychotic pharmacologic treatment is essential for these patients. Hospitalization is often indicated until the safety of mother and infant is assured.

■ Other Psychiatric Disorders

Clinicians most often focus on mood disorders during the perinatal period. However, anxiety disorders, bipolar disorders, schizophrenia, and others may also be present. Of these, bipolar disorders and schizophrenia are serious, recurrent psychiatric illnesses that require pharmacologic treatment. Treatment planning is critical with such patients, and decisions are made in collaboration with a psychiatric professional. The FDA (2011a) issued a safety communication alerting health-care providers concerning some antipsychotic medications that are associated with neonatal extrapyramidal and withdrawal symptoms similar to the neonatal behavioral syndrome seen in those exposed to SSRIs. Thus, a careful balance must be struck between minimizing medication risk to the fetus and maternal risk from untreated or undertreated disease.

■ Perinatal Loss, Trauma, and Pregnancy Interruption

When pregnancy or childbirth has a tragic outcome, a clinician's actions and words affect a woman's memory of the event and her grieving process. Health-care providers are most helpful if they speak directly, use understandable language, and share information that would provide parents a sense of control over their situation and that would address their fears. Extra time with health professionals and a perception of being a priority are also important (DiMarco, 2001; Flenady, 2014). Since grief is individual, no generalizations can be made concerning clinical treatment in these situations. Thus, a provider must ask a patient what she needs and wants. Conjoint psychotherapy may be helpful if mother and father are struggling to communicate with each other about their emotional needs and experiences of grief. Psychologic treatment may also be necessary if symptoms of posttraumatic stress disorder (PTSD) emerge in the weeks after the birth or loss. Family therapy may be indicated if other children need support to process the loss and their parents' grief. Many hospitals have pregnancy loss support services, often managed by hospital chaplaincy. In addition, online resources for information and local support groups are www.pregnancyloss.info and www.missfoundation.org.

Pregnancy interruptions due to fetal anomalies that are incompatible with life outside the womb also require enhanced caregiver sensitivity. The term "interruption" may be more acceptable than "termination." Privacy within the patient's social support system is important to understand, given that some women are more comfortable describing the loss as a "miscarriage" or "stillbirth" rather than a termination.

MENOPAUSAL TRANSITION AND MENOPAUSE

The *menopausal transition* has long been investigated as a vulnerable period for emergence of mood symptoms. Anxiety, irritable mood, and sleep problems are more likely to develop in perimenopausal women than in premenopausal counterparts (Brandon, 2008; Freeman, 2006). Moreover, data suggest that rates of new-onset depression during menopause transition are nearly twice those for premenopausal women (Cohen, 2006b). This risk persists even after adjusting for sleep disturbances and vasomotor symptoms.

Other possible risks for depression and anxiety are a prior history of depression or severe premenstrual distress, hot flashes, and disrupted sleep. Demographic predictors of higher risk during the perimenopause are lower educational status, African-American ethnicity, unemployment, and major life stressors (Bromberger, 2001; Freeman, 2006; Maartens, 2002). Developmentally, many women are transitioning from being family focused to finding new avenues in which to invest time and energy.

Mood vulnerability during menopause transition is believed to follow fluctuations in reproductive hormones. Detailed discussion of these hormones as they relate to mood changes during this transition is found in Chapter 22 (p. 500).

■ Evaluation and Treatment

Perimenopausal women with psychologic symptoms warrant a comprehensive psychosocial inventory and risk factor assessment. Since medical conditions may concurrently develop during this transition, evaluation excludes these before symptoms are considered psychosomatic. In particular, thyroid function is evaluated.

The approach to treating mood symptoms involves both pharmacotherapy and psychotherapy (Brandon, 2008). Recommended psychotropic medications are SSRIs and selective noradrenergic-reuptake inhibitors (SNRIs) such as venlafaxine (Effexor). These agents are good options for women who decline hormone therapy. Additional benefits include alleviation of vasomotor symptoms and sleep disturbance. As discussed further in Chapter 22 (p. 485), SSRIs and SNRIs may also offer significant symptom relief for those without mood disorders (Cobin, 2017; Guthrie 2015; Maki, 2018).

Studies suggest that short-term administration of estrogen is an option for perimenopausal women with depressive symptoms (Soares, 2001). However, the psychotropic role of estrogen-progesterone preparations in postmenopausal women remains unclear. Moreover, benefits are weighed against safety concerns raised by the Women's Health Initiative (WHI) Study regarding estrogen use (Chap. 22, p. 479). Of nonpharmacologic alternatives investigated for mood disturbance during menopause, yoga and moderate-intensity exercise have demonstrated benefit (Brandon, 2014). However, these studies are small.

LATE LIFE

According to the United States Census Bureau (2018), by 2035, an estimated 78 million people will be 65 years or older, whereas an estimated 77 million will be younger than 18 years. For women in later life, psychosocial issues addressed are significantly different. Stressors may include diminished mental and physical function and loss of partner, family, or friends. Erikson identified the task of this final developmental stage of life as one of consolidation and integration. In this model, women retrospectively examine their life. They may manage their last years with integrity and with satisfaction in a life well lived, or may suffer despair, feeling that all was in vain.

The prevalence rates for psychiatric disorders in older adults are understudied and are so heterogeneous that confident application of data to older women is difficult. One recent review estimates combined male and female rates of depression to be 3.3 percent; of generalized anxiety disorder, 2.3 percent; and of alcohol use disorder, 1 percent (Volkert, 2013). One review looking at gender differences and depression reported prevalence rates of at least 8.4 percent in women aged 70 and older (Luppa, 2012). Importantly, psychiatric disorders do not disappear in later life, and evaluation of older women should include considerations of mental health.

■ Evaluation and Treatment

If a psychiatric disorder is suspected, underlying medical causes for these changes are ideally excluded. For example, depression may be a comorbid disorder with or an early symptom of Alzheimer or Parkinson disease (Polidori, 2001). Alternatively, depression, anxiety, and psychosis may also result from a single medication or medication combinations.

Specific screening questionnaires for depression have been developed for the elderly, such as the Geriatric Depression Scale (Brink, 1982). This screening tool is available in various languages at: www.stanford.edu/~yesavage/GDS.html. In addition, neuropsychologic evaluation is helpful to discriminate between symptoms and cognitive impairment. Dementia screening is discussed in Chapter 1 (p. 18).

Recognizing the natural decline in serotonin levels with aging, many gerontologists prescribe SSRIs for their patients. However, communication among all treating physicians to coordinate medications and minimize interactions is particularly important.

Psychosocial treatments are often helpful for the patient and, where applicable, her caregivers. Cognitive-behavioral therapy and interpersonal therapy are both efficacious with the elderly. Moreover, family therapy can be of great value to those struggling with end-of-life issues, functional impairments, multiple losses, and caregiver burden. Social workers can often help identify additional care resources.

For depression in older adults, one metaanalysis of 89 studies found that pharmacotherapy or psychotherapy achieved comparable results. In contrast, for anxiety, another analysis of 32 studies found pharmacotherapy slightly more effective than psychotherapy (Pinquart, 2006, 2007). Thus, treatment planning is individualized and assesses patient preference, contraindications, and treatment access.

OVERVIEW OF SEXUAL HEALTH

Sexual health is an essential component of overall health and well-being. According to the World Health Organization, sexual health is defined as physical, psychologic, and sociocultural well-being related to sexuality. It reflects not only a lack of disease or dysfunction, but also the free, responsible expression of one's sexual capabilities that nurture social well-being. Sexual health requires that an individual's sexual rights be respected and that sexual experiences be safe and pleasurable, free of discrimination, violence, and coercion (World Health Organization, 2006).

Obstetric, gynecologic, and other primary care settings are a common first point of contact for patients with sexual health concerns (Gott, 2004). Unfortunately, women's sexual concerns often go unassessed. For example, patients may hesitate to initiate conversations regarding this topic (Marwick, 1999). And for clinicians, insufficient medical training can lead to a lack of confidence in their knowledge or ability to respond to a patient's sexual concerns (Kingsberg, 2006; Shindel, 2013; Solursh, 2003). Thus, an improved understanding of normal

functioning and female sexual dysfunction (FSD) would likely narrow this gap in clinical care.

FEMALE SEXUAL FUNCTIONING

■ Female Sexual Response

Female sexual functioning encompasses multiple aspects of the sexual response cycle including desire (sexual drive that can be spontaneous or responsive to sexual stimuli), arousal (sexual excitement or perception of sexual pleasure), lubrication (vaginal wetness), and orgasm (climax of sexual pleasure). FSD is characterized by a distressing impairment in a specific domain of sexual response.

The biopsychosocial model (Fig. 14-1), when applied to the female sexual response, reflects sexuality's dynamic nature and highlights its multiple variables (Althof, 2005; Kingsberg, 2015). This model underscores the importance of thorough assessment of these components and the potential benefit of a multidisciplinary approach.

■ Female Sexual Dysfunction

Prevalence estimates of FSD vary, in part, due to variations in definitions, assessment of distress, and changes in diagnostic criteria across time. In the largest FSD prevalence survey in the United States, symptoms considered distressing were measured. Approximately 10 percent of women reported low desire, 5 percent noted poor arousal, and 5 percent listed orgasm difficulties (Shifren, 2008). Pain/penetration disorders are estimated to affect 14 to 34 percent of younger women and 6.5 to 45 percent of older women (van Lankveld, 2010).

To classify FSD, the Diagnostic and Statistical Manual of Mental Health Disorders, fourth edition, text-revised (DSM-IV-TR) identified six categories (American Psychiatric Association, 2000). These were hypoactive sexual desire disorder (HSDD) (persistent lack of desire); sexual aversion disorder (persistent aversion to sexual activities); female sexual arousal disorder (FSAD) (persistent lack of lubrication-swelling in response to sexual excitement); female orgasmic disorder (persistent lack of orgasm

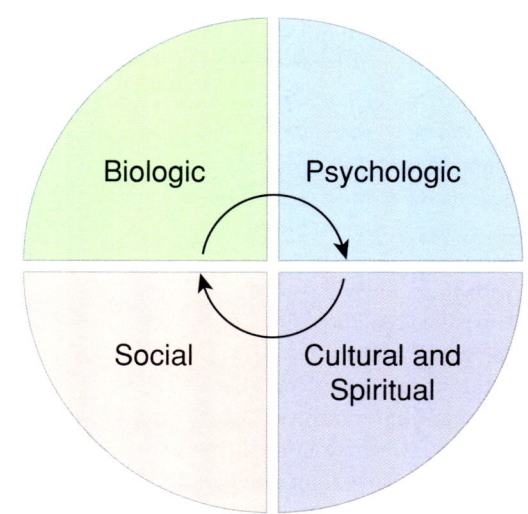

FIGURE 14-1 Biopsychosociocultural model.

following sexual excitement); dyspareunia (persistent genital pain with intercourse); and vaginismus (persistent involuntary muscle spasm in the outer third of the vagina with intercourse). FSD requires associated significant distress or impairment for diagnosis. Moreover, FSD symptoms are not better attributed to another disorder, medical condition, or effects of a substance.

The current DSM-5 describes three types of FSD (American Psychiatric Association, 2013). The first is female sexual interest/arousal disorder (FSIAD), which incorporates HSDD and FSAD. The other two are female orgasm disorder and genito-pelvic/pain or penetration disorder (GPPPD), which contains vaginismus and dyspareunia. The DSM-5 groupings remain controversial due to the combining of disorders and the lack of empirical support and validation of these combined disorders (DeRogatis, 2011; Pyke, 2015). In contrast, the International Consultation on Sexual Medicine (ICSM) Committee on Definitions and the International Society for the Study of Women's Sexual Health (ISSWSH) classifications align with the DSM-IV-TR (McCabe, 2016; Parish, 2016). The ICSM and ISSWSH recommend separation of desire and arousal disorders, noting benefits for assessment and treatment selection (Parish, 2016). Although treatment often is aimed toward addressing the primary problem, distress across more than one sexual function is common. Thus, an accurate assessment of sexual function is essential and helps to determine primary versus secondary components (Kingsberg, 2006).

ASSESSMENT OF SEXUAL FUNCTIONING

■ Brief Assessment

Providers can promote interactive discussion by establishing patient rapport and conveying comfort with the topic of female sexual health (Risen, 1995). Sitting rather than standing, relaxed but professional body language, and eye contact can increase patient ease. Moreover, knowledge and comfort with terminology can normalize the topic. Patients should be clothed, and the setting for discussion should be discreet.

A brief assessment of sexual concerns can be completed in 2 to 3 minutes using three components. First, the assessment is normalized and described as an important part of usual history taking. Questions then clarify if she is currently in a sexual relationship and determine the gender of partner(s). Third, specific patient concerns about sexual functioning are sought. For sexually inactive patients, issues that may be contributing to sexual inactivity are investigated (Kingsberg, 2006).

■ Complete Assessment

History

A complete reproductive health history can highlight components that may affect sexual response. Such information includes age at menarche, prior pregnancies or infertility, contraception use and type, and prior sexually transmitted disease. During a more systemic review, questions investigate prior gynecologic surgeries; urinary tract disease; endocrine disorders that involve sex steroid hormones, thyroid hormones, or diabetes; neurologic disorders; and cardiovascular diseases (Basson, 2000).

Many psychiatric conditions and their treatments can also negatively affect sexual response. These include mood and anxiety disorders, PTSD, substance abuse, eating disorders, and somatic symptom disorders (Atlantis, 2012; Laurent, 2009; Palha, 2008; Pinheiro, 2010; Solmaz, 2016; Yehuda, 2015). As examples, depression may decrease sexual desire and performance anxiety can affect vaginal muscle tension, creating pain or vaginismus. Other effects may stem from psychopharmacotherapy such as antiepileptics, antipsychotics, benzodiazepines, SSRIs, SNRIs, tricyclic antidepressants, and monoamine oxidase inhibitors (Basson, 2007; Kingsberg, 2007).

Partner-related variables may impair sexual functioning. The quality of the relationship, a partner's sexual functioning, and a partner's mental distress during sexual activity, such as performance anxiety, are examples. For individuals who identify as lesbian, gay, bisexual, transgender, fluid, or queer/questioning (LGBTQ), clinicians ideally are aware of specific sexual health risks and needs. Last, prior sexual victimization or physical abuse raises the risk of FSD (Luftey, 2008; Weaver, 2009).

Self-Report Measures

Validated self-report measures that assess female sexual response may help identify and qualify sexual functioning (Kingsberg, 2017). Common examples include the Female Sexual Function Index (FSFI) and the Sexual Function Questionnaire (SFQ), which both assess a range of sexual function domains. The Female Sexual Distress Scale (FSDS) assesses distress associated with impaired sexual response (DeRogatis, 2002; Quirk, 2002; Rosen, 2000). However, these measures are more commonly used in clinical research, and short screeners may be more useful in clinical settings. A single-item screener can be particularly time-efficient, and the Decreased Sexual Desire Screener (DSDS) is a five-item screener for acquired HSDD (Table 14-11) (Clayton, 2009; Flynn, 2015).

Physical Examination

To further assess physiologic components, examination may involve inspection of external genitalia and bimanual and speculum examinations (Phillips, 1998). In those with vulvodynia, significant findings and examination steps are outlined in Chapter 4 (p. 104). For those with dyspareunia, evaluation components are described in Chapter 12 (p. 266). For postmenopausal women, who may suffer from genitourinary syndrome of menopause (GSM), classic findings and treatment options are explained in Chapter 22 (p. 495).

Laboratory testing may aid diagnosis and treatment. Diagnostically, testing can help identify thyroid dysfunction, sex steroid hormone imbalance, and glucose abnormalities, which all can impair sexual function. Notably, some FSD treatments can adversely alter lipid and liver function values, and these are often assessed prior to drug initiation (Hatzichristou, 2004; Pauls, 2005).

TREATMENT

A stepped-care approach to sexual counseling allows for identification of sexual concerns and for appropriate referral. One

TABLE 14-11. The Decreased Sexual Desire Screener (DSDS)

Patient:

1. In the past was your level of sexual desire or interest good and satisfying to you?	Yes/No
2. Has there been a decrease in your level of sexual desire or interest?	Yes/No
3. Are you bothered by your decreased level of sexual desire or interest?	Yes/No
4. Would you like your level of sexual desire or interest to increase?	Yes/No

5. Please check all factors that you feel may be contributing to your current decrease in sexual desire or interest:
   A. An operation, depression, injuries, or other medical condition
   B. Medication, drugs or alcohol you are currently taking
   C. Pregnancy, recent childbirth, menopausal symptoms
   D. Other sexual issues you may be having (pain, decreased arousal or orgasm)
   E. Your partner's sexual problems
   F. Dissatisfaction with your relationship or partner
   G. Stress or fatigue

Clinician:

If the patient answers "No" to any of the questions 1 through 4, she does not qualify for a diagnosis of hypoactive sexual desire disorder (HSDD).

If she answers "Yes" to all of questions 1 through 4 and "No" to all in question 5, she does qualify for a diagnosis of HSDD.

If she answers "Yes" to all of questions 1 through 4 and "Yes" to any in question 5, decide if the answers to question 5 indicate a primary diagnosis other than HSDD. A comorbid arousal or orgasmic disorder does not exclude concurrent HSDD.

From Clayton, 2009, with permission.

example is the PLISSIT model (Annon, 1976). With it, permission (P) to discuss sexual function is first requested. Next, limited information (LI) such as genital anatomy education is provided. Last, if indicated, specific suggestions (SS) to address the concern and subsequent intensive therapy (IT) by a trained therapist are offered. This model can be implemented according to the level of training a provider has received in this area. ISSWSH has published a similar algorithm for process of care for identifying and treating HSDD (Clayton, 2018). The treatment overview presented next is artificially separated into pharmacologic and psychosocial approaches. However, given the biopsychosocial model of FSD, an interdisciplinary treatment approach may be required.

■ Pharmacologic Treatments

Neuroendocrine functions are essential to sexual response. Excitatory neurochemicals are dopamine, oxytocin, norepinephrine, and melanocortin. Inhibitory ones include serotonin, opiates, and endocannabinoids (Burnett, 2010; Kingsberg, 2015, 2017). As such, overactive inhibition or underactive excitatory mechanisms or both may contribute to lowered sexual response. Sex steroid hormones modulate response to internal and external sexual stimuli. All these factors may serve as targets for both nonhormonal and hormonal intervention (Kingsberg, 2017).

Hypoactive Sexual Desire Disorder

Flibanserin. Treatments for HSDD include nonhormonal CNS medications. Flibanserin (Addyi) is a multifunctional $5\text{-}HT_{1A}$-receptor agonist and $5\text{-}HT_{2A}$-receptor antagonist. It normalizes excitatory and inhibitory neurotransmitter levels to enhance desire. Specific central actions lower serotonin and raise dopamine and norepinephrine activities (DeRogatis, 2012; Jayne, 2012; Katz, 2013; Thorp, 2012). Currently, it is the only FDA-approved medication to treat HSDD and is approved for premenopausal women (Goldstein, 2017). Although clinical trials demonstrate efficacy within 4 weeks, 8 to 12 weeks may be required for effect.

Side effects include dizziness and sleepiness, which is countered in part by bedtime administration. Because of a risk for hypotension and syncope when combined with alcohol, prescribers are required to complete a risk evaluation and mitigation strategy (REMS) program prior to prescribing Addyi (Sprout Pharmaceuticals, 2016). Although clinical trials have demonstrated safety and efficacy in postmenopausal women, flibanserin is not FDA approved for use in this population (Portman, 2017; Simon, 2013).

Off-Label Treatments. Of other agents, off-label use of bupropion, an antidepressant that is a norepinephrine- and dopamine-reuptake inhibitor, may increase sexual excitation and improve desire (Goldstein, 2017; Segraves, 2004). The anxiolytic buspirone is a partial $5\text{-}HT_{1A}$-receptor agonist and presynaptic dopamine-receptor antagonist that can also improve desire (Clayton, 2014; Goldstein, 2017). Last, bremelanotide is a synthetic melanocortin analogue of α-melanocyte-stimulating hormone. Melanocortins are neuropeptides that modulate sexual behavior at the level of the hypothalamus and may translate sexual cues into genital response (Pfaus, 2007). In randomized trials in premenopausal women, bremelanotide improved desire and was well-tolerated (Clayton, 2016, 2018; DeRogatis, 2014; Portman, 2014). Although not currently marketed, bremelanotide is under review by the FDA for approval.

Of hormonal treatment options, large randomized trials support the efficacy of exogenous testosterone (Achilli, 2017). Testosterone influences the synthesis and storage of neurotransmitters and can improve sexual response (Goldstein, 2017; Perelman, 2007). In several RCTs, the testosterone transdermal patch (Intrinsa) demonstrated safety and efficacy for the treatment of HSDD in postmenopausal women whether they were taking estrogen therapy or not (Braunstein, 2005; Buster, 2005; Davis, 2008). However, this patch was never FDA approved and is no longer marketed in Europe.

Currently, no FDA-approved testosterone option is available for women. Therefore, off-label testosterone products in women require careful monitoring for acne or hirsutism. These side effects may stem from inconsistent dosing while titrating male products or from compounding testosterone products. In addition, data on long-term effects on breast cancer rates and cardiovascular health remain limited. Thus, if testosterone use is planned, lipid and liver function are assessed prior to initiation, and breast cancer screening is performed as described in Chapter 13 (p. 293) (Shifren, 2015).

Phase II trials indicate promise for two combination pharmacotherapies—Lybrido and Lybridos (Tuiten, 2018). These are taken as needed, and they target hyperactive inhibitory and hypoactive excitatory responses or both to improve desire (Poels, 2013; van Rooij, 2013). Lybrido is a sublingual combination of testosterone and sildenafil, which is a phosphodiesterase type 5 inhibitor (PDE5i). Lybridos is a sublingual combination of testosterone and buspirone.

Combination oral contraceptives contain a progestin, and each progestin varies in its androgenicity (Chap. 5, p. 122). Although intuitively attractive, switching COC brands to one containing a more androgenic progestin has proven largely ineffective (Davis, 2013; Wallwiener, 2010).

Systemic estrogen therapy for postmenopausal women is not typically indicated for FSD. However, local hormone therapies are helpful for the treatment of GSM-related dyspareunia. Options discussed in Chapter 22 include estrogen cream, tablets, soft-gel caps, and rings; vaginal dehydroepiandrosterone; or oral ospemifene, which is a selective estrogen-receptor modulator (SERM) (North American Menopause Society, 2017).

Female Sexual Arousal Disorder

Hormonal treatment options for FSAD with some research support include testosterone therapy, just described (Davis, 2012; Laan, 2001; Tuiten, 2002). Another is tibolone, which is a SERM (Nappi, 2015).

Of nonhormonal treatments for FSAD, bupropion, described earlier, is an option (Levin, 2014; Maravilla, 2008). Sildenafil is a PDE5i hypothesized to improve sexual function due to enhanced genital blood flow (Caruso, 2006). Evidence for sildenafil efficacy in a general premenopausal female population is conflicting. But, in specific medical populations with genital neurovascular substrate interference, for example, spinal cord injury, subjective and objective parameters of sexual response are improved (Schoen, 2009).

Pain Disorders

Several pharmacologic agents have been used to treat female sexual pain disorders. However, few randomized trials have assessed their efficacy. Treatment may include nonhormonal options such as topical lidocaine ointment, topical hormonal cream, or antidepressants. In women with vestibulodynia secondary to oral contraceptive use, application of a topical compounded preparation containing 0.03-percent estradiol and 0.01-percent testosterone to the vestibule twice daily may be helpful (Burrows, 2013).

Pelvic floor physical therapy is a widely accepted treatment for sexual pain. Various techniques incorporate breathing/relaxation training, education, local tissue desensitization, electromyographic biofeedback, manual therapy, and a graded use of vaginal dilators. However, few randomized trials demonstrate efficacy for specific physical therapy protocols (Bergeron, 2010, 2015).

Last, some data support vestibulectomy for treatment of vulvodynia in the well-selected woman. But, complication rates preclude its use as a first-line treatment (Stockdale, 2014). Fuller discussions of vulvovaginal and pelvic pain disorders and their treatment are found in Chapter 4 (p. 104) and 12 (p. 266), respectively.

■ Psychologic Treatments

Several empirically supported psychologic interventions are available to treat FSD (Kingsberg, 2017; ter Kuile, 2010). Evidence indicates they can also affect neuroplasticity and functional brain mechanisms that drive sexual response (Goldstein, 2017).

For HSDD, research provides limited support for sex therapy, cognitive-behavioral therapy (CBT), and mindfulness techniques combined with CBT (Althof, 2011; Bradford, 2014; Brotto, 2014; Nobre, 2008). Sex therapy includes psychoeducation regarding sexual functioning. Techniques include counseling and sensate focused exercises, which are a graded series of sensual touching exercises starting with nongenital touch (Althof, 2011). CBT includes psychoeducation and focuses on altering maladaptive sexual cognitions, such as unrealistic negative thoughts about sexual activity, and maladaptive behaviors, such as avoiding sexual contact (Nobre, 2008). Mindfulness-based approaches, used with CBT, enhance one's ability to be in the present moment and emphasize a nonjudgmental awareness of sexual sensation and function. Also, for FSAD, mindfulness-based techniques with CBT have some research support (Brotto, 2014).

For orgasm disorder, directed masturbation can be helpful (Andersen, 1981; McMullen, 1979; Riley, 1978). This progressive series of exercises involves self-exploration of one's body and genitals. An awareness of sexual stimulation and response is designed to achieve self-stimulated orgasm and, later, potentially partner-stimulated orgasm (Heiman, 1988).

For pain disorders, limited data support CBT, therapist-aided exposure therapy, and mindfulness-based CBT for sexual pain (Brotto, 2015; Masheb, 2009; ter Kuile, 2013). Bergeron and associates (2015) offer a review of the topic. Therapist-aided exposure therapy includes psychoeducation regarding female anatomy and function. Another component is guided, in vivo exposure exercises. During this, the patient has graded exposure to penetration by a dilator.

REFERENCES

Achilli C, Pundir J, Ramanathan P, et al: Efficacy and safety of transdermal testosterone in postmenopausal women with hypoactive sexual desire disorder: a systematic review and meta-analysis. Fertil Steril 107(2):475, 2017

Althof S: Sex therapy and combined (sex and medical) therapy. J Sex Med 8(6):1827, 2011

Althof SE, Leiblum SR, Chevret-Measson M, et al: Psychological and interpersonal dimensions of sexual function and dysfunction. J Sex Med 2(6):793, 2005

American College of Obstetricians and Gynecologists: Screening for perinatal depression. Committee Opinion No. 757, November 2018

American Psychiatric Association: Diagnostic and Statistical Manual of Mental Disorders, 4th ed., Text Revision. Washington, American Psychiatric Association, 2000

American Psychiatric Association: Diagnostic and Statistical Manual of Mental Disorders, 5th ed. Washington, American Psychiatric Association, 2013

Andersen BL: A comparison of systematic desensitization and directed masturbation in the treatment of primary orgasmic dysfunction in females. J Consult Clin Psychol 49(4):568, 1981

Anderson E, Reti I: ECT in pregnancy: a review of the literature from 1941 to 2007. Psychosom Med 71:235, 2009

Annon J: The PLISSIT model: a proposed conceptual scheme for the behavioral treatment of sexual problems. J Sex Educ Ther 2(1):1, 1976

Atlantis E, Sullivan T: Bidirectional association between depression and sexual dysfunction: a systematic review and metaanalysis. J Sex Med 9(6):1497, 2012

Bäckström T, Bixo M, Johansson M, et al: Allopregnanolone and mood disorders. Prog Neurobiol 113:88, 2014

Baller EB, Wei SM, Kohn PD, et al: Abnormalities of dorsolateral prefrontal function in women with premenstrual dysphoric disorder: a multimodal neuroimaging study. Am J Psychiatry 170(3):305, 2013

Basson R: Taking the sexual history, part 1: eliciting the sexual concerns of your patient in primary care. Med Aspects Hum Sex 1(1):13, 2000

Basson R, Schultz WW: Sexual sequelae of general medical disorders. Lancet 369(9559):409, 2007

Bergeron S, Corsini-Munt S, Aerts L, et al: Female sexual pain disorders: a review of the literature on etiology and treatment. Curr Sex Health Rep 7(3):159, 2015

Bergeron S, Morin M, Lord MJ: Integrating pelvic floor rehabilitation and cognitive-behavioral therapy for sexual pain: what have we learned and where do we go from here? Sex Relat Ther 25(3):289, 2010

Bloch M, Rotenberg N, Koren D, et al: Risk factors for early postpartum depressive symptoms. Gen Hosp Psychiatry 28(1):3, 2006

Boyce P, Hickey A: Psychosocial risk factors to major depression after childbirth. Soc Psychiatry Psychiatr Epidemiol 40(8):605, 2005

Bradford A: Inhibited sexual desire in women. In Grossman L, Walfish R (eds): Translating Psychological Research into Practice. New York, Springer, 2014, p 515

Brandon AR, Crowley SK, Gordon JL, et al: Non-pharmacologic treatments for depression related to reproductive events. Curr Psychiatr Rep 16 (12), 526, 2014

Brandon AR, Shivakumar G, Freeman MP: Perimenopausal depression. Curr Psychiatr 7(10):38, 2008

Braun DL, Sunday SR, Halmi KA: Psychiatric comorbidity in patients with eating disorders. Psychol Med 24(4):859, 1994

Braunstein GD, Sundwall DA, Katz M, et al: Safety and efficacy of a testosterone patch for the treatment of hypoactive sexual desire disorder in surgically menopausal women: a randomized, placebo-controlled trial. Arch Intern Med 165(14):1582, 2005

Brink TL, Yesavage JA, Lum O, et al: Screening tests for geriatric depression. Clin Gerontol 1(1):37, 1982

Bromberger JT, Meyer PM, Kravitz HM, et al: Psychologic distress and natural menopause: a multiethnic community study. Am J Public Health 91(9):1435, 2001

Brotto LA, Basson R: Group mindfulness-based therapy significantly improves sexual desire in women. Behav Res Ther 57:43, 2014

Brotto LA, Basson R, Smith KB, et al: Mindfulness-based group therapy for women with provoked vestibulodynia. Mindfulness 6:417, 2015

Burnett AL, Goldstein I, Andersson KE, et al: Future sexual medicine physiological treatment targets. J Sex Med 7(10):3269, 2010

Burrows LJ, Goldstein AT: The treatment of vestibulodynia with topical estradiol and testosterone. Sex Med 1(1):30, 2013

Buster JE, Kingsberg SA, Aguirre O, et al: Testosterone patch for low sexual desire in surgically menopausal women: a randomized trial. Obstet Gynecol 105(5 Pt 1):944, 2005

Caruso S, Rugolo S, Agnello C, et al: Sildenafil improves sexual functioning in premenopausal women with type 1 diabetes who are affected by sexual arousal disorder: a double-blind, crossover, placebo-controlled pilot study. Fertil Steril 85(5):1496, 2006

Centre for Maternal and Child Enquiries: Saving mothers' lives: reviewing maternal deaths to make motherhood safer: 2006–08. BJOG 118(Suppl 1): 1, 2011

Clayton A, Althof S, Kingsberg S, et al: Bremelanotide for female sexual dysfunction in premenopausal women: a randomized placebo-controlled dose-finding trial. Womens Health 12(3):325, 2016

Clayton A, Kingsberg S, Simon J, et al: Safety and efficacy of bremelanotide for HSDD in women: RECONNECT study open-label extension phase results. Presented at Annual Meeting of the American College of Obstetricians and Gynecologists, 27–30 April 2018

Clayton AH, El Haddad S, Iluonakhamhe JP, et al: Sexual dysfunction associated with major depressive disorder and antidepressant treatment. Expert Opin Drug Saf 13(10):1361, 2014

Clayton AH, Goldfischer ER, Goldstein I, et al: Validation of the Decreased Sexual Desire Screener (DSDS): a brief diagnostic instrument for generalized acquired female hypoactive sexual desire disorder (HSDD). J Sex Med 6(3):730, 2009

Clayton AH, Goldstein I, Kim NN, et al: The International Society for the Study of Women's Sexual Health process of care for management of hypoactive sexual desire disorder in women. Mayo Clin Proc 93(4):467, 2018

Cobin RH, Goodman NF, et al: American Association of Clinical Endocrinologists and American College of Endocrinology position statement on menopause-2017 update. Endocr Pract 23(7):869, 2017

Cohen LS, Altshuler LL, Harlow BL, et al: Relapse of major depression during pregnancy in women who maintain or discontinue antidepressant treatment. JAMA 295(5):499, 2006a

Cohen LS, Soares CN, Vitonis AF, et al: Risk for new onset of depression during the menopausal transition: the Harvard study of moods and cycles. Arch Gen Psychiatry 63(4):385, 2006b

Cox J, Holden J, Sagovsky R: Detection of postnatal depression: development of the 10-item Edinburgh postnatal depression scale. Br J Psychiatry 150:782, 1987

Cronje WH, Vashisht A, Studd JW: Hysterectomy and bilateral oophorectomy for severe premenstrual syndrome. Hum Reprod 19:2152, 2004

Culbert KM, Racine SE, Klump KL: Research review: what we have learned about the causes of eating disorders—a synthesis of sociocultural, psychological, and biological research. J Child Psychology Psychiatry 56(11):1141, 2015

Dashe JS, Cunningham FG: Teratology, teratogens, and fetotoxic agents. In Cunningham FG, Leveno KJ, Bloom SL, et al (eds): Williams Obstetrics, 25th ed. New York, McGraw-Hill, 2018, p 238

Davis SR, Bitzer J, Giraldi A, et al: Change to either a nonandrogenic or androgenic progestin-containing oral contraceptive preparation is associated with improved sexual function in women with oral contraceptive-associated sexual dysfunction. J Sex Med 10(12):3069, 2013

Davis SR, Braunstein GD: Efficacy and safety of testosterone in the management of hypoactive sexual desire disorder in postmenopausal women. J Sex Med 9(4):1134, 2012

Davis SR, Moreau M, Kroll R, et al: Testosterone for low libido in postmenopausal women not taking estrogen. N Engl J Med 359(19):2005, 2008

De Souza MC, Walker AF, Robinson PA, et al: A synergistic effect of a daily supplement for 1 month of 200 mg magnesium plus 50 mg vitamin B6 for the relief of anxiety-related premenstrual symptoms: a randomized, double-blind, crossover study. J Womens Health Gend Based Med 9(2):131, 2000

Deligiannidis KM, Freeman MP: Complementary and alternative medicine therapies for perinatal depression. Best Pract Res Clin Obstet Gynaecol 28(1):85, 2014

DeRogatis LR, Clayton AH, Rosen RC: Should sexual desire and arousal disorders in women be merged? Arch Sex Behav 40(2):217, 2011

DeRogatis LR, Edelson J, Jordan R, et al: Bremelanotide for female sexual dysfunctions: responder analyses from a phase 2B dose-ranging study. Obstet Gynecol 123(Suppl 1):26s, 2014

DeRogatis LR, Komer L, Katz M, et al: Treatment of hypoactive sexual desire disorder in premenopausal women: efficacy of flibanserin in the VIOLET Study. J Sex Med 9(4):1074, 2012

DeRogatis LR, Rosen R, Leiblum S et al: The Female Sexual Distress Scale (FSDS): initial validation of a standardized scale for assessment of sexually related personal distress in women. J Sex Marital Ther 28(4):317, 2002

DiMarco MA, Menke EM, McNamara T: Evaluating a support group for peri-natal loss. MCN Am J Matern Child Nurs 26(3):135, 2001

Engel GL: The need for a new medical model: a challenge for biomedicine. Science 196(4286):129, 1977

Erikson EH: Childhood and Society, 2nd ed. New York, Norton, 1963

Field T, Diego M, Hernandez-Reif M, et al: Yoga and massage therapy reduce prenatal depression and prematurity. J Body Mov Ther 16(2):204, 2012

Flenady V, Boyle F, Koopmans L, et al: Meeting the needs of parents after a stillbirth or neonatal death. BJOG 121(Suppl 4):137, 2014

Flynn KE, Tessler Lindau S, et al: Development and validation of a single-item screener for self-reporting sexual problems in U.S. adults. J Gen Intern Med 30(10):1468, 2015

Food and Drug Administration: Antipsychotic drug labels updated on use during pregnancy and risk of abnormal muscle movements and withdrawal symptoms in newborns. 2011a. Available at: http://www.fda.gov/Drugs/DrugSafety/ucm243903.htm. Accessed November 30, 2018

Food and Drug Administration: Content and format of labeling for human pre-scription drug and biological products; requirements for pregnancy and lac-tation labeling. 2014. Available at: http://federalregister.gov/a/2014-28241. Accessed November 30, 2018

Food and Drug Administration: Selective serotonin reuptake inhibitor (SSRI) antidepressant use during pregnancy and reports of a rare heart and lung con-dition in newborn babies. 2011b. Available at: http://www.fda.gov/Drugs/DrugSafety/ucm283375.htm. Accessed November 30, 2018

Food and Drug Administration: Selective serotonin reuptake inhibitors (SSRIs), selective serotonin-norepinephrine reuptake inhibitors (SNRIs), 5-hydroxytryptamine receptor agonists (triptans), 2006. Available at: http://www.fda.gov/Drugs/DrugSafety/PostmarketDrugSafetyInformationforPatientsandProviders/DrugSafetyInformationforHeathcareProfessionals/ucm085845.htm. Accessed November 30, 2018

Freeman EW, Sammel MD, Lin H, et al: Associations of hormones and meno-pausal status with depressed mood in women with no history of depression. Arch Gen Psychiatry 63(4):375, 2006

Gaynes BN, Gavin N, Meltzer-Brody S, et al: Perinatal depression: prevalence, screening accuracy, and screening outcomes. Evid Rep Technol Assess 119:1, 2005

Goldstein I, Kim NN, Clayton AH, et al: Hypoactive sexual desire disorder: International Society for the Study of Women's Sexual Health (ISSWSH) Expert Consensus Panel Review. Mayo Clin Proc 92(1):114, 2017

Gott M, Galena E, Hinchliff S, et al: "Opening a can of worms": GP and practice nurse barriers to talking about sexual health in primary care. Fam Pract 21(5):528, 2004

Gressier F, Rotenberg S, Cazas O, et al: Postpartum electroconvulsive ther-apy: a systematic review and case report. Gen Hosp Psychiatry 37(4):310, 2015

Guthrie KA, LaCroix AZ, Ensrud KE, et al: Pooled analysis of six pharmaco-logic and nonpharmacologic interventions for vasomotor symptoms. Obstet Gynecol 126(2):413, 2015

Halbreich U: The etiology, biology, and evolving pathology of premenstrual syndromes. Psychoneuroendocrinology 28(Suppl 3):55, 2003a

Halbreich U, Borenstein J, Pearlstein T, et al: The prevalence, impairment, impact, and burden of premenstrual dysphoric disorder (PMS/PMDD). Psychoneuroendocrinology 28(Suppl 3):1, 2003b

Hantsoo L, Epperson N: Premenstrual dysphoric disorder: epidemiology and treatment. Curr Psychiatry Rep 17(11):87, 2015

Hatzichristou D, Rosen RC, Broderick G, et al: Clinical evaluation and man-agement strategy for sexual dysfunction in men and women. J Sex Med 1(1):49, 2004

Heiman JR, LoPiccolo J: Becoming Orgasmic: a Sexual and Personal Growth Program for Women (revised and expanded edition). New York, Simon & Schuster, 1988

Hoek HW: Incidence, prevalence and mortality of anorexia nervosa and other eating disorders. Curr Opin Psychiatry 19(4):389, 2006

Hübel C, Leppä V, Breen G, et al: Rigor and reproducibility in genetic research on eating disorders. Int J Eat Dis 51(7):593, 2018

Jayne C, Simon JA, Taylor LV, et al: Open-label extension study of flibanse-rin in women with hypoactive sexual desire disorder. J Sex Med 9(12):3180, 2012

Kanes S, Colguhoun H, Gundez-Bruce H, et al: Brexanolone (SAGE-547 injection) in post-partum depression: a randomised controlled trial. Lancet 390(10093):480, 2017

Kaplan PS, Burgess AP, Sliter JK, et al: Maternal sensitivity and the learning-promoting effects of depressed and nondepressed mothers' infant-directed speech. Infancy 14(2):143, 2009

Katz M, DeRogatis LR, Ackerman R, et al: Efficacy of flibanserin in women with hypoactive sexual desire disorder: results from the BEGONIA trial. J Sex Med 10(7):1807, 2013

Kessler RC, Berglund P, Demler O, et al: Lifetime prevalence and age-of-onset distributions of DSM-IV disorders in the National Comorbidity Survey Replication. Arch Gen Psychiatry 62(6):593, 2005

Kingsberg SA: Taking a sexual history. Obstet Gynecol Clin N Am 33(4):535, 2006

Kingsberg SA, Althof A, Simon JA, et al: Female sexual dysfunction—medical and psychological treatments, Committee 14. J Sex Med 14(12):1463, 2017

Kingsberg SA, Clayton AG, Pfaus JG: The female sexual response: current models, neurobiological underpinnings and agents currently approved or under investigation for the treatment of hypoactive sexual desire disorder. CNS Drugs 29(11):915, 2015

Kingsberg SA, Janata J: Female sexual disorders: assessment, diagnosis, and treatment. Urol Clin North Am 34(4):497, 2007

Kolar DR, Rodriguez DL, Chams MM, et al: Epidemiology of eating disor-ders in Latin America: a systematic review and meta-analysis. Curr Opin Psychiatry 29(6):363, 2016

Laan E, van Lunsen RH, Everaerd W: The effects of tibolone on vaginal blood flow, sexual desire and arousability in postmenopausal women. Climacteric 4(1):28, 2001

Lancaster CA, Gold KJ, Flynn HA, et al: Risk factors for depressive symp-toms during pregnancy: a systematic review. Am J Obstet Gynecol 202(1):5, 2010

Laurent SM, Simons AD: Sexual dysfunction in depression and anxiety: con-ceptualizing sexual dysfunction as part of an internalizing dimension. Clin Psychol Rev 29(7):573, 2009

Levin RJ: The pharmacology of the human female orgasm—its biological and physiological backgrounds. Pharmacol Biochem Behav 121:62, 2014

Luftey KE, Link CL, Litman HJ et al: An examination of the association of abuse (physical, sexual, or emotional) and female sexual dysfunction: results from the Boston Area Community Health Survey. Fertil Steril 90(4):957, 2008

Luppa M, Sikorski C, Luck T, et al: Age- and gender-specific prevalence of depression in latest-life—systematic review and meta-analysis. J Affect Disord 136(3):212, 2012

Maartens LWF, Knottnerus JA, Pop VJ: Menopausal transition and increased depressive symptomatology: a community based prospective study. Maturitas 42(3):195, 2002

Maki PM, Kornstein SG, Joffe H, et al: Guidelines for the evaluation and treatment of perimenopausal depression: summary and recommendations. Menopause 25(10):1069, 2018

Manber R, Schnyer RN, Lyell D, et al: Acupuncture for depression during pregnancy: a randomized controlled trial. Obstet Gynecol 115(3):511, 2010

Mangweth-Matzek B, Hoek HW, Pope HG: Pathological eating and body dis-satisfaction in middle-aged and older women. Curr Opin Psychiatry 27:431, 2014

Maravilla KR, Yang CC: Magnetic resonance imaging and the female sexual response: overview of techniques, results, and future directions. J Sex Med 5(7):1559, 2008

Marjoribanks J, Brown J, O'Brien PM, et al: Selective serotonin reup-take inhibitors for premenstrual syndrome. Cochrane Database Syst Rev 6:CD001396, 2013

Marwick C: Survey says patients expect little physician help on sex. JAMA 281(23):2173, 1999

Masheb RM, Kerns RD, Lozano C, et al: A randomized clinical trial for women with vulvodynia: cognitive behavioral therapy vs. supportive psychotherapy. Pain 141(1-2):31, 2009

McCabe MP, Sharlip ID, Atalla E: Definitions of sexual dysfunctions in women and men: a consensus statement from the fourth International Consultation on Sexual Medicine 2015. J Sex Med 13(2):135, 2016

McMullen S, Rosen RC: Self-administered masturbation training in the treat-ment of primary orgasmic dysfunction. J Consult Clin Psychol 47(5):912, 1979

Meltzer-Brody S, Colguhoun H, Riesenberg R, et al: Brexanolone injection in post-partum depression: two multicentre, double-blind, randomised, placebo-controlled, phase 3 trials. Lancet 392(10152):1058, 2018

Mitchell AM, Bulik CM: Eating disorders and women's health: an update. J Midwifery Womens Health 51(3):193, 2006

Nappi RE, Cucinella L: Advances in pharmacotherapy for treating female sexual dysfunction. Expert Opin Pharmacother 16(6):875, 2015

National Institute of Mental Health: Major Depression. 2016. Available at: https://www.nimh.nih.gov/health/statistics/major-depression.shtml. Accessed November 30, 2018

Nevatte T, O'Brien PM, Bäckström T, et al: ISPMD consensus on the manage-ment of premenstrual disorders. Arch Womens Ment Health 16(4):279, 2013

Newport DJ, Wilcox MM, Stowe ZN: Maternal depression: a child's first adverse life event. Semin Clin Neuropsychiatry 7(2):113, 2002

Nobre PJ, Pinto-Gouveia J: Cognitions, emotions, and sexual response: analysis of the relationship among automatic thoughts, emotional responses, and sexual arousal. Arch Sex Behav 37(4):652, 2008

North American Menopause Society: The 2017 hormone therapy position statement of The North American Menopause Society. Menopause 24(7):728, 2017

Oral E, Kirkan TS, Yildirim A, et al: Serum brain-derived neurotrophic factor differences between the luteal and follicular phases in premenstrual dysphoric disorder. Gen Hosp Psychiatry 37(3):266, 2015

Ossewaarde L, van Wingen GA, Rijpkema M, et al: Menstrual cycle-related changes in amygdala morphology are associated with changes in stress sensitivity. Hum Brain Mapp 34:1187, 2013

Palha A, Esteves M: Drugs of abuse and sexual functioning. Adv Psychosom Med 29:131, 2008

Parish SJ, Goldstein AT, Goldstein SW: Toward a more evidence-based nosology and nomenclature for female sexual dysfunctions—Part II. J Sex Med 13(12):1888, 2016

Pauls RC, Kleeman SD, Karram MM: Female sexual dysfunction: principles of diagnosis and therapy. Obstet Gynecol Surv 60(3):196, 2005

Pearlstein TB, Bachmann GA, Zacur HA, et al: Treatment of premenstrual dysphoric disorder with a new drospirenone-containing oral contraceptive formulation. Contraception 72:414, 2005

Perelman MA: Clinical application of CNS-acting agents in FSD. J Sex Med 4(Suppl 4):280, 2007

Pfaus J, Giuliano F, Gelez H: Bremelanotide: an overview of preclinical CNS effects on female sexual function. J Sex Med 4(Suppl 4):269, 2007

Phillips NA: The clinical evaluation of dyspareunia. Int J Impot Res 10(Suppl 2): S117, 1998

Pike KM, Dunne PE: The rise of eating disorders in Asia: a review. J Eat Disord 17(3):33, 2015

Pinheiro AP, Raney TJ, Thornton LM, et al: Sexual functioning in women with eating disorders. Int J Eat Disord 43(2):123, 2010

Pinquart M, Duberstein PR: Treatment of anxiety disorders in older adults: a meta-analytic comparison of behavioral and pharmacological interventions. Am J Geriatr Psychiatry 15(8):639, 2007

Pinquart M, Duberstein PR, Lyness JM: Treatments for later-life depressive conditions: a meta-analytic comparison of pharmacotherapy and psychotherapy. Am J Psychiatry 163(9):1493, 2006

Poels S, Bloemers J, van Rooij K, et al: Toward personalized sexual medicine (part 2): testosterone combined with a PDE5 inhibitor increases sexual satisfaction in women with HSDD and FSAD, and a low sensitive system for sexual cues. J Sex Med 10(3):810, 2013

Polidori MC, Menculini G, Senin U, et al: Dementia, depression and parkinsonism: a frequent association in the elderly. J Alzheimer Dis 3(6):553, 2001

Portman DJ, Brown L, Yuan J, et al: Flibanserin in postmenopausal women with hypoactive sexual desire disorder: results of the PLUMERIA study. J Sex Med 14(6):834, 2017

Portman DJ, Edelson J, Jordan R, et al: Bremelanotide for hypoactive sexual desire disorder: analyses from a phase 2B dose-ranging study. Obstet Gynecol 123(Suppl 1):31s, 2014

Pyke RE, Clayton A: Models vs. realities in female sexual dysfunction. J Sex med 12(9):1977, 2015

Quirk FH, Heiman JR, Rosen RC: Development of a sexual function questionnaire for clinical trials of female sexual dysfunction. J Womens Health Gend Based Med 11(3):277, 2002

Reid RL, Soares CN: Premenstrual dysphoric disorder: contemporary diagnosis and management. J Obstet Gynaecol Can 40(2):215, 2018

Riley AJ, Riley EJ: A controlled study to evaluate directed masturbation in the management of primary orgasmic failure in women. Br J Psychiatry 133:404, 1978

Risen CB: A guide to taking a sexual history. Psychiatr Clin N Am 18(1):39, 1995

Rosen R, Brown C, Heiman J, et al: The Female Sexual Function Index (FSFI): a multidimensional self-report instrument for the assessment of female sexual function. J Sex Marital Ther 26(2):191, 2000

Rundgren S, Brus O, Båve U, et al: Improvement of postpartum depression and psychosis after electroconvulsive therapy: a population-based study with a matched comparison group. J Affect Disord 235:258, 2018

Rush AJ, Trivedi MH, Ibrahim HM, et al: The 16-item quick inventory of depressive symptomatology (QIDS), clinician rating (QIDS-C), and self-report (QIDS-SR): a psychometric evaluation in patients with chronic major depression. Biol Psychiatry 54(5):573, 2003

Sayil M, Gure A, Uçanok Z: First time mothers' anxiety and depressive symptoms across the transition to motherhood: associations with maternal and environmental characteristics. Women Health 44(3):61, 2007

Schoen C, Bachmann G: Sildenafil citrate for female sexual arousal disorder: a future possibility? Nat Rev Urol 6(4):216, 2009

Segraves RT, Clayton A, Croft H, et al: Bupropion sustained release for the treatment of hypoactive sexual desire disorder in premenopausal women. J Clin Psychopharmacol 24(3):339, 2004

Shah NR, Jones JB, Aperi J, et al: Selective serotonin reuptake inhibitors for premenstrual syndrome and premenstrual dysphoric disorder: a meta-analysis. Obstet Gynecol 111:1175, 2008

Sharma V, Mazmanian D: The DSM-5 peripartum specifier: prospects and pitfalls. Arch Womens Ment Health 17(2):171, 2014

Shifren JL: Testosterone for midlife women: the hormone of desire? Menopause 22(10):1147, 2015

Shifren JL, Monz BU, Russo PA: Sexual problems and distress in United States women: prevalence and correlates. Obstet Gynecol 112(5): 970, 2008

Shindel AW, Parish SJ: Sexuality education in North American medical schools: current status and future directions. J Sex Med 10(1):3, 2013

Shivakumar G, Brandon AR: Antenatal depression: a rationale for studying exercise. Depress Anxiety 28(3): 234, 2011

Shorey S, Chee CYI, Ng ED, et al: Prevalence and incidence of postpartum depression among healthy mothers: a systematic review and meta-analysis. J Psychiatr Res 104:235, 2018

Sie SD, Wennink JM, van Driel JJ, et al: Maternal use of SSRIs, SNRIs and NaSSAs: practical recommendations during pregnancy and lactation. Arch Dis Child Fetal Neonatal Ed 97(6):F472, 2012

Simon JA, Kingsberg SA, Shumel B, et al: Efficacy and safety of flibanserin in postmenopausal women with hypoactive sexual desire disorder: results of the SNOWDROP trial. Menopause 21(6):633, 2013

Soares CN, Almeida OP, Joffe H: Efficacy of estradiol for the treatment of depressive disorders in perimenopausal women: a double-blind, randomized, placebo-controlled trial. Arch Gen Psychiatry 58(6):529, 2001

Sockol LE: A systematic review and meta-analysis of interpersonal psychotherapy for perinatal women. J Affect Disord 232:316, 2018

Sockol LE: A systematic review of the efficacy of cognitive behavioral therapy for treating and preventing perinatal depression. J Affect Disord 177:7, 2015

Solmaz V, Ceviz A, Aksoy D, et al: Sexual dysfunction in women with migraine and tension-type headaches. Int J Impot Res 28(6):201, 2016

Solursh D, Ernst J, Lewis R, et al: The human sexuality education of physicians in North American medical schools. Int J Impot Res 15(Suppl 5): 41, 2003

Sprout Pharmaceuticals: Addyi (flibanserin): prescribing information. Bridgewater, Sprout Pharmaceuticals, 2016

Stockdale CK, Lawson HW: 2013 Vulvodynia guideline update. J Low Genit Tract Dis 18(2):93, 2014

Stoving RK, Hangaard J, Hagen C: Update on endocrine disturbances in anorexia nervosa. J Pediatr Endocrinol 14(5):459, 2001

Strumia R: Dermatologic signs in patients with eating disorders. Am J Clin Dermatol 6(3):165, 2005

Stuart S, Koleva H: Psychological treatments for perinatal depression. Best Pract Res Clin Obstet Gynaecol 28(1):61, 2014

Su KP, Huang SY, Chiu TH, et al: Omega-3 fatty acids for major depressive disorder during pregnancy: results from a randomized, double-blind, placebo-controlled trial. J Clin Psychiatry 69(4):644, 2008

Substance Abuse and Mental Health Services Administration: Results from the 2012 National Survey on Drug Use and Health: mental health findings. NSDUH Series H-47, HHS Publication No. (SMA) 13–4805, Rockville, 2013

ter Kuile MK, Both S, van Lankveld JJ: Cognitive behavioral therapy for sexual dysfunctions in women. Psychiatr Clin N Am 33(3): 595, 2010

ter Kuile MM, Melles R, de Groot HE: Therapist-aided exposure for women with lifelong vaginismus: a randomized waiting-list control trial of efficacy. J Consult Clin Psychol 81(6):1127, 2013

Thomas JJ, Lee S, Becker AE: Updates in the epidemiology of eating disorders in Asia and the Pacific. Curr Opin Psychiatry 29(6):354, 2016

Thorp J, Simon J, Dattani D, et al: Treatment of hypoactive sexual desire disorder in premenopausal women: efficacy of flibanserin in the DAISY study. J Sex Med 9(3):793, 2012

Thys-Jacobs S: Micronutrients and the premenstrual syndrome: the case for calcium. J Am Coll Nutr 19(2):220, 2000

Trace SE, Baker JH, Peñas-Lledó E, et al: The genetics of eating disorders. Annu Rev Clin Psychol 9:589, 2013

Tuiten A, van Honk J, Verbaten R, et al: Can sublingual testosterone increase subjective and physiological measures of laboratory induced sexual arousal? Arch Gen Psychiatry 59(5):465, 2002

Tuiten A, van Rooij K, Bloemers J, et al: Efficacy and safety of on-demand use of 2 treatments designed for different etiologies of female sexual interest/arousal disorder: 3 randomized clinical trials. J Sex Med 15(2):201, 2018

United States Census Bureau: Older people projected to outnumber children for first time in US History. 2018. Available at https://www.census.gov/newsroom/press-releases/2018/cb18-41-population-projections.html. Accessed January 5, 2019

van Lankveld JJ, Granot M, Weijmar Schultz WC, et al: Women's sexual pain disorders. J Sex Med 7(1 Pt 2):615, 2010

van Rooij K, Poels S, Bloemers J, et al: Toward personalized sexual medicine (part 3): testosterone combined with a serotonin 1A receptor agonist increases sexual satisfaction in women with HSDD and FSAD, and dysfunctional activation of sexual inhibitory mechanisms. J Sex Med 10(3): 824, 2013

VanderKruik R, Barreix M, Chou D, et al: The global prevalence of postpartum psychosis: a systematic review. BMC Psychiatry 17(1):272, 2017

Volkert J, Schulz H, Härter M, et al: The prevalence of mental disorders in older people in Western countries—a meta-analysis. Ageing Res Rev 12(1): 339, 2013

Wallwiener M, Wallwiener LM, Seeger H, et al: Effects of sex hormones in oral contraceptives on the female sexual function score: a study in German female medical students. Contraception 82(2):155, 2010

Wang M, Seippel L, Purdy RH, et al: Relationship between symptom severity and steroid variation in women with premenstrual syndrome: study on serum pregnenolone, pregnenolone sulfate, 5 alpha-pregnane-3,20-dione and 3 alpha-hydroxy-5 alpha-pregnan-20-one. J Clin Endocrinol Metab 81(3):1076, 1996

Weaver TL: Impact of rape on female sexuality: review of selected literature. Clin Obstet Gynecol 52(4): 702, 2009

Wirz-Justice A, Bader A, Frisch U, et al: A randomized, double-blind, placebo-controlled study of light therapy for antepartum depression. J Clin Psychiatry 72(7):986, 2011

Wittchen HU, Becker E, Lieb R, et al: Prevalence, incidence and stability of premenstrual dysphoric disorder in the community. Psychol Med 32(1): 119, 2002

Woody CA, Ferrari AJ, Siskind DJ, et al: A systematic review and meta-regression of the prevalence and incidence of perinatal depression. J Affect Disord 219:86, 2017

World Health Organization: Defining sexual health: report of a technical consultation on sexual health, 28–31 January 2002, Geneva, 2006. Available at: http://www.who.int/reproductivehealth/publications/sexual_health/defining_sexual_health.pdf. Accessed December 15, 2018

Wyatt KM, Dimmock PW, Ismail KM, et al: The effectiveness of GnRHa with and without "add-back" therapy in treating premenstrual syndrome: a meta-analysis. BJOG 111:585, 2004

Wyatt KM, Dimmock PW, Jones PW, et al: Efficacy of vitamin B-6 in the treatment of premenstrual syndrome: systematic review. BMJ 318:1375, 1999

Yehuda R, Lehrner A, Rosenbaum TY: PTSD and sexual dysfunction in men and women. J Sex Med 12(5):1107, 2015

Yonkers KA, Brown C, Pearlstein TB, et al: Efficacy of a new low-dose oral contraceptive with drospirenone in premenstrual dysphoric disorder. Obstet Gynecol 106:492, 2005

Yonkers KA, Wisner KL, Stewart DE, et al: The management of depression during pregnancy: a report from the American Psychiatric Association and the American College of Obstetricians and Gynecologists. Gen Hosp Psychiatry 31(5):403, 2009

Pediatric and Adolescent Gynecology

Pediatric gynecology is a unique subspecialty that encompasses knowledge from various specialties including general pediatrics, gynecology, and reproductive endocrinology, as well as pediatric endocrinology and pediatric urology. Treatment of a particular patient may thus require the collaboration of clinicians from one or more of these fields. In 1986, the North American Society for Pediatric and Adolescent Gynecology (NASPAG) was established to conduct and encourage medical education and research in the field of pediatric and adolescent gynecology (PAG). To further this mission, PAG fellowships are now available nationwide.

Gynecologic disorders in children can differ greatly from those encountered in the adult female. Even the simple physical examination of the genitalia differs significantly. A thorough understanding of these differences can aid in diagnosis.

PHYSIOLOGY AND ANATOMY

■ Hypothalamic-Pituitary-Ovarian Axis

A carefully orchestrated cascade of events unfolds in the neuroendocrine system and regulates development of the female reproductive system. In utero, gonadotropin-releasing hormone (GnRH) neurons develop in the olfactory placode. These neurons migrate through the forebrain to the arcuate nucleus of the hypothalamus by 11 weeks' gestation (Fig. 17-5, p. 378). They form axons that extend to the median eminence and to the capillary plexus of the pituitary portal system (Fig. 16-9, p. 344). GnRH, a decapeptide, is influenced by higher cortical centers and is released from these neurons in a pulsatile fashion into the pituitary portal plexus. As a result, by midgestation, the GnRH "pulse generator" stimulates secretion of gonadotropins from the anterior pituitary. The gonadotropins are follicle-stimulating hormone (FSH) and luteinizing hormone (LH). In turn, the pulsatile release of gonadotropins stimulates ovarian synthesis and release of sex steroid hormones. Concurrently, accelerated germ cell division and follicular development begins, resulting in the creation of 6 to 7 million oocytes by 5 months' gestation. By late gestation, sex steroids exert a negative feedback on secretion of both hypothalamic GnRH and pituitary gonadotropins. During this time, oocyte numbers decline through a process of gene-related apoptosis to reach a level of 1 to 2 million by birth (Vaskivuo, 2001).

At birth, FSH and LH concentrations rise abruptly in response to the fall in placental estrogen levels. Levels of these gonadotropins are highest in the first 3 months of life (Fig. 15-1). This transient rise in their levels is followed by an increase in sex steroid concentrations. This rise is thought to explain instances of neonatal breast budding, minor bleeding from endometrial shedding, short-lived ovarian cysts, and transient white vaginal mucous discharge. Following these initial months, gonadotropin levels gradually decline to reach prepubertal levels by age 1 to 2 years.

The childhood years are thus characterized by low plasma levels of FSH, LH, and estradiol. Estradiol levels typically measure <10 pg/mL, and LH values are <0.3 mIU/mL. Both may be assessed if precocious development is suspected (Neely, 1995; Resende, 2007). During childhood, ovaries undergo active follicular growth and oocyte atresia. As a result of this attrition, by puberty, only approximately 300,000 oocytes remain (Baker, 1963).

■ Anatomy

Pelvic anatomy also changes during early childhood. In the neonate, sonographically, the uterus measures approximately 3.5 to 4 cm in length and 1.5 cm in width. Because the cervix is larger than the fundus, the neonatal uterus is typically spade-shaped (Fig. 15-2) (Kaplan, 2016; Nussbaum, 1986). An echogenic central endometrial stripe is common and reflects the transiently elevated sex steroid levels described earlier. Fluid is seen within the endometrial cavity in 25 percent of female

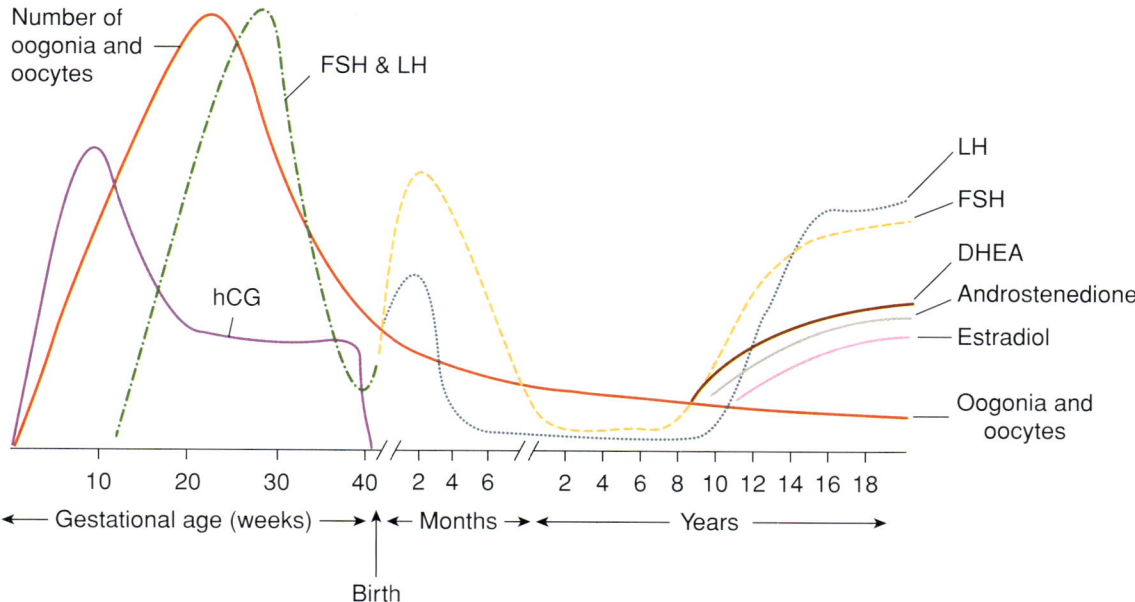

FIGURE 15-1 Variation in oocyte number and hormone levels during prenatal and postnatal periods. DHEA = dehydroepiandrosterone; FSH = follicle-stimulating hormone; hCG = human chorionic gonadotropin; LH = luteinizing hormone. (Adapted with permission from Fritz, 2011.)

newborns. Ovarian volume measures ≤1 cm³, and small cysts are frequently found (Cohen, 1993; Kaplan, 2016).

During childhood, the uterus measures 3 to 4 cm and is tubular as a result of the cervix and fundus becoming equal size. The ovaries grow in size as childhood progresses, and volumes range from 0.5 to 2 cm³ (Buzi, 1998; Herter, 2002).

■ Pubertal Changes

Puberty marks the normal physiologic transition from childhood to sexual and reproductive maturity. With puberty, the hypothalamus, pituitary, and ovaries initially undergo an intricate

maturation process. This maturation leads to a limited acceleration in body growth and to a complex development of secondary sexual characteristics involving the breast, sexual hair, and genitalia. Each landmark of hormonal and anatomic change during this time represents a spectrum of what is considered "normal."

Marshall and Tanner (1969) recorded breast and pubic hair development in schoolgirls and created the *Tanner stages* to describe pubertal development (Fig. 15-3). Initial pubertal changes begin between ages 8 and 13 years in most North American females (Tanner, 1985). Changes before or after are categorized as either precocious puberty or delayed puberty and warrant evaluation. In most girls, breast budding, termed

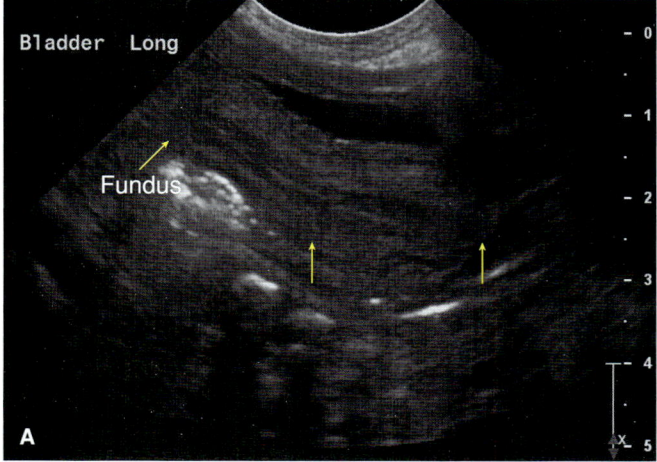

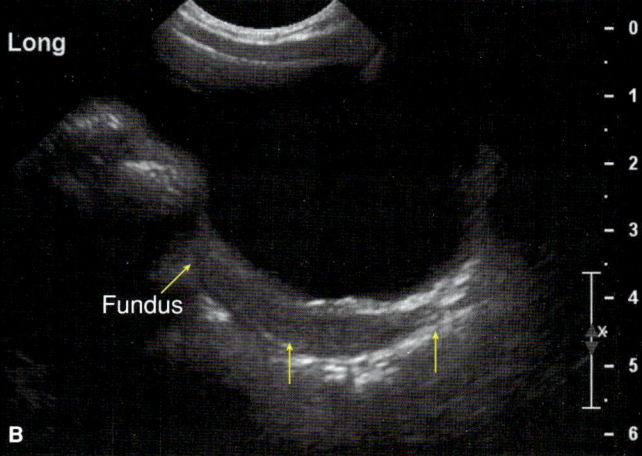

FIGURE 15-2 Transabdominal pelvic sonograms. **A.** Normal neonatal uterus. Midline longitudinal sonogram of the pelvis in this 3-day-old newborn demonstrates the uterus posterior to the bladder. Yellow arrows mark the fundus, isthmus, and cervix, respectively. The anteroposterior (AP) diameter of the cervix is greater than that of the fundus and creates a spade-shaped uterus. Due to the effect of maternal and placental hormones, a central echogenic endometrial cavity stripe is clearly visible. **B.** Normal prepubertal uterus. Midline longitudinal sonogram of the pelvis in this 3-year-old girl demonstrates the uterus posterior to the bladder. Yellow arrows mark the fundus, isthmus, and cervix, respectively. The uterus is homogeneously hypoechoic. The AP diameter of the cervix is equal to that of the fundus, and this gives the uterus a tubular shape. (Reproduced with permission by Dr. Neil Fernandes.)

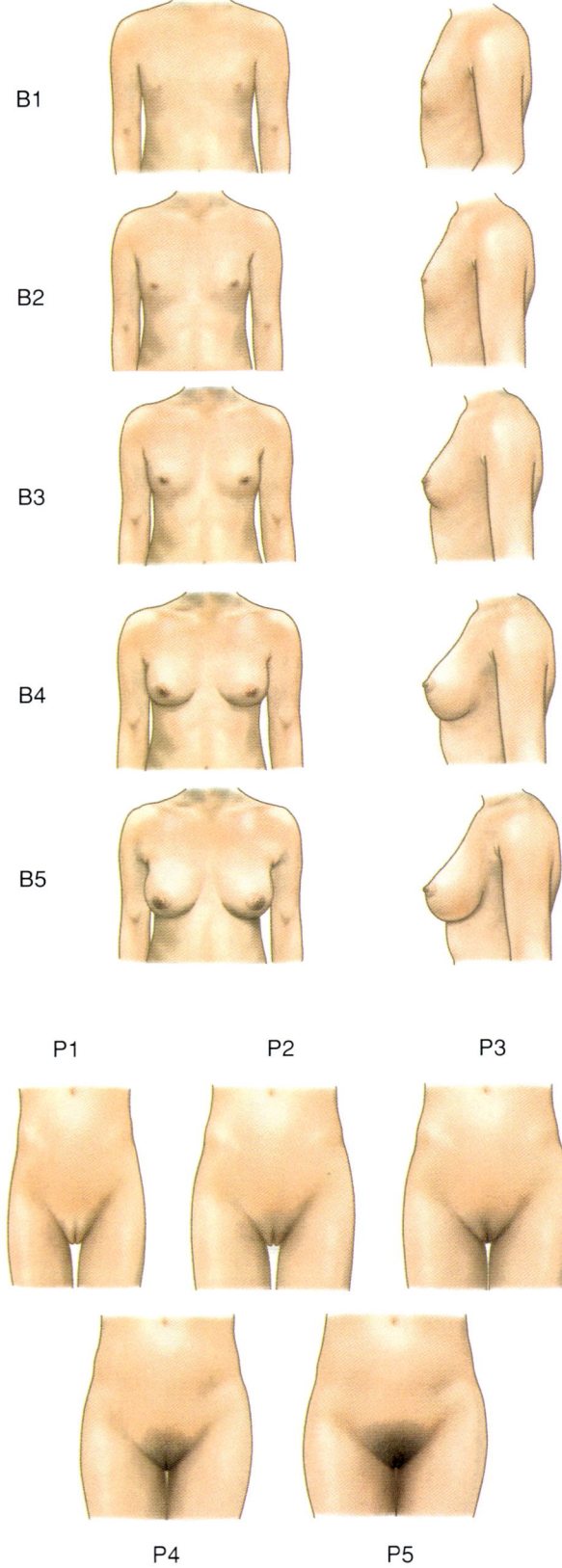

FIGURE 15-3 The Tanner stages of female breast and pubic hair development.

thelarche, is the first physical sign of puberty and begins at approximately age 10 (Aksglaede, 2009; Biro, 2006). In a minority, pubic hair growth, known as *pubarche*, develops first. Following breast and pubic hair growth, adolescents undergo an accelerated increase in height, termed a *growth spurt*, during a 3-year span from ages 10.5 to 13.5 years.

Since these original population studies, U.S. girls have trended to start thelarche and menarche earlier, although this trend has leveled off since the 1980s. Differences in onset timing are also related to race and higher body mass index (BMI) (Biro, 2013; Rosenfield, 2009). For example, higher BMI correlates with earlier pubertal development. The mean age of menarche in white girls is 12.7 years and is 6 months earlier, or 12.1 years, in black girls (Tanner, 1973).

GYNECOLOGIC EXAMINATION

An adolescent who has reached the age of 18 may consent to medical examination and treatment. Prior to this age, individual state laws govern whether minors can give their own consent for treatment of certain healthcare topics. Some examples include contraception, pregnancy care, substance abuse, mental health, and sexually transmitted diseases (STDs). Every state has laws allowing minors to consent to care if they are emancipated, living apart from their parents, or pregnant. The Guttmacher Institute (2018) and the Center for Adolescent Health & the Law offer resources (English, 2010).

A routine yearly examination of a child by her pediatrician generally includes a brief examination of the breasts and external genitalia. Congenital anomalies that are visible externally, such as imperforate hymen, may be identified. Alternatively, if parent or child has a specific complaint regarding vulvovaginal pain, rash, bleeding, discharge, or lesions, a gynecologic examination is directed toward the area of concern.

A parent or guardian should be present at the examination. This allows the child to understand that the examination is sanctioned. Moreover, clinicians can use this opportunity to inform a parent regarding findings and potential treatment. They can also emphasize the concept of inappropriate genital touching by others and parental notification if this occurs. In mid-to-late adolescence, however, a patient may prefer, for privacy reasons, not to be examined with a parent present.

"Child-friendly" objects or pictures and distracting conversation can ease fears and aid examination. Similarly, using an anatomically appropriate doll to explain the steps may decrease anxiety. The examination begins with a less-threatening approach of checking the ears, throat, heart, and lungs. Breasts are inspected. The external genital examination is best performed with the child in a frog-leg or knee-chest position to improve visualization. Occasionally, the patient may feel more comfortable sitting in a parent's lap. Sitting on a chair or examination table, the parent allows the child's legs to straddle the parent's thighs (Fig. 15-4).

Once the child is optimally positioned, each labium may be gently held with a thumb and forefinger and pulled toward the examiner and laterally. In this manner, the introitus, hymen, and lower portion of the vagina are inspected (Fig. 15-5). If a foreign body is suspected, vaginal irrigation can be performed in the office using a small feeding tube attached to a 60-mL

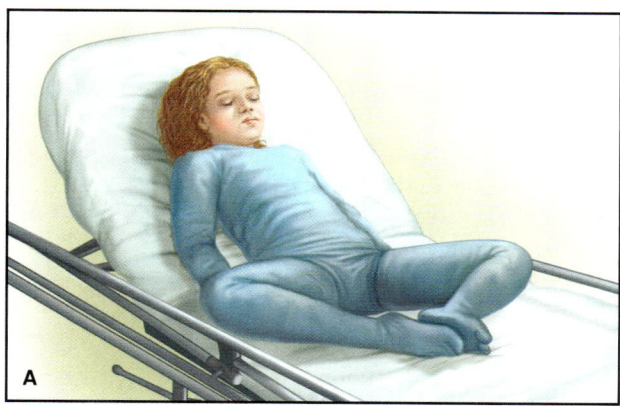

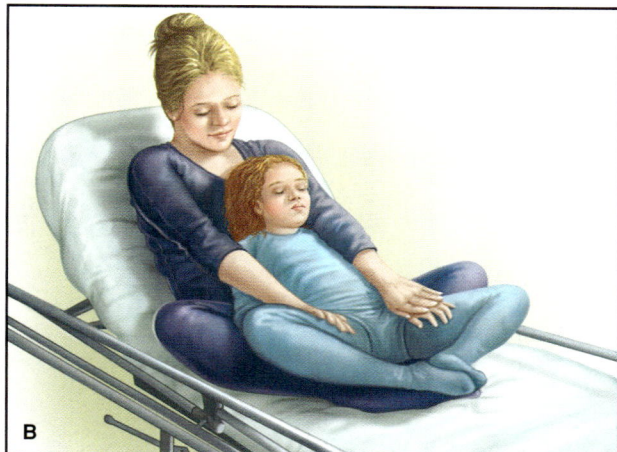

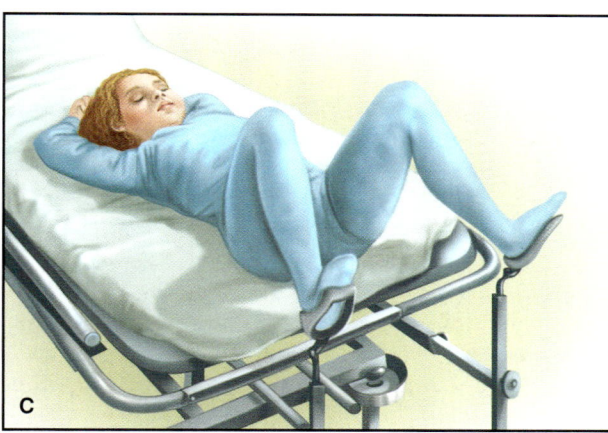

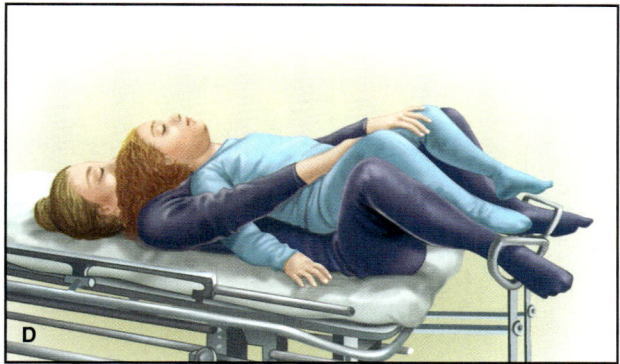

FIGURE 15-4 Various positions for examination of the pediatric patient (**A–D**).

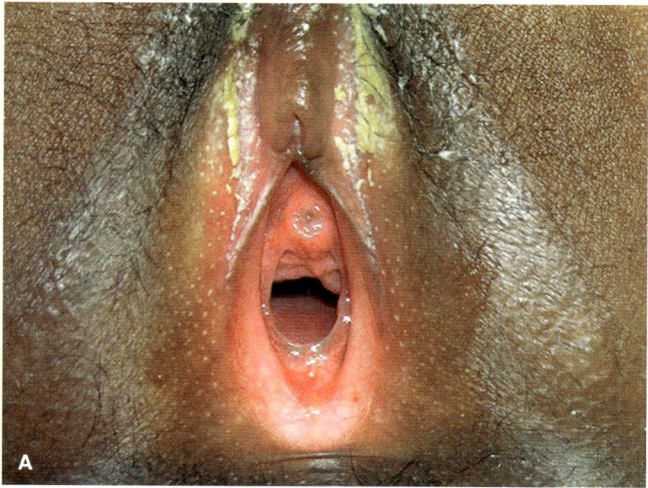

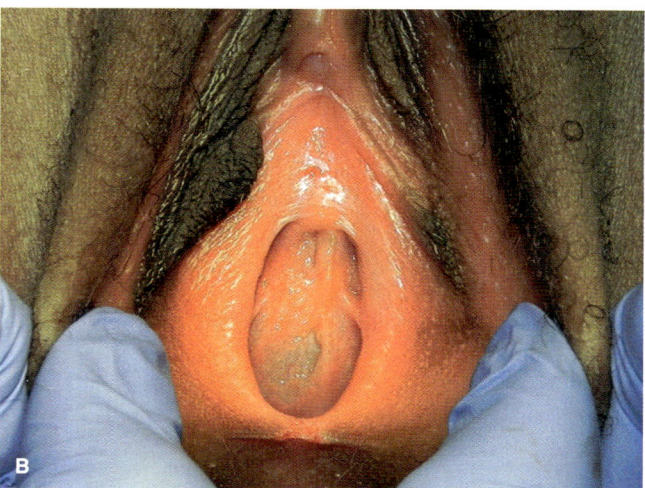

FIGURE 15-5 A. Normal prepubertal genitalia. **B.** Imperforate hymen.

syringe of saline. This will often help expel small pieces of toilet paper that may have lodged behind the hymen.

An internal examination is rarely necessary unless a persistent foreign body, tumor, or vaginal bleeding is suspected. This evaluation is best accomplished under general anesthesia.

Vaginoscopy may be performed using a small-caliber hysteroscope or cystoscope that will fit the hymeneal aperture. Warm normal saline serves as the distending media. The labia majora are manually approximated, which occludes the vagina, traps the saline, and permits vaginal distention. The endoscope is withdrawn to within approximately 1 cm of the introitus for full visualization of the vagina (Fig. 15-6). Notably, in the unestrogenized prepubertal vagina, petechiae may form with vaginal distention.

LABIAL ADHESION

Adhesion between the labia minora begins as a small posterior midline fusion, which is usually asymptomatic. This fusion may remain an isolated minor finding or may progress toward the clitoris to completely close the vaginal orifice. Also termed *labial agglutination*, this adhesion develops in 1 to 5 percent

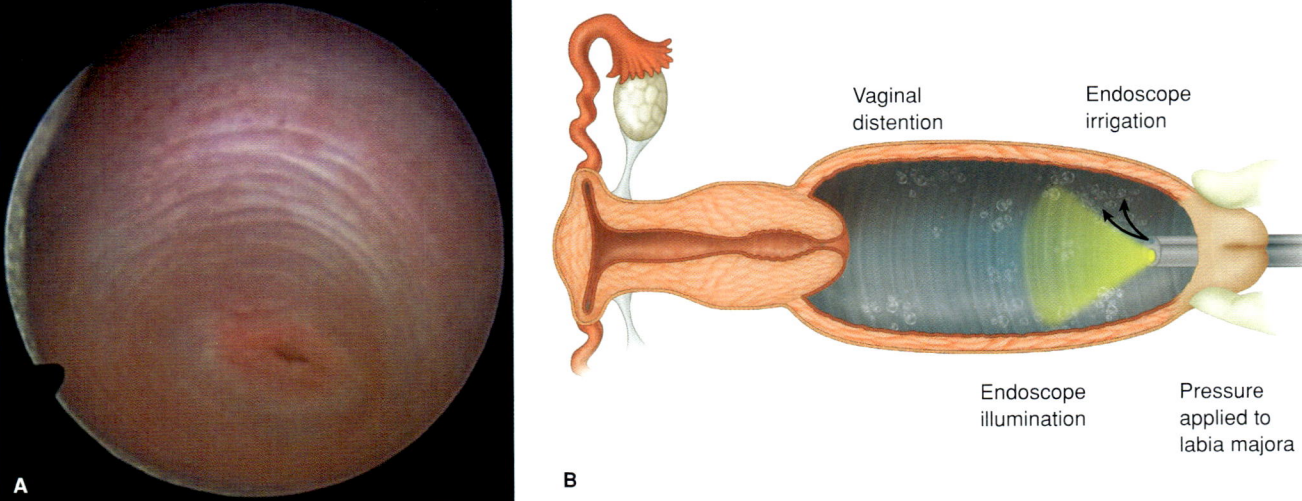

FIGURE 15-6 A. Photograph taken during vaginoscopy in an 8-year-old female. Typical for prepubertal girls, the cervix is almost flush with the proximal vagina. **B.** Drawing of vaginoscopy. The endoscope is first inserted toward the cervix to permit distention of the fornices. Next, the endoscope is retracted to within 1 cm of the hymen to allow global inspection of the vagina.

of prepubertal girls and in approximately 10 percent of female infants within the first year of life (Berenson, 1992; Christensen, 1971).

The cause of labial adhesion is unknown, although hypoestrogenism is implicated. This fusion typically develops in a low-estrogen environment. Namely, it is seen in infants and young girls and tends to undergo spontaneous resolution at puberty (Norris, 2018). Additionally, erosion of the vulvar epithelium is implicated in some cases of labial adhesion. For example, some cases of adhesion can be associated with lichen sclerosus, with herpes simplex viral (HSV) infection, and with vulvar trauma following sexual abuse.

The diagnosis is made visually. The labia majora appear normal, whereas the labia minora are fused with a distinct thin line of demarcation or *raphe* between them (Fig. 15-7). Extensive agglutination may leave only a ventral pinhole meatus between the labia. Located immediately beneath the clitoris, this small opening may lead to urinary dribbling as urine pools behind the adhesion. In these cases, urinary tract infection, urethritis, or vulvovaginitis can develop.

Treatment varies according to the degree of scarring and symptoms. In many instances, if the patient is asymptomatic, no intervention is necessary as the adhesion will typically resolve spontaneously with the rise of estrogen levels at puberty. Extensive adhesion with urinary symptoms, however, will require estrogen cream therapy. Estradiol (0.01 percent) cream (Estrace) or conjugated equine estrogen (Premarin) cream is applied to the fine, thin raphe twice daily for 2 weeks, followed by daily applications for an additional 2 to 4 weeks. A generous pea-sized amount of cream is placed with a finger or cotton-tipped applicator onto the raphe. With each application, gentle outward traction is exerted on the labia majora to help separate the adhesion. Similarly, light pressure may also be applied with the cotton applicator itself, as tolerated. After adhesion separation, a petroleum jelly (Vaseline) or vitamins A and D ointment (A&D ointment) may be applied nightly for 6 months to decrease the risk of recurrence. If the adhesion

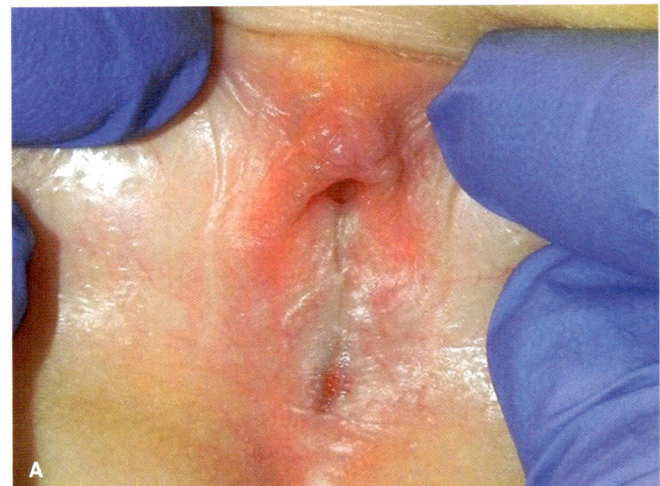

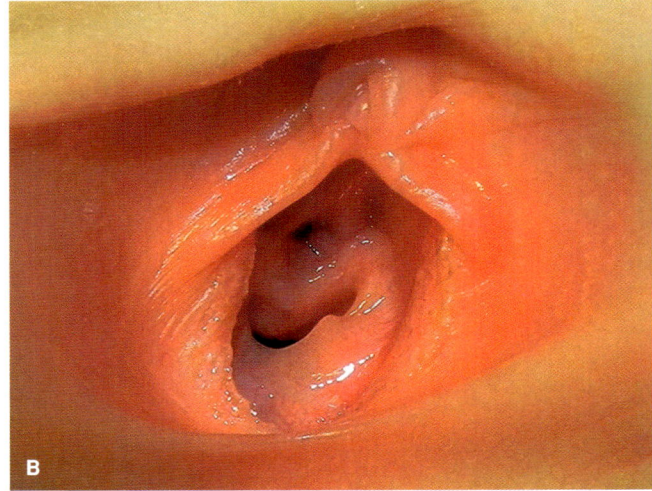

FIGURE 15-7 Labial adhesion. **A.** Labia minora are agglutinated in the midline. **B.** Resolution and restoration of normal anatomy.

reforms during the subsequent months or years, the process may be similarly repeated. Occasionally, with overuse of estrogen cream, local irritation, vulvar pigmentation, and minor breast budding may develop, at which time topical treatment is discontinued. These side effects are reversible once treatment is halted (Bacon, 2015). Alternatively, the use of 0.05-percent betamethasone cream applied twice daily for 4 to 6 weeks is another topical option (Mayoglou, 2009; Meyers, 2006).

For symptomatic patients, manual separation of labial adhesion in an outpatient setting without analgesia is painful and thus generally not advised. In addition, recurrence is much more common. However, if the adhesion persists despite consistent use of estrogen cream, then labia minora separation may be attempted several minutes after applying 5-percent lidocaine ointment to the adhesion raphe.

If manual separation is not easily accomplished or tolerated, surgical separation is best performed in an operating room under general anesthesia as an outpatient procedure. Midline division of the fused labia, also termed *introitoplasty*, uses an electrosurgical fine tip and does not require suturing.

To prevent repeated agglutination after manual separation or after surgery, an estrogen cream is applied nightly for 2 weeks. This is followed by an emollient cream nightly for at least 6 months.

CONGENITAL ANATOMIC ANOMALIES

Several anatomic and müllerian abnormalities present in early adolescence as obstructions to menstrual outflow. Described in Chapter 19, these include imperforate hymen, transverse vaginal septum, cervical and vaginal agenesis with an intact uterus, unicornuate uterus with an obstructed (noncommunicating) rudimentary horn, and the OHVIRA syndrome (obstructed hemivagina with ipsilateral renal agenesis) (Dietrich, 2014). These are often diagnosed in an adolescent with primary amenorrhea and cyclic pain. Notably, an adolescent with OHVIRA or with an obstructed rudimentary uterine horn will have menses, but these become increasingly painful over 6 to 9 months.

VULVITIS

■ Allergic and Contact Dermatitis

Vulvar inflammation may develop in isolation or in association with vaginitis. Allergic and contact dermatitis are common, whereas atopic dermatitis (eczema) and psoriasis are less frequent sources of itching and rash. With allergic and contact dermatitis the underlying pathophysiology varies, but the clinical appearance is usually similar. Vesicles or papules form on bright-red, edematous skin. However, in chronic cases, scaling, skin fissuring, and lichenification may be seen. In response, information regarding the degree of hygiene and continence and exposure to potential skin irritants is sought.

Typical offending agents include bubble baths and soaps, laundry detergents, fabric softeners and dryer sheets, bleach, and perfumed or colored toilet paper (Table 4-1, p. 93). Topical creams, lotions, and ointments used to soothe an area also may be an irritant to some children. For most, removing the offending agent and encouraging once- or twice-daily sitz baths

is sufficient. These baths consist of placing two tablespoons of baking soda in warm water and soaking for 20 minutes. If itching is severe, an oral medication may be prescribed, such as hydroxyzine hydrochloride (Atarax) 2 mg/kg/d divided in four doses. Alternatively, a 2.5-percent topical hydrocortisone ointment can be applied twice daily for 1 week. Aside from chemical irritants, children can also develop diaper dermatitis from urine and stool exposure. Corrective measures aim to keep the skin dry by more frequent diaper changes or to create a moisture barrier by application of emollient creams, such as Vaseline or A&D ointment.

■ Lichen Sclerosus

Vulvitis may also be caused by lichen sclerosus, which has a premenarchal prevalence of 1 in 900 (Powell, 2001). With this, the vulva displays hypopigmentation; atrophic, parchment-like skin; and occasional fissuring. Lesions are usually symmetrical and may form an "hourglass" appearance around the vulva and perianal areas (Fig. 15-8). Occasionally, the vulva develops dark

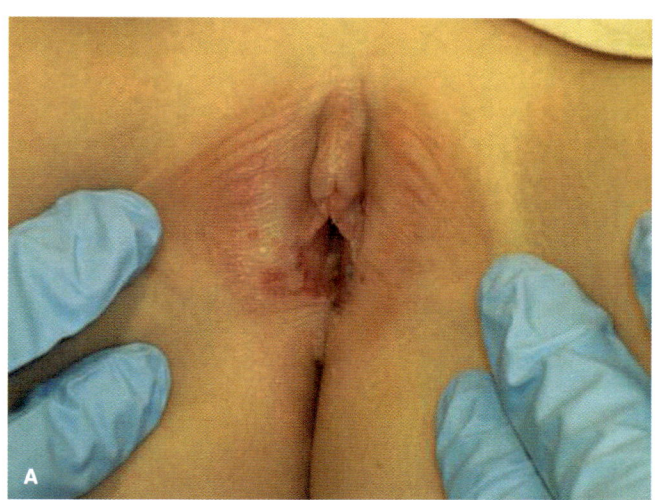

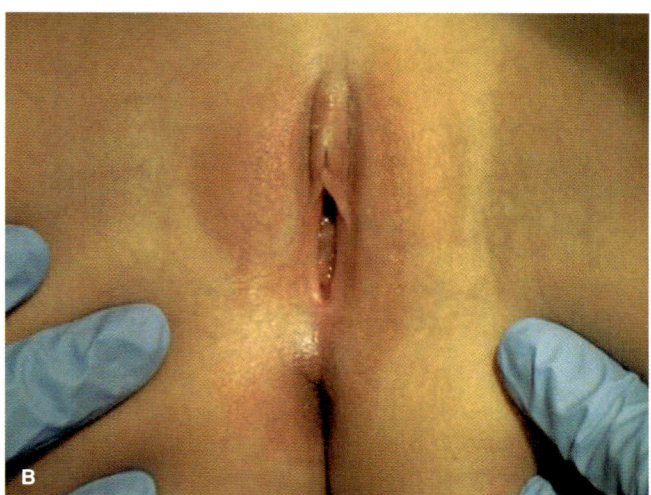

FIGURE 15-8 Lichen sclerosus before and after treatment. **A.** Findings include thin, parchment-like skin on the labia majora, ecchymoses on the labia minora and majora, and mild disease on the perianal skin. Involvement of both the vulva and perianal skin gives a figure-eight shape to affected areas. **B.** Skin texture and ecchymoses improved following treatment. (Reproduced with permission by Dr. Mary Jane Pearson.)

purple vulvar ecchymoses, which may bleed. Over time, if left untreated, the periclitoral area may scar, the labia minora may become attenuated, and the posterior fourchette may fissure and bleed.

Similar to labial adhesion, lichen sclerosus can develop concurrently with hypoestrogenism or with inflammation. Lichen sclerosus more commonly affects postmenopausal women and carries risks for vulvar malignancy. This association is not found in affected pediatric patients. The exact pathophysiology of lichen sclerosus is unknown, but a genetic susceptibility is implicated (Doulaveri, 2013; Sherman, 2010). An autoimmune process is also suspected given its association with Graves thyroiditis, vitiligo, and pernicious anemia (Meyrick Thomas, 1988). Patients may complain of intense itching, discomfort, bleeding, excoriations, and dysuria. Diagnosis typically relies on visual inspection. Rarely, a vulvar biopsy may be indicated in children if the classic skin changes are absent or if lesions are resistant to initial therapy (Bercaw-Pratt, 2014).

Treatment consists of proper hygiene and avoidance of irritants. For mild cases, topical corticosteroid ointment or cream such as 2.5-percent hydrocortisone is applied nightly to the vulva for 6 weeks. If improvement is noted, the dose may be lowered to 1-percent hydrocortisone and continued for 4 to 6 weeks. Thereafter, petroleum-based ointment use and strict attention to hygiene are recommended. Severe cases require a more potent corticosteroid such as 0.05-percent clobetasol propionate (Temovate), applied twice daily for 2 weeks. This initial dosing is followed by an individualized regimen, which slowly tapers the dose to a once-weekly bedtime application. Goals are resolution of skin atrophy, scarring, and symptoms.

The long-term prognosis for childhood lichen sclerosus is unclear. Although some cases resolve at puberty, small case series suggest that as many as 75 percent of affected children have disease that persists or recurs following puberty (Powell, 2002; Smith, 2009).

■ Infection

Some common infectious organisms that may cause prepubertal vulvitis include group A beta-hemolytic streptococcus, *Candida* species, and pinworms. With group A beta-hemolytic streptococcus, the vulva and introitus may be bright "beefy" red, and symptoms include dysuria, vulvar pain, pruritus, or bleeding. In most cases, vulvovaginal culture and clinical setting typically lead to diagnosis. Group A beta-hemolytic streptococcus is treated with an oral first-generation penicillin or cephalosporin or other appropriate antibiotic for 10 days.

Candidiasis is rare in prepubertal girls. It more often develops during the first year of life, after a course of antibiotics, or in females with juvenile diabetes or immunocompromise. A reddened, raised rash with well-demarcated borders and occasional satellite lesions is typical. Microscopic examination of a vaginal sample prepared with 10-percent potassium hydroxide (KOH) will help identify hyphae (Fig. 3-5, p. 64). For treatment, antifungal creams such as clotrimazole, miconazole, or butoconazole are applied to the vulva twice daily for 10 to 14 days or until the rash clears.

Enterobius vermicularis, also known as *pinworm*, can create intense vulvar itching. Nocturnal pruritus results from an intestinal infection with these 1-cm-long threadlike white worms that often exit the anus at night. Inspecting this area with a flashlight at night, parents may identify worms perianally. The "Scotch-tape test" entails pressing a piece of cellophane tape to the perianal area in the morning, affixing the tape to a slide, and visualizing parasite eggs by microscopy. Treatment is albendazole (Albenza) 200 to 400 mg in a single-dose chewable tablet.

VULVOVAGINITIS

Several months after birth, as estrogen levels wane, the vulvovaginal epithelium becomes thin and atrophic. As a result, the vulva and vagina are more susceptible to irritants and infections until puberty, and vulvovaginitis is a common prepubertal problem. Three fourths of vulvovaginitis cases in this age group are nonspecific, with culture results yielding "normal flora." Alternatively, several infectious agents, discussed subsequently, may be identified.

With *nonspecific vulvovaginitis*, the pathogenesis is not well defined, but known instigating factors are included in Table 15-1. Symptoms include itching, vulvar redness, discharge, dysuria, and odor. Most children and those adolescents who are not sexually active tolerate speculum examination poorly. But, a vaginal swab for bacterial culture can be comfortably obtained. In cases of nonspecific vulvovaginitis, cultures typically only isolate normal vaginal flora. Culture results that reveal bowel flora suggest contamination with fecal aerobes. Treatment attempts to correct the underlying cause. Itching and inflammation may be relieved with a low-dose topical corticosteroid ointment such as hydrocortisone, 1 or 2.5 percent. Occasionally, severe itching can lead to a secondary bacterial infection that requires oral antibiotics. Oral agents often selected are amoxicillin, an amoxicillin plus clavulanic acid combination, or a similar cephalosporin given during a 7- to 10-day course.

Infectious vulvovaginitis often presents with a malodorous, yellow or green purulent discharge, and vaginal cultures are routinely obtained in these cases. The respiratory pathogen group A beta-hemolytic streptococcus is the most common specific infectious agent found in prepubertal females. It is isolated from 7 to 20 percent of girls with vulvovaginitis (Pierce, 1992; Piippo, 2000). Treatment of group A beta-hemolytic streptococcus consists of amoxicillin, 40 mg/kg, taken orally three times daily

TABLE 15-1. Causes of Vulvovaginitis in Children

Poor vulvar hygiene
Short distance from the anus to the vagina
Inadequate front-to-back wiping after bowel movements
Lack of labial fat pads and labial hair
Nonestrogenized vulvovaginal epithelium
Vaginal foreign body
Chemical irritants such as soaps
Coexistent eczema or seborrhea
Chronic disease or altered immune status
Sexual abuse

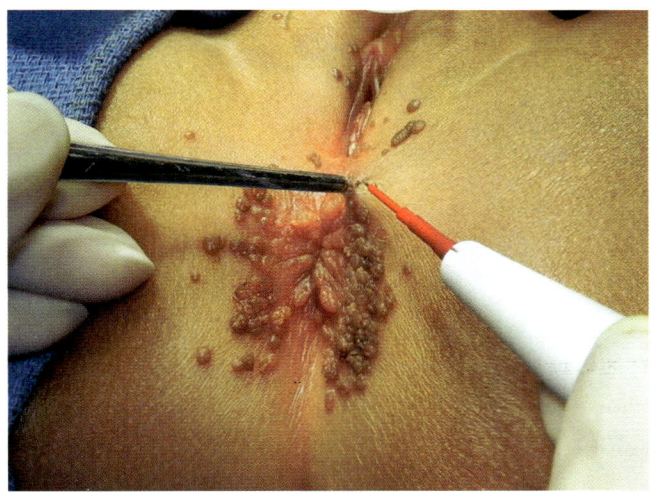

FIGURE 15-9 Surgical excision of extensive vulvar condyloma in a prepubertal girl.

for 10 days. Less frequently, other respiratory pathogens found include *Haemophilus influenzae, Staphylococcus aureus,* and *Streptococcus pneumoniae* (Zuckerman, 2016). Enteric pathogens such as *Shigella* and *Yersinia* species also may be found by culture of vaginal discharge. Classically, *Shigella* species incite a mucopurulent bloody discharge, which typically follows diarrhea caused by the same organism. Treatment is with oral trimethoprim-sulfamethoxazole, 6 to 10 mg/kg/d, divided and given every 12 hours (Bogaerts, 1992).

Sexual abuse may lead to infections including those caused by *Neisseria gonorrhoeae, Chlamydia trachomatis,* HSV, *Trichomonas vaginalis,* and human papillomavirus (HPV). The clinical presentation of each mirrors the infectious findings in adults. Perinatal vertical transmission and latency may permit some of these to persist into infancy and childhood. Long latency and several possible modes of transmission render HPV especially difficult to assign origin (Fig. 15-9) (Unger, 2011). That said, child protective services are notified of any child suspected to be the victim of sexual abuse (Chap. 1, p. 23).

Vulvar aphthous ulcers, described in Chapter 4 (p. 100) cause marked pain. Vulvar mastocytosis and histiocytosis have been also described in prepubertal girls (Jorgensen, 2018; Lawson, 2018). Last, adolescents with inflammatory bowel disease may present with vulvar pain, ulcers, and edema prior to gastrointestinal symptoms (Debiec, 2018).

GENITAL TRAUMA

The prepubertal vulva is less protected from blunt injury due to the lack of labial fat pads. In addition, children are more physically active, thereby raising the trauma risk. Fortunately, most injuries to the vulva are blunt, minor, and accidental. Sharp-object penetration, however, may cause more serious injury to the vulvovaginal area. Sexual or physical abuse is also considered. Management of vulvovaginal trauma is discussed in greater detail in Chapter 4 (p. 107).

OVARIAN TUMORS

Ovarian masses, typically cysts, are common in childhood. They may be found prenatally during maternal sonographic evaluation or during prepubertal years and adolescence. Although most are benign, approximately 1 percent of all malignant tumors in this age group are ovarian (Breen, 1977, 1981).

Fetal and neonatal ovarian cysts are typically identified incidentally during antenatal sonographic examination. Although the true incidence of fetal ovarian cysts is not known, some cystic development has been reported in 30 to 70 percent of fetuses (Brandt, 1991; Lindeque, 1988). Most fetal cysts result from maternal hormonal stimulation in utero. Those during the neonatal period and infancy usually develop from the postnatal gonadotropin surge seen with the withdrawal of maternal hormones after birth. They are usually simple, unilateral, and asymptomatic, and they usually regress spontaneously by 4 months after birth, whether they are simple or complex. The risk of malignancy is low, although rupture, intracystic hemorrhage, visceral compression, and torsion followed by autoamputation of the ovary or adnexa may be complications.

For uncomplicated fetal or neonatal cysts measuring <5 cm in diameter, appropriate management is observation and sonographic examination every 4 to 6 weeks (Bagolan, 2002; Nussbaum, 1988). For simple cysts measuring ≥5 cm, antenatal or neonatal percutaneous cyst aspiration has been described to prevent torsion (Diguisto, 2018; Papic, 2014). Large complex ovarian cysts that do not regress postnatally require surgical excision.

In children, most ovarian masses are cystic and symptoms vary. Asymptomatic cysts may be discovered incidentally during abdominal examination or during sonographic evaluation for some other indication. Enlarging cysts can increase abdominal girth or cause chronic pain. Hormone-secreting cysts may lead to isosexual or heterosexual precocious puberty, and thus evaluation for signs of early pubertal development is indicated. Moreover, rupture, hemorrhage, or torsion may precipitate acute abdominal pain, similar to that seen in adults.

For imaging, a prepubertal child will not tolerate sonographic examination with a transvaginal probe. Thus, in this age group, transabdominal pelvic sonography is most frequently used. Sonographic qualities concerning for ovarian malignancy mirror those found in adults (Renaud, 2019). These are large size; thick, vascular septations; cyst wall excrescences; and mixed cystic with solid architecture (Chap. 10, p. 221). Computed tomography (CT) is helpful if a mature cystic teratoma (dermoid cyst) is suspected, as fat is better appreciated with this modality. Although magnetic resonance (MR) imaging is preferred for congenital müllerian anomaly evaluation, it is less helpful than pelvic sonography for ovarian mass determination.

The most common complex cysts found in childhood and adolescence are germ cell tumors, specifically benign mature cystic teratoma (Panteli, 2009). Rarely, tumors may be malignant germ cell tumors, which are the most common ovarian malignancy in this age group, or may be epithelial or sex cord–stromal ovarian tumors (Baert, 2016).

As with those of the fetal and neonatal periods, small simple ovarian cysts without thick septation or internal echoes may be monitored with serial sonographic examination. Most less than 5 cm will resolve within 1 to 4 months (Thind, 1989). Persistent or enlarging cysts warrant surgery, and laparoscopy is preferred. Optimal management includes fertility-sparing ovarian cystectomy with preservation of normal ovarian tissue.

Following puberty, ovarian cysts in adolescents, as in adults, are frequent. Management mirrors that of adnexal masses found in adults as described in Chapter 10 (p. 219).

BREAST DEVELOPMENT AND DISEASE

Some newborns may have minor breast budding due to transplacental passage of maternal hormones in utero. Similarly, newborn breasts may produce *witches' milk*, which is a bilateral white nipple discharge, also a result of maternal hormone stimulation. Both effects are transient and diminish over several weeks to months.

At puberty, under the influence of ovarian hormones, the breast bud grows rapidly. The epithelial sprouts of the mammary gland branch further and become separated by increasing deposition of fat. Such breast development, termed *thelarche*, begins in most girls between the ages of 8 and 13 years. Thelarche prior to age 8 or lack of breast development by age 13 is considered abnormal and is investigated (p. 321).

Breast examination begins in the newborn period and extends through the prepubertal and adolescent years, as abnormalities can develop in any age group. Assessment includes inspection for accessory nipples, infection, lipoma, fibroadenoma, and premature thelarche.

■ Polythelia

Accessory nipples, also termed *polythelia*, are common and noted in 6 percent of patients (Göttlicher, 1986; Schmidt, 1998). Most frequently, a small areola and nipple are found along the embryonic milk line, which extends from the axilla to the mons pubis bilaterally. Accessory nipples are usually asymptomatic, and excision is not required. Rarely, however, they may contain glandular tissue that can lead to pain, nipple discharge, or development of fibroadenomas.

■ Breast Shape

Growth during early breast development in girls aged 13 to 14 years may be asymmetric. The etiology is not known. However, in some cases, sports injury or surgical trauma during early breast development may lead to asymmetry (van Aalst, 2009). Examination seeks to exclude a breast mass such as a fibroadenoma or cyst. If no mass is identified, then yearly breast examinations determine the extent and persistence of asymmetry. In most cases, asymmetry will resolve by the completion of breast maturity (Templeman, 2000). Therefore, a decision toward surgical intervention is not made until full breast growth is attained. Until that time, adolescents may be fitted with padded bras or even prosthetic inserts to ensure symmetry when fully clothed.

Extremely large breasts without concurrent large breast masses can rarely develop in adolescence. Such breast hypertrophy can incite back pain, shoulder discomfort from

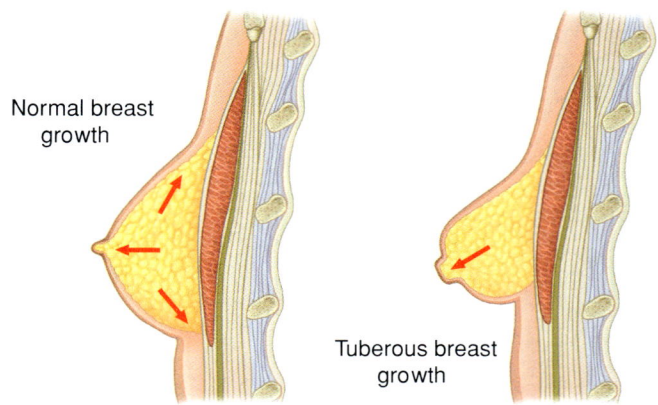

FIGURE 15-10 Comparison of normal and tuberous breast development.

bra-strap pressure, kyphosis, and psychologic distress. These young women will often seek reduction mammoplasty, but surgery is delayed until age 18 years (American College of Obstetricians and Gynecologists, 2017a). Other elements of surgical timing include attainment of breast maturity and stability of bra cup size over 6 months.

Tuberous breasts are another growth variant (Fig. 15-10). With normal development, growth on the breast's ventral surface projects the areola forward, and circumferential peripheral growth enlarges the breast base. In some adolescents, the fascia is densely adhered to the underlying muscle and prohibits peripheral breast growth. Only forward breast growth is permitted, and *tuberous breasts* form (Grolleau, 1999). This appearance can also follow exogenous hormone replacement that may be prescribed to girls with a lack of breast development from genetic, metabolic, or endocrine conditions. To avoid tuberous development in this setting, hormone replacement is initiated at small dosages and gradually increased over time. For example, transdermal estrogen (estradiol patch), 0.025 mg, may be applied twice a week for 6 months, followed by incremental dose increases every 6 months, through doses 0.05 mg and 0.075 mg, to finally reach 0.1 mg twice a week. Medroxyprogesterone acetate (Provera), 10 mg, is given orally each day for 12 days of the month to prompt withdrawal periods. Once estrogen patch dosing has reached 0.1 mg daily, the patient may alternatively be placed on a low-dose oral contraceptive pill instead.

■ Absent Breast Development

Congenital absence of breast glandular tissue, termed *amastia*, is rare. More commonly, a lack of breast development results from low estrogen levels caused by constitutionally delayed puberty, chronic disease, Poland syndrome, radiation or chemotherapy, genetic disorders such as gonadal dysgenesis, or extremes of physical activity. Treatment is based on the etiology. For example, once a competitive athlete completes her career, breast development may begin spontaneously without hormonal treatment. In contrast, to prompt breast development and prevent osteoporosis, patients with gonadal dysgenesis will require some form of hormonal replacement, such as that described in the preceding section.

Breast Mass or Infection

Breast lump complaints in an adolescent often reflect fibrocystic changes. These are characterized by patchy or diffuse, bandlike thickenings. For discrete breast masses, sonography is selected to distinguish cystic from solid masses and to define cyst qualities (Kaneda, 2013). In contrast, mammography has a limited role. Its limited sensitivity and specificity in young, dense breast tissue yields high rates of false-negative results (Williams, 1986).

Actual breast cysts are found on occasion and will usually resolve spontaneously over a few weeks to months. If a cyst is large, persistent, or symptomatic, a fine-needle aspiration may be performed using local analgesia in an office setting.

Similarly, most breast masses in children and adolescents are benign and may include normal but asymmetric breast bud development, fibroadenoma, fibrocyst, lymph node, or abscess. The most common breast mass identified in adolescence is a fibroadenoma, which accounts for 80 to 90 percent of masses (McLaughlin, 2018; Sanders, 2018). Fortunately, breast cancer in pediatric populations is rare, and cancer complicates less than 1 percent of breast masses identified in this group (Gutierrez, 2008). Primary breast cancer may develop more frequently in pediatric patients with a history of prior radiation, especially treatment directed to the chest wall. Additionally, metastatic disease is a consideration in those with a known cancer.

Treatment of breast masses includes observation, needle biopsy, and surgical excision. Observation may be appropriate for small asymptomatic lesions considered to be fibroadenomas. Masses that are symptomatic, large, or enlarging are preferably excised, and techniques mirror those in the adult (Chap. 13, p. 280). For any mass not surgically excised, clinical surveillance is recommended to ensure mass stability.

Mastitis is rare in the pediatric population. Its incidence displays a bimodal distribution that peaks in the neonatal period and again in children older than 10 years. The etiology in these cases is unclear, but the association with breast enlargement during these two periods is implicated. *Staphylococcus aureus* is the most common isolate, and abscess develops more commonly than in the adult (Faden, 2005; Montague, 2013). In adolescents, infections may be associated with lactation and pregnancy, trauma from sexual foreplay, shaving periareolar hair, and nipple piercing (Templeman, 2000; Tweeten, 1998). Infections are treated with antibiotics to cover *S aureus* and occasional drainage if an abscess has formed.

VAGINAL BLEEDING

Neonates may present with vaginal bleeding during the first week of life due to the withdrawal of maternal hormones at birth. Bleeding typically resolves after a few days. Prepubertal bleeding in a child, however, merits careful evaluation (Table 15-2). Most instances of vaginal bleeding in these girls are due to local causes such as lichen sclerosis or urethral prolapse and can be elucidated with a simple history and physical examination. Foreign body is suspected when vaginal bleeding develops in children without signs of puberty or without local findings. Vaginal irrigation can be performed as described earlier (p. 322). Occasionally, an examination under anesthesia with saline vaginoscopy is required

TABLE 15-2. Causes of Vaginal Bleeding in Children

Foreign body
Genital tumors
Urethral prolapse
Lichen sclerosus
Vulvovaginitis
Condyloma acuminata
Trauma
Precocious puberty
Exogenous hormone usage

for diagnosis, particularly if a foreign body is present in the upper vagina (Fig. 15-11).

PRECOCIOUS PUBERTY

Early pubertal development may be seen in both sexes, but females are much more commonly affected, with a sex ratio of 23:1 (Bridges, 1994). For girls, precocious puberty has historically been defined as breast or pubic hair development in those younger than 8 years. However, Herman-Giddens and colleagues (1997) noted that girls in the United States overall are undergoing normal pubertal development at younger ages than previously reported. In addition, racial differences exist. Puberty begins earliest in black girls, followed by Hispanic and white girls. Accordingly, to limit the proportion of girls requiring unneeded assessment for precocious puberty, some have suggested lowering the threshold age for evaluation (Herman-Giddens, 1997; Kaplowitz, 1999).

Premature pubertal development may result from various causes. These have been categorized based on pathogenesis and include central precocious puberty, peripheral precocious puberty, heterosexual precocious puberty, and temporal variation of normal puberty. Most girls evaluated are found to have normal pubertal development that has merely begun prior to standard temporal milestones and does not stem from identifiable

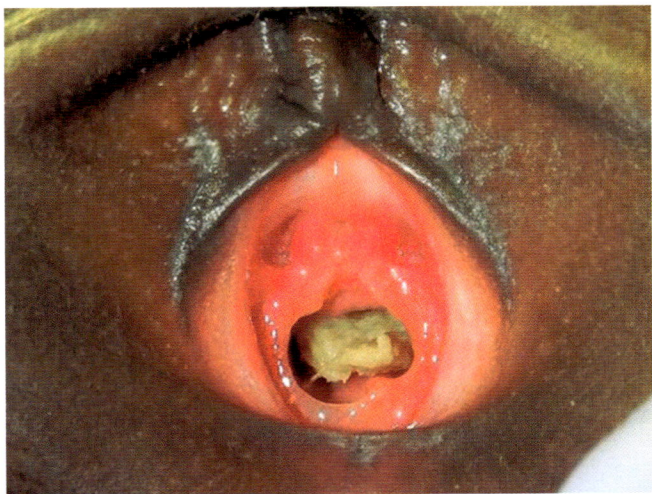

FIGURE 15-11 A clump of retained toilet paper was the foreign body found in this prepubertal girl.

pathology. However, because many of the underlying etiologies of precocious puberty carry significant sequelae, girls with early pubertal development are fully evaluated when identified.

Central Precocious Puberty (Gonadotropin Dependent)

Early activation of the hypothalamic-pituitary-ovarian axis leads to pulsatile GnRH secretion, increased gonadotropin production, and, in turn, higher sex steroid levels. Often termed *true precocious puberty* or *gonadotropin-dependent precocious puberty*, central precocious puberty is rare and affects 1 in 5000 to 10,000 individuals in the general population (Partsch, 2002). The most common cause of central precocious puberty is idiopathic, however, central nervous system lesions must be excluded (Table 15-3) (Muir, 2006; Nathan, 2005).

Symptoms of central precocious puberty are similar to those of normal puberty but at an earlier age. As outlined in Table 15-4, testing includes radiographic measurement of hand and wrist bone age. To explain bone age, as children develop, their bones change in size and shape. These changes can be seen radiographically and can be correlated with chronologic age. Thus, the radiographic "bone age" is the average age at which children in general reach a particular stage of bone maturation. Girls with early estrogen excess from precocious puberty show growth-rate acceleration, rapid bone-age advancement, and early epiphyseal closure, which leads to short stature. If the bone age is advanced by 2 or more years, puberty has begun and evaluation of precocious puberty is indicated. Also during evaluation, pelvic sonography is informative. Uterine length >3.5 cm

TABLE 15-3. Common Etiologies of Precocious Puberty

Central (GnRH-dependent)
Idiopathic[a]
CNS tumors
CNS anomaly
CNS infection
Head trauma
Ischemia
Iatrogenic: radiation, chemotherapy, surgical

Peripheral (GnRH-independent)
Estrogen- or testosterone-producing tumors (adrenal or ovarian)
Gonadotropin- or hCG-producing tumors
Congenital adrenal hyperplasia
Exogenous androgen or estrogen exposure
McCune-Albright syndrome
Ovarian follicular cysts
Primary hypothyroidism
Aromatase excess syndrome
Glucocorticoid resistance

[a]The most common cause of precocious puberty is idiopathic.
CNS = central nervous system; GnRH = gonadotropin-releasing hormone; hCG = human chorionic gonadotropin.

TABLE 15-4. Evaluation of Precocious Puberty[a]

Girls with signs of estrogen excess
Radiographic bone age
FSH, LH, estradiol, TSH
Pelvic sonography
CNS MR imaging
Leuprolide stimulation test may help differentiate premature thelarche from true central and peripheral precocious puberty.

Girls with signs of virilization
Radiographic bone age
FSH, LH, estradiol
DHEAS, testosterone
17α-Hydroxyprogesterone
Androstenedione
11-Deoxycortisol

Pelvic sonography if testosterone elevated
Adrenal imaging if DHEAS elevated

[a]Serum levels of the cited hormones.
CNS = central nervous system; DHEAS = dehydroepiandrosterone sulfate; FSH = follicle-stimulating hormone; GnRH = gonadotropin-releasing hormone; LH = luteinizing hormone; MR = magnetic resonance; TSH = thyroid-stimulating hormone.

indicates estrogen exposure, and multifollicular ovaries reflect central stimulation (Sultan, 2018). In addition, serum FSH, LH, and estradiol levels are elevated for chronologic age and typically lie in the pubertal range. Early in the process, however, FSH and LH levels may be elevated only in the evenings, and a leuprolide stimulation test can be diagnostically helpful.

During leuprolide stimulation, baseline FSH, LH, and estradiol levels are obtained. Leuprolide (Lupron), which is an initial GnRH agonist, is given as a single intravenous dose of 20 μg/kg and does not to exceed a total dose of 500 μg. FSH plus LH levels are measured at 1, 2, and 3 hours. An estradiol level is measured at 24 hours. Central precocious puberty is confirmed by a rise in serum LH levels following infusion of the GnRH agonist. In those with elevated gonadotropin levels, MR imaging of the central nervous system may identify a cerebral abnormality associated with central precocious puberty. In contrast, high estradiol levels and low gonadotropin levels during the stimulation test suggest peripheral precocious puberty, described subsequently.

Treatment goals focus on preventing short adult height and limiting the psychologic effects of early pubertal development. Epiphyseal fusion is an estrogen-dependent process. Thus, treatment consists of chronic GnRH agonist therapy with leuprolide. Although this agent acts as an initial stimulus to GnRH release, over time it desensitizes the GnRH receptor. This ultimately downregulates pituitary gonadotropes and in turn inhibits FSH and LH release. As a result, estrogen levels drop, and often breast and uterine sizes regress. If therapy is instituted after menses have begun, menstrual periods will cease. Timing for GnRH therapy discontinuation and reinitiation of pubertal development is determined by the primary therapy goals: maximizing height, synchronizing puberty with peers, and allaying psychological distress. From a review of several studies, the mean age at treatment discontinuation was approximately 11 years (Carel, 2009).

■ Peripheral Precocious Puberty (Gonadotropin Independent)

Less commonly, elevated estrogen levels may originate from a peripheral source, such as an ovarian cyst. Termed *peripheral precocious puberty* or *gonadotropin-independent precocious puberty*, this category is characterized by lack of GnRH pulsatile release and low levels of pituitary gonadotropins, yet elevated serum estrogen concentrations.

Although the originating source is variable, the most common cause is a granulosa cell tumor, which accounts for more than 60 percent of cases (Emans, 2005). Other types of ovarian cysts, adrenal disorders, iatrogenic disorders, and primary hypothyroidism are additional causes (see Table 15-3). McCune-Albright syndrome is characterized by a "triad" of polyostotic fibrous dysplasia, irregular café-au-lait spots, and endocrinopathies. Precocious puberty is a frequent finding and results from estrogen production in the ovarian cysts that are common in these girls.

Testing of girls with peripheral precocious puberty finds estrogen levels that are characteristically elevated, whereas serum levels of LH and FSH are low. Bone age determination shows advanced aging, and GnRH stimulation shows no elevation in serum LH levels. Pelvic sonography helps to identify ovarian cysts or tumors.

Treatment aims to eliminate excess estrogen. For those with exogenous exposure, halting the estrogen source, such as hormonal pills or creams, is sufficient. An estrogen-secreting ovarian or adrenal tumor will require surgical excision, and hypothyroidism is treated with thyroid hormone replacement.

■ Heterosexual Precocious Puberty

Androgen excess with signs of virilization is rare in childhood (Chap. 18, p. 397). Termed *heterosexual precocious puberty*, this condition is most commonly caused by increased androgen secretion in young females from the adrenal gland or ovary. Causes include androgen-secreting ovarian or adrenal tumors, congenital adrenal hyperplasia, Cushing syndrome, and exposure to exogenous androgens. Testing is outlined in Table 15-4. Treatment is directed at correction of the underlying etiology.

■ Variations of Normal Puberty

Although standardized age guidelines accurately reflect the timing of pubertal development in most girls, others begin development early. Premature thelarche, premature adrenarche, and premature menarche describe the premature pubertal development of breast tissue, pubic hair, and menses, respectively. Each develops in isolation and without other evidence of pubertal development.

Premature thelarche is a diagnosis of exclusion but is suggested if the bone age is normal and falls within 2 standard deviations of chronologic age. Normal prepubertal FSH and LH levels, normal or slightly elevated estradiol levels, normal pelvic sonographic findings, and normal growth are noted. Slightly elevated serum estradiol levels are seen more commonly in those who were very low-birthweight neonates (Klein, 1999; Nelson, 1983). Treatment consists of careful surveillance and reassurance that the remainder of pubertal development will progress at a normal age.

Adrenarche is the onset of dehydroepiandrosterone (DHEA) and DHEA sulfate (DHEAS) production from the adrenal zona reticularis, which can be detected around age 6 years. The phenotypic result of adrenarche is axillary and pubic hair development, termed *pubarche*, which begins in girls at approximately age 8 years (Auchus, 2004). *Premature adrenarche* is defined therefore as the growth of pubic hair prior to age 8, but other signs of estrogenization or virilization are absent. Most girls will have an elevated DHEAS level, which suggests that the adrenal gland is maturing prematurely (Korth-Schultz, 1976). Some girls with premature adrenarche are found to later develop polycystic ovarian syndrome in adolescence (Ibanez, 1993; Miller, 1996). Others have a partial deficiency of 21-hydroxylase. Therefore, girls with premature adrenarche are screened for precocious puberty. When isolated, premature adrenarche treatment includes reassurance and monitoring at 3- to 6-month intervals for other signs of puberty.

Uterine bleeding that occurs once for several days or monthly, without other signs of puberty, is termed *premature menarche*. The condition is rare, and other sources of bleeding are considered and excluded first.

DELAYED PUBERTY

Puberty is considered delayed if no secondary sexual characteristics are noted by age 13, which is more than 2 standard deviations from the mean age. It is also considered delayed if menses have not commenced by age 15 or within 3 years of thelarche. Delayed puberty affects 3 percent of adolescents. Causes include those in Table 15-5. With the exception of constitutional delay, these other abnormalities are discussed in greater detail in Chapters 17, 18, and 19.

Constitutional delay is the most common cause, and adolescents lack both secondary sexual characteristics and pubertal growth spurt by age 13 years (Albanese, 1995; Malasanoa, 1997). The probable cause is a delay in reactivation of the GnRH pulse generator (Layman, 1994). Patients may be started on low-dose estrogen until puberty progresses, at which point estrogen may be discontinued. During low-dose estrogen treatment, it is not necessary to introduce progesterone withdrawal because in early puberty there is a similar long period of unopposed estrogen prior to ovulatory cycling.

SEXUALITY

■ Gender Identity

In most cases, phenotypic gender directs rearing practices, and girls are "raised as girls" and boys are "raised as boys." Gender-appropriate clothes and behaviors are adopted by the child and reinforced by parental approval. Practices in conflict with

TABLE 15-5. Causes of Delayed Puberty

Constitutional (physiologic delay)[a]

Chronic anovulation (PCOS)

Anatomic: outlet obstruction or agenesis

Androgen insensitivity syndrome

Hypergonadotropic hypogonadism
Gonadal dysgenesis (Turner syndrome)
Pure gonadal dysgenesis (46,XX or 46,XY)
Premature ovarian failure

Hypogonadotropic hypogonadism
Central nervous system (CNS)
  CNS tumor, infection, or trauma
  Chronic disease
  GnRH deficiency (Kallman syndrome)
  Isolated gonadotropin deficiency
  Hypothyroidism
  Hyperprolactinoma
Adrenal
  Congenital adrenal hyperplasia
  Cushing syndrome
  Addison disease
Psychosocial
  Eating disorders
  Excessive exercise
  Stress, depression

[a]The most common cause of delayed puberty is constitutional delay.
GnRH = gonadotropin-releasing hormone;
PCOS = polycystic ovarian syndrome.

gender are generally discouraged. However, young children will often explore various behaviors, both masculine and feminine, which make up normal experiences in the process of sex-role socialization (Mischel, 1970; Serbin, 1980).

In cases of ambiguous genitalia in the newborn, sexual assignment is more challenging. Initially, life-threatening disease such as congenital adrenal hyperplasia is excluded. As outlined in Chapter 19, gender assignment may be best delayed until test results identify genetic gender and the underlying problem. The final gender assignment in such cases is termed the sex of rearing and reflects the pattern of gender behavior to be emphasized. The final determination for the *sex of rearing* is based not only on the individual's karyotype but also on the functional capacity of their external genitalia. Early reconstructive surgery is performed less frequently. Instead, delays allow time for intersex children to reach an age of autonomous decision making, usually 18 years, regarding gender-defining surgery and hormone replacement.

Gender dysphoria describes individuals who perceive themselves to be different from their assigned gender. In the *Diagnostic and Statistical Manual of Mental Disorders, Fifth Edition* (DSM-5), this is a recognized psychiatric diagnosis but is not considered a psychiatric disorder (American Psychiatric Association, 2013). That said, the discordance may cause depression and anxiety. At our institution, the Gender Education and Care Interdisciplinary Support (GENCIS) Clinic provides a multi-disciplinary approach to treating the psychological, social, and medical needs of this population of children. Primary care of the transgender patient is described in Chapter 1 (p. 8).

■ Adolescent Sexuality

Adolescent sexuality develops during a period of rapid change that provides opportunities for adolescents to experience both risk-taking and health-promoting behaviors. Data from a large surveys of U.S. females show the percentage of those who become sexually active rises steadily after age 14, and 55 percent have had intercourse by age 18 (Abma, 2017; Liu, 2015).

Adolescents view providers as an important resource for information and education regarding healthy sexual development. However, many parents and educators oppose sexuality education because of concerns that providing such information will encourage the onset of intercourse, termed *coitarche*, and will raise intercourse frequency. On the contrary, studies find that such education actually lowers the frequency of sexual activity, increases contraceptive use, and reduces rates of unprotected intercourse, pregnancy, and STDs (Chin, 2012).

Oral sex is now more commonplace among adolescents. The National Survey of Family Growth in 2005 reported that one in four adolescents aged 15 to 19 years who had not had vaginal intercourse reported practicing oral sex with an opposite partner. Of those adolescents who practiced sexual intercourse, 83 percent of females and 88 percent of males stated they had engaged in oral sex (Mosher, 2005). Adolescents may see oral sex as an alternative way to maintain their "virginity," prevent pregnancy, or avoid STDs, or they may perceive it as a step on the way to engaging in sexual intercourse with a dating partner.

Sexual activity and partner violence appear to have a frequent association in adolescent populations (Chap. 1, p. 24). For example, Kaestle and Halpern (2005) noted that violent victimization was more likely to occur in romantic relationships that included sexual intercourse (37 percent) compared with those that did not (19 percent). Abma and colleagues (2010) reported that among females with coitarche before age 20, 7 percent described their first intercourse as nonvoluntary.

■ Contraception

Despite wide availability of contraceptive options, nearly one half of pregnancies in the United States are unintended (Finer, 2016). Of adolescents, almost 20 percent do not use contraception at first intercourse (Patel, 2016).

The most commonly used contraceptive by adolescents is the combination oral contraceptive (COC) pill. The intrauterine device (IUD) and the etonogestrel implant are long-acting reversible contraceptives (LARC), which are safe and suitable for adolescents (American College of Obstetricians and Gynecologists, 2017b, 2018a). One study of 179 adolescents found an 85-percent continuation rate after 1 year with the levonorgestrel-releasing IUD (Paterson, 2009). Ideally, this counseling begins prior to onset of sexual activity and includes discussion of emergency contraception. Many adolescents have misperceptions about contraception, including beliefs that it may cause infertility or birth defects. Such concerns may be important topics during counseling.

Pelvic examination is not necessary when a contraceptive is prescribed if no other complaints are present. Moreover, guidelines from the American College of Obstetricians and Gynecologists (2018b) note that cervical cancer screening does not usually begin until age 21 regardless of sexual activity. HIV-positive status is an exception, and full screening recommendations are described in Chapter 29 (p. 630). Sexually active adolescents are counseled and screened for gonorrhea and chlamydial infection (U.S. Preventive Services Task Force, 2014). For adolescents, the preferred method is collection of a urine sample for nucleic acid amplification testing (NAAT). If positive, repeat testing follows 3 months after treatment. Other STDs are screened as clinically indicated.

HPV vaccination also can be offered, and the currently available vaccine in the United States is Gardasil 9. It is now approved by the Food and Drug Administration (2018) for females or males aged 9 through 45 years. Ideally at age 11 or 12 years, a series of two doses is provided. After the first dose, a second follows 6 to 12 months later. After age 15, three doses are needed (Robinson, 2017). In this instance, a second dose is administered 1 to 2 months later, and a third dose is given 6 months after the initial one. These vaccines are discussed further in Chapter 29 (p. 625).

To smooth the transition to adult care, the American College of Obstetricians and Gynecologists (2017c) has published guidelines, which include ages 18 to 26 years. Providers ideally discuss and screen for sexual and mental health, sleep disorders, nutrition, safety, and substance abuse.

REFERENCES

Abma JC, Martinez GM: Sexual activity and contraceptive use among teenagers in the United States, 2011–2015. Natl Health Stat Report 104:1, 2017

Abma JC, Martinez GM, Copen CE: Teenagers in the United States: sexual activity, contraceptive use, and childbearing, National Survey of Family Growth 2006–2008. National Center for Health Statistics. Vital Health Stat 23:30, 2010

Aksglaede L, Sørensen K, Petersen JH, et al: Recent decline in age at breast development: the Copenhagen Puberty Study. Pediatrics 123(5):e932, 2009

Albanese A, Stanhope R: Investigation of delayed puberty. Clin Endocrinol 43:105, 1995

American College of Obstetricians and Gynecologists: Breast and labial surgery in adolescents. Committee Opinion No. 686, January 2017a

American College of Obstetricians and Gynecologists: Counseling adolescents about contraception. Committee Opinion No. 710, August 2017b

American College of Obstetricians and Gynecologists: The transition from pediatric to adult health care: preventive care for young women aged 18–26 years. Committee Opinion No. 626, March 2015, Reaffirmed 2017c

American College of Obstetricians and Gynecologists: Adolescents and long-acting reversible contraception: implants and intrauterine devices. Committee Opinion No. 735, May 2018a

American College of Obstetricians and Gynecologists: Cervical cancer screening and prevention. Practice Bulletin No. 168, October 2016, Reaffirmed 2018b

American Psychiatric Association: Diagnostic and Statistical Manual of Mental Disorders, Fifth Edition, DSM-5, Washington, American Psychiatric Association, 2013

Auchus RJ, Rainey WE: Adrenarche—physiology, biochemistry and human disease. Clin Endocrinol 60(3):288, 2004

Bacon JL, Romano ME, Quint EH: Clinical recommendation: labial adhesions. J Pediatr Adolesc Gynecol 28(5):405, 2015

Baert T, Storme N, Van Nieuwenhuysen E, et al: Ovarian cancer in children and adolescents: a rare disease that needs more attention. Maturitas 88:3, 2016

Bagolan P, Giorlandino C, Nahom A, et al: The management of fetal ovarian cysts. J Pediatr Surg 37:25, 2002

Baker TG: A quantitative and cytological study of germ cells in human ovaries. Proc R Soc Lond B Biol Sci 158:417, 1963

Bercaw-Pratt JL, Boardman LA, Simms-Cendan JS, et al: Clinical recommendation: pediatric lichen sclerosus. J Pediatr Adolesc Gynecol 27(2):111, 2014

Berenson AB, Heger AH, Hayes JM, et al: Appearance of the hymen in prepubertal girls. Pediatrics 89:3878, 1992

Biro FM, Greenspan LC, Galvez MP, et al: Onset of breast development in a longitudinal cohort. Pediatrics 132(6):1019, 2013

Biro FM, Huang B, Crawford PB, et al: Pubertal correlates in black and white girls. J Pediatr 148(2):234, 2006

Bogaerts J, Lepage P, De Clercq A, et al: Shigella and gonococcal vulvovaginitis in prepubertal central African girls. Pediatr Infect Dis J 11:890, 1992

Brandt ML, Luks FI, Filiatrault D, et al: Surgical indications in antenatally diagnosed ovarian cysts. J Pediatr Surg 26:276, 1991

Breen JL, Bonamo JF, Maxson WS: Genital tract tumors in children. Pediatr Clin North Am 28:355, 1981

Breen JL, Maxson WS: Ovarian tumors in children and adolescents. Clin Obstet Gynecol 20:607, 1977

Bridges NA, Christopher JA, Hindmarsh PC, et al: Sexual precocity: sex incidence and aetiology. Arch Dis Child 70:116, 1994

Buzi F, Pilotta A, Dordoni D, et al: Pelvic ultrasonography in normal girls and in girls with pubertal precocity. Acta Paediatr 87(11):1138, 1998

Carel JC, Eugster EA, Rogol A, et al: Consensus statement on the use of gonadotropin-releasing hormone analogs in children. Pediatrics 123:e752, 2009

Chin HB, Sipe TA, Elder R, et al: The effectiveness of group-based comprehensive risk-reduction and abstinence education interventions to prevent or reduce the risk of adolescent pregnancy, human immunodeficiency virus, and sexually transmitted infections: two systematic reviews for the Guide to Community Preventive Services. Am J Prev Med 42(3):272, 2012

Christensen EH, Oster J: Adhesions of labia minora (synechia vulvae) in childhood: a review and report of fourteen cases. Acta Paediatr Scand 60:709, 1971

Cohen HL, Shapiro M, Mandel F, et al: Normal ovaries in neonates and infants: a sonographic study of 77 patients 1 day to 24 months old. AJR 160:583, 1993

Debiec KE, Lee SD, Wahbeh GT, et al: Outcomes of therapy for vulvar manifestation of inflammatory bowel disease in adolescents. J Pediatr Adolesc Gynecol 31(2):149, 2018

Dietrich JE, Millar DM, Quint EH: Obstructive reproductive tract anomalies. J Pediatr Adolesc Gynecol 27(6):396, 2014

Diguisto C, Winer N, Benoist G, et al: In-utero aspiration vs expectant management of anechoic fetal ovarian cysts: open randomized controlled trial. Ultrasound Obstet Gynecol 52(2):159, 2018

Doulaveri G, Armira K, Kouris A, et al: Genital vulvar lichen sclerosus in monozygotic twin women: a case report and review of the literature. Case Rep Dermatol 5(3):321, 2013

Emans S, Laufer M, Goldstein D: Pediatric and Adolescent Gynecology, 5th ed. Philadelphia: Lippincott Williams & Wilkins, 2005, pp 127, 159

English A, Bass L, Boyle AD, et al: State minor consent laws: a summary, 3rd ed. Chapel Hill, Center for Adolescent Health & the Law, 2010

Faden H: Mastitis in children from birth to 17 years. Pediatr Infect Dis J 24(12):1113, 2005

Finer LB, Zabin LS: Does the timing of the first family planning visit still matter? Fam Plann Perspect 30(1):30, 1998

Finer LB, Zolna MR: Declines in unintended pregnancy in the United States, 2008–2011. N Engl J Med 374(9):843, 2016

Food and Drug Administration: FDA approves expanded use of Gardasil 9 to include individuals 27 through 45 years old. 2018. Available at: https://www.fda.gov/NewsEvents/Newsroom/PressAnnouncements/ucm622715.htm. Accessed November 3, 2018

Fritz M, Speroff L: Clinical Gynecologic Endocrinology and Infertility, 8th ed. Baltimore, Lippincott Williams & Wilkins, 2011, p 393

Göttlicher S: [Incidence and location of polythelias, polymastias and mammae aberratae. a prospective one year study of 1,660 patients of a gynecologic practice]. [German]. Geburtshilfe Frauenheilkd 46(10):697, 1986

Grolleau JL, Lanfrey E, Lavigne B, et al: Breast base anomalies: treatment strategy for tuberous breasts, minor deformities, and asymmetry. Plast Reconstruct Surg 104(7):2040, 1999

Gutierrez JC, Housri N, Koniaris LG et al: Malignant breast cancer in children: a review of 75 patients. J Surg Res 147(2):182, 2008

Guttmacher Institute: An overview of minors' consent law. 2018. Available at: https://www.guttmacher.org/state-policy/explore/overview-minors-consent-law. Accessed December 26, 2018

Herman-Giddens ME, Slora EJ, Wasserman RC, et al: Secondary sexual characteristics and menses in young girls seen in office practice: a study from the Pediatric Research in Office Settings network. Pediatrics 99:505, 1997

Herter LD, Golendziner E, Flores JA, et al: Ovarian and uterine sonography in healthy girls between 1 and 13 years old: correlation of findings with age and pubertal status. AJR Am J Roentgenol 178(6):1531, 2002

Ibanez L, Potau N, Virdis R, et al: Postpubertal outcome in girls diagnosed of premature pubarche during childhood: increased frequency of functional ovarian hyperandrogenism. J Clin Endocrinol Metab 76:1599, 1993

Jorgensen EM, Chen PP, Rutter S, et al: Vulvar lesions in an 8-year-old girl: cutaneous manifestations of multisystem Langerhans cell histiocytosis. J Pediatr Adolesc Gynecol 31(2):153, 2018

Kaestle CE, Halpern CT: Sexual intercourse precedes partner violence in adolescent romantic relationships. J Adolesc Health 36(5):386, 2005

Kaneda HJ, Mack J, Kasales CJ, et al: Pediatric and adolescent breast masses: a review of pathophysiology, imaging, diagnosis, and treatment. AJR Am J Roentgenol 200(2):W204, 2013

Kaplan SL, Edgar JC, Ford EG, et al: Size of testes, ovaries, uterus and breast buds by ultrasound in healthy full-term neonates ages 0–3 days. Pediatr Radiol 46(13):1837, 2016

Kaplowitz PB, Oberfield SE: Reexamination of the age limit for defining when puberty is precocious in girls in the United States: implications for evaluation and treatment. Pediatrics 104:936, 1999

Klein KO, Mericq V, Brown-Dawson JM, et al: Estrogen levels in girls with premature thelarche compared with normal prepubertal girls as determined by an ultrasensitive recombinant cell bioassay. J Pediatr 134:190, 1999

Korth-Shcultz S, Levine LS, New M: Dehydroepiandrosterone sulfate (DS) levels, a rapid test for abnormal adrenal androgen secretion. J Clin Endocrinol Metab 42:1005, 1976

Lawson A, Mir A, Wilson EE: Vulvar nodules: a rare presentation of mastocytosis. J Pediatr Adolesc Gynecol 31(2):156, 2018

Layman LC, Reindollar RH: Diagnosis and treatment of pubertal disorders. Adolesc Med 5:37, 1994

Lindeque BG, du Toit JP, Muller LM, et al: Ultrasonographic criteria for the conservative management of antenatally diagnosed fetal ovarian cysts. J Reprod Med 33:196, 1988

Liu G, Hariri S, Bradley H, et al: Trends and patterns of sexual behaviors among adolescents and adults aged 14 to 59 years, United States. Sex Transm Dis 42(1):20, 2015

Malasanoa TH: Sexual development of the fetus and pubertal child. Clin Obstet Gynecol 40:153, 1997

Marshall WA, Tanner JM: Variations in pattern of pubertal changes in girls. Arch Dis Child 44(235):291, 1969

Mayoglou L, Dulabon L, Martin-Alguacil N, et al: Success of treatment modalities for labial fusion: a retrospective evaluation of topical and surgical treatments. J Pediatr Adolesc Gynecol 22(4):247, 2009

McLaughlin CM, Gonzalez-Hernandez J, Bennett M, et al: Pediatric breast masses: an argument for observation. J Surg Res 228:247, 2018

Meyers JB, Sorenson CM, Wisner BP, et al: Betamethasone cream for the treatment of pre-pubertal labial adhesions. J Pediatr Adolesc Gynecol 19(6):401, 2006

Meyrick Thomas RH, Ridley CM, McGibbon DH, et al: Lichen sclerosus et atrophicus and autoimmunity—a study of 350 women. Br J Dermatol 118(1):41, 1988

Miller DP, Emans SJ, Kohane I: A follow-up study of adolescent girls with a history of premature pubarche. J Adolesc Health 18(4):301, 1996

Mischel W: Sex-typing and socialization. In Mussen PH (ed): Carmichaels Manual of Child Psychology, 3rd ed. New York, Wiley, 1970, p 3

Montague EC, Hilinski J, Andresen D, et al: Evaluation and treatment of mastitis in infants. Pediatr Infect Dis J 32(11):1295, 2013

Mosher WD, Chandra A, Jones J: Sexual behavior and selected health measures: men and women 15–44 years of age, United States, 2002. Adv Data, 362:1, 2005

Muir A: Precocious puberty. Pediatr Rev 27:373, 2006

Nathan BM, Palmert MR: Regulation and disorders of pubertal timing. Endocrinol Metab Clin North Am 34(3):617, 2005

Neely EK, Hintz RL, Wilson DM, et al: Normal ranges for immuno- chemiluminometric gonadotropin assays. J Pediatr 124(1):40, 1995

Nelson KG: Premature thelarche in children born prematurely. J Pediatr 103: 756, 1983

Norris JE, Elder CV, Dunford AM, et al: Spontaneous resolution of labial adhesions in pre-pubertal girls. J Paediatr Child Health 54(7):748, 2018

Nussbaum A, Sanders R, Jones B: Neonatal uterine morphology as seen on real-time US. Radiology 160:641, 1986

Nussbaum AR, Sanders RC, Hartman DS, et al: Neonatal ovarian cysts: sonographic-pathologic correlation. Radiology 168:817, 1988

Panteli C, Curry J, Kiely E, et al: Ovarian germ cell tumours: a 17-year study in a single unit. Eur J Pediatr Surg 19(2):96, 2009

Papic JC, Billmire DF, Rescorla FJ, et al: Management of neonatal ovarian cysts and its effect on ovarian preservation. J Pediatr Surg 49(6):990, 2014

Partsch CJ, Heger S, Sippell WG: Management and outcome of central precocious puberty. Clin Endocrinol 56(2):129, 2002

Patel PR, Lee J, Hirth J, et al: Changes in the use of contraception at first intercourse: a comparison of National Survey of Family Growth 1995 and 2006–2010 databases. J Womens Health 25(8):777, 2016

Paterson H, Ashton J, Harrison-Woolrych M: A nationwide cohort study of the use of the levonorgestrel intrauterine device in New Zealand adolescents. Contraception 79(6):433, 2009

Pierce AM, Hart CA: Vulvovaginitis: causes and management. Arch Dis Child 67:509, 1992

Piippo S, Lenko H, Vuento R: Vulvar symptoms in paediatric and adolescent patients. Acta Paediatr 89:431, 2000

Powell J, Wojnarowska F: Childhood vulvar lichen sclerosus: an increasingly common problem. J Am Acad Dermatol 44(5):803, 2001

Powell J, Wojnarowska F: Childhood vulvar lichen sclerosus. The course after puberty. J Reprod Med 47(9):706, 2002

Renaud EJ, Sømme S, Islam S, et al: Ovarian masses in the child and adolescent: an American Pediatric Surgical Association Outcomes and Evidence-Based Practice Committee systematic review. J Pediatr Surg 54(3):369, 2019

Resende EA, Lara BH, Reis JD, et al: Assessment of basal and gonadotropin-releasing hormone-stimulated gonadotropins by immunochemiluminometric and immunofluorometric assays in normal children. J Clin Endocrinol Metab 92(4):1424, 2007

Robinson CL, Romero JR, Kempe A, et al: Advisory Committee on Immunization Practices recommended immunization schedule for children and adolescents ages 18 years or younger – United States, 2017. MMWR 66(5):134, 2017

Rosenfield RL, Lipton RB, Drum ML: Thelarche, pubarche, and menarche attainment in children with normal and elevated body mass index. Pediatrics 123:84, 2009

Sanders LM, Sharma P, El Madany M, et al: Clinical breast concerns in low-risk pediatric patients: practice review with proposed recommendations. Pediatr Radiol 48(2):186, 2018

Schmidt H: Supernumerary nipples: prevalence, size, sex and side predilection—a prospective clinical study. Eur J Pediatr 157(10):821, 1998

Serbin LA: Sex-role socialization: a field in transition. In Lahey BB, Kazdin AE (eds): Advances in Clinical Child Psychology, Vol 3. New York, Plenum Publishing, 1980, p 41

Sherman V, McPherson T, Baldo M, et al: The high rate of familial lichen sclerosus suggests a genetic contribution: an observational cohort study. J Eur Acad Dermatol Venereol 24(9):1031, 2010

Smith SD, Fischer G: Childhood onset vulvar lichen sclerosus does not resolve at puberty: a prospective case series. Pediatr Dermatol 26(6):725, 2009

Sultan C, Gaspari L, Maimoun L, et al: Disorders of puberty. Best Pract Res Clin Obstet Gynaecol 48:62, 2018

Tanner JM: Trend toward earlier menarche in Long, Oslo, Copenhagen, the Netherlands and Hungary. Nature 243:95, 1973

Tanner JM, Davies PWS: Clinical longitudinal standards for height and height velocity for North American children. J Pediatr 107:317, 1985

Templeman C, Hertweck SP: Breast disorders in the pediatric and adolescent patient. Obstet Gynecol Clin North Am 27(1):19, 2000

Thind CR, Carty HM, Pilling DW: The role of ultrasound in the management of ovarian masses in children. Clin Radiol 40:180, 1989

Tweeten SS, Rickman LS: Infectious complications of body piercing. Clin Infect Dis 26(3):735, 1998

Unger ER, Fajman NN, Maloney EM, et al: Anogenital human papillomavirus in sexually abused and nonabused children: a multicenter study. Pediatrics 128(3):e658, 2011

U.S. Preventive Services Task Force: The Guide to Clinical Preventive Services, 2014. Rockville, 2014

van Aalst JA, Phillips JD, Sadove AM: Pediatric chest wall and breast deformities. Plast Reconstr Surg 124(1 Suppl):38e, 2009

Vaskivuo TE, Anttonen M, Herva R, et al: Survival of human ovarian follicles from fetal to adult life: apoptosis, apoptosis-related proteins, and transcription factor GATA-4. J Clin Endocrinol Metab 86:3421, 2001

Williams SM, Kaplan PA, Peterson JC, et al: Mammography in women under age 30: is there clinical benefit? Radiology 161:49, 1986

Ziereisen F, Guissard G, Damry N, et al: Sonographic imaging of the paediatric female pelvis. Eur Radiol 15:1296, 2005

Zuckerman A, Romano M: Clinal recommendation: vulvovaginitis. J Pediatr Adolesc Gynecol 29(6):673, 2016

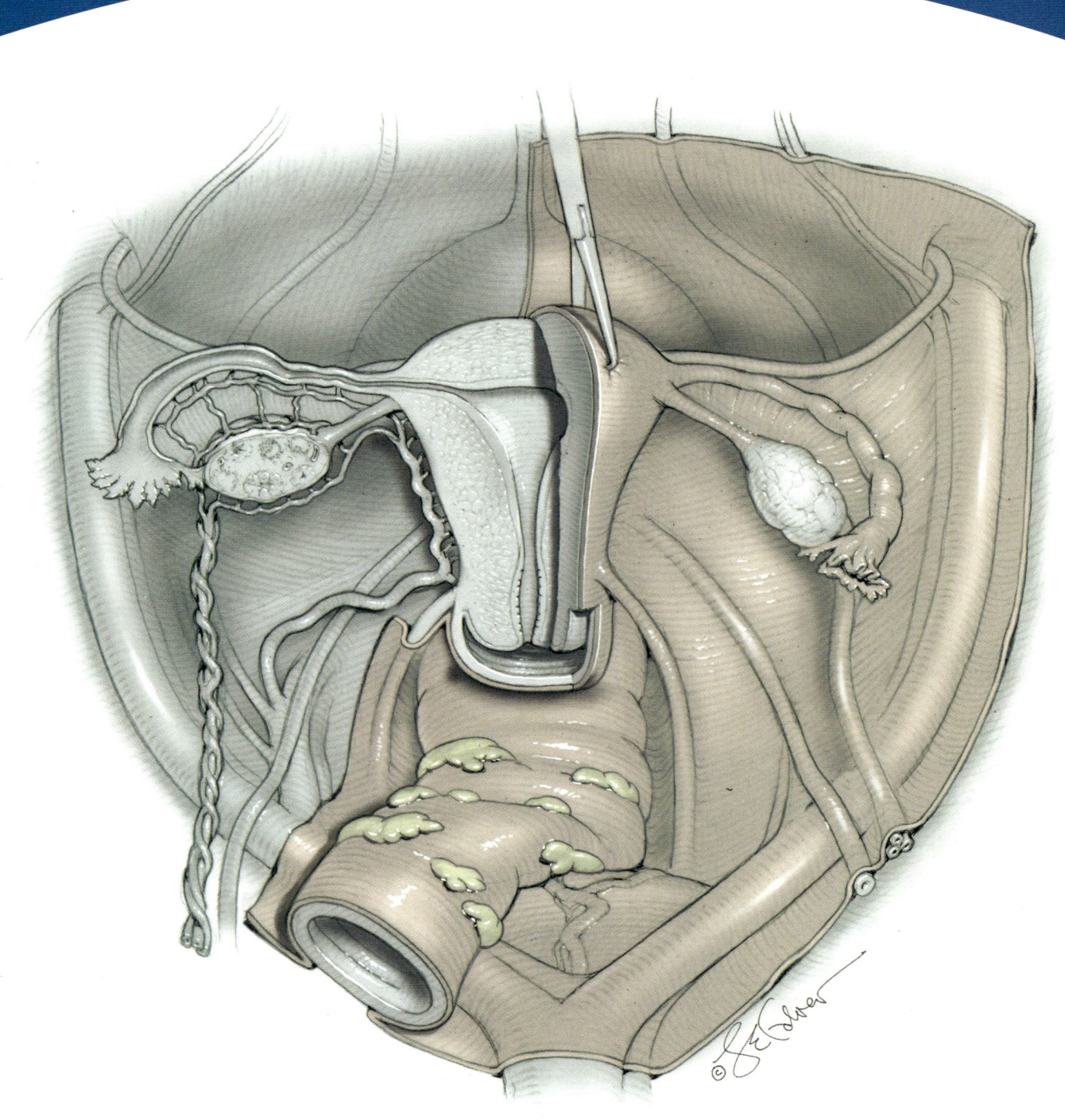

CHAPTER 16

Reproductive Endocrinology

Reproductive endocrinology is the study of hormones and neuroendocrine factors that are produced by and/or affect reproductive tissues. These tissues include the hypothalamus, anterior pituitary gland, ovary, endometrium, and placenta. A hormone is classically described as a cell product that is secreted into the peripheral circulation and that exerts its effects in distant target tissues (Fig. 16-1). This is termed *endocrine secretion*. Additional forms of cell-to-cell communication exist in reproductive physiology. *Paracrine* communication, common within the ovary, refers to chemical signaling between neighboring cells. *Autocrine* communication occurs when a cell releases substances that influence its own function. Production of a substance within a cell that affects that cell before secretion is termed an *intracrine* effect.

Neurotransmitters, in classic neural pathways, cross a small extracellular space called a synaptic junction and bind to dendrites of a second neuron (Fig. 16-2). Alternatively, these factors are secreted into the vascular system and are transported to other tissues where they exert their effects in a process termed *neuroendocrine secretion* or *neuroendocrine signaling*. One example is gonadotropin-releasing hormone (GnRH) secretion into the portal vasculature with effects on the gonadotropes within the anterior pituitary gland.

Normal reproductive function requires precise quantitative and temporal regulation of the hypothalamic-pituitary-ovarian

axis (Fig. 16-3). Within the hypothalamus, specific centers or nuclei release GnRH in pulses. This decapeptide binds to surface receptors on the gonadotrope subpopulation of the anterior pituitary gland. In response, gonadotropes secrete glycoprotein gonadotropins—namely, luteinizing hormone (LH) and follicle-stimulating hormone (FSH)—into the peripheral circulation. Within the ovary, LH and FSH bind to the theca and granulosa cells to stimulate folliculogenesis and ovarian production of steroid hormones (estrogens, progesterone, and androgens), gonadal peptides (activin, inhibin, and follistatin), and growth factors. Among other functions, these ovarian-derived

Endocrine action

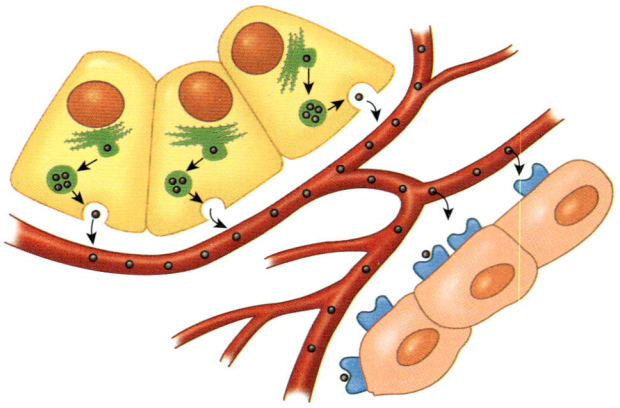

Paracrine action

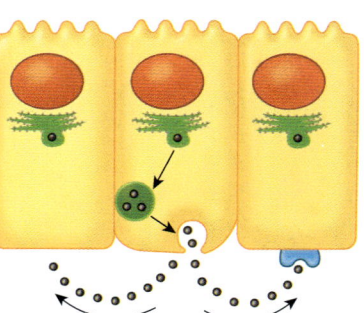

Autocrine action

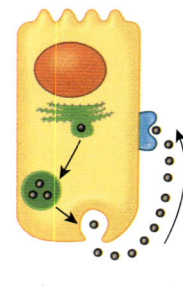

FIGURE 16-1 Different types of hormone communication. Endocrine: hormones travel through the circulation to reach their target cells. Paracrine: hormones diffuse through the extracellular space to reach their target cells, which are neighboring cells. Autocrine: hormones feed back on the cell of origin, without entering the circulation.

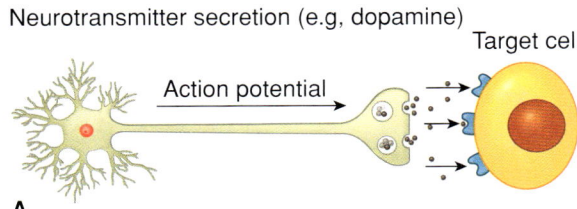

Neurotransmitter secretion (e.g, dopamine)

A

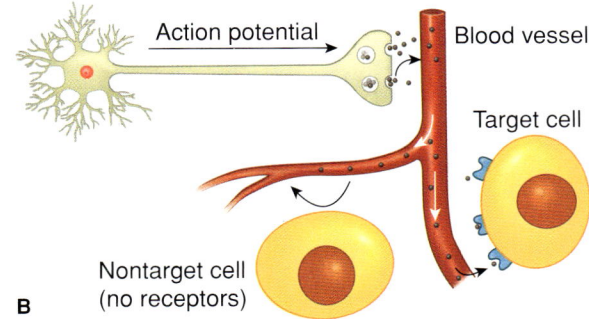

Neurohormone secretion (e.g, GnRH)

B

FIGURE 16-2 Types of neurotransmitter secretion. **A.** Classic neurotransmitter release and binding. Transmission of an action potential down a neural axon leads to release of neurotransmitters, which travel across a synaptic cleft to reach their target cell. **B.** Neurohormonal secretion. An action potential leads to release of neurotransmitters. In this instance, neurotransmitters enter into and travel through the circulation to reach their target organ.

factors feed back to the hypothalamus and pituitary gland to inhibit or, at the midcycle surge, to augment GnRH and gonadotropin secretion. The ovarian steroids are also critical for preparing the endometrium for placental implantation if pregnancy ensues.

HORMONE BIOSYNTHESIS AND MECHANISM OF ACTION

Hormones can be broadly classified as either steroids or peptides, each with their own mode of biosynthesis and mechanism of action. The receptors for these hormones can be divided into two groups. The first are receptors present on the cell surface, which in general bind water-soluble hormones, namely peptides. The second are primarily intracellular and bind lipophilic hormones such as steroids. Hormones are normally present in serum and tissues in very low concentrations. Therefore, receptors must have both high affinity and high specificity for their ligand to produce the correct biologic response.

◼ Peptide Hormones: LH, FSH, and hCG

The gonadotropins LH and FSH are biosynthesized and secreted by the gonadotrope subpopulation of the anterior pituitary gland. These hormones play a critical role in stimulating ovarian steroidogenesis, follicular development, and ovulation. The closely related peptide human chorionic gonadotropin (hCG) is produced by placental trophoblast and is important for pregnancy maintenance.

LH, FSH, and hCG are heterodimers consisting of a common glycoprotein α-subunit linked to a unique β-subunit. This β-subunit provides functional specificity. Although glycoprotein α- and β-subunits can be found in their unassociated form in the circulation, these "free" subunits lack biologic activity. Nevertheless, their measurement may be useful in screening tests for conditions such as pituitary adenomas and pregnancy.

The LH and hCG β-subunits are encoded by two separate genes within a gene grouping called the LH/CG cluster. The amino acid sequence of the human LH and CG β-subunits demonstrates approximately 80-percent similarity. However, the hCG β-subunit contains an additional 24-amino-acid extension on the carboxy terminus. The presence of these

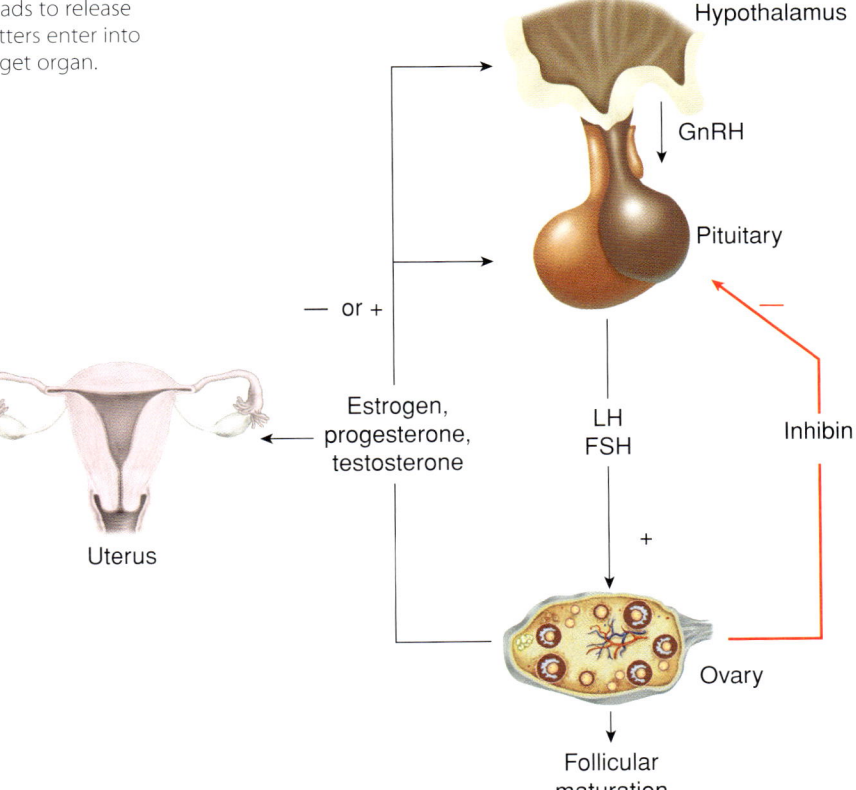

Female Reproductive Axis

FIGURE 16-3 Positive and negative feedback loops seen with the hypothalamic-pituitary-ovarian axis. Pulsatile release of gonadotropin-releasing hormone (GnRH) leads to release of luteinizing hormone (LH) and follicle-stimulating hormone (FSH) from the anterior pituitary. Effects of LH and FSH result in follicle maturation, ovulation, and production of the sex steroid hormones (estrogen, progesterone, and testosterone). Rising serum levels of these hormones exert negative feedback inhibition on GnRH and gonadotropin release. Sex steroid hormones vary in their effects on the endometrium and myometrium as discussed in the text. Inhibin, produced in the ovary, has a negative effect on gonadotropin release.

additional amino acids has allowed the development of highly specific assays that can distinguish LH from hCG.

In pituitary thyrotropes, the glycoprotein α-subunit interacts with the specific thyroid-stimulating hormone β-subunit to form thyroid-stimulating hormone (TSH). The similarity between TSH and hCG can have clinical implications. For example, molar pregnancies frequently produce very high levels of hCG, which can bind to TSH receptors, resulting in hyperthyroidism (Walkington, 2011).

Human Chorionic Gonadotropin

This glycosylated peptide hormone is produced by the placental syncytiotrophoblast. With hCG, the degree and type of glycosylated moieties attached to its peptide frame vary and may indicate pregnancy stage, placental function, or pathology (Fournier, 2015). One example is the hyperglycosylated hCG that is found more commonly in gestational trophoblastic neoplasia (GTN) (Chap. 37, p. 780).

hCG can be detected in serum as early as 7 to 9 days after the LH surge. In early pregnancy, hCG levels rise rapidly, doubling approximately every 2 days. Levels of this peptide hormone peak at approximately 100,000 mIU/mL during the first trimester of pregnancy. This is followed by a relatively sharp decline in early second-trimester concentrations and maintenance of lower levels throughout the remainder of pregnancy.

In early pregnancy, hCG binds to LH/CG receptors on corpus luteum cells and stimulates steroidogenesis in the ovary. To maintain endometrial integrity and uterine quiescence, hCG levels are critical for corpus luteum steroid production during early pregnancy before the placenta attains adequate steroidogenic capability. The transfer in production of estrogens and progesterone from the ovary to the placenta is often called the *luteal-placental shift*. In addition to effects on ovarian function, hCG exerts autocrine/paracrine effects in the placenta, promoting syncytiotrophoblast formation, trophoblast invasion, and angiogenesis.

As the placenta is the primary source for hCG production, measurement of plasma hCG levels has proved to be an effective screening tool for pregnancies with altered placental mass or function. Relatively elevated levels of hCG are observed in multifetal gestations and fetuses with Down syndrome. Markedly abnormal elevations in hCG levels are most often observed with GTN.

Lower hCG levels are observed in cases of poor placentation including ectopic pregnancy or spontaneous miscarriage. Recent efforts have focused on the development of algorithms using serial hCG levels and sonographic findings to accurately determine the status of a pregnancy of undetermined location (PUL) (Zee, 2014). Serial hCG measurements are helpful because the doubling time in normal pregnancy is relatively reliable.

hCG is also secreted by nontrophoblastic neoplasias and can serve as a useful tumor marker. Ectopic (nonplacental) production of hCG, either the intact dimer or the β-subunit, is frequently associated with germ cell tumors and has been reported in various tumors arising from the mucosal epithelium of the cervix, bladder, lung, gastrointestinal (GI) tract,

and nasopharynx. It has been postulated that hCG inhibits apoptosis in these tumors and thereby allows rapid growth.

In addition to secretion by placental syncytiotrophoblast, hCG is produced by other cell types and presumably serves other functions (Cole, 2010). For example, cytotrophoblasts secrete a hyperglycosylated variant of hCG that may prove to be a sensitive marker of early pregnancy (Chuan, 2014). The pituitary gonadotropes also make small amounts of hCG. These concentrations rise in postmenopausal women and may be a rare cause of erroneously positive hCG testing in this age group (Cole, 2008).

◼ Steroid Hormones

Classification

Sex steroids are divided into three groups based on the number of carbon atoms that they contain. Each carbon in this structure is assigned a number identifier, and each ring is assigned a letter (**Fig. 16-4**). The 21-carbon series includes progestogens, glucocorticoids, and mineralocorticoids. Androgens contain 19 carbons, whereas estrogens have 18.

Steroids are given scientific names according to a generally accepted convention in which functional groups below the plane of the molecule are preceded by the α symbol and those above the plane of the molecule are indicated by a β symbol. A Δ symbol indicates a double bond. Those steroids with a double bond between carbon atoms 5 and 6 are called Δ^5 *steroids* and include pregnenolone, 17-hydroxypregnenolone, and dehydroepiandrosterone. Those with a double bond between carbons 4 and 5 are termed Δ^4 *steroids* and include progesterone, 17-hydroxyprogesterone, androstenedione, testosterone, mineralocorticoids, and glucocorticoids.

Steroidogenesis

Sex steroid hormones are synthesized in the gonads, adrenal gland, and placenta. Cholesterol is the primary building block. All steroid-producing tissues, except the placenta, are capable of synthesizing cholesterol from the two-carbon precursor, acetate. Steroid hormone production, which involves at least 17 enzymes, primarily occurs in the mitochondria and the abundant smooth endoplasmic reticulum found in steroidogenic

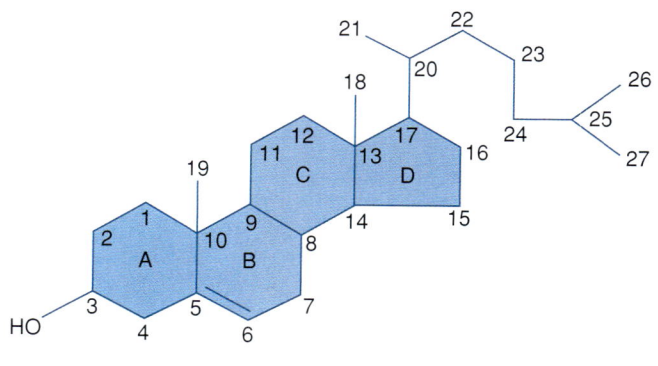

Cholesterol

FIGURE 16-4 The chemical structure of cholesterol, which is the common precursor in sex-steroid biosynthesis. All sex steroids contain the basic cyclopentanophenanthrene molecule, which consists of three 6-carbon rings and one 5-carbon ring.

TABLE 16-1. Steroidogenic Enzymes

Enzyme	Cellular Location	Reactions
P450scc	Mitochondria	Cholesterol side-chain cleavage
P450c11	Mitochondria	11-Hydroxylase 18-Hydroxylase 19-Methyloxidase
P450c17	ER	17-Hydroxylase 17,20-Lyase
P450c21	ER	21-Hydroxylase
P450arom	ER	Aromatase

ER = endoplasmic reticulum.

cells (Mason, 2002). These enzymes are members of the cytochrome P450 superfamily. As such, genes that encode these enzymes begin with *CYP*.

Steroidogenic enzymes catalyze four basic modifications of the steroid structure. These are: (1) side-chain cleavage (desmolase reaction), (2) conversion of hydroxyl groups to ketones (dehydrogenase reactions), (3) addition of a hydroxyl group (hydroxylation reaction), and (4) removal or addition of hydrogen to create or reduce a double bond (lyase reaction) (Table 16-1). The steroid biosynthesis pathway in simplified form is shown in

Figure 16-5. This pathway is identical in all steroidogenic tissues. However, the distribution of products synthesized by each tissue is determined by the presence of requisite enzymes. For example, the ovary is deficient in 21-hydroxylase and 11β-hydroxylase and thus is unable to produce corticosteroids. Of note, many steroidogenic enzymes exist as multiple isoforms, each with different precursor preferences and directional activities. As a result, specific steroids may be produced via multiple pathways in addition to the classic pathway shown in Figure 16-5 (Auchus, 2009).

Of specific hormones, estrogens are synthesized by aromatization of C19 androgens by *aromatase*. This enzyme is a cytochrome P450 enzyme encoded by the gene *CYP19*. In addition to the ovary, aromatase is expressed in significant levels in adipose tissue, skin, and brain (Boon, 2010). Importantly, sufficient estrogen can be derived from peripheral aromatization to produce endometrial bleeding in postmenopausal women, especially those who are overweight or obese.

Circulating estrogens in the reproductive-aged female include estradiol (E_2), estrone (E_1), and estriol (E_3). Estradiol is the primary estrogen produced by the ovary during reproductive years. Levels are derived both from direct synthesis in the granulosa cells of developing follicles and through conversion of the less potent estrone. Estrone, the primary estrogen during menopause, is secreted mainly by the ovary. Estriol, the predominant estrogen during pregnancy, is secreted primarily from the placenta. However, both estrone and estriol can be derived from androstenedione in the periphery.

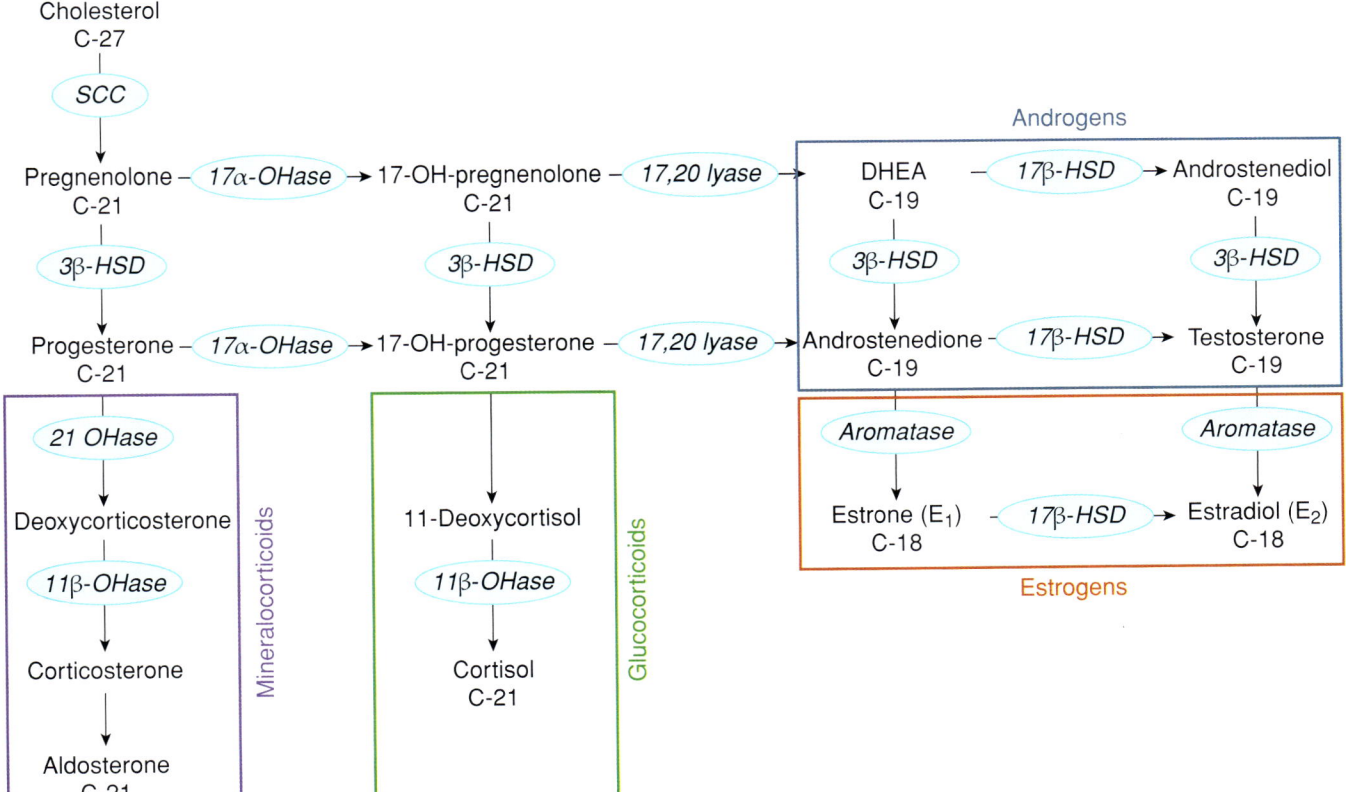

FIGURE 16-5 Steps in the steroidogenesis pathway. Enzymes are found within the blue ovals. The C18, C19, or C21 designation beneath the sex steroid reflects the number of carbon atoms it contains. Colored boxing groups these pathway products. 3β-HSD = 3β-hydroxysteroid dehydrogenase; 11β-OHase = 11β-hydroxylase; 17α-OHase = 17α-hydroxylase; 17β-HSD = 17β-hydroxysteroid dehydrogenase; 21OHase = 21-hydroxylase; DHEA = dehydroepiandrosterone; SCC = side-chain cleavage enzyme.

Within androgen synthesis, the 5α-reductase enzyme converts testosterone to dihydrotestosterone (DHT), a more potent androgen. DHT promotes transformation of vellus hair to terminal hair. Thus, medications that antagonize 5α-reductase are often effective in the treatment of hirsutism (Stout, 2010). This enzyme exists in two forms, each encoded by a separate gene. The type 1 enzyme is found in the skin, brain, liver, and kidneys. In contrast, the type 2 enzyme is expressed predominantly in male genitalia (Russell, 1994).

The ovary also produces androgens in response to LH stimulation of theca cell function. The two primary products are the relatively weak androgens androstenedione and dehydroepiandrosterone (DHEA). Smaller amounts of testosterone also are secreted. Although the adrenal cortex mainly produces mineralocorticoids and glucocorticoids, it also contributes to approximately one half of the daily production of androstenedione and DHEA and essentially all of the sulfated form of DHEA (DHEAS). In women, 25 percent of circulating testosterone is secreted by the ovary, 25 percent is secreted by the adrenal gland, and the remaining 50 percent is produced by peripheral conversion of androstenedione to testosterone (Table 16-2) (Silva, 1987).

The adult adrenal gland is composed of three zones. Each zone expresses a different complement of steroidogenic enzymes and as a result synthesizes different products. The zona glomerulosa lacks 17α-hydroxylase activity. Instead, it contains large amounts of aldosterone synthase (P450aldo) and therefore produces mineralocorticoids. The zona fasciculata and zona reticularis, both of which express the 17α-hydroxylase gene, synthesize glucocorticoids and androgens, respectively.

Steroid Hormone Transport in the Circulation

Most steroids in the peripheral circulation are bound to carrier proteins. These proteins may be specific, such as sex hormone-binding globulin (SHBG), thyroid-binding globulin, or corticosteroid-binding globulin, or nonspecific, such as albumin. Only 1 to 2 percent of circulating androgens and estrogens are unbound or free.

Only the unbound steroid fraction is believed to be biologically active. However, albumin's low affinity for sex steroids may allow steroids bound to this protein to exert some effects. The amount of free, biologically active hormone is inversely related to the amount of bound hormone, and the amount of bound hormone is a direct reflection of the levels of carrier protein. As a result, small changes in carrier protein expression can produce substantial alterations in steroid effect.

SHBG circulates as a homodimer that binds a single steroid molecule. This binding protein is synthesized primarily in the liver, although it has also been detected in the brain, placenta, endometrium, and testes. SHBG levels are increased by hyperthyroidism, pregnancy, and estrogen administration. In contrast, androgens, progestins, growth hormone (GH), insulin, and corticoids lower SHBG levels. Weight gain, particularly central body fat, can significantly blunt SHBG expression. In turn, this decreases bound hormone levels and raises active hormone levels (Hammond, 2012).

Free testosterone levels are the most commonly ordered free steroid hormone tests, but the most accurate assays are performed by only a few commercial laboratories (Rosner, 2007). Although mass spectrometry is considered the preferred measurement method, it has not been widely adopted due to complexity and cost (Kanakis, 2019). The more available *calculated* free levels are relatively inaccurate, and results should be interpreted with caution.

Fortunately, free testosterone level measurement is rarely necessary for clinical diagnosis in the female and is unlikely to add more information than the total testosterone level. For example, measurement of testosterone levels in patients with presumed polycystic ovarian syndrome (PCOS) is important to exclude an androgen-producing tumor, which will produce markedly elevated total testosterone levels. In contrast, normal or high-normal levels of total testosterone are consistent with the diagnosis of PCOS. Because testosterone lowers SHBG levels, patients with normal total testosterone levels, but with clinical evidence of hyperandrogenism (hirsutism and/or acne), invariably have either elevated free testosterone levels or increased sensitivity of the hair follicle and sebaceous glands.

Ultimately, steroids are metabolized mainly in the liver and to a lesser extent in the kidney and intestinal mucosa. Hydroxylation of estradiol results in production of estrone or catechol estrogens. These estrogens are then conjugated to glucuronides or sulfates to form water-soluble compounds for excretion in the urine. Accordingly, administration of certain pharmacologic steroid hormones may be contraindicated in those with active liver or renal disease.

RECEPTOR STRUCTURE AND FUNCTION

Steroid hormones and peptide factors differ in their specific receptor-mediated actions. Yet, both eventually lead to DNA transcription and protein production in the target cell.

■ G Protein–Coupled Receptors

These are cell membrane–associated receptors that bind peptide factors. These receptors consist of a hydrophilic extracellular domain, an intracellular domain, and a hydrophobic transmembrane domain that spans the cell membrane seven times. When bound to hormone, these receptors undergo a conformational change, activate intracellular signaling pathways, and, through a series of phosphorylation events, ultimately modulate transcription of multiple genes within the target cell (Fig. 16-6).

TABLE 16-2. Contribution of the Ovaries and Adrenal Glands to Androgen Production

Product	Ovary	Adrenal Gland
Testosterone[a]	25%	25%
Androstenedione	50%	50%
DHEA	10%	90%
DHEAS	0%	>99%

[a]Remaining testosterone derived from conversion of androstenedione to testosterone in the periphery.
DHEA = dehydroepiandrosterone; DHEAS = DHEA sulfate.

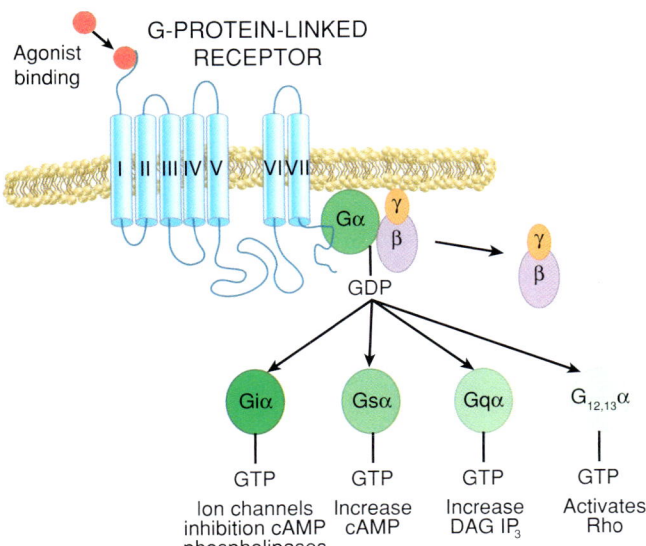

G-PROTEIN-LINKED RECEPTOR

Agonist binding

FIGURE 16-6 G protein–coupled receptors are integral transmembrane proteins that transduce extracellular signals to the cell interior. These receptors consist of seven membrane-spanning regions. Receptor occupation by an agonist promotes interaction between the receptor and the G protein on the membrane's inner surface. This induces an exchange of guanosine diphosphate (GDP) for guanosine triphosphate (GTP) on the G protein α subunit and dissociation of the α subunit from the βγ heterodimer. A large number of both activating and inhibiting α subunits exist, which allows for a wide array of responses. (From Mahendroo, 2018, with permission.)

The gonadotropin-releasing hormone receptor (GnRH-R) is a G protein–coupled receptor that has been identified in the ovary, testes, hypothalamus, prostate, breast, and placenta (Yu, 2011). Although data are still preliminary, GnRH and its receptor may form an autocrine/paracrine regulatory network in reproductive tissues including the ovaries and placenta in addition to the classic neuroendocrine hypothalamic-pituitary system (Kim, 2007; Lee, 2010).

Both LH and hCG bind to a single G protein–coupled receptor known as the LH/CG receptor. Relative to LH, hCG has a slightly higher affinity for the receptor and has a longer half-life. In contrast, FSH binds to a unique G protein–coupled receptor located on the granulosa cell membrane.

Within the ovary, the LH/CG receptor is expressed on theca cells, interstitial cells, and luteal cells. In the granulosa cells of preantral follicles, LH/CG receptor mRNA is nearly undetectable. However, in the differentiated granulosa cells found during follicular maturation, high levels of this receptor are observed. LH/CG and FSH receptors are also identified in endometrium, myometrium, and placenta (Stilley, 2014; Ziecik, 2007). The function of the receptor in these extraovarian tissues is poorly understood.

■ Steroid Hormone Receptors
Classification and Structure

Despite their structural similarities, estrogens, progestogens, androgens, glucocorticoids, and mineralocorticoids all interact with unique receptors known as *nuclear hormone receptors*. The nuclear receptor superfamily consists of three receptor groups. It contains: (1) those that bind steroidal ligands, (2) those that have affinity for nonsteroidal ligands such as thyroid hormone, and (3) orphan receptors. By definition, orphan nuclear receptors do not have an identified ligand. These are believed to be constitutively active, that is, they exhibit basal or intrinsic activity.

Free steroids diffuse into cells and combine with specific receptors (Fig. 16-7A) (Gruber, 2002). Members of this receptor superfamily exhibit a modular structure of distinct domains (Fig. 16-8) (O'Malley, 1999). Each region contributes distinct activities required for full receptor function. In general, nuclear receptors have two regions that are critical for gene activation, termed activation function 1 (AF1) and activation function 2 (AF2). AF1 is located in the A/B domain and is usually ligand independent. AF2 is in the ligand-binding domain (E) and is often hormone dependent. The highly conserved DNA-binding region (C) inserts into the DNA helix. Subsequently, steroid receptors enhance or repress gene transcription through interactions with specific DNA sequences, called *hormone response elements*, in the promoter region of target genes (Klinge, 2001).

Estrogen, Progesterone, and Androgen Receptors

Unliganded estrogen receptors (ERs) are located in the nucleus. In contrast, progesterone receptors (PRs), androgen receptor (AR), and those for mineralocorticoids and glucocorticoids are cytoplasmic in the absence of ligand. Ligand binding to these latter receptors allows translocation to the nucleus.

Two isoforms of estrogen receptors, ERα and ERβ, are encoded by separate genes (Kuiper, 1997). These receptors are differentially expressed in tissues and appear to serve distinct functions (Fig. 22-6, p. 484). For example, both ERα and ERβ are required for normal ovarian function. Mice lacking ERα are anovulatory and accumulate cystic follicles, whereas ovaries missing ERβ are normal histologically despite impaired ovulation (Couse, 2000).

The progesterone receptor also exists in multiple isoforms. Encoded from a single gene, PRA and PRB are identical except for an additional 164 amino acids at the amino terminus (Conneely, 2002). Similar to estrogen receptors, the PR isoforms are not interchangeable. For example, PRA is required for normal ovarian and uterine functions but is expendable in the breast (Lydon, 1996). In contrast to the estrogen and progesterone receptors, only one form of the androgen receptor has been identified.

Nongenomic Actions of Steroids

A subset of steroids, including estrogens and progestins, may alter cell function via nongenomic effects, that is, independent of the classic nuclear hormone receptors (see Fig. 16-7C). These nongenomic effects occur rapidly and may be mediated via cell-surface receptors, such as the G protein–coupled receptor 30 (GPR30) in the case of estrogen (Kowalik, 2013; Revelli, 1998). Pharmacologic agents under development specifically target these nongenomic effects to allow more precise therapy for steroid-sensitive reproductive disorders (Tang, 2019).

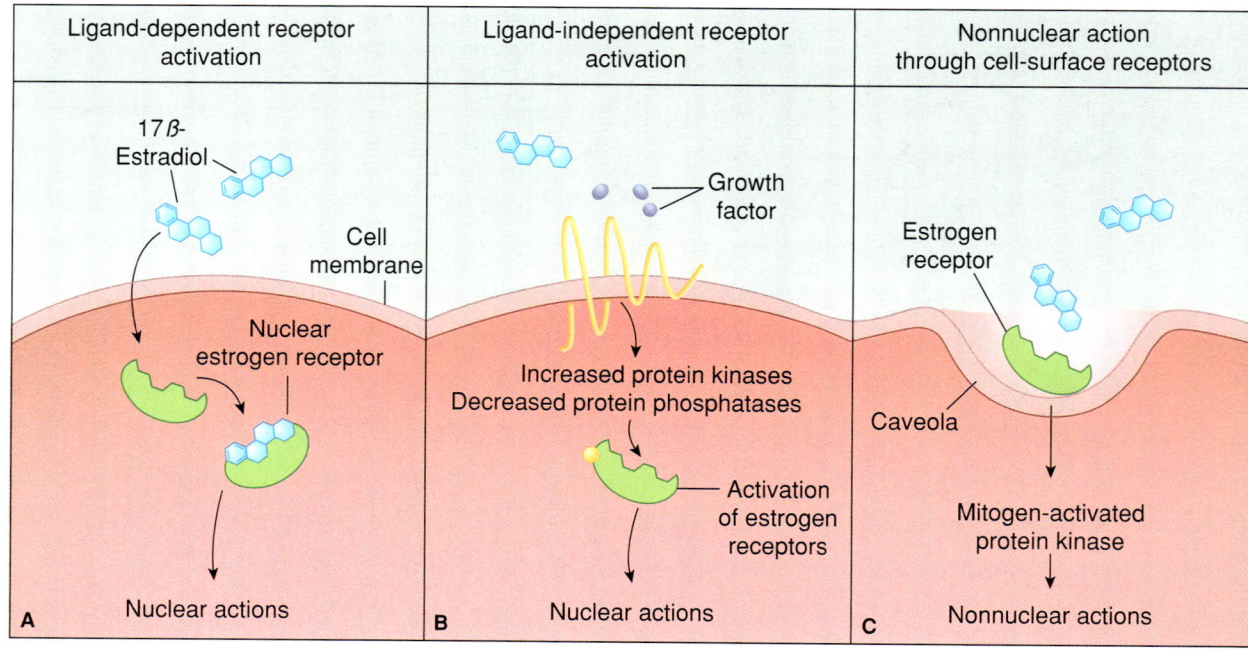

FIGURE 16-7 Estrogen receptor ligand–dependent and –independent activation. **A.** Classically, the estrogen receptor can be activated by estrogen. Unbound hormone is free to bind with empty steroid receptors found either in the cytoplasm or, more commonly, in the cell's nucleus. Hormone-bound receptors then bind to specific DNA promoter sequences. This binding typically leads to DNA transcription and eventually to specific protein synthesis. **B.** The estrogen receptor can also be activated independently of estrogen. Growth factors can increase the activity of protein kinases that phosphorylate different sites on the receptor molecule. This unbound, yet activated, receptor will then exert transcriptional effects. **C.** Nonnuclear estrogen-signaling pathways also can produce effects. Cell-membrane estrogen receptors are located in invaginations called caveolae. Estrogen binding to these estrogen receptors is linked to the mitogen-activated protein kinase pathway and results in a rapid, nonnuclear effect.

■ Receptor Expression and Desensitization

Many influences alter cellular response to sex steroids and peptide factors. The number of receptors within a cell or on the cell membrane is critical to attain maximum hormonal response.

ESTROGEN RECEPTOR

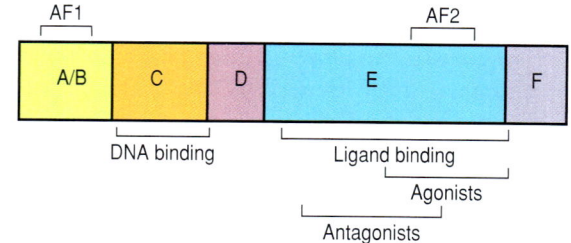

PROGESTERONE RECEPTOR

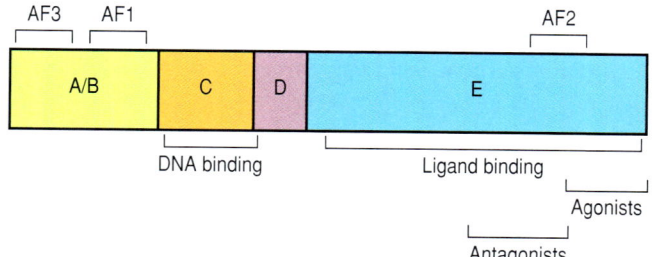

FIGURE 16-8 Functional domains within estrogen and progesterone receptors, including distinct sites for ligand and DNA binding.

Importantly, the number of receptors on a cell can be modified through gene transcription and receptor protein degradation.

Hormonally induced negative feedback of receptors is termed *homologous downregulation* or *desensitization*. Desensitization limits the duration of a hormonal response by decreasing the cell's sensitivity to a constant, prolonged level of hormone.

Within the reproductive system, desensitization is best understood for the GnRH receptor and is used clinically to produce a hypoestrogenic state. Pharmacologic agonists of GnRH, such as leuprolide acetate (Lupron), initially stimulate receptors on pituitary gonadotropes to cause a supraphysiologic release of both LH and FSH. Over a period of hours, agonists downregulate gonadotrope receptors, thus desensitizing them to further GnRH stimulation. Correspondingly, decreased gonadotropin secretion leads to suppressed estrogen and progesterone levels 1 to 2 weeks after initial GnRH agonist administration.

HORMONE IMMUNOASSAYS

■ Immunoassays

These tests use antibodies to detect most polypeptide, steroid, and thyroid hormones. They are sensitive and easily automated. Hormone concentration is usually reported as international units per volume rather than mass per volume (Table 16-3). When interpreting immunoassays, several concepts must be understood. These include reference standards, the "hook effect," biologic activity, normal ranges, and supplementary hormone levels.

TABLE 16-3. Reference Ranges for Selected Reproductive Steroids in Adult Human Serum

Steroid	Subjects	Reference Values
Androstenedione	Men	2.8–7.3 nmol/L
	Women	3.1–12.2 nmol/L
Testosterone	Men	6.9–34.7 nmol/L
	Women	0.7–2.8 nmol/L
Dihydrotestosterone	Men	1.0–3.10 nmol/L
	Women	0.07–.086 nmol/L
Dehydroepiandrosterone	Men/women	5.5–24.3 nmol/L
Dehydroepiandrosterone sulfonate	Men/women	2.5–10.4 µmol/L
Progesterone	Men	<0.3–1.3 nmol/L
	Women	
	Follicular	0.3–3.0 nmol/L
	Luteal	19.0–45.0 nmol/L
Estradiol	Men	<37–210 pmol/L
	Women	
	Follicular	<37–360 pmol/L
	Luteal	625–2830 pmol/L
	Midcycle	699–1250 pmol/L
	Postmenopausal	<37–140 pmol/L
Estrone	Men	37–250 pmol/L
	Women	
	Follicular	110–400 pmol/L
	Luteal	310–660 pmol/L
	Postmenopausal	22–230 pmol/L
Estrone sulfonate	Men	600–2500 pmol/L
	Women	
	Follicular	700–3600 pmol/L
	Luteal	1100–7300 pmol/L
	Postmenopausal	130–1200 pmol/L

Reproduced with permission from Yen SS, Jaffe RB, Barbieri RL: Reproductive Endocrinology, 4th ed. Philadelphia, Saunders, 1999.

First, to minimize assay-to-assay variability, a reference material is needed to standardize assays. Reference standards serve as anchors that can provide comparability across time and methods. Such reference preparations are produced by the World Health Organization (WHO) and the National Institutes of Health (NIH). More than 20 assay standards are available to measure LH, FSH, prolactin (PRL), and hCG. Thus, knowing which reference standard is used by a specific assay is essential, as results may differ significantly. Clinically, this can become an issue in patients with possible ectopic pregnancies when serial β-hCG levels are obtained at different health-care facilities.

Second, the hook effect can alter immunoassay result interpretation. With this, significantly elevated endogenous hormone levels saturate the assay's targeting antibody and thereby prevent required binding of the hormone to the assay. This creates a falsely low reading. One example is a negative urine pregnancy test result in a woman with a complete hydatidiform mole. When clinically suspected, specimen dilution can help resolve the hook effect.

Importantly, the amount of hormone present in a sample does not necessarily correlate with the biologic activity of that hormone. For example, PRL exists in multiple isoforms, many of which are immunologically detectable but not biologically active. Similarly, varying glycosylation patterns of gonadotropins at different times during the reproductive life span are believed to alter their biologic activity.

Another caveat is a result that lies in the "normal range." For many hormones, a stated normal range is often broad. As such, the hormone level of an individual may double, but remain within the normal range, although the result is actually abnormal for that individual.

Last, the addition of other hormone levels may be necessary to define the significance of a result. In the context of the pituitary gland and its target endocrine glands, it may be adequate to measure the pituitary hormone concentration alone. For example, high levels of circulating gonadotropins are almost invariably due to ovarian failure and loss of negative feedback. This is because pituitary overproduction of functional dimer is rare. Conversely, low gonadotropin levels can be attributed to hypothalamic-pituitary dysfunction rather than ovarian failure. Thus, the measurement of ovarian-derived products such as estrogen can clarify the condition.

At times, the measurement of both pituitary and target hormone levels may be indicated. For example, in many laboratories, an abnormal TSH value will lead to "reflex," that is, automatic testing for thyroid hormone levels. Low levels of both a stimulating-hormone and target hormone indicate an abnormality in either hypothalamic or pituitary function. High levels of a target-gland hormone coupled with low levels of its stimulating pituitary hormone suggest autonomous secretion by the target organ such as occurs in the hyperthyroidism of Graves disease.

■ Stimulation and Suppression Tests

Stimulation tests may be useful when hypofunction of an endocrine organ is suspected. These tests use an endogenous stimulating hormone to assess the reserve capacity of the tissue of interest. The trophic hormone used may be a hypothalamic releasing factor such as GnRH or thyrotropin-releasing hormone (TRH). Alternatively, a substitute hormone may be used, such as hCG as a substitute for LH or leuprolide acetate for GnRH. The ability of the target gland to respond is measured by an increase in the appropriate hormone's plasma level. One example, the leuprolide stimulation test, may be used to evaluate abnormal pubertal development and is described in Chapter 15 (p. 330). Leuprolide substitutes for GnRH, as clinical-grade GnRH is often unavailable (Rosenfield, 2013).

Suppression tests may be performed when endocrine hyperfunction is suspected. For example, a dexamethasone suppression test may be given to a patient with suspected hypercortisolism (Cushing disease or syndrome). Described in full in Chapter 18 (p. 399), this test gauges the ability of dexamethasone to inhibit adrenocorticotropic hormone (ACTH) secretion and thus cortisol production by the adrenal. The failure of glucocorticoid treatment to suppress cortisol production would be consistent with primary hyperadrenalism.

HYPOTHALAMIC-PITUITARY AXIS

■ Anatomy

The hypothalamus consists of nuclei located at the base of the brain, just superior to the optic chiasm. Neurons within the hypothalamus form synaptic connections with other neurons throughout the central nervous system (CNS). A subset of the hypothalamic neurons within the arcuate, ventromedial, and paraventricular nuclei project to the median eminence. In the median eminence, a dense network of capillaries arises from the superior hypophyseal arteries (Fig. 16-9). These capillaries drain into portal vessels that traverse the pituitary stalk and then form a capillary network within the anterior pituitary gland (adenohypophysis). The primary direction of this hypophyseal portal system is from hypothalamus to pituitary. However, retrograde flow also exists. This creates an ultrashort feedback loop between the pituitary gland and hypothalamic neurons.

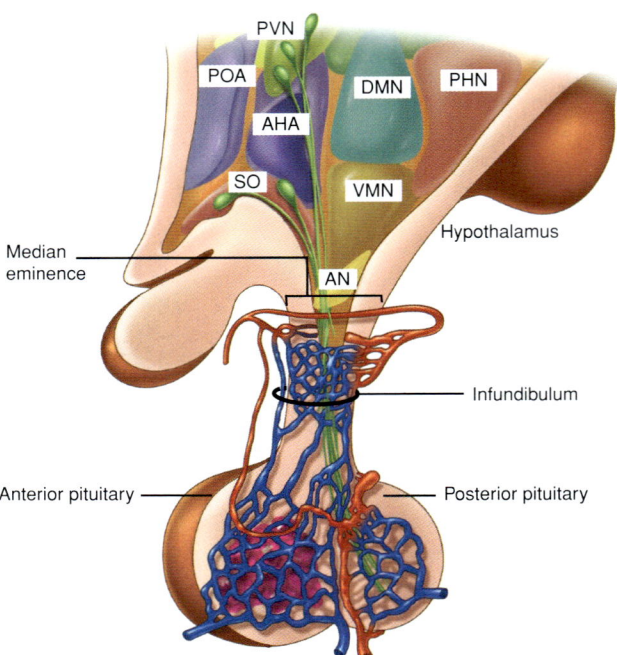

FIGURE 16-9 Sagittal section through the hypothalamus and pituitary gland with rostral structures to the left and caudal ones to the right. The hypothalamus is anatomically and functionally linked with the anterior pituitary by the portal system of blood supply. The posterior pituitary contains the axon terminals of neurons arising in the supraoptic (SO) nucleus and paraventricular nucleus (PVN) of the hypothalamus. AHA = anterior hypothalamic area; AN = arcuate nucleus; DMN = dorsomedial nucleus; PHN = posterior hypothalamic nucleus; POA = preoptic area; VMN = ventromedial nucleus. (Reproduced with permission from Mahendroo MS: Parturition. In Cunningham FG, Leveno KJ, Bloom SL, et al (eds): Williams Obstetrics, 23rd ed. New York, McGraw-Hill, 2010.)

The hypothalamus is thus a critical locus for integration of information from the environment, nervous system, and multiple organ systems.

The anterior pituitary gland consists of endocrine cells and is derived from an invagination of the Rathke pouch in the roof of the embryonic oral cavity. In contrast, the posterior pituitary gland (neurohypophysis) is neural tissue and consists of the axon terminals of magnocellular neurons arising in the supraoptic and paraventricular nuclei of the hypothalamus.

■ Hypothalamic Neuroendocrinology

The list of known neurotransmitters continues to expand as our understanding of their anatomic distribution, mode of regulation, and mechanism of action increases. Neurotransmitters can be classified as: (1) biogenic amines (dopamine, epinephrine, norepinephrine, serotonin, histamine), (2) neuropeptides, (3) acetylcholine, (4) excitatory amino neurotransmitters (glutamate, glycine, aspartic acid), (5) the inhibitory amino acid gamma-aminobutyric acid (GABA), (6) gaseous transmitters (nitric oxide, carbon monoxide), and (7) miscellaneous factors (cytokines, growth factors).

Clinically important neuropeptides within the reproductive axis include the endogenous opiates, kisspeptin, galanin, neurokinin B, neuropeptide Y, galanin, and pituitary adenylate cyclase-activating peptide. This list is expanding rapidly with ongoing study and should not be considered exhaustive.

Endogenous Opiates

Central opioidergic neurons are important mediators of hypothalamic-pituitary function. Depending on the precursor peptide from which they are derived, these neuropeptides can be categorized into three classes: endorphins, enkephalins, and dynorphins. Of these, endorphins (endogenous morphines) are cleavage products of the proopiomelanocortin *POMC* gene, which also yields ACTH and α-melanocyte stimulating hormone (α-MSH) (Taylor, 1997). The endorphins serve a wide range of physiologic functions that include regulation of temperature, cardiovascular and respiratory systems, pain perception, mood, and reproduction. Several opioid receptor subtypes exist. Within the reproductive axis, activation of the μ-opioid receptor by β-endorphins is of critical importance (Seeber, 2019).

Proopiomelanocortin is produced in highest concentration in the anterior pituitary gland but is also expressed in the brain, sympathetic nervous system, gonads, placenta, GI tract, and lungs. The primary peptide synthesized from this pathway depends on the tissue source. For example, the predominant products in the brain are the opioids, whereas pituitary biosynthesis results principally in ACTH production.

Hypothalamic opioids play a central role in menstrual cyclicity by tonically suppressing the hypothalamic release of GnRH (Funabashi, 1994). Estrogen promotes endorphin secretion, and this is increased further with the addition of progesterone (Cetel, 1985). Thus, endorphin levels rise during the follicular phase, peak during the luteal phase, and drop markedly during menses. This pattern suggests that opioid tone and progesterone both decrease GnRH pulse frequency in the luteal phase, thus stimulating FSH secretion. For reasons that are not fully understood, opioid suppression of GnRH is relieved at the time of ovulation (King, 1984). In addition, functional hypothalamic amenorrhea due to eating disorders, intensive exercise, and stress correlates positively with higher endogenous opiate concentrations (Chap. 17, p. 378).

Kisspeptin

Hypothalamic kisspeptin neurons are involved in sexual differentiation, puberty initiation, and adult reproductive function. These neurons are part of the KNDy neuronal system, named for the coexpression of <u>k</u>isspeptin with <u>n</u>eurokinin B and the opioid, <u>dy</u>norphin. Kisspeptin neurons send processes to GnRH neurons, allowing direct control of GnRH secretion. Interestingly, one group of kisspeptin neurons may mediate negative steroid feedback, whereas another may be responsible for the positive feedback observed before ovulation (Millar, 2014; Skorupskaite, 2014; Trevisan, 2018).

Kisspeptin expression has more recently been identified in numerous nonneuronal reproductive tissues. Ovarian kisspeptin is thought to play a role in follicular development, oocyte maturation, ovulation, and steroidogenesis (Hu, 2018). Uterine kisspeptin is implicated in endometrial decidualization. Kisspeptin is also expressed in the placenta throughout pregnancy (Cao, 2019).

Neurons located throughout the hypothalamus project to kisspeptin neurons, to GnRH neurons, and to other CNS areas that have roles in reproductive function. Moreover, kisspeptin neuronal activity is affected by inputs from throughout the CNS and by hormonal feedback. As such, modulation of kisspeptin and the KNDy system as therapeutic targets in pubertal disorders, hypothalamic amenorrhea, ovulation induction, and hot flashes are current investigational areas (Yang, 2016). Studies are also pursuing the use of circulating kisspeptin levels as a potential biomarker of pregnancy complications (Hu, 2019).

Other Hypothalamic Neuropeptides

Neuropeptide Y and galanin secretion varies in response to changes in energy level, such as with anorexia and obesity. Both of these neuropeptides alter GnRH pulsatility and potentiate GnRH-induced gonadotrope secretion (Lawrence, 2011; Peters, 2009). Recent interest has focused on gonadotropin-inhibitory hormone (GnIH)/RFamide-related peptide 3 (RFRP-3). Expressed in both the hypothalamus and anterior pituitary gland, this peptide is linked to gonadotropin suppression in response to stress (Iwasa, 2018).

Also secreted by hypothalamic neurons, pituitary adenylate cyclase–activating peptide (PACAP) enters the portal system. It binds to receptors on anterior pituitary cells and stimulates hormone secretion including gonadotropin secretion, albeit more weakly than GnRH. Gonadotropes themselves also secrete PACAP, suggesting an autocrine/paracrine role for this hormone within the pituitary. PACAP modulates GnRH-receptor expression and, conversely, GnRH alters PACAP-receptor expression on the gonadotrope cell surface. Furthermore, pituitary PACAP gene expression is markedly increased by GnRH (Halvorson, 2014). Thus, these two important neuropeptides are functionally linked at the level of the anterior pituitary.

Nutritional Status and Reproduction

Puberty onset and menstrual cyclicity are altered by nutritional status. As one component of this status, adipose functions as endocrine tissue and an energy storage depot and links reproductive capacity and energy homeostasis. Adipose-derived cytokine factors, termed *adipokines*, are members of the cytokine family and include *leptin* and *adiponectin*. Decreased energy reserves, which may develop with food scarcity, eating disorders, or certain types of exercise, are associated with lower circulating leptin and higher adiponectin levels.

Data suggest that a reduction in serum leptin concentrations increases activity of neuropeptide Y neurons to stimulate appetite. Conversely, a higher serum leptin level raises activity of proopiomelanocortin and kisspeptin neural networks. This in turn reduces food intake and stimulates GnRH secretion to thereby alter reproductive function (Chehab, 2014; Guzman, 2019). In addition to CNS effects, leptin likely affects reproductive function via alterations in gonadotrope GnRH receptor expression in the pituitary (Odle, 2018).

Adiponectin alters hypothalamic kisspeptin expression. Adiponectin receptor expression is documented throughout the hypothalamic-pituitary-gonadal axis and in the uterus, placenta, and developing embryo (Dobrzyn, 2018). Other metabolic signals, such as pancreatic insulin and gastric ghrelin, also likely contribute to central mediation of reproduction.

◼ Anterior Pituitary Hormones

The anterior pituitary gland contains five hormone-producing cell types: (1) gonadotropes (which produce LH and FSH), (2) lactotropes (PRL), (3) somatotropes (GH), (4) thyrotropes (TSH), and (5) adrenocorticotropes (ACTH). Of these, gonadotropes constitute approximately 10 to 15 percent of all hormonally active cells in the anterior pituitary (Childs, 1983).

With the exception of PRL, which is under tonic inhibition, pituitary hormones are stimulated by hypothalamic neuroendocrine secretion. Both of the gonadotropins, LH and FSH, are regulated by a single releasing peptide, GnRH, which acts on the anterior pituitary's gonadotrope subpopulation. Most gonadotropes contain secretory granules that contain both LH and FSH. However, a significant number of cells are monohormonal, that is, secrete only LH or only FSH.

Of the other pituitary-releasing hormones, corticotropin-releasing hormone stimulates biosynthesis and secretion of ACTH by the pituitary adrenocorticotropes. Thyrotropin-releasing hormone prompts thyrotrope secretion of TSH, also known as *thyrotropin*. Various hypothalamic secretagogues regulate expression of somatotrope-derived GH. Last, PRL expression is primarily under inhibitory regulation by dopamine. As a consequence of these regulatory mechanisms, damage to the pituitary stalk results in hypopituitarism for LH, FSH, GH, ACTH, and TSH, but an associated increase in PRL secretion.

◼ Hypothalamic-Releasing Peptides

These are small peptides with short half-lives of a few minutes due to their rapid degradation. Hypothalamic-releasing peptides are released in minute quantities and are highly diluted in the peripheral circulation. Therefore, biologically active concentrations of these factors are locally restricted to the anterior pituitary gland. Clinically, the extremely low concentrations of these hormones render them essentially undetectable in serum. Thus, levels of their corresponding pituitary factors are measured as surrogate markers.

Gonadotropin-Releasing Hormone

GnRH is a decapeptide that has a half-life <10 minutes (Fig. 16-10). Pulsatile GnRH input is required for activation and maintenance of GnRH receptors. This characteristic is exploited clinically by administering long-acting GnRH agonists to treat steroid-dependent conditions such as endometriosis, leiomyomas, precocious puberty, breast cancer, and prostate cancer. These agonists compete with endogenous pulsatile GnRH at the receptor and thereby depress gonadotropin secretion. This in turn lowers serum ovarian sex steroid levels.

Various GnRH agonists and antagonists have been created by introducing amino acid modifications within the native GnRH sequence (Padula, 2005). A change in the glycine at position 6 led to agonists with longer half-lives. In contrast, changes in positions 1, 2, and 3 prevent GnRH-receptor activation, and examples of these antagonists are cetrorelix and ganirelix. Many of these products require subcutaneous injection, although nasal agonists are available. More recently and described in Chapter 11 (p. 244), an orally active nonpeptide antagonist, elagolix, was approved in the United States for treatment of endometriosis-associated pain (Taylor, 2018).

Humans express two forms of GnRH termed GnRH I and GnRH II (Cheng, 2005). The GnRH II peptide has a different expression pattern than the classically described GnRH and differs in receptor activation (Neill, 2002). Further research is needed to determine the overlapping and divergent functions of these two forms.

Migration of the GnRH Neurons. Many hypothalamic neurons arise within the CNS, but GnRH-containing neurons have a unique embryologic origin. Progenitor GnRH neurons originate in the medial olfactory placode and migrate along the vomeronasal nerve into the hypothalamus (Fig. 17-5, p. 378). A series of soluble factors regulate GnRH neuronal migration at specific locations along their migratory route. These factors include secreted signaling molecules such as GABA, adhesion molecules, and growth factors (Wierman, 2011). Failure of normal migration may stem from various genetic defects in these signaling molecules and can lead to Kallmann syndrome, which is discussed in Chapter 17 (p. 378).

GnRH cell bodies are located primarily within the arcuate nucleus. From these neuronal cell bodies, GnRH is axonally transported along the

GnRH

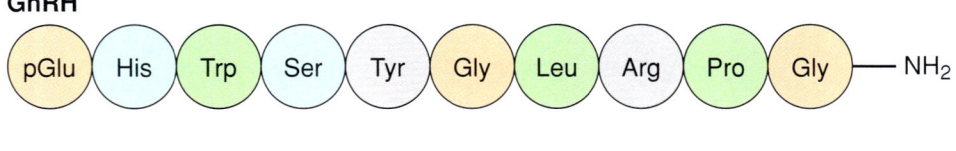

Leuprolide acetate

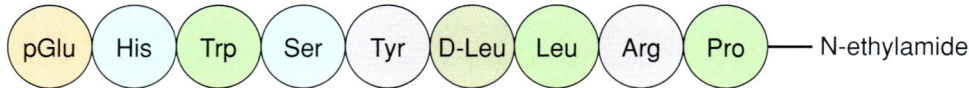

Cetrorelix acetate

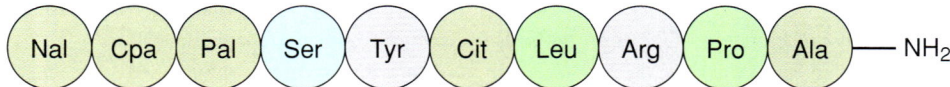

FIGURE 16-10 Amino acid composition of the decapeptide gonadotropin-releasing hormone (GnRH), the agonist leuprolide acetate, and the antagonist cetrorelix acetate. Glu = glutamic acid; His = histidine; Trp = tryptophan; Ser = serine; Tyr = tyrosine; Gly = glycine; Leu = leucine; Arg = arginine; Pro = proline; Nal = naphthylalanine; Cpa = cyanopropionic amino acid; Pal = pyridylalanine.

tuberoinfundibular tract to the median eminence. GnRH is then secreted into the portal system that drains directly to the anterior pituitary gland and stimulates gonadotropin biosynthesis and secretion. The number of GnRH neurons in the adult is strikingly low, with only a few thousand cells dispersed within the arcuate nucleus.

The olfactory origin of GnRH neurons and nasal epithelial cells suggest a link between reproduction and olfactory signals. Compounds released by one individual that affect other members of the same species are known as *pheromones*. Pheromones obtained from the axillary secretions of women in the late follicular phase accelerate the LH surge and shorten menstrual cycles of women exposed to these chemicals. Secretions from women in the luteal phase have the opposite effects. Thus, pheromones may be one mechanism by which women who are together frequently often exhibit synchronous menstrual cycles (Stern, 1998).

A subset of GnRH neurons sends projections into other areas of the CNS, including the limbic system. These projections are not required for gonadotropin secretion, but they may play a role in modulation of reproductive behavior (Nakai, 1978; Silverman, 1987).

Pulsatile GnRH Secretion. In elegant experiments, Knobil (1974) demonstrated that pulsatile delivery of GnRH to the pituitary gonadotropes is required to achieve sustained gonadotropin secretion. As shown in **Figure 16-11**, continuous infusion with GnRH rapidly diminishes both LH and FSH secretion. This effect is easily reversed with a return to pulsatile stimulation (Knobil, 1980).

Compared with the luteal phase, follicular-phase GnRH pulsatility is characterized by higher pulse frequency and lower amplitude. Higher pulse frequency preferentially stimulates LH, whereas lower frequency favors FSH secretion (Thompson, 2014). Therefore, changes in GnRH pulse frequency affect the absolute levels and the ratio of LH to FSH release.

Pulsatile activity was believed to be an intrinsic property of GnRH neurons. Although not yet definitive, more recent data suggest that kisspeptin neurons may actually drive GnRH pulsatility (Terasawa, 2019). Regardless, GnRH pulse rate and amplitude is modulated by a complex array of neurotransmitters and circulating hormones. In animal models, estrogen increases GnRH pulse frequency and therefore leads to an increase in LH levels relative to FSH levels. In contrast, progesterone decreases

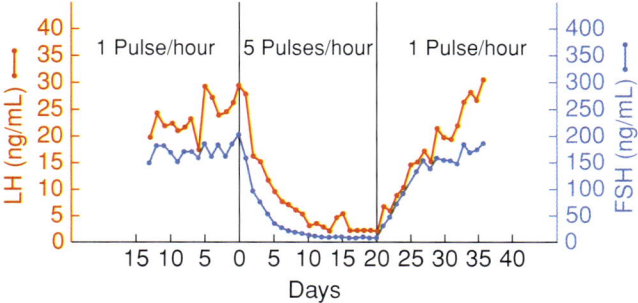

FIGURE 16-11 Changes in luteinizing hormone (LH) and follicle-stimulating hormone (FSH) levels as gonadotropin-releasing hormone (GnRH) pulsatile release varies.

TABLE 16-4. Hypothalamic-Pituitary Products and Their End Organs

Hypothalamus	Pituitary	End Organ
GnRH	LH/FSH	Gonads
Dopamine	PRL	Breast
TRH	TSH	Thyroid
CRH	ACTH	Adrenal
GHRH	GH	Somatic

ACTH = adrenocorticotropin hormone; CRH = corticotropin-releasing hormone; FSH = follicle-stimulating hormone; GH = growth hormone; GHRH = growth hormone–releasing hormone; GnRH = gonadotropin-releasing hormone; LH = luteinizing hormone; PRL = prolactin; TRH = thyrotropin-releasing hormone; TSH = thyroid-stimulating hormone.

GnRH pulsatility. The increase in progesterone during the luteal phase may explain the preferential stimulation of FSH observed toward the end of this phase. This rise in FSH is critical for the initiation of follicular recruitment.

■ Other Hypothalamic-Pituitary Axes

Dopamine and Prolactin

In contrast to the other anterior pituitary hormones, PRL release is primarily regulated via inhibition, specifically by dopamine (Table 16-4). These dopamine-containing fibers arise chiefly in the hypothalamic arcuate nucleus and project to the median eminence where dopamine enters the portal vessels. Prolactin-releasing factors, although less potent, include TRH, vasopressin, vasoactive intestinal peptide (VIP), endogenous opioids, and acetylcholine.

There are five forms of the dopamine receptor divided into two groups, D_1 and D_2. Cells in the anterior pituitary gland primarily express the D_2 subtypes. The medical treatment of prolactinomas has been improved in terms of both effectiveness and patient tolerance by the development of the D_2-specific ligands. For example, the dopamine agonist cabergoline is a D_2-specific ligand, whereas bromocriptine is nonspecific.

Thyrotropin-Releasing Hormone

As indicated by its name, thyrotropin-releasing hormone stimulates secretion of TSH from the anterior pituitary gland thyrotrope subpopulation. Of note, TRH also is a potent prolactin-releasing factor and results in a clinical link between hypothyroidism and secondary hyperprolactinemia (Messini, 2010).

TSH binds to specific receptors on the plasma cell membrane of thyroid gland cells. This stimulates thyroid hormone biosynthesis through an increase in thyroid gland size and vascularity. Thyroid hormone exerts negative feedback on TRH- and TSH-releasing cells.

Corticotropin-Releasing Hormone

This is the primary hypothalamic factor that stimulates synthesis and secretion of ACTH. Corticotropin-releasing hormone

(CRH) is distributed in multiple locations within the hypothalamus and other CNS areas. Release of CRH is stimulated by catecholaminergic input from other brain pathways and inhibited by endogenous opioids.

CRH binds to CRH receptors in the anterior pituitary gland to stimulate ACTH biosynthesis and secretion. In turn, ACTH stimulates glucocorticoid production by the adrenal gland's zona fasciculata and androgen production by its zona reticularis. CRH secretion is under negative-feedback regulation by circulating cortisol produced in the adrenal gland. In contrast, mineralocorticoid production by the zona glomerulosa is primarily regulated by the renin-angiotensin system. As a result, abnormalities in the CRH–ACTH pathway do not result in electrolyte disturbances.

Central CRH pathways are believed to mediate many stress responses (Kalantaridou, 2004). Clinically, in women with hypothalamic amenorrhea, CRH levels have been found to be elevated. Elevated levels of CRH inhibit hypothalamic GnRH secretion by direct action and by augmenting central opioid concentrations (Fig. 17-6, p. 379). This functional pathway may explain, in part, the association between hypercortisolism and menstrual abnormalities. However, recent work suggests that the link may be substantially more complex and involve multiple neural circuits and transmitters (McCosh, 2019).

Growth Hormone–Releasing Hormone

GH secretion by pituitary somatotropes is stimulated by hypothalamic growth hormone–releasing hormone (GHRH) and inhibited by somatostatin. GHRH is secreted primarily by the hypothalamus, but small quantities are released by placental and immune cells. In contrast, somatostatin is widely distributed in the CNS and in the placenta, pancreas, and GI tract.

As with GnRH, GHRH depends on pulsatile secretion to exert a physiologic effect. Exercise, stress, sleep, and hypoglycemia stimulate GH release, whereas free fatty acids and other factors related to adiposity blunt GH release. Estrogen, testosterone, and thyroid hormone also play a role in increased GH secretion.

GH stimulates skeletal and muscle growth, regulates lipolysis, and promotes the cellular uptake of amino acids. This hormone induces insulin resistance, and thus GH excess may be associated with new-onset diabetes mellitus. Most of the growth effects of GH are mediated via the insulin-like growth factors IGF-I and IGF-II. These growth factors are produced in high quantities in the liver. Many of the target tissues in which they exert local effects also synthesize IGFs. Within the ovary, IGF-I and IGF-II stimulate granulosa cell proliferation and steroidogenesis during folliculogenesis (Silva, 2009). IGFs also suppress GH secretion through negative-feedback mechanisms.

■ Posterior Pituitary Peptides

Neurons projecting to the posterior pituitary synthesize and secrete the nine-amino-acid cyclic peptides oxytocin and arginine vasopressin. Precursors for these peptides are produced in the neuronal cell body and transported down the axon in secretory granules. During transport, precursors are cleaved into mature peptides and a carrier protein—neurophysin (Verbalis, 1983). Activation of these neurons generates an axon potential that results in calcium influx and secretion of granule contents into the perivascular space. These secreted peptides then enter adjacent blood vessels for transport throughout the peripheral circulation.

Of these two peptides, oxytocin has significant roles in both parturition and lactation (Kiss, 2005). The role of oxytocin in labor initiation is disputed, as serum oxytocin levels are constant until the expulsive portion of labor (Blanks, 2003). Nevertheless, greater myometrial and decidual oxytocin-receptor expression has been noted near term, primarily due to a rise in estrogen levels.

Once labor is initiated, oxytocin is the primary mediator of myometrial contractility. Cervical and vaginal stimulation results in an acute release of oxytocin from the posterior pituitary in a process known as the *Ferguson reflex*. Clinically, oxytocin's ability to induce uterine contractions is exploited to induce or augment labor.

Vaginal distention, such as occurs with coitus, also augments oxytocin release. Based on this observation, oxytocin may be responsible for the rhythmic uterine and tubal contractions that aid sperm delivery to the oocyte. Oxytocin may also play a role in orgasm and ejaculation.

During lactation, PRL is critical for milk production in breast alveoli. The glandular cells of the alveoli are surrounded by a mesh of myoepithelial cells. Suckling triggers nerve impulses from mechanoreceptors in the nipple and areola that increase hypothalamic neuronal activity. Subsequent oxytocin release prompts the myoepithelial cells to contract and thereby express milk from the alveoli into the ducts and sinuses (Crowley, 1992). Other conditioned stimuli, such as the sight, sound, or smell of a baby or sexual arousal, can have similar effects.

Oxytocin expression has also been detected in the anterior pituitary, placenta, fallopian tubes, gonads, and corpus luteum (Williams, 1990). Its function in these tissues is unclear.

MENSTRUAL CYCLE

The "typical" menstrual cycle is 28 ± 7 days with menstrual flow lasting 4 ± 2 days and blood loss averaging 20 to 60 mL. By convention, the first day of vaginal bleeding is considered day 1 of the menstrual cycle. Menstrual cycle intervals vary among women and often for an individual woman at different times during her reproductive life. That said, cycles are least variable between the ages of 20 and 40 years. In a study of more than 2700 women, menstrual cycle intervals were most irregular in the 2 years following menarche and the 3 years preceding menopause (Treloar, 1967). Specifically, a trend toward shorter intervals followed by interval lengthening is common during the menopausal transition. In a recent study of more than 600,000 menstrual cycles, cycle length progressively shortened by 0.19 days per year for women aged 25 to 45 years (Bull, 2019).

When viewed from a perspective of ovarian function, the menstrual cycle can be defined as a preovulatory follicular phase and postovulatory luteal phase. Corresponding phases in the endometrium are termed the proliferative and secretory phases (Table 16-5). In the recent study just noted, a mean follicular-phase length of 16.9 days and mean luteal phase length

TABLE 16-5. Menstrual Cycle Characteristics

	Menstrual Cycle Phases		
Cycle day	1–5	6–14	15–28
Ovarian phase	Early follicular	Late follicular	Luteal
Endometrial phase	Menstrual	Proliferative	Secretory
Estrogen/progesterone	Low levels	Estrogen	Progesterone

of 12.4 days were found (Bull, 2019). As new data accumulate, reevaluation of the classic definition of cycle phase duration may be needed, but for now is not indicated (Fig. 16-12). For most women, the luteal phase of the menstrual cycle is stable. Thus, variations in normal cycle length generally result from variable duration of the follicular phase (Ferin, 1974).

■ The Ovary

Ovarian Morphology

The adult human ovary is oval with a length of 2 to 5 cm, a width of 1.5 to 3 cm, and a thickness of 0.5 to 1.5 cm. During the reproductive years, the ovary weighs between 5 and 10 g. It

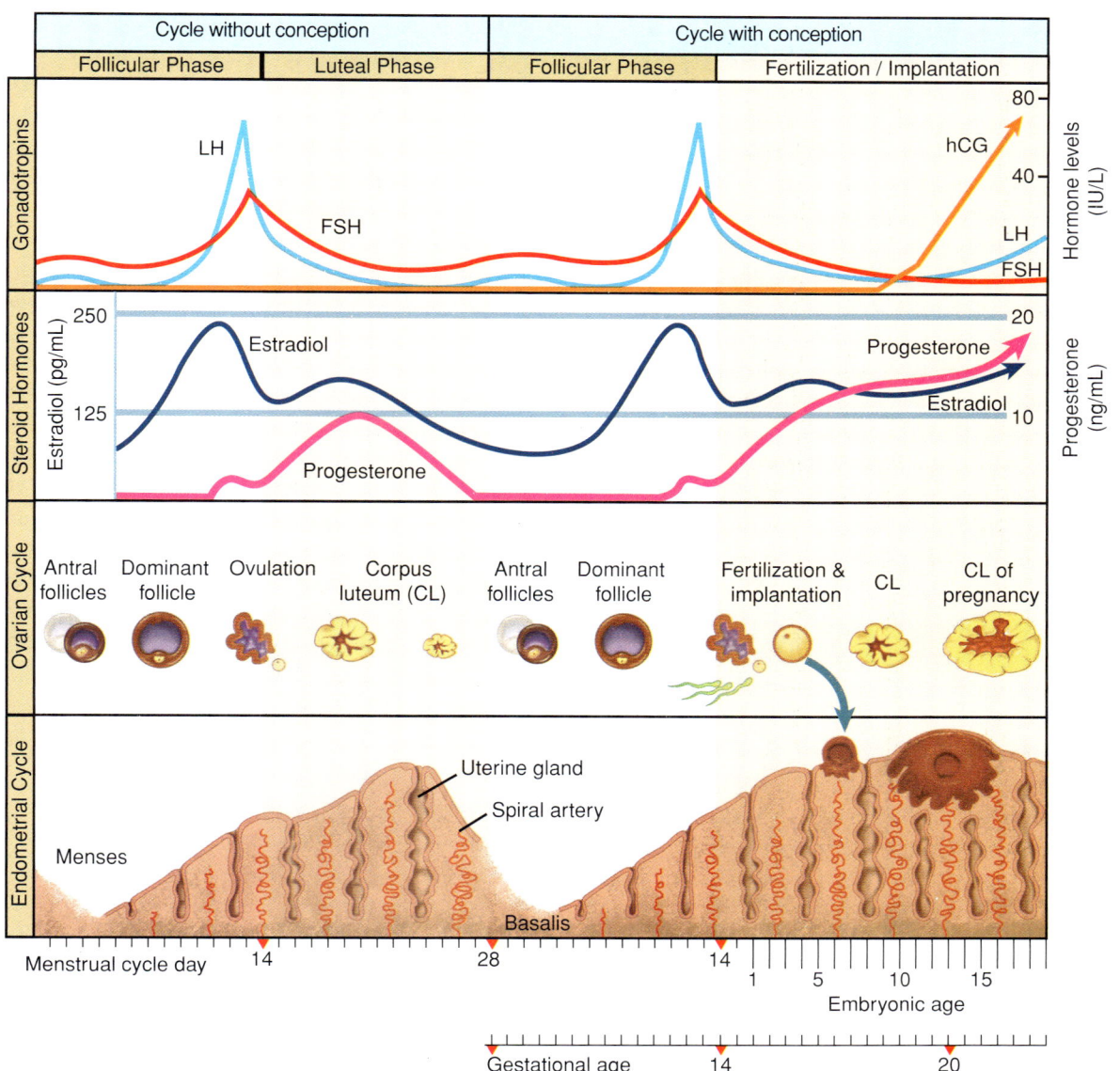

FIGURE 16-12 Gonadotropin control of the ovarian and endometrial cycles. The ovarian-endometrial cycle has been structured as a 28-day cycle. If implantation occurs, the developing blastocyst will begin to produce human chorionic gonadotropin (hCG) and rescue the corpus luteum, thus maintaining progesterone production. FSH = follicle-stimulating hormone; LH = luteinizing hormone. (Reproduced with permission from Mahendroo MS, Cunningham FG: Implantation and placental development. In Cunningham FG, Leveno KJ, Bloom SL, et al (eds): Williams Obstetrics, 25th ed. New York, McGraw-Hill, 2018a.)

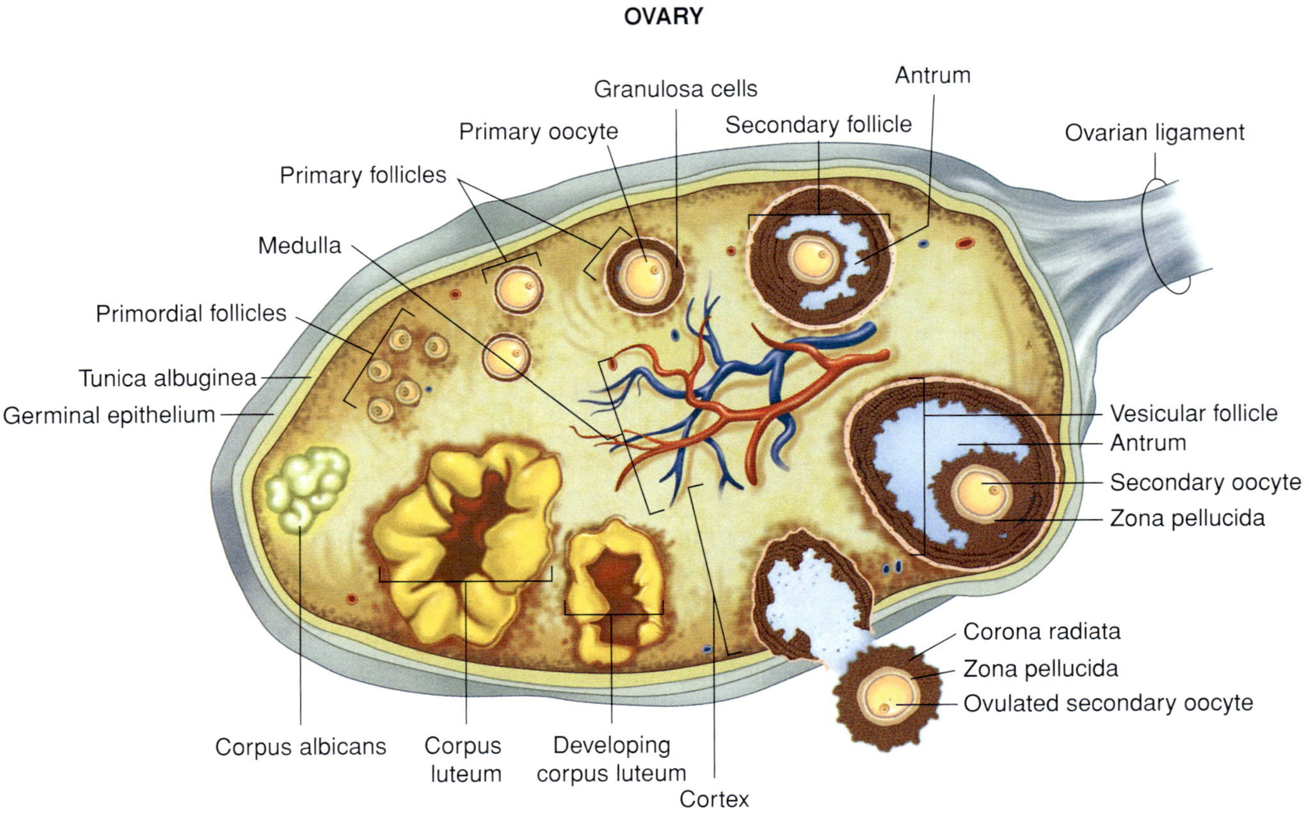

OVARY

FIGURE 16-13 Ovarian anatomy and various sequential steps of follicular development.

is composed of three parts. The outer cortical region contains both the germinal epithelium and the follicles. The medullary region consists of connective tissue, myoid-like contractile cells, and interstitial cells. Last, the hilum contains blood vessels, lymphatics, and nerves that enter the ovary (Fig. 16-13).

Ovaries have two interrelated functions. The first is generation of mature oocytes. Second, production of steroid and peptide hormones creates an environment in which fertilization and subsequent blastocyst implantation in the endometrium can occur. Within each cycle, endocrine functions of the ovary correlate closely to the morphologic appearance and disappearance of follicles and the corpus luteum.

Ovarian Embryology

The ovary develops from three major cellular sources. First, primordial germ cells, which arise from the endoderm of the yolk sac, differentiate into the primary oogonia. Coelomic epithelial cells develop into granulosa cells, which surround the oocytes. Third, mesenchymal cells from the gonadal ridge become the ovarian stroma. Additional information regarding gonadal differentiation is found in Chapter 19 (p. 406).

Primordial germ cells can be seen in the yolk sac as early as the third week of gestation (Gosden, 2013). These cells begin their migration into the gonadal ridge during the sixth week of gestation and generate primary sex cords. The ovary and testes are indistinguishable by histologic criteria until approximately 10 to 11 weeks of fetal life.

After the primordial cells reach the gonad, they continue to multiply through successive mitotic divisions. Starting at

12 weeks' gestation, a subset of oogonia will enter meiosis to become primary oocytes. Primary oocytes are surrounded by a single layer of flattened granulosa cells, creating a primordial follicle.

Oocyte Loss with Aging

All oogonia either develop into primary oocytes or become atretic. Classic teaching states that additional oocytes cannot be generated postnatally. This differs markedly from the male, in whom sperm are produced continuously throughout adulthood. However, recent studies suggest that ovarian stem cells may be able to generate mature oocytes, providing hope for future female fertility preservation. Currently, these results remain preliminary and somewhat controversial (Martin, 2019; Notarianni, 2011; Virant-Klun, 2015).

The maximal number of oogonia is achieved at the 20th week of gestation, at which time 6 to 7 million oogonia are present in the ovary (Baker, 1963). Approximately 1 to 2 million oogonia are present at birth (Fig. 15-1, p. 321). Fewer than 400,000 are present at the initiation of puberty, of which fewer than 500 are destined to ovulate. Therefore, most germ cells are lost through atresia (Hsueh, 1996). Follicular atresia is thought not to be a passive, necrotic process, but rather a precisely controlled active process, namely apoptosis, which is under hormonal control. Apoptosis begins in utero and continues throughout reproductive life.

Oocyte Maturation

As previously mentioned, primary oogonia enter meiosis in utero to become primary oocytes. These oocytes are arrested in development at prophase I during the first meiotic division. Meiotic progression resumes each month in a cohort of follicles. Meiosis I is completed in the oocyte destined for ovulation in response to the LH surge. Once again, the process is arrested, this time in the second meiotic metaphase. Meiosis II is completed only if the ovum is fertilized (Fig. 16-14).

Normal oocyte development requires cytoplasmic modifications in addition to meiotic maturation. Changes in

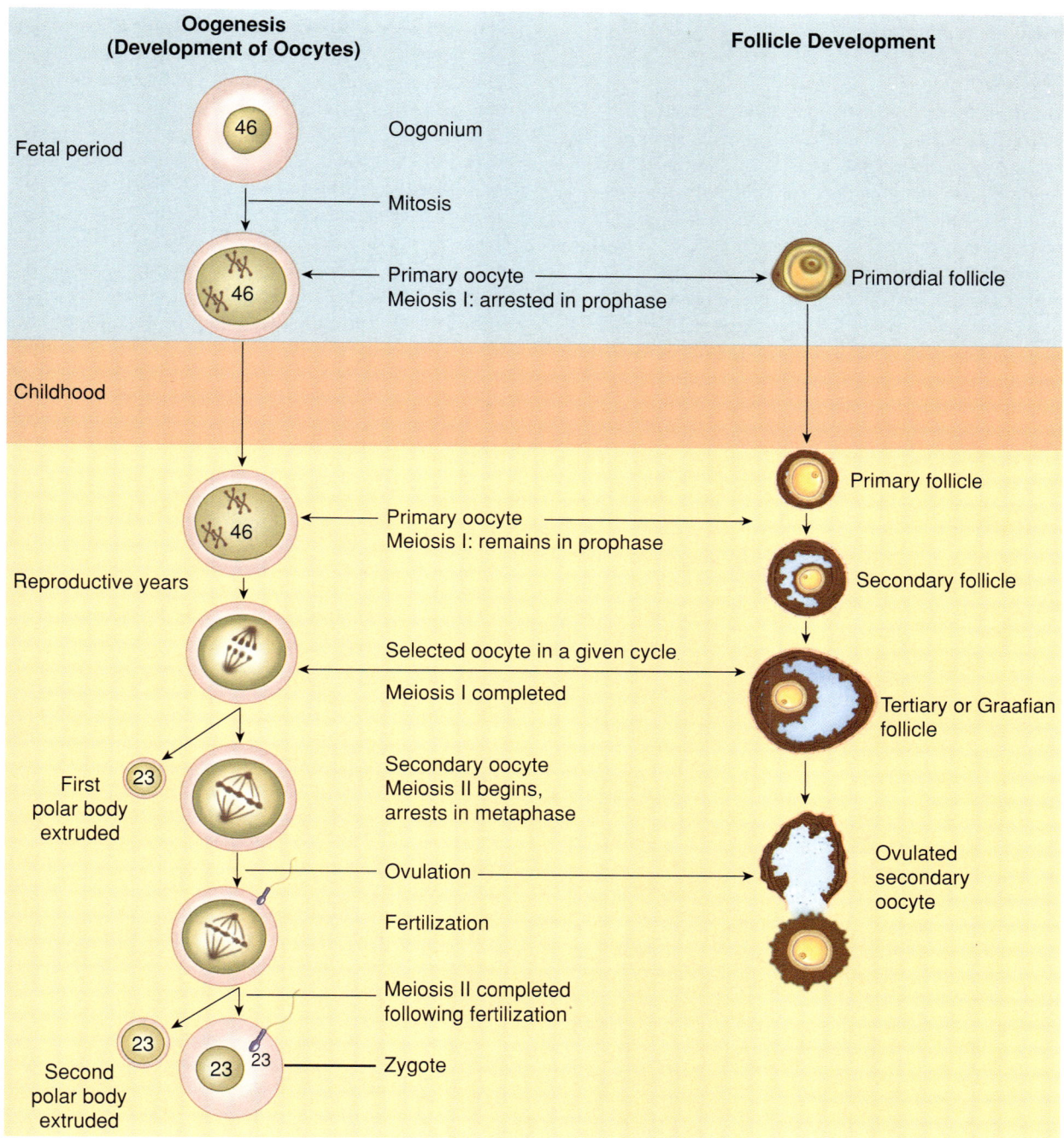

FIGURE 16-14 The steps of oocyte development and corresponding follicular maturation. In the fetal period, once the primordial germ cells arrive in the gonad, they differentiate into oogonia. Mitotic division of oogonia increases the population. Many oogonia further differentiate into primary oocytes, which begin meiosis. However, the process arrests after only prophase is completed. A primary oocyte with its surrounding epithelial cells is called a primordial follicle. In childhood, primary oocytes remain suspended in prophase I. Beginning in puberty and extending through the reproductive years, several primordial follicles mature each month into primary follicles. A few of these continue development to secondary follicles. One or two secondary follicles progress to a tertiary or graafian follicle stage. At this stage, the first meiotic division completes to produce a haploid secondary oocyte and a polar body. During this process, cytoplasm is conserved by the secondary oocyte. Consequently, the polar body is disproportionately small. The secondary oocyte halts meiosis at its second prophase. One of the secondary oocytes is then released at ovulation. If the oocyte is fertilized, completion of the second meiotic division follows. If fertilization fails to occur, then the oocyte degenerates before completion of the second meiotic division.

microtubules and actin filaments enable rearrangement of cellular organelles to allow successful polar body extrusion and fertilization (Coticchio, 2015). The critical cumulus cells that surround the oocyte modulate maturation both by cell-to-cell contact via gap junctions and by secretion of paracrine factors. Our growing understanding of these factors and processes is improving in vitro maturation protocols to aid fertility preservation and infertility treatments.

Stromal Cells

Ovarian stroma contains interstitial cells, contractile cells, and connective tissue cells. These last cells provide structural support to the ovary. The group of interstitial cells that surround a developing follicle and granulosa cells differentiates into theca cells. Under gonadotropin stimulation, theca cells grow in size and develop lipid stores, which is characteristic of steroid-producing cells (Saxena, 1972).

Another group of interstitial cells in the ovarian hilum are known as *hilus cells*. These closely resemble testicular Leydig cells, and hyperplasia or neoplastic changes in hilus cells may result in excess testosterone secretion and virilization. The normal role of these cells is unknown, but their intimate association with blood vessels and neurons suggest that they may convey systemic signals to the remainder of the ovary.

■ Ovarian Hormone Production

The normal functioning ovary synthesizes and secretes estrogens, androgens, and progesterone in a precisely controlled pattern determined, in part, by the pituitary gonadotropins, FSH and LH. The most important secretory products of ovarian steroid biosynthesis are progesterone and estradiol. However, the ovary also secretes quantities of estrone, androstenedione, testosterone, and 17α-hydroxyprogesterone. Sex steroid hormones play an important role in the menstrual cycle by preparing the uterus for implantation of a fertilized ovum. If implantation does not occur, ovarian steroidogenesis declines, the endometrium degenerates, and menstruation ensues.

Two-Cell Theory

Ovarian estrogen biosynthesis requires the combined action of LH and FSH on theca and granulosa cells. This concept is known as the two-cell theory of ovarian steroidogenesis (Fig. 16-15) (Peters, 1980). Until the late antral stage of follicular development, LH-receptor expression is limited to the theca compartment, and FSH-receptor expression is limited to granulosa cells.

Theca cells express all of the enzymes needed to produce androstenedione. This includes high levels of *CYP17* gene expression, whose enzyme product catalyzes 17-hydroxylation. This is the rate-limiting step in the conversion of progesterones to androgens (Sasano, 1989). This enzyme is absent in granulosa cells, and they are incapable of producing the androgenic precursors needed to produce estrogens. Granulosa cells therefore rely on theca cells. Namely, in response to LH stimulation, theca cells synthesize androstenedione and testosterone. These androgens are secreted into the extracellular fluid and diffuse across the basement membrane to the granulosa cells to provide precursors for estrogen production. In contrast to theca cells, granulosa cells have high levels of aromatase activity in response to FSH stimulation. Thus, granulosa cells efficiently convert androgens to estrogens and primarily to the potent estrogen estradiol. In sum, ovarian steroidogenesis is dependent on the effects of LH and FSH acting independently on the theca cells and granulosa cells, respectively.

Steroidogenesis across the Life Span

Circulating levels of the gonadotropins LH and FSH vary markedly at different ages of a woman's life. In utero, the fetal

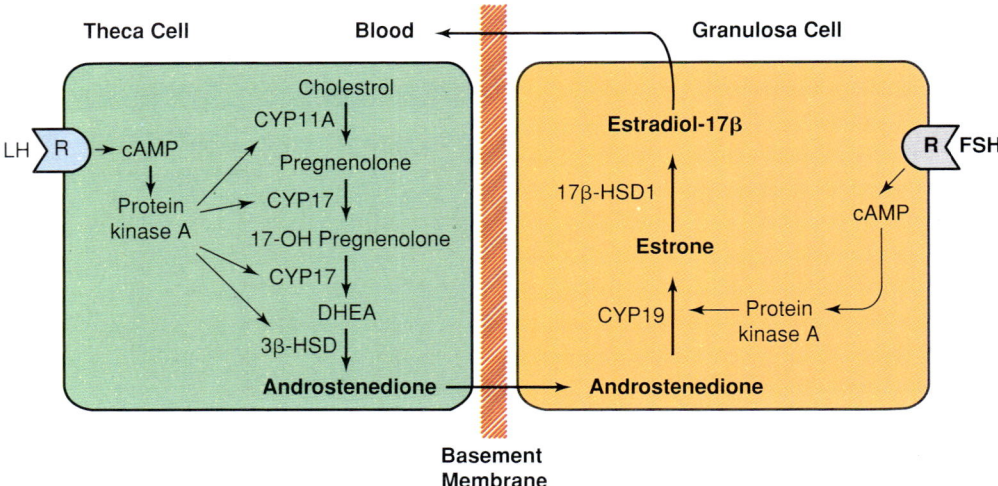

FIGURE 16-15 Diagram illustrates the two-cell theory of ovarian follicular steroidogenesis. Theca cells contain large numbers of luteinizing hormone (LH) receptors. Binding of LH to these receptors leads to cyclic AMP activation and synthesis of androstenedione from cholesterol. Androstenedione diffuses across the basement membrane of theca cells to enter granulosa cells of the ovary. Here, under the activation of follicle-stimulating hormone (FSH), androstenedione is converted by the enzyme aromatase to estrone and estradiol. cAMP = cyclic adenosine monophosphate; CYP11A = cholesterol side-chain cleavage enzyme; CYP17 = 17α-hydroxylase; CYP19 = aromatase; DHEA = dehydroepiandrosterone; 3β-HSD = 3β-hydroxysteroid dehydrogenase; 17β-HSD1 = 17β-hydroxysteroid dehydrogenase; R = receptor.

human ovary can produce estrogens by 8 weeks' gestation. However, a minimal amount of steroid is actually synthesized during fetal development (Miller, 1988). During the second trimester, the plasma levels of gonadotropins rise to levels similar to those observed in menopause (Temeli, 1985). The fetal hypothalamic-pituitary axis continues to mature during this time, becoming more sensitive to the high circulating levels of estrogen and progesterone secreted by the placenta (Kaplan, 1976). Prior to birth and in response to these high steroid levels, fetal gonadotropins fall to low levels.

After delivery, gonadotropin levels in the neonate rise abruptly due to separation from the placenta and subsequent freedom from placental steroid feedback inhibition (Winter, 1976). The elevated gonadotropin levels persist for the first few months of life and then decline to low levels in early childhood (Schmidt, 2000). Multiple etiologies may explain the low gonadotropin levels during this time. The hypothalamic-pituitary axis has increased sensitivity to negative feedback, even by the low circulating levels of gonadal steroids at this stage. Moreover, a direct CNS role may maintain low gonadotropin levels. In support of this mechanism, low levels of LH and FSH are found even in children with gonadal dysgenesis who lack negative feedback by gonadal steroids.

With puberty onset, one early sign is a sleep-associated rise in LH secretion (Fig. 16-16) (Faiman, 1976). Over time, greater gonadotropin secretion is noted throughout the day. An increased FSH to LH ratio is typical in the premenarchal girl and postmenopausal woman. During the reproductive years, LH exceeds FSH levels and inverts this ratio. These increased gonadotropin levels stimulate ovarian estradiol production. The rise in estrogen levels prompts pubertal breast enlargement, which is termed *thelarche*, and internal and external genitalia maturation.

This is accompanied by development of a female habitus, including a height growth spurt. Activation of the pituitary-adrenal axis results in greater adrenal androgen production and the associated pubertal development of axillary and pubic hair, termed *adrenarche* or *pubarche*. Increased gonadotropin levels ultimately lead to ovulation and subsequent menses. The first menstrual period defines *menarche*. This developmental process spans approximately 3 to 4 years and is discussed further in Chapter 15 (p. 321).

Following menopause, the postmenopausal ovary contains only a few follicles. As a result, plasma estrogen and inhibin levels decline markedly after cessation of ovulatory cycles. Through loss of this negative feedback, LH and FSH levels are strikingly elevated. High LH levels can stimulate production of C19 steroids (mainly androstenedione) in ovarian stromal cells. This ovarian-derived androstenedione and adrenal androgens can be converted by peripheral tissues to estrone, the principal serum estrogen in the postmenopausal women. The major site for the conversion of androstenedione to estrone is adipose tissue. Peripheral conversion of circulating androstenedione to estrone is directly correlated to body weight. For a given body weight, conversion is higher in postmenopausal women than in premenopausal women. However, these low circulating estrogen levels are usually not adequate to protect against bone loss.

■ Gonadal Peptides and the Menstrual Cycle

Of gonadal peptides, *inhibin*, *activin*, and *follistatin* modulate gonadotrope activity (de Kretser, 2002). As suggested by their names, inhibin decreases and activin stimulates gonadotrope function. Follistatin suppresses *FSHβ* gene expression, most likely by binding to and thereby preventing the interaction of activin with its receptor (Xia, 2009).

Inhibin and activin are closely related peptides. Inhibin consists of an α-subunit (unrelated to the LH and FSH glycoprotein α-subunit) linked by a disulfide bridge to one of two highly homologous β-subunits to form inhibin A ($\alpha\beta_A$) or inhibin B ($\alpha\beta_B$). Activin is composed of homodimers ($\beta_A\beta_A$, $\beta_B\beta_B$) or heterodimers ($\beta_A\beta_B$) of the same β-subunits as inhibin (Bilezikjian, 2012). In contrast, follistatin is structurally unrelated to either inhibin or activin.

Although originally isolated from follicular fluid, these peptides are expressed in the pituitary, ovary, testes, and placenta and in the brain, adrenal, liver, kidney, and bone marrow to provide diverse tissue-specific functions (Muttukrishna, 2004). Activin and follistatin most likely act as autocrine/paracrine factors in the tissues in which they are expressed, including the ovary.

In contrast, ovarian-derived inhibins circulate in significant concentrations and are believed to be critical for negative

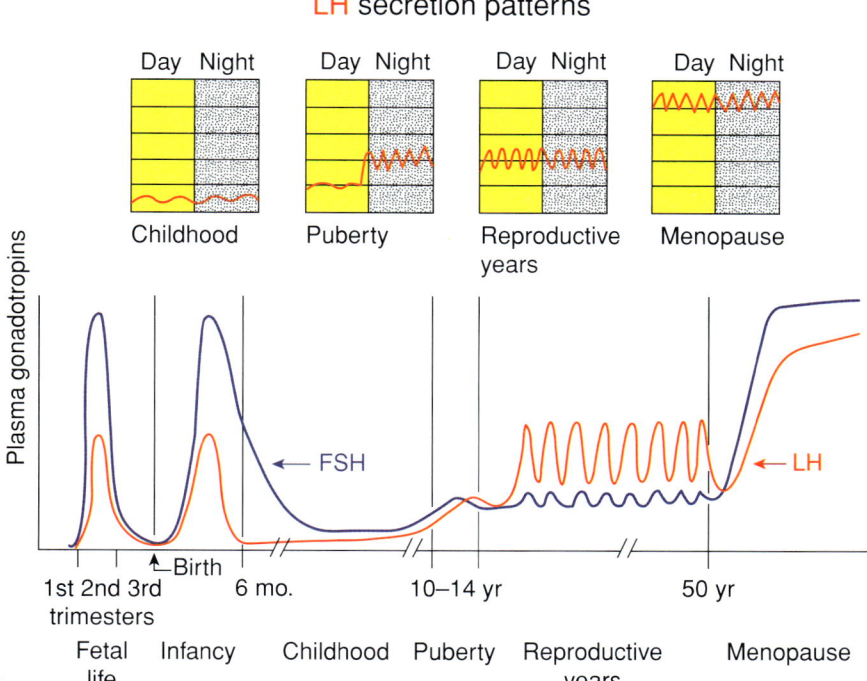

LH secretion patterns

Day Night   Day Night   Day Night   Day Night

Childhood   Puberty   Reproductive years   Menopause

Plasma gonadotropins

FSH

LH

1st 2nd 3rd trimesters   6 mo.   10–14 yr   50 yr
↑ Birth

Fetal life   Infancy   Childhood   Puberty   Reproductive years   Menopause

FIGURE 16-16 Variations in luteinizing hormone (LH) and follicle-stimulating hormone (FSH) during different life stages in the female.

feedback of gonadotropin gene expression. Specifically, during the early follicular phase, FSH stimulates the secretion of inhibin B by the granulosa cells (Fig. 16-17) (Buckler, 1989). However, increasing levels of circulating inhibin B blunt later FSH secretion in the follicular phase. During the luteal phase, regulation of inhibin production comes under the control of LH and switches from inhibin B to inhibin A (McLachlan, 1989). Inhibin B levels peak with the LH surge, whereas inhibin A levels peak a few days later, in the midluteal phase. All inhibin levels decline with the loss of luteal function and remain low during the luteal-follicular transition and early follicular phase. The inverse relationship between circulating inhibin levels and FSH secretion is consistent with a negative-feedback role for inhibin in regulating FSH secretion.

Distinct from these three peptides, insulin-like growth factors also mediate ovarian function. Only IGF-II is involved in primordial follicle development, but both IGF-I and IGF-II stimulate growth of secondary follicles. Gonadotropins stimulate IGF-II production in theca cells, granulosa cells, and luteinized granulosa cells. Receptors for IGF are expressed on the theca and granulosa cells, supporting an autocrine/paracrine action in the follicle. FSH also mediates expression of IGF-binding proteins. This system, although complex, allows additional fine-tuning of intrafollicular activity (Silva, 2009).

Follicular Development
Follicle Stages

Development begins with primordial follicles that were generated during fetal life (see Fig. 16-14). These follicles consist of an oocyte arrested in the first meiotic division surrounded by a single layer of flattened granulosa cells. The follicles are separated from the stroma by a thin basement membrane. Preovulatory follicles are avascular. As such, they are critically dependent on diffusion and on the later development of gap junctions for obtaining nutrients and clearing metabolic waste. Diffusion also allows passage of steroid precursors from the theca cell layer to the granulosa cell layer.

In the primary-follicle stage, the granulosa cells of developing follicles become cuboidal, increase in number, and form a pseudostratified layer. Intercellular gap junctions develop between adjacent granulosa cells and between granulosa cells and the developing oocyte (Albertini, 1974). Gap junctions allow cells without gonadotropin receptors to receive signals from cells with receptor expression. As a result, hormone-mediated effects can be transmitted throughout the follicle.

During this stage, the oocyte secretes products to form an acellular coat known as the *zona pellucida*. The human zona pellucida contains at least three proteins, named *ZP1, ZP2,* and *ZP3*. In current physiologic models, receptors on the acrosome head of the sperm recognize ZP3. This interaction releases acrosomal contents that permit penetration of the zona pellucida and ovum fertilization. Enzymes released from the acrosome induce alterations in ZP2 resulting in hardening of the coat, which prevents fertilization of the oocyte by more than one sperm (Gupta, 2015).

Development of a secondary, or preantral, follicle includes final oocyte growth and a further increase in granulosa cell number. The stroma around the granulosa cell layer differentiates into the *theca interna* and the *theca externa* (Eppig, 1979).

Tertiary follicles, also called *antral follicles*, form from ongoing development in selected oocytes. In these, follicular fluid collects between the granulosa cells, ultimately producing a fluid-filled space known as the *antrum*. Granulosa cells in the antral follicle are histologically and functionally divided into two groups. The granulosa cells surrounding the oocyte form the *cumulus oophorus*, whereas the granulosa cells surrounding the antrum are known as *mural granulosa cells*. Antral fluid consists of a plasma filtrate and factors secreted by the granulosa cells. These locally produced factors, which include estrogen and growth factors, are present in substantially higher concentrations in follicular fluid than in the circulation and are likely

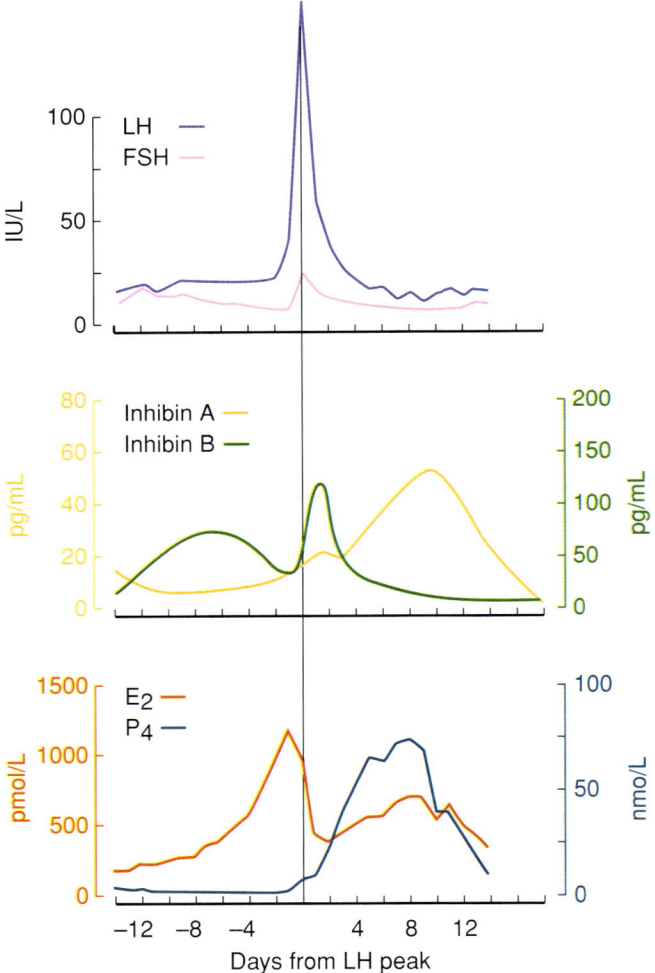

FIGURE 16-17 Gonadotropin, inhibin, and sex steroid level changes during a normal menstrual cycle. The top graph displays peaking of luteinizing hormone (LH) (purple line) and follicle-stimulating hormone (FSH) (pink line) levels. The middle graph shows changing levels of inhibin A and inhibin B. Note that inhibin B levels (green line) peak temporally near the midcycle surge in the LH level, whereas maximal elevation of inhibin A (orange line) occurs several days following this peak. In the bottom graph, elevations in estradiol levels (red line) are noted prior to the surge in LH levels and in the midluteal phase. Progesterone levels (blue line) peak in the midluteal phase. E_2 = estradiol; P_4 = progesterone.

critical for successful follicular maturation (Asimakopoulos, 2006; Silva, 2009). Further accumulation of antral fluid results in rapid follicular size growth and development of a preovulatory follicle, also called a *graafian follicle* (Hennet, 2012).

During this process, early stages of development (up to the secondary follicle) do not require gonadotropin stimulation and thus are said to be "gonadotropin-independent." Final follicular maturation requires adequate amounts of circulating LH and FSH and is therefore said to be "gonadotropin-dependent" (Butt, 1970). Data suggest that progression from gonadotropin-independent to -dependent stages is not as discrete as previously believed.

Selection Window

Follicular development is a multistep process, which proceeds over at least 3 months and culminates in ovulation from a single follicle. Each month, a group of follicles known as a *cohort* begins a phase of semisynchronous growth. The cohort size appears to be proportional to the number of inactive primordial follicles within the ovaries and ranges from 3 to 11 follicles per ovary in young women (Hodgen, 1982; Pache, 1990). Importantly, the ovulatory follicle is recruited from a cohort that began development two to three cycles prior to the current ovulatory cycle. During this time, most follicles will die as they will not be at an appropriate stage of development during the selection window.

During the luteal-follicular transition, a small rise in FSH levels is responsible for selection of the single dominant follicle that will ultimately ovulate (Schipper, 1998). As previously described, theca cells produce androgens and granulosa cells generate estrogens. Estrogen levels rise with growing follicular size, enhance the effects of FSH on granulosa cells, and create a feed-forward action on follicles that produce estrogen.

Intrafollicular levels of the insulin-like growth factors are believed to synergize with FSH to help select the dominant follicle (Son, 2011). In addition, vascular endothelial growth factor (VEGF) levels around the follicle that will be selected are elevated. VEGF-associated enhancement of vascularity would presumably expose this follicle to higher levels of circulating factors, such as FSH.

Granulosa cells also produce inhibin B, which passes from the follicle into the plasma and specifically inhibits the release of FSH, but not of LH, by the anterior pituitary gland. The combined production of estradiol and inhibin B by the dominant follicle results in the decline of follicular-phase FSH levels and may be responsible at least in part for the failure of the other follicles to reach preovulatory status during any one cycle.

Estrogen-Dominant Microenvironment

Ongoing follicular maturation requires the successful conversion from an "androgen-dominant" microenvironment to an "estrogen-dominant" one. At low concentrations, androgens stimulate aromatization and contribute to estrogen production. However, intrafollicular androgen levels will rise if aromatization in the granulosa cells lags behind androgen production by the thecal layer. At higher concentrations, androgens are converted to the more potent 5α-androgens, such as dihydrotestosterone. These androgens inhibit aromatase activity, cannot be aromatized to estrogens, and inhibit

FSH induction of LH-receptor expression on the granulosa cells (Gervásio, 2014).

This model predicts that follicles that lack adequate FSH receptor and granulosa cell number will remain primarily androgenic and will become atretic. An increased androgen-to-estrogen ratio is found in the follicular fluid of atretic follicles, and several studies demonstrate that high estrogen levels prevent apoptosis.

Insulin-like growth factor I also has apoptosis-suppressing activity and is produced by granulosa cells. This action of IGF-I is diminished by certain IGF-binding proteins that are present in the follicular fluid of atretic follicles. The action of FSH to prevent atresia may therefore result, in part, from its ability to stimulate IGF-I synthesis and suppress synthesis of IGF-binding proteins.

◼ Menstrual Cycle Phases

Follicular Phase

During the end of a previous cycle, estrogen, progesterone, and inhibin levels decline abruptly, whereas circulating FSH levels rise (Hodgen, 1982). As just described, this higher FSH level is responsible for recruitment of the follicle cohort that contains the follicle destined for ovulation. Despite general belief, sonographic studies in women demonstrate that ovulation does not alternate sides but occurs randomly from either ovary (Baird, 1987).

In women with waning ovarian function, FSH levels in the early follicular phase are elevated relative to those of younger women, presumably due to a loss of ovarian inhibin production in the prior luteal phase. Thus, measurement of cycle-day-3 FSH and estradiol levels is frequently performed in infertility clinics. The accelerated rise in serum FSH levels results in more robust recruitment of follicles and may explain both the shortened follicular phase observed in older reproductive-aged women and their increased incidence of spontaneous twinning.

During the midfollicular phase, follicles produce greater amounts of estrogen and inhibin. This leads to a decline in FSH levels through negative feedback. This drop in FSH levels is believed to aid selection of the follicle destined to ovulate, termed the *dominant follicle*. Based on this theory, remaining follicles, which will undergo atresia, express fewer FSH receptors and are unable to respond adequately to declining FSH levels. As noted earlier, decreased VEGF expression also plays a role by decreasing surrounding vascularity and delivery of circulating factors to these follicles (Ravindranath, 1992).

During most of follicular development, granulosa cells respond to FSH by raising their cell number, augmenting aromatase expression, and, in the presence of estradiol, increasing expression of LH receptors on the granulosa cells. With LH-receptor expression during the late follicular phase, granulosa cells begin to produce small amounts of progesterone. This progesterone decreases granulosa cell proliferation and thereby slows follicular growth (Chaffkin, 1992).

Ovulation

Toward the end of the follicular phase, estradiol levels increase dramatically. Although not completely understood but perhaps related to changes at the kisspeptin neurons, the rapid estradiol level rise triggers a switch from negative to positive feedback at both the hypothalamus and anterior pituitary gland. This feedback change generates a surge in LH levels. Estradiol concentrations of 200 pg/mL for 50 hours are necessary to initiate this LH surge (Young, 1976). A small preovulatory rise in progesterone concentrations generates an FSH level surge, which occurs in tandem with the LH surge (McNatty, 1979). Progesterone may also augment the ability of estradiol to trigger the LH surge. These effects may explain the occasional induction of ovulation in anovulatory amenorrheic women when given progesterone to induce menses.

The LH surge acts quickly on both the granulosa and theca cells of the preovulatory follicle to terminate the genes involved in follicular expression and turn on the genes necessary for ovulation and luteinization. In addition, the LH surge initiates reentry of the oocyte into meiosis, expansion of the cumulus oophorus, synthesis of prostaglandins, and luteinization of granulosa cells. The mean duration of the LH surge is 48 hours, and ovulation occurs 36 to 40 hours after the LH surge onset (Hoff, 1983; Lemarchand-Beraud, 1982).

The surge is abruptly terminated and is thought to follow acutely augmented steroid and inhibin secretion by the corpus luteum. Alternatively, production of a gonadotropin surge-inhibiting/attenuating factor (GnSIF/AF) by either the ovary or hypothalamus also is postulated. The identity of this factor remains unknown (Vega, 2015).

The granulosa cells surrounding the oocyte, unlike mural granulosa cells, do not express LH receptors or synthesize progesterone. These cumulus oophorus granulosa cells develop tight gap junctions between themselves and with the oocyte. The cumulus mass that accompanies the ovulating oocyte is believed to provide a rough surface and larger size to improve oocyte "pick-up" by the tubal fimbria.

Amphiregulin, epiregulin, and betacellulin are recently discovered epidermal growth factor–like factors that can be substituted to elicit the morphologic and biochemical events triggered by LH (Hsieh, 2009). Thus, these growth factors are part of the downstream cascade that begins with LH binding to its receptor and ends with ovulation.

Based on sonographic surveillance, extrusion of the oocyte lasts only a few minutes (Fig. 16-18) (Knobil, 1994). The exact mechanism of this expulsion is poorly defined but is not due to a rise in follicular pressure (Espey, 1974). The presence of proteolytic enzymes in the follicle, including plasmin and collagenase, suggests that these enzymes are responsible for follicular wall thinning (Beers, 1975). The preovulatory gonadotropin surge stimulates expression of tissue plasminogen activator by the granulosa and theca cells. The surge also lowers expression of plasminogen inhibitor and leads to a marked increase in plasminogen activity (Piquette, 1993).

Prostaglandins also reach a peak concentration in follicular fluid during the preovulatory gonadotropin surge (Lumsden, 1986). Prostaglandins may stimulate smooth muscle contraction in the ovary and thereby aid ovulation (Yoshimura, 1987). Women undergoing infertility treatment are advised to avoid prostaglandin synthetase inhibitors in the preovulatory period to avoid *luteinized unruptured follicle syndrome (LUFS)* (Smith,

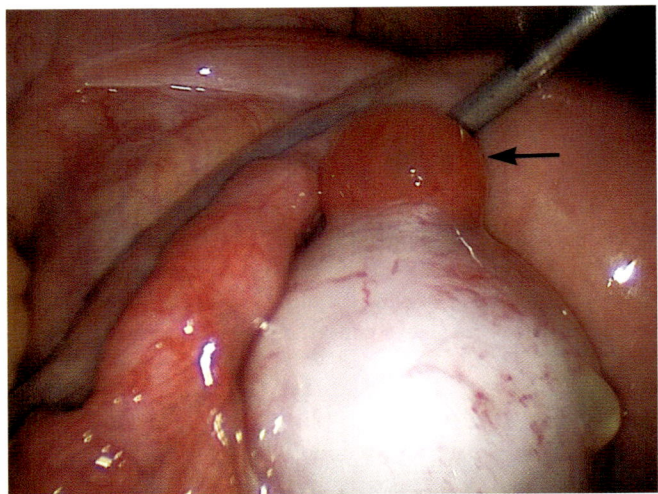

FIGURE 16-18 During laparoscopy, a stigma (*arrow*) on the ovarian surface prior to ovulation is seen. (Reproduced with permission from Dr. David Rogers.)

1996). Whether LUFS is considered pathologic or simply a sporadic event is controversial (Kerin, 1983).

Luteal Phase

Following ovulation, the remaining follicular cells differentiate into the corpus luteum, literally *yellow body* (Corner, 1956). This process, which requires LH stimulation, includes both morphologic and functional changes known as *luteinization*. The granulosa and theca cells proliferate and undergo hypertrophy to form granulosa-lutein cells and smaller theca-lutein cells, respectively (Patton, 1991).

During corpus luteum formation, the basement membrane that separated granulosa cells from theca cells degenerates and allows vascularization of the previously avascular granulosa cells. Capillary invasion begins 2 days after ovulation and reaches the center of the corpus luteum by the fourth day. This augmented perfusion provides these luteal cells with access to circulating low-density lipoprotein (LDL), which is used to provide precursor cholesterol for steroid biosynthesis. This enhanced blood supply can also have clinical implications, and pain from a hemorrhagic corpus luteum cyst is a relatively frequent diagnosis in emergency rooms.

Steroidogenesis in the corpus luteum depends on adequate serum LH levels, LH receptors on luteal cells, and a sufficient number of luteal cells. Thus, it is critical that LH receptor expression on granulosa cells was appropriately induced during the prior follicular phase. Furthermore, blunted serum LH concentrations have been correlated with a shortened luteal phase. Luteal function is also influenced by gonadotropin levels from the preceding follicular phase. Reduced LH or FSH secretion is associated with poor luteal function. Presumably, a lack of FSH leads to fewer granulosa cells. Furthermore, luteal cells in these suboptimal cycles have fewer FSH-induced LH receptors and thus will be less responsive to LH stimulation.

The luteal phase is considered progesterone dominant, which contrasts with the estrogen dominance of the follicular phase. Increased vascularization, cellular hypertrophy, and more intracellular organelles transform the corpus luteum into the most active steroidogenic tissue in the body. Maximal levels of progesterone production are observed in the midluteal phase and have been estimated at an impressive 40 mg of progesterone per day. Ovulation can be safely assumed to have occurred if the progesterone level exceeds 3 ng/mL on cycle day 21.

Although progesterone is the most abundant ovarian steroid during the luteal phase, estradiol also is produced in significant quantities. Estradiol levels drop transiently immediately after the LH surge and may explain the midcycle spotting noticed by some women. Although the reason is unknown, this estradiol decline may result from a direct inhibition of granulosa cell growth by rising progesterone levels (Hoff, 1983). Subsequent to this decline, estradiol levels steadily increase to reach a maximum during the midluteal phase.

The corpus luteum also produces large quantities of inhibin A. This coincides with a drop in circulating FSH levels in the luteal phase. If inhibin A levels decline at the end of the luteal phase, FSH levels rise once more to begin selection of an oocyte cohort for the next menstrual cycle.

If pregnancy does not occur, the corpus luteum regresses through a process called *luteolysis*. The mechanism is poorly understood, but luteal regression is presumed to be tightly regulated. Following luteolysis, the blood supply to the corpus luteum diminishes, progesterone and estrogen secretion drop precipitously, and the luteal cells undergo apoptosis and become fibrotic. This creates the *corpus albicans* (white body).

If pregnancy occurs, hCG produced by the early gestation "rescues" the corpus luteum from atresia by binding to and activating the LH receptor on luteal cells. hCG stimulation of corpus luteum steroidogenesis maintains endometrial stability until placental steroid production is adequate to assume this function late in the first trimester. For this reason, surgical removal of the corpus luteum during pregnancy should be followed by progesterone replacement as outlined in Chapter 6 (p. 139) until approximately 10 weeks' gestation.

ENDOMETRIUM

◼ Menstrual Cycle Changes

The endometrium consists of two layers: the *basalis layer*, which lies against the myometrium, and the *functionalis layer*, which is apposed to the uterine lumen. The basalis layer does not change significantly across the menstrual cycle and serves as the reserve for endometrium regeneration following menstrual sloughing. The functionalis layer is further subdivided into the more superficial *stratum compactum*, a thin layer of gland necks and dense stroma, and the underlying *stratum spongiosum* containing glands and large amounts of loosely organized stroma and interstitial tissue.

After menstruation, the endometrium is 1 to 2 mm thick. Under the influence of estrogen, the glandular and stromal cells of the functionalis layer proliferate rapidly following menses (Fig. 16-19). This period of rapid growth, the *proliferative phase*, corresponds to the ovary's follicular phase. As this phase progresses, glands become more tortuous and cells lining the glandular lumen undergo pseudostratification. The stroma remains compact. Endometrial thickness approximates 12 mm

at the time of the LH surge and does not increase significantly thereafter.

Following ovulation, the endometrium transforms into a secretory tissue. The time during and after this transformation is the *secretory phase* of the endometrium and correlates to the ovary's luteal phase. Glycogen-rich subnuclear vacuoles appear in cells lining the glands. Under further stimulation by progesterone, these vacuoles move from the glandular cells' base toward their lumen and expel their contents. This secretory process peaks on approximately postovulatory day 6 and coincides with the day of implantation. Throughout the luteal phase, glands become more tortuous, and the stroma becomes more edematous. In addition, spiral arteries that feed the endometrium increase their number and coiling.

If a blastocyst does not implant and the corpus luteum is not maintained by placental hCG, progesterone levels drop and endometrial glands begin to collapse. Polymorphonuclear leukocytes and monocytes from nearby vessels infiltrate the endometrium. The spiral arteries constrict, leading to local ischemia, and lysosomes release proteolytic enzymes that accelerate tissue destruction. Prostaglandins, particularly prostaglandin $F_{2\alpha}$, are present in the endometrium and likely contribute to arteriolar vasospasm. Prostaglandin $F_{2\alpha}$ also induces myometrial contractions, which may aid expelling the endometrial tissue.

The entire endometrial functionalis layer is thought to exfoliate with menstruation and leaves only the basalis layer to provide cells for endometrial regeneration. However, in studies, the amount of tissue shed from different levels of the endometrium varies widely. Following menstruation, reepithelialization of the desquamated endometrium is initiated within 2 to 3 days after menses onset and is completed within 48 hours.

◼ Regulation of Endometrial Function
Tissue Degradation and Hemorrhage

Within the endometrium, numerous proteins maintain a delicate balance between tissue integrity and the localized destruction required for menstrual sloughing or for trophoblast invasion during implantation. Cytokines, growth factors, and steroid hormones are believed to regulate the genes encoding these tissue proteins (Maybin, 2012). Of these proteins, tissue factor, which is a membrane-associated protein, activates the coagulation cascade upon contact with blood. In addition, urokinase and tissue plasminogen activator (TPA) increase the conversion of plasminogen to plasmin to activate tissue breakdown. TPA activity is blocked by plasminogen activator inhibitor 1, which is present in endometrial stroma (Lockwood, 1993; Schatz, 1995). Another key mediator group is the matrix metalloproteinases (MMPs). This enzyme family has overlapping substrate specificities for collagens and other extracellular matrix components. The composition of MMPs varies within different endometrial tissues and during the menstrual cycle. Endogenous MMP inhibitor levels rise premenstrually and limit MMP degradative activity.

Vasoconstriction and Myometrial Contractility

Effective menstruation depends upon appropriately timed endometrial vasoconstriction and on myometrial contraction.

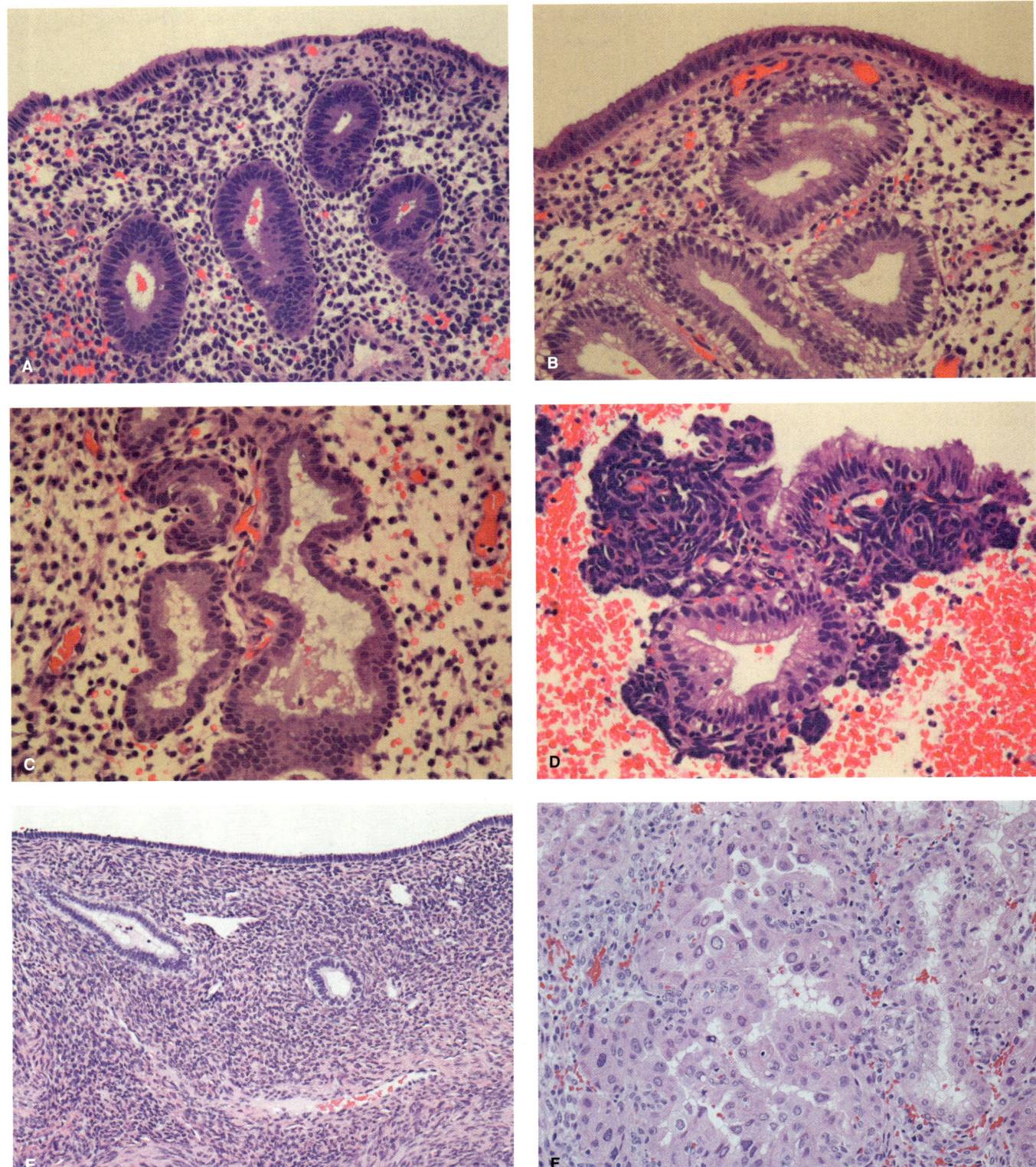

FIGURE 16-19 Endometrial changes during the menstrual cycle. **A.** Proliferative phase: straight to slightly coiled, tubular glands are lined by pseudostratified columnar epithelium with scattered mitoses. **B.** Early secretory phase: coiled glands with a slightly widened diameter are lined by simple columnar epithelium with clear subnuclear vacuoles. Stroma is variably edematous at this time. **C.** Late secretory phase: serrated, dilated glands with intraluminal secretion are lined by short columnar cells. **D.** Menstrual phase: fragmented endometrium with condensed stroma and glands with secretory vacuoles are seen in a background of blood. **E.** Atrophic endometrium: thin endometrium of the postmenopause has straight tubular glands lined by mitotically inactive, cuboidal epithelium. Stroma is dense and mitotically inactive. **F.** Gestational endometrium: hypersecretory glandular pattern featuring closely apposed glands with papillary infoldings and variable cytoplasmic vacuolization. The hypersecretory gland in the center shows the benign Arias-Stella reaction, with nuclear atypia characterized by variable nuclear enlargement, nuclear membrane irregularities, slight chromatin coarseness, nuclear vacuolization, and intranuclear pseudoinclusions. (Reproduced with permission from Dr. Kelley Carrick.)

Vasoconstriction produces ischemia, endometrial damage, and subsequent menstrual sloughing. Within the endometrium, epithelial and stromal cells secrete endothelin 1, a potent vasoconstrictor. Enkephalinase, an endothelin-degrading enzyme, is expressed at its highest levels in the midsecretory endometrium (Head, 1993). However, in the late luteal phase, the drop in serum progesterone leads to a loss of enkephalinase expression. This permits greater endothelin activity, which promotes an environment amenable to vasoconstriction.

In concert with endometrial sloughing, myometrial contractions control blood loss by compressing endometrial vessels and expelling menstrual discharge. A fall in serum progesterone levels lowers concentrations of an enzyme that degrades prostaglandins. This allows greater prostaglandin $F_{2\alpha}$ activity in the myometrium and triggers myometrial contractions (Casey, 1980).

Estrogens and Progestogens

The expression of estrogen and progesterone receptors in the endometrium is highly regulated across the menstrual cycle. This provides an additional mechanism for controlling steroid effects on endometrial development and function. Estrogen receptors are expressed in the nuclei of epithelial, stromal, and myometrial cells, and concentrations peak during the proliferative phase. However, during the luteal phase, rising progesterone levels blunt estrogen receptor expression. Endometrial progesterone receptors peak at midcycle in response to rising estrogen levels. By midluteal phase, progesterone receptor expression in the glandular epithelium is nearly absent, although expression remains strong in the stromal compartment (Lessey, 1988).

The proliferation and differentiation of the uterine epithelium is under the control of estradiol, progesterone, and various growth factors. The importance of estrogens for endometrial development is demonstrated by the predominance of endometrial hyperplasia in women receiving unopposed estrogen therapy. Estrogen interacts directly with estrogen receptors but also can indirectly induce various growth factors that include IGF-I, transforming growth factor α, and epidermal growth factor (Beato, 1989; Dickson, 1987). The effects of progesterone on endometrial growth vary among endometrial layers. Progesterone is critical for the conversion of the functionalis layer from a proliferative to a secretory pattern. Within the basalis layer, progesterone appears to promote cellular proliferation.

Growth Factors and Cell Adhesion Molecules

Numerous growth factors and associated receptors act in the endometrium. Each factor has its own pattern of expression, making it difficult to determine which factor is most critical for endometrial function (Ohlsson, 1989; Sharkey, 1995).

In addition to growth factors, cell adhesion molecules play an important role in endometrial function. These molecules fall into four classes: integrins, cadherins, selectins, and members of the immunoglobulin superfamily. Each has been implicated in endometrial regeneration and embryo implantation, discussed next.

Implantation Window

The embryo enters the uterine cavity 2 to 3 days after fertilization, and implantation begins approximately 4 days later. Normal implantation and embryonic development require synchronous development of the endometrium and the embryo (Pope, 1988). However, the human blastocyst may have less stringent implantation requirements than other species, as ectopic implantation occurs relatively frequently.

Uterine receptivity is defined as the temporal window of endometrial maturation during which trophectoderm attaches to endometrial epithelial cells and subsequently invades into endometrial stroma. The implantation window in humans is relatively broad and extends from day 20 through 24 of the menstrual cycle. Precise determination of this temporal window is critical since only those factors expressed during this time act as direct functional mediators of uterine receptivity.

Endometrial receptivity is associated with loss of surface microvilli and ciliated cells and with development of cellular protrusions, called *pinopods*, on the apical surface of the endometrium. Pinopods are considered an important morphologic marker of peri-implantation endometrium. Pinopod formation is highly progesterone dependent (Yoshinaga, 1989).

Cell adhesion molecules, immunoglobulins, and cytokines are believed to be necessary for uterine receptivity. Integrins are particularly well studied in this regard (Casals, 2010). Clinically, finding a panel of markers that would noninvasively diagnose an endometrial implantation abnormality or determine the implantation window would greatly aid infertility evaluation and treatment. However, at this time, despite substantial effort, no currently available test has demonstrated the reliability or reproducibility to warrant acceptance.

The term *luteal phase defect* describes dyssynchrony between endometrial development and menstrual cycle phase that leads to subsequent implantation failure and early pregnancy loss (Noyes, 1950; Olive, 1991). This term currently has limited utility in clinical practice, because of our inability to accurately diagnose or treat the disorder.

Following implantation, the endometrium undergoes essential remodeling by invading trophoblast. In addition, the maternal endocrine environment changes extensively because of altered maternal physiology and contributions by the placenta and fetus. A more detailed discussion of these changes is found in *Williams Obstetrics*, 25th edition (Mahendroo, 2018a).

HYPOTHALAMIC-PITUITARY AXIS ABNORMALITIES

Classically, abnormalities in this axis result in low gonadotropin and resultant low sex steroid levels. Termed *hypogonadotropic hypogonadism*, this can be developmental or acquired. Developmental lesions due to inherited genetic defects include Kallmann syndrome and idiopathic hypogonadotropic hypogonadism. Acquired abnormalities include functional disorders (eating disorders, excessive exercise, stress) and hypothalamic-pituitary lesions due to tumor, infiltrative diseases, infarction, surgery, or radiation therapy. Information regarding hypothalamic disorders and other causes of hypogonadotropic hypogonadism can be found in Chapter 17 (p. 377). Hyperprolactinemia and pituitary adenomas are discussed here.

■ Hyperprolactinemia

Etiology

Elevated circulating PRL levels can be caused by various physiologic activities including pregnancy, sleep, eating, and coitus. Increased PRL levels, which in general can lead to galactorrhea, may also be observed following chest wall stimulation such as occurs with suckling, breast examination, chest wall surgery, herpes zoster infection, or nipple piercing (Table 13-2, p. 285). PRL is primarily regulated by tonic inhibition of dopamine secretion. PRL secretion is increased by serotonin, norepinephrine, opioids, estrogen, and TRH. Therefore, medications that block dopamine-receptor action (phenothiazines) or increase catecholamine levels (monoamine oxidase inhibitors) may increase PRL levels. Moreover, hyperprolactinemia may be caused by cranial tumor, radiation, or infiltrative diseases such as sarcoid and tuberculosis. These can damage the pituitary stalk and thereby prevent dopamine-mediated inhibition of PRL secretion.

Primary hypothyroidism also is associated with mild elevations in serum PRL levels. Specifically, low circulating thyroid hormone levels produce a reflex rise in hypothalamic TRH levels due to loss of feedback inhibition. TRH can bind directly to anterior pituitary gland lactotropes and stimulate PRL production. As a rule, thyroid function tests should be performed when confirming a diagnosis of hyperprolactinemia, as a patient may require thyroid replacement rather than further evaluation for pituitary adenoma (Hekimsoy, 2010).

Prolactin-secreting adenomas, also termed *prolactinomas*, are the most common pituitary adenoma and the most common adenomas to be diagnosed by gynecologists. Affected women typically present with microadenomas and signs of PRL excess such as galactorrhea and amenorrhea.

Diagnosis

Hyperprolactinemia is, by definition, present in any patient with an elevated serum PRL level. Optimally, PRL levels are drawn in the morning, that is, at the PRL nadir. Prior to testing, breast examination is avoided to prevent false-positive results.

If a mildly elevated PRL level is found, sampling is repeated because PRL levels vary throughout the day. Moreover, many factors including the stress of venipuncture may produce false elevations.

Normal PRL levels are typically <20 ng/mL in nonpregnant women, although the upper limit of normal varies by assay. Importantly, PRL levels rise nearly 10-fold during pregnancy and make detection of a prolactinoma difficult at this time. Occasionally, the reported PRL value will be falsely low due to a "hook effect" present in the assay and discussed earlier (p. 343) (Frieze, 2002). Importantly, a mismatch between the adenoma size noted on magnetic resonance (MR) imaging and the degree of PRL level elevation should alert a clinician to either the possibility of an incorrect assay result or the likelihood that the macroadenoma is actually not primarily PRL secreting. Macroadenomas of any cell type may damage the pituitary stalk and prevent transfer of hypothalamic dopamine to the lactotropes.

Conversely, a patient may rarely have an elevated PRL level on assay despite a lack of clinical features of hyperprolactinemia. The hyperprolactinemia in these patients is thought to be secondary to alternate forms of PRL, including the so-called *big prolactin* or *macroprolactin*, which contains multimers of native PRL. Macroprolactin is not physiologically active but may be detected by PRL assays (Fahie-Wilson, 2005).

For all patients with confirmed hyperprolactinemia, MR imaging is advisable. Some advocate limiting imaging to women with a PRL level >100 ng/mL, as lower levels are most likely due to small microadenomas (Fig. 16-20). Although this is undoubtedly a safe approach in most women, mildly elevated PRL levels may also be due to pituitary stalk compression by a non-prolactin-secreting macroadenoma or a craniopharyngioma, which are diagnoses with severe potential consequences.

The availability of sensitive neuroimaging techniques now affords earlier diagnosis and intervention. Although computed tomography (CT) scanning provides useful information on tumor size, bony artifacts may limit interpretation. Therefore, MR imaging, using both T1- and T2-weighted images, has become the preferred radiologic approach due to its high sensitivity and excellent spatial resolution (Ruscalleda, 2005).

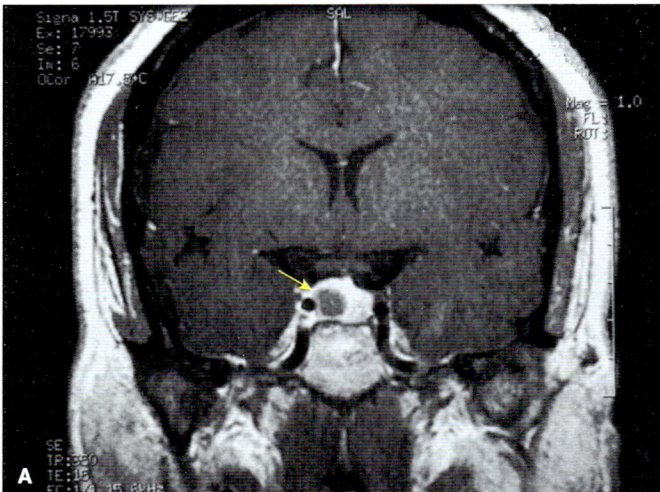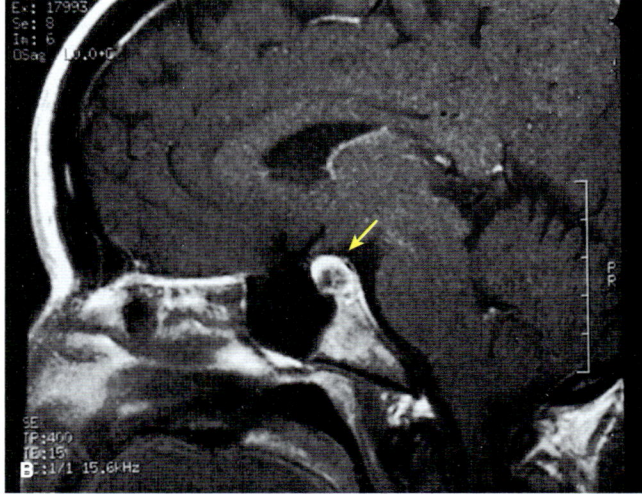

FIGURE 16-20 Magnetic resonance images of a pituitary microadenoma (*arrows*). **A.** Coronal image. **B.** Sagittal image.

Frequently, MR imaging is performed with and without gadolinium contrast to highlight anatomy.

Associated Amenorrhea

The primary mechanism linking hyperprolactinemia and amenorrhea is believed to be a reflex rise in central dopamine levels. Stimulation of the dopaminergic receptors on the GnRH neurons alters GnRH pulsatility, thereby disrupting folliculogenesis. As dopamine receptors have also been identified in the ovaries, detrimental effects on folliculogenesis also may play a role. Additional mechanisms undoubtedly exist in view of the complex interactions that influence hypothalamic function.

■ Pituitary Adenomas
Classification

Pituitary adenomas are the most common cause of acquired pituitary dysfunction and constitute approximately 15 percent of all intracranial tumors (Melmed, 2015; Pekic, 2015). Clinically, symptoms of galactorrhea, menstrual disturbances, or infertility may lead to its diagnosis. Most tumors are benign, and only an estimated 0.1 percent of adenomas develop into frank carcinoma with metastasis (Kaltsas, 2005). Nevertheless, pituitary adenomas may cause striking abnormalities in both endocrine and nervous system function.

Pituitary adenomas were historically classified as eosinophilic, basophilic, or chromophobic according to their hematoxylin and eosin staining characteristics. Tumors are now classified by their hormonal expression pattern as determined by immunohistochemistry (Fig. 16-21). Adenomas are further grouped by size into *microadenomas* (<10 mm in diameter) and *macroadenomas* (>10 mm in diameter).

Most adenomas secrete PRL, however, adenomas may release any of the pituitary hormones (Table 16-6). These may be secreted either as a single hormone (monohormonal adenoma) or in combinations (multihormonal adenoma). In the past, a subset of tumors was considered nonsecreting. However, with more sensitive assays, most have been determined to secrete the common α-subunit or the gonadotropin β-subunits and therefore are gonadotrope-derived. Rarely, both α- and β-subunits are secreted as functional dimeric hormone.

Symptoms

Pituitary adenomas may cause symptoms via excess hormone secretion and lead to hyperprolactinemia, acromegaly, or Cushing disease. Alternatively, adenomas may result in hormone deficiency due to damage of other pituitary cell types or the pituitary stalk by an expanding adenoma or following treatment of the primary lesion.

As might be predicted, pituitary microadenomas are typically diagnosed during evaluation of an endocrinopathy. Macroadenomas frequently present with patient symptoms from invasion of surrounding structures. The anterior pituitary gland neighbors both the optic chiasm and cavernous sinuses. Disruption of the optic chiasm by suprasellar growth of the pituitary mass may create bitemporal hemianopsia, in which the outer portion of the right and left visual fields is lost. The cavernous sinuses are a paired collection of thin-walled veins located on either side of the sella turcica. Pituitary tumor compression can lead to cavernous sinus syndrome. This constellation of symptoms includes headache, visual disturbances, and cranial nerve palsies, specifically of cranial nerves III, IV, and VI.

Any pituitary mass can lead to reproductive dysfunction that may include delayed puberty, anovulation, oligomenorrhea, and infertility. The exact mechanisms linking adenomas to menstrual dysfunction are not well understood for many adenoma subtypes, with the exception of prolactinomas. Macroadenomas likely affect reproductive function either by compressing the

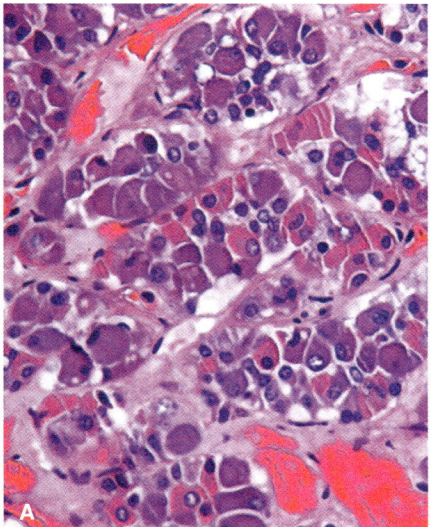 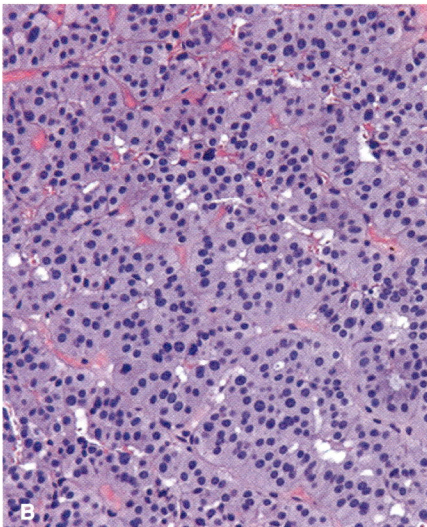 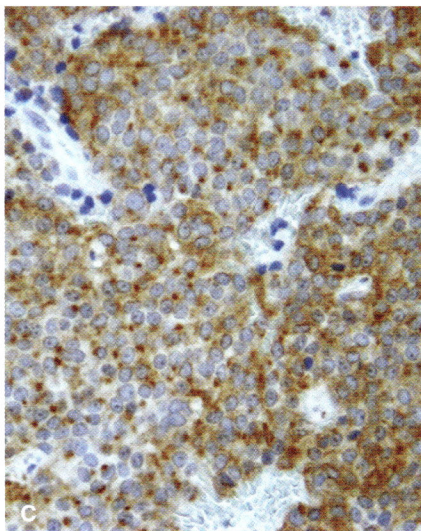

FIGURE 16-21 Photomicrographs from the anterior pituitary gland. **A.** Normal anterior pituitary gland. Secretory cells of the various types are arranged in small clusters between sinusoidal capillaries. **B.** Pituitary adenoma. In contrast to normal anterior pituitary gland, adenomas are composed of highly monomorphic cells. Note the absence of small clusters and sinusoids. **C.** Prolactin-secreting adenoma. Immunohistochemistry demonstrates expression of prolactin by many of the neoplastic cells. The dotlike pattern is characteristic of many prolactin-producing adenomas. (Reproduced with permission from Dr. Jack Raisanen.)

TABLE 16-6. Clinical Features of Pituitary Adenomas

Adenoma Cell Origin (Hormone)	Clinical Syndrome	Testing[a]	Typical Results	Treatment
Lactotrope (PRL)	Galactorrhea; hypogonadism	PRL	Elevated	Dopamine agonist; surgical excision
Gonadotrope (LH, FSH, free subunits)	Silent or hypogonadism; rarely gonadotrope excess	Free α-, FSHβ-, and LHβ-subunits	Elevated	Surgical excision
Somatotrope (GH)	Acromegaly or gigantism; menstrual irregularity	IGF-I; 100-g glucose suppression test	Elevated; no GH suppression	Surgical excision; somatostatin analogues
Corticotrope (ACTH)	Cushing syndrome; amenorrhea	ACTH; 24-hour urinary free cortisol; dexamethasone suppression	Elevated ACTH and cortisol; no suppression	Surgical excision; ketoconazole to blunt adrenal steroidogenesis
Thyrotrope (TSH)	Thyrotoxicosis; menstrual abnormalities	TSH, T$_3$, and T$_4$	All elevated	Surgical excision; PTU or methimazole; β-blockers for tachycardia

[a]All tests are serum measurements except for urinary free cortisol.
ACTH = adrenocorticotropin hormone; CRH = corticotropin-releasing hormone; FSH = follicle-stimulating hormone; GH = growth hormone; GnRH = gonadotropin-releasing hormone; IGF = insulin-like growth factor; LH = luteinizing hormone; PRL = prolactin; PTU = propylthiouracil; SHBG = sex hormone–binding globulin; TSH = thyroid-stimulating hormone; T$_3$ = triiodothyronine; T$_4$ = thyroxine.

pituitary stalk, which results in hyperprolactinemia, or, less commonly, by directly compressing gonadotropes.

Spontaneous hemorrhage into a pituitary adenoma, termed *pituitary apoplexy*, is a rare life-threatening medical emergency. Signs and symptoms include acute visual changes, severe headache, neck stiffness, hypotension, loss of consciousness, and coma. These symptoms result from: (1) leakage of blood and necrotic material into the subarachnoid space, (2) acute hypopituitarism, and (3) a rapidly expanding hemorrhagic intrasellar mass that compresses the optic chiasm, cranial nerves, or hypothalamus and internal carotid arteries. Apoplexy may lead to severe hypoglycemia, hypotension, CNS hemorrhage, and death. Nevertheless, with rapid diagnosis and management, the outcome of patients with pituitary apoplexy is excellent (Singh, 2015). Glucocorticoid replacement is a mainstay of supportive treatment. Surgical decompression is frequently but not invariably required.

Pregnancy and Pituitary Adenomas

The pituitary gland enlarges during pregnancy, primarily due to hypertrophy and hyperplasia of the lactotropes in response to elevated serum estrogen levels. Although the tumor can enlarge during pregnancy, clinical experience shows this risk is small. Tumor growth leading to significant symptoms complicates approximately 2 percent of microadenomas and 21 percent of untreated macroadenomas (Molitch, 2015). However, because significant expansion may lead to headaches or compression of the optic chiasm and blindness, visual field testing is considered in every trimester for women with macroadenomas. Although dopamine agonist therapy has been associated with a higher risk of spontaneous miscarriages, preterm deliveries, and congenital malformation, data overall suggest that most patients can be treated safely. Nevertheless, most experts advise that dopamine agonist therapy be discontinued during pregnancy when possible.

■ Treatment of Hyperprolactinemia and Pituitary Adenomas

Dopamine agonists may be considered in any patient with hyperprolactinemia in whom a large non-prolactin-producing tumor or other cause of hyperprolactinemia has been excluded. In this situation, it is likely that the patient has an undetectable microadenoma. However, the incidence of this is decreasing with the advent of highly sensitive MR imaging.

Most pituitary tumors grow slowly, and many cease growth after attaining a certain size. Thus, asymptomatic patients with a microprolactinoma may be managed conservatively with serial MR imaging and serum PRL levels every 1 to 2 years. The risk of progression to a macroadenoma is <10 percent (Schlechte, 1989). These women should be followed for even mild changes in menstrual cyclicity, as they are at risk for developing hypoestrogenism.

When tumors of any size are associated with amenorrhea or galactorrhea, therapy is considered (Fig. 16-22). Neurosurgical evaluation is mandatory when visual field defects or severe headaches are present. In general, first-line treatment is medical for both micro- and macroadenomas. Specifically, women should receive a dopamine agonist such as the nonspecific dopamine-receptor agonist bromocriptine (Parlodel) or the dopamine-receptor type 2 agonist cabergoline (Dostinex).

These dopamine agonists decrease PRL secretion and shrink tumor size. However, bromocriptine treatment is

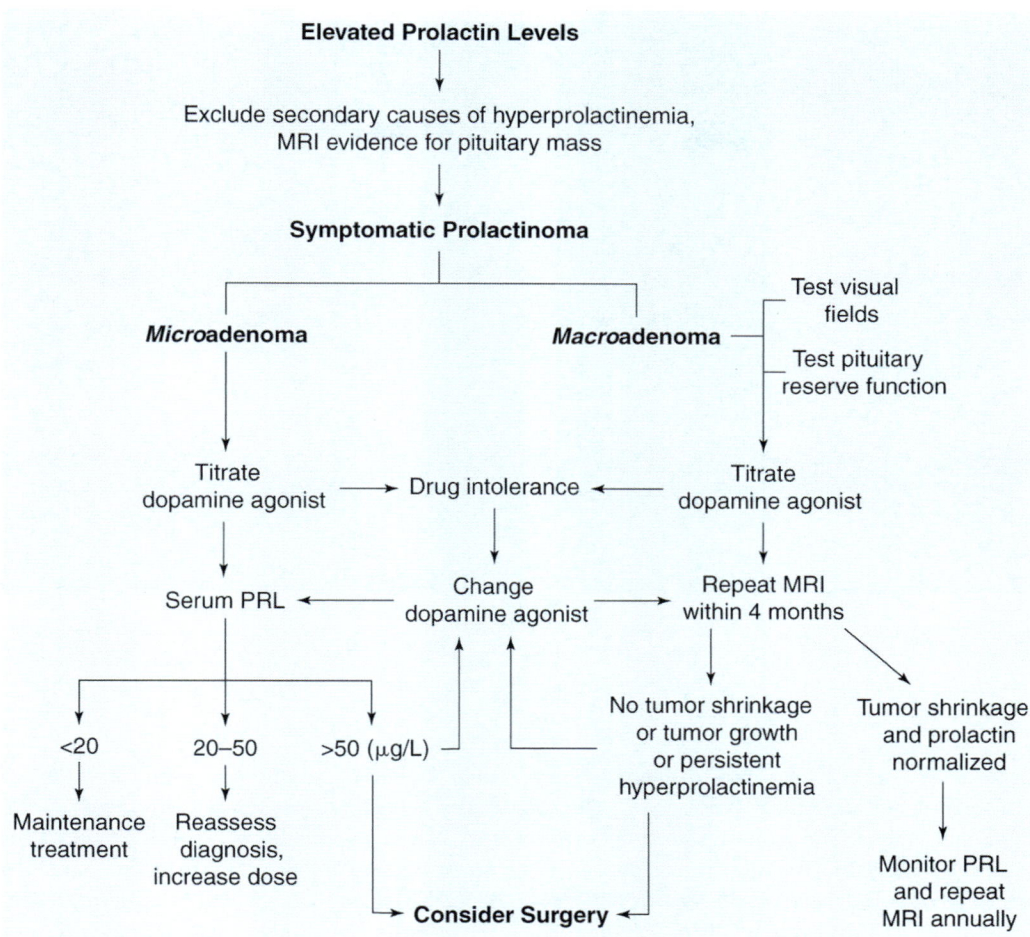

FIGURE 16-22 Algorithm describing the evaluation and treatment of pituitary adenomas. MRI = magnetic resonance imaging; PRL = prolactin. (Redrawn with permission from Melmed S, Jameson JL: Pituitary tumor syndromes. In Jameson JL, Fauci AS, Kasper DL, et al (eds): Harrison's Principles of Internal Medicine, 20th ed. New York, McGraw-Hill Education, 2018.)

associated with several common side effects, including headache, postural hypotension, blurry vision, drowsiness, and leg cramps. Most of these are attributable to activation of type 1 dopamine receptors. Due to its receptor specificity, cabergoline treatment is generally better tolerated than bromocriptine. Cabergoline also has a longer half-life, allowing once- or twice-weekly dosing. This compares favorably against the multiple daily doses that may be required for bromocriptine. Typical initial cabergoline dosages are 0.25 mg orally twice weekly. Cabergoline has been found to be more effective than bromocriptine in normalizing PRL levels (dos Santos Nunes, 2011). Nevertheless, cabergoline can be prohibitively expensive. Most patients can tolerate bromocriptine if started at a low dose—½ tab or 0.125 mg—each night to minimize associated nausea and dizziness. This dose can be slowly increased to three times daily as tolerated. Reliable measurement of posttreatment serum PRL levels can be obtained 1 month following a steady medication dose.

Neurosurgery is required for refractory tumors or those causing acutely worsening symptoms. The pituitary is approached through a transsphenoidal route whenever possible (Fig. 16-23). Complications of surgery, although rare, include intraoperative hemorrhage, a cerebrospinal fluid leak causing rhinorrhea,

diabetes insipidus, damage to other pituitary cell types, and meningitis (Miller, 2014).

Radiation therapy may be used for patients with surgically nonresectable, persistent, or aggressive tumors. The radiation dose necessary to stop tumor growth is lower than the dose necessary to achieve normalization of hormonal hypersecretion. More precise stereotactic radiosurgical approaches such as the gamma knife have improved radiation-beam focus, which significantly lessens local tissue damage and improves patient tolerance. Risks include optic nerve damage and delayed hypopituitarism (Pashtan, 2014).

DISORDERS OF PEPTIDE AND STEROID HORMONES IN REPRODUCTION

Clinical disorders may result from mutations in genes affecting hormone biosynthesis or the receptors that transduce the response. Both pituitary peptide and steroid hormones can be affected.

First, numerous mutations have been identified in the genes that encode the LH/CG and FSH receptors. Most of the identified mutations inactivate function. These produce gonadotropin

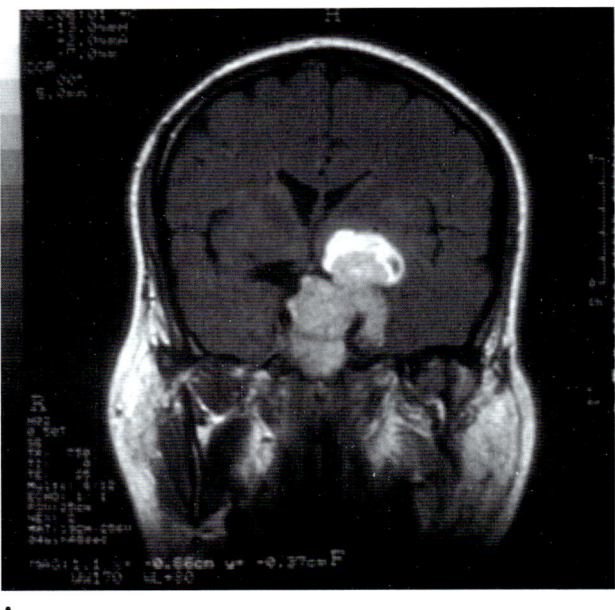 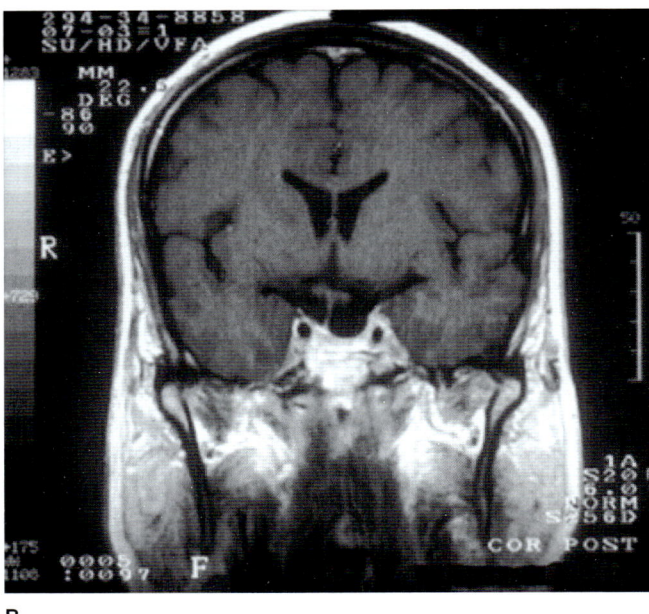

A   **B**

FIGURE 16-23 Magnetic resonance images of a pituitary macroadenoma before and after surgical resection. **A.** Preoperative coronal image reveals tumor measuring greater than 10 mm. **B.** Postoperative coronal image of the same patient following tumor excision.

resistance of variable severity that ranges from primary amenorrhea to oligomenorrhea and infertility (Latronico, 2013). Receptor mutations that activate function appear to be rare. However, a constitutively active LH/CG mutant receptor does cause a familial gonadotropin-independent precocious puberty that is limited to males (Ulloa-Aguirre, 2014). Although uncommon, mutations in the genes encoding the gonadotropin hormones themselves result in varying degrees of hypogonadism (Basciani, 2012; Kottler, 2010).

Second, gene mutation can lead to decreased function in steroid receptors. The best known is androgen insensitivity syndrome (AIS). With AIS, inactivating mutations in the androgen receptor impair the ability to respond to androgens. As a result, these 46,XY individuals haven female external genitalia and scant to absent pubic and axillary hair. However, their testes do produce antimüllerian hormone, their müllerian ducts fail to develop, and thus a blind-ending vaginal pouch without uterus or fallopian tubes results. Breasts develop in response to estrogens obtained from aromatization of circulating testicular steroids (Tadokoro-Cucaro, 2014). Phenotypes of AIS are further described in Chapter 19 (p. 414).

Last, mutations in the enzymes necessary for steroidogenesis create broad clinical effects. Phenotypes depend on the location and severity of the resulting enzymatic deficiency within the steroidogenic pathway (Miller, 2011). The most common is congenital adrenal hyperplasia (CAH), typically due to a 21-hydroxylase deficiency. With severe enzymatic deficiency, affected patients have life-threatening salt wasting and female-to-male disorder of sexual differentiation (46,XX DSD). A less severe mutation may lead to "simple virilizing CAH," in which elevated androgen levels are the primary hormonal abnormality (Auchus, 2015). The mildest abnormalities present as "nonclassic," "late-onset," or "adult-onset" CAH. In these patients, activation of the adrenal axis at puberty increases steroidogenesis and unmasks a mild 21-hydroxylase deficiency. Excess androgen provides negative feedback to GnRH receptors in the hypothalamus. These patients often have hirsutism, acne, and anovulation. Thus, late-onset CAH may mimic PCOS (McCann-Crosby, 2014). Additional discussion of CAH and disorders of sexual differentiation is found in Chapter 19 (p. 415).

ESTROGENS AND PROGESTINS IN CLINICAL PRACTICE

In gynecology, estrogen and/or progestins are used for contraception and for treating abnormal uterine bleeding, endometriosis, leiomyomas, PCOS, and menopausal symptoms. Specific uses are found in the respective chapters on these topics. Of the various estrogen and progestin preparations, each differs in its biologic efficacy, and clinicians should understand these differences.

■ Estrogens

Classic estrogens are C18 steroid compounds containing a phenolic ring (Fig. 16-24). This group contains the natural estrogens—estradiol, estrone, estriol—and their derivatives. It also contains conjugated equine estrogens (CEE). The predominant synthetic C18 estrogen is ethinyl estradiol, which is the estrogen present in most combination oral contraceptives. Synthetic nonsteroidal estrogens include diethylstilbestrol (DES) and selective estrogen-receptor modulators. Despite their variation from the classic steroid ring shape, nonsteroidal estrogens are still able to bind to the estrogen receptor.

Of the natural estrogens, 17β-estradiol is the most potent and is followed by estrone and then estriol. In comparing some pharmacologically used estrogens, ethinyl estradiol, a derivative of 17β-estradiol, is approximately 100 to 1000 times more

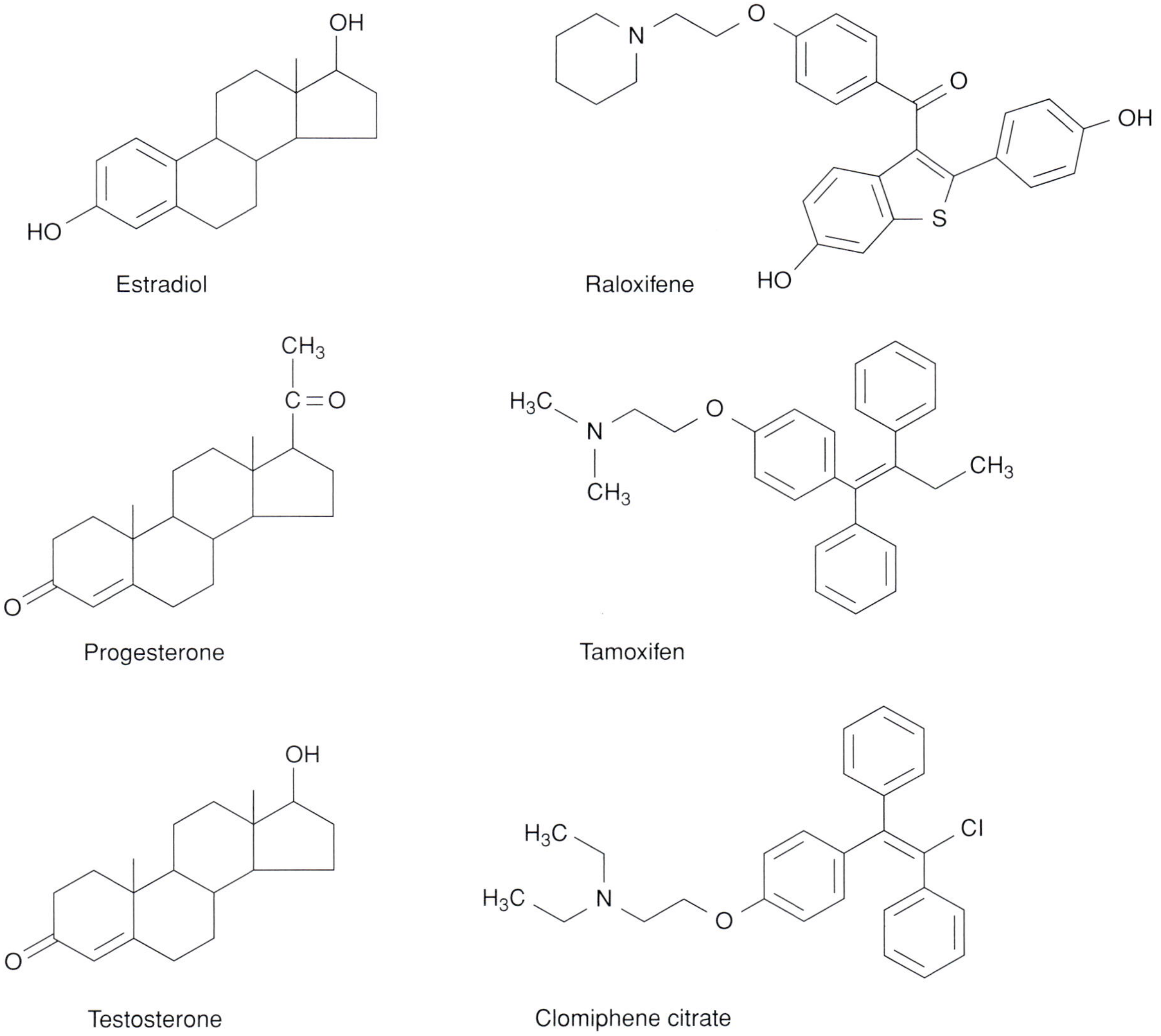

FIGURE 16-24 Chemical structures of important sex steroids and selective estrogen-receptor modulators.

potent on a per-weight basis than either micronized estradiol or CEE in increasing SHBG levels, which is one marker of estrogen potency (Kuhl, 2005; Mashchak, 1982).

■ Progestogens

Although not codified, *progestogens* include natural progesterone and synthetic progestogens, which are called *progestins*. Only progesterone can maintain human pregnancy. Progestins can be classified as derivatives of either 19-norprogesterone or 19-nortestosterone (Kuhl, 2005). Of the 19-norprogesterones, the most commonly used are medroxyprogesterone acetate and megestrol acetate.

Most progestins used in contraceptives are derived from 19-nortestosterone. These are commonly grouped as first generation (norethindrone), second generation (levonorgestrel, norgestrel), or third generation (desogestrel, norgestimate). As described in Chapter 5 (p. 121), each generation was designed to have progressively less androgenic effects. The fourth-generation progestin drospirenone is unique in that it is derived from spironolactone. Although it has no androgenic activity, drospirenone's affinity for the mineralocorticoid receptor is

approximately five times that of aldosterone. This explains its diuretic action.

■ Selective Steroid-Receptor Modulators

As indicated by their names, these synthetic compounds bind to their target receptors and exert tissue-specific effects, acting as agonists in some tissues and antagonists in others (Table 16-7). The variable activity among the selective estrogen-receptor modulators (SERMs) is attributed to differences at the molecular level. Each SERM binds to an estrogen receptor to generate a unique molecular conformation that affects the interaction of the complex with transcriptional cofactors and gene promoter regions. The response is also modified by the relative expression of ERα and ERβ receptors in the target tissue. The hormonal milieu also may affect the agonist–antagonist profile of a specific SERM. For example, a SERM may act as an estrogen agonist in a low-estrogen state, such as menopause, but as a competitive antagonist in a patient with high circulating estradiol levels.

Development of new SERMs with specific agonist/antagonist profiles continues as an active research topic. The SERM ospemifene (Osphena) may have favorable characteristics for

TABLE 16-7. Agonist or Antagonist Effects of Estradiol and Selected SERMs

Drug	Breast	Bone	Lipids	Endometrium
Tamoxifen	Antagonist	Agonist	Agonist	Agonist
Raloxifene	Antagonist	Agonist	Agonist	Antagonist
Ospemifene	Neutral	Agonist	Neutral	Partial agonist
Bazedoxifene	Antagonist	Agonist	Agonist	Antagonist
Estradiol	Agonist	Agonist	Agonist	Agonist

SERM = selective estrogen-receptor modulator.
Compiled from Archer, 2015; Miller, 2008; Ylikorkala, 2003.

long-term relief of genitourinary syndrome of menopause (Archer, 2015). The SERM bazedoxifene is combined with CEE and marketed as Duavee. This coupled approach yields a drug group categorized as *tissue-selective estrogen complexes (TSECs)*. The goal of TSECs is to provide estrogen agonist/antagonist profiles that optimize clinical efficacy and safety.

Selective progesterone-receptor modulators (SPRMs) are available for emergency contraception and in some countries for treatment of abnormal uterine bleeding, leiomyomas, and endometriosis (Wagenfeld, 2016). Of these, ulipristal acetate has been linked to possible severe liver damage and is discussed in Chapter 9 (p. 208).

Selective androgen-receptor modulators (SARMs) also are under investigation for osteopenia treatment and decreased libido. Ideally, these will avoid the virilizing effects of testosterone treatment (Solomon, 2019).

As indicated by the preceding discussion, the agonist–antagonist effect of a steroid hormone is inextricably related to the clinical tissue of interest. This concept is most frequently discussed in terms of selective steroid-receptor modulators, but all steroid hormones within a class exert differences in their pattern of action across tissues. As a result, when a steroid is chosen for treatment, each clinical end point should be considered individually.

Steroid Hormone Potency

The efficacy of estrogen and progestogen treatments is altered by numerous factors. These include: (1) receptor binding affinity, (2) formulation, (3) administration route, (4) metabolism, and (5) affinity for binding globulins. First, even small chemical modifications can substantially alter the biologic effects of steroid preparations. For example, the progestins in clinical use all exert progestogenic effects but may also act as weak androgens, antiandrogens, glucocorticoids, or antimineralocorticoids. These differences are likely explained by variations in binding affinity for each of these steroid receptors (Table 16-8) (Wiegratz, 2004).

Second, estrogens and progestogens can be administered as oral, transdermal, vaginal, or intramuscular preparations, among others. The choice of carrier molecule affects hormone bioavailability. For example, although crystalline progesterone is poorly absorbed via the intestine, dispersion of the progesterone into small particles (micronization) markedly increases surface area and uptake.

Third, oral medications pass through the intestine and the liver prior to systemic dissemination. As these tissues are sites for steroid metabolism, oral medications and their levels may be significantly altered prior to reaching their target organs. As an example, the bioavailability of orally administered micronized

TABLE 16-8. Relative Binding Affinities of Steroid Receptors and SHBG to Progestogens

Progestogen	PR	AR	ER	GR	MR	SHBG	CBG
Progesterone	50	0	0	10	100	0	36
MPA	115	5	0	29	160	0	0
Levonorgestrel	150	45	0	1	75	50	0
Etonogestrel	150	20	0	14	0	15	0
Norgestimate	15	0	0	1	0	0	0
Dienogest	5	10	0	1	0	0	0
Drospirenone	35	65	0	6	230	0	0

AR = androgen receptor; CBG = cortisol-binding globulin; ER = estrogen receptor; GR = glucocorticoid receptor; MPA = medroxyprogesterone acetate; MR = mineralocorticoid receptor; PR = progesterone receptor; SHBG = sex hormone–binding globulin.

TABLE 16-9. Relative Potency of Various Estrogens Concerning Clinical and Metabolic Parameters[a]

Estrogen	Suppression of:		Increase Serum Levels of:			
	Hot flashes	FSH	HDL	SHBG	CBG	Angiotensinogen
Estradiol-17β	100	100	100	100	100	
Estriol	30	20				
CEE	120	110	150	300	150	500
Ethinyl estradiol	12,000	12,000	40,000	50,000	60,000	35,000

[a]The values are estimated on a weight basis.

CBG = cortisol-binding globulin; CEE = conjugated equine estrogens; FSH = follicle-stimulating hormone; HDL = high-density lipoprotein; SHBG = sex hormone–binding globulin.

progesterone is <10 percent and compares poorly with the estimated 50- to 70-percent bioavailability for norethindrone and 100-percent level for levonorgestrel. This difference stems from a high level of "first pass" metabolism of micronized progesterone but not of these modified progestins (Stanczyk, 2002). As another example, the half-life of ethinyl estradiol is greatly extended relative to that of unconjugated estradiol by the presence of the ethinyl group, which impairs metabolism.

Absorption and metabolism rates may differ between individuals due to inherited or acquired differences in liver, intestinal, and renal function (Kuhl, 2005). Local metabolism also will lower steroid efficacy and can include conversion between steroids (for example, androgens to estrogens by aromatase) or within a steroid type (for example, estradiol to the weaker estrone). Diet, alcohol consumption, cigarette smoking, exercise, and stress all have been postulated to alter steroid metabolism. Thyroid disease also affects drug metabolism rates. Medications that elevate hepatic enzyme activity may increase estrogen metabolism. Best understood is the ability of some antiepileptic drugs to decrease estrogen-containing contraceptive efficacy, which is described in Chapter 5 (p. 126) (O'Brien, 2010).

Last, steroid potency depends on affinity for the various carrier proteins produced by the liver. Only unbound hormone, and to a much lesser extent the amount bound to albumin or cortisol-binding globulin (CBG), is functionally active. Steroid bound to SHBG is considered inactive. Ethinyl estradiol is bound nearly exclusively to albumin, and this enhances its bioavailability (Barnes, 2007). As shown in Table 16-8, significant differences in carrier binding are also observed for progestogens (Wiegratz, 2004).

Importantly, hormonal status affects expression of carrier proteins. Specifically, estrogens and thyroid hormone stimulate SHBG, whereas androgens blunt serum SHBG levels. To add further complexity, target cells are thought to secrete SHBG, which then acts locally as a membrane receptor to stimulate cyclic adenosine monophosphate (cAMP) intracellular signaling pathways (Rosner, 2010).

■ Steroid Bioassays

A limited number of studies have used bioassays to evaluate the efficacy of pharmacologic estrogens in women using clinical, endocrinologic, and metabolic parameters (Table 16-9)

(Kuhl, 2005). As seen in animal studies, different preparations vary markedly in their potency. Of note, estrogens also demonstrate differences in terms of their tissue specificity. For example, 17β-estradiol and CEE suppress pituitary FSH to a similar extent, whereas CEE is a more potent stimulator of liver SHBG production. Data suggest that these distinctions are likely important to assess the physiologic effects of pharmacologic, herbal, and environmental sources of steroids on health.

REFERENCES

Albertini DF, Anderson E: The appearance and structure of intercellular connections during the ontogeny of the rabbit ovarian follicle with particular reference to gap junctions. J Cell Biol 63:234, 1974

Archer DF, Carr BR, Pinkerton JV, et al: Effects of ospemifene on the female reproductive and urinary tracts: translation from preclinical models into clinical evidence. Menopause 22(7):786, 2015

Asimakopoulos B, Koster F, Felberbaum R, et al: Cytokine and hormonal profile in blood serum and follicular fluids during ovarian stimulation with the multidose antagonist or the long agonist protocol. Hum Reprod 21:3091, 2006

Auchus RJ: Management considerations for the adult with congenital adrenal hyperplasia. Mol Cell Endocrinol 408:190, 2015

Auchus RJ: Non-traditional metabolic pathways of adrenal steroids. Rev Endocr Metab Disord 10:27, 2009

Baird DT: A model for follicular selection and ovulation: lessons from superovulation. J Steroid Biochem 27:15, 1987

Baker TG: A quantitative and cytological study of germ cells in human ovaries. Proc R Soc Lond B Biol Sci 158:417, 1963

Barnes RR, Levrant SG (eds): Pharmacology of estrogens. In Treatment of the Postmenopausal Woman. New York, Columbia University, 2007, p 767

Basciani S, Watanabe M, Mariani S, et al: Hypogonadism in a patient with two novel mutations of the luteinizing hormone β-subunit gene expressed in a compound heterozygous form. J Clin Endocrinol Metab 97(9):3031, 2012

Beato M: Gene regulation by steroid hormones. Cell 56:335, 1989

Beers WH: Follicular plasminogen and plasminogen activator and the effect of plasmin on ovarian follicle wall. Cell 6:379, 1975

Bilezikjian LM, Justice NJ, Blackler AN, et al: Cell-type specific modulation of pituitary cells by activin, inhibin and follistatin. Mol Cell Endocrinol 359(1-2):43, 2012

Blanks AM, Thornton S: The role of oxytocin in parturition. BJOG 110 Suppl 20:46, 2003

Boon WC, Chow JD, Simpson ER: The multiple roles of estrogens and the enzyme aromatase. Prog Brain Res 181:209, 2010

Buckler HM, Healy DL, Burger HG: Purified FSH stimulates production of inhibin by the human ovary. J Endocrinol 122:279, 1989

Bull JR, Rowland SP, Scherwitzl EB, et al: Real-world menstrual cycle characteristics of more than 600,000 menstrual cycles. NPJ Digit Med 2:83, 2019

Butt WR, Crooke AC, Ryle M, et al: Gonadotrophins and ovarian development; proceedings of the two Workshop Meetings on the Chemistry of the Human Gonadotrophins and on the Development of the Ovary in Infancy. Birmingham, 1969, Edinburgh, Livingstone, 1970

Cao Y, Li Z, Jiang W, et al: Reproductive functions of kisspeptin/KISS1R systems in the periphery. Reprod Biol Endocrinol 17(1):65, 2019

Casals G, Ordi J, Creus M, et al: Osteopontin and αvβ3 integrin as markers of endometrial receptivity: the effect of different hormone therapies. Reprod Biomed Online 21:349, 2010

Casey ML, Hemsell DL, MacDonald PC, et al: NAD+-dependent 15-hydroxyprostaglandin dehydrogenase activity in human endometrium. Prostaglandins 19:115, 1980

Cetel NS, Quigley ME, Yen SS: Naloxone-induced prolactin secretion in women: evidence against a direct prolactin stimulatory effect of endogenous opioids. J Clin Endocrinol Metab 60:191, 1985

Chaffkin LM, Luciano AA, Peluso JJ: Progesterone as an autocrine/paracrine regulator of human granulosa cell proliferation. J Clin Endocrinol Metab 75:1404, 1992

Chehab FF: 20 years of leptin: leptin and reproduction: past milestones, present undertakings, and future endeavors. J Endocrinol 223(1):T37, 2014

Cheng CK, Leung PC: Molecular biology of gonadotropin-releasing hormone (GnRH)-I, GnRH-II, and their receptors in humans. Endocr Rev 26:283, 2005

Childs GV, Hyde C, Naor Z, et al: Heterogeneous luteinizing hormone and follicle-stimulating hormone storage patterns in subtypes of gonadotropes separated by centrifugal elutriation. Endocrinology 113:2120, 1983

Chuan S, Homer M, Pandian R, et al: Hyperglycosylated human chorionic gonadotropin as an early predictor of pregnancy outcomes after in vitro fertilization. Fertil Steril 101(2):392, 2014

Chwalisz K, Perez MC, Demanno D, et al: Selective progesterone receptor modulator development and use in the treatment of leiomyomata and endometriosis. Endocr Rev 26:423, 2005

Clayton RN, Catt KJ: Gonadotropin-releasing hormone receptors: characterization, physiological regulation, and relationship to reproductive function. Endocr Rev 2:186, 1981

Cole LA: Biological functions of hCG and hCG-related molecules. Reprod Biol Endocrinol 8:102, 2010

Cole LA, Khanlian SA, Muller CY: Detection of perimenopause or postmenopause human chorionic gonadotropin: an unnecessary source of alarm. Am J Obstet Gynecol 198(3):275.e1, 2008

Conneely OM, Mulac-Jericevic B, DeMayo F, et al: Reproductive functions of progesterone receptors. Recent Prog Horm Res 57:339, 2002

Corner GW Jr: The histological dating of the human corpus luteum of menstruation. Am J Anat 98:377, 1956

Coticchio G, Dal Canto M, Mignini Renzini M, et al: Oocyte maturation: gamete-somatic cells interactions, meiotic resumption, cytoskeletal dynamics and cytoplasmic reorganization. Hum Reprod Update 21(4):427, 2015

Couse JF, Curtis HS, Korach KS: Receptor null mice reveal contrasting roles for estrogen receptor alpha and beta in reproductive tissues. J Steroid Biochem Mol Biol 74:287, 2000

Critchley HO, Kelly RW, Brenner RM, et al: The endocrinology of menstruation—a role for the immune system. Clin Endocrinol (Oxf) 55(6):701, 2001

Crowley WR, Armstrong WE: Neurochemical regulation of oxytocin secretion in lactation. Endocr Rev 13:33, 1992

de Kretser DM, Hedger MP, Loveland KL, et al: Inhibins, activins, and follistatin in reproduction. Hum Reprod Update 8:529, 2002

Dickson RB, Lippman ME: Estrogenic regulation of growth and polypeptide growth factor secretion in human breast carcinoma. Endocr Rev 8:29, 1987

Dobrzyn K, Smolinska N, Kiezun M, et al: Adiponectin: a new regulator of female reproductive system. Int J Endocrinol 2018:7965071, 2018

dos Santos Nunes V, El Dib R, Boguszewski CL, et al: Cabergoline versus bromocriptine in the treatment of hyperprolactinemia: a systematic review of randomized controlled trials and meta-analysis. Pituitary 14(3):259, 2011

Eppig JJ: A comparison between oocyte growth in coculture with granulosa cells and oocytes with granulosa cell-oocyte junctional contact maintained in vitro. J Exp Zool 209:345, 1979

Espey LL: Ovarian proteolytic enzymes and ovulation. Biol Reprod 10:216, 1974

Fahie-Wilson MN, John R, Ellis AR: Macroprolactin; high molecular mass forms of circulating prolactin. Ann Clin Biochem 42:175, 2005

Faiman C, Winter JS, Reyes FI: Patterns of gonadotrophins and gonadal steroids throughout life. Clin Obstet Gynaecol 3(3):467, 1976

Ferin M, International Institute for the Study of Human Reproduction: Biorhythms and human reproduction; a conference sponsored by the International Institute for the Study of Human Reproduction. New York, Wiley, 1974

Fournier T, Guibourdenche J, Evain-Brion D: Review: hCGs: different sources of production, different glycoforms and functions. Placenta 36 Suppl 1:S60, 2015

Frieze TW, Mong DP, Koops MK: "Hook effect" in prolactinomas: case report and review of literature. Endocr Pract 8:296, 2002

Funabashi T, Brooks PJ, Weesner GD, et al: Luteinizing hormone-releasing hormone receptor messenger ribonucleic acid expression in the rat pituitary during lactation and the estrous cycle. J Neuroendocrinol 6:261, 1994

Gervásio CG, Bernuci MP, Silva-de-Sá MF, et al: The role of androgen hormones in early follicular development. ISRN Obstet Gynecol 2014:818010, 2014

Gosden RG: Oocyte development and loss. Semin Reprod Med 31(6):393, 2013

Gruber CJ, Tschugguel W, Schneeberger C, et al: Production and actions of estrogens. N Engl J Med 346(5):340, 2002

Guzmán A, Hernández-Coronado CG, Rosales-Torres AM, et al: Leptin regulates neuropeptides associated with food intake and GnRH secretion. Ann Endocrinol (Paris) 80(1):38, 2019

Gupta SK: Role of zona pellucida glycoproteins during fertilization in humans. J Reprod Immunol 108:90, 2015

Halvorson LM: PACAP modulates GnRH signaling in gonadotropes. Mol Cell Endocrinol 385(1-2):45, 2014

Hammond GL, Wu TS, Simard M: Evolving utility of sex hormone-binding globulin measurements in clinical medicine. Curr Opin Endocrinol Diabetes Obes 19(3):183, 2012

Haskell SG: Selective estrogen receptor modulators. South Med J 96:469, 2003

Head JR, MacDonald PC, Casey ML: Cellular localization of membrane metalloendopeptidase (enkephalinase) in human endometrium during the ovarian cycle. J Clin Endocrinol Metab 76:769, 1993

Hekimsoy Z, Kafesçiler S, Güçlü F, et al: The prevalence of hyperprolactinaemia in overt and subclinical hypothyroidism. Endocr J 57(12):1011, 2010

Hennet ML, Combelles CM: The antral follicle: a microenvironment for oocyte differentiation. Int J Dev Biol 56(10-12):819, 2012

Hodgen GD: The dominant ovarian follicle. Fertil Steril 38:281, 1982

Hoff JD, Quigley ME, Yen SS: Hormonal dynamics at midcycle: a reevaluation. J Clin Endocrinol Metab 57:792, 1983

Hsieh M, Zamah AM, Conti M: Epidermal growth factor-like growth factors in the follicular fluid: role in oocyte development and maturation. Semin Reprod Med 27(1):52, 2009

Hsueh AJ, Eisenhauer K, Chun SY, et al: Gonadal cell apoptosis. Recent Prog Horm Res 51:433, 1996

Hu KL, Zhao H, Chang HM, et al: Kisspeptin/kisspeptin receptor system in the ovary. Front Endocrinol (Lausanne) 8:365, 2018

Hu KL, Zhao H, Yu Y, et al: Kisspeptin as a potential biomarker throughout pregnancy. Eur J Obstet Gynecol Reprod Biol 240:261, 2019

Iwasa T, Matsuzaki T, Yano K, et al: The roles of kisspeptin and gonadotropin inhibitory hormone in stress-induced reproductive disorders. Endocr J 65(2):133, 2018

Kalantaridou SN, Makrigiannakis A, Zoumakis E, et al: Stress and the female reproductive system. J Reprod Immunol 62(1-2):61, 2004

Kaltsas GA, Nomikos P, Kontogeorgos G, et al: Clinical review: diagnosis and management of pituitary carcinomas. J Clin Endocrinol Metab 90:3089, 2005

Kanakis GA, Tsametis CP, Goulis DG: Measuring testosterone in women and men. Maturitas 125:41, 2019

Kaplan SL, Grumbach MM, Aubert ML: The ontogenesis of pituitary hormones and hypothalamic factors in the human fetus: maturation of central nervous system regulation of anterior pituitary function. Recent Prog Horm Res 32:161, 1976

Kerin JF, Kirby C, Morris D, et al: Incidence of the luteinized unruptured follicle phenomenon in cycling women. Fertil Steril 40:620, 1983

Kim HH, Mui KL, Nikrodhanond AA, et al: Regulation of gonadotropin-releasing hormone in nonhypothalamic tissues. Semin Reprod Med 25:326, 2007

King JC, Anthony EL: LHRH neurons and their projections in humans and other mammals: species comparisons. Peptides 5(Suppl 1):195, 1984

Kiss A, Mikkelsen JD: Oxytocin—anatomy and functional assignments: a minireview. Endocr Regul 39:97, 2005

Klinge CM: Estrogen receptor interaction with estrogen response elements. Nucleic Acids Res 29:2905, 2001

Knobil E: On the control of gonadotropin secretion in the rhesus monkey. Recent Prog Horm Res 30:1, 1974

Knobil E: The neuroendocrine control of the menstrual cycle. Recent Prog Horm Res 36:53, 1980

Knobil E: The Physiology of Reproduction. New York, Raven Press, 1994

Kottler ML, Chou YY, Chabre O, et al: A new FSHbeta mutation in a 29-year-old woman with primary amenorrhea and isolated FSH deficiency: functional characterization and ovarian response to human recombinant FSH. Eur J Endocrinol 162(3):633, 2010

Kowalik MK, Rekawiecki R, Kotwica J: The putative roles of nuclear and membrane-bound progesterone receptors in the female reproductive tract. Reprod Biol 13(4):279, 2013

Kuhl H: Pharmacology of estrogens and progestogens: influence of different routes of administration. Climacteric 8(Suppl 1):3, 2005

Kuiper GG, Carlsson B, Grandien K, et al: Comparison of the ligand binding specificity and transcript tissue distribution of estrogen receptors alpha and beta. Endocrinology 138:863, 1997

Latronico AC, Arnhold IJ: Gonadotropin resistance. Endocr Dev 24:25, 2013

Lawrence C, Fraley GS: Galanin-like peptide (GALP) is a hypothalamic regulator of energy homeostasis and reproduction. Front Neuroendocrinol 32:1, 2011

Lee HJ, Snegovskikh VV, Park JS, et al: Role of GnRH-GnRH receptor signaling at the maternal-fetal interface. Fertil Steril 94(7):2680, 2010

Lehman MN, Coolen LM, Goodman RL: Minireview: kisspeptin/neurokinin B/dynorphin (KNDy) cells of the arcuate nucleus: a central node in the control of gonadotropin-releasing hormone secretion. Endocrinology 151:3479, 2010

Lemarchand-Beraud T, Zufferey MM, Reymond M, et al: Maturation of the hypothalamo-pituitary-ovarian axis in adolescent girls. J Clin Endocrinol Metab 54:241, 1982

Lessey BA, Killam AP, Metzger DA, et al: Immunohistochemical analysis of human uterine estrogen and progesterone receptors throughout the menstrual cycle. J Clin Endocrinol Metab 67:334, 1988

Lockwood CJ, Nemerson Y, Krikun G, et al: Steroid-modulated stromal cell tissue factor expression: a model for the regulation of endometrial hemostasis and menstruation. J Clin Endocrinol Metab 77:1014, 1993

Lumsden MA, Kelly RW, Templeton AA, et al: Changes in the concentration of prostaglandins in preovulatory human follicles after administration of hCG. J Reprod Fertil 77:119, 1986

Lydon JP, DeMayo FJ, Conneely OM, et al: Reproductive phenotypes of the progesterone receptor null mutant mouse. J Steroid Biochem Mol Biol 56(1-6 Spec No):67, 1996

Mahendroo MS, Cunningham FG: Implantation and placental development. In Cunningham FG, Leveno KJ, Bloom SL, et al (eds): Williams Obstetrics, 25th ed. New York, McGraw-Hill, 2018a, p 81

Mahendroo MS, Cunningham FG: Parturition. In Cunningham FG, Leveno KJ, Bloom SL, et al (eds): Williams Obstetrics, 23rd ed. New York, McGraw-Hill, 2010, p 159

Mahendroo MS, Cunningham FG: Physiology of labor. In Cunningham FG, Leveno KJ, Bloom SL, et al (eds): Williams Obstetrics, 25th ed. New York, McGraw-Hill Education, 2018b, p 406

Mashchak CA, Lobo Ra, Dozono-Takano R, et al: Comparison of pharmacodynamic properties of various estrogen formulations. Am J Obstet Gynecol 144:511, 1982

Martin JJ, Woods DC, Tilly JL: Implications and current limitations of oogenesis from female germline or oogonial stem cells in adult mammalian ovaries. Cells 8(2):E93, 2019

Mason JI: Genetics of Steroid Biosynthesis and Function. New York, Taylor & Francis, 2002

Maybin JA, Critchley HO: Steroid regulation of menstrual bleeding and endometrial repair. Rev Endocr Metab Disord 13(4):253, 2012

McCann-Crosby B, Chen MJ, et al: Nonclassical congenital adrenal hyperplasia: targets of treatment and transition. Pediatr Endocrinol Rev 12(2):224, 2014

McCosh RB, Breen KM, Kauffman AS: Neural and endocrine mechanisms underlying stress-induced suppression of pulsatile LH secretion. Mol Cell Endocrinol September 12, 2019 [Epub ahead of print]

McLachlan RI, Cohen NL, Vale WW, et al: The importance of luteinizing hormone in the control of inhibin and progesterone secretion by the human corpus luteum. J Clin Endocrinol Metab 68:1078, 1989

McNatty KP, Makris A, DeGrazia C, et al: The production of progesterone, androgens, and estrogens by granulosa cells, thecal tissue, and stromal tissue from human ovaries in vitro. J Clin Endocrinol Metab 49:687, 1979

Melmed S: Pituitary tumors. Endocrinol Metab Clin North Am 44(1):1, 2015

Melmed S, Jameson JL: Pituitary tumor syndromes. In Jameson JL, Fauci AS, Kasper DL, et al (eds): Harrison's Principles of Internal Medicine, 20th ed. New York, McGraw-Hill Education, 2018

Messini CI, Dafopoulos K, Chalvatzas N, et al: Effect of ghrelin and thyrotropin-releasing hormone on prolactin secretion in normal women. Horm Metab Res 42(3):204, 2010

Millar RP: New developments in kisspeptin, neurokinin B and dynorphin A regulation of gonadotropin-releasing hormone pulsatile secretion. Neuroendocrinology 99(1):5, 2014

Miller BA, Ioachimescu AG, Oyesiku NM: Contemporary indications for transsphenoidal pituitary surgery. World Neurosurg 82(6 Suppl):S147, 2014

Miller PD, Chines AA, Christiansen C, et al: Effects of bazedoxifene on BMD and bone turnover in postmenopausal women: 2-yr results of a randomized, double-blind, placebo-, and active-controlled study. J Bone Miner Res 23(4):525, 2008

Miller WL: Molecular biology of steroid hormone synthesis. Endocr Rev 9:295, 1988

Miller WL, Auchus RJ: The molecular biology, biochemistry, and physiology of human steroidogenesis and its disorders. Endocr Rev 32(1):81, 2011

Molitch ME: Endocrinology in pregnancy: management of the pregnant patient with a prolactinoma. Eur J Endocrinol 172(5):R205, 2015

Muttukrishna S, Tannetta D, Groome N, et al: Activin and follistatin in female reproduction. Mol Cell Endocrinol 225:45, 2004

Nakai Y, Plant TM, Hess DL, et al: On the sites of the negative and positive feedback actions of estradiol in the control of gonadotropin secretion in the rhesus monkey. Endocrinology 102:1008, 1978

Negro-Vilar A: Selective androgen receptor modulators (SARMs):a novel approach to androgen therapy for the new millennium. J Clin Endocrinol Metab 84:3459, 1999

Neill JD: GnRH and GnRH receptor genes in the human genome. Endocrinology 143:737, 2002

Notarianni E: Reinterpretation of evidence advanced for neo-oogenesis in mammals, in terms of a finite oocyte reserve. J Ovarian Res 4:1, 2011

Noyes RW, Hertig AT, Rock J: Dating the endometrial biopsy. Fertil Steril 1:3, 1950

O'Brien MD, Guillebaud J: Contraception for women taking antiepileptic drugs. J Fam Plann Reprod Health Care 36(4):239, 2010

Odle AK, Akhter N, Syed MM, et al: Leptin regulation of gonadotrope gonadotropin-releasing hormone receptors as a metabolic checkpoint and gateway to reproductive competence. Front Endocrinol (Lausanne) 8:367, 2018

Ohlsson R: Growth factors, protooncogenes and human placental development. Cell Differ Dev 28:1, 1989

Olive DL: The prevalence and epidemiology of luteal-phase deficiency in normal and infertile women. Clin Obstet Gynecol 34:157, 1991

O'Malley BW, Strott CA: Steroid hormones: metabolism and mechanism of action. In Yen SS, Jaffe RB, Barbieri RL (eds): Reproductive Endocrinology, 4th ed. Philadelphia, Saunders, 1999, p 128

Pache TD, Wladimiroff JW, de Jong FH, et al: Growth patterns of nondominant ovarian follicles during the normal menstrual cycle. Fertil Steril 54:638, 1990

Padula AM: GnRH analogues—agonists and antagonists. Anim Reprod Sci 88(1-2):115, 2005

Pashtan I, Oh KS, Loeffler JS: Radiation therapy in the management of pituitary adenomas. Handb Clin Neurol 124:317, 2014

Patton PE, Stouffer RL: Current understanding of the corpus luteum in women and nonhuman primates. Clin Obstet Gynecol 34:127, 1991

Pekic S, Stojanovic M, Popovic V: Contemporary issues in the evaluation and management of pituitary adenomas. Minerva Endocrinol 40(4):307, 2015

Peters EE, Towler KL, Mason DR, et al: Effects of galanin and leptin on gonadotropin-releasing hormone-stimulated luteinizing hormone release from the pituitary. Neuroendocrinology 89:18, 2009

Peters H, Joint A (eds): The Ovary: A Correlation of Structure and Function in Mammals. Berkeley, University of California Press, 1980

Piquette GN, Crabtree ME, el Danasouri I, et al: Regulation of plasminogen activator inhibitor-1 and -2 messenger ribonucleic acid levels in human cumulus and granulosa-luteal cells. J Clin Endocrinol Metab 76:518, 1993

Pope WF: Uterine asynchrony: a cause of embryonic loss. Biol Reprod 39:999, 1988

Ravindranath N, Little-Ihrig L, Phillips HS, et al: Vascular endothelial growth factor messenger ribonucleic acid expression in the primate ovary. Endocrinology 131:254, 1992

Revelli A, Massobrio M, Tesarik J: Nongenomic actions of steroid hormones in reproductive tissues. Endocr Rev 19(1):3, 1998

Rosenfield RL, Bordini B, Yu C: Comparison of detection of normal puberty in girls by a hormonal sleep test and a gonadotropin-releasing hormone agonist test. J Clin Endocrinol Metab 98(4):1591, 2013

Rosner W, Auchus RJ, Azziz R, et al: Position statement: utility, limitations, and pitfalls in measuring testosterone: an Endocrine Society position statement. J Clin Endocrinol Metab 92(2):405, 2007

Rosner W, Hryb DJ, Kahn SM, et al: Interactions of sex hormone-binding globulin with target cells. Mol Cell Endocrinol 316:79, 2010

Ruscalleda J: Imaging of parasellar lesions. Eur Radiol 15:549, 2005

Russell DW, Wilson JD: Steroid 5 alpha-reductase: two genes/two enzymes. Annu Rev Biochem 63:25, 1994

Sasano H, Okamoto M, Mason JI, et al: Immunolocalization of aromatase, 17 alpha-hydroxylase and side-chain-cleavage cytochromes P-450 in the human ovary. J Reprod Fertil 85:163, 1989

Saxena BB, Beling CG, Gandy HM, et al: Gonadotropins. New York, Wiley-Interscience, 1972

Schatz F, Aigner S, Papp C, et al: Plasminogen activator activity during decidualization of human endometrial stromal cells is regulated by plasminogen activator inhibitor 1. J Clin Endocrinol Metab 80:2504, 1995

Schipper I, Hop WC, Fauser BC: The follicle-stimulating hormone (FSH) threshold/window concept examined by different interventions with exogenous FSH during the follicular phase of the normal menstrual cycle: duration, rather than magnitude, of FSH increase affects follicle development. J Clin Endocrinol Metab 83:1292, 1998

Schlechte J, Dolan K, Sherman B, et al: The natural history of untreated hyperprolactinemia: a prospective analysis. J Clin Endocrinol Metab 68:412, 1989

Schmidt H, Schwarz HP: Serum concentrations of LH and FSH in the healthy newborn. Eur J Endocrinol 143(2):213, 2000

Seeber B, Böttcher B, D'Costa E, et al: Opioids and reproduction. Vitam Horm 111:247, 2019

Sharkey AM, Dellow K, Blayney M, et al: Stage-specific expression of cytokine and receptor messenger ribonucleic acids in human preimplantation embryos. Biol Reprod 53:974, 1995

Silva JR, Figueiredo JR, van den Hurk R: Involvement of growth hormone (GH) and insulin-like growth factor (IGF) system in ovarian folliculogenesis. Theriogenology 71:1193, 2009

Silva PD, Gentzschein EE, Lobo RA: Androstenedione may be a more important precursor of tissue dihydrotestosterone than testosterone in women. Fertil Steril 48:419, 1987

Silverman AJ, Jhamandas J, Renaud LP: Localization of luteinizing hormone-releasing hormone (LHRH) neurons that project to the median eminence. J Neurosci 7:2312, 1987

Singh TD, Valizadeh N, Meyer FB, et al: Management and outcomes of pituitary apoplexy. J Neurosurg 10:1, 2015

Skorupskaite K, George JT, Anderson RA: The kisspeptin-GnRH pathway in human reproductive health and disease. Hum Reprod Update 20(4):485, 2014

Smith G, Roberts R, Hall C, et al: Reversible ovulatory failure associated with the development of luteinized unruptured follicles in women with inflammatory arthritis taking non-steroidal anti-inflammatory drugs. Br J Rheumatol 35:458, 1996

Solomon ZJ, Mirabal JR, Mazur DJ, et al: Selective androgen receptor modulators: current knowledge and clinical applications. Sex Med Rev 7(1):84, 2019

Son WY, Das M, Shalom-Paz E, et al: Mechanisms of follicle selection and development. Minerva Ginecol 63(2):89, 2011

Stanczyk FZ: Pharmacokinetics and potency of progestins used for hormone replacement therapy and contraception. Rev Endocr Metab Disord 3:211, 2002

Stern K, McClintock MK: Regulation of ovulation by human pheromones. Nature 392:177, 1998

Stilley JA, Christensen DE, Dahlem KB, et al: FSH receptor (FSHR) expression in human extragonadal reproductive tissues and the developing placenta, and the impact of its deletion on pregnancy in mice. Biol Reprod 91(3):74, 2014

Stout SM, Stumpf JL: Finasteride treatment of hair loss in women. Ann Pharmacother 44:1090, 2010

Tadokoro-Cuccaro R, Hughes IA: Androgen insensitivity syndrome. Curr Opin Endocrinol Diabetes Obes 21(6):499, 2014

Tang ZR, Zhang R, Lian ZX, et al: Estrogen-receptor expression and function in female reproductive disease. Cells 8(10):E1123, 2019

Taylor HS: Use of elagolix in gynaecology. J Obstet Gynaecol Can 40(7):931, 2018

Taylor HS, Vanden Heuvel GB, Igarashi P: A conserved Hox axis in the mouse and human female reproductive system: late establishment and persistent adult expression of the Hoxa cluster genes. Biol Reprod 57:1338, 1997

Temeli E, Oprescu M, Coculescu M, et al: LH and FSH levels in serum and cerebrospinal fluid (CSF) of human fetus. Endocrinologie 23(1):55, 1985

Terasawa E: Mechanism of pulsatile GnRH release in primates: unresolved questions. Mol Cell Endocrinol September 10, 2019 [Epub ahead of print]

Thompson IR, Kaiser UB: GnRH pulse frequency-dependent differential regulation of LH and FSH gene expression. Mol Cell Endocrinol 385(1-2):28, 2014

Treloar AE, Boynton RE, Behn BG, et al: Variation of the human menstrual cycle through reproductive life. Int J Fertil 12(1 Pt 2):77, 1967

Trevisan CM, Montagna E, de Oliveira R, et al: Kisspeptin/GPR54 system: what do we know about its role in human reproduction? Cell Physiol Biochem 49(4):1259, 2018

Ulloa-Aguirre A, Reiter E, Bousfield G, et al: Constitutive activity in gonadotropin receptors. Adv Pharmacol 70:37, 2014

Vega MG, Zarek SM, Bhagwat M, et al: Gonadotropin surge-inhibiting/attenuating factors: a review of current evidence, potential applications, and future directions for research. Mol Reprod Dev 82(1):2, 2015

Verbalis JG, Robinson AG: Characterization of neurophysin-vasopressin prohormones in human posterior pituitary tissue. J Clin Endocrinol Metab 57:115, 1983

Virant-Klun I: Postnatal oogenesis in humans: a review of recent findings. Stem Cells Cloning 8:49, 2015

Wagenfeld A, Saunders PT, Whitaker L, et al: Selective progesterone receptor modulators (SPRMs): progesterone receptor action, mode of action on the endometrium and treatment options in gynecological therapies. Expert Opin Ther Targets 20(9):1045, 2016

Walkington L, Webster J, Hancock BW, et al: Hyperthyroidism and human chorionic gonadotrophin production in gestational trophoblastic disease. Br J Cancer 104(11):1665, 2011

Wiegratz I, Kuhl H: Progestogen therapies: differences in clinical effects? Trends Endocrinol Metab 15:277, 2004

Wierman ME, Kiseljak-Vassiliades K, Tobet S: Gonadotropin-releasing hormone (GnRH) neuron migration: initiation, maintenance and cessation as critical steps to ensure normal reproductive function. Front Neuroendocrinol 32(1):43, 2011

Williams CL, Nishihara M, Thalabard JC, et al: Duration and frequency of multiunit electrical activity associated with the hypothalamic gonadotropin releasing hormone pulse generator in the rhesus monkey: differential effects of morphine. Neuroendocrinology 52:225, 1990

Winter JS, Hughes IA, Reyes FI, et al: Pituitary-gonadal relations in infancy: 2. Patterns of serum gonadal steroid concentrations in man from birth to two years of age. J Clin Endocrinol Metab 42:679, 1976

Xia Y, Schneyer AL: The biology of activin: recent advances in structure, regulation and function. J Endocrinol 202(1):1, 2009

Yang L, Dhillo W: Kisspeptin as a therapeutic target in reproduction. Expert Opin Ther Targets 20(5):567, 2016

Yen SS, Quigley ME, Reid RL, et al: Neuroendocrinology of opioid peptides and their role in the control of gonadotropin and prolactin secretion. Am J Obstet Gynecol 152:485, 1985

Ylikorkala O, Cacciatore B, Halonen K, et al: Effects of ospemifene, a novel SERM, on vascular markers and function in healthy, postmenopausal women. Menopause 10(5):440, 2003

Yoshimura Y, Wallach EE: Studies of the mechanism(s) of mammalian ovulation. Fertil Steril 47:22, 1987

Yoshinaga K, Serono Symposia USA: Blastocyst Implantation. Boston, Adams, 1989

Young JR, Jaffe RB: Strength-duration characteristics of estrogen effects on gonadotropin response to gonadotropin-releasing hormone in women. II. Effects of varying concentrations of estradiol. J Clin Endocrinol Metab 42:432, 1976

Yu B, Ruman J, Christman G: The role of peripheral gonadotropin-releasing hormone receptors in female reproduction. Fertil Steril 95:465, 2011

Zee J, Sammel MD, Chung K, et al: Ectopic pregnancy prediction in women with a pregnancy of unknown location: data beyond 48 h are necessary. Hum Reprod 29(3):441, 2014

Ziecik AJ, Kaczmarek MM, Blitek A, et al: Novel biological and possible applicable roles of LH/hCG receptor. Mol Cell Endocrinol 269(1-2):51, 2007

CHAPTER 17

Amenorrhea

Evaluation and management of a patient with amenorrhea is common in gynecology, and the prevalence of pathologic amenorrhea ranges from 3 to 4 percent in reproductive-aged populations (Bachmann, 1982). Amenorrhea has classically been defined as primary (no prior menses) or secondary (cessation of menses). Although this distinction does suggest a relative likelihood of finding a particular diagnosis, the approach to diagnosis and treatment is similar for either presentation (Tables 17-1 and 17-2). Of course, amenorrhea is a normal state prior to puberty, during pregnancy and lactation, and following menopause. Evaluation is considered for an adolescent: (1) who has not menstruated by age 15 or within 3 years of thelarche or (2) has not menstruated by age 14 and shows signs of hirsutism, excessive exercise, or eating disorder (American College of Obstetrician and Gynecologists, 2017d). Secondary amenorrhea for 3 months or fewer than nine cycles per year also is investigated (American Society for Reproductive Medicine, 2008; Klein, 2013). In some circumstances, testing reasonably may be initiated despite the absence of these strict criteria. Examples include a patient with the stigmata of Turner syndrome, obvious virilization, or a history of uterine curettage. An evaluation for delayed puberty is also considered before the ages listed above if the patient or her parents are concerned.

NORMAL MENSTRUAL CYCLE

A differential diagnosis for amenorrhea can be constructed based on requirements for normal menses. Ovarian function in a normal menstrual cycle is divided into the follicular phase (preovulatory), ovulation, and luteal phase (postovulatory). Endometrial characteristics are partitioned into the proliferative phase (preovulatory) and secretory phase (postovulatory).

Generation of a cyclic, controlled pattern of uterine bleeding requires precise temporal and quantitative regulation of several reproductive hormones (Chap. 16, p. 348). First, the hypothalamic-pituitary-ovarian axis must be functional. The hypothalamus releases pulses of gonadotropin-releasing hormone (GnRH) into the hypophyseal portal circulation at defined frequencies and amplitude. GnRH stimulates the synthesis and secretion of the gonadotropins luteinizing hormone (LH) and follicle-stimulating hormone (FSH) by the gonadotrope cells of the anterior pituitary gland. These gonadotropins enter the peripheral circulation and act on the ovary to stimulate both follicular development and ovarian hormone production. These ovarian hormones include estrogens, progesterone, and androgens. Gonadal steroids are typically inhibitory at both the pituitary and the hypothalamus. Development of a mature follicle, however, creates a rapid rise in estrogen levels, which instead

TABLE 17-1. Primary Amenorrhea: Frequency of Etiologies

Presentation	Frequency (%)
Hypergonadotropic hypogonadism	43
45,X and variants	27
46,XX	14
46,XY	2
Eugonadism	30
Müllerian agenesis	15
Vaginal septum	3
Imperforate hymen	1
AIS	1
PCOS	7
CAH	1
Cushing and thyroid disease	2
Low FSH without breast development	27
Constitutional delay	14
GnRH deficiency	5
Other CNS disease	1
Pituitary disease	5
Eating disorders, stress, excess exercise	2

AIS = androgen insensitivity syndrome; CAH = congenital adrenal hyperplasia; CNS = central nervous system; FSH = follicle-stimulating hormone; GnRH = gonadotropin-releasing hormone; PCOS = polycystic ovarian syndrome. Adapted from Reindollar, 1981, with permission.

TABLE 17-2. Secondary Amenorrhea: Frequency of Etiologies[a]

Etiology	Frequency (%)
Low or normal FSH level: various	<u>67.5</u>
Eating disorders, stress, excess exercise	15.5
Nonspecific hypothalamic	18
Chronic anovulation (PCOS)	28
Hypothyroidism	1.5
Cushing syndrome	1
Pituitary tumor/empty sella	2
Sheehan syndrome	1.5
High FSH level: gonadal failure	<u>10.5</u>
46,XX	10
Abnormal karyotype	0.5
High prolactin level	13
Anatomic	<u>7</u>
Asherman syndrome	7
Hyperandrogenic states	<u>2</u>
Nonclassic CAH	0.5
Ovarian tumor	1
Undiagnosed	0.5

[a]Excluding pregnancy diagnoses.
CAH = congenital adrenal hyperplasia; FSH = follicle-stimulating hormone; PCOS = polycystic ovarian syndrome.
Adapted from Reindollar, 1986, with permission.

act positively to generate an LH release surge. This surge is essential for ovulation.

Following ovulation, LH stimulates luteinization of the granulosa and theca cells, which had surrounded the mature oocyte, to form the corpus luteum. The corpus luteum continues to produce estrogen but also secretes high levels of progesterone. The thickened, proliferative endometrial lining produced by high circulating estrogen levels during the follicular phase is now converted to a secretory pattern by this luteal progesterone. If pregnancy occurs, the corpus luteum is "rescued" by human chorionic gonadotropin (hCG) secreted from early placental trophoblast. Structurally similar to LH, hCG binds to and signals via the same receptor and assumes the role of corpus luteum support during early pregnancy. If pregnancy does not occur, then progesterone and estrogen secretion ceases, the corpus luteum regresses, and the endometrium sloughs. The pattern of this "progesterone withdrawal bleed" varies in duration and amount among women but is relatively constant across cycles for a given individual.

Amenorrhea may follow disruption of this choreographed communication. However, menses may be absent even with normal cyclic hormonal changes due to anatomic abnormalities. The endometrium must be able to respond normally to hormonal stimulation, and the cervix, vagina, and introitus must be present and patent.

CLASSIFICATION SYSTEM

Numerous classification systems for the diagnosis of amenorrhea have been developed, and all have their strengths and weaknesses. One useful scheme is outlined in Table 17-3. This system divides causes of amenorrhea into anatomic versus hormonal etiologies, with further division into congenital and acquired disorders.

As described above, normal menses require adequate ovarian production of steroid hormones. Decreased ovarian function (hypogonadism) may result either from a lack of stimulation by the gonadotropins (*hypo*gonadotropic hypogonadism) or from primary failure of the ovary (*hyper*gonadotropic hypogonadism) (Table 17-4). Several disorders are associated with relatively normal LH and FSH levels (*eu*gonadotropic), however, appropriate cyclicity is lost.

ANATOMIC DISORDERS

■ Inherited Disorders

Anatomic abnormalities causing amenorrhea can broadly be viewed as either inherited or acquired disorders of the outflow tract (uterus, cervix, vagina, and introitus). Of these two, inherited causes will generally present at menarche in adolescents. Pelvic anatomy is abnormal in approximately 15 percent of women with primary amenorrhea (American Society for Reproductive Medicine, 2008). Figure 17-1 depicts the range of anatomic defects that may present with amenorrhea. Various classification schemes for congenital genital tract anomalies have been developed. Of these, the American Society for Reproductive Medicine (ASRM) classification is longstanding and likely the most used (American Fertility Society, 1988). However, the consensus classification more recently developed by the European Society of Human Reproduction and Embryology (ESHRE) and the European Society for Gynaecological Endoscopy (ESGE) is gaining popularity (Grimbizis, 2013). These are additionally discussed in Chapter 19 (p. 419).

Lower Outflow Tract Obstruction

Amenorrhea is associated with imperforate hymen (1 in 2000 women), a complete transverse vaginal septum (1 in 70,000

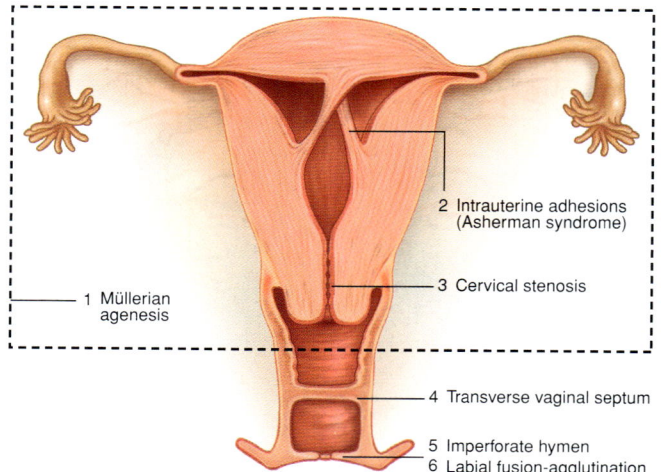

FIGURE 17-1 Anatomic defects that may lead to amenorrhea. Müllerian agenesis results in an absence of the upper reproductive tract structures contain within the dash-lined box.

TABLE 17-3. Classification Scheme for Nonphysiologic Amenorrhea

Anatomic

Congenital
Müllerian agenesis (partial or complete)
Vaginal septum
Cervical atresia
Imperforate hymen
Complete androgen resistance

Acquired
Intrauterine synechiae (Asherman syndrome)
Cervical stenosis

Hormonal/Endocrinologic

Hypergonadotropic hypogonadism (POI)
Inherited
  Chromosomal (gonadal dysgenesis)
  Single-gene disorders
Acquired
  Infectious
  Autoimmune
  Iatrogenic (chemotherapy or radiation)
  Environmental
  Idiopathic

Hypogonadotropic hypogonadism
Disorders of the hypothalamus = hypothalamic amenorrhea
Inherited
  Idiopathic hypogonadotropic hypogonadism (IHH)
  Kallmann syndrome
Acquired
  Hypothalamic amenorrhea ("functional")
    Eating disorders
    Excessive exercise
    Stress
  Destructive processes
    Tumor
    Radiation
    Trauma
    Infection
    Infiltrative disease
  Pseudocyesis

Eugonadotropic amenorrhea
Inherited
  Polycystic ovarian syndrome
  Nonclassic congenital adrenal hyperplasia
Acquired
  Hyperprolactinemia
  Thyroid disease
  Cushing syndrome
  Acromegaly
  Ovarian tumors (steroid producing)

Hypogonadotropic hypogonadism (cont'd)
Disorders of the anterior pituitary gland
Inherited/congenital
  Pituitary hypoplasia
Acquired
  Adenoma
    Prolactinoma
  Destructive processes
    Macroadenoma
    Metastases
    Radiation
    Trauma
    Infarction (Sheehan syndrome)
    Infiltrative disease
Chronic disease
  End-stage kidney disease
  Liver disease
  Malignancy
  Acquired immunodeficiency syndrome
  Malabsorption syndromes
  Drug abuse

POI = premature ovarian insufficiency.

TABLE 17-4. Categories of Amenorrhea Based on Gonadotropin and Estrogen Levels

Type of Hypogonadism	LH/FSH	Estrogen	Primary Defect
Hypergonadotropic	High	Low	Ovary
Hypogonadotropic	Low	Low	Hypothalamus/pituitary
Eugonadotropic	Normal[a]	Normal[a]	Varied

[a]Generally in normal range, but lack cyclicity.
FSH = follicle-stimulating hormone; LH = luteinizing hormone.

women), or isolated vaginal atresia (Banerjee, 1998; Parazzini, 1990). Also, although structurally normal, labia in some girls may be severely agglutinated and can lead to obstruction. Most with agglutination are treated early with topical estrogen and/or manual separation, and outflow obstruction is thereby avoided.

Patients with outflow obstruction have a 46,XX karyotype, female secondary sexual characteristics, and normal ovarian function. Thus, the amount of uterine bleeding is normal, but its normal path for egress is obstructed or absent. Patients may note moliminal symptoms, such as breast tenderness, food cravings, and mood changes, which are attributable to elevated progesterone levels. With inherited or acquired outflow obstruction, accumulation of blood behind the blockage frequently results in cyclic abdominal pain. Intrauterine trapping of fluid (hydrometra), pus (pyometra), or blood (hematometra) creates a soft, enlarged uterus. Similarly, the terms *hydrotrachelos, pyotrachelos,* and *hematotrachelos* define distention of the cervix, whereas *hydrocolpos, pyocolpos,* and *hematocolpos* describe distention of the vagina. These are seen with more distal obstructions. Importantly, in women with outflow blockage, an increase in retrograde menstruation places the patient at high risk for endometriosis development.

Müllerian Defects

During embryonic development, the müllerian ducts give rise to the upper vagina, cervix, uterine corpus, and fallopian tubes. Agenesis during these ducts' development may be partial or complete. Accordingly, amenorrhea may result from outflow obstruction or from a lack of endometrium in cases involving uterine agenesis. In complete müllerian agenesis, often called *Mayer-Rokitansky-Küster-Hauser (MRKH) syndrome,* patients fail to develop any müllerian structures, and examination reveals only a vaginal dimple. With an incidence of 1 per 5000 females, MRKH ranks second only to gonadal dysgenesis as a cause of primary amenorrhea (Aittomaki, 2001; American College of Obstetricians and Gynecologists, 2018b). Research has begun to identify gene mutations that may contribute to this disorder (Fontana, 2017).

Importantly, complete müllerian agenesis may be confused with complete androgen insensitivity syndrome. In the latter condition, the patient has a 46,XY karyotype and functioning

TABLE 17-5. Comparison of Müllerian Agenesis and Androgen Insensitivity Syndrome

Presentation	Müllerian Agenesis	Androgen Insensitivity
Inheritance pattern	Sporadic	X-linked recessive
Karyotype	46,XX	46,XY
Breast development	Yes	Yes
Axillary and pubic hair	Yes	No
Uterus	No	No
Gonad	Ovary	Testis
Testosterone	Female levels	Male levels
Associated anomalies	Yes	No

testes (Batista, 2018). However, underlying androgen receptor mutations prevent normal testosterone binding, normal male ductal system development, and virilization. These two syndromes are compared in Table 17-5 and discussed further in Chapter 19 (p. 421).

■ Acquired Disorders
Cervical Stenosis

Other abnormalities of the uterus that cause amenorrhea include cervical stenosis and extensive intrauterine adhesions. With stenosis, postoperative scarring and cervical os narrowing may follow dilatation and curettage (D & C), cervical conization, loop electrosurgical excision procedures, infection, and neoplasia. Severe atrophic or radiation changes are other sources. Stenosis involves the internal or external os, and symptoms in menstruating women include amenorrhea or abnormal bleeding, dysmenorrhea, and infertility. Management seeks to reopen the os and is discussed in Chapter 41 (p. 903).

Intrauterine Adhesions

Also known as *uterine synechiae* and, when symptomatic, as *Asherman syndrome,* the spectrum of scarring includes filmy adhesions, dense bands, or complete obliteration of the uterine cavity (Fig. 17-2). Normally, the endometrium is divided into a functional layer, which lines the endometrial cavity, and a basal

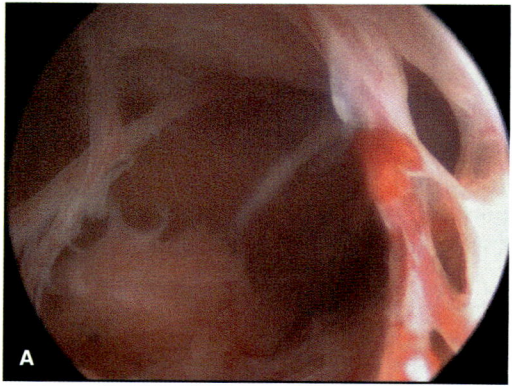 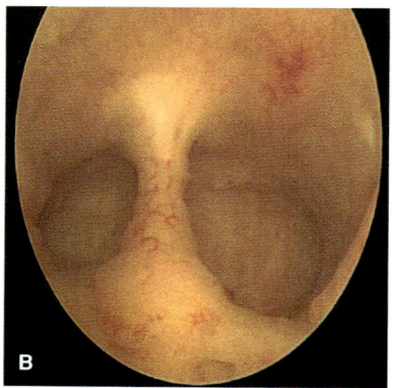 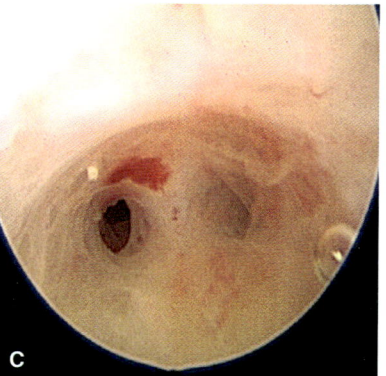

FIGURE 17-2 Hysteroscopic photographs of progressively dense intrauterine adhesions found with Asherman syndrome. **A.** Filmy. **B.** Dense. **C.** Nearly obliterating. (Reproduced with permission from Drs. David Rogers and Kevin Doody.)

layer, which regenerates the functional layer with each menstrual cycle. Destruction of the basal endometrium prevents endometrial thickening in response to ovarian steroids. Thus, no tissue is produced or subsequently sloughed when steroid hormone levels fall at the end of the luteal phase.

Endometrial damage may follow vigorous curettage, usually in association with postpartum hemorrhage, miscarriage, or elective abortion complicated by infection. In a series of 1856 women with Asherman syndrome, 88 percent followed postabortal or postpartum uterine curettage (Schenker, 1982). Risks for intrauterine adhesions rise with the number of D & Cs for spontaneous first-trimester abortion (Hooker, 2014). In one prospective study, the risk was 16 percent after a single termination. The rate rose to 32 percent and with progressively more dense adhesions observed following three or more procedures (Friedler, 1993).

Damage may also result from other uterine surgery, including metroplasty, myomectomy, or cesarean delivery, or from infection related to an intrauterine device. Although rare in the United States, tuberculous endometritis is a relatively common cause of Asherman syndrome in developing countries (Sharma, 2009). Of course, Asherman syndrome may also be an intentional outcome following uterine ablation for heavy menstrual bleeding.

Depending on the degree of scarring, patients may describe amenorrhea; in less severe cases, hypomenorrhea; or recurrent pregnancy loss due to inadequate placentation (March, 2011). In their evaluation of 292 women with intrauterine adhesions, Schenker and Margalioth (1982) noted delivery of term pregnancies in only 30 percent of 165 pregnancies. The remaining pregnancies either were spontaneously aborted (40 percent) or delivered prematurely.

If intrauterine adhesions are suspected, radiologic evaluation of the uterine cavity is often performed. If information regarding tubal patency is needed, hysterosalpingography (HSG) offers information regarding both uterine cavity and fallopian tube patency. Otherwise, saline-infusion sonography (SIS) provides an excellent alternative. Intrauterine adhesions characteristically appear as irregular, angulated filling defects within the cavity (Fig. 20-6, p. 439 and Fig. 2-23, p. 41). At times, uterine polyps, leiomyomas, air bubbles, and blood clots may masquerade as adhesions. Definitive diagnosis requires hysteroscopy. To improve fertility rates or to relieve symptomatic hematometra, hysteroscopic lysis of adhesions is the preferred surgical treatment. The procedure is described in Section 44-18 (p. 1069), and fertility advantages are discussed in Chapter 21 (p. 461). Although still experimental, recent research has proposed the use of uterine or bone marrow–derived stem cells in the treatment of Asherman syndrome and other reproductive disorders (Santamaria, 2018; Simoni, 2018).

HYPERGONADOTROPIC HYPOGONADISM

The term *hypergonadotropic hypogonadism* describes any process in which: (1) ovarian function is reduced or absent (hypogonadism) and (2) the gonadotropins, LH and FSH, have elevated serum levels (hypergonadotropic) due to absent negative

TABLE 17-6. Differential Diagnosis of Premature Ovarian Insufficiency

Genetic
  Chromosomal/Gonadal dysgenesis
    Normal karyotype
    Abnormal karyotype
  Specific gene defects
    Fragile X (*FMR1* premutation)
    Galactosemia
    Other

Iatrogenic
  Ovarian surgery
  Gonadal radiation
  Systemic chemotherapy

Autoimmune disease

Toxins

Viruses

Miscellaneous

sex-steroid and inhibin feedback. This category of disorders implies primary dysfunction within the ovary rather than hypothalamic or pituitary dysfunction (Table 17-6). This process can also be termed *premature menopause* or *premature ovarian failure (POF)*. The term *premature ovarian insufficiency* or *primary ovarian insufficiency (POI)* is currently preferred as it conveys the fact that ovarian function may fluctuate before complete oocyte depletion. This may lead to occasional transient menses resumption or even pregnancy in 5 to 10 percent of patients (Bidet, 2011). For our purposes, the term premature ovarian insufficiency will be used.

POI is defined as loss of oocytes and the surrounding support cells prior to age 40 years. The diagnosis is determined by two serum FSH levels that measure greater than a threshold range of 30 to 40 mIU/mL and are obtained at least 1 month apart. This definition distinguishes POI from the physiologic loss of ovarian function, which occurs with normal menopause. The incidence of POI has been estimated at 1 in 1000 women younger than 30 years and at 1 in 100 women younger than 40 (Coulam, 1986).

Careful evaluation is mandatory as the diagnosis and effective treatment may have significant implications for the patient's psychologic, cardiovascular, bone, and sexual health. The finding of a genetic disorder may also require evaluation of family members. Nevertheless, in most cases, an etiology for POI is not determined (American College of Obstetricians and Gynecologists, 2018c).

■ Heritable Disorders

Gonadal Dysgenesis

Gonadal dysgenesis is the most frequent cause of POI. In this disorder, a normal complement of germ cells is present in the early fetal ovary. However, oocytes undergo accelerated atresia, and the ovary is replaced by a fibrous streak—termed a *streak*

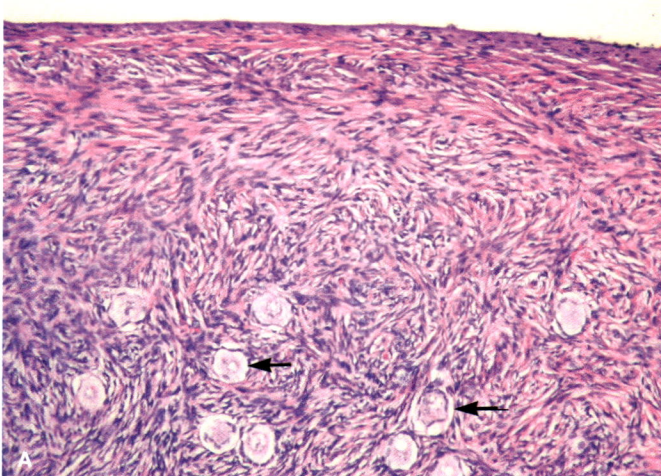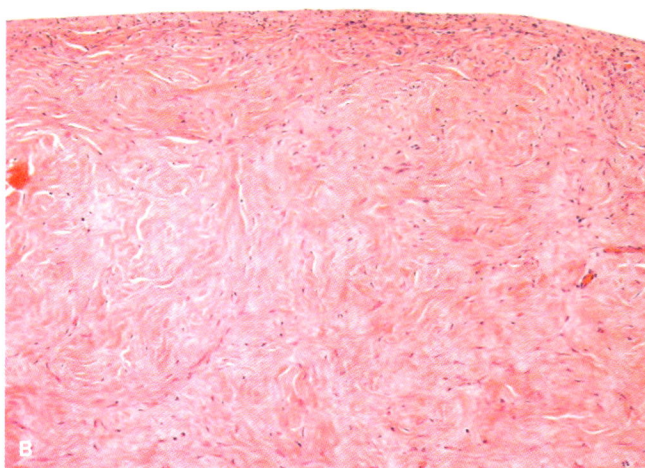

FIGURE 17-3 Photomicrographs of histologic samples. **A.** Normal premenopausal ovarian cortex with multiple primordial follicles. (Reproduced with permission from Dr. Kelley Carrick.) **B.** Ovary from a woman with gonadal dysgenesis. Streak ovary showing ovarian-type stroma with no primordial follicles (Reproduced with permission from Dr. Raheela Ashfaq.)

gonad (Figs. 17-3 and 17-4) (Singh, 1966). Individuals with gonadal dysgenesis may present with various clinical features and can be divided into two broad groups based on whether their karyotype is normal or abnormal (Rossetti, 2017). These are all discussed further in Chapter 19 (p. 412).

Those with normal karyotype (46,XX or 46,XY) are described as having "pure" gonadal dysgenesis. Patients with a 46,XY genotype and gonadal dysgenesis (Swyer syndrome) are phenotypically female due to absent testosterone and absent antimüllerian hormone (AMH) secretion by dysgenetic testes. The etiology of the gonadal failure in both genetically male and female patients is poorly understood but is likely due to single gene defects or destruction of gonadal tissue in utero, perhaps by infection or toxins (Hutson, 2014).

Those with abnormal karyotype include Turner syndrome (45,X) and chromosomal mosaics such as 45,X/46,XX or 45,X/46,XY. In general, approximately 90 percent of individuals

with gonadal dysgenesis from a loss of X genetic material never menstruate. The remaining 10 percent have sufficient residual follicles to experience menses and rarely may achieve pregnancy. However, the menstrual and reproductive lives of such individuals are invariably brief (Kaneko, 1990; Tho, 1981).

As noted, in some cases of gonadal dysgenesis, a Y chromosome is present. If Y chromosomal material is found, the streak gonads are removed because nearly 25 percent of these patients will develop a malignant germ cell tumor (Chap. 36, p. 756) (Cools, 2018; Pyle, 2017). Thus, chromosomal analysis is performed in all cases of amenorrhea associated with POI, particularly before age 30. The presence of a Y chromosome cannot be determined clinically, as only a few patients will demonstrate signs of androgen excess.

Specific Genetic Defects

In addition to chromosomal abnormalities, patients may experience POI due to single gene mutations (Cordts, 2011). First, a significant relationship is noted between fragile X syndrome and POI (American College of Obstetricians and Gynecologists, 2017a). This syndrome is caused by a triple repeat sequence mutation in the X-linked *FMR1* (fragile X mental retardation) gene. This gene is unstable, and its size can expand during parent-to-child transmission. The fully expanded mutation (>200 CGG repeats) becomes hypermethylated, resulting in silencing of gene expression. As such, this fully expanded mutation is the most common known inherited genetic cause of mental retardation and of autism. Males with the so-called premutation (50 to 200 CGG repeats) are at risk for fragile X–associated tremor/ataxia syndrome (FXTAS). Females with the premutation have a 13- to 26-percent risk of developing POI, although the mechanism is unclear. An estimated 0.8 to 7.5 percent of sporadic POI and 13 percent of familial POI cases are due to premutations in this gene. The prevalence of premutations in women approximates 1 in 129 to 300 (Wittenberger, 2007).

Less common gene defects are *CYP17* mutations. These decrease 17α-hydroxylase and 17,20-lyase activity and thereby

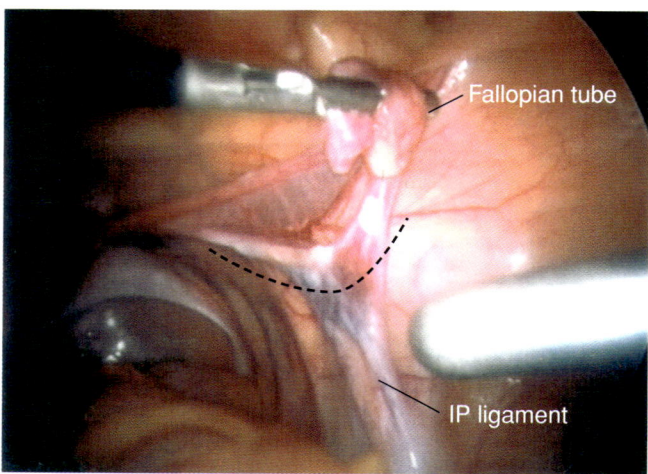

FIGURE 17-4 Photograph taken during laparoscopy of a streak gonad (*dotted line*). IP = infundibulopelvic. (Reproduced with permission from Dr. Victor Beshay.)

Fallopian tube

IP ligament

prevent production of cortisol, androgens, and estrogens (Fig. 16-5, p. 339). Affected patients have sexual infantilism and primary amenorrhea due to absent estrogen secretion. *Sexual infantilism* describes patients with a lack of breast development, absent pubic and axillary hair, and a small uterus. Mutations in *CYP17* also raise adrenocorticotropin hormone (ACTH) release, thereby stimulating mineralocorticoid secretion. This, in turn, leads to hypokalemia and hypertension (Miller, 2018).

Mutations in genes that encode LH and FSH receptors also have been reported. These defects prevent normal responses to circulating gonadotropins, a condition termed *resistant ovary syndrome* (Aittomaki, 1995; Latronico, 2013). Identification of other single-gene mutations that can cause POI is an area of active investigation. The list of implicated genes now includes those that encode both estrogen receptors (ERα and ERβ), extracellular signaling proteins (specifically, BMP15), and transcription factors FOXL2, FOX03, and SF-1 (Cordts, 2011; Goswami, 2005). These factors provide further insights into normal ovarian physiology and may lead to new infertility treatments and contraceptive options.

Perrault syndrome, which is characterized by sensorineural hearing loss and ovarian dysfunction, is gaining attention. Ovarian disturbances range from gonadal dysgenesis and primary amenorrhea to POI. Associated neurologic features include learning disabilities, developmental delay, and cerebellar ataxia (Newman, 2018).

Although frequently cited, galactosemia is a rare cause of POI. Classic galactosemia affects 1 in 30,000 to 60,000 live births. Inherited as an autosomal recessive disorder, this condition leads to abnormal galactose metabolism due to a deficiency of galactose-1-phosphate uridyl transferase, encoded by the *GALT* gene. Galactose metabolites are believed to have a direct toxic effect on many cell types, including germ cells. Potential complications include neonatal death, ataxic neurologic disease, cognitive disabilities, and cataracts (Thakur, 2018). In one large cohort study, only 68 percent of girls achieved spontaneous menarche. Of these, fewer than 15 percent were still cycling regularly after 10 years (Frederick, 2018). Treatment is lifelong dietary restriction of galactose, which is present in milk-based foods, and may not reliably prevent POI development. Galactosemia is frequently diagnosed during newborn screening programs or during pediatric evaluation of impaired growth and development. This is typically long before a patient would present to a gynecologist.

■ Acquired Abnormalities

Hypergonadotropic hypogonadism can be acquired from infection, environmental exposures, autoimmune disease, or medical treatments. Of these, infectious causes of POI are rare and poorly understood, and mumps oophoritis is the most frequently reported (Hviid, 2008). Various environmental toxins have a clear detrimental effect on follicular health. These include cigarette smoking, heavy metals, solvents, pesticides, and industrial chemicals (Budani, 2017; Mlynarcikova, 2005; Vabre, 2017).

Autoimmune disorders historically are said to account for an estimated 40 percent of POI cases. This may be an overestimate

as the data behind this statistic are limited (Hoek, 1997). Ovarian dysfunction may be one component of the inherited autoimmune polyendocrine syndromes APS-1 and APS-2. Both syndromes are characterized by circulating autoantibodies and lymphocytic infiltration of affected tissues that lead to organ failure. With an estimated prevalence of 1:1000, APS-2 is more common and is associated with Addison's disease, thyroid disease, and type 1 diabetes mellitus (Husebye, 2018). POI is associated with systemic lupus erythematosus. Ovarian effects likely stem from treatment of severe cases with alkylating chemotherapeutics from the disease process itself (Oktem, 2016). Myasthenia gravis, idiopathic thrombocytopenic purpura, rheumatoid arthritis, vitiligo, inflammatory bowel disease, and autoimmune hemolytic anemia also have been linked to POI (Silva, 2014). Although several antiovarian antibodies have been characterized, no validated serum antibody marker is currently available to aid autoimmune POI diagnosis (American Society for Reproductive Medicine, 2008).

Iatrogenic ovarian failure is relatively common. This group includes patients who have undergone surgical removal of the ovaries or cystectomy. Alternatively, a woman may experience amenorrhea following pelvic radiation for cancer or following chemotherapy for treatment of malignancies or severe autoimmune disease.

With the last two, the chance of developing POI is correlated with increasing radiation and chemotherapeutic dose. Patient age also is a significant factor, and younger patients are less likely to develop failure and more likely to regain ovarian function over time (Gradishar, 1989). With radiotherapy, ovaries are preventively repositioned using surgery (oophoropexy), if possible, out of the anticipated radiation field prior to therapy (Terenziani, 2009). Of chemotherapeutic drugs, alkylating agents are believed to be particularly damaging to ovarian function. Preventive adjuvant GnRH analogues may lower rates of chemotherapy-induced POI (Chap. 27, p. 594). Although this approach remains controversial, recent studies and metaanalyses show promising results (Chen, 2011; Lambertini, 2018). Importantly, recent advances in oocyte and ovarian tissue cryopreservation and in vitro maturation make it likely that oocyte harvest prior to treatment will become the preferred approach when feasible.

HYPOGONADOTROPIC HYPOGONADISM

The term *hypogonadotropic hypogonadism* implies that the primary abnormality lies in the hypothalamic-pituitary axis. As a result, poor gonadotropin stimulation of the ovaries leads to impaired follicular development. Generally in these patients, LH and FSH levels, although low, will still be in the detectable range (<5 mIU/mL). However, levels may be undetectable in patients with complete absence of hypothalamic stimulation, such as occurs in forms of inherited hypothalamic abnormalities. In addition, absent pituitary function due to abnormal development or severe pituitary damage may lead to similarly low levels. Thus, the group of hypogonadotropic hypogonadism disorders may be viewed as a continuum with perturbations leading to luteal dysfunction, oligomenorrhea, and, in the most severe presentation, amenorrhea.

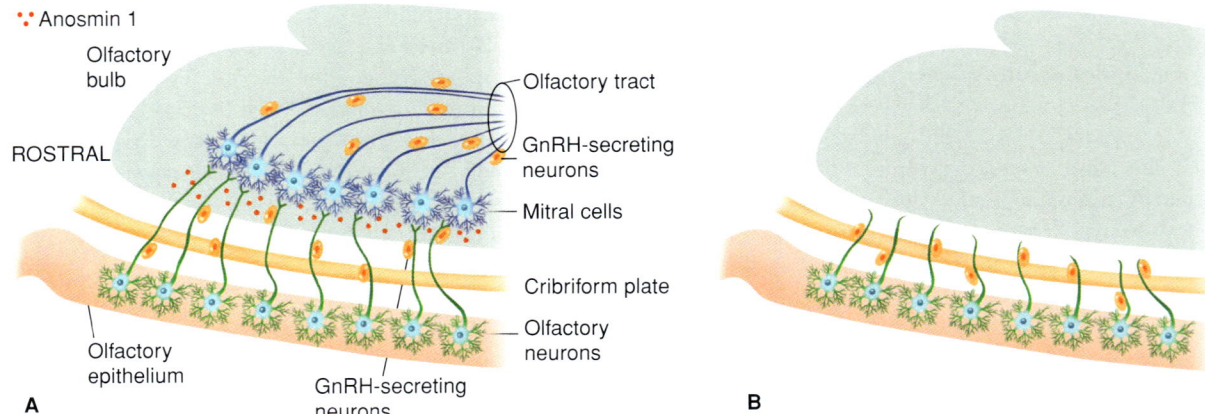

FIGURE 17-5 Normal GnRH neuron migration and the pathogenesis of Kallmann syndrome. **A.** During normal development, olfactory neurons arising in the olfactory epithelium extend their axons through the cribriform plate of the ethmoid bone to reach the olfactory bulb. Here, these axons synapse with dendrites of mitral cells, whose axons form the olfactory tract. Mitral cells secrete anosmin-1, which is the protein product of the *KAL1* gene. This protein is necessary to direct the olfactory axons to their correct location in the olfactory bulb. The GnRH-secreting neurons use this axonal path to migrate from the olfactory placode to the hypothalamus. **B.** Patients with Kallmann syndrome due to a *KAL1* mutation lack anosmin-1 expression. As a result, the axons of the olfactory neurons cannot interact properly with mitral cells, and their migration ends between the cribriform plate and olfactory bulb. As GnRH neuronal migration is dependent on this axonal trail, the GnRH secretion pathway likewise ends at this location.

Hypothalamic Disorders

Inherited Hypothalamic Abnormalities

Inherited hypothalamic abnormalities primarily consist of those patients with idiopathic hypogonadotropic hypogonadism (IHH). A subset has associated defects in the ability to smell (hyposmia or anosmia) and are said to have Kallmann syndrome. This syndrome can be inherited as an X-linked, autosomal dominant, or autosomal recessive disorder (Cadman, 2007). The X-linked form was the first to be characterized and follows mutation in the *KAL1* gene on the short arm of the X chromosome. Expressed during fetal development, this gene encodes an adhesion protein named anosmin-1. As this protein is critical for normal migration of both GnRH and olfactory neurons, loss of normal anosmin-1 expression results in both reproductive and olfactory deficits (Fig. 17-5) (Franco, 1991). Kallmann patients have a normal complement of GnRH neurons, however, these neurons fail to migrate and instead remain near the nasal epithelium (Quinton, 1997). As a result, locally secreted GnRH is unable to stimulate gonadotropes in the anterior pituitary gland to release LH and FSH. In turn, marked declines in ovarian estrogen production result in absence of breast development and menstrual cycles.

Kallmann syndrome is also associated with midline facial anomalies such as cleft palate, unilateral renal agenesis, cerebellar ataxia, epilepsy, neurosensory hearing loss, and synkinesis (mirror movements of the hands). Kallmann syndrome can be distinguished from IHH by olfactory testing. This is performed easily in the office with strong odorants such as ground coffee or perfume. Interestingly, many of these patients are unaware of their olfactory deficit.

During the past 15 years, an array of autosomal genes has been identified that contribute to normal development, migration, and secretion by GnRH neurons (Caronia, 2011; Howard, 2018; Layman, 2013). Mutations in several of these genes have

been described in patients with hypothalamic amenorrhea. Genes include *FGF8*, *KAL1*, *NELF*, *PROK2*, *PROKR2*, *CHD7*, *KISS1/KISS1R*, and *LEP/LEPR*. As a result, the percentage of patients in whom this disorder need be considered idiopathic is gradually decreasing. Of note, mutation in the *CHD7* gene may cause either normosmic IHH or Kallmann syndrome, thereby blurring the distinction between these disorders.

Acquired Hypothalamic Dysfunction

Acquired hypothalamic abnormalities are much more frequent than inherited deficiencies. Most commonly, gonadotropin deficiency leading to chronic anovulation is believed to arise from functional disorders of the hypothalamus or higher brain centers. Also called "hypothalamic amenorrhea," this diagnosis encompasses three main categories: eating disorders, excessive exercise, and stress. From a teleologic perspective, amenorrhea in time of starvation or extreme stress can be seen as a mechanism to prevent pregnancy at a time in which resources are suboptimal for raising a child. Each woman appears to have her own hypothalamic "setpoint" or sensitivity to environmental factors. For example, individual women can tolerate markedly different amounts of stress without developing amenorrhea. In addition to amenorrhea, these conditions are associated with infertility and cardiovascular, bone, and psychologic effects (Gordon, 2017; Shufelt, 2017).

Eating Disorders. Anorexia nervosa and bulimia, both described in Chapter 14 (p. 305), can lead to amenorrhea (American College of Obstetricians and Gynecologists, 2018a). Hypothalamic dysfunction is severe in anorexia and may affect other hypothalamic-pituitary axes in addition to the reproductive axis. Amenorrhea in anorexia nervosa can precede, follow, or appear coincidentally with weight loss. In addition, even with return to normal weight, not all women with anorexia will regain normal menstrual function. Patients with premenarchal

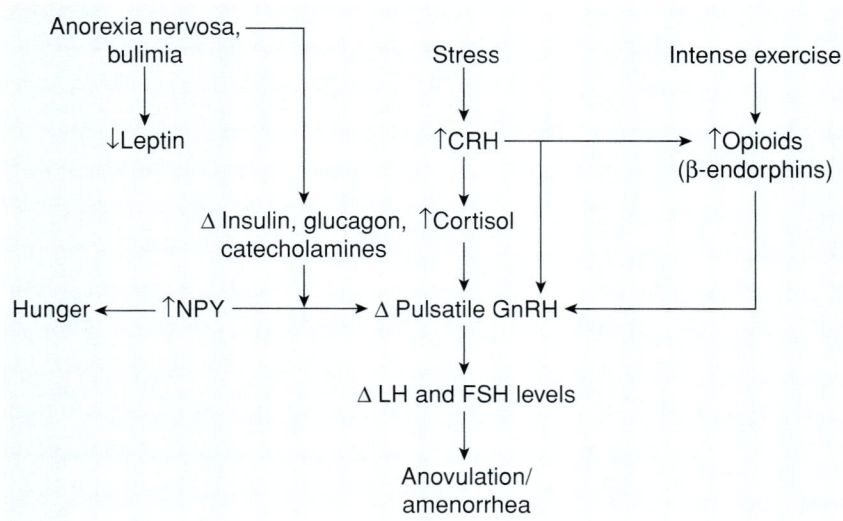

FIGURE 17-6 Diagram depicting a simplified model for the development of amenorrhea in women with eating disorders, high stress levels, or rigorous exercise. CRH = corticotropin-releasing hormone; FSH = follicle-stimulating hormone; GnRH = gonadotropin-releasing hormone; LH = luteinizing hormone; NPY = neuropeptide Y.

onset of anorexia are at particular risk for protracted amenorrhea (Dempfle, 2013).

Exercise-induced Amenorrhea. This is most common in women whose exercise regimen is associated with significant loss of fat, including ballet, gymnastics, and long-distance running. In those women who continue to menstruate, cycles are notable for their variability in cycle interval and length due to reduced ovulatory function (De Souza, 1998). Puberty may be delayed in girls who begin training before menarche (Frisch, 1981).

An appreciation for the link between exercise and reproductive health has led to the concept of the *female athlete triad,* which consists of menstrual dysfunction, low energy availability with or without disordered eating, and low bone mineral density in extreme athletes (American College of Obstetricians and Gynecologists, 2017b). Two international symposia held in this field have begun to develop risk stratification and recommendations for this population (Ackerman, 2018; Joy, 2014).

In 1970, Frisch and Revelle proposed that an adolescent girl needed to achieve a critical body weight to begin menstruating (Frisch, 1970). This mass was initially postulated to approximate 48 kilograms and was subsequently refined to a minimal body mass index (BMI) approaching normal, which is ≥19. Subsequent studies suggest that, although body fat and reproductive function show clear correlation at both ends of the weight spectrum, overall energy balance better predicts the onset and maintenance of menstrual cycles (Billewicz, 1976; Gonzales, 1996; Kaplowitz, 2008). For example, many elite athletes regain menstrual cyclicity following a decrease in exercise intensity prior to any gain in weight (Abraham, 1982). Of note, no weight or BMI has been determined to reliably predict pubertal onset.

Stress-induced Amenorrhea. This may be associated with clearly traumatic life events. Nevertheless, less severe life events and even positive events may be associated with stress. For example,

stress-related amenorrhea is frequently associated with leaving for college, test taking, or wedding planning.

Pathophysiology of Functional Hypothalamic Amenorrhea. Eating disorders, exercise, and stress may disturb menstrual function through overlapping mechanisms. This observation may be in part because these problems are often concurrent. For example, women with eating disorders frequently exercise excessively and are undoubtedly under stress as they attempt to control their eating patterns. Figure 17-6 depicts a simplified model for the development of amenorrhea in these patients. Importantly, each cause of functional hypothalamic amenorrhea may act via one or all of these pathways. Furthermore, in many cases, the factors known to affect reproductive function are likely acting indirectly on GnRH neurons through various neuronal subtypes that have synaptic connections to GnRH neurons. The kisspeptin neuronal system is likely a critical mediator between physiologic status and GnRH secretion and is discussed in Chapter 16 (Wahab, 2018).

Exercise is associated with an increase in endogenous opioid (β-endorphin) levels, producing the so-called runner's high. Opioids alter GnRH pulsatility. Opioids further alter reproduction through effects on ovarian, endometrial, and myometrial function (Böttcher, 2017).

As part of the stress response, each of these conditions may lead to greater corticotropin-releasing hormone (CRH) release by the hypothalamus, which in turn results in cortisol secretion by the adrenal gland. CRH alters the pattern of pulsatile GnRH secretion, whereas cortisol may act directly or indirectly to disrupt GnRH neuronal function.

Eating disorders are thought to disturb ovulatory function through several hormonal factors including insulin, insulin-like growth factor 1, cortisol, adiponectin, ghrelin, and leptin (Misra, 2014). First identified in 1994, leptin is a 167-amino-acid protein encoded by the *ob* gene and produced in white adipose tissue (Zhang, 1994). Leptin receptors have been identified in the central nervous system (CNS) and a wide range of peripheral tissues. Primarily produced in adipose tissue, leptin provides an important link between energy balance and reproduction, although it is one of many mechanisms (Chou, 2014; Schneider, 2004). Leptin has been termed a "satiety factor" as human leptin gene mutation results in morbid obesity, diabetes mellitus, and hypogonadism. This trio of abnormalities can be successfully reversed with recombinant human leptin treatment (Licinio, 2004).

Patients with anorexia nervosa have been found to have low circulating leptin levels (Mantzoros, 1997). It is hypothesized that a decrease in leptin production due to weight loss could secondarily stimulate neuropeptide Y, which is known to stimulate hunger and alter GnRH pulsatility. Leptin likely acts through various additional neurotransmitters and neuropeptides that include the β-endorphins and α-melanocyte-stimulating hormone.

Pseudocyesis. Although rare, this is considered in any woman with amenorrhea and pregnancy symptoms but negative pregnancy test results. Pseudocyesis exemplifies the ability of the mind to control physiologic processes. More than 500 cases of pseudocyesis are reported in the medical literature in women ranging from ages 6 to 79 years. These patients fervently believe that they are pregnant and subsequently demonstrate several pregnancy signs and symptoms, including amenorrhea.

Endocrine evaluation in a limited number of patients has suggested a pattern of hormonal derangements. These include alterations in LH pulse frequency concurrent with elevated serum androgen levels, which may explain the observed amenorrhea. Elevated serum prolactin levels and resultant galactorrhea have been noted in a subset of patients. Nocturnal growth hormone secretion also appears blunted (Tarin, 2013).

A common link in these patients is a history of severe grief, such as recent miscarriage, infant death, or longstanding infertility. Pseudocyesis may be more common in developing countries, where societal pressure to produce children may be strong (Seeman, 2014). Psychiatric treatment is generally required to treat the associated depression, which is often exacerbated when the patient is informed that she is not pregnant (Whelan, 1990).

Anatomic Destruction. Any process that destroys the hypothalamus can impair GnRH secretion and lead to hypogonadotropic hypogonadism and amenorrhea. Due to the complex neurohormonal input to the GnRH neurons, abnormalities do not need to directly interact with GnRH neurons but may operate indirectly by altering the activity of modulatory neurons.

The tumors most often associated with amenorrhea include craniopharyngiomas, germinomas, endodermal sinus tumors, eosinophilic granuloma (Hand-Schüller-Christian syndrome), gliomas, and metastatic lesions. The most common of these tumors, craniopharyngiomas, are located in the suprasellar region and frequently present with headaches and visual changes. Alternatively, impaired GnRH secretion may follow trauma, radiation, infections such as tuberculosis, or infiltrative diseases such as sarcoidosis.

■ Anterior Pituitary Gland Disorders

The anterior pituitary gland consists of gonadotropes (producing LH and FSH), lactotropes (prolactin), thyrotropes (thyroid-stimulating hormone), corticotropes (adrenocorticotropic hormone), and somatotropes (growth hormone) (Chap. 16, p. 346). Although various disorders may directly affect gonadotropes, many causes of pituitary-derived amenorrhea may also follow abnormalities in other pituitary cell types, which in turn alter gonadotrope function.

Inherited Abnormalities

Our understanding of genetic mechanisms that regulate normal pituitary development and function is rapidly advancing. First, patients with pituitary hormone deficiency combined with central facial and/or neurologic defects due to a failed midline fusion have been described. This syndrome is known as *septo-optic dysplasia*. Many of these patients carry mutations

in the *PROP1* gene (Cadman, 2007). Second, mutations in genes that encode the LH or FSH β-subunits or the GnRH receptor have also been identified as rare causes of hypogonadotropic hypogonadism. Last, mutations in genes encoding the nuclear hormone receptors SF-1 and DAX1 (NR0B1) as well as genes encoding the G protein–coupled receptor 54 (GPR54) for kisspeptin 1 are associated with hypothalamic and pituitary dysfunction (Matthews, 1993; Pallais, 2006; Seminara, 2006; Weiss, 1992).

Acquired Pituitary Dysfunction

Most pituitary dysfunction is acquired after menarche and therefore presents with normal pubertal development followed by secondary amenorrhea. Nevertheless, in rare cases, these disorders may begin prior to puberty, resulting in delayed puberty and primary amenorrhea (Howlett, 1989).

Pituitary adenomas are the most frequent cause of acquired pituitary dysfunction (Chap. 16, p. 361) (Molitch, 2017). These most commonly secrete prolactin, but excessive secretion of any pituitary-derived hormone can result in amenorrhea. Significantly elevated serum prolactin levels (>100 ng/mL) are almost always due to a pituitary mass.

Increased serum prolactin levels are found in as many as one-tenth of amenorrheic women, and more than half of women with both galactorrhea and amenorrhea have elevated prolactin levels (the "galactorrhea-amenorrhea syndrome"). Mechanistically, dopamine is released by the hypothalamus and acts on the anterior pituitary. Dopamine is the primary regulator of prolactin biosynthesis and secretion and plays an inhibitory role. Thus, elevated prolactin levels feed back to the hypothalamus and are associated with a reflex rise in central dopamine production to lower prolactin concentrations. This rise in central dopamine levels alters GnRH neuronal function.

Pituitary tumors also may indirectly alter gonadotrope function by a mass effect. First, tumor growth may compress neighboring gonadotropes. Second, damage to the pituitary stalk can disrupt dopamine's pathway to inhibit prolactin secretion. In this latter case, resulting elevated prolactin levels lead to elevated central dopamine levels that presumably interfere with menstrual function through the same mechanisms described in the previous paragraph.

As in the hypothalamus, pituitary function may also be diminished by inflammation, infiltrative disease, metastatic lesions, surgery, or radiation treatment (Dahan, 2017). Although a rare condition, peripartum lymphocytic hypophysitis can be a dangerous cause of pituitary failure. Infiltrative diseases include sarcoidosis and hemochromatosis.

Sheehan syndrome refers to panhypopituitarism. It classically follows massive postpartum hemorrhage and associated hypotension. The abrupt, severe hypotension leads to pituitary ischemia and necrosis (Kelestimur, 2003). Patients with the most severe form develop shock due to pituitary apoplexy. Pituitary apoplexy is characterized by a sudden onset of headache, nausea, visual deficits, and hormonal dysfunction due to acute hemorrhage or infarction within the pituitary. In less severe forms, loss of gonadotrope activity in the pituitary leads to anovulation and subsequent amenorrhea. Damage to the other specific pituitary cell types lead to a failure to lactate, loss of sexual and axillary hair, and hypothyroidism or adrenal insufficiency symptoms. Pituitary cell types are differentially sensitive to damage. For this reason, prolactin secretion deficiency is the most common, followed by loss of gonadotropin and growth hormone release, loss of ACTH production, and, least commonly, decreases in thyroid-stimulating hormone (TSH) secretion (Veldhuis, 1980).

■ Other Causes of Hypogonadotropic Hypogonadism

Hypogonadotropic amenorrhea may be observed in various chronic diseases including end-stage kidney disease, liver disease, malignancies, acquired immunodeficiency syndrome, and malabsorption syndromes. The mechanisms by which these disorders result in menstrual dysfunction are poorly understood. End-stage kidney disease is associated with increased serum prolactin and altered leptin levels, both of which may disrupt normal GnRH pulsatility (Ghazizadeh, 2007). Of patients with nonalcoholic chronic liver disease, the cause of the low gonadotropin levels is unknown and is observed only in a subset of those with amenorrhea (Cundy, 1991). Chronic diseases may produce amenorrhea through common mechanisms, such as stress and nutritional deficiencies. For example, patients with malabsorption due to celiac disease may have delayed menarche, secondary amenorrhea, and early menopause, which have been attributed to deficiencies in trace elements such as zinc and selenium. These are required for normal gonadotropin biosynthesis and secretion (Walker, 2019).

EUGONADOTROPIC AMENORRHEA

Several disorders that produce amenorrhea are not associated with significantly abnormal gonadotropin levels, at least as measured at a single point in time, as is done in clinical settings. Even so, gonadotropin amplitude or pulse frequency is likely disturbed in these patients. As a result, chronic sustained sex-steroid secretion interferes with the normal feedback between the ovary and the hypothalamic-pituitary axis. Normal oocyte maturation and ovulation are impaired, and menstruation fails to occur.

Due to relatively normal gonadotropin levels, these patients will secrete estrogen and therefore can also be said to have *chronic anovulation with estrogen present.* This is in contrast to patients with ovarian failure or hypothalamic-pituitary failure, in whom estrogen levels are low or absent. This distinction may be useful during evaluation and treatment.

■ Polycystic Ovarian Syndrome

This syndrome is by far the most common cause of chronic anovulation with estrogen present and is discussed fully in Chapter 18 (p. 389). Patients with PCOS may have various menstrual presentations. First, complete amenorrhea may follow anovulation. Without ovulation, progesterone is lacking, and an absent progesterone withdrawal fails to prompt menses. In some women with PCOS, however, amenorrhea may be attributable to the ability of androgens, which are elevated in PCOS patients, to atrophy the endometrium. Alternatively,

heavy menstrual or intermenstrual bleeding can result from unopposed estrogen stimulation of the endometrium. Within this unstable, thickened proliferative-phase endometrium, episodic stromal breakdown and shedding leads to irregular bleeding. Vessels may be abnormally dilated in anovulatory endometria, and bleeding may be severe. Last, women with PCOS may experience occasional ovulatory cycles, and normal withdrawal menses or pregnancy can occur.

■ Nonclassic Congenital Adrenal Hyperplasia

This condition closely mimics the presentation of PCOS with hyperandrogenism and irregular menstrual cycles. Most commonly, nonclassic congenital adrenal hyperplasia (CAH), also termed *adult-onset CAH* or *late-onset CAH*, is due to a mutation in the *CYP21A2* gene, which encodes the 21-hydroxylase enzyme. With a mild mutation, patients are asymptomatic until adrenarche, a time that requires greater adrenal steroidogenesis. Patients with CAH are unable to convert an adequate percentage of progesterone to cortisol and aldosterone, thus raising the production of androgens (Fig. 16-5, p. 339). As in PCOS, elevated androgen levels blunt oocyte maturation and thereby result in anovulation and amenorrhea.

■ Ovarian Tumor

Although uncommon, chronic anovulation with estrogen present can also be observed with ovarian tumors producing either estrogens or androgens. As discussed in Chapter 36, examples include granulosa cell tumors, theca cell tumors, and other sex cord–stromal tumors (p. 763) (Pectasides, 2008; Thomas, 2012).

■ Hyperprolactinemia and Hypothyroidism

Although hyperprolactinemia can cause hypogonadotropic hypogonadism, as described earlier, many hyperprolactinemic women may instead have relatively normal gonadotropin levels (p. 380). As a group, however, their estrogen levels will be mildly depressed. Aside from pituitary adenomas, other circumstances can significantly raise prolactin levels. First, many medications and herbs are associated with hyperprolactinemia, galactorrhea, and disrupted menstrual cycling (Table 13-2, p. 285). The antipsychotic group of medications is a frequent cause.

Second, primary hypothyroidism is the most common reason for elevated prolactin levels. One example is Hashimoto thyroiditis. In this disorder, the decline in circulating thyroid hormone levels results in a compensatory rise in hypothalamic thyrotropin-releasing hormone (TRH) secretion. TRH prompts pituitary gland thyrotropes to produce TSH. In addition, TRH also binds to pituitary lactotropes, increasing prolactin secretion. This tight link between thyroid function and prolactin levels justifies measurement of TSH and prolactin levels during evaluation of galactorrhea or amenorrhea.

Whether due to adenoma, medications, or hypothyroidism, prolactin elevation creates a compensatory rise in central levels of dopamine, the primary inhibitor of prolactin secretion. Greater central dopamine levels alter GnRH secretion, thereby disrupting normal cyclic gonadotropin secretion and preventing ovulation. With thyroid disease, additional proposed mechanisms include direct effects of thyroid hormone and prolactin on peripheral cells, as thyroid receptors are found in most cell types. Prolactin receptors have been identified in the ovary and in the endometrium. Moreover, thyroid hormone raises sex hormone–binding globulin levels, which alters the levels of unbound, and thereby active, ovarian steroids.

These potentially discordant effects are reflected in the various bleeding patterns seen with thyroid disease (Krassas, 2010). Classically, hypothyroidism is stated to cause anovulation and subsequent heavy menstrual bleeding (Chap. 8, p. 192).

Hyperthyroidism is implicated in amenorrhea. Nevertheless, these patterns are not strictly observed. As might be expected, the likelihood of menstrual abnormality correlates with the severity of the thyroid function disturbance (Kakuno, 2010).

EVALUATION

History

Figure 17-7 offers an algorithm for approaching the patient with amenorrhea. Initial questions investigate whether pubertal

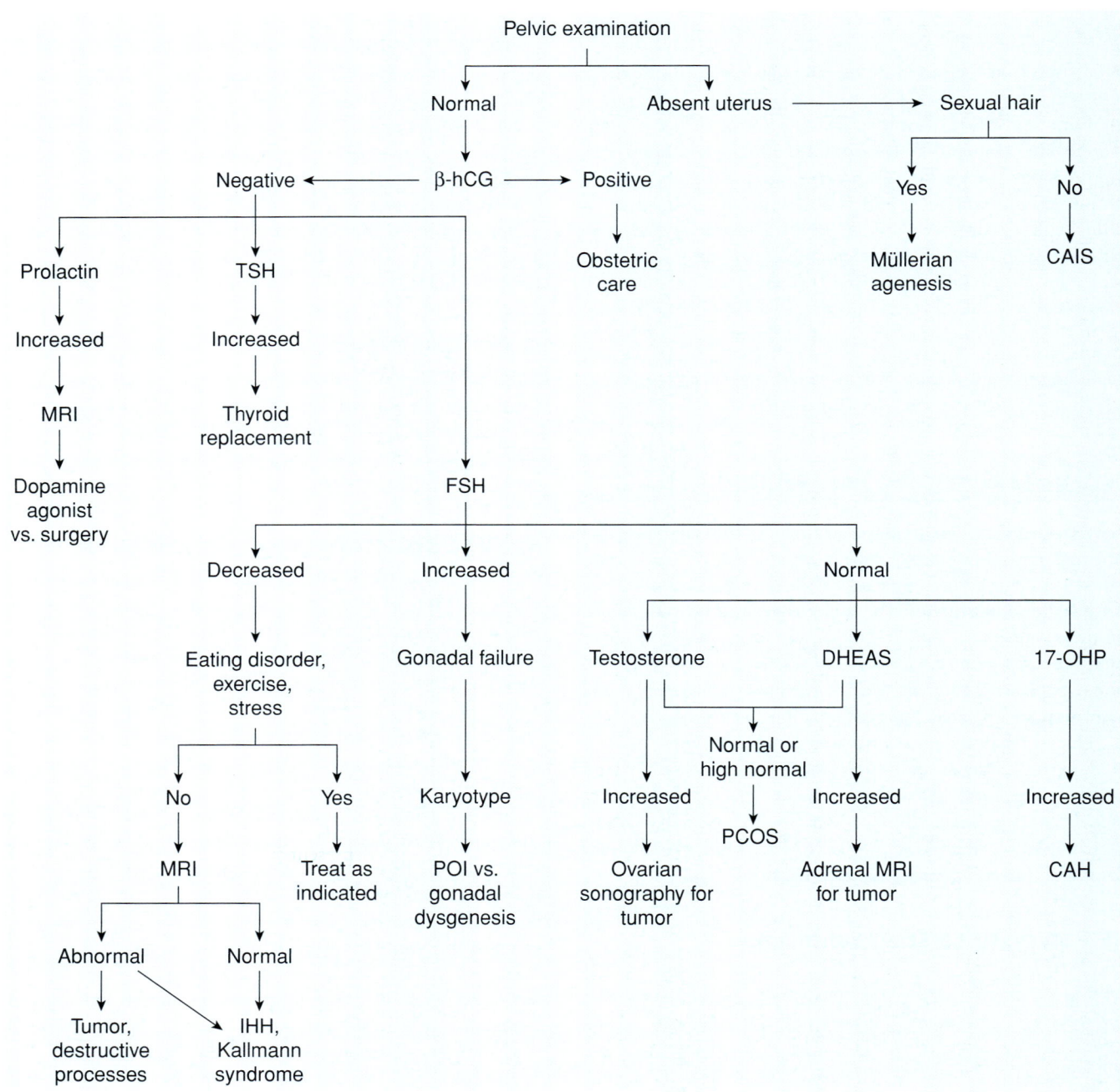

FIGURE 17-7 Diagnostic algorithm to evaluate amenorrhea. CAH = congenital adrenal hyperplasia; CAIS = complete androgen insensitivity syndrome; DHEAS = dehydroepiandrosterone sulfate; FSH = follicle-stimulating hormone; hCG = human chorionic gonadotropin; IHH = idiopathic hypogonadotropic hypogonadism; MRI = magnetic resonance imaging; 17-OHP = 17-hydroxyprogesterone; PCOS = polycystic ovarian syndrome; POI = premature ovarian insufficiency; TSH = thyroid-stimulating hormone.

Tanner stages have been reached and whether menses have begun (Fig. 15-3, p. 322). The cycle interval, duration, and amount of menstrual flow are characterized. Also, the development of amenorrhea may be temporally correlated with androgen excess, eating disorders, stress, intensive exercise, cancer therapy, or other illnesses. Surgical history focuses on prior pelvic surgery, especially intrauterine surgery. Patients are questioned regarding postoperative infection or other surgical complications.

A review of symptoms can be helpful. For example, new-onset headaches or visual changes may suggest a tumor of the CNS or pituitary gland. Pituitary tumors may impinge on the optic chiasm, resulting in bitemporal hemianopsia, that is, the loss of both right and left outer visual fields. Bilateral milky breast discharge may reflect hyperprolactinemia. Thyroid disease can be associated with heat or cold intolerance, weight changes, and sleep or bowel motility abnormalities. Hirsutism and acne are often seen with PCOS or with nonclassic CAH. Cyclic pelvic pain would suggest a reproductive tract outlet obstruction. Hot flashes and vaginal dryness point to hypergonadotropic hypogonadism, that is, POI. Of note, the range, severity, and persistence of symptoms observed in women with POI appear to exceed those experienced by women with age-appropriate menopause (Allshouse, 2015).

Important questions regarding family history include premature cessation of menses or a history of autoimmune disease, including thyroid disease, which would suggest a greater risk for POI. Sudden neonatal death may have occurred in family members carrying mutations in the *CYP21A2* gene responsible for CAH.

Any medications are inventoried, especially those such as antipsychotics that raise prolactin levels. The social history investigates exposure to environmental toxins, including cigarettes.

■ Physical Examination

General appearance can be helpful in the evaluation of amenorrhea. A low BMI, perhaps in conjunction with tooth enamel erosion from recurrent vomiting, is highly suggestive of an eating disorder. Signs of Turner syndrome are evaluated, including short stature, webbed neck, shield-shaped chest, and others listed in Table 19-3 (p. 413) (Turner, 1972). Midline facial defects, such as cleft palate, are consistent with a developmental defect of the anterior pituitary gland. Hypertension in a prepubertal girl may reflect mutation in the *CYP17* gene and shunting of the steroidogenic pathway toward aldosterone.

Visual field defects, particularly bitemporal hemianopsia, may indicate a pituitary gland or CNS tumor. Skin is inspected for acanthosis nigricans, hirsutism, or acne, which may indicate PCOS or other hyperandrogenism causes. Supraclavicular fat, abdominal striae, and hypertension may be noted in those with Cushing syndrome. Hypothyroidism can present with an abnormally enlarged thyroid gland, delayed reflexes, and bradycardia. During breast examination, bilateral galactorrhea implies hyperprolactinemia.

Examination of the genitalia starts by noting hair pattern. Sparse or absent axillary or pubic hair may reflect either lack of adrenarche or androgen insensitivity syndrome. Conversely, elevated androgen levels will result in a male pattern of genital hair growth. Markedly elevated levels of androgens can produce signs of virilization, most noticeably clitoromegaly (Chap. 18, p. 397). These women may also note voice deepening and male pattern balding.

Evidence of estrogen production includes a pink, moist vagina and cervical mucus. With estrogen present, vaginal smears demonstrate mostly superficial epithelial cells, whereas with atrophy, parabasal cell numbers increase (Fig. 22-12, p. 497). Low estrogen levels also manifest with a pale or red, thin, unrugated vagina.

Determination of müllerian anomalies by physical examination is described in Chapter 19 (p. 421). Rectal and digital vaginal examination may help identify a uterus above an obstruction at the level of the introitus or in the vagina. Hematocolpos suggests normal ovarian and endometrial function.

■ Testing

The differential diagnosis of amenorrhea is extensive, but evaluation of most women is relatively straightforward. For all disorders, testing may be modified by patient history and physical examination. All reproductive-aged women with amenorrhea and a uterus are assumed pregnant until proven otherwise. Thus, a urinary or serum β-hCG level is almost always obtained.

Progesterone Withdrawal

Classically, patients are given exogenous progesterone and monitored for a progesterone withdrawal bleed, which follows a few days after progesterone completion (progesterone challenge test). One regimen is medroxyprogesterone acetate (Provera) given as a 10-mg daily oral dose for 10 days. If bleeding ensues after cessation, a woman is assumed to produce estrogen and to have a developed endometrium and patent outflow tract. If bleeding does not follow, then a patient is given estrogen followed by progesterone treatment. A single pack of combination oral contraceptives (COCs) works nicely for this. If a woman again fails to bleed several days after completing the 21 hormone-containing pills, an anatomic abnormality is diagnosed.

Several factors can lead to an incorrect test interpretation. First, women with high androgen levels, such as occurs with PCOS and CAH, may have an atrophic endometrium and may fail to bleed. Specifically, up to 20 percent of women in whom estrogen is present will fail to bleed following progesterone withdrawal (Rarick, 1990). Second, estrogen levels may fluctuate both in hypothalamic amenorrhea and in the early stages of ovarian failure. As a result, patients with these disorders may have at least some bleeding after progesterone withdrawal. Namely, menses may be observed after progesterone administration in up to 40 percent of women with hypothalamic amenorrhea due to stress, weight loss, or exercise and in up to 50 percent of women with POI (Nakamura, 1996). This bleeding derives from endometrium that grew prior to amenorrhea onset. Due to the limitations in interpreting the results, use of this test likely is best restricted to those situations in which accurate serum hormone measurements are unavailable.

TABLE 17-7. Tests Commonly Used in the Evaluation of Amenorrhea

Primary Laboratory Tests	Diagnosis
β-hCG	Pregnancy
FSH	Hypogonadotropic versus hypergonadotropic hypogonadism[a]
Estradiol	Hypogonadotropic versus hypergonadotropic hypogonadism
Prolactin	Hyperprolactinemia
TSH ± fT4	Thyroid disease
Secondary Laboratory Tests	
Testosterone	PCOS and exclude ovarian tumor
DHEAS	Exclude adrenal tumor
17-OHP	Nonclassic CAH
2-hour glucose tolerance test	PCOS
Fasting lipid panel	PCOS
Autoimmune testing	POI
Adrenal antibodies (CYP21A2)	POI
Fragile X (FMR1 premutation)	POI
Karyotype	POI <35 years
Radiologic Evaluation	
Sonography	PCOS, uterine agenesis, or ovarian tumor
HSG or SIS	Müllerian anomaly or intrauterine synechiae
MR imaging	Müllerian anomaly or hypothalamic-pituitary disease

[a]Hypogonadotropic hypogonadism includes functional causes of hypothalamic amenorrhea (excessive exercise, eating disorders, and stress). Hypergonadotropic hypogonadism refers primarily to premature ovarian insufficiency (POI).
CAH = congenital adrenal hyperplasia; DHEAS = dehydroepiandrosterone sulfate; FSH = follicle-stimulating hormone; fT4 = free thyroxine; hCG = human chorionic gonadotropin; HSG = hysterosalpingography; MR = magnetic resonance; 17-OHP = 17-hydroxyprogesterone; PCOS = polycystic ovarian syndrome; SIS = saline-infusion sonography; TSH = thyroid-stimulating hormone.

Serum Hormone Levels

As suggested by the American Society for Reproductive Medicine (2008), it may be more reasonable to begin with hormonal evaluation in any woman found to have a normal pelvic examination (Table 17-7). First, *serum FSH levels* are typically assessed, and levels that are low suggest hypothalamic-pituitary dysfunction. An elevated FSH level is consistent with POI. FSH levels in the normal range suggest an anatomic defect or eugonadotropic hypogonadism, such as occurs in PCOS, hyperprolactinemia, or thyroid disease. Although many patients with PCOS have elevated LH to FSH level ratios >2, testing for this relationship is unnecessary as a normal ratio does not exclude this diagnosis.

If an FSH value is low, repeating this measurement and adding an LH level, which will also be low, can help confirm hypogonadotropic hypogonadism. Additional testing may include a GnRH stimulation test. Several different protocols have been employed, but one common approach provides 100 μg of GnRH as an intravenous bolus and then measures LH and FSH levels at 0, 15, 30, 45, and 60 minutes. In patients with hypogonadotropic hypogonadism or delayed puberty, although both LH and FSH levels will be blunted, FSH levels will be high relative to LH ratios during the test (Job, 1977). Although this test is informative, providers may be unable to perform it due to a lack of consistently available clinical-grade GnRH.

In contrast, an elevated FSH level strongly suggests the presence of hypergonadotropic hypogonadism, namely, POI. This diagnosis requires two FSH levels greater than a threshold range of 30 to 40 mIU/mL and obtained at least 1 month apart. At least two elevated values are required because the course of POI may fluctuate over time. This variation likely explains the occasional pregnancy that has been reported in affected women. Patients keep a menstrual calendar while testing is completed because bleeding 2 weeks following an elevated serum FSH level may simply indicate that the sample was obtained during a normal midcycle gonadotropin surge.

As adjuncts to FSH testing, ancillary markers that will increase the sensitivity and specificity of ovarian reserve testing have been investigated. Many clinicians obtain measurements for estradiol in addition to FSH, although this has not been consistently shown to increase diagnostic accuracy. Likewise, the use of circulating serum AMH levels is an attractive option but has not been shown to be helpful (Chap. 20, p. 437) (Visser, 2012).

Prolactin and *thyroid-stimulating hormone levels* are tested in most patients with amenorrhea as prolactin-secreting adenomas and thyroid disease are relatively common and require specific treatment. Because of the relationship between hypothyroidism and prolactin levels, both hormones are measured simultaneously. If present, treatment for hypothyroidism will also normalize prolactin levels. If a TSH level is elevated, an unbound thyroxine (T_4) level is drawn to confirm clinical hypothyroidism.

Serum testosterone levels are measured in women with suspected PCOS or with clinical signs of androgen excess. Hormonal evaluation includes measurement of serum total testosterone levels. Measurement of free testosterone levels is generally unwarranted as these assays are more expensive and less reliable unless sent to a specialized laboratory. Mild elevations in testosterone levels are consistent with the diagnosis of PCOS. However, values >200 ng/dL may suggest an ovarian tumor and warrant pelvic sonography.

Serum dehydroepiandrosterone sulfate (DHEAS) production is essentially limited to the adrenal gland. Levels in high-normal range or mildly above are consistent with PCOS. Adrenal adenomas may produce circulating DHEAS levels above 700 µg/dL and merit investigation with magnetic resonance (MR) imaging or computed tomography (CT) scanning of the adrenals. Measurement of 17-hydroxyprogesterone (17-OHP) aims to identify patients with nonclassic CAH. However, confirmation of this diagnosis can be difficult due to the overlapping values among normal patients and heterozygote and homozygote carriers of mutations in the 21-hydroxylase (*CYP21A2*) gene. Accordingly, adrenal stimulation with ACTH, often colloquially termed the *cort stim test*, may be required as described in Chapter 18 (p. 398).

Other Serum Testing

At times, other serum testing may be prudent. If an eating disorder is suspected, an immediate assessment of serum electrolytes is warranted as imbalances can be life-threatening. An electrocardiogram also is considered in those patients perceived to have severe disease. A reverse triiodothyronine (T_3) level is often elevated in patients with functional hypothalamic amenorrhea. Women with PCOS are screened for insulin resistance and lipid abnormalities, as these are often found in affected patients and raise risks for diabetes and cardiovascular disease (Chap. 18, p. 399). Although no consensus exists, repeating these tests every few years in those with PCOS is sound practice.

Many patients with POI will not have a clear etiology for their disorder based on medical history or genetic testing and may reasonably be assumed to have an autoimmune cause. Current recommendations focus on measurement of antiadrenal antibodies, specifically antibodies directed against 21-hydroxylase. Addition of antithyroid antibodies such as antimicrosomal/thyroid peroxidase antibodies (TPOAb) also is logical if thyroid dysfunction is suspected.

Chromosomal Analysis

Patients with gonadal dysgenesis, such as Turner syndrome, are considered for chromosomal analysis. Classic teaching suggests that this test is unnecessary after age 30. However, consideration is given to testing patients up to age 35 because a rare individual mosaicism may retain functional oocytes and thus sustain cyclic menses longer than expected. As previously indicated, a Y-containing cell line requires bilateral oophorectomy because of the higher risk for ovarian germ cell tumors. Due to the close association between stature and abnormalities in the X chromosome, many specialists advise karyotyping all women with POI who are shorter than 60 inches (Saenger, 2001). Chromosomal studies are also considered in any woman

with a family history of POI. Analysis is generally performed using classic karyotype approaches. However, with the advent of advanced sequencing methods, whole genome sequencing or other deep sequencing approaches may be considered in select circumstances.

Radiologic Evaluation

Any patient with hypogonadotropic hypogonadism is assumed to have an anatomic CNS or pituitary gland abnormality until proven otherwise by MR imaging or CT scanning. Thus, functional hypothalamic amenorrhea due to stress, exercise, or eating disorder is a diagnosis of exclusion. Imaging is highly sensitive for identification of destructive disorders such as tumors or infiltrative diseases of the hypothalamus or pituitary gland. Although fundamentally normal, a subset of patients with genetic causes for Kallmann syndrome or IHH will demonstrate developmental defects of the hypothalamus, olfactory bulbs, or pituitary gland during MR imaging (Klingmuller, 1987).

Reproductive tract anatomic disorders can be evaluated with several modalities depending on the suspected cause. Sonographic examination is frequently useful as a first screen for a uterus deemed grossly normal by physical examination. HSG or SIS is excellent for the detection of intrauterine synechiae or developmental anomalies. Changing trends favor SIS unless information on tubal patency also is required. Three-dimensional (3-D) sonography and 3-D SIS also can add information. MR imaging is frequently used for delineation of more complex uterine structures, such as a noncommunicating or hypoplastic uterine horn. Imaging of congenital reproductive tract anomalies is discussed further in Chapter 19 (p. 420).

TREATMENT

Treatment of amenorrhea depends on its etiology and patient goals such as a desire to treat hirsutism or seek pregnancy. Anatomic abnormalities often require surgical correction, if possible, and are discussed in Chapter 19 (p. 421). Hypothyroidism is treated with thyroid hormone replacement, and a suggested dosage of levothyroxine is 1.6 µg/kg of body weight per day (Baskin, 2002). For most, a common starting dose is 50 to 100 µg of levothyroxine orally daily. TSH response is slow, and levels are rechecked 6 to 8 weeks following initiation. A TSH level in the lower range of normal is the therapeutic goal. If needed, the dose may be increased by an increment of 12.5 or 25 µg (Jameson, 2012). Women with hyperprolactinemia receive a dopamine agonist, such as bromocriptine or cabergoline. Macroadenomas may require surgery if secondary deficits such as visual changes are observed. Both medical and surgical specifics of pituitary disease treatment are found in Chapter 16 (p. 362).

◾ Estrogen Replacement

This therapy is instituted in essentially every patient with hypogonadism to avoid osteoporosis. As in postmenopausal women, bone loss is accelerated in the first few years following estrogen deprivation. Thus, treatment is instituted quickly. Women with a uterus also require continuous or intermittent progesterone administration to protect against endometrial hyperplasia or cancer (Chap. 22, p. 481). There is no consensus, however, on an optimal regimen in these patients. Importantly, an escalating estrogen dose regimen is used for patients who have amenorrhea due to pubertal delay and will promote normal breast development (Chap. 15, p. 331). For women in their 20s, some experts recommend higher doses of estrogen than is routinely given to postmenopausal women as this is a time of ongoing bone deposition. Frequently, it is easiest to prescribe COCs. Younger women may prefer this treatment as their friends may also use these pills, and in their minds, hormone replacement therapy may be associated with aging. Of note, bone health may not be fully protected by estrogen in patients with ongoing energy deficits from eating disorders (Gordon, 2017). Additionally, consensus is lacking on treatment duration in those with hypogonadism. For most individuals, continuation until approximately age 50, the usual age of menopause, seems reasonable (American College of Obstetricians and Gynecologists, 2017c).

Patients who have eating disorders or who exercise excessively will require behavior modification. In a patient with an eating disorder, psychiatric intervention is imperative due to the significant morbidity and mortality associated with this diagnosis (American Psychiatric Association, 2013; Michopoulos, 2013). Elite athletes may choose not to alter their exercise regimens and will therefore require estrogen treatment.

■ Polycystic Ovarian Syndrome

Treatment of women with PCOS may include cyclic or constant progesterone treatment as outlined in Chapter 18 (p. 400). Insulin-sensitizing agents such as metformin (Glucophage) may be indicated in those with diabetes mellitus. In women with hyperandrogenism due to PCOS, COCs and/or spironolactone are often warranted.

Depending on its severity, nonclassic CAH in some women may be treated with low-dose corticosteroids to partially block ACTH stimulation of adrenal function and thereby decrease adrenal androgen overproduction.

■ Infertility

Alternative approaches may be required in a patient who desires conception. Adequate treatment of hyperprolactinemia and thyroid disease typically results in ovulation and in normal fertility for most women. If clearly linked to infertility, anatomic abnormalities are surgically corrected whenever possible. However, depending on the type and severity of the abnormality, a surrogate to carry a gestation may be needed. Although uterine transplantation followed by successful birth has been reported, this currently remains highly experimental (American Society for Reproductive Medicine, 2018). Stem cells also have been proposed for POI, but loss of ovarian reserve is best considered irreversible at present. Affected individuals can be offered in vitro fertilization using a donor oocyte to conceive. Assuming that behavioral modification is not successful, women with hypogonadotropic hypogonadism are referred to an infertility specialist for treatment with gonadotropins. Women with PCOS will frequently ovulate following treatment with the selective estrogen-receptor modulator clomiphene citrate

or with an aromatase inhibitor such as letrozole. Clomiphene citrate is believed to act by transient inhibition of estrogen feedback at the hypothalamus and pituitary gland (Fig. 21-1, p. 452). This treatment, however, is not effective in those with hypogonadotropic hypogonadism as they lack significant levels of circulating estrogen.

■ Patient Education

Patients are adequately counseled regarding their diagnosis, its long-term implications, and treatment options. All women with an intact endometrium must understand the risks of unopposed estrogen action, whether the estrogen is exogenous, such as through hormone therapy, or endogenous, such as in PCOS. For hypoestrogenic women, clinicians explain the importance of estrogen replacement to protect against bone loss. As detailed in Chapter 22 (p. 502), estrogen may have additional benefits. Last, even if not raised by the patient, the potential or lack of potential for future child-bearing is discussed.

REFERENCES

Abraham SF, Beumont PJ, Fraser IS, et al: Body weight, exercise and menstrual status among ballet dancers in training. BJOG 89(7):507, 1982

Ackerman KE, Misra M: Amenorrhoea in adolescent female athletes. Lancet Child Adolesc Health 2(9):677, 2018

Aittomaki K, Eroila H, Kajanoja P: A population-based study of the incidence of müllerian aplasia in Finland. Fertil Steril 76(3):624, 2001

Aittomaki K, Lucena JL, Pakarinen P, et al: Mutation in the follicle-stimulating hormone receptor gene causes hereditary hypergonadotropic ovarian failure. Cell 82(6):959, 1995

Allshouse AA, Semple AL, Santoro NF: Evidence for prolonged and unique amenorrhea-related symptoms in women with premature ovarian failure/primary ovarian insufficiency. Menopause 22(2):166, 2015

American College of Obstetricians and Gynecologists: Carrier screening for genetic conditions. Committee Opinion No. 691, March 2017a

American College of Obstetricians and Gynecologists: Female athlete triad. Committee Opinion No. 702, June 2017b

American College of Obstetricians and Gynecologists: Hormone therapy in primary ovarian insufficiency. Committee Opinion No. 698, May 2017c

American College of Obstetricians and Gynecologists: Menstruation in girls and adolescents: using the menstrual cycle as a vital sign. Committee Opinion No. 651, December 2015, Reaffirmed 2017d

American College of Obstetricians and Gynecologists: Gynecologic care for adolescents and young women with eating disorders. Committee Opinion No. 740, June 2018a

American College of Obstetricians and Gynecologists: Müllerian agenesis: diagnosis, management, and treatment. Committee Opinion No. 728, January 2018b

American College of Obstetricians and Gynecologists: Primary ovarian insufficiency in adolescents and young women. Committee Opinion No. 605, July 2014, Reaffirmed 2018c

American Fertility Society: The American Fertility Society classifications of adnexal adhesions, distal tubal occlusion, tubal occlusion secondary to tubal ligation, tubal pregnancies, müllerian anomalies and intrauterine adhesions. Fertil Steril 49(6):944, 1988

American Psychiatric Association: Diagnostic and Statistical Manual of Mental Disorders, Fifth Edition. Arlington, American Psychiatric Association, 2013

American Society for Reproductive Medicine: American Society for Reproductive Medicine position statement on uterus transplantation: a committee opinion. Fertil Steril 110(4):605, 2018

American Society for Reproductive Medicine: Current evaluation of amenorrhea. Fertil Steril 90(Supp 5):219, 2008

Bachmann GA, Kemmann E: Prevalence of oligomenorrhea and amenorrhea in a college population. Am J Obstet Gynecol 144(1):98, 1982

Banerjee R, Laufer MR: Reproductive disorders associated with pelvic pain. Semin Pediatr Surg 7(1):52, 1998

Baskin HJ, Cobin RH, Duick DS, et al: American Association of Clinical Endocrinologists medical guidelines for clinical practice for the evaluation and treatment of hyperthyroidism and hypothyroidism. Endocr Pract 8(6):457, 2002

Batista RL, Costa EMF, Rodrigues AS, et al: Androgen insensitivity syndrome: a review. Arch Endocrinol Metab 62(2):227, 2018

Bidet M, Bachelot A, Bissauge E, et al: Resumption of ovarian function and pregnancies in 358 patients with premature ovarian failure. J Clin Endocrinol Metab 96(12):3864, 2011

Billewicz WZ, Fellowes HM, Hytten CA: Comments on the critical metabolic mass and the age of menarche. Ann Hum Biol 3(1):51, 1976

Böttcher B, Seeber B, Leyendecker G, Wildt L: Impact of the opioid system on the reproductive axis. Fertil Steril 108(2):207, 2017

Budani MC, Tiboni GM: Ovotoxicity of cigarette smoke: a systematic review of the literature. Reprod Toxicol 72:164, 2017

Cadman SM, Kim SH, Hu Y, et al: Molecular pathogenesis of Kallmann's syndrome. Horm Res 67(5):231, 2007

Caronia LM, Martin C, Welt CK, et al: A genetic basis for functional hypothalamic amenorrhea. N Engl J Med 364:215, 2011

Chen H, Li J, Cui T, Hu L: Adjuvant gonadotropin-releasing hormone analogues for the prevention of chemotherapy induced premature ovarian failure in premenopausal women. Cochrane Database Syst Rev 11:CD008018, 2011

Chou SH, Mantzoros C: 20 years of leptin: role of leptin in human reproductive disorders. J Endocrinol 223(1):T49, 2014

Cools M, Nordenström A, Robeva R, et al: Caring for individuals with a difference of sex development (DSD): a consensus statement. Nat Rev Endocrinol 14(7):415, 2018

Cordts EB, Christofolini DM, Dos Santos AA, et al: Genetic aspects of premature ovarian failure: a literature review. Arch Gynecol Obstet 283(3):635, 2011

Coulam CB, Adamson SC, Annegers JF: Incidence of premature ovarian failure. Obstet Gynecol 67(4):604, 1986

Cundy TF, Butler J, Pope RM, et al: Amenorrhoea in women with non-alcoholic chronic liver disease. Gut 32(2):202, 1991

Dahan MH, Tan SL: A primer on pituitary injury for the obstetrician gynecologist: Simmond's disease, Sheehan's Syndrome, traumatic injury, Dahan's Syndrome, pituitary apoplexy and lymphocytic hypophysitis. Minerva Ginecol 69(2):190, 2017

Dempfle A, Herpetz-Dahlmann B, Timmesfeld N, et al: Predictors of the resumption of menses in adolescent anorexia nervosa. BMC Psychiatry 13:308, 2013

De Souza MJ, Miller BE, Loucks AB, et al: High frequency of luteal phase deficiency and anovulation in recreational women runners: blunted elevation in follicle-stimulating hormone observed during luteal-follicular transition. J Clin Endocrinol Metab 83(12):4220, 1998

Fontana L, Gentilin B, Fedele L, et al: Genetics of Mayer-Rokitansky-Küster-Hauser (MRKH) syndrome. Clin Genet 91(2):233, 2017

Franco B, Guioli S, Pragliola A, et al: A gene deleted in Kallmann's syndrome shares homology with neural cell adhesion and axonal path-finding molecules. Nature 353(6344):529, 1991

Frederick AB, Zinsli AM, Carlock G, et al: Presentation, progression, and predictors of ovarian insufficiency in classic galactosemia. J Inherit Metab Dis 41(5):785, 2018

Friedler S, Margalioth EJ, Kafka I, Yaffe H: Incidence of post-abortion intrauterine adhesions evaluated by hysteroscopy–a prospective study. Hum Reprod 8(3):442, 1993

Frisch RE, Gotz-Welbergen AV, McArthur JW, et al: Delayed menarche and amenorrhea of college athletes in relation to age of onset of training. JAMA 246(14):1559, 1981

Frisch RE, Revelle R: Height and weight at menarche and a hypothesis of critical body weights and adolescent events. Science 169(943):397, 1970

Ghazizadeh S, Lessan-Pezeshkii M: Reproduction in women with end-stage renal disease and effect of kidney transplantation. Iran J Kidney Dis 1(1):12, 2007

Gonzales GF, Villena A: Critical anthropometry for menarche. J Pediatr Adolesc Gynecol 9(3):139, 1996

Gordon CM, Ackerman KE, Berga SL, et al: Functional hypothalamic amenorrhea: an endocrine society clinical practice guideline. J Clin Endocrinol Metab 102(5):1413, 2017

Goswami D, Conway GS: Premature ovarian failure. Hum Reprod Update 11(4):391, 2005

Gradishar WJ, Schilsky RL: Ovarian function following radiation and chemotherapy for cancer. Semin Oncol 16(5):425, 1989

Grimbizis GF, Gordts S, Di Spiezio Sardo A, et al: The ESHRE/ESGE consensus on the classification of female genital tract congenital anomalies. Hum Reprod 28(8):2032, 2013

Hoek A, Schoemaker J, Drexhage HA: Premature ovarian failure and ovarian autoimmunity. Endocr Rev 18(1):107, 1997

Hooker AB, Lemmers M, Thurkow AL, et al: Systematic review and meta-analysis of intrauterine adhesions after miscarriage: prevalence, risk factors and long-term reproductive outcome. Hum Reprod Update 20(2):262, 2014

Howard SR: Genes underlying delayed puberty. Mol Cell Endocrinol 476:119, 2018

Howlett TA, Wass JA, Grossman A, et al: Prolactinomas presenting as primary amenorrhoea and delayed or arrested puberty: response to medical therapy. Clin Endocrinol (Oxf) 30(2):131, 1989

Husebye ES, Anderson MS, Kämpe O: Autoimmune polyendocrine syndromes. N Engl J Med 378(12):1132, 2018

Hutson JM, Grover SR, O'Connell M, et al: Malformation syndromes associated with disorders of sex development. Nat Rev Endocrinol 10(8):476, 2014

Hviid A, Rubin S, Mühlemann K: Mumps. Lancet 371(9616):932, 2008

Jameson JL, Weetman AP: Disorders of the thyroid gland. In Longo DL, Fauci AS, Kasper DL, et al (eds): Harrison's Principles of Internal Medicine, 18th ed. New York, McGraw-Hill, 2012

Job JC, Chaussain JL, Garnier PE: The use of luteinizing hormone-releasing hormone in pediatric patients. Horm Res 8(3):171, 1977

Joy E, De Souza MJ, Mattiv A, et al: 2014 female athlete triad coalition consensus statement on treatment and return to play of the female athlete triad. Curr Sports Med Rep 13(4):219, 2014

Kakuno Y, Amino N, Kanoh M, et al: Menstrual disturbances in various thyroid diseases. Endocr J 57(12):1017, 2010

Kaneko N, Kawagoe S, Hiroi M: Turner's syndrome—review of the literature with reference to a successful pregnancy outcome. Gynecol Obstet Invest 29(2):81, 1990

Kaplowitz PB: Link between body fat and the timing of puberty. Pediatrics 121(3 suppl):s208, 2008

Kelestimur F: Sheehan's syndrome. Pituitary 6(4):181, 2003

Klein DA, Poth MA: Amenorrhea: an approach to diagnosis and management. Am Fam Physician 87(11):781, 2013

Klingmuller D, Dewes W, Krahe T, et al: Magnetic resonance imaging of the brain in patients with anosmia and hypothalamic hypogonadism (Kallmann's syndrome). J Clin Endocrinol Metab 65(3):581, 1987

Krassas GE, Poppe K, Glinoer D: Thyroid function and human reproductive health. Endocr Rev 31(5):702, 2010

Lambertini M, Moore HCF, Leonard RC, et al: Gonadotropin-releasing hormone agonists during chemotherapy for preservation of ovarian function and fertility in premenopausal patients with early breast cancer: a systematic review and meta-analysis of individual patient-level data. J Clin Oncol 36(19):1981, 2018

Latronico AC, Arnhold IJ: Gonadotropin resistance. Endocr Dev 24:25, 2013

Layman LC: Clinical genetic testing for Kallmann syndrome. J Clin Endocrinol Metab 98(5):1860, 2013

Licinio J, Caglayan S, Ozata M, et al: Phenotypic effects of leptin replacement on morbid obesity, diabetes mellitus, hypogonadism, and behavior in leptin-deficient adults. Proc Natl Acad Sci USA 101(13):4531, 2004

Mantzoros C, Flier JS, Lesem MD, et al: Cerebrospinal fluid leptin in anorexia nervosa: relation with nutritional status and potential role in resistance to weight gain. J Clin Endocrinol Metab 82(6):1845, 1997

March CM: Asherman's syndrome. Semin Reprod Med 29(2):83, 2011

Matthews CH, Borgato S, Beck-Peccoz P, et al: Primary amenorrhoea and infertility due to a mutation in the beta-subunit of follicle-stimulating hormone. Nat Genet 5(1):83, 1993

Michopoulos V, Mancini F, Loucks TL, et al: Neuroendocrine recovery initiated by cognitive behavioral therapy in women with functional hypothalamic amenorrhea: a randomized, controlled trial. Fertil Steril 99(7):2084, 2013

Miller WL: Mechanisms in endocrinology: rare defects in adrenal steroidogenesis. Eur J Endocrinol 179(3):R125, 2018

Misra M, Klibanski A: Endocrine consequences of anorexia nervosa. Lancet Diabetes Endocrinol 2(7):581, 2014

Mlynarcikova A, Fickova M, Scsukova S: Ovarian intrafollicular processes as a target for cigarette smoke components and selected environmental reproductive disruptors. Endocr Regul 39(1):21, 2005

Molitch ME: Diagnosis and treatment of pituitary adenomas: a review. JAMA 317(5):516, 2017

Nakamura S, Douchi T, Oki T, et al: Relationship between sonographic endometrial thickness and progestin-induced withdrawal bleeding. Obstet Gynecol 87(5 Pt 1):722, 1996

Newman WG, Friedman TB, Conway GS, et al: Perrault Syndrome. In Adam MP, Ardinger HH, Pagon RA, et al (eds): GeneReviews, Seattle, University of Washington, 2018

Oktem O, Yagmur H, Bengisu H, et al: Reproductive aspects of systemic lupus erythematosus. J Reprod Immunol 117:57, 2016

Pallais JC, Bo-Abbas Y, Pitteloud N, et al: Neuroendocrine, gonadal, placental, and obstetric phenotypes in patients with IHH and mutations in the G-protein coupled receptor, GPR54. Mol Cell Endocrinol 254–255:70, 2006

Parazzini F, Cecchetti G: The frequency of imperforate hymen in northern Italy. Int J Epidemiol 19(3):763, 1990

Pectasides D, Pectasides E, Psyrri A: Granulosa cell tumor of the ovary. Cancer Treat Rev 34(1):1, 2008

Pyle LC, Nathanson KL: A practical guide for evaluating gonadal germ cell tumor predisposition in differences of sex development. Am J Med Genet C Semin Med Genet 175(2):304, 2017

Quinton R, Hasan W, Grant W, et al: Gonadotropin-releasing hormone immunoreactivity in the nasal epithelia of adults with Kallmann's syndrome and isolated hypogonadotropic hypogonadism and in the early midtrimester human fetus. J Clin Endocrinol Metab 82(1):309, 1997

Rarick LD, Shangold MM, Ahmed SW: Cervical mucus and serum estradiol as predictors of response to progestin challenge. Fertil Steril 54(2):353, 1990

Reindollar RH, Byrd JR, McDonough PG: Delayed sexual development: a study of 252 patients. Am J Obstet Gynecol 140(4):371, 1981

Reindollar RH, Novak M, Tho SP, et al: Adult-onset amenorrhea: a study of 262 patients. Am J Obstet Gynecol 155(3):531, 1986

Rossetti R, Ferrari I, Bonomi M, et al: Genetics of primary ovarian insufficiency. Clin Genet 91(2):183, 2017

Saenger P, Albertsson Wikland K, Conway GS, et al: Recommendations for the diagnosis and management of Turner syndrome. J Clin Endocrinol Metab 86(7):3061, 2001

Santamaria X, Mas A, Cervelló I, et al: Uterine stem cells: from basic research to advanced cell therapies. Hum Reprod Update 24(6):673, 2018

Schenker JG, Margalioth EJ: Intrauterine adhesions: an updated appraisal. Fertil Steril 37(5):593, 1982

Schneider JE: Energy balance and reproduction. Physiol Behav 81(2):289, 2004

Seeman MV: Pseudocyesis, delusional pregnancy, and psychosis: the birth of a delusion. World J Clin Cases 2(8):338, 2014

Seminara SB: Mechanisms of disease: the first kiss—a crucial role for kiss-peptin-1 and its receptor, G-protein-coupled receptor 54, in puberty and reproduction. Nat Clin Pract Endocrinol Metab 2(6):328, 2006

Sharma JB, Roy KK, Pushparaj M, et al: Hysteroscopic findings in women with primary and secondary infertility due to genital tuberculosis. Int J Gynaecol Obstet 104(1):49, 2009

Shufelt CL, Torbati T, Dutra E: Hypothalamic amenorrhea and the long-term health consequences. Semin Reprod Med 35(3):256, 2017

Silva CA, Yamakami LY, Aikawa NE, et al: Autoimmune primary ovarian insufficiency. Autoimmun Rev 13(4-5):427, 2014

Simoni M, Taylor HS: Therapeutic strategies involving uterine stem cells in reproductive medicine. Curr Opin Obstet Gynecol 30(3)209, 2018

Singh RP, Carr DH: The anatomy and histology of XO human embryos and fetuses. Anat Rec 155(3):369, 1966

Tarin JJ, Hermenegildo C, Garcia-Perez MA, et al: Endocrinology and physiology of pseudocyesis. Reprod Biol Endocrinol 11:39, 2013

Terenziani M, Piva L, Meazza C, et al: Oophoropexy: a relevant role in preservation of ovarian function and pelvic irradiation. Fertil Steril 91(3):935.e15, 2009

Thakur M, Feldman G, Puscheck EE: Primary ovarian insufficiency in classic galactosemia: current understanding and future research opportunities. J Assist Reprod Genet 35(1):3, 2018

Tho PT, McDonough PG: Gonadal dysgenesis and its variants. Pediatr Clin North Am 28(2):309, 1981

Thomas RL, Carr BR, Ziadie MS, et al: Bilateral mucinous cystadenomas and massive edema of the ovaries in a virilized adolescent girl. Obstet Gynecol 120(2 Pt 2):473, 2012

Turner H: Classic pages in obstetrics and gynecology by Henry H. Turner. A syndrome of infantilism, congenital webbed neck, and cubitus valgus. Endocrinology, vol 23, pp 566–574, 1938. Am J Obstet Gynecol 113(2):279, 1972

Vabre P, Gatimel N, Moreau J, et al: Environmental pollutants, a possible etiology for premature ovarian insufficiency: a narrative review of animal and human data. Environ Health 16(1):37, 2017

Veldhuis JD, Hammond JM: Endocrine function after spontaneous infarction of the human pituitary: report, review, and reappraisal. Endocr Rev 1(1):100, 1980

Visser JA, Schipper I, Laven JSE, et al: Anti-mullerian hormone: an ovarian reserve marker in primary ovarian insufficiency. Nat Rev Endocrinol 8:331, 2012

Wahab F, Atika B, Ullah F, et al: Metabolic impact on the hypothalamic kisspeptin-Kiss1r signaling pathway. Front Endocrinol 9:123, 2018

Walker MD, Zylberberg HM, Green PH, et al: Endocrine complications of celiac disease: a case report and review of the literature. Endocr Res 44(1–2):27, 2019

Weiss J, Axelrod L, Whitcomb RW, et al: Hypogonadism caused by a single amino acid substitution in the beta subunit of luteinizing hormone. N Engl J Med 326(3):179, 1992

Whelan CI, Stewart DE: Pseudocyesis—a review and report of six cases. Int J Psychiatry Med 20(1):97, 1990

Wittenberger MD, Hagerman RJ, Sherman SL, et al: The FMR1 premutation and reproduction. Fertil Steril 87(3):456, 2007

Zhang Y, Proenca R, Maffei M, et al: Positional cloning of the mouse obese gene and its human homologue. Nature 372(6505):425, 1994

Polycystic Ovarian Syndrome and Hyperandrogenism

NIH (2012) workshop emphasized the variable presentation of PCOS. Their consensus recommended the 2003 Rotterdam criteria be used to assign one of four specific patient phenotypes (see Table 18-1).

Importantly, these same criteria are not appropriate for adolescents. Guidance regarding specific criteria and thresholds are found later in those specific sections. In sum, the diagnosis of PCOS in adolescence is challenging because many symptoms of PCOS mimic the normal physiologic responses of puberty. For adolescents with incomplete criteria for a firm diagnosis of PCOS, careful surveillance is warranted as they may be diagnosed at a later time (Carmina, 2010; Witchel, 2015).

Polycystic ovarian syndrome (PCOS) is a common endocrinopathy typified by oligoovulation or anovulation, signs of androgen excess, and an excess of small ovarian cysts. These signs and symptoms vary widely between women and within individuals over time. Women with this endocrine disorder also have higher rates of obesity, dyslipidemia, and insulin resistance, which raise long-term health risks. As a result, women with PCOS may first present to various medical specialists, including pediatricians, gynecologists, internists, endocrinologists, or dermatologists.

DEFINITION

■ Polycystic Ovarian Syndrome

In 2003 in Rotterdam, The Netherlands, PCOS in adults was redefined in a consensus meeting between the European Society of Human Reproduction and Embryology (ESHRE) and the American Society for Reproductive Medicine (ASRM)—The Rotterdam ESHRE/ASRM-Sponsored PCOS Consensus Workshop Group, 2004. As shown in Table 18-1, affected individuals must meet two out of three criteria. However, because other etiologies, such as congenital adrenal hyperplasia, androgen-secreting tumors, and hyperprolactinemia, also may lead to oligoovulation and/or androgen excess, these must be excluded. Thus, PCOS currently is a diagnosis of exclusion.

The Rotterdam criteria constitute a broader spectrum than that formerly put forward by the National Institutes of Health (NIH) Conference in 1990 (Zawadzki, 1990). The prominent difference is that the NIH Conference defined PCOS without regard to ovarian sonographic appearance. A third organization—The Androgen Excess and PCOS Society (AE-PCOS)—also has defined criteria for PCOS (Azziz, 2006). Subsequently, an

TABLE 18-1. Definition of PCOS

ESHRE/ASRM (Rotterdam) 2003

Two of the three:
    Clinical and/or biochemical hyperandrogenism (HA)
    Oligo-/anovulation (OA)
    Polycystic ovarian morphology (PCOM)[a]

NIH (1990)

To include both:
    Clinical and/or biochemical hyperandrogenism
    Oligo-/anovulation

AE-PCOS (2006)

To include both:
    Clinical and/or biochemical hyperandrogenism
    Oligo-/anovulation and/or polycystic ovarian morphology

NIH (2012)

To identify one of four phenotypes using Rotterdam criteria
    HA + OA + PCOM
    HA + OA
    HA + PCOM
    OA + PCOM

[a]Polycystic ovarian morphology identified by transvaginal sonography.
AE-PCOS = Androgen Excess and PCOS Society; ASRM = American Society of Reproductive Medicine; ESHRE = European Society of Human Reproduction and Embryology; NIH = National Institutes of Health. PCOS = polycystic ovarian syndrome.
From Azziz, 2006; National Institutes of Health, 2012; The Rotterdam ESHRE/ASRM-Sponsored PCOS Consensus Workshop Group, 2004; Zawadzki, 1990.

Ovarian Hyperthecosis and HAIRAN Syndrome

Ovarian hyperthecosis, often considered a more severe form of PCOS, is a rare condition characterized by nests of luteinized theca cells distributed throughout the ovarian stroma. Affected women exhibit severe hyperandrogenism and greater degree of insulin resistance (Nagamani, 1986, 1999).

Hyperandrogenic-insulin resistant-acanthosis nigricans (HAIRAN) syndrome also is uncommon and consists of marked hyperandrogenism, severe insulin resistance, and acanthosis nigricans (Barbieri, 1983). Both conditions are exaggerated PCOS phenotypes, and their treatment mirrors that for PCOS.

INCIDENCE AND ETIOLOGY

PCOS is the most common endocrine disorder of reproductive-aged women and affects approximately 6 to 16 percent in general population studies (Li, 2013; Lizneva, 2016). Although symptoms of androgen excess may vary among ethnicities, PCOS appears to affect all races and nationalities similarly.

The underlying cause of PCOS is unknown. However, a genetic basis that is both multifactorial and polygenic is suspected, as the syndrome aggregates within families and first-degree relatives (Kahsar-Miller, 2001; Yildiz, 2003). Twin studies also implicate a prominent heritable influence (Vink, 2006).

Some have suggested an autosomal dominant inheritance with expression in both females and males. First-degree male relatives of women with PCOS have significantly higher rates of elevated circulating dehydroepiandrosterone sulfate (DHEAS) levels, early balding, and insulin resistance compared with male controls (Legro, 2000, 2002). Other metabolic alterations typical for PCOS also are found in greater frequency in male relatives (Cannarella, 2018; Liu, 2014; Torchen, 2016).

Several risk loci have been identified by genome-wide association studies in women with PCOS (Day, 2018; Zhao, 2016). Putative genes include those involved in androgen synthesis, obesity, and insulin resistance (Mykhalchenko, 2017). In addition, epigenetic modification of genetic susceptibility within the maternal-fetal environment may influence adult PCOS development (Dumesic, 2014).

PATHOPHYSIOLOGY

Gonadotropins

Anovulation in women with PCOS is characterized by inappropriate gonadotropin secretion (Fig. 18-1). Specifically, altered gonadotropin-releasing hormone (GnRH) pulsatility leads to preferential production of luteinizing hormone (LH) compared with follicle-stimulating hormone (FSH) (Hayes, 1998; Waldstreicher, 1988). It is currently unknown whether hypothalamic dysfunction is a primary cause of PCOS or is secondary to abnormal steroid feedback. In either case, serum LH levels rise, and elevated levels are observed clinically in approximately 50 percent of affected women (van Santbrink, 1997). Similarly, LH: FSH ratios are elevated and rise above 2:1 in approximately 60 percent of patients (Rebar, 1976).

TABLE 18-2. Consequences of Polycystic Ovarian Syndrome

Short-term consequences
Obesity
Infertility
Sleep apnea
Irregular menses
Depression/anxiety
Abnormal lipid levels
Non-alcoholic fatty liver disease
Hirsutism/acne/androgenic alopecia
Insulin resistance/acanthosis nigricans

Long-term consequences
Diabetes mellitus
Endometrial cancer
Cardiovascular disease

Insulin Resistance

Women with PCOS also display greater degrees of insulin resistance and compensatory hyperinsulinemia than nonaffected women. Insulin resistance is defined as a reduced glucose-uptake response to a given amount of insulin. This lower insulin sensitivity appears to stem from a postbinding abnormality in insulin receptor–mediated signal transduction (Dunaif, 1997). Both lean and obese women with PCOS are found to be more insulin resistant than nonaffected weight-matched controls (Dunaif, 1989, 1992).

Insulin resistance is associated with several disorders including type 2 diabetes mellitus (DM), hypertension, dyslipidemia, and cardiovascular disease (CVD). Therefore, PCOS is not simply a disorder of short-term consequences such as irregular menses and hirsutism, but also one of potential long-term health consequences (Table 18-2).

Androgens

Both insulin and LH stimulate androgen production by the ovarian theca cell (Dunaif, 1992). As a result, affected ovaries secrete elevated levels of testosterone and androstenedione. Specifically, elevated free testosterone levels are noted in 70 to 80 percent of women with PCOS, and 25 to 65 percent exhibit elevated levels of DHEAS (Moran, 1994, 1999; O'Driscoll, 1994). In turn, elevated androstenedione levels contribute to greater estrone levels through peripheral conversion of androgens to estrogens by aromatase.

Sex Hormone–Binding Globulin

Women with PCOS display decreased levels of sex hormone–binding globulin (SHBG). This glycoprotein, produced in the liver, binds most sex steroids. Only approximately 1 percent of these steroids are unbound and thus free and bioavailable. The synthesis of SHBG is suppressed by insulin and by androgens, corticoids, progestins, and growth hormone (Bergh, 1993). Because of suppressed SHBG production, less circulating

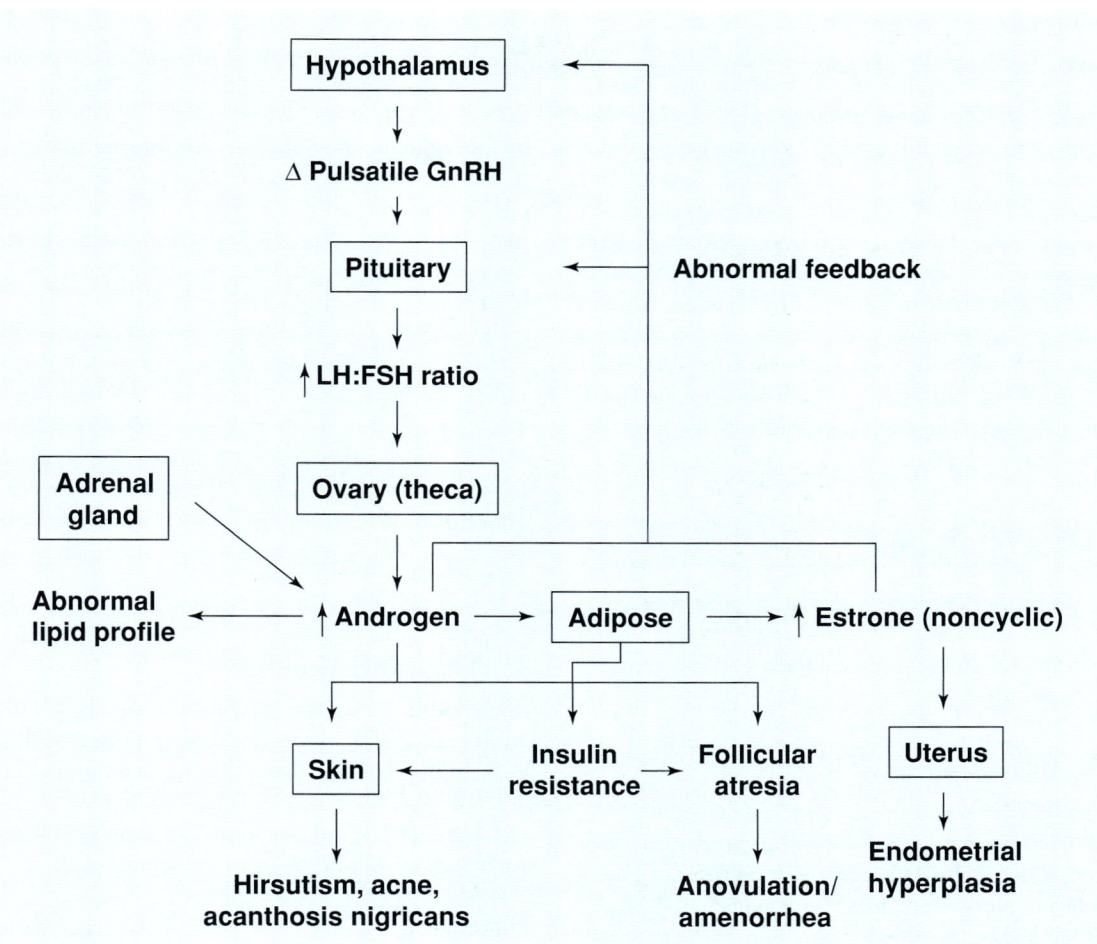

FIGURE 18-1 Model for the initiation and maintenance of polycystic ovarian syndrome (PCOS). Alterations in pulsatile gonadotropin-releasing hormone (GnRH) release may lead to a relative increase in luteinizing hormone (LH) versus follicle-stimulating hormone (FSH) biosynthesis and secretion. LH stimulates ovarian androgen production, while the relative paucity of FSH prevents adequate stimulation of aromatase activity within the granulosa cells, thereby decreasing androgen conversion to the potent estrogen estradiol.

Increased intrafollicular androgen levels result in follicular atresia. Increased circulating androgen levels contribute to abnormalities in patient lipid profiles and the development of hirsutism and acne. Increased circulating androgens can also be derived from the adrenal gland.

Elevated serum androgens (primarily androstenedione) are converted in the periphery to estrogens (primarily estrone). As conversion occurs primarily in the stromal cells of adipose tissue, estrogen production will be augmented in obese PCOS patients. This conversion results in chronic feedback at the hypothalamus and pituitary gland, in contrast to the normal fluctuations in feedback observed in the presence of a growing follicle and rapidly changing levels of estradiol. Unopposed estrogen stimulation of the endometrium may lead to endometrial hyperplasia.

Insulin resistance due to genetic abnormalities and/or increased adipose tissue contributes to follicular atresia in the ovaries as well as the development of acanthosis nigricans in the skin.

Lack of follicular development results in anovulation and subsequent oligo- or amenorrhea.

Note that this syndrome may develop from primary dysfunction of any one of a number of organ systems. For example, elevated ovarian androgen production may be due to either an intrinsic abnormality in enzymatic function and/or abnormal hypothalamic-pituitary stimulation with LH and FSH.

The common denominator is development of a self-perpetuating noncyclic hormonal pattern.

androgen is bound and thus more remains available to bind with end-organ receptors. Accordingly, some women with PCOS will have total testosterone levels in the normal range but will be clinically hyperandrogenic due to elevated free testosterone levels.

In addition to hyperandrogenism, low SHBG levels also have been linked to impaired glucose control and a risk for developing type 2 DM (Ding, 2009). The mechanism of this association is not fully understood and may reflect a role for SHBG in glucose homeostasis. For example, Veltman-Verhulst

(2010) evaluated SHBG levels in women with PCOS and found an association between low SHBG levels and subsequent development of gestational diabetes mellitus.

▪ Anovulation

The precise mechanism leading to anovulation is unclear. First, altered GnRH pulsatility and inappropriate gonadotropin secretion are implicated in menstrual irregularity.

Moreover, anovulation may result from insulin resistance, as a substantial number of anovulatory patients with PCOS may resume ovulatory cycles when treated with metformin, an insulin sensitizer (Nestler, 1998). It has been suggested that oligoovulatory women with PCOS exhibit a milder phenotype of ovarian dysfunction than anovulatory PCOS patients and have a more favorable response to ovulation induction agents (Burgers, 2010).

Last, the large antral follicle cohort and associated higher intraovarian androgen levels seen in PCOS may contribute to anovulation. This is supported by the fact that some patients who have undergone ovarian wedge resection or laparoscopic ovarian drilling have improved menstrual regularity. One study demonstrated that 67 percent of PCOS patients developed regular menses following such surgery compared with only 8 percent prior to surgery (Amer, 2002).

SIGNS AND SYMPTOMS

In women with PCOS, symptoms may include menstrual irregularities, infertility, manifestations of androgen excess, or other endocrine dysfunction. Symptoms classically become apparent within a few years of puberty.

■ Menstrual Dysfunction

In women with PCOS, menstrual dysfunction may range from amenorrhea to oligomenorrhea to episodic heavy menstrual bleeding with associated iron-deficiency anemia. In most cases, amenorrhea and oligomenorrhea result from anovulation. Namely, without ovulation and endogenous progesterone production from the corpus luteum, a normal menstrual period is not triggered.

Instead, chronic estrogen exposure results and produces constant mitogenic stimulation of the endometrium. The instability of the thickened endometrium leads to unpredictable bleeding.

Oligomenorrhea (fewer than nine menstrual periods in 1 year) or amenorrhea (absence of menses for 3 or more consecutive months) with PCOS usually begins with menarche (American Society for Reproductive Medicine, 2008). Those with PCOS fail to establish monthly ovulatory menstrual cycles

by midadolescence, and they often continue to have irregularity. Notably, many postmenarchal girls have irregular periods because of hypothalamic-pituitary-ovarian axis immaturity. However, lack of menarche by age 15 years or within 3 years of thelarche merits evaluation for delayed puberty (Chap. 15, p. 331) (American College of Obstetricians and Gynecologists, 2017). Factoring clinical context, menstrual intervals <20 days or >45 days in girls ≥2 years after menarche or menstrual interval >90 days any time after menarche merits consideration of further evaluation (Witchel, 2015).

As women with PCOS age, those with prior irregular cycle intervals may develop regular cycle patterns. A decreasing antral follicle cohort as women enter their 30s and 40s may lead to a concurrent decrease in androgen production (Elting, 2000).

Last, amenorrhea can stem from elevated androgen levels. Specifically, androgens can counteract estrogen to produce an atrophic endometrium. Thus, with markedly elevated androgen levels, amenorrhea and a thin endometrial stripe can be seen.

■ Hyperandrogenism

This condition is usually manifested clinically by hirsutism, acne, and/or androgenic alopecia. In contrast, signs of virilization such as increased muscle mass, voice deepening, and clitoromegaly are not typical of PCOS. Virilization reflects higher androgen levels and should prompt investigation for an androgen-producing tumor of the ovary or adrenal gland.

Hirsutism

In a female, hirsutism is defined as coarse, dark, terminal hairs distributed in a male pattern (Fig. 18-2). This is distinguished from hypertrichosis, which is a generalized increase in lanugo, that is, the soft, lightly pigmented hair associated with some medications and malignancies. PCOS accounts for 70 to 80 percent of cases of hirsutism, which typically begins in late adolescence or the early 20s. Idiopathic hirsutism is the second most frequent cause (Azziz, 2003). Additionally, various drugs may lead to hirsutism, and their use should be investigated (Table 18-3).

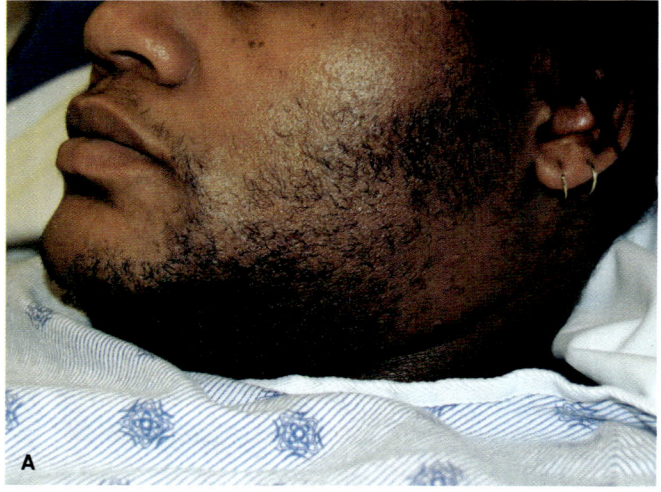
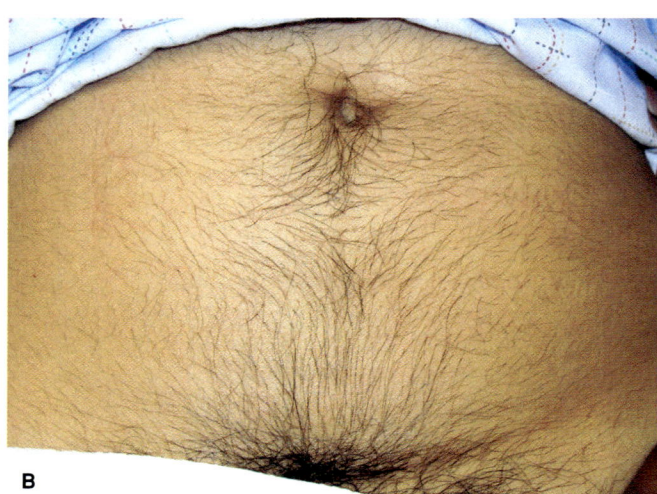

FIGURE 18-2 A. Facial hirsutism. (Reproduced with permission from Dr. Tamara Chao.) **B.** Male pattern escutcheon.

TABLE 18-3. Medications That May Cause Hirsutism and/or Hypertrichosis

Hirsutism	Hypertrichosis
Anabolic steroids	Cyclosporine
Danazol	Diazoxide
Metoclopramide	Hydrocortisone
Methyldopa	Minoxidil
Phenothiazines	Penicillamine
Progestins	Phenytoin
Reserpine	Psoralens
Testosterone	Streptomycin

Pathophysiology of Hirsutism. Elevated androgen levels play a major role in determining the type and distribution of hair. Within a hair follicle, testosterone is converted by the enzyme 5α-reductase to dihydrotestosterone (DHT) (Fig. 18-3). Although both testosterone and DHT convert short, soft vellus hair to coarse terminal hair, DHT is markedly more effective than testosterone. Conversion is irreversible, and only hairs in androgen-sensitive areas are changed in this manner to terminal hairs. As a result the most common areas affected with excess hair growth include the upper lip, chin, sideburns, chest, and

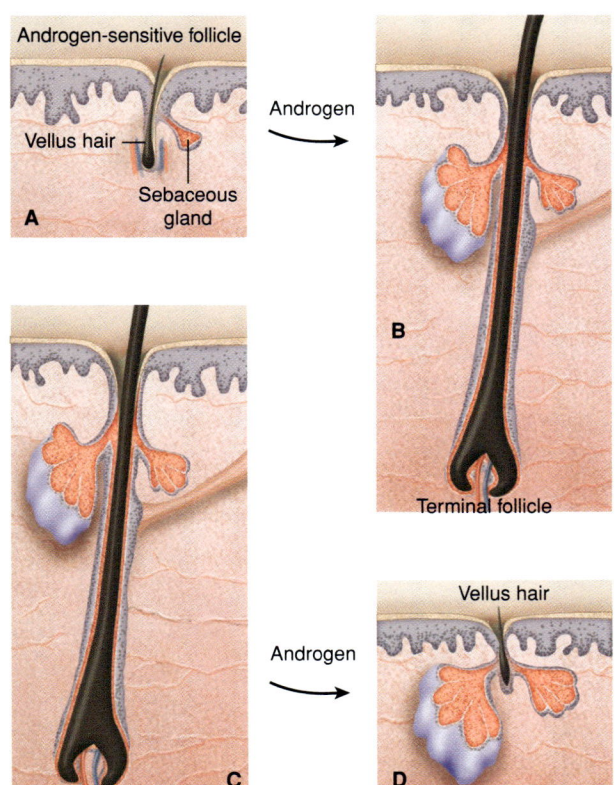

FIGURE 18-3 Androgenic effects on the pilosebaceous unit. In some hair-bearing areas, androgens stimulate sebaceous glands, and vellus follicles **(A)** are converted to terminal follicles **(B)**, leading to hirsutism. Under the influence of androgens, terminal hairs that were not previously dependent on androgens **(C)** revert to a vellus form and balding results **(D)**.

linea alba of the lower abdomen. Specifically, *escutcheon* is the term used to describe the hair pattern of the lower abdomen. In unaffected women, this pattern is triangular and overlies the mons pubis, whereas in men it extends up the linea alba to form a diamond shape.

The concentration of hair follicles per unit area does not differ between men and women, however, racial and ethnic differences do exist. Individuals of Mediterranean descent have a higher concentration of hair follicles than Northern Europeans, and a much higher concentration than Asians. For this reason, Asians with PCOS are much less likely to present with overt hirsutism than other ethnic groups. Additionally, the familial tendency for hirsutism development is strong and stems from genetic differences in 5α-reductase activity and in target tissue sensitivity to androgens.

Ferriman-Gallwey Scoring System. To quantify the degree of hirsutism for research purposes, the Ferriman-Gallwey scoring system was developed in 1961 and later modified in 1981 (Ferriman, 1961; Hatch, 1981). Within this system, abnormal hair distribution is assessed in nine body areas and scored from 0 to 4 (Fig. 18-4). Increasing numeric scores correspond to greater hair density within a given area. Many investigators define hirsutism as a score ≥4 to 6 using the modified scoring (Teede, 2019). Because of the lower follicle concentration in Far East Asians, the AE-PCOS Society suggests a threshold value ≥3 for this group (Escobar-Morreale, 2012).

The Ferriman-Gallwey scoring system is cumbersome and thus is not used frequently in clinical settings. Nevertheless, it may be useful for following treatment responses in individual patients. Alternatively, an abbreviated score that combines only the upper and lower abdomen and chin scores may be a suitable surrogate (Cook, 2011). Also, many specialists choose to classify hirsutism more generally as mild, moderate, or severe depending on the location and density of hair growth.

Acne

Mild to moderate acne vulgaris is a frequent clinical finding in adolescents. However, acne that is persistent, moderate to severe, or late onset raises concern for PCOS or other androgen excess source (Homburg, 2004; Witchel, 2015). The prevalence of acne in women with PCOS is unknown, although one study found that 50 percent of adolescents with PCOS have moderate acne (Dramusic, 1997). In addition, androgen level elevation has been reported in 80 percent of women with severe acne, 50 percent with moderate acne, and 33 percent with mild acne (Bunker, 1989). Women with moderate to severe acne have an increased prevalence (52 to 83 percent) of polycystic ovaries identified during sonographic examination (Betti, 1990; Bunker, 1989).

The pathogenesis of acne vulgaris involves four factors: blockage of the follicular opening by hyperkeratosis, sebum overproduction, proliferation of commensal *Propionibacterium acnes*, and inflammation. As in the hair follicle, testosterone is converted within sebaceous glands to its more active metabolite, DHT, by 5α-reductase. In women with androgen excess, overstimulation of androgen receptors in the pilosebaceous unit elevates sebum production that eventually leads to inflammation

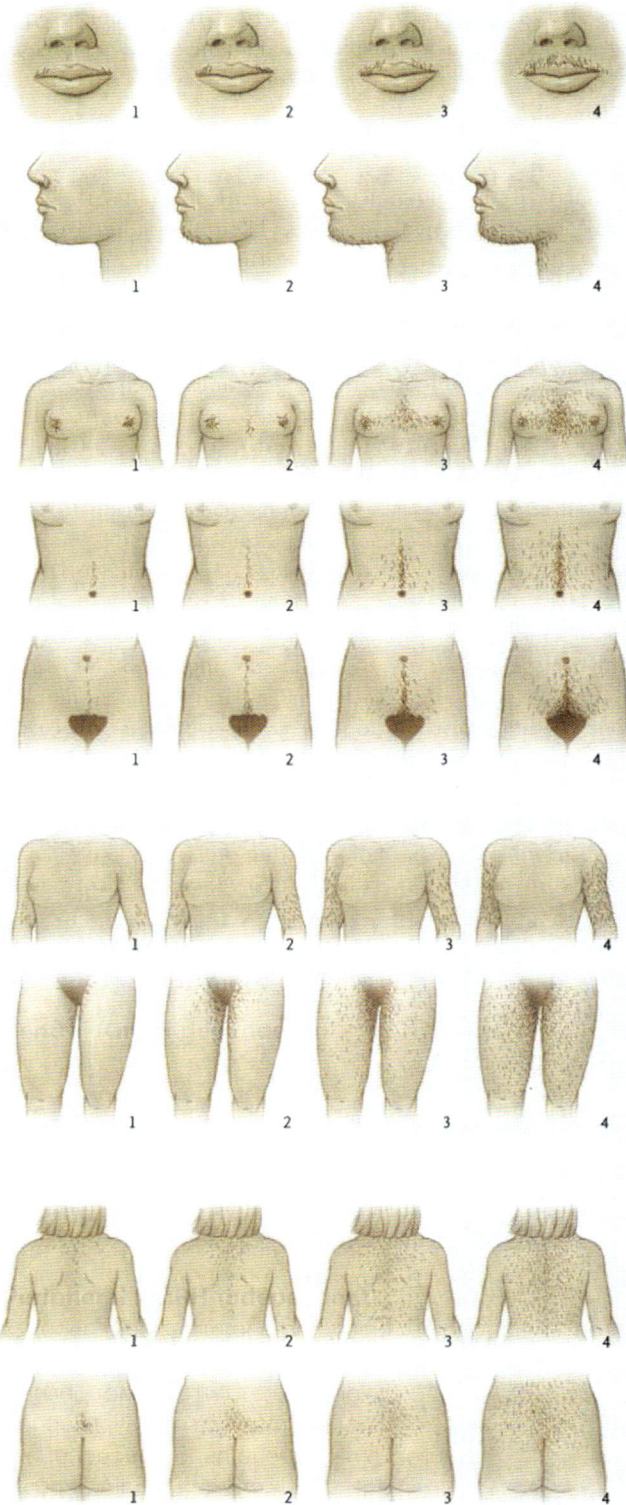

FIGURE 18-4 Depiction of the Ferriman-Gallwey system for scoring hirsutism.

and comedone formation (see Fig. 18-3). Inflammation leads to the main long-term side effect of acne—scarring. Accordingly, treatment is directed at minimizing inflammation, decreasing keratin production, lowering colonization of *P acnes*, and reducing androgen levels to diminish sebum production.

Alopecia

Female androgenic alopecia is a less common finding in women with PCOS. Hair slowly thins diffusely at the crown, but the frontal hairline is preserved (Quinn, 2014). Of the several available scoring methods, the three-grade Ludwig visual score is a recommended (Teede, 2019). The perceptible thinning of grade I progressively worsens to total balding of the crown in grade III (Gupta, 2016).

Alopecia pathogenesis involves an excess of 5α-reductase activity in the hair follicle leading to a rise in DHT levels. Moreover, androgen receptor expression in these individuals is increased (Chen, 2002). Alopecia, however, may reflect other serious disease. For this reason, affected women are also evaluated to exclude thyroid dysfunction, anemia, or other chronic illness (Levy, 2013).

■ Other Endocrine Dysfunction

Insulin Resistance

The precise incidence of insulin resistance in women with PCOS has been difficult to ascertain for lack of a simple method to determine insulin sensitivity in an office setting. Although obesity is known to exacerbate insulin resistance, one classic study demonstrated that both lean and obese women with PCOS have higher rates of insulin resistance and type 2 DM compared with weight-matched controls without PCOS (Fig. 18-5) (Dunaif, 1989, 1992).

Acanthosis Nigricans. In this skin condition, thick, gray-brown velvety plaques develop in flexure areas such as the back of the neck, axillae, inframammary creases, waist, and groin (Fig. 18-6) (Panidis, 1995). Thought to be a cutaneous marker of insulin resistance, acanthosis nigricans may be found in individuals with or without PCOS. Insulin resistance leads to hyperinsulinemia, which is believed to stimulate keratinocyte and dermal fibroblast growth, producing the characteristic skin changes (Cruz, 1992). Indeed, in one cohort of 237 women with PCOS, acanthosis nigricans was found in 70 percent of those with the metabolic syndrome and in 45 percent without metabolic syndrome (Kazemi, 2019). In another study of women with PCOS, the rate of acanthosis nigricans in obese

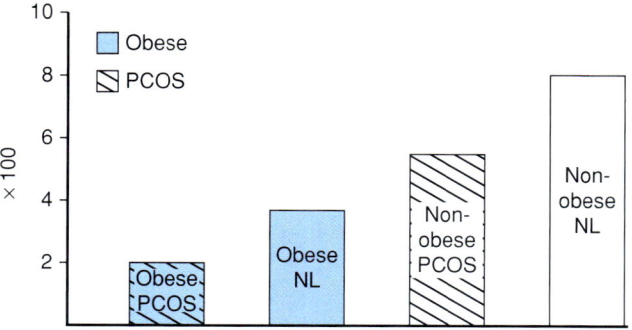

FIGURE 18-5 Insulin sensitivity is decreased in obese women with polycystic ovarian syndrome. NL = normal (those without PCOS); PCOS = polycystic ovarian syndrome. (From Dunaif, 1989, with permission.)

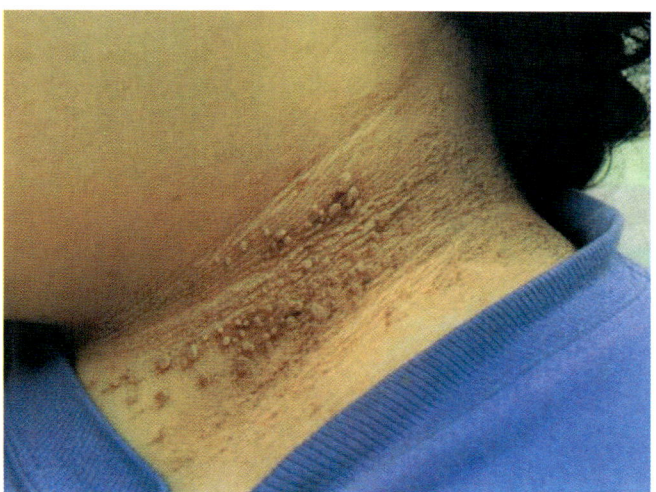

FIGURE 18-6 Acanthosis nigricans and multiple small pedunculated acrochordons (skin tags) in the neck crease. Both are dermatologic signs of insulin resistance.

woman was more than twice the rate in normal-weight women (Reyes-Muñoz, 2016).

Rarely, it is seen with genetic syndromes or gastrointestinal tract malignancy, such as adenocarcinoma of the stomach or pancreas. To differentiate, acanthosis nigricans associated with malignancy usually has a more abrupt onset, and skin involvement is more extensive (Moore, 2008).

Optimal treatment for acanthosis nigricans is directed toward decreasing insulin resistance and hyperinsulinemia. Topical retinoids are a first-line adjunct option (Patel, 2018).

Impaired Glucose Tolerance and Type 2 Diabetes Mellitus.

Women with PCOS are at increased risk for impaired glucose tolerance (IGT) and type 2 DM. Based on oral glucose tolerance testing of obese women with PCOS, the prevalence of IGT and DM approximates 30 percent and 7 percent, respectively (Legro, 1999). Even after adjusting for body mass index (BMI), women with PCOS remained more likely to have DM (Lo, 2006). Specifically, β-cell dysfunction that is independent of obesity has been reported in patients with PCOS (Dunaif, 1996). Similar findings are reported in groups of obese and normal-weight adolescent girls with PCOS (Flannery, 2013; Palmert, 2002).

Dyslipidemia

The classic atherogenic lipoprotein profile seen in PCOS shows increased low-density lipoprotein (LDL) and triglyceride levels, elevated total cholesterol:high-density lipoprotein (HDL) ratios, but depressed HDL levels (Banaszewska, 2006; Wild, 2011). Independent of total cholesterol levels, these changes may raise the cardiovascular disease risk in women with PCOS. The prevalence of dyslipidemia in PCOS approaches 70 percent (Legro, 2001; Talbott, 1998).

Obesity

Compared with age-matched controls, women with PCOS are more likely to be obese, as reflected by elevated BMIs

and waist:hip ratios (Talbott, 1995). This ratio reflects an android or central pattern of obesity, which itself is an independent risk factor for CVD and predicts insulin resistance. As noted earlier, insulin resistance is believed to play a large role in the pathogenesis of PCOS and is often exacerbated by obesity (Dunaif, 1989). For example, obesity can exacerbate hyperandrogenism by lowering SHBG levels and thereby raise bioavailable testosterone levels (Lim, 2013). Thus, obesity can have a synergistic effect on PCOS and can worsen ovulatory dysfunction, hyperandrogenism, and acanthosis nigricans.

■ Obstructive Sleep Apnea

In the general population, obstructive sleep apnea is related to central obesity (Peppard, 2000; Senaratna, 2017). Of women with PCOS, 35 percent had obstructive sleep apnea in one metaanalysis, especially obese women with PCOS (Kahal, 2019). However, some evidence suggests that some PCOS metabolic changes also may be contributory (Gopal, 2002; Tasali, 2008; Vgontzas, 2001). For example, women with PCOS have significantly higher risk of sleep apnea compared with weight-matched controls (Fogel, 2001).

■ Metabolic Syndrome and Cardiovascular Disease

The metabolic syndrome is characterized by insulin resistance, obesity, atherogenic dyslipidemia, and hypertension. It is associated with a greater risk of CVD and type 2 DM (Schneider, 2006). The prevalence of metabolic syndrome approximates 45 percent in women with PCOS compared with 4 percent in age-adjusted controls (Fig. 18-7) (Dokras, 2005). PCOS shares several endocrine features with the metabolic syndrome, although definitive evidence for an increased incidence of CVD in women with PCOS is lacking (Legro, 1999; Rebuffe-Scrive, 1989; Talbott, 1998). However, in a small group of women with PCOS, Dahlgren and colleagues (1992) predicted a relative risk of 7.4 for myocardial infarction. Another 10-year surveillance study showed an odds ratio of 6 for CVD in overweight white women with PCOS (Talbott, 1995). Thus, evidence suggests that women with PCOS should have CVD factors identified and treated (Table 1-10, p. 16) (Goodman, 2015; Teede, 2019).

■ Endometrial Neoplasia

In women with PCOS, the risk of endometrial cancer is increased three- to fourfold (Barry, 2014; Haoula, 2012; Gottschau, 2015). Endometrial hyperplasia and endometrial cancer are long-term risks of chronic anovulation, and neoplastic changes in the endometrium are felt to arise from chronic unopposed estrogen (Chap. 33, p. 699). Moreover, the effects of hyperandrogenism, hyperinsulinemia, and obesity to lower SHBG levels and raise circulating estrogen levels may add to this risk.

Few women who develop endometrial cancer are younger than 40 years, and most of these premenopausal women are

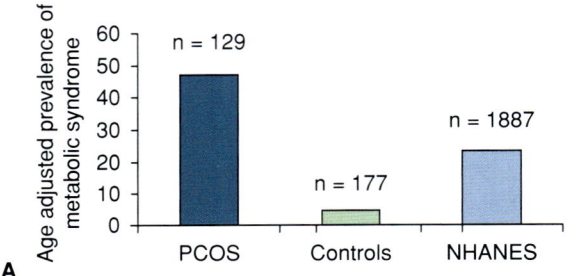

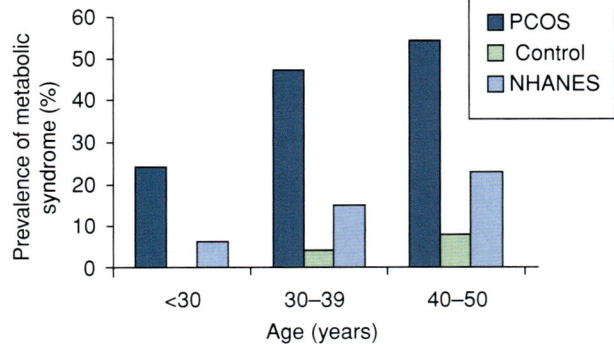

FIGURE 18-7 A. Women with polycystic ovarian syndrome (PCOS) have an increased risk of metabolic syndrome compared with age-adjusted controls and with women from the Third National Health and Nutrition Survey (NHANES III). **B.** In women with PCOS, the risk of metabolic syndrome begins earlier than in controls or those from NHANES III. NHANES III collected data from a representative sample of the noninstitutionalized civilian U.S. population from 1988 through 1994. (From Dokras, 2005, with permission.)

obese or have chronic anovulation or both (National Cancer Institute, 2019). Thus, the American College of Obstetricians and Gynecologists (2016) recommends endometrial assessment in any woman older than 45 years with abnormal uterine bleeding. In addition, those younger than 45 years with a history of unopposed estrogen exposure such as seen in obesity or PCOS, those with failed medical management, and women with persistent bleeding are ideally sampled. Steps of this procedure are found in Chapter 8 (p. 183).

■ Infertility

Infertility or subfertility is a frequent complaint in women with PCOS and results from anovulatory cycles. Moreover, in women with infertility secondary to anovulation, PCOS is a common cause. Infertility evaluation and treatment in PCOS-affected women is described in more detail in Chapter 21 (p. 453).

■ Complications in Pregnancy

Women with PCOS who become pregnant experience a higher rate (30 to 50 percent) of early miscarriage compared with a baseline rate of approximately 15 percent in the general population (Homburg, 1998; Regan, 1990; Sagle, 1988). The etiology of early miscarriage in women with PCOS is unclear. Obesity, which is commonly comorbid with PCOS, is implicated. For example, in one large longitudinal study, overweight and obese

women with PCOS suffered higher miscarriage rates, whereas a normal-weight group with PCOS did not (Joham, 2014a). Others have suggested that insulin resistance is related to miscarriage in women with PCOS. In response to this, metformin (Glucophage), an insulin level–lowering drug, has been investigated. However, a metaanalysis of 17 studies failed to show an effect of metformin administration on miscarriage risk in women with PCOS (Palomba, 2009).

Of other pregnancy complications, higher risks of gestational diabetes, pregnancy-induced hypertension, and preterm birth have been noted (Bahri Khomami, 2019; Naver, 2014; Palomba, 2015). Gestational diabetes risk persists independently of weight but is enhanced by greater BMI (Joham, 2014b). Metformin has been studied as a tool to mitigate these complications in those with PCOS but without DM. However, investigators in one study found that metformin treatment during pregnancy did not reduce rates of these complications (Vanky, 2010).

Many women with PCOS require the use of ovulation induction medications or in vitro fertilization to conceive. These practices substantially raise the risk of multifetal gestations, which are associated with elevated rates of maternal and neonatal complications (Chap. 21, p. 457).

■ Psychologic Health

Women with PCOS may present with various psychosocial problems such as anxiety, depression, eating disorders, and negative body image (Deeks, 2011; Dokras, 2011, 2012; Lee, 2017). For those diagnosed with PCOS, screening for depression and anxiety is recommended (Dokras, 2018; Teede, 2019). Screening tools are found in Chapter 14 (p. 303). Similarly, if an eating disorder is suspected, an initial screen is recommended.

DIAGNOSIS

Other potentially serious disorders may clinically appear similar to PCOS and are excluded during patient evaluation (Table 18-4). For women who present with complaints of hirsutism, the algorithm in Figure 18-8 can be used.

■ Thyroid-Stimulating Hormone and Prolactin

Thyroid disease may frequently lead to menstrual dysfunction. Thus, a serum thyroid-stimulating hormone level is typically measured during evaluation, and treatment is discussed in Chapter 17 (p. 381). Similarly, hyperprolactinemia is a well-known cause of menstrual irregularities and occasionally amenorrhea. Elevated prolactin levels lead to anovulation through inhibition of GnRH pulsatile secretion. A list of potential causes of hyperprolactinemia is found in Table 13-2 (p. 285), and treatments are described in Chapter 16 (p. 362).

■ Testosterone and Dehydroepiandrosterone Sulfate

Tumors of the ovary or adrenal are a rare but serious cause of androgen excess. Various ovarian neoplasms, both benign and malignant, may produce testosterone and lead to virilization.

TABLE 18-4. Differential Diagnoses of Ovulatory Dysfunction and Hyperandrogenism

	Evaluation	Indicative Results[a]
Causes of oligo- or anovulation		
PCOS	Total T level	Mildly increased
	DHEAS level	May be mildly increased
	LH:FSH ratio	Typically >2:1
	AMH level	Increased
Hyperthyroidism	TSH level	Decreased
Hypothyroidism	TSH level	Increased
Hyperprolactinemia	PRL level	Increased
Hypogonadotropic hypogonadism	FSH, LH, E_2 levels	All decreased
POI	FSH, LH levels	Increased
	E_2 levels	Decreased
Causes of hyperandrogenism		
PCOS		
Late-onset CAH	17-OHP level	>200 ng/dL
Androgen-secreting ovarian tumor	Total T level	>200 ng/dL
Androgen-secreting adrenal tumor	DHEAS level	>700 µg/dL
Cushing syndrome	Cortisol level	Increased
Exogenous androgen use	Toxicology screen	Increased

Summary of PCOS testing
Serum levels of FSH, LH, TSH, Total T, free T, estradiol, PRL,17-OH-P, DHEAS, 2-hr GTT, HbA_{1C}, lipid profile
Measurement of BMI, waist circumference, BP

[a]Based on reference laboratory ranges of normal.
AMH = antimüllerian hormone; BMI = body mass index; BP = blood pressure; CAH = congenital adrenal hyperplasia; DHEAS = dehydroepiandrosterone sulfate; E_2 = estradiol; FSH = follicle-stimulating hormone; GTT = glucose tolerance test; LH = luteinizing hormone; 17-OHP = 17-hydroxyprogesterone; PCOS = polycystic ovarian syndrome; POI = premature ovarian insufficiency; PRL = prolactin; T = testosterone; TSH = thyroid-stimulating hormone.

Among others, these include the stromal tumors (Chap. 36, p. 764). Importantly, an abrupt onset or sudden worsening of virilizing signs should prompt concern for a hormone-producing ovarian or adrenal tumor (Fig. 18-9). Symptoms may include those in Table 18-5. Of these, hirsutism is quantified with the Ferriman-Gallwey score, whereas clitoromegaly is assessed using the clitoral index. For the latter, clitoral length (mm) and width (mm) values are multiplied. Values greater than 35 mm^2 are abnormal (Tagatz, 1979; Verkauf, 1992).

Diagnostically, serum testosterone levels can aid ovarian tumor exclusion. Free testosterone levels are more sensitive than total testosterone levels as an indicator of hyperandrogenism. Although improving, however, current free testosterone assays lack a uniform laboratory standard. For this reason, total testosterone levels remain the best approach for identifying a possible tumor. Threshold values >200 ng/dL of total testosterone warrant evaluation for an ovarian lesion (Derksen, 1994).

Pelvic sonography is the preferred method to exclude an ovarian neoplasm in a female with very high androgen levels. Alternatively, computed tomography (CT) or magnetic resonance (MR) imaging also may be used.

DHEAS is essentially produced exclusively by the adrenal gland. Therefore, serum DHEAS levels >700 µg/dL are highly suggestive of an adrenal neoplasm, and adrenal imaging with abdominal CT or MR imaging is warranted.

■ Gonadotropins

During evaluation of amenorrhea, FSH, LH, and estradiol levels are typically measured to exclude premature ovarian insufficiency and hypogonadotropic hypogonadism (see Table 18-4). Although classically LH levels measure at least twofold higher than FSH levels, this is not found in all women with PCOS. Specifically, one third of women with PCOS have circulating LH levels in the normal range, a finding more common in obese patients (Arroyo, 1997; Taylor, 1997). Moreover, serum LH levels are affected by sample timing within a menstrual cycle, use of oral contraceptive pills, and BMI.

TABLE 18-5. Clinical Features of Virilization

Acne	Androgenic alopecia
Hirsutism	Decreased breast size
Amenorrhea	Deepening of the voice
Clitoromegaly	Increased muscle mass

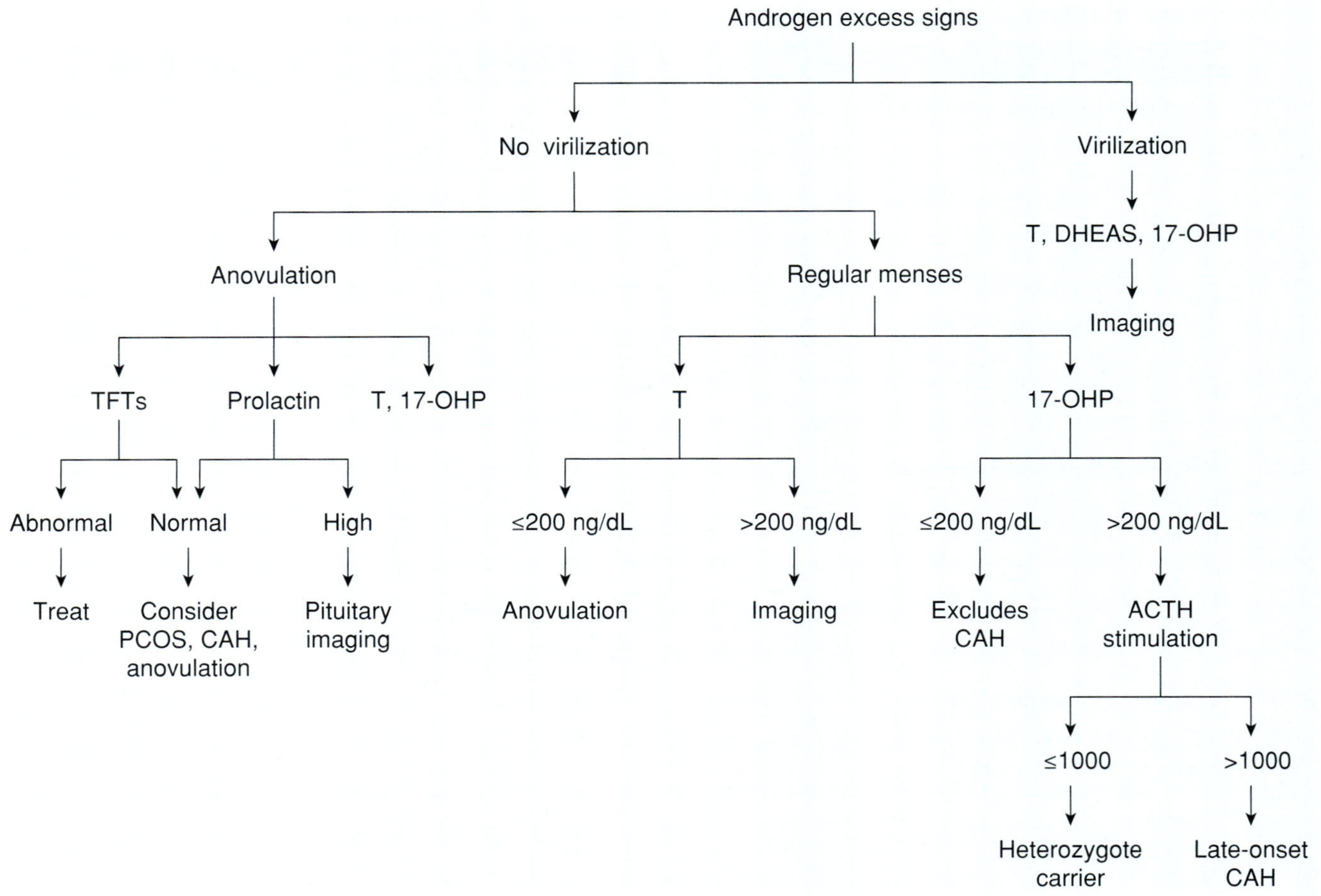

Androgen excess signs

No virilization   Virilization

Virilization → T, DHEAS, 17-OHP → Imaging

No virilization:

Anovulation   Regular menses

Anovulation:
- TFTs
- Prolactin
- T, 17-OHP

TFTs → Abnormal → Treat

TFTs → Normal → Consider PCOS, CAH, anovulation

Prolactin → Normal / High

High → Pituitary imaging

Regular menses:
- T → ≤200 ng/dL → Anovulation
- T → >200 ng/dL → Imaging

17-OHP (Virilization pathway):
- ≤200 ng/dL → Excludes CAH
- >200 ng/dL → ACTH stimulation
  - ≤1000 → Heterozygote carrier
  - >1000 → Late-onset CAH

FIGURE 18-8 Algorithm for evaluation of androgen excess. 17-OHP = 17-hydroxyprogesterone; ACTH = adrenocorticotropin hormone; CAH = congenital adrenal hyperplasia; DHEAS = dehydroepiandrosterone sulfate; PCOS = polycystic ovarian syndrome; T = testosterone; TFTs = thyroid function tests.

17-Alpha Hydroxyprogesterone

The term congenital adrenal hyperplasia (CAH) describes several autosomal recessive disorders that result from complete or partial deficiency of an enzyme involved in cortisol and aldosterone synthesis, usually 21-hydroxylase or less frequently 11-hydroxylase (Fig. 16-5, p. 339). As a result of these defects, precursors are shunted into pathways leading to androgen production. Thus, depending on the enzyme affected, CAH symptoms vary. It may present in the neonate with ambiguous genitalia and life-threatening hypotension (Chap. 19, p. 415).

Alternatively, symptoms may be milder and delayed until adolescence or adulthood. In this late-onset form of CAH, the enzyme deficiency leads to a relative cortisol deficiency. In response, adrenocorticotropic hormone (ACTH) levels rise to normalize cortisol production. Consequent to this accommodation, adrenal gland hyperplasia and elevated androgen levels develop. Therefore, symptoms of late-onset CAH reflect accumulation of precursor C_{19} steroid hormones. These precursors are converted to dehydroepiandrosterone, androstenedione, and testosterone. Thus, signs of hyperandrogenism predominate.

With late-onset CAH, the most commonly affected enzyme is 21-hydroxylase, and deficiency leads to accumulation of its substrate, 17-hydroxyprogesterone. Serum values are drawn in the morning from a fasting patient. Threshold values of 17-hydroxyprogesterone that measure >200 ng/dL should prompt an ACTH stimulation test. With this test, synthetic ACTH, 250 µg, is injected intravenously, and a serum 17-hydroxyprogesterone level is measured 1 hour later.

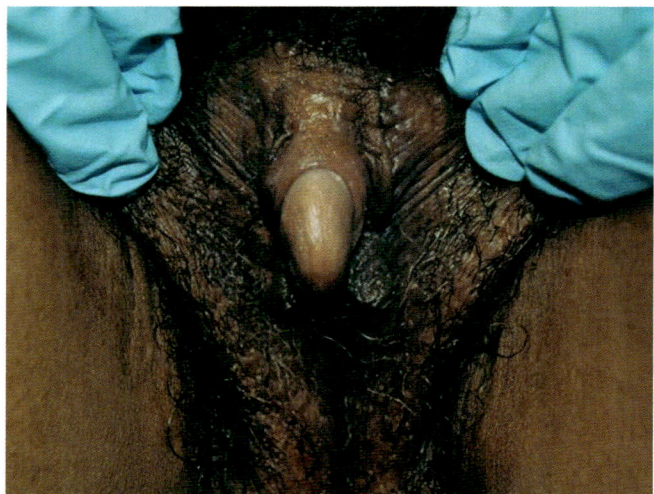

FIGURE 18-9 Woman with virilization manifest by clitoromegaly. (From Kiszka, 2019, with permission.)

To explain this test, the ACTH given during testing stimulates uptake of cholesterol and synthesis of pregnenolone. If 21-hydroxylase activity is ineffective, steroid precursors up to and including progesterone, 17-hydroxypregnenolone, and especially 17-hydroxyprogesterone accumulate in the adrenal cortex and in circulating blood. In affected individuals, serum levels of 17-hydroxyprogesterone can reach many times their normal concentrations. Levels >1000 ng/dL from blood drawn after synthetic ACTH is given are indicative of late-onset CAH.

Antimüllerian Hormone

The classic polycystic ovary contains two- to threefold more growing preantral and antral follicles than normal ovaries (Hughesdon, 1982). Within the granulosa cells of these developing follicles, the dimeric glycoprotein antimüllerian hormone (AMH) is produced. Serum AMH levels correlate closely with the number of preantral and antral follicles. Not surprisingly, AMH levels are two- to threefold higher in women with PCOS compared with nonaffected age-matched controls (Cui, 2014: Homburg, 2013). For this reason, some view AMH as a potentially useful diagnostic marker for PCOS (Iliodromiti, 2013; Pigny, 2006). That said, data regarding this marker in both PCOS and controls are incomplete and require further investigation before it can be adopted as a formal diagnostic criterion (Dewailly, 2014a; Teede, 2019).

Cortisol

Cushing syndrome results from prolonged exposure to elevated levels of either endogenous or exogenous glucocorticoids. Of these, the syndrome is most frequently caused by administration of exogenous glucocorticoids. Alternatively, the term *Cushing disease* is reserved for cases stemming from greater ACTH secretion by a pituitary tumor. Cushing syndrome shares many symptoms with PCOS such as menstrual dysfunction, physical signs of androgen excess, truncal obesity, dyslipidemia, and glucose intolerance. Classically, moon facies and purple abdominal striae also are noted. Excluding exogenous causes, Cushing syndrome is rare, and routine screening in all women with oligomenorrhea is not indicated. However, in those with classic Cushing findings, proximal muscle weakness, and easy bruising, screening is strongly considered (Nieman, 2008).

Initial laboratory testing investigates excessive glucocorticoid production, and three are endorsed by the Endocrine Society (Nieman, 2008). Of these, a 24-hour urine collection for urinary free cortisol excretion can be obtained. Alternatively, a dexamethasone suppression test administers 1 mg of dexamethasone orally at 11 PM, and a plasma cortisol level is measured at 8 AM the following morning. In women with a normal functioning feedback loop, administration of the corticosteroid dexamethasone lowers ACTH secretion and thus diminishes adrenal cortisol production. Normal testing values are <5 μg/dL (Crapo, 1979). However, if a woman has an exogenous or an ectopic endogenous source of cortisol, then cortisol levels during suppression testing will remain elevated. Last, using a late-night salivary cortisol level measurement, patients collect saliva samples between 11 PM and midnight on two separate evenings. Once identified, Cushing syndrome is treated based on the underlying source of excess glucocorticosteroid.

Measurements of Insulin Resistance and Dyslipidemia

Many women with PCOS have insulin resistance and compensatory hyperinsulinemia. The "gold standard" for evaluating insulin resistance has been the hyperinsulinemic euglycemic clamp. Unfortunately, this test and the intravenous glucose tolerance test (IV GTT) require an intravenous line and frequent sampling, are labor and time intensive, and are not practical in a clinical setting. Accordingly, other less sensitive surrogate markers that evaluate insulin resistance are used. These include: (1) a 2-hour oral glucose tolerance test (2-hr OGTT), (2) a fasting serum insulin level, (3) the homeostasis model assessment of insulin resistance (HOMA IR), (4) the quantitative insulin sensitivity check (QUICKI), and (5) calculation of serum glucose:insulin ratios.

Several organizations recommend initial DM screening and then periodic testing in obese or overweight women and adolescents diagnosed with PCOS (American Diabetes Association, 2019; Goodman, 2015; Witchel, 2015). Normal and abnormal testing level thresholds are found in Table 1-15 (p. 18). Guidelines endorsed by ESHRE and ASRM promote baseline DM screening for *all* women with PCOS and subsequent testing at 1- to 3-year intervals based on risks. Serum fasting glucose level, hemoglobin A_{1C} (HbA$_{1C}$) level, or 2-hr OGTT is suitable. Of these, 2-hr OGTT is favored for higher-risk characteristics, which are obesity (BMI >25 kg/m^2 or >23 in Asian women), a personal history of IGT or hypertension, Asian ethnicity, and family history of type 2 DM (Teede, 2019). Women with PCOS can demonstrate a worsening of glucose tolerance over time, with a reported conversion rate of approximately 2 percent per year to type 2 DM. This affirms the importance of periodic assessment of glucose tolerance with a 2-hr OGTT in women with PCOS (Legro, 1999, 2005).

In addition to assessment of insulin resistance, in overweight and obese women with PCOS, a fasting lipid profile is recommended to evaluate dyslipidemia (Teede, 2019). Subsequent testing is based on global CVD risk. Others support initial lipid screening for *all* women with PCOS (American College of Obstetricians and Gynecologists, 2018; Wild, 2011). Evaluation and treatment of dyslipidemia are further described in Chapter 1 (p. 17).

Sonography

Histologically, a polycystic ovary displays a greater number of ripening and atretic follicles, cortical stromal thickness, and number of hilar cell nests (Hughesdon, 1982). Many of these tissue changes can be seen sonographically, and pelvic sonography is commonly used to evaluate the ovaries in women with suspected PCOS. Moreover, sonography is particularly important for women with PCOS seeking fertility and in women with signs of virilization to exclude an androgen-producing ovarian cancer.

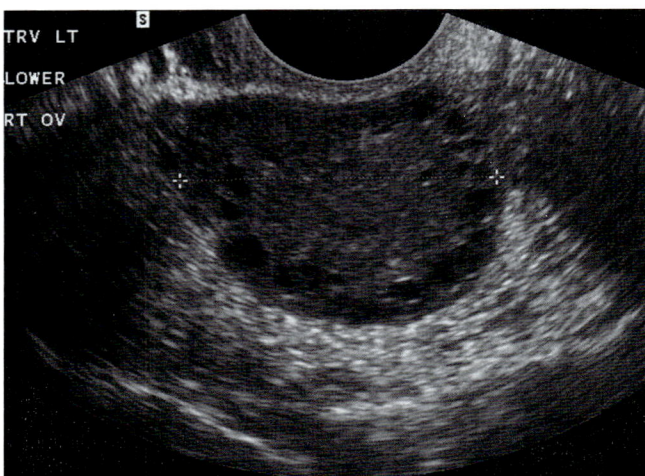

FIGURE 18-10 Transvaginal sonography displays multiple small hypoechoic cysts. (Reproduced with permission from Dr. Elysia Moschos.)

Polycystic ovarian morphology (PCOM) is one criterion for PCOS diagnosis (see Table 18-1). Earlier sonographic criteria for PCOM included ≥12 small cysts (2 to 9 mm in diameter) or an increased ovarian volume (>10 mL) or both per ovary (Fig. 18-10). More recently, follicle number per ovary (FNPO) threshold values have been raised due to improved sonographic imaging resolution (Dewailly, 2011; Lujan, 2013). Namely, an FNPO threshold of >20 follicles and/or ovarian volume >10 mL in either ovary has been adopted by ESHRE and ASRM. The AE-PCOS guidelines use the same ovarian volume value but a higher FNPO threshold of ≥25 follicles (Dewailly, 2014b). Notably, criteria do not apply to women taking combination oral contraceptive pills.

Remarkably, studies using sonography have shown that at least 23 percent of young women have ovaries that exhibit PCOM, yet many of these women have no other PCOS symptoms (Clayton, 1992; Polson, 1988). In addition, a polycystic appearance of the ovaries can often be found in other conditions of androgen excess, such as CAH, Cushing syndrome, and exogenous use of androgenic medications. For this reason, PCOM found during sonographic examination is not used solely for PCOS diagnosis.

Importantly, PCOM often reflects normal adolescent ovarian physiology (Hickey, 2011; Kristensen, 2010). Thus, sonography for PCOS evaluation is not recommended within 8 years of menarche (Teede, 2019).

TREATMENT

The treatment choice for each symptom of PCOS depends on a woman's goals and the severity of endocrine dysfunction. Thus, anovulatory women desiring pregnancy will undergo significantly different treatment than adolescents with menstrual irregularity and acne. Patients often seek treatment for a singular complaint and may see various specialists such as dermatologists, nutritionists, aestheticians, and endocrinologists prior to evaluation by a gynecologist.

■ Conservative Treatment

Women with PCOS who have fairly regular cycle intervals (8 to 12 menses per year) and mild hyperandrogenism may choose not to be treated. In these women, however, periodic screening for dyslipidemia, DM, and metabolic syndrome is reasonable.

For obese women with PCOS, important lifestyle changes focus on diet and exercise. Even modest weight loss (5 percent of body weight) can result in restoration of normal ovulatory cycles in some women. This improvement results from reductions in insulin and androgen levels, the latter mediated through increases in SHBG levels (Huber-Buchholz, 1999; Kiddy, 1992; Pasquali, 1989). Weight loss strategies are described in Chapter 1 (p. 14). Diet is one important element, and a well-balanced hypocaloric diet offers the most benefit in treating obese women with PCOS. Exercise improves weight, blood pressure, and fasting insulin and lipid levels in women with PCOS (Benham, 2018; Harrison, 2011; Jaatinen, 1993; Kite, 2019). Similarly in affected women, exercise improves cardiovascular capacity (Haqq, 2015; Vigorito, 2007).

■ Treatment of Oligo- and Anovulation

Hormonal Agents

Women with oligo- or anovulation typically have fewer than nine menses per year, often skip menses for several months at a time, or simply have amenorrhea. Flow may be scanty or may be prolonged and heavy, resulting in iron-deficiency anemia.

A first-line treatment for menstrual irregularities is combination oral contraceptive pills (COCs), which induce regular menstrual cycles, lower androgen levels, and thin the endometrium. Specifically, COCs suppress gonadotropin release, which results in decreased ovarian androgen production. Moreover, the estrogen component raises levels of SHBG, which binds free androgen. Last, the progestin component antagonizes the endometrial proliferative effect of unopposed estrogen from PCOS, thus reducing the endometrial hyperplasia risk.

Theoretically, COCs that contain progestins with fewer androgenic properties are preferred. However, no COC pill has shown superiority compared with another in reducing hirsutism (Sobbrio, 1990). Alternative combination hormonal contraceptive options include the contraceptive patch and vaginal ring.

In patients who are not candidates for combination hormonal contraception, progesterone withdrawal is recommended every 1 to 3 months. Examples of regimens used include: medroxyprogesterone acetate (MPA), 5 to 10 mg orally daily day for 12 days, or micronized progesterone, 200 mg orally each evening for 12 days. Patients are counseled that intermittent progestins will not reduce symptoms of acne or hirsutism, nor do they provide contraception. For those requiring birth control, a continuous progestin-only contraceptive pill, depot medroxyprogesterone acetate, or a progestin-releasing implant or intrauterine device may be used and will act to thin the endometrium.

Insulin Sensitizers

Metformin is a biguanide insulin sensitizer agent that is Food and Drug Administration (FDA) approved for glycemic control in type 2 DM. It is often used off-label for patients with PCOS to help restore cyclic menses, lower hyperandrogenism, and aid weight loss.

Importantly, for obese women with PCOS, weight loss and exercise are first-line strategies to reduce many of the short- and long-term side effects of PCOS, such as infertility, CVD, and DM. Thus, metformin is typically reserved for patients with PCOS and with IGT, elevated fasting insulin levels, and acanthosis nigricans. Some patients with a strong family history of DM also will benefit from metformin.

Side effects may include bloating, nausea, and diarrhea. Lactic acidosis is rare and typically develops in patients with impaired renal function. An initial 500-mg, extended-release form taken orally once daily with a meal can offset gastrointestinal side effects. This dose then can be increased slowly every 1 to 2 weeks to a final 1500-mg or 2000-mg daily dose, which can be divided across meals.

For anovulatory infertility, ESRE/ASRM guidelines recommend first-line treatment with letrozole or clomiphene citrate in women with PCOS (American Society for Reproductive Medicine, 2017; Teede, 2019). Metformin is a second-line agent. The addition of metformin to clomiphene citrate may be indicated for women with the constellation of PCOS, clomiphene citrate resistance, and anovulatory infertility. Metformin is a pregnancy category B drug.

The thiazolidinediones are another class of medications used in patients with DM. However, because of their potential for serious side effects and weight gain and their pregnancy category C status, this group is discouraged for PCOS.

Agonists of the glucagon-like peptide 1 (GLP-1) receptor make up another class of medications used for type 2 DM. One metaanalysis comparing GLP-1 agonists against metformin in women with PCOS found greater weight loss and insulin sensitivity in the GLP-1 agonist group (Han, 2019). This class is not recommended in pregnancy and should not be used in patients at risk for conceiving.

Another class of medications for patients with type 2 DM is the sodium-glucose cotransporter 2 (SGLT2) inhibitors. In patients with DM, weight loss and CVD risk factors benefit. In women with PCOS, weight loss with the SGLT2 empagliflozin was superior to that with metformin (Javed, 2019). It is pregnancy category C and not recommended in those at risk for pregnancy.

■ Hirsutism

With hirsutism treatment, a primary goal is lowering androgen levels to halt further conversion of vellus hairs to terminal ones. First, as described earlier, COCs are effective in establishing regular menses and lowering ovarian androgen production (p. 400). These are a first-line option in women who are candidates for COCs. However, medical therapies will not eliminate hair already present. Moreover, treatments may require 6 to 12 months before clinical improvement is apparent. For this reason, clinicians should be familiar with temporary hair removal methods that may be used in the interim.

Hair Removal

Both depilation and epilation are suitable techniques. In addition to hair removal, lightening hair color with bleach is a cosmetic option.

Depilation describes hair removal above the skin surface. Shaving is the most common form and does not exacerbate hirsutism, contrary to the myth that it will increase hair follicle density. Alternatively, topical chemical depilatories also are effective. Available in gel, cream, lotion, aerosol, and roll-on forms, these agents contain calcium thioglycolate. This agent breaks disulfide bonds between hair protein chains, causing hair to break down and separate easily from the skin surface.

Epilation removes the entire hair shaft and root and includes techniques such as plucking, waxing, threading, electrolysis, and laser treatment. Threading, also known as *khite* in Arabic, is a fast method for removing entire hairs and is commonly used in the Middle East and India. Hairs are snared within an outstretched strand of twisted cotton thread and pulled out.

Although waxing and plucking allow effective temporary hair removal, permanent epilation may be achieved with thermal destruction of the hair follicle. Electrolysis, performed by a trained individual, involves placement of a fine electrode and passage of electric current to destroy individual follicles. It requires repetitive treatments over several weeks to months, can be painful, and can result in scarring.

Alternatively, laser therapy directs specific laser wavelengths to permanently destroy follicles. During this process, termed *selective photothermolysis*, only target tissues absorb laser light and are heated. Surrounding tissues fail to absorb the selective wavelength and receive minimal thermal damage. For this reason, light-skinned women with dark hairs are better candidates for laser treatment due to the selective wavelength absorption by their hair. Advantageously, laser treatment can cover a wider surface area than electrolysis and therefore requires fewer treatments. It causes less pain, but is expensive and can result in dyspigmentation.

Prior to any epilation technique, topical anesthetics may be prescribed. Specifically, a topical cream combination of 2.5-percent lidocaine and 2.5-percent prilocaine (EMLA cream) can be applied as a thick layer that remains for 5 to 10 minutes and is removed just prior to epilation. Recommended adult dosing is 2.5 g for each 2 × 2-inch area of skin treated.

Eflornithine Hydrochloride

This antimetabolite topical cream is applied twice daily to affected areas and is an irreversible inhibitor of ornithine decarboxylase. This enzyme is necessary for hair follicle cell division and function, and its inhibition results in slower hair growth. Consequently, it does not permanently remove hair, and women must continue routine methods of hair removal while using this medicine.

Eflornithine hydrochloride (Vaniqa) is FDA-approved for treatment of female facial hirsutism. It may require 4 to 8 weeks of use before changes are noticed. However, approximately one third of patients have marked improvement after 24 weeks of eflornithine use compared with placebo, and 58 percent showed some overall improvement in hirsutism scores by this time (Wolf, 2007). Local burning and erythema are potential side effects.

Spironolactone

Although not FDA-approved for this indication, spironolactone (Aldactone) is the primary antiandrogen used currently in the United States for hirsutism. It is a competitive inhibitor of androgen binding to the androgen receptor. This drug also directly inhibits 5α-reductase. The typical dosage is 50 to 100 mg orally twice daily.

Spironolactone effectively treats hirsutism but carries important risks (Brown, 2009; Moghetti, 2000; Venturoli, 1999). First, as an antiandrogen, it bears a theoretical risk of interfering with external genitalia development in male fetuses of women using such medications in early pregnancy. Accordingly, it is commonly used in conjunction with COCs. Second, if used as monotherapy, intermenstrual bleeding frequently develops. Last, spironolactone is also a potassium-sparing diuretic. As such, it is not prescribed for chronic use in combination with agents that can also raise blood potassium levels, such as potassium supplements, angiotensin-converting enzyme inhibitors, nonsteroidal antiinflammatory drugs such as indomethacin, or other potassium-sparing diuretics.

Flutamide is another antiandrogen marketed for the treatment of prostate cancer. It is uncommonly used for hirsutism due to its potential hepatotoxicity. As an antiandrogen, teratogenicity again is a concern.

Finasteride

This agent is a 5α-reductase inhibitor, which blocks conversion of testosterone to DHT. Most studies have used 5-mg daily doses for women and have found finasteride to be modestly effective for hirsutism treatment (Fruzzetti, 1994; Moghetti, 1994). Side effects are few, although decreased libido has been noted. As with other antiandrogens, the risk of male fetal teratogenicity is present, and effective contraception must be used concurrently.

■ Acne

One part of acne treatment is similar to that for hirsutism and involves lowering of androgen levels. As such, therapy may include COC pills or spironolactone. In addition or alternatively, the subsequent therapies may be used.

In general, mild acne may be treated with benzoyl peroxide or topical retinoid monotherapy. If needed, benzoyl peroxide can be combined with a topical retinoid or with topical antimicrobial therapy. Moderate to severe acne may require triple therapy with the above agents. Oral retinoids or oral antibiotics are other options (Zaenglein, 2016). For this reason, women with moderate to severe acne may benefit from consultation with a dermatologist.

Topical benzoyl peroxide is bactericidal to *P acnes* by generating reactive oxygen species within the follicle. It also has weak comedolytic and antiinflammatory properties. It is the active ingredient in many over-the-counter acne products, but some prescription preparations also combine benzoyl peroxide with topical clindamycin or erythromycin.

Topical retinoids regulate the follicular keratinocyte and normalize its desquamation. In addition, these agents also have direct antiinflammatory properties and thereby target two factors linked to acne vulgaris. The most commonly used of these is tretinoin. Adapalene and tazarotene also are effective (Gold, 2006; Leyden, 2006). Initially, a pea-sized dab sufficient to cover the entire face is applied every third night and progressively increased as tolerated to nightly application. Tretinoin may cause a transient worsening of acne during the first weeks of treatment.

Tretinoin and adapalene are category C drugs and thus are not recommended for use during pregnancy or breastfeeding. However, epidemiologic studies currently do not support a link between topical retinoids and birth defects (Jick, 1993; Loureiro, 2005). Tazarotene is category X and similarly is not used during these times. It requires highly effective contraception.

Topical antibiotics typically are erythromycin and clindamycin, whereas oral antibiotics most often used for acne include doxycycline, minocycline, and erythromycin. Oral antibiotics are more effective than topical therapies but can have various side effects such as sun sensitivity and gastrointestinal upset.

Oral isotretinoin (Accutane) successfully treats severe recalcitrant acne. Despite its efficacy, oral isotretinoin is teratogenic if taken during the first trimester of pregnancy. Malformations typically involve the cranium, face, heart, central nervous system, and thymus. Therefore, isotretinoin administration is limited to women using highly effective contraception.

■ Surgical Therapy

Although ovarian wedge resection is now rarely performed, laparoscopic ovarian drilling restores ovulation in many women with PCOS that is resistant to clomiphene citrate (Section 44-7, p. 1036) (Farquhar, 2012). Rarely, GnRH agonists or oophorectomy is a viable option for women not seeking fertility who exhibit signs and symptoms of ovarian hyperthecosis and accompanying severe hyperandrogenism.

REFERENCES

Amer SA, Gopalan V, Li TC, et al: Long term follow-up of patients with polycystic ovarian syndrome after laparoscopic ovarian drilling: clinical outcome. Hum Reprod 17:2035, 2002

American College of Obstetricians and Gynecologists: Diagnosis of abnormal uterine bleeding in reproductive-aged women. Practice Bulletin No. 128, July 2012, Reaffirmed 2016

American College of Obstetricians and Gynecologists: Menstruation in girls and adolescents: using the menstrual cycle as a vital sign. Committee Opinion No. 651, December 2015, Reaffirmed 2017

American College of Obstetricians and Gynecologists: Polycystic ovarian syndrome. Practice Bulletin No. 194, June 2018

American Diabetes Association: 2. Classification and diagnosis of diabetes: standards of medical care in diabetes—2019. Diabetes Care 42(1 suppl):S13, 2019

American Society for Reproductive Medicine: Current evaluation of amenorrhea. Fertil Steril 90(5 Suppl):S219, 2008

American Society for Reproductive Medicine: Role of metformin for ovulation induction in infertile patients with polycystic ovary syndrome (PCOS): a guideline. Fertil Steril 108(3):426, 2017

Arroyo A, Laughlin GA, Morales AJ, et al: Inappropriate gonadotropin secretion in polycystic ovary syndrome: influence of adiposity. J Clin Endocrinol Metab 82:3728, 1997

Azziz R: The evaluation and management of hirsutism. Obstet Gynecol 101:995, 2003

Azziz R, Carmina E, Dewailly D, et al: Position statement: criteria for defining polycystic ovary syndrome as a predominantly hyperandrogenic syndrome: an Androgen Excess Society guideline. J Clin Endocrinol Metab 91:4237, 2006

Bahri Khomami M, Joham AE, Boyle JA, et al: Increased maternal pregnancy complications in polycystic ovary syndrome appear to be independent of obesity—a systematic review, meta-analysis, and meta-regression. Obes Rev 20(5):659, 2019

Banaszewska B, Duleba A, Spaczynski R: Lipids in polycystic ovary syndrome: role of hyperinsulinemia and effects of metformin. Am J Obstet Gynecol 194:1266, 2006

Barbieri RL, Ryan KJ: Hyperandrogenism, insulin resistance, and acanthosis nigricans syndrome: a common endocrinopathy with distinct pathophysiologic features. Am J Obstet Gynecol 147(1):90, 1983

Barry JA, Azizia MM, Hardiman PJ: Risk of endometrial, ovarian and breast cancer in women with polycystic ovary syndrome: a systematic review and meta-analysis. Hum Reprod Update 20(5):748, 2014

Benham JL, Yamamoto JM, Friedenreich CM, et al: Role of exercise training in polycystic ovary syndrome: a systematic review and meta-analysis. Clin Obes 8(4):275, 2018

Bergh C, Carlsson B, Olsson JH, et al: Regulation of androgen production in cultured human thecal cells by insulin-like growth factor I and insulin. Fertil Steril 59:323, 1993

Betti R, Bencini PL, Lodi A, et al: Incidence of polycystic ovaries in patients with late onset or persistent acne: hormonal reports. Dermatologica 181:109, 1990

Brown J, Farquhar C, Lee O, et al: Spironolactone versus placebo or in combination with steroids for hirsutism and/or acne. Cochrane Database Syst Rev 2:CD000194, 2009

Bunker CB, Newton JA, Kilborn J, et al: Most women with acne have polycystic ovaries. Br J Dermatol 121:675, 1989

Burgers JA, Fong SL, Louwers YV, et al: Oligoovulatory and anovulatory cycles in women with polycystic ovary syndrome (PCOS): what's the difference? J Clin Endocrinol Metab 95(12):E485, 2010

Cannarella R, Condorelli RA, Mongioì LM, et al: Does a male polycystic ovarian syndrome equivalent exist? J Endocrinol Invest 41(1):49, 2018

Carmina E, Oberfield SE, Lobo RA: The diagnosis of polycystic ovary syndrome in adolescents. Am J Obstet Gynecol 203(3):201.e1, 2010

Chen W, Thiboutot D, Zouboulis CC: Cutaneous androgen metabolism: basic research and clinical perspectives. J Invest Dermatol 119:992, 2002

Clayton R, Ogden V, Hodgkinson J, et al: How common are polycystic ovaries in normal women and what is their significance for the fertility of the population? Clin Endocrinol 37:127, 1992

Cook H, Brennan K, Azziz R: Reanalyzing the modified Ferriman-Gallwey score: is there a simpler method for assessing the extent of hirsutism? Fertil Steril 96(5):1266, 2011

Crapo L: Cushing's syndrome: a review of diagnostic tests. Metab Clin Exp 28:955, 1979

Cruz PD Jr, Hud JA Jr: Excess insulin binding to insulin-like growth factor receptors: proposed mechanism for acanthosis nigricans. J Invest Dermatol 98(6 suppl):82S, 1992

Cui Y, Shi Y, Cui L, et al: Age-specific serum antimüllerian hormone levels in women with and without polycystic ovary syndrome. Fertil Steril 102(1):230, 2014

Dahlgren E, Janson PO, Johansson S, et al: Polycystic ovary syndrome and risk for myocardial infarction. Evaluated from a risk factor model based on a prospective population study of women. Acta Obstet Gynecol Scand 71:599, 1992

Day F, Karaderi T, Jones MR, et al: Large-scale genome-wide meta-analysis of polycystic ovary syndrome suggests shared genetic architecture for different diagnosis criteria. PLoS Genet 14(12):e1007813, 2018

Deeks AA, Gibson-Helm ME, Paul E, et al: Is having polycystic ovary syndrome a predictor of poor psychological function including anxiety and depression? Hum Reprod 26(6):1399, 2011

Derksen J, Nagesser SK, Meinders AE, et al: Identification of virilizing adrenal tumors in hirsute women. N Engl J Med 331:968, 1994

Dewailly D, Andersen CY, Balen A, et al: The physiology and clinical utility of anti-mullerian hormone in women. Hum Reprod Update 20(3):370, 2014a

Dewailly D, Gronier H, Poncelet E, et al: Diagnosis of polycystic ovary syndrome (PCOS): revisiting the threshold values of follicle count on ultrasound and of the serum AMH level for the definition of polycystic ovaries. Hum Reprod 26(11):3123, 2011

Dewailly D, Lujan ME, Carmina E, et al: Definition and significance of polycystic ovarian morphology: a task force report from the Androgen Excess and Polycystic Ovary Syndrome Society. Hum Reprod Update 20(3):334, 2014b

Ding EL, Song Y, Manson JE, et al: Sex hormone-binding globulin and risk of type 2 diabetes in women and men. N Engl J Med 361(12):1152, 2009

Dokras A, Bochner M, Hollinrake E: Screening women with polycystic ovary syndrome for metabolic syndrome. Obstet Gynecol 106:131, 2005

Dokras A, Clifton S, Futterweit W, et al: Increased prevalence of anxiety symptoms in women with polycystic ovary syndrome: systematic review and meta-analysis. Fertil Steril 97(1):225, 2012

Dokras A, Clifton S, Futterweit W, et al: Increased risk for abnormal depression scores in women with polycystic ovary syndrome: a systematic review and meta-analysis. Obstet Gynecol 117(1):145, 2011

Dokras A, Stener-Victorin E, Yildiz BO, et al: Androgen Excess—Polycystic Ovary Syndrome Society: position statement on depression, anxiety, quality of life, and eating disorders in polycystic ovary syndrome. Fertil Steril 109(5):888, 2018

Dramusic V, Rajan U, Wong YC, et al: Adolescent polycystic ovary syndrome. Ann NY Acad Sci 816:194, 1997

Dumesic DA, Goodarzi MO, Chazenbalk GD, Abbott DH: Intrauterine environment and polycystic ovary syndrome. Semin Reprod Med 32:159, 2014

Dunaif A: Insulin resistance and the polycystic ovary syndrome: mechanisms and implication for pathogenesis. Endocr Rev 18:774, 1997

Dunaif A, Finegood DT: Beta-cell dysfunction independent of obesity and glucose intolerance in the polycystic ovary syndrome. J Clin Endocrinol Metab 81:942, 1996

Dunaif A, Segal KR, Futterweit W, et al: Profound peripheral insulin resistance, independent of obesity, in polycystic ovary syndrome. Diabetes 38:1165, 1989

Dunaif A, Segal KR, Shelley DR, et al: Evidence for distinctive and intrinsic defects in insulin action in polycystic ovary syndrome. Diabetes 41:1257, 1992

Elting MW, Korsen TJ, Rekers-Mombarg LT: Women with polycystic ovary syndrome gain regular menstrual cycles when aging. Hum Reprod 15, 24, 2000

Escobar-Morreale HF, Carmina E, Dewailly D, et al: Epidemiology, diagnosis and management of hirsutism: a consensus statement by the Androgen Excess and Polycystic Ovary Syndrome Society. Hum Reprod Update 18(2):146, 2012

Farquhar C, Brown J, Marjoribanks J: Laparoscopic drilling by diathermy or laser for ovulation induction in anovulatory polycystic ovary syndrome. Cochrane Database Syst Rev 6:CD001122, 2012

Ferriman D, Gallwey JD: Clinical assessment of body hair growth in women. J Clin Endocrinol Metab 21:1440, 1961

Flannery CA, Rackow B, Cong X, et al: Polycystic ovary syndrome in adolescence: impaired glucose tolerance occurs across the spectrum of BMI. Pediatr Diabetes 14(1):42, 2013

Fogel RB, Malhotra A, Pillar G, et al: Increased prevalence of obstructive sleep apnea syndrome in obese women with polycystic ovary syndrome. J Clin Endocrinol Metab 86:1175, 2001

Fruzzetti F, de Lorenzo D, Parrini D, et al: Effects of finasteride, a 5 alpha-reductase inhibitor, on circulating androgens and gonadotropin secretion in hirsute women. J Clin Endocrinol Metab 79(3):831, 1994

Gold LS: The MORE trial: effectiveness of adapalene gel 0.1% in real-world dermatology practices. Cutis 78(1 Suppl):12, 2006

Goodman NF, Cobin RH, Futterweit W, et al: American Association of Clinical Endocrinologists, American College of Endocrinology, and Androgen Excess and PCOS Society disease state clinical review: guide to the best practices in the evaluation and treatment of polycystic ovary syndrome – part 2. Endocr Pract 21(12):1415, 2015

Gopal M, Duntley S, Uhles M, et al: The role of obesity in the increased prevalence of obstructive sleep apnea syndrome in patients with polycystic ovarian syndrome. Sleep Med 3(5):401, 2002

Gottschau M, Kjaer SK, Jensen A, et al: Risk of cancer among women with polycystic ovary syndrome: a Danish cohort study. Gynecol Oncol 136(1):99, 2015

Gupta M, Mysore V: Classifications of patterned hair loss: a review. J Cutan Aesthet Surg 9(1):3, 2016

Haqq L, McFarlane J, Dieberg G, et al: The effect of lifestyle intervention on body composition, glycemic control, and cardiorespiratory fitness in polycystic ovarian syndrome: a systematic review and meta-analysis. Int J Sport Nutr Exerc Metab 25(6):533, 2015

Han Y, Li Y, He B: GLP-1 receptor agonists versus metformin in PCOS: a systematic review and meta-analysis. Reprod Biomed Online 39(2):332, 2019

Haoula Z, Salman M, Atiomo W: Evaluating the association between endometrial cancer and polycystic ovary syndrome. Hum Reprod 27(5):1327, 2012

Harrison CL, Lombard CB, Moran LJ, et al: Exercise therapy in polycystic ovary syndrome: a systematic review. Hum Reprod Update 17(2):171, 2011

Hatch R, Rosenfield RL, Kim MH, et al: Hirsutism: implications, etiology, and management. Am J Obstet Gynecol 140:815, 1981

Hayes FJ, Taylor AE, Martin KA, et al: Use of a gonadotropin-releasing hormone antagonist as a physiologic probe in polycystic ovary syndrome: assessment of neuroendocrine and androgen dynamics. J Clin Endocrinol Metab 83:2243, 1998

Hickey M, Doherty DA, Atkinson H, et al: Clinical, ultrasound and biochemical features of polycystic ovary syndrome in adolescents: implications for diagnosis. Hum Reprod 26(6):1469, 2011

Homburg R, Armar NA, Eshel A, et al: Influence of serum luteinising hormone concentrations on ovulation, conception, and early pregnancy loss in polycystic ovary syndrome. BMJ 297(6655):1024, 1998

Homburg R, Lambalk CB: Polycystic ovary syndrome in adolescence—a therapeutic conundrum. Hum Reprod 19:1039, 2004

Homburg R, Ray A, Bhide P, et al: The relationship of serum anti-Mullerian hormone with polycystic ovarian morphology and polycystic ovary syndrome: a prospective cohort study. Hum Reprod 28(4):1077, 2013

Huber-Buchholz MM, Carey DG, Norman RJ: Restoration of reproductive potential by lifestyle modification in obese polycystic ovary syndrome: role of insulin sensitivity and luteinizing hormone. J Clin Endocrinol Metab 84:1470, 1999

Hughesdon PE: Morphology and morphogenesis of the Stein-Leventhal ovary and of so-called "hyperthecosis." Obstet Gynecol Surv 37:59, 1982

Iliodromiti S, Kelsey TW, Anderson RA, et al: Can anti-Mullerian hormone predict the diagnosis of polycystic ovary syndrome? A systematic review and meta-analysis of extracted data. J Clin Endocrinol Metab 98(8):3332, 2013

Jaatinen TA, Anttila L, Erkkola R, et al: Hormonal responses to physical exercise in patients with polycystic ovarian syndrome. Fertil Steril 60:262, 1993

Javed Z, Papageorgiou M, Deshmukh H, et al: Effects of empagliflozin on metabolic parameters in polycystic ovary syndrome: a randomized controlled study. Clin Endocrinol (Oxf) 90(6):805, 2019

Jick SS, Terris BZ, Jick H: First trimester topical tretinoin and congenital disorders. Lancet 341:1181, 1993

Joham AE, Boyle JA, Ranasinha S, et al: Contraception use and pregnancy outcomes in women with polycystic ovary syndrome: data from the Australian Longitudinal Study on Women's Health. Hum Reprod 29(4):802, 2014a

Joham AE, Ranasinha S, Zoungas S, et al: Gestational diabetes and type 2 diabetes in reproductive-aged women with polycystic ovary syndrome. J Clin Endocrinol Metab 99(3):E447, 2014b

Kahal H, Kyrou I, Uthman OA, et al: The prevalence of obstructive sleep apnoea in women with polycystic ovary syndrome: a systematic review and meta-analysis. Sleep Breath May 20, 2019 [Epub ahead of print]

Kahsar-Miller MD, Nixon C, Boots LR, et al: Prevalence of polycystic ovary syndrome (PCOS) in first-degree relatives of patients with PCOS. Fertil Steril 75:53, 2001

Kazemi M, Pierson RA, Lujan ME, et al: Comprehensive evaluation of type 2 diabetes and cardiovascular disease risk profiles in reproductive-age women with polycystic ovary syndrome: a large Canadian cohort. J Obstet Gynaecol Can 41(10):1453, 2019

Kiddy DS, Hamilton-Fairley D, Bush A, et al: Improvement in endocrine and ovarian function during dietary treatment of obese women with polycystic ovary syndrome. Clin Endocrinol (Oxf) 36:105, 1992

Kiszka AN, Wilburn-Wren KR: Clitoromegaly (update) in Hoffman BL, Schorge JO, Bradshaw KD, et al (eds): Williams Gynecology, 3rd edition Online. Available at: https://accessmedicine.mhmedical.com/Multimedia Player.aspx?MultimediaID=7918792. New York, McGraw-Hill, 2019

Kite C, Lahart IM, Afzal I, et al: Exercise, or exercise and diet for the management of polycystic ovary syndrome: a systematic review and meta-analysis. Syst Rev 8(1):51, 2019

Kristensen SL, Ramlau-Hansen CH, Ernst E, et al: A very large proportion of young Danish women have polycystic ovaries: is a revision of the Rotterdam criteria needed. Hum Reprod 25(12):3117, 2010

Lee I, Cooney LG, Saini S, et al: Increased risk of disordered eating in polycystic ovary syndrome. Fertil Steril 107(3):796, 2017

Legro RS: Is there a male phenotype in polycystic ovary syndrome families? J Pediatr Endocrinol Metab 13(5 suppl):1307, 2000

Legro RS, Gnatuk CL, Kunselman AR, et al: Changes in glucose tolerance over time in women with polycystic ovary syndrome: a controlled study. J Clin Endocrinol Metab 90:3236, 2005

Legro RS, Kunselman AR, Demers L, et al: Elevated dehydroepiandrosterone sulfate levels as the reproductive phenotype in the brothers of women with polycystic ovary syndrome. J Clin Endocrinol Metab 87:2134, 2002

Legro RS, Kunselman AR, Dodson WC, et al: Prevalence and predictors of risk for type 2 diabetes mellitus and impaired glucose tolerance in polycystic ovary syndrome: a prospective, controlled study in 254 affected women. J Clin Endocrinol Metab 84:165, 1999

Legro RS, Kunselman AR, Dunaif A: Prevalence and predictors of dyslipidemia in women with polycystic ovary syndrome. Am J Med 111:607, 2001

Levy LL, Emer JJ: Female pattern alopecia: current perspectives. Int J Womens Health 5:541, 2013

Leyden J, Thiboutot DM, Shalita AR, et al: Comparison of tazarotene and minocycline maintenance therapies in acne vulgaris: a multicenter, double-blind, randomized, parallel-group study. Arch Dermatol 142:605, 2006

Li R, Zhang Q, Yang D, et al: Prevalence of polycystic ovary syndrome in women in China: a large community-based study. Hum Reprod 28(9):2562, 2013

Lim SS, Norman RJ, Davies MJ, et al: The effect of obesity on polycystic ovary syndrome: a systematic review and meta-analysis. Obes Rev 14(2):95, 2013

Liu DM, Torchen LC, Sung Y, et al: Evidence for gonadotrophin secretory and steroidogenic abnormalities in brothers of women with polycystic ovary syndrome. Hum Reprod 29(12):2764, 2014

Lizneva D, Suturina L, Walker W, et al: Criteria, prevalence, and phenotypes of polycystic ovary syndrome. Fertil Steril 106(1):6, 2016

Lo JC, Feigenbaum SL, Yang J, et al: Epidemiology and adverse cardiovascular risk profile of diagnosed polycystic ovary syndrome. J Clin Endocrinol Metab 91(4):1357, 2006

Loureiro KD, Kao KK, Jones KL, et al: Minor malformations characteristics of the retinoic acid embryopathy and other birth outcomes in children of women exposed to topical tretinoin during early pregnancy. Am J Med Genet A 136:117, 2005

Lujan ME, Jarrett BY, Brooks ED, et al: Updated ultrasound criteria for polycystic ovary syndrome: reliable thresholds for elevated follicle population and ovarian volume. Hum Reprod 28(5):1361, 2013

Moghetti P, Castello R, Magnani CM, et al: Clinical and hormonal effects of the 5 alpha-reductase inhibitor finasteride in idiopathic hirsutism. J Clin Endocrinol Metab 79:1115, 1994

Moghetti P, Tosi F, Tosti A, et al: Comparison of spironolactone, flutamide, and finasteride efficacy in the treatment of hirsutism: a randomized, double blind, placebo-controlled trial. J Clin Endocrinol Metab 85:89, 2000

Moore RL, Devere TS: Epidermal manifestations of internal malignancy. Dermatol Clin 26(1):17, 2008

Moran C, Knochenhauer E, Boots LR, et al: Adrenal androgen excess in hyperandrogenism: relation to age and body mass. Fertil Steril 71:671, 1999

Moran C, Tapia MC, Hernandez E, et al: Etiological review of hirsutism in 250 patients. Arch Med Res 25:311, 1994

Mykhalchenko K, Lizneva D, Trofimova T, et al: Genetics of polycystic ovary syndrome. Expert Rev Mol Diagn 17(7):723, 2017

Nagamani M, Dinh TV, Kelver ME: Hyperinsulinemia in hyperthecosis of the ovaries. Am J Obstet Gynecol 154:384, 1986

Nagamani M, Osuampke C, Kelver ME: Increased bioactive luteinizing hormone levels and bio/immuno ratio in women with hyperthecosis of the ovaries: possible role of hyperinsulinemia. J Clin Endocrinol Metab 84(5):1685, 1999

National Cancer Institute: Surveillance, Epidemiology, and End Results Program: cancer of the corpus and uterus, NOS (invasive). SEER incidence and U.S. death rates, age-adjusted and age-specific rates, by race. 2019. Available at: https://seer.cancer.gov/csr/1975_2016/browse_csr.php?sectionSEL=7&pageSEL=sect_07_table.07. Accessed June 23, 2019

National Institutes of Health: Evidence-based methodology workshop on polycystic ovary syndrome. December 3–5, 2012. Executive summary. Final report. Available at: https://prevention.nih.gov/sites/default/files/2018-06/FinalReport.pdf. Accessed June 24, 2019

Naver KV, Grinsted J, Larsen SO, et al: Increased risk of preterm delivery and pre-eclampsia in women with polycystic ovary syndrome and hyperandrogenaemia. BJOG 121(5):575, 2014

Nestler JE, Jakubowicz DJ, Evans WS, et al: Effects of metformin on spontaneous and clomiphene-induced ovulation in the polycystic ovary syndrome. N Engl J Med 338:1876, 1998

Nieman LK, Biller BM, Findling JW, et al: The diagnosis of Cushing's syndrome: an Endocrine Society Clinical Practice Guideline. J Clin Endocrinol Metab 93(5):1526, 2008

O'Driscoll JB, Mamtora H, Higginson J, et al: A prospective study of the prevalence of clearcut endocrine disorders and polycystic ovaries in 350 patients presenting with hirsutism or androgenic alopecia. Clin Endocrinol 41:231, 1994

Palmert MR, Gordon CM, Kartashov AI, et al: Screening for abnormal glucose tolerance in adolescents with polycystic ovary syndrome. J Clin Endocrinol Metab 87(3):1017, 2002

Palomba S, de Wilde MA, Falbo A, et al: Pregnancy complications in women with polycystic ovary syndrome. Hum Reprod Update 21(5):575, 2015

Palomba S, Falbo A, Orio F Jr, et al: Effect of preconceptional metformin on abortion risk in polycystic ovary syndrome: a systematic review and meta-analysis of randomized controlled trials. Fertil Steril 92(5):1646, 2009

Panidis D, Skiadopoulos S, Rousso D, et al: Association of acanthosis nigricans with insulin resistance in patients with polycystic ovary syndrome. Br J Dermatol 132:936, 1995

Pasquali R, Antenucci D, Casimirri F, et al: Clinical and hormonal characteristics of obese amenorrheic hyperandrogenic women before and after weight loss. J Clin Endocrinol Metab 68:173, 1989

Patel NU, Roach C, Alinia H, et al: Current treatment options for acanthosis nigricans. Clin Cosmet Investig Dermatol 11:407, 2018

Peppard PE, Young T, Palta M, et al: Longitudinal study of moderate weight change and sleep-disordered breathing. JAMA 284(23):3015, 2000

Pigny P, Jonard S, Robert Y, et al: Serum anti-Müllerian hormone as a surrogate for antral follicle count for definition of the polycystic ovary syndrome. J Clin Endocrinol Metab 91(3):941, 2006

Polson DW, Adams J, Wadsworth J, et al: Polycystic ovaries—a common finding in normal women. Lancet 1:870, 1988

Quinn M, Shinkai K, Pasch L, et al: Prevalence of androgenic alopecia in patients with polycystic ovary syndrome and characterization of associated clinical and biochemical features. Fertil Steril 101(4):1129, 2014

Rebar R, Judd HL, Yen SS, et al: Characterization of the inappropriate gonadotropin secretion in polycystic ovary syndrome. J Clin Invest 57:1320, 1976

Rebuffe-Scrive M, Cullberg G, Lundberg PA, et al: Anthropometric variables and metabolism in polycystic ovarian disease. Horm Metab Res 21:391, 1989

Regan L, Owen EJ, Jacobs HS: Hypersecretion of luteinising hormone, infertility, and miscarriage. Lancet 336:1141, 1990

Reyes-Muñoz E, Ortega-González C, Martínez-Cruz N, et al: Association of obesity and overweight with the prevalence of insulin resistance, prediabetes and clinical-biochemical characteristics among infertile Mexican women with polycystic ovary syndrome: a cross-sectional study. BMJ Open 6(7):e012107, 2016

Sagle M, Bishop K, Ridley N, et al: Recurrent early miscarriage and polycystic ovaries. BMJ 297:1027, 1988

Schneider JG, Tompkins C, Blumenthal RS, et al: The metabolic syndrome in women. Cardiol Rev 14:286, 2006

Senaratna CV, Perret JL, Lodge CJ, et al: Prevalence of obstructive sleep apnea in the general population: a systematic review. Sleep Med Rev 34:70, 2017

Sobbrio GA, Granata A, D'Arrigo F, et al: Treatment of hirsutism related to micropolycystic ovary syndrome (MPCO) with two low-dose oestrogen oral contraceptives: a comparative randomized evaluation. Acta Eur Fertil 21:139, 1990

Tagatz GE, Kopher RA, Nagel TC, et al: The clitoral index: a bioassay of androgenic stimulation. Obstet Gynecol 54(5):562, 1979

Talbott E, Clerici A, Berga SL, et al: Adverse lipid and coronary heart disease risk profiles in young women with polycystic ovary syndrome: results of a case-controlled study. J Clin Epidemiol 51:415, 1998

Talbott E, Guzick D, Clerici A, et al: Coronary heart disease risk factors in women with polycystic ovary syndrome. Arterioscler Thromb Vasc Biol 15:821, 1995

Tasali E, Van Cauter E, Hoffman L, et al: Impact of obstructive sleep apnea on insulin resistance and glucose tolerance in women with polycystic ovary syndrome. J Clin Endocrinol Metab 93(10):3878, 2008

Taylor AE, McCourt B, Martin KA, et al: Determinants of abnormal gonadotropin secretion in clinically defined women with polycystic ovary syndrome. J Clin Endocrinol Metab 82:2248, 1997

Teede H, Misso M, Tassone EC, et al: Anti-Müllerian hormone in PCOS: a review informing international guidelines. Trends Endocrinol Metab 30(7):467, 2019

The Rotterdam ESHRE/ASRM-Sponsored PCOS Consensus Workshop Group: Revised 2003 consensus on diagnostic criteria and long-term health risks related to polycystic ovary syndrome (PCOS). Hum Reprod 19:41, 2004

Torchen LC, Kumar A, Kalra B, et al: Increased antimüllerian hormone levels and other reproductive endocrine changes in adult male relatives of women with polycystic ovary syndrome. Fertil Steril 106(1):50, 2016

van Santbrink EJ, Hop WC, Fauser BC: Classification of normogonadotropin infertility: polycystic ovaries diagnosed by ultrasound versus endocrine characteristics of PCOS. Fertil Steril 67:452, 1997

Vanky E, Stridsklev S, Heimstad R, et al: Metformin versus placebo from first trimester to delivery in polycystic ovary syndrome: a randomized, controlled multicenter study. J Clin Endocrinol Metab 95(12):E448, 2010

Veltman-Verhulst SM, van Haeften TW, Eijkemans MJ, et al: Sex hormone-binding globulin concentrations before conception as a predictor for gestational diabetes in women with polycystic ovary syndrome. Hum Reprod (12):3123, 2010

Venturoli S, Marescalchi O, Colombo FM, et al: A prospective randomized trial comparing low dose flutamide, finasteride, ketoconazole, and cyproterone acetate-estrogen regimens in the treatment of hirsutism. J Clin Endocrinol Metab 84:1304, 1999

Verkauf BS, Von Thron J, O'Brien WF: Clitoral size in normal women. Obstet Gynecol 80(1):41, 1992

Vgontzas AN, Legro RS, Bixler EO, et al: Polycystic ovary syndrome is associated with obstructive sleep apnea and daytime sleepiness: role of insulin resistance. J Clin Endocrinol Metab 86:517, 2001

Vigorito C, Giallauria F, Palomba S, et al: Beneficial effects of a three-month structured exercise training program on cardiopulmonary functional capacity in young women with polycystic ovary syndrome. J Clin Endocrinol Metab 92(4):1379, 2007

Vink JM, Sadrzadeh S, Lambalk CB, et al: Heritability of polycystic ovary syndrome in a Dutch twin-family study. J Clin Endocrinol Metab 91(6):2100, 2006

Waldstreicher J, Santoro NF, Hall HJE, et al: Hyperfunction of the hypothalamic-pituitary axis in women with polycystic ovarian disease: indirect evidence of partial gonadotroph desensitization. J Clin Endocrinol Metab 66:165, 1988

Wild RA, Rizzo M, Clifton S, et al: Lipid levels in polycystic ovary syndrome: systematic review and meta-analysis. Fertil Steril 95(3):1073, 2011

Witchel SF, Oberfield S, Rosenfield RL, et al: The diagnosis of polycystic ovary syndrome during adolescence. Horm Res Paediatr 83:376, 2015

Wolf JE Jr, Shander D, Huber F, et al: Randomized, double-blind clinical evaluation of the efficacy and safety of topical eflornithine HCl 13.9% cream in the treatment of women with facial hair. Int J Dermatol 46(1):94, 2007

Yildiz BO, Yarali H, Oguz H, et al: Glucose intolerance, insulin resistance, and hyperandrogenemia in first degree relatives of women with polycystic ovary syndrome. J Clin Endocrinol Metab 88:2031, 2003

Zaenglein AL, Pathy AL, Schlosser BJ, et al: Guidelines of care for the management of acne vulgaris. J Am Acad Dermatol 74(5):945, 2016

Zawadzki JK, Dunaif A: Diagnostic criteria for polycystic ovary syndrome: towards a rational approach. In Dunaif A, Givens JR, Haseltine F, et al (eds): Polycystic Ovary Syndrome. Boston, Blackwell Scientific, 1990, p 377

Zhao H, Lv Y, Li L, et al: Genetic studies on polycystic ovary syndrome. Best Pract Res Clin Obstet Gynaecol 37:56, 2016

CHAPTER 19

Anatomic Disorders

Congenital anatomic disorders of the female reproductive tract develop frequently and result from insults at critical embryonic stages. Influences include genetic mutation, epigenetic factors, developmental arrest, or abnormal hormonal exposures. Disorders range from congenital absence of the vagina and uterus, to lateral or vertical fusion defects of the müllerian ducts, to external genitalia that are ambiguous. Sexual differentiation is complex and requires both hormonal pathways and morphologic development to be normal and correctly integrated. Thus, neonates with genital anomalies not surprisingly often have multiple other malformations. Associated urinary tract defects are especially frequent and are linked to the concurrent embryonic development of both reproductive and urinary tracts (Hutson, 2014).

NORMAL EMBRYOLOGY

The urogenital tract is functionally divided into the urinary system and genital system. The urinary organs include the kidney, ureters, bladder, and urethra. The reproductive organs are the gonads, ductal system, and external genitalia. Like most organ systems, the female urogenital tract develops from multiple cell types that undergo important spatial growth and differentiation. These develop during relatively narrow time windows and are governed by time-linked patterns of gene expression (Park, 2005).

Both the urinary and genital systems develop from intermediate mesoderm, which extends along the entire embryo length.

During initial embryo folding, a longitudinal ridge of this intermediate mesoderm develops along each side of the primitive abdominal aorta and is called the *urogenital ridge*. Subsequently, the urogenital ridge divides into the *nephrogenic ridge* and the *genital ridge*, also called the *gonadal ridge* (Fig. 19-1).

At approximately 60 days of gestation, the nephrogenic ridges develop into the *mesonephric kidneys* and paired *mesonephric ducts*, also termed *wolffian ducts*. These mesonephric ducts connect the mesonephric kidneys (destined for resorption) to the *cloaca*, which is a common opening into which the embryonic urinary, genital, and alimentary tracts join (Fig. 19-2A). Recall that evolution of the renal system passes sequentially through the pronephric and mesonephric stages to reach the permanent metanephric system. The ureteric bud arises from the mesonephric duct at approximately the fifth week of fetal life. It lengthens to become the metanephric duct (ureter) and induces differentiation of the metanephros, which will eventually become the final functional kidney.

The paired *paramesonephric ducts*, also termed the *müllerian ducts*, develop from invagination of the coelomic epithelium at approximately the sixth week and grow alongside the mesonephric ducts (Figs. 19-1B and 19-2B). The caudal portions of the müllerian ducts approximate one another in the midline and end behind the cloaca (Fig. 19-2C). The cloaca is divided by formation of the urorectal septum by the seventh week and is separated to create the *rectum* and the *urogenital sinus* (Fig. 19-1D). The urogenital sinus is considered in three parts: (1) the cephalad or vesicle portion, which will form the urinary bladder; (2) the middle or pelvic portion, which creates the female urethra; and (3) the caudal or phallic part, which will give rise to the distal vagina and the greater vestibular (Bartholin) glands and paraurethral glands. During differentiation of the urinary bladder, the caudal portion of the mesonephric ducts is incorporated into the trigone of the bladder wall. Consequently, the caudal portion of the metanephric ducts (ureters) penetrates the bladder with distinct and separate orifices (see Fig. 19-2D).

The close association between the mesonephric (wolffian) and paramesonephric (müllerian) ducts has important clinical relevance because developmental insult to either system is often associated with anomalies that involve the kidney, ureter, and reproductive tract. For example, Kenney and colleagues (1984) noted that up to 50 percent of females with uterovaginal malformations have associated urinary tract anomalies.

■ Gonadal Determination

Mammalian sex is determined genetically. Individuals with X and Y chromosomes usually develop as males, whereas those

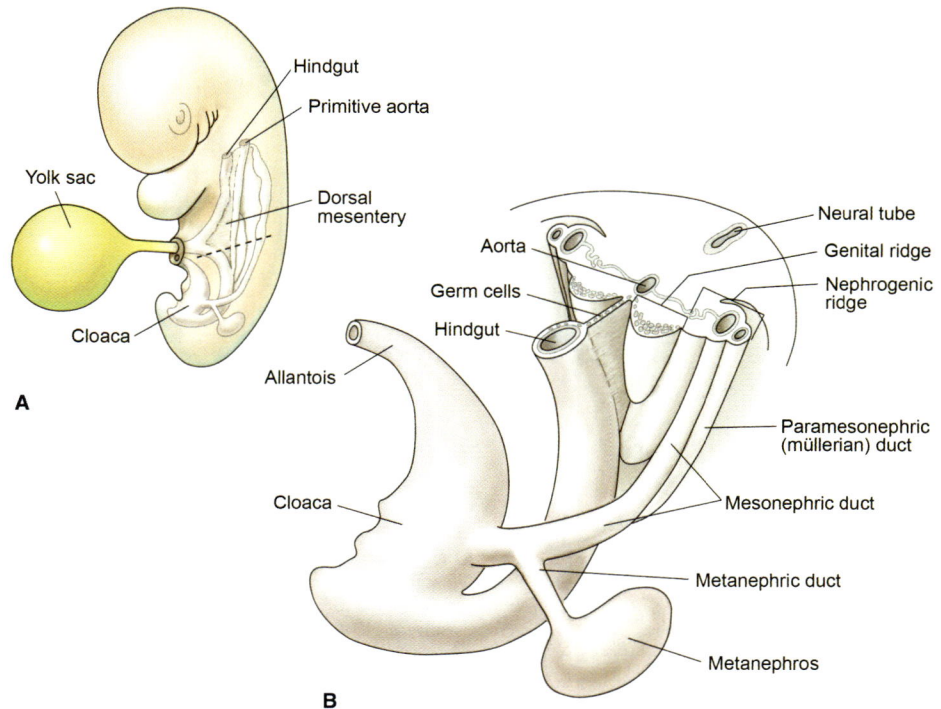

FIGURE 19-1 Early development of the embryonic genitourinary tract. **A.** In the developing embryo, the urogenital ridge forms from coelomic mesenchyme lateral to the primitive aorta. **B.** Cross section through the embryo shows division of the urogenital ridges into the genital ridge (future gonad) and nephrogenic ridge, which contains the mesonephros and mesonephric (wolffian) ducts. The mesonephros is the primitive kidney and is connected by the mesonephric ducts to the cloaca. Primordial germ cells migrate along the dorsal mesentery of the hindgut to reach the genital ridge. Paramesonephric (müllerian) ducts develop lateral to the mesonephric ducts. (Reproduced with permission from Kim Hoggatt-Krumwiede, MA.)

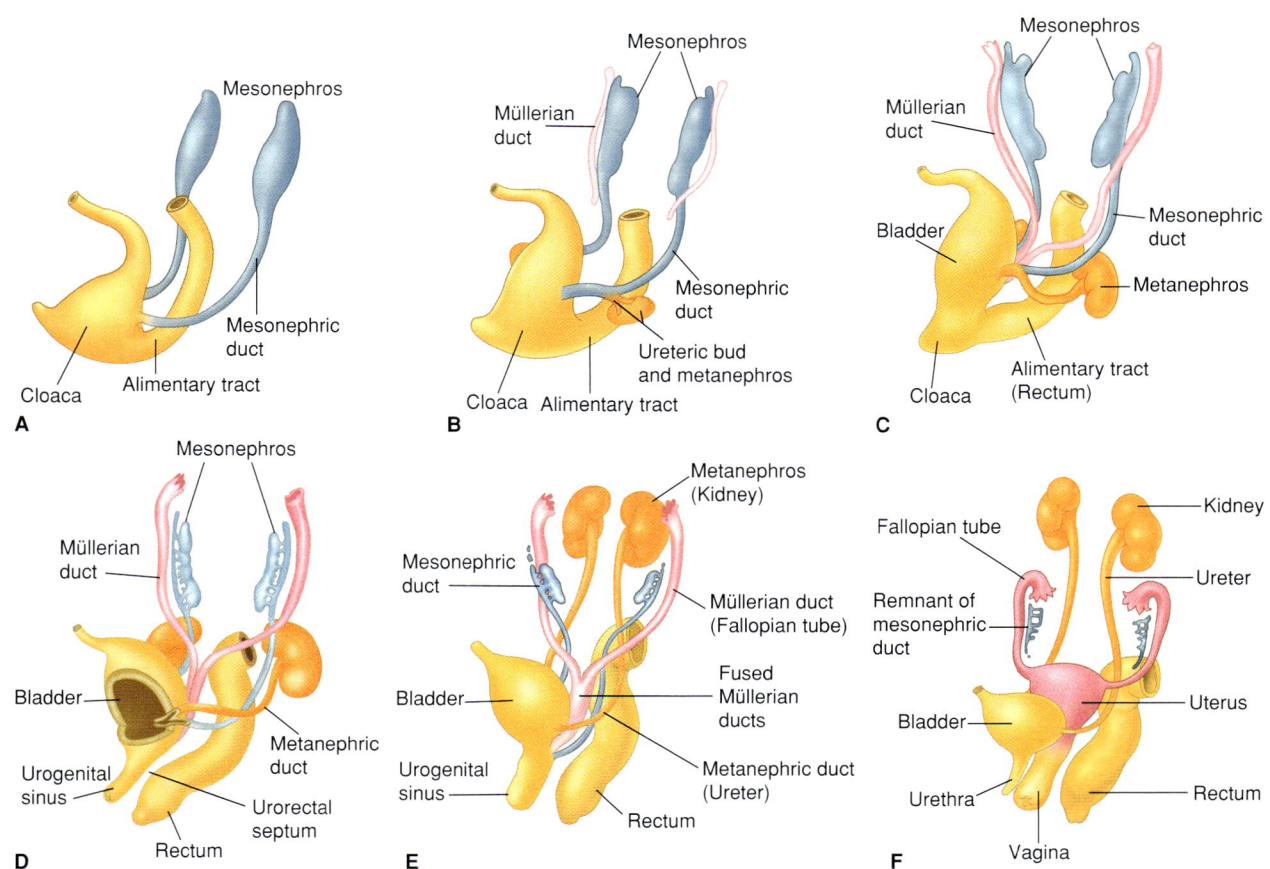

FIGURE 19-2 Embryonic development of the female genitourinary tract.

TABLE 19-1. Embryonic Urogenital Structures and Their Adult Homologues

Indifferent Structure	Female	Male
Genital ridge	Ovary	Testis
Primordial germ cells	Ova	Spermatozoa
Sex cords	Granulosa cells	Seminiferous tubules, Sertoli cells
Gubernaculum	Uteroovarian and round ligaments	Gubernaculum testis
Mesonephric tubules	Epoophoron, paroophoron	Efferent ductules, paradidymis
Mesonephric ducts	Gartner duct	Epididymis, ductus deferens, ejaculatory duct
Paramesonephric ducts	Uterus, fallopian tubes, upper vagina	Prostatic utricle, appendix of testis
Urogenital sinus	Bladder, urethra Vagina Paraurethral glands Greater (Bartholin) and lesser vestibular glands	Bladder, urethra Prostatic utricle Prostate glands Bulbourethral glands
Genital tubercle	Clitoris	Glans penis
Urogenital folds	Labia minora	Floor of penile urethra
Labioscrotal swellings	Labia majora	Scrotum

with two X chromosomes develop as females. Before 7 weeks of embryonic development, embryos of male and female sex are indistinguishable from one another (Table 19-1).

During this indeterminate time, the genital ridge begins as coelomic epithelium with underlying mesenchyme. The epithelium proliferates, and cords of epithelium invaginate into the mesenchyme to create primitive sex cords. In both 46,XX and 46,XY embryos, the primordial germ cells are first identified as large polyhedral cells in the yolk sac. These germ cells migrate by amoeboid motion along the hindgut dorsal mesentery to populate the undifferentiated genital ridge (see Fig. 19-1). Thus, the major cellular components of the early genital ridge include primordial germ cells and somatic cells.

At this point, gonadal determinant genes direct fetal gender development (Fig. 19-3) (Taylor, 2000). *Sexual determination* is the development of the genital ridge into either an ovary or testis. This depends on the genetic sex produced at fertilization, when the X-bearing oocyte is penetrated by either an X- or Y-chromosome-bearing sperm. In humans, the gene named the *sex-determining region of the Y (SRY)* is the testis-determining factor. In the presence of *SRY*, gonads typically develop as testes. Other genes are important for normal gonad development and include *SOX9, SF-1, DMRT1, GATA4, WNT4, WT1, DAX1,* and *RSPO1* (Arboleda, 2014; Blaschko, 2012). Not surprisingly, mutations in any of these genes may lead to abnormal sexual determination. Moreover, gene dosage and relative expression levels play an important role (Ocal, 2011).

In males, cells in the medullary region of the primitive sex cords differentiate into Sertoli cells, and these cells organize to form the testicular cords (Fig. 19-3A). Testicular cords are identifiable at 6 weeks and consist of these Sertoli cells and tightly packed germ cells. Early in the second trimester, the cords develop a lumen and become seminiferous tubules. Development of a testis-specific vasculature is crucial for normal testicular development (Ross, 2005).

During this early development, Sertoli cells begin secreting *antimüllerian hormone (AMH),* also called *müllerian inhibitory substance (MIS).* This gonadal hormone causes regression of the ipsilateral paramesonephric (müllerian duct) system, and this involution is completed by 9 to 10 weeks' gestation (Marshall, 1978). AMH also controls the rapid gubernacular growth necessary for the transabdominal descent of the testis. Serum AMH levels remain elevated in boys during childhood and then decline at puberty to the low levels seen in adult men.

In the testes, Leydig cells arise from the original mesenchyme of the genital ridge and lie between the testicular cords. The Leydig cells begin to secrete testosterone by 8 weeks' gestation due to stimulation of the testes by human chorionic gonadotropin (hCG). Testosterone acts in a paracrine manner on the ipsilateral mesonephric (wolffian) duct to promote virilization of the duct into the epididymis, vas deferens, and seminal vesicle. In addition, the androgens testosterone and dihydrotestosterone (DHT) are essential for male phenotype development. These androgens control differentiation and growth of the internal ducts and external genitalia and also prime male differentiation of the brain.

In the female embryo, without the influence of the *SRY* gene, the bipotential gonad develops into the ovary. The pathways regulating female sex determination have remained incompletely defined, but *WNT4, WT1, FoxL2,* and *DAX1* genes are important for normal development (Arboleda, 2014; MacLaughlin, 2004). Compared with testicular development, ovarian determination is delayed by approximately 2 weeks. Development is first characterized by the absence of testicular cords in the gonad. The primitive sex cords degenerate, and the mesothelium of the genital ridge forms secondary sex cords (Fig. 19-3B). These secondary cords become the granulosa cells that band together to form the follicular structures that surround the germ cells. Oocytes and the surrounding granulosa cells begin communication when the resting primordial

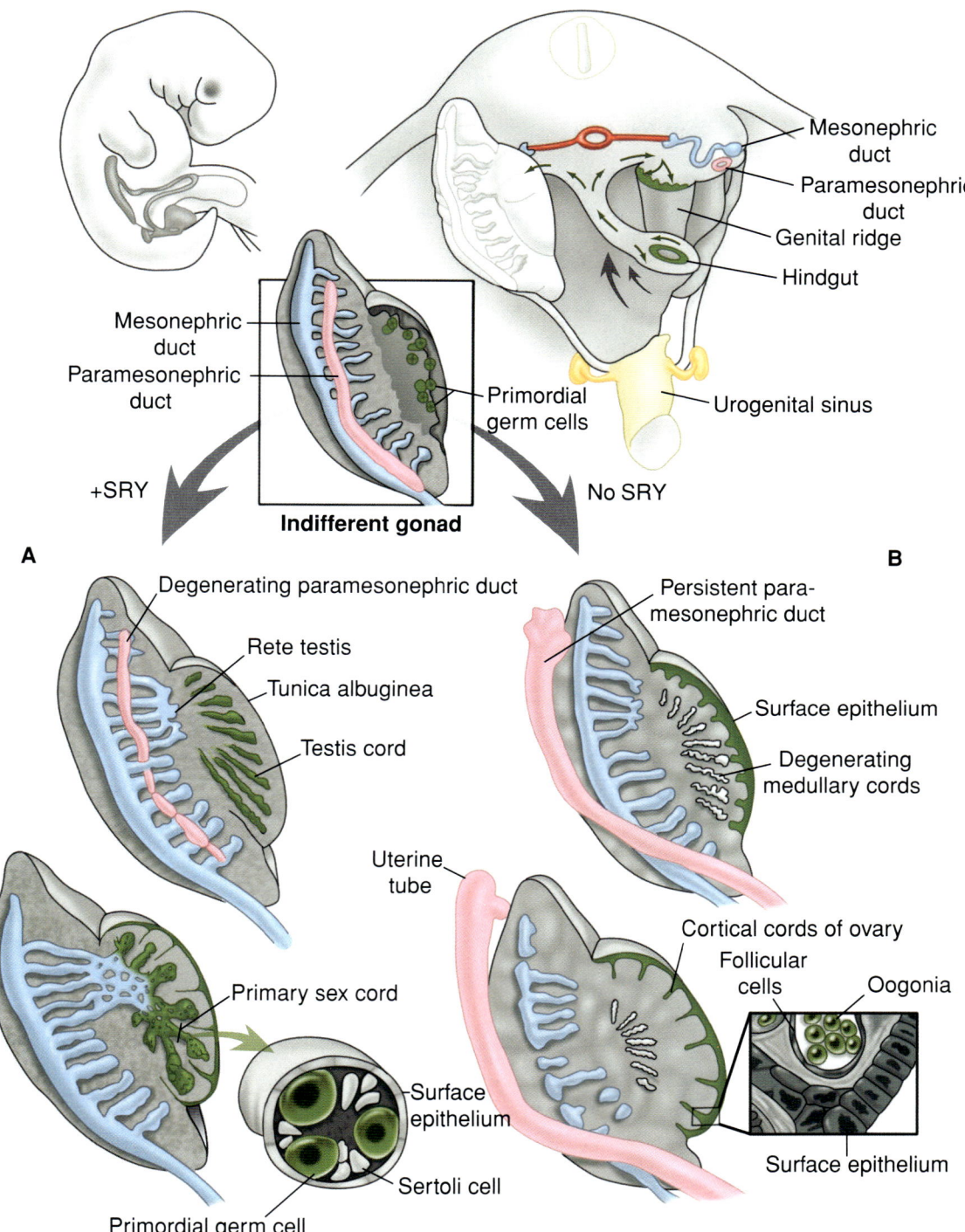

FIGURE 19-3 Development of the gonads and ductal systems in male **(A)** and female **(B)** embryos. SRY = sex-determining region of the Y. (Reproduced with permission from Hoffman, 2018.)

follicles are stimulated to grow under the influence of follicle-stimulating hormone (FSH) at puberty. The medullary portion of the gonad regresses and forms the rete ovarii within the ovarian hilum.

Germ cells that carry two X chromosomes undergo mitosis during their initial migration to the female genital ridge. They reach a peak number of 5 to 7 million by 20 weeks' gestation. At this time, the fetal ovary demonstrates mature organization of stroma and primordial follicles containing oocytes. During

the third trimester, oocytes begin meiosis but arrest during meiosis I until the oocyte undergoes ovulation after menarche. Atresia of the oocytes starts in utero, leading to a reduced number of germ cells at birth (Fig. 15-1, p. 321).

■ Ductal System Development

Sexual differentiation of the mesonephric (wolffian) and paramesonephric (müllerian) ducts begins in week 7 from the influence of gonadal hormones (testosterone and AMH) and other factors. In the male, AMH forces paramesonephric regression, and testosterone prompts mesonephric duct differentiation into the epididymis, vas deferens, and seminal vesicles.

In the female, a lack of AMH allows müllerian ducts to persist. Early, these ducts grow caudally along with the mesonephric ducts. During paramesonephric duct elongation, homeobox (Hox) genes in groups 9–13 play a role in determining positional identity along the long axis of the developing duct. For example, *HoxA9* is one such gene that is expressed at high levels in areas destined to become the fallopian tube (Park, 2005). *HoxA10* and *HoxA11* are expressed in the developing uterus and in the adult uterus. These and other ovarian determinant genes play an active role in gonadal and reproductive tract morphogenesis, but mechanisms are yet to be elucidated fully (Massé, 2009; Taylor, 2000).

During their elongation, both mesonephric and paramesonephric duct systems become enclosed in peritoneal folds that later give rise to the broad ligaments of the uterus. At approximately 10 weeks' gestation and during their caudal migration, the two distal portions of the müllerian ducts approach each other in the midline and fuse even before they reach the urogenital sinus. The fused ducts form a tube called the *uterovaginal canal*. This tube then inserts into the urogenital sinus at the Müller tubercle (Fig. 19-2E).

By 12 weeks, mesonephric ducts regress from lack of testosterone. The uterine corpus and cervix differentiate, and the uterine wall thickens. Initially, the upper pole of the uterus contains a thick midline septum that undergoes dissolution to create the uterine cavity. Dissolution of the uterine septum is usually completed by 20 weeks' gestation. The unfused cephalad portions

of the müllerian ducts become the fallopian tubes (Fig. 19-2F). Any failure of lateral fusion of the two müllerian ducts or failure to reabsorb the septum between them results in separate uterine horns or some degree of persistent midline uterine septum.

Most investigators suggest that the vagina develops under influence from the müllerian ducts and estrogenic stimulation. The vagina forms partly from the müllerian ducts and partly from the urogenital sinus (Massé, 2009). Specifically, the upper two thirds of the vagina derive from the fused müllerian ducts. The distal third of the vagina develops from the bilateral *sinovaginal bulbs*, which are cranial evaginations of the urogenital sinus.

During vaginal development, the müllerian ducts reach the urogenital sinus at the Müller tubercle (Fig. 19-4A). Here, cells in the sinovaginal bulbs proliferate cranially to lengthen the vagina and create a solid vaginal plate (Fig. 19-4B). During the second trimester, these cells desquamate, allowing full canalization of the vaginal lumen (Fig. 19-4C). The hymen is the partition that remains to a varying degree between the dilated, canalized, fused sinovaginal bulbs and the urogenital sinus (see Fig. 19-4B,C). The hymen usually perforates shortly before or after birth. An imperforate hymen represents persistence of this membrane.

■ External Genitalia

Early development of the external genitalia is similar in both sexes. By 6 weeks' gestation, three external protuberances have developed surrounding the cloacal membrane. These are the left and right cloacal folds, which meet ventrally to form the genital tubercle (Fig. 19-5A). With division of the cloacal membrane into anal and urogenital membranes, the cloacal folds become

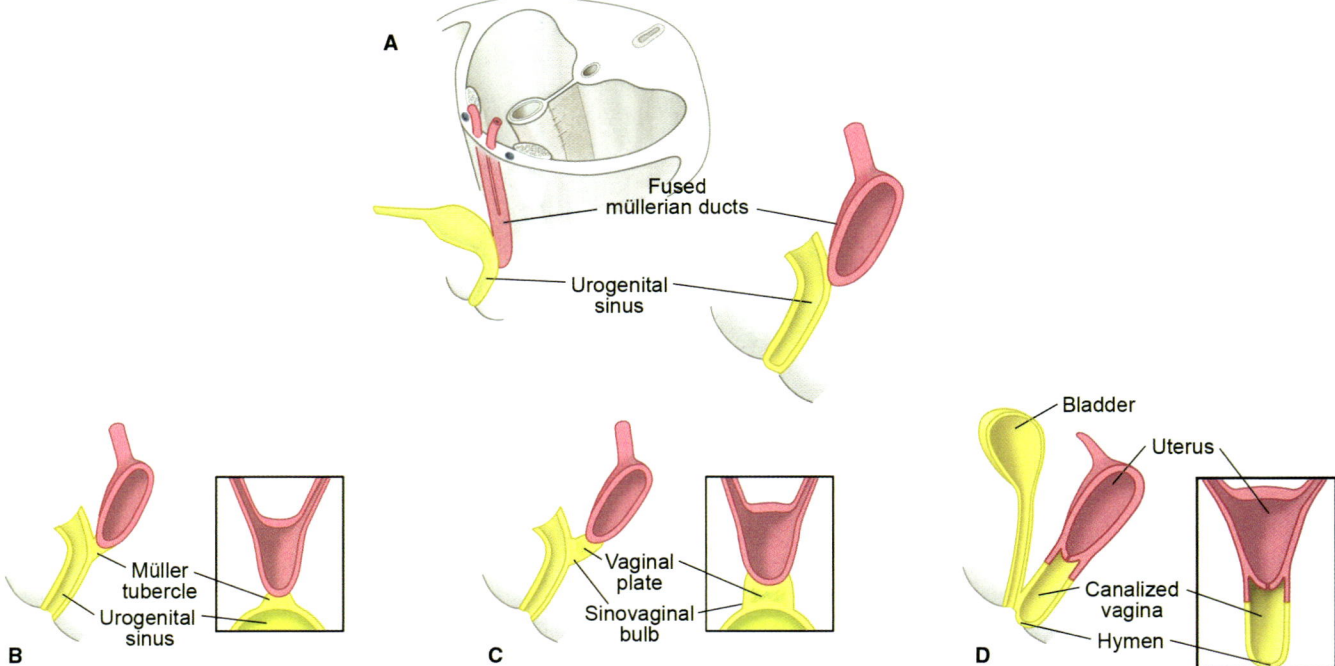

FIGURE 19-4 Development of the lower female reproductive tract. **A.** The fused müllerian ducts join the urogenital sinus at the Müller tubercle. **B.** From the urogenital sinus, the sinovaginal bulbs evaginate and proliferate cranially to create the vaginal plate **(C)**. **D.** Lengthening of the vaginal plate and canalization leads to development of the lower vagina. The upper vagina develops from the caudal end of the fused müllerian ducts. (Reproduced with permission from Kim Hoggatt-Krumwiede, MA.)

Indifferent stages

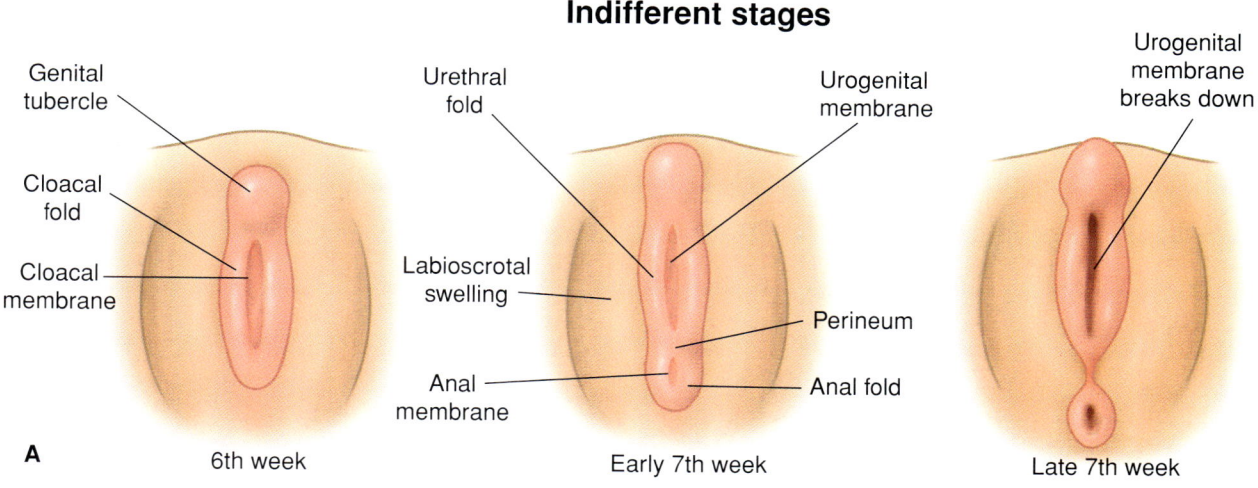

A   6th week   Early 7th week   Late 7th week

Differentiation

FIGURE 19-5 Development of the external genitalia. **A.** Indifferent stage. **B.** Virilization of external genitalia. **C.** Feminization.

the anal and urethral folds, respectively. Lateral to the urethral folds, genital swellings arise, and these become the labioscrotal folds. Between the urethral folds, the urogenital sinus extends onto the surface of the enlarging genital tubercle to form the urethral groove. By week 7, the urogenital membrane ruptures, exposing the cavity of the urogenital sinus to amnionic fluid.

The genital tubercle elongates to form the phallus in males and the clitoris in females. However, one is not able to visually differentiate between male and female external genitalia until week 12. In the male fetus, DHT forms locally by the 5α-reduction of testosterone. DHT prompts the anogenital distance to lengthen, the phallus to enlarge, and the labioscrotal folds to fuse and form the scrotum. Sonic hedgehog (*SHH*) is a gene that regulates urethral tubularization in males at 14 weeks' gestation (Shehata, 2011). Specifically, DHT and *SHH* expression promote the urethral folds to merge and enclose the penile urethra (Fig. 19-5B). In the female fetus, without DHT, the anogenital distance does not lengthen, and the labioscrotal and urethral folds do not fuse (Fig. 19-5C). The genital tubercle bends caudally to become the clitoris, and the distal urogenital sinus becomes the vestibule of the vagina. The labioscrotal folds create the labia majora, whereas the urethral folds persist as the labia minora.

DISORDERS OF SEX DEVELOPMENT

Definitions

As evident from the prior discussion, differences in sex development may involve the gonads, internal duct system, or external genitalia. Rates vary and approximate 1 in every 1000 to 4500 births (Murphy, 2011; Ocal, 2011).

Formerly, disorders or differences in sex development (DSD) were subdivided as those: (1) associated with gonadal dysgenesis, (2) associated with undervirilization of 46,XY individuals, and (3) associated with prenatal virilization of 46,XX subjects. The nomenclature used to describe atypical sexual differentiation has evolved. Instead of the terms "intersex," "hermaphroditism," and "sex reversal," consensus recommends a new taxonomy based on the umbrella term *disorder of sex development (DSD)* (Lee, 2006). Proposed classification of DSDs are: (1) sex chromosome DSDs, (2) 46,XY DSDs, and (3) 46,XX DSDs (Table 19-2) (Hughes, 2006).

Other terms describe the abnormal phenotypic findings that can be found. First, some DSDs are associated with abnormal, underdeveloped gonads, that is, *gonadal dysgenesis*. With this, if a testis is poorly formed, it is called a *dysgenetic testis*, and if an ovary is poorly formed, it is called a *streak gonad*. In affected patients, the underdeveloped gonad ultimately fails, which is indicated by elevated gonadotropin levels. Another important clinical sequela is that patients bearing a Y chromosome are at high risk of developing a germ cell tumor in the dysgenetic gonad.

A second term, *ambiguous genitalia*, describes genitalia that do not appear clearly male or female. Abnormalities may include hypospadias, undescended testes, micropenis, or enlarged clitoris, labial fusion, and labial mass.

Last, *ovotesticular* defines conditions characterized by ovarian and testicular tissue in the same individual. It was formerly

TABLE 19-2. Disorders of Sex Development (DSD) Classification

Sex Chromosome DSD
45,X Turner[a]
47,XXY Klinefelter[a]
45,X/46,XY Mixed gonadal dysgenesis
46,XX/46,XY Ovotesticular DSD

46,XY DSD
Testicular development
    Pure gonadal dysgenesis
    Partial gonadal dysgenesis
    Ovotesticular
    Testis regression
Androgen production or action
    Androgen synthesis
    Androgen receptor
    LH/hCG receptor
    AMH

46,XX DSD
Ovary development
    Ovotesticular
    Testicular
    Gonadal dysgenesis
Androgen excess
    Fetal
    Maternal
    Placental

[a]And syndrome variants.
AMH = antimüllerian hormone; hCG = human chorionic gonadotropin; LH = luteinizing hormone.

termed *true hermaphroditism*. In these cases, the morphology of the paired gonads can vary, and options that may be paired include a normal testis, a normal ovary, a streak gonad, a dysgenetic testis, or an ovotestis. In the last, both ovarian and testicular elements are combined within the same gonad. The gonadal location varies from abdominal to inguinal to scrotal. With ovotesticular DSDs, the internal ductal system structure depends on the ipsilateral gonad and its degree of determination. Specifically, the amount of AMH and testosterone determines the degree to which the internal ductal system is masculinized or feminized. External genitalia are usually ambiguous due to inadequate testosterone.

Sex Chromosome Disorders of Sex Development
Turner and Klinefelter Syndromes

Sex chromosome DSDs typically arise from an abnormal number of sex chromosomes. Of these, Turner and Klinefelter syndromes are most frequently encountered. *Turner syndrome* is caused by de novo loss or severe structural abnormality of one X chromosome in a phenotypic female. It is the most common form of gonadal dysgenesis that leads to primary ovarian insufficiency.

TABLE 19-3. Characteristic Findings of Turner Syndrome

Height 142–147 cm	High-arched palate
Micrognathia	Hearing loss
Epicanthal folds	Webbed neck
Low-set ears	Absent breast development
Shield-like chest	Widely spaced areolae
Cubitus valgus	Short fourth metacarpal
Renal abnormalities	Autoimmune disorders
Aorta coarctation	Autoimmune thyroiditis
Diabetes mellitus	

Most affected fetuses are spontaneously aborted. However, in girls with Turner syndrome who survive, phenotype varies widely, but nearly all affected patients have short stature. This results from lack of one copy of the *SHOX* gene, which resides on the short arm of the X chromosome (Hutson, 2014). The classic stigmata of Turner syndrome are listed in Table 19-3. Of these, cubitus valgus is an elbow deformity that deviates the forearm greater than 15 degrees when the arm hangs at the side. Other Turner syndrome characteristics include cardiac anomalies (especially coarctation of the aorta), renal anomalies, hearing impairment, otitis media and mastoiditis, hypertension, achlorhydria, and autoimmune links to diabetes mellitus, celiac disease, and Hashimoto thyroiditis. This syndrome may be recognized in childhood. However, some patients are not diagnosed until adolescence, when they present with short stature, prepubertal female genitalia, and primary amenorrhea. The last two stem from gonadal failure. The uterus and vagina are normal and are capable of responding to exogenous hormones.

Those with a Turner variant have a structural abnormality of the second X chromosome or have a mosaic karyotype, such as 45,X/46,XX. Indeed, more than half of the girls with this syndrome have chromosomal mosaicism. Those with a Turner variant may exhibit some or all of the syndrome signs. Patients with mosaicism are more likely to have some pubertal maturation.

For adolescents with Turner syndrome and gonadal failure, hormonal treatment is needed to induce puberty, and several protocols are acceptable. The International Turner Syndrome Consensus Group recommends estradiol initiation at ages 11 or 12 years, the use of transdermal estradiol, and gradual dose increases over 2 to 3 years. Progesterone is added after 2 years of treatment or with onset of breakthrough bleeding (Gravholt, 2017).

Women with a Turner variant and remaining ovarian function will typically have rapidly declining fertility. For these individuals, controlled ovarian hyperstimulation coupled with oocyte cryopreservation is an option (Chap. 21, p. 468) (Gravholt, 2017).

Another sex chromosome DSD is *Klinefelter syndrome* (47,XXY), which occurs in 1 in 600 births or in 1 to 2 percent of all males. These tend to be tall, undervirilized males with gynecomastia and small, firm testes. They have significantly reduced fertility from hypogonadism due to gradual testicular cell loss that begins shortly after testis determination (Nistal, 2016). These men carry higher risks for germ cell

tumors, osteoporosis, hypothyroidism, diabetes mellitus, breast cancer, and cognitive and psychosocial problems (Aksglaede, 2013). The most common genotype of Klinefelter syndrome is XXY, although variants exist with differing numbers of X chromosomes.

Chromosomal Ovotesticular DSD

Several karyotypes can create a coexistent ovary and testis, and thus ovotesticular DSD is found in all three DSD categories (see Table 19-2). In the sex chromosome DSD group, ovotesticular DSD may arise from a 46,XX/46,XY karyotype. Here, an ovary, testis, or ovotestis may be paired. The phenotype mirrors that for ovotesticular DSDs in general (p. 412).

For others in the sex chromosome DSD group, ovotesticular DSD may develop from a chromosomal mosaic such as 45,X/46,XY. With this karyotype, a picture of *mixed gonadal dysgenesis* shows a streak gonad on one side and a dysgenetic or normal testis on the other. The phenotypic appearance ranges from undervirilized male to ambiguous genitalia to Turner syndrome stigmata.

■ 46,XY Disorders of Sex Development

Insufficient androgen exposure of a fetus destined to be a male leads to 46,XY DSD, formerly called *male pseudohermaphroditism*. The karyotype is 46,XY, and testes are frequently present. The uterus is generally absent as a result of normal embryonic AMH production by Sertoli cells. These patients are most often sterile from abnormal spermatogenesis and have a small phallus that is inadequate for sexual function. As seen in Table 19-2, etiology of 46,XY DSD may stem from abnormal testis development or from abnormal androgen production or action.

46,XY Gonadal Dysgenesis

This spectrum of abnormal gonad underdevelopment includes pure or complete, partial, or mixed 46,XY gonadal dysgenesis (see Table 19-2). These are defined by the amount of normal testicular tissue and by karyotype.

Of these, *pure gonadal dysgenesis* results from a mutation in *SRY* or in another gene with testis-determining effects (*DAX1*, *SF-1*, *CBX2*) (Hutson, 2014). This leads to underdeveloped dysgenetic gonads that fail to produce androgens or AMH. Formerly named *Swyer syndrome*, the condition creates a normal prepubertal female phenotype and a normal müllerian system due to absent AMH.

Partial gonadal dysgenesis defines those with gonad development intermediate between normal and dysgenetic testes. Depending on the percentage of underdeveloped testis, wolffian and müllerian structures and genital ambiguity are variably expressed.

Mixed gonadal dysgenesis is one type of ovotesticular DSD. One gonad is streak and the other is a normal or a dysgenetic testis. Of affected individuals, a 46,XY karyotype is found in 15 percent (Nistal, 2015). The phenotypic appearance is wide ranging as with partial gonadal dysgenesis.

Last, *testicular regression* can follow initial testis development. A broad phenotypic spectrum is possible and depends on the timing of testis failure.

Because of the potential for germ cell tumors in dysgenetic gonads and intraabdominal testes, affected patients routinely have been advised to undergo gonadectomy (Chap. 36, p. 758).

Abnormal Androgen Production or Action

In some cases, 46,XY DSD may stem from abnormalities in: (1) testosterone biosynthesis, (2) luteinizing hormone (LH) receptor function, (3) AMH function, or (4) androgen receptor action. First, as evident from Figure 16-5, (p. 339), the sex steroid biosynthesis pathway can suffer enzymatic defects that block testosterone production. Depending on the timing and degree of blockade, undervirilized males or phenotypic females may result. Potential defective enzymes include steroid acute regulatory protein (StAR), cholesterol side-chain cleavage enzyme (P450scc), 3β-hydroxysteroid dehydrogenase type II, 17α-hydroxylase/17,20 desmolase (P450c17a), and 17β-hydroxysteroid dehydrogenase. The last two enzyme deficiencies can also cause congenital adrenal hyperplasia, and hypertension is a common feature in P450c17a deficiency. In addition to these central enzymatic defects, peripherally, abnormal 5α-reductase type 2 enzyme action leads to impaired conversion of testosterone to DHT. DHT is the active androgen in peripheral tissues, and undervirilization results.

Second, hCG/LH receptor abnormalities within the testes can lead to Leydig cell aplasia/hypoplasia and impaired testosterone production. In contrast, disorders of AMH and AMH receptors result in *persistent müllerian duct syndrome (PMDS)*. Affected patients appear as males but have a persistent uterus and fallopian tubes due to failed AMH action.

Last, the androgen receptor may be defective and result in androgen insensitivity syndrome (AIS). The estimated incidence of AIS ranges from 1 in 13,000 to 1 in 41,000 live births (Bangsboll, 1992; Blackless, 2000). Mutations produce a nonfunctional receptor that will not bind androgen or is unable to initiate full transcription once bound. As a result, resistance to androgens may be complete and female external genitalia are found. Alternatively, an incomplete form is associated with varying degrees of virilization and genital ambiguity. Milder forms of AIS have been described in men with severe male factor infertility and poor virilization.

Patients with complete androgen-insensitivity syndrome (CAIS) appear as phenotypically normal females at birth. They often present at puberty with primary amenorrhea. More recently, individuals may be identified when prenatal genetic testing does not match the phenotypic appearance during antenatal ultrasound or at birth. External genitalia appear normal; scant or absent pubic and axillary hair are noted; the vagina is shortened; and the uterus and fallopian tubes are absent. However, these girls develop breasts during pubertal maturation due to abundant androgen-to-estrogen conversion. Testes may be palpable in the labia or inguinal area or may be found intraabdominally.

Prior recommendation for gonadectomy after puberty in females with CAIS has now come into question. Namely, gonads of affected individuals carry a relatively low risk of tumor development (gonadoblastoma and seminoma), and these tumors tend to be easily treated (Patel, 2016). Moreover, in affected individuals, gonadectomy leads to perceived adverse symptoms. Preventively, no evidence-based protocol adequately monitors retained gonads for the development of tumor (Chavhan, 2008). If gonadectomy is undertaken, estrogen is replaced to reach physiologic levels, and a functional vagina created either by serial mechanical dilation or by surgical vaginoplasty. Adequate estrogen replacement in these patients maintains breast development and bone mass and provides relief from vasomotor symptoms.

■ 46,XX Disorders of Sex Development

As seen in Table 19-2, etiology of 46,XX DSD may stem from abnormal ovarian development or from excess androgen exposure.

Abnormal Ovarian Development

Disorders of ovarian development in those with a 46,XX complement include: (1) gonadal dysgenesis, (2) testicular DSD, and (3) ovotesticular DSD. With *46,XX gonadal dysgenesis*, streak gonads develop similar to Turner syndrome. These lead to hypogonadism, prepubertal normal female genitalia, and normal müllerian structures. However, other Turner stigmata are absent.

With *46,XX testicular DSD*, several possible genetic mutations lead to testis-like formation within the ovary (streak gonad, dysgenetic testis, or ovotestis). Defects may stem from *SRY* translocation onto one X chromosome. In individuals without *SRY* translocation, other genes with testis-determining effects are most likely present or activated. These include *WNT4, RSPO1,* or *CTNNB1* gene defects or *SOX9* gene duplication (Ocal, 2011). *SRY* guides the gonad to develop along testicular lines, and testicular hormone function is near normal. Production of AMH prompts müllerian system regression, and androgens promote development of the wolffian system and external genitalia masculinization. Spermatogenesis, however, is absent due to a lack of certain genes on the long arm of the Y chromosome. These individuals are not usually diagnosed until puberty or during infertility evaluation.

With *46,XX ovotesticular DSD*, individuals possess a unilateral ovotestis with a contralateral ovary or testis, or bilateral ovotestes. Phenotypic findings depend on the degree of androgen exposures and mirror those for other ovotesticular DSDs (p. 412).

Androgen Excess

Discordance between gonadal sex (46,XX) and the phenotypic appearance of external genitalia (masculinized) may result from excess fetal androgen exposure. This was previously termed *female pseudohermaphroditism*. In affected individuals, the ovaries and female internal ductal structures such as the uterus, cervix, and upper vagina are present. Thus, patients are potentially fertile. The external genitalia, however, are virilized to a varying degree depending on the amount and timing of androgen exposure. The three embryonic structures that are commonly affected by elevated androgen levels or ovarian development disorders are the clitoris, labioscrotal folds, and urogenital sinus. As a result, virilization may range from modest clitoromegaly to posterior labial fusion and development of a phallus with a penile urethra. Degrees of virilization can be described by the Prader score, which ranges from 0 for a normal-appearing female to 5 for a normal, virilized male.

Fetal, placental, or maternal sources may provide the excessive androgen levels. Maternally derived androgen excess may come from virilizing ovarian tumors such as luteoma and Sertoli–Leydig cell tumor or from virilizing adrenal tumors. Fortunately, these neoplasms infrequently cause fetal effects because of the tremendous ability of placental syncytiotrophoblast to convert C_{19} steroids (androstenedione and testosterone) to estradiol via the enzyme aromatase (Mahendroo, 2018). As another source, drugs such as testosterone, danazol, norethindrone, and other androgen derivatives may cause fetal virilization.

Of fetal sources, exposure can also arise from fetal congenital adrenal hyperplasia (CAH) due to 21-hydroxylase deficiency from *CYP21* mutation. This is a frequent cause of virilization, and its incidence approximates 1 in 14,000 live births (White, 2000). Early antepartum maternal dexamethasone therapy can ameliorate virilization, however, this practice is controversial (New, 2012). Namely, unless preimplantation genetic testing is undertaken, a significant number of unaffected fetuses are treated to ameliorate one case of ambiguous genitalia (Speiser, 2018). In addition, androgen excess and ambiguous genitalia can be seen with fetal 11-beta hydroxylase and 3-beta hydroxysteroid dehydrogenase deficiencies, from *CYP11B1* and *HSD3B2* gene mutations, respectively (Fig. 16-5, p. 339). Mutations of the *POR* gene also can disorder steroidogenesis. Cytochrome POR is a protein that transfers electrons to important cytochrome P450 enzymes and steroidogenic enzymes. Severely affected female neonates with *POR* gene mutations are virilized because of defective aromatase activity and because of the diversion of 17-hydroxyprogesterone to DHT by a "backdoor" androgen pathway (Fukami, 2013).

Of placental sources, placental aromatase deficiency from fetal *CYP19* gene mutation causes an accumulation of placental androgen and underproduction of placental estrogens. Consequently, both the mother and the 46,XX fetus are virilized (Murphy, 2011).

■ Gender Assignment

At birth, gender assignment of the normal newborn usually involves a simple assessment of the external genitalia. Delivery of a newborn with DSD is a potential medical emergency. It also poses a psychosocial, diagnostic, medical, and possibly surgical challenge for a multispecialty medical team. For the unprepared obstetrician in the labor room, ambiguous external genitalia in a newborn can be a stressful situation, which if poorly handled, can create possible long-lasting psychosexual and social ramifications for the individual and family. Ideally, as soon as the neonate with ambiguous genitalia is stable, parents are encouraged to hold the child. The newborn is referred to as "your baby" and not as "it" or "he/she." When discussing ambiguous development, other suggested terms used include phallus, gonads, folds, and urogenital sinus to reference underdeveloped structures. The obstetrician explains that the genitalia are incompletely formed and emphasizes the seriousness of the situation and the need for rapid consultation and laboratory testing (Fig. 19-6). During family education, the

need for accurate determination of gender and sex of rearing is emphasized.

Because similar or identical phenotypes may have several etiologies, diagnosis of a specific DSD may require several diagnostic tools (Ocal, 2011). Neonatal evaluation interrogates: (1) the ability to palpate gonads in the labioscrotal or inguinal regions, (2) the ability to palpate uterus during rectal examination, (3) phallus size, (3) genitalia pigmentation, and (4) presence of other syndromic features. The newborn's metabolic condition is assessed, and hyperkalemia, hyponatremia, and hypoglycemia may indicate CAH. The mother is examined for signs of hyperandrogenism (Thyen, 2006).

Pediatric endocrinologists or ideally a multidisciplinary DSD team that includes a pediatric endocrinologist, geneticist, pediatric gynecologist, pediatric urologist, and psychologist or therapist is consulted as soon as possible. DSD evaluation incorporates hormone level measurement, imaging, cytogenetic studies, and in some cases endoscopic, laparoscopic, and gonadal biopsy. Sonography shows the presence or absence of müllerian/wolffian structures and can locate the gonads. This imaging is ideally performed shortly after birth. With this timing, maternal hormones have already enlarged neonatal müllerian structures, which renders them easier to visualize. Sonography also can identify associated malformation such as renal abnormalities. Genetic evaluation includes karyotyping, fluorescent in situ hybridization (FISH), and, more recently, specific molecular studies to screen for mutations or gene dosage imbalances.

The psychologic and social implications of gender assignment and those relating to treatment are important and require a multidisciplinary approach. The current intense debate on the management of patients with DSD focuses on four major issues. These are etiologic diagnosis, gender assignment, indications for and timing of genital surgery, and disclosure of medical information to the patient (Daaboul, 2001; de Vries, 2007). Discussions include the need for hormonal stimulation at puberty and potential later surgical reconstruction.

DEFECTS OF THE BLADDER AND PERINEUM

The bilaminar cloacal membrane lies at the caudal end of the germinal disc and forms the infraumbilical abdominal wall. Normally, an ingrowth of mesoderm between the ectodermal and endodermal layers of the cloacal membrane leads to formation of the lower abdominal musculature and the pelvic bones. Without reinforcement, the cloacal membrane may prematurely rupture. Bladder exstrophy is a complex and severe pelvic malformation due to premature rupture of this cloacal membrane and subsequent failure of the membrane to be reinforced by an ingrowth of mesoderm. Depending on the defect size and developmental stage at rupture, possible defects are bladder exstrophy, cloacal exstrophy, or epispadias.

Of these, bladder exstrophy is characterized by an exposed bladder lying outside the abdomen. Associated findings commonly include abnormal external genitalia and a widened symphysis pubis, caused by the outward rotation of the innominate bones. Stanton (1974) noted that 43 percent of 70 females with bladder exstrophy had associated reproductive tract

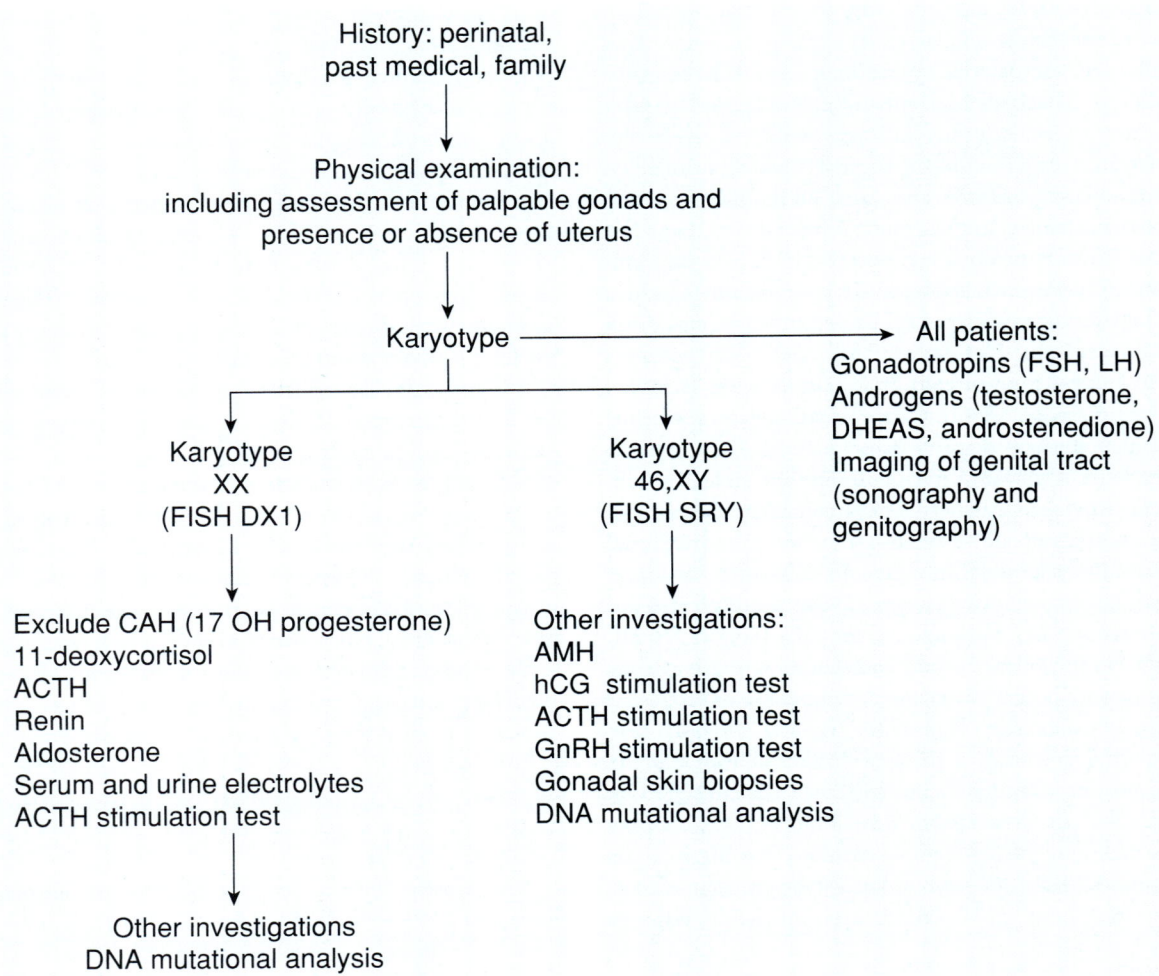

FIGURE 19-6 One algorithm for investigating disorders of sexual development. ACTH = adrenocorticotropic hormone; AMH = antimül-lerian hormone; CAH = congenital adrenal hyperplasia; DHEAS = dehydroepiandrosterone sulfate; FISH = fluorescent in situ hybridization; FSH = follicle-stimulating hormone; GnRH = gonadotropin-releasing hormone; hCG = human chorionic gonadotropin; LH = luteinizing hormone; SRY = sex-determining region of the Y.

anomalies. The urethra and vagina are typically short, and the vaginal orifice is frequently stenotic and displaced anteriorly. The clitoris is duplicated or bifid, and the labia, mons pubis, and clitoris are divergent. The uterus, fallopian tubes, and ovaries are typically normal except for occasional müllerian duct fusion defects.

A complex approach is required to achieve acceptable urinary continence and external genitalia reconstruction (Laterza, 2011). Staged surgical closure of the exstrophy is currently performed in the first 4 years of life (Massanyi, 2013). Vaginal dilation or vaginoplasty may be required to allow satisfactory intercourse in mature females (Jones, 1973). Long term, the defective pelvic floor may predispose women to uterine prolapse (Nakhal, 2012).

DEFECTS OF THE CLITORIS

Congenital abnormalities of the clitoris are unusual but include clitoral duplication, clitoral cysts, and clitoral enlargement from excess androgen exposure. Clitoral duplication, also known as

bifid clitoris, is rare and usually develops in association with bladder exstrophy or epispadias (Elder, 1992).

In those with epispadias, visibly apparent anomalies include a widened, patulous urethra; absent or bifid clitoris; flattened mons pubis; and labia that do not fuse anteriorly. Vertebral abnormalities and diastases of the pubic symphysis are also commonly associated. Female epispadias can be divided into three types—vestibular, subsymphyseal, and retrosymphyseal—which are differentiated by the type of urethral involvement (Schey, 1980). Female phallic urethra is another clitoral anomaly, and the phallic urethra opens at the clitoral tip (Sotolongo, 1983).

Epidermal cysts may be found on the clitoris, and inversion of epidermal cells beneath the dermis or subcutaneous tissue is the presumed pathogenesis. Cysts can reach 1 to 5 cm in diameter. Surgical removal of the cyst is the preferred treatment. Vasculature and nerve supply preservation during this procedure is important to sexual health (Johnson, 2013).

Clitoral enlargement noted at birth is suggestive of fetal exposure to excessive androgens. However, it simply may reflect ethnic variation (Jarrett, 2015; Phillip, 1996). In addition, in premature neonates, the clitoris may appear large, but it does not change size and appears to regress as the infant grows. Other causes of newborn clitoromegaly include breech presentation with vulvar swelling, chronic severe vulvovaginitis, and neurofibromatosis (Dershwitz, 1984; Greer, 1981).

For individuals with DSD, clitoral reduction surgery is currently very controversial and has been declared a form of torture by the United Nations (2013). Furthermore, Human Rights Watch (2017) has urged a moratorium on such surgeries. No evidence-based research supports early surgery compared with surgery performed once the individual can make an informed decision. If surgery is performed, it should be done by skilled pediatric urologists, and preservation of vasculature and nerve supply is essential.

HYMENEAL DEFECTS

The hymen is the membranous vestige of the junction between the sinovaginal bulbs and the urogenital sinus (see Fig. 19-4). It generally perforates during fetal life to establish a connection between the vaginal lumen and the perineum. Various hymeneal abnormalities include imperforate, microperforate, annular, septate, cribriform (sievelike), naviculate (boatlike), or septate types (Fig. 19-7) (Breech, 1999). Imperforate hymen follows failure of the inferior end of the vaginal plate to canalize, and its incidence approximates 1 in 1000 to 2000 females (Parazzini, 1990). Although typically sporadic, imperforate hymen in multiple family members has been reported (Stelling, 2000; Usta, 1993).

If the hymen is imperforate, blood from endometrial sloughing or mucus accumulates in the vagina. During the neonatal period, significant amounts of mucus can be secreted secondary to maternal estradiol stimulation. The newborn may have a bulging, translucent yellow-gray mass at the vaginal introitus. This condition is termed hydro/mucocolpos. Most cases are asymptomatic and resolve as the mucus is reabsorbed and estrogen levels decline. However, large hydro/mucocolpos may cause respiratory distress or may obstruct the ureters, resulting in hydronephrosis or life-threatening acute renal failure (Breech, 2009; Nagai, 2012).

After menarche, adolescents with imperforate hymen present with trapped menstrual blood behind the hymen, which creates a bluish bulge at the introitus. With cyclic menstruation, the vaginal canal greatly distends, and the cervix may dilate and allow formation of a hematometra and hematosalpinx. Cyclic pain, amenorrhea, abdominal pain mimicking acute abdomen, and difficulty with urination or defecation may be presenting symptoms (Bakos, 1999). Moreover, retrograde menstruation can lead to development of endometriosis. Other obstructive reproductive tract anomalies may present similarly. Indeed, without a bulging membrane, the clinical constellation instead may reflect a transverse vaginal septum or vaginal agenesis, which are not suitably treated by hymenectomy.

Patients with microperforate, cribriform, or septate hymen will typically complain of menstrual irregularities or difficulty with tampon placement or intercourse. Microperforate or imperforate hymen may be corrected when diagnosed and is illustrated in Section 43-17 (p. 978). Many advocate repair

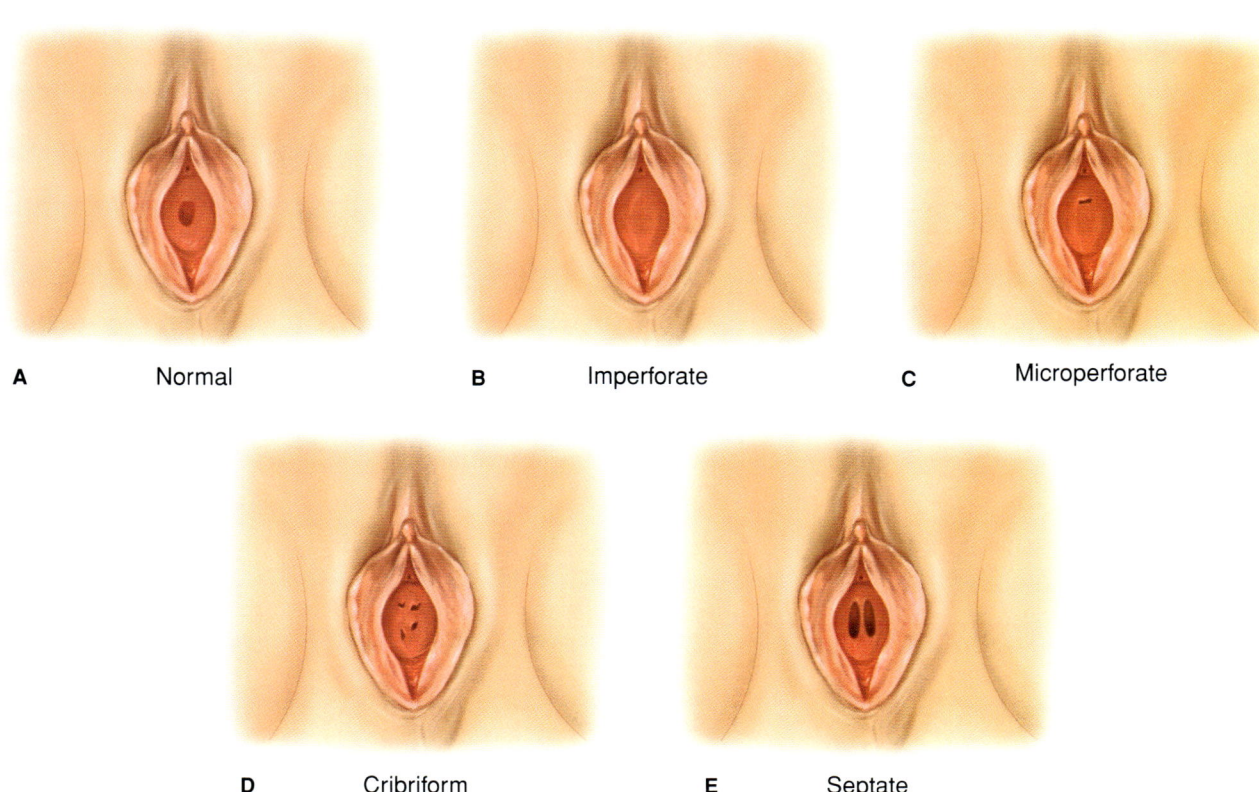

| A | Normal | B | Imperforate | C | Microperforate |

| D | Cribriform | E | Septate |

FIGURE 19-7 Types of hymens. **A.** Normal. **B.** Imperforate. **C.** Microperforate. **D.** Cribriform. **E.** Septate.

when estrogen is present to improve tissue healing, either in infancy or after thelarche, but before menarche. This timing avoids the formation of hematocolpos and possible hematometra. Importantly, clinicians should avoid needle aspiration of a hematocolpos for diagnosis or treatment. Aspiration may seed the retained blood with bacteria and raise infection risks. Moreover, recurrent hematocolpos secondary to inadequate drainage is common following needle aspiration alone.

Hymeneal cysts in the newborn must be differentiated from an imperforate hymen with hydro/mucocolpos (Nazir, 2006). These cysts typically are associated with a visible vaginal opening and may regress spontaneously (Berkman, 2004). They may also be treated by incision and drainage. Simple puncture also has been successfully performed.

TRANSVERSE VAGINAL SEPTUM

Transverse vaginal septa are believed to arise from failed müllerian duct fusion or failed canalization of the vaginal plate (Fig. 19-8) (Rock, 1982). The anomaly is uncommon, and Banerjee (1998) reported an incidence of 1 in 70,000 females. A septum may be obstructive, with mucus or menstrual blood accumulation, or nonobstructive.

Transverse vaginal septum can develop at any level within the vagina (Williams, 2014). Those in the upper vagina correspond to the junction between the vaginal plate and the caudal end of the fused müllerian ducts (see Fig. 19-4). Septal thickness may vary but typically is thin (1 cm). Thicker septa can measure 5 to 6 cm, and these tend to lie nearer the cervix (Rock, 1982).

In neonates and infants, obstructive transverse vaginal septum has been associated with fluid and mucus collection in the upper vagina. The resulting mass may be large enough to compress abdominal or pelvic organs. In addition, pyomucocolpos,

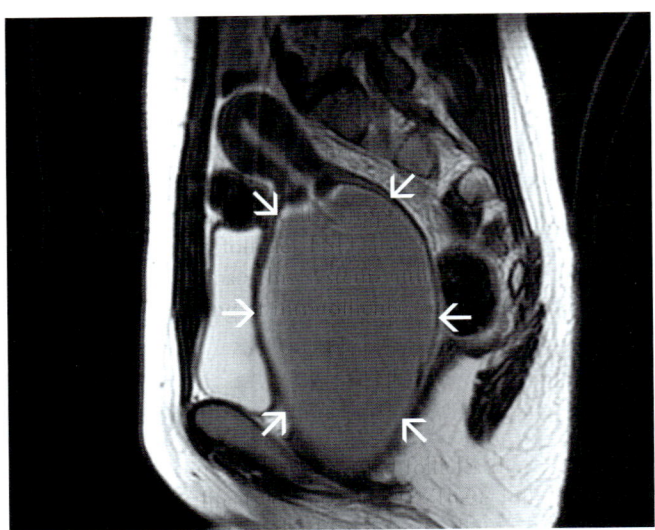

FIGURE 19-9 Magnetic resonance image of complete low transverse septum with obstruction. Marked hematocolpos is identified (*arrows*) in this 13-year-old female. The relatively low signal intensity on the T2-weighted images is consistent with subacute blood. The uterus is seen above the hematocolpos. (Reproduced with permission from Dr. Doug Sims.)

pyometria, and pyosalpinges may develop from ascension of vaginal or perineal bacteria through small septal perforations (Breech, 1999). In contrast to other müllerian duct defects, transverse vaginal septum is infrequently associated with urologic abnormalities.

Patients with transverse vaginal septum usually present with symptoms similar to those of imperforate hymen. The diagnosis is suspected when an abdominal or pelvic mass is palpated or when a foreshortened vagina and inability to identify the cervix is encountered. Diagnosis is confirmed by either sonography or magnetic resonance (MR) imaging. MR imaging is most helpful prior to surgery to determine the septal thickness and depth (Fig. 19-9). In addition, MR imaging may identify whether a cervix is present, and thereby help differentiate a high vaginal septum from cervical agenesis.

Surgical repair technique depends on septal thickness, and skin grafts or buccal mucosal grafts may occasionally be necessary to cover the defect left by excision of very thick septa. Smaller septa may be removed by excision followed by end-to-end anastomosis of the upper and lower vagina as described in Section 43-25 (p. 993).

LONGITUDINAL VAGINAL SEPTUM

A longitudinal vaginal septum results from defective lateral fusion or incomplete reabsorption of the caudal central portion of the müllerian ducts. These septa may be partial or extend the complete vaginal length. Longitudinal septa are generally seen with partial or complete duplication of the cervix and uterus. They may also accompany anorectal malformations. Renal abnormalities are common.

Affected individuals complain of difficulty with intercourse. Vaginal bleeding may occur despite placement of a tampon, because the tampon is placed in only one of the duplicated

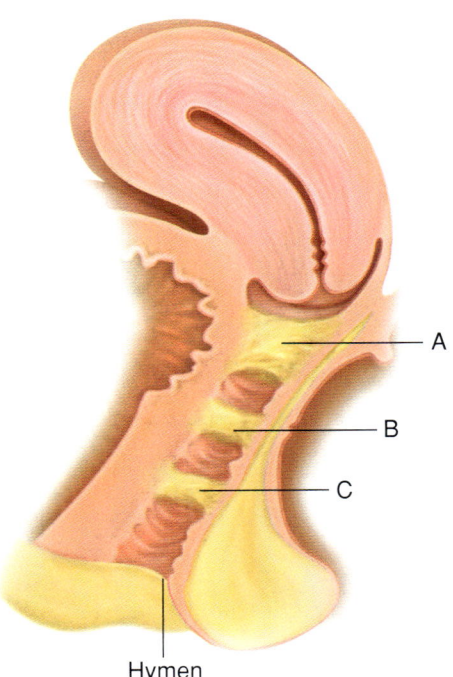

FIGURE 19-8 Potential locations of transverse vaginal septa are indicated and marked **(A–C)**.

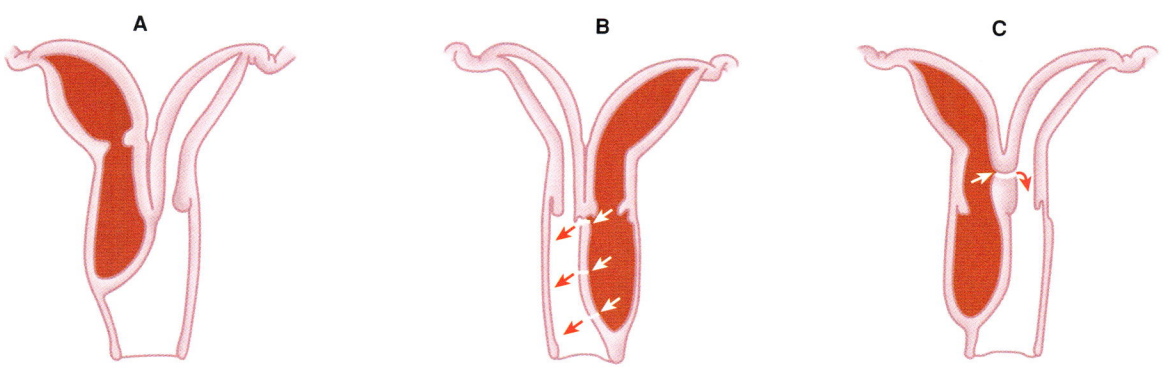

FIGURE 19-10 Uterine didelphys with obstructed hemivagina. **A.** Complete obstruction. **B.** Partial vaginal communication. **C.** Partial uterine communication.

vaginas. Nonobstructed forms can be managed conservatively unless dyspareunia develops. However, there are obstructive longitudinal vaginal septa (Fig. 19-10) (Rock, 1980). Typically, the patient presents in adolescence with normal menarche, but reports worsening, monthly unilateral vaginal and pelvic pain from outflow obstruction (Carlson, 1992). During examination, a patent vagina and cervix are noted, but a unilateral vaginal and pelvic mass can be palpated. Obstructed hemivagina is almost universally associated with ipsilateral renal agenesis. The triad of uterine didelphys, obstructed hemivagina, and ipsilateral renal anomaly is the OHVIRA syndrome, also known as *Herlyn-Werner-Wunderlich syndrome.*

Surgical correction of a longitudinal vaginal septum is described in Section 43-25 (p. 993). It consists of excision of the obstructing septum, taking precautions to avoid the urethra/bladder and rectum. With obstructive cases, sonographic guidance during excision can help identify the distended upper vagina (Breech, 2009).

CONGENITAL VAGINAL CYSTS

In each sex, the müllerian or wolffian ducts marked for degeneration normally do regress, but vestigial remnants can be found and may become clinically apparent. Thus, laterally located cysts may be mesonephric (wolffian) duct remnants. In contrast, the lower vagina derives from the urogenital sinus, which may give rise to congenital vestibular cysts (Heller, 2012).

Remnant cysts are typically located in the anterolateral wall of the vagina, although they may be found at various locations along its length. Most are asymptomatic and benign, measure 1 to 7 cm in diameter, and do not require surgical excision. Deppisch (1975) described 25 cases of symptomatic congenital vaginal cysts and reported a wide range of symptoms. These included dyspareunia, vaginal pain, difficulty with tampon use, urinary symptoms, and palpable mass. If these cysts become infected and intervention is required during the acute phase, cyst marsupialization is preferred.

Occasionally, a remnant cyst may cause chronic symptoms and warrant excision. Pelvic MR imaging can assist prior to surgery to determine the extent of the cyst and its anatomic relationship to the ureter or bladder base (Hwang, 2009). Of note, complete vaginal cyst excision may be more difficult than

anticipated, as some may extend up into the broad ligament and anatomically approximate the distal course of the ureter.

MÜLLERIAN ANOMALIES

Abnormalities of the uterus may be congenital or acquired and typically present with menstrual dysfunction, pelvic pain, infertility, or early pregnancy loss. Congenital anomalies have a heterogeneous genetic basis, and *WT1*, *Pax2*, *WNT2*, *PBX1*, and *HOX* genes are potentially involved (Hutson, 2014).

Various classification schemes for female reproductive tract anomalies exist, but the most commonly used system was proposed by Buttram and Gibbons (1979) and adapted by the American Society for Reproductive Medicine (former American Fertility Society, 1988). Within this system, six categories organize similar embryonic developmental defects (Fig. 19-11). Moreover, Acien (2009) and Rock (2010) have described types of uterovaginal and cervical malformations that do not adapt to the usual classification systems. Such anomalies are described and drawn in detail in a patient's medical record for future reference.

Most cases are diagnosed during evaluation for obstetric or gynecologic problems, but in the absence of symptoms, most anomalies remain undiagnosed. Because nearly 57 percent of women with uterine defects have successful fertility and pregnancy, the true incidence of congenital müllerian defects may be significantly understated. Nahum (1998) found that the prevalence of uterine anomalies in the general population was 1 in 201 women or 0.5 percent. Dreisler and colleagues (2014) found uterine anomalies in nearly 10 percent of 622 women from the general population undergoing saline-infusion sonography.

Anatomic uterine defects have long been recognized as a cause of obstetric complications. Recurrent pregnancy loss, preterm labor, abnormal fetal presentation, and prematurity constitute the major reproductive problems encountered. *Williams Obstetrics*, 25th edition provides a full discussion of specific müllerian abnormalities and their obstetric importance (Hoffman, 2018). Müllerian defects are also associated with renal anomalies in 30 to 50 percent of cases, and defects include unilateral renal agenesis, severe renal hypoplasia, horseshoe kidney, pelvic kidney, and ectopic or duplicate ureters (Sharara, 1998). Spinal anomalies have been reported in 10 to 12 percent of cases of müllerian anomaly and include wedge,

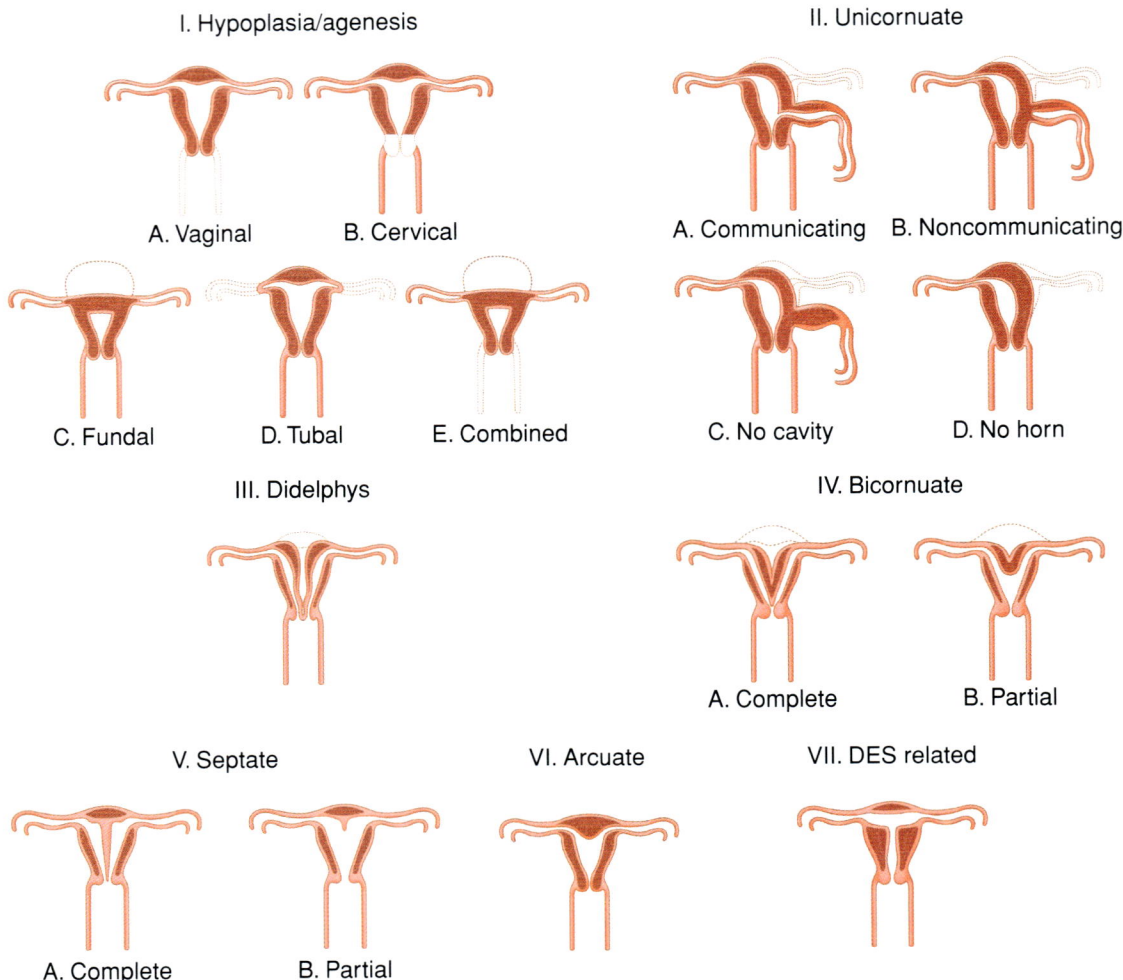

FIGURE 19-11 Classification of müllerian anomalies. (Reproduced with permission from American Fertility Society, Fertil Steril 1988 Jun;49(6):944–55.)

supernumerary, or asymmetric and rudimentary vertebral bodies (Kimberley, 2011). The combination of müllerian and renal aplasia and cervicothoracic somite dysplasia has been described as *MURCS association* (Duncan, 1979).

Depending on a woman's initial complaint, tools to diagnose müllerian anomalies may include hysterosalpingography (HSG), sonography, MR imaging, laparoscopy, and hysteroscopy. Each tool has limitations, but they may be used in combination to completely define anatomy. In women undergoing fertility evaluation, HSG is commonly selected for uterine cavity and tubal patency assessment. That said, HSG poorly defines the external uterine contour and can delineate only patent cavities.

With sonography, transabdominal views may help to maximize the viewing field, but transvaginal sonography (TVS) provides better image resolution. Saline-infusion sonography (SIS) improves delineation of the endometrium and internal uterine morphology, but only with a patent endometrial cavity. Three-dimensional (3-D) sonography can provide uterine images from virtually any angle. Thus, coronal images can be constructed and are essential in evaluating both internal and external uterine contours (Chap. 2, p. 41). Sonography is ideally completed during the luteal phase when the secretory endometrium provides contrast from its increased thickness and echogenicity (Caliskan, 2010). Investigators have reported good concordance between

3-D TVS and MR imaging of müllerian anomalies (Bermejo, 2010; Ghi, 2009).

MR imaging provides clear delineation of both the internal and external uterine anatomy and has a reported accuracy of up to 100 percent for evaluating müllerian anomalies (Fedele, 1989; Pellerito, 1992). Moreover, complex anomalies and commonly associated secondary diagnoses such as renal or skeletal anomalies can be concurrently evaluated.

Last, in some women undergoing an infertility evaluation, hysteroscopy and laparoscopy may be selected to assess for müllerian anomalies; screen for endometriosis, which is often coexistent; and exclude other tubal or uterine cavity pathologies (Puscheck, 2008; Saravelos, 2008).

■ Segmental Müllerian Hypoplasia or Agenesis

Some form of müllerian aplasia, hypoplasia, or agenesis affects 1 in every 4000 to 10,000 females and is a common cause of primary amenorrhea (American College of Obstetricians and Gynecologists, 2018). Uterine agenesis follows failed development of the lower portion of the müllerian ducts during embryogenesis and usually leads to absence of the uterus, cervix, and upper part of the vagina (Oppelt, 2006). Variants may display absence of the upper vagina but presence of the uterus. Normal ovaries are found, and affected individuals otherwise develop as phenotypically normal females and present with primary amenorrhea.

Vaginal Atresia

Females with vaginal atresia lack the lower portion of the vagina, but otherwise have normal pubertal maturation and external genitalia (see Fig. 19-11). Embryologically, the urogenital sinus fails to contribute its expected caudal portion of the vagina (Simpson, 1999). As a result, the lower portion of the vagina, usually one-fifth to one-third of the total length, is replaced by 2 to 3 cm of fibrous tissue. In some individuals, however, vaginal atresia may extend to near the cervix.

Since most affected women have normal external genitalia and upper reproductive tract organs, vaginal atresia does not often become apparent until menarche. Adolescents generally present shortly after physiologic menarche with cyclic pelvic pain due to hematocolpos or hematometra. On physical examination, the hymeneal ring is normal, and no bulging membrane is seen. Proximal to the ring, only a vaginal dimple or small pouch is found. A rectoabdominal examination confirms midline organs. Additionally, sonographic or MR imaging will display upper reproductive tract organs. Of options, MR imaging is the most accurate diagnostic tool, as length of the atresia, amount of upper vaginal dilation, and presence of a cervix can be identified. A cervix in such cases distinguishes vaginal atresia from müllerian agenesis. Laparoscopy, however, is often necessary when anatomy cannot be fully evaluated with radiographic studies. Treatment follows that for müllerian agenesis.

Cervical Agenesis

Women with congenital absence of the cervix typically also lack the upper vagina. The uterus, however, usually develops normally (see Fig. 19-11). In addition to agenesis, Rock (2010) has described various forms of cervical dysgenesis.

Women with cervical agenesis initially present similarly to patients with other reproductive tract obstructive anomalies, that is, with primary amenorrhea and cyclic pelvic pain. If a functional endometrium is present, a patient may have a distended uterus, and endometriosis may develop secondary to retrograde menstrual flow. A single midline uterine fundus is the norm, although bilateral hemiuteri have also been described (Dillon, 1979).

Radiographic studies, sonography, and MR imaging aid anatomy delineation. If imaging demonstrates an obstructed uterus, hysterectomy has been recommended by some (Rock, 1984). Niver (1980) and others report creation of an epithelialized endocervical tract and vagina. However, significant morbidity, that includes infection, recurrent obstruction requiring hysterectomy, and death due to sepsis, has been reported with establishment of such a vaginal-uterine connection (Casey, 1997; Rock, 2010). Alternatively, conservative management with a gonadotropin-releasing hormone (GnRH) agonist or with combination oral contraceptive pills may be used to suppress retrograde menses and possible endometriosis until a patient is ready for reproduction options (Doyle, 2009). Thus, the uterus

may be retained for possible reproductive potential. Thijssen and associates (1990) reported a successful pregnancy using zygote intrafallopian tube transfer in a patient with cervical agenesis. Gestational surrogacy offers another viable option for these women.

Müllerian Agenesis

Congenital absence of both the uterus and vagina is termed *müllerian aplasia, müllerian agenesis,* or *Mayer-Rokitansky-Küster-Hauser syndrome (MRKH)*. In classic müllerian agenesis, patients have a shallow vaginal pouch, measuring only 1 to 2 inches deep. In addition, the uterus, cervix, and upper part of the vagina are absent. Typically, normal ovaries persist, given their separate embryonic source, and a portion of the distal fallopian tubes is present. Most patients with müllerian agenesis have only small rudimentary müllerian bulbs without endometrial activity. However, in 2 to 7 percent of women with this condition, active endometrium develops and patients typically present with cyclic abdominal pain (American College of Obstetricians and Gynecologists, 2018). In these cases, surgical excision of symptomatic rudimentary bulbs is required. With müllerian agenesis, traditional conception is impossible, but pregnancy may be achieved using oocyte retrieval, fertilization, and gestational surrogacy. Uterine transplantation also has resulted in successful live births (Brännström, 2015, 2018).

Evaluation for associated congenital renal or other skeletal anomalies is essential in individuals with müllerian hypoplasia or agenesis. As noted, approximately 15 to 36 percent of women with uterine agenesis also have defects of the urinary system, and 12 percent may have scoliosis. Skeletal malformations observed include spina bifida, sacralization (partial fusion of L5 to the sacrum), sacral bone lumbarization (nonfusion of the first and second sacral segments), and cervical vertebral anomalies. Noted earlier, MURCS syndrome displays müllerian duct aplasia, renal aplasia, and cervicothoracic somite dysplasia (Oppelt, 2006). Cardiac and neurologic abnormalities are less common but include ventricular septal defects and unilateral hearing problems.

Treatment. One treatment goal for most affected women is creation of a functional vagina. This may be accomplished conservatively or surgically. Of the several conservative approaches, each attempts to progressively invaginate the vaginal dimple to create a canal of adequate size. Graduated hard glass dilators were initially recommended by Frank (1938). Ingram (1981) modified the Frank method by affixing the dilators to a bicycle seat mounted upon a stool. This affords patients hand mobility for other activities during the 30 minutes to 2 hours spent each day for passive dilation (American College of Obstetricians and Gynecologists, 2018). Currently, firm silicon dilators are available through several medical vendors and commercially available vibrating dilators are recommended by some providers. The involvement of a pelvic floor physical therapist may assist the patient in comfortably performing dilation herself (Patel, 2018). A vagina may also be created with repeated coitus. Overall, vaginal dilation techniques are successful in forming a functional vagina in 90 percent of cases (Croak, 2003; Roberts, 2001).

Surgical procedures are a more immediate solution to neovagina creation, and several are available. The Vecchietti procedure places a dilating sphere at the vaginal dimple. The sphere is attached to two wires, which are guided through the potential neovaginal space and subsequently follow an extraperitoneal course along the inner abdominal wall. Illustrated in Section 43-26 (p. 995), the wires then exit onto the lower abdomen. Here, they are placed on continuous tension, which is increased daily to stretch the vagina over approximately 1 week (Vecchietti, 1965).

Another method used commonly by gynecologists is the McIndoe vaginoplasty (McIndoe, 1950). Illustrated in Section 43-26 (p. 995), a canal is created within the connective tissue between the bladder and rectum. A split-thickness skin graft obtained from the patient's buttocks or thigh is then used to line the neovagina.

Modifications of the McIndoe procedure use buccal mucosa, human amnion, musculocutaneous flaps, or absorbable adhesion barriers to line the neovaginal space (Ashworth, 1986; Lin, 2003; Motoyama, 2003; Williams, 1964). Instead, Shears (1960) created the neovaginal space and allowed the space to epithelialize naturally. The Davydov procedure pulls pelvic peritoneum from the pelvis into the neovaginal space (Davydov, 1969).

All of these methods require a commitment to scheduled postoperative dilation to avoid significant vaginal stricture (Breech, 1999). Accordingly, these procedures only are considered if the patient is mature and willing to adhere to a postoperative regimen of regular intercourse or manual dilation with dilators.

To avoid these postoperative requirements, pediatric surgeons often use a segment of bowel to create the vagina. These colpoplasties use sigmoidal or ileal segments and require abdominal entry and bowel anastomosis. Many patients complain of a persistent vaginal discharge from the gastrointestinal mucosa.

■ Unicornuate Uterus

Failure of one müllerian duct to develop and elongate results in a unicornuate uterus. This anomaly is common, and Zanetti (1978) found an incidence of 14 percent in a series of 1160 uterine anomalies. With unicornuate uterus, a functional uterus, normal cervix, and normal round ligament and fallopian tube are found on one side. On the contralateral side, müllerian structures develop abnormally, and agenesis or more frequently a rudimentary uterine horn is identified (see Fig. 19-11). A rudimentary horn may communicate or more commonly not communicate with the unicornuate uterus. In addition, the endometrial cavity of the rudimentary horn may be obliterated or may contain some functioning endometrium. Active endometrium in a noncommunicating horn will eventually be symptomatic with cyclic unilateral pain and possibly with hematometra.

Women with a unicornuate uterus have a higher incidence of infertility, endometriosis, and dysmenorrhea (Fedele, 1987; Heinonen, 1983). On physical examination, the uterus is often markedly deviated, but imaging is frequently needed to further define horn anatomy (p. 420). Renal sonography is performed, because 40 percent of women with a unicornuate uterus also

have some degree of renal agenesis, usually ipsilateral to the anomalous side (Rackow, 2007). If anatomy is unclear, then MR imaging is selected to add information.

Women with unicornuate uterus have impaired pregnancy outcomes. A review of studies reveals a spontaneous abortion rate of 36 percent, a preterm delivery rate of 16 percent, and a live birth rate of 54 percent (Rackow, 2007). Other obstetric risks include malpresentation, fetal-growth restriction, fetal demise, and prematurely ruptured membranes (Chan, 2011; Reichman, 2009).

The pathogenesis of pregnancy loss associated with unicornuate uterus is incompletely understood. Reduced uterine capacity or anomalous distribution of the uterine artery is suggested (Burchell, 1978). Moreover, cervical incompetence may contribute to the risk for premature delivery and late-trimester abortion. Accordingly, a unicornuate uterus is suspected in any woman with a history of pregnancy loss, premature delivery, or abnormal fetal lie.

No surgeries are currently available to enlarge the unicornuate uterus cavity. Some obstetricians recommend prophylactic cervical cerclage, but adequate trials assessing outcome are lacking. Selection of a gestational surrogate may circumvent these anatomic limitations. Other patients, however, seem to carry their pregnancies longer with each subsequent gestation and may eventually reach fetal viability prior to labor.

Pregnancy may also occur in the rudimentary horn. In noncommunicating horns, this is thought to result from the intraabdominal transit of sperm from the contralateral fallopian tube. Pregnancy in a cavitary horn regardless of communication is associated with a high rate of uterine rupture, typically prior to 20 weeks (Rolen, 1966). Because of the high maternal morbidity secondary to intraperitoneal hemorrhage, excision of a cavitary rudimentary horn is indicated (Heinonen, 1997; Nahum, 2002). In many cases, this can be completed laparoscopically (Spitzer, 2009). Moreover, rudimentary horn pregnancy can be similarly treated in those with appropriate laparoscopic skills (Kadan, 2008).

If the rudimentary horn is obliterated, removal is not routinely recommended. Salpingectomy on the side with the obliterated rudimentary horn has been suggested to prevent ectopic pregnancy in women with a unicornuate uterus. However, the ectopic pregnancy risk is low.

■ Uterine Didelphys

A didelphic uterus results from failed fusion of the paired müllerian ducts. This anomaly is characterized by two separated uterine horns, each with an endometrial cavity and uterine cervix. A longitudinal vaginal septum runs between the two cervices in most cases. Heinonen (1984) reported that all 26 women with uterine didelphys in his series had a longitudinal vaginal septum. Occasionally, one hemivagina is obstructed by an oblique or transverse vaginal septum (see Fig. 19-10) (Hinckley, 2003). Uterine didelphys should be suspected if a longitudinal vaginal septum or if two separate cervices are discovered. Imaging is recommended to confirm the diagnosis.

Pregnancies develop in one of the two horns, and of the major uterine malformations, the didelphic uterus has a good

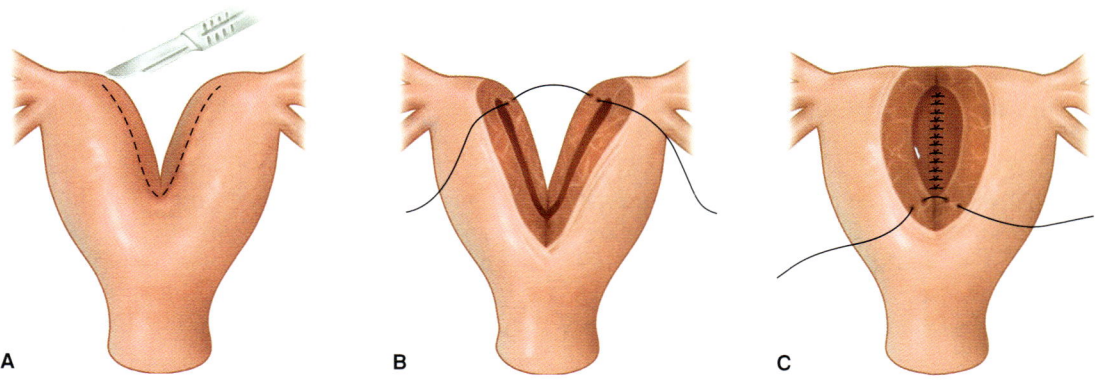

A   **B**   **C**

FIGURE 19-12 Strassman metroplasty is one of several techniques of bicornuate uterus repair. **A.** Excision of intervening uterine wall. **B.** Reapproximation of posterior uterine wall with a layer of myometrial sutures. **C.** Reapproximation of the anterior wall is closed similarly. Following placement of myometrial sutures, a layer of subserosal sutures is placed in the anterior and posterior walls.

reproductive prognosis. Compared with the unicornuate uterus, although the potential for uterine growth and capacity appears similar, uterine didelphys probably has an improved blood supply from collateral connections between the two horns. Alternatively, improved fetal survival may be secondary to earlier diagnosis, which favors more intensive prenatal care (Patton, 1994). Heinonen (2000) followed 36 women with uterus didelphys long term and found that 34 of 36 women (94 percent) who wanted to conceive had at least one pregnancy, and they produced 71 pregnancies. Of these pregnancies, 21 percent were spontaneously aborted, and 2 percent were ectopic. The rate for fetal survival was 75 percent; for prematurity, 24 percent; for fetal-growth restriction, 11 percent; for perinatal mortality, 5 percent; and for cesarean delivery, 84 percent. In this series, pregnancy located more often (76 percent) in the right horn than in the left. Because the spontaneous abortion rate mirrors that of women with normal uterine cavities, surgical procedures in response to pregnancy loss are rarely indicated. Thus, surgery is reserved for highly selected patients in whom repeated late-trimester losses or premature delivery has occurred with no other apparent etiology.

◼ Bicornuate Uterus

This anomaly is caused by incomplete fusion of the müllerian ducts. It is characterized by two separate but communicating endometrial cavities and a single uterine cervix. Failed fusion may extend to the cervix, resulting in a complete bicornuate uterus. It may be partial and cause a milder abnormality. Women with a bicornuate uterus can expect reasonable success— approximately 60 percent—in delivering a living child. As with many uterine anomalies, premature delivery is a substantial obstetric risk. Heinonen and colleagues (1982) reported a 28-percent abortion rate and a 20-percent incidence of premature labor in women with a partial bicornuate uterus. Women with a complete bicornuate uterus had a 66-percent incidence of preterm delivery and a lower fetal survival rate.

Radiologic discrimination of bicornuate and septate uteri can be challenging. However, it is important because a septate uterus is easily treated with hysteroscopic septum resection. Widely diverging horns seen during HSG may suggest a bicornuate

uterus. Namely, an intercornual angle >105 degrees suggests bicornuate uterus, whereas one <75 degrees indicates a septate uterus. However, fundal contour is not seen with HSG. Instead, 3-D sonography allows internal and external uterine assessment, and criteria for differentiating septate and bicornuate uteri are illustrated in Figure 2-25 (p. 42). Thus, sonography and HSG are acceptable imaging techniques for initial investigation. MR imaging may be indicated for complicated anatomy.

Surgical reconstruction of the bicornuate uterus may be considered in women with multiple spontaneous abortions in whom no other causative factors are identified. Strassman (1952) described the surgical technique that unified equal-sized endometrial cavities (Fig. 19-12). Two main disadvantages include required cesarean delivery to prevent uterine rupture in a subsequent pregnancy and the high rate of postoperative pelvic adhesion formation leading to subsequent infertility. Case series describe improved live-birth rates following metroplasty (Candiani, 1990; Lolis, 2005). However, in one series that had a small case-controlled group, metroplasty did not improve the live birth rate (Kirk, 1993). Given the lack of robust data and the attendant risk of uterine rupture, metroplasty is best reserved for women with recurrent pregnancy loss from no other identifiable cause.

◼ Septate Uterus

Following fusion of the müllerian ducts, failure of their medial segments to regress can create a permanent septum within the uterine cavity. Its contours can vary widely and depend on the amount of persistent midline tissue. The septum can project minimally from the uterine fundus or can extend completely to the cervical os. Septa also can develop segmentally, resulting in partial communications within the partitioned uterus (Patton, 1994). The histologic structure of septa ranges from fibrous to fibromuscular.

The true incidence of these anomalies is not known because they are usually detected only in women with obstetric complications. Although it does not predispose to higher rates of preterm labor or cesarean delivery, septate uterus is associated with a marked increase in spontaneous abortion rates

(Heinonen, 2006). Woelfer and colleagues (2001) reported a first-trimester spontaneous abortion rate for septate uterus of 42 percent. Moreover, early pregnancy loss is significantly more common with a septate than with a bicornuate uterus (Proctor, 2003).

This extraordinarily high pregnancy wastage likely results from partial or complete implantation on a largely avascular septum, from uterine cavity distortion, or from associated cervical or endometrial abnormalities. Septate uterus may rarely cause fetal malformation, and Heinonen (1999) described three newborns with a limb-reduction defect born to women with septate uterus.

Septate uterus can best be diagnosed with 3-D TVS, SIS, or MR imaging, because these display the uterine cavity and fundal contour (Chap. 2, p. 41) (American Society for Reproductive Medicine, 2016). If the presumptive diagnosis is a septate uterus, hysteroscopy can add information.

In women with recurrent pregnancy loss or infertility, hysteroscopic septum resection can improve live-birth rates and clinical pregnancy rates, respectively (Daly, 1983, 1989; DeCherney, 1983; Israel, 1984). Typically, operative hysteroscopy is combined concurrently with laparoscopic guidance or transabdominal sonographic surveillance to reduce the risk of uterine perforation (Section 44-16, p. 1065). Compared with abdominal metroplasty, hysteroscopic resection leads to higher live-birth rates, avoids mandatory cesarean delivery, and offers shorter convalescence, lower pelvic adhesion rate, and less operative morbidity (Fayez, 1986; Patton, 1994).

■ Arcuate Uterus

An arcuate uterus displays only mild deviation from normal uterine development. Anatomic hallmarks include a slight midline septum within a broad fundus, sometimes with minimal fundal cavity indentation. Most clinicians report no impact on reproductive outcomes. Conversely, Woelfer and colleagues (2001) found excessive second-trimester losses and preterm labor. Surgical resection is indicated only if excessive rates of pregnancy loss are encountered and other etiologies for recurrent spontaneous abortion have been excluded.

■ Diethylstilbestrol-Induced Reproductive Tract Abnormalities

Diethylstilbestrol (DES), a synthetic nonsteroidal estrogen, was prescribed to an estimated 3 million pregnant women in the United States from the 1940s through the early 1960s. The drug was prescribed to treat abortion, preeclampsia, diabetes, hot flashes, and preterm labor but was later found to be ineffective for these indications (Massé, 2009). Instead, Herbst and coworkers (1971) found that DES exposure in utero was linked to the development of a "T-shaped" uterus and an increased incidence of clear cell adenocarcinomas of the vagina and cervix. The risk of this vaginal malignancy approximates 1 in 1000 exposed daughters. Daughters also have higher risks of developing vaginal and cervical intraepithelial neoplasia, suggesting that DES exposure could affect gene regulation (Herbst, 2000). DES suppresses the *WNT4* gene and alters *Hox* gene expression

in mouse müllerian ducts. This provides a plausible mechanism for the uterine abnormalities, vaginal adenosis, and rarely, carcinoma observed in exposed patients (Massé, 2009).

During normal development, the vagina is originally lined by a glandular epithelium derived from the müllerian ducts. By the end of the second trimester, this layer is replaced by squamous epithelium extending up from the urogenital sinus. Failure of the squamous epithelium to completely line the vagina is termed *vaginal adenosis*. Typically appearing red and granular, its common symptoms include vaginal irritation, discharge, and intermenstrual bleeding—in particular, postcoital bleeding. Moreover, adenosis is frequently associated with vaginal clear cell adenocarcinoma.

Genitourinary malformations can follow in utero DES exposure and include those of the cervix, vagina, uterine cavity, and fallopian tubes. Transverse septa, circumferential ridges involving the vagina and cervix, and cervical collars ("cockscomb cervix") have been found. Women with cervicovaginal abnormalities are more likely to have uterine anomalies, such as smaller uterine cavities, shortened upper uterine segments, and "T-shaped" or irregularly shaped cavities (Barranger, 2002). Fallopian tube abnormalities include shortened and narrowed dimensions and absent fimbria. HSG remains the primary imaging tool for identification of these anomalies.

Males exposed to DES in utero can have structural abnormalities. Cryptorchidism, testicular hypoplasia, microphallus, and hypospadias have been reported (Hernandez-Diaz, 2002).

Women exposed to DES, in general, have impaired conception rates (Senekjian, 1988). Their reduced fertility is poorly understood but is associated with cervical hypoplasia and atresia. Of those who do conceive, the incidences of spontaneous pregnancy loss, ectopic pregnancy, and preterm delivery are higher, again particularly in those with associated structural abnormalities (Goldberg, 1999). Now, decades after DES use was halted, most affected women are past childbearing age, but higher rates of earlier menopause and breast cancer have been reported (Hatch, 2006; Hoover, 2011).

FALLOPIAN TUBE ANOMALIES

The fallopian tubes develop from the unpaired distal ends of the müllerian ducts. Congenital anomalies of the fallopian tube include accessory ostia, complete or segmental absence of the tube, and several embryonic cystic remnants. The remnants of the mesonephric duct in the female include a few blind tubules in the mesovarium, the *epoophoron*, and similar ones adjacent to the uterus, collectively called the *paroophoron* (see Fig. 19-2F) (Moore, 2013). The epoophoron or paroophoron may develop into clinically identifiable cysts. Remnants of the müllerian duct may be found along its embryologic course. The most common is a small, cystic structure attached by a pedicle to the distal end of the fallopian tube, the *hydatid of Morgagni* (Zheng, 2009).

Paratubal cysts are frequent incidental discoveries during gynecologic operations for other abnormalities or are found on sonographic examination (Chap. 10, p. 229). They may be of mesonephric, paramesonephric, or mesothelial origin. Most cysts are asymptomatic and slow growing and are discovered during the third and fourth decades of life. Large paratubal cysts found in adolescents are thought to derive from wolffian remnants and are associated with excess androgens (Dietrich, 2017).

In utero exposure to DES has been associated with various tubal abnormalities (p. 424). Short, tortuous tubes or ones with shriveled fimbria and small ostia have been linked to infertility (DeCherney, 1981).

OVARIAN ANOMALIES

A *supernumerary ovary* is an ectopic ovary that has no connection with the broad, uteroovarian, or infundibulopelvic ligaments (Wharton, 1959). This rare gynecologic anomaly may be located in the pelvis, retroperitoneum, paraaortic area, colonic mesentery, or omentum. Aberrant migration of part of the genital ridge after incorporation of germ cells describes one theory (Printz, 1973). The term *accessory ovary* describes excess ovarian tissue nearby and connected to a normally placed ovary. Wharton (1959) estimated that both accessory ovary and supernumerary ovary were rare but frequently associated genitourinary tract anomalies.

An absent ovary, with or without an associated tube, may result from congenital agenesis or from ovarian torsion with necrosis and reabsorption (Eustace, 1992; James, 1970). The incidence has been suggested to be approximately 1 in 11,240 women (Sivanesaratnam, 1986).

REFERENCES

Acien P, Acien M, Sanchez-Ferrer ML: Müllerian anomalies "without a classification": from the didelphys-unicollis uterus to the bicervical uterus with or without septate vagina. Fertil Steril 91(6):2369, 2009

Aksglaede L, Juul A: Testicular function and fertility in men and Klinefelter syndrome: a review. Eur J Endocrinol 168(4):R67, 2013

American College of Obstetricians and Gynecologists: Müllerian agenesis: diagnosis, management, and treatment. Committee Opinion No. 728, January 2018

American Fertility Society: The American Fertility Society classifications of adnexal adhesions, distal tubal occlusion, tubal occlusion secondary to tubal ligation, tubal pregnancies, müllerian anomalies and intrauterine adhesions. Fertil Steril 49(6):944, 1988

Arboleda VA, Sandberg DE, Vilain E: DSDs: genetics, underlying pathologies and psychosexual differentiation. Nat Rev Endocrinol 10(10):603, 2014

Ashworth MF, Morton KE, Dewhurst J, et al: Vaginoplasty using amnion. Obstet Gynecol 67(3):443, 1986

Ayhan A, Yücel I, Tuncer ZS, et al: Reproductive performance after conventional metroplasty: an evaluation of 102 cases. Fertil Steril 57(6):1194, 1992

Bakos O, Berglund L: Imperforate hymen and ruptured hematosalpinx: a case report with a review of the literature. J Adolesc Health 24(3):226, 1999

Banerjee R, Laufer MR: Reproductive disorders associated with pelvic pain. Semin Pediatr Surg 7(1):52, 1998

Bangsboll S, Qvist I, Lebech PE, et al: Testicular feminization syndrome and associated gonadal tumors in Denmark. Acta Obstet Gynecol Scand 71(1):63, 1992

Barranger E, Gervaise A, Doumerc S, et al: Reproductive performance after hysteroscopic metroplasty in the hypoplastic uterus: a study of 29 cases. BJOG 109(12):1331, 2002

Berkman DS, McHugh MT, Shapiro E: The other interlabial mass: hymenal cyst. J Urol 171(5):1914, 2004

Bermejo C, Martinez Ten P, et al: Three-dimensional ultrasound in the diagnosis of Müllerian duct anomalies and concordance with magnetic resonance imaging. Ultrasound Obstet Gynecol 35: 593, 2010

Blackless M, Charuvastra A, Derryck A, et al: How sexually dimorphic are we? Review and synthesis. Am J Hum Biol 12(2):151, 2000

Blaschko SD, Cunha GR, Baskin LS: Molecular mechanisms of external genitalia development. Differentiation 84(3):261, 2012

Brännström M, Dahm Kähler P, Greite R, et al: Uterus transplantation: a rapidly expanding field. Transplantation 102(4):569, 2018

Brännström M, Johannesson L, Bokström H, et al: Livebirth after uterus transplantation. Lancet 385(9968):607, 2015

Breech LL, Laufer MR: Müllerian anomalies. Obstet Gynecol Clin North Am 36(1):47, 2009

Breech LL, Laufer MR: Obstructive anomalies of the female reproductive tract. J Reprod Med 44(3):233, 1999

Burchell RC, Creed F, Rasoulpour M, et al: Vascular anatomy of the human uterus and pregnancy wastage. Br J Obstet Gynaecol 85(9):698, 1978

Buttram VC Jr, Gibbons WE: Müllerian anomalies: a proposed classification. (An analysis of 144 cases.) Fertil Steril 32(1):40, 1979

Caliskan E, Ozkan S, Cakiroglu Y, et al: Diagnostic accuracy of real-time 3D sonography in the diagnosis of congenital Mullerian anomalies in high-risk patients with respect to the phase of the menstrual cycle. J Clin Ultrasound 38(3):123, 2010

Candiani GB, Fedele L, Parazzini F, et al: Reproductive prognosis after abdominal metroplasty in bicornuate or septate uterus: a life table analysis. BJOG 97(7):613, 1990

Carlson RL, Garmel GM: Didelphic uterus and unilaterally imperforate double vagina as an unusual presentation of right lower-quadrant abdominal pain. Ann Emerg Med 21(8):1006, 1992

Casey AC, Laufer MR: Cervical agenesis: septic death after surgery. Obstet Gynecol 90(4 Pt 2):706, 1997

Chan YY, Jayaprakasan K, Tan A, et al: Reproductive outcomes in women with congenital uterine anomalies: a systematic review. Ultrasound Obstet Gynecol 38(4):371, 2011

Chavhan GB, Parra DA, Oudjhane K, et al: Imaging of ambiguous genitalia: classification and diagnostic approach. Radiographics 28(7):1891, 2008

Croak AJ, Gebhart JB, Klingele CJ, et al: Therapeutic strategies for vaginal müllerian agenesis. J Reprod Med 48(6):395, 2003

Daaboul J, Frader J: Ethics and the management of the patient with intersex: a middle way. J Pediatr Endocrinol Metab 14(9):1575, 2001

Daly DC, Maier D, Soto-Albors C: Hysteroscopic metroplasty: six years' experience. Obstet Gynecol 73(2):201, 1989

Daly DC, Walters CA, Soto-Albors CE, et al: Hysteroscopic metroplasty: surgical technique and obstetric outcome. Fertil Steril 39(5):623, 1983

Davydov SN: Colpopoeisis from the peritoneum of the uterorectal space. Akush Ginekok (Mosk) 45(12):55, 1969

DeCherney AH, Cholst I, Naftolin F: Structure and function of the fallopian tubes following exposure to diethylstilbestrol (DES) during gestation. Fertil Steril 36(6):741, 1981

DeCherney A, Polan ML: Hysteroscopic management of intrauterine lesions and intractable uterine bleeding. Obstet Gynecol 61(3):392, 1983

Deppisch LM: Cysts of the vagina: classification and clinical correlations. Obstet Gynecol 45(6):632, 1975

Dershwitz RA, Levitsky LL, Feingold M: Picture of the month. Vulvovaginitis: a cause of clitorimegaly. Am J Dis Child 138(9):887, 1984

de Vries AL, Doreleijers TA, Cohen-Kettenis PT: Disorders of sex development and gender identity outcome in adolescence and adulthood: understanding general identity development and its clinical implications. Pediatr Endocrinol Rev 4:343, 2007

Dietrich JE, Adeyemi O, Hakim J, et al: Paratubal cyst size correlates with obesity and dysregulation of the Wnt signaling pathway. J Pediatr Adolesc Gynecol 30(5):571, 2017

Dillon WP, Mudaliar NA, Wingate MB: Congenital atresia of the cervix. Obstet Gynecol 54(1):126, 1979

Doyle JO, Laufer MR: Mayer-Rokitansky-Kuster-Hauser (MRKH) syndrome with a single septate uterus: a novel anomaly and description of treatment options. Fertil Steril 92(1):391, 2009

Dreisler E, Stampe Sørensen S: Müllerian duct anomalies diagnosed by saline contrast sonohysterography: prevalence in a general population. Fertil Steril 102(2):525, 2014

Duncan PA, Shapiro LR, Stangel JJ, et al: The MURCS association: Müllerian duct aplasia, renal aplasia, and cervicothoracic somite dysplasia. J Pediatr 95:399, 1979

Elder J: Congenital anomalies of the genitalia. In Walsh PC, Retik AB, Stamey TA, et al (eds): Campbell's Urology. Philadelphia, Saunders, 1992, p 1920

Eustace DL: Congenital absence of fallopian tube and ovary. Eur J Obstet Gynecol Reprod Biol 46(2-3):157, 1992

Fayez JA: Comparison between abdominal and hysteroscopic metroplasty. Obstet Gynecol 68(3):399, 1986

Fedele L, Dorta M, Brioschi D, et al: Magnetic resonance evaluation of double uteri. Obstet Gynecol 74:844, 1989

Fedele L, Zamberletti D, Vercellini P, et al: Reproductive performance of women with unicornuate uterus. Fertil Steril 47(3):416, 1987

Frank RT: The formation of an artificial vagina without an operation. Am J Obstet Gynecol 141:910, 1938

Fukami M, Homma K, Hasegawa T, et al: Backdoor pathway for dihydrotestosterone biosynthesis: implications for normal and abnormal human sex development. Dev Dyn 242(4):320, 2013

Ghi T, Casadio P, Kuleva M, et al: Accuracy of three-dimensional ultrasound in diagnosis and classification of congenital uterine anomalies. Fertil Steril 92(2):808, 2009

Goldberg JM, Falcone T: Effect of diethylstilbestrol on reproductive function. Fertil Steril 72(1):1, 1999

Gravholt CH, Andersen NH, Conway GS, et al: Clinical practice guidelines for the care of girls and women with Turner syndrome: proceedings from the 2016 Cincinnati International Turner Syndrome Meeting. Eur J Endocrinol 177(3):G1, 2017

Greer DM Jr, Pederson WC: Pseudo-masculinization of the phallus. Plast Reconstr Surg 68(5):787, 1981

Hatch EE, Troisi R, Wise LA, et al: Age at natural menopause in women exposed to diethylstilbestrol in utero. Am J Epidemiol 164:682, 2006

Heinonen PK: Clinical implications of the didelphic uterus: long-term follow-up of 49 cases. Eur J Obstet Gynecol Reprod Biol 91(2):183, 2000

Heinonen PK: Clinical implications of the unicornuate uterus with rudimentary horn. Int J Gynaecol Obstet 21(2):145, 1983

Heinonen PK: Complete septate uterus with longitudinal vaginal septum. Fertil Steril 85(3):700, 2006

Heinonen PK: Limb anomalies among offspring of women with a septate uterus: a report of three cases. Early Hum Dev 56(2-3):179, 1999

Heinonen PK: Unicornuate uterus and rudimentary horn. Fertil Steril 68(2):224, 1997

Heinonen PK: Uterus didelphys: a report of 26 cases. Eur J Obstet Gynecol Reprod Biol 17(5):345, 1984

Heinonen PK, Saarikoski S, Pystynen P: Reproductive performance of women with uterine anomalies. An evaluation of 182 cases. Acta Obstet Gynecol Scand 61(2):157, 1982

Heller DS: Vaginal cysts: a pathology review. J Lower Genit Tract Dis 16(2):140, 2012

Herbst AL: Behavior of estrogen-associated female genital tract cancer and its relation to neoplasia following intrauterine exposure to diethylstilbestrol (DES). Gynecol Oncol 76(2):147, 2000

Herbst AL, Ulfelder H, Poskanzer DC: Adenocarcinoma of the vagina. Association of maternal stilbestrol therapy with tumor appearance in young women. N Engl J Med 284(15):878, 1971

Hernandez-Diaz S: Iatrogenic legacy from diethylstilbestrol exposure. Lancet 359(9312):1081, 2002

Hinckley MD, Milki AA: Management of uterus didelphys, obstructed hemivagina and ipsilateral renal agenesis. A case report. J Reprod Med 48(8):649, 2003

Hoffman BL: Congenital genitourinary abnormalities. In Cunningham FG, Leveno KJ, Bloom SL, et al (eds): Williams Obstetrics, 25th ed. New York, McGraw-Hill, 2018

Hoover RN, Hyer M, Pfeiffer RM, et al: Adverse health outcomes in women exposed in utero to diethylstilbestrol. N Engl J Med 365:1304, 2011

Hughes IA, Houk C, Ahmed SF, et al: Consensus statement on management of intersex disorders. J Pediatr Urol 2(3):148, 2006

Human Rights Watch: "I want to be like nature made me." Medically unnecessary surgeries on intersex children in the US. 2017. Available at: https://www.hrw.org/report/2017/07/25/i-want-be-nature-made-me/medically-unnecessary-surgeries-intersex-children-us. Accessed June 7, 2019

Hutson JM, Grover SR, O'Connell M, et al: Malformation syndromes associated with disorders of sex development. Nat Rev Endocrinol 10(8):476, 2014

Hwang JH, Oh MJ, Lee NW, et al: Multiple vaginal müllerian cysts: a case report and review of literature. Arch Gynecol Obstet 280(1):137, 2009

Ingram JM: The bicycle seat stool in the treatment of vaginal agenesis and stenosis: a preliminary report. Am J Obstet Gynecol 140(8):867, 1981

Israel R, March CM: Hysteroscopic incision of the septate uterus. Am J Obstet Gynecol 149(1):66, 1984

James DF, Barber HR, Graber EA: Torsion of normal uterine adnexa in children. Report of three cases. Obstet Gynecol 35(2):226, 1970

Jarrett OO, Ayoola OO, Jonsson B, et al: Country-based reference values and international comparisons of clitoral size in healthy Nigerian newborn infants. Acta Paediatr 104(12):1286, 2015

Johnson LT, Lara-Torre E, Murchison AM, et al: Large epidermal cyst of the clitoris: a novel diagnostic approach to assist in surgical removal. J Pediatr Adolesc Gynecol 26(2):e33, 2013

Jones HW Jr: An anomaly of the external genitalia in female patients with exstrophy of the bladder. Am J Obstet Gynecol 117(6):748, 1973

Kadan Y, Romano S: Rudimentary horn pregnancy diagnosed by ultrasound and treated by laparoscopy—a case report and review of the literature. J Minim Invasive Gynecol 15(5):527, 2008

Kenney PJ, Spirt BA, Leeson MD: Genitourinary anomalies: radiologic-anatomic correlations. Radiographics 4:233, 1984

Kimberley N, Hutson JM, Southwell BR, et al: Vaginal agenesis, the hymen, and associated anomalies. J Pediatr Adolesc Gynecol 25:54, 2012

Kirk EP, Chuong CJ, Coulam CB, et al: Pregnancy after metroplasty for uterine anomalies. Fertil Steril 59(6):1164, 1993

Laterza RM, De Gennaro M, Tubaro A, et al: Female pelvic congenital malformations. Part I: embryology, anatomy and surgical treatment. Eur J Obstet Gynecol Reprod Biol 159:26, 2011

Lee PA, Houk CP, Ahmed, et al: Consensus statement on management of intersex disorders. Pediatrics 118:488, 2006

Lin WC, Chang CY, Shen YY, et al: Use of autologous buccal mucosa for vaginoplasty: a study of eight cases. Hum Reprod 18(3):604, 2003

Lolis DE, Paschopoulos M, Makrydimas G, et al: Reproductive outcome after strassman metroplasty in women with a bicornuate uterus. J Reprod Med 50(5):297, 2005

MacLaughlin DT, Donahoe PK: Sex determination and differentiation. N Engl J Med 350(4):367, 2004

Mahendroo MM, Cunningham FG: Placentation, embryogenesis, and fetal development. In Cunningham FG, Leveno KJ, Bloom SL, et al (eds): Williams Obstetrics, 25th ed. New York, McGraw-Hill, 2018, p 103

Marshall FF: Embryology of the lower genitourinary tract. Urol Clin North Am 5(1):3, 1978

Massanyi EZ, Gearhart JP, Kost-Byerly S: Perioperative management of classic bladder exstrophy. Res Rep Urol 5:67, 2013

Massé J, Watrin T, Laurent A, et al: The developing female genital tract: from genetics to epigenetics. Int J Dev Biol 53(2-3):411, 2009

McIndoe A: The treatment of congenital absence and obliterative conditions of the vagina. Br J Plast Surg 2(4):254, 1950

Moore KL, Persaud TVN, Torchia MG: The urogenital system. In The Developing Human. Philadelphia, Saunders, 2013, p 245

Motoyama S, Laoag-Fernandez JB, Mochizuki S, et al: Vaginoplasty with Interceed absorbable adhesion barrier for complete squamous epithelialization in vaginal agenesis. Am J Obstet Gynecol 188(5):1260, 2003

Murphy C, Allen L, Jamieson MA: Ambiguous genitalia in the newborn: an overview and teaching tool. J Pediatr Adolesc Gynecol 24:236, 2011

Nagai K, Murakami Y, Nagatani K, et al: Life-threatening acute renal failure due to imperforate hymen in an infant. Pediatr Int 54(2):280, 2012

Nahum GG: Rudimentary uterine horn pregnancy. The 20th-century worldwide experience of 588 cases. J Reprod Med 47(2):151, 2002

Nahum GG: Uterine anomalies. How common are they, and what is their distribution among subtypes? J Reprod Med 43(10):877, 1998

Nakhal RS, Deans R, Creighton SM, et al: Genital prolapse in adult women with classical bladder exstrophy. Int Urogynecol J 23(9):120, 2012

Nazir Z, Rizvi RM, Qureshi RN, et al: Congenital vaginal obstructions: varied presentation and outcome. Pediatr Surg Int 22(9):749, 2006

New MI, Abraham M, Yuen T, et al: An update on prenatal diagnosis and treatment of congenital adrenal hyperplasia. Semin Reprod Med 30(5):396, 2012

Nistal M, Paniagua R, Gonzalez-Peramato P, et al: Gonadal dysgenesis. Pediatr Dev Pathol 18(4):259, 2015

Nistal M, Paniagua R, Gonzalez-Peramato P, et al: Perspectives in pediatric pathology, chapter 16. Klinefelter syndrome and other anomalies in X and Y chromosomes. Clinical and pathological entities. Pediatr Dev Pathol 19(4):259, 2016

Niver DH, Barrette G, Jewelewicz R: Congenital atresia of the uterine cervix and vagina: three cases. Fertil Steril 33(1):25, 1980

Ocal G: Current concepts in disorders of sexual development. J Clin Res Pediatr Endocrinol 3(3):105, 2011

Oppelt P, Renner SP, Kellermann A, et al: Clinical aspects of Mayer-Rokitansky-Kuster-Hauser syndrome: recommendations for clinical diagnosis and staging. Hum Reprod 21(3):792, 2006

Parazzini F, Cecchetti G: The frequency of imperforate hymen in northern Italy. Int J Epidemiol 19(3):763, 1990

Park SY, Jameson JL: Minireview: transcriptional regulation of gonadal development and differentiation. Endocrinology 146(3):1035, 2005

Patel V, Casey RK, Gomez-Lobo V. Timing of gonadectomy in patients with complete androgen insensitivity syndrome-current recommendations and future directions. J Pediatr Adolesc Gynecol 29(4):320, 2016

Patel V, Hakim J, Gomez-Lobo V, et al: Providers' experiences with vaginal dilator training for patients with vaginal agenesis. J Pediatr Adolesc Gynecol 31(1):45, 2018

Patton PE: Anatomic uterine defects. Clin Obstet Gynecol 37(3):705, 1994

Pellerito JS, McCarthy SM, Doyle MB, et al: Diagnosis of uterine anomalies: relative accuracy of MR imaging, endovaginal sonography, and hysterosalpingography. Radiology 183(3):795, 1992

Phillip M, De Boer C, Pilpel D, et al: Clitoral and penile sizes of full term newborns in two different ethnic groups. J Pediatr Endocrinol Metab 9(2):175, 1996

Printz JL, Choate JW, Townes PL, et al: The embryology of supernumerary ovaries. Obstet Gynecol 41(2):246, 1973

Proctor JA, Haney AF: Recurrent first trimester pregnancy loss is associated with uterine septum but not with bicornuate uterus. Fertil Steril 80(5):1212, 2003

Puscheck EE, Cohen L: Congenital malformations of the uterus: the role of ultrasound. Semin Reprod Med 26(3):223, 2008

Rackow BW, Arici A: Reproductive performance of women with müllerian anomalies. Curr Opin Obstet Gynecol 19(3):229, 2007

Reichman D, Laufer MR, Robinson BK: Pregnancy outcomes in unicornuate uteri: a review. Fertil Steril 91(5): 1886, 2009

Roberts CP, Haber MJ, Rock JA: Vaginal creation for müllerian agenesis. Am J Obstet Gynecol 185(6):1349, 2001

Rock JA, Jones HW Jr: The double uterus associated with an obstructed hemi-vagina and ipsilateral renal agenesis. Am J Obstet Gynecol 138(3):339, 1980

Rock JA, Roberts CP, Jones HW Jr: Congenital anomalies of the uterine cervix: lessons from 30 cases managed clinically by a common protocol. Fertil Steril 94(5):1858, 2010

Rock JA, Schlaff WD, Zacur HA, et al: The clinical management of congenital absence of the uterine cervix. Int J Gynaecol Obstet 22(3):231, 1984

Rock JA, Zacur HA, Dlugi AM, et al: Pregnancy success following surgical correction of imperforate hymen and complete transverse vaginal septum. Obstet Gynecol 59(4):448, 1982

Rolen AC, Choquette AJ, Semmens JP: Rudimentary uterine horn: obstetric and gynecologic implications. Obstet Gynecol 27(6):806, 1966

Ross AJ, Capel B: Signaling at the crossroads of gonad development. Trends Endocrinol Metab 16(1):19, 2005

Saravelos SH, Cocksedge KA, Li TC: Prevalence and diagnosis of congenital uterine anomalies in women with reproductive failure: a critical appraisal. Hum Reprod Update 14(5):415, 2008

Schey WL, Kandel G, Charles AG: Female epispadias: report of a case and review of the literature. Clin Pediatr (Phila) 19(3):212, 1980

Senekjian EK, Potkul RK, Frey K, et al: Infertility among daughters either exposed or not exposed to diethylstilbestrol. Am J Obstet Gynecol 158 (3 Pt 1):493, 1988

Sharara FI: Complete uterine septum with cervical duplication, longitudinal vaginal septum and duplication of a renal collecting system. A case report. J Reprod Med 43(12):1055, 1998

Shatzkes DR, Haller JO, Velcek FT: Imaging of uterovaginal anomalies in the pediatric patient. Urol Radiol 13(1):58, 1991

Shears BH: Congenital atresia of the vagina: a technique for tunnelling in the space between bladder and rectum and construction of a new vagina by a modified Wharton technique. J Obstet Gynaecol Br Emp 67:24, 1960

Shehata BM, Elmore JM, Bootwala Y, et al: Immunohistochemical characterization of sonic hedgehog and its downstream signaling molecules during human penile development. Fetal Pediatr Pathol 30(4):244, 2011

Simpson JL: Genetics of the female reproductive ducts. Am J Med Genet 89(4):224, 1999

Sivanesaratnam V: Unexplained unilateral absence of ovary and fallopian tube. Eur J Obstet Gynecol Reprod Biol 22(1-2):103, 1986

Sotolongo JR Jr, Gribetz ME, Saphir RL, et al: Female phallic urethra and persistent cloaca. J Urol 130(6):1186, 1983

Speiser PW, Arlt W, Auchus RJ, et al: Congenital adrenal hyperplasia due to steroid 21-hydroxylase deficiency: an Endocrine Society clinical practice guideline. J Clin Endocrinol Metab 103(11):4043, 2018

Spitzer RF, Kives S, Allen LM: Case series of laparoscopically resected noncommunicating functional uterine horns. J Pediatr Adolesc Gynecol 22(1):e23, 2009

Stanton SL: Gynecologic complications of epispadias and bladder exstrophy. Am J Obstet Gynecol 119(6):749, 1974

Stelling JR, Gray MR, Davis AJ, et al: Dominant transmission of imperforate hymen. Fertil Steril 74(6):1241, 2000

Strassman E: Plastic unification of double uterus. Am J Obstet Gynecol 64(1):25, 1952

Taylor HS: The role of HOX genes in the development and function of the female reproductive tract. Semin Reprod Med 18(1):81, 2000

Thijssen RF, Hollanders JM, Willemsen WN, et al: Successful pregnancy after ZIFT in a patient with congenital cervical atresia. Obstet Gynecol 76(5 Pt 2): 902, 1990

Thyen U, Lanz K, Holterhus PM, et al: Epidemiology and initial management of ambiguous genitalia at birth in Germany. Horm Res 66(4):195, 2006

United Nations: Report of the Special Rapporteur on torture and other cruel, inhuman or degrading treatment or punishment. 2013. Available at: https:// www.ohchr.org/Documents/HRBodies/HRCouncil/RegularSession/ Session22/A.HRC.22.53_English.pdf. Accessed June 7, 2019

Usta IM, Awwad JT, Usta JA, et al: Imperforate hymen: report of an unusual familial occurrence. Obstet Gynecol 82(4 Pt 2 Suppl):655, 1993

Vecchietti G: [Creation of an artificial vagina in Rokitansky-Kuster-Hauser syndrome]. [Italian] Actual Ostet Ginecol 11(2):131, 1965

Wharton LR: Two cases of supernumerary ovary and one of accessory ovary, with an analysis of previously reported cases. Am J Obstet Gynecol 78:1101, 1959

White PC, Speiser PW: Congenital adrenal hyperplasia due to 21-hydroxylase deficiency. Endocr Rev 21(3):245, 2000

Williams C, Nakhal R, Hall-Craggs M, et al: Transverse vaginal septae: management and long-term outcomes. BJOG 121(13):1653, 2014

Williams EA: Congenital absence of the vagina: a simple operation for its relief. J Obstet Gynaecol Br Commonw 71:511, 1964

Woelfer B, Salim R, Banerjee S, et al: Reproductive outcomes in women with congenital uterine anomalies detected by three-dimensional ultrasound screening. Obstet Gynecol 98(6):1099, 2001

Zanetti E, Ferrari LR, Rossi G: Classification and radiographic features of uterine malformations: hysterosalpingographic study. Br J Radiol 51(603):161, 1978

Zheng W, Robboy SJ: Fallopian tube. In Robboy SJ, Mutter GL, Prat J (eds): Robboy's Pathology of the Female Reproductive Tract. London, Churchill Livingstone, 2009, p 509

CHAPTER 20

Evaluation of the Infertile Couple

Infertility is defined as the inability to conceive after 1 year of unprotected intercourse of reasonable frequency. It can be subdivided into *primary infertility*, that is, no prior pregnancies, and *secondary infertility*, referring to infertility following at least one prior conception.

Conversely, fecundability is the ability to conceive, and data from large population studies show that a monthly probability of conceiving is 20 to 25 percent (Table 20-1) (Guttmacher, 1956; Mosher, 1991). In those attempting conception, more than 85 percent will be pregnant by 1 year.

Infertility is common and affects 10 to 15 percent of reproductive-aged couples. Of note, even without treatment, approximately half of women will conceive in the second year of attempting. According to the National Survey of Family Growth, the percentage of married women who reported infertility fell from 8.5 percent in 1982 to 6.0 percent in 2006 to 2010. In comparison, the percentage of women aged 15 to 44 years who had ever used infertility services rose from 9 percent

in 1982 to 12 percent in 2002 (Chandra, 2013, 2014). Rates of fertility measures for men and women remained similar from 2011 to 2015 (Martinez, 2018). Interpretation of these data is complicated by ongoing changes in marriage rates, intentional delays in childbearing, and socioeconomic and educational status changes. Nevertheless, well-publicized successes in infertility treatment now give patients greater hope that medical intervention can help them achieve their goal, and this has prompted them to seek evaluation and treatment in growing numbers.

Several factors result in substantial disparities in access to infertility care. Diagnosis of conditions in men may be delayed or missed due to social factors that hold the female primarily responsible for conception and childbearing. Also, infertility insurance coverage is unequal between the sexes (Chu, 2019; Dupree, 2016; Farland, 2016). In addition, marked disparities in access to fertility care have been noted for unmarried, homosexual, and transgender individuals. The ethical concerns raised by these discrepancies are addressed in several recent reports by the American Society for Reproductive Medicine (2013a, 2015a, d).

Most couples are more correctly considered to be *subfertile*, rather than infertile, as they will ultimately conceive if given enough time. This concept of subfertility can be reassuring. However, there are obvious exceptions, such as the woman with bilaterally obstructed fallopian tubes or the azoospermic male. In general, infertility evaluation is offered to any couple that has failed to conceive in 1 year. But, several scenarios may prompt earlier intervention. For example, delayed assessment in an anovulatory woman or a woman with a history of severe pelvic inflammatory disease (PID) may not be appropriate. Of particular note, fecundability is highly age-related. A significant decrease begins at approximately age 32 years, and a more rapid decline follows after age 37 (American Society for Reproductive Medicine, 2014a). This decline in conception rates is associated with a rise in poor pregnancy outcome rates, primarily due to higher aneuploidy rates. Thus, most experts agree that evaluation is considered after only 6 months in women older than 35 years.

Prior to initiating infertility treatment, a patient's health status is ideally optimized for an anticipated pregnancy. These issues are best addressed prior to referral to an infertility specialist whenever possible (American College of Obstetricians and Gynecologists, 2019). A complete list of preconceptional topics is provided later in this chapter and in Table 1-17 (p. 19).

Of note, accumulating data suggest that fertility status may be a marker of overall health in both men and women (Cedars, 2017). Phrased differently, the causes of infertility may be physiologically or genetically linked to somatic disorders either through association or by common pathophysiologic mechanisms. As a result, the infertility evaluation may allow early detection, prevention, and intervention for serious chronic diseases.

TABLE 20-1. Fecundity of Normal Couples Over Time

Time (months)	Couples Achieving Pregnancy (%)
1	20–36
3	57
6	72
12	85
24	93

ETIOLOGY OF INFERTILITY

Successful pregnancy requires a complex sequence that includes ovulation, ovum pick-up by a fallopian tube, fertilization, transport of a fertilized ovum into the uterus, and implantation into a receptive uterine cavity. With male infertility, sperm of adequate number and quality must be deposited at the cervix near the time of ovulation. Remembering these critical events can aid a logical evaluation and treatment strategy.

In general, infertility can be attributed to the female partner one third of the time, the male partner one third of the time, and both partners in the remaining one third. This approximation emphasizes the value of assessing both partners before instituting therapy. Although a complete investigation may not be required before instituting therapy if a clear etiology is present, strong consideration is given to finishing testing if pregnancy is not rapidly achieved. Estimates of the incidence of various causes of infertility are shown in Table 20-2 (American Society for Reproductive Medicine, 2006).

Both partners are urged to attend the initial consultation. This time provides an excellent opportunity to educate about the normal conception process and about methods to optimize their natural fertility. Such efforts may obviate the need for expensive and time-consuming interventions (American Society for Reproductive Medicine, 2017b). Couples are taught the concept of a fertile window for conception. The chance of conception is increased from the 5 days preceding ovulation through the day of ovulation (Fig. 20-1) (Wilcox, 1995). If the male partner has normal semen characteristics, a couple ideally has daily intercourse during this period to maximize the chance of conception. Although sperm concentrations will drop with greater coital frequency, this decline is generally too small to significantly lower the chance of fertilization (Stanford, 2002). Couples are also reminded to avoid oil-based lubricants, which are harmful to sperm. Many myths surround the ability to conceive. Examples, such as the importance of coital position and the need to remain horizontal following ejaculation, can add undue stress to an already stressful situation and should be dispelled.

MEDICAL HISTORY

■ Female History

Gynecologic

As with any medical condition, a thorough history and physical examination is critical (American Society for Reproductive Medicine, 2015b). Specifically, questions cover menstruation characteristics, prior contraceptive use, coital frequency, possible menopause symptoms, and infertility duration. Previous endometriosis,

TABLE 20-2. Etiology of Infertility

Male	25%
Ovulatory	27%
Tubal/uterine	22%
Other	9%
Unexplained	17%

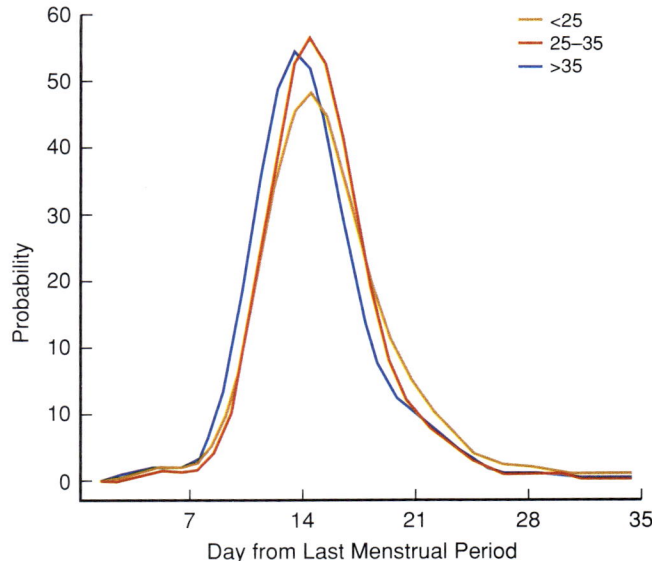

FIGURE 20-1 Day-specific probabilities of conception vary by age group. (Redrawn with permission from Stirnemann, 2013.)

recurrent ovarian cysts, leiomyomas, sexually transmitted diseases, or PID is also pertinent. Because prior conception indicates ovulation and a patent fallopian tube at some point, this history is sought. A prolonged time to conception may suggest borderline fertility and may raise the chance of determining an etiology. Pregnancy complications such as miscarriage, preterm delivery, retained placenta, postpartum dilation and curettage, chorioamnionitis, or fetal anomalies also are recorded. A coital history, including frequency and timing of intercourse, is obtained. Symptoms such as dyspareunia may point to endometriosis and a need for earlier diagnostic laparoscopy for the female partner.

Medical and Surgical

The medical history should seek symptoms of hyperprolactinemia or thyroid disease. Symptoms of androgen excess such as acne or hirsutism may point to polycystic ovarian syndrome (PCOS) or, much less commonly, congenital adrenal hyperplasia. Prior chemotherapy or pelvic irradiation may suggest ovarian failure. This is also an excellent opportunity to ensure that all indicated vaccinations are current, as several are contraindicated once pregnancy is achieved (American Society for Reproductive Medicine, 2018a).

Questions regarding medications include over-the-counter agents, such as nonsteroidal antiinflammatory drugs, that may adversely affect ovulation. In most instances, herbal remedies are discouraged. Women are encouraged to take a daily multivitamin with at least 400 µg of folic acid to lower the chance of neural-tube defects. In those with a previously affected child, 4 g is taken orally daily (American College of Obstetricians and Gynecologists, 2017d).

Previous abdominal surgeries, especially if linked to endometriosis or adhesion formation, can lower fertility. As examples, operations for ruptured appendicitis or diverticulitis raise suspicion for pelvic adhesive disease or tubal obstruction or both. Prior cervical conization can diminish cervical mucus and cervical competence. Past uterine surgery can predispose to pain, bowel obstruction, or intrauterine adhesions with resultant infertility. When planning surgery, reducing adhesion formation is a priority, and meticulous surgical technique and minimally invasive surgical approaches are favored. Surgical adhesion barriers, described in Chapter 40 (p. 855), lower postoperative adhesion rates. However, no strong evidence exists that their use improves fertility, diminishes pain, or lowers bowel obstruction rates (American Society for Reproductive Medicine, 2013b).

Social

A social history focuses on lifestyle factors such as eating habits. Of these, abnormalities in gonadotropin-releasing hormone (GnRH) and gonadotropin secretion are clearly related to body mass indices >25 or <17 (Grodstein, 1994a). An estimated 40 percent of women are obese, and most agree this incidence is rising (Hales, 2018). In these women, infertility is primarily related to a higher incidence of ovulatory dysfunction, but data also suggest that fecundity may be lowered by poorer oocyte quality and altered endometrial function (American Society for Reproductive Medicine, 2015e). Although difficult to achieve, even modest weight reduction in overweight women is correlated with normalized menstrual cycles and subsequent pregnancies. Surgically induced weight loss also has been reported to restore ovulation and menstrual regularity and chance of pregnancy, although continued study is needed (Table 20-3) (Consalvo, 2017; Pilone, 2019; Slopien, 2019).

Accumulating data suggest that cigarette smoking lowers fertility rates (American Society for Reproductive Medicine, 2018c). At least 15 percent of reproductive-aged men and women in the United States smoke cigarettes (Jamal, 2018). The prevalence of infertility is higher, and the time to conception is longer in women who smoke, or even those exposed passively to cigarette smoke. Moreover, smoking's negative effects on female fecundity do not appear to be overcome by assisted reproductive technology (ART) (Klonoff-Cohen, 2001). Toxins in the smoke can accelerate follicular depletion and increase genetic mutations in gametes or early embryos (Zenzes, 2000). Smoking has been linked to higher rates of miscarriage, abruption, fetal-growth restriction, and preterm labor (Dashe, 2018). Vasoconstrictive and antimetabolic properties of some cigarette smoke components such as nicotine, carbon dioxide, and cyanide may lead to placental insufficiency.

The effect of smoking on male fertility is more difficult to discern. Although smokers often have comparatively reduced sperm concentrations and motility, these often remain within the normal range.

Admittedly, current data do not prove causation, but only correlation, between smoking and infertility or adverse pregnancy outcomes. Nevertheless, smoking is discouraged for both male and female partners planning pregnancy. The desire for pregnancy can be a powerful motivator toward cessation (Augood, 1998). Education is the most important first step (Table 20-4). If needed, medical adjuncts such as nicotine replacement therapy, bupropion (Zyban), or varenicline (Chantix) may prove effective (Table 1-4, p. 9).

Alcohol consumption also should be limited. Heavy alcohol intake lowers fertility in women and has been associated with a decline in sperm counts and greater sexual dysfunction in men (Klonoff-Cohen, 2003; Nagy, 1986). A standardized alcoholic drink is typically defined as 12 ounces of beer, 5 ounces of wine, or 1.5 ounces of hard alcohol. Based on several studies, five to eight drinks per week negatively affects female fertility (Grodstein, 1994b; Tolstrup, 2003). As alcohol is also detrimental to early pregnancy, it is prudent to advise patients to avoid excessive alcohol consumption while trying to conceive.

Caffeine is one of the most widely used pharmacologically active substances in the world. Studies evaluating a potential relationship between caffeine and impaired fertility have varied in design and resulted in conflicting findings. One large prospective trial found no association between either total caffeine intake or coffee consumption and fecundability (Hatch, 2012). Despite this, recommendations of caffeine intake moderation in infertile women seem prudent.

Illicit drugs also may affect fecundability and pregnancy outcomes and should be strongly discouraged (American College of Obstetricians and Gynecologists, 2017c). Marijuana use has increased worldwide, and despite limited data, many in the public perceive that cannabis has no health risks (Chang, 2019; Keyhani, 2018). Reassuringly, a recent study found that time to pregnancy was not lengthened by marijuana use in either men or women (Kasman, 2018). However, in a study of 12 million births from 1999 to 2013 in the United States, neonates born to exposed mothers had a higher risk of premature rupture of membranes, prematurity, and intrauterine fetal demise (Petrangelo, 2019).

TABLE 20-3. Effects of Obesity and Environmental Factors on Fertility

Factor	Impact on Fertility
Obesity (BMI >35)	2-fold increase TTC
Underweight (BMI <19)	4-fold increase TTC
Smoking	1.6-fold increase RR
Alcohol (>2/day)	1.6-fold increase RR
Illicit drugs	1.7-fold increase RR
Toxins	1.4-fold increase RR
Caffeine (>250 mg/day)	45% decrease fecundability

BMI = body mass index; RR = relative risk of infertility; TTC = time to conception.

TABLE 20-4. Women's Awareness of Health Risks Associated with Smoking

Smoking Risk	Percentage Aware of Risk
Respiratory disease	99%
Heart disease	96%
Pregnancy complications	91%
Spontaneous abortion	39%
Ectopic pregnancy	27%
Infertility	22%
Early menopause	18%

Abbreviated from Roth, 2001, with permission.

Environmental Factors

Growing information suggests that some male and female infertility may result from environmental contaminants or toxins (Giudice, 2006). Endocrine-disrupting chemicals (EDCs) such as dioxins and polychlorinated biphenyls have been shown to be reproductive toxicants (Hauser, 2008; Mendola, 2008). Others include agricultural pesticides and herbicides, phthalates (used in making plastic materials), lead, and bisphenol A (used in the manufacture of polycarbonate plastic and resins). EDC exposure is implicated to underlie a broad range of women's reproductive disorders. Lower fecundability and lower birthweight show the most solid evidence for this correlation (Caserta, 2011). Although direct links to infertility in humans are not conclusive, clinicians should counsel patients that environmental exposures to toxic substances are avoided if possible. Currently, data should be discussed carefully to avoid alarm.

Ethnicity and Family History

The ethnic background and family history of both partners influences the need for preconceptional testing. A family history of infertility, recurrent miscarriage, or fetal anomalies may point to a genetic etiology that warrants genetic screening (p. 445). Although the inheritance pattern is complex, data suggest that both PCOS and endometriosis occur in familial clusters. For example, a woman carries an estimated sevenfold greater risk of endometriosis than that of the general population if a single first-degree family member has the disease (Moen, 1993).

■ Male History

Similar attention is paid to assessing the male partner's potential contribution to infertility (American Society for Reproductive Medicine, 2015c). Questions include pubertal development and

sexual function difficulties. Erectile dysfunction, particularly in conjunction with diminished beard growth, may suggest lower testosterone levels. Ejaculatory problems also are evaluated. This includes a search for developmental anomalies such as hypospadias, which could result in suboptimal semen deposition (Gray, 2018).

Sexually transmitted diseases or frequent genitourinary infections, including epididymitis or prostatitis, may lead to vas deferens inflammation and obstruction. Similarly, mumps in an adult can create testicular inflammation and damage spermatogenic stem cells (Beard, 1977). Moreover, prior cryptorchidism, testicular torsion, or testicular trauma may suggest abnormal spermatogenesis (Anderson, 1990; Cobellis, 2014). Compared with fertile males, males with unilateral or bilateral cryptorchidism have fertility rates of 80 percent and 50 percent, respectively (Lee, 1993). Although unclear, the relatively warm intraabdominal temperature may cause permanent stem cell damage. Alternatively, genetic abnormalities that led to the abnormal testis location may also affect sperm production.

A history of varicocele is also obtained. A varicocele consists of dilated veins of the pampiniform plexus of the spermatic cords that drain the testes. Varicoceles are believed to raise scrotal temperature, however, the negative effects of varicoceles on fertility are controversial (American Society for Reproductive Medicine, 2014b; Baazeem, 2011). Although 30 to 40 percent of men seen in infertility clinics are diagnosed with a varicocele, nearly 20 percent of men in the general population are similarly affected. If a varicocele is suspected, it should be evaluated by a urologist, preferably one with a specific interest in infertility. Current guidelines recommend against surgical repair of a nonpalpable, that is, subclinical varicocele for infertility. However, treatment for pain or other symptoms may be warranted (Kohn, 2018).

Spermatogenesis, from stem cell to mature sperm, takes nearly 90 days (Figs. 20-2 and 20-3). Thus, any detrimental event in

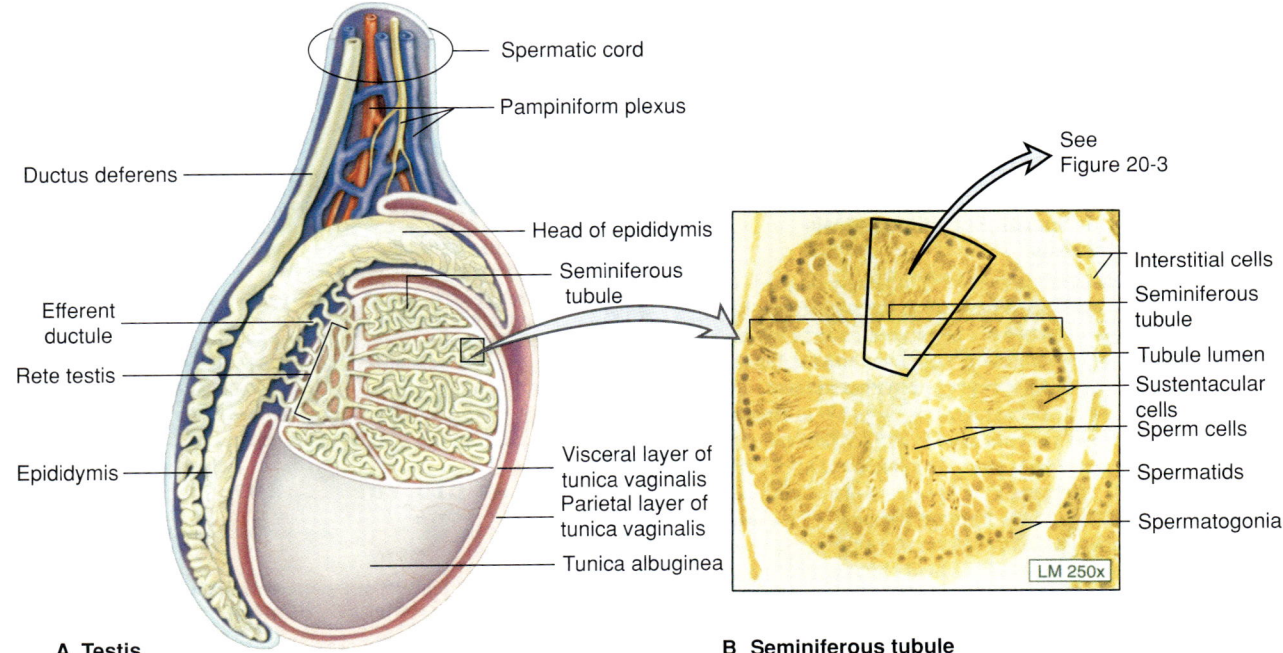

FIGURE 20-2 Male testis. **A.** Gross anatomy of a testis. **B.** Cutaway of the testis reveals the microscopic structure of a seminiferous tubule. (Reproduced with permission from McKinley, 2006.)

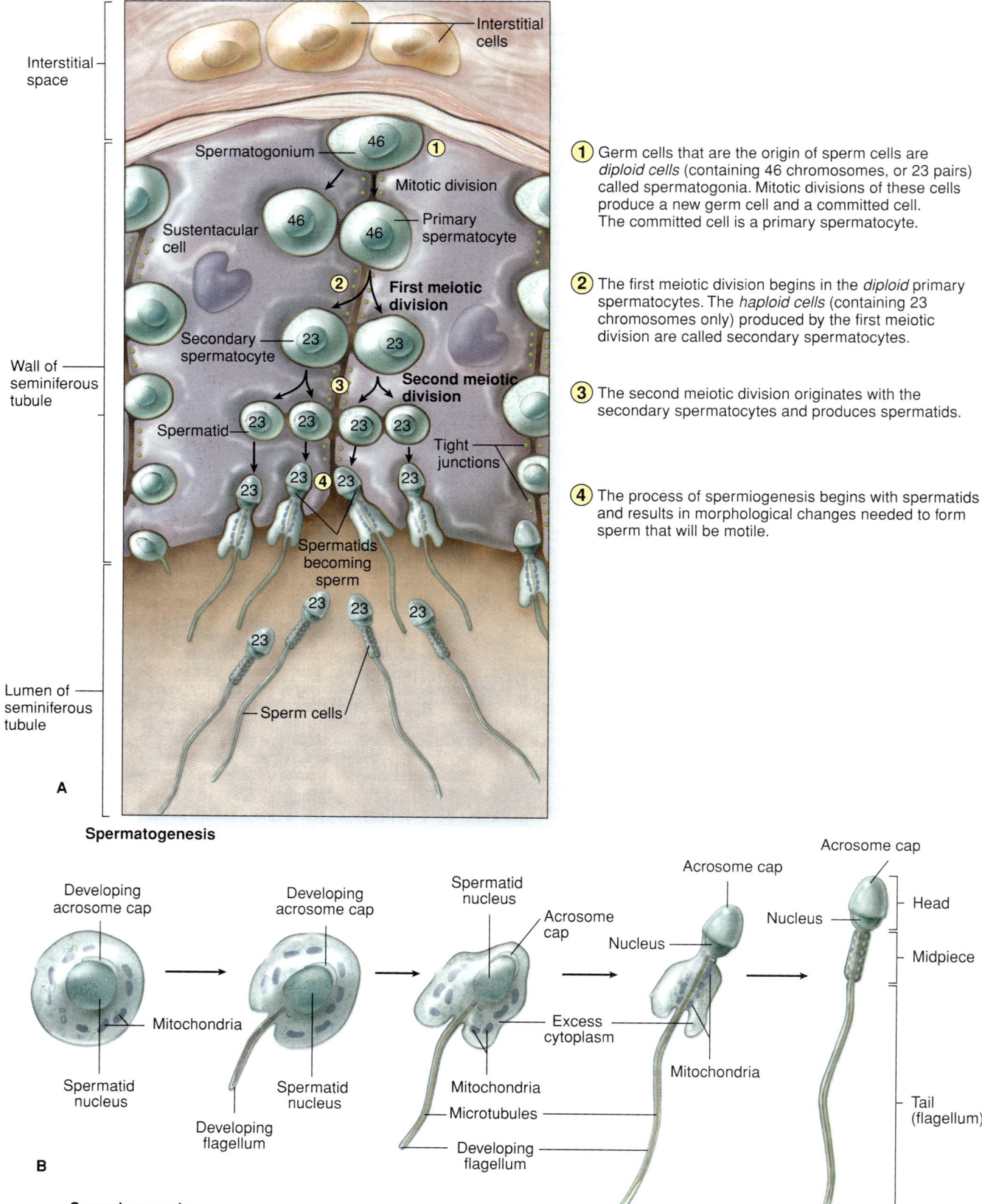

1 Germ cells that are the origin of sperm cells are *diploid cells* (containing 46 chromosomes, or 23 pairs) called spermatogonia. Mitotic divisions of these cells produce a new germ cell and a committed cell. The committed cell is a primary spermatocyte.

2 The first meiotic division begins in the *diploid* primary spermatocytes. The *haploid cells* (containing 23 chromosomes only) produced by the first meiotic division are called secondary spermatocytes.

3 The second meiotic division originates with the secondary spermatocytes and produces spermatids.

4 The process of spermiogenesis begins with spermatids and results in morphological changes needed to form sperm that will be motile.

FIGURE 20-3 Male testis. **A.** Cutaway of the seminiferous tubule shows the mitotic and meiotic divisions involved with spermatogenesis. **B.** Structural changes required during spermiogenesis, as sperm cells become spermatids. (Reproduced with permission from McKinley, 2006.)

the prior 3 months can adversely affect semen characteristics (Hinrichsen, 1980; Rowley, 1970). Spermatogenesis is optimal at temperatures slightly below body temperature, hence the location of the testes outside of the pelvis. Illness with high fevers or chronic hot tub use can temporarily impair sperm quality. But, no definitive evidence supports boxer underwear as advantageous.

Medical questions focus on prior chemotherapy or local radiation treatment that may damage spermatogonial stem cells. Hypertension, diabetes mellitus, and neurologic disorders can be associated with erectile dysfunction or retrograde ejaculation. Poor semen quality has been associated with higher rates of diabetes, ischemic heart disease, and mortality and an increased individual and familial cancer risk. These findings suggest semen quality may be a biomarker of overall health (Eisenberg, 2014, 2016; Hanson, 2018b). Excessive weight has been associated with obesity-related secondary hypogonadism, erectile dysfunction, and infertility. Similar to women, rigorous data describing the effects of bariatric surgery on male reproductive health are lacking (Di Vincenzo, 2018).

Several medications are known to worsen semen parameters, including cimetidine, erythromycin, gentamicin, tetracycline, and spironolactone (Sigman, 1997). Moreover, cigarettes, alcohol, illicit drugs, and environmental toxins all adversely affect semen quality (Bracken, 1990; Muthusami, 2005; Ramlau-Hansen, 2007). The rising use of anabolic steroids also decreases sperm production by suppressing the output of intratesticular testosterone (Gazvani, 1997). Although the effects of many medications are reversible, anabolic steroid abuse may lead to lasting or even permanent damage to testicular function.

An exercise history also is obtained. Although the evidence quality is generally low, bicycling has been associated with erectile dysfunction and decreased sperm concentration. Similar effects are suggested in long distance runners (Hwang, 2019).

PHYSICAL EXAMINATION

Examination of the Female Patient

A physical examination may provide many clues to the cause of infertility. Vital signs, height, and weight are recorded. A particularly short stature may reflect a genetic condition such as Turner syndrome. Hirsutism, alopecia, or acne indicates the need to measure androgen levels. Acanthosis nigricans is consistent with insulin resistance associated with PCOS or diabetes or, much less commonly, Cushing syndrome. Galactorrhea is often indicative of hyperprolactinemia. Additionally, thyroid abnormalities are sought. Many of these diagnoses and their management are discussed in greater detail in other chapters (Table 20-5).

A pelvic examination may be particularly informative. Inability to place a speculum through the introitus may raise doubts about coital frequency. The vagina should be moist and rugated, and the cervix should have a reasonable amount of mucus. Both indicate adequate estrogen production. An enlarged or irregularly shaped uterus may reflect leiomyomas, whereas a fixed uterus suggests pelvic scarring due to endometriosis or prior pelvic infection. Uterosacral nodularity or ovarian masses may additionally implicate endometriosis or, less commonly, malignancy.

All women should have cervical cancer screening that is up to date prior to treatment. Negative cultures for *Neisseria gonorrhoeae* and *Chlamydia trachomatis* are obtained to ensure that cervical manipulation during evaluation and treatment does not cause ascending infection. The breast examination must be normal, and when indicated by age or family history, a mammogram is obtained prior to initiating hormonal treatment.

Examination of the Male Patient

Most gynecologists will not feel comfortable performing a complete male physical examination. Nevertheless, parts of this evaluation are relatively easy to perform, and a gynecologist at minimum should understand the primary focus of the examination. Normal secondary sexual characteristics that reflect androgen production such as beard growth, axillary and pubic hair, and perhaps male pattern balding should be present. Gynecomastia or eunuchoid habitus may suggest Klinefelter syndrome (De Braekeleer, 1991).

The penile urethra should be at the glans tip for proper semen deposition in the vagina. Testicular length measures at least 4 cm

TABLE 20-5. Chapters with Relevant Information About Infertility

Etiology	Diagnosis	Chapter Title	Chapter Number
Ovulatory dysfunction	PCOS	PCOS and Hyperandrogenism	Chapter 17
	Hypothalamic-pituitary	Amenorrhea	Chapter 16
	Age-related	Menopause	Chapter 21
	POI	Amenorrhea	Chapter 16
Tubal disease	PID	Gynecologic Infection	Chapter 3
Uterine abnormalities	Congenital	Anatomic Disorders	Chapter 18
	Leiomyomas	Pelvic Mass	Chapter 9
	Asherman syndrome	Anatomic Disorders	Chapter 18
Other	Endometriosis	Endometriosis	Chapter 10

PCOS = polycystic ovarian syndrome; PID = pelvic inflammatory disease; POI = premature ovarian insufficiency.

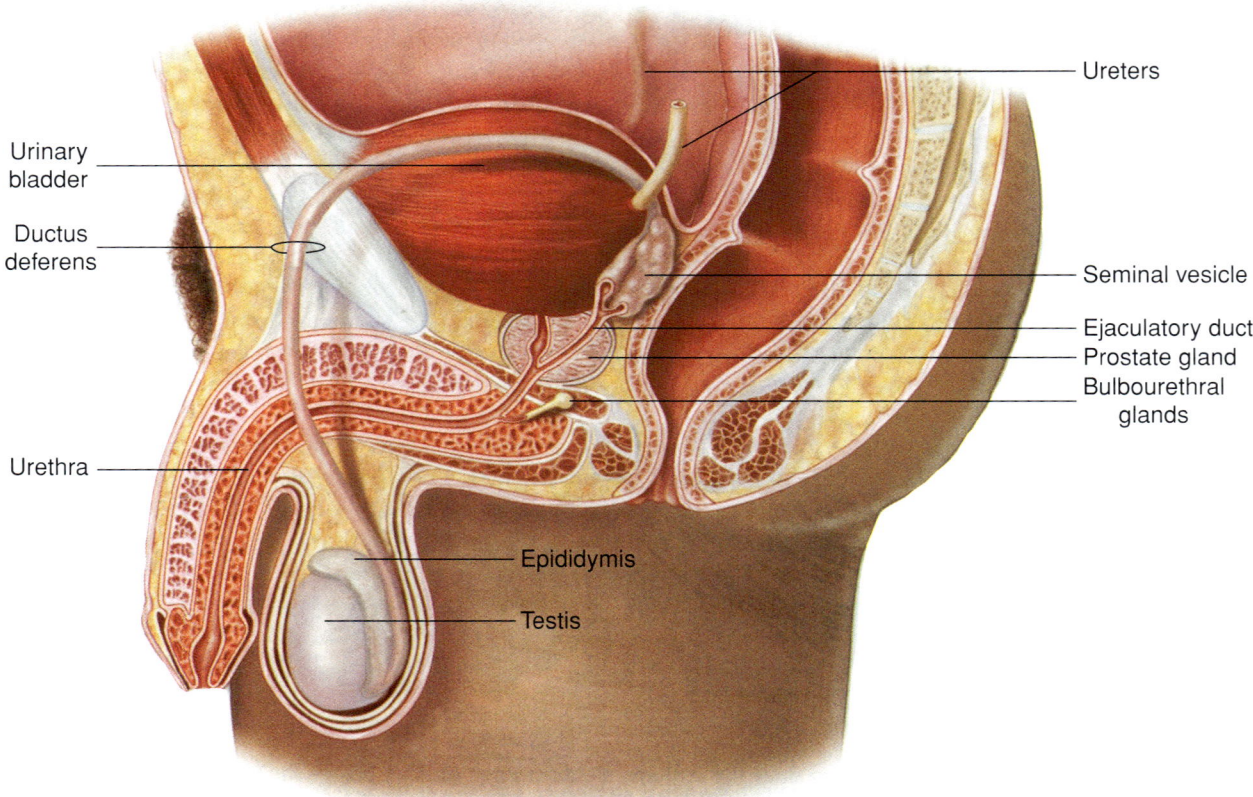

FIGURE 20-4 Male genitalia. (Reproduced with permission from McKinley, 2006.)

and a minimal testicular volume is 20 mL (Fig. 20-4) (Charny, 1960; Hadziselimovic, 2006). Small testes are unlikely to produce normal sperm numbers. A testicular mass may indicate testicular cancer, which can present as infertility. The epididymis should be soft and nontender to exclude chronic infection. Epididymal fullness may suggest vas deferens obstruction. The prostate should be smooth, nontender, and normal size. Additionally, the pampiniform plexus of veins is palpated for varicocele. Importantly, both vasa deferentia should be palpable. Congenital bilateral absence of the vas deferens is associated with mutation in the gene responsible for cystic fibrosis (Anguiano, 1992).

EVALUATION FOR ANOVULATION

The infertility evaluation can be conceptually simplified into confirmation of: (1) ovulation, (2) normal female reproductive tract anatomy, and (3) normal semen characteristics. The specifics regarding evaluation of each of these categories are detailed in the following sections and in Table 20-6.

TABLE 20-6. Infertility Testing

Etiology	Evaluation
Ovulatory function/ovarian reserve	Ovulation predictor kit Early follicular FSH ± estradiol level Antimüllerian hormone (AMH) Endocrine disorders (TSH, prolactin) Ovarian sonography (antral follicle count)
Tubal/pelvic disease	Hysterosalpingography Laparoscopy + chromotubation
Uterine factors	Hysterosalpingography Transvaginal sonography/saline-infusion sonography ± Magnetic resonance imaging Hysteroscopy ± laparoscopy
Male factor	Semen analysis

FSH = follicle-stimulating hormone; TSH = thyroid-stimulating hormone.

Of these, ovulation may be perturbed by abnormalities within the hypothalamus, anterior pituitary, or ovaries. Hypothalamic disorders may be acquired or inherited. Acquired disorders include those due to lifestyle, for example, excessive exercise, eating disorders, or stress. Alternatively, dysfunction or improper migration of the hypothalamic gonadotropin-releasing hormone neurons may be inherited, such as that which occurs in idiopathic hypogonadotropic hypogonadism (IHH) or Kallmann syndrome. Thyroid disease and hyperprolactinemia also may contribute to menstrual disturbances. Measurement of thyroid stimulating hormone (TSH) levels is considered reasonable in any infertile woman to screen for subclinical hypothyroidism, particularly in those with any question regarding menstrual regularity or with a positive family history for thyroid disease (American Society for Reproductive Medicine, 2015f). A full discussion of endocrine-related disorders that result in menstrual disturbances is found in Chapter 16 (p. 359).

Clinical Evaluation

A patient's menstrual history is an excellent predictor of regular ovulation. A woman with cyclic menses at an interval of 25 to 35 days and duration of bleeding of 3 to 7 days is most likely ovulating. Although these numbers vary widely, each woman will have her own normal pattern. Therefore, these figures typically do not vary significantly across cycles for an individual woman.

Probable ovulation is also suggested by *mittelschmerz*, which is midcycle pelvic pain associated with ovulation, or by moliminal symptoms such as breast tenderness, acne, food cravings, and mood changes. Ovulatory cycles are more likely to be associated with dysmenorrhea, although severe dysmenorrhea may suggest endometriosis.

Basal body temperature (BBT) charting has long been used to identify ovulation. This test requires that a woman's morning oral temperature be graphically charted (Fig. 20-5). Oral temperatures are usually 97.0° to 98.0°F during the follicular phase. A postovulatory rise in progesterone levels increases basal temperature by approximately 0.4° to 0.8°F. This *biphasic* temperature pattern is strongly predictive of ovulation (Bates, 1990). Nevertheless, although this test has the advantage of being inexpensive, it is insensitive in many women. Furthermore, for a couple wishing to conceive, the temperature rise follows ovulation, and therefore the window of maximal fertility has been missed (Luciano, 1990). Although this method is discussed here for completeness, most patients are better served by sensitive urinary ovulation detection kits, described next.

Ovulation Predictor Kits

These kits measure urinary luteinizing hormone (LH) concentration by colorimetric assay. They are widely available in pharmacies, are relatively easy to use, and provide clear instructions regarding interpretation. In general, a woman begins testing 2 to 3 days prior to the predicted LH surge, and testing is continued daily. No clear consensus guides the optimal time of day to test. Some specialists suggest that the concentrated first morning void is a logical time. Others are concerned that this sample may provide a false-positive result and recommend testing the second morning urine. Other clinicians reason that the serum LH peak occurs in the morning and that the greatest likelihood of detecting a urinary peak would be in the late afternoon or evening. Because the LH surge spans 48 to 50 hours, timing is probably not critical as long as the test is performed daily. In most instances, ovulation will occur the day following the urinary LH peak (Luciano, 1990; Miller, 1996).

If equivocal results are obtained, the test can be repeated in 12 hours. In one study, urine LH surge assays were estimated to have 100-percent sensitivity and 96-percent accuracy, although this is undoubtedly an overestimate of typical-use results (Grinsted, 1989; Guermandi, 2001).

Serum Progesterone

Adequate progesterone levels are required for endometrial preparation prior to implantation. This has led to the concept of *luteal phase defect (LPD)*, defined as inadequate endometrial development due to suboptimal progesterone production.

Midluteal phase serum progesterone levels have long been used to document ovulation, although the sensitivity of this test has been questioned. In a classic 28-day cycle, serum is obtained on cycle day number 21 following the first day of menstrual bleeding, or 7 days following ovulation. Levels during the follicular phase are generally <2 ng/mL. Values above

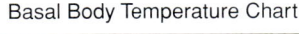

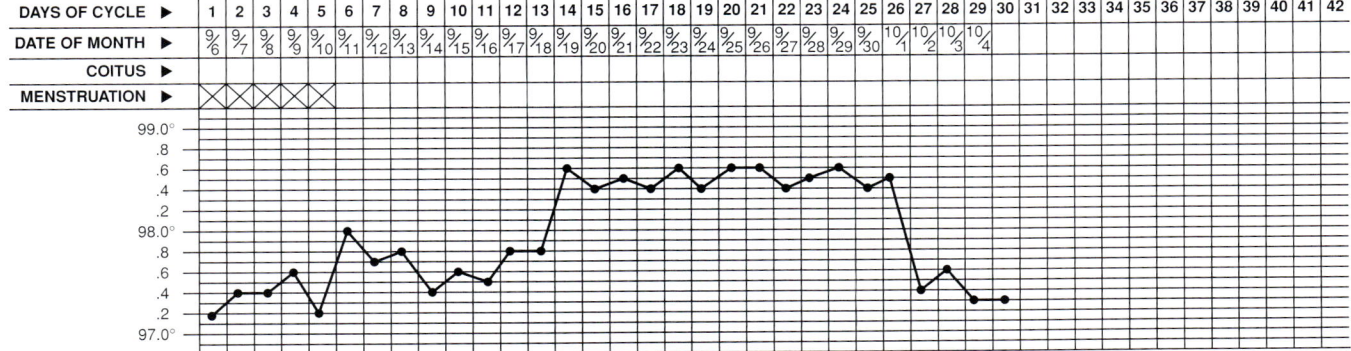

FIGURE 20-5 Biphasic pattern seen on this basal body temperature chart suggests ovulation. (Redrawn with permission from Chang, 2005.)

4 to 6 ng/mL correlate with ovulation and progesterone production by the corpus luteum (Guermandi, 2001). Progesterone is secreted as pulses, and therefore a single measurement does not indicate overall production during the luteal phase. As a result, an absolute threshold for acceptable progesterone levels has not been established. Although some clinicians empirically treat any woman with a progesterone level below approximately 10 ng/mL, the utility of this approach is unproven and is costly. Accordingly, the midluteal progesterone level is best regarded as an acceptable test for ovulation but not an absolute indicator of adequate luteal function.

Endometrial Biopsy

Luteal phase endometrial biopsy was hoped to reflect both corpus luteum function and endometrial response, and thereby provide more clinically relevant information than a serum progesterone level alone (Noyes, 1975). Unfortunately, the utility of this test is severely hampered by high intraobserver and interobserver variability during histologic evaluation (Balasch, 1992; Scott, 1993). An out-of-phase biopsy is found nearly as frequently in fertile as in infertile women, and the overlap in incidence between the two groups is large (Balasch, 1992; Scott, 1993). In its current form, the endometrial biopsy is no longer considered a routine part of infertility evaluation.

Interestingly, the timing of protein expression in the endometrial glands and stroma is being defined. Potential markers for uterine receptivity include osteopontin, cytokines, cell adhesion molecules, ion channels, and the L-selectin ligand, which has been proposed to mediate embryo attachment (Carson, 2002; Garrido-Gomez, 2014; Kao, 2003; Lessey, 1998; Petracco, 2012; Ruan, 2014). In the future, endometrial biopsy or endometrial fluid aspirates may again become part of the diagnostic evaluation if expression patterns of these proteins can predict endometrial receptivity.

Sonography

Serial ovarian sonographic evaluations can demonstrate the development of a mature antral follicle and its subsequent collapse during ovulation. This approach is time consuming, and ovulation can be missed. However, sonography is an excellent approach for supporting the diagnosis of PCOS.

EVALUATION FOR DIMINISHED OVARIAN RESERVE

Ovulatory status does not provide a complete picture of ovarian function. A woman may have regular, ovulatory menses but have reduced follicular response to ovarian stimulation compared with other women of similar age due to a smaller ovarian follicle pool. In this situation, the woman is said to have decreased or diminished ovarian reserve (DOR) and, in more severe presentations, primary ovarian insufficiency (POI). Although most often the result of advancing age, a small ovarian reserve can be linked to smoking, to genetic conditions, or to prior ovarian surgery, chemotherapy, or pelvic irradiation. A more complete discussion of accelerated follicular loss is found in Chapter 17 (p. 377).

TABLE 20-7. Female Aging and Infertility

Female Age (years)	Infertility
20–29	8.0%
30–34	14.6%
35–39	21.9%
40–44	28.7%

Reproductive Aging

Female age and fertility have a clear inverse relationship (Table 20-7) (American Society for Reproductive Medicine, 2014a). This loss is primarily attributable to a decline in oocyte quality and quantity, although accumulating risk for the development of medical disorders or uterine and pelvic abnormalities also contributes. A classic study was performed in the Hutterites, a community that eschews contraception. After ages 34, 40, and 45, the incidence of infertility was 11 percent, 33 percent, and 87 percent, respectively. The average age at last pregnancy was 40.9 years (Menken, 1986; Tietze, 1957). Another study evaluated cumulative pregnancy rates in women using donor insemination. In women younger than 31 years, 74 percent achieved pregnancy within 1 year. These rates fell to 62 percent for women between 31 and 35 years, and further declined to 54 percent in women older than 35 (Treloar, 1998).

Ongoing atresia of nondominant follicles proceeds throughout a woman's reproductive life span. In addition to declining follicular numbers, the risks of genetic abnormalities and mitochondrial deletions in the remaining oocytes substantially rise as a woman ages (Keefe, 1995; Pellestor, 2003). These factors result in lower pregnancy rates and higher miscarriage rates in both spontaneous and stimulated cycles. The overall miscarriage risk in women older than 40 years is estimated to be 50 to 75 percent (Maroulis, 1991).

The follicular loss rate and age at menopause varies between women and is likely genetically determined. For example, a family history of early menopause is correlated with a greater risk of early menopause in an individual woman. However, in most cases, it is impossible to predict the onset of menopause. Therefore, fertility testing is ideally performed starting at age 35 in all patients desiring conception. Testing is also seriously considered in any woman with an unexplained change in menstrual cyclicity, family history of early menopause, or risk factor for POI.

An array of tests has been developed to assess ovarian reserve (American Society for Reproductive, 2015g). Unfortunately, these lack sensitivity and positive predictive value for DOR, particularly if applied to patients at low risk for this process. In addition, these tests are more accurate as predictors of ovarian response to pharmacologic stimulation than as predictors of subsequent pregnancy. The optimal combination of tests and their interpretation continues to be refined. Currently, early follicular measurement of follicle-stimulating hormone (FSH) is probably the most cost-effective approach for the general practitioner. The addition of a serum antimüllerian hormone level is rapidly moving into standard practice, and this hormone is discussed subsequently. Measuring serum inhibin B levels and the clomiphene citrate challenge test have fallen out of favor.

Abnormal test findings correlate with a poorer prognosis for achieving pregnancy, and referral to an infertility specialist is advisable. Conversely, a normal test result does not negate the effect of a woman's age on her fertility status. This information may be useful in counseling a couple regarding prognosis. Poor results in an older woman can supply an impetus either to attempt donor oocyte in vitro fertilization (IVF) or to pursue alternatives such as adoption. Borderline results in a younger woman with infertility may suggest a need for more intensive treatment. However, caution is advised in using any of these tests as an impetus for immediate treatment with oocyte cryopreservation, IVF, or other treatment in the otherwise asymptomatic patient.

■ Follicle-Stimulating Hormone and Estradiol

Frequently termed a "cycle day 3" FSH, this may reasonably be drawn between days 2 and 4 following menses onset. With declining ovarian function, the support cells (granulosa cells and luteal cells) secrete less inhibin, a peptide hormone that is responsible for inhibiting FSH secretion by the anterior pituitary gonadotropes (Chap. 16, p. 353). With loss of luteal inhibin, FSH levels rise in the early follicular phase. A value >10 mIU/mL may indicate significant loss of ovarian reserve and prompt more complete evaluation.

The simultaneous measurement of an estradiol level has been thought to lower the incidence of false-negative results in FSH values alone (Buyalos, 1997). Somewhat paradoxically, despite the overall depletion of ovarian follicles, estrogen levels in older women are elevated early in the cycle due to greater stimulation of ovarian steroidogenesis by elevated FSH levels. A cycle-day-3 estradiol level >80 pg/mL is considered abnormal. However, paired FSH and estradiol measurement is no longer recommended for ovarian reserve evaluation because estradiol provides limited additional information compared with FSH testing alone (American Society for Reproductive Medicine, 2015g).

■ Antimüllerian Hormone

This is the most recent circulating factor to be analyzed as an ovarian reserve predictor (La Marca, 2009). As suggested by its name, antimüllerian hormone (AMH) is expressed by the fetal testes during male differentiation to prevent development of the müllerian system (fallopian tubes, uterus, and upper vagina) (Chap. 19, p. 408). AMH is also expressed by the granulosa cells of small preantral follicles but has limited expression in larger follicles. This suggests that AMH plays a role in dominant follicle recruitment.

Measurement of AMH levels has advantages compared with FSH and inhibin testing. First, AMH expression is gonadotropin-independent and therefore is relatively independent of cycle stage and is consistent across cycles. Second, studies suggest that AMH levels correlate with ovarian primordial follicle number more strongly than FSH or inhibin levels (Hansen, 2011). Furthermore, AMH levels may drop prior to observable changes in FSH or estradiol levels, thereby providing an earlier marker of waning ovarian function. Seifer and associates (2011) reported a steady decline in AMH serum levels across the reproductive life span. The median level approximated 3 ng/mL at age 25, and this dropped to 1 ng/mL at age 35 to 37. Of note, reference levels for FSH, estradiol, and AMH can vary between laboratories. Thus, every clinician should be familiar with their own laboratory's normal values.

Interestingly, AMH levels are under consideration as a tool for diagnosis of PCOS. Levels are raised two- to threefold in affected women compared with normal cycling women (Dumont, 2018; Hornburg, 2014). This observation is consistent with the multiple early follicles found in patients with PCOS.

■ Antral Follicle Count

Sonographic evaluation of the follicular phase antral follicle count (AFC) is commonly used as a reliable predictor for subsequent response to ovulation induction (Frattarelli, 2000; Maseelall, 2009). The number of small antral follicles reflects the size of the resting follicular pool. Antral follicles between 2 and 100 mm are counted in both ovaries. The total AFC usually ranges between 10 and 20 in a reproductive-aged woman. An AFC with <3 to 6 total antral follicles predicts poor response to gonadotropin stimulation during IVF cycles, but this measure is limited by low sensitivity.

EVALUATION FOR FEMALE ANATOMIC ABNORMALITIES

■ Tubal and Pelvic Factors

Symptoms such as chronic pelvic pain or dysmenorrhea may suggest tubal obstruction, pelvic adhesions, or both. Adhesions can prevent normal tubal movement, ovum pick-up, and transport of the fertilized egg into the uterus. Etiologies include tubal disease, especially pelvic infection; endometriosis; and prior pelvic surgery.

Of these causes, approximately one third to one fourth of all infertile women are diagnosed with tubal disease in developed countries. In the United States, the most common cause of tubal disease is infection with *C trachomatis* or *N gonorrhoeae*. With PID, tubal infertility has been estimated to follow in 12 percent, 23 percent, and 54 percent of women following one, two, or three cases of PID, respectively (Lalos, 1988). Nevertheless, an absent PID history is not overly reassuring, as nearly one half of patients who have tubal damage have no clinical history of antecedent disease (Rosenfeld, 1983).

In contrast, in developing countries, genital tuberculosis may account for 3 to 5 percent of infertility cases (Aliyu, 2004; Nezar, 2009). As a result, this diagnosis is considered in immigrant populations from countries with endemic infection. In these cases, tubal damage and endometrial adhesions are underlying causes. Genital tuberculosis typically follows hematogenous seeding of the reproductive tract from an extragenital primary infection. The likelihood of a return to fertility after antitubercular treatment is low, and IVF with embryo transfer remains the most reliable approach (Aliyu, 2004).

With endometriosis, chronic inflammation and intraperitoneal bleeding can lead to pelvic adhesions. Endometriosis is also thought to diminish fertility by an increase in peritoneal fluid inflammatory factors, alterations in endometrial immunologic function, poor oocyte or embryonic quality, or impaired implantation (American Society for Reproductive Medicine, 2012).

Salpingitis isthmica nodosa is an inflammatory condition of the fallopian tube, characterized by nodular thickening of its isthmic portion. Histologically, smooth muscle proliferation and diverticula of tubal epithelium contribute to this thickening. This uncommon condition typically develops bilaterally and progressively leads to ultimate tubal occlusion and infertility (Saracoglu, 1992). Treatment options include those for proximal tubal occlusion as discussed in Chapter 21 (p. 459).

Of note, a prior ectopic pregnancy, even if treated medically with methotrexate, implies the likelihood of significant tubal damage. Residual adhesions are common after even the most meticulous pelvic surgery. This is particularly true in cases with pelvic inflammation, due to blood, infection, or irritation caused by mature cystic teratoma (dermoid) contents.

Uterine Abnormalities

Uterine abnormalities can be either congenital or acquired. Common congenital anomalies include uterine septum, bicornuate uterus, unicornuate uterus, and uterine didelphys. With the possible exception of a large uterine septum, the fertility effects of these anomalies have been difficult to verify, although a subset are clearly associated with pregnancy complications. As a uterine septum can now be removed relatively simply and safely with hysteroscopy, most infertility specialists will proceed with surgery if this anomaly is identified. Clinical findings and management of congenital reproductive tract anomalies are fully described in Chapter 19 (p. 421).

Acquired anomalies include intrauterine leiomyomas, adenomyosis, polyps, and Asherman syndrome. Leiomyomas may diminish fertility by proposed mechanisms that include endometrial cavity distortion with associated changes in blood flow and endometrial maturation; endometrial inflammation; disordered uterine contractility that may hinder sperm or embryo transport; obstruction of the proximal fallopian tubes; or interference with ovum capture (American Society for Reproductive Medicine, 2017a; Makker, 2013; Metwally, 2012; Pritts, 2001; Samejima, 2014). Thus far, no algorithm incorporating tumor number, volume, or location accurately predicts the need to remove them, either to improve implantation rates or to lower pregnancy complications. Namely, miscarriage, placental abruption, and preterm labor are potential problems. Nevertheless, although not supported by definitive evidence, most experts suggest removal of submucosal fibroids that significantly distort the endometrial cavity. In addition, many consider surgical excision of leiomyomas larger than 4 to 5 cm or multiple smaller tumors in this range regardless of location. Importantly, surgical benefits are weighed against postoperative complications that lower subsequent fertility. These include pelvic adhesion formation, creation of Asherman syndrome following large submucous leiomyoma removal, or the need for cesarean delivery if the full myometrial thickness is transected.

The incidence of adenomyosis in the infertility population is unknown. However, improvements in imaging strongly suggest that it occurs at earlier ages than previously appreciated. Adenomyosis is thought to impact fertility and obstetric outcomes via functional and structural defects in the endometrium and myometrium (Buggio, 2018).

Endometrial polyps are found in an estimated 3 to 5 percent of infertile women (Farhi, 1995; Soares, 2000). The prevalence is higher in women with symptoms such as intermenstrual or postcoital bleeding. Although these complaints typically prompt hysteroscopic removal, most data have not clearly demonstrated an indication for removing polyps in otherwise asymptomatic women without risks for endometrial cancer (Ben-Arie, 2004; DeWaay, 2002; Jayaprakasan, 2014). Of note, however, one study suggested that removal of even small polyps (<1 cm) may improve pregnancy rates following intrauterine insemination (Perez-Medina, 2005).

The presence of intrauterine adhesions, also called *synechiae*, is termed *Asherman syndrome*. This diagnosis is discussed in Chapter 17 (p. 374). Asherman syndrome develops most frequently in women with prior uterine dilation and curettage, particularly in the context of infection and pregnancy (Schenker, 1996). The clinical history will often include an acute postsurgical decline in menstrual bleeding or even amenorrhea. A woman with an intrauterine device complicated by infection or a woman with genital tuberculosis is also at high risk for intrauterine adhesions. Treatment of Asherman syndrome involves hysteroscopic lysis of the scar tissue as described in Chapter 21 (p. 461) and Chapter 44 (p. 1069).

Anatomy Evaluation

Several approaches for evaluating pelvic anatomy are: (1) hysterosalpingography (HSG), (2) transvaginal sonography (TVS) with or without saline instillation, (3) 3-dimensional (3-D) TVS, (4) hysteroscopy, (5) laparoscopy, and (6) magnetic resonance (MR) imaging. As shown in Table 20-8, each has its own advantages and disadvantages.

Hysterosalpingography

This radiographic tool can display the shape and size of the uterine cavity and define tubal status. HSG is generally performed on cycle days 5 through 10. At this time, few intrauterine clots should remain to block tubal outflow or give the false impression of an intrauterine abnormality. Furthermore, a woman theoretically has not ovulated or possibly conceived. For this test, iodinated contrast medium is infused through a catheter placed into the uterus. With fluoroscopy, dye is followed as it fills the uterine cavity, then the tubal lumen, and finally spills out of the tubal fimbria into the pelvic cavity (Fig. 20-6).

In a large metaanalysis, HSG was demonstrated to have 65-percent sensitivity and 83-percent specificity for tubal obstruction (Swart, 1995). Tubal contractions, particularly cornual spasm, can give the incorrect impression of proximal fallopian tube obstruction (a false-positive result). A false-negative result is much less common. Many causes of tubal disease affect both tubes, and thus unilateral disease is unusual. Unilateral obstruction with a normal contralateral tube most likely reflects dye following the path of least resistance during the HSG procedure. However, laparoscopy with chromotubation is considered prior to treatment to confirm a final diagnosis.

TABLE 20-8. Advantages and Disadvantages of Various Methods for Evaluating Pelvic Anatomy

	Tubal Patency	Uterine Cavity	Developmental Defects	Endometriosis or PAD	Ovaries
HSG	+	+	–	+/–	–
TVS	–	+/–	+/–	–	+
3-D TVS	–	+	+	–	+
SIS	–	+	+	–	+
MR imaging	–	+	+	+ (endometrioma)	+
Hysteroscopy	–	+	+ (with laparoscopy)	–	–
Laparoscopy	+	–	+ (with hysteroscopy)	+	+

HSG = hysterosalpingography; MR = magnetic resonance; PAD = pelvic adhesive disease; SIS = saline-infusion sonography; TVS = transvaginal sonography.

HSG is not reliable in detecting peritubal or pelvic adhesions, although loculations of dye around the tubes may be suggestive. Thus, HSG is an excellent predictor of tubal patency but is less effective at predicting normal tubal function or pelvic adhesions. Pregnancy rates can rise after HSG and are thought to follow flushing of intratubal debris. Recent studies suggest that subsequent spontaneous pregnancy rates may be greater following oil-based dyes rather than water-based ones. Nevertheless, water-based dyes currently remain the preference in most practices as these generally carry a lower allergic reaction risk (Dreyer, 2017).

HSG also provides analysis of the intrauterine cavity contour. A polyp, leiomyoma, or adhesion within the cavity will block dye diffusion and create an intrauterine "defect" in dye

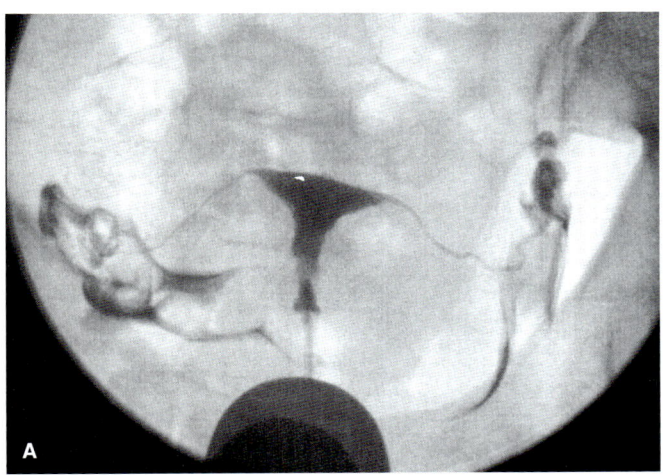

Normal

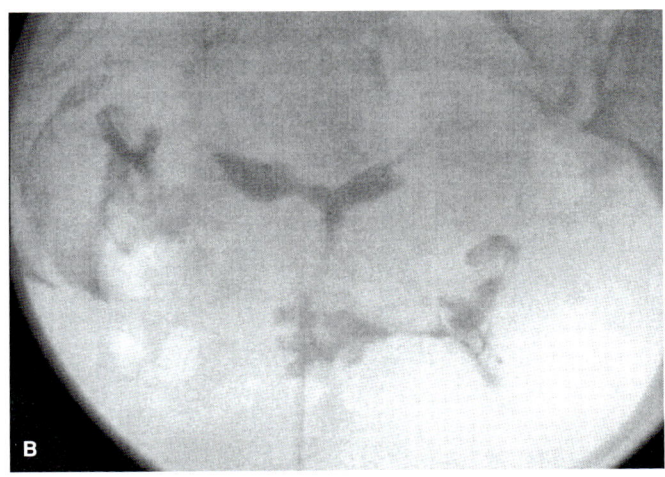

Asherman syndrome

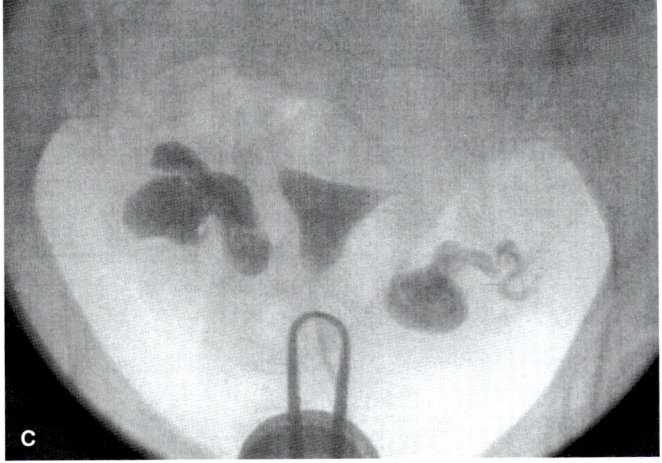

Bilateral hydrosalpinges

FIGURE 20-6 Hysterosalpingogram findings. These images are digitally reversed, causing the radiopaque contrast to appear black against a radiolucent background. **A.** Normal hysterosalpingogram. Radiopaque dye fills the uterine cavity and spills from both fallopian tubes into the peritoneal cavity. The dye catheter is seen beneath the endometrial contour. **B.** Asherman syndrome. Contrast dye fills a small and irregularly shaped endometrial cavity, often described as having a "moth-eaten" appearance. **C.** Bilateral hydrosalpinges. Note the marked tubal dilation and lack of spill of contrast medium at the fimbrial ends. (Reproduced with permission from Dr. Kevin Doody.)

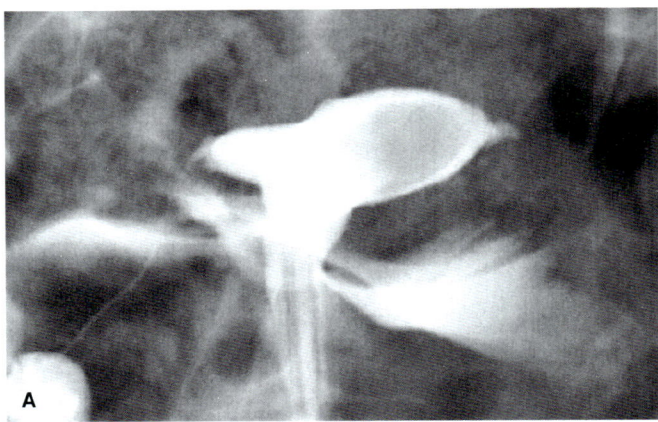

Submucous leiomyoma

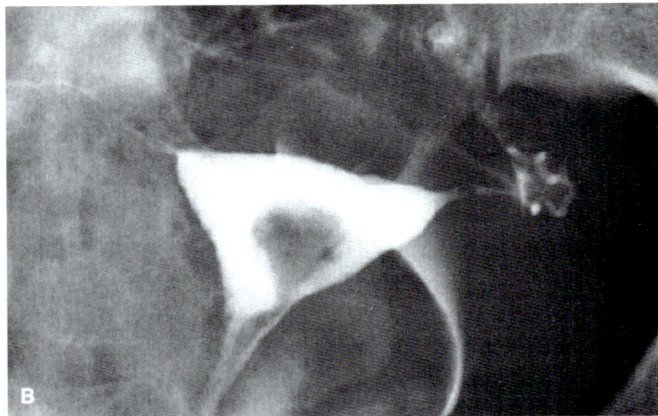

Endometrial polyp

FIGURE 20-7 Appearance of leiomyoma and endometrial polyps on hysterosalpingogram (HSG). **A.** A broad-based filling defect is formed during HSG by a submucous leiomyoma. Note distortion of the left cornu by this mass. **B.** A more irregular filling defect is created by an endometrial polyp. Note that polyps generally have a less substantial attachment to the myometrium. (Reproduced with permission from Dr. Diane Twickler.)

opacity on the radiograph (Fig. 20-7). Although false-positive results may originate from blood clots, mucus plugs, or shearing of the endometrium during placement of the intrauterine catheter, HSG accurately identifies intrauterine pathology. In one study of more than 300 women in which hysteroscopy was the gold standard, HSG was determined to be 98-percent sensitive and 35-percent specific and have a positive predictive value of 70 percent and a negative predictive value of 8 percent. Most misdiagnoses were due to an inability to distinguish polyps from submucous leiomyomas. Other studies have reported much less impressive results. For example, Soares and coworkers (2000) reported sensitivity and positive predictive values of only 50 and 30 percent, respectively, for endometrial polyp and submucous leiomyoma detection in asymptomatic patients. Nevertheless, HSG is a valuable tool for initial uterine cavity evaluation.

HSG can also define developmental uterine anomalies (Fig. 20-8). A Y-shaped uterus identified during HSG may represent either a uterine septum or bicornuate uterus. In these cases, the external contour of the uterine fundus must be evaluated using MR imaging, high-resolution sonography, 3-D TVS, or laparoscopy. With a uterine septum, a smooth fundal contour is found, whereas with a bicornuate uterus, a cleft between the two uterine horns is seen. This is an important distinction, as a septum is often resected, but a bicornuate uterus is usually not treated. In general, uterine anomalies do not cause infertility but may be associated with miscarriage, malpresentation, or preterm birth. Accordingly, it may be reasonable to surgically treat a uterine anomaly to improve pregnancy outcome. However, a couple is carefully counseled that the conception rate itself is unlikely to be affected. Fertility effects of congenital anomalies are further discussed in Chapter 19 (p. 422).

Sonography

TVS may be helpful in determining uterine anatomy, particularly during the luteal phase, when the thickened endometrium acts as contrast to the myometrium. Now more widely available, 3-D sonography is advancing discriminatory abilities and

decreasing the need for MR imaging to define uterine anatomy (Chap. 2, p. 41).

Infusion of saline into the endometrial cavity during sonography performed in the follicular phase provides another approach to create contrast between the cavity and uterine walls. This procedure has many names including hysterosonography, sonohysterography, or saline-infusion sonography (SIS). Details of this procedure are described in Chapter 2 (p. 31). SIS has a reported sensitivity of 75 percent and specificity of more than 90 percent for detecting endometrial defects. It has an acceptable positive predictive value of 50 percent and an excellent negative predictive value of 95 percent, which greatly exceeds the negative predictive value of HSG (Grimbizis, 2010; Seshadri, 2015; Soares, 2000). Moreover, SIS may be more sensitive than HSG in determining whether a cavitary defect is a pedunculated leiomyoma or a polyp (Figs. 8-5 and 9-4, pp. 186 and 206). Perhaps more importantly, SIS can help determine what portion of a submucous leiomyoma is within the cavity. Importantly, only those with less than a 50-percent intramural component are considered for hysteroscopic resection.

The primary limitation of standard SIS is that it does not provide information regarding the fallopian tubes, although rapid loss of saline into the pelvis is certainly consistent with at least unilateral patency. SIS is generally less painful than HSG and does not require radiation exposure. Thus, if information about tubal patency is not required, SIS is typically preferred. Notably, several radiologists are currently introducing air or contrast into the uterus during sonography. This permits evaluation of tubal patency and may be a broadly available alternative in the future (Groszmann, 2016).

Laparoscopy

Direct inspection provides the most accurate assessment of pelvic pathology, and laparoscopy is the gold standard approach. Chromotubation may be performed, and a dilute dye is injected through an acorn cannula placed against the cervix or through a balloon catheter positioned within the uterine cavity. Tubal

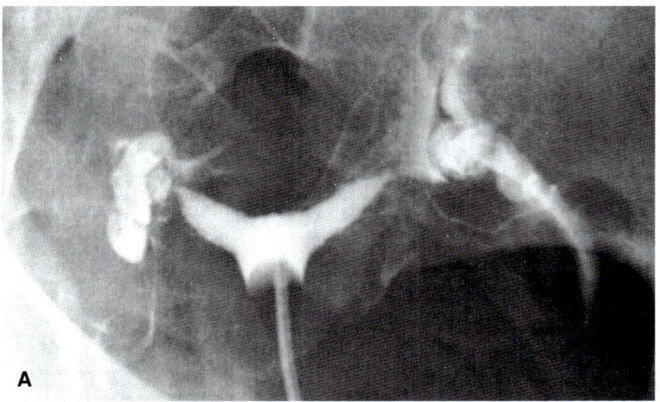

Bicornuate uterus

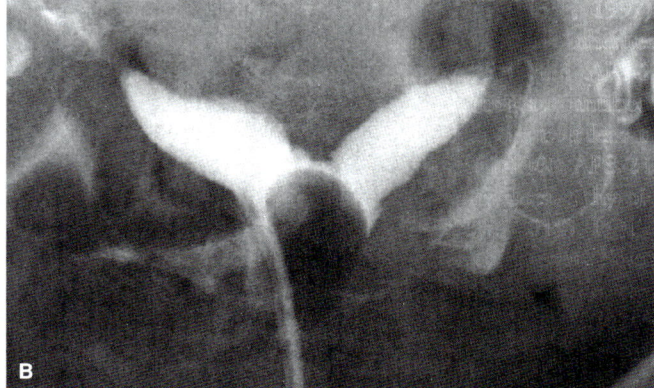

Septate uterus

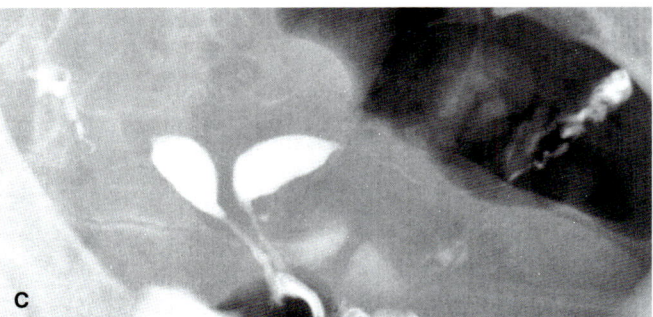

Uterine didelphys

FIGURE 20-8 Hysterosalpingogram appearance of müllerian developmental anomalies. **A.** Bicornuate uterus, due to a failure of fusion of the müllerian ducts, produces a fundal defect with wide-spaced uterine horns. **B.** Septate uterus due to a failure of resorption. This moderate septum displaces the radiopaque dye to the level of the radiolucent injector balloon. **C.** Uterine didelphys consisting of two completely separate müllerian systems including duplication of the cervix. (Reproduced with permission from Dr. Diane Twickler.)

spill is evaluated through the laparoscope (Fig. 20-9). Methylene blue is commonly used. However, methylene blue rarely may induce acute methemoglobinemia, particularly in patients with glucose-6-phosphate dehydrogenase deficiency. One 1-mL vial of methylene blue is mixed with 50 to 100 mL of sterile saline for injection through the cervical cannula. Laparoscopy allows both diagnosis and immediate surgical treatment of abnormalities such as endometriosis or pelvic adhesions.

As laparoscopy is an invasive procedure, it is not advocated in place of HSG as part of the initial infertility evaluation. Exceptions include women with a history or symptoms suggestive of endometriosis or prior pelvic inflammation. However, even in these women, a preliminary HSG may be informative (De Hondt, 2005).

If laparoscopy is clearly indicated, then hysteroscopy can also be performed to evaluate the uterine cavity. Moreover, in operative hysteroscopic cases, laparoscopy can help direct surgery and avoid perforation, for example, during septal incision.

Laparoscopy may be also considered in patients who fail to conceive with oral or gonadotropin ovulation induction. If pelvic disease is found and treated, progression to IVF may be avoided. With improvements in IVF success rates, this latter argument is becoming less justifiable, as the cost of surgery well exceeds the cost of an IVF cycle.

Hysteroscopy

Endoscopic evaluation of the intrauterine cavity is the preferred method to define intrauterine abnormalities. Hysteroscopy can be performed in an office or operating room. With improved

instrumentation, the ability to concurrently diagnose and treat abnormalities in the office is growing. However, substantially more extensive hysteroscopic surgery is possible in the operating room.

■ Cervical Factors

The cervical glands secrete mucus that is normally thick and impervious to sperm and ascending infections. High estrogen

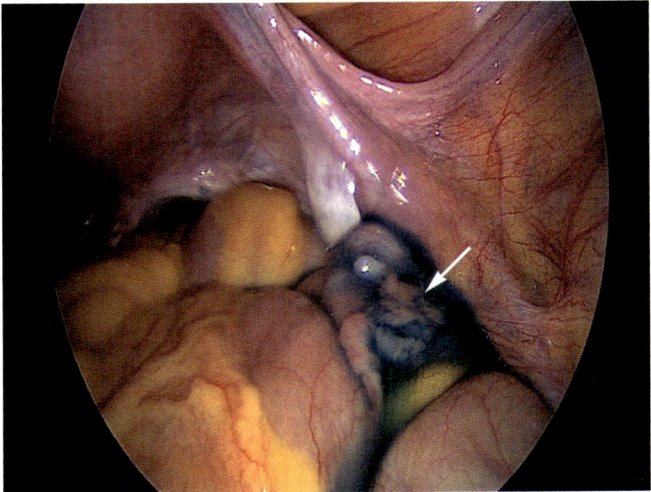

FIGURE 20-9 Chromotubation seen at laparoscopy. Note the spill of blue dye from the fimbriated end of the fallopian tube onto the ovarian surface. (Reproduced with permission from Dr. Kevin Doody.)

levels at midcycle induce mucus to become thin and stretchy and to have a higher sodium chloride concentration. Estrogen-primed cervical mucus filters out nonsperm components of semen and forms channels that help direct sperm into the uterus. Midcycle mucus also creates a reservoir for sperm. This allows ongoing release during the next 24 to 72 hours and extends the potential time for fertilization (Katz, 1997).

Abnormalities in mucus production are most frequently observed in women who have undergone cryosurgery, cervical conization, or a loop electrosurgical excision procedure (LEEP) for treatment of cervical neoplasia. Cervical infection may also worsen mucus quality, but data are conflicting. Implicated agents include *C trachomatis*, *N gonorrhoeae*, *Ureaplasma urealyticum*, and *Mycoplasma hominis* (Cimino, 1993).

The postcoital test, also known as the Sims-Huhner test, has been used historically to evaluate cervical mucus. A couple is requested to have intercourse on the day of ovulation, and a sample of the cervical mucus is evaluated for elasticity (*Spinnbarkeit*) and for the number of motile sperm per high-power field. This test has been hampered by a limited consensus on the definition of a normal test (Oei, 1995). Moreover, in a randomized trial, a normal postcoital test did not predict greater cumulative pregnancy rates (Oei, 1998).

Many infertility specialists recommend bypassing the cervix with intrauterine insemination (IUI) in any woman with prior cervical surgery, especially if she has noted a decline in midcycle mucus production. The remaining utility of the postcoital test is for the rare couple who will not consider IUI or who do not have IUI readily available. In regions in which more specific testing cannot be obtained, a postcoital test will provide basic information regarding mucus production, appropriate intercourse practices, and presence of motile sperm.

EVALUATION OF MALE INFERTILITY

Causes of male infertility can roughly be categorized as abnormalities of sperm production, sperm function, or obstruction of the ductal outflow tract. Normal sexual function with appropriate deposition of sperm during intercourse is also required (American Society for Reproductive Medicine, 2015c, 2018d).

◼ Normal Spermatogenesis

Analogous to the ovary, testes have two functions: the generation of mature germ cells (sperm) and the production of male hormones, primarily testosterone. The seminiferous tubules contain developing sperm and support cells called *Sertoli cells* or *sustentacular cells* (see Fig. 20-3). The Sertoli cells form tight junctions that produce a blood-testis barrier. This avascular space within the seminiferous tubules protects sperm from antibodies and toxins but also makes these cells dependent on diffusion for oxygen, nutrients, and metabolic precursors. Located between the seminiferous tubules are Leydig cells, also called *interstitial cells*, which are responsible for steroid hormone production. In simplistic terms, Leydig cells are similar to the theca cells of the ovary.

Unlike the ovary, testes contain stem cells that allow ongoing production of mature germ cells throughout a male's life.

In a fertile male, approximately 100 to 200 million sperm are produced each day (Sigman, 1997). The process begins with a diploid (46,XY) spermatogonial cell and results in four mature sperm with a haploid (23,X or 23,Y) karyotype (see Fig. 20-3). During this developmental process, most sperm cytoplasm is lost, mitochondria that provide energy are positioned in the sperm midpiece, and sperm flagella develop.

Production of sperm requires approximately 70 days. An additional 12 to 21 days is needed for sperm to be transported into the epididymis. Here, they further mature and develop motility (Heller, 1963; Hinrichsen, 1980; Rowley, 1970). Importantly, due to this prolonged developmental period, the results of a semen analysis reflect events during the past 3 months, not a single point in time.

To fertilize an oocyte, human sperm must undergo a process known as *capacitation*. Capacitation results in sperm hyperactivation and the ability to release acrosomal contents, which allow penetration of the ovum's zona pellucida.

High local levels of testosterone are integral to normal spermatogenesis. LH from the anterior pituitary gland stimulates production of testosterone by the Leydig cells. FSH increases LH receptor density on the Leydig cells, thus indirectly contributing to testosterone production. In addition, FSH elevates production of sex hormone–binding globulin, also called *androgen-binding protein*. Androgen-binding protein binds testosterone and maintains high concentrations of this hormone in the seminiferous tubules (Sigman, 1997).

In addition to hormone levels, testicular volume often reflects spermatogenesis, and a normal volume is between 15 and 25 mL. Most of this volume is provided by the seminiferous tubules. Thus, a small testicular volume is a strong indicator of abnormal spermatogenesis.

Spermatogenesis is directed by genes on the Y chromosome. Autosomal genes also provide important contributions, which continue to be elucidated. Therefore, genetic abnormalities may adversely affect this process, as discussed later (p. 445).

Male fertility likely diminishes modestly with aging. Pregnancy rates decline and time to conception lengthens. Studies of semen parameters across age suggest that sperm concentration is maintained, however, sperm motility and morphology progressively worsen (Levitas, 2007). The clinical significance of these changes is unclear (Kidd, 2001). Outside of semen parameters, the higher incidence of erectile and other sexual dysfunction with male aging undoubtedly contributes to lower conception rates. Data also suggest that paternal age may negatively affect reproductive outcomes in both natural and assisted pregnancies (Mazur, 2018). In sum, although advancing male age may lower fertility, it is probably insignificant compared with aging changes in women.

◼ Semen Analysis
Collection

This is a core test in male fertility evaluation. For this test, the male is asked to refrain from ejaculation for 2 to 3 days, and a specimen is collected by masturbation into a sterile cup. A proposed period of abstinence is based on the belief that this will result in a more accurate result, although this may not be true for all semen parameters (Hanson, 2018a). If masturbation is not an option, then a couple can use specially designed Silastic condoms without lubricants. Importantly, the sample should arrive in the laboratory within an hour of ejaculation to allow for optimal analysis.

The sample undergoes liquefaction, or thinning of the seminal fluid, due to enzymes from the liquid contribution of the prostate gland. This process takes 5 to 20 minutes and allows more accurate evaluation of the sperm contained in the seminal fluid. Ideally, two semen samples separated by at least a month are analyzed. In practice, frequently only a single sample is analyzed if parameters are normal.

Semen Analysis Results

The reference values for the semen analysis and frequently used terms are shown in Tables 20-9 and 20-10. Notably, semen characteristics vary across time in a single individual. Also, semen analysis results, particularly morphologic interpretation, may differ between laboratories. Thus, reference ranges for the laboratory being used should be known. Although total motile sperm count correlates with fertility, not all males with "normal" semen parameters display normal fertility (Guzick, 2001). Conversely, patients with semen analysis results outside the reference range may achieve pregnancy. The lack of absolute predictive value for this test is likely due to the fact that it does not provide information regarding sperm function, that is, the ultimate ability to fertilize an oocyte.

Most semen analysis reports will indicate semen volume, pH, and presence or absence of fructose. Nearly 80 percent of semen volume comes from the seminal vesicles. Seminal fluid is alkaline and is thought to protect sperm from acidity in prostatic secretions and in the vagina. Seminal fluid also provides fructose as an energy source for sperm. An acidic pH or lack of fructose is consistent with obstruction of the efferent ductal system (Daudin, 2000).

Low semen volume often simply reflects incomplete specimen collection or short abstinence interval. However, it may

TABLE 20-10. Semen Analysis Reference Limits

Volume	>1.5 mL[a]
Count	>15 million/mL[a]
Total Motility	>40%[a]
Morphology	>4%[a]
WBCs	<1 million/mL[b]
Round cells	<5 million/mL[b]

[a]Data from Cooper, 2010.
[b]Data from World Health Organization, 1999.
WBCs = white blood cells.

indicate partial vas deferens obstruction or retrograde ejaculation. Partial or complete vas deferens obstruction may be caused by infection, tumor, prior testicular or inguinal surgery, or trauma. Retrograde ejaculation follows failed closure of the bladder neck during ejaculation and allows seminal fluid to flow backward into the bladder. Retrograde ejaculation is suspected in men with diabetes mellitus, spinal cord damage, or prior prostate or other retroperitoneal surgery that may have damaged nerves (Hershlag, 1991). Medications, particularly β-blockers, may contribute to this problem. A postejaculatory urinalysis can detect sperm in the bladder and confirm the diagnosis. If urine is properly alkalinized, these sperm are viable and can be retrieved to achieve pregnancy.

Sperm counts may be normal, or males may have low sperm counts (oligospermia) or no sperm (azoospermia) (Sharlip, 2002). Oligospermia is defined as a concentration less than 15 million sperm per milliliter, and counts <5 to 10 million per milliliter are considered severe. The prevalence of azoospermia is approximately 1 percent of all men. Azoospermia may result from outflow tract obstruction, termed *obstructive azoospermia*, such as that which occurs with congenital absence of the vas deferens, severe infection, or vasectomy. Azoospermia may also follow testicular failure (*nonobstructive azoospermia*). In the latter case, careful centrifugation and analysis may identify a small number of motile sperm adequate for IVF use. Alternatively, this latter group may have viable sperm obtainable through either epididymal aspiration or testicular biopsy. As described later, endocrine and genetic evaluation is indicated for men with abnormal sperm counts.

Sperm movement also is assessed, and diminished motility is termed *asthenospermia*. Some laboratories will distinguish between rapid (grade 3 to 4), slow (grade 2), and nonprogressive (grade 0 to 1) movement. *Total progressive motility* is the percentage of sperm exhibiting forward movement (grades 2 to 4). Asthenospermia has been attributed to prolonged abstinence, antisperm antibodies, genital tract infections, or varicocele. To differentiate between dead and nonmotile sperm, a hypoosmotic swelling test can be completed. Unlike dead sperm, living sperm can maintain an osmotic gradient. Thus, when mixed with a hypoosmotic solution, living, nonmotile sperm with normal membrane function swell and coil as fluid is absorbed (Casper, 1996). Once identified, these viable sperm may be used for intracytoplasmic sperm injection.

Abnormal sperm morphology is termed *teratospermia* or *teratozoospermia*. Kruger and associates (1988) developed a detailed

TABLE 20-9. Semen Analysis Terminology

Term[a]	Definition[b]
Oligospermia	Sperm concentration 10–15 million sperm/mL (mild-moderate) or <5–10 million/mL (severe)
Asthenospermia	Greater proportion of immotile sperm or sperm with decreased motility
Teratospermia	Increased proportion of morphologically abnormal sperm
Azoospermia	Semen present but lacks sperm
Aspermia	Sperm and seminal plasma lacking (anejaculation)
Leukocytospermia	Increased white blood cell count
Necrospermia	All sperm nonviable or immotile

[a]Alternative terminology includes oligozoospermia, asthenozoospermia, and teratozoospermia.
[b]As compared with World Health Organization (1999) reference values.

characterization of normal sperm morphology, which showed improved correlation with fertilization rates during IVF cycles. Their criteria require careful analysis of the shape and size of the sperm head, the relative size of the acrosome in proportion to the head, and characteristics of the tail. Significantly lower fertilization rates are seen when normal morphology of the sample falls below 4 percent.

Round cells in a sperm sample may represent either leukocytes or immature sperm. White blood cells (WBCs) can be distinguished from immature sperm using various techniques, including a myeloperoxidase stain for WBCs (Wolff, 1995). True leukocytospermia is defined as greater than 1 million WBCs per milliliter and may indicate chronic epididymitis or prostatitis. In this scenario, many andrologists consider empiric antibiotic treatment prior to obtaining a repeat semen analysis. A common protocol would include doxycycline at a dosage of 100 mg orally twice daily for 2 weeks. Alternative approaches include culture of any expressible discharge or of the semen sample.

Unless a general obstetrician-gynecologist has developed expertise in male infertility, persistently abnormal semen analysis findings are an indication for referral to an infertility specialist. Although the partner may be referred directly to a urologist, it may be more reasonable to refer the couple to a reproductive endocrinologist, as the female will also require evaluation. Treatment is likely to be more complex in these couples and will typically be directed to both partners.

DNA Fragmentation

Elevated sperm DNA fragmentation as a cause of male infertility has garnered increased attention (Sakkas, 2010; Zini, 2009). Although some degree of DNA damage is likely repaired during embryogenesis, the location and extent of damage may lower fertilization and raise miscarriage rates. Greater levels of DNA damage are associated with advanced paternal age and external factors such as cigarette smoking, chemotherapy, radiation, environmental toxins, varicocele, and genital tract infections. In sperm samples with abnormal DNA fragmentation rates, higher levels of reactive oxygen species have been observed. In response to this, dietary supplementation with the antioxidants vitamin C and vitamin E has been proposed. However, data are currently lacking regarding the efficacy of this approach.

Numerous tests are currently available to analyze for DNA integrity and include the Sperm Chromatin Structure Assay (SCSA), the terminal deoxynucleotidyl transferase–mediated dUTP nick-end labeling (TUNEL) assay, the single-cell gel electrophoresis assay (COMET), and the sperm chromatin dispersion test (SCD) (American Society for Reproductive Medicine, 2013c). Each of these tests provides semiquantitative data on DNA structure. However, there is a lack of consensus regarding their appropriate threshold values and their ability to predict successful pregnancy. As a result, routine use of these is not recommended.

Additional Sperm Testing

Antisperm antibodies may be detected in as many as 10 percent of men. However, the negative fertility effects of antisperm antibodies found in semen is controversial. These antibodies may be particularly prevalent following vasectomy, testicular torsion, epididymitis, testicular biopsy, or other clinical situations in which the blood-testis barrier is breached (Lotti, 2018). Treatment historically included corticosteroids, but their efficacy to improve fertility is unclear. Moreover, significant side effects can include aseptic necrosis of the hip. Current data suggest that an antisperm antibody assay does not need to be a routine component of an infertility evaluation.

Numerous assays have been developed to test sperm function. These include the mannose fluorescence assay, hemizona assay, sperm penetration assay, and acrosome reaction test. The predictive significance of these assays is questionable, as they are based on nonphysiologic conditions and results vary among infertility centers. Most are no longer used and are not considered part of a basic infertility evaluation.

Hormonal Evaluation

Hormonal testing in the male is analogous to endocrine testing in an anovulatory female. Essentially, abnormalities may be due to central defects in hypothalamic-pituitary function or to defects within the testes. Most urologists will defer testing unless a sperm concentration is below 10 million/mL. Testing will include measurements of serum FSH and testosterone levels, and TSH and prolactin levels are considered.

Low FSH and low testosterone levels are consistent with hypothalamic dysfunction, such as idiopathic hypogonadotropic hypogonadism or Kallmann syndrome (Chap. 17, p. 378). In these patients, sperm production may be achieved with gonadotropin treatment. Although such treatment is frequently successful, at least 6 months may be required for detection of sperm production.

Elevated FSH and low testosterone levels provide evidence of testicular dysfunction, and most men with oligospermia are in this category. For men with this FSH and testosterone level pattern, the value of testosterone replacement should be determined. For example, normal spermatogenesis requires high levels of intratesticular testosterone, which cannot be achieved with exogenous testosterone. Furthermore, many of these men will lack spermatogonial stem cells. Thus, testosterone replacement will not rescue sperm production. In fact, replacement will decrease gonadotropin stimulation of remaining testicular function through negative feedback at the hypothalamus and pituitary. Unless the couple has chosen to use donor sperm, androgen supplementation is deferred during fertility treatment. However, replacement will provide other benefits, such as improved libido and sexual function, maintenance of muscle mass and bone density, and a general sense of well-being.

Imaging

Scrotal sonography is a common approach used to examine testicular morphology and identify varicocele or epididymal cysts or abscesses. Transrectal sonography provides information regarding the prostate and seminal vesicles or more central areas of obstruction in the vas deferens. More recently, MR imaging has become the preferred modality for imaging male accessory sex glands and ducts (Jurewicz, 2016; Mittal, 2017).

Testicular Biopsy

Evaluation of a severely oligospermic or azoospermic male may include either open or percutaneous testicular biopsy to determine whether viable sperm are present in the seminiferous tubules (Sharlip, 2002). For example, even men with testicular failure diagnosed by elevated serum FSH levels may have adequate sperm on biopsy for use in intracytoplasmic sperm injection. The biopsy specimen can be cryopreserved for future extraction of sperm during an IVF cycle. However, freshly biopsied specimens are generally felt to provide higher success rates. Thus, the biopsy may have diagnostic, prognostic, and therapeutic value.

GENETIC SCREENING

Testing before conception is often more straightforward and less stressful for the couple than delaying until pregnancy has been achieved. (American College of Obstetricians and Gynecologists, 2017a,b, 2018). Preconception carrier screening also allows a couple to consider the most complete range of reproductive options. Knowing the risk of having an affected child, a couple may consider preimplantation genetic diagnosis, prenatal genetic testing, or the use of donor gametes. One study demonstrated that indications for genetic screening were overlooked in approximately 25 percent of couples (McClatchey, 2018). To improve pregnancy outcomes, every attempt should be made to avoid this missed opportunity.

Traditional genotyping methods detect a limited number of mutations. These tests have been developed to be specific for the more common mutations found in a given ethnic group or clinical scenario. More recently, the cost of DNA sequencing has been greatly reduced by next-generation sequencing (NGS) techniques (Hallam, 2014). It is now possible to perform whole exome sequencing (WES) or whole genome sequencing (WGS) to obtain a full catalogue of an individual's DNA sequence.

These expanded genotyping panels hold great promise, as they allow rapid and efficient testing of many genes and thousands of mutations concurrently. However, the clinical relevance of numerous detected variants has not been determined. These are called *variants of unknown significance (VUS),* and limited data guide management once variants are identified. Thus, rigorous analytic and clinical validation is required before widespread clinical application of WES or WGS can be recommended (Prior, 2014).

Genetic Screening in the Female

Specific carrier screening is recommended by the American College of Obstetricians and Gynecologists (2017a,b) and by other advocacy groups and societies. No doubt, guidelines will continue to evolve as technology advances, costs fall, and benefits of obtaining this information become more evident. In the absence of known family history of genetic disease, it is reasonable to offer genetic carrier screening to the woman first and test the male partner only if the mother has positive results.

For all women considering pregnancy, current recommendations support offering carrier screening for cystic fibrosis, spinal muscular atrophy, thalassemias, and hemoglobinopathies. Additional testing may be indicated depending on ethnic

or racial group, for example, sickle cell screening in African Americans and multiple disorders in the Ashkenazi Jewish population. Importantly, no disorders are found uniquely in a given ethnic or racial group. Moreover, many families may be interracial, and ethnic background may be unknown.

In any patient with POI, karyotype testing for trisomy 21 mosaicism is considered. Likewise, Fragile X premutation carrier screening should be discussed with any woman with a family or personal history of POI or family history of intellectual disability. Additional information regarding genetic testing for POI is found in Chapter 17 (p. 375).

Genetic Screening in the Male

Genetic abnormalities are a relatively common cause of abnormal semen characteristics (American Society for Reproductive Medicine, 2018b). According to current World Health Organization recommendations, karyotype testing should be performed for any male with severe oligospermia ($<5 \times 10^6$ sperm/mL) or nonobstructive azoospermia (Barratt, 2017). Approximately 15 percent of azoospermic men and 5 percent of severely oligospermic men will have an abnormal karyotype. Although genetic abnormalities cannot be corrected, they may have implications for the health of the patient or their offspring. Therefore, karyotyping is pursued when indicated by these poor semen analysis results.

Klinefelter syndrome (47,XXY) will be a frequent finding. This syndrome is observed in approximately 1 in 500 men in the general population and accounts for 1 to 2 percent of male infertility cases. Classically, these men are tall, undervirilized, and have gynecomastia and small, firm testes. As the phenotype varies widely, lack of these characteristics does not preclude chromosomal evaluation. Conversely, a clinician may strongly consider obtaining karyotype testing in any male with these characteristics.

A patient with severely low sperm counts and a normal karyotype is offered testing for microdeletion of the Y chromosome. Up to 15 percent of men with severe oligospermia or azoospermia will have small deletions in a region of the Y chromosome termed the *azoospermia factor region (AZF)*. If the deletion is within the AZFa or AZFb subregions, it is unlikely that viable sperm can be recovered for use in IVF. Most men with an AZFc deletion will have viable sperm at biopsy. However, these deletions should be presumed to be inherited by their offspring. The clinical significance of microdeletions in the recently identified AZFd region is unknown, as these patients have apparently normal spermatogenesis (Hopps, 2003; Pryor, 1997).

Obstructive azoospermia may be due to congenital bilateral absence of the vas deferens (CBAVD). Approximately 70 to 85 percent of men with CBAVD will have mutations found in the cystic fibrosis transmembrane conductance regulator gene (*CFTR* gene), although not all will have clinical cystic fibrosis (Oates, 1994; Ratbi, 2007). Conversely, essentially all men with clinical cystic fibrosis will have CBAVD. Fortunately, testicular function in these men is usually normal, and adequate sperm may be obtained by epididymal aspiration to achieve pregnancy through IVF. Careful genetic counseling and testing of the female partner for carrier status is critical in these situations.

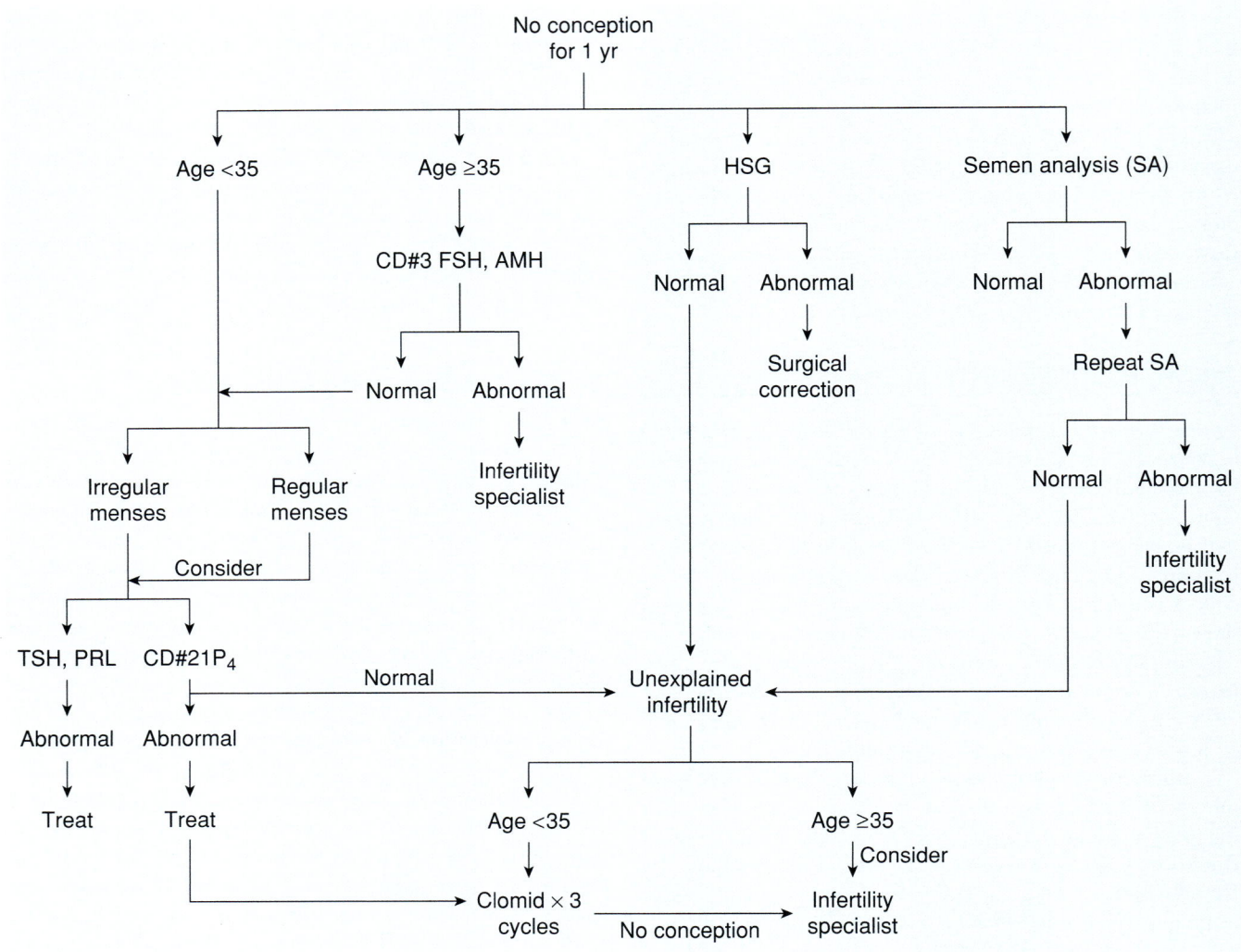

FIGURE 20-10 Diagnostic algorithm for evaluation of the infertile couple. AMH = anti-müllerian hormone; CD#3 = cycle day 3; CD#21 = cycle day 21; FSH = follicle-stimulating hormone; HSG = hysterosalpingography; P₄= progesterone; PRL = prolactin; SA = semen analysis; TSH = thyroid-stimulating hormone.

In excess of 1000 genes are believed to be required for successful sperm development. Mutations in more than 30 of these genes cause of male infertility (Okutman, 2018). Not yet standard practice, as for female infertility patients, well-validated genetic panels are expected to become available for male infertility testing in the future.

CONCLUSION

Figure 20-10 provides an algorithm for the evaluation of an infertile couple. Details will vary between practitioners and will be affected by patient presentation. In general, the female partner has some form of testing to confirm ovulation and to demonstrate normal endometrial cavity anatomy and tubal patency. In older women, evaluation of an early-follicular serum FSH level with or without AMH testing is essential to ensure adequate follicular reserves. The male partner has semen analysis performed. A subset of couples will decline HSG and semen analysis if the woman has a clear ovulatory defect. These couples are reminded that the incidence of couples having two

abnormalities is relatively high. These patients may be treated but are strongly encouraged to complete the evaluation if conception does not follow within a few months. Treatment options are discussed in Chapter 21 (p. 451).

REFERENCES

Aliyu MH, Aliyu SH, Salihu HM: Female genital tuberculosis: a global review. Int J Fertil Womens Med 49:123, 2004
American College of Obstetricians and Gynecologists: Carrier screening for genetic conditions. Committee Opinion No. 691 March 2017a
American College of Obstetricians and Gynecologists: Carrier screening in the age of genomic medicine. Committee Opinion No. 690 March 2017b
American College of Obstetricians and Gynecologists: Marijuana use during pregnancy and lactation. Committee Opinion No. 722, October 2017c
American College of Obstetricians and Gynecologists: Neural tube defects. Practice Bulletin No. 187, December 2017d
American College of Obstetricians and Gynecologists: Modern genetics in Obstetrics and Gynecology. Technology Assessment No. 14, August 2018
American College of Obstetricians and Gynecologists: Prepregnancy counseling. Committee Opinion No. 762, January 2019
American Society for Reproductive Medicine: Effectiveness and treatment for unexplained infertility. Fertil Steril 86(5) Suppl 1:S111, 2006

American Society for Reproductive Medicine: Endometriosis and infertility: a committee opinion. Fertil Steril 98(3):591, 2012

American Society for Reproductive Medicine: Access to fertility treatment by gays, lesbians, and unmarried persons: a committee opinion. Fertil Steril 100(6):1524, 2013a

American Society for Reproductive Medicine: Pathogenesis, consequences, and control of peritoneal adhesions in gynecologic surgery: a committee opinion. Fertil Steril 99(6):1550, 2013b

American Society for Reproductive Medicine: The clinical utility of sperm DNA integrity testing: a guideline. Fertil Steril 99(3):673, 2013c

American Society for Reproductive Medicine: Female age-related fertility decline. Fertil Steril 101(3):633, 2014a

American Society for Reproductive Medicine: Report on varicocele and infertility: a committee opinion. Fertil Steril 102(6):1556, 2014b

American Society for Reproductive Medicine: Access to fertility services by transgender persons: an Ethics Committee opinion. Fertil Steril 104(5):1111, 2015a

American Society for Reproductive Medicine: Diagnostic evaluation of the infertile female: a committee opinion. Fertil Steril 103(6):e44, 2015b

American Society for Reproductive Medicine: Diagnostic evaluation of the infertile male: a committee opinion. Fertil Steril 103(3):e18, 2015c

American Society for Reproductive Medicine: Disparities in access to effective treatment for infertility in the United States: an Ethics Committee opinion. Fertil Steril 104(5):1104, 2015d

American Society for Reproductive Medicine: Obesity and reproduction: a committee opinion. Fertil Steril 104(5):1116, 2015e

American Society for Reproductive Medicine: Subclinical hypothyroidism in the infertile female population: a guideline. Fertil Steril 104(3):545, 2015f

American Society for Reproductive Medicine: Testing and interpreting measures of ovarian reserve: a committee opinion. Fertil Steril 103(3):e9, 2015g

American Society for Reproductive Medicine: Removal of myomas in asymptomatic patients to improve fertility and/or reduce miscarriage rate: a guideline. Fertil Steril 108(3):416, 2017a

American Society for Reproductive Medicine: Society for Reproductive Endocrinology and Infertility. Optimizing natural fertility: a committee opinion. Fertil Steril 107(1):52, 2017b

American Society for Reproductive Medicine: Current recommendations for vaccines for female infertility patients: a committee opinion. Fertil Steril 110(5):838, 2018a

American Society for Reproductive Medicine: Evaluation of the azoospermic male: a committee opinion. Fertil Steril 109(5):777, 2018b

American Society for Reproductive Medicine: Smoking and infertility: a committee opinion. Fertil Steril 110(4):611, 2018c

American Society for Reproductive Medicine, Society for Male Reproduction and Urology: Diagnostic evaluation of sexual dysfunction in the male partner in the setting of infertility: a committee opinion. Fertil Steril 110(5):833, 2018d

Anderson J, Williamson R: Fertility after torsion of the spermatic cord. Br J Urol 65:225, 1990

Anguiano A, Oates R, Amos J, et al: Congenital bilateral absence of the vas deferens. A primarily genital form of cystic fibrosis. JAMA 267:1794, 1992

Augood C, Duckitt K, Templeton A: Smoking and female infertility: a systematic review and meta-analysis. Hum Reprod 13:1532, 1998

Baazeem A, Belzile E, Ciampi A, et al: Varicocele and male factor infertility treatment: a new meta-analysis and review of the role of varicocele repair. Eur Urol 60(4):796, 2011

Balasch J, Fabregues F, Creus M, et al: The usefulness of endometrial biopsy for luteal phase evaluation in infertility. Hum Reprod 7:973, 1992

Barratt CLR, Björndahl L, De Jonge CJ, et al: The diagnosis of male infertility: an analysis of the evidence to support the development of global WHO guidance—challenges and future research opportunities. Hum Reprod Update 23(6):660, 2017

Bates G, Garza D, Garza M: Clinical manifestations of hormonal changes in the menstrual cycle. Obstet Gynecol Clin North Am 17:299, 1990

Beard C, Benson R Jr, Kelalis P, et al: The incidence and outcome of mumps orchitis in Rochester, Minnesota, 1935 to 1974. Mayo Clin Proc 52:3, 1977

Ben-Arie A, Goldchmit C, Laviv Y, et al: The malignant potential of endometrial polyps. Eur J Obstet Gynecol Reprod Biol 115:206, 2004

Bracken M, Eskenazi B, Sachse K, et al: Association of cocaine use with sperm concentration, motility, and morphology. Fertil Steril 53:315, 1990

Buggio L, Monti E, Gattei U, et al: Adenomyosis: fertility and obstetric outcome. A comprehensive literature review. Minerva Ginecol 70(3):295, 2018

Buyalos R, Daneshmand S, Brzechffa P: Basal estradiol and follicle-stimulating hormone predict fecundity in women of advanced reproductive age undergoing ovulation induction therapy. Fertil Steril 68:272, 1997

Carson D, Lagow E, Thathiah A, et al: Changes in gene expression during the early to mid-luteal (receptive phase) transition in human endometrium detected by high-density microarray screening. Mol Hum Reprod 8:871, 2002

Caserta D, Mantovani A, Marci R, et al: Environment and women's reproductive health. Hum Reprod Update 17(3):418, 2011

Casper R, Meriano J, Jarvi K, et al: The hypo-osmotic swelling test for selection of viable sperm for intracytoplasmic sperm injection in men with complete asthenozoospermia. Fertil Steril 65:972, 1996

Cedars MI, Taymans SE, DePaolo LV, et al: The sixth vital sign: what reproduction tells us about overall health. Proceedings from a NICHD/CDC workshop. Hum Reprod Open, hox008:1, 2017

Chandra A, Copen CE, Stephen EH: Infertility and impaired fecundity in the United States, 1982–2010: data from the National Survey of Family Growth. Natl Health Stat Report 67:1, 2013

Chandra A, Copen CE, Stephen EH: Infertility service use in the United States: data from the National Survey of Family Growth, 1982–2010. Natl Health Stat Report 73:1, 2014

Chang JC, Tarr JA, Holland CL, et al: Beliefs and attitudes regarding prenatal marijuana use: perspectives of pregnant women who report use. Drug Alcohol Depend 196:14, 2019

Chang WY, Agarwal SK, Azziz R: Diagnostic evaluation and treatment of the infertile couple. In Carr BR, Blackwell RE, Azziz R (eds): Essential Reproductive Medicine. New York, McGraw-Hill, 2005, p 366

Charny C: The spermatogenic potential of the undescended testis before and after treatment. J Urol 38:697, 1960

Chu KY, Patel P, Ramasamy R: Consideration of gender differences in infertility evaluation. Curr Opin Urol 29:267, 2019

Cimino C, Borruso A, Napoli P, et al: Evaluation of the importance of Chlamydia T. and/or Mycoplasma H. and/or Ureaplasma U. genital infections and of antisperm antibodies in couples affected by muco-semen incompatibility and in couples with unexplained infertility. Acta Eur Fertil 24:13, 1993

Cobellis G, Noviello C, Nino F, et al: Spermatogenesis and cryptorchidism. Front Endocrinol 5:63, 2014

Consalvo V, Canero A, Salsano V: Bariatric surgery and infertility: a prospective study. Surg Technol Int 31:327, 2017

Cooper TG, Noonan E, von Eckardstein S, et al: World Health Organization reference values for human semen characteristics. Hum Reprod 16(3):231, 2010

Dashe JS, Cunningham FG: Teratology, teratogens, and fetotoxic agents. In Cunningham FG, Leveno KJ, Bloom SL, et al (eds): Williams Obstetrics, 25th ed. New York, McGraw-Hill, 2018, p 249

Daudin M, Bieth E, Bujan L, et al: Congenital bilateral absence of the vas deferens: clinical characteristics, biological parameters, cystic fibrosis transmembrane conductance regulator gene mutations, and implications for genetic counseling. Fertil Steril 74:1164, 2000

De Braekeleer M, Dao T: Cytogenetic studies in male infertility: a review. Hum Reprod 6:245, 1991

De Hondt A, Peeraer K, Meuleman C, et al: Endometriosis and subfertility treatment: a review. Minerva Ginecol 57:257, 2005

DeWaay DJ, Syrop CH, Nygaard IE, et al: Natural history of uterine polyps and leiomyomata. Obstet Gynecol 100:3, 2002

Di Vincenzo A, Busetto L, Vettor R, et al: Obesity, male reproductive function and bariatric surgery. Front Endocrinol (Lausanne) 9:769, 2018

Dreyer K, van Rijswijk J, Mijatovic V, et al: Oil-based or water-based contrast for hysterosalpingography in infertile women. N Engl J Med 376(21):2043, 2017

Dumont A, Robin G, Dewailly D: Anti-müllerian hormone in the pathophysiology and diagnosis of polycystic ovarian syndrome. Curr Opin Endocrinol Diabetes Obes 25(6):377, 2018

Dupree JM, Dickey RM, Lipshultz LI: Inequity between male and female coverage in state infertility laws. Fertil Steril 105(6):1519, 2016

Eisenberg ML, Li S, Behr B, et al: Semen quality, infertility and mortality in the USA. Hum Reprod 29(7):1567, 2014

Eisenberg ML, Li S, Cullen MR, et al: Increased risk of incident chronic medical conditions in infertile men: analysis of United States claims data. Fertil Steril 105(3):629, 2016

Farhi J, Ashkenazi J, Feldberg D, et al: Effect of uterine leiomyomata on the results of in-vitro fertilization treatment. Hum Reprod 10:2576, 1995

Farland LV, Collier AY, Correia KF, et al: Who receives a medical evaluation for infertility in the United States? Fertil Steril 105(5):1274, 2016

Frattarelli J, Lauria-Costab D, Miller B, et al: Basal antral follicle number and mean ovarian diameter predict cycle cancellation and ovarian responsiveness in assisted reproductive technology cycles. Fertil Steril 74:512, 2000

Garrido-Gomez T, Quinonera A, Antunez O, et al: Deciphering the proteomic signature of human endometrial receptivity. Hum Reprod 29(9):1957, 2014

Gazvani M, Buckett W, Luckas M, et al: Conservative management of azoospermia following steroid abuse. Hum Reprod 12:1706, 1997

Giudice LC: Infertility and the environment: the medical context. Semin Reprod Med 24:129, 2006

Gray M, Zilliox J, Khourdaji I, et al: Contemporary management of ejaculatory dysfunction. Transl Androl Urol 7(4):686, 2018

Grimbizis GF, Tsolakidis D, Mikos T, et al: A prospective comparison of transvaginal ultrasound, saline infusion sonohysterography, and diagnostic hysteroscopy in the evaluation of endometrial pathology. Fertil Steril 94(7):2720, 2010

Grinsted J, Jacobsen J, Grinsted L, et al: Prediction of ovulation. Fertil Steril 52:388, 1989

Grodstein F, Goldman M, Cramer D: Body mass index and ovulatory infertility. Epidemiology 5:247, 1994a

Grodstein F, Goldman M, Cramer D: Infertility in women and moderate alcohol use. Am J Public Health 84:1429, 1994b

Groszmann YS, Benacerraf BR: Complete evaluation of anatomy and morphology of the infertile patient in a single visit; the modern infertility pelvic ultrasound examination. Fertil Steril 105(6):1381, 2016

Guermandi E, Vegetti W, Bianchi M, et al: Reliability of ovulation tests in infertile women. Obstet Gynecol 97:92, 2001

Guttmacher A: Factors affecting normal expectancy of conception. JAMA 161:855, 1956

Guzick D, Overstreet J, Factor-Litvak P, et al: Sperm morphology, motility, and concentration in fertile and infertile men. N Engl J Med 345:1388, 2001

Hadziselimovic F: Early successful orchidopexy does not prevent from developing azoospermia. Int Braz J Urol 32(5):570, 2006

Hales CM, Fryar CD, Carroll MD, et al: Trends in obesity and severe obesity prevalence in US youth and adults by sex and age, 2007–2008 to 2015–2016. JAMA 319(16):1723, 2018

Hallam S, Nelson H, Greger V, et al: Validation for clinical use of, and initial clinical experience with, a novel approach to population-based carrier screening using high-throughput, next-generation DNA sequencing. J Mol Diagn 16(2):180, 2014

Hansen KR, Hodnett GM, Knowlton N, et al: Correlation of ovarian reserve tests with histologically determined primordial follicle number. Fertil Steril 95(1):170, 2011

Hanson BM, Aston KI, Jenkins TG, et al: The impact of ejaculatory abstinence on semen analysis parameters: a systematic review. J Assist Reprod Genet 35(2):213, 2018a

Hanson BM, Eisenberg ML, Hotaling JM: Male infertility: a biomarker of individual and familial cancer risk. Fertil Steril 109(1):6, 2018b

Hatch EE, Wise LA, Mikkelsen EM, et al: Caffeinated beverage and soda consumption and time to pregnancy. Epidemiology 23(3):393, 2012

Hauser R, Sokol R: Science linking environmental contaminant exposures with fertility and reproductive health impacts in the adult male. Fertil Steril 89(2 Suppl):e59, 2008

Heller C, Clermont Y: Spermatogenesis in man: an estimate of its duration. Science 140:184, 1963

Hershlag A, Schiff S, DeCherney A: Retrograde ejaculation. Hum Reprod 6:255, 1991

Hinrichsen M, Blaquier J: Evidence supporting the existence of sperm maturation in the human epididymis. J Reprod Fertil 60:291, 1980

Hopps CV, Mielnik A, Goldstein M, et al: Detection of sperm in men with Y chromosome microdeletions of the AZFa, AZFb, and AZFc regions. Hum Reprod 18(8):1660, 2003

Hornburg R, Crawford G: The role of AMH in anovulation associated with PCOS: a hypothesis. Hum Reprod 29(6):1117, 2014

Hwang K, Guo D: Sports-related male infertility. Eur Urol Focus 5(6):1143, 2019

Jamal A, Phillips E, Gentzke AS, et al: Current cigarette smoking among adults-United States, 2016. MMWR 67(2):53, 2018

Jayaprakasan K, Polanski L, Sahu B, et al: Removal of endometrial polyps prior to infertility treatment. Cochrane Database Syst Rev 8:CD009592, 2014

Jurewicz M, Gilbert BR: Imaging and angiography in male factor infertility. Fertil Steril 105(6):1432, 2016

Kao L, Germeyer A, Tulac S, et al: Expression profiling of endometrium from women with endometriosis reveals candidate genes for disease-based implantation failure and infertility. Endocrinology 144:2870, 2003

Kasman AM, Thoma ME, McLain AC, et al: Association between use of marijuana and time to pregnancy in men and women: findings from the national survey of family growth. Fertil Steril 109(5):866, 2018

Katz D, Slade D, Nakajima S: Analysis of pre-ovulatory changes in cervical mucus hydration and sperm penetrability. Adv Contracept 13:143, 1997

Keefe D, Niven-Fairchild T, Powell S, et al: Mitochondrial deoxyribonucleic acid deletions in oocytes and reproductive aging in women. Fertil Steril 64:577, 1995

Keyhani S, Steigerwald S, Ishida J, et al: Risks and benefits of marijuana use: a national survey of U.S. adults. Ann Intern Med 169(5):282, 2018

Kidd S, Eskenazi B, Wyrobek A: Effects of male age on semen quality and fertility: a review of the literature. Fertil Steril 75:237, 2001

Klonoff-Cohen H, Lam-Kruglick P, Gonzalez C: Effects of maternal and paternal alcohol consumption on the success rates of in vitro fertilization and gamete intrafallopian transfer. Fertil Steril 79:330, 2003

Klonoff-Cohen H, Natarajan L, Marrs R, et al: Effects of female and male smoking on success rates of IVF and gamete intra-fallopian transfer. Hum Reprod 16(7):1382, 2001

Kohn TP, Ohlander SJ, Jacob JS, et al: The effect of subclinical varicocele on pregnancy rates and semen parameters: a systematic review and meta-analysis. Curr Urol Rep 19(7):53, 2018

Kruger T, Acosta A, Simmons K, et al: Predictive value of abnormal sperm morphology in in vitro fertilization. Fertil Steril 49:112, 1988

Lalos O: Risk factors for tubal infertility among infertile and fertile women. Eur J Obstet Gynecol Reprod Biol 29:129, 1988

La Marca A, Broekmans FJ, Volpe A, et al: Anti-Mullerian hormone (AMH): what do we still need to know? Hum Reprod 24(9):2264, 2009

Lee P: Fertility in cryptorchidism: Does treatment make a difference? Endocrinol Metab Clin North Texas 22:479 1993

Lessey B: Endometrial integrins and the establishment of uterine receptivity. Hum Reprod 13(Suppl 3):247, 1998

Levitas E, Lunenfeld E, Weisz N, et al: Relationship between age and semen parameters in men with normal sperm concentration: analysis of 6022 semen samples. Andrologia 39(2):45, 2007

Lotti F, Baldi E, Corona G, et al: Epididymal more than testicular abnormalities are associated with the occurrence of antisperm antibodies as evaluated by the MAR test. Hum Reprod 33(8):1417, 2018

Luciano A, Peluso J, Koch E, et al: Temporal relationship and reliability of the clinical, hormonal, and ultrasonographic indices of ovulation in infertile women. Obstet Gynecol 75(3 Pt 1):412, 1990

Makker A, Goel MM: Uterine leiomyomas: effects on architectural, cellular, and molecular determinants of endometrial receptivity. Reprod Sci 20(6):631, 2013

Maroulis G: Effect of aging on fertility and pregnancy. Semin Reprod Endocrinol 9:165, 1991

Martinez GM, Daniels K, Febo-Vazquez I: Fertility of men and women aged 15–44 in the United States: national survey of family growth, 2011–2015. Natl Health Stat Report (113):1, 2018

Maseelall PB, Hernandez-Rey AE, Oh C, et al: Antral follicle count is a significant predictor of livebirth in in vitro fertilization cycles. Fertil Steril 91(4 Suppl):1595, 2009

Mazur DJ, Lipshultz LI: Infertility in the aging male. Curr Urol Rep 19(7):54, 2018

McClatchey T, Lay E, Strassberg M, et al: Missed opportunities: unidentified genetic risk factors in prenatal care. Prenat Diagn 38(1):75, 2018

McKinley M, O'Loughlin VD: Reproductive System in Human Anatomy. New York, McGraw-Hill, 2006, p 873

Mendola P, Messer LC, Rappazzo K: Science linking environmental contaminant exposures with fertility and reproductive health impacts in the adult female. Fertil Steril 89(2 Suppl):e81, 2008

Menken J, Trussell J, Larsen U: Age and infertility. Science 233(4771):1389, 1986

Metwally M, Cheong YC, Horne AW: Surgical removal of fibroids does not improve fertility outcomes. Cochrane Database Syst Rev 11:CD003857, 2012

Miller P, Soules M: The usefulness of a urinary LH kit for ovulation prediction during menstrual cycles of normal women. Obstet Gynecol 87:13, 1996

Mittal PK, Little B, Harri PA, et al: Role of imaging in the evaluation of male infertility. Radiographics 37(3):837, 2017

Moen M, Magnus P: The familial risk of endometriosis. Acta Obstet Gynecol Scand 72:560, 1993

Mosher W, Pratt W: Fecundity and infertility in the United States: incidence and trends. Fertil Steril 56:192, 1991

Muthusami KR, Chinnaswamy P: Effect of chronic alcoholism on male fertility hormones and semen quality. Fertil Steril 84(4):919, 2005

Nagy F, Pendergrass P, Bowen D, et al: A comparative study of cytological and physiological parameters of semen obtained from alcoholics and non-alcoholics. Alcohol Alcohol 21:17, 1986

Nezar M, Goda H, El-Negery M, et al: Genital tract tuberculosis among fertile women: an old problem revisited. Arch Gynecol Obstet 280(5):787, 2009

Noyes R, Hertig A, Rock J: Dating the endometrial biopsy. Am J Obstet Gynecol 122:262, 1975

Oates R, Amos J: The genetic basis of congenital bilateral absence of the vas deferens and cystic fibrosis. J Androl 15:1, 1994

Oei S, Keirse M, Bloemenkamp K, et al: European postcoital tests: opinions and practice. BJOG 102:621, 1995

Oei SG, Helmerhorst FM, Bloemenkamp KW: Effectiveness of the postcoital test: randomised controlled trial. BMJ 317(7157):502, 1998

Okutman O, Rhouma MB, Benkhalifa M, et al: Genetic evaluation of patients with non-syndromic male infertility. J Assist Reprod Genet 35(11):1939, 2018

Pellestor F, Andreo B, Arnal F, et al: Maternal aging and chromosomal abnormalities: new data drawn from in vitro unfertilized human oocytes. Hum Genet 112:195, 2003

Perez-Medina T, Bajo-Arenas J, Salazar F, et al: Endometrial polyps and their implication in the pregnancy rates of patients undergoing intrauterine insemination: a prospective, randomized study. Hum Reprod 20:1632, 2005

Petracco RG, Kong A, Grechukhina O, et al: Global gene expression profiling of proliferative phase endometrium reveals distinct functional subdivisions. Reprod Sci 19(10):1138, 2012

Petrangelo A, Czuzoj-Shulman N, Balayla J, et al: Cannabis abuse or dependence during pregnancy: a population-based cohort study on 12 million births. J Obstet Gynaecol Can 41(5):623, 2019

Pilone V, Tramontano S, Renzulli M, et al: Evaluation of anti-Müller hormone AMH levels in obese women after sleeve gastrectomy. Gynecol Endocrinol 35(6):548, 2019

Prior TW: Next-generation carrier screening: are we ready? Genome Med 6(8):62, 2014

Pritts E: Fibroids and infertility: a systematic review of the evidence. Obstet Gynecol Surv 56:483, 2001

Pryor J, Kent-First M, Muallem A, et al: Microdeletions in the Y chromosome of infertile men. N Engl J Med 336:534, 1997

Ramlau-Hansen CH, Thulstrup AM, Aggerholm AS, et al: Is smoking a risk factor for decreased semen quality? A cross-sectional analysis. Human Reprod 22(1):188, 2007

Ratbi I, Legendre M, Niel F, et al: Detection of cystic fibrosis transmembrane conductance regulator (CFTR) gene rearrangements enriches the mutation spectrum in congenital bilateral absence of the vas deferens and impacts on genetic counseling. Hum Reprod 22(5):1285, 2007

Rosenfeld DL, Scholl G, Bronson R, et al: Unsuspected chronic pelvic inflammatory disease in the infertile female. Fertil Steril 39:44, 1983

Roth LK, Taylor HS: Risks of smoking to reproductive health: assessment of women's knowledge. Am J Obstet Gynecol 184(5):934, 2001

Rowley M, Teshima F, Heller C: Duration of transit of spermatozoa through the human male ductular system. Fertil Steril 21:390, 1970

Ruan YC, Chen H, Chan HC: Ion channels in the endometrium: regulation of endometrial receptivity and embryo implantation. Hum Reprod Update 20(4):517, 2014

Sakkas D, Alvarez JG: Sperm DNA fragmentation: mechanisms of origin, impact on reproductive outcome, and analysis. Fertil Steril 93(4):1027, 2010

Samejima T, Koba K, Nakae H, et al: Identifying patients who can improve fertility with myomectomy. Eur J Obstet Gynecol Reprod Biol 185C:28, 2014

Saracoglu OF, Mungan T, Tanzer F: Pelvic tuberculosis. Int J Gynaecol Obstet 37:115, 1992

Schenker J: Etiology of and therapeutic approach to synechia uteri. Eur J Obstet Gynecol Reprod Biol 65:109, 1996

Scott R, Snyder R, Bagnall J, et al: Evaluation of the impact of intraobserver variability on endometrial dating and the diagnosis of luteal phase defects. Fertil Steril 60:652, 1993

Seifer DB, Baker VL, Leader B: Age-specific serum anti-Mullerian hormone values for 17,120 women presenting to fertility centers within the United States. Fertil Steril 95(2074), 2011

Seshadri S, El-Toukhy T, Douiri A, et al: Diagnostic accuracy of saline infusion sonography in the evaluation of uterine cavity abnormalities prior to assisted reproductive techniques: a systematic review and meta-analysis. Hum Reprod Update 21(2):262, 2015

Sharlip I, Jarow J, Belker A, et al: Best practice policies for male infertility. Fertil Steril 77:873, 2002

Sigman M, Jarow JP: Endocrine evaluation of infertile men. Urology 50(5):659, 1997

Slopien R, Horst N, Jeremek JD, et al: The impact of surgical treatment of obesity on the female fertility. Gynecol Endocrinol 35(2):100, 2019

Soares S, Barbosa dos Reis M, Camargos A: Diagnostic accuracy of sonohysterography, transvaginal sonography, and hysterosalpingography in patients with uterine cavity diseases. Fertil Steril 73:406, 2000

Stanford J, White G, Hatasaka H: Timing intercourse to achieve pregnancy: current evidence. Obstet Gynecol 100:1333, 2002

Stirnemann JJ, Samson A, Bernard JP, et al: Day-specific probabilities of conception in fertile cycles resulting in spontaneous pregnancies. Hum Reprod 28(4):1110, 2013

Swart P, Mol B, van der Veen F, et al: The accuracy of hysterosalpingography in the diagnosis of tubal pathology: a meta-analysis. Fertil Steril 64:486, 1995

Tietze C: Reproductive span and rate of reproduction among Hutterite women. Fertil Steril 8:89, 1957

Tolstrup J, Kjaer S, Holst C, et al: Alcohol use as predictor for infertility in a representative population of Danish women. Acta Obstet Gynecol Scand 82:744, 2003

Treloar S, Do K, Martin N: Genetic influences on the age at menopause. Lancet 352:1084, 1998

Wilcox A, Weinberg C, Baird D: Timing of sexual intercourse in relation to ovulation. Effects on the probability of conception, survival of the pregnancy, and sex of the baby. N Engl J Med 333:1517, 1995

Wolff H: The biologic significance of white blood cells in semen. Fertil Steril 63:1143, 1995

World Health Organization: Laboratory manual for the examination of human semen and sperm-cervical mucus interaction. Cambridge University Press, 1999

World Health Organization: WHO laboratory manual for the examination and processing of human semen, 5th ed. Geneva, WHO Press, 2010

Zenzes MT: Smoking and reproduction: gene damage to human gametes and embryos. Hum Reprod Update 6(2):122, 2000

Zini A, Sigman M: Are tests of sperm DNA damage clinically useful? Pros and cons. J Androl 30:219, 2009

CHAPTER 21

Treatment of the Infertile Couple

Infertility results from diseases of the reproductive system that impair the body's ability to perform basic reproductive function. It is defined as the failure to achieve a successful pregnancy after 12 months or more of regular unprotected intercourse. Earlier evaluation and treatment may be justified based on medical history and physical findings and is warranted after 6 months for women older than 35 (American Society for Reproductive Medicine, 2015a). Ten to 15 percent of the reproductive-aged population is infertile, and men and women are equally affected.

Infertility treatment is a complex process influenced by numerous factors. Important considerations include duration of infertility, a couple's age (especially the female's), and diagnosed cause. Additionally, the level of distress experienced by a couple is factored.

In general, initial steps strive to identify a primary cause and contributing factors. Treatment is aimed at their direct correction and is typically medication or surgery. In many cases, therapy can begin without a complete evaluation, especially if a cause is obvious. However, if pregnancy does not quickly follow, more thorough testing is prudent.

However, evaluation commonly may not yield a satisfactory explanation or may identify causes that are not amenable to direct correction. For such cases, recent advances in assisted reproduction provide effective options. Assisted reproductive technology (ART) employs procedures that at some point require extraction and isolation of an oocyte. These approaches, however, are not without disadvantages. As one example, in vitro fertilization (IVF) is linked to higher rates of some fetal

and maternal complications. Appropriate treatments may also pose ethical dilemmas for couples or their physician. For example, selective reduction of a multifetal pregnancy may improve survival chances for some fetuses but at the cost of others. Last, infertility treatment can be a financial burden, a significant source of emotional stress, or both. During consultation, an infertility specialist does not dictate treatment but offers and explains therapy options, which may include expectant management or even adoption.

LIFESTYLE THERAPIES

◼ Weight Optimization

Ovarian function is dependent on weight. Low body-fat content is linked with hypothalamic hypogonadism. In contrast, central body fat is associated with insulin resistance and contributes to ovarian dysfunction in many women with polycystic ovarian syndrome (PCOS). Lifestyle modification in overweight infertile women with PCOS leads to a reduction of central fat and improved insulin sensitivity, decreased hyperandrogenemia, lowered luteinizing hormone (LH) concentrations, and restoration of fertility in many cases (Hoeger, 2001; Kiddy, 1992). Even a 5 to 10 percent reduction in body weight can be successful in women with PCOS (Crosignani, 2003; Kiddy, 1992; Pasquali, 1989). Apart from diet, exercise can also improve insulin sensitivity. Weight loss and exercise are inexpensive and should be recommended as first-line management of obese women with PCOS.

Although pharmacologic options can effectively treat anovulation if weight cannot be lost, obesity alone is a significant risk factor for obstetric and perinatal complications. These include higher rates of gestational diabetes, cesarean delivery, preeclampsia, unexplained stillbirth, and surgical wound infection (Hawkins, 2018). Obesity also is associated with an increased risk of birth defects (American Society for Reproductive Medicine, 2015b). Thus, delaying treatments in morbidly obese women until their body mass index (BMI) can be reduced below 35 should be strongly considered. This is especially true if treatments involve surgical risks or risk of multifetal gestation.

Weight-loss options are discussed in Chapter 1 (p. 14). If bariatric surgery is selected, delaying conception for 1 to 2 years is advised (American Society for Reproductive Medicine, 2015b). Rapid weight loss during this time poses theoretical risks for fetal-growth restriction and nutritional deprivation. However, because these risks remain theoretical, any benefits of postponing pregnancy must be balanced against the risk of declining fertility with aging. It might be reasonable to consider achieving pregnancy prior to 1 year if weight has stabilized. In any case, women who have undergone bariatric surgery should be evaluated for nutritional deficiencies and the need for vitamin supplementation (American College of Obstetricians and Gynecologists, 2018b).

Undernutrition can also be problematic. The reproductive axis is closely linked to nutritional status, and inhibitory pathways suppress ovulation in subjects with significant weight loss (Chap. 17, p. 378). Anorexia nervosa and bulimia nervosa affect up to 5 percent of reproductive-aged women and may cause amenorrhea, infertility, and, in those who do conceive, an increased likelihood of miscarriage. Fortunately, recovery may follow minimal acquisition of weight because energy balance has a more important effect than body fat.

■ Exercise

Physical activity has numerous health benefits. The relationship between exercise and fertility, however, is not straightforward. Competitive female athletes often experience amenorrhea, irregular cycles or luteal dysfunction, and infertility. This may be related not specifically to physical activity itself but rather to low body-fat content or physical stress associated with competition. At this time, insufficient data exist to support or discourage physical activity in infertile women in the absence of documented ovarian dysfunction associated with obesity or low body weight.

■ Nutrition

In the absence of obesity or significant undernutrition, the role of diet in infertility is unclear. High-protein diets and gluten intolerance (celiac disease) have been investigated as underlying causes in women. However, studies sizes have been small, and conflicting results found (Collin, 1996; Jackson, 2008; Meloni, 1999). In men, dietary antioxidants have been proposed as a potential way to improve male reproductive outcomes by reducing oxidative damage in sperm DNA (Ross, 2010). Although the approach is promising, large well-designed studies to guide its clinical use are needed (Patel, 2008). The nutritional supplement carnitine also had been touted as a potential benefit for male infertility. This finding, however, has not been confirmed by a randomized trial (Sigman, 2006).

Despite a lack of conclusive benefits to supplements or diet modification in infertile couples, daily multivitamin supplementation for both is reasonable. Folic acid is contained in most multivitamins, and daily doses of 400 μg orally are recommended for women attempting pregnancy to reduce the incidence of neural-tube defects in their fetuses (American College of Obstetricians and Gynecologist, 2017).

Herbal therapies including traditional Chinese medicine (TCM) and acupuncture have been suggested to enhance fertility either alone or in conjunction with standard therapies including ART. Smith and associates (2010) found that 29 percent of infertile couples seeking pregnancy in the United States had used complementary and alternative medicine. At this time, however, current evidence does not support the benefit of TCM or acupuncture on fertility as a primary or an adjunct treatment (American Society for Reproductive Medicine, 2017).

■ Stress Management

Stress has been implicated in reproductive failure. Although severe stress can result in anovulation, less significant stress also may play a role by a yet undefined mechanism. Patients with higher stress levels have lower pregnancy rates with IVF treatments (Thiering, 1993). Accordingly, screening all infertile couples for anxiety or depression is a consideration. Although pharmacologic management of stress is not typically recommended during infertility treatments, a "mind/body" approach that combines psychological counseling and meditation may be reasonable for those patients manifesting high levels of anxiety (Domar, 1990).

CORRECTION OF OVARIAN DYSFUNCTION

■ Hyperprolactinemia

Prolactin is a pituitary hormone with important roles in various reproductive functions, and elevated levels are commonly encountered in clinical endocrinology practice. If hyperprolactinemia is found, then physiologic, pharmacologic, or other secondary causes of hormone hypersecretion are sought (Table 13-2, p. 285).

Dopamine agonists are the primary treatment of hyperprolactinemia (Chap. 16, p. 362). Surgery is only considered for prolactin-secreting adenomas that are resistant to medical therapy or that are large. During pregnancy, if hyperprolactinemia is not associated with a pituitary lesion or a lesion measures <10 mm (microadenoma), then dopamine-agonist therapy is stopped because the tumor-expansion risk is low (Molitch, 1999). If the tumor size is ≥10 mm (macroadenoma), bromocriptine (Parlodel) use is advised during pregnancy to avoid significant tumor growth.

■ Hypothyroidism

Thyroid disorders are prevalent during reproductive years and affect women four to five times more often than men. In women, oligomenorrhea and amenorrhea are frequent findings. Although ovulation and conception can still occur in those with mild hypothyroidism, treatment with thyroxine usually restores a normal menstrual pattern and enhances fertility.

Subclinical hypothyroidism may also be associated with ovarian dysfunction (Strickland, 1990). Lincoln and colleagues (1999) found a 2-percent incidence of elevated thyroid-stimulating hormone (TSH) levels in 704 asymptomatic women seeking evaluation for infertility. Correction of hypothyroidism in those with ovarian dysfunction and elevated TSH levels led to pregnancy in 64 percent. In addition, subclinical hypothyroidism may also adversely affect pregnancy outcomes, but current evidence does not support treatment of subclinical hypothyroidism during pregnancy to improve these outcomes (Casey, 2018). That said, in women seeking treatment for infertility, early detection and treatment of hypothyroidism of any degree is advised.

■ Ovulation Induction

Ovarian dysfunction is the most common indication for the use of medications to induce ovulation. These agents can also be selected for ovulatory women to enhance the likelihood of pregnancy in couples with other causes of infertility or unexplained infertility. Use of these to promote multifollicular development and prompt ovulation is called *superovulation* or *ovulation enhancement*. If these agents are administered solely to stimulate follicles and then egg harvesting is completed by ART, the termed *controlled ovarian stimulation (COS)* is used. We prefer the term *ovulation induction* to describe treatment with medications to stimulate normal (ideally monofollicular) ovulation in women with ovarian dysfunction.

Frequent causes of ovarian dysfunction include PCOS and diminished ovarian reserve. Less often, central (hypothalamic or pituitary) disorders or thyroid dysfunction can result in infertility (Table 17-3, p. 373). Rarely, ovarian tumors or adrenal abnormalities lead to abnormal ovarian function. Treatment of ovarian dysfunction is based on the identified cause and the results of any prior attempted therapy.

Clomiphene Citrate

Clomiphene citrate (CC) is the initial treatment for most anovulatory infertile women. Chemically similar to tamoxifen, CC is a nonsteroidal triphenylethylene derivative that demonstrates both estrogen agonist and antagonist properties. Antagonist properties predominate except at very low estrogen levels. As a result, negative feedback that is normally produced by estrogen in the hypothalamus is reduced (Fig. 21-1). Gonadotropin-releasing hormone (GnRH) secretion is altered and stimulates pituitary gonadotropin release. The resulting increase in follicle-stimulating hormone (FSH) levels, in turn, drives ovarian follicular activity.

Tamoxifen also has been used successfully for ovulation induction. However, it is not Food and Drug Administration (FDA) approved for this indication and does not offer significant advantage compared with CC.

CC is administered orally, typically starting on the third to fifth day after the onset of spontaneous or progestin-induced menses. Ovulation rates, conception rates, and pregnancy outcomes are similar whether treatment begins on cycle day 2, 3, 4, or 5. Prior to therapy and to avoid complications, sonography is advised to exclude significant spontaneous follicular maturation or residual follicular cysts. In general at our institution, clomiphene can be administered if no follicle is >20 mm and the endometrium is less than 5 mm. Both reflect minimal ovarian activity. Significant activity would complicate cycle stimulation. A pregnancy test is also indicated after spontaneous menses. Although not a proven teratogen, CC is classified as category X by the FDA and thus is contraindicated in suspected or documented pregnancy.

The dose required to achieve ovulation correlates with body weight. However, no reliable method accurately predicts the effective dose in an individual woman (Lobo, 1982). Consequently, CC is titrated empirically to establish the lowest productive dose for each patient. Treatment typically begins with a single 50-mg tablet taken daily for 5 consecutive days. Doses are increased by a 50-mg increment in each subsequent cycle until ovulation is induced. The dose of CC should not be increased if normal ovulation is confirmed. Thus, lack of pregnancy alone does not justify a dose increase. The effective dose of CC ranges from 50 mg/d to 250 mg/d, although doses in excess of 100 mg/d

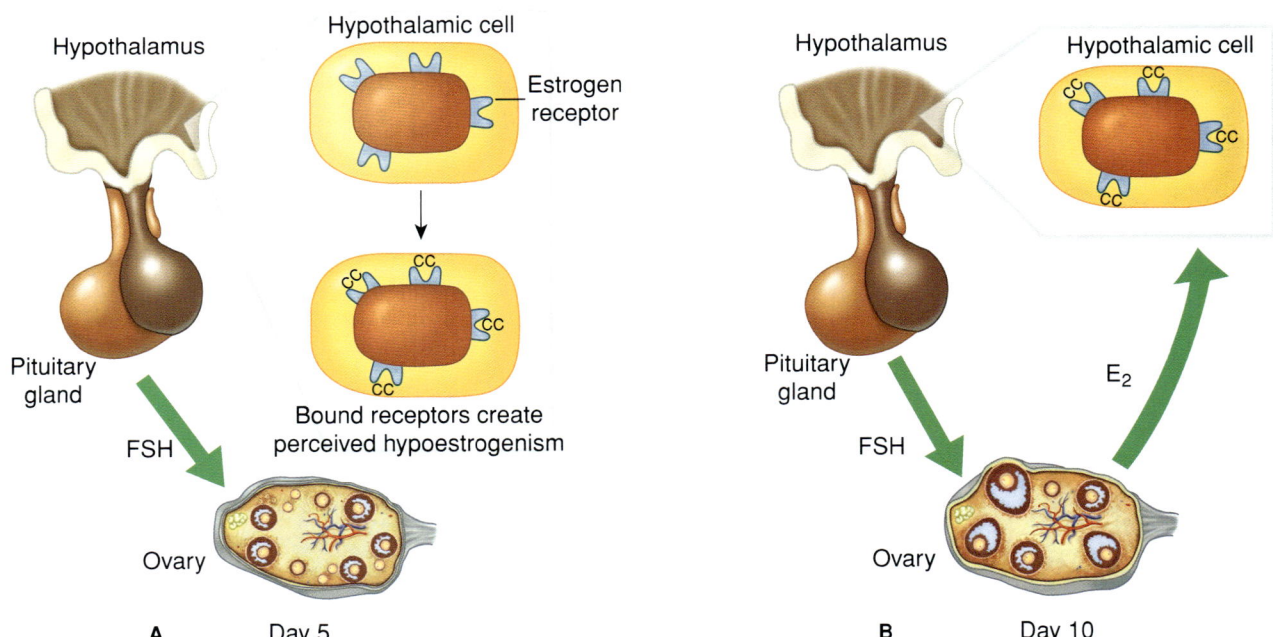

FIGURE 21-1 Effect of clomiphene citrate (CC) administration. **A.** Early in the cycle, CC binds to the estrogen receptor in the pituitary and hypothalamus. This causes an effective reduction in hypothalamic estrogen receptor number. Because of this reduced receptor number, the hypothalamus and pituitary are blinded to true circulating estrogen levels and perceived hypoestrogenism results. As a result, estrogen's negative feedback is interrupted centrally, and follicle-stimulating hormone (FSH) secretion increases from the anterior pituitary. This leads to maturation of multiple follicles. **B.** By the late follicular phase, because of CC's long retention within tissues, estrogen receptor depletion continues centrally. As a result, enhanced estradiol (E₂) secretion from the ovary is not capable of exerting normal negative feedback on FSH release. This leads to a growth of multiple dominant follicles and multiple ovulations.

TABLE 21-1. Gonadotropin Preparations Used for Ovulation Induction

Name	Product Type	Derivation	FSH Activity	LH or hCG Activity
Gonal-f or Bemfola	Follitropin alpha	Recombinant FSH	Yes	None
Follistim or Puregon	Follitropin beta	Recombinant FSH	Yes	None
Rekovelle	Follitropin delta	Recombinant FSH	Yes	None
Elonva	Follitropin gamma	Recombinant FSH	Yes	None
Menopur	Menotropin	Highly purified, urine-derived	Yes	hCG

FSH = follicle-stimulating hormone; hCG = human chorionic gonadotropin.

are not approved by the FDA and have low likelihood of success. Some studies suggest that adjunctive glucocorticoid therapy may benefit some patients not responsive to CC alone (Elnashar, 2006; Parsanezhad, 2002). The precise mechanism is unclear. This therapy may be empiric or individualized based on elevated dehydroepiandrosterone sulfate (DHEAS) levels.

In general, women failing to ovulate with a dose of 100 mg/d or failing to conceive following 3 to 6 months of ovulatory response to CC should be considered candidates for alternative treatments. In one study, 84.5 percent of pregnancies achieved with ovulation induction occurred during the first three ovulatory cycles (Gysler, 1982).

Insulin-Sensitizing Agents

Many women with PCOS exhibit insulin resistance (Chap. 18, p. 399). Insulin resistance leads to compensatory hyperinsulinemia and dyslipidemia. Given that hyperinsulinemia plays a pathogenic role in PCOS development, reduction of circulating insulin levels in women with PCOS may restore normal reproductive endocrine function. As discussed, weight loss, nutrition, and exercise clearly can lead to reduced hyperinsulinemia, resolution of hyperandrogenism, and in some cases, resumption of ovulatory function in overweight women with PCOS. However, women may be poorly compliant, and weight loss is rarely maintained over time.

Insulin-sensitizing agents have been proposed for the treatment of PCOS. In patients with insulin resistance, these compounds enhance target tissue responsiveness to insulin and thereby reduce the need for compensatory hyperinsulinemia (Antonucci, 1998). Current insulin-sensitizing agents include the biguanides and thiazolidinediones (Chap. 18, p. 401).

Of these, studies suggest that metformin (Glucophage) increases the frequency of spontaneous ovulation, menstrual cyclicity, and the ovulatory response to CC in women with PCOS (Nestler, 1998; Palomba, 2005; Vandermolen, 2001). Doses are 500 mg orally three times daily or 850 mg twice daily with meals. In contrast, a large, randomized trial failed to support the hypothesis that metformin, either alone or in combination with CC, improves the live-birth rate in women with PCOS (Legro, 2007). This study emphasizes the use of live birth as the primary endpoint for efficacy rather than intermediate or surrogate endpoints.

Gonadotropins

CC is easy to use and leads to ovulation in most patients (Hammond, 1983). However, reported cumulative pregnancy rates are disappointing and range from approximately 25 to 50 percent (Legro, 2007; Raj, 1977; Zarate, 1971). Lower than expected pregnancy rates with CC are attributed to its long half-life and peripheral antiestrogenic effects, mainly on the endometrium and cervical mucus. For such individuals, who are often classified as "clomiphene resistant," the next step is traditionally the administration of exogenous gonadotropin preparations via injections.

As with CC, the goal of ovulation induction with gonadotropins is simply to reestablish normal ovarian function. Ideally, the dose used is the minimum required to cause normal development of a single dominant follicle. Because the response to gonadotropins can differ greatly among women and even among cycles, intensive monitoring is required to adjust dosage and ovulation timing.

Gonadotropin preparations vary in terms of their source (urinary or recombinant) and by the presence or absence of LH activity (Table 21-1). Human menopausal gonadotropin (hMG) preparations were the first gonadotropin option, and agents in this class are termed *menotropins*. hMG products contain both FSH and LH activity. These medications are extracted and purified from the urine of postmenopausal women, which is a cohort with normally high FSH, LH, and human chorionic gonadotropin (hCG) levels. In the past, hMG preparations contained both LH and hCG as dual sources of LH activity (Filicori, 2002). Remember, LH and hCG both bind to the same receptor (luteinizing hormone/chorionic gonadotropin receptor [LHCGR]).

In the older, non-highly purified hMG products, significant non-gonadotropin contaminants were present. This is not true for the current generation of highly purified menopausal gonadotropin (HP-hMG) products. In currently available HP-hMG products, hCG serves as the primary/sole source of LH activity. Highly purified urinary preparations allow for administration by a subcutaneous route with minimal or no reaction at the injection site. Alternatives to hMG include purified recombinant FSH, discussed next.

Both LH and FSH activity are required for normal ovarian steroidogenesis and follicular development. In many cases, pure FSH preparations can be used because of adequate endogenous LH production. For example, ovulation induction in women with PCOS can be performed with products containing only FSH or with those containing both LH and FSH activity. At present, data do not support the superiority of one preparation compared with another. However, for ovulation induction in patients with hypogonadotropic amenorrhea, LH activity also must be provided from an exogenous source. For this, options include just-described hMG, recombinant LH, and low-dose (diluted) urinary or recombinant hCG. Pulsatile GnRH can be used to induce ovulation in these patients, although this is not yet widely available.

When used for ART, gonadotropin preparations are nearly always paired with GnRH analogues (agonist or antagonist). These analogues help avoid premature LH surge and early ovulation. However, because of the absent LH activity induced by GnRH agents, high serum FSH levels can result in elevated follicular-phase progesterone concentrations due to greater production from granulosa cells and to impaired steroid metabolism from theca cells (Fleming, 2010). As one remembers from the two-cell theory of estrogen production, progesterone is first metabolized to androgens by theca cells, and granulosa cells then convert androgens to estrogen. Thus, with impaired theca metabolism, progesterone can accumulate (Chap 16, p. 356). Progesterone levels >1.5 ng/mL in the follicular phase alter endometrial gene expression and lower pregnancy rates, most likely through poor implantation (Bosch, 2010; Laberta, 2011). Gonadotropin products containing LH/hCG activity induce *CYP17* gene expression in the theca cells and thereby promote the conversion of progesterone into androgens. These androgens are then converted into estrogen by the follicle's granulosa cells. Accordingly, HP-hMG cause fewer premature elevations in progesterone compared with recombinant FSH. In the United States, combined use of HP-hMG and recombinant FSH ("mixed protocols") for ovarian stimulation for ART is common.

Currently four different recombinant FSH products are commercially available. The first two (follitropin alpha and follitropin beta) are produced in Chinese hamster ovary (CHO) cell lines. Because they have different glycosylation structure/isoforms, they are considered different molecules. A long-acting FSH (follitropin gamma) is commercially available outside the United States. This recombinant molecule was created by adding a DNA sequence to the human gene that encodes the FSH beta subunit. This extra sequence allows for more glycosylation and hence a prolonged clearance. More recently, a novel recombinant FSH (follitropin delta) has been produced from a human embryonic retinal cell line (PER.C6) (Koechling, 2017). Low-molecular-weight molecules (nonproteins) can activate FSH and LH receptors. However, these compounds have not progressed beyond early stages of clinical development. Potential advantages of these nontraditional gonadotropins could include oral delivery.

Most clinicians begin ovulation induction attempts at a low gonadotropin dosage of 50 to 75 IU/d. This is gradually increased if no ovarian response (as assessed by serum estradiol measurements) is noted after several days (Fig. 21-2). This is referred to as a "step-up" protocol. A "step-down" protocol can also be used and offers a shorter duration of stimulation. However, the risk of excessive ovarian response, such as multiple follicle development or ovarian hyperstimulation syndrome, may be higher with this method. With either approach, if a patient fails to conceive, subsequent cycles may be started at higher doses based on prior response.

In general, gonadotropin stimulation in women with PCOS is less successful than in patients with hypogonadotropic amenorrhea (Balen, 1994). Women with PCOS have ovaries highly sensitive to gonadotropin stimulation. They have a higher risk of excessive ovarian response and of multifetal pregnancy than do those with normal ovaries (Farhi, 1995).

Aromatase Inhibitors

Gonadotropins are associated with more effective ovulation induction and higher pregnancy rates than CC. However, gonadotropins are expensive and carry higher risks for ovarian hyperstimulation syndrome and multifetal gestation. Accordingly, aromatase inhibitors have been investigated as ovulation-inducing agents (Fig. 21-3). These drugs were originally developed for breast cancer treatment and effectively inhibit *aromatase*, a cytochrome P450 hemoprotein that catalyzes the rate-limiting step in estrogen production. Aromatase inhibitors are orally administered, easy to use, relatively inexpensive, and associated with typically minor side effects (Chap. 13, p. 295).

The most widely used aromatase inhibitor to induce ovulation in anovulatory and ovulatory infertile women is letrozole (Femara). Its typical dosage is 2.5 to 5 mg orally daily for 5 days. Compared with CC, its use yields higher pregnancy rates following ovulation induction (Legro, 2014). When combined with gonadotropins (for ovulation induction), letrozole leads to lower gonadotropin requirements and may achieve pregnancy rates comparable to gonadotropin treatment alone (Casper, 2003; Mitwally, 2004). This contrasts with letrozole's lower success rate when coupled with intrauterine insemination (IUI) in patients with unexplained infertility (Diamond, 2015).

Data suggesting that letrozole use for infertility treatment might be associated with a higher risk of congenital cardiac and bone malformations in the newborn are contradictory (Biljan, 2005; Tulandi, 2006). However, in 2005, the manufacturer issued a statement to physicians worldwide advising that letrozole use in premenopausal women, specifically its use for ovulation induction, is contraindicated (Fontana, 2005). As a result, it is not likely that letrozole will gain FDA approval or widespread acceptance for ovulation induction in the near future. Larger, well-designed randomized trials are still needed (Franik, 2014).

A second aromatase inhibitor, anastrozole (Arimidex), is of the same compound class as letrozole and also is approved for breast cancer treatment. At this time, no concerns have been raised regarding its teratogenicity. However, experience with anastrozole in ovulation induction at this time is limited, and ideal dosages are currently unknown. Two trials comparing anastrozole to CC have not found it to be more effective (Tredway, 2011a,b).

Complications of Fertility Drugs

Ovarian Hyperstimulation Syndrome. This is a clinical symptom complex associated with ovarian enlargement resulting from exogenous gonadotropin therapy. Symptoms may include abdominal pain and distention, ascites, gastrointestinal problems, respiratory compromise, oliguria, hemoconcentration, and thromboembolism. These symptoms may develop during ovulation induction or in early pregnancies that were conceived through exogenous ovarian stimulation.

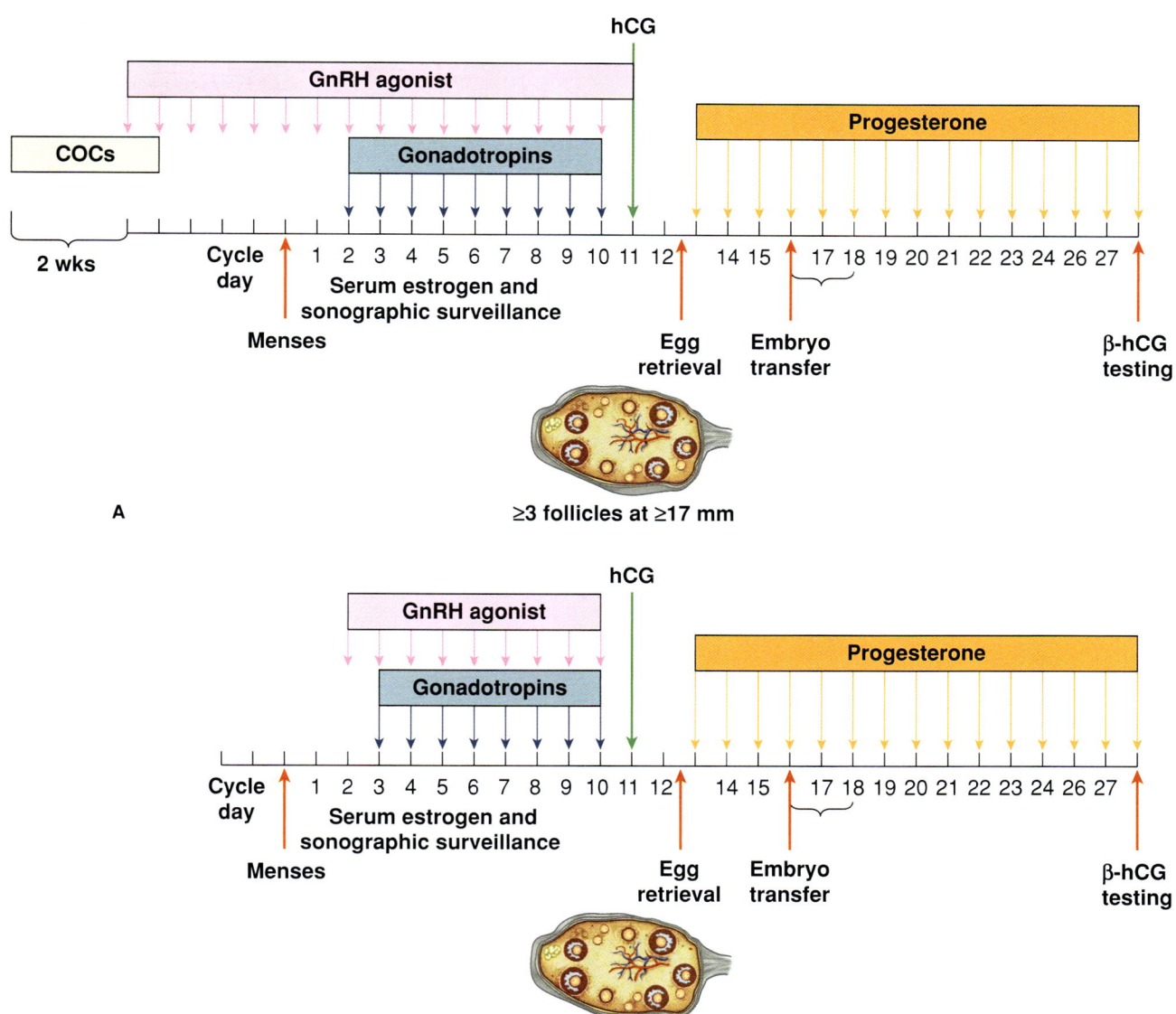

FIGURE 21-2 Drug protocols for ovulation induction. **A.** Downregulation of gonadotropin-releasing hormone (GnRH) agonist protocol. This is also known as the *long protocol*. In this diagram, the long protocol is combined with combination oral contraceptive (COC) pill pretreatment. With the long protocol, GnRH agonists are begun typically 7 days prior to gonadotropins. GnRH agonists suppress endogenous pituitary release of gonadotropins. This minimizes the risk of a premature luteinizing hormone (LH) surge and thus premature ovulation. During all protocols, serial serum estrogen levels and sonographic surveillance of follicular development accompany gonadotropin administration. Human chorionic gonadotropin (hCG) is administered to mimic the normal luteinizing hormone (LH) surge and trigger ovulation. HCG is given when sonography shows three or more follicles measuring at least 17 mm. Eggs are retrieved 36 hours later. Embryos are transfer back to the uterus 3–5 days following retrieval. Progesterone supplementation, with either vaginal preparations or intramuscular injection, follows during the luteal phase to support the endometrium. One major drawback of GnRH agonist therapy is the induction of initial transient gonadotropin release or *flare*, which may lead to ovarian cyst formation. Functional ovarian cysts can prolong the duration of pituitary suppression required prior to gonadotropin initiation and may also exert a detrimental effect on follicular development because of their steroid production. However, COC pretreatment can help prevent ovarian cyst formation. Moreover, COC pretreatment may improve induction results by providing an entire cohort of follicles synchronized at the same developmental stage that will reach maturity at the same time once stimulated by gonadotropins. **B.** GnRH flare protocol. This is also known as the *short protocol*. GnRH agonists initially bind gonadotropes and stimulate follicle-stimulating hormone (FSH) and LH release. This initial flare of gonadotropes stimulates follicular development. Following this initial surge of gonadotropins, the GnRH agonist causes receptor downregulation and an ultimately hypogonadotropic state. Gonadotropin injections begin 2 days later to continue follicular growth. As with the long protocol, continued GnRH agonist therapy prevents premature ovulation. (*Continued*)

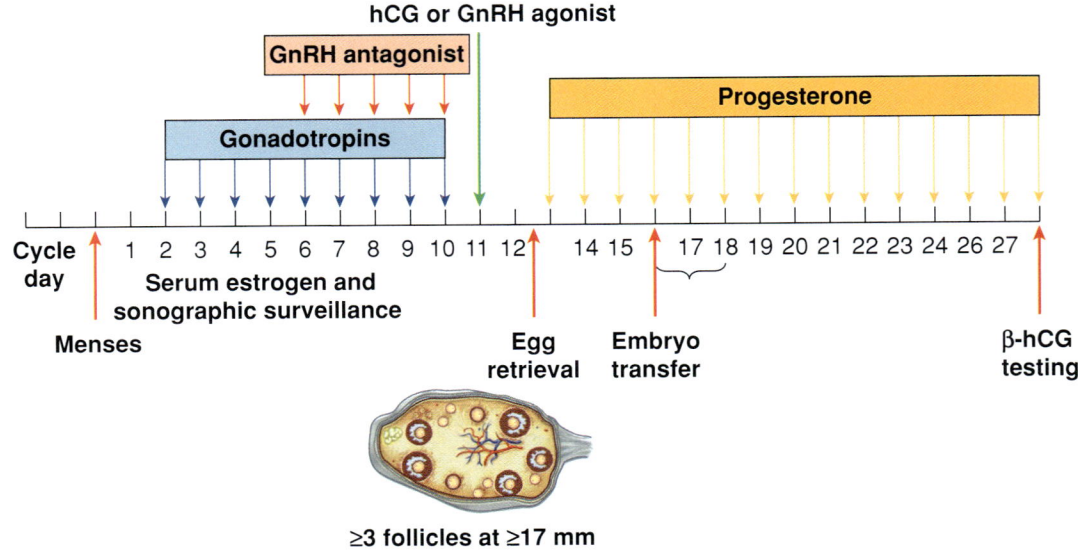

C   ≥3 follicles at ≥17 mm

FIGURE 21-2 (*Continued*) **C.** GnRH antagonist protocol. As with GnRH agonists, these agents are combined with gonadotropins to prevent premature LH surge and ovulation. This protocol attempts to minimize risk of ovarian hyperstimulation syndrome (OHSS) and GnRH side effects, such as hot flashes, headaches, bleeding, and mood changes.

The etiology of ovarian hyperstimulation syndrome (OHSS) is complex, but hCG, either exogenous or endogenous (derived from a resulting pregnancy), is believed to be an early contributing factor. Development of OHSS involves greater vascular permeability and subsequent loss of fluid, protein, and electrolytes into the peritoneal cavity, which leads to hemoconcentration. Enhanced capillary permeability is felt to result from vasoactive substances produced by the corpus luteum. Vascular endo-

thelial growth factor (VEGF) is thought to play a major role, and angiotensin II may also be involved. Hypercoagulability may be related to hyperviscosity following hemoconcentration. Alternatively, it may stem from simultaneous high estrogen levels, and these high levels can raise coagulation factor production. Predisposing factors for OHSS include multifollicular ovaries such as with PCOS, young age, high estradiol levels during ovulation induction, and pregnancy.

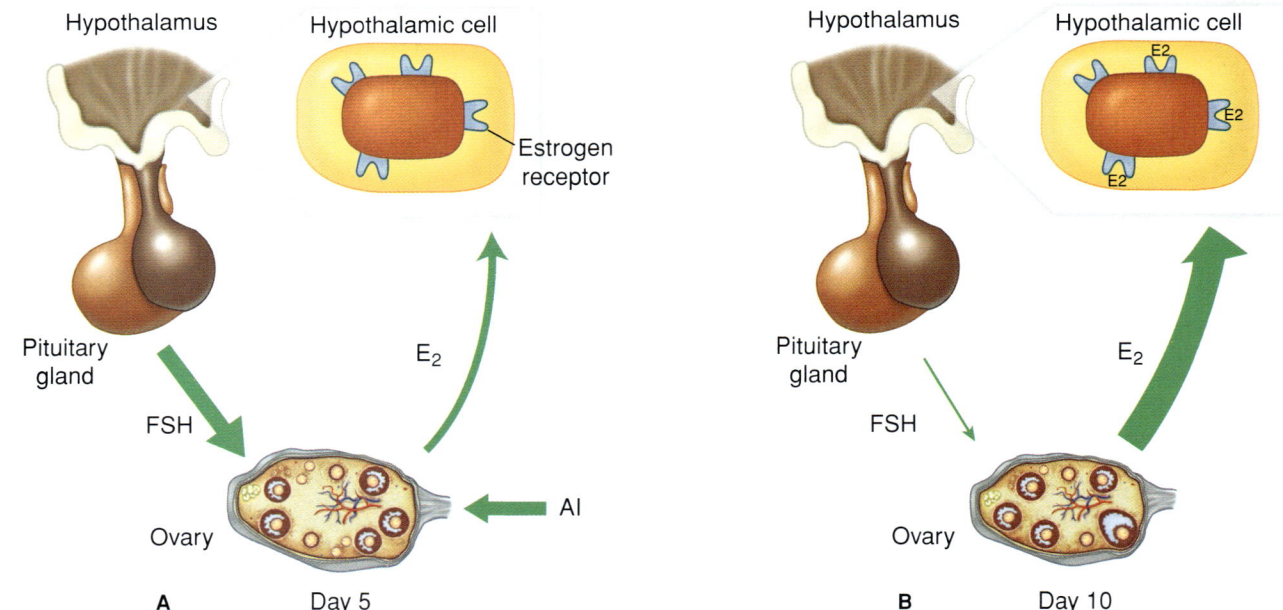

FIGURE 21-3 Effect of aromatase inhibitor (AI) administration. **A.** Administration suppresses ovarian estradiol (E_2) secretion and reduces estrogen-negative feedback at the pituitary and hypothalamus. As a result, increased follicle-stimulating hormone (FSH) secretion from the anterior pituitary stimulates growth of multiple ovarian follicles. **B.** Later in the follicular phase, the effect of the aromatase inhibitor is reduced, and E_2 levels rise as a result of follicular growth. Because AIs do not affect estrogen receptors centrally, the higher E_2 levels result in normal central negative feedback on FSH secretion. Follicles smaller than the dominant follicle undergo atresia, with resultant monofollicular ovulation in most cases.

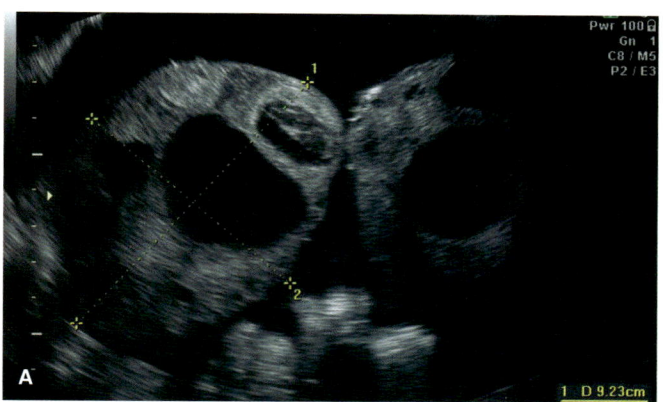 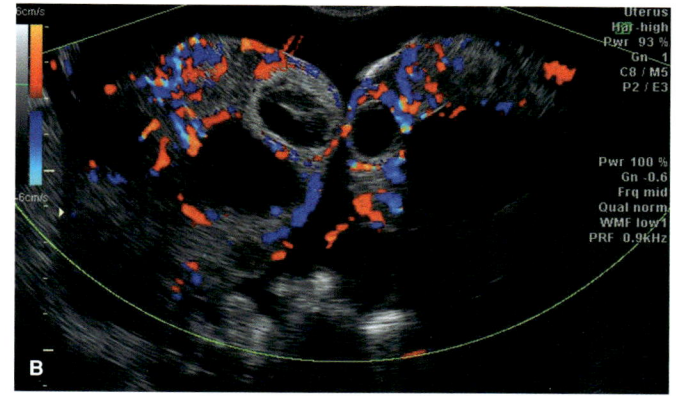

FIGURE 21-4 **A.** Transvaginal sonogram of ovaries with multiple, large cysts secondary to ovarian hyperstimulation syndrome (OHSS). Ovaries are enlarged and meet in the midline. Ascites surrounds these enlarged ovaries. **B.** Color Doppler transvaginal sonography is often performed to help exclude ovarian torsion in these patients.

Abdominal pain is prominent and caused by ovarian enlargement and accumulation of peritoneal fluid. Although sonographic examination of women with OHSS usually reveals enlarged ovaries with numerous follicular cysts and ascites, OHSS is a clinical diagnosis (Fig. 21-4). Several different classification schemes have been proposed to categorize the severity of this syndrome, and Table 21-2 lists one (Golan, 1989).

OHSS treatment is generally supportive. Paracentesis is typically performed transvaginally as an outpatient and can ameliorate abdominal discomfort and relieve respiratory distress. Reaccumulation of ascites may prompt additional paracenteses or rarely placement of a percutaneous "pigtail" catheter for continuous drainage. Untreated hypovolemia can lead to renal, hepatic, or pulmonary end-organ failure. Thus, fluid balance must be maintained by replacement with an isotonic fluid such as normal saline. Monitoring of electrolytes is critical. Because of hypercoagulability in these women, prophylaxis for thromboembolism is strongly considered with severe OHSS.

During exogenous ovulation, strategies to avoid OHSS induction include decreasing follicular stimulation (a lowered FSH dose), "coasting" (withholding FSH administration for one or more days prior to the hCG trigger injection), prophylactic treatment with volume expanders, and substitution of hCG for FSH during the final days of ovarian stimulation. With this last strategy, low-dose hCG administration can

support maturation of larger ovarian follicles but is postulated to directly or indirectly raise atresia rates of small antral follicles and thereby lower OHSS rates. However, during ovulation induction, if concern for OHSS develops, the hCG trigger can be withheld, resulting in cycle cancellation. For these patients, IVF with its egg retrieval before ovulation should often be considered rather than further attempts at inducing ovulation.

OHSS can also develop with ART therapy, and the risk can be substantially reduced with appropriate precautions. Women who are predicted to be especially sensitive to gonadotropins are those with a high number of antral follicles sonographically, a high serum antimüllerian hormone (AMH) level, or a prior robust response to ovulation induction. These individuals should be stimulated with a GnRH antagonist protocol. This allows a single GnRH agonist dose to be used for the "trigger" in place of hCG. The resulting endogenous LH surge can bring about the final stages of follicle and oocyte maturation without significant OHSS risk. As a second preempting option, prevention of pregnancy does not completely eliminate the risk of OHSS but certainly serves to limit symptom duration. Thus, in ART cycles, all embryos can be frozen and embryo transfer postponed. Last, good evidence suggests that dopamine agonists such as cabergoline started at the trigger of ovulation can reduce OHSS incidence (American Society for Reproductive Medicine, 2016).

Multifetal Gestation. From 1980 through 1997, the number of twin births rose by more than 50 percent, and the number of higher-order multifetal births increased by more than 400 percent (Fig. 21-5) (Martin, 1999). Using data from these years, the Centers for Disease Control and Prevention (CDC) (2000) estimated that approximately 20 percent of triplets and higher-order multifetal births were attributable to spontaneous events; 40 percent were related to ovulation-inducing drugs without ART; and 40 percent resulted from ART. However, further analysis of the same data indicates that most multifetal births result from spontaneously conceived twin gestations and that only approximately 10 percent result from IVF and related procedures.

Higher-order multifetal pregnancy is an adverse outcome of infertility treatment. In general, higher fetal number raises the risk of perinatal and maternal morbidity and mortality.

TABLE 21-2. Classification and Staging of Ovarian Hyperstimulation Syndrome

Grade 1:	Abdominal distention/discomfort
Grade 2:	Grade 1 plus nausea and vomiting or diarrhea Ovaries enlarged and measure 5–12 cm
Grade 3:	Sonographic evidence of ascites
Grade 4:	Clinical evidence of ascites or hydrothorax or difficulty breathing
Grade 5:	All of the above plus decreased blood volume, hemoconcentration, diminished renal perfusion and function, and coagulation abnormalities

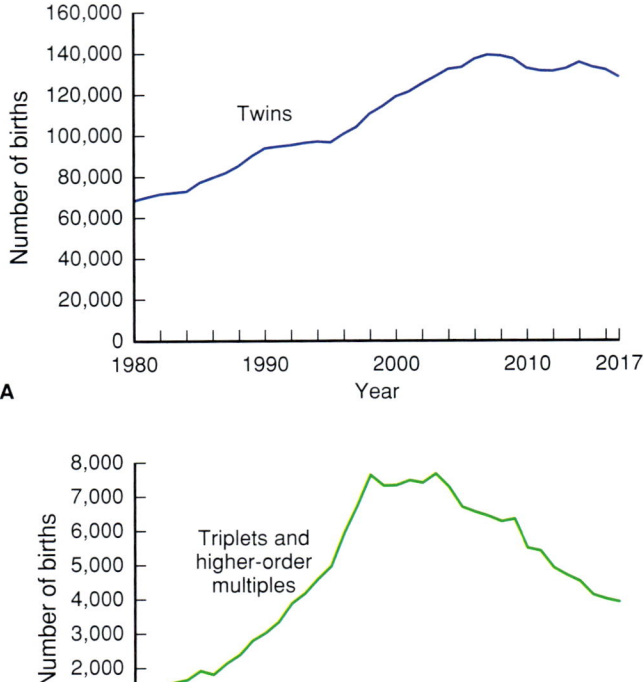

FIGURE 21-5 Trends in frequency of multifetal gestations from 1980 to 2017. **A.** Number of twin births in the United States. **B.** Number of triplet and higher-order multifetal births. (Data from Martin, 2013, 2018.)

couple's sense of urgency may lead to a preference for more aggressive strategies involving gonadotropin treatment or for more embryos to be transferred in IVF cycles. Clinicians may feel competitive pressures to achieve higher pregnancy rates and may be inclined to turn to superovulation or IVF earlier in treatment or to transfer a greater number of embryos.

Efforts to lower the multifetal gestation rates in patients undergoing ovulation induction or superovulation include serum estradiol limits and arbitrary sonographic criteria of follicular size. These, however, have been ineffective. In one randomized clinical trial involving 1255 ovulation induction cycles, hCG was withheld if the estradiol concentration rose above 3000 pg/mL or if more than six follicles greater than 18 mm in diameter were present (Guzick, 1999). Despite these limits on hCG administration, the multifetal gestation rate was still 30 percent. Although sonography and serum estradiol monitoring have not reduced the incidence of multifetal gestation or OHSS, the risk of multifetal pregnancy does correlate with the magnitude of follicular response as indicated by follicle number and serum estradiol levels. However, no consensus among centers has been reached regarding specific sonographic criteria or estradiol levels beyond which hCG should not be administered.

When the likelihood of multifetal gestation is felt to be excessive, IVF can be undertaken to reduce the risk. Because the number of embryos transferred can be strictly controlled, this strategy can minimize the risk of higher-order multifetal gestations. Guidelines set forth by the American Society for Reproductive Medicine and the Society for Assisted Reproductive Technology (2017) have significantly reduced the rates of triplet and higher-order gestations (Table 21-3).

Prematurity leads to most adverse events in these cases, but fetal-growth restriction and discordance are other potential factors.

Rates of monozygotic gestation also rise in ovulation induction and ART and are associated with greater fetal risks. These include a three- to fivefold higher perinatal mortality rate compared with that of dizygotic twins. Abnormal placentation also develops frequently. Additionally, compared with singleton neonates, monozygotic twins have congenital anomaly rates that are two- to threefold higher and that approximate 10 percent. Initially, extended embryo culture and zona manipulation were postulated to increase the risk of monozygosity. More recent, well-designed trials have refuted this contention (Franasiak, 2015; Papanikolaou, 2010).

Patients with higher-order multifetal gestations are faced with options of continuing their pregnancy with all the risks previously described, terminating the entire pregnancy, or selecting multifetal pregnancy reduction (MFPR). MFPR reduces the number of fetuses to decrease the risk of maternal and perinatal morbidity and mortality. Although MFPR lowers the risks associated with preterm delivery, it often creates profound ethical dilemmas. Moreover, multifetal reduction lowers, but does not eliminate, the risk of fetal-growth restriction in remaining fetuses. With MFPR, pregnancy loss and prematurity are primary risks. However, current data suggest that such complications have decreased as experience with the procedure has grown (Evans, 2008).

Several issues in infertility care contribute to the increased incidence of higher-order multifetal pregnancies. An infertile

TABLE 21-3. Recommended Limits on the Numbers of Embryos to Transfer

Prognosis	Age			
	<35 yr	35–37 yr	38–40 yr	41–42 yr
Cleavage-stage embryos[a]				
Euploid	1	1	1	1
Other favorable[b]	1	1	≤3	≤4
All others	≤2	≤3	≤4	≤5
Blastocysts[a]				
Euploid	1	1	1	1
Favorable[b]	1	1	≤2	≤3
All others	≤2	≤2	≤3	≤3

[a]Justification for transferring additional embryos beyond the recommended limits should be clearly documented in the patient's medical record.
[b]Other favorable = any one of these criteria. *Fresh cycle*: expectation of 1 or more high-quality embryos available for cryopreservation, or previous live birth after an IVF cycle. *FET cycle*: availability of vitrified day-5 or day-6 blastocysts, euploid embryos, 1st FET cycle, or previous live birth after an IVF cycle. FET = frozen embryo transfer; IVF = in vitro fertilization. American Society for Reproductive Medicine, 2017, with permission.

Efforts to reduce twin pregnancies through a greater use of elective single embryo transfer (eSET) are currently ongoing (Paulson 2017).

Ovarian Drilling

Surgical ovarian wedge resection was the first established treatment for anovulatory PCOS patients. It was largely abandoned because of postsurgical adhesion formation, which converted endocrinologic subfertility to mechanical subfertility (Adashi, 1981; Buttram, 1975; Stein, 1939). As a result, it was replaced by medical ovulation induction with CC and gonadotropins (Franks, 1985). However, medical ovulation induction, as discussed, has limitations. Thus, surgical therapy using laparoscopic techniques and termed *laparoscopic ovarian drilling* is an alternative in certain women resistant to medical therapies.

During laparoscopic ovarian drilling, electrosurgical coagulation, laser vaporization, or Harmonic scalpel may be used to create multiple perforations into the ovarian surface and stroma (Section 44-7, p. 1036). In many uncontrolled observational studies, drilling led to temporary, higher rates of spontaneous postoperative ovulation and conception or to improved medical ovulation induction (Armar, 1990, 1993; Farhi, 1995; Greenblatt, 1987; Kovacs, 1991).

The mechanism of action with laparoscopic ovarian drilling is thought to be similar to that of ovarian wedge resection. Both procedures destroy ovarian androgen-producing tissue and reduce peripheral conversion of androgens to estrogens. Specifically, a fall in serum levels of androgens and LH and a rise in FSH levels follow ovarian drilling (Armar, 1990; Greenblatt, 1987). Endocrine changes after surgery are thought to convert the adverse androgen-dominant intrafollicular environment to an estrogenic one and to restore the hormonal environment to normal by correcting ovarian-pituitary feedback disturbances (Aakvaag, 1985; Balen, 1993). Thus, both local and systemic effects are believed to promote follicular recruitment and maturation and subsequent ovulation.

Risks of ovarian drilling include postoperative adhesion formation and the other risks of laparoscopic surgery (Chap. 41, p. 875). Additionally, theoretical risks of diminished ovarian reserve and premature ovarian failure remain to be well investigated. As surgery is more invasive, ovarian drilling is generally not offered prior to consideration of medical therapies.

CORRECTION OF DIMINISHED OVARIAN RESERVE

Ovarian dysfunction may result from ovarian failure or from a diminished ovarian reserve, either of which may follow normal aging, disease, cancer treatment, or ovarian surgery. Even if a woman is spontaneously menstruating, a basal (day 2 or 3) FSH level above 15 IU/L predicts that medical therapies including exogenous gonadotropins will be of little benefit. For these women, the option of using donor eggs should be considered (p. 466). Expectant management also may be considered, although the likelihood of pregnancy is low. Serum AMH levels can identify patients with diminished ovarian reserve prior to the elevation of basal FSH. AMH varies little throughout the menstrual cycle and can be drawn at any time. Although patients with a low AMH level (<1 ng/mL) generally respond poorly to gonadotropins, some may benefit from ART.

CORRECTION OF ANATOMIC ABNORMALITIES

Anatomic distortions of the female reproductive tract are a major cause of infertility and may prevent ovum entry into the fallopian tube; impair transport of ova, sperm, or embryos; or interfere with implantation. The three primary types of anatomic abnormalities include tubal factors, peritoneal factors, and uterine factors. Each has differing effects and therefore may require different therapies.

■ Tubal Factors

Tubal occlusion can arise from congenital abnormality, infection, or iatrogenic causes. Additionally, a small subset of tubal infertility is idiopathic. Not only the cause of tubal damage but also the nature of an anatomic abnormality is important. For example, proximal tubal occlusion, distal tubal occlusion, and tubal absence differ markedly in their treatment.

Proximal tubal occlusion describes obstruction proximal to the fimbria and may develop at the tubal ostium, isthmus, or ampulla. *Midtubal occlusion* is considered a subset of proximal occlusion. Proximal tubal occlusion may be secondary to tubal resection, luminal obliteration, or simple plugging with mucus or debris. In contrast, *distal tubal occlusion* describes obstruction at the tube's fimbria. It typically results from prior pelvic infection and may be associated with concomitant adnexal adhesions.

Tubal Cannulation

Proximal tubal occlusion is often amenable to direct techniques. If diagnosed at the time of hysterosalpingography (HSG), consideration is given to performing concurrent selective salpingography. With this, a catheter is placed such that it wedges within the tubal ostium. This allows significant hydrostatic pressure to be applied to the tube. Such pressure will likely overcome most instances of tubal spasm or plugging by mucus or debris. If tubal patency cannot be reestablished, an inner catheter with guide wire is used to cannulate the tube. This creates patency of isolated short segmental scarring in most instances. Scarring of a longer segment or luminal obliteration, however, is not amenable to correction with tubal cannulation. In these women, surgical segmental resection with reanastomosis or IVF may be considered.

Tubal Reconstruction

Proximal Tubal Obstruction. Tubal obstruction not amenable to treatment with selective salpingography has traditionally been treated surgically, and options include hysteroscopic cannulation, surgical reanastomosis, and neosalpingostomy. Although success rates of ART have risen considerably, reproductive surgery remains an important option or complement to ART for many couples.

Some types of tubal blockage have a much better prognosis with surgical therapy than others. For example, hysteroscopic cannulation of fallopian tubes can treat some types of proximal obstruction

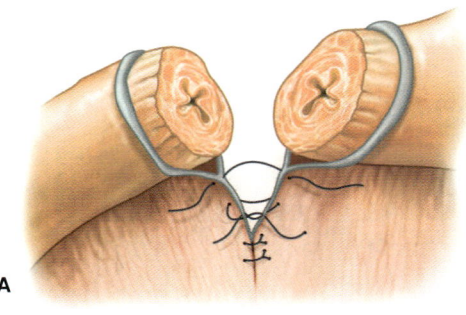

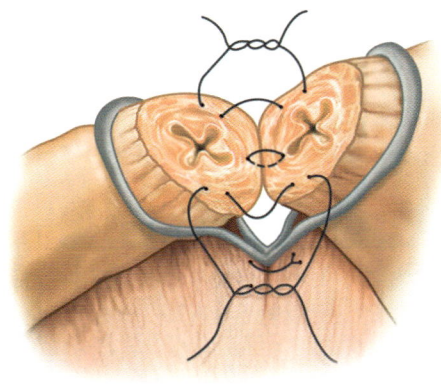

FIGURE 21-6 Surgical reanastomosis of fallopian tube segments. The scarred portion of the tube is sharply excised until nonfibrotic tubal tissues are reached. **A.** The mesosalpinx is re-approximated with interrupted stitches using 6-0 delayed-absorbable suture. **B.** The tubal muscularis is reapproximated with single stitches in each quadrant using 7-0 delayed-absorbable suture. Tubal serosa is closed with interrupted or running 6-0 delayed-absorbable suture.

in a fashion similar to selective salpingography (Section 44-17, p. 1067). Hysteroscopic cannulation is best performed with concurrent laparoscopy to verify distal tubal patency.

Proximal obstruction not amenable to cannulation techniques can be treated with segmental resection and reanastomosis (Fig. 21-6). In most cases, this can be done as an outpatient procedure through a minilaparotomy incision. However, obstruction extending into the interstitial portion of the tube is more technically challenging to repair and more prone to repeated obstruction postoperatively. Therefore, proximal occlusion extending to the interstitial segment that cannot be treated with cannulation is best treated in most instances with IVF.

Options for proximal and midtubal occlusion resulting from prior sterilization are either tubal reanastomosis or IVF. From a patient perspective, outpatient tubal reanastomosis avoids ovarian stimulation and its higher risk for multifetal gestation and provides an ability to conceive normally. In general, although the monthly probability of pregnancy following tubal reversal is likely lower than that for age-matched controls without prior sterilization, the cumulative chance of pregnancy is high. However, IVF is strongly considered if other fertility factors are present or the type of sterilization performed does not permit reconstruction. For example, in cases of sterilization completed by fimbriectomy, neosalpingostomy can be corrective.

However, the probability of pregnancy is lower, and IVF is considered. Importantly, the risk of subsequent ectopic pregnancy following reanastomosis for midtubal occlusion is 3 to 5 percent (Gordts, 2009).

The "reversibility" of sterilization can generally be determined by review of the operative report and also the pathology report if the procedure involved segmental resection. If operative records are unavailable or suggest that reanastomosis may not be feasible, laparoscopy is performed prior to laparotomy to assess chances of surgical success.

Outpatient reversal of sterilization is most commonly done by minilaparotomy. Incision size typically ranges from 3 to 6 cm depending on a patient's weight and anatomy. Some surgeons are able to complete some of these procedures laparoscopically. Robotic control may be helpful for this but may increase operating time and expense.

Distal Tubal Obstruction. Following pelvic inflammatory disorders, normal fimbrial anatomy may be destroyed, or fimbria may be encased by adnexal adhesions. In these cases, neosalpingostomy can be performed at minilaparotomy or laparoscopy (Fig. 21-7). However, women desiring neosalpingostomy for treatment of distal occlusion are counseled that the risk of ectopic pregnancy is high, the likelihood of pregnancy is 50 percent or lower, and postoperative reocclusion is common (Bayrak, 2006). Moreover, hydrosalpinges that are dilated more than 3 cm in diameter, that are associated with significant adnexal adhesions, or that display an obviously attenuated endosalpinx yield a poor prognosis. These tubes are best treated by salpingectomy. If both tubes are affected, bilateral salpingectomy is recommended prior to proceeding with IVF. This stems from data showing women with hydrosalpinges undergoing IVF have approximately half the pregnancy rate of other women with unaffected tubes (American Society for Reproductive Medicine, 2015c).

■ Uterine Factors

Various uterine factors have been implicated in infertility and include adenomyosis, leiomyomas, endometrial polyps, and intrauterine adhesions. Müllerian anomalies, especially intrauterine septum or segmental agenesis, can increase rates of

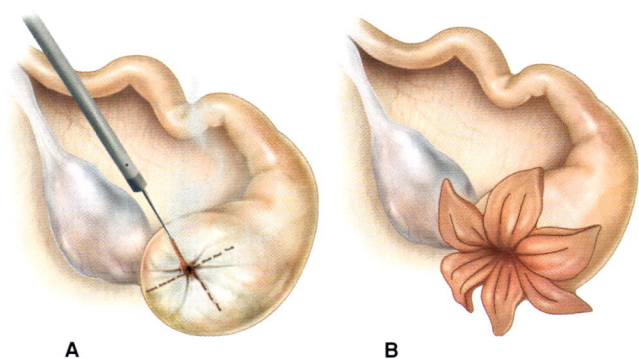

FIGURE 21-7 Neosalpingostomy. **A.** The distal end of the clubbed fallopian tube is opened sharply or with electric or laser energy. **B.** The endosalpinx is everted using Cuff or Bruhat technique.

infertility or pregnancy complications. These congenital abnormalities are described fully in Chapter 19 (p. 419). Mechanisms of infertility with these factors have not been clearly elucidated. However, the end result is diminished endometrial receptivity and reduced likelihood of embryo implantation.

Leiomyomas

These are common benign tumors of the uterus and have been associated with infertility in some women (Chap. 9, p. 205). Retrospective studies have suggested a benefit from surgically removing certain tumors to increase efficacy of both natural and assisted conception.

No randomized trials clearly demonstrate that myomectomy improves fertility (Metwally, 2012). However, in view of the many retrospective observational studies that suggest a benefit, myomectomy can be offered to well-selected infertile women, especially if tumors are large or impinge on the endometrial cavity. Leiomyomas can be removed using hysteroscopy, laparoscopy, or laparotomy, and approach selection is discussed in Chapter 9 (p. 210). Currently, for predominantly intramural or subserosal myomas, no studies validate one method compared with another in terms of efficacy. For intracavitary myomas, no data show one surgical approach to be most effective for fertility, and thus the least invasive hysteroscopic approach is reasonable. In general, clinical judgment should determine the most appropriate technique from the standpoint of safety, restoration of normal uterine anatomy, and speed of recovery.

Endometrial Polyps

These soft, fleshy endometrial growths are commonly diagnosed during infertility evaluation. Several studies suggest good pregnancy rates following polypectomy, although the mechanism by which polyps impair fertility is not established.

For management, one prospective trial of 204 women with polyps and with an additionally diagnosed cervical factor, male factor, or unexplained infertility provides some clear guidance. In this trial, women were randomly assigned to one of two groups prior to treatment with intrauterine insemination (IUI) (Pérez-Medina, 2005). The first group underwent polypectomy. The second underwent only hysteroscopic biopsy of the polyp to obtain histologic confirmation. All patients were managed expectantly for three cycles prior to proceeding with up to four cycles of IUI. The pregnancy rate in the polypectomy group was more than twice as high regardless of initial polyp size (Table 21-4). These data suggest that endometrial polyps can significantly impair infertility treatment outcome. Thus,

TABLE 21-4. Number and Percentage of Pregnancies after Hysteroscopic Polypectomy (n = 204)

	Polypectomy n = 101 (%)	Control n = 103 (%)	p-value
Subsequent pregnancy	64 (63.4)	29 (28.2)	< 0.001

RR 2.1 (95% CI 1.5–2.9).
From Pérez-Medina, 2005, with permission.

hysteroscopic polypectomy in all infertile patients if a polyp is identified seems reasonable (Section 44-13, p. 1056).

Intrauterine Adhesions

Adhesions within the endometrial cavity, also called *synechiae*, can range from asymptomatic small bands to complete or near complete obliteration of the endometrial cavity. If amenorrhea or hypomenorrhea result, the condition is termed *Asherman syndrome* (Chap. 17, p. 374).

Treatment involves surgical adhesiolysis to restore normal uterine cavity size and configuration. Dilation and curettage (D & C) and abdominal approaches were previously used. However, with the advantages of hysteroscopy, the role of these other techniques has been minimized.

Hysteroscopic adhesion resection may range from simple lysis of a small band to extensive adhesiolysis of dense intrauterine adhesions using scissors, electrosurgical cutting, or laser energy (Section 44-18, p. 1069). However, women whose uterine fundus is completely obscured and those with a markedly narrowed, fibrotic cavity present the greatest therapeutic challenge. Several techniques are described for these difficult cases, but outcome is far worse than in patients with small band adhesions. In those women with severe Asherman syndrome that is not amenable to reconstructive surgery, gestational carrier surrogacy or uterine transplantation is a valuable option (p. 466).

◼ Peritoneal Disease

Endometriosis

This condition and its effects on infertility are extensively discussed in Chapter 11 (p. 247). In women with minimal or mild disease, evidence supporting lesion ablation is limited and use of empiric general fertility boosting procedures such as ART or superovulation combined with IUI is reasonable. These treatments have been validated to increase fecundity in women with stage I and II disease (Table 21-5) (Guzick, 1999).

Moderate and severe endometriosis results in distortion of anatomic relationships of reproductive organs. In many cases, surgical treatment may improve anatomy, and pregnancy can result (American Society for Reproductive Medicine, 2012). Unfortunately, advanced disease may prevent adequate restoration of pelvic anatomy. Therefore, a surgeon's operative findings and anticipated surgical results guide postoperative strategy. If satisfactory surgical outcome is achieved, spontaneous conception can be attempted for 6 to 12 months prior to considering other options such as IVF. Notably, endometriosis in some cases may recur quickly, and unnecessary delay in attempting pregnancy postoperatively is not advised.

In women with advanced endometriosis, several studies suggest that long-term treatment with GnRH agonists before initiation of a cycle may improve fecundity (Dicker, 1992; Surrey, 2002). Currently, however, this treatment strategy is not universally accepted.

If endometriomas are noted, surgical options include cyst drainage, drainage followed by cyst wall ablation, or cyst excision. These three procedures can be performed laparoscopically in nearly all circumstances given adequate surgeon experience. Simple drainage minimizes ovarian destruction but commonly

TABLE 21-5. Cycle Fecundity with Stage I or II Endometriosis Compared with Unexplained Infertility

Treatment	Unexplained Infertility		Endometriosis-Associated Infertility		
	Guzick[a]	Deaton[a]	Chaffkin[a]	Fedele[a]	Kemmann[a]
No treatment or intracervical insemination	0.02	0.033	—	0.045	0.028
IUI	0.05[b]	—	—	—	—
Clomiphene	—	—	—	—	0.066
Clomiphene/IUI	—	0.095[b]	—	—	—
Gonadotropins	0.04[b]	—	0.066	—	0.073[b]
Gonadotropins/IUI	0.09[b]	—	0.129[b]	0.15[b]	—
IVF	—	—	—	—	0.222[b]

[a]And their colleagues.
[b]*p*<.05 for treatment vs. no treatment.
IUI = intrauterine insemination; IVF = in vitro fertilization.
From American Society for Reproductive Medicine, 2012, with permission.

results in rapid cyst recurrence. One histologic study demonstrated that a mean of 60 percent of the cyst wall surface area (range of 10 to 98 percent) was lined by endometrium to a depth of 0.6 mm (Muzii, 2007). Thus, drainage and ablation may not destroy all endometrium to this depth. Moreover, this approach is associated with significant risk of cyst recurrence and thermal damage to the ovary. For these reasons, laparoscopic excision of the cyst wall by a stripping technique is considered optimal treatment for most endometriomas (Section 44-5, p. 1030). Hart and coworkers (2008) compared ablative surgery and cyst excision. With excision, they noted more favorable rates of diminished pain, cyst recurrence, and spontaneous pregnancy. However, excision is inevitably accompanied by removal of normal ovarian tissue and often leads to decreased ovarian volume and diminished ovarian reserve (Almog, 2010; Exacoustos, 2004; Ragni, 2005).

Endometrioma recurrence is common. But, surgery for a recurrent endometrioma appears to be even more harmful to the ovarian reserve than primary surgery (Muzii, 2015). Thus, further ovarian surgery is individualized (American College of Obstetricians and Gynecologists, 2018a). If there is confidence in the diagnosis, it may be prudent in some cases to avoid surgery entirely when future fertility is desired.

Pelvic Adhesions

Pelvic adhesions may result from endometriosis, prior surgery, or pelvic infection and often vary in their density and vascularity. Adhesions may impair fertility by distorting adnexal anatomy and by interfering with gamete and embryo transport, even in the absence of tubal disease.

Surgical lysis may restore pelvic anatomy in some cases, but adhesions may recur, especially if they are dense and vascular. Adherence to microsurgical principles and minimally invasive surgery may help decrease adhesion formation. Although numerous adjuvants, such as adhesion barriers, have been used to reduce the risk of postoperative adhesion formation, currently none has been validated to improve fecundity (American Society for Reproductive Medicine, 2013b).

Among infertile women with adnexal adhesions, pregnancy rates after adhesiolysis are 32 percent at 12 months and 45 percent at 24 months of surveillance. These rates can be compared with 11 percent at 12 months and 16 percent at 24 months in those left untreated (Tulandi, 1990). As with severe endometriosis, clinical judgment regarding operative findings and results of surgery should guide the strategy postoperatively. IVF is the best option for those with a poor prognosis for normal anatomy restoration.

CORRECTION OF CERVICAL ABNORMALITIES

In response to follicular estradiol production, the cervix should produce abundant thin mucus. If present, this mucus acts as a conduit and functional reservoir for sperm. Accordingly, inadequate cervical mucus impairs sperm transport to the upper female reproductive tract.

Causes of abnormal or deficient mucus include infection, prior cervical surgery, use of antiestrogens (e.g., clomiphene citrate) for ovulation induction, and sperm antibodies. However, many women with decreased or hostile mucus have no history of predisposing factors.

Examination of cervical mucus may reveal gross evidence of chronic cervicitis that deserves treatment. Doxycycline, 100 mg orally twice daily for 10 days, is an appropriate therapy. In those with decreased mucus volume, treatments include short-term supplementation with exogenous estrogen, such as ethinyl estradiol. This can be coupled with oral doses of the mucolytic expectorant guaifenesin, which thins the mucus. However, the value of estrogen plus guaifenesin has not been confirmed. Moreover, exogenous estrogens could have a negative effect on follicular development and ovarian function.

For these reasons, most clinicians treat noninfectious, suspected cervical mucus abnormalities with IUI. Although this

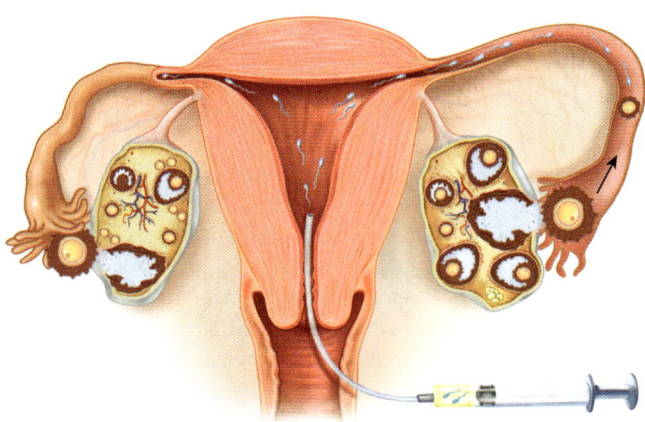

FIGURE 21-8 Intrauterine insemination (IUI). Prior to IUI, partner or donor sperm is washed and concentrated. IUI is usually combined with superovulation, and signs of impending ovulation are monitored with transvaginal sonography. At the time of suspected ovulation, a long, thin catheter is threaded through the cervical os and into the endometrial cavity. A syringe containing the sperm concentrate is attached to the catheter's distal end, and the sperm sample is injected into the endometrial cavity.

approach also has not been validated with randomized trials, the theoretical basis for this approach seems sound (Helmerhorst, 2005). Additionally, IUI is effective for treatment of unexplained infertility. As a result, many clinicians forgo cervical mucus testing and proceed directly with IUI treatments in the absence of tubal disease (Fig. 21-8).

CORRECTION OF MALE INFERTILITY

Male infertility has numerous causes and may include various sperm or semen volume abnormalities that are described subsequently. Accordingly, therapy should be planned only after thorough evaluation (Chap. 20, p. 442). In the absence of identifiable correctable cause, it is appropriate to offer IUI or ART as treatment options. The choice of whether to proceed initially with IUI therapies as opposed to the more intensive

and expensive ART treatments depends on several factors. These include duration of infertility, age of the female, and history of prior treatments. If ART is considered for male factor infertility, intracytoplasmic sperm injection (ICSI) is typically selected rather than traditional IVF (Fig. 21-9).

■ Abnormal Semen Volume

Aspermia is characterized by a complete lack of semen and results from failure to ejaculate. The physiology of ejaculation includes emission of sperm with accessory gland fluid into the urethra, simultaneous closure of the urethral sphincters, and forceful ejaculation of semen through the urethra. Emission and closure of the bladder neck are primarily alpha-adrenergically mediated thoracolumbar sympathetic reflex events with supraspinal modulation. Ejaculation is a sacral spinal reflex mediated by the pudendal nerve.

Anejaculation or anorgasmia is not rare and may stem from psychogenic factors, organic erectile dysfunction, or impaired parasympathetic sacral spinal reflex. Appropriate treatments depend on the cause and can include psychologic counseling or erectile dysfunction treatment with sildenafil citrate (Viagra) or other similar medication. Vibratory stimulation may also be effective in some instances. Electroejaculation is an invasive procedure and is generally used for men with spinal cord injuries who are unresponsive to the therapies above.

Men who always achieve orgasm but never experience prograde ejaculation or have a greatly reduced prograde volume typically have retrograde ejaculation. In these cases, oral pseudoephedrine or another alpha-adrenergic agent to aid bladder neck closure is suitable. However, for many, pharmacologic methods are ineffective, and IUI may be performed using sperm processed from a voided urine specimen collected after ejaculation. Oral sodium bicarbonate may be used prior to sperm collection to reduce the risk of harm to the sperm from a low urinary pH.

A few men who achieve orgasm, but not prograde ejaculation, have failure of emission. A trial of sympathomimetic agents is reasonable in these individuals as well, although pharmacologic therapies generally provide limited success. Alternatively, testicular or epididymal extraction of sperm via aspiration or biopsy may be used in cases refractory to medication. As with electroejaculation, this technique recovers a limited number of viable sperm and is best suited for use with ICSI.

Hypospermia, that is, low semen volume (<2 mL), impairs sperm transport into cervical mucus and can be associated with decreased sperm density or motility. Retrograde ejaculation may underlie this condition, and its treatment follows that just described for aspermia.

Alternatively, hypospermia may follow partial or complete ejaculatory duct obstruction. In these cases, transurethral excision of the ejaculatory duct obstruction has resulted in marked semen parameter improvement, and pregnancies have been achieved. However, couples are counseled that postoperative complete obstruction of the ejaculatory ducts is not rare. Thus, consideration is given to cryopreservation of sperm prior to surgical attempts in those individuals with partial obstruction.

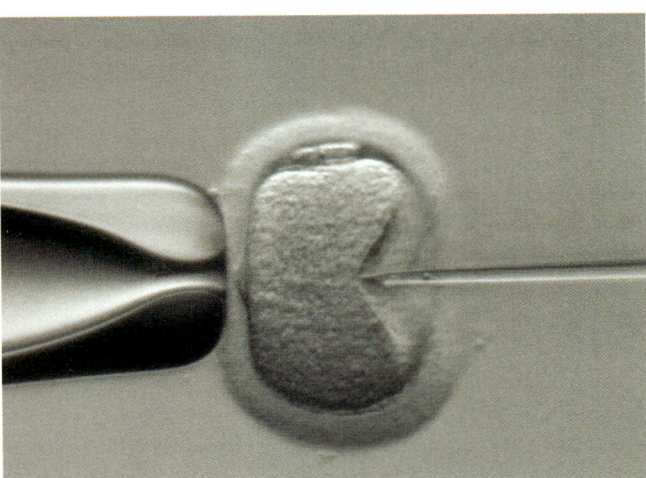

FIGURE 21-9 Photomicrograph of intracytoplasmic sperm injection.

■ Abnormal Sperm Count

Azoospermia is characterized by the total absence of sperm in semen. This may result from male reproductive tract obstruction or from nonobstructive causes.

Obstructive azoospermia, especially resulting from prior vasectomy or ejaculatory duct obstruction, may be amenable to surgical treatment. However, congenital bilateral absence of the vas deferens (CBAVD) is a common cause of azoospermia and unfortunately is not treatable surgically. In such candidates, testicular sperm extraction (TESE) may be performed in conjunction with ICSI.

Nonobstructive azoospermia may be caused by a karyotypic abnormality such as Klinefelter syndrome (47,XXY) or balanced translocation; deletion of a small portion of the Y chromosome; testicular failure; or unexplained causes. In many cases, TESE may be combined effectively with ICSI in those with Klinefelter syndrome and Y microdeletion of the AZFc region. However, in men with Y microdeletion in the AZFa or AZFb region, this ART combination has been ineffective (Choi, 2004).

Oligozoospermia is diagnosed if fewer than 15 million sperm are present per milliliter of semen. Causes are varied and include hormonal, genetic, environmental (including medications), and unexplained causes. Additionally, an obstructive cause, especially ejaculatory duct obstruction, should be considered if oligozoospermia accompanies low semen volume. If severe oligozoospermia (<5 to 10 million sperm/mL) is noted, an evaluation similar to that for azoospermia is indicated.

Oligozoospermia without decreased sperm motility not uncommonly reflects hypogonadotropic hypogonadism. In general, hypogonadotropic hypogonadism is best treated with FSH and hCG administered to the male. Alternatively, CC or aromatase inhibitors, although not FDA-approved treatment for this indication, may be considered for some males, especially if obesity and elevated serum estradiol levels are present. Spermatogenesis is a long process lasting approximately 100 days. Thus, several months may be required to identify significant improvements in sperm density with either treatment.

Environmental factors such as excessive exposure to high temperatures should be investigated. Drug and medication history also is obtained. If an environmental factor is identified, correction may improve sperm numbers (Chap. 20, p. 431).

■ Abnormal Sperm Motility or Morphology

Asthenospermia, that is, decreased sperm motility, may be seen alone or in combination with oligozoospermia or other abnormal semen parameters. In general, asthenospermia does not respond to directed treatments. Expectant management may be considered especially if the duration of infertility is short and maternal age is younger than 35 years. For treatment, IUI and ICSI are preferred, although IUI is generally not successful in severe cases (Tan, 2014). If fewer than 1 million motile sperm are available for insemination following semen processing or the couple has experienced more than 5 years of infertility, ICSI is considered as initial therapy (Ludwig, 2005).

Teratozoospermia or abnormal sperm morphology is most often seen in conjunction with oligospermia, asthenospermia, and oligoasthenospermia. Directed treatments for teratozoospermia are not available, and therapy options include IUI and ART. Because teratozoospermia may commonly be accompanied by sperm function defects that may impair fertilization, ICSI is considered if ART is selected.

■ Varicocele

This results from dilation of the pampiniform plexus of the spermatic vein and is usually left-sided (Fig. 20-2, p. 431). Traditional treatment is surgical ligation of the internal spermatic vein. Of options, retroperitoneal high ligation and trans-inguinal ligation are the most frequently performed. More recently, interventional radiographic techniques that selectively catheterize and embolize the internal spermatic vein with sclerosing solutions, tissue adhesives, or detachable balloons or coils are alternatives. Despite the widespread application of varicocele treatments, insufficient evidence demonstrates conception success with the treatment of a clinical varicocele in couples with male subfertility (Evers, 2003).

UNEXPLAINED INFERTILITY

This may represent one of the most common infertility diagnoses, and its reported prevalence reaches up to 30 percent (Dodson, 1987). The diagnosis is highly subjective and depends on the diagnostic tests performed or omitted and on their quality. Paradoxically, a diagnosis of unexplained infertility, therefore, will more often be reached if the evaluation is incomplete or poor quality (Gleicher, 2006). Nevertheless, an unexplained infertility diagnosis cannot, by definition, be directly treated. Expectant management may be considered especially with infertility of short duration and with relatively young maternal age. However, if treatment is desired, IUI, superovulation, and ART are empiric appropriate interventions to consider.

INTRAUTERINE INSEMINATION

This technique uses a thin flexible catheter to place a prepared semen sample into the uterine cavity. First, motile, morphologically normal spermatozoa are separated from dead sperm, leukocytes, and seminal plasma. This highly motile fraction is then inserted transcervically near the anticipated time of ovulation. Intrauterine insemination can be performed with or without superovulation and is appropriate therapy for treatment of cervical factors, mild and moderate male factors, and unexplained infertility.

If performed for cervical factors, IUI timed by urine LH surge is an initial strategy that achieves reasonable pregnancy rates of up to 11 percent per cycle (Steures, 2004). Although this rate is lower than that seen with superovulation combined with IUI, the side effects and expense of superovulation are avoided.

In contrast, for unexplained infertility and for male factors, IUI is most commonly performed with superovulation. A combination of CC plus IUI was evaluated against observation for unexplained infertility by Deaton and coworkers (1990) in one randomized trial. The treatment group had a significantly higher pregnancy rate (9.5 percent) compared with the observation cohort (3.3 percent). For unexplained infertility, gonadotropin treatment (FSH or hMG) alone increases the pregnancy rate, but the benefit is markedly improved with the addition of IUI (Guzick, 1999). Aromatase inhibitors do not appear to be as efficacious for IUI as conventional CC or gonadotropin treatments for unexplained infertility (Diamond, 2015).

ASSISTED REPRODUCTIVE TECHNOLOGY

ART describes clinical and laboratory techniques used to achieve pregnancy in infertile couples for whom direct corrections of underlying causes are not feasible. In principle, IUI meets this definition. By convention, however, ART procedures are those that at some point require extraction and isolation of an oocyte as described in the following paragraphs.

In Vitro Fertilization

During IVF, mature oocytes from stimulated ovaries are retrieved transvaginally with sonographic guidance (Fig. 21-10). Sperm and ova are then combined in vitro to prompt fertilization (Fig. 21-11). If successful, viable embryos are transferred transcervically into the endometrial cavity using sonographic

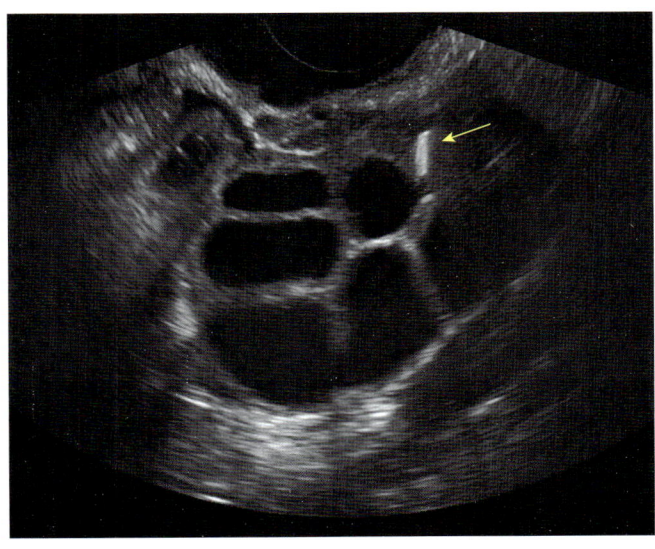

FIGURE 21-10 Transabdominal sonogram demonstrates transvaginal oocyte retrieval. The needle is seen in the upper right portion of the image as a hyperechoic line (*arrow*) entering a mature follicle.

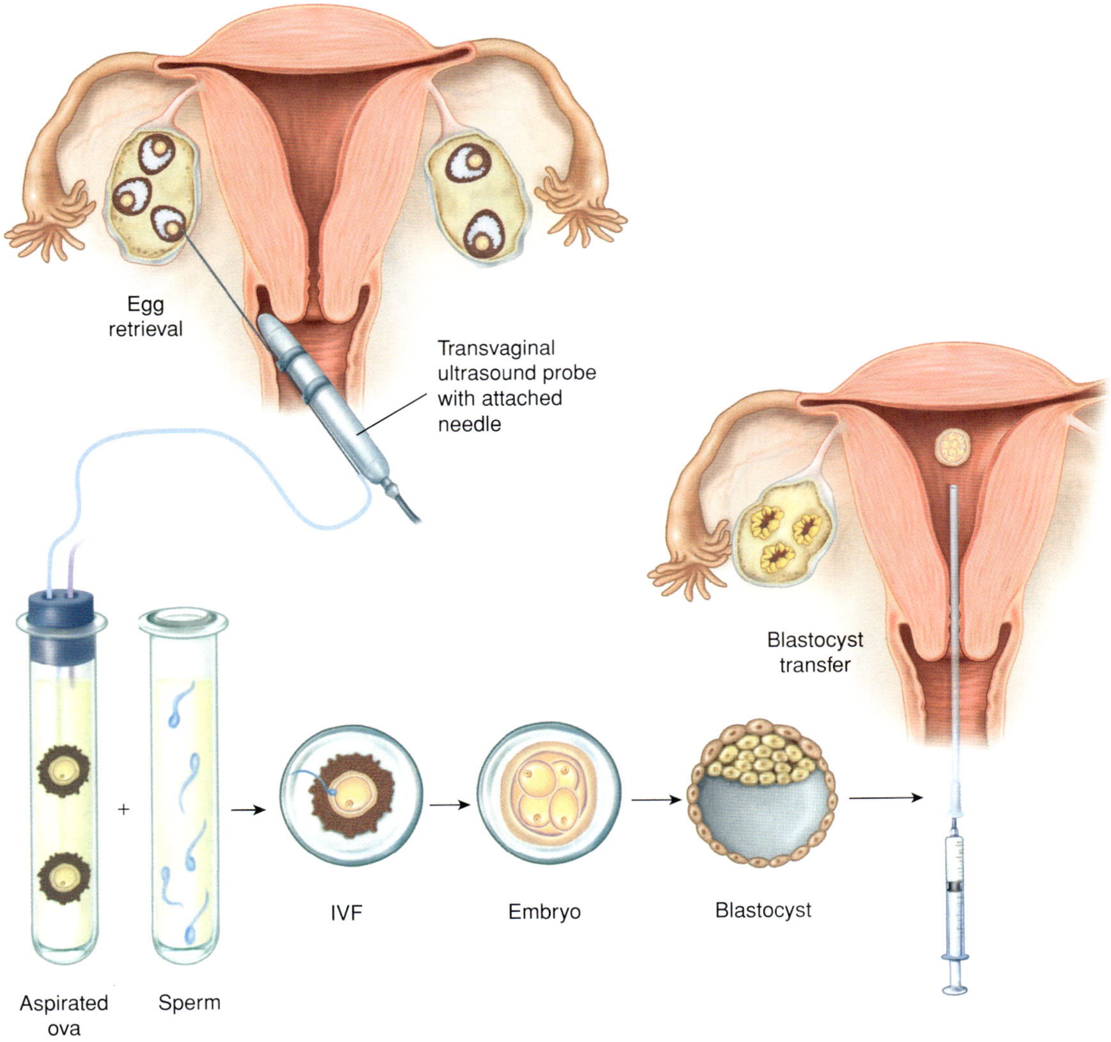

Egg
retrieval

Transvaginal
ultrasound probe
with attached
needle

Blastocyst
transfer

+

Aspirated   Sperm   IVF   Embryo   Blastocyst
ova

FIGURE 21-11 In vitro fertilization (IVF). Controlled ovarian stimulation is achieved with one of the protocols displayed in Figure 21-2, and follicle maturation is monitored over several days sonographically. Near ovulation, a transvaginal approach is used to harvest eggs from the ovaries (see Fig. 21-10). These oocytes are fertilized in vitro, and fertilized eggs develop to the blastocyst stage. Blastocysts are then drawn up into a syringe and delivered into the endometrial cavity under sonographic guidance.

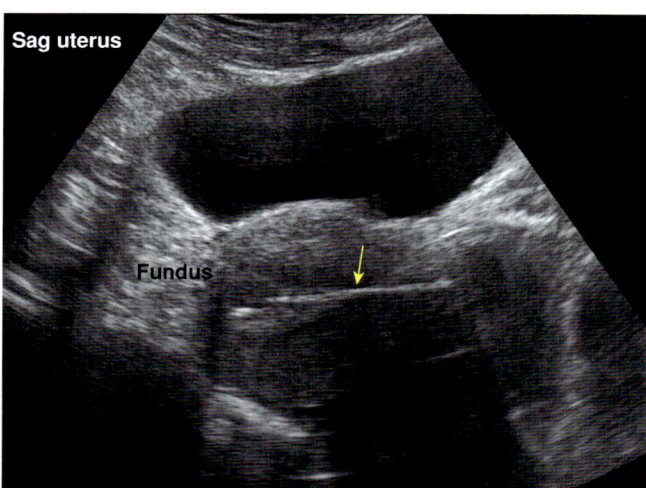

FIGURE 21-12 Embryo transfer performed using abdominal sonographic guidance for proper placement. Catheter (*arrow*) is seen within the endometrial cavity.

guidance (Fig. 21-12). Discussed earlier, prior to proceeding with IVF, hydrosalpinges are removed or tubes are interrupted to help raise implantation rates and lower miscarriage risk (p. 460).

Similar to IUI, substantial benefit is achieved using controlled ovarian stimulation prior to egg retrieval. Many ova are genetically or functionally abnormal. Thus, exposure of several ova to sperm results in a greater chance of a healthy embryo. Most often, a GnRH agonist is coupled with gonadotropins (FSH or hMG). These agonists prevent the possibility of spontaneous LH surge and ovulation prior to egg retrieval. Optimally, 10 to 20 ova are harvested, and from these, one healthy embryo is ideally transferred back to the uterus.

Unfortunately, methods to determine embryo health are imperfect. To maximize the probability of pregnancy, more than one embryo is commonly transferred to older women, which raises the multifetal gestation risk. However, advances in culture conditions now permit embryos to be cultured to the blastocyst stage. This allows transfer of fewer embryos yet maintains high pregnancy rates (Langley, 2001).

Intracytoplasmic Sperm Injection

This variation of IVF is most applicable to male factor infertility. During the micromanipulation technique of ICSI, cumulus cells surrounding an ovum are enzymatically digested, and a single sperm is directly injected through the zona pellucida and oocyte cell membrane (see Fig. 21-9). Pregnancy rates with ICSI are comparable with those achieved with IVF for other causes of infertility. For azoospermic men, ICSI has made pregnancy in their partners possible. In these cases, sperm are mechanically extracted from the testicle or epididymis.

Gestational Carrier Surrogacy

This variation of IVF places a fertilized egg into the uterus of a surrogate rather than into the "intended mother." Indications are varied, and this approach may be appropriate for women with uncorrectable uterine factors, for those in whom pregnancy would pose significant health risks, and for those with repetitive unexplained miscarriage.

Gestational carrier surrogacy has legal and psychosocial issues. In most states, a surrogate is the legal parent, and adoption must be completed after birth to give the intended mother her parental rights. However, a few states have adopted specific laws that extend protection to the intended parents.

Although still considered experimental, uterus transplantation is an alternative to gestational carrier surrogacy for women with absolute uterine factor infertility. Examples include uterine agenesis, prior hysterectomy, obliterating intrauterine adhesions, and distorting leiomyomas. In 2015, the first birth following uterine transplant was reported (Brännström, 2015). Postoperative immunosuppressive therapy and close monitoring for signs of rejection are essential. Attempts at pregnancy should be delayed until it is reasonably certain that the surgery has been successful. Initially, no attempts to achieve pregnancy were made for 12 months. IVF is required in all cases (Brännström, 2018). More recently, some transplant centers have allowed patients to undergo IVF at 6 months or earlier following surgery. Currently, uterine transplantation is done following institutional review and under strict protocols by expert transplant surgeons. A uterine transplant registry is currently being developed to follow long-term outcomes.

Egg Donation

This may be employed in cases of infertility associated with ovarian failure or diminished ovarian reserve. Fertile women whose offspring would be at risk for maternally transmitted genetic disease are other candidates. Egg donors may be known to the recipient couple or more commonly are anonymous young women recruited by an agency or IVF center.

Egg donation can be performed using "fresh" oocytes or cryopreserved eggs. Fresh egg donation cycles require synchronization of the recipient's endometrium with egg development in the donor.

To accomplish this, the egg donor completes one of the superovulation protocols outlined in Figure 21-2. Concurrently, if a recipient is not menopausal, GnRH agonists are administered to her to suppress gonadotropin production. This allows a scheduled priming of her endometrium with estrogen and progesterone. Following gonadotropin suppression, exogenous estrogen is given to the recipient. This estrogen administration begins just prior to the start of gonadotropin administration to the egg donor. After the donor receives hCG to allow the final stages of follicle and egg maturation, the recipient begins progesterone to prepare her endometrium. In the recipient, estrogen and progesterone are typically continued until late in the first trimester when placental production of these hormones is deemed to be adequate.

Gamete or Zygote Intrafallopian Transfer

Gamete intrafallopian transfer (GIFT) is similar to IVF in that egg retrieval is performed after controlled ovarian stimulation. Unlike IVF, however, fertilization and early embryo development do not take place in the laboratory. Eggs and sperm are placed via catheter through the fimbria and deposited directly into the oviduct. This transfer of gametes is most commonly performed at laparoscopy. Like IUI, GIFT is most applicable for unexplained infertility and is not considered for tubal factor causes.

This technique was most popular in the late 1980s. However, as laboratory techniques have improved, IVF has largely replaced GIFT. In general, GIFT is more invasive, provides less diagnostic information, and requires transfer of more than two eggs for optimal pregnancy chances, which raises risks for higher-order multifetal gestation. Thus, the major current indication for GIFT is to avoid the religious or ethical concerns that some patients may have with fertilization taking place outside the body.

Zygote intrafallopian transfer (ZIFT) is a variant of IVF with similarities to GIFT. Zygote transfer is not performed directly into the uterine cavity but rather into the fallopian tube at laparoscopy. If the transfer is completed after a zygote has begun to divide, the procedure is more accurately termed *tubal embryo transfer (TET)*. Although a normal fallopian tube may provide a superior environment for the early-stage embryo, improved laboratory culture methods has lessened this advantage. Accordingly, ZIFT currently is considered most appropriately in the rare case in which transcervical transfer during IVF is not technically feasible.

Intravaginal Culture

Fertilization of eggs and culture of embryos has generally required a complex and costly laboratory infrastructure to optimize the environment for the gametes/embryos. The modern IVF laboratory requires expensive air filtration systems as the embryo has no lung, kidney, or liver to act as filters (Mortimer, 2005). Incubators can provide temperature control and an optimal mix of oxygen (O_2), carbon dioxide (CO_2), and nitrogen. Those specifically designed for IVF are complex electromechanical devices and thus are prone to drift or failure. These systems require alarms, daily quality control checks, and around-the-clock monitoring.

Intravaginal culture (IVC) was proposed more than 30 years ago as a means to simplify and increase access to reproductive care (Ranoux, 1988). Initial studies, using improvised IVC devices, demonstrated that the vagina could provide an appropriate temperature and gas environment. However, adoption was limited due to instances of vaginal bacterial contamination and other device constraints.

More recently, a device specifically designed for IVC (INVOcell) has been approved by the FDA. This device is composed of polystyrene and allows maintenance of an appropriate low O_2, high CO_2 environment (Fig. 21-13). A recent prospective

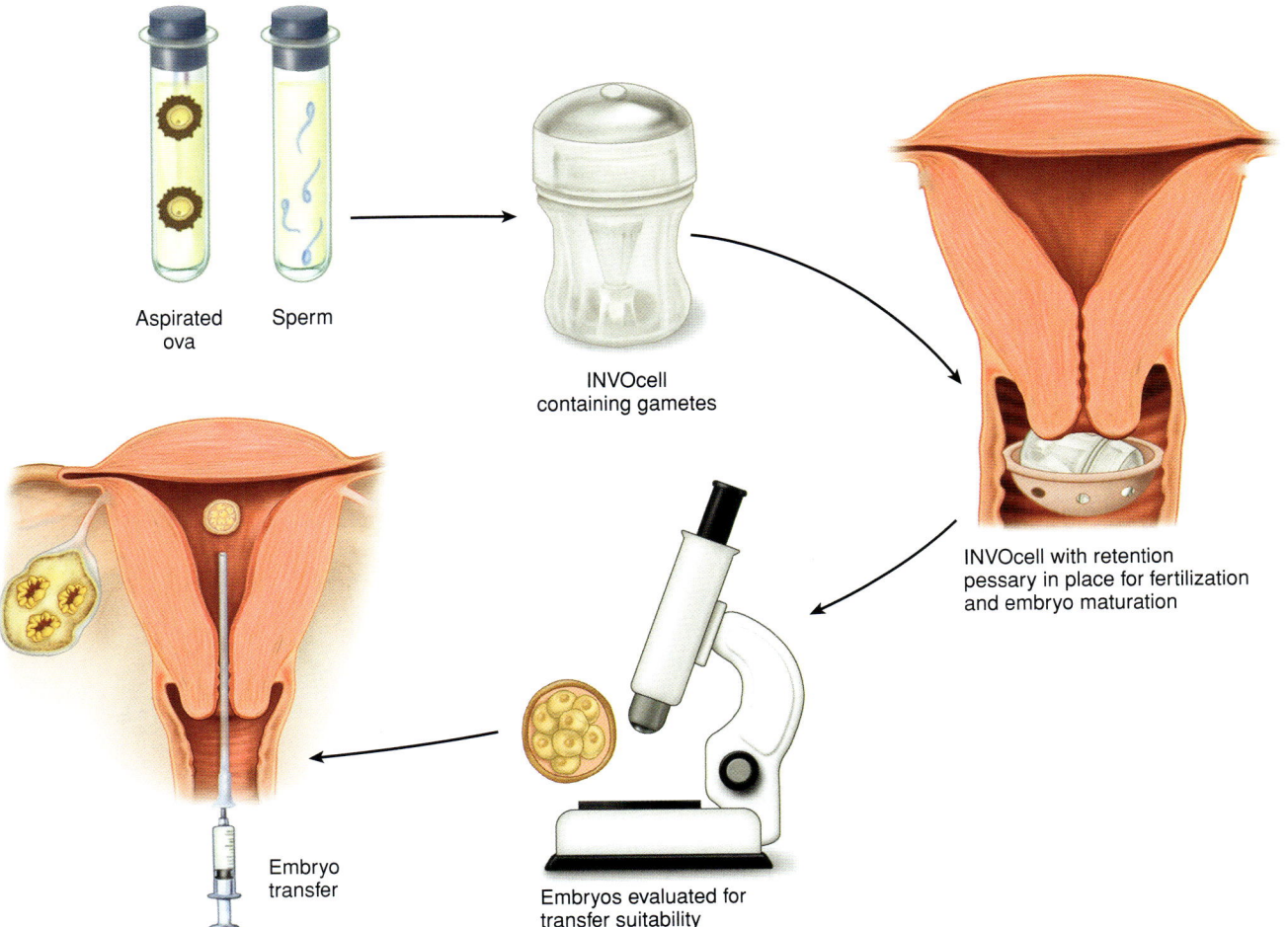

Aspirated ova

Sperm

INVOcell containing gametes

INVOcell with retention pessary in place for fertilization and embryo maturation

Embryos evaluated for transfer suitability

Embryo transfer

FIGURE 21-13 With intravaginal culture (IVC), fertilization and embryo maturation occur in vivo. First, superovulation is induced, and ova are harvested. These are then combined with sperm in the INVOcell device for fertilization within the vaginal. After several days to allow embryo maturation, the INVOcell device is removed, and embryos are inspected. One of those deemed suitable is then transferred into the endometrial cavity.

randomized trial has demonstrated live birth rates with INVOcell similar to conventional laboratory incubators when used for fertilization and extended embryo culture (day 5 blastocyst). (Doody, 2016). Further investigation will determine whether IVC will broaden access to ART care.

Embryo, Oocyte, or Ovarian Tissue Cryopreservation

With IVF, many eggs are retrieved to ultimately produce one to three healthy embryos for transfer. This frequently leads to extra embryos. Successful freezing and thawing of embryos has been possible for two decades. Moreover, advances in cryoprotectants and techniques have improved survival rates of embryos frozen at various developmental stages. With cryopreservation, these supernumerary embryos can yield pregnancies later, obviating the need for repeated ovarian stimulation and egg retrieval. For some patients, cryopreservation of all embryos avoids fresh transfer. Instead, later transfer can allow improved synchrony between the embryo and the endometrium for higher pregnancy rates (Doody, 2014).

Cryopreservation of unfertilized eggs had previously posed significant technical hurdles. These challenges have been largely overcome by ultrarapid freezing techniques (vitrification), and oocyte cryopreservation is no longer considered experimental. Egg freezing is useful for women facing gonadotoxic chemotherapy. This technique also provides greater timing flexibility to circumvent cycle synchronization during egg donation. As success improves, oocyte cryopreservation may assist women desiring to delay childbearing, although data are lacking regarding its efficacy in this patient population. Careful counseling is needed with regard to age- and clinic-specific success rates (American Society for Reproductive Medicine, 2014).

Distinct from oocyte freezing, ovarian tissue cryopreservation is another fertility-preserving option. Candidates are patients who must urgently undergo potentially gonadotoxic treatments. With this method, one or both ovaries or ovarian cortex tissue is removed during laparoscopy or minilaparotomy. Postoperatively, the ovarian cortex is cut into small tissue slivers measuring 0.3- to 2-mm thick and cryopreserved. Ovarian tissue cryopreservation by both slow freezing and vitrification has been described. Successful pregnancies have been achieved following autologous transplantation of thawed cortical tissue into a pelvic site such as a contralateral ovary or pelvic sidewall. Some pregnancies have been achieved without further intervention, whereas others have required ART. Safety concerns include the risk for reintroducing a malignancy following transplantation. This risk may be greatest with blood-borne cancers such as leukemia. Although promising, this procedure is currently considered experimental (American Society for Reproductive Medicine, 2014).

In Vitro Maturation

This technique has been used to achieve pregnancy by aspirating antral follicles from unstimulated ovaries and culturing these immature oocytes to allow resumption and completion of meiosis in vitro. In vitro maturation (IVM) may be useful in patients with PCOS in whom stimulation poses a significant risk of OHSS. Recent data suggest that success rates with standard IVF remain superior to those with IVM (Walls, 2015). Additionally, long-term outcomes are unknown, and IVM is deemed experimental (American Society for Reproductive Medicine, 2013a). In the future, refinement of this technique may make possible maturation of ova from preantral follicles. This could potentially allow preservation of fertility potential but without the need for subsequent autologous transplantation for women in whom gonadotoxic chemotherapy is required.

Preimplantation Genetic Testing

These laboratory techniques identify genetic abnormalities in eggs or embryos prior to their transfer. Preimplantation genetic testing (PGT) can analyze the DNA from oocytes (polar bodies) or embryos (cleavage stage or blastocyst) for determining genetic abnormalities or for human leukocyte antigen (HLA) typing. Options include PGT for aneuploidies (PGT-A), PGT for monogenic/single-gene defects (PGT-M), and PGT for chromosomal structural rearrangements (PGT-SR), such as balanced translocations (Zegers-Hochschild, 2017). Thus, risk for transmission of heritable disease is a well-established indication for PGT. In contrast, *PGT-A* aims to identify embryonic aneuploidy resulting from gamete meiotic errors. Its proposed indications include recurrent miscarriage, advanced maternal age, and multiple failed IVF cycles.

PGT is no longer considered experimental, and newly developed methods for genetic analysis will likely broaden its application (Society for Assisted Reproductive Technology, 2008). During PGT, cells can be removed from a developing pregnancy at various stages. Biopsy of the first and second polar body has the advantage of avoiding cell removal from the developing embryo. However, two separate micromanipulation procedures are required, and genetic abnormalities of paternal origin are not detected. Biopsy of cleavage-stage embryos (6- to 8-cell stage) allows evaluation of both maternal and paternal contribution to the genome (Fig. 21-14). However, biopsy at this stage may only partially reflect the embryo's genetic makeup if mitotic nondisjunction has occurred and embryonic mosaicism has been created. In addition, biopsied normal embryos may have a slightly lower implantation rate. Instead, biopsy of the trophectoderm at the blastocyst stage can offer several advantages (see Fig. 21-14B). The trophectoderm is the layer from which trophoblasts and thus the placenta develop. Biopsy from this layer allows evaluation of several cells but avoids removal of inner cell mass (fetal) cells. However, biopsy of embryos at this late stage generally requires embryo cryopreservation. Genetic analysis and reporting cannot be performed fast enough to allow embryo transfer in the same cycle.

Once cells are extracted, they are tested for structural aberrations and/or aneuploidy. Common testing options include single-nucleotide polymorphism (SNP) plus comparative genomic hybridization (CGH) microarrays or quantitative polymerase chain reaction. To analyze single cells for disease-specific DNA mutations, linkage analysis and DNA sequencing are generally used. Most recently, next-generation sequencing (NGS) has been used for all aspects of PGT. NGS has been rapidly adopted because of its potential to enhance efficiency and precision and lower costs (American Society for Reproductive Medicine, 2018).

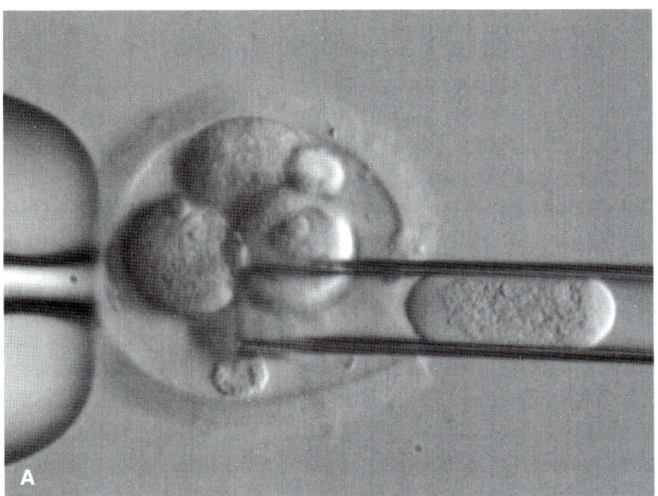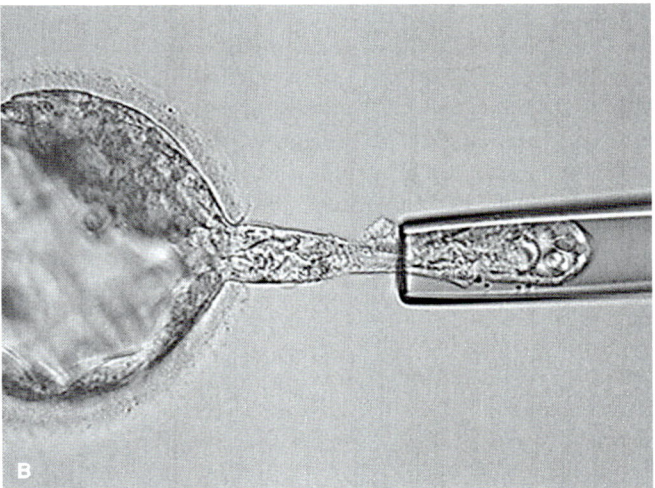

FIGURE 21-14 A. Photomicrograph of embryo biopsy. **B.** Photomicrograph of trophectoderm biopsy.

More recently, noninvasive PGT uses *spent embryo media (SEM)* to amplify cell-free DNA (cfDNA) to infer the embryo's karyotype. Of advantages, SEM collection requires no specialized training, and embryo disruption is negligible. Regarding SEM accuracy, comparisons between SEM cfDNA and "whole blastocyst" or trophectoderm biopsy show ploidy concordance rates that range from 30 to 87.5 percent (Belandres, 2019). Noninvasive PGT is unlikely to be adopted until at least 95 percent concordance rates can be achieved. This will require improvements in whole genome amplification (WGA) techniques.

Complications of Assisted Reproductive Technology

In most cases, ART leads to successful delivery of healthy singleton pregnancies. However, some pregnancy complications may develop more frequently in those conceived using ART. Of maternal risks, preeclampsia, placenta previa, and placental abruption are more common in IVF-conceived pregnancies (Table 21-6). Whether these greater risks are attributable to ART or to patient factors is unclear. One recent study found that risks for severe maternal morbidity were higher for women with conceptions achieved through infertility treatment (Luke, 2019). Specifically, in those conceived by IVF, risks were greater with pregnancy not conceived from autologous fresh cycles.

For the fetus, multifetal gestation is the most common risk. For singleton gestations, IVF has been associated with perinatal mortality, preterm delivery, low birthweight, and fetal-growth restriction. These trends persist even following adjustment for age and parity (Reddy, 2007). Other studies, however, have not confirmed this increased risk for singletons (Fujii, 2010). Additionally, congenital anomalies and epigenetic issues are concerns (see Table 21-6).

Discussions regarding the risks for congenital anomalies began shortly after the initial success of IVF and intensified following the use of ICSI. Specifically, studies do suggest a higher incidence of congenital anomalies in neonates conceived with ovulation induction, IUI, or IVF compared with those from the general population (El-Chaar, 2009; Reddy, 2007). Interpretation of

most published studies, however, is complex. For example, the patient population undergoing IVF differs from the general obstetric population with respect to age and other factors. If data are adjusted for maternal age or duration of subfertility, the risk of congenital anomalies does not appear to be increased with ART (Shevell, 2005; Zhu, 2006). This implies that much of the risk is intrinsic to the infertile couple and not related to the procedure itself. Certain rare childhood cancers, such as embryonal hepatic tumors, are more common in IVF-conceived offspring. However, the risk more likely is attributable to underlying patient factors than to the IVF process (Spector, 2019).

An increase in the risk of epigenetic issues also has been reported. Although these conditions appear to be rare, their

TABLE 21-6. Potential Risks in Singleton IVF Pregnancies

	Absolute Risk (%)	RR (95% CI)[a]
Neonatal Complications		
Preterm birth	10.3	1.70 (1.60-1.81)
Low birthweight (<2500 g)	7.7	1.65 (1.53–1.78)
Small for gestational age	7.8	1.04 (0.97–1.12)
NICU admission	7.9	1.07 (1.02–1.12)
Neonatal mortality	0.28	1.67 (1.09–2.56)
Major birth defect	2.1	1.25 (1.09–1.44)
Maternal Complications		
Pregnancy hypertension	12.6	1.22 (1.15–1.28)
Placental complications	5.2	2.81 (2.57–3.08)
Gestational diabetes	8.2	1.41 (0.85–2.34)
Prenatal hospitalization	5.3	1.81 (1.65–1.97)
Primary cesarean delivery	32.2	1.20 (1.17–1.24)

[a]Compared with pregnancies not conceived by in vitro fertilization (IVF).
CI = confidence interval; NICU = neonatal intensive care unit; RR = relative risk.
Data from Luke, 2017a,b; 2019a,b.

importance cannot be overstated. For review, each autosomal gene is represented by two copies, or alleles, and one copy is inherited from each parent. For most genes, both alleles are expressed simultaneously. However, approximately 150 human genes are *imprinted*, and with these genes, only one of the alleles is expressed. Imprinted genes are under control of an imprinting center that directs embryogenesis and viability. Alteration of the cellular environment can interfere with this regulation and may follow gamete manipulation or inadequate in vitro culture conditions. As a result, accelerated embryo growth, birth complications, placental abnormalities, and polyhydramnios have been observed in nonhuman mammalian ART pregnancies. In humans, imprinted genes may contribute to behavior and language development, alcohol dependency, schizophrenia, and bipolar affective disorders. Imprinting may also raise risks for obesity, cardiovascular disease, and cancers. Of imprinting disorders, only rates of the rare Beckwith-Wiedemann syndrome are currently suggested to be higher in human ART. Causation has not been conclusively proven. However, in view of the above increased risks, more intensive prenatal assessment in pregnancies conceived by IVF is reasonable.

Last, studies assessing cognitive development after ART are reassuring for the most part. Many studies are suboptimal due to small sample size, choice of comparison group, and confounding and mediating factors (Carson, 2010). Fortunately, currently available data suggest that the psychomotor development of preschool children conceived by IVF does not differ from that of naturally conceived children. Similarly, the socioemotional development of children conceived by IVF appears comparable with that of naturally conceived children (Ludwig, 2006).

CONCLUSION

Treatment of infertility is typically initiated only after a thorough investigation (Chap. 20, p. 434). In general, identified contributors to subfertility are addressed first. However, in many cases, no obvious cause is found. In others, the cause(s) may be discovered but not amenable to directed corrective therapies. In these circumstances, generalized fertility-boosting strategies may be recommended. These include IUI (with or without superovulation) and ART. Importantly, superovulation and ART are not without risks, and couples should be appropriately counseled. Additionally, these techniques may involve donors or gestational carriers and are associated with unique psychosocial, legal, and ethical considerations. Emerging technologies such as PGT and uterus transplantation bring additional ethical issues to be addressed and resolved.

REFERENCES

Aakvaag A: Hormonal response to electrocautery of the ovary in patients with polycystic ovarian disease. BJOG 92:1258, 1985

Adashi EY, Rock JA, Guzick D, et al: Fertility following bilateral ovarian wedge resection: a critical analysis of 90 consecutive cases of the polycystic ovary syndrome. Fertil Steril 36:30, 1981

Almog B, Sheizaf B, Shalom-Paz E, et al: Effects of excision of ovarian endometrioma on the antral follicle count and collected oocytes for in vitro fertilization. Fertil Steril 94(6):2340, 2010

American College of Obstetricians and Gynecologists: Neural tube defects. Practice Bulletin No. 187, December 2017

American College of Obstetricians and Gynecologists: Management of endometriosis. Practice Bulletin No. 114, July 2010, Reaffirmed 2018a

American College of Obstetricians and Gynecologists: Obesity in pregnancy. Practice Bulletin No. 156, December 2015, Reaffirmed 2018b

American Society for Reproductive Medicine: Endometriosis and infertility: a committee opinion. Fertil Steril 98(3):591, 2012

American Society for Reproductive Medicine: Ovarian tissue cryopreservation: a committee opinion. Fertil Steril 101(5):1237, 2014

American Society for Reproductive Medicine: Diagnostic evaluation of the infertile female: a committee opinion. Fertil Steril 103(6):e44, 2015a

American Society for Reproductive Medicine: Obesity and reproduction: a committee opinion. Fertil Steril 104(5):1116, 2015b

American Society for Reproductive Medicine: Role of tubal surgery in the era of assisted reproductive technology: a committee opinion. Fertil Steril 103(6):e37, 2015c

American Society for Reproductive Medicine: Prevention and treatment of moderate and severe ovarian hyperstimulation syndrome: a guideline. Fertil Steril 106(7):1634, 2016

American Society for Reproductive Medicine, Society for Assisted Reproductive Technology: In vitro maturation: a committee opinion. Fertil Steril 99(3): 663, 2013a

American Society for Reproductive Medicine, Society of Reproductive Surgeons: Pathogenesis, consequences, and control of peritoneal adhesions in gynecologic surgery: a committee opinion. Fertil Steril 99(6):1550, 2013b

American Society for Reproductive Medicine, Society for Assisted Reproductive Technology: Guidance on the limits to the number of embryos to transfer: a committee opinion. Fertil Steril 107(4):901, 2017

American Society for Reproductive Medicine, Society for Assisted Reproductive Technology: The use of preimplantation genetic testing for aneuploidy (PGT-A): a committee opinion. Fertil Steril 109(3):429, 2018

Antonucci T, Whitcomb R, McLain R, et al: Impaired glucose tolerance is normalized by treatment with the thiazolidinedione troglitazone. Diabetes Care 20:188, 1998

Armar N, McGarrigle H, Honour J, et al: Laparoscopic ovarian diathermy in the management of anovulatory infertility in women with polycystic ovaries: endocrine changes and clinical outcomes. Fertil Steril 53:45, 1990

Armar NA, Lachelin GC: Laparoscopic ovarian diathermy: an effective treatment for anti-oestrogen resistant anovulatory infertility in women with the polycystic ovary syndrome. BJOG 100(2):P161, 1993

Balen A, Braat D, West C, et al: Cumulative conception and livebirth rates after the treatment of anovulatory infertility: safety and efficacy of ovulation induction. Hum Reprod 9:1563, 1994

Balen A, Tan SL, Jacobs H, et al: Hypersecretion of luteinising hormone. A significant cause of infertility and miscarriage. BJOG 100:1082, 1993

Bayrak A, Harp D, Saadat P, et al: Recurrence of hydrosalpinges after cuff neosalpingostomy in a poor prognosis population. J Assist Reprod Genet 23:285, 2006

Belandres D, Shamonki M, Arrach N: Current status of spent embryo media research for preimplantation genetic testing. J Assist Reprod Genet March 36:819, 2019

Biljan MM, Hemmings R, Brassard N, et al: The outcome of 150 babies following the treatment with letrozole or letrozole and gonadotropins. Fertil Steril 84(Suppl 1):S95, 2005

Bosch E, Labarta E, Crespo J, et al: Circulating progesterone levels and ongoing pregnancy rates in controlled ovarian stimulation cycles for in vitro fertilization: analysis of over 4000 cycles. Hum Reprod 25(8):2092, 2010

Brännström M, Dahm Kähler P, Greite R, et al: Uterus transplantation: a rapidly expanding field. Transplantation 102(4):569, 2018

Brännström M, Johannesson L, Bokström H, et al: Livebirth after uterus transplantation. Lancet 385(9968):607, 2015

Buttram VC, Vaquero C: Post-ovarian wedge resection adhesive disease. Fertil Steril 26:874, 1975

Carson C, Kurinczuk JJ, Sacker A, et al: Cognitive development following ART: effect of choice of comparison group, confounding and mediating factors. Hum Reprod 25(1):244, 2010

Casey BM, Cunningham FG: Endocrinologic disorders. In Cunningham FG, Leveno KL, Bloom SL, et al (eds): Williams Obstetrics, 25th ed, New York, McGraw-Hill, 2018

Casper RF: Letrozole: ovulation or superovulation? Fertil Steril 80:1335, 2003

Centers for Disease Control and Prevention: Contribution of assisted reproductive technology and ovulation-inducing drugs to triplet and higher-order multiple births—United States, 1980–1997. MMWR 49:535, 2000

Chaffkin LM, Nulsen JC, Luciano AA, et al: A comparative analysis of the cycle fecundity rates associated with combined human menopausal gonadotropin (hMG) and intrauterine insemination (IUI) versus either hMG or IUI alone. Fertil Steril 55(2):252, 1991

Choi JM, Chung P, Veeck L, et al: AZF microdeletions of the Y chromosome and in vitro fertilization outcome. Fertil Steril 81:337, 2004

Collin P, Vilska S, Heinonen PK, et al: Infertility and coeliac disease. Gut 39(3): 382, 1996

Crosignani PG, Colombo M, Vegetti W, et al: Overweight and obese anovulatory patients with polycystic ovaries: parallel improvements in anthropometric indices, ovarian physiology and fertility rate induced by diet. Hum Reprod 18(9):1928, 2003

Deaton J, Gibson M, Blackmer K, et al: A randomized, controlled trial of clomiphene citrate and intrauterine insemination in couples with unexplained infertility or surgically corrected endometriosis. Fertil Steril 54:1083, 1990

Diamond MP, Legro RS, Coutifaris C, et al: Letrozole, gonadotropin, or clomiphene for unexplained infertility. N Engl J Med 373(13):1230, 2015

Dicker D, Goldman JA, Levy T, et al: The impact of long-term gonadotropin-releasing hormone analogue treatment on preclinical abortions in patients with severe endometriosis undergoing in vitro fertilization-embryo transfer. Fertil Steril 57:597, 1992

Dodson WC, Whitesides DB, Hughes CL, et al: Superovulation with intra-uterine insemination in the treatment of infertility: a possible alternative to gamete intrafallopian transfer and in vitro fertilization. Fertil Steril 48:441, 1987

Domar AD, Seibel MM, Benson H, et al: The mind/body program for infertility: a new behavioral treatment approach for women with infertility. Fertil Steril 54: 1183, 1990

Doody KJ: Cryopreseration and delayed embryo transfer—assisted reproductive technology registry and reporting implication. Fertil Steril 102(1):27, 2014

Doody KJ, Broome EJ, Doody KM: Comparing blastocyst quality and live birth rates of intravaginal culture using INVOcell™ to traditional in vitro incubation in a randomized open-label prospective controlled trial. J Assist Reprod Genet 33(4):495, 2016

El-Chaar D, Yang Q, Gao J, et al: Risk of birth defects increased in pregnancies conceived by assisted human reproduction. Fertil Steril 92(5):1557, 2009

Elnashar A, Abdelmageed E, Fayed M, et al: Clomiphene citrate and dexamethazone in treatment of clomiphene citrate-resistant polycystic ovary syndrome: a prospective placebo-controlled study. Hum Reprod 21(7): 1805, 2006

Evers JL, Collins JA: Assessment of efficacy of varicocele repair for male subfertility: a systematic review. Lancet 361(9372):1849, 2003

Exacoustos C, Zupi E, Amadio A, et al: Laparoscopic removal of endometriomas: sonographic evaluation of residual functioning ovarian tissue. Am J Obstet Gynecol 191(1):68, 2004

Farhi J, Soule S, Jacobs HS, et al: Effect of laparoscopic ovarian electrocautery on ovarian response and outcome of treatment with gonadotropins in clomiphene citrate-resistant patients with polycystic syndrome. Fertil Steril 64:930, 1995

Fedele L, Bianchi S, Marchini M, et al: Superovulation with human menopausal gonadotropins in the treatment of infertility associated with minimal or mild endometriosis: a controlled randomized study. Fertil Steril 58(1):28, 1992

Farhi J, West C, Patel A, et al: Treatment of anovulatory infertility: the problem of multiple pregnancy. Hum Reprod 11:429, 1996

Filicori M, Cognigni GE, Taraborrelli S, et al: Modulation of folliculogenesis and steroidogenesis in women by graded menotropin administration. Hum Reprod 17:2009, 2002

Fleming R, Jenkins J: The source and implications of progesterone rise during the follicular phase of assisted reproduction cycles. Reprod Biomed Online 21(4):446, 2010

Fontana PG, Leclerc JM: Contraindication of Femara (letrozole) in premenopausal women. 2005. Available at: http://healthycanadians.gc.ca/recall-alert-rappel-avis/hc-sc/2005/14326a-eng.php. Accessed June 3, 2019

Franasiak JM, Dondik Y, Molinaro TA, et al: Blastocyst transfer is not associated with increased rates of monozygotic twins when controlling for embryo cohort quality. Fertil Steril 103(1):95, 2015

Franik S, Kremer JA, Nelen WL, et al: Aromatase inhibitors for subfertile women with polycystic ovary syndrome. Cochrane Database Syst Rev 2: CD010287, 2014

Franks S, Adams J, Mason H, et al: Ovulation disorders in women with polycystic ovary syndrome. Clin Obstet Gynecol 12:605, 1985

Fujii M, Matsuoka R, Bergel E, et al: Perinatal risk in singleton pregnancies after in vitro fertilization. Fertil Steril 94(6):2113, 2010

Gleicher N, Barad D: Unexplained infertility: does it really exist? Hum Reprod 21:1951, 2006

Golan A, Ron-el R, Herman A, et al: Ovarian hyperstimulation syndrome: an update review. Obstet Gynecol Surv 44(6):430, 1989

Gordts S, Campo R, Puttemans P, et al: Clinical factors determining pregnancy outcome after microsurgical tubal reanastomosis. Fertil Steril 92(4):1198, 2009

Greenblatt E, Casper RF: Endocrine changes after laparoscopic ovarian cautery in polycystic ovarian syndrome. Am J Obstet Gynecol 156:279, 1987

Guzick DS, Carson SA, Coutifaris C, et al: Efficacy of superovulation and intrauterine insemination in the treatment of infertility. N Engl J Med 340:177, 1999

Gysler M, March CM, Mishell DR Jr, et al: A decade's experience with an individualized clomiphene treatment regimen including its effect on the postcoital test. Fertil Steril 37:161, 1982

Hammond M, Halme J, Talbert L, et al: Factors affecting the pregnancy rate in clomiphene citrate induction of ovulation. Obstet Gynecol 62:196, 1983

Hart RJ, Hickey M, Maouris P, et al: Excisional surgery versus ablative surgery for ovarian endometriomata. Cochrane Database Syst Rev 2:CD004992, 2008

Hawkins JS, Casey BM, Cunningham FG: Obesity. In Cunningham FG, Leveno KL, Bloom SL, et al (eds): Williams Obstetrics, 25th ed. New York, McGraw-Hill, 2018

Helmerhorst FM, Van Vliet HA, Gornas T, et al: Intra-uterine insemination versus timed intercourse for cervical hostility in subfertile couples. Cochrane Database Syst Rev 4:CD002809, 2005

Hoeger K: Obesity and weight loss in polycystic ovary syndrome. Obstet Gynecol Clin North Am 28:85, 2001

Jackson JE, Rosen M, McLean T, et al: Prevalence of celiac disease in a cohort of women with unexplained infertility. Fertil Steril 89(4):1002, 2008

Kemmann E, Ghazi D, Corsan G, et al: Does ovulation stimulation improve fertility in women with minimal/mild endometriosis after laser laparoscopy? Int J Fertil Menopausal Stud 38(1):16, 1993

Kiddy DS, Hamilton-Fairly D, Bush A, et al: Improvement in endocrine and ovarian function during dietary treatment of obese women with polycystic ovary syndrome. Clin Endocrinol (Oxf) 36:105, 1992

Koechling W, Plaksin D, Croston DE, et al: Comparative pharmacology of a new recombinant FSH expressed by a human cell line. Endocr Connect 6(5): 297, 2017

Kovacs G, Buckler H, Bangah M, et al: Treatment of anovulation due to polycystic ovarian syndrome by laparoscopic ovarian electrocautery. BJOG 98:30, 1991

Labarta E, Martínez-Conejero JA, Alamá P, et al: Endometrial receptivity is affected in women with high circulating progesterone levels at the end of the follicular phase: a functional genomics analysis. Hum Reprod 26(7):1813, 2011

Langley MT, Marek DM, Gardner DK, et al: Extended embryo culture in human assisted reproduction treatments. Hum Reprod 16:902, 2001

Legro RS, Barnhart HX, Schlaff WD, et al: Clomiphene, metformin or both for infertility in polycystic ovary syndrome. N Engl J Med 356(6):551, 2007

Legro RS, Brzyski RG, Diamond MP, et al: Letrozole versus clomiphene for infertility in the polycystic ovary syndrome. N Engl J Med 371(2):119, 2014

Lincoln SR, Ke RW, Kutteh WH: Screening for hypothyroidism in infertile women. J Reprod Med 44:455, 1999

Lobo RA, Gysler M, March CM, et al: Clinical and laboratory predictors of clomiphene response. Fertil Steril 37:168, 1982

Ludwig AK, Diedrich K, Ludwig M, et al: The process of decision making in reproductive medicine. Semin Reprod Med 23(4):348, 2005

Ludwig AK, Sutcliffe AG, Diedrich K, et al: Post-neonatal health and development of children born after assisted reproduction: a systematic review of controlled studies. Eur J Obstet Gynecol Reprod Biol 127(1):3, 2006

Luke B, Gopal D, Cabral H, et al: Adverse pregnancy, birth, and infant outcomes in twins: effects of maternal fertility status and infant gender combinations; the Massachusetts outcomes study of assisted reproductive technology. Am J Obstet Gynecol 217(3):330.e1, 2017a

Luke B, Gopal D, Cabral H, et al: Pregnancy, birth, and infant outcomes by maternal fertility status: the Massachusetts outcomes study of assisted reproductive technology. Am J Obstet Gynecol 217(3):327.e1, 2017b

Luke B, Brown MB, Wantman E, et al: Risk of prematurity and infant morbidity and mortality by maternal fertility status and plurality. J Assist Reprod Genet 36(1):121, 2019a

Luke B, Brown MB, Wantman E, et al: Risk of severe maternal morbidity by maternal fertility status: a US study in 8 states. Am J Obstet Gynecol 220(2):195.e1, 2019b

Martin JA, Hamilton BE, Osterman MJ, et al: Births: final data for 2012. Natl Vital Stat Rep 62(9):1, 2013

Martin JA, Hamilton BE, Osterman MJ, et al: Births: final data for 2017. Natl Vital Stat Rep 67(8):1, 2018

Martin JA, Park MM: Trends in twin and triplet births: 1980–97. Natl Vital Stat Rep 47:1, 1999

Meloni GF, Desole S, Vargiu N, et al: The prevalence of celiac disease in infertility. Hum Reprod 14:2759, 1999

Metwally M, Cheong YC, Horne AW: Surgical treatment of fibroids for subfertility. Cochrane Database Syst Rev 11:CD003857, 2012

Mitwally MF, Casper RF: Aromatase inhibition reduces the dose of gonadotropin required for controlled ovarian hyperstimulation. J Soc Gynecol Investig 11:406, 2004

Molitch ME: Management of prolactinomas during pregnancy. J Reprod Med 44:1121, 1999

Mortimer D, Mortimer ST: Quality and Risk Management in the IVF Laboratory. Cambridge, Cambridge University Press, 2005

Muzii L, Achilli C, Lecce F, et al: Second surgery for recurrent endometriomas is more harmful to healthy ovarian tissue and ovarian reserve than first surgery. Fertil Steril 103(3):738, 2015

Muzii L, Bianchi A, Bellati F, et al: Histologic analysis of endometriomas: what the surgeon needs to know. Fertil Steril 87(2):362, 2007

Nestler JE, Jakubowicz DJ, Evans WS, et al: Effects of metformin on spontaneous and clomiphene-induced ovulation in the polycystic ovary syndrome. N Engl J Med 338:1876, 1998

Palomba S, Orio F, Falbo A, et al: Prospective parallel randomized, double blind, double-dummy controlled clinical trial comparing clomiphene citrate and metformin as the first-line treatment for ovulation induction in nonobese anovulatory women with polycystic ovary syndrome. J Clin Endocrinol Metab 90:4068, 2005

Papanikolaou EG, Fatemi H, Venetis C, et al: Monozygotic twinning is not increased after single blastocyst transfer compared with single cleavage-stage embryo transfer. Fertil Steril 93(2):592, 2010

Parsanezhad ME, Alborzi S, Motazedian S, et al: Use of dexamethasone and clomiphene citrate in the treatment of clomiphene citrate-resistant patients with polycystic ovary syndrome and normal dehydroepiandrosterone sulfate levels: a prospective, double-blind, placebo-controlled trial. Fertil Steril 78(5):1001, 2002

Pasquali R, Antenucci D, Casmirri F, et al: Clinical and hormonal characteristics of obese amenorrheic hyperandrogenic women before and after weight loss. J Clin Endocrinol Metab 68:173, 1989

Patel SR, Sigman M: Antioxidant therapy in male infertility. Urol Clin North Am 35(2):319, 2008

Paulson RJ, Reindollar RH, Doody KJ: Toward standardizing the embryo transfer procedure: from "how to" to "how many." Fertil Steril 107(4):880, 2017

Pérez-Medina T, Bajo-Arenas J, Salazar F, et al: Endometrial polyps and their implication in the pregnancy rates of patients undergoing intrauterine insemination: a prospective, randomized study. Hum Reprod 20:1632, 2005

Ragni G, Somigliana E, Benedetti F, et al: Damage to ovarian reserve associated with laparoscopic excision of endometriomas: a quantitative rather than a qualitative injury. Am J Obstet Gynecol 193(6):1908, 2005

Raj S, Thompson I, Berger M, et al: Clinical aspects of polycystic ovary syndrome. Obstet Gynecol 49(5):552, 1977

Ranoux C, Aubriot FX, Dubuisson JB, et al: A new in vitro fertilization technique: intravaginal culture. Fertil Steril 49(4):654, 1988

Reddy UM, Wapner RJ, Rebar RW, et al: Infertility, assisted reproductive technology, and adverse pregnancy outcomes: executive summary of a National Institute of Child Health and Human Development workshop. Obstet Gynecol 109(4):967, 2007

Ross C, Morriss A, Khairy M, et al: A systematic review of the effect of oral antioxidants on male infertility. Reprod Biomed Online 20(6):711, 2010

Shevell T, Malone FD, Vidaver J, et al: Assisted reproductive technology and pregnancy outcome. Obstet Gynecol 106(5 Pt 1):1039, 2005

Sigman M, Glass S, Campagnone J, et al: Carnitine for the treatment of idiopathic asthenospermia: a randomized, double-blind, placebo-controlled trial. Fertil Steril 85(5):1409, 2006

Smith JF, Eisenberg ML, Millstein SG, et al: The use of complementary and alternative fertility treatment in couples seeking fertility care: data from a prospective cohort in the United States. Fertil Steril 93(7):2169, 2010

Society for Assisted Reproductive Technology, American Society for Reproductive Medicine: Preimplantation genetic testing: a Practice Committee opinion. Fertil Steril 90(5 Suppl):S136, 2008

Spector LG, Brown MB, Wantman E, et al: Association of in vitro fertilization with childhood cancer in the United States. JAMA Pediatr 173:e190392, 2019

Stein IF, Cohen MR: Surgical treatment of bilateral polycystic ovaries. Am J Obstet Gynecol 38:465, 1939

Steures P, van der Steeg JW, Verhoeve HR, et al: Does ovarian hyperstimulation in intrauterine insemination for cervical factor subfertility improve pregnancy rates? Hum Reprod 19:2263, 2004

Strickland DM, Whitted WA, Wians FH Jr: Screening infertile women for subclinical hypothyroidism. Am J Obstet Gynecol 163:262, 1990

Surrey ES, Silverberg KM, Surrey MW: Effect of prolonged gonadotropin-releasing hormone agonist therapy on the outcome of in vitro fertilization-embryo transfer in patients with endometriosis. Fertil Steril 78:699, 2002

Tan O, Ha T, Carr BR, et al: Predictive value of postwashed total progressively motile sperm count using CASA estimates in 6871 non-donor intrauterine insemination cycles. J Assist Reprod Genet 31(9):1147, 2014

Thiering P, Beaurepaire J, Jones M, et al: Mood state as a predictor of treatment outcome after in vitro fertilization/embryo transfer technology (IVF/ET). J Psychosom Res 37:481, 1993

Tredway D, Schertz JC, Beck D, et al: A phase II, prospective, randomized dose-finding comparative study evaluating anastrozole versus clomiphene citrate in infertile women with ovulatory dysfunction. Fertil Steril 95:1719, 2011a

Tredway D, Schertz JC, Beck D, et al: Anastrozole single-dose protocol in women with oligo- or anovulatory infertility: results of a randomized phase II dose-response study. Fertil Steril 95:1724, 2011b

Tulandi T, Collins JA, Burrows E, et al: Treatment-dependent and treatment-independent pregnancy among women with periadnexal adhesions. Am J Obstet Gynecol 162:354, 1990

Tulandi T, Martin J, Al-Fadhli R, et al: Congenital malformations among 911 newborns conceived after infertility treatment with letrozole or clomiphene citrate. Fertil Steril 85:1761, 2006

Vandermolen DT, Ratts VS, Evans WS, et al: Metformin increases the ovulatory rate and pregnancy rate from clomiphene citrate in patients with polycystic ovary syndrome who are resistant to clomiphene citrate alone. Fertil Steril 75:310, 2001

Walls ML, Hunter T, Keelan JA, et al: In vitro maturation as an alternative to standard in vitro fertilization for patients diagnosed with polycystic ovaries: a comparative analysis of fresh, frozen and cumulative cycle outcomes. Hum Reprod 30(1):88, 2015

Zarate A, Herdmandez-Ayup S, Rios-Montiel A: Treatment of anovulation in the Stein-Leventhal syndrome. Analysis of ninety cases. Fertil Steril 22:188, 1971

Zegers-Hochschild F, Adamson GD, Dyer S, et al: The international glossary on infertility and fertility care, 2017. Fertil Steril 108(3):393, 2017

Zhu JL, Basso O, Obel C, et al: Infertility, infertility treatment, and congenital malformations: Danish national birth cohort. BMJ 333(7570):679, 2006

Menopause and the Mature Woman

MENOPAUSAL TRANSITION

Menopausal transition is a progressive endocrinologic decline in hormone levels that takes a reproductive-aged woman from regular, cyclic menses to her final menstrual period, ovarian senescence, and beyond. With medical advancements, average life expectancy has risen, and most healthy women can now expect to live at least one third of their lives in the menopause. Life expectancy for women in 2014 approximated 81 years (Arias, 2019). Specifically, by 2050, approximately 47 million women will be aged 45 to 64 years (U.S. Census Bureau, 2017). Importantly, menopausal transition and years spent in the postmenopausal state bring with them issues related to quality of life and disease prevention and management.

DEFINITIONS

Menopause refers to a point in time that follows 1 year after the complete cessation of menstruation, and the *postmenopause*

describes years following that point. The average age of women experiencing their final menstrual period (FMP) is 51.5 years, but a halt to menses from ovarian failure may occur at any age. Cessation before age 40, termed *premature ovarian insufficiency*, is associated with elevated follicle-stimulating hormone (FSH) levels, and its variable causes are described in Chapter 17 (p. 375). *Menopausal transition (MT)*, often referred to as *perimenopause* or *climacteric*, refers to the late reproductive years, usually late 40s to early 50s (Harlow, 2012; Santoro, 2005). Characteristically, MT begins with menstrual cycle irregularity and extends to 1 year after permanent cessation of menses. This reproductive aging with loss of follicular activity progresses within a wide age range (42 to 58 years). The average age at its onset is 47 years, and MT length was found in the multiethnic Study of Women Across the Nation (SWAN) to range from 4 to 8 years. MT lasted longer in women who had earlier transition onset and in those who smoked (Paramsothy, 2017).

As chronologic age is an unreliable indicator, classification of reproductive aging has been proposed. The first was developed in 2001 and updated in 2012 at the Stages of Reproductive Aging Workshop +10 (STRAW) (Harlow, 2012). These staging criteria are guides rather than strictly applied diagnoses. For example, every stage may not manifest in all women, or a stage may present out of the expected sequence. Moreover, the age range and duration of each stage varies among individuals.

In the STRAW system, the anchor stage is the FMP (Fig. 22-1). Five stages precede and two stages follow the FMP. Stage +1a is the first year after FMP, stage +1b reflects years 2 to 5 postmenopause, and stage +2 refers to the ensuing later postmenopausal years, in which estrogen levels continue to decline.

INFLUENTIAL FACTORS

Environmental, genetic, and surgical influences may alter ovarian aging. Smoking advances the age of menopause by approximately 2 years (Gold, 2001; Paramsothy, 2017). Chemotherapy, pelvic radiation, hysterectomy, ovarian surgery, and autoimmune disease also may lead to earlier menopause.

During MT, more erratic fluctuations in female reproductive hormone levels lead to physical and psychological symptoms (Table 22-1) (Dennerstein, 1993; Santoro, 2016a). Diet, exercise, reproductive history, socioeconomic status, body mass index (BMI), mood, climate, and individual or cultural attitudes toward menopause may explain symptom variation (O'Neil, 2011).

FMP ▼

Stage	−5	−4	−3b	−3a	−2	−1	+1a	+1b	+1c	+2
	Early	Peak	Late		Early	Late	Early			Late
Terms	Reproductive				Menopause transition		Postmenopause			
					Perimenopause					
Stage duration	Vary				Vary	1–3 yr	2 yr	3–6 yr		Until death
Menstrual cycles	Vary or regular	Regular		Subtle Δ	≥7 d between Length varies	≥60 d between	Amenorrhea			
Endocrine										
FSH	↓	↓	↓	Vary	↓ & vary		↑ & vary	↑		↑
AMH	↑	↑	↓	↓	↓		↓	↓↓		↓↓
AFC	↑	↑	↓	↓	↓		↓↓	↓↓		↓↓

FIGURE 22-1 The stages of reproductive aging. Δ = change; AMH = antimüllerian hormone; AFC = antral follicle count; FSH = follicle-stimulating hormone. (Redrawn with permission from Harlow SD: Executive summary of the Stages of Reproductive Again Workshop + 10. Fertil Steril 97:843, 2012.)

PHYSIOLOGIC CHANGES

■ Ovary

Physiologic changes seen during MT stem from atresia of the existing pool of ovarian follicles and cessation of reproductive hormone production. Ovarian senescence is a process that begins in utero within the embryonic ovary due to programmed oocyte atresia (Fig. 15-1, p. 321). From birth onward, primordial follicles continuously are activated, mature partially, and then regress. This follicular activation continues in a constant pattern that is independent of pituitary stimulation.

A more rapid depletion of ovarian follicles starts in the late 30s and early 40s and continues until a point at which the menopausal ovary is virtually devoid of follicles (Figs. 22-2 and 22-3). The process of atresia of the nondominant cohort of follicles, largely independent of menstrual cyclicity, is the prime event that leads to the eventual loss of ovarian activity and menopause. In one study, investigators performed a quantitative histologic study of the endometrium and ovaries of women aged 44 to 55 years in MT undergoing hysterectomy for benign indications (Richardson, 1987). The women who reported regular cycles had an average of 1700 follicles in a selected ovary, but those with irregular cycles had an average of 180.

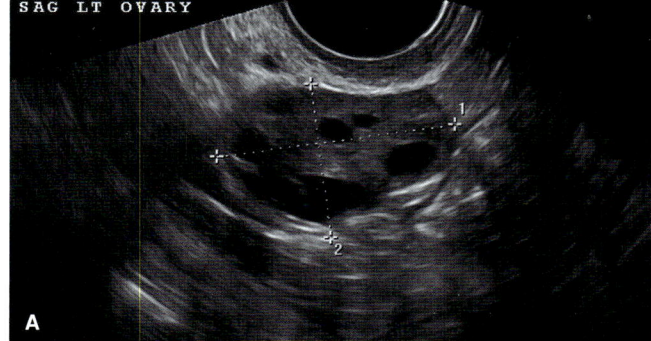

FIGURE 22-2 Transvaginal sonographic images of a pre- and postmenopausal ovary. **A.** In general, premenopausal ovaries have greater volume and contain follicles, which are seen as multiple, small, anechoic, smooth-walled cysts. **B.** In comparison, postmenopausal ovaries have smaller volume and are characteristically devoid of follicular structures. (Reproduced with permission from Dr. Elysia Moschos.)

TABLE 22-1. Symptoms Associated with Menopausal Transition

Menstrual pattern	Sexual dysfunction
Shorter cycles (typical)	Vaginal dryness
Longer cycles (possible)	Decreased libido
Irregular bleeding	Dyspareunia
Vasomotor	**Somatic**
Hot flashes	Headache
Night sweats	Dizziness
Sleep disturbances	Palpitations
Psychological/cognitive	Joint aches and back pain
Worsening PMS	**Others**
Depression	Urinary incontinence
Irritability	Dry, itchy skin
Mood swings	Weight gain
Poor concentration	
Poor memory	

PMS = premenstrual syndrome.

Reproductive-age ovary

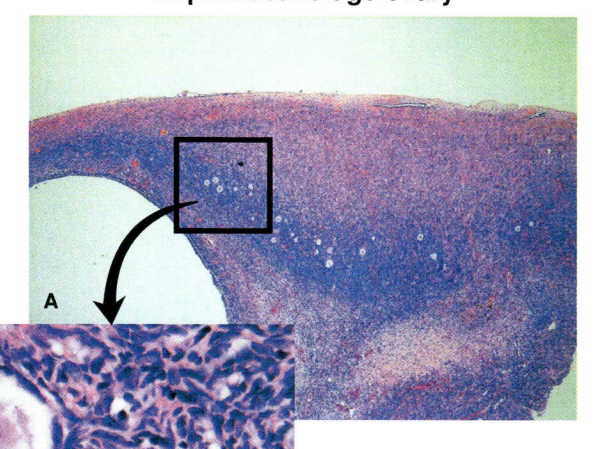

Primordial follicles

Menopausal ovary

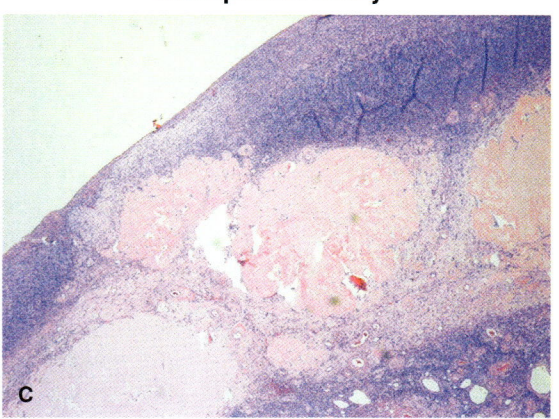

FIGURE 22-3 Microscopic differences between a reproductive-age and menopausal ovary. **A.** Reproductive-age ovary. Note preponderance of primordial follicles. **B.** High-power image of primordial follicles. **C.** The menopausal ovary shows abundance of atretic follicles and persistent corpora albicans. (Reproduced with permission from Dr. Raheela Ashfaq.)

Ovarian Reserve

During MT, the dwindling follicle pool is reflected by low inhibin B and antimüllerian hormone (AMH) levels and by low antral follicle counts measured sonographically. However, none of these measures are recognized tools to diagnose menopause. Instead, AMH is most appropriately used to evaluate ovarian reserve in women with infertility (American College of Obstetricians and Gynecologists, 2019b).

AMH is a glycoprotein secreted by the granulosa cells of secondary and preantral follicles and indirectly reflects the primordial follicle pool. Circulating AMH concentrations are highly reproducible as they remain relatively stable across the menstrual cycle in reproductive-aged women and correlate with the number of early antral follicles. AMH levels decrease markedly and progressively across MT (Hale, 2007; Kushnir, 2017). Levels are often very low, or even below detectable limits, approximately 5 years before menopause (Bertone-Johnson, 2018; Broer, 2014).

■ Hypothalamic-Pituitary-Ovarian Axis

The failing pool of ovarian follicles leads to characteristic changes in the hypothalamic–pituitary–ovarian axis. To review, during the reproductive years, gonadotropin-releasing hormone (GnRH) is released in a pulsatile fashion by the arcuate nucleus of the medial basal hypothalamus. It binds to GnRH receptors on the pituitary gonadotropes to stimulate cyclic luteinizing hormone (LH) and FSH release. These gonadotropins, in turn, stimulate ovarian production of estrogen, progesterone, and inhibin. Estrogen and progesterone exert positive and negative feedback on pituitary gonadotropin production and on the amplitude and frequency of GnRH release. Produced by granulosa cells, inhibin also exerts an important negative influence on

FSH secretion from the pituitary. This tightly regulated endocrine system leads to regular, ovulatory menstrual cycles.

In early MT (stage −2), usually beginning in the late 40s, FSH levels rise slightly to stimulate an enhanced ovarian follicular response, which raises overall estrogen levels (Jain, 2005; Klein, 1996). This FSH rise is attributed to decreased ovarian inhibin secretion rather than diminished estradiol (E_2) feedback. In perimenopausal women, E_2 production fluctuates with FSH levels and can reach concentrations even higher than those observed in women younger than 35. Generally, E_2 levels do not drop significantly until late in MT. Despite ongoing regular cyclic menstruation, progesterone levels during the early MT are lower than in mid-reproductive-aged women (Santoro, 2016a). Testosterone levels do not vary appreciably during the MT. However, sex hormone–binding globulin (SHBG) production declines after the menopause and may lead to relatively higher levels of free or unbound estrogen and testosterone.

In late MT, women exhibit impaired folliculogenesis and greater rates of anovulation compared with women in their mid-reproductive years. Also, during this time, ovarian follicles undergo an accelerated rate of loss until eventually, in late MT, the supply of follicles is depleted. These changes, including the earlier-described rise in FSH levels, reflect the reduced capability of aging follicles to secrete inhibin (Reyes, 1977; Santoro, 1996).

In stage +1a, the first year after the FMP, ovarian progesterone production ceases. Estrogen levels fluctuate and gradually decline. With ovarian failure in the menopause (stage +1b), ovarian steroid hormone release ceases, and the negative-feedback loop is opened. As a result, GnRH is released at maximal frequency and amplitude. In turn, circulating FSH and LH levels rise up to fourfold higher than those in the reproductive years (Klein, 1996).

In stage +2, which reflects the ensuing later postmenopausal years, estrogen is made primarily from conversion of androgens within adipose tissue.

Endometrium

Histologic changes in the endometrium directly represent systemic estrogen and progesterone levels and thus may change dramatically depending on the MT stage. During early MT, the endometrium may reflect ovulatory cycles, which are prevalent during this time. During later MT stages, anovulation is common, and the endometrium will display an estrogenic effect that is unopposed by progesterone. Accordingly, proliferative changes or disordered proliferative changes are frequent findings on pathologic examination of endometrial biopsy samples. After menopause, the endometrium becomes atrophic due to lack of estrogen stimulation (Fig. 16-19, p. 358).

Menstrual Disturbances

The physiologic changes described in the prior sections lead to menstrual variation and finally amenorrhea (see Fig. 22-1). In the early MT (stage −2), a woman's menstrual cycles remain regular, but the interval between cycles may be altered by ≥7 days or the woman may note that expected menses are skipped. Typically, cycle lengths become shorter.

The late MT (stage −1) is characterized by two or more skipped menses and at least one intermenstrual interval ≥60 days due to progressively higher rates of anovulation. Circulating estrogen levels are likely to be low during anovulatory cycles. The most profound hormonal changes occur during this time, and symptomatology intensifies when amenorrhea duration is prolonged (Santoro, 2016a).

Many women in their mid to late 40s do not consider themselves fertile and will cease contraception but will still have occasional ovulatory cycles. Contraception can be discontinued by all women at age 55. Some women older than 55 years may still have menstrual bleeding. However, ovulation is rare and oocytes are likely poor quality and rarely viable (Gebbie, 2010).

During MT, abnormal uterine bleeding (AUB) is common, and Treloar (1981) found that menses were irregular in more than one half of all women studied. Paramsothy (2014) reported that AUB accounted for 14 percent of all hospitalizations from 1998 to 2005 among women aged 45 to 54. Anovulation is the most common cause of erratic bleeding during MT. However, because the time interval surrounding menopause is characterized by relatively high, acyclic estrogen levels and relatively low progesterone production, women in MT are at higher risk for developing endometrial hyperplasia or carcinoma. Symptoms associated with estrogen-sensitive pathology, including endometrial polyps, uterine leiomyomas, and adenomyosis, also become more prevalent.

In all women, regardless of menopausal status, the etiology of AUB should be determined as outlined in Chapter 8 (p. 182). As noted, endometrial cancer is suspected in any woman in MT with AUB. The overall incidence of endometrial cancer approximates 0.1 percent of women in this group per year. In women with AUB in MT, however, the risk rises to 10 percent (Lidor, 1986). Thus, endometrial biopsy is done to exclude neoplasia.

Although endometrial cancer is the greatest concern during this time, endometrial biopsy frequently reveals a benign endometrium that displays estrogen effects unopposed by progesterone. In premenopausal women, this results from anovulation. In postmenopausal women, unopposed estrogen typically originates from extragonadal endogenous estrogen production. This derives from increased conversion of adrenal androgens to estrogen by the enzyme aromatase found in adipose tissue. In addition, lower SHBG levels lead to higher levels of free and therefore bioavailable estrogen (Moen, 2004). Less often, unopposed exogenous estrogen administration or an estrogen-producing ovarian tumor also can account for these effects in postmenopausal women.

Adrenal Steroid Levels

With advancing age, adrenal production of dehydroepiandrosterone sulfate (DHEAS) declines. In women aged 20 to 30 years, DHEAS concentrations peak at an average level of 6.2 μmol/L, and then decrease steadily. In women aged 70 to 80 years, DHEAS levels are diminished by 74 percent to a level of 1.6 μmol/L. Other adrenal hormone levels similarly fall with aging (Burger, 2000; Labrie, 1997). Androstenedione and pregnenolone show comparable declines. The ovary contributes to the production of these hormones during the reproductive years, but after menopause, only the adrenal gland continues this hormone synthesis.

Burger and associates (2000) prospectively studied 172 women during MT as a part of the Melbourne Women's Midlife Health Project. Analyzing hormone levels longitudinally in these women, they observed no relationship between a woman's FMP and the decline in DHEAS levels. Advancing age, regardless of menopausal status, determined DHEAS level decline.

Central Thermoregulation

Of the many menopausal symptoms that may affect quality of life, the most frequent are those related to thermoregulation dysfunction. Kronenberg (1990) tabulated all of the published epidemiologic studies and determined that *vasomotor symptoms (VMS)*, also variably termed *hot flashes*, *hot flushes*, and *night sweats*, developed in 11 to 60 percent of menstruating women during MT. In the Massachusetts Women's Health Study, the incidence rose from 10 percent during the premenopausal period to approximately 50 percent after menses cessation (McKinlay, 1992).

Hot flashes begin an average of 2 years before the FMP, and 85 percent of women who experience them will continue to experience them for more than 1 year. Of these women, 25 to 50 percent will have hot flashes for 5 years, and >15 percent may experience them for >15 years (Kronenberg, 1990). More recent studies focusing on duration of menopausal symptoms indicate that women can expect hot flashes to continue, on average, for 7 years. Black women experience the longest duration (10 years), compared with Hispanic (9 years), white (7 years), and Asian women (5 years) (Avis, 2015).

Four trajectories of hot flash onset and duration were identified in the SWAN study: early onset, late onset, low frequency, and high frequency. Those with an early, high-frequency pattern had an onset that began before the FMP and continued up to 14 years, which was the observation period length (Tepper, 2016).

Vasomotor Symptoms

Thermoregulatory and cardiovascular changes that accompany a hot flash are well documented. An individual hot flash generally lasts 1 to 5 minutes, and skin temperatures rise because of peripheral vasodilation (Kronenberg, 1990). This change is particularly marked in the fingers and toes, where skin temperature can rise 10 to 15°C. Most women sense a sudden wave of heat that spreads over the body, particularly the upper body and face. Sweating begins primarily on the upper body, and it corresponds closely in time with an increase in skin conductance (Fig. 22-4). Sweating has been observed in women during 90 percent of hot flashes (Freedman, 2001).

Elevations in both awake and sleep systolic blood pressure are noted with hot flashes (Gerber, 2007). Heart rate rises 7 to 15 beats per minute at approximately the same time as peripheral vasodilation and sweating. Heart rate and skin blood flow usually peak within 3 minutes of the hot flash onset. Simultaneously with sweating and peripheral vasodilation, the metabolic rate also significantly rises. Hot flashes can also be accompanied by palpitations, anxiety, irritability, and panic.

Starting 5 to 9 minutes after a hot flash begins, the core temperature declines 0.1 to 0.9°C due to increased peripheral vasodilation (Molnar, 1981). If heat loss and sweating are significant, a woman may experience chills. Skin temperature gradually returns to normal, sometimes taking 30 minutes or longer.

Vasomotor Symptom Pathophysiology

Although the underlying physiologic steps leading to hot flashes are not fully elucidated, dysfunction of the thermoregulatory nucleus of the hypothalamus appears relevant. This nucleus regulates perspiration and vasodilation to manage heat loss in humans. If exposed to higher temperatures, the nucleus activates these heat dissipation mechanisms. This maintains core body temperature in a regulated normal range, called the *thermoregulatory zone*. Women who experience more severe VMS are thought to have a narrower thermoregulatory zone than those without symptoms. In these women, minimal changes in core body temperature induce shivering or hot flash.

Various hormones and neurotransmitters modulate hot flash frequency. Of these, estrogens play a vital role. Although not clearly correlated, estrogen withdrawal or rapid level fluctuation rather than a chronically low estrogen concentration are associated with symptoms (Erlik, 1982; Overlie, 2002). This hypothesis is supported by the fact that women with gonadal dysgenesis (Turner syndrome), who lack normal estrogen levels, do not experience hot flashes unless first exposed to estrogen and then withdrawn from treatment.

In addition, altered neurotransmitter concentrations are believed to create a narrow thermoregulatory zone and to lower the sweating threshold (Freedman, 1998, 2014). Norepinephrine is thought to be the primary neurotransmitter responsible for lowering the thermoregulatory setpoint and triggering the heat

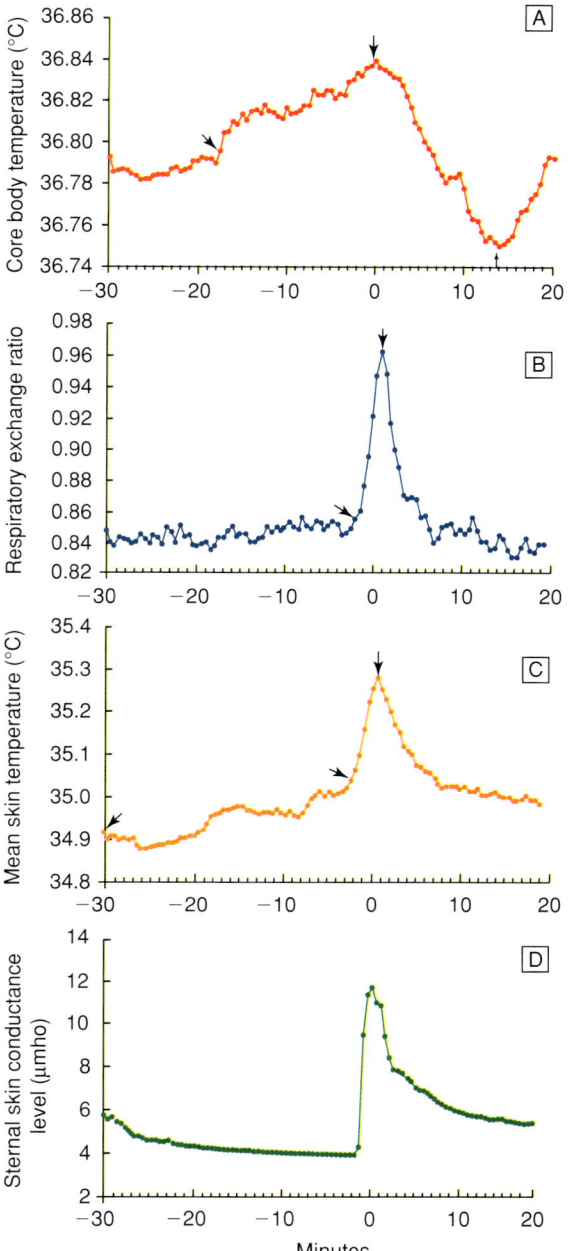

FIGURE 22-4 Physiologic changes (means) during a hot flash. **A.** Core body temperature. **B.** Respiratory exchange ratio. **C.** Skin temperature. **D.** Sternal skin conductance. Time 0 is the beginning of the sternal skin conductance response. (Reproduced with permission from Freedman RR: Biochemical, metabolic, and vascular mechanisms in menopausal hot flashes. Fertil Steril 70(2):332, 1998.)

loss mechanisms associated with hot flashes (Rapkin, 2007). Plasma levels of norepinephrine metabolites rise before and during hot flashes. Moreover, norepinephrine injections can elevate core body temperature and induce a heat loss response (Freedman, 1990). Medications that decrease norepinephrine levels, such as clonidine, may reduce VMS (Laufer, 1982).

Estrogens are known to modulate adrenergic receptors in many tissues. Freedman and colleagues (2001) suggested that menopause-related declines in estrogen levels lower hypothalamic α_2-adrenergic receptor concentrations. In turn, a decline in presynaptic α_2-adrenergic receptor levels leads to higher norepinephrine levels, thereby causing VMS.

Serotonin appears to represent another neurotransmitter involved in VMS (Slopien, 2003). Estrogen withdrawal is associated with a decreased blood serotonin level, which is followed by upregulation of serotonin receptors in the hypothalamus. Activation of specific serotonin receptors mediates heat loss (Gonzales, 1993). However, the role of serotonin in central regulatory pathways is complex because binding at some serotonin receptors can exert negative feedback on other serotonin receptor types (Bachmann, 2005). Therefore, the effect of a change in serotonin activity depends on the type of receptor activated.

Of other potential candidates, β-endorphins and other neurotransmitters affect the thermoregulatory center and make some women more prone to hot flashes (Pinkerton, 2009a). Newer studies implicate the KNDy (kisspeptin/neurokinin B/dynorphin) neuron class in the hypothalamic arcuate nucleus. KNDy neurons contain estrogen receptors and act in response to E_2 (Rance, 2013). One randomized trial of healthy women found that neurokinin B infusion induced hot flashes (Jayasena, 2015). Moreover, neurokinin B–receptor antagonists reduced self-reported hot flash rates by 45 percent during a 3-month trial (Prague, 2017).

Genetic polymorphisms and VMS prevalence and severity also may be linked. Some polymorphisms are variants of genes encoding estrogen receptor α (Crandall, 2006; Malacara, 2004). Others are single-nucleotide polymorphisms (SNPs) involved in E_2 synthesis or metabolism or in its conversion to more- or less-potent estrogens. More recently, SNPs in regions of the *tachykinin receptor 3* gene, which codes for the neurokinin B receptor (NK3R), were associated with menopausal VMS (Crandall, 2017). Another implicated neurotransmitter is *calcitonin gene–related peptide*, which raises skin temperatures in ovariectomized rats (Hay, 2009).

In sum, studies suggest that reductions and fluctuations in estrogen levels lead to a decline in inhibitory presynaptic α_2-adrenergic receptor concentrations and an increase in hypothalamic norepinephrine and serotonin release. Norepinephrine and serotonin lower the setpoint in the thermoregulatory nucleus and allow heat loss mechanisms to be triggered by subtle changes in core body temperature. The KNDy signal system also may play a role, which may lead to new nonhormonal treatment options.

Vasomotor Symptom Risk Factors

Several risk factors are associated with hot flashes. These are early or surgical menopause, race or ethnicity, BMI, sedentary lifestyle, smoking, and use of selective estrogen-receptor modulators or aromatase inhibitors. Others include premenstrual dysphoric disorder, anxiety, perceived stress, and depression (Avis, 2015; Gold, 2006; Guthrie, 2005). Moreover, women exposed to high ambient temperatures may experience more frequent and severe hot flashes (Randolph, 2005).

Among these factors, surgical menopause is associated with a 90-percent probability of hot flashes during the first year after oophorectomy. Symptoms can be more abrupt and severe than those associated with natural menopause. Both hysterectomy and unilateral oophorectomy are associated with an earlier menopause.

Among racial and ethnic groups, hot flashes appear to be more common and more bothersome in African-American than in white women and are more common among white than among Asian women (Avis, 2015; Gold, 2001; Thurston, 2008). These racial/ethnic differences in VMS persisted even after controlling for other influencing factors (Al-Safi, 2014).

The effect of BMI on hot flash frequency is unclear. Some studies find hot flashes associated with both obesity and sedentary lifestyle (Da Fonseca, 2013; Hunter, 2012; Saccomani, 2017; Wilbur, 1998).

Hot flashes and trouble sleeping may reflect posttraumatic stress disorder (PTSD) from past or ongoing intimate partner violence (IPV) or sexual assault. An observational study of 2016 healthy women assessed lifetime IPV and sexual assault rates and their effects using standardized questionnaires (Gibson, 2019). Reported rates of PTSD symptoms, emotional abuse, physical violence, and sexual assault ranged from 16 to 22 percent. Of affected women, difficulty sleeping was reported by approximately 52 percent; hot flashes, by 40 percent; and night sweats, by 34 percent. Sexual problems also were common. Rates of vaginal dryness approximated 30 percent, and painful intercourse or vaginal irritation each was noted in about 15 percent.

PATIENT EVALUATION

During MT, clinical goals aim to optimize a woman's health and well-being during and after this transition. This is an excellent time for a comprehensive health evaluation, as outlined in Chapter 1 (p. 9).

During patient visits, changes affected by aging and MT are documented. Height, weight, waist circumference, and BMI are recorded and can be used to counsel women about physical exercise and weight loss or weight gain. Height loss may be associated with osteoporosis and vertebral compression fractures and thus is recorded yearly. The remaining examination notes expected physiologic changes of MT and identify potential pathology.

The diagnosis of MT can usually be made with age-appropriate symptoms and careful physical examination. Clearly, a 50-year-old woman with menstrual irregularity, hot flashes, and vaginal dryness is considered to be in MT. Other specific genitourinary physical findings are described later (p. 495).

Measurement of serum FSH or E_2 levels, described next, can be performed to document ovarian failure. However, for those in MT, FSH levels may be normal. Even for much younger women with similar symptoms, evaluation should also include FSH level measurement. In addition, pregnancy should be excluded if applicable. If ovarian failure develops before age 40, it is usually pathologic. Thus, chromosomal abnormalities, infections, autoimmune disorders, galactosemia, cigarette smoking, or iatrogenic causes such as radiation or chemotherapy are considered (Table 17-7, p. 384).

◼ Gonadotropin and Estrogen Levels

Biochemical changes, of which a woman may be unaware, may be identified prior to cycle irregularity. For example, in the early follicular phase of the menstrual cycle in many women older than 35 years, FSH levels may rise without a concurrent LH elevation. This finding is associated with a poor prognosis for future fertility. Specifically, a cycle-day-3 FSH level greater than 10 mIU/mL is used in some in vitro fertilization programs to route patients into donor egg programs (Chap. 21, p. 459). An FSH level greater than 40 mIU/mL is used to document ovarian failure associated with menopause.

Estrogen levels may be normal, elevated, or low depending on the stage of MT. Only at menopause are serum E_2 levels extremely low or undetectable. As another use, E_2 levels may assess a woman's response to hormone treatment. Most clinicians prefer to reach a physiologic serum E_2 range of 50 to 100 pg/mL when adjusting treatment. Women who receive E_2 pellets may have elevated serum values from 300 to 500 pg/mL. Because these high levels are not uncommon with this approach, pellet use for hormone therapy is discouraged.

THE MATURE WOMAN

With ovarian senescence, declining hormone levels have specific effects. Some lead to physical symptoms, such as VMS and vaginal dryness. Metabolic and structural changes include bone loss, skin thinning, fatty replacement of the breast, lipoprotein changes, and genitourinary atrophy. As a result, postmenopausal women have unique issues associated with aging and estrogen loss that may negatively affect their individual health.

Estrogen, progestogen (a term that encompasses synthetic progestins and progesterone), and androgen therapy have been used by menopausal women for more than 100 years. Recent history surrounding menopausal hormone therapy is discussed here, as are current recommendations for symptom treatment.

HORMONE TREATMENT: HISTORY AND CONTROVERSIES

Hormone therapy (HT) has been extensively studied and evidence-based recommendations continue to evolve. The 2017 Position Statement regarding HT published by The North American Menopause Society (2017) can serve as a valuable resource. In the following discussion, HT serves as an umbrella term that encompasses both estrogen-only therapy (ET) and estrogen-progesterone therapy (EPT).

■ Evolution of Knowledge

ET for menopausal symptom relief gained popularity in the 1960s and 1970s. Proponents cited its effects to "preserve youth" and prevent chronic disease. By the mid-1970s, oral ET use was prevalent among US women. However, also in the mid-1970s, epidemiologic studies revealed that ET use among menopausal women with an intact uterus was associated with a substantially elevated risk of endometrial cancer (Smith, 1975). As a result, the U.S. Food and Drug Administration (FDA) package labeling for menopausal ET changed to reflect this risk. By the 1980s, clinicians began to prescribe progestogens concurrently with ET for menopausal women with an intact uterus.

In the late 1980s, observational study results suggested that HT prevented osteoporosis, coronary heart disease (CHD),

and dementia in menopausal women. Positive findings of these observational studies, including the large Nurses' Health Study (NHS), initially appeared discordant with those of subsequent randomized clinical trials of HT, specifically the Women's Health Initiative (WHI). However, these differences appear to derive from the mean age of HT initiation in these trials. For example, in the NHS, most participants were younger than 55 years and were within 2 to 3 years of menopause onset at the time they initiated HT. In contrast, the mean age of WHI participants at recruitment was 63 years, and most were more than 10 years beyond menopause onset. When NHS and WHI findings for participants who initiated HT at age 50 to 59 years or within 10 years of menopause onset were compared, most outcomes were similar (Bhupathiraju, 2017).

These observations support the "timing hypothesis," which postulates that estrogen has a differential effect on vascular tissue during the early and late stages of atherosclerosis progression. In younger women or those recently menopausal, estrogen appears to slow atherosclerosis progression. In contrast, if advanced atherosclerosis is present, as is common in older women, initiating HT may precipitate vascular occlusion and thrombosis.

The ELITE trial, which was designed specifically to test the timing hypothesis, found that oral E_2 slowed progression of atherosclerosis when initiated by women within 6 years of menopause but not when initiated by women 10 or more years postmenopause (Hodis, 2016; Sripasert, 2019). Evidence also suggests that early HT initiation may enhance insulin action and possibly aid Alzheimer disease prevention (Imtiaz, 2017; Pereira, 2015).

■ Women's Health Initiative

Launched in 1993, this study's goal was to evaluate the putative protective effects of HT on common chronic diseases of aging. The WHI compared the effects of a combined 0.625-mg conjugated equine estrogen (CEE)/2.5-mg medroxyprogesterone acetate (MPA) oral formulation with placebo in more than 16,000 healthy postmenopausal women aged 50 to 79 years with a uterus (EPT arm) (Rossouw, 2002). Specific end points evaluated included CHD, venous thromboembolism (VTE), breast and colon cancer, and bone fractures. Concurrently, the study also compared an oral 0.625-mg CEE dose alone against placebo in approximately 11,000 women without a uterus (ET arm).

WHI investigators selected CHD (anticipated benefit) and breast cancer (anticipated risk) as primary disease end points. After 5 years of monitoring, the EPT arm of the WHI was halted early upon recommendation of its Data and Safety Monitoring Board because overall risks exceeded benefits. In July 2002, results were released to the media. This preceded journal publication of the data and timely education of healthcare providers. As a result, widespread confusion and concern among women and clinicians followed.

In a subsequent detailed analysis of cardiovascular end points in the EPT arm, the hazard for cardiovascular death or nonfatal myocardial infarction with EPT was 1.24. This translated into 188 actual cases in the hormone group and 147

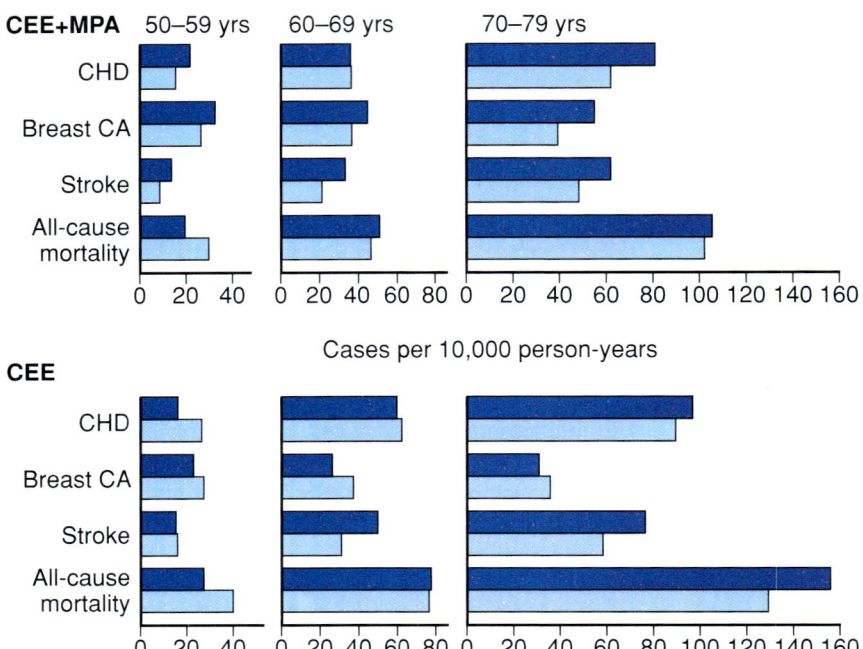

FIGURE 22-5 Graphs reflect the absolute risks of health outcomes in the Women's Health Initiative (WHI). Dark bars reflect outcomes of those administered hormones, whereas light bars reflect those women randomly assigned to placebo.

benefits were attenuated. However, a small elevated risk of breast cancer persisted over 13 years with EPT. In contrast, ET reduced the breast cancer risk (Manson, 2013). Based on these WHI data, the attributed risk of breast cancer with EPT is less than one additional case of breast cancer per 1000 users. The hazard ratio of 1.28 is slightly higher than that observed with one daily glass of wine, less than that with two daily glasses, and similar to risks associated with obesity and low physical activity (The North American Menopause Society, 2017). With respect to CHD, findings in the 2013 WHI report provide further support for the timing hypothesis (Fig. 22-5) (Manson, 2013).

In an 18-year reevaluation of WHI participants, cardiovascular, cancer, and all-cause mortality rates were essentially identical in the HT and placebo groups. Although breast cancer mortality at 18 years was elevated in the EPT group, this increase did not achieve statistical significance. A significant reduction in breast cancer mortality was noted in the ET group. Of note, a significant reduction in mortality from Alzheimer disease or dementia was also noted with HT use (Manson, 2017).

Risk of Venous Thromboembolism

In the WHI and other HT studies evaluating oral estrogen, VTE risk approximately doubles (Rossouw, 2002). No randomized trials comparing oral and transdermal estrogen are adequately powered to compare risk of VTE. However, observational and database studies have found no elevated VTE risk with transdermal HT (Canonico, 2016; Vinogradova, 2019). These risk differences likely reflect a lesser effect on coagulation parameters with a transdermal compared with an oral route (Canonico, 2014). Similarly, lower-dose transdermal E_2 (≤0.05 mg daily), in contrast with oral estrogen, does not appear to increase risk of stroke. Accordingly, the transdermal route of estrogen administration is particularly appropriate for obese women and others with cardiovascular risk factors (Shifren, 2019).

CURRENT APPROACHES TO HORMONE THERAPY

Benefits and Risks

In the shared decision-making conversation between provider and patient, treatment goals and HT risks and benefits are presented (Table 22-2). Evidence supports HT as the most effective therapy for treatment of VMS. It also effectively prevents bone loss and fractures and treats genitourinary symptoms (American College of Obstetricians Gynecologists, 2018c). As detailed earlier, when initiated soon after the onset of menopause, HT may lower CHD rates, enhance insulin's action, and prevent Alzheimer disease.

in the placebo group (Anderson, 2004). To explore the timing of HT initiation among WHI participants, Rossouw and colleagues (2007) looked specifically at HT's effect on stroke and CHD rates across categories of age and years since the menopause. Study women who initiated HT closer to menopause tended to have reduced CHD rates risk compared with a higher CHD risk seen among women more distant from menopause. Specifically, for the group aged 50 to 59 years in both study arms, the hazard ratio for CHD was 0.93, or two fewer events per 10,000 person-years. For the group aged 60 to 69 years, this ratio was 0.98 or 1 fewer event per 10,000 person-years, and for those 70 to 79 years, the ratio was 1.26 or 19 extra events per 10,000 person-years. HT increased the stroke risk—the hazard ratio was 1.32—and this risk did not vary significantly by age or time since menopause. These authors concluded, consistent with the timing hypothesis, that women who initiated HT closer to menopause tended to have reduced CHD risk compared with the greater CHD risk among women more distant from menopause. Importantly, evidence is insufficient to suggest that either ET or EPT should be initiated or continued for primary or secondary CHD prevention (American College of Obstetricians and Gynecologists, 2018b; The North American Menopause Society, 2017). Although the primary conclusion from the 2007 Rossouw article was that HT reduced CHD if initiated closer to menopause, confusion surrounding WHI findings has led providers and women, including healthy recently menopausal women with bothersome VMS, to avoid HT use (Manson, 2016).

Subsequently, a 2013 WHI report comprehensively reviewed findings from both study arms. This included extended outcome data stratified by age. Although risks and benefits of HT were observed, absolute risks in general were small. After administration of study medication stopped, most risks and

TABLE 22-2. Some Effects of Hormonal Classes Used Short Term (5-Years) for Menopausal Symptoms

Target	CEE/MPA	E$_2$P (TD)	CEE	E$_2$ (TD)	RLX	BZE/CEE	OSP	
Breast	Pot. harms	? Pot. harms	Neutral	? Neutral	Benefits	Neutral	?	?
Uterus	Neutral	Neutral	Pot. harms	Pot. harms	Neutral	Neutral	Neutral	
VMS	Benefits	Benefits	Benefits	Benefits	Pot. harms	Benefits	Pot. harms	
Vagina	Benefits	Benefits	Benefits	Benefits	Neutral	Benefits	Benefits	
Bone	Benefits	Benefits	Benefits	Benefits	Benefits	Benefits	? Benefits	
DVT/PE	Pot. harms	Neutral	Pot. harms	Neutral	Pot. harms		Pot. harms	
Lipids	Benefits	Benefits	Benefits	Benefits	Benefits	Benefits	? Benefits	

☐ Benefits   ☐ Potential harms   ☐ Neutral effects

BZE/CEE = bazedoxifene/conjugated equine estrogen; CEE = conjugated equine estrogen; DVT = deep-vein thrombosis; E$_2$ = estradiol; MPA = medroxyprogesterone acetate; OSP = ospemifene; P = progesterone; RLX = raloxifene; TD = transdermal; VMS = vasomotor symptoms.

Of risks, menopausal HT raises CHD risk if initiated in women aged ≥60 years or in those who are ≥10 years post-menopause. Across ages, HT also elevates the risk of stroke, VTE, and cholecystitis. Among women younger than 60 and those within 10 years of menopause onset, stroke is rare, and the attributed risk is <0.5 additional cases per 1000 oral HT users annually (Manson, 2013).

The breast cancer risk is modestly elevated with EPT use longer than 4 or 5 years. Detailed earlier, the attributed breast cancer risk with EPT is <1 additional case per 1000 EPT users annually (Manson, 2013) (p. 480). Short-term EPT use is not associated with an elevated breast cancer risk. ET with conjugated estrogens did not elevate the breast cancer risk in the 7 years of the WHI ET-alone arm.

■ Other Decision-Making Considerations

Based on current package labeling, HT is indicated only for treatment of bothersome VMS and genitourinary symptoms, prevention of osteoporosis, and treatment of hypoestrogenism caused by hypogonadism, surgical menopause, or premature ovarian insufficiency. Contraindications to the use of menopausal HT are listed in Table 22-3.

The appropriate type, dose, administration route, and duration guide HT selection for a given woman to achieve treatment objectives and enhance safety. Periodic changes in a woman's health status and shared decision-making will guide individual use over time (The North American Menopause Society, 2017).

For women with a uterus, ET increases the risk of endometrial neoplasia. EPT taken daily and continuously is associated with risk of endometrial cancer lower than or comparable to that observed in HT non-users. However, EPT taken as sequential progestogen therapy (e.g., 10 to 14 days each month) is associated with a slightly elevated risk of endometrial neoplasia (Anderson, 2003; Jaakola, 2009). In our practices, most patients use EPT daily and continuously, although intermittent, monthly progestogen may have less breast cancer risk.

■ Duration of Systemic Hormone Therapy

The optimal duration varies among women and relates to VMS, quality of life, osteoporosis risk, and patient comorbidities and preferences. Both the North American Menopause Society (2017) and the American College of Obstetricians and Gynecologists (2018c) recommend against arbitrary age-based

TABLE 22-3. Warnings and Precautions with Systemic Estrogen Administration

Estrogen should not be used in women with any of the following conditions:
Undiagnosed abnormal genital bleeding
Known, suspected, or history of breast cancer
Known or suspected estrogen-dependent neoplasia
Active or prior venous thromboembolism
Active or prior stroke, myocardial infarction, or TIA
Known thrombophilia
Liver dysfunction or disease
Untreated hypertension
Known hypersensitivity to the ingredients of the estrogen preparation
Known or suspected pregnancy

Estrogen should be used with caution in women with the following conditions:
Dementia
Gallbladder disease
Hypertriglyceridemia
Prior cholestatic jaundice
Hypothyroidism
Fluid retention plus cardiac or renal dysfunction
Severe hypocalcemia
Prior endometriosis
Hypothyroidism
Elevated breast cancer risk
Hepatic hemangiomas

Data from Food and Drug Administration, 2005; Kaunitz, 2015.

discontinuation and suggest a tailored approach. Although few data guide extended HT use or the method of discontinuation, the following approach is based on our clinical experience.

After several years, a patient is encouraged to try a lower HT dose, with the understanding that she can resume the prior HT dose if symptoms recur. This strategy can continue until the patient is using a low HT dose. This may be oral CEE (0.3 or 0.45 mg) or E_2 (0.5 mg) or transdermal E_2 (0.014 to 0.025 mg). After remaining VMS free on low-dose therapy, stopping HT is appropriate for many patients. However, for those with an elevated risk for osteoporosis or poor sense of well-being off systemic HT, continuing HT is reasonable.

The North American Menopause Society (2017) indicates that prevention of dementia should not be considered an indication for use of HT but also points out that some observational studies have found that HT initiation by recently menopausal women is associated with a lower risk of dementia. Accordingly, some recently menopausal women without contraindications to HT use and who do not report bothersome VMS but who have a high degree of concern regarding their future dementia risk may choose to initiate systemic HT. Before initiating HT in this context, patients should understand that prevention of dementia does not represent an established indication for HT.

VASOMOTOR SYMPTOM TREATMENT

Understanding the duration of VMS, described earlier (p. 476), allows women to make sound decisions regarding treatment. Without question, HT represents the most effective treatment. Based on the safety profile detailed previously, HT represents an appropriate choice for VMS treatment in those aged younger than 60 or those within 10 years of menopause onset (The North American Menopause Society, 2017).

■ Hormonal Therapy

Estrogen

Although estrogen injections and subdermal pellets to treat VMS are available, serum E_2 levels associated with these formulations are not well characterized. Accordingly, use of FDA-approved oral and transdermal estrogen is recommended (Table 22-4). In the United States, most prescribed systemic estrogens are oral. The most commonly prescribed oral estrogens for VMS treatment are E_2 and CEE, and standard doses are 1.0 mg and 0.625 mg, respectively (American College of Obstetricians and Gynecologists, 2018c). These estrogens are also available in higher and lower doses.

Transdermal estrogen offers the convenience of less frequent administration, with once- or twice-weekly patch changes. All transdermal estrogen formulations use E_2. Preparations in gel, emulsion, and spray are available, however, transdermal patches are most commonly prescribed in the United States. Standard-dose E_2 patches release 0.0375 mg or 0.05 mg of hormone daily, but higher and lower doses are available. All systemic HT products have FDA approval for VMS treatment. The exception is the ultra-low-dose E_2 patch Menostar, which releases 0.014 mg E_2 daily and is approved for osteoporosis prevention.

Common side effects associated with estrogen use include breast tenderness, bloating, and uterine bleeding. Lowering the estrogen dose often reduces these adverse effects, but this may also result in VMS recurrence. Some clinicians start patients on standard-dose estrogen, while others start with a lower dose. Symptom response to a given estrogen dose may not stabilize for several months. Thus, waiting 2 to 3 months before reassessing the response to a dose change is appropriate.

Monitoring serum estrogen levels should not routinely be employed when treating VMS. Occasionally, however, menopausal patients may report inadequate symptoms relief despite increasing doses of estrogen. In this setting, monitoring serum E_2 levels may help. Since serum estrogen levels fluctuate with oral estrogen use, monitoring serum E_2 levels should be reserved for women using transdermal E_2, which is associated with steady-state serum levels. A reasonable target range at menopause is 40 to 100 pg/mL, and levels below this may inadequately relieve VMS (Kaunitz, 2012, 2015).

Progestogens

Progestogens alone have efficacy in treating VMS and may be used in women for whom estrogen is contraindicated. However, most progestogen use involves EPT. In the United States, the progestogens most commonly prescribed are MPA, which is available in 2.5-mg, 5-mg, and 10-mg oral doses, and micronized progesterone, which is available in 100-mg and 200-mg oral doses. Some combined EPT therapies instead use norethindrone acetate, drosperinone, or levonorgestrel (see Table 22-4)

Among women using standard-dose estrogen, continuous progestogens therapy with a 2.5-mg MPA or a 100-mg progesterone dose is sufficient for endometrial protection. Because progesterone has a hypnotic effect, it is best taken at bedtime. Progestogens also may cause dysphoria. Changing the progestogen type, employing sequential rather than continuous progestogen therapy, or adding antidepressant therapy are options. Off-label use of a progestin-releasing intrauterine device, which protects the endometrium while exposing the central nervous system to a lower progestogen level, may be considered (Depypere, 2015; Kaunitz, 2015). Various oral and transdermal EPT formulations are available (see Table 22-4).

Bazedoxifene

Throughout the body, estrogen may bind with its receptors, estrogen receptor α (ERα) and estrogen receptor β (ERβ). These receptors vary in their distribution (Fig. 22-6). Selective estrogen-receptor modulators (SERMs) are agents that after binding to the estrogen receptor may act as an estrogen agonist or antagonist (Fig. 22-7).

Bazedoxifene (BZA) is one such SERM. It is combined with CEE as oral Duavee, which was FDA-approved in 2014 for the treatment of moderate to severe menopausal VMS and prevention of postmenopausal osteoporosis in women with an intact uterus (Lobo, 2009). This combination is called a *tissue-selective estrogen complex (TSEC)*. This TSEC offers the benefits of CEE plus the SERM's ability to offset estrogen stimulation of the endometrium and breast (Pinkerton, 2014). Accordingly, this TSEC offers a progestogen-free alternative for women with a uterus.

By itself, BZA slows bone mineral density loss, increases the number of hot flashes, and raises VTE risks. In contrast, a 20-mg BZA/0.45-mg CEE combination blunts bone mineral

TABLE 22-4. Selected Systemic Hormonal Preparations for the Treatment of Menopausal Vasomotor Symptoms

Preparation	Generic Name	Brand Name	Available Strengths
Estrogen			
Oral[a]	CEE	Premarin	0.3, 0.45, 0.625, 0.9, or 1.25 mg
	17β-Estradiol	Estrace[b]	0.5, 1.0, or 2.0 mg
	Estradiol acetate	Femtrace	0.45, 0.9, or 1.8 mg
	10 synthetic estrogens	Enjuvia	0.3, 0.45, 0.625, 0.9, or 1.25 mg
Transdermal Patch	17β-Estradiol	Alora[b]	0.025, 0.05, 0.075, or 0.1 mg/d (patch applied twice weekly to abdomen or buttock; 8 patches/box)
	17β-Estradiol	Climara[b]	0.025, 0.0375, 0.05, 0.06 0.075, or 0.1 mg/d (patch applied to abdomen or buttock weekly; 4 patches/box)
	17β-Estradiol	Menostar[b]	14 μg/d (patch applied to abdomen weekly; 4 patches/box)
	17β-Estradiol	Vivelle-Dot[b]	0.025, 0.0375, 0.05, or 0.075, 0.1 mg/d (patch applied twice weekly to abdomen; 8 patches/box)
		Minivelle[b]	(0.025, 0.0375, 0.05, 0.075 and 0.1 mg/d) (patch applied twice weekly to abdomen; 8 patches/box)
Transdermal Gel/Spray	17β-Estradiol	EstroGel[b]	1 metered dose of gel (0.06%) applied to arm daily (64 doses per 93-g can)
	17β-Estradiol	Estrasorb[b]	Gel from 2 packets applied to legs daily (56 packets/carton)
	17β-Estradiol	Divigel[b]	0.25-, 0.5-, or 1-mg packets
			Gel from 1 packet applied to thigh daily (30 packets/carton)
	17β-Estradiol	Elestrin[b]	1 metered dose of gel (0.06%) applied to arm daily (30 doses per 35-g container)
	17β-Estradiol	Evamist[b]	1 to 3 metered-dose sprays to forearm daily (56 doses per pump)
Vaginal	Estradiol acetate	Femring	0.05 or 0.1 mg/d (inserted for 90 days)
Progestogen			
Oral[a]	MPA	Provera	2.5, 5.0, or 10.0 mg
	Micronized progesterone	Prometrium[b]	100 or 200 mg (in peanut oil) (12–14 days per cycle or nightly)
Vaginal	Progesterone	Prochieve 4%[b]	45 mg
Combination preparations			
Oral sequential[a]	CEE + MPA	Premphase	0.625 mg CEE (red) plus 0.625 mg CEE/5.0 mg MPA (blue) (28 pills per pack; 14 red & 14 blue)[c]
Oral continuous[a]	CEE+ MPA	Prempro	0.3 mg CEE/1.5 mg MPA, or 0.45 mg CEE/1.5 mg MPA, or 0.625 mg CEE/2.5 mg MPA, or 0.625 mg CEE/5 mg MPA (28 pills per pack)
	17β-Estradiol + drospirenone	Angeliq	1 mg E$_2$/0.5 mg drospirenone (28 pills per pack)
	17β-Estradiol + NETA	Activella	1 mg E$_2$/0.5 mg NETA, or 0.5 mg E$_2$/0.1 mg NETA (28 pills per pack)
	Ethinyl estradiol + NETA	Femhrt	2.5 μg EE/0.5 mg NETA, or 5 μg EE/1 mg NETA (28 pills per pack)
	17β-Estradiol +100 mg progesterone	Bijuva[b]	1 mg E$_2$/100 mg progesterone (30 capsules per pack)
Transdermal continuous	17β-Estradiol + LNG	Climara Pro	0.045 mg/d E$_2$+ 0.015 mg/d LNG (patch applied weekly; 4 per carton)
	17β-Estradiol + NETA	CombiPatch	0.05 mg/d E$_2$+ 0.14 mg/d NETA, or 0.05 mg/d E$_2$+ 0.25 mg/d NETA (patch applied twice weekly to abdomen; 8 per carton)
TSEC[a]	CEE + BZA	Duavee	0.45 mg/d CEE + 20 mg BZA

[a]One pill daily.
[b]Considered a bioidentical preparation.
[c]The first 14 pills contain estrogen and the subsequent pills (15 through 28) contain estrogen with progestin.
BZA = bazedoxifene; CEE = conjugated equine estrogen; LNG = levonorgestrel; MPA = medroxyprogesterone acetate; NETA = norethindrone acetate; TSEC = tissue-selective estrogen complex.

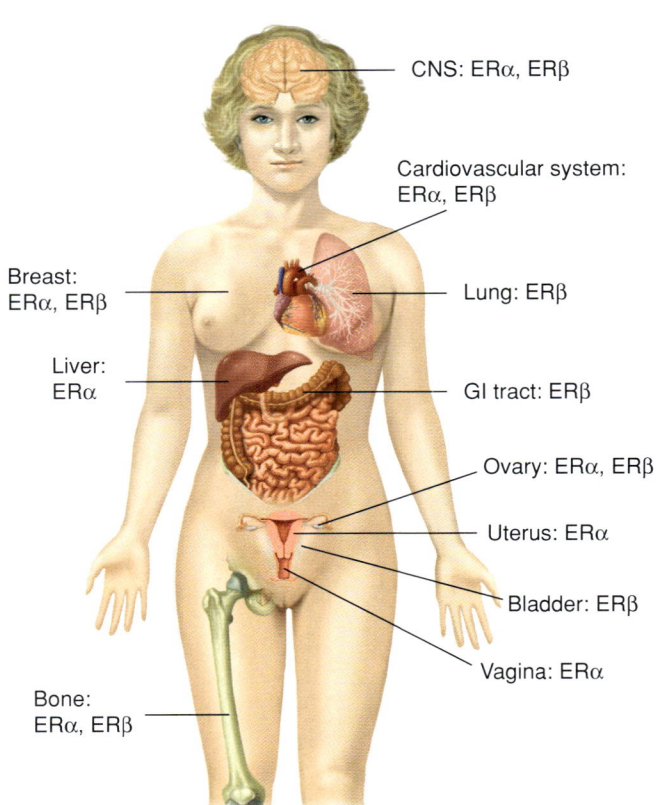

- CNS: ERα, ERβ
- Cardiovascular system: ERα, ERβ
- Breast: ERα, ERβ
- Lung: ERβ
- Liver: ERα
- GI tract: ERβ
- Ovary: ERα, ERβ
- Uterus: ERα
- Bladder: ERβ
- Vagina: ERα
- Bone: ERα, ERβ

FIGURE 22-6 The presence of estrogen receptor α and estrogen receptor β vary by organ type. Some examples are shown here.

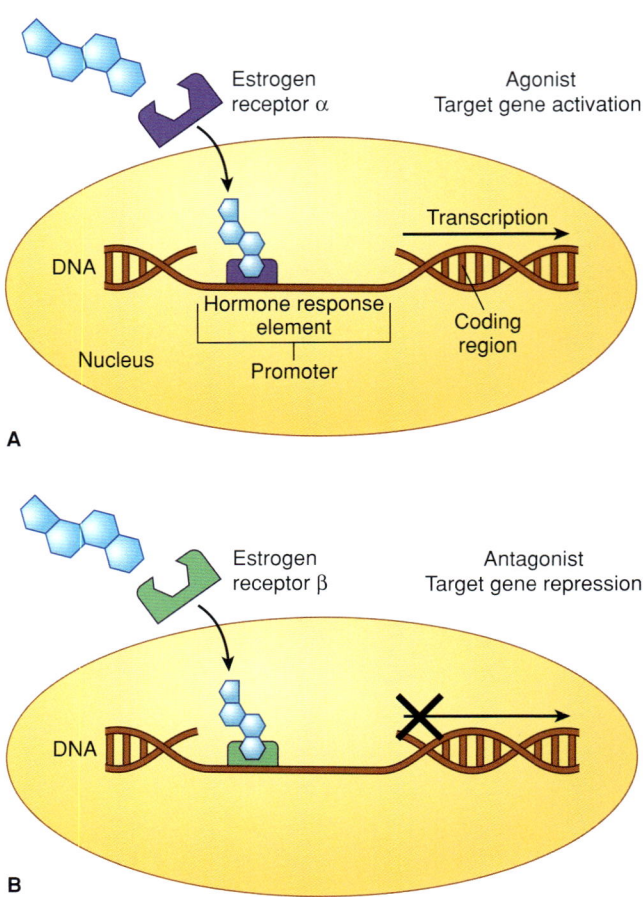

A

Estrogen receptor α — Agonist Target gene activation

DNA — Transcription

Hormone response element — Coding region

Nucleus — Promoter

B

Estrogen receptor β — Antagonist Target gene repression

DNA

FIGURE 22-7 Selective estrogen-receptor modulator (SERM) action. **A.** A given SERM may act as an agonist in one tissue type to promote DNA transcription. **B.** In a different tissue, that same SERM may act as an antagonist to block transcription of a target gene.

density loss and hot flash incidence but does not raise VTE rates compared with EPT using CEE plus MPA.

In the randomized Selective estrogens, Menopause, and Response to Therapy (SMART-2) trial, BZA/CEE reduced hot flash frequency by 74 percent at week 12 compared with a 51-percent reduction from placebo (Pinkerton, 2009b). A secondary efficacy analysis of SMART-2 data assessed sleep parameters and health-related quality of life in 318 women experiencing >7 moderate to severe hot flashes daily. Time to fall asleep, sleep disturbance, and sleep adequacy were improved with BZA/CEE compared with placebo. This dose also significantly improved the vasomotor function score and the Menopause-Specific Quality of Life (MENQOL) questionnaire score compared with placebo (Utian, 2009). In the SMART-V trial, BZA/CEE was compared with 1.5 mg MPA/0.45 mg CEE. BZA/CEE users achieved comparable relief of hot flashes and prevention of bone loss, but experienced less breast tenderness and uterine bleeding. The rates of breast tenderness, breast density changes, and uterine bleeding were similar to placebo (Pinkerton, 2013). Long-term safety and efficacy data are needed, but this TSEC appears to be neutral on the endometrium and breast in clinical trials up to 2 years.

Potential candidates for BZA/CEE include women with an intact uterus wishing to use systemic HT but concerned regarding its safety with respect to breast cancer. In addition, women who experience unpleasant mood symptoms with progestogens

or prefer to avoid bleeding may appreciate that BZA/CEE is progestogen-free.

Bioidentical Hormones

Some women believe that conventional FDA-regulated pharmaceutical estrogens and progestogens present unacceptable risks. Ironically, more is known about the absolute risks and benefits of HT than almost any other class of drugs. Although prescriptions for estrogen and progestogens have declined since publication of WHI results, the use of *bioidentical hormones* that are not FDA approved has grown. This term, invented by marketers, is often used to describe custom-compounded HT products but has no clear scientific meaning (Shifren, 2014). Custom compounding of HT may combine several hormones that include estradiol, estrone, estriol, testosterone, dehydroepiandrosterone (DHEA), and progesterone. They often use nonstandard routes of administration such as subdermal implants or creams. Some of the hormones are not FDA approved (estriol), and some compounded therapies contain nonhormonal dyes or preservatives. Moreover, these formulations have not been tested for efficacy or safety; product information is not consistently provided to women with their prescription; and batch standardization may be uncertain (Santoro, 2016b). Thus, these preparations cannot be assumed to be safer than conventional pharmaceutical estrogen or progestogens. Several organizations note that conventional FDA-approved HT products are preferred (American College of Obstetricians and Gynecologists, 2018a; The North American Menopause Society, 2017).

In conjunction with bioidentical hormones, salivary hormone testing to assist with hormone level adjustment is not recommended due to inter- and intra-patient variability (Lewis, 2002; Zava, 1998). For women who request bioidentical hormone therapy, FDA-approved bioidentical hormone therapies are noted in Table 22-4.

Nonhormonal Central Nervous System Agents

Pharmacologic therapies with supported efficacy for hot flash rate reduction include selective serotonin-reuptake inhibitors (SSRIs) and serotonin norepinephrine-reuptake inhibitors (SSNIs), gabapentinoids (gabapentin and pregabalin), and clonidine (Table 22-5). In general, these reduce hot flash frequency and severity by 50 to 60 percent (Pinkerton, 2019; Sideras, 2010).

Of these, low-dose, 7.5-mg paroxetine mesylate is the only one that is FDA-approved therapy for VMS. Paroxetine, escitalopram, and venlafaxine are the best-studied for this indication, and their doses for VMS are lower than those used for psychiatric conditions. These agents may cause dizziness, headache, and nausea, but the incidence is lower than with higher psychiatric doses. When prescribing 7.5 mg of paroxetine, initial dose escalation is not needed nor is a cessation taper. Of other caveats, fluoxetine and paroxetine are contraindicated in women taking tamoxifen due to concomitant effects on the cytochrome P450 enzyme system, the liver enzymes that metabolize them. Instead, in this setting, venlafaxine, desvenlafaxine, gabapentin,

and pregabalin are more suitable for VMS treatment, as is escitalopram, which has less effect on P450 enzymes.

Gabapentin for VMS may begin with a 100-mg oral dose three times daily and can escalate to 300 mg three times daily. For women with night-time symptoms, a 300-mg gabapentin dose at night can be increased to 600 mg after 2 weeks. For pregabalin, the recommended starting dose is 50 mg orally daily and is advanced to 75 mg twice daily. Both of these gabapentinoids may cause dizziness and sedation, which are dose-related (Sideras, 2010).

Clonidine is FDA approved for hypertension. It is used off label infrequently for VMS relief due to associated orthostatic hypotension and other side effects.

Although additional data are needed, potential new therapies include oxybutynin and neurokinin B–receptor antagonists. In the largest randomized trial of oxybutynin, 150 women were provided placebo or oral oxybutynin in 2.5-mg or 5.0-mg doses twice daily. Oxybutynin treatment at both doses lowered a hot flash composite score compared with placebo (Leon-Ferre, 2018). Prominent side effects were dry mouth and difficulty urinating, which are typical of this anticholinergic drug (Chap. 23, p. 532). With neurokinin B–receptor antagonists, both hot flash rates and sleep disturbances are improved (Pinkerton, 2019). Both agents appear to be as effective as HT and may represent a significant advance in nonhormonal treatment if safety and long-term efficacy data are positive.

Over-the-Counter Supplements

Over-the-counter herbal formulations, particularly soy, red clover, and black cohosh, are widely used to treat VMS. Unfortunately, randomized trials have not found these supplements to be more effective than placebo in treating VMS (Newton, 2006). One metaanalysis noted that phytoestrogen supplementation modestly reduces hot flash frequency but not night sweats (Franco, 2016). Another evaluating soy isoflavones found a lowered incidence and/or severity of hot flashes (Daily, 2019). That said, more robust research is needed to clearly establish benefits.

Lifestyle Changes

Practical, nonpharmacologic steps to relieve VMS include using fans, lowering ambient room temperatures, layering clothing, consuming cool beverages, and avoiding triggers such as alcohol, caffeine, and spicy foods. Weight loss, non-sweat-inducing exercise, and mindfulness stress-reducing therapies may provide quality-of-life benefits and possibly hot flash reduction. Unfortunately, the efficacy of acupuncture, exercise, yoga, paced respiration, and relaxation training in treating VMS has not been robustly documented (Kaunitz, 2015; Pinkerton, 2019). However, a recent analysis from three trials of VMS interventions found that acupuncture, yoga, and wellness education classes all provided similar relief and afforded a 35- to 40-percent reduction in hot flash frequency compared with untreated controls (Avis, 2019). In small trials, hypnosis and cognitive behavioral therapy each lowered VMS frequency. However, both interventions are limited by access to trained providers (Pinkerton, 2019; The North American Menopause Society, 2015).

TABLE 22-5. Nonhormonal Agents Used for Vasomotor Symptoms[a]

Prescription (brand name)	Dose[b]
SSRI	
Paroxetine mesylate (Brisdelle)[c]	7.5 mg
Paroxetine (Paxil)[c]	20 mg
Venlafaxine (Effexor XR)	37.5–75 mg
Citalopram (Celexa)	20 mg
Escitalopram (Lexapro)	10–20 mg
Sertraline (Zoloft)	50 mg
Fluoxetine (Prozac, Sarafem)[c]	20 mg
SNRI: Desvenlafaxine (Pristiq)	100 mg–150 mg
Clonidine (Catapres)	0.1 mg transdermal
Gabapentin (Neurontin)	600–900 mg (divided doses)
Pregabalin (Lyrica)	900 mg (divided doses)

[a]Off-label use except for paroxetine mesylate.
[b]Oral daily dosing.
[c]Avoid tamoxifen users, inhibitors of CYP2D6.
SNRI = selective norepinephrine- reuptake inhibitor;
SSRI = selective serotonin reuptake inhibitor.

BONE HEALTH

■ Bone Structure and Metabolism

The skeleton consists of two bone types. Cortical bone is more compact and is the bone of the peripheral skeleton (arms and legs). Trabecular bone is more porous and is the bone of the axial skeleton, which includes the vertebrae, pelvis, and proximal femur.

Peak bone mass is influenced by genetic and endocrine factors, and opportunity in the younger years for acquiring bone mass is brief. Almost all bone mass in the axial skeleton will be accumulated in young women by late adolescence, so the years immediately following menarche are especially important (Sabatier, 1996; Theintz, 1992). Calcium supplementation in prepubertal and pubertal girls improves bone accrual (Bonjour, 2001; Stear, 2003). Accordingly, osteoporosis prevention with weight-bearing exercise and sufficient vitamin D and calcium intake ideally begins in adolescence (Recker, 1992).

Following adolescence, bone resorption is normally coupled to bone formation such that positive bone balance is achieved when skeletal maturity is attained, typically at age 25 to 35 years. Thereafter, bone mass declines at a slow, steady rate of approximately 0.4 percent each year. During menopause, in the absence of hormone therapy, this rate rises to 2 to 5 percent per year for the first 5 to 10 years and then slows to 1 percent per year. The subsequent risk of fracture from osteoporosis will depend on bone mass at the time of menopause and the rate of bone loss following menopause (Riis, 1996).

Normal bone is a dynamic, living tissue that is in a continuous process of destruction and rebuilding. The process of bone remodeling involves a constant resorption of bone, carried out by multinucleated giant cells known as *osteoclasts*, and a concurrent process of bone formation, completed by *osteoblasts* (Fig. 22-8).

Activated osteoclasts secrete hydrochloric acid and collagen-degrading enzymes onto the bone surface, resulting in bone mineral dissolution and degradation of the organic matrix. Increased osteoclast activity in postmenopausal osteoporosis is mediated by the receptor activator of nuclear factor (RANK) ligand pathway. In this, RANK, RANK ligand, and osteoprotegerin (OPG) are three major components.

Of these, RANK ligand is expressed by osteoblasts when RANK binds to the RANK receptor on osteoclasts and osteoclast precursors (Bar-Shavit, 2007). Activation of RANK promotes osteoclast formation, function, and survival. RANK ligand is the common regulator of osteoclast activity and ultimately of bone resorption. OPG is also secreted by osteoblasts and is a natural inhibitor of RANK ligand. OPG blocks RANK ligand–mediated activation of RANK to balance bone remodeling (Kostenuik, 2005). RANK ligand is required to mediate osteoclast effects on bone resorption. Cytokines and certain hormones stimulate the expression of RANK ligand by osteoblasts and other cells. Negative regulators of this process include estrogen, which limits the expression of RANK ligand from osteoblasts. Another is OPG, a natural inhibitor of RANK ligand that sequesters and neutralizes the effects of RANK ligand. Estrogen stimulates OPG expression.

In healthy premenopausal women, estrogen limits osteoblast expression of RANK ligand. The OPG binds to RANK ligand to further limit its availability to stimulate osteoclasts. The remaining RANK ligand binds to osteoclast precursors, which fuse and form differentiated osteoclasts for bone resorption. This is followed by the appearance of osteoblasts resulting in bone formation. In sum, resorption and formation are balanced in premenopausal women.

In postmenopausal women, decreased estrogen levels lead to greater RANK ligand

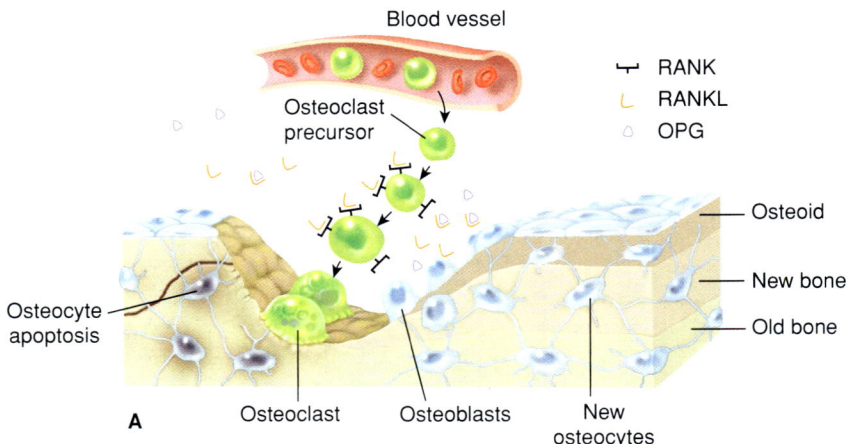

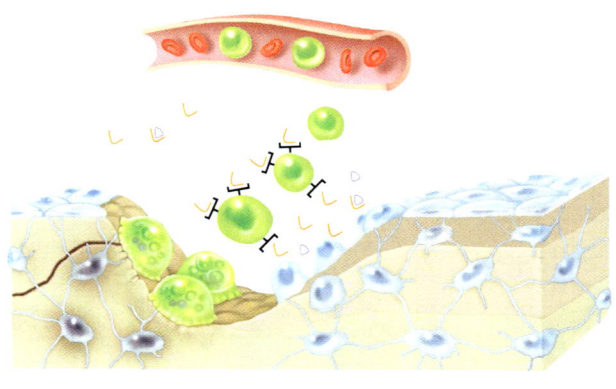

FIGURE 22-8 Bone remodeling. **A.** Osteoclasts resorb matrix, whereas osteoblasts deposit new lamellar bone. Osteoblasts that are trapped in the matrix become osteocytes. Others undergo apoptosis or form new, flattened osteoblast lining cells. Osteoblasts produce the proteins RANKL and OPG. When RANKL binds to RANK, the receptor on the surface of osteoclast progenitor cells, this promotes those cells' development, activity, and survival as osteoclasts. This leads to bone resorption. OPG serves as a counterbalance. OPG binds to RANKL and thereby, RANKL is incapable of binding with RANK to promote osteoclast development. Through this mechanism, bone resorption is limited. **B.** With hypoestrogenism, RANKL production is increased. Excessive levels of RANKL outnumber those of OPG and osteoclast development, and bone resorption is favored.

expression, which may overwhelm the natural activity of OPG. Bone resorption follows, and osteoblasts can only partially fill the resulting resorption cavities, leading to a chronic imbalance of formation and resorption resulting in bone loss. Thus, increased RANK ligand after menopause leads to excessive bone resorption and potentially to postmenopausal osteoporosis (Sambrook, 2006).

■ Osteopenia and Osteoporosis

Clinical Importance

Osteoporosis is a skeletal disorder that progressively reduces bone mass and strength (typically in trabecular bone) and leads to higher fracture rates. *Osteopenia* is a precursor to osteoporosis, and the National Osteoporosis Foundation (2014) estimates that more than 10 million Americans currently have osteoporosis and another 33.6 million have osteopenia of the femoral neck. Of postmenopausal women, 40 to 50 percent experience an osteoporosis-related fracture during their lifetime. Osteoporosis is more common in white and Hispanic women, followed by Native American, Asian, and black women (Barrett-Connor, 2005).

The vertebrae, femoral neck, and wrists are most commonly fractured, and epidemiologic studies estimate that the lifetime risk of common fragility fractures in white women after age 50 approximates 15 percent at each of these sites (Holroyd, 2008; Kanis, 1994). Following a vertebral or hip fracture, postmenopausal women are at higher risk of experiencing another fracture (Lindsay, 2001).

Fractures are associated with significant morbidity and mortality, and a clinical fracture is associated with a twofold increase in mortality risk. The overall mortality rate from femoral neck fracture alone approximates 30 percent. In addition, only 40 percent of those who sustain a femoral neck fracture are capable of returning to their prefracture level of independence. Vertebral fractures are associated with acute and chronic pain, height loss, and deformity, whereas humerus and distal forearm fractures may be associated with substantial disability. Fracture risk rises with age (FitzGerald, 2014). As such, clinicians ideally educate patients regarding bone loss prevention, screen to identify bone loss early, and work with patients to implement effective management plans.

Pathophysiology

A major proportion of bone strength is determined by bone mineral density (BMD), which is grams of mineral per area and volume of bone. However, bone quality, bone strength, and fracture risk are also affected by bone remodeling rates, bone size and geometry, microarchitecture, mineralization, damage accumulation, and matrix quality. Unlike BMD, these parameters are difficult to accurately assess (Kiebzak, 2003).

Primary osteoporosis refers to bone loss associated with aging and postmenopausal estrogen deficiency. As estrogen levels fall after menopause, this steroid's regulatory effect on bone resorption is lost. As a result, bone resorption is accelerated and is usually not balanced by compensatory bone formation. This accelerated bone loss is most rapid in the early postmenopausal years (Gallagher, 2002). If osteoporosis is caused by other diseases or medications, the term *secondary osteoporosis* is used (Stein, 2003).

The amount of bone at any point in time reflects the balance of the osteoblastic (building) and osteoclastic (resorbing) activities

(Canalis, 2007). As noted, both aging and a loss of estrogen lead to greater osteoclast activity. Also, less dietary calcium intake or impaired calcium absorption from the gut lowers the serum level of ionized calcium. This results in parathyroid hormone (PTH) secretion, which mobilizes calcium from bone by stimulation of osteoclast activity. Increased PTH levels stimulate vitamin D production. In turn, elevated vitamin D concentrations raise serum calcium levels by several effects: (1) stimulation of osteoclasts to remove calcium from bone, (2) increased intestinal calcium absorption, (3) enhanced renal calcium reabsorption, and (4) reduced PTH production by the parathyroid glands.

In healthy premenopausal women, this series of events leads to increased serum calcium levels, and PTH levels return to normal. In menopausal women, estrogen deficiency creates a greater responsiveness of bone to PTH. Thus, for any given PTH level, relatively more calcium is removed from bone, leading to bone loss and loss of microarchitecture for both trabecular and cortical bone.

Diagnosis

The primary clinical tool to identify bone loss is an assessment of BMD using dual-energy x-ray absorptiometry (DEXA) of the lumbar vertebrae, and femoral neck (Fig. 22-9) (Marshall, 1996). The lumbar vertebrae contain primarily trabecular bone, which has a faster bone remodeling rate. Therefore, early rapid bone loss can be determined by evaluation of this site. Cortical bone is denser bone and is most abundant in the long-bone shafts of the appendicular skeleton. The greater trochanter and femoral neck contain both cortical and trabecular bone, and these sites are ideal for the prediction of femoral neck fracture risk in older women (Miller, 2002). Alternatively, in those with prior back surgery or bilateral hip replacement, appendicular BMD of the radius is used.

Normative BMD values for sex, age, and ethnicity have been determined. For diagnostic purposes, results of BMD testing are reported as *T-scores*. These measure in standard deviations (SDs) the variance of an individual's BMD from that expected for a person of the same sex at peak bone mass (25 to 30 years). A T-score of −2.0 in a woman, for example, means that her BMD is two SDs below the average peak bone mass for a young woman. T-scores are used to make the diagnosis of osteoporosis in postmenopausal women. Definitions are found in Table 22-6 (National Osteoporosis Foundation, 2014). The standard criteria for diagnosing postmenopausal osteoporosis is a T-score of −2.5 or lower at the lumbar spine, femoral neck, or total hip by DEXA testing (Cosman, 2014). The fourth category, *severe osteoporosis*, describes patients who have a T-score below −2.5 and who have also suffered a fragility fracture. A

TABLE 22-6. World Health Organization Criteria for Bone Disease Based on Bone Mineral Density (BMD)

Normal BMD: T-score between +2.5 and −1.0

Osteopenia: T-score between −1.0 and −2.5

Osteoporosis: T-score at or below −2.5

Severe osteoporosis: T-score at or below −2.5 with one or more fractures

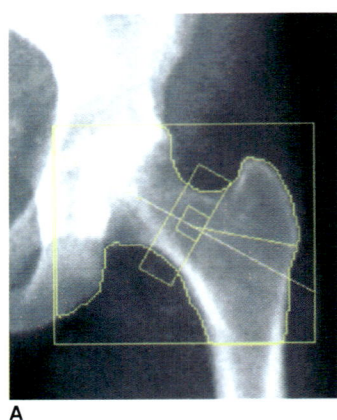

A

DXA Results Summary:

Region	Area (cm²)	BMC (g)	BMD (g/cm²)	T-Score	Z-Score
Neck	4.59	3.79	0.827	−0.2	1.0
Troch	8.57	6.65	0.775	0.7	1.5
Inter	14.62	17.48	1.196	0.6	1.2
Total	**27.79**	**27.92**	**1.005**	**0.5**	**1.3**
Ward's	1.12	0.71	0.639	−0.8	1.0

Total BMD CV 1.0%, ACF = 1.028, BCF = 0.998, TH = 6.508
WHO Classification: Normal
Fracture Risk: Not Increased

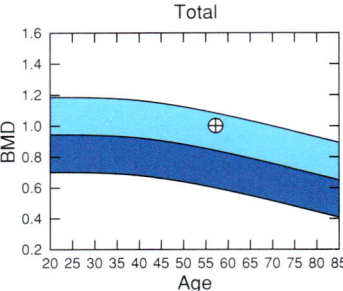

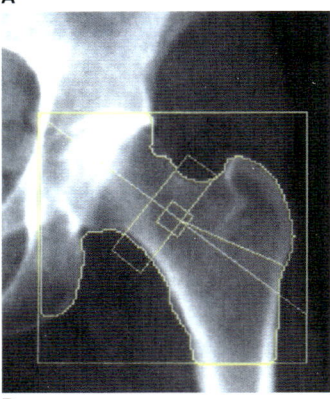

B

DXA Results Summary:

Region	Area (cm²)	BMC (g)	BMD (g/cm²)	T-Score	Z-Score
Neck	4.97	2.74	0.552	−2.7	−1.4
Troch	11.53	5.62	0.487	−2.1	−1.3
Inter	18.92	14.78	0.781	−2.1	−1.4
Total	**35.43**	**23.14**	**0.653**	**−2.4**	**−1.4**
Ward's	1.16	0.38	0.331	−3.4	−1.5

Total BMD CV 1.0%
WHO Classification: Osteopenia
Fracture Risk: Increased

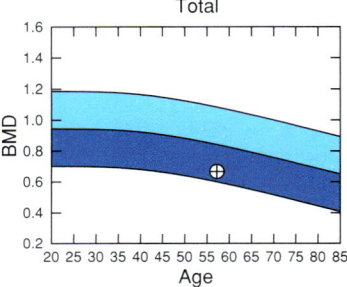

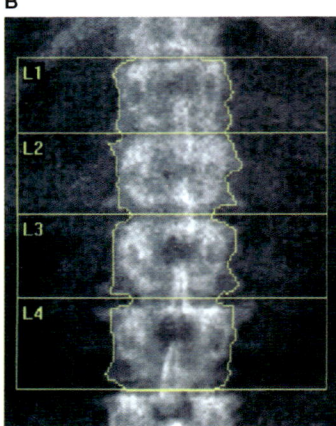

C

DXA Results Summary:

Region	Area (cm²)	BMC (g)	BMD (g/cm²)	T-Score	Z-Score
L1	12.00	12.73	1.061	1.2	2.3
L2	13.37	14.93	1.116	0.8	2.0
L3	14.03	16.56	1.181	0.9	2.1
L4	15.80	20.23	1.280	1.5	2.8
Total	**55.20**	**64.45**	**1.168**	**1.1**	**2.3**

Total BMD CV 1.0%
WHO Classification: Normal
Fracture Risk: Not Increased

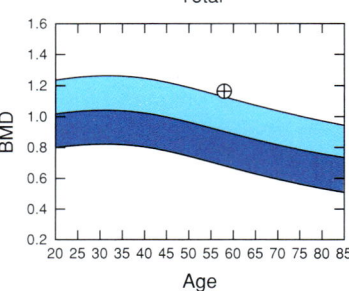

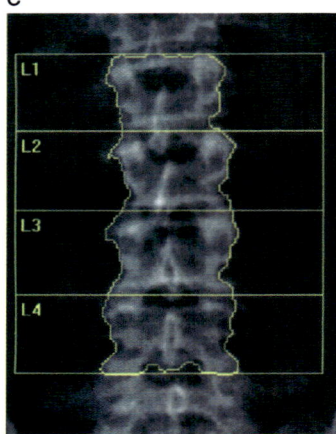

D

DXA Results Summary:

Region	Area (cm²)	BMC (g)	BMD (g/cm²)	T-Score	Z-Score
L1	11.73	8.03	0.684	−2.2	−1.0
L2	12.60	9.70	0.770	−2.3	−1.0
L3	14.59	11.70	0.802	−2.6	−1.1
L4	14.44	11.01	0.763	−3.2	−1.7
Total	**53.36**	**40.44**	**0.758**	**−2.6**	**−1.2**

Total BMD CV 1.0%, ACF = 1.028, BCF = 0.998, TH = 5.974
WHO Classification: Osteoporosis
Fracture Risk: High

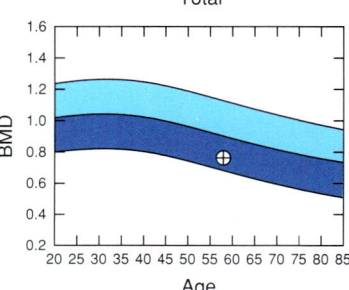

FIGURE 22-9 Dual-energy x-ray absorptiometry (DEXA) scans. **A.** DEXA report describing normal hip density. **B.** DEXA report describing osteopenia of the hip and osteoporosis of the femoral neck. **C.** DEXA report describing normal vertebral body density. **D.** DEXA report describing vertebral body osteoporosis. BMC = bone mineral content; BMD = bone mineral density.

fragility fracture is one that results from a fall from a standing or lower height and does not stem from major trauma.

Patients are also assigned a *Z-score*, which is the SD between the patient's measurement and the average bone mass for a patient with the same age and weight. The Z-score is the preferred manner of expressing BMD results in premenopausal women. Z-scores lower than −2.0 require diagnostic evaluation for *secondary osteoporosis* (Faulkner, 1999). Similarly, initial evaluation of any patient with osteoporosis should include checking for causes of secondary osteoporosis (Table 22-7).

BMD represents the most readily quantifiable fracture risk predictor for those who have not yet suffered a fragility fracture. For each SD of BMD below a baseline level (either mean peak bone mass or mean for the reference population of the person's age and sex), the fracture risk approximately doubles (National Osteoporosis Foundation, 2002).

Recognizing the difficulty in measuring bone quality accurately, the World Health Organization (WHO) developed the Fracture Risk Assessment Tool (FRAX) to assess an individual's 10-year fracture risk from age 40 to 90 years. The algorithm is applicable only for patients who have not received pharmacotherapy. The FRAX tool is accessible online and is available for multiple countries/ethnicities and in different languages (http://www.shef.ac.uk/FRAX/). This online tool incorporates 11 risk factors including prior fractures, parental hip fracture history, age, gender, BMI, ethnicity, smoking, alcohol use, glucocorticoid use, rheumatoid arthritis, and secondary osteoporosis. These are combined with the femoral neck bone density (raw or T-score) to calculate the 10-year fracture risk. This WHO site offers downloadable charts for calculating fracture risks using BMD or BMI (as a surrogate for BMD). The FRAX tool identifies patients who might benefit from pharmacotherapy and

TABLE 22-7. Common Secondary Causes of Osteoporosis and Recommended Testing

Primary hyperparathyroidism	Serum levels of: parathyroid hormone calcium phosphorus alkaline phosphatase
Secondary hyperparathyroidism from chronic renal failure	Renal function tests
Hyperthyroidism or excess thyroid hormone treatment	Thyroid function tests
Increased calcium excretion	24-hour urine collection for calcium and creatinine concentrations
Hypercortisolism, alcohol abuse, and metastatic cancer	Careful history and when indicated appropriate laboratory studies
Osteomalacia	Serum levels of: calcium phosphorus alkaline phosphatase 1,25-dihydroxyvitamin D

is most useful for assessing those with osteopenia. One screening and management algorithm from the American College of Obstetricians and Gynecologists (2019a) incorporates FRAX probability values (Fig. 22-10).

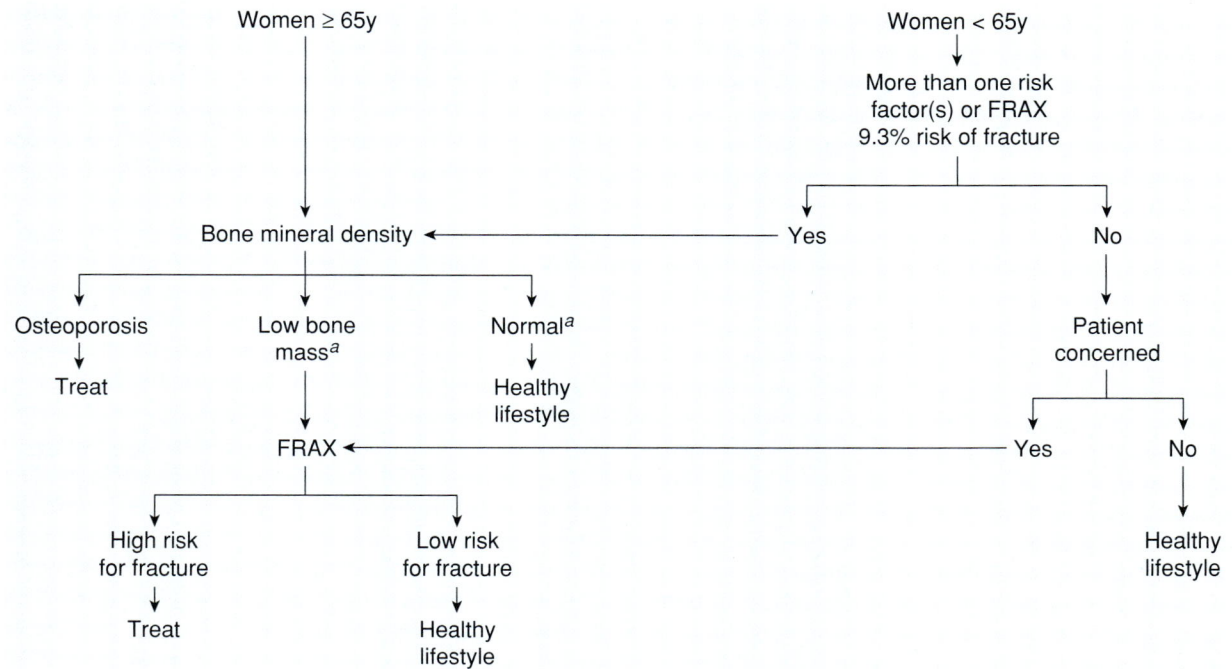

FIGURE 22-10 Screening and treatment algorithm. [a]Prior fragility fracture is an indication for treatment regardless of bone densitometry findings. Those at highest risk are ideally referred to an osteoporosis specialist. (Reproduced with permission from American College of Obstetricians and Gynecologists, 2019a.)

TABLE 22-8. Osteoporosis Risk Factors

Major Risk Factors	Minor Risk Factors
Age >65 years	Rheumatoid arthritis
Low bone mineral density	History of clinical hyperthyroidism
Vertebral compression fracture	Chronic anticonvulsant therapy
Fragility fracture after age 40	Low dietary calcium intake
Family history of osteoporotic fracture	Smoker
Systemic glucocorticoid therapy for >3 months	Excessive alcohol intake
Malabsorption syndrome	Excessive caffeine intake
Primary hyperparathyroidism	Weight <57 kg
Propensity to fall	>10 percent weight loss at age 25
Osteopenia apparent on radiography	Chronic heparin therapy
Hypogonadism	Aromatase inhibitors
Early menopause (before age 45)	

Prevention

As predictors of osteoporotic fracture, the most important factors are listed in Table 22-8. Risk factors for osteoporotic fracture are additive and are considered in the context of baseline age and sex-related fracture risk. For example, a 55-year-old woman with low BMD is at significantly less risk than a 75-year-old woman with the same low BMD. Similarly, a woman with low BMD and a prior fragility fracture is at considerably greater risk than another person with the same low BMD and no prior fracture. Any key risk factor ideally prompts further assessment and possibly active intervention, such as calcium and vitamin D therapy coupled with weight-bearing exercise or pharmacologic therapy (Table 22-9) (National Osteoporosis Foundation, 2014).

Nonmodifiable Factors. Age is a major fracture risk factor. The 10-year probability of experiencing a fracture of forearm, humerus, vertebra, or femoral neck increases as much as eightfold between ages 45 and 85 years for women (Kanis, 2001). Osteoporotic fractures occur most commonly in women older than 65 years. Medical interventions are effective only in preventing fractures in populations with an average age older than 65 years. However, most currently approved osteoporosis therapies prevent or reverse bone loss if initiated at, or soon after, age 50. Therefore, women at high risk for bone loss or with prior fragility fracture are included in those for whom BMD testing is recommended.

A prior fragility fracture places a person at a 1.5- to 9.5-fold higher risk for another fracture, depending on age at assessment, number of prior fractures, and prior fracture site (Melton, 1999). Vertebral fractures are the best studied, and a prior vertebral fracture raises the risk of a second such fracture at least fourfold. In the placebo group of a major clinical trial, 20 percent of those who experienced a vertebral fracture during the study had a second vertebral fracture within 1 year (Lindsay, 2001). Vertebral fractures also indicate vulnerability at other skeletal sites.

Persons of any ethnicity can develop osteoporosis, but data from the Third National Health and Nutrition Examination Survey (NHANES III) show the highest risk among non-Hispanic white and Asian women and lowest among non-Hispanic black women. Racial and ethnic differences are important because fracture rates do not always correlate with BMD across ethnic groups. For example, Chinese American women typically have lower BMD than white American women, but

TABLE 22-9. General Guidelines for Prevention of Osteoporosis in Postmenopausal Women

Counsel on osteoporosis risks

Check for secondary causes (Table 22-7)

For women 51 years and older, encourage diet containing calcium 1200 mg daily and vitamin D 800–1000 IU daily.
     Add supplement if diet is incomplete; emphasize dietary calcium over supplements

Recommend regular weight-bearing and muscle-strengthening exercise

Advise against tobacco smoking and excess alcohol intake

Assess for fall risks and modify as possible

Measure height annually

In women ≥65 years, recommend BMD testing

In postmenopausal women aged 50–65 years, recommend BMD testing based on the risk factor profile (Table 22-8)

In those >50 years with a new fracture, recommend BMD testing to determine degree of disease severity

For patients on pharmacotherapy, perform BMD testing 2 years after initiating therapy and every 2 years thereafter.
     However, testing frequency may be tailored to clinical situations

BMD = bone mineral density.

lower rates of femoral neck and forearm fracture (Walker, 2011). It is postulated that greater cortical density and thicker trabeculae compensate for fewer trabeculae in smaller bones. Thus, both BMD and microarchitecture appear to play distinct roles in fracture vulnerability (American College of Obstetricians and Gynecologists, 2019a).

Genetic influence on osteoporosis and BMD is important, and heredity is estimated to account for 50 to 80 percent of BMD variability (Ralston, 2002; Sigurdsson, 2008). The Study of Osteoporotic Fractures identified maternal femoral neck fracture as a predictor for similar fracture in a population of elderly women (Cummings, 1995).

Modifiable Factors. Of these, exercise and fall prevention are primary. These are discussed with other preventive steps on page 495.

Therapy with glucocorticoids lasting more than 2 to 3 months is a major risk factor for bone loss and fracture, particularly among postmenopausal women. A chronic daily dose of prednisone ≥5 mg serves as the threshold for assessment and clinical intervention to prevent or treat glucocorticoid-induced osteoporosis (National Osteoporosis Foundation, 2014). Other medications associated with bone loss include anticonvulsants (phenytoin), anticoagulants (heparin), depot MPA, chemotherapeutic drugs, gonadotropin-releasing hormone agonists, cyclosporine A, tacrolimus, and lithium.

Breast cancer survivors may be at higher risk for bone loss. Reasons include surgery- or chemotherapy-induced early menopause or the lowered estrogen levels seen with aromatase inhibitors.

Osteoporosis Screening. After risk assessment, BMD measurement helps confirm osteoporosis and determine disease severity. BMD testing by DEXA should be performed in postmenopausal women: (1) aged ≥65 years, (2) with one or more risk factors for osteoporosis, or (3) who have sustained fractures (Camacho, 2016; Cosman, 2014; The North American Menopause Society, 2010). Screening is considered for perimenopausal women if they have a specific risk factor such as prior low-trauma fracture, low BMI, or medication known to accelerate bone loss. Many vertebral fractures are asymptomatic, and vertebral imaging is recommended for women aged ≥70 years with a T-score ≤−1.0 or those 65 to 69 years with a score ≤−1.5 (National Osteoporosis Foundation, 2014).

OSTEOPOROSIS TREATMENT

■ Indications

The primary goal of osteoporosis treatment is fracture prevention in women who have low BMD or additional fracture risks (see Fig. 22-10). Toward this end, therapy aims to stabilize or increase BMD. Treatment includes lifestyle changes and often pharmacologic therapy. The key lifestyle modifications that can decrease fracture risks in postmenopausal women include regular weight-bearing exercise and a balanced diet with adequate calcium and vitamin D. Patients ideally maintain normal body weight and avoid smoking, excessive alcohol intake, and fall risks (Christiansen, 2013).

With pharmacologic therapy, several organizations recommend starting therapy for: (1) postmenopausal women with total hip, femoral neck, or lumbar spine T-scores at or below −2.5; (2) those with an osteoporotic vertebral or hip fracture; (3) those with a prior fragility fracture; and (4) those with a high FRAX fracture probability. For the last, a 10-year major osteoporotic fracture risk ≥20 percent or a hip fracture risk ≥3 percent serves as a threshold (Camacho, 2016; Cosman 2014). Prevention or treatment is consider for postmenopausal women with total hip or spine T-scores from −1.0 to −2.5 with additional fracture risk factors (see Table 22-8).

Drugs prescribed for fracture prevention are those that (1) reduce bone resorption, termed *antiresorptive agents*, or (2) stimulate bone formation, termed *anabolic agents*. Estrogen, SERMs, bisphosphonates, denosumab, vitamin D, and calcitonin each have antiresorptive properties to halt bone loss, and most also increase BMD. These act most quickly on bone that has high trabecular content and rapid turnover, such as the vertebrae. Alternatively, for the hip, therapy-related gains may be delayed because the hip contains approximately 50 percent trabecular and 50 percent cortical bone.

Anabolic agents include teriparatide and abaloparatide, which are PTH analogues that act as agonists at the PTH receptor (Miller, 2016). In contrast, romosozumab inhibits the activity of the bone protein sclerostin. In general, anabolic agents are prescribed by skeletal-health specialists, including medical endocrinologists and rheumatologists.

For osteoporosis, each agent differs in its indication for prevention, for treatment, or both. HT is indicated for the prevention of osteoporosis. Bisphosphonates and SERMs are prevention or treatment options. Calcitonin is used rarely, as other agents are more effective. Denosumab is a monoclonal antibody against RANK ligand and approved for osteoporosis treatment. PTH-receptor agonists and the new sclerostin inhibitor are approved for treatment of osteoporosis in women at high risk of fracture.

■ Hormonal Options

Estrogen and Progestogens

HT slows the bone resorption rate, which results in a BMD increase (Wells, 2002). In observational studies, HT reduces osteoporosis-related fracture rates by approximately 50 percent when started soon after menopause. Continued long term, HT significantly lowers fracture rates in women with established disease (Tosteson, 2008). Moreover, the WHI trials confirmed a significant 34-percent reduction in hip fracture rates in a healthy low-fracture-risk population of postmenopausal women receiving HT (Jackson, 2006b; The Women's Health Initiative Steering Committee, 2004).

BMD responses do not vary among estrogen preparations or administration routes. Even very low estrogen doses combined with calcium and vitamin D produce significant BMD improvement compared with placebo (Ettinger, 2004; Prestwood, 2003). Specifically, 0.5-mg doses of oral E_2; 0.3-mg doses of CEE; or a transdermal estradiol patch delivering as little as 0.014 mg/d are effective as women are further from menopause. With early menopause, higher doses may be needed.

Some study results suggest that fracture protection wanes rapidly, as significant bone loss may be seen following HT discontinuation. However, in the WHI, higher fracture rates were not seen after stopping HT (Watts, 2017). Some guidelines recommend HT to prevent bone loss for women with bothersome menopausal symptoms or for women who carry a high fracture risk but who are not candidates for alternative therapies (Camacho, 2016; The North American Menopause Society, 2017). In general and discussed earlier (p. 479), systemic HT initiation is not recommended for women older than 60 or for those 10 years beyond menopause due to associated CHD risks. Fracture risk and the potential need for an alternative therapy should be assessed before women discontinue HT.

Bazedoxifene Formulations

The 20-mg BZA/0.45-mg CEE formulation (Duavee) is indicated for VMS and postmenopausal bone loss prevention. In the randomized SMART trials noted earlier (p. 484), the adjusted mean percentage BMD change in the lumbar spine from baseline to 24 months significantly rose in those taking this BZA/CEE formulation compared with women using placebo (Lindsay, 2009). Findings were similar for total hip BMD.

Raloxifene

In postmenopausal women, this SERM is FDA approved to prevent and treat osteoporosis and to reduce the risk of invasive breast cancer. It activates estrogen receptors in the bone but does not appear to activate those in the breast or uterus.

Raloxifene appears most appropriate for prevention and treatment of vertebral disease. Raloxifene (60 mg/d) prevents vertebral fracture but does not prevent nonvertebral ones (Delmas, 2002; Ettinger, 1999). In addition to its bone effects, raloxifene reduces risk of breast cancer in high-risk women (US Preventive Services Task Force, 2019).

Of side effects, hot flashes are associated with raloxifene therapy, although the incidence is low (Cohen, 2000). Raloxifene use does raise the VTE risk and is contraindicated in patients with prior VTE (Delmas, 2002).

■ Nonhormonal Antiresorptive Agents

Bisphosphonates

Four bisphosphonates are currently available and include alendronate, risedronate, ibandronate, and zoledronate. The first three are taken orally, but zoledronate is an intravenous infusion. These agents chemically bind to calcium hydroxyapatite in bone (Fig. 22-11). They decrease bone resorption by blocking the function and survival but not the formation of osteoclasts (Diab, 2012; Russell, 2008).

The oral bisphosphonates display poor bioavailability and therefore are taken on an empty stomach with adequate water for proper dissolution and absorption. These agents have a favorable overall safety profile, and adverse event rates are comparable with placebo (Black, 1996; Harris, 1999). However, bisphosphonates may cause upper gastrointestinal inflammation, ulceration, and bleeding (Lanza, 2000). Thus, to aid delivery to the stomach and reduce esophageal irritation, dosing instructions are reinforced with each patient. First, bisphosphonates are taken in the morning after fasting and with a full glass of water. During the 30 minutes after administration, no other food or beverages are consumed. Last, for all immediate

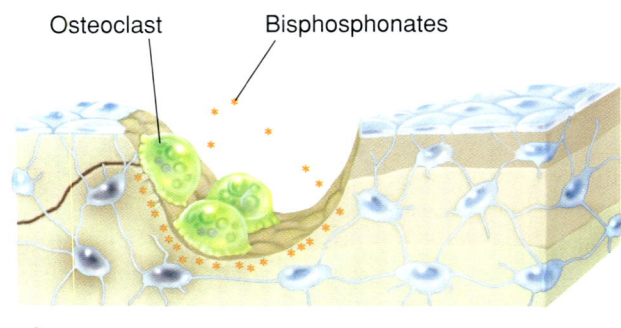

A

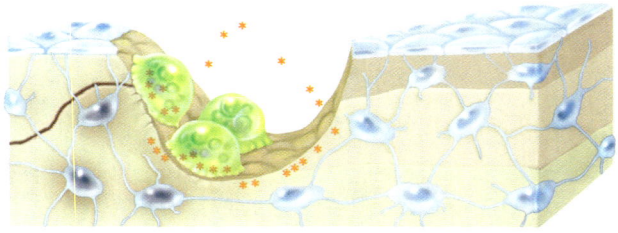

B

FIGURE 22-11 Bisphosphonates reduce fractures by suppressing bone resorption by osteoclasts. The molecular structure of the bisphosphonates is analogous to that of the naturally occurring pyrophosphates. **A.** Bisphosphonate concentration is increased eightfold at sites of active bone resorption. **B.** The bisphosphonates enter osteoclasts and reduce resorption through inhibition of farnesyl pyrophosphate synthase. Inhibition of this enzyme leads to disruption of osteoclast attachment to the bone surface. This halts resorption and promotes early osteoclast cell death.

release bisphosphonates, women must remain upright (sitting or standing) for at least 30 minutes after ingesting the drug. An enteric-coated delayed-release formulation of risedronate (Atelvia) is taken immediately after breakfast with at least 4 ounces of water, and similar upright posture is required.

In terms of long-term safety, two uncommon adverse events are osteonecrosis of the jaw (ONJ) and atypical femur fractures (AFFs) (Diab, 2013). ONJ is defined as exposed necrotic bone in the maxillofacial region that fails to heal after 8 weeks. Pain, paresthesia, soft tissue ulceration, and loose teeth are symptoms. ONJ can develop spontaneously but is generally associated with invasive dental procedures. Although described in patients with osteoporosis receiving chronic bisphosphonate therapy, ONJ is much more common in cancer patients receiving higher-dose bisphosphonates (Khosia, 2007).

AFFs are stress fractures that are frequently bilateral, are typically associated with minimal or no trauma, and are heralded by prodromal pain in the fracture region (Dell, 2012). One study found that longer bisphosphonate use (5 to 9 years) led to a greater risk of AFFs compared with shorter use (<2 years) (Meier, 2012). In one review, bisphosphonate exposure was associated with an adjusted risk ratio of 1.70 for AFFs (Gedmintas, 2013).

The risks of these adverse events may increase after 5 years of therapy, although the likelihood remains low. The FDA suggests reevaluating individually the need for continued bisphosphonate therapy beyond 3 to 5 years (Whitaker, 2012). In selected patients, a "drug holiday" may be considered because of the unique pharmacokinetics of bisphosphonates. These agents accumulate in the skeleton to create a reservoir that continues to be released for months or years after treatment. This provides some residual benefit in terms of fracture reduction after an initial 3- to 5-year therapy course. That said, continuing treatment for 10 years may be a better choice for high-risk patients. If a drug holiday is advised, risk is reevaluated sooner for drugs with lower skeletal affinity. Thus, after a drug holiday, reassessment in high-risk women may be prudent after 1 year for risedronate, 1 to 2 years for alendronate, and 2 to 3 years for zoledronate (Diab, 2014).

Alendronate.
This bisphosphonate is administered orally weekly and marketed as Fosamax or Binosto. With Fosamax, a 35-mg weekly dose is indicated for postmenopausal osteoporosis prevention, whereas a 70-mg weekly dose treats affected women. Binosto carries only the indication of osteoporosis treatment and is provided as a 70-mg weekly dose.

Alendronate reduces the risk of vertebral fractures in postmenopausal women with low BMD or osteoporosis (Black, 1996). Alendronate causes a sustained reduction in risk of nonvertebral fracture risk in women with osteoporosis. For example, women who used alendronate for 5 years and then discontinued use for a subsequent 5 years had nonvertebral fracture rates comparable to those of women using the drug for 10 years (Black, 2006; Bone, 2004).

Risedronate.
This bisphosphonate effectively treats postmenopausal osteoporosis and prevents both vertebral and hip fractures in women with osteoporosis (Cosman, 2014). Several dosages are available. Actonel is indicated for prevention or treatment, and either a 5-mg daily or a 35-mg weekly dosage is recommended. For treatment with Actonel, a 150-mg monthly dose or a 75-mg dose taken once a month on two consecutive days are other options. Atelvia is a 35-mg time-release oral tablet taken weekly and is FDA indicated solely for postmenopausal osteoporosis treatment.

Ibandronate.
This bisphosphonate is FDA approved as Boniva to prevent and treat postmenopausal osteoporosis and has been shown to prevent vertebral fractures in women with osteoporosis (Cosman, 2014). For both indications, a 150-mg oral dose is taken once monthly.

Zoledronate.
This bisphosphonate is FDA approved as Reclast to treat postmenopausal osteoporosis, and it lowers vertebral and hip fracture rates in affected women (Cosman, 2014). Zoledronate is a single, yearly intravenous infusion administered over at least 15 min. It may be a choice for women who cannot safely use oral bisphosphonates due to gastroenterologic concerns.

Denosumab
Denosumab (Prolia) is a fully human monoclonal antibody that binds and inhibits RANK ligand (see Fig. 22-8). Osteoclast development and activity is inhibited, which leads to decreased in bone resorption and greater BMD. As a result, it reduces vertebral and hip fracture rates (Cosman 2014, Bone, 2017). Rare

cases of AFFs and ONJ may complicate long-term therapy. Rapid bone loss occurs after discontinuation, and case reports describe vertebral fractures after discontinuation of denosumab (Anastasilakis, 2017). This underscores compliance with the scheduled 60-mg subcutaneous injection every 6 months. In addition, initiation of an antiresorptive agent such as a bisphosphonate is considered if denosumab therapy is stopped.

Calcitonin
The polypeptide hormone calcitonin slows bone absorption by inhibiting osteoclasts' resorptive activity. Calcitonin is delivered as an injection or nasal spray (Fortical, Miacalcin). Other available options are more effective than calcitonin in preventing bone loss and fracture. However, calcitonin appears to have an independent analgesic effect on bone, which makes it useful as an adjunct to other therapies for osteoporosis in women with painful, symptomatic fracture (Blau, 2003).

■ Parathyroid Hormone–Receptor Agonists
The PTH-receptor agonists teriparatide and abaloparatide are anabolic agents that activate osteoblastic bone formation through interactions with the PTH receptor. Teriparatide (Forteo) is given as a 20-µg daily subcutaneous injection for up to 2 years. It is FDA approved to treat postmenopausal women with established osteoporosis who are at high risk for fracture. At low daily doses, the anabolic effects of PTH predominate. This is in contrast to the catabolic effects generally associated with the long-term, higher-dose, chronic exposure to PTH seen in individuals with hyperparathyroidism.

Teriparatide improves bone microarchitecture and enhances bone quality by increasing bone density, turnover, and size (Rubin, 2002). In women with postmenopausal osteoporosis, teriparatide leads to major reductions in vertebral and nonvertebral fracture rates (Neer, 2001). Among women with prior vertebral fractures, teriparatide more effectively reduced fracture risk than risedronate in one randomized trial (Kendler, 2018). With PTH-receptor agonists, the most frequent adverse events are hypercalcemia, dizziness, leg cramps, nausea, and headache. Following therapy, switching to either bisphosphonate or denosumab therapy will preserve BMD (Ebina, 2017; Leder, 2015).

The second anabolic agent, abaloparatide (Tymlos), is a synthetic analogue of parathyroid hormone–related peptide (PTHrP) that has been modified to potentiate its anabolic effect. In one randomized trial of postmenopausal women with osteoporosis, an 80-µg daily subcutaneous abaloparatide injection reduced the relative risk of vertebral, nonvertebral, major osteoporotic, and clinical fractures compared with placebo. The PTH analogue also better lowers the risk of major osteoporotic vertebral and nonvertebral fractures compared with teriparatide (Miller, 2016). Following discontinuation of abaloparatide, substituting alendronate for an additional 6 months improved BMD and reduced fractures (Cosman, 2017).

For both PTH analogues, toxicity studies with rats have shown a higher risk of osteosarcoma. However, bone metabolism differs greatly between rats and humans, and the relevance of these data to humans is unclear. Both products have a black-box warning on their product labeling recommending avoidance of these agents in those at risk for osteosarcoma. Cumulative use for more than 2 years is not recommended due to the potential for side effects (Tashjian, 2002).

Sclerostin Inhibitor

Romosozumab, a humanized antibody that binds sclerostin, received FDA approval in 2019 to treat postmenopausal women at high risk for fracture. It binds and inhibits the activity of the protein sclerostin, which inhibits activation of osteoblast function. Thus, by blocking sclerostin, romosozumab allows osteoblasts to function. This agent increases bone formation and retards bone breakdown (McClung, 2014).

In clinical trials, romosozumab is more effective than alendronate in preventing vertebral and nonvertebral fractures among women with osteoporosis. Therapy spans 12 months, after which bone effects wane, and should be followed by either denosumab or alendronate (Cosman, 2016; Saag, 2017). Romosozumab carries a black-box warning on its product labeling that describes a potential for increased risks of myocardial infarction, stroke, and cardiovascular death. In clinical trials, ONJ and AFFs also have been reported with romosozumab use.

Therapy Recommendations

First-line therapy for postmenopausal women with osteoporosis includes antiresorptive therapy with a bisphosphonate or denosumab. Women who take bisphosphonates and who are not considered a high risk for fracture may elect a drug holiday, as bisphosphonates have relatively long-term effects in bone. For those receiving denosumab, bone effects are rapidly lost after discontinuation. Thus, a bisphosphonate is recommended after denosumab cessation to maintain BMD gains. For women at high risk for fracture, anabolic agents teriparatide, abaloparatide, and romosozumab provide transient increases in BMD and fracture reduction. These should be followed by antiresorptive treatment with a bisphosphonate or denosumab, again to maintain BMD gains.

Referral to a bone specialist for management is recommended for those at higher risk of fracture. High-risk women include those with severely low T scores (less than –3.0 SD); progressive BMD decline; new vertebral, hip, or fragility fractures; and lack of therapy response. Similarly, referral for evaluation and treatment of secondary osteoporosis or of significant idiopathic osteoporosis in premenopausal women may be considered.

Nonpharmacologic Therapy

Calcium

Nonpharmacologic interventions are cornerstones of osteoporosis prevention and include dietary modifications, exercise programs, fall prevention strategies, and education. The results of studies evaluating effects of calcium and vitamin D supplementation on fracture risk are inconsistent. However, adequate daily calcium intake is essential for bone maintenance. For women aged 31 to 50 years, the recommended dietary reference intake (DRI) is 1000 mg daily, and for those 51 years and older, 1200 mg is recommend daily. Ideally, these DRIs are obtained through diet alone, but supplementation is used to attain these levels if needed (Prentice, 2013; Ross, 2011). Few women meet these goals, and calcium deficiency is widespread. For example, more than 90 percent of women fail to consume enough dietary calcium to meet DRIs put forth by the Institute of Medicine. Although poor calcium intake is observed at all ages, it appears to be most common among older individuals, and <1 percent of women 71 years or older actually meeting recommended goals.

Calcium supplementation combined with vitamin D administration reduces bone loss and fracture risks (Chapuy, 1992; Dawson-Hughes, 1997; Larsen, 2004). Prentice and associates (2013) examined the health benefits and risk of calcium and vitamin D supplementation using WHI data. Again, a substantial hip fracture risk reduction was found. Excess calcium intake is avoided due to enhanced risk of kidney stones, milk alkali syndrome, and possibly cardiovascular events (Bolland, 2008; Jackson, 2006a). Because of concern for potentially greater atherosclerosis risk with calcium supplements, guidelines encourage *dietary* calcium sources to meet recommended amounts.

Vitamin D

The optimal daily vitamin D intake amount and appropriate target levels for serum 25-OH D are unresolved. The vitamin D DRI is 600 IU daily for a postmenopausal woman. For persons at high risk of osteoporosis or who are older than 70 years, 800 IU daily is recommended (Ross, 2011). As with calcium, the prevalence of vitamin D deficiency is high, especially in the elderly and obese. Deficiency leads to poor calcium absorption, secondary hyperparathyroidism, greater bone turnover and bone loss rates, and, if severe, impaired bone mineralization. Vitamin D deficiency also causes muscle weakness that can raise fall rates. Supplementation can reverse many of these effects and significantly lower fall and hip fracture rates (Dawson-Hughes, 1997).

The metabolite 25-hydroxyvitamin D is considered to be the best clinical measure of vitamin D stores (Rosen, 2011). Vitamin D *deficiency* is defined as a serum 25-hydroxyvitamin D level below 10 ng/mL. Vitamin D *insufficiency* is a serum level of 25-hydroxyvitamin D between 10 and 30 ng/mL. Metaanalyses do not support routine supplementation of vitamin D. Moreover, treatment with a very high dose of vitamin D once yearly has been associated with higher fall and fracture rates (Sanders, 2010). The U.S. Preventive Services Task Force (2018b) recommends against daily supplementation with >400 IU of vitamin D and with >1000 mg of calcium for the primary prevention of fractures. For women with a diagnosis of osteoporosis, adequate calcium and vitamin D intake are encouraged.

Diet

A relationship between protein intake and BMD has been reported, but a relationship with either BMD effects or fracture risk are inconsistent (Shams-White, 2017). Using data from the Third National Health and Nutrition Examination Survey (NHANES III), Kerstetter and colleagues (2000) demonstrated a significant association between protein intake and total femur

BMD among non-Hispanic white women aged 50 years and older. Moreover, protein supplementation (20 g/d) five times weekly for 6 months following hip fracture was associated with a 50-percent reduction in femoral bone loss at 1 year compared with placebo. Higher protein intake is also associated with fewer falls in at-risk elderly patients losing weight (Zoltick, 2011).

Healthy diets that provide the daily DRI of protein contain at least 46 g/d for women (Dawson-Hughes, 2002). Notably, excess urinary calcium excretion is observed with the large acid loads delivered by very-high-protein diets (Barzel, 1998).

Caffeine consumption does not appear to influence bone health in postmenopausal women who maintain an adequate daily intake of calcium and vitamin D. However, one longitudinal study showed that even moderate amounts of caffeine (two to three servings of coffee daily) may lead to bone loss in women with low calcium intake (<800 mg/d) (Harris, 1994).

Calcium reabsorption is directly proportional to sodium reabsorption in the renal tubule. Accordingly, greater dietary sodium increases urinary calcium excretion and corresponding biochemical markers of bone turnover. Specifically, a relationship between high sodium intake (>1768 mg/d) and lower BMD is described (Sellmeyer, 2002). This sodium effect appears to be independent of calcium intake and activity levels. As with caffeine, sodium intake moderation is a reasonable precautionary measure until this relationship is fully understood.

Providing magnesium supplements to patients with malabsorption may be warranted, but routine magnesium supplementation is ineffective for fracture prevention. Phytoestrogens have not shown consistent effects on bone and are not recommended for bone protection.

Physical Preventions

Small but statistically significant increases in BMD have been observed in postmenopausal women participating in exercise programs, including aerobic exercise and resistance training (heavy weight with few repetitions). One metaanalysis of 43 trials concluded that lower-limb resistance exercise was most effective for femur neck BMD, and combination-exercise programs most benefitted vertebral BMD (Howe, 2011). Another analysis that focused on walking showed advantages for femur neck BMD accrual (Ma, 2013). Strength training or resistance training is recommended for at least 30 minutes three times per week and includes free weights or resistance bands, walking or jogging, and jumping.

Although BMD may accrue, especially at exercise-directed sites, benefits also extend to lower fall rates (Carter, 2002). Namely, improved balance, stronger muscles, better muscle tone, and stronger, more flexible bone all contribute to fracture prevention.

Falls are responsible for more than 90 percent of hip fractures (Carter, 2002). Sideways falls appear to be the most detrimental and were independently associated with hip fracture in a study by Greenspan and associates (1998). Therefore, assessing women for fall risk and fall prevention are essential for women with osteopenia or osteoporosis.

Falls are associated with general frailty, such as reduced muscle strength, impaired balance, low body mass, and diminished

visual acuity (Delaney, 2006; U.S. Preventive Services Task Force, 2018a). Alcohol and sedative drug use are others.

Living conditions are modified to minimize falls by reducing clutter and implementing nonslip tiles, nonskid strips to bath and shower floor, safety bars, rugs with nonskid backing, night lights, wearing shoes with traction, and avoiding slippery or icy sidewalks. Hip protectors have been suggested for those at high risk for falling. However, these appear effective only in supervised long-term care facilities (Santesso, 2014).

GENITOURINARY SYNDROME OF MENOPAUSE

■ Terminology

High concentrations of estrogen receptors are present in the vaginal mucosa, vulva, bladder, urethra, and pelvic floor of pre- and postmenopausal women (see Fig. 22-6). Hypoestrogenism can lead to deleterious changes in this highly interdependent anatomy.

The term *vulvovaginal atrophy* has been used to describe the constellation of lower reproductive tract changes stemming from hypoestrogenism. However, midlife women may view the word *atrophy* negatively. More importantly, the term fails to adequately emphasize the global genitourinary effects. Accordingly, a consensus panel and national organizations now recommend *genitourinary syndrome of menopause (GSM)* as preferred terminology (Portman, 2014). GSM encompasses the constellation of pathophysiologic signs and symptoms listed in Table 22-10.

■ Vulvovaginal Changes

Endogenous E_2 causes the vaginal mucosa to become a thick, well-vascularized, rugated surface that supplies adequate lubrication for most premenopausal women. Low estrogen levels cause atrophic changes, in which the vagina shortens, narrows, and loses flexibility. The vaginal mucosa becomes thin and shiny, and rugae are flattened. The introitus may contract,

TABLE 22-10. Genitourinary Syndrome of Menopause Characteristics

Symptoms	Signs
Genital dryness	Labia minora resorption
Poor lubrication	Narrowed introitus
Dyspareunia	Absent hymeneal tags
Postcoital bleeding	Tissue pallor or erythema
Poor arousal, orgasm, desire	Urethral eversion
Vulvovaginal:	Urethral prolapse
irritation, burning, itching	Prominent urethral meatus
Dysuria	Absent rugae
Urinary frequency	Fragile or fissured tissue
Urinary urgency	Petechial hemorrhages
Recurrent urinary tract	Scant vaginal secretions
infection	Poor elasticity

particularly in the absence of penetrative sexual activity, and these changes can diminish lubrication during sexual stimulation. A hypoestrogenic vaginal squamous epithelium thins to only a few cell layers, and parabasal squamous cells outnumber superficial ones. The thin vaginal mucosa becomes friable and prone to bleed even with minimal trauma. Advanced changes resulting from estrogen deficiency lead to inflammation, resulting in what some clinicians refer to as *atrophic vaginitis* (The North American Menopause Society, 2013).

■ Clinical Findings

GSM symptoms are common during the MT, and the estimated prevalence among menopausal women is 50 percent (Simon, 2018). In a large observational study, vaginal dryness and dyspareunia were two of the most prevalent GSM symptoms (Palma, 2018). Surveys of menopausal women document the high prevalence of these symptoms and underscore their negative effects on sexual function, partner relationships, and quality of life (Kingsberg, 2017; Nappi 2016). Three quarters of women in the United States aged 57 to 74 are sexually active (Crawford, 2018; Lindau, 2007). Although dryness and pain with intercourse are prevalent among midlife women, few seek help. Thus, during well women visits, clinicians ideally ask about GSM symptoms to provide an opportunity for improvement.

Although a characteristic history will suggest GSM, a pelvic examination can exclude other vulvovaginal conditions that may cause similar symptoms, including chronic infections, contact dermatitis, lichen sclerosus, lichen planus, and malignancy. During menopause, the mons pubis and labia majora and minora lose bulk, whereas the urethral meatus may be prominent and erythematous. If introital or vaginal narrowing is present, use of a thin pediatric speculum with a lubricant (Fig. 1-3, p. 4) can minimize patient discomfort. The vaginal mucosa may appear smooth, shiny, and dry. Petechiae can form after minimal blunt pressure from the speculum, and sweeps with a spatula or cotton-tip swab may cause spotting. Vaginal fornices may become attenuated and result in a cervix that is flush with the vaginal apex.

Laboratory assessment is not required to diagnose GSM. However, vaginal pH and the vaginal maturation index (MI) may be informative. To assess pH, a piece of litmus paper is placed on the lateral vaginal wall until it becomes moistened. Premenopausal women without vaginal atrophy typically have a pH ≤4.5 unless they have bacterial vaginosis or trichomoniasis. A pH ≥4.6, which may be as high as 7, indicates vaginal atrophy.

A specimen to measure the MI may be collected during a vaginal speculum examination at the same time cervical cancer screening is performed. The index report is read from left to right and refers to the percentage of parabasal, intermediate, and superficial squamous cells appearing on a smear, with the total sum of all three values equaling 100 percent (Fig. 22-12) (Randolph, 2005). For example, an MI of 0:40:60 represents 0 percent parabasal cells, 40 percent intermediate cells, and 60 percent superficial cells. This MI reflects adequate vaginal estrogen influence. A shift to the left indicates an increase in parabasal or intermediate cells, which denotes low estrogen effects.

■ Treatment

Nonhormonal Options

Many women may indicate that they have few if any GSM symptoms or, if present, may choose to not treat them. However, clinicians should counsel affected women that, absent active management, this condition may worsen over time. In women without severe symptoms, over-the-counter water- or silicone-based vaginal lubricants for sexual activity and regular use of long-acting vaginal moisturizers are appropriate (Pinkerton, 2018). In this setting, women are informed that regular sexual activity including penetration by partner or device may help address symptoms and prevent progression. In some women, contraction of the introitus/vagina or vaginismus may prevent penetration. Use of graduated vaginal dilators, sometimes under the guidance of a specialized physical therapist who focuses on pelvic floor disorders, often allows these women to resume or initiate comfortable sexual activity. Initiating low-dose vaginal ET can accelerate progress.

Estrogen Options

Among women using standard-dose systemic HT to treat VMS, symptomatic GSM is uncommon. However, some women will experience vaginal dryness, dyspareunia, or other GSM symptoms during systemic HT use, particularly if lower than standard HT doses are used. In these patients, low-dose vaginal estrogen can be added to systemic HT. Alternatively, a woman using oral or transdermal systemic HT can change to the 3-month systemic vaginal ring (Femring), which releases 0.05 mg/d or 0.10 mg/d of E_2. This treats vaginal and vasomotor symptoms. Importantly, the systemic vaginal estradiol ring (Femring) differs from the 3-month local vaginal ring (Estring), which releases 7.5 μ/d of E_2. The latter is indicated solely for GSM.

Although over-the-counter lubricant and moisturizer use constitutes appropriate initial treatment for women with symptomatic GSM, prescription treatments for GSM are appropriate for inadequately addressed symptoms. Low-dose vaginal ET is highly effective in treating symptomatic GSM, and tablets, rings, and creams have comparable efficacy (Lethaby, 2016). In addition, vaginal estrogen may help prevent recurrent urinary tract infections (UTIs) and overactive bladder symptoms in menopausal women. Systemic HT, in contrast, has been found to increase urinary incontinence incidence (The North American Menopause Society, 2013).

In the United States, two low-dose estrogen creams, a ring, a tablet, and inserts are available for vaginal use (Table 22-11). Creams are applied either digitally or with graduated, plastic applicators supplied with each tube. An advantage of the creams is that they can also be applied digitally to the vaginal vestibule. Less cream may be wasted with digital vulvovaginal application, which may extend the life of each tube. One disadvantage of creams is that some women find them messy.

The 3-month low-dose vaginal ring (Estring) releases 7.5 μg/d of E_2. For users, an advantage of the ring is the convenience of placement and removal only once every 3 months. However, some women are not comfortable inserting or removing the ring. Many women, as well as their partners, choose to leave

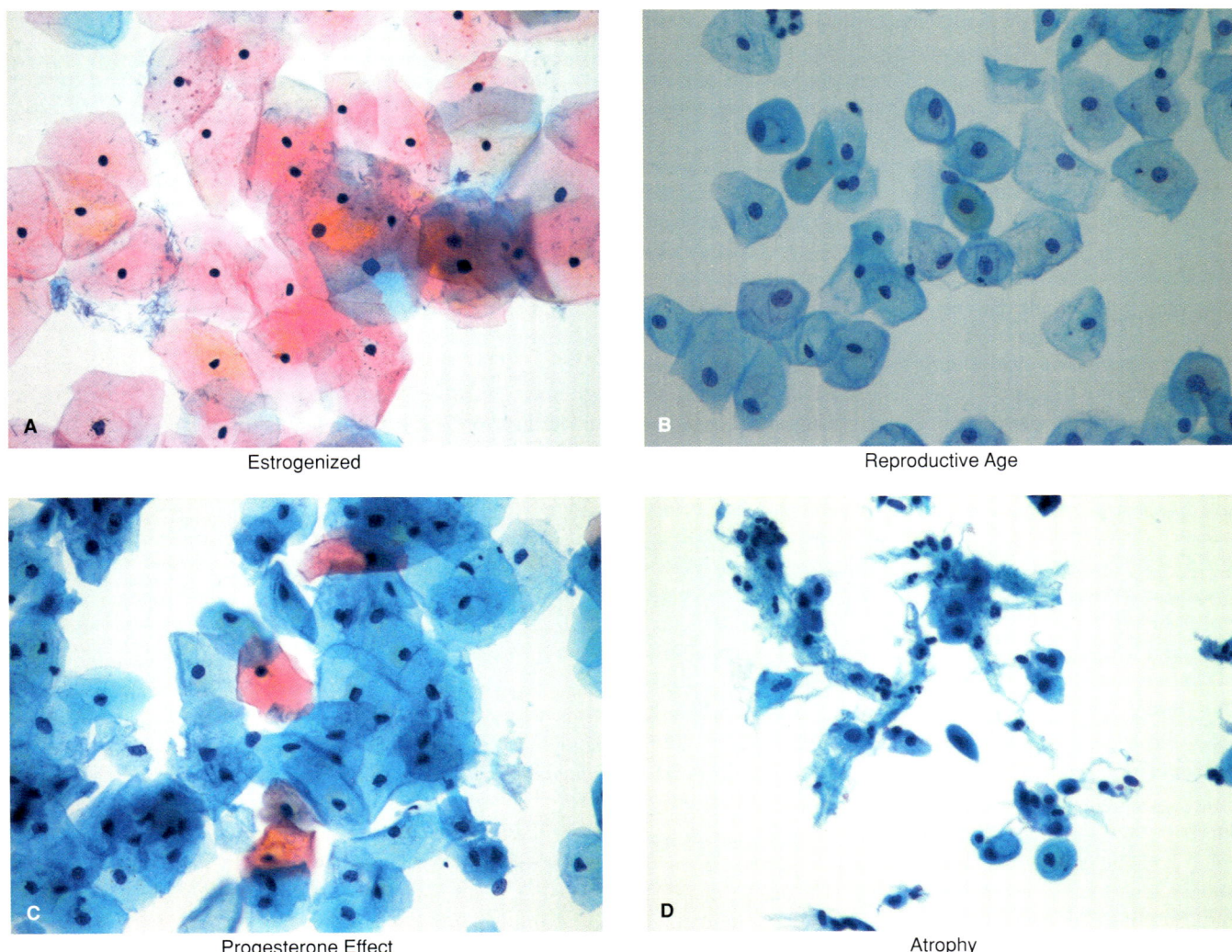

Estrogenized

Reproductive Age

Progesterone Effect

Atrophy

FIGURE 22-12 Cytologic specimens illustrate key points of the maturation index. This index provides insight into the cytohormonal status of the patient and is based on a count of parabasal, intermediate, and superficial (P:I:S) cells. Generally, a predominance of superficial or superficial and intermediate cells (**A** and **B**) is seen in reproductive-aged women. **C.** A predominance of intermediate cells is seen in the luteal phase, in pregnancy, with amenorrhea, and in newborns, premenarchal girls, and women in early menopausal transition. **D.** A predominance of parabasal cells is seen in menopausal patients with atrophy. (Reproduced with permission from Dr. Raheela Ashfaq.)

the ring in place during intercourse. If the ring is removed, it can be rinsed, avoiding detergent and hot water, and replaced as soon as possible.

Vaginal tablets (Vagifem or generic) employ a single-use plastic applicator to place one tablet nightly for two weeks and then twice weekly for maintenance therapy. Some women find the tablets less messy than creams. Another advantage is the thinner applicator compared with cream applicators.

In 2018, vaginal inserts (Imvexxy) were approved for treatment of moderate to severe dyspareunia associated with GSM. The inserts are placed digitally in the vagina without an applicator. The 4-μg insert is the lowest-dose vaginal E_2 formulation available (Constantine, 2017).

Guidance from the American College of Obstetricians and Gynecologists and the North American Menopause Society advise that low-dose vaginal ET may be used as long as needed. These groups additionally do not advise routine use of concomitant progestogen therapy for endometrial protection

during long-term vaginal ET use. However, randomized trials assessing the endometrial safety of vaginal ET for longer than 1 year are not available. Endometrial evaluation is appropriate for women reporting vaginal spotting or bleeding during use of low-dose vaginal ET, as discussed in Chapter 8 (p. 183). In women without bleeding, routine endometrial surveillance is not recommended (American College of Obstetricians and Gynecologists, 2018c; The North American Menopause Society, 2013).

Current package labelling for low-dose vaginal ET, as for all systemic HT formulations, contains a black-box warning that mentions endometrial cancer, myocardial infarction, stroke, invasive breast cancer, pulmonary embolism, and dementia. This warning relates to safety concerns resulting from findings from clinical trials of systemic HT (p. 480). However, blood steroid levels are considerably less with low-dose vaginal ET formulations than with those observed during use of systemic ET. Moreover, clinical trials do not suggest an elevated risk of

TABLE 22-11. Selected Preparations for Genitourinary Symptoms of Menopause[a]

Preparation	Generic Name	Brand Name	Dose	Generic Available
Vaginal cream	Conjugated estrogens	Premarin	0.625 mg per 1 g cream (0.5 g twice wkly or 0.5 g/d for 3 wks, then 1 wk off. May titrate up to 2 g per application) (30-g tube)	No
	17β-Estradiol	Estrace	0.1 mg per 1 g cream (2–4 g/d for 1–2 wks, then 1–2 g/d for 1–2 wks, then 1–2 g 1 to 3 times wkly) (42.5-g tube)	Yes
Vaginal tablet	Estradiol	Vagifem	0.01-mg tablet (1 tablet/d for 2 wks, then 1 tablet twice weekly)	Yes
Vaginal ring	17β-Estradiol	Estring	2-mg ring delivers 7.5 µg daily (remains for 90 d)	No
Vaginal insert	Estradiol	Imvexxy	4-µg or 10-µg insert (1 insert/d for 2 wks, then 1 insert twice wkly)	No
	Prasterone	Intrarosa	6.5-mg insert daily	No
Oral tablet	Ospemifene	Osphena	60-mg tablet daily	No

[a]Most estrogen-containing products listed in Table 22-4 for the treatment of menopausal hot flashes are also approved for the treatment of vaginal dryness.

these adverse events. As a result, revised labeling that would better educate prescribers and women to these formulations' risk and benefits was advanced by several national organizations in women's health (Manson, 2014). However, the FDA rejected proposed changes, and the boxed warning continues on all systemic *and* vaginal estrogen-containing products.

Two large observational studies provide reassuring information regarding the safety of vaginal ET. In the WHI, more than 1500 women used vaginal ET for a median duration of 2 years. This practice did not raise associated risks for CHD, VTE, or endometrial, breast, or colorectal cancer (Crandall, 2018). Similarly, in the Nurse's Health Study, almost 900 women used vaginal ET for a mean duration of 3 years, and none of these same adverse-event rates was increased (Bhupathiraju, 2018).

Dehydroepiandrosterone or Prasterone

DHEA, also known as *prasterone*, is transformed by vaginal epithelial cells to various estrogens, including E_2, and into androgens, including testosterone (Labrie, 2018). In 2016, 6.5-mg prasterone tablets (Intrarosa) were approved for GSM treatment and are administered intravaginally nightly using a single-use plastic applicator. Data have not yet been published on its effects and safety in women with breast cancer or on aromatase inhibitors.

Ospemifene

The SERM ospemifene, provided in a 60-mg oral tablet (Osphena), also is FDA approved for treatment of dyspareunia associated with GSM. Use of an oral agent may appeal to women who prefer a nonvaginal route. A large 1-year clinical trial did not identify endometrial safety concerns (see Table 22-2). However, 2 percent of those receiving placebo reported hot flashes, whereas 7 percent of those taking ospemifene reported

VMS (Simon, 2013). Other SERMs, including tamoxifen and raloxifene, can prompt VMS and raise VTE rates. The risk of similar effects with ospemifene is unknown (Simon, 2018).

Laser Therapy

GSM treatment of the vaginal wall with a carbon dioxide (CO_2) or yttrium-aluminum-garnet (YAG) laser is controversial. Minimally ablative fractional laser therapies are thought to activate cellular repair mechanisms. This in turn is suggested to enhance vascularity and collagen synthesis to thicken the vaginal wall. Histologic evaluation shows improvement similar to that from vaginal ET. Small studies have found that the fractional CO_2 laser significantly diminishes GSM symptoms after three vaginal laser treatments compared with baseline measures. YAG laser treatment has improved symptoms of GSM and stress urinary incontinence (Cruz, 2018; Rabley, 2018; Sokol, 2017). However, the FDA (2018) has not approved CO_2 laser therapy for GSM treatment and warns against its use without data from long-term, well-controlled studies. The American College of Obstetricians and Gynecologists (2016) echoes these concerns.

■ Dyspareunia

Sexual function declines with advancing menopause status, independently of age. The most frequently reported associated symptoms include low sexual desire, dyspareunia, and poor vaginal lubrication. Discussed in Chapters 4, 12, and 14, dyspareunia and sexual dysfunction are each rooted in a wide range of predisposing, precipitating, and maintaining factors, which may be biologic, psychologic, or sociocultural in origin (pp. 266, 312). In one study, 25 percent of postmenopausal women noted some degree of dyspareunia (Laumann, 1999). These same investigators found that painful intercourse correlated with lack of libido, arousal disorder, and anorgasmia. Dennerstein (2005) prospectively evaluated 438 Australian women during 6 years of their MT. Menopause was significantly associated with dyspareunia and indirectly with sexual response. Levine and colleagues (2008) studied 1480 sexually active postmenopausal women and found that the prevalence of vulvovaginal atrophy and of female sexual dysfunction each approximated 55 percent. Women with sexual dysfunction were nearly four times more likely to have vulvovaginal atrophy than women without such dysfunction.

Estrogen deficiency diminishes vaginal lubrication, blood flow, and vasocongestion with sexual activity. These changes are coupled with the structural atrophy described earlier (p. 495). Reduced testosterone levels also are implicated in genital atrophy, but the relationship between testosterone and sexuality during MT remains obscure. Circulating testosterone levels decline gradually with age from the mid-reproductive years and have dropped by 50 percent by age 45. Paradoxically, studies have not demonstrated that sexual dysfunction is related to decreased androgen levels in MT (O'Neil, 2011).

Urogenital conditions such as prolapse or incontinence correlate strongly with sexual dysfunction (Barber, 2002; Salonia, 2004). Discussed in Chapter 23, patients with urinary incontinence may have pelvic-floor hypertonicity, which may cause pain on deep penetration due to pelvic support instability (p. 519). Hypertonic or dyssynergic pelvic-floor muscles, prevalent among women with urinary frequency, constipation, and vaginismus, are often associated with superficial pain and friction during intercourse (Handa, 2004). Discussed in Chapter 24, pelvic organ prolapse may contribute to dyspareunia (p. 541). In addition, prolapse-correcting surgery may cause dyspareunia by shortening or narrowing the vagina (Goldberg, 2001). Chronic pelvic pain or abdominal and vulvar scars or adhesions also may be contributors to sexual dysfunction as discussed in Chapter 12 (p. 257).

■ Urogynecologic Changes

As part of the GSM spectrum, urinary symptoms can include dysuria, urinary urgency, urethral eversion or prolapse, and recurrent UTIs (Portman, 2014: Trutnovsky, 2014). Discussed in Chapter 23, these can be associated with urethral and bladder mucosal thinning, and thus a trial of vaginal ET is reasonable (p. 513) (Cody, 2012; Eriksen, 1999; Rahn, 2014).

The association between declining estrogen levels and incontinence is more controversial. In support of a causal link, urethral shortening associated with menopausal atrophic changes may result in stress urinary incontinence. Waetjen and coworkers (2009) evaluated women in MT and found slightly higher stress and urgency incontinence rates. In addition, they identified that these urinary symptoms were robustly associated with worsening anxiety, high baseline BMI, weight gain, and new-onset diabetes. They concluded that clinicians and women should focus first on these modifiable risk factors. Sherburn and colleagues (2001) performed a cross-sectional study of women aged 45 to 55 years to determine if MT itself was associated with incontinence. The overall incidence was 35 percent, with no increase associated with menopause.

Similarly, in a study of 382 women, stress and urgency urinary incontinence and the number of years following menopause were not significantly associated (Trutnovsky, 2014).

The effects of systemic HT on incontinence are conflicting. Bhatia and colleagues (1989) showed that systemic ET may improve or cure stress urinary incontinence in more than 50 percent of treated women, presumably by exerting a direct effect on urethral mucosa coaptation (Chap. 23, p. 528). However, two large trials noted that systemic HT users had a higher incidence of stress urinary incontinence (Hendrix, 2005; Jackson, 2006c).

With respect to vaginal ET, incontinence may be improved by enhancing periurethral and bladder-neck vascularity (Long, 2006). It also diminishes detrusor-contraction frequency and amplitude (Robinson, 2014). Thus, vaginal ET, when coupled with other strategies such as pelvic floor muscle training or pessary use, may have benefits. Evidence to support HT use for pelvic organ prolapse prevention is poor (Ismail 2010).

PSYCHOSOCIAL CHANGES

■ Libido Changes

Definitive data correlating the relationship between circulating hormone levels and libido are lacking. In the Massachusetts Women's Health Study II, sexual function in 200 women who underwent natural menopause was evaluated. None took HT, and all had sexual partners. Menopausal status significantly related to decreased sexual interest. However, after adjusting for physical and mental health, smoking, and marital satisfaction, the two were no longer associated. Indeed, many studies demonstrate that other factors besides menopause may account for libido changes (Gracia, 2007).

Some data, however, do show a link with menopause. A longitudinal study of women during MT until at least 1 year after the FMP demonstrated a significant decline in the rate of weekly coitus. Patients reported a significant drop in the number of sexual thoughts, sexual satisfactions, and vaginal lubrication after becoming menopausal (McCoy, 1985). In a study of 100 naturally menopausal women, both sexual desire and activity decreased compared with that during the premenopausal period. Women reported loss of libido, dyspareunia, and orgasmic dysfunction, and 86 percent reported no orgasms after menopause (Tungphaisal, 1991).

Estrogen can help GSM symptoms, as described on page 496. However, HT is not recommended as the sole treatment of other problems of sexual function, including diminished libido (North American Menopause Society, 2017).

Hypoactive Sexual Desire

Female sexual desire disorders include hypoactive sexual desire disorder (HSDD), female sexual arousal disorder, and orgasmic disorder/dysfunction. These may stem from neuroendocrine imbalance, ill health, interpersonal conflict, psychologic distress, and cultural or religious values. Discussed in Chapter 14 (p. 314), treatment options may include HT or other pharmacologic therapy combined with psychotherapy (Clayton, 2018; Kingsberg, 2017).

Androgen Therapy

Androgen therapy in women with HSDD is controversial. Androgen assays lack sensitivity and specificity, yielding uncertain associations between endogenous androgen concentrations and sexual function in women. Androgens can be converted in tissues, and there may be intracrine metabolism. No circulating androgen blood levels differentiate women with and without sexual dysfunction (Davis, 2019). Some studies document an association between androgen treatment and improved sexual desire, but large, quality trials with long-term surveillance are needed (Lobo, 2003; Pauls, 2005; Shifren, 2000). DHEA is an androgen precursor, and systematic reviews show no or only slightly improved sexual functioning in postmenopausal women taking this steroid systemically (Elraiyah, 2014; Scheffers, 2015). In contrast, vaginal DHEA is approved to treat GSM and improves sexual function in those women (p. 498).

Symptoms of androgen insufficiency include diminished sense of well-being, persistent fatigue, sexual function changes, and low serum free-testosterone levels. Women with these findings may be offered androgen therapy off label only, as no testosterone formulation is approved by the FDA for use in women. Therapy should be performed under close clinician supervision (Wierman, 2014).

Early effects of androgen therapy include acne and hirsutism. One study reported a 3-percent higher rate of acne in testosterone-therapy groups (Lobo, 2003). Long-term side effects such as male pattern baldness, voice deepening, and clitoral hypertrophy are infrequent within normal androgen levels. Androgen therapy may adversely affect the lipid profile, and long-term effects on cardiovascular and breast cancer risks are unknown (Braunstein, 2007; Davis, 2012, 2013).

A recent global consensus, following an extensive review and metaanalysis, concluded that testosterone therapy, *in doses that approximate physiologic testosterone concentrations for premenopausal women,* exert a beneficial effect on sexual function compared with placebo or comparator therapy. This was quantified as approximately one satisfying sexual event per month (Davis, 2019; Islam, 2019). Testosterone therapy enhances sexual desire, arousal, orgasmic function, pleasure, and sexual responsiveness and reduces sexual distress.

These doses of testosterone were noted to mildly promote acne and body and facial hair growth but not cause alopecia, clitoromegaly, or voice change. Although oral testosterone is associated with atherogenic lipid changes, non-oral, premenopausal-range doses are not associated with lipid changes, higher blood pressure, increased blood glucose or HbA_{1c} levels, or greater breast cancer risk with short-term use. The safety of physiologic doses of testosterone has been assessed for up to 2 years of use in healthy women without comorbidities. Based on expert opinion, the consensus group recommended that if an appropriate approved female testosterone preparation was not available, off-label prescribing of an approved male formulation would be reasonable. This was coupled with the provision that hormone concentrations are monitored and maintained in a physiologic female range. Supraphysiologic blood concentrations of testosterone provided by injections or pellets are not recommended.

■ Depression

Women carry a higher lifetime risk of developing depression than men. The risk of developing a major depressive disorder is 1.5 times higher in women than in men, particularly during reproductive years. A prior depressive episode, particularly if related to reproductive events, remains the strongest predictor of mood disorders or depression during midlife. VMS, anxiety, and other health-related issues can modulate depression risks (Soares, 2014).

Contemporary findings dispel myths that natural menopause itself is associated with depressed mood (Ballinger, 1990; Busch, 1994). However, a higher rate of depressive symptoms during MT is repeatedly observed in population-based studies. In the Penn Ovarian Aging Study, the risk was nearly three times higher in women in MT compared with premenopausal women. Moreover, women with no history of depression were two and a half times more likely to report depressed mood during MT than during the premenopausal period (Freeman, 2004). Other cohort studies report similar findings (Bromberger, 2011; Cohen, 2006; Dennerstein, 2004; Woods, 2008). Moreover, a high percentage of subjects suffer recurrent depression during MT (Freeman, 2007). Thus, a screen for depression is prudent for women in this transition, and tools are described in Chapters 1 (p. 18) and 14 (p. 303).

It has been suggested that significant and erratic hormonal fluctuations during early MT are in part responsible (Soares, 2005). Ballinger and colleagues (1990) showed that increased stress hormone levels and probably stress-related symptoms are physiologically linked with high estrogen levels. They also reported that women with abnormal psychometric test scores early after menopause had higher E_2 levels than women with lower scores. Spinelli and associates (2005) showed that estrogen levels correlate with menopausal symptom intensity. Moreover, in a randomized menopause-treatment study, standard CEE doses (0.625 mg/d) significantly improved sleep but also were associated with an estrogen-related increase in inward-directed hostility (Schiff, 1980).

Importantly, MT is a complex sociocultural event, and psychosocial factors may contribute to mood and cognitive symptoms. Women entering MT may face emotional stress from onset of a major illness, caring for an adolescent or aging parent, divorce or widowhood, and career change or retirement. Lock (1991) suggests that part of the stress reported by Western women is clearly culture-specific. Western culture emphasizes beauty and youth, and as women grow older, some suffer from a perceived loss of status, function, and control (LeBoeuf, 1996). For some women, the approach of menopause may also be perceived as a significant loss, both to women who have accepted childbearing and rearing as their major life roles and to those who are childless, perhaps not by choice. For these reasons, impending menopause may be perceived as a time of loss, when depression and other psychological disorders may develop (Avis, 2000). New guidelines recognize a greater risk of depression during perimenopause, and those with a prior depressive episode carry a higher risk. Women often present with classic depression symptoms and coexistent menopausal hot flashes, sleep disturbances, and psychosocial changes, making the diagnosis more challenging (Maki, 2018).

Discussed in Chapter 14 (p. 309), antidepressant medications combined with psychotherapy and counseling are principal therapeutic interventions for women with depression. HT is not considered treatment for depression. However, lesser mood symptoms may be improved concurrently with hot flash frequency and disrupted sleep (Soares, 2001; Zweifel, 1997). Fewer data are available for EPT than ET (Maki, 2018). For those with bothersome VMS and disordered mood during MT, a trial of HT may be elected. Specifically, consideration may be given to those who fail to respond to a conventional first-line intervention, those who refuse to take psychotropic agents, or those who will begin HT for other acute menopausal symptoms and who could delay antidepressant therapy until determining whether HT is sufficient.

CENTRAL NERVOUS SYSTEM

■ Sleep Dysfunction and Fatigue

Sleep quality declines with age, but MT appears to contribute. As women traverse MT, the self-reported poor-sleep rate rises, and the rate was 38 percent in the 12,603 women participating in the SWAN study (Hall, 2009). As with most menopausal symptoms, severity and prevalence both seem to peak during late MT, when women experience prolonged amenorrhea. Women may wake several times during the night and may be drenched in sweat. In one study, late-reproductive-aged women with a greater frequency of hot flashes were more likely to report poor sleep than were women with fewer VMS events (Hollander, 2001). In one study, 255 women were premenopausal at cohort enrollment, underwent natural menopause, and were followed for 16 years. The most important predictor of moderate or severe poor sleep during MT was the premenopausal sleep status. Hot flashes contributed to poor sleep regardless of baseline sleep status (Freeman, 2015). Nocturnal hot flashes are felt to be an important component, particularly in women with severe sleep difficulties (Baker, 2018).

Even women with mild VMS may experience insomnia (Erlik, 1982; Woodward, 1994). As women age, they are more likely to experience lighter sleep and are awakened more easily by pain, sound, or bodily urges. Health issues and other chronic conditions experienced by women or by their spouse or bedmate are likely to further disrupt sleep. Arthritis, carpal tunnel syndrome, chronic lung disease, heartburn, and certain medications that are known to disrupt sleep may dramatically lower the quality and quantity of restful sleep. Nocturia, urinary frequency, and urgency, all of which are more common in menopausal women, are other notable factors.

Sleep disordered breathing, which includes various degrees of pharyngeal obstruction, is common in menopausal women and their mates. Loud snoring can follow partial upper airway obstruction that ranges in severity from upper airway resistance to *obstructive sleep apnea (OSA)* (Gislason, 1993). OSA can have associated health consequences, and one screening method is found in Chapter 39 (p. 839). In women, sleep disordered breathing is often associated with higher BMI and declining estrogen and progesterone levels.

Disturbed sleep can lead to fatigue, irritability, depressive symptoms, cognitive dysfunction, and impaired daily functioning.

Common sense education components may include control of sleep timing and duration, attempts to improve the bedroom environment, or relaxation or biofeedback techniques. Importantly, although fatigue may stem from night sweats and poor sleep, other common potential etiologies, such as anemia or thyroid disease, among others, also are considered. In all these examples, treatment of underlying health conditions is the main focus to improve patient sleep. At times, short-term use of pharmacologic sleep aids is indicated, and these are listed in Table 1-16 (p. 19). HT can improve sleep disturbances and sleep quality, often along with improvement in hot flash frequency (Cintron, 2017).

■ Cognitive Dysfunction

Memory declines with advancing age. Although no direct effect of lowered estrogen levels on memory and cognition has been determined, many investigators suspect a relationship between the two. Cognitive functioning was assessed in a cohort study of reproductive-aged and postmenopausal women not using HT. In postmenopausal patients, cognitive performance declined with advancing age. This was not the case for reproductive-aged women. Premenopausal women in their 40s were less likely to exhibit cognitive decline compared with postmenopausal patients in the same decade of life. These researchers concluded that deterioration of some forms of cognitive function is accelerated after menopause (Halbreich, 1995).

In another study, 643 healthy postmenopausal women not using HT were grouped as early (<6 years after menopause) and late (>10 years after menopause) and underwent a comprehensive neuropsychologic battery (Henderson, 2013). Concurrently, serum hormone levels were measured. Cognitive outcomes included verbal memory, executive function, and global cognition scores. Endogenous sex steroid levels were unassociated with composite scores, but SHBG levels were positively associated with verbal memory. Results for early and late groups did not differ significantly, although progesterone concentrations were significantly positively associated with verbal memory and global cognition in early group women. Hormone levels were not significantly related to mood.

Factors accelerating cerebral degenerative changes represent potentially modifiable risks for cognitive decline (Kuller, 2003; Meyer, 1999). Risk factors for decreased cerebral perfusion and thinning of gray and white matter densities include prior transient ischemic attacks (TIAs), hyperlipidemia, hypertension, smoking, excess alcohol consumption, and male gender, which would imply lack of estrogen. Investigators encourage interventions to modify many of these risks.

■ Alzheimer Senile Dementia

Dementia is defined as a progressive decline in intellectual and cognitive function. Its causes can be categorized into three broad groups: (1) cases in which the brain is the target of a systemic illness; (2) primary structural causes such as tumor; and (3) primary degenerative diseases of the nervous system, such as senile dementia of the Alzheimer type (SDAT). It is estimated that up to 50 percent of women aged 85 years or older may suffer from senile dementia or SDAT. Early signs may be subtle, and testing strategies are found in Chapter 1 (p. 18).

The role of estrogen in dementia prevention is controversial. Several epidemiologic studies suggested that HT prevents SDAT development. Moreover, metaanalyses of observational studies show that HT is associated with a lower risk of dementia but does not improve established disease (Yaffe, 1998; Zandi, 2002). However, data from a large randomized trial found no preventive role. Women enrolled in the Women's Health Initiative Memory Study (WHIMS), an ancillary study of the WHI, had higher rates of dementia compared with those given placebo (Shumaker, 2003, 2004). Notably, this increased risk was statistically significant only in the group of women >75 years. This observation is concerning for its long-term implications for HT in older postmenopausal women. It is unclear whether, similar to CHD, a critical window and timing hypotheses alter HT effects on SDAT development. Unfortunately, these mixed findings leave unanswered questions regarding HT's efficacy in preventing dementia in postmenopausal women. Currently, HT is not recommended for this indication.

OTHER PHYSIOLOGIC CHANGES

■ Cardiovascular Changes

In women older than 50 years, atherosclerotic cardiovascular disease (CVD) remains the leading cause of death. Before menopause, women have a much lower risk for cardiovascular events compared with men their same age. Reasons for protection from CVD in premenopausal women are complex, but a significant contribution is assigned to greater high-density lipoprotein (HDL) levels in younger women, which is an effect of estrogen. However, after menopause, this benefit disappears over time such that a 70-year-old woman begins to have a CVD risk identical to that of a man of comparable age (Matthews, 1989). The risk of CVD increases dramatically for women as they enter menopause and as estrogen levels decline (Matthews, 1994; van Beresteijn, 1993). This becomes vitally important for women in MT, when preventive measures can significantly improve both life quality and quantity. The value of HT to alter CVD risks was described earlier on page 480. Preventive measures are outlined in Chapter 1 (p. 15).

■ Weight Gain and Fat Distribution

Weight gain is a common complaint during MT (Karvonen, 2016). On average, women gain 1.5 pounds per year during the fifth and sixth decades independent of initial body size, race, or ethnicity (Sternfeld, 2004). With aging, a woman's metabolism slows, reducing her caloric requirements. If eating and exercise habits are not altered, weight is gained (Matthews, 2001). Specifically, Espeland and associates (1997) characterized the weight and fat distribution of 875 women in the Postmenopausal Estrogen/Progestin Interventions (PEPI) trial and correlated the effects of lifestyle, clinical, and demographic factors. Women aged 45 to 54 years had significantly greater increases in weight and in hip circumference than those aged 55 to 65 years. These investigators reported that overall baseline physical activity and baseline leisure and work activities were strongly related to weight gain in the PEPI cohort. Women who reported more activity gained less weight than less active women.

Weight gain during this period is associated with fat deposition in the abdomen (central or android pattern) and increased amounts of visceral fat (Kim, 2014). In addition, older adults have higher percentages of body fat than younger adults at any age due to muscle mass loss with aging (Baumgartner, 1995).

The etiology of these changes are multifactorial, and age-related metabolism slowing, declining estrogen levels, mood disorders, sleep disturbances, and often less strenuous physical activity can be contributory (Patel, 2006; Shifren, 2014). Others include genetic factors, neuropeptides, and adrenergic nervous system activity (Milewicz, 1996; Zaitlen, 2013). Many women believe that ET at menopause causes weight gain. However, results from clinical trials and epidemiologic studies indicate that the effect of HT on body weight and girth, if any, is to slightly blunt the rate of age-related increases.

Central obesity is associated with greater insulin resistance and diabetes risks, elevated atherogenic lipid levels, hypertension, cardiovascular disease, and mortality (Dallman, 2004; Manson, 1995; Wing, 1991). Weight gain during MT and after menopause raises health risks that include cancer, osteoarthritis, mood disorders, more frequent or severe hot flashes, and sexual dysfunction (Lauby-Secretan 2016; Shifren, 2014; Thurston, 2009).

Lifestyle interventions to minimize fat mass gains and central fat distribution during MT predominantly include exercise and healthy nutrition. These are discussed fully in Chapter 1 (p. 12). Barriers to these positive changes included untreated VMS, inadequate exercise, sleep disturbances, and untreated or inadequately treated mood disorders (Grindler, 2015). HT improves menopausal symptoms and sleep disturbances. It also improves body fat distribution but is not recommended as a treatment for central obesity. Preclinical and limited clinical studies find that skeletal muscle has estrogen receptors. Unfortunately, HT does not prevent age-related loss of lean body mass (sarcopenia) (Javed, 2019).

■ Breast Changes

The breast undergoes change during MT mainly because of hormonal withdrawal. In premenopausal women, estrogen and progesterone exert proliferative effects on ductal and glandular structures, respectively. At menopause, withdrawal of these hormones leads to a relative reduction in breast proliferation. A significant reduction in volume and tissue density is seen during mammography as these areas become replaced with adipose tissue. Screening for breast cancer, including mammography, is appropriate for women using HT. Shared decision-making is used to determine screening onset and frequency. Breast imaging recommendations are fully discussed in Chapter 13 (p. 293).

The role of tissue estrogen levels in breast carcinogenesis and the levels of metabolites in healthy breast tissue remains poorly understood (Yaghjyan, 2011). The effects of HT on breast cancer risk continue to be complex. This is especially so considering the different breast effects seen with differing HT regimens and differing initiation times relative to menopause onset and may be related to underlying breast cancer risk.

■ Dermatologic Changes

As people age, their skin loses elasticity, collagen fibers, vascularity, and moisture. Approximately 30 percent of collagen may be lost within the first 5 years after menopause (Brincat, 2005; Calleja-Agius, 2009). As a result, the skin lies more loosely, and lines appear where the facial muscles attach to the skin's undersurface. Skin aging results from synergistic effects of intrinsic aging and photo-aging from sun exposure or other environmental insults (Guinot, 2005). Cosmetic changes include hyperpigmentation (age spots), wrinkling, thinning, dryness, and decreased elasticity. More seriously, wound healing can be compromised, and the susceptibility to some skin cancers is increased (Thornton, 2013).

Skin is a hormonally sensitive structure and contains both estrogen and androgen receptors (Hasselquist, 1980). Hormonal dermal changes include reduced thickness of the skin with lower collagen content, diminished sebaceous gland secretion, loss of elasticity, and decreased blood supply (Wines, 2001). However, separating hormonal deficiency from chronologic skin aging and age-related environmental insults such as smoking or photo-aging is difficult.

People with thin, dry, fair skin experience signs of facial aging earlier. Overexposure to sunlight and excessive use of tobacco and alcohol accelerate skin aging. Thus, prevention of skin aging includes protection from ultraviolet light, avoidance of tobacco, and limiting alcohol intake.

Estrogen therapy may modulate some skin changes, as its use is associated with increased epidermal and dermal thickness, greater collagen and elastin content, improved skin moisture, and fewer wrinkles (Emmerson, 2012). The predominant evidence for an estrogen effect on skin derives from observational studies using various estrogen preparations with or without cyclic progestogens. Thus, clearly assigning the effects to estrogen, progestogen, or both is challenging. Results from randomized trials show improvement in certain skin parameters, but these were inconsistent among the trials (Maheux, 1994; Sator, 2007; Sauerbronn, 2000). In the largest trial, low-dose HT (1 mg norethindrone acetate with either 5 μg or 10 μg of ethinyl estradiol) did not significantly alter age-related facial skin changes in 320 women who averaged 5 years from menopause and received treatment rather than placebo for 48 weeks (Phillips, 2008). Benefits may be greater if HT is initiated closer to menopause and prior to a significant loss of collagen. Currently, evidence is insufficient to recommend systemic HT to improve age-related skin characteristics. In small trials, topical estrogen applied to the face led to a thicker epidermis and fewer fine wrinkles (Creidi, 1994; Patriarca, 2007).

After menopause, women may experience hair loss or greater hair density. Recognized conditions include female pattern hair loss (androgenetic) and telogen effluvium. Although the characteristic low estrogen-to-androgen ratio could affect hair changes in genetically susceptible individuals, no role has been identified for HT to prevent hair loss. Antiandrogen treatments increase hair density for some women (Riedel-Baima, 2008).

■ Dental Changes

Dental problems also may develop as estrogen levels wane in late MT. Hormones influence oral health, and estrogen receptors are observed in the oral mucosa, gingiva, and salivary glands (Grover, 2014). The buccal epithelium atrophies due to estrogen deprivation and results in diminished saliva and sensation. Dysgeusia (bad taste in the mouth), higher incidence of cavities, and tooth loss also may occur (Krall, 1994). Oral alveolar bone loss is strongly positively correlated with osteoporosis and can lead to tooth loss. Even in women without osteoporosis, vertebral BMD correlates positively with the number of teeth. In turn, the beneficial effect of estrogen on skeletal bone mass is also manifested in oral bone.

REFERENCES

Al-Safi ZA, Santoro N: Menopausal hormone therapy and menopausal symptoms. Fertil Steril 101(4):905, 2014

American College of Obstetricians and Gynecologists: Fractional laser treatment of vulvovaginal atrophy and U.S. Food and Drug Administration clearance: position statement. 2016. Available at: https://www.acog.org/Clinical-Guidance-and-Publications/Position-Statements/Fractional-Laser-Treatment-of-Vulvovaginal-Atrophy-and-US-Food-and-Drug-Administration-Clearance. Accessed September 14, 2019

American College of Obstetricians and Gynecologists: Compounded bioidentical menopausal hormone therapy. Committee Opinion No. 532, August 2012, Reaffirmed 2018a

American College of Obstetricians and Gynecologists: Hormone therapy and heart disease. Committee Opinion No. 565, June 2013, Reaffirmed 2018b

American College of Obstetricians Gynecologists: Management of menopausal symptoms. Practice Bulletin No. 141, January, 2014, Reaffirmed 2018c

American College of Obstetricians and Gynecologists: Osteoporosis. Practice Bulletin No. 129, September 2012, Reaffirmed 2019a

American College of Obstetricians and Gynecologists: Use of antimüllerian hormone in women not seeking fertility care. Committee Opinion No. 773, March 2019b

Anastasilakis AD, Polyzos SA, Makras P, et al: Clinical features of 24 patients with rebound-associated vertebral fractures after denosumab discontinuation: systematic review and additional cases. J Bone Miner Res 32(6):1291, 2017

Anderson GL, Judd HL, Kaunitz AM, et al: Effects of estrogen plus progestin on gynecologic cancers and associated diagnostic procedures: the Women's Health Initiative randomized trial. JAMA 290(13):1739, 2003

Anderson GL, Limacher M, Assaf AR, et al: Effects of conjugated equine estrogen in postmenopausal women with hysterectomy: the Women's Health Initiative randomized controlled trial. JAMA 291(14):1701, 2004

Arias E, Xu J, Kochanek KD: United States Life Tables, 2016. Natl Vital Stat Rep 68(4):1, 2019

Avis NE, Crawford SL, Greendale G, et al: Study of women's health across the nation. Duration of menopausal vasomotor symptoms over the menopause transition. JAMA Intern Med 175(4):531, 2015

Avis NE, Levine BJ, Danhauer S, et al: A pooled analysis of three studies of nonpharmacological interventions for menopausal hot flashes. Menopause 26(4):350, 2019

Avis NE, Stellato R, Crawford S, et al: Is there an association between menopause status and sexual functioning? Menopause 7:297, 2000

Bachmann GA: Menopausal vasomotor symptoms: a review of causes, effects and evidence-based treatment options. J Reprod Med 50:155, 2005

Baker FC, Lampio L, Saaresranta T, et al: Sleep and sleep disorders in the menopausal transition. Sleep Med Clin 13(3):443, 2018

Ballinger CB: Psychiatric aspects of the menopause. Br J Psychiatry 156:773, 1990

Barber MD, Visco AG, Wyman JF, et al: Sexual function in women with urinary incontinence and pelvic organ prolapse. Obstet Gynecol 99:281, 2002

Barrett-Connor E, Siris ES, Wehren LE, et al: Osteoporosis and fracture risk in women of different ethnic groups. J Bone Miner Res 20(2):185, 2005

Bar-Shavit Z: The osteoclast: a multinucleated, hematopoietic-origin, bone-resorbing osteoimmune cell. J Cell Biochem 102(5):1130, 2007

Barzel US, Massey LK: Excess dietary protein can adversely affect bone. J Nutr 128(6):1051, 1998

Baumgartner RN, Heymsfield SB, Roche AF: Human body composition and the epidemiology of chronic disease. Obes Res 3:73, 1995

Bertone-Johnson ER, Manson JE, Purdue-Smithe AC, et al: Anti-Müllerian hormone levels and incidence of early natural menopause in a prospective study. Hum Reprod 33(6):1175, 2018

Bhatia NN, Bergman A, Karram MM: Effects of estrogen on urethral function in women with urinary incontinence. Am J Obstet Gynecol 160:176, 1989

Bhupathiraju SN, Grodstein F, Rosner BA, et al: Hormone therapy use and risk of chronic disease in the Nurses' Health Study: a comparative analysis with the Women's Health Initiative. Am J Epidemiol 186(6):696, 2017

Bhupathiraju SN, Grodstein F, Stampfer MJ, et al: Vaginal estrogen use and chronic disease risk in the Nurses' Health Study. Menopause 26(6):603, 2018

Black DM, Cummings SR, Karpf DB, et al: Randomised trial of effect of alendronate on risk of fracture in women with existing vertebral fractures. Fracture Intervention Trial Research Group. Lancet 348(9041):1535, 1996

Black DM, Schwartz AV, Ensrud KE, et al: Effects of continuing or stopping alendronate after 5 years of treatment: the Fracture Intervention Trial Long-term Extension (FLEX): a randomized trial. JAMA 296(24):2927, 2006

Blau LA, Hoehns JD: Analgesic efficacy of calcitonin for vertebral fracture pain. Ann Pharmacother 37(4):564, 2003

Bolland MJ, Barber PA, Doughty RN, et al: Vascular events in healthy older women receiving calcium supplementation: randomised controlled trial. BMJ 336(7638):262, 2008

Bone HG, Hosking D, Devogelaer JP, et al: Ten years' experience with alendronate for osteoporosis in postmenopausal women. N Engl J Med 350(12):1189, 2004

Bone HG, Wagman RB, Brandi ML, et al: 10 years of denosumab treatment in postmenopausal women with osteoporosis: results from the phase 3 randomised FREEDOM trial and open-label extension. Lancet Diabetes Endocrinol 5(7):513, 2017

Bonjour JP, Chevalley T, Ammann P, et al: Gain in bone mineral mass in prepubertal girls 3.5 years after discontinuation of calcium supplementation: a follow-up study. Lancet 358:1208, 2001

Braunstein GD: Safety of testosterone treatment in postmenopausal women. Fertil Steril 88(1):1, 2007

Brincat MP, Baron YM, Galea R: Estrogens and the skin. Climacteric 8(2):110, 2005

Broer SL, Broekmans FJ, Laven JS, et al: Anti-Müllerian hormone: ovarian reserve testing and its potential clinical implications. Hum Reprod Update 20(5):688, 2014

Bromberger JT, Kravitz HM, Chang YF, et al: Major depression during and after the menopausal transition: Study of Women's Health Across the Nation (SWAN). Psychol Med 41(9):1879, 2011

Burger HG, Dudley EC, Cui J, et al: A prospective longitudinal study of serum testosterone, dehydroepiandrosterone sulfate, and sex hormone-binding globulin levels through the menopause transition. J Clin Endocrinol Metab 85:2832, 2000

Busch CM, Zonderman AB, Costa PT Jr: Menopausal transition and psychological distress in a nationally representative sample: is menopause associated with psychological distress? J Aging Health 6:206, 1994

Calleja-Agius J, Brincat MP: Effects of hormone replacement therapy on connective tissue: why is this important? Best Pract Res Clin Obstet Gynaecol 23(1):121, 2009

Camacho PM, Petak SM, Binkley N, et al: American Association Of Clinical Endocrinologists and American College Of Endocrinology clinical practice guidelines for the diagnosis and treatment of postmenopausal osteoporosis—2016. Endocr Pract 22(9):1111, 2016

Canalis E, Giustina A, Bilezikian JP: Mechanisms of anabolic therapies for osteoporosis. N Engl J Med 357(9):905, 2007

Canonico M. Hormone therapy and hemostasis among postmenopausal women: a review. Menopause 21(7):753, 2014

Canonico M, Scarabin PY. Oral versus transdermal estrogens and venous thromboembolism in postmenopausal women: what is new since 2003? Menopause 23(6):587, 2016

Carter ND, Khan KM, McKay HA, et al: Community-based exercise program reduces risk factors for falls in 65- to 75-year-old women with osteoporosis: randomized controlled trial. CMAJ 167(9):997, 2002

Chapuy MC, Arlot ME, Duboeuf F, et al: Vitamin D3 and calcium to prevent hip fractures in the elderly women. N Engl J Med 327(23):1637, 1992

Christiansen C, Chesnut CH 3rd, Adachi JD, et al: Safety of bazedoxifene in a randomized, double-blind, placebo- and active-controlled Phase 3 study of postmenopausal women with osteoporosis. BMC Musculoskelet Disord 11:130, 2010

Cintron D, Lipford M, Larrea-Mantilla L, et al: Efficacy of menopausal hormone therapy on sleep quality: systematic review and meta-analysis. Endocrine 55(3):702, 2017

Clayton AH, Goldstein I, Kim NN, et al: The International Society for the Study of Women's Sexual Health process of care for management of hypoactive sexual desire disorder in women. Mayo Clin Proc 93(4):467, 2018

Cody JD, Jacobs ML, Richardson K, et al: Oestrogen therapy for urinary incontinence in post-menopausal women. Cochrane Database Syst Rev 10:CD001405, 2012

Cohen FJ, Lu Y: Characterization of hot flashes reported by healthy postmenopausal women receiving raloxifene or placebo during osteoporosis prevention trials. Maturitas 34(1):65, 2000

Cohen LS, Soares CN, Vitonis AF, et al: Risk of new onset of depression during the menopausal transition: the Harvard Study of Moods and Cycles. Arch Gen Psychiatry 63(4):385, 2006

Constantine GD, Simon JA, Pickar JH, et al: The REJOICE trial: A phase 3 randomized, controlled trial evaluating the safety and efficacy of a novel vaginal estradiol soft-gel capsule for symptomatic vulvar and vaginal atrophy. Menopause 24(4):409, 2017

Cosman F, de Beur SJ, LeBoff MS, et al: Clinician's guide to prevention and treatment of osteoporosis. Osteoporos Int 25(10):2359, 2014

Cosman F, Miller PD, Williams GC, et al: Eighteen months of treatment with subcutaneous abaloparatide followed by 6 months of treatment with alendronate in postmenopausal women with osteoporosis: results of the ACTIVExtend trial. Mayo Clin Proc 92(2):200, 2017

Cosman FN, Crittenden DB, Adachi JD, et al: Romosozumab treatment in postmenopausal women with osteoporosis. N Engl J Med 375(16):1532, 2016

Crandall CJ, Crawford SL, Gold EB: Vasomotor symptom prevalence is associated with polymorphisms in sex steroid-metabolizing enzymes and receptors. Am J Med 119:552, 2006

Crandall CJ, Hovey KM, Andrews CA, et al: Breast cancer, endometrial cancer, and cardiovascular events in participants who used vaginal estrogen in the Women's Health Initiative Observational Study. Menopause 25(1):11, 2018

Crandall CJ, Manson JE, Hohensee C, et al: Association of genetic variation in the tachykinin receptor 3 locus with hot flashes and night sweats in the women's health initiative study. Menopause 24:252, 2017

Crawford SL, Crandall CJ, Derby CA, et al: Menopausal hormone therapy trends before versus after 2002: impact of the Women's Health Initiative Study Results. Menopause 26(6):588, 2018

Creidi P, Faivre B, Agache P, et al: Effect of a conjugated oestrogen (Premarin) cream on ageing facial skin. A comparative study with a placebo cream. Maturitas 19(3):211, 1994

Cruz VL, Steiner ML, Pompei LM, et al: Randomized, double-blind, placebo-controlled clinical trial for evaluating the efficacy of fractional CO2 laser compared with topical estriol in the treatment of vaginal atrophy in postmenopausal women. Menopause 25(1):21, 2018

Cummings SR, Nevitt MC, Browner WS, et al: Risk factors for hip fracture in white women. Study of Osteoporotic Fractures Research Group. N Engl J Med 332:767, 1995

Da Fonseca AM, Bagnoli VR, Souza MA, et al: Impact of age and body mass on the intensity of menopausal symptoms in 5968 Brazilian women. Gynecol Endocrinol 29(2):116, 2013

Daily JW, Ko BS, Ryuk J, et al: Equol decreases hot flashes in Postmenopausal Women: a systematic review and meta-analysis of randomized clinical trials. J Med Food 22(2):127–139, 2019.

Dallman MF, la Fleur SE, Pecoraro NC, et al: Minireview: glucocorticoids—food intake, abdominal obesity, and wealthy nations in 2004. Endocrinology 145:2633, 2004

Davis SR: Androgen use for low sexual desire in midlife women. Menopause 20(7):795, 2013

Davis SR, Baber R, Panay N, et al: Global consensus position statement on the use of testosterone therapy for women. J Clin Endocrinol Metab 104(10):4660, 2019

Davis SR, Braunstein GD: Efficacy and safety of testosterone in the management of hypoactive sexual desire disorder in postmenopausal women. J Sex Med 9(4):1134, 2012

Dawson-Hughes B, Harris SS: Calcium intake influences the association of protein intake with rates of bone loss in elderly men and women. Am J Clin Nutr 75(4):773, 2002

Dawson-Hughes B, Harris SS, Krall EA, et al: Effect of calcium and vitamin D supplementation on bone density in men and women 65 years of age or older. N Engl J Med 337(10):670, 1997

Delaney MF: Strategies for the prevention and treatment of osteoporosis during early postmenopause. Am J Obstet Gynecol 194(2 Suppl):S12, 2006

Dell RM, Adams AL, Greene DF, et al: Incidence of atypical nontraumatic diaphyseal fractures of the femur. J Bone Miner Res 27:2544, 2012

Delmas PD, Ensrud KE, Adachi JD, et al: Efficacy of raloxifene on vertebral fracture risk reduction in postmenopausal women with osteoporosis: four-year results from a randomized clinical trial. J Clin Endocrinol Metab 87(8):3609, 2002

Dennerstein L, Guthrie JR, Clark M, et al: A population-based study of depressed mood in middle-aged, Australian-born women. Menopause 11(5):563, 2004

Dennerstein L, Hayes RD: Confronting the challenges: epidemiological study of female sexual dysfunction and the menopause. J Sex Med 2(Suppl 3):118, 2005

Dennerstein L, Smith AM, Morse C, et al: Menopausal symptoms in Australian women. Med J Aust 159:232, 1993

Depypere H, Inki P: The levonorgestrel-releasing intrauterine system for endometrial protection during estrogen replacement therapy: a clinical review. Climacteric 18(4):470, 2015

Diab DL, Watts NB: Bisphosphonates in the treatment of osteoporosis. Endocrinol Metab Clinic North Am 41:487, 2012

Diab DL, Watts NB: Postmenopausal osteoporosis. Curr Opin Endocrinol Diabetes Obes 20:501, 2013

Diab DL, Watts NB: Use of drug holidays in women taking bisphosphonates. Menopause 21(2):195, 2014

Ebina K, Hashimoto J, Kashii M, et al: The effects of switching daily teriparatide to oral bisphosphonates or denosumab in patients with primary osteoporosis. J Bone Miner Metab 35(1):91, 2017

Elraiyah T, Sonbol MB, Wang Z, et al: Clinical review: the benefits and harms of systemic dehydroepiandrosterone (DHEA) in postmenopausal women with normal adrenal function: a systematic review and meta-analysis. J Clin Endocrinol Metab 99(10):353, 2014

Emmerson E, Hardman MJ: The role of estrogen deficiency in skin ageing and wound healing. Biogerontology 13(1):3, 2012

Eriksen B: A randomized, open, parallel-group study on the preventive effect of an estradiol-releasing vaginal ring (Estring) on recurrent urinary tract infections in postmenopausal women. Am J Obstet Gynecol 180(5):1072, 1999

Erlik Y, Meldrum DR, Judd HL: Estrogen levels in postmenopausal women with hot flashes. Obstet Gynecol 59:403, 1982

Espeland MA, Stefanick ML, Kritz-Silverstein D, et al: Effect of postmenopausal hormone therapy on body weight and waist and hip girths. Postmenopausal Estrogen-Progestin Interventions Study Investigators. J Clin Endocrinol Metab 82:1549, 1997

Ettinger B, Black DM, Mitlak BH, et al: Reduction of vertebral fracture risk in postmenopausal women with osteoporosis treated with raloxifene: results from a 3-year randomized clinical trial. Multiple Outcomes of Raloxifene Evaluation (MORE) Investigators. JAMA 282(7):637, 1999

Ettinger B, Ensrud KE, Wallace R, et al: Effects of ultralow-dose transdermal estradiol on bone mineral density: a randomized clinical trial. Obstet Gynecol 104(3):443, 2004

Faulkner KG, von Stetten E, Miller P: Discordance in patient classification using T-scores. J Clin Densitom 2:343, 1999

FitzGerald G, Compston JE, Chapurlat RD, et al: Empirically based composite fracture prediction model from the global longitudinal study of osteoporosis in postmenopausal women (GLOW). J Clin Endocrinol Metab 99(3):817, 2014

Food and Drug Administration: FDA warns against use of energy-based devices to perform vaginal 'rejuvenation' or vaginal cosmetic procedures: FDA safety communication. 2018. Available at: https://www.fda.gov/medical-devices/safety-communications/fda-warns-against-use-energy-based-devices-perform-vaginal-rejuvenation-or-vaginal-cosmetic. Accessed September 14, 2019

Franco OH, Chowdhury R, Troup J, et al: Use of plant-based therapies and menopausal symptoms: a systematic review and meta-analysis. JAMA 315(23):2554, 2016

Freedman RR, Woodward S, Sabharwal SC: Alpha 2-adrenergic mechanism in menopausal hot flushes. Obstet Gynecol 76:573, 1990

Freedman RR: Biochemical, metabolic, and vascular mechanisms in menopausal hot flashes. Fertil Steril 70(2):332, 1998

Freedman RR: Menopausal hot flashes: mechanisms, endocrinology, treatment. J Steroid Biochem Mol Biol 142:115, 2014

Freedman RR: Physiology of hot flashes. Am J Hum Biol 13:453, 2001

Freeman EW, Sammel MD, Gross SA, et al: Poor sleep in relation to natural menopause: a population-based 14-year follow-up of midlife women. Menopause 22(7):719, 2015

Freeman EW, Sammel MD, Lin H, et al: Hormones and menopausal status as predictors of depression in women in transition to menopause. Arch Gen Psychiatry 61(1):62, 2004

Freeman EW, Sammel MD, Lin H, et al: Symptoms associated with menopausal transition and reproductive hormones in midlife women. Obstet Gynecol 110(2 Pt 1):230, 2007

Gallagher JC, Rapuri PB, Haynatzki G, et al: Effect of discontinuation of estrogen, calcitriol, and the combination of both on bone density and bone markers. J Clin Endocrinol Metab 87:4914, 2002

Gebbie AE, Hardman SM: Contraception in the perimenopause—old and new. Menopause Int 16(1):33, 2010

Gedmintas L, Solomon DH, Kim SC: Bisphosphonates and risk of subtrochanteric, femoral shafts, and atypical femur fracture: a systemic review and meta-analysis. J Bone Miner Res 28:1729, 2013

Gerber LM, Sievert LL, Warren K, et al: Hot flashes are associated with increased ambulatory systolic blood pressure. Menopause 14(2):308, 2007

Gibson CJ, Huang AJ, McCaw B, et al: Associations of intimate partner violence, sexual assault, and posttraumatic stress disorder with menopause symptoms among midlife and older women. JAMA Intern Med 179(1):80, 2019

Gislason T, Benediktsdottir B, Bjornsson JK, et al: Snoring, hypertension, and the sleep apnea syndrome. An epidemiologic survey of middle-aged women. Chest 103:1147, 1993

Gold EB, Bromberger J, Crawford S, et al: Factors associated with age at natural menopause in a multiethnic sample of midlife women. Am J Epidemiol 153:865, 2001

Gold EB, Colvin A, Avis N, et al: Longitudinal analysis of the association between vasomotor symptoms and race/ethnicity across the menopausal transition: Study of Women's health Across the Nation. Am J Public Health 96(7):1226, 2006

Goldberg RP, Tomezsko JE, Winkler HA, et al: Anterior or posterior sacrospinous vaginal vault suspension: long-term anatomic and functional evaluation. Obstet Gynecol 98:199, 2001

Gonzales GF, Carrillo C: Blood serotonin levels in postmenopausal women: effects of age and serum oestradiol levels. Maturitas 17:23, 1993

Gracia CR, Freeman EW, Sammel MD, et al: Hormones and sexuality during transition to menopause. Obstet Gynecol 109(4):831, 2007

Greenspan SL, Myers ER, Kiel DP, et al: Fall direction, bone mineral density, and function: risk factors for hip fracture in frail nursing home elderly. Am J Med 104(6):539, 1998

Grindler NM, Santoro NF: Menopause and exercise. Menopause 22(12):1351, 2015

Grover CM, More VP, Singh N, et al: Crosstalk between hormones and oral health in the mid-life of women: A comprehensive review. J Int Soc Prev Community Dent 4(Suppl 1):S5, 2014

Guinot C, Malvy D, Ambroisine L, et al: Effect of hormonal replacement therapy on skin biophysical properties of menopausal women. Skin Res Technol 11:201, 2005

Guthrie JR, Dennerstein L, Taffe JR, et al: Hot flushes during the menopause transition: a longitudinal study in Australian-born women. Menopause 12(4):460, 2005

Halbreich U, Lumley LA, Palter S, et al: Possible acceleration of age effects on cognition following menopause. J Psychiatr Res 29:153, 1995

Hale GE, Zhao X, Hughes CL, et al: Endocrine features of menstrual cycles in middle and late reproductive age and the menopausal transition classified according to the Staging of Reproductive Aging Workshop (STRAW) staging system. J Clin Endocrinol Metab 92(8):3060, 2007

Hall MH, Matthews KA, Kravitz HM, et al: Race and financial strain are independent correlates of sleep in midlife women: the SWAN sleep study. Sleep 32:73, 2009

Handa VL, Harvey L, Cundiff GW, et al: Sexual function among women with urinary incontinence and pelvic organ prolapse. Am J Obstet Gynecol 191:751, 2004

Harlow SD, Gass M, Hall JE, et al: Executive summary of the Stages of Reproductive Again Workshop + 10: addressing the unfinished agenda of staging reproductive aging. Fertil Steril 97:843, 2012

Harris SS, Dawson-Hughes B: Caffeine and bone loss in healthy postmenopausal women. Am J Clin Nutr 60(4):573, 1994

Harris ST, Watts NB, Genant HK, et al: Effects of risedronate treatment on vertebral and nonvertebral fractures in women with postmenopausal osteoporosis: a randomized controlled trial. Vertebral Efficacy With Risedronate Therapy (VERT) Study Group. JAMA 282(14):1344, 1999

Hasselquist MB, Goldberg N, Schroeter A, et al: Isolation and characterization of the estrogen receptor in human skin. J Clin Endocrinol Metab 50(1):76, 1980

Hay DL, Poyner DR: Calcitonin gene-related peptide, adrenomedullin and flushing. Maturitas 64(2):104, 2009

Henderson VW, St John JA, Hodis HN, et al: Cognition, mood, and physiological concentrations of sex hormones in the early and late postmenopause. Proc Natl Acad Sci USA 110(50):20290, 2013

Hendrix SL, Cochrane BB, Nygaard IE, et al: Effects of estrogen with and without progestin on urinary incontinence. JAMA 293(8):935, 2005

Hodis HN, Mack WJ, Henderson VW, et al: Vascular effects of early versus late postmenopausal treatment with estradiol. N Engl J Med 374(13):1221, 2016

Hollander LE, Freeman EW, Sammel MD, et al: Sleep quality, estradiol levels, and behavioral factors in late reproductive age women. Obstet Gynecol 98:391, 2001

Holroyd C, Cooper C, Dennison E: Epidemiology of osteoporosis. Best Pract Res Clin Endocrinol Metab 22(5):671, 2008

Howe TE, Shea B, Dawson LJ, et al: Exercise for preventing and treating osteoporosis in postmenopausal women. Cochrane Database Syst Rev 7: CD000333, 2011

Hunter MS, Gentry-Maharaj A, Ryan A, et al: Prevalence, frequency and problem rating of hot flushes persist in older postmenopausal women: impact of age, body mass index, hysterectomy, hormone therapy use, lifestyle and mood in a cross-sectional cohort study of 10,418 British women aged 54–65. BJOG 119(1):40, 2012

Imtiaz B, Tuppurainen M, Rikkonen T, et al: Postmenopausal hormone therapy and Alzheimer disease: a prospective cohort study. Neurology 88(11):1062, 2017

Islam RM, Bell RJ, Green S, et al: Safety and efficacy of testosterone for women: a systematic review and meta-analysis of randomised controlled trial data. Lancet Diabetes Endocrinol 7(10):754, 2019

Ismail SI, Bain C, Hagen S: Oestrogens for treatment or prevention of pelvic organ prolapse in postmenopausal women. Cochrane Database Syst Rev 9: CD007063, 2010

Jaakkola S, Lyytinen H, Pukkala E, et al: Endometrial cancer in postmenopausal women using estradiol-progestin therapy. Obstet Gynecol 114(6):1197, 2009

Jackson RD, LaCroix AZ, Gass M, et al: Women's health initiative investigators. Calcium plus vitamin D supplementation and the risk of fractures. N Engl J Med 354(7):669, 2006a

Jackson RD, Wactawski-Wende J, LaCroix AZ, et al: Women's health initiative investigators. Effects of conjugated equine estrogen on risk of fractures and BMD in postmenopausal women with hysterectomy: results from the women's health initiative randomized trial. J Bone Miner Res 21(6):817, 2006b

Jackson SL, Scholes D, Boyko EJ, et al: Predictors of urinary incontinence in a prospective cohort of postmenopausal women. Obstet Gynecol 108(4):855, 2006c

Jain A, Santoro N: Endocrine mechanisms and management for abnormal bleeding due to perimenopausal changes. Clin Obstet Gynecol 48:295, 2005

Javed AA, Mayhew AJ, Shea AK, Raina P. Association between hormone therapy and muscle mass in postmenopausal women: a systematic review and meta-analysis. JAMA Netw Open 2(8):e1910154, 2019

Jayasena CN, Comninos AN, Stefanopoulou E, et al: Neurokinin B administration induces hot flushes in women. Sci Rep, 2015

Kanis JA, Johnell O, Oden A, et al: Ten year probabilities of osteoporotic fractures according to BMD and diagnostic thresholds. Osteoporos Int 12:989, 2001

Kanis JA: Assessment of fracture risk and its application to screening for postmenopausal osteoporosis: synopsis of a WHO report. WHO Study Group. Osteoporos Int 4:368, 1994

Karvonen-Gutierrez C, Kim C: Association of mid-life changes in body size, body composition and obesity status with the menopausal transition. Healthcare (Basel) 4(3):1, 2016

Kaunitz AM: Transdermal and vaginal estradiol for the treatment of menopausal symptoms: the nuts and bolts. Menopause 19(6):602, 2012

Kaunitz AM, Manson JE: Management of menopausal symptoms. Obstet Gynecol 126(4):859, 2015

Kendler DL, Marin F, Zerbini CA, et al: Effects of teriparatide and risedronate on new fractures in post-menopausal women with severe osteoporosis (VERO): a multicentre, double-blind, double-dummy, randomised controlled trial. Lancet 391(10117):230, 2018

Kerstetter JE, Looker AC, Insogna KL: Low dietary protein and low bone density. Calcif Tissue Int 66(4):313, 2000

Khosia S, Burr D, Cauley J, et al: Bisphosphonate-associated osteonecrosis of the jaw: report of a task force of the American Society for Bone and Mineral Research. J Bone Miner Res 22:1479, 2007

Kiebzak GM, Miller PD: Determinants of bone strength. J Bone Miner Res 18:383, 2003

Kim JH, Cho HT, Kim YJ: The role of estrogen in adipose tissue metabolism: insights into glucose homeostasis regulation. Endocr J 61(11):1055, 2014

Kingsberg SA, Krychman M, Graham S, et al: The women's empower survey: identifying women's perceptions on vulvar and vaginal atrophy and its treatment. J Sex Med 14(3):413, 2017

Klein NA, Illingworth PJ, Groome NP, et al: Decreased inhibin B secretion is associated with the monotropic FSH rise in older, ovulatory women: a study of serum and follicular fluid levels of dimeric inhibin A and B in spontaneous menstrual cycles. J Clin Endocrinol Metab 81:2742, 1996

Kostenuik PJ: Osteoprotegerin and RANKL regulate bone resorption, density, geometry and strength. Curr Opin Pharmacol 5(6):618, 2005

Krall EA, Dawson-Hughes B, Papas A, et al: Tooth loss and skeletal bone density in healthy postmenopausal women. Osteoporos Int 4:104, 1994

Kronenberg F: Hot flashes: epidemiology and physiology. Ann NY Acad Sci 592:52, 1990

Kuller LH, Lopez OL, Newman A, et al: Risk factors for dementia in the cardiovascular health cognition study. Neuroepidemiology 22:13, 2003

Kushnir VA, Seifer DB, Barad DH, et al: Potential therapeutic applications of human anti-müllerian hormone (AMH) analogues in reproductive medicine. J Assist Reprod Genet 34(9):1105, 2017

Labrie F, Archer DF, Koltun W, et al: Efficacy of intravaginal dehydroepiandrosterone (DHEA) on moderate to severe dyspareunia and vaginal dryness, symptoms of vulvovaginal atrophy, and of the genitourinary syndrome of menopause. Menopause 25(11):1339, 2018

Labrie F, Belanger A, Cusan L, et al: Marked decline in serum concentrations of adrenal C19 sex steroid precursors and conjugated androgen metabolites during aging. J Clin Endocrinol Metab 82:2396, 1997

Lanza FL, Hunt RH, Thomson AB, et al: Endoscopic comparison of esophageal and gastroduodenal effects of risedronate and alendronate in postmenopausal women. Gastroenterology 119(3):631, 2000

Larsen ER, Mosekilde L, Foldspang A: Vitamin D and calcium supplementation prevents osteoporotic fractures in elderly community dwelling residents: a pragmatic population-based 3-year intervention study. J Bone Miner Res 19(3):370, 2004

Lauby-Secretan B, Scoccianti C, Loomis D, et al: Body fatness and cancer—viewpoint of the IARC Working Group. N Engl J Med 375(8):794, 2016

Laufer LR, Erlik Y, Meldrum DR, et al: Effect of clonidine on hot flashes in postmenopausal women. Obstet Gynecol 60:583, 1982

Laumann EO, Paik A, Rosen RC: Sexual dysfunction in the United States: prevalence and predictors. JAMA 281:537, 1999

LeBoeuf FJ, Carter SG: Discomforts of the perimenopause. J Obstet Gynecol Neonatal Nurs 25:173, 1996

Leder BZ, Tsai JN, Uihlein AV, et al: Denosumab and teriparatide transitions in postmenopausal osteoporosis (the DATA-Switch study): extension of a randomised controlled trial. Lancet 386(9999):1147, 2015

Leon-Ferre RA, Novotny PJ, Wolfe EG, et al: Oxybutynin versus placebo for hot flashes: a randomized, double-blind clinical trial (ACCRU SC1603). Presented at the 41st San Antonio Breast Cancer Symposium, December 4–8, 2018

Lethaby A, Ayeleke RO, Roberts H: Local oestrogen for vaginal atrophy in postmenopausal women. Cochrane Database Syst Rev 8:CD001500, 2016

Levine KB, Williams RE, Hartmann KE: Vulvovaginal atrophy is strongly associated with female sexual dysfunction among sexually active postmenopausal women. Menopause 15(4 Pt 1):661, 2008

Lewis JG, McGill H, Patton VM, et al: Caution on the use of saliva measurements to monitor absorption of progesterone from transdermal creams in postmenopausal women. Maturitas 41(1):1, 2002

Lidor A, Ismajovich B, Confino E, et al: Histopathological findings in 226 women with post-menopausal uterine bleeding. Acta Obstet Gynecol Scand 65:41, 1986

Lindau ST, Schumm LP, Laumann EO, et al: A study of sexuality and health among older adults in the United States. N Engl J Med 357(8):762, 2007

Lindsay R, Gallagher JC, Kagan R, et al: Efficacy of tissue-selective estrogen complex of bazedoxifene/conjugated estrogens for osteoporosis prevention in at-risk postmenopausal women. Fertil Steril 92(3):1045, 2009

Lindsay R, Silverman SL, Cooper C, et al: Risk of new vertebral fracture in the year following a fracture. JAMA 285:320, 2001

Lobo RA, Pinkerton JV, Gass ML, et al: Evaluation of bazedoxifene/conjugated estrogens for the treatment of menopausal symptoms and effects on metabolic parameters and overall safety profile. Fertil Steril 92(3):1025, 2009

Lobo RA, Rosen RC, Yang HM, et al: Comparative effects of oral esterified estrogens with and without methyltestosterone on endocrine profiles and dimensions of sexual function in postmenopausal women with hypoactive sexual desire. Fertil Steril 79(6):1341, 2003

Lock M: Medicine and culture: Contested meanings of the menopause. Lancet 337:1270, 1991

Long CY, Liu CM, Hsu SC, et al: A randomized comparative study of the effects of oral and topical estrogen therapy on the lower urinary tract of hysterectomized postmenopausal women. Fertil Steril 85(1):155, 2006

Ma D, Wu L, He Z: Effects of walking on the preservation of bone mineral density in perimenopausal and postmenopausal women: a systematic review and meta-analysis. Menopause 20(11):1216, 2013

Maheux R, Naud F, Rioux M, et al: A randomized, double-blind, placebo-controlled study on the effect of conjugated estrogens on skin thickness. Am J Obstet Gynecol 170(2):642, 1994

Maki PM, Kornstein SG, Joffe H, et al: Guidelines for the evaluation and treatment of perimenopausal depression: summary and recommendations. Menopause 25(10):1069, 2018

Malacara JM, Perez-Luque EL, Martinez-Garza S, et al: The relationship of estrogen receptor-alpha polymorphism with symptoms and other characteristics in post-menopausal women. Maturitas 49:163, 2004

Manson JE, Aragaki AK, Rossouw JE, et al: Menopausal hormone therapy and long-term all-cause and cause-specific mortality: the Women's Health Initiative randomized trials. JAMA 318(10):927, 2017

Manson JE, Chlebowski RT, Stefanick ML, et al: Menopausal hormone therapy and health outcomes during the intervention and extended post-stopping phases of the Women's Health Initiative randomized trials. JAMA 310(13):1353, 2013

Manson JE, Goldstein SR, Kagan R, et al: Why the product labeling for low-dose vaginal estrogen should be changed. Menopause 21(9):911, 2014

Manson JE, Kaunitz AM: Menopause management—getting clinical care back on track. N Engl J Med 374(9):803, 2016

Manson JE, Willett WC, Stampfer MJ, et al: Body weight and mortality among women. N Engl J Med 333(11):677, 1995

Marshall D, Johnell O, Wedel H: Meta-analysis of how well measures of bone mineral density predict occurrence of osteoporotic fractures. BMJ 312:1254, 1996

Matthews KA, Abrams B, Crawford S, et al: Body mass index in mid-life women: relative influence of menopause, hormone use, and ethnicity. Int J Obes Relat Metab Disord 25:863, 2001

Matthews KA, Meilahn E, Kuller LH, et al: Menopause and risk factors for coronary heart disease. N Engl J Med 321:641, 1989

Matthews KA, Wing RR, Kuller LH, et al: Influence of the perimenopause on cardiovascular risk factors and symptoms of middle-aged healthy women. Arch Intern Med 154:2349, 1994

McClung MR, Grauer A, Boonen S, et al: Romosozumab in postmenopausal women with low bone mineral density. N Engl J Med 370(5):412, 2014

McCoy NL, Davidson JM: A longitudinal study of the effects of menopause on sexuality. Maturitas 7:203, 1985

McKinlay SM, Brambilla DJ, Posner JG: The normal menopause transition. Maturitas 14:103, 1992

Meier RP, Perneger TV, Stern R, et al: Increasing occurrence of atypical femoral fractures associated with bisphosphonate use. Arch Intern Med 172:930, 2012

Melton LJ III, Atkinson EJ, Cooper C, et al: Vertebral fractures predict subsequent fractures. Osteoporos Int 10:214, 1999

Meyer JS, Rauch GM, Crawford K, et al: Risk factors accelerating cerebral degenerative changes, cognitive decline and dementia. Int J Geriatr Psychiatry 14:1050, 1999

Milewicz A, Bidzinska B, Sidorowicz A: Perimenopausal obesity. Gynecol Endocrinol 10:285, 1996

Miller PD, Hattersley G, Riis BJ, et al: Effect of abaloparatide vs placebo on new vertebral fractures in postmenopausal women with osteoporosis: a randomized clinical trial. JAMA 316(7):722, 2016

Miller PD, Njeh CF, Jankowski LG, et al: What are the standards by which bone mass measurement at peripheral skeletal sites should be used in the diagnosis of osteoporosis? J Clin Densitom 5(Suppl):S39, 2002

Moen MH, Kahn H, Bjerve KS, et al: Menometrorrhagia in the perimenopause is associated with increased serum estradiol. Maturitas 47:151, 2004

Molnar WR: Menopausal hot flashes: their cycles and relation to air temperature. Obstet Gynecol 57:52S, 1981

Nappi RE, Palacios S, Panay N, et al: Vulvar and vaginal atrophy in four European countries: evidence from the European REVIVE Survey. Climacteric 19(2):188, 2016

National Osteoporosis Foundation: America's bone health: the state of osteoporosis and low bone mass in our nation. Washington, The Foundation, 2002

National Osteoporosis Foundation: Clinician's Guide to Prevention and Treatment of Osteoporosis. Washington, National Osteoporosis Foundation, 2014

Neer RM, Arnaud CD, Zanchetta JR, et al: Effect of parathyroid hormone (1-34) on fractures and bone mineral density in postmenopausal women with osteoporosis. N Engl J Med 344(19):1434, 2001

Newton KM, Reed SD, LaCroix AZ, et al: Treatment of vasomotor symptoms of menopause with black cohosh, multibotanicals, soy, hormone therapy, or placebo: a randomized trial. Ann Intern Med 145(12):869, 2006

O'Neill S, Eden J: The pathophysiology of menopausal symptoms. Obstet Gynaecol Reprod Med 22(3):63, 2011

Overlie I, Finset A, Holte A: Gendered personality dispositions, hormone values, and hot flushes during and after menopause. J Psychosom Obstet Gynaecol 23(4):219, 2002

Palma F, Xholli A, Cagnacci A: As the writing group of the AGATA study. The most bothersome symptom of vaginal atrophy: Evidence from the observational AGATA study. Maturitas 108(2):18, 2018

Paramsothy P, Harlow SD, Greendale GA, et al: Bleeding patterns during the menopausal transition in the multi-ethnic Study of Women's Health Across the Nation (SWAN): a prospective cohort study. BJOG 121:1564, 2014

Paramsothy P, Harlow SD, Nan B, et al: Duration of the menopausal transition is longer in women with young age at onset: the multiethnic Study of Women's Health Across the Nation. Menopause 24(2):142, 2017

Patel SR, Malhotra A, White DP, et al: Association between reduced sleep and weight gain in women. Am J Epidemiol 164(10):947, 2006

Patriarca MT, Goldman KZ, Dos Santos JM, et al: Effects of topical estradiol on the facial skin collagen of postmenopausal women under oral hormone therapy: a pilot study. Eur J Obstet Gynecol Reprod Biol 130(2):202, 2007

Pauls RN, Kleeman SD, Karram MM: Female sexual dysfunction: principles of diagnosis and therapy. Obstet Gynecol Surv 60(3):196, 2005

Pereira RI, Casey BA, Swibas TA, et al: Timing of estradiol treatment after menopause may determine benefit or harm to insulin action. J Clin Endocrinol Metab 100(12):4456, 2015

Phillips TJ, Symons J, Menon S, et al: Does hormone therapy improve age-related skin changes in postmenopausal women? A randomized, double-blind, double-dummy, placebo-controlled multicenter study assessing the effects of norethindrone acetate and ethinyl estradiol in the improvement of mild to moderate age-related skin changes in postmenopausal women. J Am Acad Dermatol 59(3):397, 2008

Pinkerton JV, Harvey JA, Lindsay R, et al: Effects of bazedoxifene/conjugated estrogens on the endometrium and bone: a randomized trial. J Clin Endocrinol Metab 99:E189, 2014

Pinkerton JV, Harvey JA, Pan K, et al: Breast effects of bazedoxifene-conjugated estrogens: a randomized controlled trial. Obstet Gynecol 121(5):959, 2013

Pinkerton JV, Kaunitz AM, Manson JE. Not time to abandon use of local vaginal hormone therapies. Menopause 25(8):855, 2018

Pinkerton JV, Santen RJ: Managing vasomotor symptoms in women after cancer. Climacteric 13:1, 2019

Pinkerton JV, Stovall DW, Kightlinger RS: Advances in the treatment of menopausal symptoms. Womens Health (England) 5 (4):361, 2009a

Pinkerton JV, Utian WH, Constantine GD, et al: Relief of vasomotor symptoms with the tissue-selective estrogen complex containing bazedoxifene/conjugated estrogens: a randomized, controlled trial. Menopause 16:1116, 2009b

Portman DJ, Gass ML, Vulvovaginal Atrophy Terminology Consensus Conference Panel: Genitourinary syndrome of menopause: new terminology for vulvovaginal atrophy from the International Society for the Study of Women's Sexual Health and the North American Menopause Society. Maturitas 79(3):349, 2014

Prague JK, Roberts RE, Comninos AN, et al: Neurokinin 3 receptor antagonism as a novel treatment for menopausal hot flushes: a phase 2, randomised, double-blind, placebo-controlled trial. Lancet 389(10081):1809, 2017

Prentice RL, Pettinger MB, Jackson RD, et al: Health risks and benefits from calcium and vitamin D supplementation: Women's Health Initiative clinical trial and cohort study. Osteoporos Int 24:567, 2013

Prestwood KM, Kenny AM, Kleppinger A, et al: Ultralow-dose micronized 17beta-estradiol and bone density and bone metabolism in older women: a randomized controlled trial. JAMA 290(8):1042, 2003

Rabley A, O'Shea T, Terry R, et al: Laser therapy for genitourinary syndrome of menopause. Curr Urol Rep 19(10):83, 2018

Rahn DD, Carberry C, Sanses TV, et al: Vaginal estrogen for genitourinary syndrome of menopause: a systematic review. Obstet Gynecol 124(6):1147, 2014

Ralston SH: Genetic control of susceptibility to osteoporosis. J Clin Endocrinol Metab 87:2460, 2002

Rance NE, Dacks PA, Mittelman-Smith MA, et al: Modulation of body temperature and LH secretion by hypothalamic KNDy (kisspeptin, neurokinin B and dynorphin) neurons: a novel hypothesis on the mechanism of hot flushes. Front Neuroendocrinol 34(3):211, 2013

Randolph JF Jr, Sowers M, Bondarenko I, et al: The relationship of longitudinal change in reproductive hormones and vasomotor symptoms during the menopausal transition. J Clin Endocrinol Metab 90:6106, 2005

Rapkin AJ: Vasomotor symptoms in menopause: physiologic condition and central nervous system approaches to treatment. Am J Obstet Gynecol 196(2):97, 2007

Recker RR, Davies KM, Hinders SM, et al: Bone gain in young adult women. JAMA 268:2403, 1992

Reyes FI, Winter JS, Faiman C: Pituitary-ovarian relationships preceding the menopause. I. A cross-sectional study of serum follicle-stimulating hormone, luteinizing hormone, prolactin, estradiol, and progesterone levels. Am J Obstet Gynecol 129:557, 1977

Richardson SJ, Senikas V, Nelson JF: Follicular depletion during the menopausal transition: evidence for accelerated loss and ultimate exhaustion. J Clin Endocrinol Metab 65:1231, 1987

Riedel-Baima B, Riedel A: Female pattern hair loss may be triggered by low oestrogen to androgen ratio. Endocr Regul 42(1):13, 2008

Riis BJ, Hansen MA, Jensen AM, et al: Low bone mass and fast rate of bone loss at menopause: equal risk factors for future fracture: a 15-year follow-up study. Bone 19:9, 1996

Robinson D, Cardozo L, Milsom I, et al: Oestrogens and overactive bladder. Neurourol Urodyn 33(7):1086, 2014

Rosen CJ: Clinical practice. Vitamin D insufficiency. N Engl J Med 364(3):248, 2011

Ross AC, Manson JE, Abrams SA, et al: The 2011 report on dietary reference intakes for calcium and vitamin D from the Institute of Medicine: what clinicians need to know. J Clin Endocrinol Metab 96(1):53, 2011

Rossouw JE, Anderson GL, Prentice RL, et al: Risks and benefits of estrogen plus progestin in healthy postmenopausal women: principal results from the Women's Health Initiative randomized controlled trial. JAMA 288(3):321, 2002

Rossouw JE, Prentice RL, Manson JE, et al: Postmenopausal hormone therapy and risk of cardiovascular disease by age and years since menopause. JAMA 297(13):1465, 2007

Rubin MR, Cosman F, Lindsay R, et al: The anabolic effects of parathyroid hormone. Osteoporos Int 13(4):267, 2002

Russell RG, Watts NB, Ebetino FH, et al: Mechanisms of action of bisphosphonates: similarities and differences and their potential influence on clinical efficacy. Osteoporos Int 19(6):733, 2008

Saag KG, Petersen J, Brandi ML, et al: Romosozumab or alendronate for fracture prevention in women with osteoporosis. N Engl J Med 377(15):1417, 2017

Sabatier JP, Guaydier-Souquieres G, Laroche D, et al: Bone mineral acquisition during adolescence and early adulthood: a study in 574 healthy females 10–24 years of age. Osteoporos Int 6:141, 1996

Saccomani S, Lui-Filho JF, Juliato CR, et al: Does obesity increase the risk of hot flashes among midlife women?: a population-based study. Menopause 24(9):1065, 2017

Salonia A, Zanni G, Nappi RE, et al: Sexual dysfunction is common in women with lower urinary tract symptoms and urinary incontinence: results of a cross-sectional study. Eur Urol 45:642, 2004

Sambrook P, Cooper C: Osteoporosis. Lancet 367(9527):2010, 2006

Sanders KM, Stuart AL, Williamson EJ, et al: Annual high-dose oral vitamin D and falls and fractures in older women: a randomized controlled trial. JAMA 303(18):1815, 2010

Santesso N, Carrasco-Labra A, Brignardello-Petersen R: Hip protectors for preventing hip fractures in older people. Cochrane Database Syst Rev 3:CD001255, 2014

Santoro N: Perimenopause: from research to practice. J Womens Health (Larchmt) 25(4):332, 2016a

Santoro N, Braunstein GD, Butts CL, et al: Compounded bioidentical hormones in endocrinology practice: an endocrine society scientific statement. J Clin Endocrinol Metab 101:1318, 2016b

Santoro N, Brown JR, Adel T, et al: Characterization of reproductive hormonal dynamics in the perimenopause. J Clin Endocrinol Metab 81:1495, 1996

Santoro N: The menopausal transition. Am J Med 118(12 suppl):8, 2005

Sator PG, Sator MO, Schmidt JB, et al: A prospective, randomized, double-blind, placebo-controlled study on the influence of a hormone replacement therapy on skin aging in postmenopausal women. Climacteric 10(4):320, 2007

Sauerbronn AV, Fonseca AM, Bagnoli VR, et al: The effects of systemic hormonal replacement therapy on the skin of postmenopausal women. Int J Gynaecol Obstet 68(1):35, 2000

Scheffers CS, Armstrong S, Cantineau AE, et al: Dehydroepiandrosterone for women in the peri- or postmenopausal phase. Cochrane Database Syst Rev 1:CD011066, 2015

Schiff I, Tulchinsky D, Cramer D, et al: Oral medroxyprogesterone in the treatment of postmenopausal symptoms. JAMA 244:1443, 1980

Sellmeyer DE, Schloetter M, Sebastian A: Potassium citrate prevents increased urine calcium excretion and bone resorption induced by a high sodium chloride diet. J Clin Endocrinol Metab 87(5):2008, 2002

Shams-White MM, Chung M, Du M, et al: Dietary protein and bone health: a systematic review and meta-analysis from the National Osteoporosis Foundation. Am J Clin Nutr 105(6):1528, 2017

Sherburn M, Guthrie JR, Dudley EC, et al: Is incontinence associated with menopause? Obstet Gynecol 98:628, 2001

Shifren JL, Braunstein GD, Simon JA, et al: Transdermal testosterone treatment in women with impaired sexual function after oophorectomy. N Engl J Med 343(10):682, 2000

Shifren JL, Gass ML, NAMS Recommendations for Clinical Care of Midlife Women Working Group: The North American Menopause Society recommendations for clinical care of midlife women. Menopause 21(10):1038, 2014

Shumaker SA, Legault C, Kuller L, et al: Conjugated equine estrogens and incidence of probable dementia and mild cognitive impairment in postmenopausal women: Women's Health Initiative Memory Study. JAMA 291(24):2947, 2004

Shumaker SA, Legault C, Rapp SR, et al: Estrogen plus progestin and the incidence of dementia and mild cognitive impairment in postmenopausal women: the Women's Health Initiative Memory Study: a randomized controlled trial. JAMA 289(20):2651, 2003

Sideras K, Loprinzi CL: Nonhormonal management of hot flashes for women on risk reduction therapy. J Natl Compr Canc Netw 8(10):1171, 2010

Sigurdsson G, Halldorsson BV, Styrkarsdottir U, et al: Impact of genetics on low bone mass in adults. J Bone Miner Res 23(10):1584, 2008

Simon JA, Altomare C, Cort S, et al: Overall safety of ospemifene in postmenopausal women from placebo-controlled phase 2 and 3 trials. J Womens Health (Larchmt) 27(1):14, 2018

Simon JA, Lin VH, Radovich C, et al: One-year long-term safety extension study of ospemifene for the treatment of vulvar and vaginal atrophy in postmenopausal women with a uterus. Menopause 20(4):418, 2013

Slopien R, Meczekalski B, Warenik-Szymankiewicz A: Relationship between climacteric symptoms and serum serotonin levels in postmenopausal women. Climacteric 6:53, 2003

Smith DC, Prentice R, Thompson DJ, et al: Association of exogenous estrogen and endometrial carcinoma. N Engl J Med 293(23):1164, 1975

Soares CN, Almeida OP, Joffe H, et al: Efficacy of estradiol for the treatment of depressive disorders in perimenopausal women: a double-blind, randomized, placebo-controlled trial. Arch Gen Psychiatry 58(6):529, 2001

Soares CN: Menopause and mood disturbance. Psychiatric Times 12:2005

Soares CN: Mood disorders in midlife women: understanding the critical window and its clinical implications. Menopause 21(2)198, 2014

Sokol ER, Karram MM: Use of a novel fractional CO2 laser for the treatment of genitourinary syndrome of menopause: 1-year outcomes. Menopause 24(7):810, 2017

Spinelli MG: Neuroendocrine effects on mood. Rev Endocr Metab Disord 6:109, 2005

Sriprasert I, Hodis HN, Karim R, et al: Differential effect of plasma estradiol on subclinical atherosclerosis progression in early vs late postmenopause. J Clin Endocrinol Metab 104(2):293, 2019

Stear SJ, Prentice A, Jones SC, et al: Effect of a calcium and exercise intervention on the bone mineral status of 16- to 18-year-old adolescent girls. Am J Clin Nutr 77:985, 2003

Stein E, Shane E: Secondary osteoporosis. Endocrinol Metab Clin North Am 32:115, 2003

Sternfeld B, Wang H, Quesenberry CP Jr, et al: Physical activity and changes in weight and waist circumference in midlife women: findings from the Study of Women's Health Across the Nation. Am J Epidemiol 160(9):912, 2004

Tashjian AH Jr, Chabner BA: Commentary on clinical safety of recombinant human parathyroid hormone 1–34 in the treatment of osteoporosis in men and postmenopausal women. J Bone Miner Res 17(7):1151, 2002

Tepper PG, Brooks MM, Randolph JF Jr, et al: Characterizing the trajectories of vasomotor symptoms across the menopausal transition. Menopause 23(10):1067, 2016

The North American Menopause Society: Management of osteoporosis in postmenopausal women: 2010 position statement of The North American Menopause Society. Menopause 17(1):25, 2010

The North American Menopause Society: Management of symptomatic vulvovaginal atrophy: 2013 position statement of the North American Menopause Society. Menopause 20(9):888, 2013

The North American Menopause Society: The 2017 hormone therapy position statement of The North American Menopause Society. Menopause 24(7):728, 2017

The North American Menopause Society: Nonhormonal management of menopause-associated vasomotor symptoms: 2015 position statement of The North American Menopause Society. Menopause 22(11):1155, 2015

The Women's Health Initiative Steering Committee: Effects of conjugated equine estrogen in postmenopausal women with hysterectomy: The Women's Health Initiative Randomized Controlled Trial. JAMA 291:1701, 2004

Theintz G, Buchs B, Rizzoli R, et al: Longitudinal monitoring of bone mass accumulation in healthy adolescents: evidence for a marked reduction after 16 years of age at the levels of lumbar spine and femoral neck in female subjects. J Clin Endocrinol Metab 75:1060, 1992

Thornton MJ: Estrogens and aging skin. Dermatoendocrinol 5(2):264, 2013

Thurston RC, Bromberger JT, Joffe H, et al: Beyond frequency: who is most bothered by vasomotor symptoms? Menopause 5:841, 2008

Thurston RC, Sowers MR, Sternfeld B, et al: Gains in body fat and vasomotor symptom reporting over the menopausal transition: the study of women's health across the nation. Am J Epidemiol 170(6):766, 2009

Tosteson AN, Melton LJ III, Dawson-Hughes B, et al: Cost-effective osteoporosis treatment thresholds: the United States perspective. Osteoporos Int 19(4):437, 2008

Treloar AE: Menstrual cyclicity and the pre-menopause. Maturitas 3(3-4):249, 1981

Trutnovsky G, Rojas RG, Mann KP, et al: Urinary incontinence: the role of menopause. Menopause 21(4):399, 2014

Tungphaisal S, Chandeying V, Sutthijumroon S, et al: Postmenopausal sexuality in Thai women. Asia Oceania J Obstet Gynaecol 17:143, 1991

US Census Bureau: 2017 national population projections tables. 2017. Available at: https://www.census.gov/data/tables/2017/demo/popproj/2017-summary-tables.html. Accessed September 1, 2019

US Preventive Services Task Force, Grossman DC, Curry SJ, et al: Interventions to prevent falls in community-dwelling older adults: US Preventive Services Task Force recommendation statement. JAMA 319(16):1696, 2018a

US Preventive Services Task Force, Grossman DC, Curry SJ, et al: Vitamin D, calcium, or combined supplementation for the primary prevention of fractures in community-dwelling adults: US Preventive Services Task Force recommendation statement. JAMA 319(15):1592, 2018b

US Preventive Services Task Force, Owens DK, Davidson KW, et al: Medication use to reduce risk of breast cancer: US Preventive Services Task Force recommendation statement. JAMA 322(9):857, 2019

Utian W, Yu H, Bobula J, et al: Bazedoxifene/conjugated estrogens and quality of life in post-menopausal women. Maturitas 63:329, 2009

Van Beresteijn EC, Korevaar JC, Huijbregts PC, et al: Perimenopausal increase in serum cholesterol: a 10-year longitudinal study. Am J Epidemiol 137:383, 1993

Vinogradova Y, Coupland C, Hippisley-Cox J: Use of hormone replacement therapy and risk of venous thromboembolism: nested case-control studies using the QResearch and CPRD databases. BMJ 364:k4810, 2019

Waetjen LE, Ye J, Feng WY, et al: Association between menopausal transition stages and developing urinary incontinence. Obstet Gynecol 114(5):989, 2009

Walker MD, Liu XS, Stein E, et al: Differences in bone microarchitecture between postmenopausal Chinese-American and white women. J Bone Miner Res 26:1392, 2011

Watts NB, Cauley JA, Jackson RD, et al: Women's Health Initiative Investigators. No increase in fractures after stopping hormone therapy: results from the women's health initiative investigators. J Clin Endocrinol Metab 102(1):302, 2017

Wells G, Tugwell P, Shea B, et al: Metaanalyses of therapies for postmenopausal osteoporosis. V. Metaanalysis of the efficacy of hormone replacement therapy in treating and preventing osteoporosis in postmenopausal women. Endocr Rev 23:529, 2002

Whitaker M, Guo J, Kehoe T, Benson G. Bisphosphonates for osteoporosis—where do we go from here? N Engl J Med 366:2048, 2012

Wierman ME, Arlt W, Basson R, et al: Androgen therapy in women: a reappraisal: an Endocrine Society clinical practice guideline. J Clin Endocrinol Metab 99(10):3489, 2014

Wilbur J, Miller AM, Montgomery A, et al: Sociodemographic characteristics, biological factors, and symptom reporting in midlife women. Menopause 5:43, 1998

Wines N, Willsteed E: Menopause and the skin. Australas J Dermatol 42:149, 2001

Wing RR, Matthews KA, Kuller LH, et al: Weight gain at the time of menopause. Arch Intern Med 151:97, 1991

Woods NF, Smith-DiJulio K, Percival DB, et al: Depressed mood during the menopausal transition and early postmenopause: observations from the Seattle Midlife Women's Health Study. Menopause 15(2):223, 2008

Woodward S, Freedman RR: The thermoregulatory effects of menopausal hot flashes on sleep. Sleep 17:497, 1994

Yaffe K, Sawaya G, Lieberburg I, et al: Estrogen therapy in postmenopausal women: effects on cognitive function and dementia. JAMA 279(9):688, 1998

Yaghjyan L, Colditz GA: Estrogens in the breast tissue: a systematic review. Cancer Causes Control 22(4):529, 2011

Zaitlen N, Kraft P, Patterson N, Using extended genealogy to estimate components of heritability for 23 quantitative and dichotomous traits. PLoS Genet 9(5):e1003520, 2013

Zandi PP, Carlson MC, Plassman BL, et al: Hormone replacement therapy and incidence of Alzheimer disease in older women: the Cache County Study. JAMA 288(17):2123, 2002

Zava DT, Dollbaum CM, Blen M: Estrogen and progestin bioactivity of foods, herbs, and spices. Proc Soc Exp Biol Med 217(3):369, 1998

Zoltick ES, Sahni S, McLean RR, et al: Dietary protein intake and subsequent falls in older men and women: the Framingham Study. J Nutr Health Aging 15(2):147, 2011

Zweifel JE, O'Brien WH: A metaanalysis of the effect of hormone replacement therapy upon depressed mood. Psychoneuroendocrinology 22(3):189, 1997

FEMALE PELVIC MEDICINE AND RECONSTRUCTIVE SURGERY

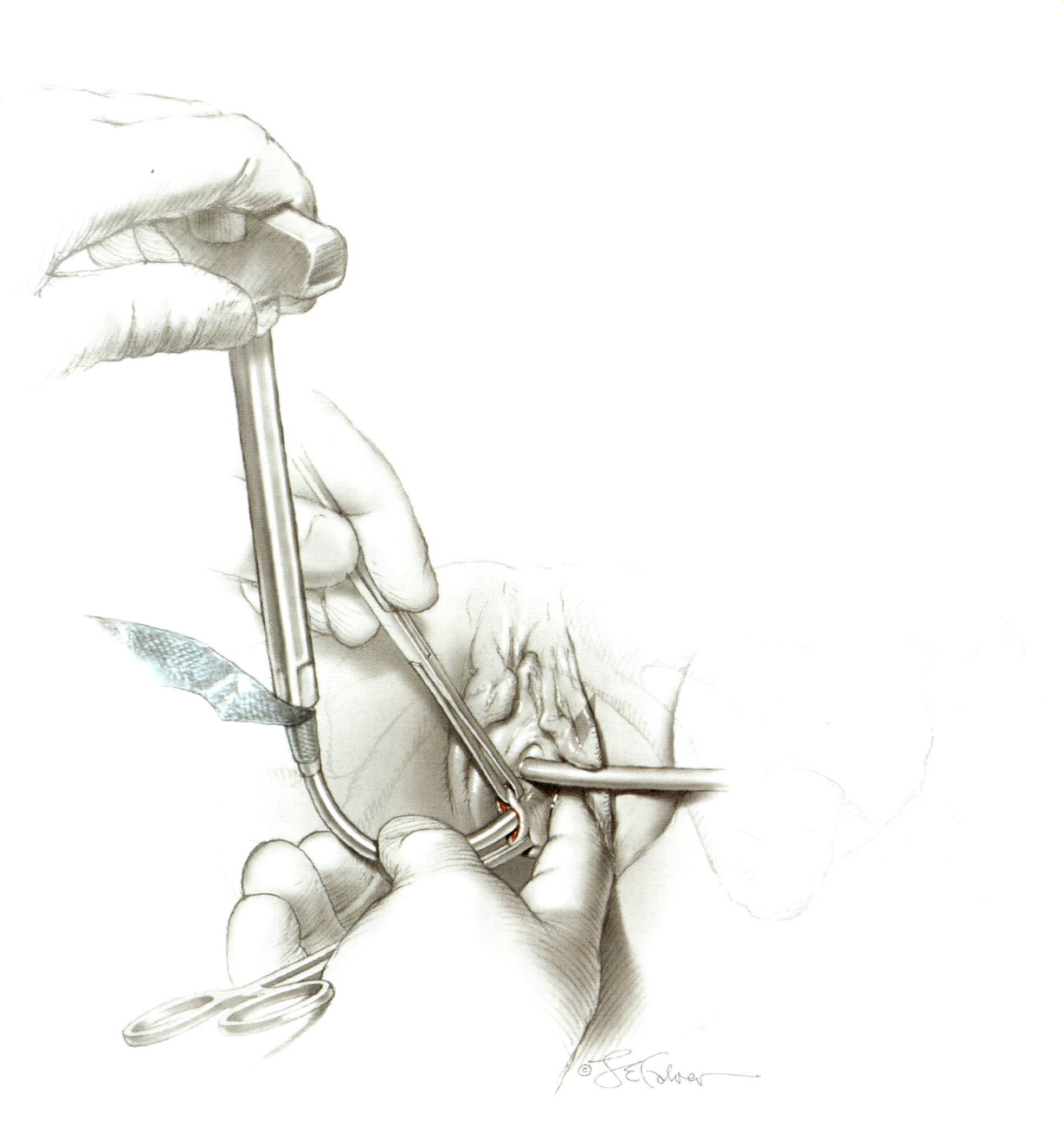

Urinary Incontinence

DEFINITIONS

Urinary incontinence is defined as involuntary leakage of urine. This contrasts with urine that leaks from extraurethral sources, such as fistulas or lower urinary tract congenital malformations. Although incontinence is categorized into several forms, this chapter focuses on the evaluation and management of stress and urgency urinary incontinence. *Stress urinary incontinence* (SUI) is the involuntary leakage of urine with increases in intraabdominal pressure. *Urgency urinary incontinence* is the involuntary leakage accompanied or immediately preceded by a perceived strong imminent need to void. A related condition, *overactive bladder*, describes urinary urgency with or without incontinence and usually with greater daytime urinary frequency and nocturia (Abrams, 2009).

According to International Continence Society guidelines, urinary incontinence is a symptom, a sign, and a condition (Abrams, 2002). For example, with SUI, a patient may complain of involuntary urine leakage with exercise or laughing. Concurrent with these symptoms, involuntary leakage from the urethra synchronous with cough or Valsalva may be observed during examination by a provider. And as a condition, SUI is objectively demonstrated during urodynamic testing if involuntary leakage of urine accompanies increased abdominal pressure and absence of detrusor muscle contraction. Under these circumstances, when the symptom or sign of SUI is confirmed with objective testing, the term *urodynamic stress incontinence* is preferred.

With urgency urinary incontinence, women have difficulty postponing urination urges and generally must promptly empty their bladder on cue and without delay. Common triggers are hand washing, running water, or exposure to cold. Urgency urinary incontinence is sometimes objectively demonstrated during urodynamic testing to correspond temporally with spontaneous detrusor muscle contractions—a condition termed *detrusor overactivity*. When both stress and urgency symptoms are present, it is called *mixed urinary incontinence*.

EPIDEMIOLOGY

In Western societies, epidemiologic studies indicate a prevalence of urinary incontinence of 25 to 51 percent and even higher among nursing home patients (Buckley, 2010; Markland, 2011). This wide range is attributed to variations in research methodologies, population characteristics, and definitions of incontinence. As part of the 2005 to 2006 National Health and Nutrition Examination Survey (NHANES), urinary incontinence characterized by participants as moderate to severe leakage was identified in 16 percent (Nygaard, 2008). A subsequent review of NHANES confirmed a similar rate of 17 percent (Wu, 2014). Among ambulatory women with urinary incontinence, SUI represents 29 to 75 percent of cases. Urgency urinary incontinence accounts for up to 33 percent, whereas the remainder is attributable to mixed forms (Hunskaar, 2000). However, current available data are limited by the fact that most women do not seek medical attention for this condition (Hunskaar, 2000). It is estimated that only one in four women will seek medical advice for incontinence, due to embarrassment, limited health-care access, or poor screening by health-care providers (Hannestad 2002; Minassian, 2012).

Urinary incontinence can significantly impair quality of life and lead to disrupted social relationships, embarrassment and frustration, and hospitalizations due to skin breakdown and urinary tract infection (UTI). As up to one third of incontinent women have urinary leakage during sexual activity, incontinence—or fear of incontinence—during intercourse may contribute to sexual dysfunction (Gray, 2018; Serati, 2009). Older women with incontinence are 2.5 times more likely to be admitted to a nursing home than continent women (Langa, 2002). Moreover, population projections from the U.S. Census Bureau forecast that the number of American women with urinary incontinence will increase 55 percent from 18.3 million to 28.4 million between 2010 and 2050 (Wu, 2009).

RISKS

◼ Age

The prevalence and severity of incontinence appears to rise gradually with age during young adult life. Data from the 2005 to 2006 NHANES demonstrated an incontinence prevalence of 7 percent in those aged 20 to 40 years, 17 percent for ages 40 to 60, 23 percent for ages 60 to 80, and 32 percent for those older than 80 (Nygaard, 2008).

TABLE 23-1. Risk Factors for Urinary Incontinence

Age
Obesity
Smoking
Pregnancy
Childbirth
Menopause
Cognitive impairment
Functional impairment
Chronically increased abdominal pressure
    Chronic cough
    Constipation
    Occupational lifting

Incontinence should not be viewed as a normal consequence of aging (Table 23-1). However, several physiologic age-related changes in the lower urinary tract may predispose to incontinence, overactive bladder, or other voiding difficulties. First, the prevalence of involuntary detrusor contractions increases with age, and detrusor overactivity is found in 21 percent of healthy, continent community-dwelling elderly (Resnick, 1995). Both total bladder capacity and the ability to postpone voiding decreases, and these declines may lead to urinary frequency. In addition, urinary flow rates are reduced in older women and are likely due to an age-associated decrease in detrusor contractility (Resnick, 1984). In women, postmenopausal drops in estrogen levels result in atrophy of the urethral mucosal seal, loss of compliance, and bladder irritation, which may predispose to both SUI and urgency urinary incontinence. Finally, renal filtration rate and diurnal levels of antidiuretic hormone and atrial natriuretic factor change with age. These shift the diurnal-predominant pattern of fluid excretion toward one with greater urine excretion later in the day (Kirkland, 1983).

■ Childbirth

Childbirth and pregnancy also play a role, and urinary incontinence prevalence is higher in parous women compared with nulliparas. The effects of childbirth may result from direct injury to pelvic muscles and connective tissue attachments. In addition, nerve damage from trauma or stretch injury can lead to pelvic muscle dysfunction. Specifically, rates of prolonged pudendal nerve latency after delivery are higher in women with incontinence compared with asymptomatic puerpera (Snooks, 1986).

Of potential obstetric factors, one large study identified that fetal birthweight >4000 g elevates the risk of all urinary incontinence types (Rortveit, 2003b). These authors also noted that cesarean delivery may offer a short-term protective effect from urinary incontinence. The adjusted odds ratio for any incontinence associated with vaginal delivery compared with that with cesarean delivery was 1.7 (Rortveit, 2003a). However, the protective effect of cesarean delivery on incontinence may dissipate after additional deliveries, declines with age, and is no longer present in older women (Nygaard, 2006).

■ Other Factors

Race may influence incontinence rates, and white women are believed to have higher SUI rates than women of other races. In contrast, urgency urinary incontinence is believed to be more prevalent among African-American women. Most reports are not population based and thus are not the best estimate of true racial differences. However, data from the Nurses' Health Study cohorts, which included more than 76,000 women, did support these racial differences (Townsend, 2010). Whether these differences are biologic, related to health-care access, or affected by cultural expectations and symptom tolerance thresholds is unclear.

Body mass index (BMI) is a significant and independent risk factor, and the prevalence of both urgency urinary incontinence and SUI rises proportionally with BMI. (Hannestad, 2003). Compared to nonobese women, obese women have an approximately threefold greater likelihood of urinary incontinence (Al-Mukhtar, 2017; Lawrence, 2007). Theoretically, the increase in intraabdominal pressure that coincides with a higher BMI results in a higher intravesical pressure. This greater pressure overcomes urethral closing pressure and leads to incontinence (Bai, 2002). Encouragingly, weight loss is considered a first-line option, and the prevalence of urinary incontinence significantly declines following weight loss achieved by behavior modification or with bariatric surgery (Burgio, 2007; Deitel, 1988; Dumoulin, 2016; Subak, 2009). Even losses of 5 to 10 percent of body weight are sufficient for significant improvement in urinary incontinence (Wing, 2010).

Menopause may have a relationship with incontinence, but studies have inconsistently demonstrated an increase in urinary dysfunction rates (Bump, 1998). In those with symptoms, separating aging changes from hypoestrogenism effects is difficult. First, high-affinity estrogen receptors are found in the urethra, pubococcygeal muscle, and bladder trigone but are infrequently found elsewhere in the bladder (Iosif, 1981). Hypoestrogenic-related collagen changes and reductions in urethral vascularity and skeletal muscle volume are factors. They are thought collectively to contribute to impaired urethral function by lowering the resting urethral pressure (Carlile, 1988). Moreover, estrogen deficiency with resulting urogenital atrophy is believed to be responsible in part for urinary sensory symptoms following menopause (Raz, 1993). Despite this evidence, it is less clear whether estrogen therapy is useful in the treatment or prevention of incontinence. Curiously, systemic estrogen replacement, compared with placebo, appears to worsen incontinence, but topical vaginal estrogen application *may improve* it (Cody, 2012; Fantl, 1994, 1996; Rahn, 2014, 2015).

Family history may alter incontinence risks, and the urinary incontinence rates—particularly for urgency urinary incontinence—may be higher in the daughters and sisters of incontinent women. In one large survey, daughters of incontinent women had an increased relative risk of 1.3 and an absolute risk of 23 percent of having urinary incontinence. Younger sisters of incontinent women also had a greater likelihood of having any urinary incontinence (Hannestad, 2004).

Chronic obstructive pulmonary disease in women older than 60 years significantly elevates urinary incontinence risks (Brown, 1996; Diokno, 1990). Similarly, cigarette smoking is identified as an independent risk factor for urinary incontinence. Both current

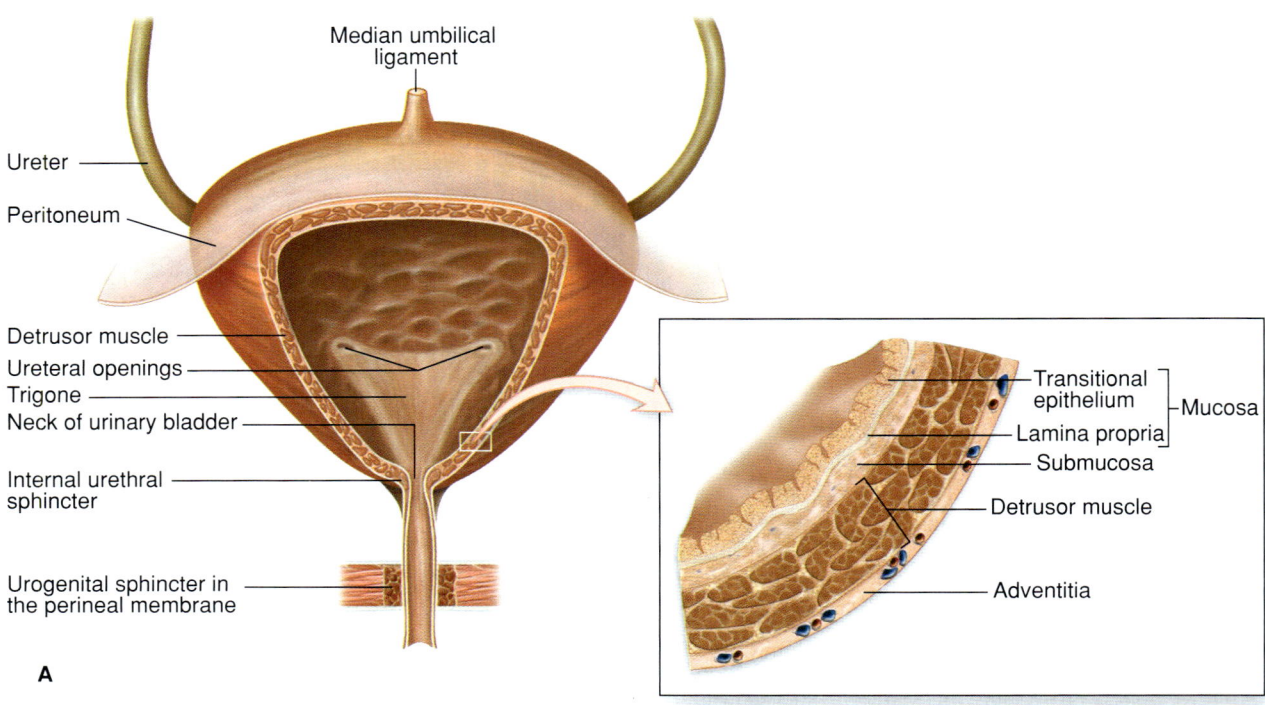

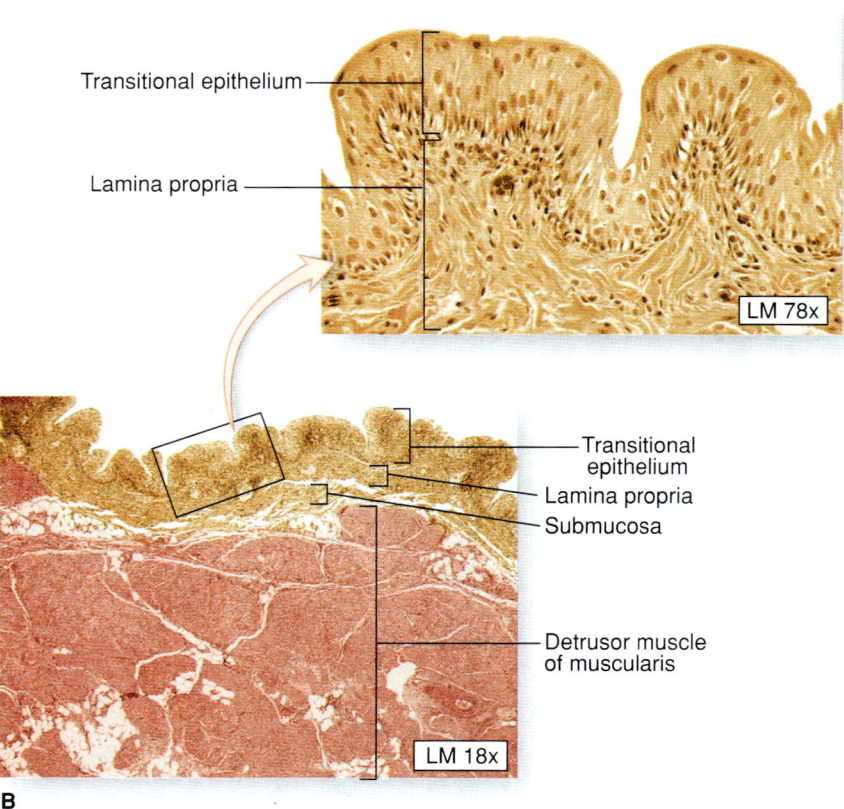

FIGURE 23-1 Bladder anatomy. **A.** Anteroposterior view of bladder anatomy. Inset: The bladder wall contains mucosal, submucosal, muscular, and adventitial layers. **B.** Photomicrograph of the bladder wall. The mucosa of an empty bladder is thrown into convoluted folds or rugae. The plexiform arrangement of muscle fibers of the detrusor muscle causes difficulty in defining its three distinct layers. (Reproduced with permission from McKinley, 2006.)

and former smokers have a two- to threefold risk of incontinence compared with nonsmokers (Brown, 1996; Bump, 1992; Diokno, 1990). In one study, current and former smoking was associated with incontinence, but only for those who smoked more than 20 cigarettes daily. Severe incontinence was weakly associated with smoking regardless of cigarette number (Hannestad, 2003). Theoretically, persistently elevated intraabdominal pressures are generated from a smoker's chronic cough, and collagen synthesis is diminished by smoking's antiestrogenic effects.

Hysterectomy does not appear to raise urinary incontinence rates. Studies that include pre- and postoperative urodynamic testing reveal clinically insignificant changes in bladder function. Moreover, evidence does not support avoidance of clinically indicated hysterectomy or the selection of supracervical hysterectomy as measures to prevent urinary incontinence (Vervest, 1989; Wake, 1980).

PATHOPHYSIOLOGY

■ Continence

The bladder has the capacity to accommodate large increases in volume with minimal or no increases in intravesical pressure. The ability to store urine coupled with convenient and socially acceptable voluntary emptying is *continence*. Continence requires the complex coordination of multiple components that include: muscle contraction and relaxation, appropriate connective tissue support, and integrated innervation and communication between these structures. Simplistically, during filling, urethral contraction is coordinated with bladder relaxation and urine is stored. During voiding, the urethra relaxes and the bladder contracts. These mechanisms can be challenged by uninhibited detrusor contractions, marked increases in intraabdominal pressure, and degradation or dysfunction of the various anatomic components of the continence mechanism.

■ Bladder Filling

Bladder Anatomy

The bladder wall is multilayered and contains mucosal, submucosal, muscular, and adventitial layers (Fig. 23-1). The bladder mucosa is composed of a transitional cell epithelium, supported by a lamina propria. With small bladder volumes, the mucosa appears as convoluted folds. However, with bladder filling, it is stretched and thinned. The bladder epithelium, termed uroepithelium, is made up of distinct cell layers. The most superficial is the umbrella cell layer, and its impermeability is thought to provide the primary urine-plasma barrier. Covering the *uroepithelium* is a glycosaminoglycan (GAG) layer. This GAG layer may prohibit bacterial adherence and prevents urothelial damage by acting as a protective barrier. Specifically, theories suggest that this carbohydrate polymer layer may be defective in patients with interstitial cystitis (Chap. 12, p. 267).

The muscular layer, termed the detrusor muscle, is composed of three smooth-muscle layers arranged in a plexiform fashion. This unique arrangement allows for rapid multidimensional expansion during bladder filling and is a key component to the bladder's ability to accommodate large volumes.

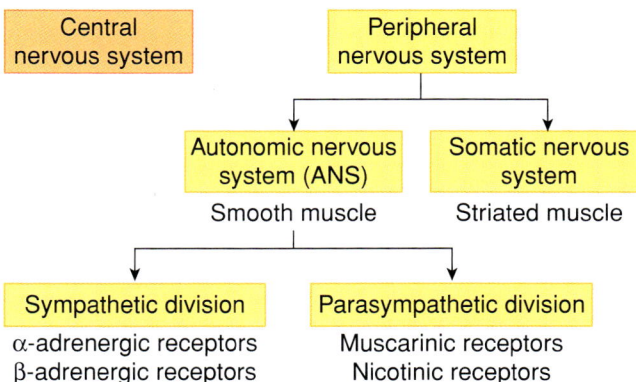

FIGURE 23-2 Divisions of the human nervous system. The peripheral nervous system includes: (1) the somatic nervous system, which mediates voluntary movements through its actions on striated muscle and (2) the autonomic nervous system, which controls involuntary motion through its actions on smooth muscle. The autonomic nervous system is further divided into the sympathetic division, which acts through epinephrine and norepinephrine binding to adrenergic receptors and (2) the parasympathetic division, which acts through acetylcholine binding to muscarinic or nicotinic receptors.

Innervation

Normal function of the lower urinary tract requires integration of peripheral and central nervous systems. The peripheral nervous system contains somatic and autonomic divisions (Fig. 23-2). Of these, the somatic component innervates striated muscle, whereas the autonomic division innervates smooth muscle.

The autonomic nervous system controls involuntary action and is categorized into sympathetic and parasympathetic divisions. The sympathetic system mediates its end-organ effects through epinephrine or norepinephrine acting on α- or β-adrenergic receptors (Fig. 23-3). The parasympathetic division acts through

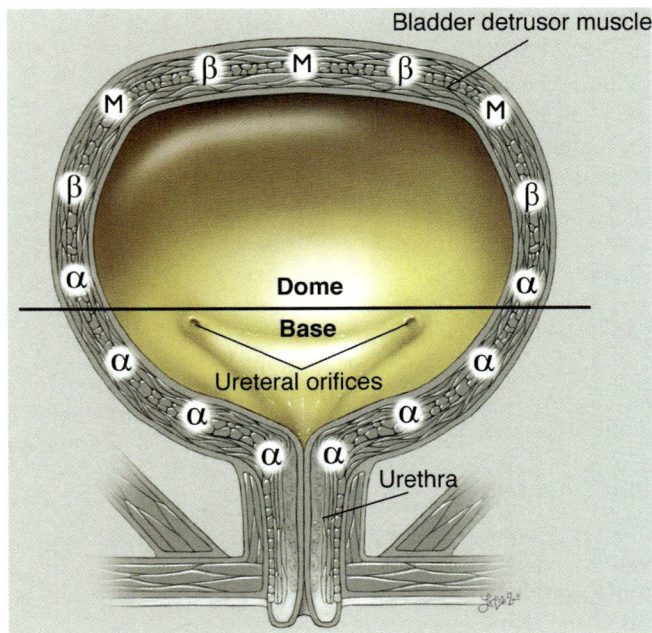

FIGURE 23-3 The bladder dome is rich in parasympathetic muscarinic receptors (M) and sympathetic β-adrenergic receptors (β). The bladder neck contains a greater density of sympathetic α-adrenergic receptors (α). (Reproduced with permission from Lindsay Oksenberg.)

acetylcholine binding to muscarinic or nicotinic receptors. In the pelvis, autonomic fibers that supply the pelvic viscera course in the superior and inferior hypogastric plexi (Fig. 23-4).

The somatic nervous system controls voluntary movement, and the portion of this system that is most relevant to lower urinary tract function originates from the Onuf somatic nucleus. This nucleus is located in the ventral horn gray matter of spinal levels S2–S4 and contains the neurons that innervate the striated urogenital sphincter complex, described next. Nerves involved with that connection include branches of the pudendal and pelvic nerves.

Urogenital Sphincter

As the bladder fills, synchronized contraction of the urogenital sphincter is integral to continence. Composed of striated muscle, this sphincter complex includes: (1) the *sphincter urethrae*, (2) the *urethrovaginal sphincter*, and (3) the *compressor urethrae*. The sphincter urethrae wraps circumferentially around the urethra. In comparison, the urethrovaginal sphincter and the compressor urethrae arch ventrally over the urethra and insert into the fibromuscular tissue of the anterior vaginal wall (Fig. 23-5).

These three muscles function as a single unit and contract to close the urethra. Contraction of these muscles circumferentially constricts the cephalad two thirds of the urethra and laterally compresses the distal one third. The sphincter urethrae is predominantly composed of slow-twitch fibers and remains tonically contracted, contributing substantially to continence at rest. In contrast, the urethrovaginal sphincter and the compressor urethrae are comprised of fast-twitch muscle fibers, which allow brisk contraction and urethra lumen closure when continence is challenged by sudden increases in intraabdominal pressure.

Innervation Important to Storage

When urine is being stored, the distention of the bladder wall stimulates low-level afferent vesical firing that, in turn, stimulates sympathetic outflow to the bladder base and urethra, and also pudendal outflow to the external urethra. This occurs by a spinal reflex pathway. The urogenital sphincter receives

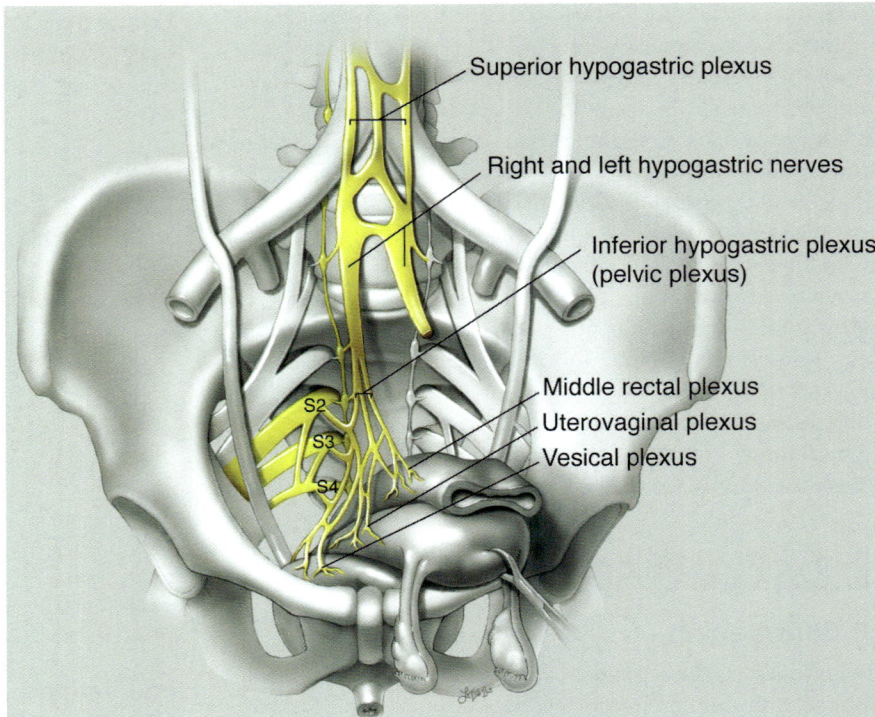

FIGURE 23-4 The inferior hypogastric plexus, also known as the pelvic plexus, is formed by visceral efferents from S2 to S4, which provide the parasympathetic component by way of the pelvic nerves. The superior hypogastric plexus primarily contains sympathetic fibers from the T10 to L2 cord segments and terminates by dividing into right and left hypogastric nerves. The hypogastric nerves and rami from the sacral portion of the sympathetic chain contribute the sympathetic component to the pelvic plexus. The pelvic plexus divides into three portions according to the course and distribution of its fibers: the middle rectal plexus, uterovaginal plexus, and vesical plexus. (Reproduced with permission from Lindsay Oksenberg.)

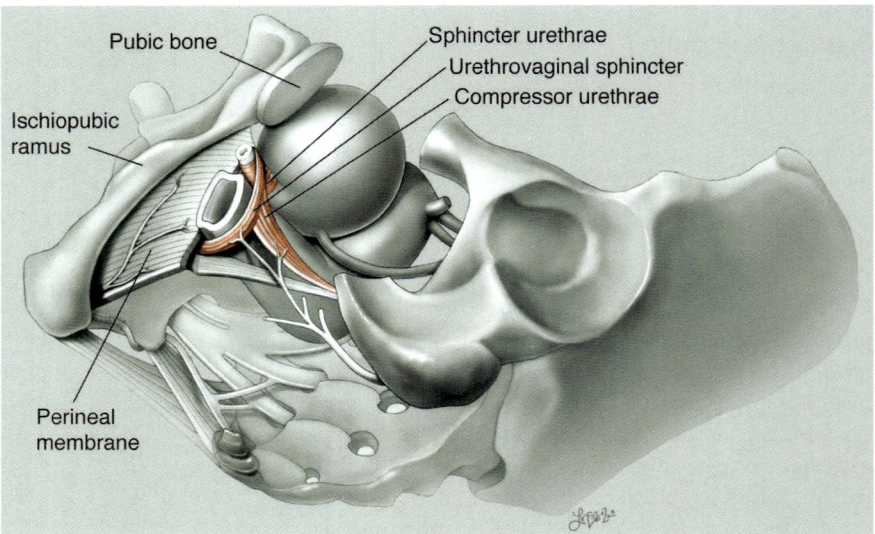

FIGURE 23-5 Striated urogenital sphincter anatomy. The perineal membrane is removed to show the three component muscles of the striated urogenital sphincter. This sphincter receives most of its somatic innervation through the pudendal nerve. (Reproduced with permission from Lindsay Oksenberg.)

somatic motor innervation through the pudendal and pelvic nerves (Fig. 23-6). Thus, pudendal neuropathy, which may follow obstetric injury, can affect normal sphincter functioning. Additionally, prior pelvic surgery or pelvic radiation therapy may damage nerves, vasculature, and soft tissue. Such injury can lead to ineffective urogenital sphincter action and contribute to incontinence. A region of the rostral pons known as the pontine storage center (or "L" region) also may increase activity of the external urethral sphincter.

Sympathetic fibers are carried through the superior hypogastric nerve plexus and communicate with α- and β-adrenergic receptors within the bladder and urethra. When norepinephrine binds to the β-adrenergic receptors in the bladder dome, it activates adenylate cyclase, which in turn raises levels of cyclic adenosine monophosphate and results in smooth-muscle relaxation and assists with urine storage (Fig. 23-7). β-Agonist medication may improve overactive

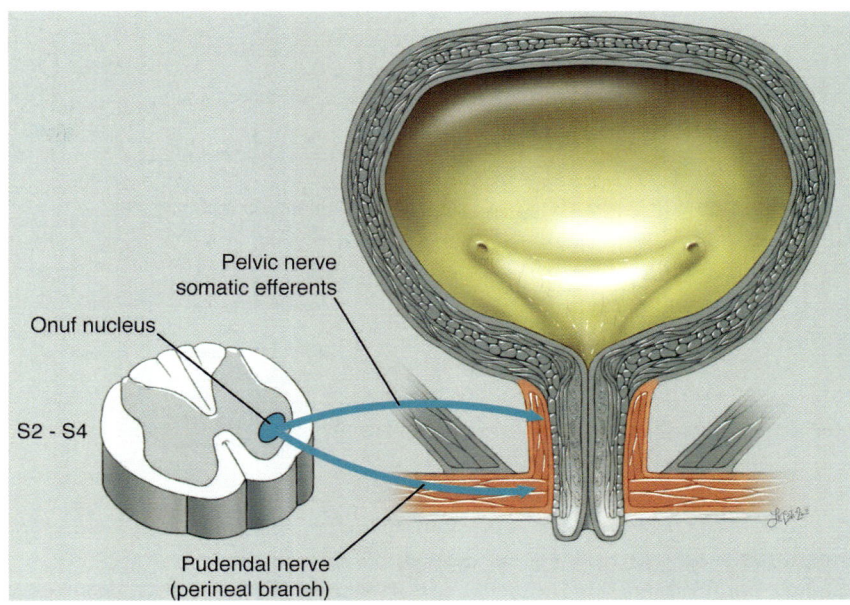

FIGURE 23-6 The Onuf nucleus is found in the ventral horn gray matter of S2 through S4. This nucleus contains the neurons whose fibers supply the striated urogenital sphincter. The urethrovaginal sphincter and compressor urethrae are innervated by the perineal branch of the pudendal nerve. The sphincter urethrae is variably innervated by somatic efferents that travel in the pelvic nerves. (Reproduced with permission from Lindsay Oksenberg.)

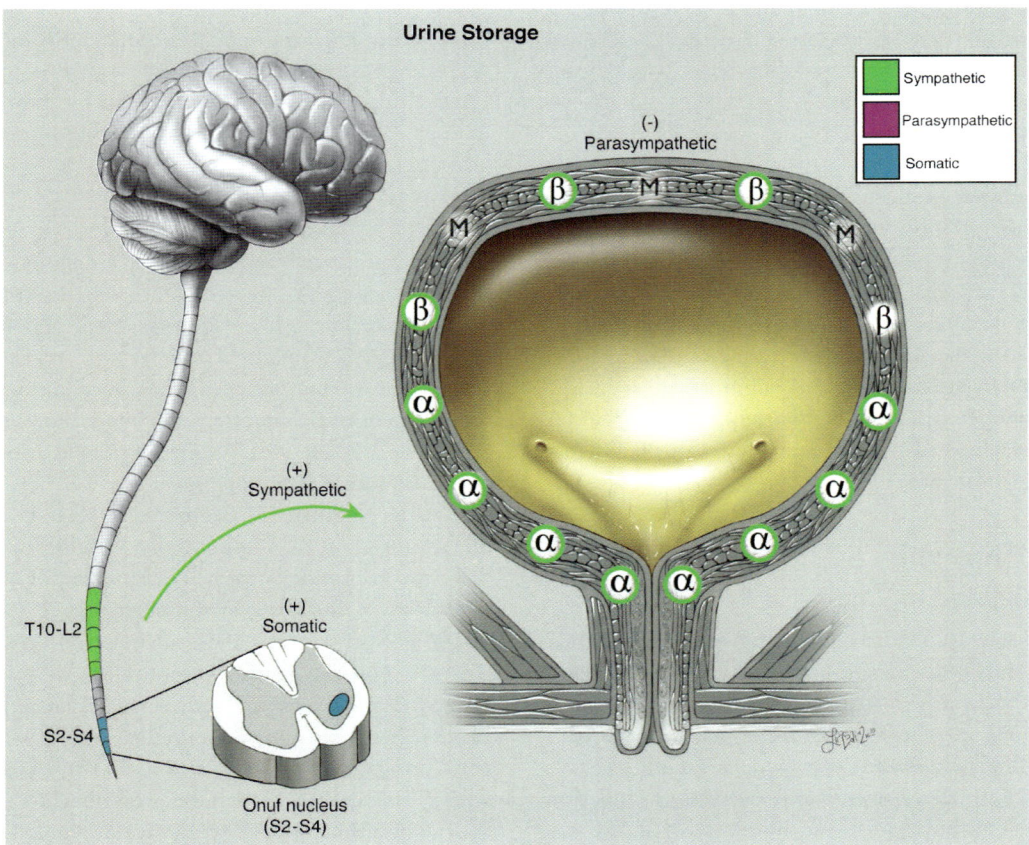

FIGURE 23-7 Physiology of urine storage. Bladder distention from filling leads to: (1) α-adrenergic contraction of the urethral smooth muscle and increased tone at the vesical neck (via the T11–L2 spinal sympathetic reflex); (2) activation of urethral motor neurons in the Onuf nucleus with contraction of striated urogenital sphincter muscles (via the pudendal nerve); and (3) inhibited parasympathetic transmission with decreased detrusor pressure. α = alpha adrenergic receptors; β = beta adrenergic; M = muscarinic (cholinergic). (Reproduced with permission from Lindsay Oksenberg.)

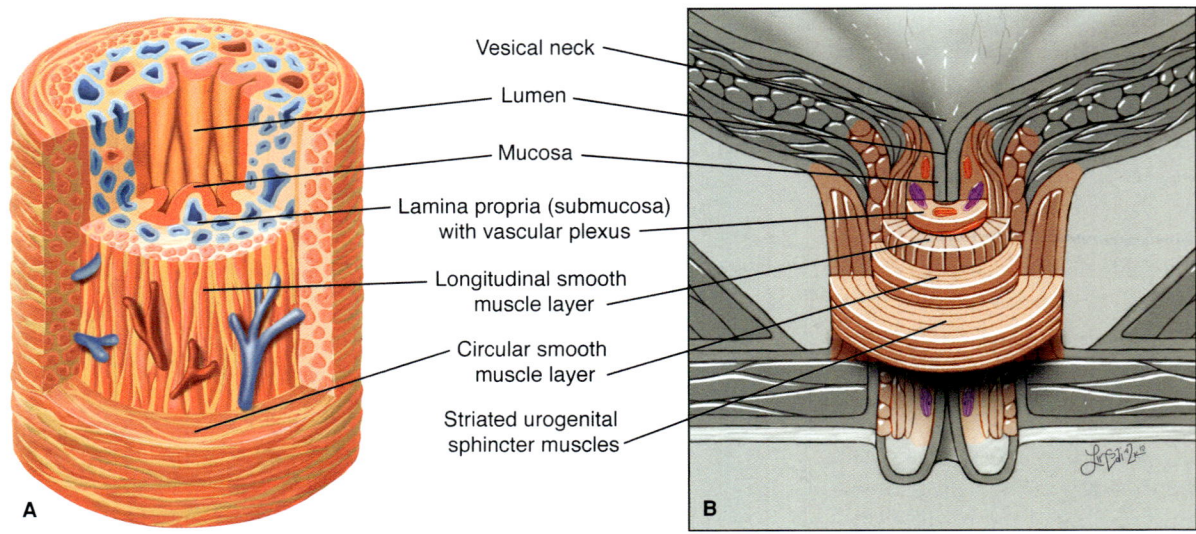

FIGURE 23-8 Drawing of urethral anatomy. **A.** Urethral anatomy in cross section. Urethral coaptation results in part from filling of the rich subepithelial vascular plexus. The urethra contains circular and longitudinal smooth muscle layers. **B.** Vesical neck and urethral anatomy. The striated urogenital sphincter lies external to the urethral smooth muscle layers. (Reproduced with permission from Lindsay Oksenberg.)

bladder symptoms through this mechanism of smooth-muscle relaxation. In contrast, α-adrenergic receptors predominate in the bladder base and urethra. These receptors are stimulated by norepinephrine, which initiates a cascade of events that preferentially leads to urethral contraction and aids urine storage and continence. These effects of α-stimulation underlie the treatment of SUI with imipramine, a tricyclic antidepressant with adrenergic agonist properties.

Urethral Coaptation

One key to continence is adequate urethral mucosal coaptation. The uroepithelium is supported by a connective tissue layer, which is thrown into deep folds, also known as *plications*. A rich capillary network runs within its subepithelial layer. This vascular network aids in urethral mucosal approximation, also termed *coaptation*, by acting like an "inflatable cushion" (Fig. 23-8). In women who are hypoestrogenic, this submucosal vasculature plexus is less prominent. In part, local hormone replacement targets this diminished vascularity and, in theory, enhances coaptation to improve continence.

▪ Bladder Emptying

Innervation Related to Voiding

When an appropriate time for bladder emptying arises, sympathetic stimulation is reduced and parasympathetic stimulation is triggered via the pontine micturition center (or "M" region). Specifically, neural impulses carried in the pelvic nerves stimulate acetylcholine release and lead to detrusor muscle contraction (Fig. 23-9). Concurrent with detrusor stimulation, acetylcholine also stimulates muscarinic receptors in the urethra and leads to outlet relaxation for voiding while sympathetic outflow through the pudendal nerve to the urethral outlet is inhibited.

Within the parasympathetic division, acetylcholine receptors are broadly defined as muscarinic and nicotinic. The

bladder is densely supplied with muscarinic receptors, which when stimulated lead to detrusor contraction. Of the muscarinic receptors, five glycoproteins designated M_1–M_5 have been identified. M_2 and M_3 receptor subtypes are predominantly responsible for detrusor smooth muscle contraction. Thus, treatment with muscarinic antagonist medication blunts detrusor contraction to improve continence. Specifically, continence drugs that target only the M_3 receptor maximize drug efficacy yet minimize activation of other muscarinic receptors and drug side effects.

Muscular Activity with Voiding

Smooth muscle cells within the detrusor fuse with one another so that a network of low-resistance electrical pathways extends from one muscle cell to the next. Thus, action potentials can spread quickly throughout the detrusor muscle to cause rapid contraction of the entire bladder. In addition, the plexiform arrangement of bladder detrusor fibers allows multidirectional contraction and is ideally suited for rapid concentric contraction during bladder emptying.

During voiding, all components of the striated urogenital sphincter relax. Importantly, bladder contraction and sphincter relaxation must be coordinated for effective voiding. Occasionally, the urethral sphincter fails to relax during contraction of the detrusor and urine retention ensues. Classically, this is a possible urinary complication of spinal cord injury termed *detrusor sphincter dyssynergia* and may lead to elevated bladder pressures and vesicoureteral reflux. Women with this condition are sometimes treated with α-blocking agents to help with sphincter relaxation and to lower bladder pressures during contraction, but these may aggravate hypotension. In women without known neurologic pathology but still with inappropriately contracted pelvic floor musculature, treatment with muscle relaxants may be appropriate. These drugs purportedly relax the urethral sphincter and levator ani muscles to improve coordinated voiding.

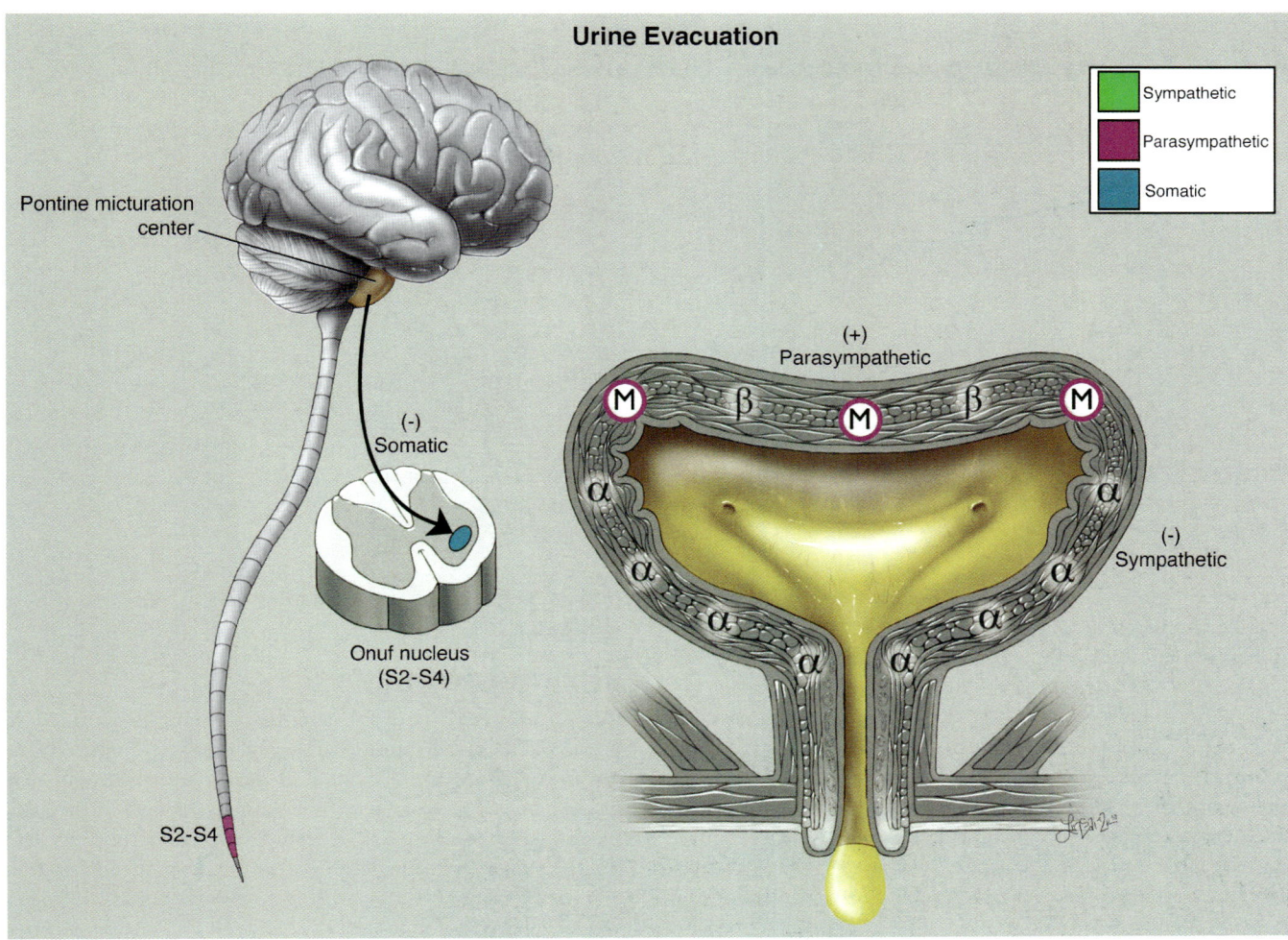

FIGURE 23-9 Physiology of urine evacuation. Efferent impulses from the pontine micturition center result in inhibition of somatic fibers in the Onuf nucleus and voluntary relaxation of the striated urogenital sphincter muscles. These efferent impulses also result in preganglionic sympathetic inhibition with opening of the vesical neck and parasympathetic stimulation, which results in detrusor muscarinic contraction. The net result is relaxation of the striated urogenital sphincter complex causing decreased urethral pressure, followed almost immediately by detrusor contraction and voiding. α = alpha adrenergic receptors; β = beta adrenergic; M = muscarinic (cholinergic). (Reproduced with permission from Lindsay Oksenberg.)

■ Incontinence Theories

Anatomic Stress Incontinence

Theories on incontinence vary in their supportive evidence but can simplistically be distilled into those that involve anatomic stress incontinence or those that describe diminished urethral integrity (sphincteric deficiency). These theories are not mutually exclusive, and both may be contributory in many women.

First, urethral and bladder neck support is integral to continence. This anatomic support derives from: (1) ligaments along the urethra's lateral aspects, termed the *pubourethral ligaments*; (2) the vagina and its lateral fascial condensation; (3) the arcus tendineus fascia pelvis; and (4) levator ani muscles. A full anatomic description of these ligaments and muscles is found in Chapter 38 (p. 808).

In an ideally supported urogenital tract, increases in intraabdominal pressure are equally transmitted to the bladder, bladder base, and urethra and are countered by supportive tissue tone provided by the levator ani muscles and vaginal

connective tissue (Fig. 23-10). With loss of support, the ability of the urethra and bladder neck to close against a firm supportive "backboard" is diminished. This results in reduced urethral closing pressures, an inability to resist increases in bladder pressure, and, in turn, incontinence. This mechanistic theory is the basis for surgical reestablishment of this support. Traditional procedures such as Burch and Marshall-Marchetti-Kranz (MMK) colposuspensions attempt to return this anatomic support to the urethrovesical junction and proximal urethra.

Sphincteric Deficiency

Another way to conceptualize SUI is to consider the urethra as providing continence through the combination of: urethral mucosal coaptation, the underlying urethral vascular plexus, the combined viscous and elastic properties of the urethral epithelium, and contraction of appropriate surrounding musculature. Taken together, these components contribute to *urethral integrity*. Defects in any or a combination of these

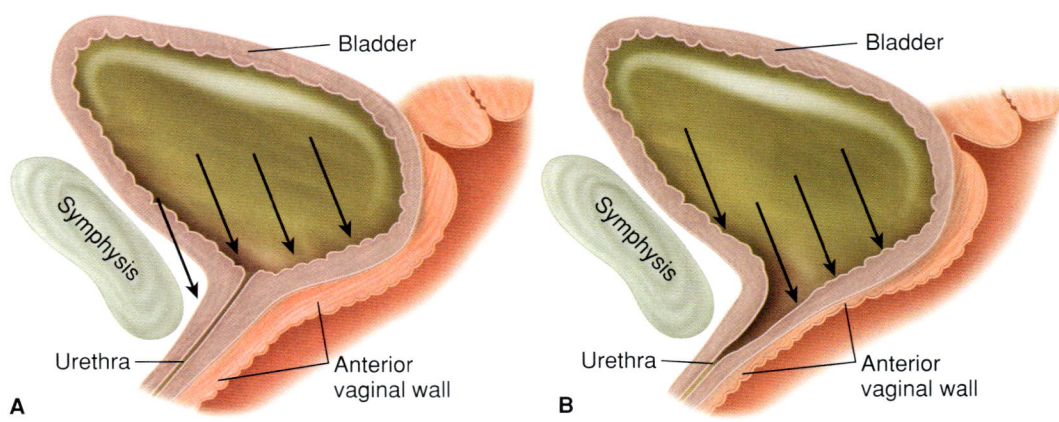

FIGURE 23-10 Drawing describes the "hammock hypothesis" theory of continence. **A.** Normal bladder neck support serves as a backboard for compression of the proximal urethra during increases in intraabdominal pressure. **B.** In those with poor urethral support, increases in intraabdominal pressure result in "funneling" of the urethra, and continence is lost.

components may lead to urine leakage and have traditionally been termed *intrinsic sphincteric deficiency (ISD)*. Prior surgery in the retropubic space may cause neuromuscular damage with denervation and scarring of the urethra and its supporting tissue. These effects subsequently prevent urethral closure and lead to incontinence. Specific causes are varied and include prior pelvic reconstructive surgeries, prior pelvic radiation therapy, diabetic neuropathy, neuronal degenerative diseases, and hypoestrogenism. With the last, women with atrophic lower genital tracts have vascular changes within the plexus surrounding the urethra that lead to poor coaptation and greater incontinence risks.

As noted earlier, nerve dysfunction following birth trauma may lead to defective urethral sphincter function (p. 513). In addition, childbirth also often injures urethral fascial support. This clinical example highlights the intimate relationship between urethral support and integrity.

Treatments to restore urethral integrity include transurethral injection of bulking agents, surgical sling procedures, and pelvic floor muscle strengthening, which are all described in later sections. In brief, bulking agents are placed at the urethrovesical junction to elevate the epithelium and promote coaptation. Sling procedures restore periurethral support anatomy or create partial urethral obstruction to enhance urethral integrity. Last, because the urethra exits through urogenital hiatus, levator ani muscle conditioning with Kegel exercises can bolster urethral integrity. These muscles can be contracted around the urethra when continence is challenged during sudden increases in intraabdominal pressures.

One concern with surgical management of patients with ISD, particularly those younger than 50 years, is that a retropubic colposuspension procedure merely elevates and stabilizes the urethra and does not promote coaptation. This may be less likely to achieve satisfactory continence than a procedure directed at both anatomic SUI and deficient urethral sphincter function and support (Sand, 1987). That said, a small trial randomizing incontinent women with ISD to Burch or sling procedures did not show differences

in postoperative voiding function or in SUI cure rates (Culligan, 2003).

Detrusor Overactivity

Detrusor overactivity (DO) describes involuntary contractions of the bladder wall during filling cystometry (Abrams, 2009). The contractions may be spontaneous or provoked and may or may not be associated with a sense of urgency or urgency incontinence. Because it is a urodynamics study finding, DO cannot be used interchangeably with the *symptom* descriptions *overactive bladder* or *urgency urinary incontinence*. Nonetheless, DO is believed to underlie these last two. DO may be defined further by the qualifiers *neurogenic* (if a relevant neurologic condition is present) or *idiopathic*.

In neurogenic DO, neurologic lesions above the sacral level of the spinal cord block the sacral reflex arcs from the cerebral cortex and other higher centers that are important to bladder inhibition. This loss in inhibition permits involuntary detrusor muscle contractions yet appropriate relaxation of the urethral sphincter, which precipitates urgency urinary incontinence. This type of DO may occur with multiple sclerosis, cerebrovascular disorders, Parkinson disease, dementia, neoplasia, and spinal cord injury.

When no neurologic pathology is suspected—as is the more common scenario—this is described as idiopathic DO. Both neurogenic and myogenic hypotheses are proposed to explain idiopathic DO. The neurogenic explanation presumes generalized nerve-mediated excitation of the detrusor muscle. The myogenic explanation suggests a combination of heightened spontaneous excitation within the bladder smooth muscle and enhanced propagation and spread of contractile signals due to cell-to-cell coupling. Another interesting hypothesis possibly linked with idiopathic DO is the existence of bacterial DNA and live bacteria in the bladders of clinically uninfected patients. This constitutes the urinary microbiome. Cohorts with and without urgency urinary incontinence have qualitatively and quantitatively different urinary microbiomes. This suggests that either pathologic microbial species or the absence of protective ones could impact female urinary health (Pearce, 2014).

TABLE 23-2. The Three Incontinence Questions (3IQ)

1. During the last 3 months, have you leaked urine (even a small amount)?
   a. Yes (continue questions)   b. No (questionnaire completed)
2. During the last 3 months, did you leak urine: (mark all that apply)
   a. When you were performing some physical activity, such as coughing, sneezing, lifting, or exercise?
   b. When you had the urge or feeling that you needed to empty your bladder, but you could not get to the toilet fast enough?
   c. Without physical activity and without a sense of urgency?
3. During the last 3 months, did you leak urine *most often*: (mark only one)
   a. When you were performing some physical activity, such as coughing, sneezing, lifting, or exercise?
   b. When you had the urge or feeling that you needed to empty your bladder, but you could not get to the toilet fast enough?
   c. Without physical activity and without a sense of urgency?
   d. About equally as often with physical activity as with a sense of urgency?

The response to question 3 with (a) or (b) indicates stress-predominant or urgency-predominant incontinence, respectively, whereas (d) indicates mixed and (c) suggests another cause of incontinence.

DIAGNOSIS

■ History

Symptom Clustering

Assessment of incontinence begins with a patient describing her urinary symptoms. These complaints may be collected through direct conversation but can be augmented with patient questionnaires. Two common forms are the Pelvic Floor Distress Inventory and the Pelvic Floor Impact Questionnaire. Both are available in long and short forms and evaluate urinary, bowel, and prolapse symptoms (Barber, 2001). Such lengthy research questionnaires may be impractical for general clinical practice. Instead, shorter validated questionnaires may easily be incorporated into the clinic setting. Shown in Table 23-2, the Three Incontinence Questions (3IQ) tool screens for incontinence and helps clarify incontinence type (Brown, 2006).

During inquiry, the number of voids and pads used per day, type of pad, frequency of pad changing, and the degree of pad saturation are important. Although these specifics alone may not establish the exact incontinence type, they do provide information regarding symptom severity and its effects on patient activities. If a woman's symptoms do not diminish her quality of life, simple observation is reasonable. Conversely, those with bothersome symptoms warrant further evaluation.

Specific to incontinence, information that describes the circumstances in which urine leaks and specific maneuvers that incite or provoke leakage are sought. With SUI, triggers may include increases in intraabdominal pressure such as coughing, sneezing, laughing, Valsalva maneuver, or deep penetration during intercourse. Alternatively, women with urgency urinary incontinence may describe urine loss after urge sensations that typically cannot be suppressed. *Overflow incontinence* was a term used in the past to refer to women who were unable to empty their bladder well but who also had involuntary, continuous urinary leakage or dribbling. Patients can sometimes have stress-like leakage when the bladder is very full or experience low-amplitude bladder contractions with symptoms more like urgency urinary incontinence. Currently, overflow

incontinence is considered by many to reflect another presentation of urgency urinary incontinence. That said, it may still be a useful concept for understanding leakage as it is associated with either bladder outlet obstruction or detrusor *under-activity*. Of these, impaired bladder muscle contractility may be a consequence of aging, smooth muscle damage, fibrosis, hypoestrogenism, peripheral neuropathy (e.g., longstanding diabetes mellitus, vitamin B_{12} deficiency), or damage to spinal detrusor efferent nerves (e.g., multiple sclerosis or spinal stenosis) (Aldamanhori, 2017; Zimmern, 2014).

During questioning, symptoms typically cluster into those most frequently seen with SUI or with urgency urinary incontinence (see Table 23-2). Alternatively, a significant overlap of complaints may reflect mixed urinary incontinence. For these reasons, pattern identification is helpful as it may direct diagnostic testing and guide initial empiric therapy.

Voiding Diary

Typically, patients may not have an entirely accurate recollection of their own voiding habits. Accordingly, to obtain a thorough record, a woman ideally completes a urinary diary (Fig. 23-11). With this, the volumes and type of each oral fluid intake, volumes of urine with each void, episodes of urinary leakage, and triggers of incontinence episodes are recorded for 3 to 7 days. During each 24-hour period, women also record times of sleep and awakening to document voluntary nocturnal

Bladder Diary			
Please record the time and amount of your oral intake, urine output, urine leakage, and pad changes FOR 3 DAYS			
Time	Oral Intake	Voided Urine	Urine Leakage or Pad Change

FIGURE 23-11 Example of a urinary diary.

voiding patterns or enuresis. Three days usually suffice to determine the general trend of incontinence. Voiding frequency is normally less than eight times a day and once at night, and total volume voided in 24 hours is typically less than 1800 mL (Lukacz, 2009).

The information gained from a voiding/urinary diary is a valuable diagnostic and sometimes therapeutic tool. The first morning void is usually the largest of the day and is a good estimate of bladder capacity. Patients often can identify patterns in intake and voiding and modify behavior. For example, a patient may recognize increased urinary frequency or more urgency urinary incontinence episodes after caffeine intake. Moreover, this diary information can serve as a baseline against which treatment effectiveness can be assessed.

Urinary Symptoms

Of these, frequent voiding without increased oral fluid intake may indicate overactive bladder, UTI, calculi, or urethral pathology and often prompts additional evaluation. In addition, urinary frequency is commonly associated with interstitial cystitis/bladder pain syndrome (IC/BPS). With IC/BPS, the numbers of voids may commonly exceed 20 per day, and treatment is discussed in Chapter 12 (p. 268). Nocturia may be noted in women with urgency urinary incontinence or in those with systemic fluid management disorders such as congestive heart failure. In the latter case, treatment of the underlying condition often leads to symptom improvement or cure of nighttime frequency.

Urinary retention may provide clues. Often incomplete emptying can result in incontinence associated with either stress or urgency. Urethral obstruction, often manifested as an inability to void or an impeded urinary stream, is uncommon in women. Its description prompts careful evaluation for pelvic organ prolapse or pelvic mass. In addition, prior trauma or pelvic or vaginal surgery could scar or obstruct the urethra.

Of other urinary symptoms, the volume of urine lost with each episode may aid diagnosis. Large volumes are typically lost following a spontaneous detrusor contraction associated with urgency urinary incontinence and may often involve loss of the entire bladder volume. In contrast, women with SUI usually describe smaller volumes lost. Moreover, these women often are able to contract the levator ani muscles to temporarily stop their urine stream. Another symptom, postvoid dribbling, is classically associated with urethral diverticulum, which may often be mistaken for urinary incontinence (Chap. 26, p. 579). Hematuria, although a common sign of UTI, may also indicate underlying malignancy or stone and can cause irritative voiding symptoms.

Symptom onset also may prove informative. Problems beginning at menopause may suggest the hypoestrogenism that underlies genitourinary syndrome of menopause (GSM). Discussed in Chapter 22 (p. 495), patients may benefit from topical vaginal estrogen or the oral selective estrogen-receptor modulator (SERM) ospemifene (Osphena). In contrast, symptoms after hysterectomy or childbirth may reflect changes in tissue support or innervation.

Past Medical History

Obstetric trauma may be associated with damage to pelvic floor support, which may lead to SUI. Thus, a prolonged labor, operative vaginal delivery, macrosomia, or postpartum catheterization for urinary retention can be informative. As noted, urinary incontinence may be linked with several medical conditions or their treatments, which could be modified to improve incontinence. To help remember these potential contributors, a useful mnemonic is "DIAPPERS": dementia/delirium, infection, atrophic vaginitis, psychological, pharmacologic, endocrine, restricted mobility, and stool impaction (Swift, 2008).

First, continence requires the cognitive ability to recognize and react appropriately to the sensation of a full bladder, motivation to maintain dryness, sufficient mobility and manual dexterity, and ready access to a toilet. Patients with dementia or significant psychological impairments often do not have the necessary cognitive ability for continence. Women with severe physical handicaps or restricted mobility may simply not have time to reach the toilet. For this so-called *functional incontinence*, simple interventions such as a bedside commode may be helpful.

UTIs cause bladder mucosal inflammation. This inflammation is thought to enhance sensory afferent activity, which contributes to an overactive bladder. Women prone to UTIs commonly experience urinary incontinence, both between UTI episodes and especially worse in the midst of an acute infection (Moore, 2008). Similarly, hypoestrogenism can lead to atrophic vaginal and urethral epithelia and may be associated with increased irritation and greater risks of UTI and overactive bladder.

A detailed medication inventory is collected. Pertinent drugs include estrogen, α-adrenergic agonists, caffeine, alcohol, and diuretics, to name a few (Table 23-3).

Of endocrinopathies, diabetes mellitus can promote osmotic diuresis and polyuria if glucose control is poor. Excessive caffeine or alcohol intake or polydipsia from diabetes insipidus can also lead to polyuria or urinary frequency. Similarly, other disorders of impaired arginine vasopressin secretion or action may cause polyuria and nocturia (Ouslander, 2004). Conditions such as congestive heart failure, hypothyroidism, venous insufficiency, and the effects of certain medications all contribute to peripheral edema, leading to urinary frequency and nocturia once a patient is supine.

Last, stool impaction resulting from poor bowel habits and constipation can contribute to overactive bladder symptoms. This is perhaps from local irritation or direct compression against the bladder wall.

■ Physical Examination

General Inspection and Neurologic Evaluation

Initially, the perineum is inspected for evidence of atrophy, which may be noted throughout the lower genital tract. In addition, a suburethral cystic mass or dilation with transurethral expression of fluid during compression suggests a urethral diverticulum (Fig. 26-7, p. 582).

Examination of an incontinent woman also includes a detailed neurologic evaluation of the perineum. Because

TABLE 23-3. Medications That May Contribute to Incontinence

Medication	Examples	Mechanism	Effect
Alcohol	Beer, wine, liquor	Decreased bladder contractility, diuretic effect, sedation, immobility	Polyuria, frequency
α-Adrenergic agonists	Midodrine, phenylephrine, various vasopressors, decongestants, diet pills	IUS contraction	Urinary retention
α-Adrenergic blockers	Prazosin, terazosin, doxazosin, alfuzosin, silodosin	IUS relaxation	Urinary leakage
Anticholinergic agents		Inhibit bladder contraction, sedation, fecal impaction	Urinary retention and/or functional incontinence
Antihistamines	Diphenhydramine, hydroxyzine, scopolamine, dimenhydrinate		
Antipsychotics	Thioridazine, chlorpromazine, haloperidol		
Antiparkinsonians	Trihexyphenidyl, benztropine mesylate		
Miscellaneous	Dicyclomine, disopyramide		
Skeletal muscle relaxants	Orphenadrine, cyclobenzaprine		
Tricyclic antidepressants	Amitriptyline, imipramine, nortriptyline, doxepin		
ACE inhibitors	Enalapril, captopril, lisinopril, losartan	Chronic cough, decreased bladder contractility	Urinary leakage
Calcium-channel blockers	Nifedipine, nicardipine, isradipine, felodipine	Relaxes bladder, fluid retention	Urinary retention, nocturnal diuresis
COX-2 inhibitors	Celecoxib	Fluid retention	Nocturnal diuresis
Diuretics	Caffeine, HCTZ, furosemide, bumetanide, acetazolamide, spironolactone	Increases urinary frequency, urgency	Polyuria
Narcotic analgesics	Opiates	Relaxes bladder, fecal impaction, sedation	Urinary retention, and/or functional incontinence
Thiazolidinediones	Rosiglitazone, pioglitazone, troglitazone	Fluid retention	Nocturnal diuresis

ACE = angiotensin-converting enzyme; COX-2 = cyclooxygenase-2; HCTZ = hydrochlorothiazide; IUS = internal urethral sphincter; NSAID = nonsteroidal antiinflammatory drug.

neurologic responses may be altered in an anxious patient who is in a vulnerable examination setting, signs elicited during evaluation may not signify true pathology and are interpreted in context and with caution. We usually begin neurologic evaluation with an attempt to elicit a *bulbospongiosus reflex*, by stroking one labium majus with a cotton swab. Generally, both labia contract at the same time. The afferent limb of this reflex is the clitoral branch of the pudendal nerve, whereas its efferent limb is conducted through the inferior hemorrhoidal branch of the pudendal nerve. This reflex is integrated at the S2–S4 spinal cord level (Wester, 2003). Thus, reflex absence may suggest central or peripheral neurologic deficits. Second, a normal circumferential anal sphincter contraction, colloquially called an *anal wink*, should follow cotton swab brushing of the

perianal skin. External urethral sphincter activity requires at least some degree of intact S2–S4 innervation, and this *anocutaneous reflex* is mediated by the same spinal neurologic level. Thus, an absent wink may indicate deficits in this neurologic distribution.

Pelvic Support Assessment

Poor urethral support commonly accompanies pelvic organ prolapse (POP). Women with significant POP are often unable to completely empty their bladder due to urethral kinking and obstruction. These women frequently must digitally elevate or reduce their prolapse to allow emptying. Thus, an external evaluation for POP, described in Chapter 24 (p. 544), is indicated for all women with urinary incontinence. Following this evaluation for vaginal compartment defects, pelvic muscle strength also is assessed. Women with mild to moderate urinary incontinence often respond well to pelvic floor therapy, and under these circumstances, a trial of this therapy is warranted and often curative (p. 527).

Lack of distal anterior vaginal wall support can lead to urethral hypermobility during increased intraabdominal pressure. In patients with descent to the level of the hymen or beyond with Valsalva, urethral hypermobility is universal (Noblett, 2005). In those with SUI and lesser anterior vaginal wall prolapse, a *Q-tip test* may provide a more objective assessment of urethral hypermobility. However, the test is now a less-essential part of pelvic floor assessment due to associated urethral pain and its poor predictive value for antiincontinence surgery success.

If performed, the soft end of a cotton swab is placed into the urethra to the urethrovesical junction. Failure to insert the swab to this depth can lead to assessment errors. An application of intraurethral analgesia may prove helpful, and 1-percent lidocaine jelly is placed on the cotton swab prior to insertion. Following placement, a Valsalva maneuver is prompted, and the swab-excursion angle at rest and with Valsalva maneuver is measured. An angle change or a resting angle >30 degrees above the horizon suggests urethral hypermobility.

Bimanual and Rectovaginal Examination

In general, these portions of the pelvic examination provide fewer diagnostic clues to underlying incontinence causes. However, bimanual examination may reveal a pelvic mass or a uterus enlarged by leiomyomas or adenomyosis. These can create incontinence through increased external pressure transmitted to the bladder. In addition, stool impaction is easily identified with rectal examination.

■ Diagnostic Testing

Urinalysis and Culture

In all women with urinary incontinence, infection or urinary tract pathology must be excluded. Urinalysis and urine culture are sent at an initial visit, and infection is treated as described in Table 3-14 (p. 77). Persistent irritative voiding symptoms, despite appropriate antibiotic treatment, warrant additional evaluation for other conditions such as IC/BPS.

Postvoid Residual Volume

This volume is routinely measured during incontinence evaluation. After a woman voids, the postvoid residual (PVR) volume may be measured by transurethral catheterization or with a handheld sonographic bladder scanner. The latter is a portable 3-dimensional ultrasound device that scans the bladder and provides numeric results (Fig. 23-12). In general, they are quick, easy to use, and more comfortable for the patient. However, if using a handheld scanner, care must be taken in women with a leiomyomatous uterus or other pelvic mass, as these may yield a falsely large PVR reading. In these instances, or if a scanner is not available, transurethral catheterization may be used to obtain the residual bladder volume.

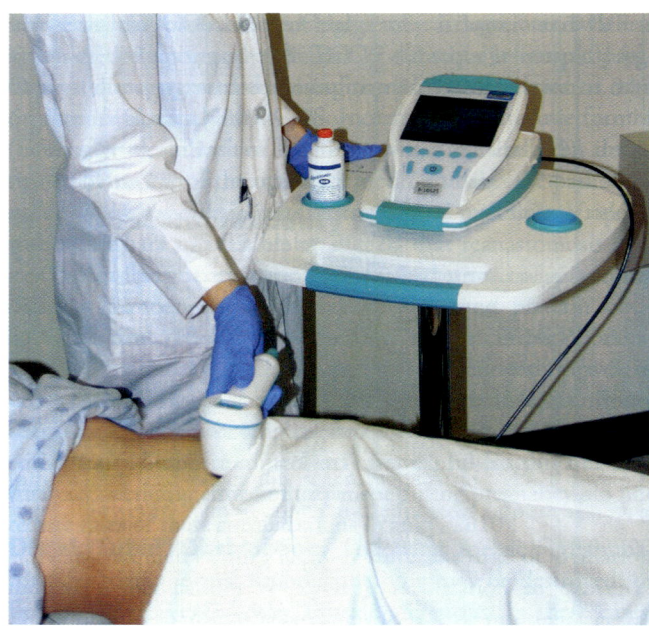

FIGURE 23-12 Handheld bladder scanner aids estimation of bladder volume.

A large PVR volume may reflect recurrent infection, urethral obstruction from a pelvic mass, or neurologic deficits. In contrast, a normal, small PVR volume is often found in those with SUI. After continence surgery, PVR measurement is a helpful indicator of a patient's ability to completely empty her bladder. Postoperative PVR volume determination and voiding trials are described in Chapter 42 (p. 919).

Urodynamic Studies

Surgical correction of incontinence is invasive and not without risk. However, the "bladder is an unreliable witness," and historical information may not always accurately indicate the true underlying type of incontinence (Blaivas, 1996). Thus, if initial conservative management is unsuccessful or surgical treatment is anticipated, objective assessment is pursued. In addition, if symptoms and physical findings are incongruous, then objective *urodynamic studies (UDS)*, using simple or multichannel cystometrics, also may be indicated. For example, in a woman with mixed urinary incontinence, who has symptoms of both stress and urgency urinary incontinence, UDS may reveal that only the urgency component is responsible for her incontinence. These cases are treated with behavioral, physical, and/or pharmacologic therapy initially. Thus, if identified by UDS, these individuals can avoid unnecessary surgery. Additionally, surgical therapy may be modified if UDS reveals parameters consistent with ISD.

Despite these indications, UDS remains controversial. Leakage noted during testing is not always clinically relevant. In addition, testing may be uninformative if the original offending maneuver or situation that led to incontinence cannot be reproduced during testing. Moreover, objective confirmation of the diagnosis is not always necessary, since empiric nonsurgical therapy in women with urgency-predominant symptoms is reasonable. Also, for women with stress-predominant urinary incontinence undergoing surgical treatment, outcomes were no different 1 year later in those screened by UDS compared with those evaluated by a simple office evaluation. Office testing included demonstrable leakage during examination, urine analysis without infection, and PVR volume <150 mL (Nager, 2012).

Simple Cystometrics. Objective measurement of bladder function, that is, UDS, combines a battery of tests termed *cystometrics*, which may be *simple* or *multichannel*. Simple cystometrics allows determination of SUI and detrusor overactivity and measurement of first sensation, desire to void, and bladder capacity. This procedure is easily performed with room-temperature sterile normal saline, 60-mL catheter-tipped syringe, and urinary catheter, either Foley or Rob-Nel. The urethra is sterilely prepared, the catheter is inserted, and the bladder is drained. A 60-mL syringe with its plunger removed is attached to the catheter and is filled upright with sterile water. Water is added in increments until a woman feels a sensation of bladder filling, urge to void, and bladder maximum capacity. A normal bladder capacity for most women ranges from 300 to 700 mL. Changes in the fluid meniscus within the syringe are monitored. In the absence of a cough or Valsalva maneuver that would raise intraabdominal pressure, an abrupt meniscus elevation indicates bladder contraction and suggests detrusor overactivity. Once bladder capacity is reached, the catheter is removed, and the woman is asked to perform a Valsalva maneuver or cough while standing. Leakage directly linked to these increases in intraabdominal pressure indicates SUI.

Simple cystometrics require inexpensive equipment and can typically be completed by most gynecologists. One limitation, however, is its inability to assess for ISD, which may preclude certain surgical options. Multichannel cystometrics can evaluate for ISD and thus may offer advantages. An interesting potential application of simple cystometrics is in the evaluation of the *continent* patient planning surgery for POP. With 300 mL of saline instilled in the bladder and vaginal prolapse reduced with large cotton swabs, some patients will demonstrate leakage with cough or Valsalva—perhaps when standing if not seen supine. In these women with "potential" or "occult" SUI, some may consider a prophylactic continence procedure. Available decision-aid tools attempt to quantify the risk of this unmasked incontinence to help patients balance concomitant continence surgery benefits and risks (Jelovsek, 2014; Wei, 2012).

Multichannel Cystometrics. This UDS type provides more information on other physiologic bladder parameters than simple cystometrics. Multichannel cystometrics more commonly is performed by urogynecologists or urologists due to the expense and limited availability of needed equipment. Testing can be performed with a woman standing or seated upright in a specialized testing chair. During evaluation, two catheters are used. One is placed into the bladder and the other into either the vagina or rectum. The vagina is preferred unless advanced POP is evident, as stool in the rectal vault may obstruct catheter sensors and lead to inaccurate readings. Additionally, vaginal placement for most women is more comfortable. From each of these two catheters, distinct

pressure readings are obtained or calculated. These include: (1) intraabdominal pressure, (2) vesicular pressure, (3) calculated detrusor pressure, (4) bladder volume, and (5) saline-infusion flow rate. Shown in Figures 23-13 and 23-14, the various incontinence forms can be differentiated.

Uroflowmetry. Initially, a woman is asked to empty her bladder into a commode connected to a flowmeter (uroflowmetry). After a maximal flow rate is recorded, the patient is catheterized to measure PVR volume and to ensure an empty bladder prior to further testing. This test provides information on a woman's ability to empty her bladder and can identify women with urinary retention and other types of voiding dysfunction. Presuming that a patient begins with a comfortably full bladder of 200 mL or greater, most patients can empty their bladder over 15 to 20 seconds with flow rates >20 mL/s. Maximum flow rates <15 mL/s, with a voided volume >200 mL, are generally considered abnormally slow. In this setting—especially if accompanied by urinary retention—voiding dysfunction is identified. This may signal obstruction from a kinked urethra, which can result from anterior vaginal wall prolapse or from postoperative antiincontinence support that is too tight. As another example, voiding dysfunction may reflect neurologic dysfunction and poor detrusor contractility, as in those with longstanding poorly controlled diabetes.

Cystometrography. Following uroflowmetry, cystometrography is performed to determine whether a woman has urodynamic stress incontinence (USI) or detrusor overactivity (DO). Additionally, this test provides information on bladder threshold volumes at which a woman senses bladder capacity. Delayed sensation or sensation of bladder fullness only with large capacities may indicate neuropathy. Conversely, extreme bladder sensitivity may suggest sensory disorders such as IC/BPS.

For the cystometrogram, a small (approximately 7F) catheter with a pressure transducer at its tip is inserted transurethrally into the bladder and a second similar catheter is inserted into the vagina or rectum (see Fig. 23-14). While the patient is seated, the bladder is filled with room-temperature sterile normal saline, and the patient is asked to cough at regular intervals. Additionally, during filling, the volumes at which a first desire to void and maximal bladder capacity is reached are noted. From pressure readings, DO and/or USI may be identified.

After cystometrography, once approximately 200 mL of saline has been instilled, an abdominal *leak point pressure* is measured. The patient is asked to perform a Valsalva maneuver, and the pressure generated by the effort is measured and evidence of urine leakage is sought. If leakage is seen when a pressure of <60 cmH$_2$O is generated, criteria have been met for a diagnosis of ISD. At our institution, abdominal leak point pressures are measured at a bladder volume of 200 mL, using the true zero of intravesical pressure as the baseline. However, the volume at which this test is performed varies among institutions, with some choosing to use bladder capacity and others choosing to use 150 mL as the testing volume.

Pressure Flowmetry. This evaluation usually follows cystometrography and is similar to the uroflowmetry conducted

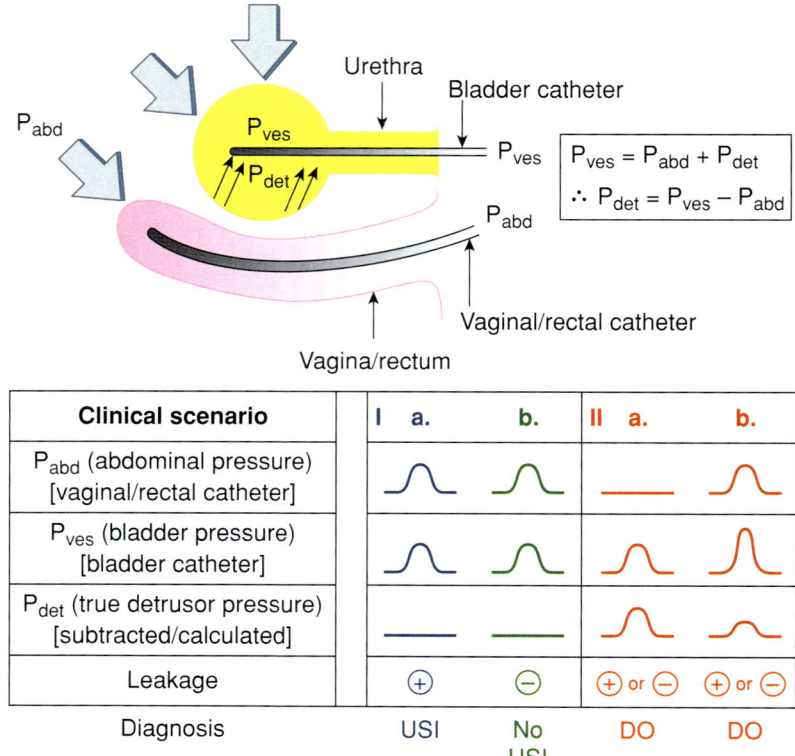

Clinical scenario	I a.	b.	II a.	b.
P$_{abd}$ (abdominal pressure) [vaginal/rectal catheter]	⌢	⌢	—	⌢
P$_{ves}$ (bladder pressure) [bladder catheter]	⌢	⌢	⌢	⌢
P$_{det}$ (true detrusor pressure) [subtracted/calculated]	—	—	⌢	⌢
Leakage	⊕	⊖	⊕ or ⊖	⊕ or ⊖
Diagnosis	USI	No USI	DO	DO

FIGURE 23-13 Interpretation of multichannel urodynamic evaluation: cystometrogram. A catheter is placed in the bladder to determine the pressure generated within it (P$_{ves}$). The pressure in the bladder is produced from a combination of the pressure from the abdominal cavity and the pressure generated by the detrusor muscle of the bladder. Bladder pressure (P$_{ves}$) = Pressure in abdominal cavity (P$_{abd}$) + Detrusor pressure (P$_{det}$). A second catheter is placed in the vagina (or rectum if advanced-stage prolapse is present) to determine the pressure in the abdominal cavity (P$_{abd}$). As room temperature water is instilled into the bladder, the patient is asked to cough every 50 mL and the external urethral meatus is observed for leakage of urine around the catheter. The volume at first desire to void and the bladder capacity is recorded. Additionally, the detrusor pressure (P$_{det}$) channel is observed for positive deflections to determine if there is detrusor activity during testing. The detrusor pressure (P$_{det}$) cannot be measured directly by any of the catheters. However, from the first equation, we can calculate the detrusor pressure (P$_{det}$) by subtracting the abdominal pressure (P$_{abd}$) from the bladder pressure (P$_{ves}$):

Detrusor pressure (P$_{det}$) = Bladder pressure (P$_{ves}$) − Pressure in abdominal cavity (P$_{abd}$)

I. Urodynamic Stress Incontinence (USI)

Urodynamic stress incontinence is diagnosed when urethral leakage is seen with increased abdominal pressure, in the *absence* of detrusor pressure.

a. +USI (Column 1): Abdominal pressure is generated with Valsalva maneuver or cough. This pressure is transmitted to the bladder and a bladder pressure (P$_{ves}$) is noted. The calculated detrusor pressure is zero. Leakage is observed and diagnosis of USI is assigned.

b. No USI (Column 2): Abdominal pressure is generated with Valsalva maneuver or cough. This pressure is transmitted to the bladder and a bladder pressure (P$_{ves}$) is noted. The calculated detrusor pressure is zero. Leakage is *not* observed. The patient is *not* diagnosed as having USI.

II. Detrusor Overactivity (DO)

Detrusor overactivity is diagnosed when the patient has involuntary detrusor contractions during testing with or without leakage.

a. +DO (Column 3): Although no abdominal pressure is observed, a vesicular pressure is noted. A calculated detrusor pressure is recorded and noted to be present. A diagnosis of DO is made regardless of whether leakage is seen or not.

b. +DO (Column 4): In this example, an abdominal pressure as well as a vesicular pressure is observed. Using only the P$_{abd}$ and the P$_{ves}$ channels, it is difficult to tell whether the detrusor muscle contributed to the pressure generated in the bladder. On subtraction, a calculated detrusor pressure is recorded. Thus, a diagnosis of DO is made, again regardless of whether leakage is seen.

In addition to these channels, occasionally a channel to detect electromyographic activity is used.

Flow rate = rate of fluid infusion (usually 100 mL/min); P$_{abd}$ = pressure in abdominal cavity; P$_{det}$ = detrusor pressure (calculated); P$_{ves}$ = bladder pressure; Vol = volume of fluid instilled in the bladder.

at the beginning of urodynamic testing. A woman is asked to void into a large beaker that rests on a calibrated weighted sensor. Maximum flow rate and postvoid residual volume are once again recorded. Similar to uroflowmetry, the output from the urodynamics instrumentation provides a graphical representation of the void. However, during voiding, a woman now has a microtip transducer catheter in her bladder, which provides an additional display of detrusor pressure during the void, including pressures at the point of maximum flow rate. This is particularly useful in women who may have incomplete bladder emptying. In this instance, pressure flowmetry may suggest either an obstructive scenario (elevated maximal detrusor

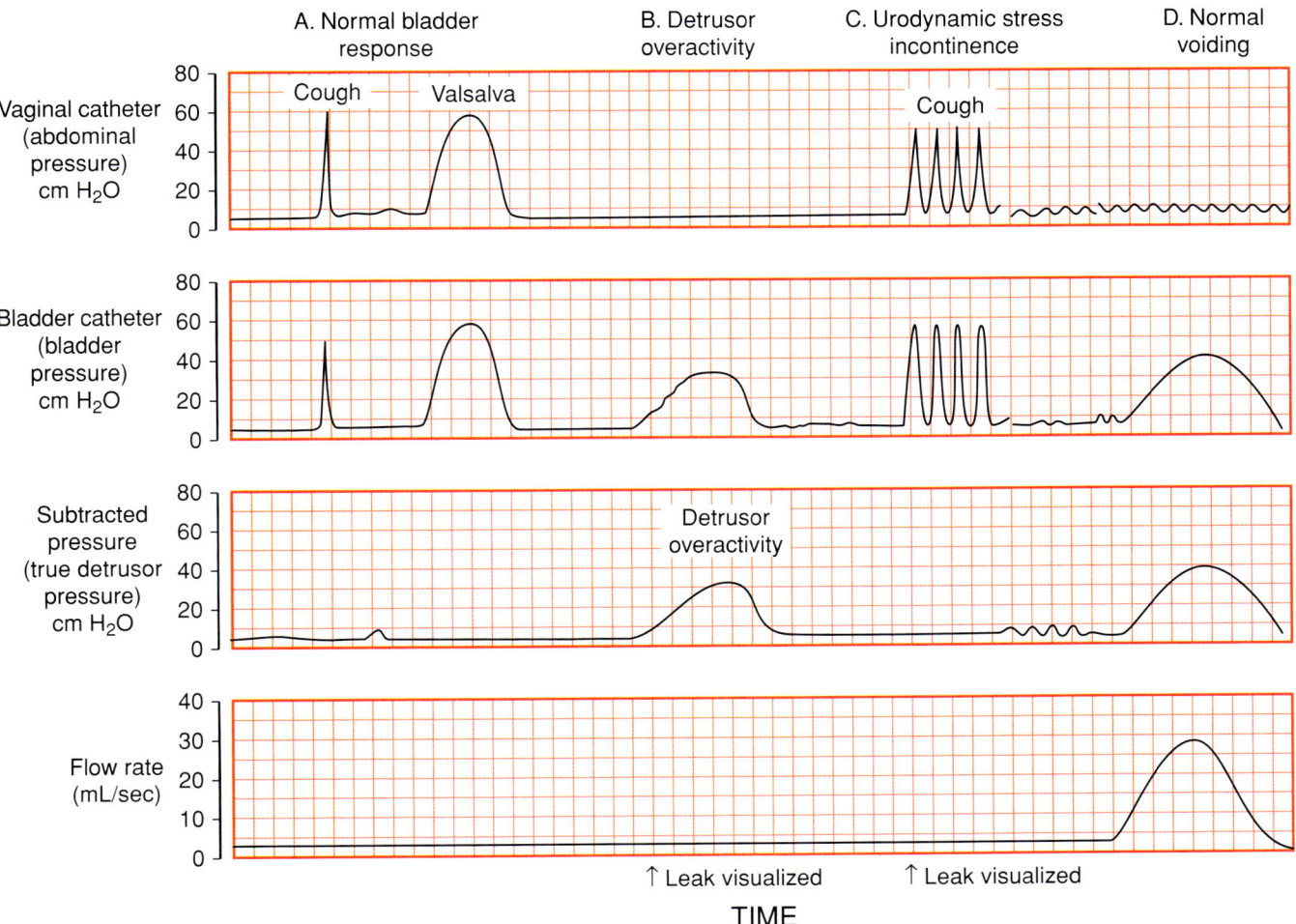

FIGURE 23-14 Multichannel cystometrics. **A.** A patient with normal function. Note that provocation by coughing or Valsalva maneuver does not provoke an abnormal rise in detrusor pressure. **B.** A patient with combined detrusor overactivity and urodynamic stress incontinence. First, spontaneous detrusor activity leads to increased bladder pressure reading in the absence of cough or Valsalva maneuver. **C.** Second, a cough alone leads to urine leakage, independent of detrusor muscle activity. **D.** At maximum capacity and on command, a detrusor contraction is generated and voiding is initiated.

pressure with slow flow rate) or poor detrusor contractility (low detrusor pressure and slow flow rate).

Urethral Pressure Profile. The final part of cystometric testing is the urethral pressure profile. At our institution, we usually perform this test in the seated patient with a volume of 200 mL instilled in the bladder. However, again, this volume is often institution dependent. A catheter transducer is positioned within the bladder, and the microtip dual-sensor catheter is pulled through the urethra with the aid of an automated puller arm at a speed of 1 mm/sec. Maximum urethral closure pressure (MUCP) is determined by averaging the pressure from three pull-throughs of the thin 7F catheter. As such, the MUCP values provide important information on the intrinsic properties of the urethra and aid in diagnosis of ISD. A diagnosis of ISD is made if the MUCP is <20 cmH$_2$O or, as described in the last section, if the leak point pressure is <60 cmH$_2$O (McGuire, 1981). These terms and concepts provide the rationale for procedures aimed at correcting stress incontinence. Importantly, the values used to define ISD are not well standardized and inconsistently predict surgical outcome (Monga, 1997; Weber, 2001).

TREATMENT

Conservative/Nonsurgical

Pelvic Floor Strengthening

Conservative management is a reasonable initial and generally recommended approach to most patients with urinary incontinence. The rationale behind conservative management is to strengthen the pelvic floor and provide a supportive "backboard" against which the urethra may close. For both SUI and urgency urinary incontinence, these fundamentals prove valuable. With SUI, pelvic floor strengthening attempts to compensate for anatomic support defects. For urgency urinary incontinence, it intensifies pelvic floor muscle contractions to provide temporary continence during waves of involuntary bladder detrusor contraction. For strengthening, options include active pelvic floor exercises and occasionally passive electrical pelvic floor muscle stimulation.

Active pelvic floor muscle training (PFMT) may lessen, if not cure, urinary incontinence in women who have mild to moderate symptoms. Also known as *Kegel (pronounced "Kay-gull") exercises*, PFMT entails voluntary contraction of the levator ani muscles.

Exercise sets are performed a number of times during the day, with some reporting up to 50 or 60 times each day. However, specific details of these exercise regimens vary according to provider preference and may be individualized according to the clinical presentation and muscle recruitment abilities of the patient.

In other PFMT protocols, a woman is asked to squeeze and hold contracted levator ani muscles. Women, however, often have difficulty isolating these muscles. Frequently, patients will erroneously contract their abdominal wall muscles. To help localize the correct muscle group, in an office setting, contraction of the levator ani muscle complex can be palpated through the vagina by the practitioner to provide direct and immediate feedback to the patient (Fig. 12-4, p. 260). Instructing the patient to identify the muscles that are tightened when snug pants are pulled up and over her hips is another suggestion that may help patients with correct muscle isolation.

At our institution, we aim to help patients achieve a sustained pelvic floor contraction of 10 seconds. A typical PFMT regimen begins with the contraction duration a patient can sustain (e.g., 3 seconds) and ask them to hold for this long and then relax for one to two times this duration (e.g., 6 seconds). This squeeze and release is repeated 10 to 15 times. Three sets are performed throughout the day for a total of approximately 45 contractions. Within weeks and with frequent follow-up visits, the contraction duration and pelvic floor muscle tone steadily increase. As a result, patients with SUI are usually able to more forcefully squeeze their muscles in anticipation of sudden increases in intraabdominal pressure.

Alternatively, a woman may be asked to rapidly contract and relax the levator ani muscles. These "quick flicks" may prove advantageous if waves of urinary urgency strike. Of note, no advantage is gained by stopping actual midstream urination, and women are counseled that this practice may worsen voiding dysfunction.

To augment exercise efficacy, weighted vaginal cones or obturators may be placed into the vagina during Kegel exercises. These provide resistance against which pelvic floor muscles can work.

PFMT for women with urinary incontinence compared with no treatment, placebo or sham treatment, or other inactive control treatment has been reviewed (Dumoulin, 2018). Although interventions vary considerably, women who performed PFMT are more likely to report cure or improved incontinence and enhanced continence-specific quality of life than women who did not use PFMT. The exercising women also objectively demonstrated less leakage during office-based pad testing. Prognostic indicators that may predict a poor response to PFMT for SUI treatment include severe baseline incontinence, prolapse beyond the hymenal ring, prior failed physiotherapy, history of prolonged second-stage labor, BMI >30 kg/m^2, high psychological distress, and poor overall physical health (Hendriks, 2010).

As an alternative to active pelvic floor contraction, a vaginal probe can deliver low-frequency electrical stimulation to the levator ani muscles. Although the mechanism is unclear, this passive electrical stimulation may improve either SUI or urgency urinary incontinence (Indrekvam, 2001; Wang, 2004). With urgency urinary incontinence, a low frequency is traditionally applied, whereas for SUI, higher frequencies are used. Electrical stimulation may be implemented alone or more commonly in combination with active PFMT.

Many behavioral techniques, often considered together as *biofeedback therapy*, measure physiologic signals such as muscle tension and then display them to a patient in real time. In general, visual, auditory, and/or verbal feedback cues are directed to the patient during these therapy sessions. Specifically, during biofeedback for active PFMT, a sterile vaginal probe that measures pressure changes within the vagina during levator ani muscle contraction is commonly used. Visual readings reflect an estimate of muscle contraction strength. Treatment sessions are individualized, dictated by the underlying dysfunction, and modified based on response to therapy. In many cases, reinforcing sessions at various subsequent intervals may also prove advantageous.

Dietary

Various food groups that may have high acidity or caffeine content can lead to greater urinary frequency and urgency. Dallosso and colleagues (2003) found consumption of carbonated drinks to be associated with development of urgency urinary incontinence symptoms. Accordingly, elimination of these dietary irritants may benefit this group. In addition, certain dietary supplements such as calcium glycerophosphate (Prelief) have been shown to decrease urgency and frequency symptoms (Bologna, 2001). This is a phosphate-based product that buffers urine acidity.

Scheduled Voiding

Women with urgency urinary incontinence may feel voiding urges as frequently as every 10 to 15 minutes. Initial goals extend voidings to half-hour intervals. Tools used to achieve this include Kegel exercises during waves of urgency or mental distraction techniques during these times. Scheduled voiding, although used primarily for urgency urinary incontinence, also may be helpful for those with SUI. For these patients, regularly scheduled urination leads to an empty bladder during a greater percentage of the day. Because some women will leak urine only if bladder volumes surpass specific volumes, frequent emptying can significantly decrease incontinence episodes.

Estrogen Replacement

Estrogen has been shown to enhance urethral blood flow and increase α-adrenergic receptor sensitivity. This thereby improves urethral coaptation and urethral closure pressure. Hypothetically, estrogen may also increase collagen deposition and promote vascularity of the periurethral capillary plexus. These also are purported to improve urethral coaptation. Thus, for incontinent women who are atrophic, administration of exogenous estrogen is reasonable.

Estrogen is commonly administered topically, and many different regimens are appropriate. At our institution, we use conjugated equine estrogen cream (Premarin cream) administered twice weekly. Although no data are available to address the duration of treatment, women may be treated chronically with topical estrogen cream. Alternatively, oral estrogen may be prescribed if other menopausal symptoms for which estrogen would be beneficial coexist (Chap. 22, p. 480). However, despite these suggested benefits, a consensus regarding estrogen's beneficial effects on the lower urinary tract has not been reached. Specifically, some studies have shown worsening or development of urinary incontinence with systemic estrogen administration (Cody, 2012; Grady, 2001; Grodstein, 2004; Hendrix, 2005; Jackson, 2006).

■ Treatment of Stress Urinary Incontinence
Medications

Pharmaceutical treatment plays a minor role for those with SUI. For women with mixed urinary incontinence, a trial of imipramine can be considered to aid urethral contraction and closure. As discussed, this tricyclic antidepressant has α-adrenergic effects, and the urethra contains a high content of these receptors. However, the efficacy of this pharmacologic intervention may not be substantial, providing only mild symptomatic improvement.

Pessary and Urethral Inserts

Certain pessaries have been designed to treat incontinence and comorbid POP. These "incontinence pessaries" are designed to reduce downward excursion or funneling of the urethrovesical junction (Fig. 24-16, p. 548). This provides bladder neck support and thereby helps reduce incontinence episodes. Pessary use success rates for urinary incontinence vary, depending on the degree of prolapse and other factors. Not all women are appropriate candidates for devices, nor will all desire long-term management of incontinence or prolapse with these.

One large prospective trial compared incontinence pessary use and behavioral therapy for women with SUI (Richter, 2010b). Those using pessary (40 percent) and women completing behavioral therapy (49 percent) were either much or very much improved at 3 months. The women randomly assigned to behavioral therapy reported greater treatment satisfaction,

and a higher percentage reported no bothersome incontinence symptoms. An over-the-counter vaginal insert called Impressa is also available to address SUI.

As an alternative to pessaries, urethral occlusive devices include *urethral inserts* (FemSoft; Reliance Urinary Control Insert) and *urethral patches* (CapSure; Re/Stor). Urethral inserts conform to the urethra and create a seal at the bladder neck to prevent accidental leakage. During routine bathroom visits, the insert is removed, discarded, and replaced with a fresh insert. Although data are limited on the effectiveness of inserts, adverse effects of mucosal irritation or superficial bacterial infection are generally minor. In an observational study of 150 women, Sirls and associates (2002) found significantly reduced rates of incontinence episodes with the FemSoft device. With urethral patches, a water-tight seal is created over the urethra after the patch adheres to surrounding periurethral skin using adhesive gel. Similarly, although success rates vary between 44 and 97 percent, these devices are associated with minimal adverse effects (Bellin, 1998; Versi, 1998).

Surgery

For those who are unsatisfied with or do not desire conservative management, surgery may be an appropriate next step for SUI. As noted earlier, urethral support is integral to continence (p. 519). Thus, surgical procedures that recreate this support often diminish or cure incontinence. In general, these surgical procedures are believed to prevent bladder neck and proximal urethra descent during increases in intraabdominal pressure and are grouped as shown in Table 23-4. General postoperative risks for continence surgeries include lower urinary tract injury, uncorrected or recurrent SUI, and creation of de novo voiding dysfunction such as urgency or retention.

TABLE 23-4. Summary of Incontinence Procedures

Procedure	Description	Indication	Comments
Midurethral slings: TVT, TOT	Midurethra supported by mesh placed: by retropubic approach or by transobturator approach	SUI; ISD SUI	Effective short-term treatment, rapid postoperative recovery; TVT with long-term efficacy data; further study required to determine effectiveness of TOT in patients with ISD
Retropubic urethropexy	Periurethral and perivesicular fibromuscular tissue attached to: Cooper ligament (Burch) or symphysis pubis (MMK)	SUI	Effective long-term treatment; requires surgeon experience; less reproducible benefits than midurethral sling procedure
Pubovaginal slings	Bladder neck supported by fascial strip attached to anterior abdominal wall	ISD; failed SUI procedure	Effective long-term treatment; may be useful when synthetic material is not desirable; requires graft isolation
Urethral injection	Bulking agent into urethral submucosa	ISD	Also for SUI in poor surgical candidates; may require several repeated injections
Needle suspension	Proximal urethra suspended by anterior abdominal wall	SUI	Low long-term success rates; no longer recommended for SUI
Paravaginal defect repair	Lateral vaginal wall attached to ATFP	Vaginal prolapse	No longer recommended for SUI

ATFP = arcus tendineus fascia pelvis; ISD = intrinsic sphincteric deficiency; MMK = Marshall-Marchetti-Krantz procedure; SUI = stress urinary incontinence; TOT = transobturator tape; TVT = tension-free vaginal tape.

Midurethral Slings. The therapeutic mechanism of these slings is based on the integral theory hypothesized by Petros and Ulmsten (1993). In brief, control of urethral closure involves the interplay of three structures: the pubourethral ligaments, the suburethral vaginal hammock, and the pubococcygeus muscle. Loss of these supports lead to urinary incontinence and pelvic floor dysfunction. Midurethral slings are believed to recreate this structural support.

These procedures vary, but all use a vaginal approach to place synthetic mesh beneath the midurethra. Recovery from midurethral sling placement is rapid, and many gynecologists provide this surgery on an outpatient basis. As such, these are often a popular surgical treatment for SUI. Simplistically, they are classified according to the route of placement and are subdivided into a retropubic or a transobturator approach.

For the retropubic approach, several commercial kits are available, and one commonly used is the tension-free vaginal tape (TVT). With this, the sling (tape) is placed through a vaginal incision to create a hammock beneath the urethra. On each side of the urethra, the sling's arms are brought out to the lower anterior abdominal wall and affixed. For this procedure, sharp trocars traverse the retropubic space as illustrated in Section 45-4 of the atlas (p. 1094). Thus, bladder puncture and retropubic space vessel laceration are specific risks. Many studies attest to this procedure's efficacy (Holmgren, 2005; Song, 2009). One prospective long-term observational study confirmed the long-term safety and efficacy of the TVT device. At 17 years, 87 percent were subjectively cured or significantly improved (Nilsson, 2013).

For the transobturator tape (TOT) approach, various kits are available, and sling material is directed bilaterally through the obturator foramen and underneath the midurethra. The entry point overlies the proximal tendon of the adductor longus muscle of the inner thigh as shown in Section 45-5 (p. 1097). This approach was introduced with the intent to reduce the vascular and lower urinary tract injury risks that can be associated with traversing the retropubic space.

The TOT procedure is indicated for primary SUI secondary to loss of urethral support. Subjective success rates range from 73 to 92 percent up to 5 years after surgery (Abdel-Fattah, 2012; Laurikainen, 2014; Wai, 2013). In patients with SUI secondary to ISD, the value of the TOT approach is unclear as results are conflicting and data are limited (Miller, 2006; O'Connor, 2006; Richter, 2010a).

Although abundant longer-term data regarding the efficacy of TOT approaches are lacking, several intermediate-term studies comparing the two types of midurethral sling procedures suggest similar efficacy with respect to the treatment of urodynamic stress incontinence. One multicenter randomized study of 597 women found no significant differences at 12 months in objective and subjective success rates between the retropubic (81 and 62 percent) and the transobturator (73 and 56 percent) routes, respectively (Richter, 2010a). The retropubic route had a significantly higher rate of postoperative voiding dysfunction that required reoperation, whereas the transobturator route resulted in more neurologic symptoms. Overall quality of life and satisfaction scores with the two procedures were similar. Others have found similar findings with respect to procedure–related complications. Namely, the retropubic route has a higher rate of bladder injury but required a decreased use of anticholinergic medication postoperatively (Barber, 2006; Brubaker, 2011).

Modification of the TVT and TOT procedure is seen with the minimally invasive slings, sometimes called "microslings" or "minislings." With this technique, an 8-cm-long strip of polypropylene synthetic mesh is placed across and beneath the midurethra through a small vaginal incision. Mesh is not threaded through the retropubic space as with TVT, nor does it perforate the obturator membrane as with TOT. That said, lower urinary tract injury is not completely averted with this method. Initial results for the minislings suggested high objective and subjective cure rates (Neuman, 2008). However, in one study, the minisling group had a higher proportion of patients with more severe incontinence 1 year after surgery than those in a retropubic sling group (Barber, 2012).

The Food and Drug Administration (FDA) (2019) has confirmed their update regarding considerations about surgical mesh for SUI. In that statement, the established safety and efficacy of mesh sling procedures for the treatment of SUI were upheld for full-length multiincision operations. They further noted that the safety and effectiveness of minislings had not yet been adequately demonstrated.

Retropubic Urethropexy. Traditionally performed via laparotomy, this group includes the Burch and Marshall-Marchetti-Krantz (MMK) colposuspension procedures. The Burch technique uses the strength of the iliopectineal ligament (Cooper ligament) to lift the anterior vaginal wall and the periurethral and perivesicular fibromuscular tissue. In contrast, during MMK surgery, the periosteum of the symphysis pubis is used to suspend these tissues. Thus, an added risk for MMK is osteitis pubis. However, with the advent of less invasive procedures for SUI, such as the midurethral sling, these techniques are less commonly performed.

Retropubic urethropexy effectively treats SUI. One-year overall continence rates range between 85 and 90 percent, and the 5-year continence rate approximates 70 percent (Lapitan, 2009). As another indication, data suggest that Burch retropubic urethropexy performed concurrently with abdominal sacrocolpopexy (ASC) may significantly reduce rates of later, postoperative de novo SUI (Chap. 24, p. 554) (Brubaker, 2008a). In support of this practice, a 7-year follow-up study showed that patients undergoing ASC and prophylactic Burch urethropexy still demonstrated lower de novo SUI rates than women receiving ASC alone (Nygaard, 2013).

Pubovaginal Slings. With this surgery, a strip of either rectus fascia or fascia lata is placed under the bladder neck and through the retropubic space. The ends are secured at the level of the rectus abdominis fascia (Section 45-6, p. 1099). This surgery has traditionally been used for SUI stemming from ISD. In addition, this procedure may also be indicated for patients with prior failed continence operations. Last, concern for potential mesh complications with surgery for incontinence and pelvic floor reconstruction has re-stimulated interest in the Burch and pubovaginal sling procedures.

Urethral Bulking Agent Injection. Using cystoscopic guidance, agents can be injected into the urethral submucosa to "bulk up" the mucosa and improve coaptation. Surgical steps and agent types are described in Section 45-7 (p. 1101). This option has traditionally been indicated for women who have stress incontinence associated with ISD. However, the FDA has broadened criteria for their use to include patients with less severe leak point pressures. Thus, those with leak point pressures <100 cmH$_2$O also may be candidates (McGuire, 2006). Additionally, this office procedure is a useful alternative for women with SUI who have multiple medical problems and are thus poor surgical candidates.

Transvaginal Needle Procedures and Paravaginal Defect Repair. In the 1960s through 1980s, needle suspension procedures such as the Raz, Pereyra, and Stamey techniques were popular operations for SUI but have now largely been replaced by other methods. In brief, these surgeries use specially designed ligature carriers to place sutures through the anterior vaginal wall and/or periurethral tissues and suspend them to various levels of the anterior abdominal wall. These rely on the strength and integrity of the periurethral tissue and abdominal wall strength to correct urethral hypermobility and prevent bladder neck and proximal urethra descent. Although initial cure rates are satisfactory, the durability of these procedures wanes with time. Success rates range from 50 to 60 percent, well below rates found with other current continence procedures (Moser, 2006). Failure stems largely from "pull-through" of sutures at the level of the anterior vaginal wall.

In addition, abdominal paravaginal defect repair (PVDR) is a surgical procedure that corrects lateral support defects of the anterior vaginal wall. The technique involves suture attachment of the lateral vaginal wall to the arcus tendineus fascia pelvis. Currently, PVDR is primarily a prolapse-correcting operation. Although previously used to correct SUI, long-term data show this to no longer be a superior method for primary treatment of SUI (Colombo, 1996; Mallipeddi, 2001).

■ Treatment of Urgency Urinary Incontinence

Anticholinergic Medications

These medications appear to work at the level of the detrusor muscle by competitively inhibiting acetylcholine at muscarinic receptors (M$_2$ and M$_3$) (Miller, 2005). These agents thereby blunt detrusor contractions to reduce the number of incontinence episodes and volume lost with each. These medications are significantly better than placebo at improving symptoms of urgency urinary incontinence and overactive bladder. However, in one systematic review, the reduction in baseline urgency incontinence episodes per day reflected only a modest benefit (Nabi, 2006).

Oxybutynin, Tolterodine, and Fesoterodine. These frequently used drugs competitively bind to cholinergic receptors (Table 23-5). As noted, muscarinic receptors are not limited

TABLE 23-5. Pharmacologic Treatment of Overactive Bladder

Drug Name	Brand Name	Drug Type	Dosage[a]	Available Doses
Oxybutynin (short-acting)	Ditropan	Antimuscarinic	2.5–5 mg three times daily	5-mg tablet, 5-mg/mL syrup
Oxybutynin (long-acting)	Ditropan XL	See above	5–30 mg daily	5-, 10-, 15-mg tablet
Oxybutynin (transdermal)	Oxytrol	See above	3.9 mg/d; change patch twice weekly	36-mg patch, 8 per carton
Oxybutynin (transdermal) 10% gel	Gelnique	See above	Gel apply 1 g daily	1-g packet, 30 per carton 1-g pump dose, 30 doses per bottle
Tolterodine (short-acting)	Detrol	See above	1–2 mg twice daily	1-, 2-mg tablet
Tolterodine (long-acting)	Detrol LA	See above	2–4 mg daily	2-, 4-mg capsule
Fesoterodine fumarate	Toviaz	See above	4–8 mg daily	4-, 8-mg tablets
Trospium chloride	Sanctura	Antimuscarinic quaternary amine	20 mg twice daily	20-mg tablet
Trospium chloride	Sanctura XR	See above	60 mg daily	60-mg tablet
Darifenacin	Enablex	M$_3$-selective antimuscarinic	7.5–15 mg daily	7.5-, 15-mg tablet
Solifenacin	Vesicare	M$_3$-selective antimuscarinic	5–10 mg daily	5-, 10-mg tablets
Imipramine hydrochloride	Tofranil	Tricyclic antidepressant, anticholinergic, α-adrenergic, antihistamine	10–25 mg one to four times daily. Begin with 10–25 mg nightly.	10-, 25-, 50-mg tablets
Mirabegron	Myrbetriq	β$_3$ adrenergic agonist	25–50 mg daily	25-, 50-mg tablets

[a]Oral dosing except for transdermal forms.

TABLE 23-6. Potential Anticholinergic Side Effects

Side Effect	Potential Clinical Consequence
Increased pupil size	Photophobia
Decreased visual accommodation	Blurred vision
Decreased salivation	Gingival and buccal ulceration
Decreased bronchial secretions	Small-airway mucus plugging
Decreased sweating	Hyperthermia
Increased heart rate	Angina, myocardial infarction
Decreased detrusor function	Bladder distention and urinary retention
Decreased gastrointestinal mobility	Constipation

to the bladder. Thus, drug side effects may be significant. Of these, dry mouth, constipation, and blurry vision are common, and dry mouth is a primary reason for drug discontinuation (Table 23-6). Importantly, anticholinergics are contraindicated in those with narrow-angle glaucoma.

Because of these side effects, the therapeutic goal of bladder M_3 blockade with these antimuscarinic agents is often limited. Thus, drug selection is tailored, and efficacy is balanced against tolerability. For example, Diokno and associates (2003) found oxybutynin to be more effective than tolterodine. However, tolterodine was associated with lower side effect rates. Tolterodine and fesoterodine have also been compared in a randomized study of 1135 patients. Fesoterodine was found to perform better than tolterodine, although once again, side effects were lowest in the tolterodine group (Chapple, 2008). A population-based study reported that only 56 percent of women felt their overactive bladder medication was effective, and half discontinued it (Diokno, 2006).

Most side effects attributed to oxybutynin stem from its secondary metabolite that follows liver metabolism. Therefore, to minimize oral oxybutynin side effects, a transdermal patch was designed to lower liver metabolism and the "first-pass" effect of this drug. Dmochowski and coworkers (2003) found fewer anticholinergic side effects with transdermal oxybutynin compared with long-acting oral tolterodine.

Transdermal oxybutynin is supplied as a 7.6 × 5.7 cm patch that is applied to the abdomen, hip, or buttock; worn continuously; and changed twice weekly. Each patch contains 36 mg of oxybutynin and delivers approximately 3.9 mg daily. Application-site pruritus is the most frequent side effect, and varying the application site may minimize skin reactions (Sand, 2007). A transdermal 3-percent oxybutynin gel is applied daily to skin of the abdomen, upper arms/shoulders, or thigh, and application sites are rotated.

Imipramine. This agent is less effective than tolterodine and oxybutynin but displays α-adrenergic and anticholinergic characteristics. Therefore, it is occasionally prescribed for those with mixed urinary incontinence. Importantly, doses of imipramine used to treat incontinence are significantly lower than those used to treat depression or chronic pain. In our experience, this minimizes the theoretical risk of drug-related side effects.

Selective Muscarinic-Receptor Antagonists. These anticholinergic medications were introduced with the aim of reducing side effects. The agents are all M_3-receptor selective antagonists and include solifenacin, trospium chloride, and darifenacin. Earlier urgency warning time and fewer muscarinic side effects have been shown in randomized studies (Cardozo, 2004; Chapple, 2005; Haab, 2006; Zinner, 2004). However, although the side-effect profiles of these drugs are potentially more attractive, they have not been proven superior in efficacy to nonselective muscarinic agents (Hartmann, 2009).

Mirabegron

This is a β_3-adrenergic–receptor agonist for the treatment of urgency urinary incontinence, urgency, and frequency. Activation of these receptors results in relaxation of the detrusor smooth muscle and greater bladder capacity. Most commonly reported adverse reactions include hypertension, nasopharyngitis, UTIs, dry mouth, and headache (Herschorn, 2013). Mirabegron is contraindicated in patients with severe uncontrolled hypertension (systolic blood pressure ≥180 mm Hg or diastolic blood pressure ≥110 mm Hg, or both).

Sacral Neuromodulation

Urine storage and bladder emptying require a complex coordinated interaction of spinal cord and higher brain centers, peripheral nerves, urethral and pelvic floor muscles, and the detrusor muscle. If any of these levels are altered, normal micturition is lost. To overcome these problems, electrical nerve stimulation, also called *neuromodulation*, has been used. InterStim is the only implantable neuromodulation system approved by the FDA for treatment of refractory urgency urinary incontinence and for treatment of anal incontinence. It may be also considered for those with pelvic pain, IC/BPS, and defecatory dysfunction, although it is not FDA-approved for these indications. Sacral neuromodulation is not considered primary therapy and is typically offered mainly to women who have exhausted pharmacologic and conservative options.

This outpatient surgically implanted device contains a pulse generator, which is connected to electrical leads that are placed into the sacral foramina. Here, it acts to modulate bladder and pelvic floor innervation. Although incompletely understood, it promotes somatic afferent inhibition that interrupts abnormal reflex arcs in the sacral spinal cord involved in the filling and evacuation phases of micturition.

Implantation is typically a two-stage process. Initially, leads are placed and attached to an externally worn generator (Section 45-12, p. 1111). After placement, frequency and amplitude of electrical impulses can be adjusted and tailored to maximize effectiveness. If a 50-percent or greater improvement in symptoms is noted, internal implantation of a permanent pulse generator is planned. This minimally invasive procedure is typically completed in a day-surgery setting. Rare complications are pain or infection at the generator insertion site.

Although its use is often reserved for those who have been unsuccessfully treated with behavioral or pharmacologic therapy, this modality is effective for urinary symptom treatment. In studies, improvement rates range from 60 to 75 percent, and cure rates approximate 45 percent (Janknegt, 2001; Schmidt, 1999; Siegel, 2000). Long-term follow-up shows sustained improvement from baseline incontinence parameters. One 3-year study reported a 57-percent reduction in incontinence episodes per day, and similar findings were found in a separate 5-year study (Kerrebroeck, 2007; Siegel, 2000). A systematic review of 17 case series at follow-up periods of 3 to 5 years similarly reported 39 percent of patients cured and 67 percent with >50-percent improvement in incontinence symptoms (Brazzelli, 2006).

Percutaneous Tibial Nerve Stimulation

Sometimes referred to as *posterior tibial nerve stimulation*, percutaneous tibial nerve stimulation (PTNS) is becoming a more common therapy for refractory urgency urinary incontinence. It involves percutaneous needle electrode placement into an area cephalic to the medial malleolus of the lower extremity. Electrical pulses are sent via a generator to the tibial nerve. This nerve originates from spinal roots L4–S3, and its stimulation leads to retrograde neuromodulation. Multicenter studies have demonstrated its efficacy compared with sham or with primary treatment with anticholinergic medication (Peters, 2009, 2010; MacDiarmid, 2010).

Botulinum Toxin A

Injection of botulinum toxin A (onabotulinumtoxinA) into the bladder wall is approved for the treatment of idiopathic detrusor overactivity. Three placebo-controlled studies showed the effectiveness of this treatment (Anger, 2010). All three used cystoscopic injection of 200 units of botulinum toxin A toxin or placebo, and each demonstrated significantly improved incontinence. Improvement occurred as early as 4 weeks after injection (Brubaker, 2008b; Flynn, 2009; Khan, 2010; Sahai, 2007). Urinary retention—defined as a postvoid residual volume measuring >200 mL—is a common side effect and developed in 27 to 43 percent of patients in these randomized trials. Most patients are asymptomatic, but patients receiving botulinum toxin A for overactive bladder or urgency urinary incontinence are counseled that temporary self-catheterization may be required after injection. More commonly, 100 units of botulinum toxin A is injected, and retention rates are lower.

A patient can expect the effects of the toxin to wane over time. In a small study describing the need for repeat injections, 20 patients from a cohort of 34 received a second injection, and nine patients received up to four injections. These repeat injections appear to be equally effective as the primary injection. Median time between injections approximates 377 days (Sahai, 2010).

One randomized trial compared oral anticholinergic therapy and botulinum toxin A injection in women with idiopathic urgency urinary incontinence. Comparable reductions in incontinence episodes were found. The botulinum toxin A group was less likely complain of dry mouth and more likely to have complete resolution of urgency urinary incontinence (Visco, 2012). Another study comparing botulinum toxin A (200 units) to sacral neuromodulation in a population of women with refractory urgency urinary incontinence found that women in the botulinum toxin A group had a modestly greater reduction in mean number of urgency incontinence episodes per day at 6 months. They also reported greater improvement in symptom bother, treatment satisfaction,

and endorsement of treatment. Conversely, the botulinum toxin A patients had a greater number of UTIs (35 percent) compared with sacral neuromodulation (11 percent) (Amundsen, 2016).

REFERENCES

Abdel-Fattah M, Mostafa A, Familusi A, et al: Prospective randomised controlled trial of transobturator tapes in management of urodynamic stress incontinence in women: 3-year outcomes from the evaluation of transobturator tapes study. Eur Urol 62(5):843, 2012

Abrams P, Artibani W, Cardozo L, et al: Reviewing the ICS 2002 terminology report: the ongoing debate. Neurourol Urodyn 28(4):287, 2009

Abrams P, Cardozo L, Fall M, et al: The standardisation of terminology of lower urinary tract function: report from the Standardisation Sub-committee of the International Continence Society. Am J Obstet Gynecol 187:116, 2002

Aldamanhori R, Chapple CR: Underactive bladder, detrusor underactivity, definition, symptoms, epidemiology, etiopathogenesis, and risk factors. Curr Opin Urol 27:293, 2017

Al-Mukhtar Othman J, Åkervall S, Milsom I, et al: Urinary incontinence in nulliparous women aged 25–64 years: a national survey. Am J Obstet Gynecol 216(2):149, 2017

Amundsen CL, Richter HE, Menefee SA, et al: OnabotulinumtoxinA vs sacral neuromodulation on refractory urgency urinary incontinence in women: a randomized clinical trial. JAMA 316:1366, 2016

Anger JT, Weinberg A, Suttorp MJ, et al: Outcomes of intravesical botulinum toxin for idiopathic overactive bladder symptoms: a systematic review of the literature. J Urol 183:2258, 2010

Bai SW, Kang JY, Rha KH, et al: Relationship of urodynamic parameters and obesity in women with stress urinary incontinence. J Reprod Med 47:559, 2002

Barber MD, Gustilo-Ashby AM, Chen CC, et al: Perioperative complications and adverse events of the MONARC transobturator tape, compared with the tension-free vaginal tape. Am J Obstet Gynecol 195:1820, 2006

Barber MD, Kuchibhatla MN, Pieper CF, et al: Psychometric evaluation of 2 comprehensive condition-specific quality of life instruments for women with pelvic floor disorders. Am J Obstet Gynecol 185(6):1388, 2001

Barber MD, Weidner AC, Sokol AI, et al: Single-incision mini-sling compared with tension-free vaginal tape for the treatment of stress urinary incontinence: a randomized controlled trial. Obstet Gynecol 119:328, 2012

Bellin P, Smith J, Poll W, et al: Results of a multicenter trial of the CapSure (Re/Stor) Continence shield on women with stress urinary incontinence. Urology 51:697, 1998

Blaivas JG: The bladder is an unreliable witness. Neurourol Urodyn 15:443, 1996

Bologna RA, Gomelsky A, Lukban JC, et al: The efficacy of calcium glycerophosphate in the prevention of food-related flares in interstitial cystitis. Urology 57(6, Suppl 1):119, 2001

Brazzelli M, Murray A, Frasier C: Efficacy and safety of sacral nerve stimulation for urinary urge incontinence. A systematic review. J Urol 175:835, 2006

Brown JS, Bradley CS, Subak KK, et al: The sensitivity and specificity of a simple test to distinguish between urge and stress urinary incontinence. Ann Int Med 144(10):715, 2006

Brown JS, Seeley DG, Fong J, et al: Urinary incontinence in older women: who is at risk? Study of Osteoporotic Fractures Research Group. Obstet Gynecol 87(5 Pt 1):715, 1996

Brubaker L, Norton PA, Albo ME, et al: Adverse events over two years after retropubic or transobturator midurethral sling surgery: findings from the Trial of Midurethral Slings (TOMUS) study. Am J Obstet Gynecol 205:498.e1, 2011

Brubaker L, Nygaard I, Richter HE, et al: Two-year outcomes after sacrocolpopexy with and without Burch to prevent stress urinary incontinence. Obstet Gynecol 112:49, 2008a

Brubaker L, Richter HE, Visco AG, et al: Refractory idiopathic urge incontinence and botulinum A injection. J Urol 180:217, 2008b

Buckley BS, Lapitan MC, Epidemiology Committee of the Fourth International Consultation on Incontinence, Paris, 2008: Prevalence of urinary incontinence in men, women, and children—current evidence: findings of the Fourth International Consultation on Incontinence. Urology 76(2):265, 2010

Bump RC, McClish DK: Cigarette smoking and urinary incontinence in women. Am J Obstet Gynecol 167:1213, 1992

Bump RC, Norton PA: Epidemiology and natural history of pelvic floor dysfunction. Obstet Gynecol Clin North Am 25:723, 1998

Burgio KL, Richter HE, Clements RH, et al: Changes in urinary and fecal incontinence symptoms with weight loss surgery in morbidly obese women. Obstet Gynecol 110(5):1034, 2007

Cardozo L, Lisec M, Millard R, et al: Randomized, double-blind placebo controlled trial of the once daily antimuscarinic agent solifenacin succinate in patients with overactive bladder. J Urol 172(5 Pt 1):1919, 2004

Carlile A, Davies I, Rigby A, et al: Age changes in the human female urethra: a morphometric study. J Urol 139:532, 1988

Chapple CR, Martinez-Garcia R, Selvaggi L, et al: A comparison of the efficacy and tolerability of solifenacin succinate and extended release tolterodine at treating overactive bladder syndrome: results of the STAR Trial. Eur Urol 48:464, 2005

Chapple CR, Van Kerrebroeck PE, Jünemann KP, et al: Comparison of fesoterodine and tolterodine in patients with overactive bladder. BJU Int 102(9):1128, 2008

Cody JD, Jacobs ML, Richardson K, et al: Oestrogen therapy for urinary incontinence in post-menopausal women. Cochrane Database Syst Rev 4:CD001405, 2012

Colombo M, Milani R, Vitobello D, et al: A randomized comparison of Burch colposuspension and abdominal paravaginal defect repair for female stress urinary incontinence. Am J Obstet Gynecol 175:78, 1996

Culligan PG, Goldberg RP, Sand PK: A randomized controlled trial comparing a modified Burch procedure and a suburethral sling: long-term follow-up. Int Urogynecol J Pelvic Floor Dysfunct 14(4):229, 2003

Dallosso HM, McGrother CW, Matthews RJ, et al: The association of diet and other lifestyle factors with overactive bladder and stress incontinence: a longitudinal study in women. BJU Int 92:69, 2003

Deitel M, Stone E, Kassam HA, et al: Gynecologic-obstetric changes after loss of massive excess weight following bariatric surgery. J Am Coll Nutr 7:147, 1988

Diokno AC, Appell RA, Sand PK, et al: Prospective, randomized, double-blind study of the efficacy and tolerability of the extended-release formulations of oxybutynin and tolterodine for overactive bladder: results of the OPERA trial. Mayo Clin Proc 78:687, 2003

Diokno AC, Brock BM, Herzog AR, et al: Medical correlates of urinary incontinence in the elderly. Urology 36:129, 1990

Diokno AC, Sand PK, MacDiarmid S, et al: Perceptions and behaviors of women with bladder control problems. Fam Pract 23(5):568, 2006

Dmochowski RR, Sand PK, Zinner NR, et al: Comparative efficacy and safety of transdermal oxybutynin and oral tolterodine versus placebo in previously treated patients with urge and mixed urinary incontinence. Urology 62:237, 2003

Dumoulin C, Cacciari LP, Hay-Smith EJ: Pelvic floor muscle training versus no treatment, or inactive control treatments, for urinary incontinence in women. Cochrane Database Syst Rev 10:CD005654, 2018

Dumoulin C, Hunter KF, Moore K, et al: Conservative management for female urinary incontinence and pelvic organ prolapse review 2013: summary of the 5th International Consultation on Incontinence. Neurourol Urodyn 35(1):15, 2016

Fantl JA, Bump RC, Robinson D, et al: Efficacy of estrogen supplementation in the treatment of urinary incontinence. The Continence Program for Women Research Group. Obstet Gynecol 88(5):745, 1996

Fantl JA, Cardozo L, McClish DK: Estrogen therapy in the management of urinary incontinence in postmenopausal women: a meta-analysis. First report of the Hormones and Urogenital Therapy Committee. Obstet Gynecol 83:12, 1994

Flynn M, Amundsen CL, Perevich M, et al: Short term outcomes of a randomized, double blind placebo controlled trial of botulinum A toxin for the management of idiopathic detrusor overactivity incontinence. J Urol 181(6):2608, 2009

Food and Drug Administration: Considerations about surgical mesh for SUI. 2019. Available at: https://www.fda.gov/medicaldevices/productsandmedicalprocedures/implantsandprosthetics/urogynsurgicalmesh/ucm345219.htm. Accessed April 21, 2019

Grady D, Brown JS, Vittinghoff E, et al: Postmenopausal hormones and incontinence: the heart and estrogen/progestin replacement study. Obstet Gynecol 97:116, 2001

Gray T, Campbell P, Jha S, et al: Evaluation of coital incontinence by electronic questionnaire: prevalence, associations and outcomes in women attending a urogynaecology clinic. Int Urogynecol J 29(7):969, 2018

Grodstein F, Lifford K, Resnick NM, et al: Postmenopausal hormone therapy and risk of developing urinary incontinence. Obstet Gynecol 103:254, 2004

Haab F, Corcos J, Siami P, et al: Long-term treatment with darifenacin for overactive bladder: results of a 2-year, open-label extension study. BJU Int 98:1025, 2006

Hannestad YS, Lie RT, Rortveit G, et al: Familial risk of urinary incontinence in women: population based cross sectional study. BMJ 329(7471):889, 2004

Hannestad YS, Rortveit G, Daltveit AK, et al: Are smoking and other lifestyle factors associated with female urinary incontinence? The Norwegian EPINCONT Study. BJOG 110:247, 2003

Hannestad YS, Rortveit G, Hunskaar S: Help-seeking and associated factors in female urinary incontinence. The Norwegian EPINCONT Study. Epidemiology of Incontinence in the County of Nord-Trøndelag. Scand J Prim Health Care 20:102, 2002

Hartmann KE, McPheeters ML, Biller DH, et al: Treatment of overactive bladder in women. Evidence report/technology assessment No. 187, Rockville, Agency for Healthcare Research and Quality, 2009

Hendriks EJ, Kessels AG, de Vet HC, et al: Prognostic indicators of poor short-term outcome of physiotherapy intervention in women with stress urinary incontinence. Neurourol Urodyn 29:336, 2010

Hendrix SL, Cochrane BB, Nygaard IE, et al: Effects of estrogen with and without progestin on urinary incontinence. JAMA 293:935, 2005

Herschorn S, Barkin J, Castro-Diaz D, et al: A phase III, randomized, double-blind, parallel-group, placebo-controlled, multicentre study to assess the efficacy and safety of the β_3 adrenoceptor agonist, mirabegron, in patients with symptoms of overactive bladder. Urology 82(2):313, 2013

Holmgren C, Nilsson S, Lanner L, et al: Long-term results with tension-free vaginal tape on mixed and stress urinary incontinence. Obstet Gynecol 106(1):38, 2005

Hunskaar S, Arnold EP, Burgio K, et al: Epidemiology and natural history of urinary incontinence. Int Urogynecol J Pelvic Floor Dysfunct 11:301, 2000

Indrekvam S, Sandvik H, Hunskaar S: A Norwegian national cohort of 3198 women treated with home-managed electrical stimulation for urinary incontinence—effectiveness and treatment results. Scand J Urol Nephrol 35:32, 2001

Iosif CS, Batra S, Ek A, et al: Estrogen receptors in the human female lower urinary tract. Am J Obstet Gynecol 141:817, 1981

Jackson SL, Scholes D, Boyko EJ, et al: Predictors of urinary incontinence in a prospective cohort of postmenopausal women. Obstet Gynecol 108:855, 2006

Janknegt RA, Hassouna MM, Siegel SW, et al: Long-term effectiveness of sacral nerve stimulation for refractory urge incontinence. Eur Urol 39:101, 2001

Jelovsek JE, Chagin K, Brubaker L, et al: A model for predicting the risk of de novo stress urinary incontinence in women undergoing pelvic organ prolapse surgery. Obstet Gynecol 123:279, 2014

Kerrebroeck PE, Voskuilen A, Heesakkers J, et al: Results of sacral neuromodulation therapy for urinary voiding dysfunction: outcomes of a prospective, worldwide clinical study. J Urol 178:2029, 2007

Khan S, Panicker J, Roosen A, et al: Complete continence after botulinum neurotoxin type A injections for refractory idiopathic detrusor overactivity incontinence: patient-reported outcome at 4 weeks. Eur Urol 57(5):891, 2010

Kirkland JL, Lye M, Levy DW, et al: Patterns of urine flow and excretion in healthy elderly people. BMJ 287: 1665, 1983

Langa KM, Fultz NH, Saint S, et al: Informal caregiving time and costs for urinary incontinence in older individuals in the United States. J Am Geriatr Soc 50:733, 2002

Lapitan MC, Cody DJ, Grant AM: Open retropubic colposuspension for urinary incontinence in women. Cochrane Database Syst Rev 4:CD002912, 2009

Laurikainen E, Valpas A, Aukee P, et al: Five-year results of a randomized trial comparing retropubic and transobturator midurethral slings for stress incontinence. Eur Urol 65(6):1109, 2014

Lawrence JM, Lukacz ES, Liu IL, et al: Pelvic floor disorders, diabetes, and obesity in women: findings from the Kaiser Permanente Continence Associated Risk Epidemiology Study. Diabetes Care 30:2536, 2007

Lukacz ES, Whitcomb EL, Lawrence JM, et al: Urinary frequency in community-dwelling women: what is normal? Am J Obstet Gynecol 200:552, 2009

MacDiarmid SA, Peters KM, Shobeiri SA, et al: Long-term durability of percutaneous tibial nerve stimulation for the treatment of overactive bladder. J Urol 183:234, 2010

Mallipeddi PK, Steele AC, Kohli N, et al: Anatomic and functional outcome of vaginal paravaginal repair in the correction of anterior vaginal wall prolapse. Int Urogynecol J Pelvic Floor Dysfunct 12:83, 2001

Markland AD, Richter HE, Fwu CW, et al: Prevalence and trends of urinary incontinence in adults in the United States, 2001 to 2008. J Urol 186(2): 589, 2011

McGuire EJ: Urethral bulking agents. Nat Clin Pract Urol 3(5):234, 2006

McGuire EJ: Urodynamic findings in patients after failure of stress incontinence operations. Prog Clin Biol Res 78:351, 1981

McKinley M, O'Loughlin VD: Urinary system. In Human Anatomy. New York, McGraw-Hill, 2006, p 843

Miller JJ, Botros SM, Akl MN, et al: Is transobturator tape as effective as tension-free vaginal tape in patients with borderline maximum urethral closure pressure? Am J Obstet Gynecol 195:1799, 2006

Miller JJ, Sand PK: Diagnosis and treatment of overactive bladder. Minerva Ginecol 57:501, 2005

Minassian VA, Yan X, Lichtenfeld MJ, et al: The iceberg of health care utilization in women with urinary incontinence. Int Urogynecol J 23:1087, 2012.

Monga AK, Stanton SL: Urodynamics: prediction, outcome and analysis of mechanism for cure of stress incontinence by periurethral collagen. BJOG 104:158, 1997

Moore EE, Jackson SL, Boyko EJ, et al: Urinary incontinence and urinary tract infection: temporal relationships in postmenopausal women. Obstet Gynecol 111:317, 2008

Moser F, Bjelic-Radisic V, Tamussino K: Needle suspension of the bladder neck for stress urinary incontinence: objective results at 11 to 16 years. Int Urogynecol J 17:611, 2006

Nabi G, Cody JD, Ellis G, et al: Anticholinergic drugs versus placebo for overactive bladder syndrome in adults. Cochrane Database Syst Rev 4:CD0003781, 2006

Nager CW, Brubaker L, Litman HJ, et al: A randomized trial of urodynamic testing before stress-incontinence surgery. N Engl J Med 366(21):1987, 2012

Neuman M: Perioperative complications and early follow-up with 100 TVT-SECUR procedures. J Minim Invasive Gynecol 15(4):480, 2008

Nilsson CG, Palva K, Aarnio R, et al: Seventeen years' follow-up of the tension-free vaginal tape procedure for female stress urinary incontinence. Int Urogynecol J 24(8):1265, 2013

Noblett K, Lane FL, Driskill CS: Does pelvic organ prolapse quantification exam predict urethral mobility in stages 0 and I prolapse? Int Urogynecol J Pelvic Floor Dysfunct 15:268, 2005

Nygaard I: Is cesarean delivery protective? Semin Perinatol 30:267, 2006

Nygaard I, Barber MD, Burgio KL, et al: Prevalence of symptomatic pelvic floor disorders in U.S. women. JAMA 300(11): 1311, 2008

Nygaard I, Brubaker L, Zyczynski HM, et al: Long-term outcomes following abdominal sacrocolpopexy for pelvic organ prolapse. JAMA 309:2016, 2013

O'Connor RC, Nanigian DK, Lyon MB, et al: Early outcomes of mid-urethral slings for female stress urinary incontinence stratified by Valsalva leak point pressure. Neurourol Urodyn 25:685, 2006

Ouslander JG: Management of overactive bladder. N Engl J Med 350(8):786, 2004

Pearce MM, Hilt EE, Rosenfeld AB, et al: The female urinary microbiome: a comparison of women with and without urgency urinary incontinence. MBio 5(4):e01283, 2014

Peters KM, Carrico DJ, Perez-Marrero RA, et al: Randomized trial of percutaneous tibial nerve stimulation versus sham efficacy in the treatment of overactive bladder syndrome: results from the SUmiT trial. J Urol 183:1438, 2010

Peters KM, MacDiarmid SA, Wooldridge LS, et al: Randomized trial of percutaneous tibial nerve stimulation versus extended-release tolterodine: results from the overactive bladder innovative therapy trial. J Urol 182:1055, 2009

Petros PE, Ulmsten UI: An integral theory of female urinary incontinence. Experimental and clinical considerations. Scand J Urol Nephrol 153(Suppl):1, 1993

Rahn DD, Carberry C, Sanses TV, et al: Vaginal estrogen for genitourinary syndrome of menopause: a systematic review. Obstet Gynecol 124(6):1147, 2014

Rahn DD, Ward RM, Sanses TV, et al: Vaginal estrogen use in postmenopausal women with pelvic floor disorders: systematic review and practice guidelines. Int Urogynecol J 26(1):3, 2015

Raz R, Stamm WE: A controlled trial of intravaginal estriol in postmenopausal women with recurrent urinary tract infections. N Engl J Med 329:753, 1993

Resnick NM: Voiding dysfunction in the elderly. In Yalla SV, McGuire EJ, Elbadawi A, et al (eds): Neurourology and Urodynamics: Principles and Practice. New York, Macmillan, 1984, p 303

Resnick NM, Elbadawi A, Yalla SV: Age and the lower urinary tract: what is normal? Neurourol Urodyn 14:577, 1995

Richter HE, Albo ME, Zyczynski HM, et al: Retropubic versus transobturator midurethral slings for stress incontinence. N Engl J Med 362(22):2066, 2010a

Richter HE, Burgio KL, Brubaker L, et al: Continence pessary compared with behavioral therapy or combined therapy for stress incontinence. A randomized controlled trial. Obstet Gynecol 115(3):609, 2010b

Rortveit G, Daltveit AK, Hannestad YS, et al: Urinary incontinence after vaginal delivery or cesarean section. N Engl J Med 348(10):900, 2003a

Rortveit G, Daltveit AK, Hannestad YS, et al: Vaginal delivery parameters and urinary incontinence: the Norwegian EPINCONT study. Am J Obstet Gynecol 189(5):1268, 2003b

Sahai A, Dowson C, Khan MS, et al: Repeated injections of botulinum toxin-A for idiopathic detrusor overactivity. Urology 75(3):552, 2010

Sahai A, Khan MS, Dasgupta P: Efficacy of botulinum toxin-A for treating idiopathic detrusor overactivity: results from a single center, randomized, double-blind, placebo controlled trial. J Urol 177(6):2231, 2007

Sand P, Zinner N, Newman D, et al: Oxybutynin transdermal system improves the quality of life in adults with overactive bladder: a multicentre, community-based, randomized study. BJU Int 99(4):836, 2007

Sand PK, Bown LW, Panganiban R, et al: The low pressure urethra as a factor in failed retropubic urethropexy. Obstet Gynecol 62:399, 1987

Schmidt RA, Jonas UD, Oleson KA, et al: Sacral nerve stimulation for treatment of refractory urinary urge incontinence. J Urol 162:352, 1999

Serati M, Salvatore S, Uccella S, et al: Female urinary incontinence during intercourse: a review on an understudied problem for women's sexuality. J Sex Med 6:40, 2009

Siegel SW, Catanzaro F, Dijkema HE, et al: Long-term results of a multicenter study on sacral nerve stimulation for treatment of urinary urge incontinence, urgency-frequency, and retention. Urology 56(6 Suppl 1):87, 2000

Sirls LT, Foote JE, Kaufman JM, et al: Long-term results of the FemSoft1 Urethral Insert for the management of female stress urinary incontinence. Int Urogynecol J 13:88, 2002

Song PH, Kim YD, Kim HT, et al: The 7-year outcome of the tension-free vaginal tape procedure for treating female stress urinary incontinence. BJU Int 104(8):1113, 2009

Snooks SJ, Swash M, Henry MM, et al: Risk factors in childbirth causing damage to the pelvic floor innervation. Int J Colorectal Dis 1:20, 1986

Subak LL, Wing R, West DS, et al: Weight loss to treat urinary incontinence in overweight and obese women. N Engl J Med 360(5):481, 2009

Swift SE, Bent AE: Basic evaluation of the incontinent female patient. In Bent AE, Cundiff GW, Swift SE (eds): Ostergard's Urogynecology and Pelvic Floor Dysfunction, 6th ed. Philadelphia, Lippincott Williams & Wilkins, 2008, p 67

Townsend MK, Curhan GC, Resnick, et al: The incidence of urinary incontinence across Asian, black, and white women in the United States. Am J Obstet Gynecol 202:378.e1, 2010

Versi E1, Griffiths DJ, Harvey MA: A new external urethral occlusive device for female urinary incontinence. Obstet Gynecol 92:286, 1998

Vervest HA, van Venrooij GE, Barents JW, et al: Non-radical hysterectomy and the function of the lower urinary tract. II: Urodynamic quantification of changes in evacuation function. Acta Obstet Gynecol Scand 68:231, 1989

Visco AG, Brubaker L, Richter HE, et al: Anticholinergic therapy vs. onabotulinumtoxinA for urgency urinary incontinence. N Engl J Med 367:1803, 2012

Wai CY, Curto TM, Zyczynski HM, et al: Patient satisfaction after midurethral sling surgery for stress urinary incontinence. Obstet Gynecol 121(5):1009, 2013

Wake CR: The immediate effect of abdominal hysterectomy on intravesical pressure and detrusor activity. BJOG 87:901, 1980

Wang AC, Wang YY, Chen MC: Single-blind, randomized trial of pelvic floor muscle training, biofeedback-assisted pelvic floor muscle training, and electrical stimulation in the management of overactive bladder. Urology 63:61, 2004

Weber AM: Leak point pressure measurement and stress urinary incontinence. Curr Womens Health Rep 1:45, 2001

Wei JT, Nygaard I, Richter HE, et al: A midurethral sling to reduce incontinence after vaginal prolapse repair. N Engl J Med 366(25):2358, 2012

Wester C, Fitzgerald MP, Brubaker L, et al: Validation of the clinical bulbocavernosus reflex. Neurourol Urodyn 22:589, 2003

Wing RR, Creasman JM, West DS, et al: Improving urinary incontinence in overweight and obese women through modest weight loss. Obstet Gynecol 116:284, 2010

Wu JM, Hundley AF, Fulton RG, et al: Forecasting the prevalence of pelvic floor disorders in U.S. women 2010 to 2050. Obstet Gynecol 114(6):1278, 2009

Wu JM, Vaughan CP, Goode PS, et al: Prevalence and trends of symptomatic pelvic floor disorders in U.S. women. Obstet Gynecol 123:141, 2014

Zimmern P, Litman HJ, Nager CW, et al: Effect of aging on storage and voiding function in women with stress predominant urinary incontinence. J Urol 192:464, 2014

Zinner N, Gittelman M, Harris R, et al: Trospium chloride improves overactive bladder symptoms: a multicenter phase III trial. J Urol 171(6 Pt 1):2311, 2004

Pelvic Organ Prolapse

Pelvic organ prolapse (POP) is a common condition that can lead to urogenital tract dysfunction and diminished quality of life. *Signs* include descent of one or more of the following: the anterior vaginal wall, posterior vaginal wall, uterus and cervix, vaginal apex, or the perineum (Haylen, 2010). S*ymptoms* include the sensation of a vaginal bulge, pelvic pressure, and pelvic organ descent. Some degree of POP is present in a large proportion of the female population (Swift, 2000). It is considered a disease state only if surgical or nonsurgical reduction relieves the symptoms, restores function, and improves quality of life.

EPIDEMIOLOGY

POP affects millions of women worldwide. In the United States, it is the third most frequent indication for hysterectomy, and in women older than 70 years, prolapse repair is the most common inpatient procedure (Oliphant, 2010). A woman has a 12- to 19-percent cumulative lifetime risk to undergo POP-corrective surgery (Smith, 2010; Wu, 2014). Considering most women with POP do not elect surgical treatment, these percentages underestimate its true prevalence. Disease estimates are also hampered by inconsistent definitions. If examination alone is used to describe pelvic organ support, 30 to 65 percent of women presenting for routine gynecologic care have stage 2 prolapse (Bland, 1999; Swift, 2000, 2005; Trowbridge, 2008). In contrast, with POP defined solely by patient symptoms, prevalence rates range from 3 to 6 percent in the United States (Bradley, 2005; Nygaard, 2008; Rortveit, 2007). As the population ages, the number of women with POP is expected to rise dramatically, with 9.2 million women predicted to be affected in 2050 (Wu, 2009).

RISK FACTORS

■ Obstetrics-Related Risks

Table 24-1 summarizes predisposing factors for POP. It usually develops gradually over a span of years, and its etiology is multifactorial. The relative importance, however, of each factor is unknown.

Vaginal childbirth is the risk factor most commonly associated with POP. Some evidence suggests that pregnancy itself predisposes to POP. However, in numerous studies, vaginal delivery is linked to a woman's propensity for developing POP. In the Pelvic Organ Support Study (POSST), the risk of POP rose 1.2 times with each vaginal delivery (Swift, 2005). Compared with nulliparas, Rortveit and colleagues (2007) found that the prolapse risk grew significantly with rising parity in woman with one, two, or three or more vaginal deliveries. In a longitudinal study of 1011 women, vaginal delivery compared with cesarean delivery without labor was associated with a significantly greater risk of vaginal prolapse to the hymen or beyond (Handa, 2011). Last, in a large prospective cohort followed for 17 years, the risk of hospital admission for POP rose fourfold with one delivery and eightfold with two deliveries (Mant, 1997).

Although vaginal delivery is implicated in a woman's lifetime risk for POP, specific obstetric risk factors remain controversial. These include fetal macrosomia, prolonged second-stage labor, episiotomy, anal sphincter laceration, epidural analgesia, forceps use, and oxytocin stimulation of labor. The individual influence of each is yet to be defined.

TABLE 24-1. Risk Factors Associated with Pelvic Organ Prolapse

Pregnancy
Vaginal childbirth
Menopause
   Aging
   Hypoestrogenism
Chronically increased intraabdominal pressure
   Chronic obstructive pulmonary disease
   Constipation
   Obesity
Pelvic floor trauma
Genetic factors
   Race
   Connective tissue disorders
Spina bifida

Currently, two obstetric interventions—elective forceps delivery to shorten second-stage labor and elective episiotomy—are not advocated. Both lack evidence of benefit and carry risks for maternal and fetal harm. First, forceps delivery is directly implicated in pelvic floor injury through its association with anal sphincter laceration and levator ani muscle avulsion. In one study of pelvic floor anatomy at a median of 11 years postdelivery, 45 percent of all levator ani muscle avulsion lesions were sonographically identified in women with prior forceps delivery. In those with recognized avulsion, prolapse beyond the hymen was more prevalent (Handa, 2019). Overall, evidence suggests that operative vaginal birth raises the odds for POP sevenfold (Handa, 2011). For these reasons, elective forceps delivery is not recommended solely to prevent pelvic floor disorders. Likewise, at least twelve randomized trials comparing elective and selective episiotomy for women not undergoing operative vaginal delivery found no benefit from routine episiotomy. Instead, an association with anal sphincter laceration, postpartum anal incontinence, and postpartum pain was identified (Jiang, 2017).

Elective cesarean delivery to prevent pelvic floor disorders such as POP and urinary incontinence is controversial. In one large study of women followed 5 to 10 years after a first delivery, the POP risk in women who delivered vaginally was five times higher than that in those who underwent cesarean delivery without labor (Handa, 2011). Theoretically, if all women underwent cesarean delivery, fewer women would have POP. However, most women do not have symptomatic POP. Thus, cesarean delivery on maternal request (CDMR) with the goal of POP prevention would subject many women who would otherwise not develop the problem to a potentially dangerous intervention. Specifically, given the 11-percent lifetime risk for POP or incontinence surgery, for every one woman who would avoid pelvic floor surgery later in life by undergoing primary elective cesarean delivery, nine women would gain no benefit yet would nevertheless assume the potential risks of the cesarean (Patel, 2006). Currently, decisions regarding CDMR to prevent pelvic floor disorders must be individualized. The American College of Obstetricians and Gynecologists (2019a) recommends vaginal delivery as safe and appropriate in the absence of recognized maternal or fetal indications for cesarean delivery. The opinion does not address POP risk as a cesarean delivery indication and cites poor-quality evidence.

Age

Data from several studies show that POP prevalence rises steadily with aging (Nygaard, 2008; Olsen, 1997; Swift, 2005). In the POSST study, in women aged 20 to 59 years, the POP incidence roughly doubled with each decade. Aging is a complex process, and separating the effects of physiologic aging and estrogen deprivation is problematic. Reproductive hormones are essential to maintain pelvic organ support, and their specific effects on pelvic support are outlined earlier (Chap. 22, p. 499).

Connective Tissue Disease

Women with connective tissue disorders may be more likely to develop POP. In a small case series, one third of women with Marfan syndrome and three fourths of those with Ehlers-Danlos syndrome reported a history of POP (Carley, 2000).

Race

POP prevalence varies by race (Schaffer, 2005). Black and Asian women show the lowest risk, whereas Hispanic and white women appear to have the highest (Hendrix, 2002; Kim, 2005; Whitcomb, 2009). Differences may derive from variable collagen content or bony pelvis shape. For instance, black women more commonly have a narrow pubic arch and an android or anthropoid pelvis. These shapes protect against POP compared with the gynecoid pelvis typical of most white women.

Intraabdominal Pressure

Elevated intraabdominal pressure from chronic constipation, chronic coughing, repetitive heavy lifting, and obesity may contribute to POP pathogenesis. In the Women's Health Initiative trial, being overweight increased the POP rate by 31 to 39 percent, and being obese raised the POP rate by 40 to 75 percent (Hendrix, 2002). Similarly, overweight and obese women were 40 to 50 percent more likely to have POP compared with normal-weight women in one metaanalysis (Giri, 2017).

With regard to lifting, Danish nursing assistants who were involved with repetitive heavy lifting had a higher rate of surgical intervention for POP compared with the general population rate (Jorgensen, 1994). Similarly, in another study, laborers had greater rates of severe POP than those with sedentary jobs (Woodman, 2006).

Cigarette smoking and chronic obstructive pulmonary disease (COPD) also are implicated in POP development (Gilpin, 1989; Olsen, 1997). In one case-control study, COPD was associated with an increased risk of future pelvic floor repair after hysterectomy (Blandon, 2009). The repetitive elevations in intraabdominal pressure resulting from chronic coughing may predispose to POP. Also, rather than the cough itself, inhaled tobacco chemicals may cause connective tissue changes that lead to POP (Wieslander, 2005).

Genetic Factors

Ongoing studies suggest a genetic basis for POP (Ward, 2014). Some studies show a fivefold higher rate of POP among siblings with severe POP compared to the general population (Jack, 2006). Likewise, concordance of POP in twins and in sister pairs is significant (Altman, 2008). Moreover, recent genome-wide linkage studies have identified specific predisposition genes (Allen-Brady, 2015). Future investigations may allow better genetic risk stratification, patient counseling, and prevention strategies.

DESCRIPTION AND CLASSIFICATION

Visual Descriptors

POP is descent of the anterior vaginal wall, posterior vaginal wall, uterus (cervix), the vaginal apex after hysterectomy, rectum, or the perineum, alone or in combination. The terms *cystocele, rectocele,* and *enterocele* have traditionally described the structures thought to be prolapsed behind the vaginal wall. However, these terms are imprecise and misleading, as they focus on what is presumed to be prolapsed rather than what is objectively seen to

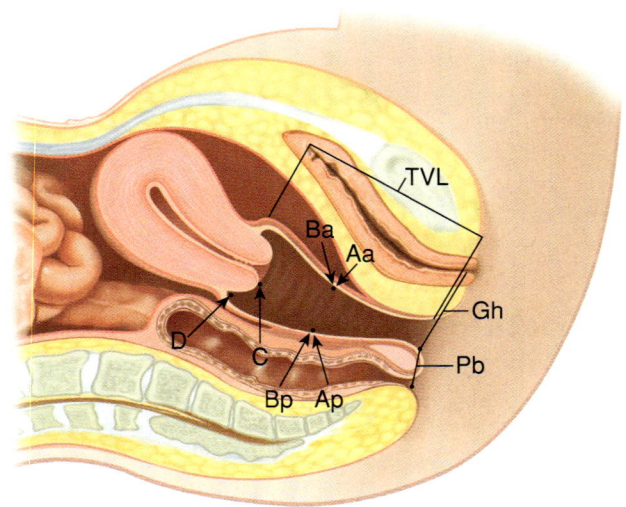

FIGURE 24-1 Anatomic landmarks used during pelvic organ prolapse quantification (POP-Q).

be prolapsed. Current preferred terms are *anterior vaginal wall prolapse, apical prolapse, cervical prolapse, posterior vaginal wall prolapse, rectal prolapse,* and *perineal descent.*

■ Pelvic Organ Prolapse Quantification

In 1996, the International Continence Society defined a system of Pelvic Organ Prolapse Quantification (POP-Q) (Bump, 1996). Demonstrating high intra- and interexaminer reliability, the POP-Q system measures the site-specific components of pelvic organ support. Prolapse in each segment is measured relative to the hymen, which is an anatomic landmark that can be identified consistently. The numeric measurement is assigned a negative sign if the prolapsed point is proximal to the hymen or is given a positive sign if it protrudes past the hymen. Six points are located with reference to the hymeneal plane: two on the anterior vaginal wall (points Aa and Ba), two at the vaginal apex (points C and D), and two on the posterior vaginal wall

(points Ap and Bp) (Fig. 24-1). The genital hiatus (Gh), perineal body (Pb), and total vaginal length (TVL) are also measured. All POP-Q points, except TVL, are measured during patient Valsalva and should reflect maximum protrusion.

The POP-Q measurements can be organized using a three-by-three grid shown in Figure 24-2. Figures 24-3 and 24-4 illustrate the use of POP-Q in evaluating different examples of POP (Bump, 1996).

The degree of prolapse can also be quantified using a five-stage ordinal system summarized in Table 24-2 (Bump, 1996). Stages are assigned according to the most severe portion of the prolapse. Used in the past and now less preferred, the Baden-Walker Halfway system uses a grading system to define POP. Normal organ positioning is grade 0, whereas organ descent that is half the distance to the hymen, at the hymen, or maximally prolapsed are grades 1, 2, and 3, respectively (Baden, 1992).

Vaginal Apex Points

With POP-Q assessment, the two apical points, C and D, which are located in the proximal vagina, represent the most

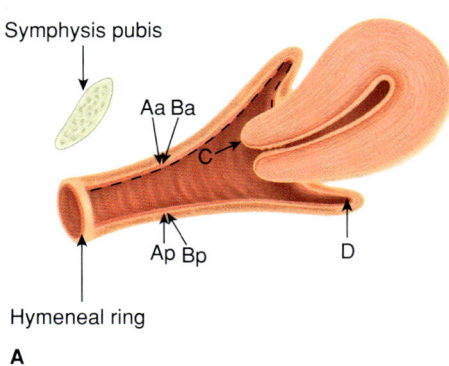

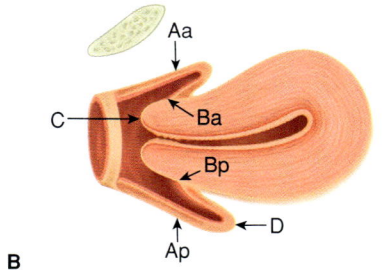

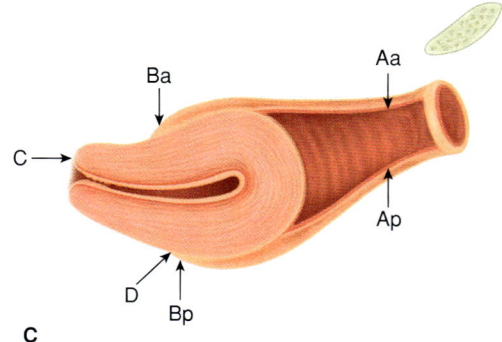

FIGURE 24-3 POP-Q depiction of varying degrees of uterine prolapse. **A.** Stage 0. **B.** Stage 2. **C.** Stage 4.

anterior wall	anterior wall	cervix or cuff
Aa	**Ba**	**C**
genital hiatus	perineal body	total vaginal length
gh	**pb**	**tvl**
posterior wall	posterior wall	posterior fornix
Ap	**Bp**	**D**

FIGURE 24-2 Grid system used for charting in pelvic organ prolapse quantification (POP-Q).

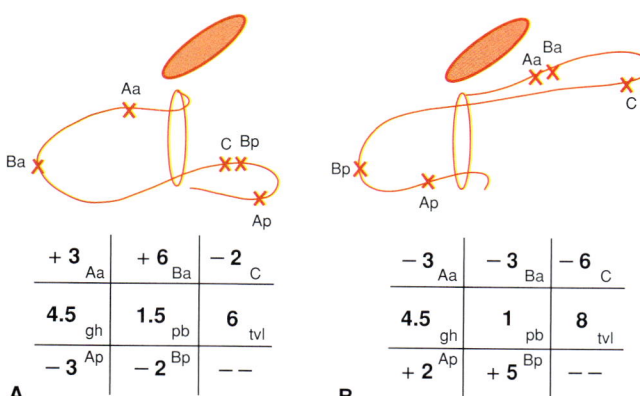

+3 Aa	+6 Ba	-2 C
4.5 gh	1.5 pb	6 tvl
-3 Ap	-2 Bp	--

A

-3 Aa	-3 Ba	-6 C
4.5 gh	1 pb	8 tvl
+2 Ap	+5 Bp	--

B

FIGURE 24-4 Grid and drawing of an anterior support defect (**A**) and posterior support defect (**B**).

cephalad locations of the vagina. Point C defines a point that reflects: (1) the most distal edge of the cervix or (2) the leading edge of the vaginal cuff after total hysterectomy. Point D defines a point that represents the posterior fornix in a woman who still has a cervix. It is omitted in the absence of a cervix. This point represents the level of uterosacral ligament attachment to the cervix and thus differentiates uterosacral ligament support failure from cervical elongation. The TVL is the greatest depth of the vagina in centimeters when point C or D is reduced to its fullest position.

Genital Hiatus and Perineal Body

The genital hiatus is measured from the middle of the external urethral meatus to the midline of the posterior hymeneal ring. The perineal body is measured from the posterior margin of the genital hiatus to the midanal opening (see Fig. 24-1).

Anterior Vaginal Wall Points

Point Aa defines a point that lies in the midline of the anterior vaginal wall and is 3 cm proximal to the external urethral meatus. This corresponds to the proximal location of the urethrovesical crease. In relation to the hymen, this point's position ranges from -3 (normal support) to +3 cm (maximum prolapse of point Aa).

Point Ba represents the most distal position of any part of the upper anterior vaginal wall, that is, the segment of vagina that normally would lie cephalad from point Aa. It is -3 cm in the absence of prolapse. In a woman with total vaginal eversion post-hysterectomy, Ba would have a positive value equal to the position of the cuff from the hymen.

Posterior Vaginal Wall Points

Point Ap defines a point in the midline of the posterior vaginal wall that lies 3 cm proximal to the hymen. Relative to the hymen, this point's range of position is by definition -3 (normal support) to +3 cm (maximum prolapse of point Ap).

Point Bp represents the most distal position of any part of the upper posterior vaginal wall. By definition, this point is at -3 cm in the absence of prolapse. In a woman with total post-hysterectomy vaginal vault eversion, Bp would have a positive value equal to the position of the cuff from the hymen.

PATHOPHYSIOLOGY

■ Levator Ani Muscle

Pelvic organ support is maintained by complex interactions among the pelvic floor muscles, pelvic floor connective tissue, and vaginal wall. These work in concert to provide support to and aid function of the vagina, urethra, bladder, and rectum.

The levator ani muscle is a pair of striated muscles composed of three regions, which are the *iliococcygeus muscle*, *pubococcygeus muscle*, and *puborectalis muscle*. These are illustrated in Chapter 38 (p. 798). Connective tissue covers the superior and inferior fascia of the levator ani muscle. Normally, its baseline resting contraction elevates the pelvic floor and compresses the vagina, urethra, and rectum toward the pubic bone (Fig. 38-10, p. 800). This narrows the genital hiatus and prevents POP. In addition, the upper vagina normally lies nearly horizontal

TABLE 24-2. The Pelvic Organ Prolapse Quantification (POP-Q) Staging System of Pelvic Organ Support

Stage 0:	No prolapse is demonstrated. Points Aa, Ap, Ba, and Bp are all at -3 cm and either point C or D is between -TVL (total vaginal length) cm and -(TVL-2) cm (i.e., the quantitation value for point C or D is ≤-[TVL-2] cm). Fig. 24-1 represents stage 0
Stage I:	The criteria for stage 0 are not met, but the most distal portion of the prolapse is >1 cm above the level of the hymen (i.e., its quantitation value is <-1 cm)
Stage II:	The most distal portion of the prolapse is ≤1 cm proximal to or distal to the plane of the hymen (i.e., its quantitation value is ≥-1 cm but ≤+1 cm)
Stage III:	The most distal portion of the prolapse is >1 cm below the plane of the hymen but protrudes no further than 2 cm less than the total vaginal length in centimeters (i.e., its quantitation value is >+1 cm but <+[TVL-2] cm). Fig. 24-4A represents stage III Ba and Fig. 24-4B represents stage III Bp prolapse
Stage IV:	Essentially, complete eversion of the total length of the lower genital tract is demonstrated. The distal portion of the prolapse protrudes to at least (TVL-2) cm (i.e., its quantitation value is ≥+[TVL-2] cm). In most instances, the leading edge of stage IV prolapse will be the cervix or vaginal cuff scar. Fig. 24-3C represents stage IV C prolapse

From Bump, 1996, with permission.

in the standing female. Thus, during periods of greater intraabdominal pressure, the upper vagina is compressed against the levator plate. One theory suggests that lost levator ani muscle tone allows the vagina to drop from a horizontal position to a semivertical one (Fig. 38-11, p. 800). This widens the genital hiatus, and the pelvic viscera are thereby predisposed to prolapse. Moreover, without adequate levator ani muscle support, visceral fascial attachments of the pelvic contents are placed on tension. These attachments stretch over time and eventually fail.

Loss of skeletal muscle volume and function develops in virtually all striated muscles during aging. Results obtained from young and older women with POP indicate that the levator ani muscle undergoes substantial morphologic and biochemical changes with time. Thus, loss of levator tone with age may contribute to pelvic organ support failure in older women, especially those with preexisting defects in connective tissue support.

Another hypothesis suggests that levator ani muscle tone may be lost following denervation. During second-stage labor, nerve injury can result from stretch or compression or both (DeLancey, 1993; Peschers, 1997; Shafik, 2000). Experimental evidence for this theory has been difficult to obtain and is contradictory (Boreham, 2009; Gilpin, 1989; Hanzal, 1993; Heit, 1996; Koelbl, 1989). In sum, denervation-induced injury is not currently implicated in POP genesis.

Connective Tissue

A continuous interdependent system of connective tissues and ligaments surrounds the pelvic organs and attaches them to the levator ani muscle and bony pelvis. Comprised of collagen, elastin, smooth muscle, and microfibers, this connective tissue network provides substantial pelvic organ support.

One component is the *arcus tendineus fascia pelvis*. It is a condensation of parietal fascia covering the medial aspects of the obturator internus and levator ani muscle (Fig. 38-7, p. 797). It provides the lateral and apical anchor sites for the anterior and posterior vagina. The arcus tendineus fascia pelvis is thus poised to withstand downward pressures against the anterior vaginal wall, vaginal apex, and proximal urethra. In one theory, loss of vaginal apex support leads to stretching or tearing of the arcus tendineus fascia pelvis. The result is apical and anterior vaginal wall prolapse.

The *uterosacral ligaments* also contribute to apical support by suspending and stabilizing the uterus, cervix, and upper vagina. The ligament contains approximately 20 percent smooth muscle. In women with prolapse, smooth muscle content in the uterosacral ligaments is diminished (Reisenauer, 2008; Takacs, 2009).

The muscular and connective tissue support of the pelvic floor is estrogen responsive, and estrogen deficiency can diminish the quality and quantity of collagen. Specifically, estrogen and progesterone receptors are identified in the connective tissue and smooth-muscle cells of both the levator ani muscle and uterosacral ligaments (Smith, 1990, 1993). In histologic studies, the ratio of collagen I to collagen III and IV is decreased in postmenopausal women not using estrogen therapy (Moalli, 2004). This relative decline in well-organized, dense collagen is believed to weaken vaginal wall tensile strength and raise vaginal wall

prolapse susceptibility. Rahn and coworkers (2014) found that vaginal estrogen application before POP surgery improved the vaginal maturation index, enhanced synthesis of mature collagen, and increased vaginal epithelial thickness. This suggests a possible role in healing and postsurgical support. Indeed, estrogen supplementation before or after prolapse surgery is considered essential by many pelvic reconstruction surgeons. Although this practice is empirically sound, evidence is yet to show improved surgical outcomes with this use of adjuvant estrogen.

Last, abnormalities of connective tissue and connective tissue repair may predispose women to POP (Norton, 1995; Smith, 1989). As noted, women with Ehlers-Danlos or Marfan syndrome are more likely to develop POP and urinary incontinence (Carley, 2000; Norton, 1995).

Vaginal Wall

The vaginal wall and its attachments to the pelvic floor muscles are integral to pelvic organ support. The vaginal wall is composed of mucosa (epithelium and lamina propria), a muscularis layer, and an adventitial layer that is made up of loose areolar tissue, abundant elastic fibers, and neurovascular bundles (Fig. 24-5). The muscularis and adventitial layers together form the *fibromuscular layer*, which was previously referred to as "endopelvic fascia." The fibromuscular layer coalesces laterally and attaches to the arcus tendineus fascia pelvis and superior fascia of the levator ani muscle. In the lower third of the vagina, the vaginal wall is attached directly to the perineal membrane and the perineal body. This suspensory system, together with the uterosacral ligaments, prevents vaginal and uterine descent.

Thus, abnormalities in the anatomy, physiology, and cellular biology of vaginal wall smooth muscle may contribute to POP. Specifically, in fibromuscular tissue taken from vaginal walls at the apex, prolapse is associated with loss of smooth muscle, myofibroblast activation, abnormal smooth muscle phenotype, and enhanced protease activity (Boreham, 2001, 2002a,b; Moalli, 2005; Phillips, 2006). Abnormal synthesis or degradation of

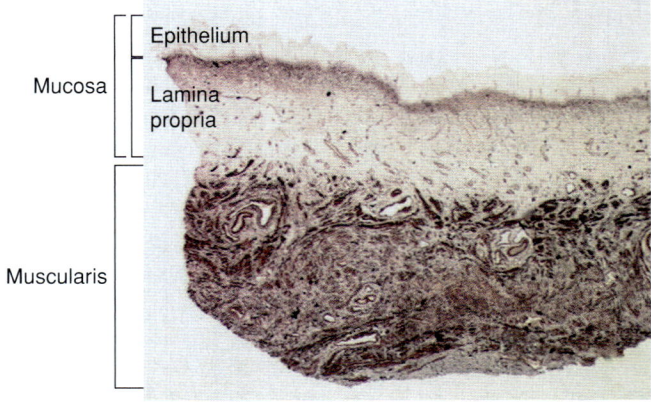

FIGURE 24-5 Photomicrograph shows a cross section of the vaginal wall. Mucosal and muscularis layers are shown here. The adventitia, which is typically seen deep to muscularis, is not shown in this section. The fibromuscular layer is comprised of muscularis and adventitial layers. (Reproduced with permission from Dr. Ann Word.)

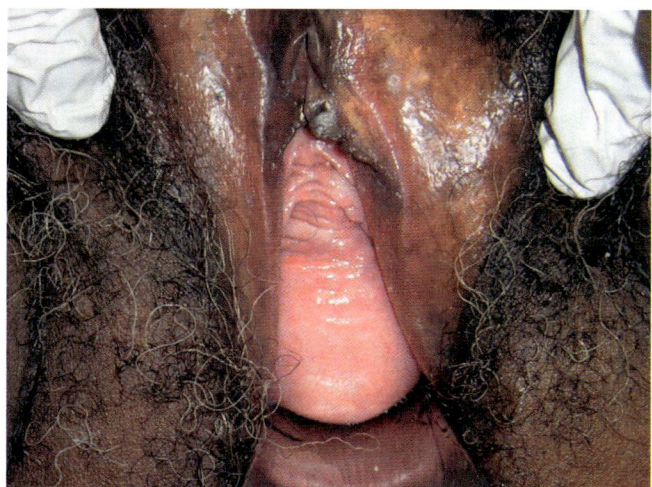

FIGURE 24-6 Midline or distension anterior vaginal wall defect. Note the characteristic loss of vaginal wall rugae.

vaginal wall collagen and elastin fibers also appears to contribute to POP.

◼ The Defect Theory of Pelvic Organ Prolapse

This theory states that tears in the fibromuscular connective tissue of the vaginal wall allow pelvic organ herniation. For example, weakness, attenuation, or tearing of the vaginal wall in the midline but without loss of lateral fascial attachments is called a *distention* or *midline* anterior vaginal wall defect (Fig. 24-6). With this defect, the vaginal wall appears smooth and without rugae, due to abdominal contents pressed against the vagina from within. In contrast, an anterior wall flaw due to connective tissue detachment of the lateral vaginal wall to the pelvic sidewall is described as a *displacement* or *paravaginal* anterior vaginal wall defect (Fig. 24-7). With

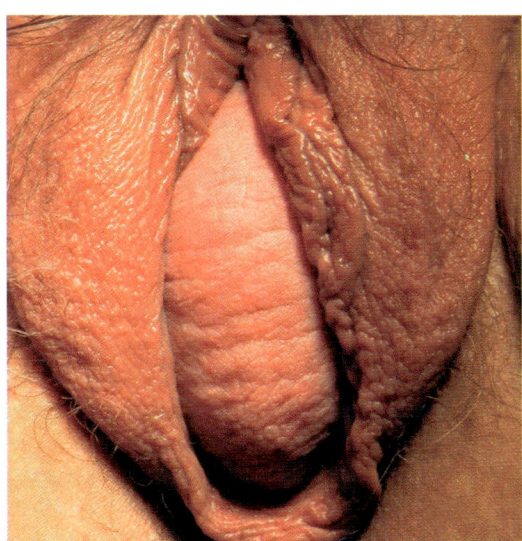

FIGURE 24-7 Lateral anterior vaginal wall defect, also termed paravaginal or displacement anterior vaginal wall defect. Rugae are present, which indicates that loss of support is lateral rather than central.

displacement-type prolapse, vaginal rugae are visible. Other defects include analogous midline and lateral defects in the posterior vaginal wall, loss of apical support, and defects at the level of the perineal body.

Many experts believe that loss of support at the vaginal apex is the most important factor in the development of POP. This loss allows the apical portions of the anterior and posterior vaginal walls to descend. As such, resuspension of the vaginal apex will restore support to both these.

◼ Levels of Vaginal Support

DeLancey (1992) has described three levels of vaginal support. Level I support suspends the upper or proximal vagina. Level II support attaches the midvagina along its length to the arcus tendineus fascia pelvis. Level III support results from fusion of the distal vagina to adjacent structures. Defects in each level of support result in identifiable vaginal wall prolapse.

Level I support is the attachment of the cardinal and uterosacral ligaments to the cervix and upper vagina (Fig. 38-15, p. 804). The cardinal ligaments fan out laterally and attach to the parietal fascia of the obturator internus and piriformis muscles, the anterior border of the greater sciatic foramen, and the ischial spines. The uterosacral ligaments are posterior fibers that attach to the presacral region at the level of S2 through S4. Together, this dense visceral connective tissue complex maintains vaginal length and horizontal axis. It allows the vagina to be supported by the levator plate and positions the cervix just superior to the level of the ischial spines. Defects in this support complex can lead to apical prolapse. This is frequently associated with small bowel herniation into the vaginal wall, that is, enterocele.

Level II support consists of the paravaginal attachments that are contiguous with the cardinal/uterosacral complex at the ischial spine. These are the connective tissue attachments of the lateral vagina anteriorly to the arcus tendineus fascia pelvis and posteriorly to the arcus tendineus rectovaginalis. Detachment of this connective tissue from the arcus tendineus fascia pelvis leads to lateral or paravaginal anterior vaginal wall prolapse.

Level III support is composed of the perineal body, superficial and deep perineal muscles, and fibromuscular connective tissue. Collectively, these support the distal one third of the vagina and introitus. The perineal body is essential for distal vaginal support and proper function of the anal canal. Damage to level III support contributes to anterior and posterior vaginal wall prolapse, gaping introitus, and perineal descent.

PATIENT EVALUATION

◼ Symptoms

POP involves multiple anatomic and functional components (Table 24-3). It rarely creates severe morbidity but can greatly diminish quality of life. In contrast, many women with mild to advanced POP lack bothersome symptoms. Thus, initial evaluation must carefully assess prolapse-related symptoms and their quality-of-life effects.

TABLE 24-3. Symptoms Associated with Pelvic Organ Prolapse

Symptoms	Other Possible Causes
Bulge symptoms	
Sensation of vaginal bulging or protrusion	Rectal prolapse
Seeing or feeling a vaginal or perineal bulge	Vulvar or vaginal cyst/mass
Pelvic or vaginal pressure	Pelvic mass
Heaviness in pelvis or vagina	Hernia (inguinal or femoral)
Urinary symptoms	
Urinary incontinence	Urethral sphincter incompetence
Urinary frequency	Detrusor overactivity
Urinary urgency	Hypoactive detrusor function
Weak or prolonged urinary stream	Bladder outlet obstruction (i.e., postsurgical)
Hesitancy	Excessive fluid intake
Feeling of incomplete emptying	Interstitial cystitis
Manual reduction of prolapse to start or complete voiding	Urinary tract infection
Position change to start or complete voiding	
Bowel symptoms	
Incontinence of flatus or liquid/solid stool	Anal sphincter disruption or neuropathy
Feeling of incomplete emptying	Diarrheal disorder
Hard straining to defecate	Rectal prolapse
Urgency to defecate	Irritable bowel syndrome
Digital evacuation to complete defecation	Rectal inertia
Splinting vagina or perineum to start or complete defecation	Pelvic floor dyssynergia
Feeling of blockage or obstruction during defecation	Hemorrhoids
	Anorectal neoplasm
Sexual symptoms	
Dyspareunia	Vaginal atrophy
Decreased lubrication	Levator ani syndrome
Decreased sensation	Vulvodynia
Decreased arousal or orgasm	Other female sexual disorder
Pain	
Pain in vagina, bladder, or rectum	Interstitial cystitis
Pelvic pain	Levator ani syndrome
Low back pain	Vulvodynia
	Lumbar disc disease
	Musculoskeletal pain
	Other causes of chronic pelvic pain

From Barber, 2005a, with permission.

During symptom inventory, two commonly used questionnaires are the Pelvic Floor Distress Inventory (PFDI) and the Pelvic Floor Impact Questionnaire (PFIQ) (Barber, 2005b). The PFDI measures urinary, colorectal, and POP symptoms, whereas the PFIQ assesses POP-related quality of life (Tables 24-4 and 24-5).

Bulge symptoms most strongly correlate with POP, and pelvic pressure or a vaginal or perineal protrusion are typical. These symptoms worsen with prolapse progression (Ellerkmann, 2001). Namely, women with prolapse beyond the hymen are more likely to report a vaginal bulge and have more symptoms than those with prolapse that stops above the hymen (Bradley, 2005; Tan, 2005; Weber, 2001a). If bulge symptoms are the primary com-

plaint, successful replacement of the prolapse with nonsurgical or surgical therapy will usually provide adequate symptom relief.

Urinary symptoms often accompany POP and may include stress urinary incontinence (SUI), urgency urinary incontinence, frequency, urinary retention, recurrent urinary tract infection, or voiding dysfunction. These symptoms may be caused or exacerbated by POP, but correction of prolapse does not guarantee a cure. For example, irritative bladder symptoms (frequency, urgency, and urgency urinary incontinence) do not always improve with prolapse replacement. Moreover, they may be unrelated to the prolapse and require alternative therapy. In contrast, urinary retention, if due to an obstructed urethra, will improve with prolapse treatment (FitzGerald, 2000).

TABLE 24-4. Short Form: Pelvic Floor Impact Questionnaire 7-Item (PFIQ-7)

Please select the best answer to each question below.
Name _____

Has your prolapse affected your:

1. Ability to do household chores (cooking, house cleaning, laundry)?
   _ Not at all   _ Mildly   _ Moderately   _ Severely

2. Physical recreation such as walking, swimming, or other exercises?
   _ Not at all   _ Mildly   _ Moderately   _ Severely

3. Entertainment activities (movies, church)?
   _ Not at all   _ Mildly   _ Moderately   _ Severely

4. Ability to travel by car or bus more than 30 minutes from home?
   _ Not at all   _ Mildly   _ Moderately   _ Severely

5. Participation in social activities outside your home?
   _ Not at all   _ Mildly   _ Moderately   _ Severely

6. Emotional health (nervousness, depression)?
   _ Not at all   _ Mildly   _ Moderately   _ Severely

7. Feeling frustrated?
   _ Not at all   _ Mildly   _ Moderately   _ Severely

From Flynn, 2006, with permission.

TABLE 24-5. Short Form: Pelvic Floor Distress Inventory 22-Item (PFDI-22)[a]

POPDI—6

Do you usually_____, and if so how much are you bothered by:
1. experience pressure in the lower abdomen
2. experience heaviness or dullness in the abdomen or genital area
3. have a bulge or something falling out that you can see or feel in the vaginal area
4. have to push on the vagina or around the rectum to have or complete a bowel movement
5. experience a feeling of incomplete bladder emptying
6. have to push up on a bulge in the vaginal area with your fingers to start or complete urination

CRADI—8

_____, and if so how much are you bothered by it
1. Do you usually feel you need to strain too hard to have a bowel movement
2. Do you usually feel you have not completely emptied your bowels at the end of bowel movement
3. Do you usually lose stool beyond your control if your stool is well formed
4. Do you usually lose stool beyond your control if your stool is loose or liquid
5. Do you usually lose gas from the rectum beyond your control
6. Do you usually have pain when you pass your stool
7. Do you usually experience a strong sense of urgency and have to rush to the bathroom to have a bowel movement
8. Does part of your bowel ever pass through the rectum and bulge outside during or after a bowel movement

UDI—8

Do you usually have _____, and if so, how much are you bothered by:
1. frequent urination
2. leakage related to feeling of urgency
3. leaking related to activity, coughing, or sneezing
4. leakage when you go from sitting to standing
5. small amounts of urine leakage (i.e., drops)
6. difficulty emptying the bladder
7. pain or discomfort in the lower abdomen or genital area
8. pain in the middle of your abdomen as your bladder fills

[a]For each question, patients fill in the blank with each phrase underneath the question. The same multiple choice responses (not at all, mildly, moderately, and severely) used for the PFIQ-7 are used for the PFDI-22.
From Flynn, 2006, with permission.

For these reasons, urodynamic testing is a valuable adjunct in women with urinary symptoms who are undergoing POP treatment (Chap. 23, p. 524). This testing attempts to determine the relationship between urinary symptoms and POP and will help guide therapy. Additionally, consideration may also be given to temporarily placing a pessary to determine if urinary symptoms improve.

Constipation is often present in women with POP, but POP generally is not the cause of constipation. An exception is a posterior vaginal wall defect that bulges as it fills with hard stool. This disrupts the normal mechanics of defecation to create obstruction-type constipation. Thus, constipation symptoms should be thoroughly assessed before proceeding with surgery. In one study of defect-directed posterior repair, constipation resolved postoperatively in only 43 percent of patients (Kenton, 1999). Thus, surgical repair or treatment with a pessary usually will not cure constipation, and it should be evaluated separately (Chaps. 12, p. 268 and 25, p. 569).

Digital decompression by the woman of her posterior vaginal wall, perineal body, or distal rectum to evacuate the rectum is the most common defecatory symptom associated with posterior vaginal wall prolapse (Burrows, 2004; Ellerkmann, 2001). Surgical approaches to this problem provide variable success, and symptom resolution rates range from 36 to 70 percent (Cundiff, 2004; Kenton, 1999).

Anal incontinence of flatus, liquid, or solid stool may also associate with POP. On occasion, prolapse may lead to stool trapping in the distal rectum with subsequent leakage of liquid stool around retained feces. If symptoms are present, a full anorectal evaluation is performed as described in Chapter 25 (p. 561). Most types of anal incontinence would not be expected to improve with surgical repair of prolapse. However, if evaluation reveals an anal sphincter defect as the cause of anal incontinence, anal sphincteroplasty may be performed concurrently with prolapse repair.

Female sexual dysfunction is frequently multifactorial and includes psychosocial factors, urogenital atrophy, aging, and male sexual dysfunction (Chap 14, p. 312). Often, sexual dysfunction also is seen in women with POP. However, study findings are inconsistent. In one study, a validated sexual function questionnaire was used to compare intercourse frequency, libido, dyspareunia, orgasmic function, and vaginal dryness in women with and without POP (Weber, 1995). No differences were seen between the two groups. In another, pelvic floor symptoms were associated with dyspareunia, reduced arousal, and infrequent orgasm (Handa, 2008). In addition, sexual dysfunction was worse in women with symptomatic prolapse versus those with asymptomatic prolapse. In one evaluation, decreased sexual activity was associated with shorter vaginal length, and one quarter of women avoided sexual activity due to pelvic floor symptoms (Edenfield, 2015). Accordingly, women with an obstructing bulge as a cause of sexual dysfunction may benefit from therapy to reduce the prolapse. Unfortunately, some prolapse procedures such as posterior repair with levator plication and vaginal placement of mesh may contribute to postoperative dyspareunia. Thus, sexual dysfunction should be factored during treatment planning (Ulrich, 2015).

Pelvic pain and back pain are common complaints in women with POP, but little evidence supports a direct association (Heit, 2002; Swift, 2003). Some suggest that low back pain in a patient with POP may be caused by altered body mechanics. However, if pain is a primary symptom, other sources should be sought (Chap. 12, p. 257). Without an identifiable etiology, temporary pessary placement may determine if prolapse reduction will improve pain symptoms. Referral to a physical therapist may also shed light on a connection among prolapse, altered body mechanics, and pain.

Importantly, although POP is associated with varied complaints, symptoms and their severity do not always correlate well with advanced-stage POP. In addition, apical, anterior, or posterior wall prolapse each can cause similar symptoms (Jelovsek, 2005; Kahn, 2005; Weber, 1998). Thus, when planning surgical or nonsurgical therapy, realistic expectations should be set with regard to symptom relief. A patient is informed that symptoms directly related to prolapse such as vaginal bulge and pelvic pressure are likely to lessen with a successful anatomic repair. However, constipation, back pain, and urinary urgency and frequency may or may not improve.

■ Physical Examination

Perineal Examination

Physical examination begins with a full body systems evaluation to identify pathology outside the pelvis. Cardiovascular, pulmonary, renal, or endocrinologic disease may affect treatment choices and are ideally identified early.

The initial pelvic examination is performed with a woman in lithotomy position. The vulva and perineum are examined for signs of vulvar or vaginal atrophy or other abnormalities. A neurologic examination of sacral reflexes is performed using a cotton swab. First, the *bulbospongiosus reflex* is elicited by tapping or sweeping lateral to the clitoris and observing contraction of the bulbospongiosus muscles bilaterally. Second, evaluation of anal sphincter innervation is completed by sweeping lateral to the anus and observing a reflexive contraction of the anus, known as the *anal wink reflex*. Intact reflexes suggest normal sacral pathways. Still, they may be absent in women with intact neurologic functioning.

POP examination begins by asking a woman to attempt a Valsalva maneuver before placing a speculum in the vagina (Fig. 24-8). Patients who are unable to adequately complete a Valsalva maneuver are asked to cough. This "hands-off" approach more accurately displays true anatomy. For example, with speculum examination, structures are artificially lifted, supported, or displaced. During assessment, the specific prolapsing vaginal compartment, its degree of descent, and changes in genital hiatus diameter are determined.

A woman is asked to describe the extent of prolapse beyond the hymen during real-life activities. This degree may be conveyed in terms of inches. Alternatively, a mirror may be placed at the perineum. Here, the patient can visually confirm that the examiner is seeing the true extent of the prolapse.

POP is a dynamic condition that responds to the effects of gravity and intraabdominal pressure. It frequently worsens over the course of a day or during physical activity. Thus, POP

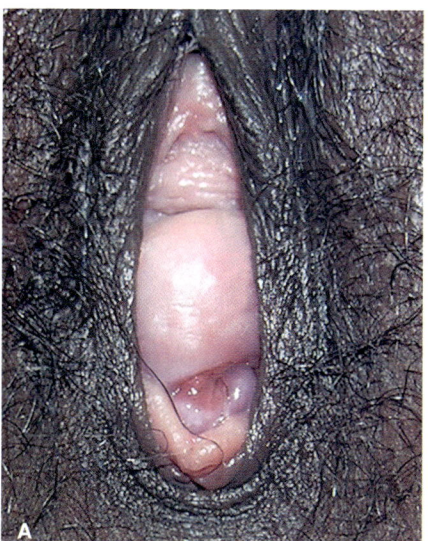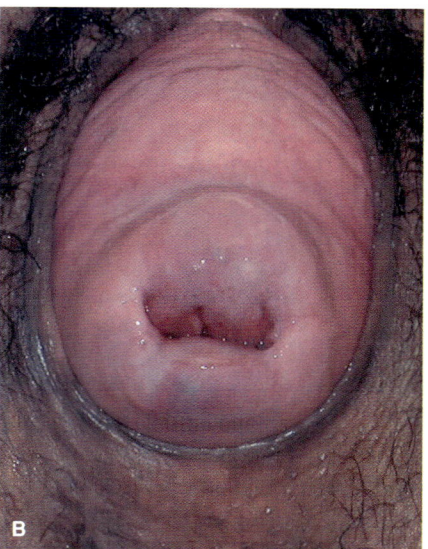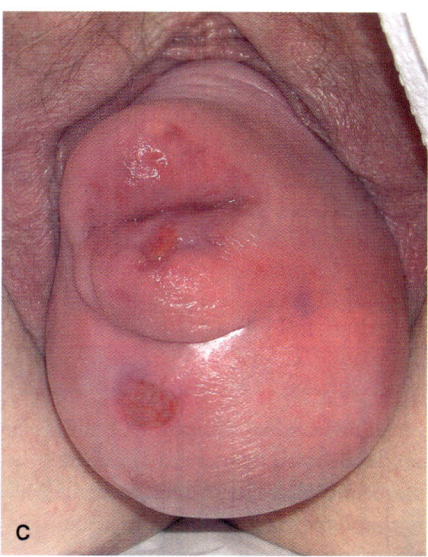

FIGURE 24-8 A. Stage 2. This stage is defined by the most distal edge of the prolapse lying within 1 cm of the hymeneal ring. **B.** Stage 3. This stage is defined by the most distal portion of the prolapse being >1 cm below the plane of the hymen, but protruding no farther than 2 cm less than the total vaginal length in centimeters. **C.** Stage 4. This stage is defined as complete or near complete eversion.

might not be evident during office examination early in the morning. If the full extent of prolapse cannot be demonstrated, a woman should be examined in a standing position and during Valsalva maneuver.

Vaginal Examination

All POP-Q points, except TVL, are measured during patient Valsalva. The genital hiatus and perineal body are measured first (Fig. 24-9). TVL is next measured by placing a marked ring forceps or a ruler at the vaginal apex and noting the distance to the hymen. This is replaced by a bivalve (Graves) speculum, which is inserted to the vaginal apex. It displaces the anterior and posterior vaginal walls, and points C and D are measured during a Valsalva maneuver. During the maneuver, the speculum is slowly withdrawn to assess descent of the apex.

A split speculum is then used to displace the posterior vaginal wall and allow viewing of the anterior wall and measurement of points Aa and Ba. Attempts are made to characterize the anterior vaginal wall defect. Sagging lateral vaginal sulci with vaginal rugae present suggest a *paravaginal defect*, that is, a lateral loss of support (Fig. 24-10). A central bulge and loss of vaginal rugae is called a *midline* or *central defect* (see Fig. 24-6). If loss of support appears to arise from detachment of the anterior vaginal wall's apical segment, it is termed a *transverse* or *anterior apical defect* (Fig. 24-11). Transverse defects are assessed by replacing the apex with a split-speculum blade and observing whether the prolapse descends during Valsalva maneuver.

The split speculum is then rotated 180 degrees to displace the anterior wall and allow examination of the posterior wall. Points

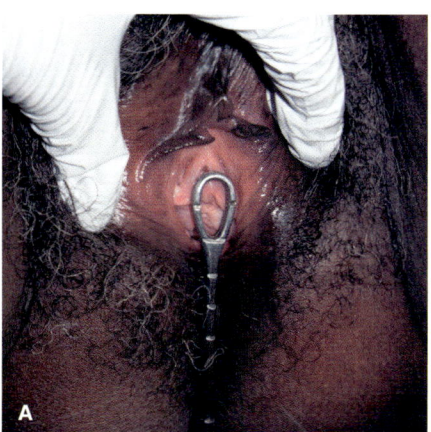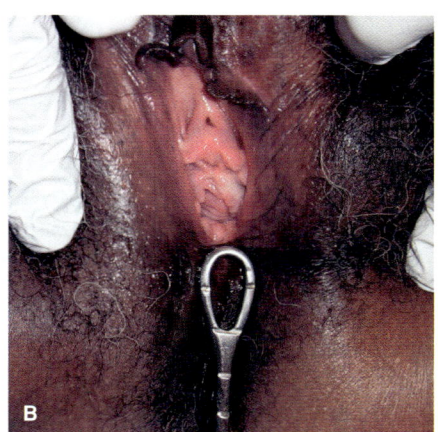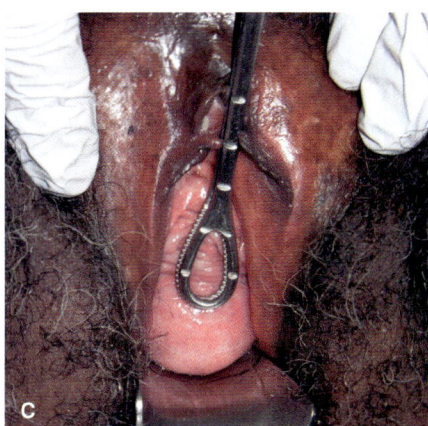

FIGURE 24-9 A. Measurement of the genital hiatus (Gh). For POP-Q evaluation, a sponge stick is marked at 1-, 2-, 3-, 4-, 5-, 7.5-, and 10-cm increments. Measurement is obtained with a woman performing maximum Valsalva maneuver. **B.** Measurement of the perineal body. **C.** Measurement of points Aa and Ba. Aa is a discrete point lying 3 cm proximal to the urethral meatus and is measured in relation to the hymen. During measurement, a split speculum displaces the posterior vaginal wall, but downward traction is avoided, as this causes artificial descent of the anterior vaginal wall.

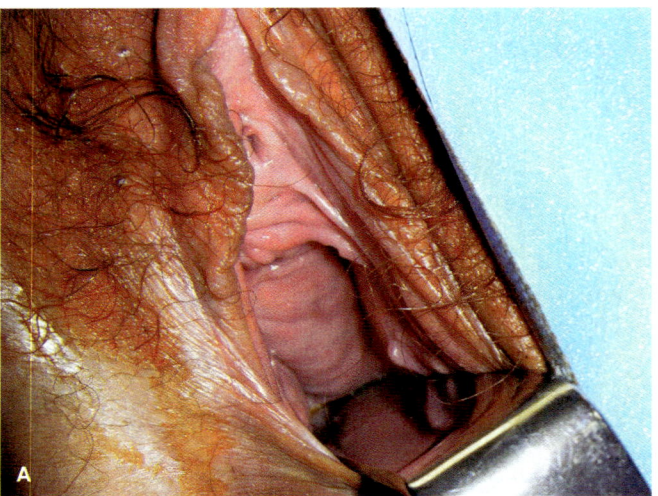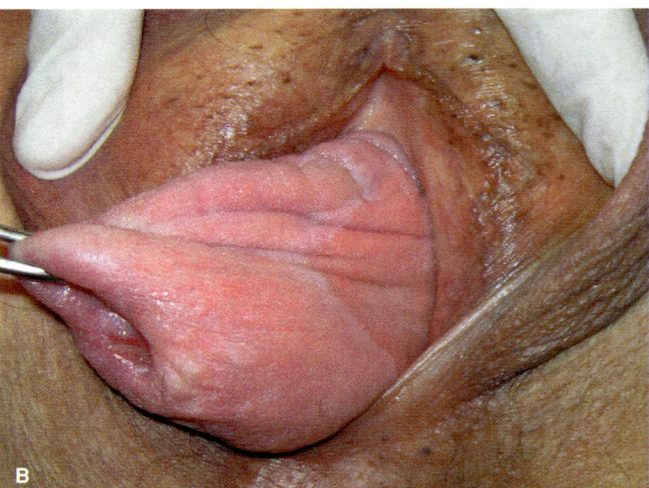

FIGURE 24-10 A. Normal lateral support as noted by normal positioning of the vaginal sulci. **B.** Complete loss of lateral support, shown as absent lateral sulci.

Ap and Bp are measured (Fig. 24-12). If the posterior vaginal wall descends, attempts are made to determine if a posterior vaginal wall defect or an enterocele is present. An enterocele can be definitively diagnosed by observing small-bowel peristalsis behind the vaginal wall (Fig. 24-13). In general, bulges at the apical segment of the posterior vaginal wall implicate enteroceles. As a further diagnostic step, a clinician's index finger is placed in the rectum and thumb on the posterior vaginal wall. Small bowel may be palpated between the rectum and vagina, confirming enterocele.

Differentiation of midline, lateral, apical, and distal defects of the anterior and posterior vaginal walls has poor inter- or intraexaminer reliability. However, individual evaluation may help assess prolapse severity and clarify anatomy if surgical correction is planned (Barber, 1999; Whiteside, 2004).

As mentioned, apical prolapse is thought to cause most anterior and posterior wall descent. Thus, the apex is replaced to its normal position during evaluation. If this maneuver restores anterior and posterior support, it can be determined

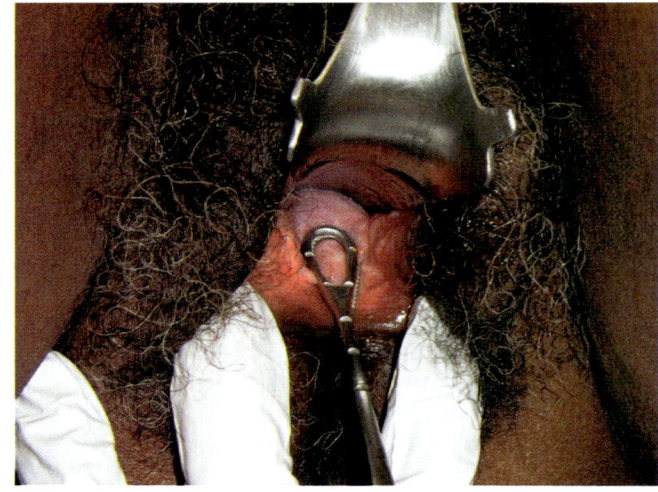

FIGURE 24-12 Split speculum displaces the anterior vaginal wall. This allows for measurement of points Ap and Bp. Ap is always defined as a discrete point lying 3 cm proximal to the hymen.

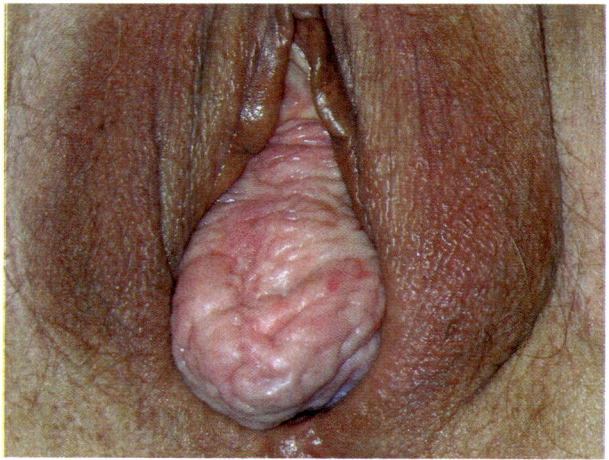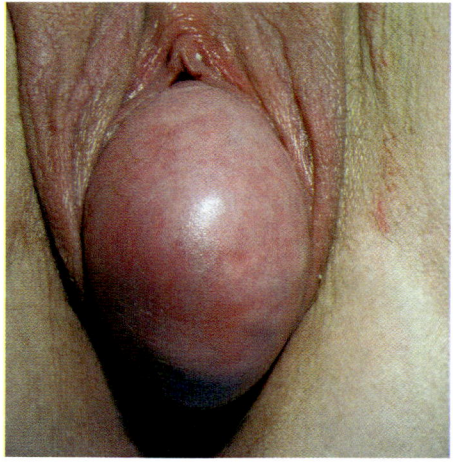

FIGURE 24-11 Transverse vaginal wall defect. Note detachment of the anterior vaginal wall from the apex and the presence of rugae, which suggests that this is not a midline or central defect.

FIGURE 24-13 During evaluation, small-bowel peristalsis may be noted behind the vaginal wall. Such enteroceles are most commonly noted at the vaginal apex, although anterior and posterior vaginal wall enteroceles may occur.

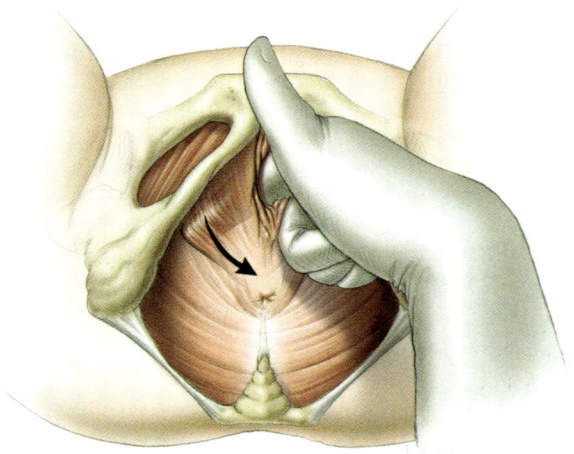

FIGURE 24-14 Pelvic floor muscle assessment. The index finger is placed 2 to 3 cm inside the hymen at 4 and 8 o'clock. Both resting and contraction tone and strength are evaluated.

that restoration of apical support will improve prolapse in all three compartments.

Bimanual examination is performed to identify other pelvic pathology. We strongly recommend assessment of pelvic floor musculature (Fig. 12-4, p. 260). This examination is essential if pelvic floor rehabilitation is considered for treatment. During part of the evaluation, an index finger is placed 1 to 3 cm inside the hymen, at 4 and then 8 o'clock (Fig. 24-14). Muscle resting tone and strength is assessed using the 0 through 5 Oxford grading scale, in which 5 represents normal tone and strength (Laycock, 2002). Muscle symmetry also is evaluated. Asymmetric muscles, with palpable defects or scarring, may be associated with a prior obstetric forceps delivery, episiotomy, or laceration.

APPROACH TO TREATMENT

For women who are asymptomatic or mildly symptomatic, expectant management is appropriate. The natural history of prolapse is unknown, and many women will never develop symptoms. Thus, invasive therapy is typically not selected for asymptomatic women, as risks likely outweigh benefits.

For women with significant POP or for those with bothersome symptoms, nonsurgical or surgical therapy is an option. Treatment choice is influenced by symptom type and severity, age, medical comorbidities, factors for recurrence, and desire for future sexual function and/or fertility. Once these are assessed, options and their success rates are discussed. In the simplest case, a patient with prolapse of the vaginal apex beyond the hymen, whose only symptom is bulge or pelvic pressure, could be offered pessary or surgical repair. In a more complex case, a woman with prolapse beyond the hymen may note a bulge, constipation, urgency urinary incontinence, and pelvic pain. Symptoms would be ranked by severity and importance of resolution. To address all complaints, therapy might involve a pessary or surgery for bulge symptoms, and nonsurgical treatment of constipation, incontinence, and pelvic pain.

NONSURGICAL TREATMENT

■ Pessary

Pessary Indications

Various vaginal devices can be inserted to support vaginal prolapse. Today's pessaries are appropriate effective options for prolapse of anterior, posterior, or apical compartments. Usually made of silicone or inert plastic, pessaries are typically safe and simple to manage. In one randomized trial, women with stage 1 through 3 POP were treated with either pelvic floor muscle training (PFMT) alone or a combination PFMT plus a vaginal pessary. At 12 months, women in both groups had improved scores on the POP distress inventory and the POP impact questionnaire. However, the mean score differences were higher in the pessary group (Cheung, 2016).

Pessaries may also help some women with prolapse and associated urinary incontinence. One randomized trial compared two pessary types for relief of prolapse symptoms and urinary complaints. Pessaries modestly improved urinary obstructive, irritative, and stress symptoms (Schaffer, 2006).

Pessaries can also aid diagnosis and treatment prognosis. First, symptoms may not correlate with prolapse type or severity. Short-term pessary use may help clarify this relationship. Even if a patient declines long-term pessary use, she may agree to a short trial to determine if her chief complaint is improved or resolved. Second, a pessary may also be placed prior to surgery to identify which women are at risk for urinary incontinence after a prolapse-correcting procedure (Chaikin, 2000; Liang, 2004).

Pessary Selection

Pessaries are divided into support and space-filling categories (Fig. 24-15). Support pessaries, such as the ring pessary, use a spring mechanism that rests in the posterior fornix and against the symphysis pubis. Vaginal support derives from elevation of the vaginal apex by the spring, which is supported by the symphysis pubis. Ring pessaries may be constructed as a simple circular ring or as a ring with support that looks like a large contraceptive diaphragm (Fig. 24-16). The diaphragm portion of a support ring can serve as a shelf to limit anterior vaginal wall descent. When properly fitted, the device should lie behind the pubic symphysis anteriorly and behind the cervix posteriorly.

In contrast, space-filling pessaries maintain their position by creating suction between the pessary and vaginal walls (cube), by creating a diameter larger than the genital hiatus (donut), or by both mechanisms (Gellhorn). The Gellhorn is often used for moderate to severe prolapse and for complete procidentia. It contains a concave disc that fits against the cervix or vaginal cuff and has a stem that is positioned just cephalad to the introitus. The concave disc supports the vaginal apex by creating suction, and the stem is useful for device removal. Of all pessaries, the two most commonly used and studied devices are the ring and the Gellhorn pessaries.

Patient Evaluation and Pessary Placement

A patient must be an active participant in the treatment decision to use a pessary. Its success depends on her ability to care for the

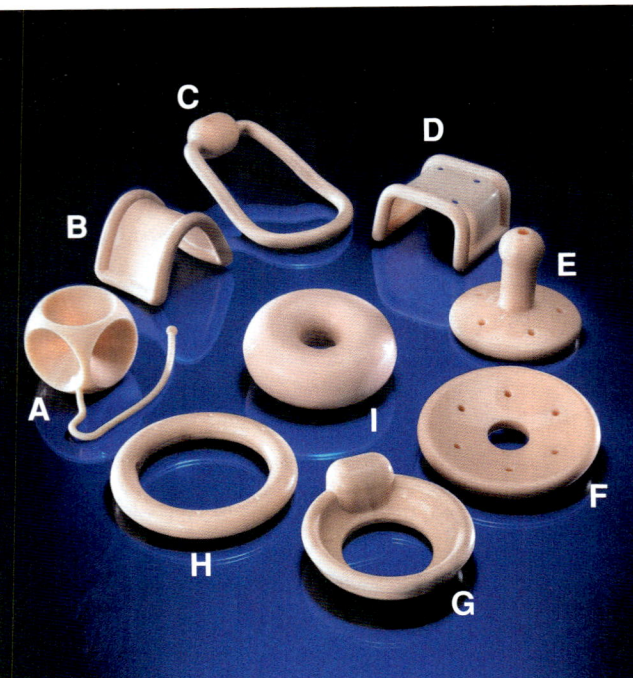

FIGURE 24-15 Types of Milex pessaries. **A.** Cube pessary. **B.** Gehrung pessary. **C.** Hodge with knob pessary. **D.** Regula pessary. **E.** Gellhorn pessary. **F.** Shaatz pessary. **G.** Incontinence dish pessary. **H.** Ring pessary. **I.** Donut pessary. (Reproduced with permission of CooperSurgical, Inc., Trumbull, CT.)

device—either alone or with the assistance of a caregiver—and her willingness and availability to come for subsequent evaluations. Vaginal atrophy is ideally treated before or concomitantly with pessary initiation, and options are found in Table 22-11 (p. 498). In women who are suitable candidates for estrogen therapy, vaginal estrogen cream is recommended. In one regimen, 1 g of conjugated equine estrogen cream (Premarin cream) is inserted nightly for 2 weeks, then two times per week thereafter. Vaginal ospemifene is another option.

Device selection integrates patient factors such as hormonal status, sexual activity, prior hysterectomy, and stage and site

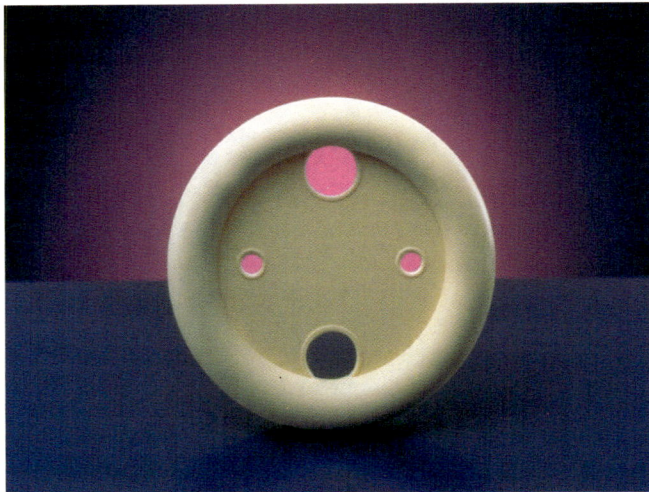

FIGURE 24-16 Milex ring pessary with support. (Reproduced with permission of CooperSurgical, Inc., Trumbull, CT.)

of POP. After a pessary is chosen, a woman is fitted with the largest size that can be comfortably worn. If a pessary is ideally fitted, a patient is not aware of it. As a woman ages and gains or loses weight, alternate sizes may be required.

Generally, a patient is fitted with a pessary while in the lithotomy position after she has emptied her bladder. A digital examination is performed to assess vaginal length and width, and an initial estimation of pessary size is made. For ring pessary placement, the device is held in the clinician's dominant hand in a folded position. Lubricant is placed on the vaginal introitus or on the pessary's leading edge. While holding the labia apart, a provider inserts the pessary by pushing it cephalad and against the posterior vaginal wall. Once the upper vagina is reached, the pessary is released and it opens. Next, an index finger is directed into the posterior vaginal fornix to ensure that the cervix is resting above the pessary. In a well-sized device, the clinician's finger should barely slide between the lateral edges of the ring pessary and the vaginal sidewall. The pessary ideally fits snugly but not tightly against the symphysis pubis and the posterior and lateral vaginal walls. Excessive pressure increases the risk for pain. Figure 24-17 shows Gellhorn pessary placement.

Following pessary placement, a woman is prompted to bear down, which might dislodge an improperly fitted pessary. She should be able to stand, walk, cough, and urinate without difficulty or discomfort. Instruction on removal and placement then follows. For removal of a ring pessary, an index finger is inserted into the vagina to hook the ring's edge. Traction is applied along the vaginal axis to bring the ring toward the introitus. Here, it may be grasped by the thumb and index finger and removed.

Ideally, a pessary is removed nightly to weekly, washed in soap and water, and replaced the next morning. Women also receive instructions describing the management of commonly encountered problems (Table 24-6). After initial placement, a return visit may follow in 1 to 2 weeks. For patients comfortable with their pessary management, return visits may be semiannual. If the patient and the provider are motivated, most women can be taught to self-manage a pessary. For those unable or unwilling to remove and replace a device themselves, a pessary may be removed and the patient's vagina inspected at the provider's office every 2 or 3 months. Delaying visits longer than this may lead to problematic discharge and odor.

Pessary Complications

Serious complications such as erosion into adjacent organs are rare with proper use and usually result only after years of neglect. At each return visit, the pessary is removed, and the vagina is inspected for erosions, abrasions, ulcerations, or granulation tissue (Fig. 24-18). Vaginal bleeding is usually an early sign and should not be ignored. *Pessary ulcers* or abrasions are treated by changing the pessary type or size to alleviate pressure points or by removing the pessary completely until sites heal. Treatment of vaginal atrophy with local estrogen is commonly required. Alternatively, water-based lubricants applied to the pessary may help prevent these complications. *Prolapse ulcers* have the same appearance as pessary ulcers, however, the former result from the prolapsed bulge rubbing against patient clothing. These are treated by replacing the prolapse either with a pessary or by surgery. Topical hormone therapy can be an interim adjunct.

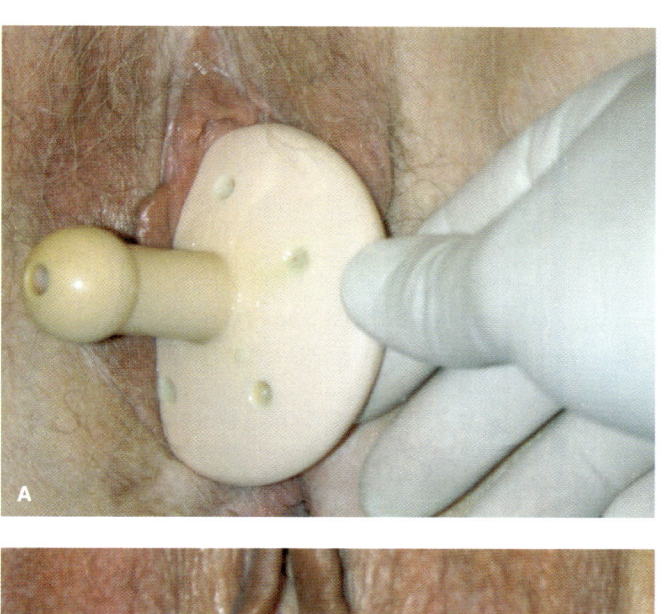
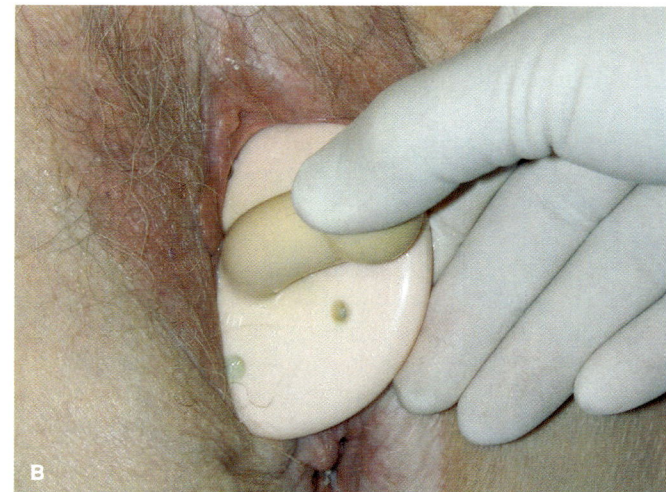
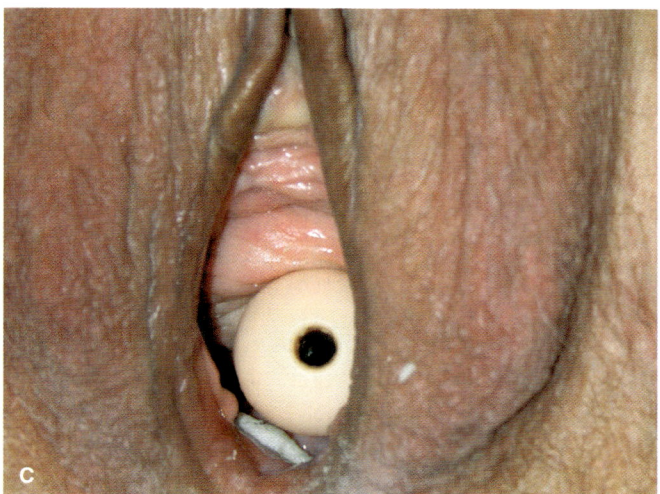
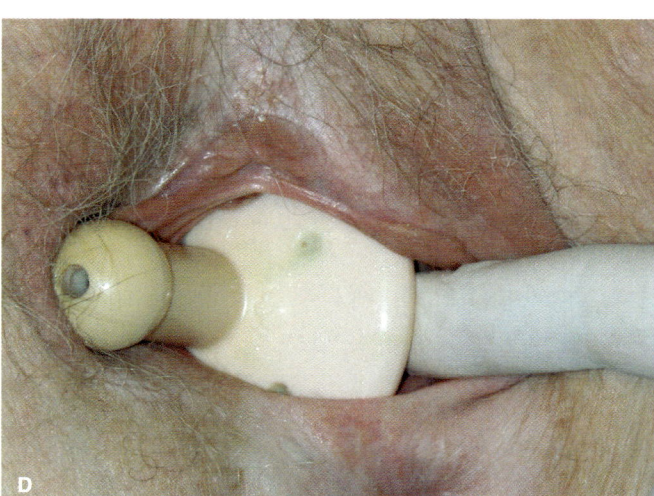

FIGURE 24-17 Technique for placement and removal of a Gellhorn pessary. Figures **A–C** show placement. **D.** To remove a Gellhorn pessary, an index finger is placed behind the disk and suction is broken prior to removal.

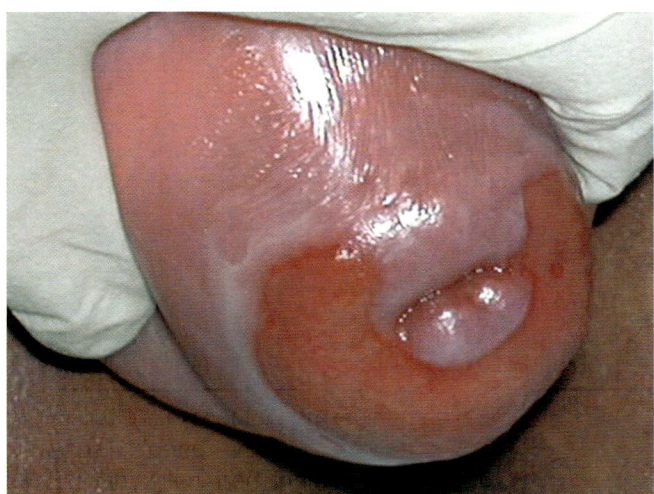

FIGURE 24-18 Granulation tissue involving the anterior and posterior vaginal wall resulting from pessary trauma.

Of other related symptoms, pelvic pain is not considered normal and usually indicates a device that is too large. Second, all pessaries tend to trap vaginal secretions and obstruct normal drainage to some degree. The resulting odor may be managed by encouraging nighttime device removal, washing, and reinsertion the next day on a more frequent basis. Alternatively, a woman may use a pH-based deodorant gel (Trimo-San gel) once or twice weekly or may douche with warm water. Trimo-San gel helps restore and maintain normal vaginal acidity that aids in reducing odor-causing bacteria.

■ Pelvic Floor Muscle Training

Also known as *Kegel exercises*, the steps of pelvic floor muscle training are described fully in Chapter 23 (p. 527). To some degree, these exercises may limit POP progression and alleviate symptoms, and two hypotheses describe their benefits (Bø, 2004). First, with PFMT, women learn to consciously contract muscles before and during increases in abdominal pressure. This prevents organ descent. Second, regular muscle strength training builds permanent muscle volume and structural support.

TABLE 24-6. Guidelines for Pessary Care

Pessary type_____
      Size_____

1. After your initial pessary fitting is successful, you will be asked to return for a follow-up appointment in about 2 weeks. The purpose of this visit is to check the pessary and examine the vagina to ensure that it is healthy. Follow-up appointments will follow this schedule:
    1st year: every 3–6 months
    2nd year and beyond: every 6 months
    You may learn to care for the pessary yourself. For those patients who can remove and insert the pessary themselves, we recommend weekly overnight removal and cleansing of the pessary with soap and warm water. These patients should see the doctor at least once per year.

2. The following is a list of problems you may encounter with the pessary and our recommendations for their management.

Problem	Management
A. The pessary falls out.	Keep the pessary and notify your doctor's office. An appointment will be made. It may be possible that a change in the size or the type of pessary is needed.
B. You experience pelvic pain.	Notify your doctor's office. If the pessary has slipped and you can remove it, do so. Otherwise, have your doctor remove the pessary. A change in pessary size or type may be needed.
C. Vaginal discharge and odor.	You can douche with warm water and you may want to try using Trimo-San vaginal gel 1–3 times a week.
D. Vaginal bleeding.	Vaginal bleeding may be a sign that the pessary is irritating the lining of the vagina. Call your doctor's office and arrange an appointment.
E. Leaking from the bladder.	Sometimes, the support provided by the pessary will cause leaking from the bladder. Notify your doctor and discuss this problem.

Trimo-San (Oxyquinoline, Milex Products, Chicago, IL) helps restore and maintain the normal vaginal acidity that helps reduce odor-causing bacteria.
From Farrell, 1997, with permission.

In one randomized trial, women with stages 1 through 3 of POP were assigned a regimen or were given a prolapse lifestyle advice leaflet (Hagen, 2017). After 2 years, prolapse symptom severity scores and bladder and bowel symptoms in the PFMT group were lower. Although differences were small, women in the PFMT group also were more likely to perceive a health-related benefit. Similarly, in a metaanalysis of 13 trials, women receiving PFMT compared with those not undergoing therapy showed greater improvement in prolapse symptoms, POP-Q stage, and bowel and bladder symptoms (Li, 2016).

PFMT has minimal risk and expense. For this reason, it may be offered to asymptomatic or mildly symptomatic women who are interested in treating symptoms and/or preventing POP progression or who decline other treatments.

SURGICAL TREATMENT

In preparing for prolapse-correcting surgery, each patient should understand anticipated results, and a surgeon should factor a patient's goals and expectations. Symptoms and quality-of-life issues, such as those in Tables 24-4 and 24-5, are ranked by the patient, and elected treatment is directed towards those highest on her list (Mamik, 2013).

All endpoints may not be obtainable, and a surgeon should provide the patient with best estimates of goal attainment based on scientific evidence and the surgeon's personal experience. Importantly, in published studies, treatment success rates vary widely based on the definition of success. Generally, patients seek long-term relief of symptoms, whereas surgeons may view surgical success as restoration of normal anatomy. Thus, the surgeon and the patient must agree on desired endpoints.

■ Reconstructive Procedures

POP surgeries are viewed as either reconstructive ones, which attempt to restore normal pelvic anatomy, or obliterative types, which permanently occlude the vagina (p. 554). Of these, reconstructive procedures are more commonly performed for POP, and multiple options are available. Some are completed from a vaginal approach, whereas others use laparotomy, laparoscopy, or robotic surgery.

With a vaginal approach, patients typically resume ambulation, diet, and routine activities early, as abdominal wall entry and bowel manipulation are avoided. Operative times are usually shorter. These qualities may be especially attractive for elderly women or those with significant comorbidities.

Abdominal options offer durable outcomes, which may offer advantages to a woman with POP recurrence after prior vaginal surgery or one believed to be at higher recurrence risk. The latter is typified by a young woman with severe prolapse or a woman with chronically increased intraabdominal pressure (Benson, 1996; Maher, 2004). Another consideration is sexual activity. Some evidence suggests lower dyspareunia rates and less vaginal shortening after sacrocolpopexy, which is one abdominal approach option.

Laparoscopic and robotic approaches to prolapse repair are becoming more common. They offer smaller incisions and shorter hospital stay than laparotomy. One randomized trial compared open and laparoscopic sacrocolpopexy and found similar anatomic and subjective outcomes after 1 year (Freeman, 2013). Perceived advantages to the laparoscopic approach such as earlier return to usual activities, however, were not seen. Several small randomized trials also have compared laparoscopic and robotic sacrocolpopexy (Anger, 2014; Paraiso, 2011). In general, these studies showed similar short-term outcomes but greater expense with robot use.

Thus, a provider should recommend an operation specific to the patient's anatomy, treatment goals, and health characteristics. *One size does not fit all.*

Surgical Plan

Reconstructive prolapse repair will often combine procedures that each address different vaginal compartments. However, the decision regarding which compartment(s) to repair is not always straightforward. In the past, a defect-directed approach to prolapse repair was preferred. With this strategy, all current or potential defects are evaluated and repaired. However, current expert opinion suggests that latent defects do not always warrant repair. Additionally, repair of one asymptomatic compartment can redirect pressure vectors and create de novo POP and symptoms. For instance, repair of an asymptomatic posterior vaginal wall prolapse may lead to dyspareunia. Or, apical prolapse correction can raise later anterior vaginal wall prolapse rates. Thus, surgery in general is planned to relieve *current* symptoms.

Vaginal Apex

Vaginal apex resuspension is a vital component of POP repair and an important focus in surgery planning (Brubaker, 2005). The vaginal apex can be resuspended with several procedures that include sacrocolpopexy, sacrospinous ligament fixation, or uterosacral ligament vaginal vault suspension. These are all illustrated in Chapter 45 (p. 1124). In one worldwide analysis of nearly 700,000 POP procedures, 70 percent of apical repairs were performed vaginally, whereas 17 percent were sacrocolpopexy procedures (Haya, 2015). Compared with vaginal options, sacrocolpopexy offers lower postoperative rates of POP recurrence, SUI, and dyspareunia but carries longer operative and recovery times (Maher, 2011, 2016). Similarly, in three large randomized trials that compared open sacrocolpopexy and vaginal repair options, sacrocolpopexy yielded a sixfold higher rate of POP resolution (Rogers, 2018). Success was defined as no bulge symptoms, no prolapse beyond the hymen, and no retreatment 2 years after surgery. Despite these data, consensus regarding the most effective approach is still lacking.

Of these, *sacrocolpopexy* suspends the vaginal vault to the sacrum using synthetic mesh. Advantages include the procedure's durability over time and conservation of normal vaginal anatomy. For example, compared with other vault suspension procedures, sacrocolpopexy offers greater vaginal apex mobility and minimizes vaginal shortening. In addition, sacrocolpopexy provides enduring correction of apical prolapse, and long-term success rates approximate 90 percent. This procedure may be used primarily or as a second surgery for women with recurrences after failure of other prolapse repairs.

Sacrocolpopexy may be performed as an abdominal, laparoscopic, or robotic procedure. When hysterectomy is performed in conjunction with sacrocolpopexy, consideration is given to performing a supracervical rather than a total abdominal hysterectomy. With the cervix left in situ, the mesh is attached to the cervical stump. The mesh is not exposed to vaginal flora, which occurs when the vagina is opened with total hysterectomy (Griffis, 2006). The risk of postoperative mesh erosion at the vaginal apex is thus diminished (McDermott, 2009). In addition, the strong connective tissue of the cervix allows for an additional anchoring point for the mesh. Other important consenting points with total or supracervical hysterectomy are found in Chapter 43 (p. 957).

Sacrospinous ligament fixation (SSLF) is one of the most popular apical suspension options. With it, the vaginal apex is suspended to the sacrospinous ligament unilaterally or bilaterally using a vaginal approach that does not enter the peritoneum (extraperitoneal). After SSLF, recurrent apical prolapse is uncommon. However, anterior vaginal wall prolapse develops postoperatively in 6 to 28 percent of patients. This is thought to develop from surgical deflection of the vagina posteriorly, which redirects abdominal forces toward the anterior vaginal wall (Barber, 2014; Benson, 1996; Morley, 1988; Paraiso, 1996). SSLF complications include neurologic and buttock pain from nerve involvement with surgical ligatures in up to 12 percent of patients and vascular injury in 1 percent (Barber, 2014; Sze, 1997a,b). Although infrequent, significant and life-threatening hemorrhage can follow injury to blood vessels located behind the sacrospinous ligament.

Uterosacral ligament vaginal vault suspension is another apical surgery. With this, the vaginal apex is attached to remnants of the uterosacral ligament at the level of the ischial spines or higher. Performed vaginally or abdominally, the uterosacral ligament suspension (USLS) is believed to replace the vaginal apex to a more anatomically correct position than SSLF (Barber, 2000; Maher, 2004; Shull, 2000). Because of this angle difference, USLS compared with SSLF was thought to reduce the rates of anterior vaginal wall prolapse (Shull, 2000). However, the randomized OPTIMAL trial, which compared the two operations, did not show a difference in anterior vaginal wall prolapse recurrence rates. Moreover, investigators found no significant differences in anatomic or functional outcomes between the two procedures at 2 years (Barber, 2014).

Hysterectomy or Uterine-Preserving Surgeries

In the United States, hysterectomy is often completed concurrently with POP surgery, whereas in many European countries, it is rarely performed during pelvic floor reconstruction. If the apex is not prolapsed, hysterectomy need not be incorporated into POP repair. However, with apical prolapse, hysterectomy readily allows the vaginal apex to be resuspended with the just-described apical suspension procedures. Otherwise, procedures must be modified or specific uterine suspension procedures selected to accommodate the retained uterus.

The rationale for hysterectomy is that resuspension of the vaginal apex can more successfully be accomplished after the uterus is removed. However, one recent systematic review concluded that uterine-preserving prolapse surgeries offer shorter operating times, less blood loss, and lower risk of mesh exposure, yet provide similar short-term prolapse outcomes compared with POP repairs coupled with hysterectomy (Meriwether, 2018). Other perceived advantages of uterus retention include faster recovery as well as maintenance of fertility, sexual function, a sense of femininity, and quality of life (Bradley, 2018). In preference studies, a uterine-preserving prolapse repair was preferred by 36 to 60 percent of patients if anticipated efficacy was equivalent whether the uterus was retained or removed (Frick, 2013; Korbly, 2013). Indeed, uterine-preserving apical prolapse procedures are gaining popularity in the United States. These made up 1.8 percent of inpatient POP procedures in 2002 and 5 percent in 2012 (Madsen, 2017). Notably, uterine or cervical conditions that may raise the risk for later hysterectomy but that are unrelated to prolapse should be factored.

Hysteropexy Types

An apical prolapse repair that preserves the uterus is called a *hysteropexy*. Variations may be completed by vaginal, abdominal, laparoscopic, and robotic approaches and may be augmented with mesh.

With *sacrospinous hysteropexy*, a vaginal approach and extraperitoneal access allows sutures to be driven through the supporting sacrospinous ligament. To recreate apical support, these sutures are then attached to the cervix or uterosacral ligament. Similar to SSLF, the vaginal axis is shifted posteriorly and thereby adds potential risk for anterior vaginal wall prolapse.

With *vaginal uterosacral hysteropexy*, vaginal culdotomy and intraperitoneal entry provide access to the uterosacral ligaments. Two sutures are placed in each ligament and then attached to the uterine cervicoisthmic junction for support (Romanzi, 2012).

With *vaginal mesh hysteropexy*, a T-shaped mesh is anchored to the sacrospinous ligaments bilaterally and attached to the cervix and anterior vaginal wall (Gutman, 2017). Previously marketed mesh kits are no longer available.

With *sacrohysteropexy*, two pieces of synthetic mesh are attached to the proximal vagina and cervix on their anterior and posterior surfaces. The mesh is then secured to the anterior longitudinal ligament at the sacrum similar to sacrocolpopexy (Gutman, 2017).

With *abdominal uterosacral hysteropexy*, sutures are placed through the uterosacral ligament and then through the cervix (Haj Yahya, 2018). For this surgery, robotic or laparoscopic approaches are described.

Pregnancy outcomes after hysteropexy are not well studied. In general, most experts believe that women with symptomatic prolapse who have not completed childbearing may be offered conservative management with a pessary as first-line therapy.

Anterior Compartment

Many procedures for anterior vaginal wall prolapse repair have been described. Historically, anterior colporrhaphy was the most common, yet long-term anatomic success rates are poor. In one randomized trial of three anterior colporrhaphy techniques, Weber and associates (2001b) found a low rate of anatomic success. Specifically, satisfactory anatomic results were obtained in only 30 percent of their traditional midline plication group, 46 percent of the ultralateral repair group, and 42 percent of the group undergoing traditional plication plus lateral reinforcement with polyglactin 910 synthetic mesh. These differences were not statistically significant. However, despite anatomic results that may appear suboptimal, symptom relief from anterior colporrhaphy can be acceptable. For example, a re-analysis of data from this trial used clinically relevant definitions of success that included no prolapse beyond the hymen, no prolapse symptoms, and no retreatment requests. With these, 88 percent of subjects met the definition of success (Chmielewski, 2011).

Anterior vaginal wall prolapse may result from central (midline), lateral, or apical fibromuscular defects. If a central defect is suspected, anterior colporrhaphy is a reasonable option (Chap. 45, p. 1114). For an anterior apical defect, in which the fibromuscular layer is detached from the vaginal apex, an apical suspension procedure described in the prior sections will resuspend the anterior vaginal wall to the apex and improve anterior wall prolapse.

Last, if a lateral defect is suspected, paravaginal repair can be performed through a vaginal, abdominal, laparoscopic, or robotic route (Chap. 45, p. 1117). Paravaginal repair is performed by reattaching the fibromuscular layer of the vaginal wall to the arcus tendineus fascia pelvis.

Mesh or biomaterial has also been used in conjunction with anterior colporrhaphy. Either is used to reinforce the vaginal wall and is frequently sutured in place laterally. Several studies show a better anatomic outcome with these compared with repair of existing tissue (native tissue repair) (Maher, 2016). However, functional or quality-of-life outcomes do not differ. Complications with mesh include vaginal erosions in 10 percent of cases, pain, and dyspareunia (Sung, 2008). For these reasons, the use of mesh for anterior vaginal wall prolapse remains controversial and is discussed further on page 553 (American College of Obstetricians and Gynecologists, 2017). Although free mesh is still available, mesh kits have been removed from the market in the United States and other countries.

Posterior Compartment

Posterior vaginal wall prolapse may be due to enterocele or a distal vaginal wall defect. Enterocele is defined as herniation of small bowel through a discontinuity in posterior vaginal wall fibromuscular layers, usually at the vaginal apex. Accordingly, enterocele repairs strive to reattach these fibromuscular layers.

Posterior vaginal wall defects without such herniation are repaired with one of several techniques, which are illustrated in Chapter 45 (p. 1119). Of these, traditional posterior colporrhaphy aims to rebuild the attenuated fibromuscular layer between the rectum and vagina by performing a midline fibromuscular plication. The anatomic cure rate is 76 to 96 percent, and most studies report a greater than 75-percent improvement rate of bulge symptoms (Cundiff, 2004). To narrow the genital hiatus and prevent recurrence, some surgeons plicate the levator ani muscle concurrently with posterior repair. However, this practice may contribute to dyspareunia rates of 12 to 27 percent (Kahn, 1997; Mellegren, 1995; Weber, 2000). Thus, it may be best avoided in women who are sexually active.

Site-specific posterior repair is an approach based on the assumption that specific tears in the fibromuscular layer can be repaired in a discrete fashion. Defects may be midline, lateral, distal, or superior. This approach is conceptually analogous to a fascial hernia, in which the fascial tear is identified and repaired. Thus, its theoretical advantage lies in its restoration of normal anatomy rather than plication of tissue in the midline. Anatomic cure rates range from 56 to 100 percent, similar to that with traditional posterior colporrhaphy (Muir, 2007). However, anatomic and functional long-term outcomes have yet to be reported.

Mesh reinforcement with allograft, xenograft, or synthetic mesh has been used in conjunction with posterior colporrhaphy and site-specific repair to help reduce prolapse recurrence. However, the efficacy and safety of graft augmentation in the posterior vaginal wall has not been established. Paraiso and coworkers (2006) randomly assigned 105 women to posterior colporrhaphy, site-specific repair, or site-specific repair plus a graft using porcine small intestine. After 1 year, those with graft augmentation had a significantly higher anatomic failure rate (46 percent) than those who received site-specific repair alone (22 percent) or posterior colporrhaphy (14 percent). More research is needed to determine the safety, efficacy, and optimal material for posterior wall graft augmentation. Until then, the use of graft in the posterior vaginal wall should generally be avoided.

Last, sacrocolpoperineopexy is a modification of sacrocolpopexy. It may be selected for correction of posterior vaginal wall descent when an abdominal approach is employed for other prolapse procedures or if treatment of perineal descent is necessary (Cundiff, 1997; Lyons, 1997; Sullivan, 2001). With this procedure, the posterior sacrocolpopexy mesh is extended down the posterior vaginal wall to the perineal body. In several case series, anatomic cure rates exceeded 75 percent.

Perineum

The perineal body provides distal support to the posterior vaginal wall and anterior rectal wall and anchors these structures to the pelvic floor. A disrupted perineal body will allow descent of the distal vagina and rectum and will contribute to a widened genital hiatus.

To recreate normal anatomy, perineorrhaphy is often done in conjunction with posterior colporrhaphy (Chap. 45, p. 1122). During surgery, the perineum is rebuilt through midline plication of the perineal muscles and connective tissue. Importantly, overly aggressive plication can narrow the introitus, create a posterior vaginal wall ridge, and lead to entry dyspareunia. However, in a woman who is not sexually active, high perineorrhaphy with intentional introital narrowing is believed to lower the risk of posterior wall prolapse recurrence.

■ Mesh in Reconstructive Pelvic Surgery

Mesh Indications

Approximately 30 percent of women undergoing surgery for POP will require a repeat operation for recurrence (Olsen,

1997). To improve long-term outcomes of primary operations, surgeons may add synthetic mesh or biologic graft. A rationale for mesh use may include the need to bridge a space, weak or absent connective tissue, high recurrence risk, or comorbid connective tissue disease.

Synthetic mesh for sacrocolpopexy and for midurethral slings has been used for years, is widely studied, appears both safe and effective, and is considered standard of care. Mesh erosion develops in a small percentage of cases but can be managed with local estrogen therapy and limited vaginal wall mesh excision. Rarely is excision of the entire mesh warranted. Moreover, pelvic pain is rare after sacrocolpopexy or midurethral sling, and mesh is generally not implicated. Surgeons have also used biologic grafts for sacrocolpopexy and midurethral slings. However, these materials are associated with high rates of prolapse recurrence (FitzGerald, 1999, 2004; Gregory, 2005).

Synthetic mesh use for prolapse repair surgery expanded rapidly after the first mesh product specifically for transvaginal repair came to market in 2001. Unfortunately, widespread adoption of transvaginal mesh procedures followed but without long-term safety and efficacy data. A systematic review of the literature in 2008 found a lack of high-quality data (Sung, 2008). More recently, a Cochrane review of 10 trials comparing transvaginal mesh with native tissue repair found that mesh reduced the risk of recurrent anterior vaginal wall prolapse and prolapse symptoms (Maher, 2016). However, the mesh erosion rate was significantly higher. Other adverse associations, which can be irreversible, included scarring, pain, and dyspareunia.

In 2011, the Food and Drug Administration (FDA) updated a public health warning to state that mesh-related complications were more serious than previously noted and were not rare. After this warning, the use of mesh for prolapse repair declined sharply (Sammarco, 2018). Subsequently, the FDA ordered mesh manufacturers to perform studies comparing transvaginal mesh–augmented repair against native tissue repair. However, prior to the conclusion of these studies, the FDA (2019) determined that it had not received sufficient evidence regarding transvaginal mesh's safety and efficacy or its superiority to native tissue. Manufacturers were required to immediately halt sales of their mesh products. Although free mesh is still available, there are no FDA-approved surgical mesh products intended for the use in the transvaginal repair of prolapse. Importantly, this does not include the use of synthetic mesh for sacrocolpopexy or midurethral sling.

As a result of the FDA action, synthetic mesh should not be routinely used in transvaginal prolapse repairs. However, for some high-risk individuals, benefits may outweigh risks. Candidates may include those with recurrent prolapse, with an unacceptable risk of failure using non-mesh approaches, or with specific medical comorbidities that preclude a lengthier alternative repair. Only experienced prolapse surgeons should perform these repairs and only after a careful discussion in which risks and benefits are presented. The American College of Obstetricians and Gynecologists (2019b) and American Urogynecologic Society (2019) echo these concerns. They recommend that transvaginal synthetic mesh for POP repair be reserved for high-risk women in whom benefits outweigh risks.

TABLE 24-7. Types of Surgical Mesh

Type I:	Macroporous. Pore size >75 μm (size required for infiltration by macrophages, fibroblasts, blood vessels in angiogenesis, and collagen fibers) *GyneMesh, Atrium, Marlex, Prolene*
Type II:	Microporous. Pore size <10 μm in at least 1 dimension *Gore-Tex*
Type III:	Macroporous patch w/multifilaments or a microporous component *Teflon, Mersilene, Surgipro, Mycro Mesh*
Type IV:	Submicronic. Pore size <1 μm. Often used in association with type I mesh for intraperitoneal adhesion prevention *Silastic, Cellgard, Preclude*

Mesh Material

Surgeons using mesh or grafts should be familiar with the different types and their characteristics. Biologic grafts may be autologous, allograft, or xenograft. *Autologous grafts* are harvested from another part of the patient's body such as rectus abdominis fascia or fascia lata of the thigh. Morbidity is low but may include longer operative time, pain, hematoma, or weakened fascia at the harvest site. *Allografts* come from a human source other than the patient and include cadaveric fascia or cadaveric dermis. *Xenografts* are biologic tissue obtained from a source or species foreign to the patient such as porcine dermis, porcine small intestinal submucosa, or bovine pericardium. Biologic materials have varying biomechanical properties and, as noted earlier, are associated with high rates of prolapse recurrence. Thus, recommendations on the appropriate clinical situations for biologic material are limited.

Synthetic mesh is classified as types I through IV, based on pore size (Table 24-7) (Amid, 1997). Pore size is the most important property of synthetic mesh. Bacteria generally measure less than 1 μm, whereas granulocytes and macrophages are typically larger than 10 μm. Thus, a mesh with pore size <10 μm may allow bacterial but not macrophage infiltration and thereby predispose to infection. Accordingly, type I mesh has the lowest rate of infection compared with types II and III. Pore size is also the basis of tissue ingrowth, angiogenesis, flexibility, and strength. Pore sizes of 50 to 200 μm allow for superior tissue ingrowth and collagen infiltration. This again favors type I. Meshes are either monofilament or multifilament. Multifilament mesh has small intrafiber pores that can harbor bacteria, therefore, monofilament mesh is recommended. From these findings, consensus suggests that if synthetic mesh is used, type I monofilament is the best choice for reconstructive pelvic surgery.

■ Concomitant Prolapse and Incontinence Surgery

Prior to POP repairs, women should be evaluated for SUI (Chap. 23, p. 521). Those with bothersome SUI symptoms are considered for concurrent antiincontinence surgery. However, in women without SUI symptoms, latent stress incontinence may be unmasked or SUI may develop de novo following prolapse repair. Therefore, preoperative urodynamic testing with the prolapse replaced is recommended. If SUI is demonstrated, these patients are also considered for a concurrent antiincontinence

operation. This has been a difficult decision for patients and surgeons because a procedure with known risks is being performed for a problem that does not currently exist and may never develop.

The CARE (Colpopexy and Urinary Reduction Efforts) trial has added clarity (Brubaker, 2006). In this randomized trial, women undergoing abdominal sacrocolpopexy for prolapse who did not exhibit symptoms of SUI were randomly assigned to undergo concurrent Burch colposuspension or not. Three months after surgery, 24 percent of women in the Burch group and 44 percent of women in the control group met one or more criteria for SUI. The incontinence was bothersome in 6 percent of the Burch group and 24 percent of the control group.

These data can be interpreted in several ways. It can be argued that all women undergoing sacrocolpopexy for stage 2 or greater anterior vaginal wall prolapse should undergo Burch colposuspension, as 44 percent will develop SUI symptoms. However, the opposing argument is that only 24 percent will develop bothersome incontinence symptoms, thus three quarters of women would be subjected to an unnecessary operation.

In a similar trial, the Outcomes Following Vaginal Prolapse Repair and Mid Urethral Sling (OPUS) trial, women undergoing vaginal surgery for POP who did not have SUI symptoms were randomly assigned to receive a midurethral sling or sham incision. Twelve months after surgery, 27 percent of women in the sling group and 43 percent of women in the sham group had incontinence (Wei, 2012).

Importantly, these studies provide high-quality evidence for a surgeon to share during patient counseling. The decision to perform a concurrent antiincontinence operation in women without SUI should be individualized and based on risks, benefits, and patient goals and expectations.

■ Obliterative Procedures

Obliterative approaches for pronounced POP include LeFort colpocleisis and complete colpocleisis (Chap. 45, p. 1145). Performed in women with or without prior hysterectomy, these procedures involve removing vaginal epithelium, suturing anterior and posterior vaginal walls together, obliterating the vaginal vault, and effectively closing the vagina. Obliterative procedures are appropriate only for elderly or medically compromised patients with no desire for future coital activity.

Obliterative procedures are technically easier, require less operative time, and offer superior success rates compared with reconstructive procedures. Success rates for colpocleisis range from 91 to 100 percent, although the quality of evidence-based studies supporting these rates is poor (FitzGerald, 2006). After colpocleisis, fewer than 10 percent of patients express regret, which is often due to loss of coital activity (FitzGerald, 2006; Wheeler, 2005). Thus, the surgical counseling process must include an honest and thoughtful discussion with the patient and her partner regarding future sexual intercourse. Latent SUI can be unmasked with colpocleisis due to downward traction on the urethra. However, the morbidity of a concurrent antiincontinence procedure may outweigh the potential incontinence risk and is considered before adding surgeries in women who may already be medically compromised.

In patients with a uterus, vaginal hysterectomy may be performed prior to colpocleisis. However, concurrent hysterectomy increases blood loss and operative time (von Pechmann, 2003). Again, in compromised patients, this can negate some of the benefits of colpocleisis. If uterine retention is planned, neoplasia is excluded preoperatively. For this, Pap testing should be current, and interrogation of the endometrium is performed.

REFERENCES

Allen-Brady K, Cannon-Albright LA, Farnham JM, et al: Evidence for pelvic organ prolapse predisposition genes on chromosomes 10 and 17. Am J Obstet Gynecol 212(6):771, 2015

Altman D, Forsman M, Falconer C, et al: Genetic influence on stress urinary incontinence and pelvic organ prolapse. Eur Urol 54(4):918, 2008

American College of Obstetricians and Gynecologists: Pelvic organ prolapse. Practice Bulletin No. 185, November 2017

American College of Obstetricians and Gynecologists: Cesarean delivery on maternal request. Committee Opinion No. 761, January 2019a

American College of Obstetricians and Gynecologists: Practice advisory: FDA orders manufacturers of surgical mesh for transvaginal repair of pelvic organ prolapse to stop selling all devices. 2019b. Available at: https://www.acog.org/Clinical-Guidance-and-Publications/Practice-Advisories/FDA-Orders-Manufacturers-of-Surgical-Mesh-to-Stop-Distributing-Products-Immediately. Accessed May 31, 2019

American Urogynecologic Society: FDA announcement on transvaginal mesh for prolapse. 2019. Available at: https://www.augs.org/fda-announcement-on-transvaginal-mesh-for-prolapse/. Accessed May 31, 2019

Amid PK: Classification of biomaterials and their related complications in abdominal wall hernia surgery. Hernia 1:15, 1997

Anger JT, Mueller ER, Tarnay C, et al: Robotic compared with laparoscopic sacrocolpopexy: a randomized controlled trial. Obstet Gynecol 123(1):5, 2014

Baden WF, Walker T: Fundamentals, symptoms and classification. In Surgical Repair of Vaginal Defect. Philadelphia, JB Lippincott, 1992, p 14

Barber MD: Symptoms and outcome measures of pelvic organ prolapse. Clin Obstet Gynecol 48:648, 2005a

Barber MD, Brubaker L, Burgio KL, et al: Comparison of 2 transvaginal surgical approaches and perioperative behavioral therapy for apical vaginal prolapse: the OPTIMAL randomized trial. JAMA 311(10):1023, 2014

Barber MD, Cundiff GW, Weidner AC, et al: Accuracy of clinical assessment of paravaginal defects in women with anterior wall prolapse. Am J Obstet Gynecol 181:87, 1999

Barber MD, Visco AG, Weidner AC, et al: Bilateral uterosacral ligament vaginal vault suspension with site-specific endopelvic fascia defect repair for treatment of pelvic organ prolapse. Am J Obstet Gynecol 183:1402, 2000

Barber MD, Walters MD, Bump RC: Short forms of two condition-specific quality-of-life questionnaires for women with pelvic floor disorders (PFDI-20 and PFIQ-7). Am J Obstet Gynecol 193:103, 2005b

Benson JT, Lucente V, McClellan E: Vaginal versus abdominal reconstructive surgery for the treatment of pelvic support defects: a prospective randomized study with long-term outcome evaluation. Am J Obstet Gynecol 175:1418, 1996

Bland DR, Earle BB, Vitolins MZ, et al: Use of the pelvic organ prolapsed staging system of the International Continence Society, American Urogynecologic Society, and the Society of Gynecologic Surgeons in perimenopausal women. Am J Obstet Gynecol 181:1324, 1999

Blandon RE, Bharucha AE, Melton LJ 3rd, et al: Risk factors for pelvic floor repair after hysterectomy. Obstet Gynecol 113(3):601, 2009

Bø K: Pelvic floor muscle training is effective in treatment of stress urinary incontinence, but how does it work? Int Urogynecol J 15:76, 2004

Boreham M, Marinis S, Keller P, et al: Gene expression profiling of the pubococcygeus in premenopausal women with pelvic organ prolapse. J Pelvic Med Surg 4:253, 2009

Boreham MK, Miller RT, Schaffer JI, et al: Smooth muscle myosin heavy chain and caldesmon expression in the anterior vaginal wall of women with and without pelvic organ prolapse. Am J Obstet Gynecol 185:944, 2001

Boreham MK, Wai CY, Miller RT, et al: Morphometric analysis of smooth muscle in the anterior vaginal wall of women with pelvic organ prolapse. Am J Obstet Gynecol 187:56, 2002a

Boreham MK, Wai CY, Miller RT, et al: Morphometric properties of the posterior vaginal wall in women with pelvic organ prolapse. Am J Obstet Gynecol 187:1501, 2002b

Bradley CS, Nygaard IE: Vaginal wall descensus and pelvic floor symptoms in older women. Obstet Gynecol 106:759, 2005

Bradley S, Gutman RE, Richter LA: Hysteropexy: an option for the repair of pelvic organ prolapse. Curr Urol Rep 19(2):15, 2018

Brubaker L: Burch colposuspension at the time of sacrocolpopexy in stress continent women reduces bothersome stress urinary symptoms: The CARE randomized trial. J Pelvic Surg 11(Suppl 1):S5, 2005

Brubaker L, Cundiff GW, Fine P, et al: Pelvic Floor Disorders Network. Abdominal sacrocolpopexy with Burch colposuspension to reduce urinary stress incontinence. N Engl J Med. 354:1557, 2006

Bump RC, Mattiasson A, Bø K, et al: The standardization of terminology of female pelvic organ prolapse and pelvic floor dysfunction. Am J Obstet Gynecol 175:10, 1996

Burrows LJ, Meyn LA, Walters MD, et al: Pelvic symptoms in women with pelvic organ prolapse. Obstet Gynecol 104:982, 2004

Carley ME, Schaffer J: Urinary incontinence and pelvic organ prolapse in women with Marfan or Ehlers Danlos syndrome. Am J Obstet Gynecol 182:1021, 2000

Chaikin DC, Groutz A, Blaivas JG: Predicting the need for anti-incontinence surgery in continent women undergoing repair of severe urogenital prolapse. J Urol 163:531, 2000

Cheung RY, Lee JH, Lee LL, et al: Vaginal pessary in women with symptomatic pelvic organ prolapse: a randomized controlled trial. Obstet Gynecol 128(1):73, 2016

Chmielewski L, Walters MD, Weber AM, et al: Reanalysis of a randomized trial of 3 techniques of anterior colporrhaphy using clinically relevant definitions of success. Am J Obstet Gynecol 205:69.e1, 2011

Cundiff GW, Fenner D: Evaluation and treatment of women with rectocele: focus on associated defecatory and sexual dysfunction. Obstet Gynecol 104:1403, 2004

Cundiff GW, Harris RL, Coates K, et al: Abdominal sacral colpoperineopexy: a new approach for correction of posterior compartment defects and perineal descent associated with vaginal vault prolapse. Am J Obstet Gynecol 177:1345, 1997

DeLancey JO: Anatomic aspects of vaginal eversion after hysterectomy. Am J Obstet Gynecol 166:1717, 1992

DeLancey JO: Anatomy and biomechanics of genital prolapse. Clin Obstet Gynecol 36:897, 1993

Edenfield AL, Levin PJ, Dieter AA, et al: Sexual activity and vaginal topography in women with symptomatic pelvic floor disorders. J Sex Med 12(2):416, 2015

Ellerkmann RM, Cundiff GW, Melick CF, et al: Correlation of symptoms with location and severity of pelvic organ prolapse. Am J Obstet Gynecol 185:1332, 2001

Farrell SA: Practical advice for ring pessary fitting and management. J SOGC 19:625, 1997

FitzGerald MP, Edwards SR, Fenner D: Medium-term follow-up on use of freeze-dried, irradiated donor fascia for sacrocolpopexy and sling procedures. Int Urogynecol J Pelvic Floor Dysfunct 15(4):238, 2004

FitzGerald MP, Kulkarni N, Fenner D: Postoperative resolution of urinary retention in patients with advanced pelvic organ prolapse. Am J Obstet Gynecol 183:1361, 2000

FitzGerald MP, Mollenhauer J, Bitterman P, et al: Functional failure of fascia lata allografts. Am J Obstet Gynecol 181:1339, 1999

FitzGerald MP, Richter HE, Sohail S, et al: Colpocleisis: a review. Int Urogynecol J 17:261, 2006

Flynn MK, Amundsen CL: Diagnosis of pelvic organ prolapse. In Chapple CR, Zimmern PE, Brubaker L, et al (eds): Multidisciplinary Management of Female Pelvic Floor Disorders. Philadelphia, 2006, p 118

Food and Drug Administration: Urogynecologic surgical mesh implants. 2019. Available at: https://www.fda.gov/medical-devices/implants-and-prosthetics/urogynecologic-surgical-mesh-implants. Accessed April 21, 2019

Food and Drug Administration: Urogynecologic surgical mesh: update on the safety and effectiveness of transvaginal placement for pelvic organ prolapse. 2011. Available at: https://www.fda.gov/media/81123/download. Accessed May 31, 2019

Freeman RM, Pantazis K, Thomson A, et al: A randomised controlled trial of abdominal versus laparoscopic sacrocolpopexy for the treatment of post-hysterectomy vaginal vault prolapse: LAS study. Int Urogynecol J 24(3):377, 2013

Frick AC, Barber MD, Paraiso MF, et al: Attitudes toward hysterectomy in women undergoing evaluation for uterovaginal prolapse. Female Pelvic Med Reconstr Surg 19(2):103, 2013

Gilpin SA, Gosling JA, Smith AR, et al: The pathogenesis of genitourinary prolapse and stress incontinence of urine. A histological and histochemical study. BJOG 96:15, 1989

Giri A, Hartmann KE, Hellwege JN, et al: Obesity and pelvic organ prolapse: a systematic review and meta-analysis of observational studies. Am J Obstet Gynecol 217(1):11, 2017

Gregory WT, Otto LN, Bergstrom JO, et al: Surgical outcome of abdominal sacrocolpopexy with synthetic mesh versus abdominal sacrocolpopexy with cadaveric fascia lata. Int Urogynecol J Pelvic Floor Dysfunct 16:369, 2005

Griffis K, Evers MD, Terry CL, et al: Mesh erosion and abdominal sacrocolpopexy: a comparison of prior, total, and supracervical hysterectomy. J Pelvic Med Surg 12(1):25, 2006

Gutman RE, Rardin CR, Sokol ER, et al: Vaginal and laparoscopic mesh hysteropexy for uterovaginal prolapse: a parallel cohort study. Am J Obstet Gynecol 216(1):38, 2017

Hagen S, Glazener C, McClurg D, et al: Pelvic floor muscle training for secondary prevention of pelvic organ prolapse (PREVPROL): a multicentre randomised controlled trial. Lancet 389(10067):393, 2017

Haj Yahya R, Chill HH, Herzberg S, et al: Anatomical outcome and patient satisfaction after laparoscopic uterosacral ligament hysteropexy for anterior and apical prolapse. Female Pelvic Med Reconstr Surg 24(5):352, 2018

Handa VL, Blomquist JL, Knoepp LR, et al: Pelvic floor disorders 5–10 years after vaginal or cesarean childbirth. Obstet Gynecol 118(4):777, 2011

Handa VL, Blomquist JL, Roem J, et al: Pelvic floor disorders after obstetric avulsion of the levator ani muscle. Female Pelvic Med Reconstr Surg 25(1):3, 2019

Handa VL, Cundiff G, Chang HH, et al: Female sexual function and pelvic floor disorders. Obstet Gynecol 111(5):1045, 2008

Hanzal E, Berger E, Koelbl H: Levator ani muscle morphology and recurrent genuine stress incontinence. Obstet Gynecol 81:426, 1993

Haya N, Baessler K, Christmann-Schmid C, et al: Prolapse and continence surgery in countries of the Organization for Economic Cooperation and Development in 2012. Am J Obstet Gynecol 212(6):755, 2015

Haylen BT, de Ridder D, Freeman RM, et al: An International Urogynecologic Association (IUGA)/International Continence Society (ICS) joint report on the terminology for female pelvic floor dysfunction. Int Urogynecol J Pelvic Floor Dysfunct 21:5, 2010

Heit M, Benson JT, Russell B, et al: Levator ani muscle in women with genitourinary prolapse: indirect assessment by muscle histopathology. Neurourol Urodyn 15:17, 1996

Heit M, Culligan P, Rosenquist C, et al: Is pelvic organ prolapse a cause of pelvic or low back pain? Obstet Gynecol 99:23, 2002

Hendrix SL, Clark A, Nygaard I, et al: Pelvic organ prolapse in the Women's Health Initiative: gravity and gravidity. Am J Obstet Gynecol 186:1160, 2002

Jack GS, Nikolova G, Vilain E, et al: Familial transmission of genitovaginal prolapse. Int Urogynecol J Pelvic Floor Dysfunct 17(5):498, 2006

Jelovsek JE, Barber MD, Paraiso MF, et al: Functional bowel and anorectal disorders in patients with pelvic organ prolapse and incontinence. Am J Obstet Gynecol 193:2105, 2005

Jiang H, Qian X, Carroli G, et al: Selective versus routine use of episiotomy for vaginal birth. Cochrane Database Syst Rev 2:CD000081, 2017

Jorgensen S, Hein HO, Gyntelberg F: Heavy lifting at work and risk of genital prolapse and herniated lumbar disc in assistant nurses. Occup Med (Lond) 44:47, 1994

Kahn MA, Breitkopf CR, Valley MT, et al: Pelvic Organ Support Study (POSST) and bowel symptoms: Straining at stool is associated with perineal and anterior vaginal descent in a general gynecologic population. Am J Obstet Gynecol 192:1516, 2005

Kahn MA, Stanton SL: Posterior colporrhaphy: its effects on bowel and sexual function. BJOG 104:82, 1997

Kenton K, Shott S, Brubaker L: Outcomes after rectovaginal fascia reattachment for rectocele repair. Am J Obstet Gynecol 181:1360, 1999

Kim S, Harvey MA, Johnston S: A review of the epidemiology and pathophysiology of pelvic floor dysfunction: do racial differences matter? J Obstet Gynaecol Cancer 27:251, 2005

Koelbl H, Strassegger H, Riss PA, et al: Morphologic and functional aspects of pelvic floor muscles in patients with pelvic relaxation and genuine stress incontinence. Obstet Gynecol 74:789, 1989

Korbly NB, Kassis NC, Good MM, et al: Patient preferences for uterine preservation and hysterectomy in women with pelvic organ prolapse. Am J Obstet Gynecol 209(5):470, 2013

Laycock J: Patient assessment. In Laycock J, Haslam J (eds): Therapeutic Management of Incontinence and Pelvic Pain. Pelvic Organ Disorders. London, Springer, 2002, p 52

Li C, Gong Y, Wang B: The efficacy of pelvic floor muscle training for pelvic organ prolapse: a systematic review and meta-analysis. Int Urogynecol J 27(7):981, 2016

Liang CC, Chang YL, Chang SD, et al: Pessary test to predict postoperative urinary incontinence in women undergoing hysterectomy for prolapse. Obstet Gynecol 104:795, 2004

Lyons TL, Winer WK: Laparoscopic rectocele repair using polyglactin mesh. J Am Assoc Gynecol Laparosc 4:381, 1997

Madsen AM, Raker C, Sung VW: Trends in hysteropexy and apical support for uterovaginal prolapse in the United States from 2002 to 2012. Female Pelvic Med Reconstr Surg 23(6):365, 2017

Maher C, Feiner B, Baessler K, et al: Surgery for women with apical vaginal prolapse. Cochrane Database Syst Rev 10:CD012376, 2016

Maher CF, Qatawneh AM, Dwyer PL, et al: Abdominal sacral colpopexy or vaginal sacrospinous colpopexy for vaginal vault prolapse: a prospective randomized study. Am J Obstet Gynecol 190:20, 2004

Maher CM, Feiner B, Baessler K, et al: Surgical management of pelvic organ prolapse in women: the updated summary version Cochrane review. Int Urogynecol J 22(11):1445, 2011

Mamik MM, Rogers RG, Qualls CR, et al: Goal attainment after treatment in patients with symptomatic pelvic organ prolapse. Am J Obstet Gynecol 209(5):488, 2013

Mant J, Painter R, Vessey M: Epidemiology of genital prolapse: observations from the Oxford Family Planning Association Study. BJOG 104:579, 1997

McDermott CD, Hale DS: Abdominal, laparoscopic, and robotic surgery for pelvic organ prolapse. Obstet Gynecol Clin N Am 36: 585, 2009

Mellegren A, Anzen B, Nilsson BY, et al: Results of rectocele repair: a prospective study. Dis Colon Rectum 38:7, 1995

Meriwether KV, Antosh DD, Olivera CK, et al: Uterine preservation vs hysterectomy in pelvic organ prolapse surgery: a systematic review with meta-analysis and clinical practice guidelines. Am J Obstet Gynecol 219(2):129, 2018

Moalli PA, Shand SH, Zyczynski HM, et al: Remodeling of vaginal connective tissue in patients with prolapse. Obstet Gynecol 106:953, 2005

Moalli PA, Talarico LC, Sung VW, et al: Impact of menopause on collagen subtypes in the arcus tendineous fasciae pelvis. Am J Obstet Gynecol 190(3):620, 2004

Morley GW, DeLancey JO: Sacrospinous ligament fixation for eversion of the vagina. Am J Obstet Gynecol 158:872, 1988

Muir TW: Surgical treatment of rectocele and perineal defects. In Walters MD, Karram MM (eds): Urogynecology and Reconstructive Pelvic Surgery, 3rd ed. Philadelphia, Mosby-Elsevier, 2007, p 254

Norton PA, Baker JE, Sharp HC, et al: Genitourinary prolapse and joint hypermobility in women. Obstet Gynecol 85:225, 1995

Nygaard I, Barber MD, Burgio Kl, et al: Prevalence of symptomatic pelvic floor disorders in US women. JAMA 300(11):131, 2008

Oliphant SS, Jones KA, Wang L, et al: Trends over time with commonly performed obstetric and gynecologic inpatient procedures. Obstet Gynecol 116(4):926, 2010

Olsen AL, Smith VJ, Bergstrom JO, et al: Epidemiology of surgically managed pelvic organ prolapse and urinary incontinence. Obstet Gynecol 89:501, 1997

Paraiso MF, Ballard LA, Walters MD, et al: Pelvic support defects and visceral and sexual function in women treated with sacrospinous ligament suspension and pelvic reconstruction. Am J Obstet Gynecol 175:1423, 1996

Paraiso MF, Barber MD, Muir TW, et al: Rectocele repair: a randomized trial of three surgical techniques including graft augmentation. Am J Obstet Gynecol 195:1762, 2006

Paraiso MF, Jelovsek JE, Frick A, et al: Laparoscopic compared with robotic sacrocolpopexy for vaginal prolapse: a randomized controlled trial. Obstet Gynecol 118(5):1005, 2011

Patel DA, Xu X, Thomason AD, et al: Childbirth and pelvic floor dysfunction: an epidemiologic approach to the assessment of prevention opportunities at delivery. Am J Obstet Gynecol 195:23, 2006

Peschers UM, Schaer GN, DeLancey JO, et al: Levator ani function before and after childbirth. BJOG 104:1004, 1997

Phillips CH, Anthony F, Benyon C, et al: Collagen metabolism in the utero-sacral ligaments and vaginal skin of women with uterine prolapse. BJOG 113:39, 2006

Rahn DD, Good MM, Roshanravan SM, et al: Effects of preoperative local estrogen in postmenopausal women with prolapse: a randomized trial. J Clin Endocrinol Metab 99(10):3728, 2014

Reisenauer C, Shiozawa T, Oppitz M, et al: The role of smooth muscle in the pathogenesis of pelvic organ prolapse—an immunohistochemical and morphometric analysis of the cervical third of the uterosacral ligament. Int Urogynecol J Pelvic Floor Dysfunct 19:383, 2008

Rogers RG, Nolen TL, Weidner AC, et al: Open sacrocolpopexy and vaginal apical repair: retrospective comparison of success and serious complications. Int Urogynecol J 29(8):1101, 2018

Romanzi LJ, Tyagi R: Hysteropexy compared to hysterectomy for uterine prolapse surgery: does durability differ? Int Urogynecol J 23(5):625, 2012

Rortveit G, Brown JS, Thom DH, et al: Symptomatic pelvic organ prolapse; prevalence and risk factors in a population-based, racially diverse cohort. Obstet Gynecol 109(6):1396, 2007

Sammarco AG, Swenson CW, Kamdar NS, et al: Rate of pelvic organ prolapse surgery among privately insured women in the United States, 2010–2013. Obstet Gynecol 131(3):484, 2018

Schaffer JI, Cundiff GW, Amundsen CL, et al: Do pessaries improve lower urinary tract symptoms? J Pelvic Med Surg 12:72, 2006

Schaffer JI, Wai CY, Boreham MK: Etiology of pelvic organ prolapse. Clin Obstet Gynecol 48:639, 2005

Shafik A, El-Sibai O: Levator ani muscle activity in pregnancy and the post-partum period: a myoelectric study. Clin Exp Obstet Gynecol 27:129, 2000

Shull BL, Bachofen C, Coates KW, et al: A transvaginal approach to repair of apical and other associated sites of pelvic organ prolapse with uterosacral ligaments. Am J Obstet Gynecol 183:1365, 2000

Smith AR, Hosker GL, Warrell DW: The role of partial denervation of the pelvic floor in the aetiology of genitourinary prolapse and stress incontinence of urine. A neurophysiological study. BJOG 96:24, 1989

Smith FJ, Holman CD, Moorin RE, et al: Lifetime risk of undergoing surgery for pelvic organ prolapse. Obstet Gynecol 116(5):1096, 2010

Smith P, Heimer G, Norgren A, et al: Localization of steroid hormone receptors in the pelvic muscles. Eur J Obstet Gynecol Reprod Biol 50: 83, 1993

Smith P, Heimer G, Norgren A, et al: Steroid hormone receptors in pelvis muscles and ligaments in women. Gynecol Obstet Invest 30:27, 1990

Sullivan ES, Longaker CJ, Lee PY: Total pelvic mesh repair: a ten-year experience. Dis Colon Rectum 44:857, 2001

Sung VW, Rogers RG, Schaffer JI, et al: Graft use in transvaginal pelvic organ prolapse repair: a systematic review. Obstet Gynecol 112:1131, 2008

Swift S, Woodman P, O'Boyle A, et al: Pelvic Organ Support Study (POSST): the distribution, clinical definition, and epidemiologic condition of pelvic organ support defects. Am J Obstet Gynecol 192:795, 2005

Swift SE: The distribution of pelvic organ support in a population of female subjects seen for routine gynecologic health care. Am J Obstet Gynecol 183: 277, 2000

Swift SE, Tate SB, Nicholas J: Correlation of symptoms with degree of pelvic organ support in a general population of women: what is pelvic organ prolapse? Am J Obstet Gynecol 189:372, 2003

Sze EH, Miklos JR, Partoll L, et al: Sacrospinous ligament fixation with trans-vaginal needle suspension for advanced pelvic organ prolapse and stress incontinence. Obstet Gynecol 89:94, 1997a

Sze HM, Karram MM: Transvaginal repair of vault prolapse: a review. Obstet Gynecol 89:466, 1997b

Takacs P, Nassiri M, Gualtieri M, et al: Uterosacral ligament smooth muscle cell apoptosis is increased in women with uterine prolapse. Reprod Sci 16:447, 2009

Tan JS, Lukaz ES, Menefee SA, et al: Predictive value of prolapse symptoms; a large database study. Int Urogynecol J Pelvic Floor Dysfunct 16:203, 2005

Trowbridge ER, Fultz NH, Patel DA, et al: Distribution of pelvis organ support in a population-based sample of middle-aged community-dwelling African American and white women in southeastern Michigan. Am J Obstet Gynecol 198:548, 2008

Ulrich D, Dwyer P, Rosamilia A, et al: The effect of vaginal pelvic organ prolapse surgery on sexual function. Neurourol Urodyn 34(4):316, 2015

von Pechmann WS, Mutone M, Fyffe J, et al: Total colpocleisis with high levator plication for the treatment of advanced pelvic organ prolapse. Am J Obstet Gynecol 189(1):121, 2003

Ward RM, Velez Edwards DR, Edwards T, et al: Genetic epidemiology of pelvic organ prolapse: a systematic review. Am J Obstet Gynecol 211(4):326, 2014

Weber AM, Abrams P, Brubaker L, et al: The standardization of terminology for researchers in female pelvic floor disorders. Int Urogynecol J Pelvic Floor Dysfunct 12:178, 2001a

Weber AM, Walters MD, Ballard LA, et al: Posterior vaginal wall prolapse and bowel function. Obstet Gynecol 179:1446, 1998

Weber AM, Walters MD, Piedmonte MR, et al: Anterior colporrhaphy: a randomized trial of three surgical techniques. Am J Obstet Gynecol 185:1299, 2001b

Weber AM, Walters MD, Piedmonte MR: Sexual function and vaginal anatomy in women before and after surgery for pelvic organ prolapse and urinary incontinence. Am J Obstet Gynecol 182:1610, 2000

Weber AM, Walters MD, Schover LR: Sexual function in women with utero-vaginal prolapse and urinary incontinence. Obstet Gynecol 85:483, 1995

Wei JT, Nygaard I, Richter HE, et al: A midurethral sling to reduce incontinence after vaginal prolapse repair. N Engl J Med 366:2358, 2012

Wheeler TL Jr, Richter HE, Burgio KL, et al: Regret, satisfaction, and symptoms improvement: analysis of the impact of partial colpocleisis for the management of severe pelvic organ prolapse. Am J Obstet Gynecol 193:2067, 2005

Whitcomb EL, Rortveit G, Brown JS, et al: Racial differences in pelvic organ prolapse. Obstet Gynecol 114(6):1271, 2009

Whiteside JL, Weber AM, Meyn LA, et al: Risk factors for prolapse recurrence after vaginal repair. Am J Obstet Gynecol 191:1533, 2004

Wieslander CK, Word RA, Schaffer JI, et al: Smoking is a risk factor for pelvic organ prolapse. J Pelvic Medicine & Surgery 26th Annual Scientific Meeting of the American Urogynecologic Society (AUGS), Atlanta, Georgia, p S16, 2005

Woodman PJ, Swift SE, O'Boyle AL, et al: Prevalence of severe pelvic organ prolapse in relation to job description and socioeconomic status: a multicenter cross-sectional study. Int Urogynecol J Pelvic Floor Dysfunct 17(4):340, 2006

Wu JM, Hundley AF, Fulton RG, et al: Forecasting the prevalence of pelvic floor disorders in U.S. Women: 2010 to 2050. Obstet Gynecol 114(6):1278, 2009

Wu JM, Matthews CA, Conover MM, et al: Lifetime risk of stress urinary incontinence or pelvic organ prolapse surgery. Obstet Gynecol 123(6):1201, 2014

Anal Incontinence, Anorectal Disorders, and Rectovaginal Fistula

ANAL INCONTINENCE

Although definitions are inconsistent, anal incontinence (AI) is most commonly defined as an involuntary loss of flatus, mucus, or fecal material that causes a social or hygienic problem (Abrams, 2018; Sultan, 2017). The definition of AI includes incontinence of flatus, whereas that of fecal incontinence (FI) does not. From a consensus workshop, a more patient-centered term "accidental bowel leakage" was suggested for communication with patients (Bharucha, 2015).

AI can lead to poor self-image and isolation, and the social and quality-of-life effects of AI are significant (Johanson, 1996). Additionally, AI raises the likelihood that an older patient will be admitted to a nursing home rather than cared for at home (Grover, 2010).

■ Epidemiology

AI is common. From one national survey, the prevalence of FI in women approximated 9 percent using 2005 through 2010 data (Wu, 2014). Of affected individuals, liquid stool incontinence was noted in 6.2 percent, mucus in 3.1 percent, and solid stool in 1.6 percent (Whitehead, 2009). The prevalence of FI rose from 2.6 percent in those aged 20 to 30 years to 15.3 percent in subjects aged 70 years or older. In older, institutionalized women, AI prevalence may reach 46 percent (Nelson, 1998). Notably, FI is also not significantly associated with race or ethnicity, education level, income, or marital status (Whitehead, 2009).

■ Physiology

Normal defecation and anal continence are complex processes that require: (1) a competent anal sphincter complex, (2) normal anorectal sensation, (3) adequate rectal capacity and compliance, and (4) conscious control. Logically, mechanisms responsible for FI include anal sphincter and pelvic floor weakness, reduced or enhanced rectal sensation, diminished rectal capacity and compliance, and diarrhea (Bharucha, 2015). In many patients, these factors are additive.

Muscular Contributions

Essential contributors to fecal continence include the internal and external anal sphincters and the puborectalis muscle (Figs. 38-9 and 38-21, p. 799). The internal anal sphincter (IAS) is the thickened distal 3- to 4-cm longitudinal extension of the colon's circular smooth-muscle layer. It is innervated by the autonomic nervous system and provides 70 to 85 percent of the anal canal's resting pressure (Frenckner, 1975). As a result, the IAS contributes substantially to the maintenance of fecal continence at rest.

The external anal sphincter (EAS) consists of striated muscle and is primarily innervated by somatic motor fibers that course in the inferior anal (rectal) branch of the pudendal nerve (Fig. 25-1A). The EAS provides the anal canal's squeeze pressure and is mainly responsible for maintaining fecal continence when continence is threatened. At times, squeeze pressure may be voluntary or may be induced by increased intraabdominal pressure. In addition, although resting sphincter tone is generally attributed to the IAS, the EAS maintains a constant state of resting contraction and may be responsible for approximately 25 percent of the anal canal's resting pressure. During defecation, however, the EAS relaxes to allow stool passage.

The puborectalis muscle is part of the levator ani muscle and is innervated from its pelvic surface by direct efferents from the third, fourth, and fifth sacral nerve roots (see Fig. 25-1B) (Barber, 2002). Although disputed, it may also be innervated from its perineal surface by the inferior rectal branch of the pudendal nerve. Its constant tone contributes to the anorectal angle, which aids in preventing rectal contents from entering the anus (Fig. 38-10, p. 800). Similar to the EAS, this muscle can be contracted voluntarily or in response to sudden increases in abdominal pressure.

The role of the puborectalis in maintaining stool continence remains controversial. However, it is best appreciated in women who remain continent of solid stool despite anal sphincter defects (Fig. 25-2). Moreover, atrophy of this muscle has been associated with FI (Bharucha, 2004). With normal puborectalis relaxation, evacuation is generally aided by the better longitudinal alignment of the rectoanal lumen. Conversely, paradoxical contraction of the puborectalis muscle during defecation may lead to impaired evacuation.

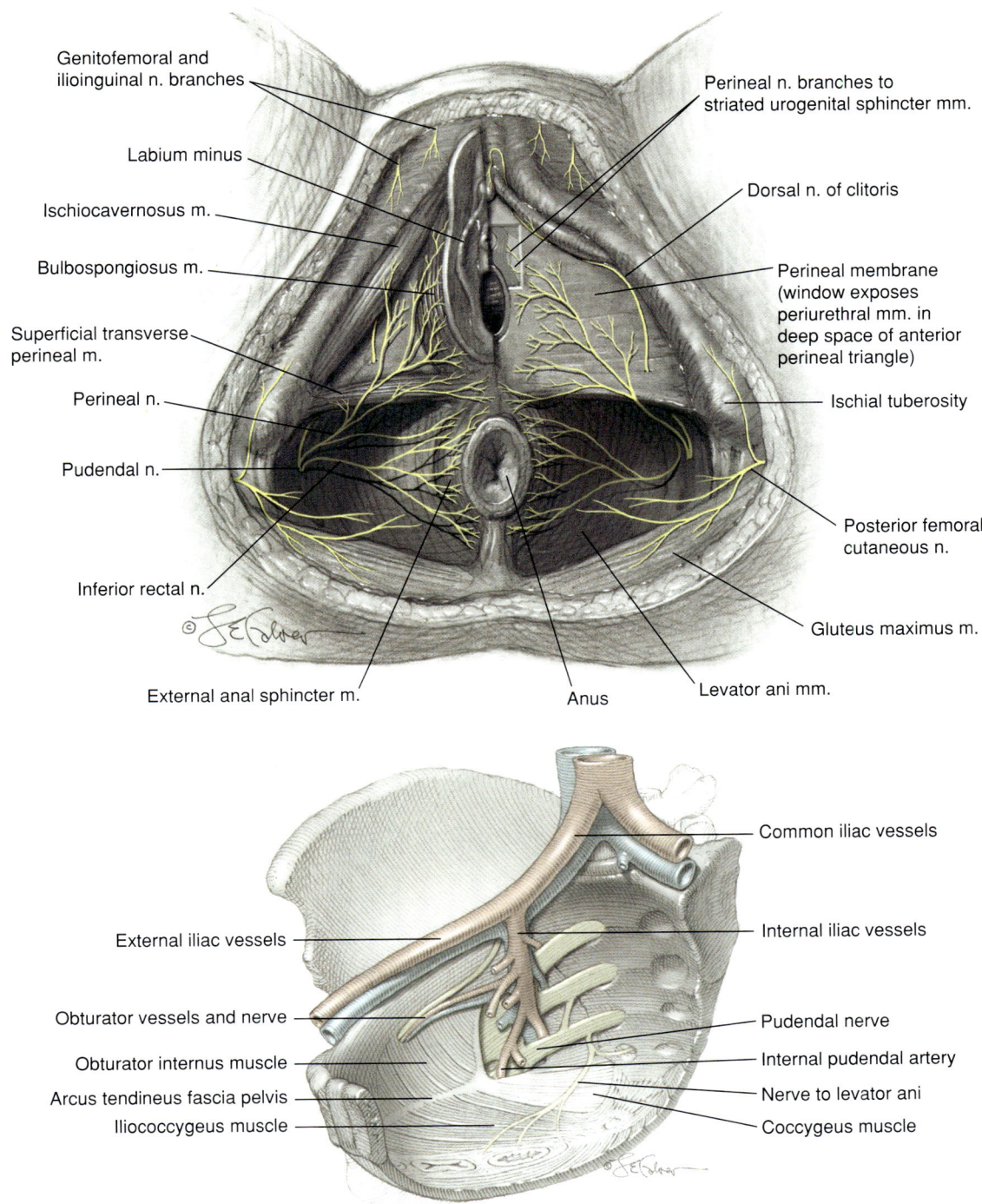

FIGURE 25-1 Innervation of the anal sphincter complex. **A.** The external anal sphincter is innervated by the inferior rectal branch of pudendal nerve. **B.** Innervation of the female pelvic floor muscles from direct branches of S3–S5.

Anorectal Sensation

Innervation to the rectum and anus is derived from intrinsic nerves present in the rectoanal wall and from the inferior hypogastric nerve plexus, which contains sympathetic and parasympathetic components (Fig. 38-13, p. 802). In addition, the inferior rectal branch of the pudendal nerve conveys sensory input from the lower anal canal and the skin around the anus. Sensory receptors within the anal canal and pelvic floor muscles can detect the presence of stool in the rectum and the degree of distention. Through these neural pathways, information regarding rectal distention and contents are transmitted and processed. With this, sphincter action can be coordinated.

The rectoanal inhibitory reflex (RAIR) refers to the transient relaxation of the IAS and contraction of EAS induced by rectal distention when stool first arrives in the rectum. This reflex is

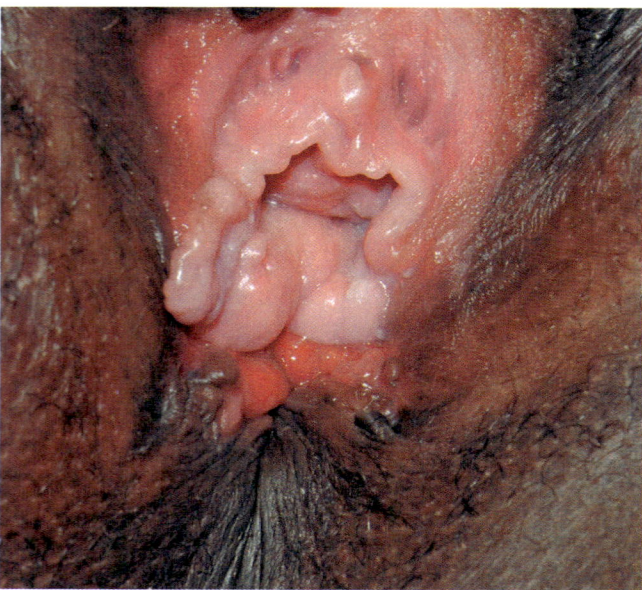

FIGURE 25-2 Chronic fourth-degree laceration with complete absence of the perineal body and the anterior portion of external anal sphincter (cloacal-like deformity).

mediated by the intrinsic nerves in the rectoanal wall and allows the sensory-rich upper anal canal to come in contact with or "sample" the rectal contents (Whitehead, 1987). Specifically, the IAS relaxes to allow the anal epithelium to ascertain whether rectal contents are gas, liquid, or solid stools (Miller, 1988).

Following integration of this neural information, defecation can ensue in the appropriate social setting. Alternatively, if required, defecation can generally be postponed, as the rectum can accommodate its contents and the EAS or puborectalis muscle or both can be voluntarily contracted. However, if rectal sensation is impaired, contents may enter the anal canal and may leak before the EAS can contract (Buser, 1986).

Evaluation of the RAIR may clarify the underlying etiology of AI in some patients. As examples, this reflex is absent in those with congenital aganglionosis (Hirschsprung disease) but preserved in patients with cauda equina lesions or after spinal cord transection (Bharucha, 2006).

Rectal Accommodation and Compliance

Following anal sampling, the rectum can relax to admit the increased rectal volume in a process known as *accommodation*. The rectum is a highly compliant reservoir that permits stool storage. As rectal volume rises, an urge to defecate is perceived. If this urge is voluntarily suppressed, the rectum relaxes to continue stool accommodation. A loss of rectal compliance may decrease the ability of the rectal wall to stretch or accommodate, and as a result, rectal pressure may remain high. This may place greater demands on the other components of the continence mechanism such as the anal sphincter complex.

Rectal compliance can be calculated by measuring the pressure sensitivity to and maximal volume tolerated from a fluid-filled balloon during anorectal manometry. Rectal compliance may be diminished in those with ulcerative and radiation proctitis. In contrast, greater compliance may be noted in certain patients with

chronic constipation. An extreme rare example is megarectum, in which the rectum can hold ≥1500 mL of stool.

■ Incontinence Risks

Obstetric

Abnormal defecation develops if components of anal continence are altered (Table 25-1). In younger, reproductive-aged women, the most common association with AI is vaginal delivery and damage to the anal sphincter muscles (Snooks, 1985; Sultan, 1993). This damage may be mechanical or neuropathic. Interestingly, the incidence of FI following vaginal delivery has declined from 13 percent of primiparas two decades ago to 8 percent in more recent series (Bharucha, 2015). This may reflect fewer instrumented vaginal deliveries and a more restricted use of episiotomy.

Rates of sphincter tear during vaginal births in the United States range from 6 to 18 percent (Fenner, 2003; Handa, 2001). In one study of primiparas delivered at term, at both 6 weeks and 6 months postpartum, women who sustained anal sphincter tears during vaginal delivery had twice the risk of FI and reported more severe FI compared with women who delivered vaginally without evidence of sphincter disruption (Borello-France, 2006). However, a retrospective study of 151 women who delivered 30 years previously reported that women with a prior sphincter disruption were more likely to have

---

TABLE 25-1. Risk Factors for Fecal Incontinence

Obstetric	
Increasing parity	Anal sphincter damage
Medical conditions	
Obesity	Diabetes mellitus
Aging	COPD
Smoking	CHTN
Postmenopausal	Stroke
Medications	Scleroderma
Decreased activity	Pelvic radiation
Urogynecologic	
Urinary incontinence	Pelvic organ prolapse
Gastrointestinal	
Constipation	Anal abscess
Diarrhea	Anal fistula
Fecal urgency	Anal surgery
Food intolerance	Cholecystectomy
IBS	Rectal prolapse
Neuropsychiatric	
Spinal cord lesion	Myopathies
Parkinson disease	Psychosis
Spinal surgery	Nerve stretch injury
Multiple sclerosis	Cognitive dysfunction
Brain tumor	

COPD = chronic obstructive pulmonary disease.
CHTN = chronic hypertension; IBD = irritable bowel disease;
IBS = inflammatory bowel disease.

"bothersome" flatal incontinence but were not at greater risk for FI compared with women who had a simple episiotomy or who underwent cesarean delivery (Nygaard, 1997). Thus, other mechanisms associated with pregnancy and with aging may contribute to AI regardless of delivery mode or anal sphincter disruption. Importantly, cesarean delivery minimizes the risk of anatomic anal sphincter injury, but it does not universally protect against later AI. The National Institutes of Health (NIH) (2006) consensus conference on cesarean delivery on maternal request concluded that evidence was insufficient to support a practice of elective cesarean delivery for the prevention of pelvic floor disorders, including FI.

Other Factors

Few epidemiologic studies have evaluated the risk factors for FI in the community. Underlying bowel disturbances, particularly diarrhea; the symptom of rectal urgency; and comorbid chronic illness are the strongest independent factors (Bharucha, 2010, 2015). Liquid stool is more difficult to control than solid, and thus FI may develop even if all components of the continence mechanism are grossly intact. Alternatively, chronic constipation with straining to defecate may damage the muscular and/or neural components of the sphincter mechanism. Similarly, other neuromuscular injury to the puborectalis and/or anal sphincter muscles, such as that associated with pelvic organ prolapse, may lead to AI.

Radiation therapy involving the rectum can result in poor compliance and loss of accommodation. Also, nervous system dysfunction in those with spinal cord injury, back surgery, multiple sclerosis, diabetes, or cerebrovascular accident may impair accommodation, sensation, reflexes, and muscle function. Finally, loss of rectal sensation and lower squeeze sphincter pressures can be seen with normal aging. One study suggests that even asymptomatic older nulliparas have anal sphincter neurogenic injury, which partly explained weak anal squeeze pressures (Bharucha, 2012).

■ Diagnosis

Barriers to care include embarrassment, perception that FI is a normal part of aging, fear that it might reflect a cancer or other serious disorder, and unfamiliarity or pessimism regarding treatment options (Brown, 2017). In one study that evaluated women presenting for benign gynecologic care, only 17 percent with FI were asked about the symptom by their health-care provider (Boreham, 2005).

No classification for FI is widely accepted. However, the type (urge, passive, or mixed), etiology, and severity provide some basis to categorize FI.

History

During this process, specific questions are posed regarding incontinence duration and frequency, stool consistency, timing of incontinent episodes, use of sanitary protection, and incontinence-related social impairment. Risk factors noted in Table 25-1 are sought. Importantly, urge-related AI is differentiated from incontinence without awareness. For example, urgency without incontinence may reflect inability of the rectal reservoir to store stool rather than a sphincteric disorder.

Validated questionnaires, stooling diaries, and the Bristol Stool Scale are objective options. Of these, a patient diary of stool habits is commonly used in research, but its utility is often limited by poor patient adherence. Instead, validated questionnaires provide objective scoring of incontinence. Four often-used symptom severity scores are the Pescatori Incontinence Score, Wexner (Cleveland Clinic) Score, St. Mark's (Vaizey) Score, and Fecal Incontinence Severity Index (FISI) (Table 25-2) (Jorge, 1993; Pescatori, 1992; Rockwood, 1999; Vaizey, 1999). All of these incorporate the type and

TABLE 25-2. St. Mark's (Vaizey) Incontinence Score

	Never[a]	Rarely[b]	Sometimes[c]	Weekly[d]	Daily[e]
Incontinence for solid stool	0	1	2	3	4
Incontinence for liquid stool	0	1	2	3	4
Incontinence for gas	0	1	2	3	4
Alteration in lifestyle	0	1	2	3	4
		No	Yes		
Need to wear a pad or plug		0	2		
Taking constipating medicines		0	2		
Lack of ability to defer defecation for 15 minutes		0	4		

[a]Never = no episodes in the past 4 weeks.
[b]Rarely = 1 episode in the past 4 weeks.
[c]Sometimes = >1 episode in the past 4 weeks but <1 a week.
[d]Weekly = 1 or more episodes a week but <1 daily.
[e]Daily = 1 or more episodes daily.
Add one score from each row: minimum score = 0 = perfect continence; maximum score = 24 = totally incontinent.
From Vaizey, 1999, with permission.

TABLE 25-3. Fecal Incontinence Quality of Life Scale Composition

Scale 1: Lifestyle

I am afraid to go out	I avoid traveling
I avoid visiting friends	I avoid traveling by plane or train
I avoid many things I want to do	I avoid staying overnight away from home
I plan my schedule around my bowel pattern	I avoid going out to eat
It is difficult for me to get out and do things	I limit how much I eat before I go out

Scale 2: Coping/Behavior

I feel I have no control over my bowels	I have sex less often than I would like to
I worry about bowel accidents	I worry about not reaching the toilet in time
The possibility of bowel accidents is always on my mind	
Whenever I go someplace new, I specifically locate where the bathrooms are	
I try to prevent bowel accidents by staying very near a bathroom	
I can't hold my bowel movement long enough to get to the bathroom	
Whenever I am away from home, I try to stay near a restroom as much as possible	

Scale 3: Depression/Self-Perception

In general, how would you say your health is?	I feel different from other people
I am afraid to have sex	I enjoy life less
I feel depressed	I feel like I am not a healthy person
During the past month, have you felt so sad, discouraged, hopeless, or had so many problems that you wondered if anything was worthwhile?	

Scale 4: Embarrassment

I leak stool without even knowing it
I worry about others smelling stool on me
I feel ashamed

Adapted from Rockwood, 2000, with permission.

frequency of leakage. The Vaizey Score and the FISI include symptom weighting. In the FISI, inclusion of patient-assigned severity scores enhances its utility compared with other scales. The ability of the Vaizey Score to incorporate a component of fecal urgency makes this scale desirable in certain clinical trials.

The patient's quality-of-life decline from AI is also characterized. The validated fecal incontinence quality-of-life (FI-QOL) questionnaire is a 29-item tool designed to estimate associated worsening lifestyle, coping behavior, depression/self-perception, and embarrassment (Table 25-3) (Rockwood, 2000). Other quality-of-life scales available include the Modified Manchester Health Questionnaire and the Gastrointestinal Quality of Life Index (Kwon, 2005; Sailer, 1998). These validated tools may be used to diagnose AI and then to follow treatment response.

Last, the Bristol Stool Scale is often selected to determine a patient's usual stool consistency (Lewis, 1997). This validated scale contains seven descriptions and pictures of stool types (Fig. 25-3) (Degen, 1996). Such stool consistency categorization correlates with objective measures of whole-gut transit time (Heaton, 1994).

Physical Examination

This begins with careful inspection of the anus and perineum to identify stool soiling, scars, perineal body length, hemorrhoids, rectal prolapse, dovetail sign, or other anatomic abnormalities (Fig. 25-4). The perianal skin is gently stroked with a cotton-tipped swab to obtain the cutaneous anal reflex. Colloquially

termed *anal wink*, circumferential contraction of the anal skin and underlying EAS is normally seen. This finding provides gross assessment of pudendal nerve integrity.

With digital rectal examination, one can assess anal resting tone, sample for gross or occult blood, palpate masses or low fecal impaction, and inspect for fistula. Squeeze pressure can subjectively be judged during voluntary patient contraction of the EAS around a gloved finger inserted into the anorectum. Last, during patient Valsalva maneuver, one observes for excessive perineal body descent, vaginal wall prolapse, rectal prolapse, or muscle incoordination (Fig. 25-5). With the last, a paradoxic contraction—that is, abnormal sphincter and/or puborectalis muscle contraction around the finger—may be elicited during patient Valsalva when an examining finger is inserted into the anorectum. To identify dyssynergia, digital rectal examination is reasonably accurate relative to manometry for assessing anal resting tone and squeeze function (Orkin, 2010; Tantiphlachiva, 2010).

Initial history and examination typically guide testing, which may include imaging and functional studies, described next. In some cases, barium enema or colonoscopy may be indicated to exclude inflammatory bowel conditions or malignancy.

Diagnostic Testing

Anorectal Manometry. Women with persistent symptoms despite conservative measures described later are best served by specialist referral and anorectal testing (p. 566). Anorectal

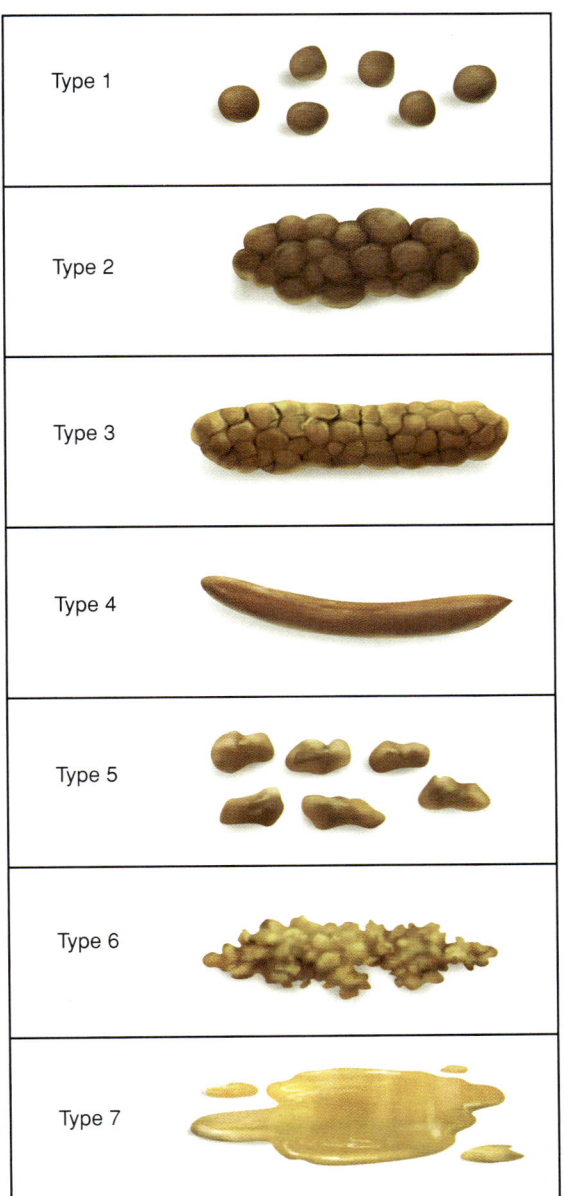

Type 1	
Type 2	
Type 3	
Type 4	
Type 5	
Type 6	
Type 7	

FIGURE 25-3 Bristol Stool Scale. Stools are categorized by their shape and texture.

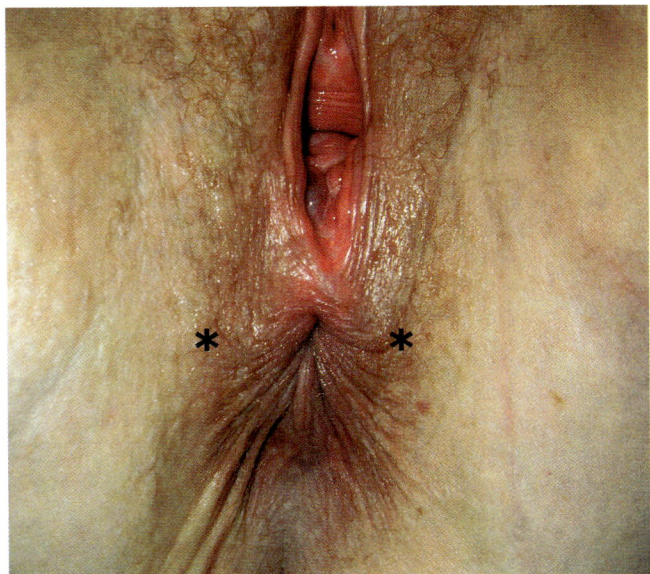

FIGURE 25-4 Photograph showing the "dovetail" sign, which is created by disruption of the anterior portion of external anal sphincter (EAS). Radial skin spikes are typically formed by attachment of skin to the EAS but are commonly absent from 10 to 2 o'clock (*asterisks*) in those with this disruption.

Second, sphincter reflexes are also assessed during pressure measurements. During balloon insufflation, relaxation of the IAS should accompany rectal distention via the RAIR, described earlier (p. 559).

Third, IAS resting pressure and EAS squeeze pressure are then measured at incremental points as the balloon is slowly withdrawn from the rectum. In general, lower pressure readings may indicate structural disruption, myopathy, or neuropathy. As an additional test, the rectal balloon expulsion test may be performed as a patient simulates defecation and expels the balloon. The balloon expulsion test is mainly used in patients with constipation, and it attempts to differentiate between obstructed constipation and functional constipation (Minguez, 2004).

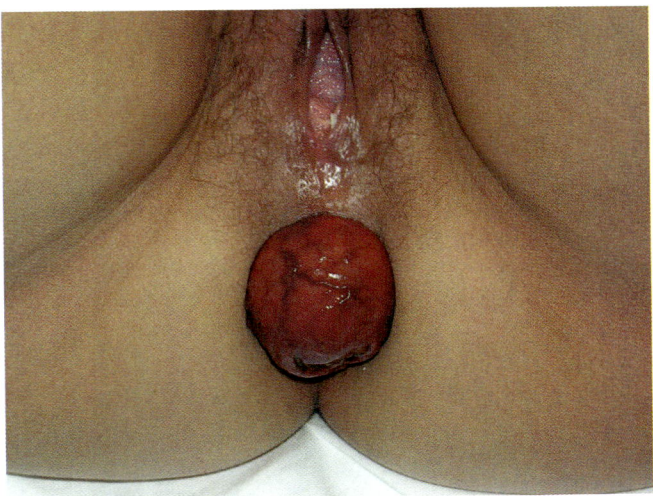

FIGURE 25-5 During patient Valsalva, a full-thickness rectal prolapse protrudes through the anal opening.

manometry is an initial step and followed, if necessary, by anorectal imaging.

Anorectal manometry is a simple test performed mainly in academic institutions with an anophysiology laboratory. Manometry provides objective assessment of: (1) rectal compliance and rectal sensation, (2) reflexes, and (3) anal sphincter function (Table 25-4). During this test, a small flexible tube containing an inflatable balloon tip and pressure transducer is inserted into the rectum (Fig. 25-6). First, rectal compliance and sensation may be determined by sequentially inflating a rectal balloon to various volumes. Poor rectal compliance may be noted by an inability to inflate a balloon to typical volumes without patient discomfort. This may indicate a rectal reservoir that is unable to appropriately store stool. In contrast, decreased perception of balloon insufflation may indicate neuropathy.

SECTION 3

TABLE 25-4. Functional Testing for Patients with Fecal Incontinence[a]

| Factors | Manometry | | | | DG | EAUS | MRI | EMG |
	Resting	Squeeze	RP	RC				
Muscle								
IAS	+					+	+	
EAS		+				+	+	+
Puborectalis					+		+	+
Rectum								
Perception			+					
Compliance				+				
Reservoir			+	+	+			
Megarectum			+		+		+	
Pelvic floor								
Perineal descent					+		+	
Anorectal angle					+		+	
Neural								
Pudendal nerve		+						+

[a]Plus sign indicates an appropriate test for a particular component of continence.
DG = defecography; EAS = external anal sphincter; EAUS = endoanal ultrasonography; EMG = electromyography; IAS = internal anal sphincter; MRI = magnetic resonance imaging; RC = rectal compliance; RP = rectal perception.

However, manometry has poor specificity. For example, high-resolution catheter manometry (HRM), introduced in 2008, demonstrates that patterns previously regarded as abnormal are also observed in most healthy patients (Basilisco, 2017). Despite this, anal manometry results can bolster results of other testing to help support a diagnosis.

Endoanal Ultrasonography. Also known as *transanal sonography*, endoanal sonography (EAUS) is now the primary diagnostic imaging technique to evaluate the integrity, thickness, and length of the IAS and EAS (Fig. 25-7). The technique uses a rotating endoprobe with a ≥10-MHz transducer, which provides a 360-degree evaluation of the anal canal. Sonographic gel is placed on the probe tip, which is sheathed with a condom prior to insertion into the anus.

This modality can also image the puborectalis muscle and perineal body. In one study of incontinent women, perineal body thickness <10 mm was associated with anal sphincter defects in 97 percent of cases, whereas perineal body thicknesses of 10 to 12 mm were associated with sphincter defects in only one third of patients (Oberwalder, 2004). Perineal body thickness >12 mm was infrequently associated with these defects.

Other techniques also may be informative. For example, dynamic endoanal or transperineal sonography can permit functional assessment of the anorectum, similar to defecography, described next (Vitton, 2011).

Evacuation Proctography. During this radiographic test, also known as barium defecography, the rectum is opacified with barium. A thick barium paste is placed in the vagina, and

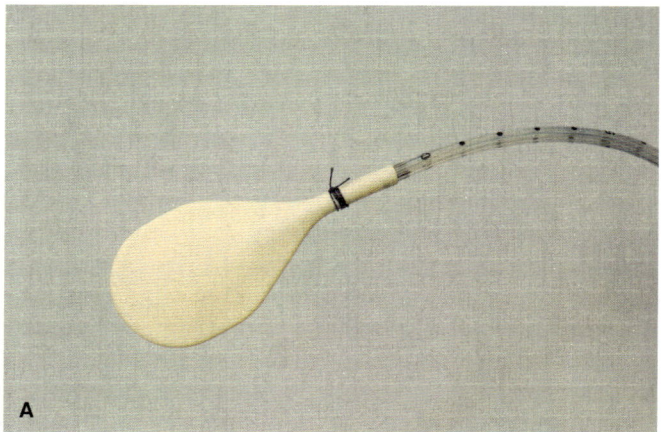
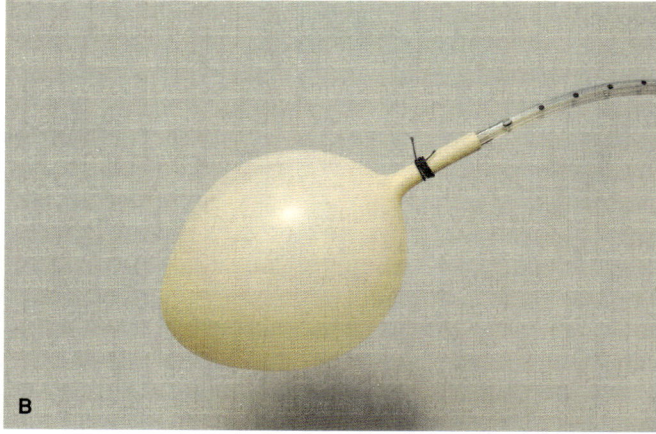

FIGURE 25-6 Manometry tube and balloon, empty **(A)** and after filling **(B)**.

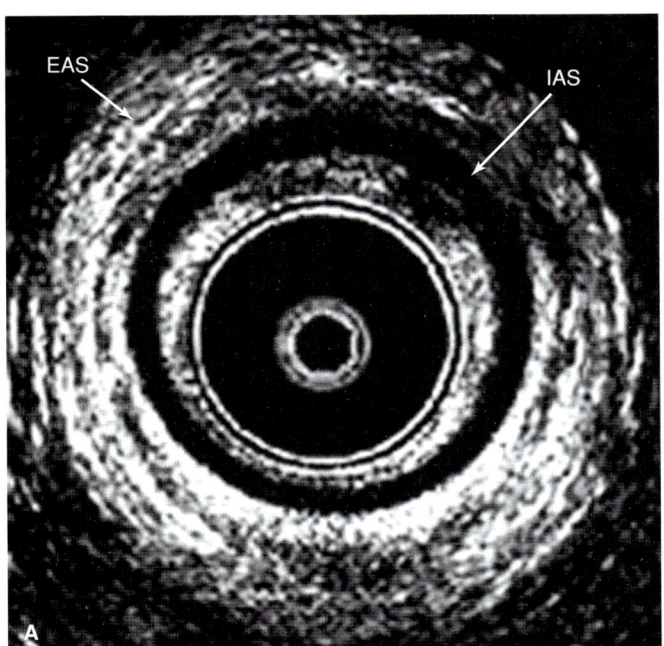 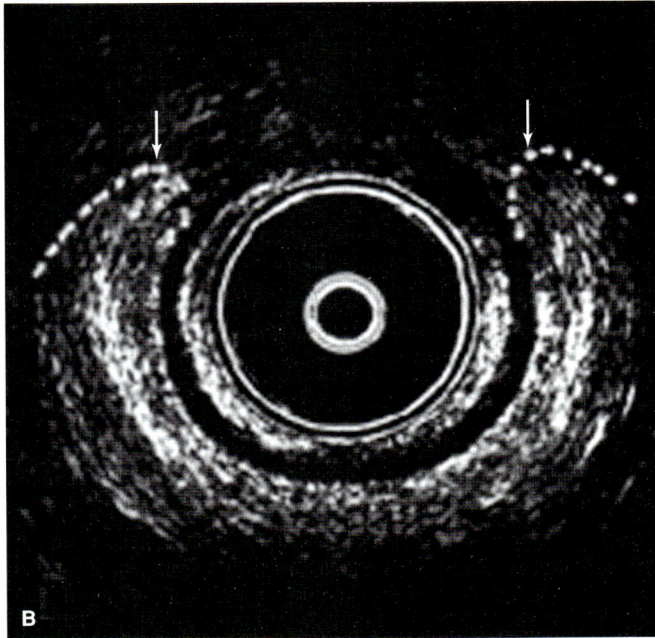

FIGURE 25-7 Cross-sectional anal endosonography images at level of mid anal canal. **A.** A woman with normal anal sphincters. **B.** Anterior defects of the external and internal anal sphincter muscles. EAS = external anal sphincter; IAS = internal anal sphincter. Dashed lines and arrows in B illustrate the ends of the torn EAS.

the small bowel is opacified by an oral barium suspension. Seated on a commode, the patient undergoes radiographic or fluoroscopic imaging while resting, contracting her sphincter, coughing, and straining to expel the barium. Both anorectal anatomy and the mechanics of defecation can be assessed. This test is not widely used to assess evacuation disorders unless obstructive causes for AI are suspected. Accordingly, it may be obtained if intussusception, internal rectal prolapse, enterocele, or failed relaxation of the puborectalis muscle during defecation is a concern.

Magnetic Resonance Imaging. Magnetic resonance (MR) imaging of the anal sphincter complex can be done either with an endoanal coil placed in the anorectum or with external phased-array coils. This latter external coil technique is preferred because physical anatomy is less distorted and the lack of an intraluminal coil aids patient comfort (Van Koughnett, 2013a). MR imaging is more expensive than EAUS, and its value for anal sphincter evaluation is controversial. First, EAUS is more sensitive in detecting IAS abnormalities, whereas MR imaging is more sensitive in defining EAS morphology, including atrophy (Beets-Tan, 2001; Rociu, 1999). This may have value preoperatively, as patients with EAS atrophy may have poorer results following anal sphincteroplasty compared with those without atrophy (Briel, 1999). Second, MR imaging results vary considerably among interpreters and their experience level. Thus, either EAUS or MR imaging can be recommended only if sufficient experience is available (Terra, 2006).

Another MR imaging modality, termed *dynamic MR imaging,* allows dynamic examination of rectal emptying and evaluation of pelvic floor muscles during rest, squeeze, and defecation (Gearhart, 2004; Kaufman, 2001). Thus, it simultaneously permits a survey of pelvic anatomy, organ prolapse, and defecatory function.

This may be particularly appealing to patients requiring multiple anorectal tests (Khatri, 2014; Van Koughnett, 2013a). However, it is technically difficult, more expensive, and again requires an experienced radiologist. Moreover, other than avoiding the ionizing radiation of evacuation proctography, this technique offers no advantage for studying rectal function. In addition, the variability of pelvic MR imaging measurements among readers is high (Lockhart, 2008). Despite these limitations, this test has been increasingly adopted in many academic settings, including our institution. Findings from a recent study provide normal values for anal sphincter and pelvic floor anatomy and function in asymptomatic healthy women (Tirumanisetty, 2018).

Electromyography. This test uses a needle or surface electrode to record electrical activity of muscles at rest and during contraction. During needle electromyography (EMG), needle electrodes are inserted through the skin into a muscle, and electrical activity detected by these electrodes is displayed graphically. Used mainly in research centers, EMG may be used to assess the neuromuscular integrity of the EAS and puborectalis muscle. Specifically, EMG can help clarify which portions of these muscles are contracting and relaxing appropriately. Additionally, following injury, muscle may be partially or completely denervated, and compensatory reinnervation may then follow. Patterns characteristic of such denervation and reinnervation can be identified with EMG.

Unlike needle electrodes, surface patch electrodes are placed on the darker-skinned area of the anus, cause little discomfort to the patient, and carry no risk of infection. However, this technique is prone to artifacts. In comparing the two, needle EMG is painful but provides useful information regarding sphincter innervation. Surface EMG may be best used during repetitive biofeedback sessions.

Pudendal Nerve Terminal Motor Latency Test. This stimulation test of the pudendal nerve measures the time delay between electrical nerve stimulation and EAS motor response. This delay, also termed *latency*, if prolonged, may indicate pudendal nerve pathology.

Although prolonged latency is a marker of idiopathic FI, this test provides little information regarding FI etiology. Moreover, pudendal nerve terminal motor latency (PNTML) results have been contradictory, and this test is not endorsed by many experts, including the American Gastroenterological Association (Diamant, 1999). Accordingly, PNTML has been replaced by more specific and sensitive tests for sphincter muscle innervation such as EMG (Barnett, 1999).

Newer and less invasive approaches for documenting neurogenic injury have been described (Carrington, 2018). The spinoanorectal pathways that govern anorectal neuronal function can be assessed using magnetic stimulation of the lumbar and sacral regions overlying these nerves. One study showed that translumbar and transsacral motor-evoked potentials of the rectum and anus provide better delineation of peripheral neuromuscular injury in individuals with fecal incontinence than PNTMLs (Rao, 2014). Although relatively easy to perform, this approach is not widely available.

■ Treatment

Nonsurgical Treatment

Treatment of FI is highly individualized. FI causes are often multifactorial, and treatments targeting only one mechanism are unlikely to benefit all patients. Moreover, because current surgical outcomes are less than optimal, most patients, even those with anatomic defects, are initially treated conservatively in a stepwise approach. This management may include patient education and normalization of stool consistency. Behavioral techniques are scheduled toileting attempts, purposeful sphincter contraction before coughing or lifting, and daily pelvic floor muscle exercises (Whitehead, 2015). Biofeedback is often recommended after conservative management fails.

Medical Management. For patients with minor incontinence, the use of bulking agents can improve stool consistency and create feces that are firmer and easier to control (Table 25-5). In support of this practice, a small randomized trial showed that fiber supplementation improved diarrhea-associated FI

(Bliss, 2001). However, evidence that fiber supplements benefit patients with constipation-associated FI is lacking. Common side effects such as abdominal distention and bloating can be improved by starting with smaller doses or switching to a different agent.

To also bulk stool, agents that slow fecal intestinal transit time can reduce overall stool volume by lengthening the time available for the colon to reabsorb fluid from stool. Loperamide hydrochloride (Imodium) also raises anal resting tone and thus may even benefit patients with FI and no diarrhea (Read, 1982). Side effects are uncommon and include dry mouth.

Diphenoxylate hydrochloride (Lomotil) is used in the same capacity as loperamide, and dosing is similar. Although diphenoxylate is a Schedule V substance, potential for physical dependence is minimal.

Of other possible medications, amitriptyline is a tricyclic antidepressant that can be used to treat idiopathic FI. Although the mechanism of action is poorly understood, some benefits may be related to its anticholinergic properties. Cholestyramine and clonidine, an α-adrenergic agonist, also have been studied, but current data are limited (Whitehead, 2015). Last, the laxative lactulose aids some nursing home residents with FI associated with fecal impaction (Omar, 2013).

Bowel Management. Many patients with fecal seepage suffer from evacuation disorders, in which a large mass of solid stool fills the rectum and loose stool leaks around the obstruction (Rao, 2004). For some, evacuation disorders stem from underlying constipation. Instead, women with an evacuation disorder may have normal stool consistency. For these, anatomic defects, such as a rectocele, may trap stool. Others may have denervation and impaired rectal sensation.

For those with an underlying rectal evacuation disorder, pelvic floor biofeedback therapy is an option. Alternatively or in addition, rectal cleansing with a small enema or tap water reduces stool trapping. Daily, timed, tap-water enemas or glycerin or bisacodyl suppositories (Dulcolax) may be used to empty the rectum after eating. Bulking agents can be used concurrently with these evacuation methods to diminish stooling between desired defecations.

Pelvic Floor Muscle Strengthening. Also known as Kegel exercises, active pelvic floor muscle training (PFMT) exercises voluntary contract the levator ani muscles. Performance

---

TABLE 25-5. Medical Management of Fecal Incontinence

Treatment	Brand Name	Oral Dosage
Bulking agents		
Psyllium	Metamucil	1 tbsp. mixed into 8 oz. of water 1–3 times daily
Psyllium	Konsyl	1 tsp. mixed into 8 oz. of water 1–3 times daily
Methylcellulose	Citrucel	1 tbsp. mixed into 8 oz. of water 1–3 times daily
Loperamide hydrochloride	Imodium	2–4 mg, 1–4 times daily to a maximum daily dose of 16 mg
Diphenoxylate hydrochloride	Lomotil	5 mg, 1–4 times daily to a maximum daily dose of 20 mg
Amitriptyline	Generic	10–25 mg at bedtime; increase by 10–25 mg weekly up to 75–150 mg at bedtime or a therapeutic drug level

of these exercises is fully described in Chapter 23 (p. 527). Exercises are safe and inexpensive and may benefit patients with mild symptoms, especially if performed in conjunction with other early conservative interventions. However, these alone are less effective than biofeedback for patients with more severe FI symptoms (Heymen, 2009).

In contrast to active PFMT, anal musculature can be passively stimulated electrically by electrodes. However, when used as sole therapy, passive electrical stimulation of the anus appears to be ineffective (Whitehead, 2015).

Biofeedback and Pelvic Floor Therapy.
Pelvic floor retraining with biofeedback therapy is recommended for patients with FI who do not respond to the conservative measures just outlined. Therapy goals aim to improve anal sphincter strength, sensory awareness of stool presence, and coordination between the rectum and the anal sphincter (Rao, 1998). The number and frequency of sessions required for improvement varies. Commonly, three to six 1-hour weekly or biweekly appointments are needed. In many cases, reinforcing sessions at various subsequent intervals are recommended.

Biofeedback is an effective treatment for FI, and up to 80 percent of treated patients show symptom improvement (Engel, 1974; Jensen, 1997; Norton, 2001). Despite this, one Cochrane review found insufficient evidence of biofeedback's benefits for FI (Norton, 2012). However, a randomized controlled trial by Heymen and coworkers (2009) offers support. These investigators initially provided education materials and instruction regarding fiber supplements and/or antidiarrheal medication. Patients who were adequately treated by these strategies (21 percent) were excluded from further study. The remaining 107 patients, who remained incontinent and dissatisfied, then progressed to treatment, either biofeedback or PFMT. Biofeedback training more effectively reduced FI severity and number of days with FI. Moreover, 3 months after training, 76 percent of biofeedback patients reported adequate relief of FI symptoms compared with only 41 percent of patients treated with PFMT. Twelve months later, biofeedback improvement persisted.

The results of this and other trials suggest that biofeedback may not be necessary for patients with milder FI symptoms. However, for those with more severe FI symptoms, instrument-assisted biofeedback is reasonable (Whitehead, 2015).

Minimally Invasive Procedures

Sacral Nerve Stimulation. In 2011, the FDA approved sacral nerve stimulation (SNS) for FI treatment. Also known as sacral neuromodulation, this surgery is typically offered to women who have failed to adequately improve with multiple other conservative therapies. A full description of the InterStim System procedure appears in Chapter 45 (p. 1111). To summarize, an electrode is placed near the S3 nerve root and is connected to a temporary pulse generator. Electrical charges to this nerve root may modulate abnormal afferent impulses (Gourcerol, 2011). Patients who show ≥50 percent improvement during the temporary test phase are eligible for a permanent pulse generator.

In one prospective trial, 90 percent of 133 patients proceeded from temporary to permanent stimulation (Wexner, 2010).

Therapeutic success was defined as a 50-percent or greater reduction of incontinent episodes per week. At 12 months, 83 percent of subjects achieved therapeutic success, and 41 percent achieved 100-percent fecal continence. At 24 months, therapeutic success was found in 85 percent. At 5 years, 89 percent were deemed a therapeutic success, and 36 percent reported complete continence (Hull, 2013). Another recent study supports the long-term durability of SNS (Janssen, 2017). However, approximately 25 percent of the patients have undergone device removal because of complications and/or loss of efficacy.

For patients with an underlying EAS defect of up to 120 degrees, limited data suggest that SNS is also effective (Tjandra, 2008, Chan, 2008; Matzel, 2011). Although unclear, efficacy in these patients may be explained by retrograde propagated contractions in the colon induced by SNS. These contractions delay colonic transit and delivery of stool to the rectum (Patton, 2013). It is unclear whether sphincteroplasty may be necessary in such patients prior to an SNS procedure.

Percutaneous Tibial Nerve Stimulation. Because of the relative invasiveness and morbidity of SNS, other less invasive modalities have been tested for FI. Of these, percutaneous tibial nerve stimulation (PTNS) was tested because of its success for overactive bladder symptoms. The posterior tibial nerve contains fibers from the sacral nerves. Stimulation of its peripheral fibers transmits impulses to the sacral nerves and reflexively neuromodulates the rectum and anal sphincters (Shafik, 2003).

Supporting evidence is contradictory. One review of 13 studies showed that 62 to 82 percent of patients reported at least a 50-percent reduction in the frequency of FI episodes (Thomas, 2013). However, one randomized trial failed to show efficacy compared with sham treatment during a 12-week course (Knowles, 2015). A smaller sham-controlled study of PTNS found similar conclusions (van der Wilt, 2017). At present, PTNS is not recommended or FDA approved for FI treatment.

Bulking Agent Injection. Injecting inert substances around the anal canal in patients with FI aims to increase resting anal canal pressure (Shafik, 1993). Although many affected patients may be candidates for injectables, the ideal candidate is one who has seepage or mild to moderate FI, has failed medical management, and yet prefers to defer surgery (Van Koughnett, 2013b).

The results of a large randomized trial support the efficacy of *nonanimal stabilized hyaluronic acid/dextranomer (NASHA Dx)* injections compared with sham injections (Graf, 2011). The primary endpoint was a ≥50-percent decline in the number of incontinence episodes and a corresponding rise in incontinent-free days. A second injection was permitted in patients who did not improve within 1 month. At 3 months, 52 percent of the dextranomer-injected patients achieved the chosen endpoint compared with 31 percent of sham-treated patients. Notably, 80 percent of patients required a second injection. A surveillance study showed that benefits persisted for 36 months (Mellgren, 2014). NASHA Dx was approved by the FDA in 2012 and is now marketed as an office-based treatment.

Subsequent studies have questioned the efficacy of bulk injections and their mechanisms of action for FI (Dehli, 2013;

Rydingen, 2017). Thus, for any perianal bulking agent, future trial design should ideally define FI clinically and include anorectal measurements and meaningful clinical endpoints (Wald, 2018).

Radiofrequency Energy Delivery to Anal Canal.
This FDA-approved outpatient procedure is currently used in some U.S. centers for refractory FI in patients without sphincter defects or pudendal neuropathy. It delivers radiofrequency energy to the IAS by means of a specifically designed anoscope. Resulting tissue heating is believed to cause collagen contraction followed by focal wound healing, remodeling, and tightening.

Small cohort studies show inconsistent or poor efficacy. Efron and colleagues (2003) found a median 70-percent resolution of symptoms in 50 patients. However, one retrospective series showed long-term benefit in only 22 percent, and most patients underwent additional treatments (Abbas, 2012). Moreover, one randomized trial of 40 patients showed no significant differences in treatment outcome, anal sphincter measurements, or quality-of-life scores at 6 months (Visscher, 2017).

Other Therapies.
Of nonsurgical options, one vaginally inserted bowel-control device contains a silicone-coated stainless steel base and posteriorly directed balloon. Using a pump, the vaginal insert is inflated to occlude the adjacent rectum. Thus, its primary limitation is that not all women are successfully fitted. In one study, the device significantly improved objective and subjective measures of FI (Richter, 2015). Approximately 86 percent of patients considered bowel symptoms "very much better" or "much better." And, no serious adverse events were reported. However, long-term outcome data are needed.

Second, anally inserted devices or anal plugs present another nonsurgical option. However, most current devices are poorly tolerated (Deutekom, 2015).

Third, magnetic beads strung on an elastic band can be inserted surgically around the anal canal and beneath the skin to increase resting pressures. Overall experience with the device has been disappointing, and it is no longer actively marketed in the United States (Bartolotti, 2015).

Lastly, stem cell therapy is a promising approach that aims to regenerate damaged sphincter muscle by injection of autologous myoblasts. One Phase II, placebo-controlled, randomized study of 24 patients with FI showed a 58-percent response rate at 12 months in patients receiving treatment compared with an 8-percent rate in those assigned placebo (Boyer, 2018). However, resting or squeeze pressures did not differ. The reasons for improvement are unclear, but additional studies of this technique are awaited.

Surgical Treatment

Available FI surgical procedures provide less than optimal results and are associated with postoperative morbidity. Thus, surgery is reserved for those with major structural abnormalities of the anal sphincter(s), those with severe symptoms, and those who fail to respond to conservative management.

Anal Sphincteroplasty.
Repair of the EAS and/or IAS is indicated for postpartum women with FI and an anterior sphincter defect from a recent obstetric injury. It may also be considered in patients with evidence of sphincter damage who present later with symptoms unresponsive to conservative measures. Others reserve sphincteroplasty for cases in which perianal bulking injection and SNS are not available or have proven unsuccessful (Bharucha, 2017).

Two methods may be used for sphincter repair and include an end-to-end technique and an overlapping method, both described in Chapter 45 (p. 1150). In patients remote from delivery, the overlapping technique is preferred by most colorectal surgeons and urogynecologists. With this, short-term continence improved 67 percent in one study (Madoff, 2004). However, during long-term postoperative surveillance, other reports show significant deterioration of continence (Bravo Gutierrez, 2004; Glasgow, 2012; Halverson, 2002). In a single, retrospective study, no patients remained completely continent to liquid and solid stool at 10 years (Zutshi, 2009). Hypotheses regarding this deterioration include aging, scarring, and progressive pudendal neuropathy related either to initial injury or to repair.

For chronic fourth-degree lacerations, also known as *cloacal-like deformities*, 46 percent of the 13 women in one study reported some form of anal incontinence at a mean of 7 years following surgery (Maldonado, 2019). The remainder was completely continent.

Patients who fail to improve after anal sphincteroplasty and who are found to have a persistent sphincter defect may be candidates for a second sphincteroplasty. However, those with an intact sphincter following repair and persistent symptoms are only considered candidates for conservative management or one of the minimally invasive surgical procedures described earlier.

At obstetric delivery, the overlapping method of anal sphincter repair does not provide superior results to those obtained with the traditional end-to-end method (Farrell, 2012; Fitzpatrick, 2000; Garcia, 2005). Moreover, overlapping repair requires greater technical skills and carries the potential for increased blood loss, operating time, and further pudendal nerve denervation injury. Thus, the end-to-end technique is likely to remain the standard method for sphincter reapproximation at delivery. Importantly, primary prevention of these lacerations should continue to be emphasized.

Bowel Diversion and Other Major Surgeries.
Diversion is reserved for patients with incapacitating FI who fail other treatments (Chap. 46, p. 1217). For these selected patients, such procedures can significantly improve their quality of life.

Of other surgeries, gracilis muscle transposition is advocated for patients who have failed sphincter repair or those with a sphincter defect too large for muscle reapproximation (Baeten, 1991). Dynamic graciloplasty separates the gracilis tendon from its point of insertion at the knee, wraps the muscle around the anus, and attaches the tendon to the contralateral ischial tuberosity. To squeeze the anus closed, the gracilis muscle is then stimulated with an electrical pulse generator that is implanted in the abdominal wall. This procedure carries significant morbidity. It is not currently performed in the United States (Cera, 2005).

Implanting an artificial anal sphincter is another option, but again, it is infrequently performed in the United States. With this, a fluid-inflated cuff is implanted around the anus, a reservoir balloon is placed within the abdominal wall, and a control pump is inserted into one labium majus. When fully inflated, the cuff occludes the anal canal. When defecation is desired, the control pump in the labia is squeezed to move fluid from the anal cuff into the reservoir balloon. The cuff, when fluid-empty, relaxes pressure around the anus and permits defecation. The fluid within the reservoir then returns to the anal cuff to restore pressure and continence (Christiansen, 1987).

ANORECTAL DISORDERS

Of functional gastrointestinal disorders, three *anorectal disorders* are described by the Rome IV Foundation expert consensus organization. These are FI, functional anorectal pain, and functional defecation disorders (Table 25-6). Anorectal disorders are defined by specific symptoms and, in the case of functional defecation disorders, also with abnormal diagnostic test results (Rao, 2016). A minimum duration of symptoms is required for diagnosis, and this avoids inclusion of self-limited conditions. Also, anorectal symptoms secondary to a neurologic or systemic disorder are not included in functional gastrointestinal disorders.

■ Fecal Incontinence

In Rome IV criteria, FI is defined as recurrent uncontrolled passage of fecal material for at least 3 months in an individual with a developmental age of at least 4 years. Stool that leaks at least two times in a 4-week period serves as a qualifying definition for research purposes. Recognized etiologies of FI, diagnostic testing, and treatment mirror those outlined earlier (p. 561).

■ Functional Anorectal Pain

Proctalgia fugax, levator ani syndrome, and *unspecified functional anorectal pain* are the three types of functional anorectal pain disorders described by Rome IV criteria. These present with chronic pain and are described fully in Chapter 12 (p. 270). The term *chronic proctalgia* is excluded from the new classification.

■ Functional Defecation Disorders

Within the *functional defecation disorders (FDD)* category, two subtypes are *inadequate defecatory propulsion* and *dyssynergic defecation* (see Table 25-6). Symptoms of excessive straining, feeling of incomplete evacuation, and digital facilitation of bowel movements are common in affected individuals. However, these symptoms do not consistently distinguish patients with FDDs from those without. Thus, FDD diagnosis relies also on

TABLE 25-6. Rome IV Categories of Anorectal Disorders

Fecal incontinence
Functional anorectal pain
Functional defecation disorder
    Inadequate defecatory propulsion
    Dyssynergic defecation

physiologic testing, and impaired evacuation must be demonstrated in two of three tests. These are the balloon expulsion test, rectal evacuation imaging (defecography), and anorectal manometry or anal surface EMG. For FDD diagnosis, the Rome IV criteria also specify that a patient must satisfy diagnostic criteria for *functional constipation* and/or for *irritable bowel syndrome with predominant constipation*. The above criteria must be fulfilled for the last 3 months, with symptom onset at least 6 months before diagnosis.

For inadequate defecatory propulsion, diagnostic criteria include insufficient propulsive forces as measured by anorectal manometry. Poor propulsion may be with or without inappropriate contraction of the anal sphincter and/or pelvic floor muscles.

Dyssynergic defecation is characterized by failed relaxation of the puborectalis muscle and EAS. This disorder is common and is thought to account for 25 to 50 percent of chronic constipation cases (Bharucha, 2014; Wald, 1990). For dyssynergic defecation, women demonstrate adequate propulsive forces during attempted defecation but display inappropriate pelvic floor muscle contraction during anal surface EMG, anorectal manometry, and defecography. Other causes of constipation should be excluded. The utility of high-resolution manometry for identifying dyssynergic defecation is unclear (Grossi, 2016; Carrington, 2018). Because a considerable proportion of healthy people exhibit dyssynergia when tested with HRM, abnormal findings with two of the three tests mentioned earlier are required to confirm FDD.

The treatment of constipation is challenging and often ineffective. Schiller and associates (1984) showed that only 53 percent of patients were satisfied with traditional medical therapies. Biofeedback interventions for dyssynergic defecation teach patients to relax their pelvic floor and anal sphincter muscles while simultaneously raising intraabdominal and intrarectal pressures (Valsalva maneuver). The efficacy of biofeedback compared with laxatives in treating dyssynergic defecation was demonstrated in a controlled trial by Chiarioni and coworkers (2006). Moreover, biofeedback benefits were sustained at 1-year follow-up. In a randomized trial by Rao and colleagues (2007), biofeedback efficacy was compared with sham feedback therapy and with standard therapy (diet, exercise, laxatives) in 77 subjects with chronic constipation and dyssynergic defecation. Subjects in the biofeedback group had an increased number of complete spontaneous bowel movements, greater bowel function satisfaction, and a lower rate of digital evacuation maneuvers than subjects receiving standard or sham therapy. In addition, colonic transit time significantly improved in biofeedback and standard therapy subjects but not in subjects who received sham feedback. This suggests that colonic transit slowing is due to dyssynergia. Based on current data, biofeedback therapy is preferred for patients with dyssynergic defecation and chronic constipation, especially for those who have failed diet, exercise, and/or laxative therapy. The effectiveness of biofeedback for inadequate defecatory propulsion is currently unknown.

SNS does not improve bowel symptoms or rectal evacuation for FDDs (Bharucha, 2017). However, for patients with intractable constipation from other diagnoses, SNS is a promising therapeutic option (p. 567). Although not yet FDA approved

TABLE 25-7. Rectovaginal Fistula Risk Factors

Obstetric complications
Third- or fourth-degree laceration repair dehiscence
Unrecognized vaginal laceration during operative
  vaginal or precipitous delivery

Inflammatory bowel disease
Most commonly Crohn disease
Ulcerative colitis less common, as it is not a transmural
  disease

Infection
Most commonly cryptoglandular abscess located in the
  anterior aspect of the anal canal
Lymphogranuloma venereum
Tuberculosis
Bartholin gland duct abscess
Human immunodeficiency virus infection
Diverticular disease

Previous surgery in the anorectal area
Hemorrhoidectomy
Low anterior resection
Excision of rectal tumors
Hysterectomy
Posterior vaginal wall repairs

Pelvic radiation therapy

Neoplasm
Invasive cervical or vaginal cancer
Anal or rectal cancer

Trauma
Intraoperative
Coital

for this indication, a prospective study showed that SNS improved idiopathic slow- and normal-transit constipation that was refractory to conservative measures (Kamm, 2010). In this study, primary end points were greater defecation frequency, less straining, and decreased sensation of incomplete evacuation. Of 62 patients who underwent temporary generator placement, 73 percent proceeded to permanent generator implantation. Of these patients, 87 percent achieved treatment success.

RECTOVAGINAL FISTULA

■ Definition and Classification

Rectovaginal fistulas (RVFs) are congenital or acquired epithelium-lined tracts between the vagina and rectum. They are classified according to their location, size, and etiology. These features aid appropriate management and help predict surgical repair outcome. The underlying cause of a fistula is the most important predictor of outcome success, as it factors tissue robustness and overall patient health (Table 25-7).

Most RVFs are related to obstetric events and develop in the distal third of the vagina just above the hymen (Fig. 25-8) (Greenwald, 1978; Lowry, 1988; Tsang, 1998). Defect diameters range from <1 mm to several centimeters, and most communicate with the rectum at or above the pectinate (dentate) line (Fig. 38-21, p. 810). In contrast, fistulas with an opening below the dentate line are also appropriately called *anovaginal fistulas.* Surgical management of these "low" RVFs depends on the condition of the EAS but a perineal (transvaginal or transanal) approach is typical. Midlevel RVFs are found in the middle third of the vagina. High RVFs have their vaginal communication close to the cervix or the vaginal cuff. In cases with high RVFs, fistulas may open into the sigmoid colon and may not be readily seen on examination. They often require contrast or endoscopic studies for diagnosis. An abdominal approach is usually needed for repair. Last, fistula-in-ano is a tract that connects the perineal skin to the anal canal. It usually involves the anal sphincter muscles and often is considered a complex fistula.

■ Diagnosis

Patients with RVF usually complain of flatus or stool leakage per vagina. They may also present with recurrent bladder or vaginal

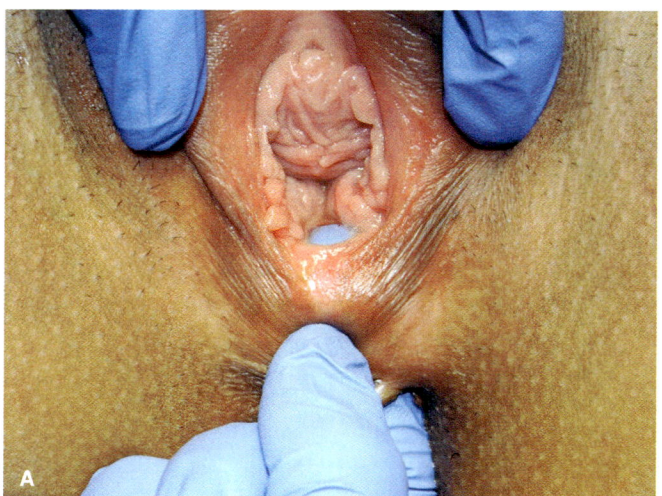
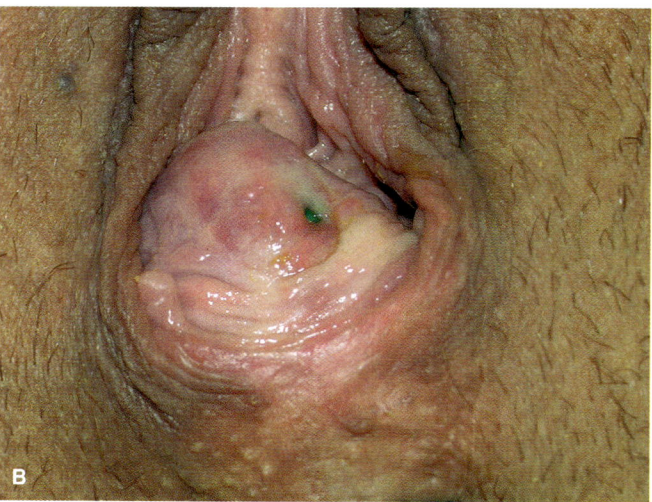

FIGURE 25-8 **A.** Gloved finger demonstrates rectovaginal fistula in the distal posterior vagina wall (Reproduced with permission of Dr. Meadow Good). **B.** The green glove of the examiner is seen through this smaller defect.

infection, rectal or vaginal bleeding, and pain. Symptoms often suggest the underlying etiology. For example, patients with obstetric injury and large defects of the anterior portion of the anal sphincters may have gross fecal incontinence. In contrast, those with an infectious or inflammatory process may complain of diarrhea, abdominal cramping, and fevers in addition to vaginal passage of stool.

During physical examination, most low RVFs can be visualized during inspection of the perineum and distal portion of the posterior vaginal wall. Rectovaginal examination assesses the thickness of the perineal body and anovaginal wall and may allow palpation and visualization of the defect. Some RVFs that are not readily seen on initial examination can be identified by noting air bubbles at the fistula's vaginal opening after filling the vagina with water during vaginoscopy (Chap. 44, p. 1055). Alternatively, methylene blue can be instilled in the rectum after a tampon is placed in the vagina. The fistula and a gross assessment of its location can be identified by inspecting the level of blue staining on the tampon following its removal.

If the fistula site is not determined by the preceding maneuvers, a contrast study is indicated. These include barium enema or computed tomography (CT) scanning that includes oral contrast.

Unless RVFs are obviously due to a prior obstetric event, a biopsy of the fistulous tract is indicated to investigate possible malignancy or inflammatory conditions. In addition, proctoscopy or colonoscopy is often warranted if inflammatory bowel disease, malignancy, or gastrointestinal infection is suspected. Anal sphincter function assessment is essential, as function plays an integral role in repair selection.

■ Treatment

Treatment of RVF depends on the underlying etiology and the defect's size and location. Some women with small RVFs following recent obstetric trauma may be followed conservatively in anticipation of spontaneous healing (Goldaber, 1993; Rahman, 2003). For small RVFs without inflammation, some data also support repair within 72 hours of trauma (Malik, 2008). If surgical repair is required, it is delayed until surrounding tissues are free of edema, induration, and infection (Wiskind, 1992). As an aid and temporizing measure, a draining seton (suture or vessel loop) can be passed through a fistulous tract to allow fistula maturation prior to more definitive repair (Rogers, 2016; Vogel, 2016).

Larger obstetric-related defects and other low RVFs are most often corrected surgically. Surgical techniques for low RVFs include a fistulotomy (surgical opening of a fistulous tract) and then transvaginal purse-string repair. Instead, a fistulectomy plus a tension-free layered closure is common and illustrated in Chapter 45 (p. 1153). Last, a transperineal approach through an episioproctotomy converts the defect into a complete perineal tear, that is, a fourth-degree laceration, which then is reconstructed. This approach only should be considered for RVFs in women with extensive anal sphincter defects and associated fecal incontinence. A promising approach for simple and complex anal fistulas is the ligation of the intersphincteric fistula tract (LIFT) procedure (Alasari, 2014). It involves suture closure and division of the fistula tract in the intersphincteric plane. The LIFT procedure results in fistula healing in 61 to 94 percent

of patients, with little morbidity and rare alterations in fecal continence (Vogel, 2016). Last, endorectal flap advancement, with or without sphincteroplasty, is a common procedure used by colorectal surgeons (MacRae, 1995; Vogel, 2016). With flap advancement, the fistulous tract is excised, a broad-based flap of rectal wall is employed to obliterate the fistula's origin, and sphincter muscle division is avoided. In patients with RVF complicated by fecal incontinence, RVF repair and anal sphincteroplasties in general provide better outcomes compared with endorectal advancement flap alone (Tsang, 1998). Thus, in patients with low RVFs, preoperative endoanal sonography of the anal sphincters is important. Namely, an episioproctotomy is avoided if the external anal sphincter is intact to reduce fecal incontinence rates (Hull, 2007).

Midlevel vaginal fistulas also are often due to obstetric trauma and are repaired transvaginally or transanally by a tension-free layered closure or an endorectal advancement flap. High fistulas are most commonly repaired by a transabdominal approach using bowel resection of the involved segment followed by primary bowel reanastomosis. An omental J flap or epiploic appendages of the colon can be used for tissue interposition during abdominal approaches.

Success rates vary depending on the underlying cause and repair method. Successful repair rates following obstetric injury vary from 78 to 100 percent (Khanduja, 1999; Tsang, 1998). Rates of 40 to 50 percent are reported with the rectal advancement flaps, and rates are more than 70 percent with episioproctotomy (Hull, 2007; Mizrahi, 2002; Sonoda, 2002). Fistulas due to other etiologies such as radiation, cancer, or active inflammatory bowel disease are more difficult to treat successfully. A labial fat interposition graft (modified Martius flap) may be considered in these cases to enhance blood supply and tissue healing. A gracilis muscle flap is another option, but data are limited. In general, success rates are highest with the first surgical attempt at repair (Lowry, 1988).).

REFERENCES

Abbas MA, Tam MS, Chun LJ: Radiofrequency treatment for fecal incontinence: is it effective long-term? Dis Colon Rectum 55:605, 2012

Abrams P, Andersson KE, Apostolidis A, et al: 6th International Consultation on Incontinence. Recommendations of the International Scientific Committee: evaluation and treatment of urinary incontinence, pelvic organ prolapse and faecal incontinence. Neurourol Urodyn 37(7):2271, 2018

Alasari S, Kim NK: Overview of anal fistula and systematic review of ligation of the intersphincteric fistula tract (lift). Tech Coloproctol 18:13, 2014

Baeten CG, Konsten J, Spaans F, et al: Dynamic graciloplasty for treatment of faecal incontinence. Lancet 338(8776):1163, 1991

Barber MD, Bremer RE, Thor KB, et al: Innervation of the female levator ani muscles. Am J Obstet Gynecol 187(1):64, 2002

Barnett JL, Hasler WL, Camilleri M: American Gastroenterological Association medical position statement on anorectal testing techniques. Gastroenterology 116(3):732, 1999

Bartolotti M: The disappointing performance of the new "magnetic sphincters": a wrong idea or a wrong realization? J Gastrointestin Liver Dis 24(2): 149, 2015

Basilisco G, Bharucha AE: High-resolution anorectal manometry: an expensive hobby or worth every penny? Neurogastroenterol Motil 29(8):1, 2017

Beets-Tan RG, Morren GL, Beets GL, et al: Measurement of anal sphincter muscles: endoanal US, endoanal MR imaging, or phased-array MR imaging? A study with healthy volunteers. Radiology 220(1):81, 2001

Bharucha AE: Outcome measures for fecal incontinence: anorectal structure and function. Gastroenterology 126(1 Suppl 1):S90, 2004

Bharucha AE: Pelvic floor: anatomy and function. Neurogastroenterol Motil 18(7):507, 2006

Bharucha AE, Daube J, Litchy W, et al: Anal sphincteric neurogenic injury in asymptomatic nulliparous women and fecal incontinence. Am J Physiol Gastrointest Liver Physiol 303:G256, 2012

Bharucha AE, Dunivan G, Goode PS, et al: Epidemiology, pathophysiology, and classification of fecal incontinence: state of the science summary for the National Institute of Diabetes and Digestive and Kidney Diseases (NIDDK) workshop. Am J Gastroenterol 110(1):127, 2015

Bharucha AE, Rao SC: An update on anorectal disorders for gastroenterologists. Gastroenterology 146:37, 2014

Bharucha AE, Rao SSC, Shin AS: Surgical interventions and the use of device-aided therapy for the treatment of fecal incontinence and defecatory disorders. Clin Gastroenterol Hepatol 15(12):1844, 2017

Bharucha AE, Zinsmeister AR, Schleck CD, et al: Bowel disturbances are the most important risk factors for late onset fecal incontinence: a population-based case-control study in women. Gastroenterology 139(5):1559, 2010

Bliss DZ, Jung HJ, Savik K, et al: Supplementation with dietary fiber improves fecal incontinence. Nurs Res 50:203, 2001

Boreham MK, Richter HE, Kenton KS, et al: Anal incontinence in women presenting for gynecologic care: prevalence, risk factors, and impact upon quality of life. Am J Obstet Gynecol 192(5):1637, 2005

Borello-France D, Burgio KL, Richter HE, et al: Fecal and urinary incontinence in primiparous women. Obstet Gynecol 108(4):863, 2006

Boyer O, Bridoux V, Giverne C, et al: Autologous myoblasts for the treatment of fecal incontinence: results of a phase 2 randomized placebo-controlled study (MIAS). Ann Surg 267(3):443, 2018

Bravo Gutierrez A, Madoff RD, Lowry AC, et al: Long-term results of anterior sphincteroplasty. Dis Colon Rectum 47(5):727, 2004

Briel JW, Stoker J, Rociu E, et al: External anal sphincter atrophy on endoanal magnetic resonance imaging adversely affects continence after sphincteroplasty. Br J Surg 86(10):1322, 1999

Brown HW, Rogers RG, Wise ME: Barriers to seeking care for accidental bowel leakage: a qualitative study. Int Urogynecol J 28(4):543, 2017

Buser WD, Miner PB: Delayed rectal sensation with fecal incontinence. Gastroenterology 91:1186, 1986

Carrington EV, Scott SM, Bharucha A, et al: Expert consensus document: advances in the evaluation of anorectal function. Nat Rev Gastroenterol Hepatol 15(5):309, 2018

Cera SM, Wexner SD: Muscle transposition: does it still have a role? Clin Colon Rectal Surg 18(1):46, 2005

Chan MK, Tjandra JJ: Sacral nerve stimulation for fecal incontinence: external anal sphincter defect vs. intact anal sphincter. Dis Colon Rectum 51:1015, 2008

Chiarioni G, Whitehead WE, Pezza V, et al: Biofeedback is superior to laxatives for normal transit constipation due to pelvic floor dyssynergia. Gastroenterology 130(3):657, 2006

Christiansen J, Lorentzen M: Implantation of artificial sphincter for anal incontinence. Lancet 2(8553):244, 1987

Degen LP, Phillips SF: How well does stool form reflect colonic transit? Gut 39(1):109, 1996

Dehli T, Stordahl A, Vatten LJ et al: Sphincter training or anal injections of dextranomer for treatment of anal incontinence: a randomized trial. Scand J Gastroenterol 48(3):302, 2013

Deutekom M, Dobben AC: Plugs for containing faecal incontinence. Cochrane Database Syst Rev 7:CD005086, 2015

Diamant NE, Kamm MA, Wald A, et al: AGA technical review on anorectal testing techniques. Gastroenterology 116:735, 1999

Efron JE, Corman ML, Fleshman J, et al: Safety and effectiveness of temperature-controlled radio-frequency energy delivery to the anal canal (Secca procedure) for the treatment of fecal incontinence. Dis Colon Rectum 46(12):1606, 2003

Engel BT, Nikoomanesh P, Schuster MM: Operant conditioning of rectosphincteric responses in the treatment of fecal incontinence. N Engl J Med 290:646, 1974

Farrell SA, Flowerdew G, Gilmour D, et al: Overlapping compared with end-to-end repair of complete third-degree or fourth-degree obstetric tears. Three-year follow-up of a randomized controlled trial. Obstet Gynecol 120(4):803, 2012

Fenner DE, Genberg B, Brahma P, et al: Fecal and urinary incontinence after vaginal delivery with anal sphincter disruption in an obstetrics unit in the United States. Am J Obstet Gynecol 189(6):1543, 2003

Fitzpatrick M, Behan M, O'Connell PR, et al: A randomized clinical trial comparing primary overlap with approximation repair of third-degree obstetric tears. Am J Obstet Gynecol 183(5):1220, 2000

Frenckner B, Euler CV: Influence of pudendal block on the function of the anal sphincters. Gut 16(6):482, 1975

Garcia V, Rogers RG, Kim SS, et al: Primary repair of obstetric anal sphincter laceration: a randomized trial of two surgical techniques. Am J Obstet Gynecol 192(5):1697, 2005

Gearhart SL, Pannu HK, Cundiff GW, et al: Perineal descent and levator ani hernia: a dynamic magnetic resonance imaging study. Dis Colon Rectum 47:1298, 2004

Glasgow SC, Lowry AC: Long-term outcomes of anal sphincter repair for fecal incontinence: a systematic review. Dis Colon Rectum 55:482, 2012

Goldaber KG, Wendel PJ, McIntire DD, et al: Postpartum perineal morbidity after fourth-degree perineal repair. Am J Obstet Gynecol 168(2):489, 1993

Gourcerol G, Vitton V, Leroi AM, et al: How sacral nerve stimulation works in patients with faecal incontinence. Colorectal Dis 13:e203, 2011

Graf W, Mellgren A, Matzel KE, et al: Efficacy of dextranomer in stabilized hyaluronic acid for treatment of faecal incontinence: a randomised, sham-controlled trial. Lancet 377:997, 2011

Greenwald JC, Hoexter B: Repair of rectovaginal fistulas. Surg Gynecol Obstet 146(3):443, 1978

Grossi U, Carrington EV, Bharucha AE, et al: Diagnostic accuracy study of anorectal manometry for diagnosis of dyssynergic defecation. Gut 65(3):447, 2016

Grover M, Busby-Whitehead J, Palmer MH, et al: Survey of geriatricians on the effect of fecal incontinence on nursing home referral. J Am Geriatr Soc 58:1058, 2010

Halverson AL, Hull TL: Long-term outcome of overlapping anal sphincter repair. Dis Colon Rectum 45(3):345, 2002

Handa VL, Danielsen BH, Gilbert WM: Obstetric anal sphincter lacerations. Obstet Gynecol 98(2):225, 2001

Heaton KW, O'Donnell LJ: An office guide to whole-gut transit time. Patients' recollection of their stool form. J Clin Gastroenterol 19(1):28, 1994

Heymen S, Scarlett Y, Jones K, et al: Randomized controlled trial shows biofeedback to be superior to pelvic floor exercises for fecal incontinence. Dis Colon Rectum 52(10):1730, 2009

Hull T, Giese C, Wexner SD, et al: Long-term durability of sacral nerve stimulation therapy for chronic fecal incontinence. Dis Colon Rectum 56:234, 2013

Hull TL, Bartus C, Bast J, et al: Success of episioproctotomy for cloaca and rectovaginal fistula. Dis Colon Rectum 50(1):97, 2007

Janssen PT, Kuiper SZ, Stassen LP, et al: Fecal incontinence treated by sacral neuromodulation: long-term follow-up of 325 patients. Surgery 161(4):1040, 2017

Jensen LL, Lowry AC: Biofeedback improves functional outcome after sphincteroplasty. Dis Colon Rectum 40(2):197, 1997

Johanson JF, Lafferty J: Epidemiology of fecal incontinence: the silent affliction. Am J Gastroenterol 91(1):33, 1996

Jorge JMN, Wexner SD: Etiology and management of fecal incontinence. Dis Colon Rectum 36:77, 1993

Kamm MA, Dudding TC, Melenhorst J, et al: Sacral nerve stimulation for intractable constipation. Gut 59(3):333, 2010

Kaufman HS, Buller JL, Thompson JR, et al. Dynamic pelvic magnetic resonance imaging and cystocolpoproctography alter surgical management of pelvic floor disorders. Dis Colon Rectum 44:1575, 2001

Khanduja KS, Padmanabhan A, Kerner BA, et al: Reconstruction of rectovaginal fistula with sphincter disruption by combining rectal mucosal advancement flap and anal sphincteroplasty. Dis Colon Rectum 42(11):1432, 1999

Khatri G: Magnetic resonance imaging of pelvic floor disorders. Top Magn Reson Imaging 23:259, 2014

Knowles CH, Horrocks EJ, Bremner SA, et al: Percutaneous tibial nerve stimulation versus sham electrical stimulation for the treatment of faecal incontinence in adults (CONFIDeNT): a double-blind, multicenter pragmatic parallel-group randomised controlled trial. Lancet 386(10004):1640, 2015

Kwon S, Visco AG, Fitzgerald MP, et al: Validity and reliability of the modified Manchester health questionnaire in assessing patients with fecal incontinence. Dis Colon Rectum 48(2):323, 2005

Lewis SJ, Heaton KW: Stool form scale as a useful guide to intestinal transit time. Scand J Gastroenterol 32(9):920, 1997

Lockhart ME, Fielding JR, Richter HE: Reproducibility of dynamic MR imaging pelvic measurements: a multi-institutional study. Radiology 249(2):534, 2008

Lowry AC, Thorson AG, Rothenberger DA, et al: Repair of simple rectovaginal fistulas. Influence of previous repairs. Dis Colon Rectum 31(9):676, 1988

MacRae HM, McLeod RS, Cohen Z, et al: Treatment of rectovaginal fistulas that has failed previous repair attempts. Dis Colon Rectum 38(9):921, 1995

Madoff RD: Surgical treatment options for fecal incontinence. Gastroenterology 126:S48, 2004

Maldonado PA, Mcintire D, Corton MM: Long-term outcomes after overlapping sphincteroplasty for cloacal-like deformities. Female Pelvic Med Reconstr Surg 25(4):271, 2019

Malik AI, Nelson RL: Surgical management of anal fistulae: a systematic review. Colorectal Dis 10:420, 2008

Matzel KE: Sacral nerve stimulation for faecal incontinence: its role in the treatment algorithm. Colorectal Dis 13(Suppl. 2):10, 2011

Mellgren AM, Matzel KE, Pollack J, et al: Long-term efficacy of NASHA Dx injection therapy for treatment of fecal incontinence. Neurogastroenterol Motil 26:1087, 2014

Miller R, Lewis GT, Bartolo DC, et al: Sensory discrimination and dynamic activity in the anorectum: evidence using a new ambulatory technique. Br J Surg 75(10):1003, 1988

Minguez M, Herreros B, Sanchiz V, et al: Predictive value of the balloon expulsion test for excluding the diagnosis of pelvic floor dyssynergia in constipation. Gastroenterology 126:57, 2004

Mizrahi N, Wexner SD, Zmora O, et al: Endorectal advancement flap: are there predictors of failure? Dis Colon Rectum 45(12):1616, 2002

National Institutes of Health: NIH state-of-the-science conference: cesarean delivery on maternal request. 2006. Available at: http://consensus.nih.gov/2006/cesareanstatement.htm. Accessed March 16, 2015

Nelson R, Furner S, Jesudason V: Fecal incontinence in Wisconsin nursing homes: prevalence and associations. Dis Colon Rectum 41(10):1226, 1998

Norton C, Cody JD: Biofeedback and/or sphincter exercises for the treatment of faecal incontinence in adults. Cochrane Database Syst Rev 7:CD002111, 2012

Norton C, Kamm MA: Anal sphincter biofeedback and pelvic floor exercises for faecal incontinence in adults—a systematic review. Aliment Pharmacol Ther 15(8):1147, 2001

Nygaard IE, Rao SS, Dawson JD: Anal incontinence after anal sphincter disruption: a 30-year retrospective cohort study. Obstet Gynecol 89(6):896, 1997

Oberwalder M, Thaler K, Baig MK, et al: Anal ultrasound and endosonographic measurement of perineal body thickness: a new evaluation for fecal incontinence in females. Surg Endosc 18(4):650, 2004

Omar MI, Alexander CE: Drug treatment for faecal incontinence in adults. Cochrane Database Syst Rev 6:CD002116, 2013

Orkin BA, Sinykin SB, Lloyd PC: The digital rectal examination scoring system (DRESS). Dis Colon Rectum 53:1656, 2010

Patton V, Wiklendt L, Arkwright JW, et al: The effect of sacral nerve stimulation on distal colonic motility in patients with faecal incontinence. Br J Surg 100(7):959, 2013

Pescatori M, Anastasio G, Bottini C, et al: New grading and scoring for anal incontinence. Evaluation of 335 patients. Dis Colon Rectum 35(5):482, 1992

Rahman MS, Al-Suleiman SA, El-Yahia AR, et al: Surgical treatment of rectovaginal fistula of obstetric origin: a review of 15 years' experience in a teaching hospital. J Obstet Gynaecol 23(6):607, 2003

Rao SS: The technical aspects of biofeedback therapy for defecation disorders. Gastroenterologist 6(2):96, 1998

Rao SS, Bharucha AE, Chiarioni G, et al: Anorectal disorders. Gastroenterology 150(6):1430, 2016

Rao SS, Coss-Adame E, Tantiphlachiva K, et al: Translumbar and transsacral magnetic neurostimulation for the assessment of neuropathy in fecal incontinence. Dis Colon Rectum 57(5):645, 2014

Rao SS, Ozturk R, Stessman M: Investigation of the pathophysiology of fecal seepage. Am J Gastroenterol 99(11):2204, 2004

Rao SS, Seaton K, Miller M, et al: Randomized controlled trial of biofeedback, sham feedback, and standard therapy for dyssynergic defecation. Clin Gastroenterol Hepatol 5(3):331, 2007

Read M, Read NW, Barber DC, et al: Effects of loperamide on anal sphincter function in patients complaining of chronic diarrhea with fecal incontinence and urgency. Dig Dis Sci 27(9):807, 1982

Richter HE, Matthews CA, Muir T, et al: A vaginal bowel-control system for the treatment of fecal incontinence. Obstet Gynecol 125:540, 2015

Rociu E, Stoker J, Eijkemans MJ, et al: Fecal incontinence: endoanal US versus endoanal MR imaging. Radiology 212(2):453, 1999

Rockwood TH, Church JM, Fleshman JW, et al: Fecal incontinence quality of life scale: quality of life instrument for patients with fecal incontinence. Dis Colon Rectum 43(1):9, 2000

Rockwood TH, Church JM, Fleshman JW, et al: Patient and surgeon ranking of the severity of symptoms associated with fecal incontinence: the fecal incontinence severity index. Dis Colon Rectum 42(12):1525, 1999

Rogers RG, Jeppson PC: Current diagnosis and management of pelvic fistulae in women. Obstet Gynecol 128:635, 2016

Rydningen M, Dehli T, Wilsgaard T, et al: Sacral neuromodulation compared with injection of bulking agents for faecal incontinence following obstetric anal sphincter injury – a randomized controlled study. Colorectal Dis 19(5):0134, 2017

Sailer M, Bussen D, Debus ES, et al: Quality of life in patients with benign anorectal disorders. Br J Surg 85(12):1716, 1998

Schiller LR, Santa Ana CA, Morawski SG, et al: Mechanism of the antidiarrheal effect of loperamide. Gastroenterology 86(6):1475, 1984

Shafik A: Polytetrafluoroethylene injection for the treatment of partial fecal incontinence. Int Surg 78:159, 1993

Shafik A, Ahmed I, El-Sibai O, et al: Percutaneous peripheral neuromodulation in the treatment of fecal incontinence. Eur Surg Res 35(2):103, 2003

Snooks SJ, Henry MM, Swash M: Faecal incontinence due to external anal sphincter division in childbirth is associated with damage to the innervation of the pelvic floor musculature: a double pathology. BJOG 92(8):824, 1985

Sonoda T, Hull T, Piedmonte MR, et al: Outcomes of primary repair of anorectal and rectovaginal fistulas using the endorectal advancement flap. Dis Colon Rectum 45(12):1622, 2002

Sultan AH, Monga A, Lee J, et al: An International Urogynecological Association (IUGA)/International Continence Society (ICS) joint report on the terminology for female anorectal dysfunction. Int Urogynecol J 28(1):5, 2017

Sultan AH, Kamm MA, Hudson CN, et al: Anal-sphincter disruption during vaginal delivery. N Engl J Med 329(26):1905, 1993

Tantiphlachiva K, Rao P, Attaluri A, et al: Digital rectal examination is a useful tool for identifying patients with dyssynergia. Clin Gastroenterol Hepatol 8:955, 2010

Terra MP, Beets-Tan RG, van der Hulst VP, et al: MRI in evaluating atrophy of the external anal sphincter in patients with fecal incontinence. AJR Am J Roentgenol 187(4):991, 2006

Thomas GP, Dudding TC, Rahbour G, et al: A review of posterior tibial nerve stimulation for faecal incontinence. Colorectal Dis 15:519, 2013

Tirumanisetty P, Prichard D, Fletcher JG, et al: Normal values for assessment of anal sphincter morphology, anorectal motion, and pelvic organ prolapse with MRI in healthy women. Neurogastroenterol Motil 30(7):e13314, 2018

Tjandra JJ, Chan MK, Yeh CH, et al: Sacral nerve stimulation is more effective than optimal medical therapy for severe fecal incontinence: a randomized, controlled study. Dis Colon Rectum 51(5):494, 2008

Tsang CB, Madoff RD, Wong WD, et al: Anal sphincter integrity and function influences outcome in rectovaginal fistula repair. Dis Colon Rectum 41(9):1141, 1998

Vaizey CJ, Carapeti E, Cahill JA, et al: Prospective comparison of faecal incontinence grading systems. Gut 44(1):77, 1999

van der Wilt AA, Giuliani G, Kubis C, et al: Randomized clinical trial of percutaneous tibial nerve stimulation versus sham electrical stimulation in patients with fecal incontinence. Br J Surg 104(9):1167, 2017

Van Koughnett JA, da Silva G: Anorectal physiology and testing. Gastroenterol Clin North Am 42(4):713, 2013a

Van Koughnett JA, Wexner SD: Current management of fecal incontinence: choosing amongst treatment options to optimize outcomes. World J Gastroenterol 19(48): 9216, 2013b

Visscher AP, Lam TJ, Meurs-Szojda MMA, et al: Temperature-controlled delivery of radiofrequency energy in fecal incontinence: a randomized sham-controlled clinical trial. Dis Colon rectum 60(8):860, 2017

Vitton V, Vignally P, Barthet M, et al: Dynamic anal endosonography and MRI defecography in diagnosis of pelvic floor disorders: comparison with conventional defecography. Dis Colon Rectum 54:1398, 2011

Vogel JD, Johnson EK, Morris AM, et al: Clinical practice guideline for the management of anorectal abscess, fistula-in-ano, and rectovaginal fistula. Dis Colon Rectum 59(12):1117, 2016

Wald A: Diagnosis and Management of Fecal Incontinence. Curr Gastroenterol Rep 20(3):9, 2018

Wald A: Surgical treatment for refractory constipation—more hard data about hard stools? Am J Gastroenterol 85(6):759, 1990

Wexner SD, Coller JA, Devroede G, et al: Sacral nerve stimulation for fecal incontinence: results of a 120-patient prospective multicenter study. Ann Surg 251(3):441, 2010

Whitehead WE, Borrud L, Goode PS, et al: Fecal incontinence in U.S. adults: epidemiology and risk factors. Gastroenterology 137(2):512.e1, 2009

Whitehead WE, Rao SC, Lowry A, et al: Treatment of Fecal Incontinence: proceedings of an NIH Conference. Am J Gastroenterol 110:138, 2015

Whitehead WE, Schuster MM: Anorectal physiology and pathophysiology. Am J Gastroenterol 82(6):487, 1987

Whitehead WE, Wald A, Norton NJ: Treatment options for fecal incontinence. Dis Colon Rectum 44(1):131, 2001

Wiskind AK, Thompson JD: Transverse transperineal repair of rectovaginal fistulas in the lower vagina. Am J Obstet Gynecol 167(3):694, 1992

Wu JM, Vaughan CP, Goode PS, et al: Prevalence and trends of symptomatic pelvic floor disorders in U.S. women. Obstet Gynecol 123:141, 2014

Zutshi M, Tracey TH, Bast J, et al: Ten-year outcome after anal sphincter repair for fecal incontinence. Dis Colon Rectum 52:1089, 2009

CHAPTER 26

Genitourinary Fistula and Urethral Diverticulum

GENITOURINARY FISTULA

A genitourinary fistula is defined as an abnormal communication between the urinary (ureters, bladder, urethra) and the genital (uterus, cervix, vagina) systems. The true incidence is unknown and varies according to whether the etiology is obstetric or gynecologic. In Asia and Africa, up to 100,000 new cases of obstetric genitourinary fistula are added each year to the estimated pool of 2 million women with unrepaired fistulas (World Health Organization, 2018). For industrialized countries, most fistulas occur iatrogenically from pelvic surgery, and the generally accepted incidence derives from data on surgeries to correct these fistulas. Numbers from the National Hospital Discharge Survey of inpatient women show that approximately 5 per 100,000 women underwent lower reproductive tract fistula repair (Brown, 2012). This likely is underestimated, as many cases are unreported, unrecognized, or treated conservatively. Of genitourinary fistulas, vesicovaginal fistula is most common (Goodwin, 1980; Shaw, 2014).

PATHOPHYSIOLOGY

The principles and phases of wound healing aid the understanding of genitourinary fistula pathogenesis. After injury, tissue damage and necrosis stimulate inflammation, and the process of cell regeneration begins (Kumar, 2015). Initially at the injury site, new blood vessels form, that is, *angiogenesis*. Three to 5 days after injury, fibroblasts proliferate and subsequently synthesize and deposit extracellular matrix, in particular collagen. This *fibrosis phase* determines the final strength of the healed wound. Collagen deposition peaks approximately 7 days after injury and continues for several weeks. Subsequent scar maturation and organization, termed *remodeling*, augments wound strength. These phases are interdependent, and any disruption of this sequence eventually may create a fistula. Most defects tend to present 1 to 3 weeks after tissue injury. This is a time during which tissues are most vulnerable to an altered healing environment that may include hypoxia, ischemia, malnutrition, radiation, and chemotherapy. Eventually, edges of the wound epithelialize, and a chronic fistulous tract is thus formed.

CLASSIFICATION

Although many classification systems exist for genitourinary fistula, no single system is considered the accepted standard nor is any one scheme superior in predicting surgical success. Fistulas can develop at any point between the genital and urinary systems, and one classification method reflects the anatomic communication (Table 26-1).

TABLE 26-1. Classification of Genitourinary Fistula Based on Anatomic Communication

	Urinary Tract		
	Ureter	**Bladder**	**Urethra**
Vagina	Ureterovaginal	Vesicovaginal	Urethrovaginal
		Vesicoureterovaginal	
Cervix	Ureterocervical	Vesicocervical	Urethrocervical
Uterus	Ureterouterine	Vesicouterine	Not reported

TABLE 26-2. Classification of Vesicovaginal Fistulas

Simple
Size <2 to 3 cm
Located near the cuff (supratrigonal)
No prior radiation or malignancy
Normal vaginal length

Complicated
Prior radiation therapy
Pelvic malignancy present
Vaginal length shortened
Size >3 cm
Located distant from cuff or has trigonal involvement

TABLE 26-3. Classification of Genitourinary Fistulas

This new classification divides genitourinary fistulas into four main types, depending on the distance of the fistula's distal edge from the external urinary meatus. These four types are further subclassified by the size of the fistula, extent of associated scarring, vaginal length, or special considerations.

Type 1: Distal edge of fistula >3.5 cm from external urinary meatus

Type 2: Distal edge of fistula >2.5–3.5 cm from external urinary meatus

Type 3: Distal edge of fistula 1.5 to >2.5 cm from external urinary meatus

Type 4: Distal edge of fistula <1.5 cm from external urinary meatus

(a) Size <1.5 cm, in the largest diameter
(b) Size 1.5–3 cm, in the largest diameter
(c) Size >3 cm, in the largest diameter

i. None or only mild fibrosis (around fistula and/or vagina) and/or vaginal length >6 cm, normal capacity
ii. Moderate or severe fibrosis (around fistula and/or vagina) and/or reduced vaginal length and/or capacity
iii. Special consideration, e.g., postradiation, ureteric involvement, circumferential fistula, or previous repair

Data from Goh, 2004, with permission.

Vesicovaginal fistulas can also be characterized by their size and location in the vagina. They are termed *high vaginal*, when found proximally in the vagina; *low vaginal*, when noted distally; or *midvaginal*, when identified centrally. For instance, posthysterectomy vesicovaginal fistulas are often proximal, or "high" in the vagina, and located at the level of the vaginal cuff.

Others classify vesicovaginal fistula based on the complexity and extent of involvement (Table 26-2) (Elkins, 1999). In this scheme, complicated vesicovaginal fistulas are those that involve pelvic malignancy, prior radiation therapy, a shortened vaginal length, or bladder trigone; those that are distant from the vaginal cuff; or those that measure >3 cm in diameter.

In one obstetric classification system, high-risk vesicovaginal fistulas are described by their size (>4 to 5 cm in diameter); involvement of urethra, ureter(s), or rectum; juxtacervical location with an inability to visualize the superior edge; and reformation following a failed repair (Elkins, 1999).

Another obstetric classification ranks urinary fistulas based on their needed surgical repairs (Waaldijk, 1995). In this system, type I fistulas are those that do not involve the urethral closure mechanism, type II fistulas do, and type III fistulas involve the ureter and include other exceptional fistulas. Type II fistulas are divided into: (A) without or (B) with subtotal or total urethra involvement. Type IIB fistulas are further subdivided as: (a) without or (b) with a circumferential configuration around the urethra.

To aid objective comparison of surgical outcomes, a more comprehensive classification system has been developed (Table 26-3). It integrates fistula distance from the external urethral meatus, fistula size, degree of surrounding tissue fibrosis, and extent of vaginal length reduction (Goh, 2004). This system has good inter- and intraobserver reproducibility and has demonstrated efficacy in predicting which patients are at risk of postfistula urinary incontinence and of failed closure (Bengtson, 2016; Goh, 2008, 2009). Despite the availability of these numerous classification systems, most clinicians will, from a practical standpoint, often describe the communicating structures and the defect's relative position in the vagina (high, mid, low).

ETIOLOGY

Congenital genitourinary fistulas are rare. If found, they are commonly associated with other renal or urogenital abnormalities.

Thus, most vesicovaginal fistulas are acquired and typically result from either obstetric trauma or pelvic surgery.

■ Obstetric Trauma

In developing countries, more than 70 percent of genitourinary fistulas arise from obstetric trauma, specifically from prolonged or obstructed labor or complicated cesarean delivery (Kumar, 2009; Raassen, 2014). Often, their development reflects social or regional obstetric practices. For example, both childbearing at a young age, before the pelvis has completely developed, and female genital mutilation may significantly narrow the vaginal introitus and obstruct labor. Prolonged obstructed labor or malpresentation of the presenting fetal part can cause pressure or ischemic necrosis of the anterior vaginal wall and bladder, subsequently resulting in fistula formation. Symphysiotomy to relieve obstructed labor also carries fistula risk (Wilson, 2016). The vagina may also be damaged by instruments used to deliver stillborn neonates or to perform abortion. Malnutrition and limited health care in many of these countries can further diminish wound healing.

In contrast, in most developed countries, fistulas uncommonly follow obstetric procedures or deliveries. Rarely, cesarean deliveries, usually those accompanied by obstetric complications, have led to complex urinary fistula (Billmeyer, 2001). Similarly, rare cases following cervical cerclage have been reported (Massengill, 2012).

■ Pelvic Surgery

In developed countries, iatrogenic injury during pelvic surgery is responsible for 90 percent of vesicovaginal fistulas, and the accepted incidence of fistula formation after pelvic surgery is 0.1 to 2 percent (Hilton, 2012a,b; Tancer, 1992). The remaining fistulas result from procedures performed by urologists and by colorectal, vascular, and general surgeons. In industrialized countries, hysterectomy is the most common surgical precursor to vesicovaginal fistula, accounting for approximately 75 percent of fistula cases (Symmonds, 1984). When all hysterectomy types are considered, vesicovaginal fistula is estimated to complicate 0.8 per 1000 procedures (Harkki-Siren, 1998). In their review of more than 62,000 hysterectomy cases, laparoscopic hysterectomies were associated with the greatest incidence (2 per 1000), followed by abdominal (1 per 1000), vaginal (0.2 per 1000), and supracervical (0 per 1000) hysterectomies. With hysterectomy for benign disease, bladder wall laceration extending into the bladder neck or ureteral orifice (trigone) significantly raised the risk of subsequent vesicovaginal fistula (Duong, 2009).

Because most genitourinary fistulas follow pelvic surgery, prevention and intraoperative recognition of lower urinary tract injury is imperative. Discussed in Chapter 40 (p. 867), intraoperative cystoscopy improves the detection rate of lower urinary tract injuries. In one study of nearly 3000 benign hysterectomies, rates of vesicovaginal fistula dropped significantly after universal cystoscopy was implemented (Chi, 2016). Thus, intraoperative cystoscopy can be a useful adjunct, particularly in cases posing greater risk for ureteral or bladder injury.

■ Other Causes

Although surgical and obstetric causes account for most urinary fistulas, other etiologies include radiation therapy, malignancy, trauma, foreign bodies, infections, pelvic inflammation, and inflammatory bowel disease.

Radiation therapy induces an endarteritis that can lead to tissue necrosis and subsequent fistula formation. This modality is a frequent cause, and some series have reported that up to 6 percent of genitourinary fistulas can result from radiation (Lee, 1988). Although most damage following this therapy develops within weeks and months, associated fistulas may present up to 20 years after the original insult (Graham, 1967; Zoubek, 1989).

Malignancy is commonly linked with tissue necrosis and may lead to genitourinary fistula. Emmert and Kohler (1996) found a 1.8-percent incidence of rectovaginal and vesicovaginal fistula in their analysis of nearly 2100 women with cervical cancer. Thus, tissue biopsy is routinely considered during diagnostic evaluation of women with a fistula and history of malignancy.

Trauma sustained during sexual activity or sexual assault can result in genitourinary fistula and has been estimated to precede 4 percent of these defects (Kallol, 2002; Lee, 1988). Foreign bodies such as a neglected pessary or vesical calculi also are documented causes (Arias, 2008; Shephard, 2017). Given that transurethral catheter placement has been linked to urethrovaginal fistula, this commonly used device should be placed, maintained, and removed with care (Dakhil, 2014). Foreign material introduced during surgery such as collagen injected transurethrally and complications resulting from synthetic mesh placement for urinary incontinence or pelvic organ prolapse are other inciting agents (Blavais, 2014; Firoozi, 2012; Pruthi, 2000). Also, during sling surgeries, excess sling tension may increase tissue stress and necrosis. Thus, initial material selection and patient evaluation for poor wound healing risk factors are important prevention steps (Giles, 2005). Mesh selection is further discussed in Chapter 24 (p. 554).

Other rare causes of fistula formation include infections such as lymphogranuloma venereum, urinary tuberculosis, pelvic inflammation, and syphilis; inflammatory bowel disease; and autoimmune disease (Ba-Thike, 1992; Monteiro, 1995). Additionally, poor wound healing is often linked to poorly controlled diabetes mellitus, smoking, peripheral vascular disease, and chronic corticosteroid therapy.

SYMPTOMS

Vesicovaginal fistula classically presents with unexplained continuous urinary leakage from the vagina after a recent operation. Depending on the size and location of the fistula, the urine amount will vary. Occasionally, small-volume, intermittent leakage is mistaken for postoperative stress urinary incontinence or a normal exudate associated with cuff healing. Thus, new-onset urinary or vaginal leakage, particularly in the setting of recent pelvic surgery, ideally prompts thorough examination to exclude fistula. Other less specific symptoms of genitourinary fistula include fever, pain, ileus, and bladder irritability.

Vesicovaginal fistula may present days to weeks after the inciting surgery, and those following hysterectomy typically present at 1 to 3 weeks. Some fistulas, however, have longer latency, and symptoms may develop several years later.

DIAGNOSIS

A thorough history and physical examination identifies most cases of vesicovaginal fistula. Accordingly, information is documented regarding obstetric deliveries, prior surgeries, previous fistula management, and malignancy treatment, especially pelvic surgery and radiation therapy.

Physical examination is equally informative, and vaginal inspection often will identify the defect (Fig. 26-1). A meticulous assessment for other fistulous tracts is performed, and their location and size are noted. Visual assistance with an endoscopic lens and translucent vaginal speculum can sometimes help identify a vaginal-apex fistula, which can be more difficult to detect.

It is essential to differentiate between "extraurethral" urinary leakage, as with a fistula, and "transurethral" leakage, that is, through the urethra, as with stress urinary incontinence. Occasionally, the vaginal fluid source is unclear, and a small amount of urine can easily be mistaken for vaginal discharge. Measurement of the vaginal fluid's creatinine content can sometimes be used to confirm its origin. Although creatinine levels in urine vary, with mean levels reaching 113.5 mg/dL, a value >17 mg/dL is consistent with urine (Barr, 2005). In contrast, fluid with a concentration <5 mg/dL is highly unlikely to be human urine.

Although a genitourinary fistula ideally is visualized directly, inspection at times is unrevealing. In these circumstances,

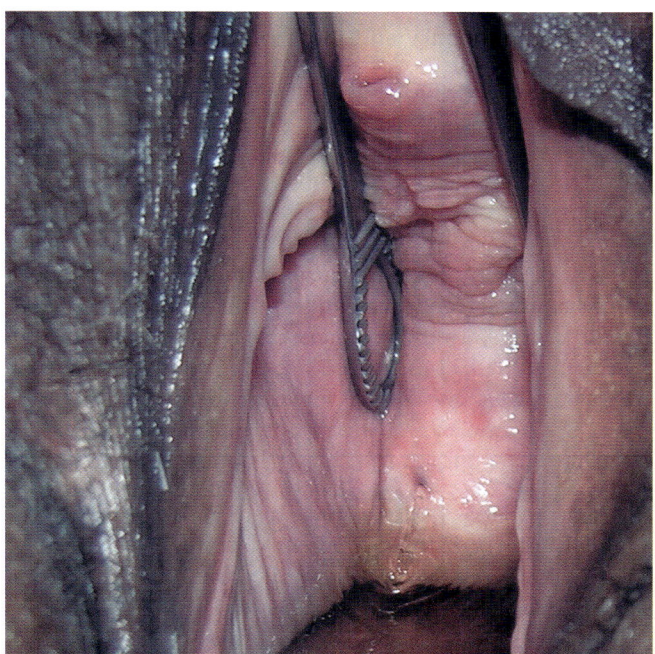

FIGURE 26-1 In this image, the anterior vaginal wall is elevated by open ring forceps. The urethra is seen between the forceps arms, and urine streams from a vesicovaginal fistula.

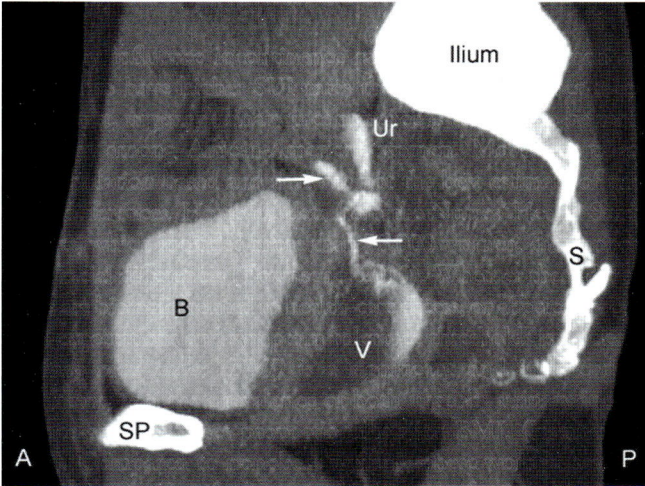

FIGURE 26-3 Ureterovaginal fistula. Both arrows show anomalous tracking of contrast. The lower arrow denotes a fistulous tract to the upper vagina. B = bladder; S = sacrum; SP = symphysis pubis; Ur = ureter; V = vagina. (Reproduced with permission from Dr. April Bailey.)

retrograde bladder instillation of visually distinct solutions such as sterile milk or dilute methylene blue can often indicate a fistula and aid in its localization.

If the presence of a urinary fistula is uncertain or its vaginal location is not identified, a *three-swab test*, commonly known as the "tampon test," is recommended (Moir, 1973). Although some literally use a tampon to perform this test, we recommend using two to four pieces of gauze sequentially packed into the vaginal canal. A diluted solution of methylene blue is instilled into the bladder using a transurethral catheter. After 15 to 30 minutes of routine activity, the gauze is removed serially from the vagina, and each is inspected for dye. The specific gauze colored with dye suggests the fistula location—a proximal or high location in the vagina for the innermost gauze

and a low or distal fistula for the outermost. If the distally placed sponge is stained with dye, urine leaking out through the urethra, as with stress urinary incontinence, must be differentiated from fistula drainage.

Cystourethroscopy is another valuable diagnostic tool (Fig. 26-2). It permits fistula localization, determination of its proximity to the ureteral orifices, inspection for multiple fistula sites, and assessment of surrounding bladder mucosa viability. In addition, cystourethroscopy and vaginoscopy used sequentially at the same visit has been described to identify vesicovaginal fistula (Andreoni, 2003).

Concomitant ureteral involvement is estimated to complicate 10 to 15 percent of vesicovaginal fistula cases and is sought during diagnostic evaluation (Goodwin, 1980). At our institution, intravenous contrast-enhanced computed tomography (CT) scanning in the excretory phase (CT urogram) is the preferred diagnostic test after initial cystourethroscopic survey is completed (Fig. 26-3). Selection of modalities other

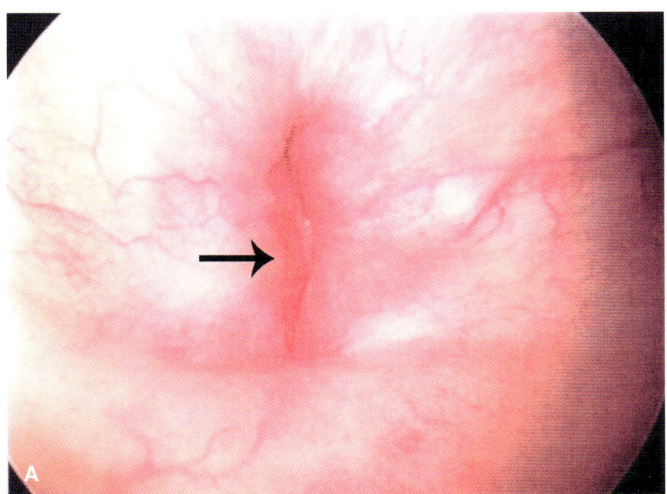

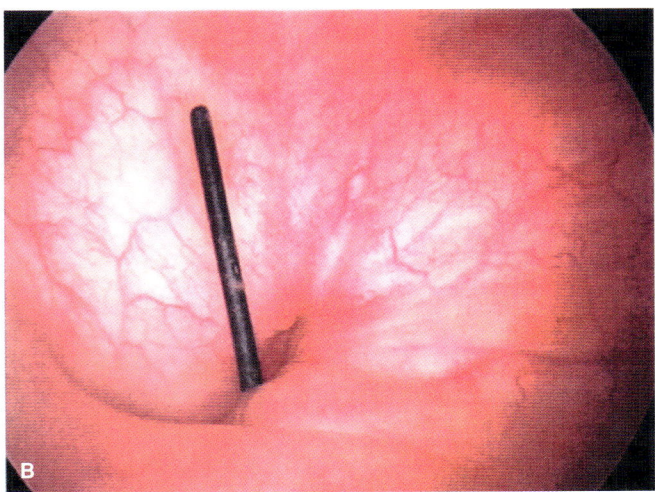

FIGURE 26-2 A. Cystoscopic view of vesicovaginal fistula (*arrow*). **B.** Probe placed through fistulous tract to aid cystoscopic visualization.

than CT for fistulous tract identification may be considered based on cost or availability. First, intravenous pyelography (IVP) can adequately confirm integrity of the upper collecting system and exclude ureteral involvement in a fistula. Second, retrograde pyelography may be used. Often carried out in conjunction with cystoscopy, it is performed by placing a small catheter into the distal ureter. Contrast material is injected through the catheter into one or both ureters. Fluoroscopic images are then obtained. Retrograde pyelography generally has been reported to have the same diagnostic value as IVP.

In some instances resources are scarce, cost may be a limitation, and access to specialized diagnostic imaging is a challenge. With some advanced planning, phenazopyridine hydrochloride (Pyridium) can be used in conjunction with the three-swab test to determine ureteral involvement, as a very rudimentary alternative to the aforementioned more sophisticated imaging. This tablet is administered orally, is excreted renally, acts as a topical bladder analgesic, and stains urine orange as a side effect. Women with suspected ureteral involvement are instructed to take a 200-mg dose a few hours before their clinic appointment. The steps of the three-swab test are then performed, as described earlier (p. 577). In this case, if the most proximal (innermost) gauze is colored with orange dye, ureteral involvement is suspected. If both orange and blue dyes are seen, then involvement of both the bladder and ureter(s) is suspected.

Voiding cystourethrography (VCUG) can help confirm the presence, location, and number of fistulous tracts. In this, the bladder is filled via catheter with contrast dye. Fluoroscopic images of the lower urinary tract are then obtained during patient micturition. However, CT has largely replaced this modality. Transabdominal sonography with applied color Doppler to identify flow through the fistula has been suggested as another diagnostic option (Volkmer, 2000). However, without color Doppler, sonography failed to identify 29 percent of vesicovaginal fistula cases in one study (Adetiloye, 2000).

TREATMENT

Conservative Treatment

Occasionally, genitourinary fistulas may spontaneously close during continuous bladder drainage using an indwelling urinary catheter. Approximately 12 percent of women treated by sustained catheterization alone had fistulas that healed spontaneously (Oakley, 2014; Waaldijk, 1994). Romics and colleagues (2002) found that in 10 percent of cases, urinary fistulas close spontaneously after 2 to 8 weeks of transurethral catheterization, especially if the fistula is small (2- to 3-mm diameter). Another series reported fistulas up to 2 cm in diameter spontaneously healed in 50 to 60 percent of patients treated with an indwelling catheter (Waaldijk, 1989).

Despite these series, data that correlate fistula size and success of conservative management are limited. Many reports of successful spontaneous closure with catheter drainage have been limited to fistulas that were 1 cm in size or smaller (Lentz, 2005; Ou, 2004). Many studies are vague regarding how fistula size is measured, and each series has potential for considerable

bias in its selection criteria. However, in general, the larger a fistula, the less likely it is to heal without surgery.

Evidence regarding the duration of catheter drainage also varies. Regardless, many agree that if a fistula has not closed within 4 weeks, it is unlikely to do so. This may be secondary to epithelialization of the fistulous tract (Davits, 1991; Tancer, 1992). Moreover, continued urinary drainage may lead to further bladder inflammation and irritation (Zimmern, 1991). Importantly, if attempting conservative treatment of a vesicovaginal fistula with catheter insertion and chronic drainage, urinary drainage ideally begins shortly after the inciting event.

Fibrin sealant (Tisseel, Evicel), also colloquially called *fibrin glue*, is formed from concentrated fibrinogen combined with thrombin to simulate the final clotting cascade stages. In gynecology, it is mainly used to control low-pressure surgical bleeding. Although fibrin sealant has been described for vesicovaginal fistula treatment, it is often selected as a surgical adjunct rather than primary surgical treatment (Evans, 2003). Data regarding fibrin sealant effectiveness are sparse, and well-designed trials are lacking. Thus, fibrin sealant monotherapy may not be the initial recommended treatment in most vesicovaginal fistula cases due to potential lack of durability and thus a risk for recurrence. However, it may provide a viable alternative in patients with multiple comorbidities that contraindicate a prolonged fistula repair surgery.

In sum, a trial of conservative therapy is usually warranted and reasonable, especially if instituted shortly after the inciting event and if the fistula is small. However, gains from a conservative approach are balanced against a patient's desire for an expedited repair to resolve the leak. Thus, the timing of intervention ideally achieves a compromise between reasonable conservative efforts and addressing the patient's immediate distress and quality of life. As noted, most urinary fistulas ultimately require surgical intervention.

Surgical Treatment

Incorporating the fundamentals of genitourinary fistula repair is essential to successful resolution. These include accurate fistula delineation; adequate assessment of surrounding tissue vascularity; timely repair; multilayer, tension-free, and watertight defect closure; and postoperative bladder drainage.

Primary surgical repair of genitourinary fistula is associated with high cure rates (75 to 100 percent) (Rovner, 2012b). Factors that support this rate include adequate vascularity of the surrounding tissue, brief fistulous tract duration, no prior radiation therapy, meticulous surgical technique, and surgeon experience. The first attempt at surgical repair is usually associated with the best chance of successful healing. Surgical repair success rates specifically for obstetric fistulas also are high. Of these, 81 percent are corrected with the first attempt, and 65 percent with the second (Elkins, 1994; Hilton, 1998).

Timing of Repair

One principle of fistula repair dictates that a repair be performed in noninfected and noninflamed tissues. Early surgical intervention of uncomplicated fistulas within the first 24 to 48 hours following the inciting surgery is possible, as it avoids the brisk postoperative inflammatory response. Such early closure does not affect success rates, and it appears to reduce social and psychologic patient distress (Blaivas, 1995; Persky, 1979).

In instances of extensive and severe inflammation, we recommend delaying operative repair for 6 weeks until inflammation subsides. During this time, a trial of catheter drainage, while the surrounding tissue has an opportunity to heal, is reasonable.

Route of Surgical Repair

Different surgical repair options are available for vesicovaginal fistula. However, data that support an optimal route are limited, and the lack of consensus may reflect variances in surgeon experience and preference. Among important surgical considerations, ability to gain access to the fistula is essential and commonly dictates the approach. Fortunately, success rates are high whether the route of repair is transvaginal or transabdominal.

Vaginal. The transvaginal approach to genitourinary fistula repair is straightforward and direct. Compared with abdominal approaches, it is associated with shorter operative times, decreased blood loss, less morbidity, and shorter hospital stays (Wang, 1990). The transvaginal route also allows easy access for ancillary equipment, such as ureteral stents. This is particularly useful if the fistula is located near ureteral orifices.

One transvaginal approach used most commonly by gynecologists, the *Latzko technique*, is illustrated in Chapter 45 (p. 1081). In this technique, likened to a partial colpocleisis, the most proximal portions of the anterior and posterior vaginal walls are surgically apposed to close the defect, without completely removing the fistulous tract. This partially obliterates the upper vagina, similar to that achieved by colpocleisis. Because of the potential for vaginal shortening, this technique may not be appropriate if vaginal depth has already been compromised or if sexual dysfunction preexists. If use of the Latzko technique is anticipated, patient counseling should specifically addresses these issues and potential sequelae. That said, recent studies evaluating sexual function show similar or higher functioning scores following vaginal repair routes compared with abdominal routes (Lee, 2014; Mohr, 2014).

The *classical technique*, in contrast to the Latzko method, involves total excision of the fistulous tract and mobilization of the surrounding anterior vaginal wall epithelium. After tract resection, the bladder mucosa is first closed, and a watertight repair is confirmed. This is followed by closure of one or two layers of fibromuscular tissue. Vaginal epithelium is then reapproximated.

Of the two approaches, some favor incomplete fistulous tract excision (Latzko repair) to avoid weakening the surrounding tissue, enlarging the defect, and thereby potentially compromising the repair. By preserving the presumptively stronger scar tissue surrounding the fistula, it theoretically permits a more secure reapproximation of surrounding tissue.

Abdominal (Transperitoneal). With this route, the fistula is accessed and excised through an intentional cystotomy on the preperitoneal side of the bladder as shown in Chapter 45 (p. 1084). This approach is used for situations in which the fistula: (1) is located proximally in a narrow vagina, (2) lies close to the ureteral orifices, (3) is complicated by a concomitant ureteric

fistula, (4) persists after prior repair attempts, (5) is large or complex in configuration, or (7) requires an abdominal interposition graft, described in the next section.

Evidence-based support for laparoscopic genitourinary fistula repair is limited to case series (Miklos, 2015). The technique requires advanced laparoscopic surgical skills. Accordingly, success with this approach appears to be highly dependent on surgeon experience.

Interposition Flaps. Surrounding tissue vascularity is essential for successful genitourinary fistula repair healing. When intervening tissues for fistula closure are thin and poorly vascularized, various tissue flaps may be placed vaginally or abdominally between the bladder and the vagina in an attempt to enhance the repair and to lend support and blood supply (Eisen, 1974; Martius, 1928). Sections 45-2 and 45-11 of the atlas illustrate the omental J-flap, which is an abdominal option, whereas a Martius bulbospongiosus fat pad flap is used during vaginal procedures (p. 1085). Although interposition flaps are useful in situations where tissue viability is in question, their utility in uncomplicated cases of vesicovaginal fistula is unclear.

■ Other Genitourinary Fistulas

Although vesicovaginal fistulas are the most common type of genitourinary fistula, other defects can develop and may be described based on their communication between anatomic structures (see Table 26-1). Urethrovaginal fistulas commonly result from surgery involving the anterior vaginal wall, in particular anterior colporrhaphy and urethral diverticulectomy (Blaivas, 1989; Scholler, 2018). In developing countries, as with vesicovaginal fistula, obstetric trauma remains the most common cause of urethrovaginal fistulas. Frequently, patients present with continuous urinary drainage into the vagina or with stress urinary incontinence. The principles of repair are similar, namely, layered closure, tension-free repair, and postoperative bladder drainage.

URETHRAL DIVERTICULUM

Along the anterior vaginal wall, paraurethral glands communicate directly with the urethra. A urethral diverticulum commonly forms from a cystic enlargement of one of these obstructed glands, which then bulges into the anterior vaginal wall. This may develop at the proximal, mid, or distal urethra. This outpouching is commonly asymptomatic but may require surgical excision for symptoms.

Urethral diverticulum is reported to develop in 1 to 6 percent of the general female population. With greater awareness and radiologic advances, diagnosis rates are increasing (Rovner, 2012a). In one population-based study, the incidence was estimated to be <0.02 percent (El-Nashar, 2014). However, the true incidence may be underestimated because diverticula are frequently asymptomatic and thus underreported. In women with lower urinary tract symptoms, the incidence dramatically rises and may reach 40 percent (Stewart, 1981).

Urethral diverticulum is diagnosed most often in the third to sixth decades of life and more commonly in females than in

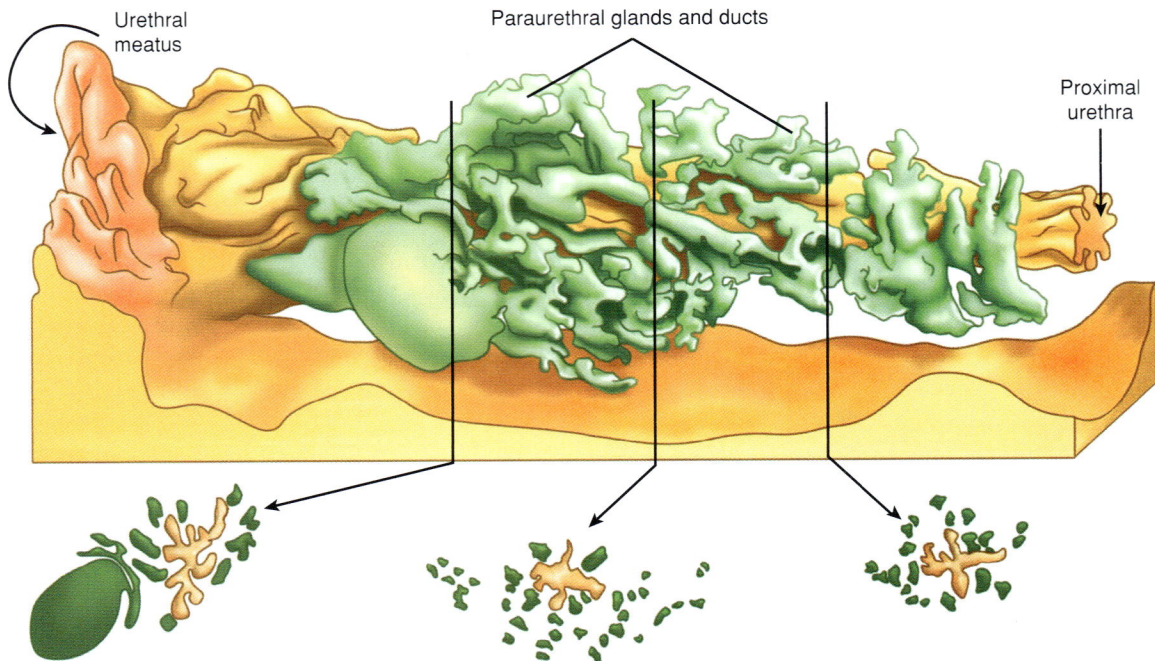

FIGURE 26-4 Complex configuration of paraurethral glands. Cross sections at the bottom show the variable gland distribution along the urethral length.

males (Aldridge, 1978; Burrows, 2005). In some studies, but not all, a greater predominance of urethral diverticula is noted in African-Americans compared with whites (Davis, 1970; Leach, 1987; Burrows, 2005).

ETIOLOGY

The cause of urethral diverticula is unclear. Most are acquired, but rare congenital diverticula have been reported. Congenital causes include persistence of embryologic remnants, defective closure of the ventral portion of the urethra, and congenital cystic dilation of paraurethral glands (Ratner, 1949). Embryology of the female genital tract, described in Chapter 19 (p. 406), contributes in part to our understanding of congenital urethral diverticulum. During female development, the müllerian ducts form the upper vagina, whereas the urogenital sinus gives rise to the distal vagina, vestibule, and female urethra (Fig. 19-4, p. 410). In the vagina, müllerian mucinous columnar epithelium is replaced by squamous epithelium of the urogenital sinus. When the process of epithelial replacement is arrested, small foci of müllerian epithelium may persist and form cysts or diverticula.

In contrast, acquired diverticula can result from infection, birth trauma, or traumatic instrumentation. The most widely held theory dates back to Routh (1890) and involves the paraurethral glands and their ducts. The paraurethral glands surround and cluster most densely along the urethra's inferolateral border (Fig. 26-4) (Huffman, 1948). Of these glands, the bilateral Skene glands are the most distal and typically the largest. Paraurethral glands connect to the urethral canal via a network of branching ducts. The arborizing pattern in portions of this network helps to explain the complexity of some urethral diverticula (Vakili, 2003).

Routh theorized that infection and inflammation obstruct individual ducts and lead to cystic dilation. If these do not spontaneously resolve or infection is not treated promptly, an abscess can form. Subsequent abscess expansion and continued inflammation may rupture the gland into the urethra. These rupture at any location along the mid to distal urethral lumen to create a fistula between the two (Fig. 26-5). As infection clears, the dilated diverticular sac and its new communicating ostium into the urethra persist. Of infectious agents, *Neisseria gonorrhoeae* and *Chlamydia trachomatis* are organisms that were once commonly associated with urethritis and severe inflammation of the paraurethral glands. However, positive identification of these organisms is no longer a prerequisite for diagnosis. More often than not, urethral cultures from women with diverticula are unrevealing.

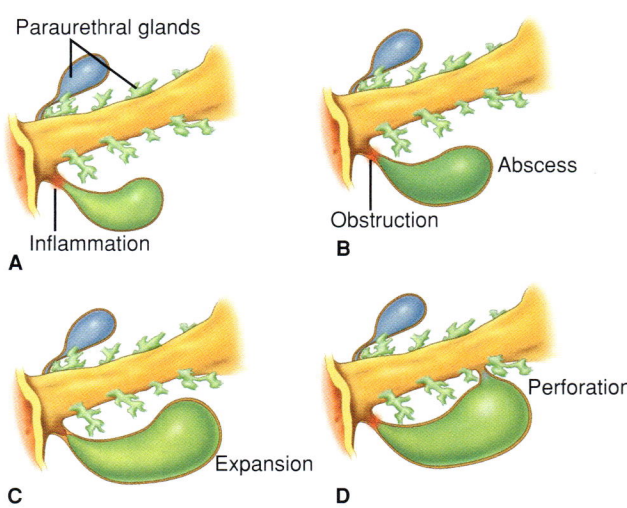

FIGURE 26-5 Mechanism of urethral diverticulum development.

In addition to infection, injured urethral tissue can swell and obstruct paraurethral ducts. Urethral trauma may stem from childbirth, urethral instrumentation, female genital mutilation, placement or removal of synthetic midurethral slings, or periurethral bulking agents (Athanasopoulos, 2008; Chan, 2015; Clemens, 2001; McNally, 1935).

CLASSIFICATION

Early classification systems organized urethral diverticula according to their radiographic complexity and described them as: (1) simple saccular, (2) multiple, or (3) compound or complex with branching sinuses (Lang, 1959). To help standardize surgical treatment and study efficacy, Ginsburg and Genadry (1983) created a preoperative classification system based on urethral location. This system organized diverticula based on their urethral location and described lesions as type 1 (proximal third), type 2 (middle third), and type 3 (distal third).

To achieve a similar end, Leach and coworkers (1993) constructed the L/N/S/C3 classification system. In this system, the diverticulum characteristics are described according to its location (L), number (N), size (S), and configuration, communication, and continence status of the patient (C3). Location describes lesions as being distal, mid-, or proximal urethral and as extending or not extending beneath the bladder neck. In Leach's series of 61 patients, most diverticula were midurethral. Logically, this distribution reflects the predominance of paraurethral glands along the middle third of the urethra. Ascertainment of the number of diverticula is important to prevent incomplete excision of multiple lesions and thus symptom persistence. Diverticulum size similarly can influence treatment. For example, some recommend concomitant interposition flaps for a large diverticulum. Moreover, urinary incontinence may develop de novo or persist if the diverticulum is extremely large and involves sphincter continence mechanisms.

Diverticula variably wrap around the urethra. As the first of the three "C"s, diverticula configuration may be described as solitary or multiloculated and as simple, saddle-shaped, or circumferential (Fig. 26-6). Preoperative delineation aids complete

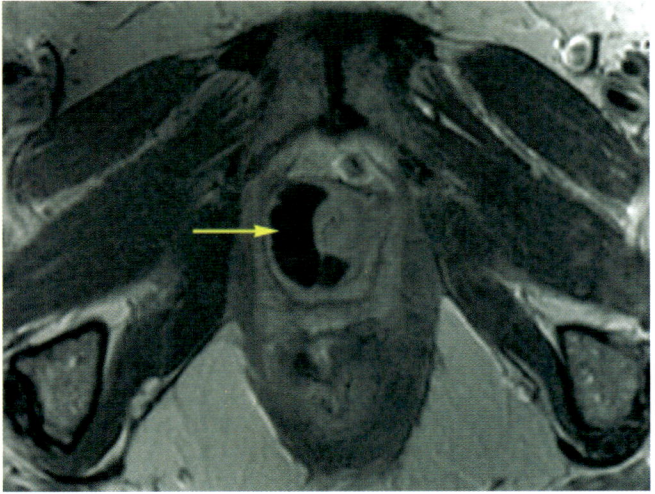

FIGURE 26-6 In this magnetic resonance image, a circumferential urethral diverticulum (*arrow*) is seen extending around the urethra.

surgical excision. It also helps identify those requiring an interposition flap or needing ureteral catheter placement to delineate anatomy during dissection (Rovner, 2003).

Second, successful repair of the urethral wall defect depends in great part on locating the diverticular opening into the urethral canal. Thus, the communication site is sought preoperatively and classified as proximal, mid-, or distal urethral. In the previously cited study, midurethral communication sites were the most common (60 percent), followed by proximal (25 percent) and distal (15 percent) sites.

Finally, in the Leach system, the continence status and urethral hypermobility of the patient are documented. Almost half of the patients in Leach's series had stress urinary incontinence, and these authors suggest that urethral hypermobility is an indication for concomitant incontinence surgery. Several studies have documented the safety of performing concurrent antiincontinence surgery, mainly pubovaginal sling. However, some still consider this approach controversial because of urethral erosion concerns, especially with synthetic sling material (Enemchukwu, 2015; Ganabathi, 1994; Swierzewski, 1993). Although consensus is lacking on this issue, repairing the diverticulum first and then considering antiincontinence surgery if urinary incontinence persists is reasonable. This staged fashion is a particularly realistic option because of the current array of effective minimally invasive surgical procedures, such as midurethral slings. If a staged approach is elected, some suggest urodynamic testing prior to diverticulum repair. This establishes a continence baseline for later comparison.

SYMPTOMS

Urethral diverticula are frequently discovered incidentally during gynecologic or urologic examination. However, symptoms may vary and reflect diverticulum size, location, and extension. The classic triad is postvoid dribbling, dysuria, and dyspareunia. In addition, finger compression of a suburethral mass elicits egress of discharge from the diverticulum and into the urethra (Fig. 26-7).

Importantly, not all women present so classically. Romanzi and coworkers (2000) found pain in 48 percent of affected women. Pain most likely stems from cystic dilation and also possibly from concurrent inflammation. Baradaran and associates (2016) noted dyspareunia, stress urinary incontinence, recurrent urinary tract infections, and vaginal mass as primary findings. Those with dyspareunia may note either entry or deep dyspareunia, depending on diverticular location along the urethra.

A large diverticulum can sometimes be mistaken for early-stage pelvic organ prolapse, especially when the presenting complaint is vaginal fullness, bulge, or pressure. In these cases, the palpable diverticular vaginal mass may mimic a cystocele or rectocele. In most, careful systematic palpation of the vaginal wall will distinguish prolapse from a discrete vaginal wall cyst or diverticulum.

As described, lower urinary tract symptoms frequently accompany urethral diverticulum. Urinary incontinence is noted by 35 to 60 percent of affected women (Gabanathi, 1994; Romanzi, 2000). In addition, during micturition, urine may enter the diverticular sac, only to later spill from the sac and present as postvoid dribble or be misinterpreted

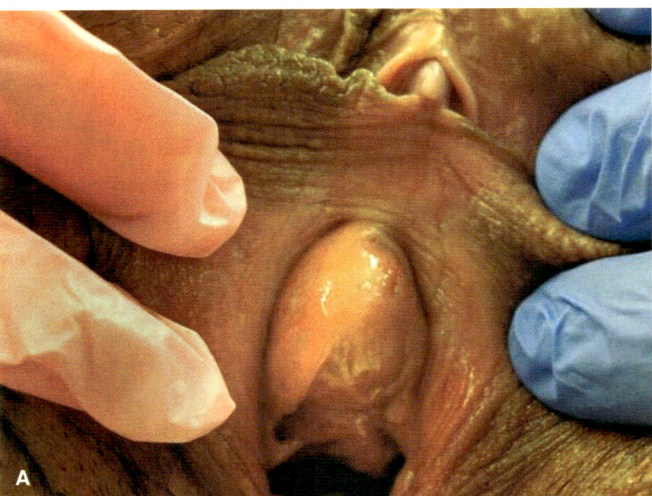
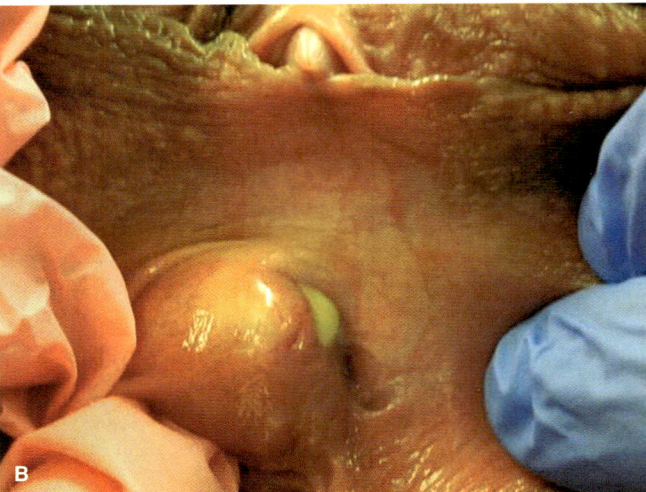

FIGURE 26-7 **A.** Urethral diverticulum seen in the anterior vaginal wall. **B.** Transurethral expression of discharge during its compression.

as urinary incontinence. Conversely, urinary retention also has been reported (Nitti, 1999). Retention frequently accompanies periurethral or diverticular sac cancers, discussed later. Urinary tract infection often complicates urethral diverticulum. In one review of 60 affected women, recurrent urinary tract infection was highly specific for urethral diverticula (Pathi, 2013).

Less frequently, stones may form from urine stagnation and salt precipitation within the diverticular sac. As such, stones may be singular or multiple and are usually composed of calcium oxalate or calcium phosphate. Approximately 10 percent of women with diverticula are affected (Perlmutter, 1993).

Malignant transformation within a urethral diverticulum is rare and accounts for only 5 percent of urethral cancers. Most of these tumors are adenocarcinomas, although transitional cell and squamous cell carcinomas have been identified (Clayton, 1992). Tumors typically present in the sixth or seventh decade of life, and hematuria, irritative voiding complaints, and urinary retention are common. Thus, palpation of an indurated or a solid, fixed periurethral mass typically prompts further diagnostic evaluation and tissue biopsy (Fig. 26-8) (von Pechmann,

2003). Given the few number of these cancers, codified treatment strategies are lacking. Currently, these malignancies are treated by anterior exenteration or by diverticulectomy, alone or with adjuvant radiation therapy (Shalev, 2002).

DIAGNOSIS

For many women, urethral diverticula may be diagnosed using a detailed history, physical examination, and high index of suspicion. Patient evaluation focuses on the common characteristics and symptoms noted earlier (p. 581). However, despite available clinical tools, the diagnosis for many women is delayed as they may initially be treated for stress or urgency incontinence, chronic cystitis, trigonitis, urethral syndrome, vulvovestibulitis, pelvic organ prolapse, and idiopathic chronic pelvic pain. Moreover, the diverticulum itself may mimic a Gartner duct cyst, müllerian remnant vaginal cyst, vaginal epidermoid inclusion cyst, ectopic ureterocele, or endometrioma.

■ Physical Examination

The most frequent physical finding, an anterior vaginal mass beneath or adjacent to the urethra, is detected in 50 to 90 percent of symptomatic patients (Ganabathi, 1994; Gerrard, 2003; Romanzi, 2000). Digital expression of purulent material during compression of the mass is not seen universally. Stenosis of the diverticular duct may obstruct sac emptying in these cases. Thus, meticulous examination and palpation is performed along the entire length of the urethra. Once diverticula are identified, their number, size, consistency, and configuration are determined.

Occasionally, physical examination alone may be insufficient to completely characterize a mass. Of ancillary tests, each has its advantages and disadvantages. Thus, familiarity with each modality's strengths aids selection of the most appropriate test for a given patient.

■ Cystourethroscopy

Of the diagnostic procedures used to detect urethral diverticula, cystourethroscopy is the only tool that allows direct inspection

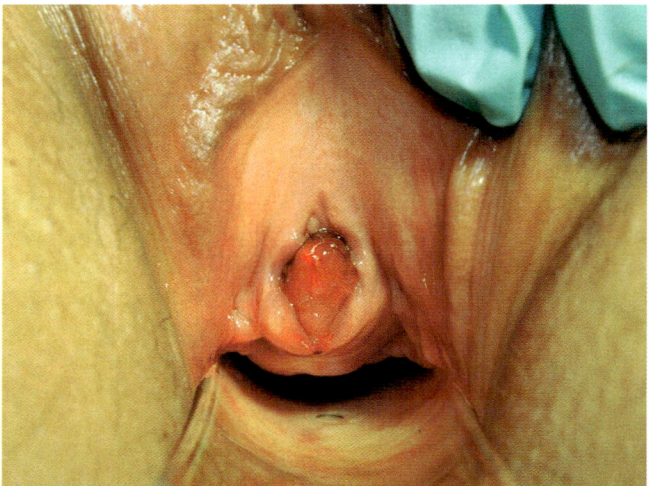

FIGURE 26-8 For this urethral mass, lidocaine was used, and directed biopsy using Tischler biopsy forceps was performed.

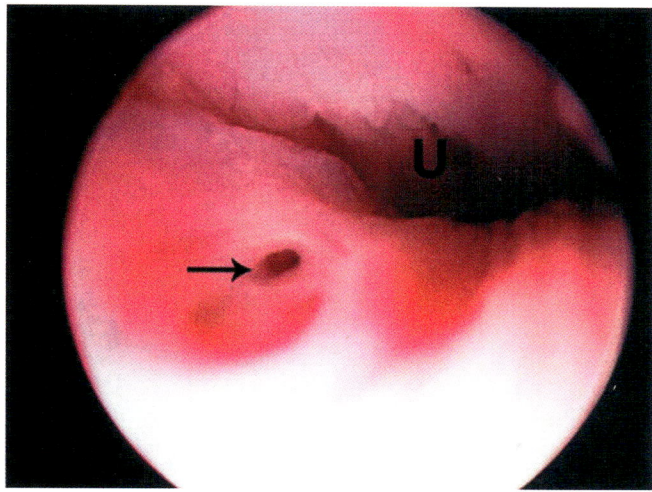

FIGURE 26-9 Diverticular opening visualized on cystourethroscopic examination (*arrow*). U = urethra.

of the urethra and bladder. During endoscopy, fingers pressed upward against the proximal anterior vaginal wall help occlude the bladder neck and allow the distending medium to create positive pressure that may open diverticular ostia (Fig. 26-9). A zero-degree cystoscope lens allows complete radial assessment of the urethra to aid identification of diverticular ostia and, at times, purulent discharge exuding from them.

A primary advantage to cystourethroscopy includes its accuracy for detecting diverticular ostia (Summitt, 1992). Moreover, in those with nonspecific lower urinary tract symptoms, other causes such as urethritis, cystitis, stones, or stenosis can be excluded. Despite these advantages and its common use by urogynecologists, gynecologic generalists employ cystourethroscopy less frequently. Obstacles include inexperience evaluating bladder and urethral mucosal anatomy, cystoscopic expertise, instrumentation costs, and credentialing challenges. Even for clinicians who are experienced with this tool, not all diverticular ostia are identified. For example, a poor seal between the cystoscope and distal urethral mucosa may lead to inadequate sac distention and failure to see very distally located diverticula. Also, narrow or stenotic diverticular ostia may not communicate with the urethral lumen and can be missed. Although cystourethroscopy is minimally invasive, patient pain and risk of postprocedural infection are additional considerations. Last, important information regarding diverticular size, number, and configuration may not be obtained with this tool.

■ Magnetic Resonance Imaging

This imaging modality has become the diagnostic standard to characterize periurethral masses because of its superior resolution of soft tissue. Specifically, for detecting urethral diverticula, magnetic resonance (MR) imaging has comparable or superior sensitivity compared with other radiologic techniques (Lorenzo, 2003; Neitlich, 1998). To improve resolution with MR imaging, an imaging coil housed inside a probe may be placed into the rectum. Instead, an external plate positioned on the lower abdomen can be used to similarly enhance resolution. Compared with the coil, the external plate is preferred by many institutions

because its diagnostic accuracy is comparable but patient comfort is superior. Despite MR imaging's advantages, procedure costs are balanced against the need for additional anatomic information. For a solitary diverticulum with clearly demarcated boundaries and no evidence of extension, costly and extensive imaging may not be necessary.

■ Other Imaging Tools

We use the two previously mentioned techniques most commonly, and other techniques traditionally performed in the past are no longer routinely used at our institution for initial evaluation. Of these, a *voiding cystourethrogram (VCUG)* relies on radiographic contrast being instilled into the bladder and filling a diverticular sac during voiding. Radiographs are then obtained. This painless, simple test has an overall reported accuracy that approximates 85 percent. However, some prefer positive-pressure urethrography as a primary diagnostic tool, since VCUG requires a diverticular communication to be patent during testing (Blander, 2001). Moreover, VCUG involves ionizing radiation exposure for the patient, although the amount is small.

Positive pressure urethrography (PPUG) also uses radiographic contrast and x-ray. With PPUG, a double-balloon, triple-lumen catheter (Trattner catheter) is inserted through the urethra, and its tip enters the bladder (Fig. 26-10). Inflating the proximal balloon in the bladder allows it to be pulled snug against and occlude the urethra at the urethrovesical junction. A distal balloon obstructs the distal urethra. A single catheter port between the two balloons allows instillation of radiopaque contrast. Pressure from the contrast within the blocked urethra distends the urethral caliber and fills the diverticulum. For accurately identifying diverticula, PPUG has a sensitivity surpassing that of VCUG (Golomb, 2003). Disadvantageously, PPUG can be time-consuming, technically difficult, and associated with patient discomfort and postprocedural infection risk. Additionally, similar to VCUG, diverticula may be missed if

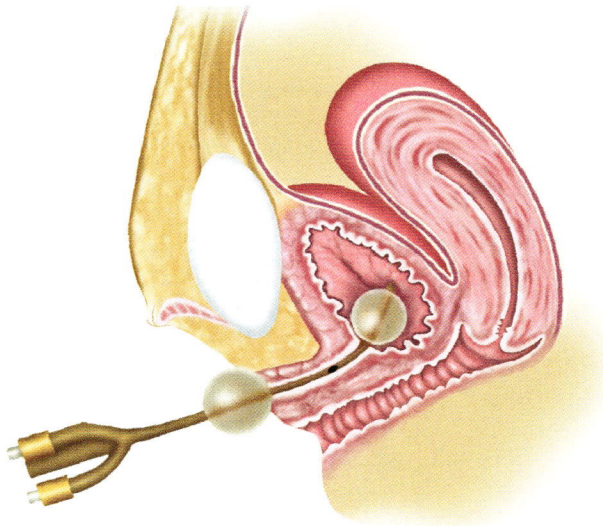

FIGURE 26-10 Trattner double-balloon catheter used to diagnose urethral diverticula.

thick exudate or debris prevents adequate filling with contrast medium or if the diverticular ostium is stenotic. Last, fewer radiologists are proficient with the technique, and Trattner catheters are not commonly not stocked in hospitals.

Sonography, especially with 3-dimensional rendering, is a relatively new modality for urethral diverticulum assessment and appears to have some efficacy (Gerrard, 2003). Suggested technical advantages include visualization of diverticula that do not fill during radiographic contrast studies and characterization of diverticular wall thickness, size, and internal architecture (Yang, 2005). Transabdominal, -vaginal, -rectal, -perineal, and -urethral sonographic techniques have been described (Keefe, 1991; Vargas-Serrano, 1997). Although the endourethral technique appears to have excellent specificity, it is expensive and may be more invasive that the other sonographic routes (Chancellor, 1995). Advantages of sonography include patient comfort, avoidance of ionizing radiation and contrast exposure, relative low cost, and reduced invasiveness. However, in addition to its learning curve, sonography's role in urethral diverticulum diagnosis has not been clearly established. Currently, it remains an academic, investigational, or adjunctive technique.

Because consensus is lacking on which primary modality is best, we begin with cystourethroscopic evaluation. If the initial evaluation is unrevealing but the diagnostic suspicion remains high or if the lesion appears more complex, then MR imaging is elected. Intravenous contrast and an external plate are added to help improve image resolution.

TREATMENT

■ Acute Treatment

A urethral diverticulum may acutely provoke pain, urinary symptoms, or focal tenderness during examination. Conservative management is initially recommended and includes sitz baths, oral analgesics, and a broad-spectrum antibiotic such as a cephalosporin or fluoroquinolone.

■ Chronic Diverticula

For a chronic diverticulum, a conservative approach may be elected by women who have few or no symptoms or who decline surgery due to its associated risks. Important surgical risks include urethrovaginal fistula, worsening or de novo urinary incontinence, altered voiding stream or pattern, and dyspareunia. For those electing observation, however, long-term data are lacking regarding rates of subsequent symptom development, diverticulum enlargement, or eventual need for surgical excision.

Many practitioners may deliberate as to whether an enlarged inflamed cystic connection with the urethra is termed an "inflamed Skene gland cyst" or a "urethral diverticulum." Pragmatically, for those with persistent bothersome symptoms the treatment is the same, with surgical intervention often indicated. Procedures include diverticulectomy, transvaginal partial ablation, and marsupialization. Each is described in Chapter 45 (p. 1106).

Of these, *diverticulectomy* is the most frequently chosen to treat diverticula at any site along the urethra. This involves excision of the entire diverticulum and closure of the ostium

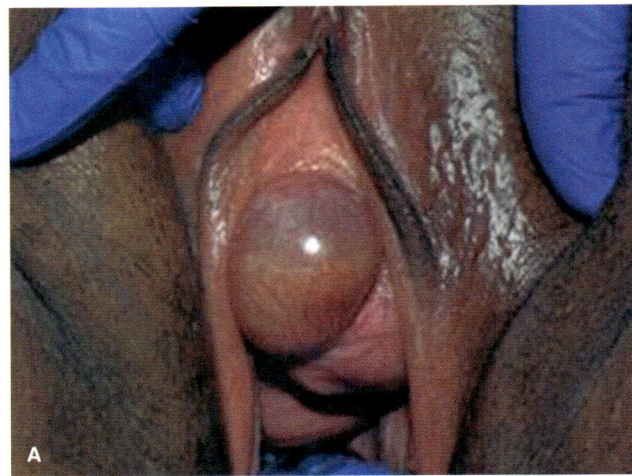

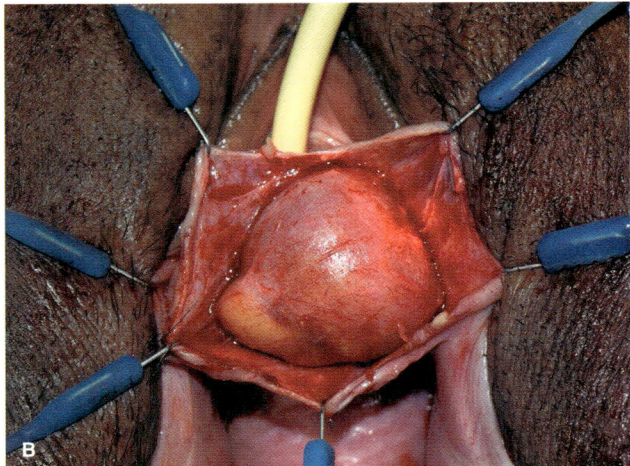

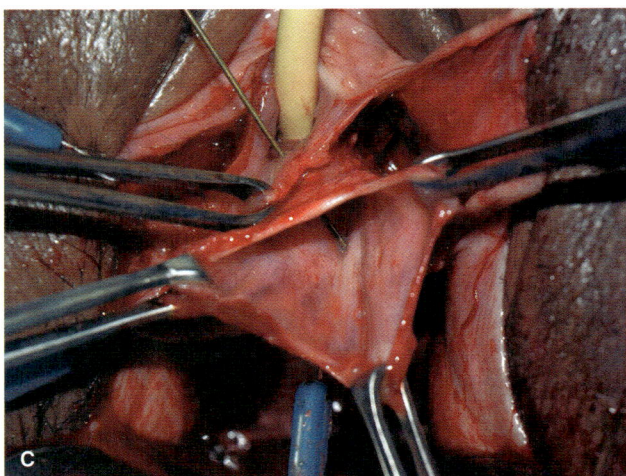

FIGURE 26-11 Diverticulectomy photographs. **A.** Urethral diverticulum. **B.** Anterior vaginal wall incised and self-retaining retractor used to expose the diverticulum. Foley catheter seen within the urethra. **C.** The diverticulum is opened. Passage of a lacrimal duct probe demonstrates the communication between the urethral lumen and the diverticular cavity.

and communication into the urethra (Fig. 26-11). The technique provides long-term correction of the urethral defect, normal urine stream, and high rates of postoperative continence. However, disadvantages include risks for postsurgical urethral stenosis, urethrovaginal fistula, injury to the urinary sphincter continence mechanism with subsequent incontinence, and recurrence. For patients who also have stress urinary incontinence, some practitioners recommend concomitant placement of either a midurethral or pubovaginal sling. As noted earlier, although this practice is supported by some studies, our preference is to approach it as a staged procedure (p. 581). We perform the defect repair first and later reassess the need for antiincontinence surgery.

Another surgery, *partial diverticular sac ablation,* may be preferred for proximal diverticula to avoid bladder entry or bladder neck injury. With this procedure, unneeded diverticular sac is excised, but the diverticular neck is not removed. Instead, the preserved diverticular sac tissue is reapproximated to close the defect (Tancer, 1983).

Last and less frequently, diverticulum marsupialization, also known as the Spence procedure, has been used for distal diverticula (Spence, 1970). The procedure is a meatotomy that when healed forms a new wider urethral meatus. Although simple to perform, this procedure alters the shape and function of the urethral meatus. Patients often note de novo spraying of their urine stream.

Other procedures described in case reports include urethroscopic transurethral electrosurgical fulguration of the diverticular sac and transurethral incision to widen the diverticular ostia (Miskowiak, 1989; Saito, 2000; Vergunst, 1996). Data are lacking, however, regarding long-term efficacy and complication rates with these techniques.

REFERENCES

Adetiloye VA, Dare FO: Obstetric fistula: evaluation with ultrasonography. J Ultrasound Med 19:243, 2000
Aldridge CW Jr, Beaton JH, Nanzig RP: A review of office urethroscopy and cystometry. Am J Obstet Gynecol 131:432, 1978
Andreoni C, Bruschini H, Truzzi JC, et al: Combined vaginoscopy-cystoscopy: a novel simultaneous approach improving vesicovaginal fistula evaluation. J Urol 170:2330, 2003
Arias BE, Ridgeway B, Barber MD: Complications of neglected vaginal pessaries: case presentation and literature review. Int Urogynecol J 19:1173, 2008
Athanasopoulos A, McGuire EJ: Urethral diverticulum: a new complication associated with tension-free vaginal tape. Urol Int 81(4):480, 2008
Baradaran N, Chiles LR, Freilich DA, et al: Female urethral diverticula in the contemporary era: is the classic triad of the "3Ds" still relevant? Urology 94: 53, 2016
Barr DB, Wilder LC, Caudill SP, et al: Urinary creatinine concentrations in the U.S. population: implications for urinary biologic monitoring measurements. Environ Health Perspect 113:192, 2005
Ba-Thike K, Than A, Nan O: Tuberculous vesico-vaginal fistula. Int J Gynaecol Obstet 37:127, 1992
Bengtson AM, Kopp D, Tang JH, et al: Identifying patients with vesicovaginal fistula at high risk of urinary incontinence after surgery. Obstet Gynecol 128(5):945, 2016
Billmeyer BR, Nygaard IE, Kreder KJ: Ureterouterine and vesicoureterovaginal fistulas as a complication of cesarean section. J Urol 165:1212, 2001
Blaivas JG: Vaginal flap urethral reconstruction: an alternative to the bladder flap neourethra. J Urol 141:542, 1989
Blaivas JG, Heritz DM, Romanzi LJ: Early versus late repair of vesicovaginal fistulas: vaginal and abdominal approaches. J Urol 153:1110, 1995
Blander DS, Rovner ES, Schnall MD, et al: Endoluminal magnetic resonance imaging in the evaluation of urethral diverticula in women. Urology 57:660, 2001
Brown HW, Wang L, Bunker CH, et al: Lower reproductive tract fistula repairs in inpatient US women, 1979–2006. Int Urogynecol J 23(4):403, 2012
Burrows LJ, Howden NL, Meyn L, et al: Surgical procedures for urethral diverticula in women in the United States, 1979–1997. Int Urogynecol J Pelvic Floor Dysfunct 16(2):158, 2005

Chan R, Rajanahally S, Hollander A, et al: Urethral diverticulum after midurethral sling erosion, excision, and subsequent management. Female Pelvic Med Reconstr Surg 21(1):e3, 2015
Chancellor MB, Liu JB, Rivas DA, et al: Intraoperative endo-luminal ultrasound evaluation of urethral diverticula. J Urol 153(1):72, 1995
Chi AM, Curran DS, Morgan DM, et al: Universal cystoscopy after benign hysterectomy: examining the effects of an institutional policy. Obstet Gynecol 127(2):369, 2016
Clayton M, Siami P, Guinan P: Urethral diverticular carcinoma. Cancer 70: 665, 1992
Clemens JQ, Bushman W: Urethral diverticulum following transurethral collagen injection. J Urol 166(2):626, 2001
Dakhil L: Urethrovaginal fistula: a rare complication of transurethral catheterization. Female Pelv Med Reconstr Surg 20: 293, 2014
Davis BL, Robinson DG: Diverticula of the female urethra: assay of 120 cases. J Urol 104:850, 1970
Davits RJ, Miranda SI: Conservative treatment of vesicovaginal fistulas by bladder drainage alone. Br J Urol 68:155, 1991
Duong TH, Gellasch TL, Adam RA: Risk factors for the development of vesicovaginal fistula after incidental cystotomy at the time of a benign hysterectomy. Am J Obstet Gynecol 201(5):512.e1, 2009
Eisen M, Jurkovic K, Altwein JE, et al: Management of vesicovaginal fistulas with peritoneal flap interposition. J Urol 112:195, 1974
Elkins TE: Surgery for the obstetric vesicovaginal fistula: a review of 100 operations in 82 patients. Am J Obstet Gynecol 170:1108, 1994
Elkins TE, Thompson JR: Lower urinary tract fistulas. In Walters MD, Karram MM (eds): Urogynecology and Reconstructive Pelvic Surgery. St. Louis, Mosby, 1999, p 355
El-Nashar SA, Bacon MM, Kim-Fine S, et al: Incidence of female urethral diverticulum: a population-based analysis and literature review. Int Urogynecol J 25(1):73, 2014
Emmert C, Kohler U: Management of genital fistulas in patients with cervical cancer. Arch Gynecol Obstet 259:19, 1996
Enemchukwu E, Lai C, Reynolds WS, et al: Autologous pubovaginal sling for the treatment of concomitant female urethral diverticula and stress urinary incontinence. Urology 85(6):1300, 2015
Evans LA, Ferguson KH, Foley JP, et al: Fibrin sealant for the management of genitourinary injuries, fistulas and surgical complications. J Urol 169:1360, 2003
Firoozi F, Ingber MS, Moore CK, et al: Purely transvaginal/perineal management of complications from commercial prolapse kits using a new prostheses/grafts complication classification system. J Urol 187(5):1674, 2012
Ganabathi K, Leach GE, Zimmern PE, et al: Experience with the management of urethral diverticulum in 63 women. J Urol 152:1445, 1994
Gerrard ER Jr, Lloyd LK, Kubricht WS, et al: Transvaginal ultrasound for the diagnosis of urethral diverticulum. J Urol 169:1395, 2003
Giles DL, Davila GW: Suprapubic-vaginocutaneous fistula 18 years after a bladder-neck suspension. Obstet Gynecol 105:1193, 2005
Ginsburg D, Genadry R: Suburethral diverticulum: classification and therapeutic considerations. Obstet Gynecol 61:685, 1983
Goh JT: A new classification for female genital tract fistula. Aust N Z J Obstet Gynaecol 44:502, 2004
Goh JT, Browning A, Berhan B, et al: Predicting the risk of failure of closure of obstetric fistula and residual urinary incontinence using a classification system. Int Urogynecol J Pelvic Floor Dysfunct 19(12):1659, 2008
Goh JT, Krause HG, Browning A, et al: Classification of female genito-urinary tract fistula: inter- and intra-observer correlations. J Obstet Gynaecol Res 35(1):160, 2009
Golomb J, Leibovitch I, Mor Y, et al: Comparison of voiding cystourethrography and double-balloon urethrography in the diagnosis of complex female urethral diverticula. Eur Radiol 13:536, 2003
Goodwin WE, Scardino PT: Vesicovaginal and ureterovaginal fistulas: a summary of 25 years of experience. J Urol 123:370, 1980
Graham JB: Painful syndrome of postradiation urinary-vaginal fistula. Surg Gynecol Obstet 124:1260, 1967
Harkki-Siren P, Sjoberg J, Tiitinen A: Urinary tract injuries after hysterectomy. Obstet Gynecol 92:113, 1998
Hilton P: Urogenital fistula in the UK: a personal case series managed over 25 years. BJU Int 110:102, 2012a
Hilton P, Cromwell DA: The risk of vesicovaginal and urethrovaginal fistula after hysterectomy performed in the English National Health Service—a retrospective cohort study examining patterns of care between 2000 and 2008. BJOG 119:1447, 2012b
Hilton P, Ward A: Epidemiological and surgical aspects of urogenital fistulae: a review of 25 years' experience in southeast Nigeria. Int Urogynecol J Pelvic Floor Dysfunct 9:189, 1998
Huffman JW: The detailed anatomy of the paraurethral ducts in the adult human female. Am J Obstet Gynecol 55:86, 1948

Kallol RK, Vaijyanath AM, Sinha A, et al: Sexual trauma—an unusual case of a vesicovaginal fistula. Eur J Obstet Gynecol 101:89, 2002

Keefe B, Warshauer DM, Tucker MS, et al: Diverticula of the female urethra: diagnosis by endovaginal and transperineal sonography. AJR Am J Roentgenol 156:1195, 1991

Kumar A, Goyal NK, Das SK, et al: Our experience with genitourinary fistulae. Urol Int 82(4):404, 2009

Kumar V, Abbas AK, Aster JC: Inflammation and repair. In Kumar V, Abbas AK, Fausto N (eds): Robbins and Cotran Pathologic Basis of Disease. St. Louis, Saunders, 2015

Lang EK, Davis HJ: Positive pressure urethrography: a roentgenographic diagnostic method for urethral diverticula in the female. Radiology 72:401, 1959

Leach GE, Bavendam TG: Female urethral diverticula. Urology 30:407, 1987

Leach GE, Sirls LT, Ganabathi K, et al: L N S C3: a proposed classification system for female urethral diverticula. Neurourol Urodyn 12:523, 1993

Lee D, Dillon BE, Lemack GE, et al: Long-term functional outcomes following nonradiated vesicovaginal repair. J Urol 191(1):120, 2014

Lee RA, Symmonds RE, Williams TJ: Current status of genitourinary fistula. Obstet Gynecol 72:313, 1988

Lentz SS: Transvaginal repair of the posthysterectomy vesicovaginal fistula using a peritoneal flap: the gold standard. J Reprod Med 50:41, 2005

Lorenzo AJ, Zimmern P, Lemack GE, et al: Endorectal coil magnetic resonance imaging for diagnosis of urethral and periurethral pathologic findings in women. Urology 61:1129, 2003

Martius H: Die operative Wiederherstellung der vollkommen fehlenden Harnrohre und des Schiessmuskels derselben. Zentralbl Gynak 52:480, 1928

Massengill JC, Baker TM, Von Pechmann WS, et al: Commonalities of cerclage-related genitourinary fistulas. Female Pelvic Med Reconstr Surg 18(6):362, 2012

McNally A: A diverticulum of the female urethra. Am J Surg 28:177, 1935

Miklos JR, Moore RD: Laparoscopic extravesical vesicovaginal fistula repair: our technique and 15-year experience. Int Urogynecol J 26(3):441, 2015

Miskowiak J, Honnens de Lichtenberg M: Transurethral incision of urethral diverticulum in the female. Scand J Urol Nephrol 23(3):235, 1989

Mohr S, Brandner S, Mueller MD, et al: Sexual function after vaginal and abdominal fistula repair. Am J Obstet Gynecol 211(1):74.e1, 2014

Moir JC: Vesico-vaginal fistulae as seen in Britain. J Obstet Gynaecol Br Commonw 80:598, 1973

Monteiro H, Nogueira R, de Carvalho H: Behçet's syndrome and vesicovaginal fistula: an unusual complication. J Urol 153:407, 1995

Neitlich JD, Foster HE Jr, Glickman MG, et al: Detection of urethral diverticula in women: comparison of a high resolution fast spin echo technique with double balloon urethrography. J Urol 159:408, 1998

Nitti VW, Tu LM, Gitlin J: Diagnosing bladder outlet obstruction in women. J Urol 161:1535, 1999

Oakley SH, Brown HW, Greer JA, et al: Management of vesicovaginal fistulae: a multicenter analysis from the Fellows' Pelvic Research Network. Female Pelvic Med Reconstr Surg 20(1):7, 2014

Ou CS, Huang UC, Tsuang M, et al: Laparoscopic repair of vesicovaginal fistula. J Laparoendosc Adv Surg Tech A 14:17, 2004

Pathi SD, Rahn DD, Sailors JL, et al: Utility of clinical parameters, cystourethroscopy, and magnetic resonance imaging in the preoperative diagnosis of urethral diverticula. Int Urogynecol J 24(2):319, 2013

Perlmutter S, Huang AB, Hon M, et al: Sonographic demonstration of calculi within a urethral diverticulum. Urology 42:735, 1993

Persky L, Herman G, Guerrier K: Nondelay in vesicovaginal fistula repair. Urology 13:273, 1979

Pruthi RS, Petrus CD, Bundrick WS Jr: New onset vesicovaginal fistula after transurethral collagen injection in women who underwent cystectomy and orthotopic neobladder creation: presentation and definitive treatment. J Urol 164:1638, 2000

Raassen TJ, Ngongo CJ, Mahendeka MM: Iatrogenic genitourinary fistula: an 18-year retrospective review of 805 injuries. Int Urogynecol J 25(12):1699, 2014

Ratner M, Siminovitch M, Ritz I: Diverticulum of the female urethra with multiple calculi. Can Med Assoc J 60:510, 1949

Romanzi LJ, Groutz A, Blaivas JG: Urethral diverticulum in women: diverse presentations resulting in diagnostic delay and mismanagement. J Urol 164:428, 2000

Romics I, Kelemen Z, Fazakas Z: The diagnosis and management of vesicovaginal fistulae. BJU Int 89:764, 2002

Routh A: Urethral diverticulum. BMJ 1:361, 1890

Rovner ES: Bladder and female urethral diverticula. In Wein AJ, Kavoussi LR, Novick AC, et al (eds): Campbell-Walsh Urology, 10th ed. Philadelphia, Saunders, 2012a

Rovner ES: Urinary tract fistulae. In Wein AJ, Kavoussi LR, Novick AC, et al (eds): Campbell-Walsh Urology, 10th ed. Philadelphia, Saunders, 2012b

Rovner ES, Wein AJ: Diagnosis and reconstruction of the dorsal or circumferential urethral diverticulum. J Urol 170:82, 2003

Saito S: Usefulness of diagnosis by the urethroscopy under anesthesia and effect of transurethral electrocoagulation in symptomatic female urethral diverticula. J Endourol 14:455, 2000

Schöller D, Brucker S, Reisenauer C: Management of urethral lesions and urethrovaginal fistula formation following placement of a tension-free suburethral sling: evaluation from a university continence and pelvic floor centre. Geburtshilfe Frauenheilkd 78(10):991, 2018

Shalev M, Mistry S, Kernen K, et al: Squamous cell carcinoma in a female urethral diverticulum. Urology 59:773, 2002

Shaw J, Tunitsky-Bitton E, Barber MD, et al: Ureterovaginal fistula: a case series. Int Urogynecol J 25(5):615, 2014

Shephard SN, Lengmang SJ, Kirschner CV: Bladder stones in vesicovaginal fistula: is concurrent repair an option? Experience with 87 patients. Int Urogynecol J 28(4):569, 2017

Spence HM, Duckett JW Jr: Diverticulum of the female urethra: clinical aspects and presentation of a simple operative technique for cure. J Urol 104:432, 1970

Stewart M, Bretland PM, Stidolph NE: Urethral diverticula in the adult female. Br J Urol 53:353, 1981

Summitt RL Jr, Stovall TG: Urethral diverticula: evaluation by urethral pressure profilometry, cystourethroscopy, and the voiding cystourethrogram. Obstet Gynecol 80:695, 1992

Swierzewski SJ 3rd, McGuire EJ: Pubovaginal sling for treatment of female stress urinary incontinence complicated by urethral diverticulum. J Urol 149:1012, 1993

Symmonds RE: Incontinence: vesical and urethral fistulas. Clin Obstet Gynecol 27:499, 1984

Tancer ML: Observations on prevention and management of vesicovaginal fistula after total hysterectomy. Surg Gynecol Obstet 175:501, 1992

Tancer ML, Mooppan MM, Pierre-Louis C, et al: Suburethral diverticulum treatment by partial ablation. Obstet Gynecol 62:511, 1983

Vakili B, Wai C, Nihira M: Anterior urethral diverticulum in the female: diagnosis and surgical approach. Obstet Gynecol 102:1179, 2003

Vargas-Serrano B, Cortina-Moreno B, Rodriguez-Romero R, et al: Transrectal ultrasonography in the diagnosis of urethral diverticula in women. J Clin Ultrasound 25:21, 1997

Vergunst H, Blom JH, De Spiegeleer AH, et al: Management of female urethral diverticula by transurethral incision. Br J Urol 77:745, 1996

Volkmer BG, Kuefer R, Nesslauer T, et al: Colour Doppler ultrasound in vesicovaginal fistulas. Ultrasound Med Biol 26:771, 2000

von Pechmann WS, Mastropietro MA, Roth TJ, et al: Urethral adenocarcinoma associated with urethral diverticulum in a patient with progressive voiding dysfunction. Am J Obstet Gynecol 188:1111, 2003

Waaldijk K: Surgical classification of obstetric fistulas. Int J Gynaecol Obstet 49:161, 1995

Waaldijk K: The immediate surgical management of fresh obstetric fistulas with catheter and/or early closure. Int J Gynaecol Obstet 45:11, 1994

Waaldijk K: The (surgical) management of bladder fistula in 775 women in northern Nigeria. Doctoral thesis, University of Utrecht, 1989, p 85

Wang Y, Hadley HR: Nondelayed transvaginal repair of high lying vesicovaginal fistula. J Urol 144:34, 1990

Wilson A, Truchanowicz EG, Elmoghazy D, et al: Symphysiotomy for obstructed labour: a systematic review and meta-analysis. BJOG 123(9):1453, 2016

World Health Organization: 10 facts on obstetric fistula. 2018. Available at: http://www.who.int/features/factfiles/obstetric_fistula/en. Accessed February 8, 2019

Yang JM, Huang WC, Yang SH: Transvaginal sonography in the diagnosis, management and follow-up of complex paraurethral abnormalities. Ultrasound Obstet Gynecol 25:302, 2005

Zimmern PE, Leach GE: Vesicovaginal fistula repair. Prob Urol 5:171, 1991

Zoubek J, McGuire EJ, Noll F, et al: The late occurrence of urinary tract damage in patients successfully treated by radiotherapy for cervical carcinoma. J Urol 141:1347, 1989

SECTION 3

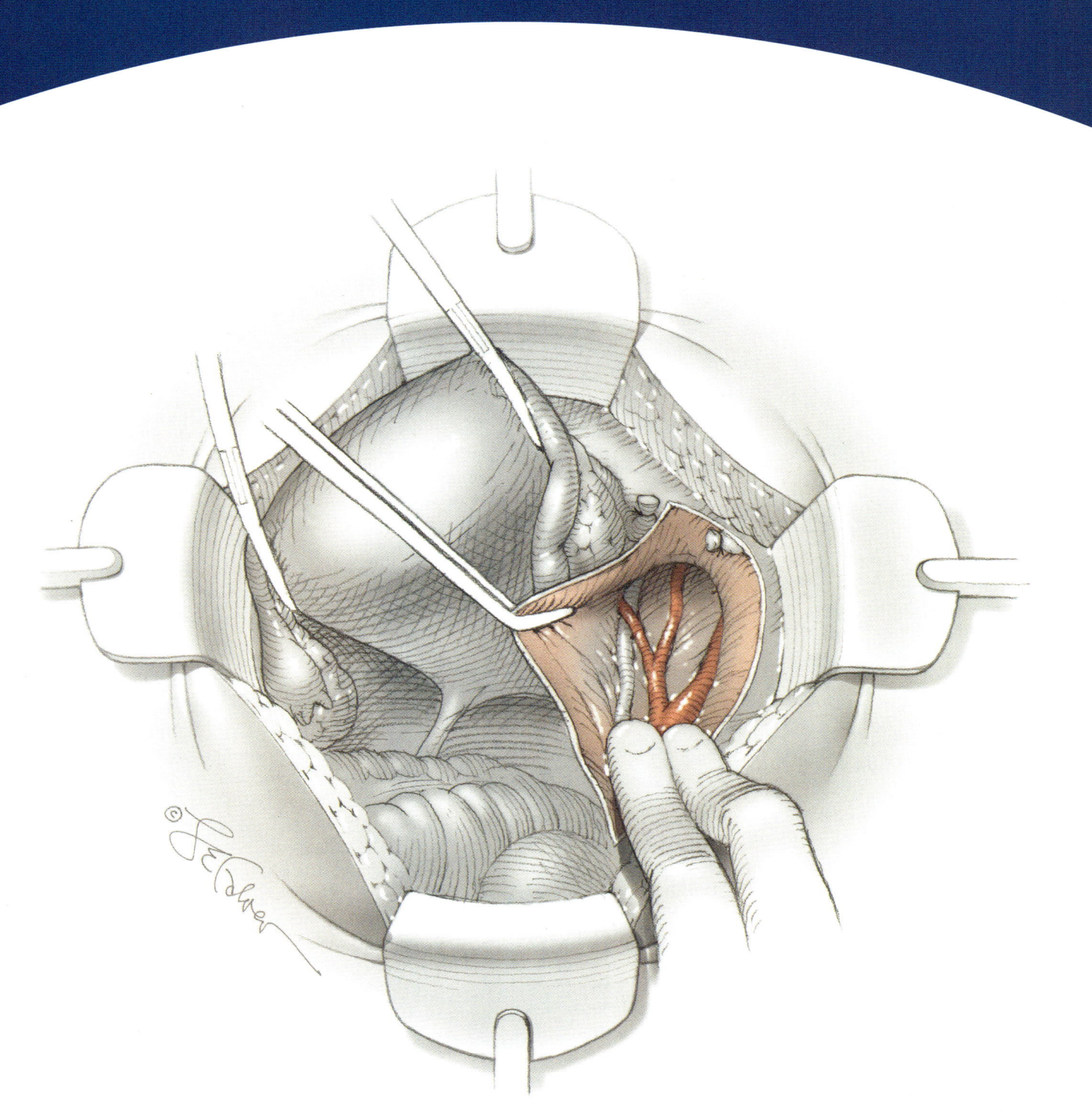

CHAPTER 27

Principles of Chemotherapy

BIOLOGY OF CANCER GROWTH

In principle, chemotherapeutic drugs are able to treat cancer and spare normal cells by exploiting inherent differences in their individual growth patterns. Each tumor type has its own characteristics, which explains why the same chemotherapy regimen is not equally effective for the whole spectrum of gynecologic cancers. Selecting appropriate drugs and limiting toxicity demands an understanding of cellular kinetics and biochemistry.

■ The Cell Cycle

All dividing cells follow the same basic sequence for replication. The *cell generation* time is the time required to complete the five phases of the cell cycle (Fig. 27-1). The G_1 phase (G = gap) involves various cellular activities, such as protein synthesis, RNA synthesis, and DNA repair. When this is prolonged, the cell is considered to be in the G_0 phase, that is, the resting phase. G_1 cells may either terminally differentiate into the G_0 phase or reenter the cell cycle after a period of quiescence. During the S phase, new DNA is synthesized. The G_2 (premitotic) phase is characterized by cells having twice the DNA content as they prepare for division. Finally, actual mitosis and chromosomal division take place during the M phase.

Tumors do not typically have faster generation times. They instead have many more cells in the active phases of replication and have dysfunctional apoptosis (programmed cell death). In contrast, normal tissues have a much larger number of cells in the G_0 phase. As a result, cancer cells proceeding through the cell cycle may be more sensitive to chemotherapeutic agents, whereas normal cells in G_0 are protected. This growth pattern disparity underlies the effectiveness of chemotherapeutic agents.

■ Cancer Cell Growth

Tumors are characterized by a *gompertzian growth* pattern. Namely, a tumor mass requires progressively longer times to double in size as it enlarges. When a cancer is microscopic and non-palpable, growth is exponential. However, as a tumor enlarges, the number of its cells undergoing replication decreases due to limitations in blood supply and increasing interstitial pressure.

When tumors are in the exponential phase of gompertzian growth, they should be more sensitive to chemotherapy because a larger percentage of cells are in the active phase of the cell cycle. For this reason, metastases should be more sensitive to chemotherapy than a large primary tumor. To capitalize on this potential benefit, advanced ovarian cancer is usually first treated with surgery to remove the primary tumor, debulk large masses, and leave only microscopic residual disease for the adjuvant chemotherapy to act on. In addition, when a tumor mass shrinks in response to treatment, the presumption is that a greater number of cells will enter the active phase of the cell cycle to accelerate growth. This larger percentage of replicating cells should also increase the sensitivity of a tumor to chemotherapy.

■ Doubling Time

The cell cycle generally refers to the activity of individual tumor cells. Instead, the *doubling time* refers to the time needed for the entire heterogeneous tumor mass to double in size. In humans, the doubling times of specific tumors vary greatly. The speed with which tumors grow and double in size is largely regulated by the number of cells that are actively dividing—known as the *growth fraction*. Typically, only a small percentage of the tumor will have cells that are rapidly proliferating. The remaining cells are in the G_0 resting phase. In general, tumors that are cured by chemotherapy are those with a high growth fraction, such as gestational trophoblastic neoplasia. When tumor volume is reduced by surgery or chemotherapy, the remaining tumor cells are theoretically propelled from the G_0 phase into the more vulnerable phases of the cell cycle, rendering them susceptible to chemotherapy.

■ Cell Kinetics

Chemotherapeutic agents typically work by first-order kinetics to kill a constant *fraction* of cells rather than a constant

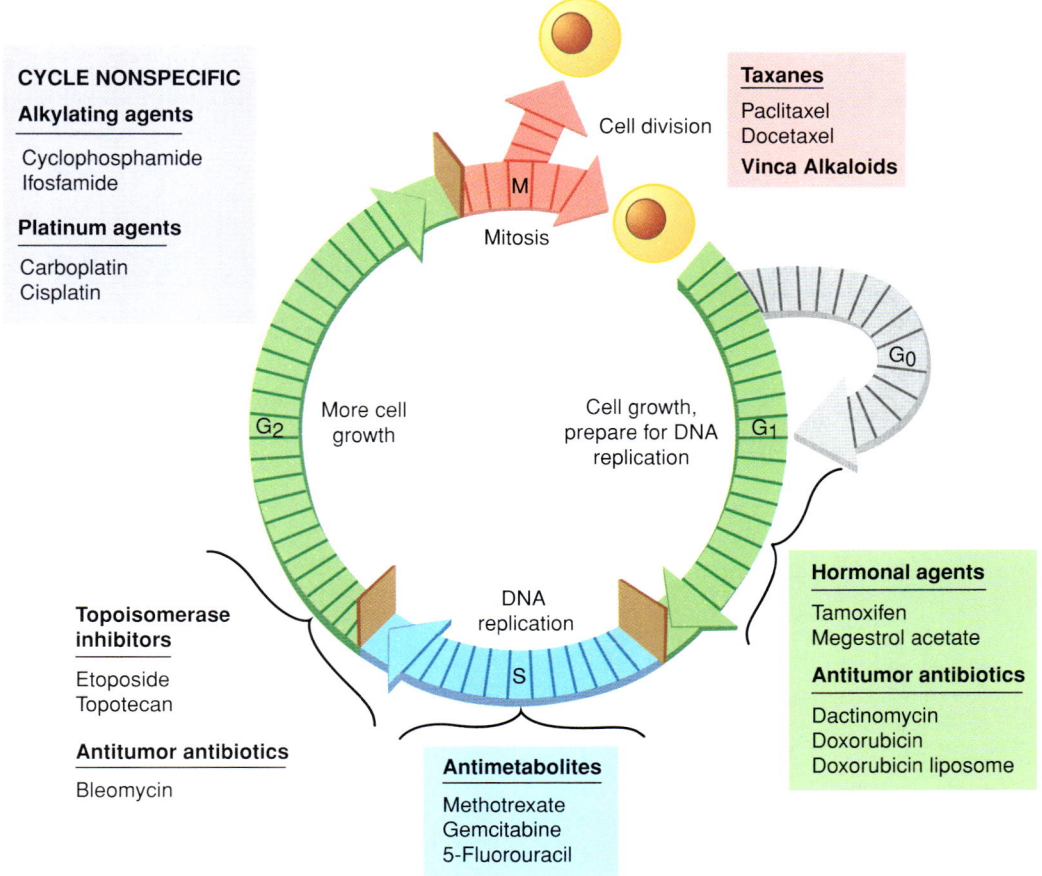

CYCLE NONSPECIFIC

Alkylating agents

Cyclophosphamide
Ifosfamide

Platinum agents

Carboplatin
Cisplatin

Taxanes

Paclitaxel
Docetaxel

Vinca Alkaloids

Hormonal agents

Tamoxifen
Megestrol acetate

Antitumor antibiotics

Dactinomycin
Doxorubicin
Doxorubicin liposome

Topoisomerase inhibitors

Etoposide
Topotecan

Antitumor antibiotics

Bleomycin

Antimetabolites

Methotrexate
Gemcitabine
5-Fluorouracil

Cell division

M

Mitosis

More cell growth

G_2

Cell growth, prepare for DNA replication

G_1

G_0

DNA replication

S

FIGURE 27-1 Diagram of the cell cycle. Agents are organized according to the cell cycle stage in which they are most effective for tumor control.

number. For example, one dose of a cytotoxic drug may result in a few logs (10^2 to 10^4) of cell kill. This, however, is not curative since tumor burden may be 10^{12} cells or more. Thus, the magnitude of cell kill necessary to eradicate a tumor typically requires intermittent courses of chemotherapy. In general, a cancer's curability is inversely proportional to the number of viable tumor cells at the beginning of chemotherapy.

Some drugs achieve cell kill at several phases of the cell cycle. These *cell cycle–nonspecific* agents act in all phases of replication from G_0 to the M phase. *Cell cycle–specific* agents act only on cells that are in a specific phase. By combining drugs that act in different phases of the cell cycle, the overall cell kill should be enhanced.

CLINICAL USE OF CHEMOTHERAPY

■ Clinical Setting

Chemotherapy may be used in at least five different ways. The term *induction chemotherapy* is defined as primary treatment for patients with an advanced malignancy when no feasible alternative treatment exists. *Adjuvant chemotherapy* is given to destroy remaining microscopic cells that may be present after the primary tumor is removed by surgery. *Neoadjuvant chemotherapy* refers to drug treatment directed at an advanced cancer to decrease preoperatively the extent or morbidity of a subsequent surgical resection. *Consolidation* (or *maintenance*) *chemotherapy*

is given after cancer has disappeared following the initial therapy and aims to prolong the duration of clinical remission or to prevent ultimate relapse. Therapy applied to recurrent disease or to a tumor that is refractory to initial treatment is termed *salvage* (or *palliative*) *chemotherapy*. In these incurable patients, the intent is to achieve tumor shrinkage or stability yet maintain quality of life.

In general, chemotherapy is used with either curative or palliative intent. When implementing chemotherapy with curative intent, the number of courses is typically predefined. Emphasis is placed on maintaining curative dosages and adhering closely to the treatment schedule. This may lead to significant toxicity and require growth-factor support to counter anemia or neutropenia. However, for the possibility of achieving cure, these side effects are typically deemed acceptable.

Chemotherapy is often not used with curative intent but is instead applied for effective, compassionate palliation. In this setting, greater importance is attached to avoiding excessive toxicity. Rather than a defined number of treatment courses, a clinician must frequently revisit treatment efficacy and alter the dosage and timing of chemotherapy administration accordingly.

■ Drug Regimens

With few exceptions, single drugs administered at clinically tolerable doses do not cure cancer. However, using two or more drugs simultaneously may greatly exacerbate toxicity. Thus, in principle, the goal of combination chemotherapy is to provide maximum cell kill with minimal or tolerable adverse patient side effects. Drugs are selected based on their proven efficacy as single agents, differing mechanisms of action, and toxicities that overlap minimally or not at all.

Combination chemotherapy is more effective in attacking heterogeneous populations of cells. Moreover, the use of multiple drugs with differing mechanisms tends to minimize the emergence of drug resistance. Typically, drugs used in combination should have clinical data indicating that their effects will be synergistic or at least additive. Drugs in combination are used at their optimal doses and schedules. Dose reductions initiated solely to allow the addition of other agents are counterproductive because most drugs must be used near their maximum tolerated dose to ensure efficacy.

Frequently, chemotherapy is combined with radiation therapy or sequenced with surgery. The goal of *chemoradiation* is to achieve local control by chemically rendering the tumor more sensitive to radiation. For example, care of locally advanced cervical cancer was transformed by adding weekly cisplatin to standard radiotherapy. In addition, concurrent chemotherapy is intended to treat micrometastases outside the radiation field.

However, patients recently treated with radiation therapy may have bone marrow, skin, or other body systems that are more susceptible to chemotherapy toxicity. As a result, dose reductions or delays are commonplace. Furthermore, chemotherapy is generally less effective in tumors that lie within a previously irradiated field due to increased fibrosis and capillary destruction.

Combining chemotherapy with surgery has many different applications. A woman with endometrial cancer may have nodal metastases detected during surgery. She may then receive pelvic radiation preceded or followed by combination chemotherapy. Alternatively, a woman with recurrent ovarian cancer may be treated by combination chemotherapy with or without preceding secondary cytoreductive surgery. Sequencing treatment in this way reduces tumor bulk and thereby augments chemotherapy effectiveness. In general, adjunctive therapy is begun within a few weeks after surgery. The short delay allows surgical healing.

■ Directing Care of the Patient

To effectively counsel a gynecologic cancer patient and then guide her chemotherapeutic treatment course requires a comprehensive understanding of the diagnosis, alternatives, and goals of care. As the intended therapy is finalized, extensive information regarding anticipated side effects and clarification of all potential logistical challenges (e.g., intravenous access) is provided to allay concerns. A consent form must be reviewed and signed by the patient.

Prior to drug infusion, a complete medical history and comprehensive physical examination are mandatory. Blood work, including a complete blood count, comprehensive metabolic panel, and tumor markers as indicated, is performed and reviewed before orders to begin infusion are signed. The setting for drug administration must provide staff that are immediately available should the need arise. Afterward, the patient is provided contact numbers in case of questions or problems.

Typically, regular office visits shortly before or on the day of treatment allow assessment of toxicity and general health. Patient examination and review of blood work results, in the context of the tumor response and overall treatment goals, will help determine whether drugs are changed or their dosages revised. Over time, the treatment strategy is continually reassessed as circumstances change.

PHARMACOLOGIC PRINCIPLES

■ Dosing and Dose Intensity

Overall, treatment effectiveness depends on drug concentration and duration of exposure to critical tumor sites. Chemotherapeutic agents typically have a narrow therapeutic range or "window." Thus, doses must be calculated accurately to achieve an optimal effect above a critical threshold yet avoid undue toxicity.

Most commonly, chemotherapy doses are calculated based on the patient's body surface area (BSA), and doses are expressed in milligrams per meter squared (mg/m^2). BSA uses height and weight and is a better indicator of metabolic mass than body weight because it is less affected by abnormal adipose mass. Although height is a fixed variable, patient weights are obtained prior to every therapy course, as they may fluctuate significantly. Rarely, tissue edema or ascites must be factored, since doses should be based on weight without this coexisting fluid. The BSA is most often calculated by using a nomogram (standard reference graph table). Consistent derivation of the BSA at each visit is important, and various calculators are routinely available via software or online. "Normal" adult BSA for women approximates $1.7\ m^2$.

The dosing of some drugs differs from the above. For example, bevacizumab is a monoclonal antibody metabolized and eliminated via the reticuloendothelial system. It is dosed only by patient weight (mg/kg). For renally excreted drugs, such as carboplatin, dosing may be based on an estimate of the glomerular filtration rate (Calvert formula).

The amount of drug administered over time is known as the dose intensity. Its primary importance is in highly responsive tumors, in which cure can be achieved with chemotherapy. However, in less-sensitive tumors, it may not be possible to increase the dose to a level sufficient to produce demonstrable benefit without producing dose-limiting toxicity. On the other hand, reducing dose intensity to lower toxicity can produce inferior therapeutic results.

■ Administration Route and Excretion

In gynecologic oncology, chemotherapy drugs are provided orally in an increasing number, rarely subcutaneously (SC), and occasionally intramuscularly (IM). Most are given by an intravenous (IV) route. During IV administration, several drugs known as *vesicants* require special care (Table 27-1). Extravasation of these into the subcutaneous tissue can result in severe pain and necrosis. These drugs require slow infusion either through a rapidly flowing peripheral IV catheter or preferably via a central venous catheter. If extravasation is suspected, the infusion is immediately stopped, the affected arm elevated, and ice packs applied. In severe cases, a plastic surgeon is consulted.

TABLE 27-1. Chemotherapeutic Agents and Their Association with Extravasation Injury

Vesicants	Exfoliants	Irritants	Inflammants	Neutral
Dactinomycin	Cisplatin	Carboplatin	Methotrexate	Bleomycin
Doxorubicin	Docetaxel	Etoposide		Cyclophosphamide
Paclitaxel	Liposomal doxorubicin			Gemcitabine
	Topotecan			Ifosfamide

Vesicant, agent capable of causing skin ulceration and tissue necrosis on extravasation; *exfoliant*, agent capable of causing skin exfoliation on extravasation; *irritant*, agent capable of causing skin irritation on extravasation; *inflammant*, agent capable of causing skin inflammation on extravasation.
Adapted with permission from Gershenson DM, McGuire WP, Gore M, et al (eds): Gynecologic Cancer Controversies in Management. Philadelphia, Elsevier, 2004.

Regional chemotherapy delivers drugs directly into the cavity in which the tumor is located. Clearance for many agents from a body cavity is slower than from systemic circulation. As a result, cancer cells are exposed longer to higher concentrations of active agents. This technique has been most extensively studied in ovarian cancer, in which tumors are usually confined to the intraperitoneal (IP) space. Clinical studies have uniformly demonstrated a pharmacologic advantage favoring administration into the IP compartment. However, penetration into peritoneal tumor nodules by passive diffusion can be limited by intraabdominal adhesions, poor fluid circulation, fibrotic tumor encapsulation, and coexisting ascites. Because of these limitations in drug penetration, IP chemotherapy is typically administered postoperatively to women with minimal residual disease. As a variation, heated chemotherapy may further improve absorption by tumors and destroy microscopic cancer cells. Hyperthermic intraperitoneal chemotherapy (HIPEC) involves heating the solution and circulating it throughout the abdomen for 1.5 hours at the completion of debulking surgery. The solution is then drained before closing the incision.

Drug inactivation, elimination, or excretion dramatically influences activity and toxicity. For the most part, this takes place primarily via the liver or kidneys. As a result, drug activity may be diminished and toxicity exacerbated when normal hepatic or renal function is impaired. In addition, drug toxicity is often more pronounced in the elderly or malnourished. For example, a low serum creatinine level in cachectic women may not accurately reflect underlying renal function. If a carboplatin dose is calculated using this falsely low value, the amount may be excessive and result in considerable morbidity. Instead, a preset creatinine level may need to be selected (0.8 or 1.0 mg/dL) to aid safer dosing in some patients.

■ Drug Interactions and Allergic Reaction

Most women who receive chemotherapy are prescribed medication for other noncancerous conditions. Moreover, women also often receive analgesics, antiemetics, and antibiotics during chemotherapy. Most drug interactions are of little consequence, but some may lead to substantially altered drug toxicity. Drugs that are metabolized in the liver are particularly at risk for such interactions. For example, using methotrexate in a woman taking warfarin (Coumadin) will usually enhance the anticoagulant effect and thus will require a warfarin dose reduction.

An anaphylactic, allergic, or hypersensitivity reaction during or after administration of chemotherapy may develop, despite patient history review and administration of prophylactic medications. Accordingly, a trained nursing staff and resources to manage these sudden, but common, issues are required. Prior to drug administration, the patient is instructed to report symptoms that may herald an anaphylactic reaction such as flushing, pruritus, dyspnea, tachycardia, hoarseness, or lightheadedness. Emergency equipment that includes supplemental oxygen, ventilatory face mask and bag, or intubation equipment must be immediately available. For a localized hypersensitivity response, administration of intravenous diphenhydramine (Benadryl) and/or corticosteroids may be sufficient. However, for a generalized hypersensitivity or anaphylactic response, chemotherapy should be stopped immediately, the emergency team notified, and emergency drugs administered, such as epinephrine (1 to 5 mL of a 0.1/mL solution [1:10,000 solution]) (Table 27-2).

■ Drug Resistance

In principle, larger tumor masses have a greater proportion of cells that have already developed intrinsic or acquired resistance to one drug or to multiple agents. Intrinsic drug resistance is seen if tumors are first exposed to an agent and fail to respond. In contrast, with acquired drug resistance, tumors no longer respond to drugs to which they were initially sensitive. Sometimes, this develops with a specific drug. More often, however, acquired resistance is "pleiotropic," meaning that a cancer is resistant to multiple chemotherapy agents. Advanced ovarian cancer is a good example. Most patients will initially achieve remission with platinum-based chemotherapy, but 80 percent will ultimately relapse and die from tumors that have become resistant to all cytotoxic therapy.

■ Evaluating Response to Chemotherapy

The effective use of chemotherapy is a dynamic process in which a treating clinician is constantly weighing toxicity to the patient against tumor response. In counseling women to continue treatment or switch to a different regimen, a clinician must have objective criteria for response (Table 27-3) (Eisenhauer, 2009).

TABLE 27-2. Management of Hypersensitivity Reactions

1. Stop the chemotherapy infusion
2. Assess the patient's airway, breathing, and circulation
3. Administer intravenous normal saline if hypotensive
4. Administer oxygen if dyspneic or hypoxic
5. Administer intravenous antihistamine (e.g., 50 mg intravenous diphenhydramine or 25–50 mg intravenous promethazine)
6. Administer 5 mg of nebulized salbutamol if the patient has bronchospasm
7. Administer intravenous corticosteroids (e.g., 100 mg of hydrocortisone); this may have no effect on the initial reaction, but may prevent rebound or prolonged allergic manifestations
8. If the patient does not promptly improve or has symptoms of persistent or severe hypotension or persistent bronchospasm or laryngeal edema, administer adrenaline or epinephrine (0.1–0.25 mg intravenous); further acute resuscitation measures may be required
9. Reassure the patient that the problem is a recognized and treatable one

Adapted with permission from Gershenson DM, McGuire WP, Gore M, et al (eds): Gynecologic Cancer Controversies in Management. Philadelphia, Elsevier, 2004.

The most important indicator is the *complete response rate*. For ovarian cancer, this would include normal CA125 levels (usually <35 U/mL), physical examination findings, and imaging test results. Ultimately, women who have any possibility of cure are those who first achieve a complete response. However, if chemotherapy results in a partial response, many women still view this as advantageous compared with supportive care, even if a survival benefit is unproven.

CHEMOTHERAPEUTIC DRUGS

■ Antimetabolites

The antimetabolites are analogues of naturally occurring components of the metabolic pathways that lead to the synthesis of purines, pyrimidines, and nucleic acids. In most cases, they are S phase–specific agents that are most effective in rapidly growing tumors associated with short doubling times and large growth fractions (Table 27-4).

Methotrexate

This antimetabolite is U.S. Food and Drug Administration (FDA)-approved for treatment of women with gestational trophoblastic neoplasia (GTN). It is also commonly used for the medical management of ectopic pregnancy. Methotrexate (MTX) tightly binds to dihydrofolate reductase, blocking the reduction of dihydrofolate to tetrahydrofolate (the active form of folic acid) (Fig. 27-2). As a result, thymidylate synthetase

and various steps in de novo purine synthesis are halted. This leads to arrest of DNA, RNA, and protein synthesis.

Most commonly, single-agent treatment of GTN involves MTX given IM as an 8-day regimen of 1 mg/kg on treatment days 1, 3, 5, and 7. Alternatively, a daily dose of 0.4 mg/kg is given for 5 days every 2 weeks. Combination therapy for high-risk disease includes 100 mg/m^2 MTX given IV over 30 minutes, followed by a 200 mg/m^2 IV dose over 12 hours. With MTX, patients are counseled to avoid folate-containing supplements unless specifically directed.

MTX causes few side effects at typical doses. However, at high doses, although used infrequently, this agent can lead to fatal bone marrow toxicity. This toxicity can be prevented by "rescue" doses of leucovorin. Leucovorin is folinic acid, has activity that is equivalent to folic acid, and thus is readily converted to tetrahydrofolate. Leucovorin, however, does not require dihydrofolate reductase for its conversion. Therefore, its function is unaffected by inhibition of this enzyme by MTX. Leucovorin administration, therefore, allows for some purine and pyrimidine synthesis. Leucovorin rescue is incorporated into the 8-day alternating MTX schedule, and a 0.1-mg/kg leucovorin dose is provided orally on treatment days 2, 4, 6, and 8.

In addition to myelosuppression, renal toxicity and acute cerebral dysfunction are typically only seen at high MTX doses. Methotrexate is predominantly excreted through the kidneys, and thus women with renal insufficiency have doses reduced. Serum MTX levels are carefully monitored in these patients, as they may require prolonged leucovorin rescue.

TABLE 27-3. Clinical End Points in Evaluating Response to Chemotherapy

End Point	Definition
Complete response (CR)	Disappearance of all measurable "target" lesions
Partial response (PR)	A decrease of ≥30% in the sum of diameters of all target lesions
Progressive disease (PD)	An increase of ≥20% in the sum of diameters of target lesions or the identification of one or more new lesions
Stable disease (SD)	Neither sufficient shrinkage to qualify for PR, nor sufficient increase to qualify for PD

TABLE 27-4. Chemotherapy Antimetabolites Used for Gynecologic Cancer

Generic Name	Brand Name	Indications	Routes	Common Dosages	Common Toxicity
Methotrexate	Trexall, Rheumatrex	GTN	PO, IM, IV, intrathecal	IM: 1 mg/kg on days 1, 3, 5, 7 or 0.4 mg/kg on days 1–5, every 2 wk IV: 100 mg/m² during 30 min, then 200 mg/m² during 12 hr	BMD, mucositis, renal toxicity, CNS dysfunction
Gemcitabine	Gemzar	Recurrent ovarian CA, uterine sarcoma	IV	600–1250 mg/m²/wk over 30 min × 2–3 wk	BMD, N/V/D, malaise and fever
5-Fluorouracil	Adrucil	Cervical CA, vulvar CA	IV	800–1000 mg/m²/d during 96 hr	Mucositis, PPE
	Efudex	VAIN	Vaginal cream	3 mL QOD × 1 wk, then weekly up to 10 wk	Vulvovaginal irritation

BMD = bone marrow depression; CA = cancer; CNS = central nervous system; GTN = gestational trophoblastic neoplasia; IM = intramuscular; IV = intravenous; N/V/D = nausea, vomiting, and diarrhea; PPE = palmar-plantar erythrodysesthesia; PO = orally; QOD = every other day; VAIN = vaginal intraepithelial neoplasia.

Gemcitabine

This antimetabolite is FDA approved to be used with other agents for treatment of recurrent ovarian cancer but is also commonly used for uterine sarcoma. Gemcitabine (Gemzar) is a synthetic nucleoside analogue that undergoes multiple phosphorylations to form the active metabolite. The resulting triphosphate is subsequently incorporated into DNA as a fraudulent base pair. Following the insertion of gemcitabine, one additional deoxynucleotide is added to the end of the DNA chain before replication is terminated, and DNA synthesis is thereby halted.

The usual administration of gemcitabine is by 30-minute infusion. Longer durations, such as those greater than 60 minutes, are associated with increased toxicity due to intracellular accumulation of the triphosphate. Depending on whether it is used as a single agent or in combination, gemcitabine is typically given at doses between 600 and 1000 mg/m² once weekly for 2 weeks, followed by a week off therapy.

Myelosuppression, especially neutropenia, is the main dose-limiting side effect. Gastrointestinal (GI) toxicity, such as nausea, vomiting, diarrhea, or mucositis, also is common. Approximately 20 percent of patients will develop a flulike syndrome, including fever, malaise, headache, and chills. Pulmonary toxicity is infrequent, but reported.

5-Fluorouracil

5-Fluorouracil (5-FU) is not FDA approved for gynecologic cancer but is occasionally paired with cisplatin during chemoradiation for cervical cancer. A topical form (Efudex) can be used for vaginal intraepithelial neoplasia (VAIN) treatment (Chap. 29, p. 642). This "false" pyrimidine antimetabolite acts principally as a thymidine synthetase inhibitor to block DNA replication.

Systemic 5-FU (Adrucil) is usually given as a 96-hour continuous IV infusion of 800 to 1000 mg/m²/d. Mucositis and/or diarrhea may be severe and dose-limiting. Hand-foot syndrome (palmar-plantar erythrodysesthesia), described later, is less common but also can be dose-limiting (p. 596). Myelosuppression, mainly neutropenia and thrombocytopenia, are less frequent. Nausea and vomiting are usually mild.

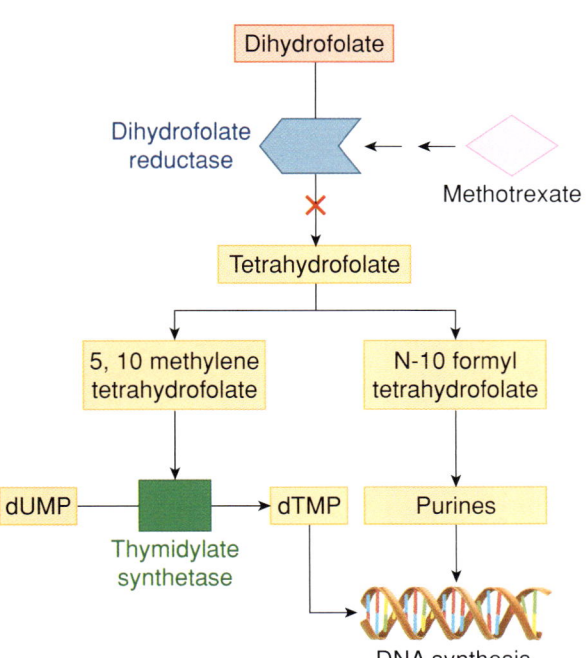

FIGURE 27-2 Methotrexate's primary target is the enzyme dihydrofolate reductase (DHFR). Inhibition of DHFR leads to partial depletion of 5,10 methylene tetrahydrofolate and N-10 formyl tetrahydrofolate, which are cofactors required for the respective synthesis of thymidylate and purines. As a result, methotrexate leads to arrested DNA, RNA, and protein synthesis. dTMP = deoxythymidine monophosphate; dUMP = deoxyuridine monophosphate.

TABLE 27-5. Chemotherapy Alkylating Agents Used for Gynecologic Cancer

Generic Name	Brand Name	Indication	Routes	Dosages	Toxicity
Cyclophosphamide	Cytoxan	GTN, recurrent ovarian CA	PO, IV	IV: 500–750 mg/m^2 over 30 min, every 3 wk PO: 50 mg/d	BMD, cystitis, N/V, alopecia
Ifosfamide	Ifex	Recurrent ovarian CA, cervical CA, uterine sarcoma	IV	1.2–1.6 g/m^2/d, days 1–3 of 3-wk cycle	BMD, cystitis, N/V, alopecia, CNS and renal toxicity

BMD = bone marrow depression; CA = cancer; CNS = central nervous system; GTN = gestational trophoblastic neoplasia; IV = intravenous; N/V = nausea and vomiting; PO = orally.

■ Alkylating Agents

Cyclophosphamide

The class of alkylating agents is characterized by positively charged alkyl groups that bind to negatively charged DNA to form adducts (Table 27-5). Binding leads to DNA breaks or cross-links and a halt to DNA synthesis. In general, these drugs are cell cycle–nonspecific agents.

Of alkylating agents, cyclophosphamide (Cytoxan) is FDA approved by itself or in combination for epithelial ovarian cancer treatment. Cyclophosphamide is the "C" of EMA-CO (etoposide, methotrexate, actinomycin D, cyclophosphamide, Oncovin [vincristine]), which is a regimen prescribed for high-risk GTN. It is also used as salvage therapy for recurrent epithelial ovarian cancer (Bower, 1997; Cantu, 2002). Cyclophosphamide is a derivative of nitrogen mustard and is activated through a multistep process by microsomal enzymes in the liver. It promotes DNA cross-linking and DNA synthesis inhibition.

It is typically given IV at doses of 500 to 750 mg/m^2 over 30 minutes every 3 weeks. Orally, a metronomic (repetitive low-dose) regimen of 50 mg daily is often used to minimize toxicity and target the tumor endothelium or stroma in combination with a biologic agent, such as bevacizumab (Chura, 2007).

Myelosuppression, mainly neutropenia, is the usual dose-limiting side effect. Cyclophosphamide is excreted exclusively by the kidneys. One of its metabolites, acrolein, can alkylate and inflame the bladder mucosa. As a result, hemorrhagic cystitis is a classic complication that may follow from 24 hours to several weeks after administration. To prevent this effect, adequate hydration is imperative to aid acrolein excretion. In addition, GI toxicity, such as nausea, vomiting, or anorexia, is common. Alopecia is typically severe. Moreover, later secondary malignancy rates are increased, particularly acute myelogenous leukemia and bladder cancer.

Of chemotherapeutic drugs, alkylating agents are believed to be particularly damaging to ovarian function. Preventatively, adjuvant gonadotropin-releasing hormone (GnRH) agonists may lower rates of chemotherapy-induced ovarian failure, although the efficacy of this approach remains controversial (Chen, 2011; Elgindy, 2013). Importantly, advances in oocyte and ovarian tissue cryopreservation make it likely that the removal of oocytes prior to treatment will become the preferred approach when feasible (Chap. 21, p. 468).

Ifosfamide

This alkylating agent is not FDA approved for gynecologic cancers but is occasionally administered for salvage treatment of cervical cancer and uterine sarcoma. Ifosfamide (Ifex) is a structural analogue of cyclophosphamide, differing only slightly. However, its metabolic activation occurs more slowly and leads to a greater production of chloracetaldehyde, a possible neurotoxin.

Ifosfamide is administered IV, usually as a short infusion. Common doses of 1.2 to 1.6 g/m^2 are given on days 1 through 3 of a 3-week cycle. As with cyclophosphamide, adequate hydration is recommended to reduce the incidence of drug-induced hemorrhagic cystitis. In addition, concurrent mesna (Mesnex) is used to prevent severe hematuria. A mesna metabolite chemically binds with acrolein, an ifosfamide metabolite, and detoxifies acrolein in the bladder. Other side effects are similar to those of cyclophosphamide. However, neurotoxicity, manifested as lethargy, confusion, seizure, ataxia, hallucinations, and occasionally coma, is more likely. These symptoms are caused by the chloracetaldehyde metabolite and are reversible with removal of the drug and supportive care. The incidence of neurotoxicity is higher in the rare patient receiving high-dose therapy and also in those with impaired renal function. With the latter, a preventive dose reduction is typically necessary.

■ Antitumor Antibiotics

Dactinomycin

The antitumor antibiotics are generally derived from microorganisms. Most antitumor antibiotics exert their cytotoxic effects by DNA intercalation during multiple phases of the cell cycle. They are considered cell cycle specific.

In this group, dactinomycin is FDA approved to treat GTN as a single agent or as part of combination chemotherapy (Table 27-6). Dactinomycin (Cosmegen), also known as actinomycin D, is the "A" of the EMA-CO chemotherapy combination. Dactinomycin becomes anchored into purine-pyrimidine DNA base pairs, resulting in DNA synthesis inhibition. It also produces toxic oxygen free radicals that cause DNA breaks. Dactinomycin is excreted mainly through the biliary system.

The usual "pulse" dosage of dactinomycin is 1.25 mg IV push every other week, but it is sometimes administered as a 0.5-mg dose on days 1 through 5 every 2 to 3 weeks. Myelosuppression is the main dose-limiting side effect and may be severe.

TABLE 27-6. Chemotherapeutic Antibiotics Used for Gynecologic Cancer

Generic Name	Brand Name	Indication	Route	Dosage	Toxicity
Actinomycin D (dactinomycin)	Cosmegen	GTN	IV	1.25 mg IV push every other wk or 0.5 mg on days 1–5, every 2–3 wk	BMD, N/V/D, alopecia, vesicant
Bleomycin	Blenoxane	Germ cell or SCST ovarian CA, GTN	IV, IM, SC, intrapleural	IV: 20 U/m^2 (maximum dose of 30 U), every 3 wk	Pulmonary toxicity, fever, skin reaction
Doxorubicin	Adriamycin	Uterine sarcoma, recurrent epithelial ovarian CA	IV	45–60 mg/m^2 every 3 wk	BMD, cardiac toxicity, alopecia, vesicant
Liposomal doxorubicin	Doxil	Recurrent epithelial ovarian CA	IV	40–50 mg/m^2 over 30 min, every 4 wk	PPE, stomatitis, infusion reaction

BMD = bone marrow depression; CA = cancer; GTN = gestational trophoblastic neoplasia; IM = intramuscular; IV = intravenous; N/V/D = nausea, vomiting, and diarrhea; PPE = palmar-plantar erythrodysesthesia; SC = subcutaneous; SCST = sex cord-stromal tumor.

Moreover, GI toxicity, including nausea, vomiting, mucositis, and diarrhea, is often significant. Alopecia is common. As with others in the antibiotic group, dactinomycin is a potent vesicant (see Table 27-1).

Bleomycin

This antitumor antibiotic is FDA approved for malignant pleural effusion treatment or for palliative therapy of recurrent squamous cervical or vulvar cancer. An off-label use includes bleomycin as the "B" in BEP (bleomycin, etoposide, cisplatin) regimens, which are used as adjuvant treatment of malignant ovarian germ cell or sex cord–stromal tumors (Park, 2012; Weinberg, 2011). Additionally, it is used in GTN salvage treatment (Alazzam, 2016). Bleomycin (Blenoxane), when complexed with iron, creates activated oxygen free radicals, which cause DNA strand breaks and cell death. It is maximally effective during the G$_2$ phase.

The usual dosage of bleomycin is 20 units/m^2 given IV every 3 weeks. Bleomycin can also be administered IM, SC, or intrapleurally. The dose is quantified by international units of "cytotoxic activity."

Pulmonary toxicity is the main dose-limiting side effect, developing in 10 percent of patients and causing death in 1 percent. Accordingly, for women prescribed bleomycin, chest radiographs and pulmonary function tests (PFTs) are performed at baseline and obtained regularly before every one or two treatment cycles. The most important PFT measurement is the diffusing capacity of the lung for carbon monoxide (DLCO). The DLCO measures the ability to transfer oxygen from the lungs to the blood stream. If the DLCO declines by 15 to 30 percent, it indicates development of restrictive lung disease. In patients receiving bleomycin, therapy may then be stopped before the onset of symptomatic pulmonary fibrosis. Fibrosis often presents clinically as pneumonitis with cough, dyspnea, dry inspiratory crackles, and infiltrates on chest radiograph. Bleomycin is not myelosuppressive. However, skin reactions are common and include hyperpigmentation or erythema.

Doxorubicin

This antitumor antibiotic is FDA approved to treat epithelial ovarian cancer, but doxorubicin (Adriamycin) is more frequently used for uterine sarcoma (Hyman, 2014; Mancari, 2014). This agent intercalates into DNA to inhibit DNA synthesis, inhibits topoisomerase II, and forms cytotoxic oxygen free radicals. The drug is metabolized extensively in the liver and eliminated through biliary excretion.

The usual dose of doxorubicin is 45 to 60 mg/m^2 IV, repeated every 3 weeks. Myelosuppression, particularly neutropenia, is the main dose-limiting side effect. However, cardiotoxicity is a classic complication. Patients are monitored with a multiple-gated acquisition (MUGA) radionuclide scan at baseline and periodically during therapy. The risk of cardiotoxicity is higher in women older than 70 and those with cumulative doses exceeding 550 mg/m^2. Ultimately, women may develop an irreversible dilated cardiomyopathy associated with congestive heart failure. Gastrointestinal toxicities are generally mild, but alopecia is universal.

Doxorubicin Liposome

This antitumor antibiotic is FDA approved and commonly used for the salvage treatment of recurrent epithelial ovarian cancer (Gordon, 2004). The liposomal encapsulation of doxorubicin (Doxil) dramatically alters the pharmacokinetic and toxicity profiles of the drug. Researchers developed liposomal doxorubicin to reduce cardiotoxicity and to selectively target tumor tissues.

Liposomal doxorubicin may be administered as an IV infusion over 30 to 60 minutes and is dosed at 40 to 50 mg/m^2 every 4 weeks. In contrast to doxorubicin, administration of the encapsulated liposome is associated with minimal nausea, vomiting, alopecia, and cardiotoxicity. Infusion-related reactions develop in less than 10 percent of patients and are most common during the first treatment course. However, an increased rate of stomatitis and palmar-plantar erythrodysesthesia (PPE) is noted.

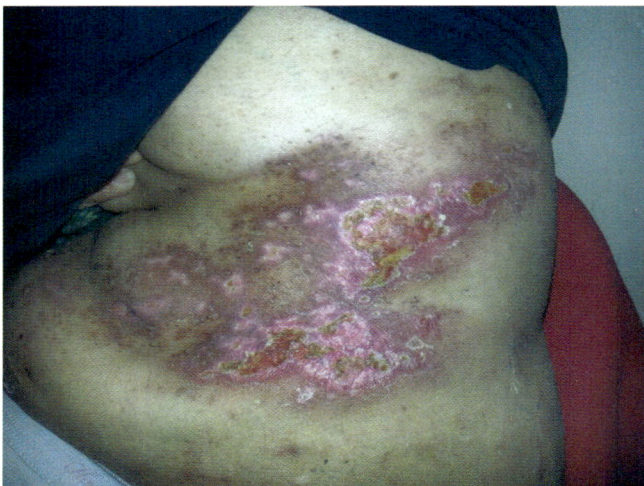

FIGURE 27-3 Erythematous plaques of palmar-plantar erythro-dysesthesia (PPE) on the lateral aspect of the abdomen.

PPE is characterized by a cutaneous reaction of varying intensity (Fig. 27-3). Patients may initially complain of tingling sensations on their soles and palms that generally progress to swelling and tenderness to touch. Erythematous plaques typically develop that can become extremely painful and often lead to desquamation and skin cracking. Symptoms result from the prolonged blood levels of this time-released cytotoxic agent and may last several weeks.

■ Plant-Derived Agents

Taxanes

The cytotoxic activity of all the plant-derived agents stems from the disturbance of normal assembly, disassembly, and stabilization of intracellular microtubules to halt cell division during mitosis (Fig. 27-4). The group includes the taxanes, vinca alkaloids, and topoisomerase inhibitors.

Of the taxanes, paclitaxel and docetaxel are both cell cycle–specific agents that have maximal activity during the M phase (Table 27-7). Derived from yew tree species, they act to "poison" the mitotic spindle by preventing depolymerization of the microtubules and inhibiting cellular replication.

Paclitaxel. This agent is FDA approved for the treatment of primary or recurrent epithelial ovarian cancer. It is also extensively used for endometrial cancer, cervical cancer, and occasionally GTN.

Paclitaxel (Taxol) is typically administered IV as a 3-hour infusion but may also be given as an intraperitoneal (IP) dose. The usual IV dosage is 135 to 175 mg/m² every 3 weeks. Weekly paclitaxel is also effective in a regimen of 80 mg/m² IV for 3 consecutive weeks on a 21-day schedule for primary disease or on a 28-day schedule for recurrent disease (Katsumata, 2009; Markman, 2006). For initial therapy of optimally debulked ovarian cancer following a day 1 IV dose, paclitaxel is usually given IP on day 8 at a dose of 60 mg/m² (Armstrong, 2006).

Myelosuppression is the usual dose-limiting side effect. Additionally, a hypersensitivity reaction occurs in approximately one third of patients due to its formulation in Cremophor-EL,

CELLULAR MITOSIS

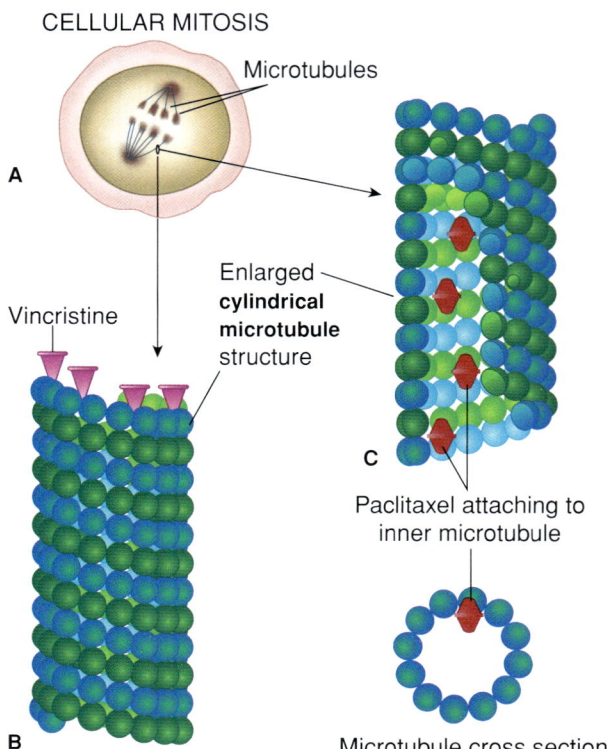

FIGURE 27-4 Diagram of taxane's and vinca alkaloid's mechanism of action. Parts B and C show magnified microtubule structure. **A.** During cellular mitosis, microtubules are essential for chromosome alignment and separation. **B.** Vincristine, one of the vinca alkaloids, attaches consistently to one end of the microtubule to inhibit microtubule assembly. **C.** Paclitaxel, one of the taxanes, binds to the inner ring of the microtubule and prohibits microtubule disassembly. In both B and C, microtubule function is impaired.

an emulsifying agent. Typically, the reaction develops within minutes of starting an initial infusion. Fortunately, the incidence can be decreased tenfold by premedication with corticosteroids, usually dexamethasone, 20 mg orally 12 and 6 hours before paclitaxel infusion. Neurotoxicity is the principal nonhematologic dose-limiting side effect. Common symptoms include numbness, tingling, and/or burning pain in a stocking-glove distribution. Peripheral neuropathy progresses with increased paclitaxel exposure and may become debilitating. Alopecia affects almost all patients and results in total body hair loss.

Docetaxel. This taxane is not FDA approved for gynecologic cancers but is often used to treat uterine sarcoma and occasionally recurrent epithelial ovarian cancer (Gockley, 2014; Herzog, 2014). In addition, patients with worsening peripheral neuropathy with paclitaxel are often switched to docetaxel, which has less neurotoxicity.

The usual dosage of docetaxel (Taxotere) is 75 to 100 mg/m² IV, repeated every 3 weeks. For recurrent ovarian cancer, weekly docetaxel is also effective at a dosage of 35 mg/m² IV for 3 consecutive weeks on a 28-day schedule (Tinker, 2007).

Myelosuppression is the main dose-limiting side effect. Fluid retention syndrome develops in approximately half of patients and manifests as weight gain, peripheral edema, pleural effusion, and ascites. Corticosteroid prophylaxis prevents most

TABLE 27-7. Chemotherapeutic Plant Alkaloids Used for Gynecologic Cancer

Generic Name	Brand Name	Indications	Routes	Dosages	Toxicity
Paclitaxel	Taxol	Recurrent epithelial ovarian CA, endometrial CA, cervical CA, GTN	IV, IP	IV: 135–175 mg/m^2 every 3 wk, or 80 mg/m^2/wk for 3 weeks IP: 60 mg/m^2 on day 8 following a day-1 IV dose	HSR, peripheral neurotoxicity, BMD, alopecia, bradycardia and arrhythmia
Docetaxel	Taxotere	Recurrent epithelial ovarian CA, uterine sarcoma	IV	75–100 mg/m^2 every 3 weeks, or 35 mg/m^2/week for 3 weeks	BMD, peripheral edema, HSR, alopecia
Vincristine	Oncovin	GTN	IV	0.8–1.0 mg/m^2 every other week	Neurotoxicity, abdominal pain, alopecia
Topotecan	Hycamtin	Recurrent epithelial ovarian CA, cervical CA	IV	1.5 mg/m^2/d, days 1–5, every 3 wk, or 4 mg/m^2/wk for 3 wk, or 0.75 mg/m^2/d, days 1–3, every 3 wk	BMD, N/V, alopecia, fever, malaise
Etoposide	VP-16	Germ cell or SCST ovarian CA; recurrent epithelial ovarian CA	IV, PO	IV: 100 mg/m^2 days 1 & 2, every 2 wk, or 75–100 mg/m^2, days 1–5, every 3 wk PO: 50 mg/m^2/day for 3 wk	BMD, alopecia, secondary cancers

BMD = bone marrow depression; CA = cancer; GTN = gestational trophoblastic neoplasia; HSR = hypersensitivity reaction; HTN = hypertension; IV = intravenous; N/V = nausea and vomiting; PO = orally; SCST = sex cord-stromal tumor.

of this toxicity, as well as dermatologic side effects and hypersensitivity reactions.

Vinca Alkaloids

Vincristine, vinblastine, and vinorelbine are cell cycle–specific drugs derived from the periwinkle plant with maximal activity in the M phase. These compounds inhibit normal microtubular polymerization by binding to the tubulin subunit at a site distinct from the taxane-binding site (see Fig. 27-4). These drugs are rarely used in gynecologic oncology. That said, vincristine is the "O" of EMA-CO combination chemotherapy for GTN treatment. The usual dosage of vincristine (Oncovin) is 0.8 to 1.0 mg/m^2 given IV every other week. The total individual dose is capped at 2 mg to prevent or delay neurotoxicity. This is the most common dose-limiting toxicity and may include peripheral neuropathy, autonomic nervous system dysfunction, cranial nerve palsies, ataxia, or seizures. Moreover, concurrent administration with other neurotoxic agents such as cisplatin and paclitaxel may increase severity. GI toxicity also is common, including constipation, abdominal pain, and paralytic ileus. However, myelosuppression is typically mild.

Topoisomerase Inhibitors

Topoisomerase (TOPO) enzymes unwind and rewind DNA to aid DNA replication. Topoisomerase inhibitors interfere with this function and halt DNA synthesis. This group is further divided into categories based on the specific topoisomerase enzyme they inhibit.

Topotecan. This TOPO I inhibitor binds to and stabilizes a transient TOPO I–DNA complex. This results in double-strand breakage and lethal DNA damage. Topotecan (Hycamtin) is FDA approved as salvage therapy of recurrent epithelial ovarian cancer and recurrent cervical cancer. It is infrequently used due to alternatives with fewer side effects (Long, 2005).

Topotecan is usually administered IV in two different schedules for recurrent ovarian cancer (see Table 27-7). When combined with cisplatin for recurrent cervical cancer, the usual dosage is 0.75 mg/m^2 on days 1 through 3, given every 3 weeks (Long, 2005).

Myelosuppression, most commonly neutropenia, is the main dose-limiting side effect. GI toxicity also is frequent and includes nausea, vomiting, diarrhea, and abdominal pain. Systemic symptoms such as headache, fever, malaise, arthralgias, and myalgias are typical. Alopecia is often as complete as that seen with paclitaxel.

Etoposide. This cell cycle–specific agent has maximal activity in the late S and G$_2$ phase. Etoposide "poisons" the TOPO II enzyme by stabilizing an otherwise transient form of the TOPO II–DNA complex. As a result, DNA cannot unwind, and double-strand DNA breaks form. This agent is not FDA approved for gynecologic cancers. However, it is most often used IV as part of combination chemotherapy. Etoposide (VP-16) represents the "E" of the EMA-CO regimen, which is used for GTN. In addition, it is a component of the BEP regimen, used for ovarian germ cell or sex cord–stromal tumors. Oral etoposide may be efficacious as a single agent for salvage treatment of recurrent epithelial ovarian cancer.

The dosage of etoposide varies. In the EMA-CO regimen, 100 mg/m² is administered IV on days 1 and 2, every 2 weeks. In the BEP regimen, it is usually prescribed in dosages of 75 to 100 mg/m² IV on days 1 through 5, given every 3 weeks. The oral dosage is 50 mg/m²/day for 3 weeks, followed by a week off during a 28-day schedule.

Up to 95 percent of etoposide is protein-bound, mainly to albumin. Thus, decreased albumin levels result in a higher fraction of free drug and potentially a higher incidence of toxicity. Myelosuppression, most commonly neutropenia, is the main dose-limiting side effect. GI symptoms of nausea, vomiting, and anorexia are usually minor, except with oral administration. Most patients will develop alopecia. With etoposide, particularly if the total dose exceeds 2000 mg/m², a later secondary malignancy is a small (approximately 1 in 1000) but significant risk. Acute myelogenous leukemia is the most common secondary cancer.

■ Miscellaneous

Carboplatin

Several antineoplastic compounds do not clearly fit into any of the preceding categories but have similarities with alkylating agents. Among these cell cycle–nonspecific drugs are carboplatin and cisplatin.

Carboplatin (Paraplatin) produces DNA adducts that inhibit DNA synthesis. This agent is one of the most widely used, particularly in adjuvant or salvage treatment of epithelial ovarian cancer, and is FDA approved for this indication. It is also frequently used off-label for endometrial cancer.

The usual IV dose of carboplatin is calculated to a target "area under the curve" (AUC) of 6, based on the glomerular filtration rate (GFR). For dose calculation, the Calvert equation is the most often used (Carboplatin total dose [mg] = AUC × [GFR + 25]). In clinical practice, the estimated creatinine clearance (CrCl) is usually substituted for the GFR and may be calculated by the Cockcroft-Gault equation (CrCl = [140 – age] × weight [kg]/0.72 × serum creatinine level [mg/100 mL]). The infusion takes 30 to 60 minutes, and dosing is repeated every 3 to 4 weeks.

Myelosuppression, most commonly thrombocytopenia, is the main dose-limiting side effect. GI toxicity and peripheral neuropathy are notably less severe than with cisplatin. Hypersensitivity reactions will eventually develop in up to 25 percent of women receiving more than six cycles.

Cisplatin

Similar to carboplatin, this agent produces DNA adducts that inhibit DNA synthesis. Cisplatin is one of the oldest and most widely used agents and is FDA approved for ovarian, cervical, and germ cell cancer. It may be given concomitantly with radiation as a radiosensitizing agent for primary treatment of cervical cancer or given as a single agent or in combination for recurrent cervical cancer. Alternatively, cisplatin is part of combination chemotherapy as the "P" of BEP, given for ovarian germ cell or sex cord–stromal tumors. However, for use in epithelial ovarian cancer, cisplatin has largely been replaced by carboplatin.

The usual dosage of cisplatin varies depending on the indication. In cervical cancer, dosages of 40 mg/m² IV weekly or 75 mg/m² every 3 weeks are given during radiation therapy. For patients with recurrent cervical disease, 50 mg/m² IV is provided every 3 weeks (Long, 2005). As part of the BEP protocol, cisplatin is administered 20 mg/m² IV on days 1 through 5 every 3 weeks. Alternatively, for ovarian cancer IP chemotherapy, cisplatin is given on day 1 or 2 of a 21-day cycle at a dose of 75 to 100 mg/m² (Armstrong, 2006; Dizon, 2011).

Cisplatin has several significant toxicities. Of these, nephrotoxicity is the main dose-limiting side effect. Accordingly, patients must be aggressively hydrated before, during, and after drug administration. Mannitol (10 g) or furosemide (20 to 40 mg) may be necessary to maintain a urine output of at least 100 to 150 mL/hour. With cisplatin, electrolyte abnormalities, such as hypomagnesemia and hypokalemia, are common. In addition, severe, prolonged nausea and vomiting can be dramatic without adequate premedication (Table 27-8). Patients often describe a metallic taste and loss of appetite following treatment. Neurotoxicity, usually in the form of peripheral neuropathy, can also be dose limiting and irreversible. Ototoxicity typically manifests as high-frequency hearing loss and tinnitus. Similar to carboplatin, hypersensitivity reactions may develop with prolonged use. Overall, cisplatin is significantly more toxic than carboplatin, except for its reduced hematologic toxicity.

■ Hormonal Agents

Tamoxifen

Due to their minimal toxicity and reasonable activity, hormonal agents are often used for palliative treatment of endometrial and ovarian cancers despite lacking formal FDA approval for these indications. Of these, tamoxifen is a selective estrogen-receptor modulator. It is a nonsteroidal prodrug and is metabolized into a high-affinity estrogen-receptor antagonist in breast tissue. It does not activate the estrogen receptor and thereby blocks breast cancer cell growth. The complex is then transported into the tumor cell nucleus, where it binds to DNA and halts cellular growth and proliferation in the G_0 or G_1 phase. Antiangiogenic effects also have been suggested. In addition to breast cancer, tamoxifen (Nolvadex) is occasionally used to treat endometrial and ovarian cancer (Fiorica, 2004; Hurteau, 2010).

Tamoxifen is orally administered and usually prescribed in doses of 20 to 40 mg for continuous daily use. Toxicity associated with tamoxifen is minimal, mainly consisting of menopausal symptoms. Moreover, some degree of fluid retention and peripheral edema develops in one third of patients. Reduced cognition and libido also may be noted during therapy.

In the endometrium, tamoxifen acts as a partial estrogen-receptor agonist. Sustained use increases the risk for endometrial polyp formation, and endometrial cancer risks triple. Moreover, thromboembolic event risks are raised, especially during and immediately after major surgery or periods of immobility. In contrast, tamoxifen prevents osteoporosis due to its partial agonist properties in bone and has beneficial effects on the serum lipid profile.

TABLE 27-8. Dose and Schedule of Antiemetics to Prevent Emesis Induced by Antineoplastic Therapy of High Emetic Risk

Antiemetics	Brand Name	Single Dose Administered before Chemotherapy	Single Dose Administered Daily
5-HT₃ serotonin-receptor antagonists			
Granisetron	Kytril	Oral: 2 mg IV: 1 mg or 0.01 mg/kg Transdermal patch: apply 1	
Ondansetron	Zofran	Oral: 8 mg twice daily IV: 8 mg or 0.15 mg/kg	
Palonosetron	Aloxi	IV: 0.50 or 0.25 mg	
Dolasetron	Anzemet	Oral: 100 mg	
Dexamethasone	Decadron	Oral: 12 mg	Oral: 8 mg, days 2–4
NK₁ receptor antagonist			
Aprepitant	Emend	Oral: 125 mg	Oral: 80 mg, days 2 and 3
Fosaprepitant	Emend	IV: 150 mg	
Olanzapine	Zyprexa	Oral: 10 mg	Oral: 10 mg, days 2–4

5-HT₃ = 5-Hydroxytryptamine-3; IV = intravenous; NK₁ = neurokinin 1.
From Hesketh, 2008, 2017.

Megestrol Acetate

This agent is a synthetic derivative of progesterone and has activity on tumors through its antiestrogenic effects. As such, megestrol acetate (Megace) is most often used to treat endometrial intraepithelial neoplasia (EIN), nonoperable endometrial cancer, and recurrent endometrial cancer, especially in those patients with grade 1 disease (Chap. 33, p. 716).

For cancer, the usual dosage is 80 mg twice daily. Megestrol acetate has minimal toxicity, but patients often gain weight from a combination of fluid retention and increased appetite. Thromboembolic events are rare. Patients with diabetes mellitus are carefully monitored because of the possibility of exacerbating hyperglycemia due to its concurrent glucocorticoid activity.

BIOLOGICAL AND TARGETED THERAPY

Differing molecular features within normal and malignant cells have led to targeted agents that exploit these differences. These advances, paired with an FDA initiative to accelerate approval, have revolutionized the availability of novel biologic agents. As a group, these targeted therapies offer the potential for improved long-term disease control with less toxicity.

■ Antiangiogenesis Agents

Angiogenesis is a normal physiologic process that forms new blood vessels and remodels vasculature for oxygen and nutrient transport to tissues. This process is usually transient and tightly regulated by various pro- and antiangiogenic factors. However, the homeostatic balance is dysregulated in malignancy. In cancers, sustained angiogenesis leads to tumor growth and metastasis and provides access to systemic lymphatic and circulatory systems. Thus, targeted inhibition of angiogenesis is an appealing therapeutic approach.

The binding of vascular endothelial growth factor (VEGF) to the VEGF receptor is a vital first step in stimulating normal angiogenesis. Many malignancies, such as ovarian cancer, are characterized by increased levels of VEGF or other proangiogenic factors. Several novel agents interfere with this process to halt tumor growth.

Bevacizumab

This agent is a monoclonal antibody that binds to VEGF to prevent VEGF interaction with its receptor (Fig. 27-5A). Currently, bevacizumab (Avastin) is FDA approved for persistent, recurrent, or metastatic cervical cancer. For advanced epithelial ovarian cancer, bevacizumab is coupled with chemotherapy after initial surgery and then used as single-agent maintenance. Last, it is suitable for relapsed platinum-resistant epithelial ovarian

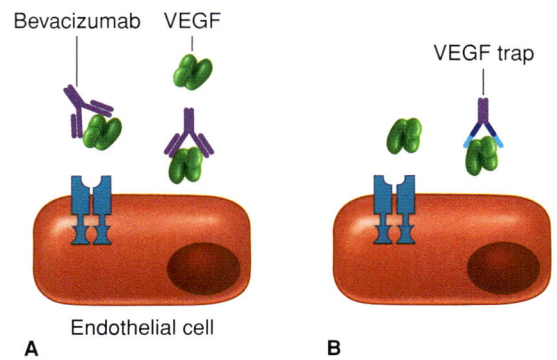

FIGURE 27-5 Mechanisms of action for two antiangiogenesis agents. **A.** Bevacizumab is a monoclonal antibody that binds vascular endothelial growth factor (VEGF). Binding prevents VEGF from combining with its endothelial-bound receptor, which is a receptor tyrosine kinase. **B.** VEGF Trap similarly binds VEGF and prevents receptor binding. In both cases, angiogenesis is inhibited, and tumor growth is halted.

cancer (Burger, 2011; Pujade-Lauraine, 2014; Tewari, 2014). Its usual dosage is 15 mg/kg given IV every 3 weeks with or without cytotoxic chemotherapy. In most cases, toxicity with bevacizumab is minimal. However, GI perforation may occur in up to 10 percent of patients (Cannistra, 2007). This complication is more likely in women with preexisting inflammatory bowel disease or in those with bowel resection at their primary surgery for advanced ovarian cancer (Burger, 2014). Elevated blood pressure is common and may lead to hypertensive crisis. Other possible toxicities include incomplete wound healing, weakness, pain, nosebleed, and proteinuria.

VEGF Trap

VEGF-A is the main isoform of VEGF. It can be bound by bevacizumab, as just described, or by a recombinant "fusion protein" named VEGF Trap (aflibercept). VEGF Trap is constructed by fusing two specific portions of the VEGF receptor and the "Fc" constant region of the IgG molecule. The receptor portions provide high-affinity binding of VEGF (see Fig. 27-5B). Clinical experience in gynecologic cancers is preliminary. Early reports suggest a risk of GI perforation similar to that for bevacizumab (Tew, 2014).

Cediranib

A receptor tyrosine kinase (RTK) inhibitor of VEGF, cediranib (Recentin), has demonstrated clinical activity in ovarian and cervical cancer. Even more promising results have been observed when this agent is combined with olaparib, a poly(adenosine diphosphate [ADP]) ribose polymerase inhibitor described later (Liu, 2014). Yet, significant toxicity that includes diarrhea and hypertension has limited more widespread drug development.

Lenvatinib

This oral agent is a multiple kinase inhibitor against all three isotypes of vascular endothelial growth factor receptor (VEGFR) and against other specific growth factor receptors. Lenvatinib (Lenvima) is FDA approved at a dose of 24 mg daily when used

with pembrolizumab at 200 mg IV every 3 weeks for the treatment of advanced endometrial cancer. Hypertension occurs in one third of patients. Diarrhea, fatigue, and PPE also are reported (Makker, 2018).

■ Poly(ADP) Ribose Polymerase Inhibitors

A very promising group of targeted therapies, poly(ADP) ribose polymerase (PARP) inhibitors, exploit the differences in DNA damage repair between normal and malignant cells. During the cell cycle, DNA is routinely damaged thousands of times. Homologous recombination (HR) is an important pathway that repairs double-strand breaks, and PARP repairs single-strand breaks. In the functioning cell, if HR does not repair the break, PARP will (Fig. 27-6).

Until recently, HR was thought to be performed almost exclusively by the *BRCA1* and *BRCA2* genes. In fact, although up to one quarter of women with ovarian cancer have a predisposing germline mutation that is usually in *BRCA1* or *BRCA2*, numerous other HR deficiency genes (e.g., *BRIP1*, *RAD51C*) also may predispose cells to loss of repair function. Moreover, an additional 5 to 7 percent of patients develop somatic (acquired) HR mutations within the tumor that also result in similar repair dysfunction. In sum, half of all high-grade serous ovarian cancers have aberrations in HR repair (Pardoll, 2012). Normal cells do not replicate their DNA as often as cancer cells. And, without a mutation in one of the HR deficiency genes, they still have functional HR, which allows them to survive PARP inhibition. Thus, only tumor cells with nonfunctioning HR are almost entirely dependent on PARP repair. If PARP repair is prevented, cancer cell DNA cannot be repaired and cells die. In contrast, normal cells are unaffected.

Because most epithelial ovarian cancers have some degree of HR deficiency, even in patients without a confirmed *BRCA1* or *BRCA2* germline mutation, PARP inhibitors have become increasingly popular. All three clinically available PARP inhibitors are now FDA approved for maintenance treatment of

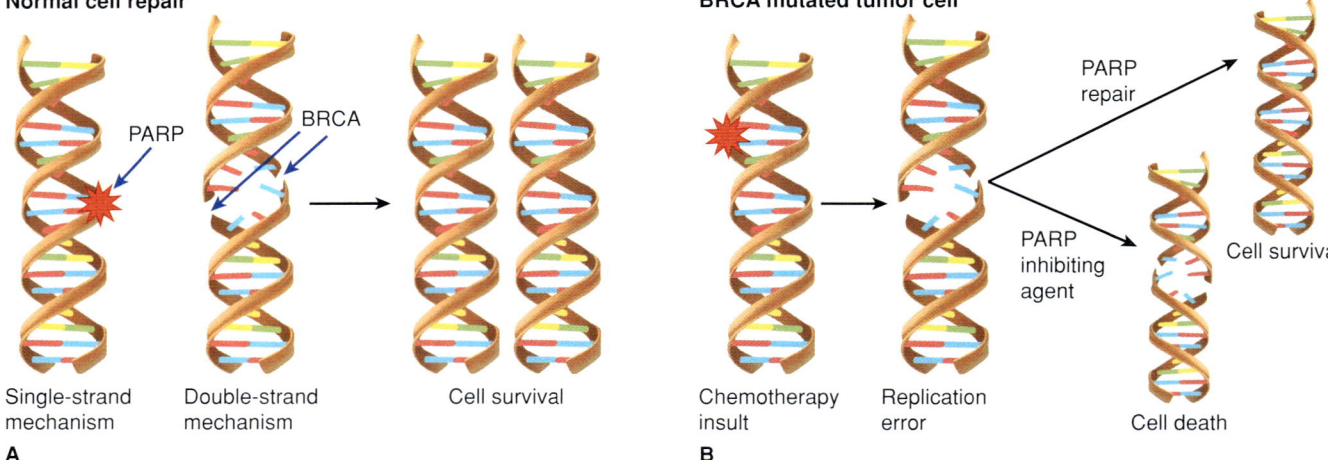

FIGURE 27-6 A. For DNA breaks, both PARP and homologous recombination (HR) pathways are important for repair and cell survival. HR is often but not exclusively performed by BRCA. **B.** With BRCA and other HR mutations, only PARP is available for DNA repair to permit cell survival. If a PARP inhibitor is administered, then DNA breaks are not repaired, and the tumor cell dies.

recurrent epithelial ovarian cancer following a complete or partial response to platinum-based chemotherapy. All three prolong survival, regardless of HR deficiency gene status, yet allow suitable quality of life during therapy (Coleman, 2017; Friedlander, 2018; Ison, 2018; Pujade-Lauraine, 2017).

Olaparib is used for *BRCA1* and *BRCA2* mutation carriers with relapsed ovarian cancer that has demonstrated resistance to platinum drugs (Kaufman, 2015). As a single agent, the usual oral dose is 300 mg twice daily. The most frequent toxicity is anemia, but other side effects are fatigue, nausea, or abdominal pain (Kaufman, 2015; Pujade-Lauraine, 2017).

Niraparib has a daily oral dose of 300 mg daily. Most significant side effects are hematologic and can be managed with dose adjustments (Mirza, 2016; Oza, 2018).

Rucaparib is used for patients with a *BRCA* mutation (germline or somatic) and with recurrent epithelial ovarian cancer treated by two or more courses of therapy. The oral dose is 600 mg twice daily. Side effects are few and include anemia, asymptomatic transaminitis, and bowel obstruction (Coleman, 2017; Swisher, 2017).

■ Immunotherapy

Another promising group of new drugs exploit the fact that cancer cells often have surface molecules, called tumor-associated antigens (TAAs), which can be detected by the body's immune system. Active immunotherapy targets TAAs, and directs the immune system to attack these tumor cells. In contrast, passive immunotherapies enhance existing antitumor responses by using monoclonal antibodies, lymphocytes, and cytokines.

Of passive immunotherapy agents, pembrolizumab (Keytruda) is the first cancer drug to be FDA approved based on tumor genetics rather than the tumor's tissue type or site of origin. Thus, it requires tumor profiling results before clinical use. Pembrolizumab is a therapeutic humanized antibody that targets and blocks the programmed cell death 1 (PD-1) receptor of T cell lymphocytes (Fig. 27-7). This receptor is an "immune checkpoint," responsible for preventing the immune system from attacking the body's own tissues. However, when a T cell's PD-1 receptor binds with the programmed cell death ligand (PD-L) on a tumor cell, it permits an attack by that lymphocyte. Cancers with microsatellite instability–high state (MSI-H) or DNA mismatch repair (MMR) deficiencies generate many mutated TAAs that bind to PD-1 and prohibit binding with the PD-L. This binding of TAAs and PD-1 thereby shuts down the ability of the host to kill the tumor on its own. By inhibiting PD-1 with pembrolizumab, the immune system is able to target and destroy these otherwise undetectable cancer cells. Yet, this same mechanism also allows the immune system to attack the body itself, and checkpoint inhibitors have immune-dysfunction side effects as a result (Pardoll, 2012).

Pembrolizumab is approved for any unresectable or metastatic solid tumor with MSI-H or MMR deficiencies and for advanced cervical cancer in PD-L1–positive patients (Frenel, 2017). In combination with lenvatinib, it is also FDA approved for advanced endometrial cancer (Makker, 2018). The dose of pembrolizumab is 200 mg IV every three weeks. In PD-L1–positive advanced cervical cancer, the response rate approximates 15 percent. Side effects are few and include rash and fever (Chung, 2018; Frenel, 2017).

■ Mammalian Target of Rapamycin Inhibitors

The *mammalian target of rapamycin (mTOR)* is a protein kinase that regulates membrane trafficking, transcription, translation, and cell cytoskeleton maintenance. Its downstream effect is to raise VEGF production. Thus, efforts to inhibit mTOR signaling also can inhibit angiogenesis. Rapamycin inhibits mTOR, and analogues of this drug, such as temsirolimus and everolimus, are currently being studied for gynecologic cancer treatment (Alvarez, 2013; Fleming, 2014; Slomovitz, 2010).

SIDE EFFECTS

Chemotherapy regimens, especially those including cytotoxic drugs, are universally toxic and display a narrow margin of safety. The Cancer Therapy Evaluation Program (CTEP) of the National Cancer Institute (NCI) has developed a detailed and comprehensive set of guidelines for the description and grading of toxicity. Termed the Common Terminology Criteria for Adverse Events (CTCAE), the most recent revision is version 5.0 and is available at http://evs.nci.nih.gov/ftp1/CTCAE/About.html.

In general, treatment modifications depend on the degree (grade) and duration of toxicity experienced. Doses are reduced if a woman experiences a severe reaction but then may be subsequently increased if tolerance improves. However, treatment is not resumed until toxicity has resolved to baseline or "Grade 1" levels and may be delayed on a week-to-week basis to permit recovery. Dose modification and supportive care are implemented to prevent delays of greater than 2 weeks, which would otherwise compromise therapeutic efficacy. Serious myelosuppression can be partially corrected

Blunted immune response   **Full immune response**

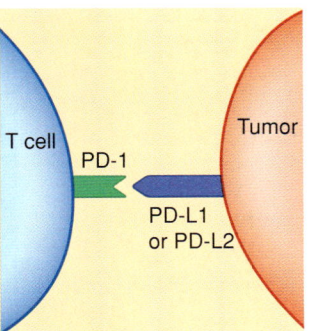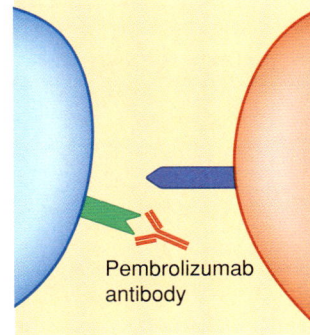

FIGURE 27-7 A. Normally, T cells recognize foreign peptides presented on cell surfaces. This recognition leads to a robust immune response. During this response, programmed cell death protein 1 (PD-1) limits T cell activity when it interacts with one of two ligands (PD-L1 or PD-L2). **B.** Action of the drug pembrolizumab. This agent is an antibody that binds to the PD-1 receptor and blocks its interaction with PD-L1 or PD-L2. This helps restore a robust immune response against a cancer cell.

with the use of hematopoietic growth factors (p. 603). Many of the common toxicities can be prevented with proper use of premedications or alleviated with supportive measures.

Bone Marrow Toxicity

Myelosuppression, especially neutropenia, is the most common dose-limiting side effect of cytotoxic drugs. The absolute neutrophil count (ANC) is the critical measure when determining patient infection risk and may reflect mild (1000–$1500/mm^3$), moderate (500–$1000/mm^3$), or severe ($<500/mm^3$) neutropenia. Frequently, patients receiving therapy will have a nadir into the neutropenic range that will recover before the next scheduled treatment course. However, if they are admitted to the hospital for fever or other condition, neutropenic precautions should be observed. Although guidelines vary, these precautions include assiduous provider hand washing; provider outer gowns, gloves, and masks; and patient isolation from potential infection carriers.

Moderate degrees of anemia often develop in cancer patients receiving chemotherapy and may contribute to chronic fatigue. Frequent transfusions are not practical or recommended, and many patients will adapt to chronic anemia with minimal symptoms. Synthetic erythropoietin is infrequently indicated and is discussed later (p. 603).

Thrombocytopenia is less common but may predispose the patient to serious bleeding if the platelet count drops below $10,000/mm^3$. No predetermined platelet value should prompt routine transfusion, but ongoing bleeding in affected patients is a warranted indication.

Gastrointestinal Toxicity

Most anticancer agents are associated with some degree of nausea, vomiting, and anorexia. Typically, the emetogenic potential of a particular drug or regimen will dictate the antiemetic regimen used (Tables 27-9 and 27-10). Mild nausea and vomiting can often be managed effectively by prochlorperazine (Compazine) with or without dexamethasone. If drugs with

TABLE 27-9. Emetic Risk of Intravenously Administered Antineoplastic Agents Used in Gynecologic Oncology

Emetic Risk	Incidence of Emesis (without Antiemetics)	Agent
High	>90%	Cisplatin Dactinomycin
Moderate	30–90%	Carboplatin Cyclophosphamide <1500 mg/m^2 Doxorubicin Ifosfamide
Low	10–30%	Etoposide Docetaxel Doxorubicin liposome Fluorouracil Gemcitabine Methotrexate Paclitaxel Temsirolimus Topotecan
Minimal	<10%	Bevacizumab Bleomycin Nivolumab Pembrolizumab Vinblastine Vincristine Vinorelbine

Items arranged alphabetically.
From Hesketh, 2008, 2017; Roila, 2006.

more severe emetogenic effects such as cisplatin are administered, then ondansetron, granisetron, or palonosetron, which are 5-hydroxytryptamine antagonists, can be given IV before chemotherapy. Ondansetron (Zofran) and granisetron (Kytril)

TABLE 27-10. Drug Regimens for the Prevention of Chemotherapy-Induced Emesis by Emetic Risk Category

Emetic Risk Category (Incidence of Emesis without Antiemetics)	Antiemetic Regimens and Schedules
High (>90%)	5-HT$_3$ serotonin receptor antagonist: day 1 NK$_1$ receptor antagonist: day 1 Olanzapine: days 1–4 Dexamethasone: days 1–4
Moderate (30% to 90%)	5-HT$_3$ serotonin receptor antagonist: day 1 Dexamethasone: days 1–3
Low (10% to 30%)	5-HT$_3$ serotonin receptor antagonist: day 1 or Dexamethasone: day 1
Minimal (<10%)	Prescribe as needed

5-HT$_3$ = 5-Hydroxytryptamine-3; NK$_1$ = neurokinin 1.
From Hesketh, 2008, 2017.

can also be provided orally to manage delayed and/or chronic nausea after chemotherapy. However, these drugs can induce significant constipation as a side effect. Chemotherapy-related diarrhea, oral mucositis, esophagitis, and gastroenteritis are treated with supportive care.

■ Dermatologic Toxicity

Drug-associated changes include hyperpigmentation, photosensitivity, nail abnormalities, rashes, urticaria, erythema, and alopecia. Many of these are drug specific and self-limited, but occasionally, they may be dose limiting. As discussed earlier, PPE is a known toxicity of liposomal doxorubicin (p. 595). In addition, changes in skin pigmentation are seen with bleomycin, whereas docetaxel can produce nail discoloration and onycholysis. Mild urticarial reactions are prevented or alleviated by premedication with diphenhydramine hydrochloride, 50 mg IV or orally.

One of the most emotionally distressing side effects of many chemotherapeutic agents is scalp alopecia. Fortunately, this is usually reversible. With some drugs such as paclitaxel, women will also experience loss of eyelashes, eyebrows, and other body hair. In general, techniques to minimize alopecia are unsuccessful. Instead, women are counseled regarding cosmetic options such as false eyelashes and wigs.

■ Neurotoxicity

Peripheral neuropathy develops commonly with cisplatin, paclitaxel, and the vinca alkaloids. Cisplatin-induced neurotoxicity usually resolves slowly, due to axonal demyelination and loss. To counter this toxicity, amifostine (Ethyol) may be administered, but substitution of carboplatin will avoid much of the toxicity. Gabapentin (Neurontin) is the usual treatment for neuropathic pain, starting at a dosage of 300 mg daily. Other options to treat symptomatic peripheral neuropathy that have shown some efficacy include oral glutamine (up to 15 g twice daily) or oral vitamin B_6 (up to 50 mg three times daily).

With chemotherapeutic agents in general, drug dosing may need to be adjusted if peripheral neuropathy becomes problematic—for example, if a patient can no longer hold a cup of coffee. More dramatic instances of acute cerebellar syndromes, cranial nerve palsies or paralysis, and occasionally acute and chronic encephalopathies are managed with supportive care and usually with discontinuation of the offending agent.

GROWTH FACTORS

■ Synthetic Erythropoietins

In some situations, hematopoietic drug factors to prompt red blood cell (RBC) or granulocyte production may have merit. Of these, epoetin alfa and darbepoetin alfa are synthetic erythropoietins that have the same biologic effects as endogenous erythropoietin to stimulate RBC production. These agents are recommended for patients with chemotherapy-associated anemia and a hemoglobin concentration that is approaching, or has fallen below, 10 g/dL. However, when used at higher hemoglobin levels, they may actually be associated with tumor progression and shorten survival (Rizzo, 2010). Moreover, several large studies have shown that despite reducing the need for RBC transfusions, erythropoiesis-stimulating agents (ESAs) increase the risk for thromboembolic events and death in cancer patients treated with epoetin alfa (Aapro, 2012; Tonia, 2012). As a result, the FDA issued a "black-box" warning stating that a higher mortality rate and/or shortened time to tumor progression were found when ESAs were dosed with the intent to achieve hemoglobin values ≥12 g/dL compared with placebo or observational controls. Once routinely used, these agents are now infrequently administered to gynecologic cancer patients due to safety concerns.

When used, epoetin alfa (Procrit, Eprex, and Epogen) is usually prescribed as 40,000 units SC weekly (Case, 2006). Beyond local pain at the injection site, this agent has minimal side effects. Possible toxicity may include diarrhea, nausea, or hypertension (Bohlius, 2006; Khuri, 2007). For darbepoetin alfa (Aranesp), the usual SC dose is 200 μg every other week or 500 μg given every 3 weeks. Darbepoetin alfa has minimal side effects beyond local pain at the injection site.

■ Granulocyte Colony-Stimulating Factors

Filgrastim and pegfilgrastim are human granulocyte colony-stimulating factors (G-CSF) produced by recombinant DNA technology. As such, these cytokines bind to hematopoietic cells and prompt proliferation, differentiation, and activation of granulocyte progenitor cells. These growth factors are mainly used to prevent episodes of febrile neutropenia (ANC <1500), particularly in patients with a greater than 20-percent risk for such an event. Fortunately, none of the common regimens used in the treatment of gynecologic cancer have a risk that exceeds 20 percent, and thus growth factors are typically not required for initial prophylaxis. Instead, growth factors are usually indicated following a neutropenic event and chemotherapy delay to permit a patient to maintain her treatment schedule.

Filgrastim (Neupogen) is given SC, and the usual SC dose is 5 μg/kg/d. However, patients typically are given either 300 μg or 480 μg, which is the content of manufactured vials. It should be administered at least 24 hours after chemotherapy completion. Therapy is terminated when the white blood count (WBC) exceeds 10,000/mm³ or when the ANC exceeds 1000/mm³ for 3 consecutive days. Toxicity with filgrastim is limited, and transient bone pain is usually mild to moderate.

Pegfilgrastim (Neulasta) acts similarly to filgrastim to stimulate production of granulocyte progenitor cells within the bone marrow. The "peg" in pegfilgrastim refers to a polyethylene glycol unit that prolongs the time it remains in the body. Pegfilgrastim is given as a single 6-mg SC injection once per chemotherapy cycle. This is usually far more convenient than daily filgrastim doses. It should not be administered during the 14 days before and within 24 hours after administration of cytotoxic chemotherapy. Transient bone pain is usually mild to moderate, but often more pronounced than with filgrastim.

TUMOR PROFILING

The ability to identify distinct molecular alterations by tumor profiling, so-called precision medicine, has led to more effective targeted treatment with biological agents. Currently, the FoundationFocus CDxBRCA test is an FDA-approved test detecting germline (inherited) and somatic (acquired) *BRCA1* and *BRCA2* gene mutations. With positive results, potential candidates for PARP inhibitor therapy are identified. To aid pembrolizumab therapy selection, the PD-L1 IHC 22C3 pharmDx test is FDA approved for cervical cancer patients. PD-L1 protein expression is significant when the Combined Positive Score (CPS) exceeds 1. The CPS is the number of PD-L1 staining cells divided by the total number of viable tumor cells, multiplied by 100.

Less rigorous chemotherapy sensitivity and resistance assays are theoretically appealing due to the possibility of tailoring treatment. Using this strategy, viable tumor tissue is collected from the patient during surgery or other intervention (e.g., paracentesis). The sample is shipped to a specialized laboratory. Here, in vitro analysis determines whether tumor growth is inhibited by a drug or panel of drugs.

The potential of selecting effective cancer treatments while sparing unnecessary ones is intriguing, and patients may even request testing. However, no current assay has demonstrated sufficient efficacy to support its use. Thus, these assays are not recommended for individual patients outside of a clinical trial (Burstein, 2011).

CANCER DRUG DEVELOPMENT

The only proven way to improve cancer treatment success rates is to test new agents, higher doses, novel combinations, or unique ways of administering treatment. Promising drugs are usually first identified by demonstrating success in cancer cell lines or in animals inoculated with tumor. After preclinical steps, novel agents traditionally proceed through four phases of clinical testing.

Phase I trials use a dose-escalating design to determine the dose-limiting toxicity, maximum tolerated dose (MTD), and pharmacokinetic parameters of the drug. In a Phase I trial, detecting a tumor response is not critical, since enrolled patients have typically completed extensive prior therapy. However, observed responses would encourage further disease-specific Phase II trials.

Phase II trials aim to define the actual response rate in patients with a specific cancer type. Typically, patients enrolled in Phase II trials have received only one prior chemotherapy regimen. This allows for a reasonable chance of response compared with subjects in Phase I studies. End points of Phase II trials include a measure of disease response, determination of the "progression-free interval," cumulative incidence of dose-limiting toxicity over multiple cycles, and overall survival rates.

Phase III randomized trials are designed to directly compare the drug with existing standard regimens in a particular stage and type of cancer. Phase III trials generally require a minimum of 150 patients per "arm" to provide adequate statistical precision. Finally, Phase IV clinical trials evaluate drugs that are already FDA approved. The goal of Phase IV trials is to study long-term drug safety and efficacy.

In general, although patients are strongly encouraged to participate in appropriate phase I, II, and III clinical trials, fewer than 5 percent do so. Doing so expands their options for treatment. In addition to expanding their options for treatment, the results of such studies are the primary method to improve the future outcomes of women diagnosed with gynecologic cancer.

REFERENCES

Aapro M, Jelkmann W, Constantinescu SN, et al: Effects of erythropoietin receptors and erythropoiesis-stimulating agents on disease progression in cancer. Br J Cancer 106(7):1249, 2012

Alazzam M, Tidy J, Osborne R, et al: Chemotherapy for resistant or recurrent gestational trophoblastic neoplasia. Cochrane Database Syst Rev 1:CD008891, 2016

Alvarez EA, Brady WE, Walker JL, et al: Phase II trial of combination bevacizumab and temsirolimus in the treatment of recurrent or persistent endometrial carcinoma: a Gynecologic Oncology Group study. Gynecol Oncol 129(1):22, 2013

Armstrong DK, Bundy B, Wenzel L, et al: Intraperitoneal cisplatin and paclitaxel in ovarian cancer. N Engl J Med 354(1):34, 2006

Bohlius J, Wilson J, Seidenfeld J, et al: Recombinant human erythropoietins and cancer patients: updated meta-analysis of 57 studies including 9353 patients. J Natl Cancer Inst 98(10):708, 2006

Bower M, Newlands ES, Holden L, et al: EMA/CO for high-risk gestational trophoblastic tumors: results from a cohort of 272 patients. J Clin Oncol 15(7):2636, 1997

Burger RA, Brady MF, Bookman MA, et al: Incorporation of bevacizumab in the primary treatment of ovarian cancer. N Engl J Med 365(26):2473, 2011

Burger RA, Brady MF, Bookman MA, et al: Risk factors for GI adverse events in a phase III randomized trial of bevacizumab in first-line therapy of advanced ovarian cancer: a Gynecologic Oncology Group Study. J Clin Oncol 32(12):1210, 2014

Burstein HJ, Mangu PB, Somerfield MR, et al: American Society of Clinical Oncology clinical practice guideline update on the use of chemotherapy sensitivity and resistance assays. J Clin Oncol 29(24):3328, 2011

Cannistra SA, Matulonis UA, Penson RT, et al: Phase III study of bevacizumab in patients with platinum-resistant ovarian cancer or peritoneal serous cancer. J Clin Oncol 25(33):5180, 2007

Cantu MG, Buda A, Parma G, et al: Randomized controlled trial of single-agent paclitaxel versus cyclophosphamide, doxorubicin, and cisplatin in patients with recurrent ovarian cancer who responded to first-line platinum-based regimens. J Clin Oncol 20(5):1232, 2002

Case AS, Rocconi RP, Kilgore LC, et al: Effectiveness of darbepoetin alfa versus epoetin alfa for the treatment of chemotherapy induced anemia in patients with gynecologic malignancies. Gynecol Oncol 101(3):499, 2006

Chen H, Li J, Cui T, et al: Adjuvant gonadotropin-releasing hormone analogues for the prevention of chemotherapy induced premature ovarian failure in premenopausal women. Cochrane Database Syst Rev 11:CD008018, 2011

Chung HC, Schellens JH, Delord JP, et al: Pembrolizumab treatment of advanced cervical cancer: updated results from the phase 2 KEYNOTE-158 study. J Clin Oncol 36(15 suppl):5522, 2018

Chura JC, Van Iseghem K, Downs LS Jr, et al: Bevacizumab plus cyclophosphamide in heavily pretreated patients with recurrent ovarian cancer. Gynecol Oncol 107(2):326, 2007

Coleman RL, Oza AM, Lorusso D, et al: Rucaparib maintenance treatment for recurrent ovarian carcinoma after response to platinum therapy (ARIEL3): a randomised, double-blind, placebo-controlled, phase 3 trial. Lancet 390(10106):1949, 2017

Dizon DS, Sill MW, Gould N, et al: Phase I feasibility study of intraperitoneal cisplatin and intravenous paclitaxel followed by intraperitoneal paclitaxel in untreated ovarian, fallopian tube, and primary peritoneal carcinoma: a gynecologic oncology group study. Gynecol Oncol 123(2):182, 2011

Eisenhauer EA, Therasse P, Bogaerts J, et al: New response evaluation criteria in solid tumours: revised RECIST guideline (version 1.1). Eur J Cancer 45:228, 2009

Elgindy EA, El-Haieg DO, Khorshid OM, et al: Gonadatrophin suppression to prevent chemotherapy-induced ovarian damage: a randomized controlled trial. Obstet Gynecol 121(1):78, 2013

Fleming GF, Filiaci VL, Marzullo B, et al: Temsirolimus with or without megestrol acetate and tamoxifen for endometrial cancer: a Gynecologic Oncology Group study. Gynecol Oncol 132(3):585, 2014

Frenel JS, Le Tourneau C, O'Neil B, et al: Safety and efficacy of pembrolizumab in advanced, programmed death ligand 1-positive cervical cancer: results from the Phase Ib KEYNOTE-028 Trial. J Clin Oncol 35(36):4035, 2017

Friedlander M, Gebski V, Gibbs E, et al: Health-related quality of life and patient-centered outcomes with olaparib maintenance after chemotherapy in patients with platinum-sensitive, relapsed ovarian cancer and a BRCA1/2 mutation (SOLO2/ENGOT Ov-21): a placebo-controlled, phase 3 randomised trial. Lancet Oncol 19(8):1126, 2018

Gockley AA, Rauh-Hain JA, Del Carmen MG: Uterine leiomyosarcoma: a review article. Int J Gynecol Cancer 24(9):1538, 2014

Gordon AN, Tonda M, Sun S, et al: Long-term survival advantage for women treated with pegylated liposomal doxorubicin compared with topotecan in a phase 3 randomized study of recurrent and refractory epithelial ovarian cancer. Gynecol Oncol 95(1):1, 2004

Herzog TJ, Monk BJ, Rose PG, et al: A phase II trial of oxaliplatin, docetaxel, and bevacizumab as first-line therapy of advanced cancer of the ovary, peritoneum, and fallopian tube. Gynecol Oncol 132(3):517, 2014

Hesketh PJ: Chemotherapy-induced nausea and vomiting. N Engl J Med 358(23):2482, 2008

Hesketh PJ, Kris MG, Basch E, et al: Antiemetics: American Society of Clinical Oncology clinical practice guideline update. J Clin Oncol 35(28):3240, 2017

Hyman DM, Grisham RN, Hensley ML: Management of advanced uterine leiomyosarcoma. Curr Opin Oncol 26(4):422, 2014

Ison G, Howie LJ, Amiri-Kordestani L, et al: FDA approval summary: niraparib for the maintenance treatment of patients with recurrent ovarian cancer in response to platinum-based chemotherapy. Clin Cancer Res 24(17):4066, 2018

Katsumata N, Yasuda M, Takahashi F, et al: Dose-dense paclitaxel once a week in combination with carboplatin every 3 weeks for advanced ovarian cancer: a phase 3, open-label, randomised controlled trial. Lancet 374(9698):1331, 2009

Kaufman B, Shapira-Frommer R, Schmutzler RK, et al: Olaparib monotherapy in patients with advanced cancer and a germline BRCA1/2 mutation. J Clin Oncol 33(3):244, 2015

Khuri FR: Weighing the hazards of erythropoiesis stimulation in patients with cancer. N Engl J Med 356(24):2445, 2007

Liu JF, Barry WT, Birrer M, et al: Combination cediranib and olaparib versus olaparib alone for women with recurrent platinum-sensitive ovarian cancer: a randomised phase 2 study. Lancet Oncol 15(11):1207, 2014

Long HJ III, Bundy BN, Grendys EC Jr., et al: Randomized phase III trial of cisplatin with or without topotecan in carcinoma of the uterine cervix: a Gynecologic Oncology Group Study. J Clin Oncol 23(21):4626, 2005

Makker V, Rasco DW, Vogelzang NJ, et al: Lenvatinib + pembrolizumab in patients with advanced endometrial cancer: updated results. J Clin Oncol 36(15 suppl):5596, 2018

Mancari R, Signorelli M, Gadducci A, et al: Adjuvant chemotherapy in stage I-II uterine leiomyosarcoma: a multicentric retrospective study of 140 patients. Gynecol Oncol 133(3):531, 2014

Markman M, Blessing J, Rubin SC, et al: Phase II trial of weekly paclitaxel (80 mg/m^2) in platinum and paclitaxel-resistant ovarian and primary peritoneal cancers: a Gynecologic Oncology Group study. Gynecol Oncol 101(3):436, 2006

Mileshkin L, Antill Y, Rischin D: Management of complications of chemotherapy. In Gershenson DM, McGuire WP, Gore M, et al (eds): Gynecologic Cancer Controversies in Management. Philadelphia, Elsevier, 2004, p 618

Mirza MR, Monk BJ, Herrstedt J, et al: Niraparib maintenance therapy in platinum-sensitive, recurrent ovarian cancer. N Engl J Med 375(22):2154, 2016

Oza AM, Matulonis UA, Malander S, et al: Quality of life in patients with recurrent ovarian cancer treated with niraparib versus placebo (ENGOT-OV16/NOVA): results from a double-blind, phase 3, randomised controlled trial. Lancet Oncol 19(8):1117, 2018

Pardoll DM: The blockade of immune checkpoints in cancer immunotherapy. Nat Rev Cancer 12(4):252, 2012

Park JY, Jin KL, Kim DY, et al: Surgical staging and adjuvant chemotherapy in the management of patients with adult granulosa cell tumors of the ovary. Gynecol Oncol 125(1):80, 2012

Pujade-Lauraine E, Hilpert F, Weber B, et al: Bevacizumab combined with chemotherapy for platinum-resistant recurrent ovarian cancer: the AURELIA open-label randomized phase III trial. J Clin Oncol 32(13):1302, 2014

Pujade-Lauraine E, Ledermann JA, Selle F, et al: Olaparib tablets as maintenance therapy in patients with platinum-sensitive, relapsed ovarian cancer and a BRCA1/2 mutation (SOLO2/ENGOT-Ov21): a double-blind, randomised, placebo-controlled, phase 3 trial. Lancet Oncol 18(9):1274, 2017

Rizzo JD, Brouwers M, Hurley P, et al: American Society of Clinical Oncology/American Society of Hematology clinical practice guideline update on the use of epoetin and darbepoetin in adult patients with cancer. J Clin Oncol 28(33):4996, 2010

Roila F, Hesketh PJ, Herrstedt J, et al: Prevention of chemotherapy- and radiotherapy-induced emesis: results of the 2004 Perugia International Antiemetic Consensus Conference. Ann Oncol 17:20, 2006

Slomovitz BM, Lu KH, Johnston T, et al: A phase 2 study of the oral mammalian target of rapamycin inhibitor, everolimus, in patients with recurrent endometrial carcinoma. Cancer 116(23):5415, 2010

Swisher EM, Lin KK, Oza AM, et al: Rucaparib in relapsed, platinum-sensitive high-grade ovarian carcinoma (ARIEL2 Part 1): an international, multicentre, open-label, phase 2 trial. Lancet Oncol 18(1):75, 2017

Tew WP, Colombo N, Ray-Coquard I, et al: Intravenous aflibercept in patients with platinum-resistant, advanced ovarian cancer: results of a randomized, double-blind, phase 2, parallel-arm study. Cancer 120(3):335, 2014

Tewari KS, Sill MW, Long HJ 3rd, et al: Improved survival with bevacizumab in advanced cervical cancer. N Engl J Med 370(8):734, 2014

Tinker AV, Gebski V, Fitzharris B, et al: Phase II trial of weekly docetaxel for patients with relapsed ovarian cancer who have previously received paclitaxel—ANZGOG 02-01. Gynecol Oncol 104(3):647, 2007

Tonia T, Mettler A, Robert N, et al: Erythropoietin or darbepoetin for patients with cancer. Cochrane Database Syst Rev 12:CD003407, 2012

Weinberg LE, Lurain JR, Singh DK, et al: Survival and reproductive outcomes in women treated for malignant ovarian germ cell tumors. Gynecol Oncol 121(2):285, 2011

Principles of Radiation Therapy

To effectively incorporate radiation treatment into cancer care, clinicians must understand the fundamental concepts and vocabulary used in radiation oncology. Clinically, radiation therapy, often combined with chemotherapy, can be used as primary treatment for many gynecologic malignancies (Table 28-1). Additionally, radiation therapy may be recommended postoperatively if the probability of tumor recurrence is high. Radiation therapy is also used frequently in the relief of symptoms caused by metastasis of any gynecologic cancer.

RADIATION PHYSICS

Radiation therapy is the focused delivery of energy in tissue to accomplish controlled biologic damage. Radiation used in this therapy can be delivered as electromagnetic waves or particles.

■ Electromagnetic Radiation

Photons (x-rays) and *gamma rays* are the two types of electromagnetic radiation used for radiation therapy. Photons, used in

TABLE 28-1. Role of Radiation Therapy in the Management of Gynecologic Cancers

Intent	Site
Curative	Cervix, vulva, vagina, uterus
Adjunctive to surgery	Cervix, vulva, vagina, uterus
Palliative	Metastasis causing symptoms: bleeding, pain, obstruction

external beam therapy, are produced when a stream of electrons collides with a high-atomic-number target (tungsten) located in the head of a linear accelerator (Fig. 28-1). In contrast, gamma rays originate from unstable atom nuclei and are emitted during decay of radioactive materials, also termed *radionuclides*, which are widely used in *brachytherapy*.

■ Particle Radiation

Whereas electromagnetic waves are defined by their wavelengths, particles are defined by their masses. For clinical use, particles include electrons, neutrons, protons, helium ions, heavy charged ions, and pi mesons. Except for electrons, which are available in all modern radiation oncology centers, and protons, other particles have limited clinical use. Proton facility numbers are expanding, with 30 facilities operating in the United States and 14 additional centers planned or under construction.

Particles are produced by linear accelerators or other high-energy generators and are usually delivered by external beam. Of clinically used particles, *electrons* are negatively charged and deposit most of their energy near the surface. In contrast, heavy charged particles, such as *protons*, deposit most of their energy in the absorbing tissues as their velocity decreases, that is, near the end of the particle path (the Bragg peak effect). Because of this, a major advantage of proton therapy is the lack of an exiting dose through normal tissues. Proton therapy use for gynecologic malignancies is primarily investigational. But as an example, proton therapy can treat affected deep pelvic and paraaortic lymph nodes, while sparing unnecessary dosing and injury to anterolateral organs, such as the bowel and kidneys (Fig. 28-2).

■ Radiation Sources
Radionuclides

Also called *radioisotopes*, radionuclides undergo nuclear decay and can emit: (1) positively charged alpha particles, (2) negatively charged beta particles (electrons), and (3) gamma rays. Radionuclides commercially available are shown in Table 28-2. Cesium and iridium are commonly used in gynecologic brachytherapy.

Linear Accelerator

One of the main types of radiation-producing units is the linear accelerator, also called a *linac*. A linac can produce both photon and electron beams (see Fig. 28-1). In the *photon-therapy mode*, indicated for deep-seated tumors, the accelerated electron beam is guided to hit a metal target to produce photons. The unit

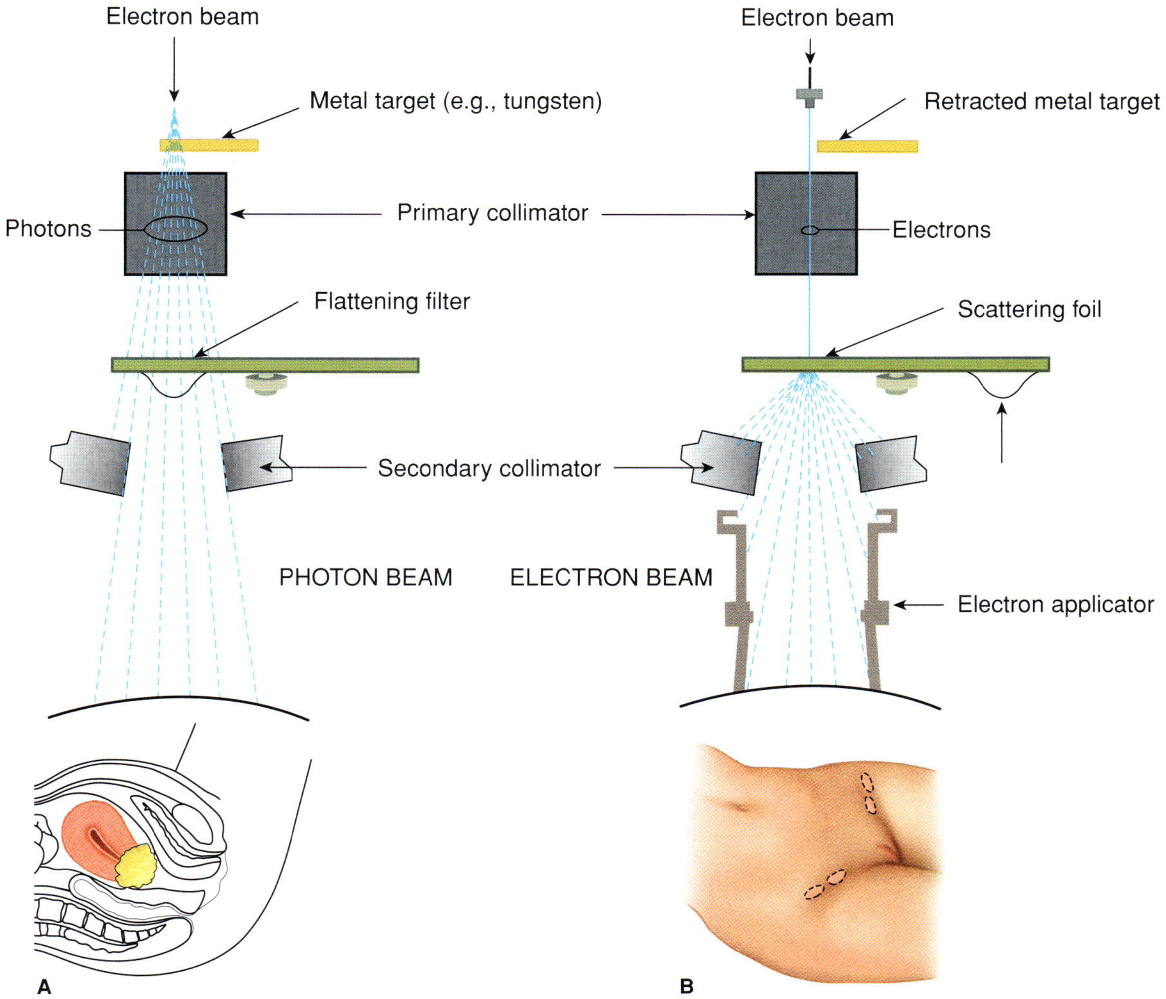

Electron beam

Metal target (e.g., tungsten)

Photons

Primary collimator

Flattening filter

Secondary collimator

PHOTON BEAM

Electron beam

Retracted metal target

Electrons

Scattering foil

Electron applicator

ELECTRON BEAM

A

B

FIGURE 28-1 Block diagram of a linear accelerator used to create external beam radiation. Either photon beams or electron beams may be produced. **A.** Photon beam therapy is suited for deep tumors such as the cervical cancer shown here. Beam energy is measured in millions of volts (MV). **B.** Electron beam therapy is indicated for superficial lesions such as inguinal lymph nodes. Beam energy is measured in millions of electron volts (MeV).

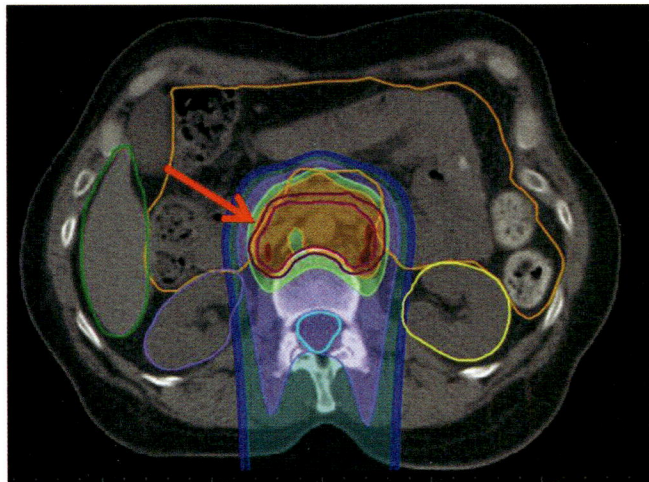

FIGURE 28-2 Proton dose distribution in a patient with cervical cancer receiving treatment to the paraaortic lymph nodes. The proton beam originates posteriorly and is directed anteriorly. The red arrow shows the target volume (*dark magenta*). The area anterior to this is bowel (*orange outline*), which is significantly spared from radiation.

used to describe the energy of a photon beam is MV (million volts). In the *electron-therapy mode,* indicated for superficial lesions, the electron beam strikes a lead scattering foil instead of the metal target. The unit for electron beam energy is MeV (million electron volts). **Figure 28-3** displays a linac with three moveable components: gantry, treatment head, and couch. These components can all rotate 360 degrees, which allows multiple fields and angles to achieve optimal dose delivery to a tumor.

■ Electromagnetic Radiation Energy Deposition

When electromagnetic radiation is used in daily clinical practice, it contacts target tissues, and energy is transferred to those tissues. This transfer creates ions by dislodging electrons from atoms within these tissues. These electrons then collide with surrounding molecules to initiate radiation damage.

Three mechanisms are involved in energy transfer: (1) photoelectric effect, (2) Compton effect, and (3) pair production

TABLE 28-2. Physical Properties and Clinical Use of Selected Radionuclides

Element	Radiation Energy (MeV)	Half-Life	Clinical Use
Cesium-137	0.6	30 years	Brachytherapy
Iridium-192	0.4	74 days	Brachytherapy
Cobalt-60	1.2	5 years	Brachytherapy
Iodine-125	0.028	60 days	Brachytherapy
Phosphorus-32	1.7	14 days	Intraperitoneal instillation
Gold-196	0.4	2.7 days	Intraperitoneal instillation
Strontium-89	1.4	51 days	Diffuse bone metastases
Samarium-153	0.6	1.9 days	Diffuse bone metastases

MeV = million electron volts.

(Fig. 28-4). Depending on the energy level of the incident radiation, one of these mechanisms will predominate. The *photoelectric effect* is dominant if the incident energy is low (less than 100 kV). The *Compton effect* dominates in mid- to high energy ranges (1 MV to 20 MV) and is the most important in clinical radiation therapy. Last, *pair production* occurs when a photon beam with very high energy (beyond 20 MV) strikes the electromagnetic field of the nucleus.

■ Depth-Dose Curve

Controlled biologic damage is accomplished by greater selective radiation dose distribution within malignant tissue than within the surrounding, "innocent bystander" normal tissues. This is achieved by using radiation beams with differing physical properties to define the spatial distribution of an absorbed dose when these beams strike tissue. Ideally, an absorbed radiation dose is as conformal as possible. Perfect conformality is achieved when the targeted malignant tissue absorbs 100 percent of the prescribed dose and the adjacent normal tissues absorb 0 percent.

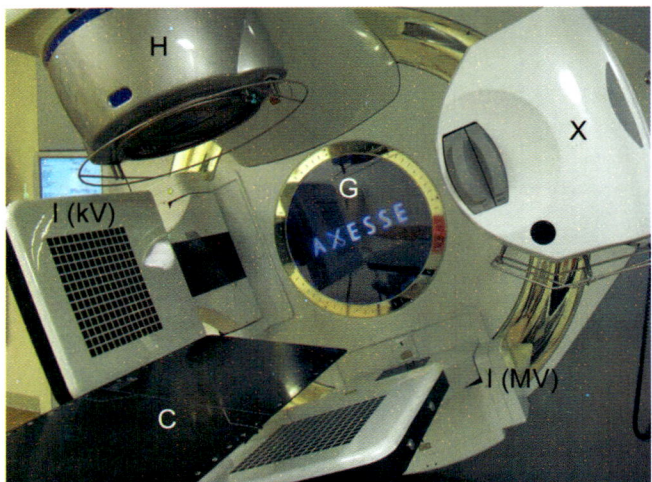

FIGURE 28-3 Linear accelerator currently in use at Tufts Medical Center. The patient lies on the treatment couch (C). The gantry (G), couch, and head (H) can all rotate and allow radiation beams to reach target tissues through different angles. A kV x-ray source (X) is used in conjunction with an image intensifier (I-kV) for image-guided radiotherapy (IGRT). Another image intensifier (I-MV) is used for standard port imaging.

In practice, this cannot be obtained. However, both acute radiation side effects and the potential for late, delayed radiation complications can be minimized as the spatial radiation dose distribution approaches this ideal.

A *depth-dose curve* specifically illustrates the dose distribution of a given radiation beam as it penetrates tissues. Radiation oncologists rely on these curves when choosing a radiation beam with an appropriate energy to reach a given tumor. With electron beam therapy, the maximum dose lies close to the surface, and therefore, electron beam therapy is indicated for targets that are close to the skin surface, such as metastatic cancer to the inguinal lymph nodes. With high-energy photons, the maximum dose is deposited well below the surface. Beyond this point, the dose gradually diminishes as energy is absorbed by the deep surrounding tissues. This explains the so-called *skin-sparing effect* of high-energy photons. A patient with a pelvic malignancy is usually treated with at least 6-MV photon beams.

Dosimetry

This is the discipline of calculating the radiation dose absorbed by the patient. Dosimetric calculations are based on the depth-dose measurements of the radiation beams used to treat an actual patient. The dose distribution is usually displayed as a colorful map overlaid on the radiologic images of the patient (see Fig. 28-2). These calculations *predict* the absorbed dose in a given situation.

■ Radiation Unit

Quantification of the absorbed radiation dose is essential, as it correlates with the biologic effect of radiation. The current Standard International unit for absorbed dose is gray (Gy). One Gy equals 100 rad or 1 joule/kg. Clinically, the radiation doses for curative and palliative treatment are 70 to 85 Gy and 30 to 40 Gy, respectively.

RADIATION BIOLOGY

■ DNA Molecule as Radiation Target

The DNA molecule is the target for the biologic effect of radiation on mammalian cells. DNA injuries involve its strands, bases, and cross-links, but the hallmark damage is breaking of single- and

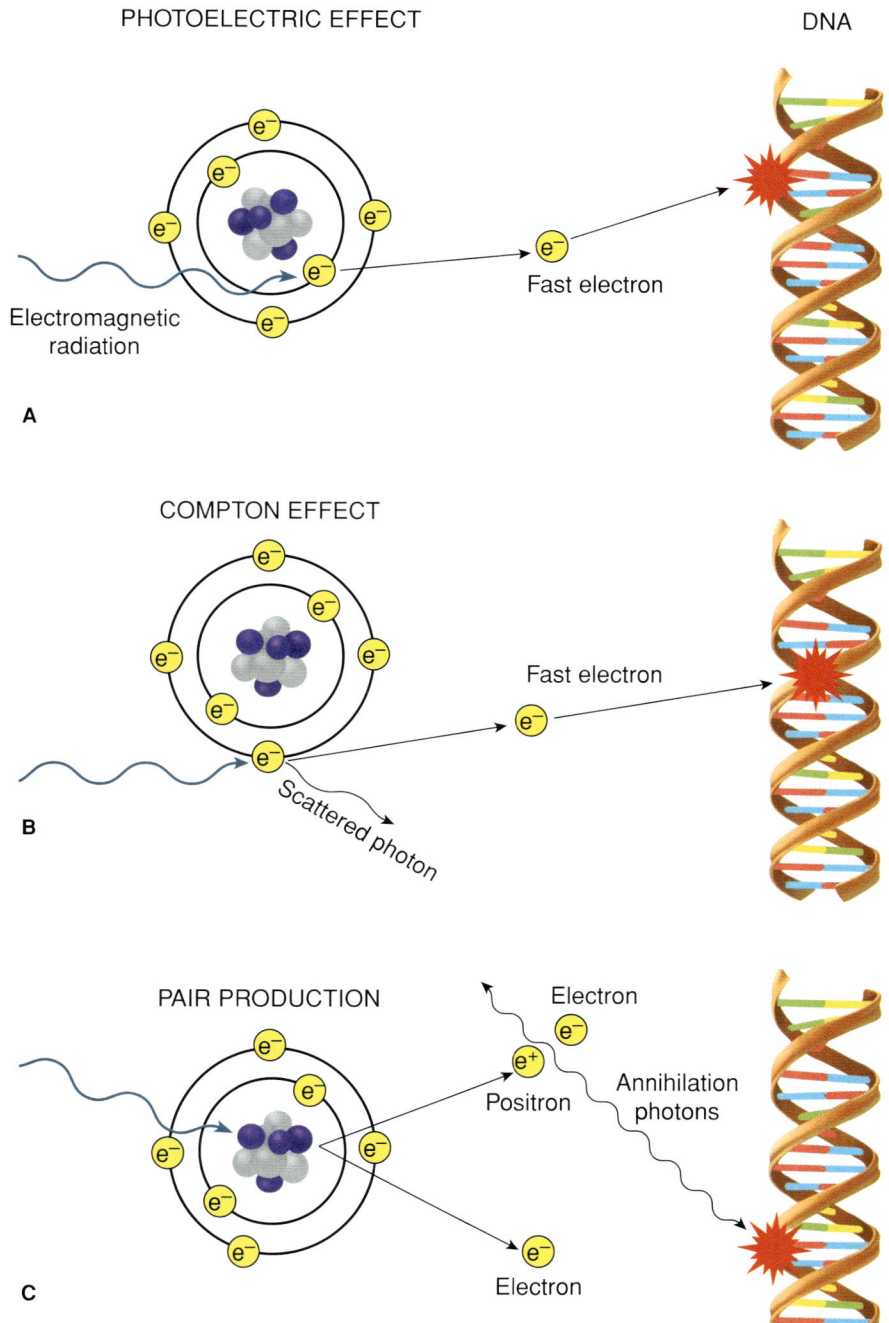

PHOTOELECTRIC EFFECT

Electromagnetic radiation

Fast electron

A

DNA

COMPTON EFFECT

Fast electron

Scattered photon

B

PAIR PRODUCTION

Electron

Positron

Annihilation photons

Electron

C

FIGURE 28-4 When electromagnetic radiation impacts target tissues, energy is transferred to those tissues. The three mechanisms involved in this energy transfer are the photoelectric effect, Compton effect, and pair production. Both photoelectric effect **(A)** and Compton effect **(B)** result in creation of fast electrons, which then initiate the biologic process of radiation damage. **A.** With photoelectric effect, radiation interacts with an inner orbital electron. **B.** With Compton effect, interaction occurs with an outer orbital electron. **C.** During pair production, impact of radiation on the atom's nuclear forces produces a positron-electron pair. When a positron later combines with a free electron in these tissues, two photons are created, which can then lead to radiation damage.

Direct versus Indirect Actions of Ionizing Radiation

Radiation can interact *directly* or *indirectly* with the atoms in the DNA molecule. Direct actions create ions that then initiate the biologic damage process. This *direct* effect is predominant with high linear energy transfer (LET) particles such as protons, fast neutrons, and heavy ions (Fig. 28-5). However, most DNA damage is caused indirectly, which is the predominant effect with low-LET particles such as photons. Indirect DNA damage occurs through an important chemical intermediate, the hydroxyl radical ($\cdot$OH), which is highly reactive because of its unpaired electron.

Cell Death

The two main cell death pathways after radiation are *apoptosis* and *mitotic catastrophe*. Mitotic catastrophe is thought to be the most common mechanism of cell death after radiation exposure. With this, cells with damaged DNA enter mitosis prematurely, before DNA can be repaired, and die attempting to complete the next two to three mitotic cycles. Apoptosis, or programmed cell death, occurs after an intracellular stress, such as radiation-induced irreparable double-strand breaks. A series of events develop rapidly within hours, leading to cell membrane blebbing, apoptotic body formation in the cytoplasm, chromatin condensation, nuclear fragmentation, and DNA laddering (Okada, 2004).

Four R's of Radiation Biology: Repair, Reassortment, Repopulation, Reoxygenation

In classic radiation biology, cells respond to radiation by four mechanisms. Cellular *repair* can be described by sublethal damage repair (SLDR) and potentially lethal damage repair (PLDR). SLDR occurs when a radiation dose is split into two or more fractions and a few hours separate the fractions. Cells have time to repair their damage, and their survival rate increases. The last process seen in SLDR is *repopulation*, which is the tissue's response to replenish the cell pool (Trott, 1999).

Following the initial repair of sublethal damage, *reassortment* begins. Within a tumor, proliferating cells are in different phases of the cell cycle (Fig. 27-1, p. 581). Cells in mitosis (M) and G_2

most importantly double-stranded DNA. Double-strand breaks lead to DNA fragmentation when two or more breaks are formed and when cells attempt to repair these strand breaks. The DNA pieces may rejoin incorrectly, leading to gene translocation, mutation, or amplification, and ultimately cell death.

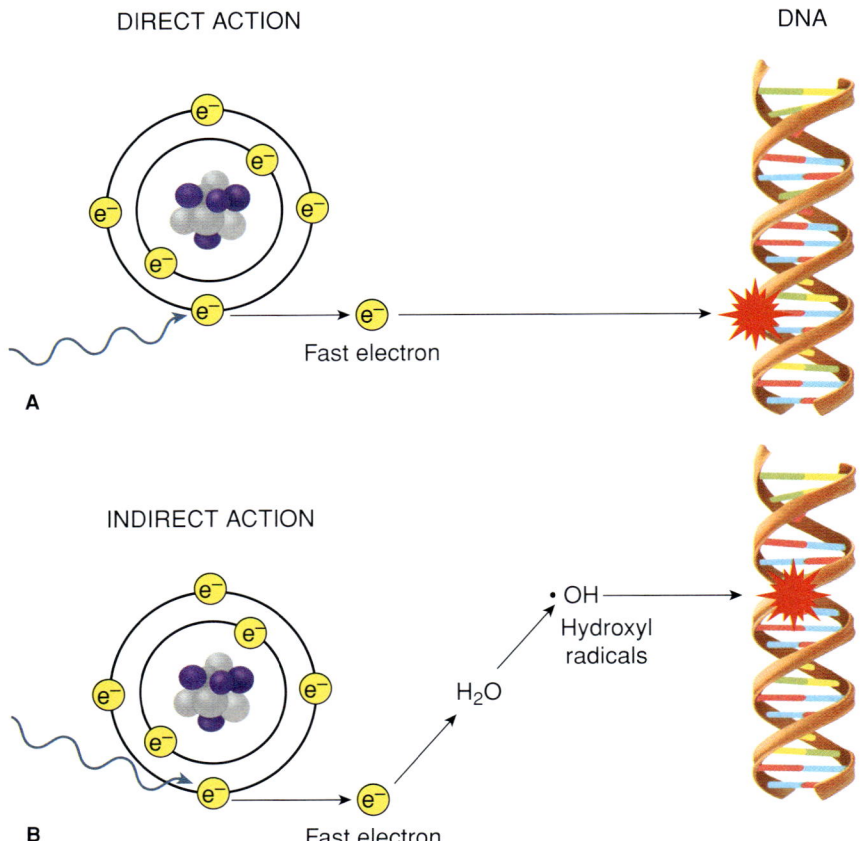

DIRECT ACTION

A

Fast electron

INDIRECT ACTION

B

Fast electron

H_2O

• OH
Hydroxyl
radicals

DNA

FIGURE 28-5 Direct and indirect actions of radiation. **A.** Fast electrons may directly strike DNA to create damage. **B.** Alternatively, a fast electron may interact with water to create a hydroxyl radical, which subsequently interacts with DNA to cause injury.

are most sensitive to radiation. Conversely, cells in G_1 and S (DNA synthesis) phases are less sensitive (Pawlik, 2004). When exposed to radiation, those cells that are in the G_2/M phase are killed. During reassortment, surviving cell populations restart their progression through the mitotic cycle.

The fourth "R" of radiation biology theory is _reoxygenation_. A tumor cell population is composed of oxygenated and hypoxic components. Cells located within 100 microns of blood capillaries are oxygenated, and beyond 100 microns, cells are hypoxic. After radiation, the oxygenated cells are killed by the hydroxyl radical described earlier. Following cell death, the tumor shrinks and allows hypoxic cells to be positioned within the oxygen diffusion range of blood capillaries. Thereby, they become oxygenated and susceptible.

■ Linear-Quadratic Theory and the Alpha/Beta Ratio

For low-LET radiation, the linear-quadratic curve has been adopted to explain the relationship between the fraction of cells surviving a given dose of radiation (Fig. 28-6). The initial linear (alpha) portion of the curve shows that the probability of cell death is proportional to the radiation dose. In the higher-dose region, the curved quadratic (beta) portion indicates that the probability of cell death is proportional to the _square_ of the dose.

The alpha/beta ratio reflects the response of normal tissues to radiation. _Early-responding tissues_ have a high alpha/beta ratio and will manifest reactions to radiation within a few days to weeks after treatment. Examples are tissues with high proliferation rates such as bone marrow, reproductive organs, and gastrointestinal tract mucosa. Preventatively, by administering multiple small radiation dose fractions, sublethal damage repair predominates, and early acute reactions can be decreased.

In contrast, _late-responding_ tissues show clinical reactions only weeks to months after completion of a radiation therapy course. Examples are the lung, kidney, spinal cord, and brain. These tissues have a low alpha/beta ratio and are slow to respond. More time is needed to repair sublethal damage, and thus high-dose-per-fraction radiation therapy can easily lead to severe late complications.

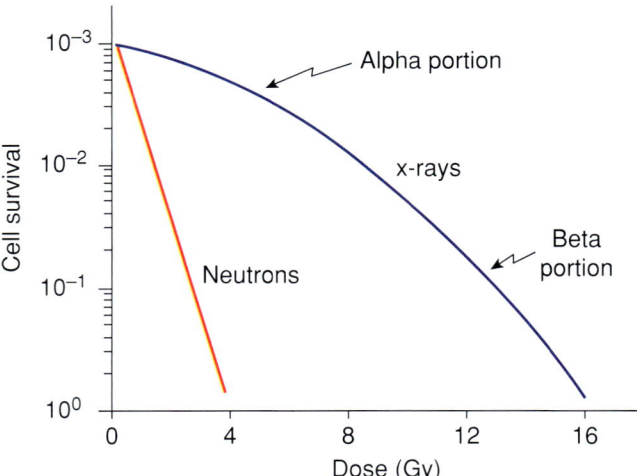

FIGURE 28-6 Linear quadratic mammalian cell survival curve. The cell survival is plotted on a logarithmic scale. The dose (in Gy) is on a linear scale. The typical cell survival curves with low-LET (linear energy transfer) (_blue curve_) and with high-LET radiation (_red line_) are shown. With low-LET x-ray doses, the alpha (linear) portion of the curve is flat and shows that cell survival is proportional to the dose. However, as the dose increases, the beta (quadratic) portion bends, which implies that cell survival is proportional to the dose squared. In contrast, with high-LET radiation, such as neutrons, the survival curve is straight.

RADIATION ONCOLOGY PRACTICE

The expertise of the radiation oncologist who is designing and monitoring a course of radiation treatment is paramount. The radiation oncologist carves out, en-bloc, a volume of cancerous tissue, its local extensions, and its regional lymphatics, while accommodating the patient's comorbidities, general health status, and surrounding normal tissue quality.

As cancer management is frequently multimodal, superior treatment outcomes are highly dependent on clear communication between radiation oncologists and their colleagues in surgical and medical oncology. Optimal integration of diagnostic imaging and histologic evaluation also is vital to planning and implementing potentially curative radiation therapy. As such, early involvement of the radiation oncologist in patient evaluation and counseling enhances the probability of effective and coordinated cancer care.

■ Radiation Fractionation Schemes

Parameters that affect the efficacy and safety of a radiation course include the total radiation dose applied, the size of each radiation "fraction" (treatment), the time between treatments ("fractionation schedule"), and the elapsed time to deliver the total prescribed dose.

Standard Fractionation

Successful eradication of a localized cancer requires that the cancer cells be killed more rapidly and efficiently than surviving cancer cells can proliferate and repopulate. Because of the inevitable exposure of some normal tissues to substantial radiation, limits are placed on the total radiation dose that can be prudently administered to a given target volume. In general, delivery of this dose over the shortest feasible elapsed time will maximize efficacy. Accomplishing this objective is limited by the known deleterious consequences of a high dose per fraction on normal tissues. As noted, this can result in delayed radiation injury expressed months or years after therapy completion. For this reason, radiation delivered with curative intent is generally administered in daily treatments (Monday through Friday) of 1.8 Gy to 2.0 Gy. Cumulative doses range from 45 Gy to treat microscopic disease to 70 Gy or more to treat gross disease. This concern for delayed injury is less when short courses of radiation are administered with palliative intent, often in dose fractions of 2.5 Gy to 4.0 Gy.

Altered Fractionation

Regimens involving treatments given more than once a day are reserved for selected cases. In such instances, increased local tumor control and decreased long-term complications may be achieved by manipulating both fraction size and overall treatment time. Two major strategies have been employed, namely, hyperfractionation and accelerated treatment.

With *hyperfractionation*, the goal is to reduce late damage to normal tissues, and accordingly, a smaller dose per fraction is given. Two or more fractions are administered each day, typically 6 hours apart to provide an interval for normal tissue repair.

Accelerated fractionation shortens the treatment duration with or without a drop in the total dose to overcome tumor cell repopulation. The usual weekend break is either shortened or eliminated. With accelerated treatment, however, severe acute reactions are frequent.

Altered fractionation has been studied in gynecologic cancers. Radiation Therapy Oncology Group (RTOG) trials 88-05 and 92-10 were Phase II trials that investigated the use of twice-daily radiation and chemoradiation, respectively, in advanced cervical cancer. RTOG 88-05 showed similar local control, survival rates, and toxicity compared with historical controls. However, when chemotherapy and larger-field twice-daily radiation were added, rates of late Grade 4 toxicity were unacceptably high (Grigsby, 2001, 2002).

■ Radiation Therapy

External Beam Radiation Therapy

External beam radiation therapy is indicated when an area to be irradiated is large. For example, the fields needed to treat a locally advanced cervical cancer may cover the whole pelvis and, occasionally, the paraaortic lymph nodes.

Conformal radiation therapy (CRT) describes a radiation treatment technique that maximizes tumor damage yet minimizes injury to the surrounding normal tissues. To achieve this goal, the radiation oncologist must know the precise extent of the cancer to be irradiated and its relationship to surrounding normal tissues. This process begins with a review of the patient's cancer imaging including computed tomography (CT), magnetic resonance (MR) imaging, and positron emission tomography (PET). Imaging, along with careful review of the patient's pathology and operative report, assists in defining the 3-dimensional (3-D) target (tumor or regions of potential microscopic tumor spread) and normal tissue volumes.

Next, a simulation is performed in a simulation suite to delineate the anticipated therapy fields prior to an actual treatment session. During this process, patient positioning, immobilization techniques, and treatment fields are defined. If feasible, radiation blocking techniques are used to shape the treatment beams to shield normal tissues. The patient is placed in the treatment position, and a CT scan of the area of interest is performed. Later, on each of the computer-based CT scan slices, the radiation oncologist carefully delineates the anatomic areas that will receive a tumoricidal dose. During this, four volumes are defined: (1) a gross tumor volume (GTV), which encompasses any gross disease; (2) a clinical target volume (CTV), which incorporates any areas at risk for microscopic tumor spread; (3) a planning target volume (PTV), which accounts for uncertainties in treatment delivery such as patient motion or daily set-up error; and (4) a volume that defines the normal organs at risk (OAR), which will be exposed, albeit to a lesser radiation dose.

Once simulation is completed, a radiation dosimetrist employs treatment planning software to develop an optimal plan, called *dose optimization*. This is often a reiterative process in which the physician and the dosimetrist will arrive at an acceptable option, which means an optimal arrangement and shaping of the radiation beams.

One tool that is particularly helpful during radiation planning and optimization is the dose-volume histogram (DVH). This is a graphic summary of the entire dose distribution to the cancer and normal structures. Thus, the DVH provides information regarding whether the cancer will be adequately treated with a tumoricidal dose and whether surrounding normal structures are minimally affected. In addition to the DVH, dose distributions are displayed as computer-generated radiation dose map images that are overlaid on the CT images. This provides a visual dose-anatomy relationship. These dose distributions are produced for

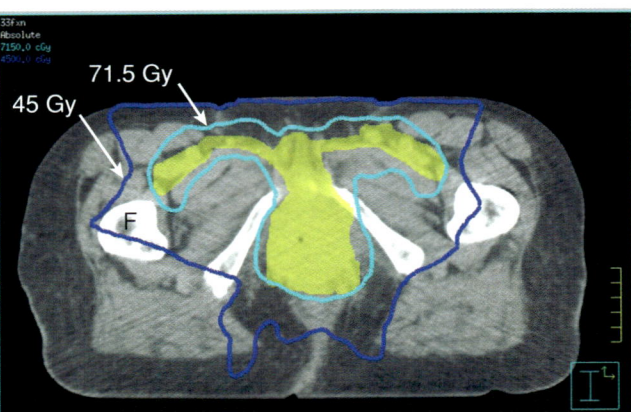

A

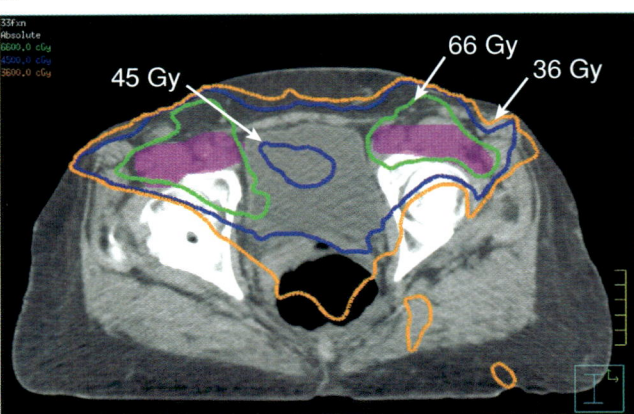

B

FIGURE 28-7 IMRT dose distribution in a patient with stage T4 N2 M0 cancer of the vulva. This technique allows for the delivery of tumoricidal doses to the vulva and inguinal nodes while minimizing that to normal tissues. **A.** The yellow area displays the actual vulvar cancer and inguinal lymph nodes. Doses to the vulva and femoral heads (F) are shown (*arrows*). The doses to the vulva and femoral heads are 71.5 Gy and 45 Gy, respectively. **B.** Pink shading displays the inguinal nodes. Doses to the inguinal nodes, bladder, and rectum are shown (*arrows*). The doses to the inguinal nodes, bladder, and rectum were 66 Gy, 45 Gy, and 36 Gy, respectively.

the radiation oncologist to review, adjust, and finally approve. The final chosen plan is reviewed by a radiation physicist who ensures that the physical and technical details can be implemented.

To further improve the conformality of the dose distribution, especially around concave targets, a more advanced 3D-CRT planning system, called *intensity-modulated radiation therapy (IMRT)*, can be used (Fig. 28-7). As a result of this improved conformality, IMRT has the potential to decrease bowel and bladder toxicity during pelvic radiation therapy (Heron, 2003). IMRT modulates the intensity of radiation beams to be used with the help of dedicated computer software. For quality assurance, weekly or sometimes even daily imaging of the treated regions is performed to verify that treatment configurations are correct.

Stereotactic Body Radiation Therapy. Over the past decade, a novel external beam radiation therapy technique, *stereotactic body radiation therapy (SBRT)*, has become commonly used in sites such as the lung, liver, and spine. It uses

a hypofractionated regimen of five or fewer fractions (10 to 20 Gy per fraction). Using *image-guided radiation therapy (IGRT)*, precise, safe SBRT and IMRT have become possible through "real-time" approaches to overcome technical factors such as patient or organ motion and tumor size and shape changes during a treatment course.

Brachytherapy

Brachytherapy means treatment at a short distance. During this therapy, sealed or unsealed radioisotopes are inserted into the cancer or its immediate vicinity. Radiation doses fall sharply with increasing distances from the radioactive source. Thus, brachytherapy is indicated only for small tumor volumes (less than 3 to 4 cm). For this reason, brachytherapy is typically practiced after external beam radiation therapy has decreased a large tumor volume.

Brachytherapy may be intracavitary or interstitial. During *intracavitary brachytherapy*, applicators that hold sealed radioactive sources such as iridium-192 (^{192}Ir) are inserted into a body cavity such as the uterus. Alternatively, *interstitial brachytherapy* requires the placement of catheters or needles directly into the cancer and surrounding tissues.

Brachytherapy may be temporary or permanent. In *temporary brachytherapy*, the radioisotopes are removed from the patient after a period of time, ranging from minutes to days. All intracavitary and some interstitial implants are temporary. In *permanent brachytherapy*, the radioisotopes are left permanently to decay within the tissues.

Equipment. For routine gynecologic intracavitary implantation, standard equipment includes an applicator, called a *tandem*, which fits into the uterine cavity, and a pair of vaginal applicators, which are known as *ovoids* (Fig. 28-8). The tandem and ovoid device (T&O) is inserted under general anesthesia or conscious sedation. Following placement, radioactive sources can then be loaded into both the tandem and ovoids. In gynecologic oncology, brachytherapy with T&O is indicated for cervical cancer. For uterine cancer, vaginal brachytherapy with a cylinder is used to treat the vaginal apex or length of the vagina, which is the most common site of disease recurrence after hysterectomy (Fig. 28-9).

For temporary interstitial implantation, flexible plastic catheters or metal needles are surgically placed into the target

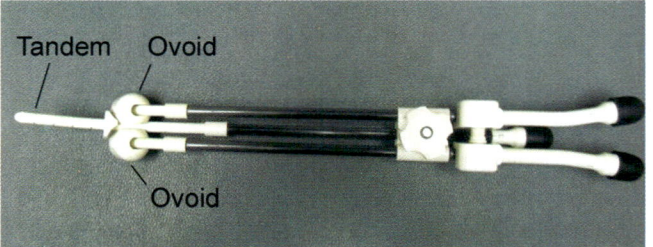

FIGURE 28-8 Computed tomography/magnetic resonance–compatible tandem and ovoids used for cervical cancer brachytherapy. The long slender portion of the device (tandem) is inserted into the endometrial cavity, and white cylinders (ovoids) are positioned in the proximal vagina. Radioactive sources can be loaded into both the tandem and ovoid reservoirs.

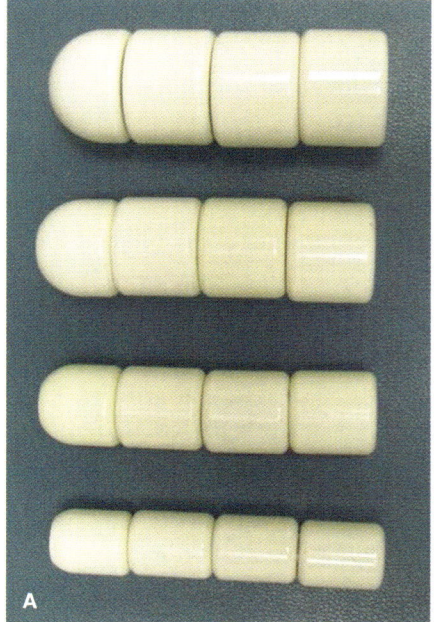
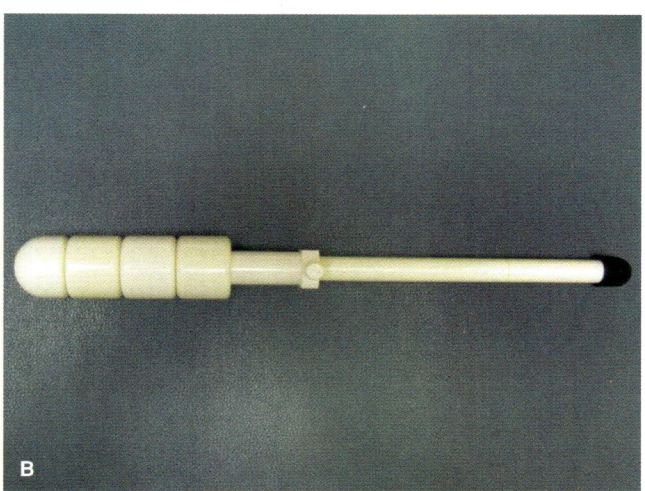

FIGURE 28-9 Computed tomography/magnetic resonance–compatible cylinders (**A**) come in different sizes to allow the most appropriate fit for the patient's anatomy. The largest possible diameter is preferred. **B.** The cylinder is used for vaginal brachytherapy after surgery for uterine cancer. It is placed in the vagina and high dose-rate brachytherapy is delivered. This treatment decreases the risk of vaginal cuff recurrences.

tissues and held in place by a perineal template. These are then afterloaded with ^{192}Ir seeds. Templates are suitable for patients with advanced cancers, suboptimal anatomy for T&O application, and selected recurrent cancers.

In addition to T&O, vaginal cylinder, and interstitial needles, physicians may choose to use a tandem and ring, split-ring, or tandem and cylinder. Appropriate brachytherapy applicator selection requires expertise, as applicator choice depends on patient anatomy and a specific device's dose distribution.

Manual versus Remote Afterloading. Once the brachytherapy instruments are in place, the radioactive sources are inserted. Historically, the sources were placed manually, however, this method increased hospital staff radiation exposure. Subsequently, a *remote afterloading* approach was developed and is commonly practiced today. This remote control system delivers a single miniaturized iridium source from a protective safe through connecting cables to the holding devices previously inserted into the patient. Following treatment, the radioactive source is automatically retracted back into the safe**.**

Low Dose-Rate versus High Dose-Rate Brachytherapy. Traditionally, low dose-rate (LDR) brachytherapy is delivered over the course of many days and requires patient hospitalization. Over the past few decades, however, high-dose-rate (HDR) brachytherapy has become more popular. With this technique, treatment is shortened to minutes. Low dose is defined as dose rates from 0.4 Gy to 2 Gy/hr, and high dose describes dose rates higher than 12 Gy/hr. For example, with an intracavitary implant for cervical cancer and an LDR technique, a dose of 30 to 40 Gy is delivered continuously over several days. In contrast, with HDR, an equivalent dose can be delivered in 3 to 5 weekly fractions. The dose per fraction is 5 to 7 Gy and can be

given in 10 to 20 minutes. Unlike LDR, HDR avoids lengthy inpatient hospitalization and minimizes patient immobility and thromboembolic events. Furthermore, long-term analysis shows similar local tumor control and late complication rates in patients treated for cervical cancer with both HDR and LDR (Arai, 1991; Hareyama, 2002; Wong, 2003).

■ Tumor Control Probability

With most epithelial cancers, the probability that radiation therapy will control a cancerous mass depends on the tumor's size and intrinsic radiosensitivity and on the radiation dose and delivery schedule. For example, within a given stage, large tumors are more difficult to control with radiation than smaller ones (Bentzen, 1996; Dubben, 1998).

Intrinsic Radiosensitivity

It is recognized that a tumor's radiosensitivity in general is determined by its pathologic type (Table 28-3). However, even cancers with a similar histology may have variable responses to radiation. This may be explained by heterogeneity within a given tumor and by the cancer cell's ability to repair radiation damage (Schwartz, 1988, 1996; Weichselbaum, 1992).

TABLE 28-3. Radiosensitivity of Some Selected Cancers

Sensitivity	Cancer Type
Highly sensitive	Lymphoma, dysgerminoma, small cell cancer, embryonal cancer
Moderately sensitive	Squamous carcinoma, adenocarcinoma
Poorly sensitive	Osteosarcoma, glioma, melanoma

Treatment Time

When protracted time intervals are required to complete a fractionated radiation therapy course, tumor control probability decreases, especially in rapidly proliferating epithelial cancers. Thus, treatment breaks or delays for any reason are minimized. In a retrospective review of 209 patients with stage I to III cervical cancer treated with radiation therapy, the 5-year pelvic control and overall survival rates were better for those who completed the treatment in less than 55 days (87 percent and 65 percent, respectively) than for those who did so in more than 55 days (72 percent and 54 percent, respectively) (Petereit, 1995).

Tumor Hypoxia

Tumor hypoxia is a major factor leading to poor local tumor control and poor survival rates in patients with cervical cancer (Brizel, 1999; Nordsmark, 1996). The close relationship between tumor hypoxia, anemia, and angiogenesis was demonstrated in a study involving 87 patients with stage II, III, and IV cervical cancer treated with radiation only. Of these, patients with hemoglobin levels <11 g/dL and a median tumor oxygen tension pO_2 <15 mm Hg had decreased 3-year survival rates (Dunst, 2003).

To overcome tumor hypoxia, many strategies have been devised and vary in efficacy. Of these, hyperbaric oxygen used in conjunction with radiation therapy in cervical cancer was not effective in clinical studies (Dische, 1999). An alternate method to increase oxygen delivery to tissues manipulates blood vessel hemodynamics with either inhaled carbogen (95 percent oxygen and 5 percent carbon dioxide) or nicotinamide (a vasoactive agent). This approach of *accelerated radiotherapy with carbogen and nicotinamide (ARCON)* improves tumor control in patients with anemia but is not commonly used (Janssens, 2014).

Another approach to minimize tumor hypoxia effects employs *bioreductive agents*. This family of hypoxic cell sensitizers selectively kills hypoxic cells. Earlier findings with one of these, tirapazamine (TPZ), was encouraging. However, results of a Gynecologic Oncology Group (GOG) Phase III trial that evaluated TPZ, cisplatin, and radiation therapy compared with cisplatin and radiation show no improvement in survival or tumor control rates for patients with cervical cancers (DiSilvestro, 2014).

Last, to ensure adequate oxygen carrying capacity, a hemoglobin level of at least 12 g/dL is desirable in patients receiving radiation therapy. To this goal, transfusion ameliorates tumor hypoxia and increases radiation response. In a study of 204 women with cervical cancer who were treated with radiation, those who were transfused to maintain a hemoglobin level >11 g/dL had a similar 5-year disease-free survival rate (71 percent) compared with a group of women who never required transfusion. The disease-free survival rate was only 26 percent for those with persistent anemia (Kapp, 2002). The use of erythropoietin to maintain hemoglobin above 12 g/dL was also tested in a randomized trial of patients with cervical cancer receiving chemotherapy and radiation. This trial closed early due to higher rates of thromboembolism with erythropoietin use (Thomas, 2008).

■ Ionizing Radiation and Chemotherapy

Radiation is often combined with chemotherapy, surgery, or both to improve local disease control and decrease distant metastasis. Radiation therapy and chemotherapy can be administered in a concurrent or alternating fashion to maximize tumoricidal effects and minimize overlapping toxicities and complications (Steel, 1979). This practice is supported by results from many controlled studies involving cervical and other cancers.

In the management of gynecologic cancers, platinum compounds are most commonly used with radiation therapy. Both radiation and cisplatin cause single- and double-strand DNA breaks and base damage. Although most lesions are repaired, if cisplatin-induced DNA damage lies close to a radiation-induced single-strand break, then the damage is irreparable and leads to cell death (Amorino, 1999; Begg, 1990). Since the late 1990s, the standard treatment for newly diagnosed locally advanced cervical cancer has been radiation therapy and cisplatin (Keys, 1999; Morris, 1999; Rose, 1999).

Nucleoside analogues such as fludarabine and gemcitabine also are used to enhance the effects of radiation-induced cell killing. These agents inhibit DNA synthesis by blocking cells at the G_1/S checkpoint. The remaining cell population is synchronized at the G_2/M junction, the most radiation-sensitive phase of the cell cycle. Clinically, in a Phase III study of cervical cancer patients, the progression-free survival and overall survival rates improved in patients randomized to receive gemcitabine, cisplatin, and radiation followed by adjuvant gemcitabine compared with cisplatin and radiation alone (Duenãs-González, 2011). However, inclusion of gemcitabine is still considered investigational for cervical cancer treatment.

Taxanes, such as paclitaxel and docetaxel, enhance the effects of radiation by causing microtubule dysfunction and blocking cells at the G_2/M junction (Mason, 1999). Taxanes have been administered with platinum agents and radiation therapy in small nonrandomized trials involving patients with locally advanced cervical cancer (Lee, 2007).

■ Radiation Therapy and Surgery

Radiation therapy can be given before, after, or at the time of surgery. With this combination, surgical resection and its associated morbidity can often be minimized.

Preoperative adjuvant radiation, which is radiation prior to surgery, may offer several advantages for tumor control. First, primary cancers tend to locally infiltrate surrounding normal tissues with microscopic extension. Accordingly, radiation can be delivered prior to surgery to decrease the potential for locoregional and distant tumor dissemination and the likelihood of positive surgical margins. To sterilize areas of subclinical infiltration, doses of 40 to 50 Gy administered over 4 to 5 weeks are required. Although preoperative radiation therapy is not expected to render the main tumor mass cancer-free at the time of surgery, it is common to find no evidence of cancer in the surgical specimen. Second, the combination of radiation and surgery in locally advanced vulvovaginal cancer can allow surgeons to avoid extensive surgery such as pelvic exenteration (Boronow, 1982). Last, in patients who present with unresectable cancers, preoperative radiation therapy can transform them into suitable candidates for a surgical attempt (Montana, 2000). Surgery is usually delayed 4 to 6 weeks after radiation completion. By then, the acute radiation reactions have subsided, and pathologic interpretation of the resected specimen is easier.

Two studies by the GOG (GOG 71 and 123) have investigated preoperative radiation and chemoradiation, respectively, in patients with bulky stage IB cervical cancer (Keys, 1999, 2003). In both trials, the pathologic complete response rate, defined as no residual disease in a resected specimen, approximated 50 percent.

Postoperatively, a high probability for local recurrence may often be predicted by factors such as positive margins, lymph node metastases, lymphovascular invasion, and high-grade disease. In these cases, postoperative radiation therapy may be beneficial and is ideally delivered 3 to 6 weeks following surgery. This delay allows initial wound healing (Sedlis, 1999). The radiation fields should encompass the operative bed due to the possibility of tumor contamination at the time of surgery and adjacent areas that are at risk for tumor dissemination.

Postoperative radiation is employed in the treatment of many gynecologic malignancies. For cervical cancer, postoperative radiation is recommended in those with lymphovascular invasion, deep stromal invasion, or large tumor size (Sedlis, 1999). Postoperative chemoradiation is offered if positive parametria, positive margins, or positive lymph nodes are found. The addition of cisplatin and 5-fluorouracil to radiation in cervical cancer patients with these high-risk features has been shown to improve survival rates and tumor control (Peters, 2000).

For uterine cancer, postoperative radiation is frequently used for patients with stage IB or greater disease. Several large randomized controlled trials have demonstrated significant improvements in local control in patients with intermediate-risk endometrial adenocarcinoma who receive adjuvant pelvic radiation (ASTEC/EN.5 Study Group, 2009; Creutzberg, 2011; Keys, 2004). Intermediate risk includes older age, lymphovascular invasion, deep myometrial invasion, or intermediate- or high-grade disease. Patients with fewer risk factors can often be treated with vaginal brachytherapy alone. Vaginal brachytherapy treats the vaginal apex, where approximately 75 percent of recurrences are located. A randomized trial showed similar vaginal and pelvic tumor control rates with fewer side effects when vaginal brachytherapy alone was compared with pelvic external beam radiation therapy (Nout, 2010).

Intraoperative radiation therapy (IORT) is infrequently elected. It may be delivered either by interstitial brachytherapy or by an electron beam produced by a dedicated linear accelerator installed in the operating room. A single dose of 10 to 20 Gy is typically directed to the area at risk for recurrence or suspected of harboring residual cancer (Gemignani, 2001).

Further information on the role of radiation therapy in the treatment of gynecological malignancies is available in guidelines prepared by the American Society for Radiation Oncology and the American Brachytherapy Society (Beriwal, 2012; Lee, 2012a; Klopp, 2014; Jones, 2016; Small, 2012; Viswanathan, 2012a,b). Additionally, the American College of Radiology has formulated guidelines regarding the use of radiotherapy in specific gynecological malignancies (American College of Radiology, 2018).

■ Normal Tissue Response to Radiation Therapy

In general, radiation therapy is less well tolerated if: (1) the irradiated tissue volume is large, (2) the radiation dose is high, (3) the dose per fraction is large, and (4) the patient's age is advanced. Furthermore, the radiation damage to normal tissues can be exacerbated by factors such as prior surgery, concurrent chemotherapy, infection, diabetes mellitus, hypertension, and inflammatory bowel disease.

In general, if tissues with a rapid proliferation rate such as epithelium of the small intestine or oral cavity are irradiated, acute clinical symptoms develop within a few days to weeks. This contrasts with muscular, renal, and neural tissues, which have low proliferation rates and may not display signs of radiation damage for months to years after treatment. To avoid serious complications, radiation oncologists must use published tolerance doses for normal tissues as a guide and rely on their own clinical experience. For example, to avoid severe rectal and bladder complications in patients with cervical cancer, doses of no more than 65 Gy and 70 Gy are recommended to the rectum and bladder, respectively (Milano, 2007).

Epithelium and Parenchyma

Atrophy is the most consistent sequela of radiation therapy. It affects all lining epithelia—including skin and the epithelia of the gastrointestinal, respiratory, and genitourinary tracts and of the endocrine glands. Additionally, necrosis and ulceration may develop. Within the submucosa and deep soft tissues, fibrosis frequently follows radiation therapy, leading to tissue contracture and stenosis (Fajardo, 2005).

Of vascular structures, the capillary is the most radiosensitive, and ischemia results from endothelial damage, capillary wall rupture, loss of capillary segments, and reduction of microvascular networks. In large arteries, atheroma-like calcifications develop (Friedlander, 2003; Zidar, 1997).

Skin

Four general types of skin reactions may follow radiation therapy. In order of increasing severity, they include erythema, dry desquamation, moist desquamation, and skin necrosis. For many women during a 6- to 7-week radiation therapy course, the first three of these reactions are common. Within 2 weeks following radiation exposure, the skin develops mild erythema. By the fourth week, the redness becomes more pronounced and dry desquamation may begin. After 5 to 6 weeks, moist desquamation may follow. This involves epidermal sloughing, followed by serum and blood oozing through denuded skin. This reaction is mostly pronounced in skin folds, such as the inguinal, axillary, and inframammary creases.

Preventatively, throughout and after a radiation course, the skin is kept clean and aerated. For dry desquamation, ointments or aloe vera–containing creams promote dermal hydration with an emollient effect. During the moist desquamation phase, skin treatment may include moisturizers (e.g., Biafine), sitz baths, and silver sulfadiazine–containing, nonadhering dressings for weeping areas. Importantly, individuals are instructed to avoid applying heating pads, soaps, or alcohol-based lotions to irradiated skin.

Regeneration of the epithelium starts soon after radiation treatment and is usually complete in 4 to 6 weeks. Months later, areas of skin hyper- and hypopigmentation can be seen. The skin may remain atrophied, thin, and dry, and telangiectasias may be visible.

Vagina

Radiation therapy directed to the pelvis frequently leads to acute vaginal mucositis. Although mucosal ulceration is rare, discharge is present in most cases. For these women, a dilute hydrogen peroxide and water solution used at the vulva provides symptomatic relief.

In contrast, delayed reactions to radiation may include atrophic vaginitis, formation of vaginal synechiae or telangiectasia, and most commonly, vaginal stricture. Less frequently, rectovaginal or vesicovaginal fistulas may develop after radiation therapy, especially with advanced-stage cancers. Of these delayed reactions, Grade 3 vaginal stricture is defined by the Common Terminology Criteria for Adverse Events (CTCAE) as "vaginal narrowing and/or shortening interfering with the use of tampons, sexual activity or physical examination" (National Cancer Institute, 2017). Preventatively, vaginal stricture or synechiae may be avoided if intercourse is resumed following treatment or if women are instructed regarding dilator use. Dilators are inserted vaginally by the patient daily for 10 seconds, and this schedule continues from radiation therapy completion until the first follow-up visit at 6 weeks. At this point, weekly insertion or intercourse is recommended. Increased severe late vaginal toxicity is associated with poor dilator compliance, concurrent chemotherapy, and age >50 (Gondi, 2012). Importantly, stricture prevention also aids the ability to complete thorough vaginal examinations for cancer surveillance.

For women who remain sexually active following radiation therapy, water-based *vaginal lubricants* (e.g., Astroglide or K-Y Jelly) may be of benefit during intercourse but have no sustained effects. For chronic vaginal dryness, *vaginal moisturizers* may prove superior. Moisturizers (e.g., Replens and K-Y Silk-E) can be used daily or several times weekly to maintain moist vaginal tissues. Alternatively, topical estrogen cream (e.g., Premarin or Estrace cream) may improve atrophic symptoms in those who are estrogen candidates (Table 22-11, p. 498).

Despite these products, persistent adverse vaginal changes affect sexual dysfunction. In a study of 118 women treated for cervical cancer, 63 percent of those who engaged in sexual activities before radiation therapy continued to do so following treatment, although less frequently (Jensen, 2003). In a comparison of women treated with radiation versus radical hysterectomy and lymph node dissection for cervical cancer, women treated with radiation reported significantly lower sexual dysfunction scores than patients who underwent surgery (Frumovitz, 2005).

Ovary

The effects of radiation on ovarian function depend on radiation dose and patient age. For example, a dose of 4 Gy may sterilize 30 percent of young women but 100 percent of those older than 40. In addition, fractionated radiation therapy appears to be more damaging. Ash (1980) noted that after 10 Gy given in 1 fraction, 27 percent of the women recovered ovarian function compared with only 10 percent of those receiving 12 Gy over 6 days. In patients with gynecologic cancers who receive pelvic radiation therapy, symptoms of ovarian failure mirror those of natural menopause. The diagnosis and symptom treatment of premature ovarian insufficiency is outlined in Chapter 17 (p. 375).

To minimize radiation exposure to the ovaries of premenopausal women, the gonads may be surgically repositioned, termed *transposition,* out of the radiation fields. A review of prepubertal and adolescent girls undergoing transposition prior to pelvic radiation demonstrated long-term ovarian preservation rates ranging from 33 to 92 percent. However, only 11 of 347 women (3 percent) achieved pregnancy (Irtan, 2013).

Pregnancy Outcomes

Exposure to radiotherapy in childhood or adulthood does not significantly raise the risk for a congenital anomaly or genetic disease in their offspring (Seppänen, 2016; Signorello, 2012; Winther, 2012). However, prior childhood abdominopelvic radiation can affect pregnancy outcomes. Adverse effects include elevated rates of abortion, low birthweight, stillbirth, and preterm birth (Reulen, 2009; Signorello, 2010; Winther, 2008). Proposed explanations include reduced uterine volume, endometrial and myometrial atrophy, fibrosis, and impaired uterine blood flow (Arrivé, 1989; Critchley, 1992).

Bladder

Most patients receiving pelvic radiation note some acute cystitis symptoms within 2 to 3 weeks of beginning treatment. Although urinary frequency, spasm, and pain develop commonly, hematuria is rare. Typically, phenazopyridine hydrochloride (Pyridium) or fluid ad lib promptly relieves symptoms. Antibiotics are prescribed when indicated. Major chronic complications following radiation therapy are infrequent and include bladder contracture and hematuria. For severe hematuria, bladder saline irrigation, transurethral cystoscopic fulguration, and temporary urinary diversion are proven techniques. Fistulas involving the bladder typically require urinary diversion.

Small Bowel

The small bowel is particularly vulnerable to acute early damage from radiation therapy. After a single dose of 5 to 10 Gy, crypt cells are destroyed, and villi become denuded. An acute malabsorption syndrome ensues to cause nausea, diarrhea, vomiting, and cramping. Adequate fluid intake and a low-lactose, low-fat, and low-fiber diet is recommended. Additionally, antinausea and antidiarrheal medications may be warranted (Tables 25-5, p. 566, and 42-9, p. 916). Bowel antispasmodics with sedatives (e.g., Donnatal) are particularly helpful.

Patients are warned about the late, chronic nature of radiation-induced enteritis. Intermittent diarrhea, crampy abdominal pain, nausea, and vomiting, which in combination may mimic a low-grade bowel obstruction, can develop. Those patients with comorbidities, such as obesity, small-vessel diseases resulting from diabetes or hypertension, prior abdominal surgeries, and inflammatory conditions of the pelvis or bowel, are at greater risk.

Preventatively, several types of devices have been surgically inserted to displace the small bowel from the pelvis. These have included saline-filled tissue expanders, omental slings, and absorbable mesh (Hoffman, 1998; Martin, 2005; Soper, 1988). Furthermore, defining the areas at risk with surgical clips and careful radiation therapy planning, including the use of IMRT, may minimize bowel toxicity (Portelance, 2001). Consideration of dose constraints can further minimize injury. Studies show that irradiating a volume larger than 15 cm^3 or a point dose greater than 55 Gy is associated with a significant risk of small bowel damage (Stanic, 2013; Verma, 2014). Radiation treatment with patients prone also can limit the small bowel dose (Adli, 2003). In contrast, trials incorporating radiation protectors, such as amifostine, have been unsuccessful (Small, 2011).

Rectosigmoid

Commonly, within a few weeks after radiation therapy initiation, patients may develop diarrhea, tenesmus, and mucoid discharge, which can be bloody. In these cases, antidiarrheal medications, low-residue diet, steroid-retention or sucralfate enemas, and hydration are management mainstays. Alternatively, rectal bleeding may be seen months to years after radiation therapy. Hemorrhage can at times be severe and require blood transfusion. Moreover, invasive procedures may be needed to control bleeding neovasculature. These include the topical application of 4-percent formalin, cryotherapy, and vessel coagulation with laser (Kantsevoy, 2003; Konishi, 2005; Smith, 2001; Ventrucci, 2001). During the evaluation of late-onset rectal bleeding, barium enema is often indicated. The study usually reveals narrowing of the rectosigmoid lumen and wall thickening. In cases of severe obstruction, resection of the involved colonic segment is necessary. In addition, rectovaginal fistulas may result from radiation therapy (Chap. 25, p. 570). Small fistulas may heal over many months following a diverting colostomy.

Brachytherapy, in addition to external beam radiation, can further escalate rectal toxicity. The D2cc metric (minimum dose to the most irradiated contiguous volume of 2 cc) is commonly used to evaluate the rectal dose in brachytherapy. Doses >62 Gy are associated with higher rates of Grade 2 to 4 rectal toxicities (Lee, 2012b). This metric was developed as part of the GEC-ESTRO (Groupe Européen de Curiethérapie—European Society of Therapeutic Radiation Oncology) guidelines, which provide dose-reporting parameters for the bladder, rectum, and sigmoid colon using 3-D image-based treatment planning (Potter, 2006).

Kidney

Manifestations of acute radiation nephropathy typically appear 6 to 12 months after radiation exposure. Affected patients develop hypertension, edema, anemia, microscopic hematuria, proteinuria, and decreased creatinine clearance (Luxton, 1964). Although deteriorating renal function is occasionally reversible, it usually worsens and leads to chronic nephropathy. Patients receiving concurrent radiation and chemotherapy require special consideration because of the nephrotoxicity associated with many chemotherapeutics (Chap. 27, p. 592).

Bone

Radiation-induced insufficiency fractures are not infrequent following pelvic radiation. They develop in weakened bone and typically manifest as pain. The sacrum is most commonly involved (Cooper, 1985). Rates are higher in patients receiving definitive radiation therapy, and in a large series of 557 patients with cervical cancer, 20 percent developed insufficiency fractures over 5 years (Oh, 2008). In a more recent series of 222 patients receiving postoperative pelvic radiation therapy, only 5 percent developed pelvic insufficiency fractures. These developed at a median time of 11.5 months after radiation therapy completion (Shih, 2013). The fracture rate was higher in patients with osteoporosis (16 percent), in those on hormone replacement therapy (15 percent), and in patients with a lower body mass index. Treatment for a pelvic insufficiency fracture is conservative and consists of pain management and rest, with most patients becoming symptom free by 20 months.

Hematologic Toxicity

Radiation therapy can significantly deplete bone marrow hematopoietic stem cells that include erythrocyte, leukocyte, and platelet precursors. These effects are exacerbated by combined chemoradiation or by irradiation of large fields that contain a significant portion of bone marrow. Accordingly, there are thresholds at which radiation is held to prevent further bone marrow suppression. For example, if platelet levels measure $<35,000 \times 10^9/L$ and leukocyte counts are $<1.0 \times 10^9/L$, then radiation may be held until these values rise. For anemia, transfusion is recommended (p. 614). To spare bone marrow injury, IMRT may be beneficial (Klopp, 2013).

■ Radiation-Induced Carcinogenesis

A secondary cancer may develop as a result of prior radiation therapy. The accepted criteria for the diagnosis of radiation-induced cancer require that the cancer be located within the previously irradiated region and that its pathology differ from that of the original malignancy. Additionally, a latent period of at least a few years should have transpired. In the updated analysis of the Post-Operative Radiation Therapy in Endometrial Carcinoma (PORTEC-1) trial, which compared postoperative adjuvant pelvic radiation against observation, the secondary cancer rates at 15 years were 22 percent in the radiation group compared with 16 percent in the observation group. However, this difference did not reach statistical significance (Creutzberg, 2011).

Development of a secondary radiation-induced cancer depends on factors such as patient age at exposure, radiation dose, and susceptibility of specific tissue types to radiation-induced carcinogenesis (Table 28-4). In general, those receiving higher radiation doses and those exposed at an earlier age have higher risks for second malignancies. The latency of secondary

TABLE 28-4. Susceptibility of Selected Tissues to Radiation-Induced Cancer

Susceptibility	Tissues
High	Bone marrow, female breast, thyroid
Moderate	Bladder, colon, stomach, liver, ovary
Low	Bone, connective tissue, muscle, cervix, uterus, rectum

tumor development also varies depending on the type of second malignancy. For example, the latent period between radiation exposure and the clinical appearance of leukemia is less than 10 years, whereas solid tumors may not develop for decades. The most common example is development of uterine sarcoma years after pelvic radiation for treatment of cervical cancer (Mark, 1996). Preventatively, irradiation of smaller fields with advanced technologies such as IMRT compared with larger-field 2-D external beam radiation may reduce the incidence of radiation-induced malignancies (Herrera, 2014).

REFERENCES

Adli M, Mayr NA, Kaiser HS et al: Does prone positioning reduce small bowel dose in pelvic radiation with intensity-modulated radiotherapy for gynecologic cancer? Int J Radiat Oncol Biol Phys 57(1):230, 2003

American College of Radiology: Appropriateness criteria. 2018. Available at: https://acsearch.acr.org/list. Accessed November 7, 2018

Amorino GP, Freeman ML, Carbone DP, et al: Radiopotentiation by the oral platinum agent, JM216: role of repair inhibition. Int J Radiat Oncol Biol Phys 44(2):399, 1999

Arai T, Nakano T, Fukuhisa K, et al: Second cancer after radiation therapy for cancer of the uterine cervix. Cancer 67(2):398, 1991

Arrivé L, Chang YC, Hricak H, et al: Radiation-induced uterine changes: MR imaging. Radiology 170(1 Pt 1):55, 1989

Ash P: The influence of radiation on fertility in man. Br J Radiol 53:271, 1980

ASTEC/EN.5 Study Group: Adjuvant external beam radiotherapy in the treatment of endometrial cancer (MRC ASTEC and NCIC CTG EN.5 randomised trials): pooled trial results, systematic review and meta-analysis. Lancet 373:137, 2009

Begg AC: Cisplatin and radiation: interaction probabilities and therapeutic possibilities. Int J Radiat Oncol Biol Phys 19(5):1183, 1990

Bentzen SM: Tumor volume and local control probability: clinical data and radiobiological interpretations. Int J Radiat Oncol Biol Phys 36(1):247, 1996

Beriwal S, Demanes DJ, Erickson B, et al: American Brachytherapy Society consensus guideline for interstitial brachytherapy for vaginal cancer. Brachytherapy 11(1):68, 2012

Boronow RC: Combined therapy as an alternative to exenteration for locally advanced vulvo-vaginal cancer: rationale and results. Cancer 49(6):1085, 1982

Brizel DM, Dodge RK, Clough RW, et al: Oxygenation of head and neck cancer: changes during radiotherapy and impact on treatment outcome. Radiother Oncol 53(2):113, 1999

Cooper KL, Beabout JW, Swee RG: Insufficiency fractures of the sacrum. Radiology 156:15, 1985

Creutzberg CL, Nout RA, Lybeert ML, et al: Fifteen-year radiotherapy outcomes of the randomized PORTEC-1 trial for endometrial carcinoma. Int J Radiat Oncol Biol Phys 81(4):631, 2011

Critchley HO, Wallace WH, Shalet SM, et al: Abdominal irradiation in childhood: the potential for pregnancy. BJOG 99(5):392, 1992

Dische S, Saunders MI, Sealy R, et al: Carcinoma of the cervix and the use of hyperbaric oxygen with radiotherapy: a report of a randomised controlled trial. Radiother Oncol 53(2):93, 1999

DiSilvestro PA, Ali S, Craighead PS, et al: Phase III randomized trial of weekly cisplatin and irradiation versus cisplatin and tirapazamine and irradiation in stages IB2, IIA, IIB, IIIB, and IVA cervical carcinoma limited to the pelvis: a Gynecologic Oncology Group study. J Clin Oncol 32(5):458, 2014

Dubben HH: Tumor volume: a basic and specific response predictor in radiotherapy. Radiother Oncol 47(2):167, 1998

Dueñas-González A, Zarbá JJ, Patel F, et al: Phase III, open-label, randomized study comparing concurrent gemcitabine plus cisplatin and radiation followed by adjuvant gemcitabine and cisplatin versus concurrent cisplatin and radiation in patients with stage IIB to IVA carcinoma of the cervix. J Clin Oncol 29(13):1678, 2011

Dunst J, Kuhnt T, Strauss HG, et al: Anemia in cervical cancers: impact on survival, patterns of relapse, and association with hypoxia and angiogenesis. Int J Radiat Oncol Biol Phys 56(3):778, 2003

Fajardo LF: The pathology of ionizing radiation as defined by morphologic patterns. Acta Oncol 44(1):13, 2005

Friedlander AH, Freymiller EG: Detection of radiation-accelerated atherosclerosis of the carotid artery by panoramic radiography. A new opportunity for dentists. J Am Dent Assoc 134(10):1361, 2003

Frumovitz M, Sun CC, Schover LR, et al: Quality of life and sexual functioning in cervical cancer survivors. J Clin Oncol 23(30):7428, 2005

Gemignani ML, Alektiar KM, Leitai M, et al: Radical surgical resection and high-dose intraoperative radiation therapy (HDR-IORT) in patients with recurrent gynecologic cancers. Int J Radiat Oncol Biol Phys 50(3):687, 2001

Gondi V, Bentzen SM, Sklenar KL et al: Severe late toxicities following concomitant chemoradiotherapy compared to radiotherapy alone in cervical cancer: an inter-era analysis. Int J Radiat Oncol Biol Phys 84(4):973, 2012

Grigsby P, Winter K, Komaki R et al: Long-term follow-up of RTOG 88-05: twice-daily external irradiation with brachytherapy for carcinoma of the cervix. Int J Radiat Oncol Biol Phys 54:51, 2002

Grigsby PW, Heydon K, Mutch DG et al: Long-term follow up of RTOG 92-10: cervical cancer with positive para-aortic lymph nodes. Int J Radiat Oncol Biol Phys 51(4):982, 2001

Hareyama M, Sakata K, Oouchi A, et al: High-dose-rate versus low-dose-rate intracavitary therapy for carcinoma of the uterine cervix: a randomized trial. Cancer 94(1):117, 2002

Heron DE, Gersztzen K, Selvaraj RN, et al: Conventional 3D conformal versus intensity-modulated radiotherapy for the adjuvant treatment of gynecologic malignancies: a comparative dosimetric study of dose-volume histograms. Gynecol Oncol 91(1):39, 2003

Herrera FG, Cruz OS, Achtari C, et al: Long-term outcome and late side effects in endometrial cancer patients treated with surgery and postoperative radiation therapy. Ann Surg Oncol 21(7):2390, 2014

Hoffman JP, Sigurdson ER, Eisenberg BL: Use of saline-filled tissue expanders to protect the small bowel from radiation. Oncology 12(1):51, 1998

Irtan S, Orbach D, Helfre S, et al: Ovarian transposition in prepubescent and adolescent girls with cancer. Lancet Oncol 14:e601, 2013

Janssens GO, Rademakers SE, Terhaard CH, et al: Improved recurrence-free survival with ARCON for anemic patients with laryngeal cancer. Clin Cancer Res 20(5):1345, 2014

Jensen PT, Groenvold M, Klee MC, et al: Longitudinal study of sexual function and vaginal changes after radiotherapy for cervical cancer. Int J Radiat Oncol Biol Phys 56(4):937, 2003

Jones E, Beriwal S, Beyer D, et al: An analysis of appropriate postoperative radiation therapy for endometrial cancer using the RAND/UCLA Appropriateness Method: Executive Summary. Advances Radiat Oncol 1(1): 26, 2016

Kantsevoy SV, Cruz-Correa MR, Vaughn CA, et al: Endoscopic cryotherapy for the treatment of bleeding mucosal vascular lesions of the GI tract: a pilot study. Gastrointest Endosc 57(3):403, 2003

Kapp KS, Poschauko J, Geyer E, et al: Evaluation of the effect of routine packed red blood cell transfusion in anemic cervix cancer patients treated with radical radiotherapy. Int J Radiat Oncol Biol Phys 54(1):58, 2002

Keys HM, Bundy BN, Stehman FB, et al: A comparison of weekly cisplatin during radiation therapy versus irradiation alone each followed by adjuvant hysterectomy in bulky stage IB cervical carcinoma: a randomized trial of the Gynecologic Oncology Group. N Engl J Med 340:1154, 1999

Keys HM, Bundy BN, Stehman FB et al: Radiation therapy with and without extrafascial hysterectomy for bulky stage IB cervical carcinoma: a randomized trial of the Gynecologic Oncology Group. Gynecol Oncol 89(3):343, 2003

Keys HM, Roberts JA, Brunetto VL, et al: A phase III trial of surgery with or without adjunctive external pelvic radiation therapy in intermediate risk endometrial adenocarcinoma: a Gynecologic Oncology Group study. Gynecol Oncol 92:744, 2004

Klopp AH, Moughan J, Portelance L, et al: Hematologic toxicity in RTOG 0418: a phase 2 study of postoperative IMRT for gynecologic cancers. Int J Radiat Oncol Biol Phys 86(1):83, 2013

Klopp AH, Smith BD, Alektiar K, et al: The role of postoperative radiation therapy for endometrial cancer: Executive Summary of an American Society for Radiation Oncology evidence-based guideline. Prac Radiat Oncol 4(1):137, 2014

Konishi T, Watanabe T, Kitayama J, et al: Endoscopic and histopathologic findings after formalin application for hemorrhage caused by chronic radiation-induced proctitis. Gastrointest Endosc 61(1):161, 2005

Lee LJ, Das IJ, Higgins SA, et al: American Brachytherapy Society consensus guidelines for locally advanced carcinoma of the cervix. Part III: low-dose-rate and pulsed-dose-rate brachytherapy. Brachytherapy 11(1):53, 2012a

Lee LJ, Viswanathan AN: Predictors of toxicity after image-guided high-dose-rate interstitial brachytherapy for gynecologic cancer. Int J Radiat Oncol Biol Phys 84(5):1192, 2012b

Lee MY, Wu HG, Kim K, et al: Concurrent radiotherapy with paclitaxel/carboplatin chemotherapy as a definitive treatment for squamous cell carcinoma of the uterine cervix. Gynecol Oncol 104(1):95, 2007

Luxton RW, Kunkler PB: Radiation nephritis. Acta Radiol Ther Phys Biol 66:169, 1964

Mark RJ, Poen J, Tran LM et al: Postirradiation sarcoma of the gynecologic tract. A report of 13 cases and a discussion of the risk of radiation-induced gynecologic malignancies. Am J Clin Oncol 19(1):59, 1996

Martin J, Fitzpatrick K, Horan G, et al: Treatment with a belly-board device significantly reduces the volume of small bowel irradiated and results in low acute toxicity in adjuvant radiotherapy for gynecologic cancer: results of a prospective study. Radiother Oncol 74(3):267, 2005

Mason KA, Kishi K, Hunter N, et al: Effect of docetaxel on the therapeutic ratio of fractionated radiotherapy in vivo. Clin Cancer Res 5:4191, 1999

Milano MT, Constine LS, Okunieff P: Normal tissue tolerance dose metrics for radiation therapy of major organs. Semin Radiat Oncol 17:131, 2007

Montana GS, Thomas GM, Moore DH, et al: Preoperative chemo-radiation for carcinoma of the vulva with N2/N3 nodes: a gynecologic oncology group study. Int J Radiat Oncol Biol Phys 48(4):1007, 2000

Morris M, Eifel PJ, Watkins EB, et al: Pelvic radiation with concurrent chemotherapy versus pelvic and para-aortic radiation for high risk cervical cancer: a randomized Radiation Therapy Oncology Group clinical trial. N Engl J Med 340:1137, 1999

National Cancer Institute: Common terminology criteria for adverse events v5.0. NCI, NIH, DHHS. November 27, 2017. Available at: https://ctep.cancer.gov/protocolDevelopment/electronic_applications/ctc.htm. Accessed November 7, 2018

Nordsmark M, Overgaard M, Overgaard J: Pretreatment oxygenation predicts radiation response in advanced squamous cell carcinoma of the head and neck. Radiother Oncol 41(1):31, 1996

Nout RA, Smit VT, Putter H, et al: Vaginal brachytherapy versus pelvic external beam radiotherapy for patients with endometrial cancer of high-intermediate risk (PORTEC-2): an open-label, non-inferiority, randomised trial. Lancet 375:816, 2010

Oh D, Huh SJ, Nam H et al: Pelvic insufficiency fracture after pelvic radiotherapy for cervical cancer: analysis of risk factors. Int J Radiat Oncol Biol Phys 70(4):1183, 2008

Okada H, Mak TW: Pathways of apoptotic and non-apoptotic death in tumour cells. Nat Rev Cancer 4(8):592, 2004

Pawlik TM, Keyomarsi K: Role of cell cycle in mediating sensitivity to radiotherapy. Int J Radiat Oncol Biol Phys 59(4):928, 2004

Pereteit DG, Sarkaria JN, Chappell R, et al: The adverse effect of treatment prolongation in cervical carcinoma. Int J Radiat Oncol Biol Phys 32(5):1301, 1995

Peters WA, Liu PY, Barrett RJ, et al: Concurrent chemotherapy and pelvic radiation therapy compared with pelvic radiation therapy alone as adjuvant therapy after radical surgery in high-risk early-stage cancer of the cervix. J Clin Oncol 18(8):1606, 2000

Portelance L, Chao KS, Grigsby PW, et al: Intensity-modulated radiation therapy (IMRT) reduces small bowel, rectum, and bladder doses in patients with cervical cancer receiving pelvic and para-aortic irradiation. Int J Radiat Oncol Biol Phys 51(1):261, 2001

Potter R, Haie-Meder C, Van Limbergen E, et al: Recommendations from gynaecological (GYN) GEC ESTRO working group (II): concepts and terms in 3D image-based treatment planning in cervix cancer brachytherapy-3D dose volume parameters and aspects of 3D image-based anatomy, radiation physics, radiobiology. Radiother Oncol 78(1):67, 2006

Reulen RC, Zeegers MP, Wallace WH, et al: Pregnancy outcomes among adult survivors of childhood cancer in the British Childhood Cancer Survivor Study. Cancer Epidemiol Biomarkers Prev 18(8):2239, 2009

Rose PG, Bundy BN, Watkins EB, et al: Concurrent cisplatin-based chemoradiation improves progression free and overall survival in advanced cervical cancer: results of a randomized Gynecologic Oncology Group study. N Engl J Med 340:1144, 1999

Schwartz JL, Mustafi R, Beckett MA, et al: DNA double-strand break rejoining rates, inherent radiation sensitivity and human tumor response to radiotherapy. Br J Cancer 74(1):37, 1996

Schwartz JL, Rotmensch J, Giovanazzi S, et al: Faster repair of DNA double-strand breaks in radioresistant human tumor cells. Int J Radiat Oncol Biol Phys 15(4):907, 1988

Sedlis A, Bundy BN, Rotman MZ, et al: A randomized trial of pelvic radiation therapy versus no further therapy in selected patients with stage IB carcinoma of the cervix after radical hysterectomy and pelvic lymphadenectomy: a Gynecologic Oncology Group study. Gynecol Oncol 73(2)177, 1999

Seppänen VI, Artama MS, Malila NK, et al: Risk for congenital anomalies in offspring of childhood, adolescent and young adult cancer survivors. Int J Cancer 139:1721, 2016

Shih KK, Folkert MR, Kollmeier MA, et al: Pelvic insufficiency fractures in patients with cervical and endometrial cancer treated with postoperative pelvic radiation. Gynecol Oncol 128(3):540, 2013

Signorello LB, Mulvihill JJ, Green DM, et al: Congenital anomalies in the children of cancer survivors: a report from the childhood cancer survivor study. J Clin Oncol 30(3):239, 2012

Signorello LB, Mulvihill JJ, Green DM, et al: Stillbirth and neonatal death in relation to radiation exposure before conception: a retrospective cohort study. Lancet 376:624, 2010

Small W, Beriwal S, Demanes DJ, et al: American Brachytherapy Society consensus guidelines for adjuvant vaginal cuff brachytherapy after hysterectomy. Brachytherapy 11(1):58, 2012

Small W, Winter K, Levenback C et al: Extended-field irradiation and intracavitary brachytherapy combined with cisplatin and amifostine for cervical cancer with positive para-aortic or high common iliac lymph nodes: results of arm II of RTOG 0116. Int J Gynecol Cancer 21(7):1266, 2011

Smith S, Wallner K, Dominitz JA, et al: Argon plasma coagulation for rectal bleeding after prostate brachytherapy. Int J Radiat Oncol Biol Phys 51(3):636, 2001

Soper JT, Clarke-Pearson DL, Creasman WT: Absorbable synthetic mesh (910-polyglactin) intestinal sling to reduce radiation-induced small bowel injury in patients with pelvic malignancies. Gynecol Oncol 29(3):283, 1988

Stanic S, Mayadev JS: Tolerance of the small bowel to therapeutic radiation: a focus on late toxicity in patients receiving para-aortic nodal irradiation for gynecologic malignancies. Int J Gynecol Cancer 23(4):592, 2013

Steel GG, Peckham MJ: Exploitable mechanisms in combined radiotherapy-chemotherapy: the concept of additivity. Int J Radiat Oncol Biol Phys 5(1):85, 1979

Thomas G, Ali S, Hoebers FJ, et al: Phase III trial to evaluate the efficacy of maintaining hemoglobin levels above 12.0 g/dL with erythropoietin vs above 10.0 g/dL without erythropoietin in anemic patients receiving concurrent radiation and cisplatin for cervical cancer. Gynecol Oncol 108(2):317, 2008

Trott KR: The mechanisms of acceleration of repopulation in squamous epithelia during daily irradiation. Acta Oncol 38(2):153, 1999

Ventrucci M, Di Simone MP, Giulietti P, et al: Efficacy and safety of Nd:YAG laser for the treatment of bleeding from radiation proctocolitis. Dig Liver Dis 33(3):230, 2001

Verma J, Sulman EP, Jhingran A et al: Dosimetric predictors of duodenal toxicity after intensity modulated radiation therapy for treatment of the para-aortic nodes in gynecologic cancer. Int J Radiat Oncol Biol Phys 88(2):357, 2014

Viswanathan AN, Beriwal S, De Los Santos JF, et al: American Brachytherapy Society consensus guideline for locally advanced carcinoma of the cervix. Part II: high-dose-rate brachytherapy. Brachytherapy 11(1):47, 2012a

Viswanathan AN, Thomadsen B: American Brachytherapy Society consensus guidelines for locally advanced carcinoma of the cervix. Part I: general principles. Brachytherapy 11(1):33, 2012b

Weichselbaum RR, Beckett MA, Hallahan DE, et al: Molecular targets to overcome radioresistance. Semin Oncol 19(4 Suppl 11):14, 1992

Winther JF, Boice JD Jr, Svendsen AL, et al: Spontaneous abortion in a Danish population-based cohort of childhood cancer survivors. J Clin Oncol 26:4340, 2008

Winther JF, Olsen JH, Wu H, et al: Genetic disease in the children of Danish survivors of childhood and adolescent cancer. J Clin Oncol 30:27, 2012

Wong FC, Tung SY, Leung TW, et al: Treatment results of high-dose-rate remote afterloading brachytherapy for cervical cancer and retrospective comparison of two regimens. Int J Radiat Oncol Biol Phys 55(5):1254, 2003

Zidar N, Ferlunga D, Hvala A, et al: Contribution to the pathogenesis of radiation-induced injury to large arteries. J Laryngol Otol 111(10):988, 1997

CHAPTER 29

Preinvasive Lesions of the Lower Anogenital Tract

Office gynecology includes the diagnosis and management of preinvasive lower anogenital tract (LAGT) disease, most often involving the uterine cervix, but also the vulvar, vaginal, perianal, and anal epithelia. An understanding of human papillomavirus (HPV) as the causative agent of most LAGT neoplasia has greatly advanced screening, diagnosis, management, and prevention efforts. Importantly, in current clinical practice, evidence-based knowledge is ever evolving and translates into rapidly changing patient-care recommendations. Although most study findings and clinical guidelines to date refer to women, these are applicable to the care of some transgender men (Hembree, 2017).

LOWER ANOGENITAL TRACT NEOPLASIA

In the LAGT, the term *intraepithelial neoplasia* refers to epithelial lesions that are potential precursors of invasive cancer. These lesions demonstrate a range of histologic abnormality from mild to severe based on cytoplasmic, nuclear, and histologic changes. The severity of squamous intraepithelial lesions is graded by the proportion of epithelium with abnormal cells. These alterations begin at the basement membrane and continue upward toward the epithelium surface. With cervical intraepithelial neoplasia (CIN), abnormal cells solely confined to the lower third of the squamous epithelium are referred to

as *mild dysplasia* or *CIN 1*. Those that extend into the middle third are *moderate dysplasia* or *CIN 2;* into the upper third, *severe dysplasia* or *CIN 3;* and full-thickness involvement, *carcinoma in situ (CIS)* (Fig. 29-1). Preinvasive squamous lesions of the vagina, vulva, perianal, and anal squamous epithelia are graded similarly to CIN. The natural history of these extracervical lesions is less understood than for CIN. In contrast, the cervical columnar epithelium does not demonstrate an analogous neoplastic disease spectrum because it is only one cell layer thick. Histologic abnormalities are therefore limited to those that are contained in the columnar epithelium, *adenocarcinoma in situ (AIS)*, or those that invade past the epithelial basement membrane, *adenocarcinoma*.

The concept of cervical neoplasia (preinvasive and invasive) as a spectrum has come under question with increasing insight into HPV infection. Mild squamous dysplasia is now recognized as evidence of HPV infection, most of which is transient and unlikely to progress. Moderate to severe dysplastic squamous lesions are considered to be true cancer precursors, especially CIN 3. Current cytologic and histologic reporting reflects this two-tiered concept (Darragh, 2012; Solomon, 2002). In 1989, the Bethesda System cytologic nomenclature replaced CIN with *squamous intraepithelial lesion (SIL)*. Because cytologic and histologic changes of HPV infection and CIN 1 are not distinguished reliably and because their natural histories are similar, they are categorized together as *low-grade squamous intraepithelial lesions (LSIL)*. Similarly, CIN 2, CIN 3, and CIS are difficult to distinguish, are truer cancer precursors, and are designated together as *high-grade squamous intraepithelial lesion (HSIL)*. The diagnostic distinction between LSIL and HSIL is more reliable, biologically plausible, and clinically meaningful than diagnoses using the CIN system. This two-tiered nomenclature is now recommended for histology as well, and guidelines for the management of these lesions are grouped accordingly (Darragh, 2012).

ANATOMIC CONSIDERATIONS

■ External Genitalia

Precancerous lesions of the female LAGT are often multifocal, can involve any of its structures, and may appear similar to benign processes. For example, *micropapillomatosis labialis* is a benign anatomic variant characterized by minute epithelial projections on the inner labia minora (Fig. 29-2). This condition can be easily mistaken for HPV-related lesions. Instead, true HPV lesions tend to be multifocal, asymmetric, and show multiple papillations arising from a single base (Ferris, 2004). Micropapillomatosis often shows spontaneous regression, and treatment is not indicated (Bergeron, 1990).

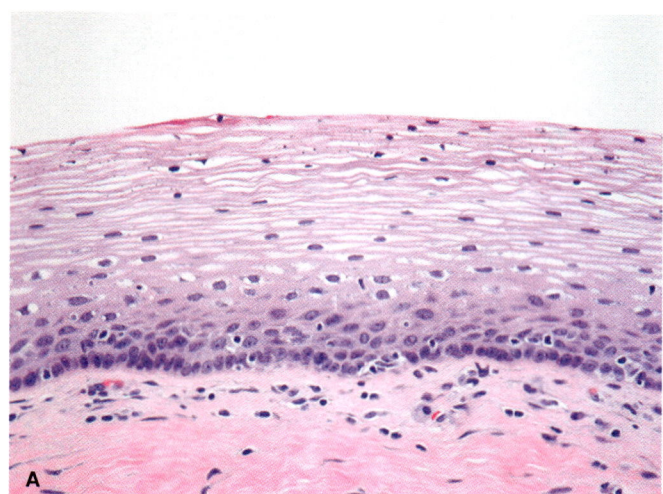

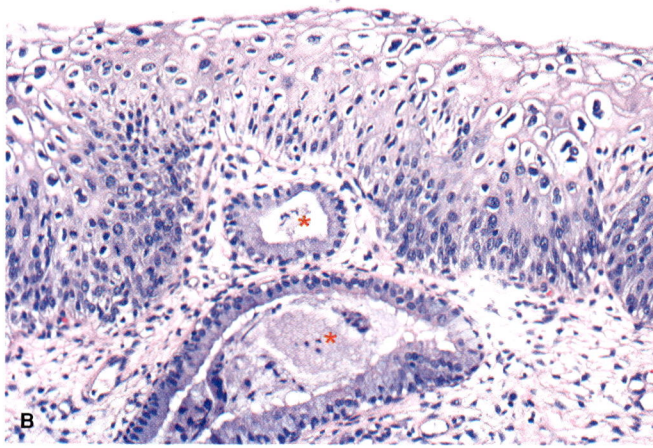

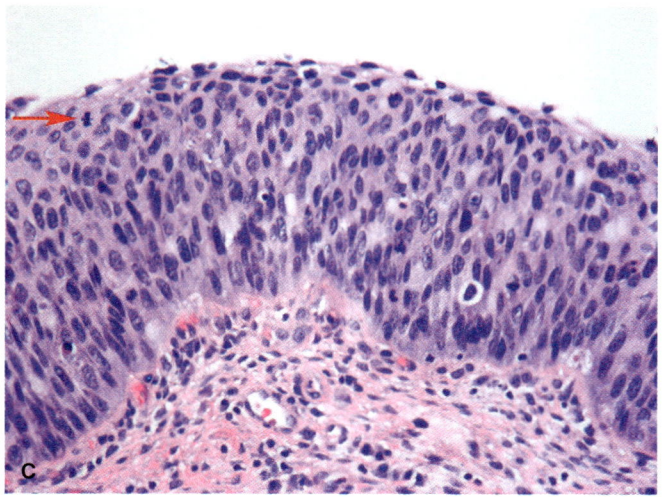

FIGURE 29-1 A. Normal ectocervical epithelium is a nonkeratinizing, stratified, squamous epithelium, which contains basal, parabasal, intermediate, and superficial layers. The epithelium matures and accumulates glycogen in its upper layers. Mitoses are usually confined to the parabasal layer. **B.** Low-grade squamous intraepithelial lesion (LSIL). This biopsy's location at the transformation zone is indicated by the presence of both mucinous columnar endocervical epithelium (*asterisks*) and squamous epithelium. LSIL has disordered squamous cell proliferation and increased mitotic activity confined to the basal one third of the epithelium. Koilocytotic atypia, indicative of proliferative human papillomavirus (HPV) infection, involves the more superficial epithelium. Koilocytosis is typified by nuclear enlargement, coarse chromatin, nuclear "wrinkling," perinuclear halos, and greater prevalence of binucleation/multinucleation. **C.** High-grade squamous intraepithelial lesion (HSIL). This example shows disordered, markedly atypical squamous cells and increased mitotic activity that involves the epithelium's full thickness. Note the mitotic figure located close to the epithelial surface (*red arrow*). (Reproduced with permission from Dr. Kelley Carrick.)

■ Vagina

The vagina is lined by nonkeratinized squamous epithelium, and glands are absent. However, islands of columnar epithelium are occasionally found within the vaginal squamous mucosa, a condition termed *adenosis*. It can result from in utero exposure to exogenous estrogen, particularly diethylstilbestrol (DES) (Trimble, 2001). Appearing as red patches within the squamous epithelium, these can be mistaken for ulcers or other lesions.

Vaginal adenocarcinoma may arise within adenosis. Of primary vaginal adenocarcinomas, the clear cell type is most closely associated with DES exposure. Thus, with DES-related adenosis, careful palpation of the vagina is warranted in addition to visual inspection, as clear cell adenocarcinoma may be palpable before becoming visible.

■ Cervix

Squamocolumnar Junction

During embryogenesis, upward migration of stratified squamous epithelium from the urogenital sinus is thought to replace müllerian epithelium (Ulfelder, 1976). This process usually terminates near the external cervical os, forming the original (congenital) squamocolumnar junction (SCJ). When visible on the

ectocervix, the SCJ is seen as a pink, smooth, squamous epithelium juxtaposed against the red, velvety, columnar epithelium surrounding the external cervical os. Rarely, this migration is incomplete, and the SCJ forms in the upper vaginal fornices. This normal variant is also seen with in utero DES exposure.

The columnar epithelium is commonly referred to as "glandular." It does produce mucus, and its deep infoldings appear histologically similar to glandular tissue (Fig. 29-3). However, true glands, which consist of acini and ducts, are not present on the cervix (Ulfelder, 1976).

The location of the SCJ varies with age and hormonal status. During the reproductive years, it everts outward onto the ectocervix in response to estrogen (especially during adolescence, pregnancy, and combination hormonal contraceptive use). It regresses into the endocervical canal with the process of squamous metaplasia and low-estrogen states like menopause, lactation, and progestin-only contraceptive use.

Squamous Metaplasia

At puberty, the rise in estrogen levels leads to greater glycogen formation within nonkeratinized cervical and vaginal squamous epithelia. In providing a carbohydrate source, glycogen allows vaginal flora to be dominated by lactobacilli, which produce lactic acid. The resultant acidic vaginal pH is the suspected

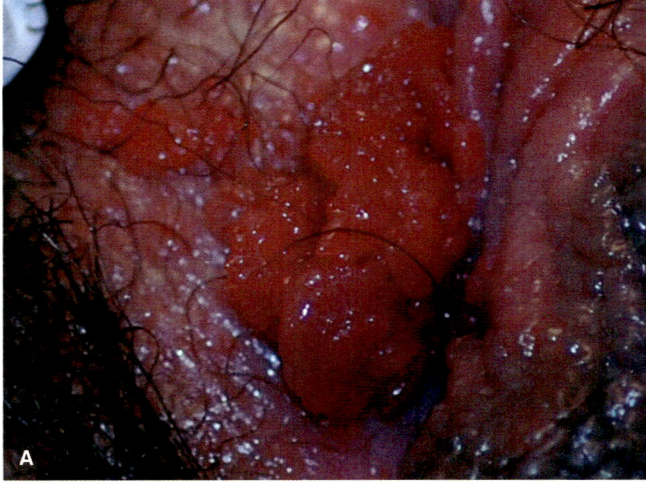

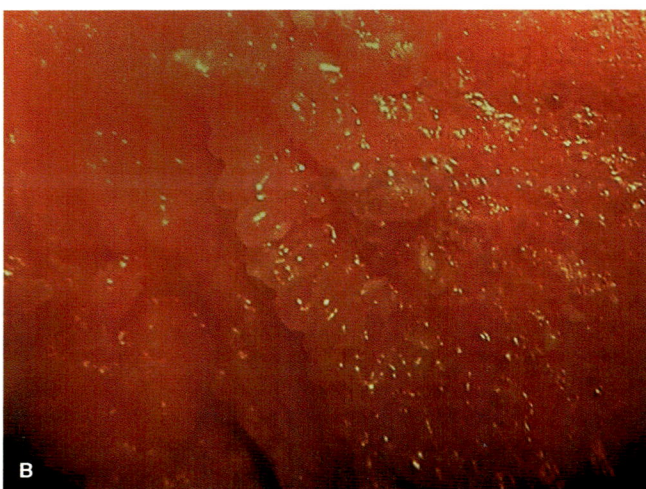

FIGURE 29-2 Benign lower genital tract lesions. **A.** Condylomata tend to be multifocal and asymmetric and have multiple papillations arising from a single base. **B.** Micropapillomatosis labialis is a normal variant of vulvar anatomy encountered along the inner labia minora and lower vagina. In contrast to condylomata, projections are uniform in size and shape and arise singly from their base attachments.

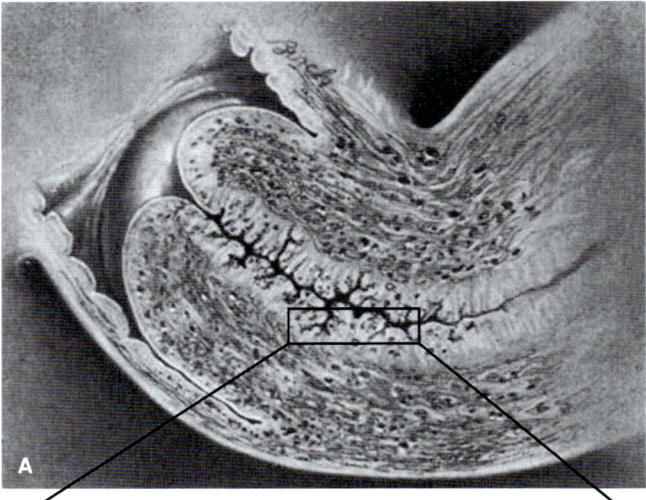

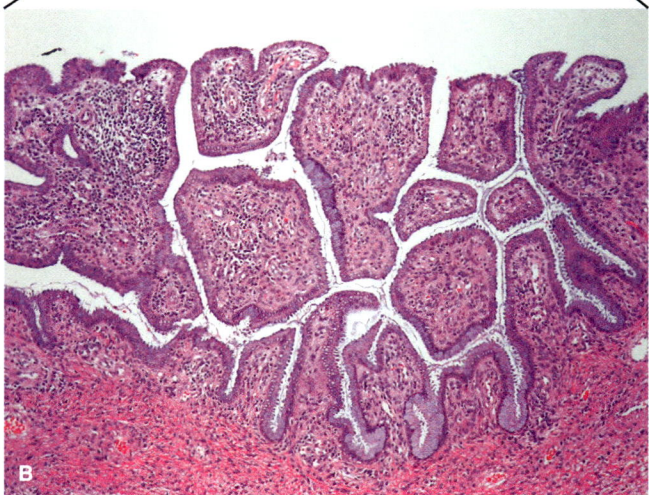

FIGURE 29-3 Endocervical anatomy. **A.** Sagittal view of the cervix. In this drawing, a portion of the endocervical canal is boxed. (Modified and reproduced with permission from Eastman, 1961.) **B.** The endocervix is lined by a simple, columnar, mucin-secreting epithelium. Crypts and small exophytic projections appear pseudo-papillary when viewed in cross section. (Reproduced with permission from Dr. Kelley Carrick.)

stimulus for *squamous metaplasia*, which is the normal replacement of columnar by squamous epithelium on the cervix. Undifferentiated reserve cells underlying the SCJ are the likely precursors of the new metaplastic cells, which differentiate further into squamous epithelium. This normal process creates a progressively widening band of newer metaplastic and maturing squamous epithelium that lies between the original squamous epithelium and the columnar epithelium and is termed the *transformation zone (TZ)* (Fig. 29-4).

Transformation Zone and Cervical Neoplasia

Nearly all cervical neoplasia, both squamous and columnar, develops within the TZ, usually adjacent to the new or current SCJ. Cervical reserve and immature metaplastic cells appear most vulnerable to the oncogenic effects of HPV and co-carcinogens (Stanley, 2010a). Squamous metaplasia is most active during adolescence and pregnancy. This may explain why

sexual activity and first pregnancy at an earlier age are cervical cancer risk factors.

HUMAN PAPILLOMAVIRUS

■ Basic Virology

The causative role of HPV in nearly all cervical neoplasia (both squamous and glandular) and in a significant proportion of vulvar, vaginal, and anal squamous neoplasias is firmly established (zur Hausen, 2009). HPV causes nearly all cervical cancers and approximately 90 percent of anal cancers, 70 percent of vaginal, and 40 percent of vulvar cancers. HPV primarily infects human squamous or metaplastic epithelial cells. It is a double-stranded DNA virus with a protein capsid unique to each viral type. More than 150 genetically distinct HPV types have been identified, and approximately 40 types infect the LAGT (Doorbar, 2012).

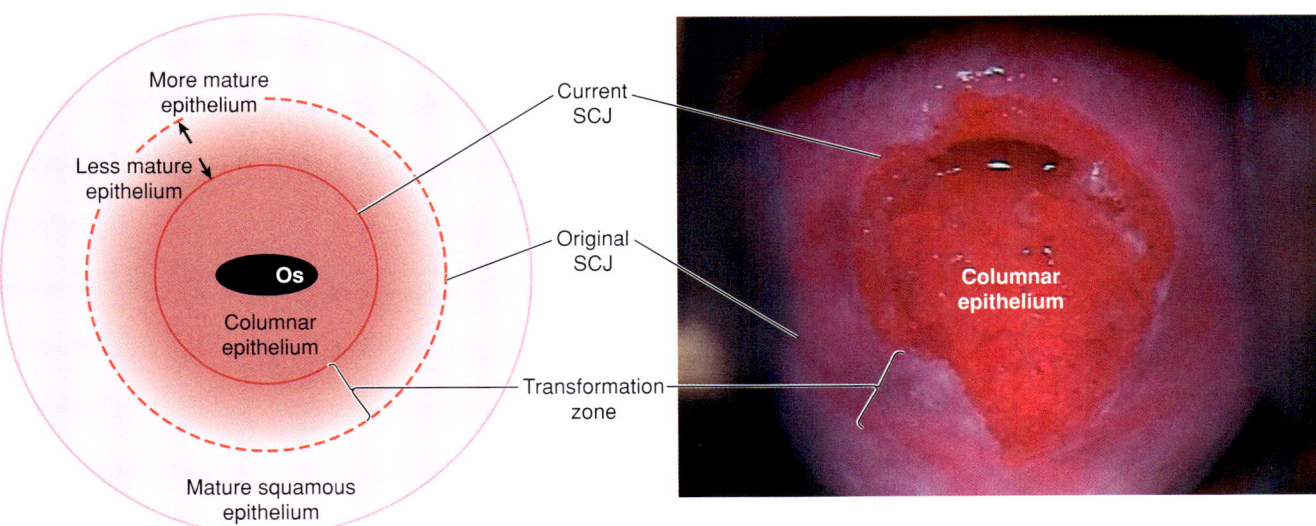

FIGURE 29-4 Relevant ectocervical landmarks depicted in a schematic drawing and corresponding photograph.

The circular HPV genome consists of only nine identified open reading frames (Stanley, 2010a). In addition to one regulatory region, the six "early" (E) genes govern functions early in the viral life cycle, including DNA maintenance, replication, and transcription. Early genes are expressed in the lower squamous epithelial layers (Fig. 29-5). The two "late" genes encode the major (L1) and minor (L2) capsid proteins. These proteins are expressed in the superficial epithelial layers late in the viral life cycle and during the assembly of new, infectious viral particles. Sequential HPV gene expression is synchronous with and dependent on squamous epithelial differentiation. Thus, completion of the viral life cycle takes place only within an intact, fully differentiating squamous epithelium (Doorbar, 2012). For this reason, HPV is not readily cultured in vitro. HPV is not released by pathogenic viral lysis, and infectiousness depends on normal desquamation of infected epithelial cells. A new infection is initiated when the L1 and L2 capsid proteins bind to the epithelial basement membrane or basal cells, which permits entry of HPV viral particles into cells of a new host (Sapp, 2009).

Clinically, HPV types are classified as high-risk (hrHPV) or low-risk (lrHPV) based on the strength of their association with cervical cancer. LrHPV types 6 and 11 cause nearly all genital warts, laryngeal papillomas, and a substantial minority of subclinical HPV infections and cytology abnormalities. LrHPV infections are rarely, if ever, oncogenic.

In contrast, persistent hrHPV infection is viewed as requisite for cervical cancer development. HrHPV types, including 16, 18, 31, 33, 35, 45, and 58, along with a few less-common types, account for approximately 95 percent of cervical cancer cases worldwide (Muñoz, 2003). HPV 16 is the most oncogenic and accounts for the largest percentage of CIN 3 lesions (45 percent) and cervical cancers (55 percent). It is also the dominant type linked to other HPV-related anogenital and oropharyngeal cancers (Schiffman, 2010; Smith, 2007). Although the prevalence of HPV 18 is much lower than that of HPV 16 in the general population, this type is found in 13 percent of cervical squamous cell carcinomas, and in an even higher proportion of cervical adenocarcinomas and adenosquamous carcinomas (approximately 40 percent) (Bruni, 2010; Smith, 2007). Together, HPVs 16 and 18 account for approximately 70 percent of cervical cancers worldwide, 68 percent of squamous cell carcinomas, and 85 percent of adenocarcinomas (Bosch, 2008). HPV type 45 is the third most common type found in cervical cancers (de Sanjose, 2019). Prior to HPV vaccination (pre-2006), HPVs 16 and 18 accounted for 1 in 5 cervical HPV infections in women. These were the most common HPVs found among low-grade lesions and in women without neoplasia (Bruni, 2010; Herrero, 2000). Thus, hrHPV infection does not cause neoplasia in most infected women, and additional host, viral, and environmental factors determine progression to LAGT neoplasia.

■ Epidemiology

Genital HPV is the most common sexually transmitted disease (STD) in the United States, and most sexually active adults are infected at some time (Dunne, 2014). U.S. women aged 14 to 59 years have a prevalence of genital HPV infection that approximates 40 percent (Hirth, 2019). Infection with HPV, predominantly high-risk types, is common soon after sexual

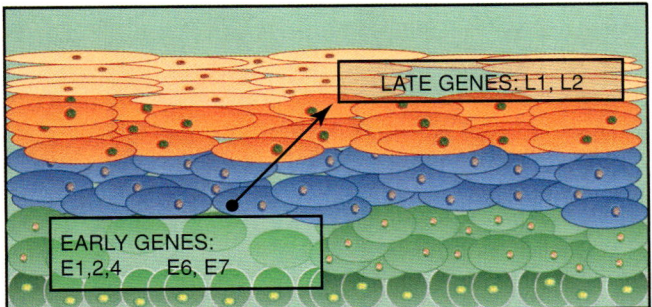

FIGURE 29-5 The human papillomavirus life cycle is completed in synchrony with squamous epithelium differentiation. Early genes, including the *E6* and *E7* oncogenes, are expressed most strongly within the basal and parabasal layers. The late genes encoding capsid proteins are expressed later in the superficial layer. Intact virus is shed during normal desquamation of superficial squames. Late genes are not strongly expressed in high-grade neoplastic lesions.

activity initiation (Brown, 2005; Winer, 2003). Infection often accompanies sexual debut and should not be equated with promiscuity (Collins, 2002). Most incident HPV infections are found in women younger than 25 years. Prevalence is highest in those aged 20 to 24 years (45 percent) and decreases with age (Dunne, 2007). Young women frequently change HPV types, and this reflects infection transience and sequential reinfection by new partners rather than persistence (Ho, 1998; Rosenfeld, 1992). Simultaneous or sequential infection with multiple HPV types is common (Schiffman, 2010).

The most important risk factors for genital HPV acquisition are number of lifetime and recent sexual partners and early age of first sexual intercourse (Burk, 1996; Fairley, 1994; Franco, 1995). Genital HPV is transmitted by direct, usually sexual contact with the genital skin, mucous membranes, or body fluids of a person with HPV infection. The infectivity of inapparent (subclinical) HPV is assumed to be high. HPV is thought to gain access to the basal cell layer and basement membrane through microabrasions of the genital epithelium during sexual contact. Once infected, the basal cells may become a viral reservoir (Stanley, 2010b).

Cervical hrHPV infection generally requires penetrative intercourse. Oral-genital and hand-genital HPV transmission are possible but are much less common than a genital-genital route (Winer, 2003). However, women who have sex with women have rates of HPV positivity, abnormal cervical cytology, and high-grade cervical neoplasia similar to those of heterosexual women, but undergo cervical cancer screening less often. Even women without past sexual experiences with men are at risk for genital HPV and its consequences. This implies that digital, oral, and perhaps object contact places them at risk of hrHPV infection (Marrazzo, 2000; McCune, 2018). Thus, all women and transgender men who retain their uterus should undergo cervical cancer screening according to current guidelines.

Genital HPV detection, including hrHPV, has been reported in apparently sexually naïve girls and young women (Doerfler, 2009; Winer, 2003). Certainly, genital warts that develop in children beyond infancy are always reason to consider the possibility of sexual abuse. However, infection by nonsexual contact, autoinoculation, or fomite transfer appears possible. This is supported by reports of nongenital HPV types in a significant minority of pediatric and adolescent genital wart cases (Cohen, 1990; Obalek, 1990; Siegfried, 1997).

Congenital HPV infection from vertical transmission (mother to fetus/newborn) beyond common, transient skin colonization is rare. Conjunctival, laryngeal, vulvar, or perianal warts that are present at birth or that develop within 1 to 3 years of birth are most likely due to perinatal exposure to maternal HPV (Cohen, 1990). Infection is not linked to presence of maternal genital warts or route of delivery (Silverberg, 2003; Syrjänen, 2010). Accordingly, cesarean delivery is not recommended solely for maternal HPV infection. Exceptions include cases of large genital warts that could obstruct delivery or avulse and bleed with cervical dilation or vaginal delivery.

■ Infection Outcomes and Natural History

Genital HPV infection causes variable physical outcomes (Fig. 29-6). These can be broadly grouped as latent or expressed

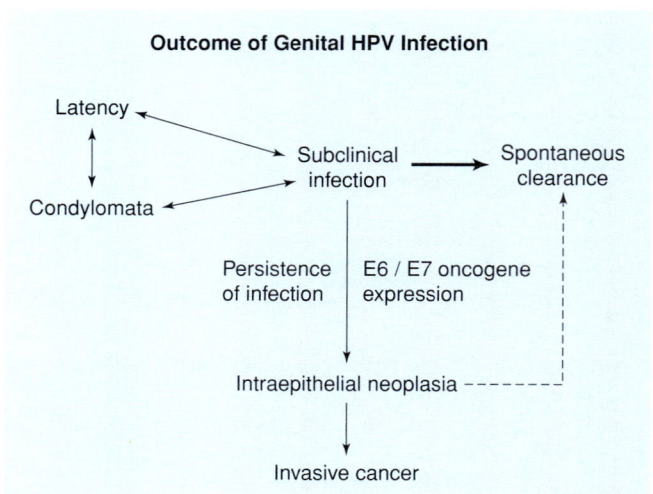

FIGURE 29-6 The natural history of genital human papillomavirus (HPV) infection varies between individuals and over time. Most infections are subclinical. Spontaneous resolution is the most common outcome. Neoplasia is the least common manifestation of HPV infection, and it develops from persistent infection and integration of HPV DNA.

infections. Infection expression may be productive, that is, creating new infectious virus particles, or it may be neoplastic, causing preinvasive disease or malignancy. Temporally, HPV infection can be transient (spontaneous resolution, clearance) or persistent. High-grade neoplasia (CIN 3, AIS, or cancer) is the least common outcome of genital HPV infection and requires HPV expression and persistence.

Latent infection theoretically occurs when cells are infected but HPV remains quiescent. No cellular or tissue effects are evident, as the virus is not actively replicating. However, HPV is present below detectable levels. Thus, it is uncertain whether apparent HPV clearance constitutes true HPV resolution or whether it reflects latency. It may be that both latency and clearance are outcomes of HPV infection. Reappearance of previously resolved HPV-related lesions after loss of immune competence is indirect evidence of latency. Clearance versus permanent immune suppression of HPV manifestations cannot be distinguished using current technology.

Productive infections are characterized by viral life-cycle completion and plentiful production of infectious viral particles (Stanley, 2010a). Viral gene expression and assemblage are completed in synchrony with terminal squamous differentiation and conclude with desquamation of infected squames. These infections have little or no malignant potential because the HPV genome remains episomal, and its oncogenes are expressed at very low levels (Durst, 1985; Stoler, 1996). Productive HPV infections cause either visible genital warts, called *condylomata acuminata*, or, much more commonly, subclinical infections, which are not readily apparent.

Neoplastic infections result in cancer precursor lesions and invasive cancers. The circular HPV genome is disrupted and integrates at random locations into a host chromosome (Fig. 30-1, p. 656). Unrestrained transcription of the *E6* and *E7* oncogenes follows (Durst, 1985; Stoler, 1996). The E6 and E7 oncoproteins produced interfere with the function of and accelerate degradation of p53 and pRb, respectively. Both are key host tumor-suppressor proteins (Fig. 30-2, p. 656). This leaves infected cells vulnerable to malignant transformation by loss of cell-cycle control, cellular proliferation, and accumulation of DNA mutations over time (Doorbar, 2012).

In resultant preinvasive lesions, normal epithelial differentiation is disrupted and incomplete. The degree of disruption is used to grade LAGT histology as low-grade or high-grade SIL. The average age at diagnosis of low-grade cervical disease is younger than that of high-grade lesions and invasive cancers. Thus, disease was thought to progress from milder- to higher-grade lesions over time. An alternative theory now proposes that low-grade lesions are generally acute, transient, and not oncogenic. High-grade lesions and cancers are likely monoclonal and arise de novo rather than from preexistent low-grade disease (Baseman, 2005; Kiviat, 1996).

Most HPV infection and related lesions, whether clinical or subclinical, spontaneously resolve, especially in adolescents and young women (Ho, 1998; Moscicki, 1998). Whether apparent clearance reflects true resolution of infection or limited testing sensitivity remains unresolved (Winer, 2011). Several studies show that lrHPV infections resolve faster than hrHPV ones (Moscicki, 2004; Schlecht, 2003; Woodman, 2001).

Persistent hrHPV infection is necessary for the development of cervical neoplasia. Few HPV infections become persistent. Most young women (65 percent) with HPV 16/18 infections lasting more than 6 months will develop SIL (Trottier, 2009). The risk of progression to high-grade neoplasia increases with age, as HPV infection in older women is more likely to reflect persistence than serial reinfection (Hildesheim, 1999). Although humoral immunity addresses initial HPV infection, cell-mediated immunity plays the larger role in HPV persistence and in progression or regression of benign and neoplastic lesions.

The pathogenesis of HPV-related neoplasia at other anogenital sites is believed to be similar to that of the cervix. Genital HPV infection is usually multifocal and involves the cervix most often. Neoplasia at one site raises the risk of neoplasia elsewhere in the LAGT (Spitzer, 1989).

■ Infection Diagnosis

HPV infection is clinically suspected based on lesions or results of cytology, histology, and colposcopy, all of which are subjective and often inaccurate. Serology is unreliable and cannot distinguish past from current infection (Dillner, 1999). As already noted, culture of HPV is not feasible. HPV testing more accurately confirms HPV infection. Clinical HPV testing involves the direct detection of HPV nucleic acids by in situ hybridization, nucleic acid amplification testing (NAAT), polymerase chain reaction (PCR), or other techniques (Molijn, 2005). Currently, four clinical hrHPV tests are approved by the Food and Drug Administration (FDA), and all use NAAT to detect any of 13 or 14 different hrHPV types. Three of these tests can report specifically the presence of HPV 16 or HPV 18 (genotyping) to aid risk stratification. A negative HPV test result does not exclude genital HPV infection because only specific oncogenic HPVs are tested for, and sensitivities are set to detect cervical neoplasia. Therefore, these tests are not approved

for routine STD screening. Testing for lrHPV has no routine clinical indication and is discouraged as it can lead to inappropriate expense, evaluation, and treatment.

The clinical role of hrHPV testing for cervical cancer screening and for surveillance of SIL continues to evolve. It is, often in combination with cytology, an important component of cervical cancer screening, management of abnormal screening-test results, and surveillance post-colposcopy and posttreatment. Numerous studies indicate that HPV self-sampling may become a useful strategy to engage more women in cervical cancer screening programs in the future (Yeh, 2019).

■ Infection Treatment

The indications to treat HPV-related LAGT disease are symptomatic warts, high-grade neoplasia, or invasive cancer. No effective treatment resolves subclinical or latent HPV infection. Harm may result from unrealistic attempts to eradicate HPV infections and LSIL, which are usually self-limited. Encouragement of positive health behaviors and optimal management of immunocompromise seem sensible. Various treatment modalities are available for genital warts and are chosen according to lesion size, location, and number (Rosales, 2014). Mechanical removal or destruction, topical immune modulators, and chemical or thermal coagulation can be used (Table 3-12, p. 73). Examination of a male partner does not benefit a female partner either by influencing reinfection or by altering the clinical course or treatment outcome of her genital warts or LAGT neoplasia (Centers for Disease Control and Prevention, 2010).

Visible lesions caused by HPV lie at either end of the disease spectrum, either condylomata or invasive cancers. They can look very similar. Intraepithelial lesions tend to be invisible to unaided inspection. Therefore, liberal use of biopsy before treatment is prudent. This is especially true for an atypical-appearing genital lesion, a visible cervical lesion, or any LAGT lesion in an immunocompromised or older patient.

■ Infection Prevention

Behavior

Sexual abstinence, delaying coitarche, and limiting the number of sexual partners are logical strategies to avoid genital HPV infection and its adverse consequences. However, evidence is lacking from trials of counseling and sexual practice modification. Condoms do not cover all anogenital skin and therefore may not be completely protective. However, condoms do appear to reduce acquisition and transmission rates of HPV, even when used inconsistently (Winer, 2003).

Vaccines

Vaccines offer the greatest promise for HPV infection prevention (prophylactic vaccines) and possibly reversal of its sequelae in those already infected (therapeutic vaccines). Although highly effective prophylactic vaccines are used worldwide, development of therapeutic vaccines for HPV-related neoplasias remains experimental at this time.

Both local and humoral immunity are thought to protect against incident HPV infection. Prophylactic vaccines elicit high levels of type-specific humoral antibody production that prevents new HPV infection by blocking its entry into host cells (Stanley, 2010b). They do not prevent transient HPV positivity or resolve preexistent infection or HPV-related neoplasia. HPV vaccination has the potential to prevent malignancy for at least six body sites that include cervix, vulva, vagina, penis, anal canal, and oropharynx if administered before vaccine-type HPV infection takes place.

Prophylactic HPV vaccines use recombinant technologies for the synthetic production of the L1 capsid proteins of each HPV type included in the vaccine. The resultant virus-like particles are highly immunogenic but not infectious, as they lack any viral DNA (Stanley, 2010b). Seroconversion rates in excess of 99 percent to vaccine viral types are typical.

Only one vaccine is currently available in the United States. Gardasil 9 is a nonavalent HPV vaccine (9vHPV) against HPV types 6, 11, 16, 18, 31, 35, 45, 52, and 58. Coverage for the latter five types was not included in earlier HPV vaccines. HPV types 6 and 11 account for at least 90 percent of genital condylomata and recurrent laryngeal papillomas, and a significant number of low-grade cervical cytologic and colposcopic abnormalities. Types 16 and 18 cause approximately 60 to 70 percent of cervical cancers; a significant number of anal, vulvar, and vaginal cancers; and many preinvasive lesions at all sites. The other five viral types in the vaccine add coverage for an additional 15 to 20 percent of cervical cancers (Petrosky, 2015). Gardasil 9 is FDA approved for the prevention of genital warts and cervical, vulvar, vaginal, and anal neoplasia caused by any of its nine HPV types. In previously uninfected individuals, it protects against at least 96 percent of incident infections and their resultant neoplasia caused by all nine HPV types.

Ideally, vaccination takes place prior to sexual activity initiation, when the potential benefit is greatest. However, a history of prior sexual activity, HPV-related disease, or HPV-test positivity should not deter vaccine administration. Moreover, HPV testing is not recommended prior to vaccination (American College of Obstetricians and Gynecologists, 2017). The Advisory Committee on Immunization Practices (ACIP) currently recommends that HPV vaccine be administered routinely to all girls and boys aged 11 to 12 years (as early as age 9 years) (Meites, 2019). Catch-up vaccination is also recommended for all 13- to 26-year-old persons. The ACIP does not recommend routine catch-up vaccination for persons aged 27 to 45 years due to limited benefit. This is despite recent FDA approval for vaccination in this age group (Food and Drug Administration, 2018). Instead, the ACIP agrees with the American College of Obstetricians and Gynecologists (2019) recommendation of shared decision-making with persons aged 27 to 45 years who have not previously received the HPV vaccine and are at risk of acquiring HPV. Strong, unequivocal advocacy for early HPV vaccination by providers is critical to vaccine uptake and effectiveness. As of 2018, U.S. HPV vaccination rates remain low. Only 51 percent of adolescents aged 13 to 17 years are up to date with the HPV vaccine series (Walker, 2019).

Gardasil 9 is administered as a three-dose series if started at or after age 15 years. The second dose is administered 1 to 2 months after the first, and the third dose is given 6 months after the first. If the vaccination schedule is interrupted for

pregnancy or other reasons, the vaccine series is continued as soon as possible with the next dose. The series is not restarted. Prolongation of the dosing schedule does not appear to diminish immunogenicity. If HPV vaccination is initiated before age 15 years, only 2 doses are needed. This is because the vaccine is more immunogenic at an earlier age. The second dose is given 6 to 12 months following the first (Meites, 2016). No data support the need for later booster dosing. Recent evidence suggests that a single dose of HPV vaccine may result in sufficient and enduring protection against HPV infection and neoplasia, and future dosing recommendations may be modified (Brotherton, 2019; Kreimer, 2018).

Vaccination that was begun with earlier two-valent (2vHPV) and four-valent HPV (4vHPV) vaccine formulations can be continued using 9vHPV. The series is not restarted. After completion of a 2vHPV or 4vHPV vaccine series, there is no ACIP recommendation for administration of 9vHPV to extend HPV coverage. The additional HPV types included in the 9vHPV vaccine mostly target cancers in women (Meites, 2016).

HPV vaccines have excellent safety profiles, are well-tolerated, and can be administered along with other recommended vaccinations. Injection-site erythema, pain, and swelling are common. These can increase in severity following subsequent doses but are usually mild to moderate. HPV vaccination is avoided during pregnancy, but pregnancy testing is not recommended prior to administration (American College of Obstetricians and Gynecologists, 2017). If inadvertently given during pregnancy, no action is needed. Vaccination can be given during lactation. Immunocompromised persons are candidates to receive the vaccine and show high seroconversion rates despite concerns for a blunted immune response. 9vHPV should be given with caution to persons who experienced an allergic reaction to a prior dose, have an allergy to yeast, or have had a recent febrile illness.

HPV vaccination prevents most, but not all, HPV-related cancers, and therefore cervical cancer screening should continue per current guidelines. Countries with high vaccination rates have dramatically lowered HPV 16 and 18 prevalence and reduced rates of anogenital warts and high-grade cervical neoplasia (Drolet, 2019). Despite suboptimal HPV vaccination rates in the United States, infections involving the HPV types in the 4vHPV (HPVs 6, 11, 16, and 18) have decreased sharply since vaccine introduction. HPV 16 and 18 prevalence has declined from 9 percent to 5.5 percent in the general population of women (Hirth, 2019). The decreased prevalence in both vaccinated and unvaccinated adolescents and women is evidence of both direct and herd immunity as a result of HPV vaccination (Markowitz, 2019). A significant drop in the diagnosis of high-grade cervical disease, including AIS, has already been observed in U.S. women aged 18 to 24 (Cleveland, 2019; McClung, 2019).

CERVICAL INTRAEPITHELIAL NEOPLASIA

■ Risk Factors

An estimated 412,000 cases of CIN are diagnosed in the United States annually (Henk, 2010). Similar to invasive cervical cancer, CIN is most strongly related to persistent genital

TABLE 29-1. Risk Factors for Cervical Neoplasia

Demographic risk factors
Ethnicity (Latin American countries, U.S. minorities)
Low socioeconomic status
Increasing age

Behavioral risk factors
Early coitarche
Multiple sexual partners
Male partner with multiple prior sexual partners
Tobacco smoking
Dietary deficiencies

Medical risk factors
Cervical high-risk human papillomavirus infection
Exogenous hormones (combination hormonal
   contraceptives)
Parity
Immunosuppression
Inadequate screening

hrHPV infection and aging (Table 29-1) (Ho, 1995; Kjaer, 2002; Remmink, 1995).

The median age of cervical cancer diagnosis in the United States (late fifth decade) is approximately a decade later than for CIN. In an older woman, HPV infection is more likely to persist than resolve. Aging is linked to waning immune competence and allows the accumulation of genetic mutations that can lead to malignant transformation. Additionally, adverse socioeconomic factors and decreased need for prenatal care or contraception cause older women to be screened less often.

Behavioral risk factors for CIN mirror those for HPV acquisition and include early sexual activity, multiple partners, and male partner promiscuity (Buckley, 1981; de Vet, 1994; Kjaer, 1991). After adjustments for HPV positivity and lower socioeconomic status, tobacco use also raises CIN risk (Castle, 2004; Plummer, 2003).

Combination oral contraceptives (COCs) have been linked to a higher risk of CIN and cervical cancer in current users (International Collaboration of Epidemiological Studies of Cervical Cancer, 2007; Roura, 2016). Possible mechanisms include increased persistence of HPV infection and oncogene expression (de Villiers, 2003). In contrast, multiple studies have not found a greater CIN risk in users of hormonal contraceptives or postmenopausal hormone therapy (Castle, 2005; Harris, 2009; Yasmeen, 2006). In addition to a known increased risk

of cervical and vaginal clear cell adenocarcinoma, DES exposure in utero appears to raise the risk of developing cervical HSIL (Hoover, 2011). However, this greater HSIL risk may be the result of higher screening rates in these women (Verloop, 2017).

Increasing parity has been correlated with cervical cancer risk, but it is unclear if this is related to earlier sexual activity, a progestin-exposure effect, or other factors. Immune suppression during pregnancy, hormonal influences on cervical epithelium, and physical trauma related to vaginal deliveries have all been suggested (Brinton, 1989; Muñoz, 2002; Roura, 2016).

Immunocompromised women in general have increased risks for CIN and for greater lesion severity, multifocal lesion patterns, and multisite LAGT disease. They also experience higher rates of treatment failure, persistence, and LAGT disease recurrence compared with those who are immune competent. Specifically, women with human immunodeficiency virus (HIV) infection have higher rates of abnormal cervical cytology and CIN compared with women without HIV. Transplant recipients have an increased risk of developing malignancy after transplantation, including neoplasms of the LAGT and anal canal (Gomez-Lobo, 2009). Women taking immune suppressive medications for other disorders show higher rates of LAGT neoplasia.

Inadequate screening is a strong cervical neoplasia risk factor. Of women with cervical cancer in the United States, approximately 50 percent had never been screened and 10 percent had not been screened during the 5 years prior to diagnosis (American College of Obstetricians and Gynecologists, 2018a). Lack of screening is a major contributor to elevated rates of cervical cancer in socioeconomically disadvantaged women (Benard, 2007).

■ Natural History

Preinvasive lesions can spontaneously regress, remain stable, or progress. The risk of progression to invasive cancer rises with CIN severity. Estimated rates of CIN progression, persistence, and regression are shown in Table 29-2 (Ostor, 1993). Low-grade lesions are thought to be manifestations of acute HPV infection, and approximately 90 percent regress within a few years. High-grade lesions are less likely to regress. Approximately 40 percent of CIN 2 cases show spontaneous regression within 2 years. This is even more frequent (>60 percent) in young, healthy women (Castle, 2009b; Moscicki, 2010). CIN 2 is thought to be a mixture of low- and high-grade lesions that are difficult to distinguish histologically, rather than an intermediate step in the progression from CIN 1 to CIN 3. The risk of progression of biopsied but untreated CIN 3 to invasive cancer approximates 30 percent over 30 years (McCredie, 2008).

TABLE 29-2. Natural History of Cervical Intraepithelial Neoplasia (CIN) Lesions

	Regression (%)	Persistence (%)	Progression to CIS (%)	Progression to Invasion (%)
CIN 1	57	32	11	1
CIN 2	43	35	22	5
CIN 3	32	<56	–	>12

CIS = carcinoma in situ.
From Ostor, 1993, with permission.

CERVICAL INTRAEPITHELIAL NEOPLASIA DIAGNOSIS

In general, LAGT preinvasive lesions are visible only with aided inspection. The exception is high-grade VIN, which is often visible, palpable, or both. Only cervical lesions at either end of the neoplastic disease spectrum are grossly visible, namely, condylomata and invasive cancers. Accordingly, grossly visible cervical lesions require prompt biopsy.

The goal of cervical cancer screening is to identify preinvasive lesions (CIN) or early-stage cervical cancer that can be treated most successfully. Abnormal test results lead to further management with repeat cytology, HPV testing, or colposcopy with biopsy of lesions. Screening previously was limited to cervical cytology. HPV testing has become an important screening tool either paired with cytology (*co-testing*) or, recently, as a stand-alone screening test.

■ Cervical Cytology

Cervical cytologic screening is one of modern medicine's great success stories (Koss, 1989). The Papanicolaou (Pap) test has never been evaluated in a randomized or controlled, prospective trial. Nonetheless, countries with organized screening programs have consistently realized dramatic declines in cervical disease. Widespread use of the Pap test since the 1950s has reduced the incidence of and mortality from invasive cervical cancer by more than 80 percent in the United States (Howlader, 2017). Approximately 7 percent of U.S. women who undergo Pap testing will have an abnormal result (Wright, 2012).

The Pap test's specificity is consistently high and approximates 98 percent. However, estimates of its sensitivity for detection of CIN 2 or worse are lower and variable, ranging from 45 to 65 percent (Whitlock, 2011). This limited sensitivity is countered by repetitive screening throughout a woman's life. Although the incidence of cervical squamous carcinoma has declined due to Pap testing, the relative and absolute incidences of cervical adenocarcinoma have increased, particularly in women younger than 50 (Herzog, 2007). Adenocarcinoma and adenosquamous carcinoma now account for at least 20 percent of cervical cancers. This rise may partly stem from the Pap test's lower sensitivity for the detection of adenocarcinoma than for squamous cancers and their precursor lesions.

False-negative Pap test results may derive from sampling errors that fail to collect abnormal cells or from screening errors where the screener overlooks or misclassifies abnormal cells (Wilkinson, 1990). Mandated quality-assurance measures and computerized slide-screening technologies can help address screening errors. Suboptimal management of abnormal results by providers and poor patient compliance also contribute to avoidable cases of cervical cancer.

Optimizing the Pap Test

Ideally, Pap tests are scheduled to avoid menstruation. Patients should abstain from vaginal intercourse, douching, vaginal tampon use, and intravaginal medicinal or contraceptive creams for a minimum of 24 to 48 hours before tested. Treatment of cervicitis or vaginitis prior to Pap testing is optimal. However, Pap testing is not deferred due to suboptimal conditions if the patient may not return. This is especially true in patients with unexplained discharge or unscheduled bleeding, as these may be signs of LAGT cancer.

As shown in Figure 22-12 (p. 497), cervical squamous cell appearance varies throughout the menstrual cycle and with hormonal status. Thus, clinical information added to pathology requisition forms aids accurate cytology interpretation. Data include date of last menstrual period, pregnancy or menopausal status, exogenous hormone use, abnormal bleeding, and prior abnormal Pap test findings, CIN, or other LAGT neoplasia. Intrauterine devices (IUDs) also can cause reactive cellular changes and are noted.

Full visualization of the cervix is essential to detect gross lesions and collect adequate specimens. Speculum placement should be as comfortable as possible. A thin coating of water-based lubricant can be smeared on the outside of the speculum blades without compromising Pap test quality or interpretation (Griffith, 2005; Harmanli, 2010). Touching the cervix prior to performing Pap testing is avoided, as dysplastic epithelium may be inadvertently removed by minimal trauma. Discharge covering the cervix may be carefully absorbed by a large swab without contacting the cervix. Vigorous blotting or rubbing can theoretically cause scant cellularity or a false-negative Pap test result. When indicated, additional cervical sampling to detect infection should follow Pap test collection.

Sampling of the transformation zone at the SCJ adds substantial sensitivity of the Pap test. Techniques are adapted and sampling devices are chosen according to SCJ location, which varies widely with age, prior obstetric laceration, and hormonal status. Women with known or suspected in utero DES exposure also may benefit from a separate Pap test of the upper vagina, because of their increased vaginal cancer risk (Chap. 32, p. 695).

Cytology Collection

Three types of plastic devices are commonly used to sample the cervix: the spatula, broom, and endocervical brush (cytobrush) (Fig. 29-7). A spatula predominantly samples the ectocervix. An endocervical brush samples the endocervical canal and is used in combination with a spatula. A broom samples both endo- and ectocervical epithelia simultaneously but can be supplemented by an endocervical brush. Wooden collection devices and cotton swabs are no longer recommended due to their inferior collection and release of cells.

A cervical Ayers spatula with its saddle-shaped end is positioned to best fit the ectocervical contour, straddle the SCJ, and sample the distal endocervical canal. It firmly scrapes the cervical surface while completing at least one full rotation. After the spatula sample is obtained, the endocervical brush is inserted into the endocervical canal until the outermost bristles remain visible just within the external os. This prevents inadvertent sampling of lower uterine segment cells, which can mimic atypical cervical cells. To minimize bleeding, the brush is used after the ectocervix has been sampled and is rotated only one-quarter to one-half turn. If the cervical canal is very wide, the brush can be directed around the canal perimeter to contact all surfaces.

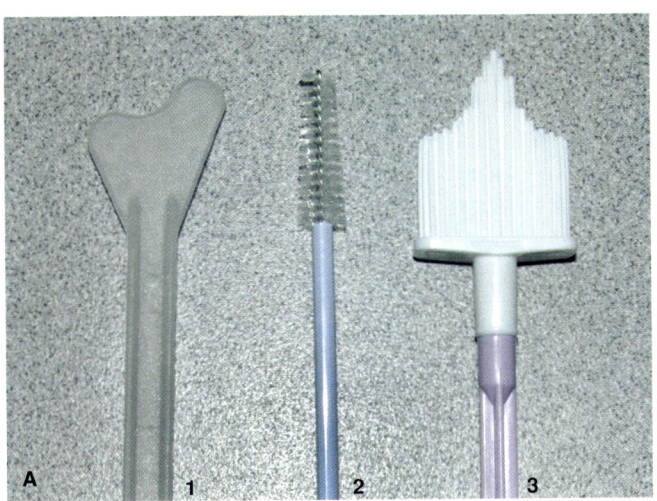

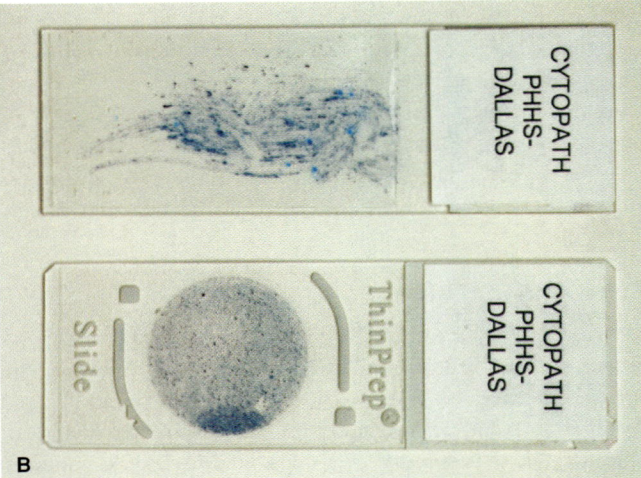

FIGURE 29-7 A. Cervical cytology collection devices: (1) Plastic spatula. (2) Endocervical brush. (3) Plastic broom. **B.** Pap test preparations. Conventional cervical cytology is prepared by smearing collected cells directly onto a glass slide with the collection device followed by immediate fixation (*upper slide*). Liquid-based cytology involves transfer of collected cells from the collection device into a liquid transport medium with subsequent processing and transfer onto a glass slide. Cells are distributed over a smaller area, and debris, mucus, blood, and cell overlap are largely eliminated (*lower slide*). (Reproduced with permission from Dr. Raheela Ashfaq.)

Broom devices have longer central bristles that are inserted into the endocervical canal and collect cells there. These long bristles are flanked by shorter ones that splay out over the ectocervix with gentle pressure during rotation. Five rotations in the same direction are recommended. Reversing direction may release and lose cellular material. Broom devices are favored for liquid-based Pap testing.

To submit collected cells to the laboratory, conventional glass slides (*Pap smear*) and liquid-based Pap tests are considered equally acceptable by all current guidelines (American College of Obstetricians and Gynecologists, 2018a; Saslow, 2012; U.S. Preventive Services Task Force, 2018).

Conventional slide preparation requires special care to avoid air drying artifact to protect slide quality. The spatula or broom sample is held, while the endocervical brush sampling immediately follows. The spatula or broom sample is then quickly spread as evenly as possible over one half to two thirds of a glass slide (see Fig. 29-7). The endocervical brush is firmly rolled over the remaining area of the slide, after which an appropriate fixative is quickly sprayed onto the slide from a distance of 10 to 12 inches or by immersing the slide completely in a container of appropriate fixative.

Currently, most cervical cytology specimens are collected into liquid-based media. Two liquid-based cytology (LBC) Pap tests are FDA approved. Sampling and cell transfer to a liquid medium is performed according to manufacturer specifications. SurePath allows for the use of all three device types but uses modified tips that are broken off and sent to the laboratory in the liquid medium. ThinPrep requires the collection device(s) to be repetitively pressed against the medium-container walls to release cells, then vigorously agitated within the medium, and finally discarded.

■ HPV Testing

HPV testing in clinical practice tests only for 13 or 14 hrHPV types. It has several indications that include cervical cancer screening, triage of lesser cytologic abnormalities to later repeat testing or immediate colposcopy, surveillance after colposcopy, or surveillance after treatment. Until recently, its use for primary cervical cancer screening was restricted to co-testing, which is a Pap test plus HPV test. However, HPV testing alone for cervical cancer screening now has approval from one oversight agency (U.S. Preventive Services task Force, 2018).

A role for HPV testing in cervical cancer screening is attractive because of its greater immediate sensitivity for CIN 3 or cervical cancer and the objectivity of its results. However, screening guidelines incorporating HPV testing must compensate for a lower specificity, particularly in young women, described in the next section.

HPV testing is usually performed from the residual LBC Pap medium after the cytology slide is prepared. Alternatively, a cervical sample for HPV can be obtained separately in a specific collection device. As noted earlier, there is no clinical role for testing for lrHPV types (p. 625) (Castle, 2014; Thomsen, 2014).

Co-testing

The combination of HPV testing with cytology (co-testing) raises the sensitivity of a single screening test for high-grade neoplasia and leads to earlier detection and management of HSIL (Ronco, 2014). The lack of sensitivity with cytology alone for cervical adenocarcinoma and its rising incidence both support HPV testing for primary screening (Castellsagué, 2006). This strategy is not recommended by current guidelines for women younger than 30 because of the high prevalence of HPV infection in this age group and the resultant lack of test specificity.

Co-testing offers a nearly 100-percent negative predictive value for high-grade neoplasia. Because of this, coupled with the slow progression of new HPV infection to high-grade neoplasia or cancer and increased cost, co-testing is repeated at 5-year intervals if both cytology and HPV test findings are negative. If cytologic results are abnormal, current cytologic-management guidelines are followed (p. 632). Cytology-negative and HPV-positive test results will occur in <10 percent of screened patients (Castle, 2009a; Datta, 2008). In such cases, co-testing is repeated 12 months later. Colposcopy is recommended for recurrent, positive HPV results or an abnormal repeat cytology.

An alternative strategy is now available for the management of normal cytologic findings but a positive HPV result. A reflex test specifically for HPVs 16 and 18, (genotyping) can be performed in many settings. If HPV 16 or 18 is found, immediate colposcopy is recommended (American College of Obstetricians and Gynecologists, 2018a; Saslow, 2012). This approach identifies those at highest risk for significant disease and shortens time to diagnosis (Khan, 2005; Wright, 2015).

Primary HPV Testing

Sufficient evidence supports HPV testing alone (without cytology) as an option for primary cervical cancer screening (Castle, 2011; Cuzick, 2006; Dillner, 2013, Ronco, 2014). HPV testing alone is approximately twice as sensitive (>90 percent) as a single Pap test and leads to earlier detection of high-grade disease. The very high negative predictive value of a single HPV test result is clinically reassuring that high-grade disease or cancer is not present. Recent evaluations show that co-testing does not perform better than HPV testing alone but adds expense (Schiffman, 2018). Specificity declines with HPV testing alone, particularly in younger women (Mayrand, 2007; Ronco, 2006, 2010). This could lead to excessive numbers of colposcopies, biopsies, and treatments of lesions that could have spontaneously regressed. Genotyping is part of primary HPV screening for cervical disease and allows the triage of women who test positive for HPV 16 or 18 to immediate colposcopy. Those with test results indicating no HPV 16 and 18 but identifying other hrHPVs receive follow-up other than immediate colposcopy. This strategy attempts to counter the lower specificity of HPV testing. In sum, primary HPV testing is expected to result in more colposcopic referrals initially but yield higher and earlier HSIL detection rates. As of 2019, two HPV tests, both providing genotyping, were approved by the FDA for primary cervical cancer screening in women aged ≥25 years. This represents a major paradigm shift in cervical cancer screening, in that Pap testing assumes a secondary role. To date, one oversight agency has approved HPV testing alone for primary cervical cancer screening in women at least 30 years old (U.S. Preventive Services Task Force, 2018). Others are expected to as well in the near future.

Interim guidelines for managing the results of primary HPV screening are published and are expected to be revised in coming years (Huh, 2015; Wentzensen, 2019). Immediate colposcopy is recommended if HPV 16 or 18 is identified. If other HPV types are found, triage to reflex cytology is proposed. Colposcopy is recommended for any cytologic abnormalities, as per current management guidelines. However, management of HPV-positive, non-HPV 16 or 18 results is not yet firmly established. Interim recommendations for reflex cytology may be replaced by other, more predictive triage tests such as p16/Ki-67 dual staining or methylation markers (Dick, 2019; Wentzensen, 2019).

■ Current Cervical Cancer Screening Guidelines

Perspectives on Guidelines

All currently approved cervical cancer screening strategies, including cytology, co-testing, and primary HPV testing, dramatically reduce an individual's lifetime risk of cervical cancer. The choice of screening strategy should be a shared decision by the provider and patient. The balance of benefits, harms, and cost-effectiveness of each screening strategy merits careful consideration by both providers and health-care policy agencies (National Cancer Institute, 2019a; U.S. Preventive Services Task Force, 2018). Evidence-based cervical cancer screening recommendations continue to evolve. All major guidelines are similar and only pertain to average-risk women, namely, immune competent women without prior HSIL, cervical cancer, or in utero DES exposure (American College of Obstetricians and Gynecologists, 2018a; Saslow, 2012; U.S. Preventive Services Task Force, 2018). All recognize the acceptability of both conventional and liquid-based cytology, the age for screening initiation and cessation, screening intervals, and continued standard screening after HPV vaccination. Importantly, patient adherence to screening guidelines or needed follow-up of abnormalities should not impede other indicated gynecologic care, especially the provision of contraception.

Screening Initiation

Cervical cancer screening begins at age 21 in average-risk women. This is true regardless of sexual history, sexual orientation, or other risk factors. In young women, most Pap test result abnormalities represent transient HPV infection, and the spontaneous regression of even high-grade lesions is common (Moscicki, 2005). Cervical cancer is rare in adolescents and less preventable by screening (Saslow, 2012). Additionally, treatment of high-grade CIN in adolescents is often followed by persistent Pap test result abnormalities and may have adverse reproductive consequences (Case, 2006; Moore, 2007).

Screening Strategies and Intervals

For women aged 21 to 29 years, all current guidelines recommend screening with cytology alone at 3-year intervals. Co-testing or primary HPV screening is not used. Women aged 30 to 65 years can continue screening with cytology alone at 3-year intervals or can begin co-testing at 5-year intervals. The American Cancer Society, American Society for Colposcopy and Cervical Pathology (ASCCP), American Society for Clinical Pathology, and American College of Obstetricians and Gynecologists (2018a) deem co-testing preferable to cytology alone in women ≥30 years (Saslow, 2012). The U.S. Preventive Services Task Force (2018) now endorses cytology alone every 3 years, co-testing every 5 years, and HPV testing alone every 5 years as equivalent, acceptable screening strategies for women aged ≥30 years or more. Co-testing and primary hrHPV testing are advantageous for individuals who desire a longer screening interval. Regardless of strategy, screening more frequently than recommended adds cost, does not significantly lower cervical cancer risk, and exposes patients to the harms of overdiagnosis and overtreatment.

Screening Discontinuation

Screening may be stopped at age 65 years in those at average risk for cervical cancer and who have undergone adequate screening, regardless of past or current sexual history. Adequate screening is defined as three consecutive, negative cytology results or two consecutive, negative co-test results in the prior 10 years, with the most recent result occurring within the past 5 years. Women with prior treatment for CIN 2, CIN 3, AIS, or cervical cancer should continue screening for at least 20 years past their diagnosis and treatment, even if this extends screening beyond age 65. These women carry increased long-term risks for cervical cancer (American College of Obstetrics and Gynecology, 2018b; Saslow, 2012; U.S. Preventive Services Task Force, 2018). Screening cessation can be considered at any age if life expectancy becomes limited to the point where the development of cervical cancer becomes unlikely.

Posthysterectomy

Primary vaginal carcinoma is rare and makes up <5 percent of all gynecologic malignancies (Siegel, 2019). All guidelines recommend against Pap test screening for women who have undergone total hysterectomy (cervix removed) for a benign-disease indication and who lack a prior high-grade CIN or cervical cancer diagnosis. The absence of a cervix should be confirmed by examination or pathology report, as many women are inaccurate in their personal reporting of hysterectomy type. Women who have undergone supracervical hysterectomy should continue routine screening. Recommendations for vaginal cytology after total hysterectomy in women with prior high-grade cervical neoplasia or cancer are less clear. Vaginal cancer is still rare in these individuals, and screening offers uncertain benefit (Saslow, 2012). The American College of Obstetricians and Gynecologists (2018b) recommends Pap testing of the vaginal cuff every 3 years for 20 years after initial posttreatment surveillance, which is traditionally a schedule of three Pap tests in the first 2 years posthysterectomy.

Vaginal cuff cytology should be collected such that the chosen collection device makes optimal contact with the upper vaginal walls. A plastic spatula or its handle end may be best suited for this. The cuff is sampled with gentle but firm pressure, drawing the device across it several times in the same direction so as not to lose cells. Deep indentations in the vaginal cuff can be sampled with an endocervical brush, and these cells are added to the transport medium. The role of HPV testing for women without a cervix is not defined or generally recommended. HPV testing is FDA approved for cervical testing only. Despite this, vaginal cuff HPV testing is common (Chappell, 2010).

Guidance for the management of vaginal cytology and HPV test results has been suggested based on only limited data (Khan, 2016). HSIL cytology or LSIL and ASC-US that are positive for HPV 16 or 18 should prompt vaginal colposcopy. Non-16/18 positive HPV test results wtih negative, ASC-US, or LSIL cytology can be followed for 2 years without colposcopy. Testing should be repeated in a year; this can be done with a co-test. Vaginal colposcopy is considered if positive HPV testing or abnormal cytology persist.

Immunocompromised Patients

Immunocompromised patients, particularly those with HIV infection and solid organ transplants, are at much greater risk of HPV-related disease, often multifocal, than the general population. As reviewed by the Panel on Opportunistic Infections in HIV-Infected Adults and Adolescents (2019), those with HIV infection have a higher risk of HPV infection and persistence, and therefore of condylomata, preinvasive disease, and cancers of the cervix, vulva, vagina, and anal canal. This risk, particularly of cervical and anal cancer, correlates with the degree of immune compromise. Due to the higher risk and poorer prognosis of cervical cancer in women with HIV infection, it was designated as an acquired immune deficiency syndrome (AIDS)-defining illness. Fortunately, women with HIV infection who receive regular screening and recommended follow-up for CIN experience the same incidence of invasive cervical cancer as women without HIV infection (Massad, 2009). Unfortunately, women with HIV infection have lower compliance rates for screening and follow-up of abnormal results, which compound their already higher risk of LAGT neoplasia (Barnes, 2018).

With HIV infection, screening should commence within 1 year of sexual activity onset and no later than age 21 years. Women aged 21 to 29 years should receive Pap testing at the time of HIV diagnosis (American College of Obstetrics and Gynecology, 2018a; Panel on Opportunistic Infections in HIV-Infected Adults and Adolescents, 2019). If an initial Pap test result is negative, testing should be repeated 6 or 12 months later and then continued every 12 months. After three consecutive, negative Pap test results, the interval of Pap testing can be extended to 3 years. For women aged ≥30 years, cytology screening can be followed as just described, or co-testing every 3 years can begin. This co-testing interval is shorter than for immune competent women. Cervical cancer screening is continued indefinitely even in those aged 65 years or older who have been adequately screened. After hysterectomy for benign disease, vaginal cuff cytology is not recommended. Those with prior high-grade cervical neoplasia or cancer should have annual vaginal cuff cytology. If the history of cervical disease preceding hysterectomy is unclear, women with HIV infection should have continued vaginal cuff cytology screening at intervals similar to cervical screening. This is because CIN is the most common indication for hysterectomy in women with HIV.

The Panel on Opportunistic Infections in HIV-Infected Adults and Adolescents (2019) recommends careful assessment of the entire LAGT with at least visual inspection as part of every routine screening examination. If cervical or vulvar lesions are found, vaginal colposcopy is indicated. No current consensus guides screening for anal cancer in persons with HIV infection. Patients should be questioned regarding anorectal pain or bleeding. A digital examination of the anal canal to detect masses is recommended routinely. Anal cytology testing is discouraged unless referral to centers that offer high-resolution anoscopy is available to address abnormal results.

For other groups of immunocompromised persons without HIV infection, guidelines have been proposed (Chin-Hong, 2019; Moscicki, 2019). The screening recommendations for women with HIV infection are extended to those with solid organ and stem-cell transplants, inflammatory bowel disease or rheumatoid arthritis treated with immune suppressants, or systemic lupus erythematosus whether or not immune suppressants are used. Solid organ transplant recipients remain at high risk of developing high-grade LAGT lesions and cancers. It is suggested they undergo thorough LAGT examinations annually (Thimm, 2019). Women with diabetes mellitus or those with rheumatoid arthritis or inflammatory bowel disease not treated with immune suppressants can be screened according to guidelines for average-risk women.

■ The Bethesda System

Cervical cytology reporting is standardized by the Bethesda System nomenclature. Clinically, the key elements reported are specimen adequacy and epithelial cell abnormalities Tables 29-3 and 29-4 (National Cancer Institute Workshop, 1989; Nayar, 2015; Solomon, 2002). Evidence-based recommendations from national organizations guide initial management of cervical cytology abnormalities for nonpregnant women

TABLE 29-3. The 2014 Bethesda System Cytology Report Components

Specimen Type
Conventional (Pap smear)
Liquid-based (Pap test)
Other

Specimen Adequacy
Satisfactory for evaluation
Unsatisfactory for evaluation (reason specified)

General Categorization (optional)
Negative for intraepithelial lesion or malignancy
Epithelial cell abnormality (see Table 29-4)
Other (see Interpretation/Results)

Interpretation/Results
Negative for intraepithelial lesion or malignancy
Epithelial cell abnormalities (see Table 29-4)
Non-neoplastic findings (optional)
   Cellular variations (atrophy, keratosis, metaplasia)
   Reactive cellular changes (inflammation, repair, radiation)
   Glandular cells status posthysterectomy
Organisms
   Trichomonas vaginalis
   Fungal organisms consistent with *Candida* spp.
   Shift in flora suggestive of bacterial vaginosis
   Cellular changes consistent with herpes simplex virus
   Cellular changes consistent with cytomegalovirus
   Bacteria consistent with *Actinomyces* spp.
   Other nonneoplastic findings (optional)
Other
   Endometrial cells in a woman ≥45 years of age
   Other malignant neoplasms (specified)

Adjunctive Testing

Computer-Assisted Interpretation

Educational Notes and Comments (optional)

TABLE 29-4. The 2014 Bethesda System: Epithelial Cell Abnormalities

Squamous cell
Atypical squamous cells (ASC):
   of undetermined significance (ASC-US)
   cannot exclude HSIL (ASC-H)
Low-grade squamous intraepithelial lesion (LSIL)
High-grade squamous intraepithelial lesion (HSIL)
Squamous cell carcinoma

Glandular cell
Atypical:
   Endocervical cells, endometrial cells, glandular cells (AGC)
Atypical, favor neoplastic:
   Endocervical, glandular (AGC)
Endocervical adenocarcinoma in situ (AIS)
Adenocarcinoma
Endocervical, endometrial, extrauterine, not otherwise specified

(American College of Obstetricians and Gynecologists, 2018b; Massad, 2013). Guidelines cannot prevent all cervical cancers. Moreover, recommendations cannot address all clinical situations and individualized management is essential. Updated, risk-based guidelines for the management of cytologic abnormalities and histologic CIN and AIS will be published in 2020 by the ASCCP. These will offer more customized management of individual patients depending on their past and current results (Castle, 2019; Demarco, 2017).

Specimen Adequacy

This is reported as *satisfactory* or *unsatisfactory* for evaluation and is based on slide cellularity and the presence of obscuring blood or inflammation. The presence or absence of TZ components, that is, endocervical cells and/or presence of squamous metaplastic cells, also is reported. A TZ component is not required for test adequacy. Although its presence is associated with increased detection of cytologic abnormalities, its absence is not associated with failure to diagnose CIN. Pap tests lacking TZ components are repeated in 3 years. For women aged ≥30 years, subsequent HPV testing is preferred and further testing is guided by results.

Unsatisfactory Pap testing samples are unreliable for the detection of cervical neoplasia and also for HPV by some tests. These samples are repeated in 2 to 4 months. If atrophy or a specific cervical or vaginal infection is present, treatment before repeat cytology may be helpful. If the sample is unsatisfactory again, colposcopy is recommended. Rarely, obscuring blood or inflammation on cervical cytology sample indicates invasive cancer. Therefore, unexplained vaginal discharge, abnormal bleeding, or abnormal physical findings should prompt immediate evaluation rather than waiting for repeat cytology or HPV results.

Epithelial Cell Abnormality Management

A cytology report interprets a screening test and does not provide a final diagnosis. Instead, a final diagnosis is determined subsequently by colposcopy and directed biopsies, as indicated. Pap tests are interpreted as either being negative for intraepithelial lesion or malignancy (NILM) or as demonstrating one or more epithelial cell abnormalities.

Atypical Squamous Cells of Undetermined Significance.
The most common cytologic abnormality is *atypical squamous cells of undetermined significance (ASC-US)*. It indicates cells suggesting but not fulfilling all the cytologic criteria for SIL. An ASC-US result often precedes the diagnosis of CIN 2 or 3, but this risk approximates only 5 to 10 percent. Cancer is found in only 1 to 2 cases per thousand (Solomon, 2002).

Management of ASC-US depends largely upon age, HPV status, and prior screening test results. If co-testing is not requested, reflex HPV testing is usually done. *Reflex HPV testing* refers to preordered HPV testing that is triggered only by specific cytology result and is not performed if cytology is negative. Approximately half of reported ASC-US cases will test positive for HPV. The combination of ASC-US cytology and positive HPV testing carries a risk profile similar to LSIL. Therefore, those with ASC-US cytology and positive HPV test results are referred for colposcopy. ASC-US cytology with negative HPV testing is followed up with a repeat co-test in 3 years. ASC-US without HPV testing calls for repeat cytology in 1 year and colposcopy if any abnormal result is obtained.

Low-Grade Squamous Intraepithelial Lesion.
LSIL encompasses the cytologic features of HPV infection and CIN 1 but carries a 10- to 15-percent risk of CIN 2 or worse. This risk is similar to the risk associated with ASC-US cytology with positive HPV test results. More than 80 percent of LSIL cases will test positive for HPV, and thus reflex HPV testing is usually not helpful. Colposcopy is generally indicated for LSIL cytology. Similar to ASC-US cytology, individualized management of LSIL is influenced by age, current HPV status if known, and past screening results.

Atypical Squamous Cells, Cannot Exclude HSIL.
Five to 10 percent of atypical squamous cell cases are designated as *atypical squamous cells, cannot exclude HSIL (ASC-H)*. This finding should not be confused with ASC-US. ASC-H describes cellular changes that do not fulfill criteria for HSIL cytology, but an underlying high-grade lesion cannot be excluded. Histologic HSIL is found in up to 25 percent of ASC-H cases, and this rate is higher than associated with ASC-US or LSIL. Thus, colposcopy is indicated regardless of age or HPV test result. Similar to LSIL, reflex HPV testing is not helpful due to a high rate of HPV positivity. If the SCJ is not fully visualized during colposcopy, a diagnostic excision procedure is recommended unless initial biopsies show invasive cancer.

High-Grade Squamous Intraepithelial Lesion.
HSIL encompasses cytologic features suggesting CIN 2 and CIN 3 (Fig. 29-8). It carries a high risk of underlying histologic HSIL (at least 70 percent) or invasive cancer (1 to 2 percent) (Kinney, 1998). Colposcopic evaluation is therefore warranted regardless of age or HPV status. Alternatively, immediate excision is acceptable in some nonpregnant patients depending on other factors such as age and concerns regarding future pregnancy.

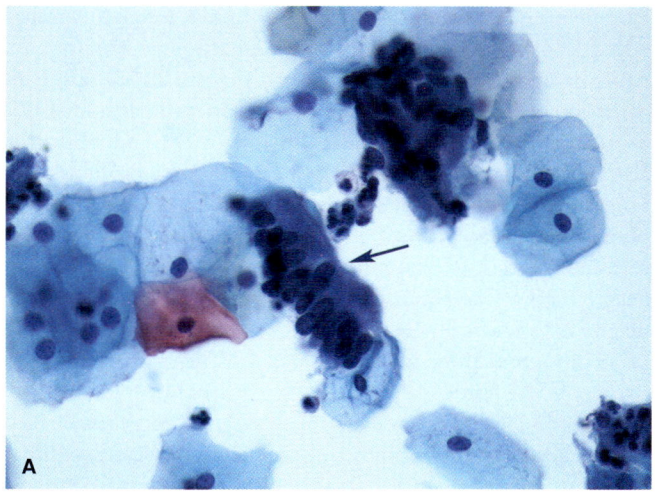

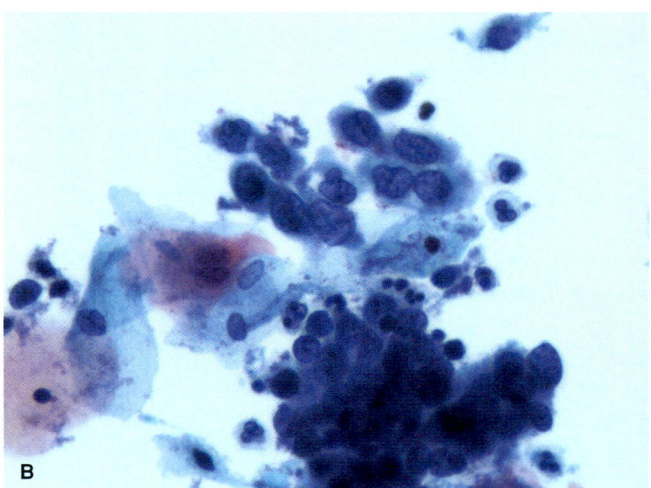

FIGURE 29-8 A. Normal Pap test findings. A fragment of benign columnar mucinous endocervical epithelium is seen (*arrow*). The endocervical cells are viewed from the side in this fragment, imparting a "picket fence" appearance. Normal squamous cells representative of the superficial epithelial layer (eosinophilic-staining cell) and intermediate cell layer (basophilic-staining cells) lie in the background. **B.** Pap smear showing a high-grade squamous intraepithelial lesion (HSIL). The dysplastic squamous cells have nuclear membrane irregularities and a high nucleus-to-cytoplasm ratio, reflecting cytologic immaturity. The greater ratio in some of these cells would classify this as severe cervical intraepithelial neoplasia (CIN 3). (Reproduced with permission from Dr. Kelley Carrick.)

This latter strategy is reasonable since colposcopy may miss small high-grade lesions, and most cases of HSIL cytology eventually result in excision for diagnosis or treatment. As with ASC-H, if the SCJ is not fully visualized during colposcopy, a diagnostic excision procedure is recommended unless initial biopsies show invasive cancer.

Glandular Cell Abnormalities.
This group includes atypical glandular cells (AGC), atypical endocervical cells, and atypical endometrial cells; atypical glandular or endocervical cells, favor neoplastic; and endocervical AIS. Similar to HSIL, this category carries a high risk of neoplasia. Adenocarcinoma cytology can be designated as endocervical, endometrial, or extrauterine.

Paradoxically, squamous neoplasia is more frequently diagnosed than glandular disease following cytology that reports AGC or atypical endocervical cells (Schnatz, 2006). The risk of endometrial and other reproductive tract cancers and risk of cancers at other sites such as breast, ovary, and colon are also elevated. In one large review of cytology results with AGC, at least CIN 2 or AIS was subsequently diagnosed in nearly 20 percent; cervical cancer, in 4 percent; and extracervical cancers, in 4 percent (Verdoodt, 2016). In this study, a concurrent negative HPV test result increased risk of extracervical disease diagnosis. Specifically, extracervical malignancy was diagnosed in 18 percent of those who were aged ≥50 years and had negative HPV test results.

Accordingly, initial evaluation of a cytologic glandular cell abnormality includes colposcopy and endocervical sampling, regardless of HPV status. It also includes endometrial sampling in patients aged ≥35 years or in younger women with risk factors for endometrial disease (Chap. 8, p. 183). If atypical endometrial cells are specified in the cytology report, initial endometrial and endocervical sampling are acceptable. These are followed by colposcopy, if initial sampling results are negative.

Reflex HPV testing is not recommended for the triage of glandular cytologic abnormalities for fear that a negative result will dissuade appropriate evaluation. However, HPV testing at time of evaluation (if not already obtained) helps distinguish cervical from endometrial disease (Castle, 2010; de Oliveira, 2006).

If initial evaluation of a glandular abnormality is negative, further management and surveillance should be guided by current clinical guidelines. Diagnostic excision is indicated for AGC, favor neoplasia or AIS cytology if initial evaluation does not reveal a cancer diagnosis.

Carcinoma. Cytology results suspicious for squamous cell carcinoma or adenocarcinoma are rare and carry the highest risk of invasive cancer. If initial evaluation fails to reveal invasive cancer, a diagnostic excision procedure is indicated.

■ Colposcopy

This outpatient procedure examines the LAGT, primarily the cervix. The colposcope provides a bright light source and variable magnification through an optical lens system or high-resolution digital imaging. Colposcopy requires special training, both didactic and clinical, that encompasses terminology, lesion identification and grading, and biopsy techniques. It is primarily indicated for the evaluation of abnormal cervical cancer screening tests, signs or symptoms of cervical cancer, and surveillance of treated or untreated CIN. Its primary goal is to identify invasive or preinvasive lesions for biopsy and subsequent management. However, sensitivity, interobserver agreement, and reproducibility of colposcopy are limited. Sensitivity estimates range between 50 and 80 percent (American College of Obstetricians and Gynecologists, 2018b; Ferris, 2005; Jeronimo, 2007). This highlights the need for further evaluation or surveillance testing when initial colposcopy fails to reveal high-grade neoplasia.

Prior to colposcopic examination, a woman's medical history is reviewed, and indications for colposcopy are confirmed

TABLE 29-5. Clinical Considerations Directing Colposcopy

Clinical objectives
Provide a magnified view of cervix, vagina
Identify cervical squamocolumnar junction
Detect lesions suspicious for neoplasia
Direct lesion biopsy

Clinical indications
Abnormal or recurrent inadequate cervical cancer screening result
Grossly visible cervical lesion
Unexplained lower genital tract bleeding
Unexplained vaginal discharge

Contraindications: none

Relative contraindications
Upper or lower reproductive tract infection
Uncontrolled, severe hypertension
Uncooperative or overly anxious patient

(Table 29-5). Urine pregnancy testing is performed if clinically indicated. Colposcopic examination is optimally timed to avoid menses but is not delayed if there is a visible cervical lesion or abnormal bleeding, or if the patient is unlikely to return. In cases of severe cervicitis or other pelvic infection, treatment may be indicated before performing biopsies or endocervical curettage. However, abnormal cervical discharge without an identified pathogen may be a cancer indicator. A Pap test performed at the time of colposcopy has questionable value, may obscure colposcopic findings, and should be performed on an individualized basis.

Examination

A bimanual examination precedes colposcopy to detect cervical enlargement or fixation suggesting malignancy, evidence of intrauterine pregnancy, or pelvic tenderness suggesting genital tract infection. Vaginal speculum selection and placement should provide optimal inspection of the cervix and upper vagina. Solutions used during colposcopy are normal saline, 3- to 5-percent acetic acid, and Lugol iodine. Because high-grade lesions are fragile, these solutions are applied by gently dabbing with a saturated swab or sponge or by spray-bottle misting. To begin, normal saline helps remove discharge and cervical mucus and allows initial assessment of vascular patterns and surface contours. A green (red-free) light filter adds contrast to aid vascular pattern visualization (Fig. 29-9).

Acetic acid 3- to 5-percent solution is mucolytic and exerts its whitening effects, termed *acetowhitening*, presumably by reversibly denaturing cellular proteins. This causes neoplastic areas to appear denser compared with the normal surrounding epithelium, and lesions assume varying hues of transient whiteness. Several minutes may be needed for this effect to fully develop.

Lugol iodine solution stains mature, glycogen-rich squamous epithelium a dark purple-brown color in reproductive-aged women with normal serum estrogen levels. Due to incomplete maturation, dysplastic epithelium has a lower glycogen content,

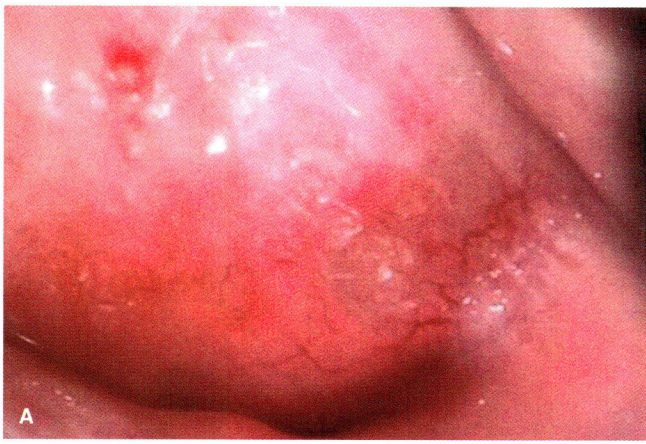

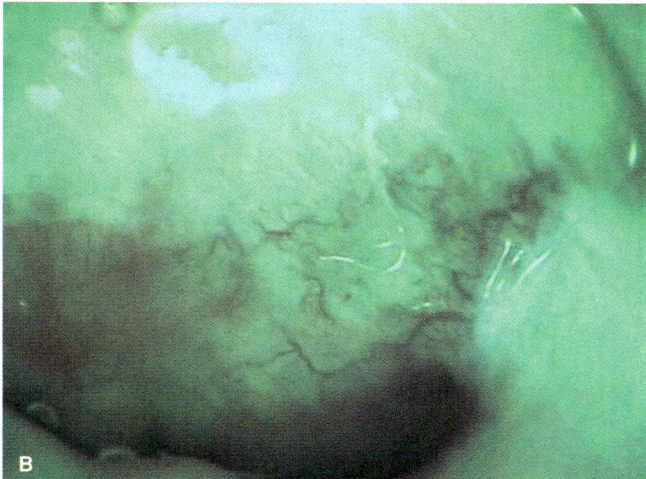

FIGURE 29-9 Evaluation of surface vessels. **A.** Benign surface vessels viewed through a colposcope using usual white light source. **B.** Use of a blue-green (red-free) light filter provides higher contrast and definition of vascular patterns.

fails to fully stain, and appears yellow (Fig. 29-10). Lugol iodine application is particularly useful when abnormal tissue is not identified using acetic acid. It is also used to define the limits of the active TZ, as cells of immature squamous metaplasia are glycogen-poor and do not stain as strongly as mature squamous epithelium. Lugol solution should not be used in patients allergic to iodine, radiographic contrast, or shellfish.

Key components of colposcopic examination include a general assessment and specific findings, described subsequently. Careful documentation of these aids neoplasia diagnosis, management, and communication between providers. Minimal and comprehensive criteria for documentation have been established by the ASCCP (Table 29-6) (Khan, 2017). Standardized colposcopic terminology used in the United States differs somewhat from that used internationally (Bornstein, 2012; Khan, 2017).

First, general assessment determines if the entire cervix and the SCJ are fully visualized. Nearly all cervical neoplasia lies within the TZ and adjacent to the SCJ. Within a dysplastic lesion, the most severe disease tends to be at its proximal (cephalad or upper) limit. Thus, complete colposcopic visualization of the cervix, SCJ, and upper limits of all lesions is essential to exclude invasive cancer and determine disease severity. When the SCJ or lesions extend into the endocervical canal, an endocervical speculum can aid in their complete visualization (Fig. 29-11).

Lesion Grading

With colposcopy, normal squamous epithelium of the cervix appears featureless, pale-pink, and smooth. Blood vessels lie below this layer and therefore are not visible or are seen as a fine capillary network. The mucin-secreting columnar epithelium appears red due to its thinness and close proximity of underlying blood vessels. Its villous appearance derives from epithelial peaks and crypts (see Fig. 29-3). Against this normal

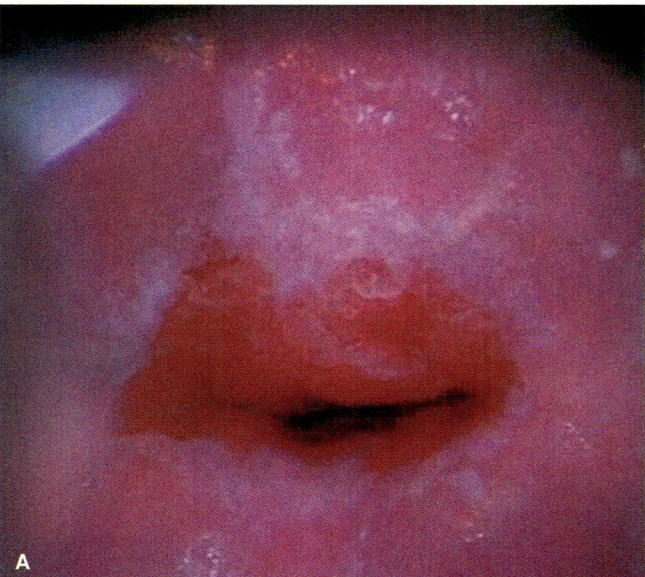

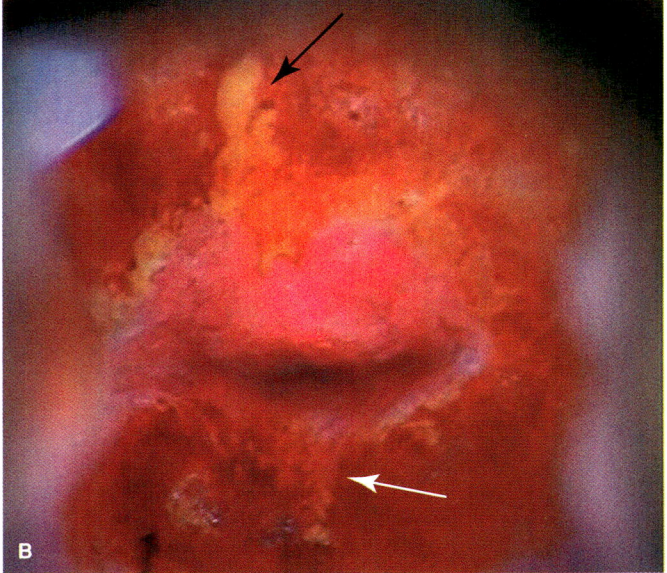

FIGURE 29-10 Solutions used for colposcopy. **A.** Cervix after application of acetic acid. Several areas of acetowhite change adjacent to the squamocolumnar junction (SCJ) are apparent. **B.** Same cervix after application of Lugol iodine solution. A nonstaining lesion at the 10 to 11 o'clock position is seen (*black arrow*), whereas an acetowhite area along the posterior SCJ (*white arrow*) shows partial iodine uptake.

TABLE 29-6. Documentation of the Colposcopic Examination

Minimum Criteria

SCJ fully visualized	yes/no
Acetowhitening	yes/no
Lesion(s) present (acetowhite or other)	yes/no
Colposcopic impression	normal/benign; low grade; high grade; cancer

Comprehensive Criteria

Cervix fully visualized	yes/no
SCJ fully visualized	yes/no
Acetowhitening	yes/no
Lesion(s) present (acetowhite or other)	yes/no
Lesion(s) fully visualized	yes/no
Location of lesions(s)	clock position, at SCJ?, satellite lesions
Size of lesion(s)	no. of quadrants, percentage of TZ area
Vascular changes	abnormal patterns (mosaic or punctuation), atypical vessels
Other features of lesion(s)	color, contour, borders, Lugol uptake
Colposcopic impression	normal/benign; low grade; high grade; cancer

SCJ = squamocolumnar junction; TZ = transformation zone.

colposcopic landscape, colposcopists discern abnormal tissue and biopsy the sites likely to represent the most severe neoplasia. A lesion's acetowhiteness, margins (borders), vascular patterns, size, and location relative to the SCJ help indicate the most abnormal epithelium (Table 29-7) (Khan, 2017).

After acetic acid application, the quality of whiteness obtained, the rapidity and duration of acetowhitening, and

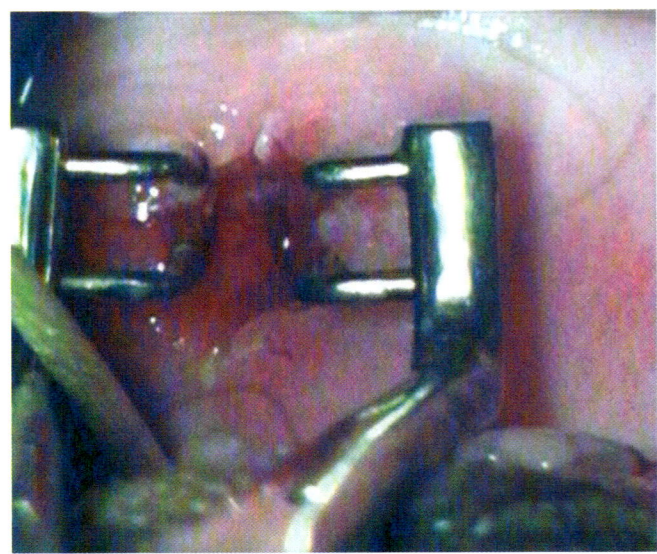

FIGURE 29-11 An endocervical speculum can aid viewing the endocervical canal.

sharpness of lesion borders are observed over several minutes. High-grade lesions demonstrate a more persistent, duller shade of white, whereas low-grade lesions are translucent or bright white, appear slowly, and fade quickly. Generally, low-grade lesions have feathery or irregular "geographic" margins, whereas high-grade lesions have straighter, sharper outlines (Figs. 29-12 and 29-13). Other lesion features that suggest high-grade dysplasia are: internal borders (inner-border sign), an opaque, rounded protuberance (ridge sign), and cuffed crypt openings. The last are round columnar crypts ringed with thick acetowhite epithelium. Satellite lesions, which are not adjacent to the SCJ on the ectocervix, tend to be low-grade. Larger, complex lesions at the SCJ tend to be higher grade.

Abnormal vascular patterns include punctation, mosaicism, and atypical vessels. Punctate and mosaic patterns are graded based on vessel caliber, intercapillary distance, and the overall uniformity of these. Fine punctation and mosaicism, with

TABLE 29-7. Colposcopic Lesion Grading

Colposcopic Feature	Low-Grade	High-Grade	Cancer
Margins/contour	Condylomatous Papillary Irregular Geographic Flat or raised	Sharp Flat contour Rolled Peeling Internal margin Ridge sign Fused columnar villi	Exophytic/gross tumor Irregular surface Necrosis/ulceration
Acetowhite change	Thin Translucent Rapid fading	Thick/dense Rapid appearance Slow fading Variegated red/white Cuffed crypts	May not be acetowhite
Vascular patterns	Fine patterns	Coarse patterns	Atypical vessels
Iodine staining	Positive/Partial	Negative	Negative

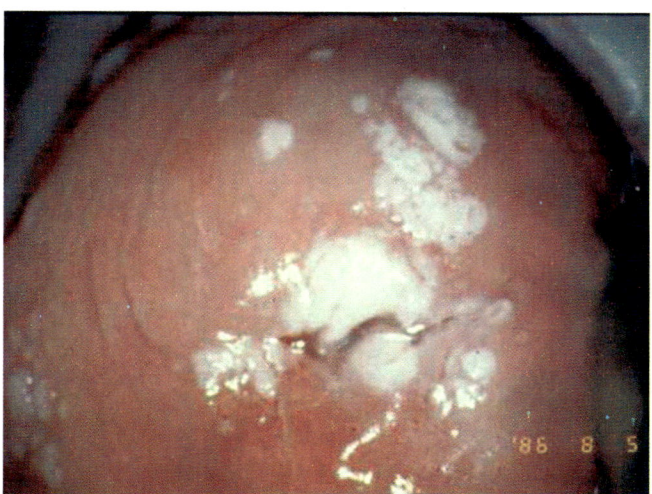

FIGURE 29-12 Low-grade squamous intraepithelial lesion (LSIL). Seen after 5-percent acetic acid application, LSIL is often multifocal and bright white with irregular borders.

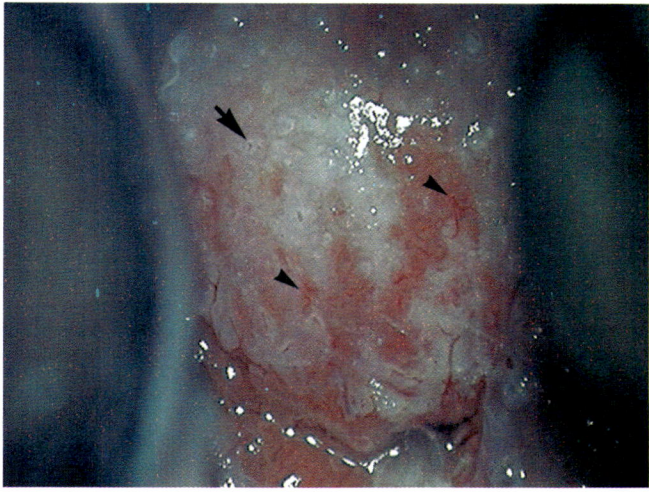

FIGURE 29-14 Colposcopy shows a large high-grade lesion with cuffed crypt openings (*arrow*) and atypical vessels (*arrowheads*) that are worrisome for invasive cancer.

narrow vessels and small, uniform intercapillary distances, typify low-grade lesions. A coarse pattern results from wide and variable vessel diameters and spacing and indicates high-grade abnormalities. Atypical vessels are irregular in caliber, shape, path, and arrangement and suggest invasive cancer (Fig. 29-14).

Importantly, malignancy often is not acetowhite due to its vascularity. Invasive cancer, especially adenocarcinoma, can create a false SCJ, and circumferential cancer mimics the redness of columnar epithelium. Thus, colposcopists should look beyond acetowhite areas to help identify invasive cancer. Moreover, areas of abnormal topography, including ulceration, should be biopsied.

■ Biopsy

Ectocervical Biopsy

All acetowhite lesions and other abnormalities are biopsied using cervical biopsy forceps under direct colposcopic visualization (Fig. 29-15). Generally, this does not require an anesthetic.

For hemostasis, pressure with or without a swab may suffice. Thickened Monsel solution (ferric subsulfate) or a silver nitrate applicator also may be applied as needed. Heavy bleeding is rare and can be controlled with direct pressure. Rarely, brief vaginal packing is needed.

Traditionally, biopsies targeted only the most severe-appearing lesion(s). However, colposcopic impression is often inaccurate and can underestimate the level of disease. Thus, limiting sampling to a single biopsy can miss a significant amount of CIN (Gage, 2006). Therefore, recommendations encourage biopsy of all acetowhite areas; two to four biopsies of abnormalities are recommended for optimal sensitivity (American College of Obstetricians and Gynecologists, 2018b; Wentzensen, 2017).

New evidence-based standards provide further biopsy guidance based on an individual's risk of high-grade CIN. Risk estimates are derived from referral screening test results and colposcopic impression (Wentzensen, 2017). For those at

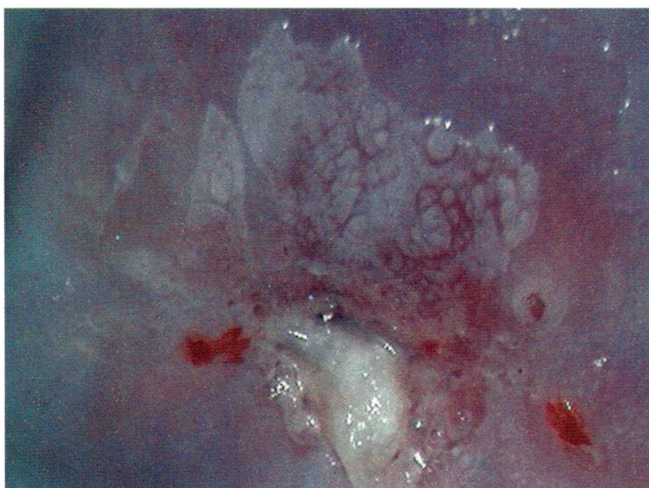

FIGURE 29-13 High-grade squamous intraepithelial lesion (HSIL). After 5-percent acetic acid application, HSIL demonstrates an off-white dull color and coarse vascular pattern.

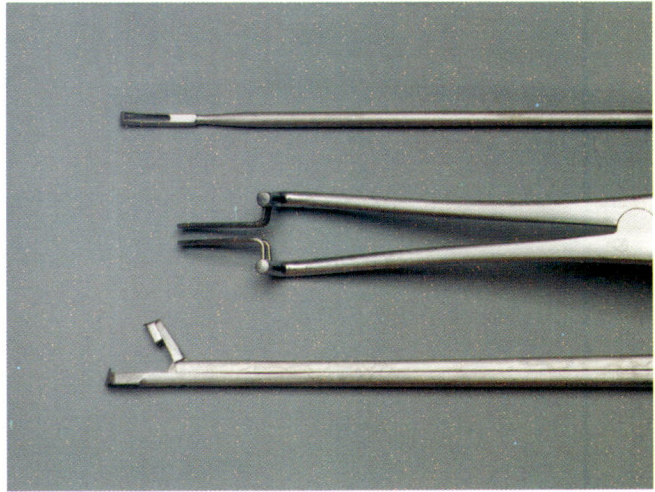

FIGURE 29-15 Tools used for cervical evaluation and biopsy. From top to bottom: endocervical curette, endocervical speculum, and cervical biopsy forceps.

lowest risk of high-grade neoplasia (cytology result less than HSIL, no positive HPV 16/18 results, normal colposcopy without acetowhitening), untargeted (random) biopsies are not recommended. At the other extreme, patients at highest risk are those with cytology reflecting HSIL or worse, positive HPV 16 or 18 testing results, and a colposcopic impression suggesting HSIL. In such patients who are aged ≥25 years and not pregnant, an immediate excision procedure or colposcopy with directed biopsies is acceptable.

Endocervical Sampling

For nonpregnant patients, endocervical sampling by curettage or brushing evaluates the endocervical canal epithelium lying beyond the colposcopist's view. Endocervical sampling is currently recommended during colposcopy for the following situations (American College of Obstetricians and Gynecologists, 2018b; Massad, 2013):

- The SCJ is not fully visualized.
- The SCJ is fully visualized, but no lesion is identified.
- Initial evaluation of ASC-H, HSIL, AGC, or AIS cytology test results.

These indications may change as evidence-based guidelines are updated.

Endocervical curettage is performed by introducing an endocervical curette 1 to 2 cm into the cervical canal (see Fig. 29-15). The length and circumference of the canal is firmly curetted, carefully avoiding sampling of the ectocervix or the lower uterine segment. Endocervical scrapings admixed with cervical mucus are then removed using a ring forceps or a cytobrush and included with the curettage specimen. Alternatively, vigorous brushing with a cytobrush may be used for endocervical sampling. Endocervical brushing is more sensitive than curettage, but grading of any dysplasia present is more difficult. It is also acceptable to perform curettage followed by a brushing to enhance sensitivity and grading of any abnormality present. Endocervical sampling is often the most uncomfortable part of a colposcopic evaluation, and cramping is common. Tissue from endocervical sampling is always sent separately from ectocervical biopsies for histologic evaluation.

■ Pregnancy

Pregnancy does not alter the natural history of cervical disease. Pregnancy is an opportunity to screen patients aged ≥21 years as indicated. Abnormal cytology is managed according to guidelines for the general population with only a few variations. When colposcopy is indicated, its primary goal during pregnancy is to exclude invasive cancer. Colposcopy and biopsy are safe and accurate during pregnancy (Economos, 1993). The number of biopsies is limited to areas of greatest concern. Endocervical and endometrial sampling are never performed during pregnancy to avoid amnionic membrane rupture, infection, or other harm to the pregnancy. CIN is reevaluated postpartum since lesion grade frequently changes after delivery and puerperal remodeling (Yost, 1999). Although cervical conization is infrequently performed during pregnancy, indications for this are discussed in Chapter 30 (p. 672).

CERVICAL INTRAEPITHELIAL NEOPLASIA MANAGEMENT

CIN management may be surveillance or treatment. Evidence-based guidelines for the management of women with biopsy-confirmed (histologic) CIN have been developed by the ASCCP and continue to evolve as new data is available (Massad, 2013). Current guidelines are found at www.asccp.org. During CIN management, the detection and prevention of invasive cervical cancer, a relatively rare outcome, must be balanced against the potential harms of excessive testing and overtreatment. Potential harms include procedure-related morbidity, psychologic stress, and possible adverse reproductive outcomes.

Special populations considered include younger and pregnant women. Despite differences in screening recommendations, immunocompromised women are no longer considered a special population for CIN management and typically are managed in accordance with general guidelines (Massad, 2013; Panel on Opportunistic Infections in HIV-Infected Adults and Adolescents, 2019). CIN severity, colposcopic findings, age, and reproductive plans play key roles in cervical disease management. Guidelines are complex and applied on an individualized basis. They cannot address all patient scenarios and cannot prevent all cases of cervical cancer.

■ CIN 1

Histologic LSIL (HPV changes or CIN 1) exhibits high rates of spontaneous regression. The LSIL diagnosis is poorly reproducible by cytology or histology and is thus unreliable. Therefore, patients should not be told they have HPV infection based upon LSIL cytology or biopsy alone. For these reasons, HPV change found by biopsy is not treated, and CIN 1 is no longer treated immediately. When diagnosed after a "lesser" cytologic abnormality such ASC-US, LSIL, or an NILM, HPV-positive screening, it can be observed indefinitely. Treatment is acceptable only if CIN 1 persists for more than 2 years. This is regardless of colposcopic examination adequacy or presence of CIN 1 in an endocervical sampling. Treatment of CIN 1 in younger women or those concerned about the possible effects of treatment on future pregnancy is discouraged. Current guidelines for surveillance without treatment and criteria that return a woman to routine screening should be followed and may involve periodic cytology or co-testing.

If deemed appropriate, persistent CIN 1 can be treated by ablation. Criteria require that the SCJ and all lesions are fully seen during colposcopy and that the endocervical sampling lacks HSIL (CIN 2/3) or ungraded CIN. If these criteria are not met and treatment is indicated, excision is recommended and ablation is unacceptable.

CIN 1 diagnosed after an ASC-H or HSIL Pap test result carries a higher risk of undiagnosed high-grade CIN. Depending on patient age and colposcopic findings, either a diagnostic excision or surveillance with colposcopy, cytology, HPV testing, or a combination of these at prescribed intervals will be recommended by current guidelines. Persistent, unexplained HSIL or AGC cytology generally warrants an excision procedure, if only CIN 1 is found with colposcopic biopsy.

HSIL: CIN 2 and CIN 3

Generally, treatment is recommended for CIN 2 or CIN 3 because of the significant malignant potential of HSIL and the efficacy of treatment to eradicate precancers. Treatment modalities include either ablation or excision of the entire TZ. Excision is greatly favored over ablation in the United States. Treatment is tailored to the individual patient, lesion, and anatomic characteristics.

An unequivocal histologic diagnosis of CIN 3 is always treated and not observed in nonpregnant patients regardless of age or reproductive history. With a CIN 3 biopsy, if HSIL or ungraded CIN is found in the endocervical sampling or if colposcopy did not fully visualize the SCJ and the upper limits of all lesions, a diagnostic excision is indicated to exclude occult invasive cervical cancer. Recurrent or persist HSIL after treatment is managed with repeat excision, not ablation. Hysterectomy as primary therapy is unacceptable. Hysterectomy may be indicated if repeat excision is needed but not anatomically feasible or if high-grade CIN recurs or persists and invasive cancer has been thoroughly excluded.

For young women, particularly of low parity, with CIN 2 or HSIL (CIN 2/3, not otherwise specified) surveillance or treatment is acceptable, if the SCJ and all lesions are fully seen during colposcopy. In this context, "young women" refers to individuals for whom the possible risk to future pregnancies from treatment outweighs the risk of progression to malignancy, although both are difficult to quantify. No upper age limit is specified for surveillance. Surveillance of specified CIN 2 is preferred in younger women, because this histologic diagnosis is less reliable and spontaneous regression of lesions over time is common. Even in younger women or those concerned with future reproduction, treatment is indicated if colposcopy does not fully visualize the SCJ and lesions present, biopsy shows CIN 3, or if CIN 2 or CIN 2/3 is persistent. Current guidelines for surveillance testing, intervals for reassessment, and acceptable upper time limits for persistence should be consulted.

Adenocarcinoma in Situ

Cervical AIS, although uncommon, is rising in incidence (Herzog, 2007). Exclusion of coexistent invasive cancer and removal of all affected tissue are primary goals. High-grade squamous lesions often accompany glandular neoplasia. However, management differs somewhat from that of HSIL, because cervical AIS and adenocarcinoma are not as easily identified colposcopically as squamous lesions. Moreover, AIS can be multifocal, lie deep within endocervical crypts, and extend high into the endocervical canal (Massad, 2013). Thus, diagnostic excision is recommended to exclude invasive cancer with maximum certainty. The choice of excision modality should favor obtaining an intact specimen with the most interpretable margins. Thus, cold-knife conization is favored over loop electrosurgical excision procedure (LEEP). If the excised specimen shows no invasive cancer, hysterectomy is recommended in women who have completed childbearing.

Women with AIS who strongly desire fertility preservation may be managed conservatively after an excision procedure. Individuals are counseled regarding the significant ongoing risk

even with negative excision margins. The risk of residual AIS is reported to be as high as 80 percent in patients with positive margins (Krivak, 2001). Accordingly, if timely hysterectomy is not planned, repeat excision is advisable for managing positive margins. Close, long-term surveillance is recommended until hysterectomy is performed (Massad, 2013).

Postcolposcopy Surveillance without Treatment

When colposcopy following abnormal screening tests fails to diagnose a high-grade precancer or there is spontaneous regression of high-grade CIN in younger women, further surveillance is indicated. Guidelines recognize the significant false-negative rate of colposcopy and the increased risk of developing CIN in the future. Surveillance involves repeat cytology, HPV testing, or colposcopy alone or in combination at specific intervals depending on the original abnormal cytology result, patient age, and current guidelines. Exceptions are AGC, favor neoplasia and AIS Pap test results. These are always followed by excision unless invasive cancer is diagnosed during initial colposcopic examination and biopsy.

CERVICAL INTRAEPITHELIAL NEOPLASIA TREATMENT

Current treatment of CIN is limited to ablation or excision procedures targeting the entire TZ. Thus, individual cervical lesions are not treated. Any treatment ideally should reach a depth of 5 to 7 mm from the surface to treat CIN adequately. Excessive depth is avoided to minimize potential complications. Treatments with topical agents or therapeutic vaccines remain investigational. Selection of treatment modality is individualized based on several factors including patient age, parity, size and severity of lesions, cervix contour and anatomy, prior CIN treatment, and coexisting medical conditions. Treatment selection also depends on provider experience and available equipment. Surgical treatments have an approximate 90-percent success rate (Martin-Hirsch, 2013). A review of clinical considerations is provided by Khan and Smith-McCune (2014).

Ablation

This involves physical destruction of tissue and is generally effective for noninvasive ectocervical disease. Before ablation, glandular neoplasia or invasive cancer are excluded with the greatest possible certainty. To this end, cytology, histology, and colposcopic impression should be concordant. Further, the entire SCJ and proximal (upper) limits of all lesions should be visualized during colposcopy and endocervical sampling should be negative for high-grade or ungraded CIN. Ablation should not be used after previous therapy, after glandular cytologic abnormalities, or for AIS.

The most commonly used ablative treatment modalities are cryosurgery and carbon dioxide (CO_2) laser. Both techniques are illustrated in Section 43-28 (p. 1004). Before the introduction of LEEP, when cold-knife conization was the only excisional option, these ablative techniques were commonly used.

However, the relative decreased morbidity and ease of performing LEEP compared with cold-knife conization has led to a decline in ablative procedures. The trend toward surveillance of CIN 1 and some CIN 2 and HSIL (CIN 2/3 lesions) in young women also is contributory.

Cryosurgery is an ablative method that delivers nitrous oxide to a metal probe that freezes tissue on contact. Cryonecrosis is achieved by crystallizing intracellular water. This treatment is most appropriate for entirely ectocervical lesions and SCJ, a smooth cervical surface without deep crevices, circumferential cervical length adequate to avoid thermal damage to the vaginal walls, and CIN limited to two quadrants of the cervix. Cryosurgery is not favored for the treatment of CIN 3 due to higher rates of disease persistence following treatment and lack of a histologic specimen to exclude undiagnosed invasive cancer (Martin-Hirsch, 2013). Moreover, cryosurgery and other ablative techniques are not favored for women with HIV infection and CIN due to higher failure rates (Spitzer, 1999).

CO_2 laser is another ablative option and is delivered using colposcopic guidance. Cervical tissue is vaporized to a depth of 5 to 7 mm. Laser ablation is appropriate for CIN if lesions and TZ are fully seen during colposcopy. It is well suited for large, irregularly shaped CIN lesions of all grades and for condylomatous and preinvasive lesions at other LAGT sites. If a cervical lesion extends onto the vagina, laser ablation may allow customized removal of the entire lesion. Laser ablation can be augmented by excision of central tissue for cases in which an ectocervical lesion extends into the endocervical canal or when the SCJ is not fully visualized (American College of Obstetricians and Gynecologists, 2018b).

■ Excision

Excision procedures are favored when the risk of invasive cancer is significant. Examples are antecedent high-grade cytologic abnormalities including ASC-H, HSIL, AGC, and AIS; cases in which the SCJ or lesions are not fully visualized during colposcopy; CIN 3 or AIS histology; or endocervical sampling that indicates ungraded or high-grade CIN or glandular neoplasia. An advantage of excision compared with ablation is provision of a histologic specimen to confirm the absence of invasive cancer and to evaluate involvement of the excised margins. With glandular cytologic abnormalities or AIS biopsy, an excision technique that provides an intact specimen with the most interpretable margins should be chosen, usually cold-knife conization (Massad, 2013). Excision is also indicated for persistence or recurrence of high-grade CIN after treatment (Paraskevaidis, 1991). *Diagnostic excision* refers to situations in which invasive cancer has not been excluded by standard colposcopic criteria. A *therapeutic excision* is performed for treatment of CIN that is fully diagnosed and criteria to exclude invasive cancer have previously been met by colposcopy and biopsy.

Excisional modalities include LEEP, also known as LLETZ (large loop excision of the transformation zone); cold-knife conization (CKC); and laser conization. These are illustrated in Section 43-27 of the atlas (p. 999). The superiority of one excision technique compared with others has not been demonstrated conclusively for any particular indication. Excisional procedures

---

TABLE 29-8. Loop Electrosurgical Excision Procedure: Clinical Characteristics

Advantages
Favorable safety profile
Ease of procedure
Outpatient procedure using local anesthesia
Low-cost equipment
Tissue specimen for histopathology evaluation

Disadvantages
Thermal damage may obscure specimen margin status
Special training required
Risk of postprocedure bleeding
Theoretical risk of vapor plume inhalation

---

have operative and long-term risks that include bleeding, cervical stenosis, and adverse pregnancy outcomes. CKC is associated with cervical incompetence and preterm birth. The relationship between preterm birth and LEEP remains uncertain. Although some studies show LEEP to be an independent risk factor for preterm birth and premature rupture of membranes, others do not. An important confounder is the greater risk of preterm birth in women with cervical neoplasia, even if they have not undergone treatment, compared with the general population. This indicates that CIN and preterm birth have overlapping risk factors, making the contribution of treatment to this already increased risk difficult to ascertain and controversial (Gatta, 2017).

LEEP involves a thin wire loop through which an electrical current passes. This can simultaneously cut and coagulate tissue, ideally during direct colposcopic visualization. As advantages, LEEP can be performed with local anesthesia, often in an office setting, and with low complication rates. Additionally, the size and shape of tissue excision can be tailored by varying loop size and the order in which loops are used. This helps conserve cervical stroma volume (Table 29-8).

Cold-knife conization uses sharp excision to remove the cervical TZ and precancerous tissue. It is performed under general or regional anesthesia. CKC may be preferred to LEEP for patients at highest risk for invasive cancer. Examples are those with cytology suggesting invasive cancer, patients older than 45 with CIN 3 or CIS, large high-grade lesions, and glandular cytologic abnormalities or AIS (Table 29-9).

CO_2 laser conization is only rarely used currently. It allows precise tailoring of the cone shape to minimize excision volume and yields less blood loss than CKC. Disadvantages are its high equipment expense, some thermal compromise of specimen margins, and special training requirements. This procedure can be performed under local, regional, or general anesthesia.

■ Surveillance after Treatment or Regression

Post-treatment surveillance with cytology, HPV testing, and/or colposcopy is required to confirm treatment success (American College of Obstetricians and Gynecologists, 2018b; Massad, 2013). After excision, surveillance will be influenced by margin status. After treatment for high-grade cervical dysplasia or invasive cancer, screening continues for at least 20 years, even if

TABLE 29-9. Cold-Knife Conization Clinical Characteristics

Advantages
Anesthetized patient
Tissue specimen without margin compromise
Enhanced patient support if hemorrhage is encountered
Variety of instruments to individualize conization

Disadvantages
Potential for hemorrhage
Lengthier procedure
Postoperative discomfort
General or regional anesthesia required
Operating room setting
High cost
Larger volume of cervical stroma removed
Increased risk of adverse reproductive outcomes

screening extends beyond age 65. This stems from a persistently higher risk of cervical neoplasia. Current guidelines should be consulted to guide long-term screening of patients based on their particular histories.

If an excision margin or endocervical curettage performed immediately after an excision is positive for HSIL (CIN 2 or CIN 3), repeat excision may be indicated. Repeat excision is indicated for special circumstances such as AIS or microinvasive carcinoma at the excision margins.

Hysterectomy

Hysterectomy is unacceptable as primary therapy for CIN (American College of Obstetricians and Gynecologists, 2018b; Massad, 2013). However, it may be considered when treating recurrent high-grade cervical disease if childbearing has been completed or if a repeat cervical excision is strongly indicated but not technically feasible. Although hysterectomy provides the lowest CIN recurrence rate, invasive cancer must always be excluded beforehand. The chosen route of hysterectomy is directed by other clinical factors. Hysterectomy is the preferred treatment of AIS, if future fertility is not desired and excision has excluded invasive cancer.

Even with negative cervical margins, hysterectomy performed for CIN 2 or worse is not completely protective. Patients, particularly those who are immunosuppressed, are at risk for recurrent disease and require postoperative periodic cytologic screening of the vaginal cuff (p. 631). This should be accompanied by palpation and visual inspection of the cuff for nodularity or lesions.

VAGINAL INTRAEPITHELIAL NEOPLASIA

Pathophysiology

Primary vaginal carcinoma is rare and makes up <5 percent of all gynecologic malignancies (Siegel, 2019). In the United States, 5350 new cases of vaginal cancer will be diagnosed in 2019 (American Cancer Society, 2019b). Nearly 50 percent of cases are diagnosed in women aged ≥70 years (Kosary, 2007). Approximately 90 percent of vaginal cancers are squamous cell carcinomas. These appear to develop slowly from precancerous epithelial changes, called *vaginal intraepithelial neoplasia (VaIN)*, in a fashion similar to cervical cancer from CIN. Due to its rarity, VaIN and its natural history, treatment efficacy, and risk of recurrence or progression are not well understood.

VaIN demonstrates histopathology similar to CIN. It is rarely found as a primary lesion and most often develops as an extension of CIN, mainly in the upper third of the vagina (Diakomanolis, 2002; Hoffman, 1992a). Unlike the cervix, the vagina lacks a TZ that is susceptible to HPV-induced neoplasia. However, HPV may gain entry from vaginal mucosal abrasions and reparative metaplastic squamous cell activity (Woodruff, 1981). In one review, HPV DNA was found in up to 98 percent of VaIN lesions and in three quarters of vaginal cancers. HPV 16 is the most common type (Alemany, 2014). Thus, HPV vaccination against oncogenic HPV types 16 and 18 has the potential to also prevent vaginal cancers (Smith, 2009).

Cervical and vulvar neoplasia raise the risk for VaIN and vaginal squamous cell cancer, especially in women aged >60 years (Strander, 2014). Moreover, one retrospective study suggests that hysterectomy for CIN is not definitive therapy for high-grade neoplasia, because the subsequent high-grade VaIN recurrence rate exceeded 7 percent (Schockaert, 2008).

Diagnosis

Generally, VaIN is asymptomatic and abnormal cytology results are often the first indication. If present, symptoms may include spotting, discharge, and odor. Subsequent examination of the vagina with a colposcope, termed *vaginoscopy*, frequently identifies a lesion for biopsy. Prior to visual evaluation, careful palpation of the vagina is advised, particularly if the patient has undergone hysterectomy for high-grade cervical neoplasia. In such cases, invasive cancer may present as a nodular lesion buried within the vaginal cuff before it becomes visible.

During vaginoscopy, inspecting the vagina using a colposcope can be challenging because of a large surface area, rugation, and surfaces that lie parallel to the colposcope's visual axis. Particular attention is paid to the upper third of the vagina due to the common etiology of VaIN as an extension of CIN. By applying 3- to 5-percent acetic acid to the vaginal mucosa, acetowhite changes consistent with HPV infection or neoplasia can be identified (**Fig. 29-16**). Vascular patterns are less common in VaIN lesions than with CIN, but coarse punctation and even atypical vessels may be seen in high-grade and invasive lesions. High-grade VaIN lesions tend to demonstrate flat, dense acetowhitening with sharply demarcated borders. Half-strength Lugol solution applied to the vagina further delineates abnormal areas. Areas with the least staining and straightest lesion margins are most suspicious.

Local anesthesia is usually not necessary for biopsy of the vagina's upper third but may be needed for more distal sites. Biopsy may be obtained by means of a cervical biopsy forceps (see Fig. 29-15), and an Emmett hook can be used to elevate and stabilize vaginal tissue if needed. The vaginal tissue is grasped and lifted to limit the biopsy depth. Menopausal

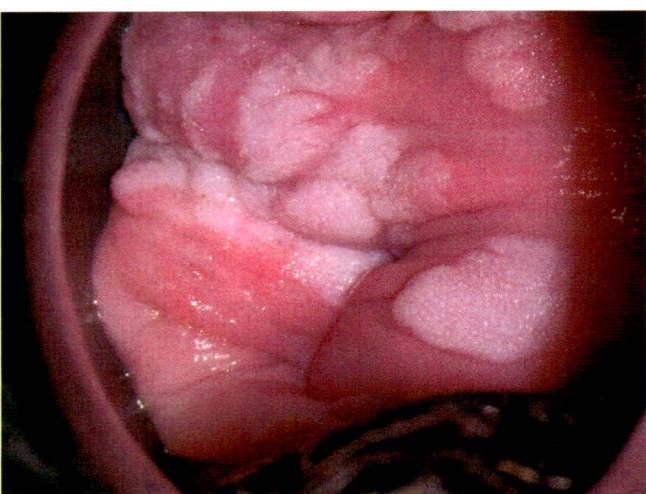

FIGURE 29-16 Vaginoscopy showing multifocal acetowhite human papillomavirus (HPV) lesions after application of 5-percent acetic acid.

women may have significant thinning of the vaginal mucosa. Thus, biopsies, possibly with a smaller biopsy forceps, are shallow to avoid vaginal wall perforation. Hemostasis is achieved using silver nitrate applicators or Monsel paste. Vaginal lesion size, location, and specific biopsy sites are carefully documented for future management and surveillance.

■ Management

Similar to high-grade CIN, high-grade VaIN is believed to be a precancerous lesion and generally warrants eradication (Punnonen, 1989; Rome, 2000). Because vaginal neoplasia is uncommon, most management strategies are derived from small, retrospective, and statistically underpowered studies. Management of VaIN is influenced by histologic diagnosis; neoplasia grade; and lesion size, number, and location. Options are observation, excision, ablation, topical antineoplastics, or, rarely, radiation therapy. Each treatment method has advantages and disadvantages and none has proven superior efficacy. Thus, comprehensive patient counseling and shared decision-making are essential.

Low-Grade VaIN

Lesions interpreted as vaginal LSIL often represent atrophy or transient HPV infection. Spontaneous regression is common. Thus, observation is preferable in most cases, and aggressive treatment is avoided. For example, in one long-term study of 132 patients with biopsy-proven VaIN, an observational approach resulted in VaIN 1 regression in seven of eight patients (88 percent) (Rome, 2000). No VaIN 1 lesion progressed to high-grade VaIN or invasive cancer. Without evidence-based guidelines, surveillance similar to that for low-grade CIN seems reasonable. Thus, cytology with or without vaginoscopy is completed every 6 to 12 months until abnormalities resolve or progress to HSIL.

High-Grade VaIN

Hodeib and colleagues (2016) reported no clear risk factors and no specific primary treatment as significantly more predictive or effective in preventing recurrence after following the clinical course of 42 patients with biopsy-proven VaIN 2/3. Observation

of VaIN 2 may be considered in selected patients, although the safety of this approach is not established. The treatment choice for patients with high-grade VaIN is influenced by the location and number of lesions, the patient's sexual activity status, vaginal length, prior radiation therapy, previous treatment modalities in patients with recurrent VaIN, and clinician experience. Potential adverse treatment effects such as pain, difficulties with sexual intercourse, and scarring are always considered.

Wide local excision of a high-grade unifocal lesion or partial vaginectomy for multifocal lesions may be selected. Hoffman (1992a) found that 9 of 32 patients (28 percent) with prior hysterectomy and VaIN 3 had occult invasive cancer in the vaginal cuff. Therefore, surgical excision is considered for high-grade lesions involving the vaginal cuff, particularly if any thickening or nodularity of the vaginal apex suggests occult invasive disease. Excisional procedures have the advantage of providing a surgical specimen for which resected-margin status can be determined and the presence of invasive vaginal cancer excluded. Partial vaginectomy is surgically challenging but has the highest cure rate and fewest recurrences for high-grade disease (Dodge, 2001).

Wide local excision carries less morbidity than vaginectomy, but both procedures may be complicated by bladder or rectal injury and hemorrhage. In addition, subsequent vaginal scarring and stenosis may compromise vaginal intercourse or cause dyspareunia. Sharp dissection is favored for wide local excision and partial vaginectomy. Laser causes significant thermal damage to the tissue specimen and generally is not recommended for excision of vaginal mucosa. Loop excision has poor depth control, carries a substantial risk of thermal damage to underlying pelvic structure, and is not recommended for vaginal surgery.

CO_2 *laser ablation* is an option for lesions not concerning for invasive disease. It is well suited to eradicate multifocal lesions and causes less scarring and blood loss than tissue excision. Rarely, hemorrhage and thermal damage to the bladder and bowel can occur. In one small case study of 21 patients undergoing CO_2 laser ablation for high-grade VaIN, 14 percent had persistent disease requiring retreatment. One patient progressed to invasive carcinoma, which underscores the importance of long-term surveillance (Perrotta, 2013). A broader explanation of laser ablation techniques is found in Section 43-28 of the atlas (p. 1005).

Topical therapy, as with ablative procedures, is suitable if invasive disease is not suspected based on findings from cytology, vaginoscopy, or histology. Persistent VaIN 2 and selected VaIN 3 lesions may be medically treated using 5-percent fluorouracil (5-FU) cream "off-label," as it is not FDA approved for this specific indication (Krebs, 1989). Although 5-FU's efficacy is unproven in large, randomized trials, Fiascone and colleagues (2017) found a 74-percent success rate and no recurrences in 47 patients with high-grade VaIN.

Treatment regimens vary widely. One dosing schedule calls for a 3-mL dose of cream placed into the vaginal vault by plastic vaginal applicator every other day during the first week of treatment and once weekly thereafter for up to 10 weeks. 5-FU cream is often associated with a robust inflammatory reaction that can include vaginal burning and vulvar irritation. To minimize leakage onto the vulva, cream is best applied intravaginally at bedtime, when a recumbent position will be maintained for hours. Additionally, an occlusive, water-resistant ointment can be spread on the vulva for protection. Protective gloves are worn when handling 5-FU cream, and measures are taken to avoid 5-FU contact by sexual partners.

Patients selected for this treatment require thorough counseling, effective contraception as needed, and consent for off-label medication use. Close monitoring observes for excessive inflammation and ulceration, which can lead to vaginal or vulvar scarring and loss of function.

Radiation therapy has a very limited role for high-grade VaIN treatment. It carries a significant risk of serious morbidity and is reserved for select cases. In a review of 136 cases of vaginal carcinoma in situ, radiation therapy was used in 27 patients, and a 100-percent cure rate was noted. However, 63 percent developed significant complications that included vaginal stenosis, adhesions, ulceration, necrosis, and fistula formation (Benedet, 1984). Furthermore, radiation treatment compromises subsequent cytologic, colposcopic, and histologic interpretation. Disease recurrence often necessitates radical surgery.

Prognosis

In a study of 132 patients treated for high-grade VaIN, excision and CO_2 laser ablation had equal cure rates of 69 percent. Topical 5-FU cream was curative in 46 percent of cases (Rome,

2000). For treatment of recurrent high-grade VaIN, a lower disease recurrence rate was associated with CO_2 laser ablation compared with medical treatment (Bogani, 2019). Patients with any grade of vaginal neoplasia require long-term monitoring, because the persistence and recurrence rate for high-grade disease is significant. Currently, no evidence-based guidelines are available for posttreatment surveillance of VaIN. Monitoring includes collection of vaginal cytology and performance of vaginoscopy approximately 2 to 4 months after treatment is completed. Continued surveillance with periodic cytology with or without vaginoscopy at 6- to 12-month intervals for several years thereafter seems prudent. Long-term cytologic screening is needed thereafter.

VULVAR INTRAEPITHELIAL NEOPLASIA

Pathophysiology

Vulvar cancer is rare, and in 2019, it is predicted to make up approximately 6 percent of all gynecologic cancers and <0.7 percent of all cancers in U.S. women (American Cancer Society, 2019c). Of vulvar cancers, 90 percent are squamous cell and in some cases may develop slowly from VIN (Fig. 29-17) (Judson, 2006).

HPV DNA has been found in up to 80 percent of VIN lesions. (Del Pino, 2013). However, vulvar cancer is not

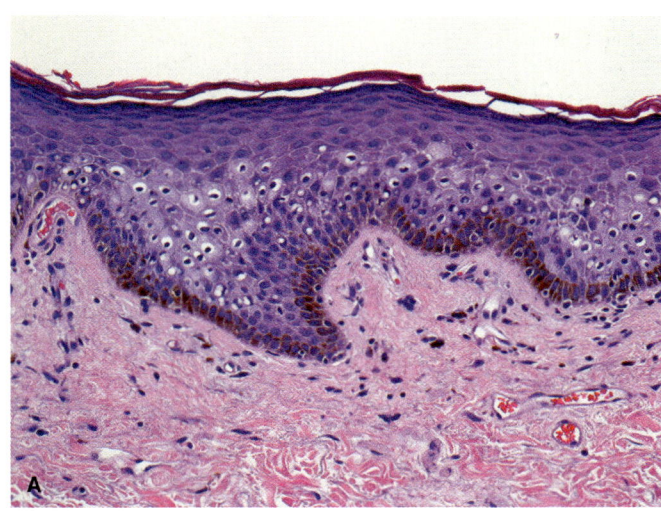

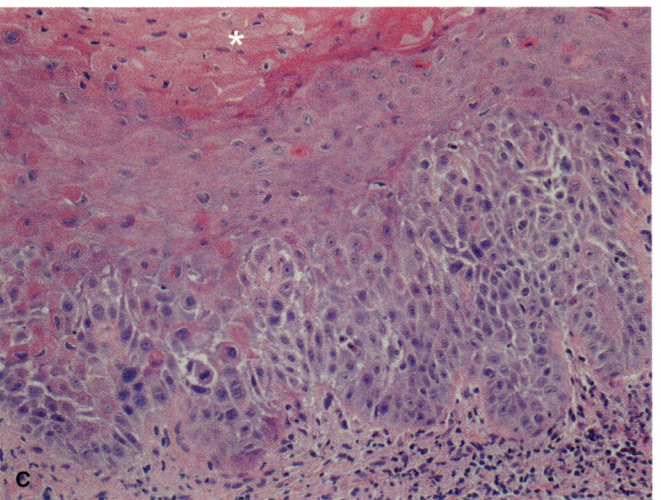

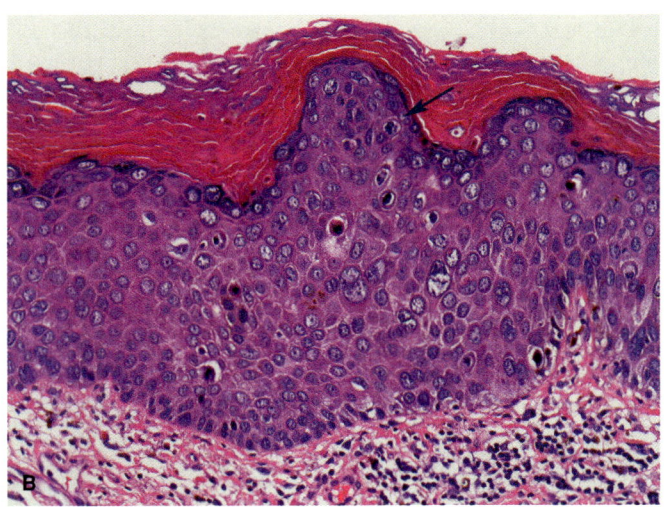

FIGURE 29-17 A. Normal vulvar histology. The keratinizing, stratified squamous epithelium is characterized by cells that have increasing cytoplasm as they mature from base to surface. Nuclei appear orderly and are devoid of atypical features. Mitoses are usually confined to the parabasal layer. **B.** Vulvar high-grade squamous intraepithelial lesion (HSIL). Cells in all epithelial layers are disordered and have nuclear pleomorphism, chromatin abnormalities, and a variably greater nucleus-to-cytoplasm ratio. An increased mitotic rate and a mitosis high in the epithelium are seen (*arrow*). This particular example has a papillomatous surface, a common finding in these lesions. **C.** Differentiated-type vulvar intraepithelial neoplasia (VIN). In this classic example, the squamous epithelium appears relatively mature but has notable cytologic atypia (nuclear pleomorphism, prominent nucleoli) involving the basal and suprabasal cell layers. Abnormal keratinocyte differentiation is evidenced by dyskeratosis and individual cell keratinization. Prominent hyperkeratosis (*asterisk*), a typical finding in differentiated-type VIN, is present at the epithelial surface. (Reproduced with permission from Dr. Kelley Carrick.)

exclusively a result of HPV infection, and rates of association range from 15 to 80 percent (Del Pino, 2013). The vulva, unlike the cervix, has no TZ, and the effect of HPV infection on the vulva's keratinized epithelium is not biologically comparable to that on the cervix or anus.

Compared with CIN, VIN less often progresses to high-grade disease and cancer. However, one study identifying trends in the incidence of vulvar carcinoma in situ found a fourfold rise from 1973 to 2000. This trend is particularly pronounced in younger women and is thought to be linked to the increased incidence of STDs, including HPV (Howe, 2001). Jones and coworkers (2005) report that the mean age of women with VIN has declined from 50 to 39 years since 1980.

Although spontaneous regression has been reported, high-grade VIN is a premalignant condition and should be treated (American College of Obstetricians and Gynecologists, 2019). In one New Zealand study, 10 of 63 patients receiving no treatment for high-grade VIN developed vulvar cancer (Jones, 2005).

■ Classification

Terminology for squamous VIN was adopted as a general category of intraepithelial squamous neoplasia by the International Society for the Study of Vulvar Disease (ISSVD) in 1986 (Wilkinson, 1986). Under this traditional classification, VIN grades 1, 2, and 3 were defined by abnormal cellular changes found to varying thicknesses within the squamous epithelium, similar to CIN. The term *differentiated-type VIN 3* was also introduced to include histologic cases exhibiting cells with prominent eosinophilic cytoplasm and keratin changes in the involved epithelium (Wilkinson, 1986).

In 2015, to recognize the 2012 Lower Anogenital Squamous Terminology (LAST) developed by the ASCCP and College of American Pathologists, the ISSVD further revised VIN terminology by incorporating a modified form of the World Health Organization classification of tumors on the vulva (Bornstein, 2016; Crum, 2014; Darragh, 2012). The rationale for the 2015 ISSVD terminology change was to provide consistent nomenclature of HPV-associated squamous lesions of the lower genital tract.

Current ISSVD terminology adopted by the American College of Obstetricians and Gynecologists (2019) is summarized in Table 29-10. VIN now has three categories of squamous intraepithelial lesions (SIL): vulvar low-grade SIL (vulvar LSIL, flat condyloma, or HPV effect); vulvar high-grade SIL (vulvar HSIL, VIN usual type); and differentiated VIN. Vulvar HSIL lesions are commonly associated with oncogenic HPV infection, particularly HPV 16 (Smith, 2009). In general, HPV-related high-grade VIN lesions histologically resemble high-grade CIN and tend to be multifocal (Feng, 2005; Haefner, 1995).

The entire lower genital tract is vulnerable to HPV infection. Risk factors for vulvar HSIL are similar to those for VaIN and CIN. Accordingly, vulvar HSIL is associated with HPV risk factors (p. 624) (Hoffman, 1992b; Jones, 2005). Tobacco smoking is strongly linked with vulvar HSIL, and cessation is encouraged (American College of Obstetricians and Gynecologists, 2019).

In contrast, differentiated VIN is less common and accounts for only 2 to 10 percent of all VIN cases (Hart, 2001). Such

TABLE 29-10. Vulvar Squamous Intraepithelial Lesion: Terminology and Characteristics

VIN Type	Clinical Presentation and Risk Factors
Vulvar LSIL	Formerly VIN 1 HPV effect Flat lesions with basal atypia and koilocytic changes such as condyloma Self-limited lesions, not precancerous
Vulvar HSIL	Formerly VIN usual type (VIN 2, VIN 3, vulvar CIS) Younger women Multicentric and multifocal disease Oncogenic HPV infection common Cigarette smoking, other STDs, immunosuppression
Differentiated VIN	Unproven but likely precursor to most vulva squamous cell carcinoma Older, postmenopausal women Unicentric and unifocal disease Oncogenic HPV infection uncommon Associated with vulvar dermatologic conditions such as lichen sclerosus

CIS = carcinoma in situ; HPV = human papillomavirus; HSIL = high-grade squamous intraepithelial lesion; LSIL = low-grade squamous intraepithelial lesion; STD = sexually transmitted disease; VIN = vulvar intraepithelial neoplasia.

lesions tend to be unifocal and are typically found in older, nonsmoking, postmenopausal women in their sixth and seventh decade. Infection with oncogenic HPV is uncommon and probably does not play a role in the genesis of these lesions. Instead, they tend to arise in a background of inflammatory dermatosis, particularly lichen sclerosus. Approximately 60 percent of vulvar squamous cell carcinoma presents independently of HPV infection, and the unproven but likely precursor may be differentiated VIN (Bigby, 2016). One study noted that progression of differentiated VIN to vulvar squamous cell carcinoma was five times higher than for vulvar HSIL (van de Nieuwenhof, 2009). Vulvar cancers arising in a background of differentiated VIN also have higher recurrence rates (Eva, 2008). The pathologic diagnosis of differentiated VIN is difficult, and interobserver agreement is low. If clinical findings warrant, review by an experienced gynecologic pathologist may be helpful (van den Einden, 2013).

Other rare intraepithelial vulvar neoplasms include melanoma and Paget disease. These remain unclassified and may require specialty consultation.

■ Diagnosis

Clinical Findings

VIN may be asymptomatic and discovered with routine gynecologic examinations or during evaluation of abnormal cervical or vaginal cytology results. No screening strategies are available for vulvar HSIL detection. When present, signs and symptoms

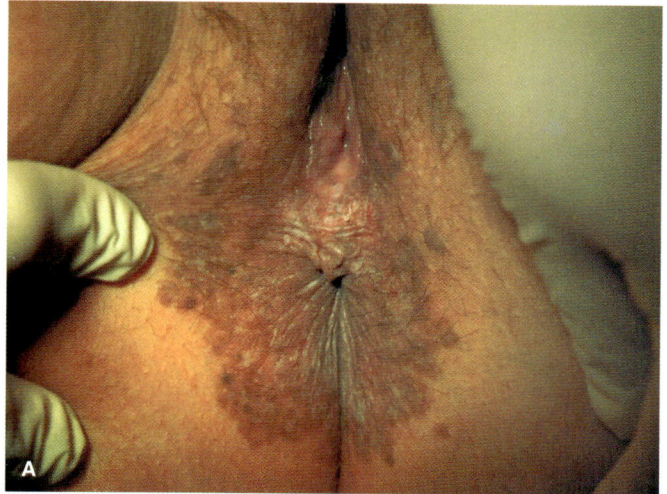
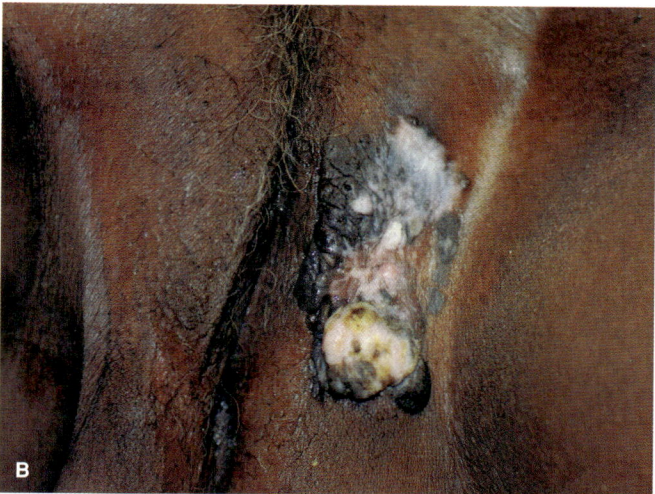

FIGURE 29-18 **A.** Extensive perineal and perianal extension of vulvar high-grade intraepithelial lesion (HSIL). **B.** Bulky lesion of differentiated vulvar intraepithelial neoplasia (VIN).

include itching, burning, and pain. Whereas high-grade lesions of the cervix and vagina are generally invisible without acetic acid application and use of a colposcope, clinically significant vulvar HSIL lesions are often visible without the aid of special techniques. Lesions vary widely in appearance but are usually sharply demarcated. They may be white, hyperkeratotic plaques; hyperpigmented lesions; or erythematous areas. Lesions may be raised or flat. Often, lesions appear bulky, resemble condylomata, and are multifocal with extensive involvement of the perineum (Fig. 29-18). Differentiated VIN is generally unifocal and may be associated with inflammatory dermatosis such as lichen sclerosis or lichen simplex chronicus of the adjacent skin. A lesion may appear as an ulcer, warty papule, or hyperkeratotic plaque.

To avoid diagnostic delay, most suspicious focal vulvar lesions are biopsied. Ulceration, surrounding induration, or inguinal adenopathy raises suspicion for invasive cancer. Other scenarios suspicious for VIN include enlarging lesions, warty lesions in postmenopausal or immune compromised women, and warts that appear atypical or persist despite topical therapies (American College of Obstetricians and Gynecologists, 2019).

Vulvoscopy

Histologic confirmation is necessary before vulvar HSIL or differentiated VIN are managed. Selection of the best location to biopsy is aided by magnification of the vulva, perineum, and perianal skin, usually with a colposcope. This examination is termed *vulvoscopy*. Alternatively, any good light source and a handheld magnifying lens can be used.

Vulvar epithelial changes are enhanced by applying a 3- to 5-percent acetic-acid-soaked gauze pad to the vulva for 5 minutes prior to vulvoscopy. Because vulvar epithelium is keratinized, application of acetic acid to achieve a useful visible effect requires longer time to develop. This is usually well tolerated but may cause pain or burning if comorbid vulvar irritation, ulceration, or fissures are present. Acetic acid accentuates surface topography and may reveal acetowhite lesions not seen grossly. Pigmented VIN lesions tend to turn a dusky gray due to hyperkeratosis, and vascular patterns are generally

not seen. Normal vulvar tissue, particularly the inner, posterior labia minora, may turn diffusely acetowhite and should not be treated based on this appearance.

As an alternative, 1-percent toluidine blue, a nuclear stain, may help define lesions (Joura, 1998). However, because its use is technically more challenging and results are fraught with both false-positive and false-negative findings, this has been largely abandoned.

The most abnormal-appearing areas are biopsied, although necrotic areas often yield nondiagnostic findings and are avoided if possible. Biopsies measuring up to 6 mm in diameter can be obtained using a Keyes punch after provision of a local anesthetic injection (Fig. 4-2, p. 94). Biopsy sites measuring 4 mm or greater occasionally require suturing for hemostasis or cosmetic closure, especially on mucosal surfaces that stretch. Topical anesthetics can be applied several minutes prior to injection of local anesthesia to decrease discomfort. If lesions are close to the clitoral hood, general anesthesia is often warranted due to greater pain with injection of local anesthesia and increased tissue vascularity. Careful documentation, mapping of vulvar biopsy sites, and photographs can aid future management.

■ Management
Vulvar LSIL

Formerly termed VIN 1, vulvar LSIL encompasses flat condyloma and changes found from HPV effect. Vulvar LSIL is self-limited and not precancerous and is not treated unless symptomatic, such as with a gross condylomatous lesion (Bornstein, 2016).

Vulvar HSIL

Vulvar HSIL is a premalignant condition that can progress to vulvar cancer. Thus, all vulvar HSIL is treated, and standard options are local destruction or excision (American College of Obstetricians and Gynecologists, 2019). If occult invasion or cancer is not suspected, vulvar HSIL can be treated with laser ablation or with off-label use of topical imiquimod. Mucosal lesions (internal to the Hart line) tend to be more superficial, whereas VIN involving hair-bearing areas of the vulva (external to the Hart line) may extend deeper into pilosebaceous units (Wright, 1992). VIN involves the pilosebaceous units in up to two thirds of cases, but it rarely exceeds 2.5 mm in depth from the epidermal surface (Shatz, 1989). This distance affects disease management, particularly if ablative procedures are considered. Regardless of the modality selected, treatment side effects are common and can include vulvar discomfort, poor wound healing, infection, and scarring that may result in chronic pain or dyspareunia. Thus, treatment objectives include: (1) excluding and preventing invasive disease, (2) preserving vulvar appearance and function, and (3) improving patient symptoms.

As allowed without damaging surrounding structures such as the clitoris or anus, *wide local excision (WLE)* with a gross surgical margin of 0.5 to 1 cm of normal tissue is preferred for large vulvar HSIL lesions, in which the possibility of invasive carcinoma cannot be excluded. Because disease recurrence is related to surgical margin status, intraoperative frozen-section histologic analysis of the specimen margins is advantageous (Friedrich, 1980; Jones, 2005). Hopkins and colleagues (2001) reported disease recurrence rates of 20 percent for cases with negative surgical margins but 40 percent for those with positive margins. Primary closure of a WLE should ideally be tension-free and may require referral to a specialist for plastic surgical techniques or skin grafting to minimize anatomic distortion, pain, and loss of function. Moreover, due to disease location, some patients are best treated by combined excisional and ablative procedures.

Laser ablation of vulvar HSIL provides good cosmetic results, but the depth of tissue destruction must be adjusted for hair-bearing areas. Laser treatment of vulvar HSIL requires full epithelial thickness cellular destruction. As CO_2 laser ablation does not allow evaluation of a surgical specimen, invasive carcinoma must be excluded by adequate biopsy beforehand. Laser is generally less disfiguring than WLE but can result in prolonged, painful healing. Preoperative counseling regarding anticipated postoperative results mirrors that for WLE. A Cochrane Review comparing surgical interventions for the treatment of vulvar HSIL concludes that surgical excision or laser vaporization is generally equally effective (Lawrie, 2016). Further, both interventions have an overall 50-percent chance of vulvar HSIL recurrence.

Cavitational ultrasonic surgical aspiration (CUSA) may be used to treat vulvar HSIL confined solely to non-hair-bearing vulvar skin. Ultrasound is used to cause cavitation and disruption of affected tissue, which is then aspirated and collected (Section 43-29, p. 1007). CUSA offers the advantages of laser, less scarring and pain than WLE, while additionally providing a pathologic specimen (von Gruenigen, 2007). However, the tissue specimen is fragmented and lacks the diagnostic accuracy of surgically excised tissue. One study evaluated CUSA in 37 patients with high-grade VIN and found an overall recurrence rate of 35 percent within a mean of 33 months (Miller, 2002).

Topical therapy can be considered if there is no concern for invasive cancer, the patient is able to self-administer the topical medication correctly, and the importance of compliance to follow-up visits is understood. No topical agent is FDA approved specifically for vulvar HSIL treatment, and use is considered off-label. Cidofovir is a cytosine analog with antiviral activity against a broad range of DNA viruses. Cidofovir cream must be specially compounded. Topical 5-FU is potentially caustic and teratogenic and is not a first-line choice for VIN treatment (National Cancer Institute, 2019b). The clinical efficacy of cidofovir and 5-FU creams has not been consistently demonstrated in clinical trials (American College of Obstetricians and Gynecologists, 2019). Topical imiquimod 5-percent has been found to be more effective than placebo in treating select vulvar HSIL lesions and has garnered the most interest for medical management (Lawrie, 2016). It has lower toxicity, and numerous case reports and two randomized trials report favorable regression rates of high-grade VIN (Mahto, 2010; van Seters, 2008). One Phase II study using imiquimod to treat high-grade VIN found a 77-percent response rate and 20-percent recurrence rate compared with a recurrence rate of 53 percent in a surgically treated cohort (Le, 2007). Currently, no studies establish the superiority of surgical or medical treatment of high-grade VIN.

■ Prognosis and Prevention

Case reports exist describing the invasive potential of untreated, high-grade VIN (Jones, 2005). Jones and associates (1994) reviewed the outcome of 113 patients with high-grade VIN. They found that 87 percent of untreated patients progressed to vulvar cancer, whereas only 3.8 percent of treated patients progressed to invasive carcinoma. Regardless of the treatment modality chosen, recurrence rates up to 50 percent are common, particularly in patients with multifocal disease or immune compromise (Lawrie, 2016). Indefinite surveillance for multifocal LAGT disease is recommended. Moreover, some consider high-grade VIN to be an indication for colposcopic evaluation of the cervix and vagina regardless of normal cervical or vaginal cytology. Although unproven, posttreatment surveillance consists of vulvar self-examination and careful office vulvar reevaluation at 6 and 12 months and annual vulvar inspection thereafter (American College of Obstetricians and Gynecologists, 2019).

For prevention, HPV vaccination lowers the risk for both vulvar LSIL and vulvar HSIL (American College of Obstetricians and Gynecologists, 2017). Smoking cessation and improving compromised immune status are others. As differentiated VIN may be found with vulvar dermatoses, treating these conditions may reduce cancer risk (Lee, 2015).

ANAL INTRAEPITHELIAL NEOPLASIA

■ Pathophysiology

In 2019, 5530 new anal cancers and 760 anal cancer deaths are predicted for U.S. women. Moreover, this relatively rare cancer's incidence and associated mortality rates have risen since 1975 (American Cancer Society, 2019a). Anal cancer is strongly associated with anal intraepithelial neoplasia (AIN) (Abbas, 2010; Palefsky, 1994). As with cervical cancer, hrHPV infection is strongly associated with and appears to be the causative agent of most anal cancer, although anal cancers are rare in healthy women with only transient HPV infection (Lamme, 2014; Mosckicki, 2015; Sehnal, 2014). The causal relationship between HPV infection and anal cancer is supported by the finding that HPV is found in 88 percent of anal cancers (Wang, 2017). As with cervical cancers, HPV types 16 and 18 are the principal etiologic agents (Zbar, 2002). Concurrent HPV infection and related disease of the cervix and anal canal are common. In one analysis, cervical and anal HPV infections were highly correlated regardless of HIV status (Lin, 2019). Santoso and associates (2010) reported a 12-percent prevalence of biopsy-proven AIN in a group of women with HPV-related disease.

Anal HPV infection and its progressive potential in women are suspected to behave similarly to cervicovaginal lesions. Cervical and anal HPV lesions generally manifest at or near their highly susceptible squamocolumnar epithelial junctions. In the anal canal, this junction is called the *transition zone* (Goldstone, 2001). Anal disease is classified by the same cytologic and histologic nomenclature used to describe cervical disease. As adopted by the American College of Obstetricians and Gynecologists (2018b), the 2012 Lower Anogenital Squamous Terminology (LAST) Project nomenclature recommendation for squamous neoplasia throughout the anogenital tract replaces AIN 1 with the term *anal LSIL*, and AIN 2/3 with *anal HSIL* (Fig. 29-19) (Darragh, 2012).

Risk factors for AIN include persistent anal HPV infection, prior abnormal cervical cytology results, receptive anal intercourse, tobacco smoking, and prior other STDs, particularly HIV. Anal cancer and its likely precursor, anal HSIL, are increasing at higher rates in populations with HIV infection compared with those without HIV (Heard, 2015; Tandon, 2010). However, in one study of 251 women with HIV infection and 68 without, those without HIV infection had an 8-percent rate of any type of AIN and a 2-percent rate of anal HSIL (Holly, 2001).

AIN progression to anal HSIL and cancer and its spontaneous regression are poorly understood. Many ongoing trials support the model of AIN progression to cancer. One 42-month surveillance study of 72 patients with AIN found that 11 percent of anal HSIL cases progressed to anal cancer (Watson, 2006).

Diagnosis

No data establish with certainty that the identification and treatment of AIN reduces anal cancer risk in the healthy woman. Currently, neither the American College of Obstetricians and Gynecologists nor the U.S. Preventive Services Task Force provides screening recommendations for AIN in women. Moscicki and associates (2015) summarized available literature on anal cancer, anal HSIL, and HPV infection in women. They proposed screening with digital anorectal examination for women at highest risk. Candidates are those with HIV infection, other immune compromising conditions, other HPV-related LAGT disease, or anal cancer symptoms (pain and bleeding). Other potential approaches for screening highest-risk women might include periodic testing with anal cytology, HPV testing, or anoscopy or with a combination of these. Some suggest that annual cervical and anal cytology should be offered to all women with HIV infection, but only if the infrastructure necessary to evaluate and manage abnormal cytology results and precancerous lesions is available (Palefsky, 2005; Panther, 2005). For the generalist, patients may be referred to tertiary care centers or colorectal surgeons.

Anal cytology as a screening test has uncertain efficacy for AIN and anal cancer (Nahas, 2009; Santoso, 2010). If used, anal cytology may be more sensitive using liquid-based preparations than conventional glass slides (Friedlander, 2004; Sherman, 1995). Sampling is obtained by inserting a Dacron swab or endocervical brush moistened with water or a small amount of water-based lubricant approximately 4 cm into the anal canal, presumably above the anal transition zone. The device is then withdrawn with a twirling motion while applying lateral pressure against the anal canal walls. The swab is then either swirled in the cytology solution to release exfoliated cells or smeared on a glass slide and fixed with isopropyl alcohol as with cervical cytology. Nothing per rectum is recommended 24 hours prior to an anal cytology test. Anal cytology may be reported using terminology and definitions of the Bethesda System for cervical cytology.

High-resolution anoscopy (HRA)-guided biopsy to identify histologic AIN uses illumination and magnification provided by a colposcope. HRA lacks general availability, is more challenging to perform than colposcopy for both patient and the provider, and requires special training. Acetic acid is applied to evaluate the anal canal in a manner similar to colposcopy (Fig. 29-20) (Jay, 1997). Anal neoplasia demonstrates colposcopic features similar to those of CIN, and analogous lesion grading and terminology are used. Biopsies are directed at the most abnormal areas. Some consider HRA to be the preferred tool for diagnosing AIN, but its role for primary screening or

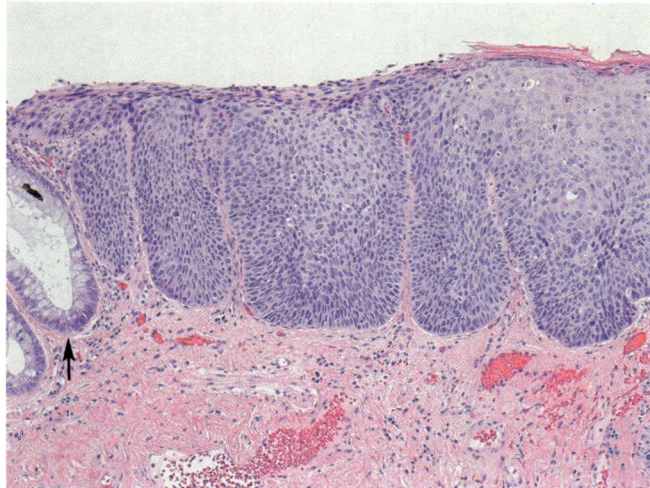

FIGURE 29-19 Anal intraepithelial neoplasia (AIN). In this example of AIN 3, the squamous epithelium has architectural disorder, nuclear pleomorphism, and markedly increased nucleus-to-cytoplasm ratios, with very little squamous maturation evident from base to surface. Mitoses are increased in number and located high in the epithelium. This biopsy was derived from the anorectal junctional area, and thus normal mucinous columnar epithelium lining rectal crypts is seen focally (*arrow*). (Reproduced with permission from Dr. Kelley Carrick.)

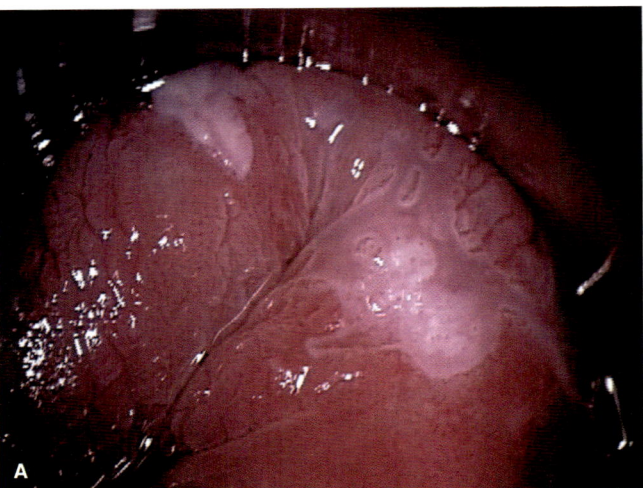

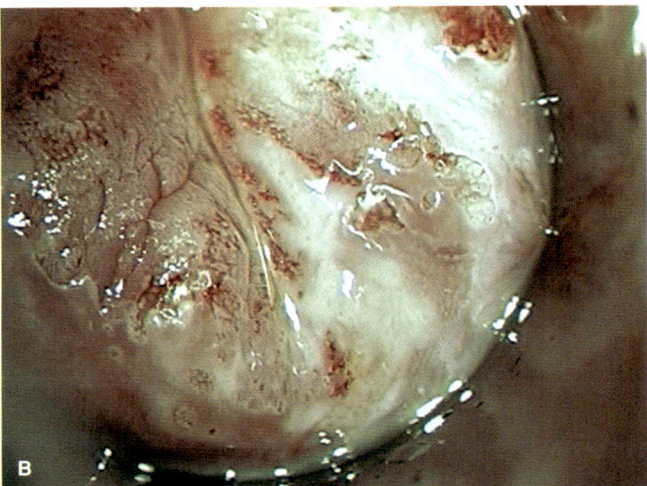

FIGURE 29-20 A. Translucent acetowhite lesion of low-grade anal intraepithelial neoplasia (AIN). **B.** Dense acetowhite lesion of high-grade AIN. (Reproduced with permission from Naomi Jay, RN NP PhD.)

for the evaluation of abnormal anal cytology results and anal cancer symptoms is not yet defined. It is presently available in a limited number of health centers.

■ Management

Some suggest that screening for and eliminating high-grade anal lesions may decrease the invasive anal cancer incidence (Santoso, 2010). However, in contrast to cervical neoplasia, the protective effect of treating anal cancer precursor lesions remains unproven. Thus, until more data are available, decisions regarding screening for and managing AIN should be shared by the provider and patient on an individual basis. Abnormal anal cytology results are best evaluated with high-resolution anoscopy. High-grade AIN lesions are referred to appropriate specialists for possible excision or ablative procedures.

Treatment is restricted to locally ablative or excisional procedures and topical therapies that eliminate individual high-grade intraepithelial lesions. Unlike the cervix, the entire anal squamocolumnar junction cannot be destroyed or removed due

to potential associated morbidity. Biopsy-proven high-grade AIN lesions have been ablated using CO_2 laser, cryoablation, electrosurgical coagulation performed under general anesthesia, or infrared coagulation as an office procedure (Chang, 2002; Goldstone, 2005). Topically applied therapies that use imiquimod, 5-FU, or trichloroacetic acid are other unproven alternatives. Last, as prevention, the FDA (2010) has approved both the quadrivalent and nonavalent HPV vaccines for the prevention of anal cancer and precancerous lesions associated with select oncogenic HPV types in both males and females.

WOMEN WITH HIV INFECTION

These individuals have a high burden of HPV-associated LAGT disease. Up to 60 percent of Pap test results are abnormal, and up to 40 percent of cases have colposcopic evidence of dysplasia. Compared with rates in uninfected women, women with HIV infection show higher rates of both CIN and VIN (Ellerbrock, 2000; Spitzer, 1999; Wright, 1994). Moreover, abnormal cervical cytology and/or cervical HPV results raise risks for anal HPV infection and anal neoplasia (Heard, 2015; Tandon, 2010). The risks of all HPV-associated cancers of the vulva, vagina, and anus appear to rise during the period from 5 years before to 5 years after HIV seroconversion (Chaturvedi, 2009).

HIV infection influences LAGT disease prognosis. For example, during the early years of the AIDS epidemic, Maiman and colleagues (1990) observed a 100-percent mortality rate in women with HIV infection and cervical cancer compared with only a 37-percent rate in women affected by this cancer but not HIV. As a result, cervical cancer was designated as an AIDS-defining condition. Fortunately, women with HIV infection who receive regular screening and recommended follow-up for CIN experience the same incidence of invasive cervical cancer as do women without HIV (Massad, 2009).

Because of a significantly higher risk of developing SIL, cervical cancer screening guidelines for women with HIV differ from those of average risk women as described earlier (p. 631) (Panel on Opportunistic Infections in HIV-Infected Adults and Adolescents, 2019). In addition, women with HIV may benefit from anal Pap screening (Palefsky, 2001). However, evidence-based screening recommendations for AIN and anal cancer are not yet available. Women with HIV infection are routinely questioned about anorectal symptoms such as pain or bleeding and are provided periodic digital rectal examinations.

The 2012 Consensus Guidelines recommend that Pap test abnormalities, including ASC-US, in women with HIV infection be managed as in the general population (Massad, 2013). However, the Centers for Disease Control and Prevention has questioned the utility of HPV testing for the triage of ASC-US in women with HIV and thus recommends that all women with ASC-US results be referred for colposcopy (Kaplan, 2009). Because women with HIV infection and CIN are often found to have extensive, multifocal dysplastic epithelial disease, any colposcopic examination includes inspection of the entire LAGT (Hillemanns, 1996; Tandon, 2010).

Women with HIV infection are at higher risk of disease persistence, recurrence, and progression after CIN or VIN treatment, and poorer outcomes correlate with degree of immune suppression. Cryotherapy for CIN has a particularly high failure rate among treatment methods (Korn, 1996; Spitzer, 1999). Additionally, ablative modalities have a greater risk of obscuring occult invasive cancer in high-grade lesions. Cervical excisional procedures that include LEEP and CKC provide histologic confirmation and margins for evaluation. Although excisional therapy is effective for eradicating CIN in immune competent patients, the same treatment may be effective only in preventing progression to cancer in women with HIV (Heard, 2005).

The therapeutic benefits of antiretroviral therapy (ART) on HPV infection are poorly understood, and results are conflicting (Heard, 2004). To date, ART does not consistently improve the natural history of HPV-related disease. In fact, anal cancer rates in individuals with HIV infection have continued to rise over the past decade (De Vuyst, 2008; Tandon, 2010). Indeed, if ART does not alter the incidence or progression of HPV-related disease, individuals on ART may gain sufficient longevity to develop HPV-related epithelial cancers (de Sanjose, 2002).

REFERENCES

Abbas A, Yang G, Fakih M: Management of anal cancer in 2010. Part 1: overview, screening, and diagnosis. Oncology (Williston Park) 24(5):417, 2010

Alemany L, Saunier M, Tinoco L, et al: Large contribution of human papillomavirus in vaginal neoplastic lesions: a worldwide study in 597 samples. Eur J Cancer 50(16):2846, 2014

American Cancer Society: Key statistics for anal cancer. 2019a. Available at: https://www.cancer.org/cancer/anal-cancer/about/what-is-key-statistics.html. Accessed September 7, 2019

American Cancer Society: Key statistics for vaginal cancer. 2019b. Available at: https://www.cancer.org/cancer/vaginal-cancer/about/key-statistics.html. Accessed September 7, 2019

American Cancer Society: Key statistics for vulvar cancer. 2019c. Available at: https://www.cancer.org/cancer/vulvar-cancer/about/key-statistics.html. Accessed September 7, 2019

American College of Obstetricians and Gynecologists: Human papillomavirus vaccination. Committee Opinion No. 704, June, 2017

American College of Obstetricians and Gynecologists: Cervical cancer screening and prevention. Practice Bulletin No. 168, October 2016, Reaffirmed 2018a

American College of Obstetricians and Gynecologists: Management of abnormal cervical cancer screening results and cervical cancer precursors. Practice Bulletin No. 140, December, 2013. Reaffirmed 2018b

American College of Obstetricians and Gynecologists: Management of vulvar intraepithelial neoplasia. Committee Opinion No. 675, October 2016, Reaffirmed 2019

Barnes A, Betts AC, Borton EK, et al: Cervical cancer screening among HIV-infected women in an urban, United States safety-net healthcare system. AIDS 32(13):1861, 2018

Baseman JG, Koutsky LA: The epidemiology of human papillomavirus infections. J Clin Virol 32(Suppl 1):S16, 2005

Benard VB, Coughlin SS, Thompson T, et al: Cervical cancer incidence in the United States by area of residence, 1998–2001. Obstet Gynecol 110:681, 2007

Benedet JL, Sanders BH: Carcinoma in situ of the vagina. Am J Obstet Gynecol 148(5):695, 1984

Bergeron C, Ferenczy A, Richart RM, et al: Micropapillomatosis labialis appears unrelated to human papillomavirus. Obstet Gynecol 76(2):281, 1990

Bigby SM, Eva LJ, Fong KL, et al: The natural history of vulvar intraepithelial neoplasia, differentiated type: evidence for progression and diagnostic challenges. Int J Gynecol Pathol 35(6):574, 2016

Bogani G, Ditto A, Ferla S, et al: Treatment modalities for recurrent high-grade vaginal intraepithelial neoplasia. J Gynecol Oncol 30(2):e20, 2019

Bornstein J, Bentley J, Bösze P, et al: 2011 colposcopic terminology of the International Federation for Cervical Pathology and Colposcopy. Obstet Gynecol 120(3):166, 2012

Bornstein J, Bogliatto F, Haefner HK, et al: The 2015 International Society for the Study of Vulvovaginal Disease (ISSVD) terminology of vulvar squamous intraepithelial lesions. Obstet Gynecol 127(2):264, 2016

Bosch FX, Burchell AN, Schiffman M, et al: Epidemiology and natural history of human papillomavirus infections and type-specific implications in cervical neoplasia. Vaccine 265:K1, 2008

Brinton LA, Reeves WC, Brenes MM, et al: Parity as a risk factor for cervical cancer. Am J Epidemiol 130:486, 1989

Brotherton JM, Budd A, Rompotis C, et al: Is one dose of human papillomavirus vaccine as effective as three? A national cohort analysis. Papillomavirus Res 8:100177, 2019

Brown DR, Shew ML, Qadadri B, et al: A longitudinal study of genital human papillomavirus infection in a cohort of closely followed adolescent women. J Infect Dis 191(2):182, 2005

Bruni L, Diaz M, Castellsagué X, et al: Cervical human papillomavirus prevalence in 5 continents: meta-analysis of 1 million women with normal cytological findings. J Infect Dis 202(12):1789, 2010

Buckley JD, Harris RW, Doll R, et al: Case-control study of the husbands of women with dysplasia or carcinoma of the cervix uteri. Lancet 2(8254):1010, 1981

Burk RD, Ho GY, Beardsley L, et al: Sexual behavior and partner characteristics are the predominant risk factors for genital human papillomavirus infection in young women. J Infect Dis 174(4):679, 1996

Case AS, Rocconi RP, Straughn JM Jr, et al: Cervical intraepithelial neoplasia in adolescent women. Obstet Gynecol 108:1369, 2006

Castellsagué X, Diaz M, de Sanjosé S, et al: Worldwide human papillomavirus etiology of cervical adenocarcinoma and its cofactors: implications for screening and prevention. J Natl Cancer Inst 98:303, 2006

Castle PE: Beyond human papillomavirus: the cervix, exogenous secondary factors, and the development of cervical precancer and cancer. J Low Genit Tract Dis 8(3):224, 2004

Castle PE, Fetterman B, Poitras N, et al: Five-year experience of human papillomavirus DNA and Papanicolaou test cotesting. Obstet Gynecol 113:595, 2009a

Castle PE, Fetterman B, Poitras N, et al: Relationship of atypical glandular cell cytology, age, and human papillomavirus detection to cervical and endometrial cancer risks. Obstet Gynecol 115:243, 2010

Castle PE, Hunt WC, Langsfeld E, et al: Three-year risk of cervical precancer and cancer after the detection of low-risk human papillomavirus genotypes targeted by a commercial test. Obstet Gynecol 123:49, 2014

Castle PE, Kinney WK, Xue X, et al: Role of screening history in clinical meaning and optimal management of positive cervical screening results. J Natl Cancer Inst 111(8):820, 2019

Castle PE, Schiffman M, Wheeler CM, et al: Evidence for frequent regression of cervical intraepithelial neoplasia-grade 2. Obstet Gynecol 113:18, 2009b

Castle PE, Stoler MH, Wright TC, et al: Performance of carcinogenic human papillomavirus (HPV) testing and HPV16 or HPV18 genotyping for cervical cancer screening of women aged 25 years and older: a subanalysis of the ATHENA study. Lancet Oncol 12:880, 2011

Castle PE, Walker JL, Schiffman M, et al: Hormonal contraceptive use, pregnancy and parity, and the risk of cervical intraepithelial neoplasia 3 among oncogenic HPV DNA-positive women with equivocal or mildly abnormal cytology. Int J Cancer 117(6):1007, 2005

Centers for Disease Control and Prevention: Sexually transmitted diseases treatment guidelines, 2010. MMWR 59(12): 1, 2010

Centers for Disease Control and Prevention: Sexually transmitted diseases treatment guidelines, 2015. MMWR 64(3):1, 2015

Chang GJ, Berry JM, Jay N, et al: Surgical treatment of high-grade anal squamous intraepithelial lesions: a prospective study. Dis Colon Rectum 45(4):453, 2002

Chappell CA, West AM, Kabbani W, et al: Off-label high-risk HPV DNA testing of vaginal ASC-US and LSIL cytologic abnormalities at Parkland Hospital. J Low Genit Tract Dis 14(4):352, 2010

Chaturvedi AK, Madeleine MM, Biggar RJ: et al: Risk of human papillomavirus-associated cancers among persons with AIDS. J Natl Cancer Inst 101(16):1120, 2009

Chin-Hong PV, Reid GE, AST Infectious Diseases Community of Practice: Human papillomavirus infection in solid organ transplant recipients: guidelines from the American Society of Transplantation Infectious Diseases Community of Practice. Clin Transplant 33(9):e13590, 2019

Cleveland AA, Gargano JW, Park IU, et al: Cervical adenocarcinoma in situ: human papillomavirus types and incidence trends in five states, 2008–2015. Int J Cancer April 13, 2019 [Epub ahead of print]

Cohen BA, Honig P, Androphy E: Anogenital warts in children. Clinical and virologic evaluation for sexual abuse. Arch Dermatol 126(12):1575, 1990

Collins S, Mazloomzadeh S, Winter H, et al: High incidence of cervical human papillomavirus infection in women during their first sexual relationship. BJOG 109(1):96, 2002

Crum CP, Herrington CS, McCluggage WG, et al: Tumours of the vulva; epithelial tumors. In Kurman RJ, Carcangiu ML, Herrington CS, et al (eds):

WHO Classification of Tumours of Female Reproductive Organs, 4th ed. Lyon, IARC Press, 2014

Cuzick J, Clavel C, Petry KU, et al: Overview of the European and North American studies on HPV testing in primary cervical cancer screening. Int J Cancer 119:1095, 2006

Darragh TM, Colga TJ, Cox JT, et al: The lower anogenital squamous terminology standardization project for HPV-associated lesions: background and consensus recommendations from the College of American Pathologists and the American Society for Colposcopy and Cervical Pathology. J Low Genit Tract Dis 16(3):205, 2012

Datta SD, Koutsky LA, Ratelle S, et al: Human papillomavirus infection and cervical cytology in women screened for cervical cancer in the United States, 2003–2005. Ann Intern Med 148:493, 2008

Del Pino M, Rodriguez-Carunchio L, Ordi J: Pathways of vulvar intraepithelial neoplasia and squamous cell carcinoma. Histopathology 62(1):161, 2013

Demarco M, Lorey TS, Fetterman B, et al: Risks of CIN 2+, CIN 3+, and cancer by cytology and human papillomavirus status: the foundation of risk-based cervical screening guidelines. J Low Genit Tract Dis 21(4):261, 2017

de Oliveira ER, Derchain SF, Sarian LO, et al: Prediction of high-grade cervical disease with human papillomavirus detect in women with glandular and squamous cytologic abnormalities. Int J Gynecol Cancer 16:1055, 2006

de Sanjose S, Palefsky J: Cervical and anal HPV infections in HIV positive women and men. Virus Res 89(2):201, 2002

de Sanjosé S, Serrano B, Tous S, et al: Burden of human papillomavirus (HPV)-related cancers attributable to HPVs 6/11/16/18/31/33/45/52 and 58. JNCI Cancer Spectr 2(4):pky045, 2019

de Vet HC, Sturmans F: Risk factors for cervical dysplasia: implications for prevention. Public Health 108(4):241, 1994

de Villiers EM: Relationship between steroid hormone contraceptives and HPV, cervical intraepithelial neoplasia and cervical carcinoma. Int J Cancer 103(6):705, 2003

De Vuyst H, Lillo F, Broutet N, et al: HIV, human papillomavirus, and cervical neoplasia and cancer in the era of highly active antiretroviral therapy. Eur J Cancer Prev 17:545, 2008

Diakomanolis E, Stefanidis K, Rodolakis A, et al: Vaginal intraepithelial neoplasia: report of 102 cases. Eur J Gynaecol Oncol 23(5):457, 2002

Dick S, Kremer WW, De Strooper LM, et al: Long-term CIN3+ risk of HPV positive women after triage with FAM19A4/miR124-2 methylation analysis. Gynecol Oncol 154(2):368, 2019

Dillner J: Primary human papillomavirus testing in organized cervical screening. Curr Opin Obstet Gynecol 25:11, 2013

Dillner J: The serological response to papillomaviruses. Semin Cancer Biol 9(6):423, 1999

Dodge JA, Eltabbakh GH, Mount SL, et al: Clinical features and risk of recurrence among patients with vaginal intraepithelial neoplasia. Gynecol Oncol 83(2):363, 2001

Doerfler D, Bernhaus A, Kottmel A, et al: Human papilloma virus infection prior to coitarche. Am J Obstet Gynecol 200:487.e1, 2009

Doorbar J, Quint W, Banks L, et al: The biology and life-cycle of human papillomaviruses. Vaccine 30(Suppl 5):F55, 2012

Drolet M, Bénard É, Pérez N, et al: Population-level impact and herd effects following the introduction of human papillomavirus vaccination programmes: updated systematic review and meta-analysis. Lancet 394(10197):497, 2019

Dunne EF, Markowitz LE, Saraiya M, et al: CDC grand rounds: reducing the burden of HPV-associated cancer and disease. MMWR 63(4):69, 2014

Dunne EF, Unger ER, Sternberg M, et al: Prevalence of HPV infection among females in the United States. JAMA 297:813, 2007

Durst M, Kleinheinz A, Hotz M, et al: The physical state of human papillomavirus type 16 DNA in benign and malignant genital tumours. J Gen Virol 66(Pt 7):1515, 1985

Economos K, Perez Veridiano N, Delke I, et al: Abnormal cervical cytology in pregnancy: a 17-year experience. Obstet Gynecol 81(6):915, 1993

Ellerbrock TV, Chiasson MA, Bush TJ, et al: Incidence of cervical squamous intraepithelial lesions in HIV-infected women. JAMA 283(8):1031, 2000

Eva LJ, Ganesan R, Chan KK, et al: Vulval squamous cell carcinoma occurring on a background of differentiated vulval intraepithelial neoplasia is more likely to recur: a review of 154 cases. J Reprod Med 53:397, 2008

Fairley CK, Chen S, Ugoni A, et al: Human papillomavirus infection and its relationship to recent and distant sexual partners. Obstet Gynecol 84(5):755, 1994

Feng Q, Kiviat NB: New and surprising insights into pathogenesis of multicentric squamous cancers in the female lower genital tract. J Natl Cancer Inst 97: 1798, 2005

Ferris DG, Cox JT, O'Connor DM: The biology and significance of human papillomavirus infection. In Haefner HK, Krumholz BA, Massad LS (eds): Modern Colposcopy. Dubuque, Kendall/Hunt Publishing Company, 2004, p 454

Ferris DG, Litaker M: Interobserver agreement for colposcopy quality control using digitized colposcopic images during the ALTS trial. J Low Genit Tract Dis 9(1):29, 2005

Fiascone S, Vitonis AF, Feldman S: Topical 5-fluorouracil for women with high-grade vaginal intraepithelial neoplasia. Obstet Gynecol 130(6):1237, 2017

Food and Drug Administration: FDA approves expanded use of Gardasil 9 to include individuals 27 through 45 years old. 2018. Available at: https://www.fda.gov/news-events/press-announcements/fda-approves-expanded-use-gardasil-9-include-individuals-27-through-45-years-old. Accessed September 6, 2019

Food and Drug Administration: Gardasil approved to prevent anal cancer. 2010. Available at: https://web.archive.org/web/20141218134237/http://www.fda.gov/NewsEvents/Newsroom/PressAnnouncements/ucm237941.htm. Accessed September 17, 2019

Franco EL, Villa LL, Ruiz A, et al: Transmission of cervical human papillomavirus infection by sexual activity: differences between low and high oncogenic risk types. J Infect Dis 172(3):756, 1995

Friedlander MA, Stier E, Lin O: Anorectal cytology as a screening tool for anal squamous lesions: cytologic, anoscopic, and histologic correlation. Cancer 102(1):19, 2004

Friedrich EG Jr, Wilkinson EJ, Fu YS: Carcinoma in situ of the vulva: a continuing challenge. Am J Obstet Gynecol 136(7):830, 1980

Frisch M, Glimelius B, van den Brule AJ, et al: Sexually transmitted infection as a cause of anal cancer. N Engl J Med 337(19):1350, 1997

Gage JC, Anson VW, Abbey K, et al: Number of cervical biopsies and sensitivity of colposcopy. Obstet Gynecol 108(2):264, 2006

Gatta LA, Kuller JA, Rhee EH: Pregnancy outcomes following cervical conization or loop electrosurgical excision procedures. Obstet Gynecol Surv 72(8):494, 2017

Goldstone SE, Kawalek AZ, Huyett JW: Infrared coagulator: a useful tool for treating anal squamous intraepithelial lesions. Dis Colon Rectum 48(5):1042, 2005

Goldstone SE, Winkler B, Ufford LJ, et al: High prevalence of anal squamous intraepithelial lesions and squamous-cell carcinoma in men who have sex with men as seen in a surgical practice. Dis Colon Rectum 44(5):690, 2001

Gomez-Lobo V: Gynecologic care of the transplant recipient. Postgrad Obstet Gynecol 29(10):1, 2009

Griffith WF, Stuart GS, Gluck KL, et al: Vaginal speculum lubrication and its effects on cervical cytology and microbiology. Contraception 72:60, 2005

Haefner HK, Tate JE, McLachlin CM, et al: Vulvar intraepithelial neoplasia: age, morphological phenotype, papillomavirus DNA, and coexisting invasive carcinoma. Hum Pathol 26(2):147, 1995

Harmanli O, Jones KA: Using lubrication for speculum insertion. Obstet Gynecol 116(No. 2, Part 1):415, 2010

Harris TG, Miller L, Kulasingam SL, et al: Depot-medroxyprogesterone acetate and combined oral contraceptive use and cervical neoplasia among women with oncogenic human papillomavirus infection. Am J Obstet Gynecol 200:489.e1, 2009

Hart WR: Vulvar intraepithelial neoplasia: historical aspects and current status. Int J Gynecol Pathol 20(1):16, 2001

Heard I, Etienney I, Potard V, et al: High prevalence of anal human papillomavirus-associated cancer precursors in a contemporary cohort of asymptomatic HIV-infected women. Clin Infect Dis 60(10):1559, 2015

Heard I, Palefsky JM, Kazatchkine MD: The impact of HIV antiviral therapy on human papillomavirus (HPV) infections and HPV-related diseases. Antivir Ther 9(1):13, 2004

Heard I, Potard V, Foulot H, et al: High rate of recurrence of cervical intraepithelial neoplasia after surgery in HIV-positive women. J Acquir Immune Defic Syndr 39(4):412, 2005

Hembree WC, Cohen-Kettenis PT, Gooren L, et al: Endocrine treatment of gender-dysphoric/gender-incongruent persons: an Endocrine Society clinical practice guideline. J Clin Endocrinol Metab 102(11):3869, 2017

Henk HJ, Insigna RP, Singhal PK, et al: Incidence and costs of cervical intraepithelial neoplasia in a US commercially insured population. Low Genit Tract Dis 4(1):29, 2010

Herrero R, Hildesheim A, Bratti C, et al: Population-based study of human papillomavirus infection and cervical neoplasia in rural Costa Rica. J Natl Cancer Inst 92(6):464, 2000

Herzog TJ, Monk BJ: Reducing the burden of glandular carcinomas of the uterine cervix. Am J Obstet Gynecol 197(6):566, 2007

Hildesheim A, Hadjimichael O, Schwartz PE, et al: Risk factors for rapid-onset cervical cancer. Am J Obstet Gynecol 180(3 Pt 1):571, 1999

Hillemanns P, Ellerbrock TV, McPhillips S, et al: Prevalence of anal human papillomavirus infection and anal cytologic abnormalities in HIV-seropositive women. AIDS 10(14):1641, 1996

Hirth JM, Kuo YF, Starkey JM, et al: Regional variations in human papillomavirus prevalence across time in NHANES (2003-2014). Vaccine 37(30):4040, 2019

Ho GY, Bierman R, Beardsley L, et al: Natural history of cervicovaginal papillomavirus infection in young women. N Engl J Med 338(7):423, 1998

Ho GY, Burk RD, Klein S, et al: Persistent genital human papillomavirus infection as a risk factor for persistent cervical dysplasia. J Natl Cancer Inst 87(18):1365, 1995

Hodeib M, Cohen JG, Mehta S, et al: Recurrence and risk of progression to lower genital tract malignancy in women with high grade VAIN. Gynecol Oncol 141(3):507, 2016

Hoffman MS, DeCesare SL, Roberts WS, et al: Upper vaginectomy for in situ and occult, superficially invasive carcinoma of the vagina. Am J Obstet Gynecol 166(1 Pt 1):30, 1992a

Hoffman MS, Pinelli DM, Finan M, et al: Laser vaporization for vulvar intraepithelial neoplasia III. J Reprod Med 37(2):135, 1992b

Holly EA, Ralston ML, Darragh TM, et al: Prevalence and risk factors for anal squamous intraepithelial neoplasia in women. J Natl Cancer Inst 93:843, 2001

Hoover RN, Hyer M, Pfeiffer RM, et al: Adverse health outcomes in women exposed in utero to diethylstilbestrol. N Engl J Med 365 (14): 1304, 2011

Hopkins MP, Nemunaitis-Keller J: Carcinoma of the vulva. Obstet Gynecol Clin North Am 28(4):791, 2001

Howe HL, Wingo PA, Thun MJ, et al: Annual report to the nation on the status of cancer (1973 through 1998), featuring cancers with recent increasing trends. J Natl Cancer Inst 93(11):824, 2001

Howlader N, Noone AM, Krapcho M, et al: SEER cancer statistics review, 1975–2014. Bethesda, National Cancer Institute, 2017

Huh WK, Ault KA, Chelmow D, et al: Use of high-risk human papillomavirus testing for cervical cancer screening: interim clinical guidance. Obstet Gynecol 125(2):330, 2015

International Collaboration of Epidemiological Studies of Cervical Cancer: Cervical cancer and hormonal contraceptives: collaborative reanalysis of individual data for 16573 women with cervical cancer and 35509 women without cervical cancer from 24 epidemiological studies. Lancet 370:1609, 2007

Jay N, Berry JM, Hogeboom CJ, et al: Colposcopic appearance of anal squamous intraepithelial lesions: relationship to histopathology. Dis Colon Rectum 40(8):919, 1997

Jeronimo J, Massad LS, Castle PE, et al: Interobserver agreement in the evaluation of digitized cervical images. Obstet Gynecol 110:833, 2007

Jones RW, Rowan DM: Vulvar intraepithelial neoplasia III: a clinical study of the outcome in 113 cases with relation to the later development of invasive vulvar carcinoma. Obstet Gynecol 84(5):741, 1994

Jones RW, Rowan DM, Stewart AW: Vulvar intraepithelial neoplasia: aspects of the natural history and outcome in 405 women. Obstet Gynecol 106(6): 1319, 2005

Joura EA, Zeisler H, Losch A, et al: Differentiating vulvar intraepithelial neoplasia from nonneoplastic epithelial disorders. The toluidine blue test. J Reprod Med 43(8):671, 1998

Judson PL, Habermann EB, Baxter NN, et al: Trends in the incidence of invasive and in situ vulvar carcinoma. Obstet Gynecol 107:1018, 2006

Kaplan JE, Benson C, Holmes KH, et al: Guidelines for prevention and treatment of opportunistic infections in HIV-infected adults and adolescents. MMWR 58(4):1, 2009

Khan MJ, Castle PE, Lorincz AT, et al: The elevated 10-year risk of cervical precancer and cancer in women with human papillomavirus (HPV) type 16 or 18 and the possible utility of type-specific HPV testing in clinical practice. J Natl Cancer Inst 97:1072, 2005

Khan MJ, Massad LS, Kinney W, et al: A common clinical dilemma: management of abnormal vaginal cytology and human papillomavirus test results. J Low Genit Tract Dis 20(2):119, 2016

Khan MJ, Smith-McCune KK: Treatment of cervical precancers: back to basics. Obstet Gynecol 123(6):1339, 2014

Khan MJ, Werner CL, Darragh TM, et al: ASCCP colposcopy standards: role of colposcopy, benefits, potential harms, and terminology for colposcopic practice. J Low Genit Tract Dis 21(4):223, 2017

Kinney WK, Manos MM, Hurley LB, et al: Where's the high-grade cervical neoplasia? The importance of minimally abnormal Papanicolaou diagnoses. Obstet Gynecol 91(6):973, 1998

Kiviat N: Natural history of cervical neoplasia: overview and update. Am J Obstet Gynecol 175(4 Pt 2):1099, 1996

Kjaer SK, de Villiers EM, Dahl C, et al: Case-control study of risk factors for cervical neoplasia in Denmark. I: Role of the "male factor" in women with one lifetime sexual partner. Int J Cancer 48(1):39, 1991

Kjaer SK, van den Brule AJ, Paull G, et al: Type specific persistence of high risk human papillomavirus (HPV) as indicator of high grade cervical squamous

intraepithelial lesions in young women: population based prospective follow up study. BMJ 325(7364):572, 2002

Korn AP, Abercrombie PD, Foster A: Vulvar intraepithelial neoplasia in women infected with human immunodeficiency virus-1. Gynecol Oncol 61:384, 1996

Kosary C: Cancer of the vagina. In Ries LAG, Young JL, Keel GE, et al (eds): SEER Survival Monograph: Cancer Survival Among Adults: U.S. SEER Program, 1988–2001, Patient and Tumor Characteristics. NIH Publication No. 07–6215, Bethesda, 2007

Koss LG: The Papanicolaou test for cervical cancer detection. A triumph and a tragedy. JAMA 261(5):737, 1989

Krebs HB: Treatment of vaginal intraepithelial neoplasia with laser and tropical 5-fluorouracil. Obstet Gynecol 73(4):657, 1989

Kreimer AR, Herrero R, Sampson JN, et al: Evidence for single-dose protection by the bivalent HPV vaccine-review of the Costa Rica HPV vaccine trial and future research studies. Vaccine 36(32 Pt A):4774, 2018

Krivak TC, Rose GS, McBroom JW, et al: Cervical adenocarcinoma in situ: a systematic review of therapeutic options and predictors of persistent or recurrent disease. Obstet Gynecol Surv 56(9):567, 2001

Lamme J, Pattaratornkosohn T, Mercado-Abadie J, et al: Concurrent anal human papillomavirus and abnormal anal cytology in women with known cervical dysplasia. Obstet Gynecol 124(2Pt 1), 242, 2014

Lawrie TA, Nordin A, Chakrabarti M, et al: Medical and surgical interventions for the treatment of usual-type vulval intraepithelial neoplasia. Cochrane Database Syst Rev 1:CD011837, 2016

Le T, Menard C, Hicks-Boucher W, et al: Final results of a phase 2 study using continuous 5% imiquimod cream application in the primary treatment of high-grade vulva intraepithelial neoplasia. Gynecol Oncol 106(3):579, 2007

Lee A, Radford J, Fischer G: Long-term management of adult vulvar lichen sclerosus: a prospective cohort study of 507 women. JAMA Dermatol 151:1061, 2015

Lin C, Slama J, Gonzalez P, et al: Cervical determinants of anal HPV infection and high-grade anal lesions in women: a collaborative pooled analysis. Lancet Infect Dis 19(8):880, 2019

Mahto M, Nathan M, O'Maony C: More than a decade on: review of the use of imiquimod in lower anogenital intraepithelial neoplasia. Int J STD AIDS 21:8, 2010

Maiman M, Fruchter RG, Serur E, et al: Human immunodeficiency virus infection and cervical neoplasia. Gynecol Oncol 38:377, 1990

Markowitz LE, Naleway AL, Lewis RM, et al: Declines in HPV vaccine type prevalence in women screened for cervical cancer in the United States: evidence of direct and herd effects of vaccination. Vaccine 37(29):3918, 2019

Marrazzo JM, Stine K, Koutsky LA: Genital human papillomavirus infection in women who have sex with women: a review. Am J Obstet Gynecol 183(3):770, 2000

Martin-Hirsch PL, Paraskevaidis E, Bryant A: Surgery for cervical intraepithelial neoplasia. Cochrane Database Syst Rev 6:CD001318, 2013

Massad LS, Einstein MH, Huh WK, et al: 2012 Updated consensus guidelines for the management of abnormal cervical cancer screening tests and cancer precursors. J Low Genit Tract Dis 17(5):S1, 2013

Massad LS, Seaberg EC, Watts DH, et al: Long-term incidence of cervical cancer in women with human immunodeficiency virus. Cancer 115:524, 2009

Mayrand MH, Duarte-Franco E, Rodrigues I, et al: Human papillomavirus DNS versus Papanicolaou screening tests for cervical cancer. N Engl J Med 357(16):1579, 2007

McClung NM, Gargano JW, Park IU, et al: Estimated number of cases of high-grade cervical lesions diagnosed among women—United States, 2008 and 2016. MMWR 68(15):337, 2019

McCredie MRE, Sharples KJ, Paul C, et al: Natural history of cervical neoplasia and risk of invasive cancer in women with cervical intraepithelial neoplasia 3: a retrospective cohort study. Lancet Oncol 9(5):425, 2008

McCune KC, Imborek KL: Clinical care of lesbian and bisexual women for the obstetrician gynecologist. Clin Obstet Gynecol 61(4):663, 2018

Meites E, Kempe A, Markowitz LE: Use of a 2-dose schedule for human papillomavirus vaccination—updated recommendations of the Advisory Committee on Immunization Practices. MMWR 65(49):1405, 2016

Meites E, Szilagyi PG, Chesson HW, et al: Human papillomavirus vaccination for adults: updated recommendations of the Advisory Committee on Immunization Practices. MMWR 68:698, 2019

Miller BE: Vulvar intraepithelial neoplasia treated with cavitational ultrasonic surgical aspiration. Gynecol Oncol 85(1):114, 2002

Molijn A, Kleter B, Quint W, et al: Molecular diagnosis of human papillomavirus (HPV) infections. J Clin Virol 32(Suppl 1):S43, 2005

Moore K, Cofer A, Elliot L, et al: Adolescent cervical dysplasia: histologic evaluation, treatment, and outcomes. Am J Obstet Gynecol 197:141.e1, 2007

Moscicki AB: Impact of HPV infection in adolescent populations. J Adolesc Health 37:S3, 2005

Moscicki AB, Darragh TM, Berry-Lawhorn JM, et al: Screening for anal cancer in women. J Low Genit Tract Dis 19(301):S26, 2015

Moscicki AB, Flowers L, Huchko MJ, et al: Guidelines for cervical cancer screening in immunosuppressed women without HIV infection. J Low Genit Tract Dis 23(2):87, 2019

Moscicki AB, Ma Y, Wibbelsman C, et al: Rate of and risks for regression of cervical intraepithelial neoplasia 2 in adolescents and young women. Obstet Gynecol 116(6):1373, 2010

Moscicki AB, Shiboski S, Broering J, et al: The natural history of human papillomavirus infection as measured by repeated DNA testing in adolescent and young women. J Pediatr 132(2):277, 1998

Moscicki AB, Shiboski S, Hills NK, et al: Regression of low-grade squamous intra-epithelial lesions in young women. Lancet 364(9446):1678, 2004

Muñoz N, Bosch FX, de Sanjose S, et al: Epidemiologic classification of human papillomavirus types associated with cervical cancer. N Engl J Med 348(6):518, 2003

Muñoz N, Franceschi S, Bosetti C, et al: Role of parity and human papillomavirus in cervical cancer: the IARC multicentric case-control study. Lancet 359:1093, 2002

Nahas CS, da Silva Filho EV, Segurado AA, et al: Screening anal dysplasia in HIV-infected patients: is there an agreement between anal Pap smear and high-resolution anoscopy-guided biopsy? Dis Colon Rectum 52:1854, 2009

National Cancer Institute: PDQ Cervical Cancer Screening. 2019a. Available at: https://www.cancer.gov/types/cervical/hp/cervical-screening-pdq. Accessed September 7, 2019

National Cancer Institute: Vulvar cancer treatment PDQ®. 2019b. Available at: https://www.cancer.gov/types/vulvar/hp/vulvar-treatment-pdq. Accessed September 11, 2019

National Cancer Institute Workshop: The 1988 Bethesda system for reporting cervical/vaginal cytological diagnoses. JAMA 262(7):931, 1989

Nayar R, Wilbur DC: The Pap test and Bethesda 2014. Cancer Cytopathol 123(5):271, 2015

Obalek S, Jablonska S, Favre M, et al: Condylomata acuminata in children: frequent association with human papillomaviruses responsible for cutaneous warts. J Am Acad Dermatol 23(2 Pt 1):205, 1990

Ostor AG: Natural history of cervical intraepithelial neoplasia: a critical review. Int J Gynecol Pathol 12(2):186, 1993

Palefsky JM: Anal human papillomavirus infection and anal cancer in HIV-positive individuals: an emerging problem. AIDS 8:283, 1994

Palefsky JM, Holly EA, Efirdc JT, et al: Anal intraepithelial neoplasia in the highly active antiretroviral therapy era among HIV-positive men who have sex with men. AIDS 19(13):1407, 2005

Palefsky JM, Holly EA, Ralston ML, et al: Prevalence and risk factors for anal human papillomavirus infection in human immunodeficiency virus (HIV)-positive and high-risk HIV-negative women. J Infect Dis 183(3):383, 2001

Panel on Opportunistic Infections in Adults and Adolescents with HIV: Guidelines for the prevention and treatment of opportunistic infections in Adults and Adolescents with HIV: recommendations from the Centers for Disease Control and Prevention, the National Institutes of Health, and the HIV Medicine Association of the Infectious Diseases Society of America. 2019. Available at: http://aidsinfo.nih.gov/contentfiles/lvguidelines/adult_oi.pdf. Accessed September 7, 2019

Panther LA, Schlecht HP, Dezube BJ: Spectrum of human papillomavirus-related dysplasia and carcinoma of the anus in HIV-infected patients. AIDS Read 15(2):79, 2005

Paraskevaidis E, Jandial L, Mann E, et al: Pattern of treatment failure following laser for cervical intraepithelial neoplasia: implications for follow-up protocol. Obstet Gynecol 78:80, 1991

Perrotta M, Marchitelli CE, Velazco AF, et al: Use of CO_2 laser vaporization for the treatment of high-grade vaginal intraepithelial neoplasia. J Low Genit Tract Dis 17(1):23, 2013

Petrosky E, Bocchini JA Jr, Hariri S, et al: Use of 9-valent human papillomavirus (HPV) vaccine: updated HPV vaccination recommendations of the advisory committee on immunization practices. MMWR 64(11):300, 2015

Plummer M, Herrero R, Franceschi S, et al: Smoking and cervical cancer: pooled analysis of the IARC multi-centric case-control study. Cancer Causes Control 14(9):805, 2003

Punnonen R, Kallioniemi OP, Mattila J, et al: Primary invasive and in situ vaginal carcinoma. Flow cytometric analysis of DNA aneuploidy and cell proliferation from archival paraffin-embedded tissue. Eur J Obstet Gynecol Reprod Biol 32(3):247, 1989

Remmink AJ, Walboomers JM, Helmerhorst TJ, et al: The presence of persistent high-risk HPV genotypes in dysplastic cervical lesions is associated with progressive disease: natural history up to 36 months. Int J Cancer 61(3):306, 1995

Rome RM, England PG: Management of vaginal intraepithelial neoplasia: a series of 132 cases with long-term follow-up. Int J Gynecol Cancer 10:382, 2000

Ronco G, Dillner J, Elfström KM, et al: Efficacy of HPV-based screening for prevention of invasive cervical cancer: follow-up of four European randomised controlled trials. Lancet 383(9916):524, 2014

Ronco G, Giorgi-Rossi P, Carozzi F, et al: Efficacy of human papillomavirus testing for the detection of invasive cervical cancers and cervical intraepithelial neoplasia: a randomized controlled trial. Lancet Oncol 11:249, 2010

Ronco G, Segnan N, Giorgi-Rossi P, et al: Human papillomavirus testing and liquid-based cytology: results at recruitment from the new technologies for cervical cancer randomized controlled trial. J Natl Cancer Inst 98(11):765, 2006

Rosales R, Rosales C: Immune therapy for human papillomavirus-related cancers. World J Clin Oncol 5(5):1002, 2014

Rosenfeld WD, Rose E, Vermund SH, et al: Follow-up evaluation of cervicovaginal human papillomavirus infection in adolescents. J Pediatr 121(2):307, 1992

Roura E, Travier N, Waterboer T, et al: The influence of hormonal factors on the risk of developing cervical cancer and pre-cancer: results from the EPIC cohort. PLoS One 11(1):e0147029, 2016

Santoso J, Long M, Crigger M, et al: Anal intraepithelial neoplasia in women with genital intraepithelial neoplasia. Obstet Gynecol 116(3):578, 2010

Sapp M, Bienkowska-Haba M: Viral entry mechanisms: human papillomavirus and a long journey from extracellular matrix to the nucleus. FEBS J 276:7206, 2009

Saslow D, Solomon D, Lawson HW, et al: American Cancer Society, American Society for Colposcopy and Cervical Pathology, and American Society for Clinical Pathology screening guidelines for the prevention and early detection of cervical cancer. CA Cancer 62(3):147, 2012

Schiffman M, Kinney WK, Cheung LC, et al: Relative performance of HPV and cytology components of cotesting in cervical screening. J Natl Cancer Inst 110(5):501, 2018

Schiffman M, Wentzensen N: From human papillomavirus to cervical cancer. Obstet Gynecol 116(1):177, 2010

Schlecht NF, Platt RW, Duarte-Franco E, et al: Human papillomavirus infection and time to progression and regression of cervical intraepithelial neoplasia. J Natl Cancer Inst 95(17):1336, 2003

Schnatz PF, Guile M, O'Sullivan DM, et al: Clinical significance of atypical glandular cells on cervical cytology. Obstet Gynecol 107:701, 2006

Schockaert S, Poppe W, Arbyn M, et al: Incidence of vaginal intraepithelial neoplasia after hysterectomy for cervical intraepithelial neoplasia: a retrospective study. Am J Obstet Gynecol 199:113.e1, 2008

Sehnal B, Dusek L, Cibula D, et al: The relationship between the cervical and anal HPV infection in women with cervical intraepithelial neoplasia. J Clin Virol 59(1):18, 2014

Shatz P, Bergeron C, Wilkinson EJ, et al: Vulvar intraepithelial neoplasia and skin appendage involvement. Obstet Gynecol 74(5):769, 1989

Sherman ME, Friedman HB, Busseniers AE, et al: Cytologic diagnosis of anal intraepithelial neoplasia using smears and cytyc thin-preps. Mod Pathol 8(3):270, 1995

Siegel RL, Miller KD, Jemal A: Cancer statistics, 2019. CA Cancer J Clin 69:7, 2019

Siegfried EC, Frasier LD: Anogenital warts in children. Adv Dermatol 12:141, 1997

Silverberg MJ, Thorsen P, Lindeberg H, et al: Condyloma in pregnancy is strongly predictive of juvenile-onset recurrent respiratory papillomatosis. Obstet Gynecol 101(4):645, 2003

Smith JS, Backes DM, Hoots BE, et al: Human papillomavirus type-distribution in vulvar and vaginal cancers and their associated precursors. Obstet Gynecol 113(4):917, 2009

Smith JS, Lindsay L, Hoots B, et al: Human papillomavirus type distribution in invasive cervical cancer and high-grade cervical lesions: a meta-analysis update. Int J Cancer 121:621, 2007

Solomon D, Davey D, Kurman R, et al: The 2001 Bethesda System: terminology for reporting results of cervical cytology. JAMA 287(16):2114, 2002

Spitzer M: Lower genital tract intraepithelial neoplasia in HIV-infected women: guidelines for evaluation and management. Obstet Gynecol Surv 54(2):131, 1999

Spitzer M, Krumholz BA, Seltzer VL: The multicentric nature of disease related to human papillomavirus infection of the female lower genital tract. Obstet Gynecol 73(3 Pt 1):303, 1989

Stanley M: Pathology and epidemiology of HPV infection in females. Gynecol Oncol 117:S5, 2010a

Stanley M: Prospects for new human papillomavirus vaccines. Curr Opin Infect Dis 23:70, 2010b

Stoler MH: A brief synopsis of the role of human papillomaviruses in cervical carcinogenesis. Am J Obstet Gynecol 175(4 Pt 2):1091, 1996

Strander B, Hällgren J, Sparén P: Effect of ageing on cervical or vaginal cancer in Swedish women previously treated for cervical intraepithelial neoplasia 3: population based cohort study of long term incidence and mortality. BMJ 348:17361, 2014

Syrjänen S: Current concepts on human papillomavirus infections in children. APMIS 118(6-7):494, 2010

Tandon R, Baranoski AS, Huang F, et al: Abnormal anal cytology in HIV-infected women. Am J Obstet Gynecol 203:21.e1, 2010

Thimm MA, Rositch AF, VandenBussche C, et al: Lower genital tract dysplasia in female solid organ transplant recipients. Obstet Gynecol 134(2):385, 2019

Thomsen LT, Frederiksen K, Munk C, et al: High-risk and low-risk human papillomavirus and the absolute risk of cervical intraepithelial neoplasia or cancer. Obstet Gynecol 123:57, 2014

Trimble EL: A guest editorial: update on diethylstilbestrol. Obstet Gynecol Surv 56(4):187, 2001

Trottier H, Mahmud SM, Lindsay L, et al: Persistence of an incident human papillomavirus infection and timing of cervical lesions in previously unexposed young women. Cancer Epidemiol Biomarkers Prev 18(3):854, 2009

U.S. Preventive Services Task Force, Curry SJ, Krist AH, et al: Screening for cervical cancer: US Preventive Services Task Force recommendation statement. JAMA 320(7):674, 2018

Ulfelder H, Robboy SJ: The embryologic development of the human vagina. Am J Obstet Gynecol 126(7):769, 1976

van de Nieuwenhof HP, Massuger LF, van der Avoort I, et al: Vulvar squamous cell carcinoma development after diagnosis of VIN increases with age. Eur J Cancer 45(5):851, 2009

van den Einden LC, de Hullu JA, Massuger LF, et al: Interobserver variability and the effect of education in the histopathological diagnosis of differentiated vulvar intraepithelial neoplasia. Mod Pathol 26:874, 2013

van Seters M, van Beurden M, ten Kate FJ, et al: Treatment of vulvar intraepithelial neoplasia with topical imiquimod. N Engl J Med 358:1465, 2008

Verdoodt F, Jiang X, Williams M, et al: High-risk HPV testing in the management of atypical glandular cells: a systematic review and meta-analysis. Int J Cancer 138(2):303, 2016

Verloop J, van Leeuwen FE, Helmerhorst TJ, et al: Risk of cervical intraepithelial neoplasia and invasive cancer of the cervix in DES daughters. Gynecol Oncol 144(2):305, 2017

von Gruenigen VE, Gibbons HE, Gibbins K, et al: Surgical treatments for vulvar and vaginal dysplasia. Obstet Gynecol 109:942, 2007

Walker TY, Elam-Evans LD, Yankey D, et al: National, regional, state, and selected local area vaccination coverage among adolescents aged 13–17 years—United States, 2018. MMWR 68(33):718, 2019

Wang CJ, Sparano J, Palefsky J: HIV/AIDS, HPV and anal cancer. Surg Oncol Clin N Am 26(1):17, 2017

Watson AJ, Smith BB, Whitehead MR, et al: Malignant progression of anal intra-epithelial neoplasia. ANZ J Surg 76(8):715, 2006

Wentzensen N, Clarke MA, Bremer R, et al: Clinical evaluation of human papillomavirus screening with p16/Ki-67 dual stain triage in a large organized cervical cancer screening program. JAMA Intern Med 179(7):881, 2019

Wentzensen N, Massad LS, Mayeaux EJ Jr, et al: Evidence-based consensus recommendations for colposcopy practice for cervical cancer prevention in the United States. J Low Genit Tract Dis 21(4):216, 2017

Whitlock EP, Vesco KK, Eder M, et al: Liquid-based cytology and human papillomavirus testing to screen for cervical cancer: a systematic review for the U.S. Preventive Services Task Force. Ann Intern Med 155:687, 2011

Wilkinson EJ: Pap smears and screening for cervical neoplasia. Clin Obstet Gynecol 33(4):817, 1990

Wilkinson EJ, Kneale B, Lynch PJ: Report of the ISSVD Terminology Committee. J Reprod Med 31:973, 1986

Winer RL, Hughes JP, Feng Q, et al: Early natural history of incident, type-specific human papillomavirus infections in newly sexually active young women. Cancer Epidemiol Biomarkers Prev 20(4):699, 2011

Winer RL, Lee SK, Hughes JP, et al: Genital human papillomavirus infection: incidence and risk factors in a cohort of female university students. Am J Epidemiol 157(3):218, 2003

Woodman CB, Collins S, Winter H, et al: Natural history of cervical human papillomavirus infection in young women: a longitudinal cohort study. Lancet 357(9271):1831, 2001

Woodruff JD: Carcinoma in situ of the vagina. Clin Obstet Gynecol 24(2):485, 1981

Wright TC, Ellerbrock TV, Chiasson MA, et al: Cervical intraepithelial neoplasia in women infected with human immunodeficiency virus: prevalence, risk factors, and validity of Papanicolaou smears. New York Cervical Disease Study. Obstet Gynecol 84(4):591, 1994

Wright TC, Stoler MH, Behrens CM, et al: Primary cervical cancer screening with human papillomavirus: end of study results from the ATHENA study using HPV as the first-line screening test. Gynecol Oncol 136(2):189, 2015

Wright TC, Stoler MH, Behrens CM, et al: The ATHENA human papillomavirus study: design, methods, and baseline results. Am J Obstet Gynecol 206:46e1, 2012

Wright VC, Chapman W: Intraepithelial neoplasia of the lower female genital tract: etiology, investigation, and management. Semin Surg Oncol 8:180, 1992

Yasmeen S, Romano PS, Pettinger M, et al: Incidence of cervical cytological abnormalities with aging in the Women's Health Initiative. Obstet Gynecol 108:410, 2006

Yeh PT, Kennedy CE, de Vuyst H, et al: Self-sampling for human papillomavirus (HPV) testing: a systematic review and meta-analysis. BMJ Glob Health 4(3):e001351, 2019

Yost NP, Santoso JT, McIntire DD, et al: Postpartum regression rates of antepartum cervical intraepithelial neoplasia II and III lesions. Obstet Gynecol 93(3):359, 1999

Zbar AP, Fenger C, Efron J, et al: The pathology and molecular biology of anal intraepithelial neoplasia: comparisons with cervical and vulvar intraepithelial carcinoma. Int J Colorectal Dis 17(4):203, 2002

zur Hausen H: Papillomaviruses in the causation of human cancers—a brief historical account. Virology 384(2):260, 2009

CHAPTER 30

Cervical Cancer

Cervical cancer is the most common gynecologic cancer in women worldwide. Most of these cancers stem from infection with the human papillomavirus (HPV), although other host factors affect neoplastic progression following initial infection. Compared with other gynecologic malignancies, cervical cancer develops in a relatively younger population. Thus, screening for this neoplasia typically begins in young adulthood.

Most early cancers are asymptomatic. Thus, diagnosis usually follows histologic evaluation of biopsies taken during colposcopic examination or from a grossly abnormal cervix. This cancer is staged clinically, and this in turn directs treatment. In general, early-stage disease is effectively eradicated surgically. For advanced disease, chemoradiation is primarily selected. As expected, disease prognosis worsens with advancing tumor stage, and stage is the most important indicator of long-term survival.

Prevention lies mainly in identifying and treating women with high-grade dysplasia, and in HPV vaccination. Detailed in Chapter 29 (p. 628), regular screening is recommended and

HPV vaccination is encouraged to lower future rates of cervical cancer.

INCIDENCE

Worldwide, cervical cancer is common, and it ranks fourth among all malignancies for women (World Health Organization, 2019). In 2018, global cervical cancer estimates include nearly 570,000 new cases and more than 311,000 deaths. In general, higher incidences are found in developing countries, and these countries contribute 85 percent of reported cases annually. In these populations, mortality rates are similarly higher (Torre, 2015). These incidence and survival disparities highlight successes achieved by long-term cervical cancer screening programs.

In the United States, cervical cancer is the third most common gynecologic cancer and the 11th most common solid malignant neoplasm among women. Women have a 1 in 132 lifetime risk of developing this cancer. In 2019, the American Cancer Society estimated 13,170 new cases and 4250 deaths from this malignancy (Siegel, 2019). Of U.S. women, black women and those in lower socioeconomic groups have the highest age-adjusted cervical cancer death rates, and Hispanic women have the highest incidence rates (Table 30-1). This trend is thought to stem mainly from financial and cultural characteristics affecting access to screening and treatment. The age at which cervical cancer develops is in general earlier than that of other gynecologic malignancies, and the median age at diagnosis is 50 years (Howlader, 2019).

RISKS

In addition to demographic differences, other risks may alter HPV acquisition or action. Notably, the greatest risk is the lack of regular cervical cancer screening (Abed, 2006; Leyden, 2005). Most communities adopting such screening have documented declines in this cancer's incidence (Jemal, 2006).

HPV is the primary etiologic infectious agent associated with cervical cancer (Ley, 1991; Schiffman, 1993). Although other sexually transmitted factors, including herpes simplex virus 2, may play a concurrent causative role, 99.7 percent of cervical cancers are associated with an oncogenic HPV subtype (Walboomers, 1999). In one study, 63 percent of invasive cervical cancer cases were attributable to HPV serotype 16. Serotype 18 was associated with 16 percent of invasive disease cases (Guan, 2012). Each of these serotypes can lead to either squamous cell carcinoma or adenocarcinoma of the cervix. However, HPV 16 is more commonly associated with squamous cell carcinoma of

TABLE 30-1. Cervical Cancer Age-Adjusted Incidence and Death Rates (per 100,000 women per year)

	All Races	White	Black	Asian American & Pacific Islander	American Indian & Alaskan Native	Hispanic
Incidence	7.3	7.2	8.7	6.4	7.9	9.3
Death	2.3	2.2	3.5	1.7	1.8	2.6

Based on cases diagnosed during 2012 through 2016 from 21 geographic areas in the Surveillance, Epidemiology and End Results (SEER) Program.
Data from Howlader, 2019.

the cervix, whereas HPV 18 is a risk factor for cervical adenocarcinoma (Bulk, 2006).

Of other risks, lower educational attainment, older age, obesity, smoking, and neighborhood poverty are independently related to lower rates of cervical cancer screening. Specifically, those living in impoverished neighborhoods have limited access to testing and may benefit from screening outreach programs (Datta, 2006).

Cigarette smoking, both active and passive, raises cervical cancer risk. Among HPV-infected women, current and former smokers have a two- to threefold greater incidence of high-grade squamous intraepithelial lesion (HSIL) or invasive cancer. Passive smoking is also associated with higher risk, but to a lesser extent (Trimble, 2005). The mechanism underlying the association between smoking and this cancer is unclear. Smoking may alter HPV infection in those who smoke. For example, "ever smoking" is associated with reduced clearance of high-risk HPV (Koshiol, 2006; Plummer, 2003). Tobacco smoke may also modify viral oncoprotein expression in cells in which the HPV is not integrated into the host genome (Wei, 2014).

Parity has a significant association with cervical cancer. Specifically, women with seven prior full-term pregnancies have an approximately fourfold risk, and those with one or two have a twofold risk compared with nulliparas (Muñoz, 2002).

Long-term combination oral contraceptive (COC) use is another factor. In women who are positive for cervical HPV DNA and who use COCs, cervical carcinoma rates rise by up to fourfold compared with women who are HPV-positive and never users (Moreno, 2002). Additionally, current COC users and women who are within 9 years of use have a significantly higher risk of developing both squamous cell and adenocarcinoma of the cervix (International Collaboration of Epidemiological Studies of Cervical Cancer, 2006). Encouragingly, the relative risk to COC users appears to decline after cessation. Data from 24 epidemiologic studies showed that by 10 or more years following COC cessation, cervical cancer risk returns to that of never users (International Collaboration of Epidemiological Studies of Cervical Cancer, 2007).

Sexual activity logically has an association because HPV is sexually transmitted. Having more than six lifetime sexual partners elevates the relative risk of cervical cancer. Similarly, an early age of first intercourse before age 20 confers a greater risk of developing this malignancy. Intercourse after age 21 only shows a trend toward an elevated risk. Moreover, abstinence from sexual activity and barrier protection during sexual intercourse lowers cervical cancer incidence (International

Collaboration of Epidemiological Studies of Cervical Cancer, 2006).

Immunosuppressed women have an increased risk of developing cervical cancer. Cervical cancer is an acquired immune deficiency syndrome (AIDS)-defining illness, and the standardized incidence ratio (SIR) of developing this cancer in women with HIV is 5.82. For transplant recipients, the SIR is 2.01 for this malignancy (Grulich, 2007). Women with autoimmune diseases who use immunosuppressants do not appear to have an greater cervical cancer risk, except for azathioprine users (Dugue, 2015).

PATHOPHYSIOLOGY

■ Tumorigenesis

Most women readily clear HPV, but those with persistent infection may develop preinvasive dysplastic cervical lesions. From such lesions, squamous cell carcinoma of the cervix typically arises at the squamocolumnar junction (Bosch, 2002). In general, progression from dysplasia to invasive cancer requires several years, although times can vary widely. The molecular alterations involved with cervical carcinogenesis are complex and not fully understood. Carcinogenesis currently is suspected to result from the interactive effects among environmental insults, host immunity, and somatic-cell genomic variations (Helt, 2002; Jones, 1997, 2006; Wentzensen, 2004).

Increasing evidence suggests that HPV oncoproteins may be a critical component of continued cancer cell proliferation (Mantovani, 1999; Munger, 2001). Unlike low-risk serotypes, oncogenic HPV serotypes can integrate into human DNA (Fig. 30-1). As a result, with infection, oncogenic HPV's early replication proteins E1 and E2 enable the virus to replicate within cervical cells. These proteins are expressed at high levels early in HPV infection. They can lead to cytologic changes detected as low-grade squamous intraepithelial (LSIL) cytologic findings from Pap testing.

Amplification of viral replication and subsequent transformation of normal cells into tumor cells may follow (Mantovani, 1999). Specifically, the viral gene products E6 and E7 oncoproteins are implicated in this transformation (Fig. 30-2). E7 protein binds to the retinoblastoma (Rb) tumor suppressor protein, whereas E6 binds to the p53 tumor suppressor protein. In both instances, binding leads to degradation of these suppressor proteins. The E6 effect of p53 degradation is well studied and linked with the proliferation and immortalization of cervical cells (Jones, 1997, 2006; Mantovani, 1999; Munger, 2001).

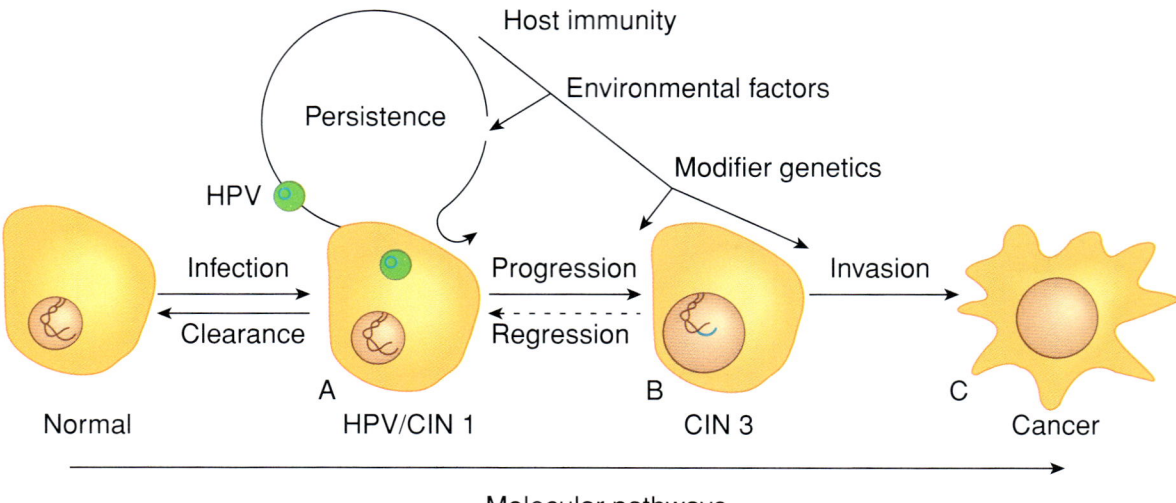

FIGURE 30-1 Critical end points lie on the spectrum of cervical dysplasia. **A.** This initial point shows the cell at risk due to active HPV infection. The HPV genome (*blue ring*) exists as a plasmid, separate from the host DNA. **B.** The clinically relevant preinvasive lesion, cervical intraepithelial neoplasia 3 (CIN 3) or carcinoma in situ (CIS), is an intermediate stage in cervical cancer development. The HPV genome has become integrated into the host DNA, resulting in increased proliferative ability. **C.** Interactive effects between environmental insults, host immunity, and somatic cell genomic variations lead to invasive cervical cancer.

■ Tumor Spread

Following tumorigenesis, the pattern of local growth may be exophytic if a cancer arises from the ectocervix, or may be endophytic if it arises from the endocervical canal (Fig. 30-3). Lesions lower in the canal and on the ectocervix are more likely to be clinically visible during physical examination. Alternatively, growth may be infiltrative, and in these cases, ulcerated lesions are common if necrosis accompanies this growth. As primary lesions enlarge and lymphatic involvement progresses, local invasion increases and will eventually become extensive.

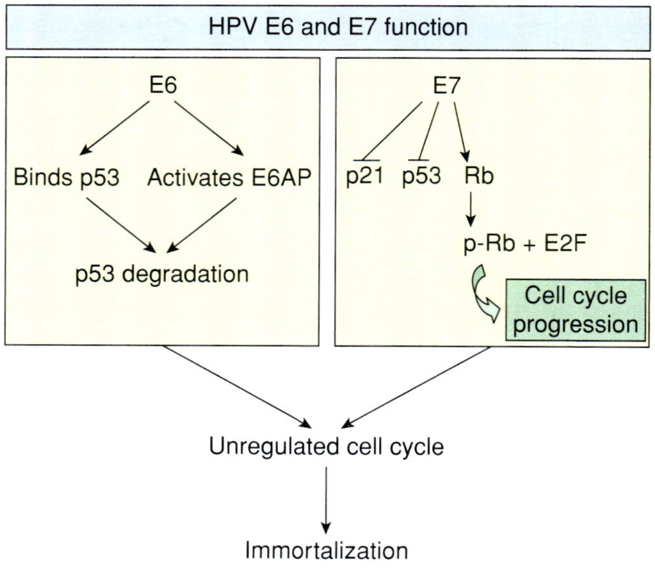

Lymphatic Spread

Lymph Node Groups. The pattern of tumor spread typically follows cervical lymphatic drainage. Thus, familiarity with this drainage aids understanding the surgical steps of radical hysterectomy performed for this cancer (Section 46-1, p. 1160). The cervix has a rich network of lymphatics, which follow the course of the uterine artery (Fig. 30-4). These channels drain principally into the paracervical and parametrial lymph nodes. These lymph nodes are clinically important and thus are removed as part of parametrial resection during radical hysterectomy. From the parametrial and paracervical nodes, lymph subsequently flows into the obturator lymph nodes and into the internal, external, common iliac lymph nodes, and ultimately the paraaortic lymph nodes. Accordingly, pelvic and paraaortic lymph nodes are also traditionally removed concurrently with radical hysterectomy. In contrast, lymphatic channels from the posterior cervix course through the rectal pillars and the uterosacral ligaments to the rectal lymph nodes. These nodes also are encountered and are removed during the extended resection of the uterosacral ligaments that is characteristic of radical hysterectomy.

Lymphovascular Space Involvement. As tumor invades deeper into the stroma, it enters blood capillaries and lymphatic channels (Fig. 30-5). Termed *lymphovascular space involvement (LVSI)*, this type of invasive growth is not included in the clinical staging of cervical cancer. However, its presence is regarded as a poor prognostic indicator, especially in early-stage cervical

FIGURE 30-2 Effects of E6 and E7 oncoproteins. On the left, viral oncoprotein E6 directly binds p53 and also activates E6AP to degrade p53 tumor suppressor protein. On the right, E7 oncoprotein phosphorylates retinoblastoma tumor suppressor protein, resulting in release of E2F transcription factors, which are involved in cell cycle progression. E7 also downregulates p21 tumor suppressor protein production and subverts p53 function. The cumulative effect of E6 and E7 oncoproteins eventually results in cell cycle alteration, promoting uncontrolled cell proliferation.

HPV E6 and E7 function

E6 — Binds p53 — Activates E6AP — p53 degradation

E7 — p21 — p53 — Rb — p-Rb + E2F — Cell cycle progression

Unregulated cell cycle

Immortalization

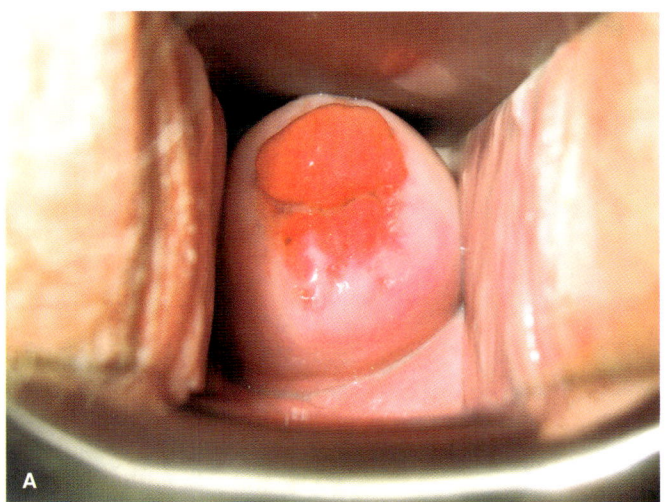
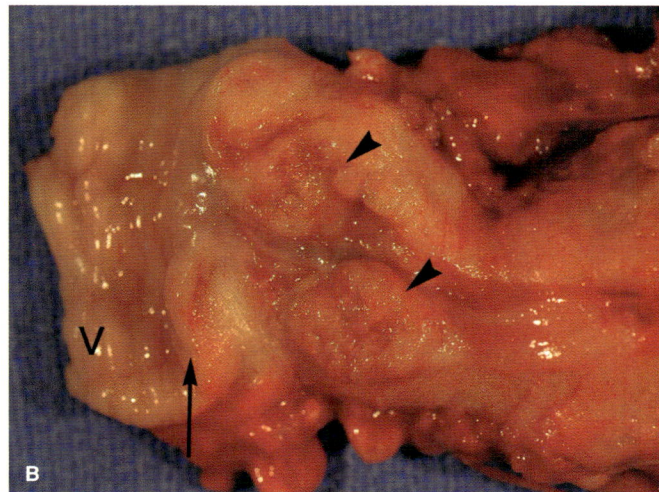

FIGURE 30-3 Cervical adenocarcinoma. **A.** Invasive cancer originating from the endocervix. (Reproduced with permission from Dr. David Miller.) **B.** Exophytic growth of cervical adenocarcinoma into the endocervical canal (*arrowheads*). In this radical hysterectomy specimen, proximal vagina (*V*) is excised with the cervix, and an arrow marks the ectocervix.

cancers. Thus, the presence of LVSI often requires tailoring the planned surgical procedure and adjuvant radiation treatment.

Local and Distant Tumor Extension

With extension through the parametria to the pelvic sidewall, ureteral blockage frequently develops, resulting in hydronephrosis (Fig. 30-6). Additionally, the bladder may be invaded by direct

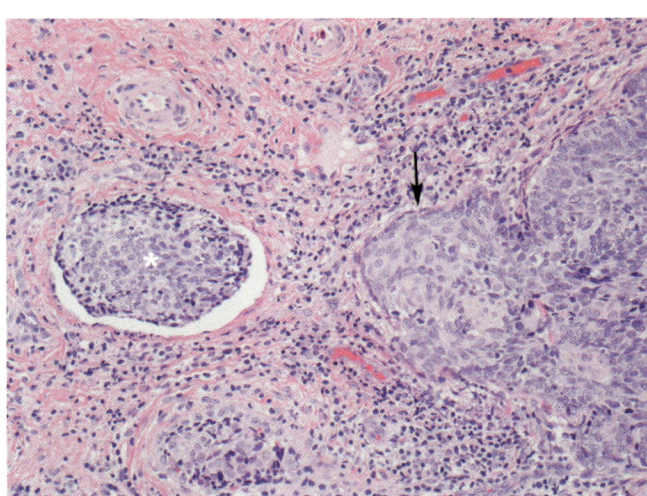

FIGURE 30-5 This poorly differentiated squamous cell carcinoma shows both stromal invasion (*arrow*) and lymphovascular space invasion (*asterisk*). With LVSI here, tumor plugs a lymphatic channel. (Reproduced with permission from Dr. Kelley Carrick.)

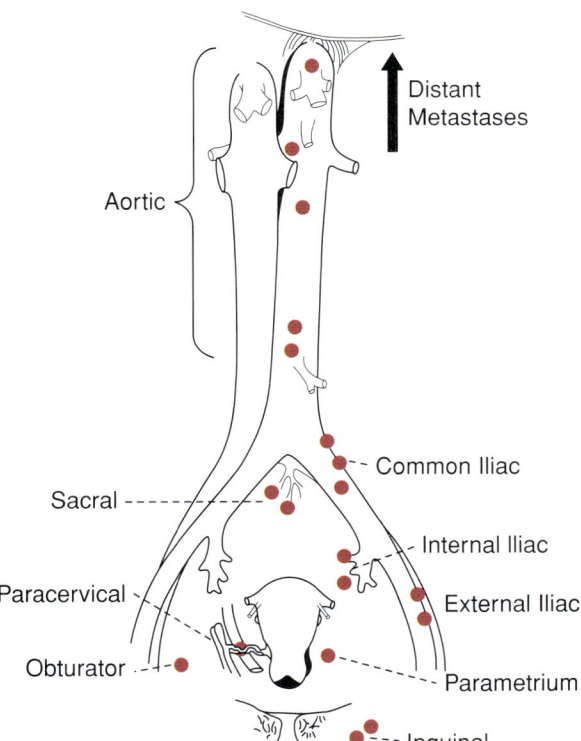

FIGURE 30-4 Lymphatic drainage of the cervix. The parametrial lymph nodes are removed during radical hysterectomy. Pelvic and paraaortic nodes also may be removed by lymphadenectomy. (Reproduced with permission from Henriksen E: The lymphatic spread of carcinoma of the cervix and of the body of the uterus; a study of 420 necropsies. Am J Obstet Gynecol 58(5):924, 1949.)

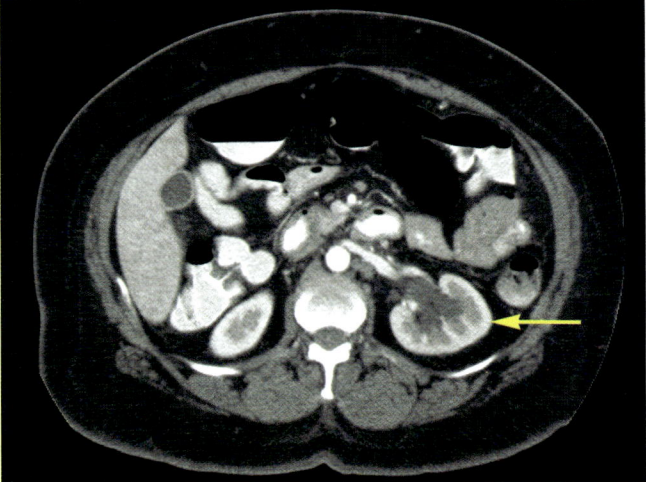

FIGURE 30-6 Computed tomography (CT) scan reveals hydronephrosis (*arrow*) caused by tumor compression of the left ureter.

TABLE 30-2. Histologic Subtypes of Cervical Cancer

Squamous cell
Keratinizing
Nonkeratinizing
Papillary

Adenocarcinoma
Mucinous
   Endocervical
   Intestinal
   Minimal deviation
   Villoglandular
Endometrioid
Serous
Clear cell
Mesonephric

Mixed cervical carcinoma
Adenosquamous
Glassy cell

Neuroendocrine cervical tumor
Large cell neuroendocrine
Small cell neuroendocrine

Others
Sarcoma
Lymphoma
Melanoma

Squamous cell carcinomas represent 70% of all cervical cancer, and adenocarcinomas account for 25% of cervical cancers. The other cell types are rare.

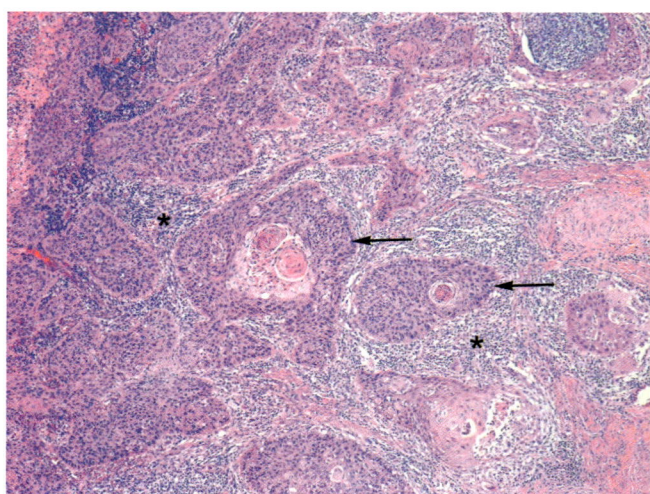

FIGURE 30-7 Invasive cervical squamous cell carcinoma. Irregular nests of malignant squamoid cells (*arrows*) invade the cervical stroma haphazardly and are accompanied by a brisk lymphocytic response (*asterisks*). Some of the tumor nests in this moderately differentiated example have eosinophilic keratin pearls at their center, a classic diagnostic feature of squamous cell carcinoma. (Reproduced with permission from Dr. Raheela Ashfaq.)

tumor extension through the vesicouterine ligaments (bladder pillars). The rectum is invaded less often because it is anatomically separated from cervix by the posterior cul-de-sac. Distant metastasis results from hematogenous dissemination, and the lungs, ovaries, liver, and bone are the most frequently affected.

HISTOLOGIC TYPES

■ Squamous Cell Carcinoma

The two most common histologic subtypes of cervical cancer are squamous cell and adenocarcinoma (Table 30-2). Of these, squamous cell tumors predominate, make up approximately 70 percent of all cervical cancers, and arise from the ectocervix. Over the past 30 years, the incidence of squamous cell cancers has declined, whereas that of cervical adenocarcinoma has risen. These changes may be attributed to an improved method of screening for early squamous lesions of the cervix (Vizcaino, 2000). Squamous cell carcinomas can be subdivided into keratinizing and nonkeratinizing carcinomas (Fig. 30-7).

■ Adenocarcinomas

Adenocarcinomas are a group of cervical cancers composed of the subtypes listed in Table 30-2. Adenocarcinomas make up

25 percent of cervical cancers and arise from the endocervical mucus-producing columnar cells. Because of this origin within the endocervix, adenocarcinomas are often occult and may be advanced before becoming clinically evident. They often give the cervix a palpable barrel shape during pelvic examination.

Adenocarcinomas exhibit various histologic patterns. Of these, *mucinous adenocarcinomas* are the most common and are subdivided as shown in Table 30-2. The mucinous endocervical type retains resemblance to normal endocervical tissue (Fig. 30-8). In

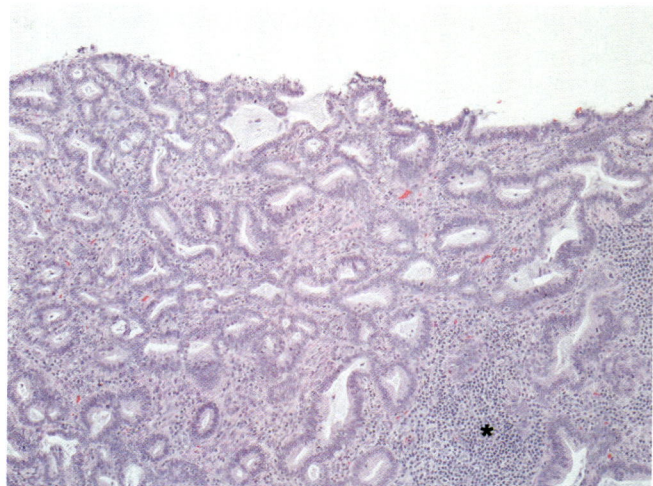

FIGURE 30-8 Invasive endocervical adenocarcinoma. This endocervical adenocarcinoma of usual (HPV-related) type is characterized by columnar, relatively mucin-poor cells with stratified, atypical nuclei and brisk mitotic activity. Tumor cells form glands that resemble native endocervical glands but invade the stroma haphazardly. A chronic inflammatory infiltrate is present at right (*asterisk*). (Reproduced with permission from Dr. Kelley Carrick.)

contrast, the intestinal type resembles intestinal cells and may include goblet cells. *Minimal deviation adenocarcinoma,* also known as *adenoma malignum,* is characterized by cytologically bland glands that are abnormal in size and shape. These tumors contain a greater number of glands positioned at a deeper level than normal endocervical glands. Women with Peutz-Jeghers syndrome are at higher risk of developing adenoma malignum. *Villoglandular adenocarcinomas* are made up of surface papillae. *Endometrioid adenocarcinomas* are the second most frequently identified and display glands resembling those of the endometrium. *Serous carcinoma* is identical to serous carcinomas of the ovaries or uterus and is rare. *Clear cell adenocarcinoma* accounts for less than 5 percent of cervical adenocarcinomas and is named for its clear cytoplasm (Jaworski, 2009). Rarely, adenocarcinomas arise in mesonephric remnants in the cervix, termed *mesonephric adenocarcinomas.*

Prognosis Comparison

Evidence describing the prognosis of squamous cell carcinoma compared with that of adenocarcinoma is contradictory. For stage IB and IIA cervical cancer, one study showed a statistically significant lower overall survival rate in those with adenocarcinoma compared with women with squamous cell carcinoma (Landoni, 1997). However, the Gynecologic Oncology Group (GOG) found in a subsequent study that overall survival rates in women with stage IB squamous and adenocarcinomas of the cervix are similar (Look, 1996). For advanced-stage (stage IIB to IVA) cancers, evidence suggests that cervical adenocarcinomas may portend a poorer overall survival rate compared with similarly staged squamous cell carcinomas (Eifel, 1990; Lea, 2002). The 2006 International Federation of Obstetricians and Gynecologists (FIGO) annual report, which reported on more than 11,000 squamous cell carcinomas and 1613 adenocarcinomas, demonstrated that women with adenocarcinomas have worse overall survival rates at every stage compared with those with squamous cell carcinoma (Quinn, 2006). In sum, evidence suggests that adenocarcinoma of the cervix is a high-risk cell type.

Other Tumor Types

Mixed cervical carcinomas are rare. Of these, *adenosquamous carcinomas* do not differ grossly from adenocarcinomas of the cervix. The squamous component is poorly differentiated and shows little keratinization. *Glassy cell carcinoma* describes a form of poorly differentiated adenosquamous carcinoma in which cells display cytoplasm with a ground-glass appearance.

Neuroendocrine tumors of the cervix include large cell and small cell tumors. These rare tumors are highly aggressive, and even early-stage cancers have a relatively low disease-free survival rate despite treatment with radical hysterectomy and adjuvant chemotherapy (Gardner, 2011; Viswanathan, 2004). Often, neuroendocrine markers, including chromogranin, synaptophysin, and CD56, are used to confirm the diagnosis. Uncommonly, endocrine and paraendocrine tumors are associated with these neuroendocrine tumors.

Of other rare types, the cervix may be the site of sarcomas, malignant lymphomas, and melanomas. Cervical leiomyosarcomas and cervical stromal sarcomas have a poor prognosis, similar to that for uterine sarcomas. Melanomas often present as ulcerated blue or black nodules and also have a poor prognosis.

DIAGNOSIS

Symptoms

Some women diagnosed with this cancer are asymptomatic. In others, early-stage cervical cancer may create a watery, blood-tinged vaginal discharge. Intermittent vaginal bleeding that follows coitus or douching also can be noted. As a malignancy enlarges, bleeding typically intensifies, and occasionally, a woman presents with uncontrolled hemorrhage from a tumor bed. In such cases, bleeding can often be controlled with a combination of Monsel paste (ferric subsulfate) and vaginal packing. Topical acetone can also be used to obtain hemostasis, especially in cases refractory to Monsel paste (Patsner, 1993). Burning from acetone makes it a less desirable choice than Monsel paste. With vaginal packing, the patient ideally remains at bed rest, and a Foley catheter is concurrently inserted to drain the bladder. The pack may interfere with normal voiding, and the catheter also allows for accurate monitoring of urine output during volume resuscitation. If bleeding continues, emergent radiation can be delivered. Alternatively, internal iliac artery embolization or ligation can be performed in cases of refractory hemorrhage. However, caution is used for these latter two options, as tumor oxygenation is impaired if the blood supply is occluded. Radiation therapy is a primary component of advanced-stage cancer, and as noted in Chapter 28 (p. 614), radiation's effects are diminished in low-oxygen environments. This can translate into worsening disease-specific survival rates (Kapp, 2005). In those with significant bleeding, hemodynamic support of the patient follows that described in Chapter 40 (p. 862).

Physical Examination

Most women with this cancer have normal general physical examination findings. In those with suspected cervical cancer, a thorough external genital and vaginal examination is performed. Because HPV is a shared risk factor for cervical, vaginal, vulvar, and anal cancers, concomitant lesions are sought. With speculum examination, the cervix can appear grossly normal if cancer is microinvasive. Visible disease displays varied appearances. Lesions may be exophytic or endophytic growth; a polypoid mass, papillary tissue, or barrel-shaped cervix; a cervical ulceration or granular mass; or necrotic tissue. A watery, purulent, or bloody discharge also can be seen. For this reason, cervical cancer may mirror the appearance of a cervical leiomyoma, cervical polyp, vaginitis, cervical eversion, cervicitis, threatened abortion, placenta previa, cervical pregnancy, condyloma acuminata, herpetic ulcer, chancre, or a prolapsing uterine leiomyoma, polyp, or sarcoma.

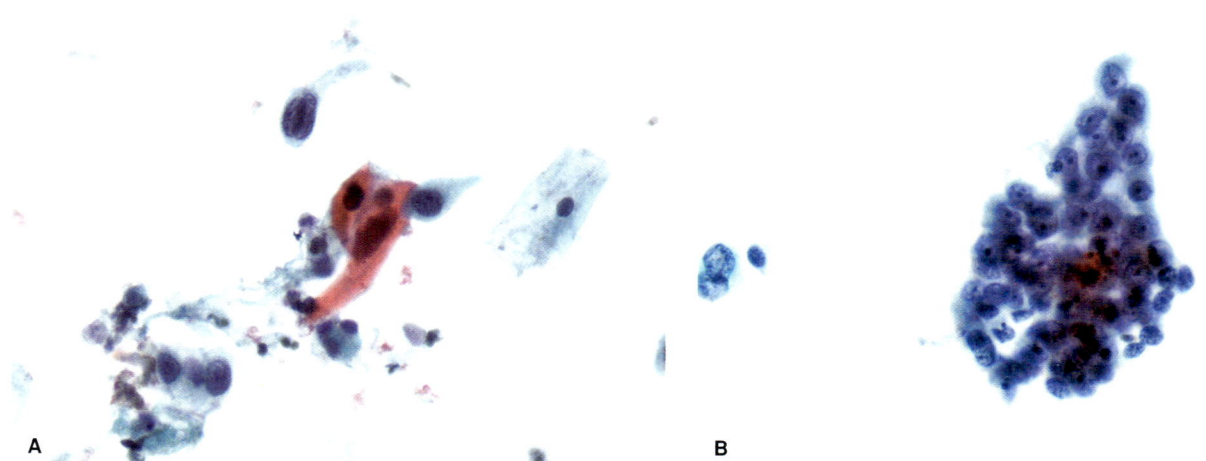

FIGURE 30-9 A. Pap smear, squamous cell carcinoma. Some show spindled tumor cells and/or cytoplasmic keratinization, as evidenced by dense orangeophilic cytoplasm. **B.** Pap smear, endocervical adenocarcinoma. This shows malignant cytologic features including nuclear pleomorphism, nuclear membrane abnormalities, and nucleolar prominence. Cytoplasm tends to be more delicate than in squamous carcinoma and may contain mucin. (Reproduced with permission from Ann Marie West, MBA, CT[ASCP].)

During bimanual examination, a clinician may palpate an enlarged uterus resulting from tumor invasion and growth. Alternatively, hematometra or pyometra may expand the endometrial cavity following obstruction of fluid egress by a primary cervical cancer. In this case, the uterus may feel enlarged and boggy. Advanced cervical cancer cases can extend into the vagina, and disease extent can be appreciated during anterior vaginal wall palpation or during rectovaginal examination. With posterior spread, palpation of the rectovaginal septum between the index and middle finger of an examiner's hand reveals a thick, hard, irregular septum. The proximal posterior vaginal wall is most commonly invaded. In addition, during digital rectal examination, parametrial, uterosacral, and pelvic sidewall involvement can be appreciated. Either one or both parametria may be invaded, and involved tissues feel thick, irregular, firm, and less mobile. A fixed mass indicates that tumor has probably extended to the pelvic sidewalls. However, a central lesion can become as large as 8 to 10 cm in diameter before reaching the sidewall.

With advancing disease, enlarged supraclavicular or inguinal lymphadenopathy suggest lymphatic tumor spread. Lower extremity edema and low back pain, often radiating down the posterior leg, may reflect compression of the sciatic nerve root, lymphatics, veins, or ureter by an expanding tumor. With ureteral obstruction, hydronephrosis and uremia can follow and may occasionally be the initial presenting finding. In these cases, ureteral stenting or percutaneous nephrostomy tube insertion are usually required. Kidney function is ideally preserved for chemotherapy. Additionally, with tumor invasion into the bladder or rectum, hematuria and/or vesicovaginal or rectovaginal fistula may be found.

■ Papanicolaou Test and Cervical Biopsy

Histologic evaluation of cervical biopsy is the primary tool to diagnose cervical cancer. Although Papanicolaou (Pap) tests are performed extensively to screen for this cancer, this test does not always detect cervical cancer. Specifically, Pap testing has only a 53- to 80-percent sensitivity for detecting high-grade lesions on any given single test (Agorastos, 2015; Benoit, 1984; Soost, 1991). Thus, the preventive power of Pap testing lies in regular serial screening (Fig. 30-9). Moreover, in women who have stage I cervical cancer, only 30 to 50 percent of single cytologic smears obtained are read as positive for cancer (Benoit, 1984). Hence, Pap testing alone for evaluation of a suspicious lesion is discouraged. Instead, these lesions are directly biopsied with Tischler biopsy forceps or a Kevorkian curette (Fig. 29-15, p. 637). When possible, biopsies are taken from the tumor periphery, as central portions often contain only necrotic tissue, which will fail to yield a histologic diagnosis. Moreover, biopsies ideally include underlying stroma, so that invasion, if present, can be assessed.

If abnormal Pap testing results are noted, colposcopy is often performed, and adequate cervical and endocervical biopsies are obtained. In some cases, cold-knife conization is needed for this. Indications for colposcopy and conization are outlined in Chapter 29, and cervical punch biopsies or conization specimens are the most accurate for allowing assessment of cervical cancer invasion. Both sample types typically contain underlying stroma and enable differentiation between invasive and in situ carcinomas. For this determination, conization specimens provide a larger tissue sample and are most helpful. However, the diagnostic value of conization is balanced against its higher short- and long-term risks compared with punch biopsy.

STAGING

The staging system widely used for cervical cancer is that developed by the International Federation of Gynecologists and Obstetricians (FIGO) in collaboration with the World Health Organization (WHO) and the International Union Against

TABLE 30-3. Clinical Stages of Cervical Cancer (FIGO, Revised 2018)

Stage	Characteristics[a]
0	**Carcinoma in situ, cervical intraepithelial lesion (CIN) 3**
I	**Carcinoma is strictly confined to cervix (extension to corpus should be disregarded)**
IA	Microscopic lesion, invasion is limited to measured stromal invasion with a maximum depth <5 mm
IA1	Measured invasion of stroma <3 mm in depth
IA2	Measured invasion of stroma ≥3 mm and <5 mm in depth
IB	Clinical lesions confined to the cervix or preclinical lesions greater than IA
IB1	Invasive carcinoma <2 cm in greatest dimension
IB2	Invasive carcinoma ≥2 cm and <4 cm in greatest dimension
IB3	Invasive ≥4 cm in greatest dimension
II	**Carcinoma extends beyond uterus but has not extended to pelvic wall; it involves vagina, but not as far as the lower third**
IIA	No obvious parametrial invasion
IIA1	Invasive carcinoma <4 cm in size
IIA2	Invasive carcinoma ≥4 cm in size
IIB	Obvious parametrial involvement
III	**Carcinoma has extended to the pelvic wall; on rectal examination there is no cancer-free space between tumor and pelvic wall; tumor involves lower third of vagina; all cases with hydronephrosis or nonfunctioning kidney should be included, unless they are known to be due to another cause; involves pelvic and/or para-aortic lymph nodes[b]**
IIIA	No extension to pelvic wall, but involvement of lower third of vagina
IIIB	Extension to pelvic wall, or hydronephrosis or nonfunctioning kidney due to tumor
IIIC1	Pelvic lymph node metastasis only
IIIC2	Paraaortic lymph node metastasis
IV	**Carcinoma has extended beyond true pelvis or has clinically involved mucosa of bladder or rectum**
IVA	Spread of growth to adjacent pelvic organs
IVB	Spread to distant organs

FIGO = International Federation of Obstetricians and Gynecologists.
[a]Histology and imaging can supplement clinical findings in all stages with respect to tumor size and extent.
[b]Adding documentation of p (pathology) and r (imaging) to indicate method of stage assignment to stage IIIC. The type of imaging modality or pathologic technique should be noted.

Cancer (UICC). Cervical cancer staging was updated in 2018 and is detailed in Table 30-3 and Figure 30-10. Historically, cervical cancer has been staged clinically. The current staging system now incorporates radiologic and surgical evaluation (Bhatla, 2019). Allowable components of clinical staging are cold-knife conization, pelvic examination under anesthesia, cystoscopy, proctoscopy, chest radiograph, and intravenous pyelogram (or this portion of the computed tomography [CT] scan can be used). Table 30-4 lists the role of these elements and also contains radiologic and surgical assessments now incorporated in current staging. The table also describes laboratory tests that are not a part of formal staging but that may contribute additional information. Bullous edema is not sufficient for the diagnosis of bladder involvement, and this involvement must be biopsy proven. Lymph node metastasis is now included in staging. In this chapter, *early-stage disease* refers to FIGO stages I through IIA. The term *advanced-stage disease* describes stages IIB and higher.

Within each gynecologic chapter in this text, staging of each cancer type (cervix, vulva, vagina, uterus, ovary) will be presented. FIGO classification is used for gynecologic cancers. In contrast, the American Joint Committee on Cancer (AJCC) developed the *TNM Staging System*, which is based on the extent of the tumor (T), the extent of spread to the lymph nodes (N), and the presence of metastasis (M).

RADIOLOGIC IMAGING

Imaging is now incorporated into FIGO staging, and accurate evaluation is critical to appropriate treatment planning. For example, early-stage tumors may be treated surgically, whereas more advanced tumors require radiation and/or chemotherapy. Imaging results can tailor treatment for an individual. Lymph node metastases worsen patient prognosis and may be identified with imaging. Thus, radiologic tools such as CT scanning, magnetic resonance (MR) imaging, or positron emission tomography (PET) scanning are commonly used as adjuncts in initial cervical cancer evaluation. PET/CT is commonly used for patients with suspected IB and higher stages.

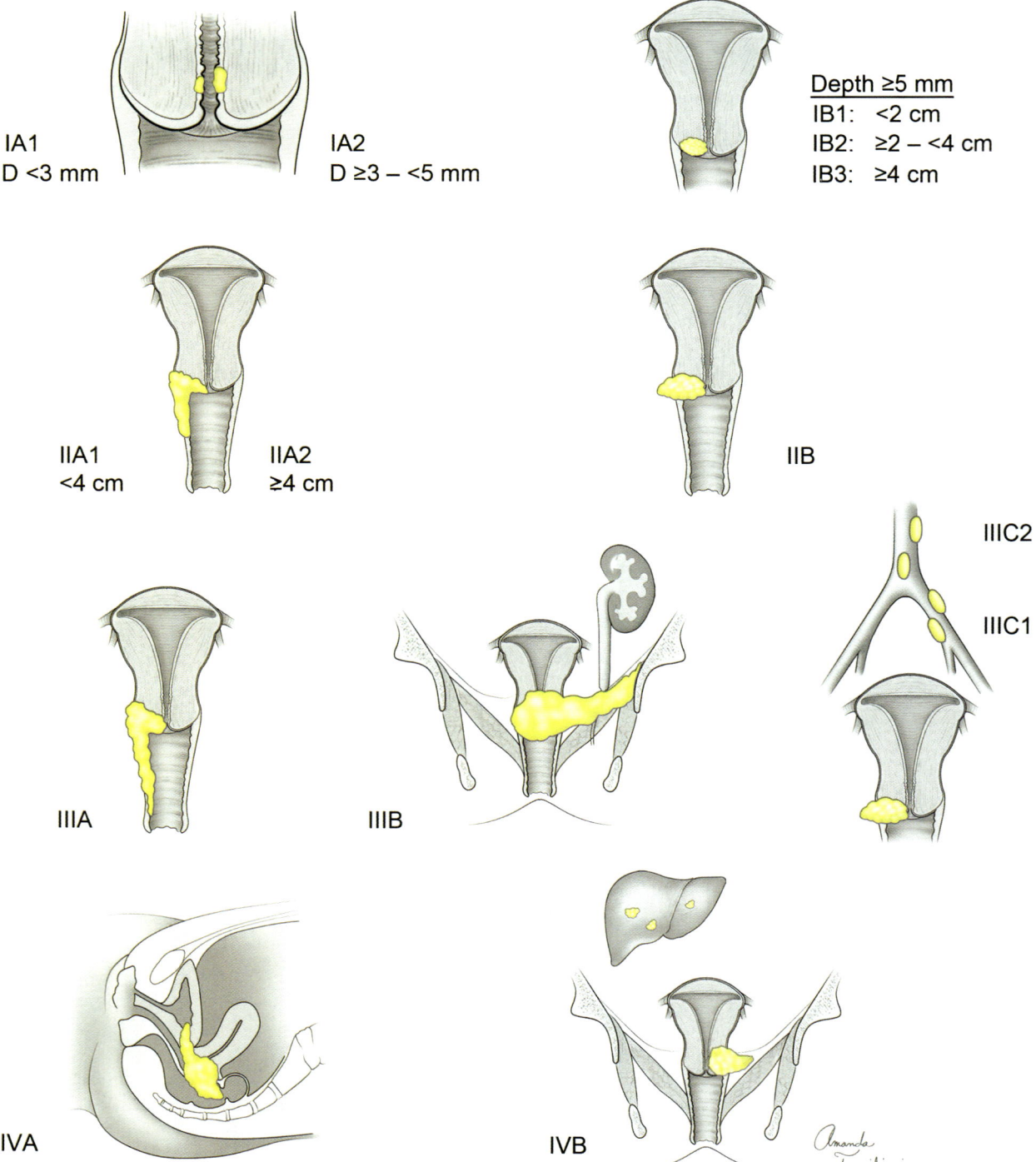

IA1
D <3 mm

IA2
D ≥3 – <5 mm

Depth ≥5 mm
IB1: <2 cm
IB2: ≥2 – <4 cm
IB3: ≥4 cm

IIA1
<4 cm

IIA2
≥4 cm

IIB

IIIA

IIIB

IIIC2

IIIC1

IVA

IVB

FIGURE 30-10 International Federation of Gynecologists and Obstetricians (FIGO) stages of cervical cancer.

Magnetic Resonance Imaging

For defining anatomy, this high-resolution imaging tool offers superior contrast resolution at soft-tissue interfaces. Thus, MR imaging effectively measures tumor size, delineates cervical tumor boundaries, and identifies surrounding bladder, rectal, or parametrial invasion. Unfortunately, MR imaging is less accurate for diagnosing microscopic or deep cervical stromal invasion or identifying minimal parametrial extension (Mitchell, 2006). These particular distinctions are important as both stromal and parametrial invasion may affect suitability for a given planned

treatment. In addition, false-negative findings occur with small volumes of disease and with tissue foci in which cancer cannot be differentiated from scar or necrosis. In these cases, PET scanning identifies metabolic rather than anatomic changes and can be a complementary tool.

For primary cervical cancer, MR imaging is superior to CT for determining carcinoma size, local tumor extension, and lymph node involvement (Bipat, 2003; Mitchell, 2006; Subak, 1995). MR imaging is often preferred for patients being considered for fertility-sparing radical trachelectomy (Abu-Rustum,

TABLE 30-4. Testing Used During Cervical Cancer Evaluation

Testing	To Identify:
Laboratory	
CBC	Anemia
Urinalysis	Hematuria
Chemistry profile	Electrolyte abnormality
Liver function	Liver metastasis
Creatinine/BUN	Renal impairment or obstruction
Radiologic	
Chest radiograph	Lung metastasis
IVP	Hydronephrosis
CT scan (abdominopelvic)	Nodal or distant organ metastasis; hydronephrosis
MR imaging	Local parametrial invasion; nodal metastasis; tumor size
PET scan	Nodal or distant organ metastasis
Procedural	
Cystoscopy	Bladder tumor invasion
Proctoscopy	Rectal tumor invasion
EUA	Extent of pelvic tumor spread; clinical staging
Lymph node evaluation	Presence of lymph node metastases

BUN = blood urea nitrogen; CBC = complete blood count; CT = computed tomography; EUA = examination under anesthesia; IVP = intravenous pyelogram; MR = magnetic resonance; PET = positron emission tomography. Lymph node evaluation can include sentinel lymph node biopsy, removal of suspicious lymph nodes, or lymphadenectomy.

2008; Olawaiye, 2009). Overall, however, both MR imaging and CT perform similarly in cervical cancer (Hricak, 2005).

■ Computed Tomography

This is the most widely used imaging tool for the assessment of nodal involvement and distant metastatic disease. It offers high-resolution depiction of anatomy, especially when used with contrast. CT scanning is obtained in many women with cervical cancer to evaluate tumor size and bulky extension beyond the cervix. CT can also aid detection of enlarged lymph nodes, ureteral obstruction, or distant metastasis (Follen, 2003).

However, CT has limitations similar to MR imaging. CT is not accurate for assessing subtle parametrial invasion or deep cervical stromal invasion because of its poor soft-tissue contrast resolution. CT is also limited by its inability to detect small-volume metastatic involvement in normal-size lymph nodes. Moreover, internal node architecture is often poorly defined. This makes distinction between reactive lymph node hyperplasia and true metastatic disease difficult.

■ Positron Emission Tomography

This nuclear medicine imaging technique creates an image of functional processes within the body. With FDG-PET, a radiolabeled analogue of glucose, fluorodeoxyglucose (FDG), is injected intravenously and is taken up by metabolically active cells such as tumor cells. PET provides a poor depiction of detailed anatomy, thus scans are frequently read side-by-side with CT scans. The combination allows correlation of metabolic and anatomic data. As a result, current PET scanners are now commonly integrated with CT scanners, and the two scans can be performed during the same session (Fig. 2-33, p. 51).

FDG-PET is superior to CT or MR imaging for lymph node metastasis identification (Belhocine, 2002; Havrilesky, 2005; Selman, 2008). However, PET is insensitive for lymphatic metastasis <5 mm. Moreover, its role in early-stage smaller, resectable tumors is limited (Sironi, 2006; Wright, 2005). PET scans can be useful in planning radiation treatment fields and also in identifying those patients who have distant metastatic disease and are candidates for palliative chemotherapy rather than curative-intent chemoradiation therapy.

LYMPH NODE DISSECTION

As a part of primary cancer staging, surgical evaluation of retroperitoneal pelvic and paraaortic lymph nodes offers accurate metastasis detection that is superior to radiologic imaging (Goff, 1999). This information is now incorporated into 2018 FIGO staging system. As a result, lymph node dissection may modify a patient's primary treatment strategy based on the level of nodal disease. For example, radiation fields may be altered to ensure that patients with negative paraaortic lymph nodes are not overtreated with extended-field radiation and that patients with positive paraaortic lymph nodes are not undertreated. Potential candidates include patients with positive or suspected positive pelvic nodes undergoing chemoradiation treatment. Supporting studies show that if positive pelvic/paraaortic nodes are identified, patients may receive a significant survival benefit from extended chemotherapy and/or extended field radiation therapy (Hacker, 1995; Holcomb, 1999; Leblanc, 2007).

In addition, tumor-laden nodes may be debulked. Several studies report similar disease-free survival rates for patients whose macroscopic nodal disease is resected compared with women with microscopic nodal disease (Cosin, 1998; Downey, 1989; Hacker, 1995). That said, there is virtually no long-term survival for patients with unresectable bulky paraaortic lymph nodes.

During lymphadenectomy, most experts recommend lymph node dissection in the common iliac and paraaortic region and resection of macroscopic lymph nodes (Querleu, 2000). Traditional laparotomy and minimally invasive surgery (MIS) approaches have been compared. Although diagnostically equivalent, laparoscopic approaches offer postoperative MIS advantages. In addition, laparoscopic lymph node dissection has been associated with significantly less radiation morbidity than that with radiation following laparotomic approaches (Vasilev, 1995).

Despite these suggested benefits, some experts argue that the benefits of surgical staging, if any, are minimal. These studies estimate only a 4- to 6-percent survival benefit after aggressive surgical debulking of retroperitoneal lymph nodes (Kupets, 2002; Petereit, 1998).

PROGNOSIS

The significance of tumor burden on survival rates is well demonstrated, whether measured by FIGO stage, centimeter size, or surgical staging (Stehman, 1991). Of these definers, FIGO stage is the most significant prognostic factor (Table 30-5). Lymph node involvement is an important prognostic feature, and modified prognosis before it was formally incorporated into the staging system. For example, in early-stage cervical cancer (stages I through IIA), nodal metastases are an independent predictor of survival (Delgado, 1990; Tinga, 1990). One GOG study demonstrated a 3-year survival rate of 86 percent for women with early-stage cervical cancer and negative pelvic lymph nodes, compared with a 3-year survival rate of 74 percent in patients who had one or more positive lymph nodes (Delgado, 1990).

In addition, the number of nodal metastases is predictive. Studies demonstrate significantly higher 5-year survival rates in those with one positive lymph node compared with rates in women with multiple involved nodes (Tinga, 1990). In advanced-stage (stage IIB through IV) cervical cancer, lymph node metastases also worsen prognosis. In general, microscopic

nodal involvement has a better prognosis than macroscopic nodal disease (Cosin, 1998; Hacker, 1995).

EARLY-STAGE PRIMARY DISEASE TREATMENT

■ Stage IA

The term *microinvasive cervical cancer* identifies this group of small tumors. By definition, these tumors are not visible to the naked eye. Specifically, criteria for stage IA tumors limit invasion depth to <5 mm (see Table 30-4). The microscopic lateral extent of the tumor is no longer factored (Bhatla, 2019). Stage IA tumors are further divided into IA1 and IA2. This subdivision reflects the greater risk for lymph node involvement with increasing depth of invasion. That said, microinvasive cervical cancer carries a minor risk of lymph node involvement and excellent prognosis following treatment.

Stage IA1

These microinvasive tumors invade <3 mm and are associated with the lowest risk for lymph node metastasis. Squamous cervical cancers with stromal invasion <1 mm have a 1-percent risk of nodal metastasis, and those with 1 to 3 mm of stromal invasion carry a 1.5-percent risk. Of 4098 women studied with this tumor stage, <1 percent died of disease following surgery (Ostor, 1995). Because of the low risk of spread into the parametrial or uterosacral nodes, these lesions may be effectively treated with cervical conization alone (Table 30-6) (Keighley, 1968; Kolstad, 1989; Morris, 1993; Ostor, 1994). However, a total extrafascial hysterectomy (type I hysterectomy) is preferred for women who have completed childbearing. Hysterectomy types are described in Table 30-7.

In stage IA1 microinvasive cancers, the presence of LVSI increases the risk of lymph node metastasis and cancer recurrence to approximately 5 percent. Accordingly, at our institution, these cases are traditionally managed with modified radical hysterectomy (type II hysterectomy) and pelvic lymphadenectomy. Radical trachelectomy with pelvic lymph node dissection can be considered in those patients desiring fertility preservation (Olawaiye, 2009).

Adenocarcinomas are typically diagnosed at a more advanced stage than squamous cell cervical cancers. Thus, microinvasive adenocarcinomas present a unique management dilemma, due to sparse data regarding this tumor stage. However, based on evaluation of Surveillance Epidemiology and End Result (SEER) data provided by the National Cancer Institute, the incidence of lymph node involvement is similar to that with squamous cancers (Smith, 2002; Spoozak, 2012). Of microinvasive cervical adenocarcinomas, 59 cases managed with uterine preservation and conization have been reported in the literature (Baalbergen, 2011; Bisseling, 2007; Ceballos, 2006; McHale, 2001; Reynolds, 2010; Schorge, 2000; Yahata, 2010). Of these cases, following conization, no recurrences were identified during surveillance in women without LVSI. According to SEER data, the 5-year overall survival rate for women with stage IA1 adenocarcinoma treated with conization is 98 percent (Spoozak, 2012).

TABLE 30-5. Cervical Cancer Survival Rates According to Stage

Stage	5-Year Survival
IA	100%
IB	88%
IIA	68%
IIB	44%
III	18–39%
IVA	18–34%

Compiled from Grigsby, 1991; Komaki, 1995; Webb, 1980.

TABLE 30-6. General Treatment for Primary Invasive Cervical Carcinoma[a]

Cancer Stage	Treatment
IA1[c]	Simple hysterectomy preferred if childbearing completed ***or*** Cervical conization
IA1[c] (with LVSI)	Modified radical hysterectomy + PLND (consider SNLB) ***or*** Radical trachelectomy + PLND (consider SNLB) for selected patients desiring fertility
IA2[b,c]	Radical hysterectomy + PLND (consider SNLB) ***or*** Radical trachelectomy + PLND (consider SNLB) for selected patients desiring fertility
IB1[b] to IIA1	Radical hysterectomy + PLND (consider SNLB if tumor <2 cm) ***or*** Radical trachelectomy + PLND for selected patients desiring fertility ***or*** Chemoradiation
Bulky IB3 to IIA2	Chemoradiation
IIB to IVA	Chemoradiation ***or*** Rarely pelvic exenteration[d]
IVB	Palliative chemotherapy ***and/or*** Palliative radiotherapy ***OR*** Supportive care (hospice)

[a]For individual patients, recommendations for treatment can vary, depending on the clinical circumstances.
[b]Some institutions perform modified (type II) radical hysterectomy + PLND for stage IA2 lesions and smaller stage IB tumors.
[c]Intracavitary brachytherapy may be selected for nonsurgical candidates.
[d]A patient with stage IVA lesion with a fistula may be a candidate for a pelvic exenteration.
PLND = pelvic lymphadenectomy; SNLB = sentinel lymph node biopsy.

Stage IA2

These microinvasive cervical lesions have stromal invasion that measures ≥3 mm to <5 mm. These cancers have a 7-percent risk of lymph node metastasis and carry a >4-percent risk of disease recurrence. In this group of women, the safety of conservative therapy is yet to be proven. Thus, for this degree of invasion, radical (or modified radical) hysterectomy and pelvic lymphadenectomy is recommended.

For fertility preservation, stage IA2 squamous cervical lesions may be treated with radical trachelectomy and lymphadenectomy. A nonabsorbable cerclage may be placed concurrently with radical trachelectomy to improve cervical competence during pregnancy. These procedures have high cure rates, and successful pregnancies have been reported. If women are carefully selected for age <45 years, smaller tumor size (<2 cm), and negative nodal involvement, then reported recurrence rates are similar to those of radical hysterectomy (Burnett, 2003; Covens, 1999a,b; Gien, 2010; Olawaiye, 2009). Some experts will offer radical trachelectomy to patients with tumors up to 4 cm (stage IB2). However, prior to surgery, approximately one third of patients with this tumor stage will instead be

found to need radical hysterectomy or adjuvant chemoradiation due to intermediate- or high-risk features (Abu-Rustum, 2008; Gien, 2010). Preoperative MR imaging to evaluate the parametria and/or CT scan to evaluate extracervical disease is recommended in these cases. If tumor has extended proximally past the internal cervical os, trachelectomy is contraindicated. Although this technique is promising, it carries a learning curve, and further studies to validate its efficacy are needed.

In addition to stage IA1 tumors, some centers are evaluating the safety of conization or extrafascial hysterectomy for a broader group of women with early-stage cervical cancer, since parametrial involvement in microinvasive cervical cancer is rare (Hou, 2011). One study, which included 51 women with stage IA1 to stage IB1 cervical cancer, demonstrated no recurrences at a median surveillance of 21 months for women treated with conization or extrafascial hysterectomy and no nodal dissection (Bouchard-Fortier, 2014). Two women received adjuvant chemoradiation based on specimen histologic analysis results. In addition, SEER data that included 3987 women with IA1 or 1A2 disease showed similar survival rates for women with adenocarcinoma treated with conization compared with hysterectomy

TABLE 30-7. Tissues Resected During Simple and Extended Hysterectomy

Procedure[b]	Type[c]	Involved Tissues[a]			
		Parametria & Paracolpos	Uterine Vessels	Uterosacral Ligament	Vagina
Simple hysterectomy	I	Preserve	Ligate at uterine isthmus	Transect at uterine insertion	Preserve
Modified radical hysterectomy	II	Removed medial to ureter	Ligate at level of ureter	Transect midway between uterus & rectum	Remove 1–2 cm
Radical abdominal hysterectomy	III	Removed medial to uterine vessel origin	Ligate at origin from internal iliac vessels	Transect near rectum[d]	Remove ≥2 cm
Type	IV[e]	Removed medial to uterine vessel origin	Ligate at origin from internal iliac vessels; ligate superior vesical artery	Transect near rectum	Remove 3/4ths
Type	V[e,f]	Removed medial to uterine vessel origin	Ligate at origin from internal iliac vessels; ligate superior vesical artery	Transect near rectum	Remove 3/4ths
Radical vaginal hysterectomy		Removed medial to ureter	Ligate at level of ureter	Partially removed	Remove ≥2 cm
Radical vaginal trachelectomy		Partially removed	Ligate descending cervicovaginal branch	Transect midway between uterus & rectum	Remove 1–2 cm
Radical abdominal trachelectomy		Removed medial to uterine vessel origin	Ligate at origin from internal iliac vessels	Transect near rectum	Remove ≥2 cm

[a]Pelvic lymph node dissection accompanies all except simple hysterectomy.
[b]Hysterectomy includes corpus and cervix removal. For all procedures, unaffected ovaries may remain in premenopausal women, but entire adnexa are usually removed in postmenopausal patients.
[c]Rutledge classification of extended hysterectomy (Piver, 1974).
[d]Although Piver, 1974, described resection of the entire uterosacral ligament, this is not done in practice today due to the high incidence of urinary retention. Instead, the uterosacral ligaments are divided near the rectum.
[e]Although described by Piver, 1974, these procedures are currently not used clinically.
[f]With Type V, the bladder and proximal ureter are removed and requires utereroileoneocystostomy.

(extrafacial or radical). However, women with squamous cell carcinoma undergoing hysterectomy had improved survival rates compared with women undergoing conization (Spoozak, 2012).

Alternatively, patients with stage IA1 and IA2 cervical cancer can be treated with intracavitary brachytherapy alone with excellent results (Grigsby, 1991; Hamberger, 1978). Potential candidates for vaginal brachytherapy include women who are elderly or who are not surgical candidates due to comorbid medical disease.

Hysterectomy

Women with FIGO stage IA2 through IIA cervical cancer, that is, those without obvious parametrial involvement, may be selected for radical hysterectomy plus pelvic lymph node dissection and with or without paraaortic lymph node dissection. Surgery is appropriate for those who are physically able to tolerate an aggressive surgical procedure, those who wish to avoid the long-term effects of radiation therapy, and/or those who

have contraindications to pelvic radiotherapy. Typical candidates include young women who desire ovarian preservation and retention of a functional, nonirradiated vagina.

Historically, five types of hysterectomy were described by Piver and colleagues (1974). However, hysterectomy techniques used clinically today vary depending on the degree of surrounding tissue that is resected and are categorized as type I, II, or III (see Table 30-7).

Type I hysterectomy is also known as an *extrafacial hysterectomy* or *simple hysterectomy*. It removes the uterus and cervix but does not require excision of the parametrium or paracolpium. It is appropriately selected for benign gynecologic pathology, preinvasive cervical disease, and stage IA1 cervical cancer.

Type II hysterectomy is also known as *modified radical hysterectomy*. With it, the cervix, proximal vagina, and parametrial and paracervical tissues are removed. This hysterectomy is well suited for tumors in patients with stage IA1 cervical cancer who have positive margins following conization and have insufficient cervix to repeat conization. This hysterectomy

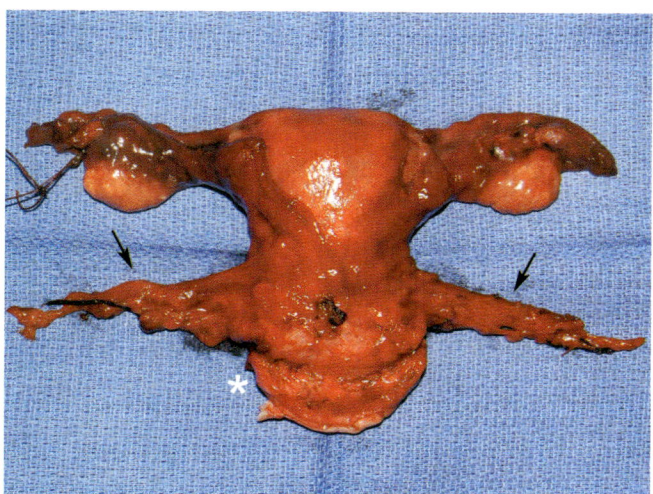

FIGURE 30-11 Gross surgical specimen following radical hysterectomy. The specimen includes the adnexa, uterus, parametria (*arrows*), and segment of proximal vagina (*asterisk*).

is also appropriate for patients with stage IA1 cervical cancer with LVSI. Some institutions perform type II hysterectomies in women with stage IA2 tumors and smaller stage IB tumors with good outcomes (Landoni, 2001).

Type III hysterectomy, also known as *radical hysterectomy*, requires greater resection of the parametria. Its goal is to remove microscopic disease that has extended into the parametrium and paracolpium, and around the uterosacral ligaments. To summarize surgical steps, the uterine arteries are ligated at their origin from the internal iliac arteries near the pelvic sidewall, and all tissue medial to this origin, that is, the parametrium, is resected (Fig. 30-11) (Section 46-1, p. 1160). The ureters are completely dissected from their beds and moved laterally for protection during wide excision of the parametrium and paracolpium. The bladder and rectum are mobilized caudally and off the vagina to permit resection of ≥2 cm of proximal vagina. The uterosacral ligaments are clamped at their midpoint. This procedure is performed for stage IA2, stage 1B2, stage IIA1; for some stage 1B3 lesions; and for patients with relative contraindications to radiation. These contraindications include diabetes, pelvic inflammatory disease, hypertension, collagen disease, inflammatory bowel disease, or adnexal masses.

Previously, the approach for type I, II, and III hysterectomies was abdominal, laparoscopic, robot-assisted, or vaginal. Selection was influenced by patient characteristics and surgeon experience. Advantages of MIS include less blood loss and shorter hospital stay. Intra- and postoperative complications are similar regardless of approach (Ramirez, 2008). However, in 2018, the results of the randomized Laparoscopic Approach to Cervical Cancer (LACC) Trial were published. In this trial, women with FIGO 2009 stage IA1 with LVSI, IA2, or IB1 cervical cancer underwent hysterectomy by a MIS or laparotomy approach. This trial was closed early because women in the MIS group compared with the laparotomy group had worse disease-free rates (86 versus 96.5 percent at 4.5 years) and overall survival rates (93.8 versus 99 percent at 3 years), respectively (Ramirez, 2018). Similarly, in a cohort study of 2461 women

with stage IA2 or IB1 cervical cancer who underwent radical hysterectomy and a median follow-up of 45 months, women who underwent MIS had a higher mortality rate (Melamed, 2018). Subgroup analysis found a higher risk for tumor size >2 cm, but the study was underpowered to detect a difference in tumors <2 cm. If MIS is considered, women should be well counseled regarding all potential risks and benefits.

Radical Trachelectomy

This surgical option can preserve fertility in selected young women with cervical cancer, and the cancer stages appropriate for radical trachelectomy mirror those for radical hysterectomy. Compared with radical hysterectomy, radical trachelectomy is less often performed.

Radical trachelectomy was originally completed vaginally, as described by Dargent (2000), but an abdominal approach is now used more commonly (Abu-Rustum, 2006). The abdominal approach allows for a larger resection of the parametria and is suitable for patients with larger tumors (>2 cm). With radical trachelectomy, steps of radical hysterectomy proceed and thus the uterine vessels are ligated, the parametria is resected, ureterolysis is completed, the bladder and rectum are mobilized, and the upper vagina is resected. To remove the cervix, the uterus is incised at or just below the level of the internal os, with the goal to leave 5 mm of endocervix still attached to the uterus. At this remaining endocervical margin, a thin tissue sample is sharply excised, termed a *shave margin*, and sent for frozen section. If cancer is absent in this specimen, reconstruction may proceed. For this, a cerclage using permanent suture is placed, and the knot is tied posteriorly. The uterus is then stitched to the vagina using absorbable sutures. From each side, the corpus ultimately retains blood supply through the uterine branch of the ovarian artery.

Following radical trachelectomy, women continue to menstruate, and conception can occur naturally. However, cervical stenosis may develop, and thus intrauterine insemination or in vitro fertilization is often needed. Pregnancies are frequently complicated by second-trimester loss and higher rates of preterm birth (Plante, 2005; Shepherd, 2008). In one review of 485 women for whom a radical abdominal trachelectomy was planned, 47 cases (10 percent) were converted to radical hysterectomy. Another 25 women required adjuvant therapy based on final pathologic specimen findings. Thus, 413 women (85 percent) retained fertility. In this fertile cohort, there were 75 pregnancies, 18 miscarriages, and 47 deliveries (19 term, 12 preterm, 16 not stated), and 10 women were pregnant at the time of publication (Pareja, 2013). Cesarean delivery with a classical incision is recommended.

■ Stage IB to IIA

Stage IB lesions are defined as those extending past the limits of microinvasion yet still confined to the cervix. This stage is now subcategorized as IB1 if tumors measure <2 cm or as IB2 if they measure ≥2 cm but <4 cm. Last, IB3 describes lesions measuring ≥4 cm (Fig. 30-12).

Stage II cancers extend outside the cervix. They may invade the upper vagina and the parametria but do not reach the pelvic

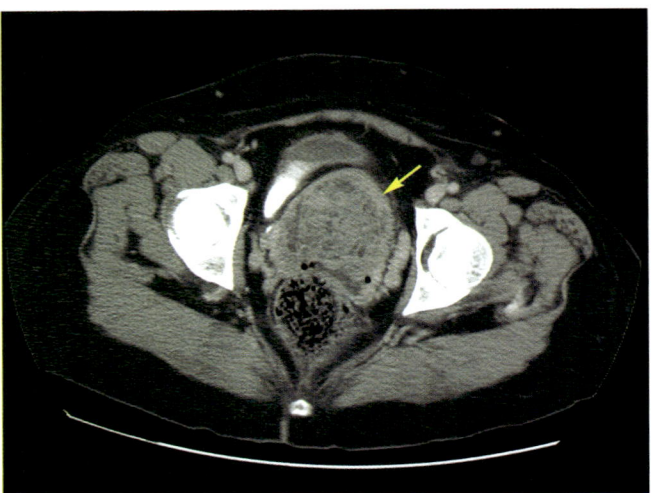

FIGURE 30-12 Computed tomography (CT) scan of stage IB3 cervical cancer (*arrow*).

sidewalls. Stage IIA tumors have no parametrial involvement but can extend vaginally as far as the proximal two thirds of the vagina. Stage IIA is further subdivided into stage IIA1 for tumor size <4 cm and IIA2 for tumor size ≥4 cm. Stage IIB cancer may invade the vagina to a similar extent and also invade the parametria.

Treatment

Stage IB to IIA cancers do not extend into the parametria and thus can be managed with either surgery or chemoradiation. In a prospective study of primary therapy, 393 women were randomly assigned to undergo radical hysterectomy and pelvic lymphadenectomy or receive primary radiation therapy. Five-year overall survival and disease-free survival rates were statistically equivalent (83 percent and 74 percent, respectively). Patients who underwent radical surgery followed by radiation had the worst morbidity (Landoni, 1997).

Because chemoradiation and surgery are both viable options, the optimum treatment for each woman ideally assesses clinical factors such as menopausal status, age, concurrent medical illness, tumor histology, and cervical diameter. For stage IB1 and IIA1 cervical cancers, it is left to the physician's discretion and patient preference as to which treatment modality is preferred. Our general approach to patients with bulky stage IB3 or stage II cervical cancers, that is, those measuring >4 cm, is to manage them primarily with chemoradiation, in a similar fashion to advanced-stage cervical cancers.

In general, radical hysterectomy for stage IB through IIA tumors is usually selected for premenopausal women who wish to preserve ovarian function and for women who have concerns about altered sexual functioning following radiotherapy. Age and weight are not contraindications to surgery. However, in general, older women may have longer hospital stays, and heavier women can have longer operative time, greater blood loss, and higher rates of wound complications. Surgery is contraindicated in patients with severe cardiac or pulmonary disease.

In those electing surgery, oophorectomy may be deferred in younger women. One GOG study evaluated tumor spread to the ovary in those with IB tumors electing radical hysterectomy without adnexectomy. Ovarian metastases were identified in only 0.5 percent of 770 women with stage IB squamous cell cancers and in 2 percent of those with adenocarcinomas (Sutton, 1992). For those electing ovarian preservation, ovarian transposition, accomplished by oophoropexy of the ovary into the upper abdomen, can be performed during radical hysterectomy. This repositioning helps preserve ovarian function, in case postoperative pelvic radiation is indicated. In addition, to reduce complications from radiotherapy that might be needed following radical hysterectomy, a surgeon may perform an omental J-flap. Namely, after surgery, the small bowel may become fixed in the pelvis by adhesions, which renders it vulnerable to radiation damage. The omental J-flap can fill the pelvis to reduce this adhesion risk and is described in Section 46-8 (p. 1186).

Systematic lymphadenectomy can lead to complications such as lymphocyst and lymphedema. Therefore, in women with cervical cancer, sentinel lymph node biopsy is an attractive option to assess lymphatic spread yet avoid extensive nodal resection. As a review, the sentinel node is the first node(s) receiving lymphatic drainage from a given tumor. To find this node, either a blue-colored vital dye or a technetium radioactive tracer or both are separately injected preoperatively into the cervix. At surgery, the sentinel node is stained blue and emits radioactivity discernible by Geiger counter. From a metaanalysis including 67 studies, the pooled sentinel node detection rate was 89 percent and sensitivity was 90 percent. Both were highest in women injected with both radiotracer and dye. Smaller tumor size (<2 cm) and early-stage disease were associated with the highest sensitivity and detection rate (Kadkhodayan, 2015). Sentinel lymph node biopsy can be considered for women with tumors <2 cm and is now included in the National Comprehensive Cancer Guidelines (Altgassen, 2008; Koh, 2019; Salvo, 2017).

Weighing Surgical and Radiotherapy Complications

Complications for early-stage cervical cancer radical surgery include ureteral stricture, vaginal fistulas, bladder dysfunction, constipation, wound breakdown, lymphocyst, and lymphedema. The risk of venous thromboembolism warrants chemoprophylaxis and/or sequential compression devices as outlined in Table 39-10 (p. 834). If radiotherapy is added as an adjuvant to surgery, the risk of many of these is increased.

On the other hand, radiation therapy also carries long-term complications described in Chapter 28 (p. 615). Of these, altered sexual function secondary to a shortened vagina, dyspareunia, psychologic factors, and vaginal stenosis are common. Late urinary and bowel complications such as fistula formation, enteritis, proctitis, and bowel obstruction also may develop following radiotherapy.

Positive Pelvic Lymph Nodes

Approximately 15 percent of patients with clinical stage I through IIA cervical cancers will have positive pelvic nodes. Risk factors for lymph node involvement include those listed in Table 30-8. Of those with involved nodes, 50 percent will have grossly positive pelvic nodes intraoperatively. In most cases involving grossly positive nodes, radical hysterectomy is

TABLE 30-8. Percentage of Cases with Positive Pelvic Lymph Nodes by Pathologic Factors[a]

Factor	(%)	p value
Histologic grade		0.01
1	9.7	
2	13.9	
3	21.8	
Keratinizing/cell size		0.6
Large cell nonkeratinizing	14.5	
Large cell keratinizing	17.2	
Small cell/other	17.6	
Depth of invasion		0.0001
≤5 mm	3.4	
6–10 mm	15.1	
11–15 mm	22.2	
16–20 mm	38.8	
21+ mm	22.6	
Stromal invasion		0.0001
Inner third	4.5	
Middle third	13.3	
Outer third	26.4	
Uterine extension		0.2
Negative	14.6	
Positive	21.6	
Surgical margins		0.4
Negative	15.2	
Positive	25.0	
Parametrial extension		0.0001
Negative	13.5	
Positive	43.2	
LVSI		0.0001
Negative	8.2	
Positive	25.4	

[a]Patients with squamous cell carcinoma, no gross disease beyond the uterus and cervix, and negative aortic nodes.
LVSI = lymphovascular space involvement.
Data from Delgado, 1990.

abandoned. After recovering from surgery, whole-pelvic radiation and brachytherapy with concomitant chemotherapy is administered. The 50 percent of patients with involved nodes not grossly identified intraoperatively are considered to be at high risk of recurrence following their radical hysterectomy. As described subsequently, these women require postoperative adjuvant chemoradiation therapy.

Recurrence Risk

For women who have completed radical surgery for early-stage cervical cancer, the GOG has defined risk factors to help identify women for tumor recurrence. *Intermediate risk* describes those who on average would have a 30-percent risk of cancer recurrence within 3 years. Factors included in this model are depth of tumor invasion, clinical tumor diameter, and LVSI.

To determine appropriate treatment, patients with these intermediate-risk factors have been studied. In one trial, women were randomly assigned to receive pelvic radiation therapy following radical hysterectomy or to undergo radical hysterectomy and observation. A nearly 50-percent reduced risk of recurrence was found in those who received postoperative adjuvant radiation therapy (Sedlis, 1999). However, this adjuvant radiation did not prolong overall survival. Notably, these patients did not receive chemotherapy coupled with their radiation. In our practice, these intermediate-risk patients are counseled regarding their recurrence risk and offered the option of adjuvant chemoradiation therapy. A GOG clinical trial (GOG #263) that is assessing chemoradiation in this patient population is ongoing.

A *high-risk* category for early-stage cervical cancer patients who underwent radical surgery also has been described. High risk is defined as a 50- to 70-percent risk of recurrence within 5 years. These women have positive lymph nodes, positive surgical margins, or microscopically positive parametria (Peters, 2000). This group is routinely offered adjuvant radiation therapy. Moreover, the GOG demonstrated that the addition of concurrent chemotherapy significantly prolongs disease-free and overall survival rates in this group of women with high-risk early-stage cancer (Peters, 2000).

Adjuvant Hysterectomy Following Primary Radiation

Treating bulky stage I (previous stage IB2, now IB3) cervical cancers with adjuvant hysterectomy after radiation therapy has been evaluated. Adjuvant hysterectomy reduces locoregional relapse but does not contribute to an overall improvement in survival rates. However, initial lesion size may affect efficacy. In one study, those with tumors measuring <7 cm who underwent postradiation hysterectomy survived longer than did women with equivalent tumors in the radiation-only regimen group. In contrast, those with lesions ≥7 cm who underwent postradiation hysterectomy fared worse than their counterparts receiving only radiotherapy (Keys, 2003).

Early-Stage Cervical Adenocarcinoma

These cancers may be more radioresistant than squamous cell cervical carcinomas. Although some prefer radical hysterectomy to radiotherapy, studies suggest equivalent survival rates with either (Eifel, 1991, 1995; Hopkins, 1988; Nakano, 1995). However, larger lesions may not regress if managed by radiation alone (Leveque, 1998; Silver, 1998). The centers of bulky tumors may be less radiosensitive due to relative cellular hypoxia. This effect underscores the advantages of radical hysterectomy for women with stage I cervical adenocarcinoma.

ADVANCED-STAGE PRIMARY DISEASE TREATMENT

■ Stages IIB to IVA

Advanced-stage cervical cancers extend past the confines of the cervix and often involve adjacent organs and retroperitoneal lymph nodes. Untreated, these tumors progress rapidly.

Management is individualized, yet most advanced-stage tumors have a poor prognosis. Five-year survival rates are <50 percent.

Radiation Therapy

This modality forms the cornerstone of advanced-stage cervical cancer management. Both external beam pelvic radiation and brachytherapy are typically delivered (Chap. 28, p. 611). Of these, external beam radiation usually precedes intracavitary radiation, which is one form of brachytherapy. External beam radiation is commonly administered in 25 fractions during 5 weeks (40 to 50 Gy). During evaluation, if paraaortic nodal metastases are found, extended field radiation can be added to treat these affected lymph nodes.

During brachytherapy, bowel and bladder are moved away from the intracavitary source using vaginal packing during tandem insertion to limit radiation to these organs. Treatment is often prescribed to point A, that is, a point 2 cm lateral and 2 cm superior to the external cervical os, and to point B, which is a point 3 cm lateral to point A. Side effects during and following radiation therapy are common, and these are discussed in Chapter 28 (p. 615).

Chemoradiation

Current evidence indicates that chemotherapy given concurrently with radiation therapy significantly improves overall and disease-free survival rates in women with cervical cancer. Chemoradiation is also associated with superior survival rates compared with pelvic and extended field paraaortic region irradiation alone (Morris, 1999).

After five trials demonstrated improved survival rates, it is now recommended that cisplatin-based chemotherapy should be considered in women undergoing radiation for cervical cancer (Keys, 1999; Morris, 1999; Peters, 2000; Rose, 1999; Whitney, 1999). The characteristics of this agent are described in Chapter 27 (p. 598), and Figure 30-13 describes its tumoricidal action. Nonplatinum regimens also have activity but have not been directly compared with cisplatin-containing regimens

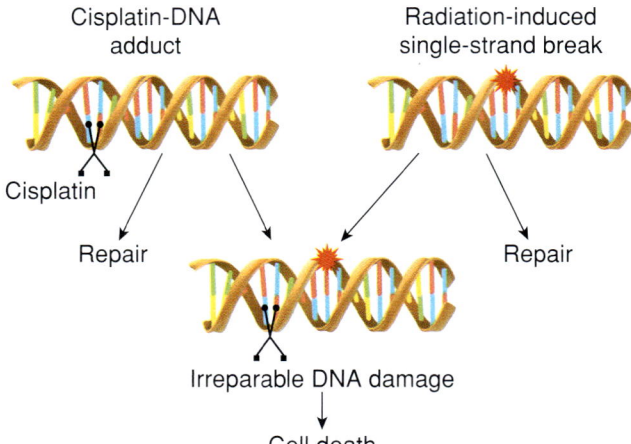

FIGURE 30-13 Cisplatin can bind covalently to DNA bases. Radiation therapy may create single-strand breaks. If occurring alone, each damaging event is likely to be repaired. However, if both occur in close proximity, irreparable damage can lead to cell death.

(Vale, 2008). At our institution, cisplatin is given weekly for 5 weeks. It is administered concurrently with external beam radiation and with brachytherapy. Unfortunately, the recurrence risk remains as high as 40 percent after chemoradiation given for curative intent (Chemoradiotherapy for Cervical Cancer Meta-Analysis Collaboration, 2008). Therefore, a large international randomized Phase III trial is currently evaluating whether the addition of adjuvant chemotherapy after completion of chemoradiation improves overall survival rates for women with stage IB1 with positive nodes and for those with stage IB2 through IVA disease.

Pelvic Exenteration for Primary Disease

This ultraradical surgery encompasses removal of the bladder, rectum, uterus, fallopian tubes and ovaries (if present), vagina, and surrounding tissues (Section 46-5, p. 1180). Primary exenteration may be considered for women with stage IVA cancer, that is, with direct tumor invasion into bladder and/or bowel but without distant spread. Exenteration is rarely performed for this indication, yet for suitable candidates, the survival rate can reach 30 percent (Million, 1972; Upadhyay, 1988).

■ Stage IVB

Patients with stage IVB disease have a poor prognosis and are treated with a goal of palliation. Pelvic radiation is administered to control vaginal bleeding and pain. Systemic chemotherapy is offered to palliate symptoms and prolong overall survival. The chemotherapy regimens used in this group of women are similar to those used in the setting of recurrent cancer (p. 671).

SURVEILLANCE

■ Following Radiotherapy

Women who receive radiotherapy are closely monitored to assess their response. Tumors may be expected to regress for up to 3 months after therapy. Pelvic examination and/or radiologic scanning should document progressive shrinkage of the cervical mass. The rectovaginal examination is used to detect nodularity in the ligaments and parametria. If disease progresses locally after this interval, prognosis is poor. Pelvic exenteration may sometimes be indicated for this clinical setting.

In general, patients are seen at 3-month intervals for 2 years, then every 6 months until 5 years have passed from treatment, and then annually. At each visit, in addition to pelvic examination, a thorough manual nodal survey includes neck, supraclavicular, axillary, and inguinal lymph nodes. A cervical or vaginal cuff Pap test also is collected annually for 20 years after treatment completion. Findings of HSIL lesions with screening should prompt colposcopic evaluation and biopsy of suspicious lesions. If recurrent cancer is diagnosed from these biopsies, then CT or PET/CT imaging is performed.

Once radiotherapy is completed, patients are encouraged to use a vaginal dilator or have vaginal intercourse three times per week. This helps keep the vagina patent, aids pelvic examination and Pap tests in the future, and ensures that the patient can remain sexually active if desired. Otherwise, radiation may result in vaginal fibrosis, which can create a shortened, nonfunctional vagina. The use of a water-based lubricant is recommended.

■ Following Surgery

After a radical hysterectomy, 80 percent of recurrences are detected within the subsequent 2 years. During patient surveillance, an abnormal pelvic mass or abnormal pelvic examination finding typically prompts CT scanning of the abdomen and pelvis. Clinical findings include cervical or vaginal lesion, rectovaginal nodularity, pain radiating down the posterior thigh, or new-onset lower extremity edema. Pelvic recurrences after radical hysterectomy, if diagnosed early, can be treated with radiation therapy. The same schedule of visits and Pap tests as outlined above for surveillance following radiotherapy is then recommended.

■ Hormone Therapy

Cervical cancer is not estrogen-dependent and thus hormone therapy is not contraindicated to treat menopausal symptoms (Chap. 22, p. 480). Moreover, hormone therapy is strongly considered for any premenopausal patient undergoing radiation treatment for cervical cancer until the average age of menopause. This is because radiation doses given for cervical cancer lead to menopause. Ovaries previously transposed out of the pelvic radiation field may be exceptions. Either systemic or vaginal forms of estrogen are suitable. Estrogen alone is used if the uterus has been surgically removed, whereas combination hormonal therapy is given if the uterus remains.

SECONDARY DISEASE

This is defined as either persistent or recurrent cancer. *Persistent disease* is cervical cancer that has not completely regressed within 3 months of finishing radiotherapy. *Recurrent disease* is defined as a new lesion after primary therapy completion and initial regression.

Treatment of persistent or recurrent disease depends on its location and extent. The intent in these cases is usually palliative. However, in certain instances, a woman may qualify for pelvic radiation if she previously had not received this treatment. Alternatively, a woman may be a candidate for curative-intent surgery. Metastatic cervical cancer is not curable. In this setting, the goal of chemotherapy is to maximize existing patient quality of life and prolong survival.

■ Pelvic Exenteration for Secondary Disease

When curative-intent surgery is contemplated, local disease should be biopsy proven. Clinically, a patient may be considered for pelvic exenteration if the triad of lower extremity edema, back pain, and hydronephrosis are absent. If present, these suggest disease extension to the pelvic sidewalls, which would contraindicate surgery. In addition, regional and distant metastasis should be excluded by both physical examination and radiologic imaging, which typically is a PET/CT scan.

Pelvic exenteration begins with exploratory laparotomy, biopsies of suspicious lesions, and paraaortic lymph node evaluation. Exenteration is completed only if no disease is found in frozen section specimens sampled at the beginning of surgery. A complete surgical description of this procedure is found in Section 46-5 (p. 1180).

Alternatively, in highly selected patients, radical hysterectomy may be considered as an alternative to pelvic exenteration (Coleman, 1994). In these circumstances, women should have small cervical recurrences measuring <2 cm and have disease-free pelvic lymph nodes both prior to and during surgery.

With either operation, intraoperative and postoperative complications can be significant. Reported 5-year survival rates approximate 50 percent. Most recurrences occur in the first 2 years postoperatively (Berek, 2005; Goldberg, 2006).

■ Radiotherapy or Chemotherapy for Secondary Disease

Patients with central or limited peripheral recurrences who are radiotherapy naïve are candidates for curative-intent chemoradiation treatment. In these groups, survival rates of 30 to 70 percent have been reported (Ijaz, 1998; Ito, 1997; Lanciano, 1996; Potter, 1990).

Antineoplastic drugs are used to palliate both disease and symptoms of advanced, persistent, or recurrent cervical cancer (Table 30-9). Cisplatin is considered the single most active cytotoxic agent in this setting (Thigpen, 1995). Overall, response duration to cisplatin is 4 to 6 months, and survival in such women only approximates 7 months (Vermorken, 1993). A four-arm prospective randomized study demonstrated that the combinations of cisplatin with topotecan, vinorelbine, or gemcitabine are not superior to the combination of cisplatin and paclitaxel (Monk, 2009). More recently, a randomized study evaluated adding bevacizumab, which is a monoclonal antibody targeting vascular endothelial growth factor (VEGF), to combination chemotherapy. This addition increased the median overall survival length by 3.7 months (see Table 30-9) (Tewari, 2014).

Pembrolizumab (Keytruda) is an immune checkpoint inhibitor against programmed cell death 1 (PD-1), described in Chapter 27 (p. 601). This was approved in 2018 for women with recurrent or persistent cervical cancer with a combined positive score (CPS) ≥1 who have cancer progression despite systemic chemotherapy (Chung, 2019). The CPS is the number of positive PD-L1 cells (tumor cells, lymphocytes, and macrophages), divided by the total number of viable tumor cells and then multiplied by 100.

PALLIATIVE CARE

Palliative chemotherapy is administered only if this treatment does not significantly lower patient quality of life and is balanced against the benefits of supportive care. Women with persistent nausea and vomiting from tumor-associated ileus may benefit from a gastrostomy tube. Bowel obstruction can be managed surgically, provided a patient is an appropriate surgical

TABLE 30-9. Combination Chemotherapy Regimens and Response Rates of Cervical Cancer

Study	Chemotherapy Agents	Response Rates (%)	Progression-Free Survival (months)	Overall Survival (months)
Moore, 2004	Cisplatin vs.	19	2.8	8.8
	Cisplatin and paclitaxel	36	4.8	9.7
Long, 2005	Cisplatin vs.	13	2.9	6.5
	Cisplatin and topotecan	27	4.6	9.4
Morris, 2004	Cisplatin and vinorelbine	30	5.5	—
Brewer, 2006	Cisplatin and gemcitabine	22	2.1	—
Monk, 2009	Cisplatin and paclitaxel vs.	29	5.8	12.9
	Cisplatin and vinorelbine vs.	26	4	
	Cisplatin and gemcitabine vs.	22	4.7	10–10.3
	Cisplatin and topotecan	23	4.6	
Tewari, 2014	Cisplatin and paclitaxel ± bevacizumab vs.	45	7.6	14.3
		50		17.5
	Topotecan and paclitaxel ± bevacizumab	27	5.7	12.7
		47		16.2

candidate. Percutaneous nephrostomy tubes may be placed for urinary fistulas or urinary tract obstruction.

Pain management forms the basis of palliation. Cervical cancer patients can experience significant pain, and this is assessed at each visit. Many will require narcotics (Table 42-3, p. 910). If a patient has been using opioids and is hospitalized for inadequate pain control, patient-controlled analgesia is considered. The total dose that controls the pain in a 24-hour period is determined. This dose can then be converted an equivalent dose of long-acting opioids. To allow for incomplete cross-tolerance between narcotics, the dose should be decreased by 25 to 50 percent. A supplemental short-acting opioid can be available for breakthrough pain and is typically prescribed at a dose that is 10 to 20 percent of the long-acting total daily dose and given at appropriate intervals.

Narcotics can constipate, and patients using these are given a bowel regimen. This can be individualized, and suitable agents are listed in Table 25-5 (p. 566). In particular, a combination of stool softeners (docusate sodium) plus laxative (senna) plus polyethylene glycol is often effective.

We recommend discussion of medical directives if a patient has adequate mental capability. Often, such discussion is conducted over time, giving a woman an opportunity to understand the severity and progression of her disease. Home hospice is an invaluable part of terminal care for most of these women, who require intensive pain management and considerable assistance with daily living activities.

MANAGEMENT DURING PREGNANCY

Survival rates between pregnant and nonpregnant women with cervical cancer do not differ when matched by age, stage, and year of diagnosis. Overall survival rates are slightly better for cervical cancer in pregnancy, because a greater proportion of patients have stage I disease.

■ Diagnosis

A Pap test is recommended for all pregnant patients older than 21 at the initial prenatal visit. Additionally, clinically suspicious lesions are directly biopsied. If Pap test results reveal HSIL, adenocarcinoma in situ (AIS), or suspected malignancy, colposcopy is performed and biopsies are obtained. However, endocervical curettage is excluded to prevent amnionic sac rupture.

If Pap testing indicates malignant cells and colposcopy-directed biopsy fails to confirm malignancy, diagnostic conization may be necessary. Many experts recommend delaying conization until the second trimester due to concern for pregnancy loss. However, median blood loss during excisional procedures increases with gestational age, especially in the third trimester. In pregnant patients, the loop electrosurgical excision procedure (LEEP) does not appear to offer an advantage compared with cold-knife conization. Moreover, one study found a surgical complication rate of 25 percent with LEEP in pregnancy, and 47 percent of the women had persistent or recurrent disease (Robinson, 1997).

■ Stages I and II Cancer in Pregnancy

Women with microinvasive squamous cell cervical carcinoma found during conization that measures <3 mm and contains no LVSI (stage IA1) may deliver vaginally and be reevaluated 6 weeks postpartum. Moreover, for those with stage IA or IB disease, studies find no greater maternal risk if treatment is intentionally delayed to optimize fetal maturity regardless of the trimester in which the cancer was diagnosed. Given the outcomes, a planned treatment delay is generally acceptable for women who are 20 or more weeks' gestational age at diagnosis with stage I disease and who desire to continue their pregnancy.

However, a patient may be able to delay from earlier gestational ages if she wishes. For women who wish to continue pregnancy, pelvic lymph node dissection can be performed in pregnancy in the first and second trimester using MIS

(Vercellino, 2014). Women with positive nodes may elect to be treated with definitive treatment, rather than delay. For definitive treatment with early-stage disease, a radical hysterectomy with the fetus in situ and lymphadenectomy can be performed. Instead, a gravida may opt for neoadjuvant chemotherapy during pregnancy or for early delivery. For patients with stage IA2 through IIA1, a cesarean section via a classical uterine incision may be performed at term, followed immediately by radical hysterectomy and lymph node dissection. Notably, a classical cesarean incision minimizes the risk of cutting through tumor in the lower uterine segment, which can cause serious blood loss and result in tumor spread.

■ Advanced Cervical Cancer in Pregnancy

Women with advanced cervical cancer diagnosed prior to fetal viability are offered primary chemoradiation. Spontaneous abortion of the fetus tends to follow whole-pelvic radiation therapy. For women who decline pregnancy termination, systemic chemotherapy can be administered. Cisplatin with vincristine or paclitaxel can be administered in pregnancy. Rates of congenital anomalies, growth restriction, and preterm delivery are not increased in fetuses of women who receive chemotherapy after the first trimester (Cardonick, 2010). If cancer is diagnosed after fetal viability is reached and a delay until fetal pulmonary maturity is elected, then a classical cesarean delivery is performed. Chemoradiation is administered after uterine involution. For patients with advanced disease and treatment delay, pregnancy may impair prognosis. A woman who elects to delay treatment, to provide quantifiable benefit to her fetus, will need to accept an undefined risk of disease progression.

REFERENCES

Abed Z, O'Leary M, Hand K, et al: Cervical screening history in patients with early stage carcinoma of the cervix. Ir Med J 99:140, 2006

Abu-Rustum NR, Neubauer N, Sonoda Y, et al: Surgical and pathologic outcomes of fertility-sparing radical abdominal trachelectomy for FIGO stage IB1 cervical cancer. Gynecol Oncol 111:261, 2008

Abu-Rustum NR, Sonoda Y, Black D, et al: Fertility-sparing radical abdominal trachelectomy for cervical carcinoma: technique and review of the literature. Gynecol Oncol 103:807, 2006

Agorastos T, Chatzistamatiou K, Katsamagkas T, et al: Primary screening for cervical cancer based on high-risk human papillomavirus (HPV) detection and HPV 16 and HPV 18 genotyping, in comparison to cytology. PLoS One 10:1, 2015

Altgassen C, Hertel H, Brandstadt A, et al: Multicenter validation study of the sentinel lymph node concept in cervical cancer: AGO study group. J Clin Oncol 26:2943, 2008

Baalbergen A, Smedts F, Helmerhorst TJ: Conservative therapy in microinvasive adenocarcinoma of the uterine cervix is justified. An analysis of 59 cases and a review of the literature. Int J Gynecol Cancer 21:1620, 2011

Belhocine T, Thille A, Fridman V, et al: Contribution of whole-body ^{18}FDG PET imaging in the management of cervical cancer. Gynecol Oncol 87:90, 2002

Benoit AG, Krepart GV, Lotocki RJ: Results of prior cytologic screening in patients with a diagnosis of stage I carcinoma of the cervix. Am J Obstet Gynecol 148:690, 1984

Berek JS, Howe C, Lagasse LD, et al: Pelvic exenteration for recurrent gynecologic malignancy: survival and morbidity analysis of the 45-year experience at UCLA. Gynecol Oncol 99:153, 2005

Bhatla N, Berek JS, Cuello Fredes M, et al: Revised FIGO staging for carcinoma of the cervix uteri. Int J Gynaecol Obstet 145(1):129, 2019

Bipat S, Glas AS, van der Velden J, et al: Computed tomography and magnetic resonance imaging in staging of uterine cervical carcinoma: a systemic review. Gynecol Oncol 91:59, 2003

Bisseling KC, Bekkers RL, Rome RM, et al: Treatment of microinvasive adenocarcinoma of the uterine cervix: a retrospective study and review of the literature. Gynecol Oncol 107:424, 2007

Bosch FX, Munoz N: The viral etiology of cervical cancer. Virus Res 89:183, 2002

Bouchard-Fortier G, Reade CJ, Covens A: Non-radical surgery for small early-stage cervical cancer. Is it time? Gynecol Oncol 132:624, 2014

Brewer CA, Blessing JA, Nagourney RA, et al: Cisplatin plus gemcitabine in previously treated squamous cell carcinoma of the cervix: a phase II study of the Gynecologic Oncology Group. Gynecol Oncol 100(2):385, 2006

Bulk S, Berkhof J, Bulkmans NW, et al: Preferential risk of HPV16 for squamous cell carcinoma and of HPV18 for adenocarcinoma of the cervix compared to women with normal cytology in the Netherlands. Br J Cancer 94:171, 2006

Burnett AF, Roman LD, O'Meara AT, et al: Radical vaginal trachelectomy and pelvic lymphadenectomy for preservation of fertility in early cervical carcinoma. Gynecol Oncol 88:419, 2003

Cardonick E, Usmani A, Ghaffar S: Perinatal outcomes of a pregnancy complicated by cancer, including neonatal follow-up after in utero exposure to chemotherapy. Am J Clin Oncol 33:221, 2010

Ceballos KM, Shaw D, Daya D: Microinvasive cervical adenocarcinoma (FIGO stage IA tumors), results of surgical staging and outcome analysis. Am J Surg Pathol 30:370, 2006

Chemoradiotherapy for Cervical Cancer Meta-Analysis Collaboration: Reducing uncertainties about the effects of chemoradiotherapy for cervical cancer: a systematic review and meta-analysis of individual patient data from 18 randomized trials. J Clin Oncol 26:5802, 2008

Chung HC, Ros W, Delord JP, et al: Efficacy and safety of pembrolizumab in previously treated advanced cervical cancer: results from the Phase II KEYNOTE-158 study. J Clin Oncol 37(17):1470, 2019

Coleman RL, Keeney ED, Freedman RS, et al: Radical hysterectomy for recurrent carcinoma of the uterine cervix after radiotherapy. Gynecol Oncol 55:29, 1994

Cosin JA, Fowler JM, Chen MD, et al: Pretreatment surgical staging of patients with cervical carcinoma: the case for lymph node debulking. Cancer 82:2241, 1998

Covens A, Kirby J, Shaw P, et al: Prognostic factors for relapse and pelvic lymph node metastases in early stage I adenocarcinoma of the cervix. Gynecol Oncol 74:423, 1999a

Covens A, Shaw P, Murphy J, et al: Is radical trachelectomy a safe alternative to radical hysterectomy for patients with stage IA-B carcinoma of the cervix? Cancer 86:2273, 1999b

Dargent D, Martin X, Saccetoni A, et al: Laparoscopic vaginal radical trachelectomy. Cancer 88:1877, 2000

Datta GD, Colditz GA, Kawachi I, et al: Individual-, neighborhood-, and state-level socioeconomic predictors of cervical carcinoma screening among U.S. black women: a multilevel analysis. Cancer 106:664, 2006

Delgado G, Bundy B, Zaino R, et al: Prospective surgical-pathological study of disease-free interval in patients with stage IB squamous cell carcinoma of the cervix: a Gynecologic Oncology Group study. Gynecol Oncol 38:352, 1990

Downey GO, Potish RA, Adcock LL, et al: Pretreatment surgical staging in cervical carcinoma: therapeutic efficacy of pelvic lymph node resection. Am J Obstet Gynecol 160:1055, 1989

Dugue P, Rebolj M, Hallas J, et al: Risk of cervical cancer in women with autoimmune diseases, in relation with their use of immunosuppressants and screening: population-based cohort study. Int J Cancer 136:E711, 2015

Eifel PJ, Burke TW, Delclos L, et al: Early stage I adenocarcinoma of the uterine cervix: treatment results in patients with tumors less than or equal to 4 cm in diameter. Gynecol Oncol 41:199, 1991

Eifel PJ, Burke TW, Morris M, et al: Adenocarcinoma as an independent risk factor for disease recurrence in patients with stage IB cervical carcinoma. Gynecol Oncol 59:38, 1995

Eifel PJ, Morris M, Oswald MJ, et al: Adenocarcinoma of the uterine cervix. Prognosis and patterns of failure in 367 cases. Cancer 65:2507, 1990

Follen M, Levenback CF, Iyer RB, et al: Imaging in cervical cancer. Cancer 98(9S):2028, 2003

Gardner G, Reidy-Lagunes D, Gehrig PA: Neuroendocrine tumors of the gynecologic tract: a Society of Gynecologic Oncology (SGO) clinical document. Gynecol Oncol 122(1):190, 2011

Gien LT, Covens A: Fertility-sparing options for early stage cervical cancer. Gynecol Oncol 117:350, 2010

Goff BA, Muntz HG, Paley PJ, et al: Impact of surgical staging in women with locally advanced cervical cancer. Gynecol Oncol 74:436, 1999

Goldberg GL, Sukumvanich P, Einstein MH, et al: Total pelvic exenteration: the Albert Einstein College of Medicine/Montefiore Medical Center experience (1987 to 2003). Gynecol Oncol 101:261, 2006

Grigsby PW, Perez CA: Radiotherapy alone for medically inoperable carcinoma of the cervix: stage IA and carcinoma in situ. Int J Radiat Oncol Biol Phys 21:375, 1991

Grulich AE, van Leeuwen MT, Falster MO, et al: Incidence of cancers in people with HIV/AIDS compared with immunosuppressed transplant recipients: a meta-analysis. Lancet 370:59, 2007

Guan P, Howell-Jones R, Li N, et al: Human papillomavirus types in 115,789 HPV-positive women: a meta-analysis from cervical infection to cancer. Int J Cancer 131:2349, 2012

Hacker NF, Wain GV, Nicklin JL: Resection of bulky positive lymph nodes in patients with cervical carcinoma. Int J Gynecol Cancer 5:250, 1995

Hamberger AD, Fletcher GH, Wharton JT: Results of treatment of early stage I carcinoma of the uterine cervix with intracavitary radium alone. Cancer 41:980, 1978

Havrilesky LJ, Kulasingam SL, Matchar DB, et al: FDG-PET for management of cervical and ovarian cancer. Gynecol Oncol 97: 183, 2005

Helt AM, Funk JO, Galloway DA: Inactivation of both the retinoblastoma tumor suppressor and p21 by the human papillomavirus type 16 E7 oncoprotein is necessary to inhibit cell cycle arrest in human epithelial cells. J Virol 76:10559, 2002

Henriksen E: The lymphatic spread of carcinoma of the cervix and of the body of the uterus; a study of 420 necropsies. Am J Obstet Gynecol 58(5):924, 1949

Holcomb K, Abulafia O, Matthews RP, et al: The impact of pretreatment staging laparotomy on survival in locally advanced cervical carcinoma. Eur J Gynaecol Oncol 20:90, 1999

Hopkins MP, Schmidt RW, Roberts JA, et al: The prognosis and treatment of stage I adenocarcinoma of the cervix. Obstet Gynecol 72:915, 1988

Hou J, Goldberg GL, Qualls CR, et al: Risk factors for poor prognosis in microinvasive adenocarcinoma of the uterine cervix (IA1 and IA2): a pooled analysis. Gynecol Oncol 121:135, 2011

Howlader N, Noone AM, Krapcho M, et al: SEER Cancer Statistics Review, 1975–2016, National Cancer Institute. 2019. Available at: https://seer.cancer.gov/statfacts/html/cervix.html. Accessed July 2, 2019

Hricak H, Gatsonis C, Chi, et al: Role of imaging in pretreatment evaluation of early invasive cervical cancer: results of the intergroup study American College of Radiology Imaging Network 6651–Gynecologic Oncology Group 183. J Clin Oncol 23:9329, 2005

Ijaz T, Eifel PJ, Burke T, et al: Radiation therapy of pelvic recurrence after radical hysterectomy for cervical carcinoma. Gynecol Oncol 70:241, 1998

International Collaboration of Epidemiological Studies of Cervical Cancer: Comparison of risk factors for invasive squamous cell carcinoma and adenocarcinoma of the cervix: collaborative reanalysis of individual data on 8,097 women with squamous cell carcinoma and 1,374 women with adenocarcinoma from 12 epidemiological studies. Int J Cancer 120:885, 2006

International Collaboration of Epidemiological Studies of Cervical Cancer, Appleby P, Beral V, et al: Cervical cancer and hormonal contraceptives: collaborative reanalysis of individual data for 16,573 women with cervical cancer and 35,509 women without cervical cancer from 24 epidemiological studies. Lancet 370(9599):1609, 2007

Ito H, Shigematsu N, Kawada T, et al: Radiotherapy for centrally recurrent cervical cancer of the vaginal stump following hysterectomy. Gynecol Oncol 67:154, 1997

Jaworski RC, Roberts JM, Robboy SJ, et al: Cervical glandular neoplasia. In Robboy SJ, Mutter GL, Prat J, et al (eds): Robboy's Pathology of the Female Reproductive Tract, 2nd ed. Churchill Livingstone Elsevier, 2009, p 273

Jemal A, Siegel R, Ward E, et al: Cancer statistics, 2006. CA Cancer J Clin 56:106, 2006

Jones DL, Munger K: Analysis of the p53-mediated G1 growth arrest pathway in cells expressing the human papillomavirus type 16 E7 oncoprotein. J Virol 71:2905, 1997

Jones EE, Wells SI: Cervical cancer and human papillomaviruses: inactivation of retinoblastoma and other tumor suppressor pathways. Curr Mol Med 6:795, 2006

Kadkhodayan S, Hasanzadeh M, Treglia G, et al: Sentinel node biopsy for lymph nodal staging of uterine cervix cancer: a systematic review and meta-analysis of the pertinent literature. Eur J Surg Oncol 41:1, 2015

Kapp KS, Poschauko J, Tauss J, et al: Analysis of the prognostic impact of tumor embolization before definitive radiotherapy for cervical carcinoma. Int J Radiat Oncol Biol Phys 62:1399, 2005

Keighley E: Carcinoma of the cervix among prostitutes in a women's prison. Br J Vener Dis 44:254, 1968

Keys HM, Bundy BN, Stehman FB, et al: Cisplatin, radiation and adjuvant hysterectomy compared with radiation and adjuvant hysterectomy for bulky stage IB cervical carcinoma. N Engl J Med 340: 1154, 1999

Keys HM, Bundy BN, Stehman FB, et al: Radiation therapy with and without extrafascial hysterectomy for bulky stage IB cervical carcinoma: a randomized trial of the Gynecologic Oncology Group. Gynecol Oncol 89:343, 2003

Koh WJ, Abu-Rustum NR, Bean S, et al: Cervical Cancer, Version 3.2019, NCCN Clinical Practice Guidelines in Oncology. J Natl Compr Canc Netw 17(1):64, 2019

Kolstad P: Follow-up study of 232 patients with stage Ia1 and 411 patients with stage Ia2 squamous cell carcinoma of the cervix (microinvasive carcinoma). Gynecol Oncol 33:265, 1989

Komaki R, Brickner TJ, Hanlon AL, et al: Long-term results of treatment of cervical carcinoma in the United States in 1973, 1978, and 1983: Patterns of Care Study (PCS). Int J Radiat Oncol Biol Phys 31:973, 1995

Koshiol J, Schroeder J, Jamieson DJ, et al: Smoking and time to clearance of human papillomavirus infection in HIV-seropositive and HIV-seronegative women. Am J Epidemiol 164:176, 2006

Kupets R, Thomas GM, Covens A: Is there a role for pelvic lymph node debulking in advanced cervical cancer? Gynecol Oncol 87:163, 2002

Lanciano R: Radiotherapy for the treatment of locally recurrent cervical cancer. J Natl Cancer Inst Monogr 21:113, 1996

Landoni F, Maneo A, Colombo A, et al: Randomised study of radical surgery versus radiotherapy for stage Ib-IIa cervical cancer. Lancet 350:535, 1997

Landoni F, Maneo A, Cormio G, et al: Class II versus class III radical hysterectomy in stage IB-IIA cervical cancer: a prospective randomized study. Gynecol Oncol 80:3, 2001

Lea JS, Sheets EE, Wenham RM, et al: Stage IIB-IVB cervical adenocarcinoma: prognostic factors and survival. Gynecol Oncol 84:115, 2002

Leblanc E, Narducci F, Frumovitz M, et al: Therapeutic value of pretherapeutic laparoscopic staging of locally advanced cervical carcinoma. Gynecol Oncol 105:304, 2007

Leveque J, Laurent JF, Burtin F, et al: Prognostic factors of the uterine cervix adenocarcinoma. Eur J Obstet Gynecol Reprod Biol 80:209, 1998

Ley C, Bauer HM, Reingold A, et al: Determinants of genital human papillomavirus infection in young women. J Natl Cancer Inst 83:997, 1991

Leyden WA, Manos MM, Geiger AM, et al: Cervical cancer in women with comprehensive health care access: attributable factors in the screening process. J Natl Cancer Inst 97:675, 2005

Long HJ III, Bundy EC Jr, Grendys EC Jr, et al: Randomized phase III trial of cisplatin with or without topotecan in carcinoma of the uterine cervix: a Gynecologic Oncology Group study. J Clin Oncol 23(21):4626, 2005

Look KY, Brunetto VL, Clarke-Pearson DL, et al: An analysis of cell type in patients with surgically staged stage IB carcinoma of the cervix: a Gynecologic Oncology Group study. Gynecol Oncol 63:304, 1996

Mantovani F, Banks L: Inhibition of E6 induced degradation of p53 is not sufficient for stabilization of p53 protein in cervical tumour derived cell lines. Oncogene 18:3309, 1999

McHale MT, Le TD, Burger RA, et al: Fertility sparing treatment for in situ and early invasive adenocarcinoma of the cervix. Obstet Gynecol 98: 726, 2001

Melamed A, Margul DJ, Chel L, et al: Survival after minimally invasive radical hysterectomy for early-stage cervical cancer. N Engl J Med 379:1905, 2018

Million RR, Rutledge F, Fletcher GH: Stage IV carcinoma of the cervix with bladder invasion. Am J Obstet Gynecol 113:239, 1972

Mitchell DG, Snyder B, Coakley F, et al: Early invasive cervical cancer: tumor delineation by magnetic resonance imaging, computed tomography, and clinical examination, verified by pathologic results, in the ACRIN 6651/GOG 183 intergroup study. J Clin Oncol 24:5687, 2006

Monk BJ, Sill MW, McMeekin DS, et al: Phase III trial of four cisplatin-containing doublet combinations in stage IVB, recurrent, or persistent cervical carcinoma: a Gynecologic Oncology Group study. J Clin Oncol 27:1, 2009

Moore DH, Blessing JA, McQuellon RP, et al: Phase III study of cisplatin with or without paclitaxel in stage IVB, recurrent, or persistent squamous cell carcinoma of the cervix: a Gynecologic Oncology Group study. J Clin Oncol 22(15):3113, 2004

Moreno V, Bosch FX, Muñoz N, et al: Effect of oral contraceptives on risk of cervical cancer in women with human papillomavirus infection: the IARC multicentric case-control study. Lancet 359:1085, 2002

Morris M, Blessing JA, Monk BJ, et al: Phase II study of cisplatin and vinorelbine in squamous cell carcinoma of the cervix: a Gynecologic Oncology Group study. J Clin Oncol 22(16):3340, 2004

Morris M, Eifel PJ, Lu J, et al: Pelvic radiation with concurrent chemotherapy compared with pelvic and para-aortic radiation for high-risk cervical cancer. N Engl J Med 340:1137, 1999

Morris M, Mitchell MF, Silva EG, et al: Cervical conization as definitive therapy for early invasive squamous carcinoma of the cervix. Gynecol Oncol 51:193, 1993

Munger K, Basile JR, Duensing S, et al: Biological activities and molecular targets of the human papillomavirus E7 oncoprotein. Oncogene 20:7888, 2001

Muñoz N, Franceschi S, Bosetti C, et al: Role of parity and human papillomavirus in cervical cancer: the IARC multicentric case-control study. Lancet 359:1093, 2002

Nakano T, Arai T, Morita S, et al: Radiation therapy alone for adenocarcinoma of the uterine cervix. Int J Radiat Oncol Biol Phys 32:1331, 1995

Olawaiye A, Del Carmen M, Tambouret R, et al: Abdominal radical trachelectomy: success and pitfalls in a general gynecologic oncology practice. Gynecol Oncol 112:506, 2009

Ostor AG: Pandora's box or Ariadne's thread? Definition and prognostic significance of microinvasion in the uterine cervix. Squamous lesions. Pathol Annu 30(Pt 2):103, 1995

Ostor AG, Rome RM: Micro-invasive squamous cell carcinoma of the cervix: a clinico-pathologic study of 200 cases with long-term follow-up. Int J Gynecol Cancer 4:257, 1994

Pareja R, Rendon GJ, Sanz-Lomana CM, et al: Surgical, oncological, and obstetrical outcomes after abdominal radical trachelectomy: a systematic literature review. Gynecol Oncol 131:77, 2013

Patsner B: Topical acetone for control of life-threatening vaginal hemorrhage from recurrent gynecologic cancer. Eur J Gynaecol Oncol 14:33, 1993

Petereit DG, Hartenbach EM, Thomas GM: Para-aortic lymph node evaluation in cervical cancer: the impact of staging upon treatment decisions and outcome. Int J Gynecol Cancer 8:353, 1998

Peters WA III, Liu PY, Barrett RJ, et al: Concurrent chemotherapy and pelvic radiation therapy compared with pelvic radiation therapy alone as adjuvant therapy after radical surgery in high-risk early-stage cancer of the cervix. J Clin Oncol 18:1606, 2000

Piver MS, Rutledge F, Smith JP: Five classes of extended hysterectomy for women with cervical cancer. Obstet Gynecol 44(2):265, 1974

Plante M, Renaud MC, Hoskins IA, et al: Vaginal radical trachelectomy: a valuable fertility-preserving option in the management of early-stage cervical cancer. A series of 50 pregnancies and review of the literature. Gynecol Oncol 98(1):3, 2005

Plummer M, Herrero R, Franceschi S, et al: Smoking and cervical cancer: pooled analysis of the IARC multi-centric case-control study. Cancer Causes Control 14:805, 2003

Potter ME, Alvarez RD, Gay FL, et al: Optimal therapy for pelvic recurrence after radical hysterectomy for early-stage cervical cancer. Gynecol Oncol 37:74, 1990

Querleu D, Dargent D, Ansquer Y, et al: Extraperitoneal endosurgical aortic and common iliac dissection in the staging of bulky or advanced cervical carcinomas. Cancer 88:1883, 2000

Quinn MA, Benedet JL, Odicino F, et al: Carcinoma of the cervix uteri. Int J Gynecol Obstet 95(suppl 1):S43, 2006

Ramirez PT, Frumovitz M, Parja R, et al: Minimally invasive versus abdominal radical hysterectomy for cervical cancer. N Engl J Med 379:1895, 2018

Ramirez PT, Soliman PT, Schmeler KM, et al: Laparoscopic and robotic techniques for radical hysterectomy in patients with early-stage cervical cancer. Gynecol Oncol 110:S21, 2008

Reynolds EA, Tierney K, Keeney GL, et al: Analysis of outcomes of microinvasive adenocarcinoma of the uterine cervix by treatment type. Obstet Gynecol 116:1150, 2010

Robinson WR, Webb S, Tirpack J, et al: Management of cervical intraepithelial neoplasia during pregnancy with LOOP excision. Gynecol Oncol 64:153, 1997

Rose PG, Adler LP, Rodriguez M, et al: Positron emission tomography for evaluating para-aortic nodal metastasis in locally advanced cervical cancer before surgical staging: a surgicopathologic study. J Clin Oncol 17:41, 1999

Salvo G, Ramirez PT, Leenback CF, et al: Sensitivity and negative predictive value for sentinel lymph node biopsy in women with early-stage cervical cancer. Gynecol Oncol 145:96, 2017

Schiffman MH, Bauer HM, Hoover RN, et al: Epidemiologic evidence showing that human papillomavirus infection causes most cervical intraepithelial neoplasia. J Natl Cancer Inst 85:958, 1993

Schorge JO, Lee KR, Sheets EE: Prospective management of stage IA(1) cervical adenocarcinoma by conization alone to preserve fertility: a preliminary report. Gynecol Oncol 78:217, 2000

Sedlis A, Bundy BN, Rotman MZ, et al: A randomized trial of pelvic radiation therapy versus no further therapy in selected patients with stage IB carcinoma of the cervix after radical hysterectomy and pelvic lymphadenectomy: a Gynecologic Oncology Group Study. Gynecol Oncol 73:177, 1999

Selman TJ, Mann C, Zamora J, et al: Diagnostic accuracy of tests for lymph node status in primary cervical cancer: a systematic review and meta-analysis. CMAJ 178:855, 2008

Shepherd JH, Milliken DA: Conservative surgery for carcinoma of the cervix. Clin Oncol 20:395, 2008

Siegel RL, Miller KD, Jemal A: Cancer statistics, 2019. CA Cancer J Clin 69(1):7, 2019

Silver DF, Hempling RE, Piver MS, et al: Stage I adenocarcinoma of the cervix: does lesion size affect treatment options and prognosis? Am J Clin Oncol 21:431, 1998

Sironi S, Buda A, Picchio M, et al: Lymph node metastasis in patients with clinical early-stage cervical cancer: detection with integrated FDG PET/CT. Radiology 238:272, 2006

Smith HO, Qualls CR, Romero AA, et al: Is there a difference in survival for IA1 and IA2 adenocarcinoma of the uterine cervix? Gynecol Oncol 85:229, 2002

Soost HJ, Lange HJ, Lehmacher W, et al: The validation of cervical cytology. Sensitivity, specificity and predictive values. Acta Cytol 35:8, 1991

Spoozak L, Lewin S, Burke WM, et al: Microinvasive adenocarcinoma of the cervix. Am J Obstet Gynecol 206:80, 2012

Stehman FB, Bundy BN, DiSaia PJ, et al: Carcinoma of the cervix treated with radiation therapy. I. A multivariate analysis of prognostic variables in the Gynecologic Oncology Group. Cancer 67:2776, 1991

Subak LL, Hricak H, Powell CB, et al: Cervical carcinoma: computed tomography and magnetic resonance imaging for preoperative staging. Obstet Gynecol 86:43, 1995

Sutton GP, Bundy BN, Delgado G, et al: Ovarian metastases in stage IB carcinoma of the cervix: a Gynecologic Oncology Group study. Am J Obstet Gynecol 166(1 Pt 1):50, 1992

Tewari KS, Sill MW, Long HJ, et al: Improved survival with bevacizumab in advanced cervical cancer. N Engl J Med 370:734, 2014

Thigpen JT, Vance R, Puneky L, et al: Chemotherapy as a palliative treatment in carcinoma of the uterine cervix. Semin Oncol 22(2 Suppl 3):16, 1995

Tinga DJ, Timmer PR, Bouma J, et al: Prognostic significance of single versus multiple lymph node metastases in cervical carcinoma stage IB. Gynecol Oncol 39:175, 1990

Torre LA, Bray F, Siegel RL, et al: Global cancer statistics, 2012. CA Cancer J Clin 65:87, 2015

Trimble CL, Genkinger JM, Burke AE, et al: Active and passive cigarette smoking and the risk of cervical neoplasia. Obstet Gynecol 105:174, 2005

Upadhyay SK, Symonds RP, Haelterman M, et al: The treatment of stage IV carcinoma of cervix by radical dose radiotherapy. Radiother Oncol 11:15, 1988

Vale C, Chemoradiotherapy for Cervical Cancer Meta-Analysis Collaboration: Reducing uncertainties about the effects of chemoradiotherapy for cervical cancer: a systematic review and meta-analysis of individual patient data from 18 randomized trials. J Clin Oncol 26:5802, 2008

Vasilev SA, McGonigle KF: Extraperitoneal laparoscopic paraaortic lymph node dissection: development of a technique. J Laparoendosc Surg 5:85, 1995

Vercellino GF, Koehler C, Erdemoglu E, et al: Laparoscopic pelvic lymphadenectomy in 32 pregnant patients with cervical cancer: rationale, description of the technique, and outcome. Int J Gynecol Cancer 24:364, 2014

Vermorken JB: The role of chemotherapy in squamous cell carcinoma of the uterine cervix: a review. Int J Gynecol Cancer 3:129, 1993

Viswanathan AN, Deavers MT, Jhingran A, et al: Small cell neuroendocrine carcinoma of the cervix: outcome and patterns of recurrence. Gynecol Oncol 93:27, 2004

Vizcaino AP, Moreno V, Bosch FX, et al: International trends in incidence of cervical cancer: II. Squamous-cell carcinoma. Int J Cancer 86:429, 2000

Walboomers JN, Jacons MV, Manos M, et al: Human papillomavirus is a necessary cause of invasive cervical cancer worldwide. J Pathol 189:12, 1999

Webb MJ, Symmonds RE: Site of recurrence of cervical cancer after radical hysterectomy. Am J Obstet Gynecol 138(7 Pt 1):813, 1980

Wei L, Griego AM, Chu M, et al: Tobacco exposure results in increased E6 and E7 oncogene expression, DNA damage and mutation rates in cells maintaining episomal human papillomavirus 16 genomes. Carcinogenesis 35:2372, 2014

Wentzensen N, Vinokurova S, von Knebel DM: Systematic review of genomic integration sites of human papillomavirus genomes in epithelial dysplasia and invasive cancer of the female lower genital tract. Cancer Res 64:3878, 2004

Whitney CW, Sause W, Bundy BN, et al: Randomized comparison of fluorouracil plus cisplatin versus hydroxyurea as an adjunct to radiation therapy in stage IIB-IVA carcinoma of the cervix with negative para-aortic lymph nodes: a Gynecologic Oncology Group and Southwest Oncology Group study. J Clin Oncol 17:1339, 1999

World Health Organization: Cancer today: estimated number of new cases in 2018, worldwide, all cancers, female, all ages. 2019. Available at: https://gco.iarc.fr/today/home. Accessed July 1, 2019

Wright JD, Dehdashti F, Herzog TJ, et al: Preoperative lymph node staging of early-stage cervical carcinoma by [18F]-fluoro-2-deoxy-d-glucose-positron emission tomography. Cancer 104:2484, 2005

Yahata T, Nishino K, Kashmima K, et al: Conservative treatment of stage IA1 adenocarcinoma of the uterine cervix with a long-term follow-up. Int J Gynecol Cancer 20:1063, 2010

CHAPTER 31

Vulvar Cancer

Cancers of the vulva are uncommon and constitute only 6 percent of all gynecologic malignancies. Most vulvar cancers are diagnosed in older women. Early-stage vulvar cancers are highly curable, and thus biopsy of any abnormal vulvar lesion is imperative to help diagnose this cancer expeditiously.

The Surveillance, Epidemiology, and End Results Program (SEER) provides online survival and incidence trends for cancers in the United States. SEER (2018) data from 2008 to 2014 show vulvar cancers carry a 5-year relative survival rate of 71 percent. Historically, treatment of vulvar cancer resulted in extensive short- and long-term morbidity, with dramatic anatomic and functional deformity. Surgery is now more conservative yet preserves oncologic efficacy. For unresectable, locally advanced disease, chemoradiation may be used either primarily or as an adjunct to surgery to aid tumor control.

RELEVANT ANATOMY

The *external vulva* includes the mons pubis, labia majora and minora, clitoris, vestibule, vestibular bulbs, Bartholin glands, lesser vestibular glands, paraurethral glands, and the urethral and vaginal openings. Lateral margins of the vulva are the labiocrural folds (Fig. 38-26, p. 815). Vulvar cancer may involve any of these external structures and typically arises within the covering squamous epithelium. Importantly, unlike the cervix, the vulva lacks an identifiable transformation zone.

However, the Hart line on the vestibule marks the border between the vulvar keratinized squamous epithelium, which lies laterally, and the nonkeratinized squamous mucosa, which lies medially. Vulvar squamous neoplasia arises predominantly along the Hart line.

Deep to the external vulva are the superficial and deep urogenital triangle compartments. The superficial space lies between Colles fascia (superficial perineal fascia) and the perineal membrane (deep perineal fascia) (Fig. 38-26 p. 815). Within this space lie the ischiocavernosus, bulbospongiosus, and transverse perineal muscles and the highly vascular vestibular bulb and clitoral crus. During radical vulvectomy, dissection is carried to the depth of the perineal membrane. As a result, contents of this superficial urogenital triangle compartment that lie beneath the mass are removed during tumor excision.

The lymphatics of the vulva and distal third of the vagina typically drain into the superficial inguinal node group (Fig. 38-31, p. 819). From here, lymph travels through the deep femoral lymphatics and the node of Cloquet to the pelvic nodal groups. Importantly, lymph can also drain directly from the clitoris and upper labia to the deep femoral nodes (Way, 1948). Vulvar lymphatics cross at the mons pubis and the posterior fourchette but do not cross the labiocrural folds (Morley, 1976). Thus, lesions found within 2 cm of the midline may spread to either lymph node. In contrast, lateral lesions rarely send metastases to contralateral nodes. This anatomy point influences the decision for ipsilateral or bilateral node dissection, discussed later.

The superficial inguinal nodes cluster within the femoral triangle formed by the inguinal ligament, sartorius muscle, and adductor longus muscle (Fig. 38-31, p. 819). The deep femoral nodes lie within the borders of the fossa ovalis and just medial to the femoral vein. An *inguinofemoral lymphadenectomy* typically refers to removal of both superficial inguinal and deep femoral lymph nodes (Levenback, 1996).

EPIDEMIOLOGY

In the United States, women have a 1 in 333 chance of developing this cancer at some point. For 2019, approximately 6070 new vulvar cancers and 1280 cancer deaths are predicted (Siegel, 2019). SEER (2018) data from 1975 to 2015 show that rates of vulvar cancer have been rising on average by 0.6 percent every year and that the death rate has been increasing yearly by 1.2 percent.

Of vulvar cancers, approximately 90 percent are squamous cell carcinoma (Fig. 31-1). Malignant melanoma is the second most common, but rare histologic subtypes also may be encountered (Table 31-1).

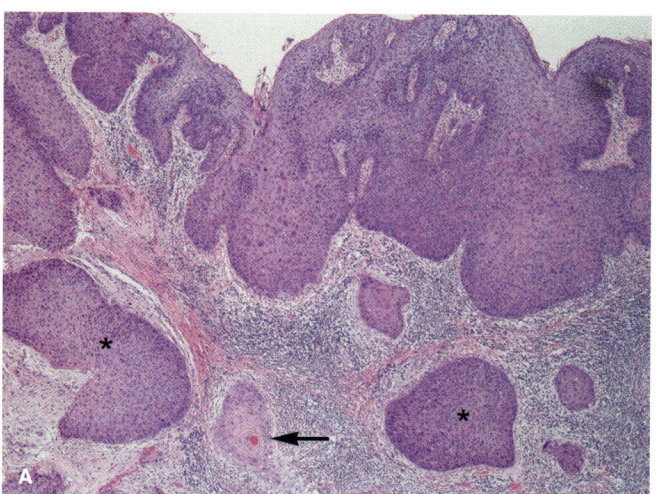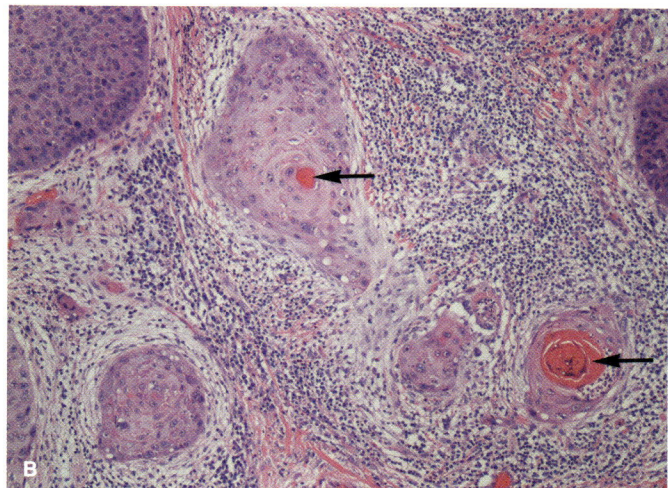

FIGURE 31-1 Vulvar squamous cell carcinoma. **A.** Low-power view. The surface epithelium shows high-grade squamous dysplasia. Nests of invasive squamous cell carcinoma (*arrow*) are present. A brisk chronic inflammatory infiltrate is present as is often the case with invasive squamous cell carcinoma. Portions of the surface epithelium extend deep and are cut tangentially (*asterisks*), giving the false impression of invasive tumor at these sites. **B.** Tumor shows classic diagnostic features of invasive squamous cell carcinoma that include a squamoid appearance, intercellular bridges, and brightly eosinophilic keratin pearls (*arrows*). Nests of invasive tumor are surrounded by chronic inflammation. (Reproduced with permission from Dr. Kelley Carrick.)

RISK FACTORS

The cause of vulvar cancer is unknown, but associated risk factors have been identified. The average age at diagnosis is 65 years, hence *age* is a prominent factor. However, vulvar cancer can develop at any age.

Women who are infected with *human papillomavirus (HPV)* have a greater risk of vulvar cancer. Specifically, 50 to 75 percent of invasive vulvar cancers are associated with high-risk HPV serotypes (Gargano, 2012). Strong correlations also can be seen between high-risk HPV infection and preinvasive

TABLE 31-1. Vulvar Cancer Histologic Subtypes

Vulvar carcinomas
Squamous cell carcinoma
Adenocarcinoma
Carcinoma of Bartholin gland
   Adenocarcinoma
   Squamous carcinoma
   Transitional cell
Vulva Paget disease
Merkel cell tumors
Verrucous carcinoma
Basal cell carcinoma

Vulvar malignant melanoma

Vulvar sarcoma
Leiomyosarcoma
Malignant fibrous histiocytoma
Epithelial sarcoma
Malignant rhabdoid tumor

Metastatic cancers to vulva

Yolk sac tumors

lesions of the vulva (Gargano, 2012). HPV becomes a stronger contributor when combined with other cofactors such as smoking or herpes simplex virus (HSV) infection (Madeleine, 1997). Women who have smoked and have a history of HPV genital warts have a 35–fold greater risk for developing vulvar cancer compared with women without these predispositions (Brinton, 1990; Kirschner, 1995).

Vulvar intraepithelial neoplasia (VIN) is considered a pre-invasive condition of the vulva and is thoroughly discussed in Chapter 29 (p. 643). VIN is categorized as *usual type VIN* and *differentiated type VIN*. Usual type VIN is associated with high-risk HPV infection and develops usually in young women. In contrast, the differentiated type VIN occurs in postmenopausal women with chronic skin conditions such as lichen sclerosis (Reyes, 2014). Of these two, differentiated type VIN has a significantly stronger association with squamous cell carcinoma compared with usual type VIN (Eva, 2009). Also with VIN, high-grade disease is more closely linked with invasive vulvar cancer. Approximately 4 percent of women with a history of high-grade VIN subsequently develop vulvar cancer (Jones 2005). And, an underlying squamous carcinoma can be found in one fifth of women initially treated for VIN 3 (Modesitt, 1998). Hence, we recommend early definitive treatment for those with high-grade vulvar dysplasia.

Vaccines against HPV have the theoretical potential to lower vulvar neoplasia rates. The nonavalent vaccine (Gardasil 9) is effective against high-risk HPV serotypes 16 and 18 (Huh, 2017). It is hoped that this vaccine will lower future rates of HPV-related invasive cancer (Garland, 2018; Saraiya, 2015).

Chronic immunosuppression can predispose to vulvar cancer. For example, transplant patients have a high incidence. In this group, vulvar cancer develops at a much younger age than in the general population, and more than 50 percent have a prior history of condyloma acuminata (Penn, 2000). With human immunodeficiency virus (HIV) infection, vulvar cancer rates also are elevated (Elit, 2005; Frisch, 2000). Indeed, HIV-infected patients make up most of the increased high-grade VIN and invasive vulvar carcinoma incidence noted in younger women (Casolati, 2003). A possible explanation is the association of HIV and high-risk HPV serotypes. However, vulvar cancer is not yet considered an acquired immunodeficiency syndrome (AIDS)-defining malignancy. Because of these links with vulvar cancer, we recommend that all immunocompromised women undergo thorough vulvar inspection and, when indicated, vulvoscopy and biopsy.

Lichen sclerosus is a chronic vulvar inflammatory disease and is described in Chapter 4 (p. 94). This condition is related to vulvar cancer development. Keratinocytes affected by lichen sclerosus show a proliferative phenotype and can exhibit markers of neoplastic progression. As such, lichen sclerosus may be a precursor lesion to differentiated type VIN and invasive squamous vulvar cancers (Halonen, 2017).

DIAGNOSIS

■ Symptoms

Women with VIN and vulvar cancer commonly present with pruritus and a visible lesion (Fig. 31-2). However, pain, bleeding, ulceration, and inguinal mass may be other complaints (Fig. 31-3). Manifestations can persist for weeks or months before diagnosis, as many patients may be embarrassed or may not recognize the significance of their symptoms.

■ Lesion Evaluation

Lesions may be raised, ulcerated, pigmented, or warty, but in younger women with multifocal disease, a well-defined mass is not always present. Importantly, other clinical entities may present similarly and include VIN, infection, chronic inflammatory disease, and granulomatous disease. Thus, the goal of evaluation is to obtain an accurate and definitive pathologic diagnosis.

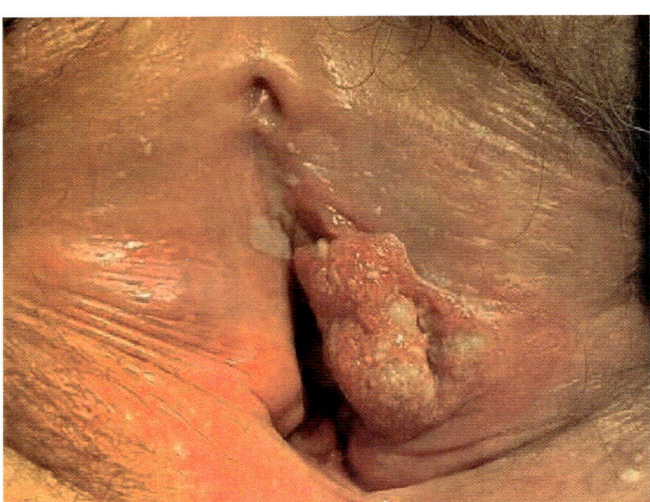

FIGURE 31-2 Early-stage (T2) squamous cell cancer of the vulva with adjacent vulvar intraepithelial neoplasia (VIN). (Reproduced with permission from Dr. Sarah Capelouto.)

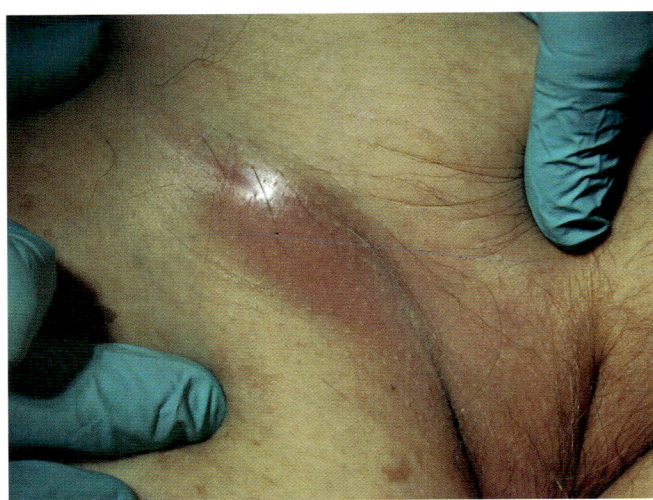

FIGURE 31-3 Enlarged inguinal lymph node containing metastatic squamous cell vulvar cancer. (Reproduced with permission from Dr. William Griffith.)

For this, colposcopic examination of the vulva, termed *vulvoscopy*, can direct biopsy site selection. To begin, the vulva is soaked with 3-percent acetic acid for 5 minutes to allow adequate penetration into the keratin layer. This aids identification of acetowhite areas and abnormal vascular patterns, which are characteristics of vulvar neoplasia (Chap. 29, p. 645). The entire vulva and perianal skin are systematically examined. We recommend obtaining multiple biopsies, as illustrated in Figure 4-2 (p. 94), from the most suspicious raised or dyspigmented skin. Specimens removed with a Keyes punch should be approximately 4 mm thick to include the surface epithelial lesion and the underlying stroma. This permits evaluation for invasion and depth of invasion. Concurrent colposcopic examination of the cervix and vagina and careful evaluation of the perianal area are recommended to diagnose any synchronous lesions or associated neoplasm of the lower genital tract.

■ Cancer Patient Evaluation

Following histologic diagnosis, a patient with vulvar cancer is assessed for the clinical extent of disease and for comorbid conditions. Thus, detailed physical examination includes measurement of the primary tumor and evaluation of cancer extension into other genitourinary compartments, the anal canal, the bony pelvis, and inguinal lymph nodes. At our institution, if a thorough physical examination is not possible because of patient discomfort or disease extent, an examination under anesthesia is performed. This may be coupled with cystourethroscopy, proctosigmoidoscopy, or both if suspicion of tumor invasion into the urethra, bladder, or anal canal is high (Fig. 31-4).

Women with small tumors and clinically negative inguinal nodes require few additional diagnostic studies other than those needed for surgical preparation (Chap. 39, p. 822). Although not a formal part of surgical tumor staging, preoperative imaging should be performed in those with larger tumors or with clinically suspected metastatic disease. In such cases, computed tomography (CT) of the chest, abdomen, and pelvis; positron emission tomography (PET); or magnetic resonance (MR) imaging of the

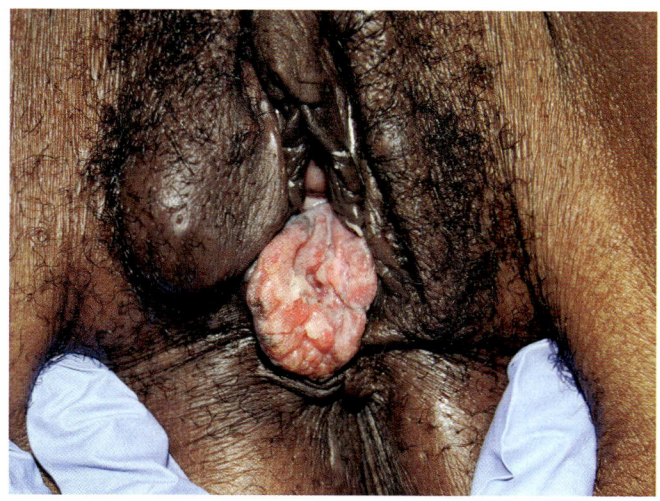

FIGURE 31-4 Photograph of invasive vulvar cancer involving midline mucosal structures.

abdomen and pelvis provide information regarding disease extent or metastases that may modify preoperative planning.

■ Staging Systems

The International Federation of Gynecology and Obstetrics (FIGO) advocates staging of patients with vulvar cancer that is based on a tumor, node, metastasis (TNM) classification. Frequently, stage is determined after definitive surgical

management. Thus, staging involves: (1) primary tumor evaluation to obtain tumor dimensions and extension and (2) sentinel lymph node biopsy or dissection of superficial and deep inguinofemoral lymph nodes to evaluate tumor spread (Pecorelli, 2009). This system is used to direct treatment and predict prognosis (Van der Steen, 2010). Table 31-2 and Figure 31-5 describe FIGO staging and American Joint Committee on Cancer (AJCC) staging criteria for all vulvar cancer types except melanoma. This cancer's staging is discussed on page 685. The general nuanced differences between FIGO and AJCC systems are described in Chapter 30 (p. 661).

PROGNOSIS

Overall survival rates of women with squamous cell carcinoma of the vulva are relatively good and approximate 65 percent (Razzaghi, 2018). SEER (2018) data from 2008 to 2014 show that a 5-year survival rate of 86 percent can be expected for local disease (stage I and II). As anticipated, 5-year survival rates for higher stages are poorer, and a rate of 54 percent can be expected for regional (stage III and IVA) disease and a rate of 16 percent for stage IVB. Apart from FIGO stage, other important prognostic factors include lymph node metastasis, lesion size, depth of invasion, resected-margin status, and lymphatic vascular space involvement (Table 31-3).

Of these, *lymph node metastasis* is the single most important vulvar cancer predictor, since inguinal node metastasis reduces long-term survival rates by 50 percent (Farias-Eisner, 1994;

TABLE 31-2. Invasive Vulvar Cancer Staging

TNM[a]	Stage[b]	Characteristics
	I	**Tumor confined to the vulva**
T1a	IA	Lesions ≤2 cm in size, confined to the vulva or perineum and with stromal invasion ≤1.0 mm[c], no nodal metastasis
T1b	IB	Lesions >2 cm in size or with stromal invasion >1.0 mm[c], confined to the vulva or perineum, with negative nodes
T2	**II**	**Tumor of any size with extension to adjacent perineal structures (1/3 lower urethra, 1/3 lower vagina, anus) with negative nodes**
	III	**Tumor of any size with or without extension to adjacent perineal structures (1/3 lower urethra, 1/3 lower vagina, anus) with positive inguinofemoral lymph nodes**
N1b	IIIA	(i) With 1 lymph node metastasis (≥5 mm), or
N1a		(ii) 1–2 lymph node metastasis(es) (<5 mm)
N2b	IIIB	(i) With 2 or more lymph node metastases (≥5 mm), or
N2a		(ii) 3 or more lymph node metastases (<5 mm)
N2c	IIIC	With positive nodes with extracapsular spread
	IV	**Tumor invades other regional (2/3 upper urethra, 2/3 upper vagina), or distant structures**
T3	IVA	Tumor invades any of the following: (i) upper urethral and/or vaginal mucosa, bladder mucosa, rectal mucosa, or fixed to pelvic bone, or (ii) fixed or ulcerated inguinofemoral lymph nodes
M1	IVB	Any distant metastasis including pelvic lymph nodes

[a]American Joint Committee on Cancer staging that reflects tumor, nodes, and metastases (TNM).
[b]International Federation of Gynecology and Obstetrics (FIGO) staging.
[c]The *depth of invasion* is defined as the measurement of the tumor from the epithelial-stromal junction of the adjacent most superficial dermal papilla to the deepest point of invasion.

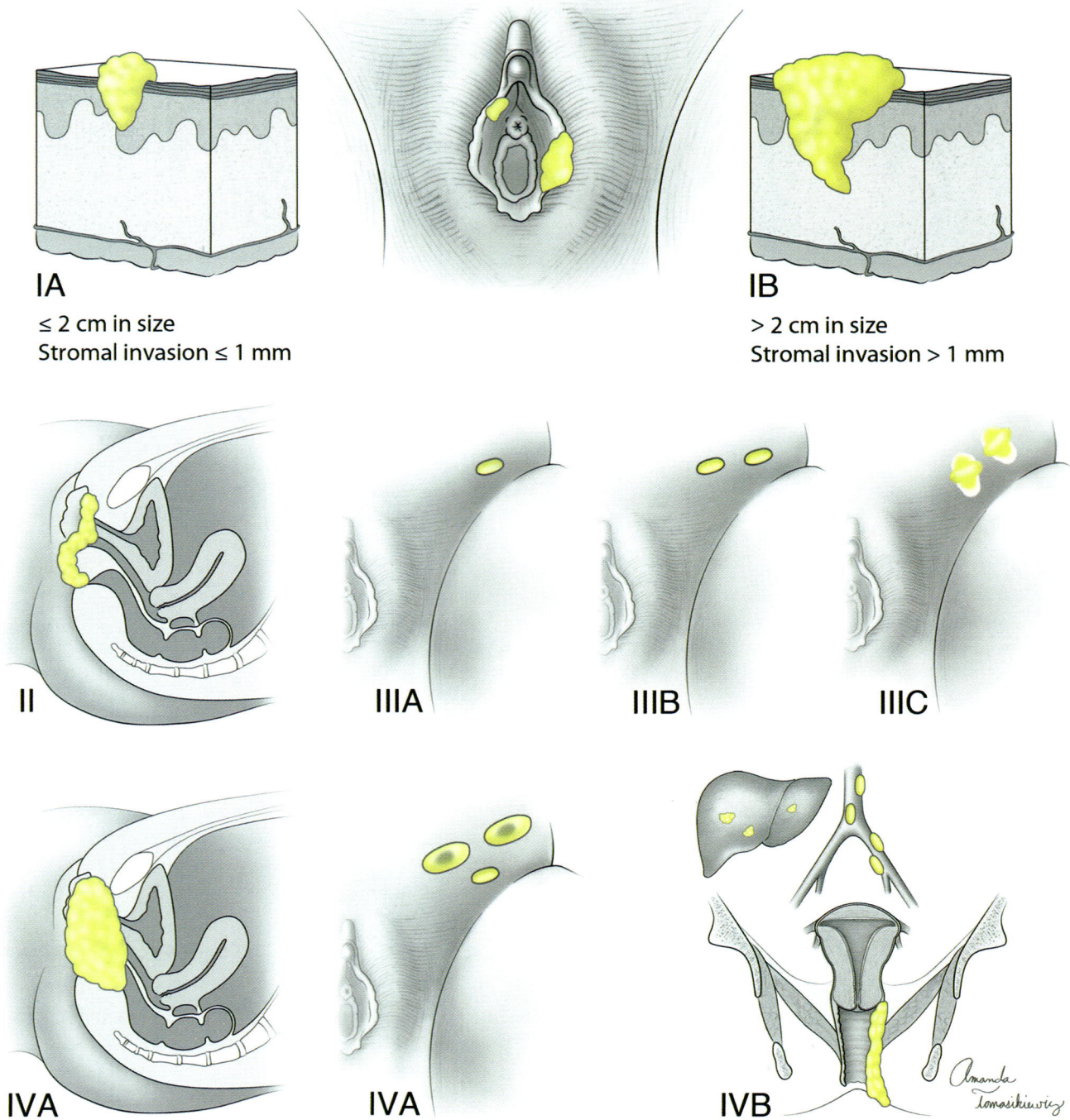

IA
≤ 2 cm in size
Stromal invasion ≤ 1 mm

IB
> 2 cm in size
Stromal invasion > 1 mm

II   IIIA   IIIB   IIIC

IVA   IVA   IVB

FIGURE 31-5 FIGO (International Federation of Gynecology and Obstetrics) staging of invasive vulvar cancer.

Figge, 1985). Nodal status is determined by sentinel lymph node biopsy or lymphadenectomy and histologic evaluation. Among patients with nodal metastasis, other factors further predict poor prognosis. These include a high number of involved lymph nodes, large nodal metastasis size, extracapsular invasion, and fixed or ulcerated nodes (Homesley, 1991; Origoni, 1992).

Tumor diameter also influences survival rates. But this stems mainly from the positive correlation between lesion size and nodal metastasis rates (Homesley, 1993).

Depth of invasion is another prognostic element. This depth is measured from the epidermis basement membrane to the deepest point of invasion into the dermis and subcutaneous layer (Kurman, 2014). Tumors with a depth of invasion <1 mm carry little or no risk of inguinal lymph node metastasis. However, depth of invasion positively correlates with increased nodal metastasis.

Surgical margins that are tumor-free lower local tumor recurrence rates. Thus, at a minimum, a 2-cm tumor-free margin is

TABLE 31-3. Prognostic Predictors

Depth of Invasion (mm)	Positive Nodes (%)
1	3
2	9
3	19
4	31
5	33
≥5	48

Tumor Diameter (cm)	5-Year Survival (%)	Groin Nodes Positive (%)
0–1	90	18
1–2	89	19
2–3	83	31
3–4	63	54
>4	44	40–52

Abbreviated from Homesley, 1993; Stehman, 2006.

desired. More specifically, two large retrospective series demonstrated that a tumor-free surgical margin ≥8 mm at final pathologic analysis yielded a high rate of local control. In contrast, if tumor was found within this 8-mm margin, the recurrence rate was 23 to 48 percent (Chan, 2007; Heaps, 1990). Other studies have failed to confirm that a minimum margin of 8 mm is necessary to reduce local recurrence (Nooij, 2016; Woelber, 2016). However, tumor-positive margin status is a consistent independent risk factor for disease recurrence. Reexcision or adjuvant radiotherapy is indicated when margins are positive for cancer. Management of patients with narrow tumor-free margins is controversial. There is no clear consensus on the prognostic value of a specific tumor-free margin threshold. Therefore, observation or adjuvant radiation can be considered for narrow tumor-free vulvar margins to prevent cancer recurrence. When lesions are close to the clitoris, anus, urethra, or vagina, we recommend aiming for margins sufficiently wide to preserve important anatomic function.

Lymphatic vascular space invasion (LVSI) describes histologic identification of tumor cells within lymphatic vessels and is a predictor of early disease recurrence (Preti, 2005). LVSI is also associated with a higher frequency of lymph node metastasis and a lower overall 5-year survival rate (Hoskins, 2000).

Perineural invasion is also a poor prognostic indicator for women diagnosed with vulvar cancer. Patients with perineural invasion have a higher likelihood of lymph node involvement, advanced cancer stage, and LVSI. They also have worse progression-free and overall survival rates (Salcedo, 2019).

TREATMENT

■ Surgery

Surgery is often an integral part of vulvar cancer treatment. Potential procedures, in increasing order of radicality, include wide local excision, radical partial vulvectomy, and radical total vulvectomy.

Wide local excision can be appropriate for preinvasive disease and microinvasive tumors (stage IA) of the vulva and some rare histologic types. With this excision, also termed *simple partial vulvectomy*, a 1-cm surgical margin is obtained around the lesion. Deep surgical margins measuring 1 cm also are preferred. This deep margin usually corresponds to Colles fascia (Fig. 38-26, p. 815).

With *radical partial vulvectomy* (Chap. 46, p. 1235), tumor-containing portions of the vulva are completely removed, wherever they are located. Skin margins are ideally 2 cm, and excision extends deep to the perineal membrane (Fig. 31-6). Radical partial vulvectomy is typically reserved for lesions that are not too large or extensive, with an otherwise normal vulva.

Radical total vulvectomy (Chap. 46, p. 1238) is a complete dissection of vulvar tissue to the level of the perineal membrane and the periosteum of the pubic rami or symphysis. Adequate

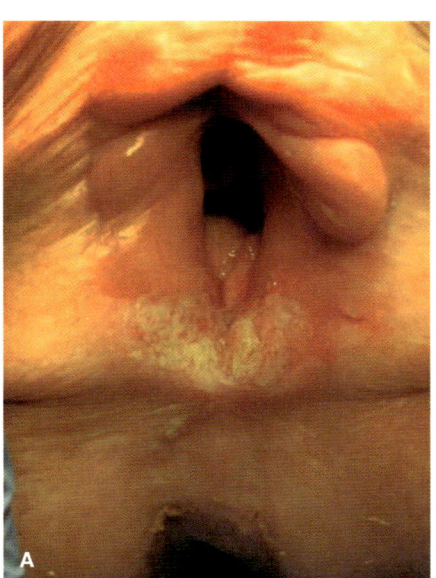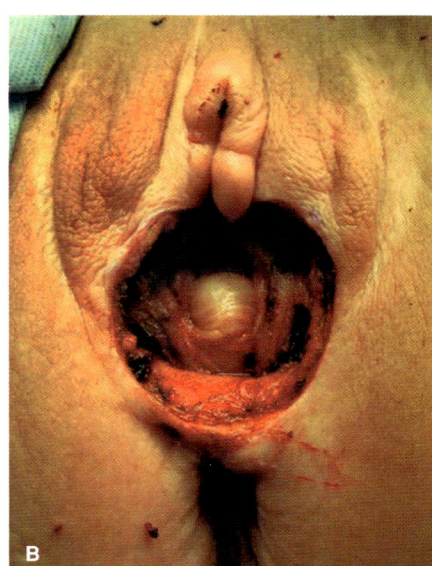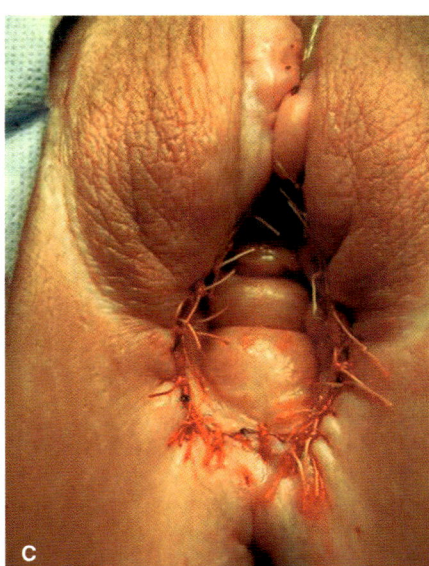

FIGURE 31-6 A. Vulvar cancer following radiation therapy and in preparation for surgical excision. **B.** Radical partial vulvectomy. **C.** Primary surgical closure. (Reproduced with permission from Dr. David Miller.)

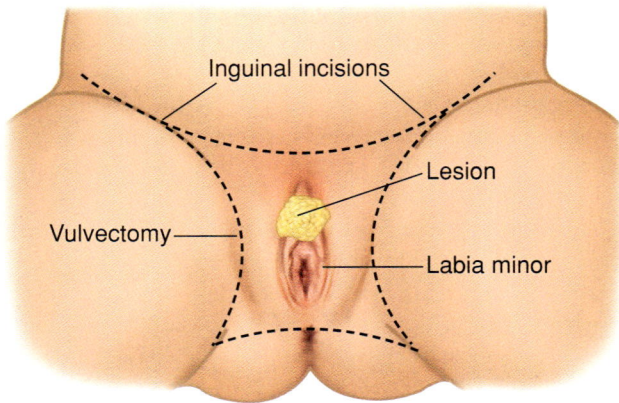

A

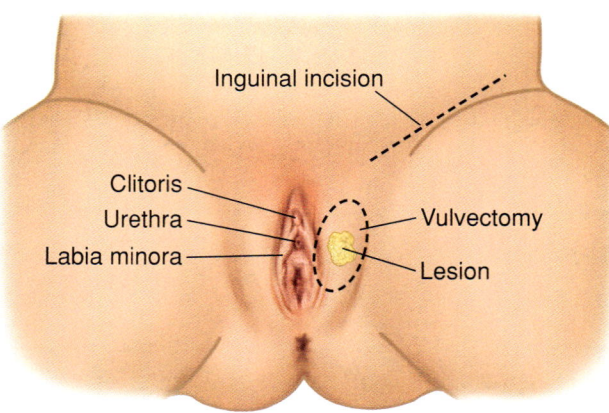

B

C

FIGURE 31-7 Types of vulvectomy used in the treatment of vulvar cancer. **A.** En bloc radical vulvectomy with bilateral inguinofemoral lymphadenectomy. **B.** Radical total vulvectomy with bilateral inguinofemoral lymphadenectomy. **C.** Radical partial vulvectomy with ipsilateral inguinofemoral lymphadenectomy.

margins will generally require an incision in the labiocrural fold that extends down to the fourchette and up over the mons pubis (Figure 31-7). All intervening subcutaneous tissue is excised. Lesions involving or adjacent to the clitoris may require wider margins cephalad to the mons. Such radical resections are performed for large midline or multifocal vulvar cancers. Flap reconstruction is occasionally needed and described in

Chap. 46, (p. 1244). Contraindications to a radical total vulvectomy include poor surgical risk, poor patient compliance, and metastatic disease beyond regional lymph nodes.

Of the three procedures shown in Figure 31-7, the en bloc incision, colloquially termed the *butterfly* or *longhorn* incision, has largely been abandoned. It has survival rates equivalent to radical total vulvectomy but carries significantly greater morbidity.

Inguinofemoral Lymphadenectomy

This procedure is usually an integral part of surgical cancer staging and accompanies radical partial or radical total vulvectomy for squamous cell carcinoma of the vulva. It is recommended for all vulvar squamous carcinomas that invade deeper than 1 mm on initial biopsy or that have a tumor diameter >2 cm regardless of invasion depth (stages IB-IVA). To maximize metastatic disease detection and staging accuracy, surgical evaluation of the inguinal nodes is recommended. Traditionally, both the superficial inguinal and deep femoral lymph nodes have been removed for evaluation of metastatic disease (Gordinier, 2003). Moreover, lymph nodes may be excised unilaterally or bilaterally. Traditionally, an ipsilateral inguinofemoral lymphadenectomy is performed for a "lateralized" vulvar lesion, namely, one that lies >2 cm beyond the midline. Bilateral node excision is recommended for all midline lesions and lesions within 2 cm of the midline. Aside from acquiring staging information, inguinofemoral lymphadenectomy may also be used to debulk large, cancerous lymph nodes.

Entire steps for lymphadenectomy are described and illustrated in Chapter 46 (p. 1241). To summarize, the superficial inguinal lymph nodes lie within the fatty tissue caudal to the inguinal ligament and superficial to the thigh's fascia lata. This node-containing tissue is dissected free to reach the fossa ovalis. Here, deep femoral nodes are excised from their location medial to and alongside the femoral vein. For these deep nodes, a modified approach preserves the cribriform fascia (portion of fascia lata overlying the fossa ovalis) by removing the deep femoral nodes through the cribriform fascia's perforations. This modification yields cancer recurrence rates comparable to those obtained following classic inguinofemoral node dissection (Bell, 2000; Hacker, 1983). Advantageously, complication rates of wound breakdown, infection, and lymphedema are significantly lower (Table 31-4). However, a classic inguinofemoral node dissection is occasionally required to reach these deep femoral lymph nodes. In such cases, the cribriform fascia is transected, lymph nodes are removed, and the sartorius muscle

TABLE 31-4. Postoperative Complications of Inguinofemoral Lymphadenectomy

Complication	No. of Events	Percent of Groins
Lymphedema	13	14.0
Lymphocele	11	11.8
Groin infection	7	7.5
Groin necrosis	2	2.2
Groin separation	7	7.5

From Bell, 2000, with permission.

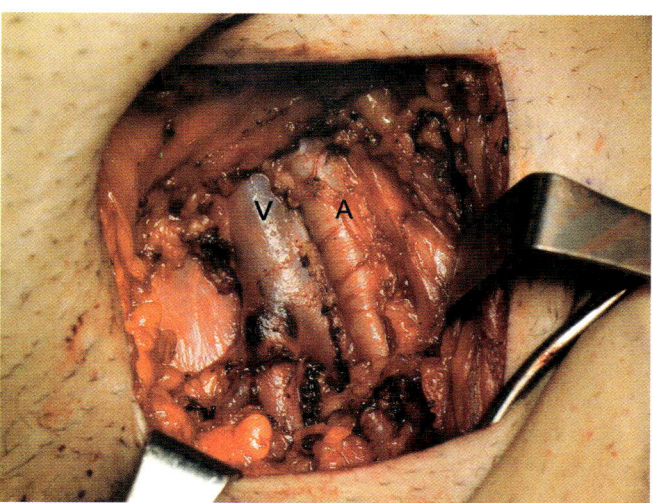

FIGURE 31-8 Surgical photography during inguinofemoral lymphadenectomy. Here, the cribriform fascia has been excised and nodes have been removed. The femoral vein (*V*) and artery (*A*) are marked. (Reproduced with permission from Dr. Matthew Carlson.)

can then be transposed over the femoral vessels (Fig. 31-8). This transposition may reduce the risk of postoperative erosion into the skeletonized and thus more exposed femoral vessels if superficial wound dehiscence occurs. However, this transposition does not reduce overall postoperative wound morbidity rates (Judson, 2004; Rouzier, 2003).

Inguinal femoral lymphadenectomy versus primary radiation therapy in patients with clinically negative nodes is controversial. Surgical evaluation of the groin nodes has been reported to confer a superior prognosis compared with primary groin irradiation in some studies. One study by the Gynecologic Oncology Group (GOG) showed that patients undergoing primary inguinal node dissection experienced significantly fewer groin recurrences and a better prognosis compared with women receiving groin irradiation (Stehman, 1992). In other studies, a higher than acceptable groin recurrence rate after primary groin irradiation has been supported but also challenged (Hallack, 2007; Manavi, 1997; Perez, 1993; Petereit, 1993). At our institution, surgical evaluation of one or both groins is performed if

the patient is a reasonable surgical candidate. In general, both deep and superficial inguinal lymph node removal is performed to allow thorough evaluation for nodal metastasis in women with tumor diameter ≥4 cm. Sentinel lymph node biopsy is used in vulvar lesions <4 cm in diameter.

Sentinel Lymph Node Biopsy

As one less morbid option, selective dissection of a solitary node or nodes, termed *sentinel lymph node biopsy (SLNB)*, dramatically reduces surgical morbidity yet adequately assesses nodal involvement. Physiologically, the first lymph node to receive tumor lymphatic drainage is termed the *sentinel lymph node*. Thus, a sentinel lymph node devoid of disease implies absent lymph node metastases within the entire lymph node basin. SLNB is not performed if groin node metastases are clinically suspected.

Currently, both lymphoscintigraphy and isosulfan blue dye techniques are recommended when performing SLNB for vulvar cancer (Levenback, 2008). To begin, intraoperative lymphatic mapping is accomplished by injecting radionuclide intradermally at the tumor border that lies closest to the ipsilateral groin. For midline tumors, both sides of the tumor are injected. A handheld gamma counter aids attempts to identify the sentinel node subcutaneously, and the skin is marked by pen over the strongest signal. Next, isosulfan blue dye is injected at the same tumor border, and the groin skin over the prior pen mark is incised approximately 5 minutes later (Fig. 31-9). The tracer and dye are taken up by the specific node that drains the tumor site first. The sentinel node may be localized by the handheld gamma counter signal, and/or it can be visually isolated by its blue color. Once identified, it is separated and excised from the other nodes within that regional group.

Several studies have confirmed the accuracy of SLNB to predict vulvar cancer metastasis in the inguinal lymph nodes in select patients. One trial by the GOG reported the sensitivity of this technique exceeded 90 percent, and the false negative predictive value was 2 percent for tumors measuring <4 cm in diameter (Frumovitz, 2005).

A second study, the GROningen International Study on Sentinel nodes in Vulvar cancer (GROINSS-V), evaluated SLNB

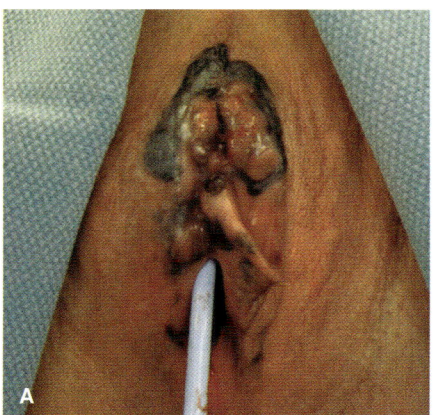 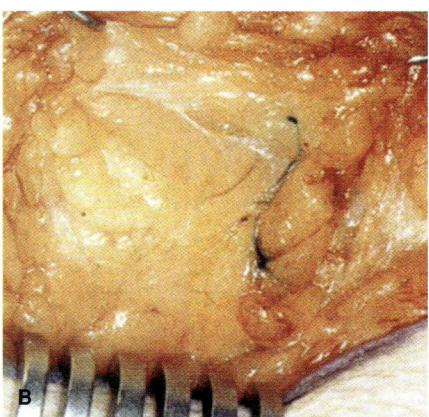 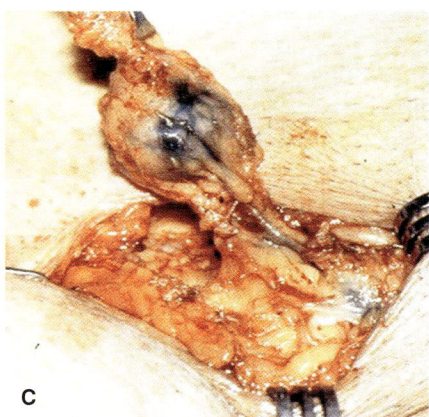

FIGURE 31-9 Sentinel lymph node evaluation. **A.** Blue dye and radiotracer are injected at the tumor periphery. **B.** Blue dye is taken up by the specific node that drains the tumor site. **C.** This sentinel node can be visually identified, separated from the other nodes within the regional group, and removed for evaluation.

for patients with unifocal squamous cell cancer of the vulva measuring <4 cm. It too confirmed the satisfactory false negative predictive value of SLNB (2.9 percent). The isolated groin recurrence rate was 2.5 percent in sentinel node–negative patients, and all groin recurrences were identified within 16 months after primary treatment (Te Grootenhuis, 2016). Last, although results are pending, the completed GROINSS-V-II study (GOG protocol 270) observed early-stage vulvar cancer patients with a sentinel node metastasis measuring ≤2 mm to see if complete inguino-femoral lymphadenectomy can be safely replaced by adjuvant radiotherapy following vulvectomy.

■ Microinvasive Tumors (Stage IA)

Within the FIGO system, stage I vulvar cancers are divided into two categories. Stage IA lesions measure ≤2 cm in diameter, are confined to the vulva or perineum, and display stromal invasion ≤1 mm. These lesions, termed *microinvasive cancers*, reflect a subpopulation in which the risk of inguinal metastasis is negligible (Binder, 1990; Donaldson, 1981; Hacker, 1984). Women with microinvasive stage IA tumors tend to be younger and have multifocal disease associated with HPV. For probable cure, these patients can undergo wide local excision with a 1-cm margin. Lymphadenectomy is not indicated because associated lymph node metastasis is rare.

■ Stage IB–II

Patients with early-stage vulvar cancer typically present with T1B and T2 lesions (stage IB and II) of the vulva and clinically negative groin nodes. For stage IB lesions, radical resection of the primary tumor and inguinofemoral lymphadenectomy is recommended. If adequate margins and dissection to the perineal membrane can be achieved, then radical partial vulvectomy offers similar recurrence rates but less morbidity than radical total vulvectomy (Tantipalakorn, 2009). Because 20 to 30 percent of women with T1 and T2 disease will have diseased nodes, SLNB and/or inguinofemoral lymphadenectomy is performed. Described earlier, lesion laterality and clinical impression regarding groin involvement guides the decision to perform ipsilateral or bilateral groin dissection (p. 682).

Stage II cancers are most often managed with a larger radical partial excision. For example, a 4-cm lesion involving the clitoral hood may be managed by an anterior hemi-vulvectomy and bilateral inguinofemoral lymphadenectomy. Again, reported experience with conservative surgery suggests identical local recurrence rates if 1- to 2-cm tumor-free surgical margins are achieved (Burke, 1995; Farias–Eisner, 1994; Tantipalakorn, 2009). Occasionally, a radical total vulvectomy may be required, depending on tumor size and location.

■ Stage III

By definition, stage III vulvar cancers include node-positive tumors. Affected patients have T1 or T2 vulvar lesions and involved regional lymph nodes that are not fixed or ulcerated. Most patients with clinically negative nodes typically undergo a radical partial or total vulvectomy and either SLNB or inguino-femoral lymphadenectomy. For cases in which groin nodes are grossly positive and resectable, inguinofemoral lymphadenectomy is performed. Most women with stage III vulvar cancer also receive postoperative adjuvant radiation directed to both groins and the pelvis. Efficacy for this was shown in a randomized GOG trial of 114 patients with invasive squamous cell carcinoma of the vulva and diseased groin nodes. Adjuvant radiation to both groins and the pelvic midplane following lymphadenectomy proved superior to extended pelvic node resection. However, 12 percent of women completing radiotherapy still relapsed in the groin and pelvis, and 8.5 percent at distant sites (Homesley, 1986; Kunos, 2009).

Evidence that nodal metastasis raises the risk of recurrence on the vulva is inconclusive. Hence, adjuvant vulvar radiation is the treating physician's decision and guided by margin status and tumor size and location.

■ Stage IVA

These locally advanced vulvar cancers involve the proximal urethra, proximal vagina, bladder or rectal mucosa, or pelvic bone and may or may not have affected inguinal lymph nodes (Fig. 31-10). With stage IVA vulvar cancers, women occasionally can be treated with radical primary surgery. Much more often, tumor size and location necessitate some form of exenterative surgical procedure to remove the entire lesion with adequate margins. Such poorly resectable, locally advanced vulvar cancers can be effectively treated with neoadjuvant chemoradiation to drastically minimize the surgical resection required. Two GOG studies GOG have demonstrated the feasibility of this approach using cisplatin regimens (Moore, 1998, 2012). An ongoing phase II trial is currently evaluating the efficacy of cisplatin, gemcitabine, and intensity-modulated radiation therapy (IMRT) for primary treatment of locally advanced squamous cell carcinoma of the vulva. Described in Chapter 28 (p. 612), IMRT offers greater sculpting of radiation delivery to minimize toxicity.

Our current practice is to offer preoperative cisplatin-based chemoradiation to women with inoperable primary tumors or with extensive lesions that would require pelvic exenteration. In

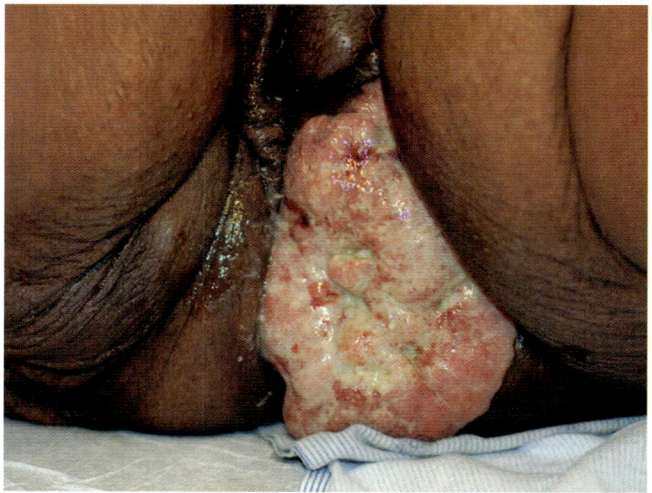

FIGURE 31-10 Locally advanced vulvar cancer that is a candidate for primary radiation therapy. (Reproduced with permission from Dr. William Griffith.)

cases without fixed groin nodes, pretreatment inguinofemoral lymphadenectomy is performed to determine the need for groin irradiation. If groin nodes are fixed or ulcerated, then primary chemoradiation is administered to treat these involved nodes.

If residual disease remains on the vulva following chemoradiation, then local resection is indicated. If the clinical response appears complete, the primary tumor site undergoes excisional biopsy to confirm pathologic response. Unresected groins that are clinically or radiographically positive 8 weeks after surgery are biopsied by fine-needle aspiration (FNA). If the FNA is positive, a targeted excision of the groin is performed.

In contrast, for stage IVB vulvar cancer, treatment is individualized. A multimodal approach that may include chemotherapy and radiation may be used for palliation.

SURVEILLANCE

After completing primary treatment, all patients receive thorough physical examination that includes inguinal lymph node palpation and pelvic examination every 3 months for the first 2 to 3 years. Surveillance examinations are then scheduled every 6 months to complete a total of 5 years. Thereafter, disease-free women may be seen annually (Salani, 2017). Biopsies are performed if concerning areas are noted. Radiologic imaging and targeted biopsies to diagnose possible tumor recurrence are completed as indicated.

RECURRENT DISEASE

■ Vulvar Recurrences

For women with local tumor recurrence, the 5-year survival rate is 67 percent. This compares with a rate >80 percent in women with no recurrence (Woelber, 2016). In a woman with suspected recurrence, careful evaluation helps define disease extent. Local vulvar recurrences are most common, and surgical reexcision is usually the best option. Radical partial vulvectomy is appropriate for smaller lesions. Patients who had SLNB during primary treatment and who have not previously received groin irradiation are candidates for concurrent inguinofemoral lymphadenectomy at the time of local recurrence resection. If a patient has received prior vulvar radiation, those with large central recurrences involving the urethra, vagina, or rectum may require a total pelvic exenteration with reconstructive surgery (Chap. 46, p. 1174).

With exenteration, to maintain sexual function, vaginal reconstruction can be completed at the time of surgery or after a short postoperative interval (Chap. 46, p. 1190). Radiated tissue often has a poor blood supply. Thus, vulvar recurrences in a previously radiated field typically require myocutaneous flaps for reconstruction after surgical resection. Last, for patients who are not surgical candidates but are radiation naïve to the vulva, external beam radiation combined with interstitial brachytherapy can be an option.

■ Distant Recurrences

Inguinal lymph node recurrences are virtually always associated with ultimately fatal disease, and few women are alive at the end of the first year following this diagnosis. Women with pelvic or distant metastases can be offered palliative chemotherapy. Combination platinum-based chemotherapy has modest activity in recurrent vulvar cancers (Cunningham, 1997; Moore, 1998). Platinum-based regimens (e.g., cisplatin/paclitaxel) might be considered for vulvar cancer if palliative chemotherapy is indicated.

MANAGEMENT DURING PREGNANCY

Squamous cell cancer of the vulva diagnosed and surgically treated during pregnancy is rare, and an incidence of 1 per 20,000 deliveries is reported (DiSaia, 1997). Nevertheless, any suspicious lesion is evaluated, even during pregnancy.

Radical total or partial vulvectomy and inguinofemoral lymphadenectomy can be performed if indicated after the first trimester. During the third trimester, markedly increased genital vasculature can raise surgical morbidity. During the late third trimester, lesions may be removed by wide local excision, and definitive surgery completed postpartum. In cases diagnosed at delivery, definitive surgery is performed typically 2 to 3 weeks postpartum.

The mode of delivery following cancer surgery is heavily influenced by the state of the postsurgical vulva. With vaginal stenosis, significant fibrosis, or tumor involvement, a cesarean delivery is recommended. Otherwise vaginal delivery is appropriate.

VERRUCOUS CARCINOMA

This rare variant of squamous cell carcinoma constitutes <1 percent of all vulvar cancers. Verrucous carcinomas can affect both younger and older women. Its etiology is unknown, but HPV genome and usual type VIN are found in association with some of these tumors. Verrucous carcinomas are locally invasive and rarely metastasize. Most women have a cauliflower-shaped vulvar mass that usually elicits pruritus or pain. Surgery is preferred, and most tumors are excised by wide local excision that ensures a 1-cm surrounding margin. Inadequate margins risk local recurrence. Verrucous carcinomas are resistant to radiotherapy and if exposed may undergo anaplastic transformation to become more aggressive and invasive. Enlarged groin lymph nodes are evaluated preoperatively by FNA because they usually are inflammatory.

MELANOMA

■ Clinical Presentation and Staging

Melanoma is the second most common vulvar cancer and accounts for 10 percent of all vulvar malignancies. Vulvar melanoma disproportionately affects the elderly and develops more often among whites. Vulvar melanoma has an overall poor prognosis, and 5-year survival rates range from 8 to 55 percent (Evans, 1994; Piura, 1992).

Malignant vulvar melanomas most frequently arise from the labia minora, labia majora, or clitoris (Fig. 31-11) (Moore, 1998; Woolcott, 1988). Some benign pigmented lesions also can be found here and include lentigo simplex, vulvar melanosis, acanthosis nigricans, seborrheic keratosis, and nevi (Chap. 4, p. 101). Last, pigmented vulvar neoplasia may be VIN, squamous cell carcinoma, or Paget disease. Thus, tissue sampling is typically needed, and immunohistochemical studies or electron microscopy can

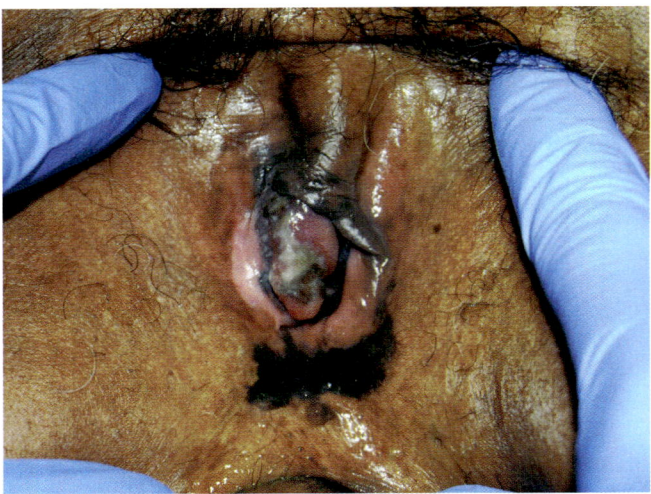

FIGURE 31-11 Vulvar melanoma. (Reproduced with permission from Dr. William Griffith.)

help clarify the diagnosis (Fig. 31-12). Three histologic subtypes of vulvar melanoma are described: superficial spreading melanoma, nodular melanoma, and acral lentiginous melanoma.

Vulvar melanomas have been staged by several microstaging systems that include the Chung, the Clark, and the Breslow systems and by the macroscopic systems published by FIGO and the American Joint Committee on Cancer (AJCC) (Table 31-5). The AJCC stage and Breslow thickness are major predictors of overall survival rates and are used most often. Breslow thickness measures in millimeters the thickest portion of the lesion from the intact epithelium's most superficial surface to the deepest point of invasion (Moxley, 2011; Verschraegen, 2001).

■ Treatment

Surgery

Vulvar melanoma has limited response to both chemotherapy and radiotherapy. Thus, excision is the single best definitive therapy.

Conservative surgery, such as wide local excision or a radical partial vulvectomy, is preferred as radical surgery appears to offer no greater survival advantage (Irvin, 2001; Verschraegen, 2001).

Nodal metastasis is a major predictor of prognosis. The incidence of occult inguinal lymph node metastases is <5 percent for thin melanomas measuring <1 mm thickness but is >70 percent for lesions >4 mm (Hoskins, 2000). Women with clinically positive groin lymph nodes should undergo inguino-femoral lymphadenectomy if possible, as surgical removal of regional disease is the most effective method of control. In patients with clinically negative groins, the decision to perform inguinofemoral lymphadenectomy or SLNB is influenced by lesion thickness. Primary lesions that warrant inguinofemoral node evaluation are those that have a Breslow thickness >1 mm. Other high-risk candidate tumors are those lesions measuring <1 mm thick but showing ulceration, a mitotic rate >1 per mm^2, or LVSI. Another high-risk lesion is that with ambiguous thickness due to a biopsy's positive deep margin (Lens, 2002b). At our institution, we encourage women with clinically negative groins to first undergo SLNB. If diseased nodes are detected, then an inguinofemoral lymphadenectomy can be considered. Primary radiation therapy can be considered as palliative for patients with advanced vulvar melanoma who are either unfit or unwilling to undergo surgery.

Adjuvant Therapy

Women may be considered for adjuvant therapy if their primary vulvar melanoma poses a great risk for disease recurrence. These risk factors include positive margins or positive inguinofemoral nodes. Although melanomas were once felt to be radioresistant, adjuvant radiation therapy can be considered for local control (Ballo, 2005; Moxley, 2011).

Previously, adjuvant alpha interferon (IFN-α) was recommended for patients with high-risk cutaneous melanoma due to an increase in both progression-free and overall survival rates (Lens, 2002a). Now, biologic antitumor agents offer superior tumor control. Of these, ipilimumab (Yervoy), a cytotoxic T

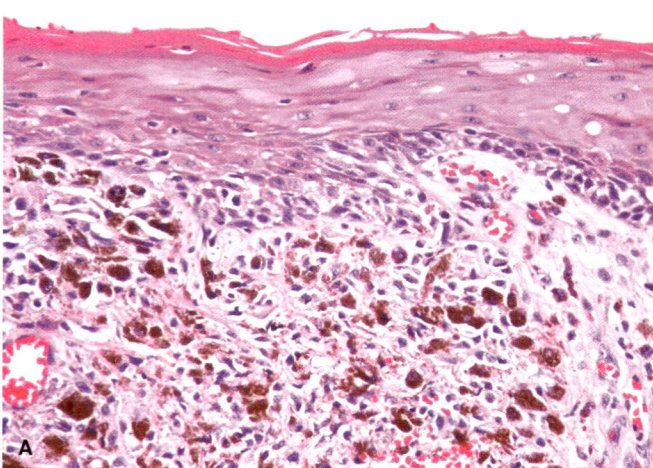

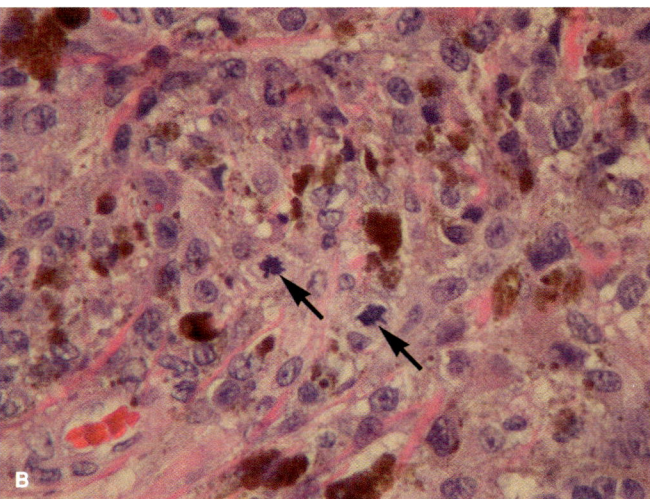

FIGURE 31-12 Vulvar melanoma. **A.** Medium-power view. Atypical, hyperchromatic melanoma cells are identified within the basal portion of the surface epithelium. Melanoma cells containing intracytoplasmic melanin pigment invade subepithelial stroma in a broad swath. **B.** High-power view. The malignant melanoma cells in this case have occasionally prominent nucleoli, abundant intracytoplasmic melanin pigment, and frequent mitoses (*arrows*) including abnormal mitoses. (Reproduced with permission from Dr. Kelley Carrick.)

TABLE 31-5. Melanoma Staging

Staging	Class	Thickness (mm)	Tumor Ulceration Status/Mitoses
IA	T1a, N0, M0	≤1	a: Without ulceration and mitosis <1/mm^2
IB	T1b, "		b: With ulceration or mitosis ≥1/mm^2
	T2a, "	1.01–2.0	a: Without ulceration
IIA	T2b, "		b: With ulceration
	T3a, "	2.01–4.0	a: Without ulceration
IIB	T3b, "		b: With ulceration
	T4a, "	>4.0	a: Without ulceration
IIC	T4b, "		b: With ulceration

		Lymph Node (No.)	Nodal Metastatic Burden
IIIA	T1-4a, N1a, M0	1	a: Micrometastasis
	T1-4a, N2a, "	2–3	a: Micrometastasis
IIIB	T1-4b, N1a, "	1	a: Micrometastasis
	T1-4b, N2a, "	2–3	a: Micrometastasis
	T1-4a, N1b, "	1	b: Macrometastasis
	T1-4a, N2b, "	2–3	b: Macrometastasis
	T1-4a, N2c, "	2–3	c: In transit metastasis only
IIIC	T1-4b, N1b, "	1	b: Macrometastasis
	T1-4b, N2b, "	2–3	b: Macrometastasis
	T1-4b, N2c, "	2–3	c In transit metastasis only
	Any T, N3, "	>4	

			Distant Metastasis Site
IV	Any T or N, M1a		Distant skin, subQ, or node
	Any T or N, M1b		Lung
	Any T or N, M1c		Other viscera

SubQ = subcutaneous.
Summarized from Balch, 2009.

lymphocyte–associated protein 4 (CTLA4) checkpoint inhibitor, was subsequently recommended instead of IFN-α due to the magnitude of overall survival benefit (Eggermot, 2015). Currently, adjuvant treatment with nivolumab (Opdivo), a programmed cell death protein 1 (PD-1) checkpoint inhibitor, can be considered in patients with stage III or IV vulvar melanoma. Its mechanism is illustrated in Chapter 27 (p. 601). Nivolumab prolonged disease-free survival compared with ipilimumab in one trial of 906 patients with acral, mucosal, or cutaneous melanoma (McDermott, 2019).

Targeting key driver mutations is another option for metastatic melanoma. Namely, *BRAF* and *c-KIT* gene mutations may be found in these tumors, and women with melanoma often have their tumors tested for these mutations. Vemurafenib (Zelboraf), a BRAF inhibitor, was approved by the Food and Drug Administration (FDA) for treatment of metastatic or unresectable melanoma that exhibits the *BRAF* mutation (Robert, 2011). Imatinib (Gleevec) may be used for tumors with the *c-KIT* mutation.

BASAL CELL CARCINOMA

Basal cell carcinoma of the vulva accounts for <2 percent of all vulvar cancers and is most commonly found in elderly women (DiSaia, 1997). Lesions typically arise on the labia majora and are characterized by poor pigmentation and pruritus. They often mimic eczema, psoriasis, or intertrigo. As a result, correct diagnosis is often delayed due to treatment for other presumed inflammatory or infectious dermatoses.

Although ultraviolet radiation is thought to be the primary risk factor for basal cell carcinoma on sun-exposed areas, its development on sun-protected areas raises the possibility of other, yet undefined, etiologies. Some suggest that local trauma and advancing age may contribute at these sites (LeSueur, 2003; Wermuth, 1970).

Basal cell carcinoma is removed by radical partial vulvectomy using a minimum surgical margin of 1 cm. Lymphatic or distant spread is rare, but inguinofemoral lymphadenectomy or SLNB is considered for clinically suspicious nodes. However, disease may locally recur, particularly in tumors removed with suboptimal margins. Most basal cell carcinomas of the vulva are indolent and locally invasive but rarely metastatic. If surgery is contraindicated, then primary radiation therapy can be considered. Local immunomodulators such as imiquimod can be selected for patients who are inappropriate surgical candidates. Because surgery is the recommended treatment, any other treatment modalities will warrant close observation to detect cancer progression.

VULVAR SARCOMA

Sarcoma of the vulva is rare, and leiomyosarcoma, malignant fibrous histiocytoma, epithelioid sarcoma, and malignant rhabdoid tumor are the more frequently encountered histologic types. Of these, leiomyosarcoma appears to be most common. Tumors typically develop as isolated masses on the labia majora, clitoris, or Bartholin gland (Fig. 31-13). Unlike squamous cell carcinoma, the age of affected women is significantly broader and varies between histologic types.

The outcome of vulvar sarcomas is influenced by tumor size, degree of mitotic activity, and level of infiltration. That is, disease associated with lesions >5 cm in diameter, with infiltrating margins, with extensive necrosis, and with more than five mitoses per 10 high-power fields is most likely to recur after surgical resection (Magné, 2011).

Hematogenous metastasis is the most frequent route of tumor dissemination. Radical partial or total vulvectomy or pelvic exenteration is recommended if total surgical resection is possible. Removal of inguinofemoral lymph nodes is performed if nodes are large and/or symptomatic. Adjuvant radiation, chemotherapy, or both can be considered depending on risk factors for recurrence. Neoadjuvant chemotherapy and/or radiotherapy are considerations for unresectable vulvar sarcomas.

BARTHOLIN GLAND CARCINOMA

Primary malignant tumors arising from the Bartholin gland can be adenocarcinomas, squamous cell carcinomas, or transitional cell carcinomas. The incidence of Bartholin gland carcinomas peaks in women in their mid-60s. Soft, distensible tissue normally surrounds these glands, and tumors may reach considerable size before patients develop symptoms. Dyspareunia is a common first complaint. Bartholin gland enlargement in a woman older than 40 years and recurrent cysts or abscesses

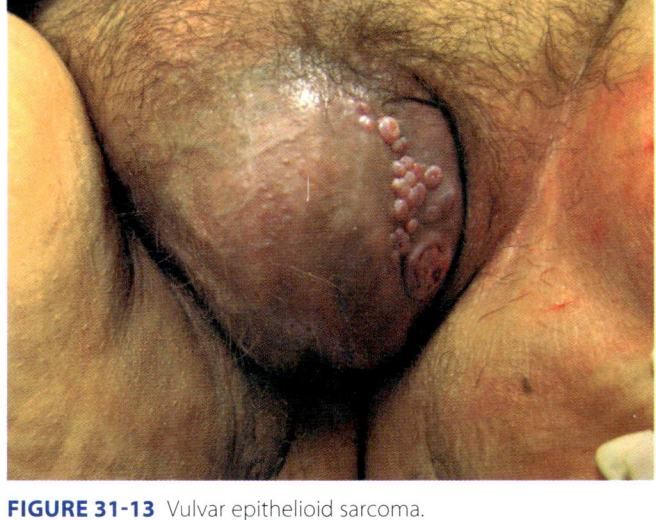

FIGURE 31-13 Vulvar epithelioid sarcoma.

warrant a biopsy or excision. Similarly, all solid masses require FNA or biopsy to establish a definitive diagnosis.

Bartholin gland carcinomas tend to spread into the ischiorectal fossa and have a propensity for lymphatic spread into the inguinal and pelvic lymph nodes. Therapy for most early cancer stages includes a radical partial vulvectomy with inguinofemoral lymphadenectomy. Decisions to perform ipsilateral or bilateral groin dissection follow the same criteria as for squamous cell tumors. Postoperative chemoradiation reduces the likelihood of local recurrence for all stages. If the initial lesion impinges on the rectum or anal sphincter, preoperative chemoradiation can be used to avoid extensive surgery.

VULVAR PAGET DISEASE

Extramammary Paget disease is a heterogeneous group of intraepithelial neoplasias and, when present on the vulva, appears as an eczematoid, red, weeping area (Fig. 31-14). These

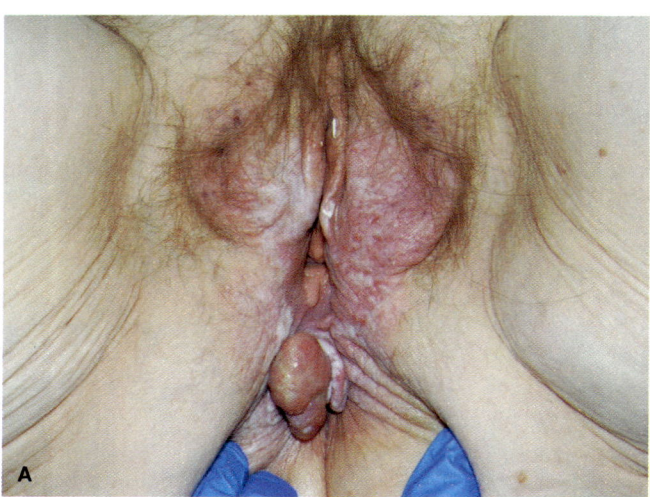

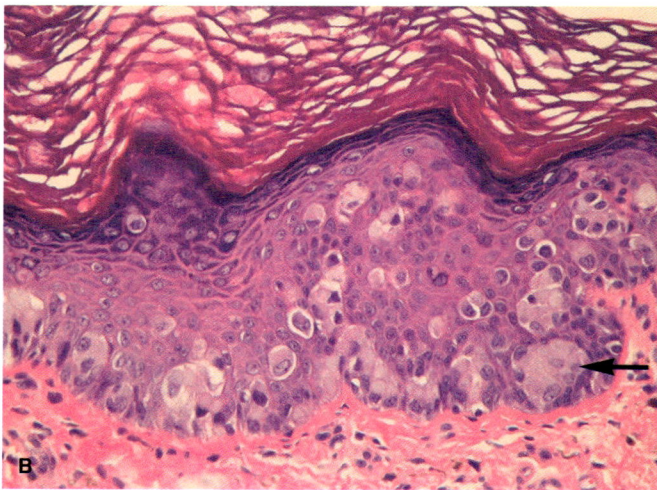

FIGURE 31-14 A. Vulvar Paget disease involving the labia bilaterally, perineum, perianus, and solid right perianal mass. (Reproduced with permission from Dr. Claudia Werner.) **B.** Photomicrograph of primary cutaneous vulvar Paget disease. This is characterized microscopically by the presence of relatively large atypical cells with prominent nucleoli and abundant delicate cytoplasm (*arrow*). These cells are disposed singly or in clusters at various levels within the epithelium. The neoplastic cells are most often confined to the epithelium and would in these instances be classified as an adenocarcinoma in situ. (Reproduced with permission from Dr. Kelley Carrick.)

are often localized to the labia majora, perineal body, or clitoris. This disease typically develops in older white women and accounts for approximately 2 percent of all vulvar tumors. Vulvar Paget disease is accompanied by invasive Paget disease or adenocarcinoma of the vulva in 10 to 20 percent of cases (Hoskins, 2000). Moreover, 20 percent of patients with extramammary Paget disease of the vulva will have a carcinoma at another nonvulvar location (Pang, 2010; Wilkinson, 2002). Screening and surveillance for tumors at nongynecologic sites is considered and includes evaluation of the breasts and the gastrointestinal and genitourinary tracts. A discussion of Paget disease of the breast is presented in Chapter 13 (p. 290).

A histologic classification proposed by Wilkinson and Brown (2002) includes: (1) primary vulvar cutaneous Paget disease, (2) Paget disease as an extension of transitional cell carcinoma of the bladder or urethra, and (3) Paget disease as an extension of an associated adjacent primary cancer such as vulvar, anal, or rectal cancers. The histologic differentiation of these Paget disease types is important because the specific diagnosis significantly influences treatment selection.

Of these, primary cutaneous vulvar Paget disease displays slow growth. Diseased areas ideally are resected by wide local excision with a 1- to 2-cm margin. In contrast to resected VIN 3, margins are often positive, and disease recurrence develops frequently regardless of the surgical margin status (Black, 2007). Long-term surveillance is prudent since repeated surgical excision is often necessary. Patients with positive margin after surgical excision of the primary tumor can be followed conservatively.

If invasive disease is suspected, radical partial vulvectomy is warranted by extending the deep margins to the perineal membrane. The latter is frequently accompanied with an ipsilateral or bilateral inguinofemoral lymphadenectomy.

CANCER METASTATIC TO THE VULVA

Metastatic tumors make up approximately 8 percent of all vulvar cancers. Tumors may extend from primary cancers of the bladder, urethra, vagina, or rectum. Less proximate cancers include those from the breast, kidney, lung, and stomach, as well as gestational choriocarcinoma (Wilkinson, 2011).

REFERENCES

Balch CM, Gershenwald JE, Soong S, et al: Final version of 2009 AJCC melanoma staging and classification. J Clin Oncol 27(36):6199, 2009

Ballo MT, Garden AS, Myers JN, et al: Melanoma metastatic to cervical lymph nodes: can radiotherapy replace formal dissection after local excision of nodal disease? Head Neck 27(8):718, 2005

Bell JG, Lea JS, Reid GC: Complete groin lymphadenectomy with preservation of the fascia lata in the treatment of vulvar carcinoma. Gynecol Oncol 77:314, 2000

Binder SW, Huang I, Fu YS, et al: Risk factors for the development of lymph node metastasis in vulvar squamous cell carcinoma. Gynecol Oncol 37:9, 1990

Black D, Tornos C, Soslow RA, et al: The outcomes of patients with positive margins after excision for intraepithelial Paget's disease of the vulva. Gynecol Oncol 104:547, 2007

Brinton LA, Nasca PC, Mallin K, et al: Case-control study of cancer of the vulva. Obstet Gynecol 75:859, 1990

Burke TW, Levenback C, Coleman RL, et al: Surgical therapy of T1 and T2 vulvar carcinoma: further experience with radical wide excision and selective inguinal lymphadenectomy. Gynecol Oncol 57:215, 1995

Casolati E, Agarossi A, Valieri M, et al: Vulvar neoplasia in HIV positive women: a review. Med Wieku Rozwoj 7(4 Pt 1):487, 2003

Chan JK, Sugiyama V, Pham H, et al: Margin distance and other clinico-pathologic prognostic factors in vulvar carcinoma: a multivariate analysis. Gynecol Oncol 104:636, 2007

Cunningham MJ, Goyer RP, Gibbons SK, et al: Primary radiation, cisplatin, and 5-fluorouracil for advanced squamous carcinoma of the vulva. Gynecol Oncol 66:258, 1997

DiSaia PJ, Creasman WT (eds): Invasive cancer of the vulva. In Clinical Gynecologic Oncology, 5th ed. St. Louis, Mosby–Year Book, 1997, pp 202, 229

Donaldson ES, Powell DE, Hanson MB, et al: Prognostic parameters in invasive vulvar cancer. Gynecol Oncol 11:184, 1981

Eggermont AM, Chiarion-Sileni V, Grob JJ, et al: Adjuvant ipilimumab versus placebo after complete resection of high-risk stage III melanoma (EORTC 18071): a randomised, double-blind, phase 3 trial. Lancet Oncol 16(5):522, 2015

Elit L, Voruganti S, Simunovic M: Invasive vulvar cancer in a woman with human immunodeficiency virus: case report and review of the literature. Gynecol Oncol 98:151, 2005

Eva LJ, Ganesan R, Chan KK, et al: Differentiated-type vulval intraepithelial neoplasia has a high-risk association with vulval squamous cell carcinoma. Int J Gynecol Cancer 19(4):741, 2009

Evans RA: Review and current perspectives of cutaneous malignant melanoma. J Am Coll Surg 179:764, 1994

Farias-Eisner R, Cirisano FD, Grouse D, et al: Conservative and individualized surgery for early squamous carcinoma of the vulva: the treatment of choice for stage I and II (T1–2N0–1M0) disease. Gynecol Oncol 53:55, 1994

Figge DC, Tamimi HK, Greer BE: Lymphatic spread in carcinoma of the vulva. Am J Obstet Gynecol 152:387, 1985

Frisch M, Biggar RJ, Goedert JJ: Human papillomavirus-associated cancers in patients with human immunodeficiency virus infection and acquired immunodeficiency syndrome. J Natl Cancer Inst 92:1500, 2000

Frumovitz M, Ramirez PT, Levenback C: Lymphatic mapping and sentinel node detection in gynecologic malignancies of the lower genital tract. Curr Oncol Rep 7(6):435, 2005

Gargano JW, Wilkinson EJ, Unger ER, et al: Prevalence of human papillomavirus types in invasive vulvar cancers and vulvar intraepithelial neoplasia 3 in the United States before vaccine introduction. J Low Genit Tract Dis 16(4):471, 2012

Garland SM, Joura EA, Ault KA, et al: Human papillomavirus genotypes from vaginal and vulvar intraepithelial neoplasia in females 15–26 years of age. Obstet Gynecol 132(2):261, 2018

Gordinier ME, Malpica A, Burke TW, et al: Groin recurrence in patients with vulvar cancer with negative nodes on superficial inguinal lymphadenectomy. Gynecol Oncol 90:625, 2003

Hacker NF, Berek JS, Lagasse LD, et al: Individualization of treatment for stage I squamous cell vulvar carcinoma. Obstet Gynecol 63:155, 1984

Hacker NF, Berek JS, Lagasse LD, et al: Management of regional lymph nodes and their prognostic influence in vulvar cancer. Obstet Gynecol 61(4):408, 1983

Hallak S, Ladi L, Sorbe B: Prophylactic inguinal-femoral irradiation as an alternative to primary lymphadenectomy in treatment of vulvar carcinoma. Int J Oncol 31(5):1077, 2007

Halonen P, Jakobsson M, Heikinheimo O, et al: Lichen sclerosus and risk of cancer. Int J Cancer 140(9):1998, 2017

Heaps JM, Fu YS, Montz FJ, et al: Surgical-pathologic variables predictive of local recurrence in squamous cell carcinoma of the vulva. Gynecol Oncol 38(3):309, 1990

Homesley HD, Bundy BN, Sedlis A, et al: Assessment of current International Federation of Gynecology and Obstetrics staging of vulvar carcinoma relative to prognostic factors for survival (a Gynecologic Oncology Group study). Am J Obstet Gynecol 164(4):997, 1991

Homesley HD, Bundy BN, Sedlis A, et al: Prognostic factors for groin node metastasis in squamous cell carcinoma of the vulva (a Gynecologic Oncology Group study). Gynecol Oncol 49(3):279, 1993

Homesley HD, Bundy BN, Sedlis A, et al: Radiation therapy versus pelvic node resection for carcinoma of the vulva with positive groin nodes. Obstet Gynecol 68:733, 1986

Hoskins WJ, Perez CA, Young RC (eds): Vulva. In Principles and Practice of Gynecologic Oncology, 3rd ed. Philadelphia, Lippincott Williams & Wilkins, 2000, p 665

Huh WK, Joura EA, Giuliano AR, et al: Final efficacy, immunogenicity, and safety analyses of a nine-valent human papillomavirus vaccine in women aged 16–26 years: a randomised, double-blind trial. Lancet 390(10108):2143, 2017

Irvin WP Jr, Legallo RL, Stoler MH, et al: Vulvar melanoma: a retrospective analysis and literature review. Gynecol Oncol 83:457, 2001

Jones RW, Rowan DM, Stewart AW: Vulvar intraepithelial neoplasia: aspects of the natural history and outcome in 405 women. Obstet Gynecol 106(6):1319, 2005

Judson PL, Jonson AL, Paley PJ, et al: A prospective, randomized study analyzing Sartorius transposition following inguinal-femoral lymphadenectomy. Gynecol Oncol 95:226, 2004

Kirschner CV, Yordan EL, De Geest K, et al: Smoking, obesity, and survival in squamous cell carcinoma of the vulva. Gynecol Oncol 56:79, 1995

Kunos C, Simpkins F, Gibbons H, et al: Radiation therapy compared with pelvic node resection for node-positive vulvar cancer: a randomized controlled trial. Obstet Gynecol 114:537, 2009

Kurman RJ, Carcangiu ML, Herrington CS, et al (eds): WHO Classification of Tumours of Female Reproductive Organs, 4th ed. Lyon, International Agency for Research on Cancer, 2014, p 231

Lens MB, Dawes M: Interferon alfa therapy for malignant melanoma: a systematic review of randomized controlled trials. J Clin Oncol 20(7):1818, 2002a

Lens MB, Dawes M, Goodacre T, et al: Excision margins in the treatment of primary cutaneous melanoma: a systematic review of randomized controlled trials comparing narrow vs wide excision. Arch Surg 137(10):1101, 2002b

LeSueur BW, DiCaudo DJ, Connolly SM: Axillary basal cell carcinoma. Dermatol Surg 29:1105, 2003

Levenback C: Update on sentinel lymph node biopsy in gynecologic cancers. Gynecol Oncol 111(2 Suppl):S42, 2008

Levenback C, Morris M, Burke TW, et al: Groin dissection practices among gynecologic oncologists treating early vulvar cancer. Gynecol Oncol 62(1):73, 1996

Madeleine MM, Daling JR, Carter JJ, et al: Cofactors with human papillomavirus in a population-based study of vulvar cancer. J Natl Cancer Inst 89:1516, 1997

Magné N, Pacaut C, Auberdiac P, et al: Sarcoma of vulva, vagina and ovary. Best Pract Res Clin Obstet Gynaecol 25(6):797, 2011

Manavi M, Berger A, Kucera E, et al: Does T1, N0-1 vulvar cancer treated by vulvectomy but not lymphadenectomy need inguinofemoral radiation? Int J Radiat Oncol Biol Phys 38(4):749, 1997

McDermott DF, Shah R, Gupte-Singh K, et al: Quality-adjusted survival of nivolumab plus ipilimumab or nivolumab alone versus ipilimumab alone among treatment-naive patients with advanced melanoma: a quality-adjusted time without symptoms or toxicity (Q-TWiST) analysis. Qual Life Res 28(1):109, 2019

Modesitt SC, Waters AB, Walton L, et al: Vulvar intraepithelial neoplasia III: occult cancer and the impact of margin status on recurrence. Obstet Gynecol 92(6):962, 1998

Moore D, Ali S, Barnes M, et al: A phase II trial of radiation therapy and weekly cisplatin chemotherapy for the treatment of locally advanced squamous cell carcinoma of the vulva: a Gynecologic Oncology Group study. Gynecol Oncol 124(3):529, 2012

Moore DH, Thomas GM, Montana GS, et al: Preoperative chemoradiation for advanced vulvar cancer: a phase II study of the Gynecologic Oncology Group. Int J Radiat Oncol Biol Phys 42:79, 1998

Morley GW: Infiltrative carcinoma of the vulva: results of surgical treatment. Am J Obstet Gynecol 124:874, 1976

Moxley KM, Fader AN, Rose PG, et al: Malignant melanoma of the vulva: an extension of cutaneous melanoma? Gynecol Oncol 122(3):612, 2011

Nooij LS, van der Slot MA, Dekkers OM, et al: Tumour-free margins in vulvar squamous cell carcinoma: Does distance really matter? Eur J Cancer 65:139, 2016

Origoni M, Sideri M, Garsia S, et al: Prognostic value of pathological patterns of lymph node positivity in squamous cell carcinoma of the vulva stage III and IVA FIGO. Gynecol Oncol 45:313, 1992

Pang J, Assaad D, Breen D et al: Extramammary Paget disease: review of patients seen in a non-melanoma skin cancer clinic. Curr Oncol 17(5):43, 2010

Pecorelli S: Revised FIGO staging for carcinoma of the vulva, cervix, and endometrium. Int J Gynaecol Obstet 105(2):103, 2009

Penn I: Cancers in renal transplant recipients. Adv Ren Replace Ther 7(2):147, 2000

Perez CA, Grigsby PW, Galakatos A, et al: Radiation therapy in management of carcinoma of the vulva with emphasis on conservation therapy. Cancer 71(11):3707, 1993

Petereit DG, Mehta MP, Buchler DA, et al: A retrospective review of nodal treatment for vulvar cancer. Am J Clin Oncol 16(1):38, 1993

Piura B, Egan M, Lopes A, et al: Malignant melanoma of the vulva: a clinicopathologic study of 18 cases. J Surg Oncol 50:234, 1992

Preti M, Rouzier R, Mariani L, et al: Superficially invasive carcinoma of the vulva: diagnosis and treatment. Clin Obstet Gynecol 48:862, 2005

Razzaghi H, Saraiya M, Thompson TD, et al: Five-year relative survival for human papillomavirus-associated cancer sites. Cancer 124(1):203, 2018

Reyes MC, Cooper K: An update on vulvar intraepithelial neoplasia: terminology and a practical approach to diagnosis. J Clin Pathol 67(4):290, 2014

Robert C, Thomas L, Bondarenko I, et al: Ipilimumab plus dacarbazine for previously untreated metastatic melanoma. N Engl J Med 364(26):2517, 2011

Rouzier R, Haddad B, Dubernard G, et al: Inguinofemoral dissection for carcinoma of the vulva: effect of modifications of extent and technique on morbidity and survival. J Am Coll Surg 196:442, 2003

Salani R, Khanna N, Frimer M, et al: An update on post-treatment surveillance and diagnosis of recurrence in women with gynecologic malignancies: Society of Gynecologic Oncology (SGO) recommendations. Gynecol Oncol 146(1):3, 2017

Salcedo MP, Sood AK, Dos Reis R, et al: Perineural invasion (PNI) in vulvar carcinoma: a review of 421 cases. Gynecol Oncol 152(1):101, 2019

Saraiya M, Unger ER, Thompson TD, et al: US assessment of HPV types in cancers: implications for current and 9-valent HPV vaccines. J Natl Cancer Inst 107(6):djv086, 2015

SEER: Surveillance, Epidemiology, and End Results Program: Cancer stat facts: vulvar cancer. 2018. Available at: https://seer.cancer.gov/statfacts/html/vulva.html. Accessed March 28, 2019

Siegel RL, Miller KD, Jemal A: Cancer statistics, 2019. CA Cancer J Clin 69(1):7, 2019

Stehman FB, Bundy BN, Thomas G, et al: Groin dissection versus groin radiation in carcinoma of the vulva: a Gynecologic Oncology Group study. Int J Radiat Oncol Biol Phys 24(2):389, 1992

Stehman FB, Look KY: Carcinoma of the vulva. Obstet Gynecol 107(3):719, 2006

Tantipalakorn C, Robertson G, Marsden DE, et al: Outcome and patterns of recurrence for International Federation of Gynecology and Obstetrics (FIGO) stages I and II squamous cell vulvar cancer. Obstet Gynecol 113(4):895, 2009

Te Grootenhuis NC, van der Zee AG, van Doorn HC, et al: Sentinel nodes in vulvar cancer: Long-term follow-up of the GROningen INternational Study on Sentinel nodes in Vulvar cancer (GROINSS-V) I. Gynecol Oncol 140(1):8, 2016

Van der Steen S, de Nieuwenhof HP, Massuger L, et al: New FIGO staging system of vulvar cancer indeed provides a better reflection of prognosis. Gynecol Oncol 119(3):520, 2010

Verschraegen CF, Benjapibal M, Supakarapongkul W, et al: Vulvar melanoma at the M. D. Anderson Cancer Center: 25 years later. Int J Gynecol Cancer 11:359, 2001

Way S: The anatomy of the lymphatic drainage of the vulva and its influence on the radical operation for carcinoma. Ann R Coll Surg Engl 3(4):187, 1948

Wermuth BM, Fajardo LF: Metastatic basal cell carcinoma: a review. Arch Pathol 90:458, 1970

Wilkinson EJ: Premalignant and malignant tumors of the vulva. In Kurman RJ, Ellenson LH, Ronnett BM (eds): Blaustein's Pathology of the Female Genital Tract, New York, Springer, 2011, p 95

Wilkinson EJ, Brown HM: Vulvar Paget disease of urothelial origin: a report of three cases and a proposed classification of vulvar Paget disease. Hum Pathol 33(5):549, 2002

Woelber L, Griebel LF, Eulenburg C, et al: Role of tumour-free margin distance for loco-regional control in vulvar cancer-a subset analysis of the Arbeitsgemeinschaft Gynäkologische Onkologie CaRE-1 multicenter study. Eur J Cancer 69:180, 2016

Woolcott RJ, Henry RJ, Houghton CR: Malignant melanoma of the vulva: Australian experience. J Reprod Med 33:699, 1988

CHAPTER 32

Vaginal Cancer

Cancer found in the vagina is most likely metastatic disease. Primary vaginal carcinoma is rare and makes up less than 5 percent of all gynecologic malignancies (Siegel, 2019). This low incidence reflects the infrequency with which primary carcinoma arises in the vagina and the strict criteria for its diagnosis. According to International Federation of Gynecology and Obstetrics (FIGO) staging criteria, a vaginal lesion that involves adjacent organs such as the cervix or vulva, by convention, is deemed primary cervical or vulvar, respectively (Pecorelli, 1999). The most common histologic type of primary vaginal cancer is squamous cell carcinoma, followed by adenocarcinoma (Platz, 1995).

RELEVANT ANATOMY

During embryogenesis, the müllerian ducts fuse caudally to form the uterovaginal canal (Chap. 19, p. 406). The canal's distal portion forms the proximal vagina, whereas the distal vagina arises from the urogenital sinus. The uterovaginal canal is lined by columnar epithelium, which is subsequently replaced by squamous cells migrating cephalad from the urogenital sinus. These squamous cells stratify, and the vaginal epithelium matures and thickens. Underlying this epithelium, muscularis and adventitial layers surround the vaginal tube.

With vaginal cancer, local extension and lymphatic invasion are common patterns of spread. The lymphatic channels that drain the vagina form extensive, complex, and variable anastomoses. As a result, any node in the pelvis, groin, or anorectal area may drain any part of the vagina. Of these, the external, internal, and common iliac lymph nodes are the primary sites of vaginal lymphatic drainage. Thus, pelvic lymphadenectomy, which samples these nodal groups, is commonly performed during primary surgical excision of proximally located vaginal cancers. Alternatively, lymphatic vessels of the posterior vagina

may empty into the inferior gluteal, presacral, or perirectal nodes, and those of the vagina's distal third may drain to the superficial and deep inguinal lymph nodes (Frank, 2005).

Hematogenous spread of vaginal cancer is less frequent, and venous drainage consists of the uterine, pudendal, and rectal veins, which drain into the internal iliac vein. Arterial blood supply to the vagina comes primarily from internal iliac artery branches, which include the uterine, vaginal, middle rectal, and internal pudendal arteries (Fig. 38-12, p. 801).

INCIDENCE

According to estimates for 2019, approximately 5000 new cases of vaginal cancer will be diagnosed in the United States, and there will be 1430 deaths (Siegel, 2019). The overall incidence is 0.45 cases per 100,000 women but is notably lower in whites (0.42 cases) compared with black and Hispanic women (0.73 and 0.56 cases, respectively) (Watson, 2009). Vaginal cancer rates rise with age and peak among women aged ≥80 years. The median age at diagnosis is 58 (Watson, 2009). Of histologic forms, squamous cell carcinoma accounts for 70 to 80 percent of all primary vaginal cancer cases (Beller, 2003; Ghia, 2011).

SQUAMOUS CELL CARCINOMA

■ Risks

Squamous cell cancer of the vagina arises within its stratified nonkeratinized epithelium (Fig. 32-1). As with other cancers of the lower reproductive tract, human papillomavirus (HPV) has been closely linked with squamous cell vaginal cancer (Chap. 30, p. 655). A systematic review found an HPV prevalence of 65 percent in samples from invasive vaginal cancer, and a 93-percent prevalence in high-grade vaginal dysplasia lesions. HPV 16 was the most common type and was present in 55 percent of vaginal cancer samplings (Smith, 2009). One retrospective study of 31 countries found similar results (Alemany, 2014).

Because of this association with HPV infection, vaginal in situ and invasive squamous cell carcinomas share risk factors similar to those for cervical cancer. Some of these include multiple lifetime sexual partners, early age at first intercourse, and current cigarette smoking. Women with a vulvar or cervical cancer history also are at greater risk. This last association may stem from the field effect of HPV affecting multiple lower genital tract epithelia or may result from direct tumor spread.

Vaginal intraepithelial neoplasia (VaIN) is a precursor to invasive vaginal cancer, and up to 3 percent of patients with

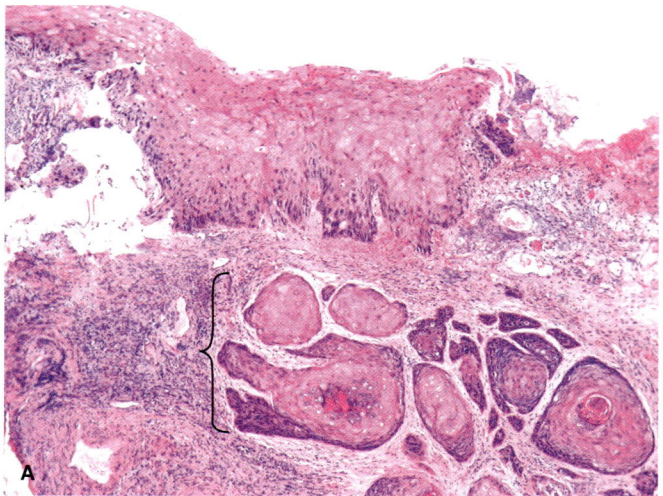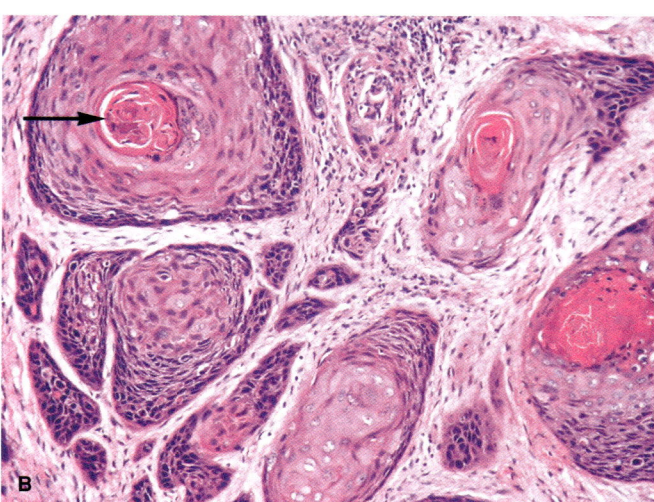

FIGURE 32-1 Sections showing invasive squamous cell carcinoma of the vagina. **A.** Invasive, well-differentiated squamous cell carcinoma of the vagina (*bracket*) invading the subepithelial stroma (×4). **B.** Invasive, well-differentiated squamous cell carcinoma of the vagina (×10). Invasive tumor is composed of irregular nests of malignant squamous cells with keratin pearls (*arrow*) and intercellular bridges. (Reproduced with permission from Dr. Kelley Carrick.)

VaIN will progress to invasive cancer (Ratnavelu, 2013; Zeligs, 2013). Gardasil 9 vaccine is effective against HPV 16 and 18 (Huh, 2017). It is possible that this vaccine will lower future rates of invasive vaginal cancer.

■ Diagnosis

Vaginal bleeding is the most common complaint associated with vaginal cancer, although pelvic pain and vaginal discharge also may be noted. Less often, lesions involving the anterior vaginal wall may lead to dysuria, hematuria, or urgency. Alternatively, constipation may result from posterior wall masses. Most vaginal cancers develop in the upper third of the vagina.

During pelvic evaluation in all women, the vagina is inspected as the speculum is inserted or removed. If a gross lesion is found, vaginal cancer usually can be diagnosed by punch biopsy in the office. Biopsy may be obtained with Tischler biopsy forceps (Fig. 29-15, p. 637). An Emmett hook, one type of skin hook, may be useful to elevate and stabilize vaginal tissue during biopsy. Monsel paste is applied as needed for hemostasis. If a gross lesion is not detectable,

a colposcope can guide directed biopsy. Bimanual examination assists in determining the tumor size, and rectovaginal examination is especially important for posterior wall lesions. Once cancer is diagnosed, no specific laboratory testing other than that used generally for preoperative preparation is required.

■ Staging and Classification

Vaginal cancer staging is completed clinically. This involves physical examination and perhaps cystourethroscopy and/or proctosigmoidoscopy depending on tumor location. If needed, general anesthesia can permit a more detailed pelvic examination for accurate staging. Proctosigmoidoscopy to a depth of at least 15 cm can detect local bowel invasion, whereas cystourethroscopy assists identification of bladder or urethral involvement. Chest radiography aids the search for metastatic disease (Table 32-1 and Table 32-2).

TABLE 32-1. Vaginal Cancer Evaluation

Vaginal biopsy
Physical examination
Endocervical curettage
Endometrial biopsy
Cystourethroscopy
Proctosigmoidoscopy
Chest radiograph
Abdominopelvic CT scan or MR imaging[a]

[a]Useful for treatment planning but not used to assign FIGO stage.
CT = computed tomography; MR = magnetic resonance.

TABLE 32-2. FIGO Staging Classification of Vaginal Cancer

Stage	Characteristics
I	The carcinoma is limited to the vaginal wall
II	The carcinoma has involved the subvaginal tissue but has not extended to the pelvic wall
III	The carcinoma has extended to the pelvic wall
IV	The carcinoma has extended beyond the true pelvis or has involved the mucosa of the bladder or rectum; bullous edema as such does not permit a case to be allotted to stage IV
IVA	Tumor invades bladder and/or rectal mucosa and/or direct extension beyond the true pelvis
IVB	Spread to distant organs

FIGO = International Federation of Gynecology and Obstetrics.

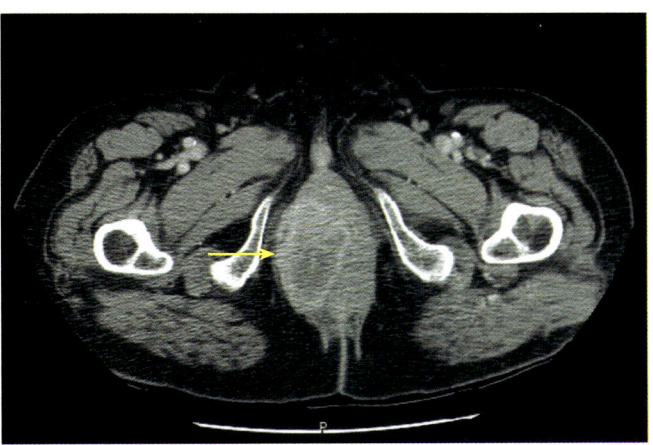

FIGURE 32-2 Computed tomography (CT) scan reveals size and extent of vaginal mass (*arrow*).

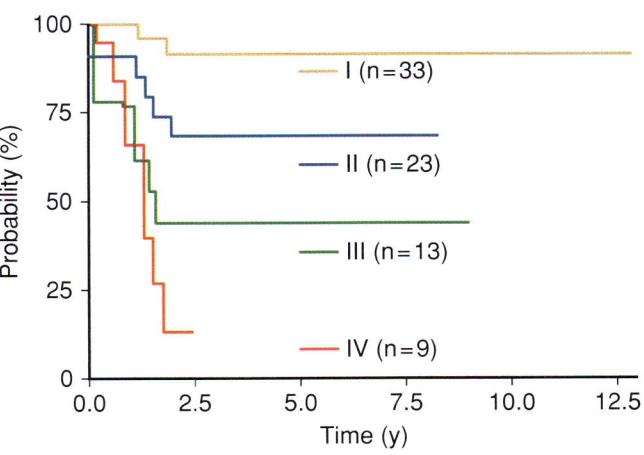

FIGURE 32-4 Disease-specific survival stratified by International Federation of Gynecology and Obstetrics (FIGO) stage. (From Tran, 2007, with permission.)

Computed tomography (CT) scanning, magnetic resonance (MR) imaging, and fluorodeoxyglucose positron emission tomography (FDG-PET) may help treatment planning but are not classically used to determine disease stage. CT scanning can delineate the size and extent of many tumors (Fig. 32-2).

However, if the extent of cancer expansion is unclear, MR imaging is the most useful radiologic tool available to visualize the vagina due to its superior soft tissue resolution. FDG-PET can be selected to evaluate lymph node involvement and distant metastases. In one study, FDG-PET was more sensitive than CT for detection of abnormal lymph nodes (Lamoreaux, 2005).

■ Prognosis

Earlier diagnosis and advances in radiation technology are largely responsible for the improved prognosis of vaginal squamous cell carcinoma. The 5-year survival rate now ranges from 45 to 68 percent for all stages (Ghia, 2011; Hellman, 2006).

The prognosis of vaginal squamous cell carcinoma depends primarily on FIGO stage (Fig. 32-3 and Table 32-2) (Frank, 2005; Rajagopalan, 2014). Other factors associated with poor prognosis include larger tumor size, adenocarcinoma cell type, older age, and tobacco use (Chyle, 1996; Gunderson, 2013; Hellman, 2006). The 5-year disease-specific survival rate is 85 to 92 percent for women with stage I disease, 68 to 78 percent for those with stage II, and 13 to 58 percent for those with stage III or IV (Fig. 32-4) (Frank, 2005; Tran, 2007).

■ Treatment

Stage I

Because of vaginal cancer's rarity, data are limited to guide evidence-based treatment. Therefore, therapy is individualized and based on factors such as tumor type, stage, location, and size.

For stage I disease, both surgery and radiotherapy are options. However, surgery is preferred for most if negative surgical margins can be achieved. Surgery includes radical vaginectomy, radical hysterectomy (for women with an intact

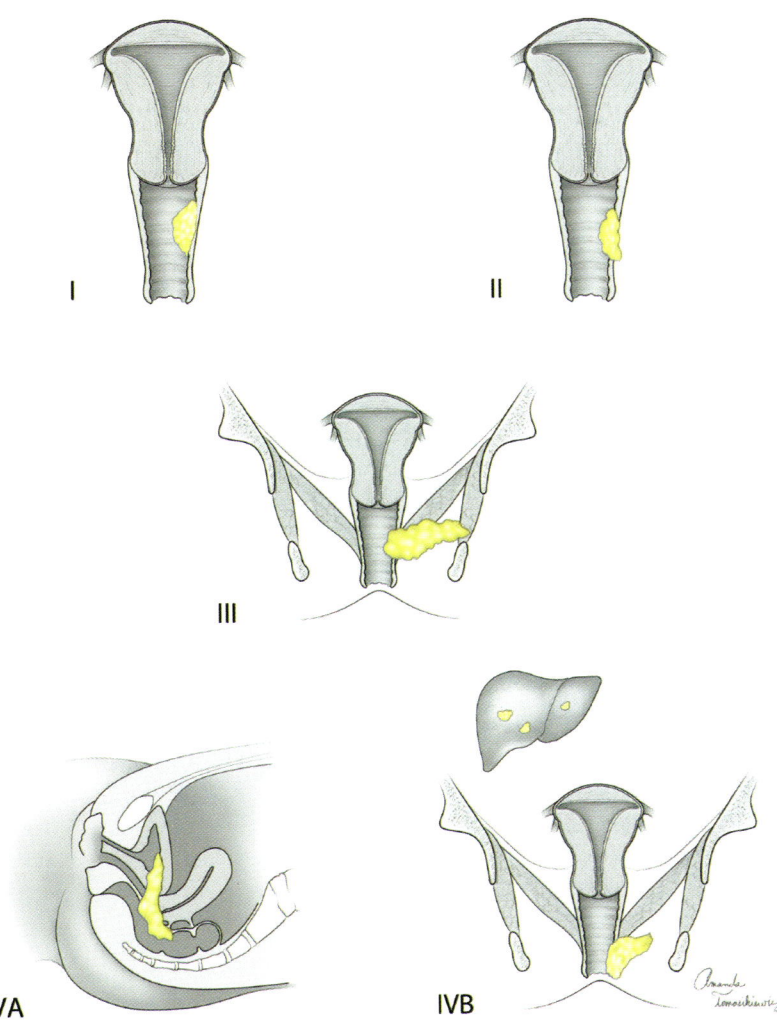

FIGURE 32-3 FIGO (International Federation of Gynecology and Obstetrics) staging of vaginal cancer.

uterus), and pelvic lymphadenectomy for most tumors located in the upper third of the vaginal vault. A review of the National Cancer Database (NCDB) showed that women with stage I disease treated with surgery alone had a significantly improved 5-year survival rate compared with those treated with radiation (90 percent versus 63 percent) (Creasman, 1998). However, other reports have found no significant difference in disease-free survival rates in women with stage I disease treated with surgery compared with radiation alone (Stock, 1995). Radiotherapy may be delivered by external beam, with or without brachytherapy. Further, brachytherapy alone has been used successfully to treat selected small stage I lesions (Nori, 1983; Perez, 1999; Reddy, 1991).

Stage II

Depending on circumstances and the treating clinician, primary surgery or radiation may be selected for stage II cancers. Stock and colleagues (1995) found a significant survival advantage at 5 years in those with stage II disease treated with surgery compared with those treated with radiation (62 percent versus 53 percent). Review of the NCDB showed that the 5-year survival rate for women with stage II disease treated with surgery alone was 70 percent; with radiotherapy alone, 57 percent; and with a combination of surgery and radiotherapy, 58 percent (Creasman, 1998). However, other researchers have found no survival advantage from surgery compared with radiotherapy in stage II disease (Davis, 1991; Rubin, 1985).

Radiation is generally recommended if negative margins cannot be achieved surgically due to tumor location or size or due to patient comorbidities that preclude surgery. If primary radiation is administered for stage II disease, a combination of external beam radiation and brachytherapy is most common. External beam radiation generally is given first, and depending on tumor response, brachytherapy is tailored to remaining disease. As discussed later, adjuvant chemotherapy is often administered during radiotherapy.

Stage III and IVA

For advanced disease, external beam radiation alone or in combination with brachytherapy is usually administered (Frank, 2005). Concurrent chemotherapy with cisplatin as a radiation adjunct is generally also recommended.

Stage IVB

Metastatic vaginal cancer is not curable, and treatment may include systemic chemotherapy or supportive hospice care. The most common sites of distant spread include liver, lung, and bone. The choice of chemotherapeutic agents is commonly extrapolated from cervical cancer data. For example, bevacizumab (Avastin) was approved by the Food and Drug Administration (FDA) in 2014 as a treatment for metastatic cervical cancer, in combination with paclitaxel and either cisplatin or topotecan. The addition of bevacizumab to these chemotherapy combinations improved overall survival length by approximately 4 months in women with metastatic cervical cancer (Tewari, 2014).

Chemoradiation

The numbers of women with vaginal cancer have been too small for prospective, randomized trials. However, concurrent chemotherapy with cisplatin can be considered to benefit those with locally advanced vaginal cancer because of its proven efficacy for cervical cancer. The characteristics of this agent are described in Chapter 27 (p. 598) and Figure 30-13 (p. 670).

In a Surveillance Epidemiology and End Result (SEER) database analysis of 326 patients with vaginal cancer treated with external beam radiation and/or brachytherapy between 1991 and 2005, a notable rise in sensitizing chemotherapy use was observed after 1999. This coincided with a National Cancer Institute announcement regarding the efficacy of chemoradiation in cervical cancer. Despite this greater use, the authors did not find a survival advantage among those vaginal cancer patients who received chemoradiation compared with radiation alone (Ghia, 2011).

However, data from the NCDB compared women with vaginal cancer treated between 1998 and 2011 with radiation therapy alone or with chemotherapy. Of 8086 women, 49 percent received chemoradiation. The median overall survival rate was 56 months in those patients receiving chemoradiation compared with 41 months for those receiving radiation alone (Rajagopalan, 2014).

Of other agents, a phase II trial, which included 22 cervical cancer patients and three with stage II–IV vaginal cancer, demonstrated a 96-percent response rate for women given weekly cisplatin, radiation, and triapine, a ribonucleotide reductase inhibitor (Kunos, 2013). Larger studies are ongoing in cervical cancer patients.

Chemotherapy

In general, chemotherapy alone is ineffective to treat vaginal cancer, although data are limited. The Gynecologic Oncology Group (GOG) performed a phase II trial evaluating 50-mg/m^2 doses of cisplatin given every 3 weeks for advanced or recurrent vaginal cancer in 26 patients. Only one woman with squamous cell carcinoma achieved a complete response. Five of 16 patients with squamous cell carcinoma had stable disease, and 10 had cancer progression. Based on this trial, single-agent cisplatin is considered to have insignificant activity (Thigpen, 1986).

Radiation Therapy

Radiation to the primary tumor usually involves pelvic external beam radiation coupled with brachytherapy. Concurrent platinum-based chemotherapy may be added in settings described in the last section. Additionally, groin radiation is effective in those with palpable nodal metastases. Moreover, elective irradiation may be delivered to clinically negative inguinal lymph nodes if the distal third of the vagina is involved. In one review, of 100 women who did not receive groin radiation, none developed groin metastases if their disease was confined to the upper two thirds of the vagina. However, 10 percent of patients with lower-third primary tumors and 5 percent with tumors involving the entire length of the vagina developed inguinal node metastases (Perez, 1999).

■ Surveillance

Treatment failures usually develop within 2 years of primary therapy completion. Patients at low risk for recurrence are usually examined every 6 months for the first 2 years and then annually. Patients at high risk of recurrence are typically examined every 3 months for the first 2 years, then every 6 months for 5 years (Pingley, 2000; Salani, 2017). After 5 years following treatment, women can be seen annually. A Pap test and pelvic examination with careful attention to the inguinal and scalene nodes are performed. Surveillance with CT or MR imaging is at a clinician's discretion.

Recurrent Disease

Disease recurrence should be confirmed by biopsy if further treatment is planned. Therapeutic options in women with central pelvic recurrence who have had prior pelvic radiation are limited. Pelvic exenteration can be considered if a patient is psychologically and medically fit to undergo radical surgery associated with high morbidity (Chap. 46, p. 1174). It is attempted only in those whose cancer is limited to the central pelvis. Therefore, clinicians are alert to the triad of sciatic pain, leg edema, and hydronephrosis, which suggests pelvic sidewall disease. These women are typically not surgical candidates but can be managed with chemoradiation or with chemotherapy alone for women previously irradiated.

Immunotherapy may be an option for recurrent or metastatic disease after chemotherapy. Pembrolizumab blocks the receptor for *programmed cell death protein 1 (PD-1)* and helps promote a robust immune response against cancer cells. This agent is now FDA-approved for women with recurrent or metastatic cervical cancer after chemotherapy. Potential candidates are those with a *combined positive score* ≥1 (Chung, 2018). This score reflects a ratio of PD-1–carrying cells versus tumor cells and is defined further in Chapter 30 (p. 671).

In general, survival after relapse is poor. In a review of 301 patients, 5-year survival rates were 20 percent for local recurrence and 4 percent for metastatic disease recurrence (Chyle, 1996).

ADENOCARCINOMA

Primary adenocarcinoma of the vagina is rare, making up only 13 percent of all vaginal cancers (Platz, 1995). Histologic types include clear cell, endometrioid, mucinous, and serous carcinomas. These may arise in endometriosis foci, in areas of vaginal adenosis, in periurethral glands, or in wolffian duct remnants. *Adenosis* in the vagina is defined by subepithelial glandular structures lined by mucinous columnar cells that resemble endocervical cells (Sandberg, 1965). These represent residual glands of müllerian origin. Clinically, adenosis appears as red granular spots or patches that do not stain following Lugol solution application. Vaginal adenosis is more common in females exposed to diethylstilbestrol (DES) (Chap. 19, p. 424).

More often, vaginal adenocarcinoma is metastatic disease, typically from the genital tract. Disease is frequently metastatic from the endometrium, although it also may originate from the cervix or ovary (Saitoh, 2005). In addition, adenocarcinoma metastases from the breast, pancreas, kidney, and colon also have been identified in the vagina.

Treatment is similar to that for squamous cell carcinoma. Thus, surgery, radiation, or a combination can be used. Primary vaginal adenocarcinoma in general is more aggressive than squamous cell carcinoma. In one series of 30 patients, it was associated with local and metastatic relapse rates that were more than double those for squamous cell carcinoma (Chyle, 1996).

Clear Cell Adenocarcinoma

Of primary vaginal adenocarcinomas, the clear cell type is most closely associated with DES exposure, described in Chapter 19 (p. 424). In 1971, clear cell adenocarcinoma of the vagina was linked to in utero DES exposure. An estimated 1 to 4 million women used this synthetic estrogen, and approximately 0.01 percent of females exposed in utero developed vaginal clear cell adenocarcinoma (Melnick, 1987). Most DES-exposed patients with vaginal cancer were born between 1951 and 1956, when the drug was prescribed most frequently. The rate of clear cell carcinoma peaked at age 19 for women exposed to DES, with a second peak at age 42 (Huo, 2017).

However, in the Netherlands, a bimodal distribution of vaginal clear cell carcinoma has been observed—the first peak occurring with a mean age of 26 years and the second at 71 years. The younger group had all been exposed in utero to DES, whereas the older group, born before 1947, had not been exposed (Hanselaar, 1997). It remains to be seen if the incidence of vaginal clear cell carcinoma will rise as the DES-exposed population ages.

Treatment is similar to that for squamous cell carcinoma of the vagina. For stage I vaginal clear cell adenocarcinoma, the 5-year survival rate for 219 patients was 92 percent and was equivalent regardless of therapy mode (Senekjian, 1987). With stage II disease, the reported 5-year survival for 76 patients was 83 percent (Senekjian, 1988). A smaller study from MD Anderson shows worse 5-year overall survival rate (34 versus 58 percent) for women with primary adenocarcinoma of the vagina not associated with DES exposure compared with squamous cell carcinoma of the vagina. Five-year survival rates for non-DES-associated vaginal adenocarcinoma were 80 percent for stage I disease, 34 percent for stage II, 26 percent for stage III, and no survivors with stage IV disease (Frank, 2007).

MESENCHYMAL TUMORS

Embryonal Rhabdomyosarcoma

This is the most common malignancy of the vagina in infants and children, and most embryonal rhabdomyosarcomas are the sarcoma botryoides subtype. This rare tumor develops almost exclusively in girls younger than 5 years, although vaginal and cervical sarcoma botryoides have been reported in female adolescents (Copeland, 1985). In infants and children, sarcoma botryoides usually involves the vagina; in reproductive-aged women, the cervix; and after menopause, the uterus. The gross specimen can exhibit multiple polyp-like structures or can be a solitary growth with a nodular, cystic, or pedunculated appearance (Fig. 32-5) (Hilgers, 1970). Although this distinctive appearance may guide diagnosis, the classic histologic finding of this tumor is the rhabdomyoblast. Typical complaints include bleeding or a vaginal mass.

Embryonal rhabdomyosarcomas have a poor prognosis, but sarcoma botryoides is the easiest to treat and has the best

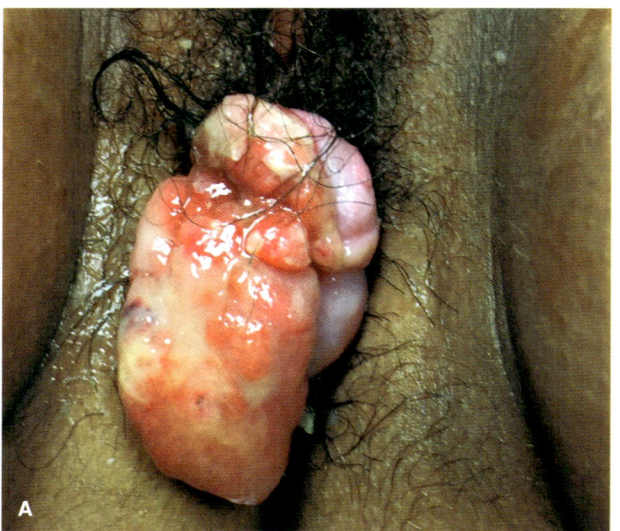

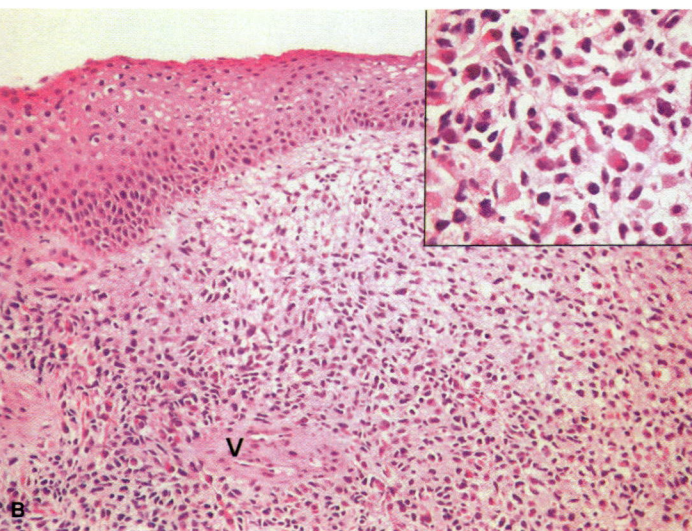

FIGURE 32-5 A. Sarcoma botryoides protruding through the vaginal introitus. (Reproduced with permission from Dr. Ellen Wilson.)
B. Embryonal rhabdomyosarcoma (×10). Tumor cells lie within a fibromyxoid stroma beneath the vaginal epithelium and cluster around blood vessels (V). Inset (×40): Some tumor cells have little discernible cytoplasm, whereas others have a round or strap-like shape and brightly eosinophilic cytoplasm consistent with rhabdomyoblastic differentiation. This example has abundant rhabdomyoblasts. (Reproduced with permission from Dr. Kelley Carrick.)

chance of cure. It may be that its superficial location allows earlier detection. Childhood sarcoma botryoides treatment has dramatically changed. It has gradually shifted away from radical pelvic exenteration surgery and toward primary chemotherapy plus radiation or adjuvant conservative surgery to excise residual tumor (Andrassy, 1995, 1999; Hays, 1985; Pommert, 2017).

■ Leiomyosarcoma

This is the most common type of vaginal sarcoma in adults. However, it makes up no more than 1 percent of vaginal malignancies, and less than 150 cases have been reported (Khafagy, 2017; Khosla, 2014). The age of affected individuals is broad, but most are older than 40 years (Zaino, 2011). Because of the small number of these tumors, few risk factors have been identified. However, patients previously treated with pelvic radiotherapy for cervical cancer carry a risk.

Affected women most often complain of an asymptomatic vaginal mass, but other symptoms mirror those of their squamous cell counterpart. Any wall of the vagina may be involved, but most tumors develop posteriorly (Ahram, 2006). Microscopically, tumors resemble uterine leiomyosarcoma (Fig. 34-2, p. 724). Tumors spread by local invasion and hematogenous dissemination.

Surgical resection with negative margins is the preferred primary treatment. The benefit of adjuvant radiation is unclear due to a lack of controlled trials. However, some clinicians recommend adjuvant radiation for those with high-grade tumor or local recurrence (Curtin, 1995).

MELANOMA

Primary malignant melanoma in the vagina is rare, accounting for less than 3 percent of all vaginal cancers. In women, only

1.6 percent of melanomas are genital. Of genital sites, the most common is the vulva (70 percent), followed by the vagina (21 percent), and the cervix (9 percent) (Miner, 2004). Using data from the SEER database, the incidence of vaginal melanoma lies between 0.26 and 0.46 per 1 million women per year (Hu, 2010; Weinstock, 1994). From U.S. and Swedish studies, the mean age at diagnosis was 66 years (Ragnarsson-Olding, 1993; Reid, 1989).

Presenting symptoms include vaginal bleeding, discharge, and vaginal mass (Fig. 32-6) (Gupta, 2002; Reid, 1989). Most are located in the distal vagina (Frumovitz, 2010; Xia, 2014). Vaginal melanoma is often detected late, and this may be largely responsible for poor treatment outcomes.

With a reported 5-year survival rate ranging from 10 to 20 percent, the prognosis is among the worst of vaginal malignancies

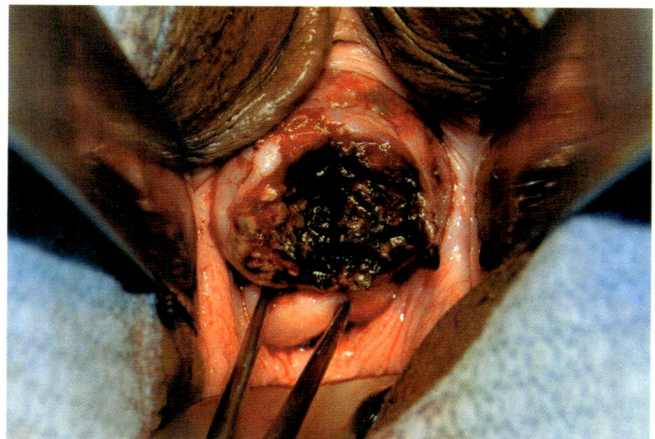

FIGURE 32-6 Vaginal melanoma of the anterior vaginal wall. Below the mass, a tenaculum can be seen on the uninvolved cervix. (Reproduced with permission from Drs. Siobhan Kehoe and Dustin Manders.)

(Ragnarsson-Olding, 1993; Xia, 2014). Although survival rates are significantly better for those with vaginal lesions measuring <3 cm, FIGO staging of vaginal melanomas does not accurately predict survival (Reid, 1989). Thus, staging criteria specific to melanoma are used. Cutaneous melanomas at other body sites use microstaging systems, including the Chung, the Clark, and the Breslow systems. These employ criteria such depth of invasion, tumor size, and tumor thickness (Chap. 31, p. 686). However, Clark levels are not applicable to vaginal melanoma because the needed microscopic skin landmarks are absent. Therefore, staging is based on tumor thickness, as described by Breslow or Chung.

Treatment is extrapolated from cutaneous melanomas, due to the rarity of vaginal melanoma. Surgery is preferred, when feasible. Although some advocate radical surgery, including exenteration, growing evidence shows that wide local excision has similar survival rates and less morbidity (Buchanan, 1998; Xia, 2014). The recommended clinical surgical margin for a melanoma with a Breslow thickness ≤1 mm is 1 cm; a thickness 1 to 2 mm warrants a 1- to 2-cm margin; and a thickness >2 mm requires a 2-cm margin (National Comprehensive Cancer Network, 2019). One study demonstrated a survival benefit to the wide local excision approach (Frumovitz, 2010). However, because of their size or location and the required margins, many vaginal melanomas are not amenable to this less radical approach.

Melanomas generally are thought to be radioresistant. However, radiotherapy in one series provided local tumor control in women who had surgically unresectable disease (Miner, 2004).

For advanced or metastatic cutaneous melanoma, several targeted biologic agents are available. B-Raf and KIT proteins are involved with directing cell growth, and mutations in their transcribing genes can lead to altered growth. Mutations in the *BRAF* and *KIT* genes are found in some cutaneous and mucosal melanomas, and vaginal melanoma tumors are tested for these mutations (Leitao, 2014). Of mutated genes in vaginal and vulvar melanomas, *BRAF* mutations make up 26 percent, and *KIT* mutations compose 22 percent (Hou, 2017). Options for those with *BRAF*^{V600E} mutations include combined BRAF and MEK inhibition by vemurafenib plus dabrafenib or by vemurafenib plus cobimetinib (Flaherty, 2012; Larkin, 2014; Long, 2014, 2015; National Comprehensive Cancer Network, 2019). Imatinib may be used for tumors with the *c-KIT* mutation (Carvajal, 2011). Ipilimumab is a monoclonal antibody that promotes T-cell activation, which in turn produces antitumor effects. Its use in melanoma patients improves overall survival rates (Hodi, 2010). Last, both PD-1 and its ligand, which is *programmed cell death ligand 1 (PD-L1)*, also are frequently expressed in vulvar and vaginal melanoma: 75 and 56 percent, respectively. Nivolumab and pembrolizumab, which are monoclonal antibodies against PD-1, are options for metastatic or unresectable cutaneous melanoma (Hamid, 2018).

REFERENCES

Ahram J, Lemus R, Schiavello HJ: Leiomyosarcoma of the vagina: case report and literature review. Int J Gynecol Cancer 16:884, 2006

Alemany L, Saunier M, Tinoco L, et al: Large contribution of human papillomavirus in vaginal neoplastic lesions: a worldwide study in 597 samples. Eur J Cancer 50(16):2846, 2014

Andrassy RJ, Hays DM, Raney RB, et al: Conservative surgical management of vaginal and vulvar pediatric rhabdomyosarcoma: a report from the Intergroup Rhabdomyosarcoma Study III. J Pediatr Surg 30:1034, 1995

Andrassy RJ, Wiener ES, Raney RB, et al: Progress in the surgical management of vaginal rhabdomyosarcoma: a 25-year review from the Intergroup Rhabdomyosarcoma Study Group. J Pediatr Surg 34:731, 1999

Beller U, Maisonneuve P, Benedet JL, et al: Carcinoma of the vagina. Int J Gynaecol Obstet 83 Suppl 1:27, 2003

Buchanan DJ, Schlaerth J, Kurosaki T: Primary vaginal melanoma: thirteen-year disease-free survival after wide local excision and review of recent literature. Am J Obstet Gynecol 178:1177, 1998

Carvajal RD, Antonescu CR, Wolchok JD, et al: KIT as a therapeutic target in metastatic melanoma. JAMA 395:2327, 2011

Chung HC, Schellens JH, Delord JP, et al: Pembrolizumab treatment of advanced cervical cancer. Updated results from the phase 2 KEYNOTE-158 study. J Clin Oncol 36(15 suppl):5522, 2018

Chyle V, Zagars GK, Wheeler JA, et al: Definitive radiotherapy for carcinoma of the vagina: outcome and prognostic factors. Int J Radiat Oncol Biol Phys 35:891, 1996

Copeland LJ, Gershenson DM, Saul PB, et al: Sarcoma botryoides of the female genital tract. Obstet Gynecol 66:262, 1985

Creasman WT, Phillips JL, Menck HR: The National Cancer Data Base report on cancer of the vagina. Cancer 83:1033, 1998

Curtin JP, Saigo P, Slucher B, et al: Soft-tissue sarcoma of the vagina and vulva: a clinicopathologic study. Obstet Gynecol 86:269, 1995

Davis KP, Stanhope CR, Garton GR, et al: Invasive vaginal carcinoma: analysis of early-stage disease. Gynecol Oncol 42:131, 1991

FIGO Committee on Gynecologic Oncology: Current FIGO staging for cancer of the vagina, fallopian tube, ovary, and gestational trophoblastic neoplasia. Int J Gynaecol Obstet 105(1):3, 2009

Flaherty KT, Infante JR, Daud A, et al: Combined BRAF and MEK inhibition in melanoma with BRAF V600 mutations. N Engl J Med 367:1694, 2012

Frank SJ, Deavers MT, Jhingran A, et al: Primary adenocarcinoma of the vagina not associated with diethylstilbestrol (DES) exposure. Gynecol Oncol 105:470, 2007

Frank SJ, Jhingran A, Levenback C, et al: Definitive radiation therapy for squamous cell carcinoma of the vagina. Int J Radiat Oncol Biol Phys 62:138, 2005

Frumovitz M, Etchepareborda M, Sun CC, et al: Primary malignant melanoma of the vagina. Obstet Gynecol 116:1358, 2010

Ghia AJ, Gonzalez VJ, Tward JD, et al: Primary vaginal cancer and chemoradiotherapy: a patterns-of-care analysis. Int J Gynecol Cancer 21:378, 2011

Gunderson CC, Nugent EK, Yunker AC, et al: Vaginal cancer: the experience from 2 large academic centers during a 15-year period. Journal of Lower Genital Tract Disease 17:409, 2013

Gupta D, Malpica A, Deavers MT, et al: Vaginal melanoma: a clinicopathologic and immunohistochemical study of 26 cases. Am J Surg Pathol 26:1450, 2002

Hamid O, Robert C, Ribas A, et al: Antitumor activity of pembrolizumab in advanced mucosal melanoma: a post-hoc analysis of KEYNOTE-001, 002, 006. Br J Cancer 119(6):670, 2018

Hanselaar A, van Loosbroek M, Schuurbiers O, et al: Clear cell adenocarcinoma of the vagina and cervix: an update of the central Netherlands registry showing twin age incidence peaks. Cancer 79:2229, 1997

Hays DM, Shimada H, Raney RB Jr, et al: Sarcomas of the vagina and uterus: the Intergroup Rhabdomyosarcoma Study. J Pediatr Surg 20:718, 1985

Hellman K, Lundell M, Silfversward C, et al: Clinical and histopathologic factors related to prognosis in primary squamous cell carcinoma of the vagina. Int J Gynecol Cancer 16:1201, 2006

Hilgers RD, Malkasian GD Jr, Soule EH: Embryonal rhabdomyosarcoma (botryoid type) of the vagina: a clinicopathologic review. Am J Obstet Gynecol 107:484, 1970

Hodi FS, O'Day SJ, McDermott DF, et al: Improved survival with ipilimumab in patients with metastatic melanoma. N Engl J Med 363:711, 2010

Hou JY, Baptiste C, Hombalegowda RB, et al: Vulvar and vaginal melanoma: a unique subclass of mucosal melanoma based on a comprehensive molecular analysis of 51 cases compares with 2253 cases of nongynecologic melanoma. Cancer 123(8):1333, 2017

Hu DN, Yu GP, McCormick SA: Population-based incidence of vulvar and vaginal melanoma in various races and ethnic groups with comparisons to other site-specific melanomas. Melanoma Res 20(2):153, 2010

Huh WK, Joura EA, Giuliano AR, et al: Final efficacy, immunogenicity, and safety analyses of a nine-valent human papillomavirus vaccine in women aged 16–26 years: a randomised, double-blind trial. Lancet 390(10108):2143, 2017

Huo D, Anderson D, Palmer JR, et al: Incidence rates and risks of diethylstilbestrol-related clear-cell adenocarcinoma of the vagina and cervix: Update after 40-year follow-up. Gynecol Oncol 146:566, 2017

Khafagy AM, Prescott LS, Mapica A, et al: Unusual indolent behavior of leiomyosarcoma of the vagina: Is observation a viable option? Gynecol Oncol Rep 21:28, 2017

Khosla D, Patel FD, Kumar R, et al: Leiomyosarcoma of the vagina: a rare entity with comprehensive review of the literature. Int J Appl Basic Med Res 4:128, 2014

Kunos CA, Radivoyevitch T, Waggoner S, et al: Radiochemotherapy plus 3-aminopyridine-2-carboxaldehyde thiosemicarbazone (3-AP, NSC #663249) in advanced-stage cervical and vaginal cancers. Gynecol Oncol 130:75, 2013

Lamoreaux WT, Grisby PW, Dehdashti F, et al: FDG-PET evaluation of vaginal carcinoma. Int J Radiat Oncol Biol Phys 62:733, 2005

Larkin J, Ascierto PA, Dreno B, et al: Combined vemurafenib and cobimetinib in BRAF-mutated melanoma. N Engl J Med 371:1867, 2014

Leitao MM: Management of vulvar and vaginal melanomas: current and future strategies. Am Soc Clin Oncol Educ Book 2014:e277, 2014

Long GV, Stroyakovskiy D, Gogas H, et al: Combined BRAF and MEK inhibition versus BRAF inhibition alone in melanoma. N Engl J Med 371:1877, 2014

Long GV, Stroyakovskiy D, Gogas H, et al: Dabrafenib and trametinib versus dabrafenib and placebo for Val600 BRAF-mutant melanoma: a multicenter, double-blind, phse 3 randomized controlled trial. Lancet 386:444, 2015

Melnick S, Cole P, Anderson D, et al: Rates and risks of diethylstilbestrol-related clear-cell adenocarcinoma of the vagina and cervix: an update. N Engl J Med 316:514, 1987

Miner TJ, Delgado R, Zeisler J, et al: Primary vaginal melanoma: a critical analysis of therapy. Ann Surg Oncol 11:34, 2004

National Comprehensive Cancer Network: NCCN guidelines version 1.2019 Melanoma. Available at https://www.nccn.org/professionals/physician_gls/recently_updated.aspx. Accessed January 27, 2019

Nori D, Hilaris BS, Stanimir G, et al: Radiation therapy of primary vaginal carcinoma. Int J Radiat Oncol Biol Phys 9:1471, 1983

Pecorelli S, Benedet JL, Creasman WT, et al: FIGO staging of gynecologic cancer. 1994–1997 FIGO Committee on Gynecologic Oncology. International Federation of Gynecology and Obstetrics. Int J Gynaecol Obstet 65:243, 1999

Perez CA, Grigsby PW, Garipagaoglu M, et al: Factors affecting long-term outcome of irradiation in carcinoma of the vagina. Int J Radiat Oncol Biol Phys 44:37, 1999

Pingley S, Shrivastava SK, Sarin R, et al: Primary carcinoma of the vagina: Tata Memorial Hospital experience. Int J Radiat Oncol Biol Phys 46:101, 2000

Platz CE, Benda JA: Female genital tract cancer. Cancer 75:270, 1995

Pommert L, Bradely W: Pediatric gynecologic cancer. Current Oncology Reports 19:44, 2017

Ragnarsson-Olding B, Johansson H, Rutqvist LE, et al: Malignant melanoma of the vulva and vagina: trends in incidence, age distribution, and long-term survival among 245 consecutive cases in Sweden 1960–1984. Cancer 71:1893, 1993

Rajagopalan MS, Xu KM, Lin JF, et al: Adoption and impact of concurrent chemoradiation therapy for vaginal cancer: a National Cancer Data Base (NCDB) study. Gynecol Oncol 135:495, 2014

Ratnavelu N, Patel A, Fisher AD, et al: High-grade vaginal intraepithelial neoplasia: can we be selective about who we treat? BJOG 120:887, 2013

Reddy S, Saxena VS, Reddy S, et al: Results of radiotherapeutic management of primary carcinoma of the vagina. Int J Radiat Oncol Biol Phys 21:1041, 1991

Reid GC, Schmidt RW, Roberts JA, et al: Primary melanoma of the vagina: a clinicopathologic analysis. Obstet Gynecol 74:190, 1989

Rubin SC, Young J, Mikuta JJ: Squamous carcinoma of the vagina: treatment, complications, and long-term follow-up. Gynecol Oncol 20:346, 1985

Saitoh M, Hayasaka T, Ohmichi M, et al: Primary mucinous adenocarcinoma of the vagina: possibility of differentiating from metastatic adenocarcinomas. Pathol Int 55:372, 2005

Salani R, Khanna N, Frimer M, et al: An update on post-treatment surveillance and diagnosis of recurrence in women with gynecologic malignancies: Society of Gynecologic Oncology (SGO) recommendations. Gynecol Oncol 146(1):3, 2017

Sandberg EC, Danielson RW, Cauwet RW, et al: Adenosis vaginae. Am J Obstet Gynecol 93:209, 1965

Senekjian EK, Frey KW, Anderson D, et al: Local therapy in stage I clear cell adenocarcinoma of the vagina. Cancer 60:1319, 1987

Senekjian EK, Frey KW, Stone C, et al: An evaluation of stage II vaginal clear cell adenocarcinoma according to substages. Gynecol Oncol 31:56, 1988

Siegel RL, Miller KD, Jemal A: Cancer statistics, 2019. CA Cancer J Clin 69:7, 2019

Smith JS, Backes DM, Hoots BE, et al: Human papillomavirus type-distribution in vulvar and vaginal cancer and their associated precursors. Obstet Gynecol 113:917, 2009

Stock RG, Chen AS, Seski J: A 30-year experience in the management of primary carcinoma of the vagina: analysis of prognostic factors and treatment modalities. Gynecol Oncol 56:45, 1995

Tewari KS, Sill MW, Long HJ, et al: Improved survival with bevacizumab in advanced cervical cancer. N Engl J Med 370(8):734, 2014

Thigpen JT, Blessing JA, Homesley HD, et al: Phase II trial of cisplatin in advanced or recurrent cancer of the vagina: a Gynecologic Oncology Group Study. Gynecol Oncol 23:101, 1986

Tran PT, Su Z, Lee P, et al: Prognostic factors for outcomes and complications for primary squamous cell carcinoma of the vagina treated with radiation. Gynecol Oncol 105:641, 2007

Watson M, Saraiya M, Wu X: Update of HPV-associated female genital cancers in the United States, 1999–2004. J Womens Health 18:1731, 2009

Weinstock MA: Malignant melanoma of the vulva and vagina in the United States: patterns of incidence and population-based estimates of survival. Am J Obstet Gynecol 171:1225, 1994

Xia L, Han D, Yang W, et al: Primary malignant melanoma of the vagina. A retrospective clinicopathologic study of 44 cases. Int J Gynecol Cancer 24:149, 2014

Zaino RJ, Nucci M, Kurman RJ: Diseases of the vagina. In Kurman RJ, Ellenson LH, Ronnett BM (eds): Blaustein's Pathology of the Female Genital Tract, 6th ed. New York, Springer, 2011, p 137

Zeligs KP, Byrd K, Tarney C, et al: A clinicopathologic study of vaginal intraepithelial neoplasia. Obstet Gynecol 122:1223, 2013

CHAPTER 33

Endometrial Cancer

In the United States, endometrial cancer is the most common gynecologic malignancy. Risk factors include obesity and advancing age. As these factors are now more prevalent, the incidence of endometrial cancer continues to rise. Fortunately, patients usually seek medical attention early due to vaginal bleeding, and endometrial biopsy leads quickly to diagnosis. The cornerstone of treatment is hysterectomy with bilateral salpingo-oophorectomy (BSO) and surgical staging that includes lymph node assessment for most women. Of affected women, 67 percent will have stage I disease that is potentially curable by surgery alone, although high-risk stage I patients often receive adjuvant therapy (Siegel, 2019). The 21 percent of patients with regional disease and 8 percent with distant disease typically require multimodality treatment that includes some combination of surgery, chemotherapy, and radiotherapy.

EPIDEMIOLOGY AND RISK FACTORS

From the Surveillance, Epidemiology, and End Results (SEER) Program (2018) database, women in the United States have a 3-percent lifetime risk of developing endometrial cancer. In 2019, an estimated 61,880 new cases and 12,160 associated deaths are expected (Siegel, 2019). Most patients are diagnosed early and subsequently cured. As a result, endometrial cancer is the fourth leading cause of cancer, but only the sixth leading cause of cancer deaths among women.

Endometrial adenocarcinomas are categorized as type I or type II based on histology. Type I, that is, endometrioid type, makes up 80 to 90 percent of all cases (Felix, 2010). The other 10 to 20 percent are type II cancers, namely, the non-endometrioid histologic types that include serous and clear cell adenocarcinomas and carcinosarcoma. Risk factors for developing endometrial cancer are numerous (Table 33-1). Risks specifically for type I cancers are associated with an excess-estrogen environment.

Of these, *obesity* is the most common cause of endogenous overproduction of estrogen. Excessive adipose tissue increases peripheral aromatization of androstenedione to estrone. In premenopausal women, elevated estrone levels trigger abnormal feedback in the hypothalamic-pituitary-ovarian axis. The clinical result is oligo- or anovulation. In the absence of ovulation, the endometrium is exposed to virtually continuous estrogen stimulation without subsequent progestational effect and without menstrual shedding.

Unopposed estrogen therapy is the next most important potential inciting factor. Fortunately, the malignant potential of continuously administered estrogen was recognized decades ago

TABLE 33-1. Factors Affecting Endometrial Cancer Risk

Raise risk

Obesity
Polycystic ovarian syndrome
Long-term, high-dose unopposed menopausal estrogens
Early age of menarche
Late age of natural menopause
Infertility
Nulliparity
Menstrual irregularities
North America or northern Europe residence
Higher education or income level
White race
Older age
Tamoxifen, high cumulative doses
DM, CHTN, or gallbladder disease

Lower risk

Long-term COC use
Cigarette smoking

CHTN = chronic hypertension; COC = combination oral contraceptive; DM = diabetes mellitus.

(Smith, 1975). Currently, it is rare to encounter a woman with a uterus who has taken unopposed estrogen for years. Instead, combined estrogen plus progestin hormonal replacement therapy (HRT) is routinely prescribed for postmenopausal women with a uterus to reduce estrogen-related endometrial cancer risk (Strom, 2006).

Menstrual and reproductive influences are commonly associated with endometrial cancer. For example, early age at menarche or late age of menopause are both associated with higher risk (Wernli, 2006). Classically, women with polycystic ovarian syndrome (PCOS) are anovulatory and thus also have an increased risk of developing this cancer (Fearnley, 2010; Pillay, 2006).

Older age is linked with endometrial cancer development. The average age at diagnosis is the early 60s, and overall, approximately 80 percent of these cancers are diagnosed in postmenopausal women older than 55 years (Madison, 2004; Schottenfeld, 1995). From the SEER database (2018), approximately 7 percent of endometrial cancers develop in patients younger than 45 years. Of note, Nevadunsky and associates (2014) found that the age at diagnosis of endometrioid cancer decreased linearly with increasing body mass index (BMI).

Family history is another risk for endometrial cancer. Endometrial cancer is the most common extracolonic manifestation of Lynch syndrome (hereditary nonpolyposis colorectal cancer [HNPCC]) (Hemminki, 2005). This autosomal-dominant syndrome results primarily from mutations in the mismatch repair genes *MLH1, MSH2, MSH6,* and *PMS2* (Bansal, 2009). Gene mutation prevents repair of base mismatches, which are commonly produced during DNA replication. Inactivity of this DNA repair system leads to mutations that can promote carcinogenesis. Mutation carriers have a risk of developing endometrial cancer that ranges from 40 to 60 percent. Among affected women, endometrial cancer often develops at a young age, and the risk for this cancer actually exceeds that for colorectal cancer (Aarnio, 1999; Delin, 2004). Of all endometrial cancer cases, 2.3 percent are attributable to Lynch syndrome, and these cases develop more than 10 years earlier than sporadic endometrial cancer (Resnick, 2009).

Tamoxifen causes a two- to threefold higher risk of developing endometrial cancer by its modest "unopposed" estrogenic effect on the endometrium (Chap. 27, p. 598). The increased risk of endometrial cancer affects postmenopausal women almost exclusively, and cancer rates rise linearly with the duration and cumulative dose of tamoxifen therapy (Fisher, 1998; van Leeuwen, 1994). Accordingly, women taking tamoxifen are counseled regarding this endometrial risk and should report vaginal spotting, bleeding, or discharge. That said, unless a tamoxifen-treated patient has such symptoms, routine endometrial surveillance does not improve early detection rates (American College of Obstetricians and Gynecologists, 2019c).

Coexisting medical conditions such as diabetes mellitus, hypertension, and gallbladder disease are more commonly associated with endometrial cancer (Morimoto, 2006; Soliman, 2005). In general, these are frequent sequelae of obesity and an excess estrogen environment and are considered epiphenomena rather than causal.

In contrast, *combination oral contraceptive* (COC) use for at least 1 year confers as much as a 30- to 50-percent reduced endometrial cancer risk. Risk reduction extends for 10 to 20 years (Dossus, 2010; Stanford, 1993). This most likely derives from a chemopreventive effect on the endometrium provided by the progestin component (Maxwell, 2006). Logically, progesterone intrauterine devices (IUDs) also confer long-term endometrial cancer protection (Tao, 2006). Of interest, similar protective effects are seen with inert and copper IUD types (Felix, 2015).

Smokers have a lower risk of endometrial cancer. The biologic mechanism is multifactorial but in part involves lower circulating estrogen levels from weight reduction, earlier age at menopause, and altered hormonal metabolism. Both current and past smoking have a long-lasting influence (Viswanathan, 2005).

ENDOMETRIAL HYPERPLASIA

Most endometrial cancers arise following progression of histologically distinguishable hyperplastic lesions. In fact, endometrial hyperplasia is the only known direct precursor of invasive disease. Endometrial hyperplasia is defined as endometrial thickening with proliferation of irregularly sized and shaped glands and an increased gland-to-stroma ratio (Fig. 33-1) (Ellenson, 2011b). In the absence of such thickening, lesions are best designated as *disorderly proliferative endometrium* or *focal glandular crowding*.

■ Classification

Endometrial hyperplasia represents a continuum of histopathologic findings. The classification system used by the World Health Organization (WHO) and International Society of Gynecological Pathologists designates two different types with varying malignant potential (Kurman, 1985, 2014). *Hyperplasia without atypia* is characterized by exaggerated endometrial gland proliferation and an increased gland-to-stroma ratio compared with normal proliferative endometrium, but without significant cytologic atypia (see Fig. 33-1). Most importantly, hyperplasias are additionally labeled as atypical if they demonstrate nuclear atypia of the endometrial gland cells. *Atypical endometrial hyperplasias* are clearly associated with the subsequent development of adenocarcinoma (Table 33-2).

Although endometrial hyperplasias are formally classified in these two different groups, they tend to be morphologically

TABLE 33-2. World Health Organization Classification of Endometrial Hyperplasia

Types	Progressing to Cancer (%)
Simple hyperplasia	1
Complex hyperplasia	3
Simple atypical hyperplasia	8
Complex atypical hyperplasia	29

Data from Kurman, 1985.

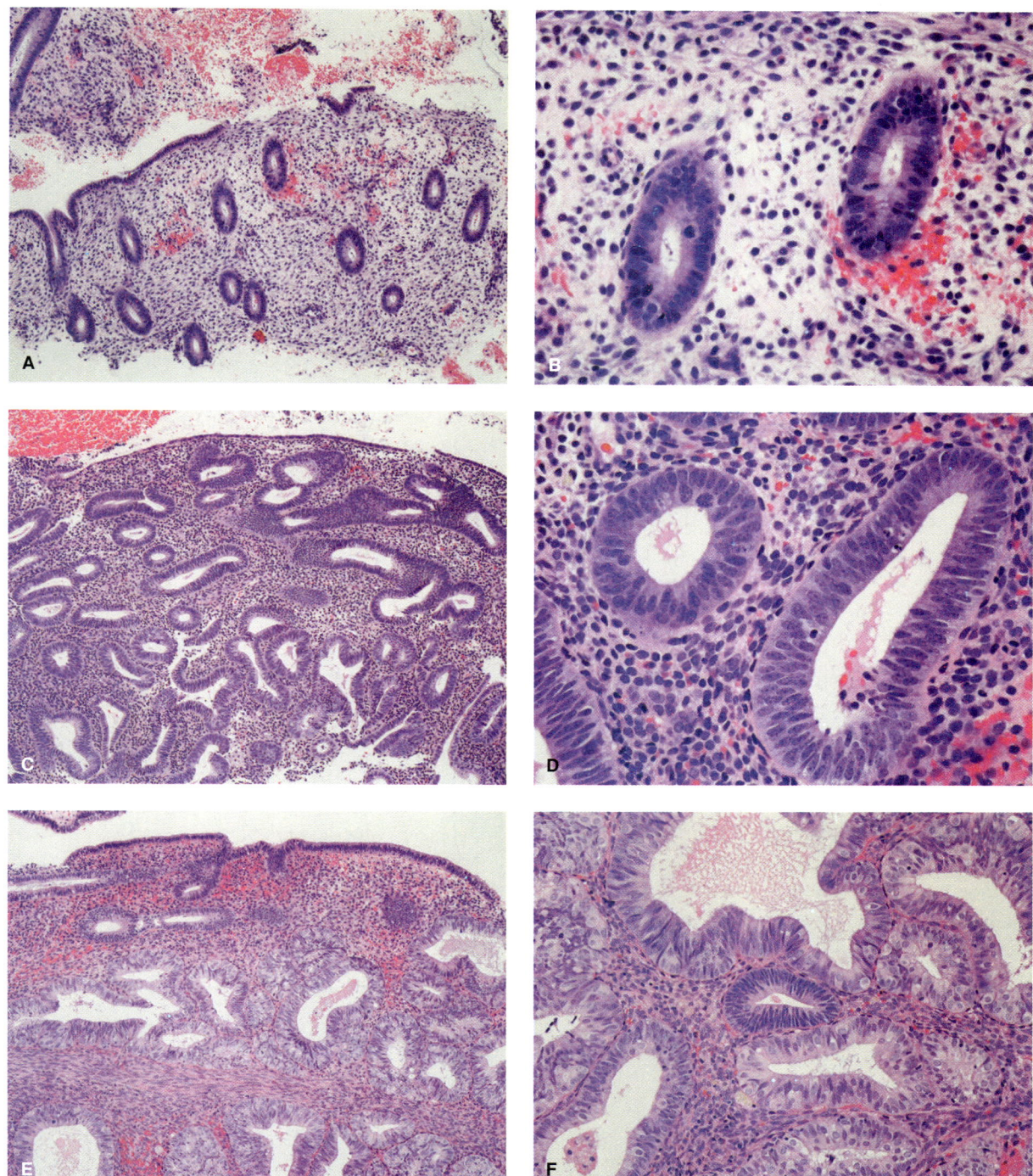

FIGURE 33-1 A. Normal proliferative endometrium shows regularly spaced, tubular endometrial glands. **B.** Normal proliferative endometrial glands have columnar lining cells with relatively bland, ovoid, mitotically active nuclei. **C.** In hyperplasia without atypia, the endometrial glands are crowded, and some have irregular shapes. **D.** In hyperplasia without atypia, glands are crowded but devoid of significant cytologic atypia. The nuclear stratification, mitotic activity, and apoptosis seen in these glands are features of normal proliferative endometrium. **E.** Hyperplasia with atypia/endometrioid intraepithelial neoplasia (EIN). The endometrial glands are crowded and complex and have nuclear atypia. **F.** Atypical hyperplasia/EIN. The atypical glandular epithelium has a tubal character in this particular example (note scattered ciliated cells). This contrasts with the single normal gland in the photograph's center (Reproduced with permission from Dr. Kelley Carrick.)

heterogeneous, both within and between individual patients. This histologic diversity explains why only a small number of conserved features are useful as diagnostic criteria. As a result, reproducible scoring of cytologic atypia is often challenging, particularly with a small amount of tissue from a biopsy sample.

Endometrial intraepithelial neoplasia (EIN) is a term introduced to more accurately distinguish the two very different clinical categories of hyperplasia. These are: (1) normal polyclonal endometria diffusely responding to an abnormal hormonal environment and (2) intrinsically proliferative monoclonal lesions that arise focally and confer an elevated risk of adenocarcinoma (Mutter, 2000). This nomenclature emphasizes the malignant potential of endometrial precancers and is in keeping with similar precedents in the cervix (CIN [cervical intraepithelial neoplasia]), vagina (VaIN), and vulva (VIN) (Chap. 29, p. 620).

Using this system, anovulatory or prolonged estrogen-exposed endometria without atypia are generally designated as *endometrial hyperplasias*. In contrast, EIN is used to describe all endometria delineated as premalignant by a combination of three morphometric features. The qualities reflect glandular volume, architectural complexity, and cytologic abnormality. The EIN classification system is a more accurate and reproducible way to predict progression to cancer and is recognized by the American College of Obstetricians and Gynecologists and Society of Gynecologic Oncology (2017a). However, it has not been universally implemented (Baak, 2005; Hecht, 2005).

■ Clinical Features and Diagnosis

The risks for developing endometrial hyperplasia generally mirror those for invasive carcinoma (Anastasiadis, 2000; Ricci, 2002). Two thirds of women present with postmenopausal bleeding (Horn, 2004). However, premenopausal women with abnormal uterine bleeding (AUB) are also evaluated as described in Chapter 8 (p. 182).

As hyperplasia is a histologic diagnosis, a Pipelle office endometrial biopsy (EMB) or outpatient dilation and curettage (D & C) are suitable choices for endometrial sampling. The American College of Obstetricians and Gynecologists (2016) recommends such a sample for women older than 45 years with AUB. EMB is also considered for those younger than 45 with chronic excess estrogen exposure (exogenous or endogenous), failed medical management, and persistent AUB.

In those with AUB, transvaginal sonography to measure endometrial thickness can also predict endometrial hyperplasia (Granberg, 1991; Jacobs, 2011). This option can be offered as an initial evaluation only to women with postmenopausal bleeding for whom no further evaluation would be needed if a thin stripe is found. For these women, endometrial stripe thickness measurements ≤4 mm are associated with bleeding that is attributed to endometrial atrophy (American College of Obstetricians and Gynecologists, 2018b). Postmenopausal women with a thicker endometrium warrant biopsy. Sonography may also identify abnormal echostructural changes in the endometrium. Cystic endometrial changes suggest polyps, homogeneously thickened endometrium may indicate hyperplasia, and a heterogeneous structural pattern is suspicious for malignancy (Figs. 33-2 and 33-3). However, these sonographic findings show great overlap and cannot be used alone.

Endometrial thickness >4 mm may be identified in postmenopausal women undergoing sonographic evaluation for reasons unrelated to postmenopausal bleeding. The positive predictive value of an "abnormal" endometrial thickness in asymptomatic women would be expected to be low, because the disease prevalence in asymptomatic patients is low. It is therefore reasonable to use a higher threshold value for these patients. The Society of Obstetrics and Gynecology of Canada suggests 11 mm as the threshold in asymptomatic women (Wolfman, 2010). This comports with a decision analysis by Smith-Bindman and colleagues (2004).

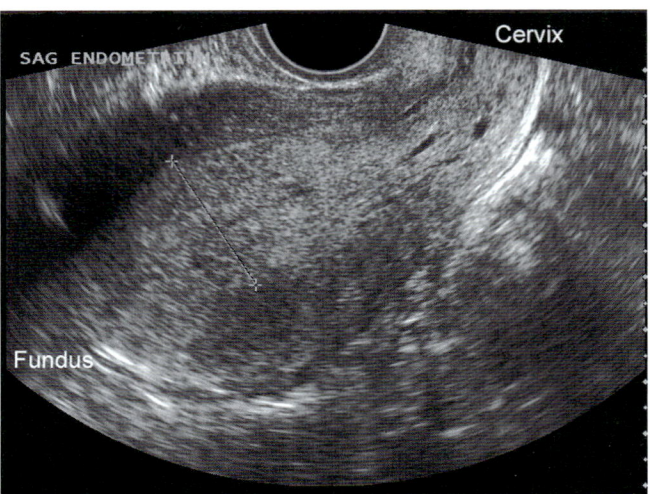

FIGURE 33-2 Transvaginal sonographic image of a uterus. In this sagittal view, the markedly thickened endometrium, which is measured by the calipers, suggests endometrial hyperplasia. (Reproduced with permission from Dr. Elysia Moschos.)

For premenopausal women, transvaginal sonography is often performed to exclude structural sources of abnormal bleeding. Similarly, researchers have attempted to create endometrial thickness guidelines. However, endometrial thicknesses can vary considerably among premenopausal women during normal menstrual cycling. From studies, suggested evidence-based abnormal thresholds range from >4 mm to >16 mm (Breitkopf, 2004; Goldstein, 1997; Shi, 2008). Thus, consensus for an endometrial thickness threshold has not been established for this group. Thus, to exclude endometrial cancer, endometrial biopsy is preferred to sonography for high-risk premenopausal women with AUB.

Of other tools, hysteroscopy is more sensitive for focal endometrial lesions. However, hyperplastic endometrium is grossly indistinct, and thus hysteroscopy has poor sensitivity for this diagnosis (Ben Yehuda, 1998; Garuti, 2006).

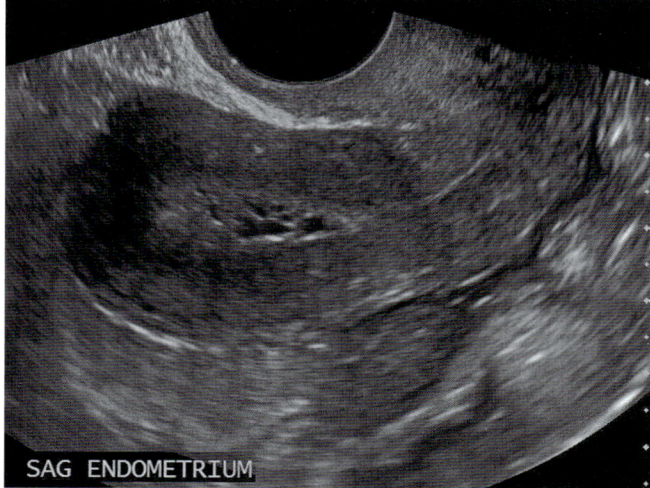

FIGURE 33-3 Transvaginal sagittal image of the endometrium from a 38-year-old woman with chronic oligomenorrhea. The abnormal endometrium is thickened, echogenic, and heterogeneous in echotexture and contains tiny cystic foci. Biopsy revealed grade 1 endometrioid adenocarcinoma, which was confirmed at surgery. (Reproduced with permission from Dr. Elysia Moschos.)

▪ Treatment

Management of women with endometrial hyperplasia mainly depends on a patient's age, comorbid risks for surgery, desire for fertility, and specific histologic features such as cytologic atypia. Hysterectomy is the most definitive treatment. Hormonal therapy is another option and includes oral or injectable progestins or the progestin (levonorgestrel-releasing) IUD.

With hyperplasia, diagnosis at times may be inconsistent due to interobserver variability among pathologists. Moreover, predicting the stability of individual lesions can be difficult. Specifically, several studies have documented low reproducibility for WHO classifications of endometrial hyperplasia (Allison, 2008; Sherman, 2008; Zaino, 2006). In addition, there is no way to anticipate which types will involute with progestin therapy. However, as long as an endometrial sample is representative and a provider has no reason to suspect a coexisting invasive carcinoma, the decision to treat endometrial hyperplasia through hormonal or surgical means relies on clinical judgment.

Nonatypical Endometrial Hyperplasia

Premenopausal Women. Nonatypical lesions may spontaneous regress without therapy. However, progestins are generally used to address the underlying etiology, that is, chronic anovulation and excess estrogen (Terakawa, 1997). Premenopausal women with nonatypical endometrial hyperplasia typically require a 3- to 6-month course of low-dose progestin therapy. Cyclic medroxyprogesterone acetate (MPA) (Provera) given orally for 12 to 14 days each month at a dose of 10 to 20 mg daily is commonly used. Continuous daily dosing with MPA 10 mg is suitable and may be more effective than cyclic administration in reversing hyperplastic changes. Another frequently used option is COC pills for those without contraindications. The levonorgestrel-releasing IUD also is effective (Gallos, 2010; Ørbo, 2014; Scarselli, 2011).

Generally, a posttreatment EMB is performed to document regression. In those with an IUD, EMB can be performed without device removal. After regression, a key point is to continue endometrial protection. Thus, once hyperplastic changes resolve, patients are continued on progestins and observed until menopause. Additional endometrial sampling is required for new bleeding.

Postmenopausal Women. Postmenopausal women with nonatypical endometrial hyperplasia may also be treated with low-dose oral cyclic MPA or a continuous 10-mg daily regimen. Importantly, in older women, providers should be confident that the sample obtained is adequate to exclude cytologic atypia. D & C may be indicated at times, especially if the tissue from Pipelle sampling is scant or if recurrent bleeding is noted.

Affected postmenopausal patients who have a contraindication to progestin therapy or who cannot tolerate the therapy can be expectantly managed. Complex hyperplasia without atypia is usually treated chronically with progestins. Office endometrial biopsy is recommended every 3 to 6 months until lesion resolution is achieved.

Response to Progestins. In cases of endometrial hyperplasia without atypia, the risk of progression to endometrial cancer is low and only 1 to 3 percent. The overall clinical and pathologic regression rates to progestin therapy range from 70 to 80 percent for nonatypical endometrial hyperplasia (Rattanachaiyanont, 2005; Reed, 2009). Patients with persistent disease on repeated biopsy may be switched to a higher-dose regimen such as MPA 40 to 100 mg orally daily. Also, megestrol acetate (Megace), 160 mg daily or 80 mg twice daily, is suitable. It can be increased even up to 160 mg twice daily if no regression is initially achieved. Again, a clinician must confirm that hormonal ablation has occurred by resampling the endometrium after a suitable therapeutic interval, usually 3 to 6 months. Hysterectomy may also be considered for lesions that are refractory to medical management.

If surgery is selected, a minimally invasive surgery (MIS) approach is considered, and options are laparoscopic, robotic, or vaginal hysterectomy. In cases in which hyperplasia has been proven or is suspected, the uterus is removed in toto and without morcellation, which might disseminate disease. Because the lesion may extend into the lower uterine segment or upper endocervix, supracervical hysterectomy is not appropriate for women undergoing hysterectomy for treatment of endometrial hyperplasia.

Atypical Endometrial Hyperplasia

Hysterectomy is the preferred treatment for women with atypical endometrial hyperplasia because the risk of progression to cancer over time approximates 29 percent. The rate of finding concurrent invasive malignancy coexistent with the atypical hyperplasia also is significant (Horn, 2004; Trimble, 2006). In postmenopausal women, a hysterectomy with removal of both tubes and ovaries is recommended.

In premenopausal women who have completed childbearing, hysterectomy is performed for hyperplasia. Risk-reducing salpingectomy is encouraged to potentially lower cancer risk that arises from the fallopian tubes (American College of Obstetricians and Gynecologists, 2019b). For premenopausal women, removal of the ovaries is optional. The deciding factors mirror those for women contemplating BSO for other benign indications and are outlined fully in Chapter 43 (p. 957).

Premenopausal women who strongly wish to preserve fertility can be treated with progestins (Trimble, 2012). High-dose progestin therapy, megestrol acetate 80 mg orally twice daily, is an option for motivated patients who will be compliant with surveillance (Randall, 1997). The IUD that releases 20 μg of intrauterine levonorgestrel daily (Mirena, Liletta) also is suitable (Ørbo, 2014). Poor surgical candidates may also warrant an attempt at hormonal ablation with progestins. Resolution of the hyperplasia must be confirmed by serial endometrial biopsies every 3 months until response is documented. Otherwise, hysterectomy is recommended. Following hyperplasia resolution, surveillance and progestins continue long-term due to the potential for eventual progression to carcinoma (Rubatt, 2005). Once fertility is complete, hysterectomy is again recommended.

The Gynecologic Oncology Group (GOG) performed a prospective cohort study of 289 patients who had a diagnosis of atypical endometrial hyperplasia. Participants underwent hysterectomy within 3 months of their biopsy, and 43 percent were found to have a concurrent endometrial carcinoma (Trimble, 2006). Suh-Burgmann and associates (2009) found a similarly high number of 48 percent. Results demonstrate the difficulty

TABLE 33-3. Type I and II Endometrial Carcinoma: Distinguishing Features

Feature	Type I	Type II
Chronic estrogen	Present	Absent
Menopause status	Pre-/peri-	Post-
Hyperplasia	Present	Absent
Race	White	Black
Grade	Low	High
Invasion[a]	Minimal	Deep
Behavior	Stable	Aggressive
Subtypes	Endometrioid	Serous
		Clear cell

[a]Myometrial invasion.

in attaining an accurate diagnosis before hysterectomy and the potential risks of conservative hormonal treatment. The high risk of coexistent endometrial cancer has prompted some surgeons to perform frozen section analysis of the endometrium at the time of hysterectomy in these cases. Surgical staging then proceeds if carcinoma is found.

ENDOMETRIAL CANCER

◼ Pathogenesis

Endometrial cancer is a biologically diverse group of neoplasms characterized by a dualistic model of pathogenesis. As noted, type I endometrioid adenocarcinomas constitute most cases. They are estrogen-dependent, low grade, and derived from atypical endometrial hyperplasia. In contrast, type II cancers are serous, carcinosarcoma, or clear cell histology; have no precursor lesion; and portend a more aggressive clinical course (Table 33-3).

From molecular studies, endometrial cancers can be broadly categorized based on genomic alterations in the tumors. The four groupings are POLE-ultramutated; microsatellite instability-high (MSI-H); copy number–low; and copy number–high (Kandoth, 2013). These categories are associated with distinct prognoses and clinical features and may help predict treatment response.

POLE-ultramutated tumors harbor mutations in the *POLE* gene, which encodes the DNA polymerase epsilon catalytic subunit. Although their associated histology is usually high-grade endometrioid or clear cell, they carry a favorable prognosis. They are heavily infiltrated with *tumor infiltrating lymphocytes (TILs)* and overexpress *programmed death 1 (PD-1)* (Bellone, 2017). The latter is an important regulator of immune response and

illustrated in Figure 27-7 (p. 601). These observations suggest that tumor immunology may play a role in their good prognosis.

Copy number–high tumors are characterized by mutations in *TP53*, which encodes the tumor suppressor protein p53. These tumors have a poor prognosis, and all serous and some high-grade endometrioid and clear cell carcinomas fall into this category.

Copy number–low tumors are generally low-grade and endometrioid type. These do not harbor *TP53* mutations but have frequent mutations in *PTEN*, which also codes for a tumor suppressor protein, and other genes. These tumors have an intermediate prognosis.

MSI-H tumors have defects in genes responsible for the repair of single base-pair mismatches. Damaged base pairs persist and lead to instability in short tandem DNA sequences, called *microsatellites*, and create genomic instability in general. In tumors, the MSI-H phenotype can be detected by direct microsatellite DNA sequence testing. Alternatively, indirect immunohistochemistry staining can test for the four proteins expressed by the mismatch repair (MMR) genes *MLH1*, *MSH2*, *MSH6*, and *PMS2*.

Although Lynch syndrome–associated endometrial cancers are MSI-H, most MSI-H tumors endometrial cancers are sporadic. MSI-H endometrial cancers have a favorable prognosis (Haruma, 2018). The MSI-H phenotype, in endometrial cancers and also other cancers, responds well to PD-1–directed immunotherapy (Ott, 2017).

◼ Prevention

Education can be effective prevention, as many endometrial cancer risks are alterable. Women with PCOS may benefit from weight loss and chronic progestin supplementation (Chap. 18, p. 400). Assessing and managing obesity may also lower risks (Chap. 1, p. 12). In a recent systematic review of five retrospective studies, patients who underwent bariatric surgery had a 68-percent endometrial cancer risk reduction compared with women who did not have this surgery (Winder, 2018).

Even for women at increased risk, routine screening of hyperplasia or endometrial cancer is not advocated. Instead, at the onset of menopause, women are counseled on the risks and symptoms of endometrial cancer and strongly encouraged to report unexpected bleeding or spotting to their provider. One screening exception is the woman with Lynch syndrome. For these individuals, EMB is recommended every 1 to 2 years beginning at age 30 to 35 years (American College of Obstetricians and Gynecologists, 2019a; Smith, 2019).

Genetic testing criteria have been published to identify the individual with Lynch syndrome (Table 33-4) (Lancaster, 2015).

TABLE 33-4. Lynch Syndrome Genetic Screening Recommendations

Patients with endometrial or colorectal cancer and tumor evidence of:
    Microsatellite instability or
    DNA mismatch repair protein loss (see Fig. 33-4)

First-degree relative with endometrial or colorectal cancer who was diagnosed:
    Before age 60 years or
    Is at risk for Lynch syndrome based on personal and medical history

First- or second-degree relative with a known DNA mismatch repair gene mutation

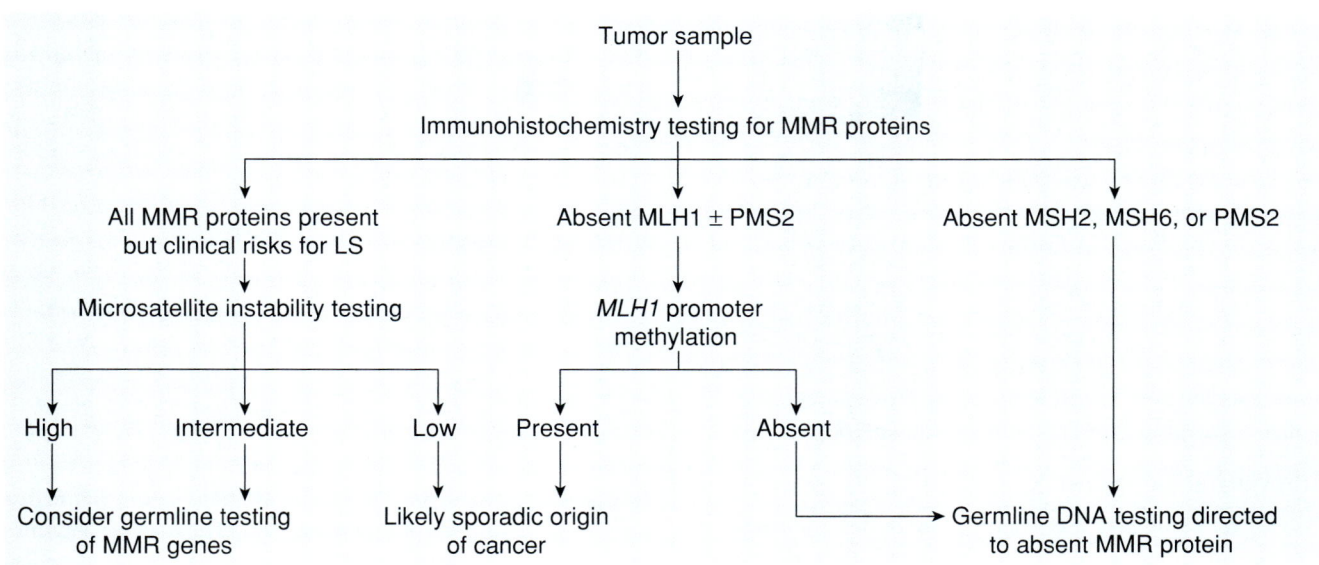

FIGURE 33-4 This algorithm begins with tumor testing for Lynch syndrome–associated proteins and genes. Immunohistochemistry staining of histologic slides is directed to the mismatch repair (MMR) proteins of interest. Right: If MSH2, MSH6, or PMS2 proteins are absent, then germline DNA testing is recommended. Center: If the MLH1 protein is absent, testing evaluates the promoter region of the *MLH1* gene. Silencing of *MLH1* by methylation reflects a sporadic, noninherited origin of the cancer. Left: If all MMR proteins are present but Lynch syndrome (LS) is still suspected, the degree of microsatellite instability in known DNA regions is evaluated. The degree of instability correlates with the risk for Lynch syndrome.

Lynch syndrome cancers include colon, endometrium, small bowel, renal pelvis and ureter, and ovary, among others (Vasen, 1999). Referral for genetic counseling based on family history can further clarify which patients may benefit from specific germline testing. For patients with endometrioid endometrial cancer, Lynch syndrome screening is performed by immunohistochemistry staining of the tumor to search for the four most important Lynch syndrome proteins, described in the last section. Intact expression of all four proteins is associated with a low risk of Lynch syndrome. These women can be counseled that formal genetic testing is unnecessary in most cases (Provenzale, 2018). For patients who have negative screening results but who are still suspected of having Lynch syndrome based on family history, further testing for microsatellite instability may be performed. The combination of intact protein expression and lack of microsatellite instability predicts a very low risk of Lynch syndrome. In these cases, formal genetic testing may be deferred, unless clinical suspicion is high. Some advocate screening all patients with endometrioid endometrial cancer. Other suggest a more selective approach, for example, screening all patients <65 years. One Lynch syndrome screening algorithm is Figure 33-4.

Because women with Lynch syndrome have such a high lifetime risk of developing endometrial cancer (40 to 60 percent), prophylactic hysterectomy is recommended once affected women reach the early to mid 40s and have completed childbearing. In a cohort of 315 Lynch syndrome patients, Schmeler and coworkers (2006) confirmed the benefit of this approach by reporting a 100-percent endometrial cancer risk reduction. In general, BSO also is performed due to the 9- to 12-percent lifetime risk of ovarian cancer. Prior to hysterectomy, colon cancer screening with colonoscopy should be up to date (American College of Obstetrician and Gynecologists, 2019a).

■ Diagnosis

Signs and Symptoms

Early diagnosis of endometrial cancer is almost entirely dependent on the prompt recognition and evaluation of irregular vaginal bleeding. In premenopausal women, a clinician must maintain a high index of suspicion for a history of prolonged, heavy menstruation or intermenstrual spotting, because many other benign disorders give rise to similar symptoms (Table 8-2, p. 182). Postmenopausal bleeding is particularly worrisome and carries a 5- to 10-percent likelihood of diagnosing endometrial carcinoma (Clarke, 2018; van Hanegem, 2017). Abnormal vaginal discharge may be another symptom in older women.

Unfortunately, some patients do not seek medical attention despite months or years of heavy, irregular bleeding. In more advanced disease, pelvic pressure and pain may reflect uterine enlargement or extrauterine tumor spread. Patients with serous or clear cell tumors often present with signs and symptoms suggestive of advanced epithelial ovarian cancer. These include pelvic pain or pressure, bloating, early satiety, and increasing abdominal girth.

Papanicolaou Test

Pap testing is a screening test for cervical cancer. However, some findings from Pap testing should prompt further investigation for endometrial cancer. Benign endometrial cells are occasionally recorded on a routine Pap test report in women 45 years or older. In premenopausal women, this is often a finding of limited importance, especially if a test is obtained following menses. However, postmenopausal women with such findings have a 3- to 5-percent risk of endometrial cancer (Simsir, 2005). In those using HRT, the prevalence of benign endometrial cells on smears is greater, and the risk of endometrial malignancy is low (1 to 2 percent) (Mount, 2002). Although endometrial biopsy is considered in asymptomatic postmenopausal women if this finding is reported, most patients ultimately diagnosed with hyperplasia or cancers also have concomitant abnormal bleeding (Ashfaq, 2001).

In contrast, *atypical glandular cells* found during Pap testing carry higher risks for underlying cervical or endometrial neoplasia. Accordingly, evaluation of a glandular abnormality includes colposcopy and endocervical curettage (ECC). It may also include endometrial sampling in nonpregnant patients older than 35 years. In those younger than 35 years, endometrial sampling is encouraged if AUB coexists, if patient risk factors for endometrial disease are present, or if the cytology report specifies that the atypical glandular cells are endometrial in origin.

Endometrial Sampling

Office Pipelle biopsy is preferred for the initial evaluation of women with bleeding suspicious for malignancy (Feldman, 1993). However, if sampling techniques fail to provide sufficient diagnostic information or if abnormal bleeding persists, D & C may be required to clarify the diagnosis.

The American College of Obstetricians and Gynecologists (2018a) considers hysteroscopy acceptable for AUB evaluation in those without advanced-stage uterine or cervical cancer. However, hysteroscopy is more sensitive for focal endometrial lesions and thus has proved less helpful in diagnosing early endometrial cancer. In those cases in which hysteroscopy is used to evaluate AUB and in which cancer is ultimately diagnosed, a higher incidence of positive peritoneal cytology has been noted during subsequent staging surgery (Obermair, 2000; Polyzos, 2010; Zerbe, 2000). Although the risk of peritoneal contamination by cancer cells may be increased by retrograde efflux of hysteroscopic media, patient prognosis overall does not appear to be worsened (Cicinelli, 2010; Revel, 2004).

Laboratory Testing

The only clinically useful tumor marker in the management of endometrial cancer is a serum CA125 level. Preoperatively, an elevated level indicates the possibility of more advanced disease (Powell, 2005). In practice, it is most useful in patients with advanced disease or serous subtypes to assist in monitoring response to therapy or during posttreatment surveillance. However, even in this setting, its utility in the absence of other clinical findings is limited (Price, 1998).

Imaging Studies

In general, for women with low-grade endometrial cancer, chest radiography may be considered. All other preoperative testing is directed toward general surgical preparation (Chap. 39, p. 822).

Computed tomography (CT) or magnetic resonance (MR) imaging is usually not necessary (American College of Obstetricians and Gynecologists, 2017b). However, CT scanning can be obtained preoperatively in cases with higher-grade lesions to assess for lymph node involvement or metastatic disease. MR imaging can occasionally help distinguish an endometrial cancer with cervical extension from a primary endocervical adenocarcinoma (Nagar, 2006). Women with serous features, carcinosarcoma, or other high-risk histology on preoperative biopsy and those with physical findings suggesting advanced disease are most appropriate for abdominopelvic CT scanning (Fig. 33-5). In these cases, advance knowledge of intraabdominal disease may help guide surgery and treatment. MR imaging is also recommended for women who are considering fertility-sparing management with hormonal therapy, because this may not be a suitable option if deep invasion is found.

■ Role of the Generalist

Although most endometrial cancers are cured by hysterectomy and BSO, primary management by gynecologic oncologists results in an efficient use of health-care resources, minimizes potential morbidity, is more likely to lead to staging, and improves the survival of patients with high-risk disease (Chan, 2011; Roland, 2004). Therefore, preoperative consultation is generally advisable for any patient with endometrial cancer who is being prepared for surgery by a generalist in obstetrics and

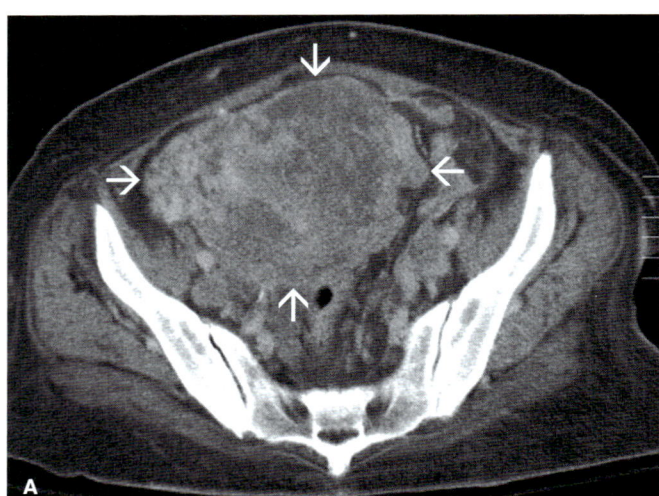
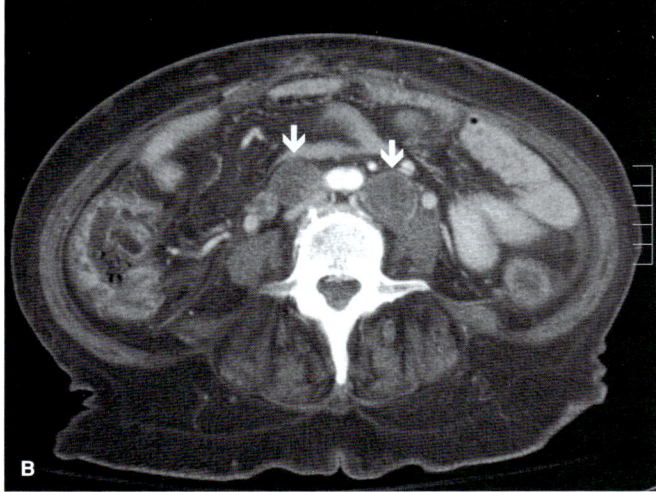

FIGURE 33-5 Computed tomographic (CT) images in the axial plane of a 61-year-old woman with endometrial cancer. **A.** Massively enlarged and inhomogeneous uterus (*arrows*) in the upper pelvis. **B.** At the level of the aortic bifurcation, enlarged lymph nodes are seen bilaterally (*arrows*), consistent with lymph node involvement. (Reproduced with permission from Dr. Diane Twickler.)

gynecology. Postoperatively, a gynecologic oncologist should be consulted if any extrauterine disease is found and if there is a question whether adjuvant therapy is indicated.

If treated by an oncologist, patients with early-stage cancer treated by surgery alone will return in many cases to their primary obstetrician-gynecologist for surveillance. Consultation is again recommended if recurrent disease is later suspected or identified.

When an endometrial cancer is unexpectedly diagnosed after hysterectomy performed by a generalist for other indications, consultation is recommended. Possible therapeutic options include no further therapy and surveillance only, reoperation to complete surgical staging, or radiotherapy to prevent local recurrence. In general, the survival advantages of staging must be weighed against the complications from another surgical procedure (American College of Obstetricians and Gynecologists, 2017b). Fortunately, the advent of laparoscopic and robotic delayed staging offers the potential for less morbidity than laparotomy (Spirtos, 2005).

Pathology

The spectrum of aggressiveness within the histopathologic types of endometrial cancer is broad (Table 33-5). Most patients have endometrioid adenocarcinomas that behave indolently. However, some will have an unfavorable histology that portends a much more aggressive tumor. In addition, the degree of tumor differentiation is an important predictor of disease spread.

Histologic Grade

The most widely used grading system for endometrial carcinoma is the three-tiered International Federation of Gynecology and Obstetrics (FIGO) system (Table 33-6). Grade 1 lesions typically are indolent with little propensity to spread outside the uterus or recur. Grade 2 tumors have an intermediate prognosis. Grade 3 cancers pose an increased potential for myometrial invasion and nodal metastasis.

Histologic grading is primarily determined by the tumor's architectural growth pattern (Zaino, 1994). However, there are exceptions, and the optimal method for determining grade is somewhat controversial. Nuclear atypia that is inappropriately

TABLE 33-5. Classification of Endometrial Carcinoma

Endometrioid adenocarcinoma
  Variant with squamous differentiation
  Villoglandular variant
  Secretory variant
  Ciliated cell variant
Mucinous carcinoma
Serous carcinoma
Clear cell carcinoma
Mixed cell carcinoma
Neuroendocrine tumor
Undifferentiated carcinoma
Squamous cell carcinoma
Carcinosarcoma
Others

TABLE 33-6. Histopathologic Criteria for Assessing Grade

Grade	Definition
1	≤5% of a nonsquamous or nonmorular solid growth pattern
2	6–50% of a nonsquamous or nonmorular solid growth pattern
3	>50% of a nonsquamous or nonmorular solid growth pattern

Summarized from Pecorelli, 1999.

advanced relative to the architectural grade raises a grade 1 or 2 tumor by one level. For example, a grade 2 lesion based on architectural features may be increased to a grade 3 lesion if significant nuclear atypia is present (Zaino, 1995). Nuclear grading based on the FIGO system is also used for all serous and clear cell adenocarcinomas (Pecorelli, 1999).

Histologic Type

Endometrioid Adenocarcinoma. This is the most common histologic type of endometrial cancer and accounts for more than 80 percent of cases. This type I tumor characteristically contains glands that resemble those of the normal endometrium (Fig. 33-6). The concomitant presence of hyperplastic endometrium correlates with a low-grade tumor and a lack of myometrial invasion. However, when the glandular component decreases and is replaced by solid nests and sheets of cells, the tumor is classified as a higher grade (Kurman, 2014). In addition, an atrophic endometrium is more frequently associated with high-grade lesions that have a greater potential to metastasize (Kurman, 1994).

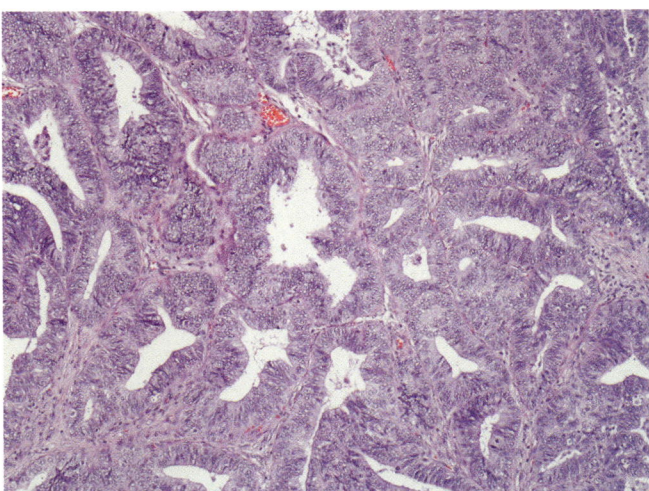

FIGURE 33-6 Endometrioid adenocarcinomas are composed of neoplastic glands resembling those of the normal endometrium. Cells are typically tall columnar with mild to moderate nuclear atypia. They form glands that are abnormally crowded or "back-to-back." Gland cribriforming, confluence, and villous structures also are common. It is these architectural forms, with the associated disappearance of intervening stroma, that distinguish well-differentiated endometrioid adenocarcinoma from atypical hyperplasia. (Reproduced with permission from Dr. Kelley Carrick.)

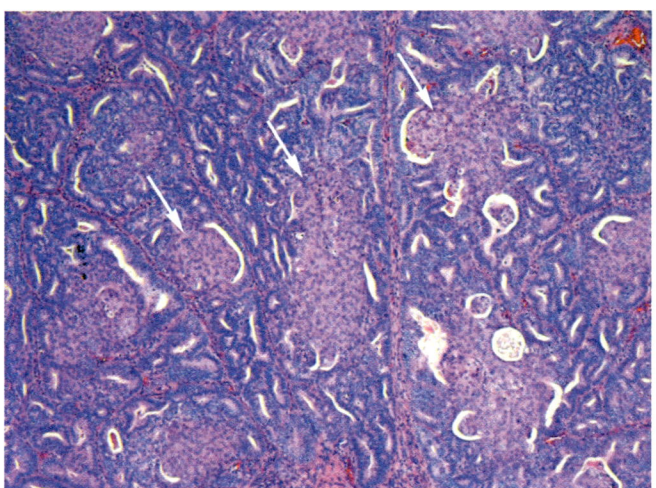

FIGURE 33-7 Endometrioid adenocarcinomas may show foci of squamous differentiation, which may be focal or relatively prominent. The squamous elements can have obvious squamous features such as keratinization or intercellular bridges or may be represented by less well-differentiated squamous morules (*arrows*), as in this example. (Reproduced with permission from Dr. Raheela Ashfaq.)

Endometrioid adenocarcinomas may also display variant forms. These include endometrioid adenocarcinoma with squamous differentiation and villoglandular, secretory, and ciliated cell types (Fig. 33-7). In general, the biologic behavior of these variant tumors reflects that of classic endometrioid adenocarcinoma.

Serous Carcinoma. Accounting for 5 to 10 percent of endometrial cancers, serous carcinoma typifies the highly aggressive type II tumors that arise from the atrophic endometrium of older women (Jordan, 2001). There is typically a complex pattern of papillary growth, and cells demonstrate marked nuclear atypia (Fig. 33-8). Commonly referred to as *uterine papillary serous carcinoma (UPSC)*, its histologic appearance resembles epithelial ovarian cancer, and psammoma bodies are seen in 30 percent of cases (Kurman, 2014).

Grossly, a papillary exophytic tumor emerges from a small, atrophic uterus. These tumors may occasionally be confined within a polyp and have no evidence for spread (Carcangiu, 1992). However, UPSC has a known propensity for myometrial and lymphatic invasion. Intraperitoneal spread, such as omental caking, which is unusual for typical endometrioid adenocarcinoma, also is common even when myometrial invasion is minimal or absent (Fig. 33-9) (Sherman, 1992). As a result, it may be impossible to distinguish UPSC from epithelial ovarian cancer during surgery. Like ovarian carcinoma, these tumors usually secrete CA125. Thus, serial serum measurements can be used to monitor disease postoperatively. UPSC is an aggressive cell type, and women with mixed endometrial cancers containing as little as 25 percent of UPSC have survival rates that mirror those with pure uterine serous carcinoma (Ellenson, 2011a).

Carcinosarcoma. Carcinosarcomas are mixed tumors demonstrating both epithelial and stromal components. These have also been known as *malignant mixed müllerian tumor (MMMT)*. In the past, carcinosarcomas were classified as a type

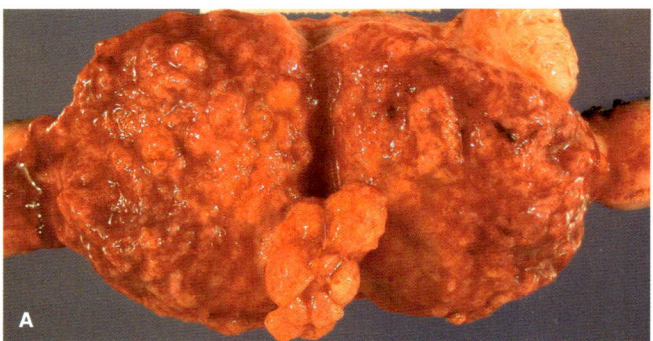

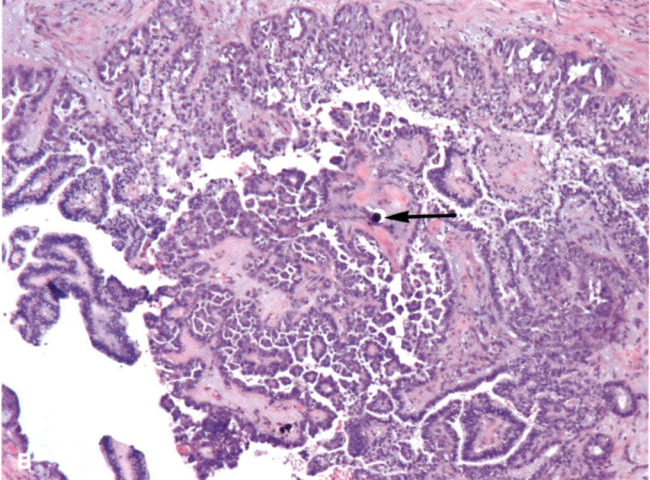

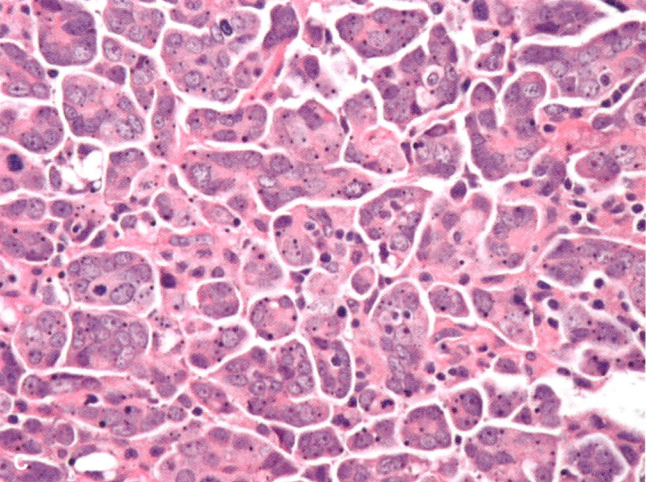

FIGURE 33-8 Uterine serous carcinoma. **A.** Uterine specimen. (Reproduced with permission from Dr. Raheela Ashfaq.) **B.** This tumor is typically characterized by a papillary architecture. Psammoma bodies, which are concentrically laminated calcifications (*arrow*), may be present. **C.** Cells are typically rounded as opposed to columnar. They have high-grade nuclear features including relatively large, pleomorphic nuclei; prominent nucleoli; and frequent, abnormal mitoses. (Reproduced with permission from Dr. Kelley Carrick.)

of uterine sarcoma, and the WHO classification still categorizes it as a mixed epithelial and mesenchymal tumor (Kurman, 2014). However, molecular studies have convincingly shown that most carcinosarcomas are monoclonal and driven by their

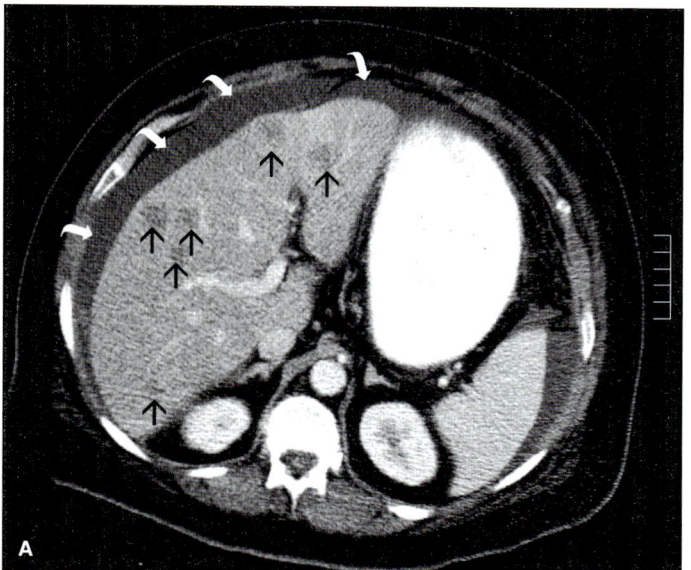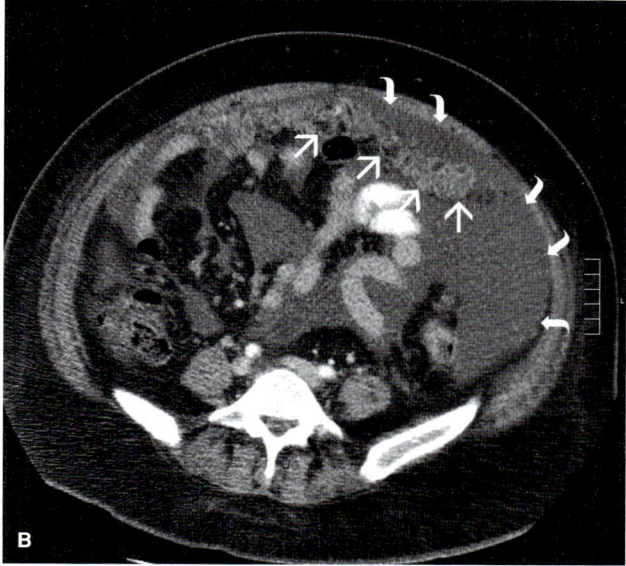

FIGURE 33-9 Computed tomographic (CT) images of liver metastases, ascites, and omental caking in a 51-year-old woman with endometrial cancer. **A.** Black arrows demarcate multiple low-density areas in the liver that are consistent with metastases, and ascites (*curved, white arrows*) surrounds the liver. **B.** A more caudal image reveals omental caking (*white arrows*) surrounded by massive ascites (*curved, white arrows*).

epithelial component (Wada, 1997). The sarcomatous element is thought to result from metaplasia of the epithelial element. Thus, these tumors generally behave like UPSC.

Grossly, the tumor is sessile or polypoid, bulky, necrotic, and often hemorrhagic (Fig. 33-10). It often fills the endometrial cavity and deeply invades the myometrium. On occasion, a large tumor protrudes through the external cervical os and fills the vaginal vault.

Microscopically, carcinosarcomas have an admixture of epithelial and mesenchymal differentiation. The malignant epithelial element is typically an adenocarcinoma of endometrioid type, but serous, clear cell, mucinous, squamous cell, and undifferentiated carcinoma also are common (Fig. 33-11). Mesenchymal components can be homologous to the uterus, usually resembling

endometrial stromal sarcomas or fibrosarcomas. Alternatively, heterologous mesenchymal differentiation can be found in association with areas of endometrial stromal or undifferentiated sarcomas. Most commonly, rhabdomyosarcoma or chondrosarcoma compose these cases of heterologous mesenchymal differentiation (Fig. 33-12). Although interesting, the homologous or heterologous designation has no clinical importance.

With carcinosarcoma, endometrial sampling will often lead to a correct diagnosis, although in many cases only the carcinomatous features are evident. The reverse is also true, and occasionally a uterine carcinosarcoma is suspected based on endometrial biopsy findings, but no sarcomatous features are found within the hysterectomy specimen.

Their pattern of spread more closely mirrors that of UPSC. In addition, metastases usually show the serous carcinomatous elements, without sarcomatous differentiation. Patients are often older and have an average age of 65 years when diagnosed. Fewer than 5 percent are discovered in women younger than 50. At the time of diagnosis, approximately 40 percent are stage I. Stage II (10 percent), stage III (25 percent), and stage IV disease (25 percent) make up the remainder (Sartori, 1997; Vaidya, 2006).

Clear Cell Carcinoma. This is another type II tumor but is rare. The microscopic appearance may be predominantly solid, cystic, tubular, or papillary. Most frequently, it consists of a mixture of two or more of these patterns (Fig. 33-13).

Endometrial clear cell adenocarcinomas are similar to those arising in the ovary, vagina, and cervix. Grossly, there are no characteristic features, but like UPSC, they tend to be high-grade, deeply invasive tumors. Patients are often diagnosed with advanced disease and have a poor prognosis (Hamilton, 2006).

Mucinous Carcinoma. Of endometrial cancers, 1 to 2 percent have a mucinous appearance that forms more than half of the

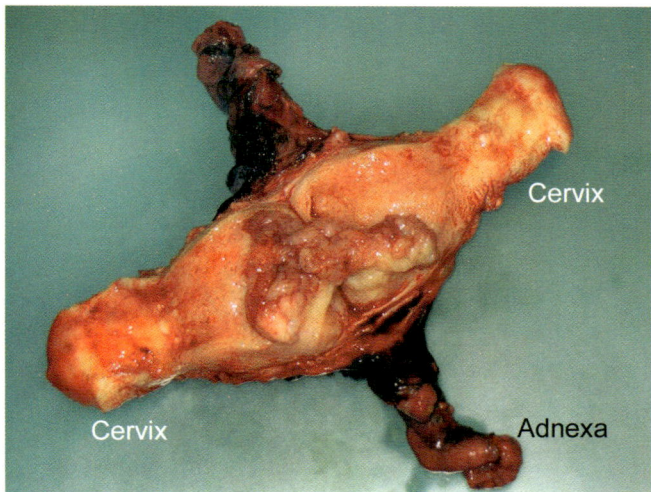

FIGURE 33-10 Carcinosarcoma. Photograph of the surgical specimen after it has been bisected and remains joined at the fundus.

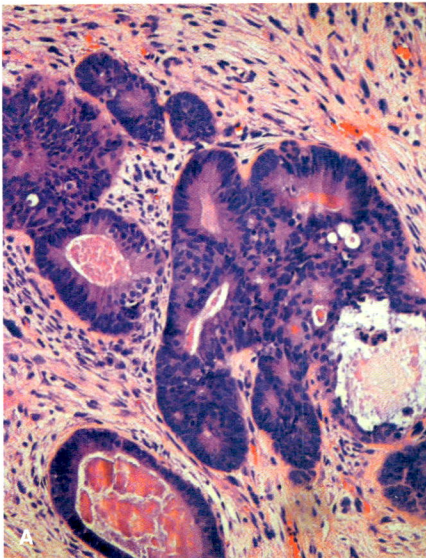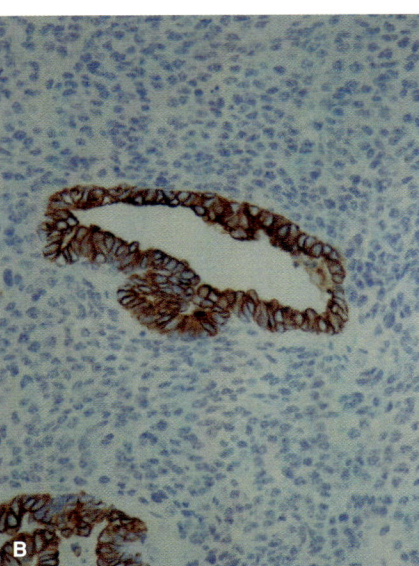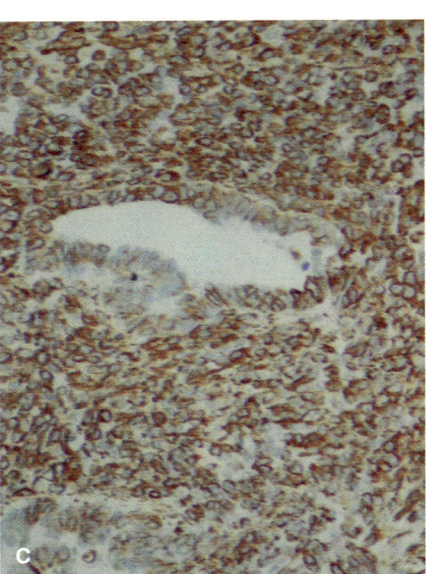

FIGURE 33-11 A. Carcinosarcoma is a biphasic malignant neoplasm composed of both carcinomatous and sarcomatous elements. In this example, malignant endometrioid-type glands are present within an atypical spindled stroma. **B.** Immunohistochemical stain for cytokeratin marks the epithelial component but not the stromal component. **C.** Conversely, an immunohistochemical stain for vimentin (a mesenchymal marker) stains the sarcomatous component. (Reproduced with permission from Dr. Raheela Ashfaq.)

tumor. However, many endometrioid adenocarcinomas will have this as a focal component (Ross, 1983). Typically, mucinous tumors have a glandular pattern with uniform columnar cells and minimal stratification (Fig. 33-14). Almost all are stage I grade 1 lesions and carry a good prognosis (Melhem, 1987). Since endocervical epithelium merges with the lower uterine segment, the main diagnostic dilemma is differentiating this tumor from a primary cervical adenocarcinoma. Immunostaining may be helpful, and MR imaging may further clarify the most likely site of origin. In general, to define anatomy, MR imaging is preferable to CT scanning as MR offers superior contrast resolution at soft-tissue interfaces.

Mixed Carcinoma, Undifferentiated Carcinoma, and Rare Types. An endometrial cancer may demonstrate combinations of two or more pure types. To be classified as a mixed carcinoma, a component must make up at least 10 percent of the tumor. Except for serous and clear cell histology, the combination of other types usually has no clinical significance. As a result, mixed carcinoma usually refers to an admixture of a type I (endometrioid adenocarcinoma and its variants) and a type II carcinoma (Kurman, 2014).

Undifferentiated carcinoma lacks architectural differentiation and is characterized by medium-sized, monotonous epithelial cells growing in solid sheets without a pattern (Silva, 2007).

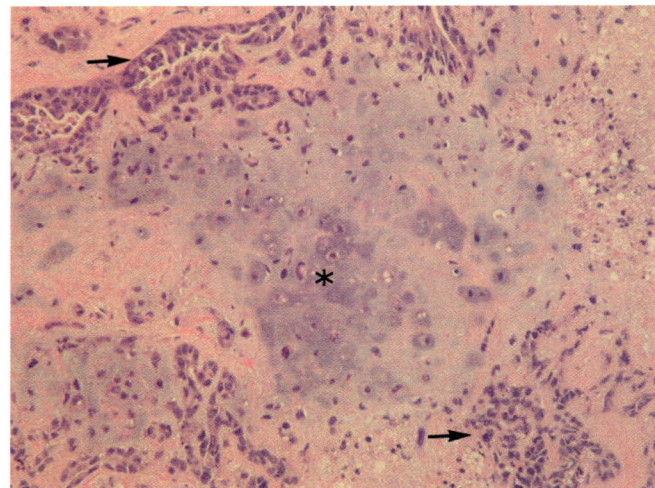

FIGURE 33-12 Carcinosarcoma with heterologous elements. In this carcinosarcoma with cartilaginous differentiation, malignant glands are present at the periphery (*arrows*). Centrally a focus of malignant cartilage (*asterisk*) is seen, with its characteristic lacunae embedded within a bluish chondroid matrix. (Reproduced with permission from Dr. Kelley Carrick.)

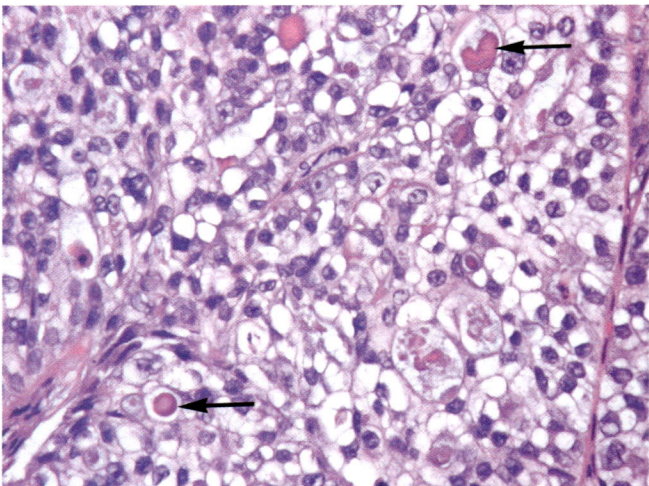

FIGURE 33-13 Clear cell adenocarcinomas are composed of cells with clear to eosinophilic granular cytoplasm. Cells are arranged in papillae, sheets, tubulocystic structures, or a combination. Eosinophilic hyaline globules (*arrows*) are a common feature. In this example, nuclei are moderately pleomorphic, with nucleolar prominence. (Reproduced with permission from Dr. Kelley Carrick.)

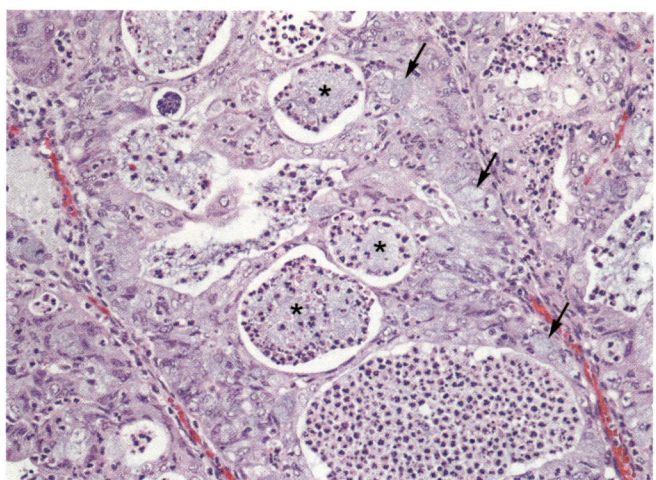

FIGURE 33-14 Mucinous adenocarcinoma of the endometrium has tumor cells containing intracytoplasmic mucin (*arrows*). Tumor cells form sheets and cribriform structures (*asterisks*), which in this example contain bluish mucin and numerous neutrophils. (Reproduced with permission from Dr. Kelley Carrick.)

TABLE 33-7. Correlation of Histologic Grade and Depth of Myometrial Invasion in Stage I Patients (*n* = 5095)

Myometrial Invasion	Grade		
	1	2	3
None	29%	11%	15%
≤50%	51%	59%	46%
>50%	20%	30%	39%

Data from Creasman, 2006.

These represent 1 to 2 percent of endometrial cancers. Overall, the prognosis is worse than in patients with poorly differentiated endometrioid adenocarcinomas (Altrabulsi, 2005). When an undifferentiated carcinoma has a component of low-grade endometrioid adenocarcinoma, these tumors are called *dedifferentiated carcinomas*.

Of rare histologic types, fewer than 100 cases of *squamous cell carcinoma* of the endometrium have been reported. Diagnosis requires exclusion of an adenocarcinoma component and no connection with the squamous epithelium of the cervix (Varras, 2002). Typically, the prognosis is poor (Goodman, 1996). *Transitional cell carcinoma* of the endometrium also is rare, and metastatic disease from the bladder or ovary must be excluded during diagnosis (Ahluwalia, 2006).

Patterns of Spread

Endometrial cancers have several different potential ways to spread beyond the uterus (Morrow, 1991). Type I endometrioid tumors and their variants most commonly spread, in order of frequency, by: (1) direct extension, (2) lymphatic metastasis, (3) hematogenous dissemination, and (4) intraperitoneal exfoliation. Type II serous and clear cell carcinomas and carcinosarcoma have a particular propensity for extrauterine disease, in a pattern that closely resembles epithelial ovarian cancer. In general, the various patterns of spread are interrelated and often develop simultaneously.

Invasion of the endometrial stroma and exophytic expansion within the uterine cavity follows initial growth of an early cancer. Over time, the tumor invades the myometrium and may ultimately perforate the serosa (Table 33-7). Tumors situated in the lower uterine segment tend to involve the cervix early, whereas those in the upper corpus tend to extend to the fallopian tubes or serosa. Advanced regional growth may lead to direct invasion into adjacent pelvic structures, including the bladder, large bowel, vagina, and broad ligament.

Lymphatic channel invasion and metastasis to the pelvic and paraaortic nodal chains can follow tumor penetration of the myometrium (Table 33-8). The lymphatic network draining the uterus is complex, and patients can have metastases to any single nodal group or combination of groups (Burke, 1996). This haphazard pattern is in contrast to cervical cancer, in which lymphatic spread usually follows a stepwise progression from pelvic to paraaortic to scalene nodal groups. Despite this, comprehensive surgical staging studies show that paraaortic nodal metastases in the absence of pelvic nodal metastases is infrequent, <2 percent (Boronow, 1984; Onda, 1997).

Hematogenous dissemination most commonly results in metastases to the lung and less commonly to the liver, brain, bone, and other sites. Deep myometrial invasion is the strongest predictor of this pattern of spread (Mariani, 2001a).

Retrograde transtubal transport of exfoliated endometrial cancer cells carries malignant cells to the peritoneal cavity. *Serosal perforation* of the tumor is another possible pathway. Most types of endometrial cancer cells found in the peritoneal cavity disappear within a short time and have low malignant potential (Hirai, 2001). Alternatively, in the presence of other high-risk features, such as adnexal metastases or serous histology, widespread intraabdominal disease may result.

TABLE 33-8. Correlation of Histologic Grade and Depth of Myometrial Invasion with Risk of Nodal Metastases

Myometrial Invasion	Pelvic Lymph Nodes			Paraaortic Lymph Nodes		
	G1	G2	G3	G1	G2	G3
None	1%	7%	16%	<1%	2%	5%
≤50%	2%	6%	10%	<1%	2%	4%
>50%	11%	21%	37%	2%	6%	13%

Data from Creasman, 2006.

Port-site metastasis is a rare but recognized method of cancer spread. Martínez and coworkers (2010) evaluated nearly 300 laparoscopic staging procedures for endometrial cancer. Port-site metastases complicated 0.33 percent of cases. Similarly, cancer dissemination following specimen morcellation has been reported (Graebe, 2015).

■ Treatment

Surgical Management

Most patients with endometrial cancer should undergo hysterectomy and BSO. The extent of surgical staging, including degree of lymph node assessment, is controversial. The National Comprehensive Cancer Network (NCCN) (2019) recently changed its guidance from recommending comprehensive pelvic and paraaortic lymphadenectomy in all patients to selective and tailored lymph node assessment, which may include sentinel lymph node biopsy.

For optimal patient management, the histopathologic description of the preoperative biopsy is carefully reviewed. Two thirds of patients are stage I at diagnosis (Fig. 33-15 and Table 33-9) (FIGO Committee on Gynecologic Oncology, 2009). Only a few circumstances contraindicate primary surgery and include a desire to preserve fertility, massive obesity, high operative risk, and clinically unresectable disease. In general, an extrafascial hysterectomy, also known as type I or simple hysterectomy, is sufficient. However, radical hysterectomy (type II or III hysterectomy) may be preferable

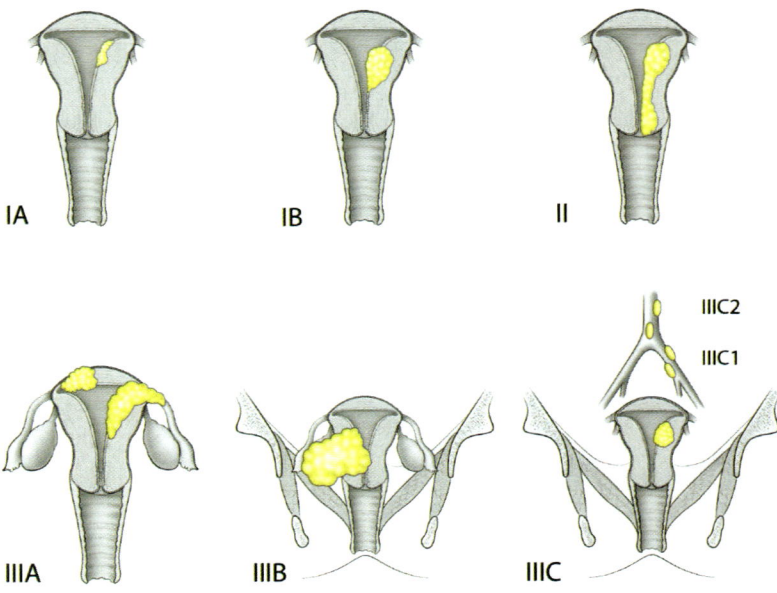

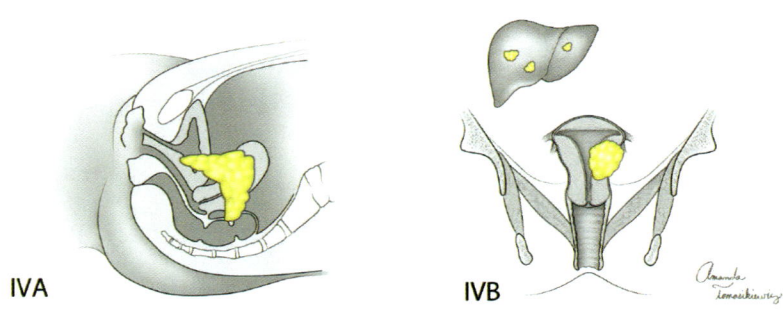

FIGURE 33-15 International Federation of Gynecology and Obstetrics (FIGO) staging of endometrial cancer.

TABLE 33-9. International Federation of Gynecology and Obstetrics (FIGO) Surgical Staging System for Endometrial Cancer

Stage[a]	Characteristics
I	**Tumor confined to the corpus uteri.**
IA	No or less than half myometrial invasion.
IB	Invasion equal to or more than half of the myometrium.
II	**Tumor invades cervical stroma but does not extend beyond the uterus[b].**
III	**Local and/or regional spread of the tumor.**
IIIA	Tumor invades the serosa of the corpus uteri and/or adnexae[c].
IIIB	Vaginal and/or parametrial involvement[c].
IIIC	Metastases to pelvic and/or para-aortic lymph nodes[c].
IIIC1	Positive pelvic nodes.
IIIC2	Positive paraaortic lymph nodes with or without positive pelvic lymph nodes.
IV	**Tumor invades bladder and/or bowel mucosa, and/or distant metastases.**
IVA	Tumor invasion of bladder and/or bowel mucosa.
IVB	Distant metastases, including intraabdominal metastases and/or inguinal lymph nodes.

[a]Either G1, G2, or G3.
[b]Endocervical glandular involvement only should be considered as stage I and no longer as stage II.
[c]Positive cytology has to be reported separately without changing the stage.

for patients with clinically obvious cervical extension of endometrial cancer (Cornelison, 1999; Mariani, 2001b). Differences in these hysterectomy types are outlined in Table 30-7 (p. 666). Vaginal hysterectomy with or without BSO is another option for women who cannot undergo systematic surgical staging due to comorbidities (American College of Obstetricians and Gynecologists, 2017b). Previously, laparotomy had been the standard approach. However, laparoscopic and robotic surgical staging are increasingly used for endometrial cancer that appears clinically confined to the uterus. Such MIS staging is safe, feasible, and now recommended (Walker, 2009).

Regardless of approach, upon entering the peritoneal cavity, a thorough intraabdominal and pelvic exploration is performed, and suspicious lesions are biopsied or excised. Ascites, if present, is collected for cytologic study. These preliminary procedures are followed by hysterectomy and BSO. If the decision to perform lymphadenectomy is contingent on depth of myometrial invasion, this may be determined by intraoperative gross examination or microscopic frozen section analysis (Sanjuan, 2006; Vorgias, 2002).

As noted, the risk of lymph node metastasis correlates with the tumor grade and depth of invasion into the myometrium. Historically, the combination of preoperative biopsy grade and intraoperative assessment of the depth of myometrial invasion were the two factors that surgeons used to determine whether to proceed with pelvic and paraaortic lymph node dissection. The inaccuracy of this approach has been reported (Eltabbakh, 2005; Leitao, 2008; Papadia, 2009). In addition, the depth of myometrial invasion determined in the operative room is often inaccurate (Frumovitz, 2004a,b).

Lymphadenectomy may allow detection of positive nodes to guide appropriate treatment. Some retrospective studies showed improved survival rates in patients who had undergone an adequate lymph node dissection (Kilgore, 1995; Todo, 2010). However, the advantage appears to be confined to those in high-risk groups. To the contrary, authors of two randomized trials reported no improvement in disease-free or overall survival rates after lymphadenectomy in patients with early-stage disease (Benedetti Panici, 2008; Kitchener, 2009). These trials were criticized because lymph node counts were low and lymph node status did not dictate treatment, as many patients received postoperative radiation regardless of their lymph node status. Moreover, concern exists that omitting lymphadenectomy may lead to missed metastatic disease and subsequent insufficient postoperative treatment. Currently, many surgeons perform complete surgical staging with pelvic and paraaortic lymphadenectomy selectively and reserve this for patients with high-risk grade 1 endometrioid cancer and any case of grade 2, grade 3 or type II cancers. Using this approach, lymphadenectomy is omitted for low-risk patients.

Distinct from the above discussion, any suspicious pelvic or paraaortic lymph nodes should be removed and histologically evaluated. Excision of grossly involved lymph nodes may lead to a survival advantage (Havrilesky, 2005).

Those patients with serous, carcinosarcoma, or clear cell features on preoperative biopsy should have extended surgical staging with an infracolic omentectomy and bilateral peritoneal biopsies of the pelvis, pericolic gutter, and diaphragm (Bristow, 2001a). As in ovarian cancer, a surgeon is also prepared to resect any metastases (Bristow, 2000).

Recently, sentinel node biopsy (SLNB) has been cited as an acceptable replacement for lymphadenectomy in endometrial cancer by NCCN (2019) and the Society of Gynecologic Oncology (Holloway, 2017). According to the sentinel node paradigm, a cancer-free sentinel node should be highly predictive of negative nodes in the remainder of that nodal basin. Thus, complete lymphadenectomy could be avoided. Unlike vulvar cancer, the best technique for SLNB is debated for endometrial cancer, because these often lack a discrete tumor around which to inject dye (Fig. 31-9, p. 683). A common approach is to inject the cervix with a vital dye (Abu-Rustum, 2009). In most cases, at least one sentinel node on each side of the pelvis can be identified. If no sentinel node is identified, a side-specific lymphadenectomy is performed. Two prospective studies have demonstrated that SLNB has high sensitivity and high negative predictive value compared with lymphadenectomy (Ballester, 2011; Rossi, 2017). Many surgeons previously have limited SLNB use to type I endometrial cancers, but evidence is accumulating to support its use for more aggressive histologies, including serous carcinomas and carcinosarcomas (Schiavone, 2016, 2017; Soliman, 2017).

As noted, an MIS approach is acceptable for suitable candidates undergoing hysterectomy and staging for endometrial cancer (Childers, 1994; Spirtos, 2005). In the GOG LAP2 study, conventional open surgery plus pelvic/paraaortic lymphadenectomy was compared with the same steps completed laparoscopically for clinical stage I and IIA endometrial carcinoma. Investigators found laparoscopic staging to be feasible and safe (Walker, 2009). Laparoscopy was completed without conversion in 74 percent of patients randomized to MIS. Advantageously, compared with those undergoing laparotomy, patients undergoing laparoscopy had similar rates of intraoperative injuries (9 versus 8 percent), fewer moderate to severe complications (14 versus 21 percent), shorter hospital stays (median 3 versus 4 days), and better quality of life at 6 weeks postoperatively. However, laparoscopic staging was linked with longer operative times (Kornblith, 2009; Walker, 2009). Importantly, long-term treatment success does not appear to be compromised with laparoscopic surgery. Overall survival and recurrence rates in early reports are similar to those for a traditional open approach (Ghezzi, 2010; Magrina, 1999; Walker, 2012; Zullo, 2009). More recently, a randomized trial compared total laparoscopic hysterectomy to laparotomy in women with early-stage endometrial cancer (Janda, 2017). Selective pelvic (with or without paraaortic) lymphadenectomy was mandated unless the patient was morbidly obese or medically unfit. Disease-free and overall survival rates did not different between the two groups.

Robot-assisted laparoscopic staging of endometrial cancer has been embraced by many gynecologic oncologists to overcome MIS technical challenges, especially in obese patients. Early evidence shows it to be feasible and safe (Hoekstra, 2009). Compared with a laparoscopic approach for endometrial cancer staging, both major complication rates and mean number of lymph nodes removed are similar.

As described in Chapter 41 (p. 873), not all women are candidates for MIS. Limiting factors can include extensive adhesive disease, a large bulky uterus, morbid obesity, cardiopulmonary disease, and other patient comorbidities. Importantly, morcellation is avoided in cancer cases to prevent disease spread.

Surveillance

Most surgically treated patients can simply be followed by pelvic examination every 3 to 6 months for the first 2 years and then every 6 to 12 months for 3 years (Salani 2017). Pap testing is not a recommended part of surveillance, as an asymptomatic vaginal recurrence is identified in <1 percent of patients (Bristow, 2006a; Cooper, 2006). Routine imaging also is not recommended. Patients should be made aware of symptoms that may indicate recurrence, particularly vaginal bleeding.

Women who have more advanced cancer that requires postoperative radiation or chemotherapy or both warrant more aggressive monitoring. Serum CA125 measurements may be valuable, particularly for UPSC, if the level was elevated prior to treatment. Intermittent imaging using CT scanning or MR imaging also may be indicated. In general, the pattern of recurrent disease depends on the original sites of metastasis and the treatment received.

Chemotherapy

Only three classes of cytotoxic drugs with definite activity for endometrial cancer have been identified, and paclitaxel (Taxol), doxorubicin (Adriamycin), and cisplatin (TAP) chemotherapy is one of the adjuvant treatment options for advanced endometrial cancer following surgery. In one GOG trial of 273 women (protocol #177), administration of seven courses of TAP was superior to doxorubicin plus cisplatin, but toxicity was increased, particularly peripheral neuropathy (Fleming, 2004). A less toxic alternative to TAP chemotherapy is paclitaxel plus carboplatin. Routinely used for ovarian cancer, this regimen is effective in advanced-stage endometrial cancer (Hoskins, 2001; Sovak, 2006, 2007). One GOG trial (protocol #209) compared TAP and the regimen of carboplatin plus paclitaxel. Results demonstrated that carboplatin plus paclitaxel was not inferior to TAP in terms of progression-free and overall survival rates. The toxicity profile favored carboplatin plus paclitaxel, and this regimen is generally used at our institution (Miller, 2012).

In practice, cytotoxic chemotherapy is frequently combined, sequenced, or sandwiched with radiotherapy in patients with advanced endometrial cancer following surgery. To reduce toxicity, directed pelvic or paraaortic radiation is usually employed rather than whole abdomen radiation (Homesley, 2009; Miller, 2009).

Radiation

Primary Radiation Therapy. This option rather than surgery is selected rarely and mainly for exceptionally poor surgical candidates. Intracavitary brachytherapy such as Heyman capsules with or without external beam pelvic radiation is the typical method (Chap. 28, p. 612). In general, the survival rate is 10 to 15 percent lower than that with surgical treatment (Chao, 1996; Fishman, 1996). These poor results suggest that a careful preoperative evaluation and appropriate consultation should be completed before any woman is denied the benefits of hysterectomy (American College of Obstetricians and Gynecologists, 2017b).

Adjuvant Radiation Therapy. In general, this option is offered after staging surgery to women at risk for endometrial cancer recurrence. Those with low-risk, early-stage cancer are typically adequately treated with surgery, may not benefit from adjuvant therapy, and usually simply begin surveillance.

In three major trials of stage I patients at intermediate risk, adjuvant radiation improved local disease control and recurrence-free survival rates. It did not decrease the rate of distant metastases or improve overall survival rates at 5 years (Aalders, 1980; Creutzberg, 2000, 2004; Keys, 2004).

However, in one of these trials, the recurrence rate reduction was particularly evident in a high-intermediate–risk subgroup of women: (1) with three risk factors (grade 2 or 3 tumors, lymphovascular invasion, and invasion of the outer third of the myometrium); (2) with age >50 years and two of these risk factors; and (3) with age >70 years and one risk factor (Keys, 2004). Therefore, adjuvant radiation is usually offered to patients with high-intermediate–risk stage I uterine cancers. The type of radiation offered is vaginal brachytherapy. The PORTEC-2 trial showed that vaginal brachytherapy compared with whole pelvic radiation offered equivalent recurrence rates but less toxicity in women with high-intermediate–risk endometrial cancer (Nout, 2010).

The aforementioned studies did not include patients with high-risk, early-stage disease, namely grade 3, deeply invasive cancers. These patients have traditionally been treated with whole pelvic radiation, and this remains a common practice. However, many patients still recur. Therefore, the PORTEC-3 trial was initiated to compare the benefit of adding chemotherapy during and after whole pelvic radiation to whole pelvic radiation alone in patients with high-risk stage I or locally advanced (stage II and III) disease. Chemotherapy consisted of cisplatin during weeks 1 and 4 of radiation, followed by four cycles of carboplatin and paclitaxel. Lymphadenectomy was optional. Preliminary results suggest that patients with high-risk stage I and stage II do not benefit from chemoradiation and are best treated with whole pelvic radiation alone (de Boer, 2017). However, women with stage III disease may benefit from the combined modality approach. For women with stage II endometrial cancer, the efficacy of postoperative radiotherapy is even harder to decipher. Most data derive from retrospective, single-institution experiences, and evidence supports external beam pelvic radiation, vaginal brachytherapy, both, or no further treatment (Cannon, 2009; Elshaikh, 2015; Rittenberg, 2005). As such, there is no standard approach, and most patients are treated individually based on coexisting risk factors (Feltmate, 1999). In general, patients who had radical hysterectomy are less likely to have pelvic radiation recommended to them postoperatively.

Chemotherapy is a treatment mainstay for patients with stage III or IV disease. This was established by GOG trial #122, in which patients with stage III or IV disease were randomly assigned following surgery to chemotherapy or whole abdomen radiation (Randall, 2006). The patients receiving chemotherapy had improved progression-free and overall survival rates.

GOG study #258 aimed to answer the important question of whether the addition of radiation to chemotherapy would result in improved outcomes compared with chemotherapy alone in patients with stage III or IV, optimally debulked disease (Matei, 2017). At a median follow up of 47 months, recurrence-free and overall survival rates did not differ, although the latter results need more time to elapse to be considered final. Local and nodal control was improved in the chemoradiation arm, but distant control was improved in the chemotherapy arm. Acute toxicities were similar in the two arms. These results do not show a clear benefit to adding radiation in this population.

Hormonal Therapy

Cancer Treatment. One of the unique characteristics of endometrial cancer is its hormonal responsiveness. Thus, for women who are not surgical candidates, continuous chronic progestin treatment or a levonorgestrel-releasing IUD can be primary treatment (Dhar, 2005; Montz, 2002). In young premenopausal patients who desire fertility, similar primary progestin therapy can help reverse pathology (p. 703).

As adjuvant therapy, single-agent, high-dose progestins also have activity in women with advanced or recurrent disease (Lentz, 1996; Thigpen, 1999). Tamoxifen upregulates progesterone-receptor expression and is postulated to thereby improve progestin therapy efficacy. Clinically, tamoxifen used adjunctively with progestin therapy provides high response rates (Fiorica, 2004; Whitney, 2004). In general, toxicity is low, but this combination is most often used for recurrent disease. Aromatase inhibitors also have activity in endometrial cancer (Altman, 2012).

Estrogen Replacement Therapy. Due to the presumed role of excess estrogen in endometrial cancer development, estrogen supplementation following endometrial cancer treatment is often met with concern for stimulating malignancy recurrence. However, this effect has not been observed (Suriano, 2001). In one GOG study, 1236 women who had undergone surgery for stage I and II endometrial cancer were randomly assigned to receive either estrogen or placebo. Although the study did not meet its enrollment goals, the low recurrence rate (2 percent) was promising (Barakat, 2006). Women should be individually counseled regarding risks and benefits before beginning post-treatment estrogen replacement for menopausal symptoms.

Uterine Papillary Serous Carcinoma Management

This most aggressive type of endometrial carcinoma is rare, and thus, randomized trials are difficult to perform. As a result, most data are single-institution, retrospective analyses. Treatment is usually individualized but is often different from that for typical endometrioid adenocarcinoma.

If a preoperative biopsy demonstrates serous features, comprehensive surgical staging for UPSC is recommended. This includes total hysterectomy, BSO, peritoneal washings, pelvic/paraaortic lymph node dissection, infracolic omentectomy, and peritoneal biopsies (Chan, 2003). Even noninvasive disease is often widely metastatic (Gehrig, 2001). Fortunately, patients tend to have a good prognosis if surgical staging confirms that disease is confined to the uterus (stage I/II) (Grice, 1998).

Occasionally, no residual UPSC is evident on the hysterectomy specimen, or the tumor minimally involves the tip of a polyp. These women with surgical stage IA can safely be observed. However, all other patients with stage I disease are considered for adjuvant treatment. For this, one common strategy is postoperative paclitaxel and carboplatin chemotherapy for three to six cycles combined with concomitant vaginal brachytherapy (Dietrich, 2005; Kelly, 2005). However, some data suggest an intrinsic radioresistance for UPSC tumors (Martin, 2005). In addition, based on the largest retrospective review of patients with stage I disease, Huh and coworkers (2003) questioned the benefit of any radiation therapy.

Women with stage II UPSC are more likely to benefit from pelvic radiotherapy with or without chemotherapy following surgery. Those with stage III disease are especially prone to have recurrent disease at distant sites. Accordingly, paclitaxel and carboplatin is considered in addition to tumor-directed radiotherapy after surgery (Bristow, 2001a; Slomovitz, 2003).

In practice, many patients will have stage IVB disease. Aggressive surgical cytoreduction is likely to be important, because one of the strongest predictors of overall survival is the amount of residual disease. Postoperatively, at least six cycles of paclitaxel and carboplatin chemotherapy are indicated (Barrena-Medel, 2009; Bristow, 2001b; Moller, 2004). Enrollment in a clinical trial is strongly considered for cases of advanced uterine cancer.

Approximately 30 percent of serous endometrial cancers overexpress human epidermal growth factor receptor 2 (HER-2) and are potentially susceptible to therapies targeting HER-2. Trastuzumab (Herceptin) is a monoclonal antibody that targets HER-2. Compared with chemotherapy alone, this agent combined with chemotherapy improved the progression-free survival rate in patients with stage III or IV or recurrent serous carcinomas that overexpressed HER-2 (Fader, 2018).

Carcinosarcoma Management

For uterine carcinosarcoma, hysterectomy and BSO are mandatory. Lymph node metastases are found in up to one third of patients with clinical stage I disease. Thus, comprehensive lymphadenectomy should be performed as that done for poorly differentiated endometrial cancers (Major, 1993; Nemani, 2008; Park, 2010; Temkin, 2007). Typically, disease spread is histologically consistent with the carcinomatous element of this tumor.

Because of the high relapse risk even with early-stage carcinosarcoma, patients often receive adjuvant therapy. In one prospective trial, 224 women with all subtypes of stage I or II uterine sarcoma were randomly assigned to receive either pelvic radiation or no further treatment. For carcinosarcomas, a reduced rate of pelvic relapse was noted with radiotherapy, although survival rates were not improved (Reed, 2008). In one phase III study of 232 patients with stage I–IV carcinosarcoma, whole abdomen radiation was compared with ifosfamide plus cisplatin chemotherapy. Although no survival advantage was demonstrated, the observed differences favored combination chemotherapy use in future trials (Wolfson, 2007).

Ifosfamide has historically been the most active single agent for carcinosarcoma. The combination of ifosfamide and paclitaxel is the current preferred treatment for advanced or recurrent uterine carcinosarcoma (Galaal, 2013). In a phase III GOG trial that randomly assigned 179 patients, this regimen demonstrated a superior response rate (45 versus 29 percent) and survival advantage compared with ifosfamide alone (protocol #161) (Homesley, 2007). The combination of carboplatin and paclitaxel also is active and is being compared with ifosfamide and paclitaxel in an ongoing GOG trial (protocol #261) (King, 2009; Powell, 2010).

Fertility-Sparing Management

Hormonal therapy without hysterectomy is an option in carefully selected young women with endometrial cancer who wish to preserve their fertility (Kim, 1997; Randall, 1997). Currently, patients considering fertility-sparing treatment are recommended to undergo a diagnostic hysteroscopy, sampling by D & C, and imaging to exclude deep myometrial invasion or extrauterine disease (Burke, 2014). Careful selection is also aided by a reproductive endocrinology consultation that clarifies the patient's posttreatment conception chances. Importantly, many of the biologic processes that lead to endometrial cancer also contribute to decreased fertility. In general, this strategy should apply only to those with grade 1 (type I tumor) adenocarcinomas and with no imaging evidence of myometrial invasion. The aim of hormonal treatment is to reverse the lesion. However, any type of medical management obviously involves inherent risk that a patient must be willing to accept (Yang, 2005).

Progestins are most commonly used for conservative treatment. Oral megestrol acetate, 160 mg daily or 80 mg twice daily, can promote cancer regression. Alternatively, oral or intramuscular MPA may be delivered at varying doses (Gotlieb, 2003). The levonorgestrel-releasing IUD is another acceptable option. Combining progestin therapy with tamoxifen or with gonadotropin-releasing hormone agonists is less frequently done (Wang, 2002). Regardless of the hormonal agent, recurrence rates are high during long-term observation (Gotlieb, 2003; Niwa, 2005).

Women receiving fertility-sparing management are carefully monitored by repeated endometrial biopsy or D & C every 3 months to assess treatment efficacy. Evidence for persistence often prompts a change in agent or a dose increase. Hysterectomy and operative staging is recommended if a lesion fails to regress with hormonal therapy or if disease progression is suspected.

Delivery of a healthy infant is a reasonable expectation for those patients who respond to treatment and have normal histologic findings in surveillance endometrial samplings. However, assisted reproductive technologies may be required to achieve pregnancy in some cases. Postpartum, patients are again regularly monitored for recurrent endometrial adenocarcinoma (Ferrandina, 2005). In general, women should undergo hysterectomy at completion of childbearing or whenever the preservation of fertility is no longer desired.

◼ Prognostic Factors

Many clinical and pathologic factors influence the likelihood of endometrial cancer recurrence and survival (Table 33-10) (Lurain, 1991; Schink, 1991). FIGO surgical stage is the most important overriding variable because it incorporates many of the most important risk factors (Table 33-11). Cases with no

TABLE 33-10. Poor Prognostic Variables in Endometrial Cancer

Advanced surgical stage
Older age
Histologic type: UPSC or clear cell adenocarcinoma or carcinosarcoma
Advanced tumor grade
Presence of myometrial invasion
Presence of lymphovascular space invasion
Peritoneal cytology positive for cancer cells
Increased tumor size

ER = estrogen receptor; PR = progesterone receptor; UPSC = uterine papillary serous carcinoma.

myometrial invasion and <50 percent invasion are considered stage IA. Stage IB includes cases with >50 percent myometrial invasion, but cancer has not spread outside the uterine corpus. Stage II now includes cases with only cervical stromal invasion, since cervical gland involvement alone does not worsen prognosis. Stage III no longer includes positive peritoneal washings since this does not appear to alter prognosis. Stage IIIC is now subdivided into IIIC1 and IIIC2, reflecting the worse prognosis associated with paraaortic lymph node involvement as opposed to pelvic only. Stage IV now includes locally advanced disease, including to the lower vagina or pelvic sidewall. One important prognostic factor not captured by FIGO stage is lymphovascular space invasion (Bosse, 2015).

◼ Recurrent Disease

Patients with recurrent endometrial cancer typically require individualized treatment. In general, the site of relapse is the most important predictor of survival. Depending on the circumstances, surgery, radiation, chemotherapy, or a combination may be used. The most curable scenario is an isolated

TABLE 33-11. Carcinoma of the Uterine Corpus 5-year Survival Rates for Each Surgical Stage

FIGO Stage	5-Year Relative Survival Rate[a]
IA	88%
IB	75%
II	69%
IIIA	58%
IIIB	50%
IIIC	47%
IVA	17%
IVB	15%

[a]Data from 21,904 cases.
FIGO = International Federation of Gynecology and Obstetrics.
Data compiled from the American Joint Committee on Cancer, 2010.

relapse at the vaginal apex in a previously unradiated patient. These women are usually effectively treated by external beam pelvic radiotherapy. In patients who were previously irradiated, exenteration is often the only curative option (Section 46-4, p. 1174) (Barakat, 1999; Morris, 1996). Nodal recurrences or isolated pelvic disease is more likely to result in further disease progression, regardless of treatment modality. However, either is often an appropriate indication for external beam radiotherapy in those not previously irradiated. Salvage cytoreductive surgery also may be beneficial in selected patients (Awtrey, 2006; Bristow, 2006b).

Widely disseminated endometrial cancer or a relapse not amenable to radiation or surgery is an indication for systemic chemotherapy (Barrena-Medel, 2009). Patients are ideally enrolled in an experimental trial due to the limited duration of response with current salvage regimens and the urgent need for more effective therapy. Paclitaxel and carboplatin is an active combination for recurrent disease and found not to be inferior to TAP (Miller, 2012). An alternative regimen, the combination of the aromatase inhibitor letrozole and the mammalian target of rapamycin (mTOR) inhibitor everolimus, has significant activity in recurrent endometrial cancer (Slomovitz, 2015). Progestin therapy with or without tamoxifen is a less toxic option that is particularly useful in selected cases (Fiorica, 2004; Whitney, 2004). Finally, the PD-1 inhibitor pembrolizumab was recently approved by the FDA for any recurrent tumor, of any origin, with high microsatellite instability (MSI-H) (Ott, 2017). This new biologic agent is more fully described in Chapter 27 (p. 601). Therefore, patients with recurrent endometrial cancer for whom systemic therapy is indicated should have their tumors tested for MSI-H. In general, effective palliation of women with incurable, recurrent endometrial cancer requires an ongoing dialogue to achieve the optimal balance between symptomatic relief and treatment toxicity.

REFERENCES

Aalders J, Abeler V, Kolstad P, et al: Postoperative external irradiation and prognostic parameters in stage I endometrial carcinoma: clinical and histopathologic study of 540 patients. Obstet Gynecol 56(4):419, 1980

Aarnio M, Sankila R, Pukkala E, et al: Cancer risk in mutation carriers of DNA-mismatch-repair genes. Int J Cancer 81(2):214, 1999

Abu-Rustum NR, Khoury-Collado F, Pandit-Taskar N, et al: Sentinel lymph node mapping for grade 1 endometrial cancer: is it the answer to the surgical staging dilemma? Gynecol Oncol 113(2):163, 2009

Ahluwalia M, Light AM, Surampudi K, et al: Transitional cell carcinoma of the endometrium: a case report and review of the literature. Int J Gynecol Pathol 25(4):378, 2006

Allison KH, Reed SD, Voigt LF, et al: Diagnosing endometrial hyperplasia: why is it so difficult to agree? Am J Surg Pathol 32(5):691, 2008

Altman AD, Thompson J, Nelson G, et al: Use of aromatase inhibitors as first- and second-line medical therapy in patients with endometrial adenocarcinoma: a retrospective study. J Obstet Gynaecol Can 34(7):664, 2012

Altrabulsi B, Malpica A, Deavers MT, et al: Undifferentiated carcinoma of the endometrium. Am J Surg Pathol 29(10):1316, 2005

American College of Obstetricians and Gynecologists: Diagnosis of abnormal uterine bleeding in reproductive-aged women. Practice Bulletin No. 128, July 2012, Reaffirmed 2016

American College of Obstetricians and Gynecologists: Endometrial intraepithelial neoplasia. Committee Opinion No. 631, May 2015, Reaffirmed 2017a

American College of Obstetricians and Gynecologists: Management of endometrial cancer. Practice Bulletin No. 149, April 2015a, Reaffirmed 2017b

American College of Obstetricians and Gynecologists: Hysteroscopy. Technology Assessment No. 13, May 2018a

American College of Obstetricians and Gynecologists: The role of transvaginal ultrasonography in evaluating the endometrium of women with postmenopausal bleeding. Committee Opinion No. 734, May 2018b

American College of Obstetricians and Gynecologists: Lynch syndrome. Practice Bulletin No. 147, November 2014a, Reaffirmed 2019a

American College of Obstetricians and Gynecologists: Opportunistic salpingectomy as a strategy for epithelial ovarian cancer prevention. Committee Opinion No. 774, March 2019b

American College of Obstetricians and Gynecologists: Tamoxifen and uterine cancer. Committee Opinion No. 601, June 2014b, Reaffirmed 2019c

American Joint Committee on Cancer: AJCC Cancer Staging Manual, 7th ed. Chicago, American Joint Committee on Cancer, 2010, p 408

Anastasiadis PG, Skaphida PG, Koutlaki NG, et al: Descriptive epidemiology of endometrial hyperplasia in patients with abnormal uterine bleeding. Eur J Gynaecol Oncol 21(2):131, 2000

Ashfaq R, Sharma S, Dulley T, et al: Clinical relevance of benign endometrial cells in postmenopausal women. Diagn Cytopathol 25(4):235, 2001

Awtrey CS, Cadungog MG, Leitao MM, et al: Surgical resection of recurrent endometrial carcinoma. Gynecol Oncol 102(3):480, 2006

Baak JP, Mutter GL, Robboy S, et al: The molecular genetics and morphometry-based endometrial intraepithelial neoplasia classification system predicts disease progression in endometrial hyperplasia more accurately than the 1994 World Health Organization classification system. Cancer 103(11):2304, 2005

Ballester M, Dubernard G, Lécuru F, et al: Detection rate and diagnostic accuracy of sentinel-node biopsy in early stage endometrial cancer: a prospective multicentre study (SENTI-ENDO). Lancet Oncol 12(5):469, 2011

Bansal N, Yendluri V, Wenham RM: The molecular biology of endometrial cancers and the implications for pathogenesis, classification, and targeted therapies. Cancer Control 16(1):8, 2009

Barakat RR, Bundy BN, Spirtos NM, et al: Randomized double-blind trial of estrogen replacement therapy versus placebo in stage I or II endometrial cancer: a Gynecologic Oncology Group study. J Clin Oncol 24(4):587, 2006

Barakat RR, Goldman NA, Patel DA, et al: Pelvic exenteration for recurrent endometrial cancer. Gynecol Oncol 75(1):99, 1999

Barrena Medel NI, Bansal S, Miller DS, et al: Pharmacotherapy of endometrial cancer. Expert Opin Pharmacother 10(12):1939, 2009

Bellone S, Eliana B, Lonardi S, et al: Polymerase ε (POLE) ultra-mutation in uterine tumors correlates with T lymphocyte infiltration and increased resistance to platinum-based chemotherapy in vitro. Gynecol Oncol 144(1):146, 2017

Ben Yehuda OM, Kim YB, Leuchter RS: Does hysteroscopy improve upon the sensitivity of dilatation and curettage in the diagnosis of endometrial hyperplasia or carcinoma? Gynecol Oncol 68:4, 1998

Benedetti Panici P, Basile S, Maneschi F, et al: Systematic pelvic lymphadenectomy vs. no lymphadenectomy in early stage endometrial carcinoma: randomized clinical trial. J Natl Cancer Inst 100:1707, 2008

Boronow RC, Morrow CP, Creasman WT, et al: Surgical staging in endometrial cancer: clinical–pathologic findings of a prospective study. Obstet Gynecol 63:825, 1984

Bosse T, Peters EE, Creutzberg CL, et al: Substantial lymph-vascular space invasion (LVSI) is a significant risk factor for recurrence in endometrial cancer—A pooled analysis of PORTEC 1 and 2 trials. Eur J Cancer 51(13):1742, 2015

Breitkopf DM, Frederickson RA, Snyder RR: Detection of benign endometrial masses by endometrial stripe measurement in premenopausal women. Obstet Gynecol 104(1):2004

Bristow RE, Asrari F, Trimble EL, et al: Extended surgical staging for uterine papillary serous carcinoma: survival outcome of locoregional (stage I–III) disease. Gynecol Oncol 81(2):279, 2001a

Bristow RE, Duska LR, Montz FJ: The role of cytoreductive surgery in the management of stage IV uterine papillary serous carcinoma. Gynecol Oncol 81(1):92, 2001b

Bristow RE, Purinton SC, Santillan A, et al: Cost-effectiveness of routine vaginal cytology for endometrial cancer surveillance. Gynecol Oncol 103(2):709, 2006a

Bristow RE, Santillan A, Zahurak ML, et al: Salvage cytoreductive surgery for recurrent endometrial cancer. Gynecol Oncol 103(1):281, 2006b

Bristow RE, Zerbe MJ, Rosenshein NB, et al: Stage IVB endometrial carcinoma: the role of cytoreductive surgery and determinants of survival. Gynecol Oncol 78(2):85, 2000

Burke TW, Levenback C, Tornos C, et al: Intraabdominal lymphatic mapping to direct selective pelvic and paraaortic lymphadenectomy in women with high-risk endometrial cancer: results of a pilot study. Gynecol Oncol 62(2):169, 1996

Burke WM, Orr J, Leitao M, et al: Endometrial cancer: a review and current management strategies: part II. Gynecol Oncol 134(2):393, 2014

Cannon GM, Geye H, Terakedis BE, et al: Outcomes following surgery and adjuvant radiation in stage II endometrial adenocarcinoma. Gynecol Oncol 113(2):176, 2009

Carcangiu ML, Chambers JT: Uterine papillary serous carcinoma: a study on 108 cases with emphasis on the prognostic significance of associated endometrioid carcinoma, absence of invasion, and concomitant ovarian carcinoma. Gynecol Oncol 47(3):298, 1992

Chan JK, Loizzi V, Youssef M, et al: Significance of comprehensive surgical staging in noninvasive papillary serous carcinoma of the endometrium. Gynecol Oncol 90(1):181, 2003

Chan JK, Sherman AE, Kapp DS, et al: Influence of gynecologic oncologists on the survival of patients with endometrial cancer. J Clin Oncol 29(7):832, 2011

Chao CK, Grigsby PW, Perez CA, et al: Medically inoperable stage I endometrial carcinoma: a few dilemmas in radiotherapeutic management. Int J Radiat Oncol Biol Phys 34(1):27, 1996

Childers JM, Spirtos NM, Brainard P, et al: Laparoscopic staging of the patient with incompletely staged early adenocarcinoma of the endometrium. Obstet Gynecol 83(4):597, 1994

Cicinelli E, Tinelli R, Colafiglio G, et al: Risk of long-term pelvic recurrences after fluid minihysteroscopy in women with endometrial carcinoma: a controlled randomized study. Menopause 17(3):511, 2010

Clarke MA, Long BJ, Del Mar Morillo A, et al: Association of endometrial cancer risk with postmenopausal bleeding in women: a systematic review and meta-analysis. JAMA Intern Med 178(9):1210, 2018

Cooper AL, Dornfeld-Finke JM, Banks HW, et al: Is cytologic screening an effective surveillance method for detection of vaginal recurrence of uterine cancer? Obstet Gynecol 107(1):71, 2006

Cornelison TL, Trimble EL, Kosary CL: SEER data, corpus uteri cancer: treatment trends versus survival for FIGO stage II, 1988–1994. Gynecol Oncol 74(3):350, 1999

Creasman W, Odicino F, Maisonneuve P, et al: Carcinoma of the corpus uteri. FIGO 26th Annual Report on the Results of Treatment in Gynecological Cancer. Int J Gynaecol Obstet 95(suppl 1):S105, 2006

Creutzberg CL, van Putten WL, Koper PC, et al: Surgery and postoperative radiotherapy versus surgery alone for patients with stage-1 endometrial carcinoma: multicentre randomised trial. PORTEC Study Group. Postoperative radiation therapy in endometrial carcinoma. Lancet 355(9213):1404, 2000

Creutzberg CL, van Putten WL, Warlam-Rodenhuis CC, et al: Outcome of high-risk stage IC, grade 3, compared with stage I endometrial carcinoma patients: the Postoperative Radiation Therapy in Endometrial Carcinoma Trial. J Clin Oncol 22(7):1234, 2004

de Boer SM, Powell ME, Mileshkin LR, et al: Final results of the international randomized PORTEC-3 trial of adjuvant chemotherapy and radiation therapy (RT) versus RT alone for women with high-risk endometrial cancer. J Clin Oncol 35(15 suppl):5502, 2017

Delin JB, Miller DS, Coleman RL: Other primary malignancies in patients with uterine corpus malignancy. Am J Obstet Gynecol 190:1429, 2004

Dhar KK, NeedhiRajan T, Koslowski M, et al: Is levonorgestrel intrauterine system effective for treatment of early endometrial cancer? Report of four cases and review of the literature. Gynecol Oncol 97(3):924, 2005

Dietrich CS III, Modesitt SC, DePriest PD, et al: The efficacy of adjuvant platinum-based chemotherapy in stage I uterine papillary serous carcinoma (UPSC). Gynecol Oncol 99(3):557, 2005

Dossus L, Allen N, Kaaks R, et al: Reproductive risk factors and endometrial cancer: the European Prospective Investigation into Cancer and Nutrition. Int J Cancer 127(2):442, 2010

Ellenson LH, Ronnett BM, Kurman RJ: Precursor lesions of endometrial carcinoma. In Kurman RJ, Ellenson LH, Ronnett BM (eds): Blaustein's Pathology of the Female Genital Tract, New York, Springer, 2011a, p 360

Ellenson LH, Ronnett BM, Soslow RA: Endometrial cancer. In Kurman RJ, Ellenson LH, Ronnett BM (eds): Blaustein's Pathology of the Female Genital Tract, New York, Springer, 2011b, p 422

Elshaikh MA, Al-Wahab Z, Mahdi H, et al: Recurrence patterns and survival endpoints in women with stage II uterine endometrioid carcinoma: a multi-institution study. Gynecol Oncol 136(2):235, 2015

Eltabbakh GH, Shamonki J, Mount SL: Surgical stage, final grade, and survival of women with endometrial carcinoma whose preoperative endometrial biopsy shows well-differentiated tumors. Gynecol Oncol 99(2):309, 2005

Fader AN, Roque DM, Siegel E, et al: Randomized phase II trial of carboplatin-paclitaxel versus carboplatin-paclitaxel-trastuzumab in uterine serous carcinomas that overexpress human epidermal growth factor receptor 2/neu. J Clin Oncol 36(20):2044, 2018

Fearnley EJ, Marquart L, Spurdle AB, et al: Polycystic ovary syndrome increases the risk of endometrial cancer in women aged less than 50 years: an Australian case-control study. Cancer Causes Control 12:2303, 2010

Feldman S, Berkowitz RS, Tosteson AN: Cost-effectiveness of strategies to evaluate postmenopausal bleeding. Obstet Gynecol 81(6):968, 1993

Felix AS, Gaudet MM, La Vecchia C, et al: Intrauterine devices and endometrial cancer risk: a pooled analysis of the Epidemiology of Endometrial Cancer Consortium. Int J Cancer 136(5):E410, 2015

Felix AS, Weissfeld JL, Stone RA, et al: Factors associated with type I and type II endometrial cancer. Cancer Causes Control 21(11):1851, 2010

Feltmate CM, Duska LR, Chang Y, et al: Predictors of recurrence in surgical stage II endometrial adenocarcinoma. Gynecol Oncol 73(3):407, 1999

Ferrandina G, Zannoni GF, Gallotta V, et al: Progression of conservatively treated endometrial carcinoma after full term pregnancy: a case report. Gynecol Oncol 99(1):215, 2005

FIGO Committee on Gynecologic Oncology: Revised FIGO staging for carcinoma of the vulva, cervix, and endometrium. Int J Gynaecol Obstet 105(2):103, 2009

Fiorica JV, Brunetto VL, Hanjani P, et al: Phase II trial of alternating courses of megestrol acetate and tamoxifen in advanced endometrial carcinoma: a Gynecologic Oncology Group study. Gynecol Oncol 92(1):10, 2004

Fisher B, Costantino JP, Wickerham DL, et al: Tamoxifen for prevention of breast cancer: report of the National Surgical Adjuvant Breast and Bowel Project P-1 Study. J Natl Cancer Inst 90(18):1371, 1998

Fishman DA, Roberts KB, Chambers JT, et al: Radiation therapy as exclusive treatment for medically inoperable patients with stage I and II endometrioid carcinoma with endometrium. Gynecol Oncol 61(2):189, 1996

Fleming GF, Brunetto VL, Cella D, et al: Phase III trial of doxorubicin plus cisplatin with or without paclitaxel plus filgrastim in advanced endometrial carcinoma: a Gynecologic Oncology Group study. J Clin Oncol 22(11):2159, 2004

Frumovitz M, Singh DK, Meyer L, et al: Predictors of final histology in patients with endometrial cancer. Gynecol Oncol 95(3):463, 2004a

Frumovitz M, Slomovitz BM, Singh DK, et al: Frozen section analyses as predictors of lymphatic spread in patients with early-stage uterine cancer. J Am Coll Surg 199(3):388, 2004b

Galaal K, van der Heijden E, Godfrey K, et al: Adjuvant radiotherapy and/or chemotherapy after surgery for uterine carcinosarcoma. Cochrane Database Syst Rev 2:CD006812, 2013

Gallos ID, Shehmar M, Thangaratinam S, et al: Oral progestogens vs levonorgestrel-releasing intrauterine system for endometrial hyperplasia: a systematic review and metaanalysis. Am J Obstet Gynecol 203(6):547.e1, 2010

Garuti G, Mirra M, Luerti M: Hysteroscopic view in atypical endometrial hyperplasias: a correlation with pathologic findings on hysterectomy specimens. J Minim Invasive Gynecol 13(4):325, 2006

Gehrig PA, Groben PA, Fowler WC Jr, et al: Noninvasive papillary serous carcinoma of the endometrium. Obstet Gynecol 97(1):153, 2001

Ghezzi F, Cromi A, Uccella S, et al: Laparoscopic versus open surgery for endometrial cancer: a minimum 3-year follow-up study. Ann Surg Oncol 17(1):271, 2010

Goldstein SR, Zeltser I, Horan CK, et al: Ultrasonography-based triage for perimenopausal patients with abnormal uterine bleeding. Am J Obstet Gynecol 177(1):102, 1997

Goodman A, Zukerberg LR, Rice LW, et al: Squamous cell carcinoma of the endometrium: a report of eight cases and a review of the literature. Gynecol Oncol 61(1):54, 1996

Gotlieb WH, Beiner ME, Shalmon B, et al: Outcome of fertility-sparing treatment with progestins in young patients with endometrial cancer. Obstet Gynecol 102(4):718, 2003

Graebe K, Garcia-Soto A, Aziz M, et al: Incidental power morcellation of malignancy: a retrospective cohort study. Gynecol Oncol 136(2):274, 2015

Granberg S, Wikland M, Karlsson B, et al: Endometrial thickness as measured by endovaginal ultrasonography for identifying endometrial abnormality. Am J Obstet Gynecol 164:47, 1991

Grice J, Ek M, Greer B, et al: Uterine papillary serous carcinoma: evaluation of long-term survival in surgically staged patients. Gynecol Oncol 69(1):69, 1998

Hamilton CA, Cheung MK, Osann K, et al: Uterine papillary serous and clear cell carcinomas predict for poorer survival compared to grade 3 endometrioid corpus cancers. Br J Cancer 94(5):642, 2006

Haruma T, Nagasaka T, Nakamura K, et al: Clinical impact of endometrial cancer stratified by genetic mutational profiles, POLE mutation, and microsatellite instability. PLoS ONE 13(4):e0195655, 2018

Havrilesky LJ, Cragun JM, Calingaert B, et al: Resection of lymph node metastases influences survival in stage IIIC endometrial cancer. Gynecol Oncol 99(3):689, 2005

Hecht JL, Ince TA, Baak JP, et al: Prediction of endometrial carcinoma by subjective endometrial intraepithelial neoplasia diagnosis. Mod Pathol 18(3):324, 2005

Hemminki K, Bermejo JL, Granstrom C: Endometrial cancer: population attributable risks from reproductive, familial and socioeconomic factors. Eur J Cancer 41(14):2155, 2005

Hirai Y, Takeshima N, Kato T, et al: Malignant potential of positive peritoneal cytology in endometrial cancer. Obstet Gynecol 97(5 Pt 1):725, 2001

Hoekstra AV, Jairam-Thodla A, Rademaker A, et al: The impact of robotics on practice management of endometrial cancer: transitioning from traditional surgery. Int J Med Robot 5(4):392, 2009

Holloway RM, Abu-Rustum NR, Backes FJ, et al: Sentinel lymph node mapping and staging in endometrial cancer: a Society of Gynecologic Oncology literature review with consensus recommendations. Gynecologic Oncology 146(2):405, 2017

Homesley HD, Filiaci V, Markman M, et al: Phase III trial of ifosfamide with or without paclitaxel in advanced uterine carcinosarcoma: a Gynecologic Oncology Group study. J Clin Oncol 25(5):526, 2007

Homesley HD, Filiaci V, Gibbons SK et al: A randomized phase III trial in advanced endometrial carcinoma of surgery and volume directed radiation followed by cisplatin and doxorubicin with or without paclitaxel: a Gynecologic Oncology Group study. Gynecol Oncol 112:543, 2009

Horn LC, Schnurrbusch U, Bilek K, et al: Risk of progression in complex and atypical endometrial hyperplasia: clinicopathologic analysis in cases with and without progestogen treatment. Int J Gynecol Cancer 14(2):348, 2004

Hoskins PJ, Swenerton KD, Pike JA, et al: Paclitaxel and carboplatin, alone or with irradiation, in advanced or recurrent endometrial cancer: a phase II study. J Clin Oncol 19(20):4048, 2001

Huh WK, Powell M, Leath CA III, et al: Uterine papillary serous carcinoma: comparisons of outcomes in surgical stage I patients with and without adjuvant therapy. Gynecol Oncol 91(3):470, 2003

Jacobs I, Gentry-Maharaj A, Burnell M, et al: Sensitivity of transvaginal ultrasound screening for endometrial cancer in postmenopausal women: a case-control study within the UKCTOCS cohort. Lancet Oncol 12(1):38, 2011

Janda M, Gebski V, Davies LC, et al: Effect of total laparoscopic hysterectomy vs total abdominal hysterectomy on disease-free survival among women with stage I endometrial cancer: a randomized clinical trial. JAMA 317(12):1224, 2017

Jordan LB, Abdul-Kader M, Al Nafussi A: Uterine serous papillary carcinoma: histopathologic changes within the female genital tract. Int J Gynecol Cancer 11(4):283, 2001

Kandoth C, Schultz N, Cherniack AD: Integrated genomic characterization of endometrial carcinoma. Nature 497:67, 2013

Kelly MG, O'Malley DM, Hui P, et al: Improved survival in surgical stage I patients with uterine papillary serous carcinoma (UPSC) treated with adjuvant platinum-based chemotherapy. Gynecol Oncol 98(3):353, 2005

Keys HM, Roberts JA, Brunetto VL, et al: A phase III trial of surgery with or without adjunctive external pelvic radiation therapy in intermediate risk endometrial adenocarcinoma: a Gynecologic Oncology Group study. Gynecol Oncol 92(3):744, 2004

Kilgore LC, Partridge EE, Alvarez RD, et al: Adenocarcinoma of the endometrium: survival comparisons of patients with and without pelvic node sampling. Gynecol Oncol 56(1):29, 1995

Kim YB, Holschneider CH, Ghosh K, et al: Progestin alone as primary treatment of endometrial carcinoma in premenopausal women: report of seven cases and review of the literature. Cancer 79(2):320, 1997

King LP, Miller DS: Recent progress: Gynecologic Oncology Group trials in uterine corpus tumors. Rev Recent Clin Trials 4(2):70, 2009

Kitchener H, Swart AM, Qian Q, et al: Efficacy of systematic pelvic lymphadenectomy in endometrial cancer (MRC ASTEC trial): a randomized study. Lancet 373:125, 2009

Kornblith AB, Huang HQ, Walker JL, et al: Quality of life of patients with endometrial cancer undergoing laparoscopic International Federation of Gynecology and Obstetrics staging compared with laparotomy: a Gynecologic Oncology Group study. J Clin Oncol 27(32):5337, 2009

Kurman RJ, Carcangiu ML, Herrington CS, et al (eds): WHO Classification of Tumours of Female Reproductive Organs, 4th ed. Lyon, International Agency for Research on Cancer, 2014

Kurman RJ, Kaminski PF, Norris HJ: The behavior of endometrial hyperplasia. A long-term study of "untreated" hyperplasia in 170 patients. Cancer 56(2):403, 1985

Kurman RJ, Norris HJ: Endometrial hyperplasia and related cellular changes. In Kurman RJ (ed): Blaustein's Pathology of the Female Genital Tract. 1994, p 411

Lancaster JM, Powell CB, Chen LM, et al: Society of Gynecologic Oncology statement on risk assessment for inherited gynecologic cancer predispositions. Gynecol Oncol 136(1):3, 2015

Leitao MM, Kehoe S, Barakat RR, et al: Accuracy of preoperative endometrial sampling diagnosis of FIGO grade 1 endometrial adenocarcinoma. Gynecol Oncol 111:244, 2008

Lentz SS, Brady MF, Major FJ, et al: High-dose megestrol acetate in advanced or recurrent endometrial carcinoma: a Gynecologic Oncology Group study. J Clin Oncol 14(2):357, 1996

Lurain JR, Rice BL, Rademaker AW, et al: Prognostic factors associated with disease recurrence in clinical stage I adenocarcinoma of the endometrium. Obstet Gynecol 78:63, 1991

Madison T, Schottenfeld D, James SA, et al: Endometrial cancer: socioeconomic status and racial/ethnic differences in stage at diagnosis, treatment, and survival. Am J Public Health 94(12):2104, 2004

Magrina JF, Mutone NF, Weaver AL, et al: Laparoscopic lymphadenectomy and vaginal or laparoscopic hysterectomy with bilateral salpingo-oophorectomy for endometrial cancer: morbidity and survival. Am J Obstet Gynecol 181(2):376, 1999

Major FJ, Blessing JA, Silverberg SG, et al: Prognostic factors in early-stage uterine sarcoma. A Gynecologic Oncology Group study. Cancer 71(4 Suppl):1702, 1993

Mariani A, Webb MJ, Keeney GL, et al: Hematogenous dissemination in corpus cancer. Gynecol Oncol 80(2):233, 2001a

Mariani A, Webb MJ, Keeney GL, et al: Role of wide/radical hysterectomy and pelvic lymph node dissection in endometrial cancer with cervical involvement. Gynecol Oncol 83(1):72, 2001b

Martin JD, Gilks B, Lim P: Papillary serous carcinoma—a less radio-sensitive subtype of endometrial cancer. Gynecol Oncol 98(2):299, 2005

Martínez A, Querleu D, Leblanc E, et al: Low incidence of port-site metastases after laparoscopic staging of uterine cancer. Gynecol Oncol 118(2):145, 2010

Matei D, Filiaci VL, Randall M, et al: A randomized phase III trial of cisplatin and tumor volume directed irradiation followed by carboplatin and paclitaxel vs. carboplatin and paclitaxel for optimally debulked, advanced endometrial carcinoma. J Clin Oncol 35(15 suppl):5505, 2017

Maxwell GL, Schildkraut JM, Calingaert B, et al: Progestin and estrogen potency of combination oral contraceptives and endometrial cancer risk. Gynecol Oncol 103(2):535, 2006

Melhem MF, Tobon H: Mucinous adenocarcinoma of the endometrium: a clinico-pathological review of 18 cases. Int J Gynecol Pathol 6(4):347, 1987

Miller D, Filiaci V, Fleming G, et al: Randomized phase III noninferiority trial of first line chemotherapy for metastatic or recurrent endometrial carcinoma: a Gynecologic Oncology Group study. Gynecol Oncol 125(3):771, 2012

Miller DS, Fleming G, Randall ME: Chemo- and radiotherapy in adjuvant management of optimally debulked endometrial cancer. J Natl Compr Cancer Netw 7(5):535, 2009

Moller KA, Gehrig PA, Van Le L, et al: The role of optimal debulking in advanced stage serous carcinoma of the uterus. Gynecol Oncol 94(1):170, 2004

Montz FJ, Bristow RE, Bovicelli A, et al: Intrauterine progesterone treatment of early endometrial cancer. Am J Obstet Gynecol 186(4):651, 2002

Morimoto LM, Newcomb PA, Hampton JM, et al: Cholecystectomy and endometrial cancer: a marker of long-term elevated estrogen exposure? Int J Gynecol Cancer 16(3):1348, 2006

Morris M, Alvarez RD, Kinney WK, et al: Treatment of recurrent adenocarcinoma of the endometrium with pelvic exenteration. Gynecol Oncol 60(2):288, 1996

Morrow CP, Bundy BN, Kurman RJ, et al: Relationship between surgical-pathological risk factors and outcome in clinical stage I and II carcinoma of the endometrium: a Gynecologic Oncology Group study. Gynecol Oncol 40(1):55, 1991

Mount SL, Wegner EK, Eltabbakh GH, et al: Significant increase of benign endometrial cells on Papanicolaou smears in women using hormone replacement therapy. Obstet Gynecol 100(3):445, 2002

Mutter GL: Endometrial intraepithelial neoplasia (EIN): will it bring order to chaos? The Endometrial Collaborative Group. Gynecol Oncol 76(3):287, 2000

Nagar H, Dobbs S, McClelland HR, et al: The diagnostic accuracy of magnetic resonance imaging in detecting cervical involvement in endometrial cancer. Gynecol Oncol 103(2):431, 2006

National Comprehensive Cancer Network: Uterine neoplasms, version 3.2019. Plymouth Meeting, National Comprehensive Cancer Network, 2019

Nemani D, Mitra N, Guo M, et al: Assessing the effects of lymphadenectomy and radiation therapy in patients with uterine carcinosarcoma: a SEER analysis. Gynecol Oncol 111:82, 2008

Nevadunsky NS, Van Arsdale A, Strickler HD, et al: Obesity and age at diagnosis of endometrial cancer. Obstet Gynecol 124(2 Pt 1):300, 2014

Niwa K, Tagami K, Lian Z, et al: Outcome of fertility-preserving treatment in young women with endometrial carcinomas. BJOG 112(3):317, 2005

Nout RA, Smit VT, Putter H, et al: Vaginal brachytherapy versus pelvic external beam radiotherapy for patients with endometrial cancer of high-intermediate risk (PORTEC-2): an open-label, non-inferiority, randomised trial. Lancet 375(9717):816, 2010

Obermair A, Geramou M, Gucer F, et al: Does hysteroscopy facilitate tumor cell dissemination? Incidence of peritoneal cytology from patients with early stage endometrial carcinoma following dilatation and curettage (D & C) versus hysteroscopy and D & C. Cancer 88(1):139, 2000

Onda T, Yoshikawa H, Mizutani K, et al: Treatment of node-positive endometrial cancer with complete node dissection, chemotherapy and radiation therapy. Br J Cancer 75:1836, 1997

Ørbo A, Vereide A, Arnes M, et al: Levonorgestrel-impregnated intrauterine device as treatment for endometrial hyperplasia: a national multicentre randomised trial. BJOG 121(4):477, 2014

Ott PA, Bang YJ, Berton-Rigaud D, et al: Safety and antitumor activity of pembrolizumab in advanced programmed death ligand 1-positive endometrial cancer: results from the KEYNOTE-028 study. J Clin Oncol 35(22):2535, 2017

Papadia A, Azioni G, Brusaca B, et al: Frozen section underestimates the need for surgical staging in endometrial cancer patients. Int J Gynecol Cancer 19(9):1570, 2009

Park JY, Kim DY, Kim JH, et al: The role of pelvic and/or para-aortic lymphadenectomy in surgical management of apparently early carcinosarcoma of uterus. Ann Surg Oncol 17:861, 2010

Pecorelli S, Benedet JL, Creasman WT, et al: FIGO staging of gynecologic cancer. 1994–1997 FIGO Committee on Gynecologic Oncology. Int J Gynaecol Obstet 64(1):5, 1999

Pillay OC, Te Fong LF, Crow JC, et al: The association between polycystic ovaries and endometrial cancer. Hum Reprod 21(4):924, 2006

Polyzos NP, Mauri D, Tsioras S, et al: Intraperitoneal dissemination of endometrial cancer cells after hysteroscopy: a systematic review and meta-analysis. Int J Gynecol Cancer 20(2):261, 2010

Powell JL, Hill KA, Shiro BC, et al: Preoperative serum CA-125 levels in treating endometrial cancer. J Reprod Med 50(8):585, 2005

Powell MA, Filiaci VL, Rose PG, et al: Phase II evaluation of paclitaxel and carboplatin in the treatment of carcinosarcoma of the uterus: a Gynecologic Oncology Group study. J Clin Oncol 28(16):2727, 2010

Price FV, Chambers SK, Carcangiu ML, et al: CA 125 may not reflect disease status in patients with uterine serous carcinoma. Cancer 82(9):1720, 1998

Provenzale D, Gupta S, Ahnen DJ, et al: NCCN guidelines insights: colorectal cancer screening, version 1.2018. J Natl Compr Canc Netw 16(8):939, 2018

Randall ME, Filiaci VL, Muss H, et al: Randomized phase III trial of whole-abdominal irradiation versus doxorubicin and cisplatin chemotherapy in advanced endometrial carcinoma: a Gynecologic Oncology Group study. J Clin Oncol 24(1):36, 2006

Randall TC, Kurman RJ: Progestin treatment of atypical hyperplasia and well-differentiated carcinoma of the endometrium in women under age 40. Obstet Gynecol 90(3):434, 1997

Rattanachaiyanont M, Angsuwathana S, Techatraisak K, et al: Clinical and pathological responses of progestin therapy for non-atypical endometrial hyperplasia: a prospective study. J Obstet Gynaecol Res 31(2):98, 2005

Reed NS, Mangioni C, Malmstrom H, et al: Phase III randomised study to evaluate the role of adjuvant pelvic radiotherapy in the treatment of uterine sarcomas stages I and II: a European Organisation for Research and Treatment of Cancer Gynaecological Cancer Group study (protocol 55874). Eur J Cancer 44:808, 2008

Reed SD, Voigt LF, Newton KM, et al: Progestin therapy of complex endometrial hyperplasia with and without atypia. Obstet Gynecol 113(3):655, 2009

Resnick KE, Hampel H, Fishel R, et al: Current and emerging trends in Lynch syndrome identification in women with endometrial cancer. Gynecol Oncol 114(1):128, 2009

Revel A, Tsafrir A, Anteby SO, et al: Does hysteroscopy produce intraperitoneal spread of endometrial cancer cells? Obstet Gynecol Surv 59:280, 2004

Ricci E, Moroni S, Parazzini F, et al: Risk factors for endometrial hyperplasia: results from a case-control study. Int J Gynecol Cancer 12(3):257, 2002

Rittenberg PV, Lotocki RJ, Heywood MS, et al: Stage II endometrial carcinoma: limiting post-operative radiotherapy to the vaginal vault in node-negative tumors. Gynecol Oncol 98(3):434, 2005

Roland PY, Kelly FJ, Kulwicki CY, et al: The benefits of a gynecologic oncologist: a pattern of care study for endometrial cancer treatment. Gynecol Oncol 93(1):125, 2004

Ross JC, Eifel PJ, Cox RS, et al: Primary mucinous adenocarcinoma of the endometrium. A clinicopathologic and histochemical study. Am J Surg Pathol 7(8):715, 1983

Rossi EC, Kowalski LD, Scalici J, et al: A comparison of sentinel lymph node biopsy to lymphadenectomy for endometrial cancer staging (FIRES trial): a multicentre, prospective, cohort study. Lancet Oncol 18(3):384, 2017

Rubatt JM, Slomovitz BM, Burke TW, et al: Development of metastatic endometrial endometrioid adenocarcinoma while on progestin therapy for endometrial hyperplasia. Gynecol Oncol 99(2):472, 2005

Salani R, Khanna N, Frimer M et al: An update on post-treatment surveillance and diagnosis of recurrence in women with gynecologic malignancies: Society of Gynecologic Oncology recommendations. Gynecol Oncol 146:3, 2017

Sanjuan A, Cobo T, Pahisa J, et al: Preoperative and intraoperative assessment of myometrial invasion and histologic grade in endometrial cancer: role of magnetic resonance imaging and frozen section. Int J Gynecol Cancer 16(1):385, 2006

Sartori E, Bazzurini L, Gadducci A, et al: Carcinosarcoma of the uterus: a clinicopathological multicenter CTF study. Gynecol Oncol 67:70, 1997

Scarselli G, Bargelli G, Taddei GL, et al: Levonorgestrel-releasing intrauterine system (LNG-IUS) as an effective treatment option for endometrial hyperplasia: a 15-year follow-up study. Fertil Steril 95(1):420, 2011

Schiavone MB, Scelzo C, Straight C, et al: Survival of patients with serous uterine carcinoma undergoing sentinel lymph node mapping. Ann Surg Oncol 24(7):1965, 2017

Schiavone MB, Zivanovic O, Zhou Q, et al: Survival of patients with uterine carcinosarcoma undergoing sentinel lymph node mapping. Ann Surg Oncol 23(1):196, 2016

Schink JC, Rademaker AW, Miller DS, et al: Tumor size in endometrial cancer. Cancer 67(11):2791, 1991

Schmeler KM, Lynch HT, Chen LM, et al: Prophylactic surgery to reduce the risk of gynecologic cancers in the Lynch syndrome. N Engl J Med 354(3):261, 2006

Schottenfeld D: Epidemiology of endometrial neoplasia. J Cell Biochem Suppl 23:151, 1995

Seamon LG, Cohn DE, Henretta MS, et al: Minimally invasive comprehensive surgical staging for endometrial cancer: robotics or laparoscopy? Gynecol Oncol 113(1):36, 2009

Sherman ME, Bitterman P, Rosenshein NB, et al: Uterine serous carcinoma. A morphologically diverse neoplasm with unifying clinicopathologic features. Am J Surg Pathol 16(6):600, 1992

Sherman ME, Ronnett BM, Ioffe OB, et al: Reproducibility of biopsy diagnoses of endometrial hyperplasia: evidence supporting a simplified classification. Int J Gynecol Pathol 27(3):318, 2008

Shi AA, Lee SI: Radiological reasoning: algorithmic workup of abnormal vaginal bleeding with endovaginal sonography and sonohysterography. AJR Am J Roentgenol 191(6 Suppl):S68, 2008

Siegel RL, Miller KD, Jemal A: Cancer statistics, 2019. CA Cancer J Clin 69(1):7, 2019

Silva EG, Deavers MT, Malpica A: Undifferentiated carcinoma of the endometrium: a review. Pathology 39(1):134, 2007

Simsir A, Carter W, Elgert P, et al: Reporting endometrial cells in women 40 years and older: assessing the clinical usefulness of Bethesda 2001. Am J Clin Pathol 123(4):571, 2005

Slomovitz BM, Burke TW, Eifel PJ, et al: Uterine papillary serous carcinoma (UPSC): a single institution review of 129 cases. Gynecol Oncol 91(3):463, 2003

Slomovitz BM, Jiang Y, Yates MS, et al: Phase II study of everolimus and letrozole in patients with recurrent endometrial carcinoma. J Clin Oncol 33(8):930, 2015

Smith DC, Prentice R, Thompson DJ, et al: Association of exogenous estrogen and endometrial carcinoma. N Engl J Med 293(23):1164, 1975

Smith RA, Andrews KS, Brooks D, et al: Cancer screening in the United States, 2019: a review of current American Cancer Society guidelines and current issues in cancer screening. CA Cancer J Clin 69(3):184

Smith-Bindman R, Weiss E, Feldstein V: How thick is too thick? When endometrial thickness should prompt biopsy in postmenopausal women without vaginal bleeding. Ultrasound Obstet Gynecol 24(5):558, 2004

Soliman PT, Oh JC, Schmeler KM, et al: Risk factors for young premenopausal women with endometrial cancer. Obstet Gynecol 105(3):575, 2005

Soliman PT, Westin SN, Dioun S, et al: A prospective validation study of sentinel lymph node mapping for high-risk endometrial cancer. Gynecol Oncol 146(2):234, 2017

Sovak MA, Dupont J, Hensley ML, et al: Paclitaxel and carboplatin in the treatment of advanced or recurrent endometrial cancer: a large retrospective study. Int J Gynecol Cancer 17(1):197, 2007

Sovak MA, Hensley ML, Dupont J, et al: Paclitaxel and carboplatin in the adjuvant treatment of patients with high-risk stage III and IV endometrial cancer: a retrospective study. Gynecol Oncol 103(2):451, 2006

Spirtos NM, Eisekop SM, Boike G, et al: Laparoscopic staging in patients with incompletely staged cancers of the uterus, ovary, fallopian tube, and primary peritoneum: a Gynecologic Oncology Group (GOG) study. Am J Obstet Gynecol 193(5):1645, 2005

Stanford JL, Brinton LA, Berman ML, et al: Oral contraceptives and endometrial cancer: do other risk factors modify the association? Int J Cancer 54(2):243, 1993

Strom BL, Schinnar R, Weber AL, et al: Case-control study of postmenopausal hormone replacement therapy and endometrial cancer. Am J Epidemiol 164(8):775, 2006

Suh-Burgmann E, Hung YY, Armstrong MA: Complex atypical endometrial hyperplasia: the risk of unrecognized adenocarcinoma and value of preoperative dilation and curettage. Obstet Gynecol 114(3):523, 2009

Suriano KA, McHale M, McLaren CE, et al: Estrogen replacement therapy in endometrial cancer patients: a matched control study. Obstet Gynecol 97(4):555, 2001

Surveillance, Epidemiology, and End Results Program: Cancer stat facts: uterine cancer. 2018. Available at: https://seer.cancer.gov/statfacts/html/corp.html. Accessed April 10, 2019

Tao MH, Xu WH, Zheng W, et al: Oral contraceptive and IUD use and endometrial cancer: a population-based case-control study in Shanghai, China. Int J Cancer 119(9):2142, 2006

Temkin SM, Hellmann M, Lee YC, et al: Early-stage carcinosarcoma of the uterus: the significance of lymph node count. Int J Gynecol Cancer 17:215, 2007

Terakawa N, Kigawa J, Taketani Y, et al: The behavior of endometrial hyperplasia: a prospective study. Endometrial Hyperplasia Study Group. J Obstet Gynaecol Res 23(3):223, 1997

Thigpen JT, Brady MF, Alvarez RD, et al: Oral medroxyprogesterone acetate in the treatment of advanced or recurrent endometrial carcinoma: a dose-response study by the Gynecologic Oncology Group. J Clin Oncol 17(6):1736, 1999

Todo Y, Kato H, Kaneuchi M, et al: Survival effect of para-aortic lymphadenectomy in endometrial cancer (SEPAL study): a retrospective cohort analysis. Lancet 375(9721):1165, 2010

Trimble CL, Kauderer J, Zaino R, et al: Concurrent endometrial carcinoma in women with a biopsy diagnosis of atypical endometrial hyperplasia: a Gynecologic Oncology Group study. Cancer 106(4):812, 2006

Trimble CL, Method M, Leitao M, et al: Management of endometrial precancers. Obstet Gynecol 120(5):1160, 2012

Vaidya AP, Horowitz NS, Oliva E, et al: Uterine malignant mixed müllerian tumors should not be included in studies of endometrial carcinoma. Gynecol Oncol 103:684, 2006

van Hanegem N, Breijer MC, Slockers SA, et al: Diagnostic workup for postmenopausal bleeding: a randomised controlled trial. BJOG 124(2):231, 2017

van Leeuwen FE, Benraadt J, Coebergh JW, et al: Risk of endometrial cancer after tamoxifen treatment of breast cancer. Lancet 343(8895):448, 1994

Varras M, Kioses E: Five-year survival of a patient with primary endometrial squamous cell carcinoma: a case report and review of the literature. Eur J Gynaecol Oncol 23(4):327, 2002

Vasen HF, Watson P, Mecklin JP, et al: New clinical criteria for hereditary nonpolyposis colorectal cancer (HNPCC, Lynch syndrome) proposed by the International Collaborative Group on HNPCC. Gastroenterology 116(6):1453, 1999

Viswanathan AN, Feskanich D, De Vivo I, et al: Smoking and the risk of endometrial cancer: results from the Nurses' Health Study. Int J Cancer 114(6):996, 2005

Vorgias G, Hintipas E, Katsoulis M, et al: Intraoperative gross examination of myometrial invasion and cervical infiltration in patients with endometrial cancer: decision-making accuracy. Gynecol Oncol 85(3):483, 2002

Wada H, Enomoto T, Fujita M, et al: Molecular evidence that most but not all carcinosarcomas of the uterus are combination tumors. Cancer Res 57(23):5379, 1997

Walker JL, Piedmonte MR, Spirtos NM, et al: Laparoscopy compared with laparotomy for comprehensive surgical staging of uterine cancer: Gynecologic Oncology Group study (LAP2). J Clin Oncol 27(32): 5331, 2009

Walker JL, Piedmonte MR, Spirtos NM, et al: Recurrence and survival after random assignment to laparoscopy versus laparotomy for comprehensive surgical staging of uterine cancer: Gynecologic Oncology Group LAP2 study. J Clin Oncol 30(7):695, 2012

Wang CB, Wang CJ, Huang HJ, et al: Fertility-preserving treatment in young patients with endometrial adenocarcinoma. Cancer 94(8):2192, 2002

Wernli KJ, Ray RM, Gao DL, et al: Menstrual and reproductive factors in relation to risk of endometrial cancer in Chinese women. Cancer Causes Control 17(7):949, 2006

Whitney CW, Brunetto VL, Zaino RJ, et al: Phase II study of medroxyprogesterone acetate plus tamoxifen in advanced endometrial carcinoma: a Gynecologic Oncology Group study. Gynecol Oncol 92(1):4, 2004

Winder AA, Kularatna M, MacCormick AD: Does bariatric surgery affect the incidence of endometrial cancer development? A systematic review. Obes Surg 28(5):1433, 2018

Wolfman W, Leyland N, Heywood M, et al: Asymptomatic endometrial thickening. J Obstet Gynaecol Can 32(10):990, 2010

Wolfson AH, Brady MF, Rocereto T, et al: A gynecologic oncology group randomized phase III trial of whole abdominal irradiation (WAI) vs. cisplatin-ifosfamide and mesna (CIM) as post-surgical therapy in stage I-IV carcinosarcoma (CS) of the uterus. Gynecol Oncol 107:177, 2007

Yang YC, Wu CC, Chen CP, et al: Reevaluating the safety of fertility-sparing hormonal therapy for early endometrial cancer. Gynecol Oncol 99(2):287, 2005

Zaino RJ, Kauderer J, Trimble CL, et al: Reproducibility of the diagnosis of atypical endometrial hyperplasia: a Gynecologic Oncology Group study. Cancer 106(4):804, 2006

Zaino RJ, Kurman RJ, Diana KL, et al: The utility of the revised International Federation of Gynecology and Obstetrics histologic grading of endometrial adenocarcinoma using a defined nuclear grading system. A Gynecologic Oncology Group study. Cancer 75(1):81, 1995

Zaino RJ, Silverberg SG, Norris HJ, et al: The prognostic value of nuclear versus architectural grading in endometrial adenocarcinoma: a Gynecologic Oncology Group study. Int J Gynecol Pathol 13(1):29, 1994

Zerbe MJ, Zhang J, Bristow RE, et al: Retrograde seeding of malignant cells during hysteroscopy in presumed early endometrial cancer. Gynecol Oncol 79(1):55, 2000

Zullo F, Palomba S, Falbo A, et al: Laparoscopic surgery vs laparotomy for early stage endometrial cancer: long-term data of a randomized controlled trial. Am J Obstet Gynecol 200(3):296.e1, 2009

CHAPTER 34

Uterine Sarcoma

Malignant tumors of the uterine corpus are broadly divided into carcinomas and sarcomas. Although sarcomas are rarely encountered, they tend to behave more aggressively and contribute to a disproportionately higher number of uterine cancer deaths. Pure sarcomas differentiate toward smooth muscle (leiomyosarcoma) or toward endometrial stroma (endometrial stromal tumors). In general, uterine sarcomas grow quickly, hematogenous or lymphatic spread occurs early, and the overall prognosis is poor. However, there are several notable exceptions among these tumors.

EPIDEMIOLOGY AND PATHOGENESIS

Sarcomas account for approximately 3 to 8 percent of all malignancies of the uterine corpus (Brooks, 2004; D'Angelo, 2010; Major, 1993). Historically, uterine sarcomas included carcinosarcomas, accounting for 40 percent of cases; leiomyosarcomas, 40 percent; endometrial stromal sarcomas, 10 to 15 percent; and undifferentiated sarcomas, 5 to 10 percent. In 2009, the International Federation of Gynecology and Obstetrics (FIGO) reclassified carcinosarcomas as a metaplastic form of endometrial carcinoma. These tumors are described in Chapter 33 (p. 708).

Because of their infrequency, uterine sarcomas have few identified risk factors. These include chronic excess estrogen exposure, tamoxifen use, African American race, and prior pelvic radiation. In contrast, combination oral contraceptive pill use and smoking appear to lower risks for some of these tumors (Felix, 2013).

In their pathogenesis, *leiomyosarcomas* have a monoclonal origin, and for the most part, they do not arise from benign leiomyomas. Instead, they appear to develop de novo as solitary lesions (Zhang, 2006). Supporting this theory, leiomyosarcomas have molecular pathways distinct from those of leiomyomas or normal myometrium (Cui, 2017). The most consistent findings across molecular studies involve functional loss of *RB1* and *PTEN*, which are tumor suppressor genes (El-Rifai, 1998; Gibault, 2011).

Endometrial stromal tumors have heterogeneous chromosomal aberrations (Halbwedl, 2005). However, the pattern of rearrangements is clearly nonrandom, and chromosomal arms 6p and 7p are frequently involved (Micci, 2006). Genetic translocations involving several chromosomes and the resultant fusion proteins are thought to be involved in endometrial stromal sarcoma pathogenesis (Lee, 2012; Panagopoulos, 2012).

DIAGNOSIS

Signs and Symptoms

As in endometrial cancer, abnormal vaginal bleeding is the most frequent symptom for uterine sarcomas (Gonzalez-Bosquet, 1997). Pelvic or abdominal pain also is common. Up to one third of women will describe significant discomfort that may result from passage of clots, rapid uterine enlargement, or prolapse of a sarcomatous polyp through an effaced cervix (De Fusco, 1989). In addition, a profuse, foul-smelling discharge may be obvious, and gastrointestinal and genitourinary complaints are frequent. Importantly, degenerating leiomyomas with necrosis can mimic these same signs and symptoms.

With rapid growth, a uterus may extend out of the pelvis into the mid- or upper abdomen (Fig. 34-1). Fortunately, the incidence of malignancy in such cases is low (<0.5 percent), and in most instances, benign enlarging leiomyomas are found (Leibsohn, 1990; Parker, 1994). Although uterine leiomyosarcomas do tend to grow quickly, no criteria define what constitutes significant growth. Despite these often-dramatic presentations, many women with uterine sarcoma will have few symptoms other than abnormal vaginal bleeding and a seemingly normal uterus on physical examination.

Endometrial Sampling

The sensitivity of an office endometrial biopsy or dilation and curettage (D & C) to detect sarcomatous elements is lower than that for endometrial carcinomas (Bansal, 2008). Specifically, with leiomyosarcoma, symptomatic women receive a correct preoperative diagnosis in only 35 to 50 percent of cases (Hinchcliff, 2016). This inability to accurately sample the tumor is probably related to the origin of these neoplasms in the myometrium rather than the endometrium. Similarly,

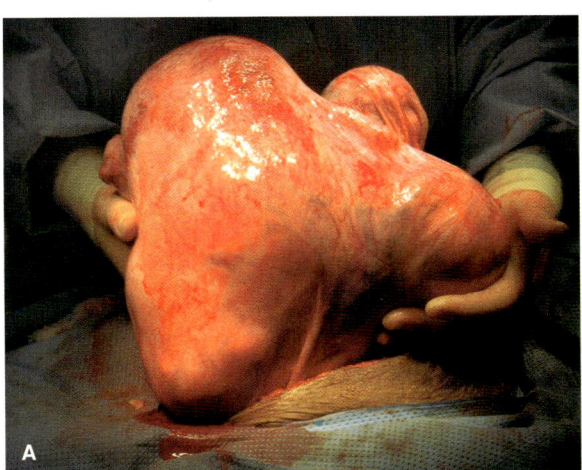 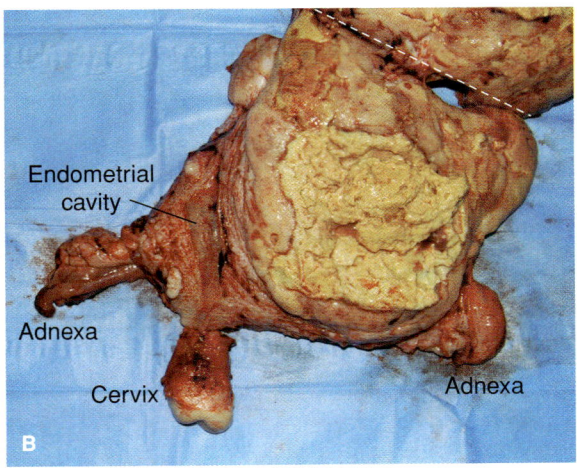

FIGURE 34-1 Leiomyosarcoma. **A.** Intraoperative photograph. **B.** Surgical specimen has been bisected and remains joined at the fundus. The other half of the specimen lies above the white dashed line and out of view. The large tumor lies to the right of the endometrial cavity. It has central necrosis seen as yellow amorphous debris within the tumor borders. (Reproduced with permission from Dr. Martha Rac.)

endometrial stromal nodules and endometrial stromal sarcoma may be undetectable by Pipelle biopsy, especially if the neoplasm is intramural (Yang, 2002).

■ Imaging Studies

These are often helpful if sarcoma is suspected before hysterectomy. In most cases, a computed tomography (CT) scan of the abdomen and pelvis is routinely performed. This serves at least two purposes. First, sarcomas often violate normal soft tissue planes in the pelvis, and therefore, unresectable tumors may be identified preoperatively. Second, extrauterine metastases may be found. In either case, treatment may be altered based on radiographic findings.

Diffusion weighted magnetic resonance (MR) imaging may be more diagnostic in distinguishing uterine sarcoma from a benign "mimic" (DeMulder, 2018; Sumi, 2015). As a diagnostic tool for sarcoma, sonography is far less helpful. Positron emission tomography (PET) scanning is most effective in the setting of recurrent uterine sarcoma but offers little advantage compared with CT or MR imaging (Sharma, 2012).

■ Role of the Generalist

Preoperative consultation with a gynecologic oncologist is recommended for any patient with a biopsy suggesting uterine sarcoma. The potential for intraabdominal metastases and disruption of tissue planes within the pelvis increases the technical difficulty and surgical risks. The approach to staging is subtly dissimilar to that of endometrial carcinomas. For example, due to the low rate of metastasis, only sampling nodes suspicious for leiomyosarcomas may be appropriate instead of performing complete pelvic and paraaortic lymphadenectomy (Nasioudis, 2019). Moreover, ovarian preservation may be suitable with certain sarcomas because of their low risk for spread to the adnexa, but not in others. In general, a treatment plan is best organized preoperatively, if possible.

Many uterine sarcomas are not diagnosed until surgery or several days later when a pathology report is available. As a result, unstaged cases are common, and a gynecologic oncologist

should be consulted at the earliest feasible time. If the diagnosis is made postoperatively, the criteria to recommend surveillance only, reoperation, or radiotherapy vary widely and depend on the sarcoma type and other clinical circumstances. Generally, these options are less straightforward than in typical endometrial carcinomas, largely due to the rarity of these tumors and the comparatively limited data supporting one strategy over another.

With adoption of minimally invasive surgery (MIS), gynecologists are faced with how best to achieve removal of bulky uteri or myomas through small incisions. Tissue fragmentation using laparoscopic power morcellation was a popular approach, until the increased concerns about dispersion of clinically occult gynecologic cancers became more evident. In particular, encountering an unexpected uterine sarcoma during surgery for presumed benign disease is rare, and rates range from 0.09 to 0.6 percent (Kho, 2016; Lieng, 2015; Multinu, 2019). These investigators also

TABLE 34-1. Histologic Classification of Mesenchymal Tumors of the Uterus

Mesenchymal tumors
Leiomyoma
   Diffuse leiomyomatosis
   Intravenous leiomyomatosis
   Metastasizing leiomyoma
Smooth muscle tumor of uncertain malignant potential
Leiomyosarcoma
Endometrial stromal tumors
   Endometrial stromal nodule
   Endometrial stromal sarcoma
   High-grade undifferentiated sarcoma

Mixed epithelial and mesenchymal tumors
Adenomyoma
Atypical polypoid adenomyoma
Adenofibroma
Adenosarcoma
Carcinosarcoma

found no clear preoperative risk factors. However, if a patient undergoes inadvertent morcellation and dispersion of an occult sarcoma, it may worsen her prognosis (Perri, 2009). In 2018, the Food and Drug Administration warned that power morcellator use should be curtailed in patients who are peri- or postmenopausal or who are candidates for en bloc removal through the vagina or a minilaparotomy. At minimum, if uncontained intraperitoneal morcellation is selected by those at low risk for cancer, patients should be aware of the risks that it poses (American College of Obstetricians and Gynecologists, 2019).

PATHOLOGY

Uterine mesenchymal tumors are classified broadly into pure and mixed tumors (Table 34-1). Also, the term *homologous* denotes tissues normally found in the uterus and *heterologous* refers to tissue foreign to the uterus. Pure sarcomas are virtually all homologous and differentiate into mesenchymal tissue that is normally present within the uterus, such as smooth muscle (leiomyosarcoma) or stromal tissue within the endometrium (endometrial stromal tumors). Pure heterologous sarcomas, such as chondrosarcoma, are rare.

Mixed sarcomas contain a malignant mesenchymal component admixed with an epithelial element. If the epithelial element is also malignant, the tumor is termed *carcinosarcoma*. If the epithelial element is benign, the term *adenosarcoma* is used.

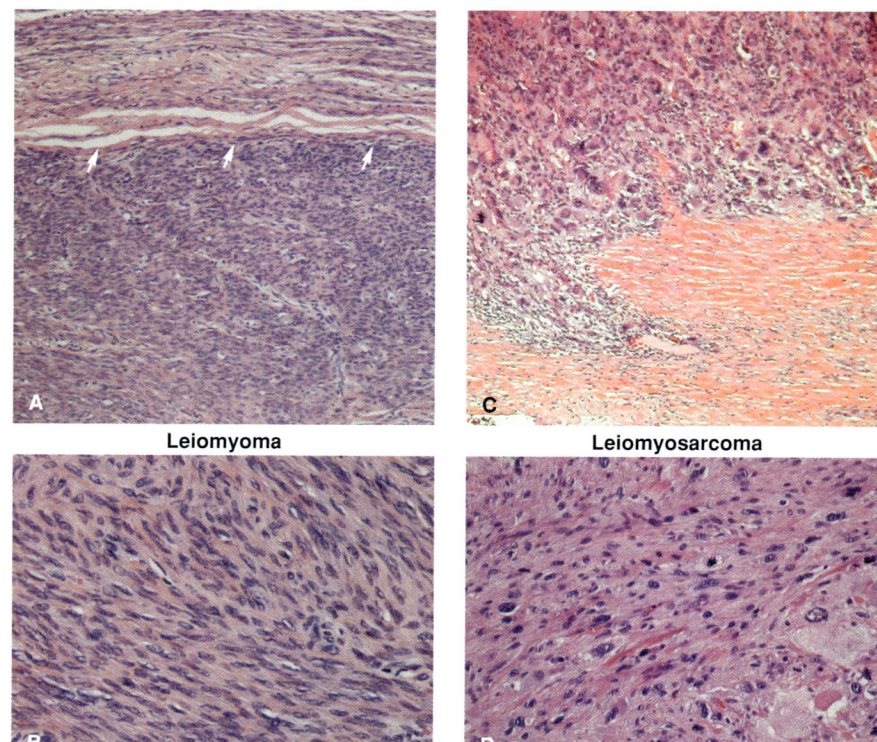

Leiomyoma / **Leiomyosarcoma**

FIGURE 34-2 Leiomyoma (**A, B**) and leiomyosarcoma (**C,D**). **A.** Leiomyomas tend to be well-circumscribed masses. This leiomyoma shows a well-demarcated interface (*arrows*) with the less cellular myometrium above it. **B.** Although leiomyomas may have variable histologic features, most are composed of bland spindled cells with blunt-ended nuclei and limited mitotic activity. **C.** Leiomyosarcoma is a malignant smooth muscle neoplasm that may differ markedly in its microscopic appearance from case to case. Generally, leiomyosarcoma shows some combination of coagulative tumor necrosis, increased mitotic activity, and/or nuclear atypia. This example has marked nuclear atypia and pleomorphism and an infiltrative growth pattern at its periphery. This differs from the usually smooth, pushing border of typical leiomyomas. **D.** This particular example has moderate to marked nuclear atypia. (Reproduced with permission from Drs. Kelley Carrick and Raheela Ashfaq.)

Leiomyosarcoma

Leiomyosarcomas account for 1 to 2 percent of all uterine malignances. In two Surveillance, Epidemiology, and End Results (SEER) database studies, the median age at presentation was 52 and 50 years, respectively (Hosh, 2016; Kapp, 2008). Most tumors were localized at the time of diagnosis, whereas 3 to 14 percent had regional disease. Distant disease composed 7 to 31 percent.

The Stanford criteria are the commonly used histologic criteria for diagnosing leiomyosarcoma. They are somewhat controversial but include the frequency of mitotic figures, extent of nuclear atypia, and presence of coagulative tumor cell necrosis (Fig. 34-2) (Bell, 1994). In reading Table 34-2, each row illustrates combinations of histologic findings that may be found in leiomyosarcomas. In most cases, the mitotic index exceeds 15 mitotic figures total when 10 high-power fields are examined, moderate to severe cytologic atypia is seen, and tumor cell necrosis is prominent (Oliva, 2014b; Zaloudek, 2011). Occasionally, a leiomyosarcoma will be reported as low-, intermediate-, or high-grade, but the overall utility of grading is controversial, and no grading system is universally accepted.

Smooth Muscle Tumor of Uncertain Malignant Potential (STUMP)

These are tumors with some worrisome histologic features, such as necrosis or nuclear atypia, but without criteria to be

TABLE 34-2. Diagnostic Criteria for Uterine Leiomyosarcoma

Coagulative Tumor Cell Necrosis	Mitotic Index[a]	Degree of Atypia
Present	≥10 MF/10 HPF	None
Present	Any	Diffuse, significant
Absent	≥10 MF/10 HPF	Diffuse, significant

[a]MF/10 HPF = the total number of mitotic figures counted when 10 high-powered fields are examined.

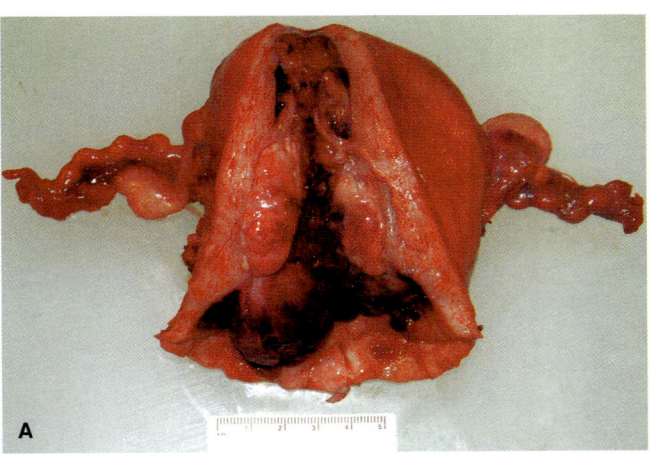 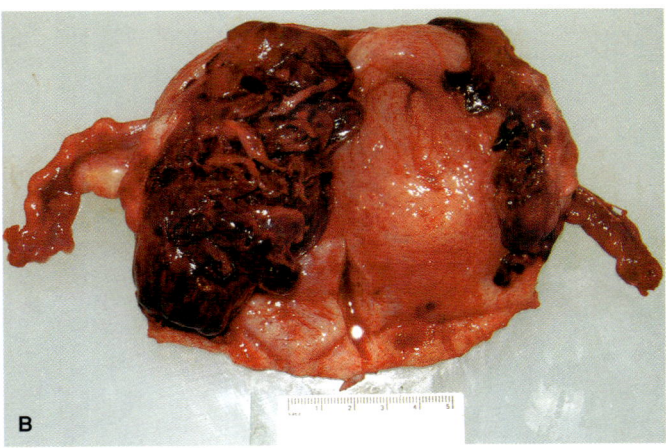

FIGURE 34-3 Gross uterine specimen with endometrial stromal sarcoma. **A.** The mass partially prolapsed through the cervix. **B.** Opened uterine specimen.

diagnosed reliably as benign or malignant. The diagnosis should be used sparingly and is reserved for smooth muscle neoplasms whose appearance is ambiguous (Oliva, 2014b).

■ Endometrial Stromal Tumors

Significantly less common than leiomyosarcomas, the group of endometrial stromal tumors represent fewer than 10 percent of all uterine sarcomas. In a SEER database study of 831 patients, the median age at diagnosis was 52 years (Chan, 2008). Although constituting a wide morphologic spectrum, endometrial stromal tumors are composed exclusively of cells that resemble the endometrial stroma.

Historically, there has been controversy in subdividing these tumors. The division of endometrial stromal sarcomas into low-grade and high-grade categories has fallen out of favor. In its place, the designation *endometrial stromal sarcoma* is now best restricted to neoplasms that were formerly referred to as low-grade. Alternatively, the term *high-grade undifferentiated sarcoma* is believed to more accurately reflect those tumors without recognizable evidence of a definite endometrial stromal phenotype. These lesions often resemble the mesenchymal component of a uterine carcinosarcoma and in this revised classification, the distinctions are not determined by mitotic count but by features such as nuclear pleomorphism and necrosis (Oliva, 2014a,b).

Endometrial Stromal Nodule

Representing less than a quarter of tumors in the endometrial stromal tumor group, these rare nodules are benign, characterized by a well-delineated margin, and composed of neoplastic cells that resemble proliferative-phase endometrial stromal cells. Grossly, the tumor is a solitary, round or oval, fleshy nodule measuring a few centimeters. Histologically, they are distinguished from endometrial stromal sarcomas by their lack of myometrial infiltration (Hoang, 2018). Because these nodules are benign, myomectomy is an appropriate option. However, because differentiation between endometrial stromal sarcoma and this benign lesion cannot be determined clinically, it is important to remove the entire nodule. Thus, for large lesions, hysterectomy may be required.

Endometrial Stromal Sarcoma

The precise frequency of these tumors is difficult to estimate because they are excluded from some reports and included in others, and the terminology used has been inconsistent. In general, endometrial stromal sarcomas are thought to be the most frequently encountered stromal tumor variant and are twice as common as high-grade undifferentiated sarcomas.

Typically, they extensively invade the myometrium and extend to the serosa in approximately half of cases (Fig. 34-3). Less often, they present as a solitary, well-delineated, predominantly intramural mass that is difficult to grossly distinguish from an endometrial stromal nodule. Microscopically, endometrial stromal sarcomas resemble the stromal cells of proliferative-phase endometrium (Fig. 34-4) (Hoang, 2018).

Metastases are rarely detected prior to the diagnosis of the primary lesion. However, permeation of the lymphatic and vascular channels is characteristic. In up to one third of cases, extrauterine extension is present, often appearing as "worm-like" plugs of tumor within the vessels of the broad ligament and adnexa. At operation, this may resemble intravenous leiomyomatosis or a broad ligament leiomyoma, but frozen section analysis can usually make the distinction.

High-Grade Undifferentiated Sarcoma

Compared with endometrial stromal sarcomas, these tumors tend to be larger and more polypoid, often filling the uterine cavity. Instead of an infiltrating pattern, high-grade undifferentiated sarcomas displace the myometrium more destructively, leading to prominent hemorrhage and necrosis.

Microscopically, the cells are larger and more pleomorphic. The presence of marked cellular atypia is characteristic. Typically, there are more than 10 mitoses per 10 high-power fields, but frequently more than 20 mitoses are seen in the most active areas. These tumors lack specific differentiation and bear no histologic resemblance to endometrial stroma (Oliva, 2014b; Zaloudek, 2011).

■ Adenosarcoma

This rare, biphasic neoplasm is characterized by a benign epithelial component and a sarcomatous mesenchymal component.

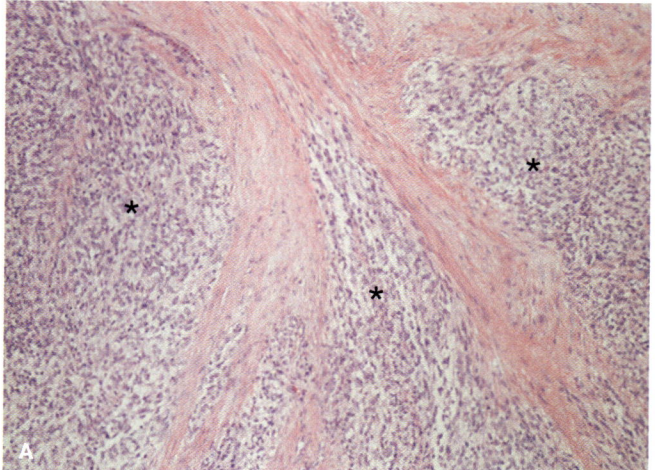

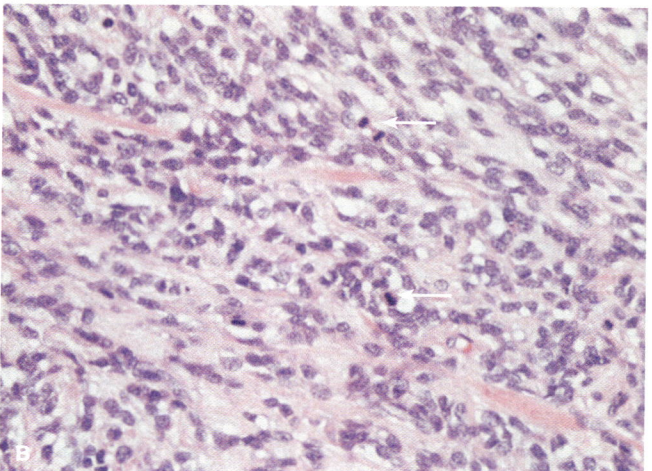

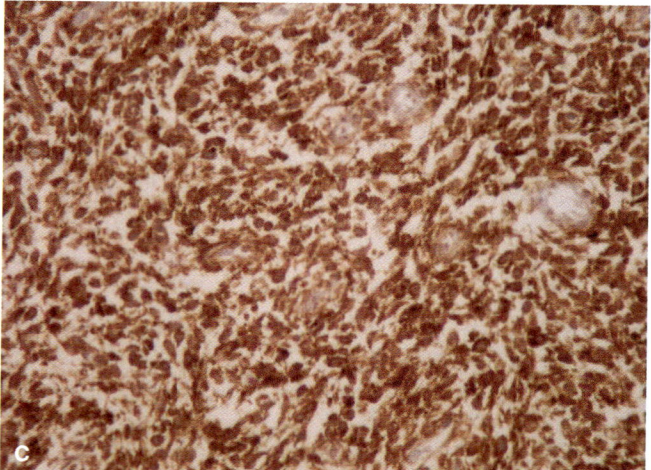

FIGURE 34-4 Endometrial stromal sarcoma (ESS). **A.** ESS is composed of cells morphologically similar to proliferative phase endometrial stromal cells. In this low-power view that involved the corpus and cervix, irregular tongues of tumor (*asterisks*) are seen dissecting into the cervical stroma. **B.** The tumor cells are spindled and relatively bland, similar to normal endometrial proliferative phase stroma. Two mitoses are identified in this single medium-power field (*white arrows*). **C.** Endometrial stroma marks positively with CD10, as does ESS. A battery of immunostains, including CD10, may be used to help distinguish ESS from other spindle cell neoplasms. (Reproduced with permission from Dr. Kelley Carrick.)

Tumors may develop in women of all ages. Grossly, adenosarcomas grow as exophytic polypoid masses that extend into the uterine cavity. Rarely, they may arise in the myometrium, presumably from adenomyosis. Microscopically, isolated glands are dispersed throughout the mesenchymal component and are often dilated or compressed into thin slits (Fig. 34-5). Typically, the mesenchymal component resembles an endometrial stromal sarcoma or fibrosarcoma and contains varying amounts of fibrous tissue and smooth muscle. In general, these are considered low-grade tumors with mild atypia and relatively few mitotic figures. However, 10 percent have a more malignant behavior due to one-sided proliferation of the sarcomatous, often high-grade, component. This subgroup of adenosarcomas is designated as having "sarcomatous overgrowth," and patients have a poor prognosis (Friedlander, 2014; Wells, 2014).

PATTERNS OF SPREAD

Uterine sarcomas generally fall into two categories of malignant behavior. Leiomyosarcomas and high-grade undifferentiated sarcomas are consistently characterized by an aggressive growth pattern and rapid disease progression despite treatment. In contrast, endometrial stromal sarcomas and most adenosarcomas have an indolent growth pattern with long disease-free intervals. All of these tumors invade, to some degree, by direct extension.

Leiomyosarcomas have a propensity for hematogenous dissemination. Lung metastases are particularly common, and more than half of patients will have distant spread if diagnosed with recurrent disease. In the absence of widespread disease, leiomyosarcomas rarely metastasize via lymphatic channels (Machida, 2017).

STAGING

Uterine sarcomas are surgically staged. Formerly, most clinicians used the FIGO surgical staging system for endometrial cancer to stage uterine sarcomas. Endometrial stromal sarcomas and adenosarcomas share new criteria, whereas leiomyosarcomas have a different system for stage I (Table 34-3 and Fig. 34-6). Stages I and II are considered early-stage disease, whereas stages III and IV reflect advanced disease.

TREATMENT OF EARLY-STAGE DISEASE

■ Surgery

The highest chance of cure is achieved by complete surgical resection of a sarcoma that is confined to the uterus (Seagle, 2017b). The staging laparotomy described for endometrial cancer in Chapter 33 (p. 712) can be revised to incorporate the unique spread patterns of uterine sarcomas. Exploration is particularly important to assess the abdomen for unresectable or widely metastatic disease that might indicate a need to abort the procedure. Some evidence shows benefit from aggressive cytoreductive surgery (Dinh, 2004; Leath, 2007; Thomas, 2009).

With *uterine leiomyosarcoma*, all patients should undergo a hysterectomy, if feasible. A modified radical or radical procedure may be occasionally required if there is parametrial infiltration. In

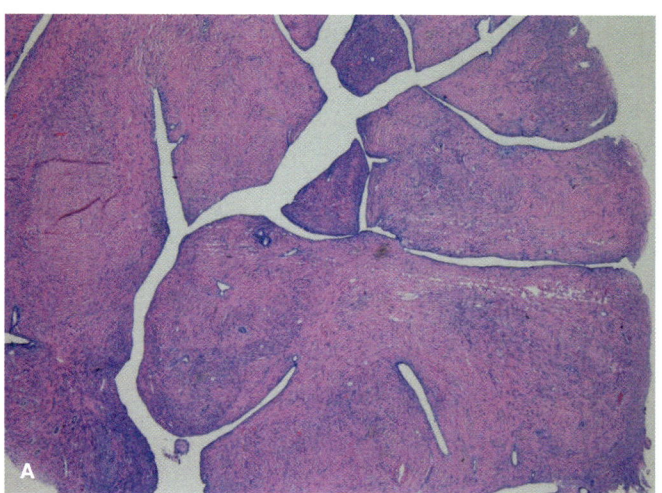 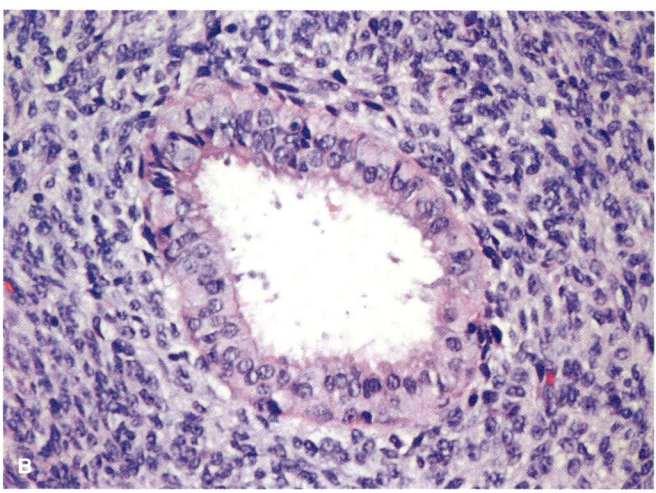

FIGURE 34-5 Adenosarcoma. **A.** A broad-based villous architecture is seen typically. **B.** Normal endometrial glands are surrounded by a cellular stroma consisting of a low-grade sarcoma. In this case, an endometrial stromal sarcoma is the sarcoma component. (Reproduced with permission from Dr. Raheela Ashfaq.)

TABLE 34-3. FIGO Staging for Uterine Sarcomas (Leiomyosarcomas, Endometrial Stromal Sarcomas, and Adenosarcomas)

Stage	Characteristics
Leiomyosarcomas	
I	**Tumor limited to uterus**
IA	<5 cm
IB	>5 cm
II	**Tumor extends to the pelvis**
IIA	Adnexal involvement
IIB	Tumor extends to extrauterine pelvic tissue
III	**Tumor invades abdominal tissues (not just protruding into the abdomen)**
IIIA	One site
IIIB	>One site
IIIC	Metastasis to pelvic and/or paraaortic lymph nodes
IV	
IVA	Tumor invades bladder and/or rectum
IVB	Distant metastasis
Adenosarcomas and endometrial stromal sarcomas[a]	
I	**Tumor limited to uterus**
IA	Tumor limited to endometrium/endocervix with no myometrial invasion
IB	Less than or equal to half myometrial invasion
IC	More than half myometrial invasion
II	**Tumor extends to the pelvis**
IIA	Adnexal involvement
IIB	Tumor extends to extrauterine pelvic tissue
III	**Tumor invades abdominal tissues (not just protruding into the abdomen)**
IIIA	One site
IIIB	>One site
IIIC	Metastasis to pelvic and/or paraaortic lymph nodes
IV	
IVA	Tumor invades bladder and/or rectum
IVB	Distant metastasis

[a]Note: Simultaneous tumors of the uterine corpus and ovary/pelvis in association with ovarian/pelvic endometriosis should be classified as independent primary tumors.
FIGO = International Federation of Gynecology and Obstetrics.

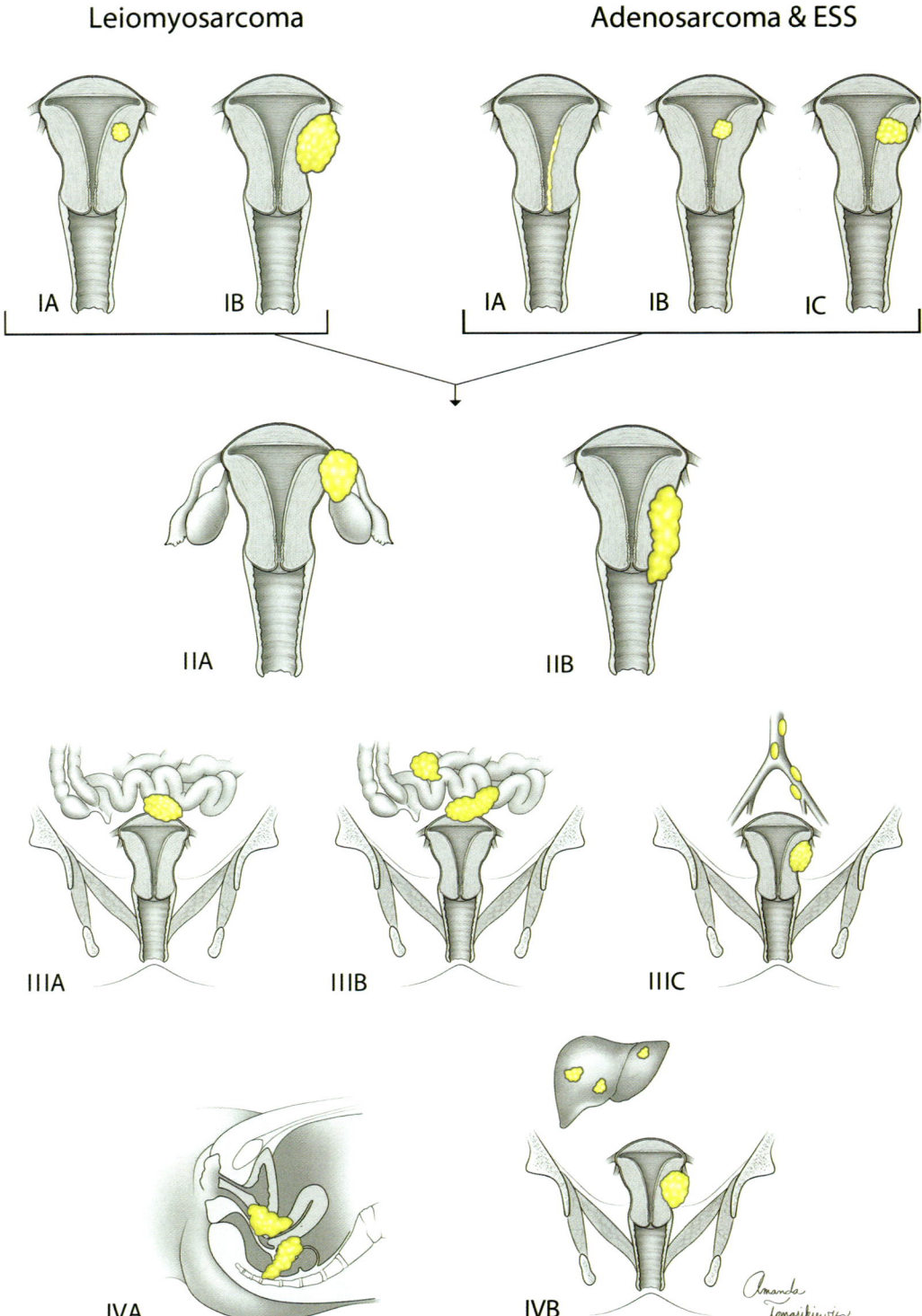

FIGURE 34-6 FIGO staging of leiomyosarcoma and that of adenosarcoma and endometrial stromal sarcoma (ESS).

the absence of other gross disease, fewer than 5 percent will have ovarian or nodal metastases. Ovarian preservation is therefore an option for premenopausal women (Seagle, 2017b). In addition, lymph node dissection is reserved for only patients with clinically suspicious nodes. For STUMP, hysterectomy alone is sufficient.

Endometrial stromal tumors and *adenosarcomas* also are best treated by hysterectomy (Seagle, 2016). Again, a more radical procedure may be required to encompass local disease. Preservation of

the ovaries is generally accepted for adenosarcomas in the absence of extrauterine disease but may result in a higher recurrence rate for endometrial stroma sarcoma (Michener, 2001; Nasioudis, 2019). However, bilateral salpingo-oophorectomy (BSO) is indicated for high-grade undifferentiated sarcomas (Meurer, 2019). Unlike leiomyosarcoma, lymph node dissection is typically more informative. Although nodal metastases are most often identified in patients with obvious extrauterine disease, they do occur in 5 to

10 percent of patients with no evidence for intraabdominal spread (Machida, 2017; Seagle, 2017a).

■ Surveillance

In women with early-stage uterine sarcoma, adjuvant treatment is routinely employed but has not been demonstrated to improve survival rates (Hensley, 2018; Koh, 2018; Reed, 2008). Thus, because the recurrence rate for the clinically aggressive types is excessive, enrollment in an experimental clinical trial should be carefully considered, if available.

After surgery, menopausal symptoms such as hot flashes may be treated as appropriate for uterine leiomyosarcomas, high-grade undifferentiated sarcomas, and adenosarcomas. However, the use of estrogen replacement therapy for endometrial stromal sarcoma has been associated with disease progression and is avoided (Chu, 2003; Nasioudis, 2019; Pink, 2006).

Surgically treated patients with uterine sarcoma should have a physical examination every 3 months for the first 2 years and then at 6- to 12-month intervals thereafter. Due to the high rates of distant recurrences, CT scanning of the chest, abdomen, and pelvis are recommended at 6- to 12-month intervals or as clinically indicated (Salani, 2017). Most recurrences will be distant, and thus Pap tests are largely irrelevant.

■ Adjuvant Radiation

Approximately half of patients with stage I disease who are observed without adjuvant therapy will relapse (Leath, 2009). Due to the rarity of these tumors and limited data to support a consistent approach, the use of postoperative therapy is usually individualized. From a prospective trial that randomly assigned 224 women over 13 years with all subtypes of surgical stage I or II uterine sarcomas to either pelvic radiation or no further treatment, no benefit was found for those with leiomyosarcomas. Unfortunately, the number of patients with endometrial stromal sarcoma was too small to permit analysis (Reed, 2008).

■ Adjuvant Chemotherapy

There is yet no proven survival benefit for using adjuvant chemotherapy in patients with stage I uterine sarcoma (Hensley, 2018; Rauh-Hain, 2014). For leiomyosarcomas, completely resected stage I and II disease treated with gemcitabine and docetaxel was not associated with significantly improved disease-free or overall survival rates (Hensley, 2018; Littell, 2017). In high-grade undifferentiated sarcomas, chemotherapy regimens used for more advanced disease may be considered. For stages I and II endometrial stromal sarcoma and adenosarcoma, observation is recommended (Koh, 2018). However, because most patients will recur distantly, adjuvant systemic treatment is frequently used for recurrences.

■ Fertility-Sparing Management

Rarely, young patients may desire to delay definitive hysterectomy after a fertility-sparing "myomectomy" demonstrates sarcomatous features on final pathology (Lissoni, 1998; Yan, 2010). Expectant management following tumor resection can result in successful pregnancies in select patients. However, it

is risky not to perform a hysterectomy, and eventually all such women should undergo this surgery. Most patients, even those with negative margins, are counseled regarding definitive surgery and ovarian preservation during surgery for clinical stage I uterine leiomyosarcomas or endometrial stromal sarcomas. Egg retrieval, assisted reproductive technologies, and pregnancy surrogacy would still be possible. For more advanced disease, fertility-sparing management is not a reasonable option.

TREATMENT OF ADVANCED OR RECURRENT DISEASE

Patients with advanced or recurrent uterine sarcoma generally have a dismal prognosis. For advanced-stage disease, upfront surgery with maximal effort to completely remove all visible disease (similar in approach to advanced ovarian cancer) is considered standard. This is generally followed by adjuvant chemotherapy. Neoadjuvant chemotherapy can be considered for patients whose disease is considered unresectable or who are medically unfit for surgery.

For recurrent disease, secondary cytoreductive surgery may be feasible in some circumstances (Giuntoli, 2007). Palliative radiation also may have a role, depending on the site and distribution of the tumor. In general, uterine sarcomas have a propensity for relapse at distant sites, and chemotherapy is more useful. Since current treatment options have only modest efficacy, patients are encouraged to enroll in experimental clinical trials.

■ Leiomyosarcoma

Doxorubicin is considered the most active single agent (Miller, 2000; Omura, 1983). However, treatment with the combination of gemcitabine and docetaxel currently has the highest proven response rate (36 percent) (Hensley, 2008). Addition of bevacizumab to this regimen was not beneficial (Hensley, 2015). Other agents are approved for leiomyosarcoma refractory to doxorubicin and include trabectedin, dacarbazine, temozolomide, and pazopanib. Response rates are generally less than 20 percent, and clinical trial participation is encouraged.

For late recurrences of leiomyosarcoma, consideration of surgery must be individualized. Five-year survival rates of 30 to 50 percent have been reported following pulmonary resection for lung metastases. Local and regional recurrences also may be amenable to surgical resection (Giuntoli, 2007).

■ Endometrial Stromal Tumors

Surgical resection may be feasible for some patients with recurrent endometrial stromal sarcoma, but hormonal therapy is particularly useful. In general, these tumors are estrogen- and progesterone-receptor (ER/PR) positive (Sutton, 1986). Progestins such as megestrol acetate and medroxyprogesterone acetate are most commonly used either postoperatively for advanced-stage disease or for relapses (Reich, 2006). Using this strategy, complete responses are often possible. Aromatase inhibitors and gonadotropin-releasing hormone (GnRH) agonists also have demonstrated activity (Burke, 2004; Leunen, 2004).

High-grade undifferentiated sarcomas do not exhibit the same level of sensitivity to hormonal agents, primarily because

TABLE 34-4. Overall Survival Rates of Women with Uterine Sarcomas (All Stages)

Type	5-Year Survival
Leiomyosarcoma	41%
Endometrial stromal tumors	
Endometrial stromal sarcoma	91%
High-grade undifferentiated sarcoma	33%
Müllerian adenosarcoma	72%

Data from Seagle, 2016; 2017a,b.

they are usually ER/PR negative. Advanced disease or recurrences of these rare tumors are also typically not amenable to surgical resection. Palliative radiation may have some utility. Systemic chemotherapy is usually the only option, and treatment decisions are often extrapolated from leiomyosarcoma studies.

SURVIVAL AND PROGNOSTIC FACTORS

In general, women with uterine sarcoma have a poor prognosis (Table 34-4). FIGO stage is the most important independent variable associated with survival (Livi, 2003). Other poor prognostic factors across all subtypes include older age, African-American race, and lack of primary surgery (Chan, 2008; Kapp, 2008; Nemani, 2008).

Tumor histology is the other main predictor of outcome. High-grade undifferentiated uterine sarcomas have the worst prognosis and are followed by the group of leiomyosarcomas (Seagle, 2017a,b). Endometrial stromal sarcomas and uterine adenosarcomas without sarcomatous overgrowth are the two notable exceptions. Patients with these tumors tend to have a good prognosis due to their indolent growth (Seagle, 2016, 2017a).

REFERENCES

American College of Obstetricians and Gynecologists: Uterine morcellation for presumed leiomyomas. Committee Opinion No. 770, March 2019

Bansal N, Herzog TJ, Burke W, et al: The utility of preoperative endometrial sampling for the detection of uterine sarcomas. Gynecol Oncol 110(1):43, 2008

Bell SW, Kempson RL, Hendrickson MR: Problematic uterine smooth muscle neoplasms. A clinicopathologic study of 213 cases. Am J Surg Pathol 18(6):535, 1994

Brooks SE, Zhan M, Cote T, et al: Surveillance, epidemiology, and end results analysis of 2677 cases of uterine sarcoma 1989–1999. Gynecol Oncol 93(1):204, 2004

Burke C, Hickey K: Treatment of endometrial stromal sarcoma with a gonadotropin-releasing hormone analogue. Obstet Gynecol 104(5 Pt 2):1182, 2004

Chan JK, Kawar NM, Shin JY, et al: Endometrial stromal sarcoma: a population-based analysis. Br J Cancer 99:1210, 2008

Chu MC, Mor G, Lim C, et al: Low-grade endometrial stromal sarcoma: hormonal aspects. Gynecol Oncol 90(1):170, 2003

Cui RR, Wright JD, Hou JY: Uterine leiomyosarcoma: a review of recent advances in molecular biology, clinical management and outcome. BJOG 124(7):1028, 2017

D'Angelo E, Prat J: Uterine sarcomas: a review. Gynecol Oncol 116:131, 2010

De Fusco PA, Gaffey TA, Malkasian GD Jr, et al: Endometrial stromal sarcoma: review of Mayo Clinic experience, 1945–1980. Gynecol Oncol 35(1):8, 1989

DeMulder D, Ascher SM: Uterine leiomyosarcoma: can MRI differentiate leiomyosarcoma from benign leiomyoma before treatment? AJR Am J Roentgenol 211(6):1405, 2018

Dinh TA, Oliva EA, Fuller AF Jr, et al: The treatment of uterine leiomyosarcoma. Results from a 10-year experience (1990-1999) at the Massachusetts General Hospital. Gynecol Oncol 92:648, 2004

El-Rifai W, Sarlomo-Rikala M, Knuutila S, et al: DNA copy number changes in development and progression in leiomyosarcomas of soft tissues. Am J Pathol 153(3):985, 1998

Felix AS, Cook LS, Gaudet MM, et al: The etiology of uterine sarcomas: a pooled analysis of the epidemiology of endometrial cancer consortium. Br J Cancer 108(3):727, 2013

Food and Drug Administration: Laparoscopic power morcellators. 2018. Available at: https://www.fda.gov/medical-devices/surgery-devices/laparoscopic-power-morcellators. Accessed April 5, 2019

Friedlander ML, Covens A, Glasspool RM, et al: Gynecologic Cancer InterGroup (GCIG) consensus review for mullerian adenosarcoma of the female genital tract. Int J Gynecol Cancer 24(9 Suppl 3):S78, 2014

Gibault L, Pérot G, Chibon F, et al: New insights in sarcoma oncogenesis: a comprehensive analysis of a large series of 160 soft tissue sarcomas with complex genomics. J Pathol 223(1):64, 2011

Giuntoli RL, Garrett-Mayer E, Bristow RE, et al: Secondary cytoreduction in the management of recurrent uterine leiomyosarcoma. Gynecol Oncol 106(1):82, 2007

Gonzalez-Bosquet E, Martinez-Palones JM, Gonzalez-Bosquet J, et al: Uterine sarcoma: a clinicopathological study of 93 cases. Eur J Gynaecol Oncol 18(3):192, 1997

Greer BE, Koh WJ, Abu-Rustum NR, et al: Uterine neoplasms. NCCN Clinical Practice Guidelines in Oncology. Version 2. 2015. Available at: www.nccn.org/professionals/physician_gls/default.aspx#uterine. Accessed April 24, 2015

Halbwedl I, Ullmann R, Kremser ML, et al: Chromosomal alterations in low-grade endometrial stromal sarcoma and undifferentiated endometrial sarcoma as detected by comparative genomic hybridization. Gynecol Oncol 97(2):582, 2005

Hensley ML, Blessing JA, Mannel R, et al: Fixed-dose rate gemcitabine plus docetaxel as first-line therapy for metastatic uterine leiomyosarcoma: a Gynecologic Oncology Group phase II trial. Gynecol Oncol 109:329, 2008

Hensley ML, Enserro D, Hatcher H, et al: Adjuvant gemcitabine plus docetaxel followed by doxorubicin versus observation for high-grade uterine leiomyosarcoma: a phase III NRG Oncology/Gynecologic Oncology Group study. J Clin Oncol 36(33):3324, 2018

Hensley ML, Miller DS, O'Malley DM, et al: Randomized phase III trial of gemcitabine plus docetaxel plus bevacizumab or placebo as first line treatment for metastatic uterine leiomyosarcoma: an NRG Oncology/Gynecologic Oncology Group study. J Clin Oncol 33(10):1180, 2015

Hinchcliff EM, Esselen KM, Watkins JC, et al: The role of endometrial biopsy in the preoperative detection of uterine leiomyosarcoma. J Minim Invasive Gynecol 23(4):567, 2016

Hoang L, Chiang S, Lee CH: Endometrial stromal sarcomas and related neoplasms: new developments and diagnostic considerations. Pathology 50(2):162, 2018

Hosh M, Antar S, Nazzal A, et al: Uterine sarcoma: analysis of 13,089 cases based on Surveillance, Epidemiology, and End Results Database. Int J Gynecol Cancer 26(6):1098, 2016

Kapp DS, Shin JY, Chan JK: Prognostic factors and survival in 1396 patients with uterine leiomyosarcomas: emphasis on impact of lymphadenectomy and oophorectomy. Cancer 112(4):820, 2008

Kho KA, Lin K, Hechanova M, et al: Risk of occult uterine sarcoma in women undergoing hysterectomy for benign indications. Obstet Gynecol 127(3):468, 2016

Koh WJ, Abu-Rustum NR, Bean S, et al: Uterine neoplasms, version 1.2018, NCCN clinical practice guidelines in oncology. J Natl Compr Canc Netw 16(2):170, 2018

Leath CA III, Huh WK, Hyde J Jr, et al: A multi-institutional review of outcomes of endometrial stromal sarcoma. Gynecol Oncol 105:630, 2007

Leath CA III, Numnum TM, Kendrick JE, et al: Patterns of failure for conservatively managed surgical stage I uterine carcinosarcoma: implications for adjuvant therapy. Int J Gynecol Cancer 19:888, 2009

Lee CH, Ou WB, Mariño-Enriquez A, et al: 14-3-3 fusion oncogenes in high-grade endometrial stromal sarcoma. Proc Natl Acad Sci USA 109(3):929, 2012

Leibsohn S, d'Ablaing G, Mishell DR, et al: Leiomyosarcoma in a series of hysterectomies performed for presumed uterine leiomyomas. Am J Obstet Gynecol 162(4):968, 1990

Leunen M, Breugelmans M, De Sutter P, et al: Low-grade endometrial stromal sarcoma treated with the aromatase inhibitor letrozole. Gynecol Oncol 95(3):769, 2004

Lieng M, Berner E, Busund B: Risk of morcellation of uterine leiomyosarcomas in laparoscopic supracervical hysterectomy and laparoscopic myomectomy, a retrospective trial including 4791 women. J Minim Invasive Gynecol 22(3):410, 2015

Lissoni A, Cormio G, Bonazzi C, et al: Fertility-sparing surgery in uterine leiomyosarcoma. Gynecol Oncol 70(3):348, 1998

Littell RD, Tucker LY, Raine-Bennett T, et al: Adjuvant gemcitabine-docetaxel chemotherapy for stage I uterine leiomyosarcoma: trends and survival outcomes. Gynecol Oncol 147(1):11, 2017

Livi L, Paiar F, Shah N, et al: Uterine sarcoma: twenty-seven years of experience. Int J Radiat Oncol Biol Phys 57(5):1366, 2003

Machida H, Nathenson MJ, Takiuchi T, et al: Significance of lymph node metastasis on survival of women with uterine adenosarcoma. Gynecol Oncol 144(3):524, 2017

Major FJ, Blessing JA, Silverberg SG, et al: Prognostic factors in early-stage uterine sarcoma. A Gynecologic Oncology Group study. Cancer 71(4 Suppl): 1702, 1993

Meurer M, Floquet A, Ray-Coquard I, et al: Localized high grade endometrial stromal sarcoma and localized undifferentiated uterine sarcoma: a retrospective series of the French Sarcoma Group. Int J Gynecol Cancer 29(4):691, 2019

Micci F, Panagopoulos I, Bjerkehagen B, et al: Consistent rearrangement of chromosomal band 6p21 with generation of fusion genes JAZF1/PHF1 and EPC1/PHF1 in endometrial stromal sarcoma. Cancer Res 66(1):107, 2006

Michener CM, Simon NL: Ovarian conservation in a woman of reproductive age with müllerian adenosarcoma. Gynecol Oncol 83(2):424, 2001

Miller DS, Blessing JA, Kilgore LC, et al: Phase II trial of topotecan in patients with advanced, persistent, or recurrent uterine leiomyosarcomas: a Gynecologic Oncology Group study. Am J Clin Oncol 23(4):355, 2000

Multinu F, Casarin J, Tortorella L, et al: Incidence of sarcoma in patients undergoing hysterectomy for benign indications: a population-based study. Am J Obstet Gynecol 220(2):179.e1, 2019

Nasioudis D, Ko EM, Kolovos G, et al: Ovarian preservation for low-grade endometrial stromal sarcoma: a systematic review of the literature and meta-analysis. Int J Gynecol Cancer 29(1):126, 2019

Nemani D, Mitra N, Guo M, et al: Assessing the effects of lymphadenectomy and radiation therapy in patients with uterine carcinosarcoma: a SEER analysis. Gynecol Oncol 111:82, 2008

Oliva E: Cellular mesenchymal tumors of the uterus: a review emphasizing recent observations. Int J Gynecol Pathol 33(4):374, 2014a

Oliva E, Carcangiu ML, Carinelli SG, et al: Mesenchymal tumours. In Kurman RJ, Carcangiu LM, Herrington CS, et al (eds): WHO Classification of Tumours of Female Reproductive Organs. Lyon, International Agency for Research on Cancer, 2014b, p 135

Omura GA, Major FJ, Blessing JA, et al: A randomized study of adriamycin with and without dimethyl triazenoimidazole carboxamide in advanced uterine sarcomas. Cancer 52(4):626, 1983

Panagopoulos I, Micci F, Thorsen J, et al: Novel fusion of MYST/ESA1-associated factor 6 and PHF1 in endometrial stromal sarcoma. PLoS One 7(6):e39354, 2012

Parker WH, Fu YS, Berek JS: Uterine sarcoma in patients operated on for presumed leiomyoma and rapidly growing leiomyoma. Obstet Gynecol 83(3):414, 1994

Perri T, Korach J, Sadetzki S, et al: Uterine leiomyosarcoma: does the primary surgical procedure matter? Int J Gynecol Cancer 19:257, 2009

Pink D, Lindner T, Mrozek A, et al: Harm or benefit of hormonal treatment in metastatic low-grade endometrial stromal sarcoma: single center experience with 10 cases and review of the literature. Gynecol Oncol 101(3):464, 2006

Rauh-Hain JA, Goodman A, Boruta DM, et al: Endometrial stromal sarcoma: a clinicopathologic study of 29 patients. J Reprod Med 59(11-12):547, 2014

Reed NS, Mangioni C, Malmstrom H, et al: Phase III randomised study to evaluate the role of adjuvant pelvic radiotherapy in the treatment of uterine sarcomas stages I and II: a European Organisation for Research and Treatment of Cancer Gynaecological Cancer Group study (protocol 55874). Eur J Cancer 44:808, 2008

Reich O, Regauer S: Survey of adjuvant hormone therapy in patients after endometrial stromal sarcoma. Eur J Gynaecol Oncol 27(2):150, 2006

Salani R, Khanna N, Frimer M, et al: An update on post-treatment surveillance and diagnosis of recurrence in women with gynecologic malignancies: Society of Gynecologic Oncology (SGO) recommendations. Gynecol Oncol 146(1):3, 2017

Seagle BL, Kanis M, Strohl AE, et al: Survival of women with mullerian adenosarcoma: a National Cancer Data Base study. Gynecol Oncol 143(3):636, 2016

Seagle BL, Shilpi A, Buchanan S, et al: Low-grade and high-grade endometrial stromal sarcoma: a National Cancer Database study. Gynecol Oncol 146(2):254, 2017a

Seagle BL, Sobecki-Rausch J, Strohl AE, et al: Prognosis and treatment of uterine leiomyosarcoma: a National Cancer Database study. Gynecol Oncol 145(1):61, 2017b

Sharma P, Kumar R, Singh H, et al: Role of FDG PET-CT in detecting recurrence in patients with uterine sarcoma: comparison with conventional imaging. Nucl Med Commun 33(2): 185, 2012

Sumi A, Terasaki H, Sanada S, et al: Assessment of MR imaging as a tool to differentiate between the major histological types of uterine sarcomas. Magn Reson Med Sci 14(4):295, 2015

Sutton GP, Stehman FB, Michael H, et al: Estrogen and progesterone receptors in uterine sarcomas. Obstet Gynecol 68(5):709, 1986

Thomas MB, Keeney GL, Podratz KC, et al: Endometrial stromal sarcoma: treatment and patterns of recurrence. Int J Gynecol Cancer 19:253, 2009

Wells M, Oliva E, Palacios J, et al: Mixed epithelial and mesenchymal tumours. In Kurman RJ, Carcangiu LM, Herrington CS, et al (eds): WHO Classification of Tumours of Female Reproductive Organs. Lyon, International Agency for Research on Cancer, 2014, p 148

Yan L, Tian Y, Zhao X: Successful pregnancy after fertility-preserving surgery for endometrial stromal sarcoma. Fertil Steril 93:269.e1, 2010

Yang GC, Wan LS, Del Priore G: Factors influencing the detection of uterine cancer by suction curettage and endometrial brushing. J Reprod Med 47(12):1005, 2002

Zaloudek C, Hendrickson MR, Soslow RA: Mesenchymal tumors of the uterus. In Kurman RJ, Ellenson LH, Ronnett BM (eds): Blaustein's Pathology of the Female Genital Tract, 6th ed. New York, Springer, 2011, p 453

Zhang P, Zhang C, Hao J, et al: Use of X-chromosome inactivation pattern to determine the clonal origins of uterine leiomyoma and leiomyosarcoma. Hum Pathol 37(10):1350, 2006

CHAPTER 35

Epithelial Ovarian Cancer

In the United States, ovarian cancer accounts for more deaths than any other gynecologic malignancy. Worldwide each year, more than 295,000 women are diagnosed, and 185,000 women die from this disease (Bray, 2018). Of these, epithelial ovarian carcinomas make up 90 percent of all cases, including the more indolent low-malignant-potential (borderline) tumors (Torre, 2018). The remainder includes germ cell and sex cord–stromal tumors, which are described in Chapter 36 (p. 756). Due to the similarities of primary peritoneal carcinomas and fallopian tube cancers, they are included within this section for simplicity.

Approximately one quarter of patients will have stage I disease and an excellent long-term survival rate. However, no test effectively screens for ovarian cancer, and early symptoms are few. As a result, two thirds of patients have advanced disease when diagnosed. Debulking surgery sequenced with platinum-based chemotherapy usually results in clinical remission. However, up to 90 percent of these women will develop a relapse that eventually leads to disease progression and death.

EPIDEMIOLOGY AND RISK FACTORS

In the United States, 1 in 78 women (1.3 percent) will develop ovarian cancer during her lifetime (Torre, 2018). Because the incidence has declined by 30 percent during the past three decades, ovarian cancer no longer resides among the top ten leading causes of cancer in women. In 2019, 22,530 new cases and 13,980 deaths are expected. Yet due to the high rate of mortality, ovarian cancer remains the fifth leading cause of cancer-related death (Siegel, 2019). Overall, the average age at diagnosis is in the early 60s.

Numerous reproductive, environmental, and genetic risk factors have been associated with ovarian cancer (Table 35-1) (Armstrong, 2019). The most important is a *family history* of breast or ovarian cancer, and up to 25 percent of patients have an inherited genetic predisposition (American College of Obstetricians and Gynecologists, 2017a). For the other 75 percent with no identifiable genetic link for their ovarian cancer, risks have traditionally been attributed to a pattern of uninterrupted ovulatory cycles during the reproductive years (Pelucchi, 2007). Repeated stimulation of the ovarian surface epithelium is hypothesized to lead to malignant transformation (Schildkraut, 1997).

Nulliparity is associated with long periods of repetitive ovulation, and patients without children have double the risk of developing ovarian cancer (Purdie, 2003). Among nulliparas, those with a history of infertility have an even higher risk. This association is thought to reflect an inherent ovarian predisposition rather than an iatrogenic effect of ovulation-inducing drugs. For example, women treated for infertility who successfully

TABLE 35-1. Risk Factors for Developing Epithelial Ovarian Cancer

Nulliparity
Early menarche
Late menopause
White race
Increasing age
Residence in North America and Northern Europe
Family history
Personal history of breast cancer
Ethnic background (European Jewish, Icelandic, Hungarian)
Postmenopausal hormone therapy
Pelvic inflammatory disease

Modified from Schorge, 2010, with permission.

achieve a live birth do not have a greater risk of ovarian cancer (Rossing, 2004). For all women, risks decrease with each live birth, eventually plateauing in women delivering five times (Hinkula, 2006).

Early menarche and *late menopause* also are associated risks. In contrast, breastfeeding has a protective effect, perhaps by prolonging anovulation (Yen, 2003). Presumably by also preventing ovulation, long-term combination oral contraceptive (COC) use reduces the risk of ovarian cancer by up to 50 percent. The duration of protection persists for more than 30 years after the last use (Collaborative Group on Epidemiological Studies of Ovarian Cancer, 2008). In contrast, hormone replacement therapy after menopause carries an elevated associated risk (Lee, 2016).

White women have the highest incidence of ovarian cancer among all racial and ethnic groups. Compared with that of black and Hispanic women, the risk is elevated by 30 to 40 percent (Torre, 2018). Racial discrepancies in parity and rates of gynecologic surgery are believed to account for some of the differences.

Tubal ligation and *hysterectomy* are each associated with a substantial reduction in risk (Rice, 2014). Theoretically, any gynecologic procedure that precludes irritants from reaching the ovaries via ascension from the lower genital tract might plausibly exert a similar protective effect. In turn, women who regularly use perineal talc may possibly have an increased risk (Cramer, 2016; Penninkilampi, 2018).

Women *residing in North America, Northern or Eastern Europe,* or *any industrialized Western country* have a higher ovarian cancer risk. Globally, the incidence varies greatly, but developing countries have approximately half the rate (Torre, 2015, 2017). Regional dietary habits may be partly responsible (Kiani, 2006). For example, consumption of foods low in fat but high in fiber, carotene, and vitamins appears protective (Zhang, 2004).

Most epithelial ovarian cancers are now believed to actually originate in the fallopian tube fimbria. This recognition makes it difficult to reconcile these listed risk factors and current theories of carcinogenesis (American College of Obstetricians and Gynecologists, 2019). New biologically plausible theories will be required.

■ Hereditary Breast and Ovarian Cancer

Genetic Screening

A family history of ovarian cancer in a first-degree relative, that is, a mother, daughter, or sister, triples a woman's lifetime risk. Two or more afflicted first-degree relatives or other individuals with premenopausal breast cancer further escalate risk. Approximately 75 percent of inherited ovarian cancers result from germline mutations in the *BRCA1*, *BRCA2*, or other homologous recombination deficiency genes. Thus, any patient with a personal history of epithelial ovarian cancer or breast cancer in certain circumstances or those from a family carrying a known deleterious mutation should undergo testing (Table 35-2) (Lancaster, 2015).

If a family history is mainly composed of colon cancer, clinicians may consider Lynch syndrome, also known as *hereditary nonpolyposis colorectal cancer (HNPCC)*. Patients with this syndrome have a high lifetime risk of colon cancer (85 percent) and ovarian cancer (10 to 12 percent). Endometrial cancer is the predominant gynecologic malignancy, and women with the syndrome have a 40 to 60 percent lifetime risk for this cancer. HNPCC is described in more detail in the endometrial cancer chapter (Chap. 33, p. 700).

Typically, an individual is referred to a certified genetic counselor, and a comprehensive pedigree is constructed first. Then, risk assessment is performed using one of several validated population models. These include the BRCAPRO and Tyrer-Cuzick programs, which are available, respectively, at http://www4.utsouthwestern.edu/breasthealth/cagene/ and by contacting the International Breast Cancer Intervention Study (IBIS) at ibis@cancer.org.uk. These models and their associated software quantify an individual's risk for carrying a germline deleterious mutation.

TABLE 35-2. Women Who Should Undergo Genetic Testing

Epithelial ovarian cancer[a] at any age
Breast cancer diagnosed at age 45 or younger
Breast cancer with two distinct and sequential primaries, first one diagnosed at age 50 or younger
Breast cancer that is triple-negative and diagnosed at age 60 or younger
Breast cancer at any age, with at least one close relative[b] diagnosed at age 50 or younger
Breast cancer diagnosed at any age, with two or more close relatives with breast cancer; one close relative with epithelial ovarian cancer; or two close relatives with pancreatic cancer or aggressive prostate cancer
Breast cancer, with a close male relative with breast cancer at any age
Breast cancer and Ashkenazi Jewish ancestry
Individuals from a family with a known deleterious mutation (see Table 35-3)

---

[a]Throughout table, peritoneal and fallopian tube cancer are considered as part of the spectrum of the Hereditary Breast/Ovarian Cancer syndrome.
[b]Throughout table, *close relative* is defined as a first-, second-, or third-degree relative (i.e., mother, sister, daughter, aunt, niece, grandmother, granddaughter, first cousin, great grandmother, great aunt).
Adapted from Lancaster, 2015 with permission.

BRCA1 and *BRCA2* Genes

These are tumor-suppressor genes whose protein products are BRCA1 and BRCA2. These two proteins provide double-stranded DNA repair through the process of *homologous recombination (HR)* to preserve intact chromosomal structure. Mutations of *BRCA1* and *BRCA2* genes lead to BRCA1 and BRCA2 protein dysfunction, which results in genetic instability and subjects cells to a higher risk of malignant transformation.

The *BRCA1* gene is located on chromosome 17q21. Patients with a proven mutation have a dramatically elevated risk of developing ovarian cancer (39 to 46 percent). *BRCA2* is located on chromosome 13q12 and in general is less likely to lead to ovarian cancer (10 to 27 percent). The estimated lifetime risk of breast cancer with a *BRCA1* or *BRCA2* mutation is 45 to 85 percent (American College of Obstetricians and Gynecologists, 2017a).

Until recently, it was thought that HR was performed almost exclusively by the *BRCA1* and *BRCA2* genes. Instead, up to one quarter of predisposing germline mutations is due to another of the HR deficiency genes (Table 35-3) (American College of Obstetricians and Gynecologists, 2017a; Ring, 2017). All of these genes are inherited in an autosomal dominant fashion but show variable penetrance. Thus, although a carrier will pass the gene to a son or daughter in 50 percent of cases, the offspring with the gene mutation may or may not actually develop breast or ovarian cancer. As a result, *BRCA1* or *BRCA2* or other HR deficiency gene mutations can appear to skip generations.

Genetic Testing

The two main genetic testing options for hereditary breast and ovarian cancer syndrome are *BRCA* mutation testing or multigene panel testing that includes *BRCA* and other genetic mutations. The choice of testing strategy will depend on whether or

TABLE 35-3. Genes Associated with Breast or Ovarian Cancer

Genetic Syndrome	Gene	Breast Cancer Risk[a]	Ovary Cancer Risk[a,b]	Other Cancer Risk	Risk-Reduction Strategy (age to consider)
HBOC	*BRCA1*	↑	↑	Prostate	RRSO (35–40 y)
HBOC	*BRCA2*	↑	↑	Melanoma, pancreas, prostate	RRSO (40–45 y)
Lynch	*MLH1, MSH2, EPCAM, MSH6, PMS2*	?	↑	Uterus, colon, renal pelvis, small bowel + others	RRSO after childbearing (35–40 y) Risk-reducing hysterectomy after childbearing
HOC	*BRIP1*	—	↑	?	Consider RRSO (45–50 y)
HOC	*RAD51C*	—	↑	?	Consider RRSO (45–50 y)
HOC	*RAD51D*	—	↑	?	Consider RRSO (45–50 y)
Peutz-Jeghers	*STK11*	↑	↑ SCST	Colorectal, stomach, small bowel, pancreas	No recommendations
Cowden	*PTEN*	↑	—	Uterus, thyroid, renal, colorectal	Discuss hysterectomy after childbearing
Li-Fraumeni	*TP53*	↑	—	Sarcomas, brain, leukemia, medulloblastoma, adrenocortical	No recommendations
Ataxia-telangiectasia	*ATM*	↑	—	—	No recommendations
Hereditary diffuse gastric cancer	*CDH1*	↑	—	Stomach	No recommendations
_____	*CHEK2*	↑	—	Colon	No recommendations
_____	*PALB2*	↑	—	?	No recommendations

[a]Legend: ↑ = increased risk; — = no increased risk; ? = insufficient evidence or unknown.
[b]Includes fallopian tube and primary peritoneal cancers.
HBOC = hereditary breast and ovarian cancer; HOC = hereditary ovarian cancer; RRSO = risk-reducing salpingo-oophorectomy; SCST = sex cord–stromal tumor.

not a specific mutation is known within the family (American College of Obstetricians and Gynecologists, 2017a). Ideally, genetic testing identifies women with deleterious mutations, leads to intervention with prophylactic surgery, and thereby prevents ovarian cancer.

Four distinct results are possible with this testing. A "true positive" test suggests the presence of a deleterious mutation. The most common are 185delAG or 5382insC in *BRCA1* and 6174delT in *BRCA2*. Each of these "frameshift" mutations significantly alters the downstream amino acid sequence, resulting in an altered BRCA1 or BRCA2 tumor suppressor protein.

Second, "variants of uncertain clinical significance" may actually be pathogenic (true mutations) or just polymorphisms (normal variants found in at least 1 percent of alleles in the general population). These unclassified variants are common, representing approximately one third of *BRCA1* test results and half of those for *BRCA2*. Most are missense mutations, which result in a single amino acid change in the protein but without a frameshift. Given the prognostic uncertainty and high rate of reclassification, individualized counseling and directing efforts toward surveillance, chemoprevention, or salpingectomy are recommended (Garcia, 2014).

The third potential and most reassuring genetic test result is "true negative." This indicates the absence of a deleterious mutation in an individual who has relatives with cancer and a known pathogenic variant in the family.

The fourth possible outcome is "uninformative negative," which indicates the absence of a deleterious mutation in an individual. However the test is inconclusive because other cancer-affected family members have not tested positive for the given mutation. In this case, the affected family members may have no high-risk mutation or it may be undetectable (American College of Obstetricians and Gynecologists, 2017a). For example, due to the large size of the *BRCA1* and *BRCA2* genes, the false-negative rate is 5 to 10 percent. To capture additional, otherwise undetected large genomic rearrangements in *BRCA* and to expand the testing for other HR deficiency genes, individuals with a negative test result 5 to 10 years ago might need to be retested.

PREVENTION

▨ Ovarian Cancer Screening

In addition to genetic testing, other screening strategies for ovarian cancer have been evaluated. However, despite enormous effort, no evidence suggests that routine screening with serum markers, sonography, or pelvic examinations lowers mortality rates. Hundreds of possible markers have been identified, yet no test currently available approaches sufficient levels of accuracy (American College of Obstetricians and Gynecologists, 2017b). Consequently, the U.S. Preventive Services Task Force (2018) recommends against screening in asymptomatic women who are not known to have a high-risk inherited syndrome.

High-Risk Women

Screening strategies are mainly directed at *BRCA1* or *BRCA2* carriers and women with a strong family history of breast and

ovarian cancer. Even so, cancer antigen 125 (CA125) serum level measurements and/or transvaginal sonography are not routinely recommended. An exception is their use in women at high-risk for short-term surveillance starting at age 30 to 35 years and continuing until risk-reducing surgery (American College of Obstetricians and Gynecologists, 2017a).

CA125 is a glycoprotein that is not produced by normal ovarian epithelium but that may be produced by both benign and malignant ovarian tumors. CA125 is synthesized within affected ovarian epithelial cells and often secreted into cysts. In benign tumors, excess antigen is released into and may accumulate within cyst fluid. Hypothetically, the abnormal tissue architecture associated with malignant tumors allows antigen release into the vascular circulation (Verheijen, 1999).

Alone, CA125 is a poor marker for ovarian cancer detection. However, a more sensitive *R*isk of *O*varian *C*ancer *A*lgorithm (ROCA) is based on the slope of serial CA125 measurements drawn at regular intervals (Skates, 2003). If a ROCA score exceeds a 1-percent risk of having ovarian cancer, patients then undergo transvaginal sonography to determine whether additional intervention is warranted. This strategy, in 3692 high-risk women, demonstrated somewhat better ability to detect ovarian cancer at an early stage. However, it still was deemed not very clinically useful (Skates, 2017).

General Population

To establish the effect of ROCA-based CA125 screening and study-directed sonography, a randomized trial of 202,638 patients was conducted. In The United Kingdom Collaborative Trial of Ovarian Cancer Screening (UKCTOCS), asymptomatic, average-risk postmenopausal women aged 50 to 74 years were randomly assigned to no treatment, to annual CA125 screening with transvaginal sonography as a second-line test if indicated by ROCA interpretation, or to annual screening with transvaginal sonography. The ROCA-directed approach demonstrated a 35-percent positive predictive value, more than 10 times higher than annual sonography (3 percent). Although ROCA-directed sonography was shown to be feasible in this study, the mortality rate reduction was not significant (Jacobs, 2016). Because no sufficiently accurate early detection tests are currently available, routine screening for women at average risk is not recommended (U.S. Preventive Services Task Force, 2018).

Physical Examination

In general, pelvic examination only occasionally detects ovarian cancer, generally when the disease is already in advanced stages. In asymptomatic women, there is no evidence that it lowers mortality or morbidity rates as a screening test (Bloomfield, 2014; U.S. Preventive Services Task Force, 2017).

Chemoprevention

Noted on page 733, COC use is associated with an up to 50-percent decreased risk of developing ovarian cancer. More than 200,000 cases of this cancer and 100,000 deaths are estimated to have been prevented by COC use (Collaborative Group on Epidemiological Studies of Ovarian Cancer, 2008). Emerging evidence suggests that intrauterine devices also may reduce the risk (Jareid, 2018). Discussed in Chapter 5 (p. 126), the slightly higher risk of breast cancer during current COC use should be presented during patient counseling (Mørch, 2017).

COCs are suitable for women with a high-risk inherited syndrome and similarly can lower later ovarian cancer rates (Friebel, 2014). Rates of breast cancer linked to COC use do not appear elevated in this group (Iodice, 2010; Moorman, 2013).

Prophylactic Surgery

The only proven way to directly prevent ovarian cancer is surgical removal. However, premenopausal oophorectomy has several negative health consequences (Chap. 43, p. 957). Moreover, with growing recognition that carcinogenesis actually originates on the fallopian tube fimbria, consideration of opportunistic salpingectomy at the time of gynecologic surgery or in place of tubal ligation has revolutionized the approach to risk-reduction in the general population (American College of Obstetricians and Gynecologists, 2019).

In women at high risk of ovarian cancer from known mutations, bilateral salpingectomy alone is not currently recommended for ovarian cancer risk reduction. However, clinical trials are underway to determine whether prophylactic salpingectomy–delayed oophorectomy (PSDO) is an effective strategy. Currently, in these high-risk women, prophylactic bilateral salpingo-oophorectomy (BSO) still is recommended.

The procedure's timing can be individualized depending on the particular genetic mutation, the patient's desires for further childbearing, and her family history. In general, prophylactic BSO should be offered to *BRCA1* carriers at age 35 to 40 years. For *BRCA2* carriers, BSO is recommended between 40 and 45, and at age 45 to 50 years for other HR deficiency (*BRIP1*, *RAD51C*) carriers (American College of Obstetricians and Gynecologists, 2017a).

In these patients, the procedure is approximately 90-percent effective in preventing epithelial ovarian cancer (Kauff, 2002; Rebbeck, 2002). Prophylactic BSO also reduces the risk of developing breast cancer by 50 percent (Rebbeck, 2002). Predictably, the protective effect is strongest among premenopausal women (Kramer, 2005). In women with HNPCC, the ovarian cancer risk reduction approaches 100 percent (Schmeler, 2006).

The term *prophylactic* implies that the tubes and ovaries are normal at the time of removal. However, approximately 5 percent of *BRCA* mutation carriers undergoing prophylactic BSO will have an otherwise undetected, often microscopic, fallopian tube cancer at the time of surgery (Manchanda, 2011; Sherman, 2014). To account for this possibility, cytologic washings should be collected during surgery. Peritoneal surfaces are thoroughly inspected, and abnormal areas are biopsied. Last, the pathology requisition should clearly state that the BSO was performed for a prophylactic indication. In these cases, the ovaries and tubes, especially the fimbria, undergo more intensive scrutiny and are serially microsectioned to identify occult disease. Using a rigorous operative and pathologic protocol such as this can significantly raise the detection rate of occult tubal or ovarian malignancy in carriers of *BRCA* mutations (American College of Obstetricians and Gynecologists, 2017a). Typically, the BSO, washings collection, and peritoneal biopsy can be completed laparoscopically.

Prophylactic BSO in young women will induce premature menopause and its associated vasomotor and urogenital symptoms, decline in sexual interest, and osteoporosis. Estrogen therapy (ET) commonly is used to alleviate these symptoms in women without prior breast cancer (American College of Obstetricians and Gynecologists, 2019). Other ET contraindications and options are found in Chapter 22 (p. 480) Overall, mainly due to the favorable reduction in cancer worries, prophylactic BSO does not adversely affect quality of life (Madalinska, 2005).

In women with HNPCC syndrome, hysterectomy is mandatory when performing prophylactic BSO because of coexisting endometrial cancer risks. In *BRCA* mutation carriers, hysterectomy should not be recommended routinely (Vyarvelska, 2014). Few reports have suggested a meaningful association between *BRCA* mutations and a greater risk of endometrial cancer. Mainly, these develop in patients taking tamoxifen for breast cancer treatment or for breast cancer chemoprevention (Beiner, 2007).

In low-risk patients who are not *BRCA* carriers, risk-reducing salpingectomy also is now considered in those undergoing hysterectomy or permanent sterilization. Ovarian cancer risk is reduced up to 65 percent (Falconer, 2015; Lessard-Anderson, 2014). This consideration has been endorsed by both the Society of Gynecologic Oncology (Walker, 2015) and the American College of Obstetricians and Gynecologists (2019). Pathologic specimen processing in low-risk women includes representative sections of the tube, any suspicious lesions, and entire sectioning of the fimbriae. Neither organization specifies pelvic washing collection in this low-risk population.

LOW-MALIGNANT-POTENTIAL TUMORS

■ Pathology

Ten to 15 percent of epithelial ovarian cancers have histologic and biologic features that are intermediate between clearly benign cysts and frankly invasive carcinomas. In general, these low-malignant-potential (LMP) tumors, also termed *borderline tumors*, are associated with risk factors that are similar to those for epithelial ovarian cancer (Huusom, 2006). Typically, they are not considered part of any of the hereditary breast-ovarian cancer syndromes. Although LMP tumors may develop at any age, on average, patients are in their mid-40s, which is 15 years younger than women with invasive ovarian carcinoma. For various reasons, their diagnosis and optimal management are frequently problematic.

Histologically, LMP tumors are distinguished from benign cysts by having at least two of the following features: nuclear atypia, epithelial stratification, microscopic papillary projections, cellular pleomorphism, or mitotic activity (Fig. 35-1). Unlike invasive carcinomas, LMP tumors lack stromal invasion. However, up to 10 percent of LMP tumors will exhibit areas of *microinvasion*, defined as foci measuring <3 mm in diameter and forming <5 percent of the tumor (Buttin, 2002). Due to the subtle nature of many of these findings, it is challenging to diagnose an LMP tumor with certainty based on intraoperative frozen section specimen analysis.

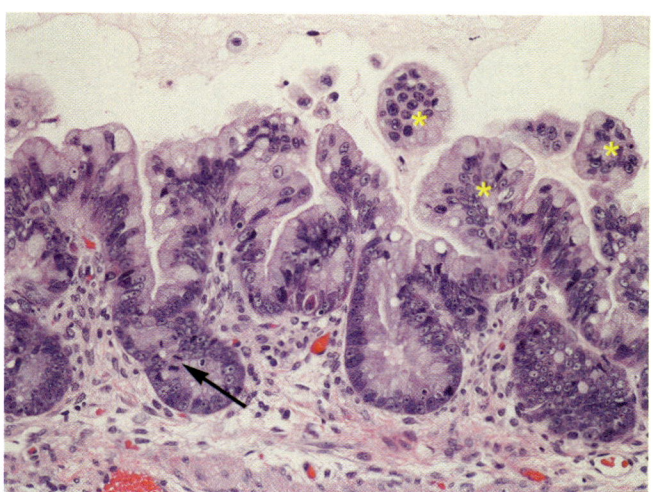

FIGURE 35-1 Mucinous borderline tumor/atypical proliferative mucinous tumor. These tumors are distinguished from benign mucinous cystadenomas by epithelial proliferation and nuclear atypia. This example of a mucinous borderline tumor has mild to moderate nuclear atypia as evidenced by limited nuclear pleomorphism and visible nucleoli. A mitotic figure also is seen (*arrow*). Epithelial proliferation is indicated by epithelial tufts (*asterisks*), which are unsupported by fibrovascular cores. (Reproduced with permission from Dr. Kelley Carrick.)

CHAPTER 35

■ Clinical Features

Ovarian LMP tumors present similar to other adnexal masses. Preoperatively, no sonographic findings are pathognomonic, and serum CA125 levels are nonspecific. Depending on the clinical setting, computed tomography (CT) scanning may be indicated to exclude ascites or omental caking, which would suggest a more typical ovarian cancer. Regardless, any woman with a suspicious adnexal mass should have it removed.

■ Treatment

LMP tumors are primarily managed surgically. The operative plan will vary, depending on circumstances, and patients are carefully counseled beforehand. All women should be prepared for complete ovarian cancer surgical staging or debulking, if necessary. In many cases, a laparoscopic approach is appropriate. If laparotomy is planned, a vertical incision is selected to allow access to the upper abdomen and paraaortic nodes, if needed, for cancer staging.

During surgery, peritoneal washings are immediately collected upon entrance into the abdomen, which is then carefully explored. The ovarian mass is removed intact and submitted for pathologic consultation and frozen section evaluation. However, differentiating a benign adnexal mass, LMP tumor, or invasive ovarian cancer is almost impossible until final histologic slides have been reviewed (Shah, 2019). Accordingly, premenopausal women who have not completed childbearing and who are intraoperatively diagnosed with an LMP tumor may undergo fertility-sparing surgery. This approach preserves the uterus and contralateral ovary (Delle Marchette, 2019). This is a reasonable approach even if the final diagnosis shows invasive stage I cancer (Fruscio, 2016). Alternatively, postmenopausal women should undergo hysterectomy and BSO.

Biopsies of the peritoneum and omentum as a part of limited ovarian cancer staging are considered. However, they rarely contain microscopic foci of metastatic LMP tumor unless the tissues appear abnormal (Kristensen, 2014). Additionally, the appendix also is examined and potentially removed, especially if the tumor has mucinous histology (Timofeev, 2010). Without enlarged lymph nodes or a frozen section suggestive of frankly invasive disease, routine pelvic and paraaortic lymph node dissection may not be necessary (Rao, 2004).

LMP tumors are staged with the same FIGO criteria used for invasive ovarian cancer (p. 747). For the most part, surgical staging has limited value in altering the prognosis of those with LMP tumors unless invasive cancer is ultimately diagnosed (Wingo, 2006). Although 97 percent of gynecologic oncologists advocate comprehensive surgical staging of LMP tumors, in current practice it is performed in only 12 percent of patients (Lin, 1999; Menzin, 2000). This disparity stems from the fact that often the diagnosis is not suspected intraoperatively, no frozen section is requested or it is inaccurate, and a clinician is alerted only when the final pathology report has been completed. In this circumstance, consultation with a gynecologic oncologist is recommended, but comprehensive surgical restaging is not necessarily required if the tumor appears confined to a single ovary (Zapardiel, 2010). However, if a cystectomy has been performed, the risk of residual disease should prompt a discussion regarding removal of the entire adnexa with washings and limited staging (Poncelet, 2006).

For patients with stage II–IV disease, usually demonstrated by noninvasive implants (Fig. 35-2) or nodal metastases, the utility of adjuvant chemotherapy is speculative (Shih, 2010; Sutton, 1991). The most worrisome finding is invasive peritoneal or omental implants. In general, these patients are treated like those with typical epithelial ovarian carcinoma and receive surgical debulking and postoperative chemotherapy (Leary, 2014).

■ Prognosis

The prognosis is excellent for patients with ovarian LMP tumors. Five-year survival rates range from 96 to 99 percent for stages I–III, whereas it reaches 77 percent for stage IV disease (Trimble, 2002). Overall, more than 80 percent have stage I disease. If treated by hysterectomy and BSO, stage I tumors rarely, if ever, recur (du Bois, 2013). In fact, such women have an overall survival rate similar to the general population (Hannibal, 2014). Fertility-sparing surgery is associated with up to a 15-percent risk of relapse, usually in the contralateral ovary, but remains highly curable by reoperation and resection (Park, 2009; Rao, 2005).

Approximately 15 percent of women with LMP tumors have stage II and III disease, which almost invariably is serous histology. Stage IV ovarian LMP tumors account for fewer than 5 percent of diagnoses and have the worst prognosis (Trimble, 2002). For these advanced-stage tumors, the most reliable prognostic indicators are the presence of invasive peritoneal implants or residual disease after primary surgery and tumor debulking (Morice, 2012; Seidman, 2000).

Due to the indolent nature of these tumors, symptomatic recurrence often follows years or even decades after the initial

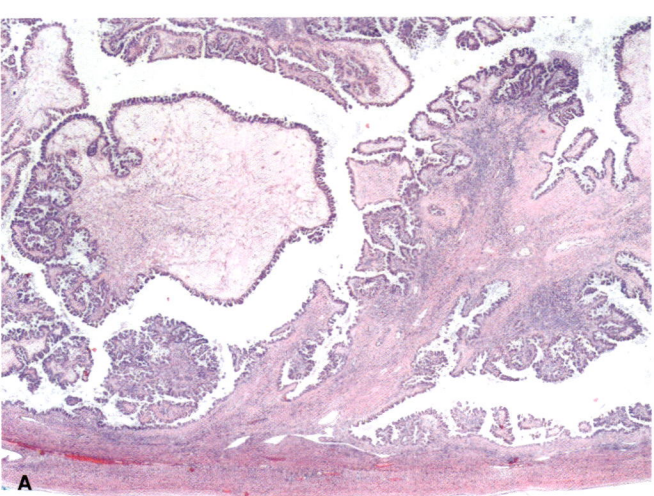
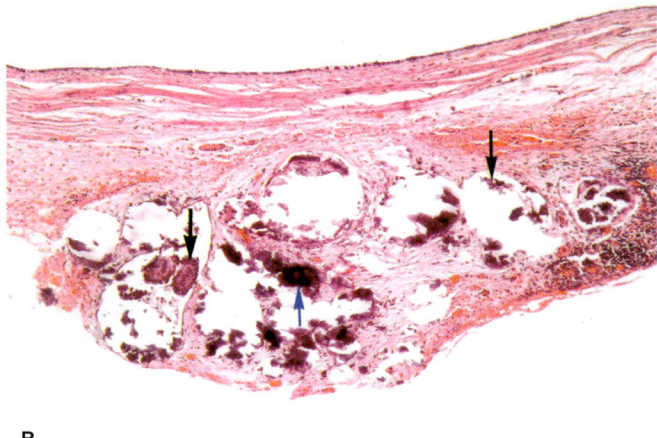

FIGURE 35-2 A. Serous borderline tumor/atypical proliferative serous tumor. These tumors are noninvasive tumors characterized by branching stromal papillae lined by cuboidal to columnar nonmucinous cells with minimal cytologic atypia. Papillae show a varying degree of epithelial proliferation, indicated by stratification or tufting. (Reproduced with permission from Dr. Kelley Carrick.) **B.** A noninvasive implant of a serous borderline tumor. Bland proliferative serous-type epithelium (*black arrows*) and associated psammoma bodies (*blue arrow*) adhere to the underlying tissue but do not invade it. The proliferative serous epithelium forms small clusters and papillary structures. Psammoma bodies, concentrically lamellated calcifications, are often associated with benign or malignant ovarian serous tumors. The artifactual shattering seen here is due to the calcified psammoma bodies. (Reproduced with permission from Dr. Raheela Ashfaq.)

diagnosis (Silva, 2006). Approximately 70 percent of relapses show only LMP histology. Malignant transformation into an invasive ovarian cancer develops in the other 30 percent. Most of these are low-grade carcinomas, but approximately one third will have high-grade features, which adversely affects prognosis (du Bois, 2013; Harter, 2014). As in primary ovarian LMP tumors, complete surgical excision is the most effective therapy for recurrent disease (Crane, 2015). Cytotoxic chemotherapy is reserved for patients with invasive features, but low-grade tumors tend to be particularly resistant to standard agents. Hormonal therapy is increasingly used with good results and much less toxicity (Gershenson, 2017; Tang, 2019).

EPITHELIAL OVARIAN CANCER

■ Pathogenesis

At least two distinct, albeit controversial, tumorigenic pathways account for epithelial ovarian cancer's heterogeneity (Table 35-4) (Kurman, 2016). The first tumor group develops either from benign extraovarian lesions that implant on the ovary and subsequently undergo malignant transformation or

from a portion of the ovarian surface epithelium that becomes entrapped within the ovarian cortex. This trapped cortical inclusion cyst undergoes müllerian metaplasia and is exposed to hormone and inflammatory stimuli that induce DNA damage and mutations. These mutations can thereby transform the metaplastic cyst into a mucinous, endometrioid, or low-grade serous carcinoma (Levanon, 2008). These tumors usually present as large, unilateral, cystic neoplasms without ascites. They are clinically indolent, are diagnosed early, and account for only 10 percent of ovarian cancer deaths. Shown in Table 35-4, this first group is divided into endometriosis-associated tumors, low-grade serous carcinomas, and mucinous carcinomas plus malignant Brenner tumors (Kurman, 2016).

The second, more common group invariably contains high-grade serous carcinomas arising from the fallopian tube fimbria. This group was formerly thought to arise spontaneously on the ovarian or peritoneal surface. Although the neoplastic transformational trigger of the fallopian tube cells is unclear, serous tubal intraepithelial carcinoma (STIC) is a precursor condition (Fig. 35-3). STIC develops several years before initiation of ovarian carcinoma, yet metastases follow rapidly thereafter (Labidi-Galy, 2017).

TABLE 35-4. Dualistic Model of Ovarian Cancer Genesis

TYPE I				TYPE II
Endometriosis	**Fallopian Tube**	**Germ Cell**	**Transitional Cell**	**Fallopian Tube**

Endometrioid
Clear cell
Seromucinous
	Low-grade serous	Mucinous	Mucinous
			Brenner tumor
				High-grade serous
				  Histologic subtype:
				    Usual type
				    Transitional cell type
				  Carcinosarcoma
				  Undifferentiated carcinoma

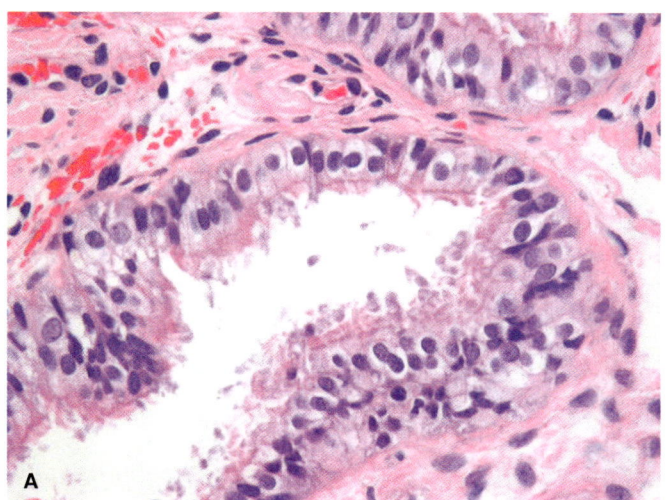 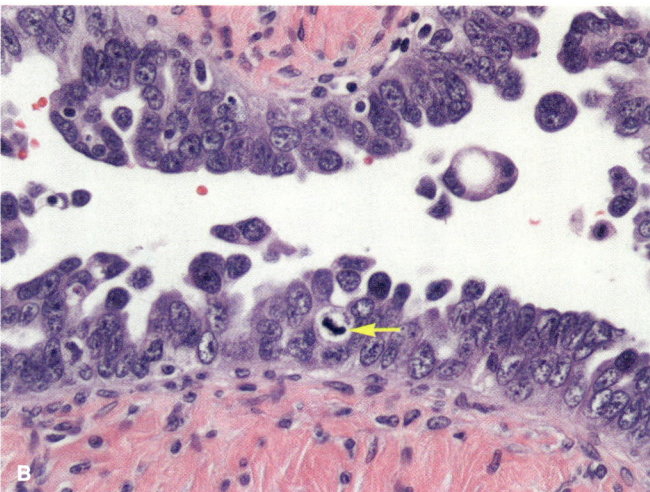

FIGURE 35-3 A. Normal fallopian tube epithelium is composed of three cell types—columnar ciliated cells, nonciliated secretory (peg) cells, and intercalary cells. **B.** Serous tubal intraepithelial carcinoma (STIC). The cells of serous carcinoma lining this fallopian tube are markedly atypical, with nuclear pleomorphism, chromatin coarseness, loss of nuclear polarity, increased nuclear/cytoplasmic ratio, and mitotic activity (*arrow*). Epithelial proliferation/tufting and loss of cell cohesion lead to cell shedding into the tubal lumen. (Reproduced with permission from Dr. Kelley Carrick.)

Approximately half of these tumors are characterized by mutations in genes involved in the HR pathway of DNA repair, especially *BRCA1* and *BRCA2* (Kroeger, 2017). Most of these mutations result from an inherited predisposition. For example, women born with a *BRCA* mutation require only one "hit" to the other normal copy (allele) to "knock out" the *BRCA* tumor-suppressor gene product. As a result, BRCA-related cancers develop approximately 15 years before sporadic cases. Alternatively, the tumor itself may develop a somatic mutation that deactivates BRCA's tumor suppression. As a result, current practice is for a woman to undergo both germline and tumor testing for *BRCA* and HR deficiency gene mutations.

High-grade serous tumors are aggressive, are diagnosed at advanced stages more than three quarters of the time, and display a greater volume of extraovarian disease and significant ascites. These tumors account for 90 percent of ovarian cancer deaths (Kurman, 2016).

■ Diagnosis

Symptoms and Physical Findings

Ovarian cancer is typically portrayed as a "silent" killer that lacks appreciable early signs or symptoms. This is a misconception. Actually, patients often are symptomatic for several months before the diagnosis, even with early-stage disease (Goff, 2000). The difficulty is distinguishing these symptoms from those that normally occur in women.

In general, persistent symptoms that are more severe or frequent than expected and have a recent onset merit further diagnostic investigation. Commonly, increased abdominal size, bloating, urinary urgency, and pelvic pain are reported. Fatigue, indigestion, inability to eat normally, constipation, and back pain also may be noted (Goff, 2004). Abnormal vaginal bleeding is rare. Occasionally, patients present with nausea, vomiting, and a partial bowel obstruction if carcinomatosis is particularly widespread. Unfortunately, women and clinicians

often attribute most symptoms to menopause, aging, dietary changes, stress, depression, or functional bowel problems, and thus diagnosis is delayed.

A pelvic or abdominopelvic mass is palpable in most patients with ovarian cancer during bimanual evaluation. Malignant tumors tend to be solid, nodular, and fixed, but no classic findings reliably distinguish these growths from benign tumors. Paradoxically, a huge mass filling the pelvis and abdomen more often represents a benign or borderline tumor. To aid surgical planning, a rectovaginal examination also is performed. For example, a woman with tumor involving the rectovaginal septum may need to be positioned in dorsal lithotomy to perform a low anterior colon resection.

An abdominal fluid wave or, less commonly, flank bulging suggests significant ascites. In a woman with a pelvic mass and ascites, the diagnosis is ovarian cancer until proven otherwise. However, ascites without an identifiable pelvic mass suggests the possibility of cirrhosis or primary malignancies from the stomach or pancreas. In advanced disease, examination of the upper abdomen usually reveals a central mass signifying omental caking. Although rare, an umbilical nodule, the "Sister Mary Joseph sign," reflects spread from an intraabdominal malignancy.

Auscultation of the chest also is important, since patients with malignant pleural effusions may not be overtly symptomatic. The remainder of the examination includes palpation of the peripheral nodes in addition to a general physical assessment.

Laboratory Testing

A routine complete blood count and metabolic panel often demonstrates a few characteristic features. Of affected women, 20 to 25 percent will present with thrombocytosis (platelet count $>400 \times 10^9$/L) (Li, 2004). Malignant ovarian cells releasing cytokines are believed to raise platelet production rates. Hyponatremia, typically ranging between 125 and 130 mEq/L, is another common finding. In these patients, tumor secretion of a vasopressin-like substance can cause a clinical picture suggesting a syndrome of inappropriate antidiuretic hormone (SIADH).

The serum CA125 level is integral to epithelial ovarian cancer management. In 90 percent of women presenting with malignant nonmucinous tumors, CA125 levels are elevated. However, there are caveats to bear in mind during adnexal mass evaluation. Half of stage I ovarian cancers will have a normal CA125 measurement (false negative). Also, an elevated value (false positive) may be associated with various common benign indications such as pelvic inflammatory disease, endometriosis, leiomyomas, pregnancy, and even menstruation. Thus, in postmenopausal women with a pelvic mass, a CA125 measurement may better predict a higher likelihood of malignancy (Table 10-1, p. 220) (Im, 2005).

Another marker, the human epididymal protein 4 (HE4) tumor marker, is approved by the U.S. Food and Drug Administration (FDA), along with CA125, when used in the Risk of Ovarian Malignancy Algorithm (ROMA). This algorithm predicts the likelihood of finding malignancy at surgery in a woman with an adnexal mass. The ROMA score is derived from the results of both blood tests plus menopausal status (Moore, 2009, 2010).

OVA1 is another biomarker blood test panel that may be used for the preoperative triage of women with an identified ovarian mass when surgery is planned (Ueland, 2011; Ware Miller, 2011). Scores ≥5.0 in premenopausal and scores ≥4.4 in postmenopausal women suggest a need for gynecologic oncologist consultation. Importantly, this test is not a screening tool and is reserved for those with a known surgical mass to aid preoperative triage (Zhang, 2010).

Validation studies evaluating ROMA and OVA1 are limited, and their role in preoperative triage is yet to be clearly defined. As a result, they are not necessarily recommended for determining the status of an identified but undiagnosed pelvic mass (Armstrong, 2019).

Similarly, the risk of malignancy index (RMI) algorithm factors menopausal status, CA125 serum level, and sonographic score. This last element is derived from ovarian appearance, and presence of ascites or intraabdominal metastases (Jacobs, 1990; Karlsen, 2012).

When a mucinous ovarian tumor is suspected or found, cancer antigen 19-9 (CA19-9) and carcinoembryonic antigen (CEA) serum tumor markers may be better indicators. Markers that more suitably reflect germ cell tumors or sex cord–stromal tumors are found in Tables 36-1 and 36-4 (p. 757).

Imaging

Transvaginal sonography is typically the most useful imaging test to differentiate benign tumors and early-stage ovarian cancers (Chap. 10, p. 221). In general, malignant tumors are multiloculated, solid or echogenic, and large (>5 cm), and they have thick septa with areas of nodularity (Fig. 35-4A). Other features may include papillary projections or neovascularization—demonstrated by adding color Doppler (Figs. 35-4B and 35-4C). Although several presumptive imaging models have been described to help distinguish benign masses from ovarian

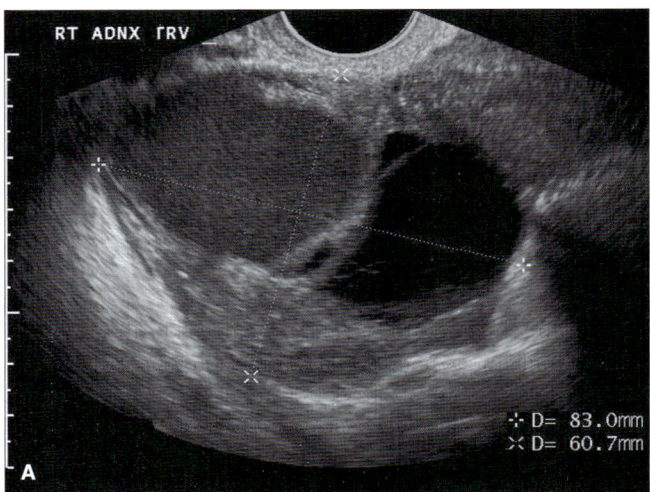

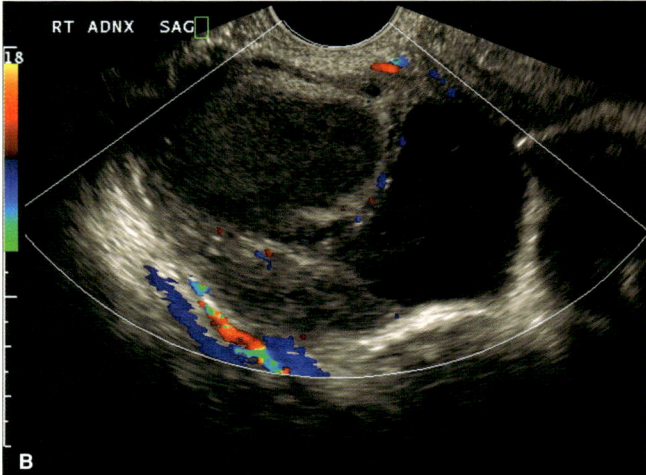

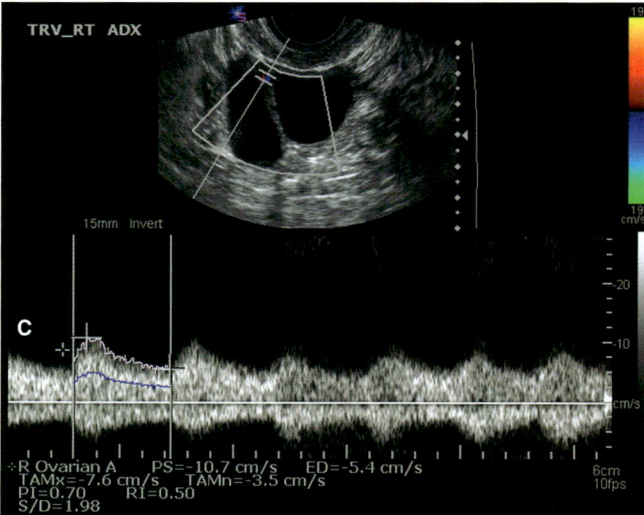

FIGURE 35-4 Sonograms of an ovarian cyst. **A.** Transvaginal sonogram depicts a complex ovarian mass. Cystic and solid components and a thick intracystic septum are seen. These findings raise clinical concern for malignancy. **B.** Color Doppler transvaginal sonogram shows neovascularization within this ovarian tumor. **C.** Transvaginal Doppler study of ovarian mass vessels reveals decreased impedance. (Reproduced with permission from Dr. Diane Twickler.)

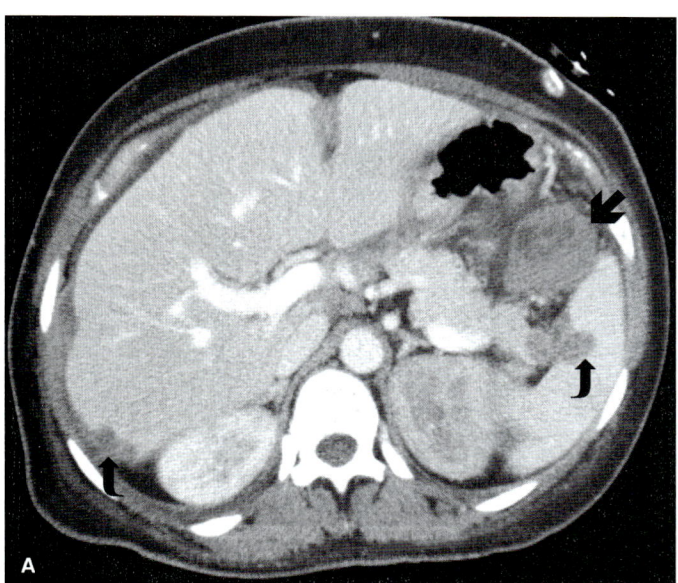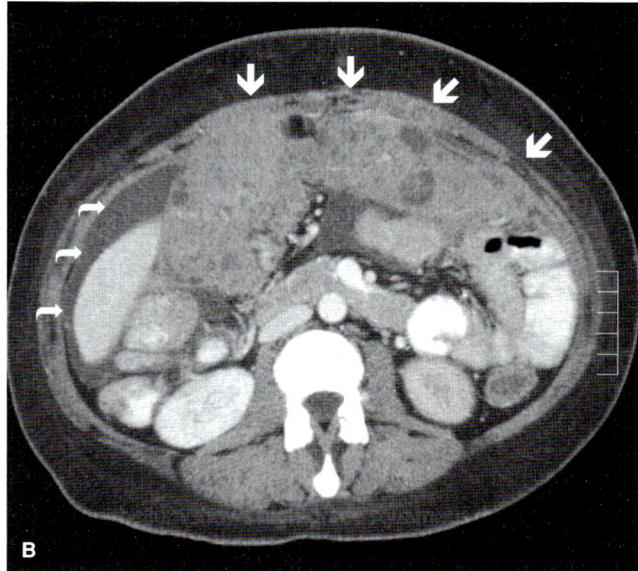

FIGURE 35-5 Computed tomographic scans in a woman with ovarian cancer **A.** Axial CT image at the level of the liver and spleen reveals metastatic lesions in the spleen and liver (*curved arrows*) and a bulky lesion at the splenorenal ligament (*arrow*). **B.** More caudal axial CT image reveals ascites (*curved arrows*) and marked omental caking (*arrows*). (Reproduced with permission from Dr. Diane Twickler.)

cancers preoperatively, none has been universally implemented (Elder, 2014; Suh-Burgmann, 2018).

In patients with advanced disease, sonography is less helpful. The pelvic sonogram may be particularly difficult to interpret if a large mass encompasses the uterus, adnexa, and surrounding structures. Ascites, if present, is easily detected, but in general, abdominal sonography has limited use.

Of *radiographic tests*, patients with suspected ovarian cancer should have a chest radiograph to detect pulmonary effusions or, infrequently, pulmonary metastases. Rarely, a barium enema is clinically helpful in excluding diverticular disease or colon cancer or in identifying ovarian cancer involvement of the rectosigmoid.

CT scanning has a primary role in treatment planning for women with advanced ovarian cancer. Preoperatively, implants in the liver, retroperitoneum, omentum, or other intraabdominal sites are detected to thereby guide surgical cytoreduction or demonstrate obviously unresectable disease (Fig. 35-5) (Suidan, 2014). However, CT is not particularly reliable in detecting intraperitoneal disease smaller than 1 to 2 cm in diameter. Moreover, CT scanning accuracy is poor for differentiating a benign ovarian mass from a malignant tumor when disease is limited to the pelvis. In these cases, transvaginal sonography is superior. Other radiologic studies such as magnetic resonance (MR) imaging, bone scans, and positron emission tomography (PET) in general provide limited additional information preoperatively.

Paracentesis

A woman with a pelvic mass and ascites usually can be assumed to have ovarian cancer until surgically proved otherwise. Thus, few patients require diagnostic paracentesis. Moreover, this procedure is typically avoided diagnostically as cytologic results are often nonspecific and abdominal wall metastases may form at the needle entry site (Kruitwagen, 1996). However, paracentesis

may be indicated for those with ascites in the *absence* of a pelvic mass.

Aside from diagnosis, paracentesis also may relieve volume-related symptoms in those with large accumulations. This may be done at the bedside, using connector tubing and vacuum bottles, or completed by an interventional radiologist. Relative dehydration is common afterward and manifest by thirst, oliguria, and short-term creatinine level rise. These all correct with normal oral intake.

■ Role of the Generalist

Using the currently available diagnostic modalities, clinicians often face tremendous difficulty in distinguishing benign from malignant. However, ascites or evidence of metastases should prompt consideration of consultation with an oncologist (American College of Obstetricians and Gynecologists, 2016, 2017b). Additionally, premenopausal women with elevated CA125 levels (>200 U/mL) or an OVA1 score ≥5.0 are at higher risk. Similarly, postmenopausal women with any CA125 level elevation or an OVA1 score ≥4.4 are concerning.

Ideally, for patients with suspicious adnexal masses, surgery is performed in a hospital with a pathologist able to reliably interpret an intraoperative frozen section. At minimum, samples for peritoneal cytology are obtained when the abdomen is entered. The mass is removed intact through an incision that permits thorough staging and resection of possible metastatic sites. Alternatively, the ovarian mass and adjacent tube may be detached laparoscopically or robotically, placed within a bag, brought to the abdominal wall trocar site, and removed by contained tissue extraction without intraabdominal spill.

If malignancy is diagnosed, surgical staging is completed. However, in a study of more than 10,000 women with ovarian cancer, almost half of those with early-stage disease did not undergo the recommended surgical procedures (Goff, 2006). Surgeons should be prepared to appropriately stage and potentially debulk ovarian cancer or have a gynecologic oncologist immediately available. This type of careful planning achieves the best surgical results and improves survival rates (Earle, 2006; Engelen, 2006; Mercado, 2010). Moreover, since broader resources are usually available, patients cared for at high-volume hospitals also tend to have better outcomes (Bristow, 2010).

For women with malignancy identified only postoperatively or intraoperatively and without adequate staging, management will vary. Women with suspected early-stage disease may be restaged laparoscopically or robotically. Those with advanced disease may undergo a second laparotomy to achieve optimal tumor debulking (Grabowski, 2012). However, if extensive disease is found at the initial surgery, chemotherapy may be selected first and followed later by interval cytoreduction.

At some point during postoperative surveillance, many women with early-stage disease, depending on the diagnosis, will return to their referring physician. Monitoring for relapse is often coordinated between the gynecologic oncologist and generalist in obstetrics and gynecology, especially if no chemotherapy is required following surgery.

Pathology

Although epithelial ovarian cancer is often considered a single entity, the different histologic types vary in their behavior (Table 35-5) (Kurman, 2014). Sometimes, two or more cell types are mixed. Within each histologic type, tumors are further categorized as benign, borderline (low malignant potential), or malignant.

Mainly in early-stage disease, grade is an important prognostic factor that affects treatment planning (Armstrong, 2019). Unfortunately, no grading system for epithelial ovarian carcinoma is universally accepted. Instead, numerous different schemes, most based on architecture and/or nuclear pleomorphism, are currently used. In general, tumors are classified as grade 1 (well differentiated), grade 2 (moderately differentiated), and grade 3 (poorly differentiated) (Pecorelli, 1999).

TABLE 35-5. World Health Organization Histological Classification of Ovarian Carcinoma

Serous adenocarcinoma
Mucinous adenocarcinoma
Endometrioid adenocarcinoma
Clear cell adenocarcinoma
Malignant Brenner tumor
Mixed epithelial and mesenchymal
   Adenocarcinoma
   Carcinosarcoma
Squamous cell carcinoma
Mixed carcinoma
Undifferentiated carcinoma
Small cell carcinoma

Adapted from Kurman, 2014, with permission.

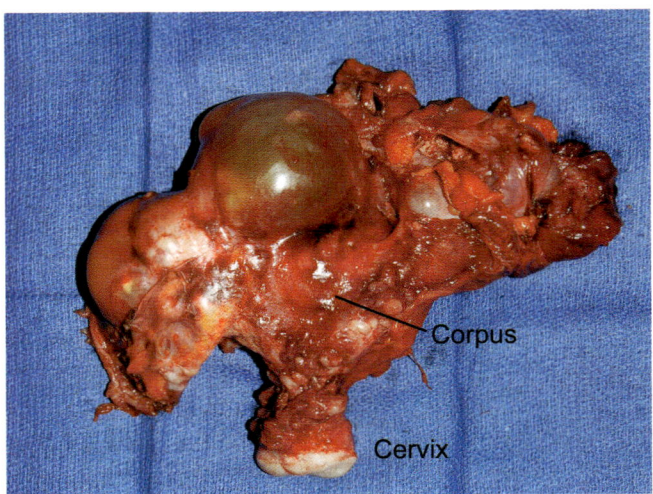

FIGURE 35-6 Hysterectomy specimen and bilateral adnexa encompassed by serous adenocarcinoma of the ovary.

Grossly, no features distinguish the different types of epithelial ovarian cancer. In general, each has solid and cystic areas of varying sizes (Fig. 35-6).

Serous Tumors

More than 50 percent of all epithelial ovarian cancers have serous histology. Microscopically, in well-differentiated tumors, cells may resemble fallopian tube epithelium, whereas in poorly differentiated tumors, anaplastic cells with severe nuclear atypia predominate (Fig. 35-7). During frozen section analysis, psammoma bodies are essentially pathognomonic of an ovarian-type serous carcinoma. These tumors often contain other cell types as a minor component (<10 percent) that may cause diagnostic problems but do not influence outcome (Lee, 2003).

Endometrioid Tumors

Endometrioid adenocarcinomas compose 15 to 20 percent of epithelial ovarian cancers and are the second most common histologic type (Fig. 35-8). The lower frequency results largely because poorly differentiated endometrioid and serous tumors cannot be easily distinguished and such cases are usually classified as serous. As a result, well-differentiated endometrioid tumors are proportionally more common, which may also explain their overall relatively good prognosis.

In 15 to 20 percent of cases, uterine endometrial adenocarcinoma coexists. This is usually regarded as a synchronous tumor, but metastasis from one site to the other is difficult to exclude (Soliman, 2004). A müllerian "field effect" is theorized to account for these independently developing, histologically similar tumors. In addition, many such patients are noted to have pelvic endometriosis.

Carcinosarcoma

Malignant mixed müllerian tumor, now preferably termed *carcinosarcoma*, is a variant of poorly differentiated epithelial ovarian cancer that contains highly aggressive malignant epithelial and mesenchymal elements (Armstrong, 2019). It represents <1 percent of ovarian cancers, has a poorer prognosis than either high-grade serous or endometrioid tumors, and is

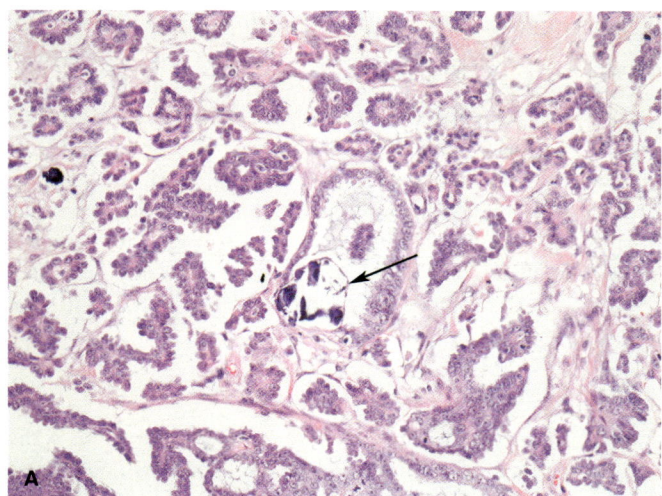

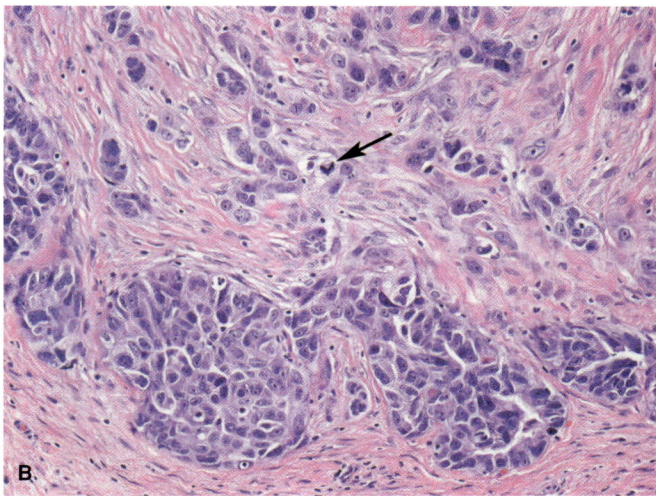

FIGURE 35-7 Tuboovarian serous carcinomas vary in their architecture, degree of nuclear pleomorphism, and mitotic rate. **A.** This low-grade serous carcinoma is characterized by well-differentiated architectural patterns (gland formation and papillae), mild to moderate nuclear atypia, and relatively low mitotic rate. Here, mildly atypical tumor cells are arranged primarily in fine papillae, with focal gland formation. An associated psammoma body is seen in the center (*arrow*). **B.** High-grade serous carcinoma has high-grade nuclear atypia with increased nuclear pleomorphism, chromatin abnormalities, and nucleolar prominence. The mitotic rate is typically high, and architectural patterns may be less well-differentiated. Tumor invades in cords and glands with ill-defined intraluminal papillation. An abnormal mitosis is seen (*arrow*). (Reproduced with permission from Dr. Kelley Carrick.)

histologically similar to uterine carcinosarcoma (Berton-Rigaud, 2014).

Mucinous Tumors

Mucinous adenocarcinomas compose 5 to 10 percent of true epithelial ovarian cancers. The frequency is usually overestimated because many are undetected primary intestinal cancers from the appendix or colon. Well-differentiated ovarian mucinous tumors closely resemble mucin-secreting adenocarcinomas of intestinal or endocervical origin (Fig. 35-9). Histologically, the distinction may be impossible without clinical correlation

(Lee, 2003). Advanced-stage mucinous ovarian carcinomas are rare, tend to be resistant to platinum chemotherapy, and have a prognosis significantly worse than that for serous tumors (Zaino, 2011).

Pseudomyxoma Peritonei. This clinical term describes the rare finding of abundant mucoid or gelatinous material in the pelvis and abdominal cavity that is surrounded by thin fibrous capsules. An ovarian mucinous carcinoma with ascites rarely develops this, and evidence suggests that ovarian mucinous tumors associated with pseudomyxoma peritonei are almost all

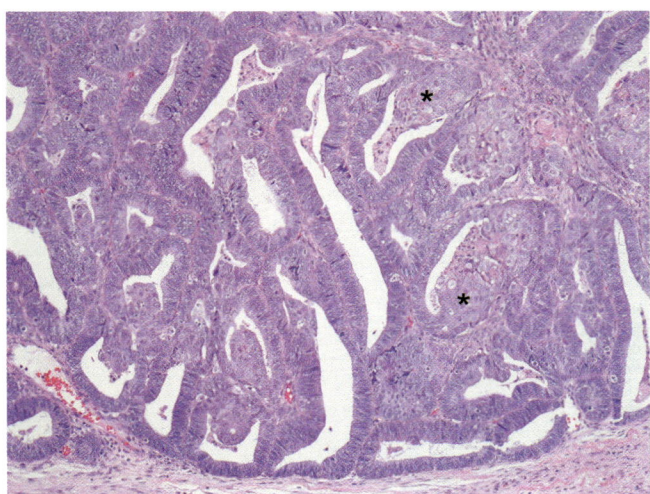

FIGURE 35-8 Ovarian endometrioid adenocarcinomas are morphologically similar to their counterparts arising in the endometrium. Better differentiated tumors like this one have glands resembling proliferative endometrial glands, which are typically disposed in a closely packed pattern. These tumors often show foci of squamous differentiation (*asterisks*). (Reproduced with permission from Dr. Kelley Carrick.)

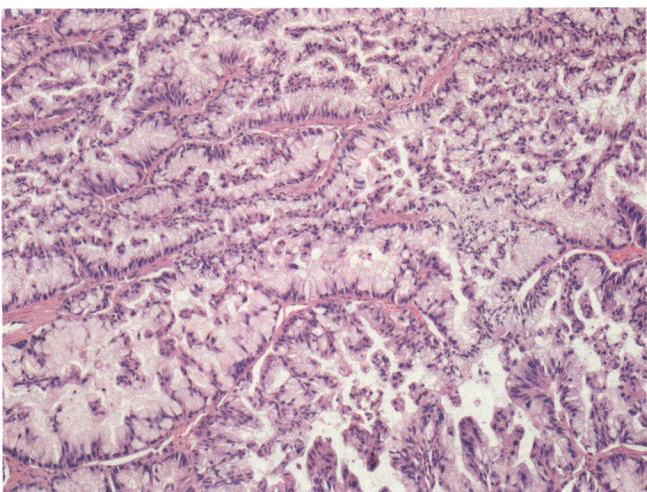

FIGURE 35-9 Ovarian mucinous adenocarcinoma is composed of cells with varying amounts of intracytoplasmic mucin. This particular invasive carcinoma has an expansile pattern and is characterized by mucinous cells with relatively low-grade nuclear atypia. These form markedly crowded, labyrinthine glands with intraglandular complexity. (Reproduced with permission from Dr. Kelley Carrick.)

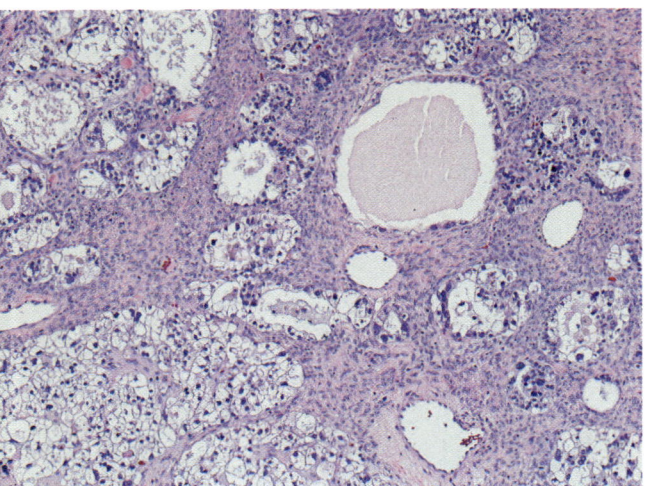

FIGURE 35-10 Ovarian clear cell adenocarcinoma has cytologic and architectural features similar to its counterparts in the endometrium, cervix, and vagina. It contains clear, eosinophilic, and/or hobnail cells. In this example, cells have strikingly clear cytoplasm and marked nuclear atypia, with nuclear pleomorphism and hyperchromasia. In the photomicrograph's upper portion, tumor has the classic tubulocystic architecture in which tumor cells form dilated glands and smaller tubules. At the bottom left, tumor has a solid, nested pattern. (Reproduced with permission from Dr. Kelley Carrick.)

metastatic rather than primary. As a result, appendiceal or other intestinal sites of origin should be excluded (Ronnett, 1997). The primary appendiceal tumor may be small relative to the ovarian tumor(s) and may not be appreciated macroscopically. Thus, removal and thorough histologic examination of the appendix is indicated in all cases of pseudomyxoma peritonei.

If the peritoneal epithelial cells are benign or borderline-appearing, the condition is referred to as *disseminated peritoneal adenomucinosis*. Affected patients have a benign or a protracted, indolent clinical course (Ronnett, 2001). If the peritoneal epithelial cells appear malignant, the clinical course is invariably fatal.

Clear Cell Adenocarcinoma

Comprising 5 to 10 percent of epithelial ovarian cancers, clear cell adenocarcinomas are most frequently associated with pelvic endometriosis. These tumors appear similar to clear cell carcinomas that develop sporadically in the uterus, vagina, and cervix. Typically, tumors are confined to the ovary and generally are cured by surgery alone. However, the 20 percent presenting with advanced disease tend to be platinum resistant and carry a worse prognosis than serous carcinoma (Al-Barrak, 2011).

Microscopically, both clear and "hobnail" cells are characteristic (Fig. 35-10). In clear cells, the visibly translucent cytoplasm results from the dissolution of glycogen as the tissue specimen is histologically prepared. Hobnail cells have bulbous nuclei that protrude far into the cystic lumen beyond the apparent cytoplasmic limits of the cell (Lee, 2003).

Transitional Cell Tumors

Transitional cell carcinoma accounts for fewer than 5 percent of ovarian cancers. Microscopically, these tumors resemble a primary bladder carcinoma, often with squamous differentiation, but have an immunoreactive pattern consistent with an ovarian origin (Lee, 2003). Thus, transitional cell carcinoma is considered a high-grade form of serous carcinoma but carries a better prognosis (Guseh, 2014).

The rare *malignant Brenner tumor* characteristically has transitional cell carcinoma coupled with foci of benign or borderline Brenner features. These tumors classically have a dense, abundant fibrous stroma with embedded nests of transitional epithelium. They carry a better prognosis than pure transitional cell carcinomas.

Other Histologic Types

Primary squamous cell carcinoma of the ovary is rare. This is the newest category to be recognized and typically carries a poor prognosis for most women with advanced disease (Park, 2010). More commonly, squamous cell carcinomas arise from mature cystic teratomas (dermoid cysts) and are classified as malignant ovarian germ cell tumors (Pins, 1996). In other cases, ovarian endometrioid variants may have extensive squamous differentiation, or alternatively, metastases from a cervical primary are present.

Mixed carcinoma describes an ovarian cancer that contains more than 10 percent of a second cell type. Common combinations include mixed clear cell/endometrioid or serous/endometrioid adenocarcinomas.

Undifferentiated carcinomas are rare epithelial ovarian tumors that are too poorly differentiated to be classified into any of the müllerian types previously described. Microscopically, the cells are arranged in solid groups or sheets with numerous mitotic figures and marked cytologic atypia. Typically, foci of müllerian carcinoma, usually serous, are found within the tumor. Overall, undifferentiated carcinomas of the ovary have a poor prognosis compared with the other histologic types (Silva, 1991).

*Small cell carcinoma*s are rare, extremely malignant, and consist of two subgroups. Most patients have a *hypercalcemic type*, which typically develops in young women. Nearly all tumors are unilateral, and two thirds are associated with elevated serum calcium levels that resolve postoperatively (Young, 1994). Recent data suggest these highly lethal tumors arise via a specific mutation in the *SMARCA4* gene (Jelinic, 2014). The *pulmonary type* resembles oat-cell carcinoma of the lung and develops in older women. Half of these women have bilateral ovarian disease (Eichhorn, 1992). In general, patients with small cell carcinoma die within 2 years from rapid disease progression.

■ Primary Peritoneal Carcinoma

Up to 15 percent of "typical" epithelial ovarian cancers are actually primary peritoneal carcinomas that develop de novo from the lining of the pelvis and abdomen. In some cases, especially among *BRCA1* mutation carriers, independent malignant transformation occurs at multiple peritoneal sites simultaneously (Schorge, 1998). However, more recent data suggest that nearly half of presumed cases actually arise in the fallopian tube fimbria (Carlson, 2008).

Clinically and histologically, these tumors are virtually indistinguishable from epithelial ovarian cancer. However, primary peritoneal carcinoma may develop in a woman years

TABLE 35-6. Criteria for Diagnosing Primary Peritoneal Carcinoma When Ovaries Are Present

Both ovaries must be normal in size or enlarged by a benign process
The involvement in the extraovarian sites must be greater than the involvement on the surface of either ovary
The ovarian tumor involvement must be either nonexistent, confined to the ovarian surface epithelium without stromal
  invasion, or involving the cortical stroma with tumor size less than 5 × 5 mm

after undergoing BSO. If ovaries are still present, several criteria are required to make the diagnosis (Table 35-6) (Prat, 2014). By far the most common variant is papillary serous, but any of the other histologic types are possible. In general, the staging, treatment, and prognosis of primary peritoneal carcinoma are the same as for epithelial ovarian cancer (Mok, 2003). The differential diagnosis mainly includes malignant mesothelioma.

■ Fallopian Tube Carcinoma

Historically, this carcinoma was assumed to be much rarer than epithelial ovarian cancer. However, the fallopian tube fimbria has recently been identified as an origin for many high-grade pelvic serous carcinomas that were previously assumed to arise from the ovary or peritoneum (Fig. 35-11) (Levanon, 2008).

Clinically, fallopian tube carcinoma is similar to epithelial ovarian cancer. For the most part, risk factors, histologic types, surgical staging, pattern of spread, treatment, and prognosis are comparable. To be considered a primary fallopian tube carcinoma, the tumor must be located macroscopically within the tube or its fimbriated end. Additionally, the uterus and ovary must not contain carcinoma, or if they do, it must be clearly different from the fallopian tube lesion (Alvarado-Cabrero, 2003).

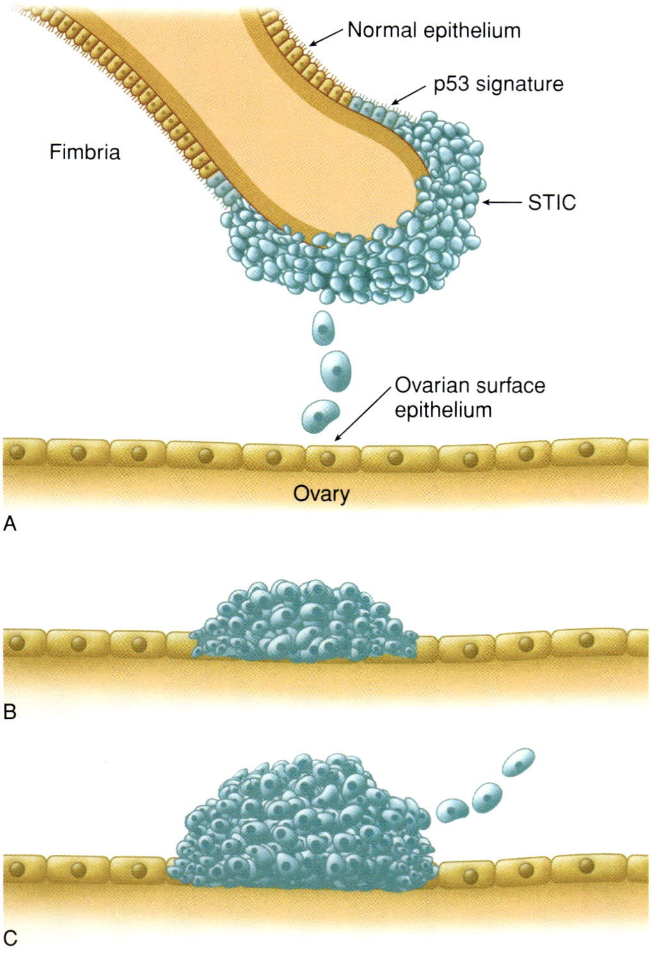

■ Secondary Tumors

Malignant tumors that metastasize to the ovary are almost invariably bilateral. The term *Krukenberg tumor* refers to a metastatic mucinous/signet ring cell adenocarcinoma of the ovaries that typically originates from primary tumors of the intestinal tract, characteristically the stomach (Fig. 35-12). Ovarian metastases often represent a late disseminated stage of the disease in which other hematogenous metastases also are found (Prat, 2003).

■ Patterns of Spread

In general, epithelial ovarian cancers—especially serous tumors—predominantly metastasize by *exfoliation*. Malignant cells are first released into the peritoneal cavity when the tumor

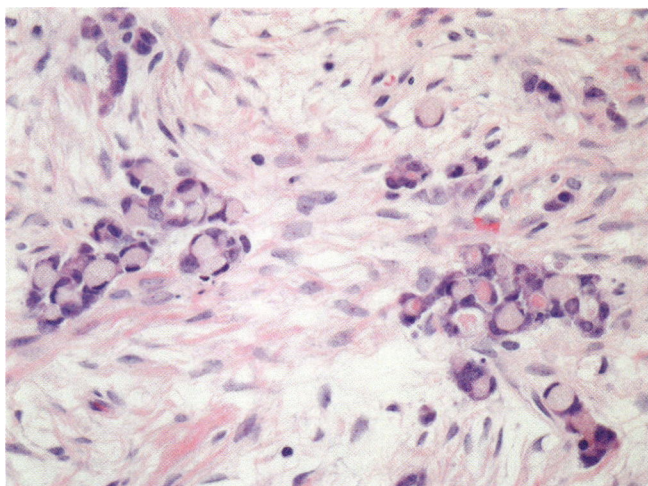

FIGURE 35-12 Krukenberg tumor refers to any adenocarcinoma with signet-ring cytology that is metastatic to the ovary. This example originated from the stomach and generated bilateral ovarian metastases. Tumor cells are arranged singly, in single file, and in small clusters. Cells are characterized by an intracytoplasmic mucin globule that displaces the nucleus to the cell periphery to produce the signet-ring morphology. (Reproduced with permission from Dr. Kelley Carrick.)

FIGURE 35-11 **A.** Normal tubal epithelium, p53 signature (a benign-appearing serous tubal intraepithelial lesion), and a serous tubal intraepithelial carcinoma (STIC) lesion at the fimbria are shown. Epithelial cells from the STIC lesion drop onto the ovarian surface epithelium. **B.** A mass forming on the surface of the ovary. **C.** Exfoliating metastatic disease to other sites.

Normal epithelium
p53 signature
Fimbria
STIC
Ovarian surface epithelium
Ovary
A
B
C

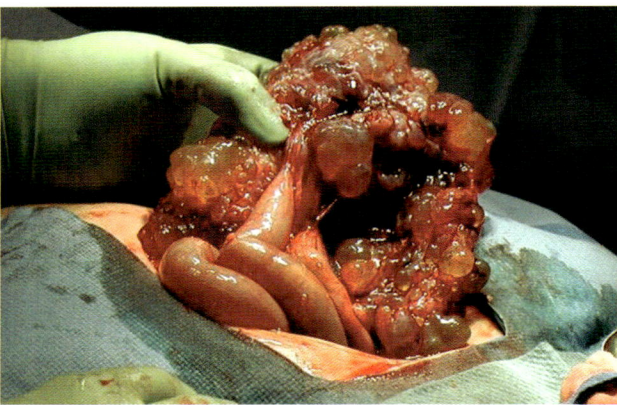

FIGURE 35-13 Omental caking caused by tumor invasion.

penetrates through the ovarian capsule surface. By following the normal circulation of peritoneal fluid, cells then may develop into implants anywhere in the abdomen. A unique characteristic of ovarian cancer is that metastatic tumors do not usually infiltrate visceral organs, but grow as surface implants. As a result, aggressive debulking is possible with acceptable morbidity.

Due to its marked vascularity, the omentum is the most frequent location to support metastatic disease and is often extensively involved with tumor (Fig. 35-13). Nodules also are commonly present on the undersurface of the right hemidiaphragm and on small bowel serosa, but all intraperitoneal surfaces are at risk.

Lymphatic dissemination is the other primary mode of spread. Malignant cells move through channels that follow the ovarian blood supply along the infundibulopelvic ligament and that terminate in paraaortic lymph nodes up to or above the level of the renal vessels. Other lymphatics pass laterally through the broad ligament and parametrium to the external iliac, obturator, and internal iliac nodal chains. Infrequently, metastases can also follow the round ligament to the inguinal nodes (Lee, 2003).

Direct extension of a progressively enlarging ovarian cancer may create confluent tumor involvement of the pelvic peritoneum and adjacent structures, including the uterus, rectosigmoid colon, and fallopian tubes. Usually, this is associated with significant induration of the surrounding tissues.

In advanced disease, several liters of ascites may collect. Either increased

production of carcinomatous fluid or decreased clearance by obstructed lymphatic channels are purported causes. Similarly, by traversing the diaphragm, a malignant pleural effusion may develop, almost invariably on the right.

Hematogenous spread is atypical. In most cases, metastases to the liver or lung parenchyma, brain, or kidneys are observed in patients with recurrent, end-stage disease and not at initial diagnosis.

■ Staging

Ovarian cancer is surgically staged, and stage is assigned according to findings before tumor removal and debulking (Fig. 35-14). The International Federation of Gynecology and

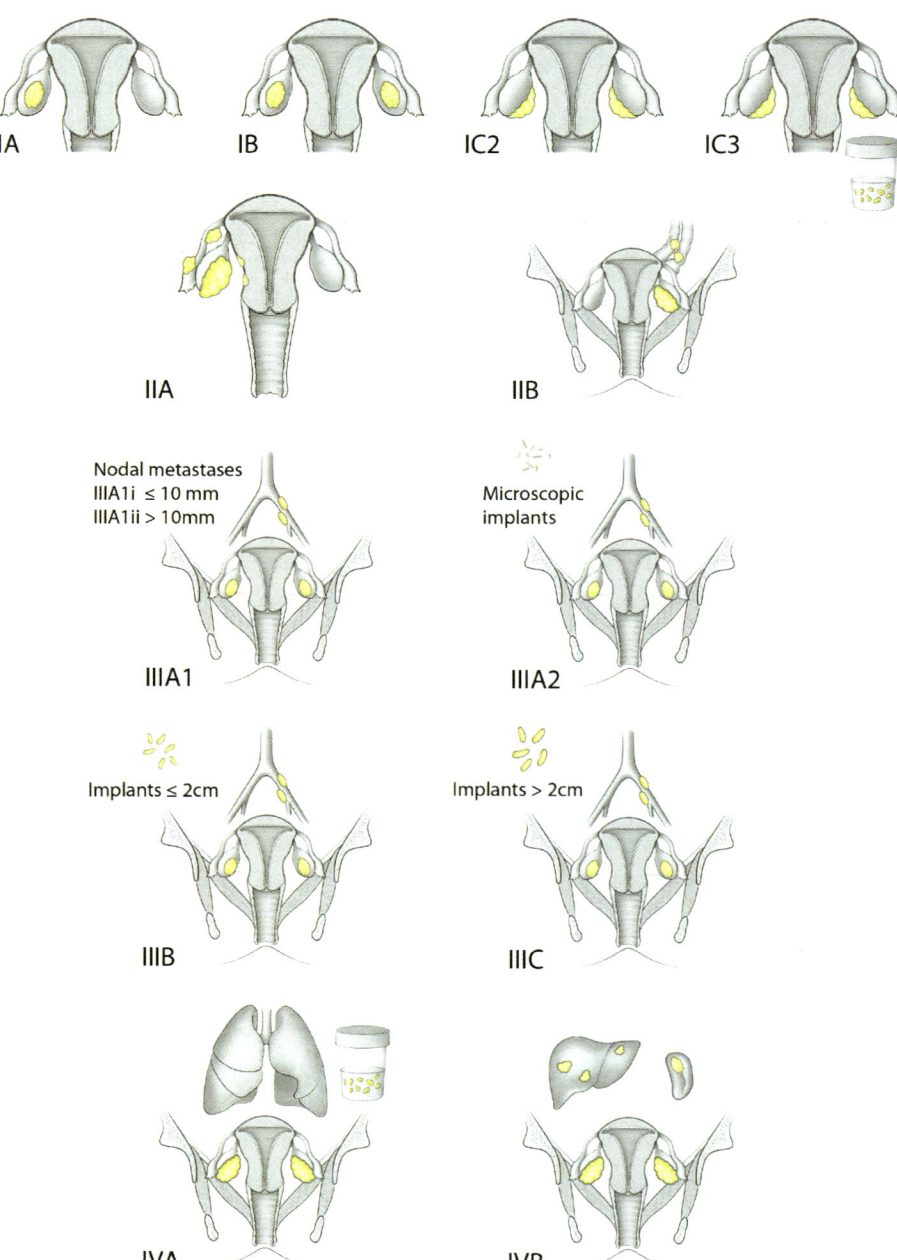

FIGURE 35-14 International Federation of Gynecology and Obstetrics (FIGO) staging for ovarian cancer.

TABLE 35-7. FIGO Staging of Carcinoma of the Ovary, Fallopian Tube, and Primary Peritoneal Carcinoma

Stage	Characteristics
I	**Tumor confined to ovaries (or to fallopian tubes)**
IA	Tumor limited to 1 ovary (or 1 tube); capsule intact, no tumor on surface, negative washings
IB	Tumor involves both ovaries (or both tubes), otherwise like IA
IC[1]	Tumor limited to 1 or both ovaries (or tubes), with surgical spill
IC[2]	Tumor limited to 1 or both ovaries (or tubes), with capsule rupture before surgery or tumor on ovarian surface
IC[3]	Tumor limited to 1 or both ovaries (or tubes), with malignant cells in ascites or peritoneal washings
II	**Tumor involves 1 or both ovaries (or 1 or both tubes) with pelvic extension (below the pelvic brim) or primary peritoneal cancer**
IIA	Extension and/or implants on uterus and/or fallopian tubes (and/or ovaries)
IIB	Extension to other pelvic intraperitoneal tissues
III	**Tumor involves 1 or both ovaries (or 1 or both tubes) with cytologically or histologically confirmed spread to the peritoneum outside the pelvis and/or metastasis to retroperitoneal lymph nodes**
IIIA1	Positive retroperitoneal lymph nodes only
(i)	Metastasis ≤10 mm
(ii)	Metastasis >10 mm
IIIA2	Microscopic, extrapelvic (above the brim) peritoneal involvement ± positive retroperitoneal nodes
IIIB	Macroscopic, extrapelvic, peritoneal metastasis ≤2 cm ± positive retroperitoneal nodes. Includes extension to capsule of liver/spleen
IIIC	Macroscopic, extrapelvic, peritoneal metastasis >2 cm ± positive retroperitoneal lymph nodes. Includes extension to capsule of liver/spleen
IV	**Distant metastasis excluding peritoneal metastasis**
IVA	Pleural effusion with positive cytology
IVB	Hepatic and/or splenic parenchymal metastasis, metastasis to extraabdominal organs (including inguinal lymph nodes and lymph nodes outside of the abdominal cavity)

FIGO = International Federation of Gynecology and Obstetrics.
Data from Prat, 2014.

Obstetrics (FIGO) stages reflect the typical patterns of ovarian cancer spread (Table 35-7) (Prat, 2014). Even if a tumor appears clinically confined to the ovary, in many cases it will have microscopically detectable metastases. Therefore, accurate surgical staging is crucial to guide treatment. Approximately one third of patients initially have surgical stage I or II disease (Table 35-8) (Heintz, 2006).

■ Management of Early-Stage Ovarian Cancer
Surgical Staging

If a malignancy appears clinically confined to the ovary, surgical removal and comprehensive staging is performed. Typically,

TABLE 35-8. Distribution of Epithelial Ovarian Cancer by FIGO Stage (*n* = 4825 patients)

FIGO Stage	Percent
I	28
II	8
III	50
IV	13

FIGO = International Federation of Gynecology and Obstetrics.
Data from Heintz, 2006.

the abdominal incision must be adequate to identify and resect any disease that may have been missed during physical examination or imaging. The operation begins by aspirating free ascitic fluid or collecting peritoneal washings. This is followed by inspection and palpation of all peritoneal surfaces. Next, an extrafascial hysterectomy and BSO are performed. In the absence of gross extraovarian disease, the infracolic omentum should be removed or at least biopsied (Section 46-14, p. 1211). Additionally, random peritoneal biopsies or scrapings are obtained, ideally near the diaphragms (Lee, 2014; Timmers, 2010). A pelvic and infrarenal paraaortic lymphadenectomy also is completed (Sections 46-10 and 46-11, p. 1194) (Chan, 2007; Cress, 2011).

Laparoscopic staging is particularly valuable as a primary treatment in women who have an apparent stage I ovarian cancer. In general, staging by minimally invasive surgery (MIS) allows all of the required procedures to be safely performed (Chi, 2005). The main putative MIS benefits are a shorter hospital stay and quicker recovery (Tozzi, 2004). However, nodal counts may be inferior, and exploration of the abdomen is unavoidably limited.

Fertility-Sparing Management

Approximately 10 percent of epithelial ovarian cancers develop in women younger than 40 years. In selected cases, fertility-sparing surgery may be an option if disease appears confined to one ovary. Although many patients will be "up-staged" as a result of the operative findings, those with surgical stage I disease have an excellent long-term survival following unilateral adnexectomy (Armstrong, 2019). In some cases, postoperative chemotherapy may be required, but patients will usually retain their ability to conceive and ultimately carry a pregnancy to term (Schilder, 2002).

Postsurgical Management

In women with stage IA or IB, grade 1 or 2 epithelial ovarian carcinoma, observation without further treatment following surgery is appropriate (Armstrong, 2019). However, one third of patients who appear to have disease confined to the ovary will be up-staged by surgical staging and require postoperative chemotherapy.

Women with stage IA or IB, grade 3 epithelial ovarian cancer and all stage IC and II tumors are treated with platinum-based chemotherapy (Armstrong, 2019). In a Phase III Gynecologic Oncology Group (GOG) trial (protocol #157), women with early-stage disease were randomly assigned to either three or six cycles of carboplatin (Paraplatin) and paclitaxel (Taxol). Overall, three cycles resulted in a relapse rate comparable to that for six cycles but caused less toxicity (Bell, 2006). However, in a subanalysis of patients in this study who had serous tumors, treatment with six cycles decreased the relapse risk (Chan, 2010a). Despite chemotherapy, more than 20 percent of women with early-stage disease develop recurrences within 5 years.

Surveillance

After treatment completion, women with early-stage ovarian cancer may be followed every 2 to 4 months for the first 2 years, twice yearly for an additional 3 years, and then annually. At each visit, complete physical and pelvic examinations are performed. In addition, a serum CA125 level may be indicated if it was initially elevated (Armstrong, 2019). However, one multi-institutional trial evaluated the utility of CA125 levels for ovarian cancer monitoring after primary therapy completion. Women with relapsed ovarian cancer did not live longer by starting chemotherapy earlier based on a rising CA125 level compared with delaying treatment until symptoms developed. The group monitored with CA125 tests received 5 more months of chemotherapy overall, whereas women who were diagnosed and treated later for clinically evident recurrence had higher quality-of-life measures (Rustin, 2010).

Whether suspected by examination, CA125 level elevation, or new symptoms, recurrent disease must be confirmed with the aid of imaging. Of modalities, CT is initially most helpful to identify intraperitoneal disease.

■ Management of Advanced Ovarian Cancer

Approximately two thirds of patients initially will have stage III–IV disease, and sequenced multimodality therapy offers the most successful outcomes (Earle, 2006). Ideally, surgical cytoreduction initially is performed to remove all gross disease and is followed by six courses of platinum-based chemotherapy. However, some women are not appropriate candidates for primary surgery due to their health status, and others will have unresectable tumor. Additionally, two randomized trials concluded that initial treatment with chemotherapy followed by

interval debulking surgery achieves equivalent results (Kehoe, 2015; Vergote, 2010). To effectively balance all clinical factors, each patient is individually assessed before initiating treatment.

Primary Cytoreductive Surgery

Residual Disease. Since the initial report by Griffiths (1975) suggested the clinical benefits of debulking, its value was largely assumed. Numerous retrospective studies subsequently supported the apparent survival advantage of this practice for women with advanced ovarian cancer. For many years, a cytoreductive effort was considered "optimal" if *≤1 cm residual disease* could be achieved. Specifically, 1 cm residual disease describes a surgical result in which no remaining areas of tumor individually measures >1 cm.

However, the assessment of gross remaining disease is entirely subjective and often inaccurate due to tissue induration or other factors (Chi, 2007). Perhaps due to the inability to reliably quantify remaining disease, a subanalysis of accumulated data from several prospective GOG trials was completed. For those with stage III ovarian cancer, 0.1 to 1.0 cm residual disease afforded only marginally improved overall survival rates compared with >1 cm residual disease. In fact, dramatic survival benefit was only achieved with complete resection (Winter, 2007). Based on these findings and other similar reports, a growing consensus supports the standard that optimal debulking should be defined as no gross residual disease (Chang, 2012; Schorge, 2014).

Because of the presumed benefits, primary surgical cytoreduction is generally performed whenever an optimal result to achieve no residual disease is clinically feasible. Yet, physical examination and imaging findings alone inherently limit the ability to accurately predict surgical success. As a result, pre-debulking laparoscopic evaluation is emerging as a more accurate, low-risk method for patient triage (Fagotti, 2005, 2013; Fleming, 2018). In this strategy, good candidates for primary cytoreduction undergo diagnostic laparoscopy. During surgery, the gynecologic oncologist assigns points to intraabdominal sites if tumor is present. Once these are totaled, laparotomy and debulking proceeds for low scores (<8). For high scores (≥8 to 10), surgery is aborted to begin neoadjuvant chemotherapy.

Surgical Approach to Cytoreductive Surgery. In general, a vertical incision is recommended to provide access to the entire abdomen. Women with advanced disease do not require peritoneal washings or cytologic assessment of fluid, but often several liters of ascites will need to be evacuated to improve visualization. The abdomen is carefully explored to quickly determine if optimal debulking is feasible. It is preferable to perform a limited surgical procedure rather than extensive debulking if it is obvious that bulky tumors will be left behind. If hysterectomy and BSO is not possible, a biopsy of the ovary and sampling of the endometrium by dilation and curettage is performed to confirm an ovarian primary and exclude the possibility of widely metastatic uterine papillary serous carcinoma. However, if disease is resectable, surgery should begin with the least complicated procedure.

Often, an infracolic omentectomy can be easily performed and extended (i.e., gastrocolic), as needed, to encompass the disease. A frozen section analysis then can be requested to confirm the presumed diagnosis of epithelial ovarian cancer. The pelvis is assessed next. Usually, an extrafascial type I abdominal hysterectomy and BSO is sufficient. However, when the tumor is confluent or invading the rectosigmoid, an en bloc resection, low anterior resection, or modified posterior pelvic exenteration may be required. These and other surgeries mentioned in this section are described and illustrated in Chapter 46 (p. 1160).

In patients with stage IV disease and those with abdominal tumor nodules at least 2 cm (already stage IIIC disease), nodal dissection is not necessarily required for staging purposes. Systematic pelvic and paraaortic lymphadenectomy in advanced ovarian cancer should not be routinely performed, as it does not extend survival and leads to a higher incidence of postoperative complications (Harter, 2019).

Optimal surgical cytoreduction also may require various other radical procedures, including splenectomy, diaphragm stripping/resection, and small or large bowel resection (Aletti, 2006; McCann, 2011). Surgically aggressive centers experienced in such techniques report higher rates of achieving minimal residual disease that correspond to better outcomes (Aletti, 2009; Chi, 2009a; Wimberger, 2007). For diagnostic purposes and since it is a frequent site of disease, an appendectomy also is commonly included (Timofeev, 2010).

Neoadjuvant Chemotherapy and Interval Cytoreductive Surgery

Many women do not undergo initial optimal surgical debulking. In some of these cases, imaging studies may suggest unresectable disease. Other patients may be too medically compromised, may not have received initial care by a gynecologic oncologist, or may have large-volume "suboptimal" residual disease despite attempted debulking. In such circumstances, three to four courses of chemotherapy are used to shrink disease before attempting an "interval" cytoreductive surgery.

Neoadjuvant chemotherapy with an interval procedure is associated with less perioperative morbidity, higher rates of optimal cytoreduction, and similar survival rates (Kehoe, 2015; Vergote, 2010). Due to the often dramatic response to treatment, MIS techniques have become more commonplace. Approximately 15 percent of interval debulking operations for stage IIIC-IV ovarian cancer are performed either laparoscopically or robotically (Melamed, 2017). In this setting, MIS offers shorter hospitalization and comparable clinical outcomes to laparotomy.

Adjuvant Chemotherapy

Intravenous Chemotherapy.
Advanced ovarian cancer is considered to be relatively sensitive to cytotoxic agents. Largely due to recent advances in identifying active drugs, survival duration among patients has lengthened over the past two decades. Despite these improvements, fewer than 20 percent of those requiring chemotherapy will be cured. This is largely due to clinically occult residual chemoresistant tumor cells.

Platinum-based chemotherapy is the foundation for systemic treatment of most epithelial ovarian cancer types. For advanced mucinous and clear cell carcinomas, alternative regimens are currently being studied because of these tumors' known chemoresistance. In two large collaborative group trials (GOG protocol #158 and Arbeitsgemeinschaft Gynäkologische Onkologie [AGO] protocol OVAR-3), the combination of carboplatin and paclitaxel was easier to administer, similarly efficacious, and less toxic than a cisplatin/paclitaxel regimen (du Bois, 2003; Ozols, 2003). As a result, the most widely used intravenous (IV) regimen in the United States is six courses of carboplatin and paclitaxel. If additional cycles are required to achieve clinical remission, this suggests relative tumor chemoresistance and usually leads to an earlier relapse. In Europe, single-agent carboplatin often is used. This preference is based on two large Phase III trials of the International Collaborative Ovarian Neoplasm (ICON) Group, which did not detect a survival advantage for combination chemotherapy (The ICON Collaborators, 1998; The ICON Group, 2002).

Although the carboplatin and paclitaxel regimen is undoubtedly effective, other modifications have been studied. For instance, the addition of a third cytotoxic agent was postulated to further improve outcome. Unfortunately, none of the experimental regimens demonstrated superiority compared with the control group (Bookman, 2009). Addition of the biologic agent bevacizumab (Avastin) during primary chemotherapy, followed by use as maintenance therapy, provides only a modest improvement in progression-free survival. This addition was most effective in poor-prognosis disease (GOG protocol #218 and ICON-7) (Burger, 2011; Perren, 2011).

Last, administering paclitaxel in a dose-dense weekly schedule may have some advantages but at the cost of additional toxicity (Katsumata, 2009). The GOG conducted a definitive Phase III trial (protocol #262) among women with poor-prognosis, advanced ovarian cancer. Patients received dose-dense weekly paclitaxel plus carboplatin or were given paclitaxel plus carboplatin every 3 weeks. Bevacizumab was optional in both arms. Weekly paclitaxel plus carboplatin provided no clinical benefit in the group opting for added bevacizumab (Chan, 2016).

Intraperitoneal Chemotherapy.
In January 2006, the National Cancer Institute (NCI) issued a rare Clinical Announcement encouraging the use of intraperitoneal (IP) chemotherapy. This coincided with the publication of results from a Phase III GOG trial (protocol #172) of optimally debulked stage III ovarian cancer patients who were randomly assigned to receive either IV or combination IV/IP paclitaxel and cisplatin chemotherapy. The median duration of overall survival was 66 months in the IV/IP group compared with 50 months in the IV group (Armstrong, 2006).

The theoretical advantages of IP chemotherapy are dramatic, and interest has waxed and waned over the past few decades. In general, epithelial ovarian cancer mainly spreads along peritoneal surfaces. In postoperative patients with minimal residual disease, a much higher dose of chemotherapy can be achieved at the tumor site by administration directly into the abdomen (Alberts, 1996; Markman, 2001).

However, toxicity is generally higher with IP therapy, catheter-related problems are common, and the true long-term survival advantage remains controversial (Walker, 2006). Despite re-emergent interest in IP chemotherapy following the NCI announcement, more recently it has again been largely discarded following results of a randomized Phase III GOG trial (protocol #252) that compared: (1) dose-dense paclitaxel and IV carboplatin, (2) dose-dense paclitaxel and IP carboplatin, and (3) a modified GOG protocol #172 IP cisplatin regimen. All groups received concurrent bevacizumab followed by maintenance bevacizumab. The dose-dense arm was much better tolerated, and neither IP regimen offered a clinical advantage (Walker, 2019).

Although conventional IP therapy has again largely faded from routine clinical practice, hyperthermic intraperitoneal chemotherapy (HIPEC) has emerged. Heating chemotherapy enhances cytotoxicity against tumor cells. HIPEC has entered mainstream practice following promising results from a Phase III trial. Following three courses of neoadjuvant IV chemotherapy, 245 patients were randomly assigned to undergo interval debulking alone or to debulking surgery followed immediately by intraoperative HIPEC with cisplatin. The overall survival rate was extended by 1 year using HIPEC (van Driel, 2018). Additional studies are underway, and it remains unclear how widely this method will be adopted.

Management of Patients in Remission

In most women with advanced ovarian cancer, the combination of surgery and platinum-based chemotherapy will lead to clinical remission (normal examination, CA125 levels, and CT scan findings). However, up to 90 percent will eventually relapse and die from disease progression. Lower CA125 levels, that is, single-digit values, are generally associated with longer time until relapse and better survival rates (Juretzka, 2007). Since most patients achieving remission still will have residual, clinically occult, drug-resistant cells, options to consider include surveillance or maintenance therapy.

First, surveillance after treatment completion may include regular examinations and CA125 levels, as in early-stage disease. In those with new symptoms, physical findings, or rising CA125 titers, imaging may be indicated. In general, clinicians should maintain a heightened suspicion for relapse.

A second option is *maintenance chemotherapy*. Traditionally, limited evidence supported an advantage for additional treatment in women who achieve clinical remission after six courses of platinum-based chemotherapy. However, due to the known high rate of recurrence, several agents have been tested as maintenance therapy, in randomized studies. Of these, monthly paclitaxel was disappointing and caused significant neuropathy (Markman, 2003, 2009). In a later Phase III trial of 1157 patients, neither lower-dose paclitaxel nor CT-2103 (paclitaxel poliglumex) reduced the death rate compared with no maintenance therapy.

Bevacizumab, an antiangiogenic agent, also has been studied as maintenance therapy in several Phase III trials. In GOG protocol #218 and the Gynecologic InterGroup Trial (ICON-7) studies noted earlier (p. 749), bevacizumab was combined with paclitaxel and carboplatin and then continued alone for a year of maintenance therapy. This regimen demonstrated only a 2- to 4-month prolongation of progression-free survival and no overall survival benefit (Tewari, 2019). Of added interest, when maintenance bevacizumab was stopped, several patients experienced relapse soon after (Burger, 2011; Perren, 2011).

TABLE 35-9. Epithelial Ovarian Cancer 5-Year Survival Rates

Stage	5-Year Survival (%)
Localized (confined to primary site)	92
Regional (spread to regional nodes)	72
Distant (cancer has metastasized)	27
Unknown (unstaged)	22

Reproduced from National Cancer Institute: Ovarian epithelial cancer treatment (PDQ), 2014b, with permission.

Therefore, current trials allow maintenance bevacizumab to be continued indefinitely or until disease progression is identified.

Pazopanib, an oral multikinase inhibitor of the vascular endothelial growth factor (VEGF) receptor, also shows some promise as maintenance therapy. In a Phase III trial, patients receiving pazopanib had a 5.6-month improvement in progression-free survival compared with placebo. Still, it was associated with significant toxicity and lack of overall survival benefit (du Bois, 2014).

A breakthrough in maintenance therapy was achieved with the use of a poly (ADP-ribose) polymerase (PARP) inhibitor for BRCA-mutated ovarian cancer (Chap 27, p. 600). In a Phase III trial, 391 women with stage III or IV ovarian cancer that displayed *BRCA1/2* mutations were randomly assigned to olaparib (Lynparza) or placebo. The risk of disease progression or death was 70 percent lower with olaparib (Moore, 2018). This substantial benefit has led to an increased urgency to conduct germline and tumor testing in all patients with epithelial ovarian cancer to allow maintenance therapy with olaparib for the 25 percent with a *BRCA* or HR deficiency gene mutation.

■ Prognostic Factors

The overall 5-year survival rate of all stages of epithelial ovarian cancer approximates 45 percent, far lower than uterine (84 percent) or cervical cancer (73 percent). Survival rates mirror the assigned FIGO stage and largely depend on disease metastasis, which worsens outcomes (Table 35-9). Additional prognostic factors are shown in Table 35-10 (National Cancer Institute, 2019). Interestingly, carriers of *BRCA* mutations have a better prognosis, chiefly due to greater associated platinum sensitivity (Alsop, 2012; Lacour, 2011). However, even with favorable prognostic factors and despite recent innovations, most patients will ultimately relapse.

TABLE 35-10. Most Important Favorable Prognostic Factors for Ovarian Cancer

No ascites
Younger age
Early-stage disease
Well-differentiated tumor
Otherwise good health status
Histologic type other than mucinous or clear cell
Small disease volume prior to surgical debulking
Small residual tumor following primary cytoreductive surgery

Adapted from National Cancer Institute: Ovarian epithelial cancer treatment (PDQ), 2014b, with permission.

Management of Recurrent Ovarian Cancer

Gradual elevation of the CA125 level is usually the first sign of relapse. Tamoxifen may be administered when only "biochemical" evidence indicates disease progression. It has some activity in treating recurrent disease, and its toxicity is minimal (Hurteau, 2010). Alternatively, patients may be offered participation in a clinical trial, started on conventional cytotoxic chemotherapy, or observed until clinical symptoms arise. Without treatment, the recurrence usually will become clinically obvious within 2 to 6 months. Almost invariably, the tumor will be located somewhere within the abdomen.

Women who progress during primary chemotherapy are classified as having "platinum-refractory" disease and have a dismal prognosis. Those who relapse within 6 months of completing chemotherapy have "platinum-resistant" ovarian cancer and a somewhat better prognosis. For these groups, participation in an experimental clinical trial should be encouraged whenever possible. Otherwise, response rates typically range from 5 to 15 percent using nonplatinum FDA-approved conventional cytotoxic drugs such as paclitaxel, pegylated liposomal doxorubicin (Doxil), docetaxel (Taxotere), topotecan (Hycamtin), or gemcitabine (Gemzar). Recently, bevacizumab in combination with weekly paclitaxel, doxorubicin, or topotecan was shown to provide a 27-percent response rate. This was more than double the rate with single-agent chemotherapy alone in patients with platinum-resistant disease (Pujade-Lauraine, 2014). As a result, bevacizumab is now FDA-approved for this indication.

Women who relapse more than 6 months after primary therapy completion are considered "platinum-sensitive." These patients, especially those in prolonged remission beyond 18, 24, or 36 months, are usually retreated with a platinum-based combination. Carboplatin combined with either paclitaxel or gemcitabine has demonstrated modest superiority compared with carboplatin alone (Parmar, 2003; Pfisterer, 2006). Moreover, in one randomized Phase III trial, the novel combination of carboplatin and pegylated liposomal doxorubicin was superior to carboplatin and paclitaxel (Pujade-Lauraine, 2010). Of interest, although patients with primary early-stage ovarian cancer have a more favorable overall prognosis, survival after relapse is comparable to those who recurred after treatment of advanced-stage disease (Chan, 2010b).

Secondary Cytoreductive Surgery

Although patient selection is somewhat arbitrary, the best candidates for secondary cytoreductive surgery have: (1) platinum-sensitive disease, (2) a prior long disease-free interval, (3) a solitary-site recurrence, and (4) no ascites (Chi, 2006; Armstrong, 2019). To achieve a maximal survival benefit, debulking must result in minimal residual disease (Harter, 2006; Schorge, 2010). However, approximately half of patients will be explored without achieving this goal.

The overall survival benefit of this approach is currently being studied in a Phase III GOG trial (protocol #213). Surgical candidates with platinum-sensitive relapsed disease were randomly assigned to secondary debulking or not, followed by carboplatin and paclitaxel with or without additional bevacizumab. Of patients enrolled in this study, only 15 to 20 percent have thus far been considered surgical candidates.

Salvage Chemotherapy

In general, most relapsed ovarian cancer patients will end up receiving multiple sequential courses of chemotherapy (Armstrong, 2019). Regardless of which regimen is selected initially, reevaluation usually follows two to four cycles of chemotherapy (depending on the agent) to determine the clinical benefit. Typically, a CA125 level decline with or without confirmation of tumor shrinkage by CT imaging provides sufficient reassurance to continue therapy. Nonresponders are changed to a different regimen. Patients with a germline *BRCA1* or *BRCA2* gene mutation who develop resistance to platinum may benefit from targeted therapy with olaparib, niraparib (Zejula), or rucaparib (Rubraca). All three PARP inhibitors are now FDA-approved for this indication (Kaufman, 2015). However, at some point, usually after multiple agents have been tried, treatment will no longer be effective, which should prompt a discussion about further goals of care.

It would seem plausible that targeting therapy for an individual patient's disease might be more effective than empiric drug selection. In vitro chemosensitivity testing is occasionally used for this purpose. In principle, different agents are tested against the patient's tumor, and the chemotherapeutic drug demonstrating the best response should result in a better outcome. Unfortunately, this approach lacks demonstrable efficacy and is not recommended outside of a clinical trial (Armstrong, 2019; Burstein, 2011).

Palliation of End-Stage Ovarian Cancer

At some point, patients with recurrent disease will develop worsening symptoms that warrant reevaluation of their overall treatment strategy. Of these, intermittent episodes of partial small and large bowel obstruction are common during treatment. Bowel obstruction that does not resolve with nasogastric suction can be managed in two very different ways. Patients at first relapse or early in their course may warrant an aggressive approach that includes chemotherapy with or without surgical intervention and incorporates total parenteral nutrition. A colostomy, ileostomy, or intestinal bypass will often relieve symptoms (Chi, 2009b). Unfortunately, a satisfactory surgical result is sometimes impossible due to disease burden and multiple sites of partial or complete obstruction. In addition, successful palliation rarely is achieved when the bowel transit time is prolonged due to diffuse peritoneal carcinomatosis or when anatomy requires a bypass that results in the short bowel syndrome. Further, recovery may be complicated by an enterocutaneous fistula, reobstruction, or other morbid event (Pothuri, 2004). For patients with a refractory bowel obstruction due to progressive disease despite multiple lines of chemotherapy, the best approach usually is placement of a palliative gastrostomy tube, IV hydration, and hospice care. The final decision should be based on a frank discussion. Topics include treatment options, the natural history of progressive ovarian cancer, and the realistic chances of further disease response by switching to a different therapy.

Another common scenario is a woman with symptomatic, rapidly reaccumulating ascitic fluid. This may be alleviated by repeated paracenteses or by placement of an indwelling peritoneal catheter (PleurX), which can be self-drained as needed. Similarly, a refractory malignant pleural effusion can usually be managed by thoracentesis, indwelling pleural catheter placement, or pleurodesis. With this last procedure, irritants are instilled into the pleural space to incite adhesions that obliterate the space. Although these procedures and others may be appropriate in selected patients, the inability to halt disease progression should be acknowledged. In addition, any intervention has the potential to result in an unanticipated, catastrophic complication. Overall, palliative procedures are most compassionately used when incorporated into the overall treatment plan. For example, in a woman with stable disease and normal renal function, tumor-induced ureteral compression and hydronephrosis does not necessarily require stent placement or a nephrostomy tube.

All patients deserve a positive, hopeful, but honest approach to the management of progressive, incurable disease. Often, expectations regarding the benefit of palliative chemotherapy are unrealistic, but emotionally it may be preferable to the idea of "giving up" (Doyle, 2001). There is no substitute for mutual trust in the doctor–patient relationship when making sound decisions aimed at improving the quality of life of women with end-stage ovarian cancer.

REFERENCES

Al-Barrak J, Santos JL, Tinker A, et al: Exploring palliative treatment outcomes in women with advanced or recurrent ovarian clear cell carcinoma. Gynecol Oncol 122(1):107, 2011

Alberts DS, Liu PY, Hannigan EV, et al: Intraperitoneal cisplatin plus intravenous cyclophosphamide versus intravenous cisplatin plus intravenous cyclophosphamide for stage III ovarian cancer. N Engl J Med 335:1950, 1996

Aletti GD, Dowdy SC, Gostout BS, et al: Quality improvement in the surgical approach to advanced ovarian cancer: the Mayo Clinic experience. J Am Coll Surg 208:614, 2009

Aletti GD, Dowdy SC, Podratz KC, et al: Surgical treatment of diaphragm disease correlates with improved survival in optimally debulked advanced stage ovarian cancer. Gynecol Oncol 100:283, 2006

Alsop K, Fereday S, Meldrum C, et al: *BRCA* mutation frequency and patterns of treatment response in *BRCA* mutation-positive women with ovarian cancer: a report from the Australian Ovarian Cancer Study Group. J Clin Oncol 30(21):2654, 2012

Alvarado-Cabrero I, Cheung A, Caduff R: Tumours of the fallopian tube and uterine ligaments [Tumours of the fallopian tube]. In Tavassoli FA, Devilee P (eds): World Health Organization Classification of Tumours. Geneva, WHO, 2003, p 206

American College of Obstetricians and Gynecologists: Evaluation and management of adnexal masses. Practice Bulletin No. 174, November 2016

American College of Obstetricians and Gynecologists: Hereditary breast and ovarian cancer syndrome. Practice Bulletin No. 182, September 2017a

American College of Obstetricians and Gynecologists: The role of the obstetrician-gynecologist in the early detection of epithelial ovarian cancer in women at average risk. Committee Opinion No. 716, September 2017b

American College of Obstetricians and Gynecologists: Opportunistic salpingectomy as a strategy for epithelial ovarian cancer prevention. Committee Opinion No. 774, March 2019

Armstrong DK, Alvarez RD, Bakkum-Gamez JN, et al: NCCN Guidelines Insights: Ovarian Cancer, Version 1.2019. J Natl Compr Canc Netw 17(8):896, 2019

Armstrong DK, Bundy B, Wenzel L, et al: Intraperitoneal cisplatin and paclitaxel in ovarian cancer. N Engl J Med 354:34, 2006

Beiner ME, Finch A, Rosen B, et al: The risk of endometrial cancer in women with *BRCA1* and *BRCA2* mutations: a prospective study. Gynecol Oncol 104(1):7, 2007

Bell J, Brady MF, Young RC, et al: Randomized phase III trial of three versus six cycles of adjuvant carboplatin and paclitaxel in early stage epithelial ovarian carcinoma: a Gynecologic Oncology Group study. Gynecol Oncol 102:432, 2006

Berton-Rigaud D, Devouassoux-Shisheboran M, Ledermann JA, et al: Gynecologic Cancer Intergroup (GCIG) consensus review for uterine and ovarian carcinosarcoma. Int J Gynecol Cancer 24(9 suppl 3):S55, 2014

Bloomfield HE, Olson A, Greer N, et al: Screening pelvic examinations in asymptomatic, average-risk adult women: an evidence report for a clinical practice guideline from the American College of Physicians. Ann Intern Med 161(1):46, 2014

Bookman MA, Brady MF, McGuire WP, et al: Evaluation of new platinum-based treatment regimens in advanced-stage ovarian cancer: a phase III trial of the Gynecologic Cancer Intergroup. J Clin Oncol 27:1419, 2009

Bray F, Ferlay J, Soerjomataram I, et al: Global cancer statistics 2018: GLOBOCAN estimates of incidence and mortality worldwide for 36 cancers in 185 countries. CA Cancer J Clin 68(6):394, 2018

Bristow RE, Palis BE, Chi DS, et al: The National Cancer Database report on advanced-stage epithelial ovarian cancer: impact of hospital surgical case volume on overall survival and surgical treatment paradigm. Gynecol Oncol 118:262, 2010

Burger RA, Brady MF, Bookman MA, et al: Incorporation of bevacizumab in the primary treatment of ovarian cancer. N Engl J Med 365(26):2473, 2011

Burstein HJ, Mangu PB, Somerfield MR, et al: American Society of Clinical Oncology clinical practice guideline update on the use of chemotherapy sensitivity and resistance assays. J Clin Oncol 29(24):3328, 2011

Buttin BM, Herzog TJ, Powell MA, et al: Epithelial ovarian tumors of low malignant potential: the role of microinvasion. Obstet Gynecol 99:11, 2002

Carlson JW, Miron A, Jarboe EA, et al: Serous tubal intraepithelial carcinoma: its potential role in primary peritoneal serous carcinoma and serous cancer prevention. J Clin Oncol 26:4160, 2008

Chan JK, Brady MF, Penson RT, et al: Weekly vs. every-3-week paclitaxel and carboplatin for ovarian cancer. N Engl J Med 374(8):738, 2016

Chan JK, Munro EG, Cheung MK, et al: Association of lymphadenectomy and survival in stage I ovarian cancer patients. Obstet Gynecol 109:12, 2007

Chan JK, Tian C, Fleming GF, et al: The potential benefit of 6 vs. 3 cycles of chemotherapy in subsets of women with early-stage high-risk epithelial ovarian cancer: an exploratory analysis of a Gynecologic Oncology Group study. Gynecol Oncol 116:301, 2010a

Chan JK, Tian C, Teoh D, et al: Survival after recurrence in early-stage high-risk epithelial ovarian cancer: a Gynecologic Oncology Group study. Gynecol Oncol 116:307, 2010b

Chang SJ, Bristow RE: Evolution of surgical treatment paradigms for advanced-stage ovarian cancer: redefining 'optimal' residual disease. Gynecol Oncol 125(2):483, 2012

Chi DS, Abu-Rustum NR, Sonoda Y, et al: The safety and efficacy of laparoscopic surgical staging of apparent stage I ovarian and fallopian tube cancers. Am J Obstet Gynecol 192:1614, 2005

Chi DS, Eisenhauer EL, Zivanovic O, et al: Improved progression-free and overall survival in advanced ovarian cancer as a result of a change in surgical paradigm. Gynecol Oncol 114:26, 2009a

Chi DS, McCaughty K, Diaz JP, et al: Guidelines and selection criteria for secondary cytoreductive surgery in patients with recurrent, platinum-sensitive epithelial ovarian carcinoma. Cancer 106:1933, 2006

Chi DS, Phaeton R, Miner TJ, et al: A prospective outcomes analysis of palliative procedures performed for malignant intestinal obstruction due to recurrent ovarian cancer. Oncologist 14:835, 2009b

Chi DS, Ramirez PT, Teitcher JB, et al: Prospective study of the correlation between postoperative computed tomography scan and primary surgeon assessment in patients with advanced ovarian, tubal, and peritoneal carcinoma reported to have undergone primary surgical cytoreduction to residual disease 1 cm or less. J Clin Oncol 25(31):4946, 2007

Collaborative Group on Epidemiological Studies of Ovarian Cancer, Beral V, Doll R, et al: Ovarian cancer and oral contraceptives: collaborative reanalysis of data from 45 epidemiological studies including 23,257 women with ovarian cancer and 87,303 controls. Lancet 371(9609):303, 2008

Cramer DW, Vitonis AF, Terry KL, et al: The association between talc use and ovarian cancer: a retrospective case-control study in two US states. Epidemiology 27(3):334, 2016

Crane EK, Sun CC, Ramirez PT, et al: The role of secondary cytoreduction in low-grade serous ovarian cancer or peritoneal cancer. Gynecol Oncol 136(1):25, 2015

Cress RD, Bauer K, O'Malley CD, et al: Surgical staging of early stage epithelial ovarian cancer: results from the CDC-NPCR ovarian patterns of care study. Gynecol Oncol 121:94, 2011

Delle Marchette M, Ceppi L, Andreano A, et al: Oncologic and fertility impact of surgical approach for borderline ovarian tumours treated with fertility sparing surgery. Eur J Cancer 111:61, 2019

Doyle C, Crump M, Pintilie M, et al: Does palliative chemotherapy palliate? Evaluation of expectations, outcomes, and costs in women receiving chemotherapy for advanced ovarian cancer. J Clin Oncol 19:1266, 2001 du Bois A, Ewald-Riegler N, de Gregorio N, et al: Borderline tumours of the ovary: a cohort study of the Arbeitsgemeinschaft Gynäkologische Onkologie (AGO) Study Group. Eur J Cancer 49(8):1905, 2013

du Bois A, Floquet A, Kim JW, et al: Incorporation of pazopanib in maintenance therapy of ovarian cancer J Clin Oncol 32(30):3374, 2014

du Bois A, Luck HJ, Meier W, et al: A randomized clinical trial of cisplatin/paclitaxel versus carboplatin/paclitaxel as first-line treatment of ovarian cancer. J Natl Cancer Inst 95:1320, 2003

Earle CC, Schrag D, Neville BA, et al: Effect of surgeon specialty on processes of care and outcomes for ovarian cancer patients. J Natl Cancer Inst 98:172, 2006

Eichhorn JH, Young RH, Scully RE: Primary ovarian small cell carcinoma of pulmonary type: a clinicopathologic, immunohistologic, and flow cytometric analysis of 11 cases. Am J Surg Pathol 16:926, 1992

Elder JW, Pavlik EJ, Long A, et al: Serial ultrasonographic evaluation of ovarian abnormalities with a morphology index. Gynecol Oncol 135(1):8, 2014

Engelen MJ, Kos HE, Willemse PH, et al: Surgery by consultant gynecologic oncologists improves survival in patients with ovarian carcinoma. Cancer 106:589, 2006

Fagotti A, Fanfani F, Ludovisi M, et al: Role of laparoscopy to assess the chance of optimal cytoreductive surgery in advanced ovarian cancer: a pilot study. Gynecol Oncol 96(3):729, 2005

Fagotti A, Vizzielli G, De Iaco P, et al: A multicentric trial (Olympia-MITO 13) on the accuracy of laparoscopy to assess peritoneal spread in ovarian cancer. Am J Obstet Gynecol 209(5):462.e1, 2013

Falconer H, Yin L, Grönberg H, et al: Ovarian cancer risk after salpingectomy: a nationwide population-based study. J Natl Cancer Inst 107(2), 2015

Fleming ND, Nick AM, Coleman RL, et al: Laparoscopic surgical algorithm to triage the timing of tumor reductive surgery in advanced ovarian cancer. Obstet Gynecol 132(3):545, 2018

Friebel TM, Domchek SM, Rebbeck TR: Modifiers of cancer risk in BRCA1 and BRCA2 mutation carriers: systematic review and meta-analysis. J Natl Cancer Inst 106(6):dju091, 2014

Fruscio R, Ceppi L, Corso S, et al: Long-term results of fertility-sparing treatment compared with standard radical surgery for early-stage epithelial ovarian cancer. Br J Cancer 115(6):641, 2016

Garcia C, Lyon L, Littell RD, et al: Comparison of risk management strategies between women testing positive for a BRCA variant of unknown significance and women with known BRCA deleterious mutations. Genet Med 16(12):896, 2014

Gershenson DM, Bodurka DC, Coleman RL, et al: Hormonal maintenance therapy for women with low-grade serous cancer of the ovary or peritoneum. J Clin Oncol 35(10):1103, 2017

Goff BA, Mandel L, Muntz HG, et al: Ovarian carcinoma diagnosis. Cancer 89:2068, 2000

Goff BA, Mandel LS, Melancon CH, et al: Frequency of symptoms of ovarian cancer in women presenting to primary care clinics. JAMA 291:2705, 2004

Goff BA, Matthews BJ, Wynn M, et al: Ovarian cancer: patterns of surgical care across the United States. Gynecol Oncol 103:383, 2006

Grabowski JP, Harter P, Hils R, et al: Outcome of immediate re-operation or interval debulking after chemotherapy at a gynecologic oncology center after initially incomplete cytoreduction of advanced ovarian cancer. Gynecol Oncol 126(1):54, 2012

Griffiths CT: Surgical resection of tumor bulk in the primary treatment of ovarian carcinoma. Natl Cancer Inst Monogr 42:101, 1975

Guseh SH, Rauh-Hain JA, Tambouret RH, et al: Transitional cell carcinoma of the ovary: a case-control study. Gynecol Oncol 132(3):649, 2014

Hannibal CG, Vang R, Junge J, et al: A nationwide study of serous "borderline" ovarian tumors in Denmark 1978–2002: centralized pathology review and overall survival compared with the general population. Gynecol Oncol 134(2):267, 2014

Harter P, Bois A, Hahmann M, et al: Surgery in recurrent ovarian cancer: the Arbeitsgemeinschaft Gynaekologische Onkologie (AGO) DESKTOP OVAR Trial. Ann Surg Oncol 13:1702, 2006

Harter P, Gershenson D, Lhomme C, et al: Gynecologic Cancer InterGroup (GCIG) consensus review for ovarian tumors of low malignant potential (borderline ovarian tumors). Int J Gynecol Cancer 24(9 Suppl 3):S5, 2014

Harter P, Sehouli J, Lorusso D, et al: A randomized trial of lymphadenectomy in patients with advanced ovarian neoplasms. N Engl J Med 380(9):822, 2019

Heintz AP, Odicino F, Maisonneuve P, et al: Carcinoma of the ovary. In FIGO annual report on the results of treatment in gynaecological cancer. Int J Obstet Gynecol 95(Suppl 1):S161, 2006

Hinkula M, Pukkala E, Kyyronen P, et al: Incidence of ovarian cancer of grand multiparous women: a population-based study in Finland. Gynecol Oncol 103:207, 2006

Hurteau JA, Brady MF, Darcy KM, et al: Randomized phase III trial of tamoxifen versus thalidomide in women with biochemical-recurrent-only epithelial ovarian, fallopian tube or primary peritoneal carcinoma after a complete response to first-line platinum/taxane chemotherapy with an evaluation of serum vascular endothelial growth factor (VEGF): a Gynecologic Oncology Group study. Gynecol Oncol 119:444, 2010

Huusom LD, Frederiksen K, Hogdall EV, et al: Association of reproductive factors, oral contraceptive use and selected lifestyle factors with the risk of ovarian borderline tumors: a Danish case-control study. Cancer Causes Control 17:821, 2006

Im SS, Gordon AN, Buttin BM, et al: Validation of referral guidelines for women with pelvic masses. Obstet Gynecol 105:35, 2005

Iodice S, Barile M, Rotmensz N, et al: Oral contraceptive use and breast or ovarian cancer risk in BRCA1/2 carriers: a meta-analysis. Eur J Cancer 46(12):2275, 2010

Jacobs I, Oram D, Fairbanks J, et al: A risk of malignancy index incorporating CA 125, ultrasound and menopausal status for the accurate preoperative diagnosis of ovarian cancer. BJOG 97(10):922, 1990

Jacobs IJ, Menon U, Ryan A, et al: Ovarian cancer screening and mortality in the UK collaborative trial of ovarian cancer screening (UKCTOCS): a randomised controlled trial. Lancet 387(10022):945, 2016

Jareid M, Thalabard JC, Aarflot M, et al: Levonorgestrel-releasing intrauterine system use is associated with a decreased risk of ovarian and endometrial cancer, without increased risk of breast cancer. Results from the NOWAC Study. Gynecol Oncol 149(1):127, 2018

Jelinic P, Mueller JJ, Olvera N, et al: Recurrent SMARCA4 mutations in small cell carcinoma of the ovary. Nat Genet 46(5):424, 2014

Juretzka MM, Barakat RR, Chi DS, et al: CA-125 level as a predictor of progression-free survival and overall survival in ovarian cancer patients with surgically defined disease status prior to the initiation of intraperitoneal consolidation therapy. Gynecol Oncol 104(1):176, 2007

Karlsen MA, Sandhu N, Høgdall C, et al: Evaluation of HE4, CA125, risk of ovarian malignancy algorithm (ROMA) and risk of malignancy index (RMI) as diagnostic tools of epithelial ovarian cancer in patients with a pelvic mass. Gynecol Oncol 127(2):379, 2012

Katsumata N, Yasuda M, Takahashi F, et al: Dose-dense paclitaxel once a week in combination with carboplatin every 3 weeks for advanced ovarian cancer: a phase 3, open-label, randomized controlled trial. Lancet 374:1331, 2009

Kauff ND, Satagopan JM, Robson ME, et al: Risk-reducing salpingo-oophorectomy in women with a BRCA1 or BRCA2 mutation. N Engl J Med 346:1609, 2002

Kaufman B, Shapira-Frommer R, Schmutzler RK, et al: Olaparib monotherapy in patients with advanced cancer and a germline BRCA1/2 Mutation. J Clin Oncol 33(3):244, 2015

Kehoe S, Hook J, Nankivell M, et al: Primary chemotherapy versus primary surgery for newly diagnosed advanced ovarian cancer (CHORUS): an open-label, randomised, controlled, non-inferiority trial. Lancet 386(9990):249, 2015

Kiani F, Knutsen S, Singh P, et al: Dietary risk factors for ovarian cancer: the Adventist Health Study (United States). Cancer Causes Control 17:137, 2006

Kramer JL, Velazquez IA, Chen BE, et al: Prophylactic oophorectomy reduces breast cancer penetrance during prospective, long-term follow-up of BRCA1 mutation carriers. J Clin Oncol 23:8629, 2005

Kristensen GS, Schledermann D, Mogensen O, et al: The value of random biopsies, omentectomy, and hysterectomy in operations for borderline ovarian tumors. Int J Gynecol Cancer 24(5):874, 2014

Kroeger PT Jr, Drapkin R: Pathogenesis and heterogeneity of ovarian cancer. Curr Opin Obstet Gynecol 29(1):26, 2017

Kruitwagen RF, Swinkels BM, Keyser KG, et al: Incidence and effect on survival of abdominal wall metastases at trocar or puncture sites following laparoscopy or paracentesis in women with ovarian cancer. Gynecol Oncol 60:233, 1996

Kurman RJ, Carcangiu ML, Herrington CS, et al (eds): WHO Classification of Tumours of Female Reproductive Organs, 4th ed. Lyon, International Agency for Research on Cancer, 2014

Kurman RJ, Shih IM: The dualistic model of ovarian carcinogenesis: revisited, revised, and expanded. Am J Pathol 186(4):733, 2016

Labidi-Galy SI, Papp E, Hallberg D, et al: High grade serous ovarian carcinomas originate in the fallopian tube. Nat Commun 8(1):1093, 2017

Lacour RA, Westin SN, Meyer LA, et al: Improved survival in non-Ashkenazi Jewish ovarian cancer patients with BRCA1 and BRCA2 gene mutations. Gynecol Oncol 121:358, 2011

Lancaster JM, Powell CB, Chen LM, et al: Society of Gynecologic Oncology statement on risk assessment for inherited gynecologic cancer predispositions. Gynecol Oncol 136(1):3, 2015

Leary A, Petrella MC, Pautier P, et al: Adjuvant platinum-based chemotherapy for borderline serous ovarian tumors with invasive implants. Gynecol Oncol 132(1):23, 2014

Lee AW, Ness RB, Roman LD, et al: Association between menopausal estrogen-only therapy and ovarian carcinoma risk. Ovarian cancer association consortium. Obstet Gynecol 127(5):828, 2016

Lee JY, Kim HS, Chung HH, et al: The role of omentectomy and random peritoneal biopsies as part of comprehensive surgical staging in apparent early-stage epithelial ovarian cancer. Ann Surg Oncol 21(8):2762, 2014

Lee KR, Tavassoli FA, Prat J, et al: Tumours of the ovary and peritoneum [Surface epithelial-stromal tumours]. In Tavassoli FA, Devilee P (eds): World Health Organization Classification of Tumours. Geneva, WHO, 2003, p 117

Lessard-Anderson CR, Handlogten KS, Molitor RJ, et al: Effect of tubal sterilization technique on risk of serous epithelial ovarian and primary peritoneal carcinoma. Gynecol Oncol 135(3):423, 2014

Levanon K, Crum C, Drapkin R: New insights into the pathogenesis of serous ovarian cancer and its clinical impact. J Clin Oncol 26:5284, 2008

Li AJ, Madden AC, Cass I, et al: The prognostic significance of thrombocytosis in epithelial ovarian carcinoma. Gynecol Oncol 92:211, 2004

Lin PS, Gershenson DM, Bevers MW, et al: The current status of surgical staging of ovarian serous borderline tumors. Cancer 85:905, 1999

Madalinska JB, Hollenstein J, Bleiker E, et al: Quality-of-life effects of prophylactic salpingo-oophorectomy versus gynecologic screening among women at increased risk of hereditary ovarian cancer. J Clin Oncol 23:6890, 2005

Manchanda R, Abdelraheim A, Johnson M, et al: Outcome of risk-reducing salpingo-oophorectomy in BRCA carriers and women of unknown mutation status. BJOG 118(7):814, 2011

Markman M, Bundy BN, Alberts DS, et al: Phase III trial of standard-dose intravenous cisplatin plus paclitaxel versus moderately high-dose carboplatin followed by intravenous paclitaxel and intraperitoneal cisplatin in small-volume stage III ovarian carcinoma: an intergroup study of the Gynecologic Oncology Group, Southwestern Oncology Group, and Eastern Cooperative Oncology Group. J Clin Oncol 19:1001, 2001

Markman M, Liu PY, Moon J, et al: Impact on survival of 12 versus 3 monthly cycles of paclitaxel (175 mg/m^2) administered to patients with advanced ovarian cancer who attained a complete response to primary platinum-paclitaxel: follow-up of a Southwest Oncology Group and Gynecologic Oncology Group phase III trial. Gynecol Oncol 114(2):195, 2009

Markman M, Liu PY, Wilczynski S, et al: Phase III randomized trial of 12 versus 3 months of maintenance paclitaxel in patients with advanced ovarian cancer after complete response to platinum and paclitaxel-based chemotherapy: a Southwest Oncology Group and Gynecologic Oncology Group trial. J Clin Oncol 21:2460, 2003

McCann CK, Growdon WB, Munro EG, et al: Prognostic significance of splenectomy as part of initial cytoreductive surgery in ovarian cancer. Ann Surg Oncol 18(10):2912, 2011

Melamed A, Nitecki R, Boruta DM II, et al: Laparoscopy compared with laparotomy for debulking ovarian cancer after neoadjuvant chemotherapy. Obstet Gynecol 129(5):861, 2017

Menzin AW, Gal D, Lovecchio JL: Contemporary surgical management of borderline ovarian tumors: a survey of the Society of Gynecologic Oncologists. Gynecol Oncol 78:7, 2000

Mercado C, Zingmond D, Karlan BY, et al: Quality of care in advanced ovarian cancer: the importance of provider specialty. Gynecol Oncol 117:18, 2010

Mok SC, Schorge JO, Welch WR, et al: Tumours of the ovary and peritoneum [Peritoneal tumours]. In Tavassoli FA, Devilee P (eds): World Health Organization Classification of Tumours. Geneva, WHO, 2003, p 197

Moore K, Colombo N, Scambia G: Maintenance olaparib in patients with newly diagnosed advanced ovarian cancer. N Engl J Med 379(26):2495, 2018

Moore RG, Jabre-Raughley M, Brown AK, et al: Comparison of a novel multiple marker assay vs the Risk of Malignancy Index for the prediction of epithelial ovarian cancer in patients with a pelvic mass. Am J Obstet Gynecol 203(3):228.e1, 2010

Moore RG, McMeekin DS, Brown AK, et al: A novel multiple marker bioassay utilizing HE4 and CA125 for the prediction of ovarian cancer in patients with a pelvic mass. Gynecol Oncol 112(1):40, 2009

Moorman PG, Havrilesky LJ, Gierisch JM, et al: Oral contraceptives and risk of ovarian cancer and breast cancer among high-risk women: a systematic review and metaanalysis. J Clin Oncol 31(33):4188, 2013

Mørch LS, Skovlund CW, Hannaford PC, et al: Contemporary hormonal contraception and the risk of breast cancer. N Engl J Med 377(23):2228, 2017

Morice P, Uzan C, Fauvet R, et al: Borderline ovarian tumour: pathological diagnostic dilemma and risk factors for invasive or lethal recurrence. Lancet Oncol 13(3):e103, 2012

National Cancer Institute: National Cancer Institute issues clinical announcement for preferred method of treatment for advanced ovarian cancer. 2006. Available at: https://www.nih.gov/news-events/news-releases/nci-issues-clinical-announcement-preferred-method-treatment-advanced-ovarian-cancer. Accessed August 12, 2019

National Cancer Institute: Ovarian epithelial, fallopian tube, and primary peritoneal cancer treatment (PDQ®)–Health Professional Version. 2019. Available at: https://www.cancer.gov/types/ovarian/hp/ovarian-epithelial-treatment-pdq. Accessed August 12, 2019

Ozols RF, Bundy BN, Greer BE, et al: Phase III trial of carboplatin and paclitaxel compared with cisplatin and paclitaxel in patients with optimally resected stage III ovarian cancer: a Gynecologic Oncology Group study. J Clin Oncol 21:3194, 2003

Park JY, Kim DY, Kim JH, et al: Surgical management of borderline ovarian tumors: the role of fertility-sparing surgery. Gynecol Oncol 113:75, 2009

Park JY, Song JS, Choi G, et al: Pure primary squamous cell carcinoma of the ovary: a report of two cases and review of the literature. Int J Gynecol Pathol 29:328, 2010

Parmar MK, Ledermann JA, Colombo N, et al: Paclitaxel plus platinum-based chemotherapy versus conventional platinum-based chemotherapy in women with relapsed ovarian cancer: the ICON4/AGO-OVAR-2.2 trial. Lancet 361:2099, 2003

Pecorelli S, Benedet JL, Creasman WT, et al: FIGO staging of gynecologic cancer, 1994–1997. FIGO Committee on Gynecologic Oncology, International Federation of Gynecology and Obstetrics. Int J Gynaecol Obstet 65:243, 1999

Pelucchi C, Galeone C, Talamini R, et al: Lifetime ovulatory cycles and ovarian cancer risk in 2 Italian case-control studies. Am J Obstet Gynecol 196(1):83.e1, 2007

Penninkilampi R, Eslick GD: Perineal talc use and ovarian cancer: a systematic review and meta-analysis. Epidemiology 29(1):41, 2018

Perren TJ, Swart AM, Pfisterer J, et al: A phase 3 trial of bevacizumab in ovarian cancer. N Engl J Med 365(26):2484, 2011

Pfisterer J, Plante M, Vergote I, et al: Gemcitabine plus carboplatin compared with carboplatin in patients with platinum-sensitive recurrent ovarian cancer: an intergroup trial of the AGO-OVAR, the NCIC CTG, and the EORTC GCG. J Clin Oncol 24:4699, 2006

Pins MR, Young RH, Daly WJ, et al: Primary squamous cell carcinoma of the ovary. Report of 37 cases. Am J Surg Pathol 20:823, 1996

Poncelet C, Fauvet R, Boccara J, et al: Recurrence after cystectomy for borderline ovarian tumors: results of a French multicenter study. Ann Surg Oncol 13:565, 2006

Pothuri B, Meyer L, Gerardi M, et al: Reoperation for palliation of recurrent malignant bowel obstruction in ovarian carcinoma. Gynecol Oncol 95:193, 2004

Prat J, FIGO Committee on Gynecologic Oncology: Staging classification for cancer of the ovary, fallopian tube, and peritoneum. Int J Gynaecol Obstet 124(1):1, 2014

Prat J, Morice P: Tumours of the ovary and peritoneum [Secondary tumours of the ovary]. In Tavassoli FA, Devilee P (eds): World Health Organization Classification of Tumours. Geneva, WHO, 2003, p 193

Pujade-Lauraine E, Hilpert F, Weber B, et al: Bevacizumab combined with chemotherapy for platinum-resistant recurrent ovarian cancer: the AURELIA open-label randomized phase III trial. J Clin Oncol 32(13):1302, 2014

Pujade-Lauraine E, Wagner U, Aavall-Lundqvist E, et al: Pegylated liposomal doxorubicin and carboplatin compared with paclitaxel and carboplatin for patients with platinum-sensitive ovarian cancer in late relapse. J Clin Oncol 28:3323, 2010

Purdie DM, Bain CJ, Siskind V, et al: Ovulation and risk of epithelial ovarian cancer. Int J Cancer 104:228, 2003

Rao GG, Skinner E, Gehrig PA, et al: Surgical staging of ovarian low malignant potential tumors. Obstet Gynecol 104:261, 2004

Rao GG, Skinner EN, Gehrig PA, et al: Fertility-sparing surgery for ovarian low malignant potential tumors. Gynecol Oncol 98:263, 2005

Rebbeck TR, Lynch HT, Neuhausen SL, et al: Prophylactic oophorectomy in carriers of BRCA1 or BRCA2 mutations. N Engl J Med 346:1616, 2002

Rice MS, Hankinson SE, Tworoger SS: Tubal ligation, hysterectomy, unilateral oophorectomy, and risk of ovarian cancer in the Nurses' Health Studies. Fertil Steril 102(1):192, 2014

Ring KL, Garcia C, Thomas MH, et al: Current and future role of genetic screening in gynecologic malignancies. Am J Obstet Gynecol 217(5):512, 2017

Ronnett BM, Shmookler BM, Sugarbaker PH, et al: Pseudomyxoma peritonei: new concepts in diagnosis, origin, nomenclature, and relationship to mucinous borderline (low malignant potential) tumors of the ovary. Anat Pathol 2197, 1997

Ronnett BM, Yan H, Kurman RJ, et al: Patients with pseudomyxoma peritonei associated with disseminated peritoneal adenomucinosis have a significantly more favorable prognosis than patients with peritoneal mucinous carcinomatosis. Cancer 92:85, 2001

Rossing MA, Tang MT, Flagg EW, et al: A case-control study of ovarian cancer in relation to infertility and the use of ovulation-inducing drugs. Am J Epidemiol 160:1070, 2004

Rustin GJ, van der Burg ME, Griffin CL, et al: Early versus delayed treatment of relapsed ovarian cancer (MRC OV05/EORTC 55955): a randomized trial. Lancet 376:1155, 2010

Schilder JM, Thompson AM, DePriest PD, et al: Outcome of reproductive age women with stage IA or IC invasive epithelial ovarian cancer treated with fertility-sparing therapy. Gynecol Oncol 87:1, 2002

Schildkraut JM, Bastos E, Berchuck A: Relationship between lifetime ovulatory cycles and overexpression of mutant p53 in epithelial ovarian cancer. J Natl Cancer Inst 89:932, 1997

Schmeler KM, Lynch HT, Chen LM, et al: Prophylactic surgery to reduce the risk of gynecologic cancers in the Lynch syndrome. N Engl J Med 354:261, 2006

Schorge JO, Clark RM, Lee SI, et al: Primary debulking surgery for advanced ovarian cancer: are you a believer or a dissenter? Gynecol Oncol 135(3):595, 2014

Schorge JO, Muto MG, Welch WR, et al: Molecular evidence for multifocal papillary serous carcinoma of the peritoneum in patients with germline *BRCA1* mutations. J Natl Cancer Inst 90:841, 1998

Schorge JO, Wingo SN, Bhore R, et al: Secondary cytoreductive surgery for platinum-sensitive ovarian cancer. Int J Gynaecol Obstet 108:123, 2010

Seidman JD, Kurman RJ: Ovarian serous borderline tumors: a critical review of the literature with emphasis on prognostic indicators. Hum Pathol 31:539, 2000

Shah JS, Mackelvie M, Gershenson DM, et al: Accuracy of intraoperative frozen section diagnosis of borderline ovarian tumors by hospital type. J Minim Invasive Gynecol 26(1):87, 2019

Sherman ME, Piedmonte M, Mai PL, et al: Pathologic findings at risk-reducing salpingo-oophorectomy: primary results from Gynecologic Oncology Group Trial GOG-0199. J Clin Oncol 32(29):3275, 2014

Shih KK, Zhou QC, Aghajanian C, et al: Patterns of recurrence and role of adjuvant chemotherapy in stage II-IV serous ovarian borderline tumors. Gynecol Oncol 119:270, 2010

Siegel RL, Miller KD, Jemal A: Cancer statistics, 2019. CA Cancer J Clin 69(1):7, 2019

Silva EG, Gershenson DM, Malpica A, et al: The recurrence and the overall survival rates of ovarian serous borderline neoplasms with noninvasive implants is time dependent. Am J Surg Pathol 30:1367, 2006

Silva EG, Tornos C, Bailey MA, et al: Undifferentiated carcinoma of the ovary. Arch Pathol Lab Med 115:377, 1991

Skates SJ, Greene MH, Buys SS, et al: Early detection of ovarian cancer using the risk of ovarian cancer algorithm with frequent CA125 testing in women at increased familial risk-combined results from two screening trials. Clin Cancer Res 23(14):3628, 2017

Skates SJ, Menon U, MacDonald N, et al: Calculation of the risk of ovarian cancer from serial CA-125 values for preclinical detection in postmenopausal women. J Clin Oncol 21:206, 2003

Soliman PT, Slomovitz BM, Broaddus RR, et al: Synchronous primary cancers of the endometrium and ovary: a single institution review of 84 cases. Gynecol Oncol 94:456, 2004

Suh-Burgmann E, Flanagan T, Osinski T, et al: Prospective validation of a standardized ultrasonography-based ovarian cancer risk assessment system. Obstet Gynecol 132(5):1101, 2018

Suidan RS, Ramirez PT, Sarasohn DM, et al: A multicenter prospective trial evaluating the ability of preoperative computed tomography scan and serum CA-125 to predict suboptimal cytoreduction at primary debulking surgery for advanced ovarian, fallopian tube, and peritoneal cancer. Gynecol Oncol 134(3):455, 2014

Sutton GP, Bundy BN, Omura GA, et al: Stage III ovarian tumors of low malignant potential treated with cisplatin combination therapy: a Gynecologic Oncology Group study. Gynecol Oncol 41:230, 1991

Tang M, O'Connell RL, Amant F, et al: PARAGON: a phase II study of anastrozole in patients with estrogen receptor-positive recurrent/metastatic low-grade ovarian cancers and serous borderline ovarian tumors. Gynecol Oncol 154(3):531, 2019

Tewari KS, Burger RA, Enserro D, et al: Final overall survival of a randomized trial of bevacizumab for primary treatment of ovarian cancer. J Clin Oncol 37(26):2317, 2019

The ICON Collaborators: ICON2: Randomised trial of single-agent carboplatin against three-drug combination of CAP (cyclophosphamide, doxorubicin, and cisplatin) in women with ovarian cancer. International Collaborative Ovarian Neoplasm Study. Lancet 352:1571, 1998

The ICON Group: Paclitaxel plus carboplatin versus standard chemotherapy with either single-agent carboplatin or cyclophosphamide, doxorubicin, and cisplatin in women with ovarian cancer: the ICON3 randomised trial. Lancet 360:505, 2002

Timmers PJ, Zwinderman K, Coens C, et al: Lymph node sampling and taking of blind biopsies are important elements of the surgical staging of early ovarian cancer. Int J Gynecol Cancer 20:1142, 2010

Timofeev J, Galgano MT, Stoler MH, et al: Appendiceal pathology at the time of oophorectomy for ovarian neoplasms. Obstet Gynecol 116:1348, 2010

Torre LA, Bray F, Siegel RL, et al: Global cancer statistics, 2012. CA Cancer J Clin 65(2):87, 2015

Torre LA, Islami F, Siegel RL, et al: Global cancer in women: burden and trends. Cancer Epidemiol Biomarkers Prev 26(4):444, 2017

Torre LA, Trabert B, DeSantis CE, et al: Ovarian cancer statistics, 2018. CA Cancer J Clin. 68(4):284, 2018

Tozzi R, Kohler C, Ferrara A, et al: Laparoscopic treatment of early ovarian cancer: surgical and survival outcomes. Gynecol Oncol 93:199, 2004

Trimble CL, Kosary C, Trimble EL: Long-term survival and patterns of care in women with ovarian tumors of low malignant potential. Gynecol Oncol 86:34, 2002

Ueland FR, Desmone CP, Seamon LG, et al: Effectiveness of a multivariate index assay in the preoperative assessment of ovarian tumors. Obstet Gynecol 117(6):1289, 2011

U.S. Preventive Services Task Force, Bibbins-Domingo K, Grossman DC: Screening for gynecologic conditions with pelvic examination: US Preventive Services Task Force recommendation statement. JAMA 317(9):947, 2017

U.S. Preventive Services Task Force, Grossman DC, Curry SJ, et al: Screening for ovarian cancer: US recommendation statement. US Preventive Services Task Force. JAMA 319(6):588, 2018

van Driel WJ, Koole SN, Sikorska K, et al: Hyperthermic intraperitoneal chemotherapy in ovarian cancer. N Engl J Med 378(3):230, 2018

Vergote I, Trope CG, Amant F, et al: Neoadjuvant chemotherapy or primary surgery in stage IIIC or IV ovarian cancer. N Engl J Med 363:943, 2010

Verheijen RH, Mensdorff-Pouilly S, van Kamp GJ, et al: CA-125: fundamental and clinical aspects. Semin Cancer Biol 9:117, 1999

Vyarvelska I, Rosen B, Narod SA: Should hysterectomy complement prophylactic salpingo-oophorectomy in *BRCA1* and *BRCA2* mutation carriers? Gynecol Oncol 134(2):219, 2014

Walker JL, Armstrong DK, Huang HQ, et al: Intraperitoneal catheter outcomes in a phase III trial of intravenous versus intraperitoneal chemotherapy in optimal stage III ovarian and primary peritoneal cancer: a Gynecologic Oncology Group study. Gynecol Oncol 100:27, 2006

Walker JL, Brady MF, Wenzel L, et al: Randomized trial of intravenous versus intraperitoneal chemotherapy plus bevacizumab in advanced ovarian carcinoma: an NRG Oncology/Gynecologic Oncology Group study. J Clin Oncol 37(16):1380, 2019

Walker JL, Powell CB, Chen LM, et al: Society of Gynecologic Oncology recommendations for the prevention of ovarian cancer. Cancer 121(13):2108, 2015

Ware Miller R, Smith A, DeSimone CP, et al: Performance of the American College of Obstetricians and Gynecologists' ovarian tumor referral guidelines with a multivariate index assay. Obstet Gynecol 117(6):1298, 2011

Wimberger P, Lehmann N, Kimmig R, et al: Prognostic factors for complete debulking in advanced ovarian cancer and its impact on survival. An exploratory analysis of a prospectively randomized phase III study of AGO-OVAR. Gynecol Oncol 106:69, 2007

Wingo SN, Knowles LM, Carrick KS, et al: Retrospective cohort study of surgical staging for ovarian low malignant potential tumors. Am J Obstet Gynecol 194:e20, 2006

Winter WE 3rd, Maxwell GL, Tian C, et al: Prognostic factors for stage III epithelial ovarian cancer: a Gynecologic Oncology Group Study. J Clin Oncol 25(24):3621, 2007

Yen ML, Yen BL, Bai CH, et al: Risk factors for ovarian cancer in Taiwan: a case-control study in a low-incidence population. Gynecol Oncol 89:318, 2003

Young RH, Oliva E, Scully RE: Small cell carcinoma of the ovary, hypercalcemic type: a clinicopathological analysis of 150 cases. Am J Surg Pathol 18:1102, 1994

Zaino RJ, Brady MF, Lele SM, et al: Advanced stage mucinous adenocarcinoma of the ovary is both rare and highly lethal: a Gynecologic Oncology Group study. Cancer 117:554, 2011

Zapardiel I, Rosenberg P, Peiretti M, et al: The role of restaging borderline ovarian tumors: single institution experience and review of the literature. Gynecol Oncol 119:274, 2010

Zhang M, Lee AH, Binns CW: Reproductive and dietary risk factors for epithelial ovarian cancer in China. Gynecol Oncol 92:320, 2004

Zhang Z, Chan DW: The road from discovery to clinical diagnostics: lessons learned from the first FDA-cleared in vitro diagnostic multivariate index assay of proteomic biomarkers. Cancer Epidemiol Biomarkers Prev 19(12):2995, 2010

Ovarian Germ Cell and Sex Cord–Stromal Tumors

Three major categories account for virtually all malignant ovarian tumors. Organization of these groups is based on the anatomic structures from which the tumors originate (Fig. 36-1). Epithelial ovarian cancers account for 90 to 95 percent of malignant ovarian tumors (Chap. 35, p. 732). Germ cell and sex cord–stromal ovarian tumors account for the remaining

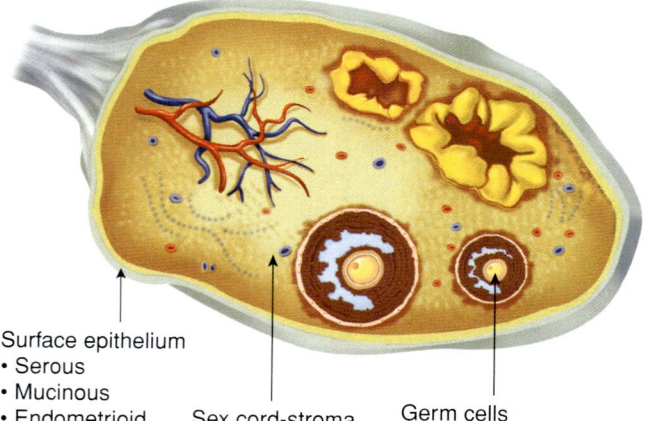

FIGURE 36-1 Origins of the three main types of ovarian tumors.

Surface epithelium
• Serous
• Mucinous
• Endometrioid
• Clear cell
• Transitional cell

Sex cord-stroma
• Granulosa cell
• Thecoma
• Fibroma
• Sertoli cell
• Sertoli-Leydig
• Steroid

Germ cells
• Dysgerminoma
• Yolk sac
• Embryonal carcinoma
• Choriocarcinoma
• Teratoma

5 to 10 percent and have unique qualities that require special management (Quirk, 2005).

MALIGNANT OVARIAN GERM CELL TUMORS

Germ cell tumors arise from the ovary's germinal elements and make up one third of all ovarian neoplasms. The mature cystic teratoma, also called *dermoid cyst*, is by far the most common subtype. This accounts for 95 percent of all germ cell tumors, is clinically benign, and discussed in Chapter 10 (p. 224). Of malignant ovarian cancers, germ cell tumors compose only 2 to 3 percent and include *dysgerminoma, yolk sac tumor, immature teratoma*, and other less common types.

Three clinical features distinguish malignant germ cell tumors from epithelial ovarian cancers. First, individuals typically are younger, usually in their teens or early 20s. Most have stage I disease at diagnosis. Last, prognosis is excellent—even for those with advanced disease—due to exquisite tumor chemosensitivity. Fertility-sparing surgery is the primary treatment for women seeking future pregnancy, although most will require postoperative chemotherapy.

■ Epidemiology

The age-adjusted incidence rate of malignant ovarian germ cell tumors in the United States is much lower (0.4 per 100,000 women) than that of epithelial ovarian carcinomas (15.5) (Quirk, 2005). Smith and associates (2006) analyzed 1262 cases of malignant ovarian germ cell tumors from 1973 to 2002 and observed that incidence rates have declined 10 percent during the past 30 years. Unlike a significant proportion of epithelial ovarian carcinomas, malignant germ cell tumors are not generally considered heritable, although rare familial cases are reported (Galani, 2005; Stettner, 1999).

These tumors are the most common ovarian malignancies diagnosed during childhood and adolescence, although only 1 percent of all ovarian cancers develop in these age groups. At age 20, however, the incidence of epithelial ovarian carcinoma begins to rise and exceeds that of germ cell tumors (Young, 2003).

■ Diagnosis
Patient Findings

The signs and symptoms associated with these tumors vary, but in general, most originate from tumor growth and the hormones they produce. Subacute abdominal pain is a symptom in 85 percent of patients and reflects rapid growth of a large, unilateral tumor undergoing capsular distention, hemorrhage, or necrosis. In 10 percent of cases, cyst rupture, torsion, or intraperitoneal hemorrhage leads to an acute abdomen (Gershenson, 2007). In more advanced disease, ascites may develop and cause abdominal distention. Because of the hormonal changes that frequently accompany these tumors, menses can become heavy or irregular. Although most individuals note one or more of these symptoms, one quarter of individuals are asymptomatic, and a pelvic mass is noted unexpectedly during physical or sonographic examination (Curtin, 1994).

Individuals typically seek care within 1 month of the onset of abdominal complaints, although some note subtle waxing and waning of symptoms for more than a year. Vague pelvic symptoms are common during adolescence due to initiation of ovulation and menstrual cramping. As a result, early symptoms may be missed. Moreover, young girls may be silent about changes to their normal pattern, fearful of their significance. Most young women with these tumors are nulligravidas with normal periods, but as discussed on page 758 dysgenetic gonads are known risk factors for development of these tumors (Brown, 2014b). Therefore, adolescents who present with pelvic masses and delayed menarche are evaluated for gonadal dysgenesis (Chap. 17, p. 375).

A palpable mass during pelvic examination is the most common physical finding. In children and adolescents, however, completing a comprehensive pelvic or transvaginal sonographic examination can be difficult and can lead to diagnostic delay. Accordingly, premenarchal patients may require examination under anesthesia to adequately assess a suspected adnexal tumor. The remainder of the physical examination searches for signs of ascites, pleural effusion, and organomegaly.

Laboratory Testing

In patients with a suspected malignant germ cell tumor, serum human chorionic gonadotropin (hCG) and alpha-fetoprotein (AFP) tumor markers, complete blood count, and liver function tests are drawn before treatment. Alternatively, the appropriate tumor markers may be ordered in the operating room if the diagnosis was not previously suspected (Table 36-1). Preoperative karyotyping of young women with primary amenorrhea and a suspected germ cell tumor can clarify whether both ovaries should be removed, as in the case of those with gonadal dysgenesis (p. 758) (Hoepffner, 2005).

TABLE 36-1. Serum Tumor Markers in Malignant Ovarian Germ Cell Tumors

Histology	AFP	hCG
Dysgerminoma	−	±
Yolk sac tumor	+	−
Immature teratoma	±	−
Choriocarcinoma	−	+
Embryonal carcinoma	+	+
Mixed germ cell tumor	±	±
Polyembryoma	±	±

AFP = alpha-fetoprotein; hCG = human chorionic gonadotropin.

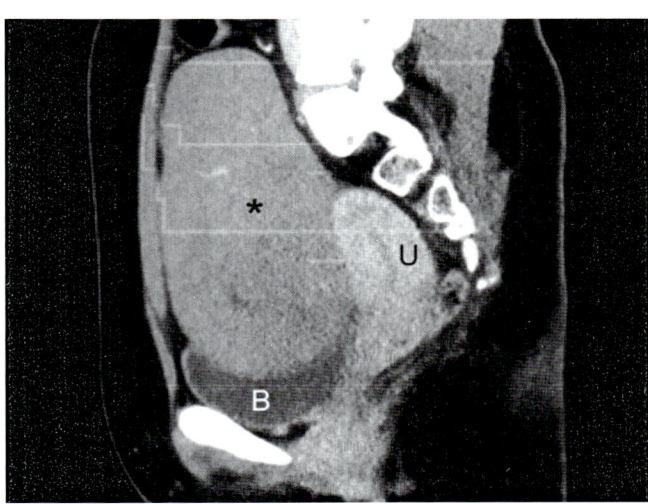

FIGURE 36-2 Computed tomographic (CT) scan of a large dysgerminoma (*asterisk*). B = bladder; U = uterus.

Imaging

In most cases, sonography can adequately display those qualities that typically characterize benign and malignant ovarian masses (Chap. 10, p. 221). Functional ovarian cysts are vastly more common in young women. Once these hypoechoic, small, smooth-walled cysts are identified sonographically, they may be observed. Mature cystic teratomas usually display characteristic features when imaged (Chap. 10, p. 226). In contrast, the appearance of malignant germ cell tumors differs, and a multilobulated complex ovarian mass is typical (Fig. 36-2). Moreover, prominent blood flow within fibrovascular septa may be seen using color flow Doppler sonography and suggests malignancy (Kim, 1995). Additional preoperative CT or magnetic resonance (MR) imaging may be indicated based on clinical suspicion. Chest radiography is warranted upon diagnosis to search for tumor metastases in the lungs or mediastinum.

Diagnostic Procedures

Surgical resection is generally required for definitive tissue diagnosis, staging, and treatment. The surgeon should request a frozen section analysis to confirm the diagnosis, but discrepancies between frozen section interpretations and the final paraffin histology are commonplace (Kusamura, 2000). In addition, specific immunostaining is often required to resolve equivocal cases. In contrast, a sonographically or CT-guided percutaneous biopsy has a very limited role in the management of select patients with an ovarian mass suspicious for malignancy.

■ Role of the Generalist

Most patients will initially be seen by a generalist gynecologist. Initial symptoms may point to the more common functional ovarian cyst. Persistent symptoms or an enlarging pelvic mass, however, should prompt sonographic evaluation. If a complex ovarian mass with solid features is noted in this young age group, then measurement of serum hCG and AFP levels and referral to a gynecologic oncologist for primary surgical management is preferred.

If a specialist is unavailable or the diagnosis is not anticipated beforehand, intraoperative decision making is crucial to adequately treat the patient without compromising future fertility. Peritoneal washings are obtained and set aside before proceeding with dissection of any suspicious adnexal mass. These can be discarded later if malignancy is excluded. Initially, the decision to perform cystectomy or oophorectomy depends on the clinical circumstances (Chap. 10, p. 222). In general, the entire adnexa is removed once a malignant ovarian germ cell tumor is diagnosed. A generalist gynecologist should request intraoperative assistance with staging from a gynecologic oncologist or refer the patient postoperatively if a specialist is not immediately available. At minimum, the entire abdomen and pelvis is inspected, with special assessment of the omentum and contralateral ovary.

Pathology

Classification and Histogenesis

The modified World Health Organization (WHO) classification of ovarian germ cell tumors is presented in Table 36-2 (Kurman, 2014). These tumors are composed of several histologically different tumor types derived from primordial germ cells of the embryonic gonad. The two major categories include the primitive malignant germ cell tumors (dysgerminomas) and the teratomas, almost all of which are accounted for by mature cystic teratomas.

During embryogenesis, primitive germ cells migrate from the wall of the yolk sac to the gonadal ridge (Fig. 19-1, p. 407). As a result, most germ cell tumors arise in the gonad. Rarely, these tumors may develop in extragonadal sites such as the central nervous system, mediastinum, or retroperitoneum (Hsu, 2002).

Ovarian germ cell tumors have a variable pattern of differentiation (Fig. 36-3). Dysgerminomas are primitive neoplasms that

---

TABLE 36-2. Modified WHO Classification of Ovarian Germ Cell Tumors

Germ cell tumors
Dysgerminoma
Yolk sac tumor (former endodermal sinus tumor)
Embryonal carcinoma
Nongestational choriocarcinoma
Mature teratoma
  Solid
  Cystic (dermoid cyst)
Immature teratoma
Mixed germ cell tumor

Monodermal teratoma and highly specialized types arising from a mature cystic teratoma
Thyroid tumors (struma ovarii: benign or malignant)
Carcinoids
Neuroectodermal tumors
Carcinomas (squamous cell or adeno-)
Sebaceous tumors

WHO = World Health Organization.

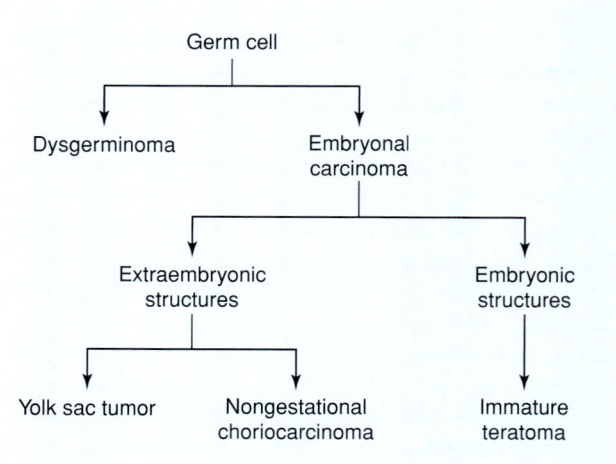

FIGURE 36-3 Differentiation pathway of malignant germ cell tumors.

do not have the potential for further differentiation. Embryonal carcinomas are composed of multipotential cells that are capable of further differentiation. This lesion is the precursor of several other types of extraembryonic (yolk sac tumor, choriocarcinoma) or embryonic (teratoma) germ cell tumors. The process of differentiation is dynamic, and the resulting neoplasms may be composed of different elements that show various stages of development (Teilum, 1965).

Dysgerminoma

Because their incidence has declined by approximately 30 percent over the past few decades, dysgerminomas currently account for only approximately one third of all malignant ovarian germ cell tumors (Chan, 2008; Smith, 2006). Dysgerminomas are the most common ovarian malignancy detected during pregnancy. This is believed to be an age-related coincidence, however, and not due to gestation.

Five percent of dysgerminomas are discovered in phenotypic females with karyotypically abnormal gonads, specifically, with a normal or abnormal Y chromosome (Morimura, 1998). Commonly, this group includes those with Turner syndrome mosaicism (45,X/46,XY) and with Swyer syndrome (46,XY, pure gonadal dysgenesis) (Chap. 19, p. 412). The dysgenetic gonads of these individuals often contain gonadoblastomas, which are benign germ cell neoplasms. These tumors may regress or alternatively may undergo malignant transformation, most commonly to dysgerminoma. Because approximately 40 percent of gonadoblastomas in these individuals undergo malignant transformation, both ovaries are removed (Brown, 2014b; Hoepffner, 2005; Pena-Alonso, 2005).

Dysgerminomas are the only germ cell malignancy with a significant rate of bilateral ovarian involvement—15 to 20 percent. Half of patients with bilateral lesions will have grossly obvious disease, whereas cancer in the remainder will only be detected microscopically. Five percent of women have elevated serum hCG levels, produced from intermingled syncytiotrophoblast. Similarly, serum lactate dehydrogenase (LDH) and the isoenzymes LDH-1 and LDH-2 may also be useful in

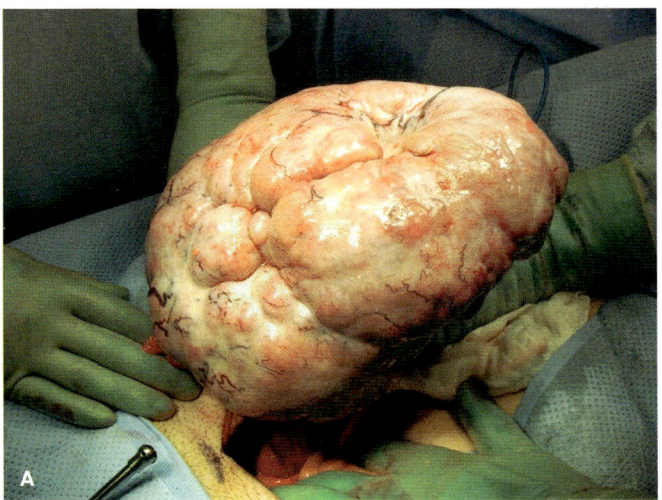
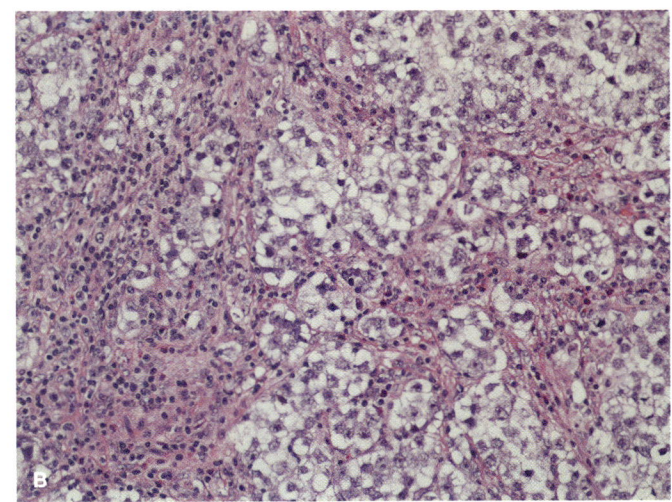

FIGURE 36-4 Dysgerminoma. **A.** Intraoperative photograph. **B.** Dysgerminoma is characterized microscopically by a relatively monotonous proliferation of large, rounded, polyhedral clear cells that are rich in cytoplasmic glycogen. These contain uniform central rounded or square-edged nuclei with one or a few prominent nucleoli. As in this case, the tumor often contains fibrous septa, which are seen here as eosinophilic strands. These septa are infiltrated by chronic inflammatory cells including lymphocytes, macrophages, and occasional plasma cells. (Reproduced with permission by Dr. Kelley Carrick.)

monitoring individuals for disease recurrence (Pressley, 1992; Schwartz, 1988).

Dysgerminomas vary, but in general they appear solid, pink to tan to cream-colored lobulated masses (Fig. 36-4). Shown in this same image, tumor cells closely resemble the primordial germ cells of the embryo and are histologically identical to seminoma of the testis.

The standard treatment of dysgerminoma usually involves fertility-sparing surgery with unilateral salpingo-oophorectomy (USO). In some extenuating circumstances, ovarian cystectomy may be considered (Vicus, 2010). Surgical staging is generally extrapolated from epithelial ovarian cancer, but lymphadenectomy is particularly important (Chap. 35, p. 747). Of the malignant germ cell tumors, dysgerminoma has the highest rate of nodal metastases, approximately 25 to 30 percent (Kumar, 2008). Although staging deviations do not adversely affect survival, comprehensive staging allows a safe observation strategy for stage IA tumors (Billmire, 2004; Palenzuela, 2008).

Preservation of the contralateral ovary leads to "recurrent" dysgerminoma in 5 to 10 percent of retained gonads during the next 2 years. This finding in many cases is thought to reflect the high rate of clinically occult disease in the remaining ovary rather than true recurrence. Indeed, at least 75 percent of recurrences develop within the first year of diagnosis (Vicus, 2010). Other common recurrence sites are within the peritoneal cavity or retroperitoneal lymph nodes. Despite this significant incidence of recurrent disease, a conservative surgical approach does not adversely affect long-term survival because of this cancer's sensitivity to chemotherapy (Liu, 2013).

Dysgerminomas have the best prognosis of all malignant ovarian germ cell tumor variants. Two thirds are stage I at diagnosis, and the 5-year disease-specific survival rate approximates 99 percent (Table 36-3). Even those with advanced disease have high survival rates following chemotherapy. For example, those with stage II–IV disease have a greater than 98-percent survival rate with platinum-based agents (Chan, 2008). As a result, carboplatin may be preferable to cisplatin in these patients due to equivalent outcomes with reduced long-term toxicity (Shah, 2018; Skalleberg, 2017).

Yolk Sac Tumors

These tumors account for 10 to 20 percent of all malignant ovarian germ cell tumors. These lesions were previously called endodermal sinus tumors, but the terminology has been revised.

TABLE 36-3. Stage at Diagnosis and 5-Year Survival of Common Malignant Ovarian Germ Cell Tumors

	Dysgerminoma	Yolk Sac Tumor	Immature Teratoma
Stage			
I	66%	50%	72%
II-IV	34%	50%	28%
Survival			
Stage I	99%	95%	98%
Stage II–IV	>98%	52–97%	73–88%

Sources for survival figures are referenced within the text.

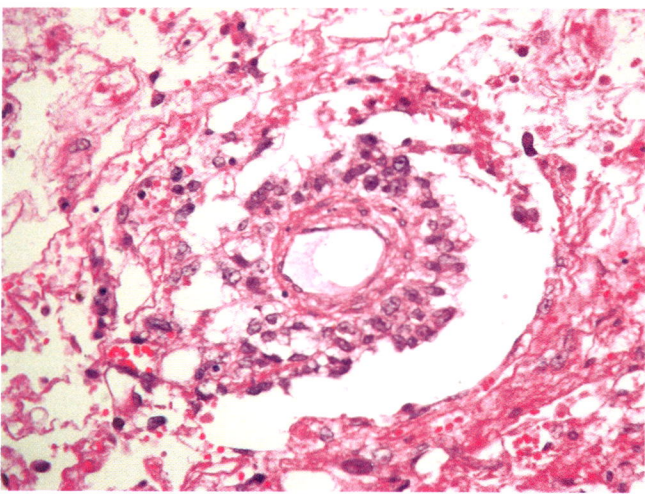

FIGURE 36-5 Schiller-Duval body. This structure consists of a central capillary surrounded by tumor cells, present within a cystic space that may be lined by flat to cuboidal tumor cells. When present, the Schiller-Duval body is pathognomonic for yolk sac tumor, although they are conspicuous in only a minority of cases. In any given case, Schiller-Duval bodies may be few in number, absent, or have atypical morphologic features. (Reproduced with permission by Dr. Kelley Carrick.)

One third of individuals are premenarchal at the time of initial presentation. Involvement of both gonads is rare, and the other ovary is usually involved with metastatic disease only when other metastases are found in the peritoneal cavity.

Grossly, these tumors form solid masses that are more yellow and friable than dysgerminomas. They are often focally necrotic and hemorrhagic, with cystic degeneration and rupture. The microscopic appearance of yolk sac tumors is often diverse. The most common appearance, the reticular pattern, reflects extraembryonic differentiation, with the formation of a network of irregular anastomosing spaces that are lined by primitive epithelial cells. *Schiller-Duval bodies* are pathognomonic when present (Fig. 36-5). These characteristically have a single papilla, which is lined by tumor cells and contains a central vessel. Yolk sac tumors usually contain cells that stain immunohistochemically for AFP, and serum AFP levels can serve as a reliable tumor marker in posttreatment surveillance.

Yolk sac tumors are the deadliest malignant ovarian germ cell tumor type. As a result, all patients are treated with chemotherapy regardless of stage. Fortunately, more than half present with stage I disease, which is associated with a 5-year overall survival rate of approximately 95 percent (Nasioudis, 2017). Disadvantageously, yolk sac tumors have a greater propensity for rapid growth, peritoneal spread, and distant hematogenous dissemination to the lungs. Accordingly, individuals with stage III–IV disease have a 5-year survival rate ranging from 52 to 97 percent. Of patients with tumor recurrence, most will do so within the first year, and treatment is usually ineffective (Cicin, 2009).

Other Primitive Germ Cell Tumors

The rarest subtypes of nondysgerminomatous tumors are typically mixed with other more common variants and are usually not found in pure form.

With *embryonal carcinoma*, patients are characteristically younger, with a mean age of 14 years, than those having other germ cell tumor. Epithelial cells resembling those of the embryonic disc form these primitive tumors. The solid disorganized sheets of large anaplastic cells, glandlike spaces, and papillary structures are distinctive and allow easy identification of these rare tumors (Ulbright, 2005). Although dysgerminomas are the most common germ cell tumor resulting from malignant transformation of gonadoblastomas in individuals with dysgenetic gonads, occasionally embryonal "testicular" tumors also may originate (LaPolla, 1990). Embryonal carcinomas typically produce hCG, and 75 percent also secrete AFP.

With *polyembryoma*, tumors characteristically contain many embryolike bodies. Each has a small central "germ disc" positioned between two cavities, one mimicking an amnionic cavity and the other a yolk sac. Syncytiotrophoblast giant cells are frequent, but elements other than the embryoid bodies should constitute less than 10 percent of the tumor for the "polyembryoma" designation to be used. Conceptually, these tumors may be viewed as a bridge between the primitive (dysgerminoma) and differentiated (teratoma) germ cell tumor types. For this reason, polyembryomas are often considered to be the most immature of all teratomas (Ulbright, 2005). Serum AFP or hCG levels or both may be elevated in these individuals due to the yolk sac and syncytial components, respectively (Takemori, 1998).

Primary ovarian choriocarcinoma arising from a germ cell appears similar to gestational choriocarcinoma with ovarian metastases (Chap. 37, p. 781). The distinction is important because nongestational tumors have a poorer prognosis (Corakci, 2005). The detection of other germ cell components indicates nongestational choriocarcinoma, whereas a concomitant or proximate pregnancy suggests a gestational form (Ulbright, 2005). Clinical manifestations are common and result from high hCG levels produced by these rare tumors. These elevated levels may induce sexual precocity in prepubertal girls or heavy, irregular menstrual bleeding in reproductive-aged women (Oliva, 1993).

Mixed Germ Cell Tumors

Ovarian germ cell tumors have a mixed pattern of cellular differentiation in 25 to 30 percent of cases, although the incidence of these tumors has also declined by approximately 30 percent over the past few decades (Smith, 2006). Dysgerminoma is the most common component and is typically seen with yolk sac tumor or immature teratoma or both. The frequency of bilateral ovarian involvement depends on the presence or absence of a dysgerminoma component and increases when it is present. However, treatment and prognosis are determined by the nondysgerminomatous component (Low, 2000). Accordingly, elevated serum hCG and particularly AFP levels in a woman with a presumed pure dysgerminoma should prompt a search for other germ cell components by a more extensive histologic evaluation (Aoki, 2003).

Immature Teratomas

Due to a 60-percent increased incidence during the past few decades, immature teratomas are now the most common variant and account for 40 to 50 percent of all malignant ovarian germ

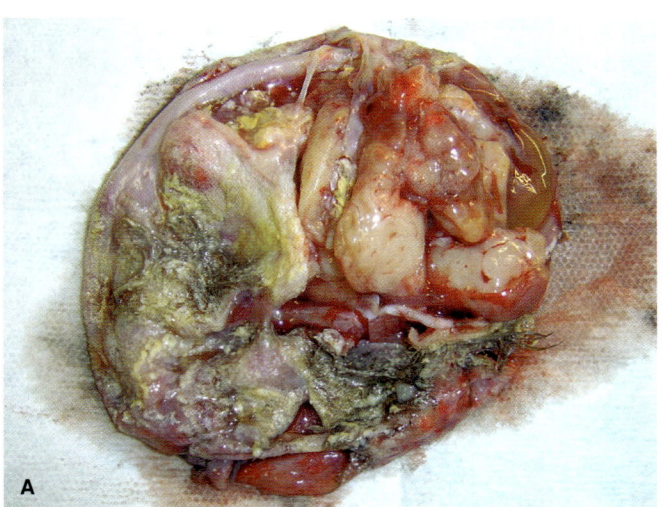
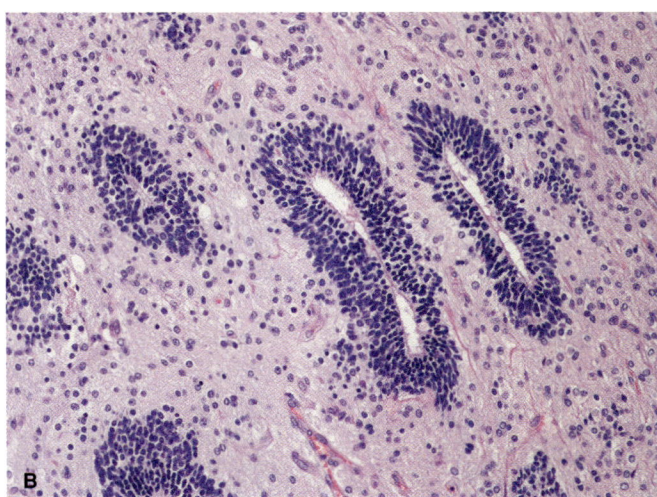

FIGURE 36-6 Immature teratoma. **A.** This opened surgical specimen shows characteristic solid and cystic architecture. As in mature teratomas, hair and other skin elements are often found. **B.** Immature teratomas contain a disorderly mixture of mature and immature tissues derived from the three germ cell layers—ectoderm, mesoderm, and endoderm. Of the immature elements, immature neuroepithelium is the most common. Here, immature neuroepithelial cells arranged in rosettes lie within a background of mature neural tissue. (Reproduced with permission by Dr. Kelley Carrick.)

cell tumors (Chan, 2008; Smith, 2006). They are composed of tissues derived from the three germ layers: ectoderm, mesoderm, and endoderm. The presence of immature or embryonal structures, however, distinguishes these tumors from the much more common and benign mature cystic teratoma (dermoid cyst). Bilateral ovarian involvement is rare, but 10 percent have a mature teratoma in the contralateral ovary. Tumor markers are often not elevated unless the immature teratoma is mingled with other germ cell tumor types. AFP, cancer antigen 125 (CA125), CA19-9, and carcinoembryonic antigen (CEA) may be helpful in some cases (Li, 2002).

With gross external inspection, these tumors are large, rounded or lobulated, soft or firm masses. They frequently perforate the ovarian capsule and invade locally. The most frequent site of dissemination is the peritoneum and much less commonly the retroperitoneal lymph nodes. With local invasion, surrounding adhesions commonly form and are thought to explain the lower rates of torsion with this tumor compared with that of its benign mature counterpart (Cass, 2001). On cut surface, the interior is typically solid with intermittent cystic areas, but occasionally the reverse is seen, with solid nodules present only in the cyst wall (Fig. 36-6). Solid parts may correspond to the immature elements, cartilage, bone, or a combination of these. Cystic areas are filled with hair and with serous fluid, mucinous fluid, or sebum.

Microscopic examination reveals a disorderly mixture of tissues. Of the immature elements, neuroectodermal tissues almost always predominate and are arranged as primitive tubules and sheets of small, round, malignant cells that may be associated with glia formation. The diagnosis is usually difficult to confirm during frozen section analysis, and most tumors are confirmed only on final pathologic review (Pavlakis, 2009). Tumors are graded 1 to 3 primarily by the amount of immature neural tissue they contain. O'Connor and Norris (1994) analyzed 244 immature teratomas and noted significant inconsistencies

in grade assignment by different observers. For this reason, they proposed changing the system to two grades: low (previous grades 1 and 2) and high (previous grade 3). This practice, however, has not been universally accepted.

In general, survival is predicted most accurately by stage and by histologic grade of the tumor. For example, almost three quarters of immature teratomas are stage I at diagnosis and have a 5-year survival rate of 98 percent (Chan, 2008). Those with stage IA grade 1 immature teratomas have an excellent prognosis and do not require adjuvant chemotherapy (Bonazzi, 1994; Marina, 1999). Patients with stage II–IV disease have a 5-year survival rate ranging from 73 to 88 percent (Chan, 2008).

Unilateral salpingo-oophorectomy is the standard care for these and other malignant germ cell tumors in reproductive-aged women. Beiner and colleagues (2004), however, treated eight women with early-stage immature teratoma with ovarian cystectomy and adjuvant chemotherapy and noted no recurrences.

Immature teratomas may be associated with mature tissue implants studding the peritoneum that do not increase the stage of the tumor or diminish the prospect of survival. However, these implants of mature teratomatous elements, even though benign, are resistant to chemotherapy and can enlarge during or after chemotherapy. Termed the *growing teratoma syndrome*, these implants require second-look surgery and resection to exclude recurrent malignancy (Bentivegna, 2015).

Malignant Transformation of Mature Cystic Teratomas

These rare tumors are the only germ cell variants that typically develop in postmenopausal women. Malignant areas are usually found as small nodules in the cyst wall or a polypoid mass within the lumen after removal of the entire mature cystic teratoma (Pins, 1996). Squamous cell carcinoma is most common and is found in approximately 1 percent of mature cystic teratomas (Fig. 36-7). Platinum-based chemotherapy

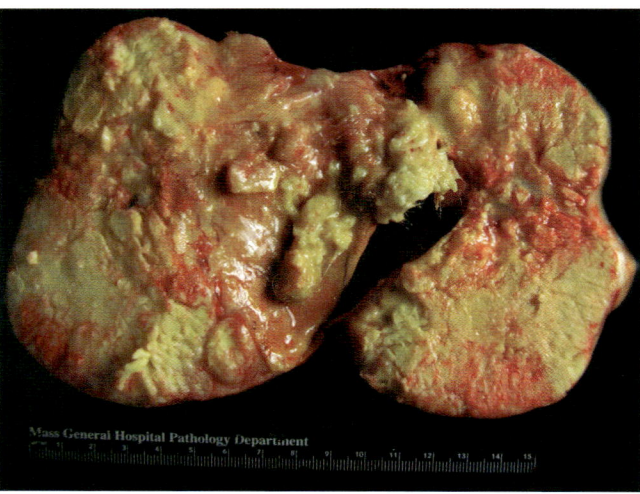

FIGURE 36-7 This opened surgical specimen reveals squamous cell carcinoma malignant transformation within a mature cystic teratoma.

with or without pelvic radiation is most often used for adjuvant treatment of early-stage disease (Dos Santos, 2007). However, regardless of treatment received, patients with advanced disease do poorly (Gainford, 2010).

Other uncommon types of malignant features may include basal-cell carcinomas, sebaceous tumors, malignant melanomas, adenocarcinomas, sarcomas, and neuroectodermal tumors. Moreover, endocrine-type neoplasms such as struma ovarii (teratoma composed mainly of thyroid tissue) and carcinoid also may be found within mature cystic teratomas.

■ Treatment

Surgery

A vertical abdominal incision is still traditionally recommended if an advanced ovarian malignancy is suspected. However, increasingly, investigators with advanced endoscopic skills have noted laparoscopy to be a safe and effective alternative for women with smaller ovarian masses and apparent stage I disease (Shim, 2013).

If present, ascites is evacuated and sent for cytologic evaluation. Otherwise, washings of the pelvis and paracolic gutters are collected for analysis prior to manipulation of the intraperitoneal contents. The entire peritoneal cavity is systematically inspected. The ovaries are assessed for size, tumor involvement, capsular rupture, external excrescences, and adherence to surrounding structures.

Fertility-sparing USO is performed in all reproductive-aged women diagnosed with malignant ovarian germ cell tumors, as this conservative approach in general does not adversely affect survival (Park, 2017). Following USO, blind biopsy or wedge resection of a normal-appearing contralateral ovary is not recommended. For the rare patient who has completed childbearing and would derive little benefit from retaining an ovary, hysterectomy with bilateral salpingo-oophorectomy (BSO) is appropriate (Brown, 2014b). In either case, following removal of the affected ovary, surgical staging by laparotomy or laparoscopy proceeds as previously described for epithelial ovarian cancer (Chap. 35, p. 747) (Gershenson, 2007). Because of

tumor dissemination patterns, lymphadenectomy is most important for dysgerminomas, whereas staging peritoneal and omental biopsies are particularly valuable for yolk sac tumors and immature teratomas (Kleppe, 2014).

Cytoreductive surgery is recommended for advanced-stage nondysgerminomatous malignant ovarian germ cell tumors if it can be accomplished with minimal residual disease (Park, 2017). Ovarian dysgerminomas are so chemosensitive they do not generally require aggressive attempts at debulking. The same general principles are applied as described for epithelial ovarian cancer (Chap. 35, p. 748). Neoadjuvant chemotherapy is a reasonable option for the atypical patient thought to have unresectable disease (Talukdar, 2014).

Many women will be referred to an oncologist after USO for a tumor that was clinically confined to the excised ovary. For such patients, if initial surgical staging was incomplete, options may include a second surgery to complete primary staging, regular surveillance, or adjuvant chemotherapy. Unfortunately, few data support a preferred approach. Because of its minimally invasive qualities, laparoscopy is a particularly attractive option for delayed surgical staging following primary excision and has been shown to accurately detect those women who require chemotherapy (Leblanc, 2004). Surgical staging following primary excision, however, is less important for scenarios in which chemotherapy will be administered regardless of surgical findings. Examples are clinical stage I yolk sac tumors and high-grade clinical stage I immature teratomas (Stier, 1996). In such patients, reassurance of no abnormalities by CT imaging is often sufficient prior to proceeding with adjuvant chemotherapy (Gershenson, 2007).

Surveillance

Patients with malignant ovarian germ cell tumors are followed by careful clinical, radiologic, and serologic surveillance every 3 months for the first 2 years after therapy completion (Morgan, 2016). Ninety percent of recurrences develop within this time frame (Messing, 1992). Second-look surgery at the completion of therapy is not necessary in women with completely resected disease or in those individuals with advanced tumor that does not contain teratoma. However, incompletely resected immature teratoma is the one circumstance among all types of ovarian cancer in which patients clearly benefit from second-look surgery and excision of chemorefractory tumor (Culine, 1996; Rezk, 2005; Williams, 1994).

Chemotherapy

Stage IA dysgerminomas and stage IA grade 1 immature teratomas do not require additional chemotherapy. More advanced disease and all other histologic types of malignant ovarian germ cell tumors have historically been treated with combination chemotherapy after surgery (Morgan, 2016). However, the feasibility of surgery followed by close surveillance in pediatric and adolescent girls is being explored (Billmire, 2014). Because chemotherapy remains effective when used at the time of relapse, some investigators are attempting to identify additional low-risk, early-stage subgroups that may be observed postoperatively to avoid treatment-related toxicity (Bonazzi, 1994; Cushing, 1999; Dark, 1997). However, before this strategy becomes general practice, additional large studies are needed.

The standard regimen is a 5-day course of bleomycin, etoposide, and cisplatin (BEP) given every 3 weeks (Gershenson, 1990; Williams, 1987). Modified 3-day BEP combinations also are safe and effective (Chen, 2014; Dimopoulos, 2004). Carboplatin and etoposide, given in three cycles, has shown promise as an alternative for selected patients (Williams, 2004). For women with incompletely resected disease, at least four courses of BEP are usually recommended (Morgan, 2016).

Radiation

Chemotherapy has replaced radiation as the preferred adjuvant treatment for all types of malignant ovarian germ cell tumors. This transition was prompted primarily by the exquisite sensitivity of these tumors to either modality, but higher likelihood of retained ovarian function using chemotherapy (Solheim, 2015). Patients treated with radiotherapy are also much more likely to develop a second cancer within 10 years (Solheim, 2014). Occasional situations may still exist in which radiotherapy is considered, such as palliation of a germ cell tumor that has demonstrated resistance to chemotherapy.

Relapse

At least four courses of BEP chemotherapy is the preferred treatment for recurrent ovarian germ cell tumors in women initially managed with surgery alone. Patients who achieved a sustained clinical remission of greater than 6 months after completing BEP or another platinum-based chemotherapy regimen may be treated again with BEP. Because their tumors are generally more responsive, these "platinum-sensitive" patients have a much better prognosis. However, women who do not achieve remission with BEP chemotherapy or relapse within a few months (fewer than 6) are considered "platinum-resistant," and treatment options are limited. Chemorefractory cases with dysgerminoma or immature teratoma appear to have a better outcome than other subtypes, and surgical salvage aimed at achieving no residual disease may benefit some patients (Li, 2007). Other palliative options for this group include vincristine, dactinomycin, and cyclophosphamide (VAC) or paclitaxel (Morgan, 2016).

■ Prognosis

Malignant ovarian germ cell tumors have an excellent overall prognosis (see Table 36-3) (Solheim, 2013, 2014). Moreover, the number of cases with distant and unstaged disease has dramatically declined, suggesting that germ cell tumors are being diagnosed earlier. In addition, the survival rates have significantly improved for all subtypes, especially with the demonstrated efficacy of platinum-based combination therapy (Smith, 2006). Histologic cell type, elevated serum marker levels, surgical stage, and the amount of residual disease at initial surgery are the major variables affecting prognosis (Murugaesu, 2006; Park, 2017). Typically, pure dysgerminomas recur within 2 years and are highly treatable (Vicus, 2010). However, for nondysgerminomatous tumors, outcome after relapse is poor, and fewer than 10 percent of patients achieve long-term survival (Murugaesu, 2006).

Most women treated with fertility-sparing surgery, with or without chemotherapy, will resume normal menses and are able to conceive and bear children (Park, 2017). In addition, none of the reported studies has noted a greater rate of birth defects or spontaneous abortion in those treated with chemotherapy (Tangir, 2003; Zanetta, 2001).

■ Management During Pregnancy

Persistent adnexal masses are detected in 1 to 2 percent of all pregnancies. These neoplasms are usually seen during routine obstetric sonographic examination. Occasionally, a dramatically elevated maternal serum alpha-fetoprotein (MSAFP) level is the presenting sign of a malignant germ cell tumor (Horbelt, 1994). Mature cystic teratomas (dermoid cysts) make up one third of tumors resected during pregnancy. In contrast, dysgerminomas account for only 1 to 2 percent of such neoplasms but still are the most common ovarian malignancy during pregnancy. Development of other germ cell tumors is rare (Shimizu, 2003).

Initial surgical management including surgical staging is the same as for the nonpregnant woman (Horbelt, 1994; Zhao, 2006). Fortunately, very few patients have advanced disease necessitating radical dissection for cytoreduction. The decision to administer chemotherapy during pregnancy is controversial. Malignant ovarian germ cell tumors have the propensity to grow rapidly, and delaying treatment until after delivery is potentially hazardous. Treatment with BEP appears to be safe during pregnancy, but some reports have speculated that fetal complications are possible (Elit, 1999; Horbelt, 1994). For this reason, some advocate postponing treatment until the puerperium (Shimizu, 2003). Unfortunately, results from large studies to resolve this dilemma are lacking. For completely resected dysgerminomas, BEP administration may be delayed until the puerperium. However, for patients with nondysgerminomatous tumors (mainly yolk sac tumors and immature teratomas) and those with incompletely resected disease, chemotherapy during pregnancy is strongly considered.

OVARIAN SEX CORD-STROMAL TUMORS

Sex cord–stromal tumors (SCSTs) are a heterogeneous group of rare neoplasms that originate from the ovarian matrix. Cells within this matrix have the potential for hormone production, and nearly 90 percent of hormone-producing ovarian tumors are SCSTs. As a result, individuals with these tumors typically show signs and symptoms of estrogen or androgen excess.

Surgical resection is primary treatment, and SCSTs are generally confined to one ovary at the time of diagnosis. Most have an indolent growth pattern and low malignant potential. For these reasons, few patients ever require platinum-based chemotherapy. Tumors infrequently relapse, and recurrences tend to be late and usually develop in the abdomen or pelvis (Abu-Rustum, 2006). Although recurrent disease often responds poorly to treatment, patients may live for many years because of characteristically slow tumor progression.

Overall prognosis for ovarian SCSTs is excellent—primarily due to early-stage disease at diagnosis and curative surgery. The scarcity of these tumors, however, limits the understanding of their natural history, treatment, and prognosis.

TABLE 36-4. Tumor Markers for Ovarian Sex Cord–Stromal Tumors with Malignant Potential

Granulosa cell tumors (adult and juvenile)	Inhibin A and B, estradiol (not as reliable)
Sertoli–Leydig cell tumors	Inhibin A and B, alpha-fetoprotein (occasionally)
Sex cord tumor with annular tubules	Inhibin A and B
Steroid cell tumors not otherwise specified	Steroid hormones elevated pretreatment

■ Epidemiology

SCSTs account for 3 to 5 percent of ovarian malignancies (Ray-Coquard, 2014). These tumors are more than twice as likely to develop in black women for reasons that are unclear (Quirk, 2005). In contrast with epithelial ovarian cancers or malignant germ cell tumors, ovarian SCSTs typically affect women of all ages. This range contains a unique bimodal distribution that reflects inherent tumor heterogeneity. For example, juvenile granulosa cell tumors, Sertoli-Leydig cell tumors, and sclerosing stromal tumors are found predominantly in prepubertal girls and women within the first three decades of life (Schneider, 2005). Adult granulosa cell tumors commonly develop in older women, at an average age in the mid-50s (van Meurs, 2013).

SCSTs have no proven risk factors. However, in a hypothesis-generating case-control study, obesity as a hyperestrogenic state was independently associated, whereas parity, smoking, and oral contraceptive use were protective (Boyce, 2009).

The etiology of SCSTs is largely unknown. However, a single, recurrent *FOXL2* gene mutation is present in virtually all adult-type granulosa cell tumors (Schrader, 2009; Shah, 2009). Also, women with a germline *DICER1* mutation are predisposed to developing SCSTs (Heravi-Moussavi, 2012). Last, ovarian SCSTs develop in association with several defined hereditary disorders at a frequency that exceeds mere chance. These include Ollier disease, which is characterized by multiple benign but disfiguring cartilaginous neoplasms, and Peutz-Jeghers syndrome, characterized by intestinal hamartomatous polyps (Stevens, 2005).

■ Diagnosis

Patient Findings

Isosexual precocious puberty is the presenting sign in more than 80 percent of prepubertal girls ultimately diagnosed with an ovarian SCST (Kalfa, 2005). Adolescents often report secondary amenorrhea. As a result, these young individuals with endocrinologic symptoms tend to be diagnosed at earlier stages. Abdominal pain and distention are other common complaints in this age group (Schneider, 2003).

In adult women, heavy, irregular menstrual bleeding and postmenopausal bleeding are the most frequent symptoms. In addition, mild hirsutism that rapidly progresses to frank virilization should prompt evaluation to exclude these tumors. The classic presentation is a postmenopausal woman with rapidly evolving stigmata of androgen excess and a complex adnexal mass. Abdominal pain or a mass palpable by the patient herself are other telling signs and symptoms (Chan, 2005).

The size of SCSTs varies widely, but most women have a palpable abdominal or pelvic mass during examination regardless of their age. A fluid wave and other physical findings suggestive of advanced disease, however, are rare.

Diagnostic Procedures

Elevated circulating levels of testosterone or androstenedione or both strongly suggest an ovarian SCST in a virilized woman. Clinical hyperandrogenism is more likely to be idiopathic or related to polycystic ovarian syndrome, but serum testosterone levels >150 ng/dL or dehydroepiandrosterone sulfate (DHEAS) levels >8000 µg/L strongly suggest the possibility of an androgen-secreting tumor (Carmina, 2006). In most instances, tumor marker studies are not obtained preoperatively, because the diagnosis of ovarian SCST is often not suspected. When the diagnosis is confirmed, the appropriate tumor markers may be drawn during or following surgery (Table 36-4).

The gross appearance of an SCSTs varies from a large multicystic to small solid mass—effectively precluding a specific radiologic diagnosis. Granulosa cell tumors often sonographically demonstrate semisolid features but are not reliably discernible from epithelial tumors (Fig. 36-8) (Sharony, 2001). In addition, the endometrium may be thickened from increased tumor estrogen production. Preoperative endometrial sampling is reasonable to exclude comorbid endometrial hyperplasia or adenocarcinoma. Although CT or MR imaging has been used to clarify indeterminate sonograms of these tumors, no definitive radiologic study allows confident diagnosis (Jung, 2005).

Surgical resection for definitive tissue diagnosis, staging, and treatment is required for patients with an ovarian mass suspicious for malignancy. Sonographically or CT-guided percutaneous biopsy has no role. Moreover, diagnostic laparoscopy or laparotomy with visual assessment of the adnexal mass alone is inadequate. Following removal, ovarian SCSTs can usually be distinguished histologically from germ cell tumors, epithelial ovarian cancers, or other spindle-cell neoplasms by immunostaining for inhibin (Cathro, 2005; Schneider, 2005).

■ Role of the Generalist

Preoperatively, patients with a potentially malignant ovarian SCST are ideally referred to a gynecologic oncologist for evaluation. Most ovarian SCSTs, however, are diagnosed by generalist gynecologists following resection of a seemingly benign but complex mass in a woman with a CA125 level that is typically normal, if known beforehand. The initial surgery is often performed in a community-based hospital and without adequate staging. In this setting, prior to referral, histologic results should be reviewed and confirmed by an experienced pathologist. Following referral to a gynecologic oncologist, surgical staging may be indicated.

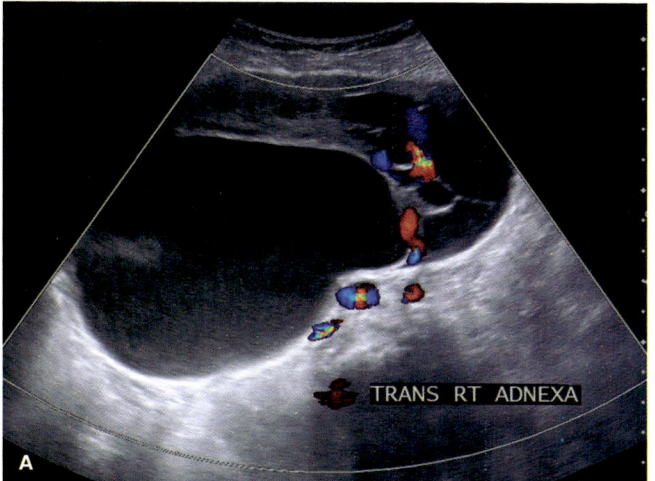

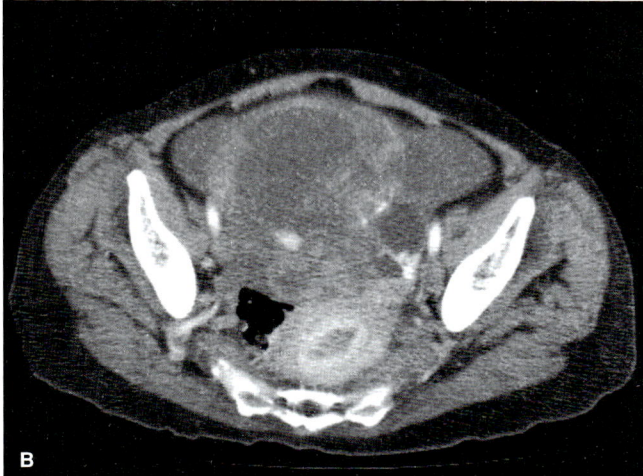

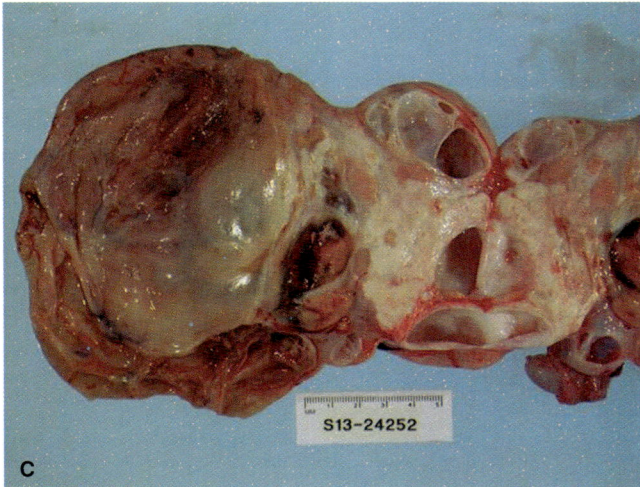

FIGURE 36-8 Adult granulosa cell tumor. **A.** Abdominal sonography displays a large adnexal mass with solid and cystic areas. With application of color Doppler, thick vascular septa are seen. **B.** Computed tomographic (CT) scan of the same tumor. **C.** The tumor was opened after excision, and again its mixed architecture is noted. (Reproduced with permission by Dr. Christa Nagel.)

TABLE 36-5. Modified WHO Classification of Ovarian Sex Cord–Stromal Tumors

Pure stromal tumors
Fibroma/fibrosarcoma
Thecoma
Sclerosing stromal tumor
Leydig cell tumor
Steroid cell tumor

Pure sex cord tumors
Granulosa cell tumor
    Adult type
    Juvenile type
Sertoli cell tumor
Sex cord tumor with annular tubules

Mixed sex cord–stromal tumors
Sertoli-Leydig cell tumors
Sex cord-stromal tumors, NOS

NOS = not otherwise specified; WHO = World Health Organization.

■ Pathology

Classification

Ovarian SCSTs arise from sex cord and mesenchymal cells of the embryonic gonad (Chap. 19, p. 409). Granulosa and Sertoli cells develop from the sex cords and thus from the coelomic epithelium. In contrast, theca cells, Leydig cells, and fibroblasts are derived from the mesenchyme. The primitive gonadal stroma possesses sexual bipotentiality. Therefore, developing tumors may be composed of a male-directed cell type (Sertoli or Leydig cell) or a female-directed cell type (granulosa or theca cell). Although distinct categories of SCSTs have been defined, mixed tumors are relatively common (Table 36-5) (Kurman, 2014). For example, ovarian granulosa cell tumors may have admixed Sertoli components. Similarly, tumors that are predominantly Sertoli or Sertoli-Leydig cells may contain minor granulosa elements. These mixed tumors are believed to arise from a common lineage with variable differentiation and do not represent two concurrent separate entities (McKenna, 2005; Vang, 2004).

Ovarian granulosa cell tumors are universally considered to have malignant potential, but most other SCST subtypes do not have definitive criteria for clearly defining benign and malignant. Attempts to grade these tumors using nuclear characteristics or mitotic activity counts have produced inconsistent results (Chen, 2003).

Granulosa Cell Tumors

Adult Granulosa Cell Tumors. Seventy percent of ovarian SCSTs are granulosa cell tumors (Colombo, 2007). These tumors are believed to arise from cells surrounding germ cells. There are two clinically and histologically distinct types: the adult form, which comprises 95 percent of cases, and the juvenile type, accounting for 5 percent.

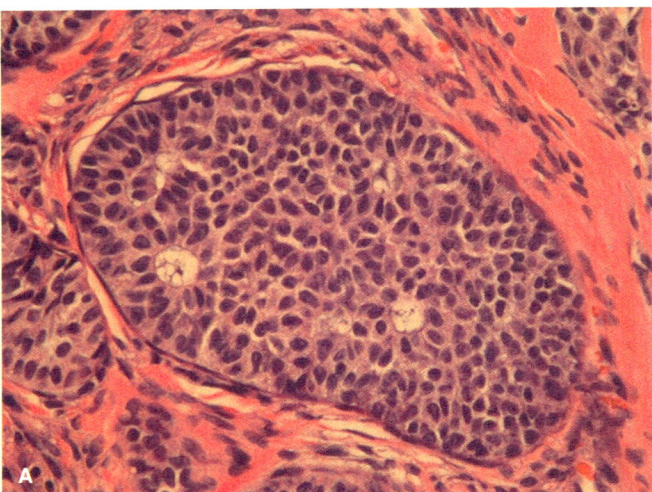
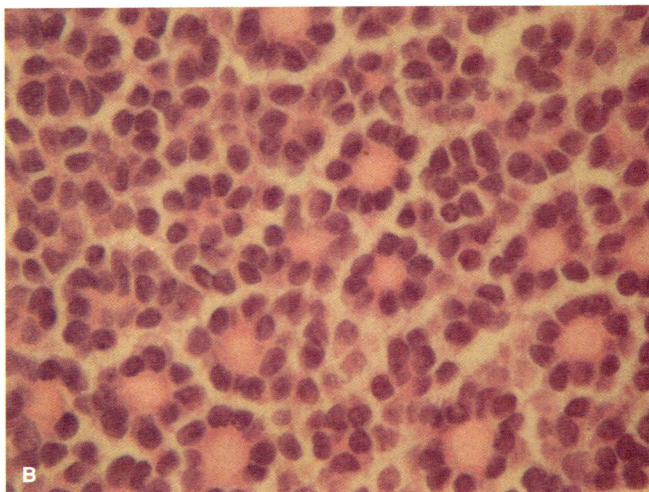

FIGURE 36-9 Adult granulosa cell tumor. **A.** Cells are typically crowded and contain scant, pale cytoplasm. Their elongated nuclei may have a longitudinal fold or groove that gives them a "coffee bean" appearance. **B.** Call-Exner bodies are identified by their rosette appearance. (Reproduced with permission by Dr. Raheela Ashfaq.)

With adult granulosa cell tumor, most women are diagnosed after age 30, and the average age approximates 55 years. Heavy, irregular menstrual bleeding and postmenopausal bleeding are common and reflect prolonged exposure of the endometrium to estrogen. Related to this estrogen excess, coexisting pathology such as endometrial hyperplasia or adenocarcinoma has been found in 25 to 30 percent of patients with adult granulosa cell tumor (van Meurs, 2013). Similarly, breast enlargement and tenderness are frequent associated complaints, and secondary amenorrhea has been reported (Kurihara, 2004). Alternatively, symptoms may stem from the mass of the ovary rather than from hormones produced (Ray-Coquard, 2014). An enlarging and potentially hemorrhagic tumor can cause abdominal pain and distention. Acute pelvic pain may suggest adnexal torsion, or tumor rupture with hemoperitoneum can mimic ectopic pregnancy.

During surgery, if an adult granulosa cell tumor is confirmed, tumor markers may be requested. Of these, inhibin B seems to be more accurate than inhibin A, frequently being elevated months before clinical detection of recurrence (Mom, 2007). The diagnostic value of these markers, however, is often hampered by their physiologically broad normal ranges (Schneider, 2005). Estradiol also has limited use in surveillance. This is particularly true for the younger patient wishing to preserve fertility and having the contralateral ovary left in situ.

Grossly, adult granulosa cell tumors are large and multicystic and often exceed 10 to 15 cm in diameter (see Fig. 36-8). The surface is frequently edematous and unusually adhered to other pelvic organs. For this reason, more extensive dissection is typically required than for epithelial ovarian cancers or malignant germ cell tumors. During excision, inadvertent rupture and intraoperative bleeding from the tumor itself is common.

The interior of the tumor is highly variable. Solid components may predominate and contain large areas of hemorrhage and necrosis. Alternatively, the mass can be cystic, with numerous locules filled with serosanguinous or gelatinous fluid (Colombo, 2007). Microscopic examination shows predominately granulosa cells with pale, grooved, "coffee bean" nuclei. The characteristic

microscopic feature is the Call-Exner body—a rosette arrangement of cells around an eosinophilic fluid space (Fig. 36-9).

Adult granulosa cell tumors are low-grade malignancies that typically demonstrate indolent growth. Ninety-five percent are unilateral, and 70 to 90 percent are stage I at diagnosis (Table 36-6). The 5-year survival for patients with stage I disease is 90 to 95 percent (Colombo, 2007; Zhang, 2007). However, 15 to 25 percent of stage I tumors will eventually relapse. The median time to recurrence is 5 to 6 years but may be several decades (Abu-Rustum, 2006; East, 2005). Advantageously, these indolent tumors usually progress slowly thereafter, and the median length of survival after relapse is another 6 years. Poor prognostic factors are advanced stage, large tumor size, and residual disease (Seagle, 2017). Patients with stage II–IV tumors have a 5-year survival rate of 50 to 80 percent (Seagle, 2017). Cellular atypia and mitotic count may help in determining the prognosis but are difficult to reproducibly quantify (Miller, 2001).

Juvenile Granulosa Cell Tumors. These rare neoplasms develop primarily in children and young adults, and approximately 90 percent are diagnosed before puberty (Colombo, 2007). The

TABLE 36-6. Stage and Survival of Common Ovarian Sex Cord–Stromal Tumors

	Adult Granulosa Cell	Sertoli-Leydig Cell
Stage at diagnosis		
I	70–90%	97%
II–IV	10–20%	2–3%
Five-year survival		
Stage I	90–95%	90–95%
Stage II–IV	50–80%	10–20%

Sources for survival figures are referenced within the text.

mean age at diagnosis is 13 years, but patient ages range from newborn to 67 years (Young, 1984). Juvenile granulosa cell tumors are sometimes associated with Ollier disease or with Maffucci syndrome, which is characterized by endochondromas and hemangiomas (Young, 1984; Yuan, 2004).

In affected females, estrogen, progesterone, and testosterone levels may be elevated and lead to suppression of gonadotropins. As a result, menstrual irregularities or amenorrhea are common. Prepubertal girls typically display isosexual precocious puberty, which is characterized by breast enlargement and development of pubic hair, vaginal secretions, and other secondary sexual characteristics. These tumors infrequently secrete androgens, but in such cases they may induce virilization. Despite these endocrinologic signs, a delayed diagnosis of juvenile granulosa cell tumors in pre- and postpubertal girls is common and associated with a higher risk of peritoneal tumor spread (Kalfa, 2005).

In addition to hormonal changes, individuals may display tumor effects. For example, older patients usually seek medical attention for abdominal pain or swelling. Preoperative rupture with resulting hemoperitoneum may create acute abdominal symptoms in 5 to 10 percent of cases (Colombo, 2007). Ascites is present in 10 percent (Young, 1984).

Juvenile granulosa cell tumors are grossly similar to the adult-type tumor and display variable solid and cystic components. They can attain significant size and have an average diameter of approximately 12 cm. Microscopically, cytologic features that distinguish these tumors from the adult type are their rounded, hyperchromatic nuclei without "coffee-bean" grooves. Call-Exner bodies are rare, but often a theca cell component is found (Young, 1984).

Prognosis is excellent, and the 5-year survival rate is 95 percent. Similar to adult-type tumors, 95 percent of juvenile granulosa cell tumors are unilateral and stage I at diagnosis (Young, 1984). However, the juvenile type is more aggressive in advanced stages, and the time to relapse and death is much shorter. Recurrences typically develop within 3 years and are highly lethal. Later recurrences are unusual (Frausto, 2004).

Thecoma-Fibroma Group

Thecomas. These are relatively common SCSTs and are rarely malignant. Thecomas are unique because they typically develop in postmenopausal women in their mid-60s and develop infrequently before age 30. These solid tumors are among the most hormonally active of the SCSTs and usually produce excess estrogen. As a result, the primary signs and symptoms are abnormal vaginal bleeding or pelvic mass or both. Many women also have concurrent endometrial hyperplasia or adenocarcinoma (Aboud, 1997). These tumors are composed of lipid-laden stromal cells that are occasionally luteinized. Half of these luteinized thecomas are hormonally inactive or are androgen-producing.

Thecomas are solid tumors whose cells resemble the theca cells that normally surround the ovarian follicles (Chen, 2003). Because of this texture, these tumors appear sonographically as solid adnexal masses and may mimic extrauterine leiomyomas.

Bilateral ovarian involvement and extraovarian spread are rare. Fortunately, ovarian thecomas are clinically benign, and surgical resection is curative.

Fibromas. Fibromas also are relatively common, hormonally inactive SCST variants that usually occur in perimenopausal and menopausal women (Chechia, 2008). These solid, generally benign ovarian neoplasms arise from the spindled stromal cells that form collagen. Most fibromas are found incidentally during pelvic or sonographic examination. They are round, oval, or lobulated solid tumors associated with free fluid or less commonly, with frank ascites and possess minimal to moderate vascularization (Paladini, 2009).

Perhaps 1 percent of women present with *Meigs syndrome*, which is a triad of pleural effusion, ascites, and a solid ovarian mass (Siddiqui, 1995). Pleural effusions are usually right-sided, and these, as well as accompanying ascites, are typically transudative and resolve after tumor resection (Majzlin, 1964). Despite this association of ascites with benign fibromas, when ascites and a pelvic mass coexist, evaluation is based on an assumption of malignancy.

The prognosis following excision of fibromas is that for any benign tumor. However, 10 percent will demonstrate increased cellularity and varying degrees of pleomorphism and mitotic activity that indicate a tumor better characterized as having low malignant potential. In 1 percent of cases, malignant transformation to *fibrosarcoma* is found.

Sclerosing Stromal Tumors. These tumors are rare and account for less than 5 percent of SCSTs. The average patient age is approximately 20 years, and 80 percent develop before age 30. Sclerosing stromal tumors are clinically benign and typically unilateral. Menstrual irregularities and pelvic pain are both frequent symptoms (Marelli, 1998). Ascites is seldom encountered (unlike fibromas), and sclerosing stromal tumors are hormonally inactive (unlike thecomas). Tumor size ranges from microscopic to 20 cm. Histologically, the presence of pseudolobulation of cellular areas separated by edematous connective tissue, increased vascularity, and prominent areas of sclerosis are distinguishing features.

Sertoli-Stromal Cell Tumors

Sertoli Cell Tumors. Ovarian Sertoli cell tumors are rare and account for less than 5 percent of all SCSTs. The mean patient age at diagnosis is 30 years, but ages range from 2 to 76 years. One quarter of patients have estrogenic or androgenic manifestations, but most tumors are clinically nonfunctional.

Sertoli cell tumors are typically unilateral, solid, and yellow and measure 4 to 12 cm. Derived from the cell type that gives rise to the seminiferous tubules, these tumor cells often organize into histologically characteristic tubules (Young, 2005). Sertoli cell tumors, however, may also mimic many different tumors, and immunostaining in these cases is invaluable to confirm the diagnosis.

More than 80 percent are stage I at diagnosis, and most are clinically benign. Moderate cytologic atypia, brisk mitotic activity, and tumor cell necrosis are indicators of greater malignant potential. These are found in 10 percent of individuals with stage I disease and most of those with stage II–IV tumors. The risk of recurrence is higher when these features are identified (Oliva, 2005).

Sertoli-Leydig Cell Tumors. Sertoli-Leydig cell tumors constitute only 5 to 10 percent of ovarian SCSTs (Zhang, 2007). Their incidence mirrors that of Sertoli cell tumors, and the average age is 25 years. Although Sertoli-Leydig cell tumors have been identified in children and postmenopausal females, more than 90 percent develop during the reproductive years.

These tumors frequently produce sex-steroid hormones, most commonly androgens. As a result, frank virilization develops in one third of women, and another 10 percent have clinical manifestations of androgen excess (Young, 1985). Menstrual disorders are also common. Accordingly, Sertoli-Leydig cell tumors are suspected preoperatively in a patient with a unilaterally palpable adnexal mass and with androgenic manifestations. For these women, an elevated serum testosterone-to-androstenedione ratio further suggests the diagnosis.

Although these hormonal effects frequently develop, one half of patients will have nonspecific abdominal mass symptoms as their only complaint. Associated ascites is infrequent (Outwater, 2000). Thyroid abnormalities also coexist with Sertoli-Leydig cell tumors at a frequency that exceeds mere chance.

These tumors tend to be large at the time of excision. In most cases, Sertoli-Leydig cell tumors appear yellow and lobulated. They can be solid, partially cystic, or completely cystic (Fig. 36-10). Microscopically, tumors contain cells resembling epithelial and stromal testicular cells in varying proportions. The five subtypes of differentiation (well, intermediate, poor, retiform, and heterologous) have considerable overlap. Well-differentiated tumors are all clinically benign (Chen, 2003; Young, 2005).

Overall, 15 to 20 percent of Sertoli-Leydig cell tumors are clinically malignant. Prognosis depends predominantly on the stage and degree of tumor differentiation in these malignant variants. For example, Young and Scully (1985) performed a clinicopathologic analysis of 207 malignant cases and identified stage I disease in 97 percent. The 5-year survival rate for patients with stage I disease exceeds 90 percent (Zaloudek, 1984). Malignant features were observed in approximately 10 percent of tumors with intermediate differentiation and in 60 percent of poorly differentiated tumors. Retiform and heterologous elements are seen only in intermediate or poorly differentiated Sertoli-Leydig cell tumors and typically are associated with poorer prognosis. Overall, the 2 to 3 percent of patients with stage II–IV disease have a dismal prognosis (Young, 1985).

Sex Cord Tumors with Annular Tubules

This tumor accounts for 5 percent of SCSTs and is characterized by ring-shaped tubules and distinctive cellular elements that are histologically intermediate between Sertoli-cell and granulosa cell tumors. Two clinically distinct types are recognized. First, one third of cases are clinically benign and develops in patients with Peutz-Jeghers syndrome (PJS). These tumors are typically small, multifocal, calcified, bilateral, and diagnosed incidentally. Fifteen percent of PJS-associated cases will also develop adenoma malignum of the cervix, which is a rare, extremely well-differentiated adenocarcinoma. In contrast, two thirds of tumors are not associated with PJS. These masses are usually larger, unilateral, and symptomatic and carry a clinical malignancy rate of 15 to 20 percent (Young, 1982).

Steroid Cell Tumors

Fewer than 5 percent of SCSTs are steroid cell tumors. The average age at diagnosis is the mid-20s, but the age range is

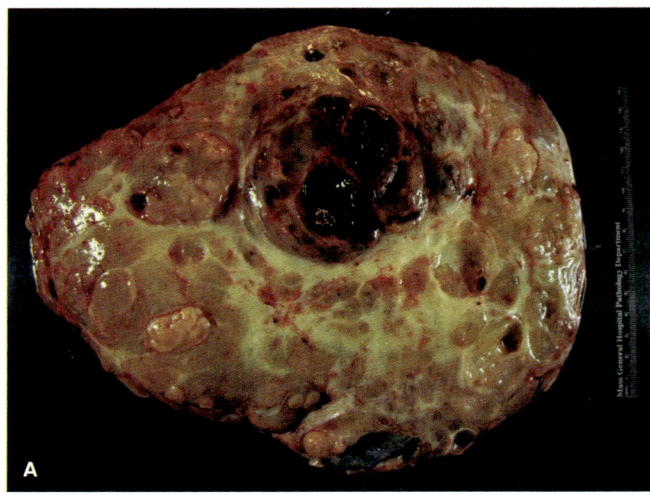

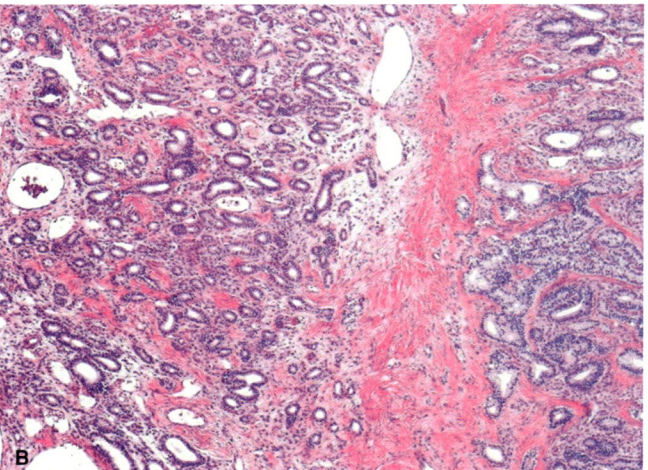

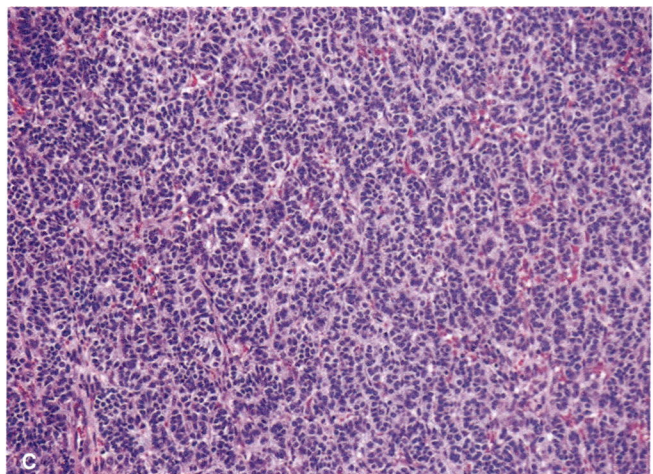

FIGURE 36-10 Sertoli-Leydig cell tumor (SLCT). **A.** SLCTs show variable gross features depending on the degree of differentiation and presence of heterologous elements. This opened surgical specimen has a predominantly solid cut surface with focal cysts, variegated yellow-brown color, and foci of hemorrhage. **B.** Well-differentiated SLCT composed of hollow tubules admixed with clusters of mature Leydig cells. **C.** This intermediate differentiated SLCT contains solid tubules, which are thought to resemble those of the fetal testis. (Reproduced with permission by Dr. Katja Gwin.)

broad. These tumors are composed entirely or predominantly of cells that resemble steroid hormone–secreting cells and are categorized according to these cell's histologic composition.

Stromal luteomas are clinically benign tumors that by definition lie completely within the ovarian stroma. They are usually seen in postmenopausal women. Estrogenic effects are common, but occasional individuals have androgenic manifestations.

Leydig cell tumors are also benign and typically are seen in postmenopausal women. They are distinguished microscopically by rectangular, crystal-like cytoplasmic inclusions, termed crystals of Reinke. Leydig cells secrete testosterone, and these tumors are usually associated with androgenic effects.

Steroid cell tumors not otherwise specified (NOS) are the most common subtype within this group and typically present in younger reproductive-aged women. Some of these cases may represent large stromal luteomas that have grown to reach the ovarian surface or Leydig-cell tumors in which Reinke crystals cannot be identified. These tumors are typically associated with androgen excess, but estrogen or cortisol overproduction (i.e., Cushing syndrome) also has been reported. One third of steroid-cell tumors NOS are clinically malignant and have a dismal prognosis (Oliva, 2005).

Unclassified Sex Cord-Stromal Tumors

Unclassified tumors account for 5 percent of SCSTs and have no clearly predominant pattern of testicular (Sertoli cells) or ovarian (granulosa cells) differentiation. These ill-defined tumors are especially common during pregnancy due to alterations in their usual clinical and pathologic features (Young, 2005). They may be estrogenic, androgenic, or nonfunctional. The prognosis is similar to that of granulosa cell tumors and Sertoli-Leydig cell tumors of similar degrees of differentiation.

Gynandroblastomas

These are the rarest type of ovarian SCST. Patients present at a mean age of 30 years and typically have menstrual irregularities or evidence of hormonal excess. The tumors are characterized by intermingled granulosa cells and tubules of Sertoli cells. Theca or Leydig cells or both also may be present in varying degrees. Gynandroblastomas have low malignant potential, and only one death has been reported (Martin-Jimenez, 1994).

■ Treatment

Surgery

The mainstay of treatment for patients with an ovarian SCST is complete surgical resection. This group shows relative insensitivity to adjuvant chemotherapy or radiation. Thus, operative goals are to establish a definitive tissue diagnosis, determine the extent of disease, and remove all grossly visible tumors in those infrequent patients with advanced-stage disease. Moreover, during

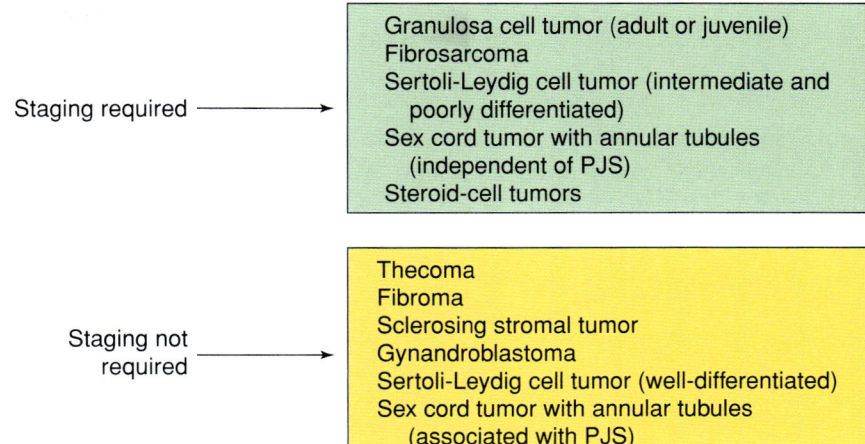

FIGURE 36-11 Staging of sex cord-stromal tumors. PJS = Peutz-Jeghers syndrome.

preoperative planning, clinicians should consider the patient's age and desire for future fertility. Hysterectomy with BSO is performed for those who have completed childbearing, whereas fertility-sparing USO with preservation of the uterus and remaining ovary may be appropriate in the absence of obvious disease spread to these organs (Zanagnolo, 2004). Endometrial sampling is performed, especially if fertility-sparing surgery is planned in women with granulosa cell tumors or thecomas. This is because many of these patients will have coexisting hyperplasia or adenocarcinoma that may affect the decision for hysterectomy.

Minimally invasive laparoscopic surgery has various relevant applications. For some, the diagnosis of SCST may not be discovered until the mass is laparoscopically removed and sent for frozen section analysis. Laparoscopic surgical staging can then proceed. If the diagnosis is not made until the final pathology report is confirmed postoperatively, laparoscopic staging may be proposed to determine whether metastatic disease is present. This can reduce the morbidity of a second operation (Shim, 2013).

Surgical staging is essential to determine the extent of disease and the need for adjuvant therapy in most individuals with potentially malignant SCST subtypes (Fig. 36-11). That said, only approximately 20 percent of cases have complete staging (Abu-Rustum, 2006; Brown, 2009). More recent data suggest that, due to surface and hematogenous routes of spread, the standard ovarian cancer procedure can be modified. Pelvic washings, exploration of the abdomen, peritoneal biopsies, and partial omentectomy remain important. However, the utility of routine pelvic and paraaortic lymphadenectomy has been increasingly challenged. In a National Cancer Database study of 2680 ovarian granulosa cell tumors, half of whom underwent lymphadenectomy, only 3 percent had positive nodes. And, those cases usually had concurrent widespread disease (Seagle, 2017). Additionally, performing a lymphadenectomy does not improve survival rates in those with SCSTs (Cheng, 2018).

Surgical removal of hormone-producing SCSTs results in an immediate drop in elevated preoperative sex-steroid hormone levels. Physical manifestations of these elevated levels, however, partially or completely resolve more gradually.

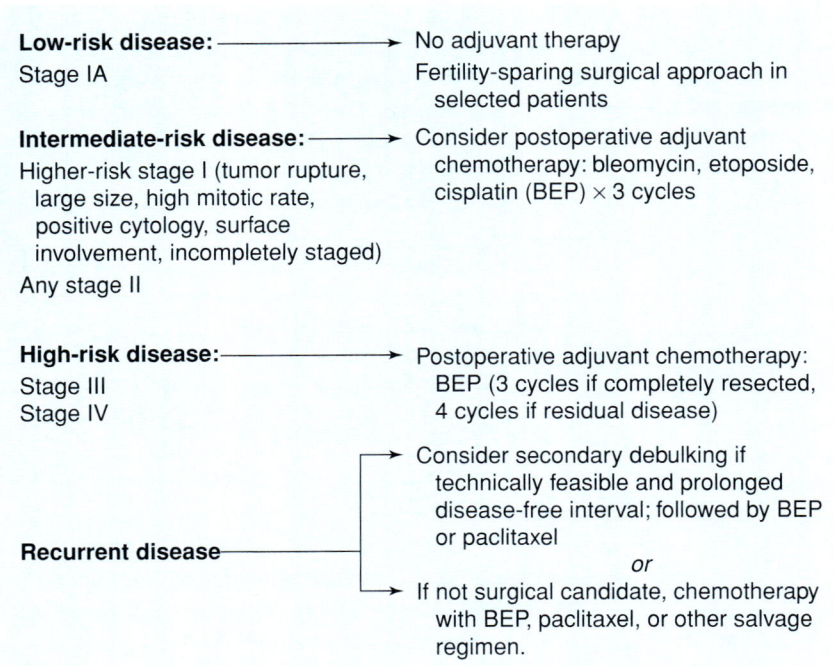

Low-risk disease: ⟶ No adjuvant therapy
Stage IA   Fertility-sparing surgical approach in
                                  selected patients

Intermediate-risk disease: ⟶ Consider postoperative adjuvant
Higher-risk stage I (tumor rupture,   chemotherapy: bleomycin, etoposide,
   large size, high mitotic rate,   cisplatin (BEP) × 3 cycles
   positive cytology, surface
   involvement, incompletely staged)
Any stage II

High-risk disease: ⟶ Postoperative adjuvant chemotherapy:
Stage III   BEP (3 cycles if completely resected,
Stage IV   4 cycles if residual disease)

                         ⟶ Consider secondary debulking if
                           technically feasible and prolonged
                           disease-free interval; followed by BEP
                           or paclitaxel
Recurrent disease ⟶   *or*
                         ⟶ If not surgical candidate, chemotherapy
                           with BEP, paclitaxel, or other salvage
                           regimen.

FIGURE 36-12 Postoperative treatment of sex cord–stromal tumors.

Surveillance

In general, women with stage I ovarian SCSTs have an excellent prognosis following surgery alone and usually can be followed at regular intervals without the need for further treatment (Morgan, 2016). Surveillance includes a general physical and pelvic examination, serum marker level testing if initially elevated, and imaging as clinically indicated.

Chemotherapy

The decision to administer postoperative therapy depends on various factors (**Fig. 36-12**). Although typically treated solely with surgery, malignant stage I ovarian SCSTs may require adjuvant chemotherapy when large tumor size, high mitotic index, capsular excrescences, tumor rupture, incomplete staging, or equivocal pathology results are noted. Women with one or more of these suspicious features carry a higher risk of relapse and are considered for platinum-based chemotherapy (Morgan, 2016). Stage II–IV disease warrants postoperative treatment. In general, SCSTs display less sensitivity to chemotherapy than other ovarian malignancies, yet adjuvant platinum-based chemotherapy is recommended (van Meurs, 2014).

The 5-day bleomycin, etoposide, and cisplatin (BEP) regimen is the most widely used first-line chemotherapy combination (Gershenson, 1996; Homesley, 1999). For completely resected disease, three courses given every 3 weeks are sufficient. Four cycles are recommended for patients with incompletely resected tumor (Homesley, 1999). In addition to BEP, taxanes have demonstrated modest activity as a single-agent against ovarian SCSTs, but the combination of paclitaxel and carboplatin chemotherapy appears more promising (Brown, 2004, 2005; Burton, 2016). To determine the most effective regimen, a prospective randomized study is currently underway, comparing paclitaxel and carboplatin against BEP in those with newly

diagnosed ovarian SCSTs (GOG protocol #264). Unfortunately, the relative scarcity of women who have ovarian SCST and then receive chemotherapy limits the ability to conduct large randomized studies.

Radiation

Postoperative radiation therapy currently has a limited role in the management of ovarian SCSTs. There is some evidence indicating a prolonged survival in at least some women with newly diagnosed disease who received whole-abdominal radiotherapy (Wolf, 1999). However, chemotherapy is usually the primary postoperative treatment because it is generally better tolerated, more widely accessible, and easier to administer. Radiation is best reserved for palliation of local symptoms (Dubuc-Lissoir, 2001).

Relapse

The management of recurrent ovarian SCST depends on the clinical circumstances. Secondary surgical debulking is strongly considered due to the indolent growth pattern, the typically long disease-free interval after initial treatment, and the inherent insensitivity to chemotherapy (Crew, 2005; Powell, 2001). Platinum-based combination chemotherapy is the primary treatment chosen for recurrent disease with or without surgical debulking (Uygun, 2003). Of regimens, BEP is most frequently administered because it has the highest known response rate (Homesley, 1999).

There is no standard treatment for women who have progressive disease despite aggressive surgery and platinum-based chemotherapy. Recently, bevacizumab (Avastin) demonstrated a 17-percent response rate in a Phase II trial (Brown, 2014a). Hormonal therapy is minimally toxic, but the clinical experience with this approach is extremely limited (Hardy, 2005). Medroxyprogesterone acetate and the gonadotropin-releasing hormone (GnRH) agonist leuprolide acetate (Lupron) have each demonstrated activity in halting the growth of recurrent ovarian SCSTs (Fishman, 1996; Homesley, 1999). GnRH antagonists, however, may not be as effective (Ameryckx, 2005).

In addition to traditional drugs, discovery of the *FOXL2* 402C>G mutation occurring exclusively in all adult granulosa cell tumors may lead to the development of targeted therapies for women with advanced or recurrent disease. Currently, FOXL2 as a transcription factor does not represent a perfect pharmacologic target. Further insights into its function and downstream effects may identify molecular alterations in these tumors that can be targeted (Kobel, 2009).

■ Prognosis

In general, ovarian SCSTs portend a much better prognosis than epithelial ovarian carcinomas chiefly because most women with SCSTs are diagnosed with stage I disease. Stage II–IV tumors are rare, but women with these cancers have a poor prognosis similar to their counterparts with epithelial disease. Unfortunately, survival rates for ovarian SCSTs have not improved during the past few decades (Chan, 2006). Of prognostic factors, younger age, surgical stage, tumor size, and residual disease are the most important (Lee, 2008; Seagle, 2017; Zanagnolo, 2004).

■ Management During Pregnancy

Ovarian SCSTs are rarely detected during pregnancy (Okada, 2004). Granulosa cell tumors are most common, but only 10 percent are diagnosed during pregnancy (Hasiakos, 2006). One third of pregnant women with SCSTs are incidentally diagnosed at cesarean delivery, one third have abdominal pain or swelling, and the remainder may present with hemoperitoneum, virilization, or vaginal bleeding (Young, 1984). Surgical management should be the same as for the nonpregnant woman. For most, conservative management with USO and staging is the primary procedure, but hysterectomy and BSO may be indicated in selected circumstances (Young, 1984). Postoperative chemotherapy is typically withheld until after delivery because SCSTs have an indolent growth pattern.

REFERENCES

Aboud E: A review of granulosa cell tumours and thecomas of the ovary. Arch Gynecol Obstet 259:161, 1997

Abu-Rustum NR, Restivo A, Ivy J, et al: Retroperitoneal nodal metastasis in primary and recurrent granulosa cell tumors of the ovary. Gynecol Oncol 103:31, 2006

Ameryckx L, Fatemi HM, De Sutter P, et al: GnRH antagonist in the adjuvant treatment of a recurrent ovarian granulosa cell tumor: a case report. Gynecol Oncol 99:764, 2005

Aoki Y, Kase H, Fujita K, et al: Dysgerminoma with a slightly elevated alpha-fetoprotein level diagnosed as a mixed germ cell tumor after recurrence. Gynecol Obstet Invest 55:58, 2003

Beiner ME, Gotlieb WH, Korach Y, et al: Cystectomy for immature teratoma of the ovary. Gynecol Oncol 93:381, 2004

Bentivegna E, Azaïs H, Uzan C, et al: Surgical outcomes after debulking surgery for intraabdominal ovarian growing teratoma syndrome: analysis of 38 cases. Ann Surg Oncol 22(3 suppl):S964, 2015

Billmire D, Vinocur C, Rescorla F, et al: Outcome and staging evaluation in malignant germ cell tumors of the ovary in children and adolescents: an intergroup study. J Pediatr Surg 39:424, 2004

Billmire DF, Cullen JW, Rescorla FJ, et al: Surveillance after initial surgery for pediatric and adolescent girls with stage I ovarian germ cell tumors: report from the Children's Oncology Group. J Clin Oncol 32(5):465, 2014

Bonazzi C, Peccatori F, Colombo N, et al: Pure ovarian immature teratoma, a unique and curable disease: 10 years' experience of 32 prospectively treated patients. Obstet Gynecol 84:598, 1994

Boyce EA, Costaggini I, Vitonis A, et al: The epidemiology of ovarian granulosa cell tumors: a case-control study. Gynecol Oncol 115:221, 2009

Brown J, Brady WE, Schink J, et al: Efficacy and safety of bevacizumab in recurrent sex cord-stromal ovarian tumors: results of a phase 2 trial of the Gynecologic Oncology Group. Cancer 120(3):344, 2014a

Brown J, Friedlander M, Backes FJ, et al: Gynecologic Cancer Intergroup (GCIG) consensus review for ovarian germ cell tumors. Int J Gynecol Cancer 24(9 Suppl 3):S48, 2014b

Brown J, Shvartsman HS, Deavers MT, et al: The activity of taxanes compared with bleomycin, etoposide, and cisplatin in the treatment of sex cord–stromal ovarian tumors. Gynecol Oncol 97:489, 2005

Brown J, Shvartsman HS, Deavers MT, et al: The activity of taxanes in the treatment of sex cord–stromal ovarian tumors. J Clin Oncol 22:3517, 2004

Brown J, Sood AK, Deavers MT, et al: Patterns of metastasis in sex cord-stromal tumors of the ovary: can routine staging lymphadenectomy be omitted? Gynecol Oncol 113:86, 2009

Burton ER, Brady M, Homesley HD, et al: A phase II study of paclitaxel for the treatment of ovarian stromal tumors: an NRG Oncology/Gynecologic Oncology Group Study. Gynecol Oncol 140(1):48, 2016

Carmina E, Rosato F, Janni A, et al: Extensive clinical experience: relative prevalence of different androgen excess disorders in 950 women referred because of clinical hyperandrogenism. J Clin Endocrinol Metab 91:2, 2006

Cass DL, Hawkins E, Brandt ML, et al: Surgery for ovarian masses in infants, children, and adolescents: 102 consecutive patients treated in a 15-year period. J Pediatr Surg 36:693, 2001

Cathro HP, Stoler MH: The utility of calretinin, inhibin, and WT1 immunohistochemical staining in the differential diagnosis of ovarian tumors. Hum Pathol 36:195, 2005

Chan JK, Cheung MK, Husain A, et al: Patterns and progress in ovarian cancer over 14 years. Obstet Gynecol 108:521, 2006

Chan JK, Tewari KS, Waller S, et al: The influence of conservative surgical practices for malignant ovarian germ cell tumors. J Surg Oncol 98:111, 2008

Chan JK, Zhang M, Kaleb V, et al: Prognostic factors responsible for survival in sex cord stromal tumors of the ovary: a multivariate analysis. Gynecol Oncol 96:204, 2005

Chechia A, Attia L, Temime RB, et al: Incidence, clinical analysis, and management of ovarian fibromas and fibrothecomas. Am J Obstet Gynecol 199:473e1, 2008

Chen CA, Lin H, Weng CS, et al: Outcome of 3-day bleomycin, etoposide and cisplatin chemotherapeutic regimen for patients with malignant ovarian germ cell tumours: a Taiwanese Gynecologic Oncology Group study. Eur J Cancer 50(18):3161, 2014

Chen VW, Ruiz B, Killeen JL, et al: Pathology and classification of ovarian tumors. Cancer 97:2631, 2003

Cheng H, Peng J, Yang Z, et al: Prognostic significance of lymphadenectomy in malignant ovarian sex cord stromal tumor: a retrospective cohort study and meta-analysis. Gynecol Oncol 148(1):91, 2018

Cicin I, Saip P, Guney N, et al: Yolk sac tumours of the ovary: evaluation of clinicopathological features and prognostic factors. Eur J Obstet Gynecol Reprod Biol 146:210, 2009

Colombo N, Parma G, Zanagnolo V, et al: Management of ovarian stromal cell tumors. J Clin Oncol 25:2944, 2007

Corakci A, Ozeren S, Ozkan S, et al: Pure nongestational choriocarcinoma of ovary. Arch Gynecol Obstet 271:176, 2005

Crew KD, Cohen MH, Smith DH, et al: Long natural history of recurrent granulosa cell tumor of the ovary 23 years after initial diagnosis: a case report and review of the literature. Gynecol Oncol 96:235, 2005

Culine S, Lhomme C, Michel G, et al: Is there a role for second-look laparotomy in the management of malignant germ cell tumors of the ovary? Experience at Institut Gustave Roussy. J Surg Oncol 62:40, 1996

Curtin JP, Morrow CP, D'Ablaing G, et al: Malignant germ cell tumors of the ovary: 20-year report of LAC-USC Women's Hospital. Int J Gynecol Cancer 4:29, 1994

Cushing B, Giller R, Ablin A, et al: Surgical resection alone is effective treatment for ovarian immature teratoma in children and adolescents: a report of the Pediatric Oncology Group and the Children's Cancer Group. Am J Obstet Gynecol 181:353, 1999

Dark GG, Bower M, Newlands ES, et al: Surveillance policy for stage I ovarian germ cell tumors. J Clin Oncol 15:620, 1997

Dimopoulos MA, Papadimitriou C, Hamilos G, et al: Treatment of ovarian germ cell tumors with a 3-day bleomycin, etoposide, and cisplatin regimen: a prospective multicenter study. Gynecol Oncol 95:695, 2004

Dos Santos L, Mok E, Iasonos A, et al: Squamous cell carcinoma arising in mature cystic teratoma of the ovary: a case series and review of the literature. Gynecol Oncol 105:321, 2007

Dubuc-Lissoir J, Berthiaume MJ, Boubez G, et al: Bone metastasis from a granulosa cell tumor of the ovary. Gynecol Oncol 83:400, 2001

East N, Alobaid A, Goffin F, et al: Granulosa cell tumour: a recurrence 40 years after initial diagnosis. J Obstet Gynaecol Can 27:363, 2005

Elit L, Bocking A, Kenyon C, et al: An endodermal sinus tumor diagnosed in pregnancy: case report and review of the literature. Gynecol Oncol 72:123, 1999

Fishman A, Kudelka AP, Tresukosol D, et al: Leuprolide acetate for treating refractory or persistent ovarian granulosa cell tumor. J Reprod Med 41:393, 1996

Frausto SD, Geisler JP, Fletcher MS, et al: Late recurrence of juvenile granulosa cell tumor of the ovary. Am J Obstet Gynecol 1:366, 2004

Gainford MC, Tinker A, Carter J, et al: Malignant transformation within ovarian dermoid cysts: an audit of treatment received and patient outcomes. An Australia New Zealand Gynaecological Oncology Group (ANZGOG) and Gynaecologic Cancer Intergroup (GCIG) study. Int J Gynecol Cancer 20:75, 2010

Galani E, Alamanis C, Dimopoulos MA: Familial female and male germ cell cancer: a new syndrome? Gynecol Oncol 96:254, 2005

Gershenson DM: Management of ovarian germ cell tumors. J Clin Oncol 25:2938, 2007

Gershenson DM, Morris M, Burke TW, et al: Treatment of poor-prognosis sex cord–stromal tumors of the ovary with the combination of bleomycin, etoposide, and cisplatin. Obstet Gynecol 87:527, 1996

Gershenson DM, Morris M, Cangir A, et al: Treatment of malignant germ cell tumors of the ovary with bleomycin, etoposide, and cisplatin. J Clin Oncol 8:715, 1990

Hardy RD, Bell JG, Nicely CJ, et al: Hormonal treatment of a recurrent granulosa cell tumor of the ovary: case report and review of the literature. Gynecol Oncol 96:865, 2005

Hasiakos D, Papakonstantinou K, Goula K, et al: Juvenile granulosa cell tumor associated with pregnancy: report of a case and review of the literature. Gynecol Oncol 100(2):426, 2006

Heravi-Moussavi A, Anglesio MS, Cheng SW, et al: Recurrent somatic DICER1 mutations in nonepithelial ovarian cancers. N Engl J Med 366(3):234, 2012

Hoepffner W, Horn LC, Simon E, et al: Gonadoblastomas in 5 patients with 46,XY gonadal dysgenesis. Exp Clin Endocrinol Diabetes 113:231, 2005

Homesley HD, Bundy BN, Hurteau JA, et al: Bleomycin, etoposide, and cisplatin combination therapy of ovarian granulosa cell tumors and other stromal malignancies: a Gynecologic Oncology Group study. Gynecol Oncol 72:131, 1999

Horbelt D, Delmore J, Meisel R, et al: Mixed germ cell malignancy of the ovary concurrent with pregnancy. Obstet Gynecol 84:662, 1994

Hsu YJ, Pai L, Chen YC, et al: Extragonadal germ cell tumors in Taiwan: an analysis of treatment results of 59 patients. Cancer 95:766, 2002

Jung SE, Rha SE, Lee JM, et al: CT and MRI findings of sex cord–stromal tumor of the ovary. AJR Am J Roentgenol 185:207, 2005

Kalfa N, Patte C, Orbach D, et al: A nationwide study of granulosa cell tumors in pre- and postpubertal girls: missed diagnosis of endocrine manifestations worsens prognosis. J Pediatr Endocrinol Metab 18:25, 2005

Kim SH, Kang SB: Ovarian dysgerminoma: color Doppler ultrasonographic findings and comparison with CT and MR imaging findings. J Ultrasound Med 14:843, 1995

Kleppe M, Amkreutz LC, Van Gorp T, et al: Lymph-node metastasis in stage I and II sex cord stromal and malignant germ cell tumours of the ovary: a systematic review. Gynecol Oncol 133(1):124, 2014

Kobel M, Gilks CB, Huntsman DG: Adult-type granulosa cell tumors and FOXL2 mutation. Cancer Res 69:9160, 2009

Kumar S, Shah JP, Bryant CS, et al: The prevalence and prognostic impact of lymph node metastasis in malignant germ cell tumors of the ovary. Gynecol Oncol 110:125, 2008

Kurihara S, Hirakawa T, Amada S, et al: Inhibin-producing ovarian granulosa cell tumor as a cause of secondary amenorrhea: case report and review of the literature. J Obstet Gynaecol Res 30:439, 2004

Kurman RJ, Carcangiu ML, Herrington CS, et al (eds): WHO Classification of Tumours of Female Reproductive Organs, 4th ed. Lyon, International Agency for Research on Cancer, 2014

Kusamura S, Teixeira LC, dos Santos MA, et al: Ovarian germ cell cancer: clinicopathologic analysis and outcome of 31 cases. Tumori 86:450, 2000

LaPolla JP, Fiorica JV, Turnquist D, et al: Successful therapy of metastatic embryonal carcinoma coexisting with gonadoblastoma in a patient with 46,XY pure gonadal dysgenesis (Swyer's syndrome). Gynecol Oncol 37:417, 1990

Leblanc E, Querleu D, Narducci F, et al: Laparoscopic restaging of early stage invasive adnexal tumors: a 10-year experience. Gynecol Oncol 94:624, 2004

Lee YK, Park NH, Kim JW, et al: Characteristics of recurrence in adult-type granulosa cell tumor. Int J Gynecol Cancer 18:642, 2008

Li H, Hong W, Zhang R, et al: Retrospective analysis of 67 consecutive cases of pure ovarian immature teratoma. Chin Med J (Engl) 115:1496, 2002

Li J, Yang W, Wu X: Prognostic factors and role of salvage surgery in chemorefractory ovarian germ cell malignancies: a study in Chinese patients. Gynecol Oncol 105:769, 2007

Liu Q, Ding X, Yang J, et al: The significance of comprehensive staging surgery in malignant ovarian germ cell tumors. Gynecol Oncol 131(3):551, 2013

Low JJ, Perrin LC, Crandon AJ, et al: Conservative surgery to preserve ovarian function in patients with malignant ovarian germ cell tumors: a review of 74 cases. Cancer 89:391, 2000

Majzlin G, Stevens FL: Meigs' syndrome. Case report and review of literature. J Int Coll Surg 42:625, 1964

Marelli G, Carinelli S, Mariani A, et al: Sclerosing stromal tumor of the ovary: report of eight cases and review of the literature. Eur J Obstet Gynecol Reprod Biol 76:85, 1998

Marina NM, Cushing B, Giller R, et al: Complete surgical excision is effective treatment for children with immature teratomas with or without malignant elements: a Pediatric Oncology Group/Children's Cancer Group Intergroup study. J Clin Oncol 17:2137, 1999

Martin-Jimenez A, Condom-Munro E, Valls-Porcel M, et al: [Gynandroblastoma of the ovary: review of the literature.] French. J Gynecol Obstet Biol Reprod (Paris) 23:391, 1994

McKenna M, Kenny B, Dorman G, et al: Combined adult granulosa cell tumor and mucinous cystadenoma of the ovary: granulosa cell tumor with heterologous mucinous elements. Int J Gynecol Pathol 24:224, 2005

Messing MJ, Gershenson DM, Morris M, et al: Primary treatment failure in patients with malignant ovarian germ cell neoplasms. Int J Gynecol Cancer 2:295, 1992

Miller BE, Barron BA, Dockter ME, et al: Parameters of differentiation and proliferation in adult granulosa cell tumors of the ovary. Cancer Detect Prev 25:48, 2001

Mom CH, Engelen MJ, Willemse PH, et al: Granulosa cell tumors of the ovary: the clinical value of serum inhibin A and B levels in a large single center cohort. Gynecol Oncol 105:365, 2007

Morgan RJ Jr, Armstrong DK, Alvarez RD, et al: Ovarian cancer, version 1.2016, NCCN clinical practice guidelines in oncology. J Natl Compr Canc Netw 14(9):1134, 2016

Morimura Y, Nishiyama H, Yanagida K, et al: Dysgerminoma with syncytiotrophoblastic giant cells arising from 46,XX pure gonadal dysgenesis. Obstet Gynecol 92:654, 1998

Murugaesu N, Schmid P, Dancey G, et al: Malignant ovarian germ cell tumors: identification of novel prognostic markers and long-term outcome after multimodality treatment. J Clin Oncol 24:4862, 2006

Nasioudis D, Chapman-Davis E, Frey MK, et al: Management and prognosis of ovarian yolk sac tumors; an analysis of the National Cancer Data Base. Gynecol Oncol 147(2):296, 2017

O'Connor DM, Norris HJ: The influence of grade on the outcome of stage I ovarian immature (malignant) teratomas and the reproducibility of grading. Int J Gynecol Pathol 13:283, 1994

Okada I, Nakagawa S, Takemura Y, et al: Ovarian thecoma associated in the first trimester of pregnancy. J Obstet Gynaecol Res 30:368, 2004

Oliva E, Alvarez T, Young RH: Sertoli cell tumors of the ovary: a clinicopathologic and immunohistochemical study of 54 cases. Am J Surg Pathol 29:143, 2005

Oliva E, Andrada E, Pezzica E, et al: Ovarian carcinomas with choriocarcinomatous differentiation. Cancer 72:2441, 1993

Outwater EK, Marchetto B, Wagner BJ: Virilizing tumors of the ovary: imaging features. Ultrasound Obstet Gynecol 15:365, 2000

Paladini D, Testa A, Van Holsbeke C, et al: Imaging in gynecological disease (5): clinical and ultrasound characteristics in fibroma and fibrothecoma of the ovary. Ultrasound Obstet Gynecol 34:188, 2009

Palenzuela G, Martin E, Meunier A, et al: Comprehensive staging allows for excellent outcome in patients with localized malignant germ cell tumor of the ovary. Ann Surg 248:836, 2008

Park JY, Kim DY, Suh DS, et al: Analysis of outcomes and prognostic factors after fertility-sparing surgery in malignant ovarian germ cell tumors. Gynecol Oncol 145(3):513, 2017

Pavlakis K, Messini I, Vrekoussis T, et al: Intraoperative assessment of epithelial and non-epithelial ovarian tumors: a 7-year review. Eur J Gynaecol Oncol 30:657, 2009

Pena-Alonso R, Nieto K, Alvarez R, et al: Distribution of Y-chromosome-bearing cells in gonadoblastoma and dysgenetic testis in 45,X/46,XY infants. Mod Pathol 18:439, 2005

Pins MR, Young RH, Daly WJ, et al: Primary squamous cell carcinoma of the ovary: report of 37 cases. Am J Surg Pathol 20:823, 1996

Powell JL, Connor GP, Henderson GS: Management of recurrent juvenile granulosa cell tumor of the ovary. Gynecol Oncol 81:113, 2001

Pressley RH, Muntz HG, Falkenberry S, et al: Serum lactic dehydrogenase as a tumor marker in dysgerminoma. Gynecol Oncol 44:281, 1992

Quirk JT, Natarajan N: Ovarian cancer incidence in the United States, 1992–1999. Gynecol Oncol 97:519, 2005

Ray-Coquard I, Brown J, Harter P, Gynecologic Cancer InterGroup (GCIG) consensus review for ovarian sex cord stromal tumors. Int J Gynecol Cancer 24(9 Suppl 3):S42, 2014

Rezk Y, Sheinfeld J, Chi DS: Prolonged survival following salvage surgery for chemorefractory ovarian immature teratoma: a case report and review of the literature. Gynecol Oncol 96:883, 2005

Schneider DT, Calaminus G, Harms D, et al: Ovarian sex cord–stromal tumors in children and adolescents. J Reprod Med 50:439, 2005

Schneider DT, Calaminus G, Wessalowski R, et al: Ovarian sex cord–stromal tumors in children and adolescents. J Clin Oncol 21:2357, 2003

Schrader KA, Gorbatcheva B, Senz J, et al: The specificity of the FLXL2 c.402G>G somatic mutation: a survey of solid tumors. PLoS One 4(11):e7988, 2009

Schwartz PE, Morris JM: Serum lactic dehydrogenase: a tumor marker for dysgerminoma. Obstet Gynecol 72:511, 1988

Seagle BL, Ann P, Butler S, et al: Ovarian granulosa cell tumor: a National Cancer Database study. Gynecol Oncol 146(2):285, 2017

Shah R, Xia C, Krailo M, et al: Is carboplatin-based chemotherapy as effective as cisplatin-based chemotherapy in the treatment of advanced-stage dysgerminoma in children, adolescents and young adults? Gynecol Oncol 150(2):253, 2018

Shah SP, Kobel M, Senz J, et al: Mutation of FOXL2 in granulosa-cell tumors of the ovary. N Engl J Med 360:2719, 2009

Sharony R, Aviram R, Fishman A, et al: Granulosa cell tumors of the ovary: do they have any unique ultrasonographic and color Doppler flow features? Int J Gynecol Cancer 11:229, 2001

Shim SH, Kim DY, Lee SW, et al: Laparoscopic management of early-stage malignant nonepithelial ovarian tumors: surgical and survival outcomes. Int J Gynecol Cancer 23(2):249, 2013

Shimizu Y, Komiyama S, Kobayashi T, et al: Successful management of endodermal sinus tumor of the ovary associated with pregnancy. Gynecol Oncol 88:447, 2003

Siddiqui M, Toub DB: Cellular fibroma of the ovary with Meigs' syndrome and elevated CA-125: a case report. J Reprod Med 40:817, 1995

Skalleberg J, Solheim O, Fosså SD, et al: Long-term ototoxicity in women after cisplatin treatment for ovarian germ cell cancer. Gynecol Oncol 145(1):148, 2017

Smith HO, Berwick M, Verschraegen CF, et al: Incidence and survival rates for female malignant germ cell tumors. Obstet Gynecol 107:1075, 2006

Solheim O, Gershenson DM, Tropé CG, Prognostic factors in malignant ovarian germ cell tumours (The Surveillance, Epidemiology and End Results experience 1978–2010). Eur J Cancer 50(11):1942, 2014

Solheim O, Kaern J, Tropé CG, et al: Malignant ovarian germ cell tumors: presentation, survival and second cancer in a population based Norwegian cohort (1953-2009). Gynecol Oncol 131(2):330, 2013

Solheim O, Tropé CG, Rokkones E, et al: Fertility and gonadal function after adjuvant therapy in women diagnosed with a malignant ovarian germ cell tumor (MOGCT) during the "cisplatin era." Gynecol Oncol 136(2):224, 2015

Stettner AR, Hartenbach EM, Schink JC, et al: Familial ovarian germ cell cancer: report and review. Am J Med Genet 84:43, 1999

Stevens TA, Brown J, Zander DS, et al: Adult granulosa cell tumors of the ovary in two first-degree relatives. Gynecol Oncol 98:502, 2005

Stier EA, Barakat RR, Curtin JP, et al: Laparotomy to complete staging of presumed early ovarian cancer. Obstet Gynecol 87:737, 1996

Takemori M, Nishimura R, Yamasaki M, et al: Ovarian mixed germ cell tumor composed of polyembryoma and immature teratoma. Gynecol Oncol 69:260, 1998

Talukdar S, Kumar S, Bhatla N, et al: Neo-adjuvant chemotherapy in the treatment of advanced malignant germ cell tumors of ovary. Gynecol Oncol 132(1):28, 2014

Tangir J, Zelterman D, Ma W, et al: Reproductive function after conservative surgery and chemotherapy for malignant germ cell tumors of the ovary. Obstet Gynecol 101:251, 2003

Teilum G: Classification of endodermal sinus tumour (mesoblastoma vitellinum) and so-called "embryonal carcinoma" of the ovary. Acta Pathol Microbiol Scand 64:407, 1965

Ulbright TM: Germ cell tumors of the gonads: a selective review emphasizing problems in differential diagnosis, newly appreciated, and controversial issues. Mod Pathol 18 (Suppl 2):S61, 2005

Uygun K, Aydiner A, Saip P, et al: Clinical parameters and treatment results in recurrent granulosa cell tumor of the ovary. Gynecol Oncol 88:400, 2003

van Meurs HS, Bleeker MC, van der Velden J, et al: The incidence of endometrial hyperplasia and cancer in 1031 patients with a granulosa cell tumor of the ovary: long-term follow-up in a population-based cohort study. Int J Gynecol Cancer 23(8):1417, 2013

van Meurs HS, Buist MR, Westermann AM, et al: Effectiveness of chemotherapy in measurable granulosa cell tumors: a retrospective study and review of literature. Int J Gynecol Cancer 24(3):496, 2014

Vang R, Herrmann ME, Tavassoli FA: Comparative immunohistochemical analysis of granulosa and Sertoli components in ovarian sex cord–stromal tumors with mixed differentiation: potential implications for derivation of Sertoli differentiation in ovarian tumors. Int J Gynecol Pathol 23:151, 2004

Vicus D, Beiner ME, Klachook S, et al: Pure dysgerminoma of the ovary 35 years on: a single institutional experience. Gynecol Oncol 117:23, 2010

Williams SD, Birch R, Einhorn LH, et al: Treatment of disseminated germ cell tumors with cisplatin, bleomycin, and either vinblastine or etoposide. N Engl J Med 316:1435, 1987

Williams SD, Blessing JA, DiSaia PJ, et al: Second-look laparotomy in ovarian germ cell tumors: the Gynecologic Oncology Group experience. Gynecol Oncol 52:287, 1994

Williams SD, Kauderer J, Burnett AF, et al: Adjuvant therapy of completely resected dysgerminoma with carboplatin and etoposide: a trial of the Gynecologic Oncology Group. Gynecol Oncol 95:496, 2004

Wolf JK, Mullen J, Eifel PJ, et al: Radiation treatment of advanced or recurrent granulosa cell tumor of the ovary. Gynecol Oncol 73:35, 1999

Young JL Jr, Wu XC, Roffers SD, et al: Ovarian cancer in children and young adults in the United States, 1992–1997. Cancer 97:2694, 2003

Young RH: Sex cord–stromal tumors of the ovary and testis: their similarities and differences with consideration of selected problems. Mod Pathol 18:S81, 2005

Young RH, Dudley AG, Scully RE: Granulosa cell, Sertoli–Leydig cell, and unclassified sex cord–stromal tumors associated with pregnancy: a clinicopathological analysis of thirty-six cases. Gynecol Oncol 18:181, 1984

Young RH, Scully RE: Ovarian Sertoli–Leydig cell tumors: a clinicopathological analysis of 207 cases. Am J Surg Pathol 9:543, 1985

Young RH, Welch WR, Dickersin GR, et al: Ovarian sex cord tumor with annular tubules: review of 74 cases including 27 with Peutz-Jeghers syndrome and four with adenoma malignum of the cervix. Cancer 50:1384, 1982

Yuan JQ, Lin XN, Xu JY, et al: Ovarian juvenile granulosa cell tumor associated with Maffucci's syndrome: case report. Chin Med J 117:1592, 2004

Zaloudek C, Norris HJ: Sertoli-Leydig tumors of the ovary: a clinicopathologic study of 64 intermediate and poorly differentiated neoplasms. Am J Surg Pathol 8:405, 1984

Zanagnolo V, Pasinetti B, Sartori E: Clinical review of 63 cases of sex cord stromal tumors. Eur J Gynaecol Oncol 25:431, 2004

Zanetta G, Bonazzi C, Cantu M, et al: Survival and reproductive function after treatment of malignant germ cell ovarian tumors. J Clin Oncol 19:1015, 2001

Zhang M, Cheung MK, Shin JY, et al: Prognostic factors responsible for survival in sex cord stromal tumors of the ovary—an analysis of 376 women. Gynecol Oncol 104:396, 2007

Zhao XY, Huang HF, Lian LJ, et al: Ovarian cancer in pregnancy: a clinicopathologic analysis of 22 cases and review of the literature. Int J Gynecol Cancer 16:8, 2006

CHAPTER 37

Gestational Trophoblastic Disease

Gestational trophoblastic disease (GTD) refers to a spectrum of interrelated but histologically distinct tumors originating from the placenta (Table 37-1) (Hui, 2014a,b). These diseases are characterized by a reliable tumor marker, which is the β-subunit of human chorionic gonadotropin (β-hCG), and have varied tendencies for local invasion and spread.

Gestational trophoblastic neoplasia (GTN) refers to the subset of GTD that develops malignant sequelae. These tumors require formal staging and typically respond favorably to chemotherapy. Most commonly, GTN develops after a molar pregnancy but may follow any gestation. The prognosis for most GTN cases is excellent, and patients are routinely cured, even with widespread metastases. The outlook for preservation of fertility and for successful subsequent pregnancy outcomes

---

TABLE 37-1. Modified WHO Classification of GTD

Molar pregnancies
Hydatidiform mole
  Complete
  Partial
Invasive mole

Trophoblastic tumors
Choriocarcinoma
Placental site trophoblastic tumor
Epithelioid trophoblastic tumor

GTD = gestational trophoblastic disease; WHO = World Health Organization.

is equally bright (Vargas, 2014; Wong, 2014). Accordingly, although GTD is uncommon, because the opportunity for cure is great, clinicians should be familiar with its presentation, diagnosis, and management.

EPIDEMIOLOGY AND RISK FACTORS

The incidence of GTD has remained fairly constant at approximately 1 to 2 per 1000 deliveries in North America and Europe (Eysbouts, 2016; Gockley, 2016; Lybol, 2011). Although historically higher incidence rates have been reported in parts of Asia, some of this disparity may reflect discrepancies between population-based and hospital-based data collection (Chong, 1999; Kim, 2004; Matsui, 2003). Improved socioeconomic conditions and dietary changes may be partly responsible as well. That said, certain Southeast Asian populations as well as Hispanics and Native Americans living in the United States do have increased incidences (Drake, 2006; Smith, 2003; Tham, 2003).

Maternal age at the upper and lower extremes carries a higher risk of GTD (Gockley, 2016). This association is much greater for complete moles, whereas the risk of partial molar pregnancy varies relatively little with age. One explanation relates to ova from older women having higher rates of abnormal fertilization. Similarly, older paternal age has been associated with a greater risk (La Vecchia, 1984; Parazzini, 1986).

A history of prior unsuccessful pregnancies also raises the risk of GTD. For example, previous spontaneous abortion at least doubles the risk of molar pregnancy (Parazzini, 1991). More significantly, a personal history of GTD increases the risk of developing a molar gestation in a subsequent pregnancy at least tenfold. The frequency in a subsequent conception is approximately 1 percent, and most cases mirror the same type of mole as the preceding pregnancy (Garrett, 2008; Sebire, 2003). Furthermore, following two episodes of molar pregnancy, 23 percent of later conceptions result in another molar gestation (Berkowitz, 1998). For this reason, women with a prior history of GTD should undergo first-trimester sonographic examination in subsequent pregnancies. Familial molar pregnancies, however, are rare (Fallahian, 2003).

Of other risk factors, combination oral contraceptive (COC) pill use has been associated with an increased risk of GTD. Specifically, prior COC use approximately doubles the risk, and longer duration of use also correlates positively with risk (Palmer, 1999; Parazzini, 2002). Moreover, women who used COCs during the cycle in which they conceived have a higher risk in some but not all studies (Costa, 2006; Palmer, 1999). Many of these associations, however, are weak and could be explained by confounding factors other than causality (Parazzini, 2002).

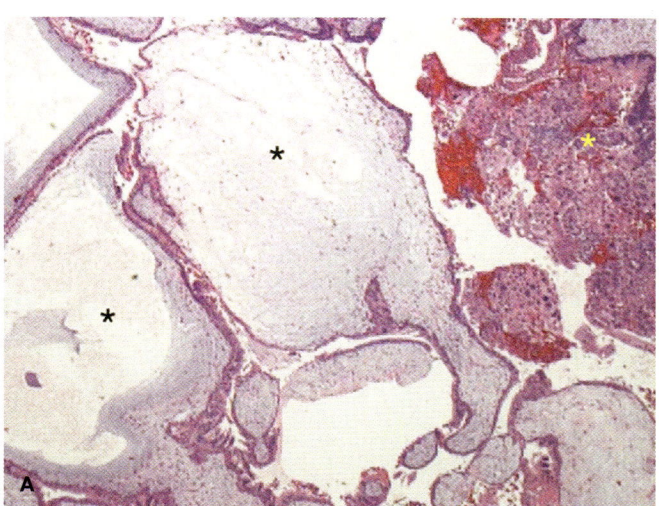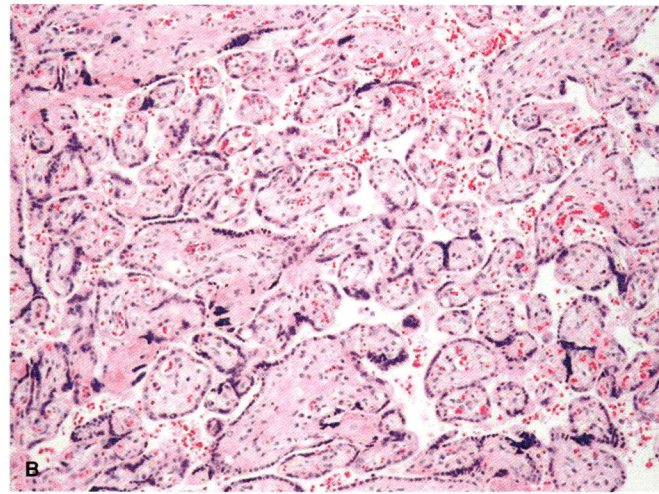

FIGURE 37-1 A. Complete hydatidiform mole. These moles are characterized by enlarged, hydropic villi, some of which have cistern formation, that is, central cavitation within the edematous villi (*black asterisks*). Seen diffusely throughout the placenta, these changes create the vesicles noted grossly in complete moles (see Fig. 37-3). Complete moles also typically show trophoblastic proliferation (*yellow asterisk*), which may be focal or widespread (Reproduced with permission from Dr. Erika Fong). **B.** This contrasts with a normal-term placenta showing smaller, nonedematous villi and absence of trophoblastic proliferation. (Reproduced with permission from Dr. Kelley Carrick).

Some epidemiologic characteristics differ markedly between complete and partial moles. For example, vitamin A deficiency and low dietary intake of carotene are associated only with a higher risk of complete moles (Berkowitz, 1985, 1995; Parazzini, 1988). Partial moles have been linked to higher educational levels, smoking, irregular menstrual cycles, and obstetric histories in which only male infants are among the prior live births (Berkowitz, 1995; Parazzini, 1986).

HYDATIDIFORM MOLE (MOLAR PREGNANCY)

Hydatidiform moles are abnormal pregnancies characterized histologically by aberrant changes within the placenta. Classically, the chorionic villi in these placenta show varying degrees of trophoblast proliferation and edema of the stroma within villi (Fig. 37-1). Hydatidiform moles are categorized as either *complete hydatidiform moles* or *partial hydatidiform moles* (Table 37-2). Chromosomal abnormalities play an integral role in hydatidiform mole development.

■ Complete Hydatidiform Mole

These molar pregnancies differ from partial moles with regard to their karyotype, their histologic appearance, and their clinical presentation. First, complete moles typically have a diploid karyotype, and 85 to 90 percent of cases are 46,XX. The chromosomes, however, in these pregnancies are entirely of paternal origin, and thus, the diploid set is described as *diandric*. Specifically, complete moles are formed by *androgenesis*, in which the ovum is fertilized by a haploid sperm that then duplicates its own chromosomes after meiosis (Fig. 37-2) (Fan, 2002; Kajii, 1977). The ovum fails to contribute chromosomes. Most of these moles are 46,XX, but dispermic fertilization of a single ovum, that is, simultaneous fertilization by two sperm, can produce a 46,XY karyotype (Lawler, 1987). Although nuclear DNA is entirely paternal, mitochondrial DNA remains maternal in origin (Azuma, 1991).

Microscopically, complete moles display enlarged, edematous villi and abnormal trophoblastic proliferation. These changes diffusely involve the entire placenta (see Fig. 37-1). Macroscopically, these changes transform the chorionic villi

TABLE 37-2. Features of Hydatidiform Moles

Feature	Complete Mole	Partial Mole
Karyotype	46,XX or 46,XY	69,XXX or 69,XXY
Pathology		
Fetus/embryo	Absent	Present
Villous edema	Diffuse	Focal
Trophoblastic proliferation	Can be marked	Focal and minimal
p57Kip2 immunostaining	Negative	Positive
Clinical presentation		
Typical diagnosis	Molar gestation	Missed abortion
Postmolar malignant sequelae	15–20%	4–6%

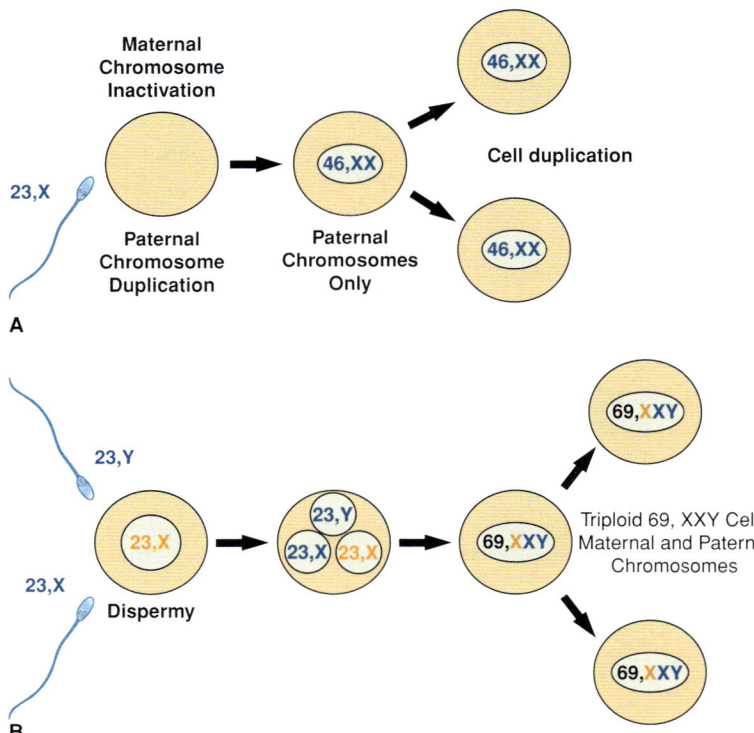

FIGURE 37-2 A. A 46,XX complete mole may be formed if a 23,X-bearing haploid sperm penetrates a 23,X-containing haploid egg whose genes have become "inactive." Paternal chromosomes then duplicate to create a 46,XX diploid chromosomal complement solely of paternal origin. Alternatively, this same type of inactivated egg can be fertilized independently by two sperm, either 23,X- or 23,Y-bearing, to create a 46,XX or 46,XY chromosomal complement, again of paternal origin only. **B.** Partial moles may be formed if two sperm, either 23,X- or 23,Y-bearing, both fertilize a 23,X-containing haploid egg, whose genes have not been inactivated. The resulting fertilized egg is triploid. Alternatively, a similar haploid egg may be fertilized by an unreduced diploid 46,XY sperm.

into clusters of vesicles with variable dimensions. Indeed, the name *hydatidiform mole* literally stems from this "bunch of grapes" appearance. In these pregnancies, no fetal tissue or amnion is produced. As a result, this mass of placental tissue completely fills the endometrial cavity (Fig. 37-3).

Clinically, the presentation of a complete mole has changed considerably. In the 1960s and 1970s, more than half of affected patients had anemia and uterine sizes in excess of that predicted for their gestational age. In addition, hyperemesis gravidarum, preeclampsia, and theca-lutein cysts developed in approximately one quarter of women (Soto-Wright, 1995). Theca-lutein cysts develop with prolonged exposure to luteinizing hormone (LH) or β-hCG (Fig. 37-4). These cysts range in size from 3 to 20 cm, and most regress with falling β-hCG titers after molar evacuation. If such cysts are present, and especially if they are bilateral, the risk of postmolar GTN is increased.

Complete moles, however, infrequently present today with these traditional signs and symptoms. As a result of β-hCG testing and sonography, the mean gestational age at evacuation currently approximates 9 weeks, compared with 12 weeks in the 1980s and 1990s and 16 to 17 weeks in the 1960s and 1970s (Sun, 2015; Soto-Wright, 1995). A large proportion of patients are asymptomatic at diagnosis. For the remainder, vaginal bleeding remains the most common presenting symptom, and β-hCG levels are often greater than expected. One quarter of women will have uterine size greater than dates, but the incidence of anemia is less than 10 percent. Moreover, hyperemesis gravidarum, preeclampsia, and symptomatic theca-lutein cysts are now rare (Sun, 2015). Currently, these sequelae typically develop chiefly in patients without early prenatal care who present with a more advanced gestational age and markedly elevated serum β-hCG levels. Last, plasma thyroxine levels are often increased in women with complete moles, but clinical hyperthyroidism is infrequent. In these

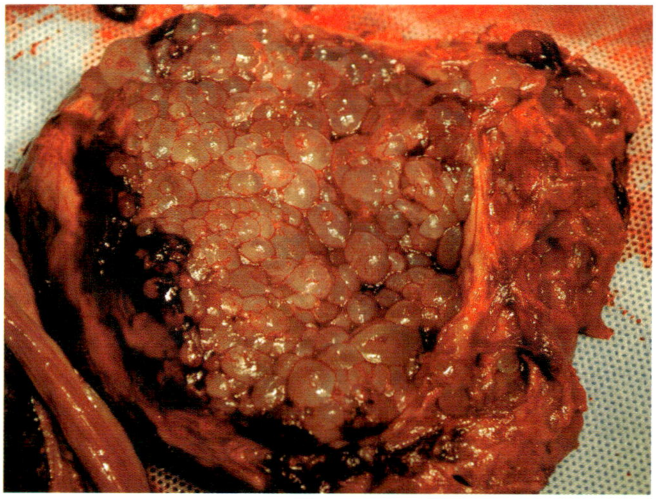

FIGURE 37-3 Photograph of a complete hydatidiform mole. Note the grape-like fluid-filled clusters of chorionic villi. (Reproduced with permission from Dr. Sasha Andrews.)

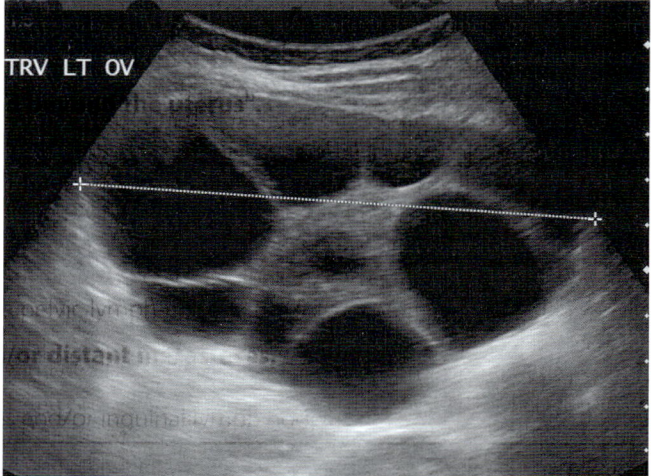

FIGURE 37-4 Transvaginal sonogram of multiple theca lutein cysts within one ovary of a woman with a complete molar pregnancy. Bilateral, multiple simple cysts are characteristic findings.

circumstances, serum free thyroxine levels are elevated as a consequence of the thyrotropin-like effect of β-hCG (Chap. 16, p. 337).

Partial Hydatidiform Mole

These moles vary from complete hydatidiform moles clinically, genetically, and histologically. The degree and extent of trophoblastic proliferation and villous edema are decreased compared with those of complete moles. Moreover, most partial moles contain fetal tissue and amnion, in addition to placental tissues.

As a result, patients with partial moles typically present with signs and symptoms of an incomplete or missed abortion. Many women will have vaginal bleeding. However, because trophoblastic proliferation is slight and only focal, uterine enlargement in excess of gestational age is uncommon. Similarly, preeclampsia, theca-lutein cysts, hyperthyroidism, or other dramatic clinical features are rare. Preevacuation β-hCG levels are typically much lower than those for complete moles and often do not exceed 100,000 mIU/mL (Sun, 2016). For this reason, partial moles are often not identified until after a histologic review of a curettage specimen.

Partial moles have a triploid karyotype (69,XXX, 69,XXY, or less commonly 69,XYY) that is composed of one maternal and two paternal haploid sets of chromosomes (see Fig. 37-2) (Lawler, 1991). The coexisting fetus present with a partial mole is nonviable and typically has multiple malformations with abnormal growth (Jauniaux, 1999).

Diagnosis

Clinical Assessment

In reproductive-aged women with vaginal bleeding, diagnoses may include gynecologic causes of abnormal bleeding and complications of first-trimester pregnancy. The trophoblast of molar pregnancies produce β-hCG, and elevated hormone levels reflect their proliferation. Accordingly, initial urine or serum β-hCG measurement and transvaginal sonography are invaluable in guiding evaluation. Because of these, first-trimester diagnosis of hydatidiform mole is now common.

Although β-hCG levels are helpful, the diagnosis of molar pregnancy is more frequently found sonographically. Most first-trimester complete moles demonstrate a complex, echogenic, intrauterine mass containing many small cystic spaces, which reflect swollen chorionic villi. Fetal tissues and amnionic sac are absent (Fig. 37-5) (Benson, 2000). In contrast, sonographic features of a partial molar pregnancy include a thickened, hydropic placenta with a concomitant fetus (Zhou, 2005).

However, there are diagnostic limitations. For example, β-hCG levels in early molar pregnancies may not always be elevated in the first trimester (Lazarus, 1999). Moreover, sonography can lead to a false-negative diagnosis if performed at very early gestational ages, before the chorionic villi have attained their characteristic vesicular pattern. Studies show that only 20 to 30 percent of patients may have sonographic evidence to indicate a partial mole (Johns, 2005; Lindholm, 1999; Sebire, 2001). Consequently, diagnosis in early gestations is usually difficult. Often, the diagnosis is not made until after histologic review of the abortal specimen. In unclear cases with a live fetus and a desired pregnancy, fetal karyotyping to identify a triploid fetal chromosomal pattern can clarify the diagnosis and management.

Histopathology

The histopathologic changes typical of hydatidiform moles are listed in Table 37-2. But, in early pregnancy, it may be difficult to distinguish among these and a hydropic abortus. Hydropic abortuses are pregnancies formed by the traditional union of one haploid egg and one haploid sperm but are pregnancies that have failed. Their placentas display *hydropic degeneration*, in which villi are edematous and swollen, and thus mimic some villous features of hydatidiform

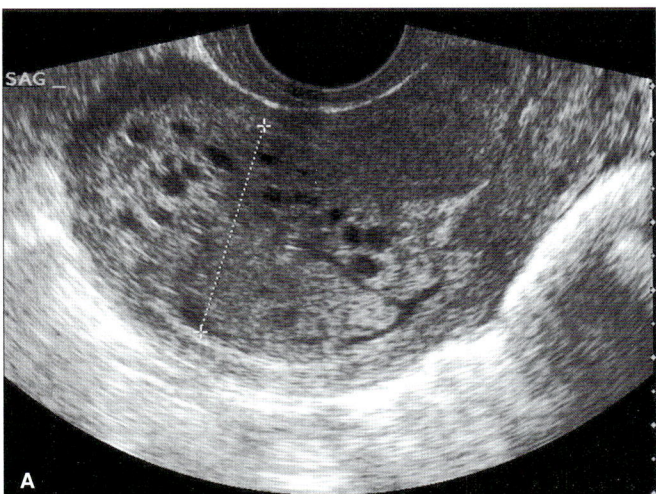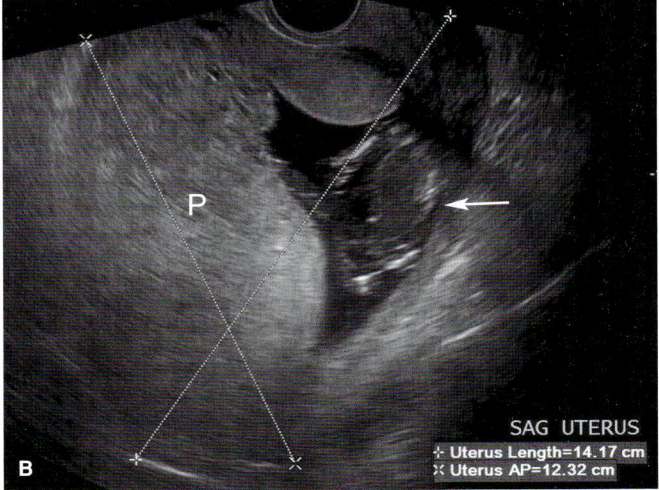

FIGURE 37-5 Sonograms of hydatidiform moles. **A.** With complete hydatidiform moles, the classic "snowstorm" appearance is created by the multiple placental vesicles. The mole completely fills this uterine cavity, and calipers measure the intrauterine contents. **B.** With partial hydatidiform mole, a fetal tissue is seen in addition to an abnormally thickened placenta with small anechoic cysts (*P*). An arrow marks the fetal torso.

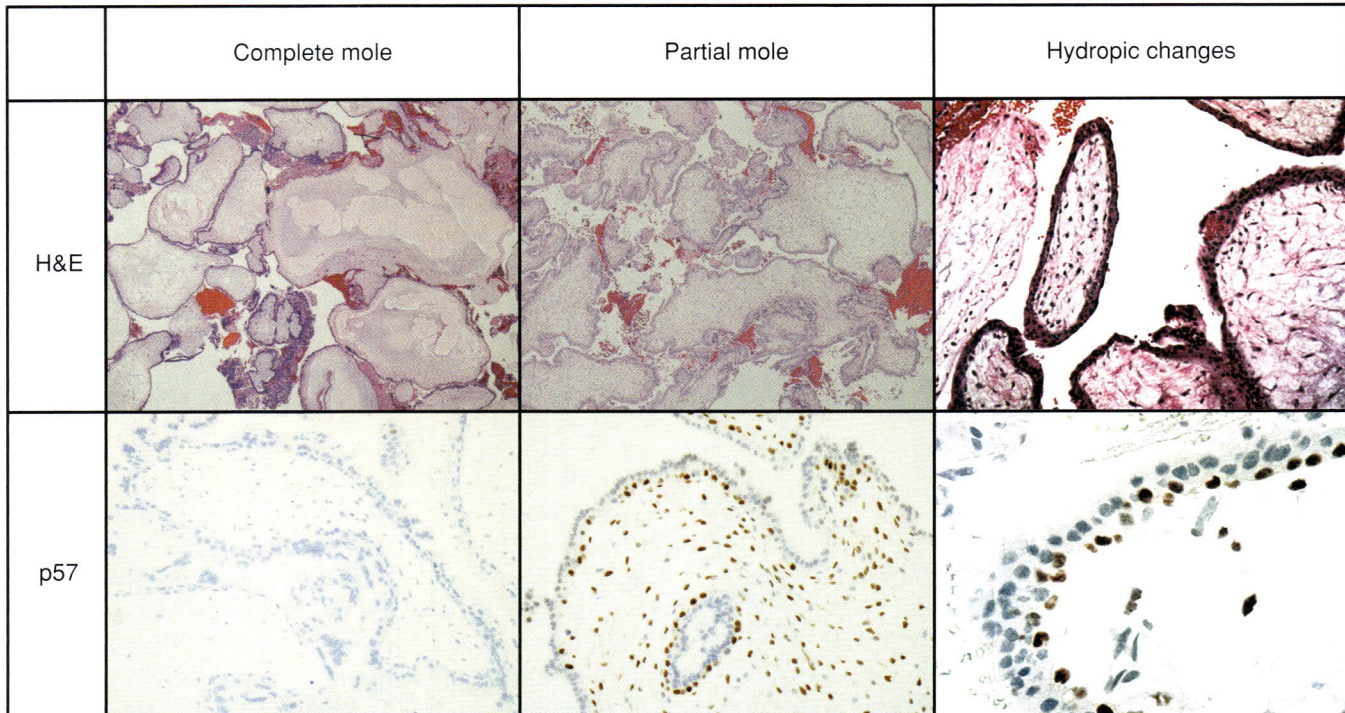

	Complete mole	Partial mole	Hydropic changes
H&E			
p57			

FIGURE 37-6 Composite showing differences among complete hydatidiform moles, partial hydatidiform moles, and nonmolar hydropic abortuses. The first row shows typical appearances of villi after hematoxylin and eosin (H & E) staining. The second row shows results with p57 staining. p57 is a nuclear protein whose gene product is produced only in tissues containing a maternal allele. After immunohisto-chemical staining for p57, note the positive (brown) staining in the villous mesenchyme and villous trophoblast of the partial hydatidiform mole and nonmolar hydropic abortus. This contrasts with the absent staining for p57 in the complete mole (only the blue counterstain is seen). (Reproduced with permission from Drs. Kelley Carrick and Raheela Ashfaq.)

moles (Fig. 37-6). Although no single criterion distinguishes these three, complete moles generally have two prominent features: (1) trophoblastic proliferation and (2) hydropic villi. In gestations younger than 10 weeks, however, hydropic villi may not be apparent, and molar stroma may still be vascular (Paradinas, 1997). As a result, identification of early complete moles must rely on more subtle histologic abnormalities, supplemented by immunohistochemical and molecular diagnostic techniques. Partial moles are optimally diagnosed when three or four major diagnostic criteria are demonstrated: (1) two populations of villi, (2) enlarged, irregular, dysmorphic villi (with trophoblast inclusions), (3) enlarged, cavitated villi ($\geq$3 to 4 mm), and (4) syncytiotrophoblast hyperplasia/atypia (Chew, 2000). Good diagnostic reproducibility can still be achieved in most circumstances using these histologic distinctions of complete and partial mole.

Ancillary Techniques

Histopathologic evaluation can be enhanced by immunohisto-chemical staining for *p57* expression and by various laboratory techniques aimed at determining ploidy. First, p57KIP2 is a nuclear protein whose gene is paternally imprinted and maternally expressed. This means that the gene product is produced only in tissues containing a maternal allele. Because complete moles contain only paternal genes, the p57KIP2 protein is absent in complete moles, and tissues do not pick up this stain (Merchant, 2005). In contrast, this nuclear protein is strongly expressed in

normal placentas, in spontaneous pregnancy losses with hydropic degeneration, and in partial hydatidiform moles (Castrillon, 2001). Accordingly, immunostaining for p57KIP2 is an effective means to isolate complete mole from the diagnostic list.

For distinction of a partial mole from a nonmolar hydropic abortus, both of which express p57, evaluation of ploidy can be used. Most partial moles are triploid or near triploid, and laboratory karyotyping to look for triploidy can be completed. Importantly, not all triploid gestations represent a partial hydatidiform mole. Thus, triploidy is not solely diagnostic of partial hydatidiform mole but serves as an informative adjunct when applied in the context of histologic findings suggestive of the mole type. Molecular genotyping is a newer technique that determines not only ploidy but also the parental source of polymorphic alleles. Thus, it can distinguish among a diploid diandric genome (complete mole), a triploid diandric-monogynic genome (partial mole), or biparental diploidy (nonmolar abortus) (Ronnett, 2011).

◼ Treatment

Suction curettage is the preferred method of evacuation regardless of uterine size in patients who wish to remain fertile. Electric vacuum aspiration is the predominant technique in North America but is not readily available throughout the world. When necessary, manual vacuum aspiration offers similar outcomes (Padron, 2018). Prostanoids to ripen the cervix are not recommended as these drugs can induce uterine contractions, which might increase the risk of trophoblastic embolization to the pulmonary vasculature (Seckl, 2010). Hysterectomy is rarely recommended unless the patient wishes surgical sterilization or is approaching menopause (Elias, 2010). Theca-lutein ovarian cysts tend not to be symptomatic and typically regress after molar evacuation. In extreme cases, these may be aspirated if symptomatic, but oophorectomy is not performed except when torsion leads to extensive ovarian infarction (Mungan, 1996).

Prior to surgery, patients are evaluated for associated medical complications. A complete blood count (CBC) and measures of liver, renal, and thyroid function tests are done. Fortunately, thyroid storm from untreated hyperthyroidism, respiratory insufficiency from trophoblastic emboli, and complications from preeclampsia are rare. Because of the tremendous vascularity of these placentas, blood products should be available prior to the evacuation of larger moles, and adequate infusion lines established. Other uterotonic agents, such as methylergonovine maleate (Methergine) and carboprost tromethamine (Hemabate), can be administered for heavy bleeding refractory to oxytocin (Pitocin) infusion alone.

At the beginning of the evacuation, the cervix is dilated to admit a 10- to 12-mm plastic suction curette. As aspiration of molar tissues ensues, intravenous oxytocin is given. At our hospital, 20 units of synthetic oxytocin are mixed with 1 L of crystalloid and infused at rates to achieve uterine contraction. If available, intraoperative sonographic guidance is preferred to help reduce the risk of uterine perforation and assist in confirming complete evacuation. Finally, a thorough, gentle curettage is performed. Following curettage, because of the possibility of partial mole and its attendant fetal tissue, Rh immune globulin is given to nonsensitized Rh D–negative women.

Postmolar Surveillance

GTN develops after evacuation in 15 to 20 percent of patients with complete moles (Braga, 2016; Sun, 2016). Despite the trend of diagnosing these abnormal pregnancies at earlier gestational ages, this incidence has not declined. Of those women who develop GTN, three quarters have locally invasive molar disease and the remaining one quarter develops metastases. In contrast, GTN develops in only 4 to 6 percent of patients with partial moles following evacuation (Sun, 2016). Malignant transformation into metastatic choriocarcinoma does occur after partial mole evacuation, but this is rare (0.1 percent) (Cheung, 2004; Seckl, 2000).

No pathologic or initial clinical features accurately predict which patients will ultimately develop GTN. Because of the trophoblastic proliferation that characterizes these neoplasms, serial serum β-hCG levels following molar evacuation can be used to effectively monitor patients for GTN development. Therefore, postmolar surveillance with serial quantitative serum β-hCG levels is the standard. Titers are monitored following uterine evacuation at least every 1 to 2 weeks until they become undetectable.

After undetectable β-hCG levels are achieved, subsequent monthly levels are drawn during 6 months of surveillance for all patients with a molar gestation (Sebire, 2007). However, poor

compliance with prolonged monitoring has been reported—especially among indigent women and certain ethnic groups in the United States (Allen, 2003; Massad, 2000). A single blood sample demonstrating an undetectable level of β-hCG following molar evacuation is sufficient to exclude the possibility of progression to GTN in the vast majority of patients. The risk of GTN after spontaneous β-hCG normalization following molar pregnancy is <0.5 percent (Braga, 2015). Thus, some women, especially those with a partial mole, may be safely discharged from routine surveillance once an undetectable value is achieved (Lavie, 2005; Wolfberg, 2004). Shortened surveillance could also enable women to attempt a subsequent pregnancy sooner.

When pregnancies occur during the monitoring period, the resulting normal β-hCG production can hinder detection of postmolar progression to GTN (Allen, 2003). But other than complicating the monitoring schedule, these pregnancies fortunately are otherwise uneventful (Tuncer, 1999). To prevent difficulties with interpretation, women are encouraged to use effective contraception until achieving a β-hCG titer <5 mIU/mL or below the individual assay's threshold. COC use decreases the likelihood of pregnancy compared with less effective barrier contraception and does not increase the risk of GTN (Braga, 2016; Dantas, 2017). Injectable medroxyprogesterone acetate is particularly useful when poor compliance is anticipated (Massad, 2000). In contrast, intrauterine devices are not inserted until the β-hCG level is undetectable because of the risk of uterine perforation if an invasive mole is present.

Prophylactic Chemotherapy

At the time of molar evacuation, chemotherapy can be administered to help prevent GTN development in high-risk patients who are unlikely to be compliant or for whom β-hCG surveillance is not available. In clinical practice, however, correctly categorizing a woman as high-risk for GTN development is difficult, as no combination of risk factors is universally accepted. Typical patients have complete moles and multiple risk factors, such as age >40 years, previous history of molar pregnancy, or an excessively high β-hCG titer prior to evacuation. That said, few women are ultimately assigned to this group. Moreover, due to the risks of increased drug resistance, delayed treatment of GTN, and toxic side effects, this practice cannot currently be recommended (Wang, 2017). Prophylactic chemotherapy is not routinely offered in the United States or Europe.

However, a single dose of dactinomycin does reduce the incidence of postmolar GTN in certain populations. For example, in one randomized trial, 60 Thai women who had high-risk complete moles were assigned to receive either prophylactic dactinomycin or placebo at the time of evacuation (Limpongsanurak, 2001). Adjuvant chemotherapy reduced the incidence of GTN from 50 percent to 14 percent, but toxicity was significant. As a result, prophylactic chemotherapy is generally used only in those countries with limited resources to reliably monitor patients after evacuation (Uberti, 2009).

Ectopic Molar Pregnancy

The true incidence of GTD developing outside the uterine cavity approximates 1.5 per 1 million births (Gillespie, 2004).

More than 90 percent of suspected cases will reflect an overdiagnosis of florid extravillous trophoblastic proliferation in the fallopian tube (Burton, 2001; Sebire, 2005b). As with any ectopic pregnancy, initial management usually involves surgical removal of the conceptus and histopathologic evaluation.

Coexistent Fetus

At times, a twin pregnancy can consist of a hydatidiform mole and a coexisting fetus. The estimated incidence is 1 per 20,000 to 100,000 pregnancies (Fig. 37-7). Lin and associates (2017) described the outcome of 72 twin pregnancies, each composed of a complete mole and a healthy co-twin. Of this group, 10 women chose to have an elective termination, 2 did not have follow-up information, and 60 continued their pregnancies. Seventeen gestations (28 percent) ended with spontaneous abortion, intrauterine demise, or extreme premature deliveries at less than 24 weeks' gestation. Seven (12 percent) were terminated due to severe maternal complications before fetal viability, and 36 viable-aged neonates (60 percent) were delivered alive. The overall risk of progression to GTN was significant at 46 percent. Because the risk of malignancy is unchanged with advancement of gestational age, pregnancy continuation may be allowed, provided that severe maternal complications are manageable and fetal growth is normal (Lin, 2017). Importantly, these cases should be distinguished early from a single partial molar pregnancy with its abnormal associated fetus. Fetal karyotyping to confirm a normal fetal chromosomal pattern is recommended (Marcorelles, 2005; Matsui, 2000).

GESTATIONAL TROPHOBLASTIC NEOPLASIA

This term primarily encompasses pathologic entities that are characterized by aggressive invasion of the endometrium and myometrium by trophoblast cells. Histologic categories include common tumors such as the invasive mole and gestational choriocarcinoma, as well as the rare placental-site trophoblastic tumor and epithelioid trophoblastic tumor. Although these histologic types have been characterized, in most cases of GTN, no tissue is available for pathologic study. Instead, GTN is diagnosed based on elevated β-hCG levels and managed clinically.

Gestational trophoblastic neoplasia typically develops with or follows some form of pregnancy. Most cases follow a hydatidiform mole. Rarely, GTN develops after a live birth, miscarriage, or termination. Occasionally, the antecedent gestation cannot be confirmed with certainty. Many of the reported nonmolar cases may actually represent disease originating from an unrecognized early mole (Sebire, 2005a).

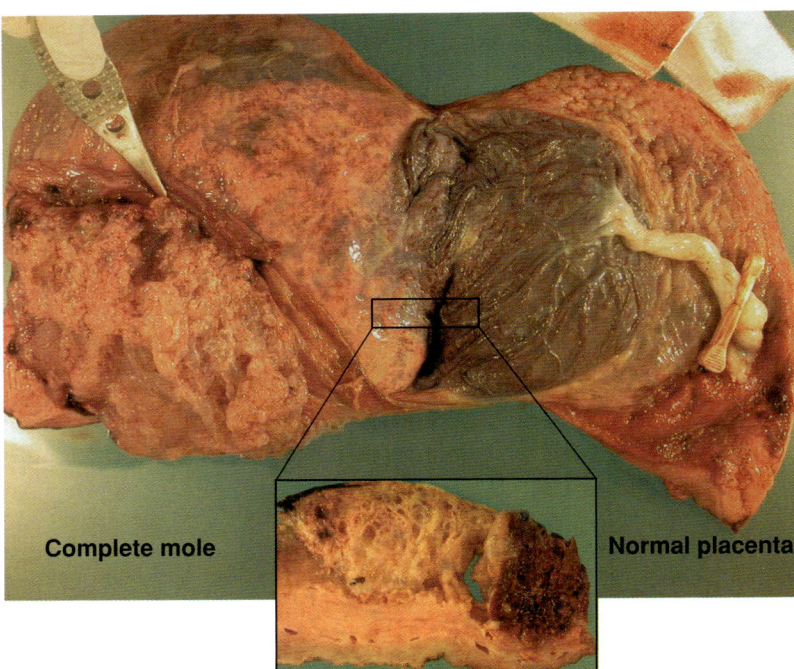

FIGURE 37-7 Photograph of placentas from a twin pregnancy with one normal twin and with a complete mole. The complete mole (*left*) shows the characteristic vesicular structure. The placenta on the right appears grossly normal. A transverse section through the border between these two is shown (*inset*). (Reproduced with permission from Drs. April Bleich and Brian Levenson.)

Histologic Classification

Invasive Mole

This common manifestation of GTN is characterized by whole chorionic villi that accompany excessive trophoblastic overgrowth and invasion (Figs. 37-8 and 37-9). These tissues penetrate deep into the myometrium, sometimes to involve the peritoneum, adjacent parametrium, or vaginal vault. Such moles are locally invasive but generally lack the pronounced tendency to develop widespread metastases typical of choriocarcinoma. Invasive moles originate almost exclusively from a complete or a partial hydatidiform mole (Sebire, 2005a).

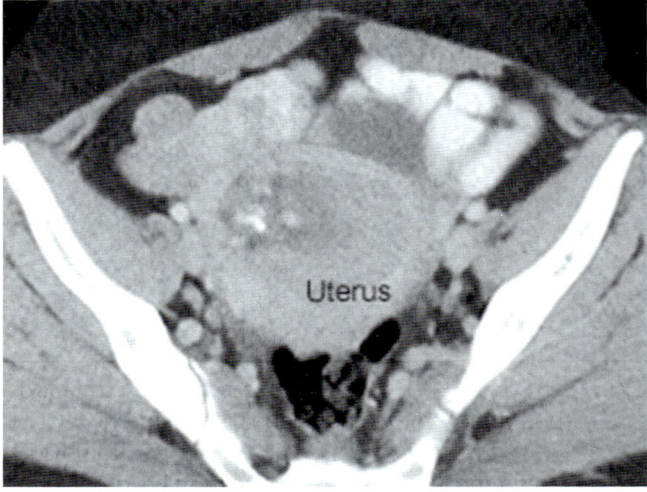

FIGURE 37-8 Computed tomography (CT) scan of gestational trophoblastic neoplasia filling and invading the uterus.

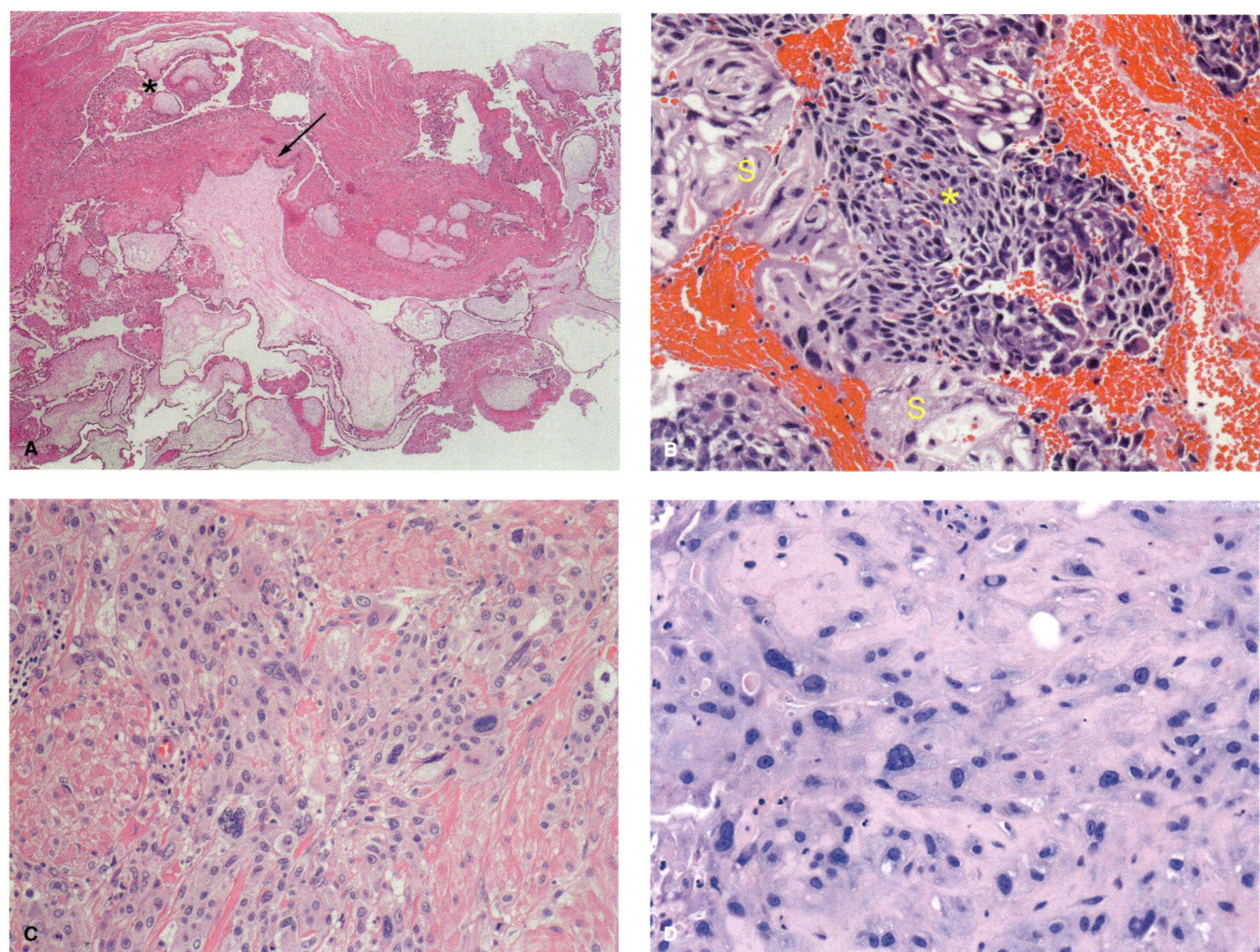

FIGURE 37-9 A. An invasive mole is a hydatidiform mole in which molar villi invade the myometrium or blood vessels. The arrow marks one enlarged villus invading the myometrium. Other invasive villi with associated trophoblast are marked by the asterisk. (Reproduced with permission from Dr. Ona Faye-Peterson.) **B.** Choriocarcinoma is a dimorphic malignant neoplasm characterized by mononucleate cytotrophoblast and intermediate trophoblast (*asterisk*), intimately admixed with multinucleate syncytiotrophoblast (*S*). Choriocarcinoma typically shows prominent hemorrhage (note blood in background) due to its extensive pseudovascular network. Central necrosis is another typical feature. **C.** Placental-site trophoblastic tumor is a trophoblastic tumor composed of neoplastic implantation site–type intermediate trophoblast. Tumor cells typically have marked nuclear atypia and relatively abundant cytoplasm, and cells spread in an infiltrative fashion. In this example, the pleomorphic tumor cells infiltrate between myometrial smooth muscle bundles (Reproduced with permission from Dr. Kelley Carrick.) **D.** Epithelioid trophoblastic tumor is composed of mononucleate or rarely multinucleate intermediate trophoblastic cells with a moderate amount of fine granular eosinophilic cytoplasm. The tumor nuclei are medium to large and show distinct nucleoli. Eosinophilic debris or hyaline-like matrix can be seen adjacent to the tumor cells (Reproduced with permission from Dr. Katja Gwin.)

Gestational Choriocarcinoma

This extremely malignant tumor contains sheets of anaplastic trophoblast and prominent hemorrhage, necrosis, and vascular invasion. However, formed villous structures are characteristically absent (see Fig. 37-9). Gestational choriocarcinoma initially invades the endometrium and myometrium but tends to develop early blood-borne systemic metastases.

Most cases develop following evacuation of a molar pregnancy, but these tumors may also follow a nonmolar pregnancy. Specifically, gestational choriocarcinoma develops in approximately 1 in 30,000 nonmolar pregnancies. One review of 100 patients with nonmolar gestational choriocarcinoma reported that 62 presented after a live birth, 6 after a live birth preceded by a molar pregnancy,

and 32 after a nonmolar abortion (Tidy, 1995). Another case series between 1964 and 1996 showed that in 89 percent of cases, the preceding pregnancy had produced an uncomplicated live birth (Rodabaugh, 1998). Hydrops, although a notable complication in the remaining fetuses in this earlier series, was not observed in a more recent cohort compiled between 1996 and 2011 (Diver, 2013). Occasionally, unanticipated choriocarcinoma is detected in an otherwise normal-appearing placenta at delivery.

More commonly, the diagnosis of choriocarcinoma is delayed for months due to subtle signs and symptoms. Most patients present with intermenstrual bleeding, and high β-hCG levels are detected (Lok, 2006). Thus, abnormal bleeding for more than 6 weeks following any pregnancy warrants evaluation with β-hCG testing to exclude a new pregnancy or GTN. Less frequently, the diagnosis is made in an asymptomatic woman by an incidental positive pregnancy test (Diver, 2013). In part because of the typical delay to diagnosis, choriocarcinomas following term pregnancies are associated with high-risk features and a higher mortality rate than GTN following nonmolar abortions. Death rates range from 10 to 15 percent (Diver, 2013; Lok, 2006; Rodabaugh, 1998; Tidy, 1995).

In contrast to this gestational choriocarcinoma, primary "nongestational" choriocarcinoma is an ovarian germ cell tumor (Chap. 36, p. 760). Although rare, ovarian choriocarcinoma has a histologic appearance identical to that of gestational choriocarcinoma. It is in part distinguished by the lack of a preceding pregnancy (Lee, 2009).

Placental-Site Trophoblastic Tumor

This tumor consists predominantly of intermediate trophoblasts at the placental site. It is a rare GTN variant with unique disease behavior. Placental-site trophoblastic tumor (PSTT) can follow any type of pregnancy but develops most commonly following a term gestation. Typically, patients have irregular bleeding months or years after the antecedent pregnancy, and the diagnosis is not entertained until endometrial sampling has been performed. PSTT tends to infiltrate only within the uterus, disseminates late in its course, and produces low β-hCG levels (van Trommel, 2013). Of interest, an elevated proportion of free β-subunit can help to discriminate it from other GTN types if the endometrial biopsy is equivocal (Cole, 2008; Harvey, 2008). In a study of 71 patients with stage I disease, the use of adjuvant chemotherapy made no significant difference in the relapse or survival rate (Zhao, 2016). For those with stage I disease but high-risk tumor features, chemotherapy can be considered. When this tumor does spread, the pattern mirrors that of gestational choriocarcinoma. Metastases often spread to the lungs, liver, or vagina (Baergen, 2006).

Hysterectomy is the primary treatment for nonmetastatic PSTT due to its relative insensitivity to chemotherapy. In particularly motivated patients, fertility-sparing procedures have mixed results (Taylor, 2013b; Zhao, 2016).

Metastatic PSTT has a much poorer prognosis than its postmolar GTN counterparts. As a result, aggressive combination chemotherapy is indicated. Regimens of etoposide, methotrexate, and dactinomycin (actinomycin D) that alternate with etoposide and cisplatin (EMA/EP) are considered the most effective (Newlands, 2000). Radiation, however, also may have a role. The overall 10-year survival is 70 percent, but patients with metastases, especially stage IV disease, have a much worse prognosis (Hassadia, 2005; Hyman, 2013; Schmid, 2009).

Epithelioid Trophoblastic Tumor

This rare trophoblastic tumor is distinct from gestational choriocarcinoma and PSTT. The preceding pregnancy event may be remote, or in some cases, a prior gestation cannot be confirmed (Palmer, 2008). Epithelioid trophoblastic tumor (ETT) develops from neoplastic transformation of chorionic-type intermediate trophoblast. Microscopically, this tumor resembles PSTT, but the cells are smaller and display less nuclear pleomorphism. Grossly, epithelioid trophoblastic tumor grows in a nodular fashion rather than the infiltrative pattern of PSTT (Shih, 1998). Hysterectomy is again the primary treatment due to presumed chemoresistance and because the diagnosis is usually confirmed in advance by endometrial biopsy. Chemotherapy options mirror that for PSTT. More than one third of patients will present with metastatic disease and demonstrable chemoresistance to multiagent therapy. This portends a poor prognosis (Davis, 2015; Frijstein, 2019).

■ Diagnosis

Most GTN cases are clinically diagnosed, using β-hCG evidence to identify persistent trophoblastic tissue. Criteria by the International Federation of Gynecology and Obstetrics (FIGO) (2002) are listed in Table 37-3. Tissue is infrequently available for pathologic diagnosis, unless a diagnosis of PSTT or ETT or nongestational tumor is being considered. As a result, most centers in the United States diagnose GTN on the basis of rising β-hCG values or a persistent plateau of β-hCG values for at least 3 weeks. Unfortunately, uniformity is lacking in the definition of a persistent plateau. Additionally, the diagnostic criteria are less stringent in the United States than in Europe. This is partly because of concern that some patients may be lost to follow-up if stricter criteria are used.

When serologic criteria for GTN are met, a new intrauterine pregnancy is excluded using β-hCG levels that are correlated with sonographic findings. This is done especially if there has been a long delay in monitoring of serial β-hCG levels or noncompliance with contraception or both.

■ Assessment

Patients with GTN undergo a thorough pretreatment assessment to determine disease extent. The initial evaluation may be limited to pelvic examination, chest radiograph, and pelvic sonography or abdominopelvic computed tomography (CT) scanning. Laboratory tests include CBC, β-hCG levels, and measure of liver, renal, and thyroid function. Although approximately 40 percent of patients will have micrometastases not

---

TABLE 37-3. FIGO Criteria for Gestational Trophoblastic Neoplasia Diagnosis

β-hCG level plateau persists in four measurements during a period of 3 weeks or longer (days 1, 7, 14, and 21)
β-hCG level rise in 3 weekly consecutive measurements or longer, over a period of 2 weeks or more (days 1, 7, and 14)
β-hCG level remains elevated for 6 months or more
Histologic diagnosis of choriocarcinoma

β-hCG = beta human chorionic gonadotropin; FIGO = International Federation of Gynecology and Obstetrics.

TABLE 37-4. FIGO Anatomic Staging

Stage I	Disease confined to the uterus
Stage II	GTN extends outside of the uterus but is limited to the genital structures (adnexa, vagina, broad ligament)
Stage III	GTN extends to the lungs, with or without known genital tract involvement
Stage IV	All other metastatic sites

FIGO = International Federation of Gynecology and Obstetrics; GTN = gestational trophoblastic neoplasia.

otherwise visible on chest radiography, chest CT is not needed because these small lesions do not affect outcome (Darby, 2009; Garner, 2004). However, pulmonary lesions identified on chest radiograph should prompt CT of the chest and magnetic resonance (MR) imaging of the brain. Fortunately, central nervous system involvement is rare in the absence of neurologic symptoms or signs (Price, 2010). Positron emission tomography (PET) may occasionally be useful to evaluate occult choriocarcinoma or relapse from previously treated GTN when conventional imaging is equivocal or fails to identify suspected metastatic disease (Dhillon, 2006; Numnum, 2005).

If no extrauterine disease is found, a second curettage or hysterectomy may be considered. β-hCG levels are then measured every 2 weeks until three consecutively lie in undetectable range. Levels are subsequently repeated monthly for 6 months. In contrast, if β-hCG levels persist after curettage or hysterectomy, patients undergo staging and chemotherapy is instituted.

■ Staging

GTN is anatomically staged based on a system adopted by FIGO (2009) and shown in Table 37-4 and Figure 37-10.

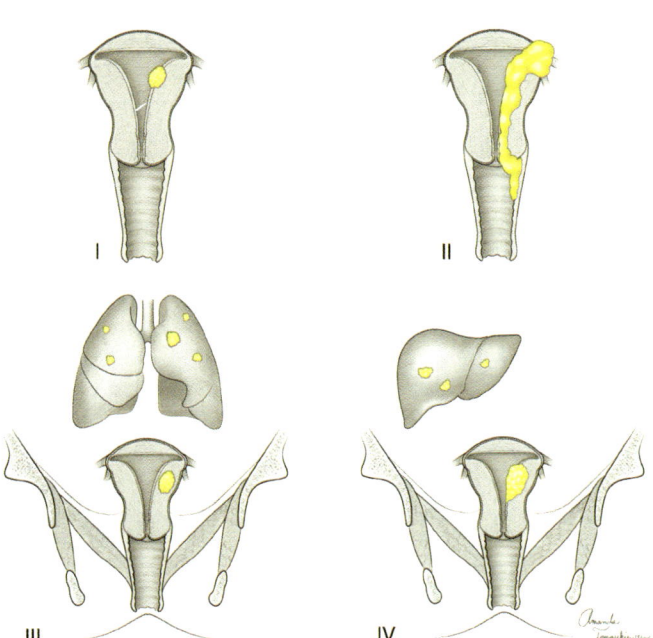

FIGURE 37-10 International Federation of Gynecology and Obstetrics (FIGO) staging of gestational trophoblastic neoplasia.

Patients at low risk for therapeutic failure are distinguished from those at high risk by using the modified prognostic scoring system of the World Health Organization (WHO) (Table 37-5). Approximately 95 percent of patients will have a WHO score of 0 to 6 and will be considered to have low-risk disease (Sita-Lumsden, 2012). The remainder will have a score of 7 or higher and be assigned to the high-risk GTN group. For the most accurate description of affected patients, the Roman numeral corresponding to FIGO stage is separated by a colon from the sum of the risk factor scores, for example, stage II:4 or stage IV:9. This description best reflects disease behavior (Ngan, 2004). Women with high-risk scores are more likely to have tumors that are resistant to single-agent chemotherapy. They are therefore treated initially with combination chemotherapy. Although patients with stage I disease infrequently have a high-risk score, those with stage IV disease invariably have a high-risk score. Women diagnosed with FIGO stage I, II, or III GTN have a survival rate approaching 100 percent (Lurain, 2010).

Nonmetastatic Disease

Invasive moles arising from complete molar gestations make up most nonmetastatic GTN cases. Approximately 12 to 16 percent of complete moles develop locally invasive disease after evacuation, compared with only 4 to 6 percent of partial moles. ETT and PSTT are other rare causes of nonmetastatic GTN. Locally invasive trophoblastic tumors may perforate the myometrium and lead to intraperitoneal bleeding (Mackenzie, 1993). Alternatively, vaginal hemorrhage can follow tumor erosion into uterine vessels, or necrotic tumor may involve the uterine wall and serve as a nidus for infection. Fortunately, the prognosis is typically excellent for all types of nonmetastatic disease despite these possible manifestations.

Metastatic Disease

Choriocarcinomas originating from complete molar gestations account for most cases of metastatic GTN. After evacuation, 3 to 4 percent of complete moles develop metastatic choriocarcinoma. This event is rare following any other type of molar or nonmolar gestation. Choriocarcinomas have a propensity for distant spread and should be suspected in any reproductive-aged woman with metastatic disease from an unknown primary (Tidy, 1995). Moreover, because of this tendency, chemotherapy has traditionally been recommended whenever choriocarcinoma is diagnosed histologically (FIGO Oncology Committee, 2002). However, more recent data suggest the FIGO guidelines may need revision. Namely, in one study of 47 women, a pathologic diagnosis of nonmetastatic gestational

TABLE 37-5. Modified WHO Prognostic Scoring System as Adapted by FIGO

Scores	0	1	2	4
Age (yr)	<40	≥40	—	—
Antecedent pregnancy	Mole	Abortion	Term	—
Interval months from index pregnancy	<4	4–6	7–12	>12
Pretreatment serum β-hCG (mIU/mL)	$<10^3$	$10^3 - <10^4$	$10^4 - <10^5$	$≥10^5$
Largest tumor size (including uterus)	<3 cm	3–4 cm	≥5 cm	—
Site of metastases	—	Spleen, kidney	GI	Liver, brain
Number of metastases	—	1–4	5–8	>8
Previous failed chemotherapy drugs	—	—	1	≥2

Low risk = WHO score of 0 to 6; high risk = WHO score of ≥ 7.
β-hCG = beta human chorionic gonadotropin; FIGO = International Federation of Gynecology and Obstetrics;
GI = gastrointestinal; WHO = World Health Organization.

choriocarcinoma was obtained by second curettage among patients with prior mole or by curettage among women with postpartum abnormal uterine bleeding, both triggered by suspicious β-hCG level elevations. These women were expectantly managed, and fewer than half ended up needing chemotherapy. Moreover, no discernable adverse effects on their prognosis were found (Braga, 2018).

Although many patients are largely asymptomatic, metastatic GTN is highly vascular and prone to severe hemorrhage either spontaneously or during biopsy. Heavy menstrual bleeding is a frequent presenting symptom. The most common sites of spread are the lungs (80 percent), vagina (30 percent), pelvis (20 percent), liver (10 percent), and brain (10 percent) (Fig. 37-11). Patients with pulmonary metastases typically have asymptomatic lesions identified on routine chest radiograph and infrequently present with cough, dyspnea, hemoptysis, pleuritic chest pain, or signs of pulmonary hypertension (Seckl, 1991). In those with early development of respiratory failure that requires intubation, the overall outcome is poor. Hepatic or cerebral involvement is encountered almost exclusively in women who have had an antecedent nonmolar pregnancy and a protracted delay in tumor diagnosis (Newlands, 2002; Savage, 2015b). These women may present with associated hemorrhagic events. Virtually all patients with hepatic or cerebral metastases have concurrent pulmonary or vaginal involvement or both. Great caution is used in attempting excision of any metastatic disease site due to the risk of profuse hemorrhage. Thus, this practice is almost uniformly avoided except in extenuating circumstances of life-threatening brainstem herniation or chemotherapy-resistant disease.

■ Treatment

Surgery

Most patients diagnosed with true postmolar GTN have persistent tumor confined to the endometrial cavity, and a second dilation and curettage may be considered to reduce the number of patients needing any further treatment (Osborne, 2016). A second evacuation followed by continued surveillance, however, is a less attractive option for poorly compliant patients than is single-agent chemotherapy (Allen, 2003; Massad, 2000). Moreover, in a randomized trial, repeat curettage did not reduce the number of chemotherapy courses required to reach β-hCG normalization and did not affect relapse rates (Hemida, 2019).

Hysterectomy may play several roles in GTN treatment. First, it may be performed to primarily treat PSTT, ETT, or other chemotherapy-resistant disease. Second, severe uncontrollable vaginal or intraabdominal bleeding may necessitate hysterectomy as an emergency procedure (Clark, 2010). Because of these more extreme indications, most women undergoing hysterectomy have elevated pretreatment risk scores, unusual pathology, and higher mortality rates (Pisal, 2002). Finally, adjuvant hysterectomy decreases the total dose of chemotherapy needed to achieve clinical remission in low-risk GTN. Patients with disease apparently confined to the uterus who do not desire future fertility should be counseled about this option (Bolze, 2018; Eysbouts, 2017). However, the risk of GTN persistence after hysterectomy remains approximately 20 to 30 percent, and these patients should be monitored postoperatively.

All patients with extrauterine disease should receive chemotherapy. Residual lung metastases may persist in 10 to 20 percent of patients achieving clinical remission of GTN after chemotherapy completion. These patients do not appear to have a greater risk of relapse compared with those having normal chest radiographs or CT scans. Thus, thoracotomy is not usually necessary unless remission cannot otherwise be achieved (Powles, 2006). In general, the optimal patient to be counseled for thoracotomy will have stage III GTN, a preoperative β-hCG level <1500 mIU/mL, and a solitary lung nodule resistant to chemotherapy (Cao, 2009; Fleming, 2008).

Chemotherapy for Low-Risk GTN

Methotrexate. Most patients with hydatidiform mole who develop GTN are at low risk of chemotherapy resistance (score 0–6) (Seckl, 2010). Single-agent methotrexate (MTX) is the most common treatment, and complete response rates range from

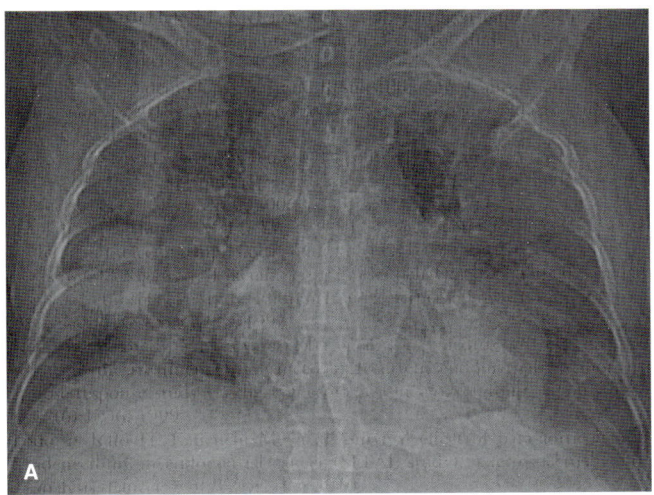

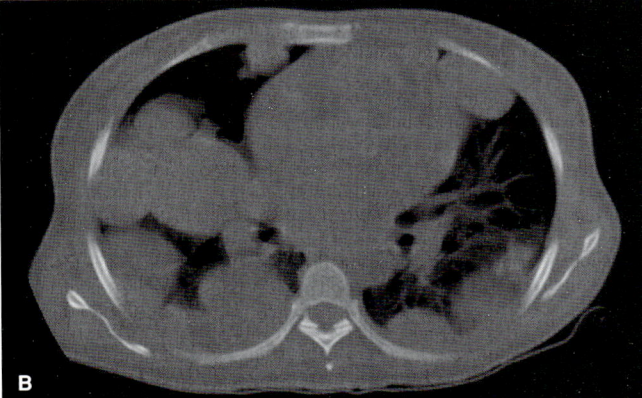

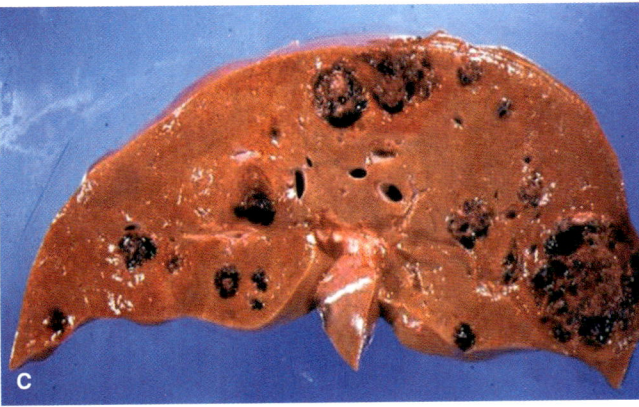

FIGURE 37-11 Common sites of gestational trophoblastic neoplasia metastasis. **A.** Chest radiography demonstrates widespread metastatic lesions. **B.** Computed tomography (CT) scan of metastatic disease to the lung. **C.** Autopsy specimen shows multiple hemorrhagic hepatic metastases. (Reproduced with permission from Dr. Michael G. Connor.)

67 to 84 percent for variations of the two most common intramuscular (IM) methotrexate regimens (Table 37-6). Although bundled as low-risk disease, the highest cure rates occur in patients with the lowest WHO scores (0–1), and rates decline proportionally as WHO scores rise (Sita-Lumsden, 2012). Thus, patients with a WHO score of 6 should at least be considered for upfront combination therapy (Taylor, 2013a). Overall, 19 to

33 percent of women develop MTX resistance and are switched to other agents, described subsequently.

With MTX, the current standard regimen is an 8-day alternating regimen of intramuscular (IM) MTX at a dose of 1 mg/kg on treatment days 1, 3, 5, and 7, and oral folinic acid, 15 mg taken orally, on days 2, 4, 6, and 8. Treatment is repeated every 2 weeks (Taylor, 2013a). Alternatively, a daily dose is given intravenously (IV) or IM for 5 days and this series is repeated every 2 weeks. MTX dosing is 0.4 mg/kg/day (National Comprehensive Cancer Network, 2018). All of these regimens are continued until β-hCG levels are undetectable, and then two or three additional weekly doses are given (Lybol, 2012).

As discussed in Chapter 27 (p. 592), MTX is a folic acid antagonist that inhibits DNA synthesis. Mild stomatitis is the most common side effect, but other serosal symptoms, especially pleurisy, develop in up to one quarter of patients treated with low-dose MTX. Pericarditis, peritonitis, and pneumonitis are infrequent (Sharma, 1999). Toxicity develops more frequently with the more intense 8-day regimens compared with weekly administration. This is despite routine folinic acid "rescue," which is provided to protect normal mucosal and serosal cells (Maesta, 2018).

Dactinomycin. Dactinomycin is less frequently used for the primary treatment of low-risk disease due to toxicity concerns, but it has superior efficacy as a single agent (Alazzam, 2016; Yarandi, 2008). In a prospective GOG trial (protocol #174) of low-risk GTN, patients were randomly assigned to biweekly "pulse" 1.25-mg dose dactinomycin or to weekly MTX, 30 mg/m². Among 215 eligible patients, a complete response was observed in 69 percent given dactinomycin and in 53 percent given MTX. However, advocates of MTX have speculated that the unexpectedly low efficacy of MTX observed in this study may be due to subtherapeutic dosing. Moreover, those randomized to dactinomycin were twice as likely to develop alopecia and were the only patients to develop grade 4 toxicity (Chap. 27, p. 594) (Osborne, 2008). As yet, no trials have directly compared pulse dactinomycin and the widely used 8-day MTX regimen. Since survival rates are so high, MTX is usually tried first because most clinicians consider it to be the least toxic (Lawrie, 2016).

Patients who do not respond to an initial single-agent chemotherapeutic regimen fail to have persistently dropping β-hCG levels. These women should have their score recalculated using the modified WHO prognostic scoring system. Most women will still be considered low-risk and may be switched to a single-agent second-line therapy. MTX-resistant GTN often responds to pulse dactinomycin, with a success rate of 71 to 74 percent (Li, 2018; Covens, 2006). Patients initially treated with pulse dactinomycin who develop resistant GTN may still be successfully treated with the 5-day course of dactinomycin (Kohorn, 2002).

Chemotherapy for High-Risk GTN

Approximately 5 percent of GTN patients present with high-risk disease and usually have numerous metastases months or years after the causative pregnancy. Such patients are likely to develop drug resistance to single-agent chemotherapy (Seckl, 2010). Etoposide, methotrexate, and dactinomycin (actinomycin D)

TABLE 37-6. Intramuscular Methotrexate Regimens for Treatment of Low-Risk GTN

Frequency	Dose	Population Studied	CR Rate (%)	Study
Weekly	30–50 mg/m^2	Nonmetastatic GTN	74–81	Homesley, 1988, 1990
	50 mg/m^2	Low-risk GTN	72	Mangili, 2018
Days 1, 3, 5, 7	50 mg/d	Low-risk GTN	67–72	Kang, 2010; Khan, 2003; McNeish, 2002
	1 mg/kg	Low-risk GTN	78–84	Maesta, 2018; Mangili, 2018

CR = clinical remission (calculated for first-line treatment without needing alternative chemotherapy); GTN = gestational trophoblastic neoplasia.

alternating with cyclophosphamide and vincristine (Oncovin) (EMA/CO) chemotherapy is a well-tolerated and highly effective regimen for high-risk GTN. It is considered the preferred treatment for most high-risk disease. Bower and associates (1997) reported a 78-percent complete remission rate in 272 consecutive women. Similarly, other investigators have observed a 71- to 78-percent complete response rate with the EMA/CO regimen (Escobar, 2003; Lu, 2008). Response rates are comparable whether patients are treated primarily or after failure of single-agent MTX and/or dactinomycin.

Patients with high-risk disease have an overall survival rate of 86 to 92 percent, although approximately one quarter become refractory to or relapse from EMA/CO (Bower, 1997; Escobar, 2003; Lu, 2008; Lurain, 2010). Secondary treatment usually involves platinum-based chemotherapy combined with possible surgical excision of resistant disease (Alazzam, 2016). Newlands and associates (2000) reported an 88-percent survival rate among 34 patients by replacing the cyclophosphamide and vincristine component with etoposide and cisplatin (EMA/EP). EMA/EP is an effective option in patients resistant to EMA/CO, but paclitaxel (Taxol) plus cisplatin alternating with paclitaxel plus etoposide (TP/TE) has comparable efficacy and appears less toxic (Patel, 2010; Wang, 2008). Bleomycin, etoposide, and cisplatin (BEP) is another potentially effective regimen (Alazzam, 2016; Essel, 2017; Lurain, 2005). Pembrolizumab, described in Chapter 27 (p. 601), also has achieved responses (Ghorani, 2017).

High-risk patients with a large disease burden are at risk for early death with standard EMA/CO due to tumor lysis–related hemorrhage and clinical deterioration. In these selected circumstances, "induction low-dose etoposide-cisplatin" appears to reduce the mortality risk tenfold (Alifrangis, 2013).

Brain Metastases

Patients with cerebral metastases may present with seizures, headaches, or hemiparesis (Newlands, 2002). Occasionally, they are moribund on arrival after not recognizing the significance of their symptoms or following an extended delay in diagnosis. In such extenuating circumstances, emergency craniotomy may help stabilize the patient and is followed by critical care support throughout the active phase of treatment (Savage, 2015b). In experienced centers, virtually all GTN-related deaths occur in stage IV patients with WHO risk scores of 12 or more (Bolze, 2016).

Fortunately, the cure rate for those with brain metastases is high if neurologic deterioration does not occur within the first weeks after diagnosis. The sequence of aggressive multimodality therapy is controversial but may include chemotherapy, surgery, and radiation. Savage and coworkers (2015b) reported an 85-percent survival rate among 27 patients treated from 1991 to 2013 by EMA/CO or EMA/EP with an enhanced intravenous dose (1 g/m^2) of MTX combined with intrathecal MTX until β-hCG levels were undetectable. Whole-brain radiation therapy also can be an efficacious adjunct to combination chemotherapy and surgery, but it can induce permanent intellectual impairment (Cagayan, 2006; Schechter, 1998).

■ Posttreatment

Surveillance

Monitoring of patients with low-risk GTN consists of weekly β-hCG measurements until the level is undetectable for 3 consecutive weeks. This is followed by monthly titers until the level is undetectable for 12 months. Patients with high-risk disease are followed for 24 months due to the greater risk of late relapse. Patients are encouraged to use effective contraception, as outlined on page 779, during the entire surveillance period.

Treatment Sequelae

Despite the favorable prognosis, patients and their partners carry pregnancy concerns for a protracted time (Wenzel, 1992). Sexual dysfunction is an underreported complication (Cagayan, 2008). These and other potential sequelae highlight the importance of a multidisciplinary approach to management (Ferreira, 2009).

Patients may expect a normal reproductive outcome after achieving remission from GTD. Data show no evidence of greater subsequent adverse maternal outcomes but inconclusive evidence of pregnancy loss or preterm birth (Cioffi, 2018; Joneborg, 2014). Women having a pregnancy affected by a histologically confirmed complete or partial mole may be counseled that the risk of a repeat mole in a subsequent pregnancy approximates 1 percent (Garrett, 2008; Joneborg, 2014). Most will be of the same type of mole as the preceding pregnancy (Sebire, 2003). Women who become pregnant within 12 months postchemotherapy for GTN can be reassured of a likely favorable outcome, although the safest option is still to delay pregnancy for the full year (Williams, 2014). Pregnancy after combination EMA/CO chemotherapy for GTN also has a high probability of success and favorable outcome (Lok, 2003). All major cytotoxic treatments except MTX increase the risk of early menopause (Cioffi, 2018; Savage, 2015a).

In some cases, secondary tumors can develop as a result of cancer treatment. Etoposide-based combination chemotherapy has been associated with an increased risk of leukemia, colon cancer, melanoma, and breast cancer up to 25 years after treatment for GTN. An overall 50-percent excess risk was observed (Rustin, 1996). Etoposide is therefore reserved to treat patients who are likely to be resistant to single-agent chemotherapy and, in particular, those with high-risk metastatic disease.

Quiescent Gestational Trophoblastic Disease

Patients with persistent mild elevations (usually ≤50 mIU/mL) of true β-hCG may have a dormant premalignant condition if no tumor is identified by physical examination or imaging studies (Khanlian, 2003). In this instance, phantom β-hCG, described next, should be conclusively excluded as a possibility. The low β-hCG titers may persist for months or years before disappearing. Chemotherapy and surgery usually have no effect. Hormonal contraception may be helpful in lowering titers to an undetectable level, but patients are closely monitored since metastatic GTN may eventually develop (Khanlian, 2003; Kohorn, 2002; Palmieri, 2007).

■ Phantom β-hCG

Occasionally, persistent mild elevations of serum β-hCG are detected and lead physicians to erroneously treat patients with cytotoxic chemotherapy or hysterectomy or both, when in reality no true β-hCG molecule or trophoblastic disease is present (Cole, 1998; Rotmensch, 2000). This "phantom" β-hCG reading results from serum heterophilic antibodies that interfere with the β-hCG immunoassay and cause a false-positive result.

Several steps can clarify the diagnosis. First, a urine pregnancy test can be performed. With phantom β-hCG, the heterophilic antibodies are not filtered or renally excreted. Thus, these test-altering antibodies will be absent from the urine, and urine testing will show true negative results for β-hCG. Importantly, to conclusively exclude trophoblastic disease by this method, the index serum β-hCG level must be significantly higher than the detection threshold of the urine test. Second, performing serial dilutions of the serum sample leads to a proportional decline in the β-hCG level if β-hCG is truly present. However, phantom β-hCG measurements will be unchanged by dilution. In addition, if phantom β-hCG is suspected, some specialized laboratories may be able to block the heterophilic antibodies. Last, heterophilic antibodies will cause interference with one assay, but they may bind poorly to another assay's antibodies. Thus, switching β-hCG assay kits to one by a different manufacturer may accurately demonstrate the absence of true β-hCG (Cole, 1998; Olsen, 2001; Rotmensch, 2000).

REFERENCES

Alazzam M, Tidy J, Osborne R, et al: Chemotherapy for resistant or recurrent gestational trophoblastic neoplasia. Cochrane Database Syst Rev 1:CD008891, 2016

Alifrangis C, Agarwal R, Short D, et al: EMA/CO for high-risk gestational trophoblastic neoplasia: good outcomes with induction low-dose etoposide-cisplatin and genetic analysis. J Clin Oncol 31(2):280, 2013

Allen JE, King MR, Farrar DF, et al: Postmolar surveillance at a trophoblastic disease center that serves indigent women. Am J Obstet Gynecol 188:1151, 2003

Azuma C, Saji F, Tokugawa Y, et al: Application of gene amplification by polymerase chain reaction to genetic analysis of molar mitochondrial DNA: the detection of anuclear empty ovum as the cause of complete mole. Gynecol Oncol 40:29, 1991

Baergen RN, Rutgers JL, Young RH, et al: Placental site trophoblastic tumor: a study of 55 cases and review of the literature emphasizing factors of prognostic significance. Gynecol Oncol 100:511, 2006

Benson CB, Genest DR, Bernstein MR, et al: Sonographic appearance of first trimester complete hydatidiform moles. Ultrasound Obstet Gynecol 16:188, 2000

Berkowitz RS, Bernstein MR, Harlow BL, et al: Case-control study of risk factors for partial molar pregnancy. Am J Obstet Gynecol 173:788, 1995

Berkowitz RS, Cramer DW, Bernstein MR, et al: Risk factors for complete molar pregnancy from a case-control study. Am J Obstet Gynecol 152:1016, 1985

Berkowitz RS, Im SS, Bernstein MR, et al: Gestational trophoblastic disease: subsequent pregnancy outcome, including repeat molar pregnancy. J Reprod Med 43:81, 1998

Bolze PA, Mathe M, Hajri T, et al: First-line hysterectomy for women with low-risk non-metastatic gestational trophoblastic neoplasia no longer wishing to conceive. Gynecol Oncol 150(2):282, 2018

Bolze PA, Riedl C, Massardier J, et al: Mortality rate of gestational trophoblastic neoplasia with a FIGO score of ≥13. Am J Obstet Gynecol 214(3):390.e1, 2016

Bower M, Newlands ES, Holden L, et al: EMA/CO for high-risk gestational trophoblastic tumors: results from a cohort of 272 patients. J Clin Oncol 15:2636, 1997

Braga A, Campos V, Filho JR, et al: Is chemotherapy always necessary for patients with nonmetastatic gestational trophoblastic neoplasia with histopathological diagnosis of choriocarcinoma? Gynecol Oncol 148(2):239, 2018

Braga A, Maestá I, Matos M, et al: Gestational trophoblastic neoplasia after spontaneous human chorionic gonadotropin normalization following molar pregnancy evacuation. Gynecol Oncol 139(2):283, 2015

Braga A, Maestá I, Short D, et al: Hormonal contraceptive use before hCG remission does not increase the risk of gestational trophoblastic neoplasia following complete hydatidiform mole: a historical database review. BJOG 123(8):1330, 2016

Burton JL, Lidbury EA, Gillespie AM, et al: Overdiagnosis of hydatidiform mole in early tubal ectopic pregnancy. Histopathology 38:409, 2001

Cagayan MS: Sexual dysfunction as a complication of treatment of gestational trophoblastic neoplasia. J Reprod Med 53:595, 2008

Cagayan MS, Lu-Lasala LR: Management of gestational trophoblastic neoplasia with metastasis to the central nervous system: a 12-year review at the Phillippe General Hospital. J Reprod Med 51:785, 2006

Cao Y, Xiang Y, Feng F, et al: Surgical resection in the management of pulmonary metastatic disease of gestational trophoblastic neoplasia. Int J Gynecol Cancer 19:798, 2009

Castrillon DH, Sun D, Weremowicz S, et al: Discrimination of complete hydatidiform mole from its mimics by immunohistochemistry of the paternally imprinted gene product p57KIP2. Am J Surg Pathol 25:1225, 2001

Cheung AN, Khoo US, Lai CY, et al: Metastatic trophoblastic disease after an initial diagnosis of partial hydatidiform mole: genotyping and chromosome in situ hybridization analysis. Cancer 100:1411, 2004

Chew SH, Perlman EJ, Williams R, et al: Morphology and DNA content analysis in the evaluation of first trimester placentas for partial hydatidiform mole (PHM). Hum Pathol 31:914, 2000

Chong CY, Koh CF: Hydatidiform mole in Kandang Kerbau Hospital: a 5-year review. Singapore Med J 40:265, 1999

Cioffi R, Bergamini A, Gadducci A, et al: Reproductive outcomes after gestational trophoblastic neoplasia. A comparison between single-agent and multiagent chemotherapy: retrospective analysis from the MITO-9 group. Int J Gynecol Cancer 28(2):332, 2018

Clark RM, Nevadunsky NS, Ghosh S, et al: The evolving role of hysterectomy in gestational trophoblastic neoplasia at the New England Trophoblastic Disease Center. J Reprod Med 5:194, 2010

Cole LA: Phantom hCG and phantom choriocarcinoma. Gynecol Oncol 71:325, 1998

Cole LA, Khanlian SA, Muller CY: Blood test for placental site trophoblastic tumor and nontrophoblastic malignancy for evaluating patients with low positive human chorionic gonadotropin results. J Reprod Med 53:457, 2008

Costa HL, Doyle P: Influence of oral contraceptives in the development of post-molar trophoblastic neoplasia—a systematic review. Gynecol Oncol 100:579, 2006

Covens A, Filiaci VL, Burger RA, et al: Phase II trial of pulse dactinomycin as salvage therapy for failed low-risk gestational trophoblastic neoplasia: a Gynecologic Oncology Group study. Cancer 107(6):1280, 2006

Dantas PRS, Maestá I, Filho JR, et al: Does hormonal contraception during molar pregnancy follow-up influence the risk and clinical aggressiveness of gestational trophoblastic neoplasia after controlling for risk factors? Gynecol Oncol 47(2):364, 2017

Darby S, Jolley I, Pennington S: Does chest CT matter in the staging of GTN? Gynecol Oncol 112:155, 2009

Davis MR, Howitt BE, Quade BJ, et al: Epithelioid trophoblastic tumor: a single institution case series at the New England Trophoblastic Disease Center. Gynecol Oncol 137(3):456, 2015

Dhillon T, Palmieri C, Sebire NJ, et al: Value of whole body 18FDG-PET to identify the active site of gestational trophoblastic neoplasia. J Reprod Med 51:979, 2006

Diver E, May T, Vargas R, et al: Changes in clinical presentation of post-term choriocarcinoma at the New England Trophoblastic Disease Center in recent years. Gynecol Oncol 130(3):483, 2013

Drake RD, Rao GG, McIntire DD, et al: Gestational trophoblastic disease among Hispanic women: a 21-year hospital-based study. Gynecol Oncol 103(1):81, 2006

Elias KM, Goldstein DP, Berkowitz RS: Complete hydatidiform mole in women older than age 50. J Reprod Med 55:208, 2010

Escobar PF, Lurain JR, Singh DK, et al: Treatment of high-risk gestational trophoblastic neoplasia with etoposide, methotrexate, actinomycin D, cyclophosphamide, and vincristine chemotherapy. Gynecol Oncol 91:552, 2003

Essel KG, Bruegl A, Gershenson DM, et al: Salvage chemotherapy for gestational trophoblastic neoplasia: utility or futility. Gynecol Oncol 146(1):74, 2017

Eysbouts YK, Bulten J, Ottevanger PB, et al: Trends in incidence for gestational trophoblastic disease over the last 20 years in a population-based study. Gynecol Oncol 140(1):70, 2016

Eysbouts YK, Massuger LF, IntHout J, et al: The added value of hysterectomy in the management of gestational trophoblastic neoplasia. Gynecol Oncol 145(3):536, 2017

Fallahian M: Familial gestational trophoblastic disease. Placenta 24:797, 2003

Fan JB, Surti U, Taillon-Miller P, et al: Paternal origins of complete hydatidiform moles proven by whole genome single-nucleotide polymorphism haplotyping. Genomics 79:58, 2002

Ferreira EG, Maesta I, Michelin OC, et al: Assessment of quality of life and psychologic aspects in patients with gestational trophoblastic disease. J Reprod Med 54:239, 2009

FIGO Committee on Gynecologic Oncology: Current FIGO staging for cancer of the vagina, fallopian tube, ovary, and gestational trophoblastic neoplasia. Int J Gynaecol Obstet 105:3, 2009

FIGO Oncology Committee: FIGO staging for gestational trophoblastic neoplasia 2000. Int J Gynaecol Obstet 77:285, 2002

Fleming EL, Garrett L, Growdon WB, et al: The changing role of thoracotomy in gestational trophoblastic neoplasia at the New England Trophoblastic Disease Center. J Reprod Med 53:493, 2008

Frijstein MM, Lok CA, van Trommel NE, et al: Management and prognostic factors of epithelioid trophoblastic tumors: results from the International Society for the Study of Trophoblastic Diseases database. Gynecol Oncol 152(2):361, 2019

Garner EI, Garrett A, Goldstein DP, et al: Significance of chest computed tomography findings in the evaluation and treatment of persistent gestational trophoblastic neoplasia. J Reprod Med 49:411, 2004

Garrett LA, Garner EI, Feltmate CM, et al: Subsequent pregnancy outcomes in patients with molar pregnancy and persistent gestational trophoblastic neoplasia. J Reprod Med 53(7):481, 2008

Ghorani E, Kaur B, Fisher RA, et al: Pembrolizumab is effective for drug-resistant gestational trophoblastic neoplasia. Lancet 390(10110):2343, 2017

Gillespie AM, Lidbury EA, Tidy JA, et al: The clinical presentation, treatment, and outcome of patients diagnosed with possible ectopic molar gestation. Int J Gynecol Cancer 14:366, 2004

Gockley AA, Melamed A, Joseph NT, et al: The effect of adolescence and advanced maternal age on the incidence of complete and partial molar pregnancy. Gynecol Oncol 140(3):470, 2016

Harvey RA, Pursglove HD, Schmid P, et al: Human chorionic gonadotropin free beta-subunit measurement as a marker of placental site trophoblastic tumors. J Reprod Med 53:643, 2008

Hassadia A, Gillespie A, Tidy J, et al: Placental site trophoblastic tumour: clinical features and management. Gynecol Oncol 99:603, 2005

Hemida R, Vos EL, El-Deek B, et al: Second uterine curettage and the number of chemotherapy courses in postmolar gestational trophoblastic neoplasia: a randomized controlled trial. Obstet Gynecol 133:1024, 2019

Homesley HD, Blessing JA, Rettenmaier M, et al: Weekly intramuscular methotrexate for nonmetastatic gestational trophoblastic disease. Obstet Gynecol 72:413, 1988

Homesley HD, Blessing JA, Schlaerth J, et al: Rapid escalation of weekly intramuscular methotrexate for nonmetastatic gestational trophoblastic disease: a Gynecologic Oncology Group study. Gynecol Oncol 39:305, 1990

Hui P, Baergen R, Cheung AN, et al: Gestational trophoblastic neoplasia. In Kurman RJ, Carcangiu LM, Herrington CS, et al (eds): WHO Classification of Tumours of Female Reproductive Organs. Lyon, International Agency for Research on Cancer, 2014a, p 155

Hui P, Baergen R, Cheung AN, et al: Molar pregnancies. In Kurman RJ, Carcangiu LM, Herrington CS, et al (eds): WHO Classification of Tumours of Female Reproductive Organs. Lyon, International Agency for Research on Cancer, 2014b, p 163

Hyman DM, Bakios L, Gualtiere G, et al: Placental site trophoblastic tumor: analysis of presentation, treatment, and outcome. Gynecol Oncol 129(1):58, 2013

Jauniaux E: Partial moles: from postnatal to prenatal diagnosis. Placenta 20:379, 1999

Johns J, Greenwold N, Buckley S, et al: A prospective study of ultrasound screening for molar pregnancies in missed miscarriages. Ultrasound Obstet Gynecol 25:493, 2005

Joneborg U, Eloranta S, Johansson AL, et al: Hydatidiform mole and subsequent pregnancy outcome: a population-based cohort study. Am J Obstet Gynecol 211(6):681.e1, 2014

Kajii T, Ohama K: Androgenetic origin of hydatidiform mole. Nature 268:633, 1977

Kang WD, Choi HS, Kim SM: Weekly methotrexate (50mg/m2) without dose escalation as a primary regimen for low-risk gestational trophoblastic neoplasia. Gynecol Oncol 117(3):477, 2010

Khan F, Everard J, Ahmed S, et al: Low-risk persistent gestational trophoblastic disease treated with low-dose methotrexate: efficacy, acute and long-term effects. Br J Cancer 89:2197, 2003

Khanlian SA, Smith HO, Cole LA: Persistent low levels of human chorionic gonadotropin: a premalignant gestational trophoblastic disease. Am J Obstet Gynecol 188:1254, 2003

Kim SJ, Lee C, Kwon SY, et al: Studying changes in the incidence, diagnosis and management of GTD: the South Korean model. J Reprod Med 49:643, 2004

Kohorn EI: Persistent low-level "real" human chorionic gonadotropin: a clinical challenge and a therapeutic dilemma. Gynecol Oncol 85:315, 2002

La Vecchia C, Parazzini F, Decarli A, et al: Age of parents and risk of gestational trophoblastic disease. J Natl Cancer Inst 73:639, 1984

Lavie I, Rao GG, Castrillon DH, et al: Duration of human chorionic gonadotropin surveillance for partial hydatidiform moles. Am J Obstet Gynecol 192:1362, 2005

Lawler SD, Fisher RA: Genetic studies in hydatidiform mole with clinical correlations. Placenta 8:77, 1987

Lawler SD, Fisher RA, Dent J: A prospective genetic study of complete and partial hydatidiform moles. Am J Obstet Gynecol 164:1270, 1991

Lawrie TA, Alazzam M, Tidy J, et al: First-line chemotherapy in low-risk gestational trophoblastic neoplasia. Cochrane Database Syst Rev 6:CD007102, 2016

Lazarus E, Hulka C, Siewert B, et al: Sonographic appearance of early complete molar pregnancies. J Ultrasound Med 18:589, 1999

Lee KH, Lee IH, Kim BG, et al: Clinicopathologic characteristics of malignant germ cell tumors in the ovaries of Korean women: a Korean Gynecologic Oncology Group Study. Int J Gynecol Cancer 19:84, 2009

Li L, Wan X, Feng F, et al: Pulse actinomycin D as first-line treatment of low-risk post-molar non-choriocarcinoma gestational trophoblastic neoplasia. BMC Cancer 18(1):585, 2018

Limpongsanurak S: Prophylactic actinomycin D for high-risk complete hydatidiform mole. J Reprod Med 46:110, 2001

Lin LH, Maestá I, Braga A, et al: Multiple pregnancies with complete mole and coexisting normal fetus in North and South America: a retrospective multicenter cohort and literature review. Gynecol Oncol 145(1):88, 2017

Lindholm H, Flam F: The diagnosis of molar pregnancy by sonography and gross morphology. Acta Obstet Gynecol Scand 78:6, 1999

Lok CA, Ansink AC, Grootfaam D, et al: Treatment and prognosis of post term choriocarcinoma in The Netherlands. Gynecol Oncol 103:698, 2006

Lok CA, van der Houwen C, ten Kate-Booji MJ, et al: Pregnancy after EMA/CO for gestational trophoblastic disease: a report from The Netherlands. BJOG 110:560, 2003

Loukovaara M, Pukkala E, Lehtovirta P, et al: Epidemiology of hydatidiform mole in Finland, 1975 to 2001. Eur J Gynaecol Oncol 26:207, 2005

Lu WG, Ye F, Shen YM, et al: EMA-CO chemotherapy for high-risk gestational trophoblastic neoplasia: a clinical analysis of 54 patients. Int J Gynecol Cancer 18:357, 2008

Lurain JR, Nejad B: Secondary chemotherapy for high-risk gestational trophoblastic neoplasia. Gynecol Oncol 97:618, 2005

Lurain JR, Singh DK, Schink JC: Management of metastatic high-risk gestational trophoblastic neoplasia: FIGO stage II-IV: risk factor score >or = 7. J Reprod Med 55:199, 2010

Lybol C, Sweep FC, Harvey R, et al: Relapse rates after two versus three consolidation courses of methotrexate in the treatment of low-risk gestational trophoblastic neoplasia. Gynecol Oncol 125(3):576, 2012

Lybol C, Thomas CM, Bulten J, et al: Increase in the incidence of gestational trophoblastic disease in The Netherlands. Gynecol Oncol 121(2):334, 2011

Mackenzie F, Mathers A, Kennedy J: Invasive hydatidiform mole presenting as an acute primary haemoperitoneum. BJOG 100:953, 1993

Maestá I, Nitecki R, Horowitz NS, et al: Effectiveness and toxicity of first-line methotrexate chemotherapy in low-risk postmolar gestational trophoblastic neoplasia: The New England Trophoblastic Disease Center experience. Gynecol Oncol 148(1):161, 2018

Mangili G, Cioffi R, Danese S, et al: Does methotrexate (MTX) dosing in a 8-day MTX/FA regimen for the treatment of low-risk gestational trophoblastic neoplasia affect outcomes? The MITO-9 study. Gynecol Oncol 151(3):449, 2018

Marcorelles P, Audrezet MP, Le Bris MJ, et al: Diagnosis and outcome of complete hydatidiform mole coexisting with a live twin fetus. Eur J Obstet Gynecol Reprod Biol 118:21, 2005

Massad LS, Abu-Rustum NR, Lee SS, et al: Poor compliance with postmolar surveillance and treatment protocols by indigent women. Obstet Gynecol 96:940, 2000

Matsui H, Iitsuka Y, Yamazawa K, et al: Changes in the incidence of molar pregnancies: a population-based study in Chiba Prefecture and Japan between 1974 and 2000. Hum Reprod 18:172, 2003

Matsui H, Sekiya S, Hando T, et al: Hydatidiform mole coexistent with a twin live fetus: a national collaborative study in Japan. Hum Reprod 15:608, 2000

McNeish IA, Strickland S, Holden L, et al: Low-risk persistent gestational trophoblastic disease: outcome after initial treatment with low-dose methotrexate and folinic acid from 1992 to 2000. J Clin Oncol 20:1838, 2002

Merchant SH, Amin MB, Viswanatha DS, et al: p57KIP2 immunohistochemistry in early molar pregnancies: emphasis on its complementary role in the differential diagnosis of hydropic abortuses. Hum Pathol 36:180, 2005

Mungan T, Kuscu E, Dabakoglu T, et al: Hydatidiform mole: clinical analysis of 310 patients. Int J Gynaecol Obstet 52:233, 1996

National Comprehensive Cancer Network: Gestational trophoblastic neoplasia, version 1.2019. Plymouth Meeting, National Comprehensive Cancer Network, 2018

Newlands ES, Holden L, Seckl MJ, et al: Management of brain metastases in patients with high-risk gestational trophoblastic tumors. J Reprod Med 47:465, 2002

Newlands ES, Mulholland PJ, Holden L, et al: Etoposide and cisplatin/etoposide, methotrexate, and actinomycin D (EMA) chemotherapy for patients with high-risk gestational trophoblastic tumors refractory to EMA/cyclophosphamide and vincristine chemotherapy and patients presenting with metastatic placental site trophoblastic tumors. J Clin Oncol 18:854, 2000

Ngan HY: The practicability of FIGO 2000 staging for gestational trophoblastic neoplasia. Int J Gynecol Cancer 14:202, 2004

Numnum TM, Leath CA III, Straughn JM Jr, et al: Occult choriocarcinoma discovered by positron emission tomography/computed tomography imaging following a successful pregnancy. Gynecol Oncol 97:713, 2005

Olsen TG, Hubert PR, Nycum LR: Falsely elevated human chorionic gonadotropin leading to unnecessary therapy. Obstet Gynecol 98:843, 2001

Osborne R, Filiaci V, Schink J, et al: A randomized phase III trial comparing weekly parenteral methotrexate and "pulsed" dactinomycin as primary management for low-risk gestational trophoblastic neoplasia: a Gynecologic Oncology Group study. Gynecol Oncol 108:S2, 2008

Osborne RJ, Filiaci VL, Schink JC, et al: Second curettage for low-risk nonmetastatic gestational trophoblastic neoplasia. Obstet Gynecol 128(3):5352016, 2016

Padrón L, Rezende Filho J, Amim Junior J, et al: Manual compared with electric vacuum aspiration for treatment of molar pregnancy. Obstet Gynecol 131(4):652, 2018

Palmer JE, Macdonald M, Wells M, et al: Epithelioid trophoblastic tumor: a review of the literature. J Reprod Med 53:465, 2008

Palmer JR, Driscoll SG, Rosenberg L, et al: Oral contraceptive use and risk of gestational trophoblastic tumors. J Natl Cancer Inst 91:635, 1999

Palmieri C, Dhillon T, Fisher RA, et al: Management and outcome of healthy women with a persistently elevated beta-hCG. Gynecol Oncol 106:35, 2007

Papadopoulos AJ, Foskett M, Seckl MJ, et al: Twenty-five years' clinical experience with placental site trophoblastic tumors. J Reprod Med 47:460, 2002

Paradinas FJ, Fisher RA, Browne P, et al: Diploid hydatidiform moles with fetal red blood cells in molar villi: 1. Pathology, incidence, and prognosis. J Pathol 181:183, 1997

Parazzini F, Cipriani S, Mangili G, et al: Oral contraceptives and risk of gestational trophoblastic disease. Contraception 65:425, 2002

Parazzini F, La Vecchia C, Mangili G, et al: Dietary factors and risk of trophoblastic disease. Am J Obstet Gynecol 158:93, 1988

Parazzini F, La Vecchia C, Pampallona S: Parental age and risk of complete and partial hydatidiform mole. BJOG 93:582, 1986

Parazzini F, Mangili G, La Vecchia C, et al: Risk factors for gestational trophoblastic disease: a separate analysis of complete and partial hydatidiform moles. Obstet Gynecol 78:1039, 1991

Patel SM, Desai A: Management of drug resistant gestational trophoblastic neoplasia. J Reprod Med 55:296, 2010

Pisal N, North C, Tidy J, et al: Role of hysterectomy in management of gestational trophoblastic disease. Gynecol Oncol 87:190, 2002

Powles T, Savage P, Short D, et al: Residual lung lesions after completion of chemotherapy for gestational trophoblastic neoplasia: should we operate? Br J Cancer 94:51, 2006

Price JM, Hancock BW, Tidy J, et al: Screening for central nervous system disease in metastatic gestational trophoblastic neoplasia. J Reprod Med 55:301, 2010

Rodabaugh KJ, Bernstein MR, Goldstein DP, et al: Natural history of postterm choriocarcinoma. J Reprod Med 43:75, 1998

Ronnett BM, DeScipio C, Murphy KM: Hydatidiform moles: ancillary techniques to refine diagnosis. Int J Gynecol Pathol 30(2):101, 2011

Rotmensch S, Cole LA: False diagnosis and needless therapy of presumed malignant disease in women with false-positive human chorionic gonadotropin concentrations. Lancet 355:712, 2000

Rustin GJ, Newlands ES, Lutz JM, et al: Combination but not single-agent methotrexate chemotherapy for gestational trophoblastic tumors increases the incidence of second tumors. J Clin Oncol 14:2769, 1996

Savage P, Cooke R, O'Nions J, et al: Effects of single-agent and combination chemotherapy for gestational trophoblastic tumors on risks of second malignancy and early menopause. J Clin Oncol 33(5):472, 2015a

Savage P, Kelpanides I, Tuthill M, et al: Brain metastases in gestational trophoblast neoplasia: an update on incidence, management and outcome. Gynecol Oncol 137(1):73, 2015b

Schechter NR, Mychalczak B, Jones W, et al: Prognosis of patients treated with whole-brain radiation therapy for metastatic gestational trophoblastic disease. Gynecol Oncol 68:183, 1998

Schmid P, Nagai Y, Agarwal R, et al: Prognostic markers and long-term outcome of placental-site trophoblastic tumors: a retrospective observational study. Lancet 374:48, 2009

Sebire NJ, Fisher RA, Foskett M, et al: Risk of recurrent hydatidiform mole and subsequent pregnancy outcome following complete or partial hydatidiform molar pregnancy. BJOG 110:22, 2003

Sebire NJ, Foskett M, Fisher RA, et al: Persistent gestational trophoblastic disease is rarely, if ever, derived from nonmolar first-trimester miscarriage. Med Hypoth 64:689, 2005a

Sebire NJ, Foskett M, Short D, et al: Shortened duration of human chorionic gonadotrophin surveillance following complete or partial hydatidiform mole: evidence for revised protocol of a UK regional trophoblastic disease unit. BJOG 114:760, 2007

Sebire NJ, Lindsay I, Fisher RA, et al: Overdiagnosis of complete and partial hydatidiform mole in tubal ectopic pregnancies. Int J Gynecol Pathol 24:260, 2005b

Sebire NJ, Rees H, Paradinas F, et al: The diagnostic implications of routine ultrasound examination in histologically confirmed early molar pregnancies. Ultrasound Obstet Gynecol 18:662, 2001

Seckl MJ, Fisher RA, Salerno G, et al: Choriocarcinoma and partial hydatidiform moles. Lancet 356:36, 2000

Seckl MJ, Rustin GJS, Newlands ES, et al: Pulmonary embolism, pulmonary hypertension, and choriocarcinoma. Lancet 338:1313, 1991

Seckl MJ, Sebire NJ, Berkowitz RS: Gestational trophoblastic disease. Lancet 376:717, 2010

Sharma S, Jagdev S, Coleman RE, et al: Serosal complications of single-agent low-dose methotrexate used in gestational trophoblastic diseases: first reported case of methotrexate-induced peritonitis. Br J Cancer 81:1037, 1999

Shih IM, Kurman RJ: Epithelioid trophoblastic tumor: a neoplasm distinct from choriocarcinoma and placental site trophoblastic tumor simulating carcinoma. Am J Surg Pathol 22:1393, 1998

Sita-Lumsden A, Short D, Lindsay I, et al: Treatment outcomes for 618 women with gestational trophoblastic tumours following a molar pregnancy at the Charing Cross Hospital, 2000–2009. Br J Cancer 107(11): 1810, 2012

Smith HO, Hilgers RD, Bedrick EJ, et al: Ethnic differences at risk for gestational trophoblastic disease in New Mexico: a 25-year population-based study. Am J Obstet Gynecol 188:357, 2003

SECTION 4

Soto-Wright V, Bernstein M, Goldstein DP, et al: The changing clinical presentation of complete molar pregnancy. Obstet Gynecol 86:775, 1995

Sun SY, Melamed A, Goldstein DP, et al: Changing presentation of complete hydatidiform mole at the New England Trophoblastic Disease Center over the past three decades: does early diagnosis alter risk for gestational trophoblastic neoplasia? Gynecol Oncol 138(1):46, 2015

Sun SY, Melamed A, Joseph NT, et al: Clinical presentation of complete hydatidiform mole and partial hydatidiform mole at a regional trophoblastic disease center in the United States over the past 2 decades. Int J Gynecol Cancer 26(2):367, 2016

Taylor F, Grew T, Everard J, et al: The outcome of patients with low risk gestational trophoblastic neoplasia treated with single agent intramuscular methotrexate and oral folinic acid. Eur J Cancer 49(15):3184, 2013a

Taylor JS, Viera L, Caputo TA, et al: Unsuccessful planned conservative resection of placental site trophoblastic tumor. Obstet Gynecol 121(2 Pt 2 Suppl 1): 465, 2013b

Tham BW, Everard JE, Tidy JA, et al: Gestational trophoblastic disease in the Asian population of northern England and North Wales. BJOG 110:555, 2003

Tidy JA, Rustin GJ, Newlands ES, et al: Presentation and management of choriocarcinoma after nonmolar pregnancy. BJOG 102:715, 1995

Tuncer ZS, Bernstein MR, Goldstein DP, et al: Outcome of pregnancies occurring within 1 year of hydatidiform mole. Obstet Gynecol 94:588, 1999

Uberti EM, Fajardo MD, da Cunha AG, et al: Prevention of postmolar gestational trophoblastic neoplasia using prophylactic single bolus dose of actinomycin D in high-risk hydatidiform mole: a simple, effective, secure and low-cost approach without adverse effects on compliance to general follow-up or subsequent treatment. Gynecol Oncol 114:299, 2009

van Trommel NE, Lok CA, Bulten H, et al: Long-term outcome of placental site trophoblastic tumor in The Netherlands. J Reprod Med 58(5-6):224, 2013

van Trommel NE, Massuger LF, Verheijen RH, et al: The curative effect of a second curettage in persistent trophoblastic disease: a retrospective cohort survey. Gynecol Oncol 99:6, 2005

Vargas R, Barroilhet LM, Esselen K, et al: Subsequent pregnancy outcomes after complete and partial molar pregnancy, recurrent molar pregnancy, and gestational trophoblastic neoplasia: an update from the New England Trophoblastic Disease Center. J Reprod Med 59(5-6):188, 2014

Wang J, Short D, Sebire NJ, et al: Salvage chemotherapy of relapsed or high-risk gestational trophoblastic neoplasia (GTN) with paclitaxel/cisplatin alternating with paclitaxel/etoposide (TP/TE). Ann Oncol 19:1578, 2008

Wang Q, Fu J, Hu L, et al: Prophylactic chemotherapy for hydatidiform mole to prevent gestational trophoblastic neoplasia. Cochrane Database Syst Rev 9:CD007289, 2017

Wenzel L, Berkowitz R, Robinson S, et al: The psychological, social, and sexual consequences of gestational trophoblastic disease. Gynecol Oncol 46:74, 1992

Williams J, Short D, Dayal L, et al: Effect of early pregnancy following chemotherapy on diseaserelapse and fetal outcome in women treated for gestational trophoblastic neoplasia. J Reprod Med 59(5-6):248, 2014

Wolfberg AJ, Feltmate C, Goldstein DP, et al: Low risk of relapse after achieving undetectable hCG levels in women with complete molar pregnancy. Obstet Gynecol 104:551, 2004

Wong JM, Liu D, Lurain JR: Reproductive outcomes after multiagent chemotherapy forhigh-risk gestational trophoblastic neoplasia. J Reprod Med 59(5-6):204, 2014

Yarandi F, Eftekhar Z, Shojaei H, et al: Pulse methotrexate versus pulse actinomycin D in the treatment of low-risk gestational trophoblastic neoplasia. Int J Gynaecol Obstet 103:33, 2008

Zhao J, Lv WG, Feng FZ, et al: Placental site trophoblastic tumor: a review of 108 cases and their implications for prognosis and treatment. Gynecol Oncol 142(1):102, 2016

Zhou Q, Lei XY, Xie Q, et al: Sonographic and Doppler imaging in the diagnosis and treatment of gestational trophoblastic disease: a 12-year experience. J Ultrasound Med 24:15, 2005

SECTION 5
ASPECTS OF GYNECOLOGIC SURGERY

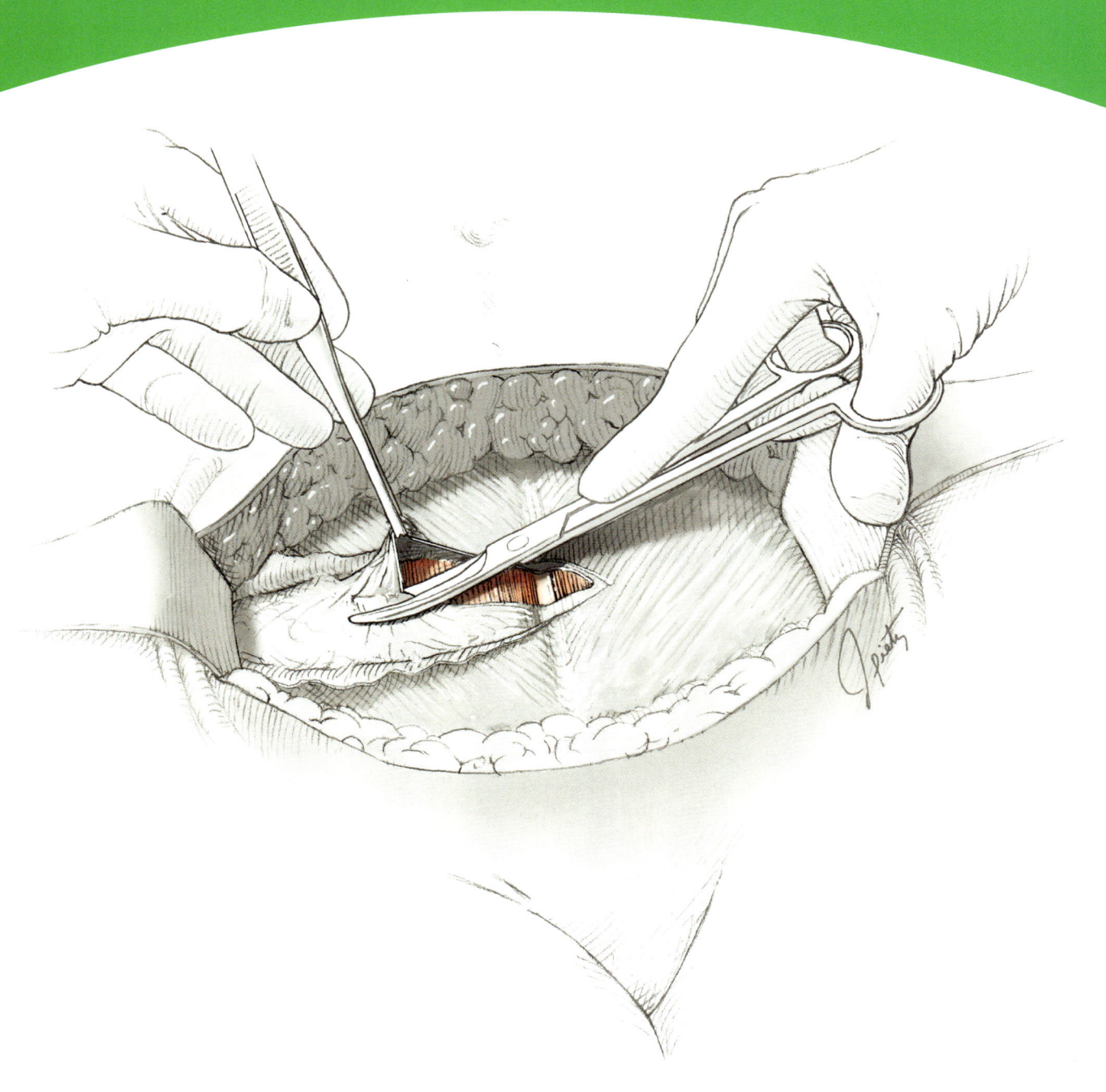

CHAPTER 38

Anatomy

ANTERIOR ABDOMINAL WALL

■ Skin and Subcutaneous Layer

Within the skin, the term *Langer lines* describes the orientation of dermal fibers. In the anterior abdominal wall, they are arranged primarily transversely (Fig. 38-1). As a result, vertical skin incisions sustain more lateral tension and thus, in general, develop wider scars compared with transverse skin incisions.

The subcutaneous tissue of the anterior abdominal wall lies between the skin and the rectus fascia. This tissue is separated into two layers. The superficial, predominantly fatty layer contains less fibrous tissue and is appropriately called the *fatty layer of the subcutaneous tissue* (formerly Camper fascia). The deeper, more fibrous layer is found closer to the rectus fascia and is named the *membranous layer of the subcutaneous tissue* (formerly Scarpa fascia) (Fig. 38-2). The fatty and membranous layers are not discrete layers but represent a continuum. If traced caudally, the membranous layer of the anterior abdominal wall is continuous with the membranous layer of the perineum, also known as Colles fascia.

■ Rectus Sheath

The *external oblique, internal oblique,* and *transversus abdominis muscles* (flank muscles) all contain a lateral muscular component and medial fibrous aponeurotic portion. All of their aponeuroses conjoin, and these united layers create the *rectus sheath,* which invests the vertical muscles of the abdomen (rectus abdominis

and pyramidalis muscles) (see Fig. 38-2). In the midline, the aponeurotic layers fuse to create the *linea alba*. The muscle fibers of the external oblique become fibrous approximately at the midclavicular line. In the lower abdomen, the muscular to the fibrous transition gradually takes place more laterally and closer to the anterior superior iliac spine. For the internal oblique and transversus abdominis muscles this same transition is seen more medially.

The anatomy of the rectus sheath changes at the *arcuate line,* which typically lies one third of the distance from the umbilicus to the pubic crest (see Fig. 38-2). Cephalad to the arcuate line, the rectus sheath lies both anterior and posterior to the rectus abdominis muscle. Here, the anterior rectus sheath is formed by the aponeurosis of the external oblique muscle and the split aponeurosis of the internal oblique muscle. The posterior rectus sheath is formed by the split aponeurosis of the internal oblique muscle and aponeurosis of the transversus abdominis muscle. Caudad to the arcuate line, all aponeurotic layers pass anterior to the rectus abdominis muscle. Thus, in the lower abdomen, the posterior surface of the rectus abdominis muscle is in direct contact with the transversalis fascia, described next.

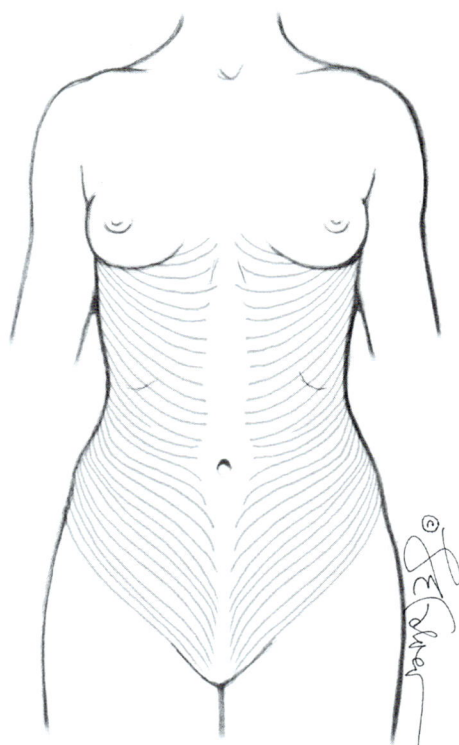

FIGURE 38-1 Langer lines of skin tension.

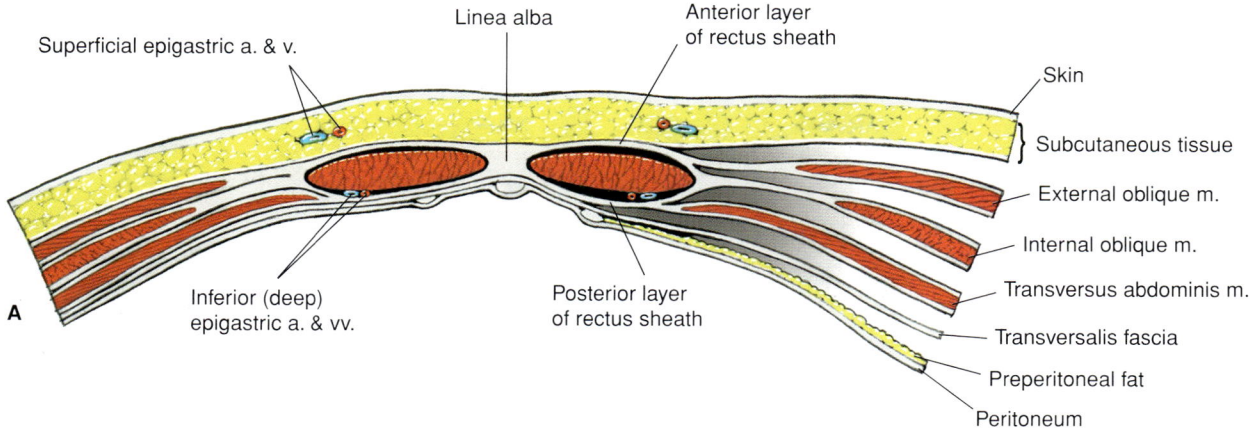

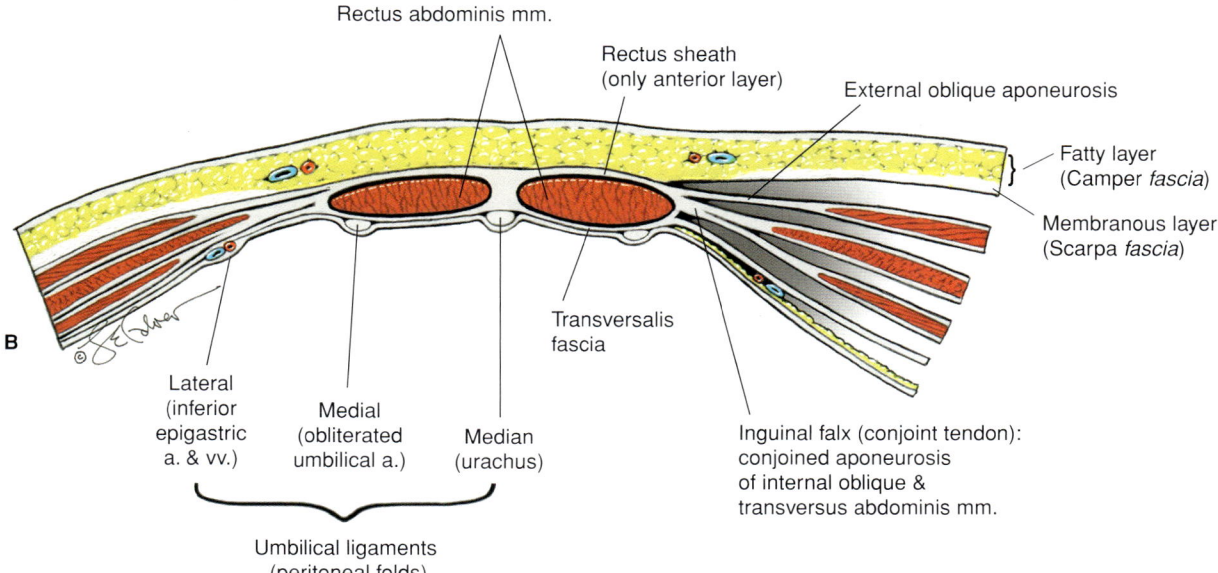

FIGURE 38-2 Transverse sections of the anterior abdominal wall above **(A)** and below **(B)** the arcuate line.

Transversalis Fascia

This thin fibrous tissue layer lies between the inner surface of the transversus abdominis muscle and the extraperitoneal fatty layer, often called the preperitoneal fat. Thus, it serves as part of the general fascial layer that lines the abdominal cavity (see Fig. 38-2) (Memon, 1999). Inferiorly, the transversalis fascia blends with the periosteum of the pubic bones.

Peritoneum

The peritoneum contains a single layer of epithelial cells and a supporting connective tissue, called the serosa. The *visceral peritoneum* densely wraps around the abdominopelvic viscera, whereas the *parietal peritoneum* lines the inner surface of the abdominal walls. In the anterior abdominal wall, five elevations of parietal peritoneum are raised by different structures (see Fig. 38-2). All five converge toward the umbilicus and are known as *umbilical ligaments*.

The single *median umbilical ligament* is formed by the urachus, an obliterated tube that extends from the apex of the

bladder to the umbilicus. In fetal life, the urachus, which is a fibrous remnant of the allantois, extends from the fetal hindgut to the umbilical cord. The paired *medial umbilical ligaments* are formed by the obliterated umbilical arteries that connected the internal iliac arteries to the umbilical cord in fetal life. The paired *lateral umbilical ligaments* contain the patent inferior epigastric vessels. The initial course of these vessels is just medial to the round ligament as the ligament enters the deep inguinal ring (Fig. 38-3).

Surgically, transection of a patent urachus can result in extravasation of urine into the abdomen. Moreover, the differential diagnosis of a midline anterior abdominal wall cyst includes urachal cyst, urachal sinus, and urachal diverticulum.

Inguinal Canal

The inguinal ligament, or Poupart ligament, is a dense connective tissue band that constitutes the inferior edge of the external oblique aponeurosis. Superior and parallel to this ligament, the inguinal canal is formed by the musculofascial layer of the

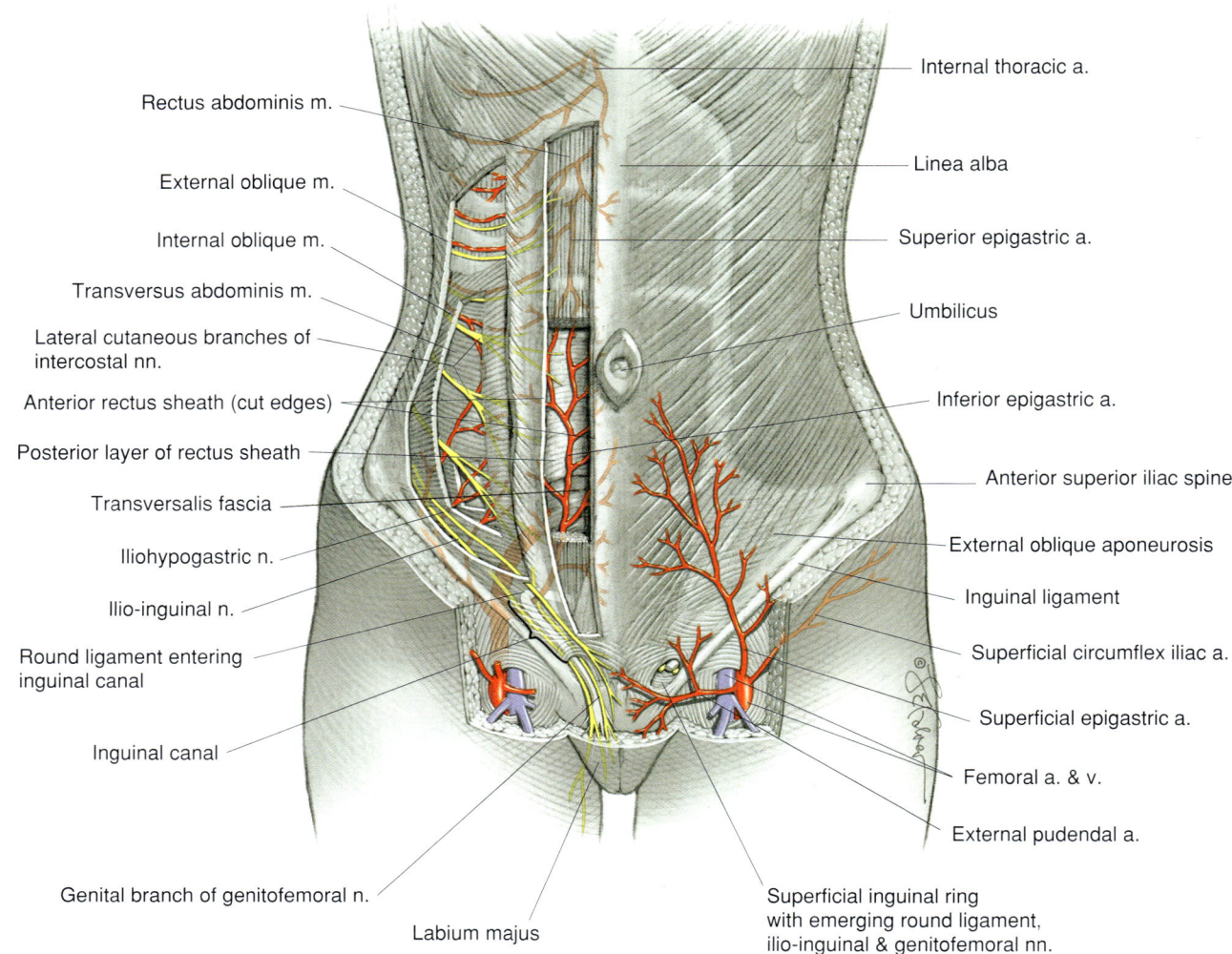

Rectus abdominis m.

External oblique m.

Internal oblique m.

Transversus abdominis m.

Lateral cutaneous branches of intercostal nn.

Anterior rectus sheath (cut edges)

Posterior layer of rectus sheath

Transversalis fascia

Iliohypogastric n.

Ilio-inguinal n.

Round ligament entering inguinal canal

Inguinal canal

Genital branch of genitofemoral n.

Labium majus

Internal thoracic a.

Linea alba

Superior epigastric a.

Umbilicus

Inferior epigastric a.

Anterior superior iliac spine

External oblique aponeurosis

Inguinal ligament

Superficial circumflex iliac a.

Superficial epigastric a.

Femoral a. & v.

External pudendal a.

Superficial inguinal ring with emerging round ligament, ilio-inguinal & genitofemoral nn.

FIGURE 38-3 Anterior abdominal wall anatomy.

abdominal wall (see Fig. 38-3). This canal has two openings, the superficial and deep inguinal rings. In the embryo, the inguinal canal is lined by an out-pocketing of the peritoneum (processus vaginalis) and abdominal musculature. Failure of the processus vaginalis to regress can lead to an indirect inguinal hernia (Chap. 12, p. 270). Through each inguinal canal, in the woman, the round ligament extends to its termination in the labium majus. In addition, the ilio-inguinal nerve and the genital branch of the genitofemoral nerve pass through the canal.

Umbilicus

The umbilicus contains the umbilical ring and coverings of skin, transversalis fascia, and peritoneum (Fig. 12-6, p. 271). The ring is a defect in the linea alba through which the fetal umbilical vessels previously passed. Following fetal life, the umbilical ring provides a window through which umbilical hernias may develop.

Of its coverings, the skin is innervated by the tenth thoracic spinal nerve (T10). The umbilical fascia is formed by a thickening in the transversalis fascia, with possible contributions from the upward extension of the bladder visceral fascia

(umbilicovesical fascia). The round ligament of the liver and the median umbilical and medial umbilical ligaments variably attach to the ring with inconstant arrangements.

The umbilicus usually lies at a vertical level corresponding to the junction between the third and fourth lumbar vertebrae. This is also the level at which the iliac veins join to form the vena cava and at which the abdominal aorta bifurcates. Thus, during initial endoscopic entry, these vessels risk laceration (Chap. 41, p. 889).

Blood Supply
Femoral Branches

The *superficial epigastric, superficial circumflex iliac,* and *external pudendal arteries* arise from the femoral artery just below the inguinal ligament in the femoral triangle (p. 820). These vessels supply the skin and subcutaneous layers of the anterior abdominal wall and mons pubis. The superficial epigastric vessels course diagonally toward the umbilicus. Surgically, during low transverse skin incision creation, the superficial epigastric vessels can usually be identified halfway between the skin and the rectus fascia, several centimeters from the midline.

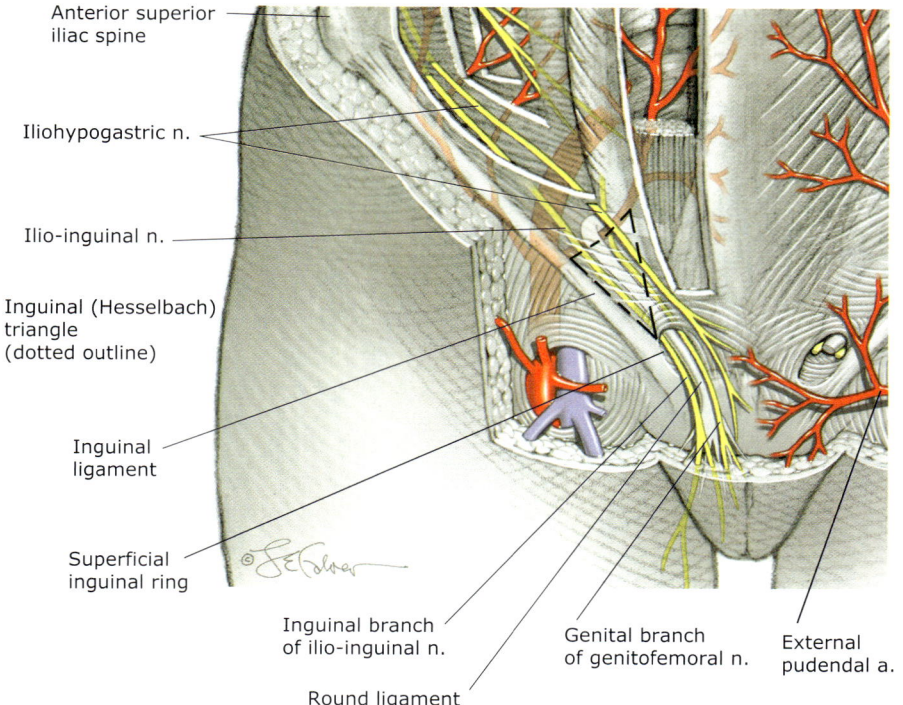

Anterior superior
iliac spine

Iliohypogastric n.

Ilio-inguinal n.

Inguinal (Hesselbach)
triangle
(dotted outline)

Inguinal
ligament

Superficial
inguinal ring

Inguinal branch
of ilio-inguinal n.

Round ligament

Genital branch
of genitofemoral n.

External
pudendal a.

FIGURE 38-4 Inguinal and upper thigh anatomy.

of the thigh through its inguinal branch (see Fig. 38-4). These two nerves enter the anterior abdominal wall at a site 2 to 3 cm medial to the anterior superior iliac spine and then course between the layers of the rectus sheath (Whiteside, 2003).

BONY PELVIS

Pelvic Bones and Joints

The hip bone, also called the *coxal bone* or *pelvic bone*, along with the *sacrum* and *coccyx* form the bony pelvis (Fig. 38-5). The hip bones consist of the *ilium*, *ischium*, and *pubis*, which all fuse at the acetabulum, a cup-shaped structure that articulates with the femoral head. The ilium articulates with the sacrum posteriorly at the sacroiliac joint, and the pubic bones articulate with each other anteriorly at the pubic symphysis. The sacroiliac joint is a synovial joint that connects the articular surfaces of the sacrum and ilium. The pubic symphysis is a cartilaginous joint that connects the articular surfaces of the pubic bones by way of a fibrocartilaginous disc. The ischial spines are clinically important bony prominences that project posteromedially from the medial surface of the ischium approximately at the level of the fifth sacral vertebra (S5).

The ligaments of the bony pelvis include the sacrospinous, sacrotuberous, and anterior longitudinal ligaments of the sacrum. These dense connective tissue condensations join bony structures and contribute significantly to bony pelvis stability (see Fig. 38-6).

The external pudendal vessels form rich anastomoses with their contralateral equivalents and with other superficial branches. These anastomoses account for the extensive bleeding often encountered with incisions made in the mons pubis area such as for retropubic midurethral sling incisions.

External Iliac Branches

The *inferior "deep" epigastric vessels* and *deep circumflex iliac vessels* are branches of the external iliac vessels (see Fig. 38-3). They supply the muscles and fascia of the anterior abdominal wall. The inferior epigastric vessels initially course lateral to, then posterior to, the rectus abdominis muscle, which they supply. They then pass anterior to the posterior rectus sheath and course between the sheath and the rectus muscles (see Figs. 38-2 and 38-3). Near the umbilicus, the inferior epigastric vessels anastomose with the superior epigastric artery and veins, which are branches of the internal thoracic vessels.

The inguinal (Hesselbach) triangle is the region in the anterior abdominal wall bounded inferiorly by the inguinal ligament, medially by the lateral border of the rectus muscles, and laterally by the inferior epigastric vessels (Fig. 38-4).

Innervation

The anterior abdominal wall is innervated by the abdominal extensions of the intercostal nerves (T7–11), the subcostal nerve (T12), and the iliohypogastric and the ilio-inguinal nerves (L1) (see Fig. 38-3). The T10 dermatome approximates the level of the umbilicus. Of these, the iliohypogastric nerve provides sensation to the skin over the suprapubic area. The ilio-inguinal nerve supplies the skin of the lower abdominal wall and upper portion of the labia majora and medial portion

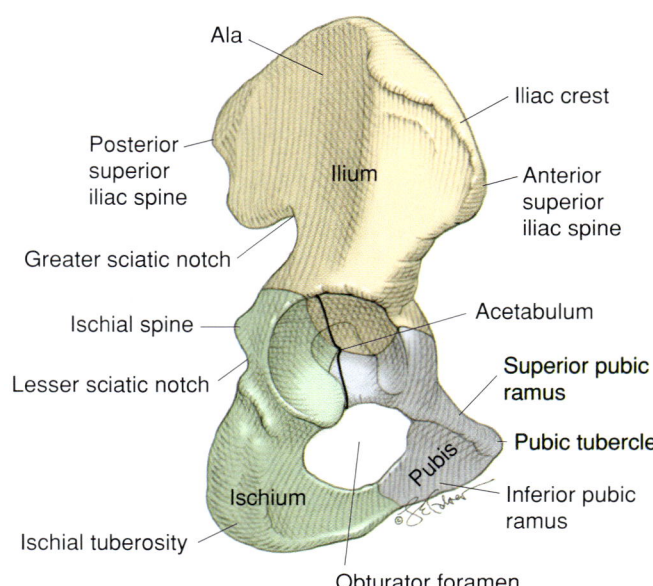

Ala

Iliac crest

Posterior
superior
iliac spine

Ilium

Anterior
superior
iliac spine

Greater sciatic notch

Ischial spine

Acetabulum

Lesser sciatic notch

Superior pubic
ramus

Pubic tubercle

Pubis

Ischium

Inferior pubic
ramus

Ischial tuberosity

Obturator foramen

FIGURE 38-5 Right hip bone.

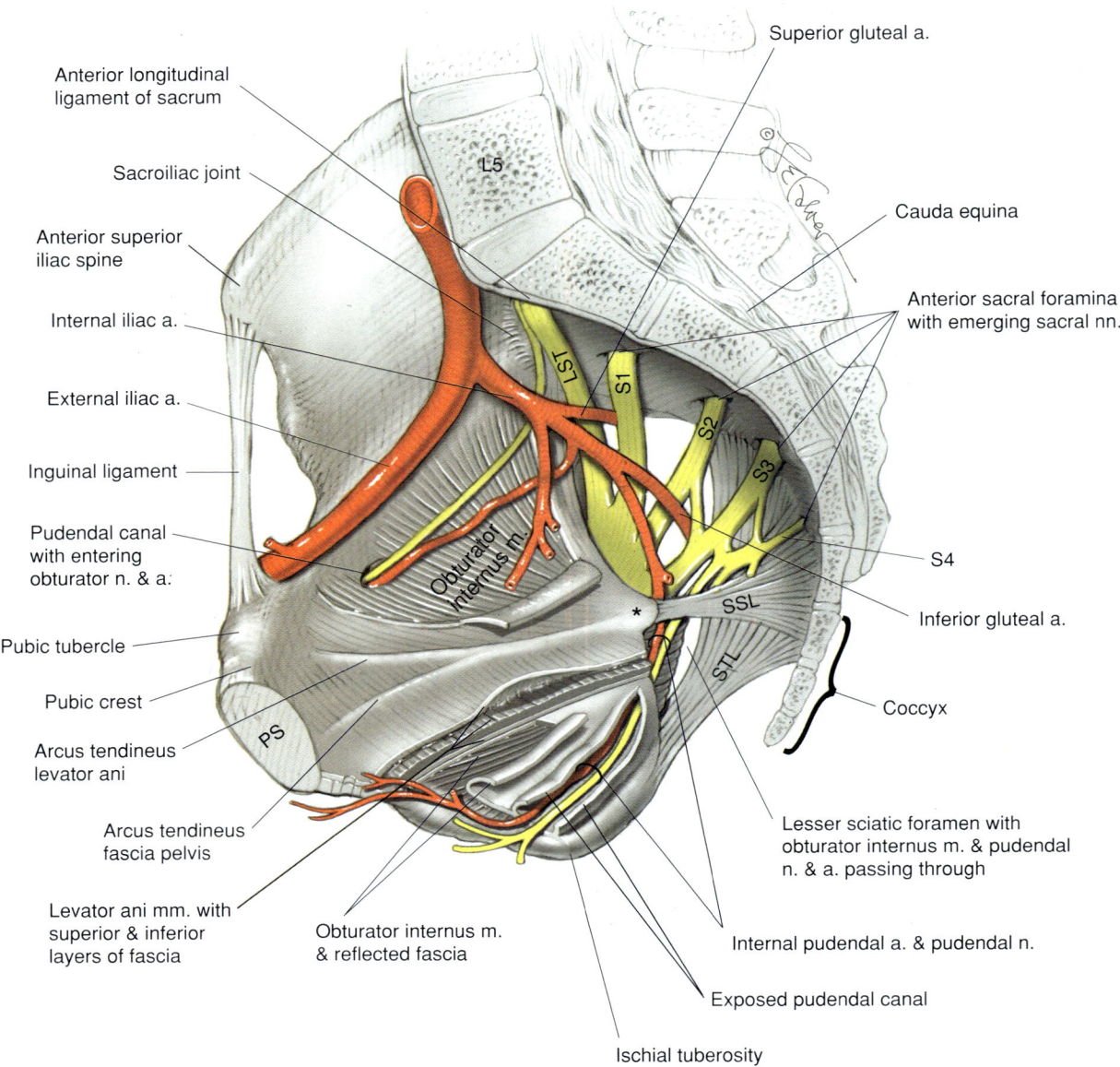

FIGURE 38-6 Bones, ligaments, and openings of the pelvic walls and associated structures. Note the obturator internus muscle extending below the levator ani muscle and then exiting through the lesser sciatic foramen to insert into the lateral femoral trochanter. Ischial spine is marked by an asterisk. L5 = fifth lumbar vertebra; LST = lumbosacral trunk; PS = pubic symphysis; S1–S4 = first through fourth sacral nerves; SSL = sacrospinous ligament; STL = sacrotuberous ligament.

■ Pelvic Openings

The posterior, lateral, and inferior walls of the pelvis have several openings through which many important structures pass. The large *obturator foramen* between the ischium and pubis is filled almost completely by the obturator membrane. In the superior portion of this membrane, a small aperture known as the *obturator canal* allows passage of the obturator neurovascular bundle into the medial compartment of the thigh (Fig. 38-6). This canal is found 5 to 6 cm from the midline of the pubic symphysis and 1 to 2 cm below the upper margin of the pectineal line (ligament) (Drewes, 2005). This ligament, also termed the Cooper ligament, is a thickening in the pubic bone periosteum, formed by the deeper and medial fibers of the inguinal ligament (Fig. 38-7).

The posterolateral walls of the pelvis are not covered by bone. Instead, two important accessory ligaments, the *sacrospinous* and *sacrotuberous ligaments*, divide the greater and lesser sciatic notches of the ischium into the *greater sciatic foramen* and *lesser sciatic foramen*. The piriformis muscle, internal pudendal vessels, superior and inferior gluteal vessels, sciatic and pudendal nerves, and other branches of the sacral nerve plexus pass through the greater sciatic foramen in close proximity to the ischial spines. Surgically, this anatomy is critical to avoid neurovascular injury during sacrospinous fixation procedures and placement of pudendal nerve blockade (Roshanravan, 2007).

The internal pudendal vessels, pudendal nerve, and obturator internus tendon pass through the lesser sciatic foramen.

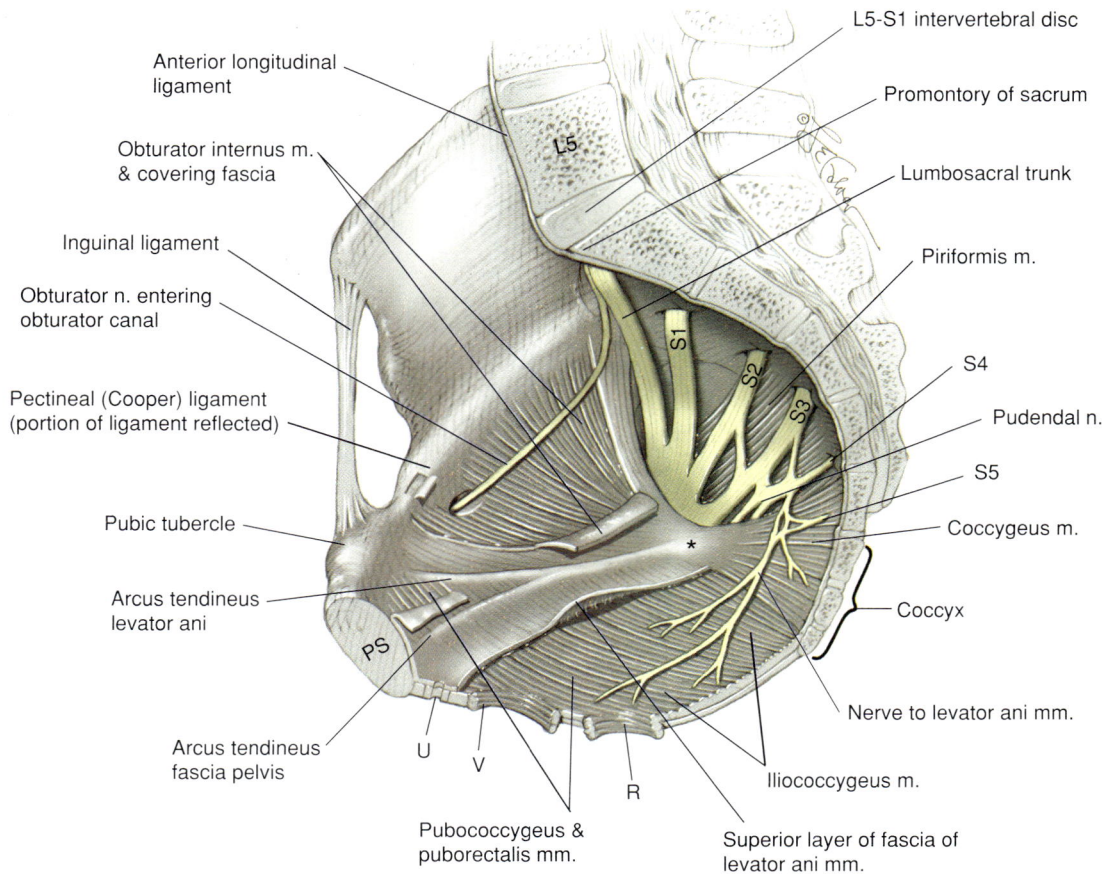

FIGURE 38-7 Muscles and fascia of the pelvic walls and pelvic floor innervation. Ischial spine is marked by an asterisk. L5 = fifth lumbar vertebra; PS = pubic symphysis; R = rectum; S1–S5 = first through fifth sacral nerves; U = urethra; V = vagina.

Posteriorly, four pairs of pelvic sacral foramina allow passage of the anterior divisions of the first four sacral nerves and lateral sacral arteries and veins.

PELVIC WALL MUSCLES AND FASCIA

◼ Pelvic Wall Muscles

The posterior, lateral, and inferior walls of the pelvis are partially covered by striated muscles and their investing layers of fasciae (see Fig. 38-7). The *piriformis muscle* arises from the anterior and lateral surface of the sacrum and partially fills the posterolateral pelvic walls. It exits the pelvis through the greater sciatic foramen, attaches to the greater trochanter of the femur, and functions as an external, that is, lateral, hip rotator.

The obturator internus muscle partially fills the sidewalls of the pelvis. This muscle arises from the pelvic surfaces of the ilium and ischium and from the obturator membrane. It exits the pelvis through the lesser sciatic foramen, attaches to the greater trochanter of the femur, and also functions as an external hip rotator.

◼ Pelvic Fascia

The three accepted names used to describe aggregations of connective tissue in the abdominopelvic cavity are parietal fascia, visceral fascia, and extraserosal fascia. Although different names are used to describe pelvic connective tissue, all layers are interconnected.

The fascia that invests striated muscles in abdomen and pelvis is termed *parietal fascia*. Examples include the rectus fascia, superior layer of fascia of levator ani muscles, and the obturator internus fascia. The *arcus tendineus levator ani* is a condensation of parietal fascia covering the medial surface of the obturator internus muscle (Figs. 38-7 and 38-8). This structure serves as the point of origin for parts of the very important levator ani muscle. Also shown is the *arcus tendineus fascia pelvis*, a condensation of parietal fascia covering the medial aspects of the obturator internus and levator ani muscles. It represents the lateral point of attachment of the anterior vaginal wall.

In contrast to parietal pelvic fascia, *visceral pelvic fascia* is intimately associated with the walls of the viscera and equates to the adventitial layer of each organ. This layer cannot be dissected in the same way that parietal fascia can be separated from skeletal muscle, such as the rectus sheath (fascia) from the rectus muscles (Table 38-1).

Extraserosal fascia is the term used to describe loose areolar tissue or condensations of connective tissue that join viscera to the pelvic sidewall. Examples include structures within broad ligaments, such as the infundibulopelvic and ovarian ligaments (p. 805). Although these connect the uterus and adnexa to the pelvic walls, they do not contribute to the support of these organs. In contrast, the cardinal and uterosacral ligaments are condensations of extraserosal fascia and do aid pelvic organ support and are discussed later (p. 804).

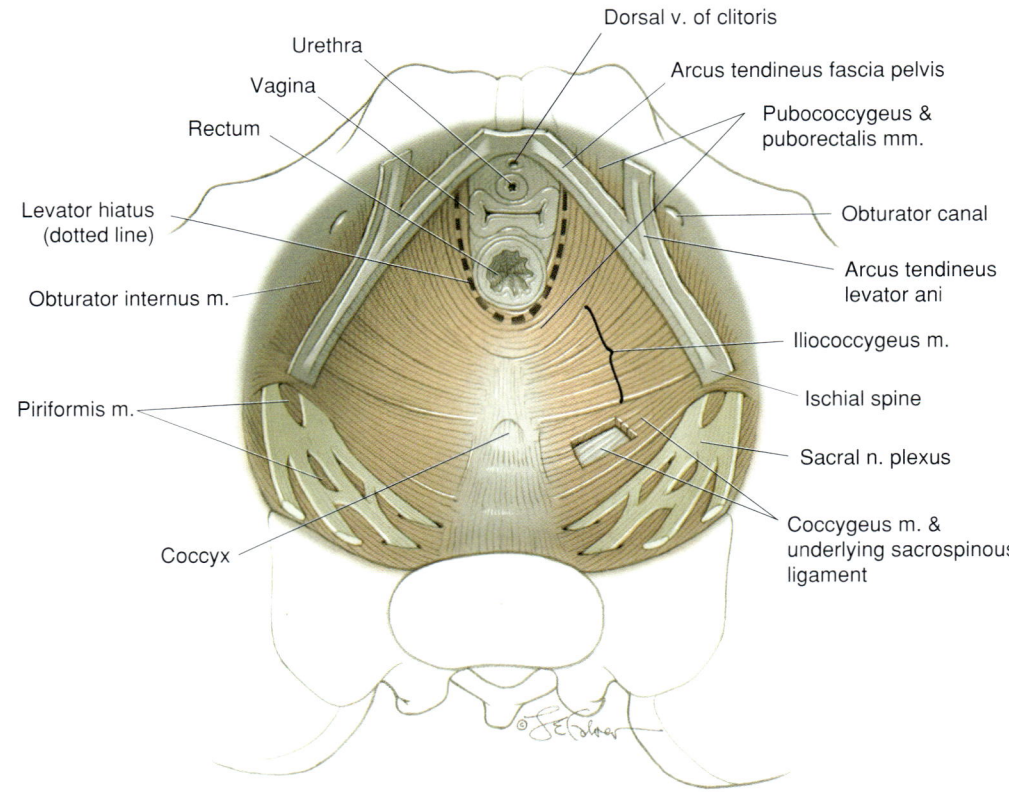

Dorsal v. of clitoris
Urethra
Vagina
Rectum
Arcus tendineus fascia pelvis
Pubococcygeus & puborectalis mm.
Levator hiatus (dotted line)
Obturator canal
Obturator internus m.
Arcus tendineus levator ani
Iliococcygeus m.
Piriformis m.
Ischial spine
Sacral n. plexus
Coccyx
Coccygeus m. & underlying sacrospinous ligament

FIGURE 38-8 Superior view of pelvic floor and pelvic wall muscles.

PELVIC FLOOR

The muscles that span the pelvic floor are collectively known as the *pelvic diaphragm* (Figs. 38-7, 38-8, and 38-9). This diaphragm consists of the levator ani and coccygeus muscles, along with their superior and inferior investing fascial layers. Inferior to the pelvic diaphragm, the perineal membrane and perineal body also contribute to the pelvic floor (p. 819). The *levator hiatus* is the U-shaped opening in the pelvic floor muscles through which the urethra, vagina, and rectum pass. The portion of the hiatus anterior to the perineal body is called the urogenital hiatus.

Levator Ani Muscles

These are the most important muscles in the pelvic floor and provide critical pelvic organ support (see Figs. 38-7 through 38-9). Physiologically, normal levator ani muscles maintain a constant state of contraction, thus providing a stable floor, which supports the weight of the abdominopelvic contents against intraabdominal forces.

The levator ani muscle consists of the *pubococcygeus, puborectalis,* and *iliococcygeus muscles.* Of these, the pubococcygeus muscle is further divided into the *pubovaginalis, puboperinealis,* and *puboanalis muscles* according to its fiber attachments. Due to the significant attachments of the *pubococcygeus muscle* to the walls of the pelvic viscera, the term *pubovisceral muscle* is often used (Kerney, 2004; Lawson, 1974).

Pubococcygeus Muscle

The anterior ends of the pubococcygeus arise on either side from the inner surface of the pubic bone. The *pubovaginalis* refers to the medial fibers that attach to the lateral walls of the vagina (see Fig. 38-9). Although the levator ani muscles have

TABLE 38-1. Differences between Visceral and Parietal Fascia of the Pelvic Floor Muscles

	Type of Fascia	
Characteristic	**Visceral or Endopelvic**	**Parietal**
Histologic	Loose arrangements of collagen, elastin, and adipose tissue	Organized collagen arrangements
Function	Allows expansion and contraction of invested structures	Provides muscle attachment to bones
Supportive role	Condensations lend some support to invested organs; encases neurovascular structures	Invests muscles to provide pelvic floor stability and function
Tensile strength	Elastic	Rigid

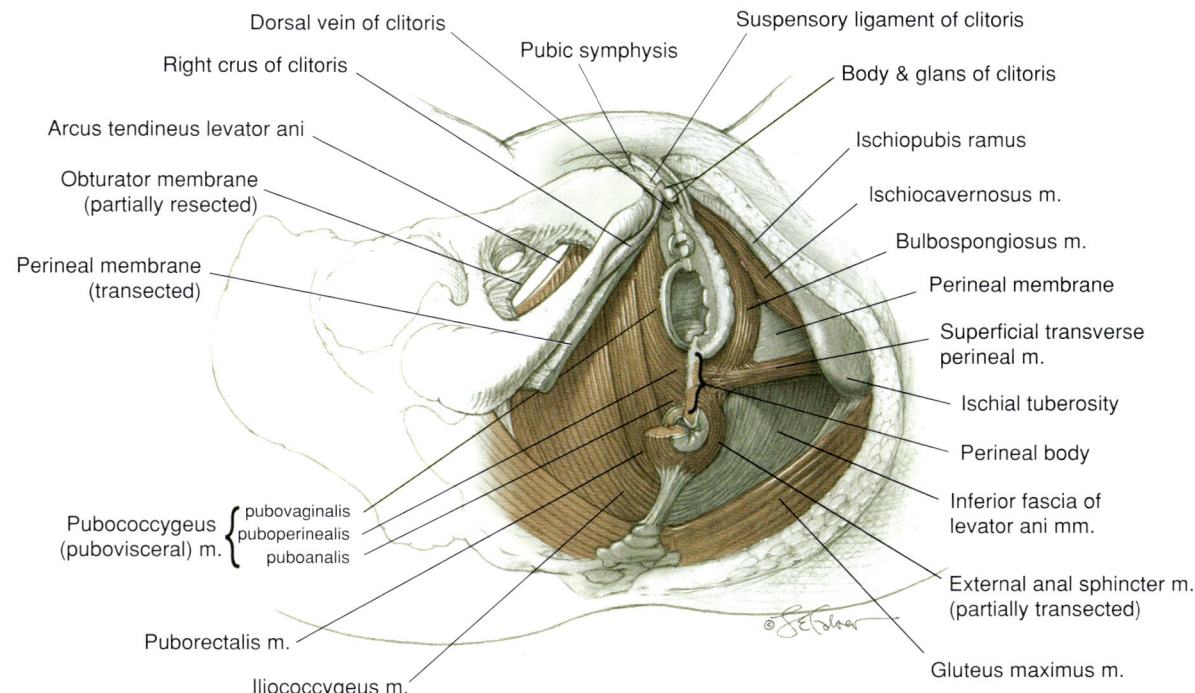

Dorsal vein of clitoris

Right crus of clitoris

Arcus tendineus levator ani

Obturator membrane
(partially resected)

Perineal membrane
(transected)

Pubococcygeus { pubovaginalis
(pubovisceral) m. { puboperinealis
{ puboanalis

Puborectalis m.

Iliococcygeus m.

Pubic symphysis

Suspensory ligament of clitoris

Body & glans of clitoris

Ischiopubis ramus

Ischiocavernosus m.

Bulbospongiosus m.

Perineal membrane

Superficial transverse
perineal m.

Ischial tuberosity

Perineal body

Inferior fascia of
levator ani mm.

External anal sphincter m.
(partially transected)

Gluteus maximus m.

FIGURE 38-9 Inferior view of pelvic floor.

no direct attachments to the urethra in females, those fibers of the muscle that attach to the vagina are responsible for elevating the urethra during a pelvic muscle contraction and hence may contribute to urinary continence (DeLancey, 1990). The *pubo-perinealis* refers to the fibers that attach to the perineal body and draw this structure toward the pubic symphysis. The *puboanalis* refers to the fibers that attach to the anus at the intersphincteric groove between the internal and external anal sphincters. These fibers elevate the anus and, along with the rest of the pubococ-cygeus and puborectalis fibers, keep the urogenital hiatus nar-rowed (see Fig. 38-8).

Puborectalis Muscle

The puborectalis represents the lateral and inferior fibers of the levator ani muscle that arise on either side from the pubic bone and form a U-shaped sling behind the anorectal junction (Figs. 38-8 through 38-10). The action of the puborectalis draws the anorectal junction toward the pubic symphysis, contributing to the anorec-tal angle. This muscle is considered part of the anal sphincter com-plex and may contribute to fecal continence (Chap. 25, p. 558).

Iliococcygeus Muscle

This muscle is the most posterior and thinnest part of the levator ani muscle and has a primarily supportive role. It arises laterally from the arcus tendineus levator ani and the ischial spines (see Figs. 38-7 through 38-10). Muscle fibers from one side join those from the opposite side in the midline between the anus and the coccyx. This meeting line is termed the *iliococcygeal raphe* and con-tributes to the *anococcygeal body*. In addition to the iliococcygeus muscle, some fibers of the pubococcygeus muscle pass behind the rectum and attach to the coccyx. These muscle fibers course cephalad to the iliococcygeus muscle and, along with attachments

of the superficial external anal sphincter, also contribute to the anococcygeal body. The *levator plate* is the clinical term used to describe the anococcygeal body (see Fig. 38-10). This portion of the levator muscles forms a supportive shelf on which the rectum, upper vagina, and uterus rest.

The levator plate in women with normal support has a mean angle of 44 degrees relative to a horizontal reference line during Valsalva (Hsu, 2006). During Valsalva, women with prolapse have a statistically greater levator plate angle com-pared with controls. This larger angle moderately correlates with larger levator hiatus length and greater downward dis-placement of the perineal body in women with prolapse com-pared with controls.

With this in mind, one theory suggests that normal levator plate support prevents excessive tension or stretching of the con-nective tissue pelvic ligaments and fasciae (Paramore, 1908). However, neuromuscular injury to the levator muscles may lead to eventual sagging or vertical inclination of the levator plate and opening of the levator hiatus. Consequently, the vaginal axis becomes more vertical, and the cervix is oriented over the opened hiatus (Fig. 38-11). The mechanical effect of this change strains the connective tissues that support the pelvic viscera. Larger hiatus size correlates with greater prolapse severity (DeLancey, 1998).

■ Pelvic Floor Innervation

The pelvic diaphragm muscles are primarily innervated by direct somatic efferents from the second through the fifth sacral nerve roots (S2-S5) (see Fig. 38-7) (Barber, 2002; Roshanravan, 2007).

Traditionally, a dual innervation has been described. The pelvic or superior surface of the muscles is supplied by direct

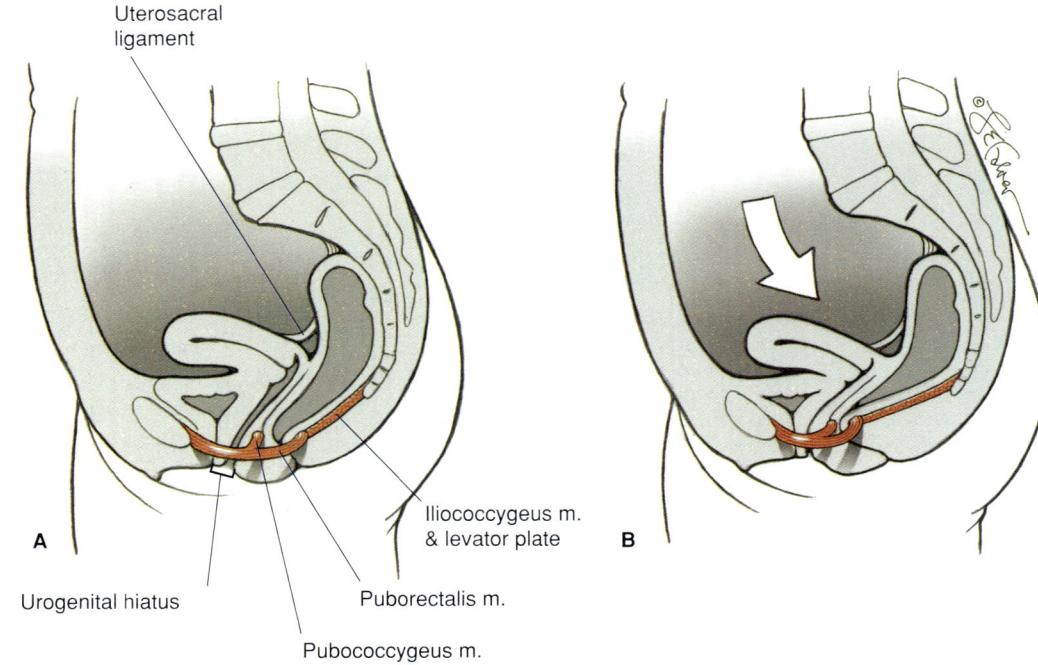

FIGURE 38-10 Pelvic organs and pelvic floor muscle and connective tissue interaction at rest **(A)** and with increasing intraabdominal pressure **(B)**.

efferents from S2–S5, collectively known as the *nerve to the levator ani muscle*. The perineal or inferior surface is supplied by pudendal nerve branches. This latter relationship has been challenged (Barber, 2002). Pudendal branches do, however, innervate parts of the striated urethral sphincter and external anal sphincter muscle (p. 818). Such separate innervation may explain why some women develop pelvic organ prolapse and others develop urinary or fecal incontinence (Heit, 1996).

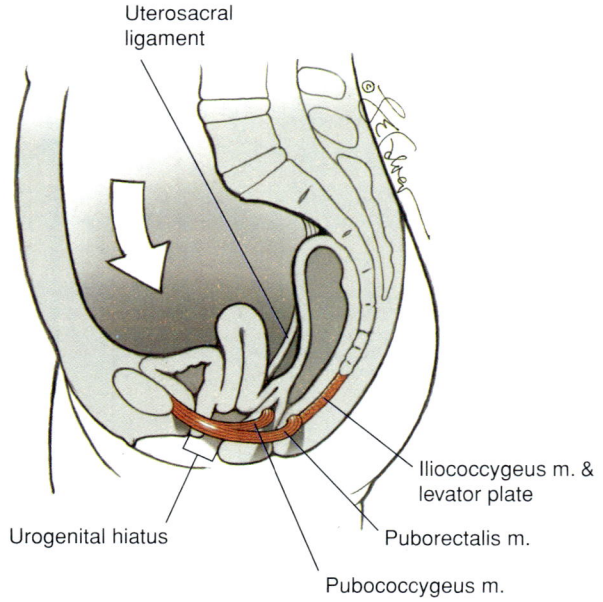

FIGURE 38-11 Pelvic floor muscles and connective tissue interaction in setting of pelvic organ prolapse.

PELVIC BLOOD SUPPLY

The pelvic organs are supplied by the visceral branches of the internal iliac (hypogastric) artery and by direct branches of the abdominal aorta (Fig. 38-12). The internal iliac artery generally divides in the area of the greater sciatic foramen into two clinically recognized divisions (see Fig. 38-6). The posterior division has the *iliolumbar, lateral sacral,* and *superior gluteal arteries.* These branches generally arise from the posterolateral wall of the internal iliac artery at a site 3 to 4 cm from its origin off the common iliac artery (Bleich, 2007). In the anterior division, the *internal pudendal, obturator,* and *inferior gluteal arteries* are parietal branches. The remaining branches of the anterior division supply pelvic viscera (uterus, vagina, rectum, and bladder). These include the *uterine, vaginal,* and *middle rectal arteries* and the *superior vesical arteries.* The superior vesical arteries commonly arise from the patent part of the umbilical arteries (Table 38-2). Internal iliac branches that supply the inferior and middle portions of the bladder are present in women, but their origins are highly variable. The middle rectal arteries are generally very small-caliber vessels and may be absent.

The two most important direct branches of the aorta that contribute to pelvic organ blood supply are the superior rectal and ovarian arteries. The *superior rectal artery,* which is the terminal branch of the inferior mesenteric artery, anastomoses with the middle rectal arteries, thus contributing blood to the rectum and vagina. The *ovarian arteries* anastomose with the ascending branch of the uterine artery and contribute blood to the uterus and adnexa. Other important anastomoses between the aorta and internal iliac arteries include anastomoses between the middle sacral and lateral sacral arteries and anastomoses between the lumbar and iliolumbar arteries.

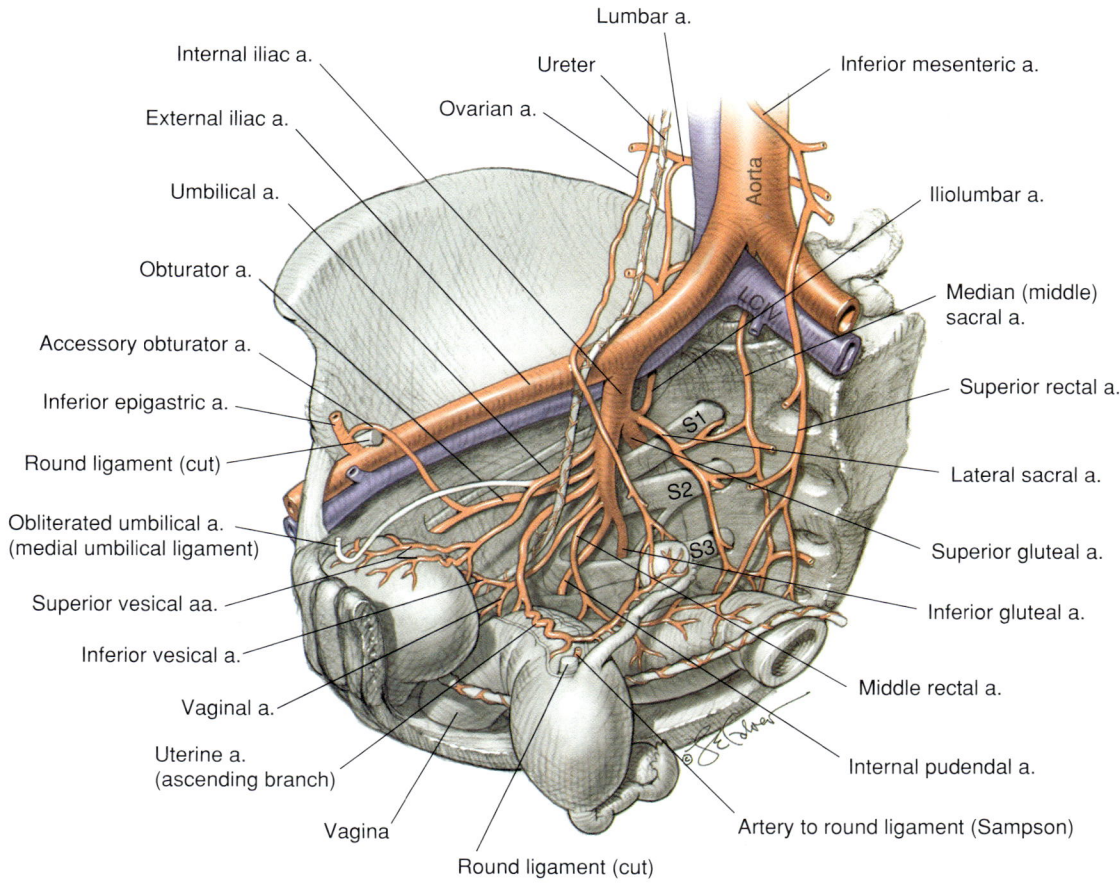

FIGURE 38-12 Pelvic arteries. In this image, the uterus and rectum are reflected to the left. LCIV = left common iliac vein; S1–S3 = first through third sacral nerves.

TABLE 38-2. Pelvic Blood Supply

Internal Iliac Artery[a]			
Anterior Division		**Posterior Division**	
Parietal Branches	**Visceral Branches**	**Parietal Branches**	**Visceral Branches**
Obturator Internal pudendal Inferior gluteal	Superior vesical (from patent segment of umbilical) Uterine Vaginal Middle rectal Middle & inferior vesicals (±)	Iliolumbar Lateral sacral Superior gluteal	None
Direct Branches of Aorta			
Parietal Branches		**Visceral Branches**	
Middle sacral		Ovarian Superior rectal (terminal branch of inferior mesenteric)	
Aortic to Internal Iliac Artery Anastomoses			
Ovarian to uterine Superior rectal to middle rectal		Middle sacral to lateral sacral Lumbar to iliolumbar	

[a]Note that great variability exists in the origin and distribution of internal iliac branches.

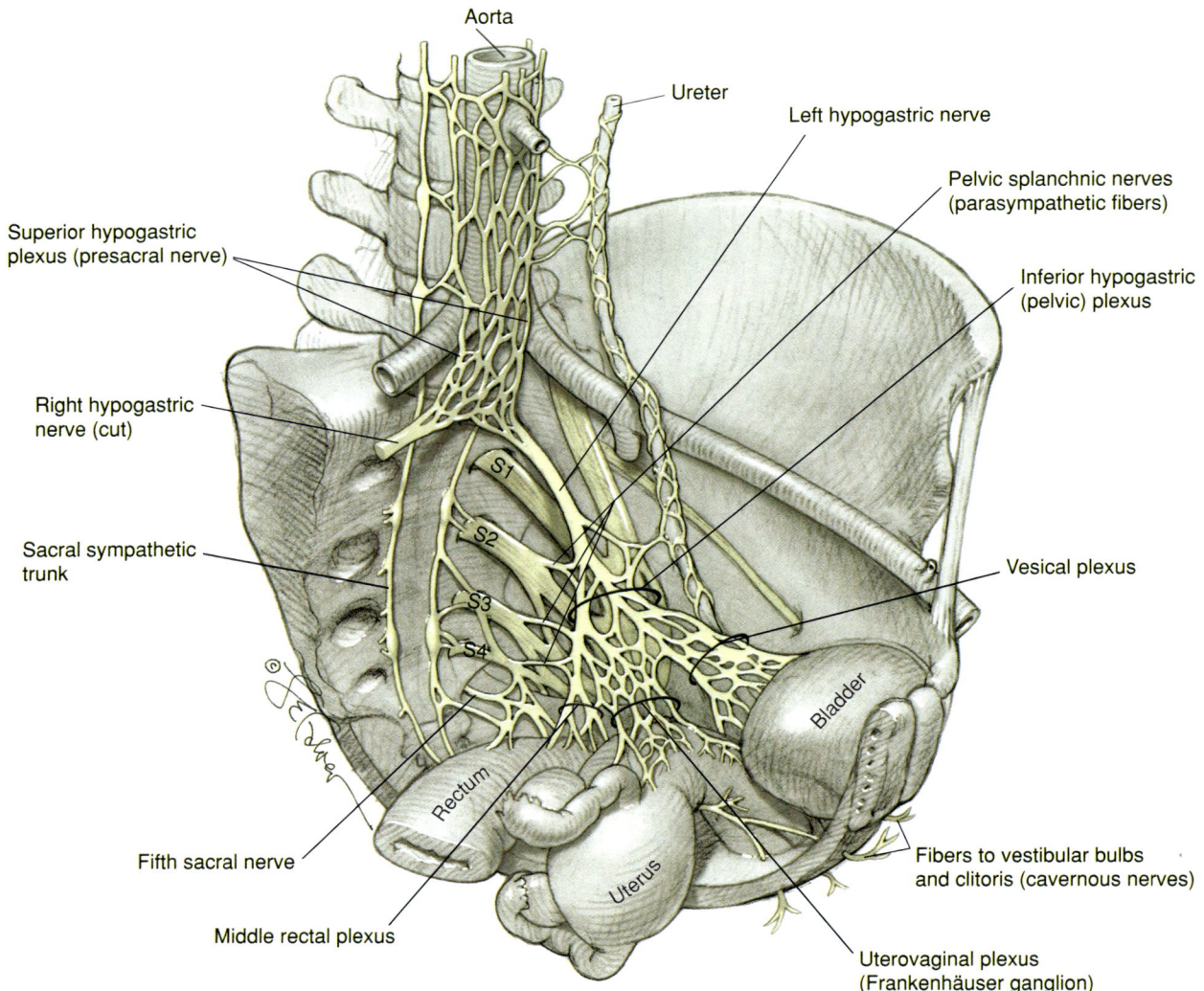

FIGURE 38-13 Pelvic autonomic nerves. Superior and inferior hypogastric plexuses and hypogastric nerves. S1–S4 = first through fourth sacral nerves.

PELVIC INNERVATION

Nerve supply to the visceral structures in the pelvis (bladder, urethra, vagina, uterus, adnexa, and rectum) arises from the autonomic nervous system. The two most important components of this system in the pelvis include the *superior* and *inferior hypogastric plexuses*. The superior hypogastric plexus, also called the *presacral nerve*, is an extension of the aortic plexus found below the aortic bifurcation (Fig. 38-13). This plexus primarily contains sympathetic fibers and sensory afferent fibers from the uterus.

The superior hypogastric plexus terminates by dividing into two trunks known as the hypogastric nerves. These nerves join parasympathetic efferents from the second through the fourth sacral nerve roots (pelvic splanchnic nerves) to form the *inferior hypogastric plexus*, also known as the *pelvic plexus*. In addition, the inferior hypogastric plexus generally receives contributions from the sacral sympathetic trunk.

With variability, fibers of the inferior hypogastric plexus accompany the distal branches of the internal iliac artery to the pelvic viscera. Accordingly, they are divided into three portions: the vesical, uterovaginal (Frankenhäuser ganglion), and middle rectal plexuses. Extensions of the inferior hypogastric plexus reach the perineum along the vagina and urethra to innervate the clitoris and vestibular bulbs via the cavernous nerves.

Clinically, the sensory afferent fibers contained within the superior hypogastric plexus are targeted in presacral neurectomy, a surgical procedure performed to treat central pelvic pain (Chap. 12, p. 265). Although visceral and sexual dysfunction may follow complete interruption of the superior hypogastric plexus, contributions from the sacral sympathetic trunk can offset interruption of this sympathetic component to the inferior hypogastric plexus. Injury to the branches of the inferior hypogastric plexus during cancer debulking, lymphadenectomy, or other extensive pelvic surgeries can lead to varying degrees of voiding, sexual, and defecatory dysfunction. Similar dysfunction is also possible during incontinence or prolapse procedures that pass sutures or trocars through the paravaginal or paraurethral tissue, which contain fiber extensions of the inferior hypogastric plexus.

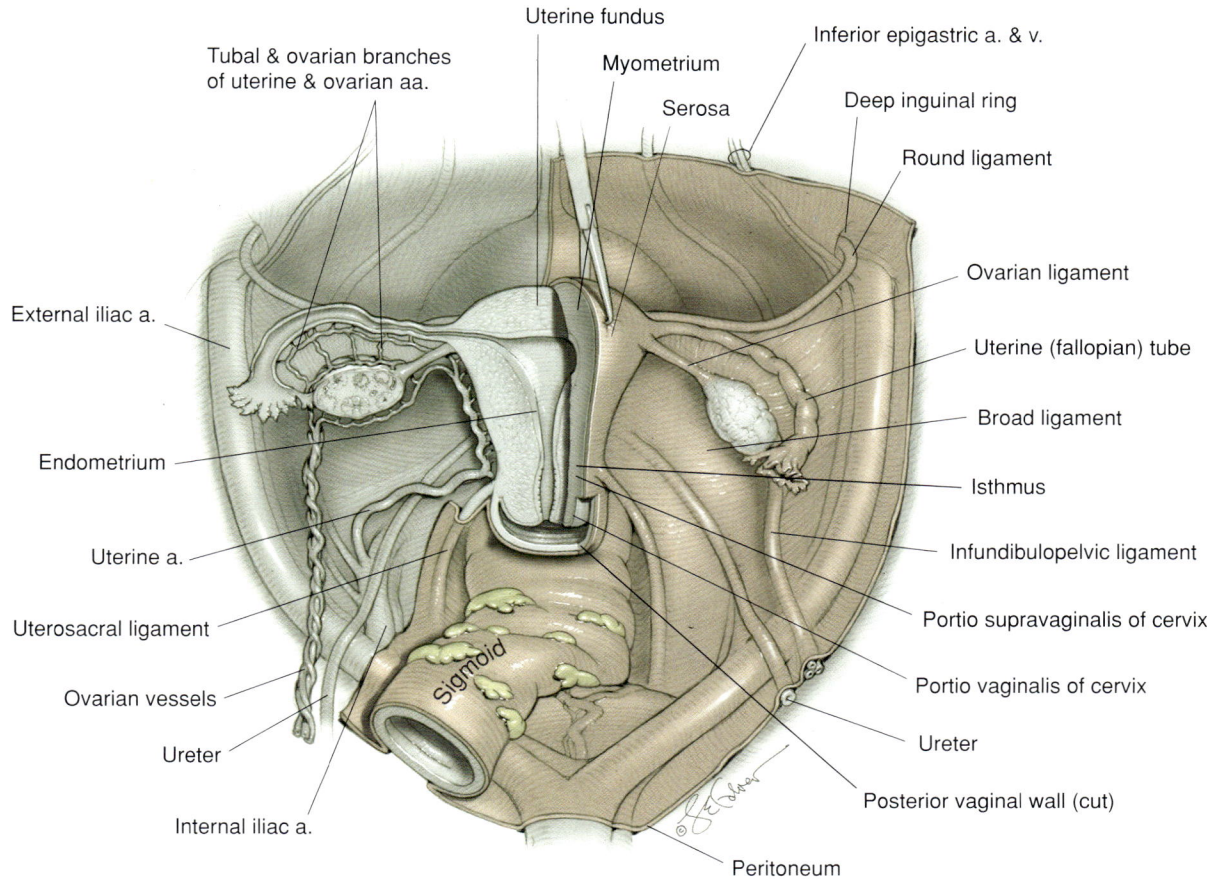

FIGURE 38-14 Uterus, adnexa, and associated anatomy.

PELVIC VISCERA AND ASSOCIATED STRUCTURES

■ Uterus

The uterus is a fibromuscular hollow organ situated between the bladder and the rectum. It is divided into two portions: an upper muscular body and a lower fibrous cervix (Fig. 38-14). The transition between the body and the cervix is known as the uterine isthmus. This also marks the transition from endocervical canal to endometrial cavity. The portion of the body that extends above the entry level of the uterine (fallopian) tubes into the endometrial cavity is known as the fundus.

The shape, weight, and dimensions of the uterus vary according to parity and estrogen stimulation. Before menarche and after menopause, the body and cervix are approximately equal in size, but during the reproductive years, the uterine body is significantly larger than the cervix. In the adult, nonpregnant woman, the uterus measures approximately 7 cm in length and 5 cm in width at the fundus.

Endometrium and Serosa

The uterus consists of an inner mucosal layer called the endometrium, which surrounds the endometrial cavity and is described in Chapter 8 (p. 180). The myometrium surrounds the endometrial cavity and contains smooth muscle bundles united by connective tissue with many elastic fibers. Interlacing myometrial fibers surround myometrial vessels and contract to compress these. Serosa overlies the myometrium, except at two sites. First, the anterior portion of the cervix is covered by the bladder. Second, the lateral portions of the body and cervix attach to the broad and cardinal ligaments.

Cervix

The uterine cervix begins caudal to the uterine isthmus and is approximately 3 cm long. The wall of the cervix, especially its distal segment, contains primarily fibrous tissue and approximately 10 percent smooth muscle. The smooth muscle is found on the cervical wall periphery and serves as the attachment point for the cardinal and uterosacral ligaments and for the fibromuscular walls of the vagina (p. 804). This smooth muscle is easily dissected from the underlying, denser fibrous cervix core and is the layer reflected during intrafascial hysterectomy.

The attachments of the vaginal walls to the outer cervix divide it into a vaginal part known as the *portio vaginalis* and a supravaginal part known as the *portio supravaginalis* (see Fig. 38-14). The portio vaginalis is covered by nonkeratinizing squamous epithelium.

The endocervical canal is lined by columnar, mucus-secreting epithelium. The lower border of the canal, called the external cervical os, contains a transition from the squamous epithelium of the portio vaginalis to the columnar epithelium of the

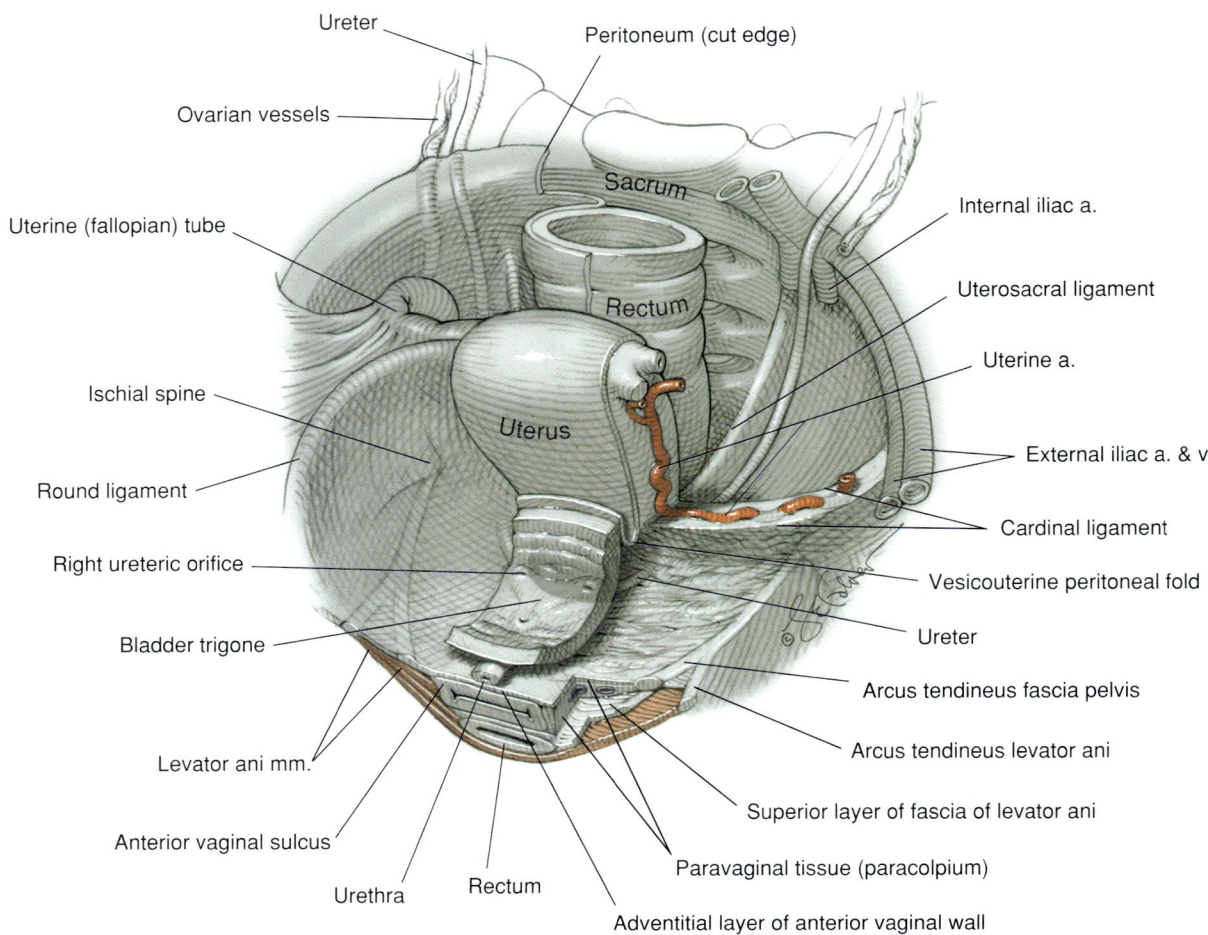

FIGURE 38-15 Pelvic viscera and their connective tissue support. Relationship of the urethra, bladder trigone, and distal ureter to the anterior vaginal wall and to the uterine cervix.

cervical canal. The exact location of this transition, termed the *squamocolumnar junction*, varies depending on hormonal status (Fig. 29-4, p. 623). At the upper border is the internal cervical os, where the narrow cervical canal becomes continuous with the wider endometrial cavity.

Uterine Support

The main support of the uterus and cervix is provided by the levator ani muscles and the connective tissue that attaches the outer cervix to the pelvic walls. This tissue that attaches lateral to the uterus and cervix on each side is called the *parametrium* and continues caudally along the vagina as the *paracolpium*. These both extend laterally to the pelvic walls and represent part of the extraserosal pelvic fascia. The parametrium consists of what is clinically known as the *cardinal ligament* and *uterosacral ligament* (Fig. 38-15).

The cardinal ligaments, also termed *transverse cervical ligaments* or *Mackenrodt ligaments*, primarily consist of vessels and connective tissue and contain some pelvic autonomic nerves in their lower portion (Ramanah, 2012; Range, 1964). They attach to the posterolateral pelvic walls near the origin of the internal iliac artery and contain the vessels supplying the uterus and vagina.

The uterosacral ligaments insert broadly into the posterior pelvic walls and sacrum and form the lateral boundaries of the posterior cul-de-sac of Douglas. These ligaments originate from

the posterior inferior surface of the cervix but may also originate, in part, from the proximal posterior vagina (Umek, 2004). They consist of a superficial and a deep section, each containing varying degrees of connective tissue, smooth muscle, pelvic autonomic nerves, and blood vessels (Campbell, 1950; Ramanah, 2012; Ripperda, 2017).

Clinically, during pelvic reconstructive surgeries that use the uterosacral ligaments as attachment sites for the vaginal apex, surrounding structures are especially vulnerable (Wieslander, 2007). Namely, the rectum lies medial to the uterosacral ligaments. The ureter, pelvic sidewall vessels, and sacral nerves run lateral to and close to these ligaments. Also, as the ligaments contain fibers of the inferior hypogastric plexus, some degrees of voiding or sexual dysfunction can follow these procedures.

Round Ligaments

These ligaments are smooth muscle extensions of the uterine body. Arising from the lateral aspect of the uterine body just below and anterior to the origin of the fallopian tubes, the round ligaments extend laterally to the pelvic sidewall (see Fig. 38-14). They enter the retroperitoneal space and pass lateral to the inferior epigastric vessels before entering the inguinal canal through the deep inguinal ring. After coursing through the inguinal canal, the round ligaments exit through their respective superficial inguinal ring to terminate in the subcutaneous tissue of each labium majus (see Fig. 38-4). The round ligaments do not significantly contribute to uterine support. They receive their blood supply from a small branch of the uterine or ovarian artery known as the *Sampson artery* (p. 801).

Broad Ligaments

These ligaments are double layers of peritoneum that extend from the lateral walls of the uterus to the pelvic walls (see Fig. 38-14). Within the upper portion of these two layers, the fallopian tube, ovarian ligament, and round ligament are found. Each of these has its separate mesentery, called the *mesosalpinx*, *mesovarium*, and *mesoteres*, respectively, which carry nerves and vessels to these structures. At the lateral border of the fallopian tube and the ovary, the broad ligament ends where the suspensory ligament of ovary (infundibulopelvic ligament), described subsequently, blends with the pelvic wall. The cardinal and uterosacral ligaments lie within the lower portion or "base" of the broad ligament.

Uterine Blood Supply

The blood supply to the uterine body arises from the ascending branch of the uterine artery and from the medial or uterine branch of the ovarian artery (see Figs. 38-14 and 38-15). The uterine artery is commonly one of the first branches of anterior division of internal iliac. (see Fig. 38-12). The uterine artery approaches the uterus at the level of the uterine isthmus. Here, the uterine artery courses over the ureter and provides a small branch to it. Several uterine veins run along the side of the artery and are variably found over or under the ureter. The uterine artery then divides into a larger ascending and a smaller descending branch that course alongside the uterus and cervix, respectively. These vessels connect on the lateral border of the uterus but form an anastomotic arterial arcade that supplies the uterine walls (Fig. 8-1, p. 180). The cervix is supplied by the descending or cervical branch of the uterine artery and by ascending branches of the vaginal artery.

Clinically, because the uterus receives dual blood supply from both ovarian and uterine vessels, some surgeons during myomectomy place tourniquets at both the infundibulopelvic ligament and uterine isthmus. This decreases blood flow from the ovarian and uterine arteries, respectively.

Uterine Lymphatic Drainage and Innervation

Lymphatic drainage is primarily to the obturator and internal and external iliac nodes (Fig. 38-16). However, some lymphatic channels from the uterine body may pass along the round ligaments to the superficial inguinal nodes, and others may extend along the uterosacral ligaments to the lateral sacral nodes.

The uterus is innervated by fibers of the uterovaginal plexus, also known as the Frankenhäuser ganglion. These fibers are found in the connective tissue of the parametria (see Fig. 38-13).

■ Ovaries and Uterine (Fallopian) Tubes

Ovaries

The ovaries and fallopian tubes constitute the *uterine adnexa*. The size and hormonal activity of the ovaries are dependent on age, stage of the menstrual cycle, and exogenous hormonal suppression.

During reproductive years, the ovaries measure 2.5 to 5 cm in length, 1.5 to 3 cm in thickness, and 0.7 to 1.5 cm in width.

The ovaries consist of an *outer cortex* and an *inner medulla*. The ovarian cortex is made up of a specialized stroma punctuated with follicles, corpora lutea, and corpora albicantia. A single layer of mesothelial cells covers this cortex as a surface epithelium. The medullary portion of the ovary primarily consists of fibromuscular tissue and blood vessels. The medial aspect of the ovary is connected to the uterus by the *ovarian (uteroovarian) ligament* (see Fig. 38-14). Laterally, each ovary is attached to the pelvic wall by the *suspensory ligament of the ovary*, clinically known as the *infundibulopelvic ligament*, which contains the ovarian vessels and nerves.

The blood supply to the ovaries comes from the *ovarian arteries*, which most commonly arise from the anterior surface of the abdominal aorta just below the origin of the renal arteries and from the ovarian branches of the uterine arteries (see Fig. 38-16). The *ovarian veins* follow an analogous retroperitoneal course as the arteries. The right ovarian vein drains into the inferior vena cava, and the left ovarian vein drains into the left renal vein.

Lymphatic drainage of the ovaries follows the ovarian vessels to the lower abdominal aorta, where they drain into the paraaortic nodes. For their innervation, the ovaries are supplied by extensions of the renal plexus that course along the ovarian vessels in the infundibulopelvic ligament. Branches of the vagus nerve form the parasympathetic contribution to this plexus.

Uterine (Fallopian) Tubes

The fallopian tubes are tubular structures that measure 7 to 12 cm in length (see Fig. 38-14). Each tube has four identifiable portions. The *uterine part*, also known as the intramural or *interstitial portion*, passes through the body of the uterus at the region known as the *cornua*. The *isthmic portion* begins adjacent to the uterine body. It consists of a narrow lumen and thick muscular wall. The *ampullary portion* begins as the lumen of the distal isthmic portion widens. The ampulla has a more convoluted mucosa. The *infundibulum* of the uterine tube is the distal continuation of the ampullary segment and contains the *fimbriated portion* at its distal end. This end has many frondlike projections that provide a wide surface area for ovum pickup. The *fimbria ovarica* is the extension that contacts the ovary.

The ovarian artery runs along the ovary's hilum and sends several branches through the mesosalpinx to supply the fallopian tubes (see Fig. 38-14). The venous plexus, lymphatic drainage, and nerve supply of the fallopian tubes follow a similar course to those of the ovaries.

■ Vagina

The vagina is a distensible hollow viscus. Its distal portion is constricted by the action of the levator ani muscles (see Fig. 38-10). Above the pelvic floor, the vaginal lumen is more capacious and expandable. In the standing or anatomic position, the apex of the vagina is directed posteriorly toward the ischial spines, and the upper two thirds of the vaginal tube lie almost parallel to the plane of the levator plate. The average length of the anterior vaginal wall is 7 to 8 cm and that of the posterior wall is 9 cm. The recesses within the vaginal lumen

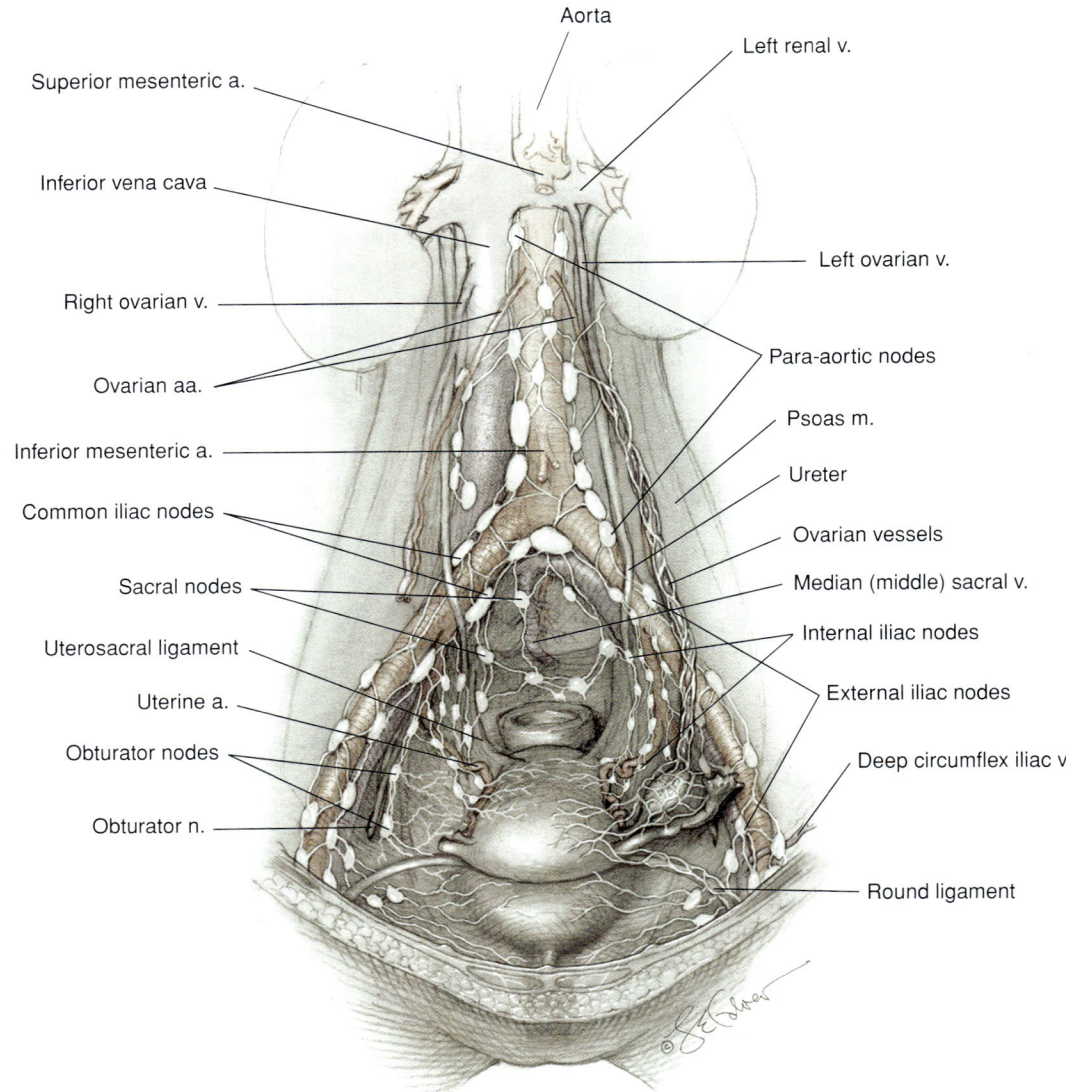

FIGURE 38-16 Pelvic lymph nodes and the course of the ureter and ovarian vessels.

in front of, behind, and lateral to the cervix are known as the *anterior fornix*, *posterior fornix*, and *lateral fornices*, respectively (Fig. 38-17).

The vaginal walls consist of three layers. A nonkeratinized squamous epithelium and its adjacent lamina propria line the vaginal lumen. This is surrounded by a muscular layer and then an outer adventitial layer, which is the visceral pelvic fascia of the vagina (Fig. 24-5, p. 540) (Weber, 1995, 1997). These latter two form the fibromuscular component of the vagina. When dissected in the operating room, this fibromuscular combination of visceral pelvic fascia and muscularis is the surgeon's "fascia."

The vagina lies between the bladder and rectum and, along with its connections to the pelvic walls, provides support to these organs (see Figs. 38-15 and 38-17). The vagina is separated from the bladder anteriorly and the rectum posteriorly by the vaginal adventitia. The continuation of this adventitial layer laterally contributes and blends into the paracolpium. The anterior fibromuscular vaginal wall and its connective tissue (paracolpium) attachments to the arcus tendineus fascia pelvis

represent the layer that supports the bladder and urethra (see Fig. 38-15).

The posterior vaginal wall's lateral attachments connect it to the parietal fascia covering the pelvic surface of the levator ani muscles. The posterior vaginal wall and this fascia contribute to support the rectum. This layer is clinically known as the *rectovaginal fascia* or *fascia of Denonvilliers*.

Similar to microscopic findings of the anterior vaginal wall, histologic studies have failed to show a separate layer between the posterior wall of the vagina and the rectum except in the distal 3 to 4 cm (Maldonado, 2019). Here, the dense fibromuscular tissue of the perineal body separates the vaginal from the anal walls (DeLancey, 1999). Because there is no true histologic "fascial" layer between the vagina and the bladder and between the vagina and the rectum, some recommend that terms such as "pubocervical/pubovesical fascia" or "rectovaginal fascia" be abandoned. They propose that these be replaced by more accurate descriptive terms such as *vaginal muscularis* or *fibromuscular layer of the anterior and posterior vaginal walls*.

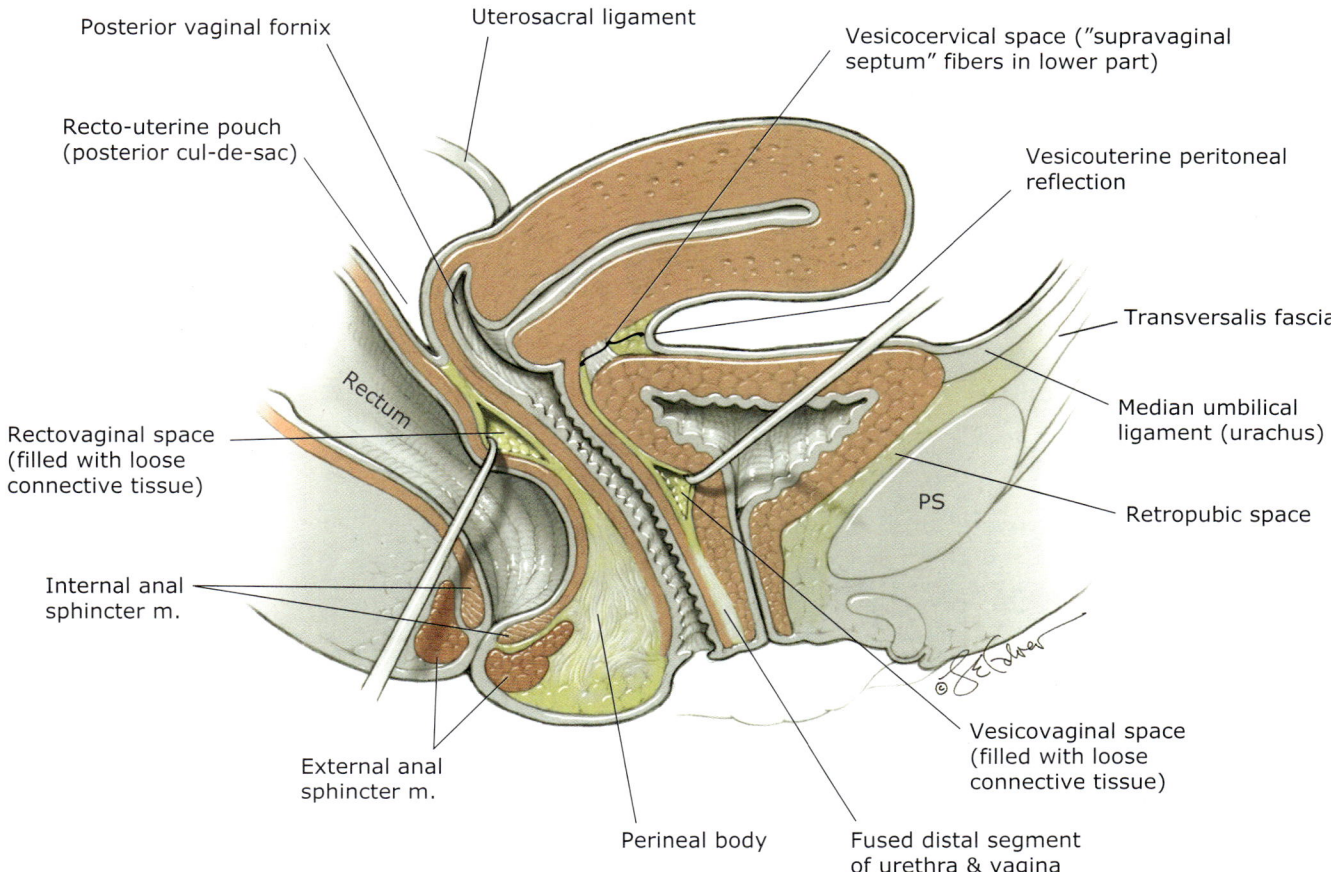

Posterior vaginal fornix

Uterosacral ligament

Vesicocervical space ("supravaginal septum" fibers in lower part)

Recto-uterine pouch (posterior cul-de-sac)

Vesicouterine peritoneal reflection

Rectum

Transversalis fascia

Median umbilical ligament (urachus)

Rectovaginal space (filled with loose connective tissue)

PS

Retropubic space

Internal anal sphincter m.

External anal sphincter m.

Perineal body

Fused distal segment of urethra & vagina

Vesicovaginal space (filled with loose connective tissue)

FIGURE 38-17 Surgical cleavage planes and spaces, peritoneal recesses, and anal sphincter complex.

Vesicocervical and Vesicovaginal "Potential" Spaces

The *vesicocervical space* begins below the vesicouterine peritoneal fold or reflection. This fold represents the loose attachments of the peritoneum in the *vesicouterine pouch*, also known as the anterior cul-de-sac (see Figs. 38-17 and 38-18). The vesicocervical space continues down as the *vesicovaginal space*, which extends to the junction of the proximal and middle thirds of the urethra. Below this point, the urethra and vagina fuse (Hamner, 2018).

Clinically, during an abdominal hysterectomy or cesarean delivery, surgeons easily lift and incise the vesicouterine peritoneal fold to create a "bladder flap" and then develop the vesicocervical and vesicovaginal spaces. Thus, to successfully enter the peritoneal cavity anteriorly, proper identification and sharp dissection of the loose connective tissue that lies within the vesicovaginal and then vesicocervical spaces is necessary (see Fig. 38-17) (Balgobin, 2016).

Rectovaginal Space

This potential space is immediately adjacent to the posterior surface of the midvagina. It extends from the rectouterine pouch, also known as the posterior cul-de-sac or pouch of Douglas, down to the superior border (apex) of the perineal body, which extends 2 to 3 cm cephalad to the hymeneal ring (see Figs. 38-17 and 38-18) (Maldonado, 2019). The posterior cul-de-sac peritoneum extends down the posterior vaginal wall 2 to 3 cm inferior to the posterior vaginal fornix (Kuhn, 1982).

The posterior cul-de-sac is bordered by the vagina anteriorly, the rectosigmoid posteriorly, and the uterosacral ligaments laterally. The inferior extensions of the uterosacral ligament fibers, also known as rectal pillars, are fibers of the posterior parametrium that extend down from the cervix and attach to the upper portion of the posterior vaginal wall. These fibers connect the vagina to the lateral walls of the rectum and to the sacrum. They also separate the midline rectovaginal space from the more lateral pararectal spaces. Clinically, the rectovaginal space contains loose areolar tissue and is easily opened with finger dissection during abdominal surgery (see Fig. 38-18).

Vaginal Support

Although the connective tissue in the pelvis is continuous and interdependent, DeLancey (1992) has described three levels of vaginal connective tissue support. First, for upper vaginal support, the parametrium continues caudally down the vagina as the paracolpium (see Fig. 38-15). This tissue attaches the upper vagina to the pelvic wall, suspending it over the pelvic floor. These attachments are known as *level I support* or *suspensory axis* and provide connective tissue support to the vaginal apex after hysterectomy. In the standing position, level I support fibers are both vertically oriented (cardinal ligaments) and posteriorly oriented (uterosacral ligaments) (Chen, 2013).

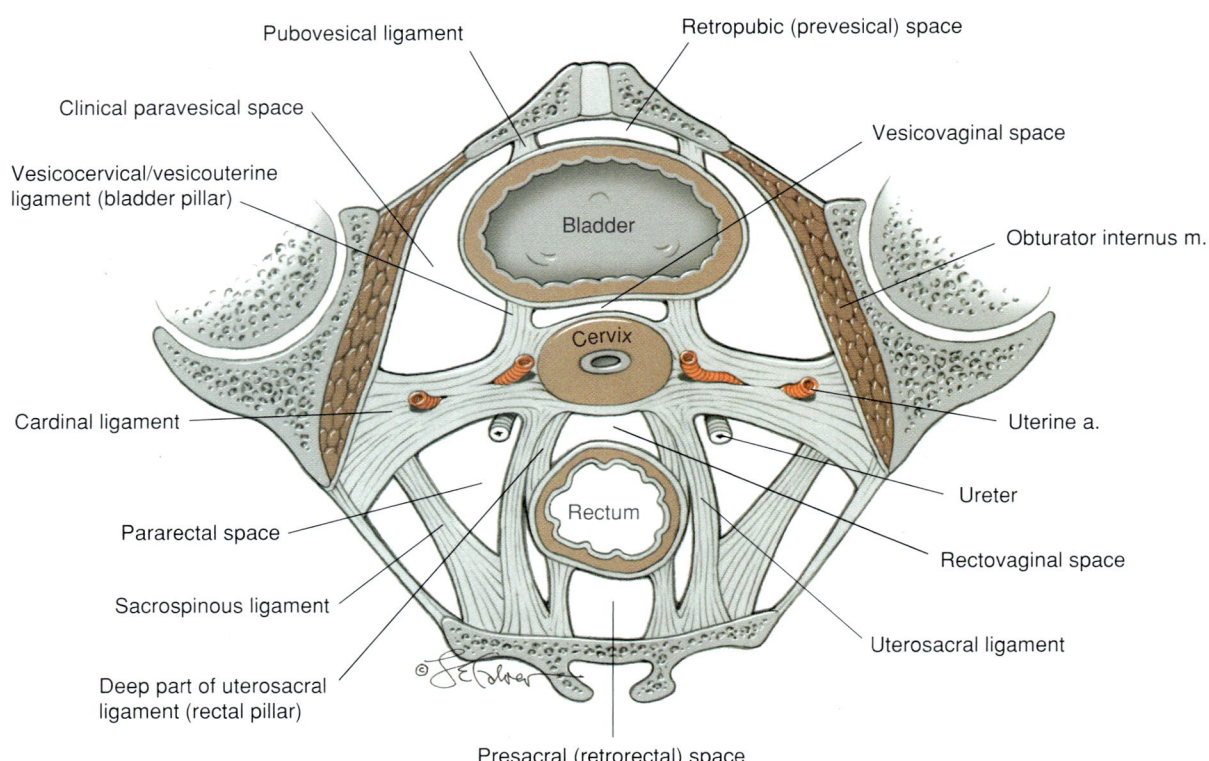

FIGURE 38-18 Connective tissue and surgical spaces of the pelvis.

For midvaginal support, the lateral walls of the vagina's mid-portion are attached to the pelvic walls on each side by the paracolpium. These lateral attachments of the vaginal walls blend into the arcus tendineus fascia pelvis and to the medial aspect of the levator ani muscles, and in doing so create the anterior and posterior lateral vaginal sulci (see Fig. 38-15). These grooves run along the vaginal sidewalls and give the vagina an "H" shape when viewed in cross section.

Attachment of the anterior vaginal wall to the levator ani muscles can aid bladder neck elevation (see Fig. 38-10). Thus, these midvaginal attachments may have significance for stress urinary continence and vaginal wall prolapse and are called *level II support* or the *attachment axis*.

For distal vaginal support, the vagina is directly attached to its surrounding structures (see Fig. 38-9). Anteriorly, the vagina is fused with the urethra (Hamner, 2018). Laterally it attaches to the pubovaginalis muscle and perineal membrane, and posteriorly to the perineal body. These vaginal attachments are *level III support* or the *fusion axis*. Failed support can lead to distal prolapse.

Vaginal Blood Supply, Lymphatics, and Innervation

The main blood supply to the vagina arises from the descending or cervical branch of the uterine artery and from the vaginal artery, a branch of the internal iliac artery (see Fig. 38-12). These vessels form an anastomotic arcade along the lateral sides of the vagina at the level of the vaginal sulci, and they anastomose with the contralateral vessels on the anterior and posterior walls of the vagina. Additionally, the middle rectal artery from the internal iliac artery contributes to the posterior vaginal wall supply. The distal walls of the vagina also receive contributions from the internal pudendal artery (p. 796). Lymphatic drainage

of the upper two thirds of the vagina is similar to that of the uterus (p. 806). The distal part of the vagina drains with the vulvar lymphatics to the inguinal nodes. A more detailed description of the vulvar lymphatics is presented later (p. 819). Last, vaginal innervation comes from inferior extensions of the uterovaginal plexus, a component of the inferior hypogastric plexus (see Fig. 38-13).

■ Lower Urinary Tract Structures

Bladder

Anteriorly, the bladder rests against the inner surface of the pubic bones and then, as it fills, also against the anterior abdominal wall (Fig. 38-19). Posteriorly, it rests against the vagina and cervix. Anteroinferiorly and laterally, the bladder contacts the loose connective and fatty tissue that fills the retropubic space, and here, the bladder lacks a peritoneal covering. The reflection of the bladder onto the abdominal wall is triangular, and the triangle apex is continuous with the median umbilical ligament.

The bladder wall consists of coarse bundles of smooth muscle known as the *detrusor muscle*, which extends into the upper part of the urethra (Fig. 23-1, p. 514). The mucosa of the bladder consists of transitional epithelium and underlying lamina propria. A submucosal layer intervenes between this mucosa and the detrusor muscle.

The bladder is divided into a *body* (dome) and a *fundus* (base) approximately at the level of the ureteric orifices. The dome is thin walled and distensible, whereas the base is thicker and undergoes less distention during filling (see Fig. 38-15). The bladder base consists of the *vesical trigone* and the *detrusor loops*. These loops are two U-shaped bands of fibers found at the

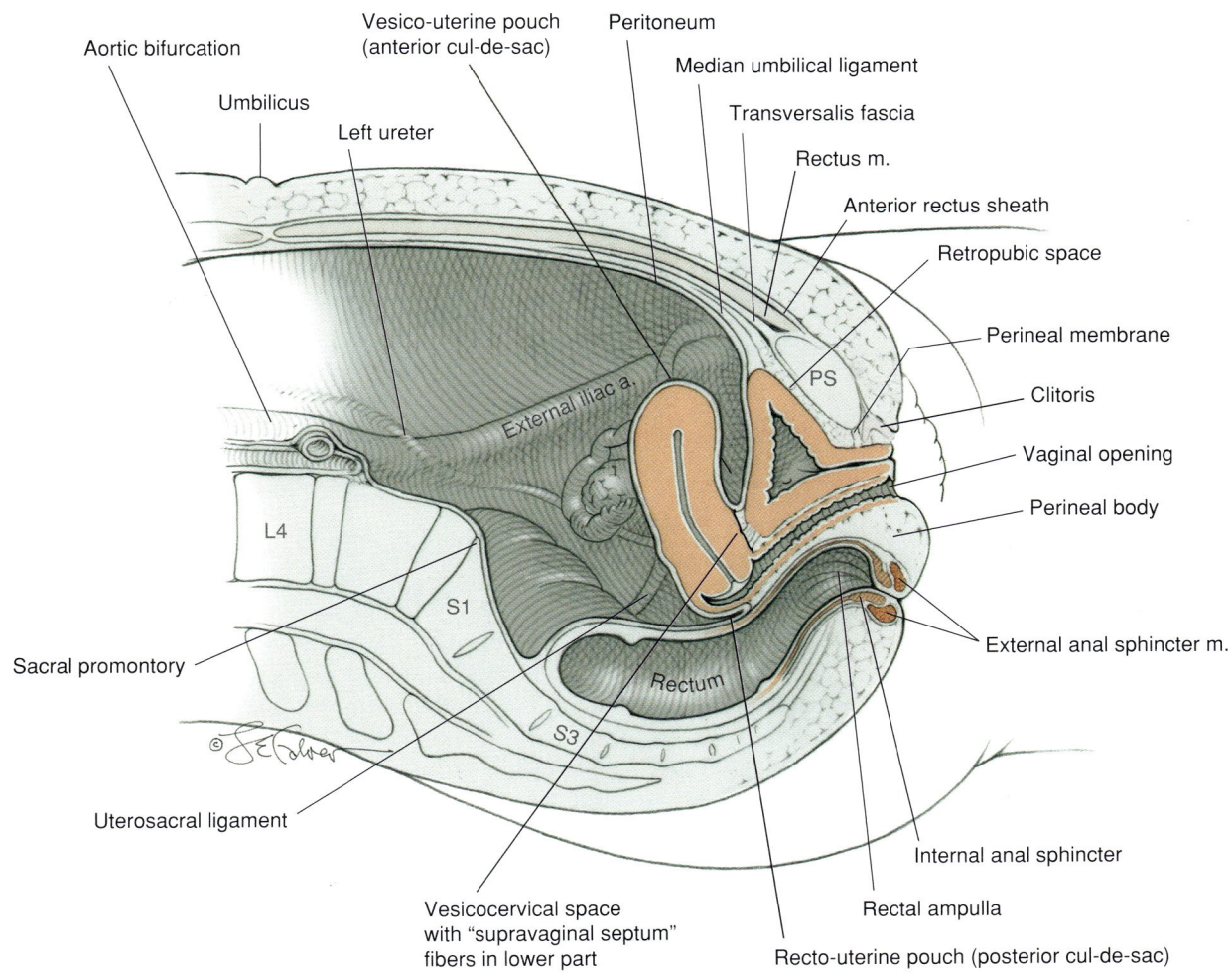

Aortic bifurcation
Umbilicus
Vesico-uterine pouch (anterior cul-de-sac)
Left ureter
Peritoneum
Median umbilical ligament
Transversalis fascia
Rectus m.
Anterior rectus sheath
Retropubic space
Perineal membrane
Clitoris
Vaginal opening
Perineal body
External iliac a.
PS
L4
S1
Sacral promontory
Rectum
S3
External anal sphincter m.
Internal anal sphincter
Rectal ampulla
Recto-uterine pouch (posterior cul-de-sac)
Vesicocervical space with "supravaginal septum" fibers in lower part
Uterosacral ligament

FIGURE 38-19 Midsagittal view of pelvic structures and associated anatomy. L4 = fourth lumbar vertebra; PS = pubic symphysis; S1, S3 = first and third sacral vertebrae.

vesical neck, where the urethra enters the bladder wall. Ureteric orifices lie within the trigone and empty here into the bladder. The pelvic ureter courses in the pelvic sidewall retroperitoneum and is discussed later (p. 811).

The blood supply to the bladder arises from the superior vesical arteries. Other contributors are the middle and inferior vesical arteries, which, when present, often arise from either the internal pudendal or the vaginal arteries (see Fig. 38-12). The nerve supply to the bladder arises from the vesical plexus, a component of the inferior hypogastric plexus (see Fig. 38-13).

Urethra

The female urethra is 3 to 4 cm long. Its proximal lumen begins at the internal urethral orifice (meatus) within the bladder. The urethra then courses through the bladder base for less than a centimeter, and this region is called the *bladder neck*. The distal two thirds of the urethra are fused with the anterior vaginal wall.

The walls of the urethra begin outside the bladder wall. They consist of two layers of smooth muscle, an inner longitudinal and an outer circular, which are in turn surrounded by a circular layer of skeletal muscle referred to as the *sphincter urethrae* or *rhabdosphincter* (Fig. 38-20). Approximately at the junction of the

middle and lower third of the urethra, and just above or deep to the perineal membrane, two strap skeletal muscles called the *sphincter urethrovaginalis* and *compressor urethrae* are found. These muscles were previously known as the *deep transverse perineal muscles* in females. Together with the sphincter urethrae, they constitute the *striated urogenital sphincter complex.* Together, these three muscles function as a unit and have an intricate innervation that is not universally agreed upon. This complex supplies constant tonus and provides emergency reflex activity mainly in the distal half of the urethra to sustain continence.

Distal to the depth of the perineal membrane, the walls of the urethra consist of fibrous tissue, serving as the nozzle that directs the urine stream. The urethra has a prominent submucosal layer that is lined by hormonally sensitive stratified squamous epithelium (Fig. 23-8, p. 518). Within the submucosal layer on the dorsal (vaginal) surface of the urethra is a group of glands known as the paraurethral glands, which open into the urethral lumen (Fig. 26-4, p. 580). Duct openings of the two most prominent glands, termed Skene glands, are seen on the inner surface of the external urethral orifice (p. 814).

The urethra receives its blood supply from branches of the inferior vesical/vaginal and internal pudendal arteries. Although still controversial, the pudendal nerve is believed to innervate

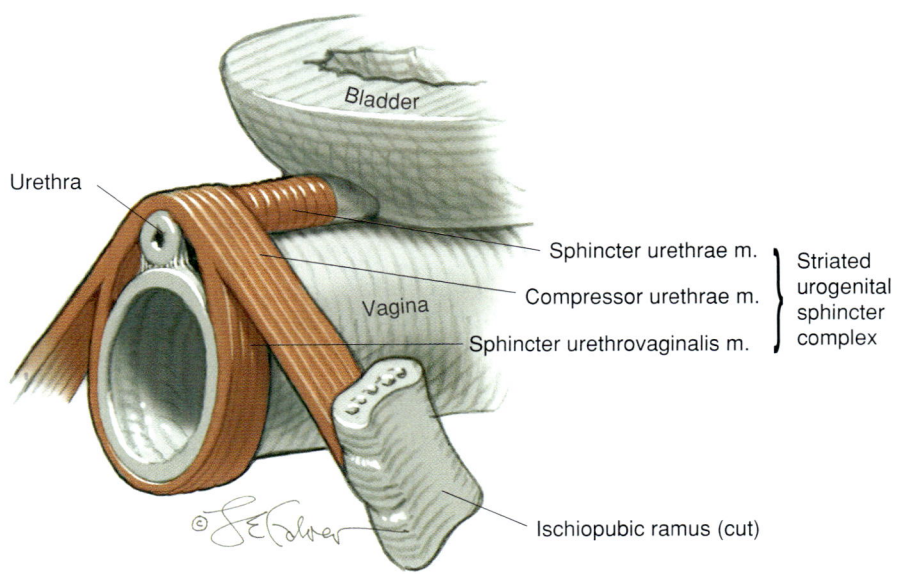

FIGURE 38-20 Urethra and associated muscles.

the most distal part of the striated urogenital sphincter complex. Somatic efferent branches from S2–S4 that course along with the inferior hypogastric plexus variably innervate the sphincter urethrae. An additional discussion of lower urinary tract innervation is found in Chapter 23 (p. 515).

■ Rectum

The rectum is continuous with the sigmoid colon on the anterior surface of the sacrum (see Fig. 38-19). Unlike other portions of the colon, the rectum lacks taeniae coli. It descends on the anterior surface of the sacrum for approximately 12 cm and ends in the anus after passing through the levator hiatus. The posterior surface of the rectum is retroperitoneal. Instead,

the anterior and lateral portions of the proximal two thirds of the rectum are covered by peritoneum. The peritoneum is then reflected onto the posterior vaginal wall to form the *rectouterine pouch.* In women, this cul-de-sac is located approximately 5 to 6 cm from the anal orifice and can be palpated manually during rectal or vaginal examination. At its commencement, the rectal wall is similar to that of the sigmoid. But, near its termination, it dilates to form the rectal ampulla, which begins below the posterior cul-de-sac peritoneal fold.

The rectum lumen contains several, usually three, transverse folds that contain a mucosa, submucosa, and circular layers of the bowel walls. These are called the *transverse folds of rectum,* also termed valves of Houston (Fig. 38-21). The largest and most constant of these folds is located anteriorly and to the right, approximately 8 cm from the anal orifice. Clinically, in the empty state, the transverse rectal folds overlap. As such, these folds may contribute to fecal continence by supporting fecal matter above the anal canal. At the distal rectum, the anorectal junction is bent at an angle of approximately 90 degrees by the anterior pulling action of the puborectalis muscle.

■ Anus

Below the anorectal junction, the gut extends as the anus, which has a series of anal valves to aid its closure. At their lower border is the pectinate (dentate) line. Here, the mucosa of the colon

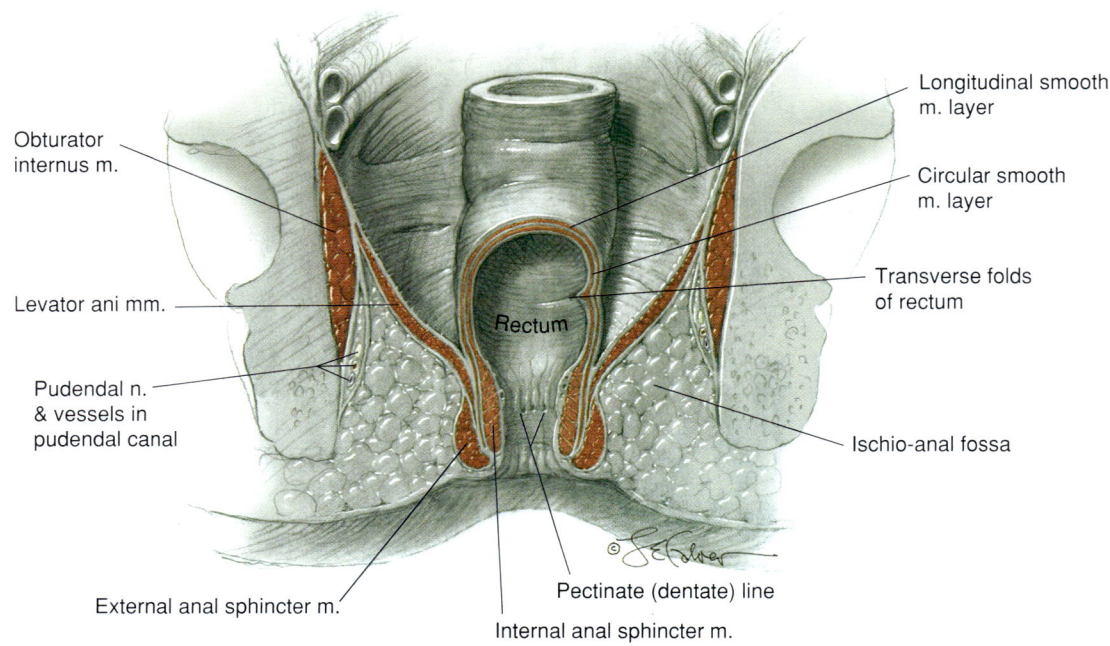

FIGURE 38-21 Ischioanal fossa and anal sphincter complex.

gives way to a transitional layer of non–hair-bearing squamous epithelium before becoming the hair-bearing perineal skin at the anocutaneous line.

The relations of the rectum and anus can be inferred from their course. They lie against the sacrum and levator plate posteriorly and against the vagina anteriorly. Inferiorly, each half of the levator ani abuts the anus's lateral wall and sends fibers to mingle with the longitudinal involuntary fibers between the internal and external anal sphincters (p. 810). Its distal portion is surrounded by the external anal sphincter.

The anorectum receives blood from several sources. The proximal rectum is served by the superior rectal branch of the inferior mesenteric artery (Fig. 38-12). Next, the rectum and ampulla above the pelvic floor receive a direct branch from the middle rectal, a branch of the internal iliac artery. Last, the anus and external sphincter receive blood from the inferior rectal branch of the internal pudendal artery (p. 818). This branch reaches the end of the gastrointestinal tract through the ischio-anal fossa.

EXTRAPERITONEAL SURGICAL SPACES

◼ Pelvic Sidewall

Several extraperitoneal spaces are important for the pelvic surgeon. Of these, the retroperitoneal space of the pelvic sidewalls contains the internal iliac vessels and pelvic lymphatics, pelvic ureter, and obturator nerve. During surgery, entering the retroperitoneum at the pelvic sidewall can be used to identify the ureter (Fig. 38-22).

The major pelvic vessels are shown in Figures 38-12, 38-14, and 38-22. The internal iliac and external iliac vessels and their corresponding lymph node groups lie within the pelvic sidewall retroperitoneal space (see Fig. 38-16).

Pelvic Ureter

As the ureter enters the pelvis, it crosses over the bifurcation of the common iliac artery or the proximal portion of the external iliac artery and passes just medial to the ovarian vessels (see Fig. 38-15). In the pelvis, it lies in a special connective tissue sheath that is attached to the peritoneum of the lateral pelvic wall and "medial leaf" of the broad ligament. This explains why the ureter remains adhered to the peritoneum and moves with it when the retroperitoneal space is entered. Along this course, the ureter lies medial to the internal iliac branches and lateral and ventral to the uterosacral ligaments (see Figs. 38-14, 38-15, and 38-22).

After passing under the uterine artery ("water under the bridge") near the level of the uterine isthmus, the ureter enters the parametrium. It lies approximately 1 to 2 cm lateral to the cervix and courses within a "ureteral tunnel" surrounded by loose areolar tissue that allows for its peristalsis. Within this tunnel, the ureter roughly separates the anterior fibers of the cardinal ligament from the posterior fibers of the uterosacral ligament. The ureter then travels anteromedially toward the bladder base (see Fig. 38-15). In this path, it runs close to the proximal third of the anterior vaginal wall (Rahn, 2007; Jackson, 2019). Finally, the ureter courses obliquely within the bladder wall for approximately 1.5 cm to terminate at the ureteric orifices.

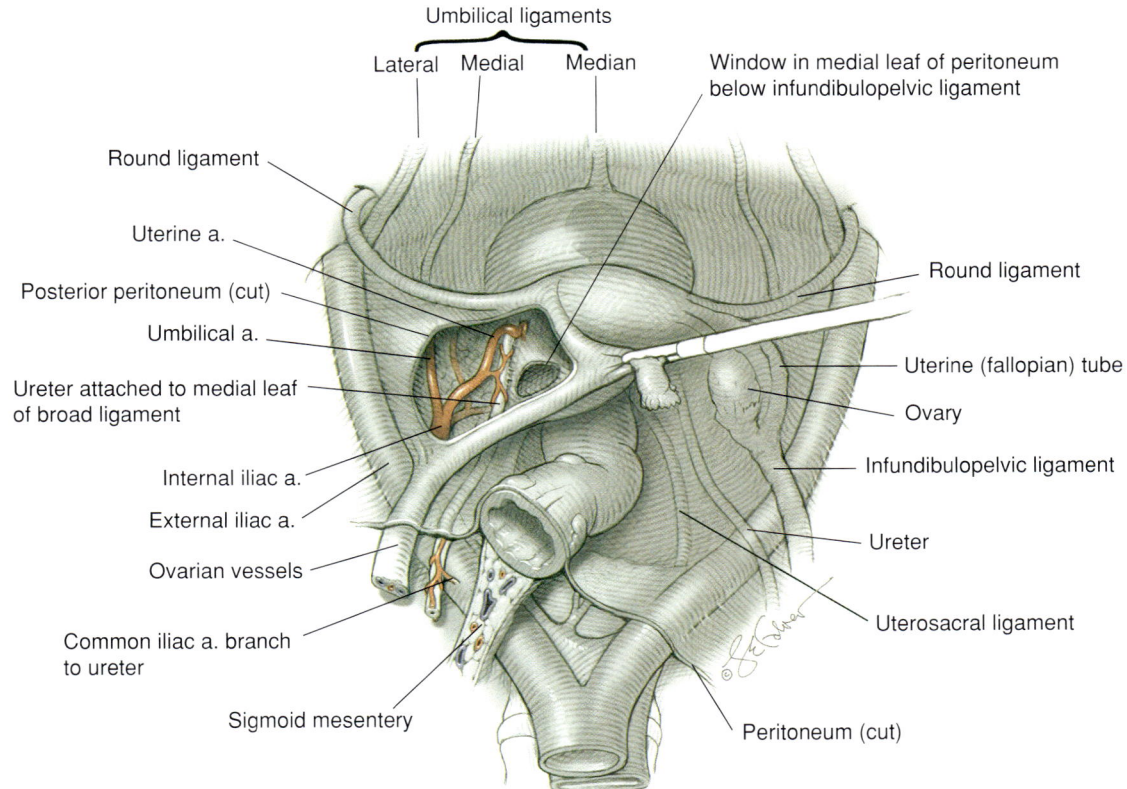

Umbilical ligaments
Lateral Medial Median

Window in medial leaf of peritoneum below infundibulopelvic ligament

Round ligament

Uterine a.

Posterior peritoneum (cut)

Umbilical a.

Ureter attached to medial leaf of broad ligament

Internal iliac a.

External iliac a.

Ovarian vessels

Common iliac a. branch to ureter

Sigmoid mesentery

Round ligament

Uterine (fallopian) tube

Ovary

Infundibulopelvic ligament

Ureter

Uterosacral ligament

Peritoneum (cut)

FIGURE 38-22 Surgical view of left pelvic sidewall retroperitoneal space showing the ureter attached to medial leaf of broad ligament.

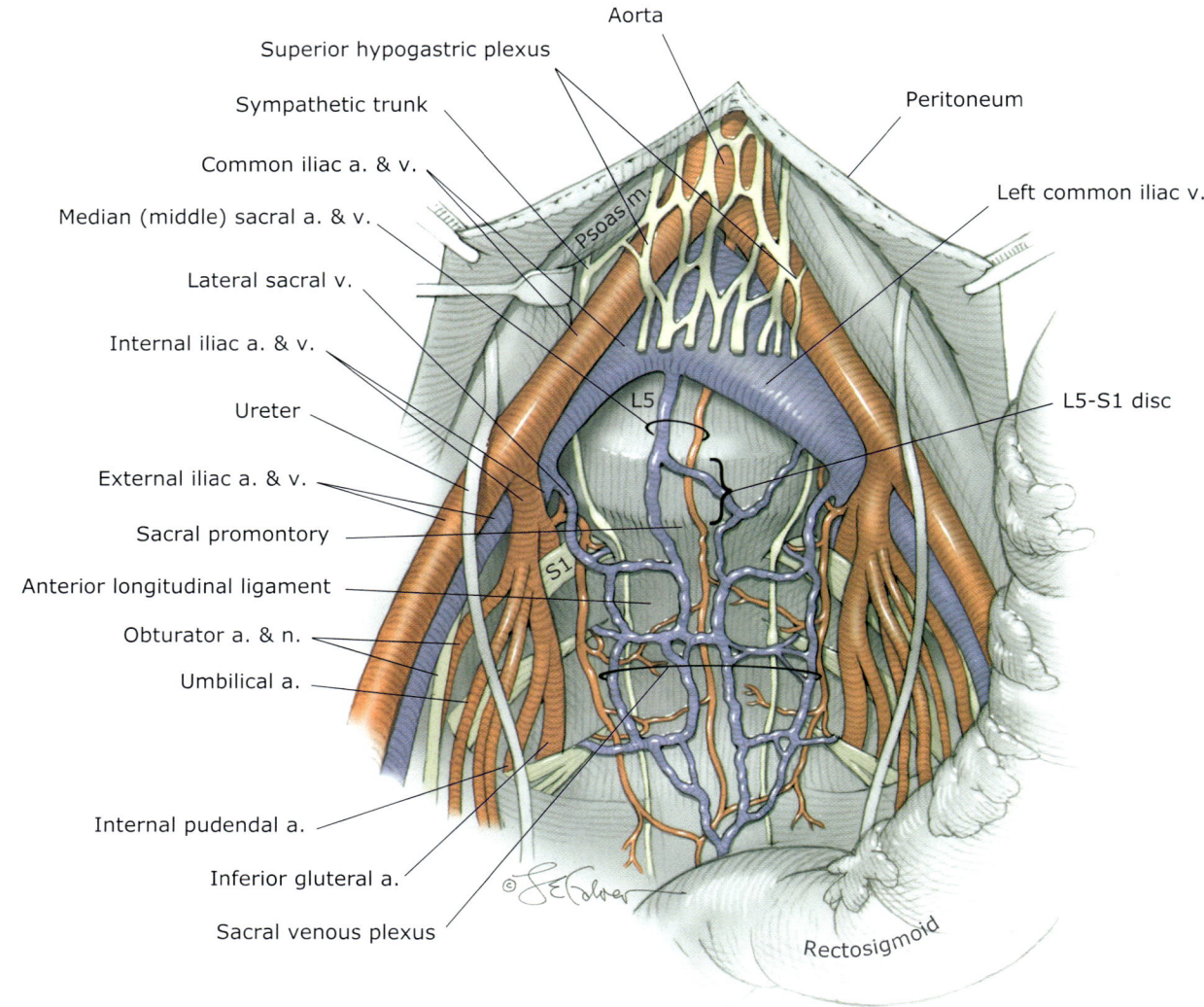

FIGURE 38-23 Presacral space. L5 = fifth lumbar vertebra; S1 = first sacral nerve.

The pelvic ureter receives blood supply from the vessels it passes: the common iliac, internal iliac, uterine, and superior vesical vessels. The ureter's course runs medial to these vessels, and thus its blood supply reaches the ureter from lateral sources. This is important during ureteral isolation to avoid its devascularization. In contrast, the abdominal part of the ureter courses lateral to major vessels and, accordingly, it receives most of its blood supply from medially located vessels. Vascular anastomoses on the connective tissue sheath enveloping the ureter form a longitudinal network of vessels. Nerve supply to the pelvic ureter stems from the pelvic autonomic nerve plexuses.

■ Presacral Space

This retroperitoneal space lies between the rectosigmoid/posterior abdominal wall peritoneum and the sacrum (Figs. 38-18 and 38-23). It begins below the aortic bifurcation and extends inferiorly to the pelvic floor. Laterally, this space is bounded by the common and internal iliac vessels and branches and by the fascia that covers the piriformis muscle and sacral nerves. Contained within the loose areolar and connective tissue of this

space are the superior hypogastric plexus, hypogastric nerves, and portions of the inferior hypogastric plexus (see Figs. 38-14 and 38-23). The sacral lymph node group also is found here (see Fig. 38-16). In addition, the sacral sympathetic trunk, a continuation of the lumbar trunk, lies against the sacrum's ventral surface and anteromedial to the sacral foramina.

The presacral space contains an extensive and intricate venous plexus, termed the *sacral venous plexus*. This plexus is formed primarily by the anastomoses of the middle and lateral sacral veins on the anterior surface of the sacrum. The *middle sacral vein* commonly drains from this plexus into the left common iliac vein, whereas each *lateral sacral vein* opens into its respective internal iliac vein. Ultimately, these vessels drain into the caval system. The sacral venous plexus also receives contributions from the *lumbar veins* of the posterior abdominal wall and from the *basivertebral veins* that pass through the pelvic sacral foramina. The *middle sacral artery*, which courses in proximity to the *middle sacral vein*, arises from the posterior and distal part of the abdominal aorta.

In studies of presacral space anatomy, the left common iliac vein was the closest major vessel identified both cephalad and

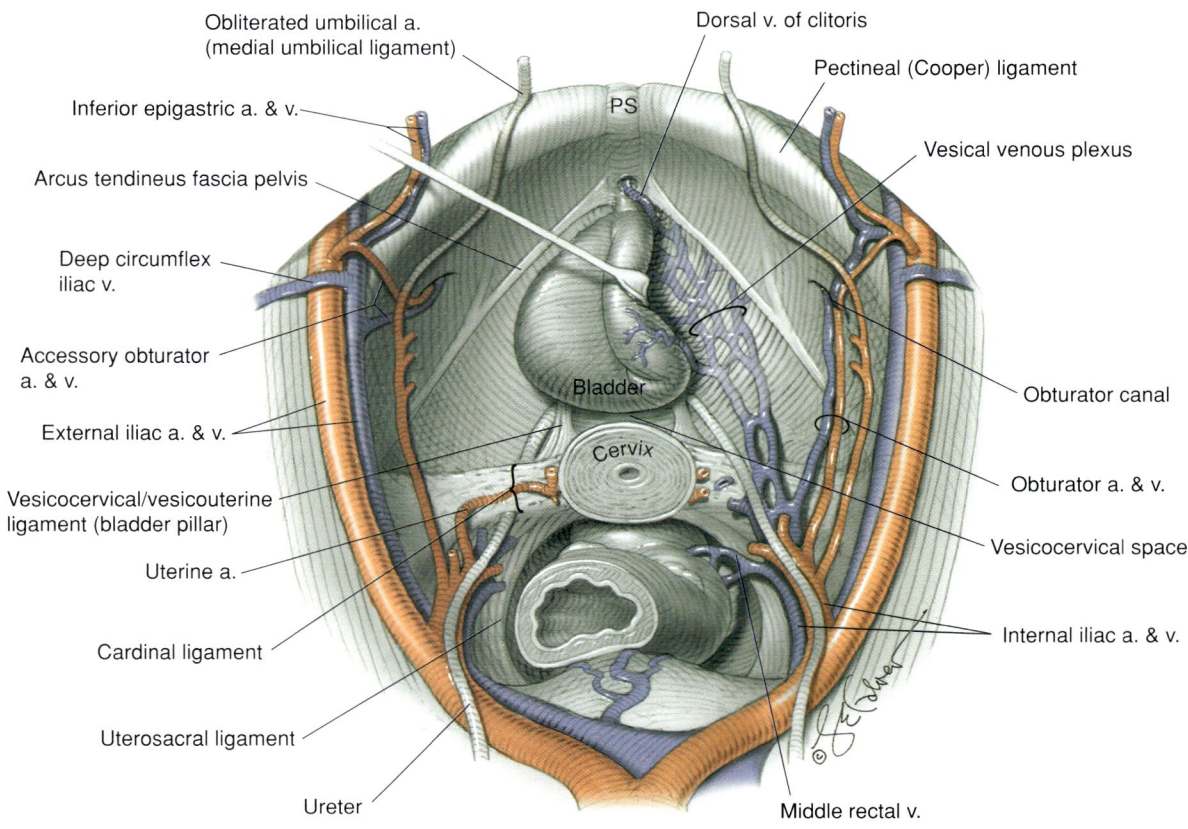

Obliterated umbilical a. (medial umbilical ligament)

Inferior epigastric a. & v.

Arcus tendineus fascia pelvis

Deep circumflex iliac v.

Accessory obturator a. & v.

External iliac a. & v.

Vesicocervical/vesicouterine ligament (bladder pillar)

Uterine a.

Cardinal ligament

Uterosacral ligament

Ureter

Dorsal v. of clitoris

Pectineal (Cooper) ligament

PS

Vesical venous plexus

Bladder

Cervix

Obturator canal

Obturator a. & v.

Vesicocervical space

Internal iliac a. & v.

Middle rectal v.

FIGURE 38-24 Retropubic space. PS = pubic symphysis.

lateral to the midsacral promontory. The average distance of the left common iliac vein from the midsacral promontory is 2.7 cm (range 0.9 to 5.2 cm) (Good, 2013b; Wieslander, 2006). Moreover, the first sacral nerve can be expected approximately 3 cm from the upper surface of the sacrum and 1.5 cm from the midline (Good, 2013b; Florian-Rodriguez, 2017). In supine women, the most prominent nonvascular presacral space structure is the L5–S1 disc, which extends approximately 1.5 cm cephalad to the "true" sacral promontory (Good, 2013a). Awareness of a 60-degree average drop between the anterior surfaces of L5 and S1 vertebrae assists intraoperative localization of the promontory.

■ Retropubic Space

Also called the *prevesical space* or *space of Retzius*, this is a potential surgical space filled with loose connective tissue that contains important neurovascular structures. The retropubic space is bounded by the bony pelvis and muscles of the pelvic wall anteriorly and laterally and by the anterior abdominal wall ventrally (Figs. 38-18, 38-19, and 38-24). The bladder and proximal urethra lie posteriorly within this space. The posterolateral limit of this space is the attachment of the bladder to the cardinal ligament and the attachment of the paravaginal tissue to the arcus tendineus fascia pelvis. These attachments separate this space from the vesicovaginal and vesicocervical spaces, described earlier (p. 808).

Several vessels and nerves are found in this space. The *dorsal vein of the clitoris* passes under the inferior border of the pubic symphysis and drains into the *vesical venous plexus*, also called the *plexus of Santorini* (Pathi, 2009). This plexus drains into the internal iliac veins. Also in this space, the inferior hypogastric plexus nerve fibers that supply the bladder, urethra, and erectile structures in the perineum run on the lateral borders of bladder and urethra. The *obturator neurovascular bundle* courses along the lateral pelvic walls and enters the obturator canal to reach the medial compartment of the thigh. Additionally, in most women, accessory obturator vessels that arise from or open into the inferior epigastric or external iliac vessels are found crossing the superior pubic rami and connecting with the obturator vessels near the each obturator canal. Clinically, the obliterated umbilical or the superior vesical arteries are used to describe the medial boundary of the clinical paravesical space.

VULVA AND PERINEUM

■ Pudendum/Vulva

The external female genitalia, collectively known as the *vulva*, lie on the pubic bones and extend posteriorly. Components of the vulva are found on the anterior perineal triangle, discussed on page 815. Structures include the mons pubis, labia majora and minora, clitoris, vestibule, vestibular bulbs, greater vestibular glands (Bartholin glands), lesser vestibular glands, Skene and paraurethral glands, and the urethral and vaginal orifices (Fig. 38-25).

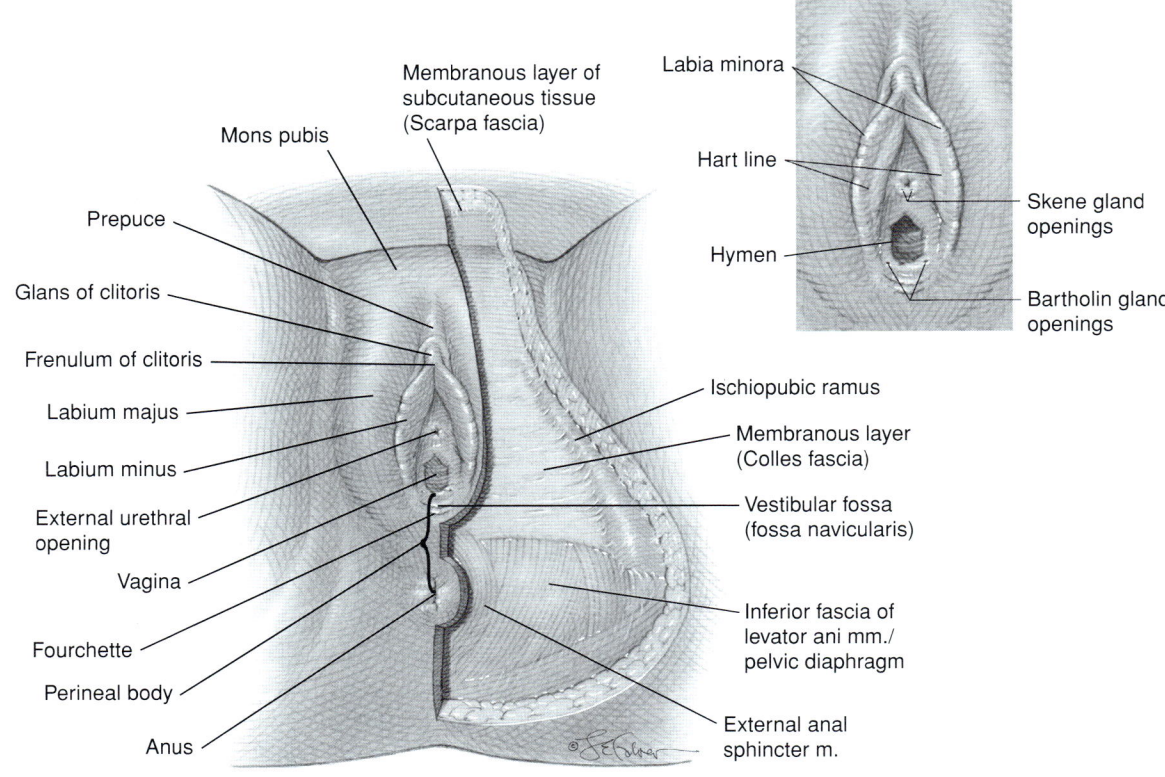

FIGURE 38-25 Vulvar structures and subcutaneous layer of anterior perineal triangle. Note the continuity of Colles and Scarpa fasciae. Inset: Vestibule boundaries and openings onto vestibule.

Mons Pubis and Labia Majora

The *mons pubis*, also called the *mons veneris*, is the rounded fat pad that lies ventral to the pubic bones. The labia majora are two prominent folds that extend from the mons pubis toward the perineal body posteriorly. Between the mons and the pudendal cleft, which is the space between separated labia majora, each labium majus join to form the anterior commissure of the labia majora. The posterior commissure represents the anterior or upper part of the skin covering the perineal body. Skin over the mons pubis and labia majora contains hair and has a subcutaneous tissue layer similar to that of the anterior abdominal wall. The subcutaneous layer contains a superficial *fatty layer of subcutaneous tissue*, which is similar to and continuous with the fatty layer of the anterior abdominal wall (Camper fascia). In the deeper part of the subcutaneous layer, there is less fat, and interconnecting fibrous connective tissue septa predominate. As it is in the abdomen, this more fibrous layer is called the *membranous layer of subcutaneous tissue* (Colles fascia). It is similar and continuous with the membranous layer of the abdominal wall (Scarpa fascia) (see Fig. 38-25). The round ligament and obliterated processus vaginalis, which is also termed the *canal of Nuck*, exit the inguinal canal and attach to the subcutaneous layer or skin of the labium majus.

Labia Minora

These two cutaneous folds lie between the labia majora (see Fig. 38-25). Posteriorly, the labia minora join in the midline to form the *frenulum of labia minora* or *fourchette*. Anteriorly, each labium minus bifurcates to form two folds that surround the

glans of the clitoris. The more anterior folds unite to form the distal end of the prepuce, which partially or completely covers the glans of clitoris and is often referred to as the hood of the clitoris. The more posterior folds insert into the underside of the glans as the *frenulum of clitoris*.

In contrast to the skin that overlies the labia majora, the skin of the labia minora lacks hair. Also, the subcutaneous tissue is devoid of fat and consists primarily of relatively dense connective tissue with interspersed nerves and small blood vessels. These attributes allows mobility of the skin during coitus and accounts for the ease of dissection with vulvectomy.

Vaginal Vestibule

This area lies between the two labia minora and is bounded laterally by the line of Hart and medially by the hymeneal ring. The Hart line represents the demarcation between the skin and mucous membrane on the inner surface of the labia minora. The vestibule extends from the clitoris anteriorly to the fourchette posteriorly (see Fig. 38-25 inset). It contains the openings of the urethra; vagina; greater vestibular glands, also known as Bartholin glands; and Skene glands, which are the largest pair of paraurethral glands. It also contains the numerous openings of the lesser vestibular glands. A shallow vestibular depression known as the vestibular (navicular) fossa lies between the vaginal orifice and the fourchette.

■ Perineum

The *perineum* is the diamond-shaped area between the thighs (see Fig. 38-25). It is bounded deeply by the inferior fascia of

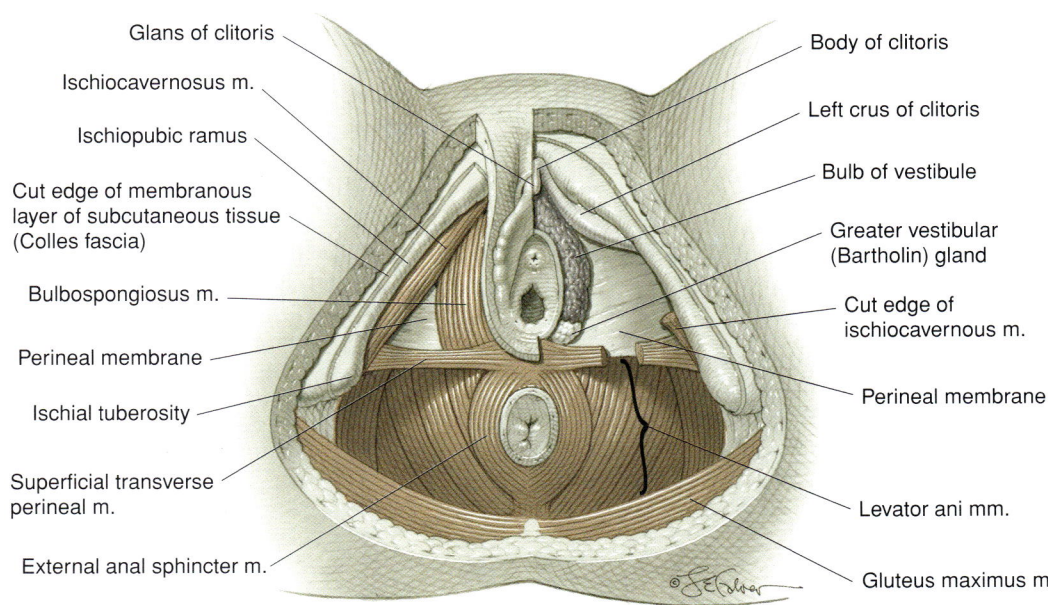

Glans of clitoris
Ischiocavernosus m.
Ischiopubic ramus
Cut edge of membranous
layer of subcutaneous tissue
(Colles fascia)
Bulbospongiosus m.
Perineal membrane
Ischial tuberosity
Superficial transverse
perineal m.
External anal sphincter m.

Body of clitoris
Left crus of clitoris
Bulb of vestibule
Greater vestibular
(Bartholin) gland
Cut edge of
ischiocavernous m.
Perineal membrane
Levator ani mm.
Gluteus maximus m.

FIGURE 38-26 Anterior (superficial space of anterior triangle) and posterior perineal triangles. On the image's left are the structures noted after removal of Colles fascia. On the image's right are the structures noted after removal of the superficial perineal muscles.

the pelvic diaphragm and superficially by the skin between the thighs. The anterior, posterior, and lateral boundaries of the perineum are the same as those of the bony pelvic outlet: the pubic symphysis anteriorly, ischiopubic rami and ischial tuberosities anterolaterally, coccyx posteriorly, and sacrotuberous ligaments posterolaterally. An arbitrary line joining the ischial tuberosities divides the perineum into the anterior or *urogenital triangle*, and a posterior or *anal triangle*.

Anterior (Urogenital) Triangle

Structures that comprise the vulva or external female genitalia lie in the anterior triangle of the perineum. The base or posterior border of this triangle is the *interischial line*, an arbitrary line drawn between the two ischial tuberosities. This line usually overlies the *superficial transverse perineal muscles* (Fig. 38-26). The anterior perineal triangle can be further divided into *subcutaneous*, *superficial*, and *deep pouches* (also called compartments or spaces), described next.

Subcutaneous Pouch

This is a potential space between the membranous layer of subcutaneous tissue on the perineum (Colles fascia) and the superficial layer of the fascia that invests the perineal muscles. Extravasations or collections in this pouch may track deep to the membranous layer of the perineum and into the abdominal wall or into the labia majora.

Superficial Pouch

This space of the anterior triangle is a fully enclosed compartment that lies between the perineal membrane and the superficial layer of fascia that invests the perineal muscles (see Figs. 38-25 and 38-26). These muscles are the ischiocavernosus, bulbospongiosus, and superficial transverse. Other contents are the Bartholin glands, the vestibular bulbs, the clitoris, and

branches of the pudendal vessels and nerve. The urethra and vagina traverse this space.

Both the membranous layer of subcutaneous tissue and the perineal membrane attach firmly to the ischiopubic rami laterally and to each other posteriorly. Furthermore, the perineal membrane has firm medial attachments to the urethra, vagina—at level of the hymen—and to the perineal body. The membranous layer of subcutaneous tissue has midline attachments to vestibular structures. These medial, lateral, and posterior attachments prevent the spread of fluid, blood, or infection from the subcutaneous perineal pouch to the thighs, posterior perineal triangle, or contralateral side. However, anteriorly, the membranous layer has no attachments to the pubic rami, and this permits communication between the area deep to this layer and the abdominal wall. This continuity may allow the spread of fluid, blood, and infection between these compartments.

Vestibular Bulbs. These are two elongated, approximately 3- to 5-cm long, richly vascular erectile masses that surround the vaginal vestibule (see Fig. 38-26). Their posterior ends contact the Bartholin glands. Their anterior ends are joined to one another and to the clitoris at the commissure of these bulbs. Their deep surfaces abut the perineal membrane, and their superficial surfaces are partially covered by the bulbospongiosus muscles.

Bartholin Glands. These glands are covered superficially by the bulbospongiosus muscle. Additionally, they contact and are often overlapped by the posterior ends of the vestibular bulbs (see Fig. 38-26). Each gland is connected to the vestibule by an approximately 2-cm-long duct. The ducts open in the groove between the hymen and the labia minora—the vestibule—at approximately 5 and 7 o'clock positions.

The glands contain columnar cells that secrete clear or white mucus with lubricant properties. These glands are stimulated by sexual arousal.

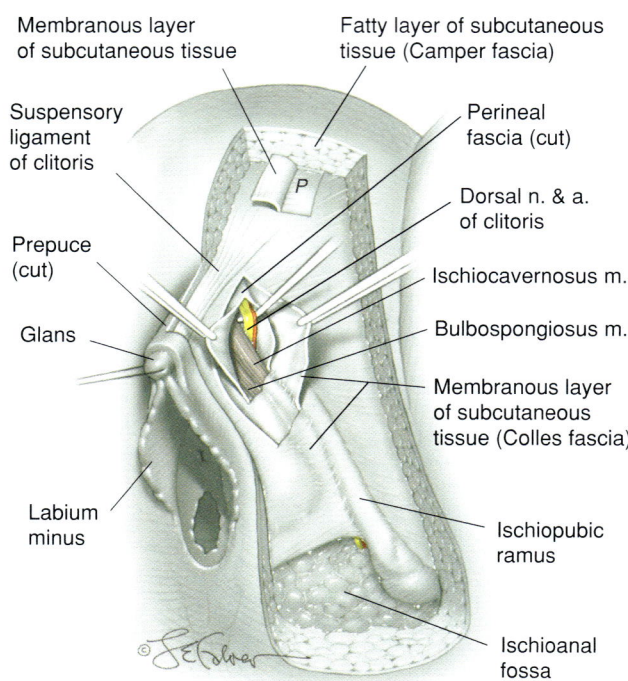

FIGURE 38-27 Dorsal nerve and artery of clitoris emerging between crus and ischiopubic ramus. The relationships of the subcutaneous connective tissue layers relative to the clitoris, dorsal nerve and artery, and superficial perineal muscles are shown. P = pubic bones.

Clitoris and Associated Structures. The clitoris is a complex erectile and highly sensitive organ, which is homologous to the penis. It is comprised of a midline body, distal glans, and paired crura (Figs. 38-27 and 38-28). The body lies on, and is suspended from, the pubic bones by the suspensory and fundiform ligaments

of the clitoris. The *fundiform ligament of clitoris* represents the fibrous condensation of the subcutaneous tissue that descends from the linea alba above the pubic symphysis. It splits and surrounds the body of the clitoris, before fusing with the fascia of the clitoris. The *suspensory ligament of the clitoris* is a more superficial condensation of membranous subcutaneous tissue. Together, these ligaments support and position the clitoral body.

The paired crura of the clitoris bend downward from the body. The pair extends posteriorly and firmly attaches to the medial aspects of each ischiopubic ramus. They join in midline to form the body of the clitoris.

The body of the clitoris consists of paired corpora cavernosa, separated in midline by a fibrous septum called the septum of corpora cavernosa. Both the corpora cavernosa and the paired crura are invested by a dense fibroconnective tissue layer called the tunica albuginea, and both are composed of relatively dense erectile tissue. The dorsal nerve and vessels of clitoris, discussed later, lie outside the tunica albuginea but within the clitoral fascia. This fascia is continuous with the fundiform ligament and deep portion of the suspensory ligament of clitoris.

The glans of clitoris is covered by a thinly keratinized stratified squamous epithelium (see Fig. 38-28). Internally, the glans contains relatively dense fibrous connective tissue with interspersed small blood vessels but lacks erectile tissue. Nerve bundles are prominent and show a paired distribution that corresponds to the paired dorsal nerves of the clitoris (Jackson, 2019). Although great variation exists, the body measures approximately 2 to 3 cm long. The glans is 0.5 to 1 cm long and 0.4 to 1 cm wide.

Superficial Space Muscles. The *ischiocavernosus muscles* attach to the medial aspect of the ischial tuberosities posteriorly and the ischiopubic rami laterally. Anteriorly, they attach to the

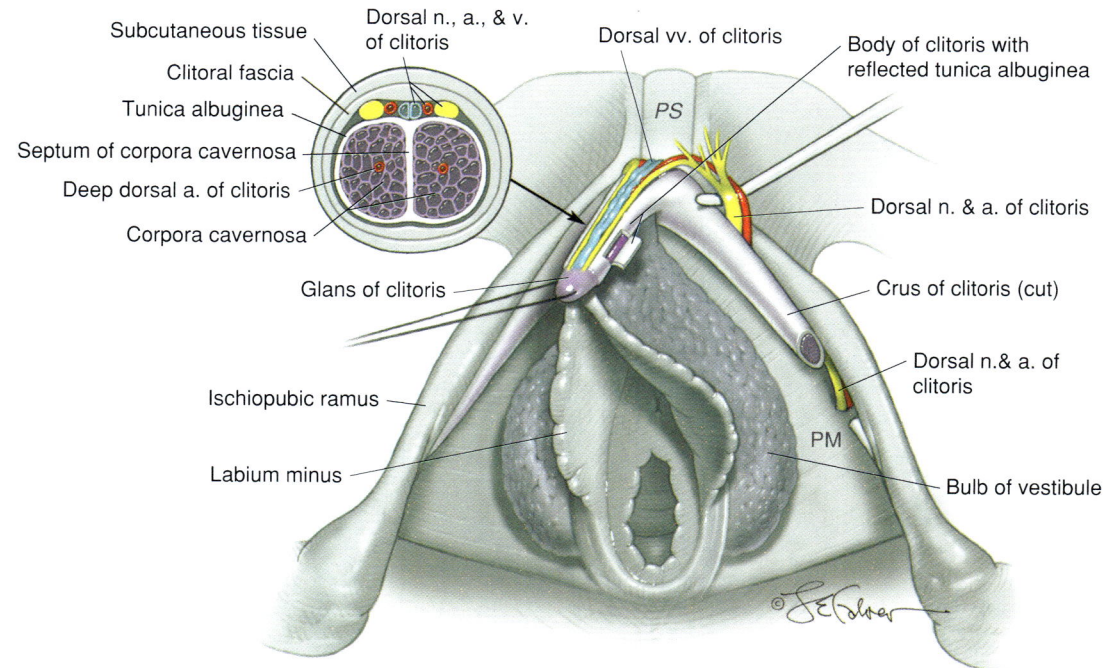

FIGURE 38-28 Clitoris and associated vulvar structures in superficial space of anterior perineal triangle. Inset: cross section through proximal body of clitoris. PM = perineal membrane; PS = pubic symphysis.

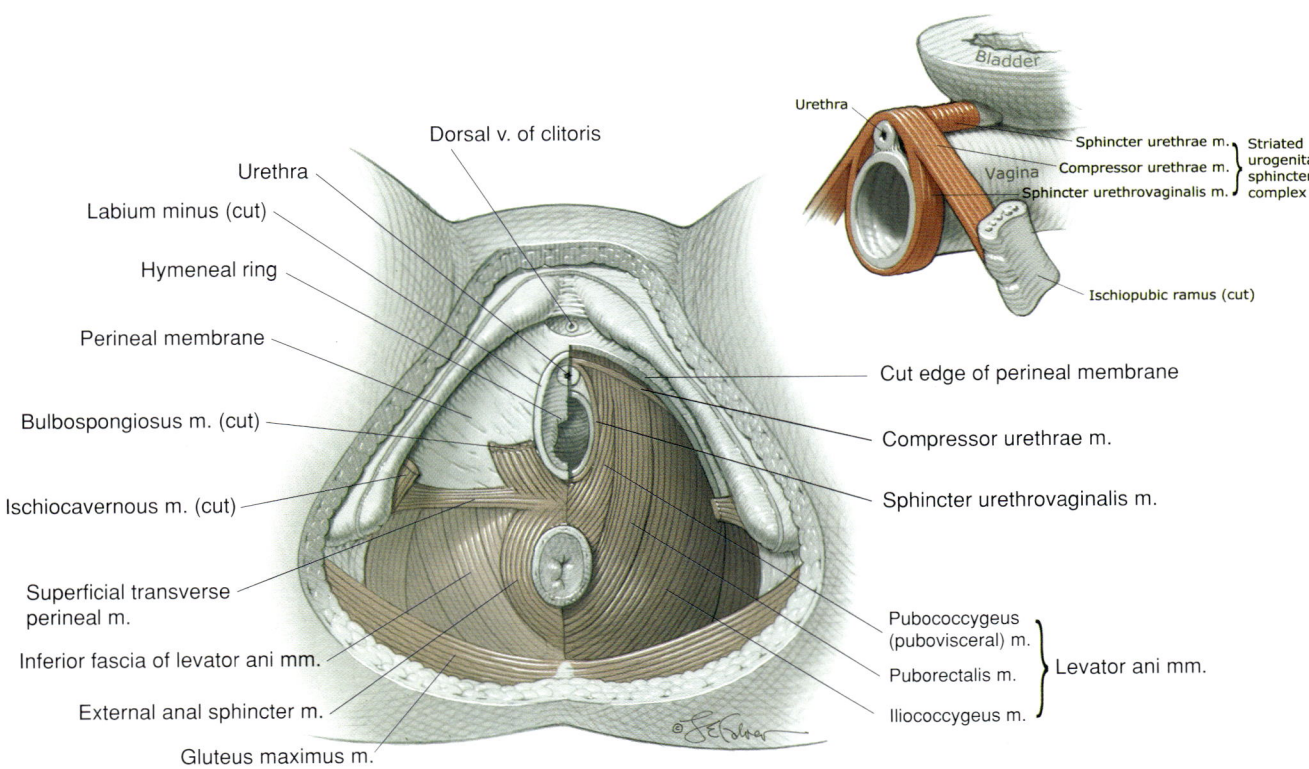

FIGURE 38-29 Deep space of anterior perineal triangle. On the image's right lie structures noted after removal of the perineal membrane. Inset: Striated urogenital sphincter muscles. Also shown are all structures that attach to perineal body: bulbospongiosus, superficial transverse perineal, external anal sphincter, and puboperinealis muscles, perineal membrane, and sphincter urethrovaginalis muscle.

crura and often to the body of the clitoris. These muscles may help maintain clitoral erection by compressing the crura of the clitoris, thus retarding venous drainage.

The *bulbospongiosus muscles* cover the superficial portion of the vestibular bulbs and Bartholin glands. The muscles act to constrict these, thereby contributing to the release of Bartholin gland secretions. These muscles attach to the body of the clitoris anteriorly and the perineal body posteriorly. They may also contribute to clitoral erection by compressing the deep dorsal vein of the clitoris and vestibular bulbs.

The *superficial transverse perineal muscles* are narrow strips that attach to the ischial tuberosity laterally and the perineal body medially. They may be attenuated or even absent, but when present, they contribute to the perineal body.

Deep Perineal Pouch

This space lies deep or superior to the perineal membrane (Fig. 38-29). In contrast to the superficial space, the deep space is an open space. It contains the compressor urethrae and urethrovaginalis muscles, parts of the urethra and vagina, branches of the internal pudendal artery, and the dorsal nerve and vein of the clitoris. It also contains the anterior recess of the ischio-anal fossa fatty tissue. Hematomas, fluid collections, and infection within this space can thus spread to the posterior perineal triangle (ischio-anal) fossa and to the contralateral side.

Perineal Membrane

The terms *urogenital diaphragm* or *inferior fascia of the urogenital diaphragm* are misnomers and have been replaced by

the anatomically correct term, *perineal membrane* (Federative International Programme on Anatomical Terminolgies, 2011; Oelrich, 1980, 1983). This membrane constitutes the deep boundary of the superficial perineal pouch (see Fig. 38-29). It attaches laterally to the ischiopubic rami, medially to the distal third of the urethra and vagina, and posteriorly to the perineal body. Anteriorly, it attaches to the arcuate ligament of the pubis.

The perineal membrane consists of two histologically and probably functionally distinct portions that span the opening of the anterior pelvic triangle (Stein, 2008). The dorsal or posterior portion is a dense fibrous sheet that attaches laterally to the ischiopubic rami and medially to the distal vagina and perineal body. The ventral or anterior portion of the perineal membrane is intimately associated with the compressor urethrae and sphincter urethrovaginalis muscles (see Fig. 38-29 inset). These muscles are part of the striated urogenital sphincter complex and lie just deep to the membrane (Oelrich, 1983). Moreover, the ventral portion of the perineal membrane is continuous with the insertion of the arcus tendineus fascia pelvis to the pubic bones (see Fig. 38-20). The deep or superior surface of the perineal membrane appears to have direct connections to the levator ani muscles. The superficial or inferior surface of the membrane fuses with the vestibular bulbs and clitoral crura. A midline gap in the anterior portion of the perineal membrane below the pubic symphysis allows passage of the dorsal vein of the clitoris and the cavernous nerves, described later (p. 816) (see Fig. 38-29).

Clinically, the perineal membrane attaches to the lateral walls of the vagina approximately at level of the hymen. It

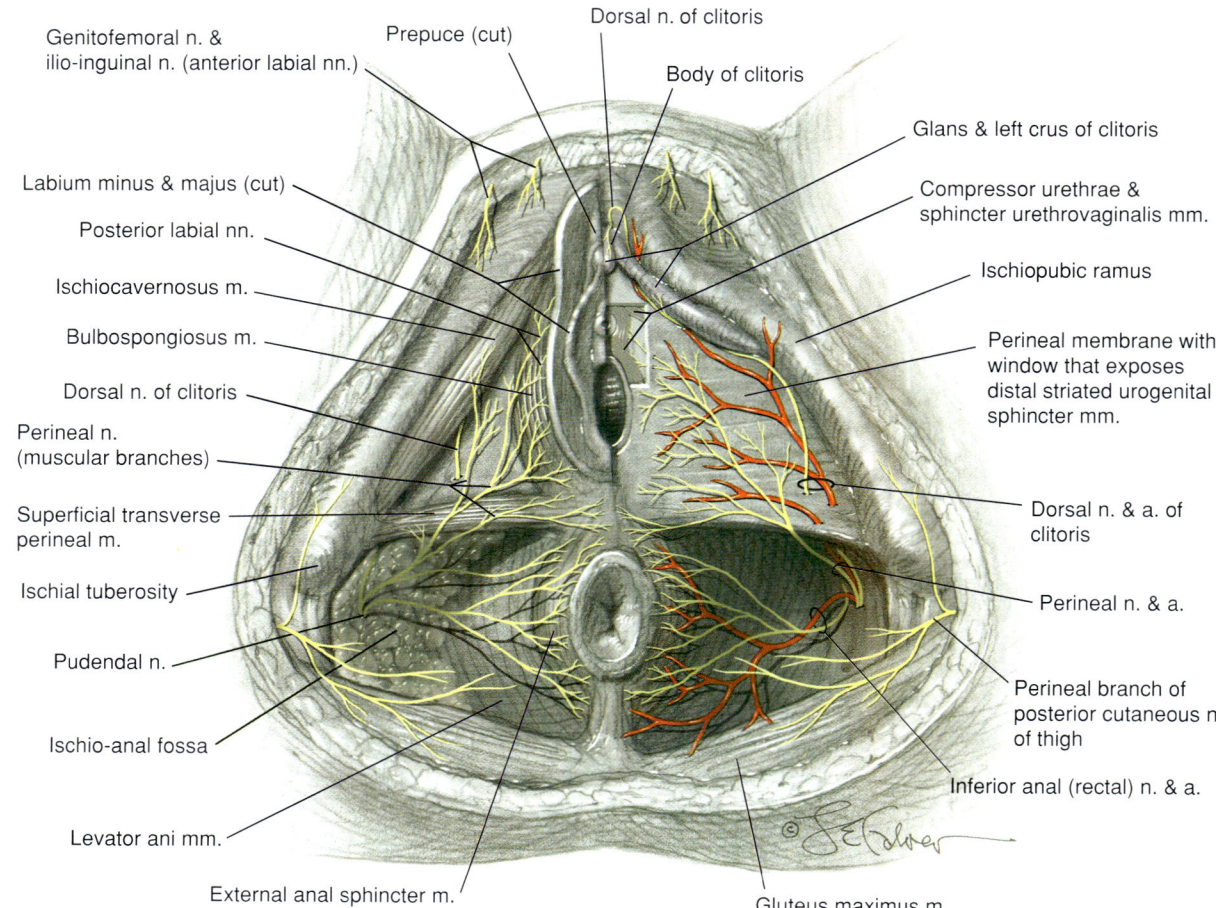

Genitofemoral n. &
ilio-inguinal n. (anterior labial nn.)

Prepuce (cut)

Dorsal n. of clitoris

Body of clitoris

Glans & left crus of clitoris

Labium minus & majus (cut)

Compressor urethrae &
sphincter urethrovaginalis mm.

Posterior labial nn.

Ischiocavernosus m.

Ischiopubic ramus

Bulbospongiosus m.

Perineal membrane with
window that exposes
distal striated urogenital
sphincter mm.

Dorsal n. of clitoris

Perineal n.
(muscular branches)

Superficial transverse
perineal m.

Dorsal n. & a. of
clitoris

Ischial tuberosity

Perineal n. & a.

Pudendal n.

Ischio-anal fossa

Perineal branch of
posterior cutaneous n.
of thigh

Levator ani mm.

Inferior anal (rectal) n. & a.

External anal sphincter m.

Gluteus maximus m.

FIGURE 38-30 Pudendal nerve and vessels. Nerve supply to striated urogenital sphincter and external anal sphincter muscles.

provides support to the distal vagina and urethra by attaching these structures to the bony pelvis. In addition, its attachments to the levator ani muscles suggest that the perineal membrane may play an active role in support.

Posterior (Anal) Triangle

This triangle contains the ischio-anal fossa, anus, anal sphincter complex, and branches of the internal pudendal vessels and pudendal nerve (see Figs. 38-21, 38-29, and 38-30). It is bounded deeply by the fascia overlying the inferior surface of the levator ani muscles, and laterally by the fascia overlying the medial surface of the obturator internus muscles. A splitting of the obturator internus fascia in this area is known as the *pudendal* or *Alcock canal* (see Figs. 38-6 and 38-21). This canal allows passage of the internal pudendal vessels and pudendal nerve before these structures split into terminal branches to supply the structures of the vulva and perineum (see Fig. 38-30).

The *ischio-anal fossa* fills most of the anal triangle (see Figs. 38-21 and 38-30). It contains adipose tissue, vessels, nerves, and the anus and anal sphincter complex. The ischio-anal fossa is bounded superomedially by the inferior fascia of the levator muscles; anterolaterally by the fascia covering the medial surface of the obturator internus muscles and the ischial tuberosities; and posterolaterally by the lower border of the gluteus maximus muscles and sacrotuberous ligaments. At a superficial

level, the ischio-anal fossa is bounded anteriorly by the superficial transverse perineal muscles. At a superior or deeper level, there is no fascial boundary between the fossa and the tissues deep to the perineal membrane. Extension of the fatty tissue into the deep pouch of the perineum is often referred to as the *anterior recess of ischio-anal fossa*. Posterior to the anus, the contents of the fossa are continuous across the midline except for the attachments of the external anal sphincter fibers to the coccyx. This continuity of the ischio-anal fossa across perineal compartments allows fluid, infection, and malignancy to spread from one side of the anus to the other. These may also spread into the anterior perineal compartment but deep to the perineal membrane (deep pouch).

The anal sphincter complex consists of two sphincters and the puborectalis muscle. The external anal sphincter consists of striated muscle that surrounds the distal anal canal. It contains a superficial and a deep portion. The more superficial fibers lie distal to the internal sphincter and are separated from the anal epithelium only by submucosa. The deep fibers blend with the lowest fibers of the puborectalis muscle. Innervated by the inferior anal branch of the pudendal nerve, the external anal sphincter provides the squeeze pressure of the anus.

The internal anal sphincter is the thickening of the circular smooth muscle layer encircling the anal canal (see Figs. 38-19 and 38-21). Under the control of the autonomic nervous system, this muscle contributes approximately 80 percent of the anal canal resting pressure. The internal sphincter lies between the anal mucosa and the external sphincter and extends more than 1 cm above the cranial margin of the external sphincter (DeLancey, 1997). The caudal margin of the internal sphincter lies approximately 3 to 4 mm cranial to the distal margin of external sphincter. Both sphincters overlap by approximately 1.5 cm, and the entire sphincter complex spans a length of 3 to 4 cm.

As noted earlier, the puborectalis muscle is the medial portion of the levator ani muscle that arises on either side from the inner surface of the pubic bones. It passes behind the rectum to form a sling behind the anorectal junction, and it contributes to the anorectal angle and possibly to fecal continence (see Figs. 38-9, 38-10, and 38-29).

■ Perineal Body

This fibromuscular tissue mass lies between the distal part of the posterior vaginal wall and the anus. It is formed by the attachment of several structures. Inferiorly or superficially, the bulbospongiosus, superficial transverse perineal, and external anal sphincter muscles contribute (see Fig. 38-26). Structures that attach at a superior or deeper level are the perineal membrane, levator ani muscles and covering fascia, sphincter urethrovaginalis muscles, and posterior vaginal wall (see Fig. 38-29). The anterior-to-posterior and the superior-to-inferior extents of the perineal body each measure approximately 2 to 4 cm (see Fig. 38-17).

■ Blood Supply, Lymphatics, and Innervation

Blood Vessels

The *external pudendal artery* is a branch of the femoral artery and supplies the skin and subcutaneous tissue of the mons pubis

(see Fig. 38-3). The *internal pudendal artery* is a terminal branch of the internal iliac artery (see Fig. 38-6). It exits the pelvis through the greater sciatic foramen, passes behind the ischial spines, and reenters the perineum through the lesser sciatic foramen. It then has a variable course through the pudendal (Alcock) canal, and ultimately divides into terminal branches. These are the inferior rectal, perineal, and clitoral arteries (see Fig. 38-30).

Additional supply to the perineum may arise from internal pudendal artery or other branches of the internal iliac artery, often the obturator, before these branches exit the pelvis. These supplemental vessels course through the retropubic space and are called accessory pudendal arteries. They reach the perineum by passing below the pubic arch, similar to the path of the dorsal vein of clitoris.

Veins that drain the vulva and perineum have courses and names similar to those of the arteries. Venous blood from the vestibular bulbs and other structures, with the exception of the erectile tissue of the clitoris, drains into the internal pudendal veins. The erectile tissue drains into the dorsal vein of the clitoris (see Fig. 38-29). This vein courses into the pelvis and terminates in the vesical venous plexus on either side of urethra or bladder (see Fig. 38-24). The venous plexus that drains the rectum and anus empties into the superior, middle, and inferior rectal veins.

Lymphatic Drainage

Structures of the vulva and perineum drain into the inguinal lymph nodes, which are located below the inguinal ligament in the upper anterior and medial thigh (Fig. 38-31). There are 10 to 20 inguinal nodes, which are divided into a superficial and a deep group. Nodes of the superficial inguinal group are more numerous and are found in the membranous layer of the subcutaneous

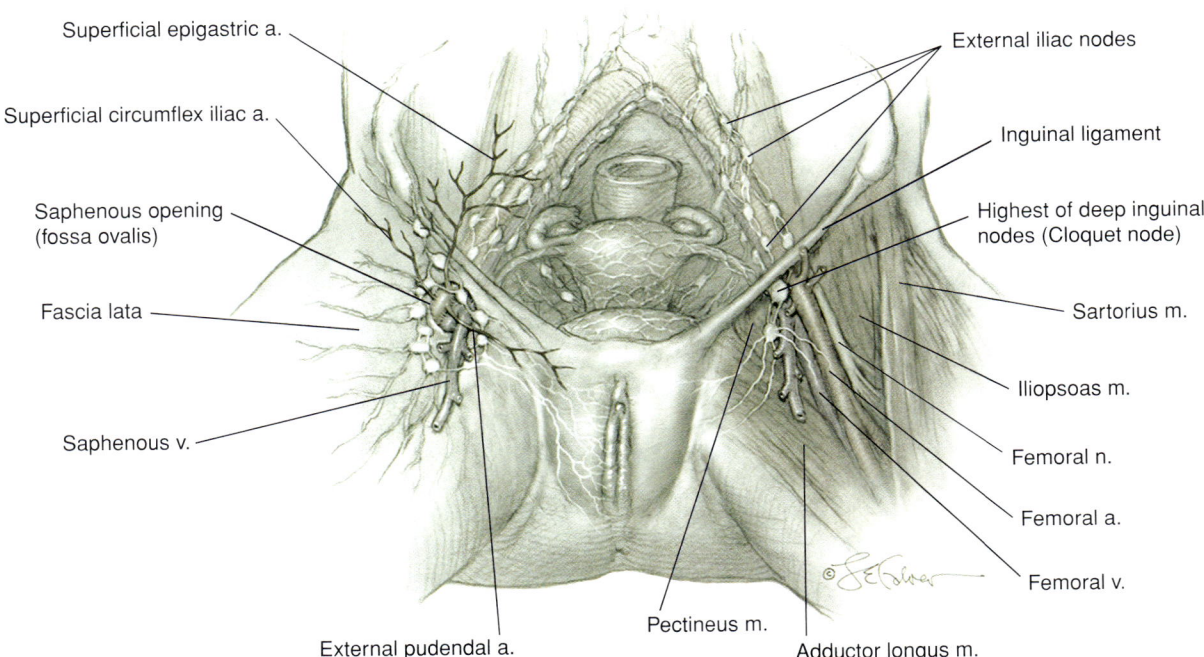

FIGURE 38-31 Inguinal lymph nodes and contents of femoral triangle. Superficial inguinal nodes are shown on the image's left, and deep inguinal nodes appear on the image's right.

tissue of the anterior thigh, just superficial to the fascia lata. The latter is fascia that invests the muscles of the thigh.

The deep inguinal nodes vary from one to three in number and are located deep to the fascia lata in the femoral triangle. This triangle is bordered superiorly by the inguinal ligament, laterally by the medial border of the *sartorius muscle*, and medially by the medial border of the *adductor longus muscle*. The *iliopsoas* and *pectineus muscles* form its floor. From lateral to medial, the structures found in this triangle are the femoral nerve, artery, vein, and deep inguinal lymphatics. On the medial side of the femoral vein, the *femoral canal* is found and contains the deep inguinal nodes. The femoral ring is the abdominal opening of this canal. The *fossa ovalis* or *saphenous opening* is an oval opening in the fascia lata and allows communication between superficial and deep inguinal nodes. Of the deep inguinal nodes, the highest one—*Cloquet node*—is located in the lateral part of the femoral ring. Efferent channels from the deep inguinal nodes pass through the femoral canal and femoral ring to the external iliac nodes. Lymphatics from the skin of the labia, clitoris, and remainder of the perineum drain into the superficial inguinal nodes. The glans and corpora cavernosa of the clitoris may drain directly to the deep inguinal nodes.

■ Innervation

The inferior anal, perineal, and dorsal nerve of the clitoris are branches of the pudendal nerve and provide sensory and motor innervation to the perineum (see Fig. 38-30). In addition, the perineal branches of the posterior cutaneous nerve of the thigh (S1–S3) supply in part the skin of the external genitalia and adjacent proximal medial surface of the thigh.

Pudendal Nerve

The pudendal nerve arises from the sacral plexus (S2–S4), and its course and distribution mirror those of the internal pudendal artery and veins. On the perineum, its three terminal branches are the dorsal nerve of clitoris, perineal nerve, and inferior anal (rectal) nerve. These branches provide sensation to the external female genitalia and motor innervation to the superficial perineal muscles, parts of the striated urethral sphincter muscles, and external anal sphincter muscle.

Dorsal Nerve of Clitoris. This nerve is the primary sensory nerve to the clitoris (see Figs. 38-27 and 38-28). After exiting the pudendal canal, this nerve remains within the deep pouch of the anterior perineal triangle firmly adhered to the inner surface of the ischiopubic ramus. It perforates the perineal membrane adjacent to the medial surface of the ramus to reach the superficial perineal pouch. Here, it courses on the deep surface of the ischiocavernous muscle and clitoral crus. In this region, the nerve is surrounded by a dense fibrous capsule that is adhered to the periosteum of the ischiopubic ramus. Approximately 2 to 3 cm lateral to the mid pubic symphysis, it emerges from the deep and lateral surface of the crus and courses toward the dorsal surface of the clitoral body. The nerve does so while tightly embedded in layers of fibroconnective tissue, including that of the suspensory and fundiform ligaments of the clitoris (see Fig. 38-28). In this region, the nerve consistently measures 2 to 4 mm in diameter.

The nerve from each side then courses along the dorsal surface of the clitoral body, at approximately the 11 o'clock and 1 o'clock positions. The nerve remains deep to the clitoral fascia but superficial to the tunica albuginea layer that invests the corpora cavernosa (Inset Fig. 38-28). Here, it gives off small branches to the prepuce and to the corpora cavernosa. It ends by perforating the glans of clitoris to which it provides sensory innervation.

Perineal Nerve. The perineal nerve is the largest branch of the pudendal nerve. It gives rise to the posterior labial nerves, which supply the labia minora and all but the anterior part of the labia majora. Its branches provide motor innervation to the muscles of the superficial perineal pouch and sensory branches to the vestibular bulbs, vestibule, and distal vagina. Although data are limited, branches of perineal nerve may provide innervation to the distal part of the striated urogenital sphincter muscles. The dorsal nerve of clitoris also may contribute branches to these structures during its course in deep perineal pouch.

Inferior Anal (Rectal) Nerve. This nerve innervates the external anal sphincter and perianal skin. The path of the inferior rectal nerve differs from that of the other pudendal nerve branches. In approximately 50 percent of cadaveric specimens, this nerve does not enter the pudendal canal (Maldonado, 2015; Montoya, 2011). Instead, the nerve passes behind the sacrospinous ligament and enters the ischio-anal fossa without entering the pudendal canal.

Autonomic Innervation to Erectile Structures

The erectile tissues of the perineum are innervated by the cavernous nerves of the clitoris. These nerves are the terminal extensions of the uterovaginal plexus (see Fig. 38-13). The cavernous nerves course within the paravaginal and paraurethral connective tissue and reach the perineum by passing under the pubic bones. Fibers join the dorsal nerve of clitoris and provide innervation to the corpora cavernosa and vestibular bulbs. In contrast to the dorsal nerve of clitoris, the cavernous nerves fibers are very small caliber, and their presence can be confirmed only by microscopy. These nerves consist of sympathetic and parasympathetic components and are critical to sexual function.

RELEVANT THIGH ANATOMY

The medial thigh compartment is one of three anatomic divisions in the thigh, and many of its more superficial muscles are relevant to gynecologic surgery. First, the pectineus muscle originates on the pectineal line of the pubis and inserts onto the femur. This muscle contributes to the floor of the femoral triangle, and its primary function is hip flexion. Medial to the pectineus muscle is the adductor longus muscle, which originates on the superior ramus of the pubis and inserts onto the femur. It forms the medial border of the femoral triangle, and it acts to adduct and flex the thigh. The gracilis muscle forms the medial border of this region and is the most superficial muscle in the medial thigh. It originates on the body of the pubis and the upper half of the inferior pubic ramus and inserts onto the proximal and medial surface of the tibia. This muscle crosses both the hip and knee joints and functions to adduct the thigh and flex the leg. The muscles of the medial thigh compartment receive blood supply from the femoral and obturator arteries, and the major source of innervation is the obturator nerve. This nerve enters the thigh through the obturator canal and promptly separates into anterior and posterior branches to supply medial compartment muscles.

In the anterior thigh compartment, the sartorius muscle originates from the anterior superior iliac spine to insert on the proximal tibia. The femoral artery and nerve supply blood and innervation, respectively. For gynecologists, it forms the lateral boundary of the femoral triangle.

REFERENCES

Balgobin S, Hamid CA, Carrick KS, et al: Distance from cervicovaginal junction to anterior peritoneal reflection measured during vaginal hysterectomy. Obstet Gynecol 128(4):863, 2016

Barber MD, Bremer RE, Thor KB, et al: Innervation of the female levator ani muscles. Am J Obstet Gynecol 187:64, 2002

Bleich AT, Rahn DD, Wieslander CK, et al: Posterior division of the internal iliac artery: anatomic variations and clinical applications. Am J Obstet Gynecol 197(6):658.e1, 2007

Campbell RM: The anatomy and histology of the sacrouterine ligaments. Am J Obstet Gynecol 59:1, 1950

Chen L, Ramanah R, Hsu Y, et al: Cardinal and deep uterosacral ligament lines of action: MRI based 3D technique development and preliminary findings in normal women. Int Urogynecol J 24(1): 37, 2013

DeLancey JO: Anatomic aspects of vaginal eversion after hysterectomy. Am J Obstet Gynecol 166:1717, 1992

DeLancey JO: Structural anatomy of the posterior pelvic compartment as it relates to rectocele. Am J Obstet Gynecol 180:815, 1999

DeLancey JO, Hurd WW: Size of the urogenital hiatus in the levator ani muscles in normal women and women with pelvic organ prolapse. Obstet Gynecol 91:364, 1998

DeLancey JO, Starr RA: Histology of the connection between the vagina and levator ani muscles: implications for the urinary function. J Reprod Med 35:765, 1990

Delancey JO, Toglia MR, Perucchini D: Internal and external anal sphincter anatomy as it relates to midline obstetric lacerations. Obstet Gynecol 90(6):924, 1997

Drewes PG, Marinis SI, Schaffer JI, et al: Vascular anatomy over the superior pubic rami in female cadavers. Am J Obstet Gynecol 193(6):2165, 2005

Federal International Programme on Anatomical Terminologies: Terminologia Anatomica, 2nd ed. Stuttgart, Thieme, 2011

Florian-Rodriguez ME, Hamner JJ, Corton MM: First sacral nerve and anterior longitudinal ligament anatomy: clinical applications during sacrocolpopexy. Am J Obstet Gynecol 217(5):607.e1, 2017

Good MM, Abele TA, Balgobin S, et al: L5-S1 discitis—can it be prevented? Obstet Gynecol 121:285, 2013a

Good MM, Abele TA, Balgobin S, et al: Vascular and ureteral anatomy relative to the midsacral promontory. Am J Obstet Gynecol 208:486.e1, 2013b

Hamner JJ, Carrick KS, Ramirez DM, et al: Gross and histologic relationships of the retropubic urethra to lateral pelvic sidewall and anterior vaginal wall in female cadavers: clinical applications to retropubic surgery. Am J Obstet Gynecol 219(6):597.e1, 2018

Heit M, Benson T, Russell B, et al: Levator ani muscle in women with genitourinary prolapse: indirect assessment by muscle histopathology. Neurourol Urodyn 15:17, 1996

Hsu Y, Summers A, Hussain HK, et al: Levator plate angle in women with pelvic organ prolapse compared to women with normal support using dynamic MR imaging. Am J Obstet Gynecol 194(5):1427, 2006

Jackson LA, Ramirez DM, Carrick KS, et al: Gross and histologic anatomy of the pelvic ureter: clinical applications to pelvic surgery. Obstet Gynecol 133(5):896, 2019

Kerney R, Sawhney R, DeLancey JO: Levator ani muscle anatomy evaluated by origin-insertion pairs. Obstet Gynecol 104:168, 2004

Kuhn RJ, Hollyock VE: Observations of the anatomy of the rectovaginal pouch and rectovaginal septum. Obstet Gynecol 59:445, 1982

Lawson JO: Pelvic anatomy: I. Pelvic floor muscles. Ann R Coll Surg Engl 54:244, 1974

Maldonado PA, Carrick KS, Montoya TI, et al: Posterior vaginal wall anatomy: implications for surgical repair. Female Pelvic Med Reconstr Surg, 2019, In press

Maldonado PA, Chin K, Garcia AA, et al: Anatomic variations of pudendal nerve within pelvis and pudendal canal: clinical applications. Am J Obstet Gynecol 213(5):727.e1, 2015

Memon MA, Quinn TH, Cahill DR: Transversalis fascia: historical aspects and its place in contemporary inguinal herniorrhaphy. J Laparoendosc Adv Surg Tech A 9:267, 1999

Montoya TI, Calver LE, Carrick KS, et al: Anatomic relationships of the pudendal nerve branches: assessment of injury risk with common surgical procedures. Am J Obstet Gynecol 205(5):504.e1, 2011

Oelrich T: The striated urogenital sphincter muscle in the female. Anat Rec 205:223, 1983

Oelrich TM: The urethral sphincter muscle in the male. Am J Anat 158:229, 1980

Paramore RH: The supports-in-chief of the female pelvic viscera. BJOG 13:391, 1908

Pathi SD, Castellanos ME, Corton MM: Variability of the retropubic space anatomy in female cadavers. Am J Obstet Gynecol 201(5):524.e1, 2009

Rahn DD, Bleich AT, Wai CY, et al: Anatomic relationships of the distal third of the pelvic ureter, trigone, and urethra in unembalmed female cadavers. Am J Obstet Gynecol 197:668.e1, 2007

Ramanah R, Berger MB, Parratte BM, et al: Anatomy and histology of apical support: a literature review concerning cardinal and uterosacral ligaments. Int Urogynecol J 23(11):1483, 2012

Range RL, Woodburne RT: The gross and microscopic anatomy of the transverse cervical ligaments. Am J Obstet Gynecol 90:460, 1964

Ripperda CM, Jackson LA, Phelan JN, et al: Anatomic relationships of the pelvic autonomic nervous system in female cadavers: clinical applications to pelvic surgery. Am J Obstet Gynecol 216(4):388.e1, 2017

Roshanravan SM, Wieslander CK, Schaffer JI, et al: Neurovascular anatomy of the sacrospinous ligament region in female cadavers: implications in sacrospinous ligament fixation. Am J Obstet Gynecol 197(6):660.e1, 2007

Stein TA, DeLancey JO: Structure of the perineal membrane in females: gross and microscopic anatomy. Obstet Gynecol 111:686, 2008

Umek WH, Morgan DM, Ashton-Miller JA, et al: Quantitative analysis of uterosacral ligament origin and insertion points by magnetic resonance imaging. Obstet Gynecol 103(3):447, 2004

Weber AM, Walters MD: Anterior vaginal prolapse: review of anatomy and techniques of surgical repair. Obstet Gynecol 89:311, 1997

Weber AM, Walter MD: What is vaginal fascia? AUGS Q Rep 13, 1995

Whiteside JL, Barber MD, Walters MD, et al: Anatomy of ilioinguinal and iliohypogastric nerves in relation to trocar placement and low transverse incisions. Am J Obstet Gynecol 189:1574, 2003

Wieslander CK, Rahn DD, McIntire DD, et al: Vascular anatomy of the presacral space in unembalmed female cadavers. Am J Obstet Gynecol 195(6):1736, 2006

Wieslander CK, Roshanravan SM, Wai CY, et al: Uterosacral ligament suspension sutures: anatomic relationships in unembalmed female cadavers. Am J Obstet Gynecol 197:672.e1, 2007

CHAPTER 39

Preoperative Considerations

As surgeons, gynecologists play a key role in preventing perioperative morbidity by assessing a patient's preoperative status. This process is often multidisciplinary and aims to identify and improve modifiable risk factors.

PREOPERATIVE PATIENT EVALUATION

A properly performed preoperative evaluation serves three important functions. It uncovers comorbidities that require further evaluation and improvement to avert perioperative complications. Second, evaluation allows effective use of operating room resources (Roizen, 2000). Last, potential problems are anticipated, and plans addressing these are devised (Johnson, 2008).

In many cases, a thorough history and physical examination averts the need for medical consultation. However, if a poorly controlled or previously undiagnosed medical condition is discovered, consultation with an internist offers benefits. Preoperative internal medicine consultation does not provide "medical clearance" but rather provides a risk assessment of a woman's current medical state. For consultation, the surgical illness and planned procedure are summarized, and clear questions are posed to the consultant (Fleisher, 2009; Goldman, 1983). A complete history and physical examination and medical records that report already completed testing should be

available to the consulting physician. This can prevent unnecessary surgical delays and cost from redundant testing.

PULMONARY EVALUATION

■ Risk Factors

Common postoperative pulmonary morbidities include atelectasis, pneumonia, and chronic lung disease exacerbation. In gynecologic surgeries performed for various indications, pulmonary complications develop in 1 to 3 percent of cases (Burks, 2017; Solomon, 2013; Wysham, 2015).

Pulmonary morbidity may arise from procedure-related or patient-related factors. Of surgery-related risks, upper abdominal incisions as they approach the diaphragm can worsen pulmonary function through mechanisms shown in Figure 39-1

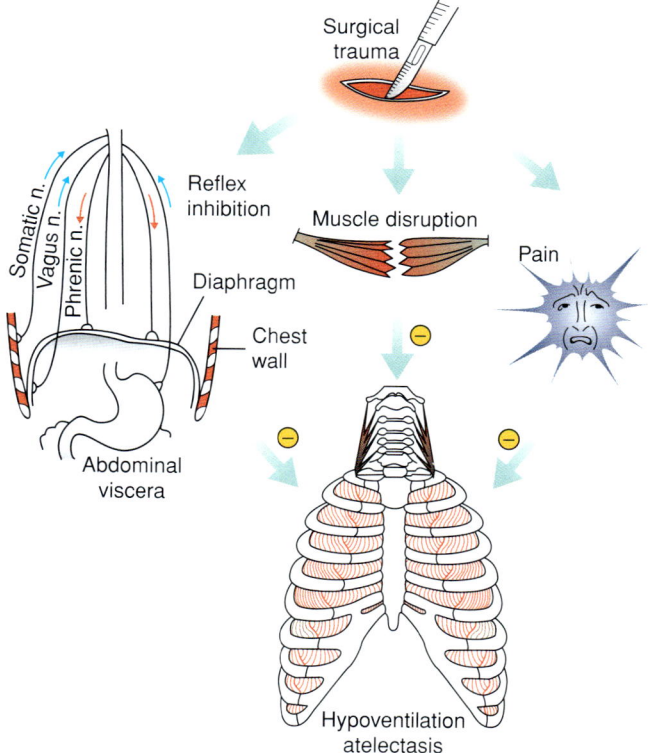

FIGURE 39-1 Surgical factors producing respiratory muscle dysfunction. These factors can reduce lung volumes and produce hypoventilation and atelectasis. (Reproduced with permission from Warner DO: Preventing postoperative pulmonary complications: the role of the anesthesiologist. Anesthesiology 92(5):1467, 2000.)

(Warner, 2000). The poor diaphragmatic movement that results from these three can produce persistent declines in vital capacity and in functional residual capacity. These diminished capacities predispose to atelectasis. Another procedure-associated factor is surgery duration. Operations in which patients receive general anesthesia for longer than 3 hours are associated with nearly double the rate of postoperative pulmonary complications. Last, emergency surgery remains a significant independent risk. Although these factors are largely unmodifiable, an appreciation of their sequelae ideally prompts greater postoperative vigilance.

Of patient-associated factors, *age* older than 65 years is linked with a higher postoperative pulmonary complication rate (Bapoje, 2007). Those between 60 and 69 have a twofold greater risk, and for those older than 70 years, the risk rises threefold (Qaseem, 2006). Functional status is another risk, and status or sensorium changes may be an early indicator of pulmonary compromise (Yang, 2015). Thus, preoperative baseline cognition is assessed and documented for at-risk patients.

Smoking, specifically a greater than 20-pack-year smoking history, confers a high incidence of postoperative pulmonary complications. Fortunately, this risk can be reduced with smoking abstinence before surgery. Preoperative cessation for at least 4 to 8 weeks offers significant improvement in lung function and reversal of smoking-related immune impairment (Akrawi, 1997; Wong, 2012). Other short-term benefits may be related to reduced nicotine and carboxyhemoglobin levels, improved mucociliary function, decreased upper airway hypersensitivity, and improved wound healing (Møller, 2002; Nakagawa, 2001). Patients with a 6-month or longer history of smoking cessation have complication risks similar to those who have never smoked. Moreover, patients often see surgery as an opportunity for positive change (Shi, 2010). Education alone may prompt successful behavior modification. For others, agents to assist with smoking cessation are found in Table 1-6 (p. 13).

In *chronic obstructive pulmonary disease (COPD)*, inflammatory mediators may account for the intra- and extrapulmonary complications observed in affected patients (Maddali, 2008). Preoperative efforts aim to optimize patient lung function but may not reduce postoperative pulmonary complication rates. However, postoperative physiotherapy and incentive spirometry with inspiratory muscle training can reduce complication rates (Agostini, 2010).

Obesity decreases chest wall compliance and functional residual capacity. Patients with a body mass index (BMI) ≥30 kg/m² are especially predisposed to intra- and postoperative atelectasis (Agostini, 2010; Zerah, 1993). Eichenberger and colleagues (2002) observed that pulmonary changes in these patients may persist for more than 24 hours and require aggressive postoperative lung expansion. Moreover, in obese patients undergoing minimally invasive surgery (MIS), these pulmonary parameters are further compromised by higher intraabdominal pressures generated by the pneumoperitoneum required for MIS (Chap. 41, p. 873). Despite these risks, pulmonary considerations related to obesity should not independently restrict needed surgical intervention (Sood, 2015; Wysham, 2015).

TABLE 39-1. Obstructive Sleep Apnea Screening (STOP-Bang)

Snoring	Snore loudly?
Tired	Tired or sleepy during the day?
Observed	Observed to stop breathing or choke/gasp while asleep?
Pressure	Treated for hypertension?
BMI	BMI >35 kg/m²?
Age	Age >50 years?
Neck size	Wear ≥16 inch shirt collar?
Gender	Male?

"Yes" replies are tallied: 0-2 = low risk; 3–4 = intermediate risk; 5–8 = high risk.
BMI = body mass index.

Obstructive sleep apnea (OSA) is another independent risk factor for pulmonary complications. Screening all patients for OSA preoperatively can identify patients previously undiagnosed. One validated screening tool for OSA is STOP-Bang (Table 39-1) (Chung, 2008). Affected women may benefit from preoperative anesthesiologist consultation to enable perioperative management (American Society of Anesthesiologists, 2014b).

Asthma, if well-controlled, is not a risk factor for postoperative pulmonary complications. Warner and coworkers (1996) reported that bronchospasm rates were <2 percent in asthmatic patients. However, patients with poorly controlled disease are best referred to an appropriate consultant to optimize airways (Woods, 2009). The level of control can be assessed as shown in Table 39-2.

■ Diagnostic Evaluation

During history taking, elements in a pulmonary review of systems that may serve as harbingers of underlying disease include poor exercise tolerance, chronic cough, and otherwise unexplained dyspnea (Smetana, 1999). During examination, decreased breath sounds, dullness to percussion, rales, wheezes, rhonchi, and a prolonged expiratory phase can carry a nearly sixfold higher rate of pulmonary complications (Straus, 2000).

Of diagnostic tests, pulmonary function tests (PFTs) in general offer little preoperative information in patients undergoing nonthoracic procedures. Outside of diagnosing COPD, PFTs are not superior to a thorough history and physical examination (Johnson, 2008; Qaseem, 2006). However, if the etiology of pulmonary symptoms remains unclear after clinical examination, PFTs may provide data to alter perioperative management.

Chest radiography is not routinely obtained preoperatively. Compared with clinical assessment, preoperative chest radiographs rarely provide evidence to modify therapy (Archer, 1993). The American College of Radiology (2015) notes that patients with new or exacerbated cardiopulmonary symptoms or those older than 70 years with chronic cardiopulmonary disease are suitable candidates. Although not exhaustive,

TABLE 39-2. Assessing Asthma Control

Components of Control	Well Controlled	Not Well Controlled	Poorly Controlled
Symptoms	≤2 days/week	>2 days/week	Throughout day
Nighttime awakenings	≤2 times/month	1–3 times/week	≥4 times/week
Interference of normal activity	None	Some limitation	Extreme limitation
Short-acting β$_2$-agonist use for symptom control[a]	≤2 days/week	>2 days/week	Several times/day
FEV$_1$ or peak flow	>80% predicted/personal best	60–80% predicted/personal best	<60% predicted/personal best

[a]Does not include use for exercise-induced bronchospasm.
FEV$_1$ = forced expiratory volume in 1 second.
Adapted from National Heart Blood and Lung Institute, 2007.

conditions for which radiography may be reasonable include acute or chronic cardiovascular or pulmonary disease, cancer, American Society of Anesthesiologist (ASA) status >3, heavy smoking, immunosuppression, recent chest radiation therapy, and new emigration from areas with endemic pulmonary disease.

Few laboratory tests are needed for those with stable chronic lung disease. One national quality improvement program found that serum albumin levels <35 mg/dL are significantly associated with increased perioperative pulmonary morbidity and mortality rates (Arozullah, 2000; Lee, 2009). This association most likely reflects confounding comorbidity, and thus albumin serves as a marker of malnutrition and disease (Goldwasser, 1997). A serum albumin level is not routinely rec-ommended for gynecologic procedures. However, in the elderly or in those with multiple comorbidities, the information may be predictive. As another marker, serum blood urea nitrogen levels >21 mg/dL similarly correlate with higher morbidity rates, but to a lesser degree (Smetana, 2006).

With all clinical components taken in sum, the ASA classification helps predict perioperative mortality rates. It also assesses risks for cardiovascular and pulmonary complications (Wolters, 1996). Table 39-3 summarizes the ASA categories and associated rates of postoperative pulmonary complications (American Society of Anesthesiologists, 2014a; Qaseem, 2006). In our institution, individuals with ASA class III or greater and women with BMI >40 kg/m^2 undergo formal anesthesiology consultation.

TABLE 39-3. American Society of Anesthesiologists (ASA) Classification

Class	Definition	Examples	PPC (%)
I	Normally healthy patient	Healthy, nonsmoking, no or minimal alcohol use	1.2
II	Mild systemic disease without substantive functional limitations	Current smoker, social alcohol drinker, pregnancy, obesity (BMI <40), well-controlled DM or HTN, mild lung disease	5.4
III	Moderate to severe systemic disease that is not incapacitating but carries substantive functional limitations	Poorly controlled DM or HTN, COPD, morbid obesity (BMI ≥40), active hepatitis, alcohol dependence or abuse, implanted pacemaker, moderately reduced ejection fraction, ESRD with regular dialysis, prior history (>3 months) of MI, CVA, TIA, or CAD/stents	11.4
IV	Incapacitating systemic disease that is a constant threat to life	Ongoing cardiac ischemia or severe valve dysfunction, severely reduced ejection fraction, sepsis, DIC, ARD or ESRD not undergoing dialysis regularly, recent history (<3 months) of MI, CVA, TIA, or CAD/stents	10.9
V	Moribund patient not expected to survive for 24 hours regardless of operation	Ruptured abdominal/thoracic aneurysm, massive trauma, intracranial bleed with mass effect, ischemic bowel with comorbid significant cardiac pathology or multiple organ/system dysfunction	NA

ARD = acute renal disease; BMI = body mass index; CAD = coronary artery disease; COPD = chronic obstructive pulmonary disease; CVA = cerebrovascular accident; DIC = disseminated intravascular coagulation; DM = diabetes mellitus; ESRD = end-stage renal disease; HTN = hypertension; MI = myocardial infarction; NA = not applicable; PPC = postoperative pulmonary complication; TIA = transient ischemic attack.

CARDIAC EVALUATION

◼ Risk Factors

Coronary artery disease (CAD) contributes significantly to perioperative cardiac complication rates (Smilowitz, 2017; Williams, 2009). Therefore, cardiac risk assessment focuses on CAD and is detailed later in this section (p. 826).

For those with *congestive heart failure (CHF),* a consulting cardiologist may employ strategies to maximize hemodynamic function. These can include perioperative medications or preoperative coronary revascularization. With CHF, diuretics are commonly used. However, restrained perioperative use will usually avoid intraoperative hypovolemia and related hypotension. But, if needed, fluid resuscitation ideally is gradual and measured to avoid volume overload.

Arrhythmias usually are symptoms of underlying cardiopulmonary disease or electrolyte abnormalities. Accordingly, preoperative management aims to correct the primary process. However, if pacemakers and implantable cardioverter-defibrillators are needed, these typically are placed for the same indications as in nonsurgical circumstances (Gregoratos, 2002). For those with pacemakers in place, electrosurgery can create electromagnetic interference even during noncardiac procedures. Although encountered less frequently with newer devices, such interference can lead to pacing failure or complete system malfunction (Cheng, 2008). Thus, current guidelines recommend that all systems be evaluated by an appropriately trained physician before and after any invasive procedure (Fleisher, 2009). In addition, as discussed in Chapter 40 (p. 857), intraoperative efforts strive to minimize the chance for electrosurgical interference. Practices include selecting bipolar electrosurgery if possible, using short intermittent bursts of electric current at the lowest possible energy levels, maximizing the distance between the current source and cardiac device, and placing the grounding pad in a position to minimize current flow toward the device.

Hypertension itself does not predict perioperative cardiac events and generally should not be a reason to postpone surgery (Crowther, 2018; Weksler, 2003). For elective procedures, exceptions might include systolic blood pressures >180 mm Hg and diastolic blood pressures >110 mm Hg. If possible, to lower hypertension-related cardiac complications, blood pressure is lowered several months prior to an anticipated procedure (Fleisher, 2002).

The day of surgery, patients using angiotensin-converting enzyme inhibitors and angiotensin-receptor antagonists hold their morning dose to reduce the risk of immediate postinduction hypotension (Roshanov, 2017). Prolonged hypotension can precipitate myocardial or kidney injury (Salmasi, 2017). Intraoperatively, all patients with hypertension are carefully monitored to avoid blood pressure extremes. Postoperatively, intravascular volume expansion, pain, and agitation may exacerbate hypertension.

Valvular heart disease is less frequently encountered. Of types, aortic stenosis, particularly when severe, carries the highest independent factor for perioperative complications (Kertai, 2004; Tashiro, 2014). Specifically, affected persons are extremely sensitive to diminished preload, which can accompany surgical blood loss or anesthetics. For other lesions, the degree of heart failure and associated cardiac arrhythmias best predict perioperative risk.

In the undiagnosed woman, cardiac sounds suggesting valvular disease should prompt echocardiography to define the abnormality. Importantly, endocarditis prophylaxis for valvular lesions during gastrointestinal (GI) or genitourinary (GU) procedures is no longer recommended by the American Heart Association unless known active infection is present (Nishimura, 2017). The transient enterococcal bacteremia associated with these procedures has not been irrefutably correlated to infective endocarditis.

◼ Diagnostic Evaluation

History and physical examination can effectively identify or characterize cardiac disease, and one questioning strategy is outlined in **Figure 39-2** (Fleisher, 2009; Hlatky, 1989). During physical examination, surgeons observe for dependent edema or jugular venous distention, whereas chest palpation searches for the point of maximum impulse and possible thrills. Auscultation of carotid arteries can exclude bruits, and listening at cardiac points investigates cardiac rate, regularity, and extra heart sounds.

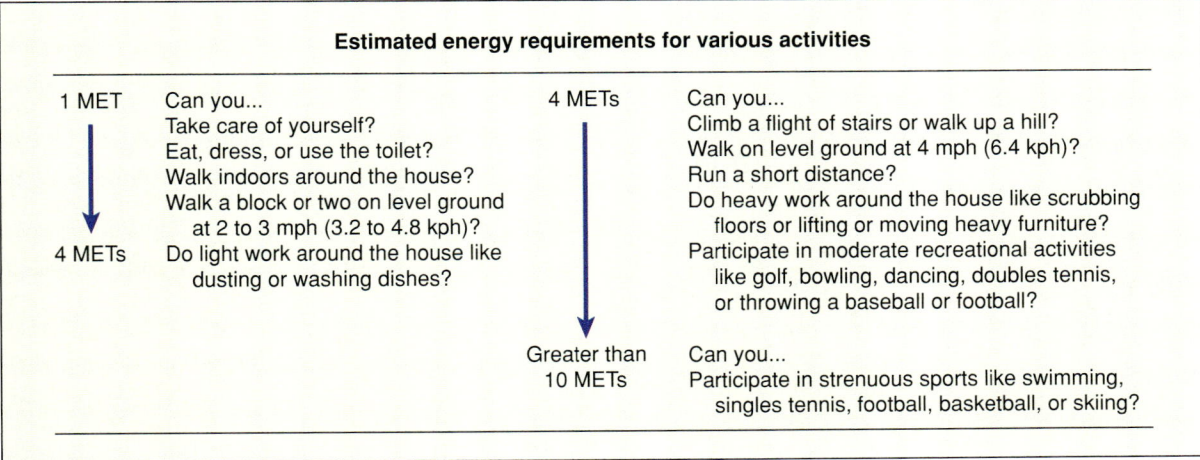

Estimated energy requirements for various activities

| 1 MET | Can you...
Take care of yourself?
Eat, dress, or use the toilet?
Walk indoors around the house?
Walk a block or two on level ground
  at 2 to 3 mph (3.2 to 4.8 kph)?
Do light work around the house like
  dusting or washing dishes? | 4 METs | Can you...
Climb a flight of stairs or walk up a hill?
Walk on level ground at 4 mph (6.4 kph)?
Run a short distance?
Do heavy work around the house like scrubbing
  floors or lifting or moving heavy furniture?
Participate in moderate recreational activities
  like golf, bowling, dancing, doubles tennis,
  or throwing a baseball or football? |
| 4 METs | | Greater than
10 METs | Can you...
Participate in strenuous sports like swimming,
  singles tennis, football, basketball, or skiing? |

FIGURE 39-2 Questions used to assess functional capacity. METs are used in the algorithm in Figure 39-3. CAD = coronary artery disease; kph = kilometers per hour; MET = metabolic equivalent; mph = miles per hour.

Of preoperative tests, 12-lead electrocardiogram (ECG) and chest radiograph are commonly considered. According to the American College of Cardiology and the American Heart Association (ACC/AHA), ECG is reasonable for patients with known coronary heart disease, significant arrhythmia, peripheral arterial disease, cerebrovascular disease, or other significant structural heart disease. ECG is not recommended for those undergoing low-risk surgeries. For asymptomatic patients without known coronary heart disease, ECG may be considered, but again is not useful in those undergoing low-risk procedures (Fleisher, 2014). Indications for preoperative chest radiography are limited and discussed on page 823. Other cardiac testing is usually ordered by a consulting cardiologist and often directed by guidelines discussed next.

■ Preoperative Cardiac Guidelines

Recommendations have been developed by several groups to help predict cardiac complications and direct perioperative care. The two most prominent are guidelines jointly developed by the ACC/AHA and the Revised Cardiac Risk Index (RCRI) (Fleisher, 2014; Lee, 1999).

Of the two, ACC/AHA guidelines provide a stepwise strategy to assess three major elements—clinical predictors,

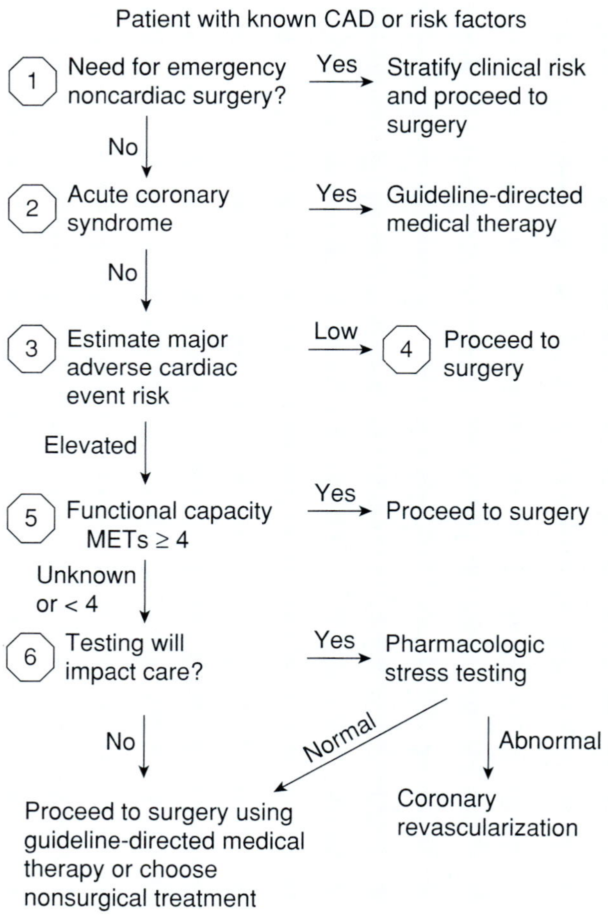

FIGURE 39-3 Stepwise approach to perioperative cardiac assessment in those with coronary artery disease (CAD). MET = metabolic equivalent.

surgery-specific risk, and functional capacity. These then direct the need for cardiac testing (Fig. 39-3) (Fleisher, 2014). In general, for gynecologic surgery, cardiac complication risks are greatest with major emergency procedures and operations associated with large intravascular fluid shifts. Lowest risks are found with planned, brief endoscopic procedures.

The RCRI is a simple assessment of clinical predictors (Lee, 1999). The major difference between the RCRI and the ACC/AHA guidelines is the incorporation of exercise capacity in the ACC/AHA tool. Creators of the RCRI suggest that cardiac risk may be overestimated by noncardiac limitations in exercise function, such as musculoskeletal pain. Thus, these investigators place greater emphasis on cardiac and vascular disease markers.

■ Prevention Strategies

Perioperative Beta Blockers

Early studies supported perioperative use of these agents to lower complication rates in patients with underlying cardiac disease (Mangano, 1996, 2004; Stone, 1988). Indeed, more recent meta-analyses of noncardiac surgery show a reduced rate of nonfatal myocardial infarctions. However, higher rates of stroke and all-cause mortality also accompany such perioperative beta blocker use (Blessberger, 2018; Bouri, 2014). These findings challenge the current AHA guidelines recommending beta blockade in targeted high-risk patients and even suggest that they may benefit the least (Poldermans, 2009). Thus, these agents usually are not recommended prior to gynecologic surgery. That said, for patients on chronic beta blocker therapy, their medication typically is continued perioperatively (Fleisher, 2014).

Coronary Revascularization

Diagnostic cardiac catheterization is considered in high-risk cardiac patients if noninvasive stress testing suggests advanced disease. In such cases, revascularization by coronary artery bypass grafting or percutaneous coronary interventions offer comparable benefits perioperatively (Hassan, 2001). Elective noncardiac surgery should be delayed by 6 months following drug-eluting stent implantation (Levine, 2016).

Anemia

This is an independent risk factor for CHF (Kannel, 1987). In one study, correcting even mild anemia (hemoglobin level <12.5 g/dL) improved cardiac function in those with varying degrees of CHF (Silverberg, 2001). Iron therapy is not a substitution for appropriate cardiac disease treatment, but extrapolated data suggest that maintaining a hemoglobin level above 10 g/dL reduces perioperative morbidity and mortality rates for those with cardiac disease. Thus, preoperative improvement of anemia in these patients is essential. In contrast, restrictive red blood cell transfusion thresholds are recommended in hemodynamically stable adults (Carson, 2016). Thus, in patients without preexisting cardiovascular disease, transfusion is considered at a hemoglobin level ≤7 g/dL. Although a hemoglobin level above 10 g/dL is beneficial, the transfusion threshold is 8 g/dL in those with cardiovascular disease. This excludes patients with acute coronary syndrome, who usually will require higher oxygen-carrying capacity.

HEPATIC EVALUATION

The liver plays a central role in drug metabolism; synthesis of proteins, glucose, and coagulation factors; and excretion of endogenous compounds. Thus, perioperative care ideally seeks to identify or address any hepatic impairment. Patients with suspected disease are queried regarding family histories of jaundice or anemia, recent travel history, exposure to alcohol or other hepatotoxins, infectious hepatitis risks, and medication use (Suman, 2006). Physical findings include jaundice, scleral icterus, spider angiomas, ascites, hepatomegaly, asterixis, and cachexia.

The liver produces many important serum proteins. If underlying liver disease is known or suspected, prothrombin time (PT), partial thromboplastin time (PTT), and serum albumin level are obtained. Additionally, a serum chemistry panel measures liver transaminases.

Of liver diseases, acute and chronic hepatitis are commonly encountered. With acute hepatitis, regardless of the cause, associated perioperative mortality rates are high. Accordingly, primary management involves supportive care and delay of elective surgery until the acute process has subsided (Patel, 1999). In those with chronic hepatitis, hepatic dysfunction varies. Compensated disease carries a low risk of perioperative complications (Sirinek, 1987). However, in patients with cirrhosis, the Child-Pugh score is a useful tool to predict survival after abdominal surgery. For score calculation, clinical measures include serum total bilirubin and albumin levels, international normalized ratio (INR) values, and severity of associated ascites and encephalopathy. Approximate mortality risks based on Child-Pugh class are class A—10 percent; class B—30 percent; class C—70 percent (Mansour, 1997).

RENAL EVALUATION

The kidney is involved with metabolic waste excretion, erythropoietin production, and fluid and electrolyte balance. Consequently, patients with known renal insufficiency typically have serum electrolytes, renal function, and complete blood count (CBC) evaluated prior to surgery.

Of specific issues, chronic anemia due to associated poor erythropoietin production will typically require preoperative administration of erythropoietin or perioperative transfusion. The procedure planned and degree of anemia will guide this choice. Dialysis patients require intensive pre- and postoperative surveillance for signs of electrolyte abnormalities and fluid overload. Ideally, dialysis the day prior to surgery will help bring these patients' volume status and electrolytes levels (potassium in particular) into optimal ranges. Additionally, further renal insult is averted by avoiding nephrotoxic agents. Pharmacokinetic consultation may be warranted to adjust medication dosages, as serum levels in these patients can be unpredictable postoperatively.

HEMATOLOGIC EVALUATION

◼ Anemia

This is frequently encountered prior to gynecologic surgery, and potentially reversible causes are sought. Queries focus on signs of symptomatic anemia that include fatigue, dyspnea with exertion, and palpitations. Inquiry also seeks to identify risk factors for underlying cardiovascular disease, as anemia is less tolerated in these individuals. Clinical evaluation incorporates thorough pelvic and rectal examination, stool guaiac screening, urinalysis, and CBC, if not already done.

With chronic iron-deficiency anemia, erythrocyte indices derived from a CBC reflect a microcytic, hypochromic anemia and show declines in mean corpuscular volume (MCV), mean corpuscular hemoglobin (MCH), and mean corpuscular hemoglobin concentration (MCHC). Moreover, an elevated platelet count and decreased reticulocyte count can be seen. In those for whom the cause of anemia is unclear, those with profound anemia, or those who fail to improve with oral iron therapy, additional testing is prudent. Iron studies coupled with vitamin B_{12} and folate levels are often indicated. Classic iron-deficiency anemia produces low serum ferritin and iron levels, elevated total iron-binding capacity, and normal vitamin B_{12} and folate levels.

Several pharmacologic options are available for preoperative iron supplementation. For oral intake, ferrous sulfate (Feosol, Slow FE), ferrous gluconate (Fergon), ferrous fumarate (Ferro-Sequels), and iron polysaccharide (Ferrex, Niferex) are available. Importantly, each of the ferrous salts has a different content of *elemental iron*. In general, therapy to correct iron deficiency aims to provide 150 to 200 mg of elemental iron daily. Thus, common and equivalent oral replacement regimens include ferrous sulfate, 325 mg tablet (contains 65 mg elemental iron), or ferrous fumarate, 200 mg tablet (contains 64 mg elemental iron), three times daily. Constipation is the primary source of preparation intolerance and can be improved with dietary changes, bulk laxatives, and stool softeners (Table 25-5, p. 566).

Several Food and Drug Administration (FDA)-approved intravenous (IV) iron preparations also are currently available. These include ferric gluconate (Ferrlecit), iron sucrose (Venofer), ferumoxytol (Feraheme), ferric carboxymaltose (Injectafer), and low-molecular-weight iron dextran (INFeD) (DeLoughery, 2014). The newer preparations have a much lower risk of anaphylactic reactions and are considered safe (Shander, 2010). The hemoglobin effects can be seen as quickly as 1 week after the first dose. For most women, iron therapy administered orally is effective to correct anemia. However, these IV forms may be most appropriate for women with poor absorption secondary to GI disease, those with chronic renal disease, or those with an intolerance or lack of response to oral iron.

In women with acute bleeding, transfusion may be required perioperatively. As noted, the decision to transfuse factors a patient's cardiac status. A full discussion of resuscitation is found in Chapter 40 (p. 862).

◼ Individuals Declining Transfusion

For Jehovah's Witnesses and other patients who decline blood transfusions, a discussion regarding permissible blood products should be part of the surgical consenting process. Accepted blood products vary widely, and a list of approved products are documented in a patient's chart. For Jehovah's Witnesses, red cells, white cells, platelets, and plasma generally are viewed as primary blood components and are eschewed. However, certain clotting factors or cell fractions may be acceptable (Lawson, 2015). Before and after surgery, iron, folate, and, if necessary, erythropoietin are accepted agents to help maximize hemoglobin levels. Perioperatively, phlebotomy is limited, and pediatric collection tubes are preferable. Intraoperative options include topical hemostatic agents, tranexamic acid, and desmopressin to promote clot formation; red blood cell salvage or acute normovolemic hemodilution to provide autologous donation; and controlled hypotensive anesthesia. Autologous transfusion options are detailed in Chapter 40 (p. 858).

Coagulopathies

These are generally grouped into two categories—inherited or acquired. Of acquired forms, a careful review of systems and complete medication list, including herbal preparations, may highlight potential causes. A personal history of easy bruising, unexpected amounts of bleeding with minor injury, or lifelong heavy menstrual bleeding are suggestive. Detailed screening for coagulopathies is outlined in Chapter 8 (p. 193), and the specifics of replacement are described in Chapter 40 (p. 865). In general, for those undergoing procedures, a transfusion threshold of ≤50,000/μL is used, and for major surgery, ≤100,000/μL (James, 2011).

Oral Anticoagulation

In patients who take anticoagulants following venous thromboembolism (VTE), surgery timing can lower the risk of a postoperative recurrence. After an acute VTE, the recurrence risk without anticoagulation lies between 40 and 50 percent.

However, the risk of recurrent disease drops significantly after 3 months of warfarin therapy. Moreover, a delay in surgery and continued warfarin therapy for an additional 2 to 3 months (6 months total) drops the recurrence risk to 5 to 10 percent (Kearon, 1997; Levine, 1995). Thus, in those with recent VTE, a surgical delay, if feasible, may be advantageous and should be considered. When surgery must proceed, protocols for anticoagulant management are described next.

Preoperative Management

Women with atrial fibrillation, mechanical heart valve, or recent VTE carry a high risk for VTE. Consequently, chronic oral warfarin therapy typically is prescribed. For these patients, a surgeon must compromise between the need for anticoagulation and risk of surgical bleeding complications. The American College of Obstetricians and Gynecologists (2019) has summarized recommendations to address this balance (Table 39-4). In general, anticoagulation is typically halted prior to surgery and started shortly postoperatively. Unfortunately, the effects of warfarin reverse slowly. Thus, patients are often transitioned or "bridged" to heparin, which can be stopped and restarting more readily. Both low-molecular-weight heparin (LMWH) and unfractionated heparin (UFH) are options (Table 39-5) (American College of Obstetricians and Gynecologists, 2019; Douketis, 2014). Of LWMH choices, enoxaparin (Lovenox) is commonly selected. During bridging, warfarin is stopped several days before surgery, and heparin is begun (Douketis, 2012; White, 1995). In those with a therapeutic INR (between 2.0 and 3.0), approximately 5 to 6 days are required for this ratio to reach 1.5. Once this is achieved, surgery can safely proceed. During bridging therapy, the last dose of LMWH is administered 24 hours prior to surgery. With UFH, therapy is halted 4 to 6 hours prior to surgery (Douketis, 2012).

TABLE 39-4. Perioperative Management of Patients on Chronic Antithrombotic Therapy

Condition	Bleeding Risk	High VTE Risk	Moderate VTE Risk	Low VTE Risk
Prior VTE	High	Protocol A	Protocol C	Protocol C
	Moderate	Protocol A	Protocol B or C Consider mechanical prophylaxis	Protocol C
Atrial fibrillation	High	Protocol A	Protocol C[a] or B	Protocol C[a] or B
	Moderate	Protocol A	Protocol A[a] or B	Protocol B or C
Mechanical heart valve	High	Protocol A	Protocol A or B	Protocol C
	Moderate	Protocol A	Protocol A	Protocol C[a] or B

Protocol A[a]: Use bridging therapy with therapeutic-dose low-molecular-weight heparin (LMWH) or unfractionated heparin (UFH). Therapeutic-dose enoxaparin is 1 mg/kg subcutaneously (SC) twice daily or 1.5 mg/kg once daily. Therapeutic-dose intravenous (IV) UFH is 80 units/kg IV push, then 18 units/kg/hr.

Protocol B[a]: Use bridging therapy with low-dose LMWH or low-dose UFH. Low-dose enoxaparin is 30 mg twice SC daily or 40 mg once SC daily. Low-dose UFH is 5000–7500 units SC twice daily.

Protocol C: Stop long-term anticoagulation therapy. Do not use bridging therapy. Restart long-term anticoagulation after surgery. Use mechanical prophylaxis with an intermittent compression device during surgery and until long-term anticoagulation is therapeutic.

[a]Protocol steps for warfarin bridging are found in Table 39-5.
VTE = venous thromboembolism.

TABLE 39-5. Anticoagulant Management

Bridging protocol for warfarin	
5 days before surgery	Stop warfarin; start LMWH or UFH
	Stop LMWH 24 hours before surgery or stop UFH at least 4–6 hours before surgery.
1 day before surgery	Check INR. If INR >1.5, give 1–2 mg of oral vitamin K
	Recheck INR
Surgery day	Start LMWH or UFH 12–24 hours after surgery, if bleeding risk is low
1 day after surgery	Start warfarin
5 days after surgery	Stop LMWH or UFH once INR is >2. Continue warfarin
Protocol for direct oral anticoagulant	
1–2 days before surgery	Stop agent: dabigatran 2 day prior; apixaban and rivaroxaban 1 day prior
1 day after surgery	Start agent
Protocol for antiplatelet agents	
7 days before surgery	Stop aspirin or clopidogrel
1 day after surgery	Start agent 12–24 hours after surgery

INR = international normalized ratio; LMWH = low-molecular-weight heparin; UFH = unfractionated heparin.

Unfortunately, emergency surgery may not allow time for bridging. In these cases, warfarin is halted, and vitamin K is provided. This vitamin promotes factor synthesis, and in urgent cases, a 5- to 10-mg IV dose is suitable (Holbrook, 2012). To minimize the anaphylactic risk, vitamin K is mixed in a minimum of 50 mL of IV fluid and administered over at least 20 minutes. Vitamin K requires 4 to 6 hours to achieve clinical effects. Thus, fresh frozen plasma (FFP) may be added at a dose of 15 mL/kg, and each FFP unit has a volume of 200 to 250 mL. Prothrombin complex concentrate is a human-derived product containing factors II, IX, and X. This product does not require thawing and may be used in place of FFP (Ageno, 2012).

Although warfarin antagonizes all vitamin K-dependent clotting factors, newer *direct oral anticoagulants (DOACs)* inhibit specific factors. The three currently licensed medications are dabigatran (Pradaxa), which targets factor IIa (thrombin), and rivaroxaban (Xarelto) and apixaban (Eliquis), which target factor Xa. Because of their recent introduction, few studies provide recommendations for their perioperative management (Kozek-Langenecker, 2014). The pharmacologic half-life is 14 hours for dabigatran and 9 hours for rivaroxaban and apixaban (Schaden, 2010). Thus, in women with normal preoperative creatinine clearance, stopping rivaroxaban and apixaban 24 hours prior to surgery and halting dabigatran 48 hours prior to surgery is reasonable. The withdrawal time is doubled if the creatinine clearance is <50 mL/min or the risk of perioperative bleeding is high (Ortel, 2012).

For the DOACs, global coagulation tests such as INR, PT, and activated partial thromboplastin time (aPTT) less reliably reflect coagulant activity. For the factor Xa inhibitors rivaroxaban and apixaban, anti–factor Xa assays can be used to measure their activity. For dabigatran, an aPTT >90 seconds and an INR >2 suggest possible overdosing (Lindahl, 2011). Also for dabigatran, thrombin time testing is more sensitive and normal values exclude significant anticoagulant effect. However, the turnaround time with this specific test can be long.

For emergent surgery or life-threatening bleeding, the factor Xa inhibitors may be reversed by andexanet alfa (Andexxa), with 80 percent of patients having hemostatic efficacy by 12 hours (Connolly, 2019). Indirect evidence suggests that recombinant factor VIIa (NovoSeven) or a prothrombin complex concentrate also can help (Ageno, 2012).

Last, antiplatelet agents such as aspirin and clopidogrel (Plavix) may increase surgical bleeding. These are generally stopped 7 days prior to surgery (American College of Obstetricians and Gynecologists, 2019).

Postoperative Management

After surgery, heparin, either UFH or LMWH, is restarted 12 to 24 hours after major surgery (see Table 39-5). Oral warfarin therapy is started concurrently as several days are required to regain therapeutic levels (Harrison, 1997; White, 1995). Once the INR ranges between 2 and 3, heparin is discontinued. DOACs are typically restarted 24 hours following surgery. Antiplatelet agents may be resumed 12 to 24 hours following surgery. In all cases, agents are begun only after surgical hemostasis is confirmed.

ENDOCRINE EVALUATION

◼ Hyperthyroidism and Hypothyroidism

The physiologic stress of surgery can exacerbate endocrine conditions such as thyroid dysfunction, diabetes mellitus, and adrenal insufficiency. Of these, both hyper- and hypothyroidism have anesthetic and metabolic derangements unique to each disease state. Nevertheless, management goals for each aim to achieve a euthyroid state before surgery.

Hyperthyroidism carries the risk of developing thyroid storm perioperatively. In those with goiter, airway compromise is a risk. Thus, during physical examination, tracheal deviation is sought. In addition to thyroid function tests, an ECG and serum electrolyte levels can help predict signs of

TABLE 39-6. Sliding-Scale Insulin Order Example[a]

Blood Glucose, mg/dL (mmol/L)[b]	Short-Acting Insulin, units		
	Low Dose	Medium Dose	High Dose
151–200 (8.4–11.0)	0	2	4
201–250 (11.1– 4.0)	2	4	6
251–300 (14.1–17.0)	4	6	8
301–350 (17.1–20.0)	6	8	10
351–400 (20.1–23.0)	8	10	12
>400 (>23.1)	Call physician	Call physician	Call physician

[a]Low dose applies to insulin naïve or sensitive patients, medium dose would be applied to most patients, and high dose applies to insulin resistant patients.
[b]For convenience, conversions of millimoles per liter to milligrams per deciliter are approximate.

preexisting metabolic stress. Patients are encouraged to maintain their usual medications at prescribed dosages until the day of surgery.

For hypothyroidism, newly diagnosed disease generally does not require preoperative therapy except in severe cases with signs of cardiac depression, electrolyte irregularities, and hypoglycemia. Typical starting levothyroxine doses and initial care are described in Chapter 17 (p. 385).

■ Diabetes Mellitus

Long-term complications of diabetes mellitus may include vascular, neurologic, cardiac, and renal dysfunction. Consequently, a vigilant preoperative risk assessment for these in affected women is completed. In addition, higher postoperative morbidity rates are linked with poor preoperative glycemic control. Specifically, glucose levels >200 mg/dL and hemoglobin A_{1c} levels >7 are both associated with wound infection (Dronge, 2006; Jehan, 2018).

Preoperatively, diabetic patients undergoing major surgical procedures benefit at minimum from three diagnostic tests—serum electrolyte levels, urinalysis, and ECG. These screen for metabolic disturbances, undiagnosed nephropathy, and unrecognized cardiac ischemia, respectively.

In general, stress induced by surgery and anesthesia elevates catecholamine levels, relative insulin deficiency, and hyperglycemia (Devereaux, 2005). Although glycemic responses vary with surgery, overt hyperglycemia is avoided to minimize postoperative complications related to dehydration, electrolyte abnormalities, diminished wound healing, and even ketoacidosis with type 1 diabetes (Jacober, 1999). However, fluctuations in oral intake and metabolic needs make optimal glycemic control labor intensive. Moreover, clear evidence for glucose targets are lacking. As a result, most providers aim for glucose readings <200 mg/dL (Table 39-6) (Finney, 2003; Garber, 2004; Hoogwerf, 2006). Table 39-7 and Figure 39-4 summarize perioperative recommendations set forth by Jacober and coworkers (1999) based on disease severity.

■ Adrenal Insufficiency

Inadequacy of the hypothalamic-pituitary-adrenal (HPA) axis due to secondary suppression from chronic corticosteroid use can lead to perioperative hypotension. In general, corticosteroid users who undergo minor surgical procedures or who use lower doses are assumed not to be at risk for adrenal suppression, and additional corticosteroid therapy is not recommended. This approach is supported by systematic reviews that find no

TABLE 39-7. Perioperative Management of Diabetes Mellitus by Disease Type

Disease	Preoperative Management	Postoperative Management
Type 2 DM treated with diet alone	No additional care with PRN subcutaneous regular insulin for AM hyperglycemia	PRN subcutaneous regular insulin
Type 2 DM treated with oral hypoglycemic agents	Discontinue all agents on the day of surgery	Supplemental subcutaneous insulin until return of normal diet, at which time preoperative therapy can be reinstituted
Type 1or 2 DM treated with insulin	See Figure 39-4	Sliding-scale insulin (Table 39-6)

DM = diabetes mellitus; PRN = as needed.

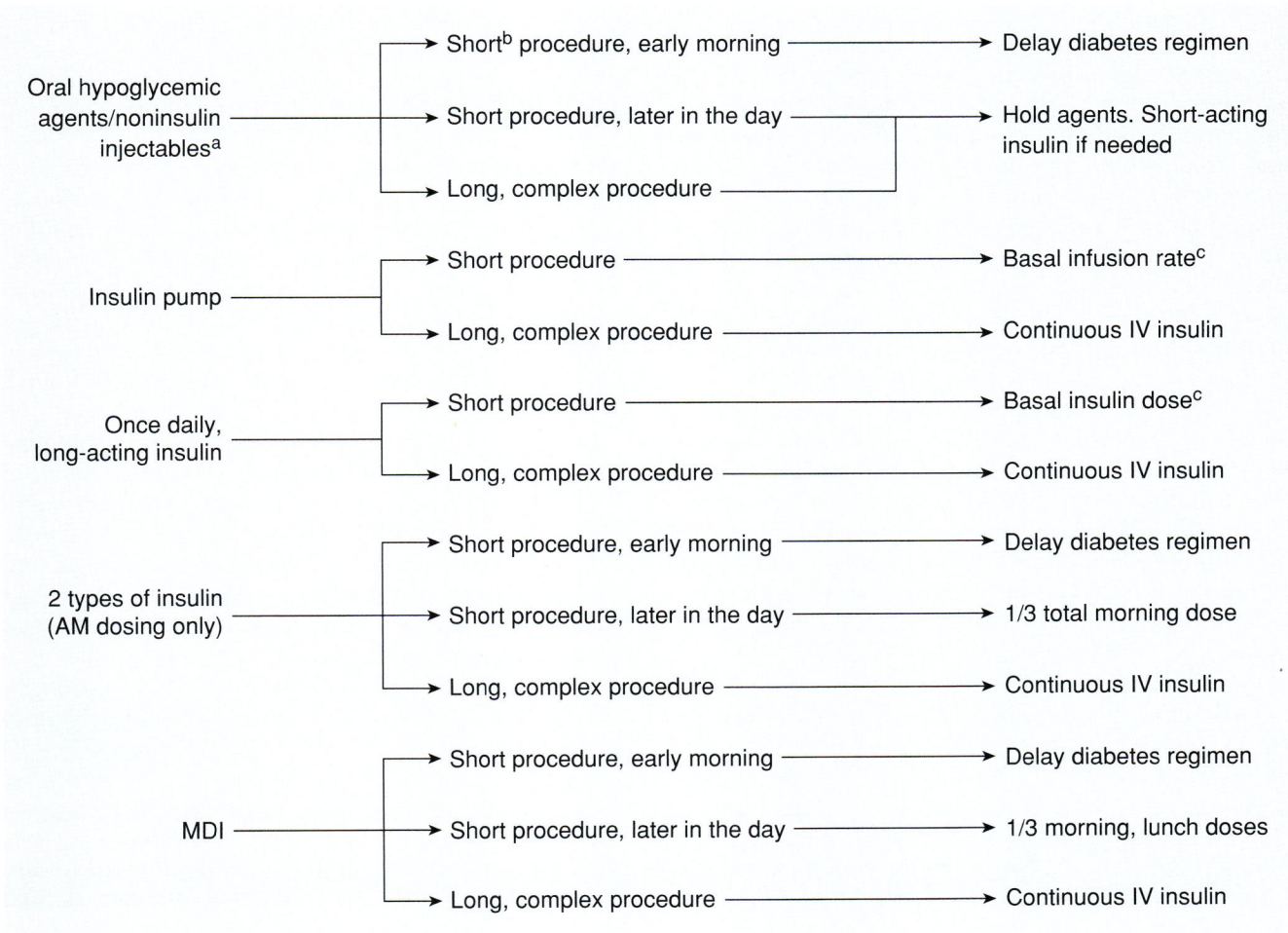

FIGURE 39-4 [a]Glucagon-like peptide-1 analogs. [b]Less than 2 hours. [c]Some authors recommend a 25-percent dose reduction. Perioperative management recommendations for surgical patients with diabetes mellitus. IV = intravenous; MDI = multiple doses of short-acting insulin.

benefit from additional supratherapeutic "stress doses." Instead, patients should continue their usual daily dose (Kelly, 2013; Marik, 2008). For patients with presumed secondary adrenal insufficiency, close hemodynamic monitoring is performed to look for volume-refractory hypotension. If this develops, stress-dose corticosteroids are initiated.

In contrast, *primary* hypothalamic-pituitary-adrenal axis disease requires stress doses in the perioperative period (Marik, 2008). One regimen is hydrocortisone, 100 mg administered IV every 8 hours and titrated to reduced doses as the patient improves.

DIAGNOSTIC TESTING GUIDELINES

Prior to elective gynecologic surgery, pregnancy is excluded in reproductive-age patients, and Pap screening should be current. Outside of these, physicians often obtain unnecessary diagnostic testing that can increase cost, delay surgery, and incite patient anxiety (Kachalia, 2015). For example, a rote panel of preoperative tests without a clear indication does not enhance the safety or quality of care. Moreover, diagnostic testing does not outperform a clinical history and physical examination

(Rucker, 1983). Thus, in the absence of changes in clinical status, diagnostic tests found to be normal 4 to 6 months prior to surgery may be used as "preoperative tests." In patients managed this way, one study found fewer than 2 percent had significant changes during the course of 4 months (MacPherson, 1990).

Codified guidelines for preoperative testing have not been crafted in the United States. However, in the United Kingdom, the National Institute for Health and Clinical Excellence (NICE) (2016) has indications for such testing at their website.

INFORMED CONSENT

Obtaining informed consent is a patient-centered process and not merely a medical record document (Nandi, 2000; Spatz, 2016). This conversation between a clinician and patient enhances a woman's awareness of her diagnosis and contains a discussion of medical and surgical care alternatives, procedure goals and limitations, and surgical risks. Multimedia decision aids, such as photographs, pamphlets, and educational videos, can augment the discussion and support shared decision-making (Coulter, 2007; Spatz, 2016; Stacey, 2017). When informed consent cannot be obtained from the patient, an independent surrogate is identified to represent the patient's best interest and wishes (American College of Obstetricians and Gynecologists, 2015). Ultimately, written documentation of the entire process serves as a historical record of a patient's understanding and agreement within the medical records. Last, pelvic examination under anesthesia is a common intraoperative practice to guide surgical decision-making. If this pelvic examination is performed solely for teaching purposes, the American College of Obstetricians and Gynecologists (2017) recommends obtaining explicit patient consent for learner participation.

Despite a clinician's recommendations, an informed patient may decline a particular intervention. A woman's decision-making autonomy must be respected, and a clinician documents informed refusal in the medical record. Appropriate documentation includes: (1) a patient's refusal of the recommended intervention, (2) notation that the intervention's value has been explained, (3) a patient's reasons for refusal, and (4) the list of subsequent health consequences described to the patient.

Preoperative informed consent also includes specific discussion regarding possible transfusion of blood products. For those

who decline transfusion, this dialogue and planning ideally begin early and are discussed on page 827.

INFECTION PROPHYLAXIS

An evidence-based approach to the prevention of surgical site infections should be consistently applied to all gynecologic surgical procedures. The Council on Patient Safety in Women's Health Care developed a consensus bundle outlining an approach that can be implemented across various clinical settings. The bundle identifies four domains important to infection prevention: readiness, recognition and prevention, response, and reporting and systems learning (Pellegrini, 2017).

Appropriate antibiotic prophylaxis is part of this bundle, and selection recommendations are summarized in Table 39-8 (Achilles, 2011; American College of Obstetricians and Gynecologists, 2018c; Morrill, 2013; Norman, 2012). Decisions regarding the choice, timing, and duration of antibiotic prophylaxis are guided by the intended procedure and the anticipated organisms (Chap. 3, p. 80). Typically, a single dose of antibiotics is given 1 hour prior to surgery. Additional doses are considered in cases with blood loss >1500 mL or with duration longer than 3 hours. For obese individuals, a

TABLE 39-8. Antimicrobial Prophylactic Regimens[a]

Procedure	Antibiotic	Single Dose
Hysterectomy Urogynecology surgeries Consider for clean laparotomy cases	1. Cefazolin[b]	2 g, 3 g IV for patients weighing >120 kg[c]
	2. Clindamycin[d] Metronidazole **PLUS** Gentamicin[e] Aztreonam	600–900 mg IV **or** 500 mg IV 5 mg/kg IV **or** 2 g IV
HSG or chromotubation	Doxycycline[f]	100 mg orally twice daily for 5 d
Surgical induced abortion	Doxycycline Metronidazole	200 mg orally **or** 2 g orally
Laparoscopy: (diagnostic or operative)	None	
Hysteroscopy: (diagnostic or operative)	None	
IUD insertion	None	
EMB	None	
Nongestational D & C	None	
Urodynamics	None	

[a]Ideally administered 1 hour prior to procedure.
[b]Acceptable alternatives include cefotetan, cefoxitin, cefuroxime, or ampicillin-sulbactam.
[c]1-g dose may be considered for patients weighing <80 kg.
[d]Antimicrobial agents of choice in women with a history of immediate hypersensitivity to penicillin.
[e]Dosage is based on patient's actual body weight. If patient's actual weight is >20% over ideal body weight (IBW) then the "dosing weight" (DW) can be calculated as follows: DW = IBW + 0.4 (actual weight − IBW).
[f]If patient has a history of pelvic inflammatory disease or procedure demonstrates dilated fallopian tubes. No prophylaxis is indicated for a study without dilated tubes.
D & C = dilation and curettage; EMB = endometrial biopsy; HSG = hysterosalpingography; IV = intravenously; IUD = intrauterine device.

higher antibiotic dose is suggested. Noted earlier, subacute bacterial endocarditis prophylaxis prior to GI or GU surgeries is not recommended (p. 825).

ENHANCED RECOVERY AFTER SURGERY

Comprehensive care that addresses the entire perioperative period has emerged to help improve outcomes. These *enhanced recovery after surgery (ERAS)* pathways flow through preadmission, preoperative, intraoperative, and postoperative periods (Fig. 39-5) (Carey, 2018). Successful implementation relies upon a team that includes patients, surgeons, anesthesiologists, and perioperative nurses and therapists.

In the preadmission phase, two key components are education and optimally controlling medical conditions. The latter has been described throughout this chapter. Education involves dedicated counseling to set expectations. Topics include postoperative pain, analgesia strategies, hospital stay duration, and ambulation benefits (American College of Obstetricians and Gynecologists, 2018a). With the last, a patient is advised that expected goals are to ambulate on the day of surgery, take all meals in a chair, and ambulate several times each day. Patient handouts can be useful support tools.

Preoperative phase goals aim to avoid dehydration and insulin resistance. Prolonged fasting longer than 12 hours may decrease liver glycogen levels, which can impair glucose metabolism and raise insulin resistance (Kehlet, 1997). The American Society of Anesthesiologists (2017) recommends perioperative feeds but high-fat meals are halted 8 hours before surgery. Light meals may be taken up to 6 hours before, and clear liquid taken up to 2 hours prior to surgery. Ingestion of a complex-carbohydrate drink in nondiabetics decreases patient thirst, anxiety, and insulin resistance (Noblett, 2006). Medications such as acetaminophen and gabapentin can assist with preoperative analgesia (Alayed, 2014; Moon, 2011). The American College of Obstetricians and Gynecologists (2018a) describes the oral trio of celecoxib, 400 mg; acetaminophen, 1000 mg; and gabapentin, 600 mg.

Intraoperative ERAS components emphasize management of pain, temperature, and fluids. An MIS route is preferred when possible and is complemented by wound infiltration with local anesthetic. Hypothermia is associated with higher rates of perioperative complications, particularly with wound healing (Sessler, 2016). Thus, normothermia is encouraged. Last, fluid management aims to maintain euvolemia. Excessive fluid administration can cause bowel edema to delay normal GI function, whereas hypovolemia may decrease cardiac output and tissue oxygenation (Miller, 2015).

Postoperative ERAS considerations such as fluid management, urinary drainage, and pain management are discussed in Chapter 42. Early ambulation and feeding are mainstays of these protocols.

GASTROINTESTINAL BOWEL PREPARATION

Mechanical bowel preparation is no longer routinely used for elective gynecologic procedures (Fanning, 2011; Nelson, 2019). This intervention was previously advocated if the risk for colon injury was high. Its purported benefit was prevention of bowel anastomotic leaks from passage of hard feces and reduction of fecal and bacterial loads to lower wound infection rates (Barker, 1971; Nichols, 1971).

Multiple studies evaluating colorectal surgery show contradictory findings (Duncan, 2009; Güenaga, 2011; Ohman, 2017; Scarborough, 2015). However, studies of laparoscopic gynecologic surgery and pelvic floor procedures do not support mechanical bowel preparation (Ballard, 2014; Siedhoff, 2014). Moreover, ERAS protocols eschew mechanical bowel preparation as its potential iatrogenic dehydration counters the goal of euvolemia.

Although routine use ideally is limited, mechanical bowel preparation may be elected for certain advanced laparoscopic surgeries or for female pelvic reconstructive procedures involving the posterior vaginal wall and anal sphincter. In these cases, rectal stool evacuation provides additional operating space and undistorted anatomy. It also permits proctosigmoidoscopy if needed to interrogate possible rectosigmoid laceration. Moreover, following sphincteroplasty, preoperative evacuation typically delays stooling and allows initial healing. If elected, regimens are: (1) low-residue or clear liquid diets the day(s) prior to surgery, (2) oral cathartics such as 240 mL of senna extract (Senokot, X-Prep) or 240 mL of magnesium citrate, (3) sodium phosphate enemas (Fleet), (4) oral phosphates (Visicol, Fleet Phospho-soda), or (5) polyethylene glycol (PEG) solutions (GoLYTELY, NuLYTELY, HalfLytely).

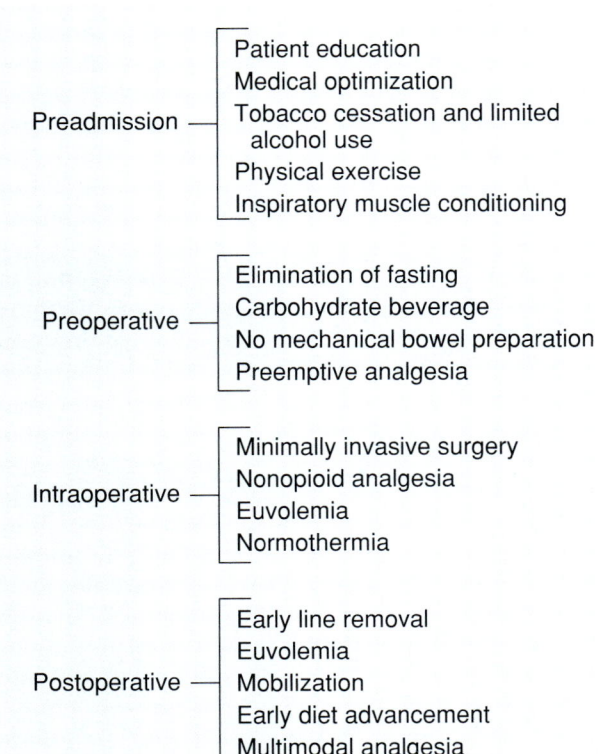

Preadmission —
- Patient education
- Medical optimization
- Tobacco cessation and limited alcohol use
- Physical exercise
- Inspiratory muscle conditioning

Preoperative —
- Elimination of fasting
- Carbohydrate beverage
- No mechanical bowel preparation
- Preemptive analgesia

Intraoperative —
- Minimally invasive surgery
- Nonopioid analgesia
- Euvolemia
- Normothermia

Postoperative —
- Early line removal
- Euvolemia
- Mobilization
- Early diet advancement
- Multimodal analgesia

FIGURE 39-5. Enhanced recovery after surgery (ERAS) phases.

TABLE 39-9. Caprini Risk Assessment Model

1 Point	2 Points	3 Points	5 Points
Age 41–60 yr	Age 61–74 yr	Age ≥75 yr	Stroke <1 month
Minor surgery	Arthroscopic surgery	Prior VTE	Elective arthroplasty
BMI >25 kg/m^2	Major laparotomy (>45 min)	Family history of VTE	Hip, pelvis, or leg fracture
Swollen legs	Laparoscopy (>45 min)	Factor V Leiden	Acute spinal cord injury
Varicose veins	Malignancy	Prothrombin 20210A	<1 month
Pregnancy or postpartum	Bed rest >72 hr	Lupus anticoagulant	
Recurrent spontaneous abortion	Immobilizing plaster cast	Anticardiolipin antibodies	
COC or HRT use	Central venous access	Elevated serum homocysteine	
Sepsis <1 month		Heparin-induced	
Serious lung disease <1 month		thrombocytopenia	
Abnormal pulmonary function		Other thrombophilia	
Acute myocardial infarction			
CHF <1 month			
IBD			
Bed rest			

BMI = body mass index; CHF = congestive heart failure; COC = combination oral contraceptive; HRT = hormone replacement therapy; IBD = inflammatory bowel disease; VTE = venous thromboembolism.
Modified from Gould, 2012, with permission.

THROMBOEMBOLISM PREVENTION

In the United States alone, the annual incidence of deep-vein thrombosis (DVT) and pulmonary thromboembolism is estimated to approach 600,000. Of those diagnosed with VTE, 10 to 30 percent die within 1 month of diagnosis (Beckman, 2010). National recommendations for prophylaxis against VTE follow a risk-based approach. The Caprini score is a tool validated using a large sample of general, vascular, and urologic surgery patients (Table 39-9) (Gould, 2012). Despite not being validated in gynecologic surgery, the patient populations are sufficiently similar to allow extrapolation. Caprini scores of 0–1 points categorize a patient as "very low risk," 2 points reflect "low risk," 3–4 points confer "moderate risk," and ≥5 points place patients at "high risk." These points are transferable to Table 39-10.

■ Thrombophilias

These are inherited or acquired deficiencies of inhibitory proteins within the coagulation cascade. Each can lead to hypercoagulability and recurrent VTE.

TABLE 39-10. Thromboprophylaxis Based on VTE and Bleeding Risks

	Risk and Consequences of Major Bleeding Complications	
Risk of VTE (Caprini Score)	**Average Bleeding Risk**	**High Bleeding Risk or Severe Consequences**
Very low (0–1)	No specific prophylaxis	
Low (2)	Mechanical prophylaxis (IPC preferred)	
Moderate (3–4)	LDUH, LMWH, *or* MP (IPC preferred)	Mechanical prophylaxis (IPC preferred)
High (≥5)	LDUH *or* LMWH *PLUS* MP (CS or IPC)	Mechanical prophylaxis (IPC preferred), until bleeding risk subsides and pharmacologic prophylaxis can be added
High risk, cancer surgery	Same as high risk *PLUS* extended LMWH prophylaxis	
High risk, heparin NA or CI	Fondaparinux or low-dose ASA *or* MP (IPC preferred) *or* both	

ASA = aspirin; CI = contraindicated; CS = compression stockings; LDUH = low-dose unfractionated heparin; LMWH = low-molecular-weight heparin; IPC = intermittent pneumatic compression; MP = mechanical prophylaxis; NA = not available; VTE = venous thromboembolism.

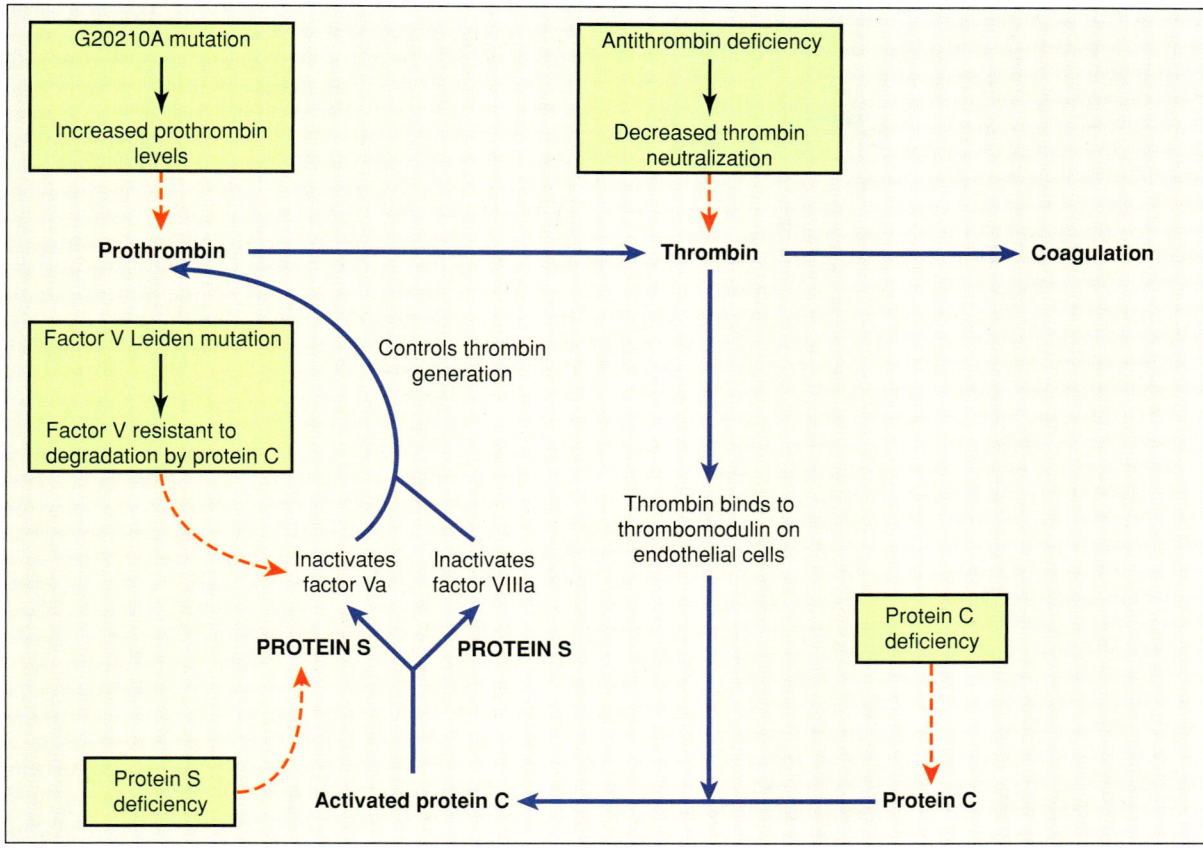

FIGURE 39-6 Points of the coagulation cascade affected by some of the thrombophilias. (Data from Seligsohn, 2001.)

Antithrombin deficiency, although rare, is the most thrombogenic. Thrombin is produced by the enzymatic cleavage of prothrombin (Fig. 39-6). Thrombin converts fibrinogen to an active form that assembles into fibrin for clot formation. Antithrombin, previously known as antithrombin III, binds to and inactivates thrombin and the activated coagulation factors IXa, Xa, XIa, and XIIa. If thrombin is not inactivated, coagulation is favored.

Protein C and *protein S deficiencies* are other thrombophilias. When thrombin is bound to thrombomodulin on intact endothelium, its procoagulant activities are neutralized. In this bound state, thrombin also activates protein C, a natural anticoagulant. Protein C and its cofactor, protein S, limit coagulation, in part, by inactivating factors Va and VIIIa.

Activated protein C resistance (Factor V Leiden mutation) is the most prevalent thrombophilia and is caused by a single mutation in the factor V gene. The mutation makes FVa resist degradation by activated protein C. The unimpeded abnormal factor V protein retains its procoagulant activity and predisposes to thrombosis.

Prothrombin G20210A mutation is a thrombophilia stemming from a prothrombin gene missense mutation that leads to excessive prothrombin accumulation. This then may be converted to thrombin to create a hypercoagulable state.

The role of thrombophilia testing is complex, because the testing can be costly and harmful if inaccurate. Guidelines to direct thrombophilia testing are lacking in the United States, and those of other international groups are incongruous (Connors, 2017; De Stefano, 2013). The American Society of Hematology recommends against thrombophilia testing in adults with VTE arising in a major transient setting such as surgery, trauma, or prolonged immobility (Hicks, 2013). Patients with these factors have a low VTE recurrence risk. With an initial surgical trigger, VTE redevelops in 0.7 percent of patients (Iorio, 2010). Moreover, testing results rarely affect clinical decisions regarding VTE treatment. The UK-based NICE guidelines (2012) recommend screening patients who have an unprovoked VTE but not those with a provoked VTE. They also recommend against screening asymptomatic first-degree relatives of a known thrombophilia patient who experienced a VTE.

■ Hormone Discontinuation

Of risks, hormone use can be modified prior to elective surgery. Combined oral contraceptive pills (COCs) induce hypercoagulable changes that are reversed if COCs are stopped at least 6 weeks prior to surgery (Robinson, 1991; Vessey, 1986). To balance the risk of unintended pregnancy in women halting COCs, a suitable alternative is recommended with clear instructions on use. In the decision to halt COCs prior to surgery, the risk of VTE in an individual is weighed against the risk of unintended pregnancy. In those undergoing major surgery and COC continuation, heparin prophylaxis is considered (American College of Obstetricians and Gynecologists, 2018b).

Postmenopausal hormone replacement therapy (HRT) may slightly raise the postsurgical VTE incidence but not to the same degree as the surgical procedure itself (Ueng, 2010). Thus, women are appropriately counseled on this additional postoperative risk, but the value and duration of HRT cessation to negate this enhanced risk is unclear.

■ Prophylaxis Options

Early ambulation, although encouraged after surgery, is not regarded as a primary strategy for VTE prophylaxis (Michota, 2006). Graded compression stockings (TED hose) prevent pooling of blood in the calves. If these are used alone and fitted properly, DVT rates are reduced 50 percent. If used in conjunction with other methods of prophylaxis, additional benefit is achieved (Amaragiri, 2000). Intermittent pneumatic compression primarily works by improving venous flow. It appears to be effective in moderate- and high-risk patients, if initiated prior to the induction of anesthesia and continued until patients are fully ambulating (Clarke-Pearson, 1993; Gould, 2012). Pharmacologic methods of VTE prophylaxis include low-dose UFH, LMWH, and DOACs. Table 39-10 summarizes appropriate treatment strategies based on risk (Gould, 2012).

REFERENCES

Achilles SL, Reeves MF, Society of Family Planning: Prevention of infection after induced abortion: release date October 2010: SFP guideline 20102. Contraception 83(4):295, 2011

Ageno W, Gallus AS, Wittkowsky A, et al: Oral anticoagulant therapy: Antithrombotic Therapy and Prevention of Thrombosis, 9th ed: American College of Chest Physicians Evidence-Based Clinical Practice Guidelines. Chest 141(2 Suppl):e44S, 2012

Agostini P, Cieslik H, Rathinam S, et al: Postoperative pulmonary complications following thoracic surgery: are there any modifiable risk factors? Thorax 65(9):815, 2010

Akrawi W, Benumof JL: A pathophysiological basis for informed preoperative smoking cessation counseling. J Cardiothorac Vasc Anesth 11(5):629, 1997

Alayed N, Alghanaim N, Tan X, et al: Preemptive use of gabapentin in abdominal hysterectomy: a systematic review and meta-analysis. Obstet Gynecol 123(6):1221, 2014

Amaragiri SV, Lees TA: Elastic compression stockings for prevention of deep vein thrombosis. Cochrane Database Syst Rev 3:CD001484, 2000

American College of Obstetricians and Gynecologists: Informed consent. Committee Opinion No. 439, August 2009, Reaffirmed 2015

American College of Obstetricians and Gynecologists: Professional responsibilities in obstetric-gynecologic medical education and training. Committee Opinion No. 500, January 2007, Reaffirmed 2017

American College of Obstetricians and Gynecologists: Perioperative pathways: enhanced recovery after surgery. Committee Opinion No. 750, September 2018a

American College of Obstetricians and Gynecologists: Prevention of deep vein thrombosis and pulmonary embolism. Practice Bulletin No. 84, August 2007, Reaffirmed 2018b

American College of Obstetricians and Gynecologists: Prevention of infection after gynecologic procedures. Practice Bulletin No. 195, June 2018c

American College of Obstetricians and Gynecologists: Chronic antithrombotic therapy and gynecologic surgery. Committee Opinion No. 610, October 2014, Reaffirmed 2019

American College of Radiology: ACR appropriateness criteria: routine admission and preoperative chest radiography. Reston, American College of Radiology, 2000, Reaffirmed 2015

American Society of Anesthesiologists: ASA Physical Status Classification System, 2014a. Available at: https://www.asahq.org/standards-and-guidelines/asa-physical-status-classification-system. Accessed July 19, 2019

American Society of Anesthesiologists: Practice guidelines for preoperative fasting and the use of pharmacologic agents to reduce the risk of pulmonary aspiration: application to healthy patients undergoing elective procedures:

an updated report by the American Society of Anesthesiologists Task Force on preoperative fasting and the use of pharmacologic agents to reduce the risk of pulmonary aspiration. Anesthesiology 126(3):376, 2017

American Society of Anesthesiologists: Practice guidelines for the perioperative management of patients with obstructive sleep apnea: an updated report by the American Society of Anesthesiologists Task Force on Perioperative Management of patients with obstructive sleep apnea. Anesthesiology 120(2):268, 2014b

Archer C, Levy AR, McGregor M: Value of routine preoperative chest x-rays: a meta-analysis. Can J Anaesth 40:1022, 1993

Arozullah AM, Daley J, Henderson WG, et al: Multifactorial risk index for predicting postoperative respiratory failure in men after major noncardiac surgery. The National Veterans Administration Surgical Quality Improvement Program. Ann Surg 232:242, 2000

Ballard AC, Parker-Autry CY, Markland AD, et al: Bowel preparation before vaginal prolapse surgery: a randomized controlled trial. Obstet Gynecol 123(2 Pt 1):232, 2014

Bapoje SR, Whitaker JF, Schulz T, et al: Preoperative evaluation of the patient with pulmonary disease. Chest 132(5):1637, 2007

Barker K, Graham NG, Mason MC, et al: The relative significance of preoperative oral antibiotics, mechanical bowel preparation, and preoperative peritoneal contamination in the avoidance of sepsis after radical surgery for ulcerative colitis and Crohn's disease of the large bowel. Br J Surg 58:270, 1971

Beckman MG, Hooper WC, Critchley SE, et al: Venous thromboembolism: a public health concern. Am J Prev Med 38(4 Suppl):S495, 2010

Blessberger H, Kammler J, Domanovits H, et al: Perioperative beta-blockers for preventing surgery-related mortality and morbidity. Cochrane Database Syst Rev 3:CD004476, 2018

Bouri S, Shun-Shin MJ, Cole GD, et al: Meta-analysis of secure randomised controlled trials of β-blockade to prevent perioperative death in non-cardiac surgery. Heart 100(6):456, 2014

Burks C, Nelson L, Kumar D, et al: Evaluation of pulmonary complications in robotic-assisted gynecologic surgery. J Minim Invasive Gynecol 24(2):280, 2017

Carey ET, Moulder JK: Perioperative management and implementation of enhanced recovery programs in gynecologic surgery for benign indications. Obstet Gynecol 132(1):137, 2018

Carson JL, Guyatt G, Heddle NM, et al: Clinical practice guidelines from the AABB: red blood cell transfusion thresholds and storage. JAMA 316(19):2025, 2016

Cheng A, Nazarian S, Spragg DD, et al: Effects of surgical and endoscopic electrocautery on modern-day permanent pacemaker and implantable cardioverter-defibrillator systems. Pacing Clin Electrophysiol 31(3):344, 2008

Chung F, Yegneswaran B, Liao P, et al: STOP questionnaire: a tool to screen patients for obstructive sleep apnea. Anesthesiology 108(5):812, 2008

Clarke-Pearson DL, Synan IS, Dodge R, et al: A randomized trial of low-dose heparin and intermittent pneumatic calf compression for the prevention of deep venous thrombosis after gynecologic oncology surgery. Am J Obstet Gynecol 168:1146, 1993

Connolly SJ, Crowther M, Eikelboom JW, et al: Full study report of andexanet alfa for bleeding associated with actor Xa inhibitors. N Engl J Med 380(14):1326, 2019

Connors JM: Thrombophilia testing and venous thrombosis. N Engl J Med 377(12):1177, 2017

Coulter A, Ellins J: Effectiveness of strategies for informing, educating, and involving patients. BMJ 335(7609):24, 2007

Crowther M, van der Spuy K, Roodt F, et al: The relationship between preoperative hypertension and intra-operative haemodynamic changes known to be associated with postoperative morbidity. Anaesthesia 73(7):812, 2018

Cunningham FG, Leveno KL, Bloom SL, et al (eds): Thromboembolic disorders. In Williams Obstetrics, 24th ed. New York, McGraw-Hill, 2014, p 1030

De Stefano V, Rossi E: Testing for inherited thrombophilia and consequences for antithrombotic prophylaxis in patients with venous thromboembolism and their relatives. A review of the Guidelines from Scientific Societies and Working Groups. Thromb Haemost 110(4):697, 2013

DeLoughery TG: Microcytic anemia. N Engl J Med 371(14):1324, 2014

Devereaux PJ, Goldman L, Cook DJ, et al: Perioperative cardiac events in patients undergoing noncardiac surgery: a review of the magnitude of the problem, the pathophysiology of the events and methods to estimate and communicate risk. CMAJ 173 (6):627, 2005

Douketis J, Bell AD, Eikelboom J, et al: Approach to the new oral anticoagulants in family practice: Part 2: addressing frequently asked questions. Can Fam Physician 60(11):997, 2014

Douketis JD, Spyropoulos AC, Spencer FA, et al: Perioperative management of antithrombotic therapy: Antithrombotic Therapy and Prevention of

Thrombosis, 9th ed: American College of Chest Physicians Evidence-Based Clinical Practice Guidelines. Chest 141(2 Suppl):e326S, 2012

Dronge AS, Perkal MF, Kancir S, et al: Long-term glycemic control and postoperative infectious complications. Arch Surg 141:375, 2006

Duncan JE, Quietmeyer CM: Bowel preparation: current status. Clin Colon Rectal Surg 22(1):14, 2009

Eichenberger A, Proietti S, Wicky S, et al: Morbid obesity and postoperative pulmonary atelectasis: an underestimated problem. Anesth Analg 95:1788, 2002

Fanning J, Valea FA: Perioperative bowel management for gynecologic surgery. Am J Obstet Gynecol 205(4):309, 2011

Finney SJ, Zekveld C, Elia A, et al: Glucose control and mortality in critically ill patients. JAMA 290:2041, 2003

Fleisher LA: Preoperative evaluation of the patient with hypertension. JAMA 287:2043, 2002

Fleisher LA, Beckman JA, Brown KA, et al: 2009 ACCF/AHA focused update on perioperative beta blockade incorporated into the ACC/AHA 2007 guidelines on perioperative cardiovascular evaluation and care for noncardiac surgery: a report of the American College of Cardiology Foundation/American Heart Association Task Force on Practice Guidelines. Circulation 120(21):e169, 2009

Fleisher LA, Fleischmann KE, Auerbach AD, et al: 2014 ACC/AHA guideline on perioperative cardiovascular evaluation and management of patients undergoing noncardiac surgery: a report of the American College of Cardiology/American Heart Association Task Force on practice guidelines. J Am Coll Cardiol 64(22):e77, 2014

Garber AJ, Moghissi ES, Bransome ED Jr, et al: American College of Endocrinology position statement on inpatient diabetes and metabolic control. Endocr Pract 10:77, 2004

Goldman L, Lee T, Rudd P: Ten Commandments for effective consultations. Arch Intern Med 143:1753, 1983

Goldwasser P, Feldman J: Association of serum albumin and mortality risk. J Clin Epidemiol 50:693, 1997

Gould MK, Garcia DA, Wren SM, et al: Prevention of VTE in nonorthopedic surgical patients: Antithrombotic Therapy and Prevention of Thrombosis, 9th ed: American College of Chest Physicians Evidence-Based Clinical Practice Guidelines. Chest 141(2 Suppl):e227S, 2012

Gregoratos G, Abrams J, Epstein AE, et al: ACC/AHA/NASPE 2002 guideline update for implantation of cardiac pacemakers and antiarrhythmia devices: summary article: a report of the American College of Cardiology/American Heart Association Task Force on Practice Guidelines (ACC/AHA/NASPE Committee to Update the 1998 Pacemaker Guidelines). Circulation 106:2145, 2002

Güenaga KF, Matos D, Wille-Jørgensen P, et al: Mechanical bowel preparation for elective colorectal surgery. Cochrane Database Syst Rev 9:CD001544, 2011

Harrison L, Johnston M, Massicotte MP, et al: Comparison of 5-mg and 10-mg loading doses in initiation of warfarin therapy. Ann Intern Med 126:133, 1997

Hassan SA, Hlatky MA, Boothroyd DB, et al: Outcomes of noncardiac surgery after coronary bypass surgery or coronary angioplasty in the Bypass Angioplasty Revascularization Investigation (BARI). Am J Med 110:260, 2001

Hicks LK, Bering H, Carson KR, et al: The ASH Choosing Wisely campaign: five hematologic tests and treatments to question. Blood 122(24):3879, 2013

Hlatky MA, Boineau RE, Higginbotham MB, et al: A brief self-administered questionnaire to determine functional capacity (the Duke Activity Status Index). Am J Cardiol 64(10):651, 1989

Holbrook A, Schulman S, Witt DM, et al: Evidence-based management of anticoagulant therapy: Antithrombotic Therapy and Prevention of Thrombosis, 9th ed: American College of Chest Physicians Evidence-Based Clinical Practice Guidelines. Chest 141(2 Suppl):e152S, 2012

Hoogwerf BJ: Perioperative management of diabetes mellitus: how should we act on the limited evidence? Cleve Clin J Med 73(Suppl 1):S95, 2006

Iorio A, Kearon C, Filippucci E, et al: Risk of recurrence after a first episode of symptomatic venous thromboembolism provoked by a transient risk factor: a systematic review. Arch Intern Med 170(19):1710, 2010

Jacober SJ, Sowers JR: An update on perioperative management of diabetes. Arch Intern Med 159:2405, 1999

James AH, Kouides PA, Abdul-Kadir R, et al: Evaluation and management of acute menorrhagia in women with and without underlying bleeding disorders: consensus from an international expert panel. Eur J Obstet Gynecol Reprod Biol 158(2):124, 2011

Jehan F, Khan M, Sakran JV, et al: Perioperative glycemic control and postoperative complications in patients undergoing emergency general surgery: what is the role of plasma hemoglobin A1c? J Trauma Acute Care Surg 84(1):112, 2018

Johnson BE, Porter J: Preoperative evaluation of the gynecologic patient: considerations for improved outcomes. Obstet Gynecol 111(5):1183, 2008

Kachalia A, Berg A, Fagerlin A, et al: Overuse of testing in preoperative evaluation and syncope: a survey of hospitalists. Ann Intern Med 162(2):100, 2015

Kannel WB: Epidemiology and prevention of cardiac failure: Framingham Study insights. Eur Heart J 8:23, 1987

Kearon C, Hirsh J: Management of anticoagulation before and after elective surgery. N Engl J Med 336:1506, 1997

Kehlet H: Multimodal approach to control postoperative pathophysiology and rehabilitation. Br J Anaesth 78(5):606, 1997

Kelly KN, Domajnko B: Perioperative stress-dose steroids. Clin Colon Rectal Surg 26(3):163, 2013

Kertai MD, Bountioukos M, Boersma E, et al: Aortic stenosis: an underestimated risk factor for perioperative complications in patients undergoing noncardiac surgery. Am J Med 116:8, 2004

Kozek-Langenecker SA: Perioperative management issues of direct oral anticoagulants. Semin Hematol 51(2):112, 2014

Lawson T, Ralph C: Perioperative Jehovah's Witnesses: a review. Br J Anaesth 115(5):676, 2015

Lee HP, Chang YY, Jean YH, et al: Importance of serum albumin level in the preoperative tests conducted in elderly patients with hip fracture. Injury 40(7):756, 2009

Lee TH, Marcantonio ER, Mangione CM, et al: Derivation and prospective validation of a simple index for prediction of cardiac risk of major noncardiac surgery. Circulation 100:1043, 1999

Levine GN, Bates ER, Bittl JA, et al: 2016 ACC/AHA guideline focused update on duration of dual antiplatelet therapy in patients with coronary artery disease: a report of the American College of Cardiology/American Heart Association Task Force on Clinical Practice Guidelines. J Thorac Cardiovasc Surg 152(5):1243, 2016

Levine MN, Hirsh J, Gent M, et al: Optimal duration of oral anticoagulant therapy: a randomized trial comparing four weeks with three months of warfarin in patients with proximal deep vein thrombosis. Thromb Haemost 74:606, 1995

Lindahl TL, Baghaei F, Blixter IF, et al: Effects of the oral, direct thrombin inhibitor dabigatran on five common coagulation assays. Thromb Haemost 105(2):371, 2011

Macpherson DS, Snow R, Lofgren RP: Preoperative screening: value of previous tests. Ann Intern Med 113:969, 1990

Maddali MM: Chronic obstructive lung disease: perioperative management. Middle East J Anesthesiol 19(6):1219, 2008

Mangano DT: Perioperative medicine: NHLBI working group deliberations and recommendations. J Cardiothorac Vasc Anesth 18:1, 2004

Mangano DT, Layug EL, Wallace A, et al: Effect of atenolol on mortality and cardiovascular morbidity after noncardiac surgery. Multicenter Study of Perioperative Ischemia Research Group. N Engl J Med 335:1713, 1996

Mansour A, Watson W, Shayani V, et al: Abdominal operations in patients with cirrhosis: still a major surgical challenge. Surgery 122(4):730, 1997

Marik PE, Varon J: Requirement of perioperative stress doses of corticosteroids: a systematic review of the literature. Arch Surg 143(12):1222, 2008

Michota FA Jr: Preventing venous thromboembolism in surgical patients. Cleve Clin J Med 73:S88, 2006

Miller TE, Roche AM, Mythen M: Fluid management and goal-directed therapy as an adjunct to enhanced recovery after surgery (ERAS). Can J Anaesth 62(2):158, 2015

Møller AM, Villebro N, Pedersen T, et al: Effect of preoperative smoking intervention on postoperative complications: a randomised clinical trial. Lancet 359:114, 2002

Moon YE, Lee YK, Lee J, et al: The effects of preoperative intravenous acetaminophen in patients undergoing abdominal hysterectomy. Arch Gynecol Obstet 284(6):1455, 2011

Morrill MY, Schimpf MO, Abed H, et al: Antibiotic prophylaxis for selected gynecologic surgeries. Int J Gynaecol Obstet 120(1):10, 2013

Nakagawa M, Tanaka H, Tsukuma H, et al: Relationship between the duration of the preoperative smoke-free period and the incidence of postoperative pulmonary complications after pulmonary surgery. Chest 120:705, 2001

Nandi PL: Ethical aspects of clinical practice. Arch Surg 135:22, 2000

National Heart Blood and Lung Institute: The expert panel report 3 (EPR—3) summary report 2007: guidelines for the diagnosis and management of asthma. NIH Publication No. 085846, 2007

National Institute for Health and Clinical Excellence: Routine preoperative tests for elective surgery. 2016. Available at: https://www.nice.org.uk/guidance/ng45. Accessed June 29, 2019

Nelson G, Bakkum-Gamez J, Kalogera E, et al: Guidelines for perioperative care in gynecologic/oncology: Enhanced Recovery After Surgery (ERAS) Society recommendations-2019 update. Int J Gynecol Cancer 29(4):651, 2019

Nichols RL, Condon RE: Preoperative preparation of the colon. Surg Gynecol Obstet 132:323, 1971

Nishimura RA, Otto CM, Bonow RO, et al: 2017 AHA/ACC focused update of the 2014 AHA/ACC guideline for the management of patients with valvular heart disease: a report of the American College of Cardiology/American Heart Association Task Force on Clinical Practice Guidelines. J Am Coll Cardiol 70(2):252, 2017

Noblett SE, Watson DS, Huong H, et al: Pre-operative oral carbohydrate loading in colorectal surgery: a randomized controlled trial. Colorectal Dis 8(7):563, 2006

Norman WV: Metronidazole prophylaxis before surgical abortion: retrospective review of 51,330 cases. J Obstet Gynaecol Can 34(7):648, 2012

Ohman KA, Wan L, Guthrie T, et al: Combination of oral antibiotics and mechanical bowel preparation reduces surgical site infection in colorectal surgery. J Am Coll Surg 225(4):465, 2017

Ortel TL: Perioperative management of patients on chronic antithrombotic therapy. Blood 120(24):4699, 2012

Patel T: Surgery in the patient with liver disease. Mayo Clin Proc 74:593, 1999

Pellegrini JE, Toledo P, Soper DE, et al: Consensus bundle on prevention of surgical site infections after major gynecologic surgery. Obstet Gynecol 129(1):50, 2017

Poldermans D, Devereaux PJ: The experts debate: perioperative beta-blockade for noncardiac surgery—proven safe or not? Cleve Clin J Med 76 Suppl 4: S84, 2009

Qaseem A, Snow V, Fitterman N, et al: Risk assessment for and strategies to reduce perioperative pulmonary complications for patients undergoing noncardiothoracic surgery: a guideline from the American College of Physicians. Ann Intern Med 144:575, 2006

Robinson GE, Burren T, Mackie IJ, et al: Changes in haemostasis after stopping the combined contraceptive pill: implications for major surgery. Br Med J 302:269, 1991

Roizen MF: More preoperative assessment by physicians and less by laboratory tests. N Engl J Med 342:204, 2000

Roshanov PS, Rochwerg B, Patel A, et al: Withholding versus continuing angiotensin-converting enzyme inhibitors or angiotensin II receptor blockers before noncardiac surgery: an analysis of the vascular events in noncardiac surgery patients cohort evaluation prospective cohort. Anesthesiology 126(1):16, 2017

Rucker L, Frye EB, Staten MA: Usefulness of screening chest roentgenograms in preoperative patients. JAMA 250:3209, 1983

Salmasi V, Maheshwari K, Yang D, et al: Relationship between intraoperative hypotension, defined by either reduction from baseline or absolute thresholds, and acute kidney and myocardial injury after noncardiac surgery: a retrospective cohort analysis. Anesthesiology 126(1):47, 2017

Scarborough JE, Mantyh CR, Sun Z, et al: Combined mechanical and oral antibiotic bowel preparation reduces incisional surgical site infection and anastomotic leak rates after elective colorectal resection: an analysis of colectomy-targeted ACS NSQIP. Ann Surg 262(2):331, 2015

Schaden E, Kozek-Langenecker SA: Direct thrombin inhibitors: pharmacology and application in intensive care medicine. Intensive Care Med 36(7):1127, 2010

Sessler DI: Perioperative thermoregulation and heat balance. Lancet 387 (10038):2655, 2016

Shander A, Spence RK, Auerbach M: Can intravenous iron therapy meet the unmet needs created by the new restrictions on erythropoietic stimulating agents? Transfusion 50(3):719, 2010

Shi Y, Warner DO: Surgery as a teachable moment for smoking cessation. Anesthesiology 112(1):102, 2010

Siedhoff MT, Clark LH, Hobbs KA, et al: Mechanical bowel preparation before laparoscopic hysterectomy: a randomized controlled trial. Obstet Gynecol 123(3):562, 2014

Silverberg DS, Wexler D, Sheps D, et al: The effect of correction of mild anemia in severe, resistant congestive heart failure using subcutaneous erythropoietin and intravenous iron: a randomized, controlled study. J Am Coll Cardiol 37:1775, 2001

Sirinek KR, Burk RR, Brown M, et al: Improving survival in patients with cirrhosis undergoing major abdominal operations. Arch Surg 122:271, 1987

Smetana GW: Preoperative pulmonary evaluation. N Engl J Med 340:937, 1999

Smetana GW, Lawrence VA, Cornell JE: Preoperative pulmonary risk stratification for noncardiothoracic surgery: systematic review for the American College of Physicians. Ann Intern Med 144(8):581, 2006

Smilowitz NR, Gupta N, Ramakrishna H, et al: Perioperative major adverse cardiovascular and cerebrovascular events associated with noncardiac surgery. JAMA Cardiol 2(2):181, 2017

Solomon ER, Muffly TM, Barber MD: Common postoperative pulmonary complications after hysterectomy for benign indications. Am J Obstet Gynecol 208(1):54.e1, 2013

Sood A, Abdollah F, Sammon JD, et al: The effect of body mass index on perioperative outcomes after major surgery: results from the National Surgical Quality Improvement Program (ACS-NSQIP) 2005–2011. World J Surg 39(10):2376, 2015

Spatz ES, Krumholz HM, Moulton BW: The new era of informed consent: getting to a reasonable-patient standard through shared decision making. JAMA 315(19):2063, 2016

Stacey D, Légaré F, Lewis K, et al: Decision aids for people facing health treatment or screening decisions. Cochrane Database Syst Rev 4:CD001431, 2017

Straus SE, McAlister FA, Sackett DL, et al: The accuracy of patient history, wheezing, and laryngeal measurements in diagnosing obstructive airway disease. CARE-COAD1 Group. Clinical Assessment of the Reliability of the Examination—Chronic Obstructive Airways Disease. JAMA 283:1853, 2000

Suman A, Carey WD: Assessing the risk of surgery in patients with liver disease. Cleve Clin J Med 73(4):398, 2006

Tashiro T, Pislaru SV, Blustin JM, et al: Perioperative risk of major non-cardiac surgery in patients with severe aortic stenosis: a reappraisal in contemporary practice. Eur Heart J 35(35):2372, 2014

Ueng J, Douketis JD: Prevention and treatment of hormone-associated venous thromboembolism: a patient management approach. Hematol Oncol Clin North Am 24(4):683, 2010

Vessey M, Mant D, Smith A, et al: Oral contraceptives and venous thromboembolism: findings in a large prospective study. Br Med J (Clin Res Ed) 292:526, 1986

Warner DO: Preventing postoperative pulmonary complications: the role of the anesthesiologist. Anesthesiology 92:1467, 2000

Warner DO, Warner MA, Barnes RD, et al: Perioperative respiratory complications in patients with asthma. Anesthesiology 85:460, 1996

Weksler N, Klein M, Szendro G, et al: The dilemma of immediate preoperative hypertension: to treat and operate or to postpone surgery? J Clin Anesth 15:179, 2003

White RH, McKittrick T, Hutchinson R, et al: Temporary discontinuation of warfarin therapy: changes in the international normalized ratio. Ann Intern Med 122:40, 1995

Williams FM, Bergin JD: Cardiac screening before noncardiac surgery. Surg Clin North Am 89(4):747, 2009

Wolters U, Wolf T, Stutzer H, et al: ASA classification and perioperative variables as predictors of postoperative outcome. Br J Anaesth 77:217, 1996

Wong J, Lam DP, Abrishami A, et al: Short-term preoperative smoking cessation and postoperative complications: a systematic review and meta-analysis. Can J Anaesth 59(3):268, 2012

Woods BD, Sladen RN: Perioperative considerations for the patient with asthma and bronchospasm. Br J Anaesth 103 (1 suppl):i57, 2009

Wysham WZ, Kim KH, Roberts JM, et al: Obesity and perioperative pulmonary complications in robotic gynecologic surgery. Am J Obstet Gynecol 213(1):33.e1, 2015

Yang CK, Teng A, Lee DY, et al: Pulmonary complications after major abdominal surgery: National Surgical Quality Improvement Program analysis. J Surg Res 198(2):441, 2015

Zerah F, Harf A, Perlemuter L, et al: Effects of obesity on respiratory resistance. Chest 103:1470, 1993

Intraoperative Considerations

Gynecologic surgery is used to treat a broad spectrum of underlying pathology. As a result, the list of procedures is extensive, but in general, techniques maximize tissue healing and patient recovery. Successful outcomes depend on appropriate patient and procedure selection, sound intraoperative technique, and preparation for possible complications.

SURGICAL SAFETY

Communication between all members of the surgical team is vital to operative success and avoidance of patient harm. The Joint Commission (2018) established the *Universal Protocol for Preventing Wrong Site, Wrong Procedure, and Wrong Person Surgery*. This protocol encompasses three components: (1) preprocedural verification of all relevant documents, (2) marking the operative site, and (3) completion of a "time out" prior to procedure initiation. The "time out" requires attention of the entire team to confirm that patient, site, and procedure are correctly identified. Important interactions also include introduction of the patient-care team members, verification of prophylactic antibiotics, estimation of procedure length, and communication of anticipated complications. Additionally, special instrumentation is requested preoperatively to prevent potential patient compromise that may accompany lacking an instrument at the time it is needed. Communication lapses are common across pre-, intra-, and postoperative phases of care and are linked to adverse events (Nagpal, 2010). Specifically, the transfer of a patient to a new care team or location is a particularly vulnerable time (Greenberg, 2007; Jones, 2018).

Checklists can enhance quality and safety. These cognitive aids standardize care, enhance teamwork, and improve communication (American College of Obstetricians and Gynecologists, 2016). The World Health Organization (WHO) Surgical Safety Checklist (2009) is widely used and lowers patient morbidity and mortality in many but not all instances (Table 40-1) (Haynes, 2009; Molina, 2016; Urbach, 2014). Checklist efficacy may be better measured by assessing associated good catches rather than solely evaluating patient harm (Putnam, 2016).

Surgical fires are a specific safety focus, and the three elements of the "fire triangle" are oxygen, ignition source, and fuel source. As prevention, surgeons ideally assess the fire risk at the procedure's start, allow adequate drying of alcohol-based skin antiseptics, and keep ignition sources off the patient or drapes when not in use (Food and Drug Administration, 2018).

SURGICAL ASSISTANT

An ideal assistant should anticipate the surgeon's needs and aid smooth progress of the operation. Therefore, an assistant must be familiar with the planned procedure's steps, relevant anatomy, and relevant patient details.

Maintaining exposure by proper retraction and keeping the operative field clear of obstruction are primary functions. Laparotomy sponge or suction use is timed to avoid interfering with the surgeon, and a sponge is used to blot rather than wipe. On bleeding surfaces, immediate pressure is placed until the situation can be assessed systematically. Clamps are released slowly to avoid tissue slippage. Attention must be fixed on the procedure. Thus, if music or conversation is distracting, they are avoided.

ANESTHESIA SELECTION

Many anesthetic options are available for patients undergoing gynecologic procedures and include general anesthesia, regional analgesia, or local paracervical blockade with or without conscious sedation. Anesthesia selection for gynecologic surgery is complex and influenced by the procedure planned, extent of disease, patient comorbidities, and personal preferences of the patient, anesthesiologist, and surgeon. Last, the providing

TABLE 40-1. Surgical Safety Checklist Modified from World Health Organization

Before Anesthesia Induction	Before Skin Incision	Before Patient Leaves Operating Room
Patient confirms her identity, site, procedure, and consent? ☐ Yes	☐ All team members state name and role	Nurse verbal confirmation: ☐ Procedure name ☐ Correct instrument, sponge, and needle counts ☐ Specimen labeling ☐ Equipment problems requiring correction
Site marked? ☐ Yes ☐ Not applicable	☐ Confirm patient name, procedure, and site	
	Antibiotic prophylaxis given in last 60 minutes? ☐ Yes ☐ Not applicable	To surgeon, anesthesia staff, nurse: ☐ Key concerns for patient recovery?
Anesthesia machine and medication check complete? ☐ Yes	Anticipated critical events: To surgeon: ☐ Critical or nonroutine steps? ☐ Case duration? ☐ Anticipated blood loss?	
Functioning pulse oximeter on patient? ☐ Yes		
Known patient allergy? ☐ No ☐ Yes	To anesthesia provider: ☐ Patient-specific concerns? To nursing team: ☐ Surgical-site sterility confirmed? ☐ Fire risk? ☐ Equipment issues or other concerns?	
Difficult airway or aspiration risk? ☐ No ☐ Yes; equipment/assistance available?		
Risk of >500 mL blood loss? ☐ No ☐ Yes; two IVs/central access and volume resuscitation planned?	Essential imaging displayed? ☐ Yes ☐ Not applicable	

IV = intravenous
Modified from World Health Organization, 2009, with permission.

hospital or clinic may further define options based on their practicing norms and availability of personnel or equipment. For example, an outpatient gynecology clinic may be equipped to provide paracervical blockade or intravenous conscious sedation, but may lack sophisticated equipment or expertise required for regional or general anesthesia.

During all cases, both the anesthesia provider and the surgeon communicate regarding patient and surgery progress and prepare for potential problems. Difficult patient intubation may complicate general anesthesia, and regional anesthetic procedures may lead to higher than anticipated levels of blockade and respiratory muscle dysfunction. Cases using paracervical blockade may be complicated by inadequate levels of anesthesia, or conversely by anesthetic toxicity. Conscious sedation may also fail to provide adequate analgesia, or alternatively may lead to respiratory depression. Thus, no procedure is free of risk, and contingency plans for each should be in place.

■ Paracervical Block

Paracervical block is used most commonly during first-trimester pregnancy evacuation but also may be selected for cervical ablative or excisional procedures, transvaginal sonographically guided oocyte retrieval, in-office hysteroscopy, and outpatient endometrial ablations (Reinders, 2017). Some studies have also described preemptive analgesia with paracervical block for vaginal hysterectomy (Long, 2009; O'Neal, 2003). Paracervical blockade is often combined with nonsteroidal antiinflammatory drugs (NSAIDs) or intravenous conscious sedation or both. Conscious sedation may be achieved with several agents, but intravenous midazolam (Versed) and fentanyl (Sublimaze) is a frequent combination (Lichtenberg, 2001).

Technique

The cervix, vagina, and uterus are richly supplied by nerves of the uterovaginal plexus (Fig. 38-13, p. 802). Also known as *Frankenhäuser plexus*, this plexus lies within the connective tissue lateral to the uterosacral ligaments. For this reason, paracervical injections are most effective if placed immediately lateral to the insertion of the uterosacral ligaments into the uterus (Rogers, 1998). Thus, divided doses are given at the 4 and 8 o'clock positions at the cervical base (Fig. 40-1).

In most cases, total doses of 10 mL of 0.25-percent bupivacaine, 1-percent mepivacaine, or 1- or 2-percent lidocaine may

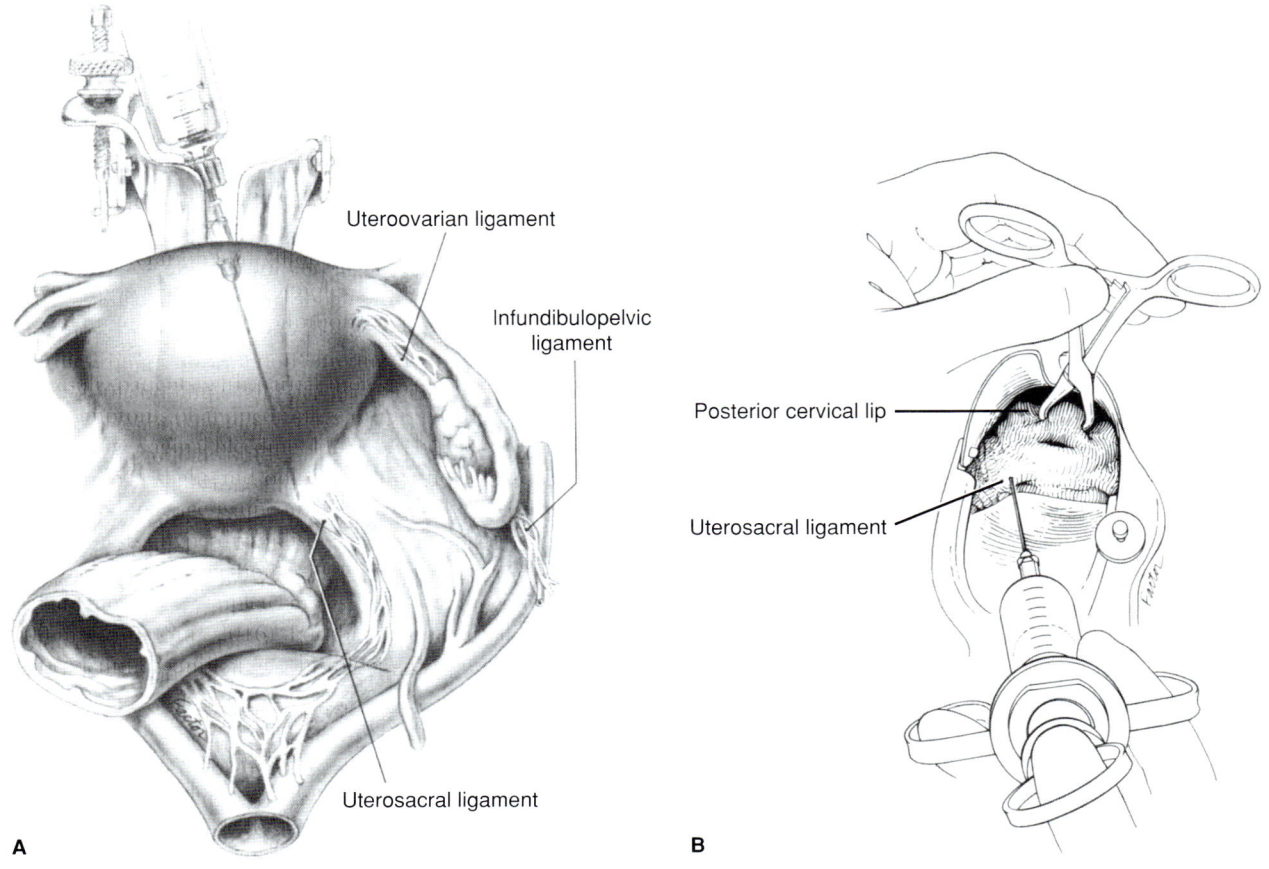

FIGURE 40-1 Paracervical blockade. **A.** Abdominal view of a paracervical block. Local anesthetic is infiltrated near sensory innervation of the cervix, which lies near the uterosacral ligament. **B.** Vaginal approach to the injection of local anesthetics into cervical base at 4 and 8 o'clock. (From Penfield, 1986, with permission.)

be administered (Cicinelli, 1998; Hong, 2006; Lau, 1999). However, specific calculation of a maximum safe dose for each patient before injection is recommended (Dorian, 2015). The toxic dose of lidocaine approximates 4.5 mg/kg (Table 40-2). For a 50-kg woman, this would equal 225 mg. Thus, if a 1-percent lidocaine solution is used, the calculated allowed amount would be: 225 mg ÷ 10 mg/mL = 22.5 mL. Of note, for any drug solution, 1-percent = 10 mg/mL. Addition of epinephrine to these solutions leads to local vasoconstriction, which enhances analgesia quality, prolongs duration of action, and lowers toxicity.

Higher doses of local anesthetics may lead to clinically significant conduction blockade within the central nervous system (CNS) and heart. Signs range from drowsiness, tinnitus, perioral tingling, and visual disturbances to confusion, seizure, coma, and ventricular arrhythmia. Monitoring patients for the subtle symptoms of CNS toxicity is important because the therapeutic-to-toxic ratios are often narrow with these agents.

When toxicity develops, cardiac effects are potentiated by acidosis, hypercapnia, and hypoxia. Thus, treatment typically includes intravenous access, adequate oxygenation, and seizure

TABLE 40-2. Characteristics of Local Anesthetics				
Drug (Brand Name)	**Available Concentrations, %**	**Maximum, mg/kg**	**Maximum Dose with Epinephrine Combined, mg/kg**	**Duration, hr**
Moderate duration				
Lidocaine (Xylocaine)	0.5, 1, 2	4.5	7	0.5–1
Mepivicaine (Carbocaine)	1, 1.5, 2	4	7	0.75–1.5
Prilocaine (Citanest)	0.5, 1	7	8.5	0.5–1.5
Long duration				
Bupivacaine (Marcaine)	0.25, 0.5, 0.75	2.5	3	2–4
Etidocaine (Duranest)	0.5, 1	4	5.5	2–3

control. A benzodiazepine such as diazepam (Valium) given intravenously is effective anticonvulsant therapy (Naguib, 1998). For treatment, diazepam, 2 mg/min, is administered until seizures stop or a total dose of 20 mg is delivered.

Intrauterine Instillation

Injection of local anesthetic solutions through a catheter into the uterine cavity can safely lower pain scores in women undergoing in-office hysteroscopy or endometrial biopsy (Api, 2010; Cicinelli, 1997; Trolice, 2000). The presumed mechanism is anesthetic blockade of nerve endings within the endometrial mucosa. Studies have used 5-mL doses of 2-percent lidocaine or of 2-percent mepivacaine. For first-trimester abortion procedures, Edelman and coworkers (2004, 2006) evaluated instillation of 5 mL of 4-percent lidocaine combined with paracervical blockade. However, for this indication, a significant number of women reported symptoms attributed to lidocaine toxicity.

Postoperative Pain

Enhanced recover after surgery (ERAS) protocols are discussed further in Chapter 42 (p. 907). As one part, anesthesiologists and gynecologic surgeons employ multimodal strategies perioperatively to reduce postoperative pain. Agents with differing actions are frequently layered, and gabapentin and ketorolac are now in common use (Alayed, 2014; De Oliveira, 2012). As a complement, presurgical or immediate postoperative transversus abdominis plane (TAP) block shows promising results with abdominal and laparoscopic hysterectomy (Carney, 2008; De Oliveira, 2014). Another method is delivery of postoperative analgesia via a suprafascial wound soaker catheter implanted after fascia closure (Iyer, 2010; Kushner, 2005). The thin catheter is later pulled out the wound's lateral aspect. Alternatively, local infiltrative analgesia, using a long-acting medication such as liposomal bupivacaine, may be injected into the incision by the surgeon (Gasanova, 2015).

NERVE INJURY PREVENTION

Anesthetized patients who undergo prolonged gynecologic procedures are at risk for peripheral neuropathy of their upper or lower extremities. These neuropathies are uncommon, and cited incidences approximate 2 percent of gynecologic cases (Bohrer, 2009). Neurologic deficits typically are mild, transient, and resolve spontaneously. Infrequently, prolonged or permanent disability may result.

During gynecologic surgery, lower extremity injuries can involve nerves of the lumbosacral plexus. Mechanisms of injury include surgical nerve transaction, rupture following increased stretch, or nerve ischemia. Ischemia may result from compression of perineural vessels during prolonged or pronounced nerve stretch or compression. Any patient may develop postoperative neuropathy, but higher rates are noted in patients who smoke, who have anatomic abnormalities, or who are thin, diabetic, or alcoholic. Use of self-retaining retractors and prolonged surgical duration are additional factors (Warner, 2000).

Symptoms reflect functional loss of the affected nerve (Fig. 40-2 and Table 40-3). Therefore, a detailed neurologic

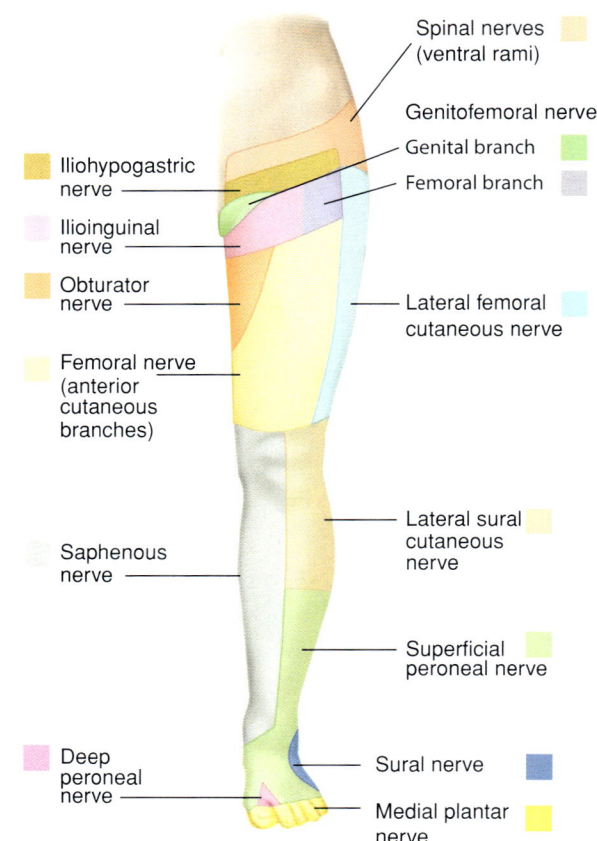

FIGURE 40-2 Peripheral nerves and their corresponding areas of sensory innervation.

examination allows clinical identification of most peripheral neuropathies. Electrodiagnostic testing is indicated if motor function is diminished (Knockaert, 1996). Generally, electromyography is most useful after a 2- to 3-week delay to permit denervational changes to fully develop within affected muscles (Winfree, 2005).

If motor function is impaired, neurologic consultation is typically indicated. Physical therapy begins immediately to minimize contracture and muscle atrophy. Alternatively, for those with only mild sensory losses, observation for return of function is reasonable. For those with pain, treatments may include oral analgesics, gabapentin, biofeedback, and serial trigger point injection with local anesthetics.

Laparotomy
Femoral Nerve

This nerve perforates the psoas muscle early in its course and passes medially beneath the inguinal ligament before exiting the pelvis. It then enters the femoral triangle to lie lateral to the femoral artery and vein. This nerve can be compressed anywhere along its course but is particularly susceptible within the body of the psoas muscle and at the inguinal ligament. Improper placement of a self-retaining retractor is the most common cause of surgical femoral nerve injury, and rates following abdominal hysterectomy may reach 10 percent (Fig. 40-3) (Goldman, 1985; Kvist-Poulsen, 1982). In affected women, the patellar reflex is usually absent in addition to impaired sensory and motor function.

TABLE 40-3. The Lumbosacral Plexus Nerve Plexus (L1–S4)

Nerve	Origin	Motor Function	Sensory Function
Iliohypogastric	L1	None	Inferior abdominal wall, upper lateral gluteal region
Ilioinguinal	L1	None	Inferior abdominal wall, mons pubis, labia majora
Genitofemoral	L1–2	None	Labia majora, anterior superior thigh
Lateral femoral cutaneous	L2–3	None	Anterolateral thigh
Femoral	L2–4	Hip flexion; knee extension	Anterior and inferomedial thigh, medial calf and foot
Obturator	L2–4	Thigh adduction, lateral rotation	Superomedial thigh
Sciatic	L4–S3		
Common fibular	L4–S2	Knee flexion; foot dorsiflexion, eversion; toe extension	Lateral calf, foot dorsum
Tibial	L4–S3	Thigh extension; knee flexion; foot plantar flexion; inversion	Foot plantar surface, toes
Pudendal	S2–4	Muscles of perineum; external anal and urethral sphincters	Perineum

In prevention, lateral retractor blades are positioned such that only the rectus abdominis muscle and not the psoas muscle is retracted (Chen, 1995). The retractor blades are evaluated when placed, to confirm that they are not resting on the psoas muscle. For thin patients, folded laparotomy towels may be placed between the retractor rim and skin to elevate blades away from the psoas muscle. Importantly, a small percentage of cases occur when a retractor has not been used.

Genitofemoral and Lateral Femoral Cutaneous Nerve

The genitofemoral nerve pierces the medial border of the psoas muscle and traverses below the peritoneum on this muscle's surface. Similar to the femoral nerve, the genitofemoral nerve may suffer injury during psoas muscle compression (Murovic, 2005). In addition, this nerve may be injured during removal of a large pelvic mass adhered to the sidewall or during pelvic lymph node dissection (Irvin, 2004).

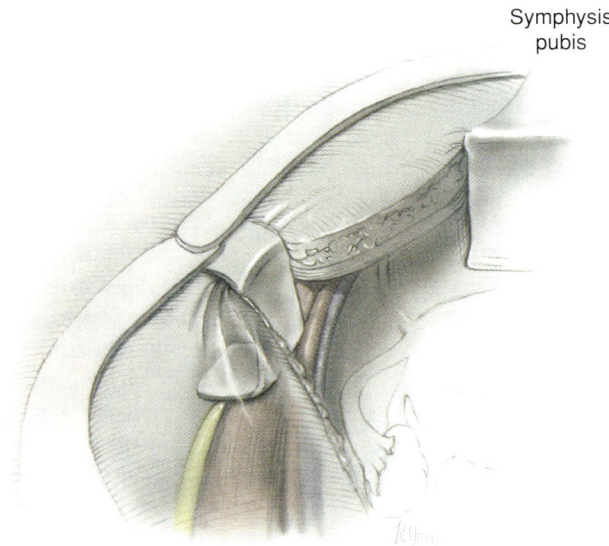

Symphysis pubis

FIGURE 40-3 If poorly positioned, the lateral blade of a self-retaining retractor can press against femoral nerve lying atop the psoas muscle.

The lateral femoral cutaneous nerve appears at the lateral border of the psoas major muscle just above the crest of the ilium. It courses obliquely across the anterior surface of the iliacus muscle and dips beneath the inguinal ligament laterally as the nerve exits the pelvis. This may be compressed along its portion that traverses the pelvic wall (Aszmann, 1997). Painful neuropathy specifically involving the lateral femoral cutaneous nerve carries the specific name *meralgia paresthetica*.

Transverse Incisions

Nerve injury during transverse abdominal entry is common and typically involves the ilioinguinal and iliohypogastric nerves or, less frequently, genitofemoral nerve branches. The ilioinguinal and iliohypogastric nerves emerge through the internal oblique muscle approximately 2 to 3 cm inferomedial to the anterosuperior iliac spine (Rahn, 2010). The iliohypogastric nerve extends a lateral branch to innervate the lateral gluteal skin. An anterior branch reaches horizontally toward the midline and runs deep to the external oblique muscle. Near the midline, this nerve perforates the external oblique muscle and becomes cutaneous to innervate the superficial tissues and skin in the region above the symphysis pubis. The ilioinguinal nerve extends medially to enter the inguinal canal and innervates the lower abdomen, labium majus, and upper thigh.

These are sensory nerves, and fortunately, most skin anesthesia or paresthesias that follow their injury resolves with time. Accordingly, injuries frequently are underreported by both patients and clinicians. Less often, pain can begin immediately or many years later and is usually sharp and episodic and radiates to the ipsilateral upper thigh, labium, or upper gluteal region. Later, sensations may become chronic and burning, as described in Chapter 12 (p. 273). To avoid compromising these nerves, a surgeon ideally avoids extending the fascial incision beyond the lateral border of the rectus muscles (Rahn, 2010).

Pelvic Sidewall Dissection

The obturator nerve pierces the medial border of the psoas muscle and extends anteriorly along the lesser wall of the pelvis. The obturator nerve exits through the obturator foramen. Lymph node dissection, tumor excision, or endometriosis resection performed at the pelvic sidewall may injure the obturator or genitofemoral nerves. Moreover, the obturator nerve also can be injured during dissection within the retropubic space during some urogynecologic procedures.

■ Dorsal Lithotomy

This surgical position is used for vaginal, laparoscopic, and hysteroscopic surgeries. It is modified and described as high, standard, or low lithotomy position (Fig. 40-4). Dorsal lithotomy may be associated with injury to several nerves derived from the lumbosacral plexus, including the femoral, sciatic, and common fibular (formerly common peroneal) nerves. For example, compression and ischemic injury of the femoral nerve beneath the rigid inguinal ligament can follow prolonged sharp flexion, abduction, and external hip rotation in dorsal lithotomy (Fig. 40-5) (Deveneau, 2017; Ducic, 2005). Ideal positioning as shown can minimize these injuries.

The sciatic nerve, derived from the lower lumbosacral plexus, exits the pelvis through the greater sciatic foramen. It extends down the posterior thigh and branches into the tibial nerve and common fibular nerve above the popliteal fossa. The sciatic and common fibular nerves are anatomically fixed at the sciatic notch and head of the fibula, respectively. For this reason, sciatic nerve injury may reflect impaired function of the entire sciatic nerve or only the common fibular division. Sciatic nerve stretch injury can develop if a patient's hips are placed in sharp flexion or pronounced external rotation or both. Moreover, even an appropriately positioned patient may be injured if a surgical assistant during vaginal surgery leans against the thigh and creates extreme hip flexion.

The common fibular nerve originates above the popliteal fossa and crosses the lateral head of the fibula before it descends down the lateral calf. At the lateral fibular head, this nerve is at risk for compression against leg stirrups. Therefore, the addition of cushioned padding or patient positioning that avoids pressure at this point can be preventive (Philosophe, 2003).

■ Brachial Plexus

This plexus derives from the ventral rami of C5–T1, traverses the neck and axilla, and supplies the arm and shoulder. Positioning injuries can follow hyperextension of the upper extremity, for example, when the arm is positioned at an angle to the body that exceeds 90 degrees. Additionally, even in situations in which the arm has been positioned appropriately, inadvertently leaning against the arm or placing the patient in steep Trendelenburg position may push the extremity into hyperextension. Shoulder braces can also apply pressure on the clavicle and stretch the brachial plexus. Braces have been used to prevent patient sliding when in steep Trendelenburg position. Instead, preferable techniques include use of gel mattress or cross-chest straps (Shveiky, 2010). With injury, either motor or sensory function can be lost

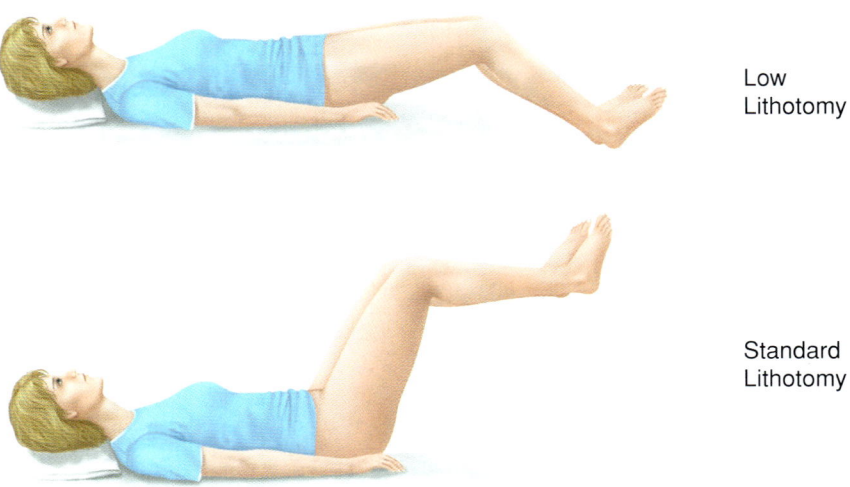

FIGURE 40-4 Lithotomy positions used in gynecologic surgery.

(Warner, 1998). Peripheral ulnar neuropathies can also develop by external compression if the arm is placed at the patient's side. Padding the elbow may help avoid this (Warner, 1998).

SURGICAL INCISIONS

In women for whom laparotomy is selected, an ideal abdominal incision allows rapid entry, affords adequate exposure, permits early ambulation, promotes strong wound healing, does not compromise pulmonary function, and maximizes cosmetic results. These criteria form the foundation in choosing the best incision for each patient. In gynecology, the abdomen typically is opened using a midline vertical incision or one of three transverse incisions, the Pfannenstiel, Cherney, or Maylard incisions.

■ Midline Vertical Incision

This incision is used frequently if access to the upper abdomen and generous operating space are required. It can be extended up and above the umbilicus and thus is preferred when the preoperative diagnosis is uncertain. Moreover, simple midline anatomy allows quick entry into the abdomen and low rates of neurovascular injury to the anterior abdominal wall (Greenall, 1980; Lacy, 1994). Because of decreased midline vascularity, Nygaard and Squatrito (1996) recommend this incision in patients who have coagulopathy, decline transfusion, or are administered systemic anticoagulation.

Its greatest disadvantage stems from greater tension on the incision when abdominal muscles contract. For this reason, compared with transverse incisions, midline vertical incisions have higher rates of fascial dehiscence and hernia formation and poorer cosmetic results (Grantcharov, 2001; Kisielinski, 2004). Additionally, patients who have repeat vertical incisions for gynecologic indications tend to develop more adhesive disease than those with transverse incisions (Brill, 1995).

■ Transverse Incisions

These incisions are used commonly in benign gynecologic surgery, provide several advantages, and are illustrated in the atlas

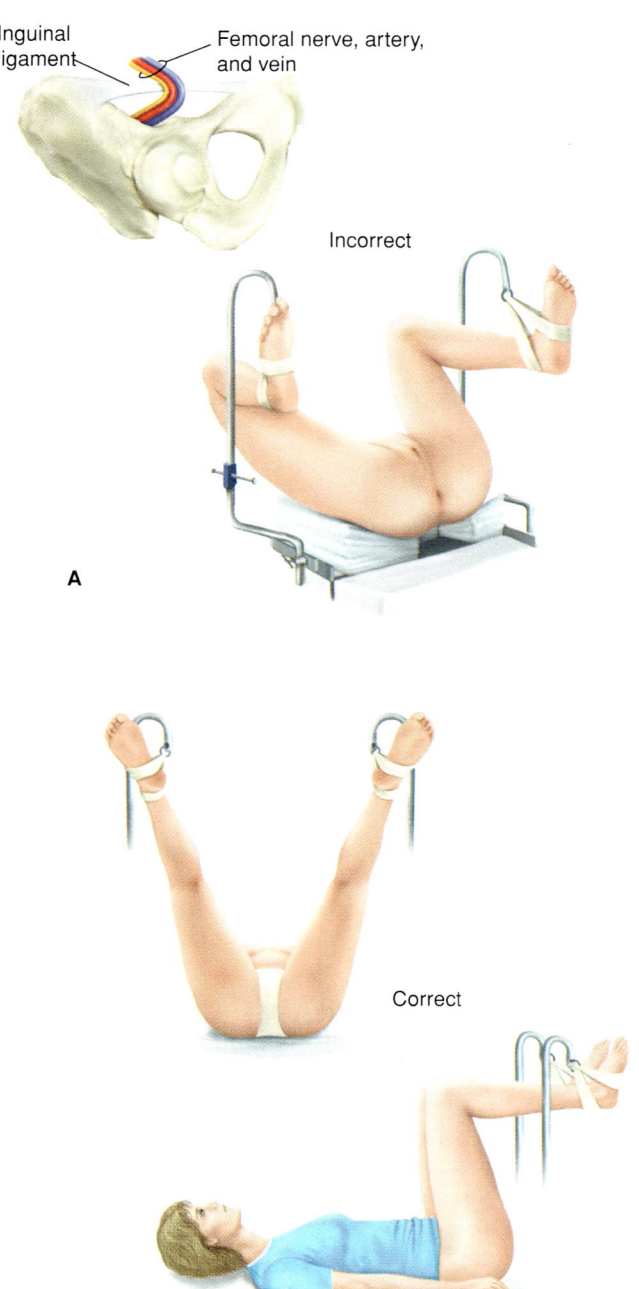

FIGURE 40-5 Lithotomy positioning. **A.** Hyperflexion of the hip can lead to compression of the femoral nerve against the inguinal ligament. **B.** Ideal dorsal lithotomy positioning with limited hip flexion, abduction, and external rotation.

(p. 933). They follow Langer lines of skin tension and thus offer superior cosmetic results. They also carry low rates of incisional hernia (Luijendijk, 1997). Moreover, their placement in the lower abdomen is associated with decreased postoperative pain and improved pulmonary function compared with midline vertical incisions. Of transverse incisions, Pfannenstiel incision is typically the simplest to perform, and for this reason, it is selected most often.

Despite these advantages, transverse incisions have limitations. These incisions limit access to the upper abdomen and offer smaller operating space compared with midline incisions.

This is especially true of the Pfannenstiel incision and results from narrowing of the surgical field by intact rectus abdominis muscle bellies, which straddle the incision.

Consequently, Cherney and Maylard incisions were developed to overcome this restriction, and to some degree, they do improve exposure. The Cherney incision releases the rectus abdominis muscle at its inferior tendinous insertion. This affords greater operating space and access to the retropubic space. The Cherney incision may also be used if a Pfannenstiel incision has already been initiated, but then additional exposure is required.

The Maylard incision transects the rectus abdominis muscle and provides substantial operative space. However, it is technically more difficult because isolation and ligation of the inferior epigastric arteries are required. The incision is used infrequently because of concerns regarding postoperative pain, decreased abdominal wall strength, longer operating times, and increased febrile morbidity. Randomized studies, however, have not supported these concerns (Ayers, 1987; Giacalone, 2002). This incision is avoided in patients whose superior epigastric vessels have been interrupted and in those with significant peripheral vascular disease who may rely on the inferior epigastric arteries for lower-extremity collateral blood supply.

■ Incision Creation

Entry into the abdomen begins with scalpel incision of the skin, and scars are excised to improve wound healing and cosmetic results. Although an electrosurgical blade may be used to incise the skin, faster healing and improved appearance in general follow scalpel incision (Hambley, 1988; Singer, 2002b).

For the remaining layers, scalpel or electrosurgical blade may be selected, with no differences in short- or long-term wound healing with either (Franchi, 2001). However, in evaluating surgical bleeding and postoperative pain, Jenkins (2003), in his review, noted an advantage with electrosurgical blade use. Regardless of the incision or instrument used, adherence to proper technique is emphasized. This incorporates obtaining meticulous hemostasis, minimizing devitalized tissue, and avoiding dead space creation.

WOUND CLOSURE

Following laparotomy, closure of a laparotomy incision must address the peritoneum, fascia, subcutaneous layer, and skin. Wound closure may be broadly categorized as either primary or secondary. With primary closure, materials are used to approximate tissue layers. In closure by secondary intention, wound layers remain open and heal by a combination of contraction, granulation, and epithelialization. Secondary closure is used infrequently in gynecologic surgery and typically is indicated if tissues planned for closure contain significant infection. The option of delayed primary closure is also available in these situations once infection has cleared.

Optimal closure of a laparotomy incision is the subject of much debate. Most data stem from general surgery and gynecologic oncology studies and from research on cesarean delivery techniques. Ideally, closure avoids wound infection, adhesion formation, dehiscence, and hernia or sinus tract formation; minimizes patient discomfort; yet preserves cosmesis to the extent possible.

■ Peritoneum and Fascia

The peritoneum provides no abdominal wall strength, and closure of this layer has been suggested to prevent adhesions between the anterior abdominal wall and adjacent organs. However, evidence is conflicting, and several studies show that nonclosure of the peritoneum compared with closure shortens operating time without increasing adhesion formation, wound complications, or infection rates (Franchi, 1997; Gupta, 1998; Tulandi, 1988). However, few well-done randomized trials have assessed long-term adhesion formation. Accordingly, closure of the visceral or parietal peritoneum is often provider dependent. Without closure, this layer typically regenerates within days following surgery (Lipscomb, 1996).

Thus in many cases, the first tissue closed is fascia. Many studies have supported the use of a continuous running-stitch closure of abdominal incisions compared with interrupted closure of the fascia (Colombo, 1997; Orr, 1990; Shepherd, 1983). Continuous closure usually is faster and associated with comparable rates of dehiscence, wound infection, and hernia formation. Suture material selection tends to favor delayed-absorbable suture compared with nonabsorbable. Delayed-absorbable sutures appear to afford adequate wound support yet lead to less pain and lower rates of sinus tract formation (Carlson, 1995; Leaper, 1977; Wissing, 1987). However, nonabsorbable suture is considered if a hernia is identified or if the incision has cut through previously placed mesh. A 0-gauge or no. 1 suture is suitable for closure of most fascial incisions. Sutures are placed approximately 1 cm apart and 1.2 to 1.5 cm from the fascial edge. Little additional security is attained beyond 1.5 cm (Campbell, 1989). Stitches ideally appose fascial edges without significant tension and allow tissues to swell postoperatively. This limits sutures from cutting through fascia or causing avascular necrosis.

■ Subcutaneous Adipose Layer and Skin

Bacterial growth can be accelerated within collections of blood and fluid. For this reason, to decrease hematoma or seroma rates, suture closure or drains are considered for the subcutaneous layer. With layers <2 cm thick, most studies find no advantage to either practice. However, wound infection and adipose thickness are the greatest risks for subcutaneous layer dehiscence (Soper, 1971; Vermillion, 2000). For subcutaneous layers ≥2 cm, closing the subcutaneous layer is effective prevention (Gallup, 1996; Guvenal, 2002; Naumann, 1995). The ideal suture and technique for closure of this layer are unknown, but efforts ideally close dead space yet minimize suture burden and inflammatory reaction. A 2-0 gauge plain gut suture is one suitable choice.

Skin may be closed effectively with staples, subcuticular suturing, wound tape, or tissue adhesive. Thus, in most instances, surgeon preference influences closure method. Technically, the incision line is approximated without skin tension, and subcutaneous adipose or deep dermal suturing ideally assists with carrying tension loads.

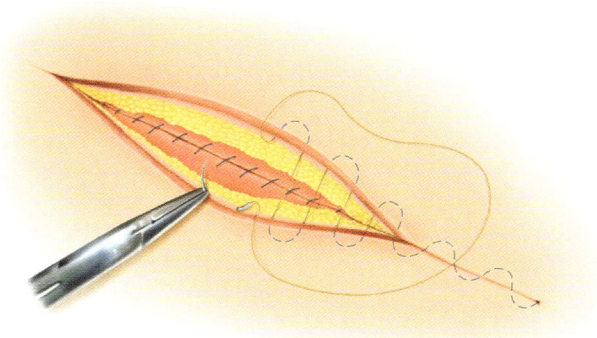

FIGURE 40-6 During subcuticular suturing, stitches are placed with a needle horizontal to the dermis. Suturing is advanced by sequentially piercing just below the dermis on alternating sides. The spot where the first stitch exits the subcutis marks the site along the wound length that the needle should enter on the opposite side.

Of options, the running subcuticular suture is placed by taking horizontal bites through the dermis on alternating sides of the wound using absorbable suture (Fig. 40-6). Delayed-absorbable material such as polyglactin (Vicryl) or poliglecaprone (Monocryl) in a fine gauge, such as 3-0 or 4-0, is suitable. Advantages include less cost, effective skin approximation, and no required suture removal. However, this method typically requires the greatest amount of time and technical expertise.

Automatic stapling devices offer fast application and secure wound closure. However, skin approximation is less accurate, and wounds requiring precise tissue apposing are less suited for stapling (Singer, 1997). Staples may be uncomfortable, may be associated with discomfort during removal, and require the patient to return for staple removal. In obese women, closure of midline vertical incisions with subcuticular suture does not reduce the risk of surgical site wound complications compared with staples (Kuroki, 2017).

Before stapling, the wound edges are everted, preferably by a second operator. If the edge(s) of a wound invert, a poorly formed, deep, noticeable scar will result. Additionally, pressing too hard against the skin surface with the stapler places the staple too deep and causes ischemia within the staple loop. When placed properly, the crossbar of the staple is elevated a few millimeters above the skin surface (Lammers, 2004). Staples are removed in a timely fashion to avoid leaving "track mark" scarring.

Of topical skin adhesives, octyl-2-cyanoacrylate (Dermabond) is applied as a liquid and polymerizes to a firm, pliable film that binds to the epithelium and bridges wound edges (Fig. 40-7). It can close skin incisions that carry minimal tension such as laparoscopy trocar or transverse laparotomy incisions or can serve as an adjunct protective layer in larger incisions. Tissue adhesives achieve results similar to those for traditional sutures (Blondeel, 2004; Singer, 2002a).

Following approximation of deeper incision layers, the adhesive is applied in three thin layers above apposed skin edges. The adhesive extends at least 0.5 cm on each side of the apposed wound edges. Placement of the liquid between skin edges is avoided because the adhesive may retard healing (Quinn, 1997).

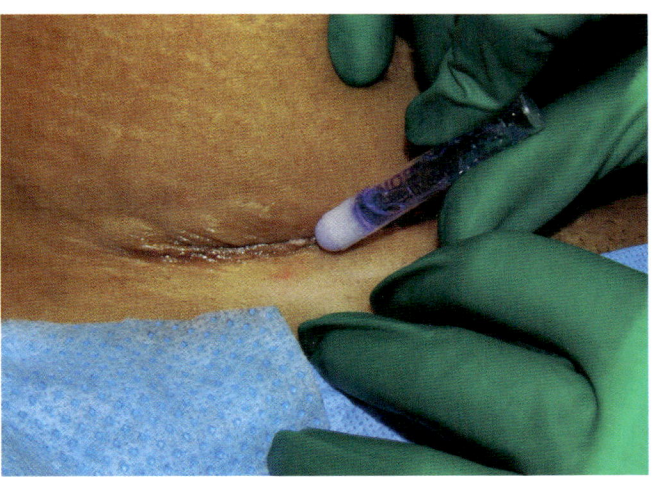

FIGURE 40-7 Application of topical skin adhesive to incision. Adhesive should be placed over apposed skin edges. Application should extend out approximately 0.5 cm laterally from the incision. (Reproduced with permission from Dr. Christine Wan.)

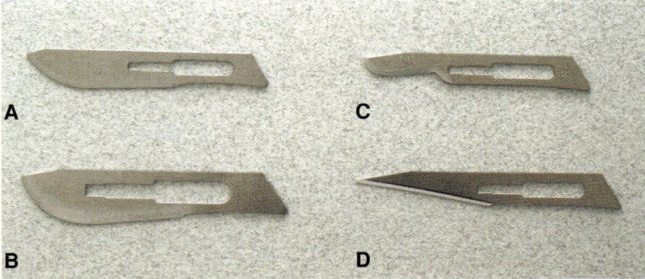

FIGURE 40-8 Photograph of surgical blades commonly used in gynecology. **A.** No. 10. **B.** No. 20. **C.** No. 15. **D.** No. 11.

Although 30 seconds between layers for drying is required, application is fast. Moreover, adhesives create their own dressing and appear to afford some antibacterial protection (Bhende, 2002). The adhesive sloughs in 7 to 10 days. Showering and gentle washing of the site are allowed, but swimming is discouraged. Petroleum-based products on the wound can decrease adhesive tensile strength and are avoided.

The primary indication for tape closure is a superficial straight laceration under little tension. Thus, closure of laparoscopy trocar sites or laparotomy incisions in which deep layer closure has brought skin edges into close proximity are suitable cases. Moreover, skin edges ideally are thoroughly dry for proper adhesion. Thus, tape may not be appropriate for a wet or oozing wound, for concave surfaces such as the umbilicus, for areas of significant tissue tension, or for areas of marked tissue laxity.

Tape closure is fast, inexpensive, and associated with high patient satisfaction scores. Tapes typically are removed by the patient 7 to 10 days following surgery. They may also be used after staple removal to provide additional strength, as wounds have regained only approximately 3 percent of their final strength at 1 week. Adhesive tape strips are applied in a parallel, nonoverlapping fashion after coating the entire application area with adjuvant adhesive such as tincture of benzoin (Katz, 1999). Importantly, skin blistering may develop if tape is stretched excessively taut across the wound (Lammers, 2004; Rodeheaver, 1983).

INSTRUMENTS

■ Scalpel and Blades

Surgical instruments extend the capability of a surgeon's hands and thus are crafted to retract, cut, grasp, and clear the operative field. Tissue types encountered in gynecologic surgery vary, and accordingly, so too do the size, fineness, and strength of the tools used.

Typical surgical blades used in gynecologic surgery are pictured in Figure 40-8 and include number 10, 11, 15, and 20 blades. Function follows form, and larger blades are used for

coarser tissues or larger incisions, whereas a no. 15 blade is selected for finer incisions. The acute angle and pointed tip of a no. 11 blade can easily incise tough-walled abscesses for drainage, such as those of the Bartholin gland duct.

With a correct scalpel grasp, a surgeon can direct blade movement. Fingers may be positioned either to straddle the scalpel, termed the "power grip," "violin grip," or "bow grip," which maximizes the use of the knife belly. Alternatively, the scalpel is held like a pencil, termed the "pencil grip" or "precision grip" (Fig. 40-9). With the no. 10 and no. 20 blades, the scalpel is held at a 20- to 30-degree angle to the skin and drawn firmly along the skin toward the surgeon using the arm, with minimal wrist and finger movement. This motion aids cutting with the full length of the scalpel belly and avoids burying the tip. The initial incision penetrates the dermis, and the scalpel remains perpendicular to the surface to prevent skin edge beveling. Firm and symmetrical lateral skin traction keeps the incision straight and helps avoid irregular skin edges and multiple tracks within the subcutaneous layer.

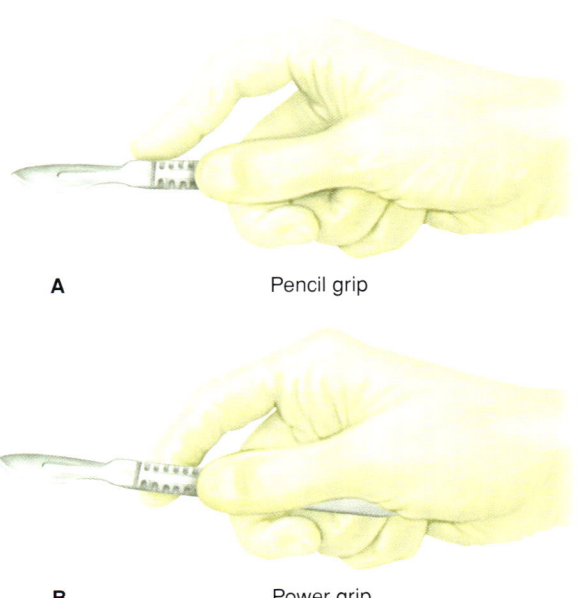

A   Pencil grip

B   Power grip

FIGURE 40-9 Scalpel grips. **A.** Scalpel is held as one would a pencil, and movement is directed by the thumb and index finger. **B.** Scalpel is held between the thumb and third finger. The end of the blade is forced up against the thenar muscles of the hand.

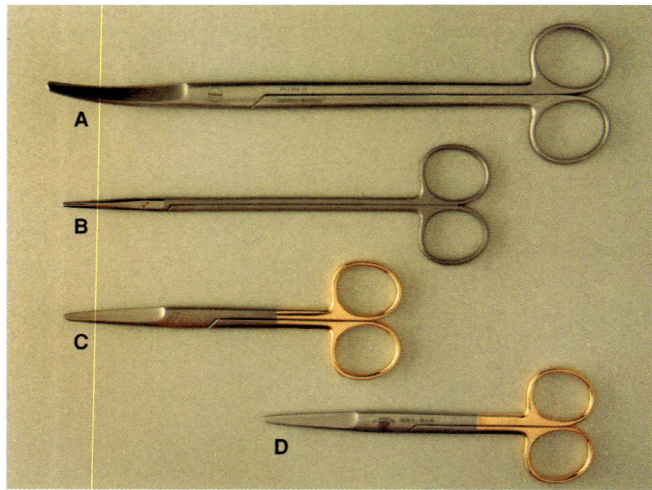

FIGURE 40-10 Scissors. **A.** Jorgenson. **B.** Metzenbaum. **C.** Curved Mayo. **D.** Straight Mayo. (Reproduced with permission from U.S. Surgitech, Inc.)

The no. 15 and 11 blades, in contrast, are typically held using the pencil grip to make fine, precise incisions. With the no. 15 blade, the scalpel is held approximately 45 degrees to the skin surface. Fine knife dissection is best controlled using the fingers, and the heel of the hand can be stabilized on adjacent tissue. The no. 11 blade scalpel is ideal for stab incisions and is held upright at nearly 90 degrees to the surface. Creating tension at the skin surface is important as it reduces the amount of force required for penetration. Omission of this can result in uncontrolled puncture of underlying structures. To lengthen the incision, a gentle, shallow, in-and-out sawing motion is used.

■ Scissors

These are used commonly to divide tissues, and modification in blade shape and size allows their use across various tissue textures (Fig. 40-10). For correct positioning, the thumb and fourth finger are placed within the instrument's rings, and the index finger is set against the crosspiece of the scissors for greater control. This "tripod" grip allows maximum shear, torque, and closing forces to be applied and provides superior stability and control. In general, surgeons cut away from themselves and from the dominant-hand side to nondominant side.

The fine blades of Metzenbaum or iris scissors are used routinely to dissect or define tissue planes. Examples are dividing thin adhesions or incising peritoneum or vaginal epithelium. During dissection, traction on opposing poles of the tissue typically simplifies the process, and a small nick is often necessary to enter the correct tissue plane. The blades are closed and inserted between planes (Fig. 40-11). The blades are stretched opened and then withdrawn. After turning both wrist and blades 90 degrees, the surgeon reinserts the lower blade, and tissues are divided. When dissecting around a curve, the scissors follow the natural curve of the structure. Dissection proceeds in the same plane to avoid burrowing into the structure or deviating away and toward unintended adjacent tissues.

For thicker tissues, sturdier scissors such as curved Mayo scissors are used. Similarly, Jorgenson scissors have thick blades and tips that are curved at a 90-degree angle. These are used commonly to separate the vagina and uterus during the final steps of hysterectomy. Suture-cutting scissors have blunt, flat blades and are reserved for this function. Repeated use of tissue scissors to cut suture dulls them unnecessarily.

■ Needle Holders

These may be straight or curved, and commonly, one with straight, blunt jaws is chosen during routine tissue approximation and pedicle ligation. Needles ideally pierce tissues perpendicularly. Thus, in most cases, the needle holder grasps a needle at a right angle and at a site approximately two thirds from the needle tip.

Alternatively, some needle holders, such as the Heaney needle holder, are curved and aid needle placement in confined or angled areas. If a curved holder is used, the needle is grasped similarly, and the inner curve of the holder typically faces the needle swage (Fig. 40-12).

Traditionally, the needle holder is held with the thumb and fourth finger in the rings. Its greatest advantage is the precision afforded. The spring tension of the handles is relieved from the lock in a controlled fashion, thereby releasing and regrasping the needle more precisely. Instead, with the "palmar grip," the needle holder is held between the ball of the thumb and the remaining fingers, and no fingers enter the instrument rings. This grip allows a simple rotating motion to drive curved needles through an arc. Its greatest advantage is the time saved during continuous suturing, as the needle can be released,

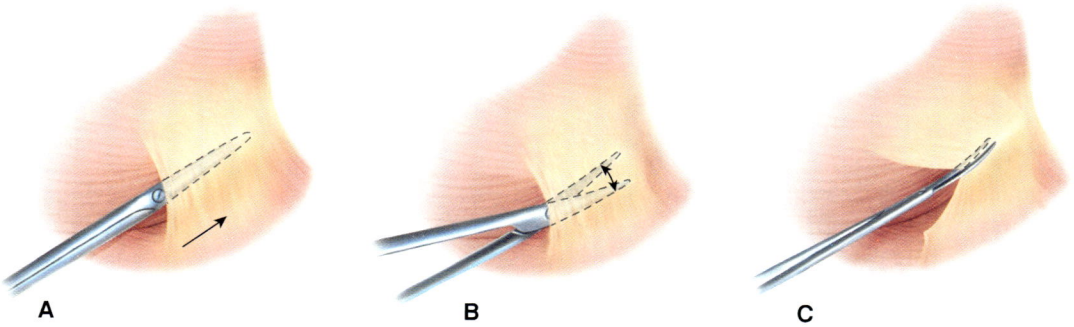

| A | B | C |

FIGURE 40-11 Plane dissection. **A.** During development of tissue planes, the tips of closed Metzenbaum scissors are placed at the border between two tissues, and forward pressure is applied to advance the tips. **B.** Scissors are spread to expand the tissue plane. **C.** The scissors are retracted and rotated 90 degrees. The lower blade is reinserted into the newly created tissue plane, and tissues are divided.

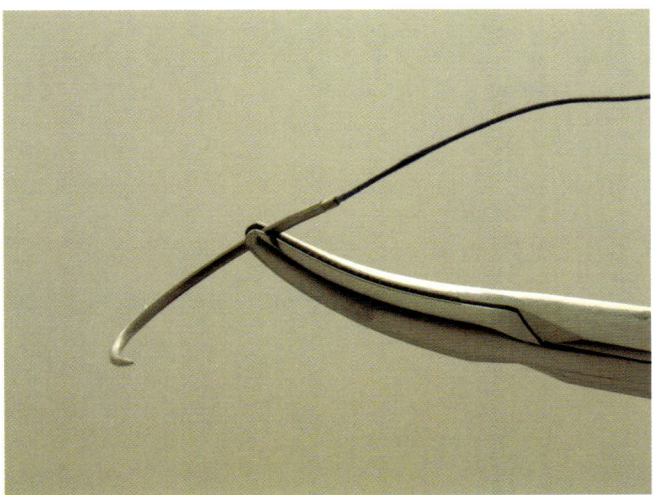

FIGURE 40-12 Correct grasp of a needle using a curved needle holder. The curve of the tip faces the needle swage. (Reproduced with permission from U.S. Surgitech, Inc.)

regrasped, and redirected without replacing fingers into the instrument rings. Disadvantageously, this grip has the potential to lack precision during needle release. When unlocking the needle driver, release of the spring lock should be smooth and gradual. This avoids an abrupt release, which may suddenly pop the handles apart with potential for awkwardness, loss of needle control, and tissue injury.

■ Tissue Forceps

Forceps function to hold tissue during cutting, retract tissue for exposure, stabilize tissue during suturing, extract needles, grasp vessels for electrosurgical coagulation, pass ligatures around hemostats, and pack sponges. Forceps are held so that one blade functions as an extension of the thumb and the other as an extension of the opposing fingers. Alternate grips can limit the full range of wrist motion, leading to suboptimal instrument use.

Heavy-toothed forceps, such as the Potts-Smith single-toothed forceps, Bonney forceps, and Ferriss-Smith forceps, are used when a firm grasp is more important than gentle tissue handling (Fig. 40-13A). These tools are often used to hold fascia for abdominal wound closure.

Light-toothed forceps, such as the single-toothed Adson, concentrate force on a tiny area and give more holding power with less tissue destruction. These are used for more delicate work on moderately dense tissue such as skin. Nontoothed forceps, also known as smooth forceps, exert their grip through fine serrations on the opposing tips (Fig. 40-13B). They are typically used for delicate tissue handling and provide some holding power with minimal injury. DeBakey forceps are another type of smooth forceps originally designed as vascular forceps but can be occasionally used for other delicate tissues. In contrast, the broader, shallow-grooved tips of Russian forceps and Singley forceps may be preferred if a broader or thicker area of tissue is manipulated.

■ Retractors

Abdominal Surgery Retractors

Clear visualization is essential during surgery, and retractors conform to body and organ angles to allow tissues to be pulled back from an operative field. In gynecology, retractors may be grouped broadly as self-retaining or handheld and as vaginal or abdominal.

During abdominal surgery, retractors that by themselves hold abdominal wall muscles apart, termed *self-retaining*, are used commonly. Styles such as the Kirschner and O'Connor-O'Sullivan contain four broad, gently curved blades and retract in four directions. Blades pull the bladder caudally and the anterior abdominal wall muscles laterally and cephalad. The Balfour retractor retracts in three directions but can be made to retract in four with the addition of an upper arm attachment. Alternatively, ring-shaped retractors such as the Bookwalter and Denis Browne styles offer greater variability in the number and positioning of retractor blades. However, these last two styles usually require more time to assemble and place. With all of these retractors, deep or shallow blades can be attached to the outer metal frame according to the abdominal cavity depth. As discussed earlier, blades should be shallow enough to avoid femoral nerve compression (p. 843).

In addition to these metal bladed styles, several disposable retractors consist of two equal-sized plastic rings connected by a cylindrical plastic sheath. One ring collapses into a canoe shape that can be threaded through the incision. Once inside the

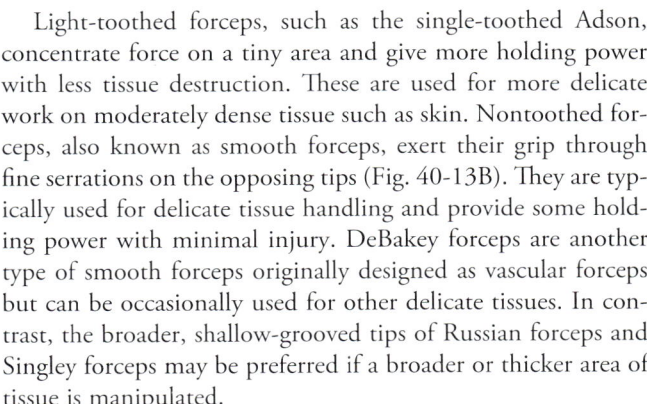

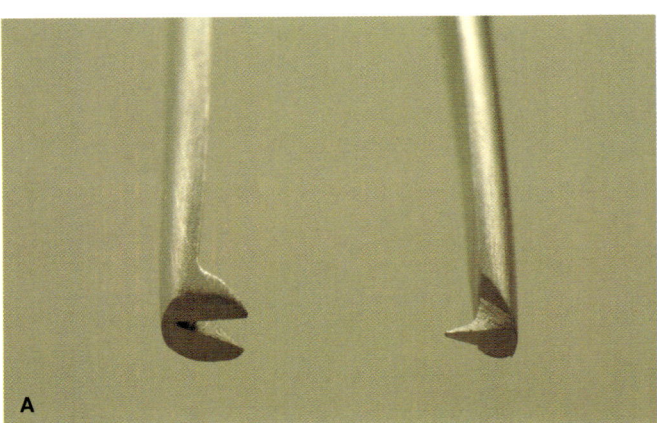

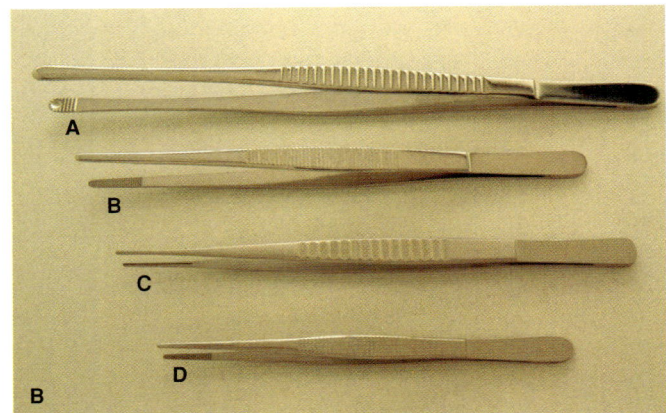

FIGURE 40-13 Forceps types. **A.** Tip of toothed forceps allows a firm tissue grasp. **B.** Smooth tissue forceps. *A*, Russian. *B*, Dressing. *C*, DeBakey. *D*, Short smooth. (Reproduced with permission from U.S. Surgitech, Inc.)

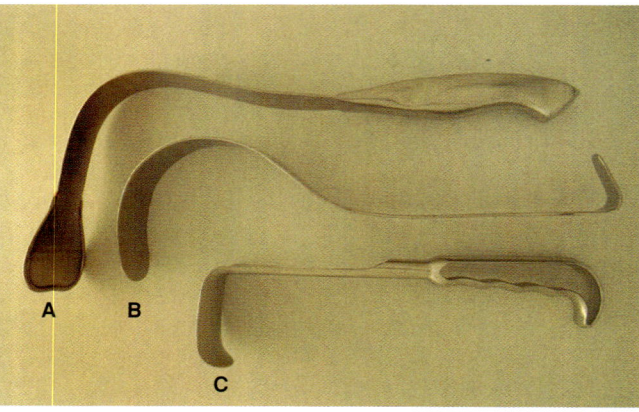

FIGURE 40-14 Long handheld abdominal retractors. **A.** Harrington. **B.** Deaver. **C.** Richardson. (Reproduced with permission from U.S. Surgitech, Inc.)

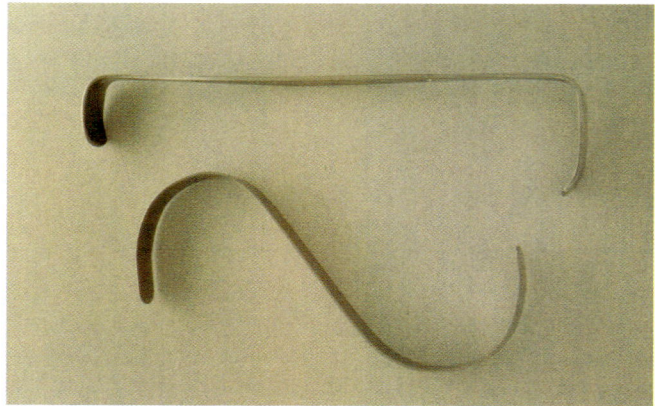

FIGURE 40-15 Short handheld abdominal retractors. Army-Navy (*above*). S-retractor (*below*). (Reproduced with permission from U.S. Surgitech, Inc.)

abdomen, it springs again to its circular form. The second ring remains outside. Between these rings, the plastic sheath spans the thickness of the abdominal wall and creates 360-degree retraction. Shown in Figure 41-13 (p. 883), Alexis or Mobius brands can be ideal for minilaparotomy, but sizes are also available for laparotomy.

Handheld retractors may be used in addition to or in place of self-retaining styles. These instruments allow retraction in only one direction but can be placed and repositioned quickly. The Richardson retractor has a sturdy, shallow, right-angled blade that can hook around an incision for abdominal wall retraction (Fig. 40-14). Alternatively, Deaver retractors have a gentle arching shape and conform easily to the curve of the anterior abdominal wall. Compared with Richardson retractors, they offer greater blade depth and are often used to retract bowel, bladder, or anterior abdominal wall muscles. A Harrington retractor, also called a *sweetheart retractor*, has a broader tip that also effectively holds back bowel.

In certain instances, such as during suturing of the vaginal cuff, a thin, deep retractor blade, termed a *malleable retractor*, may be required to retract or protect surrounding organs. Also called a *ribbon retractor*, this tool is a long, relatively flexible metal strip that can be bent to conform to various body contours for effective retraction. Narrow and wider sizes are available. These also may cover and protect underlying bowel from needle-stick injury during abdominal wall closure.

For smaller incisions, the preceding retractors are too large, and those with smaller blades such as the Army-Navy retractor or S-retractor are selected. S-retractors offer thinner, deeper blades, whereas the sturdier blades of the Army-Navy style allow stronger retraction (Fig. 40-15). A Weitlaner self-retaining retractor may also be used for minilaparotomy incisions.

Vaginal Surgery Retractors

The vaginal walls can be separated using several self-retaining models. The Gelpi retractor has two narrow teeth that are placed distally against opposing lateral vaginal walls and is most appropriate for perineal procedures (Fig. 40-16A). The Rigby retractor, with its longer blades, effectively separates lateral vaginal walls, whereas a Graves speculum holds apart anterior and posterior walls (Fig. 1-3, p. 4). An Auvard weighted speculum contains a long, single blade and ballasted end, which uses gravity to pull the posterior vaginal wall downward (Fig. 40-16B).

The degree of retraction offered by vaginal self-retaining retractors, however, at times may be limited. Therefore, handheld retractors are often required to augment or replace these instruments. Handheld retractors used in vaginal surgery include the Heaney right-angle retractor, the curved Deaver retractor, and the Breisky-Navratil retractor (Fig. 40-17).

Additionally, during vaginal procedures, the cervix often must be manipulated. A Lahey thyroid clamp or Jacobs tenaculum offers a secure grip during vaginal hysterectomy, but its several sharp teeth can cause significant trauma. These are less

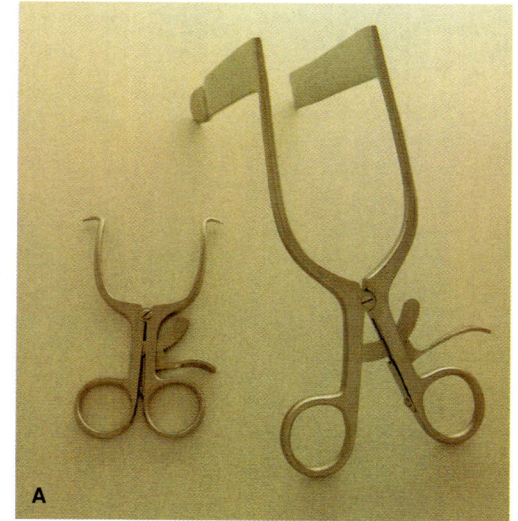
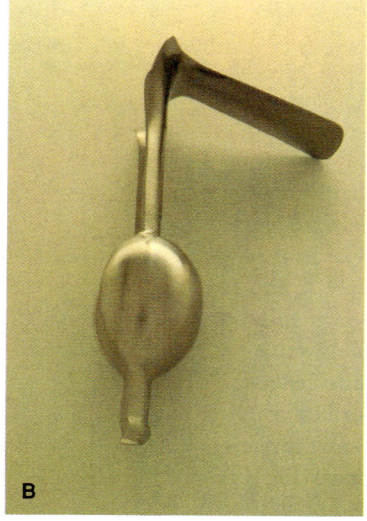

FIGURE 40-16 Vaginal self-retaining retractors. **A.** Gelpi retractor (*left*). Rigby retractor (*right*). **B.** Auvard weighted vaginal speculum. (Reproduced with permission from U.S. Surgitech, Inc.)

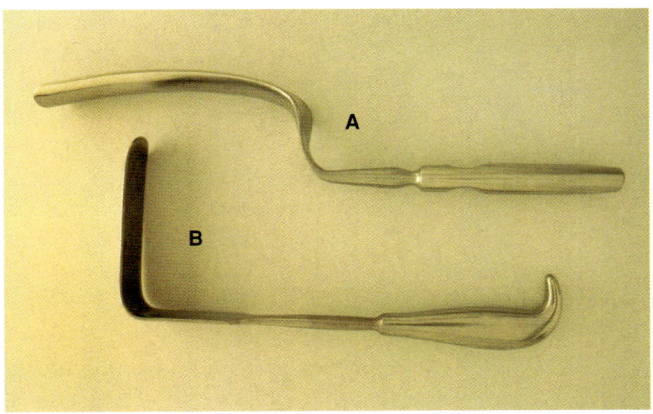

FIGURE 40-17 Vaginal handheld retractors. **A.** Breisky-Navratil retractor. **B.** Right-angle retractor. (Reproduced with permission from U.S. Surgitech, Inc.)

than ideal in patients in whom the cervix will remain. In these patients, in whom curettage or laparoscopy is performed, a single-toothed tenaculum can afford a firm grip but with less cervical damage (Fig. 40-18).

■ Tissue Clamps

Retraction is a fundamental requirement during most gynecologic surgery. As a result, various shapes, sizes, and strengths of clamps permit manipulation of differing tissues. For example, the smooth, cupped jaws of a Babcock clamp are ideal for gentle elevation of fallopian tubes, whereas the serrated teeth of the Allis and Allis-Adair clamps can provide a fine, firm grip on covering epithelia or serosa during dissection (Fig. 40-19).

Clamps are also used to occlude vascular and tissue pedicles during organ excision. Hemostats and Mixter right-angle clamps have small, slender jaws with fine, inner transverse ridges to atraumatically grasp delicate tissue (Fig. 40-20).

Heavier clamps are required to grasp and manipulate stiffer tissues such as fascia, and these include Pean (also termed Kelly) and Kocher (also termed Ochsner) clamps. These clamps have finely spaced transverse grooves along their inner jaws to minimize tissue slippage. They may be straight or curved to fit tissue contours and, like Kocher clamps, may contain a set of interlocking teeth

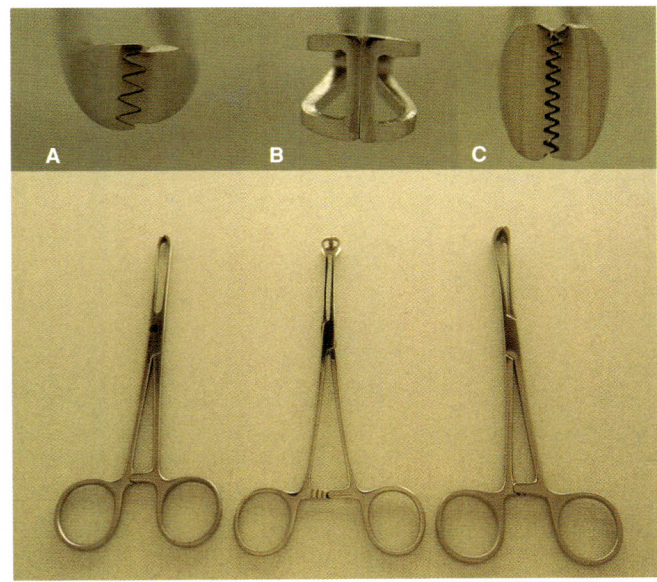

FIGURE 40-19 Tissue clamps. **A.** Allis. **B.** Babcock. **C.** Allis-Adair. (Reproduced with permission from U.S. Surgitech, Inc.)

at the tip for additional grip security. Another choice, the ring forceps, has large open circular jaws with fine transverse grooves. These effectively grasp broad, flat surfaces. Additionally, a folded gauze sponge can be placed between its jaws and used to absorb blood from the operative field or gently retract tissues.

Ligaments that support the uterus and vagina are fibrous and vascular. Thus, a sturdy clamp that resists tissue slippage from its jaws is required during hysterectomy. Several clamps, including Heaney, Ballantine, Rogers, Zeppelin, and Masterson clamps, among others, are effective (Fig. 40-21). The thick, durable jaws of these clamps carry deep, finely spaced grooves or serrations arranged either transversely or longitudinally for secure tissue grasping. Additionally, some contain a set

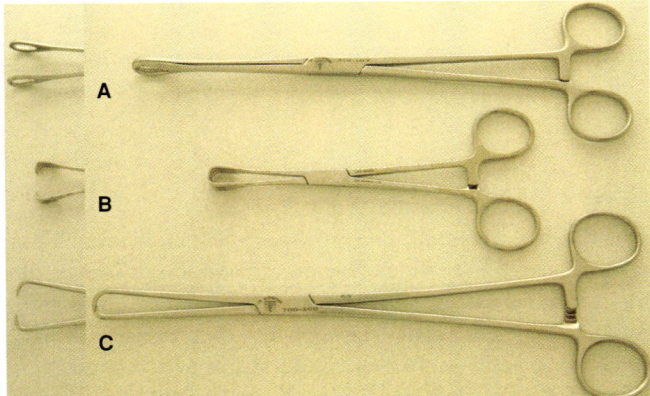

FIGURE 40-18 Clamps shown both open (*left*) and closed (*right*). **A.** Ring forceps. **B.** Lahey-thyroid clamp. **C.** Single-toothed tenaculum. (Reproduced with permission from U.S. Surgitech, Inc.)

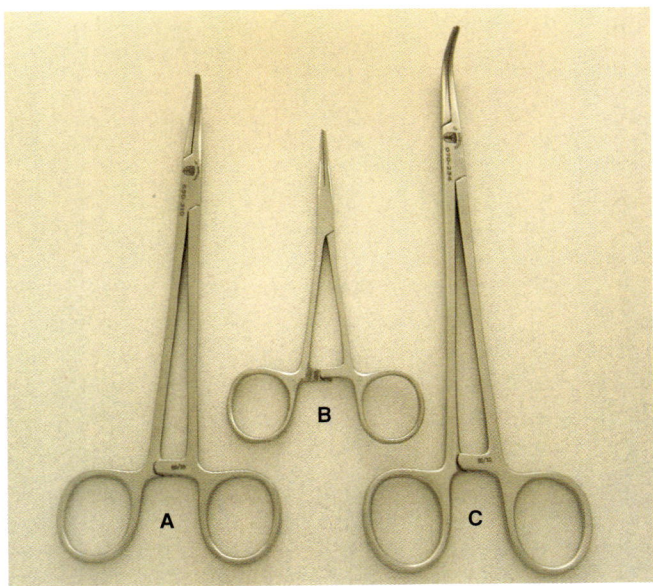

FIGURE 40-20 Vascular clamps. **A.** Tonsil. **B.** Hemostat. **C.** Mixter right-angle clamp. (Reproduced with permission from U.S. Surgitech, Inc.)

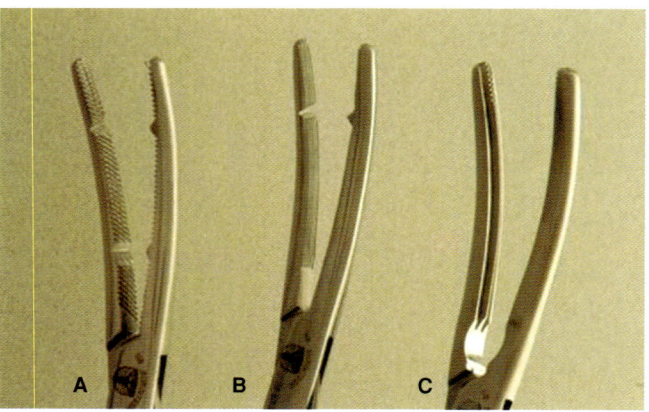

FIGURE 40-21 Heavy tissue clamps. **A.** Heaney. **B.** Heaney-Ballantine. **C.** Zeppelin. (Reproduced with permission from U.S. Surgitech, Inc.)

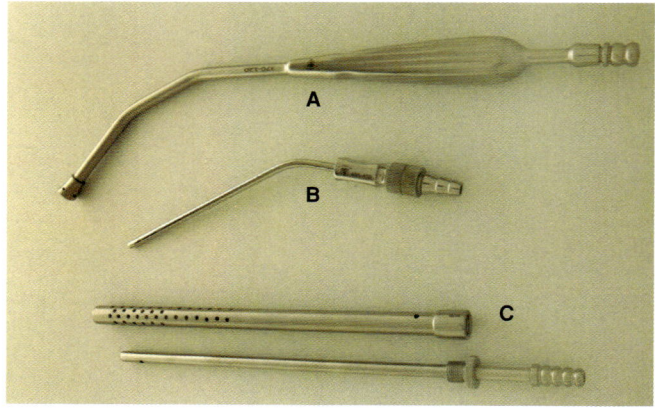

FIGURE 40-23 Suction tips. **A.** Yankauer. **B.** Frazier. **C.** Poole. (Reproduced with permission from U.S. Surgitech, Inc.)

of interlocking teeth at the tip or heel or both. Although this modification improves grip, it also may increase tissue trauma. More acutely angled clamps are typically selected when available operating space is cramped. For vaginal hysterectomy, Glenner clamps have both lateral and upward curves and may aid pedicle clamping (Glenner, 1956).

Securing tissue pedicles may be accomplished using various suturing techniques. A single tie alone may be placed around the pedicle (Fig. 40-22A). In addition, a second distal transfixing

suture can be placed to minimize dislodgement of the suture by vessel pulse pressures or pedicle manipulation.

■ Suction Tips

During gynecologic surgery, bleeding, peritoneal fluids, pus, ovarian cyst contents, and irrigants may obscure the operating field. Accordingly, choice of suction tip typically is dictated by the type and amount of fluid encountered. Adson and Frazier suction tips are fine bore and useful in shallow or confined areas and with limited bleeding (Fig. 40-23).

Alternatively, a Yankauer suction tip offers a midrange-sized tip and is often used in general gynecology. However, if a larger volume of fluid or blood is expected, then a Poole suction tip may be desired. Its multiple pores allow continued suction even if some are obstructed with clot or tissue. In addition to removing large volumes of fluid quickly, this suction tip's sieved sheath may be removed. The thinner-bore inner suction cannula can then be used for finer suctioning. Larger-bore Karman suction cannulas are used for products of conception evacuation, discussed in Section 43-15 (p. 973).

NEEDLES, SUTURES, AND KNOTS

These are foundational tools of tissue approximation, vessel ligation, and wound closure. They are crafted in various strengths, shapes, and sizes to meet surgical needs. Appropriate selection can profoundly affect wound healing and patient recovery. Thus, surgeons should be familiar with their characteristics and most appropriate applications.

■ Needles

The ideal surgical needle pierces tissue with ease, with minimal tissue damage, and without bending or breaking. Tissues differ in their density and location, and thus needles are designed with variable sizes, shapes, and tips. Needle anatomy is simple, and each contains a tip, body, and site of suture attachment (Fig. 40-24). For most gynecologic cases, the suture and needle are attached as a continuous unit, which is described as *swaged*. This contrasts with needles that have eyes for suture threading. Swaged needles may be firmly secured to the suture and require

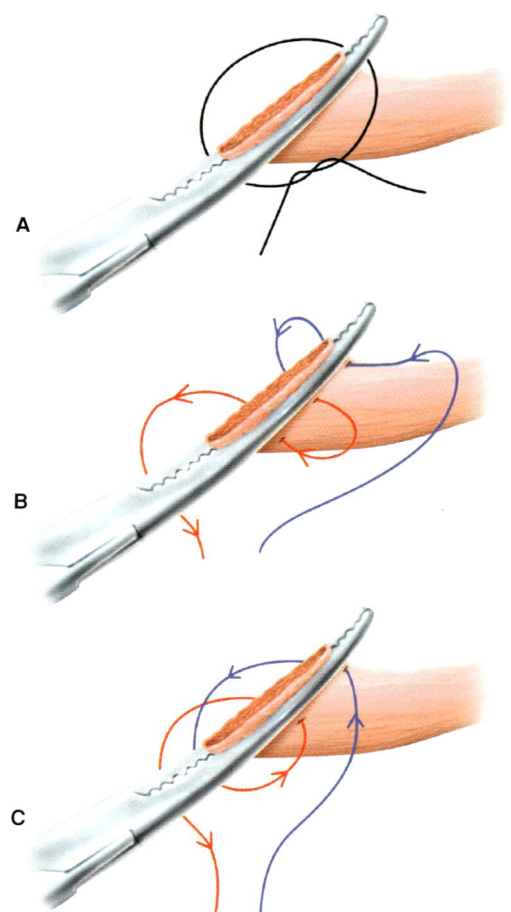

FIGURE 40-22 Different pedicle ligation techniques. All are transfixing ligatures except for **(A)**.

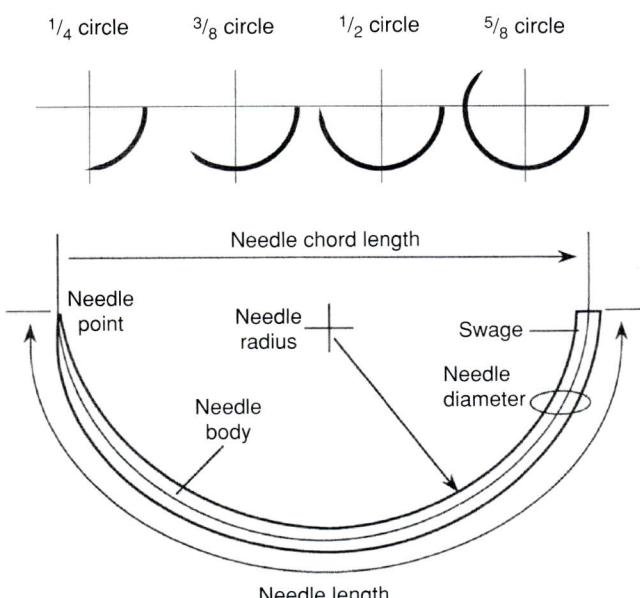

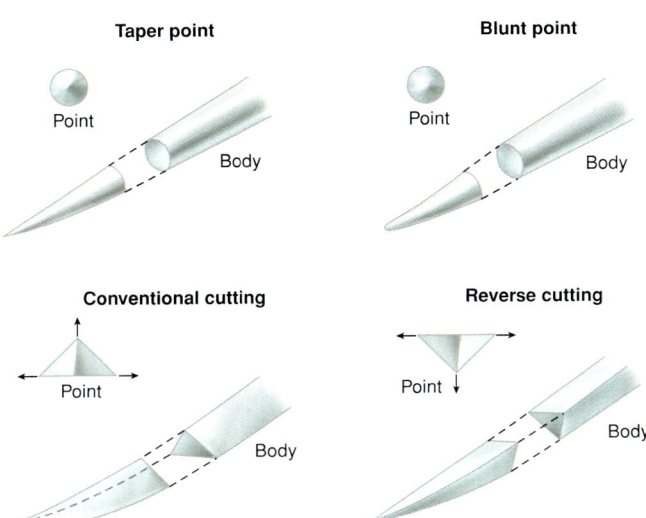

FIGURE 40-25 Configurations of various needle tips and bodies.

FIGURE 40-24 Various needle configurations and characteristics of a curved surgical needle.

cutting needles have the third cutting edge directed away from the inner curve of the needle and are used for particularly tough tissues.

■ Sutures

Sutures maximize wound healing and tissue support and are categorized by their biologic or synthetic derivation, their filamentous structure, and their ability to be degraded and reabsorbed (Table 40-4). Other qualities are described subsequently.

Sutures such as catgut, silk, linen, and cotton are derived from biologic sources. As a group, biologic sutures produce the greatest tissue reaction and have the lowest tensile strength. Accordingly, most suture materials currently used in gynecologic surgery are synthetic.

Of synthetic materials, the number of strands that make up a given suture defines it as either *monofilament* or *multifilament*. Monofilament suture is constructed as a single strand, whereas multifilament suture contains multiple strands that are braided or twisted. Monofilament sutures have lower friction coefficients and therefore pull more easily through tissues, and as a result, they create less tissue injury. As a group, they tend to incite less tissue reaction. Moreover, braid crevices are absent, and bacteria thus are less likely to adhere (Bucknall, 1983; Sharp, 1982). However, monofilament sutures are in general less pliant for knot tying and, if nicked by instruments, are more prone to break.

The diameter of a suture reflects its size and is measured in tenths of a millimeter (Table 40-5). A midpoint diameter size is designated as 0, and as suture diameter increases above this baseline, Arabic numerals are assigned. For example, no. 1 catgut is thicker than 0-gauge catgut. As suture diameter decreases from this midpoint, 0s are added. By convention, an Arabic numeral followed by a 0 may also be used to reflect the total number of 0s. For example, 3-0 suture may also be represented as 000. Moreover, 3-0 suture has a greater diameter than 4-0 (0000) suture.

Ideally, the appropriate suture caliber is fine enough to limit tissue damage during placement and minimize subsequent tissue

cutting at the end of suturing. Alternatively, *controlled-release*, or "pop-off," swaged needles detach from the suture with a brisk tug. Controlled-release needles are often used when securing vascular pedicles or placing interrupted sutures. Continuous running suturing typically requires a swaged needle without the controlled-release feature.

In certain urogynecologic procedures, such as abdominal sacrocolpopexy, a *double-armed suture* is often chosen. This suture contains identical swaged needles at each of its ends. This design enables surgeons to suture distant tissues with different ends of the suture before approximating them.

Descriptors of needle size and shape are noted in Figure 40-24. Of these, needle radius, circle configuration, and gauge more frequently influence surgical selection. For example, a needle should be large enough to pass completely through the tissue and exit far enough to allow the needle holder to be repositioned on the end of the needle at a safe distance from the tip. Repeated grasping of the needle tip leads to dulling and possible breakage of the tip. A dulled tip subsequently leads to difficult tissue penetration and greater tissue trauma.

For thicker tissues, a larger radius and gauge are warranted. For confined surgical spaces, a needle with smaller radius and greater circle configuration typically is required. Thus, for most gynecologic procedures, a three-eighths or one-half circle configuration is used. For some urogynecologic operations, a five-eighths circle configuration is preferred.

The tip should allow passage of the needle through tissue with the smallest amount of tissue damage. Those with tapered points are used for suturing thin tissues, such as peritoneum (Fig. 40-25). Alternatively, cutting needles are preferred for denser tissue such as fascia and ligaments. Cutting points have sharp edges laterally and a third sharp edge extending either toward or away from the needle's inner curve. A conventional cutting needle features the third cutting edge on the inside curve and provides shallower tissue bites. In contrast, reverse

TABLE 40-4. Specific Suture Material Characteristics

Type	Configuration	Tensile Strength	Handling	Knot Security	Reactivity
Nonabsorbable					
Silk	Braided	Good	Good	Good	High
Nylon	Monofilament	High	Fair	Fair	Low
Prolene	Monofilament	Good	Poor	Poor	Low
Mersilene	Braided synthetic	High	Good	Good	Moderate
Ethibond	Braided, coated	High	Fair	Fair	Moderate
Absorbable					
Gut (plain)	Twisted	Poor	Fair	Poor	Low
Chromic (gut)	Twisted	Poor	Fair	Poor	High
Dexon	Braided	Good	Good	Good	Low
Vicryl	Braided	Good	Good	Fair	Low
PDS II	Monofilament	Good	Fair	Poor	Low
Monocryl	Monofilament	Fair	Good	Good	Low

reaction yet provide ample tensile strength to support and approximate involved tissues. Defined as the amount of weight necessary to break a suture divided by its cross-sectional area, *tensile strength* is an important consideration during suture selection. The tensile strength of material chosen should approximate the strength of the tissues being sutured.

Tensile strength is lost at different rates among suture types. Materials that have lost most of their tensile strength by 60 days following surgery are considered to be *absorbable* (Bennett, 1988). Absorbable suture is destroyed enzymatically or hydrolyzed, whereas nonabsorbable suture persists and ultimately is encapsulated. Ideally, absorbable suture material remains throughout wound healing but no longer. Logically, individual tissue healing characteristics typically dictate whether short- or long-term sutures are required. Accordingly, nonabsorbable material plays a greater role in pelvic floor reconstruction procedures, whereas absorbable suture is used routinely in general gynecologic surgery.

All sutures, when placed within tissue, will incite inflammation. This response mirrors the total amount of suture placed

TABLE 40-5. Suture Designation

U.S.P. Designation	Synthetic Absorbable Diameter (mm)
5	0.7
4	0.6
3	0.6
2	0.5
1	0.4
0	0.35
2-0	0.3
3-0	0.2
4-0	0.15
5-0	0.1

and the suture's chemical composition (Edlich, 1973). In general, lower inflammatory responses are elicited by monofilament structure compared with multifilament, and synthetically derived compared with natural fiber (Sharp, 1982).

The ease of fluid to wick from the wet end of a suture to its dry end defines its *capillarity*. A suture's *fluid absorption ability* describes the amount of fluid it absorbs when immersed. Both properties increase absorption of contaminating bacteria (Blomstedt, 1977). In general, multifilament sutures, even those with coatings, display greater capillarity compared with synthetic monofilament sutures (Geiger, 2005).

The ability of a material to return to its prior length following stretch defines its *elasticity*. For tissues in which swelling or movement is expected postoperatively, a suture with greater elasticity is preferred because it will stretch rather than cut into approximated tissues. *Memory* defines the ability of material to return to original form following deformation. Sutures with greater memory tend to untie more easily during knot tying.

Barbed, unidirectional absorbable suture is relatively new but widely used in minimally invasive surgery (Fig. 41-32, p. 896). It does not require knotting and thus shortens operative times without raising suture complication rates (Cong, 2016; Lopez, 2019). However, rare, suture-related small bowel obstruction and volvulus have been reported (Donnellan, 2011; Lee, 2015; Sakata, 2015; Thubert 2011).

▪ Knots

The surgical knot is the weakest link in a tied suture loop, and the force necessary to break a knotted suture is less than that to break an individual suture strand. Knot failure can lead to serious complications such as bleeding, hernias, and wound dehiscence (Batra, 1993; Trimbos, 1984).

A surgical knot consists of a loop, which maintains tissue apposition, and a knot, composed of several throws snugged against each other (Fig. 40-26). A single throw is formed when one strand is wrapped around the other one time, and when wrapped twice, a double throw is created (Zimmer, 1991). This double weave forms the basis of a surgeon's knot. In characterizing

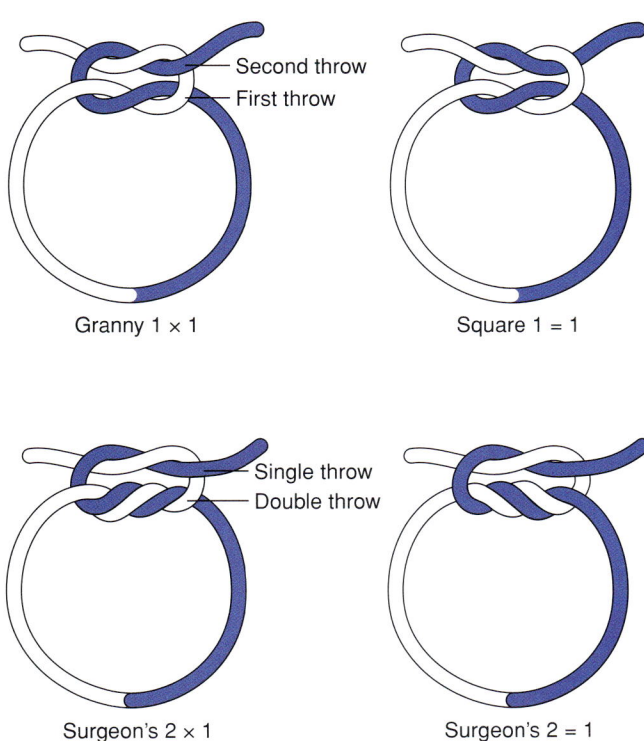

FIGURE 40-26 Surgical knots.

knots, each throw is given a numerical description, in which single throws are designated as number 1, and double throws as number 2. If successive throws are identical, a multiplication sign is placed between the numbers. If throws mirror one another, then an equal sign is used. Thus, a square knot is described as $1 = 1$; granny knot, 1×1; and square surgeon's knot, $2 = 1$. Alternative nomenclature schemes exist, but understanding the basic principles of knot construction is more clinically relevant than these descriptive definitions (Dinsmore, 1995).

Flat and Sliding Knots

Surgical knots can have flat or sliding configurations. Flat configurations include square, granny, and surgeon's knots. To construct a flat square knot, forehanded and backhanded throws are alternated, and the suture strands are pulled with equal tension in opposite directions but in the same plane. The suture strands or the hands may have to cross with each throw to ensure that the knot lies flat.

In contrast, sliding knots, also termed *slip knots*, are characterized as identical, nonidentical, and parallel. They are created when unequal tension is applied to the strands, such as during one-hand knot tying. Sliding knots are useful in situations when flat square knotting is difficult or cumbersome, such as in the limited space afforded by the deep pelvis or vagina (Ivy, 2004b). In general, sliding knots have a higher failure rate than that of flat knots (Hurt, 2005; Schubert, 2002).

Identical sliding knots are created by holding one strand constantly under tension and repeating identical tying maneuvers with the other hand. Unfortunately, these knots carry a high failure rate and are not recommended for general use (Schubert, 2002; Trimbos, 1984, 1986).

Nonidentical sliding knots are formed when a suture strand is held under constant tension, and one hand alternates forehanded and backhanded tying around this strand (Trimbos, 1986). This knot is the most frequent and practical knot used for vaginal surgery. Although these knots can unravel, additional throws can greatly improve their security (Ivy, 2004a; Trimbos, 1984; van Rijssel, 1990). A loop-to-strand variation of the nonidentical sliding knot is performed by holding the final loop of a continuous suture line taut, while alternate throws are made around the loop with the remaining single strand. Few data support the security of this loop-knot type in gynecologic surgery. When completed with monofilament suture, they carry high failure rates (Hurt, 2005).

Finally, with a *parallel sliding knot*, the suture strand under tension is alternated with each throw, causing alternate throws to slide down the other strand each time. Existing studies show this knot to be strong and reliable (Balgobin, 2013; Ivy, 2004b; Trimbos, 1986).

Surgical Knot Effectiveness

Surgical knot success depends mainly on initial loop security and knot security. *Loop security* describes the ability to maintain a tight suture loop around the tissue as the initial knot throws are placed (Lo, 2004). Loops that are initially loose will fail to secure tissues no matter how tightly the knot is tied and will result in ineffective knots, colloquially termed "air knots" (Burkhart, 1998). Three ways to optimize loop security are maintenance of tension on both strands during tying, use of an initial surgeon's throw, and slip knots (Anderson, 1980). If slip knots are placed initially, they can be converted to square knots or reinforced with a square knot once the pedicle or vessel is secured. Importantly, upward tension on both strands deep within a body cavity should be limited. Excessive force can avulse the pedicle or cause the suture loop to pull completely off.

For *knot security*, the tension with which a given throw is tied is the most important. A knot laid down tightly under great tension is less likely to slip than a knot with the same configuration but with more throws tied loosely (Gunderson, 1987).

The number and type of knots required to secure various suture materials vary. Qualities such as elasticity and memory often direct these recommendations. Multifilament sutures are generally easier to handle and display less memory, whereas synthetic monofilament suture or coated multifilament sutures have greater memory and may hold a knot poorly. For most sutures, four to six throws appears to be adequate, but the exact number depends on the type of suture and whether a flat or sliding knot is formed. Up to a point, additional throws provide more security to a knot, but this benefit must be balanced against the corresponding elevated infection risk from higher knot volume (van Rijssel, 1990).

ADHESION PREVENTION

Chronic pain, infertility, and bowel obstruction are all potential consequences of adhesion formation. These can be minimized by gentle tissue handling, meticulous hemostasis, avoidance of tissue ischemia and desiccation, and use of fine, noninflammatory suture (American Society for Reproductive Medicine, 2013).

For adhesion prevention, solid, liquid, gel, and pharmacologic agents also have been evaluated. Many have some efficacy to prevent adhesions. However, evidence fails to show benefit for clinical endpoints such as pelvic pain, fertility, quality of life, and safety (Hindocha, 2015). Of agents, both oxidized regenerated cellulose (Interceed) and sodium hyaluronate plus carboxymethylcellulose (Seprafilm) provide improved adhesion scores, whereas fibrin sheets do not (Ahmad, 2015). Data are mixed regarding the efficacy of liquid agents such as 4-percent icodextrin and 32-percent dextran compared with saline. Gel agents such as carboxymethylcellulose, polyethylene glycol, and polyethylene oxide do not improve adhesion scores but do appear to prevent scores from worsening (Ahmad, 2014). Intraperitoneal heparin and systemic promethazine are ineffective.

ELECTROSURGERY

Electrosurgery is widely used in gynecology, particularly in minimally invasive surgery. In this realm, rates of energy device–related injury approximate 1 to 2 per 1000 operations (Fuchshuber, 2018). Thus, understanding the principles of these energy forms is vital.

Semantically, *electrosurgery* differs from *electrocautery*, although the terms are often incorrectly interchanged. With electrocautery, electric current passes through a metal object, such as a wire loop, with internal resistance. Passage of current heats the loop, which then may be used surgically. The flow of current is limited to the metal being heated, and no current enters the patient. In contrast, electrosurgery directs the flow of current to the tissues themselves and produces localized tissue heating and destruction. As a result, electric current must pass through tissues to produce the desired effect (Amaral, 2005). The electrosurgical circuit contains four main parts: the generator, the active electrode, the patient, and the return electrode. Electrosurgery may be broadly categorized as monopolar or bipolar depending on the proximity of these two electrodes.

■ Monopolar Electrosurgery

Electric current is the flow of electrons through a circuit (Fig. 40-27). *Voltage* is the force that drives those charges around the circuit. *Impedance* is the combination of resistance, inductance, and capacitance that alternating current meets along the way (Morris, 2006). In monopolar electrosurgery, the return electrode in clinical use is the grounding pad. Current therefore flows (1) from the generator, which is the source of voltage, (2) through the electrosurgical tip to the patient, who is the impedance source, and then (3) onto the grounding pad, where it is dispersed. Current leaves the pad to return to the generator, and the circuit is completed (Deatrick, 2015). In electrosurgery, tissue impedance converts electric current into thermal energy that causes tissue temperatures to rise. It is these thermal increases that create electrosurgery's tissue effects.

Surgical Effects

Differing tissue effects are created by altering the manner in which current is produced and delivered. First, altering the current wave pattern can affect tissue temperatures. For example, the

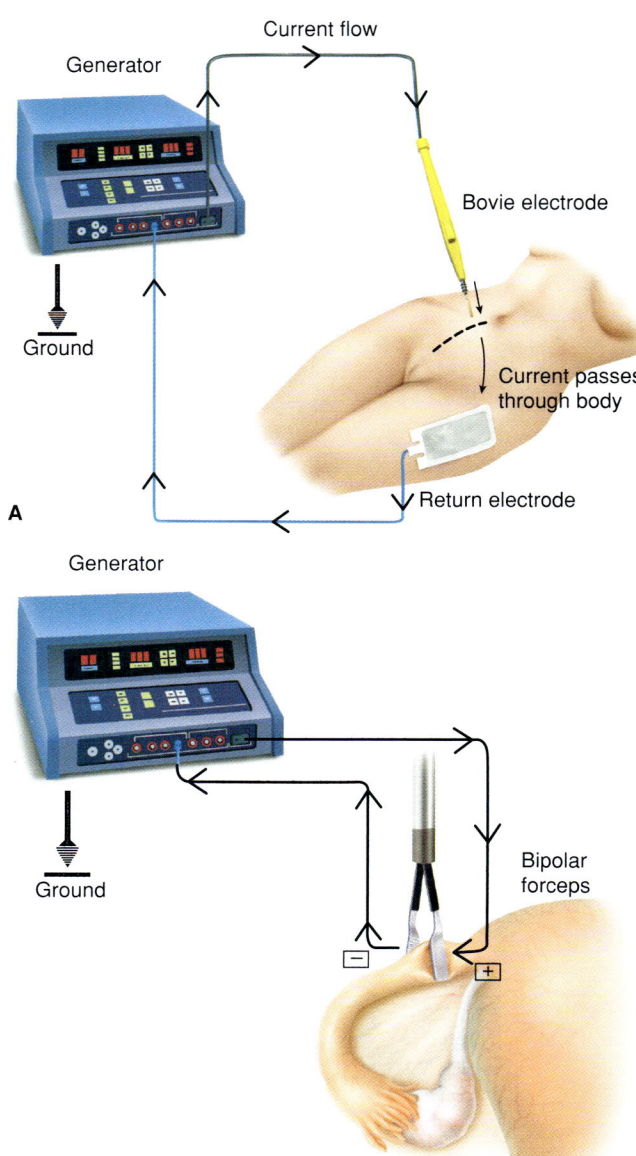

FIGURE 40-27 Circuits in electrosurgery. **A.** Monopolar electrosurgical circuit. **B.** Bipolar electrosurgical circuit.

high-frequency continuous sinusoidal waveform produced with cutting current creates higher tissue temperatures than that with coagulation current (Fig. 40-28). Second, the extent to which current is spread over an area, termed *current density*, alters the rate of heat generation (Fig. 40-29). Thus, if current is concentrated onto a small area, such as a needle-tip electrode, greater tissue temperatures are generated than if delivered over a wider area, such as an electrosurgical blade. Voltage also can alter tissue effects. As voltage increases, the degree of thermal tissue damage similarly rises. Last, the qualities and impedance of the tissues themselves affect energy transfer and heat dissipation. For example, water has low electrical impedance and liberates little heat, whereas skin with its greater impedance generates significantly higher tissue temperatures (Amaral, 2005).

With electrosurgical cutting, a continuous sine wave of current is produced. The flow of high-frequency current typically is concentrated through an electrosurgical needle or blade and

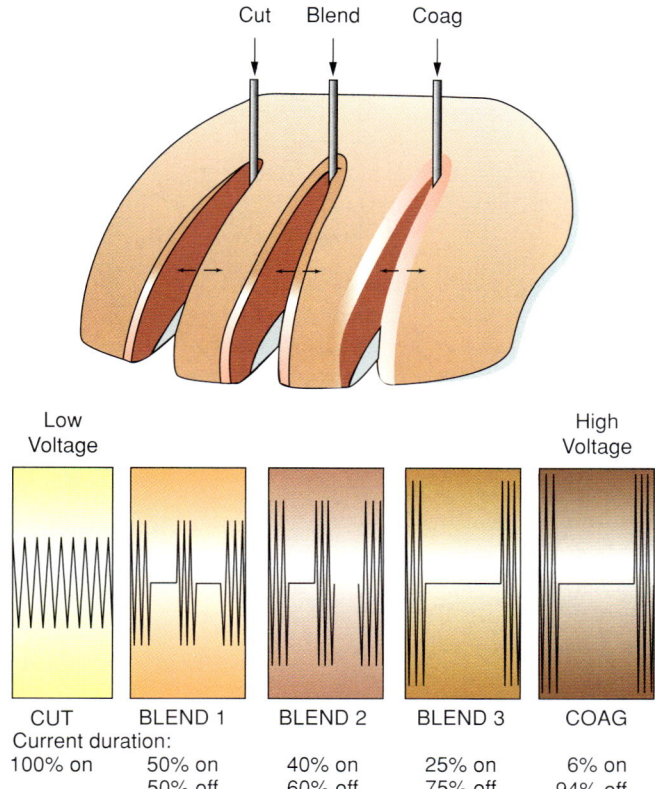

FIGURE 40-28 Tissue effects vary with cutting, blended, and coagulation currents. There is more lateral thermal damage with a pure coagulation current compared with a pure cutting or blended current. The duration of applied energy varies between current types.

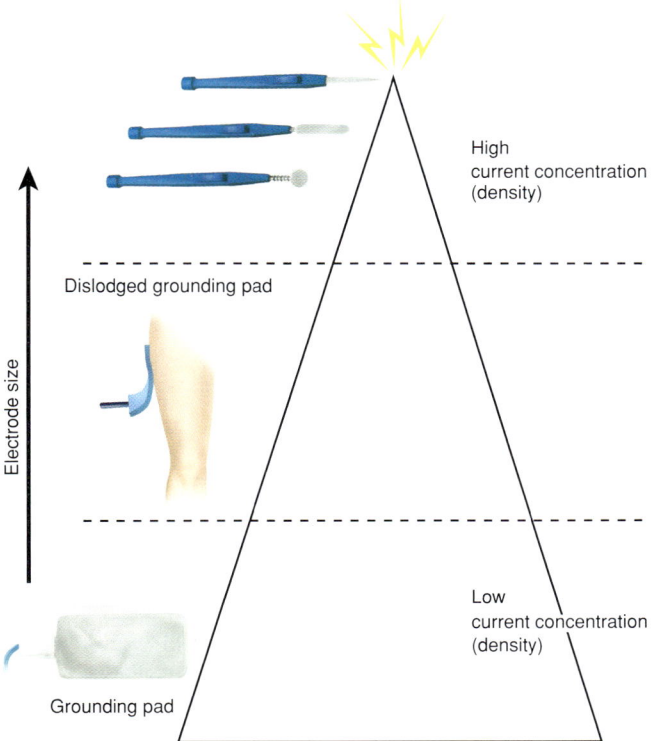

FIGURE 40-29 Current concentration and its effects. Thermal energy and risk for tissue injury diminish as current density decreases and electrode area increases.

meets tissue impedance. Sparks are created between the tissue and electrode, intense heat is produced, cellular water vaporizes, and cells in the immediate area burst. Tissues are cut cleanly, and minimal coagulum is produced. As a result, few vessels are sealed, and electrosurgical cutting provides minimal hemostasis.

In contrast, coagulation current does not produce a constant waveform. Less heat is produced than with cutting current. However, tissue temperature still rises sufficiently to denature protein and disrupt normal cellular architecture. Cells are not vaporized instantly, and cellular debris remains associated with wound edges. This coagulum seals smaller blood vessels and controls local bleeding (Singh, 2006).

Variations in the percentage of time that current is flowing can create electrosurgical effects that contain both cutting and coagulating features. Such *blended currents* are used commonly in gynecologic surgery. In most cases, specific percentages of cutting and coagulation current are selected based on surgeon preference and tissue type. Thinner vascular tissue may be best suited for a blend with less active current time, whereas denser avascular tissues may require a greater percentage of active current.

Patient Grounding

After current enters the patient, it follows the path of least resistance and exits the body through a grounding pad that has a large surface area, high conductivity, and low resistance. Dissipation across this large surface allows current to leave the body without generating significant tissue temperatures at the exit site.

However, a patient may be burned if current is concentrated through a return electrode. Clinically, this may occur if a grounding pad is partially dislodged. In this setting, the surface area is decreased, and exiting current concentration and tissue temperatures at the exit site rise. In addition, patient jewelry, metal stirrups, or other surfaces with high conductivity and low resistance may serve as a return electrode. In such cases, concentrated current exiting through these small contact sites can injure. Thus, grounding pads are ideally firmly adhered to a relatively flat body surface that is near the operative field. In most gynecologic procedures, the lateral upper thigh is used.

Patients with pacemakers, implantable cardioverter-defibrillators, or other electrical implants require special precautions. Stray electrosurgical current may be interpreted as an intracardiac signal by an implanted device and lead to pacing changes. In addition, myocardial electrical burns may result from conduction of current through the pacing electrode rather than through the grounding pad (Pinski, 2002). Accordingly, for patients with these devices, preventive recommendations include pre- and postoperative cardiology consultation; use of minimal monopolar electrosurgical current settings or substitution with bipolar electrosurgery or Harmonic scalpel; continuous cardiac monitoring; contingency plans for arrhythmias; and close proximity of active and return electrodes (Crossley, 2011).

■ Bipolar Electrosurgery

This form of electrosurgery differs from monopolar electrosurgery in that the bipolar device tip contains both an active electrode and a return electrode. For this reason, a distant grounding return pad is not required. Current is concentrated on tissues grasped between the electrodes, and tissue must remain between them. If tissue slips from between the tips, then active and return electrodes contact and create a short circuit. Current transfer will not occur (Michelassi, 1997). Bipolar electrosurgery uses only coagulation current and lacks cutting capability. However, it is useful for vessel coagulation and for fallopian tube desiccation during laparoscopic tubal sterilization (Section 44-2, p. 1021).

■ Argon Plasma Coagulation

This modality uses a stream of argon gas that has been ionized by electrical current and is then termed *plasma*. The argon plasma beam streams from a handpiece and creates noncontact monopolar coagulation. Additionally, the gas jet clears blood and tissue debris during coagulation. Argon plasma coagulation (APC) is able to coagulate broad vascular surface areas, like the liver (Beckley, 2004). It also has minimal tissue penetrance, which is particularly useful for vulnerable tissues such as ovary and bowel. In gynecologic surgery, APC is used most often during difficult endometriosis ablation over vital structures or ovarian staging cases that require extensive debulking (Cordeiro Vidal, 2017).

ULTRASONIC ENERGY

Sound waves are mechanical waves that transport energy through a medium. Those above audible range are described as *ultrasound* or *ultrasonic*. In medicine, ultrasound waves that are applied at low levels such as those used in diagnostic sonography are harmless. However, if higher power levels are used, the mechanical energy transferred to the affected tissues is sufficiently strong to produce cutting, coagulation, or tissue cavitation.

Of tools, the ultrasonic scalpel, also known as a *Harmonic scalpel*, has a tip that vibrates at high frequency. This allows the surgical device to cut or coagulate (Gyr, 2001; Wang, 2000). A balance between these two effects is controlled by the power level, tissue tension, and blade sharpness. Higher power level, greater tissue tension, and a sharp blade will lead to cutting. Lower power, decreased tissue tension, and a blunt blade will create slower cutting and greater hemostasis (Sinha, 2003). Used most commonly in laparoscopic surgery, the ultrasonic scalpel serves as an alternative to suture ligation, electrosurgical coagulation, laser, and stapling or clipping devices. However, only a few studies have compared the clinical effectiveness of this method with other methods of hemostasis (Kauko, 1998).

Cavitational ultrasonic surgical aspiration (CUSA) is another ultrasound-based tool. The ultrasonic surgical aspirator handpiece contains three main components: a high-frequency vibrator, which transfers the ultrasonic energy to tissues; irrigation tubing, which directs cooling saline to the tip; and a suction system, which draws tissue up to the tip for contact with the vibrator and which also clears away fluid and tissue fragments. The CUSA tip produces mechanical waves that create heat and vapor pockets around cells in tissues with high water content such as adipose, muscle, and carcinoma. Collapse of these pockets leads to disruption of cell architecture in a process

called *cavitation* (Jallo, 2001). Affected tissues are removed subsequently by suction aspiration. However, tissues containing less water and higher contents of collagen and elastic fibers, such as blood vessels, nerves, ureters, and serosa, are more resistant to cavitation and damage (van Dam, 1996).

In gynecology, CUSA has a limited surgical role. It may be used effectively in the treatment of vulvar intraepithelial neoplasia and bulky condyloma acuminata (Section 43-29, p. 1007). It can also speed cytoreductive ovarian cancer surgery (Aletti, 2006; Robinson, 2000).

MANAGEMENT OF HEMORRHAGE

■ Autologous Donation and Cell Salvage

Although the risk of hemorrhage accompanies most gynecologic procedures, certain factors are associated with higher rates of bleeding and are assessed prior to surgery. Specifically, obesity, large pelvic mass, dense adhesions, cancer or prior radiotherapy, and coagulation dysfunction raise hemorrhage risk. Additional consideration is given to whether the patient would accept allogeneic transfusion. For those identified to be at risk, intraoperative red cell salvage or preoperative autologous blood donation can be considered.

Red blood cell (RBC) salvage machines (autoLog; Cell Saver) collect, filter, and centrifuge blood lost during surgery. RBCs are heavier and are separated from plasma and smaller blood components during centrifugation and are then reinfused into the patient. Anticoagulants such as heparin or citrate are added to prevent clotting (Karger, 2005). Salvage efficiencies approximate 60 percent with good technique. However, vacuum levels, suction tip size, and thoroughness of salvaging efforts can affect this value. For example, turbulence destroys RBCs. Thus, suction tips with greater diameters and lower suction force can minimize hemolysis (Waters, 2005). Laparotomy sponges can be rinsed in sterile saline to maximize RBC removal. The RBC-containing saline then is suctioned into the salvage device for processing. The filtering systems in these devices have limitations. Accordingly, RBC salvage is not appropriate for contaminated cases or those in which malignancy, hemostatic agents, or amnionic fluid may be present (Waters, 2004).

Another approach for cases with expected hemorrhage involves preoperative autologous donation. With this, to avoid potential transfusion reaction or blood-borne infection, a patient may elect to donate her own blood for personal use approximately once a week for 3 to 5 weeks preceding surgery. Patient hemoglobin levels should be greater than 11.0 g/dL before each donation. Moreover, units are not collected within 72 hours before surgery. This allows intravascular volume to be replenished by the patient and units to be processed by the blood bank (Goodnough, 2005). Disadvantageously, this process has been associated with preoperative anemia secondary to donation, more liberal transfusion, transfusion reaction following clerical error, volume overload, and bacterial contamination of blood products during processing (Henry, 2002; Kanter, 1996, 1999).

Improved blood banking safety has accompanied a decline in autologous donation (Brecher, 2002). Moreover, for most gynecologic cases, the risk of transfusion is low. Thus, autologous

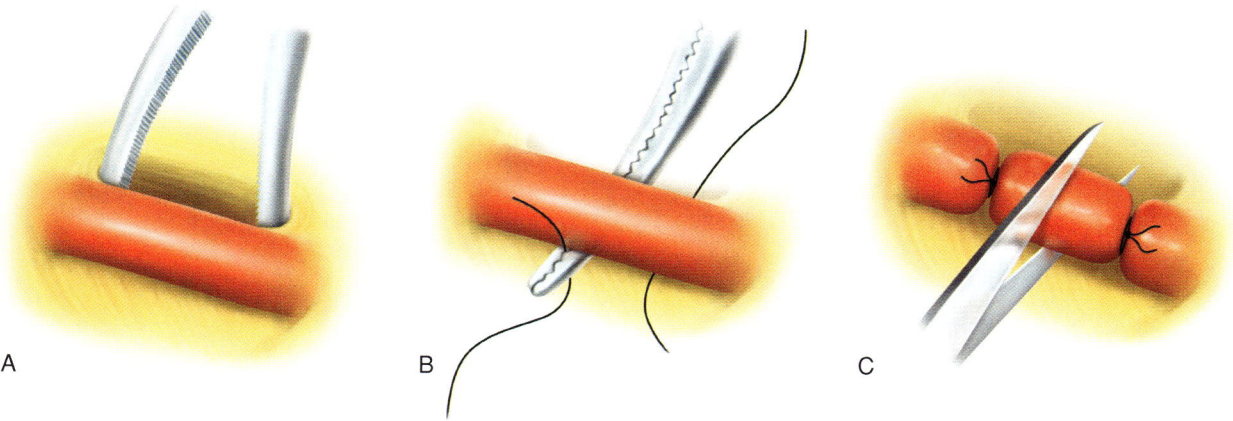

FIGURE 40-30 Steps in vessel isolation, ligation, and transection. **A.** During vessel isolation, a clamp tip can be opened and closed parallel to the side of the vessel to dissect away loose surrounding tissue. **B.** The tip of the clamp is insinuated beneath the vessel, and the jaws are opened and elevated. A suture ligature can then be grasped and pulled beneath the vessel. **C.** Two sutures are placed around the vessel, and it is transected between these ligation points.

donation typically is reserved for surgeries with a high transfusion risk or for patients with rare blood phenotypes in whom acquisition of compatible blood may be difficult.

Proper Surgical Method

In many instances, proper surgical technique can minimize vascular injury and hemorrhage. Thus, prior to ligation, vessels ideally have excess connective tissue removed sharply in a process called *skeletonizing*. Additionally, tissue clamps selected for grasping a vascular pedicle are large enough to contain the entire pedicle in the distal portion of the clamp. Large pedicles that force excess tissue toward the clamp's heel carry greater risk of tissue slippage from the heel and bleeding. Once secure, sutures placed on vascular pedicles are not be used for traction because they may be avulsed.

Tying an intact vessel at two places along its length before tissue cutting is considered in certain situations. This technique may be appropriate if a vessel is on tension or if space for a clamp is limited, such as when the ureter or bowel is nearby. A window is created below the vessel and ties are passed beneath the vessel before doubly ligating and dividing it (Fig. 40-30).

Steps of Hemorrhage Management

A methodical approach to intraoperative hemorrhage is critical. If an isolated vessel is clearly identified, grasping it with a hemostat, vascular clamp, or fine forceps may allow ligation, electrosurgical coagulation, or vascular clip application.

In contrast, venous bleeding in the pelvis is typically from a venous plexus and rarely stems from a single vessel. Vessels in these venous plexuses are thin-walled. Accordingly, indiscriminate clamping, suturing, clipping, and electrosurgical coagulation can cause further laceration and bleeding. However, if other vulnerable structures have been retracted and protected, a few shallow stitches that incorporate the bleeding area can be placed using fine absorbable suture.

If these initial efforts are unsuccessful and significant hemorrhage continues, the bleeding site is compressed with sponge stick or laparotomy sponges. Anesthesia staff is informed of

events to allow for additional monitoring. Nursing staff also is informed, as additional instruments or blood products may be required. Fluid resuscitation is individualized depending on the degree of hemorrhage and patient factors (p. 862).

Adequate exposure typically aids control of bleeding. The operative field is assessed and expanded as needed by extending a vertical incision cephalad, converting a Pfannenstiel incision to a Cherney incision, adding retractors, or converting a vaginal or laparoscopic approach to laparotomy. A second suctioning system and appropriate suture or clips may be required before removing pressure. If significant hemorrhage has already occurred and is now controlled with pressure, anesthesia is allowed time for resuscitative efforts prior to resuming surgery. Additional dissection of avascular planes around the bleeding site may improve isolation and ligation of a lacerated vessel. Furthermore, nearby vulnerable structures such as the bladder, ureter, or other vessels are identified and protected. After these steps, a surgeon may remove the tamponading pressure to assess the location, amount, and character of bleeding and to formulate the most appropriate plan to control it.

Vessel Ligation

As noted, bleeding vessels may be tied, clipped, or coagulated. Advantages to suture ligation include low cost and effectiveness over a broad range of vessel diameters. However, knot tying in general is time-consuming, is difficult in narrow spaces, and, less commonly, is associated with ligature slippage or breakage. Small vessels may be ligated by a free-tie suture placed around the heel and tip of a vascular clamp and then secured with knots (see Fig. 40-22A). Alternatively, surgeons often prefer to secure larger vascular pedicles with two separate sutures. The first ligature is a free tie placed around the toe and heel of a vascular clamp and tied. The second ligature is distal to the first and typically incorporates a bite through the tissue pedicle (see Fig. 40-22B, C). Such *transfixion* of the ligature to the pedicle decreases the risk that it will slip off the pedicle's end. Importantly, this second ligature is placed distal to the first to avert hematoma formation if a vessel is pierced during transfixion.

TABLE 40-6. Topical Hemostatic Agents

Type of Agent	Brand Name	Material
Mechanical Hemostats		
Oxidized, regenerated methylcellulose	Surgicel,	Flat loose woven fabric
	Surgicel Fibrillar,	Flat peelable layers and tufts
	Surgicel Nu-knit,	Flat loose woven fabric
	Surgicel SNoW	Flat nonwoven fabric
Porcine gelatin	Surgifoam	Powder or flat sponge
	Gelfoam	Powder or flat sponge
Bovine collagen	Avitene,	Powder, sheet, or flat sponge
	Instat	Powder
Mucopolysaccharide spheres	Arista	Powder
Active Hemostats		
Bovine thrombin	Thrombin-JMI	Liquid spray
Bovine thrombin + gelatin	Thrombi-Gel	Flat sponge
Recombinant thrombin	Recothrom	Liquid
Flowable Hemostats		
Bovine gelatin + human thrombin	FloSeal Matrix	Liquid
Porcine gelatin + Human thrombin	Surgiflo Hemostatic Matrix	Liquid
Fibrin Sealants		
Human thrombin, fibrinogen, plasminogen	Tisseel	Spray or drip application
Human thrombin, fibrinogen,	Evicel	Spray or drip application
	Evarrest	Patch

Alternatively, titanium clips seal vessels by direct compression. They are used more commonly during gynecologic oncology cases and offer the advantage of speed. However, clips are expensive, require surgical dissection of the vessel prior to application, and may dislodge from a vessel. Their use in routine gynecology is limited by these factors and surgeon preference.

Electrical and ultrasound energy can seal vessels. Ultrasonic coagulating shears (AutoSonix, Harmonic scalpel, SonoSurg) and electrosurgical bipolar vessel sealing clamps (ENSEAL, LigaSure) transfer energy that denatures vascular collagen and elastin. They seal vessels up to 7 mm in diameter (Heniford, 2001). Thermal spread for these devices is comparable and averages 2.5 mm (Harold, 2003). These tools are particularly useful for laparoscopic surgeries, in which knot tying is especially time-consuming.

Local Topical Hemostats

These topical products may be placed on bleeding sites where ligature or vessel coagulation is not possible or has been ineffective. They are most effective in controlling low-pressure bleeding, such as from veins, capillaries, and small arteries. Commercially available materials are categorized as mechanical hemostats, active hemostats, flowable hemostats, and fibrin sealants (Table 40-6). Some liquid hemostats deliver topical thrombin or thrombin plus fibrinogen and thereby induce clot formation. Others provide combined effects that, in sum, create direct pressure against wound surfaces, entrap platelets, promote platelet aggregation, and serve as a scaffold on which clot can organize.

Although effective, these agents do have disadvantages. They should not be introduced intravascularly or used with RBC salvage machines. Packing agents tightly into bony foramina is avoided because these agents can swell and cause neurologic dysfunction or pressure necrosis. Moreover, they are not placed within skin edges because they may retard edge reapproximation. They may serve as an infection nidus and thus may not be appropriate in grossly infected tissue (Anderson, 2014). Few data support the use of one agent over another. Selection typically is dictated by surgeon preference and availability in the operating room.

Tranexamic Acid

Intravenous administration of tranexamic acid, an effective antifibrinolytic, has been widely investigated in trauma surgery (Hunt, 2015). It is a synthetic lysine derivative that blocks the conversion of plasminogen to plasmin. This allows formed clots to persist (Fig. 8-12, p. 196). Massive hemorrhage may be complicated by coagulopathy and uncontrollable microvascular hemorrhage. Tranexamic acid, 1 g given intravenously, may be of benefit in this setting in concert with pelvic pressure and blood component administration.

Pelvic Artery Embolization or Pelvic Packing

Described in Chapter 9 (p. 209), embolization similar to that used to treat symptomatic leiomyomas can be used to occlude either the internal iliac artery or the uterine artery. In patients with persistent heavy bleeding despite attempts at control, pelvic packing with gauze and termination of the operation may be warranted. Rolls of gauze are packed against the bleeding site to provide constant local pressure. Typically, 24 to 48 hours later, if the patient is stable and bleeding appears to have stopped clinically, packing is removed. Some surgeons recommend leaving one end of the gauze outside the wound. After administration of general anesthesia, packing is pulled slowly through a small opening left in the incision. Alternatively, entire gauze rolls may be packed into the abdomen and removed during a second laparotomy (Newton, 1988).

Internal Iliac Artery Ligation

The internal iliac artery, also called the *hypogastric artery*, contains anterior and posterior divisions. Its anterior division supplies blood to central pelvic viscera (Fig. 38-12, p. 801). Occlusion of the internal iliac artery decreases mean blood flow by 48 percent in branches distal to ligation, which in many cases slows hemorrhage sufficiently to allow identification of specific bleeding sites (Burchell, 1968). Fortunately, the female pelvis has extensive collateral circulation, and the internal iliac artery shares arterial anastomoses with branches of the aorta, external iliac artery, and femoral artery (Table 38-2, p. 801). For this reason, ligation of the internal iliac's anterior division can be performed without compromise to pelvic organ viability. Several studies have described normal postligation fertility in these women (Demirci, 2005; Nizard, 2003).

To perform ligation, the round ligament is divided, and the pelvic sidewall peritoneum lateral to the infundibulopelvic ligament is incised cephalad. Identification of the internal iliac artery is essential because ligation of the common or external iliac arteries will have vascular consequences to the lower extremity. Once the internal iliac artery is located, a Mixter right-angle clamp is placed under the vessel at a point 2 to 3 cm distal to the bifurcation of the common iliac artery (Fig. 40-31). Two free ties of no. 1 or 0 absorbable suture are passed beneath the artery

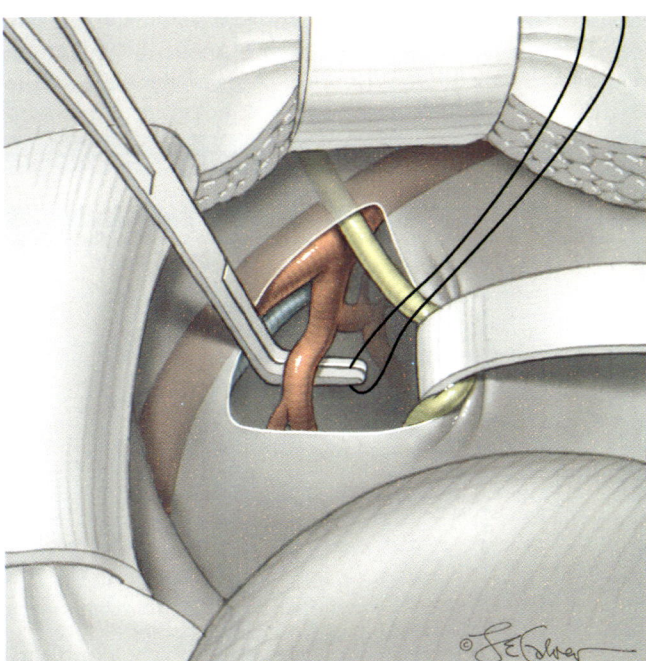

FIGURE 40-31 Internal iliac artery ligation. After opening the retroperitoneal space, the ureter is identified and retracted medially. A Mixter right-angle clamp is placed beneath the artery to receive a free tie for ligation. The artery is ligated twice but not divided. (From Gilstrap, 2017, with permission.)

and then secured. The artery is ligated but not transected. If the internal iliac is ligated at this site, its posterior division theoretically should be spared (Bleich, 2007). Care is required in passing instruments beneath the artery because the nearby thin-walled internal iliac vein is easily lacerated (Gilstrap, 2017).

■ Specific Sites of Bleeding

Infundibulopelvic Ligament

During or after ligation of this vascular pedicle, a lacerated ovarian vessel may retract into the retroperitoneum to create a hematoma. In most cases, isolation of the bleeding vessel is required to halt hematoma expansion. For this, the pelvic sidewall peritoneum lateral to the ureter and the hematoma is opened, and the incision is extended cephalad to the upper pole of the hematoma. The incision in the peritoneum may be carried up the white line of Toldt. This line, found on the right and the left, is the peritoneum's reflection over the mesenteric attachment site of the ascending or descending colon to the posterior abdominal wall. The upper pole of the hematoma is identified by a return to normal vessel caliber above the hematoma. The ovarian vessels are identified, and a closed Mixter right-angle clamp is placed beneath them. A tie on a pass then is threaded beneath and used to ligate these vessels. If large, the hematoma then is evacuated to minimize infection risk (Tomacruz, 2001). In rare cases in which vascular or ureteral anatomy is unclear, an ovarian artery may require ligation as proximal as its aortic origin below the renal arteries (Masterson, 1995).

Retropubic Space and Presacral Venous Plexus

The retropubic space, also called the *space of Retzius*, is often entered during urogynecologic procedures and contains important vascular structures. These are the obturator vessels as well as the aberrant obturator vessel and the vesical venous plexus, also called the *venous plexus of Santorini* (Fig. 38-24, p. 813). Approximately 2 percent of tension-free vaginal tape procedures are complicated by bleeding in this space (Kolle, 2005; Kuuva, 2002). In most instances, bleeding is controlled with pressure or suturing.

In contrast, the presacral venous plexus can be lacerated by dissection or suturing during sacrocolpopexy (Fig. 38-23, p. 812). Cut vessels may retract into the vertebral bone, and problematic bleeding can follow. Management is described in full in Section 45-17 (p. 1125).

Major Pelvic Vessels

High-volume pelvic vessels include the internal, external, and common iliac vessels, the inferior vena cava, and aorta. These may be lacerated during tumor removal, lymph node sampling, endometriosis excision, or laparoscopic trocar placement.

Initially following large vessel injury, pressure is applied for several minutes. If applying local pressure is unsuccessful, pressure can be applied to the abdominal aorta. Pressure is placed below the renal arteries if the bleeding is in the pelvis. Alternatively, if the bleeding is believed to originate from the abdominal aorta, such as with a primary trocar injury, pressure is applied at the level of the esophageal hiatus. Although gynecologic surgeons may attempt to repair these injuries, excessive delay in obtaining vascular surgery assistance often leads to greater blood loss (Oderich, 2004). Moreover, vessel lacerations may be made worse by a surgeon without appropriate skills. Thus, in many instances, pressure is applied, a vascular surgeon is consulted for repair, blood products are made available, and exposure is maximized. If a large vessel is punctured by a trocar or needle during laparoscopic entry, if feasible, the instrument may remain in place to act as a plug while preparations for repair are made.

Gynecologic surgery is often performed in settings in which emergent vascular surgery assistance is unavailable. In this scenario, damage-control surgery may be entertained. The pelvis is tightly packed, and the abdomen is temporarily closed. Towel clips or a running stitch using a no. 0 suture with high tensile strength can be selected for this (Sandadi, 2010). Damage-control resuscitation simultaneously is instituted, and emergency transportation to a site for definitive surgery is arranged.

Instead, if repair is undertaken, familiarity with this vascular anatomy is essential. On the left, the common and external iliac arteries remain lateral to their respective veins. On the right, however, the common iliac artery runs medial to the vein. These arteries can be repaired by placing vascular clamps 2 to 3 cm proximal and distal to the tear, then by closing the defect with a continuous suture line using monofilament synthetic 5-0 suture (Gostout, 2002; Tomacruz, 2001). The proximal clamp is removed first to allow air and debris to exit the suture line, and then the distal clamp is removed.

Parametrial and Paravaginal Vessels

During obstetric and gynecologic surgery, vessels supplying the uterus and vagina, especially venous plexuses, can be lacerated. At times, bleeding may not be easily identified or controlled by direct pressure, suturing, or clips. In these extreme situations, ligation of the internal iliac artery, which is a main source of blood supply to the pelvis, may decrease pooling of

blood and afford a better opportunity to find a bleeding source. Alternatively, if resources are available, pelvic artery embolization is effective in controlling pelvic hemorrhage. Despite these techniques, in rare persistent situations, pelvic packing and surgery termination may be indicated as described earlier (p. 860).

FLUID RESUSCITATION AND BLOOD TRANSFUSION

With acute hemorrhage, priorities include control of additional losses and replacement of sufficient intravascular volume for tissue perfusion and oxygenation. In hypoperfused areas, progressive failure of oxidative metabolism with lactate production leads to worsening systemic metabolic acidosis and eventual organ damage. To avoid these effects, resuscitation begins with an assessment of the patient's clinical status, calculation of total blood volume, and estimation of blood loss.

■ Clinical Assessment

Total blood volume for an adult approximates 70 mL/kg, and thus a 50-kg woman's calculated blood volume is 3500 mL. Of this volume, 15 percent can be lost by most patients with no changes in arterial pressure or heart rate. A 15-percent blood loss can be roughly calculated by multiplying a patient's weight in kilograms by 10. Thus, for a 50-kg woman, a 15-percent loss approximates 500 mL.

With losses of 15 to 30 percent (500 to 1000 mL for a 50-kg woman), tachycardia and narrowing of the pulse pressure are seen (Table 40-7). Peripheral vasoconstriction leads to pale, cool extremities and poor capillary refill. In unanesthetized patients, mild confusion or lethargy may develop. In most women with normal preoperative hemoglobin levels, this amount of blood loss requires fluid volume replacement, but RBC transfusion typically is not required. Greater losses, however, lead to

TABLE 40-7. Clinical Findings Associated with Increasing Severity of Hemorrhage

Hemorrhage Class	Class I	Class II	Class III	Class IV
Blood loss				
Percentage	<15	15–30	30–40	>40
Volume (mL)	750	800–1500	1500–2000	>2000
Blood pressure				
Systolic	Unchanged	Normal	Reduced	Very low
Diastolic	Unchanged	Raised	Reduced	Very low, unrecordable
Pulse (beats/min)	Slight tachycardia	100–120	120 (thready)	>120 (thready)
Capillary refill	Normal	Slow (>2 s)	Slow (>2 s)	Undetectable
Respiratory rate	Normal	Normal	Tachypnea (>20/min)	Tachypnea (>20/min)
Urinary flow rate (mL/hr)	>30	20–30	10–20	0–10
Extremities	Normal color	Pale	Pale	Pale and cold
Complexion	Normal	Pale	Pale	Ashen
Mental state	Alert	Anxious or aggressive	Anxious, aggressive, or drowsy	Drowsy, confused, or unconscious

From Baskett, 1990, with permission.

worsening perfusion, hypotension, and tachycardia. In these cases, blood transfusion in combination with intravenous fluid infusion generally is indicated (Murphy, 2001).

During surgery, blood collects in suction canisters and laparotomy sponges. Although calculations from these sources provide an approximation, blood loss estimates typically are low, and inaccuracy increases as the length and extent of a procedure increase (Bose, 2006; Santoso, 2001). Hematocrit may be measured to assess hemorrhage. However, values typically lag true losses and reflect only the degree of hemorrhage. For example, following a blood loss of 1000 mL, hematocrit levels typically fall only 3 volume percent in the first hour but usually show an 8 volume percent drop at 72 hours (Schwartz, 2006). As noted, hemorrhage leads to lactate production, and elevated serum levels can be a helpful marker. Blood gas analysis also can provide a rapid estimate of the serum base deficit. Hemorrhage severity can be stratified according to base deficits values: 2 to –5 (mild hemorrhage), –6 to –14 (moderate hemorrhage), and –15 or more (severe hemorrhage). If patients continue to have dropping base deficits despite aggressive resuscitation, ongoing hemorrhage is a concern (Davis, 1988).

■ Fluid Resuscitation

If hypovolemia is identified, fluid resuscitation begins with crystalloid solutions. If hypotension and tachycardia are present, rapid replacement is warranted, and 1 or 2 liters, as indicated, may be infused over several minutes. Normal saline and lactated Ringer solutions are the two crystalloids used commonly, and their composition is described in Chapter 42 (p. 920). For moderate hemorrhage, both perform equally well as fluid replacements (Healey, 1998).

Although crystalloids have an immediate effect to expand intravascular volume, a portion will extravasate into extracellular tissues. Thus, in the setting of moderate hemorrhage, crystalloid volume is administered in a 3:1 ratio to blood lost (Moore, 2004). Clinically, urine output of 0.5 mL/kg per hour or 30 mL or more per hour, heart rate less than 100 beats per minute, and systolic blood pressure greater than 90 mm Hg may be used as general indicators of volume improvement. If rapid crystalloid infusion fails to correct hypotension or tachycardia, then RBC transfusion usually is prudent.

In addition to or as an alternative to crystalloid solutions, colloids may be used for volume expansion. These fluids have higher molecular weights than crystalloids. As a result, a greater portion remains intravascular and is not lost to extracellular extravasation. Despite this perceived advantage, studies comparing survival rates when crystalloids or colloids are administered find no superiority with colloids but greater expense (Perel, 2013).

Damage-control resuscitation is employed for major hemorrhage, when surgical bleeding has not yet been controlled. Treatment aims to avoid coagulopathy and enhance hemostasis. For the latter, permissive hypotension (maintaining systolic blood pressure at 90 mm Hg) prevents blood pressure from rising to a level that retards fresh thrombus from forming (Sandadi, 2010). To prevent coagulopathy in patients requiring massive transfusion, component-based resuscitation is initiated early and large-volume crystalloid resuscitation is limited.

Component therapy provides plasma and platelets in equal ratios with packed RBCs (Sperry, 2018).

Intraoperative fluid management strategies broadly fall into liberal, restrictive, or goal-directed categories. Of these, evidence from colorectal and trauma surgery is now more supportive of restrictive management. Less bowel edema, quicker return of bowel function, and fewer pulmonary complications are purported benefits (Chappell, 2008; Joshi, 2005). Restrictive strategies generally use colloid to replace blood loss in a 1:1 ratio, unless RBC transfusion is indicated. Crystalloids are then used 1:1 to replace urine and insensible losses. In contrast, liberal strategies rely on large volumes of crystalloid. Last, goal-directed therapy uses a monitoring device (such as an arterial line) and administers fluids to achieve a physiologic threshold (such as stroke volume). Moderate- and high-risk surgical patients often benefit from this strategy (Hamilton, 2011).

■ Red Blood Cell Replacement
Clinical Assessment

The decision to administer RBCs is complex and must balance the risks of transfusion with needs for adequate tissue oxygenation. Assessment includes hemoglobin level, vital signs, patient age, risks for further blood loss, and underlying medical conditions, especially cardiac disease. Accordingly, no specific hemoglobin threshold dictates when RBCs are administered. Consensus guidelines suggest that in those without significant cardiac disease, transfusion to a hemoglobin level above 10 g/dL is rarely indicated (Carless, 2010). If hemoglobin levels acutely drop to 6 g/dL, transfusion almost always is required (Madjdpour, 2006). Hemoglobin levels between 6 and 10 g/dL are more problematic, and patient factors and risk for continued hemorrhage dictate therapy (American Society of Anesthesiologists, 2015).

Transfusion

When the possible need for transfusion is present, an order for a *type and screen* informs blood bank personnel that blood products may be required and initiates two tests to characterize a patient's RBCs. The first evaluation, termed *typing,* mixes commercially available standardized controls with a patient's blood sample to determine her ABO type and Rh phenotype. The second test, or *screen,* combines a patient's plasma sample with control RBCs that express clinically significant RBC antigens. If a patient has formed antibodies to any of these specific RBC surface antigens, agglutination or hemolysis of the sample is seen. However, if blood is needed immediately and a full screen is not possible, then ABO type-specific blood or O-negative blood may be used. Typing and screening require approximately 45 minutes for completion and are valid for 3 days in patients who do receive transfusion. In those who are not transfused, the validity is considerably longer and typically is determined by individual blood banks. Alternatively, an order to *type and crossmatch* blood products alerts blood bank personnel to designate specific units of blood solely for one individual's use. Those specific units are tested against the patient's for specific antigen reactions.

Previously, whole-blood transfusion was used commonly to provide RBCs, coagulation factors, and plasma proteins. This largely has been replaced by component therapy. Packed RBCs

TABLE 40-8. Characteristics of Blood Components

Component	Volume, mL	Content	Clinical Response
PRBCs	180–200	RBCs	Increases Hb 10 g/L and Hct 3%
Platelets			Increases platelet count
Random-donor unit	50–70	5.5×10^{10}	$5{-}10 \times 10^9$/L
Single-donor collection	200–400	3.0×10^{11}	$>10 \times 10^9$/L within 1 hr and $>7.5 \times 10^9$/L within 24 hr posttransfusion
FFP	200–250	Coagulation factors, including fibrinogen, proteins C and S, antithrombin	Increases coagulation factors ~2%
Cryoprecipitate	10–15	Fibrinogen, factor VIII, vWF	Increases fibrinogen level 0.1 g/L

FFP = fresh-frozen plasma; Hct = hematocrit; Hb = hemoglobin; PRBCs = packed red blood cells; RBCs = red blood cells; vWF = von Willebrand factor.

are the primary product used for most clinical situations and are prepared by removing most of the supernatant plasma during centrifugation. One unit of packed RBCs contains the same red cell mass as 1 unit of whole blood at approximately half the volume and twice the hematocrit (70 to 80 percent). One unit of packed RBCs raises the hematocrit approximately 3 volume percent in an adult or increases the hemoglobin level of a 70-kg individual by 1 g/dL (Table 40-8) (Gorgas, 2004). With severe hemorrhage that is anticipated to require ≥10 RBC units, massive transfusion protocols that combine units of packed RBCs, platelets, and plasma in 1:1:1 ratios are effective (McDaniel, 2014).

Complications

Despite numerous tests for compatibility, adverse reactions to blood products can develop (Table 40-9). First, *acute hemolytic transfusion reaction* involves immune-mediated hemolysis usually from destruction of transfused RBCs by patient antibodies. This most commonly results from ABO incompatibility. Symptoms begin within minutes or hours of transfusion and may include chills, fever, urticaria, tachycardia, dyspnea, nausea and vomiting, hypotension, and chest and back pain. In addition, these reactions can lead to acute tubular necrosis or disseminated

TABLE 40-9. Rate of RBC Transfusion-Related Adverse Event

Febrile reaction	1:950
Allergic reaction	1:1900
Delayed hemolytic reaction	1:15,000
Acute hemolytic reaction	1:63,000
TRALI	1:67,000
HIV infection	1:2 million
Hepatitis B infection	1:2 million
Hepatitis C infection	1:2 million

HIV = human immunodeficiency virus; RBC = red blood cell; TRALI = transfusion-related acute lung injury. Calculated from Busch, 2019; Harvey, 2015.

intravascular coagulopathy, and treatment is directed to these serious complications.

If acute hemolysis is suspected, transfusion is halted immediately. A sample of the patient's blood is sent with the remaining donor unit for evaluation in the blood bank. In patients with significant hemolysis, laboratory values will be altered. Specifically, serum haptoglobin levels will be lowered; serum lactate dehydrogenase and bilirubin levels will be increased; and urine and serum free hemoglobin levels will be elevated. Serum creatinine and electrolyte levels and coagulation studies additionally are ordered. To prevent renal toxicity, diuresis is prompted by administration of intravenous crystalloids and furosemide or mannitol. Alkalinization of urine may prevent precipitation of hemoglobin within the renal tubules, and thus, intravenous bicarbonate also may be given.

Delayed hemolytic transfusion reaction may develop days or weeks after transfusion. Patients often lack acute symptoms, but lowered hemoglobin levels, fever, jaundice, and hemoglobinemia may be noted. Clinical intervention typically is not required in these cases.

Febrile nonhemolytic transfusion reaction is characterized by chills and a greater than 1°C rise in temperature and is the most common transfusion reaction (Harvey, 2015). Blood transfusion typically is stopped to exclude a hemolytic reaction, and treatment is supportive. For patients with a previous history of febrile reaction, premedication with an antipyretic such as acetaminophen prior to transfusion is reasonable.

Last, an *allergic reaction* can follow an antibody-mediated response to donor plasma proteins. In U.S. Hemovigilance Module data, this was a frequent adverse event (Harvey, 2015). Urticaria alone may develop during transfusion and typically is not associated with serious sequelae. The transfusion does not need to be stopped, and treatment with an antihistamine, such as diphenhydramine (Benadryl) 50 mg orally or intramuscularly, usually suffices. Rarely, an anaphylactic reaction may complicate transfusion, and treatment follows that for classic anaphylaxis (Table 27-2, p. 592).

Infectious complications associated with packed RBC transfusion are rare. This stems mainly from routine donor-unit testing for human immunodeficiency virus (HIV); hepatitis B and C viruses; West Nile, Zika, and human lymphotropic viruses; and *Trypanosoma cruzi*. Bacterial contamination now stands as a greater infection risk (Busch, 2019).

Transfusion-related acute lung injury (TRALI) is an infrequent but serious complication of blood component therapy that is similar clinically to acute respiratory distress syndrome (ARDS). Symptoms develop within 6 hours of transfusion and may include extreme respiratory distress, frothy sputum, hypotension, fever, and tachycardia. Noncardiogenic pulmonary edema with diffuse bilateral pulmonary infiltrates on chest radiography is characteristic (Toy, 2005). Treatment of TRALI is supportive and focuses on oxygenation and blood pressure support (Silliman, 2005; Swanson, 2006).

Platelet Replacement

For patients with moderate hemorrhage, RBC transfusion typically is sufficient, but for patients with severe hemorrhage, platelet transfusion is often indicated. Platelets may be acquired from a single individual during plateletpheresis and are termed *single-donor platelets*. Alternatively, platelets may be derived from random units of whole blood and are referred to as *random-donor platelets.*

Fewer platelets are harvested from a unit of whole blood compared with the amount removed during donor plateletpheresis. Specifically, a single-donor platelet dose contains at least 3×10^{11} platelets in 250 to 300 mL of plasma, and this approximates the dose from six random-donor platelet concentrates. Each random-donor platelet concentrate contains 5.5×10^{10} platelets suspended in approximately 50 mL of plasma. Each concentrate transfused should raise the platelet count by 5 to 10×10^9/L, and the usual therapeutic dose is one platelet concentrate per 10 kg of body weight. Five to six concentrates provide a typical adult dose. Donor plasma must be compatible with recipient erythrocytes because a few RBCs are invariably transfused along with the platelets. Only platelets from D-negative donors should be given to D-negative recipients.

Surgical patients with bleeding usually require platelet transfusion if the platelet count is less than 50×10^9/L and rarely require therapy if it is greater than 100×10^9/L (American Society of Anesthesiologists, 2015). With counts between 50 and 100×10^9/L, the decision to provide platelet transfusion is based on a patient's risk for additional significant bleeding. As noted earlier, massive transfusion protocols supply equal units of platelets, RBCs, and plasma (p. 864).

Factor Replacement

Fresh-frozen plasma is one option for factor replacement and is prepared from whole blood or by plasmapheresis. It is stored frozen, and approximately 30 minutes are required for it to thaw. One unit contains all coagulation factors, including 2 to 5 mg/mL of fibrinogen in 250 mL of volume. Recommended dosing is 15 mL/kg. Fresh-frozen plasma is used commonly as first-line hemostatic therapy in massive hemorrhage because it replaces multiple coagulation factors. It is considered in a bleeding woman with a fibrinogen level below 80 to 100 mg/dL or with abnormal prothrombin and partial thromboplastin times.

Another option, cryoprecipitate, is prepared from fresh-frozen plasma and contains fibrinogen, factor VIII, von Willebrand factor, factor XIII, and fibronectin. Cryoprecipitate was developed and used originally for treatment of hemophilia A and von Willebrand disease. However, specific factor concentrates are now available for these disorders, and thus, the clinical indications for cryoprecipitate are limited. Fresh-frozen plasma provides all coagulation factors and is favored in severe hemorrhage over cryoprecipitate. However, cryoprecipitate is an excellent source of fibrinogen and may be indicated if fibrinogen levels persist below 100 mg/dL despite administration of fresh-frozen plasma, such as in disseminated intravascular coagulopathy (American Society of Anesthesiologists, 2015). The dose of cryoprecipitate is usually 2 mL/kg of body weight, and each unit contains approximately 15 mL volume. One unit should increase the fibrinogen level by 10 mg/dL (Erber, 2006).

ADJACENT ORGAN SURGICAL INJURY

Lower Urinary Tract

The lower gastrointestinal and urinary tracts are closely related to the female reproductive organs and can be damaged during gynecologic surgery. Most injuries have no antecedent risk factors, but high-risk elements are ideally sought preoperatively. These include compromised visibility from large pelvic masses, hemorrhage, pregnancy, obesity, inadequate incision size, suboptimal retraction, and poor lighting. Additionally, scarring or anatomic distortion from cervical and broad ligament leiomyomas, malignancy, endometriosis, pelvic organ prolapse, and prior pelvic infection, surgery, or radiation are risk factors (Brandes, 2004; Francis, 2002).

The overall rates of bladder and ureteral injury during benign gynecological surgery are 0.8 percent and 0.3 percent, respectively, and up to 75 percent of injuries occur during hysterectomy (Teeluckdharry, 2015; Walters, 2007). Approximately 2 percent of women undergoing hysterectomy will have a concomitant stent insertion, ureteric or bladder repair, or urinary diversion (Wallis, 2016).

Patients who sustain surgical injury to the bladder or ureter suffer significantly greater morbidity. In one case-control study, women with injury to the lower urinary tract during abdominal hysterectomy had significantly greater operative times, estimated blood loss, blood transfusion rates, febrile morbidity, and postoperative stay lengths than their respective controls (Carley, 2002).

Bladder Injury

Cystotomy is common, and approximately 0.3 to 11 cases occur per 1000 benign gynecologic surgeries (Gilmour, 2006; Mathevet, 2001; Teeluckdharry, 2015). Urogynecologic procedures and hysterectomy are disproportionately affected. During surgery, the bladder may be at greater risk during (1) initial laparotomy entry when incising the anterior parietal peritoneum, (2) dissection within the retropubic space, (3) vaginal epithelium dissection during anterior colporrhaphy, or (4) hysterectomy when dissecting in the vesicouterine space, entering the anterior vagina, or suturing the vaginal cuff. With hysterectomy, bladder injury traditionally has been associated more often with the vaginal hysterectomy, but some data suggest that endoscopic procedures pose the greatest risk (Frankman, 2010;

Sandberg, 2012; Teeluckdharry, 2015). During laparoscopy, bladder injury most often occurs during adhesiolysis or vesicouterine space dissection. Veress needle and trocar insertion are others (Wong, 2018; Yuzpe, 1990). Preventively, clear identification of the bladder, gentle retraction, meticulous surgical technique, sharp dissection, and maintenance of a drained bladder intraoperatively are standard principles.

Cystotomy is suspected if a Foley bulb, bloody urine, or urine leaking into the operative field is seen. During laparoscopy, the Foley bag may also distend with gas from the pneumoperitoneum. For diagnosis, retrograde instillation of sterile milk through a catheter confirms injury and delineates its full extent. This is superior to methylene blue dye, as infant formula does not stain surrounding tissues and is readily available. In addition, small defects can be difficult to identify and repair if the tissues surrounding the defect become dye stained. Prior to repair, cystoscopy to assess ureteral patency is indicated for any injury to the bladder base, which is where the trigone lies. More generally, cystoscopy allows the full extent of damage to be defined and additional injuries or intravesical sutures to be excluded.

Repair during the primary surgery is preferred and lowers risks of later vesicovaginal fistula formation. Suture identified in the bladder is cut, as persistence can lead to cystitis, stone formation, or both. Needle-stick and subcentimeter lacerations can be managed conservatively. Larger defects may be closed in two or three layers as described in Chapter 45 (p. 1081).

Postoperatively, continuous bladder drainage is continued for 7 to 10 days (Utrie, 1998). Evidence is conflicting regarding the use of prophylactic antibiotics for the expected duration of catheterization and thus remains at the provider's discretion. The need for computed tomography (CT) urography prior to drainage discontinuation varies. For bladder dome injuries, lacerations measuring <1 cm typically do not require postrepair imaging, whereas for longer ones it may be considered. Complicated lacerations or those in the trigone typically merit CT urography to document bladder integrity (Bochenska, 2016; Glaser, 2019).

■ Urethral Injury

The female urethra is rarely injured during gynecologic surgery, but cystoscopy, urethral diverticulum repairs, antiincontinence operations, and possibly anterior colporrhaphy are at-risk procedures. Repair is completed with 3-0 or 4-0 absorbable suture in an interrupted fashion and in multiple layers, if possible. Similar to cystotomy, a Foley catheter is typically placed postoperatively for 7 to 10 days. Antibiotic prophylaxis is provided at the surgeon's discretion (Francis, 2002).

■ Ureteral Injury

This is uncommon in benign gynecologic surgery, and the incidence approximates 0.2 to 7.3 injury cases per 1000 surgeries. For hysterectomy, the highest rate of ureteral injury is linked with laparoscopic hysterectomy, and the lowest with vaginal hysterectomy (Gilmour, 2006; Sandberg 2012; Teeluckdharry, 2015). Other associated procedures include operations for pelvic organ prolapse, urinary incontinence, malignancy, and endometriosis (Patel, 2009; Utrie, 1998).

Gynecologic ureteral injury typically occurs in the ureter's distal third and includes transection, ligation, kinking, crushing, or thermal injury (Blackwell, 2018; Brandes, 2004; Utrie, 1998; Wong, 2018). The ureter more often is transected or kinked, and each accounts for approximately 40 percent of injuries. Trauma to its outer sheath can also disrupt ureteral blood supply and devitalize it.

From anatomic studies, the ureter is vulnerable at several sites during pelvic surgery (Jackson, 2019). During hysterectomy, the ureter is prone to injury at the level of the uterine artery, and this site accounts for 80 percent of injuries (Ibeanu, 2009). The ureter is also at risk near the pelvic brim during adnexectomy and at the distal uterosacral ligaments.

Preventively, a preoperative risk evaluation and, if indicated, intravenous pyelography (IVP) or CT scanning to document the ureteral course are completed. Although prophylactic ureteral stenting does not prevent injury, it may improve intraoperative recognition and aid immediate repair (Chou, 2009). Intraoperatively, sound surgical technique and direct ureter visualization at each step in the procedure are other preventions (Findley, 2016). The ureter may also be felt to "snap" if palpated and stretched along its course on the broad ligament's medial leaf. Importantly, vessels, adipose tissue, and peritoneal folds can mimic this.

Diagnosis

Iatrogenic injury ideally is diagnosed early, as immediate repair is associated with improved outcomes and less patient morbidity (Neuman, 1991; Sakellariou, 2002). Damage may be seen directly or identified during intraoperative cystoscopy. Intravenous methylene blue, 10-percent sodium, fluorescein, or indigo carmine administration stains urine and aids cystoscopic identification of urine jets from the ureteral orifices (Doyle, 2015; Glaser, 2019). With these dyes, colored effluent is usually seen in 5 to 10 minutes, but this may take 30 to 40 minutes in a hypovolemic patient. Alternatively, phenazopyridine can be taken by mouth 1 hour prior to surgery and colors the urine reddish-orange (Propst, 2016). Nonsystemic options include retrograde bladder distension with normal saline, mannitol, or 50-percent dextrose, which all rely on viscosity differences between the urine and distending medium to identify ureteral jets (Grimes, 2017; Narasimhulu, 2016). With any of these, failure to see urine jets mandates further evaluation with either IVP or ureteral catheterization. Unfortunately, normal-appearing findings at cystoscopy do not guarantee ureteral integrity, because nonobstructive, partially obstructive, or late ureteral injuries may be unrecognized.

Diagnosing injury shortly after surgery is challenging, as patient symptoms may be attributable to other causes. Renal damage may begin 24 hours after obstruction and can be irreversible in 1 to 6 weeks (Walter, 2002). Symptoms usually develop approximately 48 hours after surgery, and fever, abdominal or flank pain, and watery vaginal or incisional discharge may be among these. Findings include hematuria, leukocytosis, elevated blood urea nitrogen level, and ileus. Prolonged skin or vaginal drainage suggests a urinary leak, and high creatinine levels in these fluids compared with patient serum levels are diagnostic of urine. Serum creatinine measurement may or may not be helpful. In one retrospective study of 187 patients, a 24-hour postoperative change <0.3 mg/dL from preoperative levels had a specificity of 98 percent and negative predictive value of 100 percent in confirming bilateral ureteral patency. Because an increase >0.2 mg/dL was associated with obstruction, the authors recommended repeating a creatinine measurement and renal imaging for persistent elevation above this level (Walter, 2002). With elevated serum creatinine levels, calculation of the fractional excretion of sodium (FENa) or assessment of urine sodium levels may help clarify the renal injury source as prerenal, intrarenal, or postrenal, as described in Chapter 42 (p. 918).

Sonography, CT, or magnetic resonance (MR) imaging will help identify hydronephrosis, urinoma, or abscess. Lack of contrast in the distal ureter on delayed CT images confirms total obstruction (Armenakas, 1999). IVP can also help localize injury. However, intravenous contrast can be nephrotoxic, and thus CT with this contrast may be a less than ideal choice for those with already elevated creatinine levels. Instead, retrograde pyelography with fluoroscopic guidance and attempted retrograde ureteral stent placement can be considered if suspicion remains high. All of these imaging modalities can be used to diagnose injury in both the early and late postoperative periods.

Treatment

The best repair method depends on the location, extent, time from surgery, and mechanism of injury. Expert assistance from a urogynecologist, gynecologic oncologist, or urologist may be prudent. The ureter can be repaired by stenting, reimplantation, or end-to-end reanastomosis. For low-grade sheath injuries from clamping or suturing, removal of the insult and stent placement may be sufficient. For incomplete obstruction or injury identified postoperatively, stenting alone can resolve injuries in up to 80 percent of cases. For more extensive injury, either reimplantation or reanastomosis is performed (Utrie, 1998).

Reimplantation, namely, *ureteroneocystotomy*, is preferred for injuries within 6 cm of the bladder. With this, if the ureter is short, tension on the repair may be relieved by a psoas hitch. The bladder is mobilized and attached to the psoas muscle. Another method to avoid repair tension is a Boari flap. In this procedure, the bladder ipsilateral to the injury is mobilized, and a pedicle of anterior bladder wall is fashioned into a tube to bridge to the ureter.

For injuries >7 cm from the bladder, ureteral reanastomosis, that is, *ureteroureterostomy*, is preferred. Rarely, transureteroureterostomy is needed for a more proximal injury or one in which the bladder cannot be mobilized. With this procedure, the injured ureter is tunneled across and connected to the healthy ureter.

Intraoperatively, tissues are their healthiest, and the likelihood for successful repair is great. However, most iatrogenic injuries are recognized after a delay and tend to be complex (Brandes, 2004). Little evidence guides the decision for reoperation in the early postoperative period. In general, reexploration within the first few days appears to be well tolerated, leads to good outcomes, and is not technically difficult (Preston, 2000; Stanhope, 1991).

For delayed diagnoses, retrograde stenting is unsuccessful in 50 to 95 percent of cases and recommended only for certain low-grade injuries (Brandes, 2004). Occasionally, an antegrade stent can be placed percutaneously, which will avoid the need for laparotomy, provided there is no ureteral leak or stricture. More extensive damage, such as complete transection, cannot be easily stented and is more appropriately repaired by definitive surgery. Reexploration 2 to 3 weeks after initial surgery is difficult due to inflammation, fibrosis, adhesions, hematoma, and distorted anatomy (Brandes, 2004). Thus, when diagnosis is significantly delayed, urinary diversion with a percutaneous nephrostomy (PCN) and later repair is preferred. For some low-grade lesions, such as ligation with absorbable suture, proximal urinary diversion by PCN may allow spontaneous healing without further surgery. In addition, PCN diversion may be used as a temporizing measure for patients temporarily unfit for surgery (Preston, 2000).

■ Universal Cystoscopy

Lower urinary tract injury is poorly detected by direct visualization, and rates of undetected injury range from 7 to 12 percent for ureteral trauma and approximate 35 percent for bladder damage (Vakili, 2005). To increase early diagnosis, universal intraoperative cystoscopy has been advocated, and detection rates near 96 percent (Ibeanu, 2009; Vakili, 2005; Visco, 2001). Proponents argue that the procedure is cost-effective, carries minimal risk, and prevents both postoperative morbidity and liability. In support of this strategy, a systematic review of benign gynecologic surgeries found that universal cystoscopy was associated with a substantial increase in urinary tract injury detection rates compared with selective use. Similar results specific to hysterectomy also have been reported (Chi, 2016; Teeluckdharry, 2015).

Opponents cite overall low rates of injury, imperfect detection rates, greater cost, credentialing problems, and a need for training (Patel, 2009; Sandberg, 2012). Interestingly, although intraoperative detection rates are improved with routine cystoscopy, postoperative detection rates have not declined (Teeluckdharry, 2015). Using a decision analysis model, one study estimated that routine cystoscopy was cost-effective when ureteral injury rates were above 1.5 percent for abdominal hysterectomy and 2 percent for vaginal and laparoscopically assisted hysterectomy (Visco, 2001).

Cystoscopy is currently indicated for urogynecologic procedures but is not strictly recommended for other routine gynecologic procedures, including hysterectomy (Patel, 2009). At present, the decision remains at the surgeon's discretion. Some prefer selective cystoscopy, in which examination is prompted by patient risk factors or by intraoperative events.

■ Bowel Injury

Injury to the bowel infrequently complicates gynecologic surgery, and rates are <1 percent (Harris, 1997; Makinen, 2001). A traumatic breach during peritoneal cavity entry, lysis of adhesions, or dissection is the most common, particularly if the bowel wall is abnormally fixed by adhesions (Mathevet, 2001; Maxwell, 2004; Krebs, 1986). In laparoscopic procedures, most injuries result during abdominal access with the Veress needle or trocars (Llarena, 2015).

The most commonly injured segment is the small intestine, followed by the colon (Krebs, 1986; Llarena, 2015). Less commonly, the stomach is punctured during laparoscopic entry, and rectal injury can complicate both vaginal and laparoscopic surgery (Hoffman, 1999; Llarena, 2015; Mathevet, 2001).

For the gynecologic surgeon, prevention includes sharp dissection for adhesiolysis, adequate exposure, gentle retraction, and sparing use of diathermy near organs. When entering through a prior abdominal incision, a surgeon ideally dissects tissue layers methodically. Alternatively, a separate incision or extension of the existing one to an area that has not been previously opened can be considered. After any extensive pelvic dissection, the bowel is systematically inspected along its entire length to detect serosal defects and unrecognized perforation. At suspected sites, the bowel is scrutinized for mucosal eversion and content leakage. Evaluation is gentle to avoid additional damage.

Enterotomy management depends on the site and size of injury, surgeon skill, blood supply compromise, and recognition timing. With the small intestines, serosal defects may be either left alone or reinforced with small-gauge absorbable suture (Maxwell, 2004). Short, small-intestine enterotomies may be repaired in layers using fine absorbable suture. During repair, rubber-shod clamps may be placed across the intestinal lumen on either side of the wound to prevent content spill. To avoid bowel lumen narrowing, the suture line should lie transverse to the normal axis of the intestine (Stanton, 1987). Postoperative antibiotics are typically not required.

Large-bowel injuries increase the risk of fecal peritonitis, sepsis, and poor wound healing. Serosal defects and small lacerations may be managed similarly to those of the small intestine. For more extensive injuries or fecal soiling that may require resection, diversion, or complicated repair, consultation with a gynecologic oncologist or colorectal surgeon is often indicated. Broad-spectrum antibiotic prophylaxis is provided for at least the next 24 hours in these cases. In general, for both small- and large-intestinal injuries, early feeding is acceptable and not associated with repair site complications (Fanning, 2001).

The rectum may be lacerated during vaginal surgery, especially when performing posterior colpotomy or posterior colporrhaphy. These injuries are typically midline, extraperitoneal, and <2 cm long. Postmenopausal status, prior posterior colporrhaphy, or pathology that obliterates the cul-de-sac or limits organ mobility raises injury risk (Hoffman, 1999; Mathevet, 2001). Prevention centers on careful examination under anesthesia to detect cul-de-sac fullness or uterine immobility, sharp dissection with the aid of a guiding rectal finger, and use of a vasoconstricting agent to reduce obscuring operative field bleeding.

Rectal injury may be extraperitoneal or intraperitoneal, and rectal examination will typically detect the injury and delineate its borders. Minor intraperitoneal injuries with minimal or no contamination can be repaired primarily in layers as described previously. Larger injuries with gross soiling may require expert consultation. Broad-spectrum antibiotic prophylaxis is provided for the next 24 hours in these cases.

Low extraperitoneal injury during vaginal surgery in a healthy patient can be repaired primarily and rarely requires a diverting colostomy or abdominal repair. Repair is accomplished transvaginally using two to three layers of fine absorbable suture. The peritoneum may be used as an additional layer for injuries near the peritoneal reflection. During repair, a digit in the rectum exposes the defect, tissues surrounding the defect are mobilized, the site is copiously irrigated, and appropriate antibiotic prophylaxis is provided for 24 hours (Hoffman, 1999). In general, small (<2 cm) rectal injuries recognized and repaired during vaginal surgery tend to heal well without complications or fistula formation (Mathevet, 2001). Diet can be advanced as tolerated, but a stool softener is recommended once the patient is taking solid foods (Hoffman, 1999).

REFERENCES

Ahmad G, Mackie FL, Iles DA, et al: Fluid and pharmacological agents for adhesion prevention after gynaecological surgery. Cochrane Database Syst Rev 7:CD001298, 2014

Ahmad G, O'Flynn H, Hindocha A, et al: Barrier agents for adhesion prevention after gynaecological surgery. Cochrane Database Syst Rev 4:CD000475, 2015

Alayed N, Alghanaim N, Tan X, et al: Preemptive use of gabapentin in abdominal hysterectomy: a systematic review and meta-analysis. Obstet Gynecol 123:1221, 2014

Aletti GD, Dowdy SC, Podratz KC, et al: Surgical treatment of diaphragm disease correlates with improved survival in optimally debulked advanced stage ovarian cancer. Gynecol Oncol 100(2):283, 2006

Amaral J: Electrosurgery and ultrasound for cutting and coagulating tissue in minimally invasive surgery. In Soper N, Swanstrom L, Eubanks W (eds): Mastery of Endoscopic and Laparoscopic Surgery. Philadelphia, Lippincott Williams & Wilkins, 2005, p 67

American College of Obstetricians and Gynecologists: The use and development of checklists in obstetrics and gynecology. Committee Opinion No. 680, November 2016

American Society for Reproductive Medicine in collaboration with Society of Reproductive Surgeons: Pathogenesis, consequences, and control of peritoneal adhesions in gynecologic surgery: a committee opinion. Fertil Steril 99(6):1550, 2013

American Society of Anesthesiologists: Practice guidelines for perioperative blood management: an updated report by the American Society of Anesthesiologists Task Force on Perioperative Blood Management. Anesthesiol 122(2):241, 2015

Anderson CK, Medlin E, Ferriss AF, et al: Association between gelatin-thrombin matrix use and abscesses in women undergoing pelvic surgery. Obstet Gynecol 124(3):589, 2014

Anderson RM, Romfh RF: Technique in the Use of Surgical Tools. New York, Appleton-Century-Crofts, 1980

Api O, Ergen B, Api M, et al: Comparison of oral nonsteroidal analgesic and intrauterine local anesthetic for pain relief in uterine fractional curettage: a randomized, double-blind, placebo-controlled trial. Am J Obstet Gynecol 203(1):28.e1, 2010

Armenakas NA: Current methods of diagnosis and management of ureteral injuries. World J Urol 17:8, 1999

Aszmann OC, Dellon ES, Dellon AL: Anatomical course of the lateral femoral cutaneous nerve and its susceptibility to compression and injury. Plast Reconst Surg 100(3):600, 1997

Ayers JW, Morley GW: Surgical incision for cesarean section. Obstet Gynecol 70(5):706, 1987

Balgobin S: Urologic and gastrointestinal injuries. In Yeomans ER, Hoffman BL, Gilstrap LC III, et al (eds): Cunningham and Gilstrap's Operative Obstetrics, 3rd ed. New York, McGraw-Hill Education, 2017, p 459

Balgobin S, Hamid CA, Brown SA, et al: Mechanical performance of surgical knots in a vaginal surgery model: J Surg Educ 70(3):340, 2013

Baskett PJ: ABC of major trauma. Management of hypovolaemic shock. BMJ 300(6737):1453, 1990

Batra EK, Franz DA, Towler MA, et al: Influence of surgeon's tying technique on knot security. J Appl Biomater 4:241, 1993

Beckley ML, Ghafourpour KL, Indresano AT: The use of argon beam coagulation to control hemorrhage: a case report and review of the technology. J Oral Maxillofacial Surg 62:615, 2004

Bennett RG: Selection of wound closure materials. J Am Acad Dermatol l18 (4 Pt 1):619, 1988

Bhende S, Rothenburger S, Spangler DJ, et al: In vitro assessment of microbial barrier properties of Dermabond topical skin adhesive. Surg Infect 3(3):251, 2002

Blackwell RH, Kirshenbaum EJ, Shah AS, et al: Complications of recognized and unrecognized iatrogenic ureteral injury at time of hysterectomy: a population based analysis. J Urol 199:1540, 2018

Bleich AT, Rahn DD, Wieslander CK, et al: Posterior division of the internal iliac artery: anatomic variations and clinical applications. Am J Obstet Gynecol 197(6):658.e1, 2007

Blomstedt B, Osterberg B, Bergstrand A: Suture material and bacterial transport. An experimental study. Acta Chirurg Scand 143(2):71, 1977

Blondeel PNV, Murphy JW, Debrosse D, et al: Closure of long surgical incisions with a new formulation of 2-octylcyanoacrylate tissue adhesive versus commercially available methods. Am J Surg 188(3):307, 2004

Bochenska K, Zyczynski HM: Utility of postoperative voiding cystourethrogram after lower urinary tract repair. Female Pelvic Med Reconstr Surg 22(5):369, 2016

Bohrer JC, Walters MD, Park A, et al: Pelvic nerve injury following gynecologic surgery: a prospective cohort study. Am J Obstet Gynecol 201(5):531.e1, 2009

Bose P, Regan F, Paterson-Brown S: Improving the accuracy of estimated blood loss at obstetric haemorrhage using clinical reconstructions. BJOG 113(8):919, 2006

Brandes S, Coburn M, Armenakas N, et al: Consensus on genitourinary trauma: diagnosis and management of ureteric injury: an evidence-based analysis. BJU Int 94(3):277, 2004

Brecher ME, Goodnough LT: The rise and fall of preoperative autologous blood donation. Transfusion 42(12):1618, 2002

Brill AI, Nezhat F, Nezhat C, et al: The incidence of adhesions after prior laparotomy: a laparoscopic appraisal. Obstet Gynecol 85:269, 1995

Bucknall TE: Factors influencing wound complications: a clinical and experimental study. Ann R Coll Surg Engl 65(2):71, 1983

Burchell RC: Physiology of internal iliac artery ligation. J Obstet Gynaecol Br Commonw 75(6):642, 1968

Burkhart SS, Wirth MA, Simonick M, et al: Loop security as a determinant of tissue fixation security. Arthroscopy 14:773, 1998

Busch MP, Bloch EM, Kleinman SH: Prevention of transfusion-transmitted infections. Blood 133(17):1854, 2019

Campbell JA, Temple WJ, Frank CB, et al: A biomechanical study of suture pullout in linea alba. Surgery 106:888, 1989

Carless PA, Henry DA, Carson JL, et al: Transfusion thresholds and other strategies for guiding allogeneic red blood cell transfusion. Cochrane Database Syst Rev 10:CD002042, 2010

Carley ME, McIntire D, Carley JM, et al: Incidence, risk factors and morbidity of unintended bladder or ureter injury during hysterectomy. Int Urogynecol J Pelvic Floor Dysfunct 13:18, 2002

Carlson MA, Condon RE: Polyglyconate (Maxon) versus nylon suture in midline abdominal incision closure: a prospective randomized trial. Am Surgeon 61(11):980, 1995

Carney J, McDonell J, Ochana A, et al: The transversus abdominis plane block provides effective postoperative analgesia in patients undergoing total abdominal hysterectomy. Anesth Analg 107:2056, 2008

Chappell D, Jacob M, Hofmann-Kiefer K, et al: A rational approach to perioperative fluid management. Anesthesiology 109:723, 2008

Chen SS, Lin AT, Chen KK, et al: Femoral neuropathy after pelvic surgery. Urology 46(4):575, 1995

Chi AM, Curran DS, Morgan DM, et al: Universal cystoscopy after benign hysterectomy: examining the effects of an institutional policy. Obstet Gynecol 127:369, 2016

Chou MT, Wang CJ, Lien RC: Prophylactic ureteral catheterization in gynecologic surgery: a 12 year randomized trial in a community hospital. Int Urogynecol J Pelvic Floor Dysfunct 20:689, 2009

Cicinelli E, Didonna T, Ambrosi G, et al: Topical anaesthesia for diagnostic hysteroscopy and endometrial biopsy in postmenopausal women: a randomised placebo-controlled double-blind study. BJOG 104(3):316, 1997

Cicinelli E, Didonna T, Schonauer LM, et al: Paracervical anesthesia for hysteroscopy and endometrial biopsy in postmenopausal women: a randomized, double-blind, placebo-controlled study. J Reprod Med Obstet Gynecol 43(12):1014, 1998

Colombo M, Maggioni A, Parma G, et al: A randomized comparison of continuous versus interrupted mass closure of midline incisions in patients with gynecologic cancer. Obstet Gynecol 89(5 Pt 1):684, 1997

Cong L, Li C, Wei B, et al: V-Loc™ 180 suture in total laparoscopic hysterectomy: a retrospective study comparing Polysorb to barbed suture used for vaginal cuff closure. Eur J Obstet Gynecol Reprod Biol 207:18, 2016

Cordeiro Vidal G, Babin G, Querleu D, et al: Primary debulking surgery of the upper abdomen and the diaphragm, with a plasma device surgery system, for advanced ovarian cancer. Gynecol Oncol 144(1):223, 2017

Crossley GH, Poole JE, Rozner MA, et al: The Heart Rhythm Society (HRS)/American Society of Anesthesiologists (ASA) Expert Consensus Statement on the perioperative management of patients with implantable defibrillators, pacemakers and arrhythmia monitors: facilities and patient management. Heart Rhythm 8(7):1114, 2011

Davis JW, Shackford SR, Mackersie RC, et al: Base deficit as a guide to volume resuscitation. J Trauma 28:1464, 1988

De Oliveira G Jr, Agarwal D, Benzon H: Perioperative single dose ketorolac to prevent postoperative pain: a meta-analysis of randomized trials. Anesth Analg 114:424, 2012

De Oliveira G Jr, Castro-Alves L, Nader A, et al: Transversus abdominis plane block to ameliorate postoperative pain outcomes after laparoscopic surgery: a meta-analysis of randomized controlled trials. Anesth Analg 118:454, 2014

Deatrick KB, Doherty GM: Power sources in surgery. In Doherty GM (ed): Current Surgical Diagnosis and Treatment, 14th ed. New York, McGraw-Hill Education, 2015

Demirci F, Ozdemir I, Safak A, et al: Comparison of colour Doppler indices of pelvic arteries in women with bilateral hypogastric artery ligation and controls. J Obstet Gynaecol 25(3):273, 2005

Deveneau NE, Forbis C, Lipetskaia L, et al: The effect of lithotomy position on nerve stretch: a cadaveric study. Female Pelvic Med Reconstr Surg 23(6):457, 2017

Dinsmore RC: Understanding surgical knot security: a proposal to standardize the literature. J Am Coll Surg 180(6):689, 1995

Donnellan NM, Mansuria SM: Small bowel obstruction resulting from laparoscopic vaginal cuff closure with a barbed suture. J Minim Invasive Gynecol 18(4):528, 2011

Dorian R: Anesthesia of the surgical patient. In Brunicardi F, Andersen D, Billiar T, et al (eds): Schwartz's Principles of Surgery, 10th ed. New York, McGraw-Hill, 2015

Doyle PJ, Lipetskaia L, Duecy E, et al: Sodium fluorescein use during intraoperative cystoscopy. Obstet Gynecol 125(3):548, 2015

Ducic I, Dellon L, Larson EE: Treatment concepts for idiopathic and iatrogenic femoral nerve mononeuropathy. Ann Plast Surg 55(4):397, 2005

Edelman A, Nichols MD, Leclair C, et al: Four percent intrauterine lidocaine infusion for pain management in first-trimester abortions. Obstet Gynecol 107(2 Pt 1):269, 2006

Edelman A, Nichols MD, Leclair C, et al: Intrauterine lidocaine infusion for pain management in first-trimester abortions. Obstet Gynecol 103(6):1267, 2004

Edlich RF, Panek PH, Rodeheaver GT, et al: Physical and chemical configuration of sutures in the development of surgical infection. Ann Surg 177(6):679, 1973

Fanning J, Andrews SA: Early postoperative feeding after major gynecologic surgery: evidence-based scientific medicine. Am J Obstet Gynecol 185(1):1, 2001

Findley AD, Solnik MJ: Prevention and management of urologic injury during gynecologic laparoscopy. Curr Opin Obstet Gynecol 28:323, 2016

Food and Drug Administration: Recommendations to reduce surgical fires and related patient injury: FDA safety communication. 2018. Available at: https://www.fda.gov/MedicalDevices/Safety/AlertsandNotices/ucm608637.htm. Accessed February 6, 2019

Franchi M, Ghezzi F, Benedetti-Panici PL, et al: A multicentre collaborative study on the use of cold scalpel and electrocautery for midline abdominal incision. Am J Surg 181(2):128, 2001

Franchi M, Ghezzi F, Zanaboni F, et al: Nonclosure of peritoneum at radical abdominal hysterectomy and pelvic node dissection: a randomized study. Obstet Gynecol 90(4 Pt 1):622, 1997

Francis SL, Magrina JF, Novicki D, et al: Intraoperative injuries of the urinary tract. J Gynecol Oncol 7:65, 2004

Frankman EA, Wang L, Bunker CH, et al: Lower urinary tract injury in women in the United States, 1979–2006. Am J Obstet Gynecol 202(5):495e1, 2010

Fuchshuber P, Schwaitzberg S, Jones D, et al: The SAGES Fundamental Use of Surgical Energy program (FUSE): history, development, and purpose. Surg Endosc 32(6):2583, 2018

Gallup DC, Gallup DG, Nolan TE, et al: Use of a subcutaneous closed drainage system and antibiotics in obese gynecologic patients. Am J Obstet Gynecol 175:358, 1996

Gasanova I, Alexander J, Ogunnaike B, et al: Transversus abdominis plane block versus surgical site infiltration for pain management after open total abdominal hysterectomy. Anesth Analg 121(5):1383, 2015

Geiger D, Debus ES, Ziegler UE, et al: Capillary activity of surgical sutures and suture-dependent bacterial transport: a qualitative study. Surg Infect 6(4):377, 2005

Giacalone PL, Daures JP, Vignal J, et al: Pfannenstiel versus Maylard incision for cesarean delivery: a randomized controlled trial. Obstet Gynecol 99(5 Pt 1):745, 2002

Gilmour DT, Das S, Flowerdew G: Rates of urinary tract injury from gynecologic surgery and the role of intraoperative cystoscopy. Obstet Gynecol 107(6):1366, 2006

Gilstrap LC III, Cunningham FG, Hoffman BL: Management of postpartum hemorrhage. In Yeomans ER, Hoffman BL, Gilstrap LC III, et al (eds): Cunningham and Gilstrap's Operative Obstetrics, 3rd ed. New York, McGraw-Hill Education, 2017, p 477

Glaser LM, Milad MP: Bowel and bladder injury repair and follow-up after gynecologic surgery. Obstet Gynecol 133(2):313, 2019

Glenner RJ: An improved vaginal hysterectomy clamp. Am J Obstet Gynecol 74(5):1016, 1956

Goldman JA, Feldberg D, Dicker D, et al: Femoral neuropathy subsequent to abdominal hysterectomy. A comparative study. Eur J Obstet Gynecol Reprod Biol 20(6):385, 1985

Goodnough LT: Autologous blood donation. Anesthesiol Clin North Am 23(2):263, 2005

Gorgas D: Transfusion therapy: blood and blood products. In Roberts J, Hedges J, Chanmugam AS, et al (eds): Clinical Procedures in Emergency Medicine. Philadelphia, Saunders, 2004

Gostout BS, Cliby WA, Podratz KC: Prevention and management of acute intraoperative bleeding. Clin Obstet Gynecol 45(2):481, 2002

Grantcharov TP, Rosenberg J: Vertical compared with transverse incisions in abdominal surgery. Eur J Surg 167(4):260, 2001

Greenall MJ, Evans M, Pollock AV: Midline or transverse laparotomy? A random controlled clinical trial. Part I: influence on healing. Br J Surg 67(3):188, 1980

Greenberg CC, Regenbogen SE, Studdert DM, et al: Patterns of communication breakdowns resulting in injury to surgical patients. J Am Coll Surg 204:533, 2007

Grimes CL, Patankar S, Ryntz T, et al: Evaluating ureteral patency in the post-indigo carmine ear: a randomized controlled trial. Am J Obstet Gynecol 217:601.e1, 2017

Gunderson PE: The half-hitch knot: a rational alternative to the square knot. Am J Surg 54:538, 1987

Gupta JK, Dinas K, Khan KS: To peritonealize or not to peritonealize? A randomized trial at abdominal hysterectomy. Am J Obstet Gynecol 178(4):796, 1998

Guvenal T, Duran B, Kemirkoprulu N, et al: Prevention of superficial wound disruption in Pfannenstiel incisions by using a subcutaneous drain. Int J Gynecol Obstet 77:151, 2002

Gyr T, Ghezzi F, Arslanagic S, et al: Minimal invasive laparoscopic hysterectomy with ultrasonic scalpel. Am J Surg 181(6):516, 2001

Hambley R, Hebda PA, Abell E, et al: Wound healing of skin incisions produced by ultrasonically vibrating knife, scalpel, electrosurgery, and carbon dioxide laser. J Dermatol Surg Oncol 14(11):1213, 1988

Hamilton MA, Cecconi M, Rhodes A: A systematic review and meta-analysis on the use of preemptive hemodynamic intervention to improve postoperative outcomes in moderate and high-risk surgical patients. Anesth Analg 112(6):1392, 2011

Harold KL, Pollinger H, Matthews BD, et al: Comparison of ultrasonic energy, bipolar thermal energy, and vascular clips for the hemostasis of small-, medium-, and large-sized arteries. Surg Endosc 17(8):1228, 2003

Harris WJ: Complications of hysterectomy. Clin Obstet Gynecol 40(4):928, 1997

Harvey AR, Basavaraju SV, Chung KW, et al: Transfusion-related adverse reactions reported to the National Healthcare Safety Network Hemovigilance Module, United States, 2010 to 2012. Transfusion 55(4):709, 2015

Haynes AB, Weiser TG, Berry WR, et al: A surgical safety checklist to reduce morbidity and mortality in a global population. N Engl J Med 360(5):491, 2009

Healey MA, Davis RE, Liu FC, et al: Lactated Ringer's is superior to normal saline in a model of massive hemorrhage and resuscitation. J Trauma 45(5):894, 1998

Heniford BT, Matthews BD, Sing RF, et al: Initial results with an electrothermal bipolar vessel sealer. Surg Endosc 15(8):799, 2001

Henry DA, Carless PA, Moxey AJ, et al: Pre-operative autologous donation for minimising perioperative allogeneic blood transfusion. Cochrane Database Syst Rev 2:CD003602, 2002

Hindocha A, Beere L, Dias S, et al: Adhesion prevention agents for gynaecological surgery: an overview of Cochrane reviews. Cochrane Database Syst Rev 1:CD011254, 2015

Hoffman MS, Lynch C, Lockhart J, et al: Injury of the rectum during vaginal surgery. Am J Obstet Gynecol 181:274, 1999

Hong JY, Kim J: Use of paracervical analgesia for outpatient hysteroscopic surgery: a randomized, double-blind, placebo-controlled study. Amb Surg 12(4):181, 2006

Hunt BJ: The current place of tranexamic acid in the management of bleeding. Anaesthesia 70(1 Suppl):50, 2015

Hurt J, Unger JB, Ivy JJ, et al: Tying a loop-to-strand suture: is it safe? Am J Obstet Gynecol 192:1094, 2005

Ibeanu OA, Chesson RR, Echols KT, et al: Urinary tract injury during hysterectomy based on universal cystoscopy. Obstet Gynecol 113:6, 2009

Irvin W, Andersen W, Taylor P, et al: Minimizing the risk of neurologic injury in gynecologic surgery. Obstet Gynecol 103(2):374, 2004

Ivy JJ, Unger JB, Hurt J, et al: The effect of number of throws on knot security with non-identical sliding knots. Am J Obstet Gynecol 191:1618, 2004a

Ivy JJ, Unger JB, Mukherjee D: Knot integrity with nonidentical and parallel sliding knots. Am J Obstet Gynecol 190:83, 2004b

Iyer C, Robertson B, Lenkovsky F, et al. Gastric bypass and on-Q pump: effectiveness of soaker catheter system on recovery of bariatric surgery patients. Surg Obes Relat Dis 6(2):181, 2010

Jackson LA, Ramirez DM, Carrick KS, et al: Gross and histologic anatomy of the pelvic ureter: clinical applications to pelvic surgery. Obstet Gynecol 133(5):896, 2019

Jallo GI: CUSA EXcel ultrasonic aspiration system. Neurosurgery 48(3):695, 2001

Jenkins TR: It's time to challenge surgical dogma with evidence-based data. Am J Obstet Gynecol 189(2):423, 2003

Jones PM, Cherry RA, Allen BN, et al: Association between handover of anesthesia care and adverse postoperative outcomes among patients undergoing major surgery. JAMA 319(2):143, 2018

Joshi G: Intraoperative fluid restriction improves outcome after major elective gastrointestinal surgery. Anesth Analg 101:601, 2005

Kanter MH, van Maanen D, Anders KH, et al: A study of an educational intervention to decrease inappropriate preoperative autologous blood donation: its effectiveness and the effect on subsequent transfusion rates in elective hysterectomy. Transfusion 39(8):801, 1999

Kanter MH, van Maanen D, Anders KH, et al: Preoperative autologous blood donations before elective hysterectomy. JAMA 276(10):798, 1996

Karger R, Kretschmer V: Modern concepts of autologous haemotherapy. Transfus Apher Sci 32(2):185, 2005

Katz KH, Desciak EB, Maloney ME: The optimal application of surgical adhesive tape strips. Dermatol Surg 25(9):686, 1999

Kauko M: New techniques using the ultrasonic scalpel in laparoscopic hysterectomy. Curr Opin Obstet Gynecol 10(4):303, 1998

Kisielinski K, Conze J, Murken AH, et al: The Pfannenstiel or so called "bikini cut": still effective more than 100 years after first description. Hernia 8(3):177, 2004

Knockaert DC, Boonen AL, Bruyninckx FL, et al: Electromyographic findings in ilioinguinal-iliohypogastric nerve entrapment syndrome. Acta Clin Belg 51(3):156, 1996

Kolle D, Tamussino K, Hanzal E, et al: Bleeding complications with the tension-free vaginal tape operation. Am J Obstet Gynecol 193(6):2045, 2005

Krebs HB: Intestinal injury in gynecologic surgery: a ten-year experience. Am J Obstet Gynecol 155(3):509, 1986

Kuroki LM, Mullen MM, Massad LS, et al: Wound complication rates after staples or suture for midline vertical skin closure in obese women: a randomized controlled trial. Obstet Gynecol 130(1):91, 2017

Kushner DM, LaGalbo R, Connor JP, et al: Use of a bupivacaine continuous wound infusion system in gynecologic oncology: a randomized trial. Obstet Gynecol 106(2):227, 2005

Kuuva N, Nilsson CG: A nationwide analysis of complications associated with the tension-free vaginal tape (TVT) procedure. Acta Obstet Gynecol Scand 81(1):72, 2002

Kvist-Poulsen H, Borel J: Iatrogenic femoral neuropathy subsequent to abdominal hysterectomy: incidence and prevention. Obstet Gynecol 60(4):516, 1982

Lacy PD, Burke PE, O'Regan M, et al: The comparison of type of incision for transperitoneal abdominal aortic surgery based on postoperative respiratory complications and morbidity. Eur J Vasc Surg 8(1):52, 1994

Lammers R, Trott A: Methods of wound closure. In Roberts J, Hedges J (eds): Clinical Procedures in Emergency Medicine. Philadelphia, Saunders, 2004, p 655

Lau WC, Lo WK, Tam WH, et al: Paracervical anaesthesia in outpatient hysteroscopy: a randomised double-blind placebo-controlled trial. BJOG 106(4):356, 1999

Leaper DJ, Pollock AV, Evans M: Abdominal wound closure: a trial of nylon, polyglycolic acid and steel sutures. Br J Surg 64(8):603, 1977

Lee ET, Wong FW: Small bowel obstruction from barbed suture following laparoscopic myomectomy-a case report. Int J Surg Case Rep 16:146, 2015

Lichtenberg ES, Paul M, Jones H: First trimester surgical abortion practices: a survey of National Abortion Federation members. Contraception 64(6):345, 2001

Lipscomb GH, Ling FW, Stovall TG, et al: Peritoneal closure at vaginal hysterectomy: a reassessment. Obstet Gynecol 87(1):40, 1996

Llarena NC, Shah AB, Milad MP: Bowel injury in gynecologic laparoscopy. Obstet Gynecol 125(6):1407, 2015

Lo IK, Burkhart SS, Chan KC, et al: Arthroscopic knots: determining the optimal balance of loop security and knot security. Arthroscopy 20:489, 2004

Long JB, Elland RJ, Hentz JG, et al: Randomized trial of preemptive local analgesia in vaginal surgery. Int Urogynecol J Pelvic Floor Dysfunct 20(1):5, 2009

López CC, Ríos JF, González Y, et al: Barbed suture versus conventional suture for vaginal cuff closure in total laparoscopic hysterectomy: randomized controlled clinical trial. J Minim Invasive Gynecol 26(6):1104, 2019

Luijendijk RW, Jeekel J, Storm RK, et al: The low transverse Pfannenstiel incision and the prevalence of incisional hernia and nerve entrapment. Ann Surg 225(4):365, 1997

Madjdpour C, Spahn DR, Weiskopf RB: Anemia and perioperative red blood cell transfusion: a matter of tolerance. Crit Care Med 34(5 Suppl):S102, 2006

Makinen J, Johansson J, Tomas C, et al: Morbidity of 10110 hysterectomies by type of approach. Hum Reprod 16(7):1473, 2001

Masterson B: Intraoperative hemorrhage. In Nichols D, DeLancey J (eds): Clinical Problems, Injuries and Complications of Gynecologic and Obstetric Surgery. Baltimore, Williams & Wilkins, 1995, p 14

Mathevet P, Valencia P, Cousin C, et al: Operative injuries during vaginal hysterectomy. Eur J Obstet Gynecol Reprod Biol 97:71, 2001

Maxwell DJ (ed): Surgical Techniques in Obstetrics and Gynecology. London, Churchill-Livingstone, 2004

McDaniel LM, Etchill EW, Raval JS, et al: State of the art: massive transfusion. Transfus Med 24(3):138, 2014

Michelassi F, Hurst R: Electrocautery, argon beam coagulation, cryotherapy, and other hemostatic and tissue ablative instruments. In Nyhus L, Baker R, Fischer J (eds): Mastery of Surgery. Boston, Little, Brown, and Company, 1997, p 234

Molina G, Jiang W, Edmondson L, et al: Implementation of the surgical safety checklist in South Carolina hospitals is associated with improvement in perceived perioperative safety. J Am Coll Surg 222(5):725, 2016

Moore FA, McKinley BA, Moore EE: The next generation in shock resuscitation. Lancet 363(9425):1988, 2004

Morris ML: Electrosurgery in the gastroenterology suite: principles, practice, and safety. Gastroenterol Nurs 29(2):126, 2006

Murovic JA, Kim DH, Tiel RL, et al: Surgical management of 10 genitofemoral neuralgias at the Louisiana State University Health Sciences Center. Neurosurgery 56(2):298, 2005

Murphy MF, Wallington TB, Kelsey P, et al: Guidelines for the clinical use of red cell transfusions. Br J Haematol 113(1):24, 2001

Nagpal K, Vats A, Ahmed K, et al: A systematic quantitative assessment of risks associated with poor communication in surgical care. Arch Surg 145(6):582, 2010

Naguib M, Magboul MM, Samarkandi AH, et al: Adverse effects and drug interactions associated with local and regional anaesthesia. Drug Safety 18(4):221, 1998

Naramsihlu DM, Prabakar C, Tang N, et al: Use of 50% dextrose as the distension medium during cystoscopy for visualization of ureteral jets. Obstet Gynecol 127(1):78, 2016

Naumann RW, Hauth JC, Owen J, et al: Subcutaneous tissue approximation in relation to wound disruption after cesarean delivery in obese women. Obstet Gynecol 85:412, 1995

Neuman M, Eidelman A, Langer R, et al: Iatrogenic injuries to the ureter during gynecologic and obstetric operations. Surg Gynecol Obstet 173(4):268, 1991

Newton M: Intraoperative complications. In Newton M, Newton E (eds): Complications of Gynecologic and Obstetric Management. Philadelphia, Saunders, 1988, p 36

Nizard J, Barringue L, Frydman R, et al: Fertility and pregnancy outcomes following hypogastric artery ligation for severe post-partum haemorrhage. Hum Reprod 18(4):844, 2003

Nygaard IE, Squatrito RC: Abdominal incisions from creation to closure. Obstet Gynecol Surv 51(7):429, 1996

Oderich GS, Panneton JM, Hofer J, et al: Iatrogenic operative injuries of abdominal and pelvic veins: a potentially lethal complication. J Vasc Surg 39(5):931, 2004

O'Neal MG, Beste T, Shackelford DP: Utility of preemptive local analgesia in vaginal hysterectomy. Am J Obstet Gynecol 189(6):1539, 2003

Orr JW Jr, Orr PF, Barrett JM, et al: Continuous or interrupted fascial closure: a prospective evaluation of No. 1 Maxon suture in 402 gynecologic procedures. Am J Obstet Gynecol 163(5 Pt 1):1485, 1990

Patel H, Bhatia N: Universal cystoscopy for timely detection of urinary tract injuries during pelvic surgery. Curr Opin Obstet Gynecol 21(5):415, 2009

Penfield JA: Gynecologic Surgery under Local Anesthesia. Baltimore, Urban and Schwarzenberg, 1986, p 48

Perel P, Roberts I, Ker K: Colloids versus crystalloids for fluid resuscitation in critically ill patients. Cochrane Database Syst Rev 2:CD000567, 2013

Philosophe R: Avoiding complications of laparoscopic surgery. Fertil Steril 80(Suppl 4):30, 2003

Pinski SL, Trohman RG: Interference in implanted cardiac devices, part II. Pacing Clin Electrophysiol 25(10):1496, 2002

Popert R: Techniques from the urologists. In Maxwell DJ (ed): Surgical Techniques in Obstetrics and Gynaecology. Edinburgh, Churchill Livingstone, 2004, pp 189, 195

Preston JM: Iatrogenic ureteric injury: common medicolegal pitfalls. BJU Int 86(3):313, 2000

Propst K, Tunitsky-Bitton E, O'Sullivan DM, et al: Phenazopyridine for evaluation of ureteral patency: a randomized controlled trial. Obstet Gynecol 128(2):348, 2016

Putnam LR, Anderson KT, Diffley MB, et al: Meaningful use and good catches: more appropriate metrics for checklist effectiveness. Surgery 160(6):1675, 2016

Quinn J, Wells G, Sutcliffe T, et al: A randomized trial comparing octylcyanoacrylate tissue adhesive and sutures in the management of lacerations. JAMA 277(19):1527, 1997

Rahn DD, Phelan JN, Roshanravan SM, et al: Anterior abdominal wall nerve and vessel anatomy: clinical implications for gynecologic surgery. Am J Obstet Gynecol 202(3):234.e1, 2010

Reinders I, Geomini P, Timmermans A, et al: Local anaesthesia during endometrial ablation: a systematic review. BJOG 124(2):190, 2017

Robinson JB, Sun CC, Bodurka-Bevers D, et al: Cavitational ultrasonic surgical aspiration for the treatment of vaginal intraepithelial neoplasia. Gynecol Oncol 78(2):235, 2000

Rodeheaver GT, Halverson JM, Edlich RF: Mechanical performance of wound closure tapes. Ann Emerg Med 12(4):203, 1983

Rogers R Jr: Basic pelvic neuroanatomy. In Steege J, Metzger D, Levy B (eds): Chronic Pelvic Pain: an Integrated Approach. Philadelphia, Saunders, 1998, p 31

Sakata S, Kabir S, Petersen D, et al: Are we burying our heads in the sand? Preventing small bowel obstruction from the V-loc® suture in laparoscopic ventral rectopexy. Colorectal Dis 17(9):O180, 2015

Sakellariou P, Protopapas AG, Voulgaris Z, et al: Management of ureteric injuries during gynecological operations: 10 years experience. Eur J Obstet Gynecol Reprod Biol 101(2):179, 2002

Sandadi S, Johannigman JA, Wong VL, et al: Recognition and management of major vessel injury during laparoscopy. J Minim Invasive Gynecol 17(6):692, 2010

Sandberg EM, Cohen SL, Hurwitz S, et al: Utility of cystoscopy during hysterectomy. Obstet Gynecol 120(6):1361, 2012

Santoso JT, Dinh TA, Omar S, et al: Surgical blood loss in abdominal hysterectomy. Gynecol Oncol 82(2):364, 2001

Schubert DC, Unger JB, Mukherjee D, et al: Mechanical performance of knots using braided and monofilament absorbable sutures. Am J Obstet Gynecol 187:1438, 2002

Schwartz D, Kaplan K, Schwartz S: Hemostasis, surgical bleeding, and transfusion. In Brunicardi F, Anersen D, Billiar T, et al (eds): Schwartz's Principles of Surgery. New York, McGraw-Hill, 2006

Sharp WV, Belden TA, King PH, et al: Suture resistance to infection. Surg 91(1):61, 1982

Shepherd JH, Cavanagh D, Riggs D, et al: Abdominal wound closure using a nonabsorbable single-layer technique. Obstet Gynecol 61(2):248, 1983

Shveiky D, Aseff JN, Iglesia CB: Brachial plexus injury after laparoscopic and robotic surgery. J Minim Invasive Gynecol 17(4):414, 2010

Silliman CC, Ambruso DR, Boshkov LK: Transfusion-related acute lung injury. Blood 105(6):2266, 2005

Singer AJ, Hollander JE, Quinn JV: Evaluation and management of traumatic lacerations. N Engl J Med 337(16):1142, 1997

Singer AJ, Quinn JV, Clark RE, et al: Closure of lacerations and incisions with octylcyanoacrylate: a multicenter randomized controlled trial. Surgery 131(3):270, 2002a

Singer AJ, Quinn JV, Thode HC Jr, et al: Determinants of poor outcome after laceration and surgical incision repair. Plast Reconst Surg 110(2):429, 2002b

Singh S, Maxwell D: Tools of the trade. Best Pract Res Clin Obstet Gynaecol 20(1):41, 2006

Sinha UK, Gallagher LA: Effects of steel scalpel, ultrasonic scalpel, CO_2 laser, and monopolar and bipolar electrosurgery on wound healing in guinea pig oral mucosa. Laryngoscope 113(2):228, 2003

Soper DE, Bump RC, Hurt WG: Wound infection after abdominal hysterectomy: effect of the depth of subcutaneous tissue. Am J Obstet Gynecol 173(2):465, 1971

Sperry JL, Guyette FX, Brown JB, et al: Prehospital plasma during air medical transport in trauma patients at risk for hemorrhagic shock. N Engl J Med 379(4):315, 2018

Stanhope CR, Wilson FO, Utz WJ, et al: Suture entrapment and secondary ureteral obstruction. Am J Obstet Gynecol 164(6 pt 1):1513, 1991

Stanton SL: Intestinal injury and how to cope. In Principles of Gynaecological Surgery, Berlin, Springer, 1987, p 159

Swanson K, Dwyre DM, Krochmal J, et al: Transfusion-related acute lung injury (TRALI): current clinical and pathophysiologic considerations. Lung 184(3):177, 2006

Teeluckdharry B, Gilmour D, Flowerdew G: Urinary tract injury at benign gynecologic surgery and the role of cystoscopy. Obstet Gynecol 126(6):1161, 2015

The Joint Commission: Universal protocol for preventing wrong site, wrong procedure, and wrong person surgery. In 2019 National Patient Safety Goals. Oakbrook Terrace, Joint Commission, 2018

Thubert T, Pourcher G, Deffieux X: Small bowel volvulus following peritoneal closure using absorbable knotless device during laparoscopic sacral colpopexy. Int Urogynecol J 22(6):761, 2011

Tomacruz RS, Bristow RE, Montz FJ: Management of pelvic hemorrhage. Surg Clin North Am 81(4):925, 2001

Toy P, Popovsky MA, Abraham E, et al: Transfusion-related acute lung injury: definition and review. Crit Care Med 33(4):721, 2005

Trimbos JB: Security of various knots commonly used in surgical practice. Obstet Gynecol 64:274, 1984

Trimbos JB, van Rijssel EJC, Klopper PJ: Performance of sliding knots in monofilament and multifilament suture material. Obstet Gynecol 68:425, 1986

Trolice MP, Fishburne C Jr, McGrady S: Anesthetic efficacy of intrauterine lidocaine for endometrial biopsy: a randomized double-masked trial. Obstet Gynecol 95(3):345, 2000

Tulandi T, Hum HS, Gelfand MM: Closure of laparotomy incisions with or without peritoneal suturing and second-look laparoscopy. Am J Obstet Gynecol 158(3 Pt 1):536, 1988

Urbach DR, Govindarajan A, Saskin R, et al: Introduction of surgical safety checklists in Ontario, Canada. N Engl J Med 370(11):1029, 2014

Utrie JW: Bladder and ureteral injury: prevention and management. Clin Obstet Gynecol 41(3):755, 1998

Vakili B, Chesson RR, Kyle BL, et al: The incidence of urinary tract injury during hysterectomy: a prospective analysis based on universal cystoscopy. Am J Obstet Gynecol 192(5):1599, 2005

van Dam PA, Tjalma W, Weyler J, et al: Ultraradical debulking of epithelial ovarian cancer with the ultrasonic surgical aspirator: a prospective randomized trial. Am J Obstet Gynecol 174(3):943, 1996

van Rijssel EJC, Trimbos JB, Booster MH: Mechanical performance of square knots and sliding knots in surgery: a comparative study. Am J Obstet Gynecol 162:93, 1990

Vermillion ST, Lamoutte C, Soper DE, et al: Wound infection after cesarean: effect of subcutaneous tissue thickness. Obstet Gynecol 95(6 Pt 1):923, 2000

Visco AG, Taber KH, Weidner AC, et al: Cost-effectiveness of universal cystoscopy to identify ureteral injury at hysterectomy. Obstet Gynecol 97(5 Pt 1):685, 2001

Wallis CJD, Cheung DC, Garbens A, et al: Occurrence of and risk factors for urological intervention during benign hysterectomy: analysis of the national surgical quality improvement program database. Urology 97:66, 2016

Walter AJ, Magtibay PM, Morse AN, et al: Perioperative changes in serum creatinine after gynecologic surgery. Am J Obstet Gynecol 186:1315, 2002

Walters MD, Karram MM (eds): Urogynecology and Reconstructive Pelvic Surgery, 3rd ed. Philadelphia, Mosby, 2007

Wang CJ, Yen CF, Lee CL, et al: Comparison of the efficacy of laparosonic coagulating shears and electrosurgery in laparoscopically assisted vaginal hysterectomy: preliminary results. Int Surg 85(1):88, 2000

Warner MA: Perioperative neuropathies. Mayo Clin Proc 73(6):567, 1998

Warner MA, Warner DO, Harper CM, et al: Lower extremity neuropathies associated with lithotomy positions. Anesthesiology 93(4):938, 2000

Waters JH: Indications and contraindications of cell salvage. Transfusion 44(12 Suppl):40S, 2004

Waters JH: Red blood cell recovery and reinfusion. Anesthesiol Clin North Am 23(2):283, 2005

Winfree CJ: Peripheral nerve injury evaluation and management. Curr Surg 62(5):469, 2005

Wissing J, van Vroonhoven TJ, Schattenkerk ME, et al: Fascia closure after midline laparotomy: results of a randomized trial. Br J Surg 74(8):738, 1987

Wong JMK, Bortoletto P, Tolentino J, et al: Urinary tract injury in gynecologic laparoscopy for benign indication. Obstet Gynecol 131(1):100, 2018

World Health Organization: WHO Surgical Safety Checklist. 2009. Available at: https://www.who.int/patientsafety/safesurgery/checklist/en/. Accessed January 30, 2019

Yuzpe AA: Pneumoperitoneum needle and trocar injuries in laparoscopy. A survey on possible contributing factors and prevention. J Reprod Med 35(5):485, 1990

Zimmer CA, Thacker JG, Powell DM, et al: Influence of knot configuration and tying technique on the mechanical performance of sutures. J Emerg Med 9:107, 1991

CHAPTER 41

Minimally Invasive Surgery Fundamentals

Minimally invasive surgery (MIS) is characteristically performed through a small incision or no incision, and visualization is provided by endoscopes. Both laparoscopy and hysteroscopy are considered in this category. With laparoscopy, small abdominal incisions provide access to introduce an endoscope and surgical instruments into the abdomen. To increase operative space, a pneumoperitoneum is created. As such, laparoscopy provides a minimally invasive option for women undergoing intraabdominal gynecologic surgery. And, with its technology improvements, almost all major intraabdominal gynecologic procedures can now be performed with MIS.

Hysteroscopy uses an endoscope and uterine cavity distention medium to provide an internal view of the endometrial cavity. This tool permits both the diagnosis and operative treatment of intrauterine pathology.

FACTORS IN CHOOSING LAPAROSCOPY

In theory, laparoscopic surgery differs from laparotomy only by its mode of access to the operative field. However, inherent qualities can make some surgical steps more difficult. These include indirect palpation of tissue, counterintuitive motion, a finite number of ports for abdominal access, restricted movement, and replacement of normal 3-dimensional (3-D) vision by 2-dimensional (2-D) video images. Development of robotic platforms addressed some of these traditional limitations of laparoscopy. In appropriately selected patients, the trade-off is a faster recovery, improved cosmesis, less postoperative pain, diminished adhesion formation, and at least equivalent surgical results (Aarts, 2015; Ellström, 1998; Falcone, 1999; Lundorff, 1991; Mais, 1996). The decision to perform laparoscopy is based on several parameters described next.

■ Patient Factors

Laparoscopy using a pneumoperitoneum is contraindicated in very few clinical conditions, but these include acute glaucoma, retinal detachment, increased intracranial pressure, and some types of ventriculoperitoneal shunts. Thus, laparoscopy is appropriate for many, although modifications are warranted for certain clinical situations.

Prior Surgeries

With laparoscopy, adhesive disease increases the risk of visceral and vascular injury during abdominal entry. Adhesions are also associated with higher conversion rates to laparotomy because long and tedious adhesiolysis may be completed by some surgeons more quickly with open surgical dissection. Thus, during preoperative physical examination, a surgeon notes the location of previous surgical scars and ascertains the risk of possible intraabdominal adhesions (Table 41-1). Similarly, a history of endometriosis, pelvic inflammatory disease, or radiation treatment may predispose to adhesions. In addition, abdominal wall hernias or hernia repairs and any reparative mesh are identified and avoided during trocar insertion. If abnormal findings are found, plans for an alternative entry site are considered (p. 892).

Laparoscopic Physiology

Compared with traditional open laparotomy, laparoscopy produces several distinct cardiovascular and pulmonary physiologic changes. These result mainly from: (1) absorption across the peritoneum and into circulation of carbon dioxide (CO_2) used for insufflation, (2) elevated intraabdominal pressure created by the pneumoperitoneum, and (3) head-down Trendelenburg positioning. These changes are typically tolerated by those with general good health but may not be by those with cardiovascular or pulmonary compromise. Thus, surgeons should be familiar with these physiologic alterations.

During laparoscopy, CO_2 absorption from the pneumoperitoneum across the peritoneum can lead to systemic CO_2 accumulation and hypercarbia. In turn, hypercarbia produces sympathetic stimulation that raises systemic and pulmonary vascular resistance and elevates blood pressure. If hypercarbia

TABLE 41-1. Frequency of Umbilical Adhesions Found at Laparoscopy in Women with and without Prior Abdominal Surgery

	Sample Size/ Prior Surgery	No Prior Surgery	Prior Laparoscopy	Prior Low Transverse Incision	Prior Vertical Midline Incision (VML)
Agarwala (2005)	918/ surgery	—	16%	22%	62%
Brill (1995)	360/ laparotomy	—	—	27%	55% with VML below umbilicus
					67% with VML above umbilicus
Audebert (2000)	814/laparoscopy	0.68%	1.6%	19.8%	51.7%
Sepilian (2007)	151/ laparoscopy	—	21%	—	—

is not cleared by compensatory ventilation, acidemia develops. From this, direct myocardial contractility depression and decreased cardiac output can follow (Ho, 1995; Reynolds, 2003; Sharma, 1996). Hypercarbia can also lead to tachycardia and arrhythmia. Less commonly, bradycardia can stem from vagal stimulation. This may follow pelvic organ manipulation, cervical stretching during uterine manipulator placement, or peritoneal stretching during pneumoperitoneum creation.

Insufflation of any gas elevates intraabdominal pressure. This raised pressure decreases flow in the inferior vena cava, causes blood pooling in the legs, and raises venous resistance. In sum, venous return to the heart is decreased, and thereby cardiac output is lowered. Increased intraabdominal pressure can also directly lower splanchnic blood flow.

Intraoperative pulmonary function may be challenged during laparoscopy. First, the diaphragm is displaced upward by intraabdominal pressure from the pneumoperitoneum. This can be accentuated by organs also being pushed cephalad against the diaphragm during Trendelenburg positioning. Moreover, insufflation pressures stiffen the diaphragm and chest wall. Together, these alterations lead to higher required airway pressures to achieve adequate mechanical ventilation. Also, as the diaphragm moves up, lung volume and functional residual capacity are diminished, which in turn reduces the reserve volume for oxygenation. Moreover, this lung volume decline favors a tendency for alveolar collapse, leading to atelectasis. This can create ventilation and perfusion mismatching and an increased alveolar-arterial oxygen gradient. In sum, all of these factors favor poorer oxygenation.

Urinary output commonly is diminished during laparoscopy. This may result from lowered cardiac output, decreased splanchnic blood flow, direct renal parenchymal compression, or release of renin, aldosterone, or antidiuretic hormone. Together, these lessen renal blood flow, reduce glomerular filtration rate, and diminish urine output. Importantly, renal function typically returns to normal following pneumoperitoneum decompression (Demyttenaere, 2007).

Health Conditions

Of these, severe cardiac and pulmonary disease, intestinal obstruction, hemoperitoneum with hemodynamic instability, and pregnancy are particularly relevant when considering laparoscopy. As just described, in those with severe cardiac or pulmonary disease, the physiologic changes during laparoscopy

may challenge cardiopulmonary reserves. In prevention, lowering intraabdominal pressures and flattening the degree of Trendelenburg may allow laparoscopic completion of a procedure.

For a clinically stable patient with hemoperitoneum, laparoscopy is not contraindicated. Thus, ruptured ectopic pregnancies or ruptured bleeding ovarian cyst may be treated via MIS. Although an unstable patient was previously considered a contraindication to laparoscopic surgery, many skilled surgeons feel they can safely and quickly enter the abdomen laparoscopically. That said, the lowered venous return and cardiac output must be factored into the decision to select laparoscopy for such patients.

Concurrent intestinal obstruction and its associated bowel distention may increase risks for bowel injury during abdominal entry. In these situations, open entry to gain initial abdominal access may be beneficial (p. 891). However, ischemic bowel may be poorly served by pneumoperitoneum-related diminished splanchnic blood flow.

Obesity

In the past, obesity had been considered a relative contraindication for gynecologic laparoscopy. First, adequate ventilation may be difficult. In general, obese patients display reduced lung compliance that is proportional to their body mass index (BMI). Moreover, abdominal wall adiposity lowers abdominal wall compliance, which in turn elevates the pneumoperitoneum pressure required for surgery. Also, fattier omentum and mesenteric fat add to the bulk forced against the diaphragm in Trendelenburg position. Other limitations include a thick subcutaneous layer that encumbers instrument motion. It can also hinder abdominal entry, and trocar tunneling is common. Just patient girth relative to surgeon arm length may limit instrument manipulation.

As possible fixes, placement of an extra ancillary port for adequate manipulation of omentum and bowel out of the operative field can be helpful. Coordination with the anesthesia team to find a comfortable degree of Trendelenburg for both successful operative manipulations and adequate ventilation is essential. Longer "bariatric" instruments can overcome many length limitations.

As a result, with a skilled surgeon, obese patients benefit generally from MIS. Healthy obese patients experience less pain, quicker recovery, and fewer postoperative complications such as wound infections and ileus after laparoscopy compared with laparotomy (Eltabbakh, 1999, 2000; Scribner, 2002). That said, certain operative parameters may be adversely affected in obese patients undergoing laparoscopy compared with normal-weight patients. Higher conversion rates to laparotomy, longer operating times, and longer hospitalizations have been noted (Chopin, 2009; Heinberg, 2004; Thomas, 2006). However, this has not been found by all investigators, and overall outcomes may be superior to an open approach (Camanni, 2010; O'Hanlan, 2003; Shah, 2015).

Pregnancy

Nonurgent conditions identified during pregnancy may often be addressed postpartum. However, laparoscopy can be performed during any trimester. Thus, familiarity with the superimposed physiologic changes of pregnancy can improve maternal and fetal safety (O'Rourke, 2006; Reynolds, 2003).

Perioperatively, left uterine displacement with a wedge for second- or third-trimester pregnancies can minimize the decreased venous return that results from pneumoperitoneum and from an enlarged uterus compressing pelvic veins and inferior vena cava. Also, rates of venous thromboembolism (VTE) are higher during pregnancy due to gestational hypercoagulability. Sequential compression stockings can help lower this risk.

Intraoperatively, steps involve avoiding placement of intracervical uterine manipulators, limiting insufflation pressures to 10 to 15 mm Hg, maintaining end-tidal CO_2 levels between 32 and 34 mm Hg, moving trocar placement appropriately cephalad to avoid puncture of the gravid uterus, and limiting uterine manipulation (Pearl, 2017). Of note, the routine use of perioperative prophylactic tocolytics is not recommended in these cases. However, pre- and postoperative fetal heart rate assessment and contraction monitoring for more advanced gestations are typically implemented.

PATIENT PREPARATION

Prophylaxis

Randomized clinical trials have demonstrated that prophylactic antibiotics significantly reduce postoperative infectious morbidity rates following abdominal or vaginal hysterectomy. During laparoscopic hysterectomy, the vagina is similarly opened. Thus, preoperative antibiotics listed in Table 39-8 (p. 832) are recommended and generally given prior to anesthesia induction. For other types of laparoscopic procedures, data do not support antibiotic prophylaxis for clean surgical cases, that is, those that do not enter the vagina, bowel, or urinary tract (Chap. 3, p. 78).

For thromboprophylaxis, the same principles used for other abdominal surgeries are currently recommended for laparoscopic cases until further data accrues (American College of Obstetricians and Gynecologists, 2018b). These are listed in Table 39-10 (p. 834). Specific to laparoscopy, pneumoperitoneum pressure may decrease venous return from the lower extremities (Caprini, 1994; Ido, 1995). Balanced against this is the rapid postoperative mobility achieved by most patients. Indeed, evidence suggests that MIS independently lowers the risk of VTE compared with laparotomy (Jorgensen, 2019).

Preoperative Bowel Preparation

Data supporting the benefits of routine mechanical bowel preparation are few, and it may cause preoperative discomfort (Arnold, 2015; Muzii, 2006). In many cases, enemas may suffice instead. Thus, plans for bowel preparation are individualized. If the risk of bowel injury and stool spillage is enhanced because of pelvic adhesions or advanced endometriosis, then bowel preparation may limit fecal contamination at the surgical site. Moreover, if proctosigmoidoscopy is planned, an appropriate bowel preparation allows adequate visualization.

Anesthesia Selection

Laparoscopy can be completed using general or regional anesthesia. In most cases, general anesthesia with endotracheal intubation is selected to provide: (1) adequate patient comfort, (2) controlled ventilation to correct hypercarbia, (3) muscle relaxation, (4) airway protection from regurgitation due to elevated intraabdominal pressures, and (5) orogastric tube placement. Evidence supporting the local anesthetic injection at port sites to diminish postoperative pain is mixed (Einarsson, 2004; Ghezzi, 2005; Tam, 2014).

Consent

Laparoscopy itself is usually associated with little associated morbidity. Of major complications, the most common is organ injury caused by puncture or by electrosurgical tools and is described next. If these occur or if surgery is hindered by bleeding or adhesions, conversion to laparotomy may be necessary. Overall, this risk of conversion is low, and logically, rates decline as surgeon experience accrues.

Minor complications of laparoscopy include port site infection or hematoma, subcutaneous emphysema from CO_2 infiltration, vulvar edema, and postoperative peritoneal irritation from retained intraabdominal CO_2. Irritation stems from conversion of CO_2 to carbonic acid, which can be a direct irritant.

Puncture Injuries

Because sharp tools are used during laparoscopic entry, vessels and abdominal organs may be punctured. Risk factors are intraabdominal adhesions, incomplete gastric emptying, full bladder, insufficient pneumoperitoneum, poor muscle relaxation, thin patient habitus, and inappropriate force of tool insertion. As discussed later, several authors advocate an open entry method as a means to lower puncture injury rates (Catarci, 2001; Hasson, 2000; Long, 2008).

Organ Injury

The organ most frequently injured during laparoscopy is bowel, and rates of 0.6 and 1.6 per 1000 cases are reported (Chapron, 1999; Harkki-Siren, 1997). Women with previous laparotomy have a higher incidence of abdominal adhesions and are at greatest risk for this complication (see Table 41-1).

Unfortunately, bowel injury sustained during laparoscopy is often missed intraoperatively. In one study, nearly 50 percent of both small and large bowel injuries were unrecognized for 24 hours or longer (Chandler, 2001). Typically, these patients present with fever, abdominal pain, nausea, and vomiting within 48 hours of surgery (Li, 1997).

In laparoscopic cases, decompression of the stomach with an orogastric tube prior to obtaining laparoscopic access can lower the stomach puncture risk. Moreover, in those with suspected abdominal adhesive disease, several preventative steps can help avoid bowel injury. These include: (1) an alternative site for primary trocar entry, for example in the left hypochondrium (Palmer point), rather than at the umbilicus; (2) introduction of a microlaparoscope to scout for adhesions; and (3) preoperative sonography using the visceral slide test to exclude bowel adhered to the anterior abdominal wall.

Bladder puncture is uncommon with laparoscopy. Bladder decompression prior to and during surgery and careful placement of secondary trocars under direct visualization will prevent many injuries. However, with increased rates of laparoscopic hysterectomy, rates of bladder and ureteral damage have concurrently risen. These occur at the same surgical steps associated with urinary tract injury during abdominal hysterectomy.

Vascular or Nerve Injury

Major vascular injury associated with laparoscopy is rare and typically results during primary trocar insertion. Puncture rates are cited as 0.09 to 5 per 1000 cases, and the terminal aorta, inferior vena cava, and iliac vessels, particularly the right common iliac artery, may be injured (Bergqvist, 1987; Catarci, 2001; Nordestgaard, 1995). Uncommonly, air embolism from gas insufflation following vessel puncture may occur.

Although rare, deaths have resulted from large vessel injury (Baadsgaard, 1989; Munro, 2002). Prevention may include use of the open entry technique or awareness of the angle and force of trocar entry. Despite these steps, if a large vessel is punctured, the wounding instrument is not removed because it may act as a vascular plug. Moreover, this tool is held stable to avoid extending the laceration. In most cases, laparotomy, direct manual pressure on the vessel, steps for hemodynamic resuscitation, and notification of a vascular surgeon should follow expeditiously.

In contrast, if the inferior epigastric artery is injured, several simple techniques can control hemorrhage. First, bipolar electrosurgical coagulation of the bleeding site may suffice. If unsuccessful, a 14F Foley catheter can be threaded through the cannula of the wounding trocar or through the defect created by this trocar. The Foley balloon then is inflated and pulled upward to create direct pressure against the posterior surface of the anterior abdominal wall. At the skin surface, a Kelly clamp is placed perpendicular across the Foley catheter and parallel to the skin to hold the balloon firmly in place. The balloon and catheter can be removed approximately 12 hours later. Alternatively, sutures can be placed that traverse the skin, abdominal wall, and peritoneum; arch under the bleeding vessel; and exit the abdomen to directly ligate the vessel (Fig. 41-1). Similarly, the Carter-Thomason tool can be used to ligate both ends of this vessel.

Nerve injury can follow in patients placed for extended periods in the dorsal lithotomy position with arms abducted. From this, injury to the common fibular (former common peroneal), femoral, lateral femoral cutaneous, obturator, sciatic, and ulnar

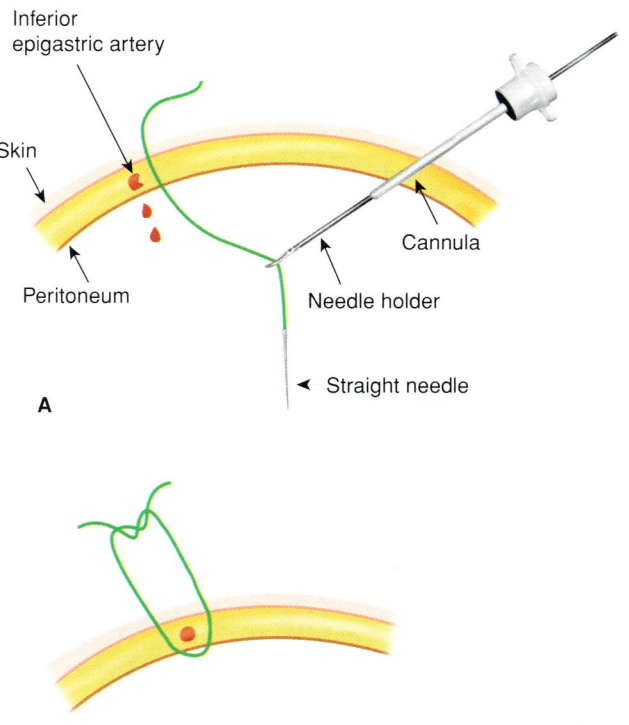

A

B

FIGURE 41-1 Ligation of lacerated inferior epigastric artery. **A.** Suture with an attached straight Keith needle is driven through the anterior abdominal wall lateral and caudal to the bleeding artery. This is performed using direct laparoscopic visualization to avoid organ injury. A laparoscopic needle driver regrasps the needle. **B.** The needle is then driven upward and through the anterior abdominal wall on the other side of the vessel. The suture loop is tied. This process is repeated cephalad to the bleeding vessel. This places sutures proximal and distal to the site of vessel laceration.

nerves and to the brachial plexus is possible (Barnett, 2007). Specific injuries and prevention are described in Chapter 40 (p. 842). Attention paid to patient position and surgery duration prevent many of these complications.

Thermal Injury

Accidental burns may follow direct instrument contact or stray electric current. Fortunately, the risk of this complication is low. Prevention steps include keeping instrument tips within the visual field when electric current is applied, strict instrument maintenance to identify insulation defects, employment of bipolar coagulation or harmonic energy for hemostasis when feasible, and use of lower-voltage (cutting) current whenever possible to reduce the applied voltage (Wu, 2000).

Incisional Hernia

Incisional hernias are a potential long-term consequence of laparoscopy, and approximately one fourth of hernias are umbilical (Lajer, 1997). Port sites hernias develop less frequently than incisional hernias after laparotomy (Schiavone, 2016). The incidence approximates 1 percent but may rise with greater use of larger trocars and single-port umbilical techniques (Clark, 2013). With the latter, hernia rates nearing 6 percent have been reported, and older age, obesity, and comorbid umbilical hernia are risk factors (Buckley, 2016).

A major risk for incisional hernia is use of large trocars measuring ≥10 mm in diameter or port sites from which larger specimens are extracted. Preventatively, smaller trocars are used when possible. Also, fascial closure is advocated at larger trocar wound sites and at port sites that may have been inadvertently extended by instrument torque or specimen extraction. The use of trocars with conical rather than pyramidal tips can lower this incidence (Leibl, 1999). Finally, peritoneal tissue is ideally not drawn into the superficial layers of the wound when removing the cannulas (Boughey, 2003; Montz, 1994).

Trocar-Site Metastasis

Rates of trocar-site cancer metastasis are low and complicate the clinical course of approximately 1 percent of patients in whom gynecologic malignancy is identified. Similarly, port-site seeding of other tissues such as endometriosis is possible. Metastases are more frequent with ovarian cancer than other malignancies, and higher rates are seen with more advanced disease (Abu-Rustum, 2004; Childers, 1994; Zivanovic, 2008). Although most trocar-site metastases are associated with advanced stages of disease, metastasis has followed surgery for tumors of low malignant potential. Suggested mechanisms include hematogenous spread or direct contamination, immune suppression, pneumoperitoneum, and surgical technique. As a result, steps of laparoscopy itself have been evaluated as a risk (Ramirez, 2004). Currently, no evidence-based consensus addresses prevention of this complication. Thus, the careful tissue extraction techniques described on page 894 are encouraged.

OPERATING ROOM ORGANIZATION

■ Operating Equipment

In laparoscopy, tool movement is limited compared with laparotomy, secondary to instrument angle restrictions and fixed ports (Berguer, 2001). Thus, room organization is essential, and equipment is positioned *before* the procedure begins. Also preoperatively, all instruments are checked and tested to confirm proper functioning.

Although equipment positioning may vary based on surgeon preference, the following is suggested to optimize efficiency and safety. The operating room table is centered in the room, and surgical lights lie directly above the operative field. Prior to surgery, the bed is checked to ensure it moves up and down and into steep Trendelenburg position. Obese patients may require a larger bariatric operating table.

Video monitors may be fixed to the ceiling with articulating arms or may be placed on portable stands. One monitor may suffice for simple procedures, however, two monitors provide easy viewing by the surgeon and assistant. When operating in the pelvis, the monitor is placed directly in front of the surgeon, and the

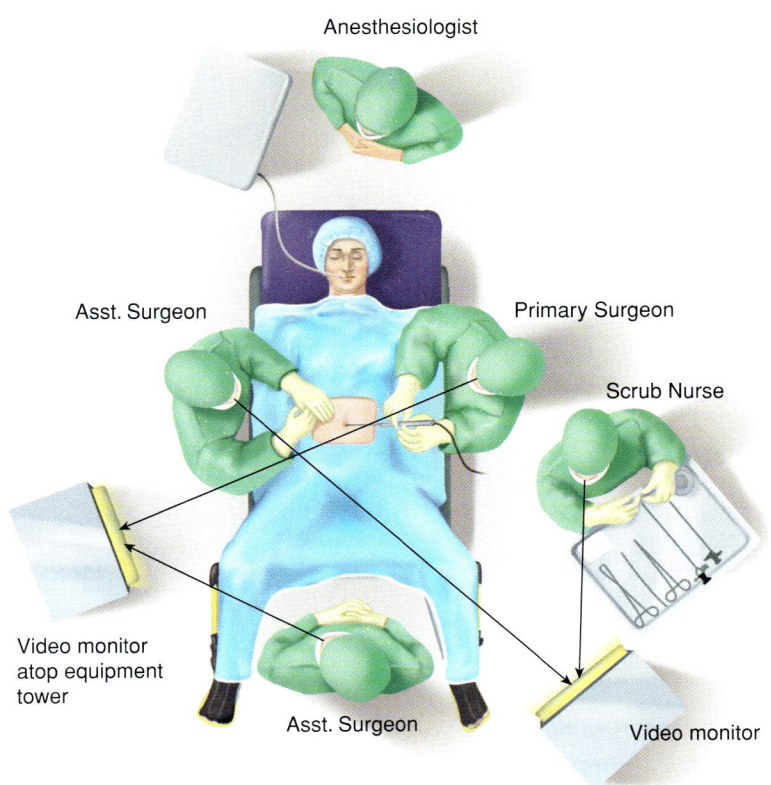

FIGURE 41-2 Operating room arrangement for laparoscopy.

surgeon, forearm-instrument axis, and video monitor are aligned in a straight line. Thus, placement of the video monitor for most gynecologic surgeries is near the patient's upper thigh (Fig. 41-2). For best surgeon ergonomics, monitor height is 10 to 20 degrees below eye level to prevent neck strain (van Det, 2009). Also, surgeons stand an appropriate distance and height relative to the operating table such that their arms are slightly abducted, their shoulders are inwardly rotated, and their elbows are extended from 90 to 120 degrees. This positioning can minimize surgeon fatigue. The scrub technician and Mayo stand generally are positioned on the side of the primary surgeon near the patient's leg. Here, instruments can be easily passed to both surgeons.

A dedicated cabinet or "tower" houses the laparoscopic light source, gas insufflator, and image capture equipment. The tower is positioned on the side opposite the primary surgeon such that he or she has an unobstructed view of equipment display panels. All insufflation tubing, camera, and light cords ideally exit the operating field from the same direction and connect to the equipment tower. Similarly, electrosurgical equipment and pedals are organized so that all these cords are aligned in one direction to reach a separate cart that houses these electrosurgical units. Pedals are oriented appropriately for the primary surgeon to comfortably reach without adjusting his body or moving his eyes from the monitor.

■ Patient Positioning

This is another essential component of safe laparoscopy. Following anesthesia induction, a patient is placed in low dorsal lithotomy position with the legs in booted support stirrups (see Fig. 41-2). To aid proper leg positioning, the stirrup brackets, which holster the stirrups, are attached to the table at the level of the patient hips. To prevent femoral nerve injury, the hips are positioned without sharp flexion or marked abduction or external hip rotation. The knees are not flexed more than 90 degrees and are positioned and padded to avoid common fibular (peroneal) nerve compression. To avert slipping when in steep Trendelenburg position and to minimize lower back pressure, a patient can be placed directly on an antiskid material such as egg-crate or gel pad. With these, patient skin directly contacts the padding for traction (Klauschie, 2010; Lamvu, 2004). If uterine manipulation is needed, the buttocks are placed slightly past the edge of the table.

Patient arms are tucked to the side in military position. This allows improved patient access and prevents upper extremity hyperextension, which can injure the brachial plexus. The arms may be tucked using an extended draw sheet, which is placed under the gel pad. This relationship limits arm slippage, which can generate pressure against the brachial plexus. Moreover, in obese patients, antiskid material and arm tucking can help prevent slippage when in Trendelenburg position (Klauschie, 2010). The arms are padded to avert compression of the ulnar and median nerves. Fingertips are facing the thighs, well-padded, and positioned away from the moving foot of the bed to prevent unintentional amputation. During arm positioning, finger oxygen monitors and intravenous access should not be dislodged.

Shoulder braces are padded brackets that are placed on the cephalic side of the operating room bed and arch around to the patient's acromion. Their goal is to brace the shoulder and prevent the head from slipping off the bed when in Trendelenburg position. If shoulder braces are required, we recommend tucking the arms in addition to using well-padded braces. However, due to the risk of nerve injury, the use of shoulder braces in general should be limited. Specifically, brachial plexus injury complicates 0.16 percent of gynecologic laparoscopic procedures. When shoulder braces are used, compression over the acromion may apply pressure that stretches the plexus. Moreover, lateral compression by braces may compress the humerus against the plexus. Both predispose to brachial plexus injury (Romanowski, 1993).

LAPAROSCOPIC INSTRUMENTS

■ Instrument Anatomy

Successful laparoscopic surgery relies on the use of appropriate surgical instruments, and many of these undergo frequent update. Most surgeons have designated preferences for certain types of graspers, dissectors, and cutting instruments.

The components of a laparoscopic instrument include the hand grip, shaft, jaw, and tip (Fig. 41-3). In general, an instrument tip's diameter is concordant with its shaft diameter, and standard sizes fit through 5-mm or 10-mm diameter cannulas. Additionally, 3-mm, 8-mm, and 15-mm instrument diameters are available for many tips. The tip defines instrument function. Jaws may be double

action or single action. With a single-action jaw, one tip is fixed, lies in the same axis as the shaft, and offers greater stability during the action performed. Double-action jaws have tips that move synchronously, and this jaw offers a wider angle in which to perform its function. Some jaws are now modified by a compression feature that allows scissor blades to secure the tissue first in the crux of the jaws and then cut tissue with greater stability and precision.

Important instrument qualities are comfort and ease of use, which stem primarily from the hand grip shape, the instrument length, and its locking capability. Most laparoscopic instruments have a standard 33-cm length. For bariatric MIS, longer instruments are now available for procedures in obese patients. Although permitting better access, these longer instruments are often more difficult to manipulate due to altered operating angles caused by the extended length.

In the hand grip, a locking feature allows a surgeon to hold tissue without maintaining constant pressure against the grip, and this decreases hand fatigue. The ability to rotate an instrument tip 360 degrees is now preferred. This versatility allows access to additional anatomic spaces and lessens the need for uncomfortable surgeon hand or arm rotation.

■ Disposable versus Reusable

Many laparoscopic instruments are available in both reusable and disposable forms, each having its own advantages. The main advantage to reusable instruments is lowered expense. Analyses demonstrate that disposable instruments add significant cost compared with reusable ones (Campbell, 2003; Morrison, 2004). The main advantage to disposable instruments is the consistent tool sharpness and avoidance of lost instrument parts. For example, dull scissors may lead to longer operating times and ineffectual surgical technique. Corson and associates (1989) showed that reusable trocars, although sharpened at regular intervals, still required twice the force for entry compared with disposable trocars. As a compromise, modified trocar systems combine the strength of these two features. Namely, the cannula is reusable, whereas a disposable inner trocar offers a consistently sharper tip.

■ Manipulators

Atraumatic Manipulators

During laparoscopic surgery, abdominopelvic organs may be elevated, retracted, or placed on tension (Fig. 41-4). Most current

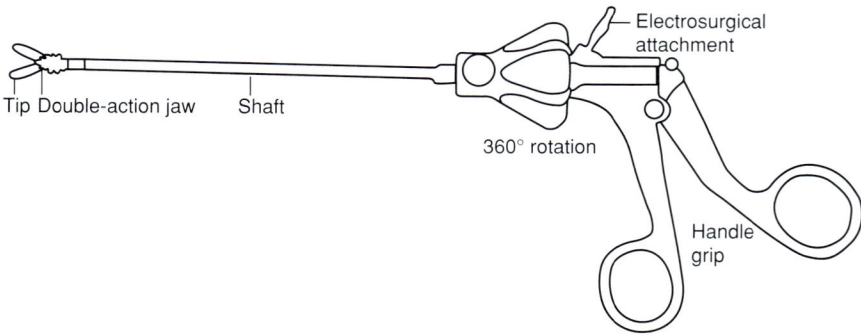

FIGURE 41-3 Parts of a typical laparoscopic instrument.

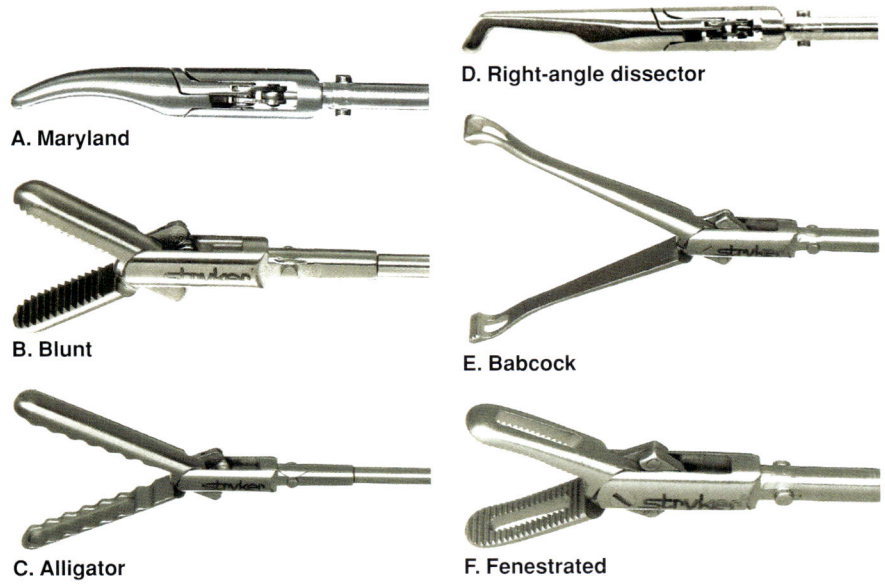

A. Maryland

B. Blunt

C. Alligator

D. Right-angle dissector

E. Babcock

F. Fenestrated

FIGURE 41-4 Laparoscopic atraumatic graspers. (Reproduced with permission from Stryker Endoscopy.)

However, its ability to retract tissues under tension is limited due to its atraumatic characteristics.

The Babcock clamp is another atraumatic tip that handles delicate tissues with minimal crushing. Its surgical role is similar to that in open techniques. However, as with the alligator clamp, its ability to retract or grasp during applied tension is poor due to slippage.

Ideally, all of these clamps are included in a general laparoscopic surgical tray for most laparoscopic procedures. Figure 41-4 shows additional tips with similar characteristics. As seen, some tips have window openings and are described as fenestrated. These are useful for tissue elevation or retraction or for passing sutures during vessel ligation.

Traumatic Graspers

Graspers with tips that are serrated or toothed are used in procedures that involve resection and tissue approximation (Fig. 41-5). Generally, such tissues are placed on tension, and a strong hold is required. In addition, a locking hand grip is typically preferred to keep grasped tissues secured. Most of these instruments have double-action jaws to allow a wide grasp around the tissue. In situations in which greater grip and tension strength is required, however, a tip with a single-action jaw and locking hand grip may be preferred.

Toothed graspers have teeth at their tip's end. These are superior for tissue manipulation but function poorly as graspers

instrument designs have incorporated safety considerations to minimize organ trauma yet allow effective manipulation. Of these, the blunt probe has an end that is modified to decrease the perforation risk to retracted tissues. It is used for exploration and retraction and is a preferred tool during diagnostic laparoscopy. Most blunt probes are stainless steel and are conductive of electric current. However, disposable probes constructed of nonconductive materials are available.

Graspers are divided into two main categories, atraumatic and those with toothed or serrated tips. Atraumatic graspers are used for exploration, gentle traction, and delicate tissue handling. The 5-mm diameter is a popular size, although 3-mm and 10-mm sizes are available. Most of these graspers have a double-action jaw, and the hand grip is typically nonlocking. Their gradually tapering curved tip permits the surgeon to define and separate tissue planes and is generally preferred for blunt dissection.

The Maryland clamp is an example of a curved blunt tip used for dissection and grasping. It compares to the Pean, hemostat, or munion, which are used in open surgery. Additionally, it can double as a needle driver if needed. Although technically considered atraumatic, this clamp may crush delicate tissues such as the fallopian tube or bowel.

The alligator clamp is a blunt grasper with a long, wide tip that handles delicate tissues with minimal crush-injury risk. It is useful for manipulating bowel, larger vessels, or reproductive organs or for exploration of vascular compartments that may be easily punctured or lacerated.

Traumatic graspers   **Scissors**

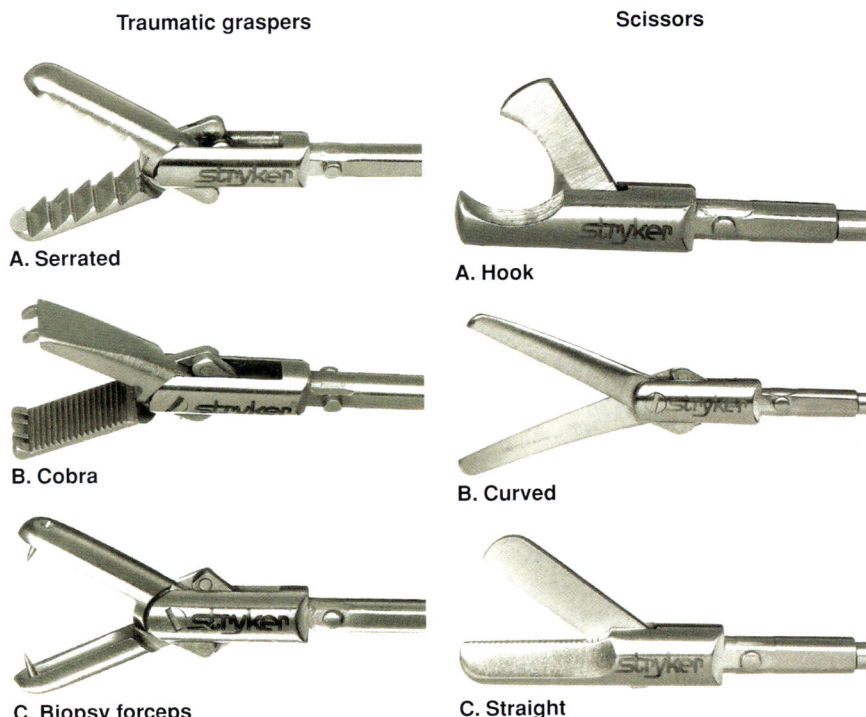

A. Serrated   **A. Hook**

B. Cobra   **B. Curved**

C. Biopsy forceps   **C. Straight**

FIGURE 41-5 Laparoscopic traumatic graspers (*left*) and scissors (*right*). (Reproduced with permission from Stryker Endoscopy.)

for sutures or needles. One example is the laparoscopic tenaculum. Single-tooth and double-tooth tenaculums are both available and effectively hold and retract dense, heavy tissue. The single-tooth tenaculum usually has a double-action jaw, whereas the double-tooth tenaculum is available with either a single- or double-action jaw. Both usually offer a locking hand grip. A tenaculum is traumatic and thus is generally used only on tissue to be resected or repaired. One common use is to grasp and remove tissue during morcellation.

The cobra grasper is a toothed instrument with a double-action jaw. It has short teeth on each side and is excellent for tissue retraction due to its strong grip strength.

Some of the toothed instruments are designed with less traumatic teeth and are selected when less tissue crushing is desired. For example, ovarian biopsy forceps provide adequate grasp with minimal tissue crushing. An appropriate setting might be ovarian cyst resection and subsequent ovarian repair. An Allis grasper has blunter teeth for grasping and holding tissue during resection. However, it provides less gripping strength than the cobra.

Serrated graspers are considered traumatic but are less damaging than toothed graspers. They offer a secure grip with minimal tissue damage and generally are used in repairs or tissue approximation. Because of their variety, a surgeon should be familiar with their grips and tissue effects to select the one that best fits the planned procedure. Serrated graspers may be fenestrated or nonfenestrated, may offer a locking hand grip, and may have single-action or double-action jaws.

A corkscrew tip probe is frequently used for marked retraction of more solid masses such as leiomyomas. It offers superior grip and strength but is limited by the trauma created as it is screwed into the tissue to be held. Additionally, surgeons are mindful of the tip location when advancing it, as the downward force required to spiral the corkscrew tip may inadvertently perforate adjacent tissues. Despite this risk, this tool can be invaluable when manipulating solid, bulky leiomyomas or uteri.

Newer, small, 2-mm and 3-mm accessory manipulators have the trocar built around the instrument shaft and eliminate the need for a dedicated port site (Fig. 41-6). These can be placed percutaneously and leave only a tiny residual abdominal wall scar. These instruments allow instrument to be removed and replaced at multiple abdominal wall sites throughout the surgical procedure. This affords flexibility and greater surgical manipulation. Of two available designs, one is fully disposable and the other is reusable.

Uterine Manipulators

These devices were originally designed for uterine manipulation to create tension, expand operating space, or improve access to specific parts of the pelvis. The Hulka and the Sargis uterine manipulators are reusable stainless steel instruments that contain the following: a stiff blunt tip for insertion into the endocervical canal, a toothed tip that affixes to the cervical lip for stabilization, and a handle for vaginal placement (Fig. 41-7). For these manipulators, the cervix should to be patent to allow entry into the lower uterine cavity.

Uterine manipulators have become increasingly versatile and offer additional functions. The Cohen cannula manipulator has

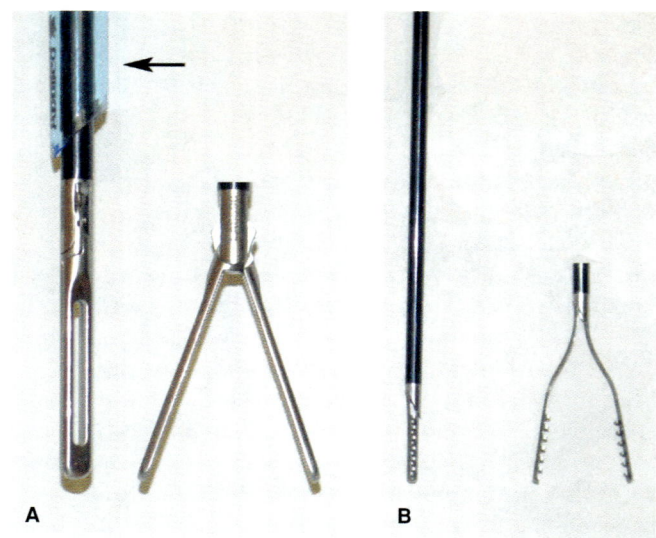

FIGURE 41-6 A. Traditional laparoscopic grasper both closed and opened. The housing cannula is blue and marked by the arrow. **B.** Percutaneous laparoscopic graspers directly pierce the abdominal wall to gain access and do not require a trocar. This MiniLap grasper has 2.4-mm diameter when closed but suitable jaw width when open. (Product provided by Teleflex, Inc.)

a hard-rubber conical tip with a patent cannula for dye injection into the uterus, such as with chromotubation (Fig. 41-8). For placement, a single-tooth tenaculum is placed on the anterior cervical lip. The manipulator's conical tip wedges firmly against the cervix and thereby minimizes retrograde dye egress back through the os. The distal end of the Cohen manipulator then articulates with the crossbar between the tenaculum's finger rings. Although commonly used, its range of motion

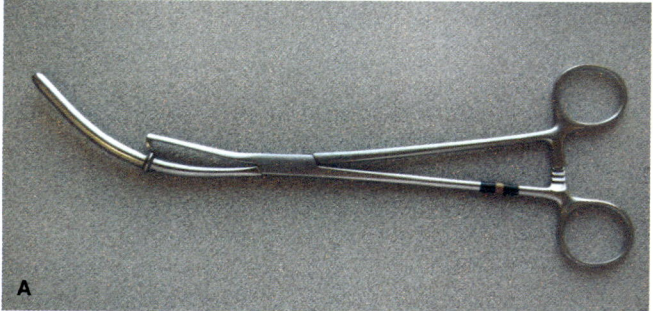

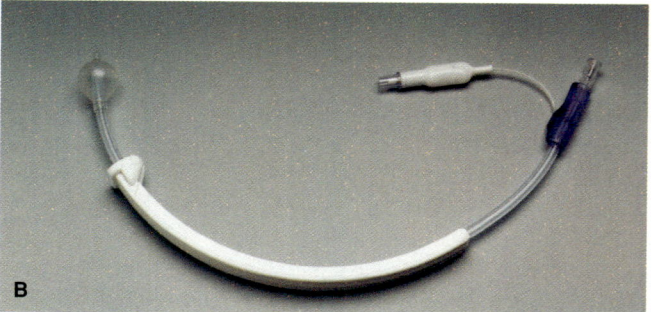

FIGURE 41-7 A. Hulka uterine manipulator. **B.** A balloon-type uterine manipulator. The deflated balloon tip is inserted into the endometrial cavity. The balloon is inflated to hold the stiff manipulator in place.

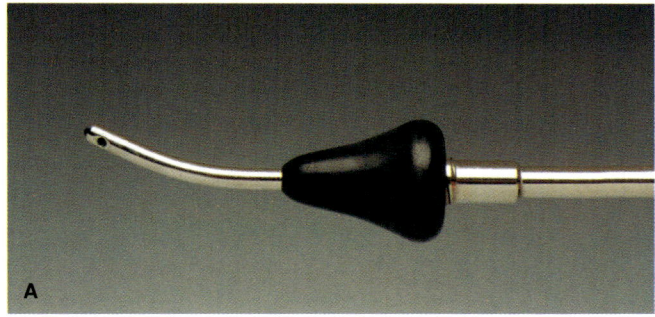

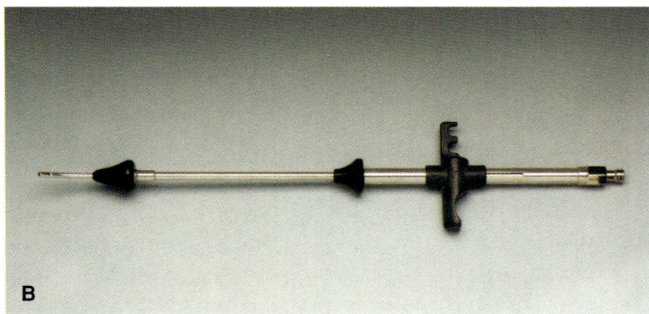

FIGURE 41-8 Cohen cannula. This device is used in conjunction with a separate tenaculum. The tenaculum is placed horizontally on the anterior cervical lip. **A.** The narrow cephalad tip of the cannula fits into the endocervical canal. The conical head abuts the external cervical os and limits insertion into the endometrial cavity. **B.** The caudal portion contains a crossbar into which the ratcheted handle of the cervical tenaculum fits.

is hindered by its straight shaft. Thus, the ability to dramatically flex a uterus anteriorly or posteriorly may be limited. The Rubin cannula manipulator is similar, with the same disadvantages. Greater flexion may be offered by the Hayden and Valtchev uterine manipulators. These have tip options, either conical or longer blunt intrauterine probes, which attach to a wristed joint at the distal end of the instrument shaft. This joint permits improved anteflexion and retroflexion. All of the manipulators just described affix to the cervical lip for stability. Thus, the risk of cervical trauma, although usually minimal, is disadvantageous.

Disposable uterine manipulators such as the Harris-Kronner Uterine Manipulator Injector (HUMI) or the Zinnanti Uterine Manipulator Injector (ZUMI) also have a cannula for introducing dye to assess uterine and tubal patency (see Fig. 41-7). Rather than affixing to the cervix, an intracavitary balloon at the manipulator's uterine end is expanded similar to a Foley balloon once the manipulator tip is placed into the uterine cavity. This prevents the device from dislodging.

More advanced MIS procedures, such as hysterectomy or myomectomy, often require manipulators that offer greater flexibility and accommodation of large uteri. These devices have longer cannulas and may have a cup that attaches to the cervix for delineation of the cervicovaginal junction. Some models are lighted, disposable, or reusable and vary in size (Fig. 41-9).

At times, a vaginal sponge stick is a practical manipulator for elevation and identification of pelvic structures. This may be selected by an advanced surgeon who wishes to eliminate

the manipulator or chosen in cases in which the uterine fundus is absent or gravid.

■ Scissors

These are integral to most laparoscopic procedures and are available in reusable and disposable models. Scissor tips vary depending on the type of dissection or resection needed (see Fig. 41-5). Scissors preferred for dissection commonly have a curved, somewhat blunted tip that tapers similar to Metzenbaum scissors. This shape allows a surgeon to use standard techniques for tissue separation and resection with minimal trauma to the surrounding tissues (Chap. 40, p. 848). These curved blades may be smooth or slightly serrated. A serrated edge tends to hold tissue and minimize slippage prior to cutting. The smooth blade is preferred for adhesiolysis.

Straight scissors are used more for cutting and are less desired for dissection. These also come with smooth or serrated blades. Many straight scissors are designed with a single-action jaw, and some surgeons feel this offers better control.

Hooked scissors have a rounded, blunt tip and hooked blades. When initially approximated, the blades close around the tissue without cutting and then cut from the tip toward the hinge. This offers a controlled transection and is useful for partial transection of tissues. Moreover, the design allows a surgeon to confirm optimum placement before cutting. This type of scissors is commonly used for suture cutting or cutting tubular structures.

■ Suction and Irrigation Devices

Successful laparoscopy requires a clear visual field. Thus, an efficient suction and irrigation system is integral to procedures that

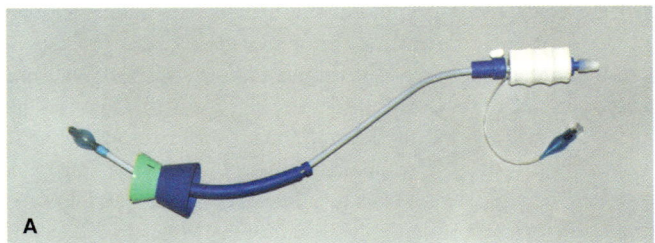

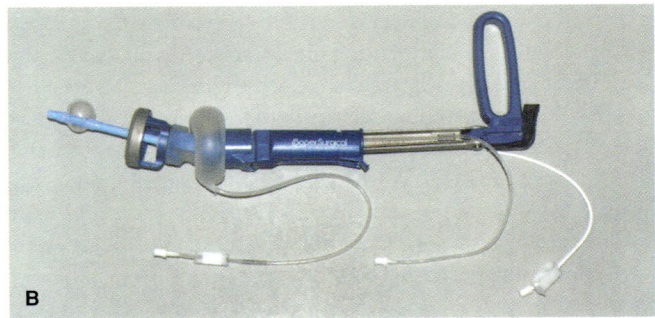

FIGURE 41-9 **A.** VCare uterine manipulator. **B.** RUMI-Koh uterine manipulator. Each has a balloon tip to secure the device tip within the uterine cavity. The cup-shaped portion toward the end of each helps to delineate the vaginal fornices during colpotomy.

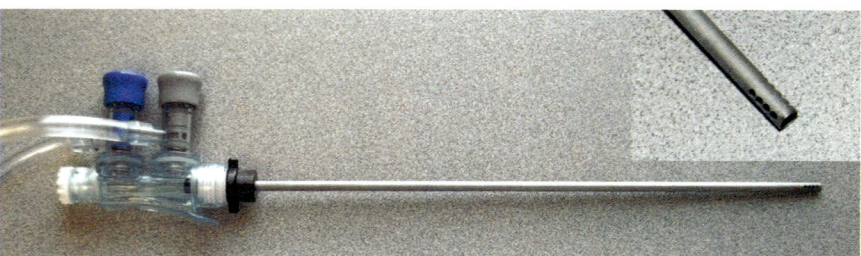

FIGURE 41-10 Suction-irrigator. Inset: Irrigator tip.

require fluid or smoke removal (Fig. 41-10). Older systems were extremely slow and thereby prolonged operative time or failed to adequately clear a field. Newer motorized systems provide faster irrigation and evacuation, and motors usually have two speeds, which can be manually adjusted. The suction tips are available in 3-, 5-, and 10-mm diameters, thereby tailoring instrument capability to the clinical setting. The latest-generation systems permit additional instruments to be placed through the hollow suction tip for concurrent monopolar electrosurgery. Newer models also have attachments to fluid management systems to monitor infused and extracted volumes.

When using a suction irrigation system, all of the suction holes are ideally submerged in the fluid to be removed. This avoids inadvertent insufflation gas removal, which then collapses the operative field. Additionally, the probe may cause suction damage to viscera, especially delicate structures such as tubal fimbria and bowel epiploica. To avoid damage, suction is used when there is a safe distance from vulnerable structures.

■ Tissue Extraction Tools
Morcellators

These instruments cut excised tissues into smaller pieces, which can then be extracted. These devices also have a self-contained grasper that pulls tissue up into the device for severing. Available morcellators use either thin cutting blades or pulsatile kinetic energy. Bladed morcellators consist of a hollow large-bore shaft that contains razorlike blades to shave tissues into thin strips. One of these, the Storz Rotocut, is reusable but houses disposable stainless steel blades that are efficient in cutting through dense masses. Although bulkier and heavier than others, it is among the fastest and most effective. The LiNa Xcise morcellator has a built-in battery pack, is slower but more ergonomic, and is disposable. The MOREsolution morcellator offers a 2-cm-diameter blade, which is currently the largest and may be helpful for large masses. Each mechanical morcellator has its advantages, and familiarity with these allows selection of the most suitable instrument for a given tissue.

Another tool, the PKS PlasmaSORD Bipolar Morcellator, is bladeless. Instead, it uses plasma kinetic energy, which is a form of pulsatile bipolar energy. Although efficient for morcellation of hysterectomy and myomectomy specimens, it produces a large smoke plume, which may reduce visibility and thereby lengthen operative time. Accordingly, cases with larger specimens may have extended operative times with this instrument compared with bladed instruments. However, no randomized studies support the superiority of one morcellator over another.

Morcellation use has evolved in recent years, and discussion of appropriate preventions to avoid tissue dissemination is found on page 894.

Endoscopic Retrieval Pouches

Endoscopic bags for tissue retrieval vary in size, material composition, and strength. Some are free-standing sacs designed for manual introduction into the abdominal cavity through cannulas and are preferred for larger and denser masses. Once loaded, the sac is simply lifted through an appropriately sized abdominal wall incision.

Other types are manufactured as pouches attached to support arms at the end of a laparoscopic shaft to create a self-contained unit. As shown in Figure 41-11, the support arms open the sac. Once the mass is bagged, the arms and shaft are retracted and removed through the port-site cannula. The cannula is then removed, bringing the bag to the incision where it is extracted. With either sac type, if a specimen does not compress or cannot be drained, the incision may require slight enlargement.

Because of concern for tissue dissemination, endoscopic bags are now available for contained morcellation. With this, the container bag is placed through a port site and into the abdomen. The specimen is placed in the bag, and the bag's sole opening is brought through and outside the designated port site. Once the bag is in position, it is insufflated. This creates a closed operative space. Both the laparoscope and morcellator

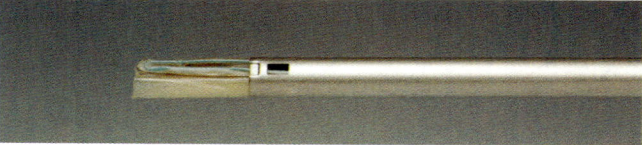
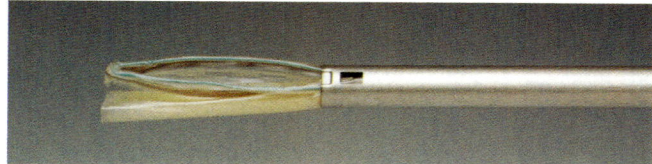
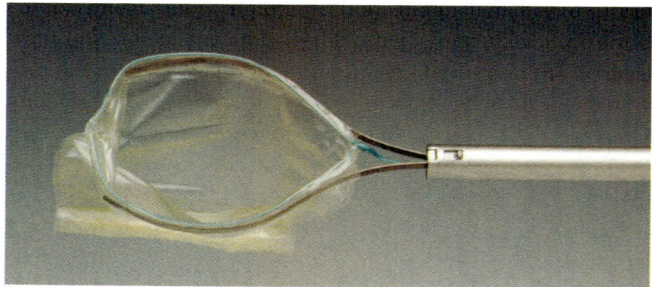

FIGURE 41-11 Endoscopic sac. With this type, the structured ring is housed within the device shaft. The top two images show gradual deployment of this ring. The final image displays the ring and attached sac. Once the specimen is bagged, the sac can be detached from the ring. The ring then retracts again into the shaft. Last, a purse string at the sac mouth is pulled closed, and the specimen bag can be removed from the abdomen.

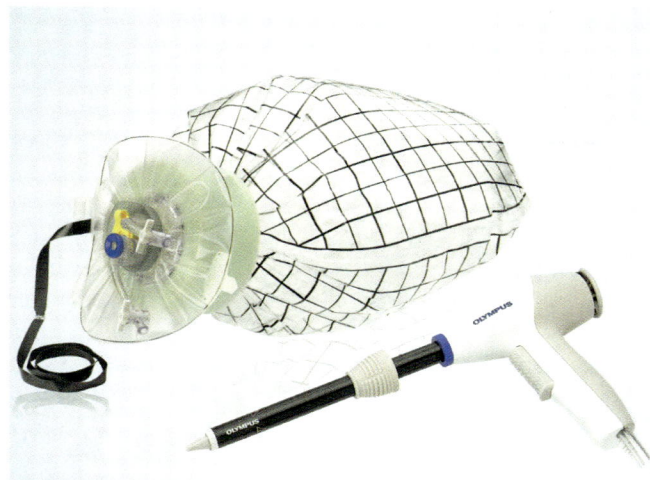

FIGURE 41-12 Enclosed morcellation. With this device (Pneumoliner), a single-incision port, which simultaneously accepts multiple instruments, is affixed to the specimen bag. Within the abdomen, the bag is insufflated and expanded to create a contained work space. The morcellator and flexible endoscope enter the bag for contained tissue morcellation under direct visualization. (Reproduced with permission from Olympus Endoscopy.)

then enter the bag through the port site to complete contained morcellation. Theoretically, this lowers the possibility of tissue dissemination and eases extraction of small tissue fragments. Some models such as the PneumoLiner use a single port to introduce all needed instruments (Fig. 41-12).

Self-Retaining Retractors

Designed to complement MIS, nonmetal self-retaining retractors consist of two equal-sized plastic rings connected by a cylindrical plastic sheath (Fig. 41-13). One ring collapses into a canoe shape that can be threaded through the incision and into the abdomen. Once inside the abdomen, it springs again into its circular form. The second ring remains exteriorized. Between these rings, the plastic sheath spans the thickness of

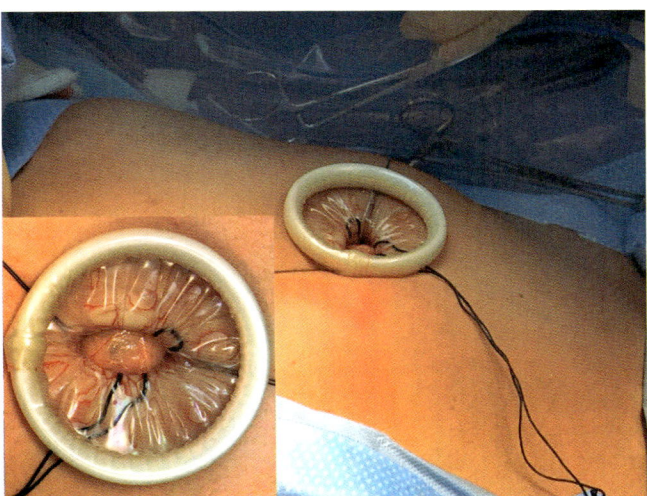

FIGURE 41-13 Nonmetal self-retaining retractor placed at the umbilicus. (Reproduced with permission from Dr. Karen Bradshaw).

the abdominal wall. To hold the retractor in place, a surgeon everts the exterior ring multiple times until the plastic sheath is tight against the skin and subcutaneous layers. This form creates 360-degree retraction. These disposable retractors maximize incision size because of their circular shape and by eliminating thick metal retractor blades within the wound opening. Brands include the Alexis and Mobius retractors, and available sizes range from extra small to extra large. In some studies, these retractors provide wound protection and lower wound infection rates (Horiuchi, 2007; Reid, 2010).

For MIS cases, these devices offer several functions. First, they retract minilaparotomy incisions to aid large specimen removal. Moreover, certain procedures, such as laparoscopic myomectomy, also can be completed through these incisions (Section 44-8, p. 1040). Second, concern about tissue dissemination has prompted development of retrieval bags that are coupled with these self-retaining retractors. For this, the retrieval bag is initially placed into the abdomen. The bag containing the excised specimen is then brought to the surface and is fanned open outside and around the minilaparotomy incision. The self-retaining circular retractor is then placed into the bag's interior and simultaneously opened within the incision. This creates a closed environment in which the specimen can be sharply morcellated manually with scissor or knife. In certain cases, the vaginal approach is preferred and the specimen bags may be brought out through a colpotomy incision (p. 895). The bag may be attached to a retraction ring to stabilize and maintain a patent orifice during the extraction. Long-term data on safety and efficacy of these enclosed approaches are not yet available.

Energy Systems in Minimally Invasive Surgery

Understanding principles and correct use of electrosurgical instruments is essential to safe laparoscopy. The same principles of electrosurgery in open surgery apply to laparoscopy (Chap. 40, p. 856). However, special considerations are necessary in a closed, MIS environment. For example, the entire length of an instrument may extend past a surgeon's visual field, thus risking unintended electrosurgical burns. Fortunately, advances in instrumentation mitigate many of the physical constraints inherent to MIS.

Monopolar Electrosurgery

Monopolar tools may be useful for tissue cutting, dissection, vaporization, and desiccation. Delivery of this energy is usually through scissors or needle point tip. Of these, monopolar scissors coagulate tissues within its jaws prior to incision. This is typically used for thin tissues and small vessels. In addition, closed blade tips can act simultaneously to cut tissue and achieve hemostasis. Monopolar energy delivered though a needle point tip is used for functions ranging from ovarian drilling to development of peritoneal planes during hydrodissection.

Unintended thermal injuries form the main risk with this energy type. With monopolar tools, shaft insulation failures, direct coupling, or capacitive coupling may each result in unintended, potentially serious electrosurgical burns. First, insulation failures are breaches in an instrument shaft's insulation.

This break provides an alternate pathway for current flow. When a monopolar instrument is activated, electric current may travel from the electrode through the insulation breach and discharge to any tissue in contact with this breach. This current flow may cause thermal damage to surrounding visceral and vascular structures without the surgeon ever being aware. Thus, before electrosurgical tools are used, systematic inspection should look for insulation cracks along their length, for aberrant or loose cord connections, and for assurance that a grounding pad is correctly placed on the patient.

Another monopolar effect is *direct coupling*, which occurs when an activated electrode contacts another metal object—either intentionally or unintentionally. This technique is frequently used during open surgery to achieve hemostasis of small vessels, such as when the electrosurgical blade tip is touched to a hemostat around a small vessel. However, in laparoscopy, unintentional direct coupling may occur when a metal instrument or object (such as a metal cannula) contacts an active monopolar instrument and thus provides an alternate and undesired current flow to surrounding viscera.

Another hazard with monopolar instruments is the risk of *capacitive coupling*. A capacitor is defined as two conductors separated by a nonconducting medium. During laparoscopy, an "inadvertent capacitor" can be created when a conductive active electrode (e.g., monopolar scissors) is surrounded by a nonconducting medium (insulation around the scissors) and is placed through another conductive medium (a metal cannula). This capacitor creates an electrostatic field between the two conductors. When current is activated through one of the conductors, this in turn will induce a current in the second conductor. Capacitive coupling occurs when this system discharges current into other surrounding conductive material. In the case of an all-metal cannula, current can be dissipated throughout the abdominal wall. With hybrid cannula systems, in which a metal cannula is anchored by a plastic sleeve or collar, the capacitor that is created has no place to discharge. Stray current can then exit to adjacent tissue that is in contact with the metal portion of the cannula, thereby damaging nearby vascular or visceral structures. This risk can be reduced by avoiding hybrid cannulas and by selecting bipolar instruments. Moreover, the addition of an integrated shield on the electrode shaft of some monopolar instruments, which monitors for stray current, can help prevent this complication.

Bipolar Energy

Bipolar energy is mainly used in laparoscopy for tissue desiccation and hemostasis. Many types of bipolar forceps are available

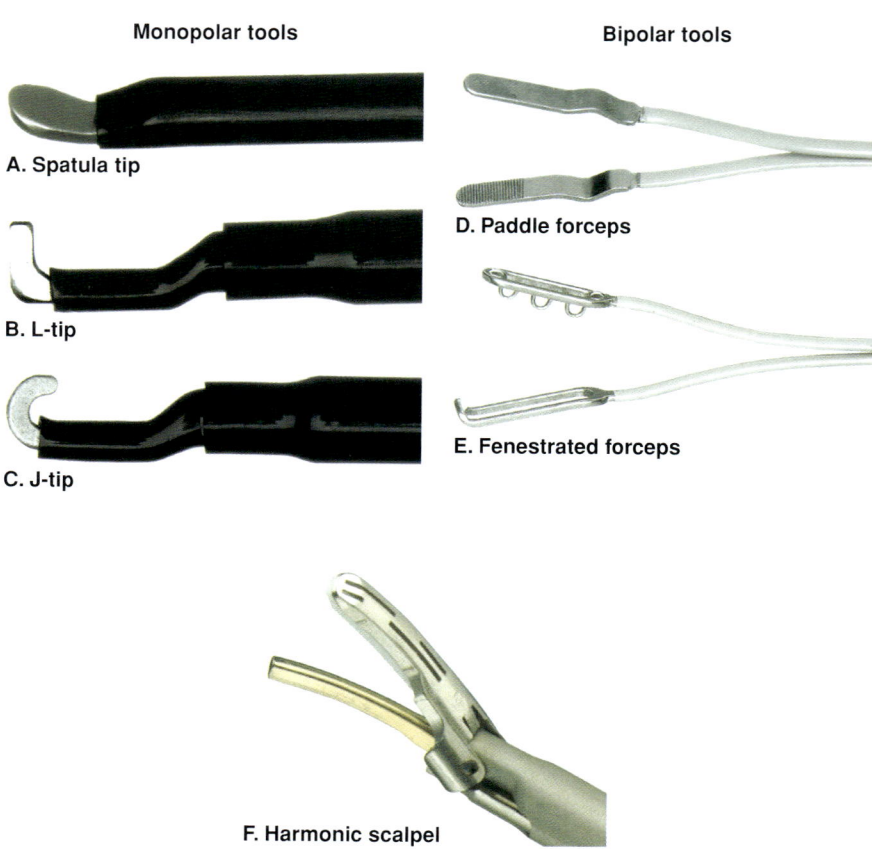

Monopolar tools

A. Spatula tip

B. L-tip

C. J-tip

Bipolar tools

D. Paddle forceps

E. Fenestrated forceps

F. Harmonic scalpel

FIGURE 41-14 A-C. Laparoscopic monopolar tools. **D, E.** Bipolar tools. (Reproduced with permission from Stryker Endoscopy.) **F.** Laparoscopic Harmonic scalpel. (Reproduced with permission from Ethicon.)

for various uses (Fig. 41-14). The paddle or Kleppinger forceps are used for tubal coagulation during sterilization procedures. Flat-tip forceps desiccate larger vessels and tissue pedicles. Fine-tip, "microbipolar" forceps aid hemostasis near or on vulnerable structures. Burns are less of a concern with bipolar energy because the currents used are typically lower. Currents, for the most part, also stay confined between the two closely approximated electrodes.

With traditional bipolar tools, an amp meter measures current flow across tissues to indicate desiccation. With these, surgeons can achieve electrosurgical effects with or without grasping tissue. For example, by slightly closing the paddles and laying the device against tissue, desiccation can be completed.

Advanced bipolar tools include the LigaSure, Plasmakinetic (PK) Gyrus, and EnSeal, which can be used for both tissue desiccation and dissection. Each of these devices employs a low voltage to deliver energy to tissue and carry impedance feedback to the electrosurgical unit to locally regulate thermal tissue effects. These adaptations allow for reduced collateral injury from thermal spread, an improved tissue seal, less plume production, and diminished tissue sticking. Whereas the LigaSure delivers a continuous bipolar radiofrequency waveform, the PK delivers energy in a pulsed waveform. The EnSeal system has a temperature-controlled feedback mechanism at its tip, which "locally" modulates energy delivery. When evaluating these devices, important considerations include thermal spread, ability to provide desired tissue effects, consistency of results, time required to achieve results, plume produced, and maximum vessel diameter that can be securely sealed (Lamberton, 2008; Newcomb, 2009).

Ultrasonic Energy

The Harmonic scalpel, also known as an ultrasonic scalpel, uses ultrasonic energy, which is converted to mechanical energy at the active blade. Seen as the lower blade in Figure 41-14, the active blade vibrates to deliver high-frequency ultrasonically generated frictional force, whereas the inactive upper arm holds tissues in apposition against the active blade. Alternatively, the active blade may be used alone. Either cutting or coagulating effects can be achieved, and a balance between these two is created by controlling several factors: power levels, tissue tension, blade sharpness, and application time. Higher power level, greater tissue tension, and a sharp blade will lead to cutting. Lower power, decreased tissue tension, and a blunt blade will create slower cutting and greater hemostasis. Limitations of the Harmonic scalpel include limited ability to coagulate vessels larger than 5 mm and the requirement for the surgeon to balance the factors listed above (Bubenik, 2005; Lamberton, 2008).

Laser Energy

Current laser forms include the CO_2, argon, KTP (potassium titanyl phosphate), and Nd-YAG (neodymium:yttrium-aluminum-garnet) lasers. These are generally used through an operative channel on the laparoscope or via a suprapubic port. These devices can cut, coagulate, and vaporize tissues and are employed for lysis of adhesions, tubal surgery, and endometriosis fulguration or resection. With a skilled surgeon, lasers offer precision and control with minimal effect on surrounding tissue. Thus, a laser is able to work near or over sensitive structures such as bowel, bladder, ureters, and vessels. Disadvantages are its learning curve, expense, lack of portability, and smoke production.

■ Laparoscopic Optics

Laparoscope Construction

Successful MIS requires excellent visualization provided by high-intensity light sources and laparoscopes with focused lenses. The modern-day rod lens system contains a series of lenses that are the diameter of the laparoscope cylinder. At the periphery of each lens are small scalloped grooves that permit light-carrying fibers to reach the endoscope end. This provides a well-lit image and minimal distortion. Uniquely, the space between lenses is filled with small, tightly packed glass rods. These rods fit exactly, which make them self-aligning to require no other structural support. Appropriate curvature and coatings to the rod ends and optimal glass quality permit superb image quality—even with cylinder tubes measuring only 1 mm in diameter.

In addition to its main cylinder, a laparoscope contains an eyepiece at one end to which a camera can be affixed. The camera usually is an attachable springed plastic cap that can be clipped onto the eyepiece. The main cylinder also has an adapter on its exterior to attach the light-source cable. Laparoscope diameters range from 0.8 mm to 15 mm. In general, greater diameters offer superior optics but require a larger incision. This trade-off typically dictates laparoscope selection for a given procedure.

Differing from traditional straight-shaft endoscopes, operative laparoscopes have an eyepiece that branches off at a 45- or 90-degree angle from the straight operative shaft. This permits tools to be placed through the operative shaft, which are then seen by the endoscope. Instruments used are generally longer than instruments typically placed in accessory ports. Most instruments are 45 cm, which is considered bariatric length. Lasers are also frequently placed through the operative shaft and can allow for precise energy application.

Angles of View

Laparoscopes vary in their angle of view. The most common are 0-, 30-, and 45-degree laparoscopes, and each offers a different view of the peritoneal cavity. A 0-degree endoscope offers a forward view and is preferred by most gynecologists. This laparoscope is used in most diagnostic procedures or simple surgeries involving biopsies, simple adhesiolysis, and excision of small masses or organs such as an ovary, fallopian tube, or appendix.

In contrast, angled-view endoscopes provide a lateral and larger field of view. These are useful during cases with more complicated pathology such as dense adhesions that obstruct the traditional forward view. For example, during difficult dissection in which multiple instruments are in action, an angled-view laparoscope offers a panoramic view at a distance. This provides a surgical field in which all instruments in use can be seen.

Angled-view endoscopes also allow a lateral view of pathology. For example, if an angled-view laparoscope is placed at one pelvic sidewall and is directed to the opposite sidewall, a surgeon is provided a large lateral visual operating space. Moreover, angled views are valuable along the sides of organs. With a large myomatous uterus, it may be challenging to identify the uterine artery and cardinal ligaments. An angled-view laparoscope permits a surgeon to "slide" along the lateral border of the uterus to reach these. Similar benefits are gained when operating in small spaces such as in the deep pelvis or retropubic space (space of Retzius).

The advantages for advanced procedures warrant the time needed to operate using an oblique view. Importantly, during orienting with an angled-view laparoscope, when the field of view is directed downward, the light cord attached to the endoscope is positioned up. Conversely, if the view is upward, the light cord will be positioned down. To maintain orientation, the camera buttons remain facing upward, while the light cord rotates in relation to it to change the viewing polarity.

Flexible Laparoscopes

The tips of these special laparoscopes are able to bend to a greater degree. As such, they can travel into smaller spaces or around corners. Whereas traditional fiberoptic laparoscopes contain fiber bundles that run the length of the endoscope, these flexible endoscopes house a camera chip at their end to transmit images as electrical signals. This results in less image distortion. The concept has also provided the option of dual camera technology, which uses two camera chips at the tip. As benefits, optics and opportunities for more advanced procedures are improved. Some newer models afford a 3-D view and are used for single-port laparoscopic approaches, in which there is traditionally less maneuverability (p. 893).

Lighting

Light is transmitted through the laparoscope from a light source via the light cable. Currently, a cold light source is used and provides a more intense beam. The term "cold light" describes the dissipation of heat along the length of the cable. Cold light sources use halogen, xenon, or halide modalities for the lamps. Despite heat dissipation, the light source still creates a hot tip at the distal laparoscope end. Thus, prolonged exposure of the tip to surgical drapes, patient skin, or internal organs is avoided. Thermal injuries have resulted from such exposure.

Light cables connect the light source to the endoscope, and fiberoptic or fluid-filled types are available. The fiberoptic cable contains multiple coaxial quartz fibers that transmit light with relatively little heat conduction. However, these cables suffer from fiber breakage and need to be serviced often. In contrast, fluid-filled cables transmit more light and conduct more heat than the fiber cables. They are stiffer and have decreased maneuverability. This coupled with difficulty in sterilization may make this type less preferred.

Once attached to a camera and light source, most laparoscopes must be adjusted to a "true white" to ensure that the colors in the viewing field are accurate. This is called *white balancing* and is performed at the procedure's beginning.

ROBOTIC SURGERY

Similar to laparoscopy, robotic surgery uses abdominal ports to introduce instruments and a pneumoperitoneum to expand the operative field. In contrast, miniaturized and wristed articulating instrument tips enable successful completion of complex procedures in tight operating spaces. Graspers, needle drivers, and cutting tips are available. Advanced video technology within an 8-mm laparoscope provides a high-definition and magnified view.

Of disadvantages, tactile feedback is lost with robotic surgery and forces a surgeon to use visual cues. This is a learned skill that carries a significant learning curve. However, surgeons experienced in advanced laparoscopic techniques adapt more quickly. Other disadvantages include extended initial set-up time needed during each case, physician training costs, and robot and instrument expenses.

When selecting a robotic approach, patient and procedure characteristics are considered. First, procedures that are currently performed efficiently by conventional laparoscopy should not be replaced by robotic surgery (American College of Obstetricians and Gynecologists, 2017). Rather, this modality is an alternative to laparotomy and thus may offer the patient a more rapid recovery and less postoperative morbidity.

Currently, the only commercially available robot is the da Vinci system. Shown in Figure 41-15, one or two surgeon consoles are used to control robot arm movement. A separate cart stands at the surgical bedside and serves as the base for the four robotic arms. Of these arms, one controls the laparoscope, whereas the other arms hold robotic instruments. Procedures are performed using two or three of the instrument arms

according to the procedure's needs and surgeon's preference. The second surgeon console is generally used for training. If port sites in addition to the basic four are needed, an assistant surgeon can also work at the patient bedside through one or two traditional laparoscopic accessory ports. These are generally placed in the right or left upper quadrants. Typically, 5- to 15-mm trocars are used for the accessory port(s), depending on the instruments required for a given procedure.

During port placement, initial abdominal entry and subsequent accessory trocars are inserted similar to laparoscopy (p. 888). Port placement for robotic surgery is unique in that ports must be placed with a minimum intervening distance of 8 cm. This keeps the robot arms from colliding with each other and with any accessory ports. Shown in Figure 41-16, the level of the laparoscope's port depends on the procedure, the complexity of the pathology, and previous patient surgeries. Importantly, a black ring around the cannula marks the depth to which a trocar is inserted. Insertion to this depth is essential to permit the robot arms the correct fulcrum to function optimally and to minimize port-site tissue stretch.

Of newer modifications, reduced-port robotic surgery uses microtip percutaneous instruments to minimize the number of 8-mm ports. Its advantage is yet to be proven with randomized trials.

Second, the Food and Drug Administration (FDA) has approved instrumentation for single-site robotic surgery, which is discussed on page 893. Last, although not FDA approved for gynecologic procedures, the newest model, the Single Port Robot is currently available. Rather than several trocar sites, it uses a solitary port to deliver multiple operative instruments through the trocar. The laparoscope and instruments are extremely flexible and allow the needed triangulation for traction and countertraction (see Fig. 41-15F). *Triangulation* describes instruments converging on a focal point from lateral angles of origin. These angles create opposing forces, which are essential for effective tissue retraction, dissection, and resection.

LAPAROSCOPIC ANATOMY

■ Anterior Abdominal Wall

The laparoscopic view of pelvic anatomy may differ slightly from laparotomy due to the effects of pneumoperitoneum, Trendelenburg positioning, and the translation of a 3-D reality into a 2-D image on the monitor. When planning abdominal entry, key structures of the anterior abdominal wall are considered to avert neurovascular complications. Key landmarks include the umbilicus, anterior superior iliac spine, and pubic symphysis. Especially in the obese patient in whom a large pannus may alter anatomic relationships, bony landmarks are used to plan safe port placement.

The umbilicus is generally located at the level of the L3–L4 vertebrae, although it may lie above or below depending on habitus. In most patients, the aorta bifurcates at the union of L4–L5 vertebrae (Nezhat, 1998). In obese patients, the umbilicus tends to be caudal to this aortic bifurcation. The left common iliac vein crosses the midline approximately 3 to 6 cm inferior to the level of the umbilicus. These structures are considered during

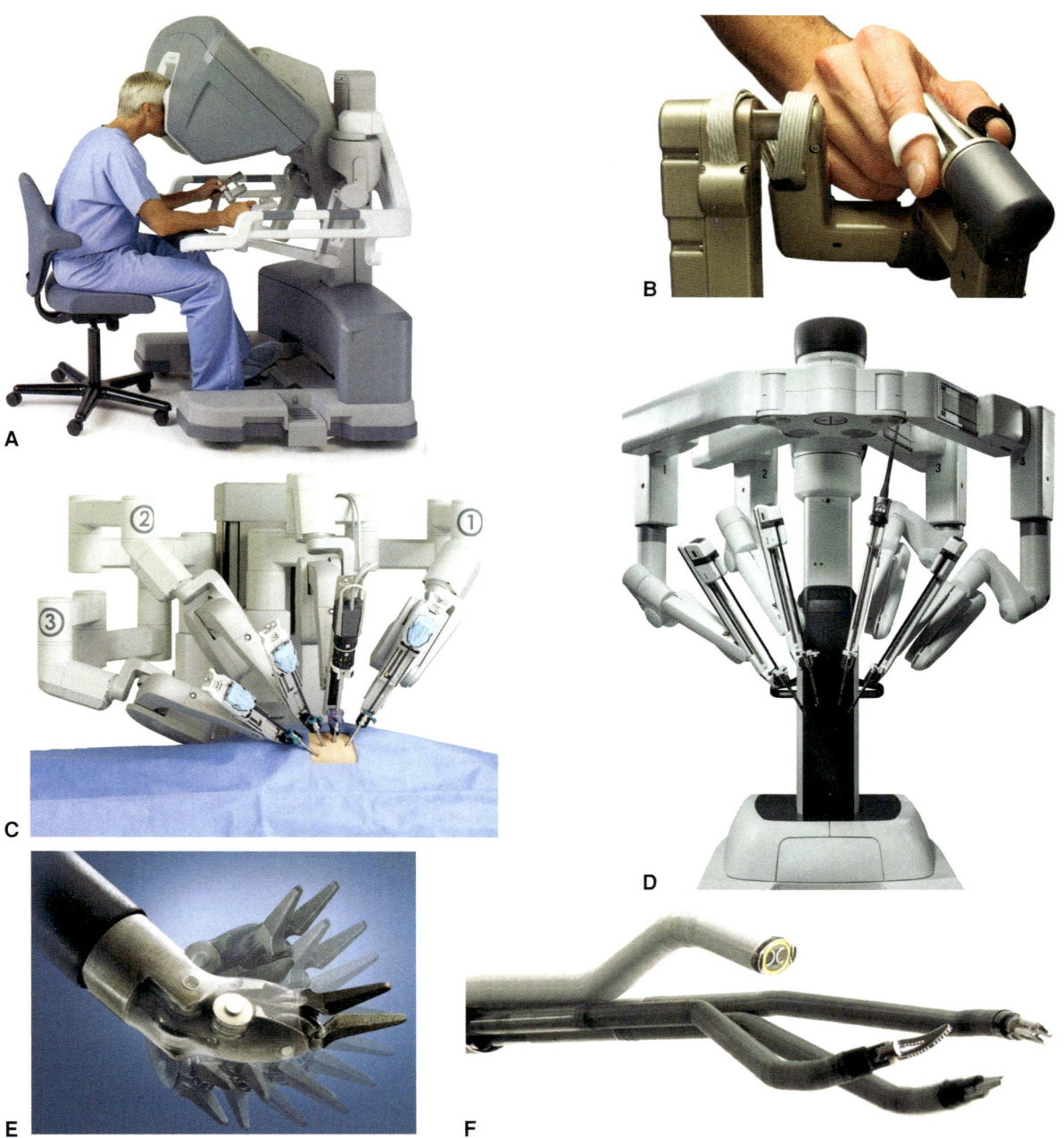

FIGURE 41-15 Da Vinci Surgical System. **A.** Operator console. **B.** A surgeon's finger movements are translated into robotic instrument movement. **C.** Robot at operative bedside. **D.** The newer Xi model has arms that extend off a central column to aid complex, multiquadrant procedures. In this model, the bed and robot arms can move simultaneously for greater surgical flexibility. **E.** Traditional wristed robotic instruments provide a wide range of motion. **F.** The Single Port cannula serves as the sole conduit for delivery of flexible instruments and laparoscope into the abdomen. (Reproduced with permission from Intuitive Surgical, Inc.)

initial trocar entry at the umbilicus as they lie approximately 6 cm deep to the base of the umbilicus in normal-sized supine patients and may be closer in thinner patients (Hurd, 1992).

Accessory ports are subsequently placed under direct visualization of important anatomic structures that include the bladder, bowel, and the inferior (deep) and superficial epigastric vessels. The inferior epigastric artery travels along the lateral third of the posterior surface of the rectus abdominis muscle and should be visualized intraperitoneally (see Fig. 41-16). This vessel also runs lateral to the medial umbilical ligaments.

The superficial epigastric artery, a branch of the femoral artery, travels in the subcutaneous tissue in a path similar to that of the inferior epigastric vessels. The superficial epigastric artery may be identified by transillumination of the anterior abdominal wall with the laparoscope. Although it cannot be visualized, nerve supply of the anterior abdominal wall also is considered to avoid trauma during trocar placement. Both the ilioinguinal and iliohypogastric nerves can be lacerated during ancillary port placement (see Fig. 41-16). Steps to limit injury to all these structures are described on the next page.

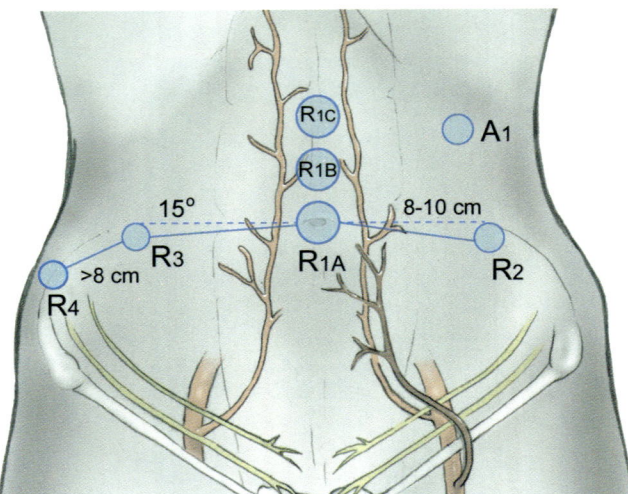

FIGURE 41-16 Typical port placements for robotic surgery. The R₁ port will house the laparoscope. Its site may be moved cephalad depending on the size of pelvic pathology as illustrated by R₁ₐ–R₁c. R₂, R₃, and R₄ mark other robot port sites. A₁ marks the assistant surgeon port site.

■ Retroperitoneal Structures

Along the anterior abdominal wall, five prominent ligaments lie beneath the peritoneum and can be easily seen laparoscopically. These intraperitoneal landmarks run cephalad to caudad and may be used to identify key anatomic structures in the retroperitoneum (Fig. 41-17). In the midline, the *median umbilical ligament* traverses from the bladder dome to the umbilicus and is the obliterated urachus.

Lateral to this lie the *medial umbilical folds*, which cover the obliterated umbilical arteries. Identification of the medial umbilical ligament is essential in the setting of a frozen pelvis and can provide access to the internal iliac artery. For this, the medial umbilical ligament is followed underneath the round ligament, through the broad ligament, to the superior vesicle artery, and finally to the internal iliac artery. Running laterally to the medial umbilical folds and to the round ligaments are the *lateral umbilical folds*. These folds are formed by peritoneum overlying

the inferior epigastric vessels before they enter the rectus sheath. Direct intraperitoneal visualization of the lateral umbilical folds will prevent injury to these vessels during port placement.

In the pelvic retroperitoneum, laparoscopy usually allows easy direct identification of the ureter and vessels of the pelvic sidewall. Moreover, the course of the pelvic ureter traveling from the pelvic brim, along the pelvic sidewall, and to the cervix routinely should be appreciated with every laparoscopy to ensure normal peristalsis and caliber. To avoid injury to the ureter, its course is confirmed repeatedly during adnexal surgery, hysterectomy, and cases with adhesive disease.

ABDOMINAL ACCESS

The choice of entry site and method is influenced by body habitus, prior surgery, risk of encountering adhesive disease, intended procedure, surgeon skill, and the site, size, and type of pathology. Nearly half of all laparoscopic complications occur during abdominal entry, and nearly one quarter of these are undetected until the postoperative period (Bhoyrul, 2001; Chandler, 2001). Thus, entry carefully factors the above variables. Each of the methods discussed below may be beneficial in different situations, but all have potential risks. It has not been established which entry method is safest (Ahmad, 2012).

■ Umbilical Entry

The umbilicus is the most frequent entry site, although the left upper quadrant and subxiphoid area are others. The umbilicus is preferred for primary trocar placement because the subcutaneous and preperitoneal tissue layers are thinnest there. Thus, the transumbilical approach is the shortest distance to the abdominal cavity, even in obese patients. From a cosmetic standpoint, the umbilical fossa also conceals the port-site scar.

Laparoscopic entry can be performed with an open or closed technique, described next. Some authors advocate an open entry method as a way to lower puncture injury rates. However, metaanalyses fail to show that any of the following techniques are superior to the others (Ahmad, 2012; Vilos, 2007).

Closed Entry

During laparoscopic entry, surgeons appropriately assess patient anatomy and their physical relationship to the supine patient. To diminish downward thrust when placing a Veress needle and trocars, a surgeon adjusts the table height and uses a short stepstool if necessary. The aorta and its bifurcation lie beneath the umbilicus. To maximize the distance between the puncturing instrument and these vessels and avert vascular injury, premature Trendelenburg positioning is avoided, and the patient should lie flat. Moreover, to minimize visceral puncture during abdominal entry, the surgeon should empty the patient's bladder and confirm with the anesthesiologist that an orogastric tube has emptied the stomach.

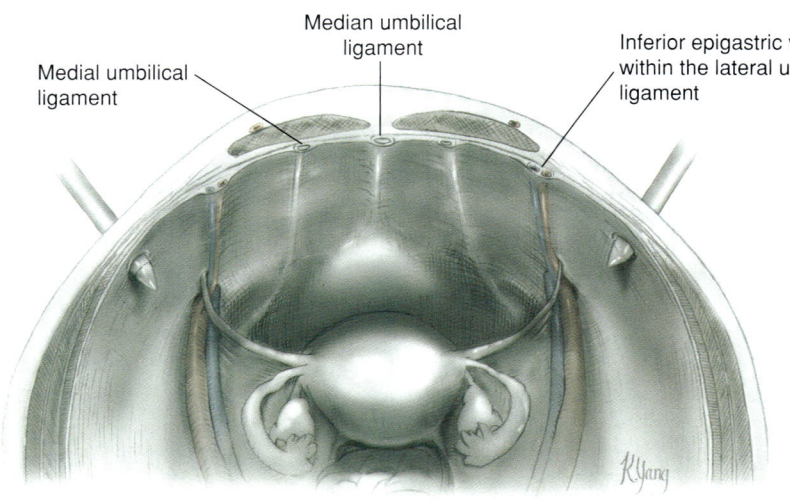

Medial umbilical ligament

Median umbilical ligament

Inferior epigastric vessels within the lateral umbilical ligament

FIGURE 41-17 Umbilical ligaments relative to trocar placement.

Palpation over these areas can confirm adequate decompression. The sacral promontory and aorta also are palpated, and a Veress needle or trocar with a length sufficient to reach the peritoneal cavity is selected. Finally, once all equipment is checked and correctly connected, the surgeon confirms with the anesthesiologist that the patient is fully paralyzed to prevent involuntary patient movement during abdominal entry.

Veress Needle Entry. The goal of this closed technique is to first create a pneumoperitoneum with a 14-gauge Veress needle. Once a pneumoperitoneum is created, the fascia and peritoneum are then secondarily punctured with a trocar. The pneumoperitoneum serves to tense the peritoneum and increases the distance of the viscera and retroperitoneal structures from the trocar entering the abdominal wall. These ideally help lower the risk of puncture injury.

With all closed methods, a skin incision appropriate to the trocar size is created, usually at the umbilicus. The incision can be either horizontal or vertical, is placed centrally within the umbilicus, and can be made with a no. 11 or 15 blade. Skin hooks or Allis clamps can aid in everting the umbilicus.

To begin, a Veress needle tip is placed through the fascia and peritoneum and into the intraabdominal cavity to allow its insufflation with CO_2. During both Veress and trocar placement, many surgeons recommend abdominal wall elevation, either manually or with instruments such as towel clips (Fig. 41-18).

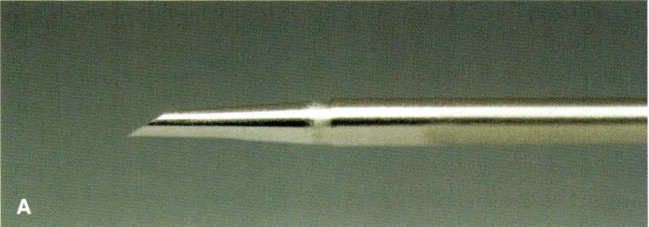

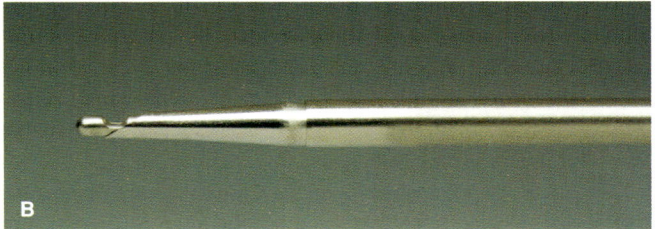

FIGURE 41-19 The Veress needle consists of a sharp outer needle **(A)**, which houses a blunt-tipped, spring-loaded inner stylet **(B)**.

A study using computed tomography images revealed that up to 8 cm can be added between the incision and retroperitoneum by elevation with towel clips (Shamiyeh, 2009). Abdominal wall elevation also provides a controlled countertension to the downward thrust of the Veress needle and subsequent trocar during insertion.

The Veress needle has a spring-loaded obturator (Fig. 41-19). As the device contacts the fascia, the obturator is pushed back, and the needle pierces the fascia and peritoneum. As soon as the tip enters the abdominal cavity, the obturator springs forward to prevent the needle from injuring abdominal viscera. Prior to insertion, the Veress needle is checked for patency by flushing saline through the needle and then withdrawing the fluid. The spring mechanism also is confirmed to function appropriately. The patient and operating table are flat, and the anterior abdominal wall is elevated. For this, we recommend using towel clips for adequate elevation. With the Veress needle angled toward the hollow of the pelvis in the midline, there is a sensation of two "pops" as the tip of the needle penetrates the fascia and then the peritoneum.

Compared with other entry methods, Veress needle access is associated with a higher incidence of failed entry and extraperitoneal insufflation. Entry failures with this method usually stem from Veress needle tip placement into the preperitoneal space (Fig. 41-20). Flow of gas through the needle creates an extraperitoneal insufflation. This gaseous dissection of the peritoneum away from the anterior abdominal wall hinders the trocar in piercing the peritoneum. Instead, the trocar further stretches and pushes the peritoneum internally. Fortunately, this problem can often be overcome by a second attempt with the Veress needle above the umbilicus or by switching to an open entry technique.

Preperitoneal insertion of the Veress needle is common and can lead to abandonment of the laparoscopic procedure. Thus, confirmation of correct needle placement in the peritoneal cavity is essential. For confirmation, a 10-mL syringe containing 5 mL of saline is attached to the hub of the inserted Veress needle. With aspiration, air bubbles should be seen in the syringe. If blood or bowel contents are aspirated, concern for vascular or

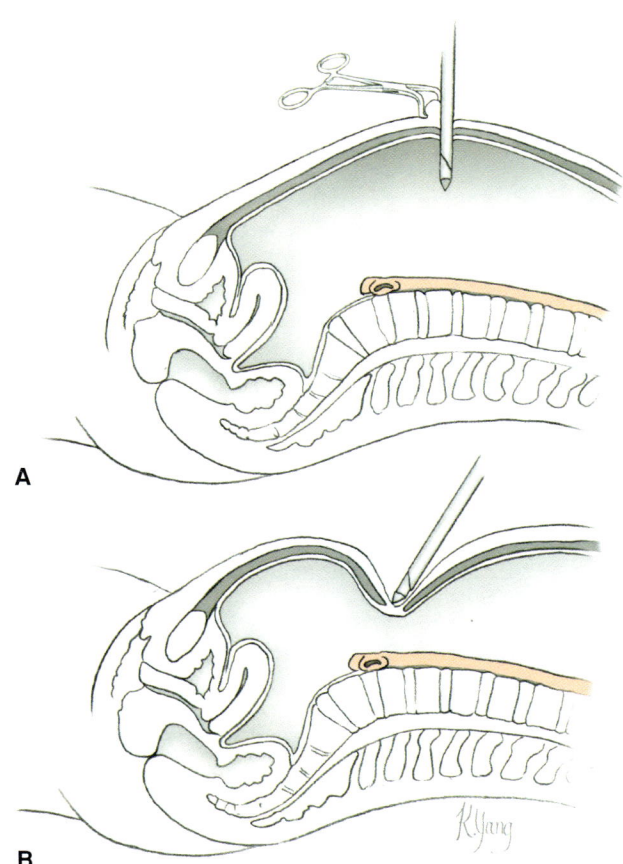

FIGURE 41-18 Primary trocar insertion. **A.** With anterior abdominal wall elevation. **B.** Without anterior abdominal wall elevation.

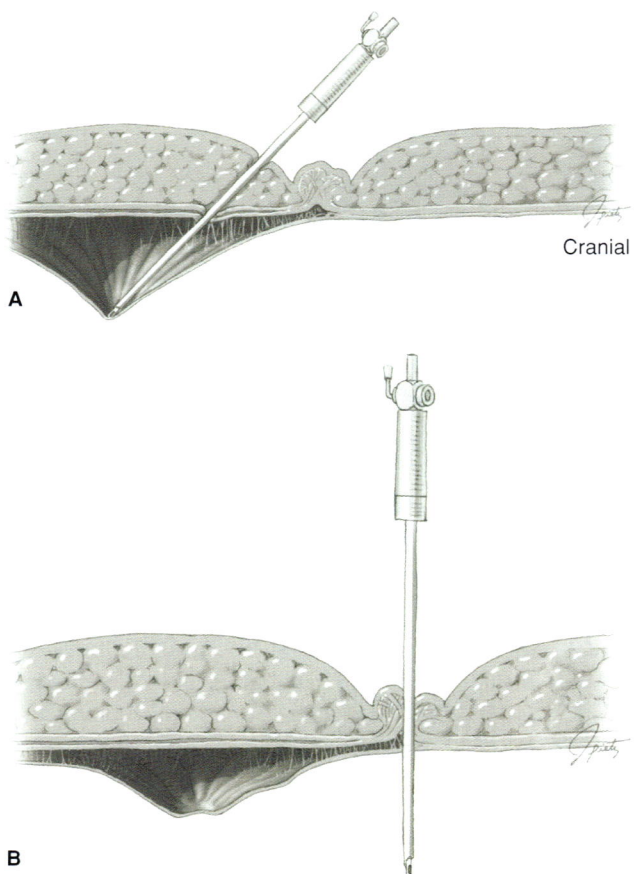

FIGURE 41-20 A. Veress needle tenting the peritoneal layer. **B.** Veress needle replaced at the umbilicus.

visceral injury should be high. In these cases, the needle is left in place to help localize the puncture site and act as a vascular plug as discussed on page 876.

With correct intraabdominal placement, after aspiration, saline is easily injected with no resistance. The surgeon should be unable to reaspirate this saline, which has dispersed into the abdominal cavity. Similarly, a hanging drop test can be used. With this, a few drops of saline are placed on the external open end of the Veress needle. If the needle tip is correctly inserted, the fluid drops disappear into the abdominal cavity. If incorrect entry is suspected, the needle is withdrawn and checked for patency. Moving the Veress needle from side to side is avoided at this stage. Such movement can create rents in the omentum or injure bowel.

Once correct placement is confirmed by these methods, the CO_2 insufflation tubing can be attached to the needle. A low-volume flow of CO_2 is selected, and initial intraabdominal pressure recordings should be <8 mm Hg while the abdominal wall is manually lifted. If the pressure is elevated, the needle is immediately removed. The initial pressure is the most sensitive measurement of correct intraperitoneal Veress needle placement (Vilos, 2007). With the needle correctly inserted, pressure and gas flow may be increased (Fig. 41-21). Simultaneously, the electronic insufflator parameters are closely monitored to ensure a steady rise in the pressure and continued flow. If the intraperitoneal pressure rises rapidly prior to insufflation

of 1.5 to 2 L of gas, one again is concerned for preperitoneal insufflation.

During insufflation, the abdomen is observed for a uniform distention and dullness to percussion over the liver. Since the total volume required to appropriately insufflate an abdomen will vary depending on patient habitus, intraperitoneal pressure, rather than total volume of gas, is used to determine adequate peritoneal insufflation. During normal insufflation, pressures should not exceed 20 mm Hg. Such elevated pressure can lead to hemodynamic and pulmonary compromise. When an intraperitoneal pressure of 20 mm Hg is achieved, the Veress needle may be withdrawn, and the pneumoperitoneum can assist safe primary trocar insertion. This transient elevated intraabdominal pressure provides a volumetric countertension for primary trocar insertion. However, once the primary trocar is inserted, the insufflation pressure is dropped to <15 mm Hg, or to the lowest pressure that allows the planned procedure to be adequately visualized and safely performed.

Although data from multiple studies are conflicting, it has been proposed that the use of humidified CO_2 for insufflation may have advantages. These include decreased postoperative pain, improved visualization from less lens fogging, and, in animal studies, less de novo adhesion formation (Farley, 2004; Ott, 1998; Peng, 2009; Sammour, 2008).

Primary Trocar Placement. Once adequate insufflation is achieved, the primary trocar may then be placed. Trocars are used to gain access to the abdominal cavity. First-generation trocars consist of a hollow, long, slender cannula that sheaths an inner obturator. Trocars typically range from 5 to 12 mm in diameter, and their tips may be conical, pyramidal, or blunt. Conical trocars are smooth except for their more pointed tip and have no cutting edges. They split the fascia rather than cut it and thus are preferred by some to lower risks of hernia formation and vessel injury (Hurd, 1995; Leibl, 1999). However, they require more penetration force to insert. In contrast, pyramidal trocars have sharp edges and tip and, as a result, cut the fascia as they are inserted into the abdomen.

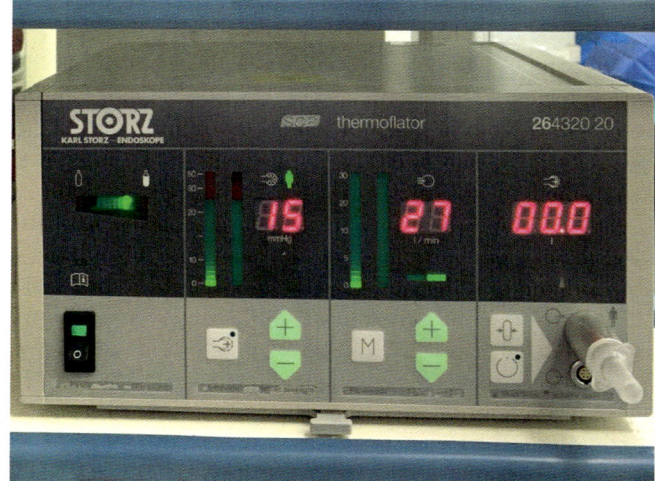

FIGURE 41-21 Most laparoscopic insufflators have monitors to display intraabdominal pressures, gas flow in liters per minute, and number of liters used. (Reproduced with permission from Dr. Lisa Chao.)

In the 1980s, trocars with retractable shields were introduced. Similar to the concept used with the Veress needle, a hollow plastic retractable shield covers the trocar tip both before and after the trocar pierces the abdominal wall. In this manner, the cutting edge is exposed only during its passage through the fascia. Despite theoretical advantages to these shielded trocars in preventing organ injury, studies have failed to show superiority of this design (Fuller, 2005).

Initial trocar entry is a blind procedure and is completed with the patient still supine and flat. The Veress needle is removed, and the trocar's tip is placed in the umbilical incision. The trocar handle is cupped in the palm of the dominant hand, and the same hand's index finger is extended along the trocar shaft to splint the trocar from inserting too deeply. The angle of trocar insertion should mirror that of the Veress needle. The anterior abdominal wall is elevated. With control and minimal downward force, the trocar punctures the fascia and underlying peritoneum and enters the abdominal cavity. After insertion, the trocar obturator is removed, and the cannula may be advanced slightly to ensure adequate placement into the peritoneal cavity. At this point, the laparoscope is inserted through the umbilical cannula to visually confirm safe and atraumatic entry.

Optical Access Trocar Entry. To reduce bowel injury risk at the time of primary trocar insertion, optical trocars were developed. These devices, in essence, combine the laparoscope and trocar into one tool. Importantly, the laparoscope should be focused once it is housed within the trocar and prior to insertion. During use, the optical trocar transmits images of the abdominal wall layers to the television monitor. These layers then are pierced under direct visualization by trocar tip advancement. If choosing a transumbilical entry, the layers visualized, in sequence, should be the subcutaneous fat, the fascia, preperitoneal fat, and peritoneum.

Optical entry methods can be used with and without the prior establishment of pneumoperitoneum. Despite the theoretical advantage of this type of trocar, major organ injury still has been reported. Moreover, no large studies have established its clinical superiority over other entry techniques (Sharp, 2002).

Direct Trocar Entry. Because of entry failures associated with preperitoneal insufflation, a direct trocar entry method may be preferred (Copeland, 1983; Dingfelder, 1978). For this, the abdominal wall is elevated and directly pierced with a trocar without prior insufflation. Comparative studies between Veress needle and direct trocar techniques show lower rates of entry failure with the direct method (Byron, 1993; Clayman, 2005; Gunenc, 2005). Moreover, investigators note comparable or lower associated minor complication rates with the direct entry method. Optical trocars may be used for a direct entry approach combining both optical and tactile feedback to the surgeon regarding anatomic placement.

Open Umbilical Entry

To lower puncture injury rates with closed entry methods, an open entry technique was described by Hasson (1971, 1974). For this, a 1- to 2-cm transverse skin incision at the lower edge

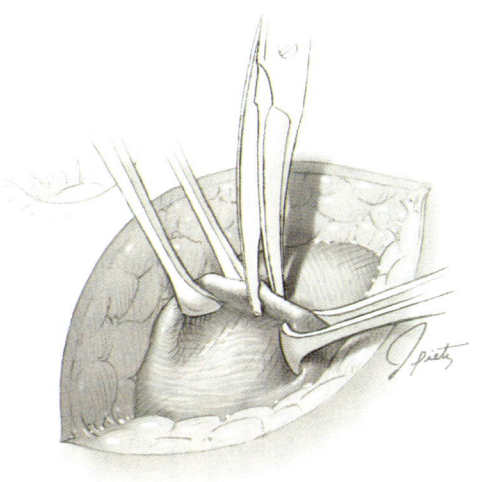

FIGURE 41-22 Fascial incision for open entry.

of the umbilicus is made while applying tension with fine-toothed forceps to its lateral borders. Skin edges are retracted laterally, and the subcutaneous layer is divided to expose the linea alba. This fascia is lifted and everted upward with two Allis clamps (Fig. 41-22). A 0.5- to 1-cm incision with scalpel or scissors then transects the fascia. The Allis clamps are repositioned, one on each free fascial edge.

A hemostat or finger is used to bluntly open the peritoneum, and the end of an S-retractor is placed into the abdomen (Fig. 41-23). The abdominal portion of the retractor is used to elevate the abdominal wall and shield underlying organs as a stitch of 0-gauge delayed-absorbable suture is placed parallel on one side of the fascial opening. This suture is not tied. This suturing step is repeated on the opposite fascial edge.

The distal, blunt end of the Hasson trocar then is inserted into the incision. The fascial tag sutures are pulled firmly upward and threaded into the suture holders found on either side of

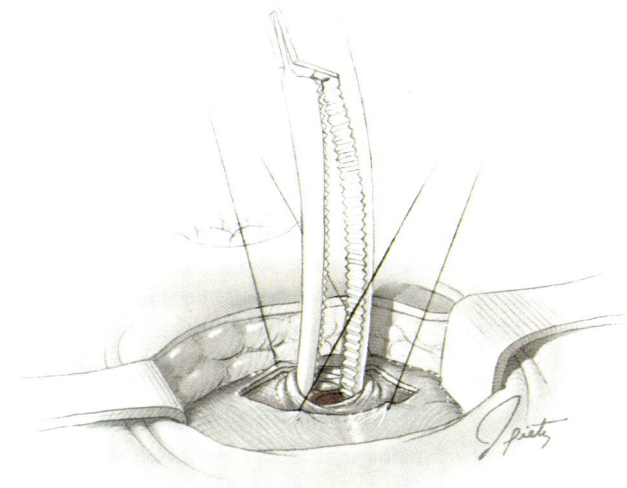

FIGURE 41-23 Peritoneal entry during open entry.

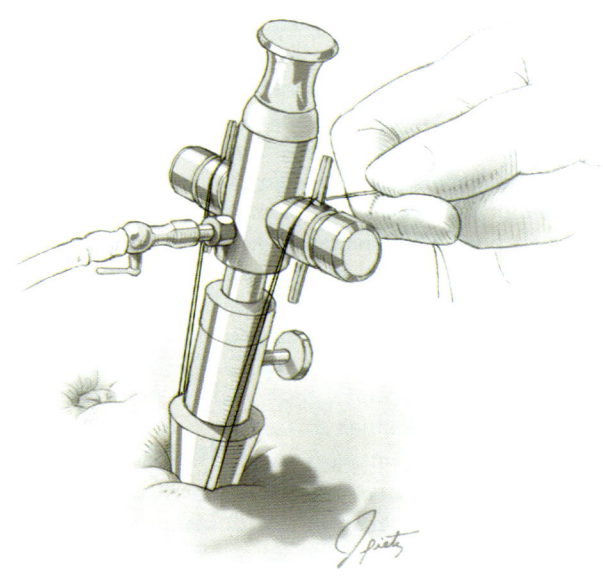

FIGURE 41-24 Primary trocar placement with open entry.

the cannula's proximal end (Fig. 41-24). The blunt obturator is removed, and the laparoscope is threaded through the cannula.

In a review of more than 5000 open entry procedures, Hasson and associates (2000) noted that minor and medium-risk complications developed at a rate of 0.5 percent. Moreover, in studies comparing open and closed techniques, open methods showed lower rates of entry failure and organ injury (Bonjer, 1997; Merlin, 2003). Open entry is recommended by many surgeons for patients with prior abdominal surgery, for those following a closed technique entry failure, for those with a large cystic mass, and for pediatric or pregnant patients (Madeb, 2004). This technique, however, is not foolproof, and organ injury, mainly bowel, has been described (Magrina, 2002). Typically, this method of entry takes longer than closed entry, and the pneumoperitoneum can be difficult to maintain in some cases due to air escape around the cannula.

■ Alternative Entry Sites
Anterior Abdominal Wall

At times, the umbilicus may be unsuitable for initial abdominal entry, and surgeons should develop comfort with entry at other sites. Of concerns, adhesive disease may tether bowel beneath the umbilicus and is suspected in women with prior intraabdominal surgery, infection, endometriosis, or malignancy (see Table 41-1). Similarly, surgical mesh placed during umbilical herniorrhaphy is linked with adhesive disease, and entry at this site may disrupt the hernia repair. Nonumbilical entry can also avoid inadvertent trauma to or rupture of a large abdominal mass or gravid uterus.

Nonumbilical anterior abdominal wall entry has been described at various locations. The left upper quadrant is most common, but the subxiphoid area is another. Both have the advantage of providing working ports at these sites once safe entry is achieved.

Of these, left upper quadrant entry is simple, has a low risk of complications, and usually is free of adhesions (Agarwala, 2005; Howard, 1997; Palmer, 1974). Although left upper quadrant access may be obtained at either the Palmer point or the ninth intercostal space, the easy accessibility of the Palmer point makes this a favored site (Fig. 41-25). The Palmer point is located 3 cm below the left costal margin in the midclavicular line. Organs in proximity to this point are the stomach, left lobe of the liver, spleen, and retroperitoneal structures, which may be as close as 1.5 cm (Giannios, 2009; Tulikangas, 2000).

For entry at the Palmer point, one ensures that the stomach is emptied using suction with an orogastric or nasogastric tube. Palpating the area will ensure adequate emptying and exclude incidental splenomegaly. A skin incision adequate for trocar insertion is made at the Palmer point. With anterior abdominal wall elevation, the Veress needle is inserted in the skin incision at an angle slightly less than 90 degrees and is directed caudad. Initial intraabdominal pressure of <10 mm Hg indicates correct intraperitoneal placement. Once adequate insufflation is obtained, the Veress needle may be removed and a trocar inserted. Alternatively, direct trocar entry may be performed at the Palmer point as well. We favor an optical access trocar to permit each layer of the anterior abdominal wall to be seen as it is penetrated (Vellinga, 2009). The trocar is directed at a 90-degree angle. During insertion, one should observe the following sequence: subcutaneous fat, outer fascial layer, muscle layer, inner fascial layer, peritoneum, and finally, abdominal organs. Remember that above the level of

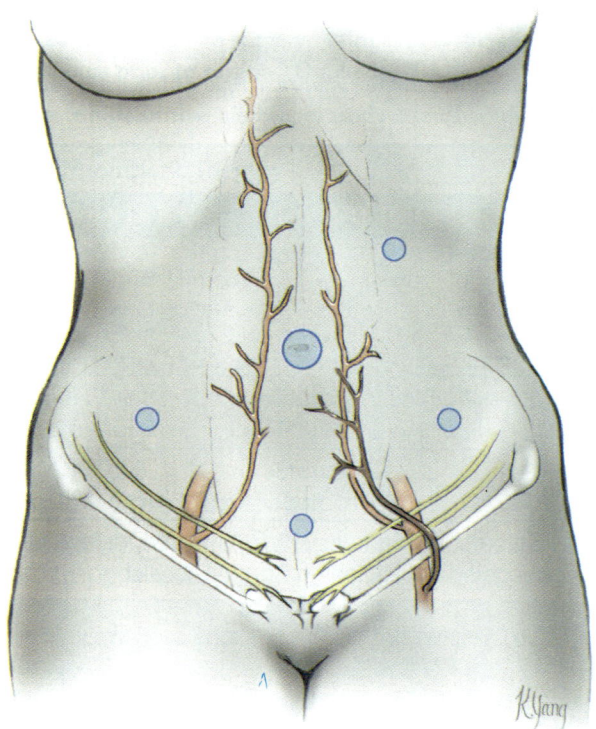

FIGURE 41-25 Common abdominal access sites include a primary entry site at the umbilicus and smaller accessory trocar sites in the lower abdomen. A frequent alternative primary entry site is the Palmer point in the left upper quadrant.

the arcuate line, posterior rectus sheath fascia is present and is the inner fascial layer.

Natural Orifice Transluminal Endoscopic Surgery

This method uses existing natural orifices such as the vagina, stomach, bladder, and rectum to access the peritoneum. In addition, a transuterine approach has been described. Although infrequently used in current practice, interest is renewed in laparoscopic access through the posterior fornix. Proposed advantages of this method are improved access to organs, better cosmesis from elimination of an external scar, shorter hospitalizations, and possibly less postoperative pain and fewer postoperative complications.

■ Single-Port Access Laparoscopy

Single-incision surgery is a laparoscopic approach in which a sole 2- to 3-cm incision accommodates a single larger port that concurrently houses multiple instruments. It is also known as single-incision laparoscopic surgery (SILS), laparoendoscopic single-site surgery (LESS), and single-port access (SPA). The proposed advantages of this method are improved cosmesis from a single port, which is usually buried in the umbilicus, and possibly faster return to normal activity. This is balanced against the longer incision that potentially has greater risks for postoperative pain, wound infection or dehiscence, and incisional hernia. Moreover, single-incision surgery is technically more challenging than conventional laparoscopy due to instrument crowding at a single port, limited visualization, and loss of instrument triangulation (Uppal, 2011). However, SPA has grown in popularity with advances in articulating instruments and flexible-tip endoscopes, which help deal with some of these challenges.

For laparoscopic SPA, several ports are popular. The SILS port (Covidien) is limited to umbilical placement and may not be suitable for large pathology that encroaches on the umbilicus. The GelPOINT (Applied Medical) may be inserted almost anywhere on the abdominal wall due to the variable depth of its self-retaining sheath attached between the two rigid loops. Moreover, the gel dome lacks preset silos for the trocars, and thus allows any size trocar to be inserted in individualized groupings.

For robotic SPA, the Single Site port (da Vinci) is placed in the umbilicus and contains cannulas for the curved trocars used in this approach (see Fig. 41-15F). However, this system can be placed only at specific abdominal wall sites. Instrument choices and movement also are more limited. For example, original robotic wristed models are not offered, but the longer curved trocars may offer sufficient instrument triangulation.

■ Gasless Laparoscopy

This variation of traditional laparoscopy addresses the physiologic disadvantages of pneumoperitoneum. With this method, an abdominal wall lift device elevates the abdominal wall to create the laparoscopic working space, and thus no gas is required. This technique affords advantages in obese patients who often poorly tolerate pneumoperitoneum combined with Trendelenburg position. For the pregnant patient, the fetal effect from CO_2 exposure and uterine pressure effect is eliminated (Akira, 2005). Additional advantages include the sustained visualization after colpotomy or with continuous suctioning. Drawbacks are a "tent-shaped" operating space, additional required incisions, and time needed for the lift device assembly. These currently limit its routine use, but gasless laparoscopy may still have value in high-risk patients with cardiorespiratory diseases (Cravello, 1999; Goldberg, 1997).

■ Accessory Port Placement

Once primary abdominal access is achieved, additional operative ports are needed to insert instruments. The number, location, and size of these cannulas will vary depending on the tools required and the laparoscopic procedure. For additional port placement, the patient is placed in Trendelenburg position to displace bowel from the pelvis and provide an unobstructed view. Ancillary trocars are always placed under direct laparoscopic visualization to minimize the puncture risk to anterior abdominal wall vessels or abdominal viscera.

Appropriate ancillary port site selection is a key step in operative planning. Correct placement permits triangulation. Poorly placed ports may create instrument angles that lead to ineffective movement, surgeon fatigue, and iatrogenic complications. Of sites, the suprapubic midline site is most frequently used. Prior to trocar insertion, the bladder is emptied, and the trocar is placed after identification of both the bladder and the urachus. For operative laparoscopy, placement of two lower quadrant ports lateral to the inferior epigastric vessels also is common. Their sites are individualized according to patient anatomy and pathology. Generally, larger pelvic masses require more cephalad placement.

During accessory port placement, transillumination of the anterior abdominal wall is useful to avoid puncture of the superficial epigastric vessels. In this process, the laparoscope, within the abdominal cavity, is placed directly against the peritoneal surface of the anterior wall. This light is seen externally as a red circular glow, and the superficial epigastric arteries are seen as dark vessels traversing it.

Unfortunately, the inferior epigastric arteries lie deep to the rectus abdominis muscle and are poorly seen with transillumination. These arteries, however, can be laparoscopically viewed directly in most cases (see Fig. 41-17) (Hurd, 2003). Also, landmarks can be used to limit vessel puncture risks. The main stem of the inferior epigastric artery can be avoided if trocars are inserted within the lateral third of the distance between the midline and anterior superior iliac spine (ASIS) (Epstein, 2004). Rahn and colleagues (2010) noted that the inferior epigastric vessels were 3.7 cm from the midline at the level of the ASIS and were always lateral to the rectus abdominis muscle at a level 2 cm superior to the pubic symphysis.

Ideally, port placement will also minimize the risk of ilioinguinal and iliohypogastric nerve injury (see Fig. 41-25). Most injuries to these nerves and to the inferior epigastric vessels can be averted by placing the accessory ports superior to the ASIS and >6 cm from the abdomen's midline (Rahn, 2010). Once all ports are positioned, the planned procedure is begun.

Newer modification of the traditional trocar now allows insufflation of a balloon incorporated into the trocar shaft.

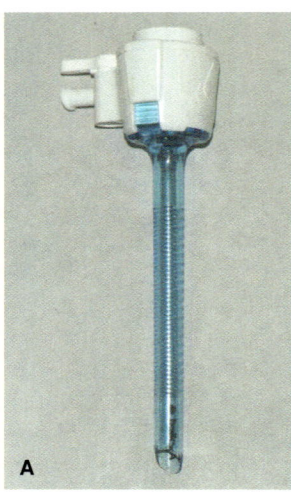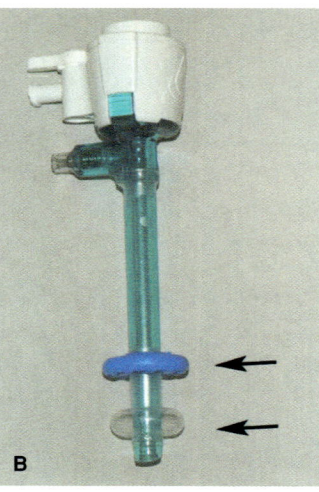

FIGURE 41-26 A. Traditional trocar. **B.** Balloon trocar. Once inserted into the abdomen, the distal balloon can be inflated (*lower arrow*) and then is pulled up tight against the peritoneum. The blue flange (*upper arrow*) is slid down and pressed against the abdominal wall skin. This apposition allows fixation of the cannula against the abdominal wall.

Shown in Figure 41-26, balloons secure the trocar at the appropriate depth and minimize the risk of the trocar being pulled out of the abdomen.

■ Tissue Extraction

Near the end of many MIS procedures, safe tissue extraction is an essential step. However, port-site seeding and inadvertent dissemination of both benign and malignant tissue during specimen fragmentation and extraction are risks. Several studies have described peritoneal leiomyomatosis, parasitic myomas, and de novo endometriosis following power morcellation of uteri and

myomas (Kho, 2009; Milad, 2014; Sepilian, 2003). Moreover, morcellation of occult cancer may worsen patient prognosis. This may be particularly likely with uterine sarcoma (Park, 2011; Pritts, 2015). That said, the risk of encountering an unexpected uterine sarcoma during surgery for presumed benign disease is rare, and rates range from 0.09 to 0.6 percent (Kho, 2016; Lieng, 2015; Multinu, 2019). Still, the FDA (2018) issued mandatory labeling that contraindicates use in those with known malignancy. Moreover, this FDA contraindication extends to peri- or postmenopausal women with myomas, in whom the cancer risk is greater. Last, it is contraindicated for those in whom tissue can be removed in toto vaginally or by minilaparotomy. The American College of Obstetricians and Gynecologists (2019) also eschews morcellation in those with known cancer. This group promotes a greater shared decision-making and discussion between patient and surgeon regarding MIS benefits and cancer risks. It recognizes a potentially greater risk versus benefit in those aged 50 years and older.

Alternatives to power morcellation are varied. First, through minilaparotomy incisions ranging from 1 to 4 cm, myomas and uteri may be brought to the anterior abdominal wall (Fig. 44-8, p. 1040). Here, they can be hand morcellated with a scalpel or scissors and extracted (Alessandri, 2006; Panici, 2005).

Second, posterior colpotomy is safe and effective to open the cul-de-sac for bulky tissue removal (Ghezzi, 2012). As shown in Figure 41-27, a posterior colpotomy is created similar to that for vaginal hysterectomy. Namely, the cervix is lifted upward, and the vagina of the posterior fornix is stretched downward to create tension. Curved Mayo scissors then incise the intervening vaginal wall and peritoneum to enter the abdomen via the posterior cul-de-sac. Once entry is confirmed, vaginal retractors can be placed for exposure. Alternatively, posterior colpotomy can be completed during laparoscopy. As Figure 41-28 illustrates,

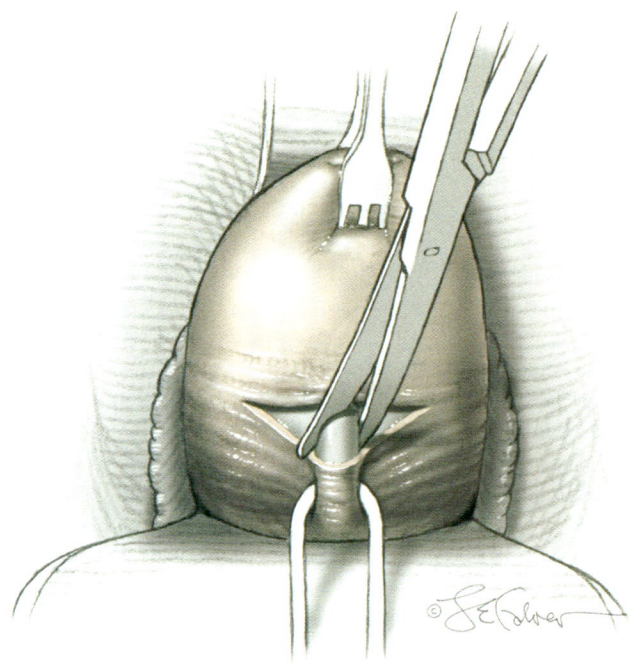

FIGURE 41-27 Posterior colpotomy incision from a vaginal approach.

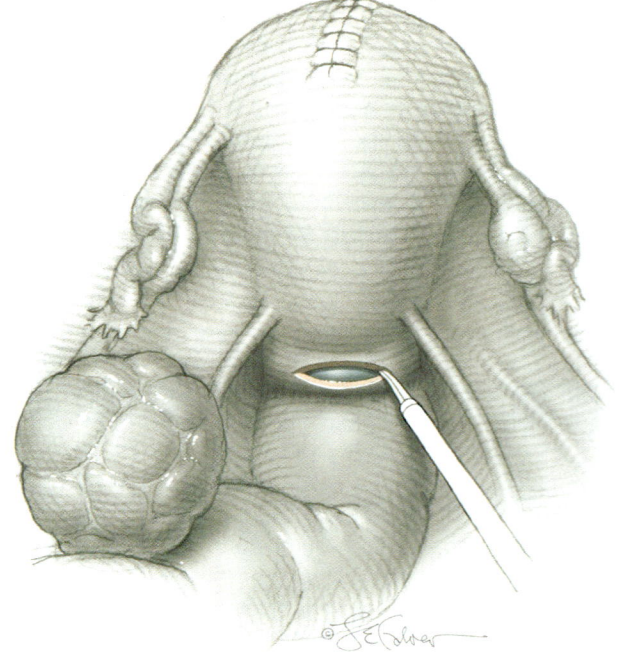

FIGURE 41-28 Posterior colpotomy incision from an abdominal approach.

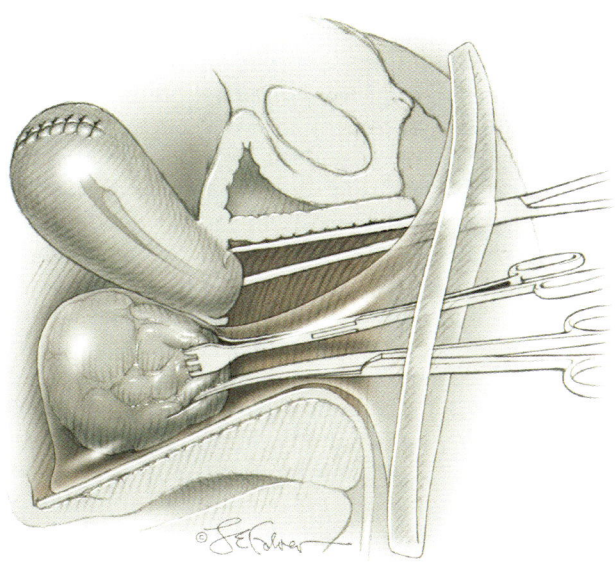

FIGURE 41-29 Through the posterior colpotomy, enclosed morcellation can be completed.

the uterosacral ligaments and ureters are first identified. A wide, blunt vaginal probe is inserted to elevate, accentuate, and stretch the posterior vaginal fornix for incision. Using an energy-based device, the vaginal wall is incised below the level of the cervix and between the uterosacral ligaments to create the posterior colpotomy incision. Whether through this opening or a mini-laparotomy, the addition of a tissue retrieval bag during tissue extraction can create a closed environment for morcellation (Fig. 41-29). This reduces the risk of inadvertent tissue dissemination during fragmentation, although long-term safety data are needed. A third method, enclosed power morcellation, is still being studied. It is described and illustrated on page 882.

Abdominal Entry Closure

The intraabdominal pressure produced by the pneumoperitoneum has an excellent hemostatic effect. Thus, at the end of cases, sites of potential bleeding are evaluated under a reduced pressure. A portion of the pneumoperitoneum is allowed to escape, and the intraabdominal pressure gauge is reset to 7 or 8 mm Hg.

With surgery completed, CO_2 insufflation is halted, and the gas tubing is disconnected from the primary cannula. The gas ports on all cannulas are opened to deflate the abdominal cavity. To prevent diaphragmatic irritation from retained CO_2, manual pressure is placed on the abdomen to help expel remaining gas. Next, cannulas are removed under laparoscopic visualization. This allows evaluation for bleeding from punctured vessels that may have been tamponaded by the cannula or the pneumoperitoneum. These sites and other potential bleeding sites are reinspected as the pneumoperitoneum diminishes. Additionally, visualization prevents herniation of bowel or omentum up through the cannula track and into the anterior abdominal wall. Once all secondary cannulas are out, the laparoscope and then the primary cannula are removed.

Many surgeons recommend reapproximation of fascial defects at port sites to prevent anterior abdominal wall hernia formation. Although closure of the fascial defect does not obviate the risk of hernia formation, in general, most surgeons close ancillary ports sites ≥10 mm. The fascia can be closed by direct visualization with the assistance of S-retractors. The fascia is grasped with Allis clamps and then reapproximated with interrupted stitches of 0-gauge delayed-absorbable suture. Also, several laparoscopic closure devices (Carter-Thomason, Endo Close, EFx Shield, and neoClose devices) are available. With these, fascial defects are reapproximated during direct laparoscopic visualization.

Skin incisions are closed with a subcuticular stitch of 4-0 delayed-absorbable suture. Alternatively, the skin may be closed with cyanoacrylate tissue adhesive (Dermabond) or with skin tape (Steri-Strip Elastic) and benzoin tincture (Chap. 40, p. 846).

For closure of an open entry incision, the sutures originally placed in the fascia are unthreaded from the cannula. Each of these sutures is brought to the midline of the incision, and square knots are tied to close the fascial defect. The skin is reapproximated in a manner similar to that just described.

SURGICAL BASICS

Tissue Approximation

Suturing Tools

Following tissue excision, reapproximation with suture is often needed. Subsequent knot tying may be performed using either inside the body, *intracorporeal*, or outside the body, *extracorporeal*, techniques. Newer devices can make these essential steps of surgery less challenging. Selection is based on the procedure planned, surgeon preference, and reapproximation goals.

Needles for MIS suturing typically pass through the placed ports. For this, the suture is grasped approximately 1 cm from the needle swage and passed through an appropriately sized cannula. Thus, the needle type chosen will depend on the size of available cannulas. One option, the ski needle, can pass through a narrow cannula (Fig. 41-30). However, its wide, flat arc prohibits suturing in tight anatomic spaces. Straight Keith needles also can be easily passed through cannulas of any size. Conventional needle shapes and sizes often require higher-diameter ports. Instead, larger needles that cannot fit directly through a cannula can be held by a grasping tool and passed through the port-site incision directly. This requires removing the cannula first.

Needle drivers are curved or straight and have either a smooth or finely serrated inner surface (Fig. 41-31). Driver tips are

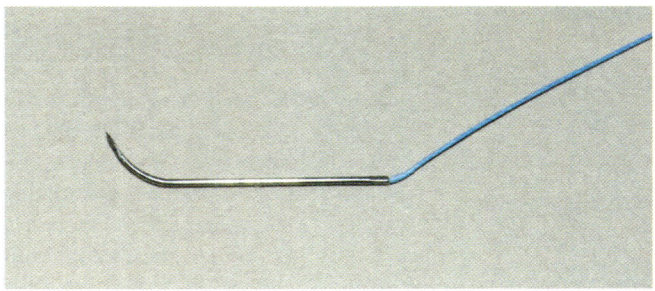

FIGURE 41-30 Ski needle.

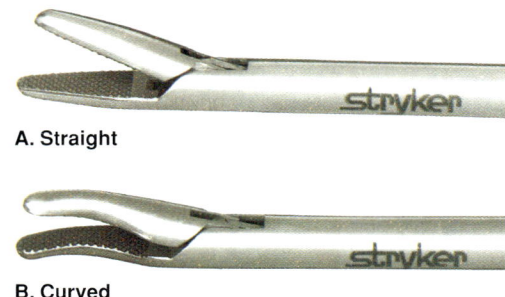

A. Straight

B. Curved

FIGURE 41-31 Laparoscopic needle driver. (Reproduced with permission from Stryker Endoscopy.)

tapered to limit tissue trauma. They also have a single-action jaw to provide a stable needle grasp. To assist with needle grasping, some driver tips are designed to guide the needle into a correct driving position. Termed *self-righting*, these drivers may be less desirable for suturing in difficult-to-reach anatomic spaces. Here, the needle may need to be grasped by the driver at an oblique angle to achieve correct suture placement. Other needle driver features include a coaxial (rotating) handle and a locking grip. These hold the needle in place yet decrease hand strain. With suturing, the needle driver is held in the dominant hand, while the nondominant hand holds a tissue grasper. Alternatively, some surgeons prefer to use a second needle driver in the nondominant hand. This assists in grasping the tissue, retrieving the needle or sutures from the dominant hand, and providing countertraction when needed.

Disposable suturing devices render needle drivers unnecessary for tissue approximation. The Endo Stitch is a 10-mm-diameter instrument with a double-action jaw. A short, straight needle juts at a right angle from the inner surface of one tip. As the instrument tips are closed, the needle passes through the desired tissue. Then, with the tips still closed and with the flip of a handle toggle, the detachable needle is released from the first tip and reanchors at a right angle into the opposite tip. Also, the RD 180 Running Device is a 5-mm instrument with a hooked tip that passes a straight needle through the tissue. These suturing tools have benefits and limitations, and familiarity is advantageous.

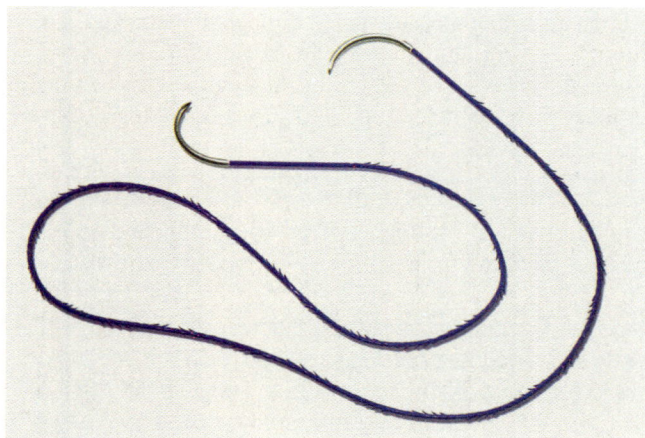

FIGURE 41-32 Barbed suture. (Reproduced with permission from Surgical Specialties Corporation.)

Suture selection depends primarily on the characteristics of tissues to be approximated and on the functional goals of reapproximation. Importantly, compared with traditional surgery, laparoscopic knot tying creates increased friction and suture fraying, and time between knot throws is longer. Thus, greater tensile strength and memory become more valued suture traits. For example, synthetic delayed-absorbable suture offers high tensile strength, less tissue reactivity, greater knot reliability, and easy handling for either intracorporeal or extracorporeal knot tying. Of filament types, although monofilament suture passes more smoothly through tissues, braided suture ties more easily and breaks less frequently. Catgut offers less tensile strength and less knot security. Accordingly, it is less popular for MIS. If used, intracorporeal knot tying is generally preferred due to the significant fraying that occurs with catgut suture during extracorporeal tying. Suture gauge selection mirrors that for open surgery (Chap. 40, p. 853).

Barbed sutures offer the unique ability to maintain tensile pressure on a continuous suture line. With this synthetic suture, multiple barbs are evenly spaced around the suture's outer surface (Fig. 41-32). These barbs flatten as they pass through the tissues to be approximated but flare out once through to the other side. These flared barbs prevent suture from slipping back through the approximated tissues. As a result, the tissues remain joined with evenly distributed tissue tension (Greenberg, 2008). By its design, this suture obviates the need for knot tying. Available barbed-suture products include Quill, Stratafix, and V-Loc sutures.

Barbed suture may be uni- or bidirectional, and these differ in the direction that suturing can proceed. *Unidirectional suture* has a small preformed loop at the tail end, which serve as the knot for that end of the suture line. Suturing moves from the looped end in the other direction. *Bidirectional suture* has needles at each end. Suturing begins at the incision midpoint and can then progress in both directions along the incision. With either suture type, the tissue is approximated by cinching the final suture line or placing a suture loop in the opposite direction. No final knot is needed to secure the suture line, which is held in place by the barbs. Alternatively, an anchoring hemostatic clip may be placed to secure the suture line end. In general, such barbed suture may be advantageous for myometrial reapproximation during laparoscopic myomectomy or for vaginal cuff closure during total laparoscopic hysterectomy. At completion of the running suture line, the suture is cut short to avoid puncture of adjacent tissue by a barb.

Knots

The length of suture will depend on the proposed suturing and knot tying. In general, 6 to 8 cm is needed for intracorporeal knot tying, and 24 to 36 cm for extracorporeal tying. Longer lengths are required for running stitches and for complex knots compared with simple interrupted stitches.

Once a stitch is completed, a knot secures the suture loop. The throws for a knot may be intracorporeal or extracorporeal. Of the two, intracorporeal tying has a steeper learning curve because the surgeon must use laparoscopic instruments rather than fingers to loop the suture (Fig. 41-33). Extracorporeal knot tying is simpler for most surgeons because the suture is looped with fingers as in traditional tying. Each formed knot

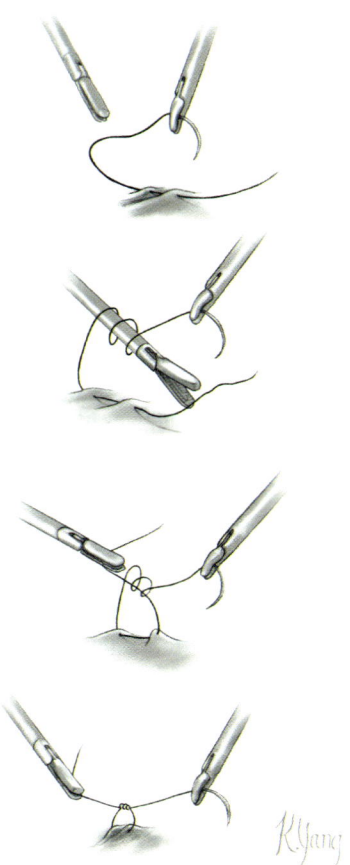

FIGURE 41-33 Intracorporeal knot tying.

throw is then guided through the laparoscopic cannula and cinched with a knot pusher to create the knot (Fig. 41-34). Of suture types, stronger braided suture is preferred if the knot pusher is used because suture fraying is a side effect of this technique. Another disadvantage of extracorporeal knot tying compared with intracorporeal methods is that it often causes more tissue tension and can tear delicate tissues.

As an alternative to manual knot tying, disposable clips can be placed at the end of a suture line for security. Specifically, a hemoclip is a titanium V-shaped clip with arms that can be squeezed together during application. These clips were originally designed to compress vessels for hemostasis and are available in various sizes. If used for this purpose, two clips are advisable. More recent developments include the Lapra-Ty. This has a locking clip made of delayed-absorbable polydioxanone. Its ability to be absorbed and its lock are advantages, whereas the applicator's need for a 11- to 12-mm port may be disadvantageous. Also, these ties are only approved to anchor suture diameters greater than 4-0. Another option is the 5-mm Ti-KNOT instrument. With this disposable device, a special titanium clip is placed around a

single or a double strand of suture. With any of these alternatives to laparoscopic knot tying, the cost may be justified by the time saved in the operating room.

Stapling

In gynecologic surgery, vascular tissue is typically ligated and then excised. Ligation is achieved with electrosurgical tools described earlier (p. 883), with stapling devices, or with suture loops. Linear staplers are mainly used for creating anastomoses as in bowel surgery and are not frequently employed for gynecologic procedures. When selected, they are chiefly used to ligate vascular pedicles, such as the infundibulopelvic ligament. Once fired, the stapler lays down three staggered double rows of staples while sharply dividing tissue in between.

Staplers are available in 35-cm or 45-cm lengths and contain an end called the "anvil," which houses the staple cartridges. *Vascular cartridges* apply staples that are 1 mm high when closed. *Tissue cartridges* apply those that are 1.5 mm when closed and are suitable for thicker pedicles. Stapling provides hemostasis with gentle handling of tissue, which ideally leads to less necrosis and better healing.

Newer models have added articulating and rotating capabilities at the jaw. These attributes permit stapling at an angle. Most staples are titanium. However, newer angled staplers for the vaginal cuff use delayed-absorbable material such as polyglactin 910 for their staples. A main limitation to stapler use is generally the price of the device and cartridges, which can be costly compared with suture. However, if operating time is reduced, these costs can be negligible.

Suture Loops

Preformed suture loops, such as the Endoloop, also may be used to ligate tissue pedicles (Fig. 41-35). This instrument has a

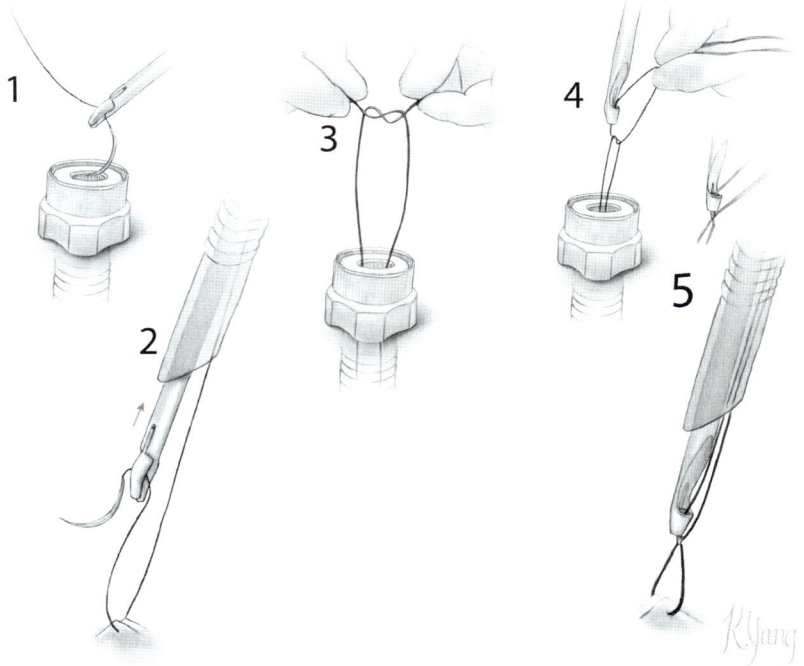

FIGURE 41-34 Extracorporeal knot tying.

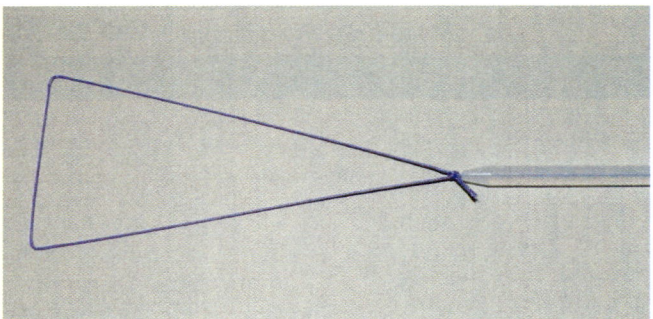

FIGURE 41-35 Laparoscopic suture loop.

length of suture housed within a stiff, 5-mm-diameter rod and has a pretied loop at the end. The loop is guided around the pedicle by the stiff rod and then is cinched like a noose. The rod tip, similar to an index finger during manual knot tying, adds pressure to secure the knot in place. Loops of absorbable, delayed-absorbable, and permanent suture are available. Other types of knots that are pretied loops include the Roeder knot, Meltzer knot, and Tayside knot. These currently are not as popular as the square knot.

■ Laparoscopic Dissection Techniques

Pelvic adhesions are often lysed to reestablish normal anatomy for planned surgery. Some situations require sharp dissection, especially if adhesions are not amenable to blunt tissue separation. For cutting fine adhesions, the tissue band may be placed on gentle stretch using an atraumatic grasper or blunt probe. Curved scissors with a dissecting tip or an energy modality (monopolar, bipolar, or harmonic) are often used.

If denser adhesions are found, they are divided in layers to prevent injury to adjacent adhered organs. The technique mirrors that for open surgery and is illustrated in Chapter 40 (p. 848). The use of energy sources in these situations is generally discouraged, as thermal injury may have a wider effect that may not be readily apparent. Conversely, a sharp cut is easier to identify and repair intraoperatively.

Hydrodissection is another method often used in MIS. With this, normal saline or other irrigation fluid is injected under pressure to separate tissue planes. For example, peritoneal endometriosis can be lifted and excised with greater ease and less trauma to retroperitoneal structures. Other uses include resection of cysts from an ovary, removal of ectopic products from a fallopian tube, or separation of tissue planes that might be obscured or in close proximity to vascular spaces or bowel. As shown in Figure 41-36, an atraumatic grasper lifts the tissue at the junction point, and a needle tip is inserted with the bevel away from the structure to be protected. Irrigation fluid is injected and creates a balloon effect. Depending on the location, 5 to 30 mL of fluid is instilled. A suction-irrigation system also is helpful for this technique. With this instrument, once the peritoneum is incised, the suction tip is insinuated into the opening. Fluid is forced to gently separate the tissue planes. Often, hydrodissection allows a surgeon to identify natural planes that might otherwise be obscured.

■ Hemostasis

As tissue planes are developed, bleeding is variably encountered. Requirements for vessel sealing differ according to vessel diameters. For small vessels, spot coagulation is suitable, and a monopolar tool is satisfactory and mimics the electrosurgical blade (Bovie) use in open procedures. For larger vessels, the bipolar or Harmonic technologies are preferred and described on page 884. When choosing a modality, the thermal spread of a device is considered. Last, microbipolar probes and needle-tip monopolar probes are useful for delicate tissues such as the fallopian tubes. The thermal spread is minimal, and the tip sizes are optimal for the small but friable vessels.

Liquid and powder topical hemostatic agents also have gained popularity and have been adapted for laparoscopic use (Table 40-6, p. 860). When using a laparoscopic adaptor, a portion of the matrix may remain in the applicator cannula. To avoid retained and thus wasted sealant, a surgeon flushes the cannula following initial matrix application. For this, a plunger is included in many sealant kits, or a syringe filled with air may be used to force matrix through the cannula and onto the desired tissue. Alternatively, an oxidized regenerated cellulose fabric sheet (Surgicel) can be applied.

HYSTEROSCOPIC CONSIDERATIONS

■ Patient Evaluation

Hysteroscopy provides an endoscopic view of the endocervical canal, endometrial cavity, and tubal ostia for both the diagnosis and operative treatment of intrauterine pathology. Development of smaller and more useful instruments permits many intrauterine procedures to now be performed in an office or outpatient setting.

Indications for hysteroscopy include evaluation and, in some cases, operative treatment of infertility, recurrent miscarriage, abnormal uterine bleeding, amenorrhea, and retained foreign bodies or products of conception. With hysteroscopic biopsy, abnormal bleeding can be accurately diagnosed and,

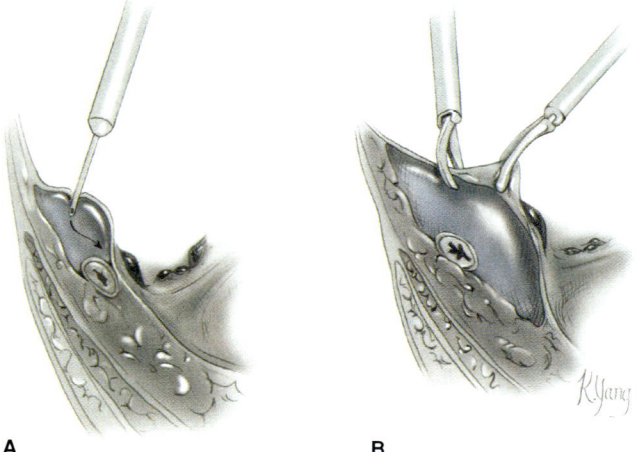

FIGURE 41-36 Hydrodissection. **A.** Needle insertion and fluid instillation to lift endometriotic implants off the adjacent ureter. **B.** Peritoneal excision of the implant.

in benign cases, treated by polypectomy, myomectomy, or endometrial ablation. Infertility may be improved with resection of a uterine septum or removal of intrauterine adhesions (synechiae). Additionally, proximal tubal obstruction can be relieved. For those seeking sterilization, Essure hysteroscopic tubal occlusion is no longer marketed due to long-term safety concerns (Chap. 5, p. 120).

Because the indications for hysteroscopy are varied, patient evaluations for specific disorders are discussed in their respective chapters. However, continuing pregnancy is an absolute contraindication to hysteroscopy and is excluded with serum or urine β-human chorionic gonadotropin testing prior to surgery. In addition, cervicitis, vaginitis, and pelvic infection are treated prior to hysteroscopy, and screening for *Neisseria gonorrhoeae* and *Chlamydia trachomatis* in those with risk factors is considered (Table 1-1, p. 4). Preoperative endometrial sampling may be completed for those with abnormal bleeding and who have additional risk factors for endometrial cancer. Although seeding of the peritoneal cavity with cancer cells has been noted following hysteroscopy, overall long-term prognosis is not negatively affected (Chap. 8, p. 187) (Kyrgiou, 2013; Soucie, 2012). Hysteroscopy is considered acceptable as part of the evaluation of abnormal uterine bleeding (American College of Obstetricians and Gynecologists, 2018a).

If diagnostic hysteroscopy is planned to locate and remove a uterine foreign body, preoperative imaging is helpful. Sonography, especially 3-D transvaginal sonography (TVS), is usually easily obtained. If a foreign body is suspected to be outside the uterus or pelvis and is radiopaque, conventional abdominal radiographs can help narrow its location. The addition of lateral or oblique views can enhance localization.

■ Patient Consenting

Complication rates for women undergoing hysteroscopy are low and cited at <1 to 3 percent (Jansen, 2000; McGurgan, 2015; Propst, 2000). Some complications mirror those associated with dilation and curettage and include false cervical pathway creation, uterine perforation, cervical laceration, hemorrhage, and postoperative endometritis. Gas venous embolism and excessive intravascular fluid absorption are uncommon risks discussed later. Last, hemorrhage or perforation with sharp or electrosurgical instruments may require immediate laparoscopy or laparotomy to evaluate surrounding organs or vessels. Thus, patients are counseled regarding the possible need for these added surgeries. In general, the complication rate rises in concert with the length and complexity of a procedure.

■ Patient Preparation

Infectious and VTE complications after hysteroscopic surgery are rare. Thus, preoperative antibiotics or VTE prophylaxis is typically not required (American College of Obstetricians and Gynecologists, 2018b,c).

Endometrial Thickness

In premenopausal women, hysteroscopy is ideally performed in the early proliferative phase of the menstrual cycle, when the endometrium is relatively thin. This allows small masses to be more easily identified and removed. Alternatively, progestins, combination oral contraceptives, danazol, and gonadotropin-releasing hormone (GnRH) agonists have preoperatively been administered individually to induce endometrial atrophy. Disadvantageously, these agents may add expense, pose side effects, alter histology, and delay surgery.

Cervical Ripening

For operative hysteroscopy, cervical dilation is typically required to insert an 8- to 10-mm hysteroscope or resectoscope. To ease dilation and lower the risk of uterine perforation, cervical preparation is considered. Misoprostol (Cytotec), a prostaglandin E_1 analogue, may be administered orally the night before and, if desired, again the morning of surgery to aid cervical softening (Al-Fozan, 2015; Salazar, 2018). Commonly used dosing options include 200 or 400 µg vaginally or 400 µg orally once 12 to 24 hours prior to surgery. Possible side effects are cramping, uterine bleeding, or nausea. Bleeding may limit endoscopic visualization, and excessive dilation can lead to media escape and poor cavity distention. Thus, the need for cervical softening is balanced against these potential side effects. Misoprostol may also be valuable for overcoming cervical stenosis, described later (p. 903).

For preoperative cervical ripening, laminaria are another option. These osmotic dilators are described and illustrated in Chapter 43 (p. 972).

HYSTEROSCOPIC INSTRUMENTS

■ Rigid Hysteroscope

Hysteroscopy requires an endoscope (hysteroscope), fiberoptic light source, uterine distention medium, and video camera. Most hysteroscopes consists of a 3- to 4-mm-diameter endoscope surrounded by an outer sheath, which directs fluid. Smaller diameter hysteroscopes are available, although their use may be limited by lower light intensity and a decreased field of view.

Hysteroscopes are broadly classified as diagnostic or operative. Diagnostic hysteroscopes may be rigid or flexible and offer a small diameter. As such, they provide an adequate endometrial cavity view yet often require no cervical dilation. Operative hysteroscopes have sheaths that increase the overall diameter and require cervical dilation in most cases. Thus, cases requiring operative hysteroscopes are most often managed in a setting in which minimal sedation or regional or general anesthesia can be administered.

Individual endoscopes offer specific angles of view. Although 0° through 70° angles are available, 0° hysteroscopes allow the easiest orientation within the uterine cavity for most procedures (Fig. 41-37). The 12° to 70° angles provide additional lateral views, which may aid complex operative procedures. Devices with views even greater than 70° are available but infrequently used.

Adequate illumination of the endometrial cavity is essential. In general, the light source system used in hysteroscopy mirrors that used for laparoscopy (p. 886). Light is delivered to the endoscope by a fiberoptic cable, which is attached directly to the endoscope during assembly.

As noted, the outer sheath surrounds the endoscope and directs the distending medium, and in some cases instruments, to the endometrial cavity. A single-channel outer sheath directs

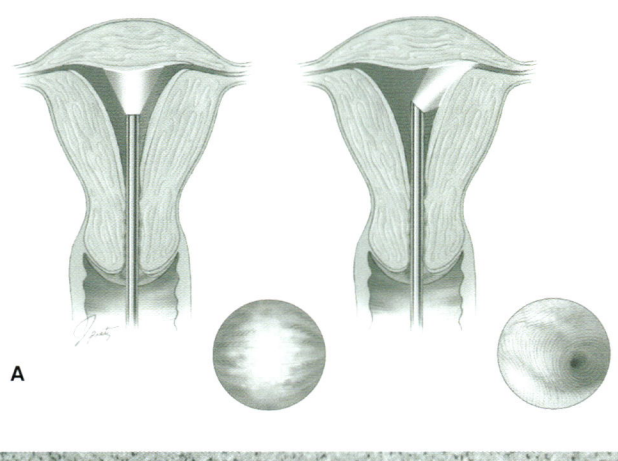

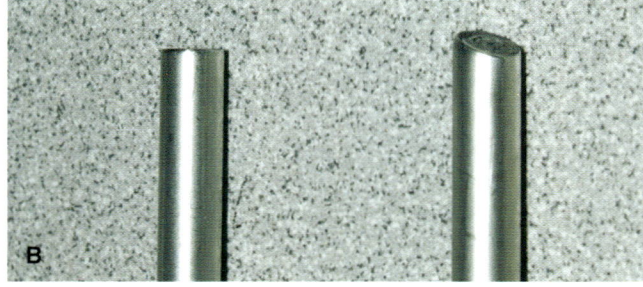

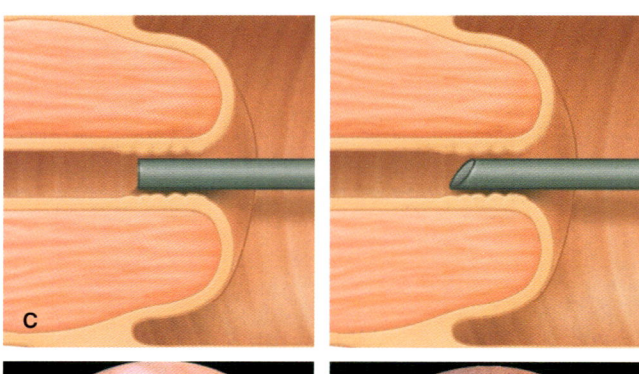

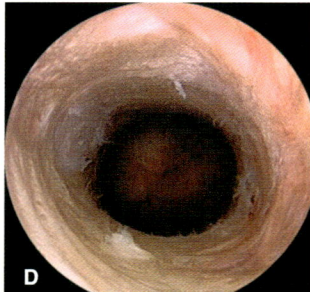
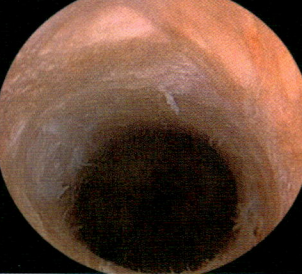

FIGURE 41-37 Differences between a 0-degree hysteroscope (*left*) and 30-degree hysteroscope (*right*). **A.** Intracavitary views. **B.** A 30-degree endoscope has an angled tip. **C.** Correct hysteroscope insertion results in each of the respective views seen in (**D**).

only inflow of distention fluid and is useful for simple diagnostic procedures. This outer sheath is 4 to 5 mm in diameter and round and thus can often successfully enter the cavity without the need for cervical dilation. This avoids causing minor trauma or bleeding in the endocervical canal.

In addition to a traditional hysteroscope, the Endosee also offers a small diameter for diagnostic viewing. This tool contains a reusable handle and a built-in 5-inch touch-screen for viewing

and documentation (Fig. 44-12.1, p. 1054). The handle attaches to a single-use, semi-rigid, hysteroscopic cannula that measures 4.3 mm at its tip. A single channel permits distention medium inflow, and the latest version features a 5F working channel for small biopsy instruments or graspers (Connor, 2015; Munro, 2015). Similarly, the LiNA Operåscope is a disposable hysteroscope and offers the advantage of an outflow channel and operative channel for use of 5.5F disposable scissors and graspers.

In general, disadvantages to all smaller, single-channel hysteroscopes are diminished illumination, poor clearing of mucus or blood from the cavity, and the need to change to a larger hysteroscope for operative procedures. However, once the architecture of the cervix and uterus are visualized and understood, cervical dilation and insertion of a larger-diameter operative endoscope may often be completed more safely.

In contrast, a larger, dual-channel outer sheath permits continuous inflow and outflow of a distention medium. This sheath, coupled with a fluid management system, allows efficient clearing of mucus and blood from the cavity and accurate fluid deficit measurement. This deficit reflects the volume of fluid that has entered or *intravasated* into the patient's vascular system.

Also in the outer sheath of an operative hysteroscope, semi-rigid, rigid, or flexible instruments can be passed through an operating channel. A basic set that suffices for most procedures includes biopsy forceps, grasping forceps, and scissors. Of these, biopsy forceps are somewhat sharp and cuplike. Grasping forceps permit removal of tissue or foreign bodies and may be toothed. Last, scissors can lyse adhesions, resect masses, or excise an intrauterine septum. Generally 5F in diameter and 34 to 40 cm long, these instruments are much smaller than those used with a resectoscope. They require no electrosurgical energy or special distention medium. Neodymium:Yttrium-Aluminum-Garnet (Nd:YAG) laser fibers for vaporization of benign tissue abnormalities also can be threaded through the operating channel. However, this technique is infrequently used today.

■ Bettocchi Hysteroscope

This small, 4- to 5-mm-diameter rigid operative hysteroscope has a 5F (1.67 mm) instrument channel that provides operative capability and bidirectional medium flow. Available in 0-degree and angled views, its main advantage is its small diameter (Bradley, 2009).

■ Flexible Hysteroscope

This is similar to the flexible laparoscopes described earlier (p. 885), but their diameter approximates that of a single-channel rigid hysteroscope. Using a thumb control, the endoscope tip will flex across a range of 120 to 160 degrees. Coupled with the rotation of the endoscope around its long axis, this flexion offers great maneuverability within irregular-shaped endometrial cavities. However, its smaller-diameter fiberoptic cable lessens illumination.

Flexible hysteroscopes are most often used diagnostically. However, a few flexible instruments are available to pass through the operating channel. This can be helpful for gaining tubal access, obtaining tissue biopsy, or lysing adhesions. Flexible hysteroscopes may cause less intraoperative pain than rigid ones and may make them better suited for office procedures (Marsh, 2004).

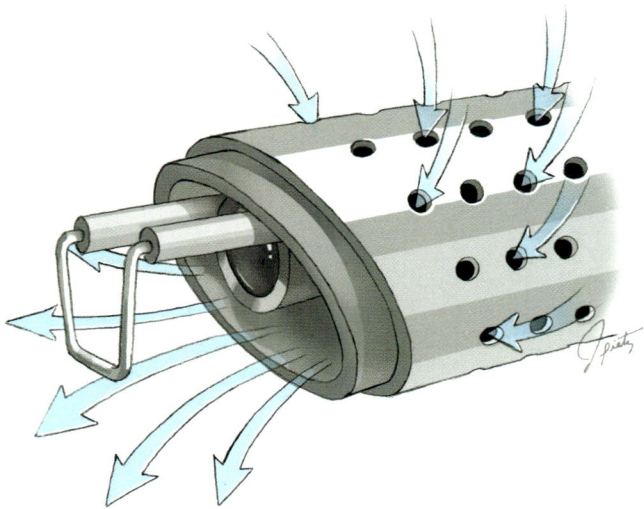

FIGURE 41-38 Resectoscope.

Resectoscope

If excision of intrauterine tissues is planned, a hysteroscopic resectoscope may be used. The 8- to 10-mm-diameter instrument contains a rigid endoscope, a working element to which various electrosurgical electrodes can be attached, and dual channels for fluid circulation. Specifically, the outflow channel allows fluid egress through a series of small holes near the distal end of the sheath (Fig. 41-38).

The working element can be extended and then retracted by means of a spring mechanism. Of electrodes that can attach to this element, the wire resection loop is used to shave off contacted tissues. Other electrodes include a roller ball or roller bar and a vaporizing electrode, which is sometimes called a twizzle tip. Both monopolar and bipolar electrosurgical modalities are available for these instruments.

During resectoscope loop tissue shaving, blood vessels in the endometrium and myometrium are opened, and fluid can thereby intravasate. Thus, fluid deficit calculations are ideally updated throughout each procedure.

Hysteroscopic Morcellator

Several morcellation devices help remove intracavitary polyps, submucous myomas, septa, retained products of conception, or intrauterine synechiae. These procedures are described in Chapter 44 (p. 1059). The morcellator tip contains a rotating or oscillating blade that shaves off contacted tissue. Compared with a resectoscope, one morcellator advantage is its ability to suction through its outflow channel. This permits simultaneous evacuation of tissue fragments. Importantly, hysteroscopic morcellation is not associated with the same risk of intraabdominal spread of endometrial, myomatous, or cancerous tissue as may occur with laparoscopic morcellation devices.

Hysteroscopic Electrosurgery

Many of the widely used hysteroscopic tissue resection or desiccation techniques rely on monopolar current. Because current is dissipated and is thus ineffective in electrolyte solutions, these techniques have typically required nonelectrolyte solutions such as sorbitol, mannitol, and glycine. However, these media can be associated with hyponatremia if fluid volume overload develops intraoperatively (p. 903). Alternatively, bipolar electrosurgical systems allow use of traditional hysteroscopic tools in a saline distention medium. Like the monopolar resectoscope, resection loop electrodes, ball electrodes, and twizzle tips are available.

DISTENTION MEDIA

Because the anterior and posterior uterine walls lie in apposition, a distending medium is required to expand the endometrial cavity for viewing. Historically, dextran and CO_2 were selected for diagnostic hysteroscopy. However, both are now infrequently used and replaced by low-viscosity fluid media that include normal saline and electrolyte-poor fluids such as sorbitol, mannitol, and glycine. Each has distinct advantages and properties (Table 41-2).

While navigating the endocervical canal during initial entry, pressures of 100 to 120 mm Hg may be required. Once inside the cavity, pressures are then lowered to a minimum that sufficiently maintains a clear endometrial cavity for viewing. Typically, to expand the cavity, intrauterine pressures of these media must reach 45 to 80 mm Hg. Simple gravity, that is, hanging the fluid bag approximately 1 meter above the patient, will yield approximately 70 mm Hg of pressure at the hysteroscope. This is suitable for many diagnostic examinations. However, for more complex and operative cases, needed hydrostatic pressures are usually generated by a formal fluid-management-system pump.

Gas Distention

If used under pressure, CO_2 tends to flatten the endometrium and provides excellent visibility. A continuous flow is necessary to replace gas lost through the tubing, and flow rates of 40 to 50 mL/min are typically adequate. Rates higher than 100 mL/min are associated with a greater risk for gas embolism and therefore discouraged. Specialized hysteroscopic insufflators, which limit maximum flow rates, must be used. *Importantly, because laparoscopic insufflating machines can permit flow rates >1000 mL/min, these machines should never be used for hysteroscopy* (American College of Obstetricians and Gynecologists, 2018a).

Disadvantages to CO_2 include its tendency, when mixed with blood or mucus, to form gas bubbles, which lower visibility. Use of CO_2 with thermal energy sources produces smoke and also prohibits adequate viewing. Because of these limitations, CO_2 is best used in cases in which minimal bleeding is anticipated, such as diagnostic hysteroscopy.

Fluid Media

Blood, mucus, and proteinaceous debris are usually present in the endometrial cavity during operative hysteroscopy. For this reason, a fluid distention medium is typically selected because of its optical clarity and ability to mix with blood. These media are characterized according to their viscosity and electrolyte status.

TABLE 41-2. Hysteroscopic Media

Medium	Properties	Indications	Risks	Safety Measures
Gas				
Carbon dioxide	Colorless gas	Diagnostic	Gas embolism	Avoid Trendelenburg Keep flow <100 mL/min Intrauterine pressure <100 mm Hg
Electrolyte fluid				
0.9% saline	Isotonic 380 mOsm/kg H_2O	Diagnostic Operative w/ bipolar tools	Volume overload	Plan to complete procedure as 2000-mL deficit approaches Stop procedure at 2.5-L deficit End earlier in patients with comorbidities or elderly
Lactated Ringer	Isotonic 273 mOsm/kg H_2O	Diagnostic Operative w/ bipolar tools	Volume overload	Same as above
Electrolyte-poor fluid				
Sorbitol 3%	Hypoosmolar 178 mOsm/kg H_2O	Operative w/monopolar tools	Volume overload Hyponatremia Hypoosmolality Hyperglycemia	Stop procedure at 1000-mL deficit End earlier in patients with comorbidities or elderly
Mannitol 5%	Isoosmolar 280 mOsm/kg H_2O	Operative w/monopolar tools	Volume overload Hyponatremia	Same as above
Glycine 1.5%	Hypoosmolar 200 mOsm/kg H_2O	Operative w/monopolar tools	Volume overload Hyponatremia Hypoosmolality Hyperammonemia	Same as above

Compiled from Cooper, 2000; American Association of Gynecologic Laparoscopists, 2013; American College of Obstetricians and Gynecologists, 2018a

Low-Viscosity Electrolyte Fluids

In general, these are preferred for modern hysteroscopy. An appropriate medium is selected based on its compatibility with electrosurgical instrumentation.

Normal saline and lactated Ringer solutions are isotonic, electrolyte-containing fluids. They are readily available in operating rooms and are frequently used for diagnostic hysteroscopy. Normal saline and lactated Ringer solutions cannot be used with monopolar electrosurgical devices. Namely, these fluids are capable of conducting electrical current; thus, dissipating instrument energy; and thereby rendering the instrument completely ineffective. Conversely, bipolar devices function regardless of the fluid electrolyte content.

The primary risk associated with isotonic, electrolyte-containing solutions is volume overload due to excess intravasation. The risk of acute hyponatremia with these is less than that with hypoosmolar fluids, described next. Still, rapid absorption of large volumes can lead to pulmonary edema.

Low-Viscosity, Electrolyte-Poor Fluids

Of other available media, 1.5-percent glycine, 3-percent sorbitol, and 5-percent mannitol are all low-viscosity, electrolyte-poor fluids. Because they are nonconductive, these media are used when monopolar electrosurgical energy devices are employed.

The primary risk associated with the use of hypotonic, hypoosmolar solutions is intravascular absorption of these media. Acute hyponatremia and hypoosmolality can develop and are associated with the potential for acute cerebral edema, seizure, respiratory arrest, and death.

Sorbitol is a six-carbon sugar and is metabolized following absorption. This effectively leaves free water in the intravascular space to lower serum sodium levels and osmolality. Sorbitol is metabolized to fructose and glucose and can also lead to hyperglycemia. Mannitol, also a six-carbon sugar, is isotonic at a concentration of 5 percent. It is not absorbed by renal tubules and thus serves as an osmotic diuretic. Because of this, serum osmolality is less affected (American Association of Gynecologic Laparoscopists, 2013; American College of Obstetricians and Gynecologists 2018a). Last, glycine, when metabolized, may create hyperammonemia due to release of amines.

Volume Management

For simple diagnostic procedures, inflow of distention media can be achieved by a gravity-fed bag of normal saline attached to the inflow port of the hysteroscope. However, for more complex or operative procedures, standard practice is to use a fluid management system, which provides continuous flow and accurate monitoring of a fluid deficit. Before the procedure and after priming the tubing and hysteroscope with the chosen medium, the fluid management system performs a series of calibrations that allow the device to closely approximate intrauterine pressure. During a procedure, measurement and documentation of the fluid deficit are performed at intervals of 15 minutes. More frequently deficit assessment may be prudent for procedure with greater risk for fluid intravasation. If a procedure has the potential for larger deficits, a Foley catheter is also reasonable to monitor urine output. In addition, ongoing communication with anesthesia staff regarding large fluid deficits is encouraged.

If a fluid deficit of a hypotonic solution approaches 1000 mL in an otherwise healthy patient, the surgeon ideally begins procedure termination. At a deficit of 1000 mL, the procedure should be terminated immediately (American Association of Gynecologic Laparoscopists, 2013). With normal saline or lactated Ringer distention medium, one should begin procedure termination at a deficit of 2000 mL. The procedure should be terminated when a deficit of 2500 mL is reached (American College of Obstetricians and Gynecologists 2018a). As discussed next, volume and electrolyte assessment are completed if these maximums are reached. At the end of every hysteroscopic procedure, a final deficit is determined, and this value is recorded in the operative note.

HYSTEROSCOPIC COMPLICATIONS

■ Volume Overload

Fluid absorption and volume overload may develop with any of the fluid media. Suggested mechanisms are: (1) absorption across the endometrium, (2) intraperitoneal absorption from fluid that has entered the abdomen through open fallopian tubes, and (3) intravascular transfer of fluid through surgically opened venous channels (intravasation). Of these, intravasation is the most closely linked to volume overload.

Most intravasation occurs through endometrial and myometrial veins exposed during tissue disruption or resection. First, thin-walled veins have lower intrinsic closing pressures and are more distensible than their arterial counterparts. Second, the venous side of the vasculature is a low-pressure system. That is, venous pressure in the pelvis of a supine patient is likely <10 to 15 mm Hg. As a result, intravasation of distention media is increased when the intrauterine pressure is elevated, when the number of disrupted blood vessels is great, and when the exposure time is long (Tuchschmid, 2008). Thus, the lowest inflow pressure that allows adequate visualization is preferably used. And, if tissue resection exposes the underlying vascular bed, procedure length is best minimized.

In the event of large fluid deficits, patients are assessed for signs of volume overload. Pulmonary auscultation, measurement of patient oxygenation with pulse oximetry, and extended observation are reasonable. Chest radiography may be indicated if pulmonary edema is suspected.

■ Acute Hyponatremia

In cases of large fluid deficits, measurement of serum electrolyte levels is reasonable. If a serum sodium level lower than 125 mEq/L is reached, care may ideally be continued in a critical care setting, in consultation with an Intensive Care or Internal Medicine specialist. Treatment includes immediate limitation of fluid intake and stimulation of diuresis with furosemide (Lasix), 20 to 40 mg given intravenously. Correction of hyponatremia is achieved with 3-percent sodium chloride, administered at a rate of 0.5 to 2 mL/kg/h. Acute neurologic symptoms and/or nausea and vomiting constitute a true medical emergency. Alternatively, 3-percent saline can instead be given in a 100 mL infusion over 30 minutes and repeated an additional two times if needed (Nagler, 2014; Verbalis, 2013). The goal of therapy is to reach a serum sodium level of 135 mEq/L within 24 hours. Rapid correction or overcorrection is avoided to prevent additional cerebral effects.

■ Cervical Stenosis

Nearly 50 percent of hysteroscopic complications are related to cervical entry (Bradley, 2002). Overcoming this obstruction can be addressed in part with preoperative misoprostol, described earlier (p. 899). Intraoperatively, cervical stenosis can also be resolved by cautious navigation of the endocervical canal by a small single-channel diagnostic hysteroscope coupled with hydrodissection. With this technique, the hydrostatic pressure of the fluid medium is increased during initial endocervical canal entry. The stenotic scar tissue can also be incised carefully with hysteroscopic shears or probed and stretched with small hysteroscopic grasping forceps (Bettochi, 2016; Suen, 2017). Last, if the stenotic cervical scar is at the external os, a shallow loop electrosurgical excision procedure (LEEP) excision of the stenotic scar is reasonable to hopefully expose the endocervical canal. The blind use of very small-caliber tools, such as a lacrimal duct probe, advocated in the past, is best avoided, as they may easily create a false passage that can lead to perforation.

Another adjunct is use of intraoperative transabdominal sonography to help guide proper instrument insertion (Christianson, 2008). In addition, intracervical injection of dilute vasopressin or dilute lidocaine plus epinephrine solutions can diminish the force required for cervical dilation (Phillips, 1997). Because the onset of action is rapid, this is especially helpful if stenosis was not anticipated preoperatively. As potent vasoconstrictors, however, both are ideally avoided in those with severe hypertension, advanced age, or cardiovascular disease.

■ Uterine Perforation

The uterus may be perforated during uterine sounding, during cervical dilation, or during hysteroscope manipulations. Risks include cervical stenosis, postmenopausal status, prior cervical or intrauterine surgery, and retroverted uterus.

The incidence of perforation is reported to be 1.4 percent (Bradley, 2002). The uterus is often perforated at the beginning of procedures, before a clear pathway into the uterus has been determined (Bradley, 2002). Creation of a false passage into the cervical stroma or myometrium during initial entry into the endocervical canal can precede perforation. Therefore, during initial instrument insertion, patience is key. In general, procedures are best halted if safe cavity entry cannot be assured. As another prevention, dilation or uterine sounding is minimized or avoided. Specifically, sounding may add little information regarding uterine size, may disrupt the endometrial architecture prior to cavity inspection, may incite visually obscuring bleeding, and can be a source of perforation.

Signs of perforation include loss of instrument resistance, a rapidly rising fluid deficit, difficulty maintaining uterine distention, or visualizing intrapelvic organs. Management varies by offending instrument and perforation site. Axial and fundal perforations created by a sound, dilator, or hysteroscope can be managed conservatively, as the myometrium will typically contract around these defects. In contrast, lateral perforation may perforate into the broad ligament or injure larger pelvic vessels; posterior perforation may injure the rectum; and those caused by sharp curettes or electrosurgical tools may cause organ laceration or burn. Diagnostic laparoscopy is indicated in these cases. Similarly, low anterior perforations prompt cystoscopy to evaluate associated bladder injury.

■ Hemorrhage

Heavy bleeding may develop during or following resection procedures. Although hysteroscopic electrosurgical electrodes can be used to contact and coagulate smaller vessels, these may be less effective for larger ones. If heavy bleeding is encountered and is refractory to electrosurgical coagulation, termination of the procedure may be indicated. Intracervical injection of dilute vasopressin can be especially helpful intraoperatively. Alternatively, a 30-mL Foley catheter balloon can be placed into the endometrial cavity and inflated incrementally with 10 to 30 mL of saline until moderate resistance to catheter tension is noted (Pasini, 2001). An attached collection bag helps document blood loss and bleeding cessation, at which point the catheter may be removed. If time permits, uterine artery embolization may be effective for cases refractory to balloon tamponade. If time is critical, emergent hysterectomy may be necessary.

■ Gas Embolization

If vessels are opened during cervical dilation or myometrial disruption, gas under pressure can be forced into the vasculature. Any undissolved portion can reach the lungs.

CO_2 is many times more soluble in plasma than is room air, and it typically dissolves sufficiently during transit from the pelvis (Corson, 1988). As a result, pulmonary embolism is rare in diagnostic hysteroscopic cases using CO_2 (Brandner, 1999).

In contrast, room air is poorly soluble in blood, and embolization can lead to rapid cardiovascular collapse. Signs and symptoms include chest pain, dyspnea, and hypotension. Anesthesia staff may note decreased end-tidal CO_2 levels, oxygen desaturation, dysrhythmias, or a "mill wheel" murmur (Groenman, 2008). In response, the patient is placed in the left lateral decubitus position with the head tilted downward. This aids movement of the air from the right outflow tract to the apex of the right ventricle, Here, the embolus may be aspirated (American College of Obstetricians and Gynecologists, 2018a).

Surgeons can minimize the risk of gas embolism by avoiding Trendelenburg positioning of the patient during hysteroscopy, ensuring that air bubbles are purged from all tubing prior to introduction of the hysteroscope into the uterus, maintaining intrauterine pressures <100 mm Hg, minimizing the effort needed to dilate the cervix, avoiding deep myometrial resections, and limiting multiple removals and reinsertions of the hysteroscope in and out of the uterine cavity.

REFERENCES

Aarts JW, Nieboer TE, Johnson N, et al: Surgical approach to hysterectomy for benign gynaecological disease. Cochrane Database Syst Rev 8: CD003677, 2015

Abu-Rustum NR, Rhee EH, Chi DS, et al: Subcutaneous tumor implantation after laparoscopic procedures in women with malignant disease. Obstet Gynecol 103(3):480, 2004

Agarwala N, Liu CY: Safe entry techniques during laparoscopy: left upper quadrant entry using the ninth intercostal space—a review of 918 procedures. J Minim Invasive Gynecol 12(1):55, 2005

Ahmad G, O'Flynn H, Duffy JM, et al: Laparoscopic entry techniques. Cochrane Database Syst Rev 2:CD006583, 2012

Akira S, Abe T, Igarashi K, et al: Gasless laparoscopic surgery using a new intra-abdominal fan retractor system: an experience of 500 cases. J Nippon Med Sch 72(4):213, 2005

Al-Fozan H, Firwana B, Al Kadri H, et al: Preoperative ripening of the cervix before operative hysteroscopy. Cochrane Database Syst Rev 4:CD005998, 2015

Alessandri F, Lijoi D, Mistrangelo E, et al: Randomized study of laparoscopic versus minilaparotomic myomectomy for uterine myomas. J Minim Invasive Gynecol 13(2):92, 2006

American Association of Gynecologic Laparoscopists, Munro MG, Storz K, et al: AAGL practice report: practice guidelines for the management of hysteroscopic distending media. J Minim Invasive Gynecol 20(2):137, 2013

American College of Obstetricians and Gynecologists: Robotic surgery in gynecology. Committee Opinion No. 628, March 2017

American College of Obstetricians and Gynecologists: Hysteroscopy. Technology Assessment No. 13, May 2018a

American College of Obstetricians and Gynecologists: Prevention of deep vein thrombosis and pulmonary embolism. Practice Bulletin No. 84, August 2007, Reaffirmed 2018b

American College of Obstetricians and Gynecologists: Prevention of infection after gynecologic procedures. Practice Bulletin No. 195, June 2018c

American College of Obstetricians and Gynecologists: Uterine morcellation for presumed leiomyomas. Committee Opinion No. 770, March 2019

Arnold A, Aitchison LP, Abbott J: Preoperative mechanical bowel preparation for abdominal, laparoscopic, and vaginal surgery: a systematic review. J Minim Invasive Gynecol 22(5):737, 2015

Baadsgaard SE, Bille S, Egeblad K: Major vascular injury during gynecologic laparoscopy: report of a case and review of published cases. Acta Obstet Gynaecol Scand 68:283, 1989

Barnett JC, Hurd WW, Rogers RM Jr, et al: Laparoscopic positioning and nerve injuries. J Minim Invasive Gynecol 14(5):664, 2007

Bergqvist D, Bergqvist A: Vascular injuries during gynecologic surgery. Acta Obstet Gynaecol Scand 66:19, 1987

Berguer R, Forkey DL, Smith WD: The effect of laparoscopic instrument working angle on surgeons' upper extremity workload. Surg Endosc 15(9):1027, 2001

Bettocchi S, Bramante S, Bifulco G, et al: Challenging the cervix: strategies to overcome the anatomic impediments to hysteroscopy: analysis of 31,052 office hysteroscopies. Fertil Steril 105(5):e16, 2016

Bhoyrul S, Vierra MA, Nezhat CR, et al: Trocar injuries in laparoscopic surgery. J Am Coll Surg 192(6):677, 2001

Bonjer HJ, Hazebroek EJ, Kazemier G, et al: Open versus closed establishment of pneumoperitoneum in laparoscopic surgery. Br J Surg 84:599, 1997

Boughey JC, Nottingham JM, Walls AC: Richter's hernia in the laparoscopic era: four case reports and review of the literature. Surg Laparosc Endosc Percutan Tech 13:55, 2003

Bradley LD: Complications in hysteroscopy: prevention, treatment and legal risk. Curr Opin Obstet Gynecol 14(4):409, 2002

Bradley LD, Falcone T: Hysteroscopy: Office Evaluation and Management of the Uterine Cavity, 1st ed. Philadelphia, Mosby, 2009, p 4

Brandner P, Neis KJ, Ehmer C: The etiology, frequency, and prevention of gas embolism during CO2 hysteroscopy. J Am Assoc Gynecol Laparosc 6:421, 1999

Buckley FP 3rd, Vassaur HE, Jupiter DC, et al: Influencing factors for port-site hernias after single-incision laparoscopy. Hernia 20(5):729, 2016

Bubenik LJ, Hosgood G, Vasanjee SC: Bursting tension of medium and large canine arteries sealed with ultrasonic energy or suture ligation. Vet Surg (3):289, 2005

Byron JW, Markenson G, Miyazawa K: A randomized comparison of Veress needle and direct trocar insertion for laparoscopy. Surg Gynecol Obstet 177:259, 1993

Camanni M, Bonino L, Delpiano EM, et al: Laparoscopy and body mass index: feasibility and outcome in obese patients treated for gynecologic diseases. J Minim Invasive Gynecol 17(5):576, 2010

Campbell ES, Xiao H, Smith MK: Types of hysterectomy: comparison of characteristics, hospital costs, utilization and outcomes. J Reprod Med 48:943, 2003

Caprini JA, Arcelus JI: Prevention of postoperative venous thromboembolism following laparoscopic cholecystectomy. Surg Endosc 8(7):741, 1994

Catarci M, Carlini M, Gentileschi P, et al: Major and minor injuries during the creation of pneumoperitoneum: a multicenter study on 12,919 cases. Surg Endosc 15:566, 2001

Chandler JG, Corson SL, Way LW: Three spectra of laparoscopic entry access injuries. J Am Coll Surg 192(4):478, 2001

Chapron C, Pierre F, Harchaoui Y, et al: Gastrointestinal injuries during gynaecological laparoscopy. Hum Reprod 14(2):333, 1999

Childers JM, Aqua KA, Surwit EA, et al: Abdominal-wall tumor implantation after laparoscopy for malignant conditions. Obstet Gynecol 84:765, 1994

Chopin N, Malaret JM, Lafay-Pillet MC, et al: Total laparoscopic hysterectomy for benign uterine pathologies: obesity does not increase the risk of complications. Hum Reprod (12):3057, 2009

Christianson MS, Barker MA, Lindheim SR: Overcoming the challenging cervix: techniques to access the uterine cavity. J Low Genit Tract Dis 12(1):24, 2008

Clark LH, Soliman PT, Odetto D, et al: Incidence of trocar site herniation following robotic gynecologic surgery. Gynecol Oncol 131(2):400, 2013

Clayman RV: The safety and efficacy of direct trocar insertion with elevation of the rectus sheath instead of the skin for pneumoperitoneum. J Urol 174:1847, 2005

Connor M: New technologies and innovations in hysteroscopy. Best Pract Res Clin Obstet Gynaecol 29(7):951, 2015

Cooper JM, Brady RM: Intraoperative and early postoperative complications of operative hysteroscopy. Obstet Gynecol Clin North Am 27:347, 2000

Copeland C, Wing R, Hulka JF: Direct trocar insertion at laparoscopy: an evaluation. Obstet Gynecol 62:655, 1983

Corson SL, Batzer FR, Gocial B, et al: Measurement of the force necessary for laparoscopic trocar entry. J Reprod Med 34:282, 1989

Corson SL, Hoffman JJ, Jackowski J, et al: Cardiopulmonary effects of direct venous CO_2 insufflation in ewes: a model for CO_2 hysteroscopy. J Reprod Med 33:440, 1988

Cravello L, D'Ercole C, Roger V, et al: Laparoscopic surgery in gynecology: randomized, prospective study comparing pneumoperitoneum and abdominal wall suspension. Eur J Obstet Gynaecol Reprod Biol 83:9, 1999

Demyttenaere S, Feldman LS, Fried GM: Effect of pneumoperitoneum on renal perfusion and function: a systematic review. Surg Endosc 21(2):152, 2007

Dingfelder JR: Direct laparoscope trocar insertion without prior pneumoperitoneum. J Reprod Med 21:45, 1978

Einarsson JI, Sun J, Orav J, et al: Local analgesia in laparoscopy: a randomized trial. Obstet Gynecol 104(6):1335, 2004

Ellström M, Ferraz-Nunes J, Hahlin M, et al: A randomized trial with a cost-consequence analysis after laparoscopic and abdominal hysterectomy. Obstet Gynecol 91(1):30, 1998

Eltabbakh GH, Piver MS, Hempling RE, et al: Laparoscopic surgery in obese women. Obstet Gynecol 94(5 Pt 1):704, 1999

Eltabbakh GH, Shamonki MI, Moody JM, et al: Hysterectomy for obese women with endometrial cancer: laparoscopy or laparotomy? Gynecol Oncol 78(3 Pt 1):329, 2000

Epstein J, Arora A, Ellis H: Surface anatomy of the inferior epigastric artery in relation to laparoscopic injury. Clin Anat 17:400, 2004

Falcone T, Paraiso MF, Mascha E: Prospective, randomized clinical trial of laparoscopically assisted vaginal hysterectomy versus total abdominal hysterectomy. Am J Obstet Gynecol 180(4):955, 1999

Farley DR, Greenlee SM, Larson DR, et al: Double-blind, prospective, randomized study of warmed, humidified carbon dioxide insufflation vs standard carbon dioxide for patients undergoing laparoscopic cholecystectomy. Arch Surg 139(7):739, 2004

Food and Drug Administration: Laparoscopic power morcellators. 2018. Available at: https://www.fda.gov/medical-devices/surgery-devices/laparoscopic-power-morcellators. Accessed April 5, 2019

Fuller J, Ashar BS, Carey-Corrado J: Trocar-associated injuries and fatalities: an analysis of 1399 reports to the FDA. J Minim Invasive Gynecol 12(4):302, 2005

Ghezzi F, Cromi A, Bergamini V, et al: Preemptive port site local anesthesia in gynecologic laparoscopy: a randomized, controlled trial. J Minim Invasive Gynecol 12(3):210, 2005

Ghezzi F, Cromi A, Uccella S, et al: Transumbilical versus transvaginal retrieval of surgical specimens at laparoscopy: a randomized trial. Am J Obstet Gynecol 207(2):112.e1, 2012

Giannios NM, Gulani V, Rohlck K, et al: Left upper quadrant laparoscopic placement: effects of insertion angle and body mass index on distance to posterior peritoneum by magnetic resonance imaging. Am J Obstet Gynecol 201(5):522.e1, 2009

Goldberg JM, Maurer WG: A randomized comparison of gasless laparoscopy and CO_2 pneumoperitoneum. Obstet Gynecol 90:416, 1997

Greenberg JA, Einarsson JI: The use of bidirectional barbed suture in laparoscopic myomectomy and total laparoscopic hysterectomy. J Minim Invasive Gynecol 15(5):621, 2008

Groenman FA, Peters LW, Rademaker BM, et al: Embolism of air and gas in hysteroscopic procedures: pathophysiology and implication for daily practice. J Minim Invasive Gynecol 15(2):24, 2008

Gunenc MZ, Yesildaglar N, Bingol B, et al: The safety and efficacy of direct trocar insertion with elevation of the rectus sheath instead of the skin for pneumoperitoneum. Surg Laparosc Endosc Percutan Tech 15:80, 2005

Harkki-Siren P, Kurki T: A nationwide analysis of laparoscopic complications. Obstet Gynecol 89:108, 1997

Hasson HM: A modified instrument and method for laparoscopy. Am J Obstet Gynecol 110:886, 1971

Hasson HM: Open laparoscopy: a report of 150 cases. J Reprod Med 12:234, 1974

Hasson HM, Rotman C, Rana N, et al: Open laparoscopy: 29-year experience. Obstet Gynecol 96:763, 2000

Heinberg EM, Crawford BL III, Weitzen SH, et al: Total laparoscopic hysterectomy in obese versus nonobese patients. Obstet Gynecol 103(4):674, 2004

Ho HS, Saunders CJ, Gunther RA, et al: Effector of hemodynamics during laparoscopy: CO_2 absorption or intra-abdominal pressure? J Surg Res 59(4):497, 1995

Horiuchi T, Tanishima H, Tamagawa K, et al: Randomized, controlled investigation of the anti-infective properties of the Alexis retractor/protector of incision sites. J Trauma 62(1):212, 2007

Howard FM, El-Minawi AM, DeLoach VE: Direct laparoscopic cannula insertion at the left upper quadrant. J Am Assoc Gynecol Laparosc (5):595, 1997

Hurd WW, Amesse LS, Gruber JS, et al: Visualization of the epigastric vessels and bladder before laparoscopic trocar placement. Fertil Steril 80:209, 2003

Hurd WW, Bude RO, DeLancey JO, et al: The relationship of the umbilicus to the aortic bifurcation: implications for laparoscopic technique. Obstet Gynecol 80(1):48, 1992

Hurd WW, Wang L, Schemmel MT: A comparison of the relative risk of vessel injury with conical versus pyramidal laparoscopic trocars in a rabbit model. Am J Obstet Gynecol 173:1731, 1995

Ido K, Suzuki T, Kimura K, et al: Lower-extremity venous stasis during laparoscopic cholecystectomy as assessed using color Doppler ultrasound. Surg Endosc 9(3):310, 1995

Jansen FW, Vredevoogd CB, van Ulzen K, et al: Complications of hysteroscopy: a prospective multicenter study. Obstet Gynecol 96:266, 2000

Jorgensen EM, Hur HC: Venous thromboembolism in minimally invasive gynecologic surgery: a systematic review. J Minim Invasive Gynecol 26(2):186, 2019

Kho KA, Lin K, Hechanova M, et al: Risk of occult uterine sarcoma in women undergoing hysterectomy for benign indications. Obstet Gynecol 127(3):468, 2016

Kho KA, Nezhat C: Parasitic myomas. Obstet Gynecol 114(3):611, 2009

Klauschie J, Wechter ME, Jacob K, et al: Use of anti-skid material and patient-positioning to prevent patient shifting during robotic-assisted gynecologic procedures. J Minim Invasive Gynecol 17(4):504, 2010

Kyrgiou M, Chatterjee J, Lyus R, et al: The role of cytology and other prognostic factors in endometrial cancer. J Obstet Gynecol 33(7):729, 2013

Lajer H, Widecrantz S, Heisterberg L: Hernias in trocar ports following abdominal laparoscopy: a review. Acta Obstet Gynaecol Scand 76:389, 1997

Lamberton GR, Hsi RS, Jin DH, et al: Prospective comparison of four laparoscopic vessel ligation devices. J Endourol 22(10):2307, 2008

Lamvu G, Zolnoun D, Boggess J, et al: Obesity: physiologic changes and challenges during laparoscopy. Am J Obstet Gynecol 191(2):669, 2004

Leibl BJ, Schmedt CG, Schwarz J, et al: Laparoscopic surgery complications associated with trocar tip design: review of literature and own results. J Laparoendosc Adv Surg Tech 9:135, 1999

Li TC, Saravelos H, Richmond M, et al: Complications of laparoscopic pelvic surgery: recognition, management and prevention. Hum Reprod Update 3:505, 1997

Lieng M, Berner E, Busund B: Risk of morcellation of uterine leiomyosarcomas in laparoscopic supracervical hysterectomy and laparoscopic myomectomy, a retrospective trial including 4791 women. J Minim Invasive Gynecol 22(3):410, 2015

Long JB, Giles DL, Cornella JL, et al: Open laparoscopic access technique: review of 2010 patients. JSLS 12(4):372, 2008

Lundorff P, Hahlin M, Källfelt B, et al: Adhesion formation after laparoscopic surgery in tubal pregnancy: a randomized trial versus laparotomy. Fertil Steril 55:911, 1991

Madeb R, Koniaris LG, Patel HR, et al: Complications of laparoscopic urologic surgery. J Laparoendosc Adv Surgical Tech A 14(5):287, 2004

Magrina JF: Complications of laparoscopic surgery. Clin Obstet Gynecol 45:469, 2002

Mais V, Ajossa S, Guerriero S, et al: Laparoscopic versus abdominal myomectomy: a prospective, randomized trial to evaluate benefits in early outcome. Am J Obstet Gynecol 174(2):654, 1996

Marsh F, Duffy S: The technique and overview of flexible hysteroscopy. Obstet Gynecol Clin North Am 31(3):655, 2004

McGurgan PM, McIlwaine P: Complications of hysteroscopy and how to avoid them. Best Pract Res Clin Obstet Gynaecol 29(7):982, 2015

Merlin TL, Hiller JE, Maddern GJ, et al: Systematic review of the safety and effectiveness of methods used to establish pneumoperitoneum in laparoscopic surgery. Br J Surg 90:668, 2003

Milad MP, Milad EA: Laparoscopic morcellator-related complications. J Minim Invasive Gynecol 21(3):486, 2014

Montz FJ, Holschneider CH, Munro MG: Incisional hernia following laparoscopy: a survey of the American Association of Gynecologic Laparoscopists. Obstet Gynecol 84:881, 1994

Morrison JE Jr, Jacobs VR: Replacement of expensive, disposable instruments with old-fashioned surgical techniques for improved cost-effectiveness in laparoscopic hysterectomy. J Soc Laparoendosc Surg 8:201, 2004

Multinu F, Casarin J, Tortorella L, et al: Incidence of sarcoma in patients undergoing hysterectomy for benign indications: a population-based study. Am J Obstet Gynecol 220(2):179.e1, 2019

Munro M: Pilot evaluation of the EndoSee hand-held hysteroscopic system for diagnostic hysteroscopy. J Minim Invasive Gynecol 20:S68, 2015

Munro MG: Laparoscopic access: complications, technologies, and techniques. Curr Opin Obstet Gynecol 14:365, 2002

Muzii L, Bellati F, Zullo MA, et al: Mechanical bowel preparation before gynecologic laparoscopy: a randomized, single-blind, controlled trial. Fertil Steril 85(3):689, 2006

Nagler EV, Vanmassenhove J, van der Veer SN, et al: Diagnosis and treatment of hyponatremia: a systematic review of clinical practice guidelines and consensus statements. BMC Med 12:1, 2014

Newcomb WL, Hope WW, Schmeltzer TM, et al: Comparison of blood vessel sealing among new electrosurgical and ultrasonic devices. Surg Endosc 23(1):90, 2009

Nezhat F, Brill AI, Nezhat CH, et al: Laparoscopic appraisal of the anatomic relationship of the umbilicus to the aortic bifurcation. J Am Assoc Gynecol Laparosc 5:135, 1998

Nordestgaard AG, Bodily KC, Osborne RW Jr, et al: Major vascular injuries during laparoscopic procedures. Am J Surg 169:543, 1995

O'Hanlan KA, Lopez L, Dibble SL, et al: Total laparoscopic hysterectomy: body mass index and outcomes. Obstet Gynecol 102(6):1384, 2003

O'Rourke N, Kodali BS: Laparoscopic surgery during pregnancy. Curr Opin Anaesthesiol 19(3):254, 2006

Ott DE, Reich H, Love B, et al: Reduction of laparoscopic-induced hypothermia, postoperative pain and recovery room length of stay by pre-conditioning gas with the Insuflow device: a prospective randomized controlled multi-center study. JSLS 2(4):321, 1998

Palmer R: Safety in laparoscopy. J Reprod Med 13(1):1, 1974

Panici PB, Zullo MA, Angioli R, et al: Minilaparotomy hysterectomy: a valid option for the treatment of benign uterine pathologies. Eur J Obstet Gynecol Reprod Biol 119(2):228, 2005

Park JY, Park SK, Kim DY, et al: The impact of tumor morcellation during surgery on the prognosis of patients with apparently early uterine leiomyosarcoma. Gynecol Oncol 122(2):255, 2011

Pasini A, Belloni C: Intraoperative complications of 697 consecutive operative hysteroscopies. Minerva Ginecol 53(1):13, 2001

Pearl JP, Price RR, Tonkin AE, et al: SAGES guidelines for the use of laparoscopy during pregnancy. Surg Endosc 31(10):3767, 2017

Peng Y, Zheng M, Ye Q, et al: Heated and humidified CO_2 prevents hypothermia, peritoneal injury, and intra-abdominal adhesions during prolonged laparoscopic insufflations. J Surg Res 151(1):40, 2009

Phillips DR, Nathanson HG, Milim SJ, et al: The effect of dilute vasopressin solution on the force needed for cervical dilatation: a randomized controlled trial. Obstet Gynecol 89(4):507, 1997

Pritts EA, Parker WH, Brown J, et al: Outcome of occult uterine leiomyosarcoma after surgery for presumed uterine fibroids: a systematic review. J Minim Invasive Gynecol 22(1):26, 2015

Propst AM, Liberman RF, Harlow BL, et al: Complications of hysteroscopic surgery: predicting patients at risk. Obstet Gynecol 96:517, 2000

Rahn DD, Phelan JN, Roshanravan SM, et al: Anterior abdominal wall nerve and vessel anatomy: clinical implications for gynecologic surgery. Am J Obstet Gynecol 202(3):234.e1, 2010

Ramirez PT, Frumovitz M, Wolf JK, et al: Laparoscopic port-site metastases in patients with gynecological malignancies. Int J Gynecol Cancer 14:1070, 2004

Reid K, Pockney P, Draganic B, et al: Barrier wound protection decreases surgical site infection in open elective colorectal surgery: a randomized clinical trial. Dis Colon Rectum 53(10):1374, 2010

Reynolds JD, Booth JV, de la Fuente S, et al: A review of laparoscopy for non-obstetric-related surgery during pregnancy. Curr Surg 60(2):164, 2003

Romanowski L, Reich H, McGlynn F, et al: Brachial plexus neuropathies after advanced laparoscopic surgery. Fertil Steril 60:729, 1993

Salazar CA, Isaacson KB: Office operative hysteroscopy: an update. J Minim Invasive Gynecol 25(2):199, 2018

Sammour T, Kahokehr A, Hill AG: Meta-analysis of the effect of warm humidified insufflation on pain after laparoscopy. Br J Surg 95(8):950, 2008

Schiavone MB, Bielen MS, Gardner GJ, et al: Herniation formation in women undergoing robotically assisted laparoscopy or laparotomy for endometrial cancer. Gynecol Oncol 140(3):383, 2016

Scribner DR Jr, Walker JL, Johnson GA, et al: Laparoscopic pelvic and para-aortic lymph node dissection in the obese. Gynecol Oncol 84(3):426, 2002

Sepilian V, Della Badia C: Iatrogenic endometriosis caused by uterine morcellation during a supracervical hysterectomy. Obstet Gynecol 102(5 Pt 2):1125, 2003

Shah DK, Vitonis AF, Missmer SA: Association of body mass index and morbidity after abdominal, vaginal, and laparoscopic hysterectomy. Obstet Gynecol 125(3):589, 2015

Shamiyeh A, Glaser K, Kratochwill H, et al: Lifting of the umbilicus for the installation of pneumoperitoneum with the Veress needle increases the distance to the retroperitoneal and intraperitoneal structures. Surg Endosc 23(2):313, 2009

Sharma KC, Brandstetter RD, Brensilver JM, et al: Cardiopulmonary physiology and pathophysiology as a consequence of laparoscopic surgery. Chest 110(3):810, 1996

Sharp HT, Dodson MK, Draper ML, et al: Complications associated with optical-access laparoscopic trocars. Obstet Gynecol 99:553, 2002

Soucie JE, Chu PA, Ross S, et al: The risk of diagnostic hysteroscopy in women with endometrial cancer. Am J Obstet Gynecol 207(1):71.e1, 2012

Suen MWH, Bougie O, Singh SS: Hysteroscopic management of a stenotic cervix. Fertil Steril 107(6):e19, 2017

Tam T, Harkins G, Wegrzyniak L, et al: Infiltration of bupivacaine local anesthetic to trocar insertion sites after laparoscopy: a randomized, double-blind, stratified, and controlled trial. J Minim Invasive Gynecol 21(6):1015, 2014

Thomas D, Ikeda M, Deepika K, et al: Laparoscopic management of benign adnexal mass in obese women. J Minim Invasive Gynecol 13:311, 2006

Tuchschmid S, Bajka M, Szczerba D, et al: Modeling intravasation of liquid distension media in surgical simulators. Med Image Anal 12(5):567, 2008

Tulikangas PK, Nicklas A, Falcone T, et al: Anatomy of the left upper quadrant for cannula insertion. J Am Assoc Gynecol Laparosc 7(2):211, 2000

Uppal S, Frumovitz M, Escobar P, et al: Laparoendoscopic single-site surgery in gynecology: review of literature and available technology. J Minim Invasive Gynecol 18(1):12, 2011

van Det MJ, Meijerink WJ, Hoff C, et al: Optimal ergonomics for laparoscopic surgery in minimally invasive surgery suites: a review and guidelines. Surg Endosc 23(6):1279, 2009

Vellinga TT, De Alwis S, Suzuki Y, et al: Laparoscopic entry: the modified Alwis method and more. Rev Obstet Gynecol 2(3):193, 2009

Verbalis JG, Goldsmith SR, Greenberg A, et al: Diagnosis, evaluation, and treatment of hyponatremia: expert panel recommendations. Am J Med 126(10 Suppl 1):S1, 2013

Vilos GA, Ternamian A, Dempster J, et al: Laparoscopic entry: a review of techniques, technologies, and complications. J Obstet Gynaecol Can 29(5):433, 2007

Wu MP, Ou CS, Chen SL, et al: Complications and recommended practices for electrosurgery in laparoscopy. Am J Surg 179:67, 2000

Zivanovic O, Sonoda Y, Diaz JP, et al: The rate of port-site metastases after 2251 laparoscopic procedures in women with underlying malignant disease. Gynecol Oncol 111(3):431, 2008

CHAPTER 42

Postoperative Considerations

Competent postoperative management requires an understanding of the patient's history, operative events, and fundamentals of the surgical stress response. Many problems after surgery can be avoided by the preoperative risk assessment and prevention strategies described in Chapter 39. However, complications can still develop despite ideal preparation, and vigilance for these adverse events can help ensure successful recovery for most patients.

POST-ANESTHESIA CARE UNIT

Patients who have received general or regional anesthesia or moderate sedation are typically transferred to a post-anesthesia care unit (PACU) after surgery for monitoring. Critically ill patients may bypass the PACU and instead recover in an intensive care unit. In either location, factors initially assessed are respiratory, cardiovascular, and neuromuscular function, temperature, pain, postoperative nausea and vomiting (PONV), mental status, fluid balance, urine output, wound drainage, and bleeding (Apfelbaum, 2013). Several scoring systems to guide discharge of the patient from the PACU are available, but none are universally recognized (Hawker, 2017). Table 42-1 presents one example (Aldrete, 1995; Marshall, 1999). Once an institution's criteria are met, the patient is either discharged home or transferred to a ward bed.

POSTOPERATIVE ORDERS

These written instructions address support of each organ system, while normal function is gradually reestablished. Although orders are customized for each woman, goals are common among all surgical patients and include fluid replacement, pain control, and resumption of daily activities. Table 42-2 offers a template for both inpatient and outpatient postoperative orders.

■ Physiologic Stress Response

Surgery has the potential to launch pathways that alter tissue perfusion, raise glucose levels, and promote inflammation. These stress responses are essential survival mechanisms, but at their extremes they can move normal functions far from the ideal steady state.

Of specific stress responses, vasopressin and aldosterone secretion expands intravascular volume by enhancing water retention by the kidney. Although this may accommodate surgical losses, aldosterone-derived hypokalemia is a potential complication. As another response, cortisol enhances liver gluconeogenesis and raises muscle catabolism to provide gluconeogenesis substrate. The resulting hyperglycemia supports recovery needs but uncontrolled hyperglycemia may impair neutrophil function and increase levels of damaging oxygen radicals (Duggan, 2017). Third, sympathetic nervous system stimulation releases catecholamines, which produce tachycardia, vasoconstriction, and catabolism to support cardiac output, maintain normotension, and create mild hyperglycemia. However, extremes can worsen cardiovascular function and glycemic control. Last, cytokines promote a local inflammatory response to aid healing (Finnerty, 2013). However, inflammation may contribute to acute renal failure or adult respiratory distress syndrome by promoting capillary leak and tissue injury. To buffer stress response extremes, enhanced recovery after surgery (ERAS) protocols are often effective to speed recovery.

■ Enhanced Recovery after Surgery

Several ERAS components pathways are presented in Chapter 39 (p. 833). Intraoperative measures are reviewed in Chapter 40 (p. 842). Postoperative ERAS elements emphasize early ambulation and feeding and judicious use of intravenous (IV) fluids (American College of Obstetricians and Gynecologists, 2018b). Pain management is multimodal and attempts to minimize opioid use (Nelson, 2016, 2019). Moreover, analgesia is ideally given proactively rather than waiting until a patient has significant pain. Discussion of each ERAS component is presented in subsequent sections.

TABLE 42-1. Postanesthetic Discharge Scoring System

Criteria	Score	
Vital signs	BP, pulse within 20% of preoperative baseline	2
	BP, pulse within 20–40% of baseline	1
	BP, pulse >40% of baseline	0
Activity	Steady gait, no dizziness, or meets preoperative level	2
	Requires assistance	1
	Unable to ambulate	0
PONV	Minimal, treated with oral medication	2
	Moderate, treated with parenteral medication	1
	Severe, continues despite treatment	0
Pain	Controlled with oral analgesics and acceptable to patient:	
	Yes	2
	No	1
Surgical bleeding	Minimal, no dressing change	2
	Moderate, up to two dressing changes	1
	Severe, more than three dressing changes	0

Score ≥9 supports discharge.
BP = blood pressure; PONV = postoperative nausea and vomiting.

■ Fluid and Electrolytes

Nearly half of the average female body's weight is water. Two thirds of this water is contained in the intracellular compartment, and the remainder is stored extracellularly. This extracellular compartment is divided into a vascular space filled with plasma and an interstitium, which is the collection of small spaces between cells. Of extracellular fluid volume, 25 percent makes up intravascular plasma, and 75 percent fills the interstitium. This 1 to 3 ratio is relevant during fluid resuscitation. Extracellular compartment osmolarity and thus the flow of fluid are controlled primarily by sodium and chloride, whereas potassium, magnesium, and phosphate are the major intracellular electrolytes. Osmotic balance is maintained by the free movement of water between the intra- and extracellular spaces.

To support these fluid volumes, the daily liquid requirement for an average adult approximates 30 mL/kg/d. Urine output and insensible losses offset these requirements (Marino, 2007). Postoperatively, crystalloid solutions are primarily used for this maintenance and in some cases for resuscitation. Sodium chloride is the main crystalloid component. Because sodium is most abundant in the extracellular space, the fluid is uniformly distributed between the interstitial areas. With crystalloid resuscitation, the primary effect is interstitial volume expansion rather than plasma volume growth. For perioperative needs, isotonic saline and lactated Ringer solution are most often used.

Colloquially called *normal saline*, isotonic saline has a higher chloride concentration compared with plasma (154 mEq/L versus 103 mEq/L) and lower pH (5.7 versus 7.4), respectively. Thus, if isotonic saline is infused in large volumes, it can create hyperchloremic metabolic acidosis (Prough, 1999). The saline-induced acidosis usually has no adverse clinical consequences, but differentiating it from lactic acidosis (a marker of tissue necrosis) can be challenging in some settings. Gastric secretions lost during vomiting or nasogastric tube suctioning are commonly replaced by a 5-percent dextrose in 0.45-percent normal saline solution with 20 mEq/L of potassium chloride (KCl) added.

Lactated Ringer solution, less often called *Hartmann solution*, contains potassium and calcium concentrations similar to plasma. However, the sodium concentration (130 mEq/L) is comparatively reduced to that of isotonic saline to maintain cationic neutrality. The addition of 28 mEq/L of lactate necessitates a reduction in chloride concentrations to a level similar to plasma. In sum, the hyperchloremic metabolic acidosis risk observed with large-volume isotonic saline infusion is avoided. In addition, lactated Ringer solution does not significantly change serum lactate levels because only 25 percent of the infused volume remains intravascular. Thus, lactated Ringer solution is preferred in cases of isotonic dehydration, such as fluid sequestration associated with bowel obstruction. Disadvantageously, lactated Ringer solution leads to greater calcium binding of certain drugs that limits their efficacy (Griffith, 1986). Moreover, calcium can bind the citrated anticoagulant found in blood products and promote clot formation in donor blood.

ERAS pathway goals strive to maintain perioperative patient euvolemia. Hypovolemia can affect cardiac output and tissue oxygenation, whereas fluid overload can result in visceral and peripheral edema and in electrolyte abnormalities (Carey, 2018). Restrictive fluid strategies have become a key component of these protocols. Purported benefits are fewer cardiopulmonary and wound healing complications, faster return of gastrointestinal (GI) function, and shorter hospital stay (Brandstrup, 2003; Lobo, 2002; Nisanevich, 2005). However, acute kidney injury from hypovolemia is one risk (Koerner, 2019; Marcotte, 2018). In one large trial that compared restrictive against liberal fluid regimens for major abdominal surgery, patients at high risk for complications showed no difference in disability-free survival rates. Rates of acute kidney injury were greater in the restrictive fluid group (Myles, 2018). Accordingly, monitoring renal function in more complex surgical patients is advisable.

TABLE 42-2. Typical Postoperative Orders

Postoperative Orders (Inpatient)

Admit to: PACU/assigned hospital floor/attending physician's name

Diagnosis: s/p what surgical procedure

Condition: stable

Allergies: NKDA

Diet: Clear liquids, advance as tolerated

IV fluids: LR at 40 mL/hr[a]; discontinue when tolerates 600 mL of oral fluids or POD#1

Activity:
POD#0: Ambulate in room and OOB to chair for all meals
POD#1 onward: OOB for 8 hr, ambulate 4 times daily

Special:
Strict I/Os
Turn, cough, deep breath hourly while awake
IS at bedside, use hourly while awake

Medications:
1. Acetaminophen 1 g every 6 hr
2. Ketorolac tromethamine 30 mg IV every 6 hr × 24 hr (only if Cr level normal) **or** meloxicam 15 mg orally once daily
3. Oxycodone 5 mg orally every 4 hr as needed for mild pain **or**
4. Oxycodone 10 mg orally every 4 hr as needed for moderate pain **or**
5. Hydromorphone 0.2 mg IV every 2 hr as needed for severe pain
6. If pain not controlled with oral meds, discontinue all other narcotics and start PCA: PCA orders: mix 30 mg morphine sulfate in 30 mL NS; load 4–6 mg, then IV every 6 min on demand; lockout 20 mg in 4 hr
7. Ondansetron 4 mg IV every 8 hr as needed[b]. Promethazine 25 mg IV every 6 hr as needed

Labs: H & H in AM (or that afternoon if necessary)

Vital signs: every 1 hr × 4; every 2 hr × 2; then every 4 hr

Notify MD for: T >101°F; BP >160/110, <90/60; P >130; RR >30, <10; UOP <120 mL/4 hr; acute changes

Discontinue Foley catheter within 24 hr of surgery
SCD hose to pump

Postoperative Orders (Outpatient)

Admit to: PACU; transfer to DSU when cleared by anesthesia

Diagnosis: s/p what surgical procedure

Condition: stable

VS per routine

Allergies: NKDA

Bed rest until A&A, then activity ad lib

NPO until after A&A, then clear liquids

IV fluids: LR at 40 mL/hr until tolerating PO, then D/C IV line

Notify MD for: T >101°F; BP >160/110, <90/60; P >130; RR >30, <10; acute changes

D/C patient home when A&A, cleared by anesthesia, taking PO, ambulating, & able to void

F/U at _____ clinic in _____ weeks

Write any necessary prescriptions

[a]Patients not euvolemic at end of surgery should receive more fluids, either by bolus or increased basal rate.
[b]Ondansetron preferred to promethazine as the latter is more sedating.
A&A = awake and alert; BP = blood pressure; BS = bedside; Cr = creatinine; D/C = discontinue, discharge; DSU = day surgery unit; F/U = follow-up; H&H = hemoglobin and hematocrit; I/Os = input and output; IM = intramuscular; IS = incentive spirometry; IV = intravenous; LR = lactated Ringer solution; MD = medical doctor; NKDA = no known drug allergies; NPO = nil per os; NS = normal saline; OOB = out of bed; P = pulse; PACU = postanesthesia care unit; PCA = patient-controlled analgesia; PO = per os; RR = respiratory rate; POD = postoperative day; SCD = sequential compression device; s/p = status post; T = temperature; UOP = urine output; VS = vital signs.

■ Pain Management

Postoperative pain management remains undervalued, and many patients continue to experience intense pain after surgery. In one survey, more than 85 percent of respondents following surgery have moderate to severe pain (Apfelbaum, 2003).

Additional evidence suggests that approximately 75 percent of patients still experience this level of pain after discharge home (Gan, 2014b). Poor pain control leads to decreased satisfaction with care, prolonged recovery time, greater use of healthcare resources, increased care-associated costs, and persistent postsurgical pain (Joshi, 2005; Kehlet, 2006; McIntosh, 2009).

Options for postoperative patient analgesia may be broadly classed as opiate-based or nonopioid, described next. This may be supplemented by local or peripheral regional anesthesia, discussed in Chapter 40 (p. 842).

Nonopioid Treatment Options

The two major classes of nonopioid therapies are acetaminophen and nonsteroidal antiinflammatory drugs (NSAIDs). Multimodal pain control postoperatively using oral or IV NSAIDs and/or acetaminophen can enhance analgesia, lower narcotic needs, reduce PONV incidence, and shorten hospital stays (Akarsu, 2004; Chan, 1996; Khalili, 2013; Mixter, 1998; Santoso, 2014). The combination of acetaminophen with NSAIDs may provide analgesia superior to either agent alone (Ong, 2010). In general, these drugs are well tolerated and carry a low risk of serious side effects. However, acetaminophen can be toxic to the liver in high doses. Thus, patients should avoid total doses exceeding 4000 mg/d and alcohol use while taking acetaminophen-containing products (Food and Drug Administration, 2011). A list of oral NSAIDs and their dosages are found in Table 11-1 (p. 242).

Opioid Treatment Options

Despite the common side effects that all opiates share—respiratory depression, nausea, and diminished GI motility—opiate therapy is the primary choice for managing moderate to severe pain. The American Pain Society recommends oral opioids rather than IV forms when possible (Chou, 2016). Common orally prescribed opiates are hydrocodone, oxycodone, codeine, and tramadol. The first three are often available in combination with acetaminophen or ibuprofen. The three most common IV opiates prescribed after gynecologic surgeries are morphine, fentanyl, and hydromorphone. Table 42-3 provides a summary of various pain medications and dosage equivalents.

TABLE 42-3. Opioid Equivalency Chart/Dosing Data for Opioids

| | Approximate Opioid Equianalgesic Dose | | | Usual Starting Dose | | | |
| | | | | Adults >50 kg Body Wt | | Children and Adults <50 kg | |
Drugs	Parenteral (mg)	Oral (mg)	Duration (hr)	Parenteral	Oral	Parenteral	Oral
Tramadol (Ultram)	—	—	4–6	—	50–100 mg	—	2 mg/kg
Codeine	130	200	3–4	60 mg (IM/SC)	60 mg	NR	1 mg/kg
Oxycodone IR (Roxicet)[a] (Percocet)[a]	—	30	3–4	NA	10 mg	NA	0.2 mg/kg
Hydrocodone (Lorcet)[a] (Lortab)[a] (Vicodin)	NA	30	6–8	NA	10 mg	NA	0.2 mg/kg
Morphine IR (Roxanol)	10	30	3–4	10 mg	30 mg	0.1 mg/kg	0.3 mg/kg
Hydromorphone (Dilaudid)	1.5	7.5	3–4	1.5 mg	6 mg	0.015 mg/kg	0.06 mg/kg
Fentanyl (Sublimaze) (Duragesic)	0.1	—	1	0.1 mg	—	—	—
Meperidine (Demerol)	75	300	2–3	100 mg	NR	0.75 mg/kg	NR
Oxycodone SR (OxyContin)	—	30	8–12	NA	10 mg	NA	0.2 mg/kg
Morphine SR (Oramorph) (MS Contin)	—	30	8–12	—	30 mg	—	0.3 mg/kg
Methadone (Dolophine)	10	20	3–4	10 mg	20 mg	0.1 mg/kg	0.2 mg/kg

[a]Narcotic/nonnarcotic combination product.

IM = intramuscular; IR = immediate release; NA = not available; NR = not recommended; SC = subcutaneous; SR = sustained release.

Meperidine, although administered in many obstetric units, is avoided in part because of neurologic side effects from its active metabolite normeperidine. Normeperidine is a cerebral irritant that can cause effects ranging from irritability and agitation to seizure.

Morphine is prescribed most frequently following gynecologic surgery and is a potent μ-opioid–receptor agonist. Action at this receptor accounts for the analgesia, euphoria, respiratory depression, and slowed GI motility seen with morphine. Its onset of action is rapid, and peak effects are seen within 20 minutes of IV administration. Benefits typically last for 3 to 4 hours. Its active metabolite, morphine-6-glucuronide, is renally excreted, and thus morphine is well tolerated in low doses in those with liver disease.

Pruritus is common after administration, although its genesis is poorly understood. Some theorize that central opiate receptors are stimulated. Others speculate that histamine is released, which creates the often comorbid urticaria, wheals, and flushing. In these cases, changing to another pain medication is logical. For pruritus treatment, most evidence-based data derive from studies of regional analgesia. Success has been found with ondansetron, 4 mg IV (George, 2009). An antihistamine, such as diphenhydramine (Benadryl) 25 mg IV, is another option. Naloxone, an opioid antagonist, can be used but may reverse the analgesia provided by morphine.

Fentanyl, a potent synthetic opiate, is more lipophilic than morphine and displays a shorter duration of action and half-life. Peak analgesia is reached within minutes of IV administration and lasts for 30 to 60 minutes. Many conscious sedation protocols used during office gynecologic procedures combine fentanyl with a sedative such as midazolam (Versed).

Hydromorphone (Dilaudid), another semisynthetic analogue of morphine, is less lipophilic than fentanyl. It is available for delivery by multiple routes that include oral, intramuscular (IM), IV, rectal, and subcutaneous (SC). Hydromorphone achieves its peak analgesia 15 minutes after IV administration, and its effects last 3 to 4 hours. Although commonly used during epidural analgesia, hydromorphone is a suitable patient-controlled analgesia (PCA) alternative in patients with a morphine allergy.

Of opioid or non-opioid options, ERAS pathways rely on non-opioids first, typically using both acetaminophen and NSAIDs in a scheduled manner. Second, on-demand opioids are administered. Scheduled opioids may then be given if pain is not yet adequately controlled. Last, PCA is employed if necessary. This strategy decreases the amount of total opioid administered (Bisch, 2018; Carey, 2018).

Urinary Drainage

Urinary catheters monitor urine output and prevent urinary retention. ERAS protocols recommend catheter removal when possible and preferably in the first 24 hours (Carey, 2018; Nelson, 2016). Removal in the operating room risks repeat catheterization, but withdrawal at 24 hours raises urinary infection risk (Zhang, 2015). One small study of 220 patients undergoing abdominal hysterectomy suggests that an intermediate time, at 6 hours, offers more advantages than immediate or late removal (Ahmed, 2014).

Ambulation

Benefits of early ambulation include lower rates of venous thromboembolism, atelectasis, and pneumonia (Cassidy, 2014; Kazaure, 2014). Overall recovery times and hospital stay also are shortened (Delaney, 2010; Lee, 2011). Thus, ERAS guidelines for gynecologic surgery strongly recommend early mobilization (Nelson, 2016, 2019). However, obstacles include poor pain control, urinary catheters, and IV poles and tubing (Liebermann, 2013). These barriers may be overcome by adherence to the other aspects of ERAS pathways described previously.

Hormone Replacement Therapy

Some women will have significant menopausal symptoms after surgical removal of both ovaries. Symptoms can range from severe hot flashes to headaches or sudden mood swings. In affected women, estrogen replacement therapy is considered in those without contraindications (Chap. 22, p. 480). For women with endometriosis and suspected residual disease, a progestin may be added to estrogen replacement (Chap. 11, 246).

Lung Expansion Modalities

Techniques to counter postoperative declines in lung volume can be simple and include deep breathing exercises, incentive spirometry (IS), and early ambulation. In conscious and cooperative patients, deep breathing effectively improves lung compliance and gas distribution (Chumillas, 1998; Ferris, 1960; Thomas, 1994). With these exercises, a woman is asked to take five sequential deep breaths every hour while awake and hold each for 5 seconds. An incentive spirometer can be added to provide direct visual feedback of her efforts. Last, early ambulation also expands lung volumes and provides some protection against venous thromboembolism. In one study, functional residual lung capacities rose up to 20 percent by simply maintaining an upright posture (Meyers, 1975). Alternatively, formal respiratory physiotherapy may include chest physical therapy in the form of percussion, clapping, or vibration; intermittent positive-pressure breathing (IPPB); and continuous positive airway pressure (CPAP).

Both simple and formal methods all effectively help prevent postoperative pulmonary morbidity, and no method is superior to another. Thomas and colleagues (1994) performed a metaanalysis to compare IS, IPPB, and deep-breathing exercises (DBE). In comparison with no therapy, IS and DBE are superior in preventing postoperative pulmonary complications, and greater than 50-percent reductions were observed. In addition, no significant differences were noted comparing IS to DBE, IS to IPPB, and DBE to IPPB. However, chest physical therapy, IPPB, and CPAP are more expensive and labor intensive (Pasquina, 2006). Accordingly, these methods are typically reserved for patients who are unable to perform simpler effort-dependent therapies (Florêncio, 2019).

PULMONARY COMPLICATIONS

Broad definitions hinder our ability to accurately assess the incidence of postoperative pulmonary complications. For gynecologic surgery, the incidence in retrospective chart reviews ranges from 1 to 3 percent (Burks, 2017; Solomon, 2013; Wysham, 2015). However, estimates are 2 to 40 percent when major abdominal surgery across surgical specialties is evaluated (Moore, 2017). Postoperative pulmonary complications include atelectasis and pulmonary embolism (PE) and, less commonly, pneumonia and acute respiratory distress syndrome (ARDS). All can potentially lead to acute respiratory failure (ARF).

■ Acute Respiratory Failure

ARF is classically divided into four subtypes defined by inadequate exchange of oxygen or carbon dioxide (CO_2) or both. Type 1 lesions exchange oxygen poorly, and examples include atelectasis, pneumonia, PE, and ARDS, all discussed in subsequent sections.

Type 2 conditions are typified by hypercapnia. It is seen with anesthesia overdose and muscle fatigue, in which ventilation suffers and CO_2 is retained. Also, heightened metabolic processes such as fever, severe sepsis, overfeeding, and hyperthyroidism can generate excess CO_2. As a result, ventilatory work rises as the body attempts to maintain appropriate arterial pCO_2 levels. This can ultimately lead to ARF.

The type 3 form is similar to type 1 but merits a distinct category because of its common occurrence following anesthesia and surgery. Physiologically, general anesthesia reduces muscle tone to decrease lung volumes and airway diameters. The resulting atelectasis and airway closure can drive abnormal gas exchange and ventilation-perfusion mismatching, which creates a lower PaO_2. This hypoxemia is further aggravated by hypoventilation, which may stem from central declines in respiratory drive, residual anesthetic effects, lung edema, or bronchospasm (Canet, 1989). Importantly, postoperative oxygen saturation levels recorded from patient pulse oximeters may significantly underestimate hypoxemia (Sun, 2015). Thus, to help circumvent type 3 ARF, important considerations include early treatment of hypoxemia, multimodal pain management, and chest physiotherapy.

The type 4 subgroup stems from shock and its associated cardiopulmonary hypoperfusion. For treatment, circulatory resuscitation, discussed in Chapter 40 (p. 862), accompanies oxygen therapy.

Treatment of ARF aims to provide adequate oxygenation and address its underlying causes. Pulse oximetry readings >92 percent reflect adequate oxygenation, however, a PaO_2 measurement by arterial blood gas most accurately assesses a patient with ARF. Of options for oxygen delivery, nasal cannula, simple masks, and nonrebreathing masks are first-line systems present on a ward. In the intensive care unit, noninvasive positive-pressure ventilation or endotracheal intubation is another.

Of choices, a nasal cannula is useful for adults with a low oxygen requirement. It will provide a low flow of 1 to 4 L/min and delivers a 25- to 40-percent oxygen concentration. Humidification to avoid drying mucous membranes is added if prolonged use of >2 L/min is anticipated. Next, simple mask supplementation can provide oxygen concentrations between 35 and 50 percent, with flow rates between 6 and 10 L/min. Both nasal cannula and simple mask allow mixing of supplemental oxygen with room air. Consequently, oxygen administration is imprecise (Bateman, 1998). Last, a nonrebreathing mask has valves that limit the mixing of exhaled gas and room air with the oxygen supply. Flow rates up to 10 to 15 L/min may be achieved and oxygen concentrations approach 95 percent (Boumphrey, 2003). Importantly, in some patients, such as those with chronic obstructive pulmonary disease (COPD), hypercapnia can worsen as hypoxemia is corrected. Affected patients are best managed in a closely monitored setting.

■ Atelectasis

This reversible closure or collapse of alveoli is seen in 90 percent of surgical patients (Lundquist, 1995). Development is associated with poor lung compliance, gas exchange abnormalities, and greater pulmonary vascular resistance. Characteristic signs are diminished breath sounds, dullness to percussion over affected lung fields, and poor oxygenation. Classically, atelectasis is associated with low-grade fevers. However, one review with nearly 1000 patients found no association between atelectasis and postoperative fever (Mavros, 2011). Chest radiographs typically shows linear densities in the lower lung fields.

Prevention using lung expansion therapies was described previously, and these also can be used for treatment. Atelectasis typically is self-limited and rarely persists past 2 days or slows a patient's hospital discharge (Platell, 1997). Its importance mainly lies in its clinical similarity to PE and pneumonia. However, in patients with severe systemic disease, atelectasis may worsen perioperative outcomes and lengthen hospital stays (Fernandez-Bustamante, 2017).

■ Hospital-Acquired and Ventilator-Associated Pneumonia

Pneumonia incidence specifically in surgical patients varies and ranges from 1 to 19 percent depending on surgical procedure and hospital surveyed (Kozlow, 2003). However, their importance is highlighted by high associated morbidity and mortality rates (Tablan, 2004).

These infections are often polymicrobial. Typically aerobic gram-negative bacilli, such as *Pseudomonas aeruginosa*, *Escherichia coli*, *Klebsiella pneumoniae*, and *Acinetobacter* species are implicated. Both methicillin-sensitive and methicillin-resistant *Staphylococcus aureus* (MRSA) also may be associated pathogens.

Clinically, pneumonia is diagnosed if chest radiographs reveal a new or progressive infiltrate and if two of three clinical features (leukocytosis, fever >38°C, or purulent secretions) are present. Empiric therapy is ideally based on an institution's distribution of pathogens. Consequently, hospitals are encouraged to periodically generate antibiograms, which are summaries of local bacterial isolates and their antimicrobial susceptibilities. However, obtaining a noninvasive sputum sample is encouraged prior to empiric therapy initiation, when possible. Patient-expectorated or endotracheal aspiration samples are suitable. A nasal swab for MRSA also is completed.

Guidelines for hospital-acquired pneumonia (HAP) treatment recommend broad-spectrum antibiotics (Table 42-4). At

TABLE 42-4. Empiric Antibiotic Therapy for Hospital-Acquired Pneumonia

No Mortality[a] and No MRSA[b] Risk	High Mortality Risk[a] or IV Antibiotics in Prior 90 Days[c]
One of the following:	**Two of the following[d]:**
Piperacillin-tazobactam 4.5 g IV every 6 hr	Piperacillin-tazobactam 4.5 g IV every 6 hr
or	*or*
Cefepime 2 g IV every 8 hr	Cefepime *or* Ceftazidime 2 g IV every 8 hr
or	*or*
Levofloxacin 750 mg IV daily	Levofloxacin 750 mg IV daily *or* Ciprofloxacin 400 mg IV q 8 hr
or	*or*
Imipenem 500 mg IV every 6 hr *or* Meropenem 1 g IV every 8 hr	Imipenem 500 mg IV every 6 hr *or* Meropenem 1 g IV every 8 hr
With MRSA Risk:	*or*
One of above **PLUS** Vancomycin 15 mg/kg IV every 8-12 hr *or* Linezolid 600 mg IV every 12 hr	Amikacin 15–20 mg/kg IV daily *or* Gentamicin 5–7 mg/kg IV daily *or* Tobramycin 5–7 mg/kg IV daily *or*
	or
	Aztreonam 2 g IV q 8h
	PLUS
	Vancomycin 15 mg/kg IV every 8–12 hr *or* Linezolid 600 mg IV every 12 hr

[a]Risk factors for mortality include need for ventilatory support or septic shock.
[b]Indications for MRSA coverage include IV antibiotic treatment in the past 90 days and/or treatment in a unit where the MRSA prevalence is unknown or >20%.
[c]If patient has factors that raise risk of gram-negative infection, two antipseudomonal agents are recommended.
[d]Avoid selection of two β-lactam antibiotics.
IV = intravenous; MRSA = methicillin-resistant *Staphylococcus aureus*.

our institution, we typically choose piperacillin-tazobactam and, if MRSA coverage is needed, add vancomycin. An agent with activity against *P aeruginosa* is included in patients who are critically ill or have received IV antibiotics in the prior 90 days. Once respiratory and blood culture results are available, antibiotic therapy is de-escalated (Kalil, 2016). Thus, if two agents with antipseudomonal activity were used initially and cultures lack pseudomonal species, one of these is discontinued. Similarly, vancomycin is stopped if MRSA is not isolated. HAP treatment is provided for 7 days. Ventilator-acquired pneumonia instead develops in patients requiring prolonged ventilator support and usually would be managed by an intensivist. Preventive measures for all pneumonias include coughing and deep-breathing exercises; elevating the head of the bed 30 to 45 degrees, particularly during feeding; and ambulation (Kazaure, 2014).

■ Acute Respiratory Distress Syndrome

This syndrome reflects acute, diffuse, and inflammatory lung injury that causes a form of severe permeability pulmonary edema plus ARF. The Berlin definition of ARDS includes onset within 1 week of the clinical insult, chest imaging demonstrating bilateral opacities, and three levels of hypoxemia (mild, moderate, and severe). Level severity correlates with mortality rates (The ARDS Definition Task Force, 2012).

The physiologic features of early postoperative ARDS are thought to stem from dysregulated coagulation, inflammation, and epithelial injury (Yadav, 2018). One theory suggests that multiple insults lead to postoperative ARDS, and this offers insight into modifiable intra- and postoperative alveolar damage prevention (Litell, 2011; Warner, 2000). Intraoperative strategies minimize lung trauma by keeping airway pressure and tidal volumes within set limits and by avoiding repeated alveolar opening and closing (Hemmes, 2013). Other measures strive to prevent infection, limit IV fluid volume, and avoid blood product transfusion (Güldner, 2013).

■ Obstructive Sleep Apnea

This repetitive collapse of the upper airway during sleep is a common chronic condition and often requires lifelong care (Epstein, 2009). Its prevalence has risen due to growing obesity rates and to greater patient and provider disease awareness (Peppard, 2013; Pickens, 2018).

Affected patients carry a higher risk of postoperative respiratory compromise, and several management strategies are implemented. First, reducing systemic opioids and avoiding concurrent administration of sedating medications helps avert respiratory depression. Supplemental oxygen is given until patients can maintain baseline oxygen saturation on room air. Patients are maintained in nonsupine positions if possible, as the supine position enhances pharynx collapse in affected individuals (Ong, 2011). Last, continuous pulse oximetry monitoring is used while patients are at risk of respiratory compromise (American Society of Anesthesiologists, 2014).

VENOUS THROMBOEMBOLISM

■ Pulmonary Embolism

If PE is suspected, evaluation begins with risk estimation and a clinical examination that especially assesses patient oxygenation and hemodynamic stability. Persistent pulse oximetry readings <92 percent despite supplemental oxygen administration for approximately 15 minutes would suggest patient instability. Systolic blood pressure <90 mm Hg persisting for 15 minutes is another indicator. Unstable patients undergo targeted resuscitation, and empiric anticoagulation is initiated in those who are deemed at high risk for PE. Most patients, however, are hemodynamically stable and diagnostic evaluation may be performed prior to anticoagulation.

PE symptoms can mirror other cardiopulmonary pathology, and chest radiography and electrocardiogram (ECG) are obtained. Radiograph findings are typically abnormal but nonspecific, and include atelectasis, elevated hemidiaphragm, cardiomegaly, and small pleural effusions (Worsley, 1993). An ECG may display tachycardia or may reflect right heart strain. Classically, this strain creates a large S wave in lead I, a Q wave in lead III, and an inverted T wave in lead III (Stein, 1991).

Wells and colleagues (2000) described one of the most widely used pretest probability assessments for PE (Table 42-5).

TABLE 42-5. Pretest Probability for Pulmonary Embolism (PE)

Criteria	Score
Clinical symptoms of DVT	3.0
Other diagnosis less likely than PE	3.0
Heart rate >100	1.5
Immobilization (≥3 days) or surgery in the previous 4 weeks	1.5
Previous DVT/PE	1.5
Hemoptysis	1.0
Malignancy	1.0

Clinical Probability Score

High	>6.0
Moderate	2.0–6.0
Low	<2.0

DVT = deep-vein thrombosis.
Modified from Wells, 2000, with permission.

TABLE 42-6. Pretest Probability for Deep-Vein Thrombosis (DVT)

Criteria	Score
Active cancer (within prior 6 months)	1
Paralysis, paresis, or immobilization of lower extremities	1
Bedridden >3 d or major surgery, either within 4 weeks	1
Localized tenderness along the distribution of the deep venous system	1
Entire leg swollen	1
Calf circumference differs >3 cm between legs (measure 10 cm below tibial tuberosity)	1
Pitting edema (greater in affected leg)	1
Collateral superficial veins (nonvaricose)	1
Alternative diagnosis equally or more likely than DVT	−2

Clinical Probability Score

High	≥3
Moderate	1 or 2
Low	0

Modified from Wells, 1997, with permission.

If probability for PE is moderate or high, computed tomographic angiography (CTA) or, less frequently, ventilation/perfusion (V/Q) scanning is ordered. Lower-extremity Doppler ultrasound usually is not the first imaging study ordered. Its sensitivity in detecting deep-vein thrombosis (DVT) is excellent but is suboptimal for diagnosing PE (Gottlieb, 1999; van Rossum, 1998).

■ Deep-Vein Thrombosis

DVT symptoms include swelling or edema, pain, and warmth of one or both lower extremities. Once DVT is suspected, a pretest probability assessment is performed, and one tool is shown in Table 42-6. Patients with a low probability score may have a D-dimer test drawn and Doppler ultrasonography ordered if the level is >500 ng/mL. Of note, patients who have undergone recent surgery may have an elevated D-dimer level and instead proceed directly to Doppler ultrasonography.

The mortality rate with a proximal DVT is higher than that with a distal DVT (Galanaud, 2009). Proximal DVTs involve the popliteal, femoral, or iliac veins. Distal thrombosis is located in the calf veins such as the peroneal or posterior tibial.

■ Management

Acute management of venous thromboembolism (VTE), either PE or DVT, involves anticoagulation with intravenous unfractionated heparin or subcutaneous low-molecular-weight heparin (Tables 42-7 and 42-8). Patients with a contraindication to anticoagulation should receive an inferior vena cava (IVC) filter (Jaff, 2011). Absolute contraindications to anticoagulation include active bleeding, severe bleeding diathesis, or recent

TABLE 42-7. Parkland Hospital Protocol for Continuous Heparin Infusion for Patients with Venous Thromboembolism

Initial Heparin Dose:
__ units IV push (recommended 80 units/kg rounded to nearest 100, maximum 7500 units), then
__ units/hr by infusion (recommended 18 units/kg/hr rounded to nearest 50).

Infusion Rate Adjustments—based on partial thromboplastin time (PTT):

PTT (sec)[a]	Intervention[b]	Baseline Infusion Rate Change[c]
<45	80 units/kg bolus	↑ by 4 units/kg/hr
45–54	40 units/kg bolus	↑ by 2 units/kg/hr
55–84	None	None
85–100	None	↓ by 2 units/kg/hr
>100	Stop infusion 60 minutes	↓ by 3 units/kg/hr

[a]PTT goal 55–84.
[b]Rounded to nearest 100.
[c]Rounded to nearest 50.

intracranial hemorrhage. Relative contraindications are thrombocytopenia with platelet counts <50,000, recent or planned surgery, intracranial or spinal tumors, and large abdominal aortic aneurysm.

Patients who develop a VTE 1 to 2 days after surgery are assessed for continued postoperative bleeding. If findings are reassuring, anticoagulation is begun. Elective surgery is typically postponed with acute VTE, but more urgent surgery would warrant consideration of IVC filter placement.

After achieving adequate anticoagulation, an oral vitamin K antagonist such as warfarin is initiated. To avoid paradoxical hypercoagulability, heparin is continued for at least 5 days after warfarin initiation (Houman Fekrazad, 2009). Once the international normalized ratio (INR) reaches a therapeutic range of 2 to 3, heparin is stopped.

Long term, anticoagulation therapy duration is dictated by clinical and patient circumstances. For those with a provoked first DVT or PE, anticoagulants are recommended for 3 months. Provocateurs include surgery, exogenous estrogen, or local trauma. Extended therapy is preferred for both those with unprovoked VTE or those with second VTE, unless the risk of bleeding is high. In this case, treatment is halted at 3 months. For those with concurrent cancer, therapy is extended regardless of bleeding risk (Kearon, 2012). Of note, thrombophilia screening is of limited utility in the setting of a first provoked episode of VTE (Goldman-Mazur, 2019).

TABLE 42-8. Characteristics of Some Low-Molecular-Weight Heparins

Name (Brand Name)	Dose
Enoxaparin (Lovenox)	1 mg/kg every 12 hr 1.5 mg/kg daily
Tinzaparin (Innohep)	175 IU/kg daily
Dalteparin (Fragmin)	100 IU/kg every 12 hr 200 IU/kg daily

IU = international units.

CARDIOVASCULAR COMPLICATIONS

Myocardial Infarction

Postoperatively, myocardial infarction (MI) is rare, and its reported incidence ranges from nearly 1 percent to as high as 37 percent among patients with surgery within 3 months of an MI (Mangano, 1990; Tinker, 1978). Coronary ischemia classically stems from declines in oxygen supply and greater myocardial demands. Events that decrease oxygen supply include hypotension, lowered coronary perfusion, or poor carrying capacity caused by anemia. Those that raise myocardial oxygen demands are greater afterload, tachycardia, and increased cardiac contractility.

Most patients with postoperative MI lack classic chest pain or pressure, which may be masked by postoperative analgesia (Muir, 1991). Dyspnea is the most common complaint and may be accompanied by acute cardiac failure and hemodynamic instability. ECG changes of postoperative MI tend to be less well defined, and most ECGs demonstrate a non–Q wave variant (Badner, 1998). Serial troponin levels are obtained and are highly specific for MI (Thygesen, 2018). Screening patients at high risk by obtaining preoperative baseline troponin levels and ECG may be considered and is an area still under study.

Postoperative MI treatment differs from that in nonsurgical patients. Namely, ischemia stems from a supply–demand mismatch rather than from a coronary plaque rupture or a thrombotic occlusion (Fleisher, 2014). Thus, correcting hypotension, anemia, and arrhythmia is essential. Ideally, these patients are cared for in a unit that provides intense monitoring, cardiopulmonary support, and cardiology consultation.

Hypertension

Patients with poorly controlled chronic hypertension before surgery tend to have greater perioperative blood pressure lability compared with normotensive patients or those with well-controlled hypertension. In general, a diastolic blood pressure >110 mm Hg preoperatively best predicts those who will have perioperative hypertension issues.

TABLE 42-9. Commonly Used Medications for Nausea and Vomiting

Medication (Brand Name)	Usual Dosage	Route(s)
Antihistamines	**Every 6 hr**	
Diphenhydramine (Benadryl)	25–50 mg	IM, IV, PO
Hydroxyzine (Atarax, Vistaril)	25–100 mg	IM, PO
Meclizine (Antivert)	25–50 mg	PO
Benzamides	**Every 6 hr**	
Metoclopramide (Reglan)	5–15 mg	IM, IV, PO
Trimethobenzamide (Tigan)	250 mg	IM, PO, PR
Phenothiazines	**Every 6 hr**	
Prochlorperazine (Compazine)	5–10 (25 PR) mg	IM, IV, PO, PR
Promethazine (Phenergan)	12.5–25 mg	IM, IV, PO, PR
Serotonin Antagonists		
Ondansetron (Zofran)	8 mg every 8 hr	IV, PO, ODT
Granisetron (Kytril)	2 mg daily	IV, PO
Dolasetron (Anzemet)	100 mg daily	IV, PO
Anticholinergics		
Scopolamine (Transderm-Scop)	1 patch, remove 24 hr postop	TD

IM = intramuscular; IV = intravenous; ODT = orally disintegrating tablet; PO = orally; PR = per rectum; TD = transdermal.

Several possible triggers may raise blood pressures in the first 24 hours after surgery. First, abrupt withdrawal of β-blocker or of centrally acting sympatholytic agents such as clonidine can cause rebound hypertension. Pain and bladder distention also may contribute. Later during recovery, sympathetic hyperactivity may stem from inadequate pain management or, less often, from alcohol withdrawal. Last, return of excess interstitial fluid back into the vascular space can create fluid overload and hypertension.

Two approaches to blood pressure treatment address either *fixed thresholds* or *relative changes from baseline*. Charlson and colleagues (1990) demonstrated higher rates of postoperative cardiac and renal complications when the mean blood pressure rose ≥20 percent above preoperative levels. If mean blood pressure readings rise by this percentage, acute management is instituted but ideally does not lower mean blood pressures by >20 percent. Instead, with a fixed threshold approach, the blood pressure target with acute management is not below 160/100 mm Hg in the first 24 hours. Thereafter, as in the general population, a target less than 130/80 mm Hg is desirable (Whelton, 2018). In patients not previously diagnosed with hypertension and now with normal-range pressures, discontinuation of therapy after 24 hours can be considered.

GASTROINTESTINAL COMPLICATIONS

■ Postoperative Nausea and Vomiting

This is one of the most common complaints following surgery, and its incidence ranges from 30 to 70 percent in high-risk patients (Møller, 2002). Those at risk for PONV include females, nonsmokers, those with prior motion sickness or prior PONV, and those with extended surgeries (Apfelbaum, 2003).

A multimodal approach to prevention is recommended (Apfel, 2004). Currently, combinations of 4 to 8 mg of dexamethasone prior to anesthesia induction are followed, toward the end of surgery, by less than 1 mg of droperidol (Inapsine) and 4 mg of ondansetron (Zofran). However, if symptoms develop within 6 hours of surgery, antiemetics from a different pharmacologic class than previously administered are selected (Gan, 2014a). Persistent nausea may benefit from combining agents from different classes (Table 42-9).

■ Bowel Function and Diet Resumption

Normal GI function requires synchronized motility, mucosal transport of nutrients, and evacuation reflexes (Nunley, 2004). However, following intraabdominal surgery, dysfunction of enteric neural activity typically disrupts normal propulsion. Activity first returns in the stomach and is noted typically within 24 hours. The small intestine also exhibits contractile activity within 24 hours after surgery, but normal function may be delayed for 3 to 4 days (Condon, 1986; Dauchel, 1976). Rhythmic colonic motility resumes last, at approximately 4 days following intraabdominal surgery (Huge, 2000). Passage of flatus characteristically marks this return of function, and stool passage usually follows in 1 to 2 days.

Postoperative feeding is most effective when started early. In most ERAS protocols, clear liquids are offered first, and diet is advanced as tolerated. Early feeding improves wound healing, promotes gut motility, decreases intestinal stasis, raises splanchnic blood flow, and stimulates reflexes that elicit GI hormone secretion to shorten postoperative ileus duration (Anderson, 2003; Braga, 2002; Correia, 2004; Lewis, 2001). Early feeding promotes faster return of bowel function, shortens hospital stays, improves patient satisfaction, and does not raise complication rates (Charoenkwan, 2014).

Ileus

Postoperative ileus (POI) is a transient impairment of GI activity from multiple factors. First, bowel manipulation during surgery leads to contributory factors involved in the surgical stress response. Second, as noted earlier, perioperative opioid use also disrupts normal GI function (p. 910). Last, bowel edema from excess IV fluid administration may play a role. This is part of the rationale for limiting IV fluids in ERAS pathways.

In sum, these lead to abdominal distention, hypoactive bowel sounds, nausea and vomiting related to GI gas and fluid accumulation, and delayed passage of flatus or stool (Livingston, 1990). POI diagnosis is often one of exclusion. In those with suspected ileus, radiography with an acute abdominal series is reasonable and displays uniform gaseous distension of the large and small bowel. In patients with a greater concern for bowel obstruction, described next, computed tomography (CT) scanning with oral contrast is selected. In addition, intraoperative urinary tract and bowel injuries are often not recognized until after surgery and may present with ileus. Thus, CT with oral and IV contrast provides greater diagnostic information. Electrolyte imbalances may contribute to ileus or may be a sequela of associated vomiting. Moreover, creatinine levels also are ideally assessed prior to IV CT contrast.

For POI management, electrolyte repletion and IV fluids to reestablish euvolemia are traditional. Routine use of nasogastric tube (NGT) decompression to promote bowel rest is inferior to its selective use. Specifically, patients without a routine NGT had significantly earlier return of normal bowel function and lower risks for wound infection and ventral hernia (Nelson, 2007). Additionally, tube-related discomfort, nausea, and hospital stays were reduced. However, with selective use, an NGT can benefit patients with abdominal bloating and recurrent vomiting.

Gum chewing after laparotomy as a preventive modality for POI was studied in several small randomized trials. In these, sugarless gum is usually chewed 15 to 30 minutes at least three times daily. In evaluations, this practice is associated with earlier improvement in bowel motility markers (Ertas, 2013; Jernigan, 2014). However, compared with placebo, gum chewing achieves these goals on average only several hours earlier (Li, 2013).

Bowel Obstruction

Obstruction of the small intestines may be partial or complete and can result from adhesions following intraabdominal surgery, infection, or malignancy. Of these, surgical adhesions are the most common (Krebs, 1987; Monk, 1994). Small bowel obstruction (SBO) develops following 1 to 2 percent of total abdominal hysterectomies, and nearly 75 percent of obstructions are complete (Al-Sunaidi, 2006). When performed for benign indications, hysterectomy route does not seem to alter the SBO risk (Muffly, 2012). Obstruction may be remote from surgery, and the mean interval between primary intraabdominal procedure and SBO approximates 5 years (Al-Took, 1999).

During SBO, the bowel lumen dilates proximal to the obstruction, and decompression may develop distally. Bacterial overgrowth in the proximal small bowel can promote bacterial fermentation and worsening dilation. The bowel wall also becomes edematous and dysfunctional (Wright, 1971). Progressive bowel pressure compromises intestinal-segment perfusion and can ultimately lead to ischemia or rupture (Megibow, 1991).

Clinical signs that may help distinguish SBO from POI include tachycardia, oliguria, and fever. Physical examination may reveal abdominal distention, high-pitched bowel sounds, and an empty rectal vault during digital examination. Last, leukocytosis with a neutrophil dominance can alert to possible coexistent bowel ischemia.

CT scanning is the primary imaging tool to identify SBO. Water-soluble contrast can safely help identify the cause and obstruction severity. Gastrografin, the most commonly used oral water-soluble dye, is a mixture of sodium amidotrizoate and meglumine amidotrizoate. Its composition can aid resolution of small bowel edema due to its high osmotic pressure and also may enhance smooth muscle contractility (Assalia, 1994). However, data supporting the therapeutic benefits of Gastrografin administration in adhesion-related SBO are conflicting (Abbas, 2007; Scotté, 2017; Zielinski, 2017).

Initial SBO management is similar to that for POI, but subsequent care varies with the degree of obstruction. For partial obstruction, feedings are held, IV fluids and antiemetics are initiated, electrolyte imbalances are corrected, and an NGT is reserved for significant nausea and vomiting. Continued surveillance monitors for signs of bowel ischemia. Symptoms in most cases of partial SBO improve within 48 hours. Those who fail to improve typically require surgical evaluation. With complete bowel obstruction, surgery to relieve the obstruction typically is indicated.

Colonic obstruction is rare following gynecologic surgery but carries a high mortality rate (Krstic, 2014). The colon can be obstructed by intrinsic lesions such as colon cancer or diverticulitis-related strictures or can be compressed by a pelvic mass or retained foreign body. An enlarged cecum found on an abdominal radiograph requires further evaluation by either a barium enema or colonoscopy. Immediate surgical intervention is necessary when the cecal diameter exceeds 10 to 12 cm to minimize perforation risks.

Diarrhea

Transient episodes of postoperative diarrhea are not uncommon after major gynecologic surgery as normal GI tract function returns. Protracted episodes and excessive amounts of diarrhea almost always stem from infection and warrant further evaluation. Stool samples are examined for ova and parasites, cultured for bacteria, and screened for *Clostridium difficile*.

Of potential etiologies, broad-spectrum antibiotics can impair normal GI flora growth and thereby promote *C difficile* toxin-associated pseudomembranous colitis. Testing for this organism and its toxin vary depending on clinical context. For best use of resources, tool sample submission for *C difficile* ideally is reserved for patients with ≥3 unformed stools within 24 hours. In this setting, a nucleic acid amplification test (NAAT) for *C difficile* toxin genes is performed on the stool sample. Other testing algorithms are provided by the Infectious Diseases Society of America (McDonald, 2018).

TABLE 42-10. Postoperative Nutritional Requirements

Nutritional Requirements	Recommendations
BEE in women	65.5 + 1.9 (height in cm) + 9.6 (weight in kg) − 4.7 (age in years)
Total calories	100% to 120% BEE
Glucose	50–70% total caloric intake Maintain blood glucose level <200 mg/dL
Protein	1.5 g/kg/d of current weight (BMI <25) 2.0 g/kg/d of ideal weight (BMI >25)

BEE = basal energy expenditure; BMI = body mass index.

For *C difficile* treatment, either oral vancomycin or fidaxomicin for 10 days is preferred to metronidazole (Gupta, 2018). Contact isolation precautions are instituted and continued for at least 48 hours after diarrhea resolution. Regardless of the pathogen, aggressive fluid and electrolyte replacement is critical to prevent further aberrations that can delay recovery.

Nutrition

Appropriate postoperative nutrition ideally improves immune function, promotes wound healing, and minimizes metabolic disturbances. Table 42-10 offers a summary of basic immediate postoperative metabolic needs (Nehra, 2002). Despite the additional stress in the immediate postoperative period, underfeeding is accepted for a brief period (Seidner, 2006). However, extended protein calorie restriction in a surgical patient can impair wound healing, diminish cardiac and pulmonary function, promote bacterial overgrowth within the GI tract, and create other complications that increase hospital stays and patient morbidity rates (Elwyn, 1975; Kinney, 1986; Seidner, 2006). If substantial oral caloric intake is delayed for 7 to 10 days, nutritional support is warranted.

In the absence of contraindications, enteral nutrition is preferred to a parenteral route. Foremost, enteral options carry fewer infectious complications compared with intravenous forms (Worthington, 2017). Its other advantages include fewer metabolic disturbances and lower cost (Nehra, 2002).

URINARY COMPLICATIONS

Oliguria

Prerenal Oliguria

Postoperative oliguria is defined as urine production <0.5 mL/kg/hr. Oliguria can be caused by a prerenal, intrarenal, or postrenal insult, and a systematic approach typically allows differentiation among these.

Prerenal oliguria is a physiologic response to hypovolemia, and coexistent tachycardia and orthostatic hypotension usually reflect this volume depletion. Causes of postoperative hypovolemia include acute hemorrhage, vomiting, severe diarrhea, and inadequate intraoperative volume replacement. In response to hypovolemia, the renin-angiotensin system is activated, and antidiuretic hormone (ADH) is released to prompt reabsorption of sodium and water by the renal tubules. Prerenal oliguria results.

Treatment focuses on volume replacement. Thus, an accurate assessment of the patient's fluid deficit is primary. Tallying estimated surgical blood loss and data from the intraoperative fluid logs kept by the anesthesiologist will help begin the calculations. Insensible loss during laparotomy approximates 150 mL/hr. That during laparoscopy is negligible (Biegner, 1999).

Intrarenal Oliguria

Ischemic injury can lead to necrosis of the renal tubules and decreased filtration. This damage may be more common in a prerenal setting, in which the renal tubules are more vulnerable to insult from nephrotoxic agents such as NSAIDs, aminoglycosides, and IV contrast media. In many cases, intrarenal and prerenal oliguria can be differentiated by calculating the fractional excretion of sodium (FENa). Using sodium (Na^+) and creatinine (Cr) levels from both serum and urine, FENa is defined as:

$$(\text{Urine } Na^+/\text{plasma } Na^+) \div (\text{Urine Cr}/\text{plasma Cr}).$$

A ratio <1 suggests a prerenal source, whereas a ratio >3 indicates an intrarenal insult. Another difference is urine sodium levels. In prerenal oliguria, the level is typically <20 mEq/L, whereas in intrarenal states, it usually is >80 mEq/L.

Postrenal Oliguria

The most common cause of postrenal oliguria is urinary catheter obstruction. In those without a catheter, urinary retention is most likely. More seriously, the ureter or bladder may be ligated or lacerated, and evaluation of these is found in Chapter 40 (p. 865). Importantly, partial or unilateral obstruction may exist despite adequate urine output. With this, associated findings may include hematuria, flank or abdominal pain, or ileus.

For diagnosis, renal sonography is highly sensitive and specific for confirming hydronephrosis. Additional diagnostic tools to identify ureteral obstruction include CT with IV contrast or retrograde pyelography. Importantly, IV contrast can be nephrotoxic, and thus CT with contrast may be a less than ideal choice for those with already elevated serum creatinine levels. Obstruction may be relieved with ureteral stenting alone or may require surgical repair (Chap. 40, p. 867).

Urinary Retention

Inability to void with a full bladder is common after gynecologic surgery, and incidences range from 2.5 to 43 percent depending on the definition used and surgical procedure

(Geller, 2014). In addition to patient discomfort, recatheterization to treat retention raises the risk of urinary tract infection and may extend hospitalization. Less often, overdistention can lead to prolonged difficulty with micturition and even permanent detrusor damage (Mayo, 1973).

Early postoperative urinary retention is most common with pelvic floor reconstructive surgeries. Other independently associated risks are age >50 years, intraoperative IV fluid administration >750 mL, and bladder urine volume >270 mL when measured upon entry to the recovery room (Keita, 2005). In one review, the risk was higher after robotic hysterectomy compared with a laparoscopic approach (Smorgick, 2012).

Despite identifiable risks, all patients are advised to notify providers for absent or difficult voiding. Clinical markers include pain, tachycardia, urgency, and bladder enlargement by palpation or percussion. These clues are diagnostically equivalent to evaluation using bedside bladder sonography (Bodker, 2003).

Once retention is identified, catheterization and bladder drainage should follow. Lau and Lam (2004) sought to determine the best catheterization strategy for managing postoperative urinary retention. Compared with overnight bladder decompression with an indwelling catheter, episodic in-and-out catheterization is equally effective. Moreover, infectious morbidity rates do not significantly differ between the two.

Voiding Trials

Normal urination requires appropriate bladder contractility in the absence of significant urethral resistance (Abrams, 1999). Objective criteria that define normal function postoperatively vary and may be assessed using either active or passive voiding trials.

With an *active voiding trial*, the bladder is filled with a set volume, and following patient voiding, residual bladder urine volumes are calculated. To begin, the bladder is completely emptied by catheterization. It may be helpful for a woman to stand upright to clear the most dependent portions of her bladder. Next, sterile water infused under gravity is instilled into the bladder through the same catheter until approximately 300 mL is used or until a subjective maximum capacity is reached. A patient is then given up to 30 minutes to void spontaneously into a urine collection device. The difference between volume infused and volume retrieved is recorded as the *postvoid residual*.

The only published study evaluating the effectiveness of this strategy was reported by Kleeman and associates (2002). They evaluated women following surgery for incontinence and prolapse. In their study, a postvoid residual of less than 50 percent carried a recatheterization rate of 8 percent. If patients could spontaneously void greater than 70 percent of the instilled volume, there were no failures.

A *passive voiding trial* serves as an alternative, and residuals may be assessed following passive, physiologic filling of the bladder. To begin, the Foley catheter is removed, and a woman is encouraged to drink increased amounts of liquid. She is encouraged to void spontaneously at her first urge to urinate or after 4 hours, whichever is first. Urine volumes in a collection device are measured. An in-and-out catheterization or bladder sonogram is then performed to measure the postvoid residual (Fig. 23-12, p. 524).

An easy rule to remember for evaluating either active or passive voiding trials is the "75/75 rule." This describes spontaneously voiding greater than 75 mL *and* voiding greater than 75 percent of the total bladder volume. These criteria constitute a successful voiding trial and obviate the need for Foley catheter reinsertion. Alternatively, on the Urogynecology Service at Parkland Hospital, a postvoid residual of less than 100 mL constitutes a success.

PSYCHIATRIC COMPLICATIONS

Brief periods of confusion are common after general anesthesia. Delirium is estimated to complicate approximately 10 to 60 percent of all surgical cases (Ganai, 2007). Elderly patients have an elevated risk, which is associated with longer hospital stays, greater hospital costs, and even risk of death (Bilotta, 2013).

Delirium is diagnosed by five psychiatric criteria. These are altered cognition, disturbed attention and awareness, a fluctuating time course, changes unrelated to a neurocognitive disorder, and a direct physiologic cause that underlies the delirium (American Psychiatric Association, 2013). In postoperative cases, delirium typically develops between 24 and 72 hours after surgery. For assessment, the Confusion Assessment Method (CAM) is a simple four-question tool, which has a sensitivity of 94 percent and specificity of 89 percent (Table 42-11) (Inouye, 2014).

Preventive strategies are typically nonpharmacologic and begin with identifying delirium predisposition. Characteristics can be categorized as modifiable or nonmodifiable. Alterable risks include infection, pain, sodium and potassium electrolyte abnormalities, anemia, hypoxia, polypharmacy, sleep-wake cycle disruption, and certain medications (American Geriatric Society, 2015; Sanders, 2011). Notable groups are opiates, antihistamines, anticholinergics, benzodiazepines, and dihydropyridines, which include calcium-channel blocking agents. Patients with impaired hearing and vision are provided with appropriate aids (Inouye, 1999). Nonmodifiable factors are older age, preexisting cognitive deficits, poor preoperative functional status, and comorbid disease.

As treatment, oxygenation, electrolyte, and fluid imbalances first are corrected. Second, pain and potential infection are assessed. In addition, all nonessential medications are halted

TABLE 42-11. Confusion Assessment Method Short Form Questionnaire

Feature 1: Acute Onset and Fluctuating Course
  Acute change in mental state from baseline?
  Did this behavior fluctuate during interview?

Feature 2: Inattention
  Did the patient have difficulty focusing attention?

Feature 3: Disorganized Thinking
  Was the patient's thinking disorganized or incoherent?

Feature 4: Altered Level of Consciousness
  Hyperalert, lethargic, stuporous, *or* unarousable

Delirium is diagnosed if the following are present: Feature 1 *and* feature 2 PLUS either feature 3 *or* 4.

to minimize confounding effects. Other strategies incorporate greater activity through physical therapy, establishment of distinct sleep-wake cycles, and even light therapy (de Jonghe, 2011; Ono, 2011).

FLUID AND ELECTROLYTE ABNORMALITIES

■ Hypovolemic Shock

Circulatory dysfunction lowers tissue oxygenation and results in multiorgan failure if not recognized and treated promptly. In gynecology, the most frequent cause of shock is hemorrhage-related hypovolemia, although cardiogenic, septic, and neurogenic sources are considered. Hypovolemic shock may develop before, after, or during surgery, and a full discussion is found in Chapter 40 (p. 858).

■ Hyponatremia

This common imbalance is defined as a serum sodium level <135 mEq/L and may produce symptoms as levels drop below 125 mEq/L. Of causes, hypotonic fluid administration is often implicated. Aggressive IV crystalloid resuscitation with comparatively hypotonic fluids is one example. Another is venous absorption of large volumes of certain distending media during long operative hysteroscopy cases (Chap. 41, p. 903). In addition, extrarenal sodium losses may follow profuse diarrhea, vomiting, or nasogastric suctioning. Less often, pain or drugs can induce water retention through a syndrome of inappropriate ADH (SIADH) (Steele, 1997). Similarly uncommon, excessive renal excretion of sodium may accompany diuretic overuse or adrenal insufficiency.

Severe hyponatremia can lead to metabolic encephalopathy and associated cerebral edema, seizures, increased intracranial pressure, and even respiratory arrest. Symptoms are not related to the specific serum sodium level as much as to the rate of change in these levels.

Treatment strategies incorporate the patient's extracellular volume balance and neurologic status. The speed of correction ideally does not exceed 0.5 mEq/L/hr or a serum sodium goal of 130 mEq/L. Overaggressive correction can result in a specific demyelination disorder known as *central pontine myelinolysis*. In those without symptoms, careful replacement with isotonic fluids and treatment of underlying conditions will correct most cases. Frequent serum sodium levels are drawn to direct care. With associated hypervolemia, furosemide (Lasix) may be added. In those with acute neurologic symptoms, 3-percent saline can be given in a 100-mL infusion over 30 minutes and repeated an additional two times if needed (Nagler, 2014; Verbalis, 2013).

■ Hypernatremia

Hypernatremia is defined as a serum sodium concentration >145 mEq/L. Common causes are loss of hypotonic body fluids such as diarrhea, gastric secretions, and sweat. The resulting plasma hypertonicity draws water out of cells to maintain intravascular fluid compartment volume. Brain cell shrinkage can cause vascular bleeds and permanent neurologic damage. To restore brain cell volume, the brain metabolically generates compensatory compounds, termed idiogenic osmoles, which

pull water back into its cells. Therefore, aggressive treatment with hypotonic fluids can overcorrect to cause cerebral edema, seizure, coma, and even death (Adrogué, 2000).

As treatment, volume replacement to correct hemodynamic instability is initiated with isotonic fluids or colloid fluids. Hypernatremia then is corrected using hypotonic solutions.

Diabetes insipidus is a condition of renal water wasting, and an excessive amount of urine devoid of solutes is produced. Central diabetes insipidus stems from a failure to release ADH, whereas nephrogenic diabetes insipidus is caused by a deficit in the renal responsiveness to ADH. For treatment, the free water deficit is replaced over 2 to 3 days. In cases of central diabetes insipidus, the addition of ADH (vasopressin) prevents ongoing free water loss (Blevins, 1992).

■ Hypokalemia

This imbalance is defined as serum potassium <3.5 mEq/L. Hypokalemia is usually caused by diarrhea or by abnormal renal losses secondary to metabolic alkalosis. Mild hypokalemia is often asymptomatic, but nonspecific symptoms seen with progression include generalized weakness and constipation. When serum levels fall below 2.5 mEq/L, muscle necrosis can begin, and an ascending paralysis can develop with levels below 2.0 mEq/L. Hypokalemia in isolation does not produce cardiac arrhythmia, but it can promote dysfunction in combination with magnesium depletion, myocardial ischemia, and digitalis use (Schaefer, 2005).

Potassium replacement is corrective. Compared with IV replacement, oral potassium is safer because it enters the circulation more slowly and reduces the risk of iatrogenic hyperkalemia. The maximum rate of IV potassium replacement is 20 mEq/L, and the patient's cardiac rhythm is concurrently monitored (Kruse, 1990). Magnesium depletion can cause hypokalemia refractory to replacement efforts, and magnesium may need to be concomitantly replenished (Whang, 1985).

■ Hyperkalemia

This imbalance is defined as a serum potassium concentration >5.0 to 5.5 mEq/L. Pseudohyperkalemia can result from traumatic hemolysis, released from muscles distal to a tourniquet, or from cellular release in a clotted specimen tube. If hypokalemia is an unsuspected finding in an asymptomatic patient, repeat measurement is sound.

Medication-induced renal excretion impairment is a leading cause of hyperkalemia. The most commonly implicated medication classes are angiotensin-converting enzyme inhibitors, potassium-sparing diuretics, and NSAIDs (Palmer, 2004; Perazella, 2000). Instead, digitalis and β-receptor antagonists can cause transcellular shifts in potassium.

Clinically, hyperkalemia can slow electrical conduction in the heart. The earliest ECG findings are narrowing and tenting of the T waves. As hyperkalemia progresses, the PR interval lengthens, P waves disappear, and QRS intervals ultimately widen.

With management, basic principles emphasize protecting myocardium, shifting potassium intracellularly, and enhancing potassium excretion. Intravenous calcium gluconate administered as 10 mL of a 10-percent solution over 2 to 3 minutes antagonizes the effect of potassium on myocardial repolarization and the conduction system. If ECG changes fail to improve, calcium administration can be repeated 5 to 10 minutes later. Additionally, a combination of IV insulin (10 units) and 50 mL of 50-percent dextrose can temporarily shift potassium to the intracellular compartment. Alternatively, a β2-agonist, such as inhaled albuterol, can drive a similar potassium shift. Last, potassium excretion can be augmented. Namely, potassium can be cleared across the GI mucosa using sodium polystyrene sulfonate (Kayexalate), cleared renally using loop diuretics, or cleared with dialysis for those with impaired renal function.

ENDOCRINE COMPLICATIONS

■ Thyroid Storm

Severe clinical manifestations of thyrotoxicosis characterize *thyroid storm*, which is rare but life threatening. The yearly incidence in hospitalized patients approximates 5 cases per 100,000 persons (Galindo, 2019). An acute event, such as surgery, trauma, or parturition may precipitate thyroid storm. Findings include hyperpyrexia (temperature >103°F or 39.4°C), tachycardia, congestive heart failure, and altered mental status. Hypotension, arrhythmias, and cardiovascular collapse resulting in death are others. Severe symptoms and laboratory tests that confirm hyperthyroidism are diagnostic.

Typically, patients are managed in an intensive care unit. A β-blocking agent and a thionamide, such as propylthiouracil or methimazole are provided. An iodine solution may be administered to block the release of thyroid hormone, and glucocorticoids are given to reduce the conversion of thyroxine (T4) to triiodothyronine (T3) (Ross, 2016).

■ Diabetes Mellitus

Postoperative hyperglycemia is a well-recognized risk factor for surgical site infection (Hopkins, 2017). Other undesired hyperglycemia effects are dehydration, electrolyte abnormalities, and possibly ketoacidosis in patients with type 1 diabetes. Thus, maintaining random blood glucose levels <200 mg/dL is advocated (Jacober, 1999). Recommendations regarding perioperative management of oral hypoglycemic agents and insulin can be found in Tables 39-6 and 39-7 (p. 830). Care is taken to avoid hypoglycemia, which may develop especially during oral intake changes.

POSTOPERATIVE FEVER

■ Pathophysiology

Fever is a response to inflammatory mediators, termed pyrogens. The inflammatory cascade also produces several cytokines in response to surgery, cancer, trauma, and infection (Wortel, 1993). Thus, fever is common after surgery and is self-limited in most cases (Garibaldi, 1985). However, for those with persistent symptoms, a systematic approach to patient evaluation helps differentiate inflammatory from infectious etiologies.

Fevers that develop more than 2 days after surgery are more likely to be infectious. More broadly, causes are categorized by the mnemonic "five Ws," which represent wind, water, walking, wound, and "wonder" drug. First, pneumonia is considered, and women at greatest risk are those who have been mechanically ventilated for a prolonged period, have an NGT in place, or have preexisting COPD. Atelectasis is common but is more likely a coincidental rather than causal finding (Mavros, 2011). Second, catheterization places women at risk for urinary tract infection. Logically, catheterization duration correlates positively with this infection risk. Third, VTE may present with low-grade fever and other disease-specific symptoms. For example, women with DVT often complain of unilateral lower-extremity edema and erythema. Those with PE may note dyspnea, cough with blood-tinged sputum, chest pain, tachycardia, and symptoms of hypotension. As for wounds, fever related to surgical site infection usually develops 5 to 7 days after the procedure. These infections may involve the pelvis or abdominal wall layers. Last, medications commonly used postoperatively—such as heparin and various antibiotics—may cause a rash, eosinophilia, or drug fever.

■ Clinical Evaluation

In multiple studies, fever evaluations that rotely include complete blood count, urinalysis, blood cultures, and chest radiographs are reported to be ineffective (Badillo, 2002; de la Torre, 2003; Schey, 2005). Thus, initial assessment of a woman with postoperative fever is individualized and begins with a focused history and physical examination. The simple diagnostic algorithm presented in Figure 42-1 can be used as one high-yield, cost-effective strategy (de la Torre, 2003). Wound and urinary tract infections are described in Chapter 3 (p. 75), whereas management of pulmonary complications and VTE is found on pages 911 and 914.

POSTOPERATIVE WOUND

■ Acute Wound Healing

Wound healing has three phases—inflammatory reaction, proliferation, and remodeling (Li, 2007). Hemostasis by coagulation initiates the first step in the *inflammatory phase*. The infiltration of leukocytes and release of cytokines helps initiate the *proliferative phase* of wound repair. During this, two activities happen simultaneously–the growth of granulation tissue to fill the wound and the formation of epithelium to cover the wound. The final stage, *remodeling*, restores the structural integrity and functional aptitude of the new tissue.

■ Wound Dehiscence

Classification and Incidence

The depth to which a wound may open varies and may involve only the subcutaneous and skin layers. Such superficial separation can result solely from a hematoma or seroma, but more commonly it is a consequence of wound infection. The reported incidence of superficial separations ranges from 3 to 15 percent (Owen, 1994; Taylor, 1998).

More seriously, separation can include the abdominal wall fascia. Fascial dehiscence occurs less frequently and is associated with greater morbidity (Carlson, 1997). Infection or sutures held under too much tension are notorious causes and lead to

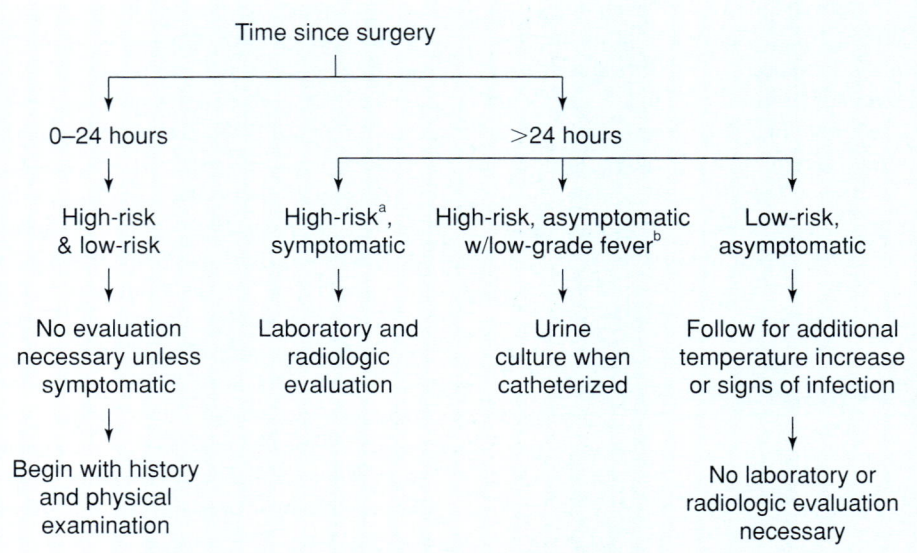

Time since surgery

0–24 hours → High-risk & low-risk → No evaluation necessary unless symptomatic → Begin with history and physical examination

>24 hours:
- High-risk[a], symptomatic → Laboratory and radiologic evaluation
- High-risk, asymptomatic w/low-grade fever[b] → Urine culture when catheterized
- Low-risk, asymptomatic → Follow for additional temperature increase or signs of infection → No laboratory or radiologic evaluation necessary

[a]High risk: (1) Cancer, with more advanced stage of disease; (2) Immunosuppressed; (3) Bowel resection; (4) Temperature > 38.5 °C or 101.3 °F, later in postoperative course than postoperative day 2.
[b]Low-grade fever = temperature < 38.4 °C or 101.1 °F.

FIGURE 42-1 Algorithm for evaluation of postoperative fever. (Redrawn from de la Torre, 2003, with permission.)

fascial necrosis. Sutures remain poorly anchored in necrotic fascia (Bartlett, 1985). These layers then separate with only minimal increases in intraabdominal pressure.

Prevention

Rates of wound dehiscence are affected by general patient health, surgical technique, and risks associated with wound infections. Of these, patient health factors may or may not be modifiable. These include age older than 65 years, pulmonary disease, malnutrition, obesity, malignancy, immune compromise, diabetes mellitus, and hypertension (Hodges, 2014; Riou, 1992).

Using proper surgical technique, a surgeon has multiple opportunities to lower wound disruption rates. Described in greater detail in Chapter 40 (p. 845), ideal technique advocates hemostasis, gentle tissue handling, removal of devitalized tissue, closure of dead space, monofilament suture use, judicious placement of closed-suction drains, and sustained normothermia (Mangram, 1999). Skin and subcutaneous disruption rates in obese women do not differ between wounds closed with staples and those closed with subcuticular sutures (Kuroki, 2017; Zaki, 2018).

Last, infection is a common underlying cause of wound disruption. Risk factors for infection are numerous and are listed in Table 3-18 (p. 85). Of these, many conditions can be improved preoperatively (Table 42-12) (American College of Obstetricians and Gynecologists, 2018a; Berríos-Torres, 2017).

Diagnosis

Superficial wound separations usually present 3 to 5 days after surgery, with wound erythema and new drainage. A delay in evacuating inflammatory exudates from this space can lead to fascial weakening. Fascial dehiscence can result and generally presents within the first 10 days postoperatively. Superficial disruption of the subcutaneous layer and extensive leakage of peritoneal fluid or purulent drainage are indicative. Given the high

mortality risk associated with fascial dehiscence and bowel evisceration, examination under anesthesia to estimate the extent of separation is often warranted. In unclear cases, CT scanning may be elected preoperatively. General surgery consultation is considered if bowel ischemia or difficult abdominal wall closure is anticipated.

Superficial Wound Dehiscence Treatment

Wet-to-dry Dressing Changes. With initial wound management, all hematomas, seromas, or pus are evacuated, and necrotic tissue is debrided. If needed, underlying infection is treated with antibiotics. Discussed in Chapter 3 (p. 83), most abdominal wound infections that follow clean cases originate from *Staphylococcus aureus*. In contrast, those after clean-contaminated cases have a greater chance of being polymicrobial, but anaerobes play a lesser role. Suitable broad-spectrum antibiotic regimens are listed in Table 3-16 (p. 82). Importantly, the number of infections caused by MRSA has grown dramatically, and coverage for this pathogen is considered.

After evacuation, wounds in the subcutaneous layer are typically gently filled with fluffed-out gauze to provide continued wound drainage and access for additional debridement. This dressing is usually removed once or twice daily, and replaced with new moist gauze. Solutions used in this dressing remove surface bacteria without disrupting normal healing components. Thus, povidone iodine, iodophor gauze, dilute hydrogen peroxide, and Daikin solution, which are cytotoxic to white blood cells, should play a limited role in wound care (Bennett, 2001; O'Toole, 1996). In very necrotic wounds, allowing gauze to dry and pulling tissue adherent to the gauze with each change is acceptable. More frequent dressing changes are avoided as they lead to aggressive debridement of vital tissues and slow wound healing. Table 42-13 lists products used in modern wound care (Sarsam, 2005).

TABLE 42-12. Selected Interventions for Surgical Site Infection Prevention

Preoperative
Maintain blood glucose levels <180–200 mg/dL
Stop smoking 30 d before operation (Table 1-6, p. 13)
Administer specialized nutritional supplements or enteral nutrition for severe malnutrition for 7–14 d preoperatively
Adequately treat preoperative infections, such as UTI or cervicitis; postpone elective surgery until remote site infections are treated
Advise patients to shower or bathe (full body) with soap or an antiseptic agent the night before surgery

Perioperative
Remove interfering hair immediately before surgery by clipping or depilatories; no perioperative shaving
Use an antiseptic surgical scrub or alcohol-based hand antiseptic for preoperative cleansing of the operative team members' hands and forearms
Prepare the skin around the operative site with an alcohol-based antiseptic agent unless contraindicated
Vaginal cleansing with either 4% chlorhexidine gluconate or povidone–iodine should be performed before hysterectomy or vaginal surgery
Administer prophylactic antibiotics for most clean-contaminated, contaminated, and dirty procedures (Table 39-8, p. 832).
Administer prophylactic antibiotics within 1 hr before incision (2 hr for vancomycin and fluoroquinolones)
Use higher dosages of prophylactic antibiotics for morbidly obese patients
Use vancomycin as a prophylactic agent only when there is a significant MRSA infection risk
Provide adequate ventilation, minimize operating room traffic, and clean instruments and surfaces with approved disinfectants
Avoid flash sterilization

Intraoperative
Carefully handle tissue, eradicate dead space, and adhere to standard principles of asepsis
Avoid use of surgical drains unless absolutely necessary
Leave contaminated or dirty-infected wounds open
Redose prophylactic antibiotics with short half-lives intraoperatively if operation is prolonged (for cefazolin if operation is >3 hr) or if there is extensive blood loss (>1500 mL)
Maintain intraoperative normothermia

Postoperative
Maintain serum glucose levels <180–200 mg/dL in patients with and without diabetes
Monitor for wound infection

MRSA = methicillin-resistant *Staphylococcus aureus*; SSI = surgical site infection; UTI = urinary tract infection.

TABLE 42-13. Wound Care Products

Product	Description
Calcium alginate	Solid sheets or ribbons that exchange ions with wound fluids to form a nonadhesive, nonocclusive, conformable gel. Indicated for moderate to high draining wounds
Silver dressing	Available in varied forms and used in wounds at risk for infection or not healing due to infection
Enzymatic debrider	Topical solution that breaks down necrotic tissue by directly digesting the collagen holding necrotic tissue to the wound bed
Film	Thin, transparent polyurethane sheets coated on one side with acrylic, hypoallergenic adhesive. The adhesive will not stick to moist surfaces, and the film is impermeable to fluids and bacteria, but semipermeable to oxygen and water vapor. Indicated in superficial wounds with little or no exudate
Foam	Available in varied forms and provide absorbency to create an insulated, moist wound environment. Indicated in light to moderate draining wounds
Gauze	Woven or nonwoven cotton or synthetic blends are ideally moistened with placement into and removal from wounds
Hydrogel	Formulated in sheets or gels. Glycerin-, saline-, or water-based to hydrate the wound. Indicated in dry or minimally draining wounds
Silver nitrate	Used to treat overgrown granulation tissue. Apply stick to hypergranulation tissue

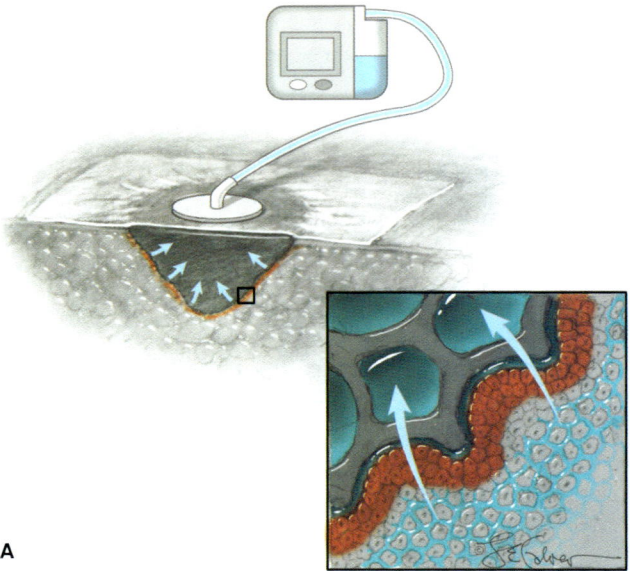

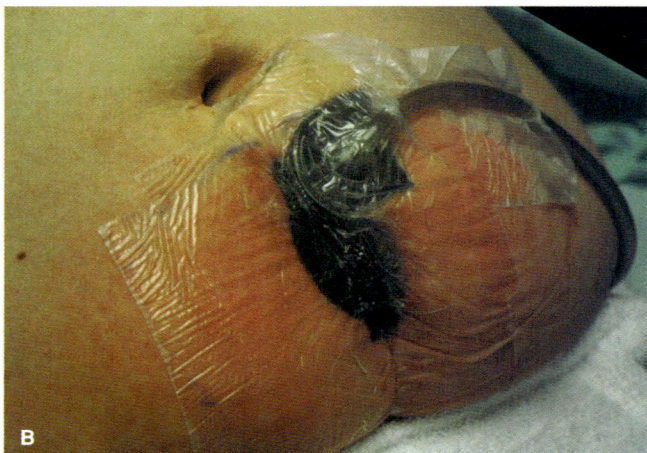

FIGURE 42-2 A. Negative-pressure wound therapy helps evacuate wound drainage and promotes wound healing. **B.** Wound vacuum in place. Porous synthetic sponge fills the wound. (Reproduced with permission from Hoffman BL, Cunningham FG: Surgical instruments. In Yeomans ER, Hoffman BL, Gilstrap LC 3rd, et al (eds): Cunningham and Gilstrap's Operative Obstetrics, 3rd ed. New York, McGraw-Hill Education, 2017.)

Negative-Pressure Wound Therapy. This is primarily used for acute wounds to minimize scarring or for chronic wounds that are resistant to other forms of wound care. Prophylactic use of negative-pressure wound therapy (NPWT) in obese patients may be considered (Hyldig, 2019; O'Leary, 2017).

The negative pressure generated by such devices evacuates wound drainage to reduce bacterial colonization. Negative pressure also promotes release of cytokines that are helpful in wound healing and enhances tissue blood flow and oxygenation. Its effects lead to uniformly reduced wound size and improve angioneogenesis (Fabian, 2000; Morykwas, 1997; Sullivan, 2009).

For NPWT, foam or moistened cotton gauze fills the wound, and evacuation tubing runs through this dressing. The wound then is covered with an adhesive film to maintain suction pressure. The tubing's other end attaches to a vacuum pump, which offers continuous or intermittent negative pressure. Exudates collect in a drainage canister (Fig. 42-2). After initial application, the dressing is typically changed within 48 hours and then two to three times weekly thereafter.

Delayed Primary Closure. Approximately 4 days after wound disruption and resolution of subcutaneous infection, a superficial vertical mattress closure with delayed-absorbable suture may be used to reapproximate tissue edges (Wechter, 2005). Depending on wound depth and patient tolerances, this can be completed in the operating room or at the bedside using a local anesthetic complemented by systemic analgesia. Overall, this strategy reduces healing time by 5 to 8 weeks and significantly lowers the number of postoperative visits.

Fascial Dehiscence Treatment

Fascial dehiscence is a surgical emergency, and a gynecologist must first determine if abdominal contents have eviscerated. If so, sterile towels soaked in saline and an outer abdominal binder can be used to cover and gently replace bowel or omentum. Broad-spectrum antibiotics are generally recommended to minimize ensuing peritonitis.

The final goal of treatment is fascial closure. For critically ill patients with significant edema, temporarily maintaining anterior abdominal wall integrity with retention sutures until a patient is clinically able to tolerate a definitive operative closure is reasonable. For those stable for surgery, debridement of necrotic or infected tissue is completed under general anesthesia. If a tension-free fascial closure is possible an interrupted mass closure using a no. 2 permanent suture is recommended typically. However, if primary fascial closure is under significant tension, a synthetic mesh bridge between the fascial edges may be required. The subcutaneous layer is considered a dirty wound and is left open. Wet-to-dry dressing changes are performed until the decision is made to proceed with delayed primary closure or allow secondary intention to compete the process (Cliby, 2002).

REFERENCES

Abbas S, Bissett IP, Parry BR: Oral water soluble contrast for the management of adhesive small bowel obstruction. Cochrane Database Syst Rev 3:CD004651, 2007

Abrams P: Bladder outlet obstruction index, bladder contractility index and bladder voiding efficiency: three simple indices to define bladder voiding function. Br J Urol Int 84:14, 1999

Adrogué HJ, Madias NE: Hypernatremia. N Engl J Med 342(20):1493, 2000

Ahmed MR, Sayed Ahmed WA, Atwa KA, et al: Timing of urinary catheter removal after uncomplicated total abdominal hysterectomy: a prospective randomized trial. Eur J Obstet Gynecol Reprod Biol 176:60, 2014

Akarsu T, Karaman S, Akercan F, et al: Preemptive meloxicam for postoperative pain relief after abdominal hysterectomy. Clin Exp Obstet Gynecol 31:133, 2004

Aldrete JA: The post-anesthesia recovery score revisited. J Clin Anesth 7(1):89, 1995

Al-Sunaidi M, Tulandi T: Adhesion-related bowel obstruction after hysterectomy for benign conditions. Obstet Gynecol 108:1162, 2006

Al-Took S, Platt R, Tulandi T: Adhesion-related small-bowel obstruction after gynecologic operations. Am J Obstet Gynecol 180:313, 1999

American College of Obstetricians and Gynecologist: Prevention of infection after gynecologic procedures. Practice Bulletin No. 195, June 2018a

American College of Obstetricians and Gynecologist: Perioperative pathways: enhanced recovery after surgery. Committee Opinion No. 750, September 2018b

American Geriatrics Society: Postoperative delirium in older adults: best practice statement from the American Geriatrics Society. J Am Coll Surg 220(2):136, 2015

American Psychiatric Association: Diagnostic and Statistical Manual of Mental Disorders, Fifth Edition. Arlington, American Psychiatric Association, 2013

American Society of Anesthesiologists Task Force on Perioperative Management of Patients with Obstructive Sleep Apnea: Practice guidelines for the perioperative management of patients with obstructive sleep apnea: an updated report by the American Society of Anesthesiologists Task Force on Perioperative Management of Patients with Obstructive Sleep Apnea. Anesthesiology 120(2):268, 2014

Anderson AD, McNaught CE, MacFie J, et al: Randomized clinical trial of multimodal optimization and standard perioperative surgical care. Br J Surg 90:1497, 2003

Apfel CC, Korttila K, Abdalla M, et al: A factorial trial of six interventions for the prevention of postoperative nausea and vomiting. N Engl J Med 350:2441, 2004

Apfelbaum JL, Chen C, Mehta SS, et al: Postoperative pain experience: results from a national survey suggest postoperative pain continues to be undermanaged. Anesth Analg 97:534, 2003

Apfelbaum JL, Silverstein JH, Chung FF, et al: Practice guidelines for postanesthetic care: an updated report by the American Society of Anesthesiologists Task Force on Postanesthetic Care. Anesthesiology 118(2):291, 2013

ARDS Definition Task Force, Ranieri VM, Rubenfeld GD, et al: Acute respiratory distress syndrome: the Berlin definition. JAMA 307(23):2526, 2012

Assalia A, Schein M, Kopelman D, et al: Therapeutic effect of oral Gastrografin in adhesive, partial small-bowel obstruction: a prospective, randomized trial. Surgery 115:433, 1994

Badillo AT, Sarani B, Evans SR: Optimizing the use of blood cultures in the febrile postoperative patient. J Am Coll Surg 194:477, 2002

Badner NH, Knill RL, Brown JE, et al: Myocardial infarction after noncardiac surgery. Anesthesiology 88(3):572, 1998

Bartlett LC: Pressure necrosis is the primary cause of wound dehiscence. Can J Surg 28:27, 1985

Bateman NT, Leach RM: ABC of oxygen. Acute oxygen therapy. BMJ 317(7161):798, 1998

Bennett LL, Rosenblum RS, Perlov C, et al: An in vivo comparison of topical agents on wound repair. Plast Reconstr Surg 108:675, 2001

Berríos-Torres SI, Umscheid CA, Bratzler DW, et al: Centers for Disease Control and Prevention guideline for the prevention of surgical site infection, 2017. JAMA Surg 152(8):784, 2017

Biegner AR, Anderson D, Olson RL, et al: Quantification of insensible water loss associated with insufflation of nonhumidified CO2 in patients undergoing laparoscopic surgery. J Laparoendosc Adv Surg Tech A 9(4):325, 1999

Bilotta F, Lauretta MP, Borozdina A: Postoperative delirium: risk factors, diagnosis, and perioperative care. Minerva Anestesiol 79(9):1066, 2013

Bisch SP, Wells T, Gramlich L, et al: Enhanced recovery after surgery (ERAS) in gynecologic oncology: system-wide implementation and audit leads to improved value and patient outcomes. Gynecol Oncol 151(1):117, 2018

Blevins LS Jr, Wand GS: Diabetes insipidus. Crit Care Med 20(1):69, 1992

Bodker B, Lose G: Postoperative urinary retention in gynecologic patients. Int Urogynecol J 14:94, 2003

Boumphrey SM, Morris EA, Kinsella SM: 100% inspired oxygen from a Hudson mask-a realistic goal? Resuscitation 57(1):69, 2003

Braga M, Gianotti L, Gentilini O, et al: Feeding the gut early after digestive surgery: results of a nine-year experience. Clin Nutr 21:59, 2002

Brandstrup B, Tønnesen H, Beier-Holgersen R, et al: Effects of intravenous fluid restriction on postoperative complications: comparison of two perioperative fluid regimens: a randomized assessor-blinded multicenter trial. Ann Surg 238(5):641, 2003

Burks C, Nelson L, Kumar D, et al: Evaluation of pulmonary complications in robotic-assisted gynecologic surgery. J Minim Invasive Gynecol 24(2):280, 2017

Canet J, Ricos M, Vidal F: Early postoperative arterial oxygen desaturation. Determining factors and response to oxygen therapy. Anesth Analg 69(2):207, 1989

Carey ET, Moulder JK: Perioperative management and implementation of enhanced recovery programs in gynecologic surgery for benign indications. Obstet Gynecol 132(1):137, 2018

Carlson MA: Acute wound failure. Surg Clin North Am 77:607, 1997

Cassidy MR, Rosenkranz P, McAneny D: Reducing postoperative venous thromboembolism complications with a standardized risk-stratified prophylaxis protocol and mobilization program. J Am Coll Surg 218(6):1095, 2014

Chan A, Dore CJ, Ramachandra V: Analgesia for day surgery: evaluation of the effect of diclofenac given before or after surgery with or without bupivacaine infiltration. Anaesthesia 51:592, 1996

Charlson ME, MacKenzie CR, Gold JP, et al: Intraoperative blood pressure. What patterns identify patients at risk for postoperative complications? Ann Surg 212(5):567, 1990

Charoenkwan K, Matovinovic E: Early versus delayed oral fluids and food for reducing complications after major abdominal gynaecologic surgery. Cochrane Database Syst Rev 12:CD004508, 2014

Chou R, Gordon DB, de Leon-Casasola OA, et al: Management of postoperative pain: a clinical practice guideline from the American Pain Society, the American Society of Regional Anesthesia and Pain Medicine, and the American Society of Anesthesiologists' Committee on Regional Anesthesia, Executive Committee, and Administrative Council. J Pain 17(2):131, 2016

Chumillas S, Ponce JL, Delgado F, et al: Prevention of postoperative pulmonary complications through respiratory rehabilitation: a controlled clinical study. Arch Phys Med Rehabil 79:5, 1998

Cliby WA: Abdominal incision wound breakdown. Clin Obstet Gynecol 45:507, 2002

Condon RE, Frantzides CT, Cowles VE, et al: Resolution of postoperative ileus in humans. Ann Surg 203:574, 1986

Correia MI, da Silva RG: The impact of early nutrition on metabolic response and postoperative ileus. Curr Opin Clin Nutr Metab Care 7:577, 2004

Dauchel J, Schang JC, Kachelhoffer J, et al: Gastrointestinal myoelectrical activity during the postoperative period in man. Digestion 14:293, 1976

de Jonghe A, van Munster BC, van Oosten HE, et al: The effects of melatonin versus placebo on delirium in hip fracture patients: study protocol of a randomised, placebo-controlled, double blind trial. BMC Geriatr 11:34, 2011

de la Torre SH, Mandel L, Goff BA: Evaluation of postoperative fever: usefulness and cost-effectiveness of routine workup. Am J Obstet Gynecol 188:1642, 2003

Delaney CP, Senagore AJ, Gerkin TM, et al: Association of surgical care practices with length of stay and use of clinical protocols after elective bowel resection: results of a national survey. Am J Surg 199(3):299, 2010

Duggan EW, Carlson K, Umpierrez GE: Perioperative hyperglycemia management: an update. Anesthesiology 126(3):547, 2017

Elwyn DH, Bryan-Brown CW, Shoemaker WC: Nutritional aspects of body water dislocations in postoperative and depleted patients. Ann Surg 182:76, 1975

Epstein LJ, Kristo D, Strollo PJ Jr, et al: Clinical guideline for the evaluation, management and long-term care of obstructive sleep apnea in adults. J Clin Sleep Med 5(3):263, 2009

Ertas IE, Gungorduk K, Ozdemir A, et al: Influence of gum chewing on postoperative bowel activity after complete staging surgery for gynecological malignancies: a randomized controlled trial. Gynecol Oncol 131(1):118, 2013

Fabian TS, Kaufman HJ, Lett ED, et al: The evaluation of subatmospheric pressure and hyperbaric oxygen in ischemic full-thickness wound healing. Am Surg 66:1136, 2000

Fernandez-Bustamante A, Frendl G, Sprung J, et al: Postoperative pulmonary complications, early mortality, and hospital stay following noncardiothoracic surgery: a multicenter study by the perioperative research network investigators. JAMA Surg 152(2):157, 2017

Ferris BG Jr, Pollard DS: Effect of deep and quiet breathing on pulmonary compliance in man. J Clin Invest 39:143, 1960

Finnerty CC, Mabvuure NT, Ali A, et al: The surgically induced stress response. JPEN J Parenter Enteral Nutr 37(5 Suppl):21S, 2013

Fleisher LA, Fleischmann KE, Auerbach AD, et al: 2014 ACC/AHA guideline on perioperative cardiovascular evaluation and management of patients undergoing noncardiac surgery: a report of the American College of Cardiology/American Heart Association Task Force on practice guidelines. J Am Coll Cardiol 64(22):e77, 2014

Florêncio RB, Aliverti A, Fagundes ML, et al: Acute effects of three pulmonary reexpansion modalities on thoracoabdominal motion of healthy subjects: randomized crossover study. PLoS ONE 14(3):e0213773, 2019

Food and Drug Administration: FDA drug safety communication: prescription acetaminophen products to be limited to 325 mg per dosage unit; boxed warning will highlight potential for severe liver failure. Silver Springs, U.S. Food and Drug Administration, 2011

Galanaud JP, Sevestre-Pietri MA, Bosson JL: Comparative study on risk factors and early outcome of symptomatic distal versus proximal deep vein thrombosis: results from the OPTIMEV study. Thromb Haemost 102(3):493, 2009

Galindo RJ, Hurtado CR, Pasquel FJ, et al: National trends in incidence, mortality, and clinical outcomes of patients hospitalized for thyrotoxicosis with and without thyroid storm in the United States, 2004–2013. Thyroid 29(1):36, 2019

Gan TJ, Diemunsch P, Habib AS, et al: Consensus guidelines for the management of postoperative nausea and vomiting. Anesth Analg 118(1):85, 2014a

Gan TJ, Habib AS, Miller TE, et al: Incidence, patient satisfaction, and perceptions of post-surgical pain: results from a US national survey. Curr Med Res Opin 30(1):149, 2014b

Ganai S, Lee KF, Merrill A, et al: Adverse outcomes of geriatric patients undergoing abdominal surgery who are at high risk for delirium. Arch Surg 142(11):1072, 2007

Garibaldi RA, Brodine S, Matsumiya S, et al: Evidence for the non-infectious etiology of early postoperative fever. Infect Contr 6:273, 1985

Geller EJ: Prevention and management of postoperative urinary retention after urogynecologic surgery. Int J Womens Health 6:829, 2014

George RB, Allen TK, Habib AS: Serotonin receptor antagonists for the prevention and treatment of pruritus, nausea, and vomiting in women undergoing cesarean delivery with intrathecal morphine: a systematic review and meta-analysis. Anesth Analg 109(1):174, 2009

Goldman-Mazur S, Wypasek E, Karpiński M, et al: High detection rates of antithrombin deficiency and antiphospholipid syndrome in outpatients aged over 50 years using the standardized protocol for thrombophilia screening. Thromb Res 176:67, 2019

Gottlieb RH, Widjaja J, Tian L, et al: Calf sonography for detecting deep venous thrombosis in symptomatic patients: experience and review of the literature. J Clin Ultrasound 27:415, 1999

Griffith CA: The family of Ringer's solutions. NITA 9(6):480, 1986

Güldner A, Pelosi P, de Abreu MG: Nonventilatory strategies to prevent postoperative pulmonary complications. Curr Opin Anaesthesiol 26(2):141, 2013

Gupta A, Cifu AS, Khanna S: Diagnosis and treatment of clostridium difficile infection. JAMA 320(10):1031, 2018

Hawker RJ, McKillop A, Jacobs S: Postanesthesia scoring methods: an integrative review of the literature. J Perianesth Nurs 32(6):557, 2017

Hemmes SN, Serpa Neto A, Schultz MJ: Intraoperative ventilatory strategies to prevent postoperative pulmonary complications: a meta-analysis. Curr Opin Anaesthesiol 26(2):126, 2013

Hodges KR, Davis BR, Swaim LS: Prevention and management of hysterectomy complications. Clin Obstet Gynecol 57(1):43, 2014

Hoffman BL, Cunningham FG: Surgical instruments. In Yeomans ER, Hoffman BL, Gilstrap LC 3rd, et al (eds): Cunningham and Gilstrap's Operative Obstetrics, 3rd ed. New York, McGraw-Hill Education, 2017, pp 25, 26

Hopkins L, Brown-Broderick J, Hearn J, et al: Implementation of a referral to discharge glycemic control initiative for reduction of surgical site infections in gynecologic oncology patients. Gynecol Oncol 146(2):228, 2017

Houman Fekrazad M, Lopes RD, Stashenko GJ, et al: Treatment of venous thromboembolism: guidelines translated for the clinician. J Thromb Thrombolysis 28(3):270, 2009

Huge A, Kreis ME, Zittel TT, et al: Postoperative colonic motility and tone in patients after colorectal surgery. Dis Colon Rectum 43:932, 2000

Hyldig N, Vinter CA, Kruse M, et al: Prophylactic incisional negative pressure wound therapy reduces the risk of surgical site infection after caesarean section in obese women: a pragmatic randomised clinical trial. BJOG 126(5):628, 2019

Inouye SK, Bogardus ST Jr, Charpentier PA, et al: A multicomponent intervention to prevent delirium in hospitalized older patients. N Engl J Med 340(9):669, 1999

Inouye SK, Kosar CM, Tommet D, et al: The CAM-S: development and validation of a new scoring system for delirium severity in 2 cohorts. Ann Intern Med 160(8):526, 2014

Jacober SJ, Sowers JR: An update on perioperative management of diabetes. Arch Intern Med 159(20):2405, 1999

Jaff MR, McMurtry MS, Archer SL, et al: Management of massive and submassive pulmonary embolism, iliofemoral deep vein thrombosis, and chronic thromboembolic pulmonary hypertension: a scientific statement from the American Heart Association. Circulation 123(16):1788, 2011

Jernigan AM, Chen CC, Sewell C: A randomized trial of chewing gum to prevent postoperative ileus after laparotomy for benign gynecologic surgery. Int J Gynaecol Obstet 127(3):279, 2014

Joshi GP, Ogunnaike BO: Consequences of inadequate postoperative pain relief and chronic persistent postoperative pain. Anesthesiol Clin North Am 23:21, 2005

Kalil AC, Metersky ML, Klompas M, et al: Management of adults with hospital-acquired and ventilator-associated pneumonia: 2016 clinical practice guidelines by the Infectious Diseases Society of America and the American Thoracic Society. Clin Infect Dis 63(5):e61, 2016

Kazaure HS, Martin M, Yoon JK, et al: Long-term results of a postoperative pneumonia prevention program for the inpatient surgical ward. JAMA Surg 149(9):914, 2014

Kearon C, Akl EA, Comerota AJ, et al: Antithrombotic therapy and prevention of thrombosis, 9th ed: American College of Chest Physicians evidence based clinical practice guidelines. Chest 141:e419S, 2012

Kehlet H, Jensen TS, Woolf CJ: Persistent postsurgical pain: risk factors and prevention. Lancet 367(9522):1618, 2006

Keita H, Diouf E, Tubach F, et al: Predictive factors of early postoperative urinary retention in the postanesthesia care unit. Anesth Analg 101:592, 2005

Khalili G, Janghorbani M, Saryazdi H, et al: Effect of preemptive and preventive acetaminophen on postoperative pain score: a randomized, double-blind trial of patients undergoing lower extremity surgery. J Clin Anesth 25(3):188, 2013

Kinney JM, Weissman C: Forms of malnutrition in stressed and unstressed patients. Clin Chest Med 7:19, 1986

Kleeman S, Goldwasser S, Vassallo B, et al: Predicting postoperative voiding efficiency after operation for incontinence and prolapse. Am J Obstet Gynecol 187:49, 2002

Koerner CP, Lopez-Aguiar AG, Zaidi M, et al: Caution: increased acute kidney injury in enhanced recovery after surgery (ERAS) protocols. Am Surg 85(2):156, 2019

Kozlow JH, Berenholtz SM, Garrett E, et al: Epidemiology and impact of aspiration pneumonia in patients undergoing surgery in Maryland, 1999–2000. Crit Care Med 31:1930, 2003

Krebs HB, Goplerud DR: Mechanical intestinal obstruction in patients with gynecologic disease: a review of 368 patients. Am J Obstet Gynecol 157:577, 1987

Krstic S, Resanovic V, Alempijevic T, et al: Hartmann's procedure vs loop colostomy in the treatment of obstructive rectosigmoid cancer. World J Emerg Surg 9(1):52, 2014

Kruse JA, Carlson RW: Rapid correction of hypokalemia using concentrated intravenous potassium chloride infusions. Arch Intern Med 150(3):613, 1990

Kuroki LM, Mullen MM, Massad LS, et al: Wound complication rates after staples or suture for midline vertical skin closure in obese women: a randomized controlled trial. Obstet Gynecol 130(1):91, 2017

Lau H, Lam B: Management of postoperative urinary retention: a randomized trial of in-out versus overnight catheterization. Aust N Z J Surg 74(8):658, 2004

Lee TG, Kang SB, Kim DW, et al: Comparison of early mobilization and diet rehabilitation program with conventional care after laparoscopic colon surgery: a prospective randomized controlled trial. Dis Colon Rectum 54(1):21, 2011

Lewis SJ, Egger M, Sylvester PA, et al: Early enteral feeding versus "nil by mouth" after gastrointestinal surgery: systematic review and meta-analysis of controlled trials. BMJ 323:773, 2001

Li J, Chen J, Kirsner R: Pathophysiology of acute wound healing. Clin Dermatol 25(1):9, 2007

Li S, Liu Y, Peng Q, et al: Chewing gum reduces postoperative ileus following abdominal surgery: a meta-analysis of 17 randomized controlled trials. J Gastroenterol Hepatol 28(7):1122, 2013

Liebermann M, Awad M, Dejong M, et al: Ambulation of hospitalized gynecologic surgical patients: a randomized controlled trial. Obstet Gynecol 121(3):533, 2013

Litell JM, Gong MN, Talmor D, et al: Acute lung injury: prevention may be the best medicine. Respir Care 56(10):1546, 2011

Livingston EH, Passaro EP Jr: Postoperative ileus. Dig Dis Sci 35:121, 1990

Lobo DN, Bostock KA, Neal KR, et al: Effect of salt and water balance on recovery of gastrointestinal function after elective colonic resection: a randomised controlled trial. Lancet 359(9320):1812, 2002

Lundquist H, Hedenstierna G, Strandberg A, et al: CT assessment of dependent lung densities in man during general anaesthesia. Acta Radiol 36:626, 1995

Mangano DT, Browner WS, Hollenberg M, et al: Association of perioperative myocardial ischemia with cardiac morbidity and mortality in men undergoing noncardiac surgery. The Study of Perioperative Ischemia Research Group. N Engl J Med 23(26):1781, 1990

Mangram AJ, Horan TC, Pearson ML, et al: Guideline for prevention of surgical site infection, 1999. Centers for Disease Control and Prevention (CDC) Hospital Infection Control Practices Advisory Committee. Am J Infect Control 27(2):97, 1999

Marcotte JH, Patel K, Desai R, et al: Acute kidney injury following implementation of an enhanced recovery after surgery (ERAS) protocol in colorectal surgery. Int J Colorectal Dis 33(9):1259, 2018

Marino PL, Sutin KM (eds): The ICU Book. Philadelphia, Lippincott Williams & Wilkins, 2007, p 1065

Marshall SI, Chung F. Discharge criteria and complications after ambulatory surgery. Anesth Analg 88(3):508, 1999

Mavros MN, Velmahos GC, Falagas ME: Atelectasis as a cause of postoperative fever: where is the clinical evidence? Chest 140(2):418, 2011

Mayo ME, Lloyd-Davies RW, Shuttleworth KE, et al: The damaged human detrusor: functional and electron microscopic changes in disease. Br J Urol 45:116, 1973

McDonald LC, Gerdin DN, Johnson S, et al: Clinical practice guidelines for Clostridium difficile infection in adults and children: 2017 update by the

Infectious Diseases Society of America (IDSA) and Society for Healthcare Epidemiology of America (SHEA). Clin Infect Dis 66(7):987, 2018

McIntosh CA, Macario A: Managing quality in an anesthesia department. Curr Opin Anaesthesiol 22(2):223, 2009

Megibow AJ, Balthazar EJ, Cho KC, et al: Bowel obstruction: evaluation with CT. Radiology 180:313, 1991

Meyers JR, Lembeck L, O'Kane H, et al: Changes in functional residual capacity of the lung after operation. Arch Surg 110:576, 1975

Mixter CG III, Meeker LD, Gavin TJ: Preemptive pain control in patients having laparoscopic hernia repair: a comparison of ketorolac and ibuprofen. Arch Surg 133:432, 1998

Møller AM, Villebro N, Pedersen T, et al: Effect of preoperative smoking intervention on postoperative complications: a randomised clinical trial. Lancet 359:114, 2002

Monk BJ, Berman ML, Montz FJ: Adhesions after extensive gynecologic surgery: clinical significance, etiology, and prevention. Am J Obstet Gynecol 170:1396, 1994

Moore JA, Conway DH, Thomas N, et al: Impact of a peri-operative quality improvement programme on postoperative pulmonary complications. Anaesthesia 72(3):317, 2017

Morykwas MJ, Argenta LC, Shelton-Brown EI, et al: Vacuum-assisted closure: a new method for wound control and treatment: animal studies and basic foundation. Ann Plastic Surg 38:553, 1997

Muffly TM, Ridgeway B, Abbott S, et al: Small bowel obstruction after hysterectomy to treat benign disease. J Minim Invasive Gynecol 19(5):615, 2012

Muir AD, Reeder MK, Foëx P, et al: Preoperative silent myocardial ischaemia: incidence and predictors in a general surgical population. Br J Anaesth 67(4):373, 1991

Myles PS, Bellomo R, Corcoran T, et al: Restrictive versus liberal fluid therapy for major abdominal surgery. N Engl J Med 378(24):2263, 2018

Nagler EV, Vanmassenhove J, van der Veer SN, et al: Diagnosis and treatment of hyponatremia: a systematic review of clinical practice guidelines and consensus statements. BMC Med 12:1, 2014

Nehra V: Fluid electrolyte and nutritional problems in the postoperative period. Clin Obstet Gynecol 45:537, 2002

Nelson G, Altman AD, Nick A, et al: Guidelines for postoperative care in gynecologic/oncology surgery: Enhanced Recovery After Surgery (ERAS®) Society recommendations—part II. Gynecol Oncol 140(2):323, 2016

Nelson G, Bakkum-Gamez J, Kalogera E, et al: Guidelines for perioperative care in gynecologic/oncology: Enhanced Recovery After Surgery (ERAS) Society recommendations-2019 update. Int J Gynecol Cancer 29(4):651, 2019

Nelson R, Edwards S, Tse B: Prophylactic nasogastric decompression after abdominal surgery. Cochrane Database Syst Rev 3:CD004929, 2007

Nisanevich V, Felsenstein I, Almogy G, et al: Effect of intraoperative fluid management on outcome after intraabdominal surgery. Anesthesiology 103(1):25, 2005

Nunley JC, FitzHarris GP: Postoperative ileus. Curr Surg 61:341, 2004

O'Leary DP, Peirce C, Anglim B, et al: Prophylactic negative pressure dressing use in closed laparotomy wounds following abdominal operations: a randomized, controlled, open-label trial: the P.I.C.O. trial. Ann Surg 265(6):1082, 2017

Ong CK, Seymour RA, Lirk P, et al: Combining paracetamol (acetaminophen) with nonsteroidal antiinflammatory drugs: a qualitative systematic review of analgesic efficacy for acute postoperative pain. Anesth Analg 110(4):1170, 2010

Ong JS, Touyz G, Tanner S, et al: Variability of human upper airway collapsibility during sleep and the influence of body posture and sleep stage. J Sleep Res 20(4):533, 2011

Ono H, Taguchi T, Kido Y, et al: The usefulness of bright light therapy for patients after oesophagectomy. Intensive Crit Care Nurs 27(3):158, 2011

O'Toole EA, Goel M, Woodley DT: Hydrogen peroxide inhibits human keratinocyte migration. Dermatol Surg 22:525, 1996

Owen J, Andrews WW: Wound complications after cesarean sections. Clin Obstet Gynecol 37:842, 1994

Palmer BF: Managing hyperkalemia caused by inhibitors of the renin-angiotensin-aldosterone system. N Engl J Med 351(6):585, 2004

Pasquina P, Tramer MR, Granier JM, et al: Respiratory physiotherapy to prevent pulmonary complications after abdominal surgery: a systematic review. Chest 130:1887, 2006

Peppard PE, Young T, Barnet JH, et al: Increased prevalence of sleep-disordered breathing in adults. Am J Epidemiol 177(9):1006, 2013

Perazella MA: Drug-induced hyperkalemia: old culprits and new offenders. Am J Med 109(4):307, 2000

Pickens AW, Forest DJ, Wyderski RJ, et al: Identifying risk of sleep apnea and major hospital events in an older inpatient population. J Am Geriatr Soc 66(9):1847, 2018

Platell C, Hall JC: Atelectasis after abdominal surgery. J Am Coll Surg 185:584, 1997

Prough DS, Bidani A: Hyperchloremic metabolic acidosis is a predictable consequence of intraoperative infusion of 0.9% saline. Anesthesiology 90(5):1247, 1999

Riou JP, Cohen JR, Johnson H Jr: Factors influencing wound dehiscence. Am J Surg 163:324, 1992

Ross DS, Burch HB, Cooper DS, et al: 2016 American Thyroid Association guidelines for diagnosis and management of hyperthyroidism and other causes of thyrotoxicosis. Thyroid 26(10):1343, 2016

Sanders RD, Pandharipande PP, Davidson AJ, et al: Anticipating and managing postoperative delirium and cognitive decline in adults. BMJ 343:d4331, 2011

Santoso JT, Ulm MA, Jennings PW, et al: Multimodal pain control is associated with reduced hospital stay following open abdominal hysterectomy. Eur J Obstet Gynecol Reprod Biol 183:48, 2014

Sarsam SE, Elliott JP, Lam GK: Management of wound complications from cesarean delivery. Obstet Gynecol Surv 60:462, 2005

Schaefer TJ, Wolford RW: Disorders of potassium. Emerg Med Clin North Am 23(3):723, 2005

Schey D, Salom EM, Papadia A, et al: Extensive fever workup produces low yield in determining infectious etiology. Am J Obstet Gynecol 192:1729, 2005

Scotté M, Mauvais F, Bubenheim M, et al: Use of water-soluble contrast medium (Gastrografin) does not decrease the need for operative intervention nor the duration of hospital stay in uncomplicated acute adhesive small bowel obstruction? A multicenter, randomized, clinical trial (adhesive small bowel obstruction study) and systematic review. Surgery 161(5):1315, 2017

Seidner DL: Nutritional issues in the surgical patient. Cleve Clin J Med 73:S77, 2006

Smorgick N, DeLancey J, Patzkowsky K, et al: Risk factors for postoperative urinary retention after laparoscopic and robotic hysterectomy for benign indications. Obstet Gynecol 120(3):581, 2012

Solomon ER, Muffly TM, Barber MD: Common postoperative pulmonary complications after hysterectomy for benign indications. Am J Obstet Gynecol 208(1):54.e1, 2013

Steele A, Gowrishankar M, Abrahamson S, et al: Postoperative hyponatremia despite near-isotonic saline infusion: a phenomenon of desalination. Ann Intern Med 126(1):20, 1997

Stein PD, Terrin ML, Hales CA, et al: Clinical, laboratory, roentgenographic, and electrocardiographic findings in patients with acute pulmonary embolism and no pre-existing cardiac or pulmonary disease. Chest 100(3):598, 1991

Sullivan N, Snyder DL, Tipton K, et al: Negative pressure wound therapy device. Technology assessment report. ECRI Institute. 2009. Available at: http://archive.ahrq.gov/research/findings/ta/negative-pressure-wound-therapy/. Accessed July 15, 2019

Sun Z, Sessler DI, Dalton JE, et al: Postoperative hypoxemia is common and persistent: a prospective blinded observational study. Anesth Analg 121(3):709, 2015

Tablan OC, Anderson LJ, Besser R, et al: Guidelines for preventing health-care—associated pneumonia, 2003: recommendations of CDC and the Healthcare Infection Control Practices Advisory Committee. MMWR 53:1, 2004

Taylor G, Herrick T, Mah M: Wound infections after hysterectomy: opportunities for practice improvement. Am J Infect Control 26:254, 1998

Thomas JA, McIntosh JM: Are incentive spirometry, intermittent positive pressure breathing, and deep breathing exercises effective in the prevention of postoperative pulmonary complications after upper abdominal surgery? A systematic overview and meta-analysis. Phys Ther 74:3, 1994

Thygesen K, Alpert JS, Jaffe AS, et al: Fourth universal definition of myocardial infarction (2018). J Am Coll Cardiol 72(18):2231, 2018

Tinker JH, Tarhan S: Discontinuing anticoagulant therapy in surgical patients with cardiac valve prostheses: observations in 180 operations. JAMA 239:738, 1978

van Rossum AB, van Houwelingen HC, Kieft GJ, et al: Prevalence of deep vein thrombosis in suspected and proven pulmonary embolism: a meta-analysis. Br J Radiol 71(852):1260, 1998

Verbalis JG, Goldsmith SR, Greenberg A, et al: Diagnosis, evaluation, and treatment of hyponatremia: expert panel recommendations. Am J Med 126(10 Suppl 1):S1, 2013

Warner DO: Preventing postoperative pulmonary complications: the role of the anesthesiologist. Anesthesiology 92:1467, 2000

Wechter ME, Pearlman MD, Hartmann KE: Reclosure of the disrupted laparotomy wound: a systematic review. Obstet Gynecol 106:376, 2005

Wells PS, Anderson DR, Bormanis J, et al: Value of assessment of pretest probability of deep-vein thrombosis in clinical management. Lancet 350(9094):1795, 1997

Wells PS, Anderson DR, Rodger M, et al: Derivation of a simple clinical model to categorize patients probability of pulmonary embolism: increasing the models utility with the SimpliRED D-dimer. Thromb Haemost 83(3):416, 2000

Whang R, Flink EB, Dyckner T, et al: Magnesium depletion as a cause of refractory potassium repletion. Arch Intern Med 145(9):1686, 1985

Whelton PK, Carey RM, Aronow WS, et al: 2017 ACC/AHA/AAPA/ABC/ACPM/AGS/APhA/ASH/ASPC/NMA/PCNA guideline for the prevention, detection, evaluation, and management of high blood pressure in adults: a report of the American College of Cardiology/American Heart Association Task Force on Clinical Practice Guidelines. Hypertension 71(6):e13, 2018

Worsley DF, Alavi A, Aronchick JM, et al: Chest radiographic findings in patients with acute pulmonary embolism: observations from the PIOPED Study. Radiology 189(1):133, 1993

Wortel CH, van Deventer SJ, Aarden LA, et al: Interleukin-6 mediates host defense responses induced by abdominal surgery. Surgery 114:564, 1993

Worthington P, Balint J, Bechtold M, et al: When is parenteral nutrition appropriate? JPEN J Parenter Enteral Nutr 41(3):324, 2017

Wright HK, O'Brien JJ, Tilson MD: Water absorption in experimental closed segment obstruction of the ileum in man. Am J Surg 121:96, 1971

Wysham WZ, Kim KH, Roberts JM, et al: Obesity and perioperative pulmonary complications in robotic gynecologic surgery. Am J Obstet Gynecol 213(1):33.e1, 2015

Yadav H, Bartley A, Keating S, et al: Evolution of validated biomarkers and intraoperative parameters in the development of postoperative ARDS. Respir Care 63(11):1331, 2018

Zaki MN, Wing DA, McNulty JA: Comparison of staples vs subcuticular suture in class III obese women undergoing cesarean: a randomized controlled trial. Am J Obstet Gynecol 218(4):451.e1, 2018

Zhang P, Hu WL, Cheng B, et al: A systematic review and meta-analysis comparing immediate and delayed catheter removal following uncomplicated hysterectomy. Int Urogynecol J 26(5):665, 2015

Zielinski MD, Haddad NN, Cullinane DC, et al: Multi-institutional, prospective, observational study comparing the Gastrografin challenge versus standard treatment in adhesive small bowel obstruction. J Trauma Acute Care Surg 83(1):47, 2017

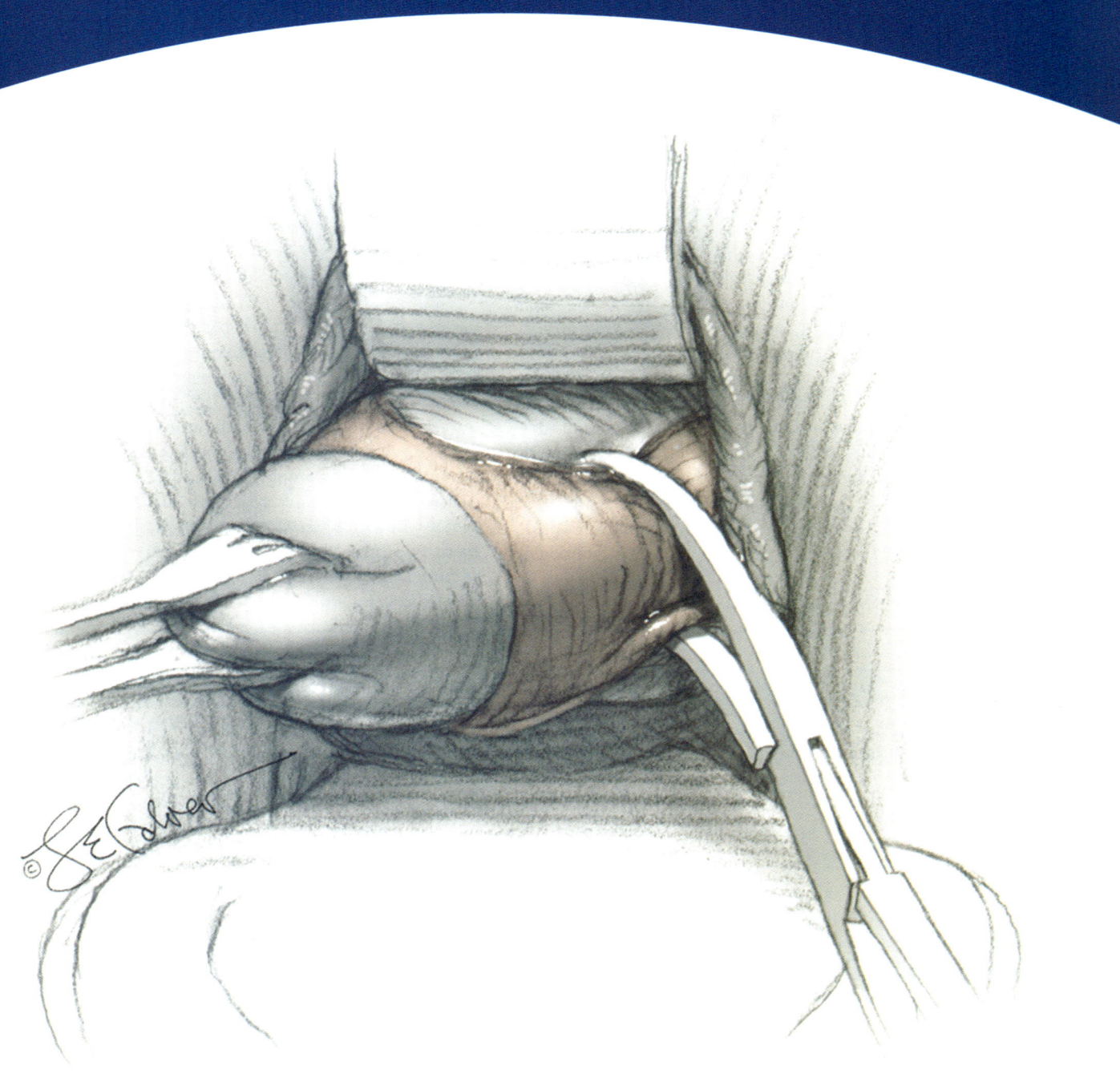

CHAPTER 43

Surgeries for Benign Gynecologic Disorders

43-1

Midline Vertical Incision

Abdominal entry is the first step for many gynecologic surgeries. Incisions are vertical or transverse, and each offers particular advantages. Vertical incisions may be midline or paramedian, but of the two, the midline is predominantly chosen. This incision offers quick entry, minimal blood loss, superior access to the upper abdomen, generous operating room, and the flexibility for easy wound extension if greater space or access is needed. No important neurovascular structures traverse this incision. Thus, it may be favored for patients using anticoagulation agents. Despite advantages, midline incisions are more frequently associated with greater postoperative pain, poorer cosmetic results, and higher risk of wound dehiscence or incisional hernia compared with low transverse incisions (Bewö, 2019; Grantcharov, 2001). For those with prior laparotomy, the incision type is typically repeated for subsequent surgeries.

PREOPERATIVE

Consent

Specific to abdominal entry, the risks of wound infection and later dehiscence are discussed. In addition, the bowel or bladder may be injured during any abdominal entry, especially when extensive adhesions are encountered.

Prophylaxis

When weighing intraoperative contamination and infection risk, laparotomy itself is considered a clean procedure. Despite this, based on some evidence, antibiotic prophylaxis listed in Table 39-8 (p. 832) may be considered solely for the indication of laparotomy (American College of Obstetricians and Gynecologists, 2018b; Morrill, 2013). Bowel preparation is infrequently needed and is dictated by the planned procedure. Prevention for venous thromboembolism (VTE) is warranted and described in Chapter 39 (p. 834).

INTRAOPERATIVE

Surgical Steps

❶ **Anesthesia and Patient Positioning.** After administration of adequate regional or general anesthesia, the patient is supine or in low lithotomy position. If needed, hair in the path of the planned incision is clipped; a Foley catheter is placed; and abdominal preparation is completed.

❷ **Skin and Subcutaneous Layer.** The skin is incised vertically in the midline beginning 2 to 3 cm above the symphysis pubis and extending cephalad to within 2 cm of the umbilicus. If less space is required, this incision may be shortened. For greater space or access, the incision may arch around the umbilicus and then continue cephalad in the upper abdominal midline. This extension passes to the left of the umbilicus to avert transection of the ligamentum teres. This remnant of the umbilical vein courses in the free border of the falciform ligament. The umbilicus itself contains attenuated fascia. Thus, the periumbilical incision arches sufficiently lateral to provide quality fascia on either side of the incision for a secure final closure.

The more superficial *fatty layer of the subcutaneous tissue* (formerly Camper fascia) and then the deeper *membranous layer of the subcutaneous tissue* (formerly Scarpa fascia) are incised either sharply with long, even strokes or with electrosurgical blade to reach the fascia. Ideally, the number of blade strokes is minimized to avoid hatch marking the tissue, which increases tissue damage and wound infection risks.

❸ **Fascia.** Tendinous fibers from the anterior abdominal wall aponeuroses merge in the midline of the abdomen to form the *linea alba*. This fascial layer is sharply entered near the midpoint of the incision to help prevent cystotomy (Fig. 43-1.1). This incision is extended first cephalad and then caudally to mirror the length of the skin incision. To minimize injury to viscera during this extension, the linea alba is elevated by index fingers of the surgeon and assistant or by the open tips of a Pean clamp (Fig. 43-1.2).

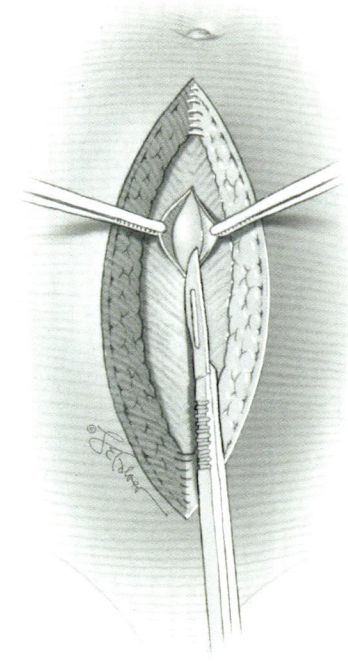

FIGURE 43-1.1 Fascial incision.

Once the fascia is incised, the right and left rectus abdominis muscle bellies are bluntly separated. Nearing the symphysis pubis, sharp incision may be required to complete this. To avert injury to organs below, the rectus muscles are elevated during this division. Each half of the pyramidalis muscle lies atop its respective rectus belly, and this muscle is similarly divided sharply at the midline.

❹ **Peritoneum.** For entry into the abdomen, the peritoneum is identified between the rectus abdominis muscle bellies. It is grasped with two hemostats and in the upper portion of the incision to avoid cystotomy. The interposed peritoneum should be palpated or visually examined to exclude intervening viscera. Only then is it sharply cut (Fig. 43-1.3). Next, an index finger sweeps directly beneath the entry point to identify adhered bowel or omentum. If free, the peritoneum is elevated by fingers of the surgeon and assistant to protect viscera beneath. As the incision is extended cephalad above the arcuate line, the transverse fibers of the posterior rectus sheath are seen and are cut along with the peritoneum. As the incision is extended caudally, the transversalis fascia is found superficial to the peritoneum. To prevent bladder dome injury, this thin fascia layer is elevated by fingers insinuated beneath it and is cut. This incisional layer is extended caudally. Next, the peritoneum beneath it is similarly incised (Fig. 43-1.4). The bladder

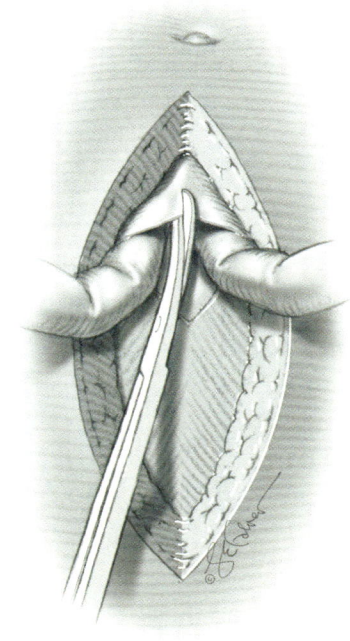

FIGURE 43-1.2 Fascial incision extended cephalad.

dome is identified by increasing tissue vascularity and thickness. Of note, the urachus, which is the remnant of the allantois, may be seen as a white cord extending from the bladder dome toward the umbilicus.

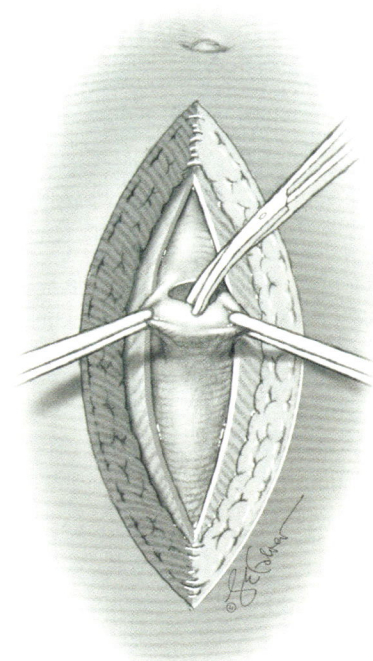

FIGURE 43-1.3 Peritoneal incision.

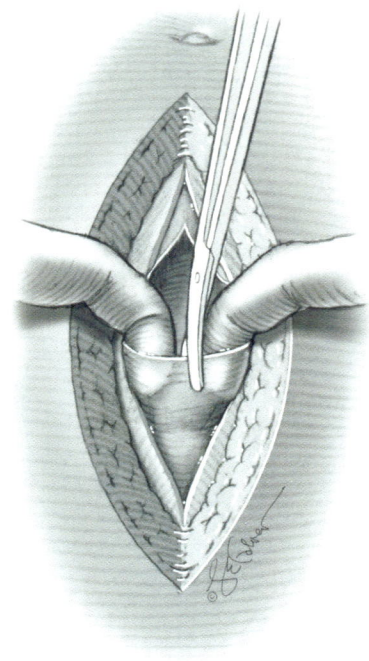

FIGURE 43-1.4 Peritoneal incision extended caudad.

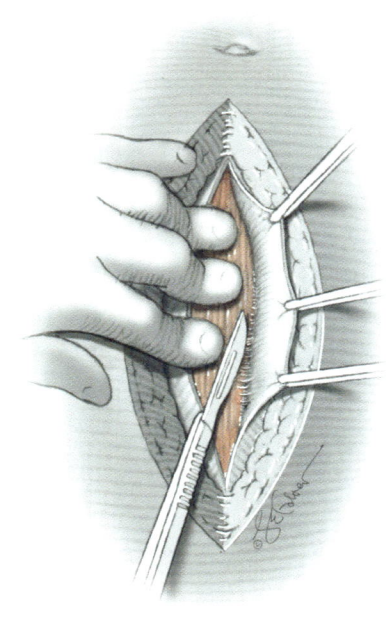

FIGURE 43-1.5 Lateral subfascial dissection.

During abdominal entry, prior surgery may blur clear tissue planes. For example, the true midline may be deviated laterally, and after fascial incision, only rectus fibers may be seen. To find the midline, fibers of the pyramidalis muscles can be followed as they angle toward the midline. Also, visually recreating a mental line between the symphysis and umbilicus can aid orientation. To reach the midline, the fascial edge closest to the presumed midline is grasped both cephalad and caudad along its length with Kocher clamps to create upward tension (Fig. 43-1.5). Simultaneously, downward manual pressure atop the ipsilateral rectus belly accentuates fibers between the fascia and underlying rectus belly. These fibers are then cut to permit lateral dissection of the fascia away from the rectus belly. This is continued until the midline is identified. If the midline is not identified after some dissection on one side, the same steps can be repeated on opposite side.

Also with prior surgery, planes between the fascia and peritoneum may be poorly defined. In these cases, a gradual layered entry is required to avoid organ injury. One technique uses Metzenbaum scissors. Scissor tips are insinuated between tissue layers such that the tips are seen each time prior to cutting. This minimizes the risk that thicker-appearing bowel or bladder wall will be cut.

⑤ Operative Field. After entry into the abdomen, a self-retaining retractor is commonly placed to retract the bowel, omentum, and abdominal wall muscles. Moist laparotomy sponges are placed around the bulk of bowel and gently directed cephalad. Adhesiolysis may be required to adequately free intestines for this repositioning. Mild Trendelenburg positioning also can aid displacement. Upper blades of the retractor assist in holding bowel loops up and away from the pelvis and operating field. The shortest blades possible are preferred for lateral retraction. This reduces the risk of femoral or genitofemoral nerve compression by a blade resting atop the psoas major muscle.

Once pelvic organs are adequately exposed, the planned abdominal surgery can proceed.

⑥ Wound Closure. Closure of the visceral or parietal peritoneum is not required and is individualized (Chap. 40, p. 846). Starting from each end of the incision, the fascia is closed to its midpoint using a continuous running suture with a 0-gauge delayed-absorbable suture. Sutures are placed approximately 1 cm apart and 1.2 to 1.5 cm from the fascial edge. Stitches ideally appose fascial edges without significant tension and allow tissues to swell postoperatively. This limits sutures from cutting through fascia or causing avascular necrosis. The suture ends are then tied together.

If the subcutaneous layer measures <2 cm, no closure is typically necessary. For deeper wounds, interrupted stitches of 2-0 to 4-0 gauge delayed-absorbable suture are used to close this layer. The skin is closed with a subcuticular stitch using 4-0 gauge delayed-absorbable suture, staples, or other suitable method (Chap. 40, p. 846).

POSTOPERATIVE

For most gynecologic surgeries, recovery from the abdominal incision constitutes the greatest portion of postsurgical healing. Midline incisions lead to significant pain during ambulating, coughing, and deep breathing. As a result, laparotomy poses a greater risk of postoperative VTE and pulmonary complications than minimally invasive surgery (MIS). In addition, return of normal bowel function is commonly slowed, and signs of ileus should be monitored. Prevention of these complications is warranted, and enhanced recovery after surgery (ERAS) approaches are described in Chapters 39 and 42. Hospitalization typically varies from 1 to 3 days, and return of normal bowel function usually dictates this course. Postoperative activity in general can be individualized, although vigorous abdominal exercise is delayed for 6 weeks to allow fascial healing. Driving can be resumed when pain does not limit the ability to brake quickly and when narcotic medications are not in use. Return to work is variable, although 6 weeks is commonly cited.

43-2

Pfannenstiel Incision

The Pfannenstiel, Cherney, and Maylard incisions are transverse abdominal incisions used for gynecologic procedures. Of these, the Pfannenstiel incision is most commonly used. Because the transverse incision follows Langer lines of skin tension, excellent cosmetic results can be achieved. Additionally, rates of postoperative pain, fascial wound dehiscence, and incisional hernia are lower than with vertical incisions (Kisielinski, 2004). The Pfannenstiel incision, however, is often less suitable for cases in which greater operating space or upper abdominal access is anticipated. Last, purulent fluid can collect between the incised internal and external oblique aponeuroses. Thus, cases involving abscess or peritonitis favor use of a midline incision, which instead divides the fused linea alba.

PREOPERATIVE

Consent

General risks associated with transverse laparotomy incisions are similar to those for vertical ones. Moreover, transverse incisions can damage the iliohypogastric and ilioinguinal nerves. These injuries frequently involve only transient sensory loss but rarely can lead to debilitating, chronic neuropathic pain.

INTRAOPERATIVE

Surgical Steps

❶ Anesthesia and Patient Positioning. After administration of adequate regional or general anesthesia, the patient is supine or in low lithotomy position. If needed, hair in the path of the planned incision is clipped; a Foley catheter is placed; and abdominal preparation is completed.

❷ Skin and Subcutaneous Layer. Two to 3 cm above the symphysis pubis, an 8- to 10-cm transverse incision is made with its lateral margins arching slightly cephalad. If less space is required, this length can be shortened. The incision is deepened sharply with scalpel or electrosurgical blade until the anterior rectus sheath is reached. The superficial epigastric vessels typically lie several centimeters from the midline and halfway between the skin and fascia. Coagulation of these vessels, if identified, will limit incisional blood loss.

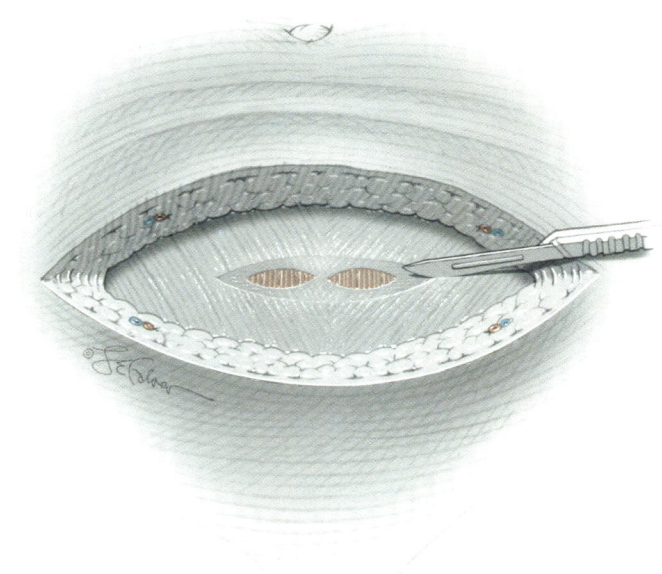

FIGURE 43-2.1 Fascial incision.

❸ Fascia. The anterior rectus sheath is sharply incised transversely in the midline (Fig. 43-2.1). The incision lies well below the arcuate line. Here, the anterior rectus sheath is composed of two visible layers, the aponeuroses from the external oblique muscle and a fused layer containing aponeuroses of the internal oblique and transversus abdominis muscles. Lateral extension of the anterior rectus sheath incision requires cutting each of these two layers individually (Fig. 43-2.2). This practice can help identify and avoid cutting the iliohypogastric and ilioinguinal nerves as they run between these two fascial layers.

Of note, the inferior epigastric vessels typically lie at the lateral border of the rectus abdominis muscle and beneath the fused aponeuroses of the internal oblique and transversus abdominis muscles. Thus, lengthening the incision farther may cut these vessels. If significant lateral extension is required, these vessels are ideally identified, clamped, and ligated. In addition, iliohypogastric and ilioinguinal nerve injury risk also rises as the incision is carried lateral to the rectus abdominis muscle borders (Rahn, 2010).

The superior edge of the fascial incision is grasped with a Kocher clamp on either side of the midline. Traction is directed cephalad and slightly outward. In the area superior to the initial incision, the anterior rectus sheath is then bluntly or sharply separated

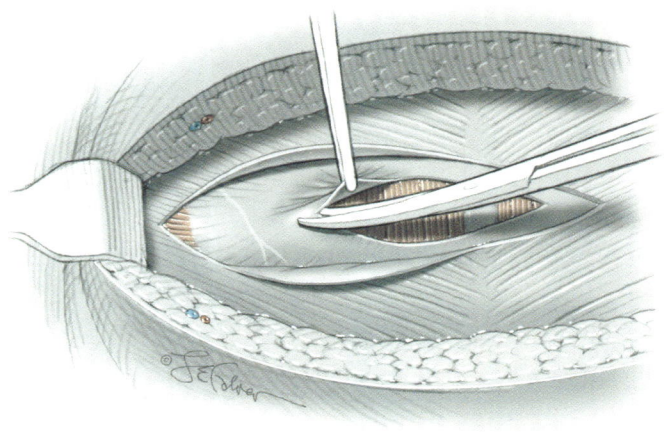

FIGURE 43-2.2 Incision extended laterally.

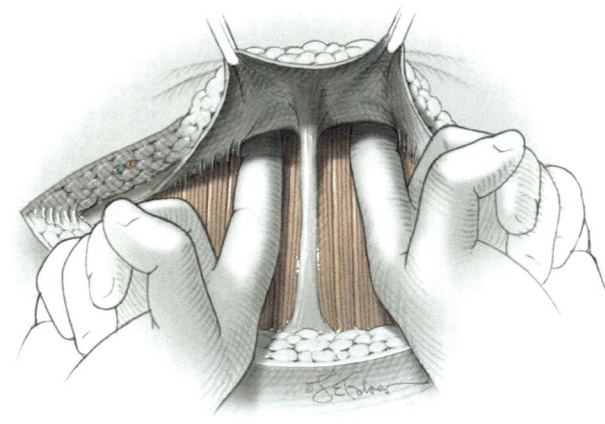

FIGURE 43-2.3 Blunt separation of anterior rectus sheath from underlying rectus abdominis muscle.

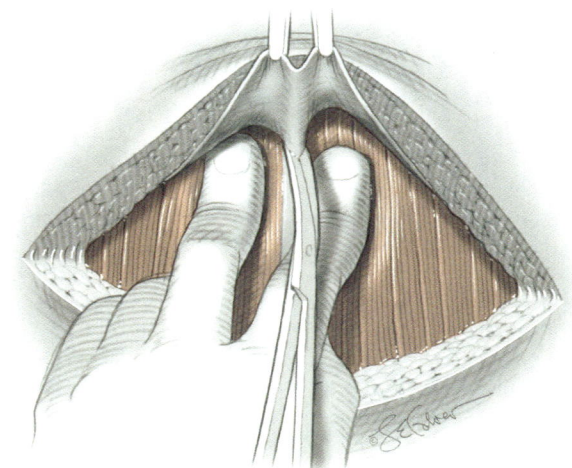

FIGURE 43-2.4 Sharp separation in the midline.

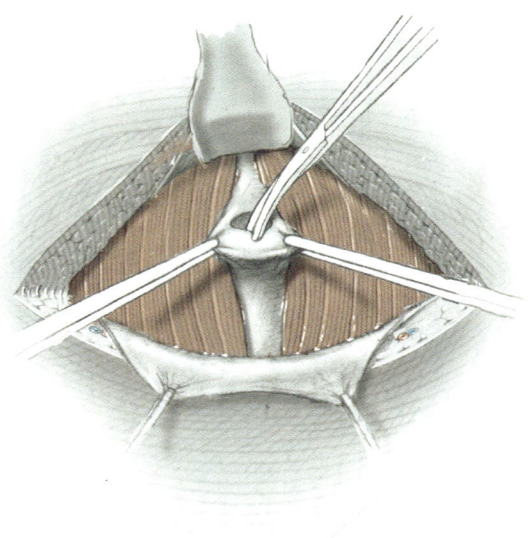

FIGURE 43-2.5 Peritoneal incision. (From Gilstrap, 2017, with permission.)

from the underlying rectus abdominis muscle (Fig. 43-2.3). The fascia separates easily from the bellies of the rectus muscle, but it may be densely adhered along the midline and require sharp dissection (Fig. 43-2.4). Several small perforating nerves and vessels traverse the space between the anterior rectus sheath and rectus muscle. These vessels are coagulated to avoid laceration and bleeding. Upon completion of this dissection, a semicircular area with a radius of 6 to 8 cm has been created. A similar separation is performed in the area inferior to the initial fascial incision.

The rectus abdominis muscle bellies are then bluntly or sharply separated and moved laterally. The pyramidalis muscle, located superficial to the rectus muscle, usually requires sharp division at the midline.

❹ **Peritoneum.** Peritoneal entry is fully described in Section 43-1, Step 4 (p. 931). To summarize, upon separation of the rectus muscle bellies, the thin, filmy peritoneum is identified, grasped with two hemostats, and sharply incised (Fig. 43-2.5). The peritoneal incision is then extended superiorly and inferiorly (Fig. 43-2.6). Once the abdominal cavity has been entered and clear visualization established, the surgeon can proceed with the planned operation.

❺ **Wound Closure.** Closure of the visceral or parietal peritoneum is not required and is individualized. Starting from each end of the incision, the fascia is closed to its midpoint using a continuous running suture with a 0-gauge delayed-absorbable suture (Fig. 43-2.7). These sutures are then tied together. The subcutaneous layer and skin are closed as with the midline vertical incision (p. 932).

POSTOPERATIVE

The postoperative course for low transverse incisions follows that described for midline incisions (p. 932).

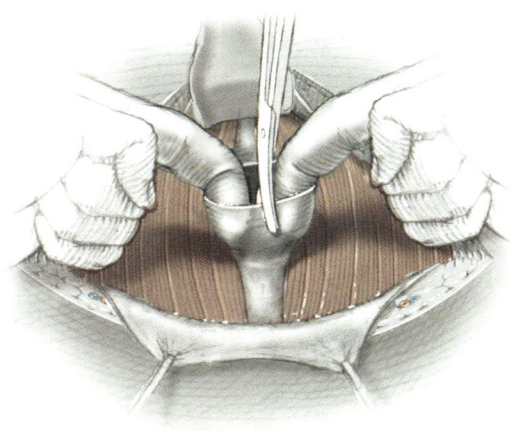

FIGURE 43-2.6 Peritoneal incision extended caudad. (From Gilstrap, 2017, with permission.)

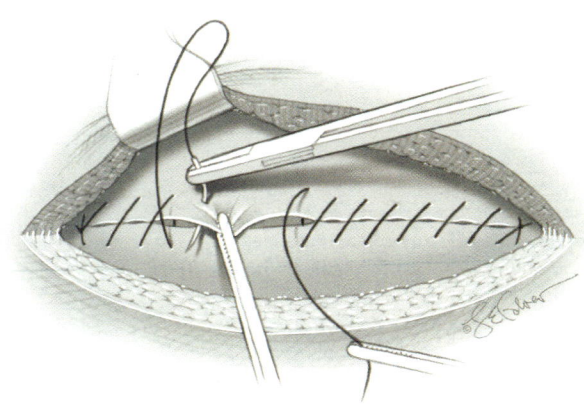

FIGURE 43-2.7 Fascial closure.

43-3

Cherney Incision

The Cherney incision is a transverse abdominal incision that is similar to the Pfannenstiel incision in its early steps. After the anterior rectus sheath is opened, however, the tendons of the rectus abdominis and pyramidalis muscles are transected 1 to 2 cm above their insertion into the symphysis pubis (Cherney, 1955). These muscles are then lifted cephalad to provide access to the peritoneum. At this more caudal level, the inferior epigastric vessels run well lateral to the rectus bellies and typically are spared. However, if additional lateral extension is required, these vessels are ligated and transected.

This incision offers generous operating space and access to the retropubic space (space of Retzius). Thus, it may be a primary choice when these requirements are anticipated (DeLia, 1995; Maher, 1999). Additionally, Pfannenstiel incisions may be converted to Cherney incisions when an unexpected need for additional space arises.

PREOPERATIVE

Preparation and consenting prior to Cherney incision are similar to that for Pfannenstiel incision (p. 933).

INTRAOPERATIVE

Surgical Steps

❶ **Initial Steps.** The initial steps mirror that of the Pfannenstiel incision (Steps 1–3, p. 933). Thus, the skin is incised transversely beginning 2 to 3 cm above the symphysis, the fascia is divided transversely, and the rectus sheath is dissected off the rectus abdominis muscle bellies. After these steps, however, the techniques diverge.

❷ **Fascia.** The fascial opening reveals the rectus abdominis and pyramidalis muscles. Cephalad to the symphysis pubis, fingers are insinuated beneath the rectus muscle tendons. This blunt dissection begins laterally and extends toward the midline. During insinuation, fingers exert pressure dorsally and against the bladder to protect it during tendon division. The tendons of both muscles are then transected 1 to 2 cm above the symphysis pubis (Fig. 43-3.1). The muscles are flipped up and cephalad.

The peritoneum is grasped at a level cephalad to the bladder dome and is sharply incised (Fig. 43-3.2). This incision

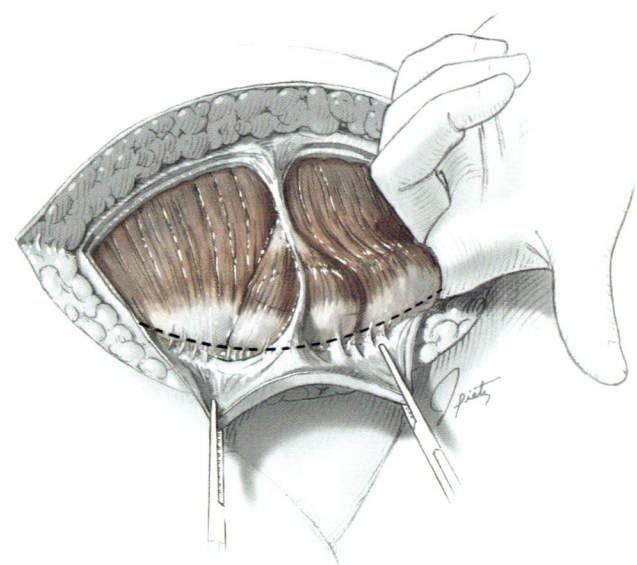

FIGURE 43-3.1 Tendon transection.

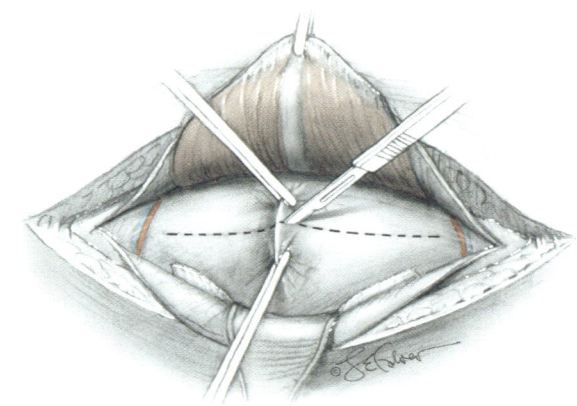

FIGURE 43-3.2 Peritoneal incision. (From Gilstrap, 2017, with permission.)

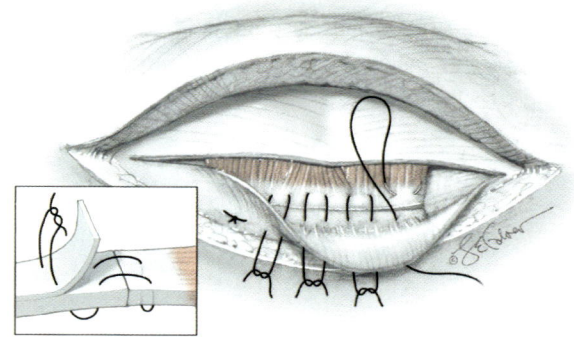

FIGURE 43-3.3 Wound closure. (From Gilstrap, 2017, with permission.)

is extended laterally. Once the abdominal cavity has been accessed, the planned surgery can proceed. Importantly, the risk of injury, particularly to the femoral and genitofemoral nerves, is heightened when self-retaining retractors are used with this generally wider incision. Thus, lateral retractor blades should fit just under the edges of the incision and not rest atop the psoas major muscle.

❸ **Wound Closure.** During wound closure, the cut ends of the rectus muscle tendons are joined and affixed to the undersurface of the inferior portion of fascia (Fig. 43-3.3). Interrupted sutures of 0-gauge delayed-absorbable sutures are suitable. To avoid osteitis pubis or osteomyelitis, tendons are not affixed directly to the symphysis pubis.

After this, starting from each end of the incision, the surgeon closes the fascia to its midpoint using a continuous running suture with a 0-gauge delayed-absorbable suture. These sutures are then tied together. The subcutaneous layer and skin are closed as with the midline vertical incision (p. 932).

POSTOPERATIVE

The postoperative course for low transverse incisions follows that described for midline incisions (p. 932).

43-4

Maylard Incision

The Maylard incision differs mainly from the Pfannenstiel incision in that the rectus sheath is not dissected away from the rectus abdominis muscle and that the bellies of the rectus abdominis muscle are transected. Transection affords extensive access to the pelvis (Helmkamp, 1990). However, it is technically more difficult due to its required isolation and ligation of the inferior epigastric vessels. Moreover, the Maylard incision has been used infrequently because of concerns regarding greater postoperative pain, decreased abdominal wall strength, longer operating times, and increased febrile morbidity. Randomized studies, however, have not supported these concerns (Ghanbari, 2009; Mathai, 2013). The Maylard incision should be avoided in those patients in whom the superior epigastric vessels have been interrupted, as this leaves the rectus abdominis muscles with inadequate blood supply. Also, patients with significant peripheral vascular disease may rely on the inferior epigastric vessels for collateral blood supply to their lower extremities (Salom, 2007).

PREOPERATIVE

Preparation and consenting prior to Maylard incision are similar to that for Pfannenstiel incision (p. 933).

INTRAOPERATIVE

Surgical Steps

❶ **Initial Steps.** The initial steps mirror that of the Pfannenstiel incision (Steps 1 and 2, p. 933). Thus, the skin is incised transversely beginning 2 to 3 cm above the symphysis, and the fascia is divided transversely. After these steps, the techniques diverge, and in contrast to the Pfannenstiel incision, the anterior rectus sheath is not dissected away from the underlying rectus muscle.

The inferior epigastric vessels lie posterolateral to the rectus abdominis muscle bellies. Bilaterally, these vessels are identified, ligated, and transected. This step avoids their laceration and hemorrhage when the rectus abdominis muscle is transected.

❷ **Rectus Abdominis Muscle.** The rectus abdominis muscle is bluntly dissected away from the underlying transversalis fascia and peritoneum. These latter are the encountered layers beneath the rectus bellies, because the posterior rectus sheath ends

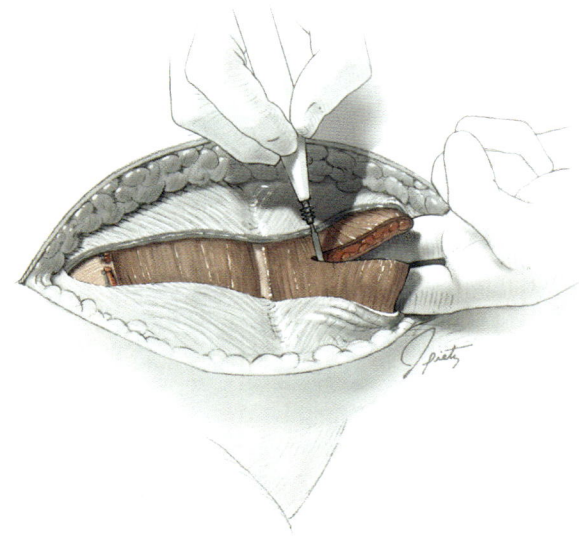

FIGURE 43-4.1 Rectus abdominis muscle transection.

at the arcuate line and is absent caudal to this line. The surgeon's fingers slide behind the rectus muscle bellies, and this muscle is then transected using an electrosurgical blade (Fig. 43-4.1).

❸ **Peritoneum.** The peritoneum is elevated by two hemostats and sharply incised at a point cephalad to the bladder dome. This is then extended laterally (Fig. 43-4.2). After access is obtained to the abdominal cavity, planned surgery can proceed. As with Cherney incisions, careful self-retaining retractor placement is necessary to lessen the risk of femoral or genitofemoral nerve injury at the psoas major muscle.

❹ **Wound Closure.** Closing the fascia adequately reapproximates the transected muscle fibers, and therefore the divided muscle bellies are not directly sutured together. This is because stitches placed through the skeletal muscle would simply tear through during later rectus abdominis muscle contraction.

For facial closure, the surgeon begins at each end of the incision. The fascia is closed to its midpoint using a continuous running suture with a 0-gauge delayed-absorbable suture. These sutures are then tied together. The subcutaneous layer and skin are closed as with the midline vertical incision (p. 932).

POSTOPERATIVE

The postoperative course for low transverse incisions follows that described for midline incisions (p. 932).

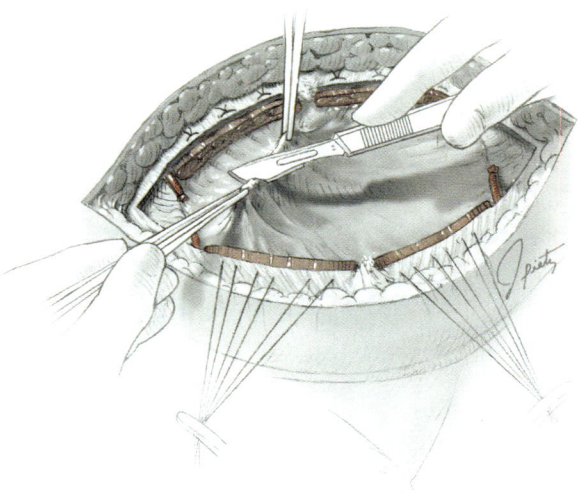

FIGURE 43-4.2 Suture placement through rectus abdominis muscle and fascia, and also peritoneal incision.

43-5

Ovarian Cystectomy

Ovarian cyst excision is typically prompted by bothersome patient symptoms and is suitable for cysts that lack qualities of ovarian malignancy. Removal of the cyst alone can offer those with ovarian pathology an opportunity to preserve hormonal function and reproductive capacity. Accordingly, ovarian cystectomy goals include gentle tissue handling to limit postoperative adhesions and reconstruction of normal ovarian anatomy to aid the transfer of ova to the fallopian tube.

In many women, a cystectomy may be performed laparoscopically rather than with laparotomy. Several studies support the safety and efficacy of MIS for this purpose (Chap. 10, p. 222). However, in some settings, a role for MIS is limited. In general, if a cyst is large, adhesive disease limits access and mobility, or the risk of malignancy is greater, then laparotomy is preferred.

PREOPERATIVE

Consent

In addition to general surgical risks of laparotomy, the major risk of cystectomy is extensive bleeding from or injury to the ovary that, in turn, necessitates removal of the entire ovary. Also, a variable degree of ovarian reserve may be lost with ovarian cystectomy. If ovarian cancer is suspected prior to surgery, patients are educated regarding the possibility of surgical staging, including the need for hysterectomy and removal of both ovaries (Chap. 35, p. 747).

Many patients undergoing cystectomy for ovarian pathology have associated pain. In most cases, cystectomy will be curative, but in other instances, pain may persist despite cyst excision. This is especially true in those with coexistent endometriosis. Thus, patients are counseled that cystectomy may not relieve chronic pain in all cases.

Patient Preparation

Ovarian cystectomy is considered a clean case. Despite this, based on some evidence, antibiotic prophylaxis listed in Table 39-8 (p. 832) may be considered solely for the indication of laparotomy (American College of Obstetricians and Gynecologists, 2018b; Morrill, 2013). Bowel preparation is typically not required. If hysterectomy is required during ovarian staging, antibiotics may be given intraoperatively, if not already

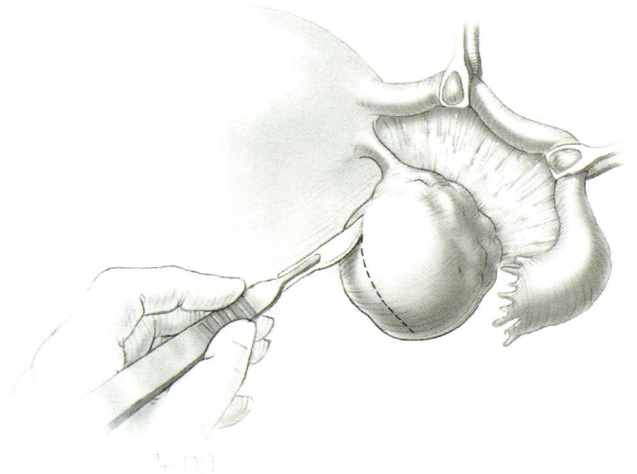

FIGURE 43-5.1 Ovarian incision.

given. Laparotomy dictates VTE prophylaxis, and options are found in Table 39-10 (p. 834).

INTRAOPERATIVE

Surgical Steps

❶ Anesthesia and Patient Positioning. Because of the potential for cancer staging in the upper abdomen if malignancy is found, general anesthesia is typically indicated for this inpatient procedure. The patient is supine or in low lithotomy position. After anesthesia induction, hair in the planned incision path is clipped if needed; a Foley catheter is inserted; and abdominal preparation is completed. Because hysterectomy may be needed if malignancy is found, the vagina is also surgically prepared.

❷ Abdominal Entry. Most ovarian cysts can be removed through a Pfannenstiel incision. Extremely large cysts or those with a greater concern for malignancy usually require a vertical incision. This latter incision provides generous operating space and adequate upper abdomen access for cancer staging. In cases with a low malignancy risk but with a cyst size that requires a long incision, cyst decompression is considered (p. 940). Importantly, the risk of advancing the stage of an occult cancer must be balanced against the benefits of a smaller incision.

Described in Chapter 35 (p. 747), cell washings from the pelvis and upper abdomen are collected prior to ovarian manipulation and are saved if cancer is found. The upper abdomen and pelvis are explored, and excrescences or suspicious areas are sampled and sent for intraoperative frozen-section analysis.

A self-retaining retractor is placed within the incision, and the bowel and omentum are packed from the operating field. The ovary is brought into view, and moist laparotomy sponges are placed in the cul-de-sac and beneath the ovary. This helps to minimize contamination of the pelvis if the cyst ruptures during excision.

❸ Ovarian Incision. The ovary is held between the surgeon's thumb and opposing fingers. The ovarian capsule that overlies the dome of the cyst is then cut with either scalpel or electrosurgical needle tip. This incision is ideally placed on the antimesenteric surface of the ovary to minimize dissection into vessels at the ovarian hilum. The incision is deepened to reach the cyst wall without entering and rupturing the cyst (Fig. 43-5.1). Allis clamps are then placed on the incised edges of the ovarian capsule to aid traction and countertraction during dissection.

❹ Cyst Dissection. Blunt dissection with fingertip or knife handle or sharp dissection with Metzenbaum scissor tips is used to develop the cleavage plane between the cyst wall and the remaining ovarian stroma (Fig. 43-5.2). If adhesions obliterate the cleavage plane, sharp dissection is preferred. As an assistant gently pulls the Allis clamps in a direction away from the cyst wall, the surgeon places fingers proximate to the advancing cleavage plane and pulls the cyst in the direction opposite the Allis clamps. Such traction and countertraction across the cleavage plane aid dissection. Because the surface of the cyst wall is often smooth and slippery, the surgeon may place an unfolded, thin gauze sponge between fingers and the cyst wall to afford a better grip.

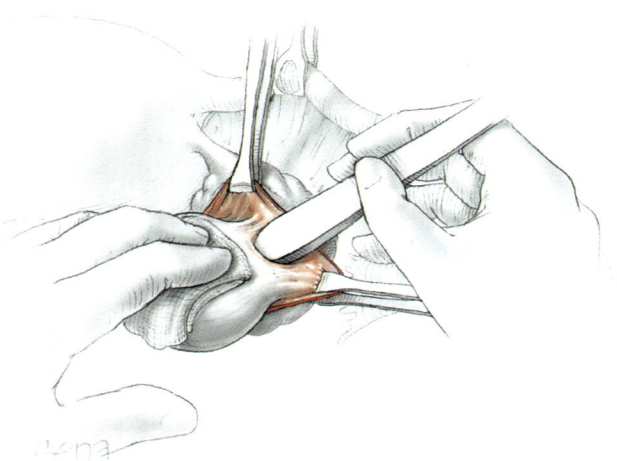

FIGURE 43-5.2 Cyst dissection.

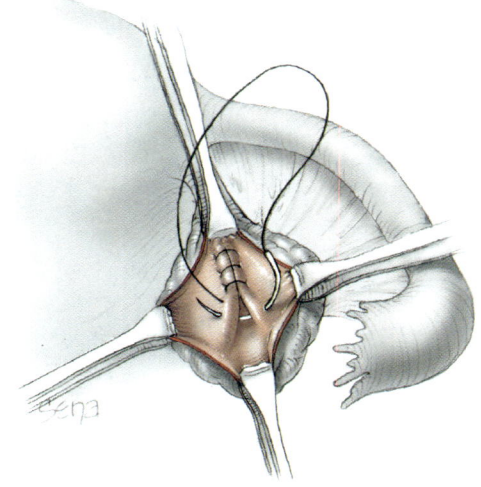

FIGURE 43-5.3 Ovarian closure.

As dissection approaches completion, the highly vascular ovarian hilum is reached. If possible, a hemostat or Pean clamp is placed across the small remaining tissue bridge between the cyst and normal ovary. The clamp is positioned closer to the ovary to allow space for scissors to cut the tissue pedicle and free the cyst without rupture. The pedicle is suture ligated with a fine absorbable suture. The ovarian bed is then examined, and bleeding points are coagulated or ligated.

❺ Cyst Excision. Once the cyst is removed, it may be sent to the pathology department for intraoperative frozen-section analysis. In benign cases, excess capsule can be sharply removed from ovaries in which large cysts have stretched and thinned the ovarian surface. This excision is performed to help restore normal ovarian anatomy. But because ovarian follicles are contained within even extremely thinned capsules, this tissue is preserved whenever possible.

❻ Ovarian Closure. The ovarian bed is then closed in layers using 3-0 or 4-0 gauge delayed-absorbable suture. These sutures reapproximate the ovarian tissue that previously surrounded the cyst on both sides (Fig. 43-5.3). With a thinned ovarian cortex, the needle tip is ideally not driven through the capsule. Exposed suture on the ovarian surface may enhance adhesion formation.

The ovarian incision is closed with a running subcortical stitch (similar to subcuticular stitch) using 5-0 gauge delayed-absorbable suture. At completion, laparotomy sponges are removed from the cul-de-sac.

❼ Large Cyst Decompression. For this variation, a minilaparotomy low transverse or midline incision is created, pelvic washings are collected, and the abdomen is explored to the degree possible. A small self-retaining retractor or hand-held retractors are positioned, and Trendelenburg positioning uses gravity to move bowel from the operative field.

The ovary is manually guided to the incision, and moist laparotomy sponges surround the opening to absorb any spill of cyst contents. A drainage site far from the ovarian hilum is determined, and here, a purse-string stitch of 3-0 silk is placed. The needle ideally passes superficially through only the ovarian cortex to avoid deeper penetration and cyst rupture. Suture tails are left long and not tied until after cyst drainage. In the middle of the purse string, the cyst is sharply entered, and a suction tip enters the defect. After cyst drainage, the purse string is tied to avoid content spill. If needed, cyst fluid may be collected and held for cytologic evaluation. The laparotomy sponges surrounding the incision are removed from the field, and the suction tip is changed. Cystectomy is now performed as in Step 4.

To complete thorough abdominal exploration, a laparoscope can be placed in the incision. For exposure, the abdominal wall is elevated with retractors rather than by pneumoperitoneum.

❽ Incision Closure. The pelvis is copiously irrigated with an isotonic solution such as lactated Ringer solution. Irrigation assumes an even greater importance with ovarian cyst rupture. For example, spill from a mature cystic teratoma (dermoid), if neglected, may induce a chemical peritonitis. Depending on the surgeon's preference and the patient's anatomy, an adhesion barrier may be placed around the ovary (Chap. 40, p. 855). The remaining packs and retractor are removed, and the abdominal incision is closed. In cases without suspected malignancy, initially gathered pelvic washings may be discarded.

POSTOPERATIVE

After surgery, care in general follows that described for laparotomy (p. 932).

43-6

Salpingo-oophorectomy

Removal of the ovary and fallopian tube is more commonly performed by laparoscopy. However, laparotomy is typically indicated if the potential for malignancy is great, if the ovary is too large to be manipulated by laparoscopic instruments, or if extensive adhesions are anticipated. With either approach, the essential steps of salpingo-oophorectomy (SO) are to identify the ipsilateral ureter, ligate the infundibulopelvic (IP) ligament, together ligate the proximal fallopian tube and uteroovarian ligament, and transect the intervening broad ligament.

Indications vary and include suspicion for ovarian malignancy, ovarian cancer prevention for at-risk women, large symptomatic ovarian cysts in postreproductive females, and for reproductive-aged women, large, symptomatic ovarian cysts that are not suitable for cystectomy. If SO is performed for cancer-risk reduction in those with a pathogenic mutation, pelvic washings are collected and sent for evaluation. Fallopian tube and uteroovarian ligament transection should snug the uterus. On the other end, excision extends 2 cm past the end of identifiable ovarian tissue. Last, to prompt more thorough tubal specimen sectioning and evaluation, the pathology requisition form should state the patient's genetic information (American College of Obstetricians and Gynecologists, 2017b).

PREOPERATIVE

Patient Evaluation

This surgery is typically performed to remove ovarian pathology that has been evaluated sonographically. If anatomy is unclear, magnetic resonance (MR) imaging may add information. As listed in Chapters 35 and 36 (pp. 740 and 757), tumor markers are selectively drawn prior to surgery if malignancy is suspected, and computed tomography (CT) imaging may help evaluate for adenopathy or extraovarian disease.

Consent

In general, serious complications with SO are infrequent but include organ injury, especially to the ureter; hemorrhage; wound infection or dehiscence; and anesthesia complications. Ovarian pathology is the most common indication for SO. Thus, the

possibility of cancer staging and a description of its steps are explained. Moreover, malignant cyst rupture and spillage are risks, and patients are informed that this will advance the cancer stage (Chap. 35, p. 747). Many women undergoing SO for ovarian pathology have associated pain. Although removal of the ovary in most cases will be curative, in other instances, pain may persist despite SO. Last, if performed bilaterally, SO dramatically curtails estrogen production. Thus, a preoperative discussion of consequences, described on page 957, is required.

Patient Preparation

Isolated SO is considered a clean case. Despite this, based on some evidence, antibiotic prophylaxis listed in Table 39-8 (p. 832) may be considered solely for the indication of laparotomy. Bowel preparation is typically not helpful. If hysterectomy is required during ovarian staging, antibiotics may be given intraoperatively, if not already provided. Laparotomy dictates VTE prophylaxis, and options are found in Table 39-10 (p. 834).

INTRAOPERATIVE

Surgical Steps

❶ **Anesthesia and Patient Positioning.** SO performed by laparotomy typically requires general anesthesia to allow staging of the upper abdomen if malignancy is found. The patient is positioned supine or standard lithotomy position. In cases with anticipated dense adhesions, which raise ureteral injury concerns, lithotomy position can permit cystoscopy. After anesthesia induction,

hair in the planned incision path is clipped if needed; a Foley catheter is inserted; and abdominal preparation is completed. Because of possible hysterectomy if malignancy is found, the vagina is also surgically prepared.

❷ **Abdominal Entry.** Either a transverse or vertical incision may be used for SO. Clinical factors such as ovarian size and risk of malignancy influence this selection (Chap. 10, p. 222).

Following abdominal entry, cell washings from the pelvis and upper abdomen are collected prior to ovarian manipulation. These are sent for pathologic evaluation if cancer is found. The upper abdomen and pelvis are explored. Suspicious peritoneal or omental implants are sampled and sent for intraoperative frozen-section analysis.

❸ **Exposure.** A self-retaining retractor is placed, and the bowel is packed from the operating field. The affected adnexa is grasped and elevated from the pelvis. If extensive adhesions are found, normal anatomic relationships are restored.

❹ **Ureter Location.** Because of its close proximity to the IP ligament, the ureter is identified prior to clamp placement. In many instances, the ureter is seen beneath the posterior pelvic sidewall peritoneum. Here, it enters the pelvis and crosses over the common iliac artery bifurcation just medial to the ovarian vessels.

In other cases, retroperitoneal isolation of the ureter is required. For this, the peritoneum within the area bounded by the round and IP ligaments and the external iliac vessels is tented with tissue forceps and incised. This first peritoneal incision is extended cephalad toward the pelvic brim (Fig. 43-6.1). The

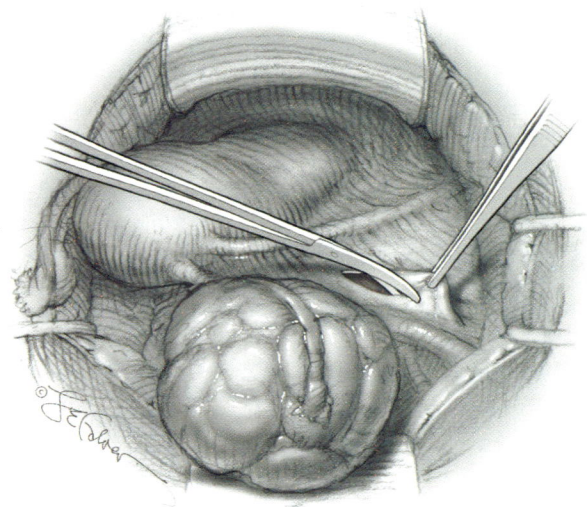

FIGURE 43-6.1 Retroperitoneal entry.

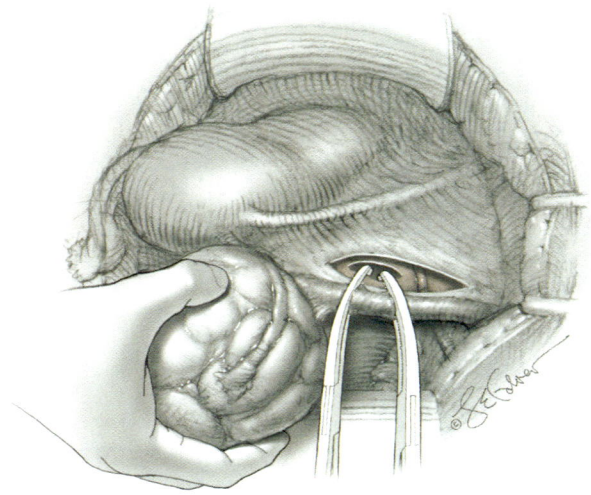

FIGURE 43-6.2 Infundibulopelvic ligament ligation.

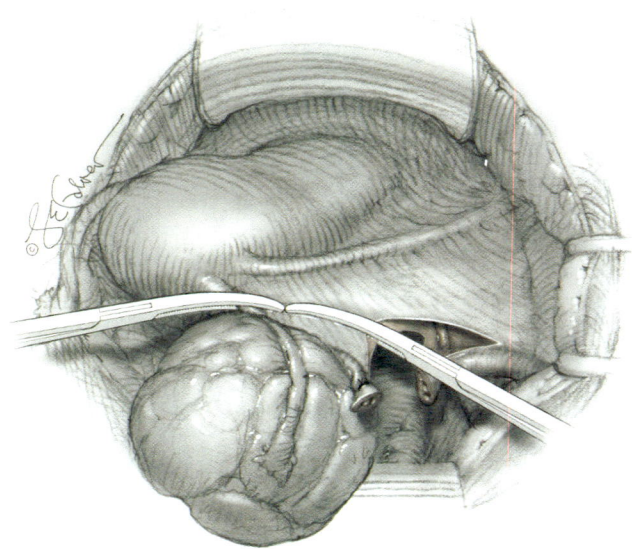

FIGURE 43-6.3 Ligation of uteroovarian ligament, fallopian tube ligation, and proximal adjacent mesovarium and mesosalpinx.

incision also later assists in isolating the IP ligament for ligation. Once this peritoneal window is open, blunt dissection is directed deep, cephalad, and slightly medially through gauzy areolar connective tissue, as shown later in Step 6 of abdominal hysterectomy (p. 959). The ureter is typically found attached to the medial leaf of the incised peritoneum.

❺ **Infundibulopelvic Ligament.** The adnexa is lifted from the pelvis and inspected. To isolate the IP ligament, a second peritoneal opening is sharply created with Metzenbaum scissors or electrosurgical blade. It is made in the posterior leaf of the broad ligament below the IP ligament but above the ureter. This incision is extended medially beneath the fallopian tube and uteroovarian ligament and toward the uterus. While remaining parallel to the IP ligament, it is also extended laterally and cephalad towards the pelvic brim. Ideally, the ureter is in view during this entire incision.

As a result of both peritoneal incisions, the IP ligament is isolated. This vascular ligament is then clamped with a Heaney or other sturdy clamp, and the clamp curve faces upward (Fig. 43-6.2). Of note, if SO is performed for cancer risk reduction, the clamp is brought across the IP close to the sidewall. A single Kelly (Pean) clamp is placed across the IP at a distance medial to the Heaney clamp. During completion of adnexectomy, this medial clamp prevents "back-bleeding" and is removed with the specimen.

The IP ligament is then transected between the Heaney and Kelly clamps. To ligate the IP pedicle, a free tie of 0-gauge delayed-absorbable suture is placed around the Heaney clamp. As the knot is secured, this clamp is opened and closed quickly, that is, "flashed." Next, a transfixing suture is placed around the Heaney clamp (Fig. 40-22, p. 852). This suture is placed below the clamp yet distal to the first free tie to avoid hematoma formation by needle puncture of ovarian vessels. As this knot is cinched in place, the Heaney clamp is removed.

If the IP ligament lies sufficiently close to the ureter to prohibit safe clamp placement, the vessel instead may be solely suture ligated. For this, a Babcock clamp grasps and elevates the IP ligament. Three strands of 0-gauge, delayed-absorbable suture are passed through the peritoneal window and below the IP ligament. Around the IP ligament, two suture ties lie in tandem proximally and are secured. A third tie is then placed 1 to 2 cm distally and is also tied around the IP ligament. Metzenbaum scissors transect the tissue between the two more distal ties. This ultimately leaves the proximal IP pedicle doubly ligated.

❻ **Fallopian Tube and Uteroovarian Ligament.** With the adnexa elevated, a Heaney or similar clamp is placed across both the uteroovarian ligament and fallopian tube. It also incorporates some of the broad ligament. The clamp's curve faces the ovary.

Next, another clamp enters laterally and is directed medially to close around the remaining broad ligament beneath the ovary. Again, the clamp curve faces the ovary. Ideally, the tips of both clamps touch beneath the adnexa (Fig. 43-6.3). Above both of these clamps are stacked second clamps, which lie a distance above their partners and closer to the ovary. Tissue between the stacked clamps is cut with curved Mayo scissors to free the adnexa.

The freed adnexa is removed from the operative site and sent to pathology for evaluation. If malignancy is suspected, an intraoperative frozen section is requested. Tissue within each of the remaining two clamps is individually suture ligated with 0-gauge delayed-absorbable suture.

❼ **Wound Closure.** The retractor and packing sponges are removed from the abdomen. The abdominal incision is then closed as described for vertical or Pfannenstiel incisions (pp. 932 and 934). In cases without suspected malignancy, initially gathered pelvic washings may be discarded.

POSTOPERATIVE

Patient recovery is similar to that described for laparotomy (p. 932). In reproductive-aged women, if only one ovary is removed, hormonal and reproductive function is preserved. However, if both are excised, surgical menopause follows, and hormone replacement is considered (Chap. 22, p. 480).

Interval Partial Salpingectomy

Interval partial salpingectomy is similar to puerperal midsegment salpingectomy and differs mainly in procedure timing and in abdominal entry. In contrast to postpartum or postabortal sterilization, the term *interval* designates performance unrelated in time to pregnancy. Accordingly, for most women undergoing interval sterilization, the uterus is small and lies within the confines of the pelvis. Thus, fallopian tubes are reached either laparoscopically or through a low transverse incision.

In general with interval partial salpingectomy, a midtubal segment of fallopian tube is excised, and the severed ends seal by fibrosis and reperitonealization. Commonly used methods of interval sterilization include the Parkland and Pomeroy techniques.

Of tubal sterilization methods, interval partial salpingectomy is infrequently selected for U.S. women who elect sterilization (Peterson, 1996). More commonly, MIS techniques are employed, mainly because of laparoscopy's postsurgical advantages (Chap. 41, p. 873). Accordingly, interval partial salpingectomy is typically selected for cases in which laparoscopy may not be indicated. Examples include women with physiologic contraindications to laparoscopy, other concurrent pelvic pathology dictating laparotomy, or extensive adhesions or settings in which laparoscopic equipment or surgical skills are lacking. Moreover, new recommendations advocate for consideration of risk-reducing total salpingectomy when feasible (p. 945). Thus, the opportunities for open interval salpingectomy may be few.

PREOPERATIVE

Patient Evaluation

As with any sterilization procedure, pregnancy should be excluded prior to the procedure by means of either urine or serum β-human chorionic gonadotropin (hCG) testing. Similarly, to limit the possibility of an early, undetected luteal-phase conceptus, sterilization is ideally performed during the follicular phase of the menstrual cycle, and an effective contraceptive method is used until surgery.

Consent

Partial salpingectomy is an effective method of sterilization. Cumulative pregnancy rates at 10 years postsurgery range from 1 to 3 percent (Peterson, 1996). Failures accrue over time and may result from tubal recanalization or technical errors, such as ligation of the wrong structure.

Tubal sterilization is a safe surgical procedure, and complication rates are <2 percent (Pati, 2000). Of these, anesthesia complications, organ injury, and wound infection are the most frequent. In addition, although pregnancy is uncommon following sterilization, when pregnancy does occur, the risk of ectopic pregnancy is high and approximates 30 percent (Peterson, 1996; Ryder, 1999). However, because tubal sterilization is highly effective contraception, the overall risk of pregnancy is low, and thus also is the risk of ectopic pregnancy.

Aside from physical risks, some women experience regret following sterilization. Rates are highest in those 30 years or younger (Curtis, 2006; Hillis, 1999). Accordingly, prior to surgery women are counseled regarding the risk of regret, the permanence of the procedure, and alternative effective long-term contraceptive methods. That said, a woman's autonomy to choose sterilization should be supported (American College of Obstetricians and Gynecologists, 2017c, 2019b). Also, consideration of risk-reducing total salpingectomy is offered and counseling points are found on page 945.

INTRAOPERATIVE

Surgical Steps

❶ Anesthesia and Patient Positioning. Interval partial salpingectomy is usually an outpatient procedure, performed under general or regional anesthesia. Following administration of anesthesia, the patient is placed supine or in low lithotomy position, the abdomen surgically prepared, and the bladder drained.

❷ Minilaparotomy. For most patients, a 4- to 6-cm transverse Pfannenstiel incision is sufficient. Small Richardson or army-navy retractors provide adequate intraabdominal visualization in most cases. A disposable self-retaining ring is another option (Fig. 41-13, p. 883). As another aid, a vaginally placed sponge stick or uterine manipulator can elevate the uterus to help bring fallopian tubes into view.

❸ Tubal Identification. A common reason for sterilization failure is ligation of the wrong structure, usually the round ligament. Identification and isolation of the fallopian tube prior to ligation and submission of tubal segments for pathologic confirmation is therefore required. In some cases, especially those with associated tubal adhesions, this step may be challenging. Lateral extension of the incision may be needed to improve exposure.

Initially, the uterine fundus is identified. At the cornu, insertion of the fallopian tube lies posterior to that of the round ligament, and this orientation can initially guide the surgeon to the correct structure. A primary Babcock clamp is used to elevate the fallopian tube proximally, while a second clamp grasps the tube more distally. The primary clamp is then moved again and is placed distal to the second. The second is then removed and again placed distal to the first. In this manner, the surgeon "marches" down the length of the tube to reach the ampulla and identify fimbria.

❹ Parkland Method. At the midpoint of the fallopian tube, an avascular space in the mesosalpinx is identified, and a hemostat is placed directly beneath the tube. The selected site should allow excision of a 2-cm tubal segment that does not incorporate the fimbria. Ligation of the fimbrial portion leads to a greater risk of tubal recanalization and higher failure rate.

The hemostat is bluntly advanced through the mesosalpinx as counterpressure is applied with the index finger. Once advanced through the defect, the hemostat tips are gently opened to expand the aperture (Fig. 43-7.1). The end of a 0-gauge chromic free tie is placed in the tip of the hemostat and guided through the opening. This is repeated, bringing another tie through the rent. The midsegment is lifted with the Babcock clamp, and the distal suture tied. The second tie is then secured around the proximal fallopian tube.

❺ Tubal Excision. Metzenbaum scissor tips are inserted through the mesosalpingeal defect, and the proximal portion of the fallopian tube is cut. A 0.5-cm pedicle is left to ensure that the tube will not slip through its ligature (Fig. 43-7.2). The tube is sharply dissected from the mesosalpinx toward the distal ligature, thereby freeing the tubal segment from the mesosalpinx. The distal part of the segment is excised to leave a 0.5-cm pedicle, and an adequate 2-cm tubal segment is obtained. The pedicles and mesosalpinx are inspected for hemostasis. The procedure is then repeated on the other side. For histologic confirmation of complete transection, each tubal segment is sent independently and marked as to its laterality.

❻ Pomeroy Method. This technique involves grasping and elevating a 2-cm midsegment of tube, ligating the tubal loop with a 2-0 plain catgut suture, and then excising the distal portion of the loop (Fig. 43-7.3). Prompt absorption of the suture following surgery causes the ligated ends to fall away, creating a resulting 2- to 3-cm gap.

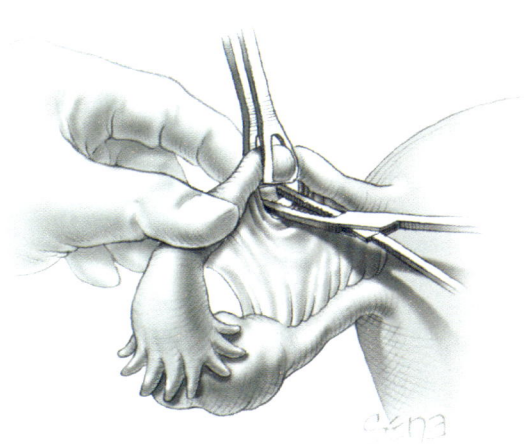

FIGURE 43-7.1 Parkland method: tubal ligation.

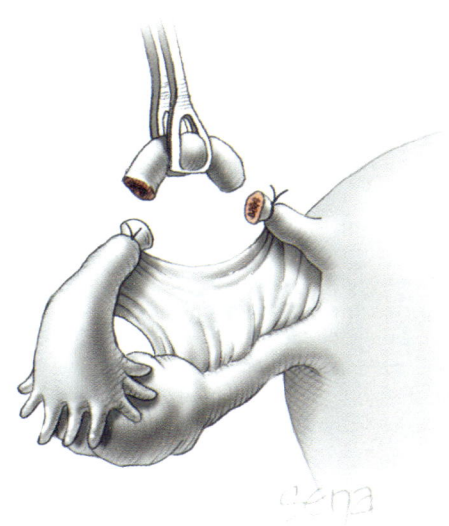

FIGURE 43-7.2 Parkland method: tubal excision.

❼ Wound Closure. The wound is closed as that for other transverse abdominal incisions (p. 934).

POSTOPERATIVE

The recovery following minilaparotomy is typically rapid and without complication, and women may resume regular diet and activities as tolerated. Sterilization is immediate following surgery, and intercourse may resume at the patient's discretion. Aside from regret, the risk of long-term physical or psychologic sequelae is low as described in Chapter 5 (p. 119). Peterson and coworkers (2000) found that women who had undergone tubal sterilization were no more likely than those without this surgery to have menstrual abnormalities. Moreover, interval tubal ligation is unlikely to negatively affect sexual interest or pleasure (Costello, 2002).

If pathologic analysis fails to document complete bilateral tubal transection, patients are counseled to use an alternative contraceptive method. Hysterosalpingography is subsequently performed to assess tubal patency.

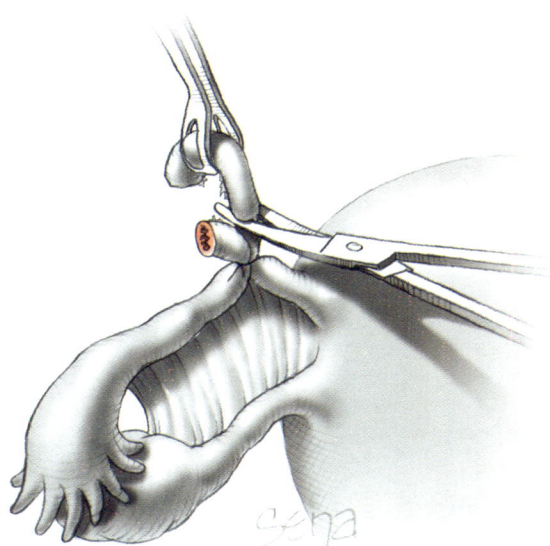

FIGURE 43-7.3 Pomeroy method.

43-8

Salpingectomy and Salpingostomy

Salpingostomy describes a lengthwise linear incision of the fallopian tube and is used to remove intraluminal ectopic pregnancy contents. In contrast, *salpingectomy* removes the fallopian tube while sparing the ovary. Indications vary, and salpingectomy may be selected for ectopic pregnancy removal, for sterilization, or for hydrosalpinx removal to improve in vitro fertilization success rates. Rarely, a fallopian tube may undergo ischemic necrosis alone from torsion and require excision. Last, the Society of Gynecologic Oncology now recommends consideration of salpingectomy instead of tubal interruption for female sterilization (Walker, 2015). For any of these indications, subsequent tubal surgery may be avoided in those undergoing salpingectomy.

MIS offers patients the advantages of shorter hospitalizations, quicker recoveries, and less postoperative pain. Accordingly, laparoscopic treatment of ectopic pregnancy is generally preferred. As a result, laparotomic approaches for salpingectomy and salpingostomy are now reserved typically for patients with ruptured ectopic pregnancies who are hemodynamically unstable or in those with contraindications to laparoscopy. Laparotomy offers fast entry into the abdomen for control of bleeding.

PREOPERATIVE

Consent

Most complications associated with salpingectomy and salpingostomy stem from ectopic pregnancies and tubal rupture–related bleeding. Regardless of the indication, injury to the ipsilateral ovary, however, is another risk. In certain cases, if severe, this damage can demand concurrent ovary removal. Additionally, involvement of the ovary with tubal pathology may necessitate oophorectomy.

Persistent Trophoblastic Tissue

Following any surgical treatment of ectopic pregnancy, trophoblastic tissue can persist. Remnant implants typically involve the fallopian tube, but extratubal trophoblastic implants have been found on the omentum and on pelvic and abdominal peritoneum. Peritoneal implants typically measure 0.3 to 2.0 cm and appear as red-black nodules. As expected, the risk of persistent trophoblast tissue is lower with salpingectomy compared with salpingostomy (Farquhar, 2005a).

Preservation of Fertility

With ectopic pregnancy, most, but not all, studies show comparable subsequent fertility rates whether salpingectomy or salpingostomy is performed. This is detailed in Chapter 7 (p. 170). Thus, with a healthy contralateral tube, neither salpingostomy nor salpingectomy offers a distinct fertility advantage. However, salpingostomy is considered a preferred option for tubal ectopic pregnancy if there is contralateral tubal disease and a desire for fertility. Unfortunately, in some cases of rupture, the extent of tubal damage or bleeding may limit tubal salvage, and salpingectomy may be required.

If salpingectomy is performed for sterilization, consenting should mirror that for interval tubal sterilization (p. 943). Because the entire tube is removed, later reanastomosis is not possible. However, all women should enter into sterilization with an understanding of its permanence.

Risk-Reducing Salpingectomy

Although currently theoretical, bilateral salpingectomy may lower ovarian cancer rates (Falconer, 2015; Lessard-Anderson, 2014). Discussed in Chapter 35 (p. 736), this may be especially relevant for women with *BRCA1* or *BRCA2* mutation, who have enhanced ovarian cancer risks. If risk-reducing salpingectomy is elected in women with a pathogenic mutation, special surgical steps are described in the introduction of Section 43-6.

In low-risk women, because the ovarian cancer risk is less than 2 percent, the risks and benefits of salpingectomy for sterilization are best assessed individually. First, data from epidemiologic studies find that bilateral tubal interruption alone offers an approximate 30-percent decline in ovarian cancer rates (Rice, 2012; Sieh, 2013). From similar studies, bilateral salpingectomy may reduce the risk by 42 to 78 percent (Gockley, 2018). Retrospective studies of laparoscopic sterilization show similar blood losses and complication rates for both salpingectomy and tubal interruption (Kim, 2019a; Powell, 2017; Westberg, 2017). However, no prospective studies of sufficient size or duration are yet available to demonstrate the true risk-benefit ratio for women with a low ovarian cancer risk. Last, with total salpingectomy, few data describe the potential effects on ovarian reserve from blood supply disruption. In one small study comparing tubal interruption or salpingectomy for sterilization, no differences in the antimüllerian hormone level, which is a measure of ovarian reserve, were found (Findley, 2013; Ganer Herman, 2017).

Patient Preparation

If performed for ectopic pregnancy, either of these procedures may be associated with substantial bleeding. Baseline complete blood count (CBC) and β-human chorionic gonadotropin (β-hCG) level are obtained. Patients undergo type and screen to establish blood type. Those with significant bleeding also require a type and crossmatch for blood products as indicated. If performed for interval sterilization, then preparation follows that for interval tubal sterilization (p. 943).

Salpingectomy and salpingostomy are associated with low infection rates. Accordingly, preoperative antibiotics are usually not required, but as noted earlier, prophylaxis can be considered for the indication of laparotomy alone (p. 931). Laparotomy dictates VTE prophylaxis, and options are found in Table 39-10 (p. 834).

INTRAOPERATIVE

Surgical Steps

❶ Anesthesia and Patient Positioning. In most cases of ectopic pregnancy managed by laparotomy, surgery is an urgent inpatient procedure and requires general anesthesia. For other indications, regional analgesia may be an option. The patient is supine. After anesthesia induction, a Foley catheter is placed; hair in the planned incision path is clipped unless time dictates against this; and abdominal preparation is completed.

❷ Abdominal Entry. Most salpingectomy or salpingostomy procedures can be managed through a Pfannenstiel incision (p. 933). However, with a hemodynamically unstable patient and large hemoperitoneum, vertical incision may offer quicker entry.

The pelvis is initially explored. With ectopic pregnancy, if the affected tube is unruptured, assessment of the contralateral tube aids the decision for salpingostomy or total tube excision.

❸ Salpingectomy. Once access to the pelvic organs is achieved, the adnexum is elevated. Distal and proximal Babcock clamps are placed around the fallopian tube and direct the tube away from the uterus and ovary. This extends the mesosalpinx (Fig. 43-8.1).

Beginning at the distal, fimbriated end of the tube, one Kelly clamp or hemostat is placed across a 2-cm-long segment of the mesosalpinx, close to the fallopian tube. The clamp's curve faces the tube. Another clamp is similarly placed but lies closer to the ovary. These clamps occlude vessels that traverse the mesosalpinx. Scissors then cut the interposed mesosalpinx.

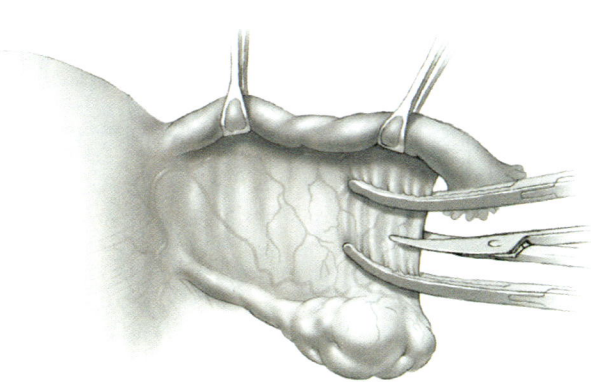

FIGURE 43-8.1 Mesosalpinx is serially clamped and cut. (From Gilstrap, 2017, with permission.)

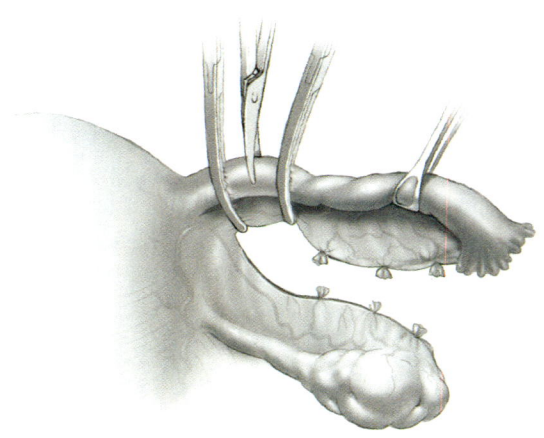

FIGURE 43-8.2 The proximal mesosalpinx and tube are clamped and cut. (From Gilstrap, 2017, with permission.)

The severed tissue pedicle that is closer to the ovary is tied with 2-0 or 3-0 gauge delayed-absorbable suture, and the clamp is removed. The clamp closer to the tube remains and leaves with the final specimen. Such clamping, cutting, and ligating are repeated serially, with each clamp incorporating a 2-cm length of mesosalpinx. Progression is directed from the ampullary end of the fallopian tube toward the uterus.

The last clamp is placed across the proximal mesosalpinx and fallopian tube (Fig. 43-8.2). Scissors then cut the mesosalpinx and tube and free these from the uterus. This pedicle is similarly ligated.

Although significantly more costly, the same steps can be performed with disposable bipolar coagulating devices (LigaSure, ENSEAL). These coagulate vessels within the mesosalpinx prior to its division. The main advantage is speed.

4 Salpingostomy. Surgical steps for salpingostomy mirror those used in laparoscopic salpingostomy and can be reviewed in Chapter 44 (p. 1028). To summarize, the affected fallopian tube is elevated with Babcock clamps. At the ectopic pregnancy site, the tube is sharply incised lengthwise on its antimesenteric border. The incision, usually 1 to 2 cm long, varies based on pregnancy size. The products of conception are grasped and gently extracted or are delivered by hydrodissection. Bleeding sites are made hemostatic with electrosurgical coagulation, and the tubal incision is left to heal by secondary intention.

5 Wound Closure. The pelvis is irrigated and rid of blood and tissue debris. The abdominal incision is closed as previously described for vertical or Pfannenstiel incision (pp. 932 and 934).

POSTOPERATIVE

In cases performed for ectopic pregnancy, salpingectomy or salpingostomy represents pregnancy termination. Accordingly, the Rh status of the patient should be evaluated. Intramuscular (IM) administration of 50 or 300 μg (250 or 1500 IU) of anti-D immune globulin within 72 hours after pregnancy termination in Rh-negative women can dramatically lower the risk of alloimmunization in future pregnancies.

Because of the higher risk of persistent trophoblastic tissue in patients undergoing salpingostomy, serial weekly serum β-hCG levels are measured until undetectable levels are reached. During this time, contraception should be used to avoid confusion between persistent trophoblastic tissue and a new pregnancy.

For elective sterilization, postoperative instructions follow those for interval tubal sterilization (p. 944). For all indications, resumption of activity and diet follow that for laparotomy (p. 932).

Cornuostomy and Cornual Wedge Resection

Interstitial pregnancy develops in a distensible portion of the tube surrounded by myometrium (Fig. 43-9.1). This location often permits pregnancies to attain greater size than ectopic pregnancy at other sites. Also, uterine rupture at the cornu, where uterine and ovarian arteries anastomose, can lead to brisk and significant hemorrhage. Fortunately, transvaginal sonography, β-hCG testing, and use of established diagnostic criteria have led to earlier diagnosis of interstitial pregnancy. This averts rupture in many circumstances.

In selected cases, this unusual type of ectopic pregnancy may be managed medically, but it is more frequently managed by various operations. *Cornuostomy* is analogous to linear salpingostomy for tubal ectopic pregnancy, and the involved fallopian tube is preserved. With *cornual wedge resection*, the interstitial pregnancy and its surrounding myometrium and fallopian tube are removed (Moawad, 2010). Few evidenced-based data guide selection of one over the other, although significant rupture usually requires wedge excision. Other factors that guide surgical route and procedure selection are gestational age, degree of rupture, hemodynamic stability, future fertility desires, and surgeon's preference and skill.

Cornual wedge resection, often performed by laparotomy, has remained a cornerstone of therapy. For a hemodynamically unstable patient or with significant anatomic rupture, laparotomy offers fast entry and avoids the vascular effects of pneumoperitoneum.

However, many less urgent cases are now managed laparoscopically. From early comparative series, blood loss and operative times are similar yet hospital stays and recovery times are shorter with laparoscopic wedge resection than with laparotomy. Persistent trophoblastic tissue is uncommon with laparotomy, but rates are significantly higher with laparoscopy (Baumann, 1991; Hwang, 2011; Tulandi, 2004).

PREOPERATIVE

Consent

With interstitial ectopic pregnancies, the risk of tubal rupture–associated bleeding is prominent. A patient is counseled regarding the possible need for blood products, which includes anti-D immune globulin for those with Rh-negative blood. Injury to the ipsilateral ovary is another surgical risk and, if severe, may require concurrent oophorectomy. Rarely, uncontrolled bleeding can mandate hysterectomy.

In the event that the patient has completed her childbearing, contralateral tubal ligation or bilateral salpingectomy may be acceptable at the time of surgery. A discussion of risk-reducing salpingectomy is found on page 945.

Patient Evaluation

In some cases, particularly those in which the cornu has ruptured and the woman is hemodynamically unstable, fluid resuscitation, blood transfusion, and plans for surgical intervention are initiated simultaneously. In unruptured cases, excessive intraoperative bleeding is still possible, and a patient is typed and crossmatched for blood products. To guide care, baseline CBC and β-hCG and electrolyte levels are obtained.

Patient Preparation

Other than optimizing hemodynamic stability of the patient and ensuring blood availability, no special preparation is required. Prophylactic antibiotics or bowel preparation are generally not required. That said, antibiotics may be considered solely for the indication of laparotomy, as noted earlier (p. 931). Laparotomy dictates VTE prophylaxis, and options are found in Table 39-10 (p. 834).

INTRAOPERATIVE

Surgical Steps

❶ **Anesthesia and Patient Positioning.** Cornual wedge resection and cornuostomy are usually performed under general anesthesia, particularly if cornual rupture is suspected. The patient is supine. After anesthesia induction, hair in the planned incision path is clipped if needed; a Foley catheter is inserted; and abdominal preparation is completed.

❷ **Abdominal Entry.** Either a transverse or vertical incision may be used depending on the clinical urgency as discussed earlier (p. 945).

❸ **Exposure.** In the absence of cornual rupture and massive bleeding, the bowel is packed away to provide adequate exposure of the pelvis. A self-retaining retractor may then be placed.

If significant hemoperitoneum is encountered upon abdominal entry, the operator can attempt to remove obscuring blood with suction and laparotomy sponges. Failing this, the surgeon can manually lift the uterus out of the pelvis to identify the rupture site. The uterus can be compressed between the operator's thumb and fingers to tamponade bleeding from the pregnancy's dual blood supply. Two heavy clamps are then placed across the base of the cornu. In rare cases, temporary compression of the aorta may be helpful if bleeding is torrential and poorly controlled in a hypotensive patient.

❹ **Inspection of the Pelvis.** In less urgent cases, the ectopic pregnancy is identified. Additional information including cornual rupture, pregnancy size, amount of bleeding, and appearance of the contralateral (unaffected) fallopian tube is needed before deciding on the exact procedure to perform.

❺ **Vasopressin Injection.** For either cornuostomy or cornual wedge resection, dilute vasopressin (20 units in 30 to 100 mL of normal saline) may be injected into the

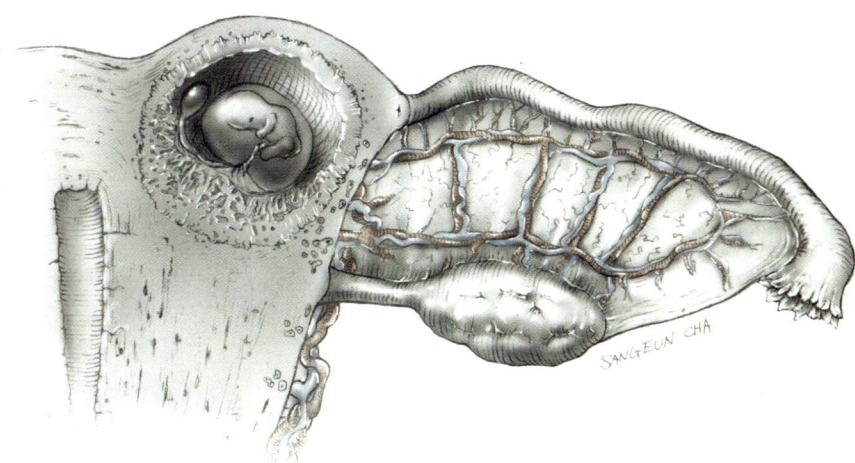

FIGURE 43-9.1 Interstitial pregnancy.

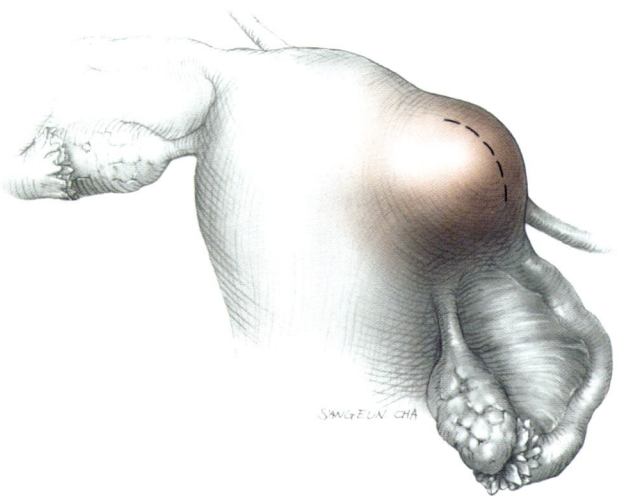

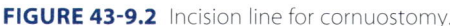

FIGURE 43-9.2 Incision line for cornuostomy.

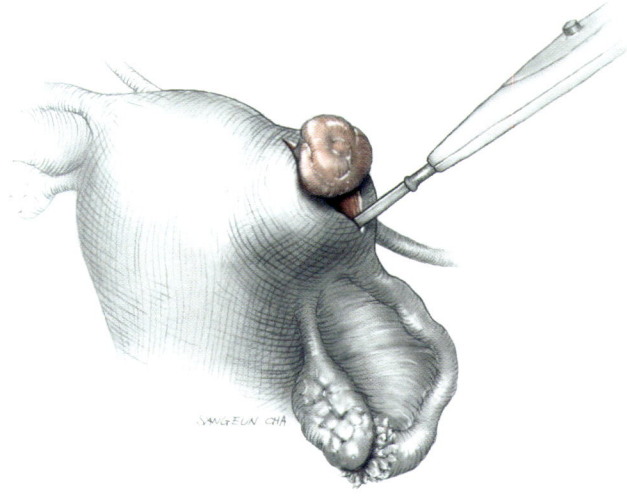

FIGURE 43-9.3 Cornuostomy with extrusion of products of conception.

myometrium surrounding the interstitial pregnancy to aid hemostasis. Needle aspiration prior to injection is imperative to avoid intravascular injection of this potent vasoconstrictor. The anesthesiologist is concurrently informed of vasopressin injection because a sudden rise in patient blood pressure may follow injection. Blanching at the injection site is expected.

❻ Cornuostomy. A linear incision is made through the uterine serosa and myometrium overlying the interstitial pregnancy (Fig. 43-9.2). As the incision is carried downward, some products of conception may extrude through the incision (Fig. 43-9.3). Products of conception may be removed by means of blunt, sharp, suction, or hydrodissection (Fig. 43-9.4). All visible placental fragments are ideally removed to help avoid persistent trophoblast tissue. Despite vasopressin, bleeding from the myometrium is common and is best managed with electrosurgical coagulation or individual figure-eight stitches with 2-0 absorbable or delayed-absorbable suture.

❼ Incision Closure. The myometrial incision is usually closed with absorbable or delayed-absorbable suture in an interrupted or continuous running fashion (Fig. 43-9.5). A gauge of sufficient strength to prevent breakage during muscle approximation is selected, typically 2-0 or 0-gauge. For this, chromic suture may be preferred due to its slight elasticity that provides tensile strength and minimal tissue cutting. Closure may be completed with one layer of sutures or may require two to three layers to aid hemostasis, avert hematoma formation, and reapproximate the myometrium. Additionally, some prefer a subserosal closure, similar to a subcuticular running stitch, as a final layer. This theoretically minimizes the amount of exposed suture and thereby limits adhesion formation.

❽ Cornual Wedge Resection. With this approach, the pregnancy, surrounding myometrium, and ipsilateral fallopian tube are excised en bloc. The fallopian tube is

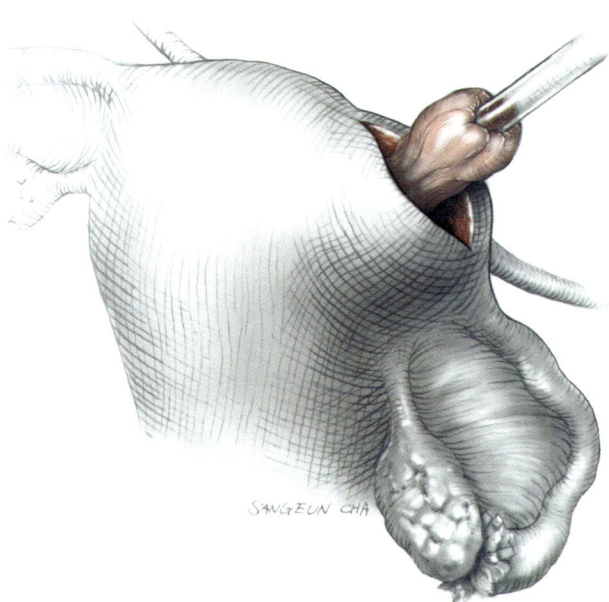

FIGURE 43-9.4 Suction removal of products of conception.

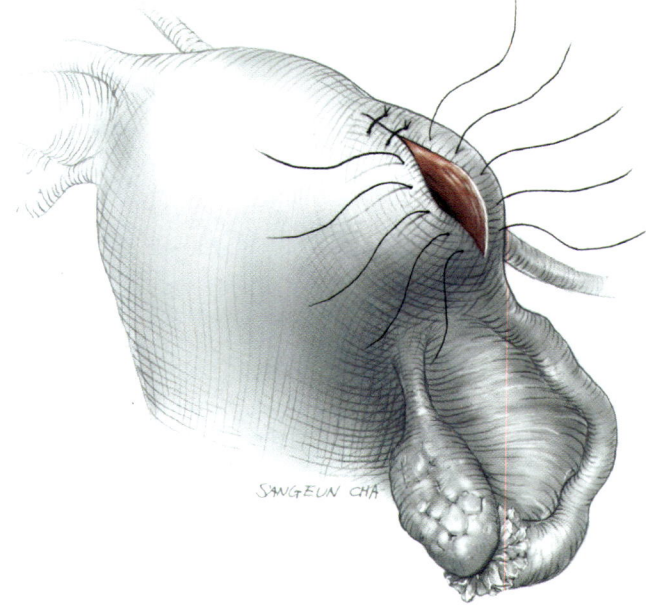

FIGURE 43-9.5 Myometrial incision closure.

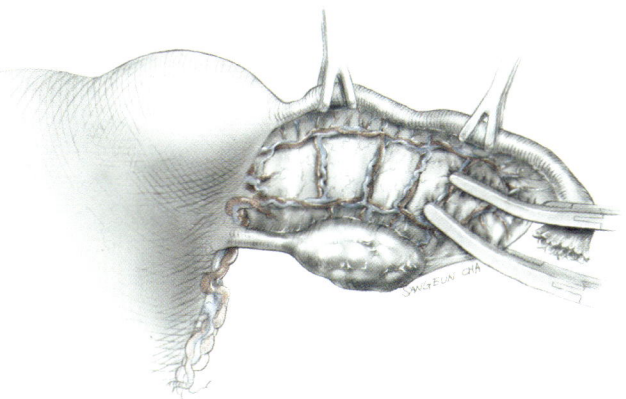

FIGURE 43-9.6 Mesosalpinx serially clamped and ligated.

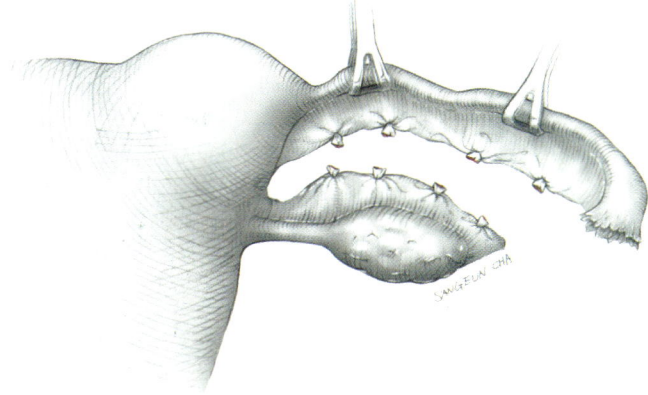

FIGURE 43-9.7 Salpingectomy completed.

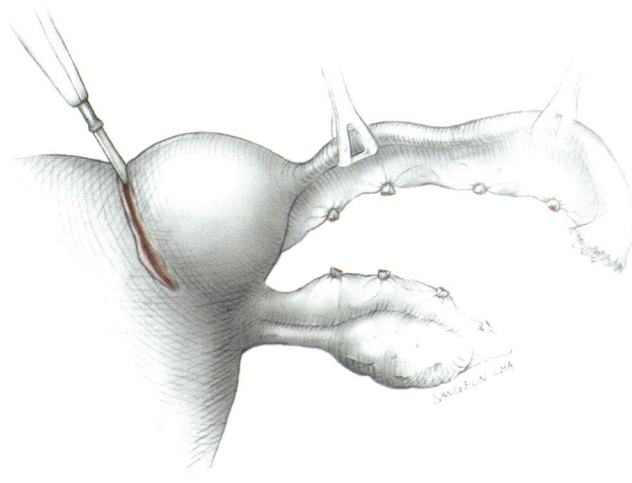

FIGURE 43-9.8 Myometrial incision.

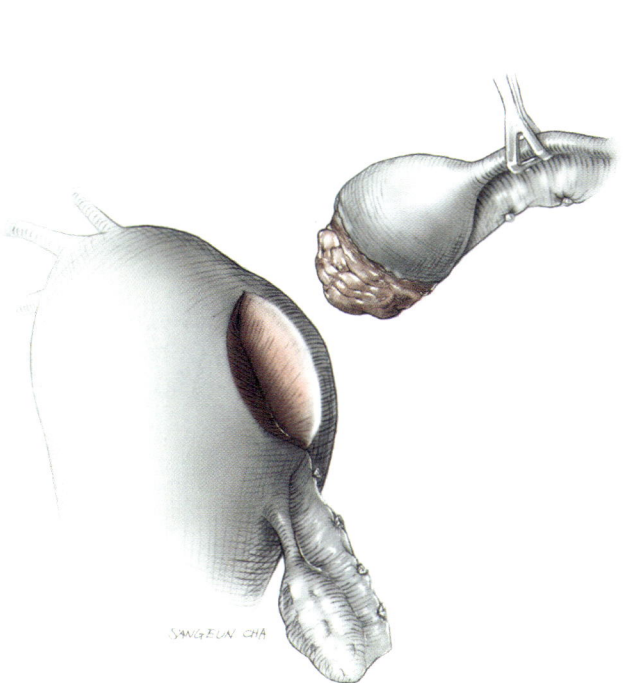

FIGURE 43-9.9 En bloc excision of interstitial pregnancy.

removed to avoid future ectopic pregnancy in this tube. Such pregnancies form when the ipsilateral ovary's eggs are fertilized by sperm that travel out the contralateral tube and are transported by peritoneal fluid to the isolated ovary and tube.

Initially, salpingectomy is completed as described in Section 43-8 (p. 945). To summarize, the mesosalpinx is serially clamped and ligated across its length (Fig. 43-9.6). This separates the tube from its mesosalpinx and ipsilateral ovary (Fig. 43-9.7).

❾ **Myometrial Incision.** Following vasopressin injection, the cornual serosa surrounding the pregnancy is incised with an electrosurgical blade (Fig. 43-9.8). This incision is angled inward as it is deepened. This creates a wedge into the myometrium (Fig. 43-9.9). Hemostasis can be achieved with electrosurgical blade coagulation or with sutures.

❿ **Incision Closure.** The myometrial incision is usually closed in two to three layers

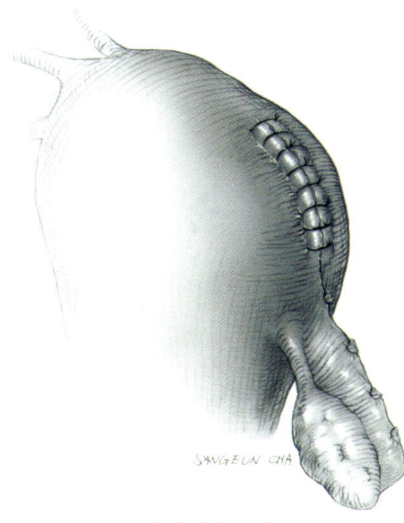

FIGURE 43-9.10 Incision closure.

with absorbable or delayed-absorbable suture in a simple interrupted or continuous running fashion. Imbricating stitches may help to close layers without undue tension. As with cornuostomy, some recommend a final subserosal layer closure. However, depending on the degree of wound tension created by the contracted myometrium, this suture may pull through the serosa, and a simple interrupted or running suture line may be required to approximate the serosa (Fig. 43-9.10).

In contrast, in cases with rupture and brisk bleeding, two clamps may have been placed across the base of the cornu. Following salpingectomy, the cornual myometrium above these clamps is sharply removed. The myometrium within each clamp is then suture ligated with a transfixing stitch.

POSTOPERATIVE

After surgery, care in general follows that described for laparotomy (p. 932). To address the greater risk of persistent trophoblastic tissue following cornuostomy, serial β-hCG levels are followed postoperatively until a negative test result is obtained. Persistent levels may warrant methotrexate therapy (Chap. 7, p. 171). For Rh-negative women, 50 or 300 μg (250 or 1500 IU) of anti-D immune globulin is given IM within 72 hours after pregnancy termination to lower the risk of alloimmunization in future pregnancies. Patients are also counseled that a higher risk of ectopic pregnancy in general follows an interstitial pregnancy. Last, as is the case with other myometrial surgeries, the uterine rupture rate in subsequent pregnancies and particularly during labor is increased. For this reason, delivery by cesarean at term before labor onset is considered.

43-10

Abdominal Myomectomy

Myomectomy involves surgical removal of leiomyomas from their surrounding myometrium. Indications can include abnormal uterine bleeding, pelvic pain, infertility, and recurrent miscarriage. Hysterectomy is chosen to treat many of these indications. However, myomectomy may be selected by those desiring organ preservation for childbearing or those wishing to avoid hysterectomy.

Myomectomy often requires laparotomy. However, laparoscopic excision may be performed by those with skills in laparoscopic suturing and is described in Chapter 44 (p. 1037) (Bhave Chittawar, 2014; Seracchioli, 2000).

PREOPERATIVE

Patient Evaluation

Because of their influence on pre- and intraoperative planning, leiomyoma size, number, and location are evaluated prior to surgery with sonography and perhaps with MR imaging or hysteroscopy. For example, submucous tumors are more easily removed hysteroscopically, whereas intramural and serosal types typically require laparotomy or laparoscopy. Leiomyomas may be small and buried within the myometrium. Thus, accurate information as to leiomyoma number and location aids excision of all masses. Last, multiple large tumors or those that are located in the broad ligament, that encroach on the tubal ostia, or that involve the cervix may raise the risk of conversion to hysterectomy.

Consent

Myomectomy has several risks including significant bleeding and need for transfusion. Larger tumors, intramural location, and greater myoma number increase this risk. Infrequently, uncontrolled hemorrhage or extensive myometrial injury during tumor removal may force hysterectomy. Fortunately, conversion rates to hysterectomy during myomectomy are low and range from 0 to 2 percent (Iverson, 1996; LaMorte, 1993; Sawin, 2000). Postoperatively, the risk of pelvic adhesion formation is significant. Also, leiomyomas can recur with time, and rates after 5 years approximate 60 percent. Some but not all recurrences lead to additional surgery (Hanafi, 2005; Kotani, 2018; Yoo, 2007).

Patient Preparation

Hematologic Status. Abnormal uterine bleeding is a common indication for myomectomy. As a result, many women who elect to undergo this surgery are anemic. In addition, significant intraoperative blood loss during myomectomy is possible. Accordingly, attempts to resolve anemia and heavy menstrual bleeding prior to surgery are pursued. Toward this goal, oral iron therapy, gonadotropin-releasing hormone (GnRH) agonists, and progesterone antagonists may have benefits.

GnRH Agonists. In addition to preoperative control of abnormal uterine bleeding, these agents significantly shrink uterine volume after several months of use (Benagiano, 1996; Friedman, 1991). Decreased uterine size following treatment may allow a less invasive surgical procedure. For example, myomectomy may be completed through a smaller laparotomy incision or by laparoscopy or hysteroscopy (Lethaby, 2002; Mencaglia, 1993). These agents also diminish leiomyoma vascularity and uterine blood flow (Matta, 1988; Reinsch, 1994).

The use of preoperative GnRH agonists, however, may also have disadvantages. Within leiomyomas, GnRH agonists can incite hyaline or hydropic degeneration, which may obliterate the pseudocapsule connective tissue interface between the tumor and the myometrium. Such obliterated cleavage planes may lead to tedious and lengthy tumor enucleation (Deligdisch, 1997). Moreover, rates of leiomyoma recurrence in women treated with GnRH agonists prior to myomectomy are higher (Fedele, 1990; Vercellini, 2003). Leiomyomas treated with these agents may shrink in volume and be missed during surgical removal.

Thus, GnRH agonists are not used routinely in all patients undergoing myomectomy. They can be recommended for preoperative use in women with greatly enlarged uteri or preoperative anemia or in cases in which a decrease in uterine volume would allow a less invasive approach. Similar to GnRH agonists, the new GnRH antagonists elagolix and relugolix may be used in the future following sufficient study and U.S. Food and Drug Administration (FDA) approval for myoma treatment.

The selective progesterone-receptor modulator (SPRM) agonists also shrink myoma volume and diminish menstrual bleeding (Donnez, 2012a,b). Available outside the United States, ulipristal acetate (Esmya, Fibristal) in oral dosages of 5 mg daily may be used during the 3 months prior to surgery to help correct anemia and shrink myomas. However, as discussed in Chapter 9 (p. 208), rare liver failure has been reported even with short-term use. Moreover, data on SPRM-associated myoma changes and their hindrance on tumor enucleation are limited (Murji, 2018). Both factors likely limit current use of this SPRM for this indication.

Other Preoperative Methods. The risk of blood transfusion varies among studies and ranges from <5 percent to nearly 40 percent (Darwish, 2005; LaMorte, 1993; Sawin, 2000; Smith, 1990). Thus, in women with large uteri, especially those with multiple leiomyomas, cell-saver blood scavenger and reuse techniques may be selected (Son, 2014; Yamada, 1997).

Also with large leiomyomas, tourniquets or vasopressin may fail to adequately limit bleeding. With this concern, preoperative uterine artery embolization (UAE) on the morning of surgery can help limit blood loss. And unlike GnRH agonist use, UAE allows tissue planes to be preserved (Ngeh, 2004; Tixier, 2010). Disadvantages of UAE include risks for subsequent pregnancy complications, collateral ovarian infarction, and formation of uterine synechiae. Thus, preoperative UAE may best be limited to patients with large uteri in whom excessive blood loss is a concern.

Prophylaxis. In assessing surgical infection risks, myomectomy is considered a clean case unless the endometrial cavity is breached. Few studies address the benefits of preoperative antibiotic use specifically for open myomectomy. Iverson and coworkers (1996), in their analysis of 101 myomectomy cases, found that although 54 percent of cases received prophylaxis, infectious morbidity was not lowered compared with cases in which antibiotics were not used. However, in cases performed for infertility, because of the potential for tubal adhesions associated with pelvic infection, antibiotic prophylaxis has been advocated (Milton, 2013). Studies of antibiotic prophylaxis practice patterns show high usage rates for this indication (Kim, 2019b; Wright, 2013a). For those in whom prophylaxis is planned, selection can follow that for hysterectomy (Table 39-8, p. 832). For all cases, because the risk of conversion to hysterectomy is present, vaginal preparation immediately prior to surgical draping is warranted.

With myomectomy, the risk of bowel injury is low. Thus, bowel preparation typically is not required. Last, laparotomy dictates VTE prophylaxis, and options are found in Table 39-10 (p. 834).

INTRAOPERATIVE

Surgical Steps

❶ Anesthesia and Patient Positioning. Myomectomy performed through a laparotomy incision is typically an inpatient procedure performed under general or regional anesthesia. The patient is supine. After anesthesia induction, hair in the planned incision path is clipped, a Foley catheter is inserted, and abdominal and vaginal preparation is completed.

❷ Abdominal Entry. The choice of Pfannenstiel incision is typically appropriate for uteri 14 weeks' size or smaller. Larger uteri usually require a midline vertical abdominal incision.

❸ Leiomyoma Identification. Following abdominal entry, the surgeon inspects the serosal surface to identify leiomyomas to be removed. Additionally, squeezing palpation of the myometrium before and during the surgery will help identify firm buried intramural or submucous leiomyomas.

❹ Use of Uterine Tourniquet. Tourniquets have been used for years to temporarily occlude blood flow through the uterine arteries. Because the uterus receives collateral flow through the ovarian arteries, some tourniquet techniques include occlusion of both uterine and ovarian vessels. First, bilateral windows are created in the leaves of the broad ligament at the level of the internal cervical os. A Penrose drain or pediatric Foley catheter is threaded through the opening to encircle the uterine isthmus. Once in place, the Penrose drain is tied or the ends of the Foley catheter are clamped to compress the uterine vessels. Additionally, temporary occlusion of the uteroovarian ligaments or infundibulopelvic ligaments with suture or a short broad clamp (bulldog clamp) to compress the ovarian arteries has been described (Al-Shabibi, 2009; Ginsburg, 1993). Last, the uterine arteries can be permanently ligated bilaterally (Sanders, 2019). Fertility outcomes following this permanent step, however, need further review.

❺ Use of Vasopressin. 8-Arginine vasopressin (Pitressin) is a sterile, aqueous solution of synthetic vasopressin. Its ability to cause vascular spasm and uterine muscle contraction effectively limits uterine blood loss during myomectomy. Compared with placebo, vasopressin injection significantly lowers blood loss during myomectomy (Frederick, 1994). Compared with tourniquet techniques, vasopressin injection is associated with comparable or less intraoperative blood loss (Fletcher, 1996; Ginsburg, 1993).

Each vial of Pitressin is standardized to contain 20 pressor units/mL, and doses used for myomectomy are 20 U diluted in 30 to 100 mL of saline (Frishman, 2009). Vasopressin is typically injected along the planned serosal incision(s). The plasma half-life of this agent is 10 to 20 minutes. For this reason, injection of vasopressin is ideally discontinued 20 minutes prior to uterine repair to allow evaluation of bleeding from myometrial incisions (Hutchins, 1996).

Local vasopressin injection can lead to inadvertent intravascular infiltration and transient increases in blood pressure, bradycardia, atrioventricular block, and pulmonary edema (Deschamps, 2005; Tulandi, 1996). Thus, patients with a history of cardiovascular disease, uncontrolled hypertension, migraine, asthma, and severe chronic obstructive pulmonary disease may not be candidates for vasopressin use. Other less-robust evidence supports vaginal misoprostol, intravenous (IV) tranexamic acid, and IV oxytocin infusion for this indication (Aslan Çetin, 2019; Atashkhoei, 2017; Fusca, 2018; Kongnyuy, 2014).

❻ Serosal Incision. Because of postoperative adhesion formation risks, surgeons ideally minimize the number of serosal incisions and attempt to place incisions on the anterior uterine wall. Tulandi and colleagues (1993) found that posterior wall incisions result in a 94-percent adhesion formation rate compared with a 55-percent rate for anterior incisions.

For most patients, a midline vertical uterine incision allows removal of the greatest number of leiomyomas through the fewest incisions. The length should accommodate the approximate diameter of the largest tumor. The incision depth should afford access to all leiomyomas (Fig. 43-10.1). To reach lateral tumors, a surgeon may create lateral myometrial incisions within the initial central incision. However, at times, separate incision may be required to excise tumors from these locations. In these instances, a horizontal incision minimizes the number of arcuate vessels transected.

❼ Tumor Enucleation. The first leiomyoma is grasped with a Lahey tenaculum or towel clip (Fig. 43-10.2). Applying traction on the leiomyoma aids in the development of a tissue plane between myometrium and leiomyoma. Sharp and blunt dissection of the pseudocapsule surrounding the leiomyoma frees the tumor from the adjacent myometrium.

❽ Bleeding. Hemorrhage during myomectomy primarily develops during tumor enucleation. Approximately two to four main arteries feed each leiomyoma and enter the tumor at unpredictable sites. Accordingly, surgeons should watch for these vessels, ligate them prior to transection when possible, and be ready to immediately grasp them with hemostats for ligation or fulguration if lacerated during tumor excision (Fig. 43-10.3).

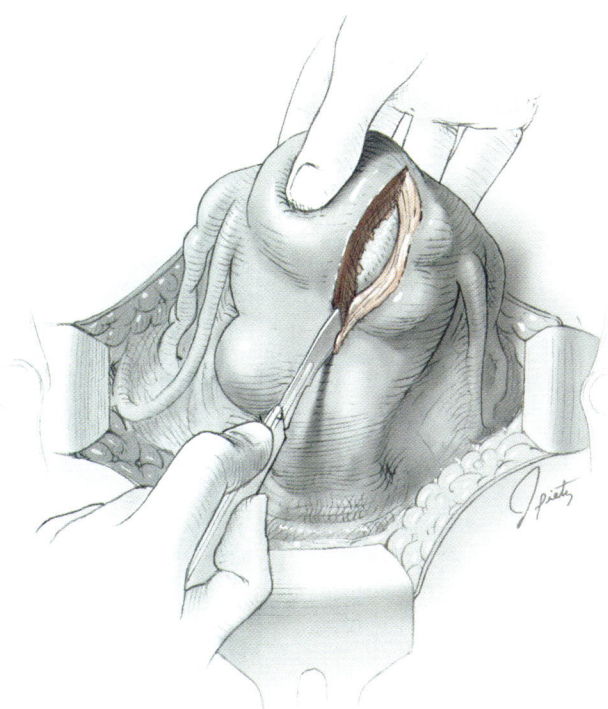

FIGURE 43-10.1 Uterine incision.

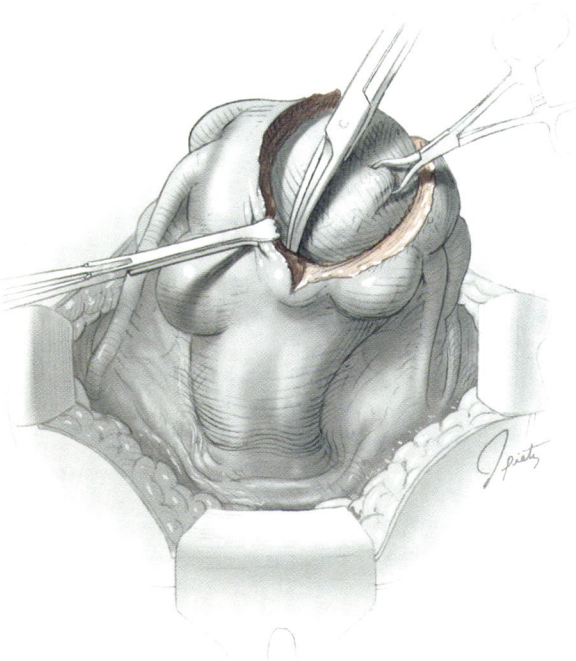

FIGURE 43-10.2 Tumor enucleation.

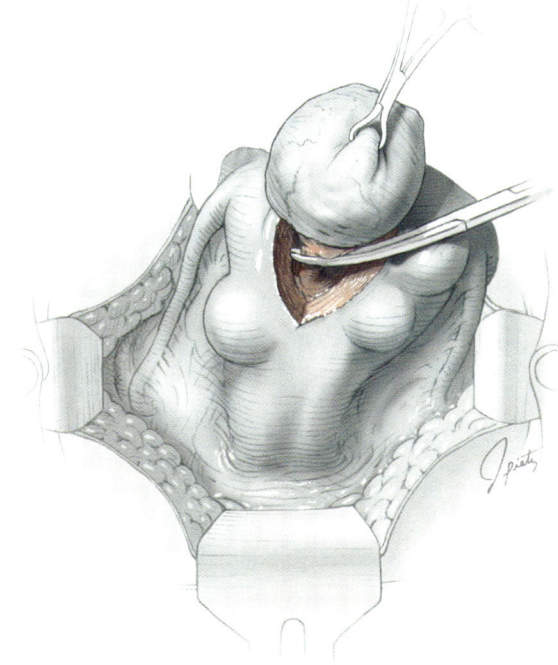

FIGURE 43-10.3 Vessel ligation.

⑨ Myometrial Closure. Following removal of all tumors, redundant serosa may be excised. If the endometrial cavity is entered, it should be closed with a running stitch of 4-0 or 5-0 gauge delayed-absorbable suture. Smaller internal myometrial incisions are closed with delayed-absorbable suture (Fig. 43-10.4). The myometrium is then closed in several layers to improve hemostasis and prevent hematoma formation. A gauge of sufficient strength to prevent breakage during muscle approximation is selected, typically 2-0 to 0-gauge.

⑩ Serosal Closure. Closure of the serosal incision using a running baseball stitch or a subserosal running closure, similar to a running subcuticular closure, may help limit adhesion formation. For this, 4-0 or 5-0 monofilament, delayed-absorbable suture may be selected. Moreover, absorbable adhesion barriers may help reduce the incidence of adhesion formation following myomectomy (Ahmad, 2015; Canis, 2014; Tinelli, 2011).

POSTOPERATIVE

After surgery, care in general follows that described for laparotomy (p. 932). Febrile morbidity of greater than 38.0°C is a common event following myomectomy (Iverson, 1996; Rybak, 2008). Purported causes include atelectasis, myometrial incisional hematomas, and factors released with myometrial destruction. Although fever is common following myomectomy, pelvic infection is not. For example, LaMorte and colleagues (1993) noted only a 2-percent rate of pelvic infection in their analysis of 128 myomectomy cases.

Following myomectomy, no clear guidelines direct the timing of pregnancy attempts. Darwish and associates (2005) performed sonographic examinations on 169 patients after myomectomy. Following myometrial indicators, they concluded that wound healing is usually completed within 3 months. No clinical trials address uterine rupture and route of pregnancy delivery after myomectomy (American College of Obstetricians and Gynecologists, 2019a). Management of these cases requires sound clinical judgment and individualized decision-making.

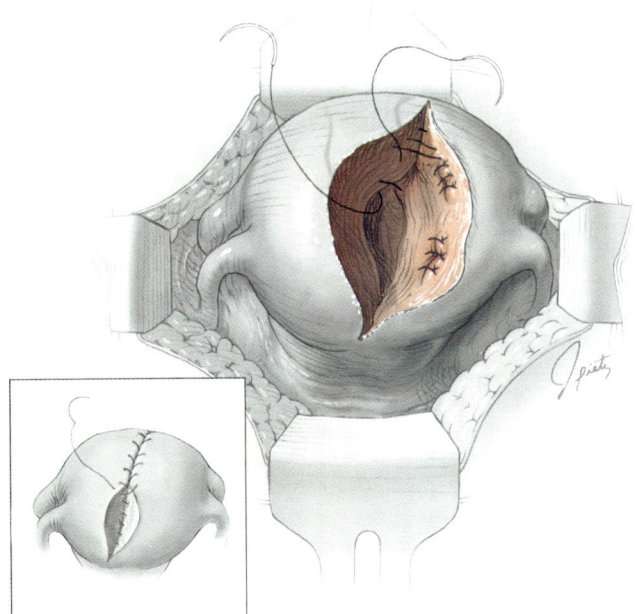

FIGURE 43-10.4 Uterine incision closure.

43-11

Vaginal Myomectomy

Prolapse of a pedunculated submucosal leiomyoma is unusual but certainly not rare. Vaginal myomectomy is usually a simple procedure and is frequently curative for the patient. Myoma and stalk size and patient discomfort are the most important variables for management. With a thin stalk, simply twisting the leiomyoma slowly off its stalk may be sufficient for removal. With larger stalk diameter or greater patient discomfort, removal in the operating room is typically preferred. Last, for those with a large obstructive myoma on a thick, short stalk, hysterectomy may be necessary (Caglar, 2005; Golan, 2005).

PREOPERATIVE

Patient Evaluation

In many cases, diagnosis of a prolapsed pedunculated submucosal leiomyoma will be obvious, as will the size of the prolapsed leiomyoma. However, as many of these patients present with abnormal uterine bleeding, evaluation for other less obvious causes of abnormal bleeding is appropriate. In other cases, only partial prolapse of a leiomyoma through the cervix may preclude assessment of total leiomyoma and stalk size, or the mass may be of unclear etiology. Accordingly, imaging studies, particularly pelvic sonography, may yield additional information beyond examination. Specifically, uterine size, shape, and degree of involvement with additional leiomyomas or other pathology can be seen. Biopsy of any mass of uncertain etiology is considered, and Tischler biopsy forceps may be selected (Fig. 29-15, p. 637). If required, Monsel solution can be applied to control bleeding from the biopsy site similar to that following colposcopic biopsy.

Consent

Except for significant uterine bleeding, complication rates with vaginal myomectomy are low. Still, the possibility of hysterectomy and its consequences are presented. Rarely, tension from the prolapsed mass may invert the uterine body. In this event, severing a stalk on great tension may concomitantly resect the attached uterine wall and injure intraabdominal organs.

Patient Preparation

Uterine bleeding with leiomyoma prolapse is common, and hypovolemia and acute blood loss anemia are corrected as needed. The benefits of VTE prophylaxis will vary by patient age and anticipated length of surgery, as outlined in Table 39-10 (p. 834). The risk of infection is low, and antibiotic prophylaxis is typically not needed in uncomplicated cases.

INTRAOPERATIVE

Surgical Steps

❶ **Anesthesia and Patient Positioning.** The patient is placed in standard lithotomy position. For vaginal myomectomy, suitable anesthesia varies mainly by myoma stalk size and patient comfort. It may include general or regional anesthesia, conscious sedation, or simple IM analgesia. For those women who are taken to the operating room at our institution, we usually prefer general anesthesia for several reasons. First, hysteroscopy is often done following vaginal myomectomy to further evaluate the uterine cavity and status of the stalk. Secondly, many leiomyomas are bulky and require at least a moderate amount of manipulation and vaginal retraction for removal.

An examination is done once the patient is relaxed to additionally assess the prolapsed leiomyoma size and the stalk length and thickness. The vagina is then surgically prepared, and the bladder is drained.

❷ **Leiomyoma Stalk Ligation.** An Auvard weighted vaginal speculum is positioned to retract the posterior vaginal wall. Heaney retractors are used as needed for sidewall and anterior vaginal wall retraction.

The initial step aims to devascularize the leiomyoma. With a narrow stalk, this can be achieved by grasping the myoma with a toothed instrument and repeatedly twisting the stalk circumferentially about itself. The myoma will avulse from the stalk as it narrows with the twisting.

With thicker stalks, a preformed endoscopic knotted loop (EndoLoop) works well (Fig. 41-35, p. 898). The loop is guided with forceps around the myoma. A tenaculum then grasps the myoma to create gentle outward tension (Fig. 43-11.1). The loop is positioned proximally around the stalk and cinched. Either single or double ligation may be preferred.

At times, loop manipulation or knot tying may be technically difficult given the size of the obstructing leiomyoma, the stalk length

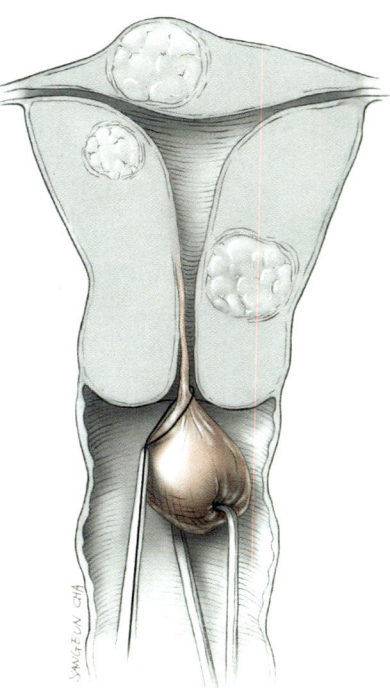

FIGURE 43-11.1 Suture loop surrounding leiomyoma stalk placed on tension.

(or lack thereof), and the cramped vaginal operating space. In such cases, tips of a Heaney right-angle clamp can be maneuvered past the myoma and then across the stalk.

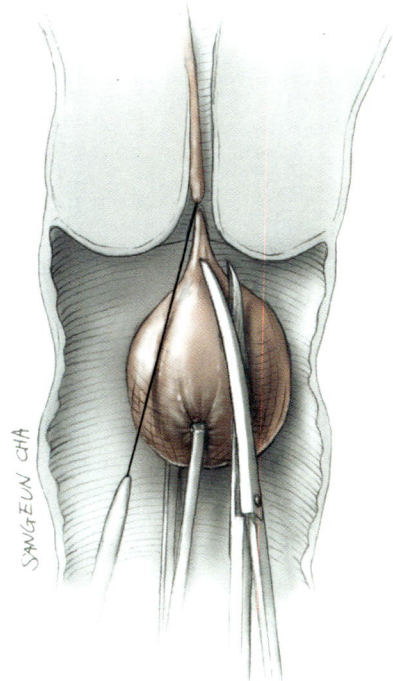

FIGURE 43-11.2 Suture loop cinched and tumor stalk transected.

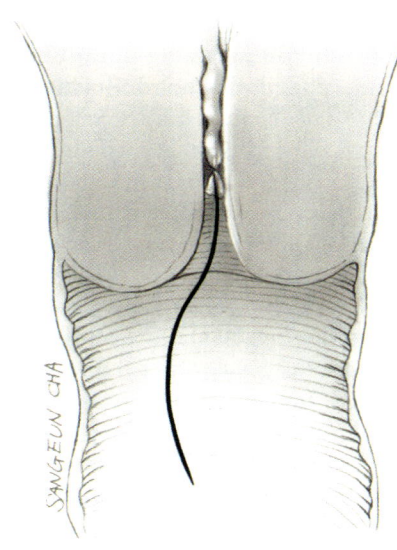

FIGURE 43-11.3 Leiomyoma excision completed.

❸ **Leiomyoma Removal.** The stalk is then sharply incised at an appropriate point distal to the ligature or clamp (Fig. 43-11.2). Because of cramped operating space, the sharp angle of Jorgenson scissors may be useful. With complete stalk transection, the prolapsed leiomyoma is freed for removal, and the ligated stalk retracts into the uterine cavity (Fig. 43-11.3).

If a Heaney clamp has been placed, the stalk is severed and the mass is removed. A simple or transfixing ligature is placed around the proximal stalk. As the suture is tied, the clamp is removed. After leiomyoma removal, hysteroscopy may optionally be performed to assess hemostasis and the uterine cavity.

POSTOPERATIVE

No special care beyond routine postoperative surveillance is necessary. Regular diet and activities are resumed quickly and can be individualized.

Abdominal Hysterectomy

Hysterectomy is one of the most frequently performed gynecologic procedures, and more than 500,000 women undergo this procedure for benign disease annually in the United States (Jacoby, 2009). Of benign indications, symptomatic leiomyomas and pelvic organ prolapse are the most frequent. Adenomyosis, endometriosis, chronic pelvic pain, and premalignant uterine or cervical disease also are common.

PREOPERATIVE

Patient Evaluation

To reach the preoperative diagnosis, testing varies and is discussed within chapters covering those etiologies. Prior to hysterectomy, all patients require cervical cancer screening. With abnormal findings, further evaluation is completed to exclude invasive cancer, which is treated instead with radical hysterectomy or chemoradiation. Similarly, women at risk for endometrial cancer and whose indication includes abnormal bleeding are also usually screened before surgery (Chap. 8, p. 183). Last, concurrent cervical infection or bacterial vaginosis is sought for preoperative eradication to lower postoperative infection risks.

Decision-Making for Approach Selection

Hysterectomy may be completed using an abdominal, vaginal, laparoscopic, or robotic approach, and selection is influenced by many factors. Shape and size of the uterus and pelvis, surgical indication, adnexal pathology, extensive pelvic adhesive disease, surgical risks, hospitalization and recovery length, hospital resources, and surgeon expertise are all weighed once hysterectomy is planned. Each approach carries distinct advantages and disadvantages, discussed subsequently. In sum, vaginal hysterectomy is preferred when feasible (American College of Obstetricians and Gynecologists, 2017a).

Vaginal Hysterectomy. Surgeons usually choose this approach if the uterus is relatively small, extensive adhesions are not anticipated, no significant adnexal pathology is expected, and some degree of pelvic organ descent is present. Compared with an abdominal approach, vaginal hysterectomy usually offers faster recovery and reductions

in hospital stay length, expense, and postoperative pain (Johnson, 2005; Nieboer, 2009). Compared with a laparoscopic approach, vaginal hysterectomy typically provides shorter operating time and lower urinary tract injury risk (Aarts, 2015).

Abdominal Hysterectomy. Despite the advantages of vaginal hysterectomy, most uteri in the United States are removed through an abdominal incision (Wright, 2013b). Either a transverse or vertical incision may be selected depending on the clinical setting (p. 930).

Abdominal hysterectomy allows the greatest ability to manipulate pelvic organs. Thus, it may be preferred if large pelvic masses or extensive adhesions are anticipated. Additionally, an abdominal approach affords access to the ovaries if oophorectomy is desired, to the space of Retzius or presacral space if concurrent urogynecologic procedures are planned, or to the upper abdomen for cancer staging. However, for surgeons with advanced skills in MIS, most of these limitations are overcome, and their indications for abdominal hysterectomy may be few. That said, abdominal hysterectomy typically requires less operating time than laparoscopic or robotic hysterectomy and requires no advanced MIS expertise or instrumentation. Moreover, as discussed in Chapter 41 (p. 894), the U.S. Food and Drug Administration (FDA) (2018) and American College of Obstetricians and Gynecologists (2019e) discourage laparoscopic power morcellation in those with known cancer or higher risk of potentially occult cancer. While data are being collected to stratify this risk, many surgeons and patients may forego MIS hysterectomy for larger uteri. Since the initial FDA warning, the rate of abdominal hysterectomy for women with leiomyomas rose 8 percent (Clark, 2017).

Disadvantages of abdominal hysterectomy include longer patient recovery and hospital stays, increased incisional pain, and greater risk of postoperative fever and wound infection (Marana, 1999; Nieboer,

2009). Compared with a vaginal approach, abdominal hysterectomy is also associated with greater risk for ureteral injury, but lower rates of bladder injury (Frankman, 2010; Gilmour, 2006).

Laparoscopic Hysterectomy. This hysterectomy group uses laparoscopic techniques to complete some or all steps of hysterectomy (Turner, 2013). Although criteria vary depending on surgeon skill, this approach is often selected if the uterus is not excessively large, extensive adhesions are not expected, and some limitation deters vaginal hysterectomy. Patient recovery, hospital stays, and postoperative pain scores are comparable with those of vaginal hysterectomy, but a laparoscopic approach allows greater visualization and access to the abdomen and pelvis. However, laparoscopy typically requires longer operating times, expensive equipment, and MIS expertise. In addition, in most studies, laparoscopic hysterectomy is associated with greater rates of ureteral injury than either abdominal or vaginal hysterectomy (Frankman, 2010; Gilmour, 2006; Mamik, 2014).

Approach Selection. If all factors are equal, vaginal hysterectomy should be considered. However, with large pelvic masses or large uteri, with risk of gynecologic cancer, with extensive adhesions, or with poor uterine descent, either abdominal or laparoscopic hysterectomy may be selected. Of note, surgical expertise is factored and strongly influences approach selection.

Total versus Supracervical Hysterectomy. Prior to hysterectomy, the decision to concurrently remove the cervix is discussed with the patient. Hysterectomy may include removal of the uterus and cervix, termed *total hysterectomy*, or may involve only the uterine corpus, called *supracervical hysterectomy (SCH)* (Fig. 43-12.1). The term *subtotal hysterectomy* is ambiguous and is not a preferred term.

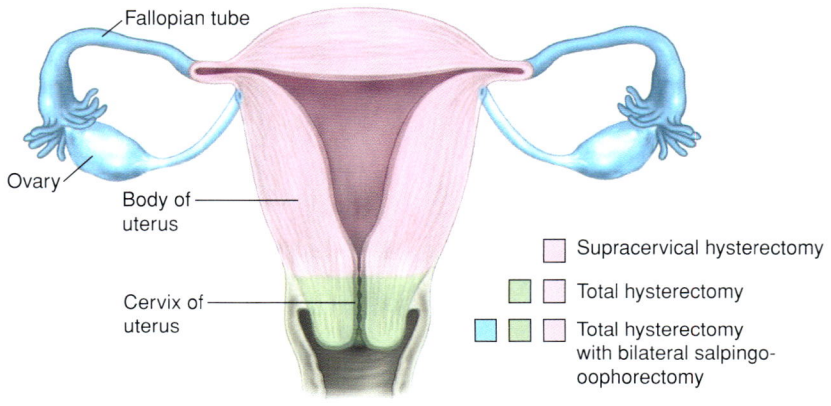

Fallopian tube

Ovary

Body of uterus

Cervix of uterus

☐ Supracervical hysterectomy

☐ ☐ Total hysterectomy

☐ ☐ ☐ Total hysterectomy with bilateral salpingo-oophorectomy

FIGURE 43-12.1 Hysterectomy classification.

Most hysterectomies performed are total, but SCH may be selected preoperatively. For example, SCH is purported to reduce the risk of mesh erosion at the cuff if concurrent hysterectomy and sacrocolpopexy are planned (Osmundsen, 2012; Tan-Kim, 2011). At one point, SCH was also suggested to improve urinary, bowel, or sexual function compared with total abdominal hysterectomy. But, several studies have shown no short- or long-term differences in these functions between total abdominal or supracervical hysterectomy (Andersen, 2015; Lethaby, 2012). Frequently, SCH may be an intraoperative decision during cases in which excision of the cervix risks greater bleeding, surrounding organ damage, or longer operating time.

As a disadvantage, 10 to 20 percent of women following SCH will still note cyclic vaginal bleeding, presumably from retained isthmic endometrium in the cervical stump. Procedures that ablate or core out the endocervical canal can help prevent this complication (Schmidt, 2011). Also, pelvic organ prolapse may develop (Hilger, 2005). For either complication, cervical stump excision, termed *trachelectomy*, may be required. Last, critics note the persistent risk for cancer in the conserved stump. However, the risk for cervical cancer in these women is comparable with that in women without hysterectomy. Moreover, the prognosis for cervical stump cancer mirrors that in women with a complete uterus (Hannoun-Levi, 1997; Hellstrom, 2001).

In sum, SCH alone offers no distinct long-term advantages compared with total abdominal hysterectomy (American College of Obstetricians and Gynecologists, 2017a). The risk of persistent bleeding following surgery may deter many women and clinicians from its use. Moreover, although data are limited, trachelectomy following SCH may be surgically challenging due to scarring of bowel or bladder to the stump. Despite these disadvantages, if concurrent sacrocolpopexy is planned, SCH may lower mesh erosion rates (Chap. 45, p. 1125).

Consent

For most women with indications, hysterectomy is a safe and effective treatment that typically leads to an improved postoperative quality of life and psychologic outcome (Hartmann, 2004; Kuppermann, 2013). However, pelvic organs may be injured during surgery, and vascular, bladder, ureteral, and bowel injury are most common. Accordingly, these and the risks of wound infection, blood loss, and transfusion are discussed with the patient before surgery. Infrequently, unintended adnexectomy may

be required and, if bilateral, will create iatrogenic menopause. Importantly, patients should understand the sterilizing effects of hysterectomy.

Concurrent Adnexal Surgery. Hysterectomy is frequently performed with other operations. Pelvic reconstructive surgeries and bilateral salpingo-oophorectomy (BSO) or salpingectomy are among the most frequent.

For adnexal surgery, distinguishing between prophylactic BSO and indicated BSO is a first step. Thus, comorbid ovarian pathology is sought preoperatively. Described in Chapter 10 (p. 220), ovarian imaging and selective serum CA125 testing are primary tools. Once indicated procedures are excluded, the risks and benefits of BSO to lower ovarian cancer risks, that is *prophylactic BSO*, are weighed. Both adnexa are prophylactically removed in approximately 40 percent of hysterectomy cases performed for benign indications in the United States (Asante, 2010).

Broadly, decisions regarding prophylactic BSO balance benefits of ovarian cancer risk reduction against the adverse, long-term health consequences of surgical menopause. Proponents of BSO note that future ovarian cancer rates are reduced by 94 percent in women after BSO compared with those patients who retain their ovaries (Parker, 2013). However, hysterectomy alone may decrease this cancer risk by 40 to 50 percent (Chiaffarino, 2005; Rice, 2014). In addition, patients with retained ovaries may require future surgery for subsequent benign ovarian disease. This risk approximates 3 percent at 10 years posthysterectomy (Casiano, 2013). Specifically, women with endometriosis, pelvic inflammatory disease, and chronic pelvic pain are at greater risk for reoperation. And, if later oophorectomy is required, the risk of ureteral or bowel injury due to adhesions encasing the ovary is increased from that with primary BSO. Last, the duration of significant ovarian estrogen production for many will be shortened following hysterectomy. For example, Siddle and coworkers (1987) noted that the mean age of ovarian failure in a group undergoing hysterectomy was 45 years. This was significantly lower than the mean age of 49 years in a control group not receiving surgery.

Arguments for ovarian conservation are convincing as well. First, conservation delays the long-term effects of hypoestrogenism (Chap. 22, p. 473). However, hysterectomy alone is associated with earlier menopause by approximately 4 years (Farquhar, 2005b). That said, Parker and colleagues (2013) noted higher ovarian and slightly elevated breast cancer rates but a lower all-cause mortality rate in women after hysterectomy with

ovarian conservation compared with those electing BSO without estrogen replacement therapy (ERT). Specifically, evidence suggests a 40-percent greater risk of all-cause mortality in women who do not use ERT and undergo BSO prior to age 45 to 50 (Mytton, 2017; Parker, 2013). Although these rates became nearly equal in those electing BSO and then receiving postoperative ERT, concerns regarding ERT compliance have been noted. Castelo-Branco and coworkers (1999) found that after 5 years following hysterectomy and BSO, only one third of patients still continued their ERT. Most stopped due to cancer concerns. In addition, ovarian androgen production is removed, and its importance in later life has not been entirely delineated (Olive, 2005). More recent trends in the United States show a significant decline in BSO rates for those younger than 55 (Karp, 2015; Novetsky, 2011; Perera, 2013).

Even if ovaries are conserved, the Society of Gynecologic Oncology encourages consideration of concurrent bilateral salpingectomy during hysterectomy (Walker, 2015). The American College of Obstetricians and Gynecologists (2019d) endorses this stance but recommends that plans for a vaginal approach should not be changed solely to complete salpingectomy. Salpingectomy is hoped to lower rates of some ovarian cancer types (Chap. 35, p. 736). That said, the degree of ovarian blood supply compromise and effects on long-term function by this resection is unknown. A fuller discussion of risk-reducing salpingectomy is found in Chapters 5 (p. 118) and 35 (p. 736).

Patient Preparation

Because of the risk of postoperative wound and urinary tract infection following hysterectomy, patients typically receive antibiotic prophylaxis with either a first- or second-generation cephalosporin (American College of Obstetricians and Gynecologists, 2018b). Suitable options are found in Table 39-8 (p. 832). Preoperative mechanical bowel preparation may be implemented selectively. Fortunately, the risk of bowel injury with hysterectomy in general is low, and thus many forego evacuation measures for their patients. Laparotomy dictates VTE prophylaxis, and options are found in Table 39-10 (p. 834).

INTRAOPERATIVE

Surgical Steps

❶ Anesthesia and Patient Positioning. Abdominal hysterectomy is typically performed under general or regional anesthesia.

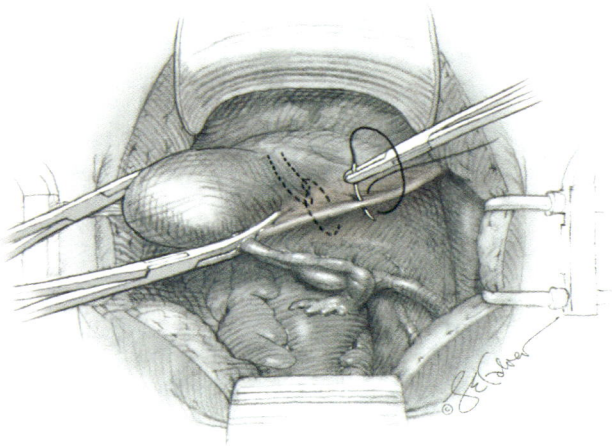

FIGURE 43-12.2 Round ligament ligation.

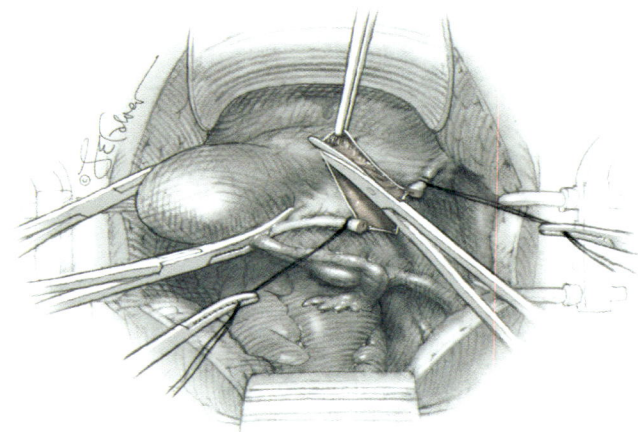

FIGURE 43-12.3 Opening of broad ligament anterior leaf.

The patient is often supine. But if concomitant vaginal procedures or cystoscopy are planned, the patient is placed in low lithotomy position in adjustable booted stirrups. After anesthesia induction, hair in the planned incision path is clipped if needed; a Foley catheter is inserted; and abdominal and vaginal preparation is completed.

❷ Abdominal Entry. Either a transverse or a vertical incision may be used for hysterectomy, and clinical factors influence selection (p. 930).

❸ Exposure. Following entry into the abdomen, a self-retaining retractor is placed. The pelvis and abdomen are visually and manually explored, the patient is placed in the Trendelenburg position to aid bowel displacement, and the bowel is packed from the operating field. The uterus is grasped and elevated from the pelvis. If extensive adhesions are present, normal anatomic relationships are restored. Hysterectomy may be performed by one surgeon, but commonly two surgeons are present, with each typically operating on his or her side of the uterus.

❹ Round Ligament Transection. Curved Kelly (Pean) clamps are placed immediately lateral to each uterine cornu to permit uterine manipulation. Hysterectomy typically begins with division of one round ligament at its midpoint (Fig. 43-12.2). This provides entry into the retroperitoneal space for ureter identification and access to the uterine artery and cardinal ligament for later transection. The round ligament is grasped with tissue forceps and elevated. A transfixing stitch using 0-gauge delayed-absorbable suture is placed approximately 1 cm lateral to the planned division site. The first bite of this stitch passes through an avascular site of the mesoteres beneath the round ligament, whereas the transfixing bite pierces the round ligament

medial to first bite. This prevents hematoma formation between the transfixing stitch and pelvic sidewall. A second simple stitch of similar suture is placed 1 cm medial to the first and through an avascular site in the mesoteres and beneath the round ligament. These sutures prevent bleeding from Sampson artery or veins within the mesoteres and aid tissue manipulation. Once secured, sutures are held by hemostats and directed outward to create tension along the interposed ligament. The round ligament is then divided, and the incision line is directed deeply into the first 1 to 2 cm of the broad ligament.

❺ Anterior Broad Ligament Leaf. With this last step, the broad ligament separates to create anterior and posterior leaves. Between them, loose areolar connective tissue with multiple small vessels is seen. To incise the anterior leaf, the round ligament sutures are placed on tension. Metzenbaum scissors are

introduced between the anterior leaf and underlying loose connective tissue. Both scissor tips are directed upward to be seen through the peritoneum as they advance. Gentle opening and closing of scissor blade tips during advancement separates the peritoneum from the underlying connective tissue and uterine vessels. The tented anterior leaf is then incised sharply or with electrosurgery tip. The line of incision curves inferiorly and medially to the level of the vesicouterine fold, which generally lies just below the uterine isthmus (Fig. 43-12.3). The incision stops well above the bladder to avoid cystotomy.

To further open the retroperitoneal space, the drape of peritoneum lying between the round ligament and infundibulopelvic (IP) ligament is grasped with smooth forceps and placed on tension. This peritoneum is incised with Metzenbaum scissors and with the same undermining technique used for the anterior leaf (Fig. 43-12.4). Lateral and parallel to the

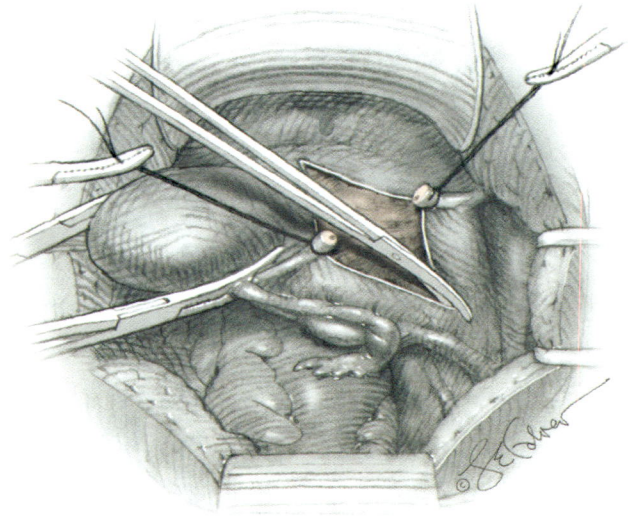

FIGURE 43-12.4 Peritoneal incision extension.

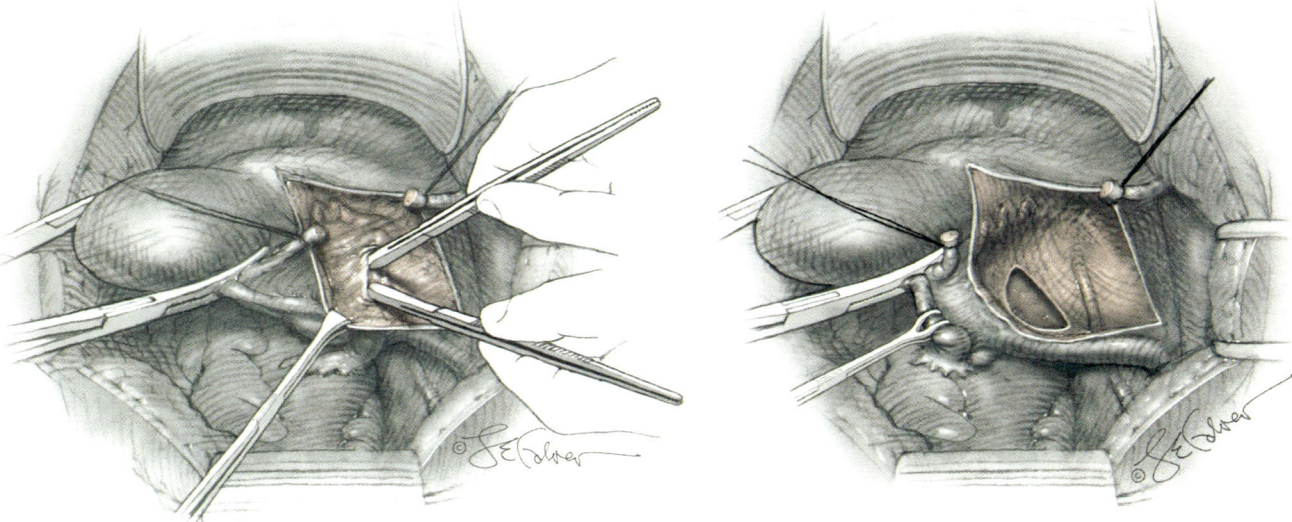

FIGURE 43-12.5 Ureter identification.

FIGURE 43-12.6 Posterior peritoneal window.

IP, the incision is extended cephalad toward the pelvic sidewall and to approximately the level of the pelvic brim.

❻ **Ureter Identification.** The ureter is most easily identified within the pararectal space, close to the pelvic brim, and at the common iliac artery bifurcation. It can then be traced deeper into the pelvis. This is accomplished by localized blunt retroperitoneal dissection that is advanced downward with gentle cephalad and caudad strokes into gauzy retroperitoneal tissue above the presumed ureter path (Fig. 43-12.5). Small vessels are coagulated as they are found. Dissection is directed downward, medially, and slightly cephalad toward the medial aspect of the posterior peritoneal leaf, along which the ureter courses.

❼ **Posterior Broad Ligament Leaf.** With the ureter directly visualized, the posterior leaf is incised to create a window. This allows isolation of the next pedicle and moves the ureter from the operative field. If ovarian preservation is planned, this window is made solely beneath the uteroovarian ligament and near the uterine body. If oophorectomy is planned, the posterior leaf is incised parallel to the IP ligament. The incision is extended toward the pelvic brim and medially toward the uterus just below the uteroovarian ligament. This delineates the IP for ligation (Fig. 43-12.6).

❽ **Adnexectomy.** If the adnexa are to be removed, the fallopian tube and ovary are grasped with a Babcock or other atraumatic clamp and elevated medially to place the IP ligament on mild tension for improved

delineation (Fig. 43-12.7). With the ureter visualized, a curved Zeppelin clamp can be placed around this ligament with its arc curving upward. The tips of the clamps are placed through the previously created peritoneal window. A Kelly clamp is placed medial to this and closer to the adnexa.

With clamps secured, the IP ligament is sharply transected above the Zeppelin clamp. A free tie of 0-gauge delayed-absorbable suture is placed around the Zeppelin clamp to ligate ovarian vessels. As the knot

of this suture is secured, the Zeppelin clamp is quickly opened and closed, that is, "flashed." A transfixing stitch is then sutured below the clamp but above and distal to the first free tie. As the knot is cinched, the Zeppelin clamp is removed.

The adnexum is thereby freed from the pelvic sidewall, and its greater mobility may obstruct the surgeon's view. Accordingly, the adnexa can be tied to the Kelly clamp still located on the cornu or can be simply excised and removed.

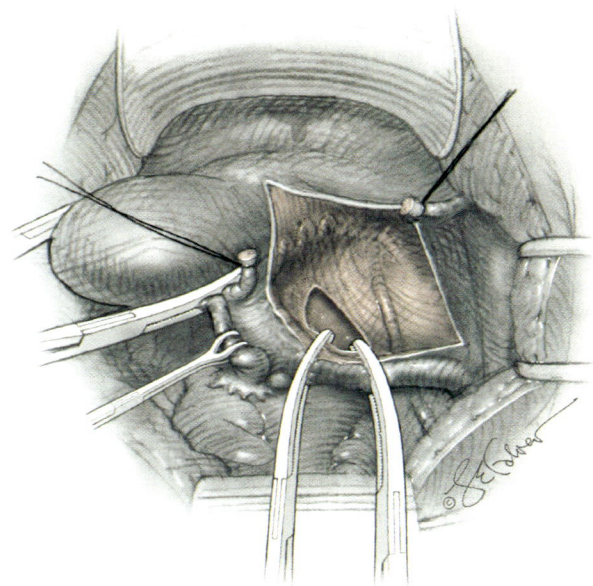

FIGURE 43-12.7 Infundibulopelvic ligament transection during oophorectomy.

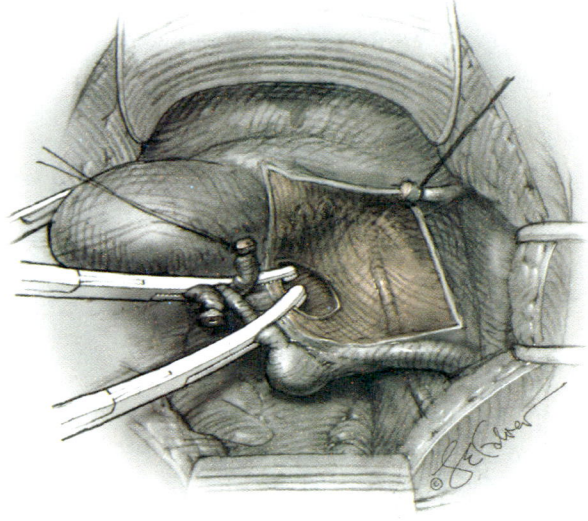

FIGURE 43-12.8 Uteroovarian ligament transection for ovarian conservation.

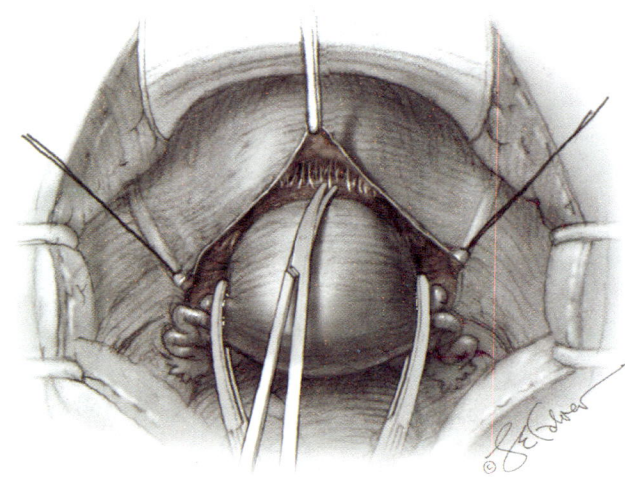

FIGURE 43-12.9 Dissection within vesicouterine space.

❾ Ovarian Conservation. With the leaves of the broad ligament now open, if the ovary is to be preserved, salpingectomy alone now can be completed. This is fully described in Section 43-8 (p. 945). In summary, the mesosalpinx is serially clamped, cut, and ligated. Each clamp incorporates approximately 2 cm of mesosalpinx, and resection progresses from the fimbria to its union with the uterus.

To preserve the ovary, one Kelly clamp is already positioned at the cornu and across the uteroovarian ligament. A Zeppelin clamp is positioned lateral to this, and its arc faces the uterus (Fig. 43-12.8).

The intervening segment of uteroovarian ligament is incised between the Zeppelin and Kelly clamps. Ligation of the ligament is carried out as in Step 8. That is, a free tie of 0-gauge delayed-absorbable suture is placed around the Zeppelin clamp. As the knot is secured, the clamp is flashed. A transfixing stitch is then placed around the same clamp but distal to the first free tie. As the knot is cinched, the Zeppelin clamp is removed. The ovary is thereby freed from the uterus and can be placed laterally near the pelvic sidewall. The Kelly clamp is left in place at the cornu to prevent bleeding and allow uterine manipulation.

❿ Bladder Flap. Steps 4 through 9 are completed bilaterally, and attention is next turned to the bladder. To avoid urinary tract injury, the bladder is moved caudad and away from the cervix. This is accomplished by first opening the vesicouterine space, the potential space between the bladder and cervix. Several techniques may be used, and at our institution, sharp dissection is preferred (Fig. 43-12.9). This method is particularly beneficial for patients with prior cesarean deliveries who may have scarring between the bladder and cervix. Alternatively, gentle blunt pressure from fingers or sponge stick can be used. Such pressure is directed beneath the bladder, against the cervix, and caudad. With either dissection method, taut uterine elevation creates helpful tension across the tissue planes to be separated. Tension is created by pulling upward on the Kelly clamps, previously placed at the cornua.

The peritoneum at the vesicouterine fold was previously incised bilaterally in Step 5. During dissection in the vesicouterine space, this peritoneum is grasped with atraumatic tissue forceps and elevated to create tension between it and the underlying cervix. Only loose connective tissue strands lie in this space, and they are easily cut with Metzenbaum scissors. Incision of these bands is kept close to the cervix to avoid cystotomy. Dissection in the midline minimizes laceration of vessels that course within the vesicocervical ligaments, colloquially termed *bladder pillars*. Once the correct plane is entered, the pearly white cervix and anterior vaginal wall are clearly differentiated from reddish bladder fibers.

The bladder is ideally dissected off the anterior vaginal wall at least 1 to 2 cm below

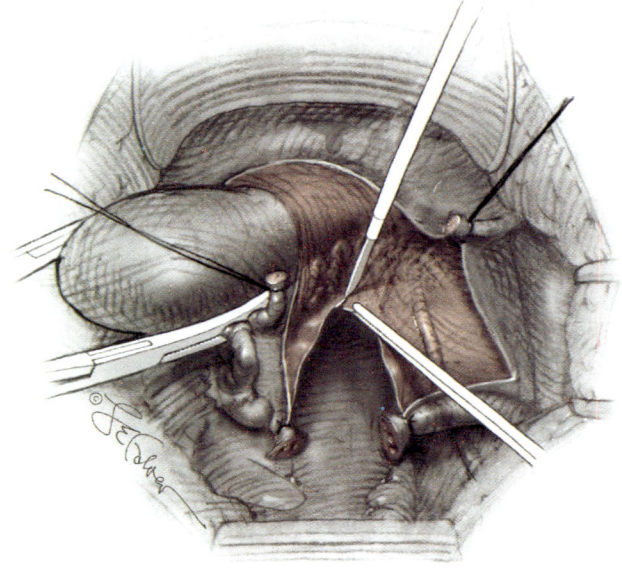

FIGURE 43-12.10 Uterine artery skeletonization.

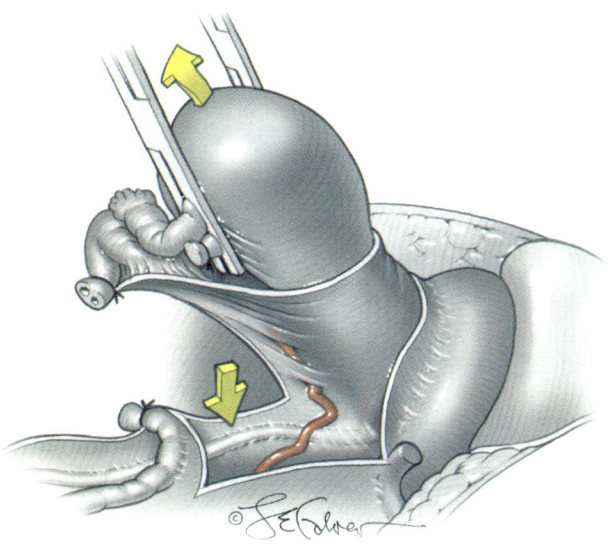

FIGURE 43-12.11 Maneuvers to protect ureter.

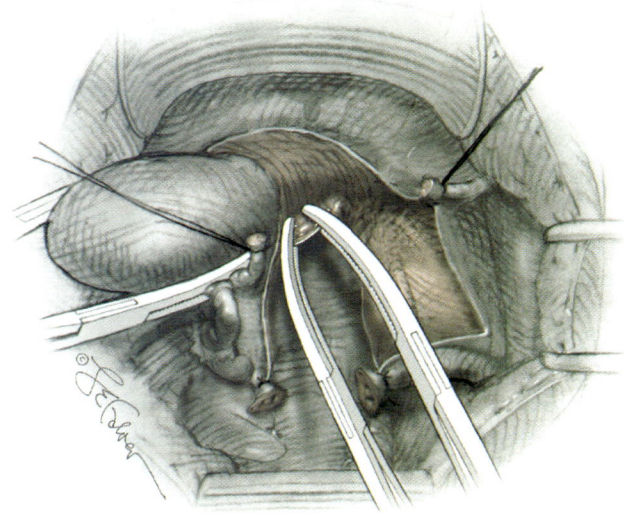

FIGURE 43-12.12 Clamps across uterine artery.

the lower margin of the cervix. This averts incorporating bladder fibers within sutures or clamps placed during cuff closure. Thereby, risks of bladder and distal ureteral injury and later genitourinary fistula are lowered.

⓫ Uterine Arteries. The uterine vessels are identified laterally along the uterus. At the level of the isthmus, some posterior peritoneum and loose areolar tissue still surrounds these. Incising and removing such tissue from around any vessel is termed *skeletonizing*. This ultimately creates a smaller vascular pedicle and minimizes risks for vessel retraction and escape during ligation.

To skeletonize, a surgeon individually grasps excess strips of perivascular connective tissue with fine smooth forceps and gently retracts them laterally and away from the vessel. Metzenbaum scissors or electrosurgery tip incise this tissue close to and parallel to the vessel, beginning superiorly and proceeding inferiorly. During this process, the remaining posterior broad ligament peritoneum is similarly incised parallel and close to the uterus

(Fig. 43-12.10). Importantly, this step further "drops" the ureter away from the path of subsequent clamps. Cephalad traction on the uterus, in combination with bladder mobilization and dissection of the posterior broad ligament peritoneum, increases the distance of the uterine vessels from the ureter (Fig. 43-12.11). Steps that may help prevent ureteral injury are summarized in Table 43-12.1.

Once skeletonized, the uterine vessels are secured by a curved Zeppelin clamp at the uterine isthmus. The clamp tips are placed horizontally across the vertical uterine vessels (Fig. 43-12.12). A Kelly clamp is placed medial and vertical to the first clamp and hugs the lateral uterus to prevent bleeding from severed vessels. Tissue between the clamps is then cut.

A simple stitch of 0-gauge delayed-absorbable suture is placed below the Zeppelin clamp's tip, and the suture ends are wrapped to the clamp's heel. As the knot is cinched, the Zeppelin clamp is slowly opened and removed. The Kelly clamp remains. A large pedicle may be tied twice to ensure ligation.

The simple stitch is placed as described, but the clamp is flashed rather than removed. The second stitch is placed above the first and prior to removal of the clamp.

⓬ Fundal Amputation. After bilateral uterine artery ligation, if the uterus is large and bulky, the uterine fundus may be sharply severed from the cervix. After removal of the corpus, Kocher clamps are placed on the anterior and posterior walls of cervix for manipulation.

If supracervical hysterectomy is planned, no further transection is required. In premenopausal women, the upper endocervical canal is coagulated or removed by sharp wedge resection to help avoid postoperative cyclic bleeding.

If the cervical stroma is hemostatic, no suturing is required. If not, the cervical stump is closed and rendered hemostatic with figure-eight stitches using 0-gauge delayed-absorbable suture. Each stitch passes through the posterior peritoneum, the posterior wall of the cervix, and then the anterior wall of the cervix before ligation.

⓭ Cardinal and Uterosacral Ligament Transection. These ligaments lie lateral to the uterus and inferior to the uterine vessels. A straight Zeppelin clamp is positioned across the cardinal ligament adjacent to the cervix and medial to the uterine artery pedicle (Fig. 43-12.13). As the Zeppelin clamp initially grasps the ligament, it is oriented parallel to the lateral side of the uterus. As the clamp is slowly closed, it is angled slightly away from the vertical axis of the cervix. Angling allows a narrow span of tissue to lie medial to the clamp. A scalpel then transects the portion of the cardinal ligament medial to the clamp. Ideally, the surgeon cuts close

TABLE 43-12.1. Sequential Steps to Help Prevent Ureteral Injury During Abdominal Hysterectomy

Trace the ureter from the pelvic brim to the cardinal ligament
Maintain upward uterine traction throughout the procedure
Create a window below the IP or uteroovarian ligaments prior to their division
Dissect the posterior leaf of the broad ligament to the level of the uterine isthmus
Mobilize the bladder caudally off the cervix and upper vagina
Skeletonize the uterine vessels
Clamp the parametrium medial to each previously created parametrial pedicle
Avoid suturing and electrosurgical energy lateral to parametrial pedicles

IP = infundibulopelvic ligament.

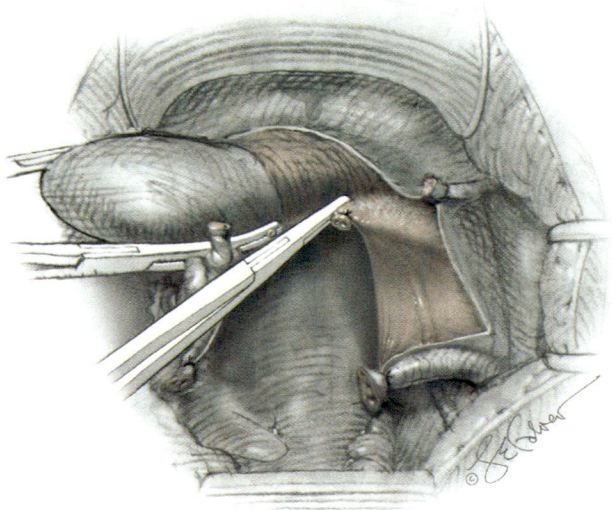

FIGURE 43-12.13 Clamp across cardinal ligament.

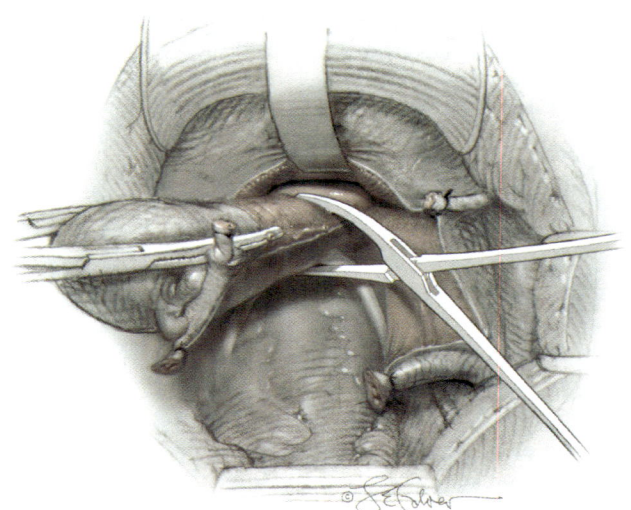

FIGURE 43-12.14 Clamp incorporating uterosacral ligament and proximal vagina.

to the uterus, and this leaves the small tissue span above the clamp. Instead, cutting flush on the clamp raises the risk of tissue slippage during clamp removal.

A transfixing stitch of 0-gauge delayed-absorbable suture is placed below the clamp, and the clamp is removed as the knot is cinched. For smaller bites through the cardinal ligament, a simple stitch without transfixion may suffice.

Depending on the ligament length, the above step may be repeated several times. In this manner, the cardinal ligament is transected and ligated from its superior to inferior extent down the lateral aspect of the cervix to the level of the upper vagina.

When this is near completion, the uterosacral ligaments remain as final support structures attached to the cervix. These ligaments are more easily felt and seen by placing upward traction on the uterus. In most benign cases, these ligaments are incorporated within instruments used to clamp across the lower cardinal ligament. The suture tails of the uterosacral ligament pedicles may be left long for identification, to allow later incorporation of these pedicles into the vaginal cuff closure.

⑭ **Vagina Transection.** For this, the surgeon's hand palpates through the anterior and posterior vaginal walls to identify the most inferior level of the cervix. Here, a curved Zeppelin clamp is placed across the anterior and posterior vaginal walls just below the cervix on one side. This is repeated on the other side, and the tips often meet in the midline (Fig. 43-12.14). Importantly, the bladder must be sufficiently mobilized away from this point to prevent injury.

The vaginal tissue above the level of these clamps is then transected. This procedure frees the uterus from the pelvis. Transfixing sutures are placed below the Zeppelin clamps, and the clamps are removed (Fig. 43-12.15).

⑮ **Vaginal Entry.** In some cases, the cervix may be poorly appreciated between the vaginal walls. To avoid shortening the vagina or leaving cervix behind, the vagina can be entered to identify the cervix. For this, a

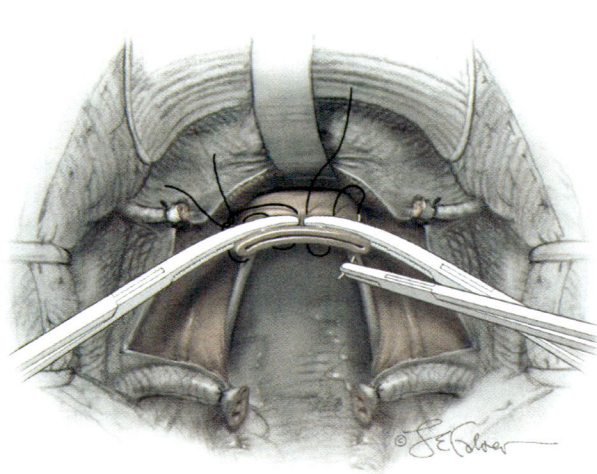

FIGURE 43-12.15 Clamps across proximal vagina. Transfixing stitch for cuff closure.

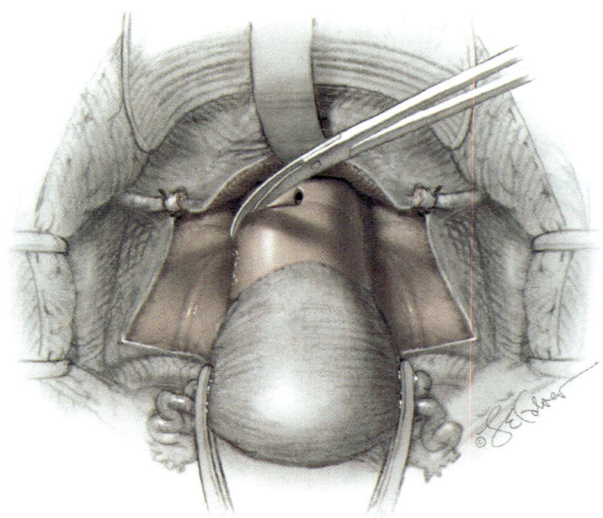

FIGURE 43-12.16 Circumferential vaginal incision.

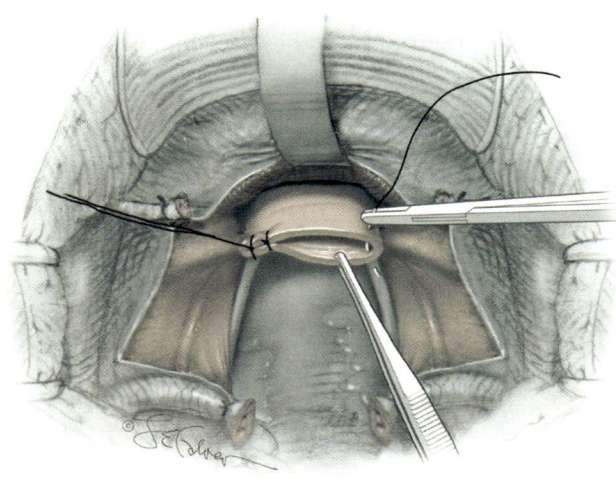

FIGURE 43-12.17 Vaginal cuff closure incorporating uterosacral ligament.

longitudinal incision is made in the midline of the upper anterior vaginal wall. A finger is inserted to palpate the cervical margin. Once this level is known, one blade of Jorgenson scissors is inserted into the vagina and positioned just below the cervix (Fig. 43-12.16). At this level, the vagina is then circumferentially cut. Kocher or Allis clamps are placed along the free cut vaginal edge as it forms.

⑯ **Vaginal Cuff Closure.** A 0-gauge delayed-absorbable suture may be placed to suspend the vaginal apex to the uterosacral ligament pedicle on either side (Fig. 43-12.17). This stitch incorporates the anterior and posterior vaginal walls with the distal portion of the uterosacral ligament and helps prevent vaginal cuff prolapse following surgery.

These sutures are kept long and held by hemostats. Upward and lateral traction elevates the vaginal cuff. The full thicknesses of the incised anterior and posterior vaginal walls are then reapproximated with a running suture line using 0-gauge delayed-absorbable suture or with several figure-eight sutures. Importantly, omitting portions of the vaginal epithelium in the closure can lead to significant postoperative bleeding. The peritoneum adjacent to the posterior vaginal cuff should be included in this closure to lessen the risk of postoperative oozing. Anteriorly, the bladder should be kept clear of the suture line. Once the vaginal cuff is hemostatic, the lateral suspending cuff sutures are cut.

⑰ **Broad Ligament Leiomyoma.** Infrequently, a leiomyoma extends laterally and between the leaves of the broad ligament. In this case, the round ligament must be divided closer to the pelvic sidewall as the myoma

obstructs its typical division point. In addition, a large myoma may stretch and attenuate the round ligament, making it difficult to isolate and divide. Instead, the retroperitoneum can be entered at a more-cephalad site. Specifically, the sigmoid on the left or the cecum on the right is retracted medially. The white line of Toldt, which represents the lateral peritoneal reflection, is grasped and entered sharply. Dissection of the peritoneum then proceeds caudally along the pelvic sidewall and aims for the round ligament. The round ligament is noticeably thicker than the peritoneum, and once reached, the ligament is divided as in Step 4.

Now with access into the retroperitoneum, dissection moves to identify the ureter and its course as in Step 6. This permits the IP or uteroovarian pedicles to be more safely divided as in Steps 8 and 9.

Uterine artery ligation is the next hindered step, and the myoma frequently obstructs viewing and the Zeppelin clamp's path. The assistant applies upward traction with a toothed clamp in the myoma. Clamps at the cornu lift the uterus. Both aid tension across connective tissues that tether the myoma to the pelvis. Sharp dissection to free the mass from its surrounding loose areolar tissue progresses methodically and with clear inspection of adjacent anatomy. Notably, aberrant vessels that provide parasitic blood supply to the myoma may be encountered. Vessels are ideally identified, clamped, cut, and suture ligated. As the mass is freed from the retroperitoneum, uterine vessel access is typically improved, and standard hysterectomy steps may resume.

⑱ **Cervical Leiomyoma.** Infrequently, a leiomyoma develops within the cervical

stroma, and this anatomy places each ureter at significant risk during parametrium division. Thus, ureterolysis and retraction of each ureter laterally with a vessel loop is one option. Ureterolysis along the ureter's posterior aspect near the uterus is ideally minimized. This theoretically helps preserve important nerves associated with bladder function (Jackson, 2019).

As alternative option, myoma excision can diminish cervical bulk. First, the posterior cul-de-sac peritoneum is sharply incised transversely in the midline at the uterine isthmus. The retrocervical potential space is then opened with blunt or sharp dissection. This exposes the posterior cervix surface. Here, vasopressin is injected to minimize bleeding. Following tissue blanching, a large, central wedge through the cervical myoma is cut and removed to decompress the cervix. A hemostatic, running stitch with 0-gauge suture quickly closes the defect. With more normal anatomy restored, standard hysterectomy steps can then be completed.

⑲ **Obliterated Posterior Cul-de-Sac.** At times, dense adhesions may obscure normal tissue planes between the cervix/vagina, rectum, and ureter and prohibit safe parametrium division. One option is downward intrafascial dissection along the posterior cervix. With this, the posterior surface of the isthmus at a level above the cul-de-sac adhesions is sharply scored transversely to enter the superficial cervical stroma. Pearly white, fibrous tissue is noted a few millimeters from the serosal surface and signifies a suitable plane. Dissection then continues caudally along the entire posterior cervix and stops at the level of the intended posterior colpotomy. This method essentially isolates the parametrium without entering the obliterated cul-de-sac and its distorted anatomy. Once isolated, the parametrium can be divided as in Step 13. Of note, this method leaves a thin mantle of cervix within the cul-de-sac, which may be undesirable in cases with cervical dysplasia or endometriosis.

A second option involves *retrograde hysterectomy*. For this, a transverse incision is made in the upper midline of the anterior vaginal wall. The incision is extended bilaterally to the paracolpium. The posterior cervical lip is grasped through this incision with a toothed clamp and is lifted upward. This provides access to the posterior vaginal fornix.

Here, a transverse, midline incision into the posterior vaginal wall allows a finger to enter the retrocervical space. Sharp dissection then progresses cephalad between the cul-de-sac peritoneum and posterior cervical aspect. Dissection ideally reaches the level of the uterine isthmus.

This dissection essentially isolates the parametrium without entering the obliterated cul-de-sac. Division of the parametrium can then progresses retrograde. Namely, one arm of a straight Zeppelin clamp advances cephalad through the anterior vaginal-wall incision, into the posterior vaginal-wall incision, and into the developed retrocervical space. The upper clamp arm lies outside the vagina and across the lowermost portion of the anterior parametrial surface. The clamp is snugged close to the uterus and is closed, which isolates the parametrium. This tissue between the clamp and cervix is then cut and ligated. The process is serially repeated and moves cephalad on both sides of the uterus. This allows complete division of the parametrium and then uterine artery ligation.

❷⓿ Wound Closure. The pelvis and tissue pedicles are inspected to assure hemostasis. The abdominal incision is closed as described in Section 43-1 or 43-2 (p. 932).

POSTOPERATIVE

Postoperative care follows that for laparotomy, although sexual intercourse is usually delayed until 6 weeks after surgery to permit satisfactory vaginal cuff healing (p. 932).

Febrile morbidity is common following abdominal hysterectomy and exceeds that seen with vaginal or MIS approaches (Peipert, 2004). Frequently, fever is unexplained. But, pelvic infections are common, and other sources of postoperative fever should be evaluated (Chap. 42, p. 921). Because of the high rate of unexplained fever, which resolves spontaneously, observation for 24 to 48 hours for mild temperature elevations is reasonable. Alternatively, antibiotics may be initiated, and appropriate choices are found in Table 3-16 (p. 82). Additional testing, including transvaginal sonography or CT scanning, may be indicated if a hematoma, abscess, or other pelvic source is suspected.

43-13

Vaginal Hysterectomy

In general, this approach is chosen by surgeons if the uterus is relatively small, extensive adhesions are not anticipated, no significant adnexal pathology is expected, and some degree of pelvic organ descent is present. Compared with abdominal hysterectomy, patients undergoing vaginal hysterectomy usually benefit from faster recovery and from reduced hospital stays, costs, and postoperative pain. During approach selection (p. 956), if all factors are equal, vaginal hysterectomy is preferred.

PREOPERATIVE

Patient evaluation, consenting, and patient preparation mirror that for abdominal hysterectomy (p. 956). With vaginal hysterectomy, although uncommon, a surgeon may be unable to safely complete scheduled adnexal surgery due to unanticipated anatomy. First, for ovarian pathology and indicated BSO, options include laparoscopic assistance or conversion to abdominal approach. Second, women affected by *BRCA* mutation and undergoing recommended adnexectomy are better served by an approach that allows pelvic washings and complete salpingectomy or BSO. Last, for women at low cancer risk undergoing

risk-reducing salpingectomy or prophylactic BSO, contingency plans and patient desires are ideally delineated before surgery. As noted, the American College of Obstetricians and Gynecologists (2019d) recommends against abandoning a vaginal approach solely to complete prophylactic salpingectomy.

INTRAOPERATIVE

Surgical Steps

❶ **Anesthesia and Patient Positioning.** After adequate general or regional anesthesia is administered, the patient is placed in standard lithotomy position (Fig. 40-4, p. 844). The vagina is surgically prepared, and the bladder is drained. Some surgeons may prefer to wait until the anterior peritoneum is entered before inserting a Foley catheter. This permits a gush of urine to signal inadvertent bladder laceration. Along the posterior vaginal wall, a short Auvard weighted vaginal speculum is placed, and a right-angle or other suitable retractor is placed anteriorly.

❷ **Vaginal Wall Incision.** A Lahey thyroid clamp is used to grasp the anterior cervical lip, while a second one holds the posterior lip. For a smaller cervix, one clamp may easily grasp both lips together. The junction between the cervix and the anterior and posterior vaginal walls can be seen and palpated by in-and-out displacement of the cervix. Just proximal to this junction, a circumferential incision is

made around the cervix and is guided by anatomy (Fig. 43-13.1). For example, if the cervix is flush with the vagina, then incision lies close to the remaining cervix to avoid rectal or bladder injury. Based on surgeon's preference this incision is made with electrosurgical blade or scalpel. In general, the incision is kept at a depth superficial to the cervical stroma to avert dissection into the cervix. To reduce blood loss during dissection, 10 to 15 mL of a dilute saline solution containing vasopressin (20 U diluted in 30 to 100 mL of saline) or 0.5-percent lidocaine and epinephrine (5 μg/mL) in a manufactured 1:200,000 dilution may be injected circumferentially along the incision path (Jeppson, 2017).

❸ **Posterior Peritoneal Entry.** Although described first here, the sequence of anterior and posterior entry is based on surgeon preference and intraoperative findings. The Lahey thyroid clamp and cervix are lifted anteriorly to expose the posterior vaginal vault, and an Allis clamp is placed below the circumcised edge of the posterior vaginal wall. Some additional sharp or blunt dissection is generally done to separate the posterior vaginal wall from the cervical stroma to expose the cul-de-sac peritoneum. Downward traction on the Allis clamp creates tension across the incision. Curved Mayo scissors positioned across the incision line cut through the exposed peritoneum to enter the cul-de-sac of Douglas (Fig. 43-13.2). Correct entry into the peritoneal cavity is suggested by

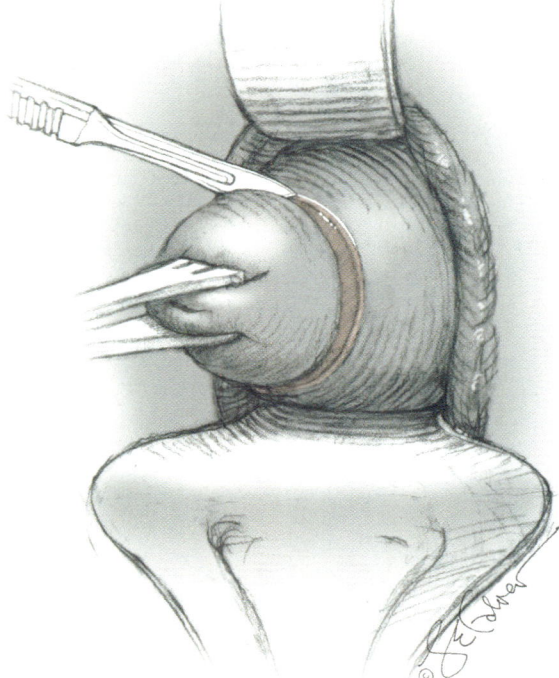

FIGURE 43-13.1 Circumferential cervical incision.

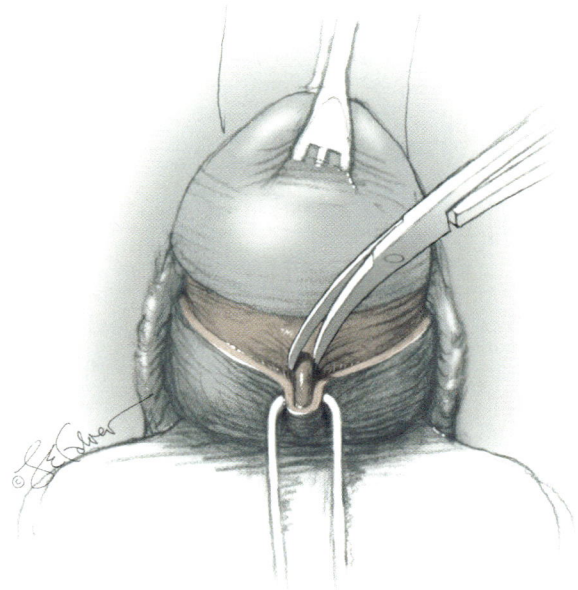

FIGURE 43-13.2 Entry into the cul-de-sac of Douglas.

palpation of uterine serosa or confirmed by visualizing small bowel or rectosigmoid.

The posterior peritoneum may be affixed centrally to the posterior vaginal wall incision with a single stitch of delayed-absorbable suture. This approximation will assist with closure of the peritoneum at the procedure's end. The short Auvard speculum is replaced by one with a longer blade, which enters the cul-de-sac.

❹ Anterior Peritoneal Entry. This is generally considered the most challenging step of vaginal hysterectomy. Whereas the peritoneum in the posterior cul-de-sac lies directly over the upper portion of the vaginal wall and direct posterior entry is possible, the anterior cul-de-sac peritoneum lies several centimeters above the cervicovaginal junction. Thus, the vesicocervical space is entered and carefully developed prior to anterior peritoneal entry. A median dissection distance of 3.4 cm (range 1.8 to 4.6 cm) can be expected from the initial circumferential incision to the peritoneal reflection during anterior colpotomy (Balgobin, 2016).

To begin, the anterior vaginal wall is grasped in the midline at the circumferential incision edge and elevated with an Allis clamp. Tension is concurrently created by outward traction on the cervical Lahey thyroid clamp. This traction reveals fibrous connective tissue bands connecting the bladder and cervix. Although the proximal part of the vesicocervical space contains easily dissected, loose areolar tissue, the distal portion contains thicker fibers, sometimes referred to as *supravaginal septum* fibers (Balgobin, 2019). These fibers require sharp dissection. Knowledge of this anatomy permits precise dissection through this dense tissue rather than premature dissection reorientation, which risks "digging" into the cervix.

At our institution, sharp dissection is preferred (Fig. 43-13.3). This method is particularly beneficial for patients with prior cesarean deliveries, who may have scarring between the bladder and cervix. With traction established, the septum fibers are incised in the midline with scissors. Tips are kept close and almost parallel to the cervix as dissection is extended cephalad. Dissection is not extended further lateral than 11 and 1 o'clock positions to avoid cervical vessel laceration. Small bleeding vessels are frequently encountered during initial dissection and are coagulated. After the initial septum fibers are transected, gentle palpation with the index finger should indicate whether the loose areolar tissue in the upper part of the vesicocervical space has been reached. In the absence of scar tissue, these fibers are easily separated by fingertip, and gentle blunt

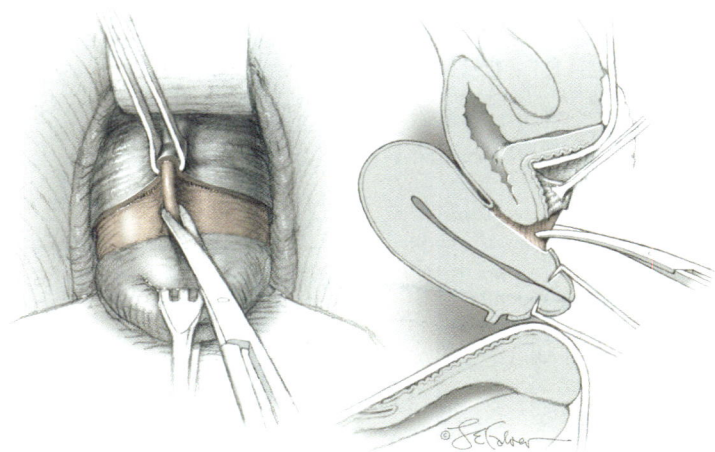

FIGURE 43-13.3 Sharp dissection of vesicouterine septum from two views.

dissection advances cephalad until the vesicouterine fold is palpated. Once in the vesicocervical space, the index finger is able to palpate the entire length of the anterior cervix. If not, dissection is likely in a plane that is too deep and is redirected more superficially. Intermittent palpation during anterior dissection can help guide dissection depth.

Alternatively, the entire vesicocervical space dissection can be completed with gentle blunt pressure from an index finger. Such pressure is directed against the cervix and cephalad toward the vesicouterine fold. However, this method often proves ineffective and poses greater risk of bladder injury, especially if significant scarring is present from prior surgery, such as cesarean delivery.

The vesicouterine fold is a thin and transparent transverse peritoneal fold at the upper border of the cervix. With palpation, this smooth layer glides against the uterine serosa. This peritoneum is grasped with atraumatic tissue forceps or clamp, placed on tension, and incised. In cases with difficult anterior entry, if the uterus is small, the surgeon may enter the posterior cul-de-sac and wrap an index finger anteriorly to palpate and accentuate the vesicouterine fold for anterior entry.

Following vesicouterine fold incision, an index finger explores the opening to confirm peritoneal entry, exclude cystotomy, and identify unanticipated pelvic pathology. Digital exploration allows direct palpation of the uterine serosa posteriorly and base of the bladder anteriorly. This finger then guides a curved Deaver retractor into the opening to elevate the bladder and anterior vaginal wall. The small bowel is generally seen after retractor placement, which further confirms correct entry into the peritoneal cavity.

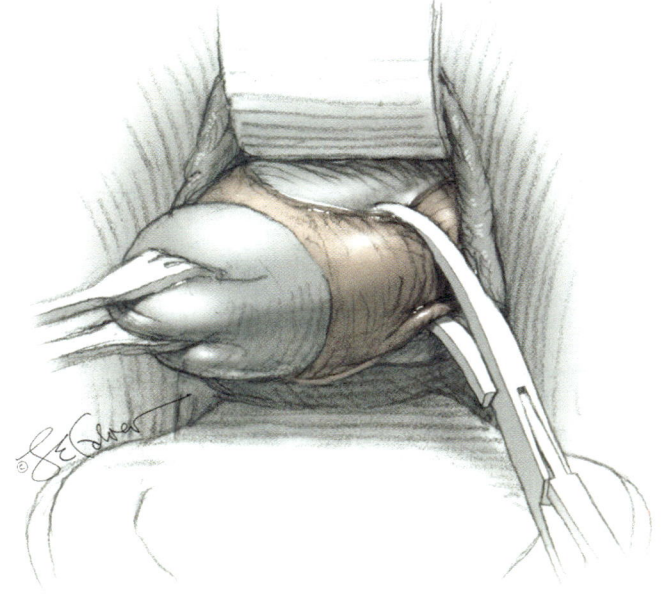

FIGURE 43-13.4 Clamp incorporating uterosacral and cardinal ligaments.

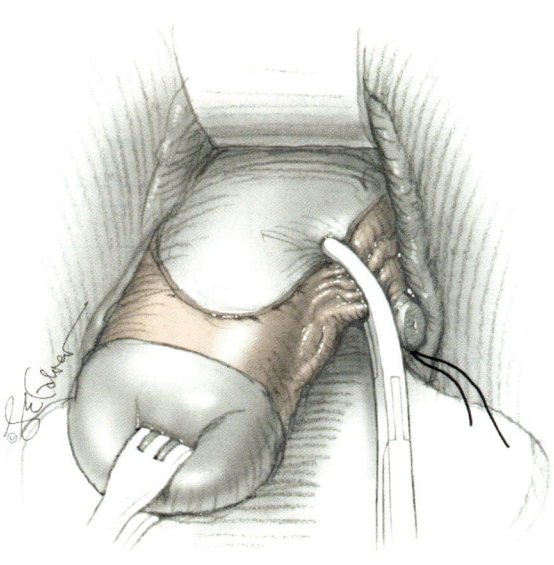

FIGURE 43-13.5 Clamp across uterine artery.

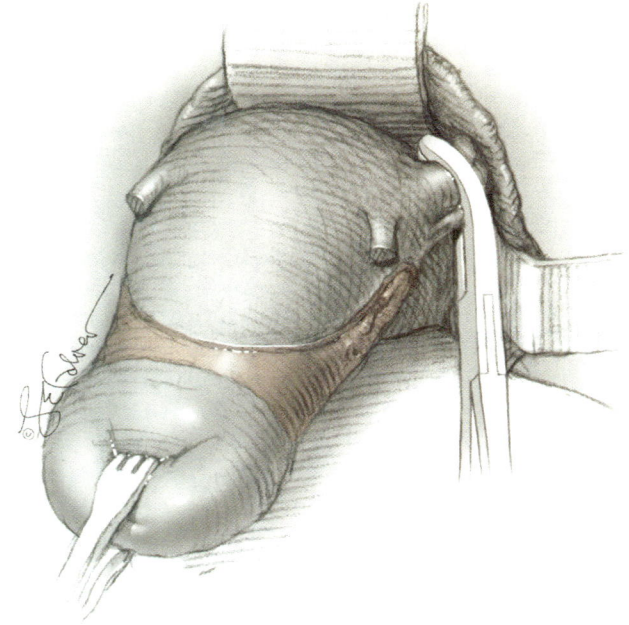

FIGURE 43-13.6 Clamp across uteroovarian and round ligaments and fallopian tube.

❺ Transection of Uterosacral and Cardinal Ligaments. Outward traction on the Lahey thyroid clamp pulls the supporting uterine ligaments into view. Such traction, along with upward bladder displacement, aids in ureteral injury prevention. If both posterior and anterior peritoneal entries have been accomplished, the uterosacral and distal cardinal ligaments are identified, clamped with a curved Heaney or similar clamp, transected, and ligated with 0-gauge delayed-absorbable suture using a transfixing stitch (Fig. 43-13.4). The posterior and, if possible, the anterior peritoneum as it joins the uterine serosa is incorporated in the clamp to minimize oozing around the pedicle. Once the knot is tied, the suture ends are not cut but are kept long for later identification. This entire step is then repeated on the opposite side.

Depending on the cardinal ligament length, similar clamping, cutting, and suturing is repeated. The anterior peritoneum can generally be incorporated into the clamp after a second purchase of uterosacral-cardinal ligament complex tissue. Advancement moves cephalad along each side of the cervix. Each sequential clamp is placed medial to the prior pedicle to reduce ureteral injury risk.

❻ Uterine Arteries. The uterine artery is identified on one side and clamped with a curved Heaney clamp. The clamp is placed nearly perpendicular to the long axis of the uterus and medial to the prior cardinal ligament pedicle (Fig. 43-13.5). The tips should firmly abut the uterus to ensure enclosure of uterine vessels within the clamp. A more laterally placed clamp may not completely enclose the artery and may also risk ureter injury. Following pedicle transection, a simple stitch is placed beneath the clamp and is secured at the clamp heel as the instrument is slowly released and removed. Uterine arteries are ligated bilaterally.

❼ Cornua. Progressing cephalad, curved Heaney clamps are next placed across the round ligament, which is transected and suture ligated. The uteroovarian ligaments and fallopian tubes together are similarly clamped, cut, and ligated. Instead, all three structures can be incorporated within

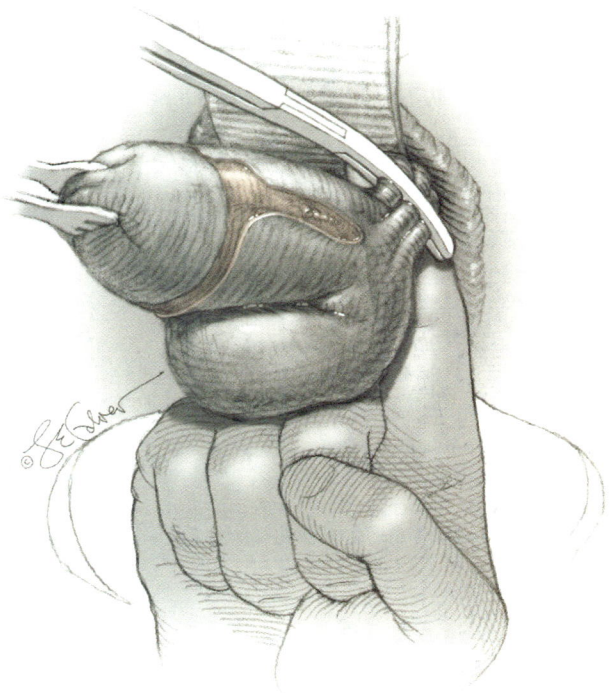

FIGURE 43-13.7 Fundal inversion to permit cornual structure clamping.

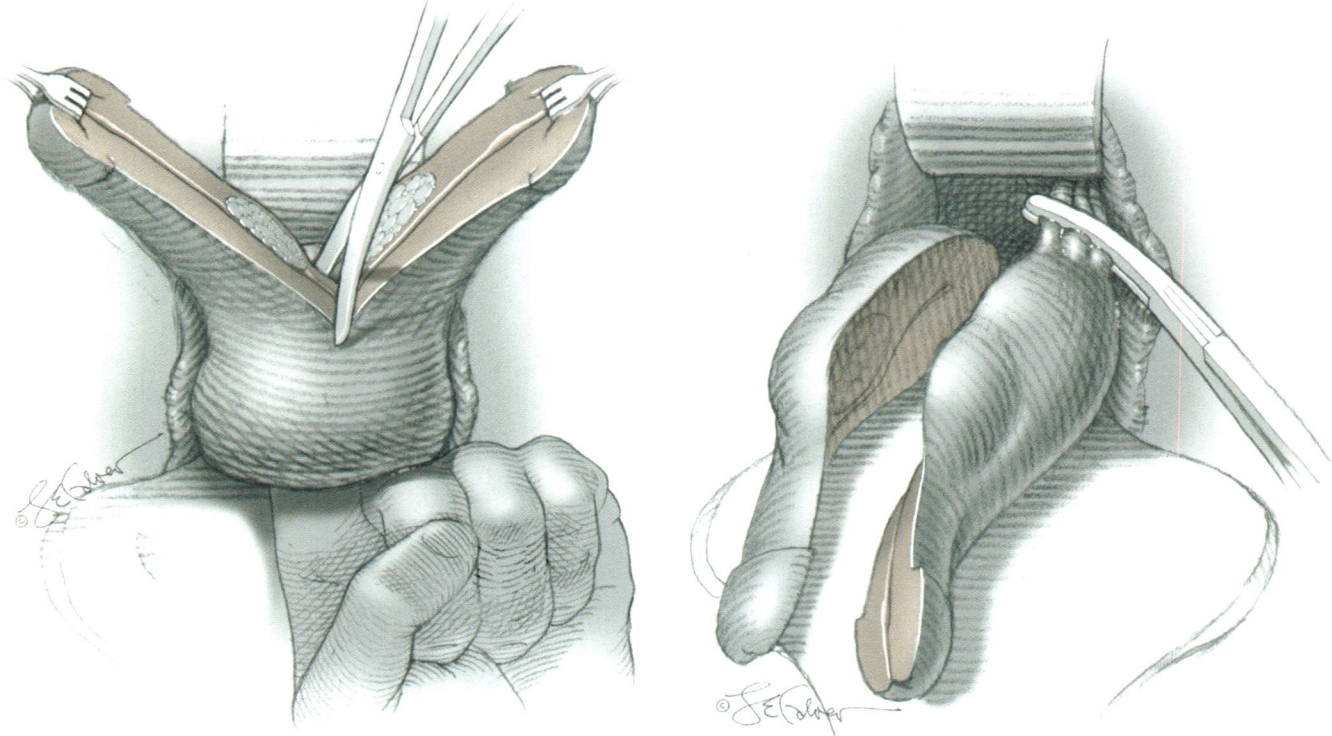

FIGURE 43-13.8 Uterus bivalved.

FIGURE 43-13.9 Clamp across cornual structures.

one clamp depending on their diameter (Fig. 43-13.6). After transection, a simple ligature of 0-gauge delayed-absorbable suture is placed proximally around the clamp. As the knot is secured, the Heaney clamp is quickly flashed. A transfixing stitch is then sutured around the clamp and positioned distal to the first stitch. As this knot is cinched, the Heaney clamp is removed. This transection is repeated bilaterally. With ovarian preservation, these sutures are cut short after confirming pedicle hemostasis. However, with adnexectomy, the transfixing suture tails may be kept long to allow gentle traction to bring the adnexa toward the vagina.

For the above step, if the uterus is larger, the uteroovarian ligament and tube may be difficult to reach and clamp. For this, the uterine corpus may be delivered through the posterior colpotomy incision to better expose these (Fig. 43-13.7). To deliver the fundus, a toothed clamp is placed on the upper posterior uterine wall, and it gently pulls the fundus into the vagina. Excessive traction may result in tissue avulsion and bleeding.

8 Morcellation. In some cases, the uterine fundus may be too large to deliver, and uterine debulking is required prior to ligation of the cornual attachments. This is preferably performed after both uterine vessel pedicles have been ligated to reduce intraoperative bleeding.

One technique bivalves the uterus using curved Mayo scissors, beginning at the cervix and moving toward the fundus. Near completion, fingers placed through the posterior colpotomy incision and behind the fundus help prevent scissor injury to adjacent organs (Fig. 43-13.8). Once completed, one half is elevated out of the operating field and into the pelvic cavity, whereas the other is brought into view for clamp placement across the uteroovarian and round ligaments and fallopian tube (Fig. 43-13.9).

Other methods strive to excise central uterine bulk. A first method involves cervix-to-fundus central coring to remove volume (Fig. 43-13.10). Instead of coring, a large central wedge can be excised. Wedge resection can be sequentially repeated until sufficient debulking is completed. Last and perhaps less preferably, a surgeon may enucleate individual large leiomyomas. The drawback with this method is the greater

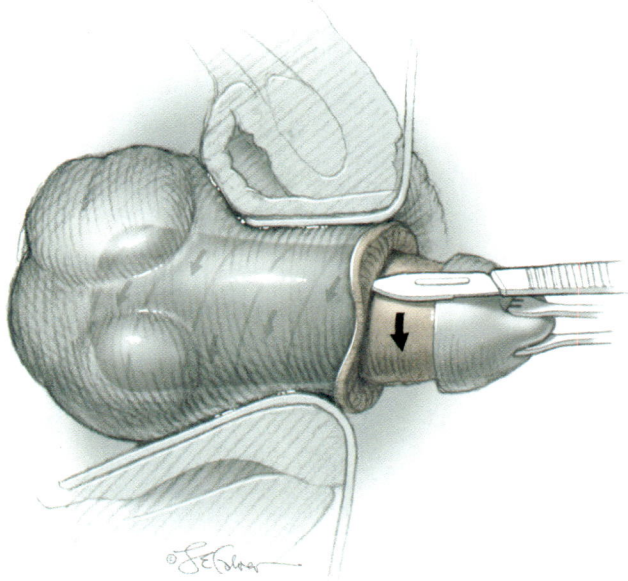

FIGURE 43-13.10 Coring of central uterine bulk.

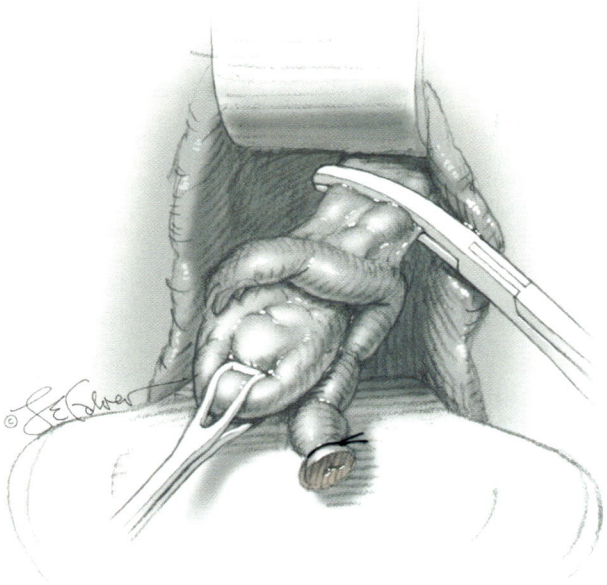

FIGURE 43-13.11 Clamp across infundibulopelvic ligament.

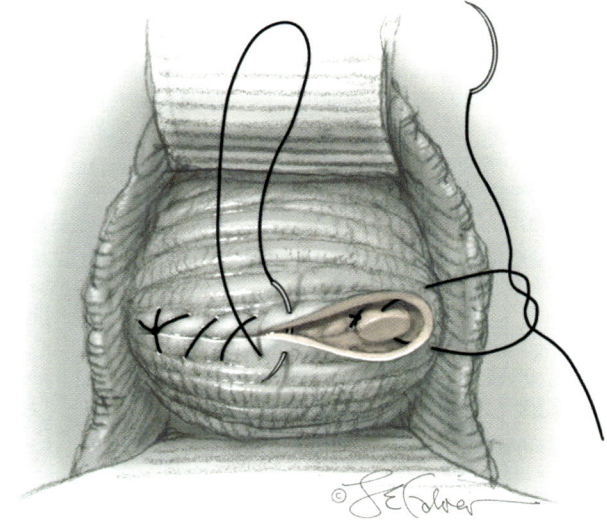

FIGURE 43-13.12 Vaginal cuff closure.

theoretical spread of myoma fragments. For any of these techniques, once bulk is diminished, a Heaney clamp is placed around the cornual structures as described in Step 7.

❾ Adnexectomy. For this, the adnexa is grasped with a Babcock clamp and gently pulled inferiorly and toward the contralateral side of the incision. This creates mild tension on the infundibulopelvic (IP) ligament for improved delineation. To expand the operating field, a right-angle or similar retractor is positioned deep into the incision and into peritoneal cavity for vaginal, pelvic sidewall, and ureter retraction. This is coupled with upward traction from the originally placed anterior wall Deaver retractor.

A curved Heaney or similar clamp is placed around the IP ligament, and its blades cover the entire pedicle width. For difficult angles, the surgeon's contralateral hand can push the ligament into correct position within the clamp. Prior to clamp closure, the surgeon confirms that no bowel or omentum is incorporated and that the entire ovary lies distal to the clamp. A moist sponge stick and slight Trendelenburg positioning can help position the bowel away.

The IP ligament is then clamped and transected (Fig. 43-13.11). First, a free tie of 0-gauge delayed-absorbable suture is placed around the Heaney clamp. As the knot is secured, the clamp is flashed. A transfixing stitch is then placed around the same clamp but distal to the first free tie. As the knot is cinched, the Heaney clamp is removed. Excess traction on this pedicle is avoided to prevent avulsion or retraction of

the ligament from the clamp. In such cases, resultant retroperitoneal bleeding may be difficult to control vaginally. Once hemostasis is ensured, the suture is cut. The contralateral IP ligament is similarly clamped and transected.

As one alternative ligation technique, two Heaney clamps and double ligatures on the IP ligament can be elected. Yet another option is a preformed endoscopic suture loop (EndoLoop) placed around the IP ligament and then cinched.

❿ Risk-Reducing Salpingectomy. Following uterine vessel ligation, the broad ligament is incised cephalad until the round ligament is reached. A finger sweep or Babcock clamp guides the fimbriated tubal end posteriorly into the operative field. Beginning at the end and progressing medially to the uterine body, the mesosalpinx is serially clamped, incised, and suture ligated. A bipolar vessel-ligating device can add speed but also expense. Following mesosalpinx division, the tube can be pressed manually against the lateral aspect of the uterine specimen for removal with it. Next, the round and utero-ovarian ligaments are secured together with a Heaney clamp, transected, and suture ligated.

⓫ Evaluation of Hemostasis. Following removal of the uterus, the surgical pedicles are inspected for bleeding. Electrosurgical coagulation or figure-eight sutures will typically control bleeding from discrete points. If indicated or preferred, a McCall culdoplasty may be performed (Section 45-22, p. 1143).

⓬ Vaginal Cuff Closure. The anterior and posterior vaginal walls are usually reapproximated by a horizontal suture line with interrupted or continuous running stitches of 0-gauge delayed-absorbable material. If short vaginal length is a concern, walls can be closed by a vertical suture line (Jeppson, 2017).

To help prevent later vaginal apex prolapse, the uterosacral ligament pedicles are incorporated within the cuff closure. For this, the initial interrupted or continuous running closure suture is passed through the anterior vaginal wall, through the previously tagged ligament, through the posterior peritoneum, and finally through the posterior vaginal wall on one side (Fig. 43-13.12). This is repeated on the other side. Suturing then progresses from each side to the midline, or a single running suture may close the entire cuff. During cuff closure, full-thickness bites through the vaginal muscularis and epithelium are taken. Also, the posterior peritoneum is incorporated with closure to minimize risks of bleeding and cuff hematoma.

POSTOPERATIVE

In general, patients who undergo vaginal hysterectomy compared with abdominal hysterectomy typically have faster return of normal bowel function, easier ambulation, and decreased analgesia requirements. Although diet and most activities are advanced quickly, intercourse is delayed for 6 weeks to permit vaginal cuff healing. Evaluation and treatment of postoperative complications mirrors that for abdominal hysterectomy.

43-14

Trachelectomy

During the 1920s through 1950s, most abdominal hysterectomies were supracervical due to inadequate antibiotic therapy and blood banking. For many women who had supracervical hysterectomy, later surgical removal of the cervix, termed *trachelectomy*, was often indicated for complaints of vault prolapse, persistent cyclic bleeding, or preinvasive cervical lesions (Pasley, 1988). Hilger and associates (2005) reported on 335 women who underwent trachelectomy between 1974 and 2003. In half of them, trachelectomy was performed, on average, 26 years after supracervical hysterectomy. Of surgical indications, prolapse and pelvic mass are the most frequent, and bleeding accounts for nearly 10 percent (Hilger, 2005; Kho, 2011).

The cervix may be removed either vaginally or abdominally, but for most women without concurrent pelvic pathology, vaginal trachelectomy is preferred (Pratt, 1976). Trachelectomy for benign indications is described here. Radical trachelectomy for invasive cervical cancer is gaining acceptance and is described in Chapter 30 (p. 667).

PREOPERATIVE

Patient Evaluation

As with hysterectomy, women require preoperative Pap testing to exclude cervical cancer. Cervical or vaginal infections are ideally cleared before surgery.

Consent

As with vaginal hysterectomy, patients are at risk for urinary tract and bowel injury. Similarly, postsurgical vaginal cuff complications may include hematoma, abscess, and cellulitis. Fortunately, complications are infrequent for most. Although Pratt and Jeffries (1976) noted complications in 91 of 262 patients, complication rates in several series range below 10 percent (Riva, 1961; Welch, 1959).

Patient Preparation

Entry into the peritoneal cavity is common during trachelectomy. Accordingly, as with vaginal hysterectomy, prophylaxis against infection and VTE is warranted, and appropriate choices are found in Tables 39-8 and 39-10 (p. 832). Prior to surgery, enemas to evacuate the rectum to improve operating space can be considered.

INTRAOPERATIVE

Surgical Steps

❶ **Anesthesia and Patient Positioning.** Trachelectomy is performed usually as a day-surgery procedure under general or regional anesthesia. The patient is placed in a standard lithotomy position, the vagina is surgically prepared, and a Foley catheter is placed.

❷ **Incision and Extraperitoneal Dissection.** The beginning steps of trachelectomy mirror those for vaginal hysterectomy (Step 2, p. 965). However, unlike vaginal hysterectomy, because the cervical stump lies outside the peritoneum, entry into the peritoneal cavity is not required for trachelectomy. Accordingly, once circumcision of the vaginal wall around the cervix is completed, dissection proceeds to the vesicouterine fold but without peritoneal entry.

In many cases, the bladder is more densely adhered to the anterior cervix, and the clear tissue planes often encountered during vaginal hysterectomy are absent. Moreover, if, at completion of the original hysterectomy, the peritoneum was reapproximated to cover the cervical stump, the bladder may be draped over and scarred to the apex of the stump as well. For this reason, dissection of the vaginal wall, bladder, and rectum from the surface of the cervix typically requires sharp rather than blunt dissection (Fig. 43-14.1). As with vaginal hysterectomy, outward traction on the cervix in combination with counter traction of the vaginal wall aids dissection. To avoid cystotomy and proctotomy, scissor blades and dissecting pressure are directed against the cervix.

❸ **Transection of Uterosacral and Cardinal Ligaments.** Once dissected free from the vaginal wall, the uterosacral and cardinal ligaments are clamped and ligated as with vaginal hysterectomy (Fig. 43-14.2). The cervical branches of the uterine artery are typically clamped and ligated with the cardinal ligament. Depending on cervical length, serial transection and ligation of the cardinal ligament is continued until the stump apex is reached.

❹ **Stump Excision and Cuff Closure.** Once the apex is reached, sharp dissection across the top of the stump will free it from the pelvis (Fig. 43-14.3). Next, incorporation of the uterosacral ligaments and reapproximation of the vaginal walls follows that for vaginal hysterectomy (Step 12, p. 969).

❺ **Intraperitoneal Entry.** This may be preferred if a vaginal apical suspension procedure or BSO is planned. Steps 1 and 2 mirror those for vaginal hysterectomy (p. 965). However, anterior peritoneal fold incision is delayed until better cervical stump descent is achieved.

Incision into the posterior vagina and peritoneum is carried out distal to the apex

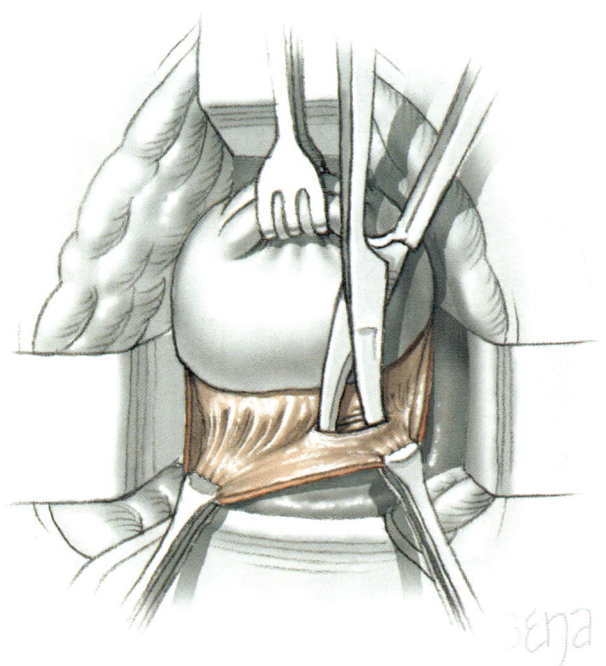

FIGURE 43-14.1 Extraperitoneal dissection.

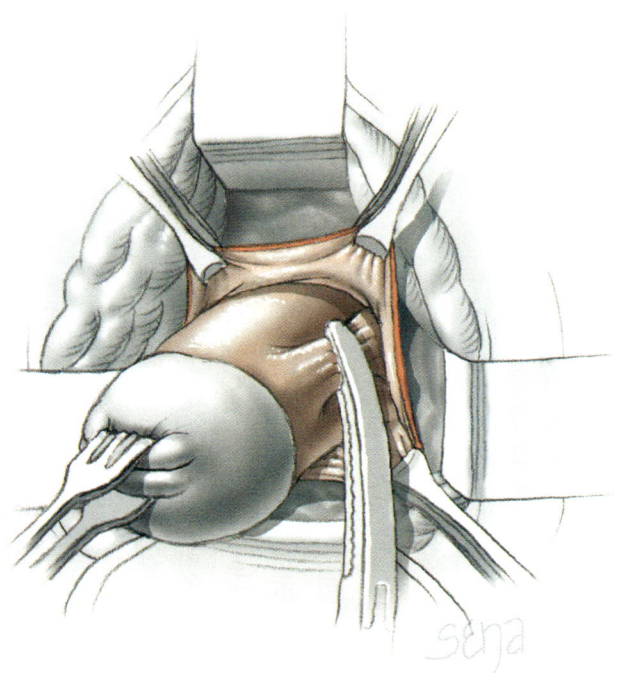

FIGURE 43-14.2 Uterosacral and cardinal ligament transection.

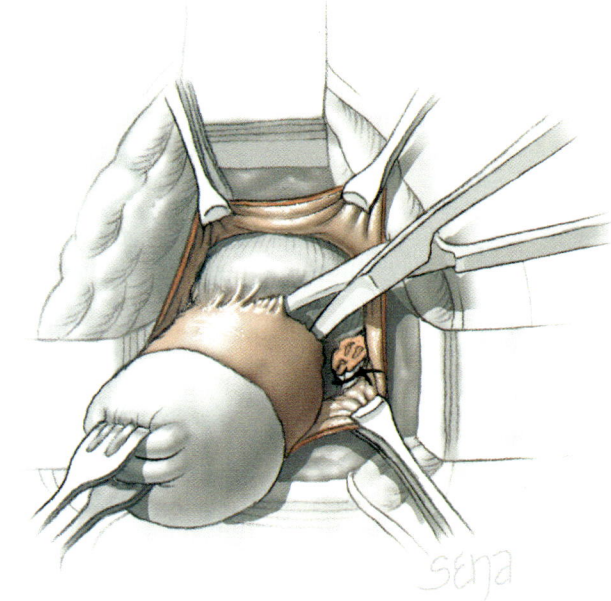

FIGURE 43-14.3 Stump excision.

of the cervical stump to avoid injury to bladder or bowel, which may be adhered to the stump. The uterosacral ligaments and distal remaining cardinal ligaments are then clamped, transected, and suture ligated to aid with downward displacement of the stump.

The upper part of the stump and peritoneum are then palpated with an index finger inserted through the posterior cul-de-sac to assess for bowel or bladder adhesions.

Adhesions to the superior aspect of the cervix can be bluntly or sharply dissected off. Direct entry into the anterior cul-de-sac can then be achieved by sharply transecting the peritoneum overlying the inserted index finger. Any remaining cardinal ligament can now be clamped, transected, and suture ligated to remove the entire cervix. Cuff closure mirrors that for vaginal hysterectomy.

POSTOPERATIVE

As with hysterectomy, women often will have unexplained febrile morbidity following trachelectomy. In his series of 55 cases, Pasley (1988) noted a rate of 9 percent. Similar to hysterectomy, patients with persistent or high-degree fevers require evaluation and possible antibiotic treatment (Chap. 42, p. 921).

43-15

Suction Dilation and Curettage

Suction dilation and curettage (D & C) is frequently used to treat incomplete or missed abortion, molar pregnancy, and elective pregnancy termination. It can also sample the endometrial cavity for trophoblastic tissue in those with a failing or a persisting pregnancy of unknown location (Insogna, 2017; Rubal, 2012). For each, patient education regarding surgical alternatives and sequelae vary and are discussed in their respective chapters.

Electric vacuum aspiration (EVA) is the most common form of suction curettage. It requires a rigid plastic cannula attached to an electric-powered vacuum source. Manual vacuum aspiration (MVA) uses a similar cannula that attaches to a handheld syringe for its vacuum source. MVA is commonly used for early first-trimester evacuation (Lichtenburg, 2013).

PREOPERATIVE

Patient Evaluation

For most women, D & C is preceded by transvaginal sonography. This imaging delineates pregnancy size and location and uterine inclination. These will guide selection of instruments and their sizes, anesthesia type, preparations for potential blood loss, and procedure venue. In addition, complete blood count and blood typing results are assessed. For women with significant preoperative bleeding, resuscitation steps described in Chapter 40 (p. 862) are initiated. For Rh-negative women, administration of 50 or 300 μg (250 or 1500 IU) anti-D immune globulin IM within 72 hours of pregnancy termination can lower the risk of alloimmunization in future pregnancies. Last, for those with risk factors for *Neisseria gonorrhoeae* or *Chlamydia trachomatis* listed in Table 1-1 (p. 4), screening is completed.

Ovulation may resume as early as 2 weeks after an early pregnancy ends. Thus, if contraception is desired, any method in a suitable candidate can be initiated that same day (Roe, 2019). This includes long-acting reversible contraception (LARC) placement. Also, despite the theoretical risk from mild hypercoagulability, combination oral contraceptive pills may be started the same day (Curtis, 2016; Lähteenmäki, 1981).

Consent

First-trimester suction D & C is a safe and effective method of uterine evacuation (Tunçalp, 2010). Short-term complication rates approximate 1 to 2 percent (Hakim-Elahi, 1990; Roberts, 2018; Upadhyay, 2015). These typically rise with gestational age and include retained products of conception, hemorrhage, uterine perforation, and infection. Of these, the need for repeat aspiration is ≤3 percent (Ireland, 2015; White, 2015). Hemorrhage requiring minor intervention or transfusion complicates ≤1 percent of cases (White, 2015). Atony, abnormal placentation, and coagulopathy are frequent causes, whereas surgical trauma is an uncommon source (Kerns, 2013). Although rare, the possibility of hysterectomy also is discussed.

Of traumas, the incidence of uterine perforation varies from 0.1 to 0.4 percent (Kaali, 1989; Zhou, 2002). Risk factors include operator inexperience, prior cervical surgery or anomaly, multiparity, and advanced gestational age (Allen, 2016; Grimes, 1984). Perforation usually is recognized when the instrument passes without resistance deep into the pelvis. Observation may be sufficient if the puncture site is small, such as that produced by a uterine sound or dilator. Considerable intraabdominal damage, however, can be caused by instruments—especially suction cannulas and sharp curettes. Because unrecognized bowel injury can lead to severe peritonitis and sepsis, laparoscopy or laparotomy to examine the abdominal contents is often the safest course in these cases.

The cervix also may be lacerated by greater tenaculum traction coupled with cervical softening. Rates approximate 0.3 percent (Cates, 1983). Direct pressure, electrosurgical coagulation, Monsel paste, or hemostatic suturing is a suitable option.

Antibiotic prophylaxis specifics are outlined in the next section. One review of surgical abortion found a cumulative infection rate of 0.5 percent in those given prophylaxis compared with 2.6 percent in those given placebo (Achilles, 2011).

Last, uterine synechiae may form, and the risk rises with the number of procedures, uterine size, and curettage for retained products (Gilman, 2014, 2016; Mentula, 2018). Most cases are mild and pose unclear reproductive significance (Hooker, 2014). However, of Asherman syndrome cases, first-trimester curettage is a common antecedent (Schenker, 1982).

Patient Preparation

Suction D & C may be performed for cases of incomplete abortion and requires no cervical dilation for procedure completion. However, in cases with a closed internal os,

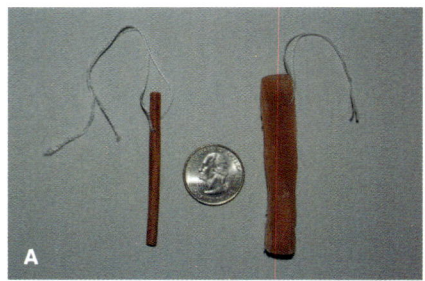

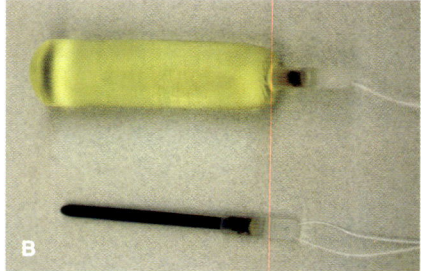

FIGURE 43-15.1 Hygroscopic dilators, dry and expanded. **A.** Laminaria. **B.** Dilapan-S.

metal dilators may be used for physical dilation, a procedural step closely associated with uterine perforation and patient discomfort. To minimize dilation forces, hygroscopic dilators can be placed in the endocervical canal to the level of the internal os. These dilators draw water from cervical proteoglycan complexes, which dissociate and thereby allow the cervix to soften and dilate. Cervical preparation may most benefit adolescents or those with late first-trimester pregnancy or mild cervical stenosis (Allen, 2016).

Of the two dilator types available in the United States, one originates from the stems of *Laminaria digitata* or *Laminaria japonica,* a seaweed. The stems are dried, sterilized, and packaged according to their hydrated size—small, 3 to 5 mm diameter; medium, 6 to 8 mm; and large, 8 to 10 mm (Fig. 43-15.1). Another, Dilapan-S, is an acrylic-based hydrogel rod, available in 3- and 4-mm diameters. Each type expands to an ultimate diameter three to four times that of its dry state. Dilapan-S achieves this in 4 to 6 hours, which is faster than the 12 to 24 hours needed for laminaria (Fox, 2014).

For dilator placement, the cervix is cleansed with povidone-iodine or similar solution and grasped anteriorly with a tenaculum. Using a uterine packing forceps, a laminaria of appropriate size is then inserted so that the tip rests at the level of the internal os (Fig. 43-15.2). Cramping frequently accompanies expansion of the device.

Alternatively, the prostaglandin E_1 analogue misoprostol (Cytotec) can serve to "ripen" the cervix. The typical dose is 400 μg administered sublingually, buccally, or placed into the posterior vaginal fornix 3 to 4 hours prior to surgery. Instead, oral administration proves less effective

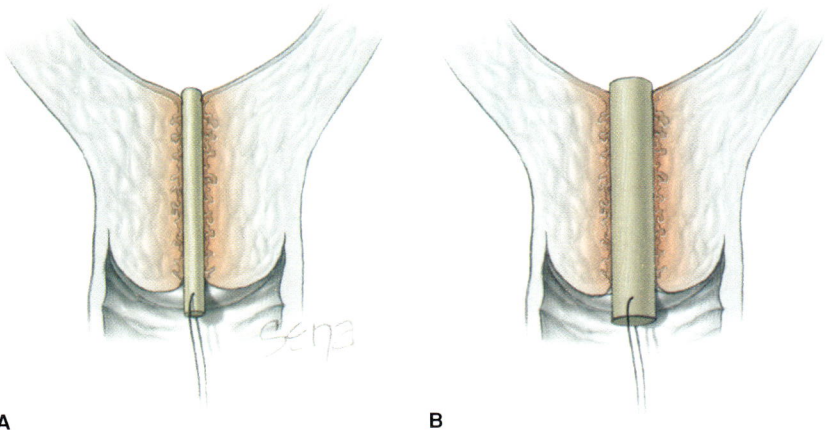

FIGURE 43-15.2 A. Correct laminaria placement. **B.** Expanded laminaria.

and may take longer (Allen, 2016). Comparing hygroscopic dilators and misoprostol for ripening, randomized studies show equal or slightly greater dilation with hygroscopic dilators. Other surgical parameters do not vary significantly (Bartz, 2013; Burnett, 2005). Of side effects, hygroscopic dilators can be uncomfortable, whereas misoprostol can induce fever, bleeding, or gastrointestinal symptoms.

Antibiotic prophylaxis is provided 1 hour before first-trimester surgical evacuation, and doxycycline, 200 mg once orally, is suitable (American College of Obstetricians and Gynecologists, 2018b). One systematic review of 11 randomized trials showed that perioperative antibiotics lowered the infection risk by 40 percent (Sawaya, 1996).

INTRAOPERATIVE

Instruments

Suction D & C requires an electric suction unit; stiff, translucent, large-bore sterile suction tubing; and sterile Karman suction cannulas (Fig. 43-15.3). Plastic suction cannulas are available in varying diameters, and size selection balances competing factors. Small cannulas risk postoperative retention of intrauterine tissue, whereas large cannulas risk cervical injury and greater discomfort. For most first-trimester evacuations, a no. 8 to 12 Karman cannula is sufficient. Intraoperatively, the suction machine, tubing, and attached cannula should be activated to confirm that the desired suction pressures can be attained. The cannula is occluded during this pressure test.

For a larger fetus or for unusual uterine anatomy, an intraoperative sonography machine and transabdominal probe can aid instrument guidance and complete evacuation. Last, the risk of hemorrhage rises with greater uterine size, leiomyomas, abnormal placentation, molar pregnancy, and evacuation of septic abortion. Uterotonics should be available and include those in Table 43-15.1 (Kerns, 2013).

Surgical Steps

❶ Anesthesia and Patient Positioning. In the absence of maternal systemic disease, abortion procedures do not require hospitalization (Guiahi, 2012). When abortion is performed outside a hospital setting, capabilities for cardiopulmonary resuscitation and for immediate transfer to a hospital must be available (American College of Obstetricians and Gynecologists, 2014).

Anesthesia or analgesia used varies and includes general or spinal anesthesia, IV sedation alone, or paracervical block plus IV or oral sedation (Allen, 2018; O'Connell, 2009). After delivery of anesthesia or analgesia, the patient is placed in standard lithotomy position.

Bimanual examination to determine uterine size and inclination is performed prior to introduction of vaginal instruments. Information obtained from this examination helps avoid uterine perforation. The vulva and vagina are then surgically prepared, and the bladder is drained.

❷ Uterine Sounding and Cervical Dilation. A Graves speculum or other suitable vaginal retractor(s) is positioned in the vagina to allow cervical access. A single-tooth tenaculum is placed on the cervical lip to provide gentle countertension during instrument passage. First, a Sims uterine sound is placed through the cervical os and into the uterine cavity to measure the depth and inclination of the uterine cavity prior to dilation (see Fig. 43-15.3). Once gentle resistance is met at the fundus, the distance from the fundus to the external os is measured by score marks along the length of the sound. Knowledge of the depth to which dilators and curettes can safely be inserted may help lower perforation risk.

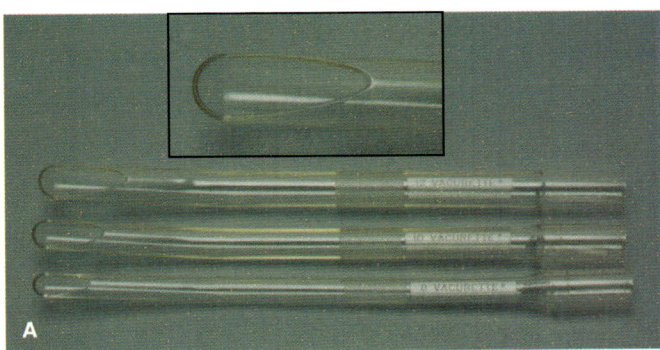

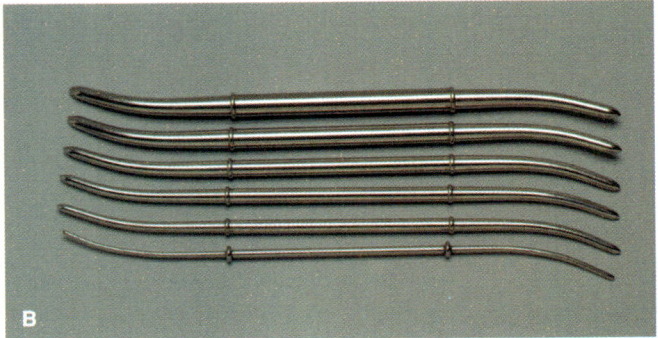

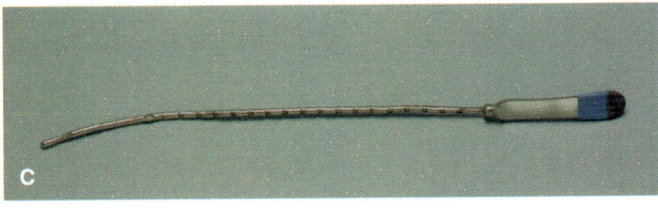

FIGURE 43-15.3 A. Karman cannulas (sizes 8 mm to 12 mm). Inset: Cannula tip. **B.** Hank dilators of serially increasing diameter. **C.** Sims uterine sound.

TABLE 43-15.1. Uterotonic Agents

Oxytocin (Pitocin): 20 units in 1000 mL LR for continuous IV infusion
One or more other uterotonic agents may be added as needed (prn):
    Methylergonovine (Methergine): 0.2 mg = 1 mL = 1 ampul IM every 2–4 hr prn
    Carboprost tromethamine ($PGF_{2\alpha}$) (Hemabate): 250 μg = 1 mL = 1 ampul IM every 15–90 min prn
    Misoprostol (PGE_1) (Cytotec): 200-mg tablets for rectal administration, 800–1000 mg once

IM = intramuscularly; IV = intravenous; LR = lactated Ringer solution.

If the cervix is closed or incompletely dilated, Pratt, Hegar, or Hank dilators of sequentially increasing diameter are placed through the external and internal os to gently open the cervix (see Fig. 43-15.3). The uterus is especially vulnerable to perforation during this step. Accordingly, the dilator is grasped as one would a pencil. The heel of the hand and fourth and fifth fingers rest on the perineum and buttock. Gentle pressure from only the thumb and first two fingers is used to guide the dilator through the cervical os (Fig. 43-15.4). If the dilator fits snugly in the canal, resting it there for 10 to 20 seconds will help the canal to stretch and accommodate.

Goals for dilation vary, but one method directly correlates millimeters of dilation to gestation age. Thus, the cervical os is dilated to an 8-mm diameter to evacuate an 8-week-sized gestation (Yonke, 2013). Hegar sizes reflect their diameter in millimeters. Pratt and Hank dilators are sized in French units, which can be converted to millimeters by dividing the French number by three.

❸ **Uterine Evacuation**. Through the now opened cervix, the cannula is inserted into the endometrial cavity (Fig. 43-15.5). The suction unit is then turned on. The cannula is moved toward the fundus, then back toward the os, and is slowly turned circumferentially to cover the entire surface of the uterine cavity (Fig. 43-15.6). A gush of clear fluid into the tubing often heralds entry of the cannula into the gestational sac. This collapses the sac and draws the placenta and membranes closer to the cannula for more expedient removal. Uterine contents are thereby removed (Fig. 43-15.7).

Tissue is collected in an attached container at the distal end of the tubing and is sent for pathologic evaluation. Occasionally, the Karman cannula may become obstructed with excess tissue. For this, the suction unit is turned off prior to cannula removal. Once the cannula opening is cleared of obstructing tissue, it may be reinserted, suction reestablished, and curettage completed.

Routine oxytocin infusion during first-trimester evacuation to limit procedural blood loss has support from many small studies but not all (Ali, 1996; Lauritz, 1980; Nygaard, 2011). Fewer oxytocin receptors are found in first-trimester myometrium compared with late pregnancy, and this may lower drug efficacy (Fuch, 1984). At our institution, we infuse oxytocin at concentrations shown in Table 43-15.1.

❹ **Sharp Curettage**. Although no more tissue is aspirated, a gentle sharp curettage is often completed to remove remaining placental or fetal fragments (Fig. 43-15.8). This is fully described next in Section 43-16.

For late first-trimester gestations following evacuation, fetal anatomic inventory can limit the risk of retained tissue. With early gestations, a small pregnancy can be missed. For confirmation, aspirated contents are rinsed in a strainer to remove blood, and

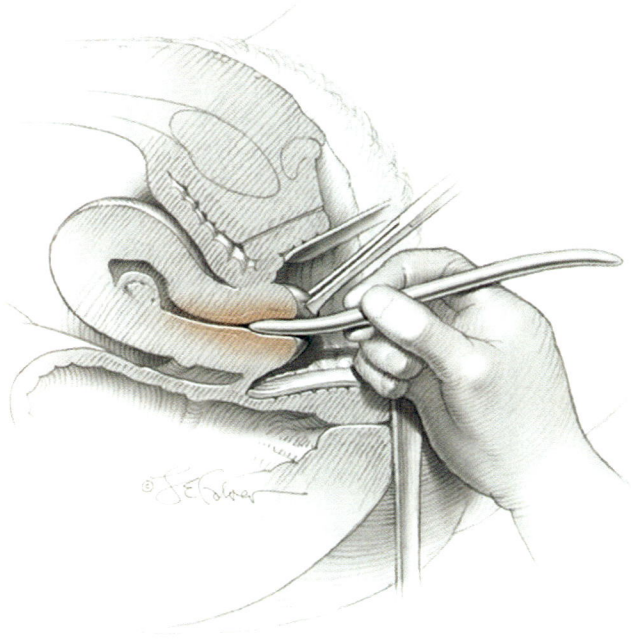

FIGURE 43-15.4 Uterine dilation.

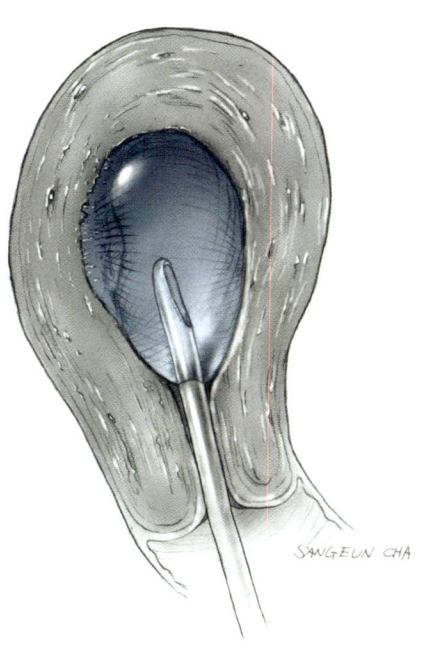

FIGURE 43-15.5 Suction cannula inserted into cavity and amnionic sac.

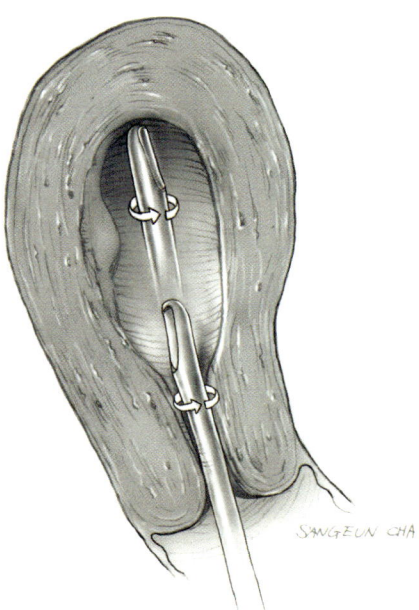

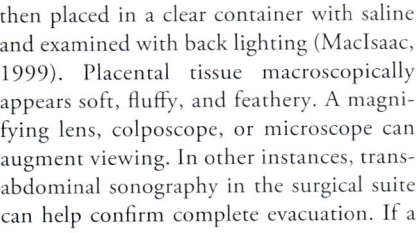

FIGURE 43-15.6 Suction cannula movement during curettage.

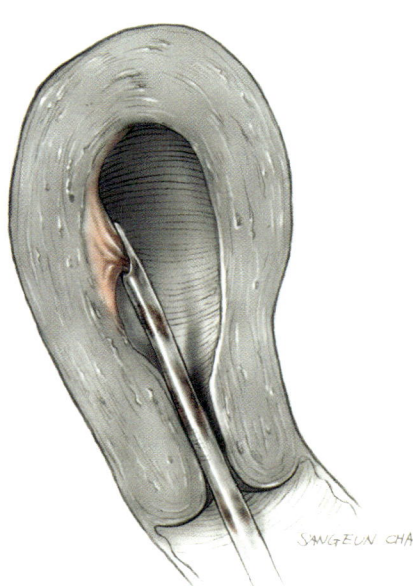

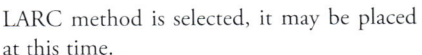

FIGURE 43-15.7 Removal of uterine contents.

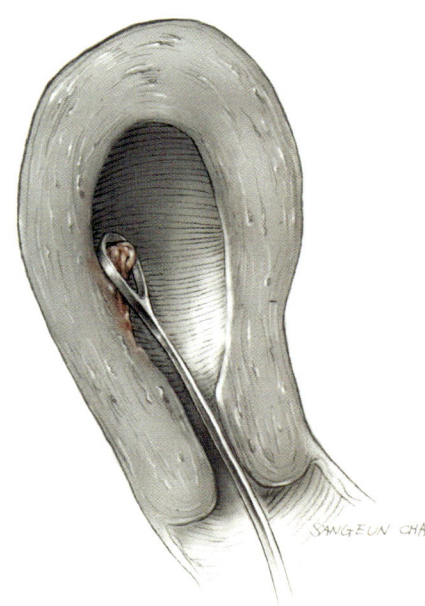

FIGURE 43-15.8 Sharp curettage.

then placed in a clear container with saline and examined with back lighting (MacIsaac, 1999). Placental tissue macroscopically appears soft, fluffy, and feathery. A magnifying lens, colposcope, or microscope can augment viewing. In other instances, transabdominal sonography in the surgical suite can help confirm complete evacuation. If a LARC method is selected, it may be placed at this time.

POSTOPERATIVE

Recovery from suction D & C is typically fast and without complication. Nonsteroidal antiinflammatory drugs (NSAIDs) are suitable for pain control. Patients may resume normal activities as they desire, but abstinence from coitus is usually encouraged during the first week following surgery.

43-16

Sharp Dilation and Curettage

This procedure is a primary tool for diagnostic evaluation and treatment of abnormal uterine bleeding. However, the indications for dilation and sharp curettage have decreased with the development of less invasive methods such as plastic endometrial samplers and transvaginal sonography (Chap. 8, p. 183).

For evaluation of abnormal uterine bleeding, sharp curettage may be used alone or more commonly in combination with hysteroscopy for those women with persistent bleeding despite normal findings with sonography and endometrial biopsy. In some, mechanical cervical dilation followed by curettage may be required to gain access to the uterine cavity when a stenotic cervical os prohibits in-office endometrial sampling. Also, if uterine neoplasia is suspected and initial biopsy is incomplete, D & C may permit a more thorough removal and interrogation of endometrial tissue.

For treatment of severe acute uterine bleeding, D & C may be used to remove hypertrophic endometrium if bleeding must be stopped promptly or if bleeding is refractory to medical management. In women with suspected ectopic pregnancy, D & C is sometimes used to document the absence of intrauterine trophoblastic tissue. Notably, sharp D & C is not recommended for pregnancy evacuation due to its greater blood loss, pain, and procedural time compared with suction D & C (National Abortion Federation, 2018; World Health Organization, 2012).

PREOPERATIVE

Consent

For most women, sharp D & C poses only a small risk of complication, and rates are typically below 1 percent (Radman, 1963; Tabata, 2001). Infection and uterine perforation are among the most frequent. With uterine perforation, concern for adjacent organ injury may require diagnostic laparoscopy or laparotomy for injury exclusion or repair. Management of these is found in Section 43-15 (p. 972). Although rare, the possibility of hysterectomy also is discussed.

Patient Preparation

Because the indications for sharp D & C are diverse, diagnostic testing prior to evacuation will vary and is discussed in their respective chapters. Sonography is often used, and images are reviewed preoperatively to reorient the surgeon to uterine inclination and pathology.

Prophylactic antibiotic administration is typically not required when sharp D & C is performed for gynecologic indications. The VTE risk with this procedure is low, and prophylaxis is reserved for those with risk factors (Table 39-9, p. 834).

INTRAOPERATIVE

Instruments

Metal curettes scrape endometrium or placenta products from the cavity. These are variably sized to accommodate differing cavity sizes. Sims curettes offer a uniform, sharp-edged tip (Fig. 43-16.1). Instead, Greene or Heaney curettes provide finely spaced transverse grooves or serrated edges, respectively. Selection is typically driven by provider preference.

Surgical Steps

❶ **Anesthesia and Patient Positioning.** D & C is typically performed as an outpatient procedure under general or regional anesthesia or with paracervical blockade combined with IV sedation. The patient is placed in standard lithotomy position, the vagina is surgically prepared, and the bladder drained.

A bimanual examination to determine uterine size and inclination is performed prior to introduction of vaginal instruments.

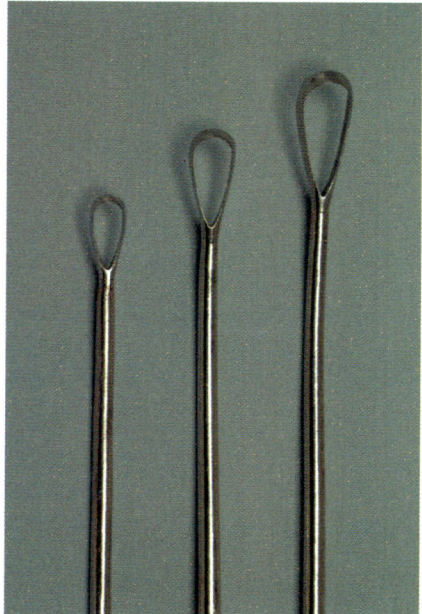

FIGURE 43-16.1 Uterine curette.

Information obtained from this examination helps avoid uterine perforation. With insertion of instruments along the long axis of the uterus, the injury risk is lessened.

❷ **Uterine Sounding.** Suitable vaginal exposure can be achieved with either a Graves speculum or individual vaginal retractors. The anterior lip of the cervix is grasped with a single-tooth tenaculum to stabilize the uterus during D & C. A Sims uterine sound is held like a pencil with the thumb and first two fingers (Fig. 43-15.3C, p. 973). The sound is slowly guided through the cervical os, into the uterine cavity, and to the fundus. To minimize perforation risks, instruments are not forced and are kept in the midline.

At times, cervical stenosis may preclude easy access to the endocervical canal. If suspected preoperatively, pretreatment with misoprostol may allow adequate cervical softening for instrument passage. Commonly used dosing options include 200 or 400 µg vaginally or 400 µg orally or sublingually once 12 to 24 hours prior to surgery. Song and coworkers (2014) noted equal efficacy but a patient preference for oral administration. Common side effects include cramping, uterine bleeding, or nausea. Instead, intracervical injection of dilute vasopressin or dilute lidocaine plus epinephrine solutions can diminish the force required for cervical dilation (Phillips, 1997). Because the onset of action is rapid, this is especially helpful if stenosis was not anticipated preoperatively. Intraoperatively, the blind use of very small-caliber tools, such as a lacrimal duct probe, is controversial. Some fear they can create a false passage and lead to perforation. If used, sonography may help visualize and guide instruments as they are being passed to help assure proper placement (Christianson, 2008). Alternatively, if the stenotic cervical scar is at the external os, a shallow loop electrosurgical excision procedure (LEEP) excision of the stenotic scar is reasonable to hopefully expose the endocervical canal.

❸ **Uterine Dilation.** After the uterus is sounded, dilators of sequentially increasing caliber are inserted to stretch the endocervical canal and internal cervical os. Shown earlier in Figure 43-15.3B a Hegar, Hank, or Pratt dilator is held by the thumb and first two fingers, while the fourth and fifth fingers and heel of the hand rest on the perineum and buttock. Each dilator is gently and gradually advanced through the internal cervical os. Serial dilation continues until the cervix will admit the selected curette.

❹ **Uterine Curettage.** Prior to curettage, a sheet of nonadherent wound dressing material (Telfa pad) is spread out in the vagina

After reaching the os, the curette is redirected to the fundus and positioned immediately adjacent to the path of the first curettage pass. After several passes, tissue accumulated in the isthmic region is scraped out onto the Telfa pad. In this fashion, the entire uterine cavity is sequentially and circumferentially curetted. The collected specimen is sent for pathologic evaluation.

❺ Uterine Exploration. Uterine polyps, both large and small, may be missed with sharp curettage. Described in Chapter 44 (p. 1054), hysteroscopy is a more accurate means to diagnose and remove focal lesions and is often coupled with D & C. In areas without these resources or expertise, uterine exploration with Randall kidney stone forceps can be used to secure and remove polyps. For this, closed forceps are inserted into the endometrial cavity. Upon reaching the fundus, forceps are opened against the uterine walls, closed, and then pulled away from the endometrium. With this technique, anterior, posterior, proximal, and distal cavity surfaces are explored. With capture of a polyp within the jaws, a tug against the closed forceps is felt as they are pulled away from the uterine wall. Firm traction typically frees the polyp. Removed tissue is sent for pathologic evaluation.

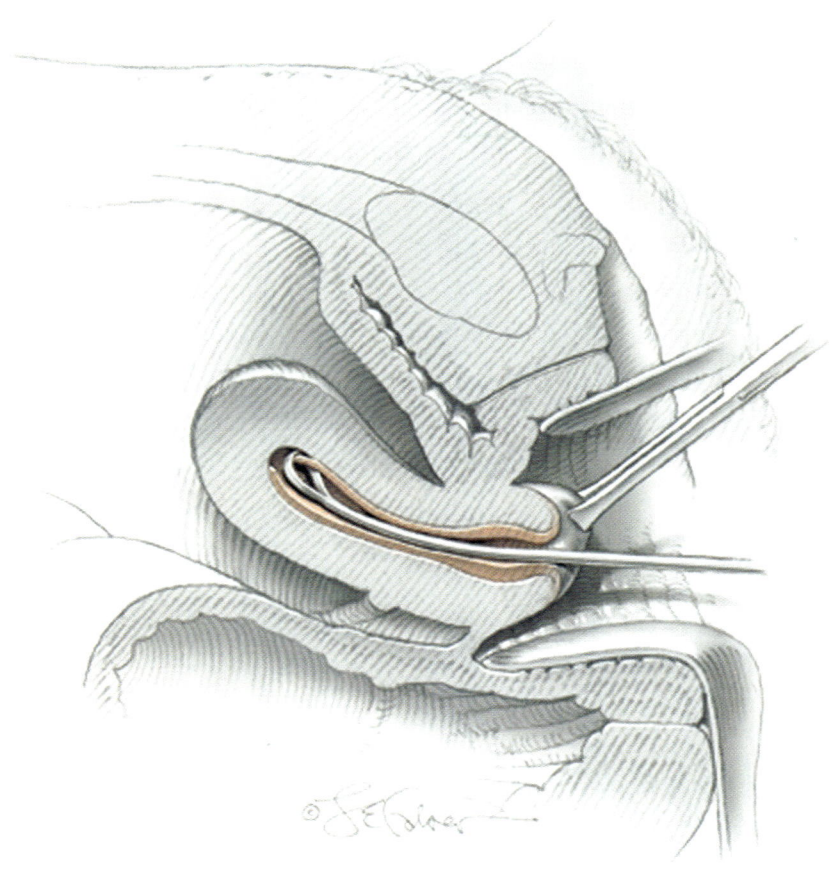

FIGURE 43-16.2 Uterine curettage.

beneath the cervix. The uterine curette is then inserted and advanced to the fundus, following the long axis of the corpus. On reaching the fundus, the sharp surface of the curette is positioned to contact the adjacent endometrium (Fig. 43-16.2). Pressure is exerted against the endometrium as the curette is pulled toward the internal cervical os.

POSTOPERATIVE

Recovery from sharp D & C is typically fast and without complication. Light bleeding or spotting is expected, and patients may resume normal activities at their own pace.

43-17

Hymenectomy

Imperforate hymen results from failure of the hymen to canalize during the perinatal period. Many cases are diagnosed after patients have become symptomatic, usually during adolescence. Accordingly, the indications for hymenectomy may include complaints of amenorrhea, pain, abdominal mass, and urinary and defecation dysfunction (Chap. 19, p. 417).

An asymptomatic imperforate hymen may also be found early, during childhood. If there is no associated large mucocele, lesions can be managed expectantly. Elective hymenectomy can then be performed during puberty, when tissues are estrogenized, but prior to menarche to avoid hematometra or hematocolpos. The presence of estrogen aids surgical repair and healing.

PREOPERATIVE

Consent

Hymenectomy is a simple gynecologic procedure, and most patients recover with no short- or long-term complications. Uncommonly, the hymeneal edges may reepithelialize, and a repeat procedure may be required (Liang, 2003).

Patient Preparation

Bowel preparation and antibiotic or VTE prophylaxis are not required for this brief surgery.

INTRAOPERATIVE

Surgical Steps

❶ Anesthesia and Patient Positioning. Hymenectomy is typically performed as a day-surgery procedure using general anesthesia. The patient is placed in the standard lithotomy position, the bladder is drained, and a sterile perineal prep is performed.

❷ Hymen Incision. To avert injury to the urethra anteriorly and to the rectum posteriorly, the surgeon avoids creating pure vertical and horizontal incisions. Instead, a cruciate incision is made anteroposteriorly from 10 to 4 and from 2 to 8 o'clock into the hymeneal membrane (**Fig. 43-17.1**). Immediately, a stream of dark menstrual blood in the case of hematocolpos or mucoid fluid with mucocolpos will follow. The hymeneal leaflets are

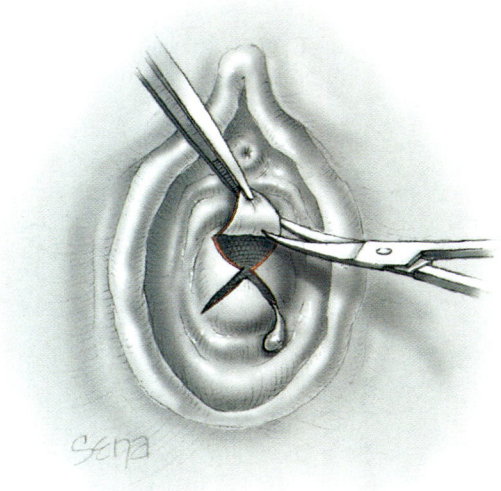

FIGURE 43-17.1 Hymenal leaflet trimming.

then sharply trimmed from the hymeneal ring. These are not excised too closely to the vaginal epithelium to avoid increased scarring at the hymeneal ring.

❸ Irrigation. The vagina is copiously irrigated using a sterile saline solution with either a red rubber catheter or bulb syringe. Intraoperative evaluation or manipulation of the upper vagina, cervix, and uterus is discouraged, as the walls of these organs may have been greatly thinned by hematocolpos or hematometra and are at risk for perforation.

❹ Suturing. The cut edges of the leaflet bases are then oversewn with interrupted stitches using 3-0 or 4-0 gauge delayed-absorbable suture to create a suture ring (**Fig. 43-17.2**). A running interlocking suture line is avoided to minimize circumferential narrowing of the introitus.

Some use an alternative method to trim leaflets. Hemostats are placed across each

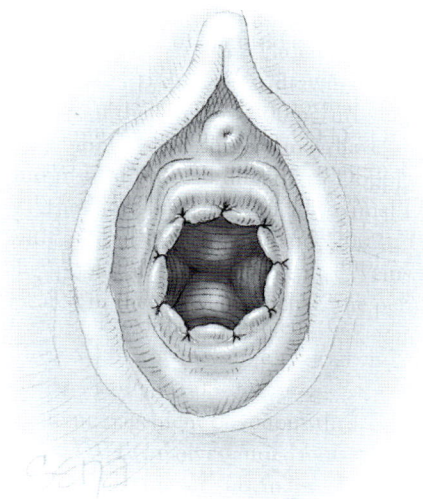

FIGURE 43-17.2 Suturing of leaflets' bases.

leaflet base for approximately a minute to crush and seal fine vessels. After clamp removal, an incision with electrosurgical blade or scissors is carried through the crush line, excises distal leaflet tissue, and eliminates the need for suturing.

POSTOPERATIVE

Following surgery, the patient may use oral analgesics and topical anesthetics such as lidocaine ointment. Local wound care includes twice-daily sitz baths. The patient is counseled that retained fluid may continue to drain from the uterus and vagina for several days following the procedure. The patient is seen 1 to 2 weeks following surgery, at which time the introitus is inspected for patency and assessment of healing.

43-18

Bartholin Gland Duct Incision and Drainage

Bartholin gland duct cysts and abscesses are vulvar masses encountered routinely in office gynecology. Bartholin duct cysts typically measure 1 to 4 cm in diameter and are frequently asymptomatic. Patients with larger cysts, however, may complain of vaginal pressure or dyspareunia. In contrast, patients with gland duct abscesses typically note rapid unilateral vulvar enlargement, significant pain, and perhaps fever. Classically, a fluctuant mass is found on one side of the introitus, external to the hymenal ring, and at the lower aspects of the vulva.

Bartholin cysts or abscesses result from ductal opening obstruction followed by accumulation of mucus or pus within the gland duct. Bartholin gland abscesses are polymicrobial infections. Anaerobic *Bacteroides* and *Peptostreptococcus* species and aerobic *Escherichia coli*, *Staphylococcus aureus*, *Streptococcus* species, and *Enterococcus faecalis* are common (Kessous, 2013; Krissi, 2016). Also, *N gonorrhoeae* and *C trachomatis* may be identified (Bleker, 1990).

Incision and drainage (I & D) alone may give immediate but sometimes only temporary relief. Often, unless a new duct ostium is created, the incised edges following I & D will seal and mucus or pus will reaccumulate. Thus, surgical goals are I & D and then subsequent steps to create a new ostium, which is sometimes referred to as *fistulization*.

Permanent resolution of the cyst or abscess is the norm following either marsupialization or I & D with Word catheter placement. Recurrence rates range from 5 to 10 percent for either procedure (Kroese, 2017; Wechter, 2009). If obstruction recurs, repeating either of these procedures is preferable to gland excision for most cases. Bartholinectomy, described on page 984, carries significantly greater morbidity than either of these two less invasive procedures.

PREOPERATIVE

Consent

Repeated obstruction of the Bartholin gland duct following initial incision and drainage (I & D) is not uncommon during the weeks and months following drainage. Patients are informed of the possible need to repeat the procedure should the duct obstruct again. Dyspareunia is an infrequent long-term sequela, but patients are counseled regarding

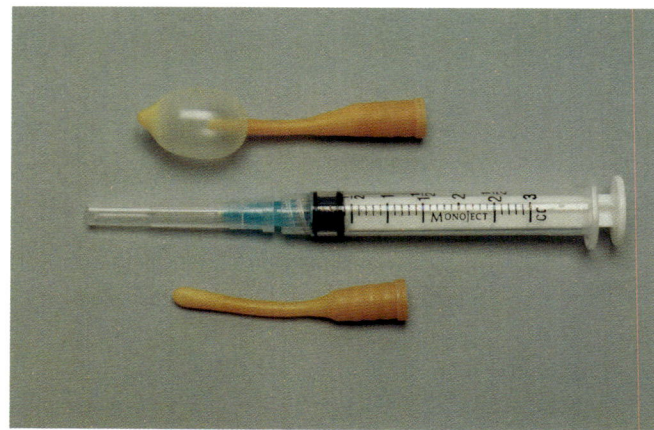

FIGURE 43-18.1 Word catheter.

this potential. Rarely, deep tissue infection or rectovaginal fistula may develop postoperatively (Zoulek, 2011).

INTRAOPERATIVE

Instruments

The goal of Bartholin gland duct I & D is to empty the cystic cavity and create a new epithelialized tract for gland drainage. For the latter, a Word catheter is typically used (Word, 1964). This is constructed of a 1-inch-long latex tube stem that has an inflatable balloon at one end and a saline-injection hub at the other (Fig. 43-18.1).

Surgical Steps

❶ Analgesia and Patient Positioning. Most procedures are performed as an outpatient procedure in the office or emergency room. Rarely, if the abscess is large or if adequate patient analgesia cannot be

obtained, I & D in the operative room may be required. The patient is placed in standard lithotomy position, and the ipsilateral labial skin is cleaned with a povidone-iodine solution or other suitable antiseptic agent. Local analgesia is sufficient for most cases and can be obtained by infiltrating the skin overlying and adjacent to the planned incision with a 1-percent lidocaine solution. This may be augmented with mild IM or IV centrally acting analgesia.

❷ Drainage. A 1-cm incision is made using a scalpel with a no. 11 blade to pierce the skin and underlying cyst or abscess wall (Fig. 43-18.2). The incision is placed on the cyst bulge, just outside and parallel to the hymen at 5 or 7 o'clock (depending on the side involved), and medial to Hart line. This position mimics the normal anatomy of the gland duct opening and avoids creation of a fistulous tract to the outer labium majus (Hill, 1998). Some use a small Keyes biopsy punch to create a hole simultaneously through the skin and cyst wall.

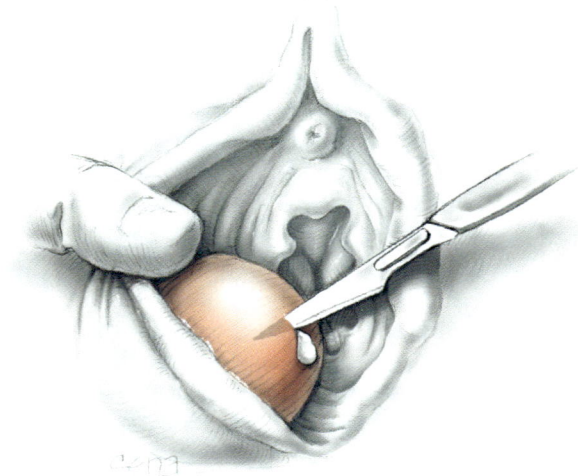

FIGURE 43-18.2 Abscess or cyst incision.

General bacterial culture and samples specific for *N gonorrhoeae* and *C trachomatis* testing can be obtained from the spontaneously extruded pus. In contrast, mucus drained from a Bartholin cyst need not be cultured. Following drainage, the cavity is explored with a small cotton swab tip to open potential pus or mucus loculations. Probing is gentle to avoid perforation through the attenuated duct wall and into the nearby and highly vascular vestibular bulb (Fig. 38-26, p. 815). Cyst wall biopsy following cavity drainage to exclude rare Bartholin gland carcinoma is considered for at-risk cases. Cysts in women older than 40 years, with solid components, or with multiple recurrences are candidates.

❸ Word Catheter Placement. A deflated Word catheter tip is placed into the empty cyst cavity. A syringe is used to inject 2 to 3 mL of sterile saline through the catheter hub to inflate the balloon. Inflation should reach a diameter sufficient to keep the catheter from falling out of the incision (Fig. 43-18.3). Alternatively, a non–latex 14F Foley catheter is a suitable substitute for those with latex allergy or in settings without a Word catheter. In either case, insufflation with saline rather than air is preferred, as the latter is associated with premature balloon deflation. The hub end of the catheter is then tucked inside the vagina to prevent it from being dislodged by perineal movement.

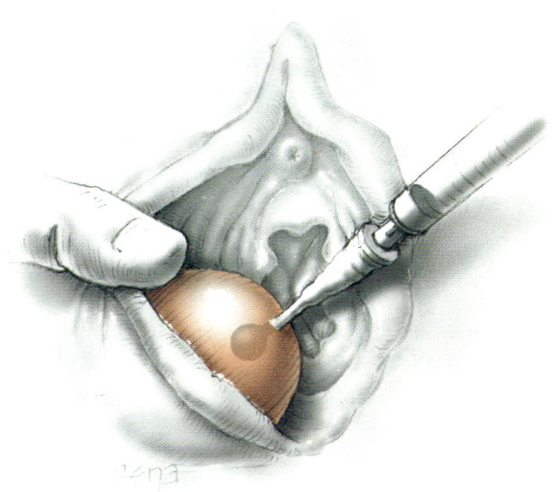

FIGURE 43-18.3 Word catheter in place.

POSTOPERATIVE

Bartholin gland duct cyst drainage does not require antibiotic treatment. In contrast, abscesses are typically surrounded by significant cellulitis, and in such cases, antibiotics are indicated. Suitable choices include trimethoprim-sulfamethoxazole (Bactrim DS, Septra DS), doxycycline, or cephalexin (Keflex), prescribed for 7 days. At our institution, affected immunocompromised women are admitted for IV antibiotic therapy until fever or erythema improves.

Patients are encouraged to soak in warm tub baths twice daily. Coitus is avoided for patient comfort and to prevent Word catheter displacement. Ideally, the catheter is left in place for 4 to 6 weeks. Often, however, a catheter will be dislodged before this time. There is no need to try and replace the catheter if displaced, and attempts to reinsert it are typically futile due to cavity closure.

43-19

Bartholin Gland Duct Marsupialization

Noted on page 980, a new duct ostium must be created following I & D of a Bartholin duct abscess to prevent the incised edges from adhering and allowing pus to reaccumulate. For this reason, marsupialization was developed as a means to create a new accessory tract for gland drainage.

With introduction of the Word catheter, however, use of marsupialization for cyst or abscess drainage has declined. Word catheter placement offers several advantages over marsupialization, and recurrence rates are equal (Blakely, 1966; Jacobson, 1960; Kroese, 2017). Marsupialization requires a greater degree of analgesia, a larger incision, placement of sutures, and longer procedure time. That said, this procedure may be selected for those with large abscesses/cysts, those with recurrences after Word catheter failures, or those with latex allergy.

PREOPERATIVE

Consent

The consenting discussion before marsupialization mirrors that for Bartholin gland duct I & D (p. 980).

INTRAOPERATIVE

Surgical Steps

❶ **Anesthesia and Patient Positioning.** Marsupialization is an outpatient procedure typically performed in an operating suite using a unilateral pudendal nerve block or general or regional anesthesia. Some authors, however, have described procedure performance in an emergency room setting (Downs, 1989). The patient is placed in standard lithotomy position, and the vulva and vagina are surgically prepared.

❷ **Skin Incision.** A vertical or elliptical incision measuring 2 cm is made across the skin overlying the cystic bulge using a scalpel with a no. 15 blade. The incision is placed just outside and parallel to the hymen at 5 or 7 o'clock (depending on the side involved) and is positioned medial to Hart line. This position mimics the normal gland duct opening anatomy and avoids creation of a fistulous tract to the outer labium majus (Fig. 43-19.1).

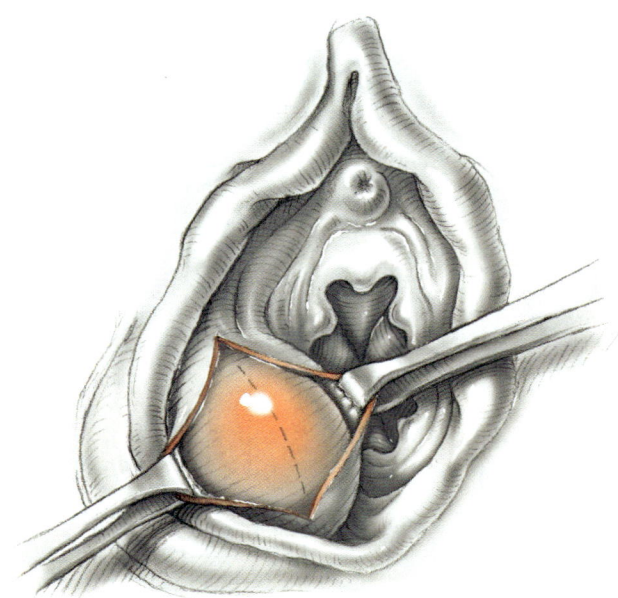

FIGURE 43-19.1 Skin incision.

❸ **Cyst Incision.** A second vertical incision then opens the underlying cyst wall, and pus or mucus under pressure spills out. Pus may be cultured as described on page 981. Allis clamps are then placed on the superior, inferior, right, and left lateral cyst wall edges and fanned out.

Following drainage, the cavity is explored with a small cotton swab tip to open potential fluid loculations. Probing is gentle to avoid perforation through the attenuated duct wall and into the nearby and highly vascular vestibular bulb. In addition, cyst wall biopsy following cavity drainage to exclude rare Bartholin gland adenocarcinoma is considered if the patient is older than 40 years or if solid components accompany the cyst.

❹ **Wound Closure.** The edges of the cyst wall are sutured to adjacent skin edges with interrupted sutures using 2-0 or 3-0 gauge delayed-absorbable suture (Fig. 43-19.2).

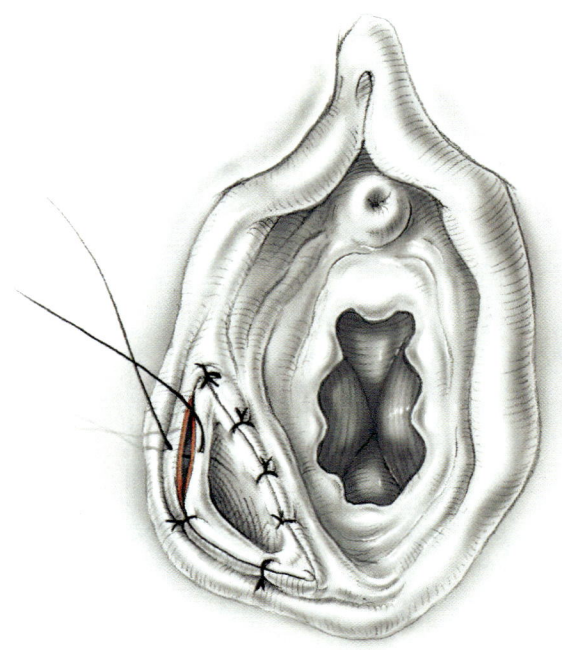

FIGURE 43-19.2 Cyst wall sutured open.

POSTOPERATIVE

Bartholin gland duct cyst drainage does not require antibiotic treatment. However, abscesses are typically surrounded by significant cellulitis, and antibiotics are warranted. Suitable choices include trimethoprim-sulfamethoxazole, doxycycline, or cephalexin, prescribed for 7 days. At our institution, affected immunocompromised women are admitted for intravenous antibiotic therapy until fever or erythema improves.

Cool packs during the first 24 hours following surgery can minimize pain, swelling, and hematoma formation. After this time, warm sitz baths, one or two times daily, aid pain relief and wound hygiene. Activities are resumed quickly, although intercourse is delayed until healing is complete.

Patients may be seen within the first week following surgery to ensure that ostium edges have not adhered to each other (Novak, 1978). Within 2 to 3 weeks, the wound shrinks to create a duct opening typically 5 mm or less.

43-20

Bartholin Gland Duct Excision

Most Bartholin gland duct cysts can be managed with I & D and Word catheter placement or with marsupialization. Symptomatic cysts, however, which repeatedly recur and refill following I & D or marsupialization, are typical candidates for excision. Others best managed with excision are cysts with solid components, which raise the concern for malignancy and multilocular cysts, which may be incompletely drained by I & D. Bartholin gland duct abscesses are not suitable for excision and instead should undergo I & D.

In the past, many excised *all* Bartholin gland cysts in women older than 40 to exclude cancer. However, a study by Visco and Del Priore (1996) suggests that the morbidity of gland excision may not be justified for this rare cancer (Chap 4, p. 103). Instead, they recommend cyst I & D with cyst wall biopsy, and this is current practice.

PREOPERATIVE

Consent

Complications are usually not encountered during bartholinectomy, but if the rich venous plexus of the nearby vestibular bulb is entered, bleeding can be significant (Fig. 38-26, p. 815). Additionally, gland excision can be associated with other morbidities such as postoperative wound cellulitis, hematoma formation, or pain from postoperative scarring. Rarely, recurrence from failure to remove the entire cyst wall, rectal injury, or rectovaginal fistula has been described.

Patient Preparation

No special antibiotic or VTE prophylaxis is typically needed for this brief day surgery. Digital rectal examination may be done during surgery to guide dissection and avoid rectal laceration. An empty rectal vault may minimize wound contamination.

INTRAOPERATIVE

Surgical Steps

❶ **Analgesia and Patient Positioning.** Excision of most Bartholin gland duct cysts is performed as an outpatient procedure, in an operative suite, and under general anesthesia. The patient is placed in standard lithotomy position, and the vagina and perineum are surgically prepared.

❷ **Skin Incision.** A gauze sponge held by a ring forceps is placed inside the vagina by an assistant, and pressure is directed outward along the back wall of the cyst. This pushes the full extent of the cyst forward. The surgeon's fingers retract the labium minus laterally to expose the medial surface of the cyst.

A vertical incision that extends the length of the cyst is made on the medial surface of the labium minus. The skin is incised but avoids puncture of the underlying cyst wall. Allis clamps are placed on the medial incision edge, which is fanned out medially toward the contralateral labium.

❸ **Cyst Dissection.** To summarize the steps as an overview, dissection begins along the cyst's medial border, then along the lateral border, and finally deep vessels are ligated and transected to free the cyst. The greatest vascular supply to these cysts is located at their posterosuperior aspect. Accordingly, dissection of each border begins at the lower cyst pole and is directed superiorly.

To begin, medial traction on the Allis clamps and lateral fingertip traction against the cyst creates tension across connective tissue bands between the cyst wall and surrounding tissue. These bands are divided, and in this fashion, the inferomedial cyst wall is bluntly and sharply dissected free. Dissection planes are kept close to the cyst wall to avoid bleeding from the vestibular bulb and to avoid incision into the rectum (Fig. 43-20.1). Because the lowermost pole of a Bartholin gland cyst may extend to lie adjacent to the rectum, the rectum can be entered accidentally during dissection. Placing a finger at times into the rectum can help orient the surgeon to the spatial relationship between the two. Bleeding from the vestibular bulb can be troublesome. Most cases can be managed with ligation of individual vessels (if identified), placement of hemostatic sutures within the general bleeding area, closure of dead space, or a combination of these techniques.

Following medial border dissection, Allis clamps are next placed on the lateral skin edges and fanned out laterally. Dissection begins near the inferolateral cyst wall and moves superiorly.

❹ **Vessel Ligation.** As dissection is completed superiorly, the main deep vascular bundle to the cyst is identified and clamped with a hemostat. The bundle is cut and ligated with 3-0 gauge delayed-absorbable or chromic suture (Fig. 43-20.2).

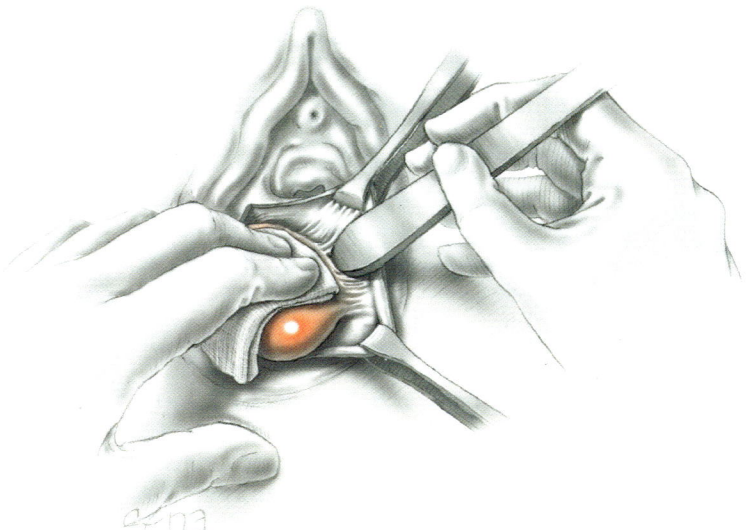

FIGURE 43-20.1 Cyst dissection.

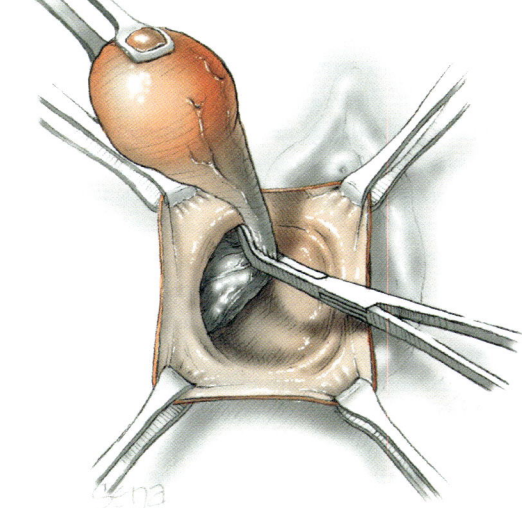

FIGURE 43-20.2 Vessel ligation.

❺ **Wound Closure.** The remaining cyst bed is closed in layers with running or interrupted sutures of 3-0 gauge delayed-absorbable suture. Typically, two layers are required prior to skin closure. However, with large or vascular cyst beds, additional layers may be required. The skin is approximated with a running subcuticular suture of 4-0 gauge delayed-absorbable suture.

POSTOPERATIVE

Cool packs during the first 24 hours following surgery can minimize pain, swelling, and hematoma formation. After this time, warm sitz baths, one or two times each day, are suggested for pain relief and wound hygiene. Intercourse is delayed for several weeks to permit wound healing, and then resumption is typically dictated by patient comfort.

43-21

Vulvar Abscess Incision and Drainage

A patient with a vulvar abscess may typically present with pain, vulvar edema and erythema, and a fluctuant mass that should be differentiated from Bartholin gland duct abscess (Fig. 43-21.1). In some cases, the abscess may be draining spontaneously, and antibiotics are added to resolve surrounding cellulitis. Similarly, for small, nondraining abscesses measuring <2 cm, local warm compresses or baths and oral antibiotics are suitable. Larger abscesses typically require incision and drainage (I & D).

PREOPERATIVE

Patient Evaluation

In most cases, this is a visual diagnosis, and for those without comorbidities, no specific laboratory testing or imaging is needed. In obese patients, a serum glucose level is considered. Immediate debridement should follow clear cases of necrotizing fasciitis. In suspicious but not convincing cases of fasciitis, computed tomography scanning, if it can be completed expeditiously, can help clarify the diagnosis (Chap. 3, p. 84).

Consent

Incomplete drainage and persistence of the abscess may follow initial incision and drainage, particularly if the abscess contains loculations. The abscess may also reform after drainage. Although uncommon, progression to or already coexisting necrotizing fasciitis may complicate the infection course.

Patient Preparation

For large abscesses or in the immunosuppressed, IV antibiotics are given preoperatively, and coverage for methicillin-resistant *Staphylococcus aureus* (MRSA) is considered. Thurman (2008) and Kilpatrick (2010) and their coworkers found MRSA to be a common pathogen in vulvar abscesses (43 and 64 percent, respectively).

INTRAOPERATIVE

Surgical Steps

❶ **Anesthesia and Patient Positioning.** Many patients with smaller abscesses can undergo I & D in an ambulatory setting. In contrast, to attain adequate analgesia, larger abscesses often require drainage in the operating room under regional or general anesthesia.

The patient is placed in standard lithotomy position, and the involved area of the vulva is cleaned with povidone-iodine solution or other suitable antiseptic. If local analgesia is planned, the skin overlying the abscess is injected with a 1-percent lidocaine solution to achieve a field effect.

❷ **Drainage.** A 1- to 2-cm incision is made with a no. 11 scalpel blade into the site where the abscess wall is most thinned and likely attempting to drain spontaneously. The incision penetrates into the abscess cavity, and extrusion of abundant pus follows. Wound cultures are obtained at this time.

The abscess cavity is explored to bluntly dissect loculations within the cavity (Fig. 43-21.2). In large abscesses, the incision may be extended to allow sufficient exploration, pus evacuation, and devitalized tissue debridement. Digital or gentle cotton swab exploration is preferred to that with a pointed surgical instrument. The latter may tear vestibular bulb veins to create significant bleeding or hematoma or may inadvertently perforate the vagina or rectum to risk fistula formation.

❸ **Procedure Completion.** The wound may be packed with iodoform or plain gauze, or the incision may simply be left open to spontaneously heal. After 24 hours, iodoform gauze is typically exchanged for plain gauze to avoid the deleterious effect of iodoform on surrounding healthy tissue.

Alternatively, depending on surgeon preference, a drain may be placed in the abscess cavity and brought out through a separate incision. The edges of the primary incision are then reapproximated with delayed-absorbable suture (Fig. 43-21.3). The drain should exit below the abscess to allow for dependent drainage.

POSTOPERATIVE

For small abscesses, the patient may be discharged following I & D, and reevaluation or wound repacking in 48 to 72 hours is reasonable. Appropriate antibiotic coverage is continued for several days, and

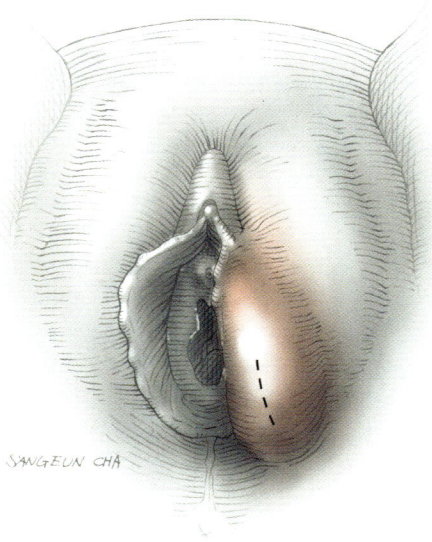

FIGURE 43-21.1 Vulvar abscess incision.

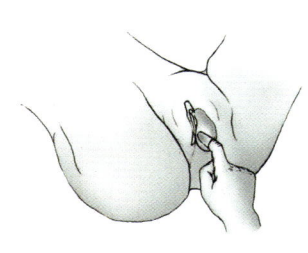

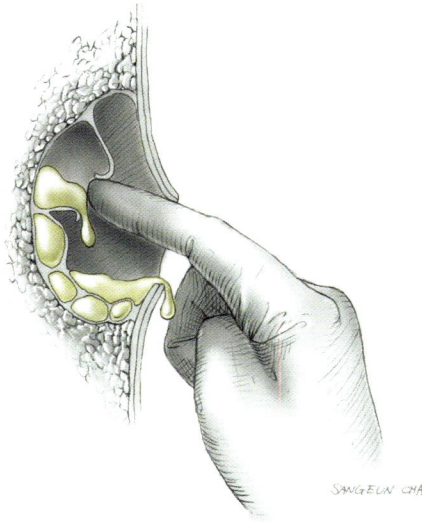

FIGURE 43-21.2 Digital exploration and disruption of abscess loculations.

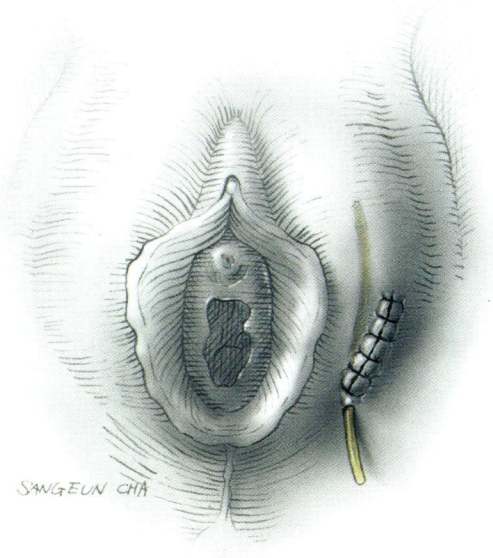

FIGURE 43-21.3 Drain placement and incision closure.

trimethoprim-sulfamethoxazole (Bactrim, Septra) is a first-line oral agent against MRSA. Women with larger abscesses or greater surrounding cellulitis often warrant admission for pain control and IV antibiotic therapy. For MRSA, clindamycin or vancomycin is an effective intravenous choice. Most women with significant immunosuppression or diabetes also require hospital admission for antibiotic administration and comorbidity management. Specifically, Kilpatrick and colleagues (2010) noted that coexistent diabetes was significantly related to hospitalization for more than 7 days, reoperation, and progression to necrotizing fasciitis.

In those without gauze packing, warm sitz baths, one or two times each day, may aid pain relief and wound hygiene. With resolving fever and surrounding cellulitis, the drain is removed. For those with gauze packing, it may be changed once or twice daily until the cavity is nearly closed and cleared of infection. Select patients with large abscess cavities may benefit from negative-pressure wound therapy. In all cases, long-term perineal hygiene and avoidance of labial shaving is emphasized.

43-22

Vestibulectomy

Anatomically, the vestibule extends along the inner labia minora, from the clitoris to the fourchette (Fig. 38-25, p. 814). Its medial border is the hymeneal ring, and its lateral aspect is the Hart line. The Hart line lies along the inner labia minora and demarcates the boundary between keratinized and non-keratinized epithelium. For some women, this region can be a source of vulvodynia or dyspareunia.

Most cases of vulvodynia are managed conservatively and options are discussed in Chapter 4 (p. 105). But, for persistently refractory cases, surgical options are vestibulectomy and perineoplasty (Edwards, 2003).

Vestibulectomy involves excision of vestibular tissue (Fig. 43-22.1). Incisions extend from the periurethral area down to the superior edge of the perineum and include the fourchette. The lateral incisions are carried along the Hart line, and the medial incisions are placed so as to excise the hymen. In sum, mucous membrane, hymen, and minor vestibular glands are removed, and Bartholin ducts are transected. Following excision, the vaginal mucosa is mobilized and pulled distally to cover the defect. In certain cases, a modified vestibulectomy is sufficient and extends only partially up the inner labia minora, well short of the periurethral area (Lavy, 2005).

Perineoplasty is the more extensive procedure and extends from just below the urethra to the perineal body, usually terminating above the anal orifice (see Fig. 43-22.1). Similarly, following tissue resection, the vaginal epithelium is advanced to cover the defect. Although used to treat vulvodynia, perineoplasty may also treat fissuring and associated pain caused by refractory lichen sclerosus (Kennedy, 2005; Rouzier, 2002).

PREOPERATIVE

Patient Evaluation

The most important factor for surgical success in treating vulvar pain is identifying the proper candidate (Chap. 4, p. 105). For example, vaginismus coexists in approximately half of patients with vulvodynia and is associated with lower rates of postsurgical pain relief (Goldstein, 2005).

Prior to anesthesia administration, the patient undergoes testing with a cotton swab to map areas of pain. These are marked with permanent marker prior to surgery to delineate the extent of excision (Haefner, 2005). Importantly, all sensitive areas are removed, even those adjacent to the urethra. If not, tender foci that should have been resected as part of the primary operation may remain (Bornstein, 1999).

Consent

Vestibulectomy provides pain resolution in 60 to 90 percent of women, and rates of improved *or* resolved pain range from 80 to 90 percent (Goldstein, 2006; Swanson, 2014; Tommola, 2010; Traas, 2006). Perineoplasty offers pain resolution in 55 to 80 percent, and rates of improved *or* resolved pain range from 80 to 97 percent (Bornstein, 1997; Foster, 1995; Marinoff, 1991). In the series by Foster and associates (1995), symptoms worsened in 4 percent after surgery. Importantly, these data derive from small case series, and robust randomized trials are lacking.

Complications are generally infrequent. These include bleeding, infection, wound separation, surgical-site granulation tissue, Bartholin duct cyst formation, anal sphincter weakness, vaginismus, and vaginal stenosis (Goetsch, 2009; Haefner, 2000).

Patient Preparation

No special antibiotic or VTE prophylaxis is typically needed for this brief day surgery. A preoperative enema may be considered to avoid immediate postoperative stool and thereby improve wound hygiene.

INTRAOPERATIVE

Surgical Steps

❶ **Anesthesia and Patient Positioning.** In most cases, vestibulectomy is a day-surgery procedure, conducted using general or regional anesthesia. The patient is placed in standard lithotomy position, and the vulvovaginal area is surgically prepared.

❷ **Surgical Excision.** The primary incision, which is the lateral border, is made to a depth of 2 to 5 mm along the Hart line. Traditionally, it begins in the periurethral area, and it extends from the openings of the Skene ducts to the fourchette. But, the amount of tissue removed anteroposteriorly is best tailored to sensitivity mapping. The medial incision is placed just proximal to the hymeneal ring.

❸ **Vaginal Mucosal Advancement.** Following vestibular tissue excision, the incised edge of the vaginal mucosa is undermined 1 to 2 cm cephalad and then pulled distally to cover the defect (Fig. 43-22.2). To prevent hematoma and wound separation, hemostasis is achieved prior to final suturing.

❹ **Wound Closure.** A deep closure layer using interrupted 3-0 gauge delayed-absorbable sutures approximates the vaginal wall to its new site covering the vestibular defect. The superficial incision between the skin and vaginal epithelium is closed in an interrupted fashion with 4-0 gauge delayed-absorbable suture.

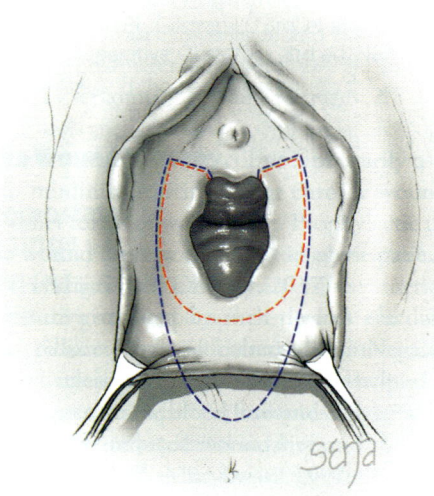

FIGURE 43-22.1 Incisions for vestibulectomy (*red line*) and for perineoplasty (*blue line*).

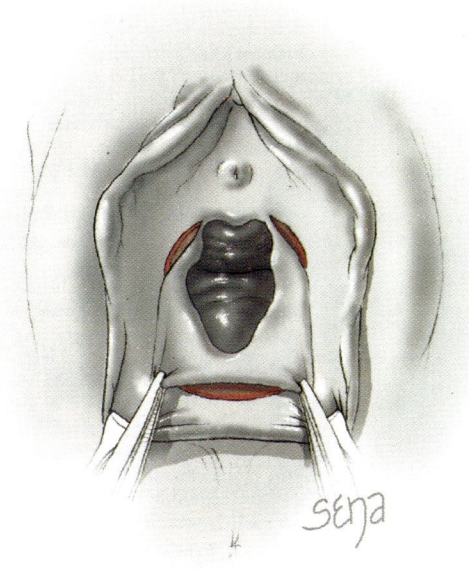

FIGURE 43-22.2 Vaginal mucosal advancement.

POSTOPERATIVE

Cool packs are used to relieve immediate discomfort, and sitz baths are initiated after the first 24 hours. Recovery is typically fast and without complications, and wound healing takes 4 to 8 weeks. Patients usually meet with their surgeon during this time and are instructed to gradually resume intercourse 6 to 8 weeks following surgery (Bergeron, 2001).

43-23

Labia Minora Reduction

When outstretched, the normal labia minora can span several centimeters from their base to their most distal edge. Shape and size varies, and currently no criteria provide a definition of labia minora hypertrophy (Özer, 2018). In some women, the extent or appearance of the labia minora, including asymmetry may cause aesthetic dissatisfaction, discomfort with tight clothing, pain with exercise, and insertional dyspareunia. As a result, some elect labia minora reduction, also known as *labiaplasty*. The American College of Obstetricians and Gynecologists (2019f) recommends labial alteration for medical indications. These include repair of female genital mutilation and treatment of labial hypertrophy or asymmetric labial growth that stems from congenital conditions or chronic irritation. Although most labial reduction operations are performed for the combined indication of discomfort plus cosmetic dissatisfaction, up to 13 percent of labial reductions in 2008 were solely cosmetic procedures (Alter, 2008). Of note, many women seeking this surgery solely for aesthetic improvement have labial lengths well within normal standards (Crouch, 2011; Gulia, 2017).

In appropriately counseled adult women, goals of surgery include reduction in labial size and maintenance of normal vulvar anatomy and function. Early reductive procedures involved anteroposterior excision along the base of the labia and reapproximation of the surgical edges. Drawbacks to this approach include a marked color contrast at the suture line, where the labia minora's dark outer surface abuts the lighter inner surface. In addition, some data suggest a greater nerve density in the distal labia than the proximal portion. This may lead to decreased labial sensation, chronic pain, and sexual dysfunction (Jackson, 2019). Moreover, the labial edge is often replaced by a stiff suture line. To reduce these effects, alternate techniques have incorporated labial V-, S-, Z- or W-plasty incisions, and surgeries are increasingly performed by plastic surgeons (Mirzabeigi, 2012). Some experts prefer V-shaped wedge resection. However, limited long-term outcomes data among the various techniques hamper robust comparison and assembly of clear safety and efficacy guidelines (Iglesia, 2013; Özer, 2018; Royal College of Obstetricians and Gynaecologists, 2013).

Unilateral or bilateral partial resection of the prepuce, a procedure known as *prepuce reduction* or *clitoral hood reduction* is sometimes combined with central wedge resection of the labia minora (Alter, 2008; Iglesia, 2013). No consensus criteria defines prepuce enlargement, and recognized indications typically mirror those listed earlier for labia minora reduction.

PREOPERATIVE

Consent

Current but limited data suggest that V-shaped wedge resection labiaplasty improves satisfaction and self-esteem in many women (Lista, 2015; Placik, 2014; Rouzier, 2000). Women are appropriately educated on the great variation in normal female external genitalia. Counseling also offers nonsurgical strategies to circumvent symptoms such as discomfort with tight clothing and hygiene. As with any aesthetic procedure, women who are seeking cosmetic correction should have realistic expectations as to the final size, shape, and color of the labia. Wound complications such as hematoma, cellulitis, asymmetry or incisional dehiscence are uncommon but should be discussed. Similarly, risks for postoperative dyspareunia, skin retraction, and delayed local pain are presented. Excision of distal labia during reduction can lead to decreased sensation and chronic pain requiring reconstruction (Kelishadi, 2016; Lista, 2015).

If concomitant prepuce reductions are planned, patients are counseled regarding the risk of overexposure of the glans of clitoris, which may lead to hypersensitivity, and injury to dorsal nerves of clitoris, which can lead to decreased glans sensation and potentially to anorgasmia (Jackson, 2019). The dorsal nerves of the clitoris have a consistent and reproducible path on the dorsal surface of the clitoral body (Figs. 38-27 and 38-28, p. 816). Surgeons should be appropriately trained to perform these procedures.

Patient Preparation

No specific radiologic imaging is needed for this condition or surgery. Antibiotic or VTE prophylaxis is not required for this brief procedure in those without specific risks.

INTRAOPERATIVE

Surgical Steps

❶ Anesthesia and Patient Positioning. Labia minora reduction may be performed as an outpatient procedure using general or regional anesthesia. The patient is placed in standard lithotomy position, and the vulva is surgically prepared.

❷ Labial Marking. Excessive tissue removal is avoided, and aggressive reduction may

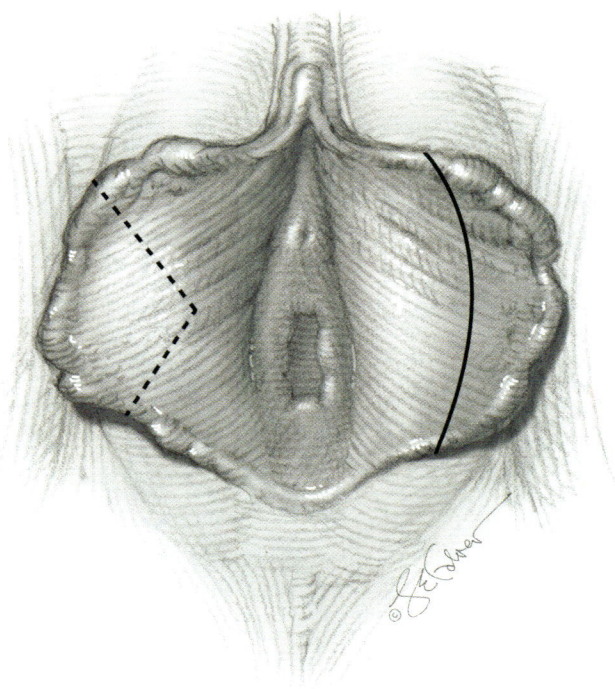

FIGURE 43-23.1 Incision lines. Wedge excision technique (*left*). Distal trimming technique (*right*).

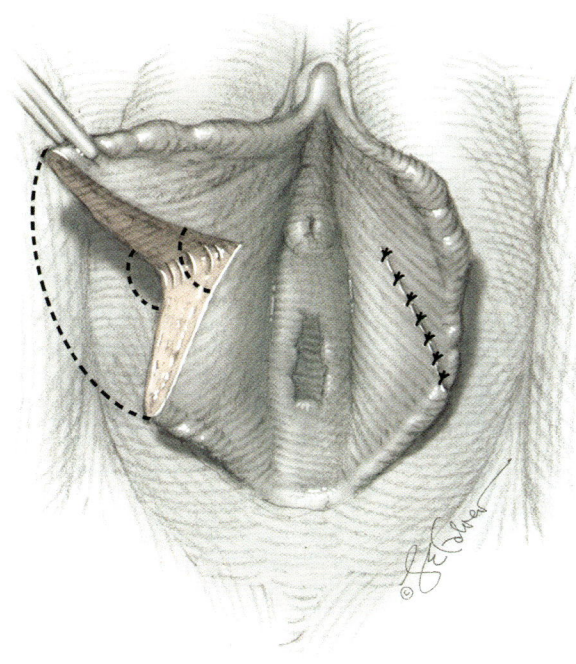

FIGURE 43-23.2 Incision closure (*left*) and final suture line (*right*).

create anteroposterior narrowing and discomfort during subsequent intercourse. For this reason, during surgical marking, the surgeon may choose to place several fingers into the vagina to distend its caliber. The labia minora are then gently outstretched laterally.

The desired lateral span of the labia will vary between women, but most surgeons strive to create a final span of 1 to 2 cm. Asymmetry between labia is common, and surgical marking helps to even this difference. With a surgical marker, the surgeon draws a V-shaped wedge on the ventral and dorsal surfaces of the labia minora, demarcating the tissue for excision (Fig. 43-23.1, *left*). In other cases, a simple curved incision that extends from the upper to lower labium is

performed (*right*). However, as noted above, this is a less-preferred method.

❸ **Wedge Excision.** The labia minora have a rich blood supply. To minimize bleeding, the incision may be infiltrated with a solution of 1-percent lidocaine and epinephrine (5 µg/mL) in a manufactured 1:200,000 dilution. The tissue wedge or line is then sharply excised. Hemostasis may be achieved using electrosurgical coagulation and is important to help avoid hematoma formation.

❹ **Incision Closure.** For wedge incisions, the subcutaneous layers of the labia are reapproximated beginning proximally at the tip of the wedge (Fig. 43-23.2, *left*). Interrupted stitches of 4-0 gauge delayed-absorbable suture are then added outward toward the wedge's base to close the remainder of the wound. For linear incisions, dead space between skin edges is closed with interrupted stitches of similar suture. With either incision, the skin is reapproximated with 4-0 or 5-0 gauge delayed-absorbable suture in a running subcuticular or interrupted fashion (see Fig. 43-23.2, *right*).

POSTOPERATIVE

Cool packs are used to relieve immediate discomfort, and sitz baths are initiated after the first 24 hours. Perineal hygiene is emphasized during the initial weeks following surgery. Exercise and intercourse may resume after wound healing in approximately 6 weeks.

Defibulation

Female genital mutilation (FGM) involves cutting or excising portions of the external genitalia to varying degrees, and specific definitions are found in Table 1-21 (p. 25). With type III lesions, also known as *infibulation*, the labia minora and/or labia majora are cut and apposed to narrow the introitus. Clitoral excision may accompany this.

In affected women, altered anatomy can lead to infertility, chronic vulvar pain, diminished sexual satisfaction, propensity for urogenital infection, and difficulty passing menstrual blood (Almroth, 2005; Andersson, 2012; World Health Organization, 2018). To help resolve these, *defibulation* incises the midline infibulation scar to expose the vestibule. *Partial defibulation* uncovers the vagina and urethra, and *total defibulation* extends the incision to reveal the clitoris, if present. The procedure is often performed during labor to allow vaginal delivery but may be completed in the nonpregnant woman desiring defibulation.

Preoperative counseling ideally discusses expected anatomic and physiologic changes. First, women with infibulation often have a slow urine stream, and they perceive menses and urine to originate from the same opening. Both will change after scar incision. Affected women also may be unfamiliar with the pink tones of normal vaginal mucosa, which will be visible following surgery. Patients are importantly reassured that defibulation does not affect virginity. Last, the length of defibulation is discussed. Some women request only the introitus and urethra to be unsheathed, whereas others prefer total defibulation to also uncover the clitoris. One excellent review is provided by Abdulcadir and coworkers (2018).

These same authors emphasize that postoperative pain may trigger symptoms of posttraumatic stress disorder, which can be present in women with prior FGM (Abdulcadir, 2017; Behrendt, 2005; Köbach, 2018). Also, in some participating cultures, blunt defibulation by the partner during coitus is a consummation custom. And, a narrow introitus is valued for male sexual pleasure. Thus, sensitivity to changes in the couple's sexuality is important (Johansen, 2017). Last, FGM is linked in many instances to culture and religion (Berg, 2013; Dehghankhalili, 2015). For all these reasons, current World Health Organization (2016) guidelines recommend psychologic support to patients undergoing surgical treatment of FGM.

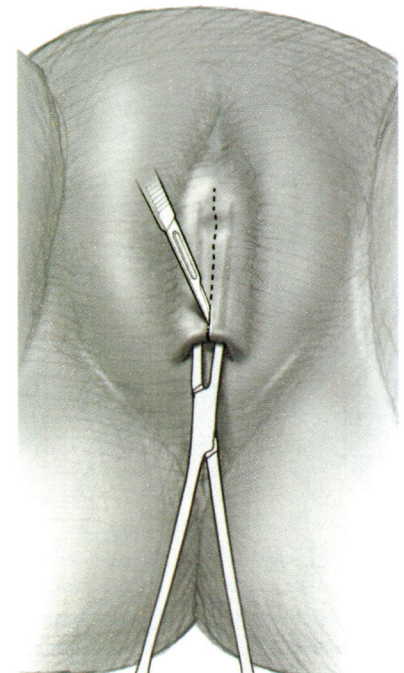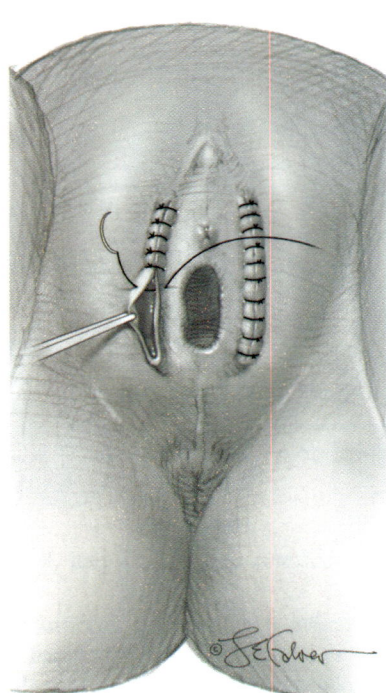

FIGURE 43-24.1 Midline scar division (*left*). Separated-edge suturing (*right*).

PREOPERATIVE

Consent

Women should have realistic and knowledgeable expectations as to the final size, shape, and color of the labia and vestibule. Wound complications such as hematoma, cellulitis, or incisional dehiscence are rare but are discussed during counseling. Postoperative dyspareunia is uncommon but should be noted. In most studies, female sexual functioning scores improve postoperatively (Berg, 2018; Krause, 2011; Nour, 2006).

Patient Preparation

Antibiotic or VTE prophylaxis is not required for this brief procedure in those without specific risks.

INTRAOPERATIVE

Surgical Steps

❶ Anesthesia and Patient Positioning. Defibulation is often performed as a day-surgery procedure using general or regional anesthesia. In-office procedures with local injection of anesthesia have been described. After anesthesia is delivered, the patient is placed in standard lithotomy position, and the vulva is surgically prepared.

❷ Midline Scar Division. To protect underlying structures, a tonsil clamp, hemostat, or other narrow clamp is insinuated while closed beneath the fused labia (Johnson, 2007). It is positioned beneath the planned incision path and then partially opened. Subsequent gentle outward tension pulls the fused labia away from the vagina, urethra, and clitoris as protection (Fig. 43-24.1, *left*). The scarred labia are then sharply divided in the midline. Scar tissue usually has poor vascularity, but hemostasis may be achieved as needed using electrosurgical coagulation to help avoid hematoma formation.

❸ Incision Closure. Skin edges on each side are reapproximated with interrupted stitches of 4-0 gauge delayed-absorbable (see Fig. 43-24.1, *right*).

❹ Examination under Anesthesia. If not previously accessible, the vaginal and cervix can be examination under anesthesia by placing a Graves speculum or other vaginal retractors. Pap testing or other needed testing also can be performed.

POSTOPERATIVE

Cool packs are used to relieve immediate discomfort during the first 24 hours. Mild oral analgesics may be required for the first few days. Perineal hygiene is emphasized during the initial weeks following surgery. Exercise may resume after wound healing. A 6-week abstinence period from intercourse is typical.

43-25

Vaginal Septum Excision

Described in Chapter 19 (p. 418), incorrect embryologic development may lead to transverse or longitudinal septa at various levels of the vagina. Some septa have small fenestrations to allow menstrual blood egress. Those without openings may lead to menstrual blood accumulation and distention of the vagina and uterus, that is, *hematocolpos* and *hematometra*, respectively. Symptoms include amenorrhea and pelvic pain. Obstructed cases also are accompanied by a high rate of comorbid endometriosis (Deligeoroglou, 2012; Smith, 2007; Williams, 2014).

Vaginal septum excision is best performed in a postpubertal adolescent or young adult. First, estrogen production following puberty can improve healing. Moreover, transverse septum excision requires some degree of postoperative vaginal dilation to avoid stricture, and regimen compliance may be limited in young girls. Unfortunately, not all cases can be delayed.

PREOPERATIVE

Patient Evaluation

Septa are frequently associated with other müllerian defects. Thus, anatomy and anomalies are usually defined preoperatively with three-dimensional sonography or more commonly with MR imaging (Chap. 19, p. 418).

Consent

Short-term risks are few, but wound separation or vaginal agglutination can complicate thicker septum excisions. The latter can be limited in part by use of a postoperative vaginal mold. Long term, vaginal stricture following excision is not infrequent (Joki-Erkkilä, 2003; Williams, 2014). Depending on the stricture severity, treatment ranges from self-applied vaginal dilator use to surgical reexcision. Dyspareunia also is a common potential long-term risk.

Patient Preparation

Antibiotic prophylaxis similar to that for hysterectomy is usually administered (Table 39-8, p. 832). VTE prophylaxis is typically not required unless a longer or more complex surgery is anticipated (Table 39-10, p. 834). Enema bowel preparation aids rectal

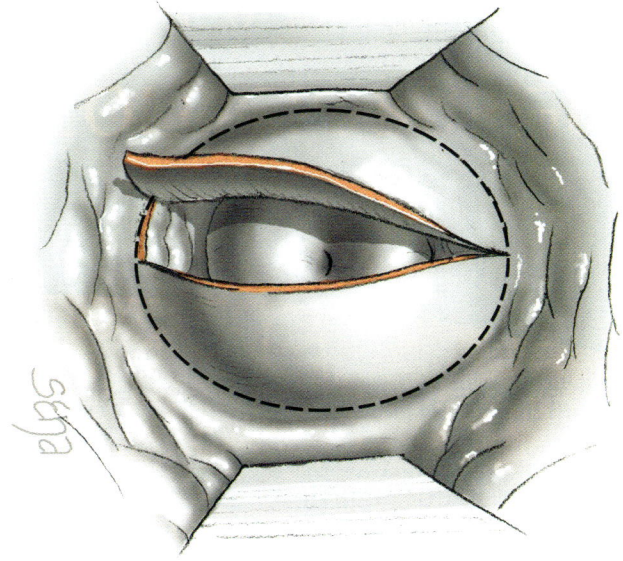

FIGURE 43-25.1 Transverse septum excision.

decompression to permit greater vaginal retraction for visualization. Also, digital rectal examination may be needed at times during surgery to direct septum excision and avoid rectal laceration. Accordingly, an empty rectal vault may minimize wound contamination.

INTRAOPERATIVE

Surgical Steps

❶ **Anesthesia and Patient Positioning.** After administration of general anesthesia, the patient is placed in standard lithotomy position, and the perineum and vagina are surgically prepared. A Foley catheter serves as a guide to avoid urethral injury during septum excision.

❷ **Transverse Septum Incision.** Retractors are placed to reveal the upper extent of the vagina. The septum is then incised transversely at its center to avoid laceration of the urethra, bladder, or rectum. A finger is placed through the transverse incision and is directed cephalad to delineate the upper vaginal walls and the circumferential margins of the septum. Similarly, the Foley catheter or a finger in the rectum may assist with orientation.

❸ **Excision.** Once the septum's perimeter and thickness is defined, the initial transverse incision is extended laterally to the vaginal wall margins. The septum is widely excised circumferentially along its base to minimize postoperative stricture (Fig. 43-25.1). Others surgeons prefer to create cruciate incisions similar to those with hymenectomy (p. 978). The four wedges are then trimmed close to the vaginal wall.

❹ **Wound Closure.** If the septum was thin, a simple circumferential ring of interrupted stitches is constructed using 2-0 gauge delayed-absorbable suture to reapproximate vaginal mucosal edges (Fig. 43-25.2). For thicker septa, the span between cephalad and caudad vaginal mucosal edges is greater. To permit mucosal edge reapproximation without suture-line tension, the vaginal mucosa is mobilized by undermining it both cephalad and caudad (Quint, 2010). Alternatively, vaginoplasty techniques to cover the exposed vaginal walls can be used (Arkoulis, 2017; Garcia, 1967; Wierrani, 2003). Last, if the vaginal septum is thick and mucosal reapproximation is not possible, a tissue graft can be applied in a manner similar to that described in the neovagina section (p. 997).

❺ **Unobstructed Longitudinal Septum.** With this septum, a pliable tissue sheet attaches to and extends between the anterior and posterior vaginal walls. This divides the vagina into right and left cylinders. Surgery starts distally and moves proximally to cut the septum's anterior and posterior vaginal wall attachments. Initial division of the anterior wall attachment is followed by initial severing of the posterior wall one. Proximal progress thus alternates between the anterior and posterior walls.

To excise the vaginal wall attachment, use of an electrosurgical blade may simultaneously achieve division and hemostasis (Brucker, 2011; Quint, 2010). A simple line of interrupted stitches of 2-0 gauge delayed-absorbable suture is placed to reapproximate incised vaginal mucosal edges. Instead, serial clamping of the septum, sharp incision, and suture ligation can be used to progress proximally (Fedele, 2012). With either method, some tissue retraction is expected, but the

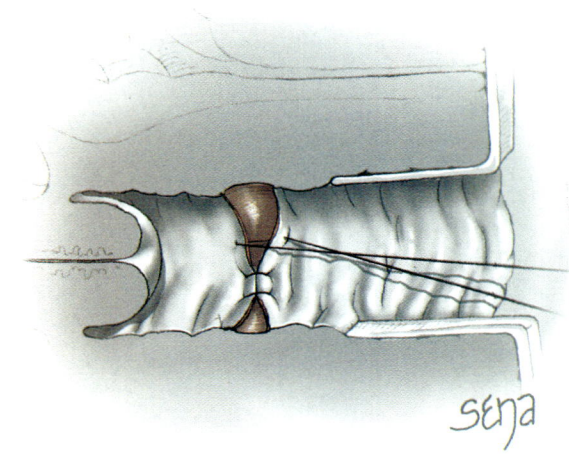

FIGURE 43-25.2 Vaginal mucosa reapproximation.

incision is kept near the union line of the septum and vaginal wall. This practice averts creation of a tissue ridge and potential later dyspareunia. The Foley catheter can act as a guide to avoid urethral or bladder neck laceration. A finger in the rectum prior to excision can define its proximity to the septum.

For a distal septum, these sequential steps will free it. For septa that extend further proximally and end between two cervices, the division should stop short of the cervix to avoid its injury. A final anteroposterior incision across the septa and in front of the cervices will release it proximally.

❻ Obstructive Longitudinal Septum. With an obstructive septum, its proximal end often originates between the two cervices of a uterine didelphys or other bicollis anomaly. Specifically, it may be part of the obstructed hemivagina and ipsilateral renal anomaly (OHVIRA) syndrome (Chap. 19, p. 419). The caudal end attaches to the right or left lateral vaginal wall to block outflow. With complete obstruction, the hemivagina distends with menstrual blood.

For excision, a longitudinal incision is made centrally along the septum, and old blood is suctioned to clear the surgical field. A finger is then placed through the incision to delineate the wall boundaries of the obstructed hemivagina and identify the occult cervix. Foley catheter tubing and a finger in the rectum may help delineate anterior and posterior vaginal wall limits, respectively. Once the septal perimeter is defined, the initial longitudinal incision is extended outward. In sum, an ellipse of tissue is excised to reach the anterior, posterior, and ipsilateral vaginal wall margins (Candiani, 1997; Dietrich, 2014; Smith, 2007). A simple line of interrupted stitches of 2-0 gauge delayed-absorbable suture is placed to reapproximate incised vaginal mucosal edges.

POSTOPERATIVE

Following septum excision, the Foley catheter is removed that day, and diet and daily activities can resume as tolerated. Vaginal discharge is expected and may last for days to a few weeks. Intercourse is delayed for 6 weeks postsurgery.

With excision of a thick transverse septum that requires graft interposition, a cylindrical vaginal stent or mold is placed, and care follows that for the McIndoe procedure, described next (p. 998).

43-26

Neovagina Creation

Creation of a functional vagina is the treatment goal for most individuals with congenital vaginal agenesis. Discussed in Chapter 19 (p. 421), passive serial vaginal dilation over time is successful in more than 90 percent of cases and is preferred (American College of Obstetricians and Gynecologists, 2018a). However, after appropriate counseling, several surgical and nonsurgical approaches may be suitable for those who fail serial dilation or who prefer surgical intervention.

Of options, the Vecchietti procedure uses upward pressure against the vaginal dimple to lengthen the vagina gradually over several days (Vecchietti, 1965). In overview, surgery places a bead-shaped "olive" at the vaginal dimple on the vestibule. Two sutures threaded through the bead traverse the vaginal remnant to enter the abdomen. Each suture then travels within an ipsilateral extraperitoneal tunnel to reach the anterior abdominal wall. Attached here to a traction plate, the sutures are sequentially tightened to increase upward pressure by the olive against the dimple. This lengthens and creates the neovaginal space.

Instead, with the McIndoe procedure, sharp dissection between the urethra/bladder and the rectum creates the neovaginal space (McIndoe, 1938). The space is then lined by a skin graft. Other variations use graft materials that include buccal mucosa, peritoneum, myocutaneous flaps, amnionic membrane, absorbable adhesion barrier, and autologous vaginal tissue (Creatsas, 2010; Davydov, 1974; Li, 2014; Motoyama, 2003; Sabatucci, 2019; Vatsa, 2017). The Shears procedure uses no graft material (Kuhn, 2013; Shears, 1960).

Vaginal stricture or shortening can be a significant complication. Thus, adherence to a postoperative regimen of vaginal dilation is mandatory. For this reason, surgery may be postponed until the patient has reached the level of maturity needed for compliance.

PREOPERATIVE

Patient Evaluation

Vaginal agenesis may be an isolated anomaly but is frequently associated with other müllerian defects. Thus, anatomy and anomalies are usually preoperatively defined with sonography or more commonly with MR imaging (Chap. 19, p. 421).

Consent

Prior to surgery, patients are informed of overall success rates of a given surgery. With the Vecchietti procedure, functional success rates range from 83 to 96 percent in systematic reviews (Callen, 2014; McQuillan, 2014). A laparoscopic technique appears to afford an equivalent vaginal outcome but also MIS advantages (Borruto, 1999). Rates of major complications approximate 1 to 2 percent, and these include bladder or rectal injury or infection (Brucker, 2008; Callen, 2014). Less common issues are hematoma, fistula, granulation tissue, dyspareunia, and need for subsequent vaginal dilation. Later pelvic organ prolapse appears infrequently (Huebner, 2018).

The McIndoe procedure provides a functional vagina to afford "satisfactory" intercourse in 90 to 97 percent of patients (Callens, 2014; Panici, 2011). From larger case series, complication rates approximate 10 to 20 percent and included vaginal stricture, dyspareunia, pelvic organ prolapse, graft failure, postcoital bleeding, fistulas involving either the bladder or rectum, and surgical reintervention for these (Alessandrescu, 1996; Cali, 1968; Klingele, 2003). Complications also can develop at the skin graft harvest site.

Patient Preparation

Antibiotic prophylaxis similar to that for hysterectomy is typically administered, and VTE prophylaxis is planned (Tables 39-8 and 39-10, p. 832). Bowel preparation aids rectal decompression to permit greater room for blunt neovagina development. Also, digital rectal examination is intermittently done during surgery to guide dissection and avoid rectal laceration. An empty rectal vault may minimize wound contamination.

INTRAOPERATIVE

Instruments

For the Vecchietti procedure, two options can serve as the olive. One is a 2-cm acrylic bead. The other is a segmented, dilator-shaped "dummy" that measures 2.5 × 10 cm. The latter's centipede-like segmentation gives flexibility to this device's length. Another needed tool is the thin 16 × 6 cm traction plate that will ultimately lie across the lower abdomen and will secure the traction sutures. To carry traction sutures through the vaginal remnant, some use a specific Vecchietti suture-carriage needle. An Endo Close or Carter-Thomason laparoscopic suture-carriage needle device also is suitable. Last, cystoscopy equipment is needed to help guide intraoperative needle passage and exclude bladder perforation.

With the McIndoe procedure, skin grafts for the neovagina are harvested from the donor site with the aid of an electrodermatome. This device can shave grafts of varying size and depth.

Following graft harvesting and creation of the neovaginal space, a stent applies the graft to the vaginal walls and holds it in place. Soft stents are preferred, and inflatable rubber stents or condoms filled with foam rubber or other soft compressible materials are examples (Adamson, 2004; Barutcu, 1998). The vagina graft produces abundant exudates, and poor drainage may lead to graft maceration, sloughing, and detachment. Accordingly, suction is attached to the soft stents to aid drainage of the neovaginal space (Yu, 2004).

Surgical Steps—Vecchietti Procedure

❶ **Anesthesia and Patient Positioning.** General anesthesia is administered. The patient is placed in standard lithotomy position in booted support stirrups, and perineal and abdominal cleansing is performed.

❷ **Abdominal Entry.** Initially, laparoscopic access at the umbilicus is gained as described in Chapter 41 (p. 888). After inspection of the pelvis, a 5-mm laparoscopic port is placed in each lower abdominal quadrant at the site intended for exit of each traction suture.

❸ **Tunnel Creation.** To begin, an extraperitoneal tunnel is created bilaterally along the inner surface of the lower anterior abdominal wall. Each tunnel will house one of the two traction suture strands and guide it outside the abdomen. On each side, the tunnel extends from the trocar port site to a point just lateral to the vaginal remnant.

On the first side, the peritoneum medial to the port is tented outward by a laparoscopic grasper. It is incised to create a 1-cm rent in the peritoneum. Through this rent, a narrow-tipped laparoscopic grasper is insinuated beneath the peritoneum. This grasper advances beneath the peritoneum to the pelvis, and thereby, a narrow extraperitoneal tunnel is created in its path. In the pelvis and near the vaginal remnant, the grasper tip dissects through the peritoneum to re-enter the abdomen proper. During tunnel creation, dissection remains superficial to avoid laceration of the inferior epigastric and external iliac vessels.

❹ **Traction Suture Tunneling.** Next, a long, large-gauge, delayed-absorbable or

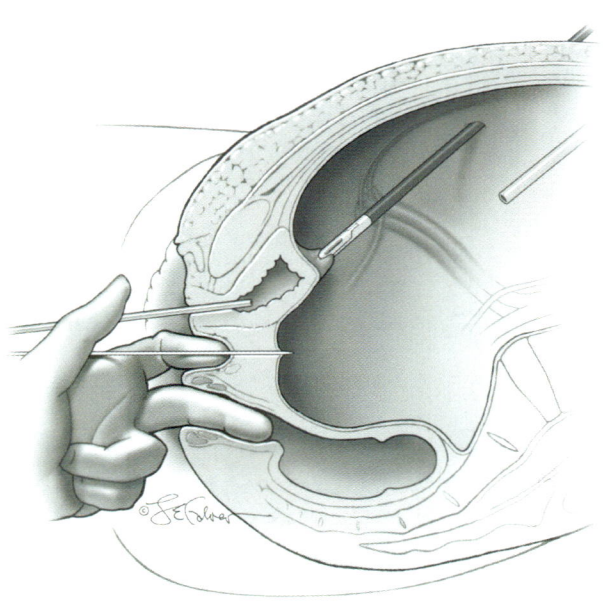

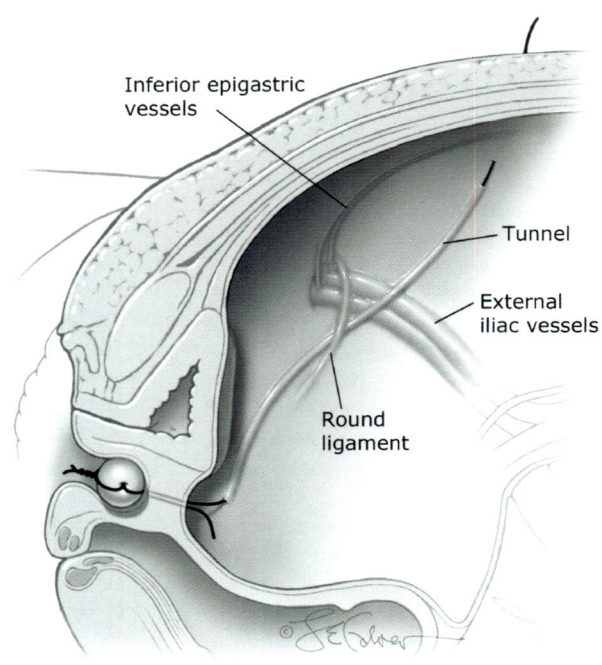

FIGURE 43-26.1 Needle passage through neovagina space.

FIGURE 43-26.2 Traction sutures extend from the olive device through the extraperitoneal tunnels to reach the abdomen.

permanent suture is grabbed outside the abdomen by the initial tunneling grasper and introduced though the laparoscopic port. Once within the abdomen, the grasper follows its previous course through the extraperitoneal tunnel. At the distal tunnel opening, the suture strand is passed to another grasper, and the initial grasper retreats through the tunnel and out the port. At this point, the strand has one end in the abdomen and one end outside the abdomen. This tunneling process is repeated on the opposite side.

❺ Needle Passage. To retrieve the abdominal end of the traction suture, a vaginal surgeon first places the suture-carriage needle at the vaginal dimple and directs it upward through the potential space between the urethra/bladder and rectum. Concurrent cystoscopy and downward pressure from a finger in the rectum help avoid organ puncture (Fig. 43-26.1). Simultaneously, a laparoscopic surgeon elevates and retracts the bladder dome laparoscopically with graspers to avert cystotomy. The needle traverses the vaginal remnant and enters the abdomen.

Here, a laparoscopic grasper delivers the intraabdominal end of the traction strand to the carriage needle. The carriage needle is then removed and carries the traction suture with it. At this point, the strand has one end outside the abdomen and one end at the vaginal dimple.

This process then is repeated again. With this, the second dimple puncture is moved

a bit lateral to the first to accommodate the olive's diameter.

This just-described pathway of suture passage guides the traction strands from a sterile starting point to the more bacteria-rich vaginal dimple. However, other descriptions of the procedure describe a reversed path and an upward ascent of traction sutures through the remnant and to the abdominal wall (Brucker, 2008; Fedele, 2000).

❻ Securing the Traction Sutures. At the vaginal dimple, both traction strands are threaded through the olive and secured to the olive with multiple knots (Fig. 43-26.2). Laparoscopic port site are next closed as described in Chapter 41 (p. 895). Last, the

extraabdominal ends of the traction sutures are threaded into the traction plate, which now lies across the lower abdomen. This plate will allow the traction sutures to be tightened gradually during the next 6 to 8 days.

Surgical Steps—McIndoe Procedure

❶ Anesthesia and Patient Positioning. General anesthesia is administered, and the patient is initially positioned prone for skin graft harvesting from the buttock. Alternatively, skin may be obtained from the thigh or hip. Choosing a location that has minimal hair growth and is cosmetically

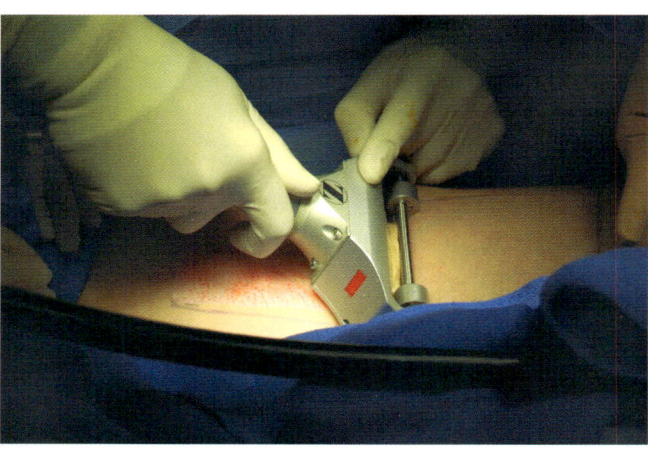

FIGURE 43-26.3 Skin graft harvest.

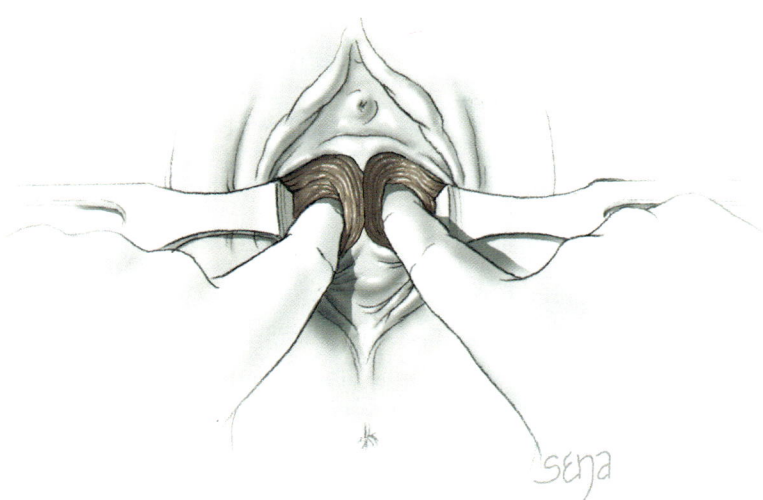

FIGURE 43-26.4 Neovaginal dissection.

discreet is desired. The assistance of a plastic surgeon can be enlisted for skin graft procurement.

❷ Skin Graft. The surgeon first marks the outline of the wound on the donor-site skin, enlarging it by 3 to 5 percent to allow for skin shrinkage immediately after excision. The surgeon uses the electrodermatome to remove a single strip of skin that is typically 0.018 inch thick, 8 to 9 cm wide, and 18 to 20 cm long (Fig. 43-26.3). Alternatively, two smaller strips of 5 cm × 10 cm can be obtained from each buttock.

Following excision, the graft is placed in a pan of sterile saline. The harvest sites are sprayed with a topical hemostatic agent and dressed with a clear occlusive dressing (Tegaderm).

❸ Perineal Incision. The patient is then placed in standard lithotomy position, perineal cleansing is performed, and a Foley catheter inserted. The lower edge of each

labia minora is grasped with Allis clamps and extended laterally. A third Allis clamp is placed on the vestibular skin below the urethra and is lifted superiorly. A dimple in the vestibule is typically identified below the urethra, and a 2- to 3-cm transverse incision is made across the depression. Allis clamps are then placed on the superior and inferior edges of this incision and are retracted.

❹ Neovaginal Dissection. With neovagina development, the goal is to create a canal that is bounded anteriorly by the connective tissue that supports the urethra and bladder, posteriorly by the tissue supporting the rectum, and laterally by the puborectalis muscles. Initially, two canals are created on either side of the median raphe, which is a midline collection of dense connective tissue bands that stretch between the urethra/bladder above

and the rectum below (Fig. 43-26.4). The canals are initially formed using a spreading and gentle pushing motion with blunt-tipped scissors. Fingers are then insinuated into the forming tunnels, and pressure is exerted cephalad to extend the tunnel depth. To widen the canals, finger pads are rolled outward, and lateral pressure is applied. Posterior pressure is avoided to prevent entering the rectum. Each canal is extended to reach near the rectouterine pouch (cul-de-sac of Douglas).

During dissection, several points are noteworthy. First, with initial caudal dissection, the surgeon may meet greater resistance than with the more cephalad tissues. Second, remaining in the correct dissection plane can be difficult. Accordingly, the surgeon's finger may be placed into the rectum to identify its location and avert perforation. Similarly, the Foley catheter tubing may serve as an orienting tool anteriorly.

To expand the space, retractors can be placed along the lateral walls of the forming tunnels and stretched outward. Cephalad, the tunnel is extended to within 2 cm of the cul-de-sac of Douglas. This leaves a layer of connective tissue affixed to the peritoneum. The skin graft will attach more effectively to this connective tissue than to a smooth peritoneal surface. Rates of subsequent enterocele formation are also lowered by this technique.

❺ Cutting the Median Raphe. Once the two tunnels are developed, the median raphe is cut. The final single canal measures

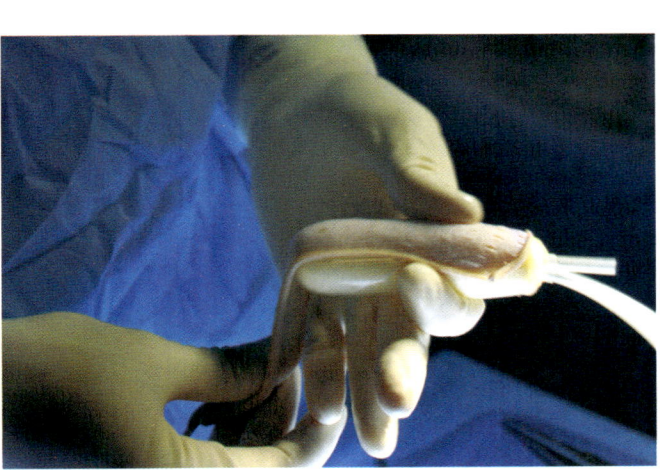

FIGURE 43-26.5 Mold creation.

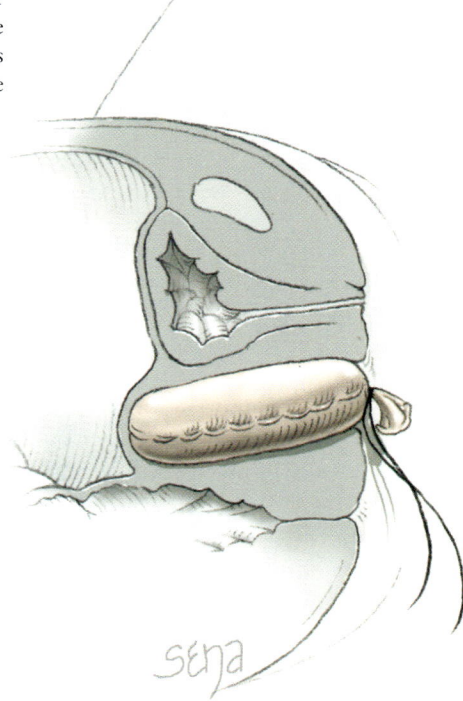

FIGURE 43-26.6 Skin graft and mold in place.

approximately 10 cm deep and three finger-breadths wide. As collections of blood can separate the skin graft from the canal bed, hemostasis is required prior to mold insertion.

6 Mold Preparation. The vaginal mold may now be covered with the harvested skin. The graft is removed from the saline bath. One end of the graft is placed at the base of one side of the mold with the skin's keratinized surface facing the mold. The long axis of the graft is laid parallel to the long axis of the mold. The graft is then draped up and over the mold tip (Fig. 43-26.5). Last, the lateral edges of the skin graft are approximated on either side of the mold using interrupted stitches of 3-0 catgut.

Adapting the mold to the size of the created neovaginal canal is essential. If the mold width is too large, pressure necrosis or inadequate drainage may result. Moreover, at the time of postoperative mold removal, a mold

that is too large and snuggly fitted into the neovagina may pull the graft loose. Once appropriately sized and constructed, the mold is then inserted (Fig. 43-26.6).

7 Perineal Sutures. The edges of the skin graft at the distal end of the mold are then reapproximated to the distal opening of the neovagina using interrupted stitches of 4-0 or 5-0 gauge delayed-absorbable suture. An elastic compression dressing is placed on the perineum.

POSTOPERATIVE

With the Vecchietti procedure, the traction sutures are tightened daily for 7 to 8 days. For this, suitable analgesia is provided. Foley catheter drainage is not required after the first day. VTE prophylaxis is generally used until patients are fully ambulating.

Once home, the patient must maintain and widen the neovaginal space by daily application for 8 to 10 hours of progressively enlarging dilators. This practice continues until regular vaginal coitus is resumed. Vaginal estrogen-based cream is used initially to promote neovaginal epithelization. Intercourse can be resumed as early as 3 weeks postprocedure and as tolerated.

With the McIndoe procedure, the soft stent is left in place for 7 days following surgery. To minimize mold dislodgement and wound contamination, a low-residue diet and loperamide is used to limit defecation. Following mold removal, a plastic dilator is worn continuously except during defecation during the first 6 weeks. During the subsequent 6 weeks, it is used only at night. Following these initial 3 months, patients are then instructed to either wear the dilator at night or engage in intercourse at least twice each week.

43-27

Excision of Preinvasive Cervical Lesions

LOOP ELECTROSURGICAL EXCISION PROCEDURE

In the United States, use of LEEP for cervical intraepithelial neoplasia (CIN) is popular and often preferred over cryotherapy or laser ablation. This procedure, also known as *large loop excision of the transformation zone (LLETZ)*, uses electric current through a monopolar wire electrode to either cut or coagulate cervical tissues. As such, these thin, semicircular electrodes allow clinicians to excise cervical lesions with minimal patient discomfort, expense, and complication. Moreover, unlike ablative procedures, LEEP permits submission of a surgical specimen for additional evaluation. Last, the procedure can be tailored to treat ectocervical lesions or to perform more extensive conization procedures.

PREOPERATIVE

Patient Evaluation

In the United States, women typically receive colposcopic evaluation and histologic interpretation of cervical biopsies prior to LEEP. Less commonly, a "see and treat" approach, in which immediate treatment rather than biopsy is initiated during colposcopy, is also acceptable for specific settings outlined in Chapter 29 (p. 634) (Ebisch, 2016).

For LEEP, patient evaluation includes her suitability for an in-office procedure. Office procedures offer lower expense and fewer anesthetic risks, however, markedly relaxed vaginal sidewalls may require significant and potentially uncomfortable retraction for adequate visualization. Also, a lesion or transformation zone that lies near the cervix periphery may risk vaginal or bladder injury during electrode-pass completion, especially if the patient moves unexpectedly. Last, patient comorbidities or anxiety may hinder her ability to remain relatively motionless. All three favor greater anesthesia in a surgical suite.

Consent

This procedure has overall complication rates that approximate 10 percent (Dunn, 2004). However, major complications are rare (0.5 percent) and may include bowel or bladder injury and hemorrhage (Dunn, 2003; Kurata, 2003). Short-term complications such as abdominal pain, heavier vaginal bleeding,

and bladder spasm are treated symptomatically. Light vaginal bleeding or discharge is expected, and patients are so counseled.

Long-term complications include cervical stenosis and failure to completely treat the neoplasia. However, failure rates are low (approximately 5 percent) and positively correlate with initial lesion size (Mitchell, 1998). Persistent disease is typically diagnosed by the first postoperative surveillance testing following LEEP. Cervical stenosis is estimated to complicate <6 percent of cases. Risk factors include endocervical disease, excision of a large tissue volume, and menopausal status (Baldauf, 1996; Kiuchi, 2016; Suh-Burgmann, 2000).

The effects of LEEP on obstetric outcomes are unclear. Several studies show that pregnancy is not adversely affected by LEEP, whereas others note higher risks of premature labor and premature rupture of membranes (Conner, 2014; Heinonen, 2013; Werner, 2010).

Patient Preparation

Ideally, LEEP is performed after completion of menses. This decreases the chance of a coexistent early pregnancy and allows cervical healing prior to the next menstrual cycle. With surgery prior to menses, abnormal postprocedural bleeding may be masked, and postsurgical swelling can block menstrual flow and intensify cramping. A normal bimanual examination is confirmed prior to surgery. If there is a possibility of pregnancy, β-hCG testing precedes treatment.

Perioperatively, LEEP excision in general does not require antibiotic or VTE prophylaxis. Bowel preparation is not needed.

INTRAOPERATIVE

Instruments

Tissue excision during LEEP requires an electrosurgical unit, wire loop electrodes, insulated speculum, and smoke evacuation system. Electrosurgical units used in LEEP procedures generate high-frequency (350 to 1200 kHz), low-voltage (200 to 500 V) electric current. Because of the risk for electric burns to the patient from stray current, grounding pads are placed on conductive tissue that is close to the operative site (Chap. 40, p. 857).

Similarly, an insulated speculum is used to limit the risk of stray current conductance to the patient. Insulation should be inspected prior to use, as small breaks can concentrate current if the active loop contacts the speculum. The insulated speculum has a port for smoke evacuation tubing, which assists in clearing smoke from the operating field to improve visualization and lower inhalation risks. Surgical smoke plumes can contain benzene, hydrogen cyanide, formaldehyde, and viruses, and thus local smoke evacuation systems are recommended (National Institute for Occupational Safety and Health, 1999). That said, transmission of infectious disease through surgical smoke has not been documented (Mowbray, 2013).

Electric current is directed to tissue via a 0.2-mm stainless steel or tungsten wire-loop electrode. These are available in various sizes to customize treatment according to lesion dimensions (Fig. 43-27.1). These instruments are disposable and discarded after each patient procedure.

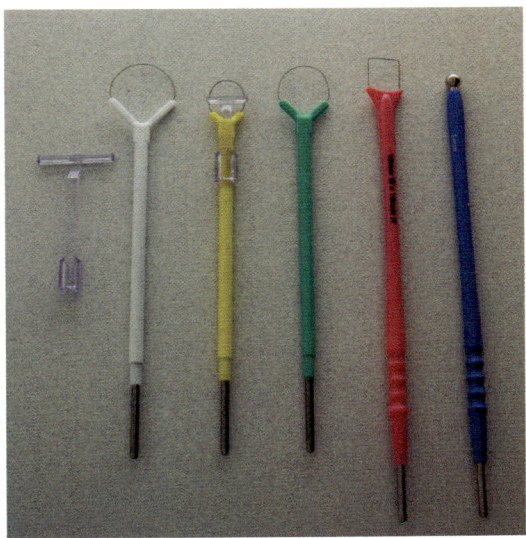

FIGURE 43-27.1 Various loop electrosurgical excision procedure (LEEP) electrodes.

SECTION 6

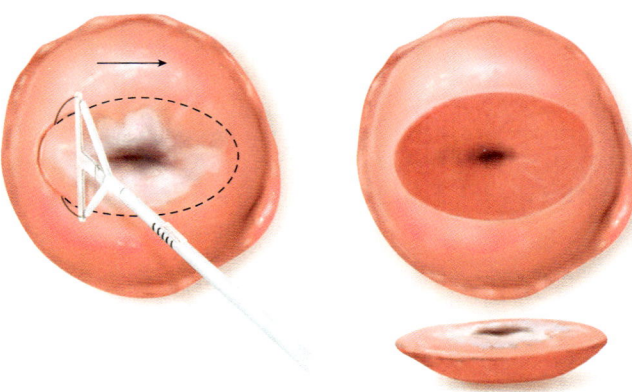

FIGURE 43-27.2 Single-pass loop electrosurgical excision.

Surgical Steps

❶ Anesthesia and Patient Positioning.
The patient's bladder should be empty at the procedure's start. The patient is placed in standard lithotomy position, and the electrosurgical grounding pad is placed on the upper thigh or buttock. The insulated speculum is inserted into the vagina, and smoke evacuation tubing is attached. The application of Lugol solution outlines lesion margins before starting the procedure (Chap. 29, p. 634).

For in-office anesthesia, vasoconstricting solutions of either: (1) vasopressin in a 1-percent lidocaine solution (10 units Pitressin in 30 mL of lidocaine) or (2) 1-percent lidocaine with epinephrine (10 µg/mL) in a manufactured 1:100,000 dilution may be selected. A 25- to 27-gauge spinal needle is used to circumferentially inject 5 to 10 mL of either solution 1 to 2 cm deep into the cervix outside the area to be excised. Cervical blanching usually follows. Alternatively, application of 4 puffs (40 mg) of 10-percent lidocaine spray to the ectocervix provides effective analgesia (Limwatanapan, 2018; Vanichtantikul, 2013).

❷ Single-Pass Excision. Ideally, the cervical transformation zone and CIN lesion is excised, and the appropriately sized loop is selected for this goal. If colposcopy is satisfactory, the correct loop diameter incorporates the transformation zone to a depth of 5 to 8 mm. The electrosurgical unit is set to cutting mode, and typically 30 to 50 W is used depending on the loop size. Larger loops require higher wattage.

To excise the transformation zone, a loop is positioned 3 to 5 mm outside the lateral perimeter of the area (Fig. 43-27.2). Current through the loop is activated prior to tissue contact, and electric sparks at the loop tip may be seen. The loop is introduced to the cervix at a right angle to ectocervix. Once a 5- to 8-mm depth is reached, the loop is then drawn parallel to the surface until a point 3 to 5 mm outside the opposite border of the transformation zone and CIN lesion is reached. The loop is then withdrawn slowly, positioning it again at right angles to the surface. Current is stopped as soon as the loop exits the tissue. Following excision, the specimen is placed in formalin for pathologic evaluation.

❸ Multiple-Pass Excision. Less commonly, bulky lesions may require multiple passes using a combination of loop electrode sizes (Fig. 43-27.3).

❹ Hemostasis. Despite use of vasoconstrictors, bleeding following LEEP is common. Sites of active bleeding may be controlled using a 3- or 5-mm ball electrode, and the electrosurgical unit switched to coagulation mode. Alternatively, Monsel paste can be applied with direct pressure to bleeding sites.

POSTOPERATIVE

A watery vaginal discharge that develops after treatment usually requires light sanitary pad use, but tampons are discouraged. Vaginal spotting is expected and can persist for weeks. During the first few days following LEEP, patients may complain of diffuse mild lower abdominal pain or cramping for which NSAIDs typically provide relief. Patients abstain from intercourse during the 4 weeks following surgery. Depending on patient symptoms, work and exercise may resume following treatment.

CERVICAL CONIZATION

Cervical conization removes ectocervical lesions and a portion of the endocervical canal by means of a conical tissue biopsy (Fig. 43-27.4). It is a safe, effective means to treat CIN, carcinoma in situ (CIS), and adenocarcinoma in situ (AIS). Moreover, cervical conization is a standard treatment for women with inadequate colposcopy and biopsies that suggest high-grade CIN. Last, it is used to investigate those with discordant cytologic and histologic findings.

Excision may be completed with a scalpel, termed *cold-knife conization*. Alternatively, laser or LEEP conization may be performed. Success rates for these excisional methods

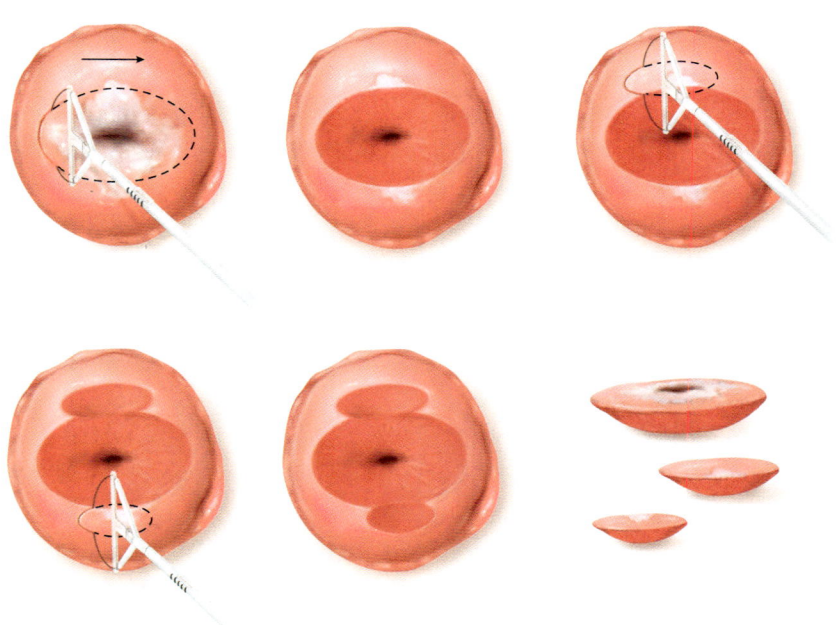

FIGURE 43-27.3 Multiple-pass excision.

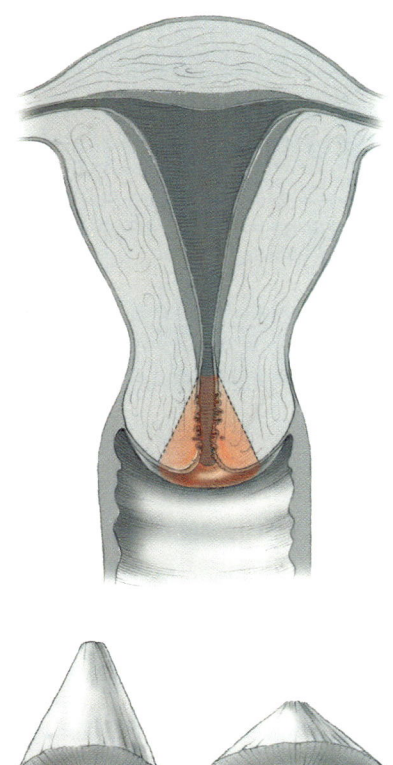

FIGURE 43-27.4 Cone-shaped tissue biopsies.

in the treatment of CIN are equivalent. However, LEEP conization has gained popularity because of its ease of use and lower cost.

PREOPERATIVE

Patient Evaluation

Prior to conization, patients will have undergone colposcopic examination and histologic evaluation of biopsies. β-hCG testing is warranted prior to conization if pregnancy is suspected. If pregnancy is confirmed and invasion is not suspected colposcopically, postpartum patient management is reasonable. Conization during pregnancy has great morbidity because of increased vascularity and subsequent cone-bed bleeding.

Consent

Risks associated with conization mirror those for LEEP excision of ectocervical lesions. However, cold-knife conization has a higher risk of bleeding compared with laser or LEEP conization. Moreover, cold-knife and laser conizations carry greater risks of cervical stenosis compared with LEEP conization (Baldauf, 1996; Houlard, 2002). Increasing age and depth of endocervical excision are significant cervical stenosis risks. Penna and

coworkers (2005) noted a lower risk of stenosis in postmenopausal women using estrogen replacement therapy compared with postmenopausal nonusers.

Cervical conization for CIN treatment is associated with a risk of adverse outcomes in subsequent pregnancies. These include preterm delivery, low-birthweight neonates, incompetent cervix, and cervical stenosis (Bjørge, 2016; Kristensen, 1993a,b; Kyrgiou, 2017). Although obstetric outcomes do not differ among the three techniques, increased cone biopsy size positively correlates with rates of preterm delivery and premature membrane rupture (Mathevet, 2003; Sadler, 2004). Cold-knife conization generally removes more cervical stroma than other excisional methods. Additionally, a short conization-to-pregnancy interval has been associated with a higher miscarriage risk (Ciavattinni, 2015; Conner, 2014). This association may partly be explained by incomplete regeneration of the cervix, as the process is not complete until 6 months postprocedure. In patients who have undergone LEEP conization, cervical dimensions attain approximately 90 percent of their baseline measurements (Song, 2016).

COLD-KNIFE CONIZATION

Surgical Steps

❶ Anesthesia and Patient Positioning. For most women, cold-knife conization is a day-surgery procedure performed under general or regional anesthesia. Following administration of anesthesia, the patient is placed in the standard lithotomy position. The vagina is surgically prepared, the bladder emptied, and vaginal sidewalls retracted to reveal the cervix. Areas of planned excision may be more easily identified following Lugol solution application.

❷ Vasoconstrictor Injection. Bleeding during cold-knife conization can be brisk and obscure the operating field. Accordingly, preventative steps can be taken perioperatively. First, vasoconstrictors described for LEEP are injected circumferentially into the cervix (p. 1000). Additionally, descending cervical branches of the uterine arteries, which supply the cervix, can be ligated with figure-eight stitches using nonpermanent suture. These are placed along the lateral aspects of the cervix at 3 and 9 o'clock. After the knots are secured, the sutures are kept long and held by hemostats to manipulate the cervix.

❸ Atrophic Cervix. If the cervix is flush with the vagina, altered anatomy raises the risk of bladder or rectal injury. First, the

bladder may be inadvertently grasped by the tenaculum. Second, deviation away from the endocervical canal during cone excision may lacerate the bladder or rectum. As an aid, stay sutures are anchored at 12 and 6 o'clock at the cervicovaginal junction in addition to those at 3 and 9 o'clock. Outward traction helps delineate cervical margins during excision. Discussed next, a uterine sound can help guide a symmetric circumferential excision.

❹ Conization. A uterine sound or small-caliber uterine dilator is placed into the endocervical canal to orient the surgeon as to the depth and direction of the canal. Using a no. 11 blade, the surgeon initiates the incision on the lower lip of the cervix. This limits blood from running downward and obscuring the planned incision path. Alternatively, a Beaver blade, which is a triangular-shaped knife blade with a 45-degree bend, may be used (Fig. 43-27.5). With either blade, a circumscribing incision creates a 2- to 3-mm border around the entire lesion (Fig. 43-27.6). The 45-degree angle of the blade is directed centrally and cephalad to excise a conical specimen. Toothed forceps or tissue hooks may be used to retract the ectocervix during cone creation. After incision of the ectocervix, a scalpel or Mayo scissors cuts the deep tip of the cone and releases the specimen. A suture is placed on the site of the specimen that corresponds to its 12 o'clock position in situ. The location of this suture is noted on the pathology requisition form and allows the pathologist to report positive and negative margin sites relative to their clock position.

❺ Endocervical Curettage. Following removal of the cone specimen, endocervical curettage is performed to evaluate for presence of residual disease distal to the excised cone apex. This is sent as a separate specimen for evaluation.

❻ Hemostasis. With excision of the specimen, bleeding is common and can be controlled with individual suturing of isolated vessels, with electrosurgical coagulation, or with Sturmdorf sutures. In

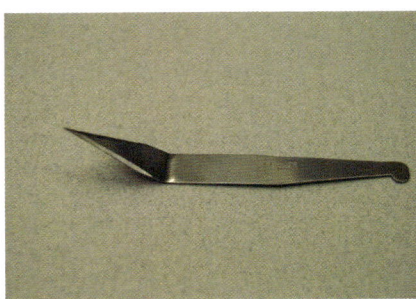

FIGURE 43-27.5 Beaver blade.

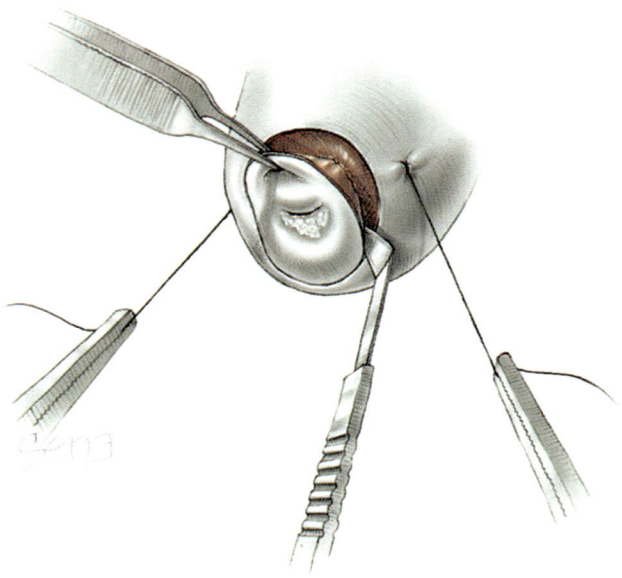

FIGURE 43-27.6 Conization incision.

addition, a topical hemostatic agent such as absorbable methylcellulose mesh can be placed in the cone bed. Last, Monsel paste is often placed in the cone bed to address minor bleeding.

With placement of Sturmdorf sutures, a running locked suture line closes the cone bed by circumferentially folding the cut ectocervical edge inward toward the endocervix.

This technique is less favored due to increased rates of postoperative dysmenorrhea, unsatisfactory postoperative surveillance Pap testing, and concerns that the flap might conceal residual disease (Kristensen, 1990; Trimbos, 1983). In contrast, a running, circumferential locked suture line may be placed at the incision edge without inverting the ectocervix.

LOOP ELECTROSURGICAL EXCISION PROCEDURE CONIZATION

Surgical Steps

The surgical steps for this more extensive LEEP mirror those used for excision of ectocervical lesions (p. 1000). However, to remove a portion of the endocervical canal, a deeper pass is made through the cervical stroma. This may be accomplished with a single, deep pass using one large loop.

Alternatively, to minimize the volume of tissue excised, a tiered or *top hat technique* can be selected. With this method, an initial pass is made to remove ectocervical lesions as previously described (see Fig. 43-27.2, p. 1000). To remove endocervical canal tissue, a second smaller loop is passed more deeply into the cervical stroma (Fig. 43-27.7). As a result, the tissue is excised in two pieces, and both are sent for evaluation. Similar to cold-knife conization, the specimen is marked with suture to note its 12 o'clock position in situ.

LASER CONIZATION

Excision of a laser cone biopsy specimen uses techniques similar to those described for laser ablation (p. 1005). However, rather than ablating the involved tissue, laser energy

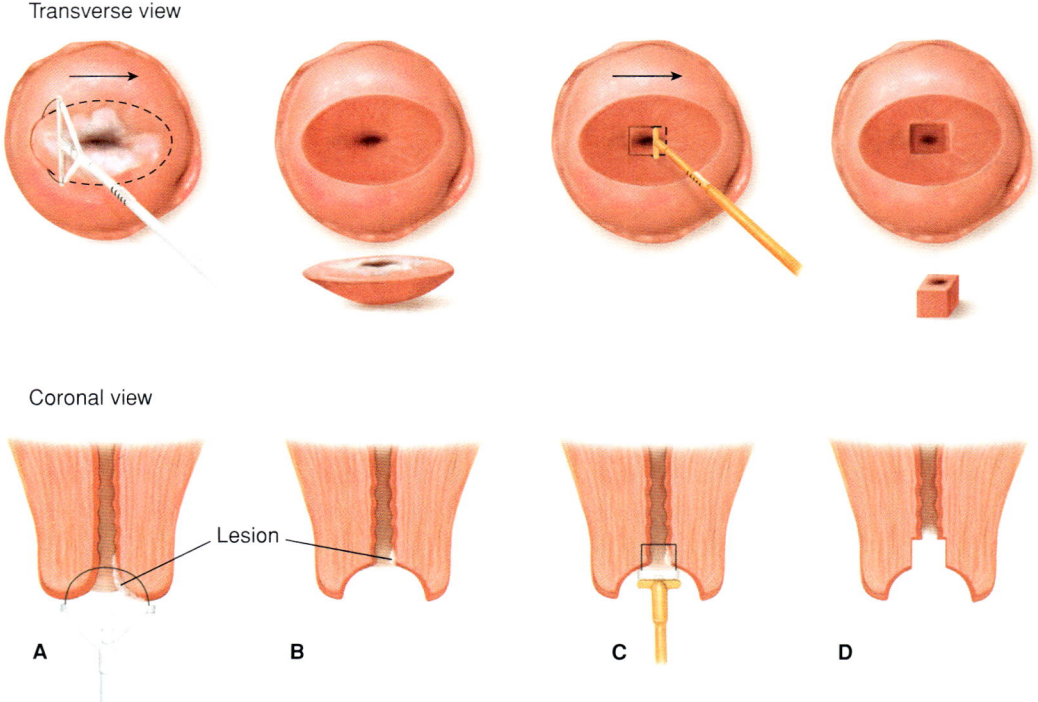

Transverse view

Coronal view

Lesion

A   B   C   D

FIGURE 43-27.7 Loop electrosurgical excision procedure (LEEP) "top hat" cervical conization procedure transverse (*upper row*) and coronal (*lower row*) views. **A.** Excision of ectocervical portion of lesion. **B.** Appearance of cervix following ectocervical excision. **C.** Excision of endocervical portion of lesion. **D.** Appearance of cervix upon procedure completion.

is directed to cut and remove the cone-biopsy specimen. A higher power density is used to create a cutting effect, for example, 25 W with a 1-mm spot size (power density = 2500 W/cm^2). A cone-shaped specimen is then excised. During excision of the cone specimen, nonreflective tissue hooks may be needed to retract the ectocervical edge away from the laser beam path and to create tissue tension along the plane of incision.

POSTOPERATIVE

Recovery following all excisional methods is rapid and follows that for other surgeries of the cervix previously described (p. 1000). However, due to the greater incision, postoperative bleeding can develop more commonly and is treated with Monsel paste or other topical hemostat. Patients require postoperative surveillance for disease persistence or recurrence, and this is described in detail in Chapter 29 (p. 640).

43-28

Ablation of Preinvasive Cervical Lesions

CERVICAL CRYOTHERAPY

For appropriate patients, cryotherapy can safely and effectively ablate the cervix's transformation zone and CIN lesion. This method uses compressed gas to create extremely cold temperatures that necrose cervical epithelium. For this, the *cryoprobe*, a tip made of silver or copper, allows contact with and conduction of extreme cold across the cervix surface. When nitrous oxide gas is used, probe temperatures can reach –65°C. Cell death occurs at –20°C (Gage, 1979).

As the cervical epithelium is cooled, an expanding layer of ice, called the *iceball*, forms beneath the center of the cryoprobe and grows circumferentially outward and past the probe margins. The expanding iceball grows in depth as well as circumference during treatment. The portion of the iceball in which temperatures fall below –20°C is termed the *lethal zone*. This zone spans from the center of the cryoprobe to a perimeter 2 mm *inside* the outer iceball edge. Past this perimeter, tissue temperatures are warmer, and necrosis may be incomplete. Thus, when cryotherapy is performed, the iceball is allowed to enlarge until it reaches a mark 7 mm distal to the probe margin, that is, a 5-mm lethal zone and a 2-mm zone of indeterminate tissue death (Ferris, 1994).

Although some use these iceball dimensions to direct therapy, the World Health Organization (2014) recommends a double-freeze method for cryotherapy, described in the steps below. Importantly, a single-freeze method is insufficient, and dysplasia recurs frequently in the first year following this treatment (Creasman, 1984; Schantz, 1984).

The specific indications and long-term rates of success for cryotherapy are discussed in Chapter 29 (p. 640). Randomized trials comparing different CIN treatment modalities show similar efficacy (Massad, 2013). In general, cryotherapy is appropriate for squamous CIN that does not extend into the endocervical canal, does not span more than two quadrants of the ectocervix, is not associated with unsatisfactory colposcopic examination or abnormal glandular cytology, and is covered by the selected cryoprobe. Anatomically, a short cervix that becomes flush with the vaginal vault under moderate pressure is a concern, as the iceball may injure the vaginal fornices. Moreover, cryosurgery is generally not favored for CIN 3 treatment due to higher rates of disease persistence following treatment and lack of a histologic specimen to exclude occult invasive cancer (Martin-Hirsch, 2013). Last, cryosurgery and other ablative techniques are not favored for women with CIN and human immunodeficiency virus (HIV) infection due to high failure rates (Spitzer, 1999).

PREOPERATIVE

Patient Evaluation

As with LEEP, women in the United States undergo colposcopy and histologic review of colposcopic biopsies prior to cryotherapy. Presurgical patient preparation mirrors that for LEEP (p. 999).

Consent

Intraoperative complications are uncommon, and hemorrhage is rare (Denny, 2005). Infrequently, women may experience a vasovagal reaction during treatment, and care is supportive. Perioperatively, patients are counseled that spotting, watery discharge, or cramping are typical, but infection is not. Long-term risks include cervical stenosis, squamocolumnar junction (SCJ) retraction into the endocervical canal, and treatment failure (Benedet, 1981, 1987; Jacob, 2005; Ostergard, 1980). Last, infertility and pregnancy complications are not associated with this treatment modality (Weed, 1978).

INTRAOPERATIVE

Instruments

Cryotherapy typically requires a tank of refrigerant gas plus a cryogun, connecting tubing, pressure gauge, and cryoprobe. Nitrous oxide and carbon dioxide are frequently used refrigerant gases. Gas moves through connecting tubing, into the barrel of the cryogun, and then to the cryoprobe. Circumferential grooves at the cryoprobe base allow it to be screwed securely to the end of the cryogun.

Selection of an appropriate cryoprobe is individualized but should cover the transformation zone and lesion. Flat-faced cryoprobes are used for lesions located on the cervical portio. Advantageously, this shape has a lower tendency to push the resulting SCJ toward the endocervical canal. Thus, it decreases the risk of unsatisfactory colposcopic examination following treatment.

❶ **Analgesia and Patient Positioning.** Cryotherapy may be performed in an office setting and requires no significant analgesia. However, to help attenuate associated uterine cramping, women are often given an NSAID prior to therapy.

The patient is asked to void and is positioned in standard lithotomy position. No vaginal cleansing is required, and a vaginal speculum is placed. The appropriate-sized cryoprobe is attached onto the end of the cryogun barrel. A water-based lubricant jelly is applied to the end of the cryoprobe to ensure even tissue contact.

❷ **Iceball Formation.** The cryoprobe is pressed firmly against the cervix (Fig. 43-28.1). The cryogun trigger is squeezed, a light hissing sound is typically heard, and frost begins to cover the cryoprobe. The trigger is held for 3 minutes as the iceball extends past the outer margin of the cryoprobe.

The cryoprobe should not contact the vaginal sidewalls. If this is identified, gas delivery is stopped to allow cryoprobe warming. The cryoprobe is gently teased away from the wall, after which the procedure is continued.

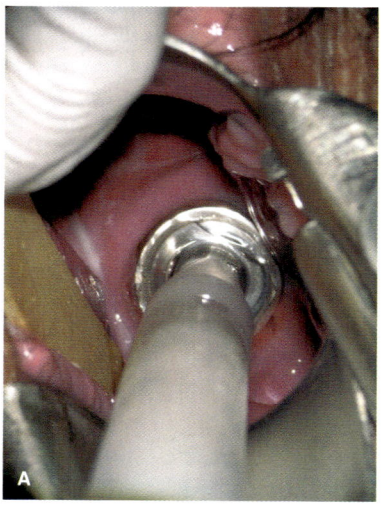 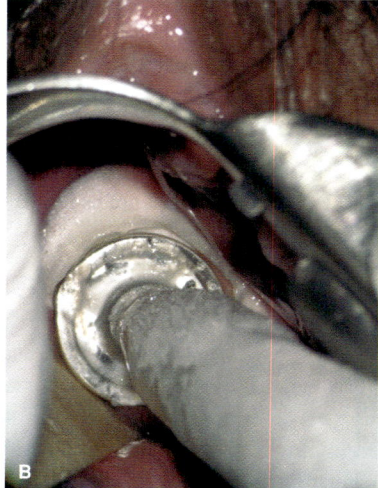

FIGURE 43-28.1 Cryotherapy. **A.** Cryoprobe applied to cervix. **B.** Creation of advancing iceball. (Reproduced with permission from Dr. Claudia Werner.)

3 First Thaw. After the first freeze, the trigger is released. The cryoprobe quickly warms and can be removed from the cervix. Attempts to remove it prior to complete defrosting can cause patient discomfort and bleeding. The surface of the cervix is allowed to thaw during the following 5 minutes.

4 Second Cycle. Subsequently, the freezing cycle is repeated for an additional 3 minutes. At completion of the second cycle, the cryoprobe and speculum are removed.

POSTOPERATIVE

As noted, watery vaginal discharge that can persist for weeks, vaginal spotting, and cramping that responds to NSAIDs are expected. Infrequently, severe pain and cramping may result from necrotic tissue obstructing the endocervical canal. Removal of the obstructing tissue typically resolves symptoms.

Because a large area of the cervix is denuded after cryotherapy, the potential for infection is increased. Accordingly, patients abstain from intercourse during the 4 weeks following surgery. If abstinence is not feasible, then condom use is encouraged. Depending on patient symptoms, work and exercise may resume quickly following treatment.

CARBON DIOXIDE LASER CERVICAL ABLATION

The carbon dioxide (CO_2) laser produces a beam of infrared light that produces heat at its focal point sufficient to boil intracellular water and vaporize tissue. Indications and success rates are discussed more fully in Chapter 29 (p. 640). In general, laser ablation may be used for cases in which the entire transformation zone can be seen with satisfactory colposcopy. There should be no evidence of microinvasive, invasive, or glandular disease, and cytology and histology should positively correlate.

Although research supports laser ablation as an effective tool in treating CIN, its popularity has declined. Laser units are significantly more expensive than those used for cryotherapy and LEEP. Moreover, lesions are destroyed with ablation, and unlike LEEP, the opportunity for additional pathologic evaluation of surgical margins is lost. Last, physician and staff training and maintenance of certification are typically required for safe, effective use of laser equipment.

PREOPERATIVE

Consent

Laser ablation is considered a safe and effective means to treat CIN. As with any

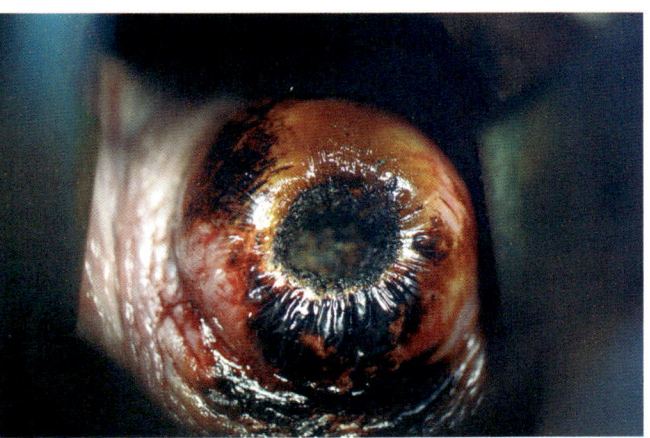

FIGURE 43-28.2 Cervical bed following laser ablation. (Reproduced with permission from Dr. Eddie McCord.)

treatment of cervical dysplasia, patients should be counseled regarding the risks of disease persistence and recurrence following treatment. These risks and surgical complications are low and comparable with those for LEEP (Nuovo, 2000).

INTRAOPERATIVE

Instruments

CO_2 lasers suitable for cervical ablation are mobile, self-contained units. Tissue effects vary depending on the interval at which energy bursts are released. As a result, continuous waves (cutting) or pulsed energy (coagulation) can be released. Laser guidance is accomplished through attachment to a colposcope.

Because laser light is reflective, protective eyewear is required for the patient and all participants, and a sign is posted on the suite door warning that a laser procedure is in progress. For this same reason, a matte-surface speculum is necessary. As with LEEP, noxious smoke is generated, and a smoke evacuation system is required.

Surgical Steps

1 Anesthesia and Patient Positioning. Laser ablation for many women is an outpatient procedure and performed in either an operating suite or an office, depending on laser equipment location and patient characteristics. In most cases, local analgesia combined with a vasoconstrictor is sufficient, and administration mirrors that used for LEEP (p. 1000). After emptying her bladder, the patient is placed in standard lithotomy position. A matte-surfaced speculum is inserted, and smoke evacuation tubing is attached to a port on the speculum. Misdirected laser energy can burn surrounding tissues and

ignite paper drapes. Therefore, moistened cloth towels are draped outside the vulva to absorb misdirected energy. To delineate the area of excision, Lugol solution is applied.

2 Laser Settings. The colposcope-laser assembly is brought into position and focused on the ectocervix. The laser is set to achieve a power density (PD) of 600 to 1200 W/cm^2 in a continuous wave mode. Average PD $= 100 \times W/D^2$; D = spot diameter in mm at 10 W at 0.1-s pulse. Thus, a power of 10 W with a spot diameter of 1 mm will yield a PD of 1000 W/cm^2.

3 Ablation. Initially, four dots are ablated at 12, 3, 6, and 9 o'clock positions on the perimeter of the cervix to surround the entire lesion. These dots serve as landmarks and are connected in an arching pattern to create a circle. Once encircled, the area is ablated to a depth of 5 to 7 mm (Fig. 43-28.2).

4 Endocervical Eversion. To help prevent postoperative retraction of the SCJ cephalad into the endocervical canal, the tissue immediately surrounding the endocervix is ablated less deeply. This allows an apparent eversion of the endocervical lining and retention of the SCJ on the ectocervix.

5 Hemostasis. Bleeding is common during CO_2 laser vaporization. A defocused laser beam and a lower power setting in a super pulse wave mode will coagulate vessels and aid hemostasis. Bleeding present at the end of surgery may also be controlled with an application of Monsel paste.

POSTOPERATIVE

Cramping is common following surgery, and light bleeding may persist for a week. Postoperative patient counseling is similar to that for LEEP (p. 1000).

43-29

Treatment of Vulvar Intraepithelial Neoplasia

WIDE LOCAL EXCISION

With high-grade vulvar intraepithelial neoplasia (VIN), treatment goals are prevention of invasive vulvar cancer and, when possible, preservation of normal vulvar anatomy and function. Wide local excision of lesions, ablative methods, and medical treatments are effective and commonly selected (Chap. 29, p. 645) (Lawrie, 2016; van Seters, 2008). If malignancy is suspected, wide local excision is performed to identify or exclude occult invasion (American College of Obstetricians and Gynecologists, 2019c). In cases that involve the clitoris, urethra, or anus, a combined surgical excision and laser ablation approach is sometimes helpful. This combined technique uses CO_2 laser vaporization at sites where excision might lead to dysfunction or poor cosmesis (Cardosi, 2001). For more widespread disease, simple vulvectomy may be appropriate and is described in Section 46-24 (p. 1233).

PREOPERATIVE

Patient Evaluation

Prior to excision, full evaluation of the lower reproductive tract for evidence of invasive disease is completed as outlined in Chapter 29 (p. 620). Importantly, vulvar biopsies are obtained during this evaluation in an attempt to exclude invasive disease, which would warrant more extensive excision (Chap. 31, p. 681).

Consent

Wide local excision of high-grade VIN successfully treats disease, and progression to invasive vulvar cancer is low (3 to 5 percent) (Jones, 2005; Rodolakis, 2003). However, disease frequently recurs, and even in those patients with tissue margins negative for disease, recurrence ranges from 15 to 40 percent (Modesitt, 1998; Satmary, 2018).

Local infection or wound separation is common. In one large series, the combined rate of both neared 30 percent (Mullen, 2019). Less frequent complications are chronic vulvodynia, dyspareunia, and scarring or altered vulvar appearance. Any vulvar operation requires thorough preoperative counseling regarding expectations for anatomic outcome and for sexual function.

Patient Preparation

This is a clean contaminated procedure and antibiotic prophylaxis may be considered, especially for those with greater risks for wound infection (American College of Obstetricians and Gynecologists, 2018b). Mullen and coworkers (2019) found no advantage to prophylaxis, mainly with cefazolin, in their large series. Patients usually ambulate quickly after this procedure, and VTE prophylaxis is reserved for those with enhanced risks (Chap. 39, p. 834). Special bowel preparation is not required.

INTRAOPERATIVE

Surgical Steps

❶ **Anesthesia and Patient Positioning.** The choice of anesthesia or analgesia will vary depending on the location and size of the treated lesion. Whereas smaller labial or perineal lesions may easily be excised using local analgesia in an office setting, larger lesions or those involving the urethra and/or clitoris may require general or regional anesthesia. The patient is placed in standard lithotomy position, pubic hair at the surgical site is clipped, and the vulva is surgically prepared.

❷ **Lesion Identification.** The area for excision should be well demarcated. For this, colposcopic examination following application of 3- to 5-percent acetic acid to the vulva will aid identification of lesion margins. Most recommend a 5- to 10-mm circumferential surgical margin surrounding the lesion (Joura, 2002; American College of Obstetricians and Gynecologists, 2019c). In the past, toluidine blue has been used to stain nuclear chromatin and enhance vulvar lesions. However, normal tissue can also absorb the stain and distort true disease margins, and use of toluidine blue is thus not recommended.

❸ **Incision.** A scalpel with a no. 15 surgical blade is used to incise smaller lesions, whereas a no. 10 blade may be suitable for larger excisions (Fig. 43-29.1). An elliptical incision is preferred and aids wound reapproximation. Most preinvasive lesions fail to extend deeper than 1 mm on non-hair-bearing areas such as the labia minora. However, in hair-bearing areas of the vulva, VIN may extend to the deepest hair follicles. This is generally deeper than 2 mm, but not more than 4 mm. Thus, incision depth will vary depending on lesion location (Shatz, 1989). Once the incision is completed, Adson forceps or skin hooks can elevate and retract the skin margin away from the incision line. Dissection beneath the lesion begins at the incision periphery and progresses toward the center of the proposed excision area and then to the opposite incision margin.

Disease recurrence is related to the presence or absence of disease-free surgical margins. Thus, frozen sections of the specimen margins can be evaluated intraoperatively if needed.

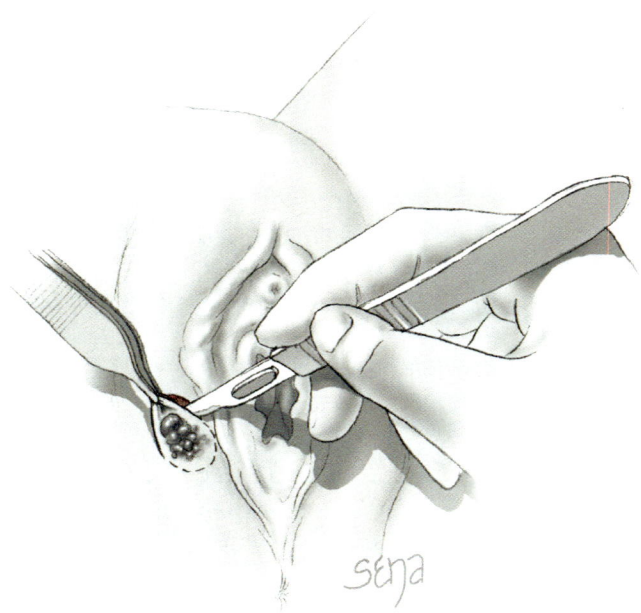

FIGURE 43-29.1 Vulvar incision.

❹ Margin Undermining. Reapproximation of the wound edges without tension decreases the risk of postoperative superficial separation. Accordingly, a surgeon may need to sharply undermine the wound margins with fine scissors to mobilize the skin and immediate underlying subcutaneous tissue. Alternatively, a few imbricating interrupted stitches of 3-0 gauge delayed-absorbable sutures may be placed in the subcutaneous layer to decrease wound tension.

❺ Wound Closure. Prior to edge reapposition, the wound bed is rendered hemostatic to minimize hematoma formation and subsequent wound separation. The edges of the skin are then reapproximated with interrupted stitches using 3-0 or 4-0 gauge delayed-absorbable sutures.

POSTOPERATIVE

Without complication, recovery from wide local excision is typically rapid, and patients may resume normal activities as desired. Oral analgesics are usually needed for the first days following surgery. Vulvar hygiene is emphasized. Intercourse is delayed until wounds have fully healed, and this time will vary depending on wound site and size. Superficial wound separation is common, and sites of separation will heal by secondary intention.

Because of the significant risk for VIN recurrence, postprocedural surveillance is essential. At our institution, patients undergo colposcopic vulvar examination every 6 months for 2 years and annually thereafter.

CAVITATIONAL ULTRASONIC SURGICAL ASPIRATION

Indications for use and mechanism of action of cavitational ultrasonic surgical aspiration (CUSA) are discussed more fully in Chapter 40 (p. 858). Briefly, cavitation causes fragmentation and disruption of tissue, which is then aspirated and collected. Thus, the tissue, although fragmented, can be sent for histologic or cytologic evaluation.

Treatment of high-grade VIN with CUSA usually produces excellent cosmetic results, which is a main advantage. Complications such as scarring and dyspareunia are rare. However, the recurrence rate is high, as it is with other treatment modalities for VIN, and especially in treated hair-bearing areas (Miller, 2002). Thus, it is generally reserved for vulvar skin without hair. Although the procedure allows for tissue evaluation, tissue disruption may preclude adequate examination of all parts of the specimen and their

associated relationships. Associated expense is greater than with excisional therapy and is similar to that with laser therapy. Depending on lesion size, CUSA can be more time consuming compared with excision or laser ablation. However, compared with laser therapy, CUSA lacks a smoke plume and avoids the risks associated with radiant energy.

In addition to VIN treatment, CUSA works well for condyloma acuminata, particularly bulky or multifocal condyloma or condyloma that are refractory to topical treatment. Information regarding cavitational therapy for condyloma acuminata is included in this section due to the similarity of treatment for VIN.

PREOPERATIVE

Patient Evaluation

The same principles apply as for excisional treatment of VIN. Specifically, a full evaluation of the lower genital tract is indicated to exclude an invasive process. Although condyloma acuminata are often diagnosed and treated on the basis of clinical appearance, a complete evaluation of the lower genital tract should likewise be undertaken preoperatively.

Consent

Risks of CUSA for VIN or condyloma are few and are similar to those of wide local excision. Postoperative healing is by secondary intention and may take several weeks.

INTRAOPERATIVE

Instruments

The CUSA unit consists of a console, an operative hand piece, and a foot pedal by which the system is activated (Fig. 43-29.2). The console allows control of amplitude or intensity, irrigation, and aspiration. Amplitude determines the relative amount of tissue fragmentation. A setting at 1 will produce cellular fragmentation to a depth of 30 µm, whereas a setting at 10 will produce cellular fragmentation to a depth of 300 µm. Fragmentation of a specific tissue is dependent on its water content. Therefore, less power is required for tissues with high water content such as skin and condyloma. Irrigation is used to control the considerable heat generated by the vibrating titanium tip (23 kHz) of the hand piece and to suspend the fragmented tissue for suction removal. The tip has a hollow 2-mm diameter and will remove tissue within a 1- to 2-mm radius of the tip. Vaporized and fragmented tissue is aspirated through the hollow tip of the hand piece and collected in a tissue trap. Each

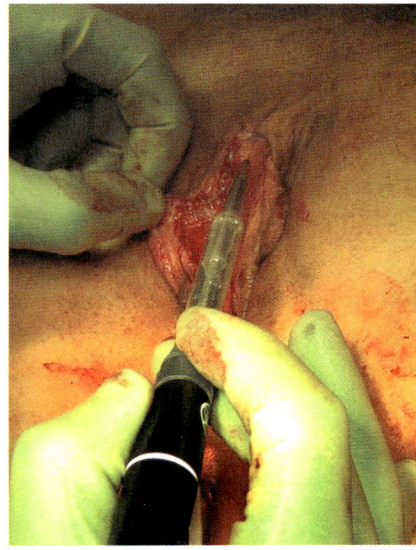

FIGURE 43-29.2 Operative handpiece of the cavitational ultrasonic surgical aspiration (CUSA) unit.

console setting may be varied depending on the needs of the operator.

Surgical Steps

❶ Anesthesia and Patient Positioning. CUSA is performed in the operating room under regional or general anesthesia. The patient is placed in standard lithotomy position. The vulva and the perianal region, if involved with disease, are surgically prepped.

❷ Lesion Identification. The same colposcopic identification techniques used prior to wide local excision apply for CUSA (p. 1006). In Figure 43-29.3A, two areas of VIN are evident even prior to application 3- to 5-percent acetic acid. The larger of the two is located in the midportion of the right labium minus, and the smaller is more anterior and toward the clitoris.

❸ Console Settings. For treatment of VIN and condyloma acuminata, an amplitude setting of 5 to 6 produces cellular fragmentation to a tissue depth of 150 µm to 180 µm and should allow adequate removal of tissue without significant thermal injury. However, some studies have used amplitude settings at 6 to 8 for treatment of VIN (Miller, 2002). Irrigation and aspiration rates may be varied depending on the need of the operator. For example, if tissue fulguration is desired, a decrease in the irrigation rate will permit additional heat production at the hand-piece tip. Aerosolization can be minimized with proper balance of irrigation and aspiration rates.

❹ **Ablation.** As with wide local excision, the area of treatment should extend at least 5 mm beyond the identified lesion(s). The hand-piece tip is moved over the vulva in a back-and-forth motion. Only close contact with the skin of the vulva is required; no pressure is necessary. Repeat movements of the tip over the involved area dictate the depth of tissue removal. However, depth of destruction is often difficult to assess. Collagen bundles and elastic fibers become visible in the reticular dermis (Reid, 1985). Tissue destruction beyond this point increases the likelihood of scarring. For treatment of VIN, depth of treatment may vary between 1.5 and 2.5 mm (Miller, 2002; Rader, 1991). For condyloma acuminata, depth of treatment need not extend beyond the basement membrane (Ferenczy, 1983). Bleeding, if any, is usually minor and is controlled with local pressure. Figure 43-29.3B shows the end result for the same patient shown in part A.

POSTOPERATIVE

A 1-percent silver sulfadiazine cream may be applied to the vulva immediately following ablative therapy and continued once or twice daily for a short time. Oral analgesics and sitz baths are helpful in pain management following therapy. Patients may be reevaluated 2 to 4 weeks postoperatively.

CARBON DIOXIDE LASER VAPORIZATION

The CO_2 laser has been used for decades for VIN treatment (Baggish, 1981). Success rates vary, however, and depend on factors such as length of patient surveillance, number of therapy courses, specific area of treatment, and total area of treated disease. In theory, the CO_2 laser is an ideal means to treat VIN. When used with the colposcope, the laser can accurately eradicate disease while preserving normal tissue structure and function. Associated bleeding is scant, healing is usually excellent, and scarring is minimal. Rates of significant complications are generally low. CO_2 laser vaporization may also be considered as an addition to an excisional procedure. One example is if multifocal disease involves both hair-bearing and non-hair-bearing areas, such as the clitoris, where excision may not be ideal. That said, Reid and colleagues (1985) recommend that only those surgeons experienced with CO_2 lasers attempt VIN vaporization by this method. Indeed, the margin between the therapy depth needed to eradicate disease and a depth that may produce delayed healing, scarring, and a poor cosmetic result is thin.

As with other destructive techniques, before laser vaporization is performed, invasive disease must be excluded. Since VIN is often multifocal, a thorough examination of the vulva and the lower genital tract with biopsy of any abnormal-appearing area is imperative. No tissue sample will be available for analysis following CO_2 laser vaporization.

PREOPERATIVE

Consent

As with other VIN treatment methods, recurrence or persistence following CO_2 laser vaporization is possible, and a patient is counseled on the need for postoperative surveillance. Pain, infection, fever, skin depigmentation, alopecia, scarring, and dyspareunia may result from treatment. Healing is generally complete in 4 to 6 weeks but may be delayed if treatment extends significantly into the dermis (Wright, 1987).

INTRAOPERATIVE

Instruments

A general description of the CO_2 laser is found on page 1005. Recommendations regarding its use for cervical ablation of CIN are likewise appropriate for treatment of VIN.

Surgical Steps

❶ **Anesthesia and Patient Positioning.** Laser ablation of VIN is nearly always performed as an outpatient procedure either in an office setting or in an operative suite depending on laser availability. The procedure may be performed under general, regional, or local anesthesia. Ferenczy and associates (1994) used disease greater than 6 cm^2 as a criterion for general anesthesia. The patient is placed in standard lithotomy position. To lessen the risk of injury from misdirected laser energy to tissues beyond those being treated, wet towels are positioned around the operative field. Paper drapes are avoided due to risk of fire. A moistened sponge is placed inside the rectum to prevent passage of flatus into the surgical field and possible gas ignition.

❷ **Laser Settings.** The laser is coupled to the colposcope, and the assembly is brought

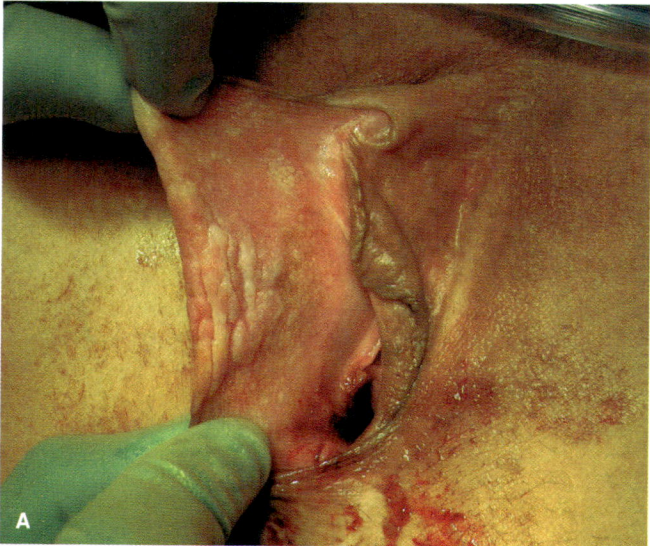
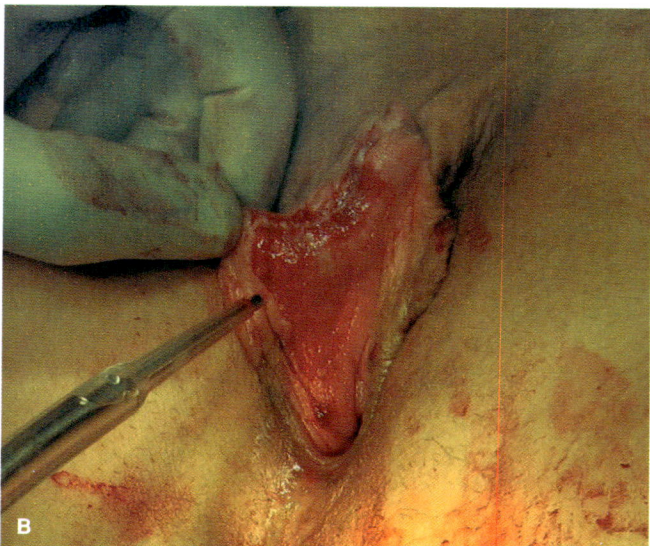

FIGURE 43-29.3 A. Vulvar intraepithelial neoplasia (VIN) involving the right labium minor. **B.** Cavitational ultrasonic surgical aspiration (CUSA) treatment of VIN completed.

into focus on the vulva. A power density (PD) of 600 to 1200 W/cm^2 delivered in continuous mode is sufficient for therapy. However, Reid and associates (1985) caution that PD >600 W/cm^2 may be difficult to control on the vulva. Calculation of power density is described on page 1005.

❸ Examination of Treatment Area. After a soaking application of 3- to 5-percent acetic acid solution is applied to the vulva, the area to be treated is examined colposcopically to delineate the zone of vaporization. This may be marked with the laser beam, incorporating a margin of 3 to 5 mm or upward to 1 cm of normal-appearing tissue (Helmerhorst, 1990; Hoffman, 1992).

❹ Ablation. The location of VIN will determine the needed depth of laser beam penetration for treatment. As hair root

sheaths may harbor VIN up to a depth of 2.5 mm, involved hairy areas of the vulva will require laser penetration into the reticular dermis (Mene, 1985). Wright and Davies (1987) recommend a depth of 3 mm for hair-bearing areas and consider this depth to correspond well with destruction into the third surgical plane as described by Reid and coworkers (1985). Non-hair-bearing areas contain no adnexal structures and therefore, if laser is used, do not require deeper treatment. One millimeter or less of laser penetration is adequate for treatment of VIN in these areas, that is, no deeper than the basement membrane.

❺ Reexamination. Carbonized debris is removed, and 3- to 5-percent acetic acid solution applied to the vulva, which is again examined colposcopically to confirm no remaining areas of disease.

POSTOPERATIVE

Care is taken to avert labial coaptation and adhesion of treated areas. Restrictive clothes are avoided, and the labia are manually separated at least daily. Sitz bath two to three times per day aids hygiene and frequently gives temporary relief of postoperative vulvar discomfort. Other measures that may be helpful include application of 1-percent silver sulfadiazine cream two to three times daily and oral analgesics. The patient should refrain from sexual activity until healing is complete.

The first postoperative visit may be scheduled at 4 to 6 weeks following the laser vaporization procedure. An acceptable schedule for surveillance of persistent or recurrent VIN is examination at 6 and 12 months and then yearly thereafter. More frequent visits, particularly in the first year after treatment, may be warranted depending on individual patient characteristics.

REFERENCES

Aarts JW, Nieboer TE, Johnson N, et al: Surgical approach to hysterectomy for benign gynaecological disease. Cochrane Database Syst Rev 8:CD003677, 2015

Adulcadir J, Bianchi Demicheli F, Willame A, et al: Posttraumatic stress disorder relapse following clitoral reconstruction after female genital mutilation: a case report. Obstet Gynecol 129(2):371, 2017

Abdulcadir J, Marras S, Catania L, et al: Defibulation: a visual reference and learning tool. J Sex Med 15(4):601, 2018

Achilles SL, Reeves MF, Society of Family Planning: Prevention of infection after induced abortion: release date October 2010: SFP guideline 20102. Contraception 83(4):295, 2011

Adamson CD, Naik BJ, Lynch DJ: The vacuum expandable condom mold: a simple vaginal stent for McIndoe-style vaginoplasty. Plast Reconstr Surg 113:664, 2004

Ahmad G, O'Flynn H, Hindocha A, et al: Barrier agents for adhesion prevention after gynaecological surgery. Cochrane Database Syst Rev 4:CD00047, 2015

Alessandrescu D, Peltecu GC, Buhimschi CS, et al: Neocolpopoiesis with split-thickness skin graft as a surgical treatment of vaginal agenesis: retrospective review of 201 cases. Am J Obstet Gynecol 175(1):131, 1996

Ali PB, Smith G: The effect of Syntocinon on blood loss during first trimester suction curettage. Anaesthesia 51(5):483, 1996

Allen RH, Goldberg AB: Cervical dilation before first-trimester surgical abortion (<14 weeks' gestation). Contraception 93(4):277, 2016

Allen RH, Singh R: Society of Family Planning clinical guidelines pain control in surgical abortion part 1 – local anesthesia and minimal sedation. Contraception 97(6):471, 2018

Almroth L, Elmusharaf S, El Hadi N, et al: Primary infertility after genital mutilation in girlhood in Sudan: a case-control study. Lancet 366:385, 2005

Alter GJ: Aesthetic labia minora and clitoral hood reduction using extended central wedge resection. Plast Reconstr Surg 122(6):1780, 2008

Al-Shabibi N, Chapman L, Madari S, et al: Prospective randomized trial comparing gonadotrophin-releasing hormone analogues with triple tourniquets at open myomectomy. BJOG 116(5):681, 2009

American College of Obstetricians and Gynecologists: Induced abortion. In Guidelines for Women's Health Care, 4th ed. Washington, 2014

American College of Obstetricians and Gynecologists: Choosing the route of hysterectomy for benign disease. Committee Opinion No. 701, June 2017a

American College of Obstetricians and Gynecologists: Hereditary breast and ovarian cancer syndrome. Practice Bulletin No. 182, September 2017b

American College of Obstetricians and Gynecologists: Sterilization of women: ethical issues and considerations. Committee Opinion No. 695, April 2017c

American College of Obstetricians and Gynecologists: Müllerian agenesis: diagnosis, management, and treatment. Committee Opinion No. 728, January 2018a

American College of Obstetricians and Gynecologists: Prevention of infection after gynecologic procedures. Practice Bulletin No. 195, June 2018b

American College of Obstetricians and Gynecologists: Alternatives to hysterectomy in the management of leiomyomas. Practice Bulletin No. 96, August 2008, Reaffirmed 2019a

American College of Obstetricians and Gynecologists: Benefits and risks of sterilization. Practice Bulletin No. 208, February 2019b

American College of Obstetricians and Gynecologists: Management of vulvar intraepithelial neoplasia. Committee Opinion No. 675, October 2016, Reaffirmed 2019c

American College of Obstetricians and Gynecologists: Opportunistic salpingectomy as a strategy for epithelial ovarian cancer prevention. Committee Opinion No. 774, March 2019d

American College of Obstetricians and Gynecologists: Uterine morcellation for presumed leiomyomas. Committee Opinion No. 770, March 2019e

American College of Obstetricians and Gynecologists: Vaginal "rejuvenation" and cosmetic vaginal procedures. Committee Opinion No. 378, September 2007, Reaffirmed 2019f

Andersen LL, Ottesen B, Alling Møller LM, et al: Subtotal versus total abdominal hysterectomy: randomized clinical trial with 14-year questionnaire follow-up. Am J Obstet Gynecol 212(6):758, 2015

Andersson SH, Rymer J, Joyce DW, et al: Sexual quality of life in women who have undergone female genital mutilation: a case-control study. BJOG 119(13):1606, 2012

Arkoulis N, Kearns C, Deeny M et al: The interdigitating Y-plasty procedure for the correction of transverse vaginal septa. BJOG 124(2):331, 2017

Asante A, Whiteman MK, Kulkarni A, et al: Elective oophorectomy in the United States: trends and in-hospital complications, 1998–2006. Obstet Gynecol 116(5):1088, 2010

Aslan Çetin B, Aydoğan Mathyk B, Köroğlu N, et al: Oxytocin infusion reduces bleeding during abdominal myomectomies: a randomized controlled trial. Arch Gynecol Obstet 299(1): 151, 2019

Atashkhoei S, Fakhari S, Pourfathi H, et al: Effect of oxytocin infusion on reducing the blood loss during abdominal myomectomy: a double-blind randomised controlled trial. BJOG 124(2): 292, 2017

Baggish MS, Dorsey JH: CO$_2$ laser for the treatment of vulvar carcinoma in situ. Obstet Gynecol 57:371, 1981

Baldauf JJ, Dreyfus M, Ritter J, et al: Risk of cervical stenosis after large loop excision or laser conization. Obstet Gynecol 88:933, 1996

Balgobin S, Hamid CA, Carrick KS, et al: Distance from cervicovaginal junction to anterior peritoneal reflection measured during vaginal hysterectomy. Obstet Gynecol 128(4):863, 2016

Balgobin S, Jeppson PC, Wheeler T II, et al: Standardized terminology of the female pelvic apical structures based on a structured medical literature review. Am J Obstet Gynecol, 2019, In press

Bartz D, Maurer R, Allen RH, et al: Buccal misoprostol compared with synthetic osmotic cervical dilator before surgical abortion: a randomized controlled trial. Obstet Gynecol 122(1):57, 2013

Barutcu A, Akguner M: McIndoe vaginoplasty with the inflatable vaginal stent. Ann Plast Surg 41:568, 1998

Baumann R, Magos AL, Turnbull A: Prospective comparison of videopelviscopy with laparotomy for ectopic pregnancy. BJOG 98(8):765, 1991

Behrendt A, Moritz S: Posttraumatic stress disorder and memory problems after female genital mutilation. Am J Psychiatry 162(5):1000, 2005

Benagiano G, Kivinen ST, Fadini R, et al: Zoladex (goserelin acetate) and the anemic patient: results of a multicenter fibroid study. Fertil Steril 66:223, 1996

Benedet JL, Miller DM, Nickerson KG, et al: The results of cryosurgical treatment of cervical intraepithelial neoplasia at one, five, and ten years. Am J Obstet Gynecol 157:268, 1987

Benedet JL, Nickerson KG, Anderson GH: Cryotherapy in the treatment of cervical intraepithelial neoplasia. Obstet Gynecol 58:725, 1981

Berg RC, Denison E: A tradition in transition: factors perpetuating and hindering the continuance of female genital mutilation/cutting (FGM/C) summarized in a systematic review. Health Care Women Int 34(10):837, 2013

Berg RC, Taraldsen S, Said MA, et al: The effectiveness of surgical interventions for women with FGM/C: a systematic review. BJOG 125(3):278, 2018

Bergeron S, Binik YM, Khalife S, et al: A randomized comparison of group cognitive-behavioral therapy, surface electromyographic biofeedback, and vestibulectomy in the treatment of dyspareunia resulting from vulvar vestibulitis. Pain 91:297, 2001

Bewö K, Österberg J, Löfgren M, et al: Incisional hernias following open gynecological surgery: a population-based study. Arch Gynecol Obstet 299(5):1313, 2019

Bhave Chittawar P, Franik S, Pouwer AW, et al: Minimally invasive surgical techniques versus open myomectomy for uterine fibroids. Cochrane Database Syst Rev 10:CD004638, 2014

Bjørge T, Skare GB, Bjørge L, et al: Adverse pregnancy outcomes after treatment for cervical intraepithelial neoplasia. Obstet Gynecol 128(6):1265, 2016

Blakely DH, Dewhurst CJ, Tipton RH: The long term results after marsupialization of Bartholin cysts and abscesses. J Obstet Gynaecol British Commonw 73:1008, 1966

Bleker OP, Smalbraak DJ, Schutte MF: Bartholin's abscess: the role of *Chlamydia trachomatis*. Genitourin Med 66:24, 1990

Bornstein J, Zarfati D, Goldik Z, et al: Vulvar vestibulitis: physical or psychosexual problem? Obstet Gynecol 93:876, 1999

Bornstein J, Zarfati D, Goldshmid N, et al: Vestibulodynia—a subset of vulvar vestibulitis or a novel syndrome? Am J Obstet Gynecol 177(6):1439, 1997

Brucker SY, Gegusch M, Zubke W, et al: Neovagina creation in vaginal agenesis: development of a new laparoscopic Vecchietti-based procedure and optimized instruments in a prospective comparative interventional study in 101 patients. Fertil Steril 90(5):1940, 2008

Brucker SY, Rall K, Campo R, et al: Treatment of congenital malformations. Semin Reprod Med 29(2):101, 2011

Burnett MA, Corbett CA, Gertenstein RJ: A randomized trial of laminaria tents versus vaginal misoprostol for cervical ripening in first trimester surgical abortion. J Obstet Gynaecol Can 27(1):38, 2005

Caglar GS, Tasci Y, Kayikcioglu F: Management of prolapsed pedunculated myomas. Int J Gynaecol Obstet 89(2):146, 2005

Cali RW, Pratt JH: Congenital absence of the vagina. Long-term results of vaginal reconstruction in 175 cases. Am J Obstet Gynecol 100(6):752, 1968

Candiani GB, Fedele L, Candiani M: Double uterus, blind hemivagina, and ipsilateral renal agenesis: 36 cases and long-term follow-up. Obstet Gynecol 90(1):26, 1997

Canis MJ, Triopon G, Daraï E, et al: Adhesion prevention after myomectomy by laparotomy: a prospective multicenter comparative randomized single-blind study with second-look laparoscopy to assess the effectiveness of PREVADH. Eur J Obstet Gynecol Reprod Biol 178:42, 2014

Cardosi RJ, Bomalaski JJ, Hoffman MS: Diagnosis and management of vulvar and vaginal intraepithelial neoplasia. Obstet Gynecol Clin North Am 28:685, 2001

Casiano ER, Trabuco EC, Bharucha AE, et al: Risk of oophorectomy after hysterectomy. Obstet Gynecol 121(5):1069, 2013

Castelo-Branco C, Figueras F, Sanjuan A, et al: Long-term compliance with estrogen replacement therapy in surgical postmenopausal women: benefits to bone and analysis of factors associated with discontinuation. Menopause 6:307, 1999

Cates W Jr, Schulz KF, Grimes DA: The risks associated with teenage abortion. N Engl J Med 309(11):62, 1983

Cherney LS: Transverse low abdominal incision with detachment of the recti from the pubis: follow-up study of eight hundred cases. JAMA 157(1):23, 1955

Chiaffarino F, Parazzini F, Decarli A, et al: Hysterectomy with or without unilateral oophorectomy and risk of ovarian cancer. Gynecol Oncol 97:318, 2005

Christianson MS, Barker MA, Lindheim SR: Overcoming the challenging cervix: techniques to access the uterine cavity. J Low Genit Tract Dis 12(1):24, 2008

Ciavattini A, Clemente N, Delli Carpini G, et al: Loop electrosurgical excision procedure and risk of miscarriage. Fertil Steril 103(4):1043, 2015

Clark NM, Schembri M, Jacoby VL: Change in surgical practice for women with leiomyomas after the U.S. Food and Drug Administration morcellator safety communication. Obstet Gynecol 130(5):1057, 2017

Conner SN, Frey HA, Cahill AG, et al: Loop electrosurgical excision procedure and risk of preterm birth: a systematic review and meta-analysis. Obstet Gynecol 123(4):752, 2014

Costello C, Hillis SD, Marchbanks PA, et al: The effect of interval tubal sterilization on sexual interest and pleasure. Obstet Gynecol 100:511, 2002

Creasman WT, Hinshaw WM, Clarke-Pearson DL: Cryosurgery in the management of cervical intraepithelial neoplasia. Obstet Gynecol 63:145, 1984

Creatsas G, Deligeoroglou E, Christopoulos P: Creation of a neovagina after Creatsas modification of Williams vaginoplasty for the treatment of 200 patients with Mayer-Rokitansky-Kuster-Hauser syndrome. Fertil Steril 94(5):1848, 2010

Crouch NS, Deans R, Michala L, et al: Clinical characteristics of well women seeking labial reduction surgery: a prospective study. BJOG 118(12):1507, 2011

Cundiff GW: Incisions and closures. In Yeomans ER, Hoffman BL, Gilstrap LC III, et al (eds): Cunningham and Gilstrap's Operative Obstetrics, 3rd ed. New York, McGraw-Hill Education, 2017

Curtis KM, Mohllajee AP, Peterson HB: Regret following female sterilization at a young age: a systematic review. Contraception 73(2):205, 2006

Curtis KM, Tepper NK, Jatlaoui TC, et al: U.S. Medical Eligibility Criteria for Contraceptive Use, 2016. MMWR 65(3):1, 2016

Darwish AM, Nasr AM, El Nashar DA: Evaluation of postmyomectomy uterine scar. J Clin Ultrasound 33:181, 2005

Davydov SN, Zhvitiashvili OD: Formation of vagina (colpopoiesis) from peritoneum of Douglas pouch. Acta Chir Plast 16(1):35, 1974

Dehghankhalili M, Fallahi S, Mahmudi F, et al: Epidemiology, regional characteristics, knowledge, and attitude toward female genital mutilation/cutting in southern Iran. J Sex Med 12(7):1577, 2015

Deligdisch L, Hirschmann S, Altchek A: Pathologic changes in gonadotropin-releasing hormone agonist analogue treated uterine leiomyomata. Fertil Steril 67:837, 1997

Deligeoroglou E, Iavazzo C, Sofoudis C, et al: Management of hematocolpos in adolescents with transverse vaginal septum. Arch Gynecol Obstet 285(4):1083, 2012

Denny L, Kuhn L, De Souza M, et al: Screen-and-treat approaches for cervical cancer prevention in low-resource settings: a randomized, controlled trial. JAMA 294:2173, 2005

Deschamps A, Krishnamurthy S: Absence of pulse and blood pressure following vasopressin injection for myomectomy. Can J Anesth 52:552, 2005

Dietrich JE, Millar DM, Quint EH: Obstructive reproductive tract anomalies. J Pediatr Adolesc Gynecol 27(6):396, 2014

Donnez J, Tatarchuk TF, Bouchard P, et al: Ulipristal acetate versus placebo for fibroid treatment before surgery. N Engl J Med 366(5):409, 2012a

Donnez J, Tomaszewski J, Vázquez F, et al: Ulipristal acetate versus leuprolide acetate for uterine fibroids. N Engl J Med 366(5):421, 2012b

Downs MC, Randall HW Jr: The ambulatory surgical management of Bartholin duct cysts. J Emerg Med 7:623, 1989

Dunn TS, Killoran K, Wolf D: Complications of outpatient LLETZ procedures. J Reprod Med 49:76, 2004

Dunn TS, Woods J, Burch J: Bowel injury occurring during an outpatient LLETZ procedure: a case report. J Reprod Med 48:49, 2003

Ebisch RM, Rovers MM, Bosgraaf RP, et al: Evidence supporting see-and-treat management of cervical intraepithelial neoplasia: a systematic review and meta-analysis. BJOG 123(1):59, 2016

Edwards L: New concepts in vulvodynia. Am J Obstet Gynecol 189:S24, 2003

Falconer H, Yin L, Grönberg H, et al: Ovarian cancer risk after salpingectomy: a nationwide population-based study. J Natl Cancer Inst 107(2), 2015

Farquhar CM: Ectopic pregnancy. Lancet 366:583, 2005a

Farquhar CM, Sadler L, Harvey SA, et al: The association of hysterectomy and menopause: a prospective cohort study. BJOG 112(7):956, 2005b

Fedele L, Bianchi S, Zanconato G, et al: Laparoscopic creation of a neovagina in patients with Rokitansky syndrome: analysis of 52 cases. Fertil Steril 74(2):384, 2000

Fedele L, Frontino G, Motta F, et al: A uterovaginal septum and imperforate hymen with a double pyocolpos. Hum Reprod 27(6):1637, 2012

Fedele L, Vercellini P, Bianchi S, et al: Treatment with GnRH agonists before myomectomy and the risk of short-term myoma recurrence. BJOG 97:393, 1990

Ferenczy A: Using the laser to treat condyloma acuminata and intradermal neoplasia. Can Med Assoc J 128:135, 1983

Ferenczy A, Wright JR, Richart RM: Comparison of CO_2 laser surgery and loop electrosurgical excision/fulguration for the treatment of vulvar intraepithelial neoplasia (VIN). Int J Gynecol Cancer 4:22, 1994

Ferris DG: Lethal tissue temperature during cervical cryotherapy with a small flat cryoprobe. J Fam Pract 38:153, 1994

Findley AD, Siedhoff MT, Hobbs KA, et al: Short-term effects of salpingectomy during laparoscopic hysterectomy on ovarian reserve: a pilot randomized controlled trial. Fertil Steril 100(6):1704, 2013

Fletcher H, Frederick J, Hardie M, et al: A randomized comparison of vasopressin and tourniquet as hemostatic agents during myomectomy. Obstet Gynecol 87:1014, 1996

Food and Drug Administration: Laparoscopic power morcellators. 2018. Available at: https://www.fda.gov/medical-devices/surgery-devices/laparoscopic-power-morcellators. Accessed April 5, 2019

Foster DC, Butts C, Shah KV, et al: Long term outcome of perineoplasty for vulvar vestibulitis. J Women's Health 4(6):669, 1995

Fox MC, Krajewski CM: Cervical preparation for second-trimester surgical abortion prior to 20 weeks' gestation: SFP Guideline #2013–4. Contraception 89(2):75, 2014

Frankman EA, Wang L, Bunker CH, et al: Lower urinary tract injury in women in the United States, 1979–2006. Am J Obstet Gynecol 202(5):495.e1, 2010

Frederick J, Fletcher H, Simeon D, et al: Intramyometrial vasopressin as a haemostatic agent during myomectomy. BJOG 101:435, 1994

Friedman AJ, Hoffman DI, Comite F, et al: Treatment of leiomyomata uteri with leuprolide acetate depot: a double-blind, placebo-controlled, multicenter study. The Leuprolide Study Group. Obstet Gynecol 77:720, 1991

Frishman G: Vasopressin: if some is good, is more better? Obstet Gynecol 113(2 Pt 2):476, 2009

Fusca L, Perelman I, Fergusson D, et al: The effectiveness of tranexamic acid at reducing blood loss and transfusion requirement for women undergoing myomectomy: a systematic review and meta-analysis. J Obstet Gynaecol Can 41:1185, 2019

Gage AA: What temperature is lethal for cells? J Dermatol Surg Oncol 5:459, 1979

Ganer Herman H, Gluck O, Keidar R, et al: Ovarian reserve following cesarean section with salpingectomy vs tubal ligation: a randomized trial. Am J Obstet Gynecol 217(4):472, 2017

Garcia RF: Z-plasty for correction of congenital transverse vaginal septum. Am J Obstet Gynecol 99(8):1164, 1967

Ghanbari Z, Baratali BH, Foroughifar T, et al: Pfannenstiel versus Maylard incision for gynecologic surgery: a randomized, double-blind controlled trial. Taiwan J Obstet Gynecol 48(2):120, 2009

Gilman AR, Dewar KM, Rhone SA, et al: Intrauterine adhesions following miscarriage: look and learn. J Obstet Gynaecol Can 38(5):453, 2016

Gilman AR, Rhone SA, Fluker MR: Curettage and Asherman's syndrome—lessons to (re-) learn? J Obstet Gynaecol Can 36(11):997, 2014

Gilmour DT, Das S, Flowerdew G: Rates of urinary tract injury from gynecologic surgery and the role of intraoperative cystoscopy. Obstet Gynecol 107(6):1366, 2006

Ginsburg ES, Benson CB, Garfield JM, et al: The effect of operative technique and uterine size on blood loss during myomectomy: a prospective, randomized study. Fertil Steril 60:956, 1993

Gockley AA, Elias KM: Fallopian tube tumorigenesis and clinical implications for ovarian cancer risk-reduction. Cancer Treat Rev 69:66, 2018

Goetsch MF: Incidence of Bartholin's duct occlusion after superficial localized vestibulectomy. Am J Obstet Gynecol 200(6):688.e1, 2009

Golan A, Zachalka N, Lurie S, et al: Vaginal removal of prolapsed pedunculated submucous myoma: a short, simple, and definitive procedure with minimal morbidity. Arch Gynecol Obstet 271(1):11, 2005

Goldstein AT, Klingman D, Christopher K, et al: Surgical treatment of vulvar vestibulitis syndrome: outcome assessment derived from a postoperative questionnaire. J Sex Med 3(5):923, 2006

Goldstein AT, Marinoff SC, Haefner HK: Vulvodynia: strategies for treatment. Clin Obstet Gynecol 48:769, 2005

Grantcharov TP, Rosenberg J: Vertical compared with transverse incisions in abdominal surgery. Eur J Surg 167(4):260, 2001

Grimes DA, Schulz KF, Cates WJ Jr: Prevention of uterine perforation during curettage abortion. JAMA 251(16):2108, 1984

Guiahi M, Davis A, Society of Family Planning: First-trimester abortion in women with medical conditions: release date October 2012 SFP guideline #20122. Contraception 86(6):622, 2012

Gulia C, Zangary A, Briganti V, et al: Labia minora hypertrophy: causes, impact on women's health, and treatment options. Int Urogynecol J 28:1453, 2017

Haefner HK: Critique of new gynecologic surgical procedures: surgery for vulvar vestibulitis. Clin Obstet Gynecol 43:689, 2000

Haefner HK, Collins ME, Davis GD, et al: The vulvodynia guideline. J Low Gen Tract Dis 9:40, 2005

Hakim-Elahi E, Tovell HM, Burnhill MS: Complications of first-trimester abortion: a report of 170,000 cases. Obstet Gynecol 76:129, 1990

Hannoun-Levi JM, Peiffert D, Hoffstetter S, et al: Carcinoma of the cervical stump: retrospective analysis of 77 cases. Radiother Oncol 43:147, 1997

Hartmann KE, Ma C, Lamvu GM, et al: Quality of life and sexual function after hysterectomy in women with preoperative pain and depression. Obstet Gynecol 104:701, 2004

Heinonen A, Gissler M, Riska A, et al: Loop electrosurgical excision procedure and the risk for preterm delivery. Obstet Gynecol 121(5):1063, 2013

Hellstrom AC, Sigurjonson T, Pettersson F: Carcinoma of the cervical stump: the Radiumhemmet series 1959–1987. Treatment and prognosis. Acta Obstet Gynaecol Scand 80:152, 2001

Helmerhorst TJ, van der Vaart CH, Dijkhuizen GH, et al: CO$_2$-laser therapy in patients with vulvar intraepithelial neoplasia. Eur J Obstet Gynecol Repro Biol 34(1-2):149, 1990

Helmkamp BF, Krebs HB: The Maylard incision in gynecologic surgery. Am J Obstet Gynecol 163(5 Pt 1):1554, 1990

Hilger WS, Pizarro AR, Magrina JF: Removal of the retained cervical stump. Am J Obstet Gynecol 193:2117, 2005

Hill DA, Lense JJ: Office management of Bartholin gland cysts and abscesses. Am Fam Physician 57:1611, 1998

Hillis SD, Marchbanks PA, Tylor LR, et al: Poststerilization regret: findings from the United States Collaborative Review of Sterilization. Obstet Gynecol 93:889, 1999

Hoffman MS, Pinelli DM, Finan M, et al: Laser vaporization for vulvar intraepithelial neoplasia. J Reprod Med 37(2):135, 1992

Hooker AB, Lemmers M, Thurkow AL, et al: Systematic review and meta-analysis of intrauterine adhesions after miscarriage: prevalence, risk factors and long-term reproductive outcome. Hum Reprod Update 20(2):262, 2014

Houlard S, Perrotin F, Fourquet F, et al: Risk factors for cervical stenosis after laser cone biopsy. Eur J Obstet Gynaecol Reprod Biol 104:144, 2002

Huebner M, DeLancey JO, Reisenauer C, et al: Magnetic resonance imaging of vaginal support structure before and after Vecchietti procedure in women with Mayer-Rokitansky-Küster-Hauser syndrome. Acta Obstet Gynecol Scand 97(7):830, 2018

Hutchins FL Jr: A randomized comparison of vasopressin and tourniquet as hemostatic agents during myomectomy. Obstet Gynecol 88:639, 1996

Hwang JH, Lee JK, Lee NW, et al: Open cornual resection versus laparoscopic cornual resection in patients with interstitial ectopic pregnancies. Eur J Obstet Gynecol Reprod Biol 156(1):78, 2011

Iglesia CB, Yurteri-Kaplan L, Alinsod L: Female genital cosmetic surgery: a review of techniques and outcomes. Int Urogynecol J 24:1997, 2013

Insogna IG, Farland LV, Missmer SA, et al: Outpatient endometrial aspiration: an alternative to methotrexate for pregnancy of unknown location. Am J Obstet Gynecol 217(2):185, 2017

Ireland LD, Gatter M, Chen AY: Medical compared with surgical abortion for effective pregnancy termination in the first trimester. Obstet Gynecol 126(1):22, 2015

Iverson RE Jr, Chelmow D, Strohbehn K, et al: Relative morbidity of abdominal hysterectomy and myomectomy for management of uterine leiomyomas. Obstet Gynecol 88:415, 1996

Jackson LA, Hare AM, Carrick KS, et al: Anatomy, histology, and nerve density of clitoris and associated structures: clinical applications to vulvar surgery. Am J Obstet Gynecol 221(5):519.e1, 2019

Jackson LA, Ramirez DM, Carrick KS, et al: Gross and histologic anatomy of the pelvic ureter: clinical applications to pelvic surgery. Obstet Gynecol 133(5):896, 2019

Jacob M, Broekhuizen FF, Castro W, et al: Experience using cryotherapy for treatment of cervical precancerous lesions in low-resource settings. Int J Gynaecol Obstet 89:S13, 2005

Jacobson P: Marsupialization of vulvovaginal (Bartholin) cysts. Am J Obstet Gynecol 79:73, 1960

Jacoby VL, Autry A, Jacobson G, et al: Nationwide use of laparoscopic hysterectomy compared with abdominal and vaginal approaches. Obstet Gynecol 114(5):1041, 2009

Jeppson PC, Balgobin S, Rahn DD, et al: Comparison of vaginal hysterectomy techniques and interventions for benign indications: a systematic review. Obstet Gynecol 129(5):877, 2017

Johansen RE: Virility, pleasure and female genital mutilation/cutting. A qualitative study of perceptions and experiences of medicalized defibulation among Somali and Sudanese migrants in Norway. Reprod Health 14(1):25, 2017

Johnson C, Nour NM: Surgical techniques: defibulation of type III female genital cutting. J Sex Med 4(6):1544, 2007

Johnson N, Barlow D, Lethaby A et al: Methods of hysterectomy: systematic review and meta-analysis of randomised controlled trials. BMJ 330(7506):1478, 2005

Joki-Erkkilä MM, Heinonen PK: Presenting and long-term clinical implications and fecundity in females with obstructing vaginal malformations. J Pediatr Adolesc Gynecol 16:307, 2003

Jones RW, Rowan DM, Stewart AW: Vulvar intraepithelial neoplasia: aspects of the natural history and outcome in 405 women. Obstet Gynecol 106:1319, 2005

Joura EA: Epidemiology, diagnosis and treatment of vulvar intraepithelial neoplasia. Curr Opin Obstet Gynecol 14:39, 2002

Kaali SG, Szigetvari IA, Bartfai GS: The frequency and management of uterine perforations during first-trimester abortions. Am J Obstet Gynecol 161(2):406, 1989

Karp NE, Fenner DE, Burgunder-Zdravkovski L, et al: Removal of normal ovaries in women under age 51 at the time of hysterectomy. Am J Obstet Gynecol 213(5):716, 2015

Kelishadi SS, Omar R, Herring N, et al. The safe labiaplasty: a study of nerve density in labia minora and its implications. Aesthet Surg J 36:705, 2016

Kennedy CM, Dewdney S, Galask RP: Vulvar granuloma fissuratum: a description of fissuring of the posterior fourchette and the repair. Obstet Gynecol 105:1018, 2005

Kerns J, Steinauer J: Management of postabortion hemorrhage: release date November 2012 SFP Guideline #20131. Contraception 87(3):331, 2013

Kessous R, Aricha-Tamir B, Sheizaf B, et al: Clinical and microbiological characteristics of Bartholin gland abscesses. Obstet Gynecol 122(4):794, 2013

Kho RM, Magrina JF. Removal of the retained cervical stump after supracervical hysterectomy. Best Pract Res Clin Obstet Gynaecol 25(2):153, 2011

Kilpatrick CC, Alagkiozidis I, Orejuela FJ, et al: Factors complicating surgical management of the vulvar abscess. J Reprod Med 55:139, 2010

Kim AJ, Barberio A, Berens P, et al: The trend, feasibility, and safety of salpingectomy as a form of permanent sterilization. J Minim Invasive Gynecol 26(7):1363, 2019a

Kim AJ, Clark NV, Jansen LJ, et al: Perioperative antibiotic use and associated infectious outcomes at the time of myomectomy. Obstet Gynecol 133(4):626, 2019b

Kisielinski K, Conze J, Murken AH, et al: The Pfannenstiel or so called "bikini cut": still effective more than 100 years after first description. Hernia 8(3):177, 2004

Kiuchi K, Hasegawa K, Motegi E, et al: Complications of laser conization versus loop electrosurgical excision procedure in pre- and postmenopausal patients. Eur J Gynaecol Oncol 37(6):803, 2016

Klingele CJ, Gebhart JB, Croak AJ, et al: McIndoe procedure for vaginal agenesis: long-term outcome and effect on quality of life. Am J Obstet Gynecol 189:1569, 2003

Köbach A, Ruf-Leuschner M, Elbert T: Psychopathological sequelae of female genital mutilation and their neuroendocrinological associations. BMC Psychiatry 18(1):187, 2018

Kongnyuy EJ, Wiysonge CS: Interventions to reduce haemorrhage during myomectomy for fibroids. Cochrane Database Syst Rev 11:CD005355, 2014

Kotani Y, Tobiume T, Fujishima R, et al: Recurrence of uterine myoma after myomectomy: Open myomectomy versus laparoscopic myomectomy. J Obstet Gynaecol Res 44(2): 298, 2018

Krause E, Brandner S, Mueller MD, et al: Out of eastern Africa: defibulation and sexual function in woman with female genital mutilation. J Sex Med 8(5):1420, 2011

Krissi H, Shmuely A, Aviram A, et al: Acute Bartholin's abscess: microbial spectrum, patient characteristics, clinical manifestation, and surgical outcomes. Eur J Clin Microbiol Infect Dis 35(3):443, 2016

Kristensen GB, Jensen LK, Holund B: A randomized trial comparing two methods of cold knife conization with laser conization. Obstet Gynecol 76:1009, 1990

Kristensen J, Langhoff-Roos J, Kristensen FB: Increased risk of preterm birth in women with cervical conization. Obstet Gynecol 81:1005, 1993a

Kristensen J, Langhoff-Roos J, Wittrup M, et al: Cervical conization and preterm delivery/low birth weight: a systematic review of the literature. Acta Obstet Gynaecol Scand 72:640, 1993b

Kroese JA, van der Velde M, Morssink LP, et al: Word catheter and marsupialisation in women with a cyst or abscess of the Bartholin gland (WoMan-trial): a randomised clinical trial. BJOG 124(2):243, 2017

Kuhn A, Neukomm C, Dreher EF, et al: Prolapse and sexual function 8 years after neovagina according to Shears: a study of 43 cases with Mayer-von Rokitansky-Küster-Hauser syndrome. Int Urogynecol J 24(6):1047, 2013

Kuppermann M, Learman LA, Schembri M, et al: Contributions of hysterectomy and uterus-preserving surgery to health-related quality of life. Obstet Gynecol 122(1):15, 2013

Kurata H, Aoki Y, Tanaka K: Delayed, massive bleeding as an unusual complication of laser conization: a case report. J Reprod Med 48:659, 2003

Kyrgiou M, Athanasiou A, Kalliala IE, et al: Obstetric outcomes after conservative treatment for cervical intraepithelial lesions and early invasive disease. Cochrane Database Syst Rev 11:CD012847, 2017

LaMorte AI, Lalwani S, Diamond MP: Morbidity associated with abdominal myomectomy. Obstet Gynecol 82:897, 1993

Lauritz JB, Paull JD, McInnes M: Oxytocin: oxytocic of choice in first trimester. Med J Aust 2(6):319, 1980

Lavy Y, Lev-Sagie A, Hamani Y, et al: Modified vulvar vestibulectomy: simple and effective surgery for the treatment of vulvar vestibulitis. Eur J Obstet Gynaecol Reprod Biol 120:91, 2005

Lawrie TA, Nordin A, Chakrabarti M, et al: Medical and surgical interventions for the treatment of usual-type vulval intraepithelial neoplasia. Cochrane Database Syst Rev 1: CD011837, 2016

Lessard-Anderson CR, Handlogten KS, Molitor RJ, et al: Effect of tubal sterilization technique on risk of serous epithelial ovarian and primary peritoneal carcinoma. Gynecol Oncol 135(3): 423, 2014

Lethaby A, Mukhopadhyay A, Naik R. Total versus subtotal hysterectomy for benign gynaecological conditions. Cochrane Database Syst Rev 4:CD004993, 2012

Lethaby A, Vollenhoven B, Sowter M: Efficacy of pre-operative gonadotrophin hormone–releasing analogues for women with uterine fibroids undergoing hysterectomy or myomectomy: a systematic review. BJOG 109:1097, 2002

Li FY, Xu YS, Zhou CD, et al: Long-term outcomes of vaginoplasty with autologous buccal micromucosa. Obstet Gynecol 123(5):951, 2014

Liang CC, Chang SD, Soong YK: Long-term follow-up of women who underwent surgical correction for imperforate hymen. Arch Gynecol Obstet 269:5, 2003

Limwatanapan N, Chalapati W, Songthamwat S, et al: Lidocaine spray versus paracervical block during loop electrosurgical excision procedure: a randomized trial. J Low Genit Tract Dis 22(1):38, 2018

Lista F, Mistry BD, Singh Y, et al: The safety of aesthetic labiaplasty: a plastic surgery experience. Aesthet Surg J 35(6):689, 2015

MacIsaac L, Grossman D, Balistreri E, et al: A randomized controlled trial of laminaria, oral misoprostol, and vaginal misoprostol before abortion. Obstet Gynecol 93(5 Pt 1):766, 1999

Maher C, Dwyer P, Carey M, et al: The Burch colposuspension for recurrent urinary stress incontinence following retropubic continence surgery. BJOG 106(7):719, 1999

Mamik MM, Antosh D, White DE, et al: Risk factors for lower urinary tract injury at the time of hysterectomy for benign reasons. Int Urogynecol J 25(8):1031, 2014

Marana R, Busacca M, Zupi E, et al: Laparoscopically assisted vaginal hysterectomy versus total abdominal hysterectomy: a prospective, randomized, multicenter study. Am J Obstet Gynecol 180:270, 1999

Marinoff SC, Turner ML: Vulvar vestibulitis syndrome: an overview. Am J Obstet Gynecol 165(4 Pt 2):1228, 1991

Martin-Hirsch PL, Paraskevaidis E, Bryant A: Surgery for cervical intraepithelial neoplasia. Cochrane Database Syst Rev 6:CD001318, 2013

Massad LS, Einstein MH, Huh WK, et al: 2012 updated consensus guidelines for the management of abnormal cervical cancer screening tests and cancer precursors. J Low Genit Tract Dis 17(5 Suppl 1):S1, 2013

Mathai M, Hofmeyr GJ, Mathai NE: Abdominal surgical incisions for caesarean section. Cochrane Database Syst Rev 5:CD004453, 2013

Mathevet P, Chemali E, Roy M, et al: Long-term outcome of a randomized study comparing three techniques of conization: cold knife, laser, and LEEP. Eur J Obstet Gynaecol Reprod Biol 106:214, 2003

Matta WH, Stabile I, Shaw RW, et al: Doppler assessment of uterine blood flow changes in patients with fibroids receiving the gonadotropin-releasing hormone agonist Buserelin. Fertil Steril 49:1083, 1988

McIndoe AH, Banister JB: An operation for the cure of congenital absence of the vagina. J Obstet Gynaecol Br Empire 45:490, 1938

McQuillan SK, Grover SR: Systematic review of sexual function and satisfaction following the management of vaginal agenesis. Int Urogynecol J 25(10):1313, 2014

Mencaglia L, Tantini C: GnRH agonist analogs and hysteroscopic resection of myomas. Int J Gynaecol Obstet 43:285, 1993

Mene A, Buckley CH: Involvement of the vulvar skin appendages by intraepithelial neoplasia. Br J Obstet Gynaecol 92:634, 1985

Mentula M, Männistö J, Gissler M, et al: Intrauterine adhesions following an induced termination of pregnancy: a nationwide cohort study. BJOG 125(11):1424, 2018

Miller BE: Vulvar intraepithelial neoplasia treated with cavitational ultrasonic surgical aspiration. Gynecol Oncol 85:114, 2002

Mirzabeigi MN, Moore JH Jr, Mericli AF, et al: Current trends in vaginal labioplasty: a survey of plastic surgeons. Ann Plast Surg 68(2):125, 2012

Mitchell MF, Tortolero-Luna G, Cook E, et al: A randomized clinical trial of cryotherapy, laser vaporization, and loop electrosurgical excision for treatment of squamous intraepithelial lesions of the cervix. Obstet Gynecol 92:737, 1998

Moawad NS, Mahajan ST, Moniz MH, et al: Current diagnosis and treatment of interstitial pregnancy. Am J Obstet Gynecol 202:15, 2010

Modesitt SC, Waters AB, Walton L, et al: Vulvar intraepithelial neoplasia III: occult cancer and the impact of margin status on recurrence. Obstet Gynecol 92:962, 1998

Morrill MY, Schimpf MO, Abed H, et al: Antibiotic prophylaxis for selected gynecologic surgeries. Int J Gynaecol Obstet 120(1):10, 2013

Motoyama S, Laoag-Fernandez JB, Mochizuki S, et al: Vaginoplasty with Interceed absorbable adhesion barrier for complete squamous epithelialization in vaginal agenesis. Am J Obstet Gynecol 188:1260, 2003

Mowbray N, Ansell J, Warren N, et al: Is surgical smoke harmful to theater staff? A systematic review. Surg Endosc 27(9):3100, 2013

Mullen MM, Merfeld EC, Palisoul ML, et al: Wound complication rates after vulvar excisions for premalignant lesions. Obstet Gynecol 133(4):658, 2019

Murji A, Wais M, Lee S, et al: A multicenter study evaluating the effect of ulipristal acetate during myomectomy. J Minim Invasive Gynecol 25(3):514, 2018

National Abortion Federation: 2018 Clinical policy guidelines for abortion care. Washington, National Abortion Federation, 2018

National Institute for Occupational Safety and Health: Control of smoke from laser/electric surgical procedures. Appl Occup Environ Hyg 14:71, 1999

Ngeh N, Belli AM, Morgan R, et al: Pre-myomectomy uterine artery embolisation minimises operative blood loss. BJOG 111:1139, 2004

Nieboer TE, Johnson N, Lethaby A, et al: Surgical approach to hysterectomy for benign gynaecological disease. Cochrane Database Syst Rev 3:CD003677, 2009

Nour NM, Michels KB, Bryant AE: Defibulation to treat female genital cutting: effect on symptoms and sexual function. Obstet Gynecol 108(1):55, 2006

Novetsky AP, Boyd LR, Curtin JP: Trends in bilateral oophorectomy at the time of hysterectomy for benign disease. Obstet Gynecol 118(6):1280, 2011

Nuovo J, Melnikow J, Willan AR, et al: Treatment outcomes for squamous intraepithelial lesions. Int J Gynaecol Obstet 68:25, 2000

Nygaard IH, Valbø A, Heide HC, et al: Is oxytocin given during surgical termination of first trimester pregnancy useful? A randomized controlled trial. Acta Obstet Gynecol Scand. 90(2):174, 2011

O'Connell K, Jones HE, Simon M, et al: First-trimester surgical abortion practices: a survey of National Abortion Federation members. Contraception 79(5):385, 2009

Olive DL: Dogma, skepsis, and the analytic method: the role of prophylactic oophorectomy at the time of hysterectomy. Obstet Gynecol 106:214, 2005

Osmundsen BC, Clark A, Goldsmith C, et al: Mesh erosion in robotic sacrocolpopexy. Female Pelvic Med Reconstr Surg 18(2):86, 2012

Ostergard DR: Cryosurgical treatment of cervical intraepithelial neoplasia. Obstet Gynecol 56:231, 1980

Özer M, Mortimore I, Jansma EP, et al: Labiaplasty: motivation, techniques, and ethics. Nat Rev Urol 15(3):175, 2018

Panici PB, Ruscito I, Gasparri ML, et al: Vaginal reconstruction with the Abbè-McIndoe technique: from dermal grafts to autologous in vitro cultured vaginal tissue transplant. Semin Reprod Med 29(1):45, 2011

Parker WH, Feskanich D, Broder MS, et al: Long-term mortality associated with oophorectomy compared with ovarian conservation in the Nurses' Health Study. Obstet Gynecol 121(4):709, 2013

Pasley WW: Trachelectomy: a review of fifty-five cases. Am J Obstet Gynecol 159:728, 1988

Pati S, Cullins V: Female sterilization: evidence. Obstet Gynecol Clin North Am 27:859, 2000

Peipert JF, Weitzen S, Cruickshank C, et al: Risk factors for febrile morbidity after hysterectomy. Obstet Gynecol 103:86, 2004

Penna C, Fambrini M, Fallani MG, et al: Laser CO_2 conization in postmenopausal age: risk of cervical stenosis and unsatisfactory follow-up. Gynecol Oncol 96:771, 2005

Perera HK, Ananth CV, Richards CA, et al: Variation in ovarian conservation in women undergoing hysterectomy for benign indications. Obstet Gynecol 121:717, 2013

Peterson HB, Jeng G, Folger SG, et al: The risk of menstrual abnormalities after tubal sterilization. U.S. Collaborative Review of Sterilization Working Group. N Engl J Med 343:1681, 2000

Peterson HB, Xia Z, Hughes JM, et al: The risk of pregnancy after tubal sterilization: findings from the U.S. Collaborative Review of Sterilization. Am J Obstet Gynecol 174:1161, 1996

Placik OJ, Arkins JP: Plastic surgery trends parallel Playboy magazine: the pudenda preoccupation. Aesthet Surg J 34(7):1083, 2014

Powell CB, Alabaster A, Simmons S, et al: Salpingectomy for sterilization: change in practice in a large integrated health care system, 2011–2016. Obstet Gynecol 130(5):961, 2017

Pratt JH, Jefferies JA: The retained cervical stump: a 25-year experience. Obstet Gynecol 48:711, 1976

Quint EH, McCarthy JD, Smith YR: Vaginal surgery for congenital anomalies. Clin Obstet Gynecol 53(1):115, 2010

Rader JS, Leake JF, Dillon MB, et al: Ultrasonic surgical aspiration in the treatment of vulvar disease. Obstet Gynecol 77(4):573, 1991

Radman HM, Korman W: Uterine perforation during dilatation and curettage. Obstet Gynecol 21:210, 1963

Rahn DD, Phelan JN, Roshanravan SM, et al: Anterior abdominal wall nerve and vessel anatomy: clinical implications for gynecologic surgery. Am J Obstet Gynecol 202(3):234.e1, 2010

Reid R, Elfont EA, Zirkin RM, et al: Superficial laser vulvectomy. II. The anatomic and biophysical principles permitting accurate control over the depth of dermal destruction with carbon dioxide laser. Am J Obstet Gynecol 152(3):261, 1985

Reinsch RC, Murphy AA, Morales AJ, et al: The effects of RU 486 and leuprolide acetate on uterine artery blood flow in the fibroid uterus:

a prospective, randomized study. Am J Obstet Gynecol 170:1623, 1994

Rice MS, Hankinson SE, Tworoger SS: Tubal ligation, hysterectomy, unilateral oophorectomy, and risk of ovarian cancer in the Nurses' Health Studies. Fertil Steril 102(1):192, 2014

Rice MS, Murphy MA, Tworoger SS: Tubal ligation, hysterectomy and ovarian cancer: a meta-analysis. J Ovarian Res 5(1):13, 2012

Riva HL, Hefner JD, Marchetti AA, et al: Prophylactic trachelectomy of cervical stump: two hundred and twelve cases. South Med J 54:1082, 1961

Roberts SC, Upadhyay UD, Liu G, et al: Association of facility type with procedural-related morbidities and adverse events among patients undergoing induced abortions. JAMA 319(24):2497, 2018

Rodolakis A, Diakomanolis E, Vlachos G, et al: Vulvar intraepithelial neoplasia (VIN): diagnostic and therapeutic challenges. Eur J Gynaecol Oncol 24:317, 2003

Roe AH, Bartz D: Society of Family Planning clinical recommendations: contraception after surgical abortion. Contraception 99(1):2, 2019

Rouzier R, Haddad B, Deyrolle C, et al: Perineoplasty for the treatment of introital stenosis related to vulvar lichen sclerosus. Am J Obstet Gynecol 186:49, 2002

Rouzier RM, Louis-Sylvestre C, Paniel BJ, et al: Hypertrophy of labia minora: experience with 163 reductions. Am J Obstet Gynecol 182(1 Pt 1):35, 2000

Royal College of Obstetricians and Gynaecologists: Ethical opinion paper: ethical considerations in relation to female genital cosmetic surgery (FGCS). 2013. Available at: https://www.rcog.org.uk/globalassets/documents/guidelines/ethics-issues-and-resources/rcog-fgcs-ethical-opinion-paper.pdf. Accessed May 31, 2019

Rubal L, Chung K: Do you need to definitively diagnose the location of a pregnancy of unknown location? The case for "yes." Fertil Steril 98(5):1078, 2012

Rybak EA, Polotsky AJ, Woreta T, et al: Explained compared with unexplained fever in postoperative myomectomy and hysterectomy patients. Obstet Gynecol 111(5):1137, 2008

Ryder RM, Vaughan MC: Laparoscopic tubal sterilization: methods, effectiveness, and sequelae. Obstet Gynecol Clin North Am 26:83, 1999

Sabatucci I, Palaia I, Marchese C, et al: Treatment of the Mayer-Rokitansky-Küster-Hauser syndrome with autologous in vitro cultured vaginal tissue: descriptive study of long-term results and patient outcomes. BJOG 126(1):123, 2019

Sadler L, Saftlas A, Wang W, et al: Treatment for cervical intraepithelial neoplasia and risk of preterm delivery. JAMA 291:2100, 2004

Sanders AP, Chan WV, Tang J, et al: Surgical outcomes after uterine artery occlusion at the time of myomectomy: systematic review and meta-analysis. Fertil Steril 111(4):816, 2019

Satmary W, Holschneider CH, Brunette LL, et al: Vulvar intraepithelial neoplasia: risk factors for recurrence. Gynecol Oncol, 148(1): 126, 2018

Sawaya GF, Grady D, Kerlikowske K, et al: Antibiotics at the time of induced abortion: the case for universal prophylaxis based on a meta-analysis. Obstet Gynecol 87:884, 1996

Sawin SW, Pilevsky ND, Berlin JA, et al: Comparability of perioperative morbidity between abdominal myomectomy and hysterectomy for women with uterine leiomyomas. Am J Obstet Gynecol 183:1448, 2000

Schantz A, Thormann L: Cryosurgery for dysplasia of the uterine ectocervix: a randomized

study of the efficacy of the single- and double-freeze techniques. Acta Obstet Gynaecol Scand 63:417, 1984

Schenker JG, Margalioth EJ: Intrauterine adhesions: an updated appraisal. Fertil Steril 37(5):593, 1982

Schmidt T, Eren Y, Breidenbach M, et al: Modifications of laparoscopic supracervical hysterectomy technique significantly reduce postoperative spotting. J Minim Invasive Gynecol 18(1):81, 2011

Seracchioli R, Rossi S, Govoni F, et al: Fertility and obstetric outcome after laparoscopic myomectomy of large myomata: a randomized comparison with abdominal myomectomy. Hum Reprod 15(12):2663, 2000

Shatz P, Bergeron C, Wilkinson EJ, et al: Vulvar intraepithelial neoplasia and skin appendage involvement. Obstet Gynecol 74(5):769, 1989

Shears BH: Congenital atresia of the vagina: a technique for tunnelling in the space between bladder and rectum and construction of a new vagina by a modified Wharton technique. J Obstet Gynaecol Br Emp 67:24, 1960

Siddle N, Sarrel P, Whitehead M: The effect of hysterectomy on the age at ovarian failure: identification of a subgroup of women with premature loss of ovarian function and literature review. Fertil Steril 47:94, 1987

Sieh W, Salvador S, McGuire V, et al: Tubal ligation and risk of ovarian cancer subtypes: a pooled analysis of case-control studies. Int J Epidemiol 42(2):579, 2013

Smith DC, Uhlir JK: Myomectomy as a reproductive procedure. Am J Obstet Gynecol 162:1476, 1990

Smith NA, Laufer MR: Obstructed hemivagina and ipsilateral renal anomaly (OHVIRA) syndrome: management and follow-up. Fertil Steril 87(4):918, 2007

Son M, Evanko JC, Mongero LB, et al: Utility of cell salvage in women undergoing abdominal myomectomy. Am J Obstet Gynecol 211(1):28.e1, 2014

Song T, Seong S, Kim BG: Regeneration process after cervical conization for cervical intraepithelial neoplasia. Obstet Gynecol 128(6):1258, 2016

Spitzer M: Lower genital tract intraepithelial neoplasia in HIV-infected women: guidelines for evaluation and management. Obstet Gynecol Surv 54(2):131, 1999

Stuart GS: Puerperal sterilization. In Yeomans ER, Hoffman BL, Gilstrap III, et al (eds): Cunningham and Gilstrap's Operative Obstetrics, 3rd ed. New York, McGraw-Hill Education, 2017

Suh-Burgmann EJ, Whall-Strojwas D, Chang Y, et al: Risk factors for cervical stenosis after loop electrocautery excision procedure. Obstet Gynecol 96:657, 2000

Swanson CL, Rueter JA, Olson JE, et al: Localized provoked vestibulodynia: outcomes after modified vestibulectomy. J Reprod Med 59(3-4):121, 2014

Tabata T, Yamawaki T, Ida M, et al: Clinical value of dilatation and curettage for abnormal uterine bleeding. Arch Gynecol Obstet 264:174, 2001

Tan-Kim J, Menefee SA, Luber KM, et al: Prevalence and risk factors for mesh erosion after laparoscopic-assisted sacrocolpopexy. Int Urogynecol J Pelvic Floor Dysfunct 22(2):205, 2011

Thurman AR, Satterfield TM, Soper DE: Methicillin-resistant *Staphylococcus aureus* as a common cause of vulvar abscesses. Obstet Gynecol 112:538, 2008

Tinelli A, Malvasi A, Guido M, et al: Adhesion formation after intracapsular myomectomy with or without adhesion barrier. Fertil Steril 95(5):1780, 2011

Tixier H, Grevoul J, Loffroy R, et al: Preoperative embolization or ligature of the uterine arteries in preparation for conservative uterine fibroma surgery. Acta Obstet Gynecol Scand 89(10):1310, 2010

Tommola P, Unkila-Kallio L, Paavonen J: Surgical treatment of vulvar vestibulitis: a review. Acta Obstet Gynecol Scand 89(11):1385, 2010

Traas MA, Bekkers RL, Dony JM, et al: Surgical treatment for the vulvar vestibulitis syndrome. Obstet Gynecol 107(2 Pt 1):256, 2006

Trimbos JB, Heintz AP, van Hall EV: Reliability of cytological follow-up after conization of the cervix: a comparison of three surgical techniques. BJOG 90:1141, 1983

Tulandi T, Al-Jaroudi D: Interstitial pregnancy: results generated from the Society of Reproductive Surgeons Registry. Obstet Gynecol 103(1):47, 2004

Tulandi T, Beique F, Kimia M: Pulmonary edema: a complication of local injection of vasopressin at laparoscopy. Fertil Steril 66:478, 1996

Tulandi T, Murray C, Guralnick M: Adhesion formation and reproductive outcome after myomectomy and second-look laparoscopy. Obstet Gynecol 82:213, 1993

Tunçalp O, Gülmezoglu AM, Souza JP: Surgical procedures for evacuating incomplete miscarriage. Cochrane Database Syst Rev 9: CD001993, 2010

Turner LC, Shepherd JP, Wang L, et al: Hysterectomy surgical trends: a more accurate depiction of the last decade? Am J Obstet Gynecol 208(4):277.e1, 2013

Upadhyay UD, Desai S, Zlidar V, et al: Incidence of emergency department visits and complications after abortion. Obstet Gynecol 125(1): 175, 2015

van Seters M, van Beurden M, ten Kate FJ, et al: Treatment of vulvar intraepithelial neoplasia with topical imiquimod. N Engl J Med 358(14):1465, 2008

Vanichtantikul A, Charoenkwan K: Lidocaine spray compared with submucosal injection for reducing pain during loop electrosurgical excision procedure: a randomized controlled trial. Obstet Gynecol 122(3):553, 2013

Vatsa R, Bharti J, Roy KK, et al: Evaluation of amnion in creation of neovagina in women with Mayer-Rokitansky-Kuster-Hauser syndrome. Fertil Steril 108(2):341, 2017

Vecchietti G: [Creation of an artificial vagina in Rokitansky-Küster-Hauser syndrome]. [Italian] Attual Ostet Ginecol 11(2):131, 1965

Vercellini P, Trespidi L, Zaina B, et al: Gonadotropin-releasing hormone agonist treatment before abdominal myomectomy: a controlled trial. Fertil Steril 79:1390, 2003

Visco AG, Del Priore G: Postmenopausal Bartholin gland enlargement: a hospital-based cancer risk assessment. Obstet Gynecol 87:286, 1996

Walker JL, Powell CB, Chen LM, et al: Society of Gynecologic Oncology recommendations for the prevention of ovarian cancer. Cancer 121(13):2108, 2015

Wechter ME, Wu JM, Marzano D, et al: Management of Bartholin duct cysts and abscesses: a systematic review. Obstet Gynecol Surv 64(6):395, 2009

Weed JC Jr, Curry SL, Duncan ID, et al: Fertility after cryosurgery of the cervix. Obstet Gynecol 52:245, 1978

Welch JS, Cousellor VS, Malkasian GD Jr: The vaginal removal of the cervical stump. Surg Clin North Am 39:1073, 1959

Werner CL, Lo JY, Heffernan T, et al: Loop electrosurgical excision procedure and risk of preterm birth. Obstet Gynecol 115(3):605, 2010

Westberg J, Scott F, Creinin MD: Safety outcomes of female sterilization by salpingectomy and tubal occlusion. Contraception 95(5):505, 2017

White K, Carroll E, Grossman D: Complications from first-trimester aspiration abortion: a systematic review of the literature. Contraception 92(5):422, 2015

Wierrani F, Bodner K, Spängler B, et al: "Z"-plasty of the transverse vaginal septum using Garcia's procedure and the Grünberger modification. Fertil Steril 79(3):608, 2003

Williams CE, Nakhal RS, Hall-Craggs MA, et al: Transverse vaginal septae: management and long-term outcomes. BJOG 121(13):1653, 2014

Word B: New instrument for office treatment of cysts and abscesses of Bartholin's gland. JAMA 190:777, 1964

World Health Organization: Care of women and girls living with female genital mutilation: a clinical handbook. Geneva, World Health Organization, 2018

World Health Organization: Safe abortion: technical and policy guidance for health systems, 2nd ed. Geneva, World Health Organization, 2012

World Health Organization: WHO Guidelines for treatment of cervical intraepithelial neoplasia 2–3 and adenocarcinoma in situ: cryotherapy, large loop excision of the transformation zone, and cold knife conization. Geneva, World Health Organization, 2014

World Health Organization. WHO Guidelines on the management of health complications from female genital mutilation. 2016. Available at: https://apps.who.int/iris/bitstream/handle/10665/206437/9789241549646_eng.pdf

Wright JD, Hassan K, Ananth CV, et al: Use of guideline-based antibiotic prophylaxis in women undergoing gynecologic surgery. Obstet Gynecol 122(6):1145, 2013a

Wright JD, Herzog TJ, Tsui J, et al: Nationwide trends in the performance of inpatient hysterectomy in the United States. Obstet Gynecol 122(2 Pt 1):233, 2013b

Wright VC, Davies E: Laser surgery for vulvar intraepithelial neoplasia: principles and results. Am J Obstet Gynecol 156(2):374, 1987

Yamada T, Yamashita Y, Terai Y, et al: Intraoperative blood salvage in abdominal uterine myomectomy. Int J Gynaecol Obstet 56: 141, 1997

Yonke N, Leeman LM: First-trimester surgical abortion technique. Obstet Gynecol Clin North Am 40(4):647, 2013

Yoo EH, Lee PI, Huh CY, et al: Predictors of leiomyoma recurrence after laparoscopic myomectomy. J Minim Invasive Gynecol 14(6):690, 2007

Yu KJ, Lin YS, Chao KC, et al: A detachable porous vaginal mold facilitates reconstruction of a modified McIndoe neovagina. Fertil Steril 81:435, 2004

Zhou W, Nielsen GL, Moller M, et al: Short-term complications after surgically induced abortions: a register-based study of 56,117 abortions. Acta Obstet Gynaecol Scand 81:331, 2002

Zoulek E, Karp DR, Davila GW: Rectovaginal fistula as a complication to a Bartholin gland excision. Obstet Gynecol 118(2 Pt 2):489, 2011

CHAPTER 44

Minimally Invasive Surgery

44-1

Diagnostic Laparoscopy

Diagnostic laparoscopy provides a minimally invasive surgery (MIS) option for thorough evaluation of the peritoneal cavity and pelvic organs. It often is performed to evaluate pelvic pain or causes of infertility, to diagnose endometriosis, or to ascertain the qualities of a pelvic mass. Importantly, systematic evaluation of the peritoneal cavity is performed during every laparoscopy, either diagnostic or operative.

PREOPERATIVE

Consent

During the informed consent process for diagnostic laparoscopy, a surgeon reviews procedure goals, including diagnosis and possible treatment of identified pathology. Among others, this includes permission for lysis of adhesions, peritoneal biopsy, and excision or ablation of endometriosis. A patient also is informed that diagnostic laparoscopy may reveal no apparent pathology.

Laparoscopy typically is associated with few complications. Of these, organ injuries caused by puncture or by electrosurgery burn are the most common major complications and are summarized in Chapter 41 (p. 875). The possible need to complete the diagnostic evaluation via laparotomy also is discussed. Reasons for conversion include failure to gain abdominal access, organ or vessel injury during entry, or extensive adhesions. In general, such conversion during diagnostic laparoscopy is uncommon.

Patient Preparation

Compared with laparotomy, laparoscopy usually is associated with lower rates of postoperative infection and venous thromboembolism (VTE). Thus, for diagnostic laparoscopy, antibiotics generally are not required, and VTE prophylaxis is implemented for those with risk factors (Table 39-10, p. 834). For most patients, bowel preparation also is not administered. However, if extensive adhesiolysis is anticipated and the risk of colorectal injury is thereby increased, bowel preparation can be considered. An empty rectum can aid intraoperative proctosigmoidoscopy and bowel manipulation needed for repair.

INTRAOPERATIVE

Instruments

Several instruments are especially helpful during diagnostic evaluation, and most are found in a standard laparoscopy instrument set. Of these, atraumatic graspers move abdominal organs gently but precisely. A uterine manipulator that allows chromopertubation also is considered if performing diagnostic laparoscopy for infertility evaluation. If this is planned, 10 mL of methylene blue is mixed with 100 to 150 mL of sterile saline for injection through the cervical cannula of the manipulator. On rare occasion, methylene blue may induce acute methemoglobinemia, particularly in patients with glucose-6-phosphate dehydrogenase deficiency.

Surgical Steps

❶ Anesthesia and Patient Positioning. Most laparoscopic surgery is performed in an operating room with general anesthesia. Peritoneal pain created by the intraabdominal pneumoperitoneum merits this degree of anesthesia. Following anesthesia induction, the patient is placed in low lithotomy position to permit access to the cervix and allow uterine manipulation. The patient's arms are tucked at her sides. Even for anticipated short procedures, correct patient positioning is critical to help avoid patient nerve injury and to optimize surgeon ergonomics and access. Positioning is described in Chapter 41 (p. 877).

A bimanual examination is completed to determine uterine inclination, which will direct uterine manipulator positioning, if used. The vagina and abdomen are surgically prepared, and the bladder is drained. For longer procedures, a Foley catheter may be required as a full bladder can obstruct the operating view or increase the risk of bladder injury.

❷ Uterine Manipulator Placement. Although not mandatory, a uterine manipulator may be placed to move the uterus during evaluation of the pelvis. Examples are shown in Chapter 41 (p. 880). For its placement, a surgeon is gowned and doubly gloved. A Graves speculum or vaginal retractors are used to display the cervix. To stabilize the cervix, a single-tooth tenaculum is placed on the anterior cervical lip. A Cohen or other uterine manipulator then is inserted into the external os (Fig. 41-8, p. 881).

Alternatively, a balloon-tip intracavitary manipulator can be used (Fig. 41-7, p. 880). For this, a Sims uterine sound first is placed through the cervical os and into the uterine cavity to measure its depth and inclination (Fig. 43-15.3C, p. 973). Once gentle resistance is met at the fundus, the distance from the fundus to the external os is measured by score marks along the length of the sound. Knowledge of the depth to which the manipulator can safely be inserted helps lower uterine perforation risk. The balloon end of an intracavitary manipulator may be threaded through the external cervical os and into the endometrial cavity. Once here, the balloon is inflated. The outer pair of surgical gloves is removed, and the surgeon moves to either side of the patient.

❸ Primary Trocar Entry. Abdominal access may be attained by any of the four basic techniques described in Chapter 41 (p. 888). These include Veress needle insertion, direct trocar insertion, optical-access insertion, or open entry methods. For diagnostic laparoscopy, no one method is superior to the others. The umbilicus is usually chosen as the site for abdominal entry. However, if a patient's history suggests periumbilical adhesions or mesh, entry at the Palmer point usually is preferred.

A 5-mm or 10-mm umbilical port will house a suitable laparoscope for diagnostic examination. Generally, starting with a 5-mm incision and 5-mm laparoscope allows adequate viewing of the abdominopelvic cavity. If improved optics are desired, these two are easily changed to 10-mm diameters. Once safe initial entry is confirmed, the abdomen is insufflated to reach an intraabdominal pressure of 15 mm Hg or less.

❹ Additional Port Site Selection. During diagnostic laparoscopy, additional operative cannulas are needed. If minimal tissue manipulation is required, a suprapubic port may suffice. However, bilateral lower quadrant locations may be desired if lysis of adhesions or greater tissue manipulation is required. Additional ports are placed under direct laparoscopic guidance, as described in Chapter 41 (p. 893).

❺ Upper Abdomen Evaluation. All laparoscopic procedures begin with a systematic and thorough diagnostic inspection of the entire peritoneal cavity, including the pelvis and upper abdomen. Once safe initial entry is confirmed, the area directly below the primary trocar entry site is evaluated for bleeding or other signs of entry trauma. Prior to Trendelenburg positioning, the upper abdomen is examined. Specifically, the liver surface, gallbladder, falciform ligament, stomach, omentum, and right and left hemidiaphragms are inspected. The ascending, transverse, and descending colon also are viewed. During inspection of the ascending portion, the appendix is identified.

After Trendelenburg positioning, bowel and omentum fall toward the upper abdomen to expose the retroperitoneal structures. Now free of intestines, the area directly beneath the initial entry site is examined again. Previously unappreciated trauma to this area from initial abdominal entry might then be seen.

❻ Examination of Pelvis. Following examination of the upper abdomen, attention is turned to the pelvis. First, the uterus is retroflexed with the aid of the uterine manipulator to provide clear viewing of the anterior cul-de-sac. Next, the manipulator tilts the uterus up and to the right to permit left pelvic sidewall inspection. The uterus then is anteflexed to provide access to the posterior cul-de-sac. Last, the uterus is tilted to the left, and the right pelvic sidewall is viewed. Peritoneal surfaces are thereby sequentially and methodically inspected. During this, endometriotic implants, peritoneal defects or windows, studding concerning for malignancy, adhesions, and fibrosis are sought.

Of pelvic organs, both ureters are found coursing from the pelvic brim, along the lower pelvic sidewall, and to the cervix. Both peristalsis and caliber are assessed. Uterine size, shape, and texture also are noted. To examine both fallopian tubes and ovaries, a surgeon places a blunt probe into the cul-de-sac and sweeps the probe forward and laterally. In doing so, the tubes and ovaries are lifted from the posterior cul-de-sac or ovarian fossa for inspection.

❼ Indicated Laparoscopic Procedures. After visual assessment of pathology, indicated procedures are performed. If adhesions are encountered, they may be divided as described in Chapter 41 (p. 898).

❽ Abdomen Deflation and Port Removal. At laparoscopy completion, carbon dioxide (CO_2) insufflation is halted, and the gas tubing is disconnected from the primary cannula. The gas valves on all cannulas are opened to deflate the abdominal cavity. To prevent diaphragmatic irritation from retained CO_2, manual pressure against the abdominal wall helps expel remaining gas.

During this process, all secondary cannulas are removed using laparoscopic visualization. This allows exclusion of bleeding from punctured vessels that may have been tamponaded by these cannulas. Additionally, it prevents herniation of bowel or omentum up through the cannula track and into the anterior abdominal wall. Of note, the pneumoperitoneum also can act as an intraoperative tamponade. Accordingly, potential bleeding sites are reinspected as the pneumoperitoneum is released. Next, the primary cannula is removed while leaving the laparoscope in the abdomen. Last, the laparoscope is slowly removed to visualize the abdomen and primary entry site for any evidence of bleeding and to prevent viscera from being pulled into the port site.

❾ **Incision Closure.** Depending on their size, incisions may require deep fascial stitches. To prevent incisional hernia formation, fascial closure often is recommended whenever trocars measuring ≥10 mm are employed (Lajer, 1997; Lambertz, 2017; Wells, 2019). Nonbladed trocars may decrease this risk (Liu, 2000). If open entry was used, the sutures originally placed in the fascia are unthreaded from the Hasson cannula. Each of these sutures is brought to the midline of the incision, and square knots are tied to close the fascial defect.

Skin incisions are closed with a subcuticular stitch of 4-0 gauge delayed-absorbable suture. Alternatively, the skin may be closed with cyanoacrylate tissue adhesive (Dermabond Topical Skin Adhesive) or skin tape (Steri-Strips) (Chap. 40, p. 846). After incision closure, the uterine manipulator is removed.

POSTOPERATIVE

Depending on the procedure performed, most patients can be discharged home on the same day as surgery. For most, physical activities and diet are resumed according to patient comfort.

Laparoscopic Sterilization and Essure Removal

Approximately 650,000 tubal sterilization procedures are performed annually in the United States. About half follow pregnancy delivery or termination, but the others are performed independent of pregnancy and are termed *interval sterilization* (Chan, 2010). Most interval procedures are performed laparoscopically, and common options achieve tubal occlusion by electrosurgical coagulation, by mechanical clips, by Silastic bands, or by suture ligation. Selection typically is directed by provider preference or by equipment availability.

Current sterilization practices will likely change with recommendations now encouraging consideration of prophylactic salpingectomy for women at average risk of ovarian cancer at the time of sterilization, abdominal or pelvic surgery, or hysterectomy (American College of Obstetricians and Gynecologists, 2019c). The goal of risk-reducing salpingectomy aims to decrease rates of certain epithelial ovarian cancers. Currently theoretical, suggested advantages are fully described in Chapters 5 and 35 (pp. 188 and 736). In sum, tubal interruption itself lowers later ovarian cancer rates by 30 percent, and salpingectomy may offer a 40- to 80-percent reduction. Salpingectomy lengthens surgery time by less than 10 minutes. If advanced bipolar coagulation devices are employed, surgical speed and ease are balanced against cost, which may be higher than with tubal interruption techniques. Blood loss and complication rates are comparable between the two (Kim, 2019a; Powell, 2017; Westberg, 2017). Few data describe the potential effects on ovarian reserve from blood supply disruption. In two small studies comparing the two surgeries, no short-term differences in antimüllerian hormone level, which is a measure of ovarian reserve, were found (Ganer Herman, 2017; Findley 2013).

In contrast to laparoscopic sterilization, the Essure Permanent Birth Control System is a microinsert made of a stainless steel inner coil that is enclosed in polyester fibers. These fibers are surrounded by an expandable outer coil made of nitinol—a nickel and titanium alloy (Fig. 5-5, p. 120). One device is inserted hysteroscopically into each proximal fallopian tube. Fibroblastic proliferation and ingrowth between the device fibers causes tubal occlusion.

Increasingly, these devices are being removed in symptomatic patients. Chronic pelvic pain after hysteroscopic sterilization may develop in 2 to 6 percent of those with inserts (Chudnoff, 2015; Kamencic, 2016; Yunker, 2015). Pain may stem from tubal perforation, device migration, or the device itself (Adelman, 2014). For those desiring removal, one method is described here. Importantly, device removal is not curative in all symptomatic patients (Clark, 2017; Maassen, 2019).

PREOPERATIVE

Patient Evaluation

Prior to sterilization, several preventive steps can avoid procedures in women with early, undiagnosed pregnancies. Namely, providing contraception well in advance of surgery, scheduling surgery in the follicular phase of the menstrual cycle, and preoperative serum β-human chorionic gonadotropin (β-hCG) level testing are effective methods to prevent or detect early pregnancy (American College of Obstetricians and Gynecologists, 2019b). Patients who require treatment of advanced cervical epithelial abnormalities and who desire sterilization may choose hysterectomy rather than tubal occlusion as a means to serve both needs. For this reason, women ideally have cervical cancer screening results reviewed prior to surgery.

For Essure removal, preoperative imaging can guide surgical planning. Essure confirmation in the United States requires hysterosalpingography (HSG), and if available, these images are reviewed prior to surgery. Pain is a common indication for removal. Thus, transvaginal sonography (TVS) or

three-dimensional TVS often is selected to image implants and to seek other potential sources of pain. If implants are not seen sonographically, plain abdominal radiographs can help identify devices that may have perforated the fallopian tube and migrated into the abdominal cavity (Djeffal, 2018). If identified here, adding a lateral radiograph view can help define device location.

Consent

Prior to sterilization, patients are counseled regarding other reversible contraceptive methods; other permanent methods, such as male sterilization; and the possibility of future regret (American College of Obstetricians and Gynecologists, 2017c). Tubal sterilization is effective and should be considered permanent by the patient.

Complications associated with tubal sterilization are few. In general, the risks of laparoscopic sterilization mirror those of laparoscopy (Chap. 41, p. 875).

Sterilizing clips and bands routinely fall from around the tube once occluded ends undergo necrosis and fibrosis (Fig. 44-2.1). Most ectopic clips are incidental findings without untoward patient effects, but less commonly they can incite local foreign body reactions. Rare cases of clip migration to sites such as the bladder, uterine cavity, and anterior abdominal wall have been reported (Dey, 2010; Gooden, 1993; Kesby, 1997).

Contraceptive failure and pregnancy rates related to each procedure are discussed with the patient and are listed in Chapter 5 (p. 119). Overall, these rates are low, and tubal sterilization is an effective method of contraception. If pregnancy does occur, however, the risk of ectopic pregnancy is greater.

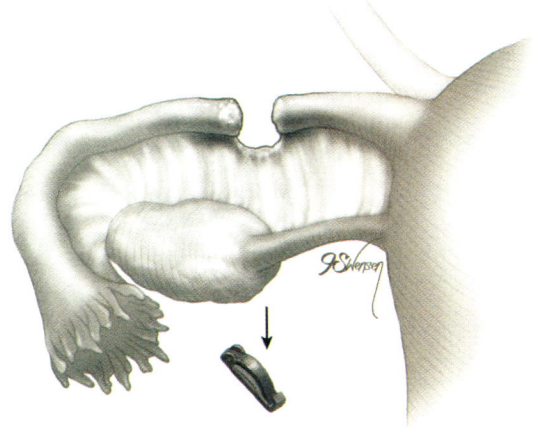

FIGURE 44-2.1 Filshie clip may fall away following fibrosis of fallopian tube ends.

Bipolar coagulation has the highest risk for this complication compared with that of clips or bands (Malacova, 2014; Peterson, 1996). Amenorrhea following any sterilization procedure should prompt serum β-hCG testing to aid in identifying ectopic pregnancies.

For Essure removal, a main potential complication is tubal bleeding that might prompt salpingectomy. Oophorectomy or hysterectomy would be rare. Other risks mirror those for diagnostic laparoscopy, which in general carries low complication rates.

Although devices are typically removed laparoscopically, device fragmentation may necessitate hysteroscopic retrieval of a portion embedded in a tubal ostium. For this reason, women are counseled regarding the steps and potential risks of operative hysteroscopy. Patients are consented for this possible addition (p. 1054). Last, women with pain should understand that all symptoms may not resolve despite device removal.

Patient Preparation

For these procedures, antibiotics and bowel preparation typically are not administered. VTE prophylaxis is implemented only for those at higher risk as listed in Table 39-10 (p. 834).

INTRAOPERATIVE

Surgical Steps

❶ Anesthesia and Patient Positioning. Most laparoscopic tubal sterilization procedures are performed using general anesthesia.

To reduce postoperative pain, investigators have evaluated the adjunctive use of bupivacaine solution injected or dripped onto the tubal serosa or delivered transcervically through balloon uterine manipulators into the fallopian tube lumen (Brennan, 2004; Schytte, 2003; Wrigley, 2000). Although results have varied, one metaanalysis suggests some benefit in diminishing immediate postoperative pain with these practices (Harrison, 2014).

For sterilization, the patient is placed in the low lithotomy position, and patient arms are tucked at the side. A bimanual examination is completed to determine uterine size and inclination. Uterine size will affect placement of the accessory trocar, and inclination will direct positioning of the uterine manipulator, if used. The vagina and abdomen are surgically prepared, and the bladder is drained. Most procedures are brief, and a Foley catheter is seldom required. Often, a uterine manipulator or instead a sponge stick is placed to provide uterine anteflexion or retroflexion during evaluation of the pelvis.

❷ Abdominal Entry and Accessory Ports. For all of the procedures described, the initial steps of laparoscopic abdominal entry are performed as described in Chapter 41 (p. 888). In most instances, one accessory port is required and is placed suprapubically in the midline to provide an equal reach to both fallopian tubes. For a normal-sized uterus, this port is placed 2 to 3 cm above the symphysis pubis. However, for a larger uterus, this position is moved cephalad as needed to access both tubes.

For Essure removal, two accessory ports are used to provide suitable instrument triangulation for device removal. Once cannulas are in place, inspection of the abdomen and pelvis is completed prior to the planned procedure.

Surgical Steps—Filshie Clip Application

❶ Filshie Clip. This titanium clip is applied with the aid of a customized metal applicator that houses the clip within its single-action jaw. The applicator requires an 8-mm cannula for insertion into the abdominal cavity. As the jaw is closed, the shorter upper rim of the clip is forced beneath the longer lower clasp. The clip thereby is locked into place around the fallopian tube.

❷ Positioning the Fallopian Tube. To begin, a blunt probe or atraumatic grasping forceps is placed through the accessory port. Using the tool, the surgeon stretches the fallopian tube out horizontally and laterally. Concurrently, a uterine manipulator can be used to tilt the uterus laterally and in the opposite direction. The blunt probe is removed from the operative port and replaced by the clip applicator.

❸ Applicator Insertion. At the beginning of clip application, a Filshie clip is held within its applicator and inserted through the accessory cannula into the abdomen. A surgeon half closes the applicator's upper jaw to insert the applicator and its clip through the cannula. The handle of the applicator is

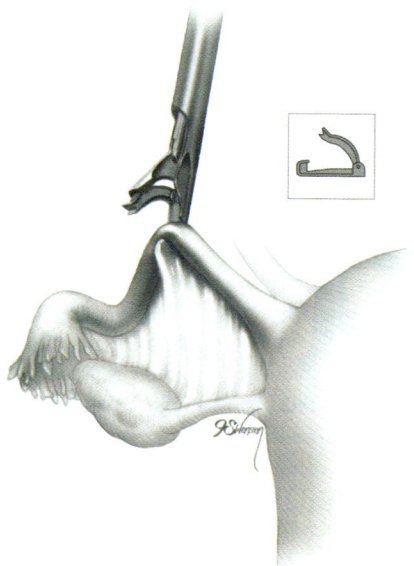

FIGURE 44-2.2 Open Filshie clip within applicator.

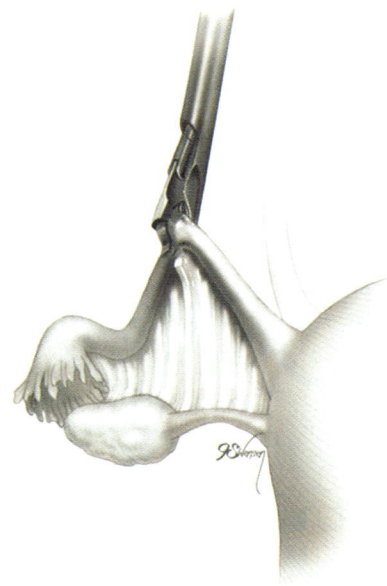

FIGURE 44-2.3 Clip application around fallopian tube.

not gripped tightly, as this may prematurely close and lock the clip (Penfield, 2000).

Once the Filshie clip emerges through the cannula tip, the applicator is opened slowly. The jaw of the applicator has the potential to spring open more quickly than the clip can open. With this, the clip can fall off the applicator and into the abdomen. Fallen clips are preferably retrieved, but if an open clip becomes lost and hidden by loops of bowel, laparotomy is not required typically for retrieval.

4 Clip Placement. After the clip is completely open, the clip and applicator are positioned with one jaw above and one below the fallopian tube at a site along the isthmic portion of the tube and 2 to 3 cm from the uterine cornu (Fig. 44-2.2). The entire diameter of the tube should lie across the base of the clip. The distal hooked end of the lower jaw should be visible through the mesosalpinx.

5 Clip Application. Once satisfied that the clip is positioned correctly, a surgeon slowly squeezes the finger bar handle toward the handle backstop and to its full limit. With this action, the upper ridge of the clip is slowly compressed and locked under the lower hooked end of the clip (Fig. 44-2.3). This flattens the entire tube within the clip (Fig. 44-2.4). As the applicator jaws are slowly opened, the clip releases automatically from the applicator as it has locked onto the tube. These steps are repeated on the opposite fallopian tube. If proper clip placement is questioned, a second clip is applied correctly to the same tube.

Rarely, a clip may transect a fallopian tube. This usually is associated with a large fallopian tube, which has been clipped too quickly. For sterilization completion, a clip is applied to both ends of the transected tube.

Surgical Steps—Bipolar Coagulation

1 Site Selection. For this method, the fallopian tube is identified and grasped in the isthmic region at least 2 to 3 cm lateral to the cornu (Fig. 44-2.5). Placement here is important as pressure from retrograde menstrual flow against a coagulated stump that has been placed too close to the cornu can risk stump recanalization and fistula formation. Leaving a 2- to 3-cm segment allows ample space for absorption of intrauterine fluid without creating excess pressure against the stump.

2 Electrocoagulation. The coagulating paddles of the bipolar forceps should span the tube. Overextending their grasp may lead to partial coagulation of the mesosalpinx and incomplete coagulation of the entire tube diameter. Before current is applied, the tube is slightly elevated and pulled away from other adjacent structures to prevent thermal injury to these. As current is applied, the tube swells and fluid often bubbles and pops from the tissue.

Current is delivered until the tube is completely desiccated. Failure to reach this end point is linked with higher contraceptive failure rates (Soderstrom, 1989). Because visual

inspection of the tube is inadequate to assess complete desiccation, an ammeter is incorporated with most bipolar generators. Water conducts current through tissues. Thus, completely desiccated tissues are unable to conduct current. For this reason, current is maintained during coagulation until zero current flow across the tube is registered by the ammeter. The tube then is released.

A second site that is lateral but contiguous with the first coagulated segment is grasped and similarly coagulated. A total of two to three contiguous sites are serially coagulated. This occludes a total span of 3 cm along the tube's length (see Fig. 44-2.5). Coagulation of shorter distances along the tube can lead to recanalization and contraceptive failure (Peterson, 1999). These steps are repeated on the opposite fallopian tube.

Occasionally following coagulation, the tube may stick to the bipolar paddles. To free the tube, the paddles are slowly opened and gently twisted to the right and then the left. Additionally, gentle fluid irrigation of the desiccated area may help release the tube.

Surgical Steps—Falope Ring Application

1 Falope Ring (Silastic Band). With this method, a Silastic Falope ring is applied with the aid of a custom metal applicator. To summarize the process, applicator tongs draw a portion of tube up into an inner sheath, and an outer sheath then pushes a Silastic band off the inner sheath and onto the fallopian tube loop.

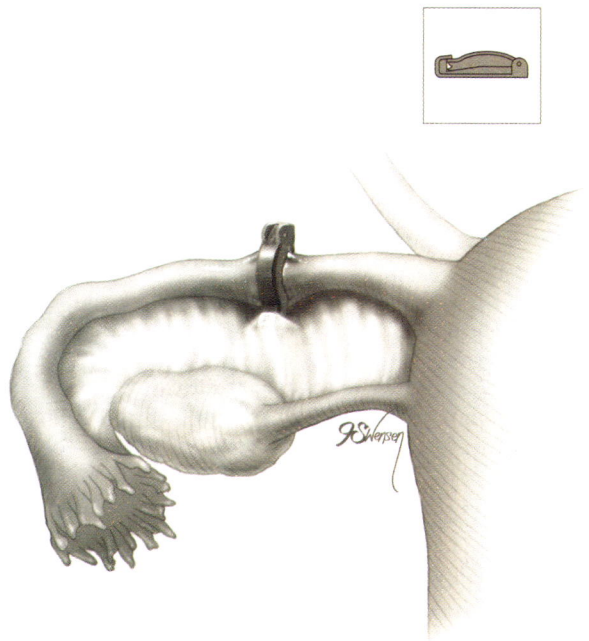

FIGURE 44-2.4 Closed clip around the tube.

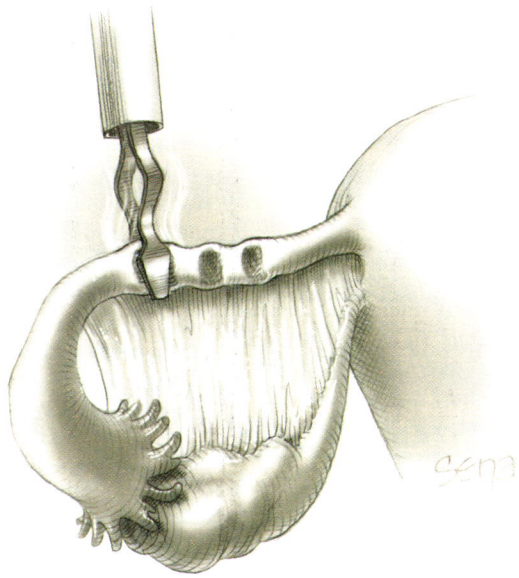

FIGURE 44-2.5 Bipolar electrosurgical coagulation.

SECTION 6

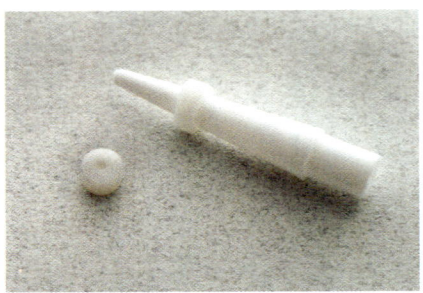

FIGURE 44-2.6 Falope ring (*left*) and ring stretched around applicator (*right*).

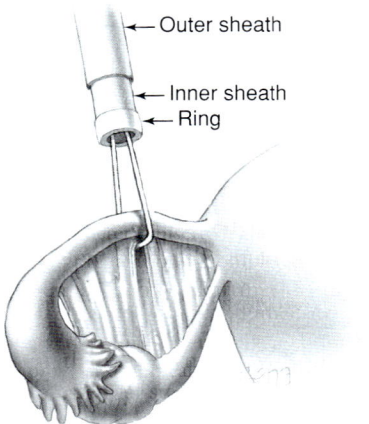

← Outer sheath

← Inner sheath
← Ring

FIGURE 44-2.7 Falope ring applicator placement.

❷ **Ring Loading.** Prior to its insertion into the abdomen, a Falope ring is stretched around the distal tip of the inner applicator sheath by means of a special ring loader and ring guide (Fig. 44-2.6).

❸ **Ring Placement.** Once inserted through the accessory port, the applicator's tongs are opened and placed completely around the fallopian tube approximately 3 cm from the cornu. Tongs grasp the mesosalpinx directly at its attachment to the tube. This prevents excess mesosalpinx from being drawn into the inner sheath (Fig. 44-2.7).

❹ **Ring Application.** A trigger on the applicator retracts the tongs and draws a loop of tube approximately 1.5 cm into the inner sheath. The total length of tube contained within the inner sheath thus is 3 cm (Fig. 44-2.8).

The outer sheath is advanced toward the loop's base. This outer sheath pushes the Silastic band off the inner sheath and onto the loop base (Fig. 44-2.9). The loop base will blanch from ischemia following band placement (Fig. 44-2.10). These steps are repeated on the opposite fallopian tube.

Tubal transection is uncommon, and a Falope ring can be applied to each of the divided segments. Vessels of the mesosalpinx can occasionally tear and bleed as the tongs and tube are drawn into the inner sheath.

The Silastic band, once applied to the loop base, will control bleeding in most instances. Thus, electrosurgical coagulation to achieve hemostasis is infrequently needed.

Surgical Steps—Hulka Clip Application

❶ **Required Instruments.** The plastic Hulka clip is also generically known as a spring clip because of the stiff outer metal spring that locks the clip into place. Required equipment includes the clips themselves and a custom metal applicator, which holds the clip during application.

❷ **Positioning the Fallopian Tube.** To begin, a blunt probe or atraumatic grasping forceps is placed through the accessory cannula. With the tool, the fallopian tube is outstretched horizontally and laterally to aid clip application. Concurrently, a uterine manipulator can be used to tilt the uterus laterally and in the opposite direction.

❸ **Clip Loading.** Before the applicator and its clip are inserted through the accessory trocar, the trigger of the applicator is gently squeezed by the surgeon's thumb. This action advances the outer rod of the

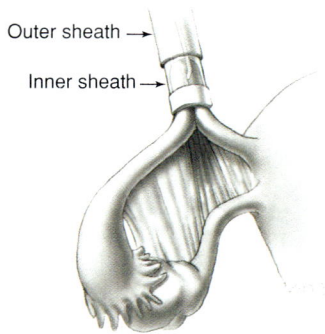

Outer sheath →

Inner sheath →

FIGURE 44-2.8 Tube drawn into inner sheath.

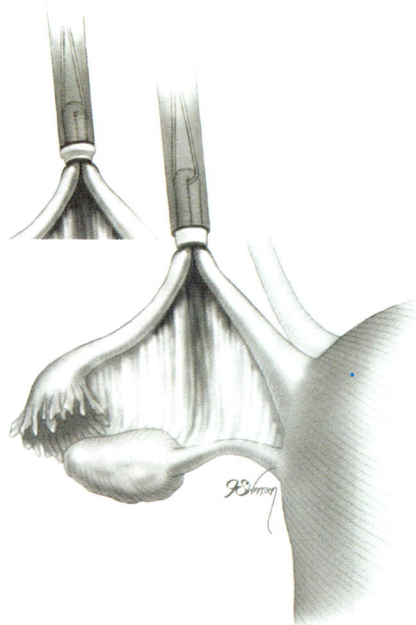

FIGURE 44-2.9 Outer sheath forces the Falope ring off the inner sheath (*Inset*) and onto the fallopian tube.

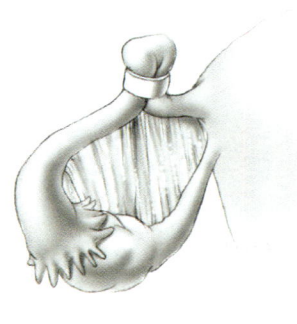

FIGURE 44-2.10 Falope ring in place.

applicator down and over the top of the clip. This closes the jaws of the clip to within 1 mm of each of other. This is an unlocked position yet allows the clip and applicator to be threaded down the accessory cannula.

❹ **Clip Application.** Once inside the abdomen, the applicator trigger is drawn backward, the outer rod retracts, and the upper jaw of the clip reopens. Held within the applicator jaws, the open clip is positioned across the narrow isthmic portion of the fallopian tube, 2 to 3 cm from the cornu, and perpendicular to the long axis of the tube (Fig. 44-2.11). The jaws are positioned around the tube in a manner that directs the tube deeply into the crux of the clip jaws. This aids in total occlusion of the tube as it is flattened across the base of the closing clip. Additionally, the applicator tip and clip are positioned such that when closed, the clip incorporates a small portion of adjacent mesosalpinx.

❺ **Clip Closure.** Once the applicator jaws are appropriately positioned, the thumb-action trigger is slowly squeezed to push forward the outer rod of the applicator and close the clip around the tube (Fig. 44-2.12). The clip application is inspected to ensure that it has completely encompassed the tube.

If placement is deemed correct, the trigger is fully depressed. This forces the center rod of the applicator forward against the butt of the clip's stiff metal spring (Fig. 44-2.13). The spring is pushed out and around the plastic frame of the clip to compress and lock the upper and lower clip jaws in place. One clip is placed on each tube. If a clip is misapplied, a second clip can be placed lateral to the first.

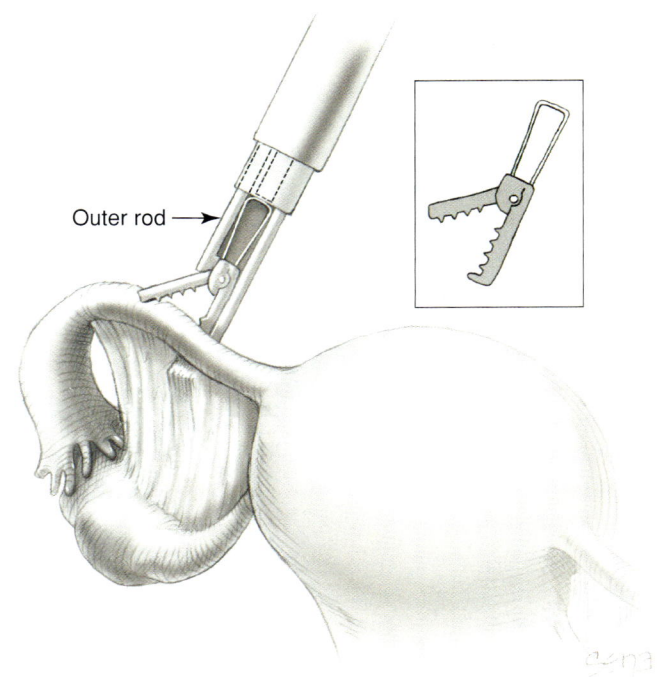

FIGURE 44-2.11 Hulka clip application.

Surgical Steps—Pomeroy Technique

❶ **Endoscopic Loop.** This procedure can be used as a sterilization technique but more commonly is used to excise fallopian tube ectopic pregnancies. A description and figures can be found in Section 44-3 (p. 1026).

Surgical Steps—Essure Device Removal

❶ **Tubal Incision.** Initially, laparoscopic ports are placed in the right and left lower abdomen. The affected fallopian tube is lifted and held with atraumatic grasping forceps (Fig. 44-2.14). The tips of monopolar dissecting scissors ideally incise the tubal wall

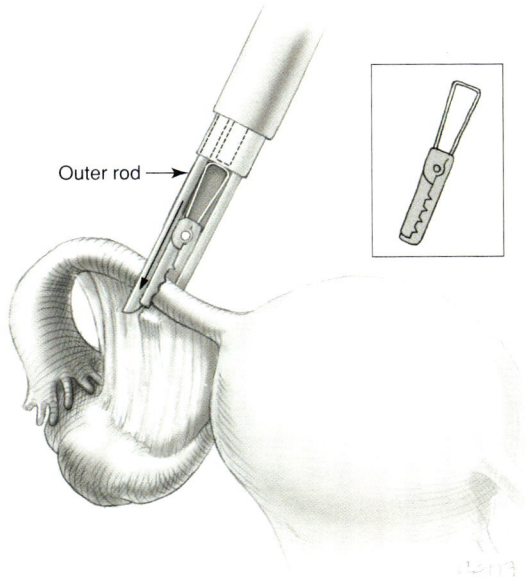

FIGURE 44-2.12 Hulka clip closure.

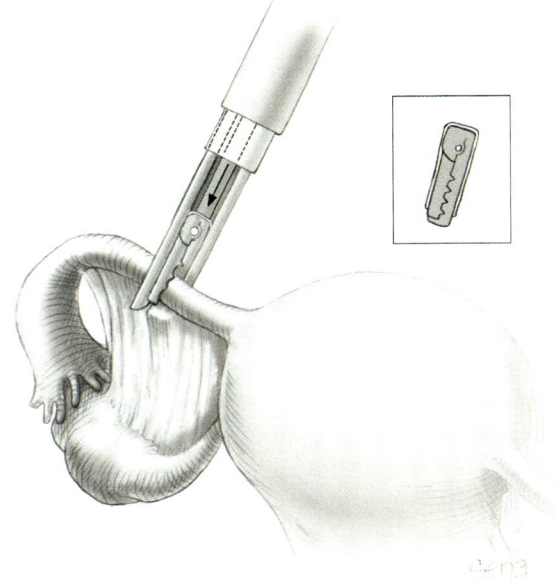

FIGURE 44-2.13 Hulka spring secured.

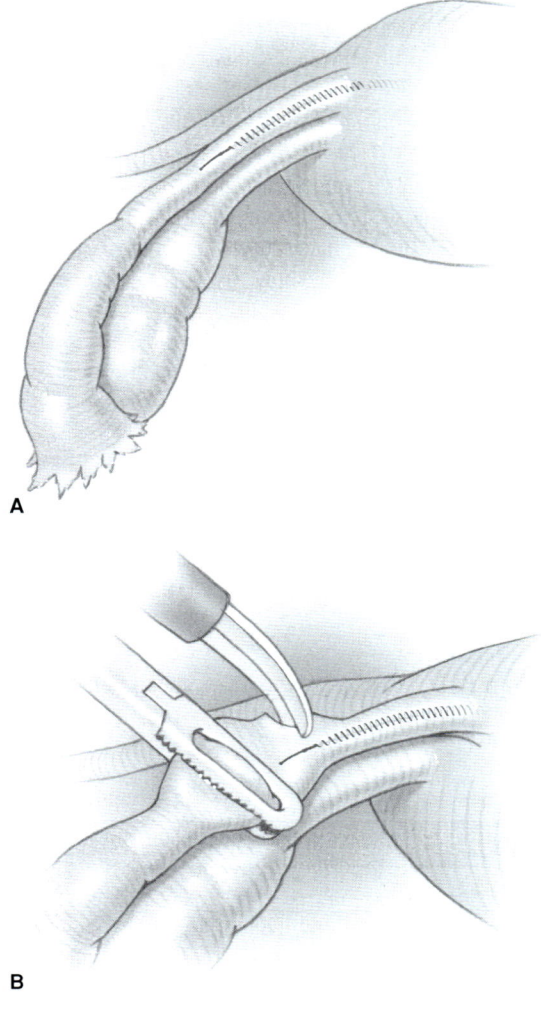

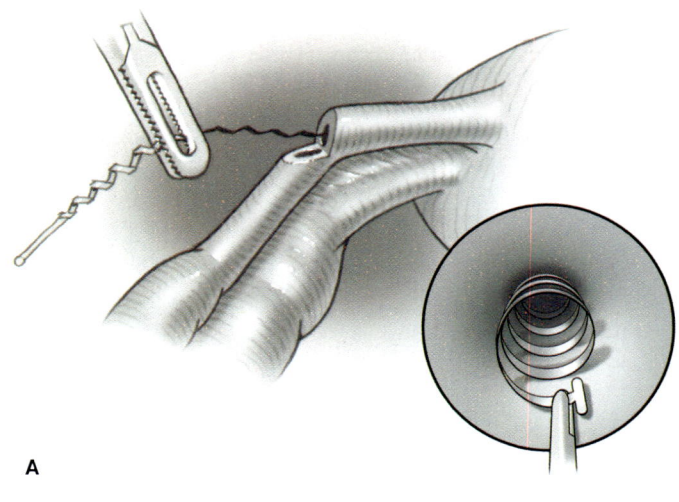

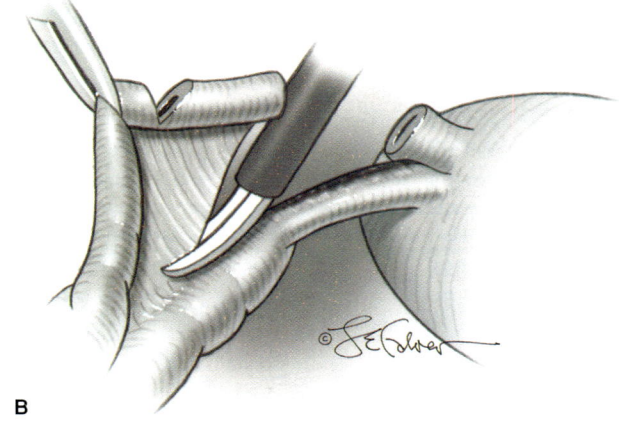

FIGURE 44-2.14 A. Essure device in place. **B.** Fallopian tube incised.

FIGURE 44-2.15 A. Device grasped and extracted. Inset: A fractured device may require hysteroscopic removal of the proximal piece. **B.** Salpingectomy performed following device removal.

on its antimesenteric surface. This avoids the extensive vascularity of the mesosalpinx. Once the tubal lumen is entered, delicate dissection with blunt forceps or scissor tips will uncover the Essure device.

❷ **Device Removal.** Once isolated, the device is held by the initial atraumatic graspers, and gentle traction is applied to remove it from the lumen (Fig. 44-2.15). Slight uncoiling of the device is common. Shown in the figure inset, in cases compli-

cated by device fragmentation, a hysteroscopic grasper can extract remaining coils. Following Essure removal, salpingectomy is completed as described on page 1025. Subsequently, the contralateral tube's device is extracted.

❸ **Wound Closure.** For sterilization or Essure removal, subsequent surgery completion steps follow those of diagnostic laparoscopy (p. 1018).

POSTOPERATIVE

Postoperatively, patients are given instructions similar to those following diagnostic laparoscopy. Sterilization is immediate, and intercourse may resume at the patient's discretion.

44-3

Laparoscopic Salpingectomy

This procedure is commonly performed for ectopic pregnancy. Goals include hemodynamic support of the patient, removal of all trophoblastic tissue, repair or excision of the damaged tube, and preservation of fertility in those who desire it. For most women, the preferred surgical approach for ectopic pregnancy management is laparoscopic rather than laparotomy. The former provides a safe and effective treatment of the affected fallopian tube while offering the advantages of laparoscopy.

For some, laparoscopic salpingostomy is desired to treat and retain the affected tube. However, if the contralateral tube is normal, data suggest that subsequent fertility is similar whether salpingectomy or salpingostomy is performed (Chap. 7, p. 170) (Fernandez, 2013; Mol, 2014). If fertility is not a consideration or if tubal damage or bleeding does not permit fallopian tube salvage, laparoscopic salpingectomy may be selected due to its lower risk of persistent trophoblastic tissue.

Of other indications, salpingectomy may also be used to remove hydrosalpinges in women undergoing in vitro fertilization (IVF). In this case, pregnancy rates are improved if such tubes are excised (Chap. 21, p. 460).

In women with *BRCA* gene mutations, early bilateral salpingectomy followed by later oophorectomy is one strategy to lower epithelial ovarian cancer and breast cancer risks yet provide extended estrogen benefits (Chap. 35, p. 736) (American College of Obstetricians and Gynecologists, 2017b, 2019c). In women at low risk for ovarian cancer, salpingectomy alone and solely for ovarian risk reduction is not recommended at this time.

Last, total salpingectomy can be used as a method of sterilization. This may be especially attractive if a primary sterilization technique has failed. For women who have a low risk for ovarian cancer and who desire sterilization, salpingectomy also can be considered as part of a risk-reducing strategy, discussed in the last section (p. 736).

PREOPERATIVE

Consent

The general risks of laparoscopic surgery are discussed in Chapter 41 (p. 875). With salpingectomy, injury to the ipsilateral ovary is possible. Thus, the potential for oophorectomy and its effects on fertility and hormone function are discussed. Prior to cases for ectopic pregnancy, a patient's desire for future fertility is investigated. If she has completed her childbearing or has failed a prior sterilization procedure, contralateral tubal ligation or bilateral salpingectomy may be acceptable at the time of surgery.

Following any surgical treatment of ectopic pregnancy, trophoblastic tissue can persist. The risk of this is lower with salpingectomy compared with salpingostomy and is discussed more fully on page 1028.

Patient Preparation

Baseline complete blood count (CBC), β-hCG level, and Rh status routinely are assessed. If salpingectomy is performed in the setting of an ectopic pregnancy, substantial bleeding may be encountered. Thus, the patient is typed and crossmatched for packed red blood cells and other blood products as indicated. For those undergoing laparoscopic salpingectomy for ectopic pregnancy, VTE prophylaxis is typically indicated due to the hypercoagulability associated with pregnancy (Table 39-10, p. 834). For prophylaxis in those with active bleeding, intermittent pneumatic compression devices are preferred. For salpingectomy performed for other indications, VTE prophylaxis typically is not required. Salpingectomy is associated with low infection rates. Thus, preoperative antibiotics usually are not administered.

INTRAOPERATIVE

Instruments

Most instruments required for salpingectomy are found in a standard laparoscopy instrument set. However, a suction irrigation system is commonly needed during salpingectomy to remove blood from a ruptured ectopic pregnancy. Depending on the size of the ectopic pregnancy or hydrosalpinges, an endoscopic retrieval bag also may be needed. For salpingectomy, the fallopian tube and mesosalpinx require ligation and excision. This may be accomplished using bipolar instruments, Harmonic scalpel, or laparoscopic suture loop (ENDOLOOP). These may not be readily available in all operating suites, and desired tools are requested prior to surgery.

Surgical Steps

❶ **Anesthesia and Patient Positioning.** The patient is prepared and positioned for laparoscopic surgery (Chap. 41, p. 877).

❷ **Abdominal Entry.** The abdomen is entered with laparoscopic techniques, and typically two or three accessory port sites are added (Chap. 41, p. 888). Depending on the size of the ectopic pregnancy, at least one 10-mm or larger accessory cannula may be needed to allow specimen removal at surgery's end. Once cannulas are in place, inspection of the abdomen and pelvis is completed prior to the planned procedure.

❸ **Mesosalpingeal Incision.** The affected fallopian tube is lifted and held with an atraumatic grasping forceps. Kleppinger bipolar electrode forceps are placed across a proximal portion of the fallopian tube. A cutting current at 25 W should suffice (**Fig. 44-3.1**). When zero amperage of flow is noted, scissors can cut the desiccated, blanched tube (**Fig. 44-3.2**).

The Kleppinger forceps are next advanced across the adjacent proximal portion of mesosalpinx. Similarly, current is applied, and the desiccated tissue is cut. This process serially moves from the proximal mesosalpinx to its

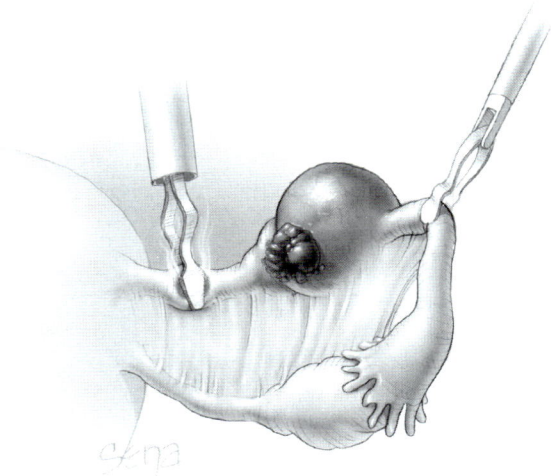

FIGURE 44-3.1 Fallopian tube desiccation.

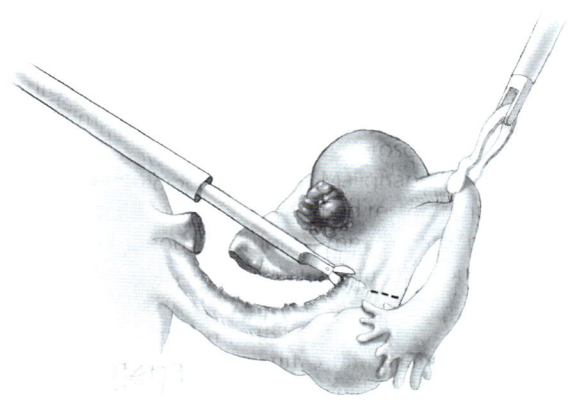

FIGURE 44-3.2 Mesosalpinx incision.

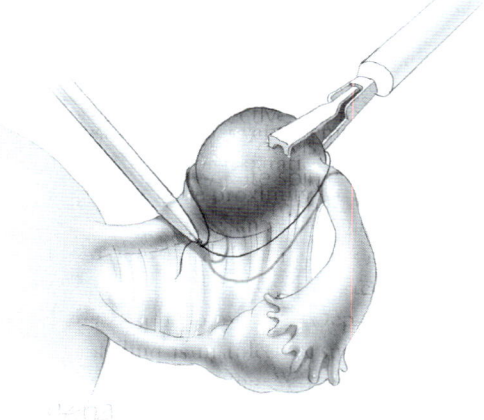

FIGURE 44-3.3 Endoscopic loop ligation.

distal extent under the tubal ampulla. As the most distal mesosalpinx segment is cut, the tube is freed.

Other energy sources also work well. Monopolar scissors themselves may be attached to current. In this technique, vessels within the mesosalpinx are first electrosurgically coagulated and then cut. Advanced bipolar technologies (LigaSure, ENSEAL), laser energy, and Harmonic scalpel are suitable options. A surgeon's expertise with a particular modality typically dictates selection. One or more of these may be preferred based on the surrounding pelvic pathology or adhesions. The major concern with any of these tools is the

amount of thermal spread to surrounding tissues. With bleeding, device efficiency and speed also can influence selection.

④ Endoscopic Loop Ligation. Alternatively, the vascular supply to the fallopian tube within the mesosalpinx can be ligated. Figure 44-3.3 shows an endoscopic suture loop encircling a loop of fallopian tube that contains an ectopic pregnancy. Absorbable and delayed-absorbable suture loops are available, and either is suitable. Two or three suture loops are sequentially placed, and the tube distal to these ligatures is cut free with scissors (**Fig. 44-3.4**).

⑤ Risk-Reducing Salpingectomy. For women with high-risk genetic mutations, posterior cul-de-sac (pelvic) washings are obtained once the abdomen is entered. Fallopian tube excision begins at its insertion into the uterine cornu and continues to its distal-most end. Excised tubes are removed in endoscopic bags.

⑥ Tissue Removal. Most tubal ectopic pregnancies are small and pliant. They can be held firmly by grasping forceps and drawn up into one of the accessory cannulas. The cannula, grasping forceps, and ectopic tissue then can be removed together. Larger tubal ectopic pregnancies may be placed in an endoscopic sac to prevent fragmentation as they are removed through the laparoscopic port site. Alternatively, larger ectopic pregnancies can be morcellated with scissors within an enclosed bag. Tissue removal techniques are presented on page 1032 and are illustrated in Chapter 41 (p. 894).

⑦ Irrigation. To remove all trophoblastic tissue, the pelvis and abdomen are irrigated and suctioned free of blood and tissue debris. Slow and systematic movement of the patient from Trendelenburg positioning to reverse Trendelenburg also can dislodge stray tissue and fluid, which then is suctioned and removed from the peritoneal cavity.

⑧ Wound Closure. Subsequent surgery completion steps follow those of diagnostic laparoscopy (p. 1018).

POSTOPERATIVE

As with most laparoscopic surgeries, patients can resume their presurgical diet and activity levels according to their comfort and typically within days. If salpingectomy is

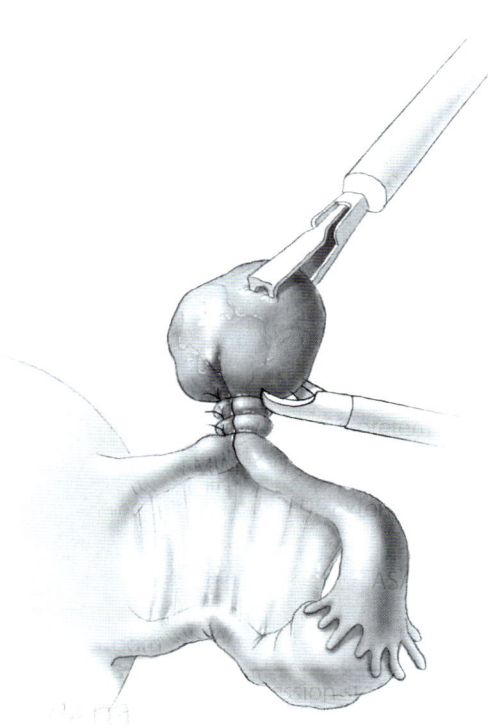

FIGURE 44-3.4 Looped portion of tube excised.

performed for ectopic pregnancy, Rh-negative patients are given a single 300-µg (1500 IU) $Rh_0(D)$ immune globulin dose intramuscularly within 72 hours. To identify patients in whom trophoblastic tissue may persist, serial serum β-hCG levels are monitored until undetectable (Seifer, 1997). Spandorfer and associates (1997) compared serum β-hCG levels 1 day postoperatively with those drawn prior to surgery. They found a significantly

lower percentage of persistent trophoblastic tissue if the β-hCG level fell more than 50 percent and noted no cases if the level declined by more than 77 percent. Until levels are undetectable, contraception is used to avoid confusion between persistent trophoblastic tissue and a new pregnancy. Ovulation may resume as early as 2 weeks after an early pregnancy ends. Therefore, if contraception is desired, methods are initiated soon after

surgery. Last, patients are counseled regarding their increased risk of future ectopic pregnancy.

If risk-reducing salpingectomy is performed for a woman at greater risk of ovarian cancer, pertinent genetic information, such as *BRCA* mutation status, should be noted on the pathology requisition form. This prompts more thorough tubal specimen sectioning and evaluation.

44-4

Laparoscopic Salpingostomy

For patients with ectopic pregnancy, laparoscopic linear salpingostomy offers the surgical advantages of laparoscopy and an opportunity to retain fertility by preserving the involved fallopian tube. Discussed in Chapter 7 (p. 170), this is most germane for those with a damaged contralateral tube. Consequently, suitable candidates are women with an unruptured isthmic or ampullary ectopic pregnancy and desiring future pregnancies. Success of the affected tube is mainly influenced by the amount of bleeding, by the ability to control it, and by the degree of tubal damage.

PREOPERATIVE

Consent

Risks of laparoscopic salpingostomy mirror those for laparoscopic salpingectomy (p. 1025). Importantly, with salpingostomy, a patient is counseled regarding the possible need for salpingectomy if the tube is irreparably damaged or bleeding from the tube cannot be controlled. Also, rates of persistent trophoblastic disease are higher with salpingostomy compared with removal of the entire affected tubal segment.

Bleeding. Because trophoblastic tissue is vascular, disruption during ectopic pregnancy removal can lead to hemorrhage. The ability of tubal muscularis to contract is minimal, and thus, bleeding during salpingostomy must be controlled with external modalities such as electrosurgical coagulation. Many devices are appropriate, and the microbipolar device can achieve hemostasis while creating minimal thermal spread. At times, bleeding may be extensive and persistent and require salpingectomy.

To improve hemostasis, vasoconstrictive agents such as vasopressin have been evaluated. Dilutions of 20 U of vasopressin in 30 to 100 mL of saline are suitable. The mesosalpinx is infiltrated with approximately 10 mL of solution. Because of the potential systemic vasoconstrictive effects of vasopressin, intravascular injection is avoided. Another approach is to inject the solution into the portion of the tube to be incised. This is dictated by surgeon preference. Additional complications and contraindications to vasopressin use are discussed on page 1039. Benefits to vasopressin include less frequent use of electrosurgery, shorter operating time, and lower conversion rates to laparotomy for surgery completion.

To avoid vasopressin's cardiovascular effects, Fedele and colleagues (1998) diluted 20 U of oxytocin in 20 mL of saline and similarly injected the mesosalpinx. Oxytocin is purported to contract the smooth muscle fibers of the tube and cause vasoconstriction of mesosalpinx vessels. Although used less often, these researchers noted easier pregnancy enucleation, less bleeding, and less frequent use of electrosurgery.

Persistent Trophoblastic Tissue. During treatment of ectopic pregnancy, trophoblastic tissue can persist in as many as 3 to 20 percent of cases. Remnant implants typically involve the fallopian tube, but extratubal trophoblastic implants have been found on the omentum and on pelvic and abdominal peritoneum. Implants typically measure 0.3 to 2.0 cm and appear as red-black nodules (Doss, 1998). Severe postoperative bleeding is the most serious complication of this persistent tissue (Giuliani, 1998).

The risk of persistent trophoblast tissue is highest following laparoscopic salpingostomy, especially in women in whom small, early pregnancies are removed. In these pregnancies, the cleavage plane between the invading trophoblast and tubal implantation site is poor. This may lead to a more difficult dissection and failure to completely remove all products of conception. For all cases, preventive recommendations include irrigation and complete suctioning of the abdomen, limited degree of Trendelenburg position to minimize blood and tissue flow to the upper abdomen, and use of endoscopic bags for removal of larger ectopic pregnancies (Ben-Arie, 2001).

INTRAOPERATIVE

Instruments

Specific tools needed for salpingostomy mirror those for salpingectomy and should be available if salpingectomy is required (p. 1025).

Surgical Steps

❶ Anesthesia and Patient Positioning. The patient is prepared and positioned for laparoscopic surgery as described in Chapter 41 (p. 877).

❷ Abdominal Entry. The abdomen is accessed with laparoscopic techniques, and typically two or three accessory port sites are used. Depending on the ectopic pregnancy size, at least one 10-mm accessory cannula may be necessary to allow specimen removal at surgery's end. Once cannulas are in place, systematic inspection of the abdomen and pelvis is completed prior to the planned procedure.

❸ Salpingostomy. The fallopian tube is lifted and held with atraumatic grasping forceps. By means of a 22-gauge needle through one of the accessory ports or through a separate abdominal wall needle puncture, a solution of vasopressin is injected into the mesosalpinx beneath the ectopic pregnancy. If the serosal layer overlying the ectopic tissue is injected instead, then a smaller 25-gauge needle may be used.

A monopolar needle tip electrode is set at a cutting voltage and used to create a 1- to 2-cm longitudinal incision (Fig. 44-4.1). The incision is positioned opposite the mesosalpinx and on the maximally distended

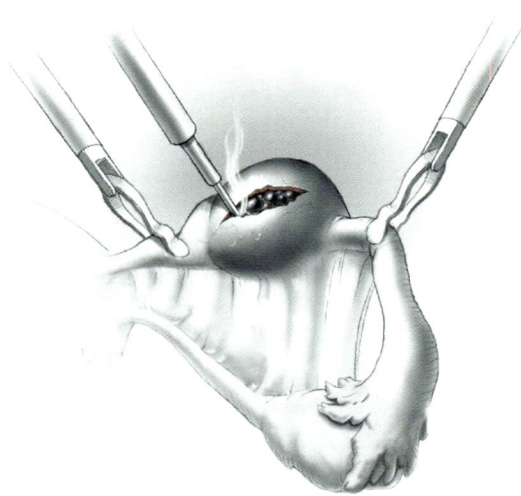

FIGURE 44-4.1 Salpingostomy.

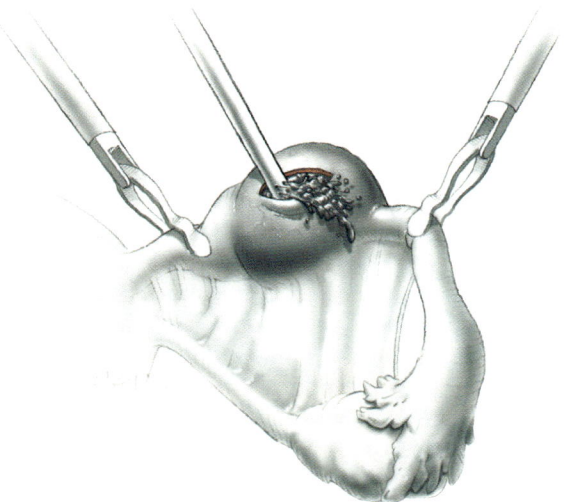

FIGURE 44-4.2 Hydrodissection.

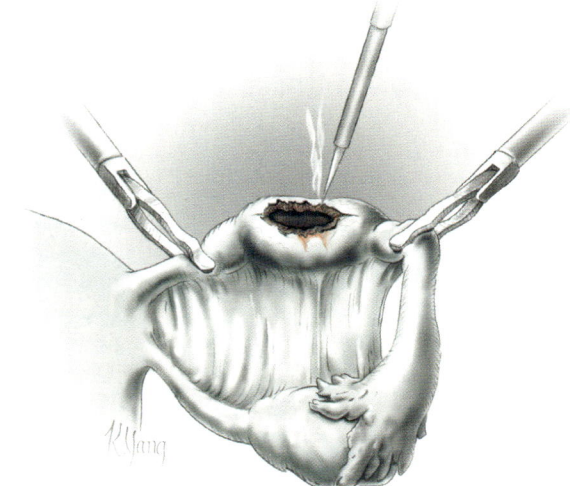

FIGURE 44-4.3 Coagulation of incision edges.

portion of the tube that overlies the pregnancy. Laparoscopic scissors, CO_2 laser, bipolar needle, and Harmonic scalpel also have been used.

❹ **Pregnancy Removal.** Atraumatic grasping forceps hold one edge of the incision while a suction-irrigation probe tip is insinuated into the tissue plane between the tubal wall and ectopic pregnancy (Fig. 44-4.2). Hydrodissection is performed on one side of the tube and then the other. A combination of high-pressure hydrodissection and gentle blunt dissection with the suction irrigator tip removes the entire conceptus from the tube. Alternatively, the pregnancy or its fragments may require extraction by smooth grasping forceps.

❺ **Hemostasis.** Bleeding points can be controlled with monopolar or bipolar electrosurgical coagulation (Fig. 44-4.3). The tubal incision is left open to heal by secondary intention. Tulandi and Guralnick (1991) found no differences in subsequent fertility and adhesion formation between salpingotomy with or without tubal suturing.

❻ **Specimen Extraction.** Most ectopic pregnancies are small and pliant. Accordingly, they can be held firmly by grasping forceps and drawn up into one of the accessory cannulas. The cannula, grasping forceps, and ectopic tissue can then be removed together. Larger ectopic pregnancies may be placed in an endoscopic sac to prevent fragmentation as they are removed through the laparoscopic trocar site.

❼ **Irrigation.** To prevent persistent trophoblastic tissue postoperatively, the pelvis and abdomen are irrigated and suctioned free of blood and tissue debris.

❽ **Adhesion Prevention.** Adjuvants are available that can be used for the prevention of postoperative adhesion formation. However, no substantial evidence documents that their use improves fertility, decreases pain, or prevents bowel obstruction (American Society for Reproductive Medicine, 2013).

❾ **Wound Closure.** Subsequent surgery completion steps follow those of diagnostic laparoscopy (p. 1018).

POSTOPERATIVE

As with most laparoscopic surgeries, patients can resume presurgical diet and activity levels according to their comfort, typically within days. Postoperative topics specific to ectopic pregnancy include Rh_0 [D] immune globulin administration, surveillance for persistent trophoblastic disease, provision of contraception if desired, and counseling on future ectopic pregnancy risk as described on page 1027.

44-5

Laparoscopic Ovarian Cystectomy

Many studies have attested to the efficacy and safety of laparoscopic cystectomy for the management of ovarian cysts. Moreover, because of recovery-associated benefits, a laparoscopic technique is advocated by many as the preferred approach in women with ovarian cysts and a low risk of malignancy. Ovarian cyst characteristics and their influence on decisions regarding laparotomy or MIS approach and regarding ovarian conservation or oophorectomy are discussed fully in Chapter 10 (p. 222).

PREOPERATIVE

Patient Evaluation

Sonography is the primary tool used to diagnose ovarian pathology, and the sonographic characteristics of a cyst aid in determining preoperatively the malignant potential of a given lesion (Chap. 10, p. 221). In those patients with indeterminate ovarian cysts following sonography, magnetic resonance (MR) imaging may enhance discrimination. In those with suspected endometrioma, some also recommend sonographic exclusion of associated hydronephrosis on the affected side (Saridogan, 2017).

The serum tumor marker cancer antigen 125 (CA125) usually is obtained preoperatively in postmenopausal patients and in any woman whose tumor displays other elements suggesting ovarian epithelial cancer (Chap. 35, p. 740). Other markers may be measured to exclude germ cell or sex cord–stromal ovarian neoplasms, if these are suspected (Chap. 36, p. 757). If future fertility is a concern, some also recommend measuring preoperative levels of antimüllerian hormone (AMH), which is a marker of ovarian reserve (Saridogan, 2017). Multiple studies show declines in AMH levels following cystectomy (Kostrzewa, 2019; Kwon, 2014; Salihoğlu, 2016).

Consent

Prior to surgery, patients are informed of the unique complications associated with laparoscopy itself (Chap. 41, p. 875). Specific to ovarian cystectomy, the risks of oophorectomy due to bleeding or extreme ovarian damage are discussed. Depending on the amount of oocyte-containing ovarian stroma that is stripped away with the cyst, diminished

ovarian reserve also is a risk and discussed in Chapter 11 (p. 245). Obviously, because many cysts are removed due to concerns of potential malignancy, patients should be familiar with the steps involved in the surgical staging if ovarian cancer is found.

Patient Preparation

Rates of pelvic and wound infection following ovarian cystectomy and laparoscopy are low, and antibiotic prophylaxis generally is not required. Bowel preparation is not required but may be considered if extensive adhesions are suspected. For this, an empty rectum can aid intraoperative proctosigmoidoscopy and bowel manipulation needed for laceration repair. VTE prophylaxis is not recommended for laparoscopic cystectomy. However, women with a greater risk of malignancy, with known VTE risks, or with an increased chance for conversion to laparotomy may benefit from these measures (Table 39-10, p. 834).

INTRAOPERATIVE

Instruments

Most instruments required for ovarian cystectomy are found in a standard laparoscopy instrument set. A suction irrigation system often is needed to remove cyst contents if rupture occurs. An endoscopic retrieval bag also is frequently used. Once contained in the sac, the cyst in some cases may be decompressed with a laparoscopic aspiration needle.

If oophorectomy is required, the infundibulopelvic (IP) ligament is ligated. This may

be accomplished using bipolar instruments, Harmonic scalpel, laparoscopic suture loop, or stapler. These may not be readily available in all operating suites, and desired tools are best requested prior to surgery.

Surgical Steps

❶ Anesthesia and Patient Positioning. The patient is prepared and positioned for laparoscopic surgery (Chap. 41, p. 877). A bimanual examination is completed to determine ovarian size and position and uterine inclination. Ovarian information will affect placement of the accessory ports, and uterine inclination will direct positioning of the uterine manipulator, if used. A uterine manipulator can help move the uterus and adnexa. In anticipation of possible hysterectomy as a part of ovarian cancer staging, the vagina and abdomen are surgically prepared, and a Foley catheter is inserted. The patient is draped to allow sterile access to the vagina and abdomen.

❷ Abdominal Entry. Primary and secondary trocars are placed as described in Chapter 41 (p. 888). For insertion of most endoscopic sacs, at least one 10-mm or larger accessory cannula may be necessary to allow specimen removal at surgery's end. Typically, two or three accessory cannulas are required for cystectomy.

Once the abdomen is entered, diagnostic laparoscopy allows inspection of the pelvis and upper abdomen for signs of malignancy such as ascites and peritoneal implants. Cellular washings from these areas are obtained and

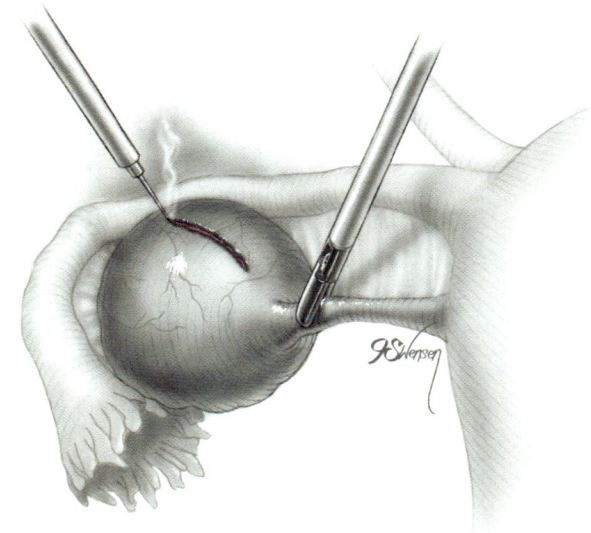

FIGURE 44-5.1 Ovarian incision.

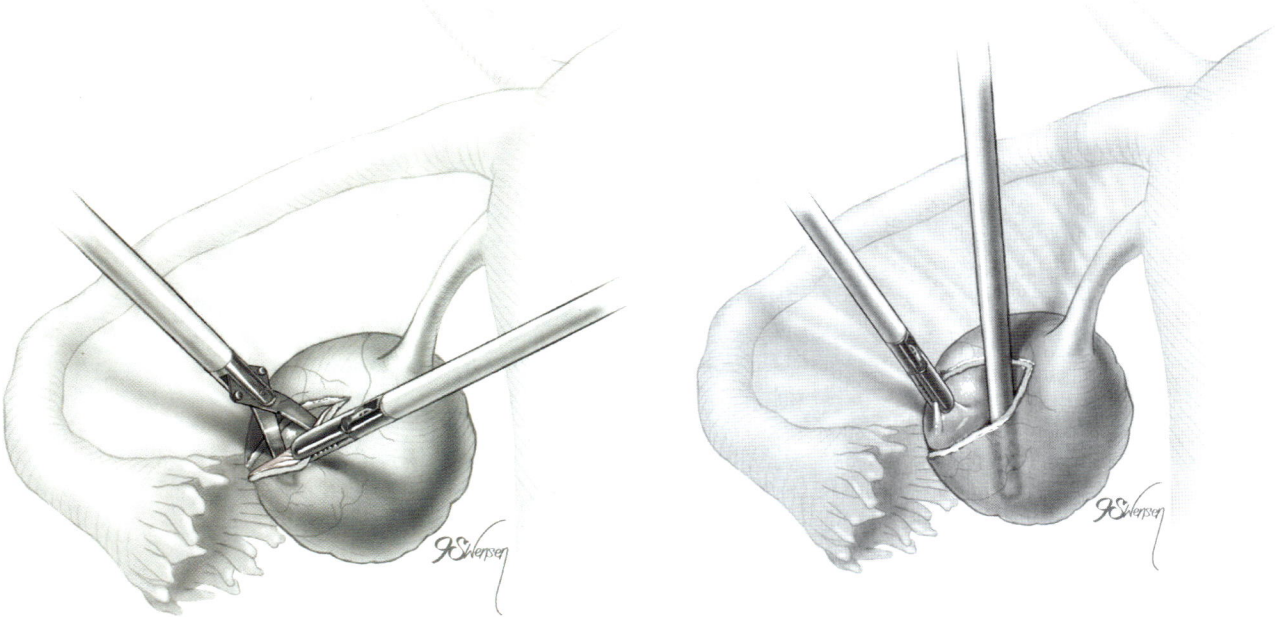

FIGURE 44-5.2 Dissection initiated.

FIGURE 44-5.3 Hydrodissection.

saved until frozen section analysis of the specimen has excluded malignancy. Similarly, identified peritoneal implants from suspicious areas are biopsied and sent for intraoperative analysis. Prior to ovarian cystectomy, adhesions are divided to restore proper anatomic relationships.

❸ **Ovarian Incision.** A blunt probe is placed under the uteroovarian ligament and posterior ovarian surface to elevate the ovary. An atraumatic grasping forceps then steadies the ovary (Fig. 44-5.1). A monopolar needle tip electrode set at a cutting voltage is used to incise the ovarian capsule that overlies the cyst. Other suitable devices for incision include a monopolar scissor blade or Harmonic scalpel. This incision is ideally on the antihilar surface of the ovary to minimize dissection into extensive vascularity at the ovarian base. The incision is extended into the ovarian stroma to the level of the cyst wall but ideally does not rupture the cyst.

❹ **Cyst Dissection.** A plane between the ovary and cyst wall is created and expanded using blunt forceps or dissecting scissors (Fig. 44-5.2). Atraumatic grasping forceps are used to hold one edge of the incision, while a blunt grasping forceps or suction-irrigation probe tip is insinuated in this space. Once the correct plane is entered, the tool bluntly is advanced inward and laterally to continue cyst separation (Fig. 44-5.3).

Blunt or hydrodissection is performed on one side of the cyst and then the other. If the cyst is adhered at points to its surrounding ovarian tissue, cystectomy may at times require sharp dissection with scissors. During dissection, points of bleeding can be coagulated, or isolated vessels may be grasped and coagulated (Fig. 44-5.4). This is especially true at the ovarian hilum.

❺ **Cyst Removal.** Following enucleation from the ovary, the cyst is placed into an

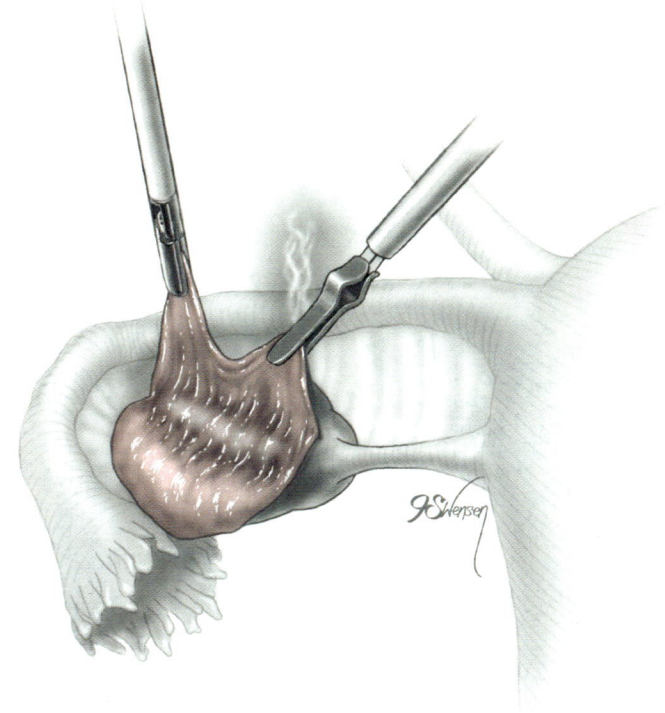

FIGURE 44-5.4 Following cyst enucleation, ovarian capsule edges are coagulated.

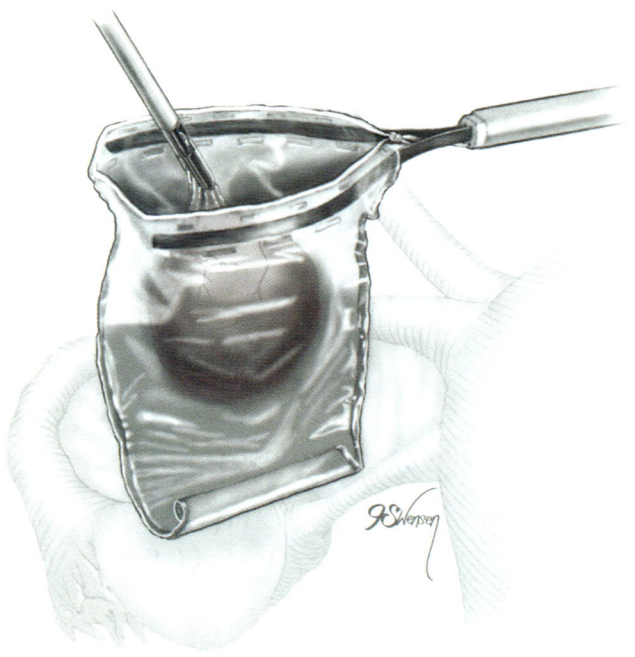

FIGURE 44-5.5 Cyst placed in endoscopic bag.

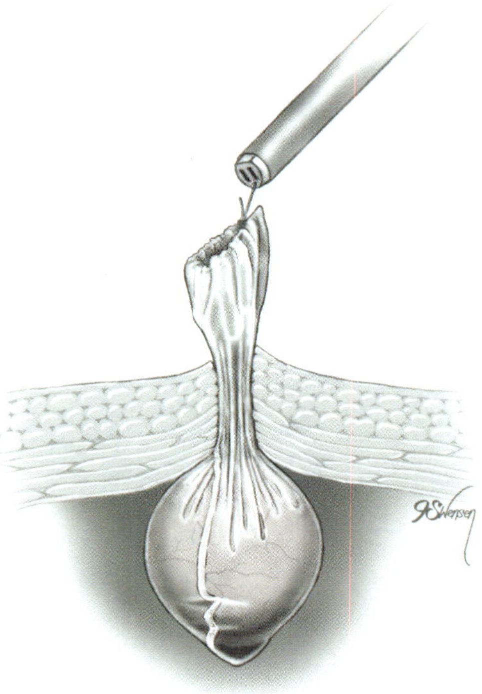

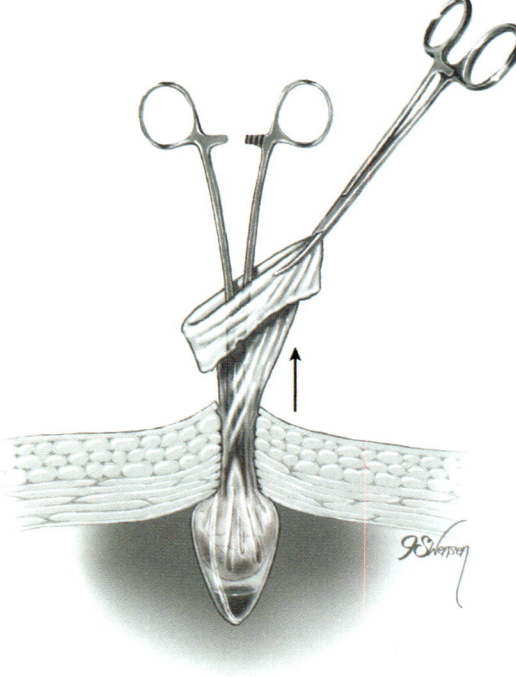

FIGURE 44-5.6 Endoscopic bag cinched and brought up to anterior abdominal wall.

endoscopic bag (Fig. 44-5.5). The opening of the sac is closed and brought up to the anterior abdominal wall (Fig. 44-5.6). Depending on its size, the cyst and endoscopic bag may be removed in toto. In this instance, the laparoscopic cannula is removed first and is followed by the cyst contained within the sac.

With larger cysts, the cannula is removed, and the entire pursed opening of the bag is drawn up through the trocar incision. The bag opening is fanned out onto the skin surface. The outer edges of the bag then are pulled upward to lift and press the cyst up against the incision. A needle tip is directed

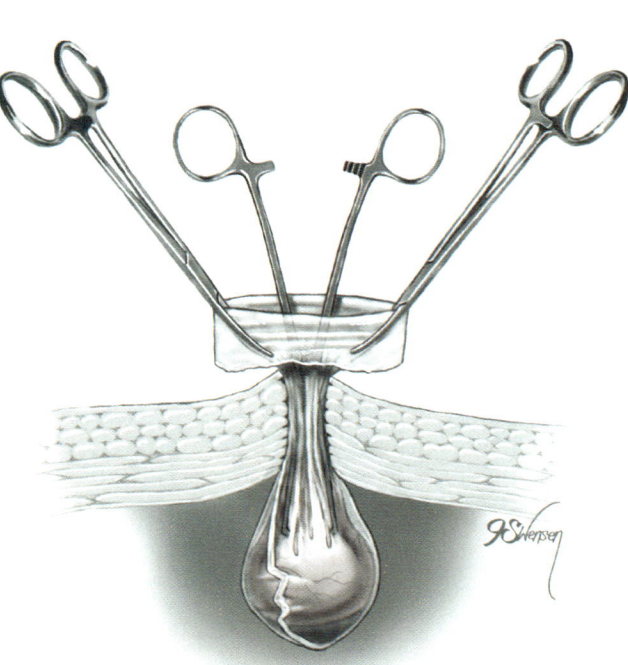

FIGURE 44-5.7 Cyst ruptured by toothed Kocher clamp within the endoscopic bag.

FIGURE 44-5.8 Bag and collapsed cyst are removed together.

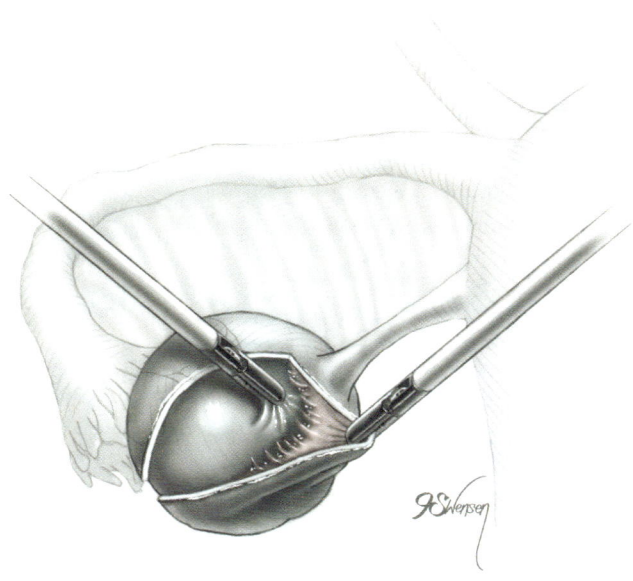

FIGURE 44-5.9 Stripping of collapsed cyst from ovarian capsule.

into the endoscopic sac and pierces the contained cyst. An attached syringe can aspirate contents. Alternatively, the cyst may be ruptured by a toothed Kocher clamp placed through the skin incision and into the sac (Fig. 44-5.7).

In either case, cyst fluid is retained within the endoscopic sac. The endoscopic bag and decompressed cyst wall are then removed together through the incision (Fig. 44-5.8). During removal, the sac should not be inadvertently punctured or torn, and all measures are used to prevent spill of cyst contents into the abdomen or port site.

❻ **Cyst Rupture.** Not uncommonly during the dissection of the cyst wall away from the ovary, the cyst may rupture. The cyst wall then is removed using a "stripping" technique (Fig. 44-5.9). With this, both the cyst wall and cyst capsule can be grasped near the dissection plane by atraumatic forceps. Traction and countertraction can separate filmy connective tissue between these to advance the dissection plane. As a result, the grasping forceps strip the cyst wall away from the underlying ovarian stroma. To prevent damage to the underlying healthy ovary, the dissection plane between the cyst and stroma should be clearly delineated by traction on each side to prevent tearing. To minimize this tissue trauma, frequent grasping and regrasping of the cyst wall and normal ovarian tissue along the dissection plane may be required. Injection of dilute vasopressin into this space also may help delineate the dissection plane and minimize bleeding. Histologically, Muzii and colleagues (2002) showed that this technique in nonendometriotic lesions spared ovarian tissue and did not strip away normal ovarian tissue and follicles. Small randomized studies also describe this

for endometriomas as a means to minimize electrosurgical coagulation and thermal tissue injury (Ghafarnejad, 2014; Saeki, 2010).

❼ **Ovary Closure.** Because of increased adhesion formation risk, the ovarian capsule usually is not sutured closed following cyst removal. Several studies show that leaving the capsule open does not promote greater adhesion formation (Marana, 1991; Wiskind, 1990).

However, if bleeding is encountered, site-specific suturing appears to preserve greater ovarian reserve than electrosurgical coagulation (Pergialiotis, 2015; Peters, 2017). Topical hemostats similarly are helpful (Chung, 2019; Song, 2014). Importantly, excess hemostat should be removed by gentle irrigation to avoid inflammatory complications and pelvic adhesions (Suzuki, 2010).

Application of an adhesion barrier such as oxidized regenerated cellulose may be considered to prevent adhesion formation (Franklin, 1995; Wiseman, 1999). However, no substantial evidence documents that their use improves fertility, decreases pain, or prevents bowel obstruction (American Society for Reproductive Medicine, 2013).

❽ **Wound Closure.** If concerning for malignancy, the specimen is submitted in most cases for immediate frozen section analysis. If benign findings are noted, steps toward surgical closure begin. If malignancy is found, surgical staging should ensue. Of note, if a large mass was removed and the port site was likely extended during cyst removal, the abdominal wall fascia is sutured closed to prevent port-site hernias. The finishing laparoscopic steps are found on page 1018.

POSTOPERATIVE

Following laparoscopic ovarian cystectomy, instructions similar to those for diagnostic laparoscopy are given (p. 1018).

Laparoscopic Salpingo-oophorectomy

Laparoscopy can be used to safely remove many adnexa and, in most cases, offers a faster recovery and less postoperative pain compared with laparotomy. As discussed in Chapter 10 (p. 222), indications for adnexectomy vary but may include torsion, ovarian cyst rupture, suspicion of ovarian malignancy, and symptomatic ovarian remnant. In addition, prophylactic adnexectomy is often considered in women with or at risk for cancers associated with specific pathogenic mutations (Chap. 35, p. 736).

Laparoscopy is a preferred approach when possible and can be safely performed in pregnancy, preferably in the early second trimester. However, for all patients, laparotomy may be preferred in certain clinical settings. These include a high suspicion of cancer, anticipation of extensive pelvic adhesions, and large ovarian size, which may preclude adequate laparoscopic manipulation or optics.

PREOPERATIVE

Patient Evaluation

Salpingo-oophorectomy is typically performed to remove ovarian pathology, and sonography is the primary tool used for diagnosis. In cases in which anatomy may be unclear, MR imaging can add additional information. Tumor markers discussed in Chapters 35 and 36 may be drawn prior to surgery if malignancy is suspected. For risk-reducing salpingo-oophorectomy in patients with hereditary breast and ovarian cancer syndromes, chance of finding occult malignancy at surgery or during final pathologic analysis approximates 5 percent (Finch, 2006; Manchanda, 2011). Thus, preoperative serum CA125 level and pelvic sonography should evaluate for malignancy.

Consent

Prior to surgery, patients are informed of the unique complications associated with laparoscopy (Chap. 41, p. 875). Specific to salpingo-oophorectomy, the risk of ureteral injury is discussed. Many adnexa are removed due to concerns of potential malignancy, and patients should be familiar with the steps involved in the surgical staging of ovarian cancer.

Patient Preparation

Unless an ovarian abscess is identified, laparoscopic salpingo-oophorectomy does not require antibiotic prophylaxis (American College of Obstetricians and Gynecologists, 2018a). VTE prophylaxis is not recommended for laparoscopic cystectomy. However, women with a greater risk of malignancy, with underlying VTE risks, or with a higher chance for conversion to laparotomy may benefit from these measures (Table 39-10, p. 834).

INTRAOPERATIVE

Instruments

Most instruments required for salpingo-oophorectomy are found in a standard laparoscopy instrument set. However, a suction irrigation system commonly is needed to remove cyst contents if rupture occurs. An endoscopic retrieval bag also is frequently used. During oophorectomy, the IP ligament is ligated. This may be accomplished using bipolar instruments, Harmonic scalpel, laparoscopic suture loop, or stapler. These may not be readily available in all operating suites, and desired tools are requested prior to surgery.

Surgical Steps

❶ Anesthesia and Patient Positioning. The patient is prepared and positioned for laparoscopic surgery as described in Chapter 41 (p. 877). A bimanual examination is completed to determine ovarian size and position and uterine inclination. Ovarian information will affect placement of the accessory ports, and uterine inclination will direct positioning of the uterine manipulator, if used. Because of possible hysterectomy as a part of ovarian cancer staging, the vagina and abdomen are surgically prepared, and a Foley catheter is inserted. A uterine manipulator may be placed to assist with manipulation of the uterus and adnexa.

❷ Abdominal Access. Primary and secondary trocars are placed as described in Chapter 41 (p. 888). Typically, two or three accessory ports are required. For insertion of most endoscopic sacs, at least one 10-mm or larger accessory cannula may be required to allow specimen removal at surgery's end.

❸ Pelvic Inspection and Washings. Once the abdomen is entered, diagnostic laparoscopy allows inspection of the pelvis and upper abdomen for signs of malignancy such as ascites and peritoneal implants (p. 1017). Cellular washings from these areas are obtained and saved until frozen section analysis of the specimen has excluded malignancy. Similarly, identified peritoneal implants from these areas are biopsied and sent for intraoperative evaluation. Prior to adnexectomy, adhesions are divided to restore proper anatomic relationships.

❹ Ureter Location. The ureter lies close to the IP ligament, and its course should be noted. If the location of the ureter is not clear, the peritoneum lateral to the ureter is incised, and retroperitoneal isolation of the ureter is completed.

❺ Infundibulopelvic Ligament Coagulation. Ligation of the ovarian vessels within the IP ligament can be completed with endoscopic loop ligatures, electrosurgical coagulating devices, Harmonic scalpel, or stapler depending on surgeon preference (Fig. 44-6.1). Once these vessels are occluded, the IP is severed.

In patients undergoing risk-reducing procedures, the IP ligament should be isolated and ligated 2 cm past the end of the ovary. This ensures that all ovarian and tubal tissue is removed (American College of Obstetricians and Gynecologists, 2017b). In other cases of endometriosis or adhesive disease, extensive retroperitoneal dissection may be required to prevent development of an ovarian remnant.

❻ Opening the Broad Ligament. After transection of the IP, the fallopian tube and ovary are gently elevated with atraumatic forceps. Incision of the broad ligament's posterior leaf then is extended medially (Fig. 44-6.2).

❼ Uteroovarian Ligament Coagulation. The uteroovarian ligament and proximal fallopian tube are identified posterior to the round ligament. Similarly to the IP, these may be coagulated, stapled, or ligated (Fig. 44-6.3). Lateral to this occlusion, the uteroovarian ligament and fallopian tube are transected, and the adnexum is freed. For risk-reducing procedures, the fallopian tube should be ligated at its insertion into the uterine cornu.

❽ Adnexum Removal. Various endoscopic bags are available for tissue removal (Chap. 41, p. 882), and removal steps are illustrated in Section 44-5. The specimen is placed into the sac, which is closed and brought up to the anterior abdominal wall. Depending on its size, the adnexum and endoscopic bag may be removed in toto. In this instance, the laparoscopic cannula is removed first, followed by the specimen contained within the sac. Our preference is to remove larger masses through a midline port (such as the primary optical port). This aims to avoid nerve or vascular injury if a lateral port site is intentionally or inadvertently extended during removal.

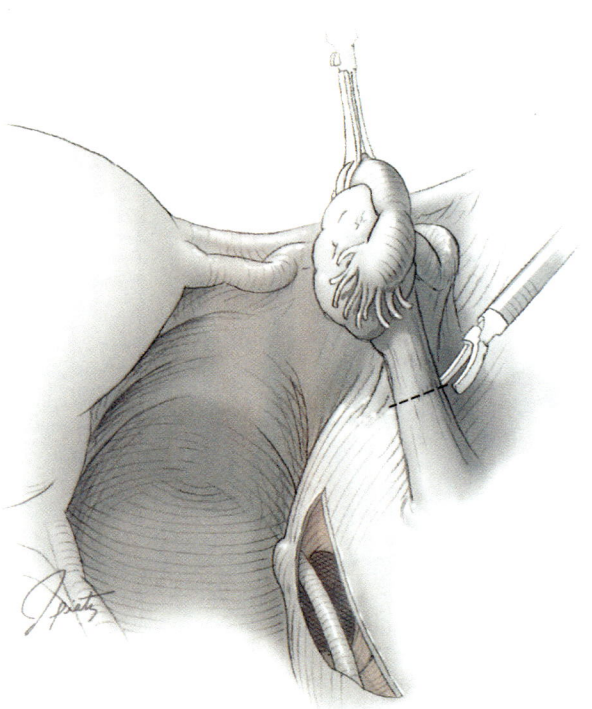

FIGURE 44-6.1 Infundibulopelvic ligament coagulation.

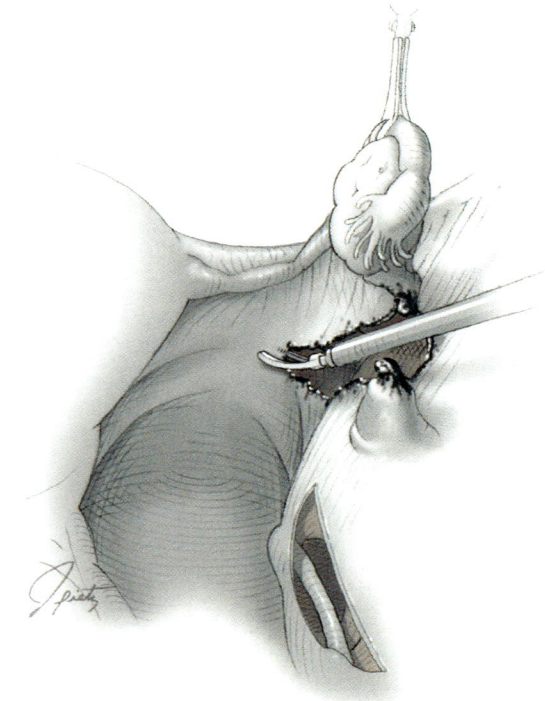

FIGURE 44-6.2 Opening of the broad ligament.

With larger cystic ovaries, the cannula is removed, and the entire pursed opening of the bag is drawn up through the incision and fanned out onto the skin surface. The open edges of the bag are pulled upward to lift and press the ovary against the incision. A needle tip is directed through the incision and into the sac. The ovary is pierced and aspiration drainage is completed by an attached syringe. Alternatively, the cyst may be ruptured by a toothed Kocher clamp placed through the skin incision and into the sac.

With either decompression method, cyst fluid is retained in the endoscopic sac. The endoscopic sac and decompressed cyst wall are removed together through the incision.

During removal, the endoscopic bag should not be inadvertently punctured or torn, and all measures are used to prevent spill of cyst contents into the abdomen or port site.

As a final method to prevent spill or to remove a larger solid mass, a minilaparotomy incision or a colpotomy incision can be made for specimen extraction. These two are described on page 1048 and illustrated in Chapter 41 (p. 894).

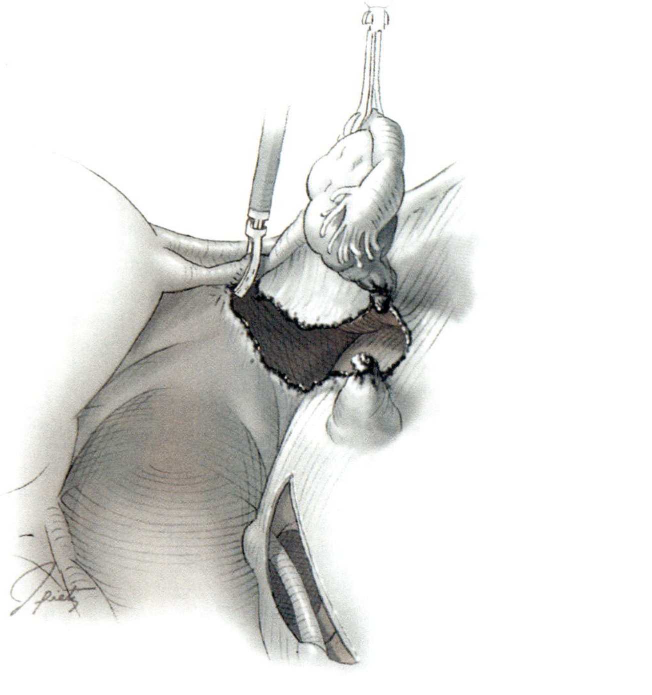

❾ Wound Closure. If malignancy is suspected, the specimen is submitted for immediate frozen section analysis. If benign findings are noted, steps toward surgical closure begin. If malignancy is found, surgical staging should ensue. Of note, if a large mass was removed and the port site was likely extended during the removal, the abdominal wall fascia is sutured closed to prevent port-site hernias.

POSTOPERATIVE

Advantages to laparoscopy include a rapid return to normal diet and activities, and postoperative complication rates are low. If both adnexa are removed, hormone replacement therapy is considered in appropriate candidates (Chap. 22, p. 479).

If risk-reducing adnexectomy is performed for a woman at greater risk of ovarian cancer, pertinent genetic information, such as *BRCA* mutation status, should be noted on the pathology requisition form. This prompts more thorough specimen sectioning and evaluation.

FIGURE 44-6.3 Fallopian tube and uteroovarian ligament coagulation to free the specimen.

44-7

Ovarian Drilling

Ovarian drilling is a technique of puncturing the ovarian capsule with an electrosurgical needle or a laser beam. Similar to ovarian wedge resection, this procedure's end goal is to reduce the amount of androgen-producing tissue in women with polycystic ovarian syndrome (PCOS). However, in wedge resection, a long cortical incision is required for the degree of resection. Thus, infertility secondary to adhesions complicates many postoperative courses (Buttram, 1975; Toaff, 1976). To minimize this risk and avoid the need for laparotomy, ovarian drilling techniques using laparoscopy were developed.

Compared with gonadotropin stimulation, ovarian drilling has lower rates of ovarian hyperstimulation syndrome (OHSS) and of multifetal gestation (Farquhar, 2012). Disadvantages include the surgical risks and cost of laparoscopy, risks of pelvic adhesion formation, and concerns regarding long-term effects on ovarian reserve. Accordingly, ovarian drilling is viewed as a second-line therapy (Teede, 2018). It can be useful in patients who fail to ovulate with clomiphene citrate, who are at risk for OHSS, or who desire to minimize their risk for multifetal gestation. To limit ovarian adhesions and spare ovarian reserve, some advocate drilling into only one ovary rather than both. However, data showing superior or comparable conception and birth rates with unilateral treatment are conflicting (Abu Hashim, 2018; Rezk, 2016; Zahiri Sorouri, 2015).

PREOPERATIVE

Consent

There appear to be relatively few complications that arise immediately after ovarian drilling. Hemorrhage, infection, and thermal bowel injury are infrequent. Similarly, ovarian atrophy following drilling is rare but has been reported (Dabirashrafi, 1989). More commonly, a decline in AMH levels has been noted. However, remember that PCOS is associated with high AMH levels (Giampaolino, 2017; Kandil, 2018). Thus, AMH declines may reflect loss of ovarian reserve or may signify improved PCOS endocrinopathy (Amer, 2017).

Adhesion formation following this procedure, however, is common. Most of these adhesions at second-look laparoscopy

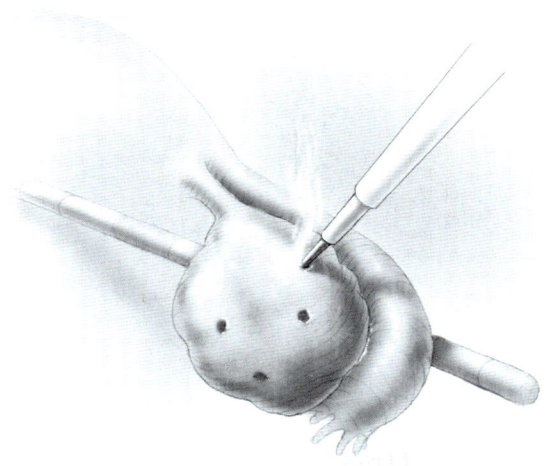

FIGURE 44-7.1 Ovarian drilling.

typically have been graded as minimal or mild (Giampaolino, 2016; Gürgan, 1991). Moreover, researchers have described only a minimal, if any, decline in fertility from these adhesions (Gürgan, 1992; Naether, 1993). This risk, however, is discussed with the patient prior to surgery.

INTRAOPERATIVE

Instruments

Ovarian drilling can be completed with monopolar or bipolar electrosurgical energy or various lasers. The goal is focal damage to the ovarian stroma and cortex. Currently, no studies support the superiority of one modality (Strowitzki, 2005).

Surgical Steps

❶ **Anesthesia and Patient Positioning.** Patient positioning and anesthesia mirror those for other laparoscopic procedures (Chap. 41, p. 877).

❷ **Abdominal Entry.** Three incisions are used for this laparoscopic procedure. In addition to a primary umbilical incision, two bilateral lower abdominal ports are established. These lower sites serve as entry ports for the electrosurgical needle tip and grasping forceps.

❸ **Ovarian Drilling.** The ovary is elevated with a blunt grasper. Monopolar electrosurgical current is set at 30 W cutting current. Some strive for a set dose per ovary of 600 joules, which can be calculated as watts × time × puncture number (Amer, 2003). An example is 30 W × 5 s × 4 punctures. Others suggest a dose of 60 J/cm^3 of ovarian

volume (Zakherah, 2011). Remember that one criteria for PCOS is an ovarian volume >10 cm^3 (American College of Obstetricians and Gynecologists, 2018d).

A electrosurgery needle tip is used to puncture the ovary perpendicular to the cortical surface and to pierce the follicular cysts that are characteristic of PCOS. Four to five punctures are placed symmetrically on the antimesenteric surface of the ovary (Fig. 44-7.1). Fewer or greater punctures may be ineffective or yield excess tissue destruction, respectively (Selim, 2011). Drilling is avoided on the lateral surfaces of the ovaries to minimize adhesions to the pelvic sidewall and is avoided at the ovarian hilum to limit bleeding risks. The needle is inserted to a depth of 4 to 10 mm. Electrical current is applied for 3 to 5 seconds. The ovarian surface can be irrigated with saline or lactated Ringer solution to cool it.

❹ **Adhesion Barriers.** Because of the risk for adhesion formation, most trials describe leaving 200 to 500 mL of saline or lactated Ringer solution in the pelvis following ovarian drilling. Greenblatt and Casper (1993) showed no improvement in adhesion prevention using Interceed adhesion barrier. No other studies have addressed the efficacy of other adhesion prevention products.

❺ **Wound Closure.** Subsequent surgery completion steps follow those of diagnostic laparoscopy (p. 1018).

POSTOPERATIVE

Postoperatively, patients are given instructions similar to those following diagnostic laparoscopy (p. 1018).

44-8

Laparoscopic Myomectomy and Leiomyoma Ablation

Myomectomy surgically excises leiomyomas from their surrounding myometrium. In contrast, myometrial ablation uses radiofrequency energy to heat and incite myoma necrosis. Either may be selected for women with symptomatic myomas who wish to preserve fertility or who decline hysterectomy. Appropriate indications include heavy menstrual bleeding, bulk symptoms, or pelvic pain attributed to myomas. Data linking myomas to infertility and recurrent miscarriage are less robust. These conditions are more closely associated with submucous myomas, which are best treated hysteroscopically (p. 1058). In general, subserosal and intramural leiomyoma myomectomies are most appropriate for a laparoscopic approach.

Historically, removal of serosal and intramural tumors required laparotomy. However, laparoscopic myomectomy may be performed by those with advanced skills in MIS and in laparoscopic suturing. Robotic myomectomy rates for this indication also have increased (Gingold, 2018). Laparoscopic-assisted myomectomy is another MIS approach and is completed through a minilaparotomy incision (Dubin, 2017). Last, myoma ablation does not require myometrial suturing skills and has significantly lower associated blood loss.

The choice of open myomectomy, MIS myomectomy, or myoma ablation is based on various factors that include tumor number, size, and location. For MIS myomectomy, comfort with laparoscopic dissection, morcellation, and suturing are other requisites.

PREOPERATIVE

Patient Evaluation

Leiomyoma size, number, and location are evaluated prior to surgery with sonography and, if needed, with MR imaging and/or hysteroscopy. For example, leiomyomas may be small and buried within the myometrium. With a laparoscopic or robotic approach, the ability to palpate and appreciate these small, deep tumors may be compromised. Thus, if multiple tumors are suspected, preoperative MR imaging may best provide accurate information to ensure complete excision. Last, multiple large masses or those that are

located in the broad ligament, are near the cornua, or involve the cervix may increase the risk of conversion to hysterectomy, and patients are so counseled. In one series of more than 2000 laparoscopic myomectomies, complications rose with more than three leiomyomas, tumor size >5 cm, and intraligamental location (Sizzi, 2007). In other large series, women selected for laparoscopic myomectomy typically had tumors numbering ≤3 and measuring <7 cm in diameter (Kumakiri, 2008; Saccardi, 2014). Accounting for these factors, a surgeon's expertise is the most important factor in determining approach to myomectomy.

Less experience is available regarding patient selection for the newer Acessa device. From case series data, radiofrequency ablation (RFA) may be best suited for women with myomas <7 cm and uterine sizes <16 weeks. From research studies, myomas >10 cm have been excluded. Because data are limited, this procedure currently is not recommended by the manufacturer for those desiring pregnancy. However, promising pregnancy data have been reported (Berman 2014; Keltz, 2017).

Consent

Myomectomy can cause significant bleeding that requires transfusion. Moreover, uncontrolled hemorrhage or extensive myometrial injury during tumor removal may necessitate hysterectomy. Patients also are counseled regarding the risk of conversion to an open procedure, which mainly is prompted by heavy intraoperative bleeding. Conversion rates ranges from 1 to 5 percent (Bean, 2017; Buckley, 2015). In contrast, conversion to laparotomy during myoma ablation is rare.

MIS myomectomy requires extraction of the enucleated myomas. Techniques include minilaparotomy, colpotomy, and tissue morcellation. These are fully described on page 1048. Concerns continue regarding electric tissue morcellation and a full discussion on which to base patient counseling is found in Chapter 41 (p. 894).

In most series, the risk of leiomyoma recurrence after laparoscopic myomectomy appears to be higher than in conventional myomectomy (Fauconnier, 2000; Kotani, 2018). As one explanation, with laparoscopic myomectomy, small, deep intramural leiomyomas may be missed because a surgeon's tactile sensation is diminished. Recurrence accrues with time from surgery, and rates at 5 years range from 25 to 50 percent. Reoperation rates for recurrence range from 5 to 35 percent (Doridot, 2001; Nezhat, 1998; Yoo, 2007). Greater myoma number and preoperative gonadotropin-releasing hormone (GnRH) agonist

use seem to be predisposing factors for this recurrence. Fewer data are available for RFA ablation, but one series showed a nearly 30 percent reintervention rate at 5 years for myoma-related symptoms (Iversen, 2017).

Postoperatively, serosal adhesions can form and lead to pain or diminished fertility. During a subsequent pregnancy, heightened concerns for potential uterine rupture stem from the challenges of laparoscopic multilayer hysterotomy closure and from extensive use of electrosurgical energy in the myometrium (Hurst, 2005; Parker, 2010). Women undergoing myomectomy who do plan to have future pregnancies are counseled regarding the possible need for cesarean delivery based on the extent of myometrial disruption during the myomectomy. Data from large series show that rupture is fortunately rare following laparoscopic myomectomy (Koo, 2015; Sizzi, 2007). For unintended pregnancy following RFA ablation, data are limited but do not indicate an elevated rupture risk (Galen, 2014; Keltz, 2017).

Patient Preparation

Hematologic Status and Tumor Size

Many preparatory steps prior to myomectomy address associated patient anemia, anticipated intraoperative blood loss, and tumor size. First, many women who undergo this surgery are often anemic secondary to associated heavy menstrual bleeding. Correction prior to surgery may include oral iron therapy and GnRH agonist administration. In anticipation of blood loss, a CBC and type and crossmatch for packed red blood cells are obtained. Autologous blood donation or cell saver devices may be considered if significant hemorrhage is expected. In addition, uterine artery embolization may be performed the morning of surgery for large uteri to minimize blood loss. However, this is most often used prior to laparotomy for significantly sized uteri.

GnRH agonists may be considered to shrink leiomyoma size, decrease uterine vascularity, lower intraoperative blood loss, and minimize adhesion rates. However, loss of pseudocapsule planes around the tumors and greater recurrence risk due to missed smaller leiomyomas is the trade-off. A fuller evidence-based discussion of these same preoperative options is found in Section 43-10 (p. 951).

Prophylaxis. Antibiotic prophylaxis is not recommended for laparoscopic cases in which bowel or vaginal entry is not anticipated (American College of Obstetricians and Gynecologists, 2018a). In cases of myomectomy performed for infertility, because of the potential for tubal adhesions associated with pelvic infection, antibiotic prophylaxis commonly is used. For those in whom prophylaxis is planned, 1 g of a first- or second-generation cephalosporin is appropriate (Iverson, 1996; Kim, 2019b).

The risk of bowel injury with this procedure is low, and bowel preparation is typically not required. With laparoscopic gynecologic surgery, the decision to provide VTE prophylaxis factors patient- and procedure-related VTE risks (Gould, 2012). Thus, if longer operating times are anticipated or preexisting VTE risks are present, prophylaxis as outlined in Table 39-10 (p. 834) is reasonable.

INTRAOPERATIVE

Instruments

Many instruments required for laparoscopic myomectomy are found in a standard laparoscopy instrument set. However, for MIS myomectomy, a laparoscopic injection needle may be required for vasopressin injection, and a suction irrigation system frequently is needed to remove blood following tumor enucleation. A myoma screw or tenaculum is helpful to create needed tissue tension and countertension for enucleation. After excision, the myoma can be extracted by several

techniques described on page 1048. Thus, required endoscopic bags or morcellators are assembled preoperatively.

In contrast, RFA with the Acessa system requires specific components. First, a special ultrasound transducer is used through a 10-mm lower abdominal laparoscopic cannula and directly contacts the uterus to localize myomas. Real-time sonographic images are displayed on a dedicated screen that is positioned directly next to the laparoscopic viewing screen. A second tool is the RFA needle, which punctures each tumor individually. Once within the myoma, a deployable electrode array housed within the needle is expanded to deliver the ablative energy. As its energy source, the RFA needle is connected to a generator. The generator display screen shows real-time energy levels being delivered to the myoma.

Surgical Steps— Laparoscopic Myomectomy

❶ Anesthesia and Patient Positioning. As with most laparoscopic procedures, the patient is placed in low lithotomy position in booted support stirrups after adequate general anesthesia has been delivered. A bimanual examination is completed to determine uterine size to aid port placement. Because of the risk of hysterectomy and because

colpotomy may be used for tumor removal, both the vagina and abdomen are surgically prepared. A Foley catheter is inserted. A uterine manipulator also may be placed, including one that will allow chromotubation at the procedure's end. If planned, 10 mL of methylene blue is mixed with 100 to 150 mL of sterile saline for injection through the cervical cannula.

❷ Trocar and Laparoscope Insertion. Primary and accessory trocars are placed as described in Chapter 41 (p. 888). For MIS myomectomy, port placement is customized to allow uterine manipulation and access to all leiomyomas. Positioning ideally provides sufficient instrument triangulation. This allows tools to create tension for myoma enucleation and pass a needle for hysterotomy repair. Depending on uterine height, the primary port may need to be placed supraumbilically. In general, this port lies at least 4 cm above the level of the fundus to provide a global view of the uterus. Typically, at least three accessory ports are required.

For RFA ablation, once optical access is obtained, an additional 10-mm port is used to introduce the laparoscopic ultrasound transducer. The diameter of the RFA needle is sufficiently small that a dedicated port is unnecessary. Instead, the device is placed percutaneously through a small stab incision and then advanced directly through the

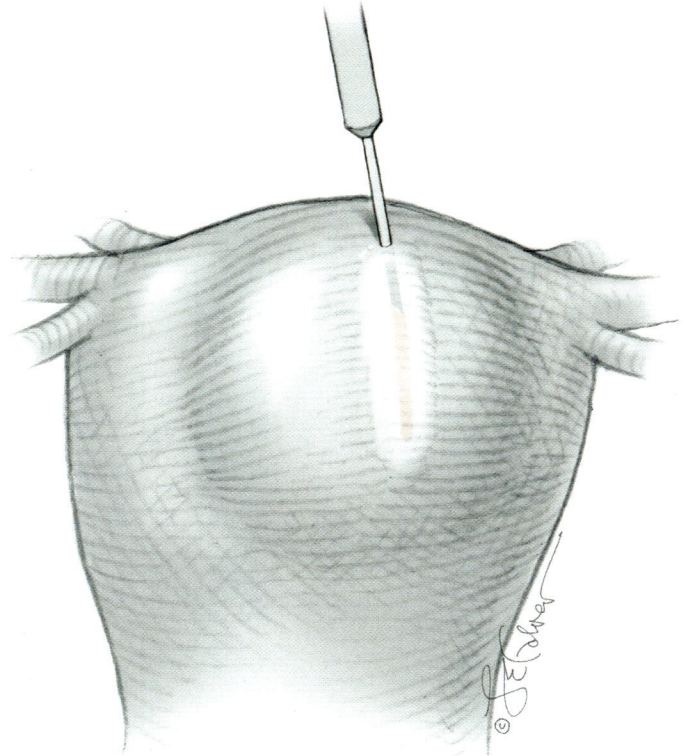

FIGURE 44-8.1 Vasopressin injection beneath serosa.

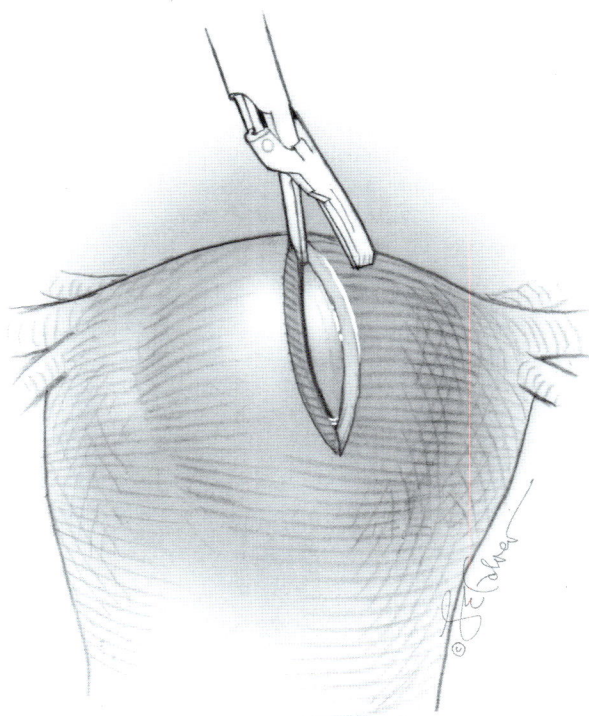

FIGURE 44-8.2 Serosal incision overlying leiomyoma.

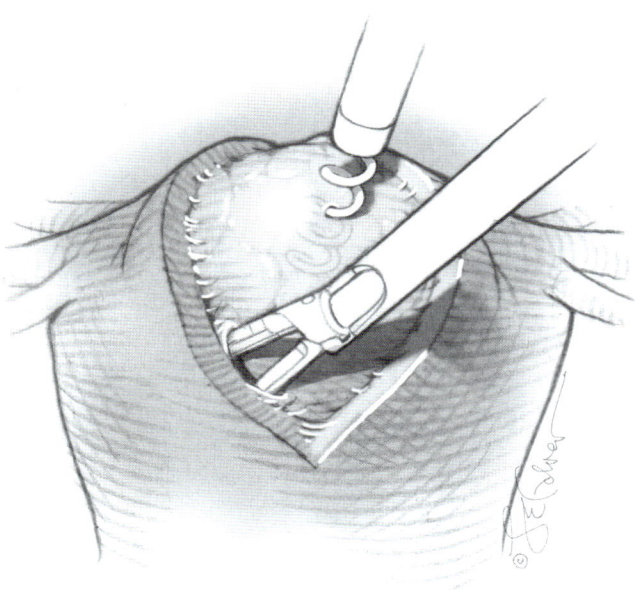

FIGURE 44-8.3 Tumor enucleation.

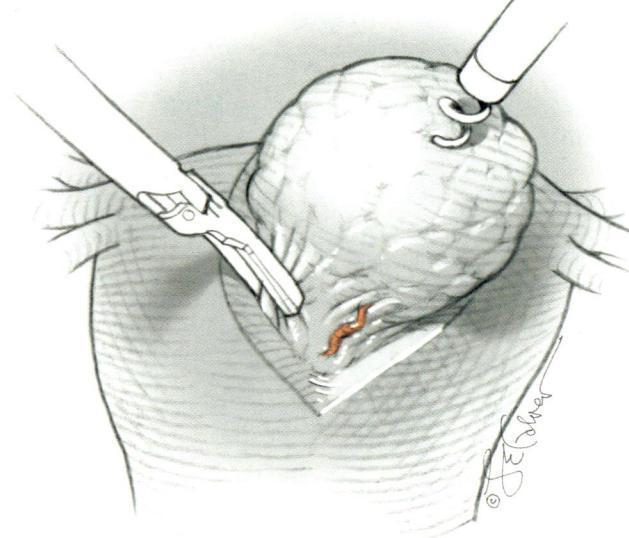

FIGURE 44-8.4 Coagulation of vascular attachments between the leiomyoma and the myometrium.

anterior abdominal wall to enter the peritoneal cavity. Its narrow diameter allows the needle to be moved to different abdominal wall sites to access each myoma, yet cumulative abdominal wall injury is minor.

③ Incision Placement. The serosal uterine surface should be inspected to identify leiomyomas to be removed. Correlating with preoperative imaging, the surgeon selects the optimal uterine incision to minimize myometrial disruption and remove the maximum number of tumors thorough one incision.

④ Vasopressin Use. 8-Arginine vasopressin (Pitressin) is a sterile, aqueous solution of synthetic vasopressin. It is effective in limiting uterine blood loss during myomectomy because of its ability to cause vascular spasm and uterine muscle contraction. Compared with placebo, vasopressin injection significantly decreases blood loss during myomectomy (Frederick, 1994).

Each vial of vasopressin is standardized to contain 20 pressor units/mL. Suitable doses for myomectomy include 20 U diluted in 30 to 100 mL of saline (Fletcher, 1996; Iverson, 1996). Vasopressin is typically injected along the planned serosal incision(s) in a plane between the myometrium and leiomyoma capsule (Fig. 44-8.1). A laparoscopic needle placed through one of the accessory cannulas or a 22-gauge spinal needle placed directly through the abdominal wall is suitable for injection. Needle aspiration prior to injection is imperative to avoid intravascular injection of this potent vasoconstrictor. The anesthesiologist is informed of vasopressin injection,

as a sudden increase in patient blood pressure may potentially occur following injection. Blanching at the injection site is expected. The plasma half-life of this agent is 10 to 20 minutes. For this reason, injection of vasopressin is discontinued 20 minutes prior to uterine repair to allow evaluation of bleeding from myometrial incisions (Hutchins, 1996).

The main risks associated with local vasopressin injection result from inadvertent intravascular infiltration and include transient blood pressure elevation, bradycardia, atrioventricular block, and pulmonary edema (Hobo, 2009; Tulandi, 1996). Patients with a significant medical history of cardiac or pulmonary disease are poor candidates for vasopressin.

⑤ Serosal Incision. Because of postoperative adhesion formation risks, surgeons minimize the number of serosal incisions and attempt to place incisions on the anterior uterine wall. Tulandi and colleagues (1993) found that posterior wall incisions result in a 94-percent adhesion formation rate compared with a 55-percent rate for anterior incisions.

After vasopressin injection, hysterotomy may be performed using a Harmonic scalpel, monopolar electrode, or laser. For most patients, an anterior midline vertical uterine incision allows removal of the greatest number of leiomyomas through the fewest incisions. The length should accommodate the approximate diameter of the largest tumor. The incision depth should afford access to all leiomyomas (Fig. 44-8.2).

⑥ Tumor Enucleation. Once the hysterotomy is created, the myometrium will

generally retract, and the first leiomyoma may be grasped with a laparoscopic single-toothed tenaculum. Alternatively, a leiomyoma screw also can manipulate the myoma to create tension between the myometrium and mass (Fig. 44-8.3). Using a blunt-tipped tool, blunt dissection of the pseudocapsule surrounding the leiomyoma frees the tumor from the adjacent myometrium. Areas requiring sharp dissection from the myometrium may be freed with any of the electrosurgical instruments that were used for the uterine incision.

⑦ Bleeding. During myomectomy, bleeding primarily develops during tumor enucleation and positively correlates with preoperative uterine size, total weight of leiomyomas removed, and operating time (Ginsburg, 1993). Approximately two to four main arteries feed each leiomyoma and enter the tumor at unpredictable sites. For this reason, surgeons must watch for these vessels, coagulate them prior to transection when possible, and be ready to immediately fulgurate remaining bleeding vessels (Fig. 44-8.4). To avoid myometrial damage, the surgeon applies electrosurgical energy only when necessary.

⑧ Myometrial Closure. Following removal of all tumors, redundant serosa may be excised. Laparoscopic suturing techniques described in Chapter 41 (p. 895) are used during incision reapproximation. The same general principles of myometrial closure for abdominal myomectomy are employed during laparoscopic myomectomy. In one method, for deep myometrial closure, a needle driver can be used with 0-gauge delayed-

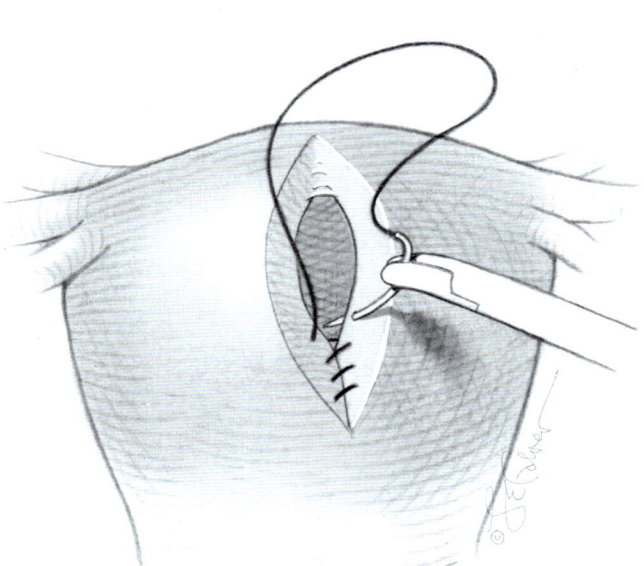

FIGURE 44-8.5 Myometrial closure.

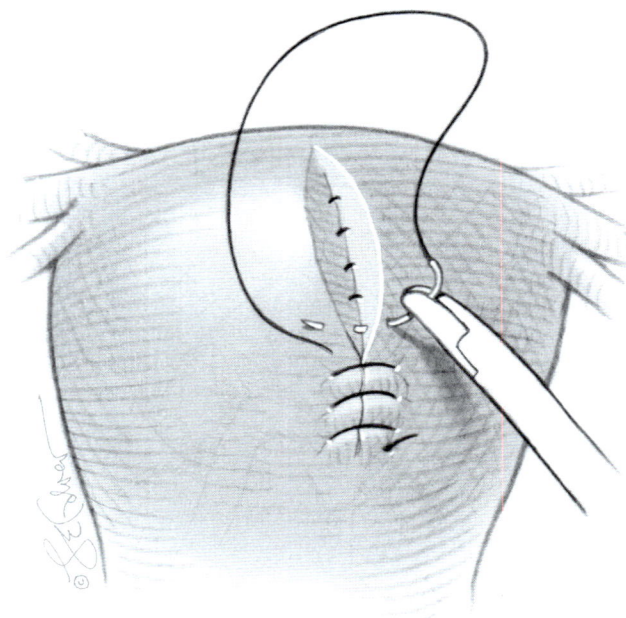

FIGURE 44-8.6 Serosal closure.

absorbable suture on a CT-2 needle in a continuous running fashion. Smaller internal myometrial incisions are closed first. The primary incision(s) then is closed in layers to improve hemostasis and prevent hematoma formation (Fig. 44-8.5). A gauge of sufficient strength to prevent breakage during muscle approximation is selected, typically 0 to 2-0 gauge. Alternatively, barbed sutures can close myometrial defects during laparoscopic myomectomy (Fig. 41-32, p. 896). These obviate the need for knot tying and yield consistent wound opposition (Einarsson, 2010; Greenberg, 2008).

❾ Serosal Closure. Closure of the serosal incision using a running baseball suture with

4-0 or 5-0 gauge monofilament delayed-absorbable suture may help to limit adhesion formation. A simple, running suture line also is suitable (Fig. 44-8.6). Absorbable adhesion barriers reduce the incidence of adhesion formation following myomectomy and may be introduced through laparoscopic cannulas (Ahmad, 2015). However, no substantial evidence documents that adhesion barrier use improves fertility, decreases pain, or prevents bowel obstruction (American Society for Reproductive Medicine, 2013).

❿ Tissue Extraction. Once amputated, the myomas must be removed, and options include minilaparotomy, colpotomy, and tissue morcellation (p. 1048).

Surgical Steps— Laparoscopically Assisted Myomectomy

❶ Minilaparotomy. Another MIS technique that may allow for safe and efficient myomectomy is laparoscopically assisted myomectomy (LAM). The procedure is initiated as described in steps 1 through 5. Abdominal cavity assessment, uterine inspection, and incision of the serosa and myometrium are performed laparoscopically. To aid in the laparoscopically challenging steps of myomectomy, LAM offers a hybrid approach. Specifically, tumor enucleation and uterine closure are completed through a 2- to 4-cm low transverse

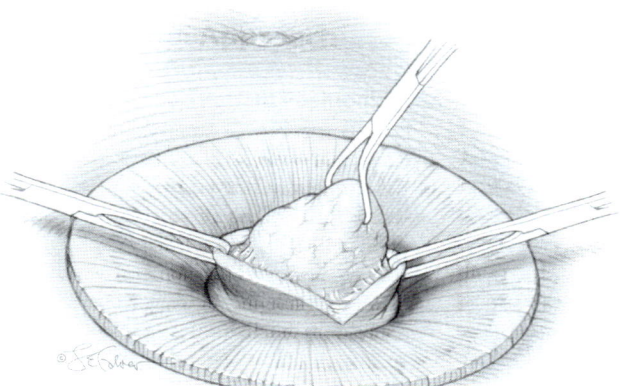

FIGURE 44-8.7 Tumor enucleation during laparoscopically assisted myomectomy.

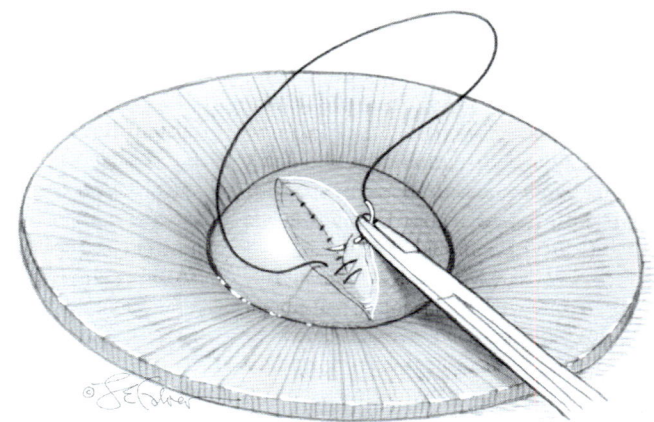

FIGURE 44-8.8 Myometrial closure during laparoscopically assisted myomectomy.

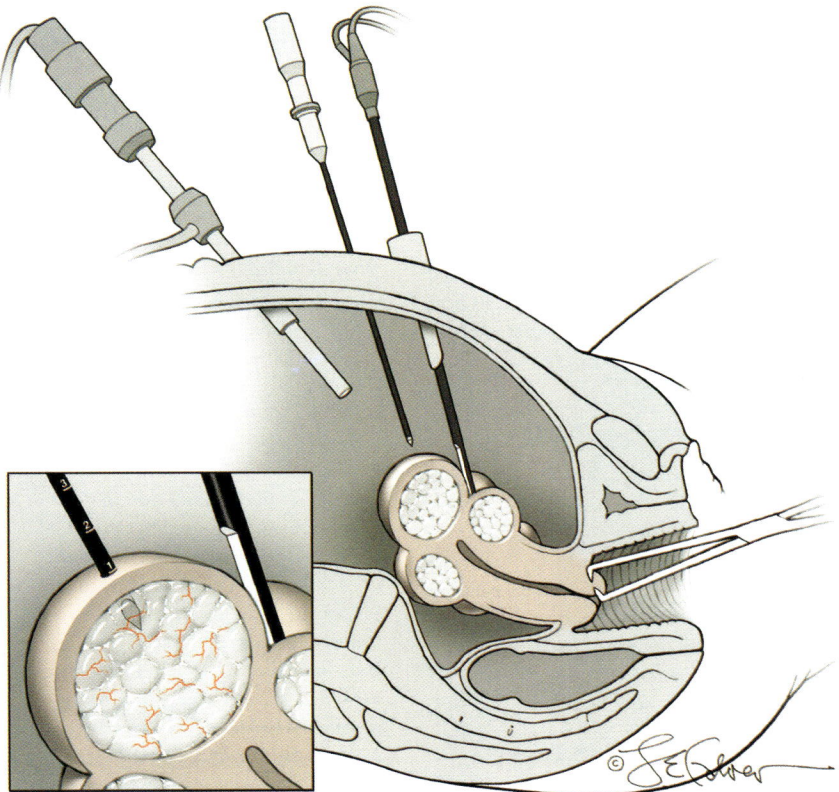

FIGURE 44-8.9 Radiofrequency ablation requires laparoscopy to guide the sonographic transducer and ablation trocar. Inset: Trocar driven into myoma under direct sonographic guidance.

and easier removal of very large tumors (Prapas, 2009; Wen, 2010). Disadvantages stem mainly from the larger abdominal wall incision.

Surgical Steps— Radiofrequency Ablation

❶ Instrument Insertion. The procedure is initiated as described in steps 1 and 2. After this, the laparoscopic ultrasound probe is placed through a 10-mm lower abdominal cannula to directly contact the uterus (Fig. 44-8.9). This allows better sonographic imaging of the myoma by permitting views from several angles.

Once the initial myoma is localized, the RFA needle punctures through the anterior abdominal wall and is guided to the desired tumor. Here, the needle pierces the uterine serosa and is driven 1 to 2 cm into the selected myoma (see Fig. 44-8.9, inset).

❷ Tumor Ablation. The fan-shaped electrode from within the needle is deployed, and the span of the array is customized to the myoma's characteristics (Fig. 44-8.10). Ideally, energy is deposited to maximize myolysis yet minimize thermal injury to surrounding tissues. As seen in the second image, radiofrequency energy is deployed to devascularize the myoma.

Once heating parameters are reached, the array is retracted and the RFA needle is removed. During its removal, monopolar energy is applied to coagulate bleeding from the initial needle puncture (see Fig. 44-8.10C). For additional myomas, the process is repeated. If needed, the narrow RFA needle can be removed from the abdomen and placed at a different abdominal wall site to provide superior access to the next selected tumor.

minilaparotomy incision. With this, the pneumoperitoneum and laparoscope viewing are lost. Instead, application of a wound retraction system such as the Alexis or Mobius retractor provides visual access to the operative field (Fig. 41-13, p. 883). The uterus and leiomyoma are brought to the surface of the anterior abdominal wall and through the laparotomy incision.

❷ Myomectomy. The tumors are then enucleated and divided through this incision (Fig. 44-8.7). This open incision also allows for conventional suturing techniques and aids suturing of large defects that require a multilayer myometrial closure (Fig. 44-8.8). Advantages include shorter operating time, technical simplicity, improved tactile sensation to detect deep intramural leiomyomas,

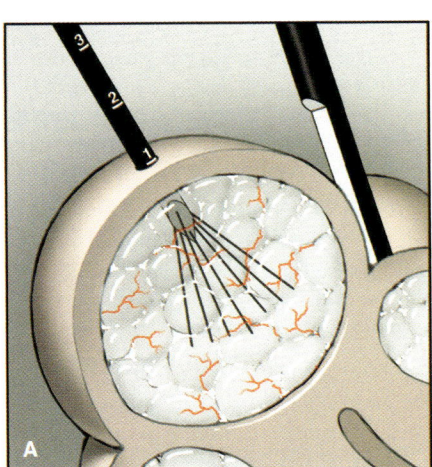
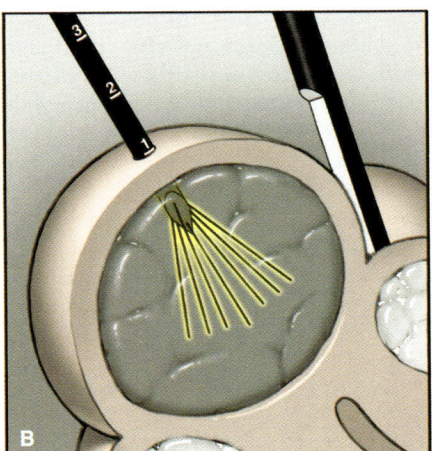
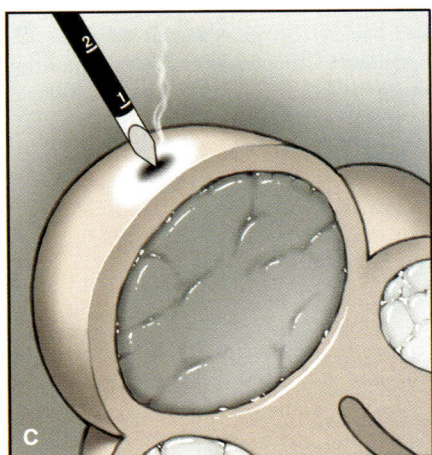

FIGURE 44-8.10 A. Device array deployed. **B.** Array activation ablates the myoma. **C.** Uterine puncture site is coagulated as trocar removed.

POSTOPERATIVE

Following myomectomy, postoperative care follows that for any major laparoscopic surgery. A patient is typically discharged home on the first postoperative day. Hemodynamic status and return of early bowel function usually dictate this course. Postoperative activity in general is advanced as tolerated, although vigorous exercise is usually delayed until 4 weeks after surgery.

Febrile morbidity of greater than 38.0°C is common following myomectomy (Iverson, 1996; LaMorte, 1993; Rybak, 2008). Purported causes include atelectasis, myometrial hematomas, and factors released with myometrial destruction. Although fever is common following myomectomy, pelvic infection is not.

Following RFA ablation, postoperative care mirrors that for minor laparoscopic surgery. A patient is typically discharged home the same day. Pain control and oral intake are usual limiting factors. For most, physical activities and diet can be resumed according to patient comfort.

No consensus guides the timing of pregnancy attempts after myomectomy. Imaging studies suggest that wound healing is usually completed within 3 months (Chang, 2009; Darwish, 2005; Tsuji, 2006). Moreover, no clinical trials specifically address the issue of uterine rupture or the route of pregnancy delivery after myomectomy (American College of Obstetricians and Gynecologists, 2019a). Management of these cases requires sound clinical judgment and individualization of care. In general, large incisions or those entering the endometrial cavity favor cesarean delivery.

44-9

Laparoscopic Hysterectomy

Several laparoscopic techniques have been developed for hysterectomy and vary depending on the degree of laparoscopic dissection versus vaginal surgery required to remove the uterus (Garry, 1994). These include:

- Diagnostic laparoscopy prior to vaginal hysterectomy (VH)
- Vaginal hysterectomy assisted by laparoscopy, that is, lysis of adhesions and/or excision of endometriosis prior to VH
- Laparoscopically assisted vaginal hysterectomy (LAVH): laparoscopic dissection down to, but not including, uterine artery transection
- Laparoscopic hysterectomy (LH): laparoscopic dissection, including uterine artery transection, but completion of hysterectomy vaginally
- Total laparoscopic hysterectomy (TLH): complete laparoscopic excision of the uterus

The laparoscopic approach offers advantages over traditional total abdominal hysterectomy (TAH). These include significant lower analgesia requirements, shorter hospital stays, rapid recovery, greater patient satisfaction, and lower rates of wound infection and hematoma formation (Kluivers, 2007; Schindlbeck, 2008). Disadvantageously, surgical time is lengthened, although the learning curve may be a factor. TLH offers fewer advantages compare with vaginal hysterectomy. Thus, in most cases, TLH should be an alternative to TAH (Aarts, 2015; American College of Obstetricians and Gynecologists, 2017a; Marana, 1999).

For all the hysterectomy types described in the following sections, plans for concurrent bilateral salpingo-oophorectomy or for prophylactic salpingectomy are individualized. A detailed discussion of the risks and benefits of surgical adnexectomy is found in Chapter 43 (p. 957). Risk-reducing salpingectomy advantages were summarized earlier (p. 1019) and fully described elsewhere (Chaps. 5 and 35, pp. 118 and 736). Notably, the American College of Obstetricians and Gynecologists (2019c) has emphasized that the planned route of hysterectomy should not be changed to complete prophylactic salpingectomy.

PREOPERATIVE

Patient Evaluation

Prior to hysterectomy, all patients require cervical cancer screening. With abnormal findings, further evaluation is completed to exclude invasive cancer, which is treated instead with radical hysterectomy or chemoradiation. Similarly, for endometrial cancer, women at risk and whose indication includes abnormal bleeding also are screened before surgery (Chap. 8, p. 182). Other required testing is dictated by hysterectomy indication and discussed in the respective topic's chapter. Last, concurrent cervical infection or bacterial vaginosis is sought for preoperative eradication to lower surgical site infection rates.

A thorough pelvic examination and history reveal factors that help determine the optimal surgical route. Poor candidates for a vaginal approach include patients with minimal uterine descent, extensive abdominal or pelvic adhesions, a large uterus not amenable to tissue manipulation or extraction methods, adnexal pathology, and a restricted vaginal vault or contracted pelvis. Patients with these findings are generally considered for TAH or TLH (Schindlbeck, 2008).

Of factors, uterine size and mobility are important. No agreed-upon size precludes LH. However, a wide bulky uterus with minimal mobility may make it difficult to visualize vital structures, to manipulate the uterus during surgery, and to remove it vaginally. A fuller discussion of hysterectomy route decision making is described in Chapter 43 (p. 956).

Consent

Similar to an open approach, possible risks of hysterectomy include increased blood loss and need for transfusion, unplanned adnexectomy, and injury to other pelvic organs, especially bladder, ureter, and bowel. The ureters are at greater risk during LH compared with other hysterectomy approaches (Harkki-Siren, 1997, 1998; Teeluckdharry, 2015). Kuno and colleagues (1998) evaluated ureteral catheterization to prevent such injury but found no benefit. Complications related specifically to laparoscopy include injury to the major vessels, bladder, and bowel during trocar placement. These and their treatment are outlined in Chapters 41 and 45 (pp. 875 and 1080).

The risk of conversion to an open procedure also is discussed. In general, factors include a large, poorly manipulated uterus; severe adhesive disease; and uncontrolled bleeding (Lim, 2016). In large series of hysterectomy for benign disease, rates approximate 5 percent. Rates are typically lower with experienced, high-volume surgeons (Keurentjes, 2018; Tunitsky 2010). Last, candidates for prophylactic adnexectomy or salpingectomy are counseled regarding associated risks.

Patient Preparation

A blood sample is typed and crossmatched for potential transfusion. Antibiotic prophylaxis is administered within the hour prior to skin incision, and appropriate antibiotic options are listed in Table 39-8 (p. 832). Overall, the likelihood of VTE during laparoscopic hysterectomy is significantly reduced compared with abdominal hysterectomy (Barber, 2015). Thus, the decision to provide VTE prophylaxis factors patient- and procedure-related VTE risks (Gould, 2012). If longer operating times are anticipated, conversion to laparotomy is a concern, or preexisting VTE risks are present, prophylaxis as outlined in Table 39-10 (p. 834) is reasonable. Although not routinely elected, bowel preparation prior to laparoscopy in specific cases may assist with colon manipulation and pelvic anatomy visualization by evacuating the rectosigmoid. If extensive cul-de-sac adhesions and potential colorectal injury is a concern, bowel preparation also can aid intraoperative proctosigmoidoscopy and bowel manipulation needed for its repair. Enemas prior to surgery may be effective for this goal.

INTRAOPERATIVE

Instruments

Vessel occlusion is an important component of any hysterectomy. For this, suitable instruments include monopolar or bipolar electrosurgical instruments, Harmonic scalpel, stapling devices, traditional sutures, and suturing devices. Several of these can be used dually for dissection and hemostasis. The Harmonic scalpel is frequently selected for its ability to cut with minimal smoke plume and little surrounding thermal tissue damage. Notably, it only is used to seal vessels up to 5 mm. Several advanced bipolar devices also offer improved vessel sealing. With various instruments, vessels measuring up to 5 mm (LigaSure, Gyrus Plasma Kinetic) and up to 7 mm (ENSEAL) can be coagulated with minimal thermal spread (Lamberton, 2008; Landman, 2003; Smaldone, 2008).

Surgical Steps

❶ **Anesthesia and Patient Positioning.** For most women, these procedures are performed in an inpatient setting under general anesthesia. The patient is placed in a low lithotomy position in booted support stirrups. A bimanual examination is completed to determine uterine size and shape to aid port placement. The abdomen and vagina are surgically prepared, a Foley catheter is inserted, and orogastric or nasogastric tube is

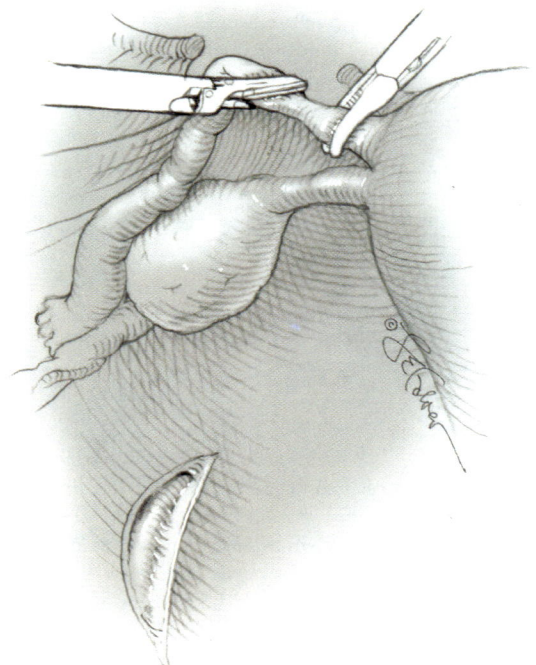

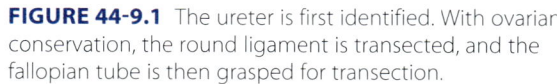

FIGURE 44-9.1 The ureter is first identified. With ovarian conservation, the round ligament is transected, and the fallopian tube is then grasped for transection.

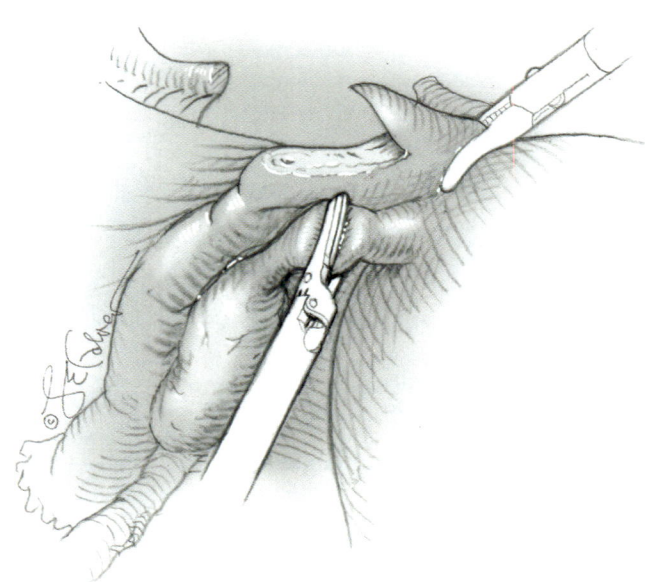

FIGURE 44-9.2 Uteroovarian ligament transection.

placed. Uterine manipulators can assist with visualization. These are considered in cases in which anatomic distortion is anticipated or the uterus large.

❷ Initial Steps. The introductory steps for laparoscopic hysterectomy mirror that for other laparoscopic procedures (Chap. 41, p. 888). The number of ports and their caliber may vary, but in general, this surgery requires a 5- to 12-mm optical port placed at the level of the umbilicus or higher for larger uteri. Two or three accessory ports are inserted at the lower abdomen. Specifically, two ports are positioned beyond the lateral borders of the rectus abdominis muscle, whereas a third may be positioned centrally and cephalad to the uterine fundus. Left upper quadrant entry is considered in cases of suspected periumbilical adhesions. For larger uteri, if the uterine fundus is close to or above the level of the umbilicus, the optical port is placed approximately 3 to 4 cm above the fundus for optimal viewing.

❸ Pelvic Evaluation. With the ports and laparoscope inserted and the patient in Trendelenburg position, a blunt laparoscopic probe can aid organ manipulation. The pelvis and abdomen are visually explored. At this point, the decision is made whether to continue with MIS or convert to laparotomy. If needed, adhesions are lysed to restore normal anatomy. The bowel is gently displaced from the pelvis into the abdomen to expand available operating space and viewing.

❹ Ureter Identification. Irrigating fluids and CO_2 used for insufflation can, with time, create peritoneal edema, which can hinder viewing of retroperitoneal structures. For this reason, the ureters are identified early. The ureters often can be seen easily beneath the pelvic peritoneum, or the retroperitoneum may be entered and explored to identify them. In such situations, the peritoneum medial to the IP ligament is grasped and tented using atraumatic forceps and incised with scissors. Hydrodissection techniques may be employed. The opening in the peritoneum then is extended caudally and cephalad along the expected axis of the ureter. Through this peritoneal window, the ureter is identified, and peristalsis should be noted (Fig. 44-9.1) (Parker, 2004).

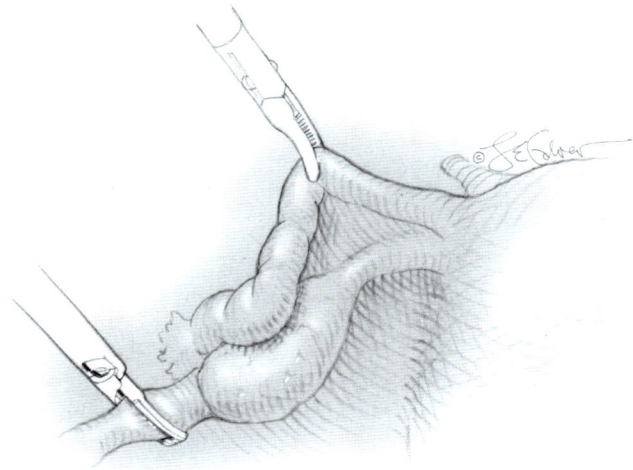

FIGURE 44-9.3 Infundibulopelvic ligament transection.

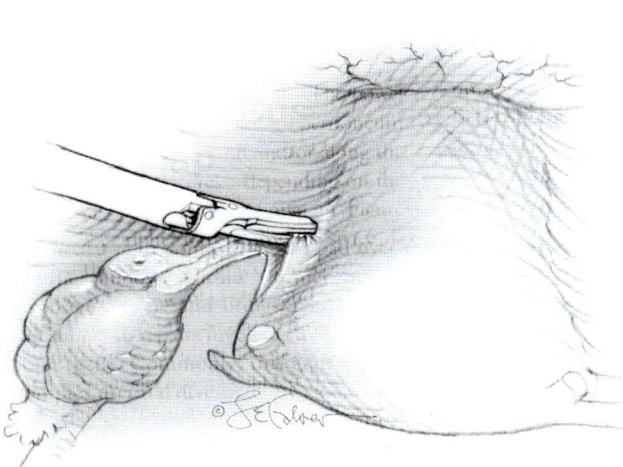

FIGURE 44-9.4 Anterior leaf of broad ligament incised caudally.

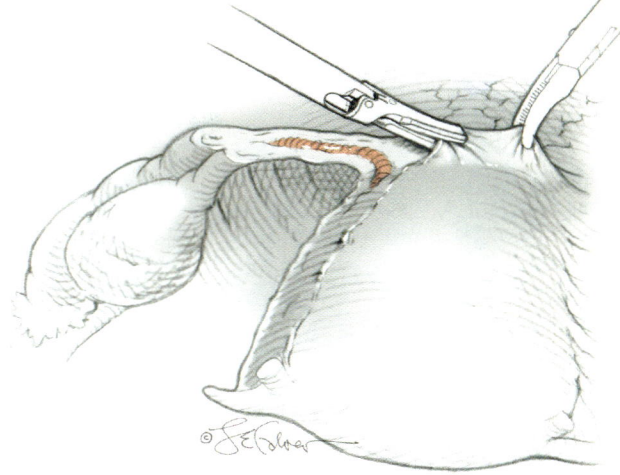

FIGURE 44-9.5 Vesicouterine fold incised.

❺ Round Ligament Transection. The proximal round ligament is grasped and divided. This also provides entry into the retroperitoneal space and is another method to identify the ureter. Entering this space also allows access later to the uterine artery and cardinal ligament for transection.

❻ Ovarian Conservation. If ovarian preservation is planned, proximal portions of the fallopian tube and uteroovarian ligament are desiccated and transected (Figs. 44-9.1 and 44-9.2). With this, the tube and ovary are freed from the uterus and can be placed in the ovarian fossa.

❼ Oophorectomy. For removal of one or both ovaries, the IP ligament is grasped and pulled up and away from retroperitoneal structures. The presence and path of the ureter is identified. The IP ligament is isolated and dissected away from the ureteral course. The pedicle is coagulated, desiccated, or stapled, and then divided (Fig. 44-9.3). For risk-reducing adnexectomy in women with a high-risk hereditary mutation, the IP is divided 2 cm past the ovary, and the fallopian tube is transected at the uterine cornu.

❽ Broad Ligament Incision. Following transection of the round ligament, the leaves of the broad ligament fall open and loose gauzy connective tissue is found between these leaves. The anterior leaf is incised sharply (Fig. 44-9.4). This incision is directed caudally and centrally to the midline above the vesicouterine fold. The posterior leaf requires incision caudally to the level of the uterosacral ligament. The loose areolar tissue separating the anterior and posterior leaves is dissected as well. Ultimately, opening the broad ligament provides access to lateral uterine anatomy, which is important for subsequent uterine artery ligation, and helps drop the ureter away from the uterus.

❾ Bladder Flap Development. After broad ligament incision bilaterally, the vesicouterine fold is grasped with atraumatic forceps, elevated away from the underlying bladder, and incised (Fig. 44-9.5). This exposes connective tissue between the bladder and underlying uterus in the vesicouterine space. Loosely attached connections can be bluntly divided by gently pushing against the cervix and caudally to move the bladder off the cervix and upper vagina (Fig. 44-9.6). Creating cephalad traction on the uterus with the uterine manipulator also may help with this dissection. Denser tissue in the vesicouterine space is better divided sharply. With this, the tissue is elevated, and the scissors are kept close to the surface of the cervix to minimize inadvertent cystotomy risk. As this tissue is dissected, the

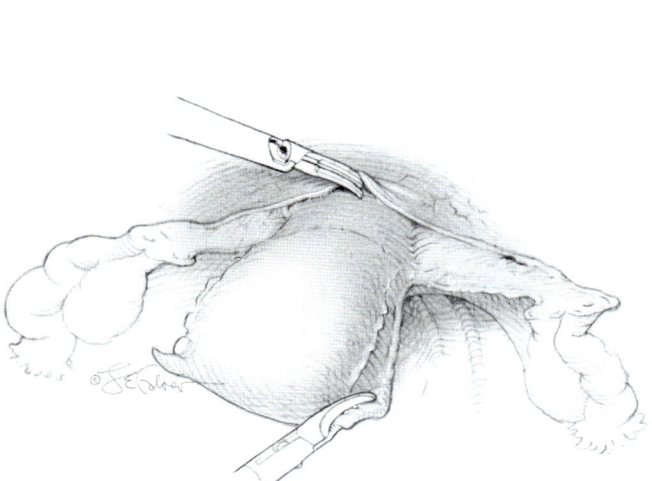

FIGURE 44-9.6 Bladder moved caudally.

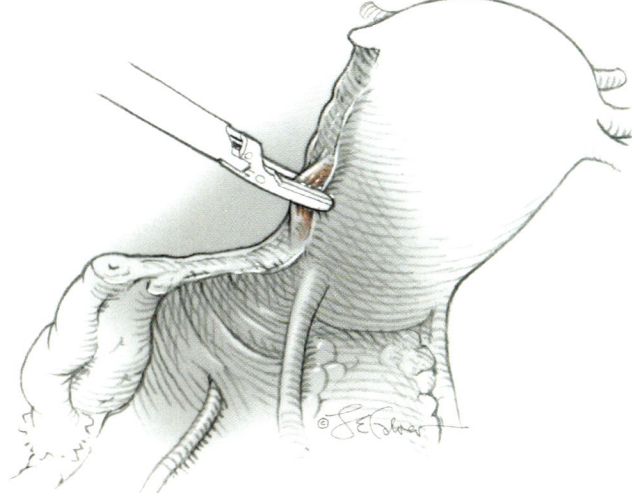

FIGURE 44-9.7 Uterine artery coagulation.

vesicouterine space is opened. Electrosurgery may be needed to coagulate small bleeding vessels.

Development of this space allows the bladder to be moved caudally and off the lower uterus and upper vagina. This repositioning is necessary for final colpotomy and uterus removal. Of the hysterectomy types, MIS approaches have the highest risk of bladder injury (Frankman, 2010; Teeluckdharry, 2015). Cystotomy occurs most frequently to the dome during this sharp or blunt dissection (Harkki, 2001). Scarring within the vesicouterine space from prior cesarean delivery or endometriosis can raise this risk.

⑩ Uterine Artery Transection. After the uterine arteries are identified, the areolar connective tissue surrounding them is grasped, placed on tension, and incised. This skeletonizing of the vessels leads to superior occlusion of the uterine artery and vein. The arteries then are coagulated and transected (Fig. 44-9.7). Alternatively, surgeons may elect to terminate the laparoscopic portion prior to uterine artery transection and complete artery ligation from a vaginal approach (LAVH).

⑪ Vaginal Hysterectomy. With laparoscopic hysterectomy, after the uterine arteries are transected, the surgical approach is converted to that for vaginal hysterectomy and is completed as outlined in Section 43-13 (p. 965). In this transition, the patient is repositioned from low lithotomy to standard lithotomy position within the same booted support stirrups.

⑫ Abdominal Inspection. After vaginal completion of the hysterectomy, attention is redirected to laparoscopic inspection of the pelvis for signs of bleeding. Before returning to the abdomen, surgeons will replace their surgical gloves.

Copious irrigation of the abdominopelvic cavity and confirmation of hemostasis is performed. During this inspection, intraabdominal pressures are lowered to better identify sources of bleeding. The laparoscopic procedure is terminated as outlined in Section 44-1 (p. 1018).

POSTOPERATIVE

Following laparoscopic hysterectomy, patient recovery mirrors that for vaginal hysterectomy. In general, compared with those undergoing abdominal hysterectomy, patients undergoing MIS have faster return of normal bowel function, easier ambulation, and decreased analgesia requirements. A clear liquid diet can be initiated the day of surgery and advanced quickly as tolerated. Postoperative complications in general mirror those for abdominal hysterectomy with the exception that superficial surgical site infection rates are lower.

44-10

Laparoscopic Supracervical Hysterectomy

Laparoscopic supracervical hysterectomy (LSH) differs from total laparoscopic hysterectomy (TLH) in that the uterine corpus is amputated, but the cervix remains. Once freed, the corpus either is delivered through a posterior colpotomy or minilaparotomy incision or undergoes enclosed morcellation. Advantageously, the uterosacral and cardinal ligaments, which are important to pelvic support, are retained.

It also is an excellent alternative for cases complicated by extensive scarring. Specifically, adhesions between the bladder and the lower uterine segment in the vesicouterine space or those in the posterior cul-de-sac may make removal of the cervix difficult. Related to this, ureteral and bladder injury rates are lowered by avoiding difficult dissection.

Last, to minimize later vaginal mesh erosion, cervical stump retention may be elected in cases with planned concurrent sacrocolpopexy. Advantages are described in Chapter 45 (p. 1125).

Certain contraindications to preserving the cervix are sought prior to selecting supracervical hysterectomy. Examples include preinvasive or invasive lesions of the cervix or uterine corpus. Patients at risk for noncompliance with routine cervical cancer screening may pose a relative contraindication.

PREOPERATIVE

Patient Evaluation

A thorough pelvic examination and history reveal factors that help determine the optimal surgical route. Uterine size and mobility are important, although no agreed-upon size precludes LSH. That said, a large bulky uterus with minimal mobility may be difficult to adequately manipulate, may limit exposure during surgery, and may be challenging to extract. Once a patient is deemed eligible for a laparoscopic approach, preoperative evaluation mirrors that for laparoscopic hysterectomy, described in the last section.

Consent

Similar to an open approach, possible risks of LSH include blood loss and need for transfusion, unplanned adnexectomy, and injury to other pelvic organs, especially bladder, ureter, and bowel. Complications related specifically to laparoscopy include injury to the major vessels, bladder, and bowel during trocar placement (Chap. 41, p. 875).

Postoperatively, endometrium within the lower uterine segment may be retained with LSH. As a result, the risk of cyclic long-term bleeding is a potential consequence. Rates quoted in early studies reach 24 percent but are lower in more recent investigations and range from 5 to 10 percent (Okaro, 2001; Sasaki, 2014; van der Stege, 1999). Techniques that ablate or resect more of the lower uterine and proximal endocervical tissue appear to decrease these long-term bleeding risks (Nouri, 2013; Schmidt, 2011; Wenger, 2005).

In some case, later secondary excision of the cervical stump may be required. Termed *trachelectomy*, this excision may be indicated if refractory long-term bleeding or significant subsequent cervical neoplasia develops postoperatively. Overall, rates of trachelectomy appear to mimic long-term bleeding rates and show a downward trend.

The risk of conversion to an open procedure also is discussed. The SCH-associated rate is lower than that with laparoscopic hysterectomy and ranges from 1 to 3 percent (Bojahr, 2006; Grosse-Drieling, 2012; Wallwiener, 2013). In general, conversion to laparotomy may be necessary if exposure and organ manipulation are limited or if bleeding is encountered that cannot be controlled with laparoscopic techniques.

Patient Preparation

A blood sample is typed and crossmatched for potential transfusion. If considered, bowel preparation prior to laparoscopy may assist with colon manipulation and pelvic anatomy visualization by evacuating the rectosigmoid. Enemas prior to surgery may be as effective for this goal. Antibiotic prophylaxis is administered within the hour prior to skin incision, and appropriate antibiotic options are listed in Table 39-8 (p. 832). With laparoscopic gynecologic surgery, the decision to provide VTE prophylaxis factors patient- and procedure-related VTE risks (Gould, 2012). Thus, if longer operating times are anticipated, conversion to laparotomy is a concern, or preexisting VTE risks are present, prophylaxis as outlined in Table 39-10 (p. 834) is reasonable.

INTRAOPERATIVE

Instruments

During cervical amputation, blunt scissors, Harmonic scalpel, laser, or monopolar needle or scissors may be used to excise the corpus. Vessel occlusion is an important component of any hysterectomy. For this, suitable instruments include monopolar or bipolar electrosurgical instruments, Harmonic scalpel, stapling devices, traditional sutures, and suturing devices. Many of these instruments may not be readily available in all operating suites, and desired tools should be requested prior to surgery. After tumor excision, removal may be accomplished by several techniques described in steps 3, 4, and 5. Thus, required endoscopic bags or morcellators are assembled preoperatively.

Surgical Steps

❶ **Initial Steps.** The initial surgical steps for LSH in general mirror those for laparoscopic hysterectomy, including coagulation of the uterine vessels. These are described in Section 44-9 steps 1 through 10 (p. 1043). With LSH, opening of the vesicocervical space

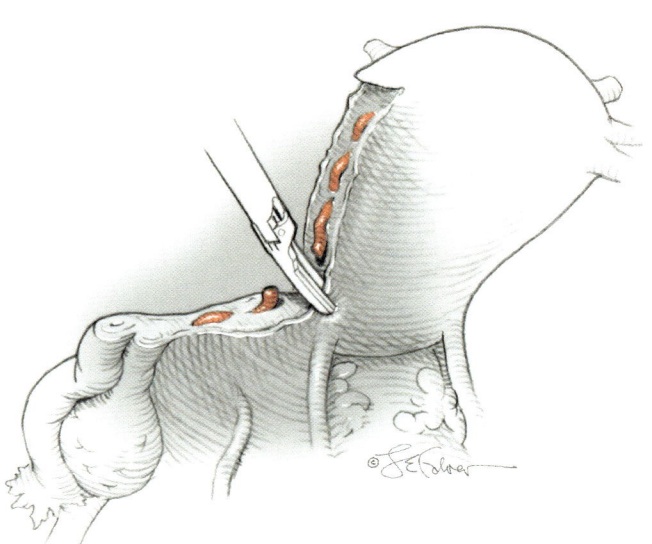

FIGURE 44-10.1 Incision initiated above uterosacral ligaments.

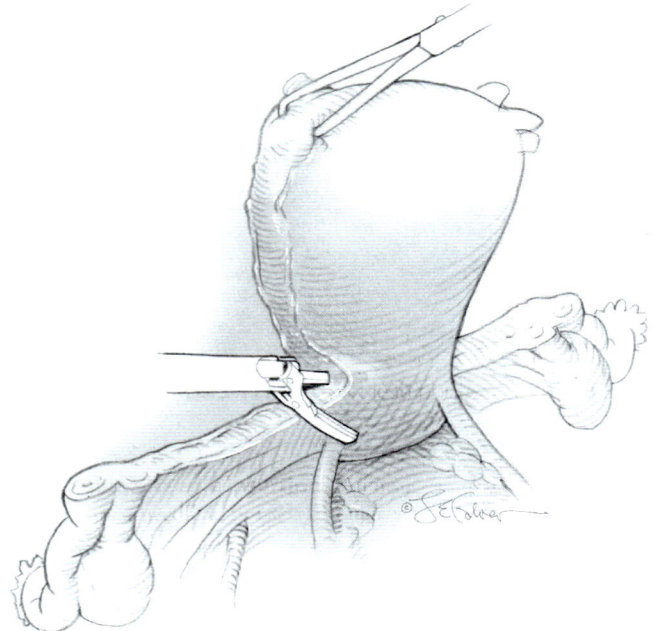

FIGURE 44-10.2 Incision extended posteriorly.

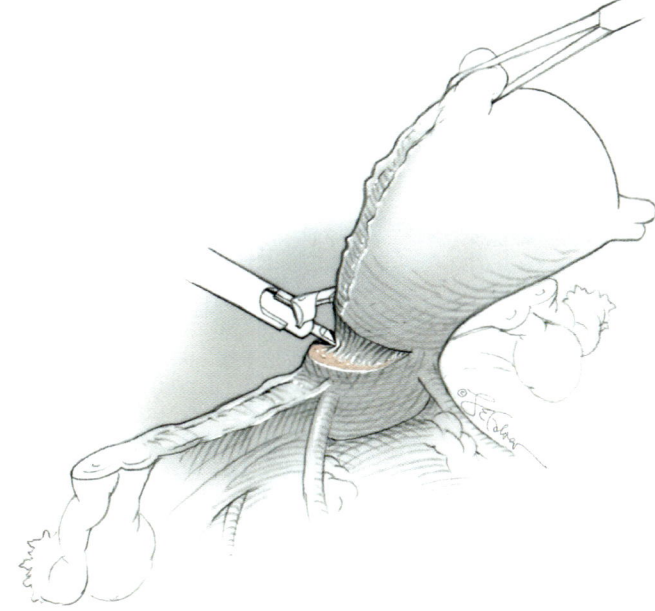

FIGURE 44-10.3 Cone-shape incision extended anteriorly.

and caudal mobilization of the bladder may be less extensive because the cervix remains.

❷ **Uterine Amputation.** The corpus is amputated from the cervix at a point just below the internal cervical os and superior to the uterosacral ligaments (Fig. 44-10.1). To limit the possibility of residual endometrium, the incision is conical and extends down into the cervix (Figs. 44-10.2 through 44-10.4). Following amputation, adjunctive coring or ablation of the endocervical canal also may be performed to decrease the risk of postoperative cyclic bleeding (Fig. 44-10.5).

❸ **Tissue Extraction.** Once amputated, the uterine corpus must be removed. Options are minilaparotomy, colpotomy, and enclosed morcellation. Although described here for the uterine corpus, these methods translate to surgical removal of other specimens.

First, for smaller specimens, a minilaparotomy incision ranging from 3 to 4 cm can be made to extract the corpus. Typically, a small Pfannenstiel incision is made, although a small midline vertical incision also is

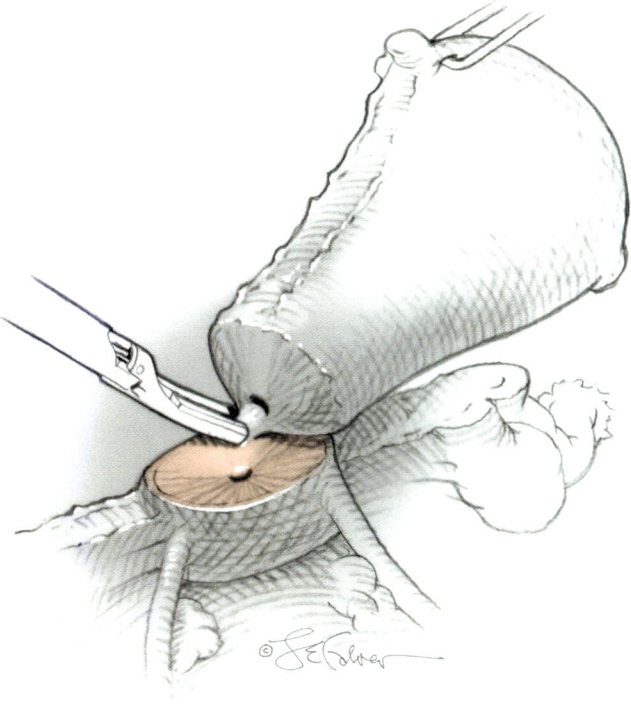

FIGURE 44-10.4 Excision completion.

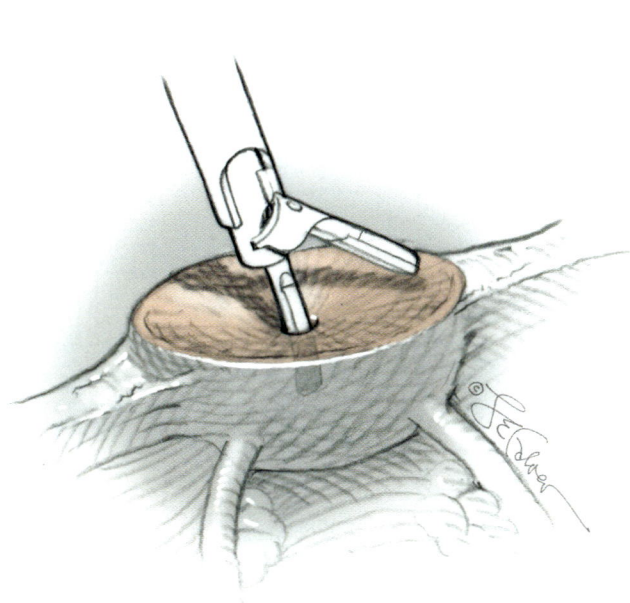

FIGURE 44-10.5 Endocervical canal coagulated.

suitable. Both incisions are illustrated in Chapter 43 (p. 930).

For larger uteri, the addition of a tissue retrieval bag can create a closed environment for scissor morcellation (Clark, 2018; Siedhoff, 2017). For this, a retrieval bag is initially placed into the abdomen. The bag containing the excised specimen is brought to the surface and is fanned open outside and around the minilaparotomy incision. A self-retaining, disposable circular retractor is placed into the bag's opening and simultaneously opened within the incision (see Fig. 44-8.7). This creates a closed environment in which the specimen can be sharply divided manually with scissors or knife.

④ Colpotomy. As another option, a posterior colpotomy can be created similar to that for vaginal hysterectomy. To enter the posterior cul-de-sac, attention is turned to the vagina, and handheld retractors are placed to expose the cervix and posterior fornix. The uterine manipulator is lifted anteriorly, and an Allis clamp is placed on the posterior vaginal wall 2 to 3 cm from the posterior cervicovaginal junction. The Allis clamp is pulled downward to create tension across the posterior vaginal wall, as shown in Figure 41-27 (p. 894). The posterior vaginal vault then is cut with curved Mayo scissors, and the posterior cul-de-sac is entered.

Alternatively, a colpotomy may be created laparoscopically by incising the posterior cul-de-sac with a monopolar instrument, a Harmonic scalpel, or Endo Shears near the cervicovaginal junction. A uterine manipulator is used to reflect the uterus anteriorly to create space for the colpotomy. A sponge stick may be used vaginally to help delineate the space. As Figure 41-28 illustrates, the rectosigmoid and ureters, which lie near the planned colpotomy, are avoided. With colpotomy, pneumoperitoneum is lost immediately. If a laparoscopic instrument is already holding the specimen, this can be passed through the colpotomy and removed vaginally.

For larger uteri, the addition of a tissue retrieval bag during tissue extraction through a colpotomy incision can create a closed environment for scissor morcellation (Fig. 41-29, p. 895) (Cohen, 2019; Kliethermes, 2017). This reduces the risk of inadvertent tissue dissemination during fragmentation, although long-term safety data are needed. Following extraction, a colpotomy incision is closed with interrupted stitches or a running suture line using 0-gauge delayed-absorbable suture.

⑤ Morcellation. A third method, enclosed power morcellation, uses a large endoscopic

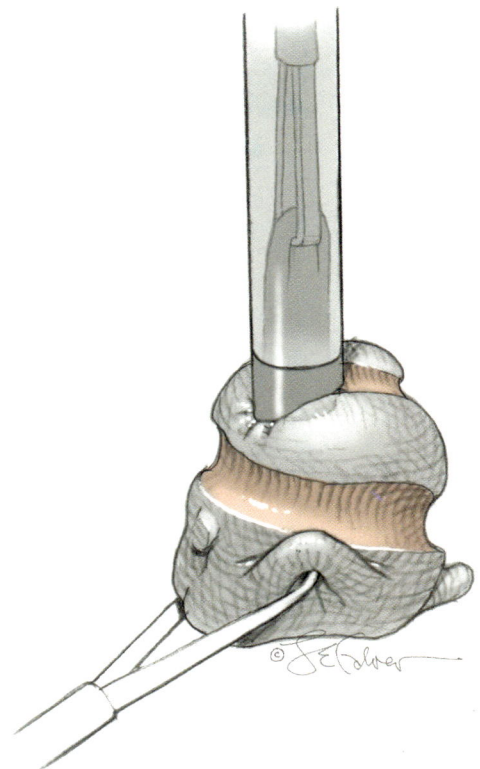

FIGURE 44-10.6 Uterine corpus morcellation.

bag that houses the insufflation gas and conforms to the abdominal cavity (Fig. 41-12, p. 883). Once inside the abdomen, the bag is unfolded to allow the specimen and gas to be contained. Depending on the pathology, the bag may be exteriorized through one abdominal port or incision or may function simply as a liner that catches disseminated tissue during power or manual morcellation (Cohen, 2014; Einarsson, 2014; Srouji, 2015).

During power morcellation, the corpus specimen is grasped securely with a toothed instrument such as a tenaculum and brought to the anterior abdominal wall. Because of the potential for surrounding organ injury, morcellators should not be moved toward the grasped tissue, but rather, those tissues should be brought to it (Fig. 44-10.6) (Milad, 2003). Importantly, the morcellator tip always is kept in laparoscopic view.

A peeling rather than coring technique is used to pare down the mass. During this, the tenaculum holding the corpus is drawn up into the morcellator cylinder and well past the edge of the morcellating blade. This avoids metal-to-metal contact, which dulls the blade. In cases of prolonged morcellation, such as with large uteri, the blade may dull. For this, the generator allows a reverse in the blade's rotary direction. Improved cutting is usually

restored with this step and generally offers enough blade life to complete the procedure.

Following morcellation, the gas is released, and the bag and its contents are removed. Limitations of currently available retrieval bags involve pouch size, working aperture diameter, tensile strength of the bag, and bag permeability (Cohen, 2016).

⑥ Hemostasis. Bleeding points are coagulated, and the surgeon may elect to reapproximate the anterior vesical and posterior cul-de-sac peritoneum to cover the cervical stump using 2-0 or 0-gauge delayed-absorbable suture. Alternatively, absorbable adhesion barriers (Interceed, Seprafilm) can be placed at the hemostatic surgical site.

⑦ Laparoscopy Final Steps. Completion of the procedure follows that for general laparoscopic procedures (p. 1018).

POSTOPERATIVE

Advantages of laparoscopy include a rapid return to normal diet and activity. With supracervical hysterectomy, there is no vaginal cuff that requires extended healing. Sexual intercourse, however, is delayed for 2 weeks following surgery to allow adequate internal healing.

44-11

Total Laparoscopic Hysterectomy

With TLH, the procedure is completed entirely from a laparoscopic approach. After detachment, the specimen is removed vaginally or by tissue extraction techniques described on page 1048.

If all factors are equal, traditional vaginal hysterectomy is considered for women undergoing hysterectomy. Ideal TLH candidates are those not suitable for vaginal hysterectomy (American College of Obstetricians and Gynecologists, 2017a). As such, TLH is viewed as a less invasive alternative to TAH. Compared with TAH, TLH benefits include quicker recovery, shorter hospitalizations, fewer minor complications of the wound or abdominal wall, and less blood loss (Walsh, 2009). These benefits are dependent on a learning curve and may not be readily apparent (Schindlbeck, 2008). Also, rates of lower urinary tract injuries are higher with TLH (Packiam, 2016; Teeluckdharry, 2015).

PREOPERATIVE

Patient Evaluation

A thorough pelvic examination and history reveal factors that help determine the optimal surgical route. Uterine size and mobility are important, although no agreed-upon size precludes TLH. That said, a wide bulky uterus with minimal mobility may be difficult to adequately manipulate, may limit exposure during surgery, and may be challenging to extract. Once a patient is deemed eligible for a laparoscopic approach, preoperative evaluation mirrors that for LH, described on page 1043.

Consent

Similar to an open approach, possible risks of this procedure include significant blood loss and need for transfusion, unplanned adnexectomy, and injury to other pelvic organs, especially bladder, ureter, and bowel. Complications related to laparoscopy include injury to the major vessels, bladder, ureter, and bowel (Chap. 41, p. 875).

The risk of conversion to an open procedure also is discussed. In general, conversion to laparotomy may be necessary if exposure and organ manipulation is limited or if bleeding is encountered that cannot be controlled with laparoscopic techniques. In large series of hysterectomy for benign disease, rates

rate from 1 to 5 percent (Harmanli, 2009; McDonnell, 2018; Wallwiener, 2013).

Patient Preparation

A blood sample is typed and crossmatched for potential transfusion. If considered, bowel preparation prior to laparoscopy may assist with colon manipulation and pelvic anatomy visualization by evacuating the rectosigmoid. Alternatively, enemas prior to surgery may be as effective for this goal. Antibiotic prophylaxis is administered within the hour prior to skin incision, and appropriate antibiotic options are listed in Table 39-8 (p. 832). With laparoscopic gynecologic surgery, the decision to provide VTE prophylaxis factors patient and procedure-related VTE risks (Gould, 2012). Thus, if longer operating times are anticipated, conversion to laparotomy is a concern, or preexisting VTE risks are present, then prophylaxis as outlined in Table 39-10 (p. 834) is indicated.

PREOPERATIVE

Instruments

The same instruments that are used for the laparoscopic hysterectomy or LSH can be used for this procedure. In addition, a uterine manipulator that has a cupping device for delineating the cervicovaginal junction is helpful for colpotomy and for final tissue extraction (Fig. 41-9, p. 881). If these are not available, a low-cost alternative is a right-angle retractor to delineate the anterior and posterior fornices for colpotomy.

Surgical Steps

❶ **Anesthesia and Patient Positioning.** For most women, TLH is performed as an inpatient procedure under general anesthesia. The patient is placed in low lithotomy position in booted support stirrups. A bimanual examination is completed to determine uterine size and shape to aid port placement. The abdomen and vagina are surgically prepared, a Foley catheter is inserted, and an orogastric or nasogastric tube is placed.

❷ **Uterine Manipulator.** A uterine manipulator with its attached cervical cup (VCare or Koh Cup with RUMI manipulator) is placed vaginally to assist uterine manipulation and delineate the cervicovaginal junction for colpotomy. To accomplish placement, the cervical diameter and thickness are assessed. From this information, the manipulator-cup size (small, medium, or large) is selected. To permit manipulator insertion, the cervical os is dilated to accept a no. 8 cervical

dilator. The uterus also is sounded to determine cavity depth for correct manipulator placement.

The surgeon tests the balloon at the manipulator's tip for patency by filling it with air via a port at the opposite end. Once again deflated, the tip is passed through the cervical os, into the endometrial cavity, and to the fundus. Here, the balloon is reinflated to hold the manipulator in place (Fig. 44-11.1A).

Two stay sutures of 0-gauge delayed-absorbable suture are placed at 6 and 12 o'clock or at 3 and 9 o'clock, depending on surgeon preference. To securely anchor the cup and cervix, stitches enter the ectocervix and exit just lateral to the endocervix. Each suture end then is passed through openings in the cup base (see Fig. 44-11.1B). They are tied firmly to the cervix on the outside face of the cup (see Fig. 44-11.1C). Once in position, the proximal rim of the cup will delineate the cervicovaginal junction. With the VCare, the blue vaginal cup is then advanced to join the interior cup and is locked in place by a locking knob at the manipulator's external end (see Fig. 44-11.1D). If the Koh Cup is used, a pneumo-occluding balloon is positioned behind the colpotomy cup.

❸ **Initial Laparoscopic Steps.** The introductory steps for TLH mirror those for other laparoscopic procedures (Chap. 41, p. 888). The number of trocars and their caliber may vary, but in general, TLH requires a 5- to 12-mm optical port, usually at the umbilicus, and two or three accessory ports placed through the lower abdominal wall. Specifically, two trocars are placed beyond the lateral borders of the rectus abdominis muscle, whereas a third may be positioned centrally and cephalad to the uterine fundus. Left upper quadrant entry is considered in cases of suspected periumbilical adhesions.

❹ **Pelvic Evaluation.** With the cannulas and laparoscope inserted and the patient in Trendelenburg position, a blunt laparoscopic probe aids bowel displacement. The pelvis and abdomen are thoroughly explored. At this point, the decision to continue with TLH or convert to laparotomy is made. If necessary, adhesions are lysed to restore normal anatomy.

❺ **Ureter Identification.** Irrigating fluids and CO_2 used for insufflation can with time create edema of the peritoneum and hinder visualization of structures beneath it. For this reason, the ureters are identified early. The ureters are often easily seen retroperitoneally, or the peritoneum may be opened to locate them. In such situations, the peritoneum medial to the IP ligament is grasped and

10 (p. 1045). These steps include transection of the round ligament, conservation or excision of the adnexa, caudad displacement of the bladder, and coagulation of the uterine vessels.

❼ Cardinal Ligament Transection. Following uterine artery coagulation, the cardinal ligaments are transected on each side to reach the level of the uterosacral attachments (Fig. 44-11.2).

❽ Colpotomy. This incision at the cervicovaginal junction may be performed with Harmonic scalpel, monopolar scissors, monopolar hook, or plasma kinetic needle point. Prior to incision, the uterine manipulator is pushed cephalad to allow the cervical cupping device to displace the ureters laterally and expose the optimal location for colpotomy. Additionally, dissection within the vesicouterine space should be sufficient to mobilize the bladder caudally and away from the planned colpotomy site.

With these preparatory steps completed, colpotomy is begun by placing the incising tool at the posterior cervicovaginal junction, which is delineated by the cervical cup. If a colpotomy cup is not used, a simple tool such as a right-angle retractor or sponge on a stick placed vaginally in the posterior fornix also can delineate the cervicovaginal junction. The posterior vaginal wall is opened first (Fig. 44-11.3). By extending this incision, the uterosacral ligament is

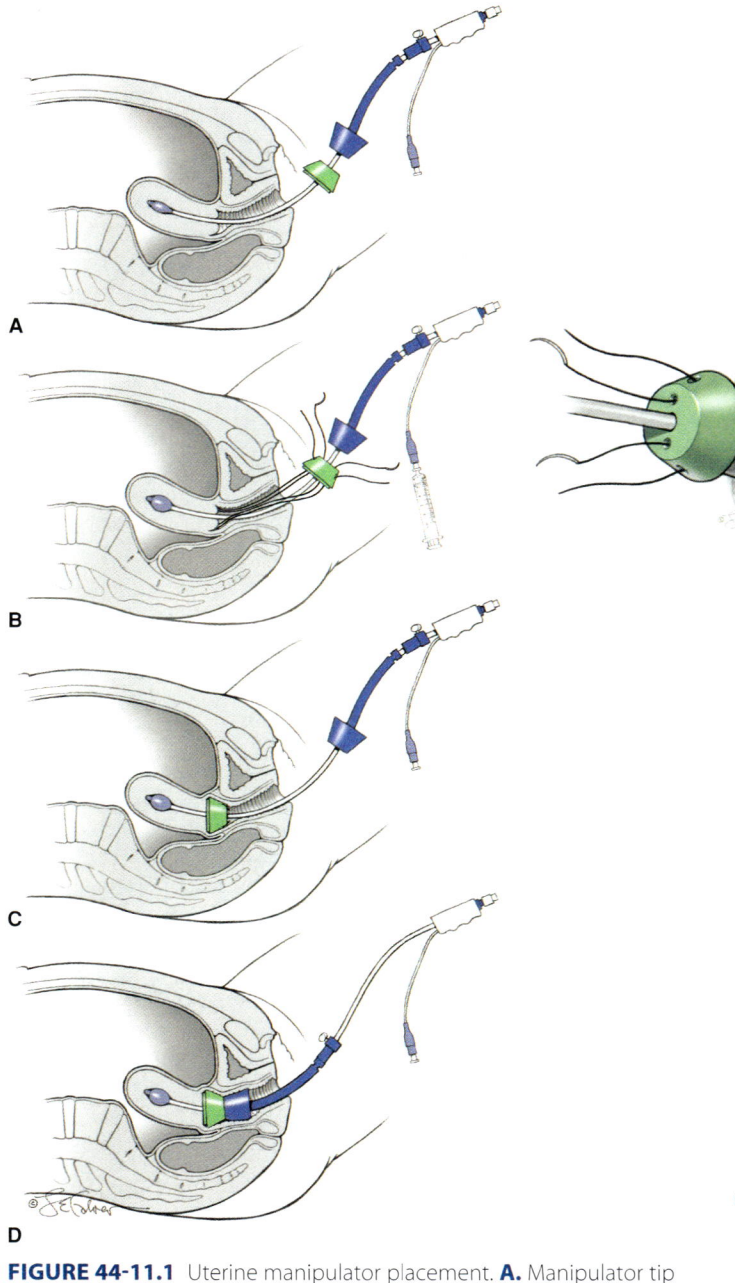

FIGURE 44-11.1 Uterine manipulator placement. **A.** Manipulator tip inserted into uterine cavity. **B.** Balloon tip inflated (*left*). Colpotomy cup sutured to cervix (*right*). **C.** Colpotomy cup sutured in place. **D.** Pneumo-occluding cup advanced and locked in place.

tented using atraumatic forceps and incised with scissors. An irrigating probe can be used to force water beneath and elevate the peritoneum for easier incision. The opening in the peritoneum then is extended a short distance caudally and cephalad over the suspected path of the ureter. Through this peritoneal window, the ureter is identified (Fig. 44-9.1, p. 1044) (Parker, 2004).

❻ Round Ligament, Adnexa, and Uterine Artery. The initial steps for TLH mirror those for laparoscopic hysterectomy, described in Section 44-9, steps 5 through

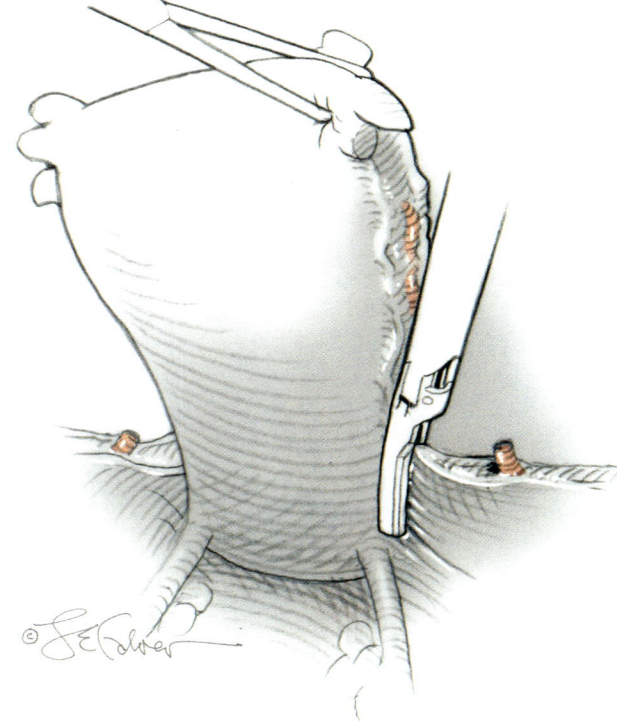

FIGURE 44-11.2 Cardinal ligament incised.

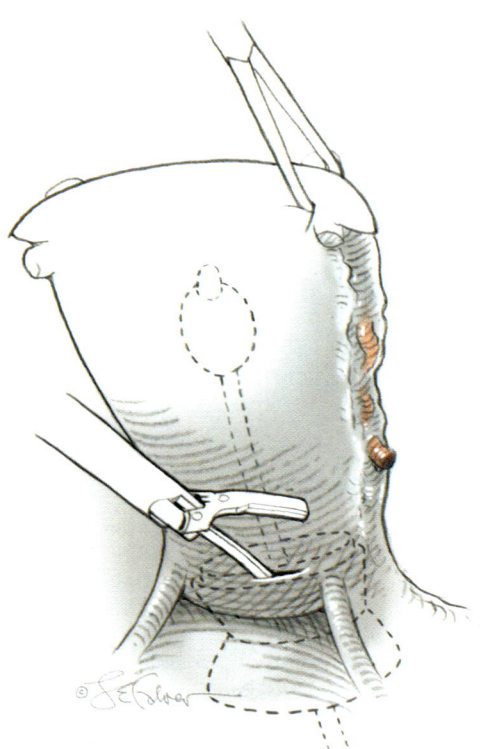

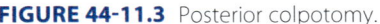

FIGURE 44-11.3 Posterior colpotomy.

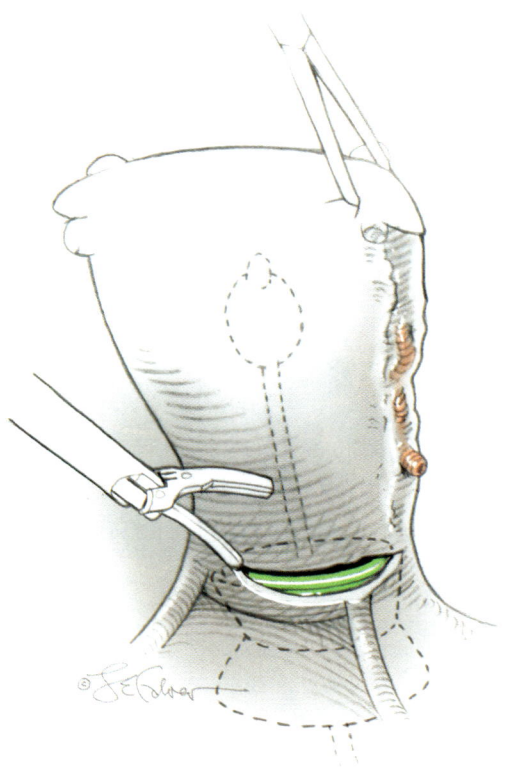

FIGURE 44-11.4 Right uterosacral ligament transected, and colpotomy extended toward the left.

next transected (Fig. 44-11.4). The opposite uterosacral ligament then is divided close to the cervix. Last, the anterior colpotomy incision is created (Fig. 44-11.5). To minimize twisting and specimen disorientation, the lateral vaginal cuff points are transected last (Fig. 44-11.6). Hemostasis is generally maintained using this technique. To prevent vaginal tissue thermal damage and subsequent cuff dehiscence, surgeons use the minimum necessary amount of electrosurgery on the vaginal cuff.

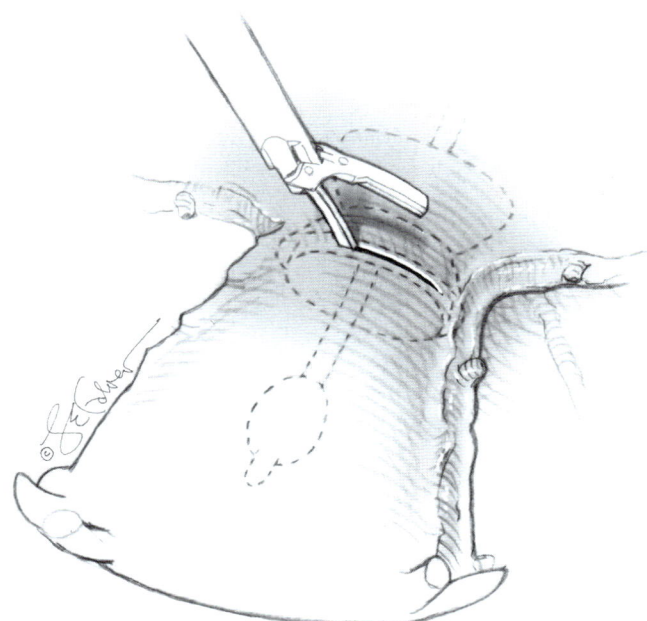

FIGURE 44-11.5 Anterior colpotomy.

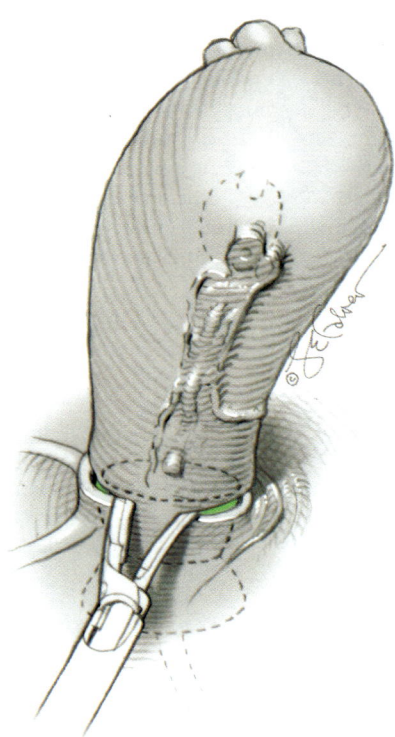

FIGURE 44-11.6 Joining anterior and posterior colpotomy incisions.

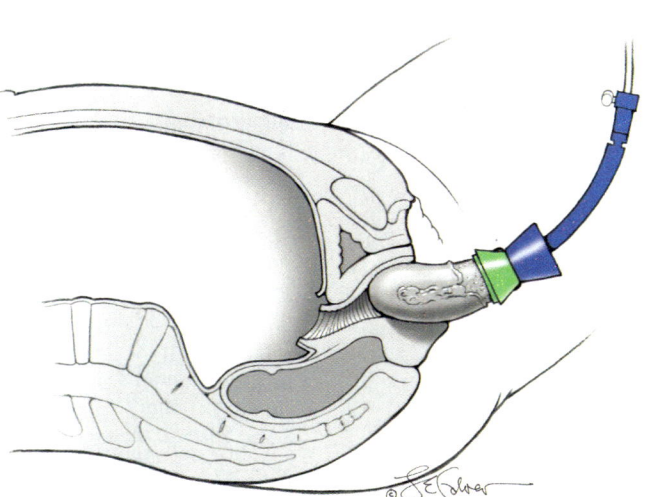
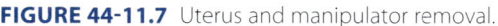

FIGURE 44-11.7 Uterus and manipulator removal.

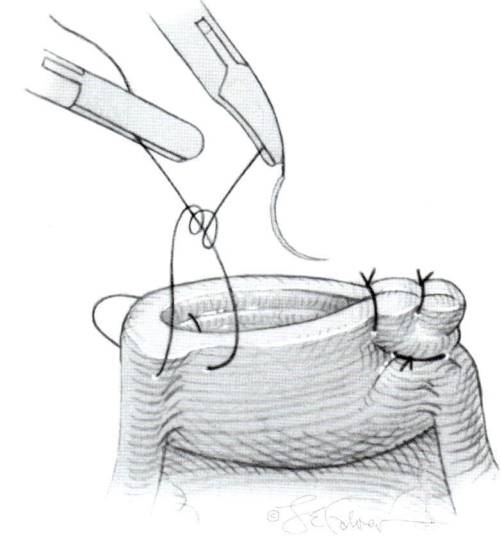

FIGURE 44-11.8 Vaginal cuff closure.

❾ Removal of Uterus. The uterus is removed intact through the vaginal vault using the manipulator, unless uterine size limits this (Fig. 44-11.7). In the case of large uteri, the uterus is removed using tissue extraction techniques described on page 1048.

❿ Repair of the Vaginal Cuff. The cuff is closed laparoscopically with a running closure of absorbable suture, with interrupted figure-of-eight sutures, or with a suturing device. For this, delayed-absorbable material is preferred, and the uterosacral ligament is incorporated into the closure for vaginal cuff support (Fig. 44-11.8). If traditional suture is used, one must maintain tension to sufficiently close the cuff.

If using barbed suture, the procedure is modified by manufacturer's recommendations to loosen stitch tension between the approximated cuff tissues. Also, if barbed suture is used, it is recommended to throw at least two final bites in the opposite direction to the original direction of closure to maintain tissue tension. For example, if closure is performed from right to left, the surgeon will reach the far left end and then will place two additional stitches in the left-to-right direction prior to final suture line cutting. It is advisable to cut the suture flush with the tissue to decrease bowel damage risk from the barbed end.

Confirmation of full-thickness closure is necessary to prevent later cuff dehiscence. Alternatively, for those less proficient with laparoscopic suturing, the cuff may be closed vaginally after removal of the uterus as described in Section 43-13 (p. 969).

After cuff closure, irrigation and confirmation of hemostasis is performed. Intraabdominal pressures are lowered during this inspection to better identify sources of bleeding.

⓫ Laparoscopy Final Steps. Completion of this operation follows that for diagnostic laparoscopy (p. 1018).

POSTOPERATIVE

The advantages of a laparoscopic approach include a rapid return to normal diet and activities. Generally, the evening of the surgery, the Foley catheter is removed, diet is advanced, and the patient is allowed to ambulate. Oral analgesics are quickly adopted in place of parenteral options. The usual precautions for abdominal hysterectomy in regard to limitation of stress on the abdominal cavity by heavy lifting are followed. Delay of sexual activity mirrors that for abdominal hysterectomy, which is typically 6 weeks.

Vaginal cuff dehiscence is a serious postoperative complication that more frequently follows laparoscopic hysterectomy approaches compared with vaginal hysterectomy or TAH (Sandberg, 2017; Uccella, 2012). From large TLH series, rates approximate 1 percent (Hur, 2016). Precipitating factors include coitus, conditions that chronically raise intraabdominal pressure, poor surgical technique, and factors linked to poor wound healing (Fuchs Weizman, 2015; Nezhat, 2018). Patients present with vaginal bleeding or evisceration. Typical treatment includes debridement of vaginal cuff edges, reapproximation with delayed-absorbable suture, and administration of antibiotic prophylaxis. However, compromised bowel may require more extensive surgeries to repair.

Preventatively, sound initial surgical technique strives to minimize electrosurgical damage during colpotomy creation and limit undue desiccation of the vaginal cuff. Approximation of all tissue planes, particularly full-thickness closure of the vaginal wall, also should be ensured. Reapproximation includes an adequate amount of viable tissue that is free of thermal effect. Of suture types, delayed-absorbable is preferred to absorbable suture. In addition, a laparoscopic two-layer closure may have an advantage over a single-layer, figure-of-eight closure (Jeung, 2010). Last, the route of cuff closure is likely less important than the above-listed clinical points. Data support both laparoscopic and vaginal approaches to cuff closure (Stevens, 2013; Uccella, 2012, 2018).

44-12

Diagnostic Hysteroscopy

Hysteroscopy provides an endoscopic view of the endometrial cavity and tubal ostia. Indications are varied and include abnormal uterine bleeding evaluation, infertility assessment, interrogation of sonographically identified intracavitary mass, or localization of a lost intrauterine device (IUD).

Contraindications to hysteroscopy include pregnancy and genital tract infections, including herpes virus infection. In addition, advanced uterine or cervical cancer may pose undue risks for hemorrhage or tumor cell dissemination. With the latter, cells reflux through the fallopian tubes and enter the peritoneal cavity. That said, hysteroscopy is acceptable as part of the evaluation of abnormal uterine bleeding (American College of Obstetricians and Gynecologists, 2018c).

PREOPERATIVE

Consent

Risks with diagnostic hysteroscopy are infrequent. Those described in Chapter 41 (p. 903) include uterine perforation and volume overload. Gas embolism is rare.

Patient Preparation

Prior to hysteroscopy, urine or serum hCG level testing excludes pregnancy in reproductive-aged women. Active cervicovaginal infection is sought during physical examination and is resolved prior to surgery. For women with risk factors for gonorrhea or chlamydial infection (Table 1-1, p. 4), organism-specific nucleic acid amplification testing (NAAT) is indicated (Chap. 3, p. 66).

If the external cervical os is small or stenotic, cervical ripening is helpful. Options are described in Chapter 41 (p. 899). Routine use of agents, however, is not recommended and can lead to bleeding that obscures the hysteroscopic view (Choksuchat, 2010; Salazar, 2018). Infection and VTE following hysteroscopic surgery are rare. Accordingly, prophylaxis typically is not required (American College of Obstetricians and Gynecologists, 2018a,e).

INTRAOPERATIVE

Instruments

Diagnostic hysteroscopy is performed using small endoscopes with diameters of 3 to 5 mm. These may be rigid, semi-rigid, or flexible. Described in Chapter 41 (p. 900), hysteroscopes usually feature a channel for the distention medium. Many offer a working channel, into which small operative instruments are threaded. For most diagnostic procedures, we use a Bettocchi hysteroscope with normal saline media or the Endosee digital handheld system (Fig 44-12.1).

Surgical Steps

❶ **Anesthesia and Patient Positioning.** Diagnostic hysteroscopy can be performed in an office or outpatient setting. Purely diagnostic procedures often require no anesthesia, however, an oral nonsteroidal anti-inflammatory drug (NSAID) administered preoperatively may reduce discomfort. In addition, intracervical or paracervical injection of a local anesthetic is associated with less pain during and after the procedure. In contrast, topical agents applied to the cervix or within the uterine cavity are not beneficial (Munro, 2010). Intravenous sedation is another option. For patients who might poorly tolerate the needed manipulation of a given examination, a day-surgery setting and general anesthesia may be preferred.

The patient is placed in standard lithotomy position and the vagina is surgically prepared. The bladder is drained, unless the patient recently voided. Because diagnostic hysteroscopy is a short procedure with little if any blood loss, saline is typically selected for uterine distention. CO_2 is rarely used today, but if chosen, steep Trendelenburg positioning is avoided to help prevent gas embolism.

❷ **Hysteroscope Assembly.** If a standard, single-channel, rigid hysteroscope is selected, the endoscope is placed within the outer sheath and locked into place. The light cord attaches to a lamp post on the outer hysteroscope. Distention media tubing is affixed to the hysteroscope's inflow channel.

❸ **Hysteroscope Introduction.** Discomfort associated with a vaginal speculum may be avoided by introducing the hysteroscope directly into the vagina using a *no-touch method* or *vaginoscopic technique* (Cooper, 2010; Di Spiezio Sardo, 2015). For this, the labia are held in gentle apposition by fingertip pressure once the hysteroscope is introduced. The flow of saline then slowly distends the vagina to expose the cervix for direct entry (Fig 44-12.2).

Instead, a vaginal speculum may be inserted with or without the application of a single-toothed tenaculum to the cervix. The tenaculum steadies the cervix and provides light countertraction to permit hysteroscope passage through a potentially snug endocervical canal. Dilation of the endocervical canal usually is not required to admit the hysteroscope's 4- to 5-mm diameter. Moreover, uterine sounding is not recommended because information regarding uterine depth and cavity inclination is provided by direct visual guidance during hysteroscope insertion. The uterine sound also may traumatize the endocervix or endometrium, which alters mucosal anatomy prior to inspection or causes obscuring bleeding.

Once the hysteroscope is introduced into the endocervical canal and distention medium flow is begun, the hydrostatic pressure serves as a gentle fluid obturator. With the endocervical canals thereby distended, the surgeon can directly view the canal to guide the hysteroscope's tip forward. With correct insertion of

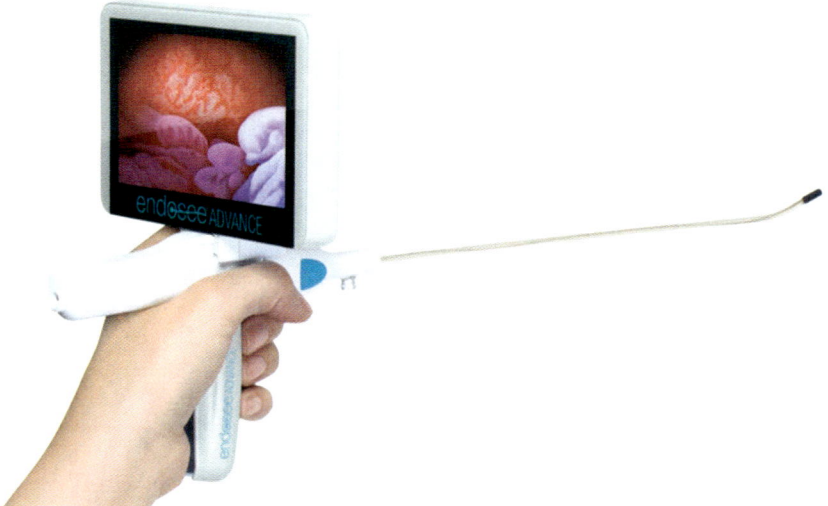

FIGURE 44-12.1 The Endosee portable cordless hysteroscopic system. (Reproduced with permission from Cooper Surgical, Inc.)

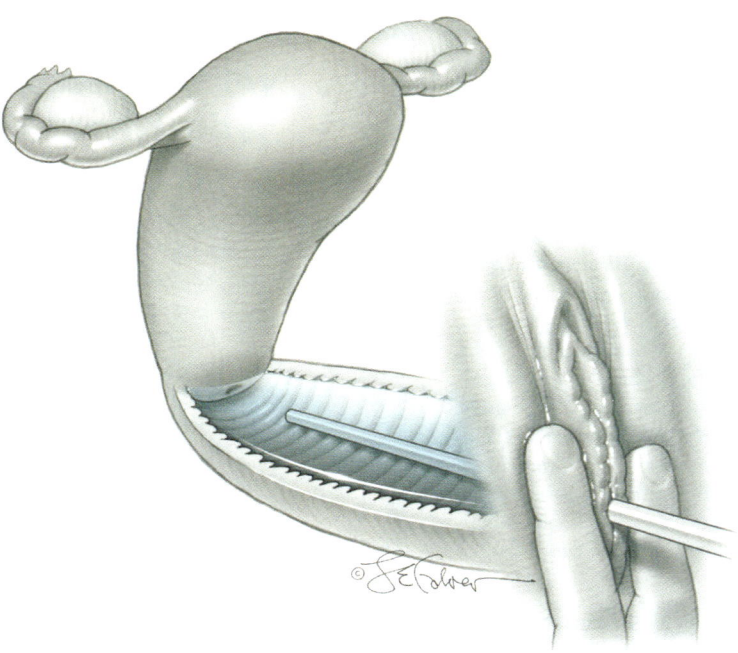

FIGURE 44-12.2 Vaginoscopy.

the hysteroscope, its long axis aligns with the endocervical canal.

For diagnostic purposes, a hysteroscope equipped with a 0-, 12-, or 30-degree forward-oblique-view lens is suitable. With a 0-degree lens, the endocervical canal should be centered in the field of view. With an angled lens, the light cord is directed downward, and the lens angle faces upward. Importantly, with this orientation, the endocervical canal should not appear in the field-of-view's center. Instead and as illustrated in Figure 41-37 (p. 900), the dark, circular canal should be seen at the field-of-view's bottom, which reflects an appropriately aligned hysteroscope.

❹ **Hysteroscopic Evaluation.** During hysteroscope insertion, the endocervical canal is examined for abnormalities. Once inside the endometrial cavity, the hysteroscope is held at the distal portion of the cavity to allow a panoramic evaluation. Systematically, the hysteroscope is moved to the fundus and then to the left and right to permit inspection of the tubal ostia (Fig. 44-12.3). If an angled lens is employed, the hysteroscope may remain in the midline and simply is rotated clockwise and

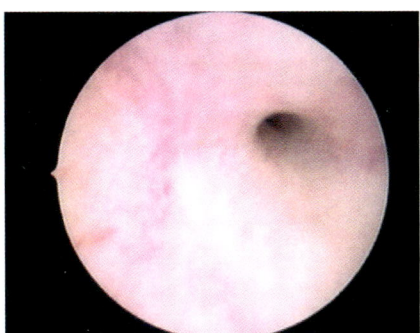

FIGURE 44-12.3 Hysteroscopic photograph of normal tubal ostia. (Reproduced with permission from Dr. Kevin Doody.)

counterclockwise to obtain lateral views. If necessary, reducing the distention medium flow can help identify lesions that may have been obliterated or flattened by greater hydrostatic pressure.

❺ **Specific Procedures.** After complete cavity inspection, if specific lesions are identified, they typically are biopsied while in view by hysteroscopic forceps. The biopsy forceps and specimen are retracted together through the operating channel. The forceps are reintroduced through the channel for additional biopsies, if needed. If diagnostic curettage is planned, it follows hysteroscopy and cavity inspection.

If IUD removal is planned, its location within the endometrial cavity, uterine wall, or peritoneal cavity is determined preoperatively as described in Chapter 5 (p. 116). Most within the endometrial cavity are grasped by the string or stem with hysteroscopic grasping forceps and are easily extracted as the entire hysteroscope is removed. Embedded or fragmented devices may require removal in pieces. Occasionally, an arm is embedded and its tip points caudad. In this case, the arm is grasped and controlled pressure is directed toward the fundus to dislodge it. Deeply embedded IUDs may require concurrent laparoscopy to help identify uterine perforation and determine whether the device is best removed hysteroscopically or laparoscopically.

❻ **Procedure Completion.** Once the procedure has ended, distending medium flow is stopped, and the hysteroscope and then tenaculum are removed. A critical step at this point, and throughout the procedure, is to note the amount of distention fluid used and the amount retrieved. These values are used to calculate the fluid deficit, which is included in the operative report.

POSTOPERATIVE

Patient recovery typically is rapid and mirrors that following dilation and curettage. Diet and activities may be resumed as desired by the patient. Spotting or light bleeding is not uncommon and typically stops within days.

44-13

Hysteroscopic Polypectomy

Indications for endometrial polyp removal include abnormal uterine bleeding, infertility, and risk of malignant transformation (Chap. 8, p. 189). Hysteroscopically, the polyp base can be incised with hysteroscopic scissors or a resectoscope loop. Alternatively, a polyp can be morcellated (Salim, 2011). Both options offer the versatility to manage small polyps or large ones with a wide base. These same polypectomy steps also can be used to remove chronic, retained products of conception (Capmas, 2019).

PREOPERATIVE

Patient Evaluation

Prior to polypectomy, preoperative transvaginal sonography or saline-infusion sonography typically has been completed to define cavity anatomy. Thus, information describing the size, number, and location of polyps is reviewed prior to surgery. Rarely, MR imaging may be indicated to fully distinguish a presumed polyp from a submucous leiomyoma. This often helps determine if myomectomy instead is required.

Consent

The complication rates for this procedure are low and mirror that for hysteroscopy in general (Chap. 41, p. 903). Thus, bleeding, infection, uterine perforation, fluid overload, and gas embolism are discussed with the patient.

Patient Preparation

As with most hysteroscopic procedures, polypectomy ideally is performed during the follicular phase of the menstrual cycle. At this time, the endometrial lining is thinnest, and polyps are most easily identified. Preoperative endometrial biopsy may be completed as part of a standard abnormal uterine bleeding evaluation for those with endometrial cancer risks (Chap. 8, p. 183). Instead, diagnostic curettage can follow polypectomy for these at-risk patients. Preoperative antibiotics or VTE prophylaxis typically is not required (American College of Obstetricians and Gynecologists, 2018a,e).

INTRAOPERATIVE

Instruments

A resectoscope with a 90-degree loop electrode is ideal to excise or shave down polyps

(p. 1059). In contrast, an intrauterine morcellator can be used. This is a hollow cannula attached to suction, which draws the polyp into the cannula aperture. Here, the device's sharp blade quickly morcellates large or small growths. The same suction pressure then draws the tissue fragments out of the cavity for collection. Last, for smaller polyps, polyp forceps or ureteral stone retrieval baskets may be threaded through the 5F operative channel to remove the polyp (Casey, 2017).

Surgical Steps

❶ **Anesthesia and Patient Positioning.** For simple in-office polypectomy, an oral NSAID, a local anesthetic injection, or intravenous sedation is suitable (p. 1054). However, many still are performed as day-surgery cases under general or regional anesthesia. Distending medium management, particularly with hypotonic fluid, warrants a degree of safety that may be best provided in an operating suite. In addition, some patients may better tolerate a procedure in this venue.

Following adequate anesthesia administration, the patient is placed in standard lithotomy position, the vagina is surgically prepared, and the bladder is drained. Less often, a Foley catheter may be inserted.

❷ **Medium Selection.** Hysteroscopic morcellation can be performed with a physiologic saline solution. However, if a monopolar resectoscopic electrode is used, a nonelectrolyte solution is required, and the risks for hyponatremia must be considered. Alternatively, a

bipolar resectoscopic electrode allows surgery in an isotonic electrolyte medium such as normal saline. This medium is associated with a lower risk of fluid overload or hyponatremia (Chap. 41, p. 903). As with any hysteroscopic procedure, fluid volume deficits are calculated and noted regularly during surgery.

❸ **Cervical Dilation.** Depending on the chosen hysteroscope's size, the cervix may require dilation to a diameter ≥8 mm. However, overdilating the cervix can allow fluid to leak out around the hysteroscope, which leads to inadequate uterine distention and poor visualization. This similarly can follow cervical ripening with misoprostol, and this agent is used judiciously (Salazar, 2018).

❹ **Resection.** Medium flow is begun, and the resectoscope is inserted into the endocervical canal with direct hysteroscopic guidance. Upon entering the cavity, a panoramic inspection is completed to identify the location and number of polyps. The resectoscope loop then is extended to reach behind each polyp. Electrosurgical current is applied only when the loop is being retracted toward the cervix to cut the polyp base. Advancing an electrosurgical cutting loop when current is active risks perforating the uterus and damaging adjacent pelvic structures. The freed polyp then is grasped and easily extracted as the entire hysteroscope is removed through the cervical os.

With a large polyp, several passes with the loop electrode may be required for complete excision. Passes begin at the polyp tip and progress until the base is reached. Polyp fragments need not be removed after each

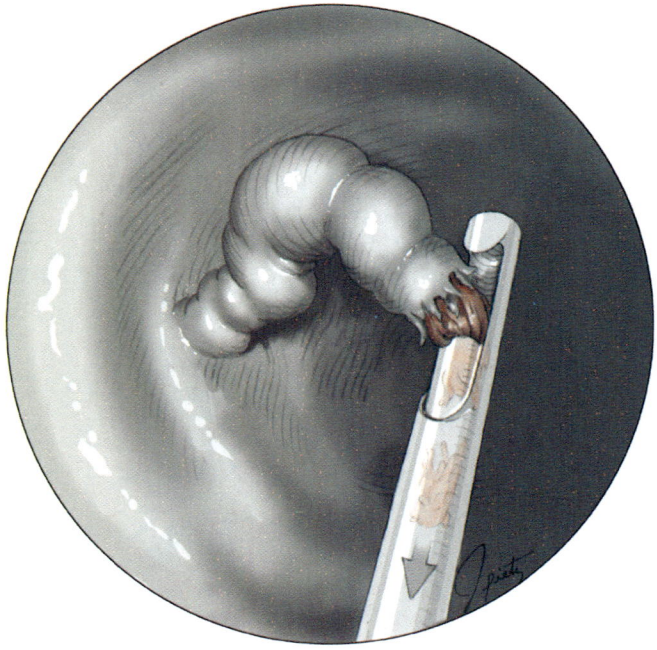

FIGURE 44-13.1 Hysteroscopic polypectomy.

pass. Instead, resected fragments are allowed to float within the cavity as resection continues. Once the entire polyp is excised, the fragments are collected on a Telfa sheet as they flow out of the cavity along with the distention medium. This practice maintains visualization of the polyp. It also minimizes gas embolism and perforation risks that are associated with numerous reinsertions of instruments into the cavity. For larger polyps, the number of floating fragments will accrue. Thus, the cavity may need to be emptied prior to complete resection to permit an unobstructed view during resection.

❺ Morcellation. As with loop resection, distention medium flow is begun. The hysteroscope and the morcellation device housed within its operating channel are inserted. During morcellation, excision proceeds from the polyp tip toward the base (Fig. 44-13.1). Moreover, the mass is kept between the morcellator opening and the optics of the camera.

The morcellator also provides suction, which can clear blood, tissue debris, and clots during resection of large growths. Better visual acuity and the continuous retrieval of tissue fragments are two advantages to this approach.

❻ Control of Bleeding. Bleeding sites may be coagulated with the same resection loop using a coagulating current. If heavy or persistent bleeding ensues, a Foley catheter with a 30-mL balloon can be introduced into the uterine cavity and inflated to tamponade vessels.

❼ Instrument Removal. At the procedure's end, the flow of distending medium is stopped, and the hysteroscope and then tenaculum are removed. A critical step at this point, and throughout the procedure, is to note the amount of distending medium used and retrieved to calculate the fluid deficit. The surgical specimen is sent for pathologic evaluation.

POSTOPERATIVE

Recovery following polypectomy typically is rapid and follows that for other hysteroscopic procedures (p. 1055). Spotting or light bleeding is common and typically stops within days.

44-14

Hysteroscopic Myomectomy

For symptomatic women with submucous leiomyomas, hysteroscopic resection of these tumors may provide symptom relief in many cases. Candidates include those with abnormal uterine bleeding, with dysmenorrhea, or with infertility in which leiomyomas are suspected to be contributory. Tumors selected for resection should be either submucous or intramural but with a predominantly submucous component. During surgery, pedunculated submucous leiomyomas may be excised similarly to polyps (p. 1056). However, tumors with an intramural component require excision with a resectoscope, morcellator, or laser.

PREOPERATIVE

Patient Evaluation

For hysteroscopic myomectomy, contraindications include pregnancy, current reproductive tract infection, potential endometrial cancer or uterine sarcoma, and medical conditions that render the patient more sensitive to fluid volume overload.

Specific leiomyoma characteristics help predict which leiomyomas are suitable for hysteroscopic resection and which instead raise the clinical failure rate (Di Spiezio Sardo, 2008). Thus, prior to resection, women typically undergo transvaginal sonography, saline-infusion sonography, or diagnostic hysteroscopy to determine these characteristics. MR imaging also can accurately depict myoma and uterine anatomy, but its expense and availability may limit its routine use.

Imaging helps describe myoma location within the uterus. This is the basis of the International Federation of Gynecologists and Obstetricians (FIGO) leiomyoma classification system described and illustrated in Chapter 9 (p. 205) (Munro, 2018). A different system by Lasmar and coworkers (2005, 2011) similarly considers the degree of tumor penetration into the myometrium. In addition, larger tumor size, wider tumor base, tumors in the upper portion of the cavity, or those found along the lateral wall receive higher scores (Table 9-3, p. 211). Higher scores raise technical difficulty, clinical failure rates, surgical risks, and need for additional surgical session to complete resection (Mazzon, 2015). Thus, for higher scores, a non-hysteroscopic technique may be the safest and most successful.

Consequently, many choose to resect only type 0 and I tumors and those measuring less than 3 cm (Vercellini, 1999; Wamsteker, 1993). Resection of larger leiomyomas may be undertaken, although this may require multiple surgical sessions to complete and require a longer recovery (Camanni, 2010).

Consent

Complications of this procedure mirror that for hysteroscopy in general, and rates of 2 to 3 percent have been reported. Hysteroscopic myomectomy is associated with a greater risk of uterine perforation. This complication may follow cervical dilation, but more frequently results during aggressive resection into the myometrium. Because of this risk, women also are consented for laparoscopy to assess and treat uterine or abdominal organ damage if perforation occurs.

Additionally, patients planning to seek pregnancy are informed of possible intrauterine adhesion formation following resection and of rare uterine rupture during subsequent pregnancies (Batra, 2004; Howe, 1993).

During hysteroscopic myomectomy, distention medium can pass into open vasculature channels, primarily venous channels, within the myometrium. Termed *intravasation*, this potentially can lead to intravascular volume overload in the patient. Thus, resection of type I or II tumors or removal of large leiomyomas may be halted due to advancing fluid volume deficits. Poor operative field visualization due to myoma-bed bleeding is another potential hindrance. Consequently, patients are counseled that more than one surgical session may be required to finish these resections. Fortunately, development of newer bipolar resectoscopes and hysteroscopic morcellating tools has helped reduce operating times and thus fluid deficits.

Last, myomectomy is effective treatment, but 15 to 20 percent of patients will eventually require reoperation. This may be hysterectomy or repeat hysteroscopic resection at a later time for either persistent or recurrent symptoms (Derman, 1991; Hart, 1999).

Patient Preparation

GnRH agonists can preoperatively shrink leiomyomas to enable resection of large tumors and decrease tumor vascularity. These agents also allow patients to rebuild their red cell mass before surgery (Chap. 9, p. 208). Disadvantages include vasomotor side effects, difficulty in cervical dilation, greater risk of uterine laceration or perforation, and reduced intracavitary volume, which limits instrument mobility. Thus, GnRH agonist use is individualized.

To allow easier cervical dilation and resectoscope insertion, misoprostol can aid cervical softening (Chap. 41, p. 899). Another alternative is dilute vasopressin (0.05 units/mL). This solution can be injected in divided doses intracervically at 4 and 8 o'clock. This method works rapidly at the time of surgery if the need for preoperative preparation was not anticipated (Phillips, 1997).

Although the risk of postoperative infection is low, because pelvic infections can have devastating effect on future fertility, antibiotic prophylaxis prior to extensive hysteroscopic resections, as with myomectomy, is reasonable. Suitable agents are found in Table 39-8 (p. 832).

Concurrent Ablation

In those women with heavy menstrual bleeding and with no desire for future fertility, endometrial ablation may be concurrently performed (p. 1061) (Loffer, 2005). In one retrospective cohort of women with submucosal leiomyomas, endometrial ablation coupled with myomectomy improved symptom outcome and lower treatment failure rates compared with hysteroscopic myomectomy alone (Shazly, 2016). However, because myomectomy alone often resolves abnormal bleeding, we do not routinely perform concomitant endometrial ablation.

INTRAOPERATIVE

Instruments

Hysteroscopic myomectomy may be performed using a resectoscope. With morcellator use, a specialized hysteroscopic morcellator can be threaded into and housed in the hysteroscope's operative channel before uterine cavity insertion. Both procedures are described.

Surgical Steps

❶ Anesthesia and Patient Positioning. In many cases, hysteroscopic myomectomy is a day-surgery procedure completed under general anesthesia. Less often and for a well-selected patient, smaller-tumor myomectomy can be performed in an office equipped and certified to provide minimal sedation. The patient is placed in standard lithotomy position, the vagina is surgically prepared, and usually a Foley catheter is inserted.

❷ Medium Selection. The choice of distention medium is dictated by the resecting tool. A morcellator, bipolar electrosurgical loop, or laser will perform in normal saline solution. However, a resectoscope's monopolar electrosurgical loop requires an electrolyte-free

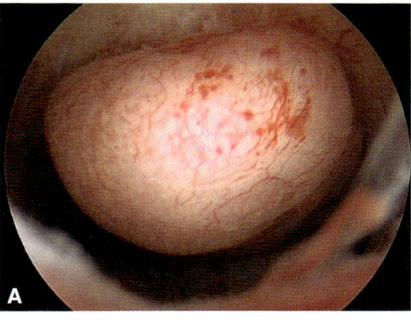

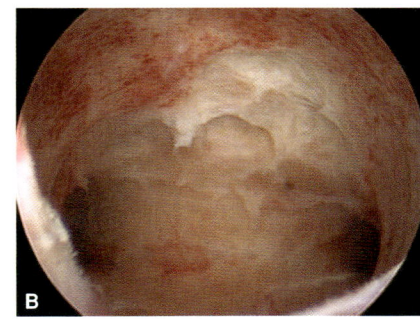

FIGURE 44-14.2 A. Type 0 submucous leiomyoma. **B.** Intracavitary view postresection.

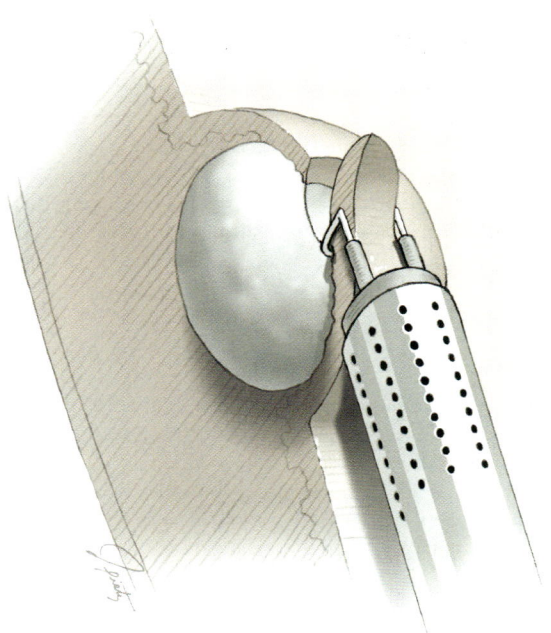

FIGURE 44-14.1 Hysteroscopic resection.

solution. Solution differences are discussed in Chapter 41 (p. 902).

❸ Cervical Dilation. Small resection devices with 5- to 6-mm diameters may not require cervical dilation. If needed, Pratt dilators or other suitable type are judiciously used (Chap. 43, p. 973). As noted, overdilating the cervix risks poor uterine cavity distention.

❹ Instrument Insertion. The distention medium flow is begun, and the selected device is inserted into the endocervical canal under direct endoscopic guidance. Upon entering the endometrial cavity, a panoramic inspection is first performed to identify and assess leiomyomas.

❺ Resection. The resectoscope loop is advanced to lie behind the leiomyoma, and electric current is applied before the loop contacts the tissue. For this procedure, the electrosurgical unit is set to a continuous-wave (cutting) mode. To minimize thermal injury and perforation, current is applied only as the loop is retracted and not when it is extended. Upon contact, the loop electrode is retracted toward the resectoscope (Fig. 44-14.1). To ensure a clean cut and complete excision of the shaved strip, current is not stopped until the entire loop is retracted. The shaved strip of smooth muscle floats within the endometrial cavity.

This shaving process is repeated serially toward the myoma's base until the tumor is excised (Fig. 44-14.2). Although strips can be removed from the cavity after each pass, this results in a repetitive loss of uterine distention. Repeated removal and reinsertion of a resectoscope also raises the risk of uterine perforation, gas embolism, and fluid intravasation. Thus in most cases, resected fragments float freely within the cavity. However, if the view becomes obstructed, resection is paused to remove these strips using endometrial polyp forceps. These fragments ultimately are sent for pathologic analysis.

❻ Morcellation. Hysteroscopic morcellators currently available include Hologic's MyoSure, Smith & Nephew's TruClear system, and Boston Scientific's Symphion system. In general, sharp moving blades are contained within a hollow, rigid tube. By means of a vacuum source connected to the hollow tube, tissue is suctioned into the window opening at the device tip (Fig 44-14.3). Here, it is shaved off by the moving blade. Suction also removes morcellated tissue fragments through the device cylinder and allows collection for pathologic analysis.

In retrospective comparisons, hysteroscopic morcellation is faster than resectoscopy and appears easier to perform. It is associated with fewer fluid-related complications and has a shorter learning curve compared with conventional resectoscopy (Emanuel, 2005). However, these devices may be less effective for removing very dense or calcified leiomyomas compared with an electrosurgical resectoscope loop.

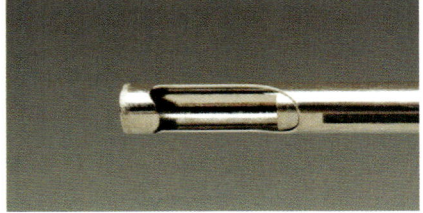

A

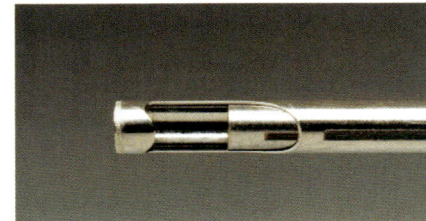

B

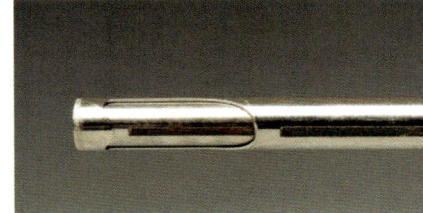

C

FIGURE 44-14.3 Hysteroscopic morcellator. **A.** Morcellator blade retracted. **B.** Blade partially advanced. The blade rapidly rotates as it is advanced and retracted. **C.** Blade is fully advanced and slices tissue drawn into the opening.

❼ Intramural Leiomyomas. During removal of leiomyomas with an intramural component, uterine perforation risks rise if resection extends below the level of the normal myometrium. Therefore, when resection reaches this level, the surgeon pauses and often the surrounding myometrium will contract around the residual tumor. This delivers deeper portions of the tumor up into the cavity for resection. Diminishing the intrauterine pressure by briefly decreasing the fluid inflow rate also can help promote extrusion of the remaining myoma.

❽ Fluid Volume Deficit. Because of the hypervolemia risk during hysteroscopic myomectomy, fluid volume deficits are carefully monitored throughout the procedure. The final fluid deficit is noted in the operative report.

❾ Hemostasis. Bleeding is common during myomectomy but often will cease as myometrial fibers contract around vessels. The reduced intracavitary volume that results from tumor resection promotes this. Thus, electrosurgical coagulation usually is not necessary, but vessels that are actively bleeding may be coagulated with the edge of the resecting loop. The electrosurgical unit is set to a modulating (coagulating) current. At times, a ball electrode may be required to expand the surface area over which current is delivered. Most current morcellation devices are mechanical, and thus, for significant bleeding, a separate electrosurgical coagulating device can be introduced. Rarely, bleeding may be poorly controlled with electrosurgical tools. In such cases, mechanical pressure applied to bleeding vessels by a Foley balloon inflated with 30 mL of saline may be required. For persistent significant bleeding, global endometrial ablation offers a similar treatment for multiple bleeding sites but is not suitable for patients desiring fertility.

POSTOPERATIVE

Recovery following myomectomy is quick and typically without complication. Patients may resume diet and activities as tolerated. Spotting or light bleeding may follow surgery for 1 to 2 weeks.

For patients desiring pregnancy, conception may be attempted in the menstrual cycle after the resection, unless the leiomyoma was broad-based or had a significant intramural component. In these patients, barrier contraception is advised for three cycles. For women who fail to conceive or continue to have abnormal bleeding following resection, postoperative HSG or hysteroscopy is recommended to evaluate for de novo synechiae.

Endometrial Ablation Procedures

Endometrial ablation broadly describes a group of hysteroscopic procedures that destroys or resects the endometrium to reduce or eliminate menstrual flow. However, establishing *normal* menstrual flow is the anticipated goal. For many women, ablation serves as a minimally invasive and effective treatment of heavy menstrual bleeding.

First-generation endometrial ablation tools and techniques require advanced hysteroscopic skills and longer operating times. Methods can be associated with distention medium complications, such as volume overload or acute hypernatremia. However, new bipolar resectoscopes and electrodes help reduce these risks. This first-generation group includes rollerball electrosurgical desiccation, endometrial resection by resectoscope, and endometrial vaporization by the neodymium:yttrium-aluminum-garnet (Nd-YAG) laser.

Comparing first-generation methods, all three produce similar bleeding and patient satisfaction outcomes (Bofill Rodriguez, 2019). However, resection methods are associated with more surgical complications, and thus desiccation methods may be preferred for women without intracavitary lesions (Overton, 1997). Specifically, rollerball endometrial ablation provides shorter operating time, less fluid absorption, and lower perforation rates than transcervical resection of the endometrium (TCRE). As such, rollerball ablation is the standard to which all new ablation techniques are compared with when seeking regulatory approval.

To reduce the risks and required specialized training of these early ablative tools, second-generation methods were developed and are now mainstream options. These tools use various modalities to destroy the endometrium but without the requirement of hysteroscopic guidance in most cases. Specifically, these *global endometrial ablation* methods employ hydrothermal energy, cryosurgery, or radiofrequency (electrosurgical) energy (Table 44-15.1).

PREOPERATIVE

Patient Evaluation

Patient selection is the most important factor determining endometrial ablation success. Preoperatively, thorough evaluation of abnormal uterine bleeding should be completed, and pregnancy, endometrial neoplasia, and active pelvic infection are first excluded. Many second-generation ablation techniques require a relatively normal endometrial cavity, and transvaginal sonography, saline-infusion sonography, and hysteroscopy may be used solely or in combination to define uterine anatomy (Chap. 8, p. 185). Of these, transvaginal sonography provides poor sensitivity to diagnose focal intracavitary lesions. Thus, saline-infusion sonography or diagnostic hysteroscopy offer superior sensitivity for focal abnormalities and may be preferred for preoperative evaluation. In addition, several second-generation techniques are not considered appropriate for large endometrial cavities. Thus, uterine depth also is assessed preoperatively by uterine sounding or sonography.

Myometrial thinning from prior uterine surgery may allow destructive ablative energy to reach surrounding viscera. Therefore, women with prior transmural uterine surgery are evaluated for type and location of uterine scar. A history of prior classical cesarean delivery or of abdominal or laparoscopic myomectomy may be considered a relative contraindication to ablation. Some experts advocate the sonographic evaluation of myometrial thickness to determine whether a patient is a candidate for ablation, although no specific thickness has been established (American College of Obstetricians and Gynecologists, 2018b).

Consent

Patients selecting ablation should be aware of success rates and treatment durability relative to other options for abnormal uterine bleeding (Chap. 8, p. 197). In general, rates of decreased menstrual flow range from 70 to 80 percent and of amenorrhea, from 15 to 35 percent (Sharp, 2006). Eumenorrhea, rather than amenorrhea, is considered a more reasonable treatment goal. Therefore, a patient should not undergo ablation if guaranteed amenorrhea is desired.

Because endometrial ablation effectively destroys the endometrium, it is contraindicated in those who desire future fertility. Despite this, endometrial tissue has tremendous regenerative capacity, and premenopausal women should institute contraception postoperatively. If pregnancy does occur, complications after ablation include prematurity, abnormal placentation, and perinatal morbidity. Thus, many providers recommend concomitant tubal sterilization at the time of endometrial ablation (American College of Obstetricians and Gynecologists, 2018b).

However, in women with tubal sterilization, either postablation tubal sterilization syndrome (PATSS) or cornual hematometra can develop due to bleeding from regenerated or remnant endometrium. With PATSS, blood collects between the occluded proximal tubal stump and postablation synechiae to cause proximal hematosalpinx and hematometra. With cornual hematometra, blood is trapped between postoperative synechial bands at one cornu. Both conditions cause associated cyclic pain. Surgical resection of synechiae or more commonly hysterectomy may be required for resolution (McCausland, 2002).

Following ablation, later evaluation of the endometrium for recurrent abnormal bleeding can be challenging (AlHilli, 2011). Namely, a Pipelle may not reach remnant endometrium, and endometrial stripe measurements can be less accurate. Endometrial ablation rarely is performed in postmenopausal women because excluding malignancy in these women can be more difficult postablation. Women who carry a greater risk for endometrial cancer development pose similar sampling challenges.

Complications associated with ablation mirror those with operative hysteroscopy, although the risk of fluid volume overload is avoided with second-generation techniques. As noted, defects in the myometrium can bring the ablative energy in contact with adjacent organs. Affected patients typically present with symptoms of delayed bowel or bladder thermal injury, described in Chapter 41 (p. 875). With hydrothermal endometrial ablation, leakage of superheated saline

TABLE 44-15.1. Second-Generation Global Endometrial Ablation Devices

Energy	Brand	Device Diameter (mm)	Uterine Length (cm)	
			Min.	Max.
Hydrothermal	Genesys HTA	7.8	4	10.5
RFA	NovaSure	7.2	6	10
RFA	Minerva	6	4	10
Cryoablation	Her Option	4.5	NS	10

HTA = hydrothermal ablation; Min. = minimum; Max. = maximum; NS = not specified; RFA = radiofrequency ablation.

may burn the vagina or perineum. Thus, many methods have safe-guard steps to minimize this risk.

Patient Preparation

During hysteroscopic surgeries, bacteria in the vagina may gain access to the upper reproductive tract and peritoneal cavity. However, postablation infection is rare, and preoperative prophylactic antibiotics generally are not indicated. Because the endometrium can thicken from only a few millimeters in the early proliferative phase to deeper than 10 mm in the secretory phase, endometrial ablation is ideally performed in the early proliferative phase. Otherwise, drugs that induce endometrial atrophy such as GnRH agonists, combination oral contraceptives, or progestins may be used for 1 to 2 months prior to surgery. Alternatively, uterine curettage may be performed immediately prior to ablation.

INTRAOPERATIVE

Surgical Steps

❶ Anesthesia and Patient Positioning. Endometrial ablation typically is a day-surgery procedure performed under general anesthesia. Some studies state that second-generation techniques may be satisfactorily completed in an outpatient setting with intravenous sedation, local anesthetic blockade, or both (Sambrook, 2010; Varma, 2010). The patient is placed in standard lithotomy position, and the perineum and vagina are surgically prepared. The bladder is emptied prior to surgery.

❷ Distention Medium Selection. With first-generation procedures, distention medium is required and selected based on the destructive energy used as described in Chapter 41 (p. 902). In general, saline may be used for laser and bipolar electrical current, whereas monopolar tools require nonelectrolyte solutions.

❸ Neodymium: Yttrium-Aluminum-Garnet Laser. Introduced in the 1980s, the Nd-YAG laser was the first ablative tool. Under direct hysteroscopic observation and uterine distention with saline, a Nd-YAG laser fiber touches the endometrium and is dragged across the endometrial surface. This creates furrows of photocoagulated tissue that are 5 to 6 mm deep (Garry, 1995; Goldrath, 1981). Laser endometrial ablation rarely is used today due to global endometrial ablation techniques, which are technically

less demanding and have lower complication risks.

❹ Transcervical Resection of the Endometrium. Because of the larger loop diameter, TCRE can be completed more quickly and less expensively than laser fiber ablation. The shorter procedure duration can reduce the risk of excess medium absorption.

TCRE uses a resectoscope with monopolar or bipolar electrical current to excise strips of endometrium and superficial myometrium. The resection technique is similar to that described for hysteroscopic myomectomy (p. 1058). The excised tissue strips are sent for pathologic evaluation. In cases with concurrent intrauterine pathology such as endometrial polyps or submucous leiomyoma, TCRE can excise these lesions in addition to the endometrium.

However, TCRE is associated with higher rates of perforation, especially at the cornua, where the myometrium is thinner. For this reason, many use a rollerball electrosurgical electrode in combination with TCRE. Rollerball ablation is completed at the cornua (Oehler, 2003). Similar to laser ablation, TCRE rarely is used today.

❺ Rollerball. A 2- to 4-mm ball-shaped or barrel-shaped electrosurgical electrode is introduced as the active element of a traditional hysteroscopic resectoscope. Ablation uses a pure or blended coagulating current at a setting of 70 to 100 W. Energy is applied only when the electrode is in view.

After thorough inspection of the cavity, the electrode is rolled across the endometrium in a systematic fashion. The goal is coagulation of the entire endometrial cavity. Treatment begins lightly at the tubal ostia and progresses to the fundus (Fig. 44-15.1A). The rollerball then moves to ablate the anterior, posterior, and lateral cavity walls. On each wall, ablation starts near the fundus and

progresses to the internal cervical os. Average ablation time is 45 minutes.

During initial coagulation, tissue may adhere to the electrode, but as the procedure nears completion, debris no longer collects. The normally pink endometrium ultimately is replaced by flattened gray tissue with scattered flecks of char (see Fig. 44-15.1B).

❻ Hysteroscopic Hydrothermal Ablation. Several second-generation ablation procedures require a normal uterine cavity. However, the Genesys HTA System allows treatment of the endometrium and coexistent small submucous leiomyomas or polyps. As another advantage, this method allows direct hysteroscopic viewing of endometrial destruction. One distinct disadvantage is the small risk of vaginal or perineal burns from circulating hot water that leaks from the cervix. In response, a now redesigned hysteroscopic sheath has added concentric Silastic rings to help prevent this leakage.

In overview, this tool ablates the endometrial lining by heating an uncontained saline solution to a temperature of 90°C and recirculating it through the uterus for 10 minutes (Fig. 44-15.2). Spill through the fallopian tubes is avoided because hydrostatic pressure during the procedure remains below 55 mm Hg, which is well below pressures needed to open the tubes to the peritoneal cavity. Similarly, the water seal created between the hysteroscope and internal cervical os prevents leakage of fluid into the vagina. For this reason, the cervix is not dilated to a diameter greater than the device itself.

To begin the procedure, a hysteroscope is inserted into the 7.8-mm diameter disposable Genesys HTA sheath. This combination is introduced into the endometrial cavity to enable viewing while room-temperature saline is instilled into the uterine cavity. The fluid flow is gradually heated and circulated to treat the endometrium. At the completion

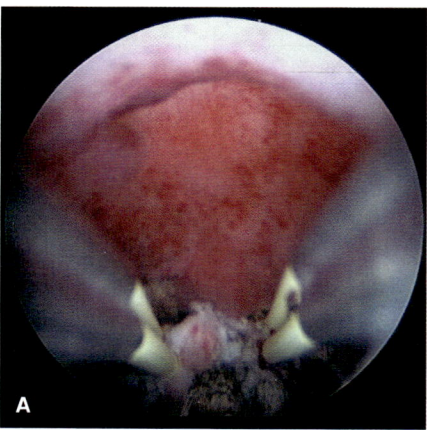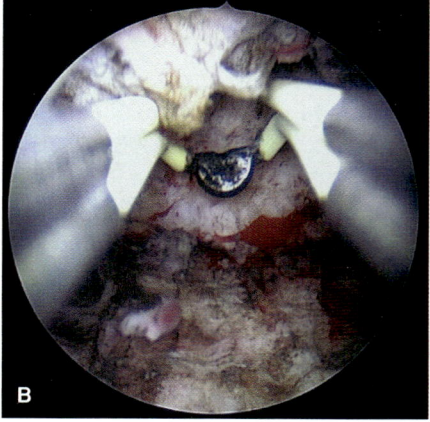

FIGURE 44-15.1 **A.** Rollerball ablation at the fundus. **B.** Cavity at ablation completion.

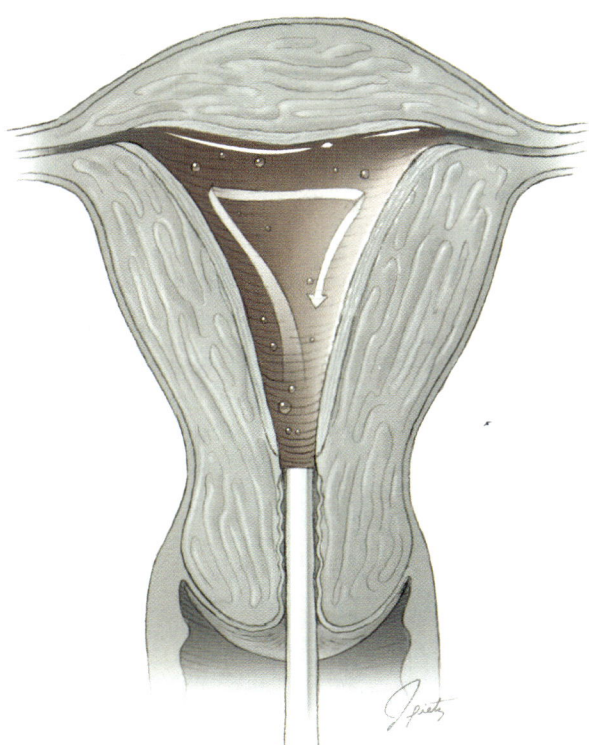

FIGURE 44-15.2 Hysteroscopic thermal ablation.

of the treatment phase, cool saline replaces the heated fluid. The instrument then is removed (Glasser, 2003).

❼ Radiofrequency Electrocoagulation. The NovaSure endometrial ablation system contains an electrode array that conforms to the uterine cavity to deliver destructive bipolar radiofrequency energy (Fig. 44-15.3). The array is a porous metallic fabric that allows continuous removal of blood, moisture, and steam and provides a uniform desiccation depth (Scordalakes, 2018).

The Minerva Endometrial Ablation System is another bipolar radiofrequency ablation device. With this, electric current ionizes argon gas that is contained within a flat triangle-shaped silicone balloon. Once ionized, the gas is termed *plasma*, which delivers its thermal energy to the adjacent endometrial lining.

Both systems use an intraoperative preprocedural uterine integrity test to identify any uterine wall defects. Treatment time is 2 minutes for both. Neither requires endometrial preparation, although in selected patients, it still may be highly advantageous. Although Food and Drug Administration (FDA) approval studies evaluated the NovaSure system in normal uterine cavities, it has been used successfully in patients with small submucosal leiomyomas and polyps (Sabbah, 2006).

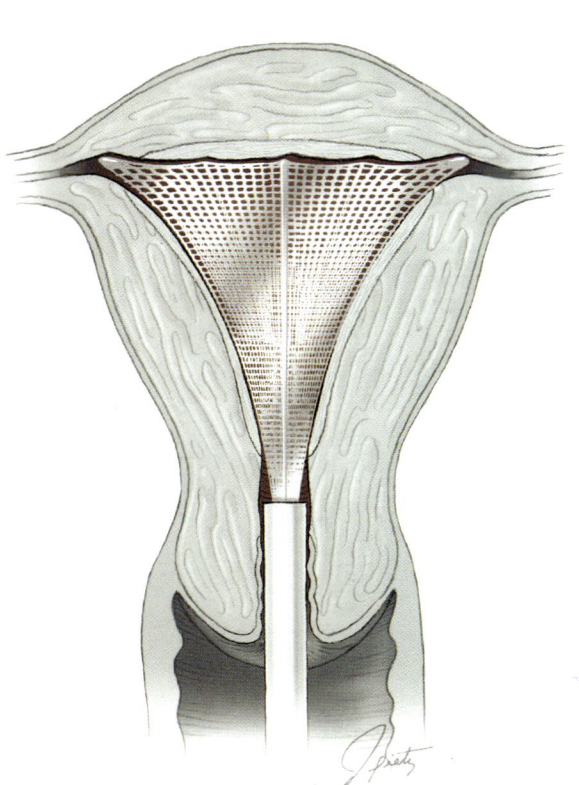

FIGURE 44-15.3 Impedance-controlled radiofrequency ablation.

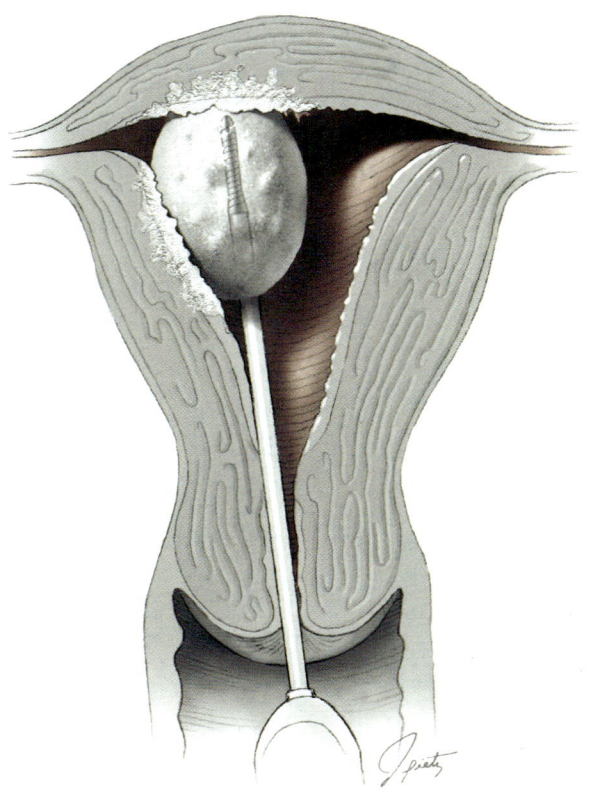

FIGURE 44-15.4 Cryoablation.

8 Cryoablation. In addition to thermal damage, endometrial ablation can be achieved with extreme cold using the Her Option cryoablation system. Similar to the physics of cervical cryotherapy, gases compressed under pressure by the base unit can generate temperatures of $-100°$ to $-120°C$ at the cryoprobe tip to produce an iceball. As an iceball grows, its leading edge advances through tissue, and cryonecrosis develops in those tissues reaching temperatures below $-20°C$ (Chap. 43, p. 1004). Notably, the manufacturer is no longer selling the base unit, but continues to supply disposable cryoprobes for those with existing units.

The Her Option cryoablation system contains a metal probe, which is covered by a 5.5-mm disposable cryoprobe. After dilation of the cervix, the cryoprobe's 1.4-inch cryotip is placed against one side of the endometrial cavity and advanced to one uterine cornu (Fig. 44-15.4). Concurrent transabdominal sonography is required to ensure accurate cryotip placement and surveillance of the increasing iceball diameter, which is seen as an enlarging hypoechoic area. The first freeze is terminated after 4 minutes or sooner, if the advancing iceball reaches to within 3 mm of the uterine serosa. The cryotip is allowed to warm, is moved from the cornu, and is redirected into the contralateral cornu. A second freeze is performed for 6 minutes or less based on iceball advancement.

9 Thermal Balloon Ablation. Outside the United States, the Cavaterm Plus system and the Thermablate Endometrial Ablation System are available thermal balloon ablation systems. The Thermachoice III Uterine Balloon Therapy System is no longer marketed in the U.S.

The Cavaterm Plus system is designed to destroy endometrial tissue using thermal energy from superheated fluid within an inflatable silicone balloon at the device tip. When inflated, it conforms to the cavity contour, and the balloon size can be tailored to a specific cavity size. For this, the sleeve on the outer device can be adjusted to shorten or lengthen the balloon.

After cervical dilation to 6 mm, the collapsed balloon tip is inserted into the uterine cavity. Here, 30 mL of a 5-percent dextrose and water solution is instilled into the balloon and heated to coagulate the endometrium. During the treatment, the fluid within the balloon is circulated to maintain a temperature of 78°C for 10 minutes. After ablation, the saline is reaspirated to collapse the balloon, which then is removed.

All hot-liquid balloon devices require no advanced hysteroscopic skills, and complication rates are low (Gurtcheff, 2003; Vilos, 2004). Disadvantages include the requirement for pharmacologic thinning prior to thermal ablation and for an anatomically normal uterine cavity. Some studies, however, have demonstrated successful use in patients with submucosal leiomyomas (Soysal, 2001). Alternatively, mechanical thinning can be accomplished with dilation and curettage prior to ablation.

POSTOPERATIVE

Advantages to endometrial ablation include rapid patient recovery and low incidence of complications. Patients may resume normal diet and activities as tolerated. Light bleeding or spotting during the first postoperative days is expected as necrotic endometrial tissue is shed. A thin serosanguinous discharge also is common and may continue for several weeks.

44-16

Hysteroscopic Septoplasty

Most uterine septa form from incomplete regression of the medial portion of the müllerian ducts during their fusion (Fig. 44-16.1) (Chap. 19, p. 406). These septa rarely result in infertility. However, they are associated with malpresentation and higher rates of first- and second-trimester pregnancy loss, which may be responsive to surgical correction.

Before the technical advances of operative hysteroscopy, septoplasty was performed abdominally and with a hysterotomy incision. Fortunately, hysteroscopic septoplasty affords MIS with significantly less morbidity to the patient and uterus. *Septoplasty* sharply divides a septum at its vertical midpoint. Bleeding is minimal due to the relative avascularity of the septum's fibroelastic tissue, which retracts upon incision. *Septum resection* is performed for broader, larger septa that have wider bases. A loop resectoscope or morcellator may be preferred for this.

PREOPERATIVE

Patient Evaluation

Diagnosis of a septate uterus follows guidelines outlined in Chapter 2 (p. 41) and includes saline-infusion sonography, three-dimensional transvaginal sonography, or MR imaging. Because of the frequent association between renal and müllerian anomalies, intravenous pyelography also is performed. Finally, although a septate uterus is associated with infertility and recurrent pregnancy loss, evaluation for other causes of these two conditions is completed prior to septum excision. Contraindications to septoplasty include pregnancy and active pelvic infection, and these should be excluded.

Consent

For the indication of recurrent pregnancy loss, postoperative live birth rates approximate 85 percent following septoplasty (Fayez, 1987). In general, complications mirror those for operative hysteroscopy, although the risk of uterine perforation appears higher. Consequently, concurrent sonography or laparoscopy may help inform a surgeon regarding the uterine serosa's proximity (Budden, 2018). Namely, as the hysteroscope nears the fundal serosa, transillumination of the hysteroscopic light indicates the potential for uterine perforation.

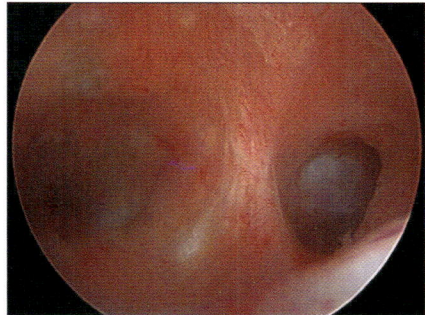

FIGURE 44-16.1 Uterine septum.

Accordingly, a patient also is consented for concurrent diagnostic laparoscopy (p. 1016).

Patient Preparation

Infectious and VTE complications following hysteroscopic surgery are rare. Thus, preoperative antibiotic or VTE prophylaxis is typically not required (American College of Obstetricians and Gynecologists, 2018a,e). In appropriately selected cases, misoprostol may be used preoperatively to ease cervical dilation (Chap. 41, p. 899).

INTRAOPERATIVE

Instruments

Septum incision or resection may be completed using hysteroscopic scissors, resectoscope loop, Nd-YAG laser, or mechanical morcellator. Selection is guided by septum dimensions and surgeon preference.

Surgical Steps

❶ Anesthesia and Patient Positioning. Hysteroscopic septoplasty typically is a day-surgery procedure performed under general anesthesia. A woman is placed in standard lithotomy position, the vagina is surgically prepared, and a Foley catheter inserted. If

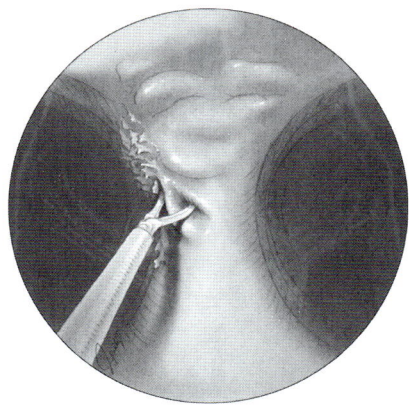

FIGURE 44-16.2 Septum incision.

surveillance laparoscopy is planned, the abdomen also is prepared.

❷ Medium Selection. The choice of distention medium is dictated by the incising tool. Sharp incision with scissors, Nd:YAG laser, or bipolar instrument is commonly selected and can be performed in any liquid medium. Monopolar technology will require a hypotonic nonconductive medium.

❸ Concurrent Laparoscopy. If planned concurrently, placement of the laparoscope follows the steps described in Chapter 41 (p. 888).

❹ Cervical Dilation. A tenaculum is placed on the anterior cervical lip. Using a Pratt or other suitable dilator, the surgeon dilates the cervix as needed.

❺ Instrument Insertion. The distention medium flow is begun, and the operative hysteroscope is inserted into the endocervical canal with direct endoscopic guidance. Upon entering the endometrial cavity, a panoramic inspection is first performed to identify the septum.

❻ Septum Incision. If scissors are used, a surgeon attempts to keep the line of incision in the anteroposterior midline. Transection begins distally, at the septum apex, and continues cephalad toward the fundus. Scissors snips are taken bilaterally and are directed toward the horizontal midline (Fig. 44-16.2). During incision of the septum, drifting from the vertical midline is common. Incisions typically drift posteriorly in an anteverted uterus and anteriorly in a retroverted one. Thus, a surgeon may pause and reorient periodically.

During septoplasty, incision rather than complete resection of the septum is sufficient. Septal stumps retract into the myometrium as the septum is transected. In most cases, the septum is relatively avascular, and cutting at its midpoint causes little bleeding. Signs that septum transection is complete include increasing tissue vascularity, serosal transillumination of the hysteroscope at the uterine fundus, and reaching a level in line with the tubal ostia.

❼ Septum Resection. In some cases, the septum is broad, wide, and difficult to simply incise. Thus, to achieve the desired uterine cavity, a surgeon must completely excise or resect the septum. In general, scissors are suitable. In other instances, vaporizing electrodes, loop electrodes, or morcellators are more useful. Instruments are selected according to surgeon skill and preference.

❽ Procedure Completion. After incision, the hysteroscope and tenaculum are removed. The final fluid deficit is noted in the operative report. Completion of laparoscopy, if performed, follows the steps outlined in Chapter 41 (p. 895).

POSTOPERATIVE

Recovery following septoplasty is rapid and typically without complication. Light bleeding or spotting may last 1 week or more. Patients may resume normal diet and activities as desired. Following resection, symptoms such as dysmenorrhea ultimately are greatly diminished.

To stimulate endometrial proliferation and prevent adhesion reformation, oral estrogen administration is effective. Although several regimens can be used, we prescribe 2 mg of oral estradiol for 30 days.

Attempts at conception are delayed for 2 to 3 months following surgery. If septum resection appeared incomplete at the time of surgery or if recurrent miscarriage or amenorrhea develops, postoperative HSG or a second hysteroscopy may be performed. Complete removal of the septum or adhesiolysis may be required (p. 1069). With subsequent pregnancy, if the myometrium was not entered, cesarean delivery is required only for obstetric indications.

44-17

Proximal Fallopian Tube Cannulation

Proximal fallopian obstruction may result from pelvic inflammatory disease, intratubal debris, congenital malformations, tubal spasm, endometriosis, tubal polyps, and salpingitis isthmica nodosa. It is generally diagnosed during evaluation of infertility when documentation of tubal patency is sought. Therapeutic options have the goal of a successful pregnancy. Therefore, approaches to occlusion in this portion of the tube include tubal cannulation, surgical tubocornual anastomosis, and IVF (Kodaman, 2004). During cannulation, attempts are made to flush debris from within the tubes and perform chromotubation.

Proximal fallopian tube cannulation may be used to treat up to 85 percent of proximal tubal obstructions, but the occlusion may recur following the surgery. Cannulation may be performed as an outpatient radiologic procedure using fluoroscopy (Papaioannou, 2003). Alternatively, cannula placement may be completed with hysteroscopic guidance (Confino, 2003). If a hysteroscopic approach is selected, laparoscopy is typically used concurrently. This allows evaluation and treatment of both proximal and distal tubal disease and provides identification of tubal perforation by the cannulating guide wire if this occurs.

PREOPERATIVE

Patient Evaluation

Proximal tubal occlusion is typically identified with HSG during evaluation of female infertility. To avoid disrupting an early pregnancy, preoperative β-hCG testing is warranted in most patients. Although this procedure may be performed at any time during the menstrual cycle, the early proliferative phase offers the advantage of a thinner endometrium to allow easy identification of tubal ostia and avoids disruption of an undiagnosed early luteal-phase pregnancy.

Consent

In addition to general complications associated with hysteroscopy and laparoscopy, patients undergoing proximal tubal cannulation are informed of the small risk of tubal perforation. Fortunately, because the guide wire measures only 0.5 mm in diameter, tubal damage is rarely significant and can be assessed by concurrent laparoscopic examination of the perforated tube.

In most cases, patients with combined proximal and distal tubal disease are best managed with IVF. As discussed in Chapter 10 (p. 230), hydrosalpinges, when present, can lower IVF success rates and are typically removed. Thus, consideration of and consent for salpingectomy can accompany plans for proximal tubal cannulation.

Patient Preparation

The risk of pelvic infection is low. However, because adhesions following such infection can have damaging effects on fallopian tube health, patients are given either a first- or second-generation cephalosporin prior to surgery. In addition, misoprostol may be used preoperatively if needed to aid cervical softening and hysteroscope insertion.

INTRAOPERATIVE

Instruments

Fallopian tubes may be cannulated with a catheter system displayed in Figure 44-17.1. This system contains an outer cannula, inner cannula, and inner guide wire. The preset bend of the outer cannula aids placement of both the inner cannula and guide wire into the tubal ostium. Once the inner cannula has been threaded into the proximal fallopian tube, the guide wire is removed. The inner cannula, now emptied of the guide wire, can be used to flush debris from the fallopian tube and allow chromotubation, which is visualized laparoscopically (Fig. 20-9, p. 441).

Surgical Steps

❶ Anesthesia and Patient Positioning. Hysteroscopic tubal cannulation with concurrent laparoscopy typically is a day-surgery procedure performed under general anesthesia. The patient is placed in standard lithotomy position, the abdomen and vagina are surgically prepared, and a Foley catheter is inserted.

❷ Medium Selection. No electrosurgery is required for tubal cannulation, thus saline is the preferred medium.

❸ Laparoscopy. The laparoscope is inserted as described in Chapter 41 (p. 888).

❹ Cervical Dilation. Because a smaller diameter operative hysteroscope is required for tubal cannulation, cervical dilation may not be required. If needed, it is performed as described in Chapter 43 (p. 973).

❺ Hysteroscope Insertion. The flow of saline is begun, and a 0- or 30-degree hysteroscope is inserted. A panoramic inspection of the entire cavity is performed, and the tubal ostia are identified (p. 1055).

❻ Tubal Cannulation. The catheter system is threaded through an operating port of the hysteroscope. Under direct endoscopic guidance, the outer catheter is advanced and placed at one of the tubal ostia. The inner catheter is then threaded approximately 2 cm into the proximal fallopian tube (Fig. 44-17.2). The guide wire is removed.

❼ Tubal Flushing. The inner catheter is flushed with water-soluble dye. Dilute methylene blue, 10 mL mixed with 100 to 150 mL of sterile saline, is commonly used. Rarely, it may induce acute methemoglobinemia, particularly in patients with glucose-6-phosphate dehydrogenase deficiency. The laparoscope is positioned to allow inspection of the distal tube to note the presence or absence of dye spill.

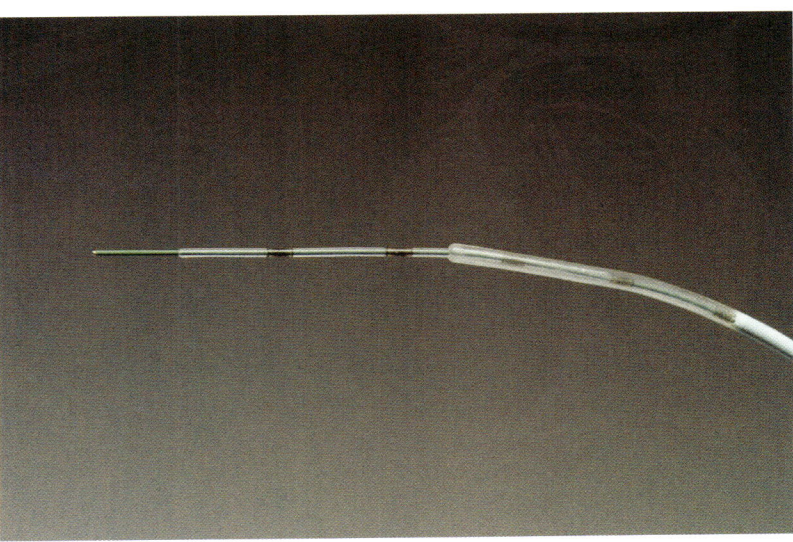

FIGURE 44-17.1 Hysteroscopic tubal cannulation catheter.

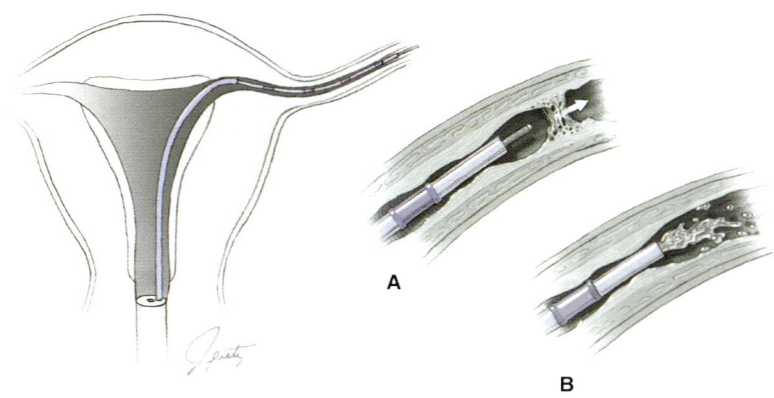

FIGURE 44-17.2 Tubal cannulation. **A.** The inner cannula and guide wire enter the proximal fallopian tube to the point of obstruction. **B.** After guide wire removal, fluid pressure flushes away obstructing debris.

❽ Concurrent Procedures. If distal tubal adhesions are noted, laparoscopic lysis of adhesions may be concurrently performed.

❾ Procedure Completion. Following cannulation, the hysteroscope and cervical tenaculum are removed. Laparoscopy is completed as described in Chapter 41 (p. 895).

POSTOPERATIVE

Recovery from hysteroscopic tubal cannulation and laparoscopy is typically quick and uncomplicated. Patients may resume diet, activity, and attempts at conception as desired.

44-18

Lysis of Intrauterine Adhesions

Intrauterine adhesions, also called *synechiae*, may develop following uterine curettage (**Fig. 44-18.1**). Less commonly, they may result from pelvic radiation, tuberculous endometritis, or endometrial ablation. The presence of these adhesions, also termed *Asherman syndrome*, may lead to hypo- or amenorrhea, pelvic pain, and infertility or pregnancy loss.

Goals of treatment include surgical re-creation of normal intrauterine anatomy and prevention of adhesion reformation. Surgery involves hysteroscopic transection rather than excision of adhesions. Thus, thin adhesions usually can be lysed using only gentle blunt force from the hysteroscopic sheath. Dense adhesions typically require hysteroscopic division with scissors or a resectoscope.

Postsurgical pregnancy and live delivery rates are markers of surgical success, and these rates vary depending on the thickness of adhesions and degree of cavity obliteration. For this reason, various adhesion classification systems are useful to help predict the success of adhesiolysis for a given woman (Al-Inany, 2001).

PREOPERATIVE

Patient Evaluation

Although hysteroscopy and saline-infusion sonography both can accurately identify adhesions, HSG is preferred initially, because it allows concurrent assessment of tubal patency. However, after adhesions have been noted, diagnostic hysteroscopy is recommended to assess the thickness and density of these bands (Fayez, 1987). Additionally, completion of fertility assessment, including semen analysis and assessment of ovulation, is recommended

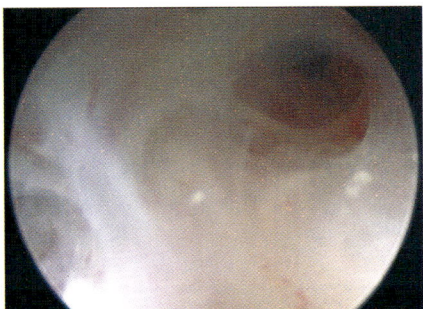

FIGURE 44-18.1 Filmy intrauterine adhesions.

prior to surgery to help predict chances of conception following the procedure.

Consent

In general, hysteroscopic adhesiolysis is an effective tool to correct menstrual disorders and improve fertility in women with uterine adhesions (Valle, 2003). Although overall cumulative delivery rates in those with no other fertility factors range from 60 to 70 percent, lower rates generally are associated with more severe disease (Pabuccu, 1997; Zikopoulos, 2004). In addition, pregnancies following surgery may be complicated by placental implantation abnormalities or by preterm labor (Dmowski, 1969; Pabuccu, 2008).

The complications mirror those for operative hysteroscopy. However, the risk of uterine perforation may be increased. For this reason, patients should also be consented for diagnostic laparoscopy.

Patient Preparation

Infections and VTE complications following hysteroscopic surgery are rare. Accordingly, preoperative antibiotic or VTE prophylaxis is typically not required (American College of Obstetricians and Gynecologists, 2018a,e). Additionally, intracervical vasopressin or preoperative misoprostol may be used to soften the cervix and ease dilation.

INTRAOPERATIVE

Surgical Steps

❶ **Anesthesia and Patient Positioning.** Hysteroscopic lysis of adhesions is typically a day-surgery procedure performed under general anesthesia. The patient is placed in standard lithotomy position, the vagina is surgically prepared, and a Foley catheter inserted.

❷ **Medium Selection.** The choice of distending medium is dictated by the tool used. Sharp transection with scissors, Nd:YAG laser, or bipolar instrument can be performed in any liquid medium. However, thick adhesions often require resection rather than division, and they are severed close to the myometrium. Thus, the potential for creation of large denuded areas and fluid intravasation is significant. Accordingly for many surgeons, 0.9-percent saline is preferred because hyponatremia is less likely if fluid overload does develop.

❸ **Concurrent Laparoscopy.** Because of the increased risk of uterine perforation

in those with more severe obliteration of the cavity, adjunctive laparoscopy may guide surgeons as to instrument proximity to the uterine serosa. The decision to use a laparoscope is individualized, and its placement follows the steps described in Chapter 41 (p. 888).

❹ **Cervical Dilation.** Using Pratt or other suitable dilators, the surgeon dilates the cervix in the standard fashion.

❺ **Instrument Insertion.** The distending medium flow is begun, and the operative hysteroscope is inserted into the endocervical canal with direct endoscopic guidance. Upon entering the endometrial cavity, a panoramic inspection is first performed to identify adhesions.

❻ **Approach to Lysis.** In general, a systematic approach to adhesiolysis begins with either blunt or sharp disruption of the most central adhesions and moves gradually to reach the most lateral ones (Khan, 2018). The size and qualities of adhesions will vary. Thin endometrial adhesions can usually be disrupted with gentle blunt force from the hysteroscopic sheath alone. Similarly, a resectoscopic wire loop without electric current can disrupt the adhesions with little trauma to the remaining endometrial cavity. However, myofibrous and fibrous adhesions are denser and may require complete sharp resection.

Adhesiolysis is continued until the endometrial cavity is restored to normal, and the tubal ostia are seen. Importantly, procedures may require termination prior to this, if significant fluid volume deficits are reached.

❼ **Chromotubation.** At completion of adhesiolysis, transcervical chromotubation is performed to document tubal patency. Chromotubation may be performed by injecting dye into the uterine cavity through a uterine manipulator during simultaneous laparoscopy. Alternatively, tubal cannulation as described previously (p. 1067) may be performed to assess tubal patency.

❽ **Mechanical Uterine Distention.** Mechanical endometrial cavity distention has been used to prevent treated areas from adhering following surgery. Either a copper IUD, placed for 3 months, or an 8F pediatric Foley catheter balloon, used for 10 days, may be chosen. In a comparison of the two, Orhue and colleagues (2003) noted fewer new adhesions and greater pregnancy rates in women using the balloon. If a Foley balloon is placed, antibiotic prophylaxis with either doxycycline 100 mg orally twice daily or other appropriate antibiotic is recommended.

POSTOPERATIVE

Recovery from hysteroscopic resection is rapid and typically without complication. Patients may resume normal activities and diet as tolerated.

To stimulate endometrial proliferation and prevent reformation of adhesions, oral estrogen administration has proved effective. Although several regimens are suitable, we prescribe 2 mg of oral estradiol for 30 days following adhesiolysis. Conjugated equine estrogen (Premarin) 1.25 mg also may be used. If an IUD is inserted, 6 to 8 weeks of oral estrogen supplementation is given.

New adhesions can form following adhesiolysis. In their early stages, these bands are thinner and thus more amenable to successful resection. For this reason, another hysteroscopy or HSG is typically performed at 3 months following the initial resection. If significant new adhesions are found, a second surgical lysis of adhesions is planned. To allow adequate uterine healing, attempts at pregnancy by the patient are delayed for 2 to 3 months.

REFERENCES

Aarts JW, Nieboer TE, Johnson N, et al: Surgical approach to hysterectomy for benign gynaecological disease. Cochrane Database Syst Rev 8: CD003677, 2015

Abu Hashim H, Foda O, El Rakhawy M: Unilateral or bilateral laparoscopic ovarian drilling in polycystic ovary syndrome: a meta-analysis of randomized trials. Arch Gynecol Obstet 297(4):859, 2018

Adelman MR, Dassel MW, Sharp HT: Management of complications encountered with Essure hysteroscopic sterilization: a systematic review. J Minim Invasive Gynecol 21(5):733, 2014

Ahmad G, O'Flynn H, Hindocha A, et al: Barrier agents for adhesion prevention after gynaecological surgery. Cochrane Database Syst Rev 4:CD000475, 2015

Al-Inany H: Intrauterine adhesions: an update. Acta Obstet Gynaecol Scand 80:986, 2001

AlHilli MM, Hopkins MR, Famuyide AO: Endometrial cancer after endometrial ablation: systematic review of medical literature. J Minim Invasive Gynecol 18(3):393, 2011

Amer SA, Li TC, Cooke ID: A prospective dose-finding study of the amount of thermal energy required for laparoscopic ovarian diathermy. Hum Reprod 18(8):1693, 2003

Amer SA, Shamy TTE, James C, et al: The impact of laparoscopic ovarian drilling on AMH and ovarian reserve: a meta-analysis. Reproduction 154(1):R13, 2017

American College of Obstetricians and Gynecologists: Choosing the route of hysterectomy for benign disease. Committee Opinion No. 701, June 2017a

American College of Obstetricians and Gynecologists: Hereditary breast and ovarian cancer syndrome. Practice Bulletin No. 182, September 2017b

American College of Obstetricians and Gynecologists: Sterilization of women: ethical issues and considerations. Committee Opinion No. 695, April 2017c

American College of Obstetricians and Gynecologists: Antibiotic prophylaxis for gynecologic procedures. Practice Bulletin No. 195, June 2018a

American College of Obstetricians and Gynecologists: Endometrial ablation. Practice Bulletin No. 81, May 2007, Reaffirmed 2018b

American College of Obstetricians and Gynecologists: Hysteroscopy. Technical Assessment No. 13, 2018c

American College of Obstetricians and Gynecologists: Polycystic ovary syndrome. Practice Bulletin No. 194, June 2018d

American College of Obstetricians and Gynecologists: Prevention of deep vein thrombosis and pulmonary embolism. Practice Bulletin No. 84, August 2007, Reaffirmed 2018e

American College of Obstetricians and Gynecologists: Alternatives to hysterectomy in the management of leiomyomas. Practice Bulletin No. 96, August 2008, Reaffirmed 2019a

American College of Obstetricians and Gynecologists: Benefits and risks of sterilization. Practice Bulletin No. 208, February 2019b

American College of Obstetricians and Gynecologists: Opportunistic salpingectomy as a strategy for epithelial ovarian cancer prevention. Committee Opinion No. 774, March 2019c

American Society for Reproductive Medicine: Pathogenesis, consequences, and control of peritoneal adhesions in gynecologic surgery: a committee opinion. Fertil Steril 99(6):1550, 2013

Barber EL, Neubauer NL, Gossett DR: Risk of venous thromboembolism in abdominal versus minimally invasive hysterectomy for benign conditions. Am J Obstet Gynecol 212(5):609, 2015

Batra N, Khunda A, O'Donovan PJ: Hysteroscopic myomectomy. Obstet Gynecol Clin North Am 31:669, 2004

Bean EM, Cutner A, Holland T, et al: Laparoscopic myomectomy: a single-center retrospective review of 514 patients. J Minim Invasive Gynecol 24(3):485, 2017

Ben-Arie A, Goldchmit R, Dgani R, et al: Trophoblastic peritoneal implants after laparoscopic treatment of ectopic pregnancy. Eur J Obstet Gynecol Reprod Biol 96(1):113, 2001

Berman JM, Guido RS, Garza Leal JG, et al: Three-year outcome of the Halt trial: a prospective analysis of radiofrequency volumetric thermal ablation of myomas. J Minim Invasive Gynecol 21(5):767, 2014

Bofill Rodriguez M, Lethaby A, Grigore M, et al: Endometrial resection and ablation techniques for heavy menstrual bleeding. Cochrane Database Syst Rev 1:CD001501, 2019

Bojahr B, Raatz D, Schonleber G, et al: Perioperative complication rate in 1706 patients after a standardized laparoscopic supracervical hysterectomy technique. J Minim Invasive Gynecol 13(3):183, 2006

Brennan MC, Ogburn T, Hernandez CJ, et al: Effect of topical bupivacaine on postoperative pain after laparoscopic tubal sterilization with Filshie clips. Am J Obstet Gynecol 190:1411, 2004

Buckley VA, Nesbitt-Hawes EM, Atkinson P, et al: Laparoscopic myomectomy: clinical outcomes and comparative evidence. J Minim Invasive Gynecol 22(1):11, 2015

Budden A, Abbott JA: The Diagnosis and surgical approach of uterine septa. J Minim Invasive Gynecol 25(2):209, 2018

Buttram VC Jr, Vaquero C: Post-ovarian wedge resection adhesive disease. Fertil Steril 26:874, 1975

Camanni M, Bonino L, Delpiano EM, et al: Hysteroscopic management of large symptomatic submucous uterine myomas. J Minim Invasive Gynecol 17(1):59, 2010

Capmas P, Lobersztajn A, Duminil L, et al: Operative hysteroscopy for retained products of conception: efficacy and subsequent fertility. J Gynecol Obstet Hum Reprod 48(3):151, 2019

Casey J, De S, Harvey LF: Endoscopic retrieval baskets: a novel technique for hysteroscopic polypectomy. J Minim Invasive Gynecol 24 (7 suppl):S162, 2017

Chan LM, Westhoff CL: Tubal sterilization trends in the United States. Fertil Steril 94(1):1, 2010

Chang WC, Chang DY, Huang SC, et al: Use of three-dimensional ultrasonography in the evaluation of uterine perfusion and healing after laparoscopic myomectomy. Fertil Steril 92(3):1110, 2009

Choksuchat C: Clinical use of misoprostol in nonpregnant women: review article. J Minim Invasive Gynecol 17(4):449, 2010

Chudnoff SG, Nichols JE Jr, Levie M: Hysteroscopic Essure inserts for permanent contraception: extended follow-up results of a phase III multicenter international study. J Minim Invasive Gynecol 22(6):951, 2015

Chung J, Law T, Chung C, et al: Impact of haemostatic sealant versus electrocoagulation on ovarian reserve after laparoscopic ovarian cystectomy of ovarian endometriomas: a randomised controlled trial. BJOG 126(10):1267, 2019

Clark NV, Cohen SL: Tissue extraction techniques during laparoscopic uterine surgery. J Minim Invasive Gynecol 25(2):251, 2018

Clark NV, Rademaker D, Mushinski AA, et al: Essure removal for the treatment of device-attributed symptoms: an expanded case series and follow-up survey. J Minim Invasive Gynecol 24(6):971, 2017

Cohen SL, Clark NV, Ajao MO, et al: Prospective evaluation of manual morcellation techniques: minilaparotomy versus vaginal approach. J Minim Invasive Gynecol 26(4):702, 2019

Cohen SL, Einarsson JI, Wang KC, et al: Contained power morcellation within an insufflated isolation bag. Obstet Gynecol 124(3):491, 2014

Cohen SL, Morris SN, Brown DN, et al: Contained tissue extraction using power morcellation: prospective evaluation of leakage parameters. Am J Obstet Gynecol 214(2):257.e1, 2016

Confino E: Tubal Catheterization and falloposcopy. In Bieber EJ, Loffer FD (eds): Hysteroscopy, Resectoscopy, and Endometrial Ablation. Boca Raton, Parthenon Publishing Group, 2003, p 113

Cooper NA, Smith P, Khan KS, et al: Vaginoscopic approach to outpatient hysteroscopy: a systematic review of the effect on pain. BJOG 117(5):532, 2010

Dabirashrafi H: Complications of laparoscopic ovarian cauterization. Fertil Steril 52:878, 1989

Darwish AM, Nasr AM, El Nashar DA: Evaluation of postmyomectomy uterine scar. J Clin Ultrasound 33:181, 2005

Derman SG, Rehnstrom J, Neuwirth RS: The long-term effectiveness of hysteroscopic treatment of menorrhagia and leiomyomas. Obstet Gynecol 77:591, 1991

Dey M, Morgan M, Bonduelle M: Filshie clip migration and retention. J Fam Plann Reprod Health Care 36(1):44, 2010

Di Spiezio Sardo A, Calagna G, Di Carlo C: Tips and tricks in office hysteroscopy. Gynecol Minim Invasive Ther 4(1):3, 2015

Di Spiezio Sardo A, Mazzon I, Bramante S, et al: Hysteroscopic myomectomy: a comprehensive review of surgical techniques. Hum Reprod Update 14(2):101, 2008

Djeffal H, Blouet M, Pizzoferato AC, et al: Imaging findings in Essure-related complications: a pictorial review. Br J Radiol 91(1090):20170686, 2018

Dmowski WP, Greenblatt RB: Asherman's syndrome and risk of placenta accreta. Obstet Gynecol 34:288, 1969

Doridot V, Dubuisson JB, Chapron C, et al: Recurrence of leiomyomata after laparoscopic myomectomy. J Am Assoc Gynecol Laparosc 8(4):495, 2001

Doss BJ, Jacques SM, Qureshi F, et al: Extratubal secondary trophoblastic implants: clinicopathologic correlation and review of the literature. Hum Pathol 29:184, 1998

Dubin AK, Wei J, Sullivan S, et al: Minilaparotomy versus laparoscopic myomectomy after cessation of power morcellation: rate of wound complications. J Minim Invasive Gynecol 24(6):946, 2017

Einarsson JI, Cohen SL, Fuchs N, et al: In-bag morcellation. J Minim Invasive Gynecol 21(5): 951, 2014

Einarsson JI, Vellinga TT, Twijnstra AR, et al: Bidirectional barbed suture: an evaluation of safety and clinical outcomes. JSLS 14(3):381, 2010

Emanuel MH, Wamsteker K: The Intra Uterine Morcellator: a new hysteroscopic operating technique to remove intrauterine polyps and myomas. J Minim Invasive Gynecol 12:62, 2005

Farquhar C, Brown J, Marjoribanks J, et al: Laparoscopic drilling by diathermy or laser for ovulation induction in anovulatory polycystic ovary syndrome. Cochrane Database Syst Rev 6:CD001122, 2012

Fauconnier A, Chapron C, Babaki-Fard K, et al: Recurrence of leiomyomata after myomectomy. Hum Reprod Update 6:595, 2000

Fayez JA, Mutie G, Schneider PJ: The diagnostic value of hysterosalpingography and hysteroscopy in infertility investigation. Am J Obstet Gynecol 156:558, 1987

Fedele L, Bianchi S, Tozzi L, et al: Intra-mesosalpingeal injection of oxytocin in conservative laparoscopic treatment for tubal pregnancy: preliminary results. Hum Reprod 13:3042, 1998

Fernandez H, Capmas P, Lucot JP, et al: Fertility after ectopic pregnancy: the DEMETER randomized trial. Human Reprod 28(5):1247, 2013

Finch A, Shaw P, Rosen B, et al: Clinical and pathologic findings of prophylactic salpingo-oophorectomies in 159 BRCA1 and BRCA2 carriers. Gynecol Oncol 100(1):58, 2006

Findley AD, Siedhoff MT, Hobbs KA, et al: Short-term effects of salpingectomy during laparoscopic hysterectomy on ovarian reserve: a pilot randomized controlled trial. Fertil Steril 100(6):1704, 2013

Fletcher H, Frederick J, Hardie M, et al: A randomized comparison of vasopressin and tourniquet as hemostatic agents during myomectomy. Obstet Gynecol 87:1014, 1996

Franklin RR: Reduction of ovarian adhesions by the use of Interceed. Ovarian Adhesion Study Group. Obstet Gynecol (3):335, 1995

Frankman EA, Wang L, Bunker CH, et al: Lower urinary tract injury in women in the United States, 1979–2006. Am J Obstet Gynecol 202(5):495.e1, 2010

Frederick J, Fletcher H, Simeon D, et al: Intra-myometrial vasopressin as a haemostatic agent during myomectomy. BJOG 101:435, 1994

Fuchs Weizman N, Einarsson JI, Wang KC, et al: Vaginal cuff dehiscence: risk factors and associated morbidities. JSLS 19(2):e2013.00351, 2015

Galen DI, Pemueller RR, Leal JG, et al: Laparoscopic radiofrequency fibroid ablation: phase II and phase III results. JSLS 18(2):182, 2014

Ganer Herman H, Gluck O, Keidar R, et al: Ovarian reserve following cesarean section with salpingectomy vs tubal ligation: a randomized trial. Am J Obstet Gynecol 217(4):472, 2017

Garry R, Reich H, Liu CY: Laparoscopic hysterectomy: definitions and indications. Gynaecol Endosc 3:1, 1994

Garry R, Shelley-Jones D, Mooney P, et al: Six hundred endometrial laser ablations. Obstet Gynecol 85:24, 1995

Ghafarnejad M, Akrami M, Davari-Tanha F, et al: Vasopressin effect on operation time and frequency of electrocauterization during laparoscopic stripping of ovarian endometriomas: a randomized controlled clinical trial. J Reprod Infertil 15(4):199, 2014

Giampaolino P, Morra I, Della Corte L, et al: Serum anti-Mullerian hormone levels after ovarian drilling for the second-line treatment of polycystic ovary syndrome: a pilot-randomized study comparing laparoscopy and transvaginal hydrolaparoscopy. Gynecol Endocrinol 33(1):26, 2017

Giampaolino P, Morra I, Tommaselli GA, et al: Post-operative ovarian adhesion formation after ovarian drilling: a randomized study comparing conventional laparoscopy and transvaginal hydrolaparoscopy. Arch Gynecol Obstet 294(4):791, 2016

Gingold JA, Gueye NA, Falcone T: Minimally invasive approaches to myoma management. J Minim Invasive Gynecol 25(2):237, 2018

Ginsburg ES, Benson CB, Garfield JM, et al: The effect of operative technique and uterine size on blood loss during myomectomy: a prospective, randomized study. Fertil Steril 60:956, 1993

Giuliani A, Panzitt T, Schoell W, et al: Severe bleeding from peritoneal implants of trophoblastic tissue after laparoscopic salpingostomy for ectopic pregnancy. Fertil Steril 70:369, 1998

Glasser MH, Zimmerman JD: The HydroThermAblator system for management of menorrhagia in women with submucous myomas: 12- to 20-month follow-up. J Am Assoc Gynecol Laparosc 10:521, 2003

Goldrath MH, Fuller TA, Segal S: Laser photovaporization of endometrium for the treatment of menorrhagia. Am J Obstet Gynecol 140:14, 1981

Gooden MD, Hulka JF, Christman GM: Spontaneous vaginal expulsion of Hulka clips. Obstet Gynecol 81:884, 1993

Gould MK, Garcia DA, Wren SM, et al: Prevention of VTE in nonorthopedic surgical patients: Antithrombotic Therapy and Prevention of Thrombosis, 9th ed: American College of Chest Physicians Evidence-Based Clinical Practice Guidelines. Chest 141(2 suppl):e227S, 2012

Greenberg JA, Einarsson JI: The use of bidirectional barbed suture in laparoscopic myomectomy and total laparoscopic hysterectomy. J Minim Invasive Gynecol 15(5):621, 2008

Greenblatt EM, Casper RF: Adhesion formation after laparoscopic ovarian cautery for polycystic ovarian syndrome: lack of correlation with pregnancy rate. Fertil Steril 60:766, 1993

Grosse-Drieling D, Schlutius JC, Altgassen C, et al: Laparoscopic supracervical hysterectomy (LASH), a retrospective study of 1,584 cases regarding intra- and perioperative complications. Arch Gynecol Obstet 285(5):1391, 2012

Gürgan T, Kisnisci H, Yarali H, et al: Evaluation of adhesion formation after laparoscopic treatment of polycystic ovarian disease. Fertil Steril 56(6):1176, 1991

Gürgan T, Urman B, Aksu T, et al: The effect of short-interval laparoscopic lysis of adhesions on pregnancy rates following Nd:YAG laser photo-coagulation of polycystic ovaries. Obstet Gynecol 80(1):45, 1992

Gurtcheff SE, Sharp HT: Complications associated with global endometrial ablation: the utility of the MAUDE database. Obstet Gynecol 102:1278, 2003

Harkki P, Kurki T, Sjoberg J, et al: Safety aspects of laparoscopic hysterectomy. Acta Obstet Gynaecol Scand 80:383, 2001

Harkki-Siren P, Sjoberg J, Makinen J, et al: Finnish national register of laparoscopic hysterectomies: a review and complications of 1165 operations. Am J Obstet Gynecol 176:118, 1997

Harkki-Siren P, Sjoberg J, Tiitinen A: Urinary tract injuries after hysterectomy. Obstet Gynecol 92:113, 1998

Harmanli OH, Tunitsky E, Esin S, et al: A comparison of short-term outcomes between laparoscopic supracervical and total hysterectomy. Am J Obstet Gynecol 201(5):536.e1, 2009

Harrison MS, DiNapoli MN, Westhoff CL: Reducing postoperative pain after tubal ligation with rings or clips: a systematic review and meta-analysis. Obstet Gynecol 124(1):68, 2014

Hart R, Molnar BG, Magos A: Long-term follow-up of hysteroscopic myomectomy assessed by survival analysis. BJOG 106:700, 1999

Hobo R, Netsu S, Koyasu Y, et al: Bradycardia and cardiac arrest caused by intramyometrial injection of vasopressin during a laparoscopically assisted myomectomy. Obstet Gynecol 113 (2 Pt 2):484, 2009

Howe RS: Third-trimester uterine rupture following hysteroscopic uterine perforation. Obstet Gynecol 81:827, 1993

Hur HC, Lightfoot M, McMillin MG, et al: Vaginal cuff dehiscence and evisceration: a review of the literature. Curr Opin Obstet Gynecol 28(4):297, 2016

Hurst BS, Matthews ML, Marshburn PB: Laparoscopic myomectomy for symptomatic uterine myomas. Fertil Steril 83:1, 2005

Hutchins FL Jr: A randomized comparison of vasopressin and tourniquet as hemostatic agents during myomectomy. Obstet Gynecol 88:639, 1996

Iversen H, Dueholm M: Radiofrequency thermal ablation for uterine myomas: long-term clinical outcomes and reinterventions. J Minim Invasive Gynecol 24(6):1020, 2017

Iverson RE Jr, Chelmow D, Strohbehn K, et al: Relative morbidity of abdominal hysterectomy and myomectomy for management of uterine leiomyomas. Obstet Gynecol 88:415, 1996

Jeung IC, Baek JM, Park EK, et al: A prospective comparison of vaginal stump suturing techniques during total laparoscopic hysterectomy. Arch Gynecol Obstet 282(6):631, 2010

Kamencic H, Thiel L, Karreman E, et al: Does Essure cause significant de novo pain? A retrospective review of indications for second surgeries after Essure placement. J Minim Invasive Gynecol 23(7):1158, 2016

Kandil M, Rezk M, Al-Halaby A, et al: Impact of ultrasound-guided transvaginal ovarian needle drilling versus laparoscopic ovarian drilling on ovarian reserve and pregnancy rate in polycystic ovary syndrome: a randomized clinical trial. J Minim Invasive Gynecol 25(6):1075, 2018

Keltz J, Levie M, Chudnoff S: Pregnancy outcomes after direct uterine myoma thermal ablation: review of the literature. J Minim Invasive Gynecol 24(4):538, 2017

Kesby GJ, Korda AR: Migration of a Filshie clip into the urinary bladder seven years after laparoscopic sterilisation. BJOG 104:379, 1997

Keurentjes JH, Briët JM, de Bock GH, et al: Surgical volume and conversion rate in laparoscopic hysterectomy: does volume matter? A multicenter retrospective cohort study. Surg Endosc 32(2):1021, 2018

Khan Z, Goldberg JM: Hysteroscopic management of Asherman's syndrome. J Minim Invasive Gynecol 25(2):218, 2018

Kim AJ, Barberio A, Berens P, et al: The trend, feasibility, and safety of salpingectomy as a form of permanent sterilization. J Minim Invasive Gynecol 26(7):1363, 2019a

Kim AJ, Clark NV, Jansen LJ, et al: Perioperative antibiotic use and associated infectious outcomes at the time of myomectomy. Obstet Gynecol 133(4):626, 2019b

Kliethermes C, Walsh T, Guan Z, et al: Vaginal tissue extraction made easy. J Minim Invasive Gynecol 24(5):726, 2017

Kluivers KB, Hendriks JC, Mol BW, et al: Quality of life and surgical outcome after total laparoscopic hysterectomy versus total abdominal hysterectomy for benign disease: a randomized, controlled trial. J Minim Invasive Gynecol 14(2):145, 2007

Kodaman PH, Arici A, Seli E: Evidence-based diagnosis and management of tubal factor infertility. Curr Opin Obstet Gynecol 16:221, 2004

Koo YJ, Lee JK, Lee YK, et al: Pregnancy outcomes and risk factors for uterine rupture after laparoscopic myomectomy: a single-center experience and literature review. J Minim Invasive Gynecol 22(6):1022, 2015

Kostrzewa M, Wilczyński JR, Głowacka E, et al: One-year follow-up of ovarian reserve by three methods in women after laparoscopic cystectomy for endometrioma and benign ovarian cysts. Int J Gynaecol Obstet 146(3):350, 2019

Kotani Y, Tobiume T, Fujishima R, et al: Recurrence of uterine myoma after myomectomy: open myomectomy versus laparoscopic myomectomy. J Obstet Gynaecol Res 44(2):298, 2018

Kumakiri J, Takeuchi H, Itoh S, et al: Prospective evaluation for the feasibility and safety of vaginal birth after laparoscopic myomectomy. J Minim Invasive Gynecol 15(4):420, 2008

Kuno K, Menzin A, Kauder HH, et al: Prophylactic ureteral catheterization in gynecologic surgery. Urology 52:1004, 1998

Kwon SK, Kim SH, Yun SC, et al: Decline of serum antimüllerian hormone levels after laparoscopic ovarian cystectomy in endometrioma and other benign cysts: a prospective cohort study. Fertil Steril 101(2):435, 2014

Lajer H, Widecrantz S, Heisterberg L: Hernias in trocar ports following abdominal laparoscopy: a review. Acta Obstet Gynaecol Scand 76:389, 1997

Lamberton GR, Hsi RS, Jin DH, et al: Prospective comparison of four laparoscopic vessel ligation devices. J Endourol 22(10):2307, 2008

Lambertz A, Stüben BO, Bock B, et al: Port-site incisional hernia—a case series of 54 patients. Ann Med Surg (Lond) 14:8, 2017

LaMorte AI, Lalwani S, Diamond MP: Morbidity associated with abdominal myomectomy. Obstet Gynecol 82:897, 1993

Landman J, Kerbl K, Rehman J, et al: Evaluation of a vessel sealing system, bipolar electrosurgery, harmonic scalpel, titanium clips, endoscopic gastrointestinal anastomosis vascular staples and sutures for arterial and venous ligation in a porcine model. J Urol 169(2):697, 2003

Lasmar RB, Barrozo PR, Dias R, et al: Submucous myomas: a new presurgical classification to evaluate the viability of hysteroscopic surgical treatment—preliminary report. J Minim Invasive Gynecol 12(4):308, 2005

Lasmar RB, Xinmei Z, Indman PD, et al: Feasibility of a new system of classification of submucous myomas: a multicenter study. Fertil Steril 95(6):2073, 2011

Lim CS, Mowers EL, Mahnert N, et al: Risk factors and outcomes for conversion to laparotomy of laparoscopic hysterectomy in benign gynecology. Obstet Gynecol 128(6):1295, 2016

Liu CD, McFadden DW: Laparoscopic port sites do not require fascial closure when nonbladed trocars are used. Am Surg 66(9):853, 2000

Loffer FD: Improving results of hysteroscopic submucosal myomectomy for menorrhagia by concomitant endometrial ablation. J Minim Invasive Gynecol 12(3):254, 2005

Maassen LW, van Gastel DM, Haveman I, et al: Removal of Essure sterilization devices: a retrospective cohort study in the Netherlands. J Minim Invasive Gynecol 26(6):1056, 2019

Malacova E, Kemp A, Hart R, et al: Long-term risk of ectopic pregnancy varies by method of tubal sterilization: a whole-population study. Fertil Steril 101(3):728, 2014

Manchanda R, Abdelraheim A, Johnson M, et al: Outcome of risk-reducing salpingo-oophorectomy in BRCA carriers and women of unknown mutation status. BJOG 118(7):814, 2011

Marana R, Busacca M, Zupi E, et al: Laparoscopically assisted vaginal hysterectomy versus total abdominal hysterectomy: a prospective, randomized, multicenter study. Am J Obstet Gynecol 180:270, 1999

Marana R, Luciano AA, Muzii L, et al: Reproductive outcome after ovarian surgery: suturing versus nonsuturing of the ovarian cortex. J Gynecol Surg 7:155, 1991

Mazzon I, Favilli A, Grasso M, et al: Predicting success of single step hysteroscopic myomectomy: a single centre large cohort study of single myomas. Int J Surg 22:10, 2015

McCausland AM, McCausland VM: Frequency of symptomatic cornual hematometra and postablation tubal sterilization syndrome after total rollerball endometrial ablation: a 10-year follow-up. Am J Obstet Gynecol 186(6):1274, 2002

McDonnell RM, Hollingworth JL, Chivers P, et al: Advanced training of gynecologic surgeons and incidence of intraoperative complications after total laparoscopic hysterectomy: a retrospective study of more than 2000 cases at a single institution. J Minim Invasive Gynecol 25(5):810, 2018

Milad MP, Sokol E: Laparoscopic morcellator-related injuries. J Am Assoc Gynecol Laparosc 10:383, 2003

Mol F, van Mello NM, Strandell A, et al: Salpingotomy versus salpingectomy in women with tubal pregnancy (ESEP study): an open-label, multicentre, randomised controlled trial. Lancet 383(9927):1483, 2014

Munro MG, Brooks PG: Use of local anesthesia for office diagnostic and operative hysteroscopy. J Minim Invasive Gynecol 17(6):709, 2010

Munro MG, Critchley HO, Fraser IS, et al: The two FIGO systems for normal and abnormal uterine bleeding symptoms and classification of causes of abnormal uterine bleeding in the reproductive years: 2018 revisions. Int J Gynaecol Obstet 143(3):393, 2018

Muzii L, Bianchi A, Croce C, et al: Laparoscopic excision of ovarian cysts: is the stripping technique a tissue-sparing procedure? Fertil Steril 77:609, 2002

Naether OG, Fischer R, Weise HC, et al: Laparoscopic electrocoagulation of the ovarian surface in infertile patients with polycystic ovarian disease. Fertil Steril 60:88, 1993

Nezhat C, Kennedy Burns M, Wood M, et al: Vaginal cuff dehiscence and evisceration: a review. Obstet Gynecol 132(4):972, 2018

Nezhat FR, Roemisch M, Nezhat CH, et al: Recurrence rate after laparoscopic myomectomy. J Am Assoc Gynecol Laparosc 5(3):237, 1998

Nouri K, Demmel M, Greilberger U, et al: Prospective cohort study and meta-analysis of cyclic bleeding after laparoscopic supracervical hysterectomy. Int J Gynaecol Obstet 122(2):124, 2013

Oehler MK, Rees MC: Menorrhagia: an update. Acta Obstet Gynaecol Scand 82:405, 2003

Okaro EO, Jones KD, Sutton C: Long term outcome following laparoscopic supracervical hysterectomy. BJOG 108:1017, 2001

Orhue AA, Aziken ME, Igbefoh JO: A comparison of two adjunctive treatments for intrauterine adhesions following lysis. Int J Gynaecol Obstet 82:49, 2003

Overton C, Hargreaves J, Maresh M: A national survey of the complications of endometrial destruction for menstrual disorders: the MISTLETOE study (minimally invasive surgical techniques—laser, endothermal or endoresection). BJOG 104:1351, 1997

Pabuccu R, Atay V, Orhon E, et al: Hysteroscopic treatment of intrauterine adhesions is safe and effective in the restoration of normal menstruation and fertility. Fertil Steril 68:1141, 1997

Pabuccu R, Onalan G, Kaya C, et al: Efficiency and pregnancy outcome of serial intrauterine device-guided hysteroscopic adhesiolysis of intrauterine synechiae. Fertil Steril 90(5):1973, 2008

Packiam VT, Cohen AJ, Pariser JJ, et al: The impact of minimally invasive surgery on major iatrogenic ureteral injury and subsequent ureteral repair during hysterectomy: a national analysis of risk factors and outcomes. Urology 98:183, 2016

Papaioannou S, Afnan M, Girling AJ, et al: Diagnostic and therapeutic value of selective salpingography and tubal catheterization in an unselected infertile population. Fertil Steril 79:613, 2003

Parker WH: Total laparoscopic hysterectomy and laparoscopic supracervical hysterectomy. Obstet Gynecol Clin North Am 31:523, 2004

Parker WH, Einarsson J, Istre O, et al: Risk factors for uterine rupture after laparoscopic myomectomy. J Minim Invasive Gynecol 17(5):551, 2010

Penfield AJ: The Filshie clip for female sterilization: a review of world experience. Am J Obstet Gynecol 182:485, 2000

Pergialiotis V, Prodromidou A, Frountzas M, et al: The effect of bipolar electrocoagulation during ovarian cystectomy on ovarian reserve: a systematic review. Am J Obstet Gynecol 213(5):620, 2015

Peters A, Rindos NB, Lee T: Hemostasis during ovarian cystectomy: systematic review of the impact of suturing versus surgical energy on ovarian function. J Minim Invasive Gynecol 24(2):235, 2017

Peterson HB, Xia Z, Hughes JM, et al: The risk of pregnancy after tubal sterilization: findings from the U.S. Collaborative Review of Sterilization. Am J Obstet Gynecol 174:1161, 1996

Peterson HB, Xia Z, Wilcox LS, et al: Pregnancy after tubal sterilization with bipolar electrocoagulation. U.S. Collaborative Review of Sterilization Working Group. Obstet Gynecol 94:163, 1999

Phillips DR, Nathanson HG, Milim SJ, et al: The effect of dilute vasopressin solution on the force needed for cervical dilatation: a randomized controlled trial. Obstet Gynecol 89(4):507, 1997

Powell CB, Alabaster A, Simmons S, et al: Salpingectomy for sterilization: change in practice in a large integrated health care system, 2011–2016. Obstet Gynecol 130(5):961, 2017

Prapas Y, Kalogiannidis I, Prapas N: Laparoscopy vs laparoscopically assisted myomectomy in the management of uterine myomas: a prospective study. Am J Obstet Gynecol 200(2):144.e1, 2009

Rezk M, Sayyed T, Saleh S: Impact of unilateral versus bilateral laparoscopic ovarian drilling on ovarian reserve and pregnancy rate: a randomized clinical trial. Gynecol Endocrinol 32(5):399, 2016

Rybak EA, Polotsky AJ, Woreta T, et al: Explained compared with unexplained fever in postoperative myomectomy and hysterectomy patients. Obstet Gynecol 111(5):1137, 2008

Sabbah R, Desaulniers G: Use of the NovaSure Impedance Controlled Endometrial Ablation System in patients with intracavitary disease: 12-month follow-up results of a prospective, single-arm clinical study. J Minim Invasive Gynecol 13:467, 2006

Saccardi C, Gizzo S, Noventa M, et al: Limits and complications of laparoscopic myomectomy: which are the best predictors? A large cohort single-center experience. Arch Gynecol Obstet 290(5):951, 2014

Saeki A, Matsumoto T, Ikuma K, et al: The vasopressin injection technique for laparoscopic excision of ovarian endometrioma: a technique to reduce the use of coagulation. J Minim Invasive Gynecol 17(2):176, 2010

Salazar CA, Isaacson KB: Office operative hysteroscopy: n update. J Minim Invasive Gynecol 25(2):199, 2018

Salihoğlu KN, Dilbaz B, Cırık DA, et al: Short-term impact of laparoscopic cystectomy on ovarian reserve tests in bilateral and unilateral endometriotic and nonendometriotic cysts. J Minim Invasive Gynecol 23(5):719, 2016

Salim S, Won H, Nesbitt-Hawes E, et al: Diagnosis and management of endometrial polyps: a critical review of the literature. J Minim Invasive Gynecol 18(5):569, 2011

Sambrook AM, Jack SA, Cooper KG: Outpatient microwave endometrial ablation: 5-year follow-up of a randomised controlled trial without endometrial preparation versus standard day surgery with endometrial preparation. BJOG 117(4):493, 2010

Sandberg EM, Twijnstra AR, Driessen SR, et al: Total laparoscopic hysterectomy versus vaginal hysterectomy: a systematic review and meta-analysis. J Minim Invasive Gynecol 24(2):206, 2017

Saridogan E, Becker CM, Feki A, et al: Recommendations for the surgical treatment of endometriosis-part 1: ovarian endometrioma. Gynecol Surg 14(1):27, 2017

Sasaki KJ, Cholkeri-Singh A, Sulo S, et al: Persistent bleeding after laparoscopic supracervical hysterectomy. JSLS 18(4):e2014.002064, 2014

Schindlbeck C, Klauser K, Dian D, et al: Comparison of total laparoscopic, vaginal and abdominal hysterectomy. Arch Gynecol Obstet 277(4):331, 2008

Schmidt T, Eren Y, Breidenbach M: Modifications of laparoscopic supracervical hysterectomy technique significantly reduce postoperative spotting. J Minim Invasive Gynecol 18(1):81, 2011

Schytte T, Soerensen JA, Hauge B, et al: Preoperative transcervical analgesia for laparoscopic sterilization with Filshie clips: a double-blind, randomized trial. Acta Obstet Gynaecol Scand 82:57, 2003

Scordalakes C, delRosario R, Shimer A, et al: Efficacy and patient satisfaction after NovaSure and Minerva endometrial ablation for treating abnormal uterine bleeding: a retrospective comparative study. Int J Womens Health 10:137, 2018

Seifer DB: Persistent ectopic pregnancy: an argument for heightened vigilance and patient compliance. Fertil Steril 68:402, 1997

Selim MF: The optimal number of ovarian punctures to be applied during laparoscopic ovarian diathermy in women with Polycystic Ovarian syndrome. J Gynecol Surg 27(4):217, 2011

Sharp HT: Assessment of new technology in the treatment of idiopathic menorrhagia and uterine leiomyomata. Obstet Gynecol 108(4):990, 2006

Shazly SA, Green IC, Laughlin-Tommaso SK, et al: Concomitant hysteroscopic myomectomy and endometrial ablation for heavy menstrual bleeding. J Minim Invasive Gynecol 23(7 suppl):S43, 2016

Siedhoff MT, Cohen SL: Tissue Extraction techniques for leiomyomas and uteri during minimally invasive surgery. Obstet Gynecol 130(6):1251, 2017

Sizzi O, Rossetti A, Malzoni M, et al: Italian multicenter study on complications of laparoscopic myomectomy. J Minim Invasive Gynecol (4):453, 2007

Smaldone MC, Gibbons EP, Jackman SV: Laparoscopic nephrectomy using the EnSeal Tissue Sealing and Hemostasis System: successful therapeutic application of nanotechnology. JSLS 12(2):213, 2008

Soderstrom RM, Levy BS, Engel T: Reducing bipolar sterilization failures. Obstet Gynecol 74:60, 1989

Song T, Lee SH, Kim WY: Additional benefit of hemostatic sealant in preservation of ovarian reserve during laparoscopic ovarian cystectomy: a multi-center, randomized controlled trial. Hum Reprod 29(8):1659, 2014

Soysal ME, Soysal SK, Vicdan K: Thermal balloon ablation in myoma-induced menorrhagia under local anesthesia. Gynecol Obstet Invest 51:128, 2001

Spandorfer SD, Sawin SW, Benjamin I, et al: Postoperative day 1 serum human chorionic gonadotropin level as a predictor of persistent ectopic pregnancy after conservative surgical management. Fertil Steril 68:430, 1997

Srouji SS, Kaser DJ, Gargiulo AR: Techniques for contained morcellation in gynecologic surgery. Fertil Steril 103(4):e34, 2015

Stevens A, Parsa MA, Paka C, et al: Vaginal cuff dehiscence in a series of 12,398 hysterectomies: effect of different types of colpotomy and vaginal closure. Obstet Gynecol 121(1):189, 2013

Strowitzki T, von Wolff M: Laparoscopic ovarian drilling (LOD) in patients with polycystic ovary syndrome (PCOS): an alternative approach to medical treatment? Gynecol Surg 2:71, 2005

Suzuki Y, Vellinga TT, Istre O, et al: Small bowel obstruction associated with use of a gelatin-thrombin matrixsealant (FloSeal) after laparoscopic gynecologic surgery. J Minim Invasive Gynecol 17(5):641, 2010

Teede HJ, Misso ML, Costello MF, et al: Recommendations from the international evidence-based guideline for the assessment and management of polycystic ovary syndrome. Fertil Steril 110(3):364, 2018

Teeluckdharry B, Gilmour D, Flowerdew G: Urinary tract injury at benign gynecologic surgery and the role of cystoscopy. Obstet Gynecol 126(6):1161, 2015

Toaff R, Toaff ME, Peyser MR: Infertility following wedge resection of the ovaries. Am J Obstet Gynecol 124:92, 1976

Tsuji S, Takahashi K, Imaoka I, et al: MRI evaluation of the uterine structure after myomectomy. Gynecol Obstet Invest 61(2):106, 2006

Tulandi T, Beique F, Kimia M: Pulmonary edema: a complication of local injection of vasopressin at laparoscopy. Fertil Steril 66:478, 1996

Tulandi T, Guralnick M: Treatment of tubal ectopic pregnancy by salpingotomy with or without tubal suturing and salpingectomy. Fertil Steril 55:53, 1991

Tulandi T, Murray C, Guralnick M: Adhesion formation and reproductive outcome after myomectomy and second-look laparoscopy. Obstet Gynecol 82:213, 1993

Tunitsky E, Citil A, Ayaz R, et al: Does surgical volume influence short-term outcomes of laparoscopic hysterectomy? Am J Obstet Gynecol 203(1):24.e1, 2010

Uccella S, Ceccaroni M, Cromi A, et al: Vaginal cuff dehiscence in a series of 12,398 hysterectomies: effect of different types of colpotomy and vaginal closure. Obstet Gynecol 120(3):516, 2012

Uccella S, Malzoni M, Cromi A, et al: Laparoscopic vs transvaginal cuff closure after total laparoscopic hysterectomy: a randomized trial by the Italian Society of Gynecologic Endoscopy. Am J Obstet Gynecol 218(5):500.e1, 2018

Valle RF: Intrauterine adhesion. In Bieber EJ, Loffer FD (eds): Hysteroscopy, Resectoscopy, and Endometrial Ablation. Boca Raton, Parthenon Publishing Group, 2003, p 93

van der Stege JG, van Beek JJ: Problems related to the cervical stump at follow-up in laparoscopic supracervical hysterectomy. JSLS 3(1):5, 1999

Varma R, Soneja H, Samuel N, et al: Outpatient Thermachoice endometrial balloon ablation: long-term, prognostic and quality-of-life measures. Gynecol Obstet Invest 70(3):145, 2010

Vercellini P, Zaina B, Yaylayan L, et al: Hysteroscopic myomectomy: long-term effects on menstrual pattern and fertility. Obstet Gynecol 94:341, 1999

Vilos GA: Hysteroscopic and nonhysteroscopic endometrial ablation. Obstet Gynecol Clin North Am 31:687, 2004

Wallwiener M, Taran FA, Rothmund R, et al: Laparoscopic supracervical hysterectomy (LSH) versus total laparoscopic hysterectomy (TLH): an implementation study in 1,952 patients with an analysis of risk factors for conversion to laparotomy and complications, and of procedure-specific re-operations. Arch Gynecol Obstet 288(6):1329, 2013

Walsh CA, Walsh SR, Tang TY, et al: Total abdominal hysterectomy versus total laparoscopic hysterectomy for benign disease: a meta-analysis. Eur J Obstet Gynecol Reprod Biol 144(1):3, 2009

Wamsteker K, Emanuel MH, de Kruif JH: Transcervical hysteroscopic resection of submucous fibroids for abnormal uterine bleeding: results regarding the degree of intramural extension. Obstet Gynecol 82:736, 1993

Wells A, Germanos GJ, Salemi JL, et al: Laparoscopic surgeons' perspectives on risk factors for and prophylaxis of trocar site hernias: a multispecialty national survey. JSLS 23(2):e2019.00013, 2019

Wen KC, Chen YJ, Sung PL, et al: Comparing uterine fibroids treated by myomectomy through traditional laparotomy and 2 modified approaches: ultraminilaparotomy and laparoscopically assisted ultraminilaparotomy. Am J Obstet Gynecol 202(2):144.e1, 2010

Wenger JM, Spinosa JP, Roche B, et al: An efficient and safe procedure for laparoscopic supracervical hysterectomy. J Gynecol Surg 21(4):155, 2005

Westberg J, Scott F, Creinin MD: Safety outcomes of female sterilization by salpingectomy and tubal occlusion. Contraception 95(5):505, 2017

Wiseman DM, Trout JR, Franklin RR, et al: Metaanalysis of the safety and efficacy of an adhesion barrier (Interceed TC7) in laparotomy. J Reprod Med 44(4):325, 1999

Wiskind AK, Toledo AA, Dudley AG, et al: Adhesion formation after ovarian wound repair in New Zealand White rabbits: a comparison of ovarian microsurgical closure with ovarian non-closure. Am J Obstet Gynecol 163:1674, 1990

Wrigley LC, Howard FM, Gabel D: Transcervical or intraperitoneal analgesia for laparoscopic tubal sterilization: a randomized, controlled trial. Obstet Gynecol 96:895, 2000

Yoo EH, Lee PI, Huh CY, et al: Predictors of leiomyoma recurrence after laparoscopic myomectomy. J Minim Invasive Gynecol 14(6):690, 2007

Yunker AC, Ritch JM, Robinson EF, et al: Incidence and risk factors for chronic pelvic pain after hysteroscopic sterilization. J Minim Invasive Gynecol 22(3):390, 2015

Zahiri Sorouri Z, Sharami SH, Tahersima Z, et al: Comparison between unilateral and bilateral ovarian drilling in clomiphene citrate resistance polycystic ovary syndrome patients: a randomized clinical trial of efficacy. Int J Fertil Steril 9(1):9, 2015

Zakherah MS, Kamal MM, Hamed HO: Laparoscopic ovarian drilling in polycystic ovary syndrome: efficacy of adjusted thermal dose based on ovarian volume. Fertil Steril 95(3):1115, 2011

Zikopoulos KA, Kolibianakis EM, Platteau P, et al: Live delivery rates in subfertile women with Asherman's syndrome after hysteroscopic adhesiolysis using the resectoscope or the VersaPoint system. Reprod Biomed Online 8:720, 2004

CHAPTER 45

Surgeries for Pelvic Floor Disorders

45-1

Diagnostic and Operative Cystoscopy and Cystourethroscopy

Diagnostic cystoscopy often is indicated following procedures that carry risks of bladder and ureteral injury. Additionally, operative cystoscopy is within the scope of many gynecologists for the passage of ureteral catheters or stents, bladder biopsy, and foreign-body removal.

Both rigid and flexible cystoscopes are available, although in gynecology, a rigid scope offers advantages. First, viewing is enhanced by its capability for higher irrigation flow rates. Rigid scopes also have larger working channels, which allow a wider variety of instruments to pass.

Of components, a cystoscope contains an outer sheath, bridge, endoscope (optical lens), and obturator. The sheath contains one port for fluid infusion and a second port for fluid egress. For office cystoscopy, a sheath measuring 17F affords greater patient comfort. However, for operative cases, a 21F or wider-diameter sheath is preferred to allow rapid fluid infusion and easier instrument and stent passage. The end of the sheath tapers, and in women with a narrow urethral meatus, an obturator can be placed inside the sheath to create a rounded tip for smooth introduction. In selected instances, gentle dilation of the external urethral opening using narrow cervical dilators is needed prior to sheath introduction.

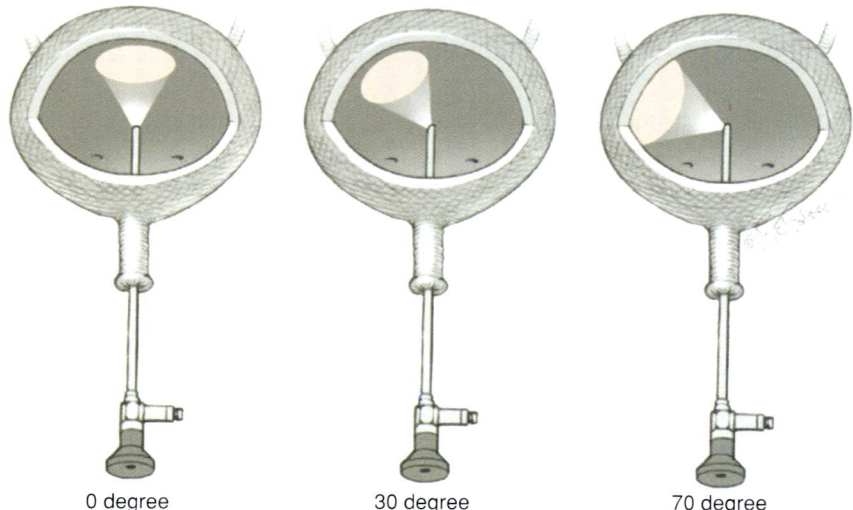

0 degree	30 degree	70 degree

FIGURE 45-1.1 Cystoscopic optical views.

The bridge attaches to the proximal portion of the sheath and connects the optical lens to the sheath. A diagnostic bridge has no working channels. For therapeutic cases, a bridge that has one to two working channels is preferred. In addition, the specialized Albarran bridge contains a lever, which can deflect wires and catheters that pass through its working channels. This aids the angling needed to cannulate ureteral orifices.

Several endoscope viewing angles are available and include 0-, 30-, and 70-degree optical views (Fig. 45-1.1). Zero-degree endoscopes are used for urethroscopy. For cystoscopy, a 70-degree endoscope is superior for providing the most comprehensive view of the lateral, anterior, and posterior walls; trigone; and ureteral orifices. To achieve a comparable view, a 30-degree endoscope requires additional manipulation. However, a 30-degree endoscope does offer advantages and allows surgeons greater flexibility, as it can be used for either urethroscopy or cystoscopy during a given examination. For operative cystoscopic cases in which instruments are passed down the sheath, a 30-degree endoscope should be used. With 0- and 70-degree endoscopes, operative instruments generally lie outside the optical field of view.

Direct viewing through the endoscope's eyepiece is feasible. However, a camera system usually is coupled to the endoscope during both office and operating room cases. Images are projected to a video screen.

PREOPERATIVE

Prior to office cystoscopy, urinary tract infection (UTI) is excluded to avoid upper tract infection. If diagnostic cystoscopy is performed properly, complications are rare. Of these, infection is the most common and results from significant bacteriuria following cystoscopy. Routine use of antibiotic prophylaxis to prevent the less than 5-percent mean risk of symptomatic UTI after diagnostic cystoscopy is controversial (Zeng, 2019). The American College of Obstetricians and Gynecologists (2018b) and others recommend against prophylaxis for routine diagnostic cystoscopy in healthy adults at low risk for surgical site infections (Wolf, 2008). At our institution, we prescribe a single perioperative antibiotic dose to cover common urinary tract pathogens.

For operative procedures, a single-dose fluoroquinolone or cephalosporin given within 1 hour of the procedure is sufficient (Christiano, 2000). During cystoscopy, if an undiagnosed UTI is suspected based on visual findings, the urine is sent for analysis, and treatment can be initiated pending culture results.

INTRAOPERATIVE

Surgical Steps

❶ Anesthesia and Patient Positioning. Cystoscopy may be performed in low or standard lithotomy position with the legs positioned in stirrups. For office cystoscopy, a lubricating gel is applied to the endoscope tip or 2-percent lidocaine gel is instilled into the urethra 5 to 10 minutes prior to cystoscope insertion. For operative procedures, an additional 50 mL of 4-percent lidocaine solution may be instilled via catheter into the bladder. The perineum and urethral meatus are surgically prepared prior to urethral manipulation.

❷ Distention Media. The bladder must be adequately distended to fully visualize all surfaces, and for diagnostic purposes, saline or sterile water is suitable. To ensure adequate media flow, an infusion bag is elevated significantly above the level of the symphysis pubis. The volume needed may vary but is reached when bladder walls are not collapsing inward. Overdistending the bladder is avoided, because temporary urinary retention can follow. If the bladder is distended beyond its capacity, excess fluid will leak out the urethral meatus and around the cystoscope rather than rupture the bladder, which is rare.

❸ Intravenous Dye. When intraoperative cystoscopy is performed to document lower urinary tract patency, intravenous dye administration colors the urine and aids cystoscopic identification of urine jets from the ureteral orifices. In addition, leakage of dye into the operative field confirms a lower urinary tract defect. However, nonvisualization of dye does not exclude injury. For example, dye may leak and collect retroperitoneally or a thermal injury may cause delayed necrosis and defect.

Of vital-dye options, indigo carmine shortages have prompted a search for safe alternatives. Ten-percent sodium fluorescein given intravenously in doses ranging from 0.25 to 1 mL leads to yellow ureteral jets minutes after injection. It has few adverse effects (Grimes, 2017). Less commonly, methylene blue is used but carries the risk of methemoglobinemia in patients with glucose-6-phosphate dehydrogenase deficiency.

Instead, some prefer intravesical instillation of certain fluids. The viscosity difference between the selected solution and urine enhances ureteral jet discrimination. Of media, the clarity provided by 50-percent dextrose solution compared with normal saline was preferred in one randomized trial. However, higher postoperative UTI rates were observed in the dextrose group (Narasimhulu, 2016). Another study compared bladder distention with a 20-percent mannitol solution against oral phenazopyridine (Pyridium), intravenous sodium fluorescein, and normal saline. The mannitol solution provided the best visualization, ease of use, and overall satisfaction but no adverse events (Grimes, 2017).

❹ Cystoscopy. Prior to cystoscope insertion, the angle of the urethra is noted. In women, this angle is directed slightly upward but is more pronounced with anterior vaginal wall prolapse. In this setting, digitally correcting the prolapse prior to insertion or during examination is helpful.

Lubricant gel is applied to the tip of the cystoscope sheath. Fluid inflow is begun and distends the meatus, which aids direct lumen visualization. This practice also limits trauma from the sheath tip. The cystoscope is

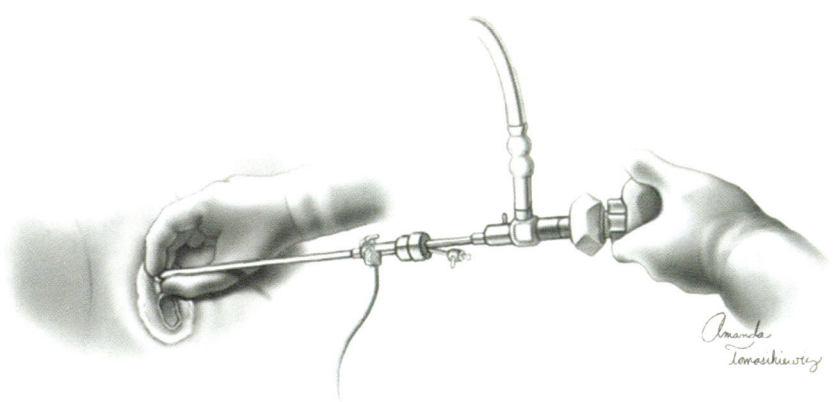

FIGURE 45-1.2 Cystoscope steadied during procedure.

inserted with the lens angle directed toward the ceiling.

The cystoscope is advanced toward the bladder, while the provider views the video screen. During the procedure, the cystoscope can be steadied with one hand holding the sheath near the urethral meatus (Fig. 45-1.2).

5 Bladder Inspection. Upon entry into the bladder, the cystoscope, oriented with the light-source cable pointing down, is slowly withdrawn until the air bubble is seen on the anterior bladder dome. Introduced into the bladder by the cystoscope, this air bubble provides orientation for the remainder of the examination. When a 70- or 30-degree cystoscope is used, it is angled upward to view this bubble. To maintain orientation during rotation, the camera is held static, while the light cord and cystoscope are rotated (Fig. 45-1.3).

As the distended bladder assumes a spherical shape, it is systematically inspected on each side from apex to internal urethral opening. First, to view the entire left side of the bladder, the cystoscope and light cable are rotated approximately 90 degrees in a clockwise fashion. The surgeon's left hand

is used to prevent awkward hand crossing. To examine the bladder wall from 12 to 3 o'clock positions, the cystoscope is initially angled upward and then pans down to the 3 o'clock position, at which point the cystoscope is parallel to the floor. Next, inspection from 3 to 6 o'clock requires gradual downward angling of the cystoscope. The left ureteral orifice is generally found at the 5 o'clock position and approximately 3 to 4 cm proximal to the internal urethral opening. Once the left orifice is noted, further subtle clockwise rotation of the cystoscope along the interureteric ridge permits identification of the right orifice.

The cystoscope is again rotated so that the light-source cable is again pointing downward and the bubble at the dome is identified. For the right side, counterclockwise movement of the cystoscope and light cord with the surgeon's right hand averts awkward hand crossing. The right wall of the bladder then is similarly examined.

While horizontal to the floor, the cystoscope is withdrawn to the bladder neck and then angled downward to provide a second view of the trigone and both ureteral orifices.

Brisk urine flow should be seen from each opening. Peristalsis of the orifice alone, without flow, is insufficient to document patency. Moreover, scant flow may indicate partial ureteral obstruction and merits further evaluation.

The average time to efflux approximates 10 minutes but can be longer. After 20 minutes, absent jets bilaterally more often reflect hypovolemia and resolve with fluid bolus. Following this bolus, 10 to 20 mg of furosemide (Lasix) can be added as needed to promote diuresis. Underlying renal disease also can delay efflux. During inspection, a unilateral jet is more concerning for ureteral injury. To evaluate, the surgeon can attempt to thread a ureteral catheter, as described in Step 8.

6 Operative Cystoscopy. For this, biopsy or grasping forceps or scissors are tool options. The instrument is introduced through the operating port until viewed within the bladder and at the cystoscope's tip. Prior to instrument insertion, a rubber adapter cap is positioned over the operating port to create a watertight seal with the operative instrument. Once in view, the tool and cystoscope are moved together as a unit toward the area of interest.

7 Ureteral Stenting. Semantically, most *stents* are designed to remain indwelling for prolonged ureteral drainage. Stents are used to relieve obstruction, treat ureteral injury, or protect a ureteral anastomosis. Instead, *ureteral catheters* typically are inserted and removed in the same therapeutic intervention. Both are hollow to permit radiopaque medium injection and to allow urine egress through or around it.

Ureteral catheters can be introduced at several points during surgery. First, these straight narrow tubes may be inserted at the beginning of surgery and left through its duration to define ureteral anatomy. Second, during surgery, catheters may be threaded to document ureteral patency. They also can be placed to perform retrograde pyelography, which can localize obstruction or transection. Last, urologists may use catheters to collect selective ureteral urine for cytology.

Ureteral catheter examples include the whistle-tip, open-ended, and cone tip. Generally, open-ended or whistle-tip types are used to delineate anatomy or exclude obstruction. The cone tip type commonly is selected for retrograde pyelography. Its conical shape occludes the ureteral orifice, prevents backflow of injected opaque medium, and thus fully fills the ureter to allow spill through a defect. A Rutner catheter also can be employed for retrograde pyelography.

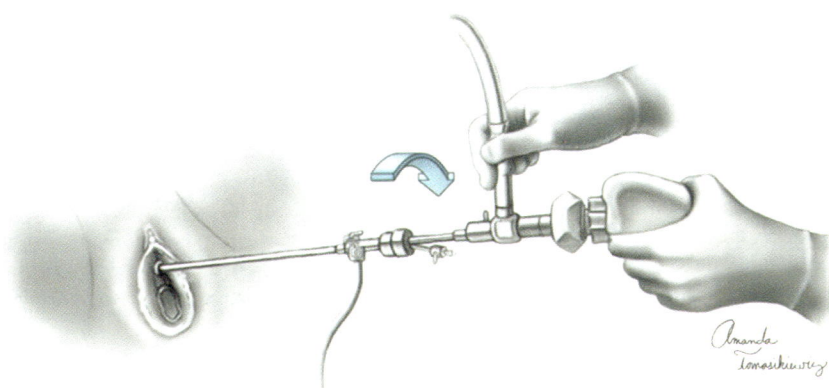

FIGURE 45-1.3 Orientation during cystoscopy is maintained by holding the camera steady while the light cord and cystoscope are rotated.

8 To Exclude Ureteral Obstruction. For this, a 4 to 6F open-ended or whistle-tip catheter is threaded through the operating channel of a 30-degree cystoscope and into the field of view. In one study, a 5F whistle-tip catheter was associated with less ureteral trauma compared with a 5F open-ended catheter (Abu-Rustum, 2006). By advancing both the catheter and cystoscope toward the ureteral orifice, the catheter is passed into the opening.

Once inserted, the catheter is advanced to the level of suspected obstruction. If the tool threads easily up toward the renal pelvis, obstruction is unlikely. In most gynecologic surgery, ureteral injury occurs at or below the pelvic brim. The corresponding catheter distance from the ureteral orifice to the brim approximates 13 cm (Jackson, 2019). Once the renal pelvis is reached, the length of the ureter can be measured and is reflected by the catheter marking seen at the ureteric orifice. Later, this may be valuable in selecting an appropriate stent length, if needed.

When passing a catheter, gentle pressure is used to avoid ureteral perforation. If resistance is encountered, catheter advancement is stopped, and retrograde pyelography is completed to guide catheter placement. In addition, the catheter can be passed over a guidewire. After catheter removal, ureteral orifice urine jets should be documented.

If ureteral transection or stricture is suspected from the just-described steps, a cone tip ureteral catheter is inserted. Through it, radiographic contrast is injected into the distal ureter to locate extravasation or point of narrowing. This is done intraoperatively with fluoroscopic guidance. If contrast flows easily up to the renal pelvis and no extravasation noted, ureteral injury is unlikely. Still, if thermal-injury concerns persist, a double-J stent is placed for 2 to 4 weeks to maintain ureteral patency while the edema and inflammation of normal healing subside.

If gross blood issues from an orifice prior to ureteral manipulation, the ureter may be partially transected, severely crushed, or coagulated. Even if suitable urine efflux from a ureteral orifice is noted, many insert and maintain a double-J stent for approximately 2 to 4 weeks. Computed tomography (CT) urography may be performed prior to stent removal to exclude extravasation. In addition, a CT urogram or renal sonogram is completed 4 to 6 weeks after stent removal to exclude stricture.

After these interrogations, persistently absent efflux from one orifice may uncommonly reflect a long-standing unilateral nonfunctioning kidney. For this, postoperative CT and nuclear scan can be performed.

9 To Delineate Anatomy. For this purpose, a ureteral catheter is advanced until gentle resistance is met, which indicates that the renal pelvis has been reached. The ureteral catheter is tied securely to the transurethral catheter and drains into the cystoscopy drape. At the conclusion of surgery, the catheter is removed if there are no concerns for ureteral injury. If concerns for injury are present, a guide wire can be placed through the catheter, the catheter is removed, and a double-J stent is threaded over the wire.

10 Ureteral Stenting. Ureteral stents range from 4 to 7F. The most common size is 6F, in which French ÷ 3 = diameter in mm. Stents vary in length from 20 to 30 cm, and a 24-cm or 26-cm length is appropriate for most adults. Double-pigtail or double-J stents describe their tip shape, and the ends coil within the renal pelvis and bladder, respectively, to prevent stent migration. Thus, insertion requires a guide wire to straighten these curls.

For placement, a guide wire is first threaded into the ureteral orifice and passed to the renal pelvis with fluoroscopic guidance. Although not essential, a 5F ureteral catheter can be threaded over the guide wire to the renal pelvis. The wire is removed, and retrograde pyelography is performed to obtain a nephrostogram (Linder, 2019). After this study, some of the radiopaque deposited contrast remains in the renal pelvis. This retention helps highlight the pelvis during stent-positioning confirmation.

This catheter also aids ureteral length measurement and thereby stent length selection. For this, markings on the catheter at the level of the ureteral orifice are noted. Other methods for stent length selection include patient's height and radiographic findings. After this, the guide wire is replaced, and the catheter removed.

Next, the double-pigtail stent is threaded over the same guide wire and advanced by a pusher device until its distal end enters the bladder. The guide wire is partially removed, allowing the upper curl to form in the renal pelvis. Correct upper coil positioning, indicated by a full curl of at least 180°, is confirmed intraoperatively using fluoroscopy or plain film radiography. Evaluation of the distal coil or curl, which also should be at least 180°, is done cystoscopically. To help avoid patient discomfort and irritative voiding symptoms, the coil should not cross the sagittal midline of the bladder (Al-Kandari, 2007).

Depending on their indication, stents usually remain 2 to 8 weeks. Longer duration may lead to greater patient discomfort, pyelonephritis, and stent encrustation. Ureteral stenting does not require antibiotic prophylaxis. However, pyelonephritis may occur in patients with stents, and diagnosis requires prompt initiation of intravenous antibiotics (Table 3-14, p. 77). Although not generally recommended, we then continue daily antibiotic prophylaxis after treating pyelonephritis until the stent is removed.

Stent-related suprapubic pain or bladder spasm is common and can be treated with an anticholinergic agent (Table 23-5, p. 531) or an alpha-adrenergic antagonist. One example of the latter is tamsulosin hydrochloride (Flomax), which is prescribed as a 0.4-mg oral dose nightly. The physiologic rationale for these both drug groups is outlined in Chapter 23 (p. 531). In addition to spasm, hematuria is a frequent finding.

Notably, pain or obstructive symptoms may reflect stent migration, which is reported in approximately 4 percent of cases (Breau, 2001). Symptoms may also stem from a distal stent coil that has crossed the bladder's sagittal midline (Al-Kandari, 2007; Giannarini, 2011). If displacement is suspected, a plain abdominal radiograph will display stent position. In this study, the symphysis pubis serves as a general marker of the midsagittal plane. In pregnant patients, coil position can be verified sonographically to avoid radiation exposure. For malpositioning, the stent can be exchanged over a guide wire in an outpatient setting.

Stents generally are removed in the office with cystoscopic guidance, and fluoroscopy or patient analgesia is not required. The lower pigtail of the stent is identified, grasped, and pulled out concurrently with the cystoscope.

11 Biopsy and Foreign Body Removal. Small mucosal lesions can be biopsied with minimal risk or discomfort to the patient. Large lesions highly suspicious for bladder cancer should be referred to a urologic oncologist.

A biopsy instrument is introduced into the cystoscope's operating port. With the instrument in view, the cystoscope is moved directly to the lesion. Biopsy is performed, and the cystoscope and instrument are withdrawn through the urethra together. In this way, a biopsy specimen is not pulled through the sheath and possibly lost. Bleeding is usually minor and will stop by itself. For brisk bleeding, electrosurgical coagulation can be used if a nonconducting solution such as water or glycine was selected as the distention medium. Electrolyte solutions such as saline cannot be used with monopolar electrosurgery. These solutions conduct current, dissipating the energy, and thereby rendering the instrument useless.

Foreign bodies, such as small stones that can pass transurethrally, are removed using the same technique as biopsy. The instrument is used to grasp the foreign body and then removed together with the cystoscope.

2-0 absorbable suture then is created at the bladder dome, with stitches placed deeply into the bladder muscularis (Fig. 45-1.4). The two suture ends are elevated but held loosely. A small stab incision is made in the purse-string's center. This incision is preferably made in the retropubic or extraperitoneal portion of the bladder dome to minimize fistula formation risk. An endoscope is introduced into the bladder, and for suprapubic teloscopy, a 30-degree lens is most effective.

The two suture ends are pulled upward and held tightly to prevent distending fluid escape. To allow visualization of the trigone and ureteral orifices, the Foley bulb is deflated but left in place. An intravenous dye is given if necessary to document ureteral efflux. If the ureteral orifices still cannot be visualized, the bladder incision is extended inferiorly into the retropubic portion to allow direct trigone visualization. At the conclusion of teloscopy, the lens is removed, and the purse-string suture is tied to close the cystotomy.

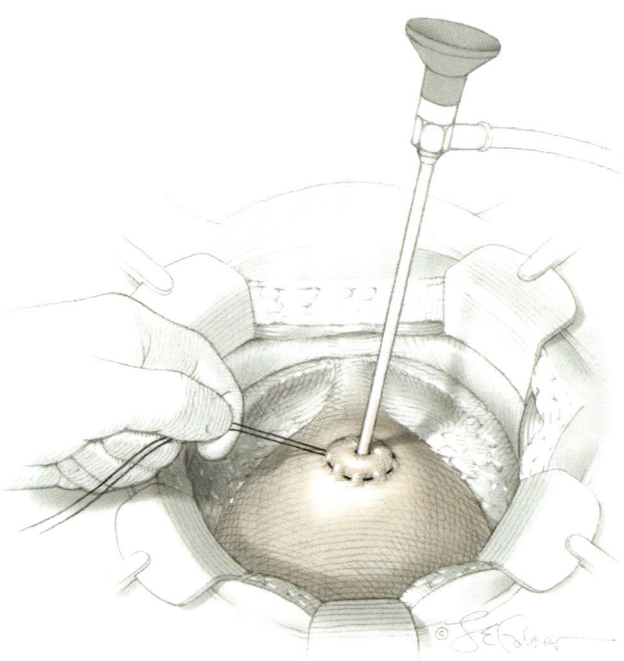

FIGURE 45-1.4 Suprapubic teloscopy.

⑫ **Suprapubic Teloscopy.** This is a technique used to visualize the bladder through an abdominal approach. It often is valuable when the ureters must be assessed during a difficult cesarean delivery or during a laparotomy case in which a woman has not been positioned to allow easy access to the urethra.

The bladder is distended using the transurethral Foley catheter until the bladder wall is distended. A wide purse-string using

POSTOPERATIVE

Office cystoscopy does not require specific postoperative management. With operative cystoscopy, hematuria may develop. It generally clears within a few days and is considered significant only if associated with symptomatic anemia.

45-2

Lower Urinary Tract Injury Repair

The bladder and ureters are especially vulnerable to injury during hysterectomy and other major gynecologic surgery. The urethra, instead, is particularly vulnerable with antiincontinence operations, urethral diverticulum excision, or a large cystotomy that extends into the bladder trigone. A description of the epidemiology and prevention of these injuries is presented in Chapter 40 (p. 865). Although these may not be identified until after surgery, primary repair intraoperatively lowers risks of later urogenital fistula formation and other serious complications.

BLADDER INJURY

The optimal bladder repair method depends on location, extent, and mechanism of injury. Smaller lacerations in the bladder dome are suitable for repair by most gynecologists. However, complex injuries benefit from the expert assistance of a urogynecologist, gynecologic oncologist, or urologist. Complex injuries are those that approximate or involve the bladder trigone, are multifocal, or occur in tissue that is anticipated to heal poorly.

The route of repair varies depending on injury severity, its timing, and minimally invasive surgery (MIS) skills. For those with suitable training, cystotomy repairs often can be completed using an MIS approach.

PREOPERATIVE

Patient Evaluation

Discussed in Chapter 40 (p. 865), intraoperative cystotomy is suspected if a Foley bulb, bloody urine, or urine leaking into the operative field is seen. During laparoscopy, the Foley bag also may distend with gas from the pneumoperitoneum. For diagnosis, sterile milk or vital dye such as diluted methylene blue, instilled retrograde through a catheter, confirms injury if the solution is noted in the operative field. Prior to repair, cystoscopy to assess ureteral patency is indicated for any injury to the bladder base. Similarly, midline laparoscopic suprapubic trocar injuries mandate cystoscopy, because through-and-through punctures can involve the bladder's posterior wall. In other cases, cystoscopy may be elected at the surgeon's discretion to fully assess potential injuries.

The bladder is divided into a body (dome) and a fundus (base) approximately at the level of the ureteric orifices. The base contains the vesical trigone. The upper part of the dome is the only part of the bladder covered by peritoneum. Instead, anteroinferiorly and laterally, the bladder abuts the loose connective tissue that fills the retropubic space, and here, the bladder lacks a peritoneal covering. An injury in this relatively sequestered retropubic portion carries the lowest risk of fistula formation, because it does not contact abdominopelvic organs.

Posteriorly, the bladder rests against the vagina and cervix. Injuries below the vesicouterine peritoneal fold and thus in the vesicovaginal space carry risk of fistula formation. Moreover, injuries here may approximate or extend into the trigone, which raises repair complexity and postoperative complication rates.

Bladder dome cystotomy management depends on the defect size and location. Overall, small defects measuring <2 mm in diameter, such as those from a Veress needle, can be managed expectantly.

Small dome injuries measuring ≤1 cm in diameter, such as those from a 5-mm laparoscopic trocar or a midurethral-sling needle, may be repaired or may be managed conservatively. For the latter, transurethral catheterization for 1 to 3 days is sufficient. For small laceration in the portion of dome covered by peritoneum, cystography can be performed prior to catheter removal to confirm bladder integrity. This practice generally is advised because of greater urine extravasation risk at this site. For midurethral-sling trocar injuries into the retropubic part of the bladder, cystography typically is not required prior to catheter removal due to the enclosed anatomy describe earlier.

For a bladder dome laceration measuring ≤1 cm and noted during abdominal or laparoscopic/robotic surgery, we prefer one-layer closure using 2-0 or 3-0 delayed-absorbable suture and interrupted stitches. Cystotomies >1 cm should be repaired in a layered fashion described next. Cystography can be done prior to catheter removal for the reason just discussed.

If bladder injury is diagnosed postoperatively but within 5 days from the primary procedure, early repair may be considered. Determining factors include lesion size and location and patient's overall condition. For example, postoperatively diagnosed injuries measuring <1 cm at the dome can be managed by prolonged bladder drainage and then later cystography. Otherwise, a delay of approximately 6 weeks and bladder drainage is recommended to permit tissue inflammation resolution. For either management, the entire urinary tract is evaluated using cystoscopy and either bilateral retrograde pyelography or CT urography (Chap. 2, p. 46). These tests help exclude concomitant ureteral injury or complex bladder injuries, defined earlier.

Consent

Risk of bladder and ureteral injury are discussed with patients during the primary procedure's consenting process. For delayed repair, counseling also explains possible stent placement, ureteral surgery, and prolonged bladder or ureteral drainage. Risk of urinary tract or wound infection, irritative voiding symptoms, hematuria, and suprapubic pain from the repair or the indwelling catheter(s) are reviewed. Although rare, repair breakdown, fistula formation, and reoperation are other risks.

Patient Preparation

Immediately prior to primary surgery, intravenous antibiotic and venous thromboembolism (VTE) prophylaxis are commonly administered. Thus, if an injury is diagnosed intraoperatively, no further antibiotics are indicated solely for cystotomy repair. However, antibiotics may be redosed for cases lasting >3 hours or associated with >1500 mL blood loss.

For delayed repairs, the American College of Obstetricians and Gynecologists (2018b) recommends antibiotic prophylaxis prior to urogynecologic surgery, and appropriate broad-spectrum choices mirror those for hysterectomy (Table 39-8, p. 832). VTE prophylaxis is recommended (Table 39-10, p. 834). Bowel preparation generally is not required.

INTRAOPERATIVE

Surgical Steps

❶ **Patient Positioning.** Women usually can remain positioned from their primary surgery if it permits cystoscopy. If supine for laparotomy, a patient is repositioned to low lithotomy position in booted support stirrups. Many cystotomies occur during hysterectomy, which serves as a reference during several of the subsequently described steps. For delayed repairs, the abdomen and vagina are surgically prepared.

❷ **Cystotomy Delineation.** Most cystotomies at time of hysterectomy are supratrigonal. However, injuries that extend laterally can involve ureters directly or during repair. Thus, to begin, cystoscopy evaluates injury location and complexity. If needed, ureteral catheters are inserted for damage near or within the trigone. Insertion technique is outlined on page 1078. Catheters delineate and later may be replaced by stents, which remain for several weeks during healing to avoid ureteral scarring and obstruction.

❸ Mucosal Layer Closure. Because additional injuries may ensue, repair is usually delayed until the hysterectomy and all other surgical dissection is completed. Moreover, the cystotomy can allow a surgeon's finger placed into the bladder to guide dissection of the bladder off the cervix or anterior vagina. Once hysterectomy is completed, the bladder is mobilized off the upper anterior vaginal wall for 1.5 to 2 cm below the planned cuff-closure suture line. The vaginal cuff is then closed as described in Chapter 43 (p. 969).

Depending on size and location, a cystotomy is repaired in two to three layers. If multiple small cystotomies lie adjacent to each other and away from the bladder trigone, sharp incision of the intervening bladder wall segments creates a single, linear, larger one for sole closure. For repair, the bladder mucosa edges are reapposed with 3-0 delayed-absorbable suture in a running fashion. Each suture incorporates the submucosa and deep detrusor fibers but does not enter the lumen (Fig. 45-2.1A). Although absorbable suture can be placed into bladder lumen, we prefer to avoid potential calculus formation around remnant suture. The initial and final suture ends are cut long to aid repair line identification.

The mucosal layer closure then is tested by retrograde instillation of 200 mL of water or saline through a Foley catheter or through the cystoscope. Cystoscopy permits repair line inspection and confirmation of ureteral integrity by urine efflux. Overdistention, which may tear the suture line, is avoided. However, if fluid leaks are noted, additional interrupted sutures are placed until a watertight repair is confirmed.

❹ Detrusor Layer Closure. The next layer incorporates the bladder muscle and imbricates the submucosal layer using 2-0 delayed-absorbable suture in a running or interrupted fashion (see Fig. 45-2.1B). This covers the first suture line and relieves tissue tension. An additional layer may be placed depending on detrusor thickness. Importantly, large tissue purchases that may tear the bladder wall or compromise ureteral patency are avoided. Cystoscopy is again performed to document ureteral patency and inspect suture line integrity.

❺ Omental Interposition. If the closed vaginal cuff and cystotomy repair site appose one another, the expected inflammatory response that attends normal healing may risk fistula formation. Infected, radiated, or friable tissue is a similar risk factor. In such cases, an interposition graft may be used. For this, the omentum is freed from its upper abdominal attachments to create a J-flap (Chap. 46, p. 1211). The omentum then is sutured to the anterior vaginal wall at a site distal to the cuff and thereby covers the cuff incision (p. 1085). This tissue interface increases vascular flow to the area with the hope to improve healing and prevent fistula formation.

❻ Incision Closure. The abdominal incision or laparoscopic incisions are closed as described in Chapters 43 (p. 932) and 41 (p. 895), respectively.

POSTOPERATIVE

The bladder is drained postoperatively to prevent the domino of overdistention, suture disruption, and fistula formation. Cystotomy size and location guides drainage duration, which ranges from 7 to 14 days. Either transurethral or suprapubic catheter placement ensures adequate drainage. At our institution, we use a transurethral catheter for 10 to 14 days following supratrigonal posthysterectomy cystotomy repairs. For injuries approximating the trigone or ureteric orifice, the bladder generally is drained for 2 to 3 weeks.

Concurrent antibiotic suppression is not required, but UTI is excluded if symptoms are present. Anticholinergic agents indicated for urgency urinary incontinence can treat bladder spasms, and options are found in Table 23-5 (p. 531). Cystography prior to catheter removal can be individualized according to injury size and location, as described on page 1080. A voiding trial and postvoid residual volume measurement after catheter removal are reasonable and described in Chapter 42 (p. 919). Some women have transient bladder dysfunction and urinary retention.

VESICOVAGINAL FISTULA REPAIR

Vesicovaginal fistulas may be repaired either vaginally or abdominally. A vaginal approach is preferred for most fistulas seen in the United States, which are posthysterectomy, apical fistulas. This approach offers comparable success rates, lower morbidity, and faster patient recovery. Of vaginal methods, the one most commonly performed by gynecologists is the Latzko technique. With this, surrounding vaginal epithelium is reflected away from the fistulous tract. The tract then is resected, but the portion opening into the bladder is not excised. This avoids a large bladder defect, which can develop with resection of even relatively small fistulas. Following excision, layered closure of the vaginal incision seals the leak. If performed for fistulas at the vaginal apex, then both anterior and posterior vaginal wall epithelia are reflected for tract access. In this location, the final layered closure simulates the steps of colpocleisis, and thus the Latzko technique for apical fistulas is often likened to a partial colpocleisis (p. 1145).

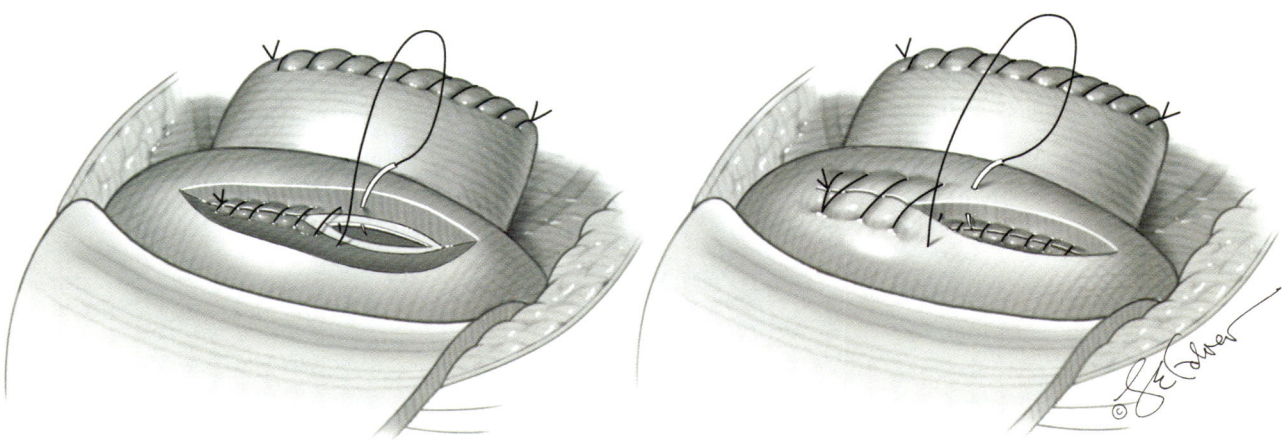

A   **B**

FIGURE 45-2.1 Cystotomy repair after hysterectomy completion. **A.** Mucosa closure. **B.** Detrusor muscle closure.

In other cases, the fistulous tract can be completely excised vaginally, and a layered repair of the bladder and then vaginal wall follows. This is preferred by many if the fistulous opening is <5 mm in diameter and lies away from ureteral orifices.

At times, an abdominal approach may be necessary for women in whom fistula location prohibits effective surgical access or in whom prior vaginal repairs have failed. The most commonly described abdominal approach, termed the *O'Conor technique*, is outlined here and involves bisecting the bladder wall to enter the fistulous tract. Modifications to this and an extravesical approach have been described, especially during MIS routes to fistula repair (Miklos, 2015). With any abdominal approach, omentum or peritoneum can be partially freed and interposed between the bladder and vagina in an attempt to prevent recurrence.

One principle of fistula repair dictates that repair is performed in noninfected and noninflamed tissues. A second rule states that tissue must be approximated without excess tension. Last, a multilayer, watertight closure aids reestablishment of bladder integrity. If these guidelines are followed, success rates are typically good and approximate 95 percent (Rovner, 2012). In the United States, most fistulas follow hysterectomy for benign causes, and their repair is associated with high cure rates. In contrast, fistulas associated with gynecologic cancer and radiation therapy may require adjunctive surgical procedures such as vascular or myocutaneous flaps. These flaps provide supportive blood supply to defects that develop in poorly vascularized or fibrotic tissue. Even with these measures, success rates are lower.

PREOPERATIVE

Patient Evaluation

Prior to repair, a fistula should be well characterized. Complex fistulas with multiple tracts or a concomitant ureterovaginal fistula should be identified. Proper evaluation typically includes cystoscopy and imaging that displays the upper and lower urinary tract such as CT urography (pyelography) or intravenous pyelography (IVP) (Fig. 26-3, p. 577).

Ureterovaginal fistulas usually are associated with upper tract abnormalities such as hydroureter and hydronephrosis. Thus, normal IVP or CT findings reassure that ureteral involvement is absent. Additionally, this imaging complements cystoscopy in ascertaining the proximity of ureters relative to a fistula for surgical planning. In general, routine posthysterectomy vesicovaginal fistulas develop midline at the vaginal apex and usually 1 to 2 centimeters above the trigone. This is away from the ureters, which enter the bladder at the midlength of the vagina. However, lateral fistulas raise concern for ureteral involvement or proximity.

Whether surgery can be performed vaginally largely depends on the ability to adequately expose the fistula. Thus, during physical examination, a surgeon assesses if a fistula can be brought down into the surgical field and if a patient's pelvis affords adequate space. Some degree of prolapse of the vaginal apex is helpful for fistula repair. However, a final decision on the repair route is sometimes made intraoperatively, when muscle relaxation from anesthesia allows better assessment. Placing a pediatric Foley through the fistula and into the bladder may allow sufficient traction (Cardenas-Trowers, 2018; Kieserman-Shmokler, 2019).

Preoperatively, tissue infection or inflammation also is sought. If it is identified, fistula repair is delayed approximately 6 weeks until resolution. However, fistulas recognized within the few days following hysterectomy may be repaired immediately and prior to the brisk inflammatory response associated with cuff healing.

Consent

Fistulas may redevelop following repair, and patients are counseled that initial surgery may not be curative. With the Latzko procedure, the vagina may be shortened. Thus, the risk of postoperative dyspareunia is included during surgical counseling. However, a recent study showed that fistula repair improves sexual function and quality of life, with no attributed difference between vaginal and abdominal routes (Mohr, 2014).

Patient Preparation

Just prior to surgery, intravenous broad-spectrum antibiotic and VTE prophylaxis are commonly administered (Tables 39-8 and 39-10, p. 832). The necessity of bowel preparation for this procedure is unclear, and administration is individualized.

INTRAOPERATIVE

Surgical Steps—Vaginal Repair

❶ Anesthesia and Patient Positioning. In most cases, repair is performed with general or regional anesthesia, and postoperative hospitalization is individualized. The patient is placed in standard lithotomy position, and the vagina is surgically prepared.

❷ Cystoscopic Survey. This is performed to delineate the location of the fistulous opening and assess its proximity to the ureteral orifices. Later, cystoscopy is repeated at different stages to document ureteral patency and assess bladder integrity. If ureters lie close to a fistula, ureteral catheters are placed. If needed, catheters later can be replaced by stents (p. 1078).

❸ Delineating a Fistulous Tract. During inspection, if a tract is wide enough to accept a pediatric Foley catheter, the tube is threaded through the fistulous tract, and the balloon is inflated within the bladder. If a tract cannot be delineated in this manner, lacrimal duct probes, ureteral stents, or other suitable narrow dilators are used to trace the tract course and direction. Subsequently, attempts are made to dilate the tract and then place the pediatric catheter.

❹ Surgical Exposure. For repair, the fistula is brought into the operative field. If catheterization of the tract is possible, tension on the pediatric catheter will allow this. Alternatively or in addition, four sutures can be placed in the vaginal wall surrounding the fistula and used to pull the fistula into the operative field (Fig. 45-2.2).

❺ Vaginal Incision. A circumferential vaginal incision is made with a 2-cm radius from the fistulous tract (Fig. 45-2.3). Vaginal epithelium within this boundary is sharply mobilized away from the vaginal fibromuscular layer and then excised with Metzenbaum scissors.

❻ Tract Excision. The fistula tract may or may not be totally excised to the level of the bladder. As noted earlier, complete tract excision creates a larger bladder defect for repair. We prefer not to excise a fistulous tract lying near a ureteral orifice to avert potential ureteral injury and need for reimplantation (Blaivas, 1995). In cases in which the fistulous tract is not excised at the bladder, a purse-string suture can be placed just outside the epithelialized tract using 3-0 absorbable suture. The suture ends are cinch and tied to close the defect.

❼ Fistula Closure. If a tract is totally excised, the bladder mucosa is reapproximated with 3-0 gauge delayed-absorbable suture in an interrupted or running fashion. Following this closure, the bladder is retrograde filled with 200 mL of fluid to exclude leaks. If a defect is found, additional reinforcing sutures are placed until a watertight repair is achieved.

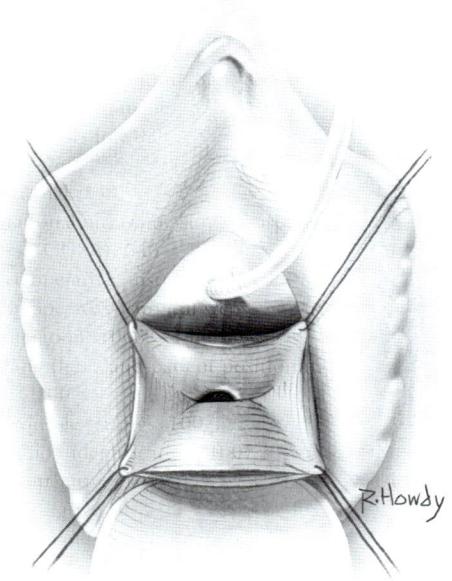

FIGURE 45-2.2 Stay sutures in the vaginal wall improve fistula access.

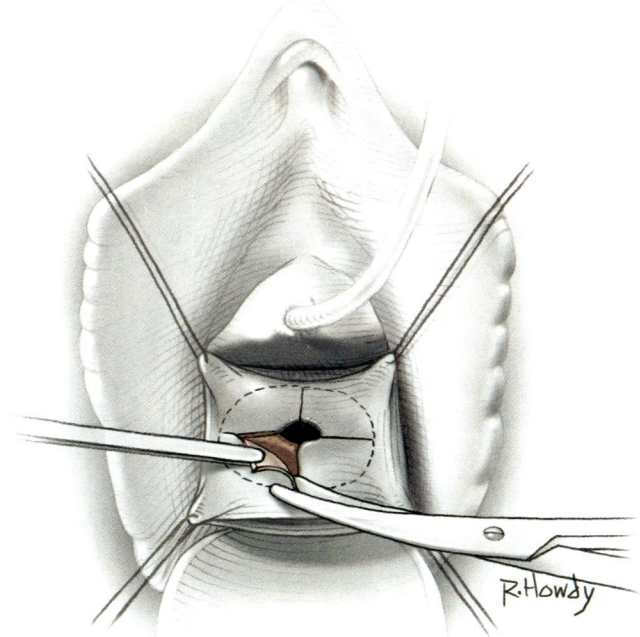

FIGURE 45-2.3 Vaginal epithelium incision.

Regardless of whether the tract is completely or partially excised, bladder and vaginal muscular layers on either side of the tract are approximated over the fistula site. For this, an interrupted or running suture line of 3-0 or 2-0 gauge delayed-absorbable sutures is created (Fig. 45-2.4). Beginning proximally and adding distally, sequential suture lines are layered (Fig. 45-2.5).

After muscular layers of the bladder and vaginal walls are closed, the vaginal epithelium is closed in a continuous running fashion using 3-0 or 2-0 gauge delayed-absorbable suture.

8 Cystoscopy. Cystoscopy is again performed to document ureteral patency and to inspect the incision site.

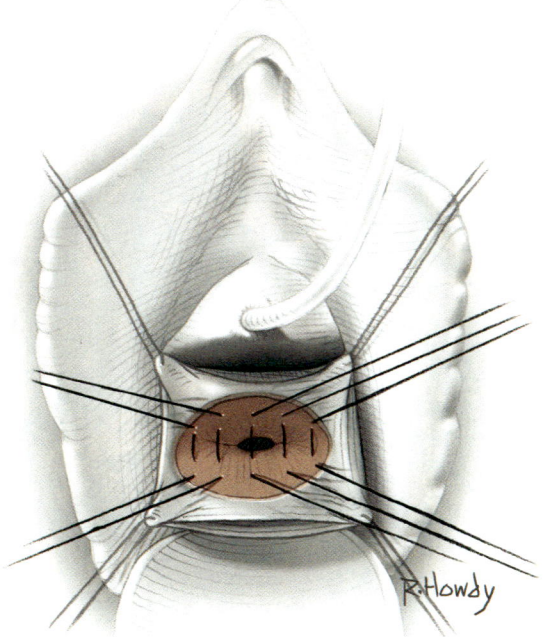

FIGURE 45-2.4 First-layer closure over fistula.

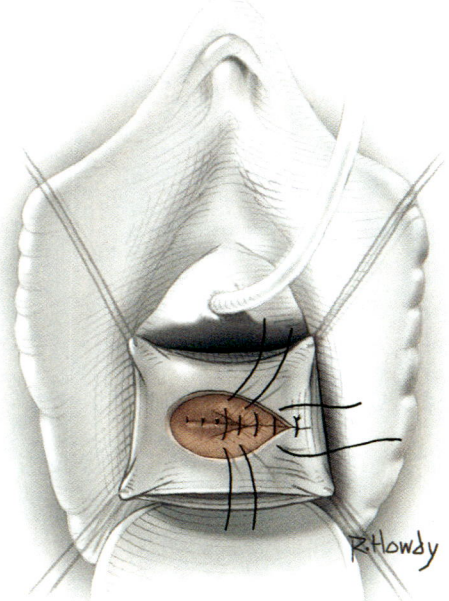

FIGURE 45-2.5 Second fibromuscular layer closure over fistula and vaginal epithelium reapproximation.

Surgical Steps— Abdominal Repair

❶ Anesthesia and Patient Positioning. In most cases, abdominal repair is performed under general anesthesia. The patient is placed in low lithotomy position within booted support stirrups. With the patient's thighs parallel to the ground and the legs separated, access to the vagina is maximized. The abdomen and vagina are surgically prepared.

❷ Cystoscopic Survey. This is first performed to delineate fistulous opening location and assess its proximity to ureteral orifices. Later, cystoscopy is repeated at different stages to document ureteral patency and assess bladder integrity. If ureters lie close to a fistula, ureteral catheters are placed. If needed, catheters later can be replaced by stents (p. 1078). A Foley catheter is inserted prior to abdominal incision.

❸ Abdominal Incision and Bladder Entry. A low transverse or vertical midline laparotomy incision is suitable. If mobilization of the omentum is anticipated, a vertical incision provides greater access to the upper abdomen. However, a Pfannenstiel incision usually is selected (Section 43-2, p. 933). Alternatively, this procedure can be performed endoscopically, preferably with robotic assistance by those with suitable skills.

After the peritoneum is entered, the abdomen is explored, bowel is packed from the operating field, and a self-retaining abdominal wall retractor is placed. The retropubic space is opened using the technique described on page 1091. Next, a vertical midline extraperitoneal incision is made into the bladder dome. Prior to this incision, filling the bladder helps avoid cutting the posterior bladder wall.

❹ Fistulous Tract Delineation and Excision. After cystotomy, the fistula and ureteral orifices are seen from within the bladder. From the dome, the cystotomy incision is extended over the top and then back of the bladder to reach the fistulous opening (Fig. 45-2.6). A lacrimal probe or pediatric catheter may be placed into the fistulous tract to delineate its course. The tract is then totally excised.

In contrast and less commonly, if a fistula tract lies close to the trigone, extension of the bladder incision to the fistulous tract may not be desired, as the resulting bladder defect would be extensive. Instead, the entire fistulous tract is directly excised using only the bladder dome incision. As a disadvantage to this approach, vascular flap interposition is limited, because the bladder wall is not significantly dissected off the vaginal wall.

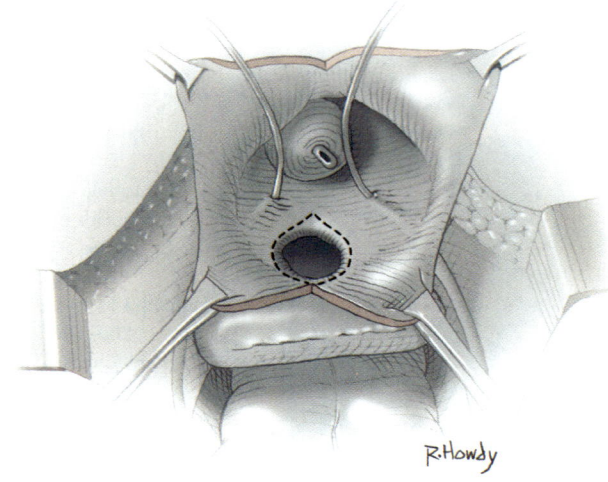

FIGURE 45-2.6 Bladder incision.

❺ Separating the Bladder and Vagina. In cases with bladder bisection, sharp dissection separates the vagina away from the bladder in the area of the fistula (Fig. 45-2.7). Scarring may be extensive, and sharp rather than blunt dissection is preferred. To assist, the rounded tip of an end-to-end anastomosis (EEA) sizer can be placed in the vagina to manipulate and accentuate the dissection plane (Fig. 46-21.4, p. 1225). The vagina is widely separated from the bladder to allow omentum or peritoneal flap placement between the two.

❻ Vaginal Closure. The vagina is closed in one or two layers with 2-0 gauge delayed-absorbable suture and running or interrupted stitches (Fig. 45-2.8). The EEA sizer or fingers within the vagina can accentuate the vaginotomy margins to aid closure.

❼ Bladder Closure. The entire bisecting bladder incision is closed in two or three layers using running sutures of 2-0 gauge delayed-absorbable suture (Fig. 45-2.9). As with the vaginal approach, after the first layer, the bladder is retrograde filled with at least 200 mL, and incision-line leaks are sought. If defects are noted, additional reinforcing sutures are placed to achieve a watertight repair. During bladder closure, each subsequent layer is imbricated such that the

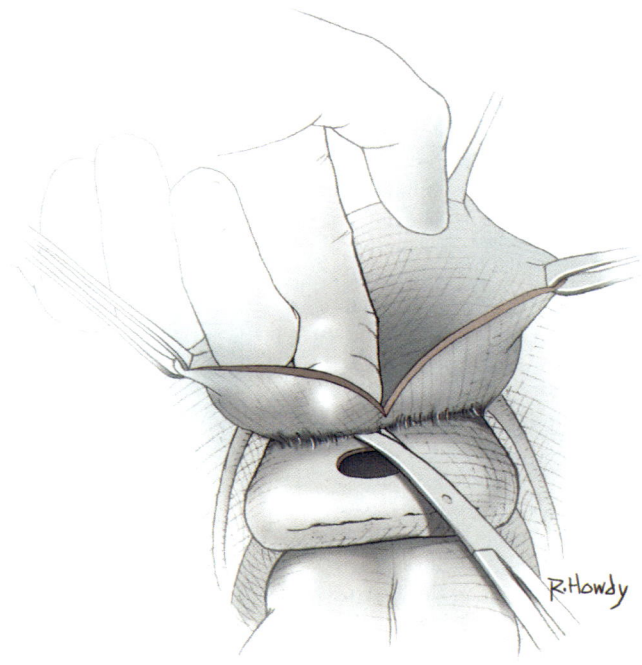

FIGURE 45-2.7 Separation of the bladder and vagina.

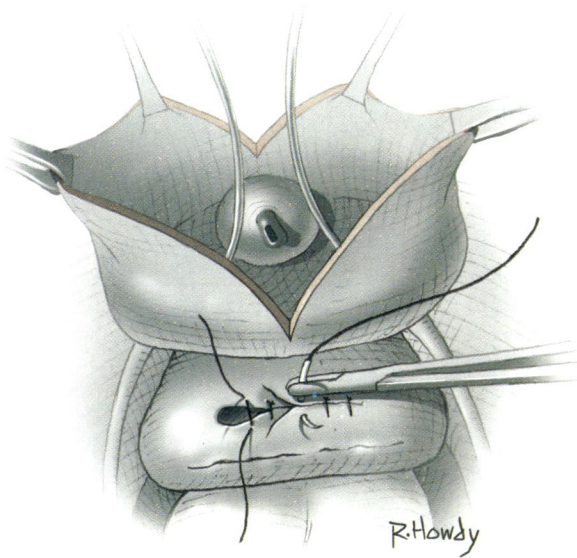

FIGURE 45-2.8 Vaginal closure.

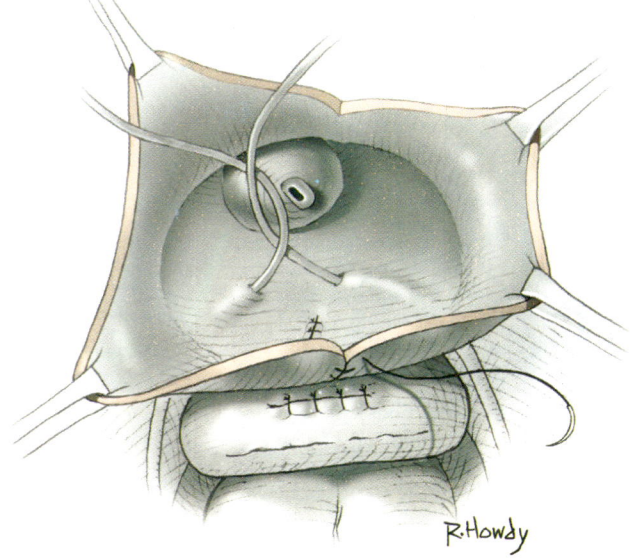

FIGURE 45-2.9 First-layer bladder closure.

preceding suture line is covered, and tension is released (Fig. 45-2.10).

If the bladder is not bisected and the fistulous tract is directly excised solely through the bladder dome cystotomy, the muscular wall of vagina is first repaired in one or two layers as in Step 6. Second, the bladder wall at the fistula excision site is closed in one or two layers using a running stitch of 2-0 gauge delayed-absorbable suture. Next, the bladder mucosa is reapproximated with a single-layer running stitch of 2-0 or 3-0 absorbable suture. Last, the entry bladder dome incision

is closed similarly, except the bladder mucosa is reapproximated first and followed by bladder wall closure in layers.

8 Omental or Peritoneal Interposition. Described in Section 46-9 (p. 1190), the omentum can be partially freed to create a J-flap. The omentum then is sutured to the anterior vaginal wall at a point distal to the fistula repair site. This covers the incision line to provide an intervening tissue layer between vagina and bladder. It also increases vascular flow to the area to aid

healing (Fig. 45-2.11). If the omentum cannot be sufficiently mobilized, the peritoneum, although less vascular, instead can be interposed to create a barrier layer.

9 Cystoscopy. Cystoscopy is again performed to document ureteral patency and inspect the incision site.

10 Incision Closure. The abdominal incision is closed as described in Chapter 43 (p. 934).

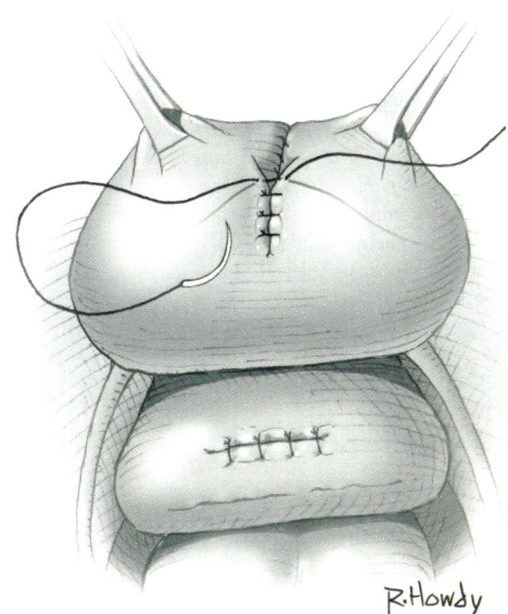

FIGURE 45-2.10 Second-layer bladder closure.

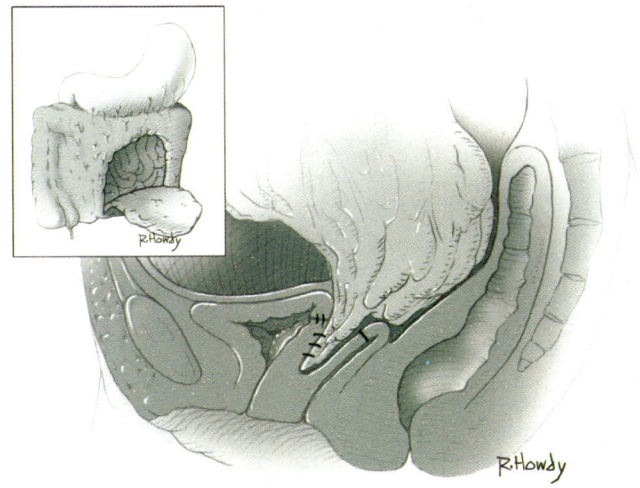

FIGURE 45-2.11 Omentum interposition.

POSTOPERATIVE

The bladder is drained postoperatively to prevent overdistention and suture disruption. Either transurethral or suprapubic catheter placement will ensure adequate drainage in the immediate postoperative period. At our institution, we generally continue catheterization for at least 2 weeks following vesicovaginal fistula repair. Antibiotic suppression is not required with this catheter use. Anticholinergic drugs listed in Table 23-5 (p. 531) may help associated bladder spasms.

URETERAL INJURY

The optimal ureteral repair method depends on location, extent, and mechanism of injury as well as patient condition and available surgical expertise. Removal of stitches that kink the ureter or management of a mild crush injury is feasible for most gynecologists. However, complex injuries that include transection, severe crush, or thermal trauma benefit from the expert assistance of a urogynecologist, gynecologic oncologist, or urologist. For those with suitable skills, repairs using an MIS approach are reasonable.

Repairs are ideally made intraoperatively at the primary surgery. With diagnosis delayed by more than a few days, surgical correction often is deferred for 6 to 8 weeks for inflammation and tissue edema to subside. However, some data suggest that immediate repairs following a delayed diagnosis do not worsen outcomes (Ahn, 2001). Importantly, if delayed correction is planned, renal function can be preserved by adequate drainage via retrograde stenting or percutaneous nephrostomy drainage with or without antegrade stenting.

PREOPERATIVE

Patient Evaluation

Discussed in Chapter 40 (p. 866), ureteral trauma is suspected if urine leaks into the operative field or if cystoscopy reveals absent or sluggish efflux from a ureteral orifice. If injury is suspected, the ureter first is identified through meticulous dissection. Retrograde passage of ureteral catheters can further help isolate the injury site. Specifically, if catheter resistance or dye extravasation is noted approximately 13 cm from the ureteric orifice, the injury likely lies near the pelvic brim. Resistance at 4 to 5 cm reflects injury during uterine vessels ligation and that at 1 to 2 cm indicates trauma near the vaginal cuff (Jackson, 2019).

Injuries, such as ureteral kinking, may be managed by simply removing the involved suture. Instead, ureteral ligation or small partial transection requires prolonged ureteral stenting. Last, complete transection or extensive crushing or thermal damage warrants either ureter reanastomosis or reimplantation. Specifically, proximal or midlength injuries generally are managed with ureteroureterostomy (end-to-end reanastomosis). For injuries in the lower-third, ureteroneocystostomy (ureter reimplantation) typically is preferred for several reasons. First, reimplantation requires less ureterolysis than reanastomosis and thus can preserve the neurovascular integrity in this vulnerable portion of the ureter. Second, the ureter is narrower at the ureterovesical junction, and end-to-end anastomosis here may increase stricture risks.

With reimplantation, an *extravesical approach* may be selected, and the ureter is reintroduced at the external surface of the bladder. In one subtype of this approach, the ureter directly enters the bladder, and urine does reflux from the bladder into the distal ureter. In another subtype, the ureter instead is tunneled a short distance within detrusor fibers before entering the bladder. This tunneling helps prevent urine reflux. That said, neither technique has a damaging effect on renal function or increases ureteral stenosis risk in adults (Pantuck, 2000; Stefanovic, 1991). Instead, reimplantation can be performed by an *intravesical approach,* which requires opening of the bladder to reintroduce the ureter. With all three techniques, the ureter is reimplanted on the posterior or anterior dome of the bladder and not on its lateral aspect. This helps avoid ureter kinking with bladder filling.

Consent

For a given primary surgery, patients are initially counseled regarding the relative risk of ureteral injury. In high-risk cases, further topics may include stenting or ureteral repair methods.

With a delayed diagnosis, surgical reconstruction procedures are vulnerable to anastomotic dehiscence and to ureteral stricture, fistula, or necrosis. Bleeding complications and surgical site infection are additional concerns (Selzman, 1996).

Patient Preparation

Immediately prior to primary surgery, intravenous antibiotic and VTE prophylaxis commonly are administered. Thus, if an injury is diagnosed intraoperatively, no further antibiotics are indicated solely for ureteral repair. However, antibiotics may be redosed for cases lasting >3 hours or those associated with >1500 mL blood loss.

For delayed repairs, the American College of Obstetricians and Gynecologists (2018b) recommends antibiotic prophylaxis prior to urogynecologic surgery, and appropriate broad-spectrum choices mirror those for hysterectomy (Table 39-8, p. 832). VTE prophylaxis is recommended (Table 39-10, p. 834). Bowel preparation generally is not required.

INTRAOPERATIVE

Surgical Steps—Extravesical Reimplantation

❶ **Patient Positioning.** Most of these injuries require abdominal inspection, either with laparotomy or laparoscopy. Thus, low lithotomy in booted support stirrups is preferred to permit concurrent cystoscopy, and patients are repositioned as needed. Instead, if the patient is supine for abdominal hysterectomy, cystotomy may replace cystoscopy for trigone inspection and retrograde ureteral catheter passage. Guided by the initial surgical route, additional abdominal or vaginal sterile preparation may be completed. A Foley catheter is placed or remains to allow retrograde bladder filling at certain steps.

For delayed repairs, the abdomen and vagina are surgically prepared. A Foley catheter is placed.

❷ **Intraabdominal Access.** For an MIS approach, additional ports may be needed for repair steps. Port placement to maximize instrument manipulation yet minimize trocar injury is outlined in Chapter 41 (p. 888). Alternatively, laparotomy using a low transverse or midline vertical incision is suitable, and steps are described in Chapter 43 (p. 930).

❸ **Ureter Mobilization.** To begin, the affected ureter is identified as it crosses either the common iliac bifurcation or the external iliac artery (Jackson, 2019). The ureter is circumferentially dissected from its connections to peritoneum and surrounding loose connective tissue. Dissection aims to provide sufficient mobility yet preserve the periadventitial tissue that encircles the ureter and that carries its blood supply. After initial freeing of the ureter, a vessel loop is placed around it to intermittently apply gentle traction during dissection. In total, dissection generally extends from the pelvic brim to a point just above the damaged segment.

❹ **Ureteral Transection.** Once fully mobilized, the ureter is sharply transected above the previously identified injury site. A segment from the distal damaged ureter may be resected and sent to pathology for injury confirmation.

The distal end then is tied, clipped, or coagulated (Fig. 45-2.12).

The proximal ureter's wall and lumen are inspected to ensure tissue that appears viable and free of stricture. Urine should easily flow from its lumen. If no flow is noted, a ureteral catheter can be threaded retrograde up into the proximal lumen to identify the true obstruction point. Here, the ureter is transected again, and lumen inspection is repeated. Ultimately, the satisfactory proximal end is brought to the intended cystotomy site in a bladder that is empty. This step confirms the ability to create a tension-free anastomosis. Usually, some degree of bladder mobilization is needed to achieve this goal.

❺ Bladder Mobilization. The bladder is freed from the abdominal wall and pubic bone attachments. First, the retroperitoneal space of the lower abdominal wall is entered by transverse incision of the peritoneum (see Fig. 45-2.12). With this, one or both obliterated umbilical arteries (medial umbilical ligaments) are transected above the bladder apex for optimal mobility. Once the retroperitoneum is entered, blunt dissection in the midline proceeds to the retropubic space. Further dissection within the retropubic space mirrors that described for the Burch colposuspension (p. 1091). With the bladder now mobile, the proximal end of the transected ureter is brought to the intended reimplantation site in the dome. If tension is still noted, a vesicopsoas hitch is required.

❻ Vesicopsoas Hitch. For this, the peritoneum overlying the psoas major muscle's anterior surface is opened at the level of common iliac artery bifurcation. Permanent sutures are placed in psoas minor muscle's tendon (see Fig. 45-2.12). This tendon may be anatomically absent, and sutures instead are placed through psoas major muscle fibers (Maldonado, 2014). For this, sutures ideally are anchored in the midline to avert puncture of the external iliac vessels and the femoral nerve, which border the psoas major muscle. With suturing, the small-caliber genitofemoral nerve, which courses atop the psoas major and minor muscles, is ideally identified and avoided. If the genitofemoral nerve is not clearly seen, sutures are placed vertically along the psoas muscle's long axis to avoid nerve entrapment. With suturing, the needle should travel no deeper than 3 to 4 mm to avoid the femoral nerve, which courses behind the psoas major muscle before moving to the muscle's lateral border.

These same sutures are placed through the cephalad portion of the posterior bladder wall on the reimplantation side. Stitches incorporate the bladder serosa and superficial detrusor muscle fibers but do not enter the bladder

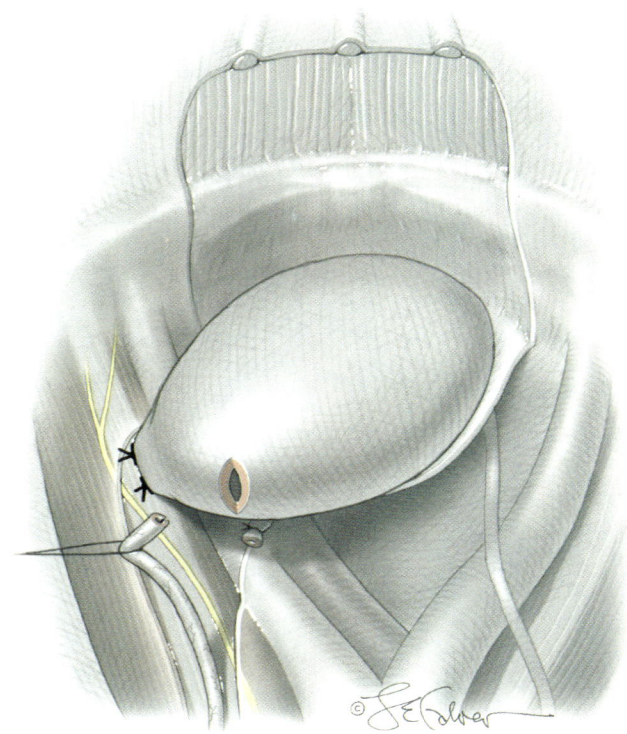

FIGURE 45-2.12 Extravesical reimplantation initial steps.

lumen. For this, retrograde bladder filling can better delineate the posterolateral wall. If a cystotomy has been made, sutures can be placed under direct visualization or with the aid of a surgeon's finger placed within the bladder.

❼ Boari Flap. In rare cases, the above steps still may fail to allow tension-free anastomosis, and a Boari flap can be created. Briefly, a proximal flap of bladder on the affected side is mobilized and fashioned into a funneled tip. This funneling bridges the gap between the bladder and the ureter. Importantly, blood supply to the flap, which stems from the superior vesical arteries, must be preserved. Again to help relieve suture-line tension, the flap usually is sutured to the psoas muscle as described in the last section.

❽ Ureteral Reimplantation. To begin, the bladder is retrograde filled with approximately 250 mL of water. For the direct technique, an approximately 1-cm full-thickness cystotomy is made with scalpel or endoscopic scissors coupled with monopolar cutting energy (Fig. 45-2.13). Bleeding vessels within the detrusor muscle are coagulated as encountered.

For the tunneling technique, a 3-cm incision is made sharply into the detrusor muscle but not the mucosa. In the most cephalad part of this incision, the detrusor muscle is carefully dissected off the mucosa. This undermining dissection extends outward

laterally from the original incision to create a loosened detrusor muscle layer. This layer is later reapproximated over the tunneled part of the ureter, and the layer's slight laxity avoids ureteral lumen obstruction. Next, a 1-cm incision is made sharply through the distal part of bladder mucosa within the original tunnel incision (Fig. 45-2.14A). This serves as the anastomosis site.

❾ Ureter Spatulation. The term *spatulation* describes a cut along the ureter's long axis. This incision ultimately allows creation of a new ureteral orifice with a diameter wider than the original one to help avert significant orifice stricture during healing.

To begin, a fine suture can be placed through the ureter's outer adventitial layer to aid manipulation and avoid forceps trauma. Beginning at its lumen, the ureter is cut longitudinally 1 cm on its posterior surface by fine scissors.

❿ Anastomosis Initiation. The posterior spatulated end of the ureter is reapproximated to the bladder defect to ensure mucosa-to-mucosa alignment between the bladder and ureter. All suture knots ideally remain outside the lumen or mucosal surfaces to prevent knot disruption during stent placement. This may also prevent mineral encrustation within the ureter's narrow lumen during healing. For repair, 4-0 gauge delayed-absorbable suture is suitable. If available, we use two differently

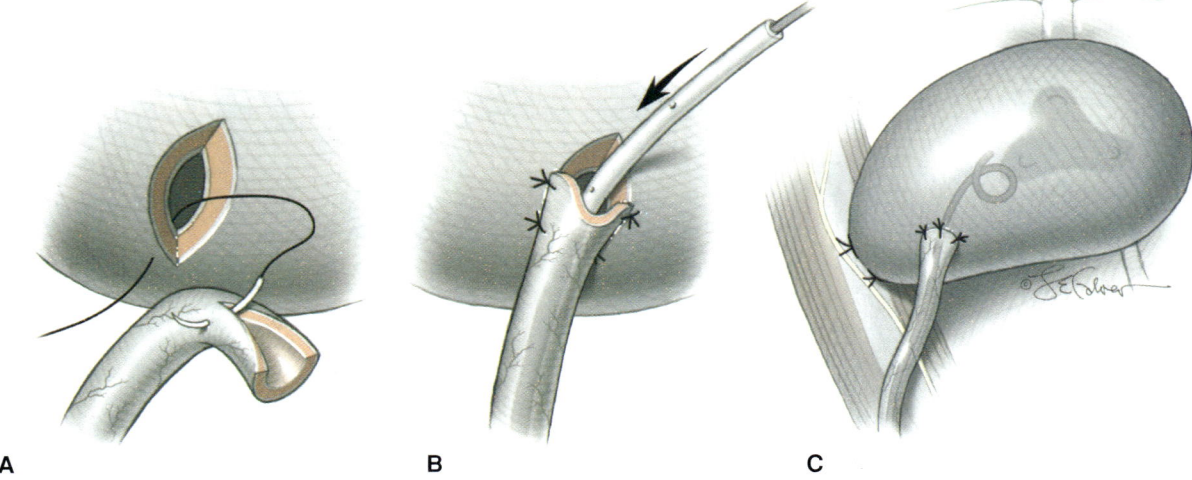

FIGURE 45-2.13 **A.** Direct extravesical reimplantation. **B.** Stent placement. **C.** Correct stent positioning.

colored sutures, such as dyed and undyed. This avoids suture tangling at the posterior part of the repair, especially in MIS cases.

The first suture is placed adjacent to the 6 o'clock position on the cystotomy site (see Fig. 45-2.13A and 45-2.14A). On the bladder, the needle passes out to in (detrusor to mucosa). The suture then traverses the apex of the V-shaped spatulation. Here, the needle path is in to out (ureteral mucosa to muscle/adventitia). This pathway ensures that knots remain outside both bladder and ureteral lumens.

These steps are repeated with a second suture, preferably of a different color. This suture is placed 1 to 2 mm from the prior one around both the cystotomy site and spatulation apex. Again, the same needle orientation ensures extraluminal knots. These interrupted sutures continue circumferentially around the reimplantation orifice until the 3 and 9 o'clock positions around the cystotomy are reached. At this time, the stent is placed over a guide wire (see Fig. 45-2.13B).

⑪ **Stent Placement.** Generally, a 6F, 22- or 24-cm stent is selected for most cases. Given that several centimeters of ureter length is lost with reimplantation, a longer stent rarely is needed. The appropriate length required may be checked by passing a 5F whistle-tip ureteral catheter prior to stent placement. Steps to placement are fully delineated in Section 45-1 (p. 1078).

⑫ **Anastomosis Completion.** With the stent in place, the remaining circumference of the anastomosis is closed, as was done in Step 10 (see Fig. 45-2.13C). To test repair integrity, the bladder is retrograde filled through a Foley catheter with approximately 250 mL of water or saline. If leaks are noted, additional sutures are placed around the anastomosis until a watertight repair is confirmed.

⑬ **Tunnel Closure.** With the tunneling technique, the detrusor muscle is now reapproximated over the tunneled part of the

ureter using 3-0 gauge delayed-absorbable interrupted sutures (see Fig. 45-2.14B).

⑭ **Drains.** A Jackson Pratt or Blake drain is typically placed near the repair site to measure postoperative output. The drain is removed once output falls below 50 mL in 24 hours. High output of clear fluid suggests an anastomotic leak or repair breakdown and warrants further evaluation with CT urography.

⑮ **Stent Positioning.** Prior to closing the abdominal incision, anteroposterior abdominal radiographs are obtained to ensure proper positioning of stent loops into the renal pelvis and bladder, respectively. If available, fluoroscopy is a suitable surrogate.

Surgical Steps— Intravesical Ureteral Reimplantation

❶ **Cystotomy.** Intravesical repairs typically involve a modified tunneling technique to prevent reflux (Fig. 45-2.15). The ureter and bladder are mobilized as in Steps 3 and 5 of the last section. A large, several-centimeter cystotomy is made sharply in the retropubic part of the dome to enter the bladder.

❷ **Ureteral Tunneling.** The site for ureteral anastomosis usually is selected at a spot medial and superior to the native ureteric orifice. However, if ureteral length and repair tension are concerns, the site is moved closer to the dome.

For this site, a 1-cm longitudinal incision is made sharply inside the bladder and through its mucosa. A 3- to 4-cm tunnel is created between the mucosa and detrusor muscle and progresses cephalad by

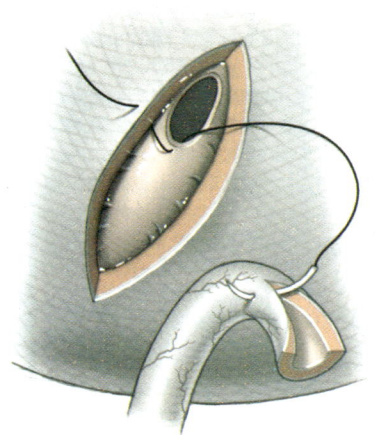
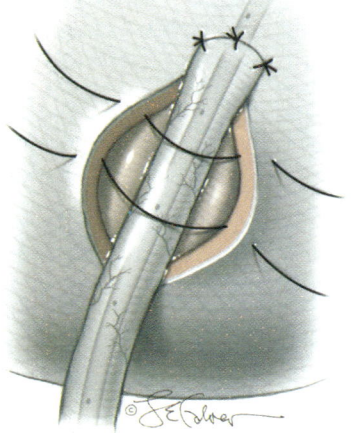

FIGURE 45-2.14 **A.** Tunneling extravesical reimplantation. **B.** Tunnel closure.

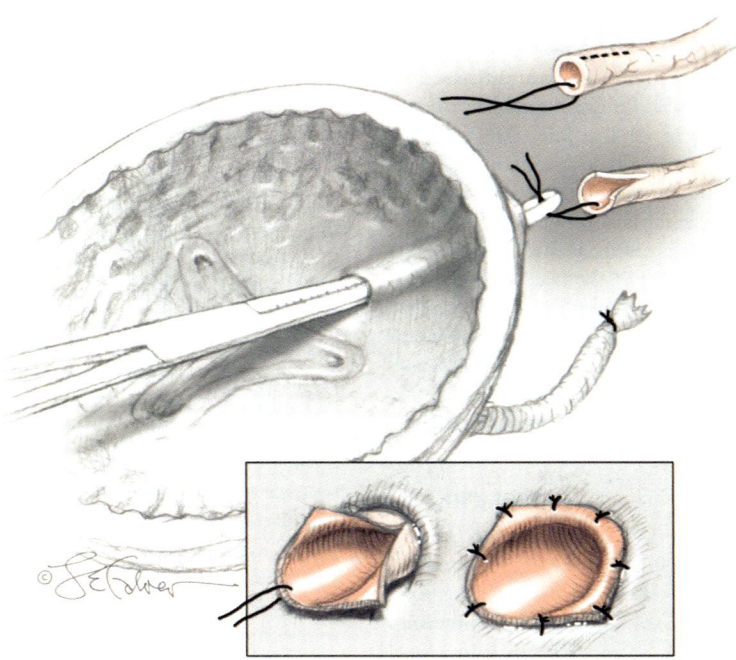

FIGURE 45-2.15 Intravesical reimplantation. (From Gilstrap, 2017, with permission.)

gently opening and closing of Pean clamp tips. This undermining dissection extends outward laterally from the original incision to create a loosened detrusor muscle layer. This layer's slight laxity avoids ureteral lumen obstruction.

Starting externally, the detrusor muscle over the opened clamp tip then is sharply incised, and the clamp tips are thereby exteriorized (see Fig. 45-2.15). The clamp is kept within the tunnel with tips outside the bladder in preparation for ureter passage.

❸ **Ureter Spatulation.** To create a sufficiently wide new orifice, the ureter is widely spatulated on its anterior surface, as described in Step 9 of Extravesical Reimplantation (p. 1087).

The suture ends are grasped by the Pean clamp tips, and ureter is passed through the tunnel. Once within the bladder, the ureter's mucosa is circumferentially reapproximated to the bladder mucosa to create a mucosal-mucosal alignment (see Fig. 45-2.15, Inset). With each interrupted stitch of 3-0 or 4-0 gauge delayed-absorbable suture, some detrusor muscle is incorporated to better anchor each stitch.

Outside the bladder, additional interrupted sutures can be placed through the bladder serosa and ureter's adventitial layer to reinforce and decrease tension on the mucosal repair. Ureteral kinking or narrowing ideally is avoided with these sutures. A stent then is placed and extends between the bladder and renal pelvis, as described in Section 45-1 (p. 1078).

❹ **Cystotomy Repair.** The retropubic cystotomy is closed in layers (p. 1081).

Surgical Steps— Ureteroureterostomy

❶ **Indication.** For 1- to 3-cm injuries in the ureter's midlength, which spans between pelvic brim and cardinal ligament, end-to-end reanastomosis is an ideal option in experienced hands. Compared with reimplantation, benefits of this technique include preservation of bladder integrity and the ureter's natural antireflux mechanism (Paick, 2006).

❷ **Ureter Mobilization.** To begin, the affected ureter is freed from the surround connective tissue and peritoneum. Importantly, the periadventitial tissue that surrounds the ureter and carries its blood supply is preserved. Dissection usually extends several centimeters above and below the damaged site. Long segments may require freeing the entire ureteral length.

❸ **Ureter Resection.** Once freed, the injured portion is transected. Remaining proximal and distal ends are further cut or debrided until healthy vascular tissue is reached. The damaged ureter segment can be sent for pathologic analysis.

❹ **Ureter Spatulation.** To avoid anastomotic stricture, the proximal and distal ureter ends are spatulated, typically on opposite sides of ureter to increase lumen diameter. The length of the spatulation approximates 1 cm (Fig. 45-2.16A).

❺ **Anastomosis Construction.** To join the two ends, several interrupted stitches of 4-0 or 5-0 gauge delayed-absorbable suture are placed across the posterior wall of the constructed anastomosis (see Fig. 45-2.16B). The first suture is passed through the apex of the posteriorly spatulated proximal ureter.

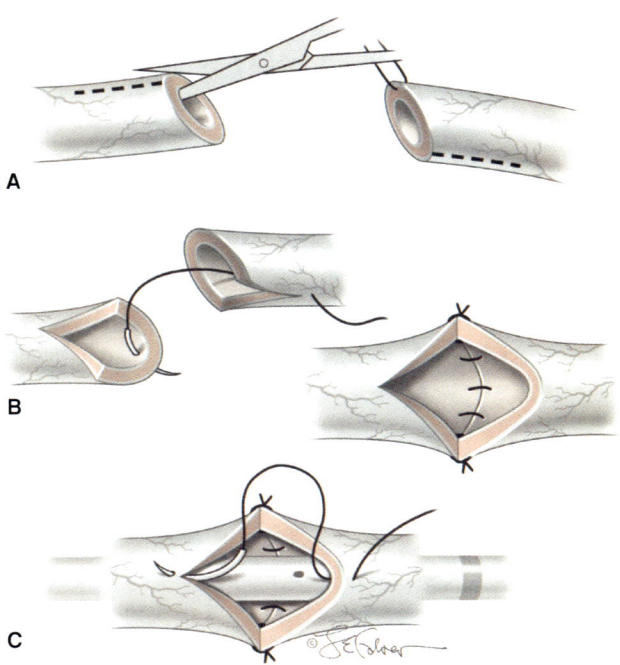

FIGURE 45-2.16 A. Ureteral spatulation. **B.** Posterior wall suturing. **C.** Anterior wall suturing over ureteral stent.

The needle travels from the adventitia toward the mucosa. It then passes through the midline of the distal ureter's posterior wall, which is not spatulated. Here, it travels from the mucosa to adventitia. The suture then is tied. This practice ensures mucosa-to-mucosa alignment between the two ureter ends and places suture knots outside the lumen. An additional adjacent two to three sutures are placed similarly through the posterior walls of ureter ends to close the posterior wall. This posterior union leaves an anterior window to view the stent as it traverses the anastomosis site.

❻ Stent Placement. A ureteral catheter is introduced cystoscopically and advances to the anastomosis site. The role of a catheter aids ultimate stent placement and is described in Section 45-1 (p. 1078). At the anastomosis site, the catheter is viewed abdominally and guided through the anastomosis. A guide wire then is introduced cystoscopically through the ureteral catheter up into the renal pelvis. With the wire held in place, the catheter is removed, and it is gently exchanged with a 6F or 7F double-J stent.

❼ Anastomosis Closure. The anterior portion of the anastomosis is then completed over the stented ureter (see Fig. 45-2.16C. Suturing mirrors that in Step 5. If possible, the anastomosis site is covered with peritoneum or omentum, and an abdominal or retroperitoneal drain typically is placed. Prior to closing surgical incisions, anteroposterior abdominal radiographs are obtained to ensure proper positioning of stent coils within the renal pelvis and bladder, respectively. If available, fluoroscopy is a suitable surrogate.

POSTOPERATIVE

Foley Catheter and Stent Duration

For reimplantation, Foley catheter bladder drainage continues for 7 to 14 days. This reduces retrograde urine reflux through the anastomosis and stented kidney during the initial healing. For reanastomosis surgery, the Foley instead is removed on the first postoperative day.

No consensus guides ureteral stent removal. In general, at 6 to 8 weeks postrepair, these are removed in the office with cystoscopic guidance. Associated stent symptoms and prophylaxis are described in Section 45-1 (p. 1078).

Surveillance Imaging

No consensus directs appropriate testing following stent removal after repair. A primary concern is ureteral stricture and subsequent renal compromise. Early diagnosis may avoid this renal loss. Accordingly, CT urography is performed at 2 to 4 weeks after stent removal and then again at 3 to 4 months and at one year. If found, strictures are increasingly being treated with ureteral dilation by endourologists and/or interventional radiologists. Less frequently, ureteral strictures refractory to above management can be treated with reimplantation.

Instead, if imaging is normal at the year mark, annual renal sonography is recommended for up to 3 years to exclude delayed stricture formation. However, asymptomatic patients often are lost to follow-up.

The role of serum creatinine as a surrogate marker of renal function in unilateral injuries is unclear. With severe hydronephrosis prior to ureteral repair or with concern for declining renal function, a nuclear medicine Lasix renal scan can assess function of the ipsilateral kidney.

45-3

Burch Colposuspension

Abdominal antiincontinence procedures attempt to correct stress urinary incontinence (SUI) by stabilizing the anterior vaginal wall and urethrovesical junction in a retropubic location. Specifically, the Burch procedure, also known as *retropubic urethropexy*, uses the strength of the pectineal ligament (Cooper ligament) to stabilize the anterior vaginal wall and anchor the wall to the skeletal framework of the pelvis (Fig. 38-24, p. 813). This is performed in the retropubic space.

The Burch colposuspension traditionally has been performed through a low transverse abdominal incision (Section 43-2, p. 933). Instead, laparoscopic approaches use suture to affix the paravaginal tissues to Cooper ligament (Ankardal, 2004; Zullo, 2004). Compared with open Burch colposuspension, a laparoscopic approach offers similar postoperative rates of subjective cure, despite some evidence for poorer objective outcomes (Carey, 2006; Dean, 2017). Safety and longer-term efficacy rates will further define its role. Data are few regarding robotic Burch colposuspension outcomes.

Recent surgical mesh concerns have led to resurgence of Burch colposuspension. However, with greater use of midurethral slings, pelvic surgeons have grown increasingly less familiar with the three-dimensional anatomy of the retropubic space.

PREOPERATIVE

Patient Evaluation

Prior to surgery, patients undergo complete urogynecologic evaluation. Although not required for uncomplicated demonstrable SUI, urodynamic testing can help differentiate stress and urgency urinary incontinence and assess bladder capacity and voiding patterns (Chap. 23, p. 524). Instead, some use physical examination findings such as a positive supine cough stress test, which is highly predictive of intrinsic urethral dysfunction (Lobel, 1996). Limited data suggest that patients with evidence of intrinsic sphincteric deficiency have better continence outcomes with retropubic midurethral slings or pubovaginal slings with autologous fascia (Koonings, 1990; Sand, 1987).

Many women with SUI may have associated pelvic organ prolapse. Consequently, other indicated pelvic reconstructive surgeries commonly accompany Burch colposuspension. A required hysterectomy does not appear to improve or worsen Burch procedure success rates (Bai, 2004; Meltomaa, 2001).

Consent

For most women with SUI, Burch colposuspension offers a safe, effective long-term treatment for incontinence. In one systematic review, overall continence rates ranged from 85 to 90 percent at 1 year and declined to 70 percent by 5 years (Lapitan, 2017). Surgical risks compare similarly with other surgeries for SUI (Green, 2005). Intraoperative complications are rare and may include ureteral injury, bladder or urethral perforation, and hemorrhage (Galloway, 1987; Ladwig, 2004).

Complications following surgery, however, are not uncommon and can include urinary tract or wound infection, voiding dysfunction, de novo urinary urgency, and pelvic organ prolapse—primarily enterocele formation (Alcalay, 1995; Demirci, 2000, 2001; Norton, 2006). However, colposuspension performed via laparotomy is associated with a lower risk of voiding dysfunction compared with pubovaginal sling surgery (Lapitan, 2017). Overcorrection of the urethrovesical angle is implicated in these late urinary and prolapse complications.

Patient Preparation

The American College of Obstetricians and Gynecologists (2018b) recommends antibiotic prophylaxis prior to urogynecologic surgery, and appropriate choices mirror those for hysterectomy (Table 39-8, p. 832). For all patients undergoing major gynecologic surgery, thromboprophylaxis also is recommended (Table 39-10, p. 834). Bowel preparation is based on surgeon preference and on other planned surgeries.

INTRAOPERATIVE

Surgical Steps

❶ Anesthesia and Patient Positioning. Burch colposuspension may be performed under general or regional anesthesia as a day-surgery procedure, unless other concurrent surgeries dictate longer stays. The patient is placed in low lithotomy position with legs in booted support stirrups. The abdomen and vagina are surgically prepared, and a Foley catheter is inserted.

For laparoscopic or robotic approaches, endoscopic ports are positioned as for laparoscopic hysterectomy (Chap. 44, p. 1044). At least one 8- to 10-mm lower abdominal port is needed for suture introduction.

❷ Abdominal Incision. A Pfannenstiel incision is performed, and surgery in the retropubic space is easier if the incision is placed low and approximately 2 cm above the symphysis pubis' upper border. If hysterectomy, culdoplasty, or other intraperitoneal procedure is planned, the peritoneum is entered and concurrent surgery completed prior to colposuspension. If the procedure is done in isolation, the anterior abdominal wall fascia and then transversalis fascia are incised, but entry into the peritoneal cavity is not required to reach the retropubic space.

❸ Retropubic Space Entry. Between the lower anterior abdominal wall peritoneum and pubic bones lies an avascular plane. To enter this retropubic space, the fingers of one hand gently dissect along the cephalad surface of the pubic bones. Alternatively, gentle sponge dissection can be used to open this space (Fig. 45-3.1). Loose areolar and fatty tissues fill this space and easily separate from the bone and the medial surfaces of levator ani muscle and obturator internus muscle fascia. However, entry into the wrong tissue plane risks bleeding and bladder injury. As an aid, direct exposure of the symphysis pubis, pectineal line of the pubis, and inner surface of the pubic bones as well as visualization of the obturator internus and levator ani muscles ensures correct entry.

In those with prior surgery, sharp dissection is generally required. Dissection begins with the curved tips of Metzenbaum scissors placed directly on the pubic bone close to the pectineal line and progresses dorsally until the space is exposed.

To avoid neurovascular injuries, dissection ideally is contained between the 10 and 2 o'clock positions relative to the symphysis pubis' midline. The obturator canal is identified early to avoid the obturator vessels and nerves traversing there. This canal is typically found 1.5 to 2.5 cm below the upper border of the pectineal ligament and approximately 5 to 7 cm from the midline of the upper border of the symphysis pubis (Drewes, 2005). Accessory obturator vessels arise from external iliac or inferior epigastric vessels and pass over the pectineal ligament also to enter the obturator canal. These can be lacerated during pronounced retraction to expose the pectineal ligament. As further orientation, the external iliac vein is found approximately 8 cm lateral to the upper border of the pectineal ligament, a short distance lateral to the level of obturator canal. Last, midline dissection over the urethra is limited to avoid laceration of the dorsal vein of the clitoris. In the midline, this vessel enters the retropubic space from the perineum by passing under the pubic arch.

❹ Paraurethral Tissue Exposure. In the retropubic space, blunt dissection of its loose tissue is coupled with sharp division

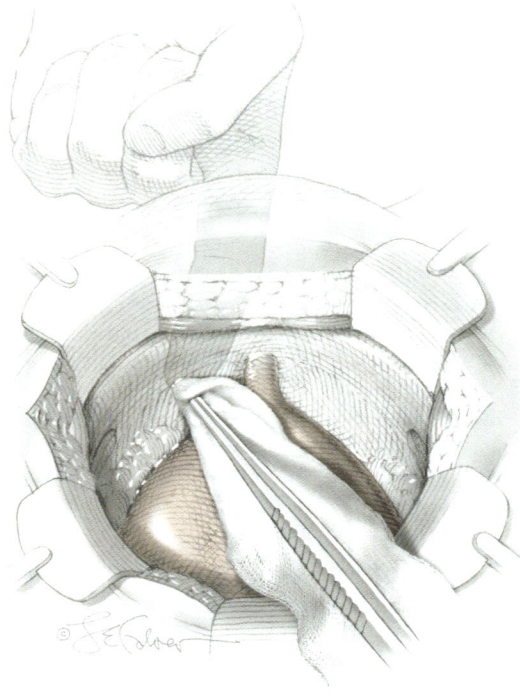

FIGURE 45-3.1 Entry into the retropubic space.

of connective tissue septa to expose the paraurethral tissue. Specifically, once the arcus tendineus fascia pelvis (ATFP) is identified on the lateral pelvic wall, gentle blunt dissection from this level toward the urethra further exposes the glistening white paraurethral tissues. If necessary, a surgeon can use a Kittner (peanut) sponge or gauze sponge stick. Importantly, to protect the delicate urethral musculature, this dissection remains lateral to the urethra.

Aggressive dissection or Burch sutures may lacerate vessels within the vesical venous plexus (plexus of Santorini) and risk significant bleeding (Fig. 38-24, p. 813). This is easily controlled with upward pressure from vaginally placed fingers. Identified vessels can be ligated.

❺ Identification of the Urethrovesical Junction. This step aids correct suture placement. The index or middle finger of the surgeon's nondominant hand is placed intravaginally at the vagina's lower length and just behind the pubic bone. To isolate the urethrovesical junction, the surgeon's vaginal hand positions the Foley catheter balloon at the bladder neck. Undue tension on the Foley catheter is avoided as this can drag the bladder into the operative field and increase the risk of sutures entering the bladder.

❻ Suture Placement. For exposure, the surgeon's vaginal finger presses upward, and

the bladder neck is gently displaced by an assistant to the contralateral side by a narrow abdominal retractor.

The more distal suture is placed first to aid later placement of the more proximal suture at the bladder neck. A double-armed suture of 2-0 gauge nonabsorbable material is placed lateral to the proximal third of the urethra—approximately 1 cm distal to the urethrovesical junction. The spot also should

lie 1.5 cm lateral to the urethral wall and thus just medial to the ATFP.

Each suture passes through the paraurethral connective tissue and anterior vaginal wall muscularis but excludes the epithelium. The surgeon's vaginal finger ensures the needle has not penetrated the vaginal lumen. The needle point is directed toward the vaginal finger, and a thimble may help avoid needlestick injury.

We pass these sutures in a helical or double-bite fashion to secure a greater surface area. Sutures are not tied unless significant bleeding is encountered. This practice may reduce entrapment of autonomic nerve fibers that course within the paravaginal tissue.

Both ends of the double-armed suture then are placed through their nearest point of the ipsilateral pectineal ligament. Thus, each stitch is positioned 4 to 5 mm apart. Slack is removed from the suture, and a knot is tied above the ligament. With knot securing, suture bridges are expected, and these stabilize but do not significantly elevate the anterior vaginal wall and urethrovesical junction. The vaginal wall ideally is stabilized just above the level of the distal portion of the ATFP and not significantly higher. Greater bladder neck elevation risks postoperative voiding dysfunction.

A second suture then is placed similarly but at a site 1.5 to 2 cm lateral to the urethrovesical junction. The same steps are repeated on the opposite side of the urethra with care to maintain suture symmetry (Fig. 45-3.2).

❼ Cystoscopy. Following suture ligation, cystoscopy is performed. This allows identification and removal of any errant sutures that may traverse the bladder or urethral mucosa.

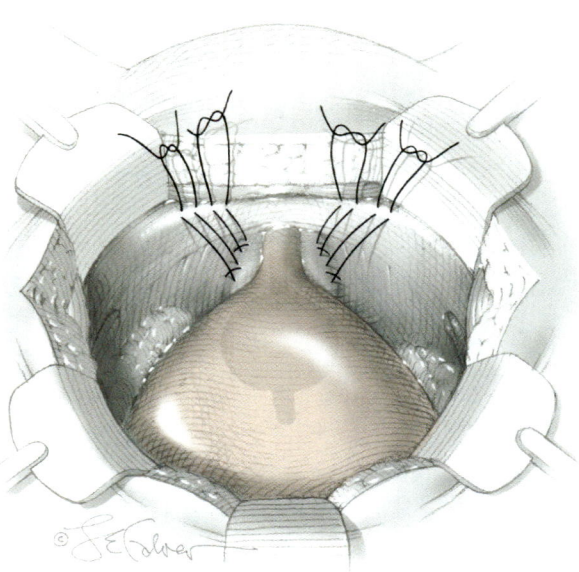

FIGURE 45-3.2 Suture placement.

Moreover, it enables a surgeon to inspect the ureteral orifices and document efflux.

❽ Catheterization. After the colposuspension, the Foley catheter may remain to drain the bladder. Alternatively, a suprapubic catheter may be placed. Investigators comparing the two have found no differences in anti-incontinence procedure success rates, length of hospitalization, or rates of infection.

However, urethral drainage was linked with a shorter duration of catheterization (Dunn, 2005; Theofrastous, 2002).

❾ Incision Closure. The anterior abdominal wall peritoneum is generally closed to prevent displacement of small bowel into the retropubic space. The remaining abdominal wall incision is closed as described in Section 43-2 (p. 934).

POSTOPERATIVE

In general, recovery follows that associated with laparotomy or laparoscopic procedures. Concurrent surgeries and incision size or number are contributing factors. A voiding trial is performed prior to hospital discharge (Chap. 42, p. 919).

45-4

Retropubic Midurethral Sling

Midurethral sling (MUS) operations are a recognized MIS option for SUI. These surgeries pass a small strip of tape mesh through either the retropubic or obturator space.

The original retropubic bottom-to-top approach or tension-free vaginal tape (TVT) procedure is the most commonly performed operation worldwide for SUI. Cure rates up to 17 years approximate 80 percent (Holmgren, 2005; Nilsson, 2013; Song, 2009). Modifications of the TVT have yielded the TOT (transobturator tape), TVT-O (tension-free vaginal tape obturator), and single-incision midurethral slings ("mini-slings"). All are part of the MUS group and are based on the concept that midurethral support is vital to continence.

The TVT procedure is indicated for SUI that is secondary to urethral hypermobility or intrinsic sphincteric deficiency (Chap. 23, p. 519). It is used for primary cases and for women with prior antiincontinence procedures. For subjective cure, one systematic review found that a bottom-to-top route is more effective than a top-to-bottom route during tape placement (Ford, 2017).

During TVT, a permanent sling material is placed underneath the midurethra, traverses the periurethral tissue, passes behind the pubic bone through the retropubic space, and exits through the anterior abdominal wall. Once positioned, tissue ingrowth ultimately holds the mesh in place. During placement, the TVT needle is directed blindly through the retropubic space and can lacerate vessels there to create significant bleeding. A modification of the TVT, the TOT was developed to avoid hemorrhage in this space and to decrease bladder and bowel perforation risks (p. 1097). However, the TVT remains the primary standard operation for SUI.

The TVT device consists of a permanent polypropylene mesh covered with a plastic sheath that is removed after the mesh is positioned. The plastic sheath is believed to prevent bacterial contamination of the mesh as it passes through the vagina and to protect the mesh from being damaged during passage. Once these plastic sheaths are removed, the mesh remains fixed in position. During placement, the mesh is attached to two disposable metal needles that are connected to a reusable metal introducer. A metal catheter guide is used to displace the urethra away from the needle during the procedure.

PREOPERATIVE

Patient Evaluation

Prior to TVT procedures, SUI is diagnosed as described in Chapter 23 (p. 521). Importantly, in some women, SUI can be occult and masked by pelvic organ prolapse that kinks and partially obstructs the urethra. Accordingly, prolapse replacement to reestablish more normal anatomy during urodynamic testing may help unmask this potential SUI. Caution also is exercised in patients who are *Valsalva voiders*. Affected women void with abdominal straining rather than with detrusor contraction and urethral relaxation. Most incontinence procedures prevent leakage by closing the urethra during cough or Valsalva maneuver. Therefore, these surgeries, when performed in women who rely on the Valsalva maneuver to urinate, will often result in voiding dysfunction. This tenet applies to all MUS procedures.

Consent

The counseling process for TVT includes an honest discussion of outcomes. At best, the 5-year cure rate is 85 percent, and an additional 10 percent is considered significantly improved. However, some patients will develop postoperative urgency urinary incontinence or bothersome voiding dysfunction. Additionally, with time and aging, incontinence may recur secondary to factors not related to urethral support.

As for all antiincontinence procedures, prior to surgery, the patient is provided surgical success rates from the literature and those of the individual surgeon. Moreover, the definition of "outcome success" varies from woman to woman. For example, in a patient with severe incontinence and 20 leakage episodes per day, improvement to one leakage episode every other day would be considered successful. However, in a woman with rare leakage, it may be more difficult to achieve an outcome considered satisfactory. Therefore, the patient's expectations are discussed prior to surgery.

Surgical complications can include hemorrhage, bladder perforation, and rarely, bowel injury. Major vessels are injured in <1 percent of cases.

After surgery, short-term, incomplete bladder emptying may require Foley catheter drainage or intermittent self-catheterization for several days. A small percentage of patients will develop long-term urinary retention that warrants reoperation for tape division or excision (p. 1103). In these women, continence rates decline. The TVT procedure is associated with a learning curve, and urinary retention rates drop as the number of cases a physician performs accrues.

Vaginal mesh erosion may develop as an early or late complication. This is managed by simple excision of the piece of eroding

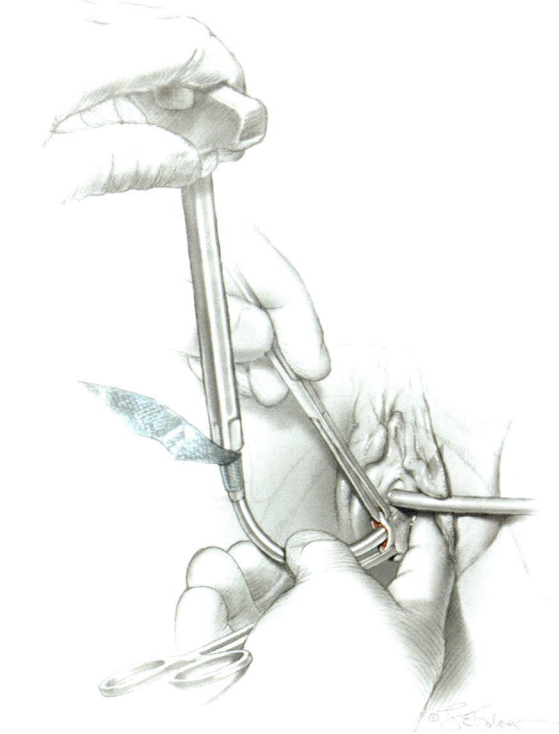

FIGURE 45-4.1 Needle placed through periurethral tunnel.

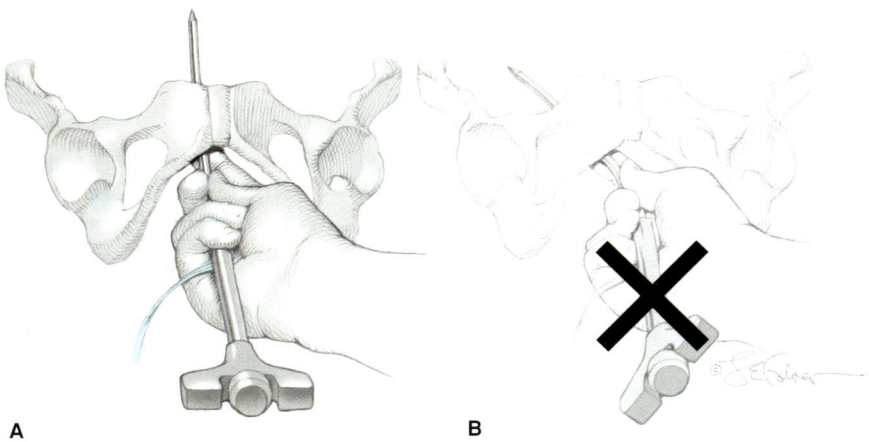

A

B

FIGURE 45-4.2 Correct and incorrect introducer positioning. **A.** Dark drawing, correct position. The tip is directed in the midline to a position behind the pubic bone. The handle is parallel to the ground. **B.** Lighter drawing, incorrect position. The tip is directed laterally.

tape and vaginal wall revision. Of note, the American Urogynecologic Society (2018) and U.S. Food and Drug Administration (FDA) (2019) consider the mesh used for this sling to be safe and effective.

Patient Preparation

The American College of Obstetricians and Gynecologists (2018b) recommends antibiotic prophylaxis prior to urogynecologic procedures, and appropriate choices mirror those for hysterectomy (Table 39-8, p. 832). For all patients undergoing major gynecologic surgery, thromboprophylaxis is recommended (Table 39-10, p. 834). Bowel preparation is based on surgeon preference and on other planned surgeries.

INTRAOPERATIVE

Surgical Steps

❶ **Anesthesia and Patient Positioning.** The procedure was initially described as an ambulatory surgical procedure performed under local anesthesia. However, it can also be performed with regional or general anesthesia. If performed solely, TVT in most cases is a day-surgery operation. The procedure is performed in standard lithotomy position. The vagina and lower abdomen are surgically prepared, and an 18F Foley catheter, which allows passage of a rigid catheter guide, is inserted to assist in deflection of the urethra during needle passage.

❷ **Abdominal Incisions.** Two 0.5-cm skin incisions are made at the level of the upper border of the symphysis pubis, and each lies no further than 2 cm from the midline. More lateral placement risks ilioinguinal nerve injury (Geis, 2002).

❸ **Vaginal Incisions.** A midline incision is made sharply in the vaginal epithelium and superficial vaginal muscularis beginning 1 cm proximal to the external urethral opening and is extended 1.5 to 2 cm cephalad. Allis clamps are placed on the edges of the vaginal incision for traction. Using Metzenbaum scissors, bilateral periurethral tunnels are created beneath the vaginal epithelium on either side of the urethra. These tunnels extend several centimeters toward

the inferior pubic rami to allow placement of the TVT needle just behind the pubic bone.

❹ **Catheter-Guide Placement.** A rigid guide is placed through the 18F Foley catheter. During TVT needle passage, a surgical assistant uses the catheter guide to deflect the urethra to the contralateral side to lower urethral injury risks.

❺ **Mesh Placement.** The TVT needle and mesh are attached to the introducer. The needle is placed through one of the periurethral tunnels so that its point touches the front surface of the ipsilateral inferior pubic ramus (Fig. 45-4.1). A hand placed in the vagina carefully guides the needle around the back of the ramus. The needle is curved upward toward the ipsilateral abdominal incision, perforates the periurethral tissue just behind the pubic bone, and enters the retropubic space (Rahn, 2006). During this, the needle is always directly behind the pubic bone. Pressure is applied to the introducer handle with the other hand, but the vaginal hand controls the needle's direction. The handle of the introducer always remains parallel to the ground to avoid lateral excursion into major vessels and obturator nerve (Fig. 45-4.2). Additionally, after the needle passes around the pubic ramus and behind the symphysis pubis, its tip is always directed toward the abdominal wall incisions. The bladder may be perforated if excessive pressure is applied and if the needle is aimed cephalad rather than toward the abdominal wall (Fig. 45-4.3).

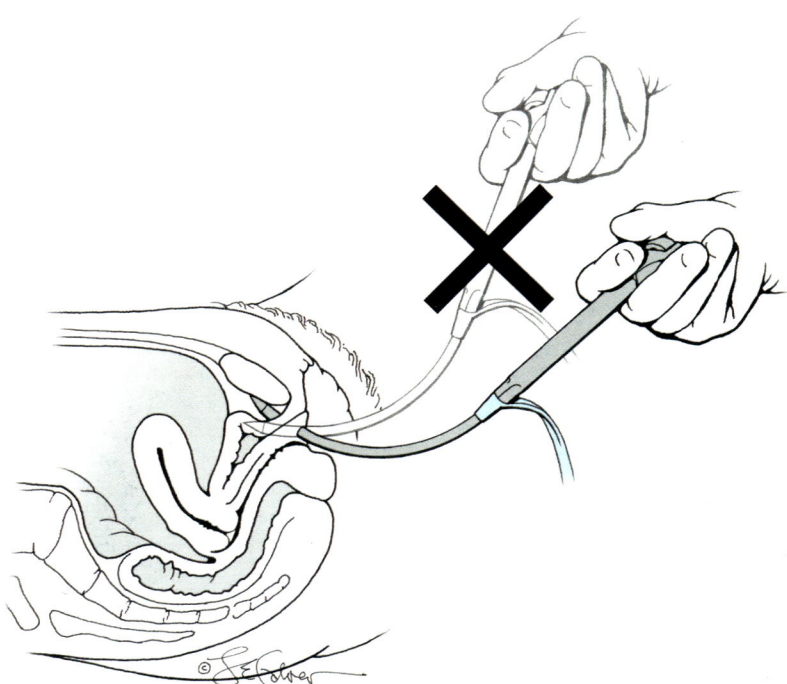

FIGURE 45-4.3 Correct (*dark introducer*) and incorrect (*light introducer*) hand and introducer positioning.

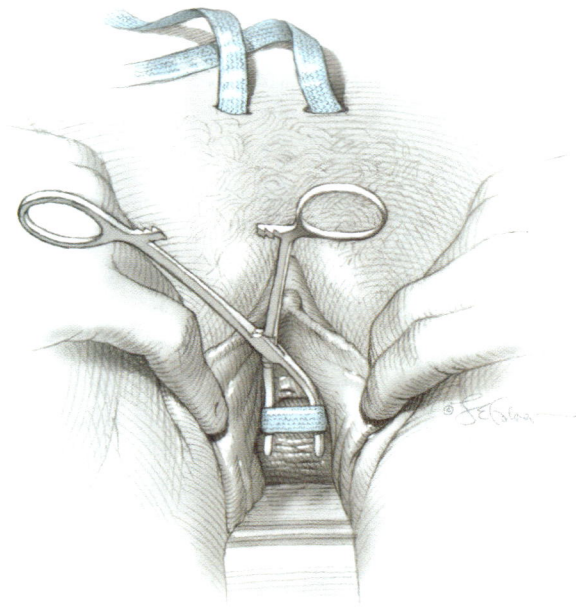

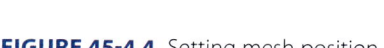

FIGURE 45-4.4 Setting mesh position.

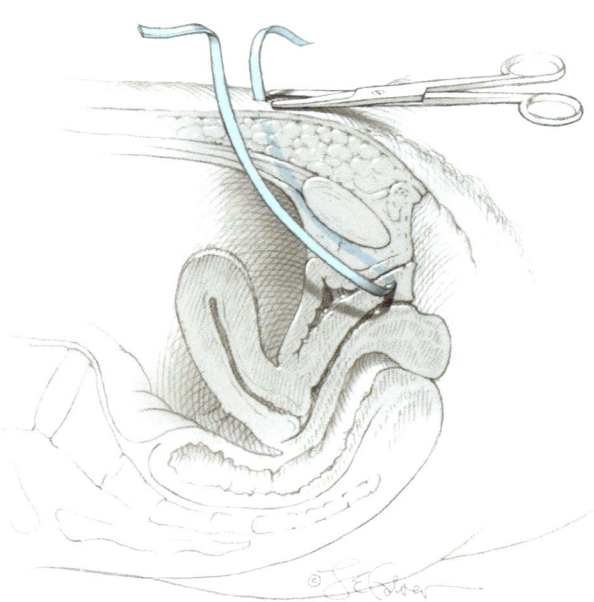

FIGURE 45-4.5 Sheath removal and tape trimming.

Small changes in the position of the hand applying handle pressure can lead to bladder perforation.

❻ Cystourethroscopy. After the needle perforates the abdominal wall, the Foley and catheter guide are removed, and cystourethroscopy is performed with a 70-degree cystoscope. The bladder is distended with 200 to 300 mL of fluid, and inspection for cystotomy is completed. Generally, perforation will be obvious, and the TVT needle will be seen entering and exiting the bladder. In this situation, the needle is removed and redirected, and correct placement is confirmed by cystoscopy. Inspection of the urethra is essential and can be performed with the same 70-degree angle scope. Alternatively, a 0-degree or 30-degree endoscope may be used. Iatrogenic trocar bladder injury, if identified intraoperatively, does not appear to influence continence outcomes or raise postoperative voiding dysfunction or infection rates (Zyczynski, 2014).

In contrast to bladder perforation, urethral perforation theoretically carries a risk of urethrovaginal fistula. Thus, if urethral perforation is noted, most surgeons abort the procedure and postpone until several months later.

Following cystoscopy, the introducer is unscrewed from the needle. The needle is brought through the abdominal wall. The needle is then cut from the mesh, and the mesh is held with a hemostat. Next, the other TVT needle is attached to the introducer and is placed on the other side of the urethra in a similar fashion. Cystourethroscopy is then repeated.

❼ Setting Mesh Position. The widest part of Mayo scissors, a partially opened hemostat, or similar instrument is placed between the suburethral tissue and the tape. The tool acts as a spacer and creates distance between the mesh and urethra (Fig. 45-4.4). This spacing avoids excessive mesh tension and lowers the risk for postoperative urinary retention and voiding dysfunction. Prior to mesh sheath removal, the vaginal sulci are inspected to exclude perforation of the vaginal epithelium during needle guidance. If perforated mesh is seen, the tape is removed and the TVT needle is again passed through a newly created periurethral tunnel that lies slightly medial to the original. The vaginal perforation defect is repaired with one or two simple interrupted delayed-absorbable sutures.

❽ Sheath Removal. Once the tape is satisfactorily positioned, an assistant removes the plastic sheath covering around the mesh, while the surgeon holds the mesh at the desired distance from the urethra using the spacer. The plastic covering is lifted away from both sides with minimal tension to avoid mesh stretching or undue urethral elevation.

With ideal positioning, a few millimeters of free space separate the suburethral tissue and mesh. The mesh is trimmed just below the skin at the abdominal incisions (Fig. 45-4.5).

❾ Wound Closure. The vaginal incision is closed in a running fashion with 2-0 gauge delayed-absorbable suture. The abdominal incisions may be closed with Dermabond or with a single interrupted 4-0 gauge delayed-absorbable skin suture.

POSTOPERATIVE

Prior to discharge from a day-surgery unit, an active voiding trial is performed (Chap. 42, p. 919). If the patient fails this trial, a Foley catheter is replaced and kept for 2 to 3 days prior to a second voiding trial. Alternatively, a patient can be taught self-catheterization. This is continued until postvoid residual volumes fall below approximately 100 mL.

Normal diet and activity can resume during the first postoperative days. Intercourse, however, is postponed until the vaginal incision is healed, usually at 6 weeks. The time to resumption of exercise and strenuous physical activity is controversial. A standard recommendation has been to delay these at least 2 months. Although no data support this, it seems reasonable for adequate healing.

45-5

Transobturator Midurethral Sling

The transobturator tape (TOT) sling procedure is one type in the MUS group. With the TOT operation, a permanent sling material is inserted bilaterally through the obturator foramen and extends underneath the midurethra. As a result, the retropubic space is avoided and thereby minimizes the potential for associated bladder, vessel, and bowel injuries. Additionally, in patients who have had a prior antiincontinence procedure and have scarring in the retropubic space, bladder perforation may be averted by avoiding repeat dissection here.

The TOT procedure differs from TVT and also has several modifications itself. The two major TOT procedure types are defined by needle direction. One begins inside the vagina and is directed outward, termed an *in-to-out* or *medial-to-lateral approach*. The other starts outside the vagina and is directed inward, called an *out-to-in* or *lateral-to-medial approach*. Existing data do not show one to be superior (Debodinance, 2007; Ford, 2017). Currently, the out-to-in technique is more commonly performed and is described here.

Generally, TOT is indicated for primary SUI secondary to urethral hypermobility (Chap. 23, p. 530). In patients with SUI secondary to intrinsic sphincteric deficiency, the effectiveness of TOT is unclear, and results are conflicting (Rechberger, 2009; Richter, 2010). If the retropubic MUS surgery (TVT) is compared with the transobturator MUS (TOT) procedure, evidence suggests the TVT results in higher subjective and objective cure rates than the latter (Ford, 2016; Kim, 2019).

PREOPERATIVE

Patient Evaluation

Evaluation and preparation prior to TOT mirrors that for TVT (p. 1094).

Consent

As with other antiincontinence surgeries, major risks are voiding dysfunction, urinary retention, urgency urinary incontinence, and failure to correct SUI. Groin and thigh pain are other potential postoperative problems. Long-term complications can be associated with the supporting mesh and include mesh erosion (Schimpf, 2014).

Intraoperatively, bladder or urethral perforation can occur, but the risk is believed to be significantly less than that with TVT. Inappropriate TOT trocar placement rarely can lead to significant hemorrhage or neurologic deficits if obturator nerve and vessel branches are damaged in the thigh compartment.

INTRAOPERATIVE

Instruments

A TOT kit will contain two TOT needles and synthetic mesh tape. The TOT needle is designed to navigate the path from the entry point, around the pubic rami, and to the midurethral vaginal wall incision. A plastic sheath surrounds the mesh tape and allows the mesh to be pulled into position smoothly. However, once these plastic sheaths are removed, the mesh remains fixed in position.

Surgical Steps

❶ Anesthesia and Patient Positioning. If performed solely, a TOT procedure in most cases is a day-surgery procedure. It is performed in standard lithotomy position under general, regional, or local anesthesia. The vagina is surgically prepared, and a Foley catheter is placed to assist in determination of urethra location and length.

❷ Vaginal Incisions. A midline incision is made sharply in the vaginal epithelium and superficial muscular layer beginning 1 cm proximal to the external urethral opening and is extended 2 to 2.5 cm cephalad. Allis clamps are placed on the edges of the vaginal incision for traction. Using Metzenbaum scissors and blunt finger dissection, bilateral periurethral tunnels are created beneath the vaginal epithelium on either side of the urethra. These tunnels extend up to and behind the inferior pubic rami.

❸ Thigh Incisions. A 0.5- to 1-cm entry incision is made bilaterally in the thigh-crease skin (labiocrural fold), 4 to 6 cm lateral to the glans clitoris, and at the point where the adductor longus insertion can be palpated.

❹ Mesh Placement. The TOT needle is grasped, and the tip is placed in one of the thigh incisions (Fig. 45-5.1). The tip is directed cephalad until the obturator membrane is perforated, and a "popping" sensation is felt. A vaginal finger is placed in the ipsilateral vaginal tunnel and is positioned up to and behind the inferior pubic ramus. Using the curve of the TOT needle, the surgeon then directs the needle tip to the end of his finger and passes the needle through the periurethral tissue and into the vagina (Fig. 45-5.2). At this time, the vaginal sulcus is inspected to

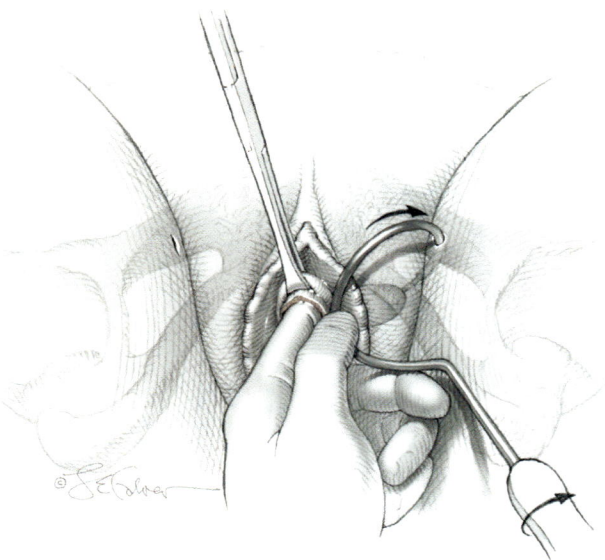

FIGURE 45-5.1 Needle introduction.

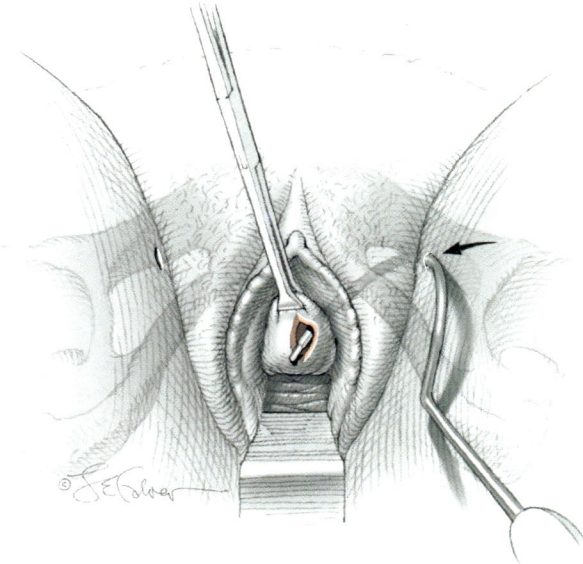

FIGURE 45-5.2 Needle passage.

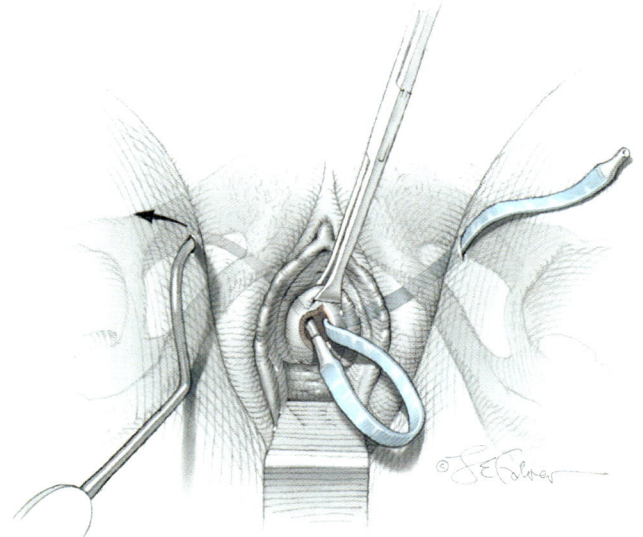

FIGURE 45-5.3 Tape placement.

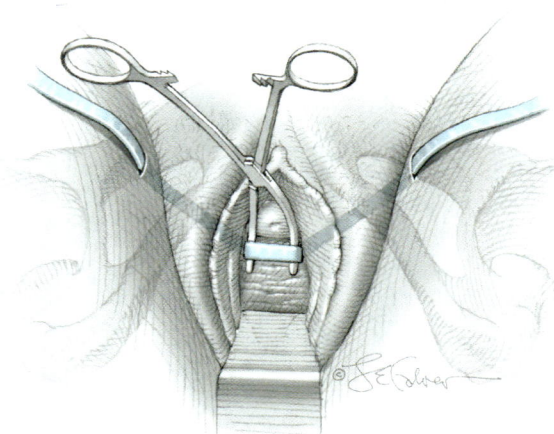

FIGURE 45-5.4 Setting mesh position.

exclude perforation. If the needle has perforated the sulcus epithelium, it is removed and reinserted correctly. At this time, the TOT covered mesh is attached to the needle end, and the needle retraces its original path as it is withdrawn back through the thigh incision. With this, the covered mesh is threaded with it and into position. The mesh is removed from the needle. The procedure is repeated on the other side (Fig. 45-5.3).

❺ **Setting Mesh Position.** A hemostat or similar instrument is placed and opened between the urethra and mesh to act as a spacer and create distance between the mesh and the urethra (Fig. 45-5.4). This spacing avoids excessive urethral elevation and lowers postoperative urinary retention risks. Prior to sheath removal, the vaginal sulci are again inspected to exclude perforation. If mesh is seen in a sulcus, the tape is removed and reinserted on the affected side.

❻ **Sheath Removal.** An assistant then removes the plastic covering of the mesh from each of the thigh incisions. Concurrently, the surgeon holds the mesh at the desired distance from the urethra using the spacer instrument. The plastic covering is removed with minimal tension to avoid mesh stretching. The mesh is trimmed just inside the thigh incisions.

❼ **Wound Closure.** The vaginal incision is closed in a running fashion with 2-0 gauge delayed-absorbable suture. The thigh incisions may be closed with a single interrupted subcuticular suture with 4-0 gauge delayed-absorbable suture or with other suitable skin closure methods (Chap. 40, p. 846).

❽ **Cystourethroscopy.** This procedure was initially marketed as one in which cystoscopy was not necessary. However, because the bladder and urethra can be injured, postprocedural cystoscopy is recommended now. In contrast to bladder perforation, urethral perforation theoretically carries a risk of urethrovaginal fistula. Thus, if urethral

perforation is noted, most surgeons abort the procedure and postpone until several months later.

POSTOPERATIVE

Prior to discharge from a day-surgery unit, an active voiding trial is performed (Chap. 42, p. 919). If significant residuals persist, a Foley catheter remains. A second voiding trial can be repeated in a few days or at the surgeon's discretion. Alternatively, a patient can be taught self-catheterization. This is continued until postvoid residuals fall below approximately 100 mL.

Normal diet and activity can resume during the first postoperative days. Intercourse, however, is delayed until the vaginal incision is healed. The time to resumption of exercise and strenuous physical activity is controversial. A standard recommendation delays these at least 2 months. Data to support this are lacking, however, logic would suggest that this is reasonable to allow adequate healing.

45-6

Pubovaginal Sling

Pubovaginal sling is a standard procedure for SUI. It has traditionally been used for SUI stemming from intrinsic sphincteric deficiency (Chap. 23, p. 519). In addition, this procedure may also aid patients with prior failed antiincontinence operations. It is generally not employed as a first antiincontinence surgery.

Autologous fascia is currently preferred for the sling. This fascia generally is obtained from the patient's rectus sheath, although fascia lata from the thigh can be harvested. During this surgery, a strip of fascia is placed at the proximal urethra through the retropubic space, and ends are secured either to each other or to the rectus fascia above the rectus abdominis muscle. If a shorter fascial strip is planned, polypropylene (Prolene) sutures are placed at each end as extenders. These ends are similarly secured either to each other or to the rectus fascia above the rectus abdominis muscle.

Unlike the standardized steps of midurethral sling procedures, the technical aspects of autologous fascia pubovaginal sling placement have greater variability. These include size and location of harvested tissue, sling anchoring method, and mesh tension determination.

PREOPERATIVE

Patient Evaluation

As with other antiincontinence procedures, patients require urogynecologic evaluation, including urodynamic testing to confirm SUI and intrinsic sphincteric deficiency. Additionally, SUI often accompanies pelvic organ prolapse. Thus, the need for concurrent repair of associated prolapse is assessed prior to surgery (Chap. 24, p. 541).

Consent

In addition to general surgical risks, patients are counseled regarding the risk of recurrent incontinence, urinary retention, and voiding dysfunction following surgery (Albo, 2007). Compared with midurethral sling operations, pubovaginal slings overall offer similar efficacy but have higher adverse effect rates (Rehman, 2011).

Patient Preparation

Antibiotic and VTE prophylaxis are given as outlined in Tables 39-8 and 39-10 (p. 832). Bowel preparation is based on surgeon preference and on other planned surgeries.

INTRAOPERATIVE

Surgical Steps

❶ Anesthesia and Patient Positioning. Pubovaginal sling may be performed under general or regional anesthesia and as an inpatient or day-surgery procedure. The patient is placed in standard lithotomy position, with the lower extremities positioned in booted support stirrups. The abdomen and vagina are surgically prepared, and a Foley catheter is inserted.

❷ Graft Harvest. A transverse skin incision is made 2 to 4 cm above the symphysis pubis and is large enough to allow removal of a transverse fascial strip that measures, at minimum, 1.5 cm wide × 6 cm long. The incision is carried down through subcutaneous tissue to the fascia.

The fascia to be harvested is outlined with a marking pen and then incised. It is sharply dissected away from the underlying rectus abdominis muscle bellies, removed, and cleaned of attached fat. A helical stitch using 0-gauge polypropylene suture then is placed through the fascia at each end of the strip. These sutures are not tied. The fascial incision is closed in a running fashion with 0-gauge delayed-absorbable suture.

❸ Vaginal Incision. At a point 2 cm proximal to the external urethral orifice, a 3- to 5-cm midline vertical incision is made sharply in the anterior vaginal wall and is extended cephalad. Alternatively, a U-shaped incision is made at the level of the bladder neck. Sharp and blunt dissection separates the vaginal epithelium from the underlying fibromuscular layer.

Next, the retropubic space is entered with a combination of sharp and blunt dissection bilaterally by penetrating the periurethral connective tissue (Fig. 45-6.1). Entry into this space is confirmed by the surgeon's finger palpating the dorsal surface of the pubic bone (Fig. 45-6.2). During entry, veins within the vesical venous plexus can be lacerated, and bleeding is controlled with compression or with stitches of 2-0 gauge absorbable suture.

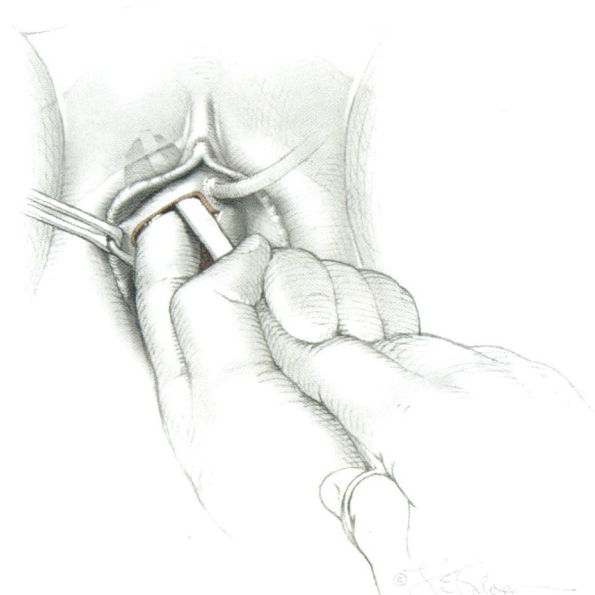

FIGURE 45-6.1 Entry into the retropubic space.

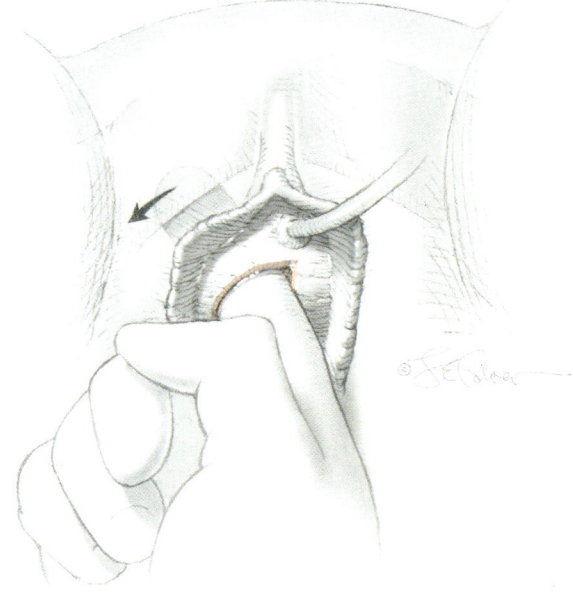

FIGURE 45-6.2 Palpation of pubic bone.

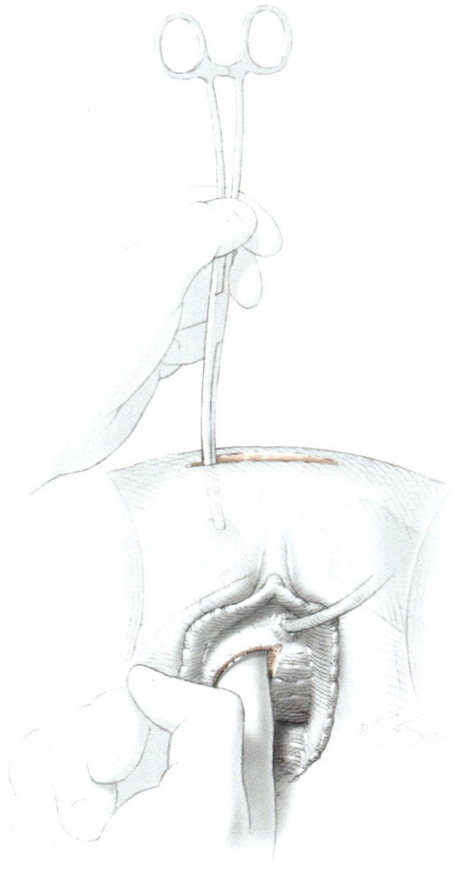

FIGURE 45-6.3 Passing of dressing forceps.

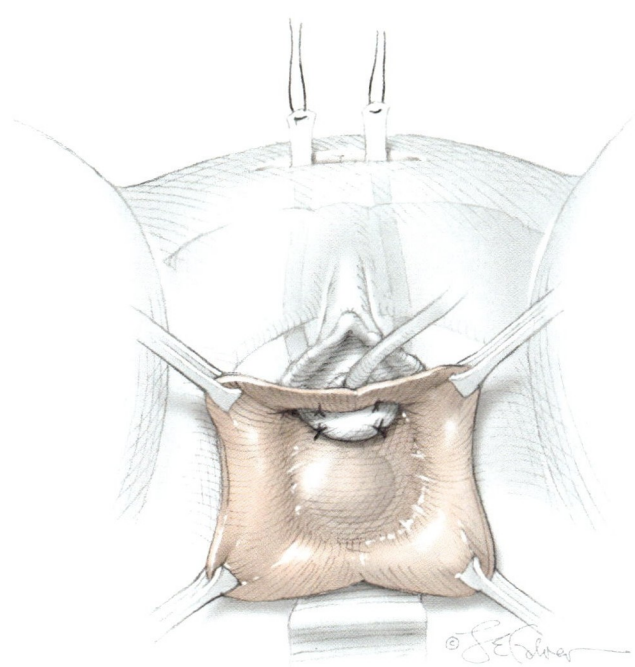

FIGURE 45-6.4 Fascial sling placed and sutured in place on vaginal side.

❹ **Fascia Placement.** Two 0.5- to 1-cm fascial incisions are made transversely in the lower abdomen, and each lies no further than 2 cm from the midline. These are placed caudal to the prior harvest incision and just above the pubic bones. A long dressing or packing forceps or a needle ligature carrier is inserted into one of these incisions and, from above, perforates the rectus abdominis muscle tendon. The instrument is placed against the back of the pubic bone and advanced toward the vagina. Concurrently, the surgeon guides the instrument to his finger within the retropubic space and advances it into and through the vaginal incision (Fig. 45-6.3). At this time, cystourethroscopy is performed to exclude bladder or urethral perforation.

The sutures at one end of the fascial strip are grasped with the perforating forceps and threaded up through the abdominal wall incision on one side of the urethra. With the other end of the sling, this step is repeated on the other side of the urethra. As a result, the fascial sling lies positioned below the bladder neck and proximal urethra (Fig. 45-6.4). Usually four 2-0 gauge delayed-absorbable

stitches may be used to fix the sling beneath the bladder neck to prevent displacement. Sutures are placed lateral to the urethra.

❺ **Setting Sling Position.** Within the abdominal wall incision, sutures attached to the sling ends from each side meet and are tied together above the rectus sheath. During knot tying, a space of two to three fingerbreadths is left between the knot and fascia to prevent bladder neck obstruction and urinary retention. In addition, a hemostat or similar instrument is placed between the suburethral tissue and the fascial sling to create distance between the sling and urethra (see Fig. 45-4.4). After the knot is secured, the urethra or bladder neck should not angle upward, and a few millimeters of free space should be noted between the fascial sling and the bladder neck.

❻ **Cystourethroscopy.** This again is performed to exclude bladder or urethral perforation. In addition, excessive resistance noted during passage of the cystoscope into the bladder may suggest undue sling tension, which can lead to postoperative obstructive voiding

symptoms. If such resistance is noted, the sling is loosened.

❼ **Vaginal Incision.** The vaginal incision is closed with 2-0 gauge delayed-absorbable suture in a running fashion. A Foley catheter is left in place. In the past, suprapubic tube insertion was common practice. However, with a trend toward tying the fascial sling with less tension, the risk of prolonged urinary retention is lowered, and suprapubic drainage typically is not required.

❽ **Abdominal Incision.** Each of the two prior 1-cm abdominal wall fascial incisions is closed with an interrupted stitch of delayed-absorbable suture. The remaining abdominal incision is closed as described in Section 43-2 (p. 934).

POSTOPERATIVE

In general, recovery follows that associated with laparotomy and is heavily dependent on incision size. Prior to hospital discharge, a voiding trial is performed as described in Chapter 42 (p. 919).

Urethral Bulking Injections

Injection of bulking agents into the urethral submucosa is one method available to treat SUI that results from intrinsic sphincter deficiency (ISD) (Chap. 23, p. 519). Some evidence suggests it can treat SUI resulting from combined ISD and urethral hypermobility (Bent, 2001; Herschorn, 1997; Steele, 2000). Although mechanisms are not completely clear, effectiveness may result from expansion of the urethral walls, which allows them to better approximate or *coapt*. As a result, intraluminal resistance to flow is increased and continence is improved or restored. Alternatively, injections elongate the functional urethra, and this may allow a more even distribution of abdominal pressures across the proximal urethra to resist opening during stress (Monga, 1997).

Urethral injection offers a cystoscopically assisted, minimally invasive treatment of SUI. It can be performed in an office under local anesthesia and is associated with a low risk of complications. Consequently, it is often chosen for women who wish to avoid surgery or who are not surgical candidates due to comorbid conditions.

Urethral injections can be performed both peri- and transurethrally. The transurethral approach is more often used and allows for more accurate placement of the bulking agent (Faerber, 1998; Schulz, 2004). Currently, several synthetic agents are approved for use in the United States and described later. Autologous myoblast injection is another promising injectable but requires further study (Kirchin, 2017).

PREOPERATIVE

Patient Evaluation

Complex urodynamic testing with assessment of urethral structure and function is completed prior to candidate selection. To initially assess for ISD, severe symptoms and a supine stress test that demonstrates incontinence are sought. Next, urodynamic parameters such as maximum urethral closure pressure or leak point pressure specifically are evaluated (Chap. 23, p. 527). However, evidence suggests these tests have poor reproducibility (Weber, 2001a,b). Additionally, urethral mobility is assessed with Q-tip testing or similar evaluation, although this may be less predictive of surgical benefits.

Consent

Procedure efficacy is discussed, and success rates in general are lower than those for surgery. Specifically, 1-year rates of curing or improving SUI range from 60 to 80 percent (Bent, 2001; Corcos, 2005; Lightner, 2002, 2009; Monga, 1995). Continence rates diminish with time, as would be intuitive, with the breakdown of collagen and fat. However, Chrouser (2004) found similar rates of decline with time even when synthetic material was compared with collagen. Accordingly, these injections are viewed as a nonpermanent treatment of SUI, and sustained continence is found in only 25 percent of patients at 5 years following injection (Gorton, 1999).

One major advantage to urethral injection is its low associated risk of complications. Side effects of injection are generally transient and may include vaginitis, acute cystitis, local pain, and voiding symptoms. Of these, urinary retention for a few days postprocedure is the most frequent. Long-term retention, however, is not a significant risk. A more serious complication is de novo urgency, which may develop in as many as 10 percent of women following injection (Corcos, 1999, 2005). Rare cases of pseudo-abscess formation and urethral erosion are reported (Kirchin, 2017).

Patient Preparation

Prior to urethral injection, UTI and anatomic pathology such as urethral diverticula are excluded. Anecdotally, we have seen bulking agent migration into such diverticula. As noted, UTI commonly can follow urethral injection. A single antibiotic dose to cover uropathogens is administered orally after procedure completion. Thromboprophylaxis typically is not required for this office procedure.

INTRAOPERATIVE

Choice of Bulking Agent

In the United States, currently used agents for urethral injection are carbon-coated synthetic microspheres (Durasphere), calcium hydroxylapatite particles (Coaptite), and polydimethylsiloxane (Macroplastique). These synthetic agents are effective. However, no randomized trials compare results among these three, and long-term data are lacking (Kirchin, 2017; Shah, 2012).

Of agents no longer used, autologous fat provided limited success for SUI due to rapid degradation and reabsorption (Haab, 1997; Lee, 2001). A bovine collagen product (Contigen) was commonly selected, but manufacturing ceased due to an inadequate supply of medical-grade collagen. Ethylene vinyl alcohol copolymer (Uryx/Tegress) was withdrawn due to urethral erosion complications.

Surgical Steps

1 Anesthesia and Patient Positioning. Urethral injection for most patients can be performed in an office setting with cystoscopic capability. The patient is placed in low lithotomy position, the vulva is prepared and draped, and the bladder drained. Two-percent lidocaine jelly is instilled into the urethra 10 minutes prior to the procedure. If necessary, topical 20-percent benzocaine can be used as an analgesic on the vulva, and 4 mL of 1-percent lidocaine can be injected in divided doses at the 3 and 9 o'clock positions of the external urethral orifice.

2 Transurethral Approach Needle Placement. A 0-degree cystoscope is positioned within the distal urethra, so that the midurethra, proximal urethra, and bladder neck are viewed simultaneously. A 22-gauge spinal needle attached to a syringe carrying the bulking agent is introduced through the cystoscopic sheath. With the bevel pointing toward the urethral lumen, the needle is directed at a 45-degree angle to the lumen and inserted through the urethral wall at the 9 o'clock position and at the level of the midurethra.

After the needle tip penetrates the urethral wall, the bevel is no longer seen. The needle then is advanced parallel to the urethral lumen for 1 to 2 cm. This positions the needle at the level of the proximal urethra.

3 Injection. The bulking agent is injected under constant pressure, and the submucosal lining begins to rise (Fig. 45-7.1). The needle is withdrawn slowly to bulk the proximal to midurethra. Bulking agent is administered until coaptation of the mucosa has developed (Fig. 45-7.2). These steps are then repeated at the 3 o'clock position. In general, 1 to 2 syringes (2.5 to 5 mL) of agent are used per procedure.

Ideally, the number of needle holes made into the urethral wall is minimized to avoid leakage of bulking agent through these punctures. Thus, if a second syringe of agent is required to achieve coaptation, the originally positioned needle remains in place, and a second syringe of agent is attached.

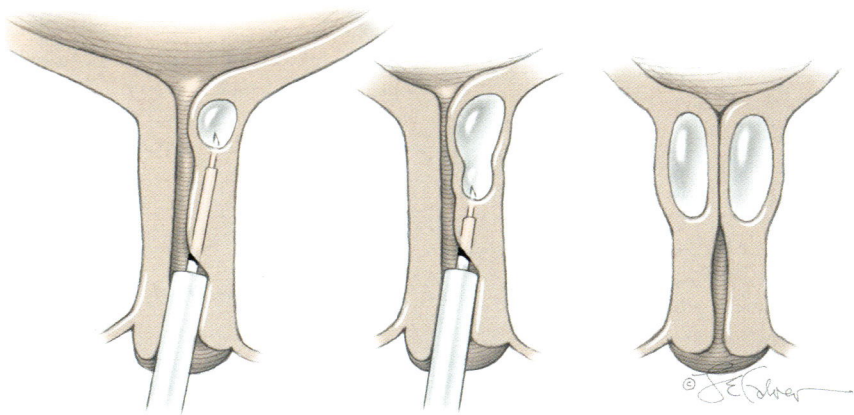

FIGURE 45-7.1 Injection of bulking agent.

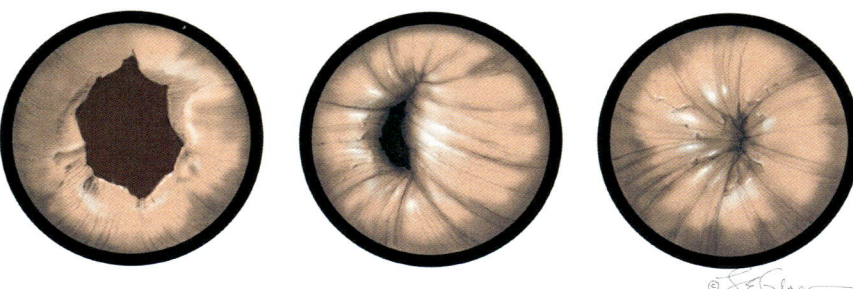

FIGURE 45-7.2 Corresponding cystoscopic views of urethral coaptation as bulking agent is injected, as shown in Figure 45-7.1.

❹ **Cystoscope Removal.** Once coaptation of the mucosa is achieved, the cystoscope is removed, taking care not to advance forward and proximal to the injection site. This avoids forceful compression of the deposited agent by the cystoscope tip and loss of coaptation.

POSTOPERATIVE

Women are discharged home following their first postinjection void, and single-dose oral antibiotic prophylaxis is prescribed. Women abstain from intercourse for approximately 10 days following injection but may otherwise resume usual activities.

If urinary retention develops, intermittent self-catheterization is begun and continued until retention resolves. For those unable to catheterize themselves, a temporary Foley catheter is placed. However, catheter placement can potentially compress deposited bulking agent and diminish urethral coaptation.

Two weeks following injection, we assess treatment success. If a patient fails to achieve desired degrees of continence, additional injections are planned to improve urethral coaptation.

Urethrolysis

Urethrolysis is the loosening or release of a prior urethral suspension procedure. This surgery is indicated for women with significant urethral obstructive symptoms, such as urinary retention and voiding dysfunction, following suspension. Performed either vaginally or abdominally, a vaginal approach is used predominantly. An abdominal approach, however, may afford a better opportunity to mobilize the bladder from the symphysis pubis. It also may be selected in instances in which the initial surgery was performed via laparotomy.

Whether a concurrent antiincontinence procedure is needed to compensate for lost urethral support with urethrolysis is debatable. However, in many cases, residual scarring prevents SUI. Thus, our belief is to avoid repeating a second potentially obstructing procedure.

PREOPERATIVE

Patient Evaluation

In women with bladder neck obstruction, symptoms usually begin soon after the primary suspension. Urodynamic testing is performed to objectively determine the cause of voiding dysfunction and to differentiate between a hypotonic bladder and obstruction. Obstruction may result from bladder neck obstruction or pelvic organ prolapse. Thus, a thorough search for prolapse is completed.

Consent

In addition to usual surgical risks, bleeding may be a significant complication due to vascularity in the retropubic space. Additionally, dissection of dense scarring around the urethra and bladder may place these structures at risk of laceration.

Following urethrolysis, initial improvement can worsen over time, because obstructive scar tissue may variably reform. In contrast, postoperative incontinence may follow deconstruction of the prior antiincontinence support or result from denervation injury during extensive periurethral dissection.

Patient Preparation

As with all genitourinary procedures, UTI is excluded prior to surgery. Antibiotic prophylaxis is administered prior to surgery to decrease risks of postoperative wound infection and UTI (Table 39-8, p. 832). Thromboprophylaxis is provided as outlined in Table 39-10 (p. 834).

INTRAOPERATIVE

Surgical Steps—Vaginal Approach

❶ Anesthesia and Patient Positioning. Urethrolysis may be performed under general or regional anesthesia. The patient is placed in standard lithotomy position with lower extremities in candy-cane or booted support stirrups. The vagina is surgically prepared, and a Foley catheter is inserted into the bladder.

❷ Vaginal Incision. Traction is placed on the Foley catheter to identify the bladder neck and assess the degree of scarring and mobility. A 2- to 3-cm-long incision, either vertical midline or U-shaped, is made in the anterior vaginal wall. The incision site will vary along the vaginal length depending on the location of the original sling or sutures (Fig. 45-8.1). Sharp dissection is used to separate the vaginal epithelium from underlying fibromuscular tissue and is extended bilaterally toward the inferior edge of each pubic ramus.

Dissection frees the urethra by dividing tethering bands that lie between the urethra and pubic rami (Fig. 45-8.2). This may be scar tissue or previous sling material or sutures. These materials may be incised or excised. Bleeding is frequently encountered

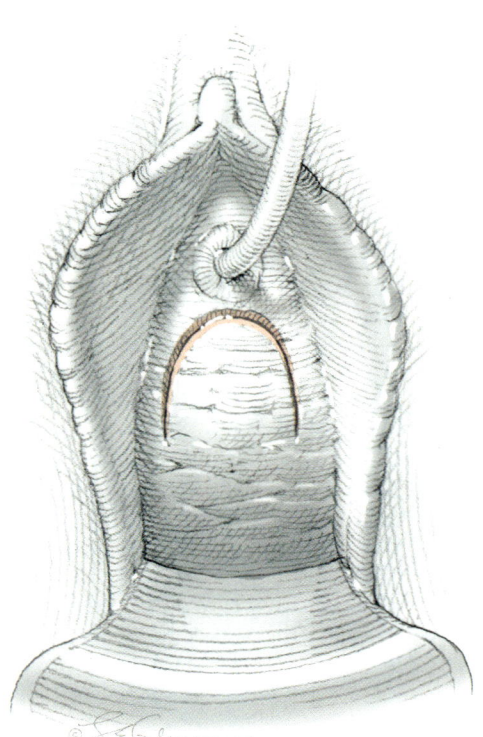

FIGURE 45-8.1 Vaginal incision.

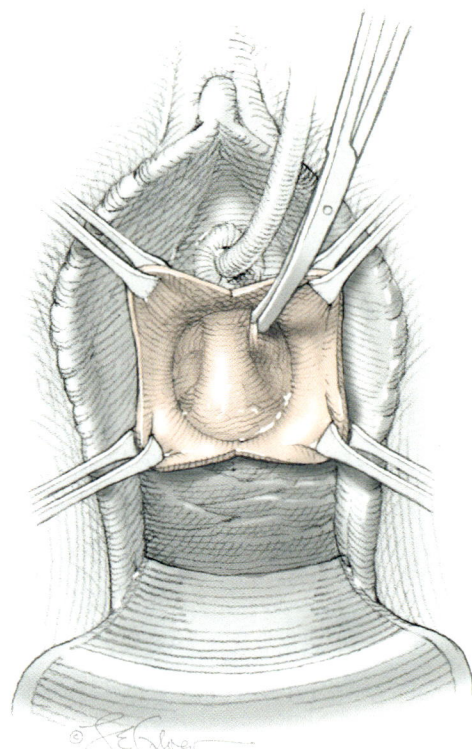

FIGURE 45-8.2 Periurethral dissection.

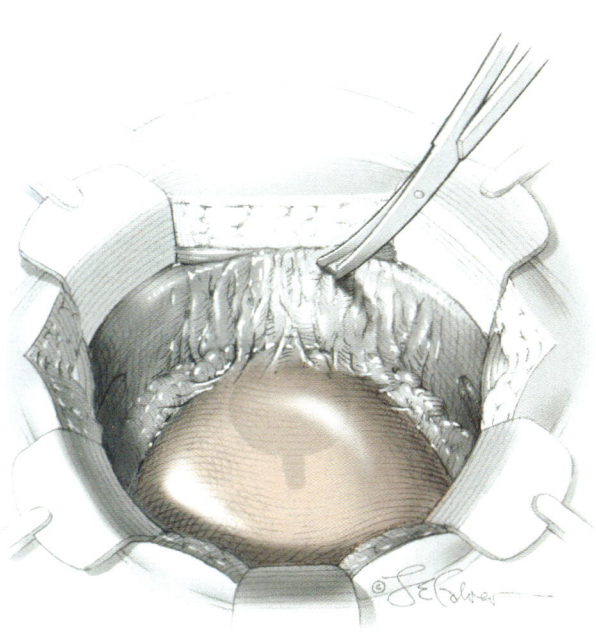

FIGURE 45-8.3 Dissection in the retropubic space.

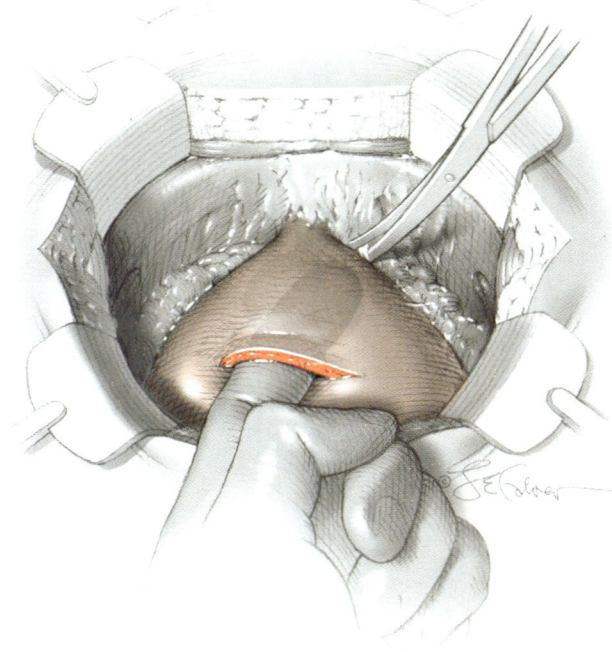

FIGURE 45-8.4 Intentional cystotomy to aid bladder and urethral dissection.

and can be controlled with direct pressure or vessel ligation.

After this lateral dissection, the periurethral tissue is perforated, and the retropubic space is entered as in Section 45-6, Step 3. Blunt dissection within this space and at the back of the symphysis pubis will additionally mobilize the proximal urethra. Dissection is kept close to the dorsal surface of the pubic bone to avoid cystotomy in a bladder that is generally densely adhered to the pubic bones.

❸ **Incision Closure.** Once the urethra is adequately freed, the vaginal incision is reapproximated with a running closure using 2-0 gauge delayed-absorbable suture.

Surgical Steps— Abdominal Approach

❶ **Anesthesia and Patient Positioning.** Again, urethrolysis may be completed under general or regional anesthesia. For an abdominal approach, booted support stirrups and low lithotomy positioning are preferred. This positioning allows vaginal access for the surgeon's hand during dissection and for cystoscopy. The abdomen and vagina are surgically prepared, and a Foley catheter is inserted into the bladder.

❷ **Abdominal Incision.** Typically, a low transverse incision is preferred to permit easy

access to the retropubic space. If the procedure is done in isolation, fascia of the anterior abdominal wall muscles and then transversalis fascia are incised, but entry into the peritoneal cavity is not necessary to reach the retropubic space. This procedure may be performed similarly by an MIS approach.

❸ **Retropubic Space Entry.** The correct plane of dissection to enter the retropubic space lies directly behind the pubic bone. Loose areolar tissue is gently dissected downward in a mediolateral fashion with fingers or sponge, beginning immediately behind the pubic bone. If the correct plane is entered, this potential space opens easily. However, women requiring urethrolysis typically have dense adhesion within the retropubic space from prior surgery. Thus, sharp downward dissection along the dorsal surface of the symphysis pubis aids entry into this space (Fig. 45-8.3).

❹ **Bladder Dissection and Urethrolysis.** The bladder also typically is densely adhered to the back of the symphysis pubis. Sharp dissection with the curved surface of scissors facing the symphysis pubis is directed against the symphysis to minimize cystotomy risk. At times, however, an intentional cystotomy may be made so that a finger can be placed inside the bladder to aid dissection (Fig. 45-8.4).

Sharp dissection is continued inferiorly and laterally down the inner surface of the

symphysis pubis and pubic bones to free the bladder and eventually also the proximal urethra.

Bleeding is common during dissection and may be controlled with electrosurgical coagulation or interrupted absorbable sutures. As the symphysis pubis' inferior surface is approached, dissection ideally avoids the dorsal vein of the clitoris. This vessel courses atop the urethra along its retropubic segment.

❺ **Abdominal Closure.** The abdomen is closed in a standard fashion (Sections 43-1 or 43-2, p. 932).

POSTOPERATIVE

An active bladder test is performed following catheter removal. If large residual volumes are found, intermittent self-catheterization or Foley catheter replacement is required. Antibiotic suppression is not required with this catheter use. If cystotomy was performed, the duration of catheterization depends on cystotomy size and location (p. 1081).

Normal diet and activity can resume during the first postoperative days. With a vaginal approach, however, intercourse is postponed until the vaginal incision is well healed. Recovery from an abdominal approach follows that for laparotomy (Section 43-1, p. 932).

Midurethral Sling Release

Symptoms of voiding obstruction may develop following MUS procedures, specifically TVT and TOT procedures. For most patients, postoperative urinary retention resolves within 2 weeks. However, voiding dysfunction requiring surgery develops in up to 3 percent and generally is identified days to weeks after surgery (Jonsson Funk, 2013; Nguyen, 2012; Richter, 2010). If obstruction is diagnosed soon after the index procedure, surgical release is performed and involves simple transection of the sling material, either in the midline or along the urethra's lateral surface (American College of Obstetricians and Gynecologists, 2017).

PREOPERATIVE

Patient Evaluation and Preparation

Inability to fully empty the bladder may stem from urethral obstruction or a hypotonic bladder. New-onset urinary retention after a MUS procedure (TVT or TOT) usually stems from sling tightness. However, other factors can be involved, such as preexisting or de novo bladder hypotonia. Thus, prior to MUS release, urodynamic testing often is performed to prove that symptoms are due to obstruction rather than to bladder hypotonicity. If urodynamic study was performed preoperatively, it is reviewed.

Sling tape may erode into the bladder or urethra in cases of obstruction, and cystoscopy allows this to be excluded. In select cases in which suburethral mesh is not palpated, three-dimensional sonography can be completed. Postprocessing digital reconstruction of the urethra can define mesh location, which aids surgery planning and patient counseling.

Other specific patient preparation usually is not required, as MUS release is considered a relatively minor surgery. The American College of Obstetricians and Gynecologists (2018b) recommends antibiotic prophylaxis prior to urogynecologic surgery, and appropriate choices mirror those for hysterectomy (Table 39-8, p. 832).

Consent

Associated with MUS release, the risks of incontinence recurrence, inadequate retention relief, fistula formation, and intraoperative bladder or urethral injury are discussed during consenting.

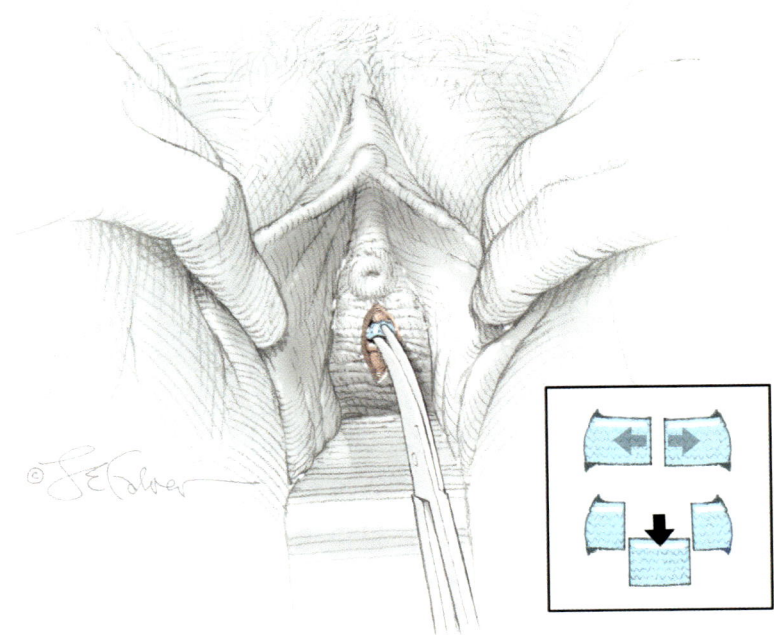

FIGURE 45-9.1 Mesh transection through vaginal incision. Inset top: Mesh incision and retraction. Inset bottom: Partial mesh excision.

INTRAOPERATIVE

Surgical Steps

❶ Anesthesia and Patient Positioning. This surgery can be performed with local, regional, or general anesthesia as an outpatient procedure. A patient is placed in standard lithotomy position with lower extremities in candy-cane or booted support stirrups. The vagina is surgically prepared, and a Foley catheter is inserted.

❷ Vaginal Incision and Tape Identification. A midline suburethral incision that follows the prior primary surgical incision is made sharply. Careful dissection is used to expose the sling material and to define the urethral borders. Alternatively, with prior TOT, tight tissue bands may be palpated in the sulci. In this case, the vagina can be incised at one sulcus, and the tape transected or partially excised here.

Often because of increased sling tension, sling material is stretched and measures only half its expected width. Moreover, tissue ingrowth into the sling material is usually extensive, and thus identification and mobilization can be difficult. Occasionally, a sling may migrate to the proximal urethra. In these instances, the vaginal incision may require cephalad extension.

❸ Sling Material Incision. After mobilization and full isolation of the sling, a hemostat is opened between the sling and urethra. Metzenbaum scissors are used to transect the entire width of sling material. In general, incision leads to immediate retraction of sling ends (Fig. 45-9.1, top inset).

If retraction does not follow, a 1-cm segment of material is excised (see Fig. 45-9.1, bottom inset). After excision, if the sling was deeply embedded and near the urethral lumen, the defect is reinforced. For this, one or two imbricating layers are placed through the vaginal muscularis using 2-0 or 3-0 gauge delayed-absorbable suture.

❹ Incision Closure. After vigorous irrigation, the vaginal epithelium is closed in a continuous running fashion using 2-0 gauge delayed-absorbable suture.

POSTOPERATIVE

Prior to discharge, an active voiding trial is performed (Chap. 42, p. 919). If a Foley catheter remains, a second voiding trial can be repeated in a few days or at the surgeon's discretion. If a woman is performing self-catheterization, this is continued until postvoid residuals fall below approximately 100 mL. Normal diet and activity can resume during the first postoperative days. Coitus, however, is postponed until the vaginal incision is healed.

45-10

Urethral Diverticulum Repair

The approach to urethral diverticulum repair varies and depends on diverticular sac location, size, and configuration. For those near the bladder neck, partial resection of the diverticular sac is often chosen to avoid damage to the bladder neck and continence mechanism. For midurethral diverticula, simple diverticulectomy is typically performed. For those located at the external urethral orifice, again, simple diverticulectomy is preferred to the Spence procedure, which is rarely performed due to its distortion of normal anatomy. Specifically, with the Spence marsupialization, a distal diverticulum and urethral orifice are sharply opened together to form a large single orifice. A spraying urination pattern may result. Last, for those with a complex diverticulum that may surround the urethra, a combination of techniques may be necessary. Of these options, complete vaginal excision of the urethral diverticulum is preferred (Antosh, 2011).

PREOPERATIVE

Patient Evaluation

As described in Chapter 26 (p. 581), urethral diverticula can be difficult to diagnose due to their often varied and nonspecific presentations. Once identified, accurate information regarding diverticular anatomy is essential to surgical planning and patient counseling. Compared with transvaginal sonography or voiding cystourethrography, magnetic resonance (MR) imaging is a superior radiographic study to delineate diverticular configuration, especially with complex diverticula (Ockrim, 2009).

Cystoscopy is a valuable adjunct in locating sac openings along the urethral length. It offers high specificity, as transurethral visualization of an ostium is unlikely to be associated with other diagnoses. However, urethral diverticulum detection (sensitivity) was only 39 percent in one study at our university (Pathi, 2013).

Women with a diverticulum can present with urinary incontinence. In such cases, we generally defer antiincontinence procedures until after postoperative reevaluation.

Consent

With diverticular repair, damage to the urethral continence mechanism may lead to postoperative incontinence. In contrast, urethral stricture or stenosis or urinary retention may develop depending on the extent and location of surgery. Urethrovaginal fistula and bladder injury are other risks. Moreover, urethral pain or recurrent UTI can persist or arise after diverticulectomy (Ockrim, 2009). Rarely, neoplasia coincides with diverticula.

Recurrence rates of 10 to 25 percent are reported. Cases with a horseshoe or circumferential configuration, proximal location, prior surgical attempt, or multiple diverticula are predisposing factors (Antosh, 2011; Ingber, 2011; Zhou, 2017). Failure is thought to stem from incomplete diverticulum excision.

Patient Preparation

Any acute diverticular infection or UTI is treated prior to surgery. Preventatively, antibiotic and VTE prophylaxis are given as outlined in Tables 39-8 and 39-10 (p. 832).

INTRAOPERATIVE

Surgical Steps—Diverticulectomy

❶ Anesthesia and Patient Positioning. Diverticulum excision can be performed as a day-surgery or inpatient procedure under general or regional anesthesia. A patient is placed in standard lithotomy position with lower extremities in candy-cane or booted support stirrups. The vagina is surgically prepared, and a Foley catheter containing a 10-mL balloon is placed in the bladder to assist in identifying the bladder neck.

❷ Cystourethroscopy. This procedure is performed at the procedure's onset with a 0-degree cystoscope to attempt diverticular ostia identification and exclude other abnormalities.

❸ Vaginal Incision. A midline or U-shaped incision is made on the anterior vaginal wall over the diverticulum, and the vaginal epithelium is dissected sharply off the fibromuscular layer of the vaginal wall (Fig. 45-10.1). Ample epithelium is freed to allow adequate exposure and to permit final tissue approximation without suture-line tension.

❹ Diverticulum Exposure. Next, the fibromuscular layer of the vagina and urethra is incised with a longitudinal or transverse incision to reach the diverticular sac. Anatomically, the distal vaginal and urethral walls are fused, and it may be difficult or impossible to separate tissue planes. Thus, sharp dissection is needed to completely mobilize the diverticular sac away from the vaginal and urethral fibromuscular layer and to the level of the diverticular sac neck (Fig. 45-10.2). During dissection, the sac may be inadvertently or intentionally

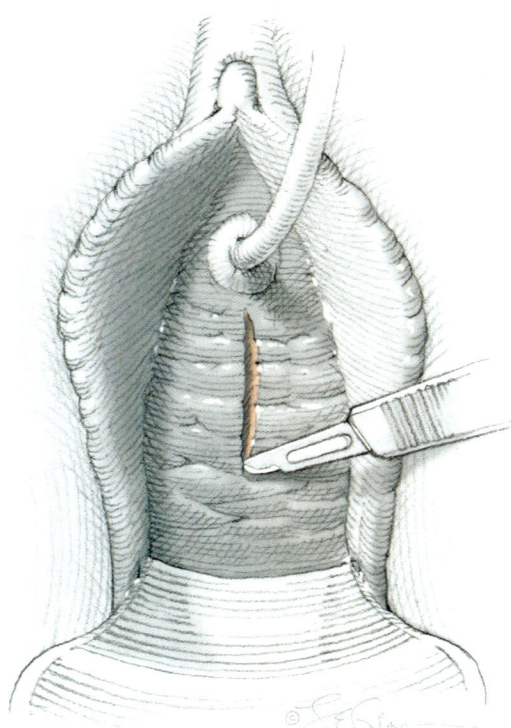

FIGURE 45-10.1 Vaginal incision.

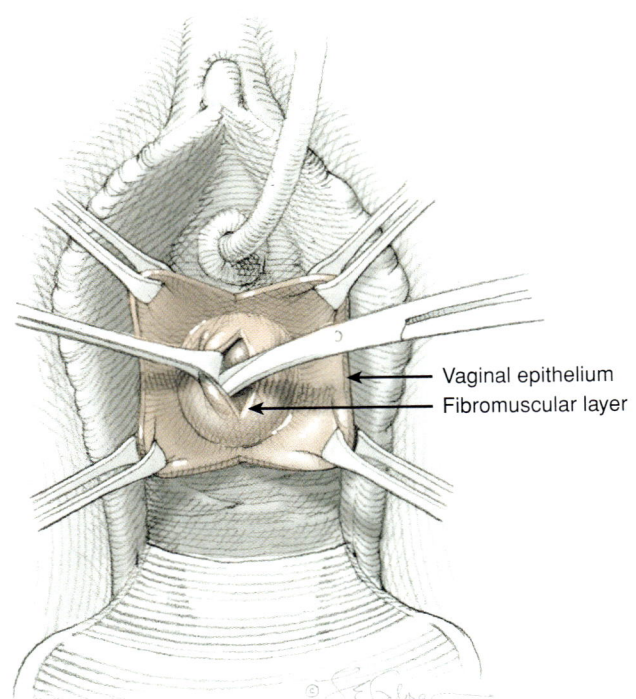

FIGURE 45-10.2 Diverticular sac dissection.

Vaginal epithelium
Fibromuscular layer

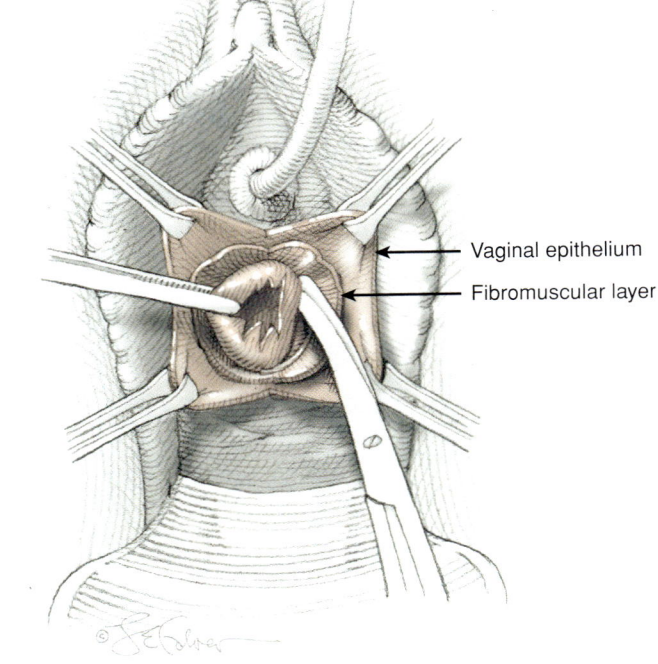

FIGURE 45-10.3 Diverticulum excision.

Vaginal epithelium
Fibromuscular layer

entered. With this, the diverticular walls can be grasped with Allis clamps to create tension across the connective tissue fibers between the diverticular walls and the vaginal fibromuscular layer to aid dissection. Similarly, an index finger placed within the sac can recreate sac fullness to stretch these same connective tissue fibers. Dissection is then continued until the diverticulum's communication with the urethra is isolated. Caution and awareness of urethral location are essential to avoid damage.

❺ **Diverticulum Excision.** At its neck, the diverticulum is excised from the urethra (Fig. 45-10.3).

❻ **Urethral Closure.** The urethral defect is closed with interrupted 4-0 gauge delayed-absorbable sutures over the Foley catheter (Fig. 45-10.4). Fibromuscular layers of the urethra and vagina are then reapproximated off tension in two or more layers. For this closure, a vest-over-pants method with 2-0 gauge delayed-absorbable suture is preferred when possible to avoid overlapping suture lines (Fig. 45-10.5). Redundant vaginal epithelium is trimmed, and the epithelium is closed in a running fashion with 2-0 gauge delayed-absorbable suture.

Surgical Steps—Partial Diverticular Ablation

If extensive dissection is required around the trigone, consideration is given to leaving the proximal portion of the sac in place to avoid direct injury or denervation injury. In addition, ureteral stents may be beneficial during the dissection.

❶ **Vaginal Incision and Diverticulum Exposure.** These early steps mirror those in Steps 3 and 4 in the prior description. However, to avoid injury to the proximal urethra and bladder neck, the diverticular sac, but not the neck of the diverticulum, is sharply excised. As much of the sac as can be accessed is resected.

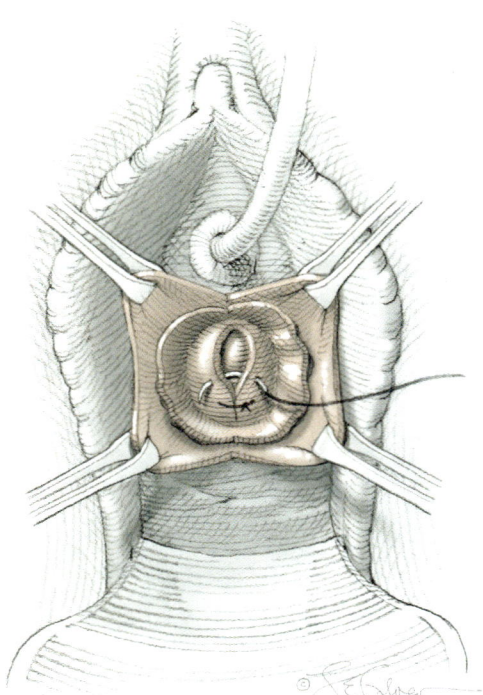

FIGURE 45-10.4 Urethral defect closure.

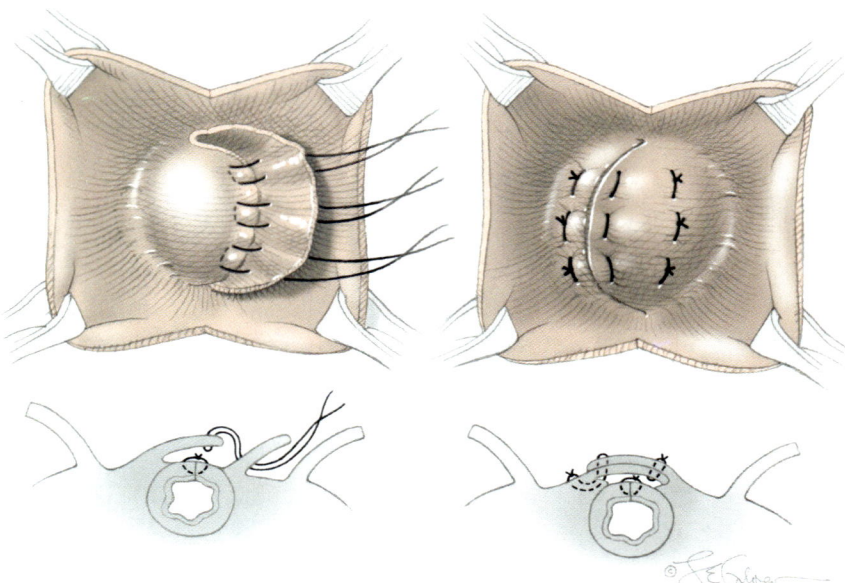

FIGURE 45-10.5 Fibromuscular layer reapproximation.

❷ Sac Closure. The base of the sac then is sutured side to side with 3-0 or 4-0 gauge delayed-absorbable suture to cover the urethral defect. A second, and possibly a third, imbricating layer using the vaginal muscularis is created with 3-0 gauge delayed-absorbable suture. Excess vaginal epithelium that had previously covered the diverticulum is trimmed. The vaginal epithelium is closed in a running fashion with a 2-0 gauge delayed-absorbable suture.

POSTOPERATIVE

Catheter management is an important aspect of postoperative care. Although no consensus guidelines exist, most experts recommend catheterization for 7 to 14 days. Surgeries of increasing complexity may require longer duration. Antibiotic suppression is not required with this catheter use. Normal diet and activity can resume during the first postoperative days. Intercourse, however, is postponed until the vaginal incision is well healed.

45-11

Martius Bulbospongiosus Fat Pad Flap

This vascular graft contains the fat pad overlying the bulbospongiosus (former bulbocavernosus) muscle and brings a supportive blood supply to repairs involving avascular or fibrotic tissue. Commonly, this graft is used in complex urethral diverticulum excisions or in complex rectovaginal or vesicovaginal fistula repairs. However, some evidence shows successful repair of certain recurrent fistulas without vascular graft interposition (Miklos, 2015; Pshak, 2013).

During graft placement, one end of the bulbospongiosus fat pad is dissected free and subsequently brought to the repair site through the primary vaginal incision. Thus, due to its anatomic origin and limited length, this fat pad, when indicated, is selected for defects involving the low to mid vagina.

PREOPERATIVE

Patient Evaluation

Often, graft placement is anticipated for those with prior radiation or fistula recurrence. Thus, preoperative planning includes assessment of tissue vascularity, connective tissue strength, and ability to adequately mobilize vaginal tissues to create a multilayered repair closure. For this procedure, a woman also must have adequate labial fat.

Consent

During consenting, women are informed of the potential for postoperative vulvar numbness, pain, paresthesias, or hematoma. Because one of the labia majora is repositioned as the graft, patients are counseled regarding the cosmetic consequences.

Patient Preparation

Because of the risk for poor wound healing in these complicated repairs, antibiotic prophylaxis listed in Table 39-8 (p. 832) is warranted. Thromboprophylaxis is given as outlined in Table 39-10 (p. 834). The necessity of bowel preparation for this procedure is unclear, and administration is individualized based on other planned procedures.

INTRAOPERATIVE

Surgical Steps

❶ Anesthesia and Patient Positioning. In most cases, fistula or diverticula repair with interposition Martius flap graft can be performed with general or regional anesthesia, and the need for postoperative hospitalization is individualized. The patient is positioned in standard lithotomy position, the vagina and perineum are surgically prepared, and a Foley catheter is inserted.

❷ Fistula or Diverticulum Repair. The specific defect is repaired as outlined in its respective section of this chapter.

❸ Labial Incision. After repair completion, the lateral margin of one labium majus is incised (Fig. 45-11.1). The length of the incision is tailored to specific labial anatomy and graft size needed. In many cases, a 6- to 8-cm incision is made beginning below the level of the clitoris and is extended inferiorly.

❹ Fat Pad Mobilization. The vulvar incision edges are retracted laterally, and sharp dissection is used to free the labial fat pad (Fig. 45-11.2). This tissue is vascular, and vessels ideally are ligated or coagulated prior to transection. For rectovaginal fistulas, a broad base is left inferiorly, and the fat pad is detached superiorly. In these cases, the blood supply to the graft mainly stems from the perineal branch of the internal pudendal artery.

The same steps can be used for vesicovaginal and urethrovaginal fistulas or urethral diverticula. However, the labial incision is extended more anteriorly and close to the anterior labial commissure. This allows the free edge of the mobilized labial fat pad to better reach the anterior vaginal wall without tension. Instead, the broad base of the pad can be maintained superiorly, while the fat pad is detached inferiorly. In these cases, the blood supply to the graft stems from the external pudendal artery, a branch of the femoral artery. In each instance, releasing the pad with this specific polarity anatomically permits the largest possible graft to cover the repair site. Occasionally, bilateral fat pads are needed.

❺ Graft Placement. After the pad is freed, a tunnel is created by bluntly dissecting with a hemostat that travels from the vulvar incision, underneath the vaginal epithelium, and to the vaginal incision at the repair site. The tunnel must be sufficiently broad to

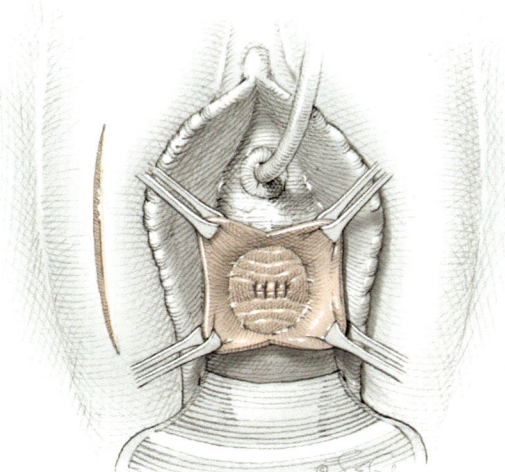

FIGURE 45-11.1 Labial incision.

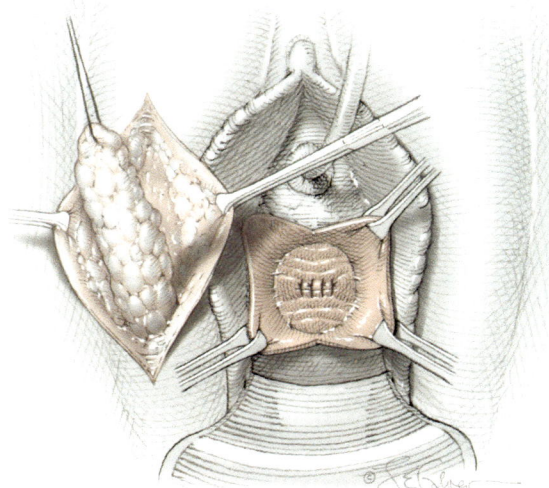

FIGURE 45-11.2 Mobilization of the fat pad.

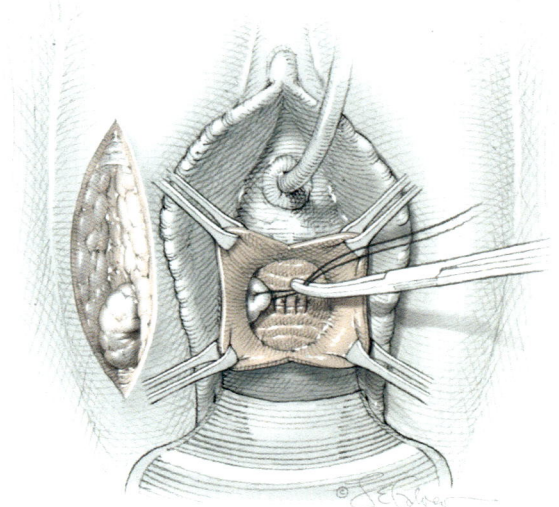

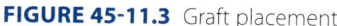

FIGURE 45-11.3 Graft placement.

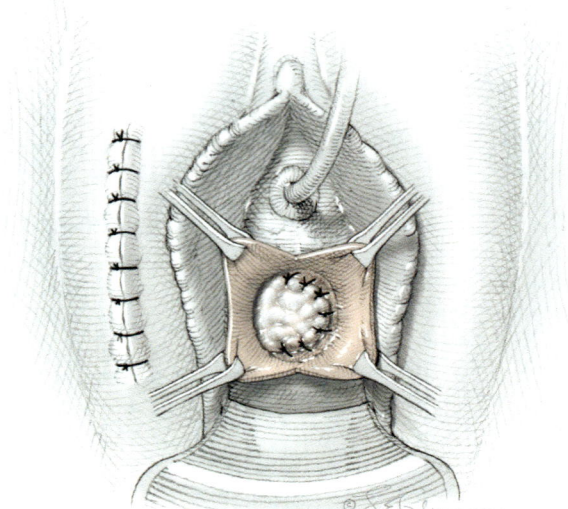

FIGURE 45-11.4 Graft fixation, and harvest-site closure.

avoid vascular compression and graft necrosis. A suture is placed at the graft tip and used to pass the graft through the tunnel and into the vagina (Fig. 45-11.3).

⑥ Graft Fixation. The graft is secured to the vaginal muscularis overlying the repair site with several interrupted stitches using 3-0 gauge delayed-absorbable suture (Fig. 45-11.4).

⑦ Incision Closure. With hemostasis established, the vulvar incision is closed along its length with continuous or interrupted stitches of 3-0 gauge delayed-absorbable sutures. A subcuticular suture line with 4-0 gauge absorbable suture also is suitable. For a deep cavity at the harvest site, fatty tissue may be reapproximated in layers to close this space with several interrupted 2-0 or 3-0 gauge delayed-absorbable sutures. Alternatively, a drain may be placed in the cavity. The vaginal epithelium overlying the defect repair is closed in a continuous running fashion using 3-0 gauge delayed-absorbable suture.

POSTOPERATIVE

Care after surgery is predominantly dictated by the associated defect repair. Ideally, the vaginal and perineal sites are kept dry rather than wet, and baths are avoided during the first 6 weeks. After each void or stool, patients rinse with a water-filled squirt bottle and gently pat dry.

45-12

Sacral Neuromodulation

Sacral neuromodulation (SNM) or sacral nerve stimulation electrically stimulates the sacral nerves to modulate reflexes that influence the bladder, sphincters, and pelvic floor (Noblett, 2014). Currently, the InterStim System is FDA-approved for the following primary indications: urgency-frequency, urgency urinary incontinence, nonobstructive urinary retention, and fecal incontinence (FI). Although not FDA-approved for chronic pelvic pain, interstitial cystitis/bladder pain syndrome, or chronic idiopathic constipation, it sometimes may be used if these symptoms coexist with the previously listed primary indications. SNM is typically offered to women who have failed to adequately improve with multiple other conservative therapies. In 2019, the Axionics SNM system was FDA-approved for FI treatment. Approval for other indications is pending (Blok, 2019).

Its mechanism of action is unclear, but one explanation describes modulation of reflex neural pathways involved with bladder storage and emptying and with innervation of the pelvic floor. Of these, pudendal afferent somatic fibers are thought to be important (deGroat, 1981; Gourcerol, 2011).

SNM generally is completed in two phases. First, during a test or trial phase, a slender, 30-cm-long, permanent (tined) lead that conducts electrical impulses to its tip is placed into one posterior sacral foramen. Here, it lies adjacent to a sacral nerve root, most commonly S3. This lead is connected to a temporary external pulse generator, which permits an efficacy trial lasting 1 to 2 weeks. If symptoms decline by at least 50 percent, the patient is deemed a suitable candidate for permanent generator implantation. The trial phase is considered the single most valuable tool for predicting the potential therapeutic success of SNM for urinary indications (Goldman, 2018).

In the implantation phase, the lead instead is connected to a permanent implantable pulse generator (IPG). The IPG is tucked within a pocket created in the buttock.

A variation of these classic steps, termed *peripheral nerve evaluation (PNE)*, inserts a *temporary* lead through the S3 foramen in the office, under local anesthesia. Despite advantages, the trial period with PNE is brief (3 to 7 days), and the less securely anchored temporary lead more easily migrates away from the target nerve.

PREOPERATIVE

Patient Evaluation

Preoperative testing will vary depending on the indication. For urinary symptoms, women undergo full evaluation including urodynamic testing, voiding diary, cystoscopy, and other selected tests described in Chapter 23 (p. 521). For fecal incontinence, colonoscopy, endoanal sonography, manometry, and possibly neurophysiologic testing, described in Chapter 25 (p. 562), are completed.

Consent

Absolute contraindications for SNM include inadequate clinical response during the therapeutic trial, inability to operate the device, and pregnancy (Goldman, 2018). Failure to significantly improve symptoms may follow either SNM phase. However, approximately 70 percent of those who undergo permanent IPG implantation achieve >50-percent symptom improvement (Van Kerrebroeck, 2012). Pain at the IPG site and superficial wound infection can complicate either phase. Long-term adverse changes include altered bowel or bladder function, undesirable sensations, neurostimulator site numbness, lead migration, and surgical device revision, replacement, or required removal. The IPG device is a relative contraindication for MR imaging, although certain IPG models permit head imaging.

Patient Preparation

A single prophylactic antibiotic dose is administered according to surgeon preference. Although not rigorously studied, prophylaxis is recommended due to needle passage from skin to perineural tissue. Thromboprophylaxis typically is not required.

INTRAOPERATIVE

Surgical Steps

❶ **Anesthesia and Patient Positioning.** The procedure usually is performed with local anesthesia and intravenous sedation, although general anesthesia can be used for the test-phase tine placement. Neuromuscular blockade prohibits adequate motor response evaluation and is contraindicated.

For easier access to the sacrum, the patient is positioned prone on a Wilson frame or with a pillow under the lower abdomen to flex the hip 30 degrees. Pillows also are placed under the shins to allow the toes to move freely during test stimulation. The drape is positioned to permit inspection of the pelvic floor and the soles for muscle responses. The area from the lower back to the perineum is surgically prepared. A Foley catheter is typically not required due to the surgery's brevity.

❷ **S3 Foramina Identification.** The landmark for lead placement is located approximately 9 cm above the coccyx and 1 to 2 cm lateral to the midline. Fluoroscopy is currently the most common method of identifying the necessary bony landmarks intraoperatively. The fluoroscopic C-arm is draped and moved into the anteroposterior (AP) position to allow mapping of the sacral region and foramina. With this, the skin overlying the S3 foramina is outlined with a surgical marker.

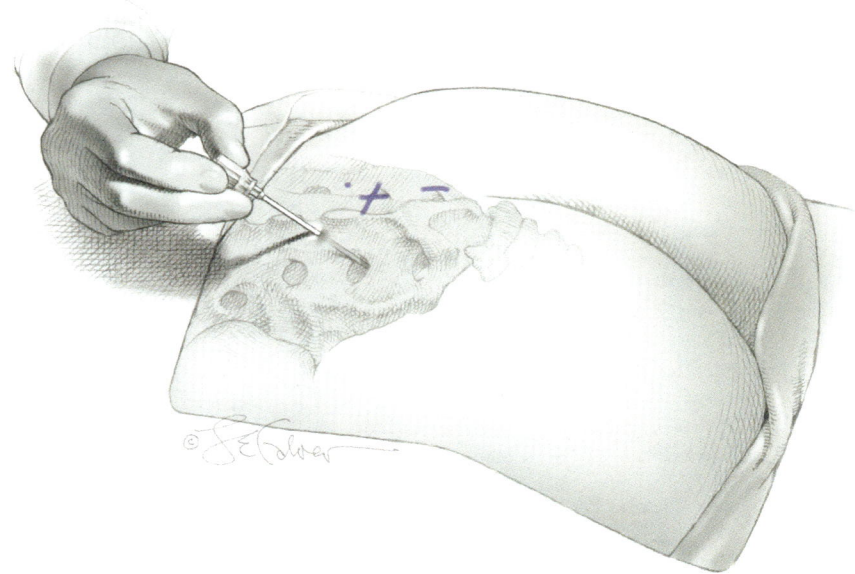

FIGURE 45-12.1 Foramen needle insertion.

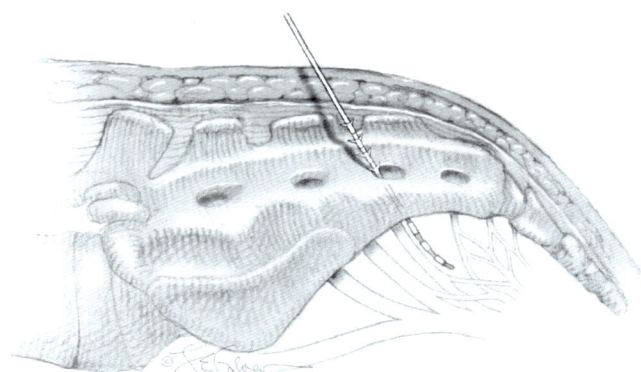

FIGURE 45-12.2 Correct lead positioning.

❸ Foramina Needle Insertion. An insulated foramen needle is inserted through the skin at a site approximately 2 cm lateral to the midline, 2 cm superior to the sciatic notch, and cephalad to the inked outline of the foramen. The needle is guided at a 60-degree angle caudally until the S3 foramen is penetrated (Fig. 45-12.1). Optimally, the needle is placed into the medial and superior aspect of the S3 foramen. The needle penetrance depth, which is usually 2.5 to 4.0 cm, is confirmed and adjusted with fluoroscopic guidance by a laterally positioned C-arm.

Once in place, the needle is used to conduct electrical test impulses to the S3 nerve. This nerve stimulates levator ani muscle contraction to create an inward retraction or "bellows" movement. S3 stimulation also causes the great toe to flex downward, that is, plantar flexion. In anesthetized patients, a sensory response cannot be elicited. However, evidence suggests that motor responses may be more or at least as predictive of success (Cohen, 2006; Govaert, 2009; Peters, 2011). The typical patient sensation with S3 stimulation is a tapping or vibration in the vagina, rectum, or perineum. Once the desired S3 motor reflexes are obtained ("bellows and toe") preferably in that order, lead placement is initiated. If these are absent, needle depth or angle is adjusted to achieve the desired responses. Instead, a needle in the contralateral foramen or in a foramen up or down one vertebral space may be tried.

❹ Lead Placement. Once positioned, the stylet present within the foramen needle is removed and replaced with a guide wire to the appropriate depth. The foramen needle is then removed while holding the guide wire in place. A small incision is made on either side of the guide wire. Next, a combined introducer sheath/hollow dilator tool is then slid over the guide wire to occupy the foramen needle's former position. The hollow dilator is unscrewed from the introducer sheath, and the dilator and guide wire are removed together. This leaves only the introducer sheath in place.

Using fluoroscopy, the long, flexible lead is passed down the introducer sheath into the S3 foramen. To aid threading, the lead contains a temporary stiff inner stylet. The curved stylet better follows anatomic contours to position the lead close to the nerve root (Jacobs, 2014). The lead also contains four circumferential electrode bands arranged in series at its tip, and proximal to these lie four plastic barbs or tines to ultimately anchor the lead within soft tissues (Fig. 45-12.2).

With correct lead positioning as shown, the most proximal of the four electrode bands are fluoroscopically visible just anterior to the sacrum (Goldman, 2018). All four electrodes on the lead should conduct pulses and elicit S3 motor responses. If necessary, the lead can be repositioned within the foramen. Once correctly positioned, the introducer sheath and then the curved lead stylet are removed. As the introducer sheath is removed, the four tines lock into place. Thus, the lead cannot be retracted after this point. All four electrodes are again tested to confirm the previously observed responses.

If lead advancement is needed, its stylet is replaced and the lead advanced. Retraction is more problematic. The lead is removed using gentle traction, and Steps 3 and 4 are repeated. The desired range of stimulation amplitude to achieve desired motor responses is 1 to 2 milliamps. Responses at lower amplitudes may indicate that the lead lies too close to the nerve, whereas requisite higher amplitudes can decrease battery longevity.

❺ Pulse Generator Incision and Lead Passage. Several centimeters below the iliac crest, a 4-cm incision is made over the lateral portion of the buttock that is ipsilateral to the selected foramen. Sharp and blunt dissection is used to create a deep pocket that can house the extension device for the temporary external pulse generator and, eventually, the permanent IPG. The pocket should remain above the gluteal muscle fascia but is made sufficiently deep to accommodate the final IPG.

After the pocket is created, a pointed passing device is used to create a narrow tunnel between the lead and the pocket (Fig. 45-12.3). The core of the passing device

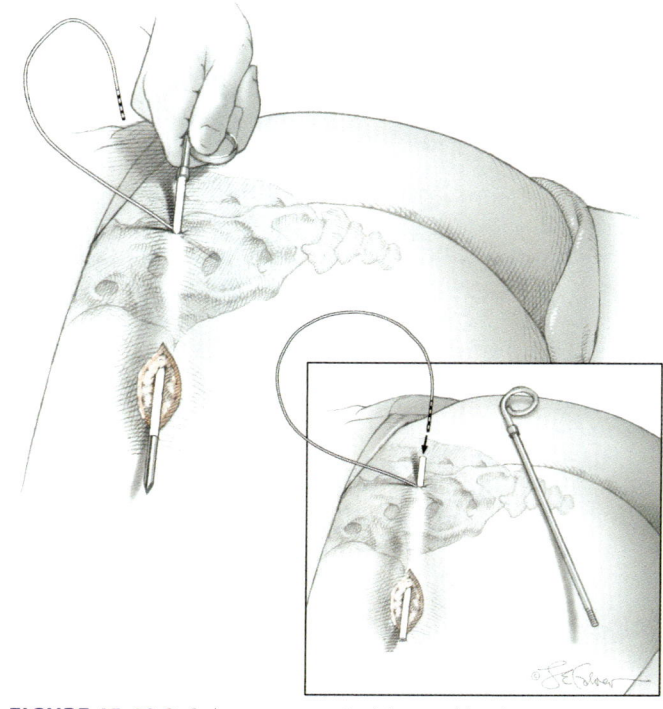

FIGURE 45-12.3 Pulse generator incision and lead passage.

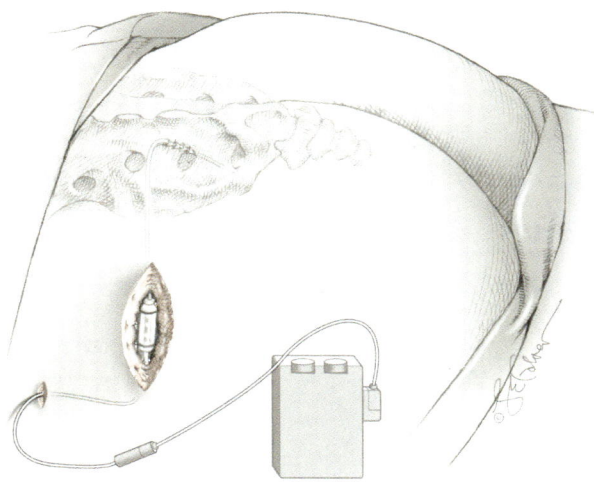

FIGURE 45-12.4 Within pocket, lead joins extension wire that extends to temporary pulse generator.

is removed, leaving a hollow straw within the tunnel (Inset). The lead is manually threaded laterally through this straw and into the pocket. The straw is then removed laterally.

❻ Extension Device Placement (Test Phase). Within the subcutaneous pocket, the lead is next connected to an extension wire that serves to join the lead to the temporary pulse generator (Fig. 45-12.4). A stab incision is created lateral to the pocket. The passing device is again used and, this time, guides the extension wire through a second tunnel between the pocket and lateral stab incision.

The subcutaneous tissue is then closed over the connector in the pocket with 2-0 gauge delayed-absorbable suture in an interrupted or running fashion. The skin is closed with a subcuticular stitch using 4-0 gauge delayed-absorbable suture or with other suitable skin closure methods. Similarly, the stab incision is closed. Last, the extender wire is joined to a temporary external pulse generator, which is used for 1 to 2 weeks (see Fig. 45-12.4). To minimize infection risk, surgical dressings are not removed during the test phase, unless deemed necessary by the surgeon. Vigorous activity is avoided for several weeks to allow the tined lead to scar in place and prevent lead migration (Goldman, 2018).

❼ IPG Placement (Implantation Phase). If significant symptom relief is obtained, the permanent IPG is placed 1 to 2 weeks after initial surgery. The procedure is performed with the patient prone, and either local anesthesia plus intravenous sedation or general anesthesia is provided.

The buttock incision is opened down to the connector. The connector and extension wire are removed. The permanent IPG is connected to the lead, and then placed into the subcutaneous pocket (Fig. 45-12.5). The incision is closed as in Step 6.

POSTOPERATIVE

After surgery, typical initial SNM settings include low-frequency stimulation of 10 to 20 Hz and pulse width of 180 to 210 microseconds. Primary symptoms are continually assessed, and the IPG is reprogrammed as needed. Namely, lowering voltage, decreasing frequency, or changing the lead configuration will often improve symptoms. If not, radiographic imaging searches for lead breakage or migration, which may necessitate lead replacement. Impedances >4000 ohms also implicate a lead fracture or microfracture, which may not be visible on imaging but likely requires lead replacement (Goldman, 2018).

Of potential complications, pain or erythema at the incision site suggests cellulitis, abscess, or seroma. These symptoms are evaluated promptly, and antibiotics are instituted if needed. Infection not responding to initial antibiotics may require full permanent device explantation and a longer oral or intravenous antibiotic course. Unusual pain also is evaluated immediately, as this could suggest lead malfunction. A woman can turn the device off by herself if necessary.

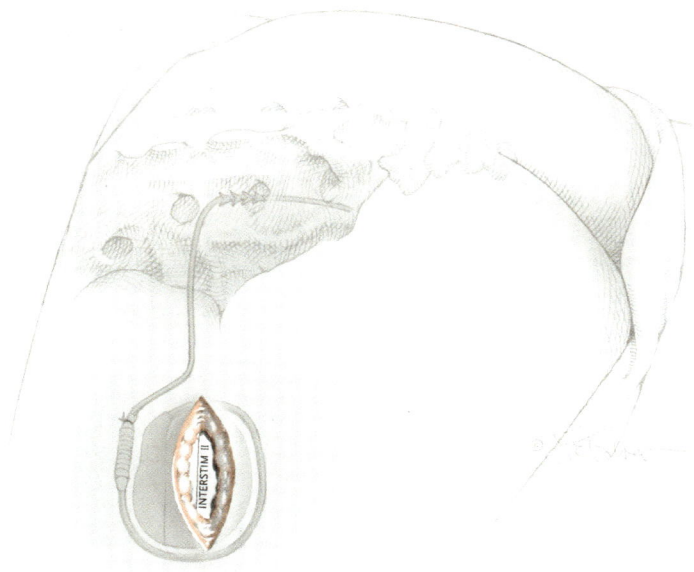

FIGURE 45-12.5 Final implanted pulse generator.

45-13

Anterior Colporrhaphy

The anterior vaginal wall is the most frequent site of clinically recognized prolapse (Brincat, 2010). One method to correct this is anterior colporrhaphy, which reapproximates attenuated fibromuscular tissue between the vagina and bladder to elevate the bladder to a more anterior and anatomically normal position. Anatomic success rates following this surgery are modest at 1 year (Altman, 2011; Weber, 2001). Thus, strategies to improve prolapse correction outcomes with colporrhaphy include: (1) concurrent vaginal paravaginal defect repair (PVDR), (2) concurrent apical support surgeries, or (3) synthetic or biologic mesh placement instead of or in addition to colporrhaphy.

Of these, PVDR attempts to provide lateral support to the anterior vaginal wall. However, a vaginal PVDR approach often is less favored as its required dissection creates a large defect within tissue that carries significant nerves and vessels. Robust efficacy data also are lacking.

Synthetic mesh placement improves anterior prolapse *anatomic* outcomes (61 versus 35 percent) compared with colporrhaphy alone, which is considered a native tissue repair (Altman, 2011). This disparity in anatomic success, however, does not always reflect the more equivalent *symptom* success rates of these two (Chmielweski, 2011). Such rates for mesh range from 75 to 96 percent compared with ranges of 62 to 100 percent for native tissue (Lee, 2012).

Moreover, mesh use significantly raises risks of mesh erosion, vaginal lumen narrowing, and pelvic abscess (Maher, 2013). These may be associated with dyspareunia, urinary complaints, and chronic pelvic pain (Food and Drug Administration, 2019a). Currently, few data guide patient selection for mesh placement, which may be best reserved for those with recurrent prolapse or those with medical comorbidities that preclude alternative procedures (American College of Obstetricians and Gynecologists, 2017b). Moreover, surgeons using mesh need adequate training and experience, and patients are educated regarding risks and benefits. The FDA (2019b) has ordered manufacturers of surgical mesh products indicated for the transvaginal repair of pelvic organ prolapse to halt distribution of their products in the United States. Alternatively, cadaveric fascia has been similarly used, but surgical success using this tissue is not significantly improved (Gandhi, 2005).

Last, growing data suggest that vaginal apex support plays a critical role in anterior vaginal wall suspension (Lowder, 2008; Summers, 2006). Thus, anterior colporrhaphy now is often complemented by apical support procedures.

PREOPERATIVE

Patient Evaluation

As stated, women with anterior wall prolapse often have other compartment defects, and a complete pelvic organ prolapse assessment aids surgical planning (Chap. 24, p. 544). Anterior vaginal wall prolapse also is frequently associated with SUI (Borstad, 1989). However, even continent women may have occult SUI that is later unmasked following prolapse correction. Thus, preoperative urodynamic evaluation is recommended. During this evaluation, the prolapse is reduced to its anticipated postoperative position to mimic corrected pelvic floor anatomy and dynamics following surgery (Chaikin, 2000; Yamada, 2001). Anterior colporrhaphy is an ineffective treatment for SUI. Thus, the decision to perform a concurrent prophylactic anti-incontinence procedure then is dictated by individual urodynamic findings and adequate patient counseling.

Consent

For most women, anterior colporrhaphy has low complication rates. Of these, defect recurrence is among the most frequent. De novo SUI described earlier, urinary retention, and voiding dysfunction are other discussion points. Although infrequent with native tissue repair, postoperative dyspareunia is another cited complication. Instead, preoperative symptoms related to sexual function generally improve with anterior colporrhaphy (Weber, 2001c). Uncommonly, serious hemorrhage, cystotomy, or ureteral injury may occur intraoperatively.

If mesh is used, these latter risks may be increased, and bowel or ureteral injury is possible. Accordingly, intraoperative cystoscopy is recommended. Less common short-term postoperative mesh complications include wound infection or hematoma. Long-term data from randomized trials show mesh erosion rates that range from 5 to 19 percent; chronic pain, up to 10 percent; and dyspareunia, 8 to 28 percent (American College of Obstetricians and Gynecologists, 2011).

Patient Preparation

Bowel preparation is generally not indicated for isolated anterior colporrhaphy but may be recommended at the surgeon's discretion

if other compartmental repairs are planned. Antibiotic prophylaxis with a first- or second-generation cephalosporin is recommended immediately prior to surgery (Table 39-8, p. 832). Thromboprophylaxis is given as outlined in Table 39-10 (p. 834).

INTRAOPERATIVE

Surgical Steps

❶ Anesthesia and Patient Positioning. After adequate general or regional anesthesia is administered, a patient is placed in standard lithotomy position, the vagina is surgically prepared, and a Foley catheter inserted. A short Auvard weighted speculum may be positioned to retract the posterior vaginal wall.

❷ Concurrent Surgery. Anterior colporrhaphy can be performed with the uterus in situ or following hysterectomy. If other reconstructive surgeries are required, they may precede or follow anterior colporrhaphy.

❸ Vaginal Incision. In those with prior hysterectomy and adequate apical support, two Allis clamps are placed on each side of the midline, 1 to 2 cm distal to the vaginal apex or at the upper extent of the anterior vaginal wall prolapse (Fig. 45-13.1) Clamps are gently pulled laterally to create tension, and the vaginal wall between them is incised transversely. If hysterectomy precedes the repair, the two Allis clamps are placed at the opened cuff edge on either side of midline.

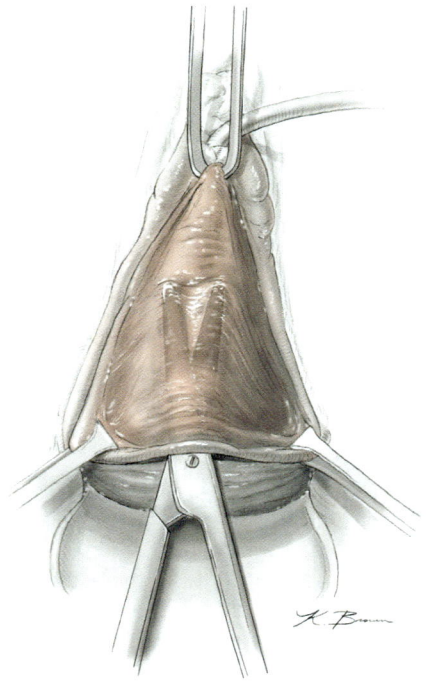

FIGURE 45-13.1 Vaginal epithelium incision and undermining dissection.

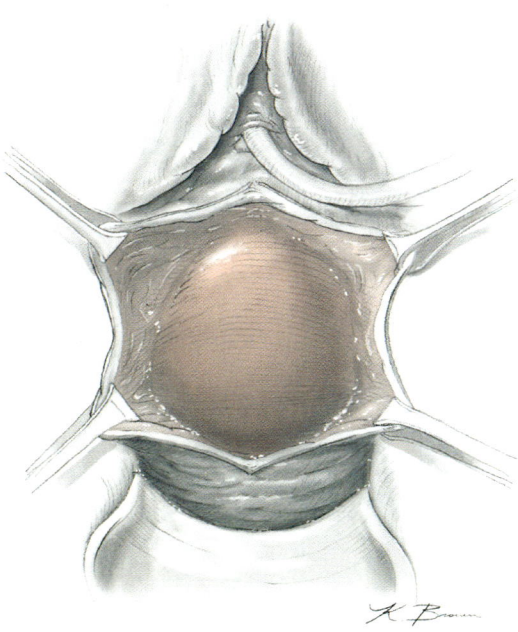

FIGURE 45-13.2 Vaginal wall incision and exposed fibromuscular layer.

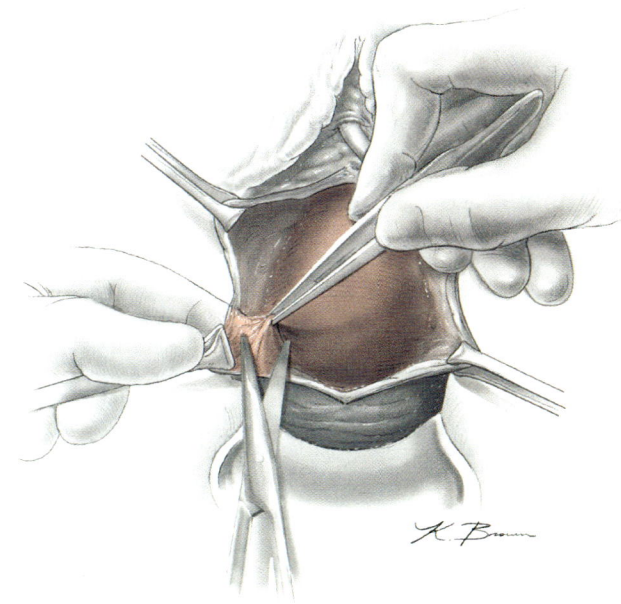

FIGURE 45-13.3 Separation of epithelium from fibromuscular layer.

A third clamp is placed in the midline vaginal wall, 3 to 4 cm distal to the apical transverse incision. All three clamps are held to create gentle outward tension. Metzenbaum scissors tips are insinuated beneath the epithelium in the midline of the previously made transverse incision and directed away from the vaginal apex. Scissor blades are opened and closed, while the surgeon exerts gentle forward pressure that is parallel to and within the plane beneath the vaginal epithelium. This technique allows separation of the epithelium from the fibromuscular layer. This dissection continues caudad to reach the distal, midline Allis clamp. The undermined vaginal wall then is incised in the midline longitudinally.

The midline Allis clamp is replaced more distally, and the process continues until the vaginal epithelium has been divided to within 2 to 3 cm of the external urethral opening (Fig. 45-13.2). This ending spot corresponds to a midpoint along the length of the urethra. If the anterior wall prolapse does not extend distally beyond the bladder neck, the distal epithelial incision terminates at the neck. If a concurrent midurethral sling procedure is planned, the colporrhaphy incision terminates just proximal to the bladder neck to allow a separate incision for sling placement.

❹ Lateral Dissection. Along the freed epithelial edges, additional Allis or Allis-Adair clamps are placed to create gentle outward tension, while the vaginal epithelium is dissected laterally off the vagina's fibromuscular wall (Fig. 45-13.3). This is accomplished with one finger placed behind the epithelium to accentuate the dissection plane. Simultaneously, scissors are held parallel to the vagina and cut connective tissue fibers between the epithelium and fibromuscular layer. Once the desired tissue plane is entered, a combination of sharp and blunt dissection readily separates the layers. Concurrent countertraction on the fibromuscular layer by an assistant using tissue forceps or a gauze-covered finger can aid dissection. This separation is extended laterally toward the pelvic walls until substantial fibromuscular tissue is exposed to permit its midline plication. The steps are repeated on the contralateral side.

❺ Traditional Anterior Colporrhaphy. Next, plication of the fibromuscular layer to the midline is begun. For this, interrupted stitches of 2-0 gauge delayed-absorbable suture are placed on either side of the midline along the length of the vaginal wall. To plicate tissue, each stitch is placed a generous

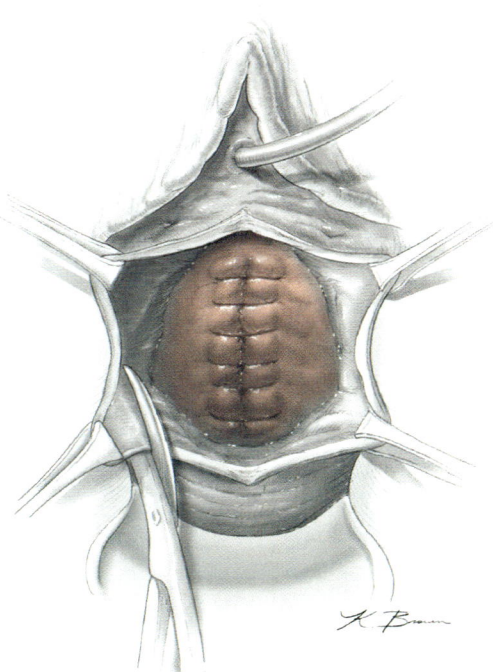

FIGURE 45-13.4 Midline plication completed.

distance from the midline to bring together the wide span of attenuated tissue. However, excessive tension is avoided to prevent sutures from pulling through the fibromuscular tissue or from significantly narrowing the vagina. As sutures are tied, the midline bladder bulge is elevated by the surgeon gently upward and away from the incision line. Such plication creates a firm fibromuscular wall layer to support the bladder and, if indicated, the urethra (Fig. 45-13.4).

❻ Vaginal Paravaginal Defect Repair.

If vaginal PVDR is planned, the vaginal dissection described above is extended laterally to the pelvic side walls at the level of the arcus tendineus fascia pelvis. Dissection also generally extends from the dorsal surface of the pubic bones to the ischial spines. Blunt dissection is typically used to enter the retropubic space. If a paravaginal defect is present, the space is easily entered.

Visualization of the pelvic sidewall is aided by Breisky-Navratil and lighted retractors. If present, the ATFP appears as a white line running from the pubic bone's dorsal surface to the ischial spine. In some cases, the ATFP is attenuated and indistinct, and stitches are instead anchored to the obturator internus muscle's investing fascia. For this, a series of four to six 2-0 gauge permanent sutures are placed in the ATFP or obturator fascia and attached to the paravaginal connective tissue (Fig. 45-13.5).

❼ Incision Closure.

Depending on the size of the original anterior wall defect, some redundant vaginal wall will likely be present and require trimming (see Fig. 45-13.4). Liberal trimming, however, can place the vaginal wall incision on excessive tension, affect wound healing, and narrow the vagina. Last, the vaginal epithelium is reapproximated in a running fashion with a 2-0 gauge delayed-absorbable suture.

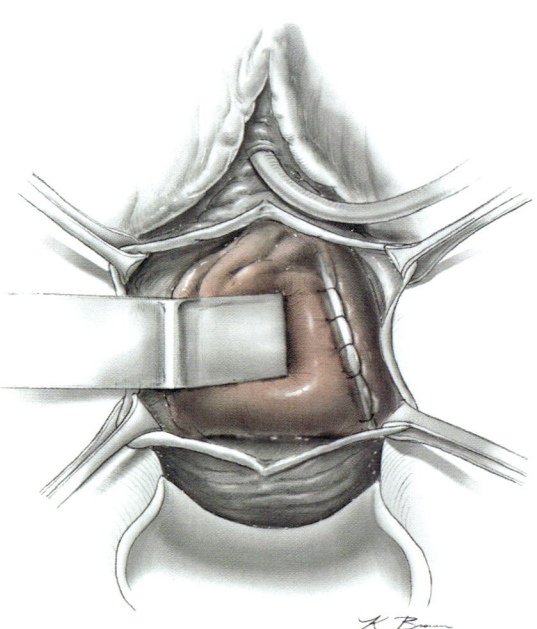

FIGURE 45-13.5 Vaginal paravaginal defect repair.

❽ Mesh Placement.

Various marketed mesh kits were previously available in the United States and still may be in situ from prior procedures. In general, broad mesh slings support the proximal anterior vaginal wall, while mesh arms extend and anchor to the sacrospinous ligaments (SSLs) to provide apical support. The recommended fixation point on this ligament was 2 to 3 cm medial to the ischial spine, which is similar to the fixation point for the traditional SSL fixation procedure (p. 1140).

❾ Cystoscopy.

Following 346 anterior colporrhaphy procedures, Kwon and colleagues (2002) performed cystoscopy and found unexpected injury in 2 percent of cases. These each required suture removal and replacement. Consequently, cystoscopy is indicated to document integrity of the ureteral orifices, bladder, and urethral lumen.

POSTOPERATIVE

For most women, recovery following anterior colporrhaphy is rapid and associated with few complications. Urinary retention or UTI, however, is common. Prior to discharge, an active voiding trial is performed. If a Foley catheter remains, a second voiding trial can be repeated in a few days or at the surgeon's discretion.

Similar to other vaginal surgeries, diet and activities advance as tolerated. However, patients abstain from intercourse until wound healing is complete, which typically is 6 to 8 weeks following repair.

Abdominal Paravaginal Defect Repair

Paravaginal defect repair (PVDR) is a prolapse procedure that aims to correct lateral defects in the anterior vaginal wall. The procedure involves attachment of the lateral vaginal wall to the ATFP (Fig. 38-8, p. 798). This procedure is rarely performed alone and is more often combined with other prolapse-correcting procedures, especially abdominal sacrocolpopexy. PVDR is an ineffective treatment for SUI. That said, abdominal PVDR may be performed in conjunction with the antiincontinence Burch colposuspension if a lateral anterior wall defect and prolapse complaints coexist with SUI. PVDR can also be performed laparoscopically or robotically in those with suitable skills.

PREOPERATIVE

Patient Evaluation

Demonstration of lateral vaginal wall defects on physical examination is required prior to surgery (Fig. 24-7, p. 541). If significant anterior wall prolapse is identified, evaluation for SUI or occult SUI is pursued. In women with a paravaginal defect, other pelvic support defects such as apical or posterior vaginal prolapse commonly coexist. Thus, attempts to identify these defects precede surgery.

Consent

PVDR provides support to the lateral vaginal walls, but as with other prolapse procedures, long-term success rates diminish with time. The procedure involves surgery in the retropubic space, which has the potential for significant blood loss. This and the risk of bladder injury are generally greater in patients with prior retropubic space surgery, because dense adhesions here between bladder and pubic bone are common. Less often, inaccurate suture placement can injure the bladder or ureters.

Patient Preparation

As with most abdominal urogynecologic surgeries, antibiotic prophylaxis is given to prevent wound infection (Table 39-8, p. 832). Bowel preparation is implemented at the surgeon's discretion and mainly indicated if additional procedures are planned. Thromboprophylaxis is given as outlined in Table 39-10 (p. 834).

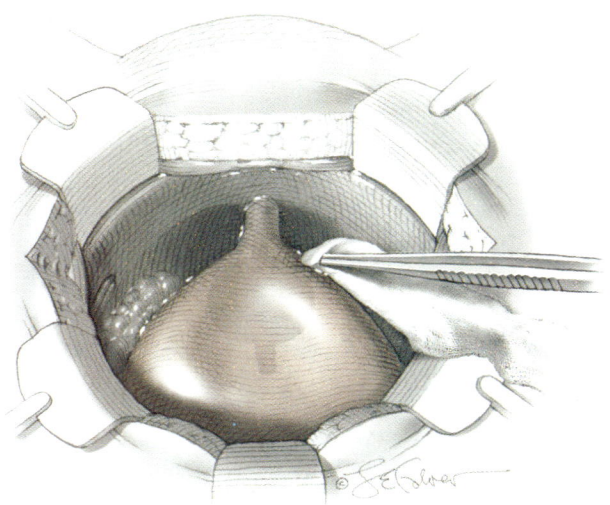

FIGURE 45-14.1 Dissection in the retropubic space.

INTRAOPERATIVE

Surgical Steps

❶ Anesthesia and Patient Positioning. When performed in conjunction with apical or other repairs, this surgery typically is performed as an inpatient procedure under general anesthesia. Following administration of anesthesia, the patient is placed in low lithotomy position in booted support stirrups. Adequate exposure to the vagina is vital because a vaginal hand is used to elevate and dissect the paravaginal/paravesical space. The abdomen and vagina are surgically prepared, and a Foley catheter with a 10-mL balloon is inserted.

❷ Abdominal Incision. A low transverse incision is placed 2 cm cephalad to the symphysis pubis to afford the best exposure into the retropubic space. PVDR is typically done in conjunction with abdominal sacrocolpopexy, and for this, the abdominal cavity is entered. If performed in isolation or with a Burch colposuspension, entry into the peritoneal cavity is not necessary to open the retropubic space.

❸ Retropubic Space Entry. After incision of the fascia, the rectus abdominis muscle bellies are separated, and retractors hold them apart. To open the retropubic space, the correct dissection plane lies directly behind the pubic bone, deep to the transversalis fascia but superficial to the peritoneum. Loose areolar tissue is gently dissected in a lateral-to-medial fashion with fingers or scissors beginning immediately behind the pubic bone (Fig. 45-14.1). If the correct plane is entered, this avascular potential space opens

easily and without significant hemorrhage. If bleeding does occur, the wrong tissue plane likely has been entered. From prior surgery in this space, the bladder often adheres both to the pubic bone and anterior abdominal wall, and thus sharp dissection is indicated.

After the medial portion of the retropubic space is opened, the obturator canal is identified bilaterally so that its associated vessels and nerve can be avoided. The canal is generally found 5 to 6 cm lateral from the symphysis pubis' midline and 1 to 2 cm below the pectineal line (Fig. 38-24, p. 813). The ischial spine then is palpated 4 to 6 cm below and posterior to the obturator canal.

The remainder of the paravaginal space is opened with gentle blunt dissection using a gauze sponge. This dissection is generally directed lateromedially, that is, from obturator fascia toward the lateral bladder border. This exposes the ATFP, obturator internus fascia, and paravaginal tissue. To assist, a vaginal hand pushing up into the space creates a firm surface to dissect against. In addition, a malleable retractor gently displaces the bladder to the contralateral side.

Small vessels within the loose areolar tissue are coagulated as encountered. Large paravaginal blood vessels (vesical venous plexus) often are noted along the lateral vaginal wall. Bleeding from these vessels can be controlled by upward pressure of the vaginal hand while hemostatic sutures are placed.

❹ Identifying the Arcus Tendineus Fascia Pelvis. The ATFP runs along the pelvic sidewall between the pubic bone and the ischial spine as a white connective tissue condensation (Fig. 45-14.2). In those with defects, it may be attenuated, torn in the middle, or completely avulsed from the

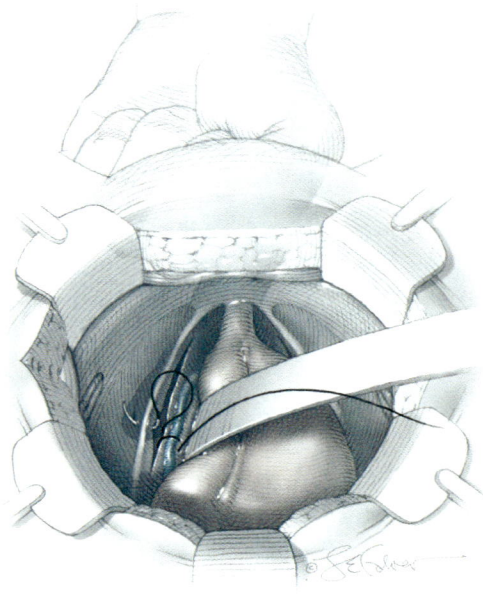

FIGURE 45-14.2 Placement of paravaginal sutures.

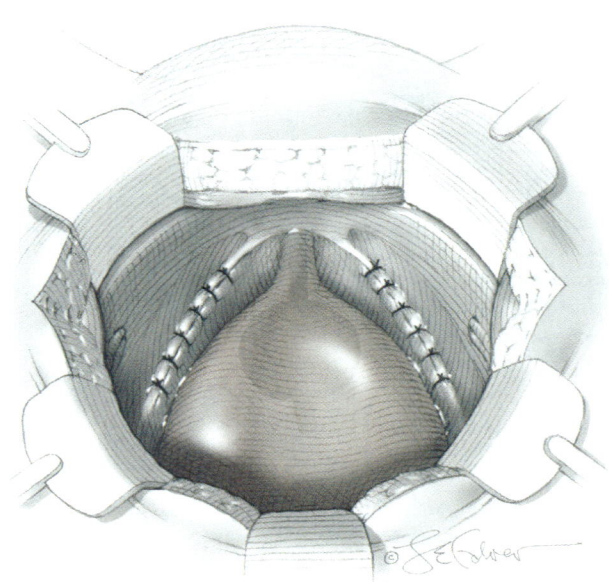

FIGURE 45-14.3 Final suture placement.

sidewall. Even in these cases, the distal third of the ATFP is generally preserved and easily identified.

⑤ Paravaginal Suture Placement. One or two fingers of the surgeon's nondominant hand are placed in the vagina to elevate the lateral vaginal wall on the planned side of defect repair. At the same time, a medium-sized malleable retractor is used to reflect the bladder medially and protect it and the ureter from inadvertent suture placement or entrapment.

Usually four to six interrupted 2-0 gauge permanent sutures placed approximately 1 cm apart are needed to obliterate the paravaginal defect (see Fig. 45-14.2). The ultimate suture line extends from the level of the ischial spine to the level of the bladder neck or proximal urethra. Each suture passes

through the paravaginal tissue just lateral to the bladder wall and through the ATFP or obturator internus fascia and is tied. A vaginal finger covered by a thimble for protection presses upward against the lateral vaginal wall to help isolate the paravaginal tissue and assess suture penetration. If a suture punctures the vaginal lumen, it is removed, discarded, and replaced by a more superficial stitch. If bleeding follows, the suture may be tied to constrict involved vessels. Prior to suture placement, the obturator canal and neurovascular bundle are identified and avoided. After all sutures are placed, the procedure is repeated on the other side of the vagina (**Fig. 45-14.3**).

⑥ Cystoscopy. Next, this is performed to note efflux from both ureteral orifices and to exclude bladder-perforating sutures. A

misplaced suture might be seen as a dimple in the bladder wall. If found, sutures entering the bladder are removed abdominally and properly placed.

⑦ Incision Closure. After vigorous irrigation of the retropubic space, the abdomen is closed in a standard fashion (Section 43-2, p. 934). If the peritoneum was opened, closure is recommended to prevent small bowel adhesions within the retropubic space.

POSTOPERATIVE

In general, recovery follows that associated with laparotomy or laparoscopy and varies depending on concurrent surgeries and incision size. Prior to hospital discharge, a voiding trial is performed (Chap. 42, p. 919).

45-15

Posterior Colporrhaphy

Posterior colporrhaphy, also colloquially termed *posterior repair*, traditionally is used to repair prolapse of the posterior vaginal compartment. Specifically, posterior colporrhaphy techniques attempt to reinforce the fibromuscular tissue layer between the vagina and rectum to prevent prolapse of the rectum into the vaginal lumen. The tissue plicated in the midline often is reapproximated distally to the level of the hymen, and here it includes the perineal body. This is especially important for women who display perineal descent and a widened genital hiatus during preoperative evaluation. For these women, perineorrhaphy usually is carried out concurrently.

Often, the vaginal wall apex also must be resuspended to obtain successful repair and prevent recurrence. The apex may be suspended vaginally to the uterosacral or sacrospinous ligament or abdominally to the anterior longitudinal ligament of the sacrum. Thus, a careful preoperative evaluation is essential to restore anatomy.

There are three current transvaginal repairs of posterior wall prolapse. First, *midline vaginal wall plication without levator myorrhaphy* brings together the vaginal wall muscularis and adventitial layers in the midline. Second, midline plication of levator ani muscles, also known as *levator myorrhaphy* or *levatorplasty*, plicates the puborectalis muscle in the midline (Francis, 1961). Last, *defect-directed repair*, also called *site-specific repair*, reapproximates attenuated vaginal wall at specific bulge sites rather than rotely in the midline.

Evidence suggests that midline plication without levator myorrhaphy has superior objective outcomes compared with site-specific repair and has lower dyspareunia rates than levator myorrhaphy (Karram, 2013). For these reasons, midline plication without levator myorrhaphy is the procedure of choice for posterior compartment prolapse. An exception might be a woman with a large genital hiatus undergoing colpocleisis. Importantly, a biologic or synthetic graft in the posterior compartment does not improve anatomic or functional outcomes (Maher, 2013; Paraiso, 2006; Sung, 2012).

PREOPERATIVE

Patient Evaluation

A detailed discussion of symptoms begins every patient evaluation prior to colporrhaphy.

Symptoms most likely to be cured or improved by posterior repair include the sensation of vaginal bulge and the need to digitally compress the rectal vault for defecation.

Posterior wall prolapse commonly accompanies other support defects, and patients undergo a complete pelvic organ prolapse examination (Chap. 24, p. 544). If concurrent anterior vaginal wall or vaginal apex prolapse is present, these also are repaired.

Consent

In addition to standard surgical risks, this procedure can be associated with failure to correct symptoms or anatomy. Thus, a patient and surgeon identify treatment goals and clarify expectations. In the few completed randomized studies, current techniques give a less than optimal anatomic repair, and success rates approximate 70 percent. Another frequent postoperative risk is dyspareunia, which is more common following the levator ani muscle plication discussed earlier. Accordingly, levator plication is not recommended in women who desire to preserve coital function. Injury to the rectum or rectovaginal fistula is another rare but potential complication.

Patient Preparation

Depending on surgeon preference, patients may be instructed to consume only clear liquids the day prior to surgery and complete one or two enemas that night or the morning of surgery. Ballard and associates (2014), however, noted no distinct advantage to this. Antibiotics and VTE prophylaxis are given as outlined in Tables 39-8 and 39-10 (p. 832).

INTRAOPERATIVE

Surgical Steps

❶ **Anesthesia and Patient Positioning.** If done in isolation, posterior colporrhaphy is typically a day-surgery procedure and performed under general or regional anesthesia. A patient is placed in standard lithotomy position in candy-cane or booted support stirrups. The vagina is surgically prepared, and a Foley catheter inserted.

❷ **Concurrent Surgery.** Posterior colporrhaphy can be performed with the uterus in situ or following hysterectomy. If other reconstructive surgeries are required, they may precede or follow posterior colporrhaphy. Notably, completion of the posterior repair prior to vaginal apex suspension permits the plicated and thus more substantial tissue to be anchored to selected ligaments during apical suspension.

❸ **Vaginal Incision and Dissection.** Two Allis clamps are placed on the posterolateral wall of the distal vagina on either side of the midline. Clamps are gently pulled laterally to create tension, and the vaginal wall between them is incised transversely at or just proximal to the level of the hymen and superficial to the perineal body. A third Allis clamp is placed in midline and 3 to 4 cm proximal to the introitus. All three clamps are held to create gentle outward tension.

Metzenbaum scissors tips are insinuated beneath the epithelium in the midline of the previously made transverse incision and directed cephalad (Fig. 45-15.1). Scissor blades are opened and closed, while the surgeon exerts gentle forward pressure that is parallel to and within the plane beneath the vaginal epithelium. This technique allows separation of the epithelium from the fibromuscular layer. This dissection continues cephalad to reach the proximal midline Allis clamp. The undermined vaginal epithelium then is incised in the midline longitudinally.

Next, the midline Allis clamp is replaced further cephalad, and the process continues until the vaginal epithelium has been divided to the level of the vaginal apex. If concurrent hysterectomy has been performed, the colporrhaphy incision generally extends to the cuff incision. In either case, if only a simple discrete distal to mid-vaginal defect exists, the midline colporrhaphy incision stops just cephalad to that defect's proximal border.

❹ **Lateral Dissection.** Along the freed epithelial edges, additional Allis or Allis-Adair clamps are placed to create gentle outward tension, while the vaginal epithelium is dissected laterally off the vagina's fibromuscular layer. This is accomplished with one finger placed behind the epithelium to accentuate the dissection plane. Scissors are held parallel to the vagina and cut connective tissue fibers between the epithelium and fibromuscular layer.

During this early lateral dissection, the perineal body is fused with the vaginal wall's fibromuscular layer, and scarring may be present from prior episiotomy or perineal lacerations. Thus, clear tissue planes often are not present, and sharp dissection is required. Cephalad to the perineal body and once the desired tissue plane is entered, a combination of sharp and blunt dissection readily separates the layers. Simultaneous countertraction on the fibromuscular tissue by an assistant using tissue forceps or a gauze-covered finger can aid dissection.

Separation in the correct tissue plane is essential. Deep dissection can enter the rectum, whereas superficial dissection can create holes in the vaginal epithelium.

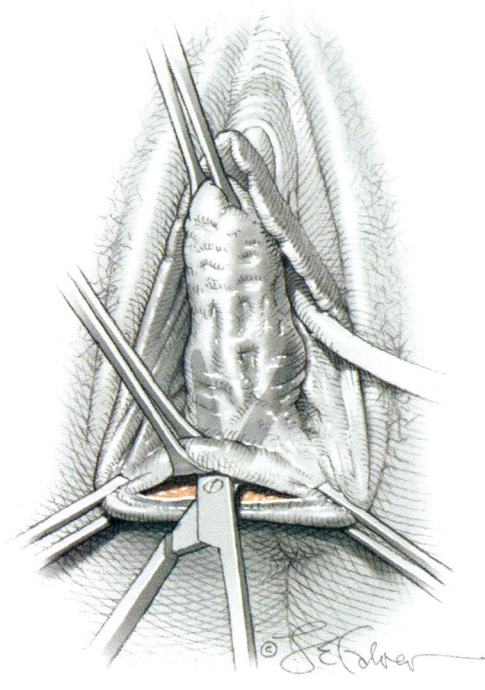

FIGURE 45-15.1 Vaginal epithelium incision and undermining dissection.

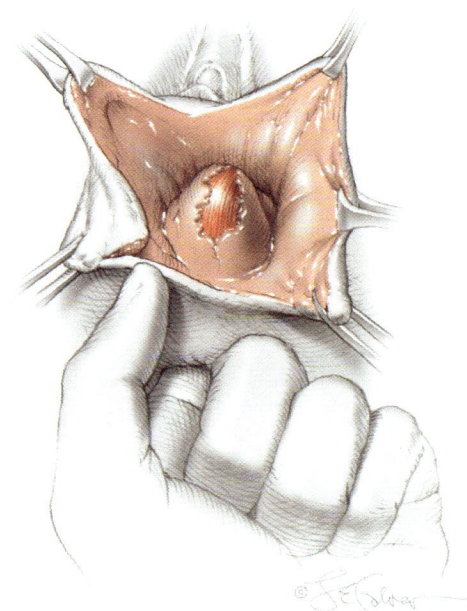

FIGURE 45-15.2 Rectal examination.

Tissue separation is extended laterally toward the pelvic walls until substantial fibromuscular tissue is exposed to permit midline plication. The steps then are repeated on the contralateral side.

❺ **Rectal Examination.** Rectal examination is performed to exclude rectal injury and to help identify the edges of the fibromuscular wall to be plicated (Fig. 45-15.2).

❻ **Midline Plication.** A series of interrupted 2-0 gauge delayed-absorbable or permanent sutures are used to plicate the vaginal muscularis and perineal body tissue along the length of the posterior vaginal wall (Figs. 45-15.3 and 45-15.4). To plicate tissue, each stitch is placed a generous distance from the midline to bring together the wide span of attenuated tissue. Such plication creates a firm fibromuscular wall layer

to support the rectum and, if indicated, the perineal body. However, excessive tension is avoided to prevent sutures from pulling through the fibromuscular tissue or from significantly narrowing the vagina. As sutures are tied, the midline rectal bulge is gently pushed downward by the surgeon and away from the incision line.

Rectal examination is again performed after all sutures are placed to exclude inadvertent

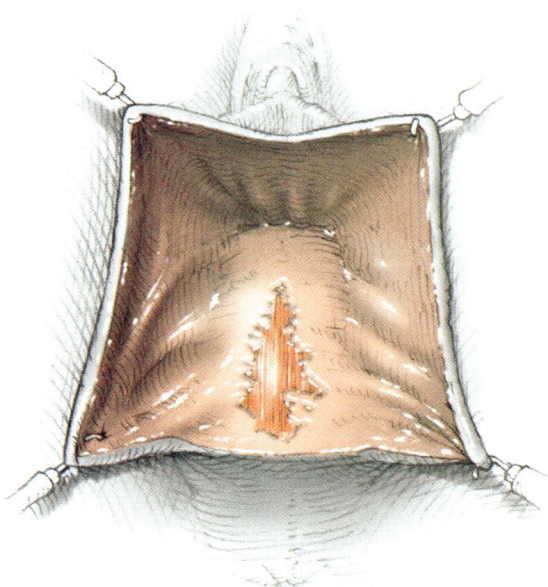

FIGURE 45-15.3 Midline defect.

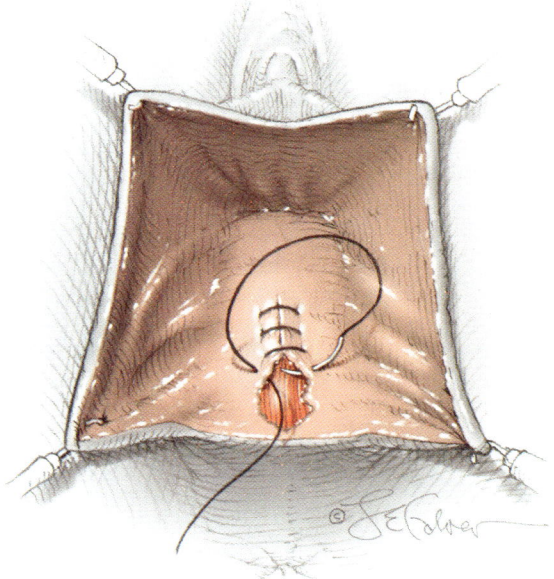

FIGURE 45-15.4 Midline plication.

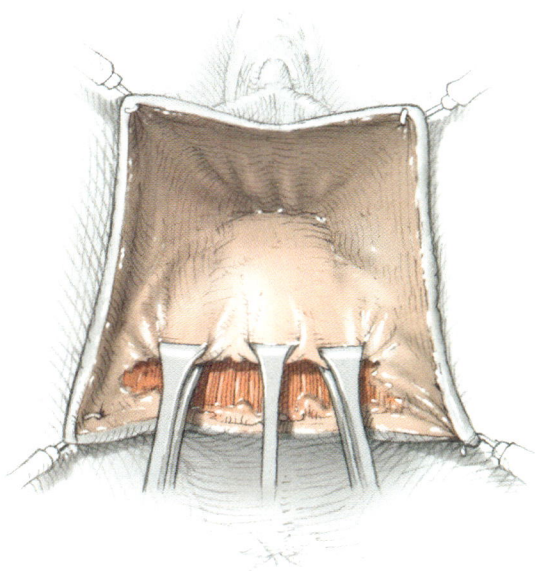

FIGURE 45-15.5 Distal defect.

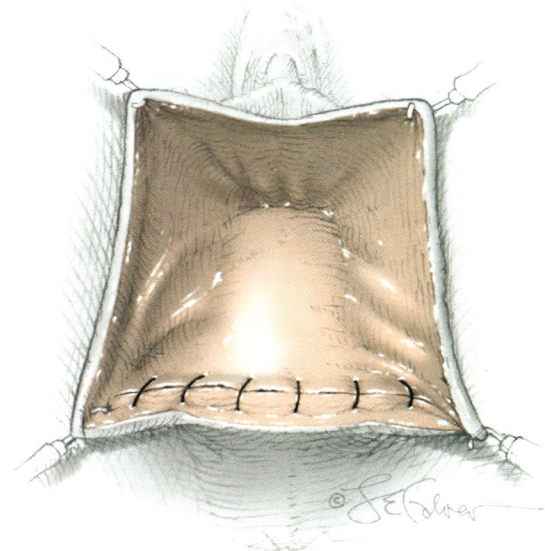

FIGURE 45-15.6 Defect-directed repair.

suture placement into the rectum. If identified, these are removed and correct suture placement completed.

❼ **Defect Assessment.** In some instances, a discrete defect is identified in the posterior fibromuscular layer after the initial dissection. Defects may be lateral, midline, apical, or perineal (Figs. 45-15.5 and 45-15.6). Repair focuses solely on the defect, which is closed by interrupted stitches of 2-0 gauge permanent or delayed-absorbable sutures. This is generally a one-layer closure. This repair may be complemented by a midline plication if significant tissue attenuation is still noted.

❽ **Indicated Apical Suspension.** If indicated, apical suspension is performed after vaginal wall plication. The proximal posterior vagina is affixed to either the uterosacral or sacrospinous ligament, described later (p. 1133). If perineorrhaphy is planned, it also is completed prior to incision closure.

❾ **Incision Closure.** Following plication, redundant vaginal epithelium often remains and requires trimming. Liberal trimming, however, can narrow the vagina and can place the vaginal wall incision on excessive tension that impairs wound healing. The vaginal epithelium is reapproximated in a running fashion using a 2-0 gauge delayed-absorbable suture. Widely positioned sutures are avoided as they can create accordion-type bunching of the vaginal epithelium and subsequent vaginal shortening when the final suture is tied.

POSTOPERATIVE

Patients are instructed on perineal hygiene. Constipation and straining are avoided, and stool softeners are usually prescribed. Similar to other vaginal surgery, diet and activity are advanced as tolerated. Women, however, abstain from intercourse until wound healing is complete, typically at 6 to 8 weeks following repair. Some women have urinary retention after posterior repairs, even without an antiincontinence procedure. If unable to void spontaneously by the time of discharge, a catheter may remain for a week or the woman may self-catheterize.

45-16

Perineorrhaphy

The perineal body serves as core support of the distal vagina, rectum, and pelvic floor. Therefore, a damaged or weakened perineal body may contribute to distal vaginal prolapse. Reinforcement of this structure, that is, *perineorrhaphy*, often is performed in conjunction with other reconstructive procedures, such as posterior colporrhaphy. To reestablish distal support, perineorrhaphy lengthens the anteroposterior dimension of a shortened perineal body, while the genital hiatus is concurrently narrowed.

PREOPERATIVE

Patient Evaluation

During prolapse assessment, both the length of the genital hiatus and the perineal body are measured (Chap. 24, p. 544). With perineorrhaphy planning, the degree to which the perineal body is lengthened can be tailored to patient symptoms, surgical goals, and clinical findings. With typical perineorrhaphy, the degree of perineal body lengthening is minimized to create or maintain a genital hiatus wide enough to preserve comfortable intercourse. Moreover, in sexually active postmenopausal women whose partners have decreased erectile tone, entry into the vagina may be difficult if the introitus is too narrow. Thus, following perineorrhaphy, 2 to 3 fingers ideally comfortably pass through the introitus.

For women with distal defects and attenuated perineal body tissue, perineorrhaphy may be coupled with posterior colporrhaphy. During the latter, the distal extent of the plicated rectovaginal wall can be reattached to the perineal body. This reestablishes continuity of connective tissue support in the posterior vaginal compartment.

In some women, pelvic support takes precedence, and coital function also is not desired. With "high" perineorrhaphy, the superior-to-inferior extent of the perineal body is lengthened and generally accompanied by plication of the levator ani muscle fascia at the superior aspect of the perineal body. The result of this extensive perineorrhaphy is a shorter genital hiatus length and narrower introitus and vaginal lumen. This may be an advantageous adjunct to colpocleisis. In contrast, data showing improved colpocleisis outcomes by adding levator myorrhaphy are limited (Gutman, 2009).

Consent

A patient preparing for perineorrhaphy is counseled regarding risks of postoperative dyspareunia, prolapse recurrence, or wound complications, such as separation or stitch abscess. Bleeding from perineal skin tearing during intercourse also may result and can require minor surgical revision.

Patient Preparation

Because of the surgical site's close proximity to the anus and because bowel injury is possible, antibiotic prophylaxis is administered prior to surgery to minimize wound infection risks (Table 39-8, p. 832). Bowel preparation mirrors that for posterior repair. Thromboprophylaxis is given as outlined in Table 39-10 (p. 834).

INTRAOPERATIVE

Surgical Steps

❶ **Anesthesia and Patient Positioning.** Perineorrhaphy is typically performed under general or regional anesthesia, and this choice is often dictated by concurrent surgeries. The patient is placed in standard lithotomy position in candy-cane or booted support stirrups. A vaginal and rectal examination under anesthesia is first performed to assess the size of the perineal body and defects of the posterior vaginal wall, which also may require repair. The vagina is surgically prepared, and a Foley catheter inserted.

❷ **Concurrent Surgery.** If concurrent surgeries have been included, perineorrhaphy is the final procedure in most cases.

❸ **Incision.** To determine the approximate appearance of the final repair, Allis clamps are placed on the posterolateral walls of the vagina at or just proximal to the hymen. These are brought together in the midline, and 2 or 3 fingers should easily pass through the intended genital hiatus. If the resulting opening is too narrow, both Allis clamps are moved closer to the midline, and the above steps are repeated. With this technique, a surgeon can judge the final size of the introitus and perineal body. Because scarring and retraction can develop, it is prudent to err on the side of leaving the genital hiatus larger rather than smaller.

To begin, a diamond-shape incision is made with its cephalad tip extending 2 to 3 cm into the vagina. The caudal tip extends to a point approximately 2 cm above the anus.

❹ **Skin and Epithelium Removal.** For traction, Allis clamps are placed at each corner of the diamond. Metzenbaum scissors are used to excise the perineal skin and vaginal epithelium within the diamond away from the underlying tissue. During dissection, the scissor tips are held parallel to the perineal and vaginal tissues, respectively.

Sharp dissection must be performed over the perineal body. This area contains a normal condensation of tissue, and scarring also may be present. As a result, development of good tissue planes is often not possible. Large veins are ligated or coagulated as needed. Frequent rectal examination during dissection may be required to assess the amount of tissue present between the anal and vaginal epithelium to prevent entry into the rectum.

❺ **Suture Placement.** Starting 1 cm caudal to the hymeneal ring, a 0-gauge delayed-absorbable suture on a CT-1 needle approximates the connective tissue surrounding the perineal muscles (bulbospongiosus and superficial transverse perineal muscles) in the midline. With suturing, a wide lateral stitch is taken, and the suture first travels in to out but on the opposite side move out to in (Fig. 45-16.1). This suture technique ultimately buries knots below the plicated tissue. However, initially, the first suture is held and not tied.

Downward traction is applied, and a second suture is placed approximately 1 cm cephalad. This suture ideally reapproximates the separated ends of the perineal membrane. As with the first, this suture is not tied. A third suture can be placed 1 cm further cephalad to this, if necessary. In a similar fashion, one to two stitches are placed 1 cm apart and caudad to the primary suture. These lower stitches plicate the connective tissue surrounding the superficial transverse perineal muscles and upper extent of the external anal sphincter muscle in the midline.

The sutures then are progressively tied. In some cases, a second, more superficial layer is placed in the perineal body for additional support.

❻ **Vaginal and Perineal Closure.** Starting at the vaginal apex, the vaginal epithelium is closed in a running fashion using 2-0 gauge delayed-absorbable suture (Fig. 45-16.2). When creating a running suture line in the vagina, stitches are placed close together. If suture bites are placed far apart during epithelial closure, the vagina can be shortened.

The running suture reapproximates the hymeneal ring and then is brought into the

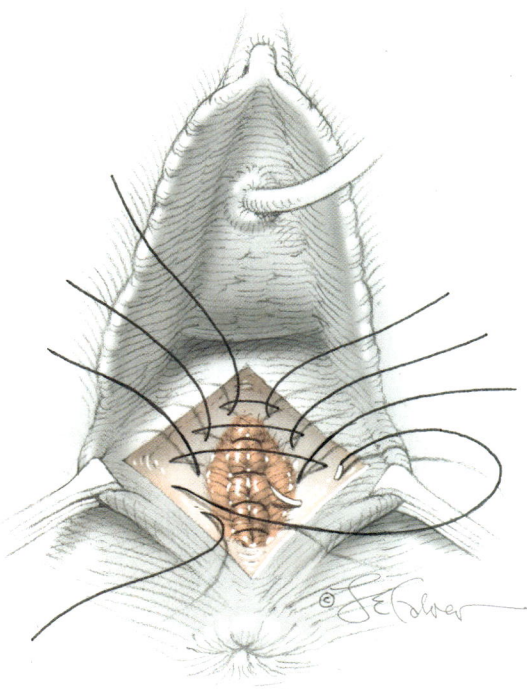

FIGURE 45-16.1 Suture placement.

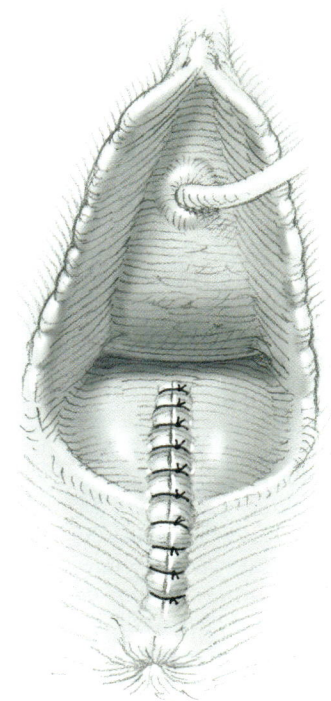

FIGURE 45-16.2 Wound closure.

perineal area. The same suture may be used in a running mattress method to reapproximate the subcutaneous tissue to the end of the incision, near the anus. Last, perineal skin is reapproximated in an interrupted or running fashion using 3-0 gauge delayed-absorbable suture.

POSTOPERATIVE

Patients are instructed on perineal hygiene. Constipation is avoided and stool softeners are usually prescribed. Similar to other vaginal surgery, diet and activity are advanced as tolerated. Women, however, abstain from intercourse until wound healing is complete, typically at 6 to 8 weeks following repair. Some women have urinary retention after perineorrhaphy, even without an antiincontinence procedure. If unable to void spontaneously by the time of discharge, a catheter may remain for a week or the woman may self-catheterize.

45-17

Abdominal Sacrocolpopexy

Abdominal sacrocolpopexy (ASC) using graft material is a widely accepted transabdominal prolapse-correcting operation. Many consider it the preferred procedure to correct advanced apical prolapse. Grafts of autologous, cadaveric, or synthetic materials may be used, but permanent (synthetic) mesh has the best success rate and is selected unless otherwise contraindicated (Culligan, 2005). The graft augments native tissue and suspends the upper third of the vagina to the anterior longitudinal ligament of the sacrum. In addition to correcting apical prolapse, the graft also covers proximal portions of the anterior and posterior vaginal walls. As such, ASC also corrects apical segment prolapse of the anterior vagina wall and of the posterior vaginal wall. A modification of the procedure, *sacrocolpoperineopexy*, is used if concomitant perineal descent is present and believed to contribute to patient symptoms (Cundiff, 1997).

One advantage to ASC is its durability, and long-term success rates for apical suspension approximate 90 percent. It may be used as a primary procedure or alternatively as a repeat surgery for patients with recurrences after other prolapse-repair failures. ASC often is chosen for women believed to be at high risk for recurrence and for whom mesh would augment their own tissue. Abdominal synthetic mesh aids durability, but its use is balanced against the potential for complications, discussed later.

The vaginal apex can be successfully suspended with vaginal approach procedures such as sacrospinous ligament fixation (p. 1138) and uterosacral ligament suspension (p. 1133), but ASC offers distinct advantages. First, ASC maintains or lengthens the vagina, in contrast to vaginal approaches, which may shorten it. Second, the use of synthetic mesh with multiple attachment sites to the vagina has a very low risk of apical failure. Last, unlike vaginal approaches, in which the vaginal apex is directly affixed to a structure such as the uterosacral or sacrospinous ligament, ASC repositions the vaginal apex to its nearly normal anatomic position. Thus, the apex typically remains mobile, which possibly lowers dyspareunia rates.

Sacrocolpopexy can be performed by laparotomy, by conventional laparoscopy, and with robotic assistance. If minimally invasive sacrocolpopexy is performed in the same manner as the open operation, similar results can be expected (p. 1129). However,

only limited data are currently available on long-term success rates with these MIS approaches (Freeman, 2013; Maher, 2013; Paraiso, 2011).

PREOPERATIVE

Patient Evaluation

Prolapse of the vaginal apex often coexists with other prolapse sites. If necessary, ASC can be completed concurrently with paravaginal defect repair, posterior colporrhaphy, or other prolapse surgeries. One review found that approximately 70 percent of ASC procedures were performed with other pelvic reconstructive operations (Beer, 2005). With the technique described here, a concurrent enterocele will be repaired by the colpopexy, and other enterocele repairs are thus unnecessary.

Prior to ASC, patients with symptoms of urinary incontinence undergo simple or complex urodynamic testing to clarify the type of incontinence and determine if an antiincontinence procedure adds benefits. For those with SUI, a concurrent antiincontinence operation generally is performed. Because prolapse correction can unmask occult SUI incontinence in some women, clinicians also test those without incontinence while manually reducing the prolapse. Last, apical suspension can predispose to later development of anterior vaginal wall prolapse and SUI. Thus, stress-continent women undergoing ASC may elect a prophylactic SUI procedure.

To evaluate this practice, investigators found that continent women undergoing ASC *plus* a prophylactic urethropexy had a 2-year postoperative SUI incidence of 32 percent. Without preventive urethropexy, SUI rates following ASC were 45 percent (Brubaker, 2006, 2008). Importantly, adding an antiincontinence procedure decreases, but does not eliminate, the risk of later de novo SUI.

Consent

Recurrent prolapse is common following any corrective surgery. Thus, a surgeon should be aware of recurrence rates quoted in the literature and his or her own personal rates. Although apical prolapse recurrence is infrequent, later prolapse of the anterior and posterior vaginal walls is more common. In one study, nearly one third of women by 5 years met the composite definition of failure (Nygaard, 2013). However, 95 percent had no retreatment for their prolapse.

Mesh erosion develops in 2 to 10 percent of cases. It is generally found at the apex and develops more often if hysterectomy is performed concurrent with ASC. Erosion

may arise soon after surgery or years later (Beer, 2005; Nygaard, 2004, 2013). Many technical points described in the following steps aim to prevent this complication.

Intraoperative, surgical findings described in the next steps may preclude ASC completion without significant risk for later mesh erosion. Thus, patients are presented the option to consent for intraoperative completion of an alternative apical suspension procedure if needed.

Patient Preparation

Bowel preparation will vary depending on surgeon preference. Patients can be instructed to consume only clear liquids the day prior to surgery and complete one or two enemas that night or the morning of surgery. Alternatively, a mechanical bowel preparation using agents listed in Chapter 39 (p. 833) may be preferred. Ballard and associates (2014), however, noted no distinct advantage to this for urogynecologic operations performed vaginally. Antibiotic and VTE prophylaxis are given as outlined in Tables 39-8 and 39-10 (p. 832).

For postmenopausal patients, vaginal estrogen cream use during the 6 to 8 weeks prior to surgery has been routinely recommended. Estrogen treatment is thought to enhance vascularity and thereby enhance tissue strength and promote healing. Although commonly practiced, no data suggest that preoperative estrogen cream decreases mesh erosion or prolapse recurrence rates.

INTRAOPERATIVE

Instruments and Materials

The upper vagina must be elevated and distended by a vaginal manipulator to allow adequate dissection and delineation of the vaginal wall fibromuscular layers for mesh placement. The manipulator may be a cylindrical stainless steel vaginal stent or a large round-tipped EEA sizer, which is present in most operating rooms.

The ideal bridging material for this procedure is permanent, nonantigenic, easily cut or customized, and readily available. The ideal mesh has a large pore size to allow host tissue ingrowth, is monofilament to decrease bacterial adherence, and is flexible (Table 24-7, p. 554). Currently for ASC, type I synthetic meshes (monofilament with large pore size), such as polypropylene mesh, are the most common synthetic grafts used. For ASC, two separate mesh strips can be fashioned as described in this section. A commercially preformed Y-shaped mesh is available as well.

Surgical Steps

1 Anesthesia and Patient Positioning. Following administration of general anesthesia, the patient is positioned in a low lithotomy position with thighs parallel to the ground and legs in booted support stirrups. Correct positioning prevents nerve injury and allows access to the vagina for manipulation and examination, to the bladder for cystoscopy, and to the abdomen for proper self-retaining retractor placement. The buttocks are positioned at the table edge or slightly distal to allow full range of vaginal manipulator motion. The vagina and abdomen are surgically prepared, and a Foley catheter is inserted.

2 Incision. A midline vertical or low transverse abdominal incision may be used, and selection is directed by a woman's body habitus and by planned concurrent procedures. A Pfannenstiel incision generally provides adequate access to the sacrum and deep pelvis. If a Burch colposuspension, paravaginal defect repair, or other surgery in the retropubic space is planned, a low transverse incision that is positioned closer to the symphysis may be preferred.

3 Bowel Packing. A self-retaining retractor is placed, and the bowel is packed up and out of the pelvis with moist laparotomy sponges. Bowel packing attempts to shift the sigmoid colon farther to the patient's left, thereby enhancing access to the sacrum.

4 Concomitant Hysterectomy. Some data suggest that hysterectomy at the time of ASC leads to higher mesh erosion rates (Culligan, 2002; Griffis, 2006). Thus, some surgeons advocate supracervical hysterectomy and allow the cervical stump to act as a barrier to infection and erosion (McDermott, 2009). If a total abdominal hysterectomy is performed, the vaginal apex is closed with absorbable suture such as 0-gauge polyglactin 910 (Vicryl) in a running or interrupted fashion. A second imbricating layer using the same suture may be placed to reduce potential mesh erosion. Another preventive measure is avoiding mesh fixation near the cuff suture line. Specifically, a 1- to 1.5-cm margin from this suture line may avert early mesh erosion during the cuff's healing phase.

5 Pelvic Anatomy Delineation. Important boundaries during presacral space dissection are identified beneath the peritoneum prior to the posterior peritoneal incision. These include the aortic bifurcation, iliac vessels, right ureter, right uterosacral ligament, medial border of the rectosigmoid colon, and sacral promontory, which is the upper anterior surface of the S1 vertebra. An understanding that the right ureter, right common iliac artery, and left common iliac vein all lie within 3 cm of the sacral promontory's midline may lower rates of their injury during surgery in the presacral space (Good, 2013b; Wieslander, 2006). Moreover, both ureters are threatened during dissection of the bladder off the anterior vaginal wall and during suturing of the anterior mesh strip.

6 Peritoneal Incision. The rectosigmoid colon is gently retracted to the left with a malleable ribbon or similar retractor. The peritoneum overlying the sacral promontory, between the rectosigmoid colon's medial border and the right ureter, is elevated with tissue forceps and incised sharply. The incision is extended caudally into the posterior cul-de-sac. As the incision approaches the deeper portion of the cul-de-sac, it is kept between the medial border of the rectum and the right uterosacral ligament. A vaginal manipulator directed ventrally creates tension to aid dissection. The incision then may be continued to the posterior vaginal wall and toward the vaginal apex.

Maintaining proper orientation is critical during this step, as inadvertent deviation can cause ureteral or iliac vessel injury on the right, or colon injury on the left. Similarly, if the initial peritoneal incision is extended above the sacral promontory, the left common iliac vein should be identified and avoided. This vessel can lie less than 1 cm from the promontory and is generally difficult to visualize or palpate due to its lack of pulsatility and decreased tone.

7 Identifying the Anterior Longitudinal Ligament. Following peritoneal incision, the loose connective tissue overlying the L5–S1 disc is removed by sharp and blunt dissection to expose the white, glistening lower part of the disc. Next, within the presacral space, fatty tissue that contains portions of the superior hypogastric plexus and right hypogastric nerve is bluntly dissected off the sacrum to expose the anterior longitudinal ligament lying along the sacrum's vertical midsection. Generally, this presacral space dissection is started at the promontory and continued 3 cm inferiorly to the upper extent of the S2 vertebra.

Within the connective tissue of the presacral space, fibers of the superior hypogastric nerve plexus, right and left hypogastric nerves, and the inferior mesenteric and superior rectal artery and vein are embedded (Fig. 38-23, p. 812). Of these, the right hypogastric nerve is the most common structure identified during dissection. Below the aortic bifurcation, this midline cordlike nerve courses laterally and, at the mid to lower sacral levels, reaches the right pelvic sidewall. Transection of this nerve is ideally avoided.

Of seminal importance, the middle sacral vessels typically also adhere to the anterior surface of the ligament. These can be avoided, ligated, or coagulated depending on surgeon's preference and operative findings. The middle sacral vein forms anastomoses with the lateral sacral veins that contribute to the sacral venous plexus. This plexus can be extensive, especially in the lower part of the sacrum.

8 Presacral Space Hemorrhage. Despite preventive steps, the sacral venous plexus can be lacerated and can lead to rapid and substantial blood loss. First, pressure is applied immediately and held for several minutes, while anesthesia staff and entire team are informed. Pressure may be particularly effective for venous bleeding. Sutures and clips may be useful, but tearing of small veins frequently worsens with suturing. Additionally, as vessels retract into the bone, isolation and ligation becomes difficult. Sterile thumbtacks directed through lacerated vessels and pushed into the sacrum can effectively compress such vessels. Unfortunately, these tacks are not routinely found in many operating rooms.

Alternatively, various topical hemostatic agents have been used to control bleeding refractory to these initial steps (Table 40-6, p. 860). Of these, the fibrin sealant family allows conformation to irregular wounds, which is a distinct advantage for presacral space hemorrhage. In refractory cases, vascular surgery consultation may be prudent. Injury to the iliac vessels or aorta necessitates immediate consultation.

9 Sacral Suture Site Selection. We prefer to affix mesh to the anterior longitudinal ligament overlying S1, with the most cephalad suture placed at or just below the sacral promontory. For promontory identification, the steep angle of descent between L5 and S1 can be used. Even correct suture placement at S1 and the sacral promontory still risks middle sacral vessel laceration. However, at S1, the middle sacral vessels are visible and can be easily isolated and avoided or, when necessary, clipped or coagulated. Additionally at S1, the anterior longitudinal ligament is thicker and stronger than at lower sacral levels (White, 2009). Affixing sutures here minimizes suture avulsion risks. Last, attachment of the mesh at S1 may result in a more anatomic suspension of the vaginal apex (Balgobin, 2013).

If safe suture placement over the S1 vertebra is prohibited, the level of the L5–S1 disc is an alternative. However, suture placement above the promontory risks left common iliac vein injury and penetration of the L5-S1 disc, which may lead to painful discitis or osteomyelitis (Good, 2013a; Wieslander, 2006). Thus, because the anterior longitudinal ligament is only 1 to 2 mm thick, shallow suturing is needed here to avoid the disc.

⑩ Sacral Suture Placement. Typically, three or four serial permanent sutures affix mesh to the anterior longitudinal ligament. These stitches can be placed first or later after vaginal mesh attachment. Needle passage moves from right to left with each stitch, and sutures are aligned vertically. Starting with the lowest suture, they are spaced approximately 0.5 to 1 cm apart. With suturing, 2-0 gauge permanent material, each double-armed with SH needles, is passed through the full thickness of the anterior longitudinal ligament (Fig. 45-17.1). During this, based on findings, stitches either encompass or avoid vessels. Once completed, sutures are held by a hemostat and not tied. Their needles are covered with a surgical towel to avoid stick injuries.

⑪ Anterior Vaginal Wall Dissection. Prior to mesh attachment, the peritoneum and bladder must be dissected off the proximal vagina. Dissection of the bladder from the upper third of the anterior vaginal wall is aided by the vaginal manipulator. The cervical stump or vaginal apex is displaced cephalad and dorsally, and its covering peritoneum is incised transversely and proximal to the bladder's cephalad margin. With prior hysterectomy, careful identification of the

vaginal apex and superior extent of bladder is critical to avoid cystotomy. This is especially important in women with short vaginal lengths or vesicovaginal adhesions. In these cases, retrograde bladder filling and Foley bulb identification may help delineate the upper bladder margin.

With cystotomy, several options are possible. If the cystotomy is small and close to the bladder dome, a two- to three-layered bladder closure, followed by an interposition flap (omental or peritoneal), may be considered. For large cystotomy or one near the trigone, an alternative approach to vault suspension may be considered to minimize mesh erosion into the bladder or fistula formation. Alternatively, the cystotomy can be repaired, and only the posterior strip of mesh can be placed.

Correct entry into the vesicovaginal space is suggested by white, glistening, vaginal wall adventitia and by loose areolar tissue between the vagina and bladder. Once this space is entered, the bladder is sharply dissected from the anterior vaginal wall for 4 to 6 cm caudally to create an extensive surface for mesh fixation (Fig. 45-17.2). Dissection progresses at a depth above the vaginal wall's fibromuscular layer. Entry into this proper plane lowers the rate of incidental entry into the vagina, which can raise future mesh erosion risks. If the vaginal lumen is entered, the opening is irrigated copiously and closed in two imbricated layers using 2-0 or 3-0 gauge delayed-absorbable suture.

⑫ Posterior Vaginal Wall Dissection. Next, the rectovaginal space is entered, and

the rectum is separated from the posterior vaginal wall. For this, the vaginal manipulator now displaces the vaginal apex ventrally. The reflection of the rectum against the posterior vaginal wall is identified, and the peritoneum is incised transversely 2 to 3 cm proximal to this reflection line. The right and left uterosacral ligaments are used as lateral dissection boundaries.

With gentle outward traction on the peritoneum, the rectovaginal space is developed with a combination of sharp and blunt dissection. In the absence of adhesions or fibrosis, the rectovaginal space easily opens inferiorly to the superior margin of the perineal body, which lies 3 to 4 cm above the hymen. Identification of loose gauzy connective tissue fibers usually indicates dissection in the correct plane. The white, glistening posterior vaginal wall provides another visual clue, and dissection is kept close to this tissue to avoid inadvertent rectal entry.

Fatty tissue or excessive bleeding generally indicates incorrect plane dissection and potential proximity to the rectum. If encountered, full-thickness rectal injury is repaired in layered fashion using 2-0 and 3-0 delayed-absorbable suture. The ASC procedure should be abandoned. For a suitably counseled patient, an alternative approach to vault suspension may be considered.

⑬ Graft Principles. Whether two separate strips of self-cut mesh or a commercially preformed Y-shaped mesh is used, several surgical principles are followed. First, depending on the extent of dissections, 6 to 12 sutures on the anterior and a similar number on the

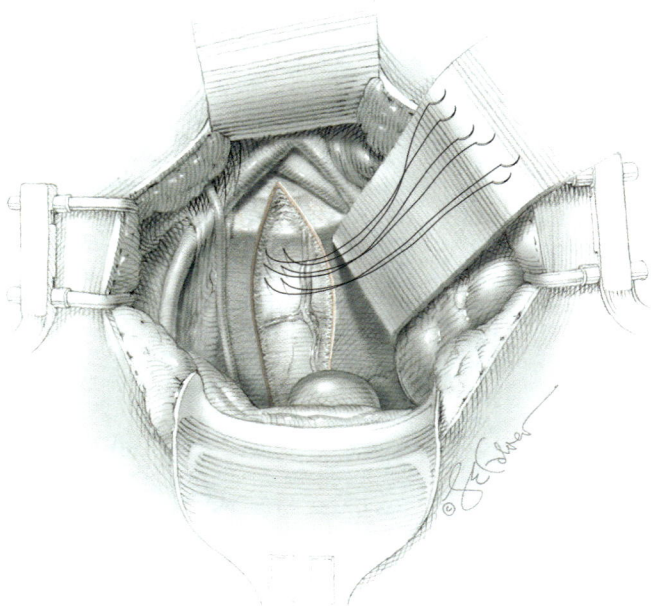

FIGURE 45-17.1 Placement of sacral sutures.

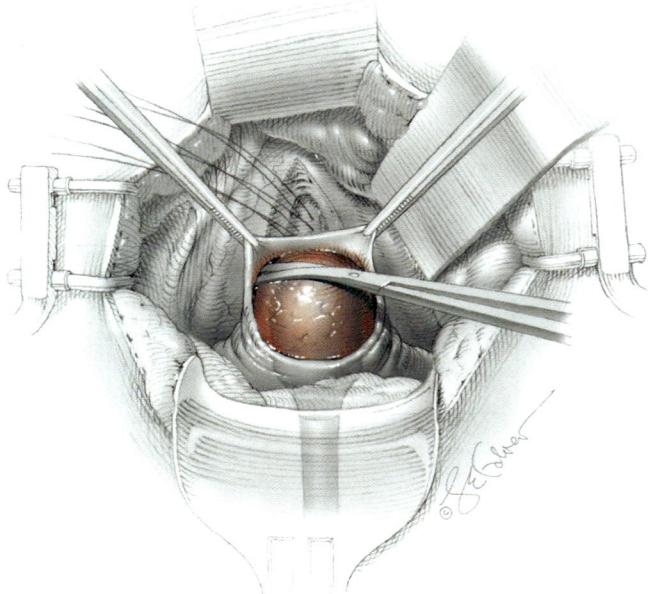

FIGURE 45-17.2 Dissection of the anterior vaginal wall.

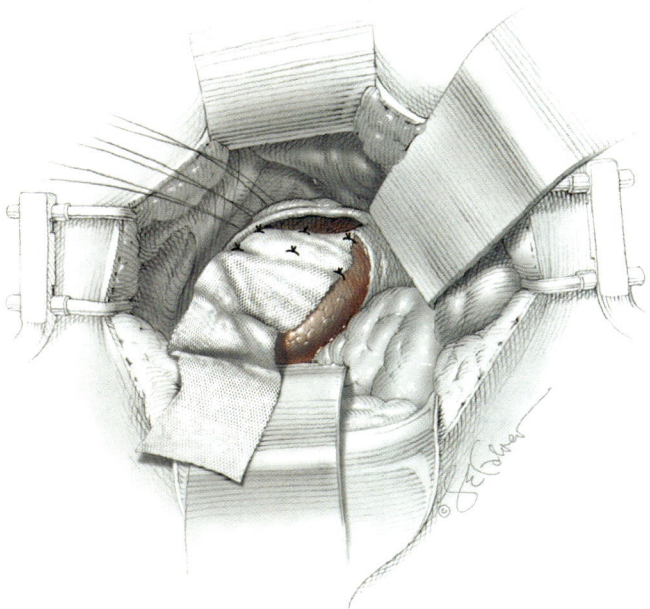

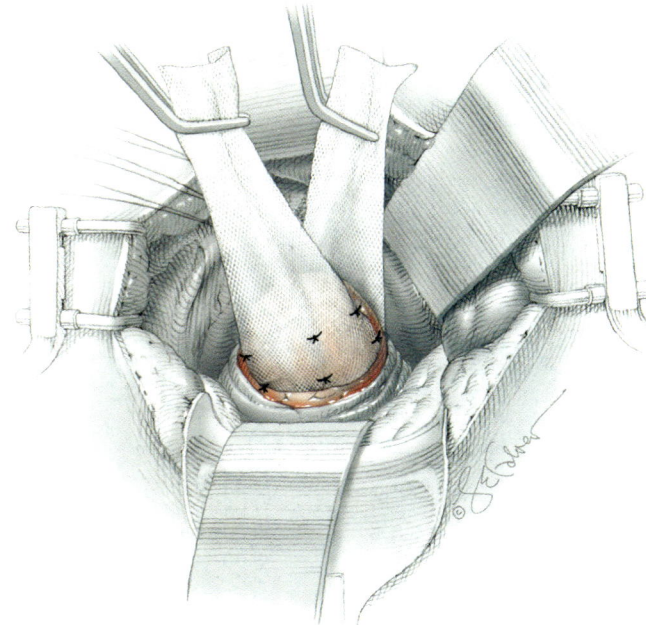

FIGURE 45-17.3 Posterior mesh secured and draped forward. Initially placed sacral sutures are seen in the background.

FIGURE 45-17.4 Anterior and posterior mesh in place.

posterior vaginal wall are placed through the mesh and the vaginal wall muscularis. Sutures ideally do not enter the vaginal lumen because epithelial healing over the stitches may be incomplete, especially with braided suture. If the fibromuscular layer is thin, this may not be possible. In this setting, many select monofilament, delayed-absorbable suture, which has a greater propensity for postoperative epithelialization.

Second, sutures are tied loosely to avoid tissue strangulation and vaginal wall necrosis, which may lead to mesh or suture erosion. Third, the lower extent of the mesh does not abut the bladder or rectal reflections to minimize potential risks of pelvic organ dysfunction or mesh erosion into these organs. Last, mesh is positioned symmetrically across the width of both the anterior and posterior vaginal walls.

At our institution, we fashion the two mesh strips only after vaginal dissection is completed. The broader area of each strip will cover the dissected anterior vaginal surface and posterior vaginal surface, respectively. Each strip also has a narrowed portion that will extend to the sacrum and be affixed to the anterior longitudinal ligament. This narrowed portion reduces mesh bulk, especially near the rectum on the left and the iliac vessels and ureter on the right, to lower mesh erosion rates. However, excessive narrowing may compromise overall repair strength (Balgobin, 2011). Generally, the narrow portion of mesh measures approximately 2 cm. Lengthwise, the proximal end of mesh is initially left long to allow correct positioning to the sacrum and later is trimmed.

⓮ **Mesh Placement.** To begin, the vaginal manipulator is pushed cephalad and ventrally to fully expose the dissected posterior vaginal wall and stabilize the vagina for suturing. The mesh commonly is attached to the posterior vaginal wall with two to four rows of 2-0 gauge permanent or delayed-absorbable sutures, and rows are placed approximately 1.5 cm apart (Fig. 45-17.3). Depending on the vaginal width and the lateral extent of dissection, each row consists of two to three sutures spaced 1 to 1.5 cm apart. The inferior and lateral extents of the dissected vagina are adequately exposed prior to suture placement to avoid incorporation of the rectum into a stitch.

For the anterior vaginal wall, mesh is sutured in exactly the same fashion as was performed on the posterior wall (Fig. 45-17.4). The bladder is protected similarly.

⓯ **Mesh Sizing and Sacral Attachment.** For this step, the prior sacral dissection is again exposed, and the portions of mesh are held by a right-angle clamp for maneuvering. The vaginal manipulator may be removed and replaced by surgeon fingers. Then, by digital pressure directed cephalad, the cuff is gently elevated, and the proximal portions of mesh are extended to the earlier placed sacral sutures. Instead, the cuff can be gently elevated by the vaginal manipulator.

With correct positioning, apical suspension reduces prolapse of the apex and the apical segments of the anterior and posterior vaginal walls. Moreover, the mesh segment between the vagina and sacrum should be tension free. Once the desired mesh position

and length are determined, the excess mesh above the most cephalad sacral suture is trimmed off. This avoids mesh contact with the right ureter, iliac vein, and other vascular structures that all lie within 1 to 2 cm of the fixation site (Kohli, 1998; Nygaard, 2004).

The six needles of the three double-armed sacral sutures are passed through the proximal portions of both mesh strips (Fig. 45-17.5). Each of the three sutures then is tied to secure the proximal mesh to the anterior longitudinal ligament (Fig. 45-17.6). To prevent air knots while the lowest sacral suture is secured, the surgeon gently pushes the vaginal apex against the lower part of the sacrum with the vaginal manipulator.

⓰ **Peritoneal Closure.** Reapproximation of the peritoneum over the mesh can be accomplished in a running or interrupted fashion using 2-0 or 3-0 gauge absorbable suture (Fig. 45-17.7). Placing this mesh retroperitoneally theoretically may lower the risk of bowel obstruction, but this complication has been reported despite peritoneal reapproximation (Pilsgaard, 1999). During closure, the right ureter is kept in constant view to avoid kinking or direct injury.

⓱ **Cystoscopy.** Cystoscopy is routinely performed prior to laparotomy closure to document ureteral integrity and absence of bladder sutures or injury. Urethral examination is important if an antiincontinence procedure is performed.

SECTION 6

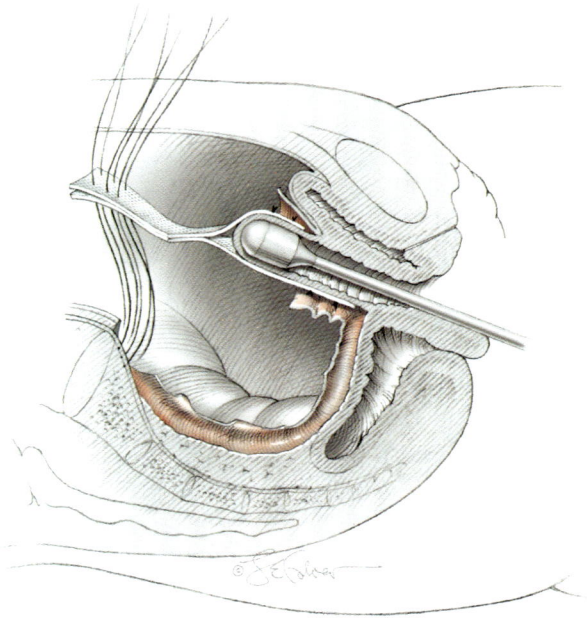

FIGURE 45-17.5 Mesh attachment to the sacrum.

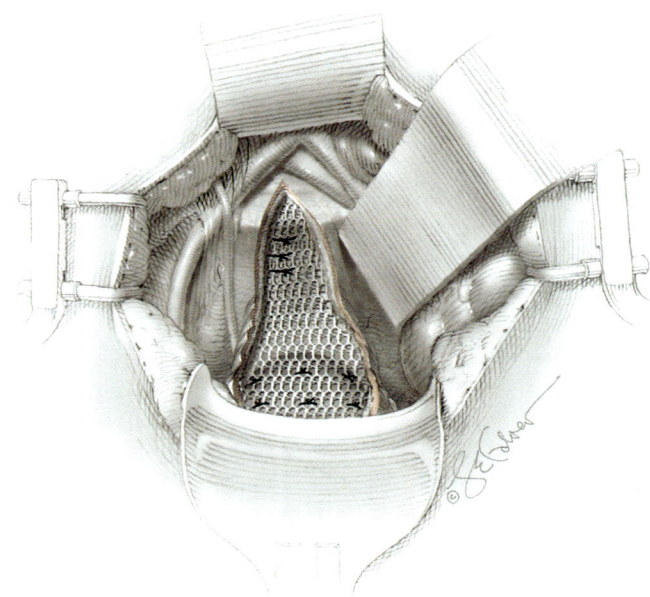

FIGURE 45-17.6 Final mesh placement.

⑱ Abdominal Closure. The abdomen is closed in a standard fashion (Section 43-1 or 43-2, p. 932).

POSTOPERATIVE

Patient Care

Postoperative hospital management is similar to that for other intraabdominal surgeries. Specific to ASC, a passive or active voiding trial can be performed on postsurgical day 1, depending on the patient's condition and extent of dissection. Some women have urinary retention after apical suspension, even without an antiincontinence procedure. If unable to void spontaneously by the time of discharge, a patient can go home with a catheter and be seen again within a week for removal. A stool softener is prescribed when regular diet is tolerated, and constipation and straining are ideally avoided.

At routine postoperative visits, the patient is evaluated for prolapse recurrence and mesh or suture erosion. Symptoms of pelvic floor dysfunction are sought. Anatomic success does not always correlate with functional success, and vice versa. Thus, continual evaluation of surgical results is based on anatomy and on symptoms such as urinary incontinence, defecatory dysfunction, pelvic pain, and sexual dysfunction.

Complications

Following ASC, the graft material or its attaching sutures can erode through the vaginal epithelium. On average, symptoms develop 14 months following surgery, and vaginal bleeding and discharge are classic symptoms (Kohli, 1998). The diagnosis is generally straightforward, as mesh or sutures can be seen directly during speculum examination.

Mesh erosion through the vaginal mucosa may initially be treated with a 6-week or longer course of intravaginal estrogen cream (American College of Obstetricians and Gynecologists, 2017a). For those with exposed mesh and symptoms, surgical removal in an operating suite may be performed vaginally. Epithelium around the erosion site is sharply dissected from the mesh and undermined. The mesh is grasped, placed on gentle tension, dissected off the adjacent tissue, and as much mesh as can be identified is resected. The vaginal epithelial edges are trimmed to freshen edges and are reapproximated in a running or interrupted fashion using 2-0 gauge delayed-absorbable suture. Failure of these wounds to heal is interpreted as a sign of graft or tissue infection, and more extensive or complete removal of the graft is considered. Sutures that are eroding into the vagina may be cut and removed in the office. Fortunately, removal of sutures or portions of eroding mesh does not generally compromise prolapse correction.

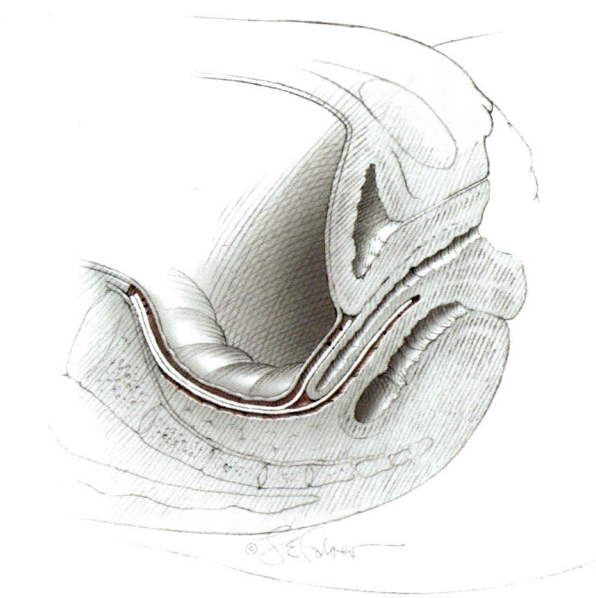

FIGURE 45-17.7 Peritoneal closure.

45-18

Minimally Invasive Sacrocolpopexy

Sacrocolpopexy is increasingly being performed with a minimally invasive approach using conventional laparoscopy or robotic-assisted laparoscopy. The basic procedural steps mirror those for ASC, described in the last section, but differ by abdominal entry method and instrumentation. For ASC, two separate mesh strips can be fashioned. A commercially preformed Y-shaped mesh also is available and is described in this section.

Compared with ASC, limited data suggest that the minimally invasive procedure has similar short-term functional and anatomic results, shorter hospitalization, but longer operating times and greater cost (Judd, 2010; Siddiqui, 2012). Comparing with laparoscopic sacrocolpopexy (LSC), robotic sacrocolpopexy (RSC) carries greater cost, longer operative time, and higher pain scores. Short-term anatomic and functional outcomes and complication rates between the two are similar (Anger, 2014; Paraiso, 2011).

PREOPERATIVE

Patient Evaluation

Candidates for minimally invasive sacrocolpopexy undergo the same prolapse and incontinence evaluation as for ASC (p. 1124). Discussed in Chapter 41 (p. 873), factors influencing selection of MIS include patient overall health, restrictions to prolonged anesthesia, body habitus, intraabdominal adhesions, and surgeon skill.

Consent

Consent considerations mirror those for ASC. Additionally, patients are counseled and consented for laparotomy if surgery cannot be completed by an MIS route.

Complications more unique to laparoscopy are discussed (Chap. 41, p. 875). These include puncture injury to organs and vessels during abdominal entry, positioning neuropathies, and delayed thermal injury to intraabdominal organs from electrosurgical tools.

Patient Preparation

This mirrors preparation for ASC and covers antibiotic and VTE prophylaxis and bowel preparation options (p. 1124).

INTRAOPERATIVE

Surgical Steps

❶ **Anesthesia and Patient Positioning.** Following administration of general anesthesia, the patient is positioned for laparoscopy as fully described in Chapter 41 (p. 877). The buttocks are positioned slightly distal to the table edge to compensate for mild upward patient migration that often occurs in the steep Trendelenburg position needed for laparoscopy. Correct positioning decreases nerve injury rates, provides access to the vagina, and allows full rotation of vaginal manipulator and laparoscopic instruments. The vagina and abdomen are surgically prepared, and a Foley catheter is inserted.

❷ **Incision and Trocar Placement.** MIS abdominal access steps are found in Chapter 41 (p. 888). For LSC, four ports are generally used (Fig. 45-18.1). A 10-mm umbilical port houses the laparoscope. One 5-mm port is placed subcostally and lateral to the rectus abdominis muscle for tissue manipulation. This can be placed on either side. Two 8- to 10-mm ports, one in each lower quadrant, allow needle-bearing sutures to be threaded into the abdomen. Knots are tied using an extracorporeal technique (Fig. 41-34, p. 897).

For RSC, five ports are placed in a shallow "W" formation. A 12-mm umbilical port houses the laparoscope. One 8- or 10-mm assistant port is placed subcostally lateral to the rectus abdominis muscle on the right. Three 8-mm robotic ports are positioned in bilateral lower quadrants, with two on the left and one on the right. We dock the robotic cart on the patient's left to permit manipulation of the vagina. Knots are tied

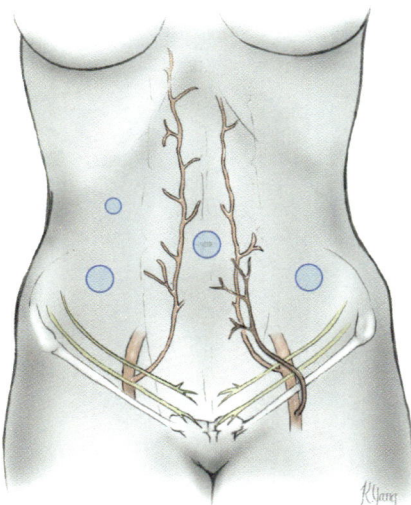

FIGURE 45-18.1 Port placement sites.

using intracorporeal knot-tying techniques (Fig. 41-33, p. 897).

❸ **Concomitant Hysterectomy.** The same considerations described for ASC apply to minimally invasive sacrocolpopexy. In addition, use of electrosurgery to amputate the uterus raises potential for cuff dehiscence and mesh erosion rates (Tan-Kim, 2011). Thus, in appropriately selected patients, supracervical hysterectomy is preferred. During the final steps of supracervical hysterectomy, to prepare for subsequent sacrocolpopexy, the serosal edges of the cervix are reapproximated over the exposed endocervical canal using three to five interrupted 2-0 or 0-gauge polyglactin 910 (Vicryl) sutures.

❹ **Pelvic Anatomy Delineation.** First, the bowel is gently swept out of the pelvis and above the pelvic brim. With LSC, the rectosigmoid epiploicae may be sutured to the left pelvic sidewall to aid presacral space visualization. With RSC, to accomplish the same goal, an atraumatic grasper used through the third robotic port gently displaces the rectosigmoid laterally.

Next, the aortic bifurcation and iliac vessels are identified, and the sacral promontory is visualized and probed in the midline. With RSC, promontory palpation using conventional laparoscopic instruments prior to robot docking is important. This provides tactile anatomic information that is not obtainable robotically. Last, other structures and boundaries are identified as described for ASC.

❺ **Peritoneal Incision.** The peritoneum overlying the sacral promontory in the midline is elevated with tissue forceps and incised sharply with endoscopic scissors (Fig. 45-18.2). The incision is extended caudally into the posterior cul-de-sac and then to the vaginal apex (Fig. 45-18.3). Upward and outward traction on the right and left peritoneal edges aids with dissection. Monopolar energy delivered through the scissors is intermittently used for peritoneal dissection and to control small-vessel bleeding.

❻ **Identifying the Anterior Longitudinal Ligament.** Following peritoneal incision, the loose connective tissue between the peritoneum and the sacrum is sharply and bluntly dissected to expose presacral space anatomy similar to that for ASC. Gentle dissection with scissors or atraumatic tissue forceps displaces the fat and areolar tissue from the sacrum. Beneath these tissues, the shiny, white, anterior longitudinal ligament is seen overlying the bone in the midline. A gauze sponge introduced through the assistant port or a laparoscopic Kittner can assist this dissection.

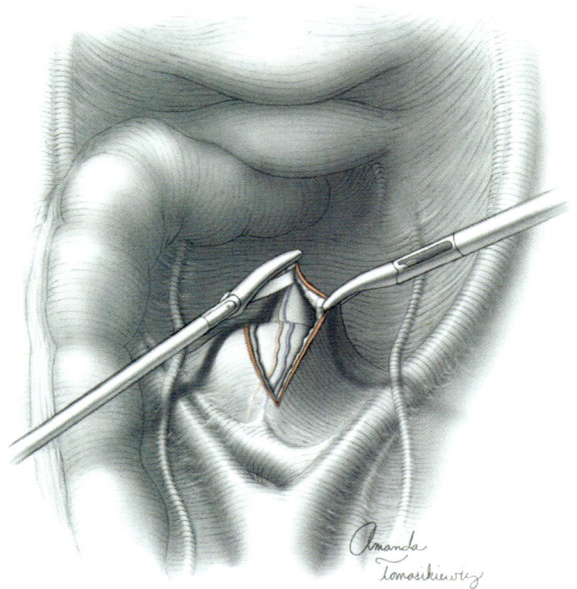

FIGURE 45-18.2 Peritoneal incision overlying the sacrum.

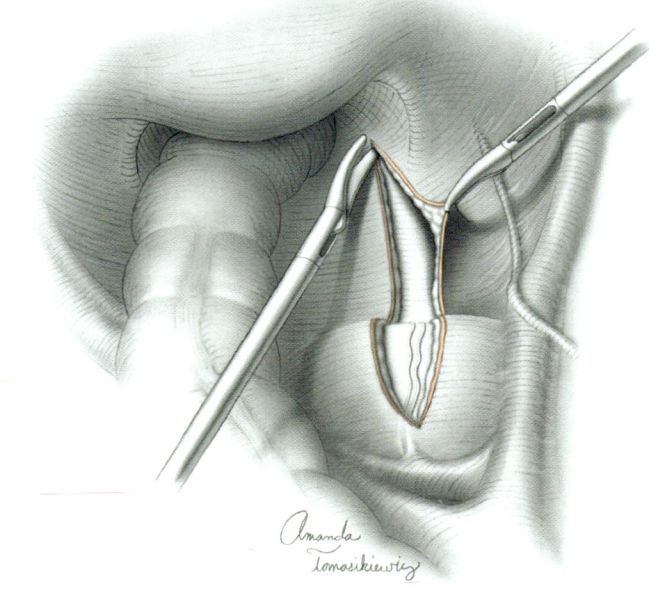

FIGURE 45-18.3 Peritoneal incision extended caudad.

During dissection, significant hemorrhage can occur. To apply bleeding site pressure, a gauze sponge and atraumatic forceps can be introduced through an assistant port. Bleeding management otherwise follows that during ASC (Step 8, p. 1125).

❼ Sacral Suture Site Selection. This is completed in a similar manner to that described for ASC. The anterior surface of S1 may be poorly seen with a 0-degree laparoscope due to this vertebral surface's steep angle of descent. In these cases, switching from a 0-degree to a 30-degree scope and directing it downward improves viewing.

❽ Anterior Vaginal Wall Dissection. A vaginal manipulator is placed to elevate the vaginal apex, and the peritoneum covering it is incised transversely. Sharp and blunt dissection is used to separate the peritoneum and bladder from the anterior vaginal wall in a manner similar to that for ASC (Fig. 45-18.4). The use of electrosurgery during dissection is limited in attempts to minimize delayed thermal injury to the bladder or ureters.

❾ Posterior Vaginal Wall Dissection. The cervical stump or vaginal apex is directed cephalad and ventrally. The peritoneum covering the posterior vaginal wall is incised transversely at a level proximal to the reflection of the rectum against the posterior vaginal wall (Fig. 45-18.5). The right and left uterosacral ligaments are used as lateral dissection boundaries. With gentle outward traction on the peritoneum, the rectovaginal space is entered

and developed with a combination of sharp and blunt dissection similar to that for ASC.

During minimally invasive procedures, with patients positioned in steep Trendelenburg, angling a straight vaginal manipulator may be difficult and thus limit posterior wall exposure. Access can be improved by instead using

a medium-sized Deaver retractor in the vagina with its tip directed anteriorly.

❿ Mesh Placement. Posterior mesh placement mirrors that in ASC. The Y-shaped mesh is threaded into the peritoneal cavity through one of the 8- or 10-mm assistant

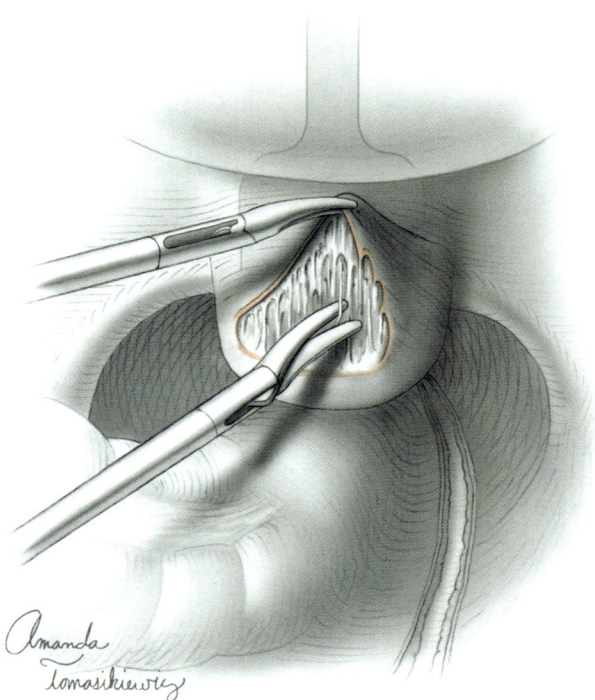

FIGURE 45-18.4 Dissection of the anterior vaginal wall.

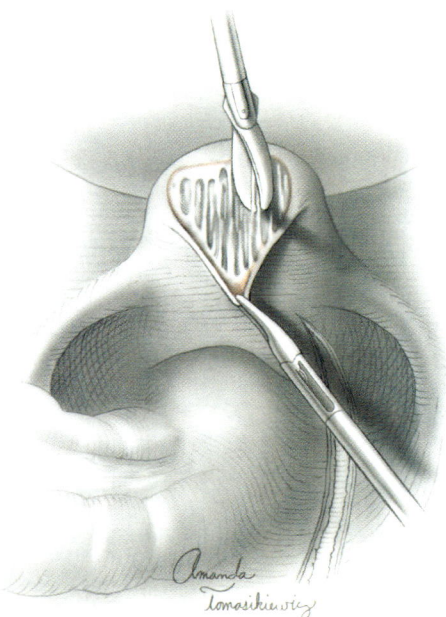

FIGURE 45-18.5 Dissection of the posterior vaginal wall.

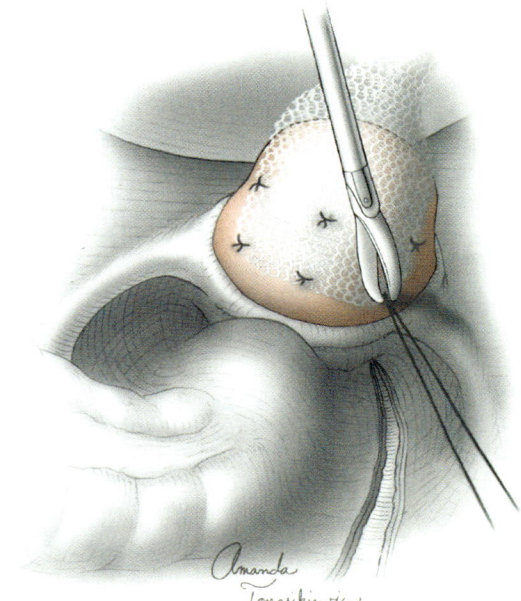

FIGURE 45-18.6 Posterior mesh placement.

cannulas. With graspers placed through a contralateral operating port, one arm of the Y is guided into place and held against the dissected portion of posterior vaginal wall. The same sutures and suturing principles used for ASC are used for minimally invasive sacrocolpopexy (Fig. 45-18.6). Sutures are placed through the mesh and the vaginal wall using laparoscopic or robotic needle drivers. However, with LSC, the knots are secured using the extracorporeal knot tying technique, but with RSC, the intracorporeal technique is used. Accordingly, long sutures, usually 30 to 36 inches, are used for LSC. Short sutures, approximately 6 inches, are used for RSC.

With the vaginal manipulator serving as a support, the other arm of the Y-shaped mesh is sutured to the anterior vaginal wall in the same manner as on the posterior vaginal wall (Figs. 45-18.7 and 45-18.8).

⓫ Mesh Sizing and Sacral Attachment.
For this step, the prior sacral dissection is again exposed, and the single part of the Y-shaped mesh is held by an atraumatic tissue forceps for maneuvering. Using the vaginal manipulator, the cuff is gently elevated, and the proximal portion of mesh is extended to the earlier exposed ligament over the S1 vertebra. With correct positioning, apical suspension reduces prolapse of the apex and the apical segments

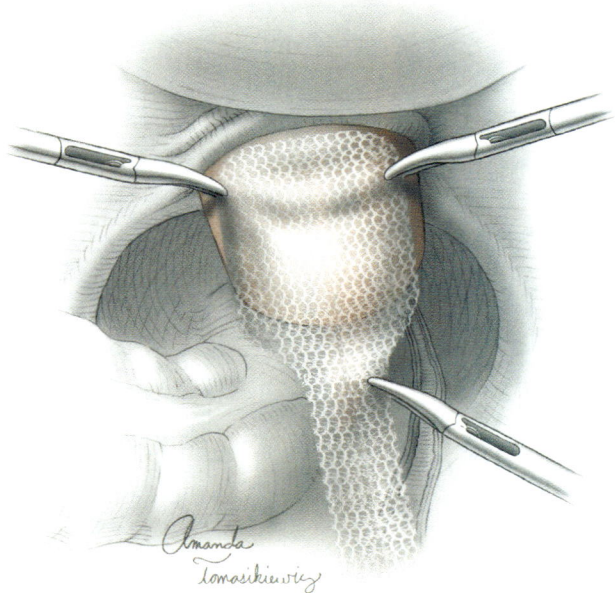

FIGURE 45-18.7 Anterior mesh placement.

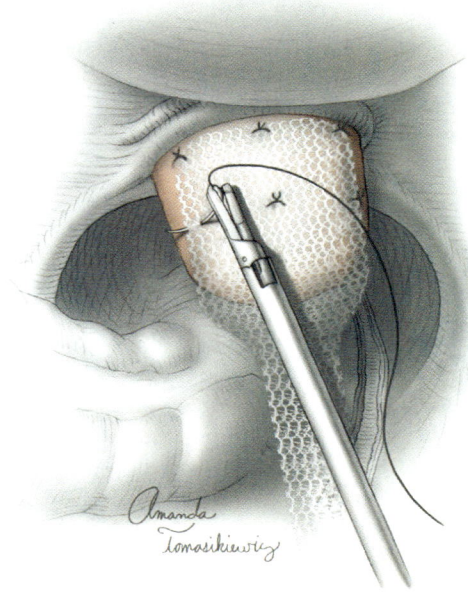

FIGURE 45-18.8 Anterior mesh sutured.

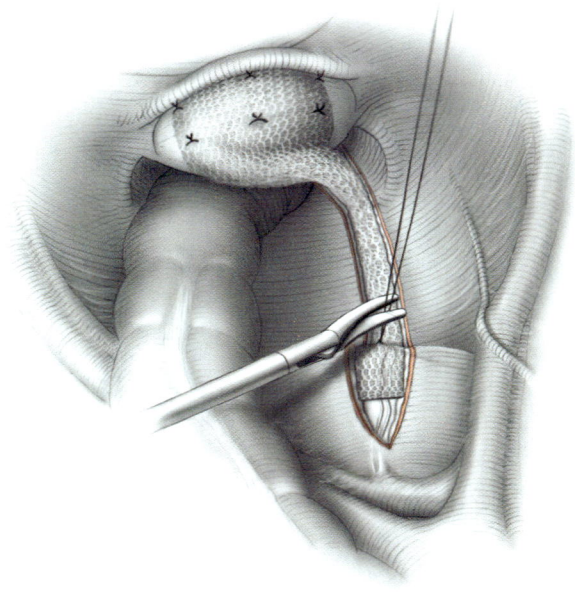
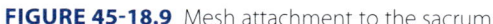

FIGURE 45-18.9 Mesh attachment to the sacrum.

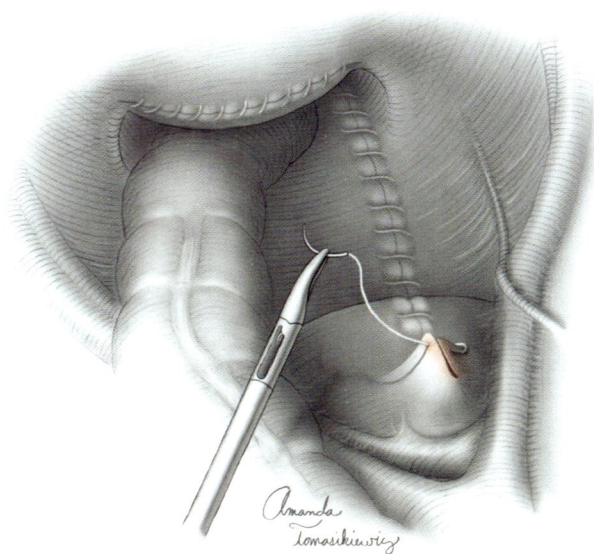

FIGURE 45-18.10 Peritoneal closure.

of the anterior and posterior vaginal walls. Moreover, the mesh segment between the vagina and sacrum should be tension free.

⑫ Sacral Suture Placement. Once desired mesh position and length are determined, excess fabric above the planned most cephalad sacral suture is trimmed off. The sacral portion of the mesh then is secured to the anterior longitudinal ligament with three to four stitches aligned vertically. For this, the mesh portion is held against the sacrum. The lowest stitch is placed first, and the needle enters on the right side of the mesh, drives through the longitudinal ligament under direct visualization, and exits on the mesh's left side. To prevent air knots as the lowest sacral suture is secured, the surgeon elevates the vaginal manipulator to gently push the vaginal apex closer to and against the lower

part of the sacrum. The tip of manipulator is displaced toward the sacrum hollow.

Two or three additional sutures are placed in the same fashion, each at a more cephalad level. Ideally, each suture lies approximately 0.5 cm from the previous one, and the most cephalad suture is at or just below the level of the promontory (Fig. 45-18.9).

⑬ Peritoneal Closure. The peritoneum is closed over the intervening and sacral portions of the mesh with 2-0 delayed-absorbable suture in a running fashion (Fig. 45-18.10). If desired, the peritoneum over the vaginal apex is closed over the exposed mesh in a similar fashion.

⑭ Return to Supine Position. With RSC, the robot is undocked at this point. With both RSC and LSC, the patient is returned

to a supine position, and the abdomen is deflated prior to cystoscopy.

⑮ Cystoscopy. This is routinely performed prior to port closure to document ureteral integrity and exclude bladder sutures or injury. Urethral examination is important if an antiincontinence procedure was performed.

⑯ Wound Closure. Subsequent surgery completion steps follow those of laparoscopy (Chap. 41, p. 895).

POSTOPERATIVE

Patients are usually discharged from the hospital the same or next day. Diet is advanced as desired, and early ambulation is encouraged. Other postoperative management specific to sacrocolpopexy mirrors that for ASC.

45-19

Vaginal Uterosacral Ligament Suspension

The vaginal apex can be effectively suspended with various vaginal or abdominal surgeries. Suturing the apex to the high (proximal) portion of each uterosacral ligaments (USL), that is, uterosacral ligament suspension (USLS), more commonly is performed vaginally, although abdominal and laparoscopic approaches are suitable. The ultimate USLS goal is vaginal apex support restoration by affixing the anterior and posterior vaginal walls to the USLs at and above the level of the ischial spines. The steps described here outline our preferred approach, which is a modification described by Shull and associates (2000).

Another vaginal apical suspension procedure, sacrospinous ligament fixation (SSLF), also strives to correct apical prolapse. However, if USLS and SSLF are compared, USLS maintains the normal vaginal axis orientation and was thought to lower rates of dyspareunia and anterior vaginal wall prolapse. However, the Operations and Pelvic Muscle Training in the Management of Apical Support Loss (OPTIMAL) trial compared outcomes of these two and found equal composite success scores that neared 60 percent after 2 years (Barber, 2014). These rates are lower than the 70- to 90-percent success rates generally reported for these apical suspension procedures, but retreatment rates remained low at 5 percent (Margulies, 2010). By 5 years, the percentage of women undergoing surgical retreatment for prolapse was 8.5 percent and 4.6 percent for USLS and SSLF, respectively (Jelovsek, 2018). Of complications in the original OPTIMAL trial, neurologic pain persisted in 4 percent of SSLF cases, but ureteral obstruction was more frequent after USLS and approximated 3 percent. The 5-year data showed higher rates of vaginal granulation tissue with USLS.

In addition to apical prolapse correction, vaginal USLS effectively repairs apical enteroceles, and thus other enterocele repairs are unnecessary. However, prolapse of the vaginal apex commonly is comorbid with prolapse in the anterior and posterior compartments. Thus, vaginal USLS often is combined with other surgeries such as colporrhaphy and perineorrhaphy.

PREOPERATIVE

Patient Evaluation

All prolapsed compartments are identified for treatment planning. Prior to vaginal USLS, patients with urinary incontinence symptoms also undergo simple or complex urodynamic testing to clarify the type of incontinence. For those with SUI, a concurrent antiincontinence operation generally is performed. Because prolapse correction can unmask occult incontinence, clinicians also test continent women while manually reducing the prolapse with a moderately full bladder. Women with occult SUI are carefully counseled and may elect to undergo concurrent antiincontinence surgery. Last, fully continent women undergoing vaginal prolapse surgery also are at risk for later development of postoperative SUI.

To evaluate whether a prophylactic midurethral sling placed during apical and anterior vaginal prolapse surgery reduces this risk in stress-continent women, the OPUS (Outcomes Following Vaginal Prolapse Repair and Midurethral Sling) trial was conducted. Investigators concluded that a prophylactic MUS procedure in these asymptomatic women leads to a 27-percent postoperative SUI incidence at 1 year compared with a 43-percent rate without concomitant MUS surgery (Wei, 2012). These results mirror the benefit of a prophylactic antiincontinence procure prior to ASC (p. 1124). However, adding an antiincontinence procedure lowers, but does not eliminate, the risk of de novo SUI.

As another preoperative step, some suggest that vaginal estrogen cream may increase vaginal wall thickness for easier dissection and suture placement. Robust data analyzing this practice for reducing suture erosion or prolapse recurrence are lacking.

Consent

Recurrent prolapse is common following any corrective surgery. Thus, a surgeon should be aware of recurrence rates quoted in the literature and his or her own personal rates. As noted, urinary incontinence or voiding or defecatory dysfunction may follow USLS. Also, USLS fixes the upper vagina to the USLs and can shorten the vagina. Accordingly, dyspareunia is another postoperative risk.

Sacral plexus nerve injury and subsequent neuropathy ensue in up to 7 percent of women following vaginal USLS (Barber, 2014; Montoya, 2012). Thus, women are counseled regarding the possible need for suture release if severe buttock pain that radiates to the posterior thigh develops postoperatively. Mild buttock pain without associated radiation and without motor deficits generally resolves during several weeks of expectant management that incorporates analgesics. Last, apical suspension suture erosion and vaginal granulation tissue are frequently reported complications (Barber, 2014; Jelovsek, 2018).

Patient Preparation

Bowel preparation will vary depending on surgeon preference. Patients can be instructed to consume only clear liquids the day prior to surgery and complete one or two enemas the night prior to or the morning of surgery. Alternatively, a mechanical bowel preparation, listed in Chapter 39 (p. 833), may be preferred. Ballard and associates (2014), however, noted no distinct advantage to this for urogynecologic operations. Antibiotic and VTE prophylaxis are given as outlined in Tables 39-8 and 39-10 (p. 832).

❶ **Anesthesia and Patient Positioning.** Vaginal USLS is typically performed under general anesthesia. The patient is placed in standard lithotomy position using candy-cane or booted support stirrups. Examination under anesthesia assesses the degree of prolapse and confirms the need for planned surgeries. The vagina is surgically prepared, and a Foley catheter is inserted.

❷ **Vaginal Apex Incision.** The initial incision can be made in various ways. If complementing vaginal hysterectomy, the vaginal cuff is already open, and each USL transfixing suture is already held by a hemostat. However, if the patient has previously undergone hysterectomy, the vaginal apex is grasped with Allis clamps, and the overlying epithelium is incised vertically or horizontally depending on circumstances. For example, for concurrent colporrhaphy, a midline vertical apical incision that extends distally along the anterior and/or posterior vaginal wall is preferred.

Alternatively, in patients with large apical enteroceles and redundant apical tissue, a diamond-shaped portion of epithelium can be excised and a new apex created. However, excessive tissue excision that may result in vaginal shortening is avoided. Stitches are placed at the lateral boundaries of the intended new apex for later identification. With enterocele, epithelial dissection at the apex typically reveals a peritoneal sac, which is incised to allow peritoneal cavity entry. Last, if a clear dissection plane is not identified, USLS can be performed by an extraperitoneal approach, or SSLF may be performed instead.

❸ **Packing, Retraction, and Identification.** Bowel must be adequately packed away for proper USL visualization to avoid bowel injury when high ligament sutures are placed. First, a Deaver retractor displaces the bladder upward. A right-angle retractor or two

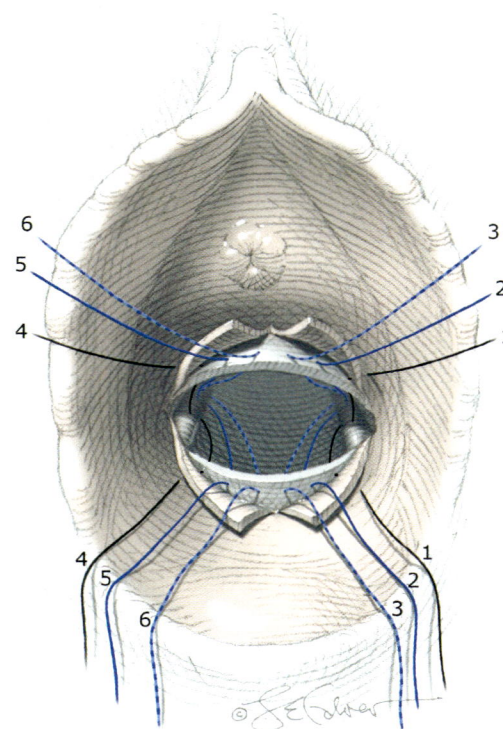

FIGURE 45-19.1 Vaginal view of sutures placed into uterosacral ligaments.

fingers in the posterior cul-de-sac gently displace the posterior peritoneum and underlying rectum downward to avoid peritoneum tearing, which creates bleeding and difficult USL identification. Two moist laparotomy sponges tied together then are gently threaded into the posterior cul-de-sac to pack bowel into the upper pelvis. The Deaver retractor is repositioned to cover the laparotomy sponges. Gentle upward retractor traction exposes the mid and proximal USL portions.

Two Allis clamps are placed at approximately 5 and 7 o'clock positions on the posterior vaginal wall and incorporate the posterior peritoneum. Gentle downward Allis clamp traction tenses the USLs, which are traced with the contralateral index finger. Concurrently, the ischial spines, which protrude from the lateral pelvic walls and lie anterolateral to the USLs, are palpated. Ureters are usually indistinct to touch, but they course anterolateral to the USLs. A lighted Breisky-Navratil retractor is useful for retracting the rectum medially to further expose the USLs. A second similar retractor is often positioned on the opposite side for improved visualization of the USL's proximal segment.

❹ Uterosacral Ligament Suture Placement.
Following adequate exposure, two to three sutures are placed through one USL. Sutures are equally spaced along the mid to proximal length of each ligament. Long,

straight needle drivers are useful for this. The sutures are individually tagged as they are placed, preferably with labeled clamps numbered 1 through 3 for one side and 4 through 6 for the other. Sutures are then loosely secured to the ipsilateral surgical drape. For the most distal stitch, we use a 2-0 gauge delayed-absorbable suture (*black*) with a swaged-on SH needle. For the more proximal stitches, a similar-gauge permanent material (*blue*) is selected (**Fig. 45-19.1**). Instead, 2-0 gauge delayed-absorbable monofilament suture can be used for all.

To begin, the distal absorbable suture perforates the USL at its midlength, which lies at approximately the level of the ischial spine. The subsequent, more proximal sutures are placed approximately 0.5 cm to 1 cm cephalad from each prior suture. Two or three sutures are placed on each side, and this number is guided by surgeon preference, the extent of USL exposed, and vaginal cuff width.

With each stitch placement, the needle tip ideally passes through the most medial portion of the ligament in a lateral-to-medial direction. These specifics attempt to minimize ureteral entrapment or kinking risks. Moreover, to lower rectal injury rates, an assistant retracts the rectum to the contralateral side, and suture purchases do not extend too medial, that is, beyond the ligament width. Similarly, stitches placed too deep risk injury to internal iliac vessels or sacral

nerves (Wieslander, 2007). At completion, gentle traction on each suture should confirm correct placement and incorporation of adequate USL tissue. Excess laxity during such USL traction usually indicates insufficient tissue to provide adequate apical support, and the suture is replaced.

Hematomas form occasionally following inadvertent laceration of pelvic sidewall veins. Application of pressure with a sponge stick typically will control bleeding.

❺ Other Procedures.
Once all the suspensory sutures are placed through each USL, colporrhaphy is completed if indicated. If a perineorrhaphy or midurethral sling procedure is planned, we defer these until the USLS operation is completed.

❻ Vaginal Wall Suture Placement.
Vaginal packing is first removed, and ultimately, four to six sutures (two or three from each USL) are placed along the vaginal cuff width. If one begins on the patient's left side, the free end of the left distal absorbable USLS suture (suture 1) is threaded into a Mayo needle. The needle and suture then pierce the left lateral anterior vaginal wall at the apex. The other end, which is needle-bearing, similarly penetrates the posterior wall (see Fig. 45-19.1). Each suture strand traverses the full vaginal wall thickness, including the epithelium.

❼ Additional Sutures.
Next, one end of the proximal (permanent) USLS suture(s) is directed anteriorly, and the other is directed posteriorly. To lower suture erosion rates, permanent sutures traverse the full thickness of the vaginal fibromuscular layer but not the epithelium (**Figs.** 45-19.1 and **45-19.2**). However, a substantial thickness of fibromuscular wall is incorporated to prevent tissue tearing, which can create suture bridges that are a bowel obstruction risk. Each successive proximal suture is placed medial to the previous suture.

The same steps are then repeated on the right. If delayed-absorbable suture is used for all suspension sutures, these all traverse the full vaginal wall thickness, including the epithelium.

Ultimately, on each side, the most cephalad USLS sutures (sutures 3 and 6) are placed most medially on the vaginal cuff. The most distal USLS sutures (sutures 1 and 4) are placed most laterally on the vaginal cuff. For organization, all completed sutures are held within numbered clamps on their respective sides.

At this point, an intravenous vital dye can be given in preparation for cystoscopy that follows knot tying (p. 1077). However, dye is not essential as urine efflux generally is easily seen. Next, knots are secured starting with

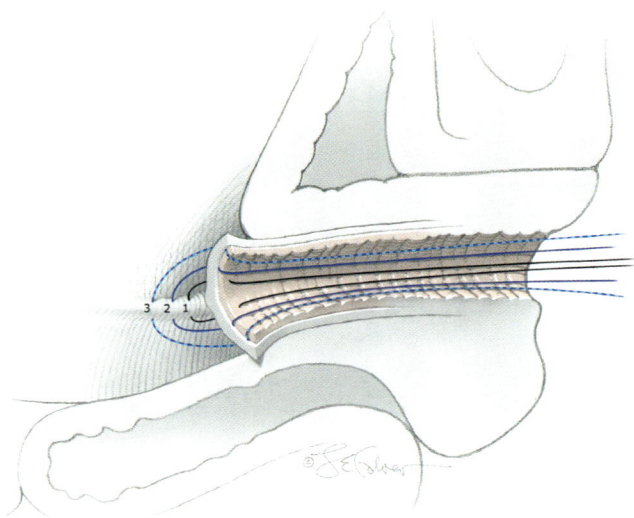

FIGURE 45-19.2 Lateral view of sutures placed into the left utero-sacral ligament.

most medial cuff sutures (sutures 3 and 6) and ending with the most lateral (sutures 1 and 4). The vaginal wall is confirmed to approximate the ULSs. Both this approximation and the order in which sutures are tied may prevent suture bridges. All sutures are held with their corresponding numbered clamps after tying until cystoscopy is completed.

8 Cystoscopy. This is performed to document ureteral patency and exclude bladder sutures or cystotomy. The ureter lies closest to the lower portion of the USL. Thus, if ureteral obstruction is suspected, the most distal USLS suture on the ipsilateral side is released first, and cystoscopy is repeated. If no flow is noted, the next most proximal suture is released, and this is continued cephalad in a stepwise fashion until efflux is seen.

9 Rectal Examination. The rectum is digitally explored to confirm approximation of the cuff against the USLs and exclude sutures entering the rectum.

10 Vaginal Cuff Closure. The suspension suture ends are now cut. If remaining defects between suspension sutures are noted, the vaginal cuff is reapproximated in a running fashion with 2-0 gauge delayed-absorbable suture. Alternatively, two to four interrupted 2-0 absorbable sutures are placed through the full thickness of the anterior and posterior vaginal cuff prior to tying of the USL sutures and held for later cuff closure. This practice aids cuff closure with high suspensions, in which vaginal edges may be inaccessible without pulling that in turn disrupts the repair.

POSTOPERATIVE

Following vaginal USLS, postoperative care mirrors that for vaginal surgery. Postoperative activity in general can be individualized, although intercourse usually is delayed until after 6 weeks following surgery. A voiding trial can be completed on the same or next day, depending on concomitant surgeries and the patient's condition. Some patients have urinary retention after apical suspension, even without an antiincontinence procedure. If unable to void spontaneously by the time of discharge, the patient can be discharged with a catheter and followed up within a week for removal. Patients are screened for lower extremity neuropathy prior to discharge. Suture erosion with granulation tissue can be a short- or long-term complication and is managed as described on page 1128.

45-20

Abdominal Uterosacral Ligament Suspension

USLS is more commonly performed vaginally (p. 1133). But for some situations, an abdominal approach, either via laparotomy or laparoscopy, offers advantages. For example, with advanced apical prolapse, many consider ASC the preferred procedure. However, limited data suggest that total hysterectomy concurrent with ASC leads to higher mesh erosion rates. Thus, with total abdominal hysterectomy, abdominal USLS represents an ASC alternative to reduce graft erosion. A second possible indication is the setting of iatrogenic cystotomy or bowel injury during ASC. In this case, to minimize mesh erosion into the bladder or bowel or fistula formation, ASC can be aborted and USLS then performed instead. Last, although not evidence-based, for women with concurrent pelvic cancer, mesh placement may not be ideal, and thus, USLS may be preferred.

During abdominal USLS, the mid to proximal span of both USLs is sutured to the anterior and posterior vaginal walls at the vaginal apex. Because of this suspension, enteroceles are effectively closed. Abdominal USLS is effective, and limited data show that success rates for the apical suspension approximate 90 percent (Lowenstein, 2009; Rardin, 2009). However, as with other apical procedures, subsequent anterior or posterior compartment defects are later risks.

PREOPERATIVE

Before surgery, patients are examined to identify other prolapsed sites, which could be concurrently repaired. Similarly, overt or occult SUI is excluded. Consenting also includes a discussion regarding prophylactic antiincontinence surgery. As with other apical suspension procedures, and as described fully on page 1124, even stress-continent women may benefit in many cases from a prophylactic antiincontinence procedure performed concurrently. However, for abdominal USLS, data on this prophylactic practice must be extrapolated from ASC and vaginal USLS studies. Last, as another preoperative step, some suggest that vaginal estrogen cream thickens the vaginal wall to aid dissection and suture placement (Rahn, 2014, 2015). However, no trials have analyzed this treatment's ability to improve dissection or to reduce suture erosion or prolapse recurrence risks.

Consenting mirrors that for vaginal USLS (p. 1133). Antibiotic and VTE prophylaxis are given as outlined in Tables 39-8 and 39-10 (p. 832). Bowel preparation is selected according to surgeon preference as for vaginal USLS.

INTRAOPERATIVE

Surgical Steps

❶ Anesthesia and Patient Positioning. Following administration of general anesthesia, the patient is positioned in a low lithotomy position with thighs parallel to the ground and legs in booted support stirrups. The vagina and abdomen are surgically prepared, and a Foley catheter is inserted.

❷ Incision. A midline vertical or low transverse abdominal incision is suitable, and a self-retaining retractor and bowel packing clears the operative field. With a laparoscopic approach, port placement is similar to that described for laparoscopic sacrocolpopexy (p. 1129).

❸ Ureter Identification. The ureters are identified early, as these can be trapped during suture placement through the USL and can be kinked with suture tying. Thus, ureter location is frequently confirmed, and cystoscopy is completed after suspension suture tying.

❹ Uterosacral Ligament Identification. Prior to hysterectomy, the surgeon identifies each USL by applying contralateral and upward uterine traction. With this technique, the USLs are stretched and more easily seen or palpated. In women with prior hysterectomy, the vaginal cuff is similarly elevated and deviated by a vaginal manipulator. The USLs run medial and posterior to the ureters, and their proximity explains the significant ureteral injury rate, which can reach 11 percent with vaginal USLS (Barber, 2000). The USL midpoint generally lies at the level of the ischial spines, which are located anterolateral to the USLs. In women with normal support, the cervix and upper vagina are located roughly at the level of these spines. Thus, this bony landmark is generally chosen as the site for the most distal USL suture. However, this site may be modified according to vaginal length and intraoperative findings.

❺ Uterosacral Ligament Suture Placement. Following adequate exposure, two to three sutures are placed through one USL. Sutures are equally spaced along the mid to proximal length of each ligament. During suture placement, the vaginal cuff is elevated to accentuate the USLs. For the most distal stitch, we use a 2-0 gauge delayed-absorbable suture (*black*) with a swaged-on SH needle. For the more proximal stitches, a similar-gauge permanent material (*blue*) is selected instead (Fig. 45-20.1).

To begin, the distal absorbable suture perforates the USL at its midlength, which lies approximately at the level of the ischial spine. The subsequent, more proximal sutures are placed approximately 0.5 cm to 1 cm cephalad from each prior suture. Two or three sutures may be placed on each side, and this number is guided by surgeon preference, the extent of USL exposed, and vaginal cuff width.

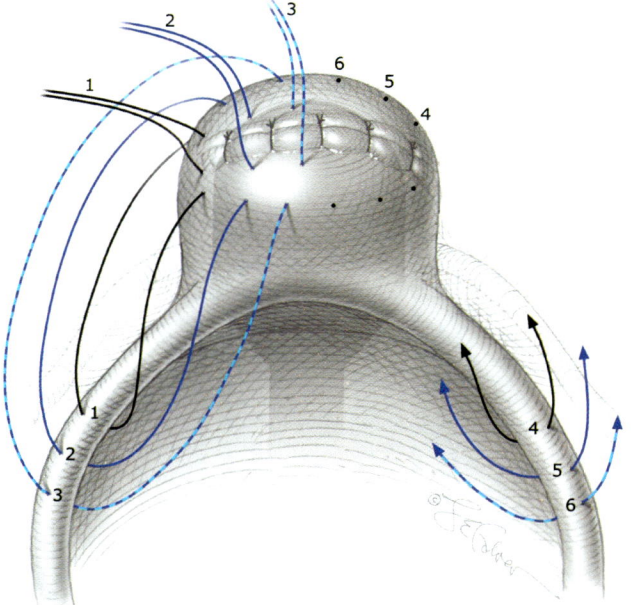

FIGURE 45-20.1 Uterosacral ligament and vaginal cuff suture placement.

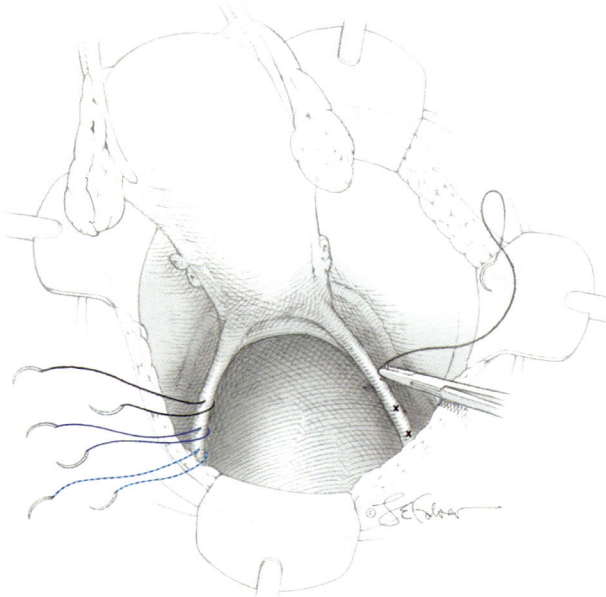

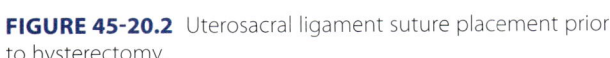

FIGURE 45-20.2 Uterosacral ligament suture placement prior to hysterectomy.

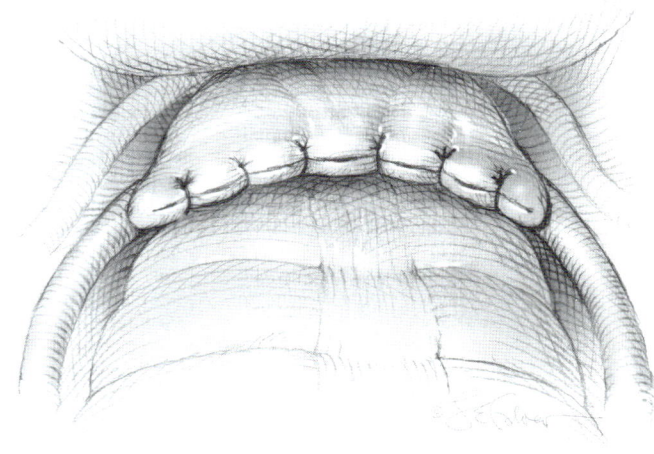

FIGURE 45-20.3 All sutures secured.

With stitch placement, each needle tip ideally passes through the most medial portion of the ligament in a lateral-to-medial direction. Moreover, the assistant retracts the rectum to the contralateral side, and suture purchases do not extend too medial, that is, beyond the ligament width. Similarly, stitches placed too deep risk injury to internal iliac vessels or sacral nerves (Wieslander, 2007). At completion, gentle traction on each suture should confirm correct placement and adequate incorporation of USL tissue. If not, the suture is replaced.

Following each placement, sutures with needles still attached are then individually tagged, preferably with labeled clamps, and are loosely secured to the ipsilateral surgical drape. This series is repeated on the other side. During endoscopic cases, the sutures are usually tied after placement to avoid entanglement.

❻ Hysterectomy. These suspensory sutures may be placed through the USL before or after abdominal hysterectomy based on surgeon preference and intraoperative findings (Fig. 45-20.2). If sutures are placed prior to hysterectomy, they are held by numbered hemostats and not tied. Their needles are covered with a surgical towel to avoid stick injuries. Hysterectomy then is completed, and the cuff is closed. During endoscopic cases, sutures are typically placed after hysterectomy and cuff closure to avoid suture tangling.

❼ Vaginal Wall Suture Placement. Ultimately, four to six sutures (two or three from each USL) are placed along the vaginal cuff width. An EEA sizer or similar blunt

manipulator is placed in the vagina for cuff movement. If one begins on the patient's left side, the free end of the left distal absorbable USLS suture (suture 1) is threaded into a Mayo needle. The needle and suture then pierce the left lateral anterior vaginal wall at the apex. The other suture end, which is needle-bearing, similarly penetrates the posterior wall (see Fig. 45-20.1). Each suture strand may traverse the full vaginal wall thickness, including the epithelium.

Next, each end of the proximal (permanent) USLS suture(s) is similarly directed anteriorly and posteriorly, respectively. Each successive proximal suture is placed medial to the previous suture. To lower suture erosion rates, permanent sutures traverse the full thickness of the vaginal fibromuscular layer but not the epithelium. However, a substantial thickness of fibromuscular wall should be incorporated to prevent tissue tearing, which can create suture bridges that are a bowel obstruction risk. The same steps are repeated on the right. As with vaginal USLS procedures, surgeons may prefer delayed-absorbable material for all suspension sutures.

Ultimately on each side, the most cephalad USLS suture (suture 3 or 6) is placed most medially along the vaginal cuff width. The most distal USLS suture (suture 1 or 4) is placed most laterally on the vaginal cuff. For organization, all completed sutures are held within numbered clamps on their respective sides.

At this point, knots are secured starting with the most medial sutures (sutures 3 and 6) and ending with the most lateral (sutures 1 and 4). The vaginal wall is confirmed to approximate the ULSs (Fig. 45-20.3). Both

this approximation and the order in which sutures are tied may prevent suture bridges. All sutures are held with their corresponding numbered clamps after tying until cystoscopy is completed. During endoscopic cases, each USLS suture is tied and cut after placement.

❽ Cystoscopy. Cystoscopy is performed after all suspension sutures are tied but prior to abdominal closure to document ureteral patency and exclude bladder sutures or cystotomy. The ureter lies closest to the lower portion of the USL. Thus, if ureteral obstruction is suspected, the most distal USLS suture on the ipsilateral side is released first, and cystoscopy is repeated. If no flow is noted, the next most proximal suture is released, and this is continued cephalad in a stepwise fashion until efflux is seen.

❾ Rectal Examination. This confirms approximation of the cuff to the USLs and excludes sutures entering the rectum.

❿ Concurrent Procedures. If necessary, a paravaginal defect repair or Burch colposuspension may be performed prior to incision closure. The abdomen is closed in a standard fashion (Chap. 43, p. 934). If posterior colporrhaphy or vaginal antiincontinence surgery is required, these will follow incision closure.

POSTOPERATIVE

Following abdominal USLS, postoperative care mirrors that for ASC (p. 1128).

45-21

Sacrospinous Ligament Fixation

Extending between the ischial spine and lower sacrum, the sacrospinous ligament (SSL) lies deep to the coccygeus muscle and adds significant stability to the bony pelvis. Sacrospinous ligament fixation (SSLF) attaches the vaginal apex to this coccygeus-sacrospinous ligament (C-SSL) complex and often is selected for apical prolapse repair. Of its modifications, apex fixation to the right ligament is most often described, likely due to the left-sided location of the rectosigmoid (Goldberg, 2001; Kearney, 2003).

Gaining access to the SSL also varies. In a more traditional approach, the pararectal space and SSL are accessed through a posterior colporrhaphy incision, and only the right aspect of the apical posterior vaginal wall is attached to the ligament. In the *Michigan four-wall modification*, the SSL instead is accessed through an apical incision. Dissection to the SSL remains extraperitoneal, and both anterior and posterior vaginal walls are directly affixed to the SSL by four points that span the vaginal apex width. Advantageously, this technique may avoid anterior enterocele, contralateral vaginal wall descent, and the need for bilateral suspension (Larson, 2013). A modification of the original Michigan approach is described here (Morley, 1988).

Success rates are comparable to those for other vaginal approaches for vault suspension (Barber, 2014; Jelovsek, 2018; Maher, 2013). However, SSLF compares less favorably with ASC. But, SSLF averts abdominal surgery and is associated with shorter operating times and quicker recovery. For these reasons, it often is preferred for women with comorbidities. This approach allows other concurrent support defects also to be repaired vaginally.

PREOPERATIVE

Patient Evaluation

Before surgery, patients are examined to identify other prolapsed sites, which could be concurrently repaired. Similarly, overt or occult SUI is excluded. Consenting also includes a discussion regarding prophylactic antiincontinence surgery. As with other apical suspension procedures, and as described fully on page 1124, even stress-continent women may benefit in many cases from a prophylactic antiincontinence procedure performed

concurrently. Last, as another preoperative step, some suggest that vaginal estrogen cream aids vaginal dissection and suture placement, as the vaginal wall thickness is increased (Rahn, 2014, 2015). However, no trials have analyzed this treatment's ability to improve dissection or reduce suture erosion or prolapse recurrence risks.

Consent

Because the vagina is fixed and laterally deviated with SSLF, dyspareunia is one postoperative risk. Recurrent prolapse also is common following any corrective surgery. Although the apical prolapse rate following SSLF is <10 percent, anterior vaginal wall prolapse rates can approach 30 percent (Barber, 2009). This anterior prolapse is attributed to the exaggerated posterior deflection of the vaginal axis, which exposes the anterior vaginal wall to greater intraabdominal stresses than other apical suspensions (Weber, 2005). Despite this theoretical vulnerability, the OPTIMAL trial, cited earlier (p. 1133), compared SSLF and vaginal USLS 2-year outcomes and found equal composite success scores nearing 60 percent (Barber, 2014). However, surgical failure increased during the follow-up period, with approximately two thirds of original trial participants meeting a priori study definitions of failure at 5 years. However, study participants maintained clinically meaningful improvements in symptoms and quality of life (Jelovsek, 2018). These percentages are lower than the 70- to 90-percent success rates generally reported for these procedures, but surgical retreatment rates remained low at 5 percent (Margulies, 2010; Jelovsek, 2018).

SSLF has low associated risks for serious complications, but neurovascular injuries can occur. Of these, low-pressure vessel bleeding encountered during dissection and exposure of the pararectal space is generally attributed to retractor or needle injury of the extensive venous plexus that drains the rectum and vagina. This bleeding usually can be controlled with sustained pressure from pararectal space packing. Second, arterial bleeding may follow retraction in the pararectal space and subsequent middle rectal artery avulsion or laceration. The internal pudendal and inferior gluteal arteries also are at risk if a needle inadvertently extends past the proximal or upper SSL border. Arterial bleeding is best controlled by vessel ligation or clipping. An internal iliac ligation for such bleeding is ineffective due to extensive collateral circulation in the pelvis.

The pudendal nerve and lower sacral nerves such as S3 and S4 can be damaged if the needle exits or enters past the ligament's proximal (upper) margin. Sutures placed too

close to the sacrum risk injury to S4 or the nerve to the coccygeus or levator ani muscles (Katrikh, 2017; Roshanravan, 2007). Even sutures that are placed in the recommended mid and lower aspect of the SSL can entrap or lacerate the nerve to the levator ani muscles. Pelvic floor muscle spasms, buttock pain, and dyspareunia may be manifestations.

Moreover, sacral plexus nerve injury with subsequent neuropathy has followed vaginal SSLF. Noted earlier, persistent neurologic pain was noted in 4 percent of SSLF cases in the OPTIMAL trial. Accordingly, women are counseled that additional surgery for suture release may be needed if severe buttock pain that radiates to the posterior thigh persists postoperatively. Mild buttock pain without associated radiation or without motor deficits is common and generally resolves within several weeks with expectant management that incorporates analgesics. This buttock pain is attributed to entrapment of the nerve to the levator ani or coccygeus muscles or to ensnaring of branches from S3 and/or S4 that course between the sacrospinous and sacrotuberous ligaments to supply the gluteus maximus muscle (Florian-Rodriguez, 2016).

Ureteral and rectal injuries and ileus are rare, mainly because this procedure is extraperitoneal. However, as with any apical suspension procedure, voiding and defecatory dysfunction can develop. If rectal injury is noted intraoperatively, the defect is closed using 2-0 gauge delayed-absorbable suture in a layered fashion. Although limited data are available, the SSLF still can be completed following this rectal repair.

Patient Preparation

Bowel preparation will vary depending on surgeon preference. Patients can be instructed to consume only clear liquids the day prior to surgery and complete one or two enemas that night or the morning of surgery. Alternatively, a mechanical bowel preparation using agents listed in Chapter 39 (p. 833) may be preferred. Ballard and associates (2014), however, noted no distinct advantage to this for urogynecologic operations. As with most vaginal surgery, because of the risk posed by the normal vaginal flora for postoperative wound cellulitis and abscess, preoperative antibiotics are warranted. Typical agents are found in Table 39-8 (p. 832). Additionally, thromboprophylaxis is provided as outlined in Table 39-10 (p. 834).

INTRAOPERATIVE

Surgical Instruments

Suture placement into the SSL can be performed with various ligature carriers and

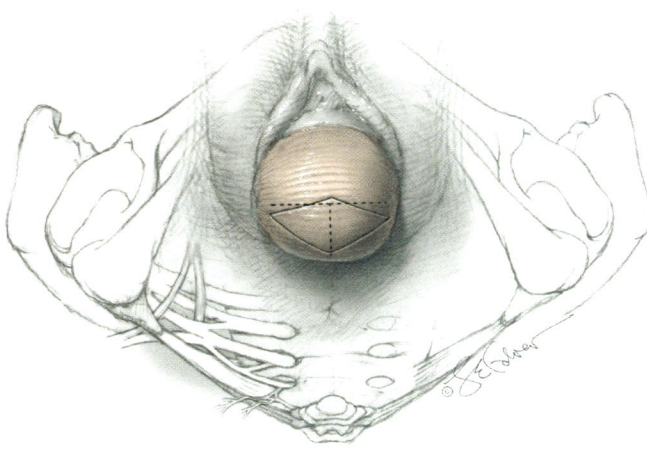

FIGURE 45-21.1 Coccygeus-sacrospinous ligament complex and surrounding pelvic anatomy. Vaginal apex diamond or "T" incisions.

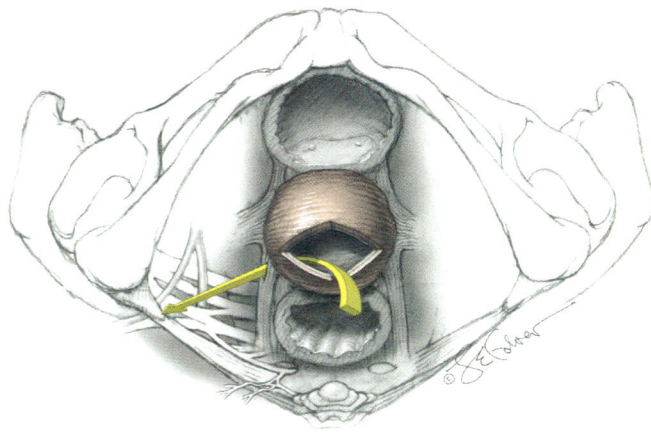

FIGURE 45-21.2 Entry into right pararectal space through rectal pillar.

include the Deschamps ligature carrier, Miya hook, Capio ligature carrier, and Endo Stitch. Alternatively, a Mayo needle and long, straight needle driver can be used.

Using the Deschamps ligature carrier, a surgeon threads the suture through an eye at the needle-shaped carrier tip. Arcs and curves constructed into the instrument aid ease of suture placement. Once the tip of the Deschamps carrier passes through the ligament, the suture is retrieved with a nerve hook, as shown in atlas Step 4. Disadvantages to this device, however, include the relative thickness of the needle tip, which may be difficult to drive through the ligament.

Alternatively, disposable devices have become popular, in particular the Capio ligature carrier. This device is easier to manipulate than the Miya hook. Its design aids placement of sutures using ligament palpation and thus obviates the need for extensive dissection.

Surgical Steps

❶ Anesthesia and Patient Positioning.
After general anesthesia has been administered, a woman is placed in standard lithotomy position. The vagina is surgically prepared, and a Foley catheter is inserted. Initially, vaginal vault prolapse is reduced to place the vagina in a normal anatomic position. Enterocele repair or anterior colporrhaphy, if planned, precedes SSLF completion.

❷ Vaginal Wall Incision. *In the setting of vaginal cuff prolapse,* the apex is grasped and brought to the level of the ligament to confirm adequate vaginal length or need for redundant tissue excision. With advanced prolapse, a new apex site is required and most often lies posterior to the former hysterectomy scar (Kearney, 2003). When indicated,

excess vaginal tissue will be excised. At the planned apex, four points in a diamond configuration are grasped with Allis clamps and individually brought to lie against the SSL. This ensures fixation off tension and correction of any anterior and posterior vaginal wall redundancy. These points include one midline anterior and posterior point and two lateral ones. Once determined, the diamond-shaped redundant vaginal wall within these four Allis clamps is incised to a depth reaching the underlying loose preperitoneal connective tissue (Fig. 45-21.1). If this diamond lies posterior to the prior cuff scar, the peritoneum is generally easily identified and the enterocele sac entered without difficulty, if needed. If this diamond lies anterior to the prior cuff, then dissection proceeds more superficially to avoid bladder entry.

If vaginal shortening is a concern, then a transverse incision is made at the new apex site and no tissue is excised. Next, a vertical incision that extends several centimeters posteriorly from this transverse incision's midpoint creates a "T" incision that aids access into the pararectal space (see Fig. 45-21.1, dotted line). With either incision configuration, the intended apex site is marked with sutures or clamps to maintain proper orientation during fixation.

In the setting of concomitant vaginal hysterectomy, after hysterectomy completion, the lateral edges of the anterior and posterior vaginal walls are grasped with Allis clamps and brought into direct contact with the SSL to similarly assess for excess tension or redundancy. A vertical incision, if needed for access, then is made through the midline posterior vaginal wall at the open cuff and extended 2 to 3 cm distally. The extraperitoneal space between the vaginal wall and the peritoneum is entered. Then, the pararectal space is entered as described next.

❸ Right Sacrospinous Ligament Access.
Whether the SSL is accessed through the apex (Michigan modification) or through the posterior vaginal wall (traditional approach), the same extraperitoneal spaces are entered. Namely, the rectovaginal space and then the pararectal space are entered sequentially to reach the SSL (Fig. 45-21.2). Following entry into the rectovaginal space, traction on the vaginal epithelium with an Allis clamp and countertraction on peritoneum with tissue forceps are applied. Sharp or blunt dissection is directed toward the right ischial spine. Important anatomic structures during entry into the right pararectal space include the rectum, which lies medially and is retracted leftward to avoid injury; blood vessels within the cardinal ligament and peritoneum, which lie ventrally and superiorly; and the levator ani muscles, which are found dorsally and laterally. To enter the pararectal space, the deep uterosacral ligament fibers, also known as *rectal pillars*, are perforated as shown by the arrow in Figure 45-21.2. This tissue is typically attenuated in women with advanced prolapse and thus easier to perforate. In some cases, perforation with a hemostat or similar instrument is needed. Once in the pararectal space, the ischial spine tip is palpated, and the index finger moves gently medially toward the lower, lateral border of the sacrum to delineate the C-SSL complex (Fig. 45-21.3). This step also allows blunt digital dissection of loose connective tissue from the ligament's midportion. If the ischial spine is blunted and difficult to palpate by vaginal examination, a rectal examination allows easier palpation of both the spine and the coccyx. These bony landmarks are palpated intermittently throughout the procedure to reconfirm anatomy.

❹ Retractor Positioning. Two to three retractors are positioned to adequately expose

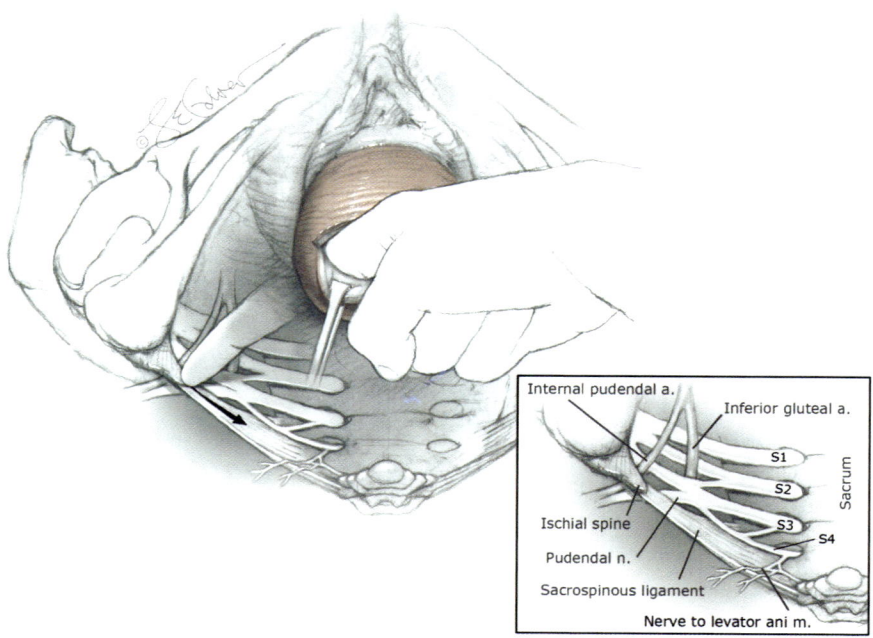

Internal pudendal a.
Inferior gluteal a.
S1
S2
Sacrum
Ischial spine
S3
S4
Pudendal n.
Sacrospinous ligament
Nerve to levator ani m.

FIGURE 45-21.3 Anatomy delineated.

the C-SSL complex (Fig. 45-21.4). We prefer a small Deaver to displace the peritoneum and blood vessels superiorly, a Breisky-Navratil retractor to displace the rectum medially, and a second Breisky-Navratil retractor to displace the levator muscles inferiorly and further expose the ligament's lower portion. Retraction is gentle to avoid vessel or rectal injury. A rectal examination at this point aims to exclude rectal laceration. During dissection and retractor positioning, vessels in the area may be lacerated, and hemostasis is obtained with direct pressure, electrosurgical coagulation, or ligatures.

❺ Placing SSL Sutures. Once the C-SSL complex is delineated, sutures are placed approximately two fingerbreadths or 2 to 3 cm medial to the ischial spine, which roughly corresponds to the SSL midportion (Roshanravan, 2007). Sutures placed too close to the spine risk injury to the pudendal nerves or vessels. Needle entry or exit points ideally remain within the lower portion of the ligament. This lowers injury risk to the inferior gluteal vessels and pudendal or sacral nerves, which course in close proximity to the upper SSL margin.

We use the Deschamps ligature carrier or a tapered Mayo needle with a half-circle radius to ultimately pass four sutures through the ligament (see Fig. 45-21.4). These can be two monofilament delayed-absorbable and two permanent sutures or, instead, can be four monofilament delayed-absorbable sutures.

To begin, two long sutures, one delayed-absorbable (*black*) and one permanent (*blue*) are threaded through the carrier eye. For the absorbable sutures we select either 2-0 or 0-gauge polydioxanone (PDS II), and for the permanent sutures we use similar-gauge polypropylene (Prolene). Thus, with a single ligament penetration, four sutures ends are available.

When the Deschamps ligature carrier is used, sutures are retrieved using a nerve hook (see Fig. 45-21.4). Once the suture ends are retrieved, suture traction is applied to test their anchorage. Firm resistance during traction confirms proper placement. Laxity indicates superficial placement through the coccygeus muscle or overlying fascia, and the sutures are replaced deeper into C-SSL. Digital palpation of the suture placement site relative to the ischial spine and upper border of the SSL is done after each needle pass and suture retrieval. At this point, the four suture ends are paired by color, tagged by individually numbered hemostats, and loosely secured to the surgical drape.

The second carrier pass then is completed approximately 1 cm medial to the first. Based on intraoperative findings, the order of the carrier passes may be reversed, that is, the lateral suture is placed second. Adequate anchorage is similarly confirmed, and these sutures are paired and tagged. Ultimately, these two carrier passes result in four suture pairs that will later be passed through the anterior and posterior vaginal walls of the new cuff.

Adequate suture labeling (1 through 4) and tagging of the suture ends loosely to the upper and lower aspects of the surgical drape avoids suture tangling and later suture bridging at the fixation site. The delayed-absorbable suture (*black*), which is placed most laterally on the ligament, is labeled "1" and will be placed through the right lateral aspect of the vaginal cuff. The delayed-absorbable suture (*black*) placed most medial on the ligament is labeled "4" and will be placed through the left lateral aspect of the vaginal cuff. Sutures 2 and 3 correspond to the permanent sutures (*blue*). These ultimately will be placed through the medial portion of the cuff.

If indicated, anterior colporrhaphy is performed at this time. If performed, the anterior vaginal wall is reapproximated with 2-0 or 3-0 gauge absorbable suture to the level of the cuff. Rectoceles are often corrected with SSLF, and posterior colporrhaphy is not

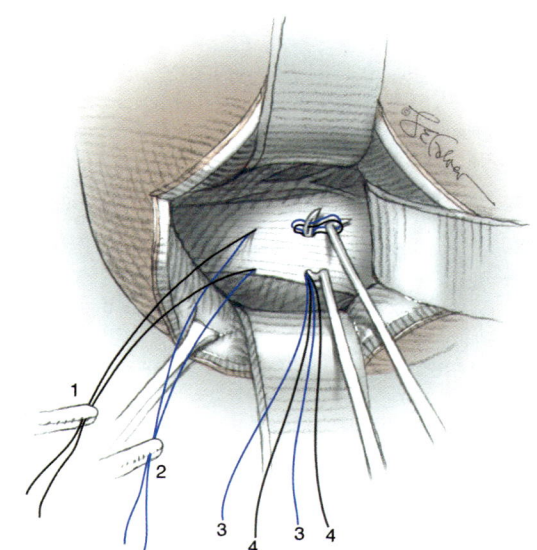

1
2
3 3 4
4

FIGURE 45-21.4 Retractor exposure and ligature placement.

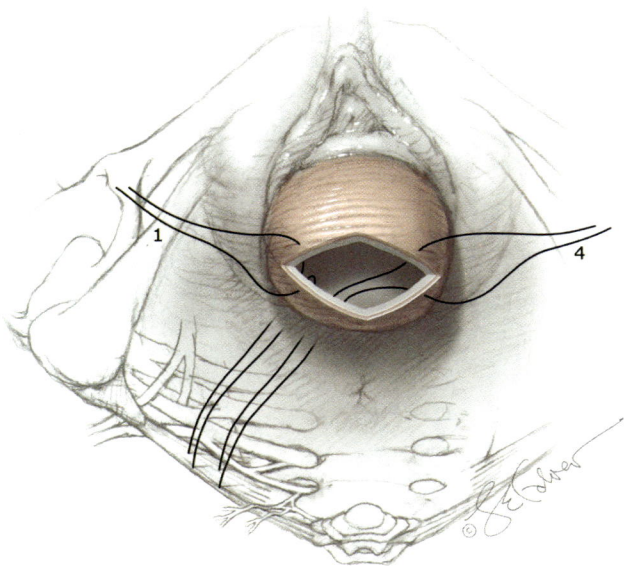

FIGURE 45-21.5 Lateral apex suturing.

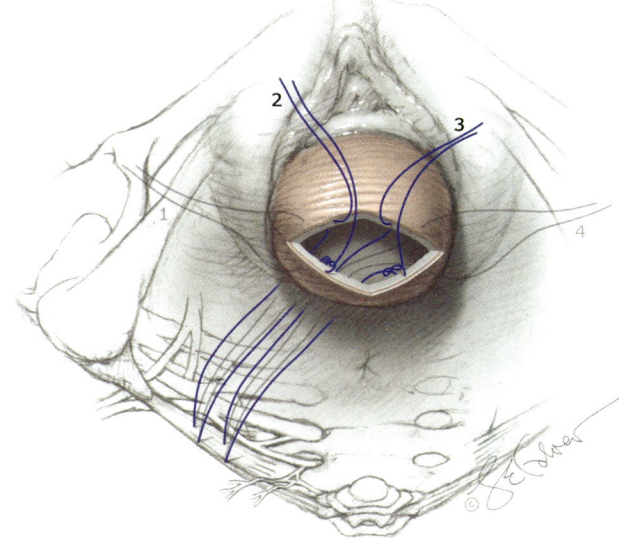

FIGURE 45-21.6 Permanent suture placement (*blue*).

frequently required. If a distal posterior midline plication, perineorrhaphy, or midurethral sling is planned, we prefer to complete this after apical suspension.

6 Suturing of the Vaginal Apex. The SSL sutures are sequentially anchored to the anterior and posterior fibromuscular walls of the vagina apex along the vaginal cuff width. To begin, the two ends of suture 1 are grasped. The end that is most cephalad on the ligament is threaded through the Mayo needle eye. This is then driven through the full thickness of the lateral right anterior vaginal wall including the epithelium, at the site of the initial intended-apex marking

suture. The other end of suture 1 is similarly threaded through the Mayo needle eye and then driven through the lateral right posterior wall. Similar steps are subsequently repeated with delayed-absorbable suture 4 on the left side of the vagina apex (Fig. 45-21.5). Suture ends are not tied but instead held on their respective sides by a hemostat.

Attention is then directed to the permanent sutures (2 and 3). First and medial to those of suture 1, the ends of suture 2 are driven through the anterior and posterior fibromuscular vaginal walls at a point right of the cuff midline. To lower suture erosion rates, permanent sutures traverse the full thickness of the fibromuscular walls but

not the epithelium. However, a substantial fibromuscular wall thickness is incorporated to prevent tissue tearing, which can create suture bridges and incomplete healing of the vaginal wall to the ligament. Second and medial to those of suture 4, the ends of suture 3 are driven through the anterior and posterior fibromuscular vaginal walls at a point left of the cuff midline. If delayed-absorbable monofilament material was chosen for all suspension sutures, as we now prefer, all suture ends can be passed through the full thickness of the vaginal wall.

7 Suspension of the Vaginal Vault. At this point, knots are secured starting with suture 4 and ending with suture 1. Order may be reversed depending on surgeon preference. We prefer to tie the most medial suture along the SSL first (suture 4) to avoid excessive suture traction and breakage from tying the most lateral one first, which is slightly further from the midline axis.

A pulley stitch may be used for the permanent sutures. With this stitch, a knot is secured on the vaginal wall (posterior wall in this case) (Fig. 45-21.6). As shown in Figure 45-21.7, traction on the other suture end (anterior dashed strand) pulls the tied wall (posterior) to the SSL. However, with the four-wall modification, this type of stitch is not necessary. This technique was described and is more useful with the traditional approach, in which permanent sutures are attached to the posterior apical section of vagina.

Each suture is tied down to ensure direct apposition of the vaginal walls to the SSL. Both this snug approximation and the order in which sutures are tied may prevent suture bridges (Fig. 45-21.8). All sutures are held

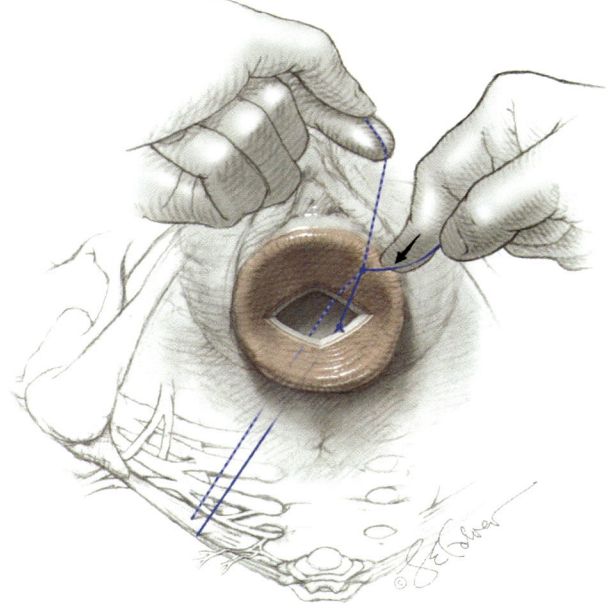

FIGURE 45-21.7 Pulley stitch.

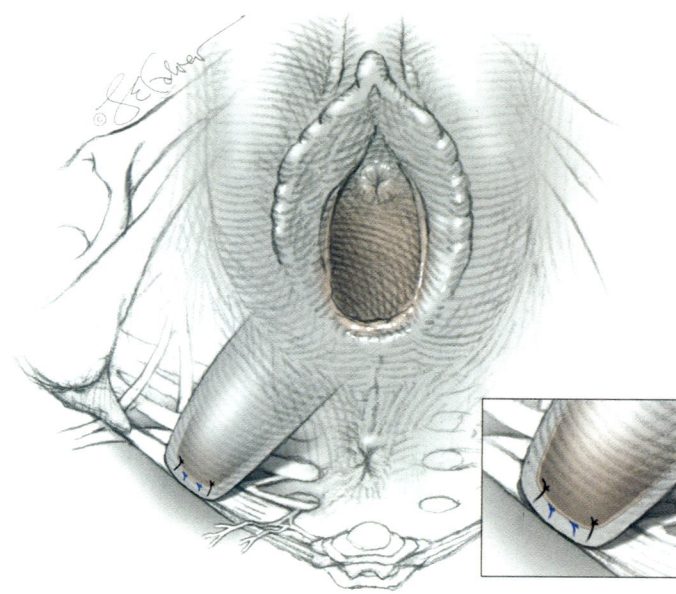

FIGURE 45-21.8 Vaginal apex approximated to ligament.

with their corresponding numbered clamps after tying until cystoscopy is completed. Rectal examination confirms apposition of the vaginal cuff to the SSL and excludes rectal injury.

❽ Cuff Closure. If gaps remain after all four suture pairs are tied, the vaginal cuff may be closed in a running or interrupted fashion using 2-0 gauge delayed-absorbable suture. If gaps measure >1 cm between suture pairs, these may be approximated using interrupted sutures to avoid disruption of the fixation from pulling on vaginal walls.

POSTOPERATIVE

Following SSLF, postoperative care mirrors that for vaginal surgery. Postoperative activity in general can be individualized, although intercourse is usually delayed until after 6 weeks following surgery. A voiding trial can be completed on the same or next day, depending on concomitant procedures and the patient's condition. Some patients have urinary retention after apical suspension, even without an antiincontinence procedure. If unable to void spontaneously by the time of discharge, the patient can be discharged with a catheter and followed up within a week for removal.

Patients are screened for lower extremity neuropathy prior to discharge. Mild gluteal pain is common and typically resolves within several weeks. Severe gluteal pain that radiates down the posterior thigh and leg is a sign of sacral nerve entrapment and is generally treated by prompt suture release. Dyspareunia is commonly attributed to the posterolateral deflection of the vaginal axis. However, given the anatomic position of the nerves to the coccygeus and levator ani muscles, entrapment of these nerves may possibly lead to transient or sustained muscle spasm and dysfunction (Roshanravan, 2007). If levator muscle tenderness is identified, physical therapy may be helpful.

McCall Culdoplasty

Culdoplasty techniques are used to obliterate the posterior cul-de-sac and prevent herniation of small bowel into the vaginal wall, that is, enterocele. Thus, culdoplasty usually complements procedures that further expose the posterior cul-de-sac to enterocele, such as retropubic urethropexy procedures. However, evidence-based studies have not borne out these benefits, and current concepts of specific pelvic-support defect repair have decreased the popularity of culdoplasty. Nevertheless, this procedure is still performed and may have value when completed in conjunction with other prolapse procedures.

Of these, McCall culdoplasty is most commonly performed during vaginal hysterectomy to close the cul-de-sac, add support to the posterior vaginal apex, and possibly prevent enterocele formation. With traditional McCall culdoplasty, two to three horizontal *internal* rows using permanent sutures are placed from one USL to the other to obliterate the posterior cul-de-sac (McCall, 1957). The term *internal* denotes that these sutures remain totally intraabdominal and do not penetrate into the vaginal lumen. In addition, one to two rows of absorbable *external* sutures are similarly placed through the USLs, but these pass through the posterior vaginal cuff.

Several modifications aim to provide better vaginal apex support. These include the Mayo/McCall culdoplasty and the modified McCall culdoplasty. The steps described next outline our approach. Importantly, if significant vaginal apex prolapse or enterocele is already present, we prefer an apical suspension procedure such as ASC, SSLF, or vaginal USLS, because more data support their efficacy.

PREOPERATIVE

Patient Evaluation

McCall culdoplasty is generally performed following vaginal hysterectomy in patients with enterocele or preventively in those without. Because the degree of pelvic organ prolapse will dictate reconstructive surgeries planned, a thorough prolapse evaluation is performed preoperatively.

Consent

As with any pelvic reconstructive surgery to correct prolapse, the risk of enterocele formation or recurrence is discussed. In addition,

because this procedure involves placement of sutures through the USLs, risks similar to USLS procedures are addressed and include dyspareunia, ureteral or bowel injury, and sacral plexus nerve damage (p. 1133). Suture erosion risks are low.

Patient Preparation

Bowel preparation will vary depending on surgeon preference and is typically dictated by concurrent surgery planned. Antibiotic and VTE prophylaxis are given as outlined in Tables 39-8 and 39-10 (p. 832).

INTRAOPERATIVE

Surgical Steps

❶ **Anesthesia and Patient Positioning.** McCall culdoplasty typically is performed under general anesthesia. The patient is placed in standard lithotomy position using candy-cane or booted support stirrups. The vagina is surgically prepared, and a Foley catheter is inserted. Vaginal hysterectomy is completed as described in Section 43-13 (p. 965), but the vaginal cuff is left open for culdoplasty completion. Excess peritoneum or vaginal wall may be excised at this time if indicated.

❷ **Packing.** After vaginal hysterectomy, a moist pack is placed into the posterior

cul-de-sac to prevent bowel or omentum descent.

❸ **Uterosacral Ligaments and Ureter Identification.** This mirrors that described for the vaginal USLS procedure (p. 1134). Briefly, a Deaver retractor displaces the bladder upward, and gentle upward retractor traction exposes the distal to mid portions of the USLs. Two Allis clamps are next placed at approximately 5 and 7 o'clock positions on the posterior vaginal wall and incorporate the posterior peritoneum. Gentle downward Allis clamp traction tenses the USLs, which are then traced with the contralateral index finger from their distal attachments in the vagina toward the sacrum. Ureters are usually indistinct to touch, but they course anterolateral to the USLs. Lighted Breisky-Navratil retractors are useful on either side to further expose the USLs.

❹ **Suture Placement.** For the internal McCall sutures, we use a 2-0 gauge permanent suture with a swaged-on SH needle. For the external McCall sutures, a similar-gauge delayed-absorbable material is selected. The number of suture rows placed is guided by cul-de-sac depth, vaginal cuff width, and surgeon preference. Generally, two to three internal and one to two external rows are placed (Fig. 45-22.1).

Of the internal sutures, the first suture row is the most distal of these, and each subsequent row is placed progressively cephalad

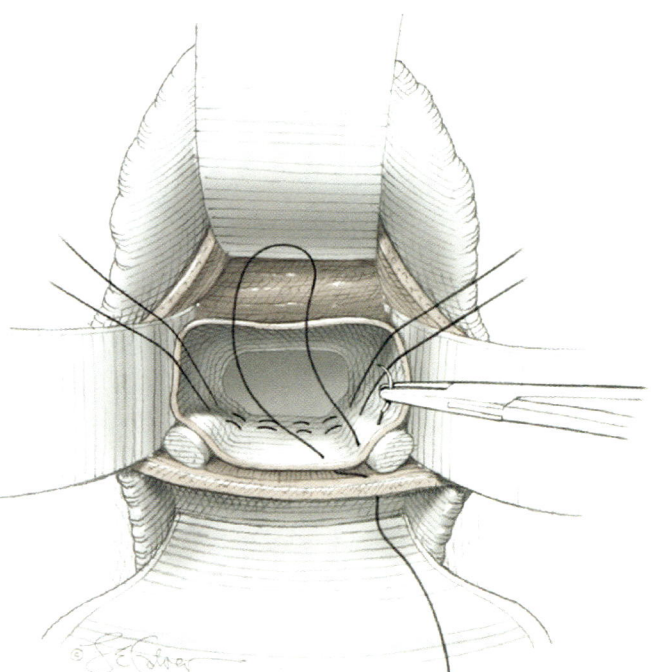

FIGURE 45-22.1 Uterosacral ligament and peritoneal suture placement.

across the posterior cul-de-sac. Each row begins with a stitch into one USL. The needle tip pierces the most medial portion of the left or right USL and travels in a lateral-to-medial direction. As with other USL suspension procedures, these specifics attempt to minimize ureteral entrapment risks. Moreover, to reduce rectal injury rates, the rectum is retracted to the contralateral side, and suture purchases do not extend too medial, that is, beyond the ligament width.

Subsequent stitches course laterally to the opposite USL. With each, the needle is passed through the cul-de-sac peritoneum or rectal serosa and finally through the USL. Each row is spaced approximately 0.5 cm to 1 cm cephalad from the previous one. The internal McCall sutures are tagged, held, and tied only after placement of the external McCall sutures.

Following these internal rows, the first external suture is placed through the full thickness of the posterior vaginal wall and incorporates the posterior peritoneum and USL (see Fig. 45-22.1). Progressive left-to-right stitches are then taken serially through the rectal serosa or peritoneum to reach the opposite uterosacral ligament (Fig. 45-22.2). Finally, the suture enters the opposite uterosacral ligament, passes through the posterior peritoneum, and exits through the full vaginal wall thickness to reenter the vagina.

❺ Suture Tying. The internal sutures are tied first. These sutures are sequentially tied beginning with the most proximal sutures and progressing caudad. The external sutures are then tied, and again the most cephalad of these is tied first.

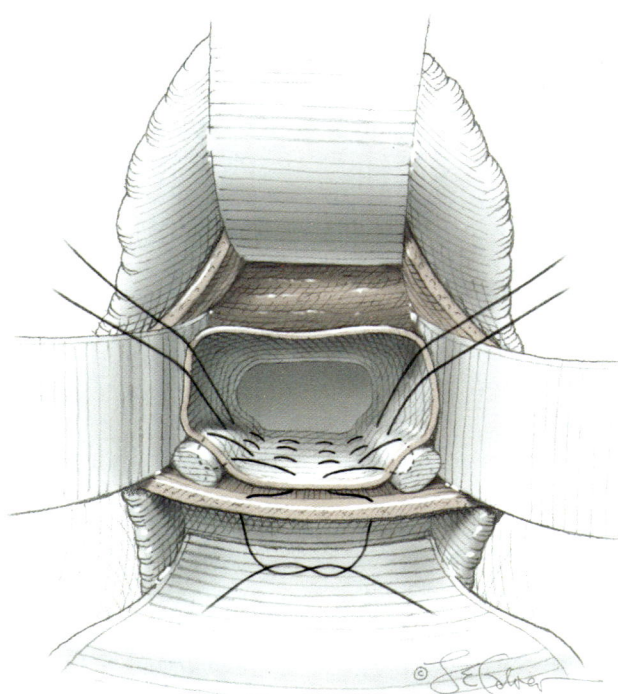

FIGURE 45-22.2 Suture reenters the vagina prior to securing.

❻ Rectal Examination. The rectum is digitally explored to exclude sutures entering the rectum.

❼ Cystoscopy. This is performed after all McCall culdoplasty sutures are tied to document ureteral patency and exclude bladder sutures or cystotomy.

❽ Vaginal Cuff Closure. Upon completion of McCall culdoplasty, the remaining steps of vaginal hysterectomy will follow as described in Section 43-13 (p. 969).

POSTOPERATIVE

Following vaginal hysterectomy and McCall culdoplasty, postoperative care mirrors that for vaginal surgery. Activity in general is individualized, although intercourse is usually delayed until 6 weeks. As with other USLS procedures, patients are screened for lower extremity neuropathy prior to discharge. Suture erosion with granulation tissue can be a short- or long-term complication and is managed as described on page 1128.

45-23

Colpocleisis

Pelvic organ prolapse surgery can broadly be grouped as reconstructive or obliterative. Complete colpocleisis, also known as *colpectomy*, *vaginal extirpation*, and *vaginectomy*, is an obliterative surgery for advanced vaginal or uterovaginal eversion. To correct prolapse, all obliterative procedures close the vaginal canal and thus are only indicated in women who do not desire to preserve vaginal anatomy or coital function or who are medically unsuitable for reconstructive surgery. Specifically, this operation may be performed quickly with general, regional, or local anesthesia.

The two main obliterating surgeries are partial colpocleisis and complete colpocleisis. With the partial procedure, also called *LeFort colpocleisis*, central rectangular sections of vaginal epithelium are dissected from the anterior and posterior vaginal walls, and the denuded fibromuscular layers are apposed and sewn together. This effectively elevates the prolapse back into the pelvic cavity and closes the vagina (Fig. 45-23.1). The remaining lateral epithelial strips are fashioned into drainage tracts on either side for genital tract fluid egress. Thus, this surgery is appropriate for women with or without a uterus.

In contrast, with total or complete colpocleisis, the entire circumference of vaginal epithelium in the upper two thirds of the vagina is resected before vaginal walls are approximated. Drainage tracts are lacking, thus, it typically is used for posthysterectomy vault prolapse. If the uterus is present, concurrent total vaginal hysterectomy and closure of the peritoneum is performed prior to complete colpocleisis.

Obliterative procedures are effective, and success rates range from 91 to 100 percent (Abassy, 2010; Fitzgerald, 2006; Weber, 2005). However, these rates are interpreted in the context of patients' shorter life expectancies, limited activity levels, and variable outcome definitions. Anatomic success following colpocleisis is likely due to the amount of vaginal tissue sutured together to create a shelf of support. Several studies evaluating symptom improvement also have found high rates of patient satisfaction and functional improvement yet low rates of regret for sexual function loss (Barber, 2007; Fitzgerald, 2008; Gutman, 2009; Hullfish, 2007).

SUI following colpocleisis is common, thus prophylactic antiincontinence surgery is considered. Additionally, high perineorrhaphy or levator myorrhaphy (p. 1122) is recommended to narrow the genital hiatus and potentially decrease the recurrent prolapse risk. Last, concurrent hysterectomy eliminates the risk of uterine or cervical cancer and of

postoperative hemato- or pyometra. However, patient morbidity, including greater blood loss, increased transfusion risk, and longer procedure time, is increased with hysterectomy (Bochenska, 2017). Support success rates following colpocleisis are similar whether or not the uterus is removed (Abassy, 2010; Fitzgerald, 2006; Weber, 2005). Thus, hysterectomy is selected based on a woman's general health, surgical goals, and risk for later comorbid genital tract disease.

PREOPERATIVE

Patient Evaluation

Because access to the cervix and endometrial cavity is not possible following this procedure, preinvasive lesions are excluded. Specifically, a normal cervical cancer screening is documented prior to surgery, and evaluation of the endometrium with either endometrial biopsy or sonography is recommended (Elkattah, 2014).

The full extent of prolapse is defined prior to surgery. Importantly, colpocleisis is difficult in women with good distal support of either the anterior or posterior vaginal walls.

Women with advanced prolapse often do not display SUI because the urethra is kinked by prolapsing organs. However, with replacement of the prolapse, many with occult SUI do manifest symptoms. Thus, preoperative cough stress test or urodynamic testing is performed with the prolapse elevated and replaced to search for occult SUI. Urinalysis and a postvoid residual measurement also are evaluated. For those who demonstrate SUI or occult SUI, antiincontinence surgery is recommended. However, even without SUI, a prophylactic antiincontinence procedure is considered to prevent later de novo SUI. Still, benefits of an additional procedure are weighed against the potential risk of urinary retention. For SUI, midurethral sling procedures or urethral bulking agents are suitable options.

Last, women with global prolapse frequently have some degree of ureteral kinking and obstruction. Thus, preoperative pyelography, CT urography, or renal sonography may be elected to identify or exclude ureteral obstruction and associated renal injury. Alternatively, preoperative or intraoperative cystoscopy prior to the colpocleisis can be used to document ureteral patency. Known preexisting obstruction will assist with interpretation of cystoscopy findings performed at the procedure's end. Also, with known ureteral obstruction, preoperative catheter placement is considered to assist with ureter identification during surgery. Colpocleisis ideally will unkink the ureter, and this can be documented during intraoperative cystoscopy after prolapse correction.

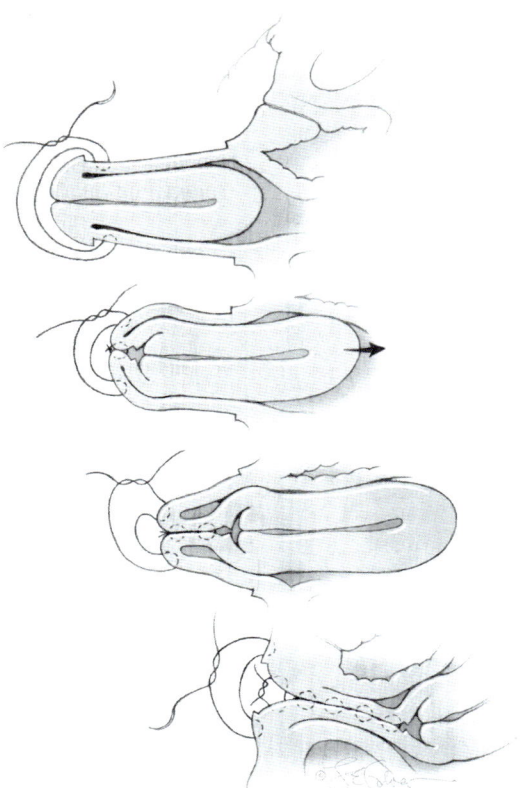

FIGURE 45-23.1 Prolapse correction following placement of serial sutures.

Consent

Women considering this procedure must be fully aware that future vaginal intercourse is not possible. Thus, a patient's partner is ideally included in the decision and consenting process. Patients expressing hesitation or doubt are excluded as candidates. As with all pelvic organ prolapse surgeries, a patient's perception of her desired outcomes is essential.

First, as with any prolapse surgery, prolapse recurrence risk is discussed, although this risk is low with colpocleisis. Of note, later de novo rectal prolapse is disproportionately prevalent, and this unique complication was reported in 4 percent of women in one study (Collins, 2007). Second, as discussed, urinary incontinence may develop postoperatively. In addition, ureteral injury has been described. Third, in the unlikely situation that cervical or uterine malignancy develops after LeFort partial colpocleisis, the diagnosis may be potentially delayed. Last, perioperative morbidity and mortality are especially pertinent in the elderly, and risks for cardiac, thromboembolic, pulmonary, or cerebrovascular events approximate 5 percent (Fitzgerald, 2006; Hill, 2016).

Patient Preparation

Bowel preparation, if any, will vary depending on surgeon preference. Patients can be instructed to consume only clear liquids the day prior to surgery and complete one or two enemas the night prior to or the morning of surgery. Alternatively, a mechanical bowel preparation, listed in Chapter 39 (p. 833), may be elected. Antibiotic and VTE prophylaxis is given as outlined in Tables 39-8 and 39-10 (p. 832).

INTRAOPERATIVE

Anesthesia and Patient Positioning

General or regional anesthesia is preferred, although colpocleisis can be performed under local anesthesia. A patient is placed in standard lithotomy position using candy-cane or booted support stirrups, the vagina is surgically prepared, and a Foley catheter is inserted.

Surgical Steps—LeFort Partial Colpocleisis

As noted, LeFort partial colpocleisis may be performed in women with or without a uterus, but the following description outlines steps in women without prior hysterectomy. In women with posthysterectomy prolapse, a partial colpocleisis may be performed to decreased operative time and

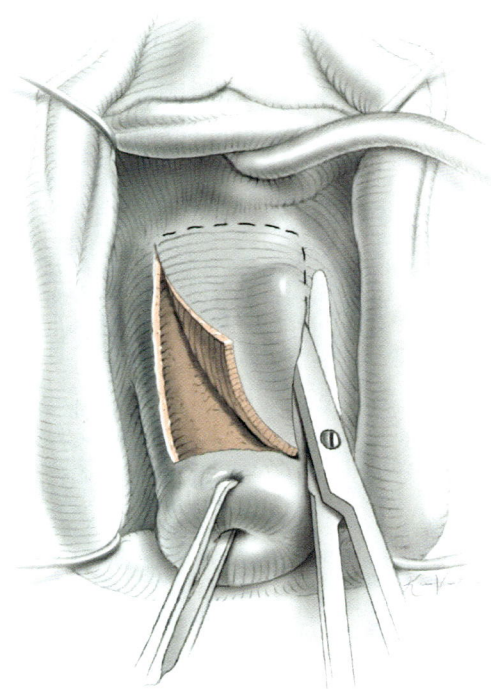

FIGURE 45-23.2 Anterior vaginal wall incision.

blood loss, especially in a setting of massive vault eversion.

❶ Marking the Vagina. Throughout the descriptions of both colpocleisis procedures, *proximal* and *distal* will describe prolapsed anatomy rather than final prolapse-corrected anatomy. To begin, the rectangular areas of vaginal mucosa on the anterior and posterior vaginal walls are outlined with a surgical marker or electrosurgical blade. The size of these areas to be removed is determined by the length and width of vaginal walls. Anteriorly, the proximal edge of the rectangle extends to within 1 to 2 cm of the bladder neck and posteriorly to within 2 to 3 cm of the posterior hymeneal ring. The distal edge reaches to within 1 to 2 cm of the cervicovaginal junction both anteriorly and posteriorly. The lateral edges of each rectangle are drawn to leave approximately 2-cm-wide lateral epithelial borders on either side. These will be fashioned into lateral channels of adequate caliber to conduct drainage.

❷ Vaginal Infiltration. The rectangular areas of the vaginal wall to be removed may be thoroughly infiltrated with 50 mL of a dilute hemostatic solution. One example is 20 units of synthetic vasopressin (Pitressin) in 60 mL of saline. This infiltration extends beyond the anticipated incision boundaries. Without infiltration, bleeding can be significant during epithelial excision.

Needle aspiration prior to injection is imperative to avoid intravascular injection

of this potent vasoconstrictor. The anesthesiologist is informed of vasopressin administration, as patient blood pressure may suddenly rise following injection. Blanching at the injection site is expected.

Due to the vasoactive effects of vasoconstrictors, patients with certain comorbidities may not be suitable candidates for their use. These can include a history of angina, myocardial infarction, cardiomyopathy, congestive heart failure, uncontrolled hypertension, migraine, asthma, and severe chronic obstructive pulmonary disease.

❸ Vaginal Dissection. Previously outlined areas are sharply incised down to the fibromuscular layer. If the anterior dissection is performed first, the vaginal wall epithelium within the previously marked anterior rectangle is dissected off the underlying vaginal wall fibromuscular layer using both sharp and blunt dissection (Fig. 45-23.2). Dissection in the correct plane will prevent inadvertent bladder or bowel entry. One effective technique places a finger behind the vaginal epithelium flap, while cephalad dissection with Metzenbaum scissors advances parallel to this epithelium. Bleeding during dissection can generally be controlled with pressure and electrosurgical coagulation. Occasionally, figure-eight stitches of 2-0 gauge absorbable suture are needed if large venous sinuses are cut. Next, the vaginal wall epithelium within the previously marked posterior rectangle is similarly dissected off the fibromuscular layer on the posterior vaginal

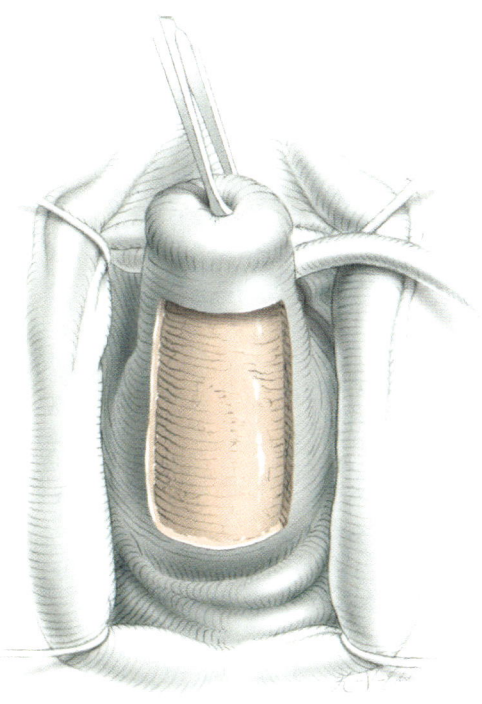

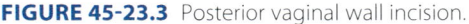

FIGURE 45-23.3 Posterior vaginal wall incision.

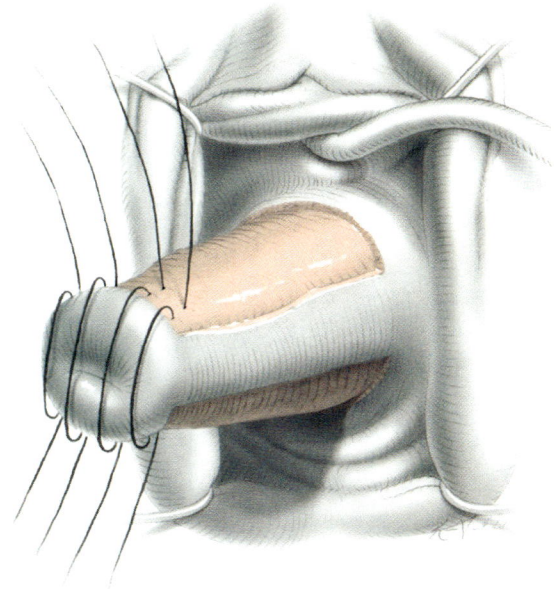

FIGURE 45-23.4 Initial suture placement imbricates cervix.

wall (Fig. 45-23.3). Of note, some prefer to dissect posteriorly first to avoid obscuring blood from the anterior wall that may ooze into the surgical field.

❹ **Apical and Lateral Channels.** After these rectangles are removed, a row of interrupted stitches using 2-0 gauge delayed-

absorbable suture are placed through the anterior and posterior distal transverse epithelium edges (Fig. 45-23.4). These will effectively close the fibromuscular layer over the cervix and create the apical channel. Next, lateral channels on each side are formed and connect with this apical channel. For this, the lateral anterior and poste-

rior epithelial edges are approximated along their full length (Fig. 45-23.5). This lateral row of sutures begins distally and progresses proximally to the original proximal transverse incision near the bladder neck. The lateral channels can be created in a stepwise fashion, alternating from one side to the other.

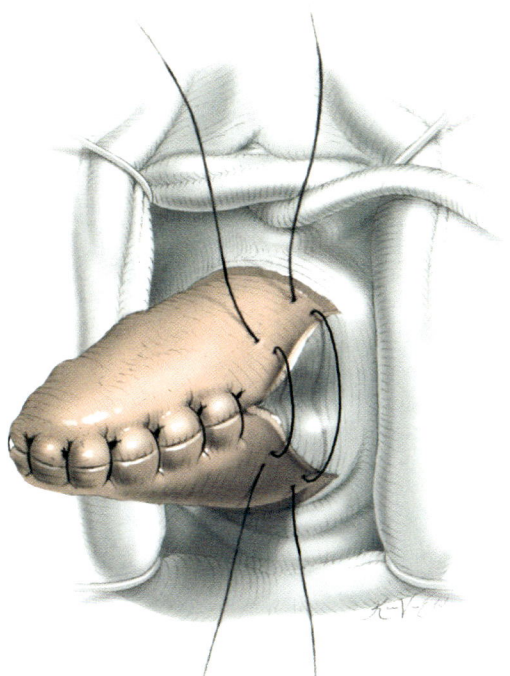

FIGURE 45-23.5 Creation of lateral drainage channels.

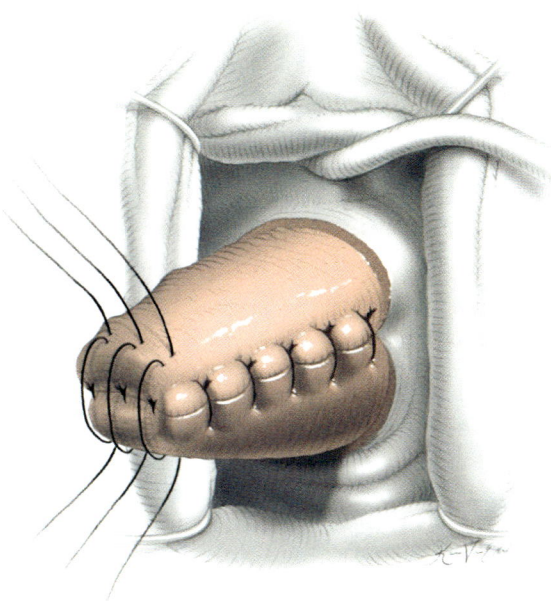

FIGURE 45-23.6 Second row of sutures.

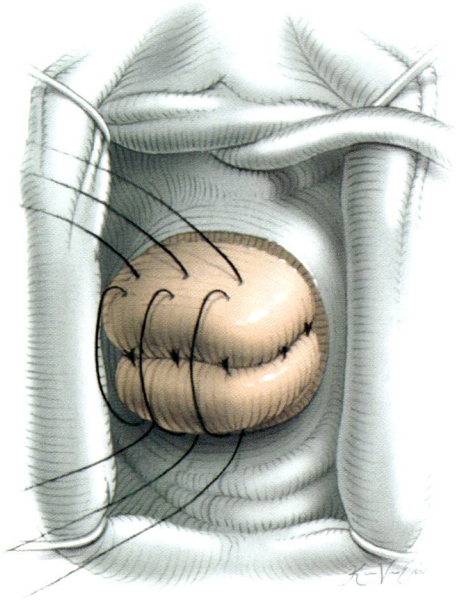

FIGURE 45-23.7 Subsequent row of sutures.

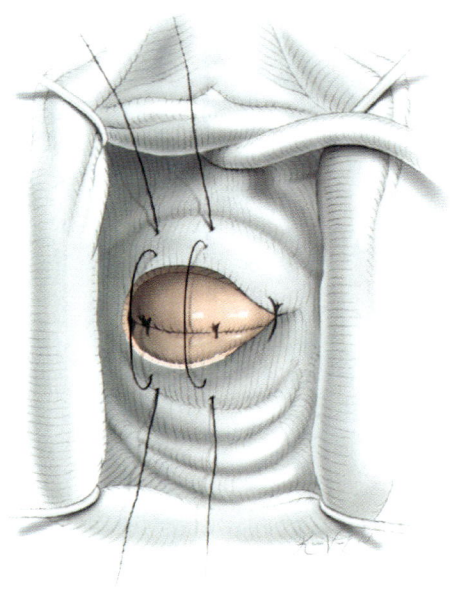

FIGURE 45-23.8 Vaginal epithelium closure.

❺ Anterior-to-Posterior Vaginal Wall Approximation. With the lateral canals now fashioned, the uterus can be sequentially elevated into the pelvic cavity. For this, a surgeon places progressive rows of interrupted 2-0 gauge permanent or delayed-absorbable sutures that approximate the anterior and posterior fibromuscular layers along the distal prolapsed-tube width (Fig. 45-23.6). Successive transverse tiers of sutures are placed approximately 1 cm apart until the proximal transverse incision is reached (Fig. 45-23.7). These rows create a tissue septum that elevates and supports the uterus (see Fig. 45-23.1).

❻ Cystoscopy. Following either colpocleisis procedure, cystoscopy is performed to exclude urinary tract injury and document ureteral patency.

❼ Closing the Vaginal Epithelium. This layer is then reapproximated in a running fashion with 2-0 or 3-0 gauge delayed-absorbable suture (Fig. 45-23.8). Importantly, the ostium of each drainage tract remains patent.

❽ Concurrent Surgery. At this point, an antiincontinence procedure may be completed as needed. Perineorrhaphy may be performed before or after vaginal wall closure (p. 1122).

Surgical Steps—Complete Colpocleisis

❶ Vaginal Infiltration. The vaginal cuff is placed on traction, and a vasoconstrictive agent may be injected in a similar fashion to that described for the LeFort partial colpocleisis.

❷ Vaginal Incision and Dissection. The borders of planned dissection are marked circumferentially with a pen or scored with electrosurgical cutting. When redundant tissue is present, marking three to four smaller rectangles over the entire prolapsed vaginal tube helps maintain orientation during dissection.

To begin, the vaginal epithelium is incised anteriorly at a point 1 to 2 cm distal to the bladder neck. Ultimately, this will be a point that lies approximately 1 cm proximal to the neck. Incision placement here will prevent downward displacement of the bladder neck

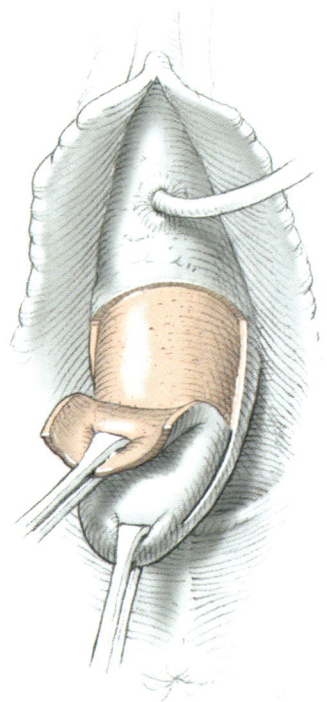

FIGURE 45-23.9 Anterior vaginal wall incision.

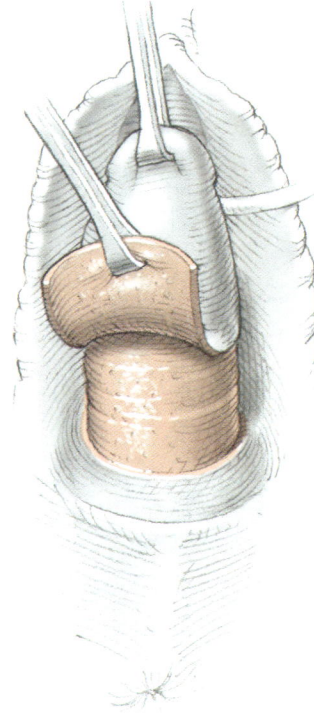

FIGURE 45-23.10 Posterior vaginal wall incision.

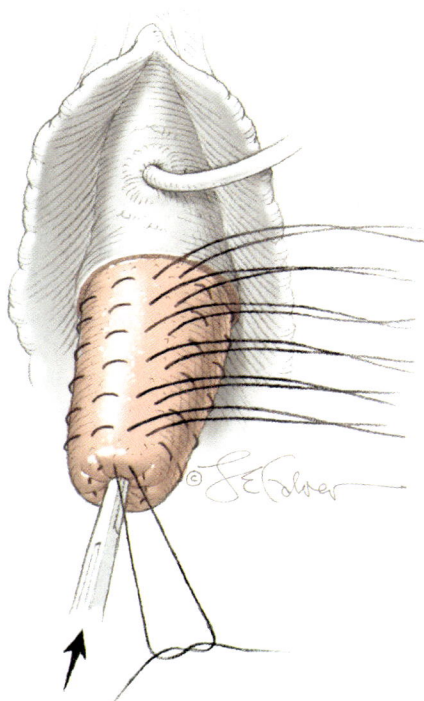

FIGURE 45-23.11 Circumferential suturing.

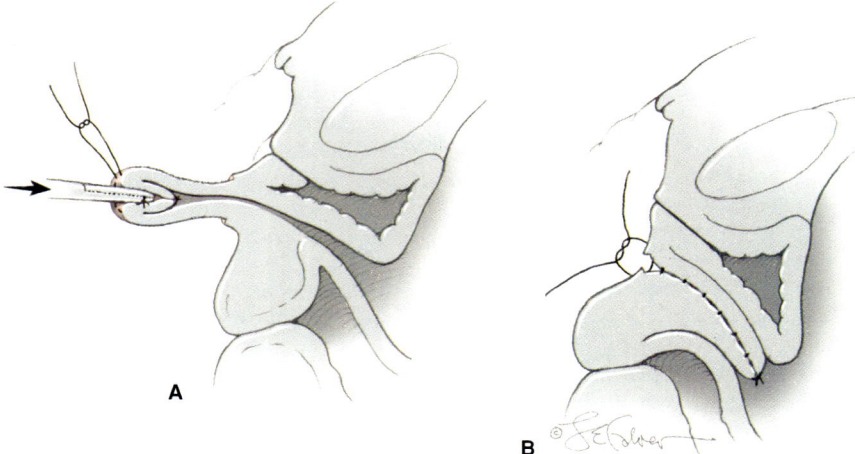

FIGURE 45-23.12 A. Cephalad pressure against telescoping vaginal tube as serial sutures are secured. **B.** Completely inverted vaginal tube.

and the proximal urethra during apposition of the anterior and posterior vaginal walls. Additionally, it will allow room for the midurethral sling if one is planned. As the incision is swept circumferentially around the prolapse tube, a 1- to 2-cm distance is maintained distal to the hymeneal ring.

The vaginal epithelium is sharply and bluntly dissected off the underlying fibromuscular layer (Figs. 45-23.9 and 45-23.10). Dissection is kept close to the epithelium to avoid inadvertent bladder or rectal entry. Once the desired plane is identified, sharp and blunt dissection can proceed quickly until the entire vaginal epithelium is removed. One technique for sharp dissection involves positioning a finger behind the vaginal epithelium flap and dissecting with Metzenbaum scissors parallel to the vaginal wall and close to the epithelium.

After entry into the correct plane, blunt dissection with a gauze-covered index finger may allow rapid and wide development of this avascular space. The entire vaginal epithelium is removed from the prolapsed vaginal tube. However, because of extensive scarring,

dissection may be difficult at the prolapsed vaginal apex, the uterosacral ligament remnants, or areas with previous or current ulcers. Here, sharp dissection may be required.

❸ **Suture Placement.** Next, to plicate the vaginal walls together and elevate the everted vagina, a surgeon places a series of circumferential purse-string sutures around the vaginal tube. With 2-0 gauge permanent or delayed-absorbable suture, stitches incorporate the fibromuscular layer but avoid deep penetration into the bladder, ureter, or rectum (Fig. 45-23.11).

The first purse-string suture is placed approximately 1 cm from the cuff, and tied while the cuff is inverted with atraumatic forceps or an Allis clamp (Fig. 45-23.12). The cut suture tails are held with a hemostat, and the second suture is placed 1 cm proximally. The hemostat inverts the vagina, while the second suture is tied, and is used again to tag the second suture. Progressive purse-string sutures are placed similarly 1 cm apart until the proximal edge of cut vaginal epithelium is reached. These serial steps telescope the prolapsed vaginal tube cephalad and toward the pelvic cavity. Depending on the size of the prolapse, approximately six to eight suture rings are needed to completely invert the prolapsed vaginal tube.

❹ **Finishing Steps.** Final steps are similar with both colpocleisis procedures. First,

cystoscopy is performed to exclude urinary tract injury and document ureteral patency. The vaginal epithelium then is reapproximated in a running fashion with 2-0 or 3-0 gauge delayed-absorbable suture. At this point, an antiincontinence procedure may be performed. Perineorrhaphy may be performed before or after vaginal wall closure (p. 1122).

POSTOPERATIVE

Hospital admission is often prudent given the usual older age and comorbidities of these patients. A normal diet can be given immediately. Oral analgesics are usually sufficient. A voiding trial is performed prior to discharge as all patients can experience urinary retention from concurrent levator myorrhaphy or perineorrhaphy. Patients with urinary retention can return within a week for a subsequent voiding trial and catheter removal.

In general, recovery with colpocleisis is quick and typically without complication. Postoperative bleeding is not anticipated, save for spotting from the surgical site. As with any prolapse procedure, constipation is avoided to protect repair strength during healing. Thus, stool softeners are recommended. Resumption of normal activities is encouraged with the exception of heavy lifting for several months.

45-24

Anal Sphincteroplasty

External anal sphincter (EAS) and/or internal anal sphincter (IAS) repair is most commonly performed in patients with acquired fecal incontinence (FI) and an anterior sphincter defect. One of two methods may be selected for sphincter repair: an end-to-end technique or an overlapping method. The end-to-end technique is most often used by obstetricians at delivery to reapproximate torn anal sphincter ends. However, in women remote from delivery, the overlapping technique is often selected, and with this, disrupted ends are overlapped and then sutured.

In cases remote from delivery, the overlapping method is preferred. However, the optimal technique or suture material for repair and the effects of pudendal neuropathy on treatment outcome are not well known (Madoff, 2004). With the overlapping method, short-term continence rates up to 85 percent were previously reported (Fleshman, 1991; Sitzler, 1996). However, newer reports show significant deterioration of FI during long-term postoperative surveillance (Bravo Gutierrez, 2004; Zutshi, 2009).

In cases at delivery, no evidence shows that either method yields superior results (Fitzpatrick, 2000; Garcia, 2005). Moreover, overlapping repair requires increased technical skills and carries the potential for increased blood loss, operating time, and pudendal neuropathy. Accordingly, the end-to-end technique is likely to remain the standard method for sphincter reapproximation at delivery until further data from randomized controlled trials are available.

PREOPERATIVE

Patient Evaluation

Because the etiology of FI in patients with documented sphincter defects may be multifactorial, careful preoperative evaluation attempts to distinguish underlying sources. Evaluation for structural gastrointestinal tract pathology typically involves colonoscopy and/or barium enema. Additionally, radiographic bowel transit studies can be used to diagnose slow transit time, which may be related to defecatory dysfunction.

Specific to the anorectum, endoanal sonography accurately defines structural disruption of the EAS and IAS (Fig. 25-7, p. 565) and is generally performed prior to sphincter repair. Exceptions are cloacal-like defects or chronic fourth-degree lacerations.

In these, the absent anterior portion of the sphincter(s) is easily identified clinically.

Anal manometry and pudendal nerve conduction studies may identify physiologic dysfunction such as neuropathy. Although these tests provide additional information and can be used during counseling, they are not necessary in patients with FI and a documented sphincter defect. In fact, the relationship of pudendal nerve function, typically assessed by determining pudendal nerve terminal motor latency, to sphincteroplasty outcome remains controversial (Madoff, 2004). One study found no association between pudendal nerve status and long-term postrepair anal continence (Malouf, 2000).

Clinicians have attempted to improve success rates by selecting only those women who may benefit most from surgery. Patient age, preoperative anal manometry readings, and pudendal nerve motor function have been evaluated as possible outcome predictors. However, research findings are conflicting, and none of these consistently predicts outcome (Bravo Gutierrez, 2004; Buie, 2001; El-Gazzaz, 2012; Gearhart, 2005).

Consent

Although many women may have improved FI immediately following anal sphincteroplasty, repair durability is poor. For example, 3 to 5 years following correction, only approximately 10 percent of women are fully continent of solid and liquid stool (Halverson, 2002; Malouf, 2000). Retrospective data show that no patients are continent 10 years following sphincteroplasty (Zutshi, 2009). However, despite FI based on validated questionnaires, the quality of life in these patients notably did not decline. In a more recent study that focused on overlapping sphincteroplasty for chronic fourth-degree lacerations, long-term subjective fecal continence rates of 54 percent were reported (Maldonado, 2019).

Reasons for worsening continence following initial improvement remain unknown but may include aging, scarring, and progressive pudendal neuropathy either from initial injury or from the sphincter repair (Madoff, 2004). In addition, skeletal muscle repair is thought to have poor success because resting muscle tone places incision lines on constant tension. Thus, preoperative counseling informs that most individuals will improve after the procedure, but continence is rarely perfect and deteriorates over time.

In addition to persistent FI, sphincteroplasty is associated with other surgical risks. More common serious complications are wound dehiscence and fistula formation. Ha and coworkers (2001) noted a wound

complication in 12 percent and fistula formation in 4 percent. Dyspareunia is a risk, especially if levator myorrhaphy (p. 1122) is concomitantly performed in sexually active women. We believe levator myorrhaphy is a nonanatomic repair and do not perform it with sphincteroplasty.

Patient Preparation

Because of the high associated risk of wound complications, antibiotic prophylaxis is warranted to minimize wound infection following surgical contamination from vaginal and rectal flora. In our division, we often continue oral antibiotics for approximately 7 days postoperatively to sustain broad antibacterial coverage, although limited evidence supports this practice (Maldonado, 2019). Although benefits from mechanical bowel preparation have not been demonstrated, some form of bowel preparation is typically administered the day or night before surgery. Options are listed in Chapter 39 (p. 833). Thromboprophylaxis is provided as outlined in Table 39-10 (p. 834).

INTRAOPERATIVE

Surgical Steps

❶ **Anesthesia and Patient Positioning.** After administration of either general or regional anesthesia, a woman is placed in standard lithotomy position using candy-cane or booted support stirrups. The vagina and perineum are surgically prepared, and a Foley catheter is inserted.

❷ **Incision and Dissection.** A downward-arching curvilinear incision is placed between the fourchette and anus, and this connects with a midline posterior vaginal wall incision (Fig. 45-24.1). The vaginal incision edges are placed on tension with Allis clamps. Along the distal 3 to 4 cm of the posterior vaginal wall, the vaginal epithelium is then sharply dissected off its underlying fibromuscular layer and off the perineal body.

On the perineum, dissection continues distally and laterally with Metzenbaum scissors. Advancement is kept just deep to the perianal skin and progresses until the scarred and usually retracted edges of the EAS are identified within the ischioanal fossa. Dissection proceeds until the EAS muscle is sufficiently mobile to ensure a tension-free overlapping repair.

As the inner arch of the EAS is sharply separated from the anal submucosa, care is taken to avoid entry into the anal lumen. To assist, a surgeon's index finger within the anus can guide dissection depth, and

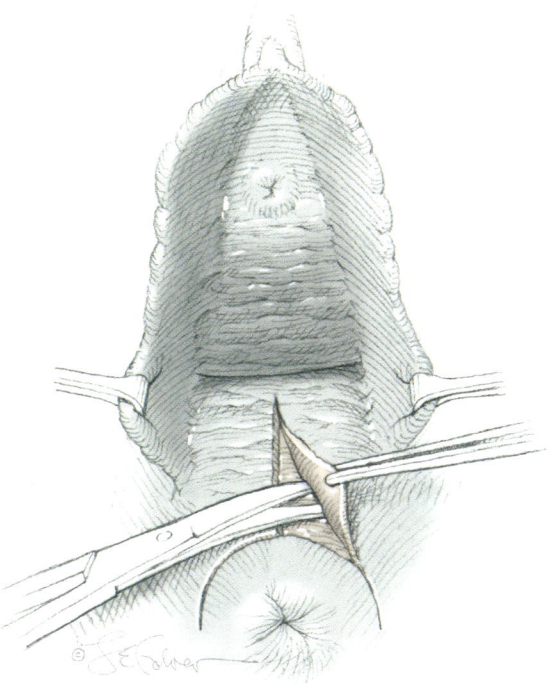

FIGURE 45-24.1 Vaginal dissection.

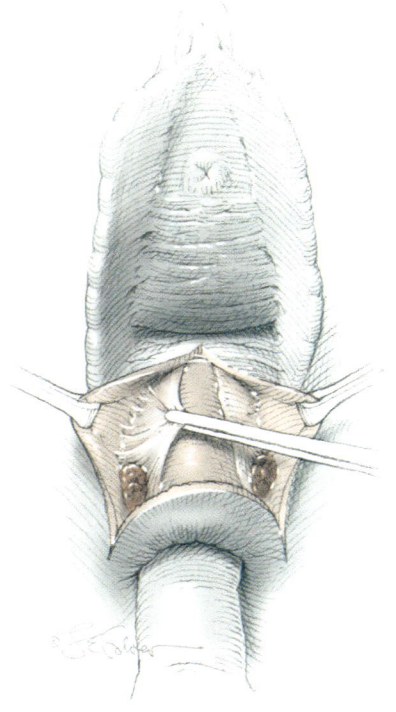

FIGURE 45-24.2 Internal anal sphincter identification.

concomitant upward traction by an assistant on the sphincter's scarred ends helps accentuate the best dissection plane. Internal pudendal vessels can be lacerated or inferior rectal nerve injured, especially if lateral dissection extends beyond the 3 o'clock and 9 o'clock positions. Thus, if extensive lateral dissection is anticipated, the end-to-end method of repair is preferred.

Scarring of EAS in the midline may be cut but is not excised. This fibrous tissue adds strength to the sphincter muscle approximation. However, with extensive scarring, sphincter muscle fibers may be difficult to isolate. A nerve stimulator or a needle-tip electrosurgical blade can assist in delineating these fibers. Electric current will contract them.

❸ **Suture Placement in the Internal Anal Sphincter.** The IAS contributes significantly to the anal canal resting tone, and its reapproximation is included in the repair. Grasped in **Figure 45-24.2**, the IAS is a smooth, rubbery, thickened white sheet lying deep to the EAS and superficial to the anal mucosa and submucosal layers. This muscle usually retracts laterally when severed.

For suturing, we prefer monofilament, delayed-absorbable suture. First, because both the IAS and EAS muscles are under constant contraction, direct tissue reapproximation by these longer-acting sutures in theory allows adequate scar formation during the critical first 3 months of postoperative healing. Second, use of permanent suture

for sphincteroplasty has been associated with high rates of suture erosion and wound dehiscence (Luck, 2005).

With suturing, the disrupted IAS edges are approximated in a continuous or interrupted fashion using 2-0 or 3-0 gauge monofilament,

delayed-absorbable sutures such as polydioxanone (PDS II) (**Fig. 45-24.3**). Sutures are spaced approximately 0.5 cm apart. As the distal extent of the IAS is generally several millimeters cephalad to the distal extent of the EAS, reapproximation of this muscle

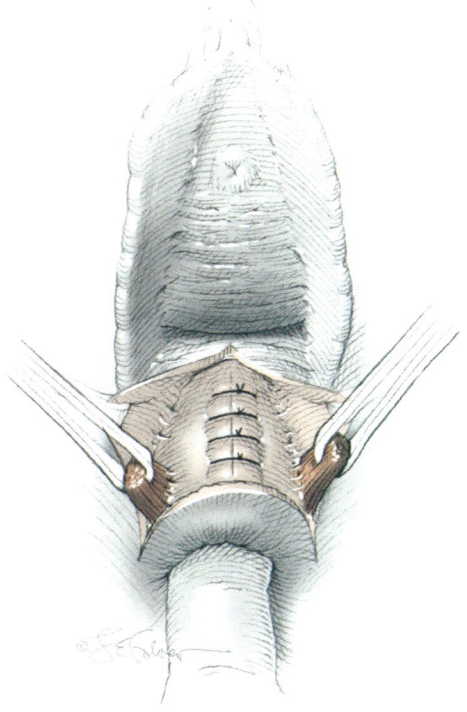

FIGURE 45-24.3 Following internal anal sphincter reapproximation, the external anal sphincter is identified and grasped.

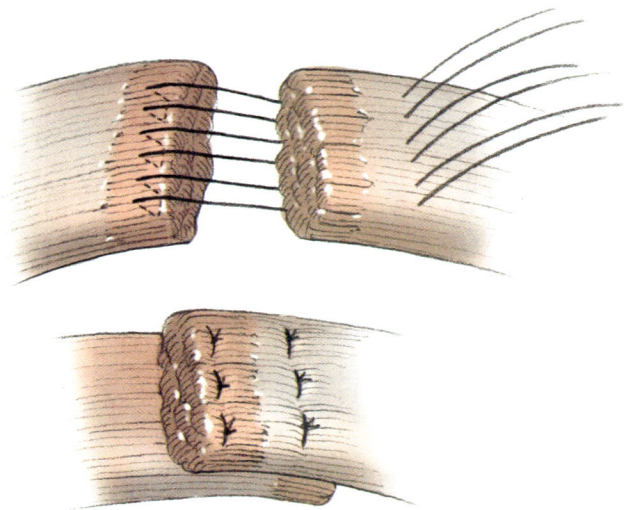

FIGURE 45-24.4 Overlapping sphincteroplasty.

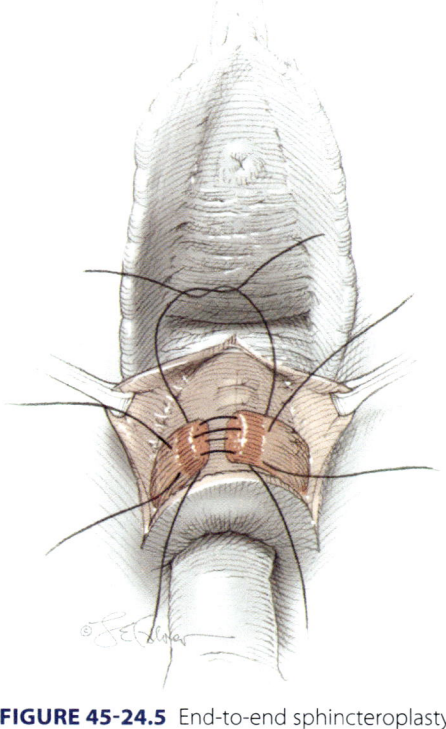

FIGURE 45-24.5 End-to-end sphincteroplasty.

ends above the anal verge. Suture placement and exposure of the IAS is aided by a finger in the rectum.

In many cases when an IAS defect is diagnosed remote from delivery, both the IAS and the EAS are usually identified as a unit. This unit is repaired en-bloc as described next.

❹ Overlapping External Anal Sphincteroplasty. The overlapping repair of the EAS or EAS/IAS muscle unit is accomplished by placing two rows of mattress stitches using 2-0 or 3-0 gauge monofilament, delayed-absorbable suture. Within each row, the first stitch is the most cephalad, and more caudal stitches are added sequentially. The first row of mattress sutures begins at a distance (1 to 1.5 cm) from the severed edge of the overlying muscle. These then travel through the distal end of the underlying muscle (Fig. 45-24.4). A final upward pass again through the overlying muscle completes the stitch. To aid viewing, the suture ends in this row are held until the second suture row is placed. The second row of stitches then traverses through and through to secure the free end of the overlying muscle to the underlying muscle.

With the overlapping method, either the right or left dissected end of the muscle can be used as the overlying muscle based on intraoperative findings. If significant mobilization cannot be achieved due to scarring or missing sphincter, an end-to-end repair is performed instead.

❺ End-to-End External Anal Sphincteroplasty. When performed for FI remote

from delivery, each end of the disrupted EAS and surrounding scar tissue is identified and grasped with an Allis clamp (see Fig. 45-25.3). The ends of the EAS are brought to the midline and reapproximated using three to four interrupted stitches of delayed-absorbable, monofilament suture (Fig. 45-24.5).

❻ Perineal Body Reconstruction. Patients with anal sphincter defects generally have a deficient perineal body. In these cases, perineal body reconstruction is performed following reapproximation of the IAS and EAS muscles. For this, the connective tissue surrounding the separated ends of the bulbospongiosus and superficial transverse perineal muscles are identified and reapproximated. A combination of 2-0 and 0-gauge absorbable sutures is used for this repair. Deep suture bites at the level of the hymen also reunite the perineal membrane, which attaches to both the vaginal walls and the perineal body at this level.

❼ Incision Closure. Excision of excess perineal skin and/or vaginal epithelium may be required prior to closing the incision. Vaginal epithelium and then perineal skin is reapproximated in a running or interrupted

fashion using 2-0 or 3-0 gauge absorbable suture.

POSTOPERATIVE

Pain varies postoperatively, and some women can be discharged home on postoperative day 2, whereas others require longer hospitalization. The Foley catheter is removed on postoperative day 1 or 2. An active voiding trial is performed, and some women may have difficulty voiding due to pain, inflammation, and levator ani muscle spasm. To limit trauma to the healing repair, we try to delay defecation for several days. Although data are lacking, we encourage patients to forego food and drink on day 1. They are subsequently advanced to clear liquids for 3 or 4 days. Stool softeners are given when a solid diet is begun and are continued for at least 6 weeks. Diet or agents that add bulk to the stool are discouraged as this may increase the repair breakdown risk. Local wound care involves perineal cleansing with a plastic water bottle following urination or defecation. Ambulation is encouraged, but physical exercise and sexual intercourse are delayed for 8 weeks. The first postoperative visit is typically 4 weeks following surgery.

45-25

Rectovaginal Fistula Repair

In general, rectovaginal fistulas (RVFs) that are encountered by gynecologists are those complicating obstetric events and develop in the distal third of the vagina just above the hymen. Surgical management of these "low" or distal RVFs varies by the condition of the external anal sphincter. These are usually corrected by a transvaginal or transanal approach, based on surgeon's training and preference. Midlevel RVFs are found in the middle third of the vagina and are usually due to obstetric trauma. These often can be repaired transvaginally or transanally by a tension-free layered closure. High RVFs may follow hysterectomy or radiation therapy and lie close to the cervix or the vaginal cuff, and these are most commonly repaired abdominally.

RVFs identified during or shortly after delivery are suitable for immediate repair. However, fistulas are not repaired in the setting of inflammation, induration, or infection. Moreover, fistulas that are associated with radiation therapy or fistula recurrence often require interposition of a vascular flap due to poor tissue vascularity.

Outcomes vary depending on the underlying cause and repair method. Success rates following obstetric injury repair range from 78 to 100 percent (Khanduja, 1999; Tsang, 1998). However, in cases with episioproctotomy, the reported success rate is 74 percent, and in those repaired by rectal advancement flap, rates reach only 40 to 50 percent (Mizrahi, 2002; Sonoda, 2002). RVFs stemming from radiation, cancer, or active inflammatory bowel disease are more difficult to treat successfully. In general, success rates are highest with the first surgical attempt at repair (Lowry, 1988).

PREOPERATIVE

Patient Evaluation

As outlined in Chapter 25 (p. 570), a thorough evaluation is necessary to assess the etiology and delineate the full fistula extent. Unless RVFs are obviously from a prior obstetric event, fistulous tract biopsy is indicated to exclude malignancy or inflammatory conditions. Proctoscopy or colonoscopy is warranted if inflammatory bowel disease, malignancy, or gastrointestinal infection is suspected. If questions exist regarding the etiology, complexity, or number of fistulas, imaging may be needed. At times, pinpoint fistulas are difficult to identify and may require examination under anesthesia with lacrimal duct probing.

Coexisting anal incontinence is assessed, as this may be related to sphincter damage or other etiologies and is likely to persist after RVF repair. With distal RVFs, endoanal or transperineal sonography can assist with evaluation of anal sphincter integrity and fistula localization. Concurrent repair of a disrupted sphincter at the time of RVF repair may decrease the incidence of persistent fecal incontinence symptoms (Rogers, 2016). However, postoperative anal incontinence can occur even if the fistula is successfully closed and sphincter repaired.

Consent

Specific risks following RVF repair include fistula recurrence, dyspareunia, and vaginal narrowing or shortening. Fecal incontinence can follow some repairs if the anal sphincter is disrupted during surgery, as with episioproctotomy, or if coexistent sphincter defects are not recognized and repaired.

Patient Preparation

A mechanical bowel preparation the day prior to surgery typically is done to clear stool from the rectal vault, and options are listed in Chapter 39 (p. 833). However, bowel preparation can lead to anal incontinence and perioperative perineal skin maceration. Additionally, recent systematic reviews find no clear benefit to mechanical bowel preparation prior to elective abdominal bowel reanastomosis (Dahabreh, 2015; Güenaga, 2011; Rollins, 2018). Although still incomplete, data challenge this practice before RVF repair (Rogers, 2016). Instead, patients can complete a single rectal enema the morning of surgery. If stool is still present in the rectum at the beginning of surgery a povidone-iodine (Betadine) flush with a Malecot drain can clear the operative field of stool.

Antibiotic prophylaxis is given concurrent with surgery, however, additional doses during the days before or following surgery are not indicated. We use a combination of a cephalosporin and metronidazole to obtain broad antibacterial coverage. Additionally, thromboprophylaxis is provided as outlined in Table 39-10 (p. 834).

INTRAOPERATIVE

Surgical Steps

1 Anesthesia and Patient Position. Rectovaginal fistula repair typically is an inpatient procedure, performed under general or regional anesthesia. A patient is placed in standard lithotomy position in candy-cane or booted support stirrups. The vagina is surgically prepared, and a Foley catheter is inserted.

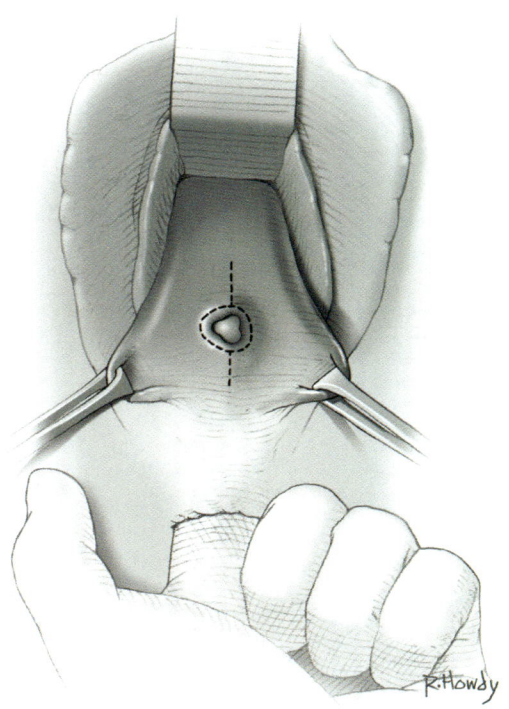

FIGURE 45-25.1 Vaginal incision.

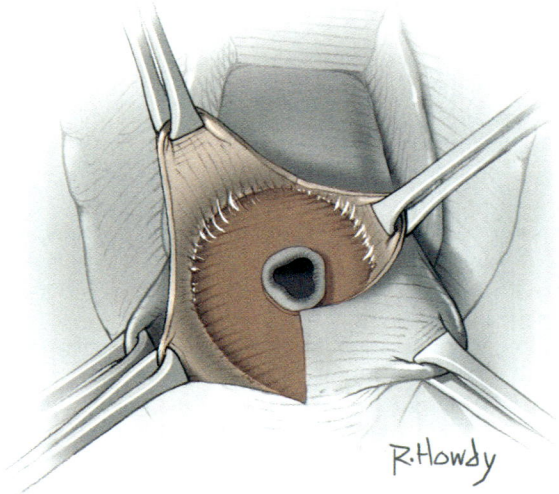

FIGURE 45-25.2 Mobilization of surrounding vaginal epithelium.

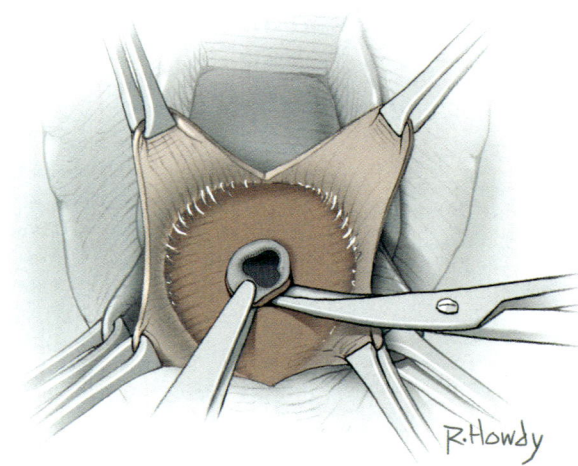

FIGURE 45-25.3 Fistulous tract excision.

❷ Fistula Identification. The fistula is identified and its course is traced with a probe or dilator. Small fistulas may be dilated to improve identification of the tract.

❸ Vaginal Incision. For a midlevel or distal RVF not involving the external anal sphincter, a circular incision is made in the vaginal epithelium surrounding the fistula (Fig. 45-25.1). The incision is made sufficiently wide to permit tract excision and generous mobilization of surrounding tissues for closure without excess suture-line tension

(Fig. 45-25.2). Remember that tenets of proper fistula repair emphasize wide tissue mobilization; tension-free, multilayered closure; and excellent hemostasis. The entire fistula tract is then excised (Fig. 45-25.3). This creates an anal or rectal opening that often is significantly larger than that found preoperatively.

❹ Closure of the Rectal Wall. Using 3-0 gauge delayed-absorbable suture, the edges of the anal mucosal defect are reapproximated in a running or interrupted fashion. Each

suture is spaced no more than 5 mm apart (Fig. 45-25.4). Although absorbable sutures can be placed into the rectal lumen, we prefer to reapproximate the submucosal tissue without needle or suture entering the rectum. One or two additional layers of the same gauge suture are placed in the anal or rectal wall muscularis to reinforce the submucosal closure. If the internal anal sphincter but not the EAS is involved, the above additional layers incorporate the torn IAS edges. This step ideally reduces the postoperative anal incontinence risk. Some recommend 3-0 monofilament polydioxanone sutures for repair of the IAS (American College of Obstetricians and Gynecologists, 2018a).

Alternatively, with very small RVFs, a purse-string suture can be placed to encircle

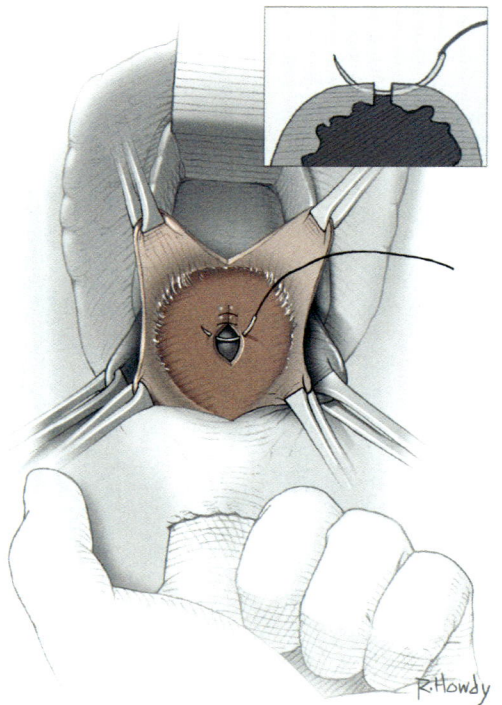

FIGURE 45-25.4 Closure of the rectal wall.

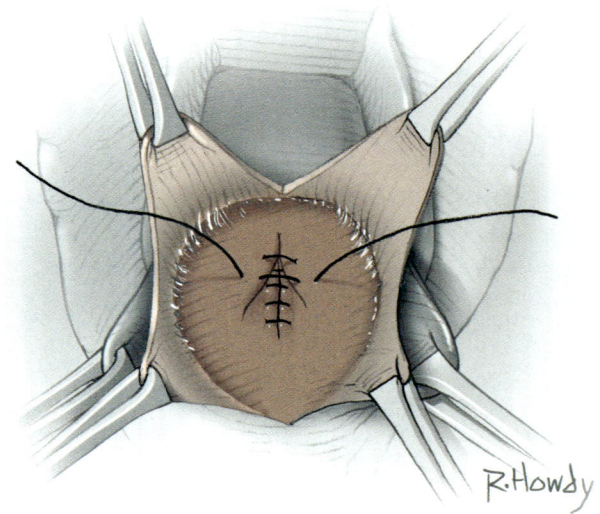

FIGURE 45-25.5 Closure of the fibromuscular layer.

the anal defect, and its perimeter lies a few millimeters from the resected fistulous tract rim. This suture is tied and inverts the defect's edges into the bowel lumen. Additional reinforcing layers then are placed as described above. Other methods used for complex fistulas involving the anal sphincters are described in Chapter 25 (p. 571).

❺ **Vaginal Fibromuscular Layer Closure.** The fibromuscular layer of the vagina is next reapproximated with 2-0 gauge delayed-absorbable sutures in a running or interrupted fashion (Fig. 45-25.5). If possible, two layers are completed to minimize incision tension and reinforce the repair. With anovaginal fistulas, these additional layers also reapproximate perineal body tissue.

If the fistula involves the EAS, an episioproctotomy—that is, conversion of the defect into a fourth-degree laceration—can be elected. Following excision of the fistulous tract and mobilization of surrounding tissue, repair of the episioproctotomy is similar to the layered repair of an obstetric fourth-degree laceration. Briefly, the anal submucosa is reapproximated with 3-0 gauge absorbable suture in a running or interrupted fashion. Repair of the IAS, EAS, and perineal body reconstruction mirror that for anal sphincteroplasty (p. 1150). This approach should be considered only for distal RVF in women with EAS defects and associated fecal incontinence.

❻ **Martius Bulbospongiosus Fat Pad Graft.** In cases in which avascular or fibrotic tissue is extensive, a Martius graft may be placed between the fibromuscular layer and vaginal epithelium (p. 1109). For RVF repair, the labial fat graft is detached anteriorly and the graft retains blood supply from perineal and inferior rectal arteries, which are internal pudendal artery branches.

❼ **Vaginal Wall Closure.** Excess vaginal mucosa is trimmed, and the vaginal mucosa is closed in a continuous running fashion using 3-0 gauge absorbable or delayed-absorbable suture.

POSTOPERATIVE

Normal activity can resume during the first postoperative days. Intercourse, however, is delayed at least 6 weeks or until the vaginal incision is healed. To limit trauma to the healing repair, dietary modifications are instituted similar to those for sphincteroplasty (p. 1152).

CHAPTER 45

REFERENCES

Abassy S, Kenton K: Obliterative procedures for pelvic organ prolapse. Clin Obstet Gynecol 53: 86, 2010

Abu-Rustum NR, Sonoda Y, Black D, et al: Cystoscopic temporary ureteral catheterization during radical vaginal and abdominal trachelectomy. Gynecol Oncol 103(2):729, 2006

Ahn M, Loughlin KR: Psoas hitch ureteral reimplantation in adults—analysis of a modified technique and timing of repair. Urology 58: 184, 2001

Albo ME, Richter HE, Brubaker L, et al: Burch colposuspension versus fascial sling to reduce urinary stress incontinence. N Engl J Med 356: 2143, 2007

Alcalay M, Monga A, Stanton SL: Burch colposuspension: a 10–20 year follow up. BJOG 102: 740, 1995

Al-Kandari AM, Al-Shaiji TF, Shaaban H, et al: Effects of proximal and distal ends of double-J ureteral stent position on postprocedural symptoms and quality of life: a randomized clinical trial. J Endourol 21:698, 2007

Altman D, Väyrynen T, Engh ME, et al: Anterior colporrhaphy versus transvaginal mesh for pelvic-organ prolapse. N Engl J Med 364(19): 1826, 2011

American College of Obstetricians and Gynecologists: Vaginal placement of synthetic mesh for pelvic organ prolapse. Committee Opinion No. 513, December 2011

American College of Obstetricians and Gynecologists: Management of mesh and graft complications in gynecologic surgery. Committee Opinion No. 694, April 2017a

American College of Obstetricians and Gynecologists: Pelvic organ prolapse. Practice Bulletin No. 185, November 2017b

American College of Obstetricians and Gynecologists: Prevention and management of obstetric lacerations at vaginal delivery. Practice Bulletin No. 198, August 2018a

American College of Obstetricians and Gynecologists: Prevention of infection after gynecologic procedures. Practice Bulletin No. 195, June 2018b

American Urogynecologic Society; Society of Urodynamics, Female Pelvic Medicine and Urogenital Reconstruction: Position statement on mesh midurethral slings for stress urinary incontinence. 2018. Available at: https://www.augs.org/assets/1/6/AUGS-SUFU_MUS_Position_Statement.pdf. Accessed July 20, 2019

Anger JT, Mueller ER, Tarnay C, et al: Robotic compared with laparoscopic sacrocolpopexy: a randomized controlled trial. Obstet Gynecol 123(1):5, 2014

Ankardal M, Ekerydh A, Crafoord K, et al: A randomised trial comparing open Burch colposuspension using sutures with laparoscopic colposuspension using mesh and staples in women with stress urinary incontinence. BJOG 111:974, 2004

Antosh DD, Gutman RE: Diagnosis and management of female urethral diverticulum. Female Pelvic Med Reconstr Surg 17(6):264, 2011

Bai SW, Kim BJ, Kim SK, et al: Comparison of outcomes between Burch colposuspension with and without concomitant abdominal hysterectomy. Yonsei Med J 45:665, 2004

Balgobin S: Urologic and gastrointestinal injuries. In Yeomans ER, Hoffman BL, Gilstrap LC III, et al (eds): Cunningham and Gilstrap's Operative Obstetrics, 3rd ed. New York, McGraw-Hill Education, 2017, p 459

Balgobin S, Fitzwater JL, White AB, et al: Effect of mesh width on vaginal apical support after abdominal sacrocolpopexy. Female Pelvic Med Reconstr Surg 17:S9, 2011

Balgobin S, Good MM, Dillon SJ, et al: Lowest colpopexy sacral fixation point alters vaginal axis and cul-de-sac depth. Am J Obstet Gynecol 208(6):488.e1, 2013

Ballard AC, Parker-Autry CY, Markland AD, et al: Bowel preparation before vaginal prolapse surgery: a randomized controlled trial. Obstet Gynecol 123(2 Pt 1):232, 2014

Barber MD, Amundsen CL, Paraiso MF, et al: Quality of life after surgery for genital prolapse in elderly women: obliterative and reconstructive surgery. Int Urogynecol J Pelvic Floor Dysfunct 18(7):799, 2007

Barber MD, Brubaker L, Burgio KL, et al: Comparison of 2 transvaginal surgical approaches and perioperative behavioral therapy for apical vaginal prolapse: the OPTIMAL randomized trial. JAMA 311(10):1023, 2014

Barber MD, Brubaker L, Menefee S, et al: Operations and pelvic muscle training in the management of apical support loss (OPTIMAL) trial: design and methods. Contemp Clin Trials 30: 178, 2009

Barber MD, Visco AG, Weidner AC, et al: Bilateral uterosacral ligament vaginal vault suspension with site-specific endopelvic fascia defect repair for treatment of pelvic organ prolapse. Am J Obstet Gynecol 183:1402, 2000

Beer M, Kuhn A: Surgical techniques for vault prolapse: a review of the literature. Eur J Obstet Gynecol Reprod Biol 119:144, 2005

Bent AE, Foote J, Siegel S, et al: Collagen implant for treating stress urinary incontinence in women with urethral hypermobility. J Urol 166: 1354, 2001

Blaivas JG, Heritz DM, Romanzi LJ: Early versus late repair of vesicovaginal fistulas: vaginal and abdominal approaches. J Urol 153(4):1110, 1995

Blok B, Van Kerrebroeck P, de Wachter S, et al: A prospective, multicenter study of a novel, miniaturized rechargeable sacral neuromodulation system: 12-month results from the RELAX-OAB study. Neurourol Urodyn 38(2):689, 2019

Bochenska K, Leader-Cramer A, Mueller M, et al: Perioperative complications following colpocleisis with and without concomitant vaginal hysterectomy. Int Urogynecol J 28:1671, 2017

Borstad E, Rud T: The risk of developing urinary stress-incontinence after vaginal repair in continent women: a clinical and urodynamic follow-up study. Acta Obstet Gynaecol Scand 68:545, 1989

Bravo Gutierrez A, Madoff RD, Lowry AC, et al: Long-term results of anterior sphincteroplasty. Dis Colon Rectum 47:727, 2004

Breau RH, Norman RW: Optimal prevention and management of proximal ureteral stent migration and remigration. J Urol 166:890, 2001

Brincat CA, Larson KA, Fenner DE: Anterior vaginal wall prolapse: assessment and treatment. Clin Obstet Gynecol 53(1):51, 2010

Brubaker L, Cundiff GW, Fine P, et al: Abdominal sacrocolpopexy with Burch colposuspension to reduce urinary stress incontinence. N Engl J Med 354:1557, 2006

Brubaker L, Nygaard I, Richter HE, et al: Two-year outcomes after sacrocolpopexy with and without Burch to prevent stress urinary incontinence. Obstet Gynecol 112 (1):49, 2008

Buie WD, Lowry AC, Rothenberger DA, et al: Clinical rather than laboratory assessment predicts continence after anterior sphincteroplasty. Dis Colon Rectum 44:1255, 2001

Carey M, Goh J, Rosamilia A, et al: Laparoscopic versus open Burch colposuspension: a randomised controlled trial. BJOG 113:999, 2006

Cardenas-Trowers O, Heusinkveld J, Hatch K: Simple and effective: transvaginal vesico-vaginal fistula repair with a modified Latzko technique. Int Urogynecol J 29(5):767, 2018

Chaikin DC, Groutz A, Blaivas JG: Predicting the need for anti-incontinence surgery in continent women undergoing repair of severe urogenital prolapse. J Urol 163:531, 2000

Chmielewski L, Walters MD, Weber AM, et al. Reanalysis of a randomized trial of 3 techniques of anterior colporrhaphy using clinically relevant definitions of success. Am J Obstet Gynecol 205:69.e1, 2011

Christiano AP, Hollowell CM, Kim H, et al: Double-blind randomized comparison of single-dose ciprofloxacin versus intravenous cefazolin in patients undergoing outpatient endourologic surgery. Urology 55(2):182, 2000

Chrouser KL, Fick F, Goel A, et al: Carbon coated zirconium beads in β-glucan gel and bovine glutaraldehyde cross-linked collagen injections for intrinsic sphincter deficiency: continence and satisfaction after extended follow-up. J Urol 171:1152, 2004

Cohen BL, Tunuguntla HS, Gousse A: Predictors of success for first stage neuromodulation: motor versus sensory response. J Urol 175:2178, 2006

Collins SA, Jelovsek JE, Chen CC, et al: De novo rectal prolapse after obliterative and reconstructive vaginal surgery for urogenital prolapse. Am J Obstet Gynecol 197(1):84e1, 2007

Corcos J, Collet JP, Shapiro S, et al: Multicenter randomized clinical trial comparing surgery and collagen injections for treatment of female stress urinary incontinence. Urology 65:898, 2005

Corcos J, Fournier C: Periurethral collagen injection for the treatment of female stress urinary incontinence: 4-year follow-up results. Urology 54:815, 1999

Culligan PJ, Blackwell L, Goldsmith LJ, et al: A randomized controlled trial comparing fascia lata and synthetic mesh for sacral colpopexy. Obstet Gynecol 106:29, 2005

Culligan PJ, Murphy M, Blackwell L, et al: Long-term success of abdominal sacral colpopexy using synthetic mesh. Am J Obstet Gynecol 187:1473, 2002

Cundiff GW, Harris RL, Coates K, et al: Abdominal sacral colpoperineopexy: a new approach for correction of posterior compartment defects and perineal descent associated with vaginal vault prolapse. Am J Obstet Gynecol 177(6):1345, 1997

Dahabreh IJ, Steele DW, Shah N, et al: Oral Mechanical Bowel Preparation for Colorectal Surgery: Systematic Review and Meta-Analysis. Dis Colon Rectum 58(7):698, 2015

Dean NM, Ellis G, Herbison GP, et al: Laparoscopic colposuspension for urinary incontinence in women. Cochrane Database Syst Rev 7:CD002239, 2017

Debodinance P: Trans-obturator urethral sling for the surgical correction of female stress urinary incontinence: outside-in (Monarc) versus inside-out (TVT-O). Are the two ways reassuring? Eur J Obstet Gynecol Reprod Biol 133(2):232, 2007

deGroat WC: Changes in the organization of the micturition reflex pathway of the cat after transection of the spinal cord. Exp Neurol 71:22, 1981

Demirci F, Petri E: Perioperative complications of Burch colposuspension. Int Urogynecol J 11:170, 2000

Demirci F, Yucel O, Eren S, et al: Long-term results of Burch colposuspension. Gynecol Obstet Invest 51:243, 2001

Drewes PG, Marinis SI, Schaffer JI, et al: Vascular anatomy over the superior pubic rami in female cadavers. Am J Obstet Gynecol 193(6):2165, 2005

Dunn TS, Figge J, Wolf D: A comparison of outcomes of transurethral versus suprapubic catheterization after Burch cystourethropexy. Int Urogynecol J 16:60, 2005

El-Gazzaz G, Zutshi M, Hannaway C, et al: Overlapping sphincter repair: does age matter? Dis Colon Rectum 55: 256, 2012

Elkattah R, Brooks A, Huffaker RK: Gynecologic malignancies post-LeFort colpocleisis. Case Rep Obstet Gynecol 2014:846745, 2014

Faerber GJ, Belville WD, Ohl DA, et al: Comparison of transurethral versus periurethral collagen injection in women with intrinsic sphincter deficiency. Tech Urol 4:124, 1998

Fitzgerald MP, Richter HE, Bradley CS, et al: Pelvic support, pelvic symptoms, and patient satisfaction after colpocleisis. Int Urogynecol J Pelvic Floor Dysfunct 19(12):1603, 2008

Fitzgerald MP, Richter HE, Siddique S, et al: Colpocleisis: a review. Int Urogynecol J 17:261, 2006

Fitzpatrick M, Behan M, O'Connell PR, et al: A randomized clinical trial comparing primary overlap with approximation repair of third-degree obstetric tears. Am J Obstet Gynecol 183(5):1220, 2000

Fleshman JW, Peters WR, Shemesh EI, et al: Anal sphincter reconstruction: anterior overlapping muscle repair. Dis Colon Rectum 34(9):739, 1991

Florian-Rodriguez ME, Hare A, Chin K, et al: Inferior gluteal and other nerves associated with sacrospinous ligament: a cadaver study. Am J Obstet Gynecol 215:646.e1, 2016

Food and Drug Administration: Considerations about surgical mesh for SUI. 2019a. Available at: https://www.fda.gov/medical-devices/urogynecologic-surgical-mesh-implants/considerations-about-surgical-mesh-sui. Accessed April 21, 2019

Food and Drug Administration: Urogynecologic surgical mesh implants. 2019b. Available at: https://www.fda.gov/medical-devices/implants-and-prosthetics/urogynecologic-surgical-mesh-implants. Accessed July 22, 2019

Ford AA, Ogah JA: Retropubic or transobturator mid-urethral slings for intrinsic sphincter deficiency-related stress urinary incontinence in women: a systematic review and meta-analysis. Int Urogynecol J 27(1):19, 2016

Ford AA, Rogerson L, Cody JD, et al: Mid-urethral sling operations for stress urinary incontinence in women. Cochrane Database Syst Rev 7:CD006375, 2017

Francis WJ, Jeffcoate TN: Dyspareunia following vaginal operations. J Obstet Gynaecol Br Commonw 68:1, 1961

Freeman RM, Pantazis K, Thomson A, et al: A randomised controlled trial of abdominal versus laparoscopic sacrocolpopexy for the treatment of post-hysterectomy vaginal vault prolapse: LAS study. Int Urogynecol J 24(3):377, 2013

Galloway NT, Davies N, Stephenson TP: The complications of colposuspension. Br J Urol 60:122, 1987

Gandhi S, Goldberg RP, Kwon C, et al: A prospective, randomized trial using solvent dehydrated fascia lata for the prevention of recurrent anterior vaginal wall prolapse. Am J Obstet Gynecol 192:1649, 2005

Garcia V, Rogers RG, Kim SS, et al: Primary repair of obstetric anal sphincter laceration: a randomized trial of two surgical techniques. Am J Obstet Gynecol 192(5):1697, 2005

Gearhart S, Hull T, Floruta C, et al: Anal manometric parameters: predictors of outcome following anal sphincter repair? J Gastrointest Surg 9:115, 2005

Geis K, Dietl J: Ilioinguinal nerve entrapment after tension-free vaginal tape (TVT) procedure. Int Urogynecol J Pelvic Floor Dysfunct 13(2):136, 2002

Giannarini G, Keeley FX Jr, Valent F, et al: Predictors of morbidity in patients with indwelling ureteric stents: results of a prospective study using the validated Ureteric Stent Symptoms Questionnaire. BJU Int 107:648, 2011

Goldberg RP, Tomezsko JE, Winkler HA, et al: Anterior or posterior sacrospinous vaginal vault suspension: long-term anatomic and functional evaluation. Obstet Gynecol 98(2):199, 2001

Goldman HB, Lloyd JC, Noblett KL, et al: International Continence Society best practice statement for use of sacral neuromodulation. Neurourol Urodyn 37(5):1823, 2018

Good MM, Abele TA, Balgobin S, et al: L5-S1 discitis—can it be prevented? Obstet Gynecol 121(2 Pt 1):285, 2013a

Good MM, Abele TA, Balgobin S, et al: Vascular and ureteral anatomy relative to the midsacral promontory. Am J Obstet Gynecol 208(6):486.e1, 2013b

Gorton E, Stanton S, Monga A, et al: Periurethral collagen injection: a long-term follow-up study. Br J Urol Int 84:966, 1999

Gourcerol G, Vitton V, Leroi AM, et al: How sacral nerve stimulation works in patients with faecal incontinence. Colorectal Dis 13(8):e203, 2011

Govaert B, Melenhorst J, van Gemert WG, et al: Can sensory and/or motor reactions during percutaneous nerve evaluation predict outcome of sacral nerve modulation? Dis Colon Rectum 52:1423, 2009

Green J, Herschorn S: The contemporary role of Burch colposuspension. Curr Opin Urol 15: 250, 2005

Griffis K, Evers MD, Terry CL, et al: Mesh erosion and abdominal sacrocolpopexy: a comparison of prior, total, and supracervical hysterectomy. J Pelvic Med Surg 12(1): 25, 2006

Grimes CL, Patankar S, Ryntz T, et al: Evaluating ureteral patency in the post-indigo carmine era: a randomized controlled trial. Am J Obstet Gynecol 217:601.e1, 2017

Güenaga KF, Matos D, Wille-Jørgensen P: Mechanical bowel preparation for elective colorectal surgery. Cochrane Database Syst Rev 9: CD001544, 2011

Gutman RE, Bradley CS, Ye W, et al: Effects of colpocleisis on bowel symptoms among women with severe pelvic organ prolapse. Int Urogynecol J 21(4):461, 2009

Ha HT, Fleshman JW, Smith M, et al: Manometric squeeze pressure difference parallels functional outcome after overlapping sphincter reconstruction. Dis Colon Rectum 44:655, 2001

Haab F, Zimmern PE, Leach GE: Urinary stress incontinence due to intrinsic sphincteric deficiency: experience with fat and collagen periurethral injections. J Urol 157:1283, 1997

Halverson AL, Hull TL: Long-term outcome of overlapping anal sphincter repair. Dis Colon Rectum 45:345, 2002

Herschorn S, Radomski SB: Collagen injections for genuine stress urinary incontinence: patient selection and durability. Int Urogynecol J 8:18, 1997

Hill AJ, Walters MD, Unger CA: Perioperative adverse events associated with colpocleisis for uterovaginal and posthysterectomy vaginal vault prolapse. Am J Obstet Gynecol 214:501.e1, 2016

Holmgren C, Nilsson S, Lanner L, et al: Long-term results with tension-free vaginal tape on mixed and stress urinary incontinence. Obstet Gynecol 106(1):38, 2005

Hullfish KL, Bovbjerg VE, Steers WD: Colpocleisis for pelvic organ prolapse: patient goals, quality of life, and satisfaction. Obstet Gynecol 110 (2 Pt 1):341, 2007

Ingber MS, Firoozi F, Vasavada SP, et al: Surgically corrected urethral diverticula: long-term voiding dysfunction and reoperation rates. Urology 77(1):65, 2011

Jacobs SA, Lane FL, Osann KE, et al: Randomized prospective crossover study of interstim lead wire placement with curved versus straight stylet. Neurourol Urodyn 33(5):488, 2014

Jackson LA, Ramirez DM, Carrick KS, et al: Gross and histologic anatomy of the pelvic ureter: clinical applications to pelvic surgery. Obstet Gynecol 133(5):896, 2019

Jelovsek JE, Barber MD, Brubaker L: Effect of uterosacral ligament suspension vs sacrospinous ligament fixation with or without perioperative behavioral therapy for pelvic organ vaginal prolapse on surgical outcomes and prolapse symptoms at 5 years in the OPTIMAL randomized clinical trial. JAMA 319(15):1554, 2018

Jonsson Funk M, Siddiqui NY, Pate V, et al: Sling revision/removal for mesh erosion and urinary retention: long-term risk and predictors. Am J Obstet Gynecol 208:73.e1, 2013

Judd JP, Siddiqui NY, Barnett JC, et al: Cost-minimization analysis of robotic-assisted, laparoscopic, and abdominal sacrocolpopexy. J Minim Invasive Gynecol 17(4):493, 2010

Karram M, Maher C: Surgery for posterior vaginal wall prolapse. Int Urogynecol J 24:1835, 2013

Katrikh AZ, Ettarh R, Kahn MA: Cadaveric nerve and artery proximity to sacrospinous ligament fixation sutures placed by a suture-capturing device. Obstet Gynecol 130:1033, 2017

Kearney R, DeLancey JO: Selecting suspension points and excising the vagina during Michigan four-wall sacrospinous suspension. Obstet Gynecol 101(2): 325, 2003

Khanduja KS, Padmanabhan A, Kerner BA, et al: Reconstruction of rectovaginal fistula with sphincter disruption by combining rectal mucosal advancement flap and anal sphincteroplasty. Dis Colon Rectum 42(11):1432, 1999

Kieserman-Shmokler C, Sammarco AG, English EM: The Latzko: a high-value, versatile vesicovaginal fistula repair. Am J Obstet Gynecol; 221(2):160.e1, 2019

Kim A, Kim MS, Park YJ, et al: Retropubic versus transobturator mid urethral slings in patients at high risk for recurrent stress incontinence: a systematic review and meta-analysis. J Urol 202(1): 132, 2019

Kirchin V, Page T, Keegan PE: Urethral injection therapy for urinary incontinence in women. Cochrane Database Syst Rev 7:CD003881, 2017

Kohli N, Walsh PM, Roat TW, et al: Mesh erosion after abdominal sacrocolpopexy. Obstet Gynecol 92:999, 1998

Koonings PP, Bergman A, Ballard CA: Low urethral pressure and stress urinary incontinence in women: risk factor for filed retropubic surgical procedure. Urology 36:245, 1990

Kwon CH, Goldberg RP, Koduri S, et al: The use of intraoperative cystoscopy in major vaginal and urogynecologic surgeries. Am J Obstet Gynecol 187:1466, 2002

Ladwig D, Miljkovic-Petkovic L, Hewson AD: Simplified colposuspension: a 15-year follow-up. Aust N Z J Obstet Gynaecol 44:39, 2004

Lapitan MC, Cody JD, Mashayekhi A: Open retropubic colposuspension for urinary incontinence in women. Cochrane Database Syst Rev 7:CD002912, 2017

Larson KA, Smith T, Berger MB, et al: Long-term patient satisfaction with Michigan four-wall sacrospinous ligament suspension for prolapse. Obstet Gynecol 122(5):967, 2013

Lee PE, Kung RC, Drutz HP: Periurethral autologous fat injection as treatment for female stress urinary incontinence: a randomized, double-blind controlled trial. J Urol 165:153, 2001

Lee U, Wolff EM, Kobashi KC: Native tissue repairs in anterior vaginal prolapse surgery: examining definitions of surgical success in the mesh era. Curr Opin Urol 22(4):265, 2012

Lightner D, Rovner E, Corcos J, et al: Randomized controlled multisite trial of injected bulking agents for women with intrinsic sphincter deficiency: mid-urethral injection of Zuidex via the Implacer versus proximal urethral injection of Contigen cystoscopically. Urology 74(4):771, 2009

Lightner DJ, Itano NB, Sweat SD, et al: Injectable agents: present and future. Curr Urol Rep 3:408, 2002

Linder BJ, Occhino JA: Cystoscopic ureteral stent placement: techniques and tips. Int Urogynecol J 30(1):163, 2019

Lobel RW, Sand PK. The empty supine stress test as a predictor of intrinsic urethral sphincter dysfunction. Obstet Gynecol 88:128, 1996

Lowder JL, Park AJ, Ellison R, et al: The role of apical vaginal support in the appearance of anterior and posterior vaginal prolapse. Obstet Gynecol 111: 152, 2008

Lowenstein L, Fitz A, Kenton K, et al: Transabdominal uterosacral suspension: outcomes and complications. Am J Obstet Gynecol 200(6):656e1, 2009

Lowry AC, Thorson AG, Rothenberger DA, et al: Repair of simple rectovaginal fistulas. Influence of previous repairs. Dis Colon Rectum 31(9):676, 1988

Luck AM, Galvin SL, Theofrastous JP: Suture erosion and wound dehiscence with permanent versus absorbable suture in reconstructive posterior vaginal surgery. Am J Obstet Gynecol 192:1626, 2005

Madoff RD: Surgical treatment options for fecal incontinence. Gastroenterology 126:S48, 2004

Maher C, Feiner B, Baessler K, et al: Surgical management of pelvic organ prolapse in women. Cochrane Database Syst Rev 4:CD004014, 2013

Maldonado PA, Mcintire D, Corton MM: Long-term outcomes after overlapping sphincteroplasty for cloacal-like deformities. Female Pelvic Med Reconstr Surg 25(4):271, 2019

Maldonado PA, Slocum PD, Chin K, et al: Anatomic relationships of psoas muscle: clinical applications to psoas hitch ureteral reimplantation. Am J Obstet Gynecol 211(5):563.e1, 2014

Malouf AJ, Norton CS, Engel AF, et al: Long-term results of overlapping anterior anal-sphincter repair for obstetric trauma. Lancet 355:260, 2000

Margulies RU, Rogers MA, Morgan DM: Outcomes of transvaginal uterosacral ligament suspension: systematic review and metaanalysis. Am J Obstet Gynecol 202(2):124, 2010

McCall ML: Posterior culdeplasty; surgical correction of enterocele during vaginal hysterectomy; a preliminary report. Obstet Gynecol 10(6):595, 1957

McDermott CD, Hale DS: Abdominal, laparoscopic, and robotic surgery for pelvic organ prolapse. Obstet Gynecol Clin North Am 36:585, 2009

Meltomaa SS, Haarala MA, Taalikka MO, et al: Outcome of Burch retropubic urethropexy and the effect of concomitant abdominal hysterectomy: a prospective long-term follow-up study. Int Urogynecol J 12:3, 2001

Miklos JR, Moore RD: Laparoscopic extravesical vesicovaginal fistula repair: our technique and 15-year experience. Int Urogynecol J 26(3):441, 2015

Mizrahi N, Wexner SD, Zmora O, et al: Endorectal advancement flap: are there predictors of failure? Dis Colon Rectum 45(12):1616, 2002

Mohr S, Brandner S, Mueller MD, et al: Sexual function after vaginal and abdominal fistula repair. Am J Obstet Gynecol 211:74.e1, 2014

Monga AK, Robinson D, Stanton SL: Periurethral collagen injections for genuine stress incontinence: a 2-year follow-up. Br J Urol 76:156, 1995

Monga AK, Stanton SL: Urodynamics: prediction, outcome and analysis of mechanism for cure of stress incontinence by periurethral collagen. BJOG 104:158, 1997

Montoya TI, Luebbehusen HI, Schaffer JI, et al: Sensory neuropathy following suspension of the vaginal apex to the proximal uterosacral ligaments. Int Urogynecol J 23(12):1735, 2012

Morley GW, DeLancey JO: Sacrospinous ligament fixation for eversion of the vagina. Am J Obstet Gynecol 158:872, 1988

Narasimhulu DM, Prabakar C, Tang N, et al: 50% dextrose versus normal saline as distension media during cystoscopy for assessment of ureteric patency. Eur J Obstet Gynecol Reprod Biol 199:38, 2016

Nguyen JN, Jakus-Waldman SM, Walter AJ, et al: Perioperative complications and reoperations after incontinence and prolapse surgeries using prosthetic implants. Obstet Gynecol 119(3):539, 2012

Nilsson CG, Palva K, Aarnio R, et al: Seventeen years' follow-up of the tension-free vaginal tape procedure for female stress urinary incontinence. Int Urogynecol J 24(8):1265, 2013

Noblett KL, Cadish LA: Sacral nerve stimulation for the treatment of refractory voiding and bowel dysfunction. Am J Obstet Gynecol 210(2):99, 2014

Norton P, Brubaker L: Urinary incontinence in women. Lancet 367:57, 2006

Nygaard I, Brubaker L, Zyczynski HM, et al: Long-term outcomes following abdominal sacrocolpopexy for pelvic organ prolapse. JAMA 309(19):2016, 2013

Nygaard IE, McCreery R, Brubaker L, et al: Abdominal sacrocolpopexy: a comprehensive review. Obstet Gynecol 104:805, 2004

Ockrim JL, Allen DJ, Shah PJ, et al: A tertiary experience of urethral diverticulectomy: diagnosis, imaging and surgical outcomes. BJU Int 103(11):1550, 2009

Paick JS, Hong SK, Park MS, et al: Management of postoperatively detected iatrogenic lower ureteral injury: should ureteroureterostomy really be abandoned? Urology 67, 237, 2006

Pantuck AJ, Han KR, Perrotti M, et al: Ureteroenteric anastomosis in continent urinary diversion: long-term results and complications of direct versus nonrefluxing techniques. J Urol 163(2):450, 2000

Paraiso M, Barber M, Muir T, et al: Rectocele repair: a randomized trial of three surgical techniques including graft augmentation. Am J Obstet Gynecol 195:1762, 2006

Paraiso MF, Jelovsek JE, Frick A, et al: Laparoscopic compared with robotic sacral colpopexy for vaginal prolapse. A randomised controlled trial. Obstet Gynecol 118(5):1005, 2011

Pathi SD, Rahn DD, Sailors JL, et al: Utility of clinical parameters, cystourethroscopy, and magnetic resonance imaging in the preoperative diagnosis of urethral diverticula. Int Urogynecol J 24(2):319, 2013

Peters KM, Killinger KA, Boura JA: Is sensory testing during lead placement crucial for achieving positive outcomes after sacral neuromodulation? Neurourol Urodynam 30:1489, 2011

Pilsgaard K, Mouritsen L: Follow up after repair of vaginal vault prolapse with abdominal colposacropexy. Acta Obstet Gynecol Scand 78:66, 1999

Pshak T, Nikolavsky D, Terlecki R, et al: Is tissue interposition always necessary in transvaginal repair of benign, recurrent vesicovaginal fistulae? Urology 82(3):707, 2013

Rahn DD, Good MM, Roshanravan SM, et al: Effects of preoperative local estrogen in postmenopausal women with prolapse: a randomized trial. J Clin Endocrinol Metab 99(10):3728, 2014

Rahn DD, Marinis SI, Schaffer JI: Anatomical path of the tension-free vaginal tape: reassessing current teachings. Am J Obstet Gynecol 195(6):1809, 2006

Rahn DD, Ward RM, Sanses TV, et al: Vaginal estrogen use in postmenopausal women with pelvic floor disorders: systematic review and practice guidelines. Int Urogynecol J 26(1):3, 2015

Rardin CR, Erekson EA, Sung VW, et al: Uterosacral colpopexy at the time of vaginal hysterectomy: comparison of laparoscopic and vaginal approaches. J Reprod Med 54(5):273, 2009

Rechberger T, Futyma K, Jankiewicz K, et al: The clinical effectiveness of retropubic (IVS-02) and transobturator (IVS-04) midurethral slings: randomized trial. Eur Urol 56:24, 2009

Rehman H, Bezerra CA, Bruschini H, et al: Traditional suburethral sling operations for urinary incontinence in women. Cochrane Database Syst Rev 7:CD001754, 2017

Richter HE, Albo ME, Zyczynski HM, et al: Retropubic versus transobturator midurethral slings for stress incontinence. N Engl J Med 362(22):2066, 2010

Rollins KE, Javanmard-Emamghissi H, Lobo DN: Impact of mechanical bowel preparation in elective colorectal surgery: a meta-analysis. World J Gastroenterol 24(4):519, 2018

Rogers RG, Jeppson PC: Current diagnosis and management of pelvic fistulae in women. Obstet Gynecol 128(3):635, 2016

Roshanravan SM, Wieslander CK, Schaffer JI, et al: Neurovascular anatomy of the greater sciatic foramen and sacrospinous ligament region in female cadavers: implications in sacrospinous ligament and iliococcygeal fascia vaginal vault suspension. Am J Obstet Gynecol 197(6):660.e1, 2007

Rovner ES: Urinary tract fistulae. In Kavoussi LR, Novick AC, Partin AW, et al (eds): Wein: Campbell-Walsh Urology, 10th ed. Philadelphia, Saunders, 2012

Sand PK, Bowen LW, Panganiban R, et al: The low pressure urethra as a factor in failed retropubic urethropexy. Obstet Gynecol 69:399, 1987

Schimpf MO, Rahn DD, Wheeler TL, et al: Sling surgery for stress urinary incontinence in women: a systematic review and metaanalysis. Am J Obstet Gynecol 211(1):71.e1, 2014

Schulz JA, Stanton SL, Baessler K, et al: Bulking agents for stress urinary incontinence: short-term results and complications in a randomized comparison of periurethral and transurethral injections. Int Urogynecol J Pelvic Floor Dysfunct 15:261, 2004

Selzman AA, Spirnak JP: Iatrogenic ureteral injuries: a 20-year experience in treating 165 injuries. J Urol 155:878, 1996

Shah SM, Gaunay GS: Treatment options for intrinsic sphincter deficiency. Nat Rev Urol 9(11):638, 2012

Shull BL, Bachofen C, Coates KW, et al: A transvaginal approach to repair of apical and other associated sites of pelvic organ prolapse with uterosacral ligaments. Am J Obstet Gynecol 183(6):1365, 2000

Siddiqui NY, Geller EJ, Visco AG: Symptomatic and anatomic 1-year outcomes after robotic and abdominal sacrocolpopexy. Am J Obstet Gynecol 206:435.e1, 2012

Sitzler PJ, Thomson JP: Overlap repair of damaged anal sphincter. A single surgeon's series. Dis Colon Rectum 39(12):1356, 1996

Song PH, Kim YD, Kim HT, et al: The 7-year outcome of the tension-free vaginal tape procedure for treating female stress urinary incontinence. BJU Int 104(8):1113, 2009

Sonoda T, Hull T, Piedmonte MR, et al: Outcomes of primary repair of anorectal and rectovaginal fistulas using the endorectal advancement flap. Dis Colon Rectum 45(12):1622, 2002

Steele AC, Kohli N, Karram MM: Periurethral collagen injection for stress incontinence with and without urethral hypermobility. Obstet Gynecol 95:327, 2000

Stefanovic K, Bukurov N, Marinkovic J: Nonantireflux versus antireflux ureteroneocystostomy in adults. Br J Urol 67: 263, 1991

Summers A, Winkel LA, Hussain HK, et al: The relationship between anterior and apical compartment support. Am J Obstet Gynecol 194:1438, 2006

Sung VW, Rardin CR, Raker CA, et al: Porcine subintestinal submucosal graft augmentation for rectocele repair: a randomized controlled trial. Obstet Gynecol 119(1):125, 2012

Tan-Kim J, Menefee SA, Luber KM, et al: Prevalence and risk factors for mesh erosion after laparoscopic-assisted sacrocolpopexy. Int Urogynecol J 22(2):205, 2011

Theofrastous, Cobb DL, Van Dyke AH, et al: A randomized trial of suprapubic versus transurethral bladder drainage after open Burch urethropexy. J Pelvic Surg 872, 2002

Tsang CB, Madoff RD, Wong WD, et al: Anal sphincter integrity and function influences outcome in rectovaginal fistula repair. Dis Colon Rectum 41(9):1141, 1998

Van Kerrebroeck PE, Marcelissen TA: Sacral neuromodulation for lower urinary tract dysfunction. World J Urol 30(4):445, 2012

Weber AM: Is urethral pressure profilometry a useful diagnostic test for stress urinary incontinence? Obstet Gynecol Surv 56(11):720, 2001a

Weber AM: Leak point pressure measurement and stress urinary incontinence. Curr Womens Health Rep 1(1):45, 2001b

Weber AM, Richter HE: Pelvic organ prolapse. Obstet Gynecol 106: 615, 2005

Weber AM, Walters MD, Piedmonte MR, et al: Anterior colporrhaphy: a randomized trial of three surgical techniques. Am J Obstet Gynecol 185:1299, 2001c

Wei JT, Nygaard I, Richter HE, et al: A midurethral sling to reduce incontinence after vaginal prolapse repair. N Engl J Med 366:2358, 2012

White AB, Carrick KS, Corton MM, et al: Optimal location and orientation of suture placement in abdominal sacrocolpopexy. Obstet Gynecol 113(5):1098, 2009

Wieslander CK, Rahn DD, McIntire DD, et al: Vascular anatomy of the presacral space in unembalmed female cadavers. Am J Obstet Gynecol 195:1736, 2006

Wieslander CK, Roshanravan SM, Schaffer JI, et al: Uterosacral ligament suspension sutures: anatomic relationships in unembalmed female cadavers. Am J Obstet Gynecol 197(6):672.e1, 2007

Wolf JS Jr, Bennett CJ, Dmochowski RR, et al: The best practice policy statement of urologic surgery antimicrobial prophylaxis. J Urol 179(4):1379, 2008

Yamada T, Ichiyanagi N, Kamata S, et al: Need for sling surgery in patients with large cystoceles and masked stress urinary incontinence. Int J Urol 8:599, 2001

Zeng S, Zhang Z, Bai Y, et al: Antimicrobial agents for preventing urinary tract infections in adults undergoing cystoscopy. Cochrane Database Syst Rev 2:CD012305, 2019

Zhou L, Luo DY, Feng SJ: Risk factors for recurrence in female urethral diverticulectomy: a retrospective study of 66 patients. World J Urol 35(1):139, 2017

Zullo F, Palomba S, Russo T, et al: Laparoscopic colposuspension using sutures or Prolene meshes: a 3-year follow-up. Eur J Obstet Gynaecol Reprod Biol 117:201, 2004

Zutshi M, Hull T, Bast J, et al: Ten-year outcome after anal sphincter repair for fecal incontinence. Dis Colon Rectum 52:6, 2009

Zyczynski HM, Sirls LT, Greer WJ, et al: Findings of universal cystoscopy at incontinence surgery and their sequelae. Am J Obstet Gynecol 210(5):480.e1, 2014

CHAPTER 46

Surgeries for Gynecologic Malignancies

46-1

Radical Abdominal Hysterectomy (Type III)

The five "types" of hysterectomy are defined in Chapter 30 (p. 666). Of these, radical hysterectomy differs from simple hysterectomy in that the parametrial, paracervical, and paravaginal tissues and their lymphatics are widely resected to achieve negative tumor margins. Described in this section, type III (radical) hysterectomy is chiefly indicated for stage IB1 to IIA1 cervical cancer or small central recurrences following radiation therapy. It may be suitable for clinical stage II endometrial cancer when tumor has extended to the cervical stroma (Koh, 2018a, 2019).

Most women with cervical cancer are treated with laparotomy and radical hysterectomy. Although type III radical hysterectomy may be performed with minimally invasive surgery (MIS), recent prospective and epidemiologic studies suggest lower disease-free and overall-survival rates in those treated for cervical cancer with an MIS approach compared with an open abdominal radical hysterectomy (Melamed, 2018; Ramirez, 2018). Speculations for these survival differences include insertion of a uterine manipulator, tumor handling during paracervical resection, and pneumoperitoneum during colpotomy. Until further work is completed to identify the true cause for this inferior survival rate, we offer open radical hysterectomy as the preferred modality for surgical management of cervical cancer. Some physicians continue to offer type III radical hysterectomy performed by MIS approaches in select cases and after careful discussion and shared decision-making with the patient.

PREOPERATIVE

Patient Evaluation

Radical hysterectomy is discouraged for women with higher-stage cancers (stage IIB through IV). Thus, accurate clinical staging is critical prior to selection of this surgery. Pelvic examination under anesthesia with cystoscopy and proctoscopy is not mandatory for smaller cervical cancer lesions, but the clinical staging described in Chapter 30 (p. 660) should be completed before proceeding surgically. To refine patient selection, for most patients with grossly visible cervical tumors, abdominopelvic computed tomography (CT) or magnetic resonance (MR) imaging is also performed to identify nodal metastases or undetected local tumor extension. The soft-tissue resolution offered by MR imaging may be especially helpful to exclude parametrial invasion, which would instead benefit from primary radiotherapy (Kong, 2016). That said, there are limitations on what can be reliably detected preoperatively (Chou, 2006).

Consent

Women undergoing hysterectomy are specifically counseled regarding the loss of fertility. In those considering bilateral salpingo-oophorectomy (BSO), a discussion of menopause and hormone replacement is included and detailed in Chapter 43 (p. 957). The tone of the consenting process should reflect the extent of the operation required to hopefully cure or at least begin treatment of the malignancy. Moreover, a patient must be advised that the procedure may be aborted if metastatic disease or pelvic tumor extension is found (Leath, 2004).

Radical abdominal hysterectomy can result in significant morbidity from short- and long-term complications. Surgery may be more difficult and complication rates higher in women with obesity or with prior pelvic infections, abdominal surgery, or pelvic radiation (Cohn, 2000). Of potential intraoperative complications, the most common is acute hemorrhage. Blood loss may reach 500 to 1000 mL, and transfusion rates are variable but high (Estape, 2009; Naik, 2010). Subacute postoperative complications may include significant postoperative bladder or bowel dysfunction from surgical denervation (20 percent), symptomatic lymphocyst formation (3 to 5 percent), and ureterovaginal or vesicovaginal fistula (1 to 2 percent) (Franchi, 2007; Hazewinkel, 2010; Likic, 2008). With any cancer surgery, risk

for venous thromboembolism (VTE) also is increased. Additionally, long-term effects on sexual function and other body functions are candidly reviewed and are detailed on page 1165 (Jensen, 2004; Serati, 2009).

Patient Preparation

For this, a blood sample is typed and cross-matched for potential transfusion. Pneumatic compression devices and prophylactic-dose unfractionated heparin (UFH) or low-molecular-weight heparin (LMWH) are planned because of the typically longer surgery and postoperative recovery times and the increased VTE risk associated with cancer (Table 39-10, p. 834) (Gould, 2012; Key, 2019; Martino, 2006).

Oral bowel preparation is excluded from Enhanced Recovery After Surgery (ERAS) Society guidelines (Nelson, 2016b, 2019). Inadvertent bowel injury is rare unless extenuating circumstances are identified. However, it may be helpful to empty the colon to limit fecal spill if extensive pelvic adhesions are anticipated due to prior infection, endometriosis, or radiation therapy.

Suitable perioperative antibiotic prophylaxis to prevent most surgical site infection is found in Table 39-8 (p. 832). Typically, a first-generation cephalosporin is given intravenously at spaced intervals. Compared with simple hysterectomy, the high-volume blood loss during radical hysterectomy clears antibiotics more rapidly from the operative site, and longer surgery may extend past the antibiotic half-life. Both necessitate the additional doses (Bouma, 1993; Sevin, 1991).

Concurrent Surgery

Early-stage cervical cancer most frequently spreads via the lymphatics. Thus, adjunctive lymph node removal seeks to identify occult metastases. Pelvic lymphadenectomy is typically completed just before or immediately after radical hysterectomy, and paraaortic lymphadenectomy may also be indicated in some cases (p. 1194) (Angioli, 1999).

Spread to the adnexa is much less common than via the lymphatics. Thus, the decision for BSO depends on histology (adenocarcinoma versus squamous), a woman's age, and her potential for developing metastatic disease (Hu, 2013; Shimada, 2006). Ovarian removal should be considered in women with cervical adenocarcinoma since the rate of metastasis to the ovary is 2 percent compared with 0.5 percent for squamous cell histology (Sutton, 1992). If ovaries are preserved, salpingectomy alone is considered to potentially reduce future risk of some epithelial ovarian cancers (Walker, 2015). In candi-

dates for ovarian preservation, transposition of ovaries out of the pelvis may be considered in young women if postoperative radiation is anticipated. However, ovarian function may be short-lived. Also, in transposed ovaries, symptomatic periadnexal cysts are commonplace (Buekers, 2001). Oocyte and ovarian cryopreservation have advanced, and the former is a more widespread option (Chap. 21, p. 468).

INTRAOPERATIVE

Surgical Steps

❶ **Anesthesia and Patient Positioning.** General anesthesia is mandatory, but transverse abdominis peripheral nerve block or epidural placement may be considered for postoperative pain control (Leon-Casasola, 1996). Bimanual examination is performed in the operating room before surgical scrubbing. Thus, in a fully anesthetized patient, parametrial, uterosacral ligament, or vaginal extension of tumor that may not have been appreciated during office examination may be found. The patient is positioned in low lithotomy. For VTE prophylaxis, lower-extremity pneumatic compression devices are placed. Hair in the path of the planned incision is clipped if needed; a Foley catheter is placed; and abdominal preparation is completed.

❷ **Abdominal Entry.** A midline vertical abdominal incision provides excellent exposure. Alternatively, Cherney or Maylard incisions offer the postoperative advantages found with transverse incisions and allow access to the lateral pelvis (p. 1162). However, upper paraaortic nodes are not readily accessible through these transverse incisions. A Pfannenstiel incision offers limited exposure and is reserved only for selected patients (Orr, 1995; Scribner, 2001).

❸ **Exploration.** Following abdominal entry, a surgeon first thoroughly explores the abdomen for obvious metastatic disease. Firm, enlarged lymph nodes and any other suspect lesions are removed or biopsied. Confirmation of metastases or pelvic tumor extension leads to a decision on whether to proceed or abort an operation based on overall intraoperative findings and clinical situation (Leath, 2004).

❹ **Entering the Retroperitoneal Space.** The uterus is placed on traction with curved Kelly clamps at the cornua. The round ligament may be divided with an electrosurgical blade or may be sutured with 0-gauge delayed-absorbable suture. This is done as laterally as possible to aid excision of the

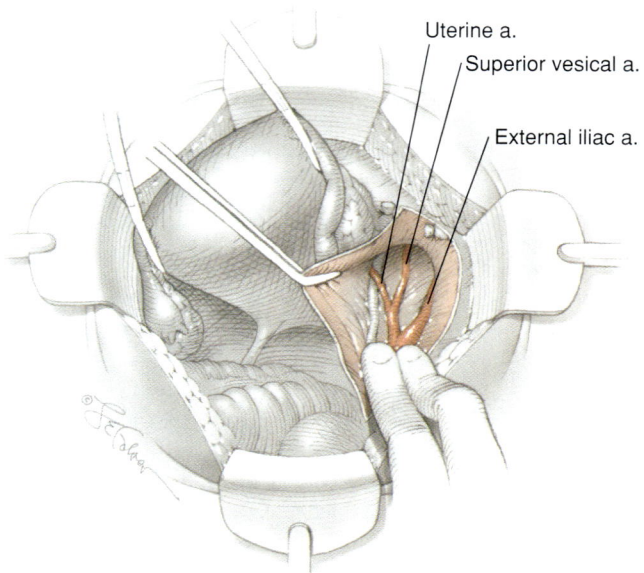

FIGURE 46-1.1 Finding the ureter.

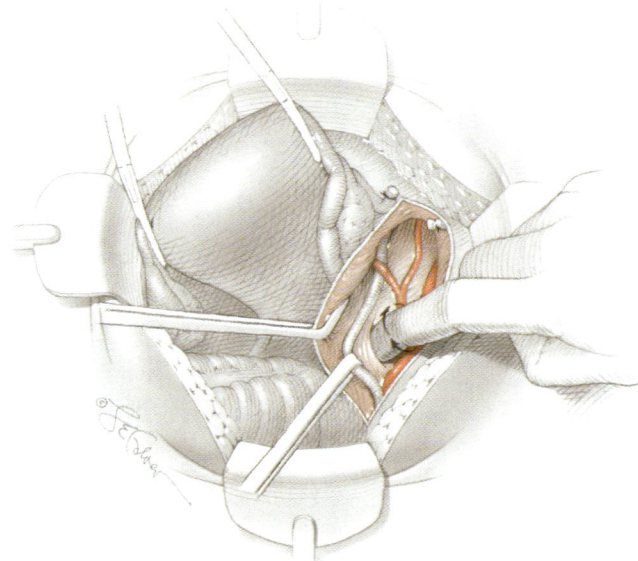

FIGURE 46-1.2 Opening the pararectal space.

parametrium out to the pelvic sidewall. Once the round ligament is divided, the broad ligament beneath it separates into thin anterior and posterior leaves that contain loose areolar connective tissue between.

The anterior leaf of the broad ligament is placed on traction and is sharply dissected to the vesicouterine fold. The posterior leaf of the broad ligament is then placed on traction and sharply dissected along the pelvic sidewall parallel to the infundibulopelvic (IP) ligament.

5 Ureter Isolation. Loose areolar connective tissue of the retroperitoneal space is bluntly dissected in the area lateral to the IP ligament until the external iliac artery is palpated just medial to the psoas major muscle. The index and middle fingers are placed on either side of the artery, and the areolar connective tissue is bluntly finger dissected toward the patient's head using a backward "walking" motion (Fig. 46-1.1).

To permit further cephalad inspection, the medial portion of the broad ligament's posterior leaf is elevated. This permits direct identification of the common iliac artery bifurcation and origins of the external and internal iliac arteries. Here, the ureter crosses over the bifurcation or over the proximal portion of the external iliac artery (Jackson, 2019). To isolate the ureter at this site, the surgeon bluntly dissects with a finger or suction tip in a sweeping motion from top to bottom along the medial peritoneal leaf to identify and sufficiently mobilize the lateral surface of the ureter.

To free the ureter's medial surface, tips of a Mixter right-angle clamp are opened and closed parallel to the ureter to develop

an avascular space between it and its medial peritoneal attachment. Through this space, clamp tips are then passed beneath the ureter to grasp a quarter-inch-wide Penrose drain. The drain is pulled through this space to surround and isolate the ureter. This assists in identifying its location throughout the remainder of surgery.

6 Creating Spaces. The parametrium that will be removed with the hysterectomy specimen lies between the paravesical and pararectal spaces (Fig. 38-18, p. 808). Thus, creation of these spaces is needed to exclude the possibility of parametrial tumor extension before proceeding. If elected, development also isolates the parametrium for transection.

The pararectal space is developed by gently opening the avascular space lateral to the ureter and medial to the internal iliac vessels, approximately 2 cm from the bifurcation of the common iliac artery. Developing this avascular space can be performed with blunt dissection using a suction catheter tip or fingertip. The path tracks in a gentle swirling motion at a 45-degree angle downward toward the midline and aiming for the coccyx (Fig. 46-1.2). Once formed, this space is bordered by the rectum and ureter medially, internal iliac artery laterally, cardinal ligament caudally, and the sacrum cephalad.

In contrast, the paravesical space is formed by dissection of the areolar tissue medial and caudal to the external iliac vessels in the direction of the pubic ramus. The index and middle finger of the opposite hand then sweep intervening avascular areolar tissue deeply and medially toward the midline. The developed paravesical space is bounded by the bladder and superior vesical artery

medially, the external iliac vessels laterally, the symphysis pubis caudally, and the cardinal ligament cephalad. Once paravesical and pararectal spaces are created, the parametrium is now isolated between these two openings.

7 Adnexa. With hysterectomy, ovaries may be retained or removed (Section 43-12, p. 959). If ovarian preservation is planned, the surgeon performs salpingectomy by serially clamping, cutting, and ligating the mesosalpinx. The uteroovarian ligament is then clamped, cut, and ligated close to the uterus. The ovary is tucked laterally during hysterectomy completion. Alternatively, if BSO is planned, the IP ligament is clamped, cut, and ligated. The uteroovarian ligament is left intact and the adnexa are ultimately removed with the uterine specimen.

8 Uterine Artery Ligation. For this step, a surgeon's left hand is inserted into the pelvis with the middle finger placed in the paravesical space and the index finger in the pararectal space. The uterus and attached Kelly clamps are cupped in the palm. The uterus is held on firm medial traction to expose the lateral pelvic sidewall.

The internal iliac artery is visualized on the lateral border of the pararectal space and traced caudally towards the superior vesical artery. The superior vesical artery is bluntly dissected to better define its location. It may be grasped with a Babcock clamp or lifted by a narrow Deaver retractor and placed on lateral traction. This traction on the superior vesical artery prevents its inadvertent ligation and aids in identification of the uterine artery (Fig. 46-1.3).

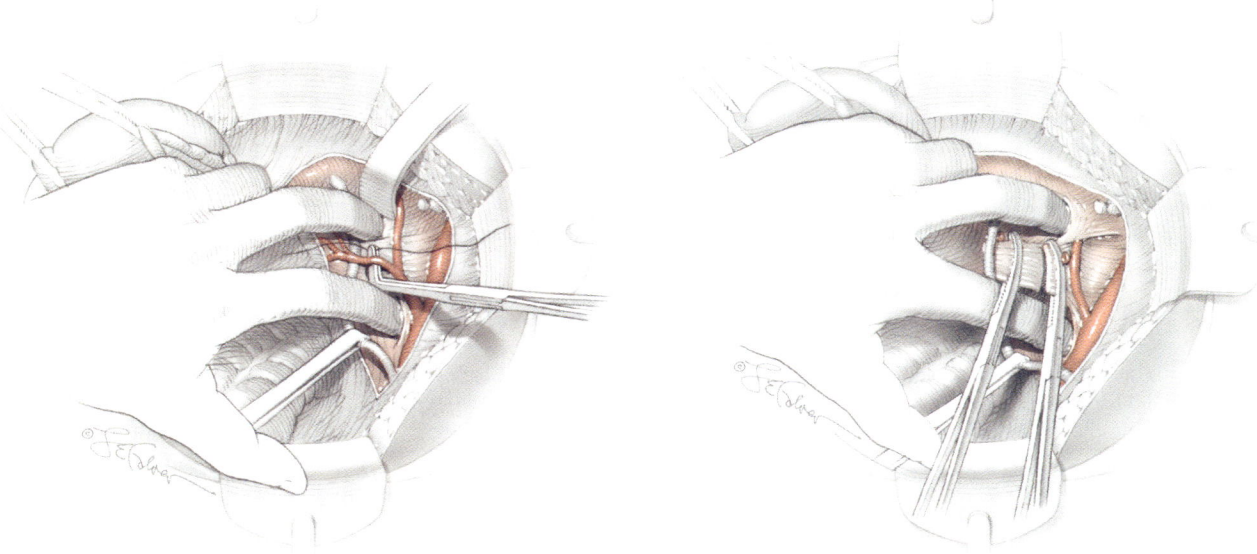

FIGURE 46-1.3 Ligating the uterine artery.

FIGURE 46-1.4 Uniting the spaces by parametrial resection.

Next, to visualize the uterine artery, a surgeon sharply dissects parametrial attachments and intervening areolar connective tissue overlying the presumed uterine artery course. The origin of the uterine artery is found during this caudal dissection.

Tissues surrounding the uterine artery are bluntly dissected, and a right-angle clamp is placed beneath this artery to retrieve a 2-0 gauge silk suture. The uterine artery tie is placed as close as possible to its origin from the internal iliac artery. The process is repeated to place a separate silk suture sufficiently medial to enable vessel transection. Black silk ties help identify the proximal and distal portions of the uterine artery throughout the remainder of the operation. A small vascular clip (Hemoclip) also can be placed lateral to the silk tie on the proximal uterine artery for additional security of hemostasis. The uterine artery is then cut. The underlying uterine vein also may then be isolated, clipped or tied, and cut.

⑨ Uniting Paravesical and Pararectal Spaces. The parametrial tissues have been pressed together by development of the paravesical and pararectal spaces. Parametrial resection to unite the upper (ventral) portion of these spaces begins near the pelvic sidewall, moves medially, and can be performed by several methods. These include: (1) clamping, cutting, and suturing, (2) electrosurgical blade dissection in which a right-angle clamp elevates and isolates parametrial tissue, or (3) use of an electrosurgical bipolar device (LigaSure, ENSEAL) (Fig. 46-1.4). Dissection continues medially until the parametrium overlying the ureter is mobile.

⑩ Ureter Mobilization. In this same area of the pelvis, tips of a right-angle clamp are positioned just superolateral to the ureter to dissect it from its attachment to the medial peritoneal leaf. As previously described, opening and closing the tips downward and parallel to the ureter develops an avascular plane to bluntly dissect it from the peritoneum. The ureter is again placed on gentle lateral traction by grasping the previously placed Penrose drain with the left hand.

The right index finger carefully sweeps the ureter downward and laterally until a "tunnel" through the paracervical tissue can be palpated ventromedially as the ureter enters this tissue (Fig. 46-1.5). Additional parametrial dissection is often required to ensure

that the uterine artery and surrounding soft tissue has been lifted medially over and off the ureter.

⑪ Bladder Dissection. To help avoid urinary tract injury, the bladder is moved caudad and away from the cervix and upper vagina. This is accomplished by first opening the vesicouterine space, the potential space between the bladder and uterine isthmus/cervix. Several techniques may be used, and at our institution, sharp dissection is preferred (Fig. 43-12.9, p. 960). This method is particularly beneficial for patients with potential scarring between the bladder and cervix.

During dissection in the vesicouterine space, this peritoneum is grasped with atraumatic

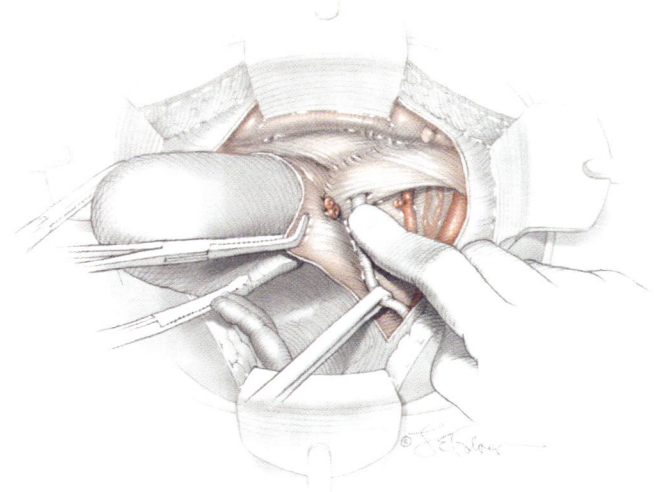

FIGURE 46-1.5 Mobilizing the ureter.

tissue forceps and elevated to create tension between it and the underlying cervix. Only loose connective tissue strands lie in this space, and they are easily cut with Metzenbaum scissors. Incision of these bands is kept close to the cervix to avoid cystotomy. Dissection in the midline minimizes laceration of vessels that course within the vesicouterine ligaments, colloquially termed *bladder pillars*. Once the correct plane is entered, the pearly white cervix and anterior vaginal wall are clearly differentiated from reddish bladder fibers.

This dissection may need to be advanced as the tunnel is progressively unroofed, described next, and the ureter is more directly visible. This ultimately allows adequate vaginal specimen margins. The bladder will eventually need to be dissected so that it lies several centimeters distal to the cervical portio and onto the upper vagina.

⑫ Unroofing the Ureteral Tunnel. The uterus is placed on lateral traction, and the proximal ureter is held on traction to straighten it by gently pulling on the Penrose drain. The roof of the ureteral "tunnel" is formed by the anterior leaf of the vesicouterine ligament. This ligament contains the cervicovesical vessels that cross from the bladder to the cervix (Fujii, 2007). The remaining tissue within the roof of the ureteric tunnel is avascular.

A right-angle clamp is inserted with its tips directed upward, while direct visualization of the underlying ureter is confirmed. The tips are directed medially toward the cervix. The tips "pop" through the paracervical tissue and create a new distal opening (Fig. 46-1.6). One tip of a second clamp is placed through the tunnel and then through

the new distal opening. The clamp closes around the paracervical tissue that lies above the ureter.

Within the tunnel, the ureter is bluntly dissected and pushed posteriorly toward the tunnel floor, which contains the posterior leaf of the vesicouterine ligament. The ureter should be visible below before cutting the overlying paracervical tissue. Delayed-absorbable 3-0 gauge suture ties are used to secure the paracervical tissue pedicles that are held by the right-angle clamps. During these steps, significant bleeding can be avoided by identifying the just-described vascular anatomic landmarks. Ureteral dissection should be performed with direct visualization of the ureter at all times to prevent injury.

After being unroofed, the ureter is retracted upward, and filmy attachments between the it and tunnel bed (posterior leaf of vesicouterine ligament) are sharply divided. The connective tissue within and beneath the vesicouterine ligament contains the middle and inferior vesical veins, which connect to the deep uterine vein. Division of the posterior leaf is avoided in most cases to preserve the inferior hypogastric plexus and help prevent bladder dysfunction (Ripperda, 2017).

⑬ Uterosacral Resection. Posterior radical dissection is often best performed near the operation's end because exposed retroperitoneal tissues typically ooze until the vaginal cuff is closed. The cervical external os is palpated, and at this level, the electrosurgical blade is used to superficially incise or "score" the peritoneum between the uterosacral

ligaments. This score line joins the incision line of the previously cut peritoneum of the broad ligament's posterior leaf.

Between the uterosacral ligaments, a plane is developed by gently pressing a finger toward the vaginal wall without poking through and into the vaginal vault. This rectovaginal plane is developed by gentle pressure toward the sacrum and enlarged laterally until three fingers can be comfortably inserted. This maneuver frees the rectosigmoid from the uterosacral ligaments and helps prevent inadvertent bowel injury.

The exposed uterosacral ligaments can be visualized, palpated, and clamped at the pelvic sidewall. Ligaments are cut and ligated with 0-gauge delayed-absorbable suture (Fig. 46-1.7). This procedure may need to be repeated to complete transection of the uterosacral ligament and adjacent supportive tissues.

⑭ Vaginal Resection. At this point in the operation, the radical hysterectomy specimen is held in place only by the paracolpium and vagina. The bladder and ureters are further bluntly and sharply dissected free until at least 3 cm of upper vagina can be included with the resected specimen. Curved clamps are placed on the lateral paracolpium. The ureter should be lateral and directly visible. Tissue is cut and suture ligated with 0-gauge delayed-absorbable suture.

The upper vagina can then be: (1) clamped, cut, and suture ligated, (2) stapled, or (3) sharply transected with electrosurgical blade and suture ligated (Fig. 46-1.8). The specimen

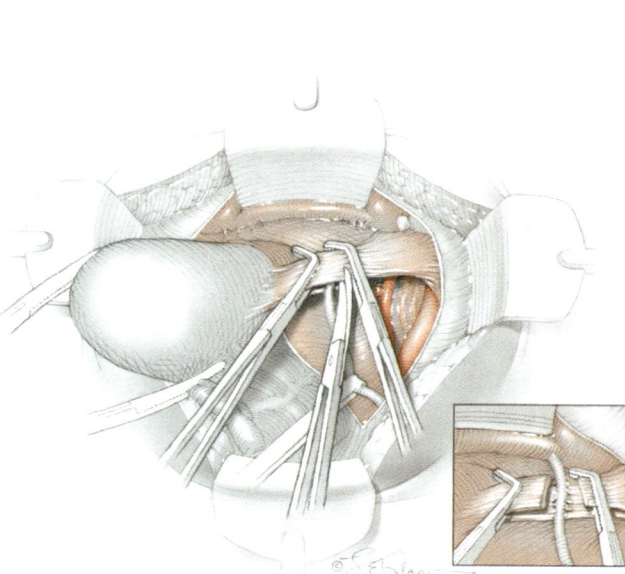

FIGURE 46-1.6 Unroofing the ureteral tunnel.

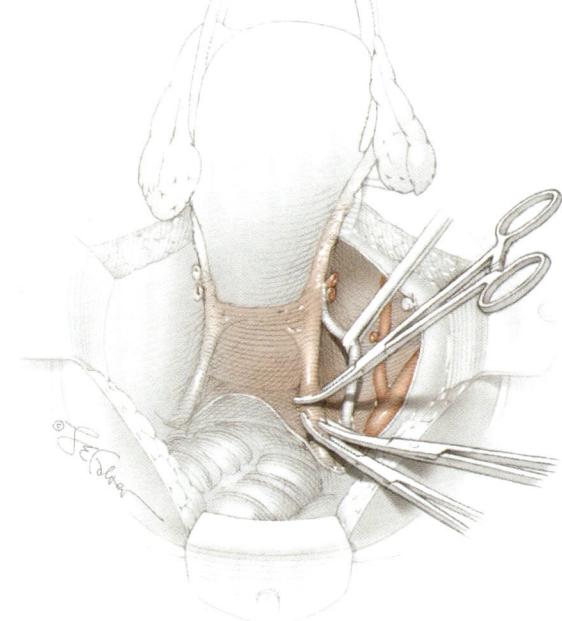

FIGURE 46-1.7 Uterosacral ligament transection.

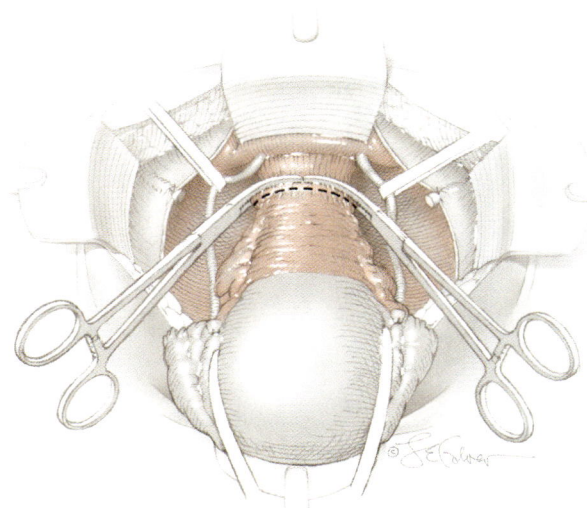

FIGURE 46-1.8 Vaginal transection.

is carefully examined to ensure an adequate upper vaginal segment and grossly negative margins.

⑮ Ovarian Transposition. For those in whom ovarian function preservation is desired, transposing ovaries out of the anticipated pelvic radiation field is an option. A distal portion of the previously freed ovary is grasped. Using traction, dissection is performed to mobilize the IP ligament so that the ovary can be lifted into the upper abdomen. For future radiography or CT interpretation, a large vascular clip is placed on the residual uteroovarian ligament stump to serve as an ovarian location marker. For transposition, a 0-gauge silk suture is placed at this stump site and tied. Its needle is covered but remains attached to the suture.

A handheld abdominal retractor is then used to expose an area of the lateral posterior peritoneum as high as possible in the abdomen. The silk suture needle is uncovered and placed through the peritoneum, and the ovary is elevated by this "pulley-stitch" and tied. The lateral pelvic defect is closed with a continuous running stitch using 0-gauge delayed-absorbable suture to prevent internal herniation, that is, entrapment of bowel within the peritoneal defect. Ovaries are inspected before abdominal closure to exclude vascular compromise by transposition.

⑯ Final Steps. Active bleeding should be immediately controlled when the radical hysterectomy specimen has been removed. A dry laparotomy sponge may be held firmly deep in the pelvis for several minutes to tamponade raw surfaces. Topical hemostatic agents may be employed (Table 40-6, p. 860). With bleeding controlled, a surgeon then assesses the vascular support to the ureter and other sidewall structures. To structures that appear particularly devascularized, an omental J-flap may provide additional blood supply (Section 46-14, p. 1211) (Fujiwara, 2003; Patsner, 1997). Routine pelvic suction drainage and closure of the peritoneum are not necessary (Charoenkwan, 2014; Franchi, 2007).

POSTOPERATIVE

Immediate postoperative care following radical hysterectomy in general follows that for laparotomy. Early ambulation after radical hysterectomy is especially important to prevent VTE complications. ERAS protocols also note fewer pulmonary complications, less muscle atrophy, and shorter stays (Nelson, 2016a). Moreover, following laparotomy for cancer, anticoagulants are continued for 4 weeks postoperatively (Gould 2012; Key, 2019). Early feeding, including rapid initiation of a clear liquid diet, may shorten the

hospital stay and lower ileus rates (Boitano, 2018; Minig, 2009).

Bladder tone returns slowly, and a major cause is thought to be partial sympathetic and parasympathetic denervation during radical dissection (Chen, 2002). Thus, Foley catheter drainage is commonly continued until a patient is passing flatus because improving bowel function typically accompanies resolving bladder hypotonia. Removal of the catheter or clamping of the suprapubic tube should be followed by a successful voiding trial (Chap. 42, p. 919). A voiding trial may be attempted prior to hospital discharge or at the first postoperative visit. Patients with adequate function are instructed to press gently on the suprapubic area for several days afterward to help completely empty the bladder and prevent retention. Successful voiding may take several weeks to achieve. In the 3 percent of women who develop long-term bladder hypotonia or atony, intermittent self-catheterization is preferred to indwelling urinary catheterization (Chamberlain, 1991; Naik, 2005).

In addition to urinary retention, tenesmus and constipation are frequent immediate symptoms that should improve significantly over months or years (Butler-Manuel, 1999; Sood, 2002). Postoperative stool softeners are often prescribed.

For cervical cancer patients undergoing BSO, estrogen replacement therapy is not contraindicated and may be initiated at the discretion of the treating oncologist. Cervical cancer survivors treated with radical hysterectomy have much better sexual functioning than those who receive radiation therapy. Despite this, more than half of surgical patients postoperatively report a worse sex life (Butler-Manuel, 1999). Severe orgasmic problems, uncomfortable intercourse due to reduced vaginal length, and severe dyspareunia may develop but often resolve within 6 to 12 months. However, persistent lack of sexual interest and poor lubrication may be long-term or permanent changes (Jensen, 2004). Disturbed vaginal blood flow response during sexual arousal may account for much of the reported constellation of symptoms (Maas, 2004). Eventually, patients treated by surgery alone can expect a quality of life and overall sexual function similar to peers without a history of cancer (Frumovitz, 2005).

SECTION 6

46-2

Modified Radical Abdominal Hysterectomy (Type II)

Four procedural differences distinguish a modified radical hysterectomy (type II) hysterectomy from the more radical type III procedure (Section 46-1, p. 1160). First, the uterine artery is transected at the point it crosses the ureter (rather than at its origin from the internal iliac artery). Second, only the medial half of the cardinal ligament is resected (instead of division at the sidewall). Additionally, the uterosacral ligament is divided halfway between the uterus and sacrum (rather than at the sacrum). And last, a smaller margin of upper vagina is removed. These modifications serve to reduce surgical time and associated morbidity, while still enabling complete resection of smaller cervical tumors (Cai, 2009; Landoni, 2001).

Clear indications for modified radical hysterectomy are few and controversial (Rose, 2001). Stage IA1 (with lymphovascular space invasion) or IA2 cervical cancer are the most common diagnoses (Koh, 2019). Type II hysterectomy is also performed on occasion for: (1) preinvasive or microinvasive disease when a more invasive lesion cannot be excluded, (2) selected stage IB1 disease with <2-cm lesions, and (3) small central postirradiation recurrences (Cai, 2009; Coleman, 1994; Eisenkop, 2005). In addition, a variation of this operation may be performed if more extensive dissection is required for known benign disease. Anatomic landmarks that distinguish a type II hysterectomy are somewhat vague and thereby allow a surgeon to sculpt the procedure to a patient's specific situation (Fedele, 2005).

PREOPERATIVE

Preparation for surgery should proceed with the same care and discretion that is essential for the success of radical (type III) abdominal hysterectomy (Section 46-1, p. 1161).

INTRAOPERATIVE

Surgical Steps

❶ Anesthesia and Patient Positioning. Modified radical hysterectomy is performed under general anesthesia with the patient supine or in low lithotomy. For VTE prophylaxis, lower-extremity pneumatic compression devices are placed. Bimanual examination is performed in the operating room before surgical scrubbing to reorient a surgeon to a patient's individual anatomy. The abdomen is surgically prepared, and a Foley catheter is placed.

❷ Abdominal Entry. Modified radical hysterectomy may be safely performed through a midline vertical or transverse incision (Fagotti, 2004).

❸ Retroperitoneal Dissection. The initial steps of modified radical (type II) hysterectomy mirror those of the type III procedure. The retroperitoneum is opened to identify structures, the ureter is mobilized, and the paravesical and pararectal spaces are developed to exclude the possibility of parametrial tumor extension before proceeding with this less radical operation (Scambia, 2001). As with radical hysterectomy, ovaries may be spared or removed (p. 1161).

❹ Uterine Artery Ligation. At this point, type II hysterectomy begins to differ from the radical type III procedure. The superior vesical artery does not have to be identified, nor does the entire extent of the internal iliac artery need to be dissected free of adventitial tissue. The ureteral tunnel opening is palpated and the uterine vessels divided at that location (Fig. 46-2.1). Ligation of the uterine artery as it crosses the ureter allows preservation of distal ureteral blood supply.

❺ Cardinal Ligament Resection. The bladder is mobilized distally off the cervix and onto the upper vagina. Parametrial tissue at the sidewall does not require mobilization over the ureter (as in a type III hysterectomy). Posterolateral attachments of the ureter remain intact, and only the medial halves of the cardinal ligaments are resected by successive clamping, cutting, and suture ligation of the paracervical tissue medial to the ureter (Fig. 46-2.2). In contrast to the type III hysterectomy, the ureter is not dissected out of the tunnel bed, but instead is rolled laterally to expose the medial cardinal ligament.

❻ Uterosacral Resection. Posterior dissection also is modified. Uterosacral ligaments are only clamped halfway to the pelvic sidewall (instead of *at* the pelvic sidewall) and transected (Fig. 46-2.3). The uterus and

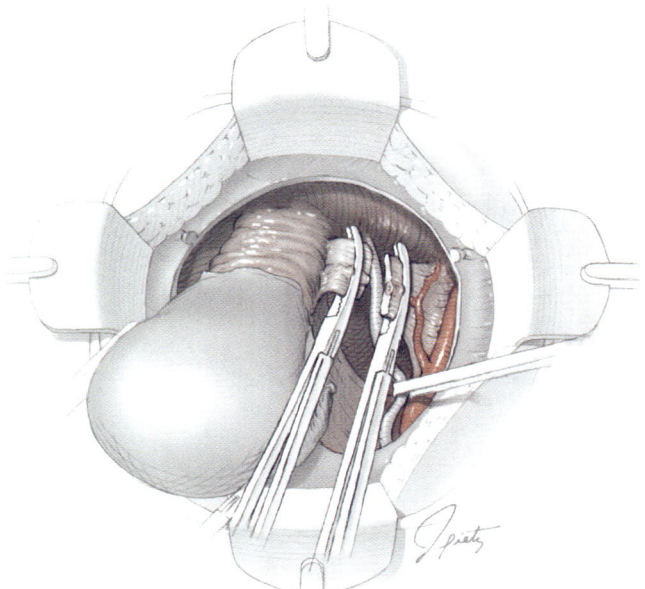

FIGURE 46-2.1 Uterine artery ligation.

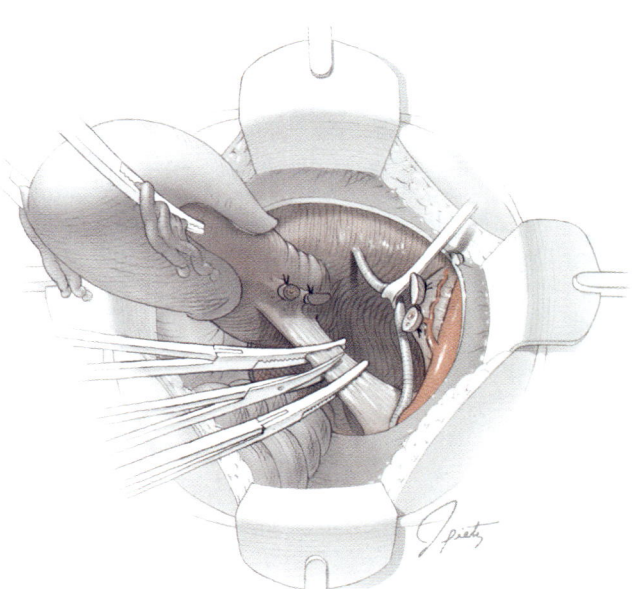

FIGURE 46-2.2 Cardinal ligament transection.

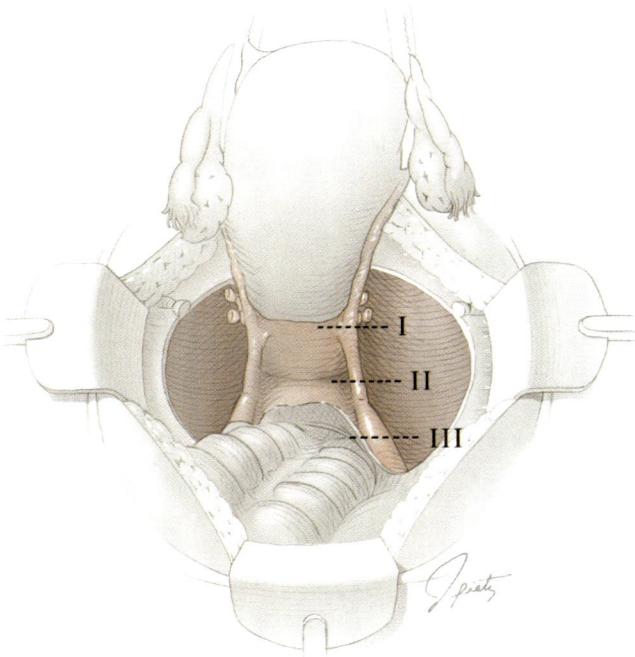

FIGURE 46-2.3 Uterosacral ligament transection.

adjacent parametrium can then be lifted well out of the pelvis and any additional tissues also clamped, cut, and ligated.

❼ **Vaginal Resection.** At this point, the modified radical hysterectomy specimen is held in place only by the paracolpium and vagina. The bladder and ureters are further bluntly and sharply dissected away until at least 2 cm of upper vagina will be included in the specimen (instead of 3 to 4 cm). Curved clamps are placed on the lateral paracolpium, cut, and suture ligated.

The upper vagina can then be: (1) clamped, cut, and suture ligated, (2) stapled, or (3) sharply transected with electrosurgical blade and suture ligated. The specimen is carefully examined to ensure an adequate upper vaginal segment and grossly negative margins.

POSTOPERATIVE

In general, postoperative care follows that for radical hysterectomy, but the incidence of complications is lower (Cai, 2009). Partial sympathetic and parasympathetic denervation should be much less extensive with a modified radical hysterectomy. Thus, bladder dysfunction is less likely than following a type III radical hysterectomy, and successful voiding begins much earlier (Landoni, 2001; Yang, 1999). Foley catheter drainage may be discontinued on the second postoperative day and is followed by a voiding trial (Chap. 42, p. 919). In addition, bowel and sexual dysfunction also should be less pronounced.

46-3

Minimally Invasive Radical Hysterectomy

Newer data on cervical cancer survival rates after MIS radical hysterectomy (type III) are discussed on page 1160. If selected, it has the same surgical steps as that via laparotomy. Thus, compared with simple hysterectomy (type I), greater resection of parametrium and paracolpium and associated lymphatics is essential to help ensure tumor-free surgical margins. This degree of resection requires significantly more retroperitoneal dissection, during which the ureter and major vessels must be identified to avoid injury.

PREOPERATIVE

Patient Evaluation

Thorough preoperative pelvic examination reveals factors that help determine the optimal surgical approach for a given patient. For example, a large broad or bulky uterus may be difficult to manipulate during MIS, may block views, and may be too large for vaginal removal. Importantly, morcellation is avoided with any gynecologic malignancy.

General challenges to MIS, such as obesity, are described in Chapter 41 (p. 873). That said, laparoscopy can be a successful option for many obese patients and offers lower rates of postoperative wound infection, which is often a major complication after laparotomy in these patients (Park, 2012). With MIS, less intraoperative blood loss and shorter hospital stays are noted, but operative times can be longer depending on surgeon proficiency (Soliman, 2011). Once a patient is deemed eligible for an MIS approach, the same preoperative evaluation as for an open procedure applies (p. 1161).

Consent

Risks of MIS radical hysterectomy mirror those listed for radical abdominal hysterectomy (p. 1161). Patient factors that contribute include older age, previous abdominal surgery, and prior radiotherapy (Chi, 2004).

General complications related to MIS are discussed in Chapter 41 (p. 875). With MIS radical hysterectomy specifically, concerns for nerve injury from a longer operation in lithotomy and steep Trendelenburg position are increased. Additionally, the risk of conversion to an open procedure is discussed. This risk may be greater if exposure and organ manipulation are limited.

Patient Preparation

Preoperative preparation is the same as for an open procedure (p. 1161). Thus, antibiotics and VTE prophylaxis are warranted (Tables 39-8 and 39-10, p. 832). Benefits of mechanical bowel preparation can be debated and are individualized. If considered, an evacuated rectosigmoid may improve colon manipulation and pelvic anatomy visualization. Options are found in Chapter 39 (p. 833).

Concurrent Surgery

Pelvic lymphadenectomy is typically completed just before or immediately after radical hysterectomy, and paraaortic lymphadenectomy also may be indicated in some circumstances. An MIS approach to lymph node removal in these areas is described in Section 46-12 (p. 1201).

Planned oophorectomy should depend on tumor histology (squamous cell or adenocarcinoma), a woman's age, and potential for metastases (Hu, 2013). Ovarian metastasis is rare with early-stage cervical cancer, and particularly with squamous cell carcinoma. Thus, if preservation is chosen, the ovary can be transposed with MIS techniques to the upper abdomen. This is done to help extend ovarian function if later radiotherapy is required. However, ovarian longevity may be shortened postoperatively, and symptomatic ovarian cysts are common. Moreover, advancements in ovarian cryopreservation and especially oocyte preservation are suitable alternatives.

Regardless of ovarian preservation, salpingectomy is now considered for all women undergoing hysterectomy (Walker, 2015). As explained in Chapter 35 (p. 736), this practice is hoped to lower rates of high-grade ovarian and peritoneal serous carcinomas.

INTRAOPERATIVE

Instruments

Basic MIS tools for laparoscopic or robotic surgery are required. Important instruments for radical hysterectomy include 5- and 12-mm trocars, combined irrigation/suction device, vaginal probe, and energy devices for cutting and vessel sealing. For the latter, several electrosurgical and ultrasonic energy-based devices are adapted for either laparoscopic or robotic cases. These include Harmonic scalpel, electrosurgical monopolar instruments, and electrosurgical bipolar coagulator devices (LigaSure, ENSEAL, PK Dissecting Forceps). For laparoscopy, the argon-beam coagulator is another option. While operating in the pelvis, a 30-degree laparoscope may be advantageous to provide superior lateral views.

Surgical Steps

❶ Anesthesia and Patient Positioning. The patient is initially supine for general endotracheal anesthesia induction. For VTE prophylaxis, lower-extremity compression devices are placed. Legs are then positioned in adjustable booted support stirrups in low lithotomy to permit adequate perineal access. Positioning should permit a transvaginal uterine manipulator to move easily in all directions. As described in Chapter 41 (p. 877), appropriate positioning of legs within the stirrups and arms at the side is crucial to reduce nerve injury risks.

Bimanual examination is performed in the operating room before surgical scrubbing to reorient a surgeon to the patient's individual anatomy. The abdomen, perineum, and vagina are then surgically prepared, and a Foley catheter is inserted. To avoid stomach puncture by a trocar during primary abdominal entry, an orogastric or nasogastric tube is placed to decompress the stomach. During MIS radical hysterectomy, a blunt vaginal probe in the vaginal fornix can be inserted.

❷ Port Placement. An illustrated description of MIS entry into the abdominal cavity is found in Chapter 41 (p. 888). Suitable entry methods include the open technique, direct trocar insertion, or transumbilical insertion of a Veress needle. For gynecologic oncology cases, the open technique is often used to minimize vascular or bowel puncture risk. For the primary port, an umbilical or supraumbilical site is preferred. Following entry, a 10- or 12-mm Hassan trocar with a blunt obturator is placed into the abdominal cavity and is secured to the fascia. Through the trocar, the obturator is removed and replaced by a 10-mm laparoscope.

After abdominal insufflation, the abdomen and pelvis are thoroughly inspected to assess the extent of disease and adhesions. At this point, confirmation of metastatic disease or pelvic tumor extension should prompt a surgeon to decide whether to proceed or abort the operation based on intraoperative findings and clinical situation. Moreover, the decision is made to proceed laparoscopically or convert to laparotomy.

For laparoscopy, the surgeon stands on one side of the patient, whereas one assistant occupies the opposite side and another stands between the patient's legs. To proceed, other ports are placed under direct laparoscopic visualization. Anatomic landmarks are identified to guide port placement and avert vascular puncture injuries. For complex MIS gynecologic procedures, four port sites are preferred (Fig. 46-3.1). Additional ports are placed according to surgeon preference. For

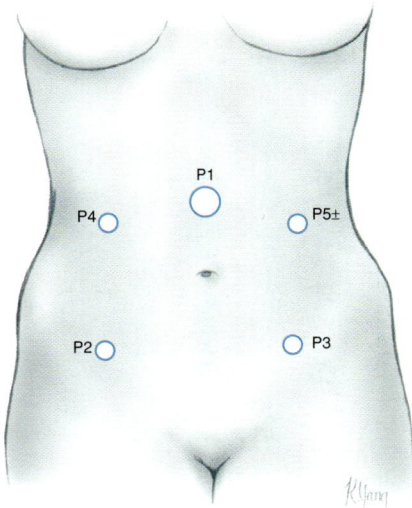

FIGURE 46-3.1 Port placement for minimally invasive radical hysterectomy.

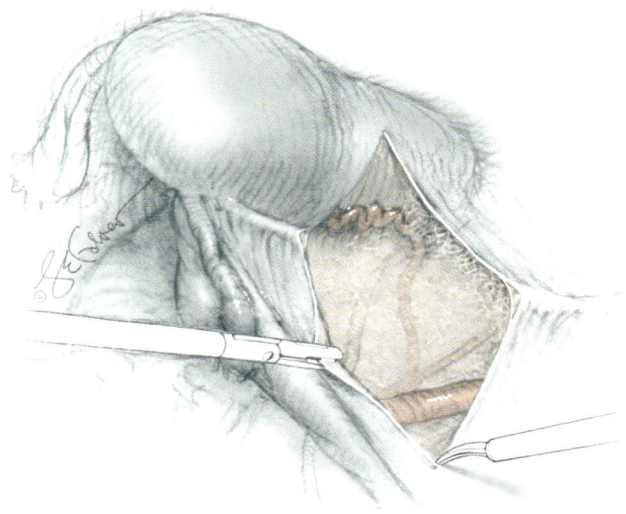

FIGURE 46-3.2 Opening the broad ligament leaf.

robotic cases, these ideally have a minimum of 8 cm between them to allow ample range of motion and to avoid robot arm collision.

❸ Opening the Retroperitoneum. This is the initial step to opening the paravesical and pararectal spaces bilaterally and identifying the ureter. Development of these spaces allows the parametrial tissue to be isolated and later resected.

First, the assistant angles the uterus to the contralateral side of dissection using a grasper holding one cornu. This creates tension across the round ligament, which is divided at its midpoint. Transection may be accomplished using any of the energy-based devices previously listed.

Once the round ligament is transected, the broad ligament beneath it separates into thin anterior and posterior leaves, with loose areolar connective tissue between them. The anterior leaf is tented upward by graspers and sharply incised with monopolar scissors or other energy-based device. Incision extends caudally and medially toward the vesicouterine fold and halts near the midline.

To further expand the retroperitoneal opening, the drape of peritoneum lying between the divided round ligament and IP ligament is elevated with smooth graspers. Incision of this tented peritoneum is extended cephalad toward the pelvic brim but remains lateral and parallel to the IP ligament (Fig. 46-3.2). This exposes the external iliac vessels and provides access to the ureter.

❹ Ureteral Identification. This is accomplished by precise sharp and blunt dissection just lateral to the medial leaf of the opened peritoneum. For this, a blunt probe

or the closed tips of a grasper may be selected. Dissection is advanced downward, medially, and slightly cephalad with gentle back-and-forth cephalad-caudad strokes into the gauzy retroperitoneal tissue and over the presumed ureter path (Fig. 46-3.3). The ureter is identified and traced along the medial leaf of the posterior peritoneum.

❺ Creating Spaces. The uterus remains deviated to the contralateral side to develop the pararectal space. This avascular space is bounded by the rectum and ureter medially, the internal iliac artery laterally, the cardinal ligament and uterine artery caudally, and sacrum cephalad. Within these borders,

the tips of closed scissors or other blunt tip push downward and medially through loose connective tissue (Fig. 46-3.4). The surgeon directs dissection downward toward the midline, aims for the pelvic floor, and stops once the levator ani muscles are reached.

For the paravesical space, boundaries are the external iliac vessels laterally, the bladder and obliterated umbilical ligament medially, the symphysis pubis caudally, and the cardinal ligament cephalad. To open this space, the previously incised edge of the broad ligament's anterior leaf is lifted at a point between the bladder and pelvic sidewall. Superficial loose connective tissue lies medial to the external iliac vessels and is bluntly dissected with closed

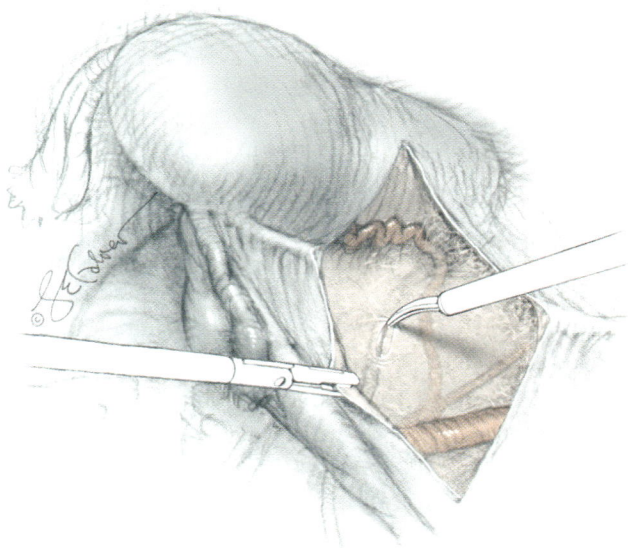

FIGURE 46-3.3 Locating the ureter.

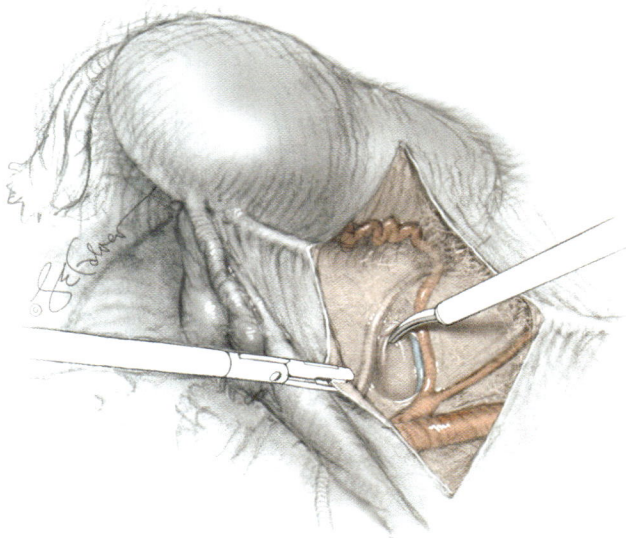

FIGURE 46-3.4 Opening the pararectal space.

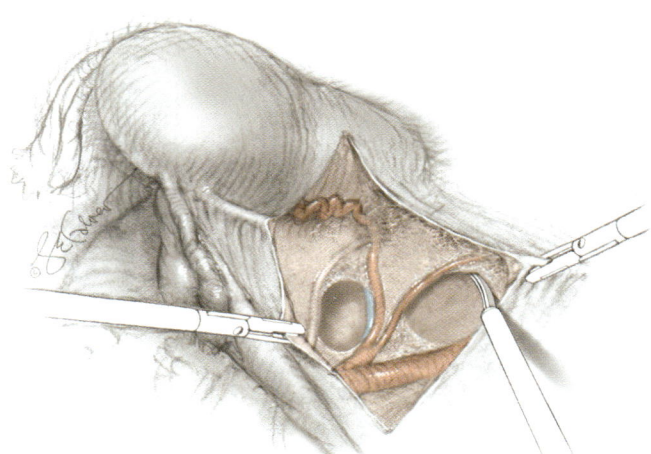

FIGURE 46-3.5 Opening the paravesical space.

scissors or grasper (Fig. 46-3.5). Staying medial to the external iliac vein and lateral to the superior vesicle/obliterated umbilical artery, dissection is directed caudally until the curve of the pubic ramus is reached.

Once the paravesical and pararectal spaces are opened, the parametria are now isolated between these two spaces for later resection. This dissection also helps to mobilize the bladder, discussed next, and to expose the external iliac vessels, which will aid later pelvic lymphadenectomy.

❻ Bladder Mobilization. During radical hysterectomy, the bladder is dissected free from the cervix and upper vagina. The mobile bladder is moved caudad and protected during final vaginal transection. To mobilize the bladder, the peritoneum at the vesicouterine fold is grasped with atraumatic graspers and elevated to create tension between it and the underlying cervix (Fig. 46-3.6). The vesicouterine space, the potential space between the bladder and cervix, is opened using sharp and blunt dissection. Only loose connective tissue fibers lie in this space and are easily cut. Incision of these bands is kept close to the cervix to avoid cystotomy. Dissection in the midline minimizes laceration of vessels that course within the vesicocervical ligaments, colloquially termed *bladder pillars*. Once the correct plane is entered, the pearly white cervix and anterior vaginal wall below are clearly differentiated from the more opaque bladder.

Ultimately, the bladder is moved sufficiently caudad to permit excision of up to 3 cm of proximal vagina at the procedure's end. This aids acquisition of tumor-free surgical margins. Generous dissection also avoids incorporating bladder fibers into the cuff

closure, which could lead to bladder injury or to later genitourinary fistula.

❼ Uterine Artery Ligation. For this step, the pelvic sidewall vessels are exposed. By visually moving from the common iliac artery toward its bifurcation, a surgeon can identify the internal iliac artery. The first anterior branch of the internal iliac artery is the umbilical artery. The uterine artery is typically the second branch and courses medially and over the ureter.

Alternatively, to isolate the uterine artery, the superior vesical artery is identified by blunt dissection on the medial border of the

paravesical space. The vessel is followed cephalad to identify the uterine artery origin. In most instances, the uterine artery originates from the internal iliac artery and is identified by its medial course toward and over the ureter.

To isolate the uterine artery for ligation at its origin from the internal iliac artery, tips of a grasper are positioned beneath the vessel. Opening and closing the grasper tips, while directing dissection downward, develops an avascular plane around the artery. Importantly, the uterine vein lies just beneath the artery, and its injury can compromise visibility from brisk bleeding. Once isolated, the uterine

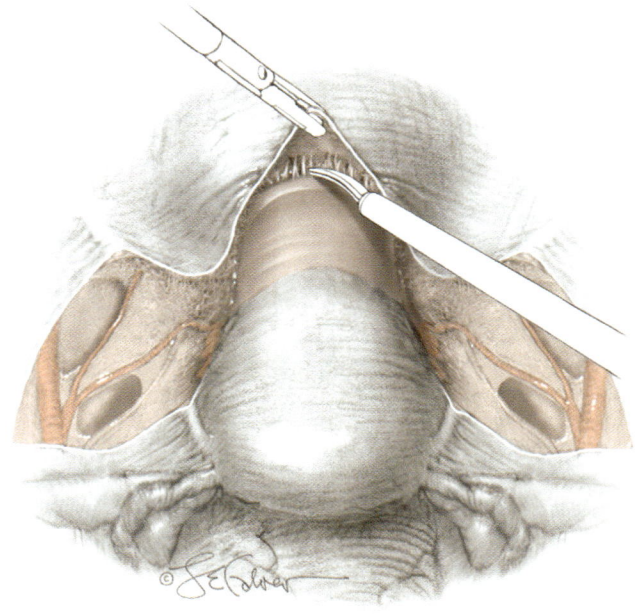

FIGURE 46-3.6 Dissection in the vesicovaginal space.

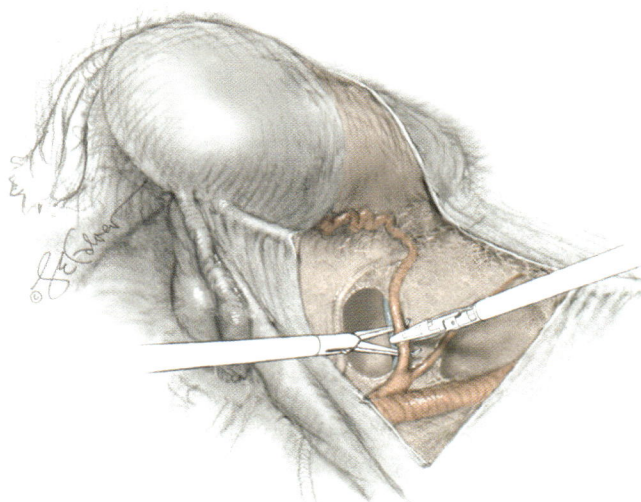

FIGURE 46-3.7 Uterine artery ligation.

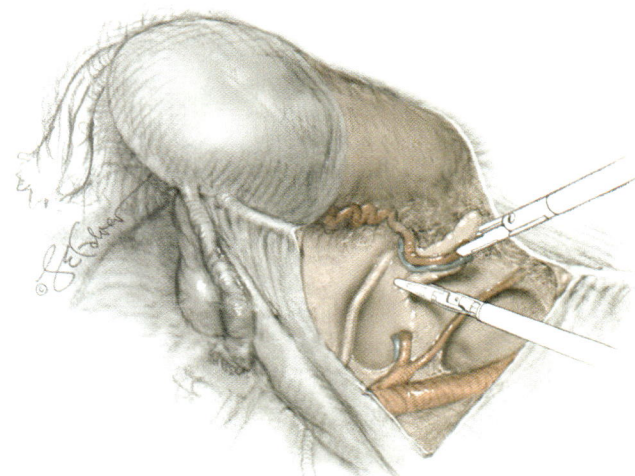

FIGURE 46-3.8 Lifting the parametrium off the ureter.

artery is coagulated using a vessel-sealing device and divided (Fig. 46-3.7). The artery ends are then elevated to identify the uterine vein, which is similarly isolated, coagulated, and divided.

❽ Ureteral Mobilization and Parametrial Dissection. Ultimately, in a radical procedure, the ureter is freed in stages from surrounding tissue until its insertion into the bladder is reached. This dissection allows the ureter to be reflected laterally and protected during the wide parametrial excision required for radical hysterectomy.

During early dissection, atraumatic graspers tent up the medial posterior peritoneal leaf to which the ureter is attached. The tips of a right-angle grasper are positioned just superolateral to the ureter and between the ureter and peritoneum. Opening and closing the tips downward and parallel to the ureter develops an avascular plane to dissect the ureter free.

Such dissection continues caudally until parametrial tissue surrounding the ureter is met. This tissue is confined between the paravesical and pararectal spaces, contains the divided uterine vessels, and will be dissected medially and up and off the ureter. For this, connective tissue around the medial coagulated end of the uterine artery is grasped laterally and then lifted up and medially (Fig. 46-3.8). Loose connective tissue bands holding the artery and vein and surrounding parametria to the pelvic floor are coagulated and sharply transected. Dissection is continued medially until the lateral border of the ureter is reached.

For ureterolysis, caudally directed tips of a Maryland grasper are insinuated and opened within the avascular space overlying the ureter. This exposes tissue pedicles

on the ureter's lateral aspect, which are then coagulated and cut. The uterine vessels and parametrium are then pulled medially and reflected off the ureter. They will be removed with the final specimen.

During continued caudal ureterolysis, the ureter is seen to enter a "tunnel" within the vesicouterine ligament. To open this tunnel and free the ureter, the ureter is retracted downward and laterally. Within the tunnel, caudally directed grasper tips are insinuated and opened within the space overlying the ureter (Fig. 46-3.9). Tips of an energy-based tool then elevate the tunnel roof above and away from the ureter. This vesicouterine ligament roof and the veins within it are then

transected. The roof is divided in small increments caudally until completely opened. At this point, the ureteral insertion into the bladder can be identified. The areolar tissue holding the ureter to the bed of the ureteric tunnel is then cut. The ureter is moved laterally with an atraumatic tool to allow later cardinal ligament transection without ureteral injury.

❾ Adnexectomy or Ovarian Preservation. The IP ligament or the uteroovarian ligament will be transected depending on whether the ovary is removed or retained, respectively. Steps for both mirror those with benign hysterectomy and are fully illustrated

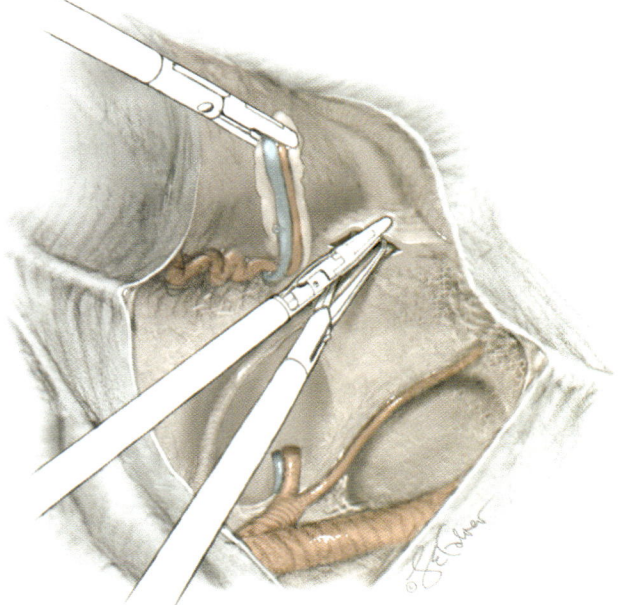

FIGURE 46-3.9 Unroofing the ureter.

in Section 44-9 (p. 1044). For these steps, a window is made in the posterior broad ligament below the IP ligament. The window can be made bluntly or with an energy-based tool, and the window is then enlarged. The incision is opened parallel to the IP ligament and is extended cephalad toward the pelvic brim and medially toward the uterosacral ligament. The ureter should be clearly identified to avoid its injury.

For adnexectomy, the IP ligament is divided with a vessel-sealing device followed by cutting. In contrast, if the ovary is to be preserved, then salpingectomy alone is first completed. For this, the mesosalpinx is divided with a vessel-sealing and cutting device, and resection progresses from the fimbria to its union with the uterus. Next, the uteroovarian ligament is transected with the same device, and the ovary is tucked over to the sidewall until hysterectomy completion.

If ovarian preservation is chosen, the ovary can be transposed laparoscopically. With this, the IP ligament is further dissected cephalad by extending the peritoneal incision on both the medial and lateral sides of the IP ligament. This mobilizes the ovary, whose uteroovarian ligament stump is then sutured to the lateral peritoneum in the upper abdomen as described on page 1165. Importantly, following transposition, the ovary is inspected to confirm adequate blood supply. A clip can be placed at the uteroovarian stump so that it can be delineated on future imaging studies.

At this point, steps 3 through 9 are completed on the contralateral side.

⑩ **Rectovaginal Space.** Developing this potential space moves the rectum downward to isolate the uterosacral ligaments for wide resection. It also permits adequate excision of the proximal vagina for tumor-free margins without rectal injury. First, the uterus is retracted upward in the midline, and the peritoneum between the uterosacral ligaments is incised at the level of the external cervical os (Fig. 46-3.10). The peritoneal edge closer to the rectum is then grasped and tented outward with atraumatic graspers, and the rectovaginal space is opened with sharp dissection with scissors or electrosurgical blade. This exposes connective tissue bands and small vessels between the rectum and vagina. These bands are coagulated and transected close to the vagina with an energy-based device (Fig. 46-3.11). Dissection continues 4 cm caudally to ultimately allow a 3-cm vaginal resection.

⑪ **Uterosacral Ligament Transection.** The uterosacral ligaments, which are now isolated, can then be ligated as close to the sacrum as possible with an energy-based

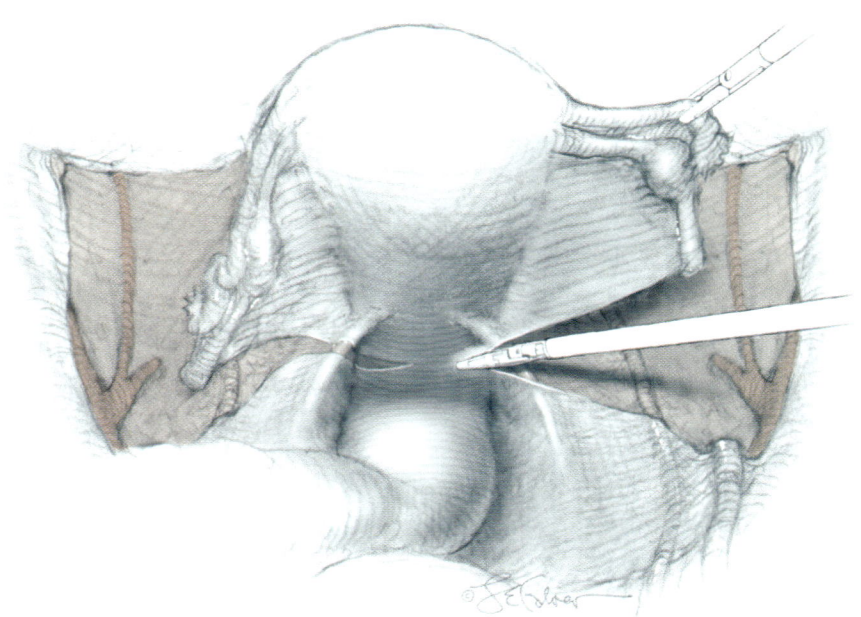

FIGURE 46-3.10 Incising the posterior peritoneum.

tool (Fig. 46-3.12). Before division of the ligament, the ureter is retracted laterally for protection.

⑫ **Cardinal Ligament Division.** Next, the lateral attachments of the cervix to the pelvic sidewalls are coagulated and transected with an energy-based device in a caudal direction (Fig. 46-3.13). During this step, the deep uterine vein is usually encountered and should be sufficiently sealed and divided. Also, the plane of transection stays at or slightly below the level of the ureter. This avoids extensive autonomic pelvic plexus

damage, which exacerbates bladder and possibly bowel and sexual dysfunction.

⑬ **Vaginal Resection.** With complete mobilization of the bladder and rectum, the anterior and posterior vagina should be easily identified. The radical hysterectomy specimen is now held in place only by the paracolpium and vagina. With the base of the bladder and ureter in clear view, the paracolpium is divided on each side using an electrosurgical bipolar coagulating device.

The goal of radical hysterectomy resection is to remove approximately 3 cm of the

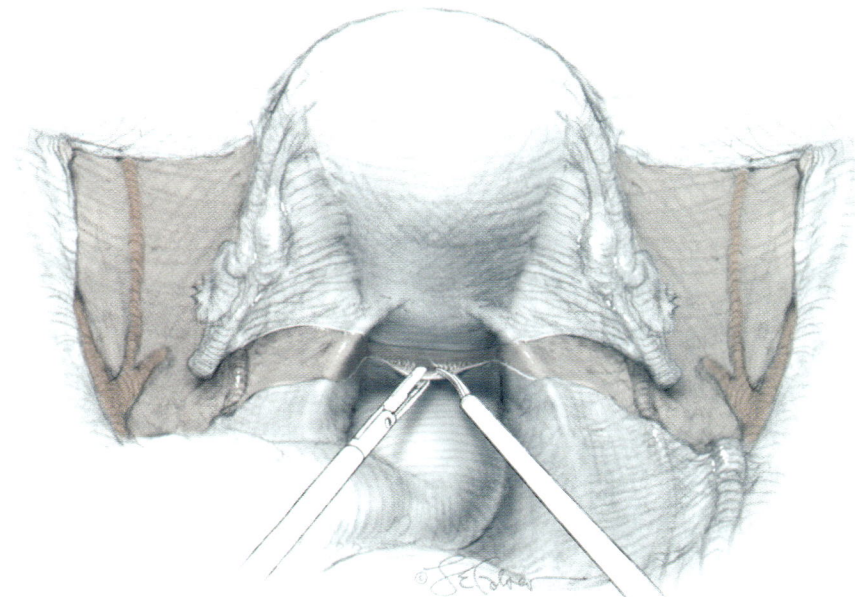

FIGURE 46-3.11 Opening the rectovaginal space.

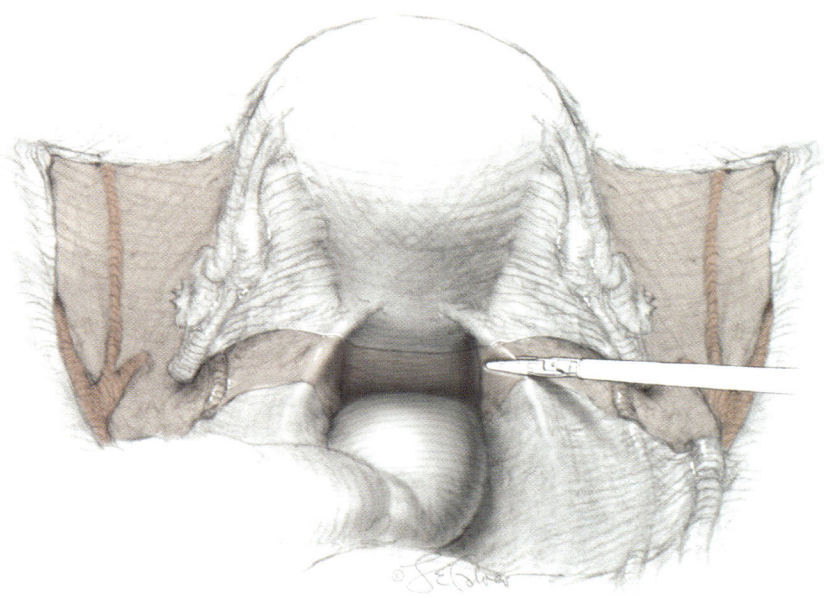

FIGURE 46-3.12 Uterosacral ligament transection.

upper vagina. For this, transverse anterior and posterior colpotomy incisions are made and extended circumferentially around the cervix.

The uterus, cervix, vaginal margin, and parametrial tissue are then freed. The specimen is removed intact through the vagina. The final specimen is labeled "radical hysterectomy specimen" and includes cervix, uterus, vaginal margin, parametrial tissue, and perhaps adnexa (Fig. 46-3.14).

⓮ Vaginal Cuff Closure. Closure of the vaginal cuff can be performed by multiple methods. As noted earlier, one option is cuff closure from a vaginal approach as done during simple vaginal hysterectomy (Section 43-13, p. 969). Alternatively, suitable endoscopic closure techniques are described and detailed in Section 44-11 (p. 1053). Following cuff closure, lymphadenectomy is begun and is described in Section 46-12 (p. 1201).

Both the ureters and bladder can be injured during these procedures. If injury is suspected, cystoscopy at the end of the procedure can aid injury recognition (Section 45-1, p. 1075).

⓯ Port Removal and Fascial Closure. Once procedures have been completed, an inspection for hemostasis is performed. Ports are then removed under direct visualization. All fascial defects ≥10 mm are closed with 0-gauge delayed-absorbable suture to avoid hernia development at the site. Various methods of skin closure are described in Chapter 41 (p. 895).

POSTOPERATIVE

Immediate postoperative care following MIS radical hysterectomy in general mirrors that for other MIS procedures. Diet is advanced more quickly than with open procedures, and most patients will tolerate a regular diet early on postoperative day 1. Patients are often discharged home on postoperative day 1 or 2 since their pain is well controlled. As with open radical procedures, the same principles for retaining a Foley catheter do apply. Therefore, many patients will be sent home with the Foley catheter and return to clinic for a voiding trial (Chap. 42, p. 919). Other postoperative care points are similar to those for open radical hysterectomy (p. 1165).

Following MIS radical hysterectomy, patients may be at higher risk for vaginal cuff dehiscence compared with an open approach. In one series, the rate was 1.7 percent and was similar whether surgery was completed laparoscopically or robotically (Nick, 2011). Preventatively, sound initial surgical technique strives to minimize electrosurgical damage during colpotomy creation. Full-thickness closure of the viable vaginal wall should be ensured, and delayed-absorbable suture is preferred to absorbable. The route of cuff closure is likely less important than these clinical points. Data support both laparoscopic and vaginal approaches to cuff closure (Stevens, 2013; Uccella, 2012, 2018).

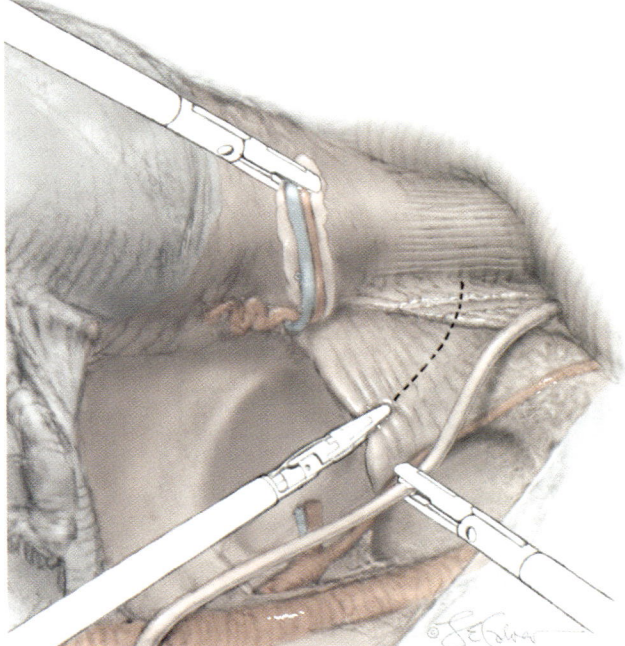

FIGURE 46-3.13 Paracolpium transected.

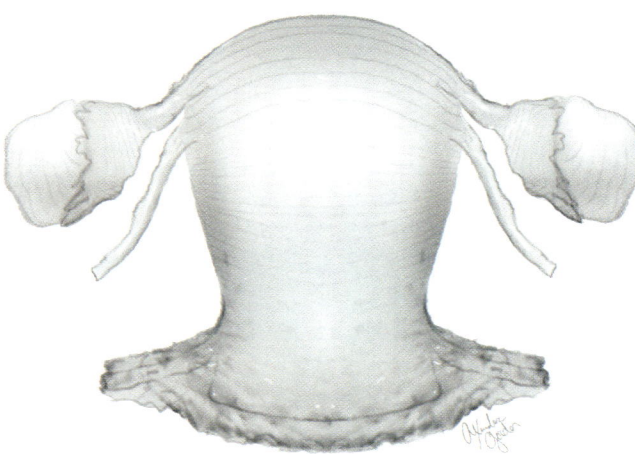

FIGURE 46-3.14 Anterior view of a radical hysterectomy specimen including uterus, cervix, proximal vagina, and parametria.

46-4

Total Pelvic Exenteration

Total pelvic exenteration removes the bladder, rectum, uterus (if present), and surrounding tissues. As such, creation of a urinary conduit and colostomy or low rectal anastomosis is required. Vaginal reconstruction may be elected and performed concurrently.

Because of the extreme radicality of this procedure, it is generally indicated for curative situations when less radical surgery, chemotherapy, or radiation options have been exhausted. The most common indication is centrally persistent or recurrent cervical cancer after radiation therapy. Less frequent indications include some instances of recurrent endometrial adenocarcinoma, uterine sarcoma, or vulvar cancer; locally advanced carcinoma of the cervix, vagina, or endometrium when radiation is contraindicated such as prior radiotherapy or malignant fistula; and melanoma of the vagina or urethra (Berek, 2005; Goldberg, 2006; Maggioni, 2009). Palliative exenterations may be of benefit on rare occasions when selected patients have severe, unrelenting symptoms (Guimarães, 2011).

Exenteration commonly follows radiation therapy, and the uterus and cervix usually have lost their distinct tissue architecture and boundaries. As a result, traditional hysterectomy steps and anatomic landmark identification are typically not possible. Minimally invasive exenterative procedures have been reported and may rarely be indicated in highly selected patients (Bizzarri, 2019; Martinez, 2011; Puntambekar, 2006).

Total pelvic exenterations are subclassified based on the extent of pelvic floor muscle and vulvar resection (Table 46-4.1) (Magrina, 1997). Supralevator (type I) exenteration may be indicated when a lesion is relatively small and does not involve the lower half of the vagina. Most total pelvic exenterations will be infralevator (type II). This type is selected if vaginal contracture, prior hysterectomy, or the inability to otherwise achieve adequate margins is present. Rarely, tumor extension warrants an infralevator exenteration with vulvectomy (type III).

PREOPERATIVE

Patient Evaluation

Initially, biopsy confirmation of recurrent invasive disease is performed. With confirmation, the single most important preoperative challenge is to search for metastatic disease that would abort plans for surgery. A positron emission tomography (PET) scan is particularly helpful in this role (Chung, 2006; Husain, 2007; Kim, 2019). Hydroureter and hydronephrosis are not absolute contraindications unless they are due to obvious pelvic sidewall disease.

Patients often initially reject the entire concept of this operation even when faced with the knowledge that it represents their only chance for cure. Counseling is essential, and overcoming denial may take several visits. Regardless, not all eligible women will wish to proceed.

Consent

The consenting process is the ideal time to finalize plans for the type and location of urinary conduit, plans for colostomy or low rectal anastomoses, and need for vaginal reconstruction or other ancillary procedures. A patient is also advised that the procedure may need to be aborted based on intraoperative findings.

For those who undergo exenteration, the perioperative mortality rate approaches 2 percent (Matsuo, 2019). However, the mortality rate from progressive cancer would otherwise be 100 percent. Patients should be prepared for admission to an intensive care unit (ICU) postoperatively. Infection, wound breakdown, bowel obstruction, and venous thromboembolic events are common short-term complications. Additionally, intestinal fistulas or anastomotic leaks or strictures may develop. Reoperation may be required. Most women will experience significant morbidity and unforeseen complications (Berek, 2005; Goldberg, 2006; Maggioni, 2009). Preexisting medical problems, morbid obesity, and malnutrition raise these risks (Matsuo, 2019; Tortorella, 2019).

Long-term effects on sexual function and other body functions are candidly reviewed. Patients with two ostomies have a lower quality of life and poorer body image. However, in those who retain vaginal capacity, quality of life and sexual function is reportedly improved compared with those without reconstruction. Thus, counseling regarding vaginal reconstruction is part of the preoperative dialogue (Section 46-9, p. 1190). In general, a woman returns to baseline functioning within a year postoperatively, but quality of life is often affected by worries regarding tumor progression (Hawighorst-Knapstein, 1997; Rezk, 2013). Patients should be aware that more than half will develop recurrent disease despite exenterative surgery (Benn, 2011; Westin, 2014).

Patient Preparation

Prior to surgery, stoma sites are marked, the consent form is reviewed, and final questions are answered. To minimize fecal contamination during bowel excision, oral bowel preparation such as with a polyethylene glycol with electrolyte solution (GoLYTELY) is mandatory. Ileus is common following exenteration, and nutritional demands are increased. Thus, total parenteral nutrition (TPN) is often initiated as early as possible when needed. In addition, routine antibiotic prophylaxis decreases infectious complications (Goldberg, 1998). Pneumatic compression devices and prophylactic-dose LMWH or UFH heparin is particularly important due to the anticipated long operation and extended postoperative recovery (Gould, 2012; Key, 2019). Patients are typed and crossmatched for potential blood product replacement. Critical care team consultation may be indicated, and an ICU bed is requested.

TABLE 46-4.1. Differences among Pelvic Exenteration Types

Pelvic Structure	Type I Supralevator	Type II Infralevator	Type III Infralevator with Vulvectomy
	Degree of Resection		
Viscera	Above levator	Below levator	Below levator
Levator ani muscles	None	Limited	Complete
Perineal membrane (Urogenital diaphragm)	None	Limited	Complete
Vulvoperineal tissues	None	None	Complete

INTRAOPERATIVE

Instruments

To prepare for complicated resections, a surgeon should have access to all types and sizes of bowel staplers. These include end-to-end anastomosis (EEA), gastrointestinal anastomosis (GIA), and transverse anastomosis (TA) staplers. Additionally, an electrosurgical bipolar coagulation device (LigaSure, ENSEAL) can speed pedicle ligation while decreasing blood loss (Slomovitz, 2006).

Surgical Steps

❶ Anesthesia and Patient Positioning. General anesthesia with or without epidural placement for postoperative pain management is mandatory. An arterial line for monitoring is typically added as a necessary precaution. Bimanual examination is performed to reorient a surgeon to a patient's individual anatomy. The abdomen, perineum, and vagina are surgically prepared, and a Foley catheter is inserted. For VTE prophylaxis, lower-extremity pneumatic compression devices are placed. Legs should be positioned in low lithotomy in booted support stirrups to permit adequate perineal access.

❷ Abdominal Entry. The type of abdominal entry may be dictated by an intended rectus abdominis flap, which requires a low transverse incision. Otherwise, a midline vertical incision is ideal. A less commonly employed option is to initially assess by laparoscopy a patient's suitability for exenteration. This minimally invasive approach may avoid unnecessary laparotomy in up to half of candidate patients (Kohler, 2002; Plante, 1998).

❸ Exploration. The most common reason that exenterations are aborted is the presence of metastatic peritoneal disease (Miller, 1993). Thus, following positioning of an abdominal self-retaining retractor, a surgeon thoroughly explores for disseminated disease that may not have been suspected preoperatively. Typically, numerous adhesions must be lysed to inspect and palpate abdominal contents. Suspicious lesions are removed or biopsied.

❹ Lymph Node Dissection. A significant number of exenterations will be aborted intraoperatively due to identification of lymph node metastases (Miller, 1993). For this reason, pelvic and paraaortic node sampling and frozen section analysis is performed to exclude metastatic disease before proceeding. Additionally, retroperitoneal dissection provides a surgeon with a sense of the degree of pelvic sidewall fibrosis, which may render the vessels, ureters, and other important structures virtually indistinguishable from the surrounding soft tissue.

❺ Pelvic Sidewall Exploration. As described in Section 46-1 (p. 1162), the retroperitoneum is entered and the external iliac and internal iliac artery bifurcation is bluntly dissected free of overlying areolar connective tissue. The ureter is identified at the pelvic brim and dissected off the medial leaf of the posterior peritoneum. A Penrose drain is looped around the ureter for later identification. The paravesical and pararectal spaces are developed.

Parametrial tumor extension is the third most common reason for aborting exenteration (Miller, 1993). Thus, the pelvic sidewall should be verified to be clinically free of disease. For this, one finger is inserted into the paravesical space, another is in the pararectal space, and intervening tissue is palpated down to the levator plate. There must be a grossly negative margin at the pelvic sidewall to proceed. Tissues may be biopsied and frozen section analysis performed to confirm this impression. Often, it is difficult to know with absolute certainty whether the margins are clear due to the varying extent of retroperitoneal fibrosis encountered.

❻ Bladder Mobilization. The bladder blade is removed from the self-retaining retractor to permit entry into the retropubic space (space of Retzius) and allow blunt reflection of the bladder from the back of the symphysis pubis. To achieve this, downward traction on the bladder and urethra will expose filmy attachments that may be electrosurgically incised (Fig. 46-4.1). Laterally positioned false ligaments of the bladder are divided between clamps or transected with an electrosurgical bipolar coagulation device. This joins the retropubic and paravesical spaces. The bladder should be floppy in the pelvis from loss of its supporting pelvic attachments and is completely freed ventrally. However, the urethra is still attached to the bladder.

❼ Rectal Mobilization. Following mobilization of the bladder, the ureters are held laterally, and the overlying peritoneum at the pelvic brim is divided on each side in a medial direction up to the sigmoid colon mesentery. By inserting a finger into each pararectal space and sweeping medially, it should be possible to develop the avascular plane between the rectosigmoid and the sacrum (retrorectal space).

A surgeon should be confident that no tumor has invaded the sacrum and that they will be able to lift the rectosigmoid out of the pelvis to achieve a posterior margin that is tumor free. This is the last decision to be made before dividing the bowel and beginning steps of the operation that are irreversible.

Once all the tumor boundaries have been assessed, exenteration proceeds by dividing the sigmoid colon with a GIA stapler and dividing the intervening mesenteric tissue and superior rectal vessels (Section 46-21, p. 1226). The proximal sigmoid colon is then packed into the upper abdomen. The distal rectosigmoid is held ventrally and cephalad while a hand is inserted posteriorly to bluntly

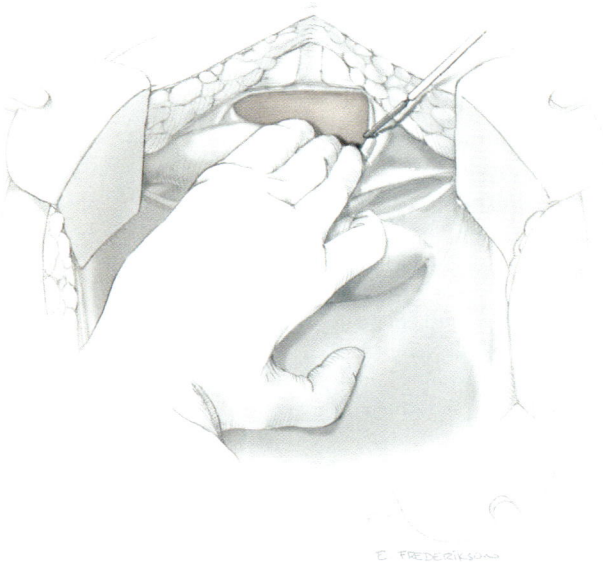

FIGURE 46-4.1 Mobilizing the bladder.

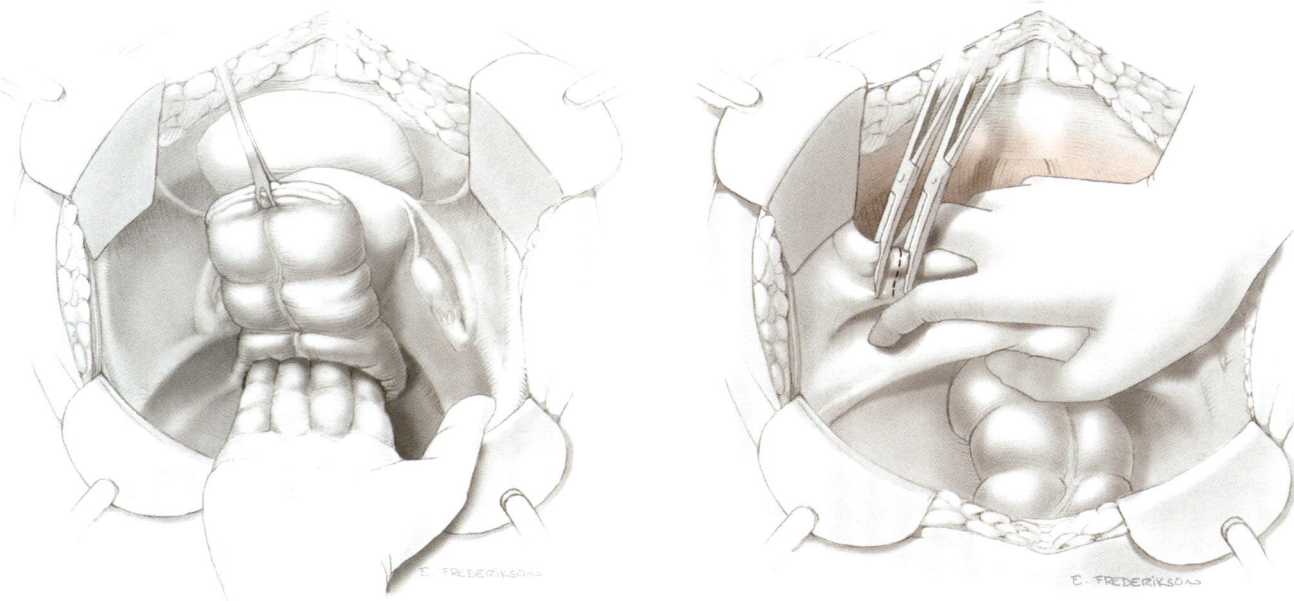

FIGURE 46-4.2 Mobilizing the rectum.

FIGURE 46-4.3 Dividing the cardinal ligaments.

dissect the adventitial tissue between the rectum and sacrum in the midline (Fig. 46-4.2). This maneuver is continued distally to the coccyx to develop the retrorectal space and isolate the laterally located rectal pillars.

❽ Cardinal Ligament Division. The mobilized bladder and distal rectum with uterus (if present) are held together on contralateral traction, while a hand is placed with one finger in the paravesical space and the other in the pararectal space to isolate the lateral pelvic attachments. The cardinal ligaments, internal iliac vessels, and ureter are often not distinguishable in a typically radiated field, but they lie within this tissue. Beginning anteriorly, these fibrous attachments are serially divided at the pelvic sidewall (Fig. 46-4.3). Vascular clips should be available in case of tissue slippage or inadvertent bleeding.

❾ Internal Iliac Vessels and Ureter Division. As the pelvic sidewall dissection continues dorsally, the anterior branches of the internal iliac artery, venous channels, and distal ureter ideally are individually located and ligated to optimize hemostasis (Fig. 46-4.4). However, blood vessels and ureters frequently will lie within fibrous tissue and may be relatively indistinguishable. Thus, clamps or electrosurgical bipolar coagulation device are placed around smaller pedicles to minimize the possibility of inadvertent blood loss. At minimum, the ureter is located, isolated, and divided as distally as possible to provide extra length for reaching the urinary conduit. Later, any damage at the

distal tip can be trimmed as needed to ensure healthy tissue for urinary conduit creation. A large vascular clip is placed on the proximal end of the ureter to distend the lumen and aid later anastomosis into the planned conduit. Dissection is repeated on the contralateral side, and any remaining lateral attachments along the levator ani muscles are divided as the pelvic floor curves toward the perineum.

❿ Rectal Pillar Division. The exenteration specimen is now chiefly tethered by the

rectal stalks and distal mesenteric attachments posteriorly. These can be skeletonized with a right-angle clamp and divided along the pelvic floor (Fig. 46-4.5). This maneuver is continued distally to expose the entire posterior pelvic floor. The exenteration specimen is then circumferentially inspected and additional dissection is performed to completely release it from all attachments leading through the levator ani muscles. At this point, steps diverge depending on whether supralevator or infralevator exenteration is planned.

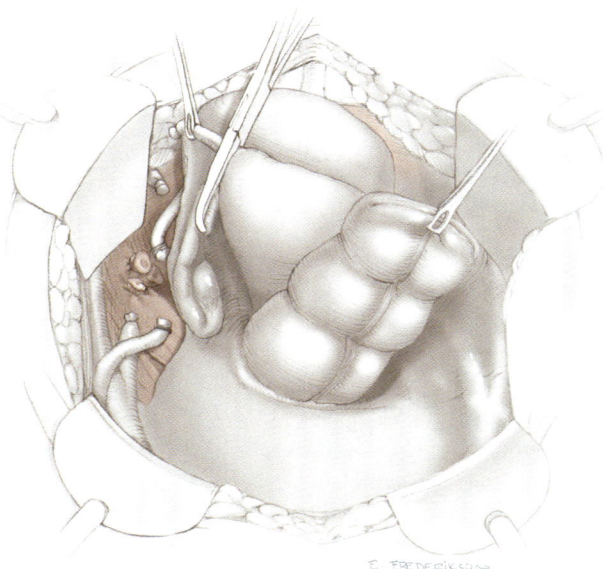

FIGURE 46-4.4 Dividing the hypogastric vessels and ureter.

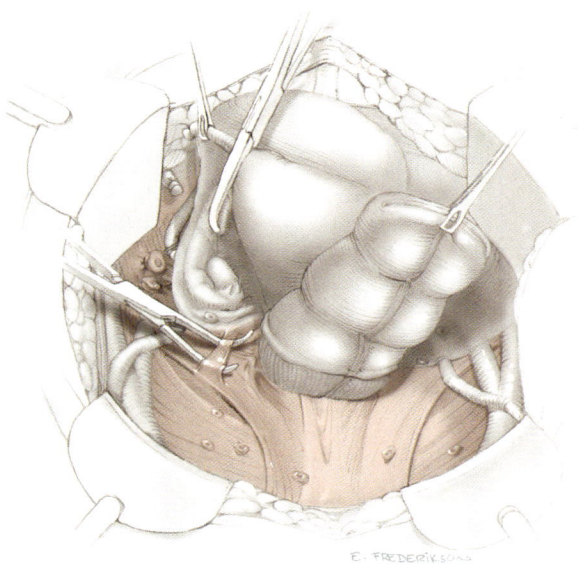

FIGURE 46-4.5 Dividing the rectal pillars.

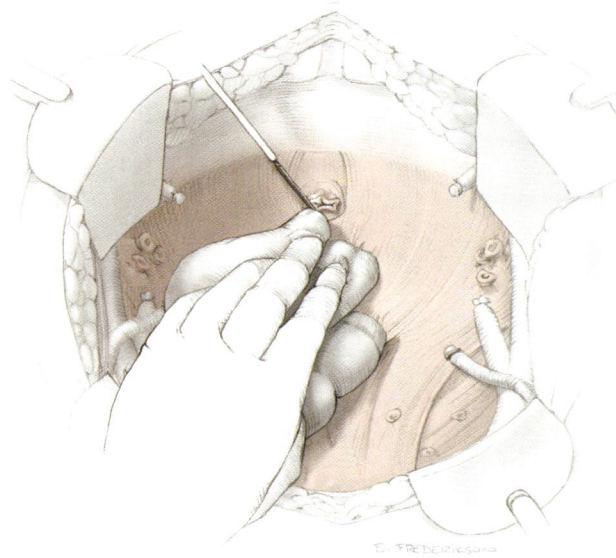

FIGURE 46-4.6 Supralevator exenteration: dividing the urethra.

⑪ Supralevator Exenteration: Final Steps. Removal of the specimen above the levator muscles begins by posterior traction on the bladder. The Foley catheter should be palpable within the urethra, and all surrounding tissue should already be dissected away. An electrosurgical blade is used to transect the distal urethra (Fig. 46-4.6). The distal opening does not require closure and may function as a natural-orifice drain postoperatively. Next, the vagina is transected and closed with 0-gauge delayed-absorbable suture in a running fashion. The transverse anastomosis (TA) or curved cutter stapler

(Contour) is placed across the distal rectum and fired (Fig. 46-4.7). This completes detachment of the specimen, which includes bladder, uterus, rectum, and surrounding tissue. The pelvic floor is then carefully assessed to identify bleeding points (Fig. 46-4.8). A laparotomy pad is packed firmly into the pelvis to tamponade any surface oozing, while the exenteration specimen is inspected to confirm grossly negative margins.

⑫ Infralevator Exenteration: Perineal Phase. With infralevator exenteration, once abdominal dissection reaches the levator muscles,

a second surgical team begins the perineal phase. The use of two teams typically shortens operative time and reduces bleeding. The planned perineal resection is outlined to encompass the tumor. As shown in Figure 46-4.9, resection may require infralevator exenteration with or without vulvectomy.

The perineal incision ideally begins concomitantly with division of the levator muscles by the abdominal team. At the perineum, a skin incision is first performed, followed by use of an electrosurgical blade to dissect through the subcutaneous tissues surrounding the urethra, vaginal opening, and anus.

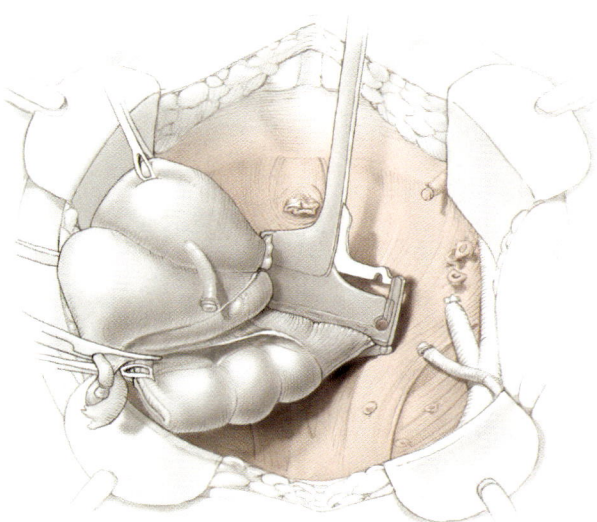

FIGURE 46-4.7 Supralevator exenteration: dividing the rectum.

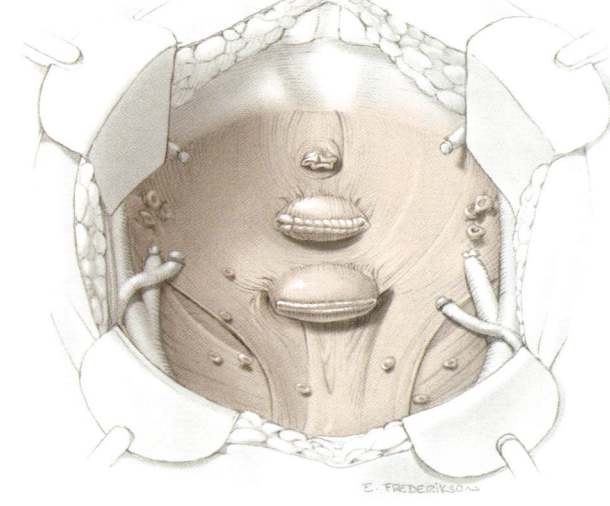

FIGURE 46-4.8 Supralevator exenteration: appearance of the pelvic floor.

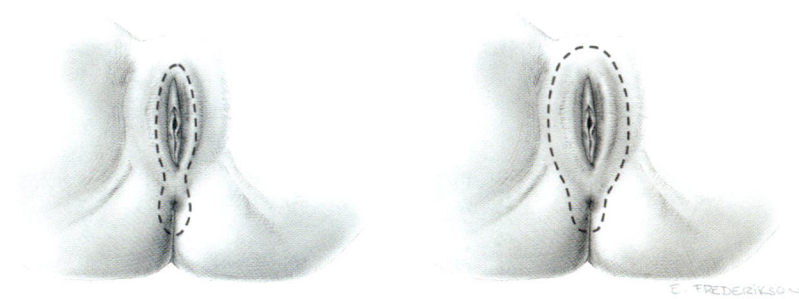

FIGURE 46-4.9 Infralevator exenteration: perineal phase incisions.

⓭ Infralevator Exenteration: Partial Resection of the Levator Muscles. Within the abdomen, the primary surgical team places the specimen on traction. Electrosurgical blade dissection is used to circumferentially incise the levator muscles lateral to the area of tumor extension (Fig. 46-4.10). The dissection proceeds distally toward the perineum.

⓮ Infralevator Exenteration: Connecting the Perineal and Abdominal Spaces. After the perineal incision has reached the fascial plane, four spaces are developed: subpubic space, left and right vaginal spaces, and retrorectal space. It is helpful to have the abdominal surgeon place a hand deep into the pelvis and guide the electrosurgical dissection by the perineal team (Fig. 46-4.11). Five pedicles are identified that separate these avascular spaces: two pubourethral pedicles, two rectal pillar pedicles, and the midline posterior anococcygeal pedicle. Electrosurgical dissection that is directed by the abdominal surgeon's finger

is performed to open the intervening spaces. From below, the five vascular pedicles are divided and ligated using the electrosurgical bipolar coagulation device.

⓯ Infralevator Exenteration: Removal of the Specimen. Circumferential dissection will result in complete detachment of the specimen that can be removed either vaginally or abdominally (Fig. 46-4.12). Hemostasis is then achieved with a series of sutures, vascular clips, or clamps and ties. Finally, the pelvic floor and pedicle sites are carefully reinspected (Fig. 46-4.13).

⓰ Infralevator Exenteration: Simple Closure. The most straightforward and quickest way to close the perineum is for the second team to perform a layered closure of the deep tissues with 0-gauge delayed-absorbable suture (Fig. 46-4.14). The perineal skin is closed with the same type of delayed-absorbable suture in a running fashion.

⓱ Final Steps. A dry laparotomy pad may be held firmly deep in the pelvis to tamponade surface oozing, while the conduit, colostomy or bowel anastomosis, other surgical procedures, or vaginal reconstruction are performed. In some instances, intraoperative radiation therapy can be a useful adjunct for an obviously positive or clinically suspicious resection margin (Backes, 2014; Foley, 2016). An omental J-flap may provide additional blood supply to the irradiated, denuded pelvic floor (Section 46-14, p. 1211). The type of postoperative suction drainage may be dictated by these ancillary procedures but should be used judiciously (Goldberg, 2006).

POSTOPERATIVE

The morbidity of total pelvic exenteration depends on various factors, which include preoperative health of the patient, intraoperative events, extent of the procedure, ancillary procedures, and postoperative vigilance. Hospitals that treat a relatively high volume of such patients report lower surgical in-hospital mortality rates (Maggioni, 2009). However, unlike a few decades ago, few institutions perform this operation on a regular basis.

The immediate life-threatening concerns are massive bleeding, acute respiratory distress syndrome, pulmonary embolism, and myocardial infarction (Fotopoulou, 2010). Every effort is made to encourage early ambulation as soon as the patient is stable. A prolonged ileus or partial small bowel obstruction will

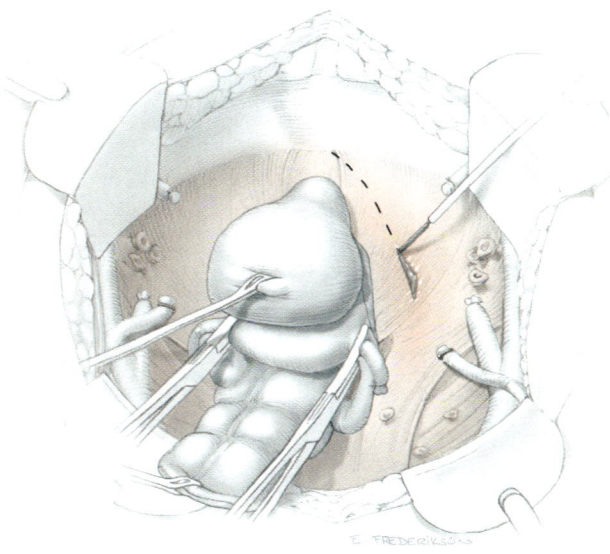

FIGURE 46-4.10 Infralevator exenteration: partial resection of the levator muscles.

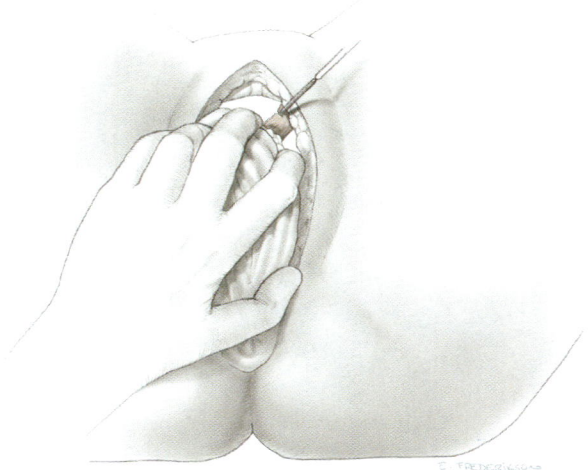

FIGURE 46-4.11 Infralevator exenteration: connecting the perineal and abdominal spaces.

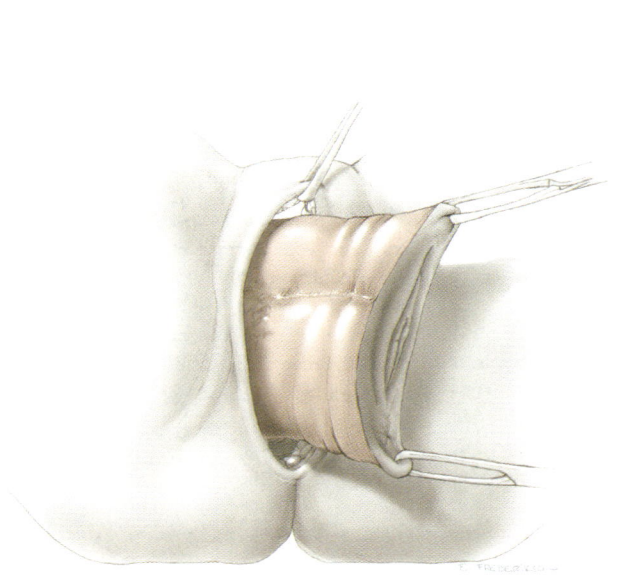

FIGURE 46-4.12 Infralevator exenteration: removal of the specimen.

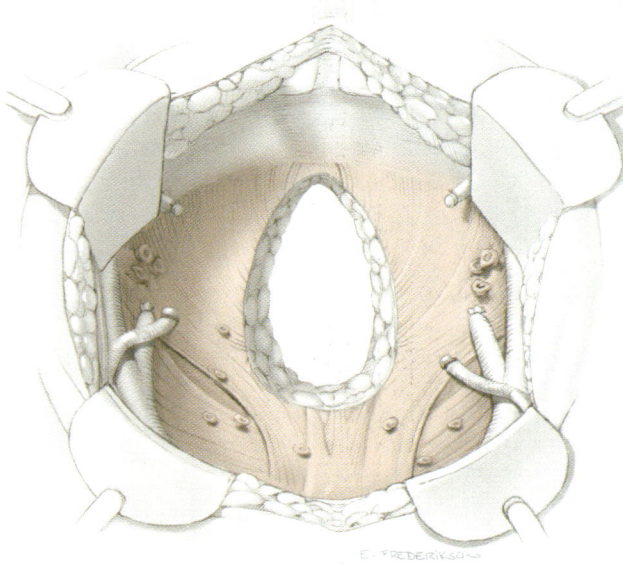

FIGURE 46-4.13 Infralevator exenteration: pelvic floor.

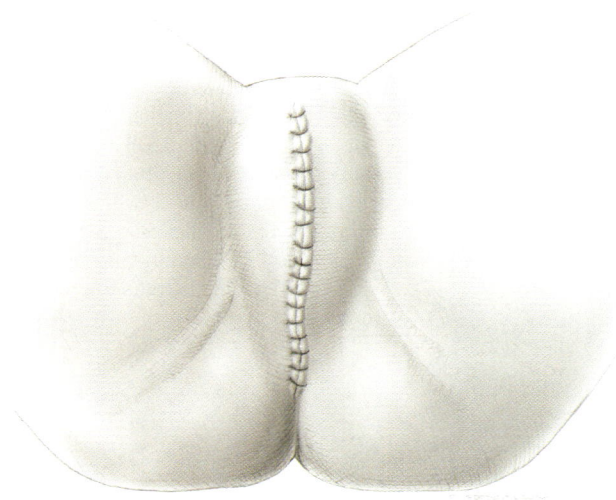

FIGURE 46-4.14 Infralevator exenteration: simple perineal closure.

typically respond to expectant management but may require TPN for weeks. Intestinal fistulas and leaks are more common when using mesh to cover the pelvic floor or when performing low rectal anastomosis. Omental pedicle grafts and rectus abdominis or gracilis myocutaneous flaps may prevent such complications. Pelvic abscess and septicemia are additional subacute complications that develop commonly (Berek, 2005; Goldberg, 2006; Maggioni, 2009). Urinary complications associated with a urinary conduit are discussed in Sections 46-7 and 46-8 (pp. 1182 and 1186). Those associated with low rectal anastomosis are described in Section 46-21 (p. 1228).

46-5

Anterior Pelvic Exenteration

Removal of the uterus, vagina, bladder, urethra, distal ureters, and parametrial tissues with preservation of the rectum is meant to be a less morbid operation than total pelvic exenteration (Section 46-4, p. 1174). That said, construction of a urinary conduit is still required. Either continent or incontinent conduit types are suitable (Uhr, 2013).

Patients are carefully selected for this more limited procedure to still achieve negative surgical margins. Women who have previously had a hysterectomy are not usually good candidates, because a complete resection of a central recurrence involving the vaginal cuff would typically require removal of both bladder and rectosigmoid colon. The most common indications include small recurrences confined to the cervix or anterior vagina after pelvic radiation. In gynecologic oncology, up to half of all exenterations performed are anterior (Berek, 2005; Maggioni, 2009).

PREOPERATIVE

The preoperative evaluation is similar to that described for total pelvic exenteration (Section 46-4, p. 1174). Although preservation of the rectum is planned, patients are advised that potentially unforeseen clinical circumstances may dictate bowel resection and colostomy or low rectal anastomosis. Accordingly, complete oral bowel preparation is still mandatory. Moreover, the patient's abdomen is marked preoperatively for a urinary conduit as well as a descending colostomy.

INTRAOPERATIVE

Surgical Steps

❶ Initial Steps. Anterior exenteration is technically similar to total pelvic exenteration, described earlier. Patients are positioned in low lithotomy in booted support stirrups, and for VTE prophylaxis, lower-extremity pneumatic compression devices are placed. The appropriate skin incision is made, the abdomen is explored, lymph nodes are removed, and spaces are developed to exclude metastatic or unresectable disease. The procedure begins to differ after the bladder has been mobilized. A surgeon then makes the final decision to leave the rectum intact and proceed with anterior pelvic exenteration.

❷ Developing the Rectovaginal Space. Instead of mobilizing the rectum and dividing the sigmoid colon, the rectovaginal space is developed much as in a type III radical hysterectomy (Step 13, p. 1164). The uterosacral ligament and the entire length of the rectal pillars are divided to free the exenteration specimen posteriorly.

❸ Lateral Pelvic Attachments. The mobilized bladder and uterus are held medially to aid in isolation of the cardinal ligaments, internal iliac vessels, and ureter. These structures are successively divided with an electrosurgical bipolar coagulation device (LigaSure, ENSEAL) or are clamped, cut, and individually ligated.

❹ Removal of the Specimen. After the anterior pelvic exenteration specimen has been completely mobilized, the urethra and vagina are divided (Fig. 46-5.1). The urethra is left open, and the vaginal cuff is closed with 0-gauge delayed-absorbable suture in a running fashion (Fig. 46-5.2).

❺ Final Steps. Typically, the lesion is small and lies above the levator ani muscles, thus a perineal phase is not required. For this reason, placement of a myocutaneous flap for vaginal reconstruction may be more problematic in these patients due to limited space in the pelvis.

POSTOPERATIVE

Morbidity of anterior pelvic exenteration is comparable with that of total pelvic exenteration (Section 46-4, p. 1178) (Sharma, 2005). Ideally, the operation is shorter and restoration of bowel function is more rapid. Some patients will experience tenesmus or long-term rectal symptoms that likely stem from interruption of the autonomic nervous system in surrounding tissue.

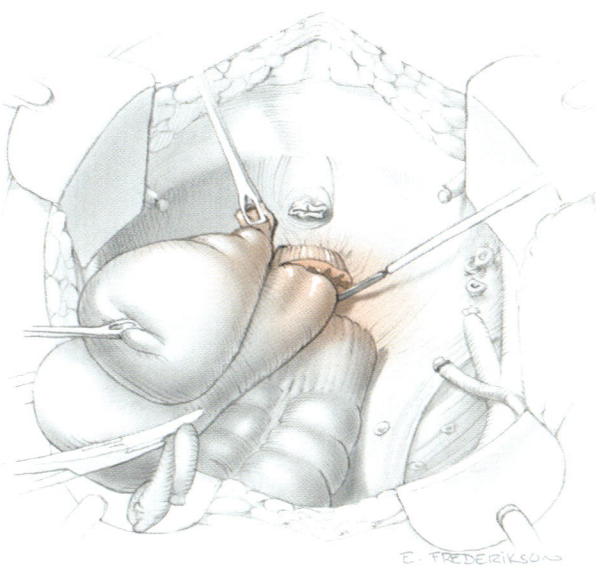
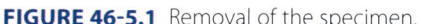

FIGURE 46-5.1 Removal of the specimen.

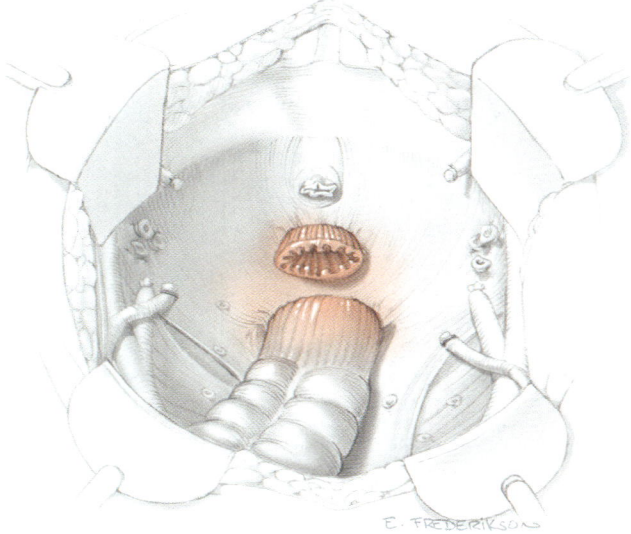

FIGURE 46-5.2 Appearance of the pelvic floor.

Posterior Pelvic Exenteration

Removal of the uterus, vagina, rectum, and parametrial tissues with preservation of the ureters and bladder is meant to be a less morbid operation than total pelvic exenteration (Section 46-4, p. 1174). However, construction of a colostomy or low rectal anastomosis is still required. Vaginal reconstruction may be elected and performed concurrently.

Patients are carefully selected for this more limited procedure to still achieve negative surgical margins. For this reason, women who have previously had a hysterectomy are not usually good candidates. The most common indication is a small postirradiation recurrence primarily involving the posterior vaginal wall or coexisting with a rectovaginal fistula. In gynecologic oncology, fewer than 10 percent of exenterations are posterior (Berek, 2005; Maggioni, 2009).

PREOPERATIVE

Preoperative evaluation is largely identical to that described for total pelvic exenteration (Section 46-4, p. 1174). A surgeon's judgment and experience are critical in deciding to proceed with a more limited operation. However, patients are advised that potentially unforeseen clinical circumstances may dictate resection of the ureters and bladder and formation of a urinary conduit.

INTRAOPERATIVE

Surgical Steps

1 **Initial Steps.** Posterior pelvic exenteration is technically similar to a type III radical hysterectomy but with the addition of rectosigmoid resection and a more extended vaginectomy (Section 46-1, p. 1161). The operation begins as a total pelvic exenteration. Patients are positioned in low lithotomy in booted support stirrups, and for VTE prophylaxis, lower-extremity pneumatic compression devices are placed. The appropriate skin incision is made, the abdomen is explored, lymph

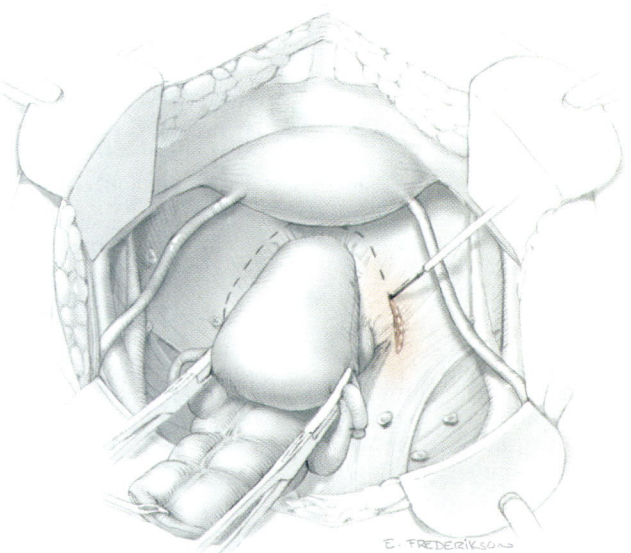

FIGURE 46-6.1 Incising the levator muscles.

nodes are removed, and spaces are developed to exclude metastatic or unresectable disease (Section 46-4, p. 1175). A surgeon then makes the final decision to leave the bladder intact and proceed with posterior exenteration.

2 **Ureteral Dissection.** As with type III radical hysterectomy, the retroperitoneum is entered, ureters are mobilized, uterine arteries are ligated at their internal iliac artery origin, and parametrial tissue is divided at the pelvic sidewall. The bladder is then mobilized away from the cervix and vagina, and ureters are unroofed from the paracervical tunnels. The paracolpium's lateral attachments are then divided all the way to the levator ani muscles. However, typically these steps are much more tedious in a previously irradiated field because of tissue fibrosis and scarring.

3 **Mobilizing the Rectum.** The sigmoid colon is divided with the mesentery and peritoneal attachments, as earlier described for a total pelvic exenteration. The retrorectal space is bluntly dissected to mobilize the rectum and enable transection of the rectal pillars and uterosacral ligaments.

4 **Removal of the Specimen.** The entire specimen may then be placed on traction to

aid placement of the transverse anastomosis (TA) or curved cutter stapler (Contour) and division of the rectum. The rectum is divided below the tumor to leave grossly negative margins.

To encompass the tumor for removal, dissection is continued circumferentially to (or through) the levator ani muscles (Fig. 46-6.1). The distal vagina is transected and sewn closed in a running fashion with 0-gauge delayed-absorbable suture. The specimen is removed.

5 **Final Steps.** Typically, the lesion is small and lies above the levator ani muscles, and thus a perineal phase is usually not required. As a result, placement of a myocutaneous flap for vaginal reconstruction may be more problematic in such patients due to limited space in the pelvis.

POSTOPERATIVE

Morbidity of posterior pelvic exenteration is comparable with that of total pelvic exenteration (Section 46-4, p. 1178) (Sharma, 2005). Ideally, the operation is shorter and urinary complications are less frequent. However, posterior exenteration in a previously irradiated patient frequently results in a contracted bladder and intractable urinary incontinence.

46-7

Incontinent Urinary Conduit

Removal of the bladder during total or anterior exenteration is the main indication for an incontinent urinary conduit. Less commonly, an otherwise irreparable postirradiation vesicovaginal fistula may warrant urinary diversion. Following cystectomy, an isolated resected segment of bowel that maintains its mesenteric connection and vascular supply is used as the new urine reservoir. A stoma is crafted using one end of the bowel segment and an opening in the anterior abdominal wall. Ureters are reimplanted into the opposite end of this isolated bowel segment.

Various techniques are available to create such urinary conduits, and these are categorized as *incontinent diversions* or *continent diversions*. An incontinent diversion is the simplest to create, but postoperatively a patient must continuously wear an ostomy bag. These conduits are often preferable for medically compromised patients, the elderly, and anyone with a short life expectancy. Alternatively, a continent urinary reservoir can be created that is emptied by intermittent patient self-catheterization of the bowel stoma.

Of incontinent diversions, an *ileal conduit* has historically been the most common urinary diversion used in gynecologic oncology (Goldberg, 2006). However, this bowel segment and distal ureters invariably lie within a previously irradiated field. Conduit construction with radiation-damaged bowel may lead to higher rates of stenosis or leakage at the ureteral anastomotic sites (Pycha, 2008). The *transverse colon conduit* is a successful alternative for previously irradiated patients (Segreti, 1996; Soper, 1989). *Sigmoid conduits* are generally less desirable due to preexisting radiation damage and proximity to a concurrent colostomy site. Electrolyte abnormalities such as chronic metabolic acidosis and hypokalemia are an associated risk. The *jejunal conduit* is another rarely used option that typically lies outside the radiation field. However, jejunal absorption of potassium and resulting hyperkalemia make this a less-desired option (Eskandar, 2008).

The basic principles of constructing an incontinent urinary conduit are the same, regardless of the intestinal segment used. First, healthy-appearing bowel with a good blood supply is selected. Second, wide-caliber ureterointestinal anastomoses and ureteral stenting are essential to minimize the risk of anastomosis stenosis. Third, sufficient mobility of the ureters and bowel segment help avoid tension that might lead to anastomotic leaks. Last, creation of a straight tunnel through the abdominal wall helps prevent bowel kinking and obstruction.

PREOPERATIVE

Patient Evaluation

The preoperative evaluation is usually dictated by the preceding exenterative procedure. The specific decision is whether to plan for an incontinent or continent urinary conduit. Patients are extensively counseled regarding the differences. The type of conduit selected should be considered permanent, although later conversions are possible (Benezra, 2004).

Consent

Patients are advised that intraoperative findings may dictate revision of an original surgical plan. Postoperatively, urinary infections with or without pyelonephritis are common with any type of conduit. Anastomotic leaks are less frequent with routine postoperative ureteral stenting but can contribute to a prolonged ileus, the need for CT-guided urinoma drainage, or potentially, surgical reexploration with revision. Episodes of small bowel obstruction are possible and often develop at the site where the bowel segment was harvested and the remaining bowel ends were reanastomosed. In the long term, ureteral strictures or stenosis may compromise renal function. Infrequently, reoperation is necessary for complications that do not respond to conservative management (Houvenaeghel, 2004).

Patient Preparation

Oral bowel preparation is mandatory, but other preparation steps are typically dictated by the preceding exenterative surgery (Section 46-4, p. 1174). Ideally, an enterostomal therapist is available to mark a conduit stoma site, typically on the abdomen's right side, that is unobstructed in the supine, sitting, and standing positions.

INTRAOPERATIVE

Surgical Steps

❶ Initial Steps. To avoid unnecessary traction on its anastomoses, the incontinent urinary conduit is constructed as the last major intraabdominal step during exenterative surgery. Hemostasis is achieved before beginning the conduit. Anesthesia, patient positioning, and skin incisions are typically dictated by the preceding operation.

❷ Exploration. The bowel segment for the planned conduit is carefully inspected. It must appear healthy, be untethered, and lie close to the distal ureters. The final decision is then made regarding which type of incontinent conduit is best for the circumstances. If the distal ileum has the typical leathery, pale, mottled appearance of radiation injury, a conduit should be prepared from the transverse colon. Overlooking the importance of this decision can lead to various otherwise preventable complications intraoperatively and postoperatively.

❸ Ileal Conduit: Preparing the Bowel Segment. The ileocecal junction is located, and the ileum is elevated to identify a bowel segment with the most mobility to reach the stoma site on the right side of the anterior abdominal wall. Ideally, the proximal end of the segment lies 25 to 30 cm from the ileocecal valve, which is a watershed area and necessary for absorption of bile salts and fat-soluble vitamins. *Watershed regions* in general receive dual blood supply from the very distal branches of two arteries and thereby are vulnerable to ischemia. At the selected site, the mesentery is scored on each side with an electrosurgical blade to aid insertion of a hemostat directly beneath the bowel loop. A Penrose drain is then pulled through. This will mark the proximal end along the ileum that will eventually become the distal part of the conduit and will form the abdominal wall stoma.

The conduit length depends on subcutaneous tissue depth and ileum mobility but should measure approximately 15 cm. The conduit's internal or butt end will house the ureteral anastomoses and is selected by measuring the ileum that lies distal to the Penrose drain, and again the mesentery is scored. The gastrointestinal anastomosis (GIA) stapler is then inserted to divide the distal bowel segment (Fig. 46-7.1). The point of division ideally is at least 15 cm from the ileocecal valve. The conduit is remeasured prior to dividing the proximal ileum, to account for possible shrinkage of the intervening segment and to again ensure sufficient length.

Once the bowel is stapled and divided, the conduit mesentery also is carefully divided on each end of the segment. This tissue division is angled inward and toward the base of the mesentery near its insertion to the posterior abdominal wall. This provides adequate mobility. The vasculature may be compromised if too much mesentery is divided, whereas too little will result in tension on the conduit. A perfect balance is required.

When convenient, intestinal continuity, minus the excised segment, is reestablished anterior to the conduit. This is completed by side-to-side small-bowel reanastomosis

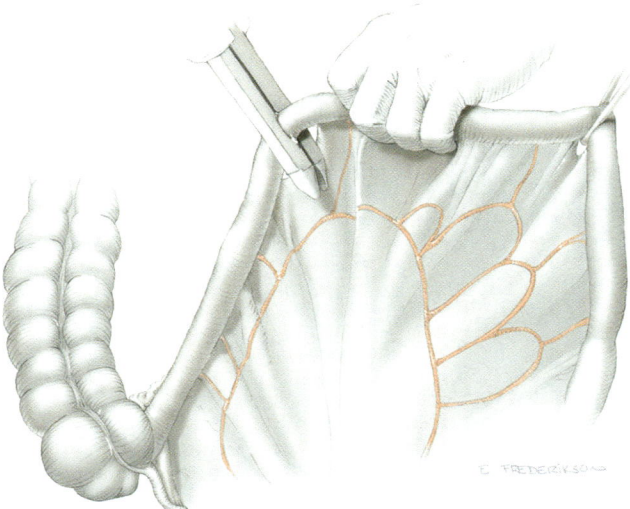

FIGURE 46-7.1 Ileal conduit: preparing the bowel segment.

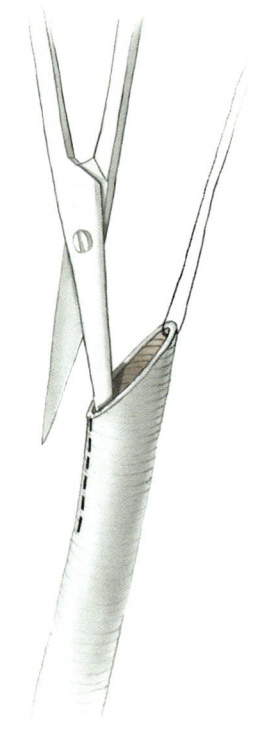

FIGURE 46-7.2 Ileal conduit: spatulating the ureter.

using the GIA and TA staplers as described in Section 46-20 (p. 1223).

④ Ileal Conduit: Preparing the Ureters. The staple line is excised from the stomal end of the conduit, and the conduit is irrigated into a basin. The ureters should now be engorged from the vascular clips placed earlier during exenteration. The distal end of each ureter should have a stay suture placed for traction. To prevent focal necrosis that may impede successful anastomosis, ureters are never directly grasped with forceps or roughly handled. They are sharply freed from their retroperitoneal attachments so that they easily reach past the point of their planned anastomosis into the conduit. The left ureter is brought *under* the inferior mesenteric artery (IMA) to prevent acute angulation and kinking. This ureter ultimately exits from beneath the base of the sigmoid colon mesentery to reach the conduit.

⑤ Ileal Conduit: Ureteral Anastomoses. The distal tip of the left ureter is cut at a 45-degree angle just behind the vascular clip placed during exenteration. If the distal ends of the ureters exhibit fibrosis, they are trimmed to reach healthy-appearing tissue. The prior distal stay-suture is removed with this trimming. Urine will drain into the abdomen while a 4-0 delayed-absorbable stay suture is placed outside-to-in through the ureter's distal tip. This leads to final knots that will lie outside the anastomosis lumen. The needle is left on this traction stitch since it will be the final suture in the anastomosis.

Fine-tip scissors are used to spatulate the ureter for approximately 1 cm, but the length is customized depending on the caliber of the ureteral lumen (Fig. 46-7.2). This maneuver increases the anastomosis diameter to

help reduce the possibility of future ureteral stricture. A 6F or 7F single-J ureteral stent is inserted into the ureter and advanced into the left renal pelvis until resistance is met. A 4-0 gauge absorbable suture, which will later dissolve, is used to secure the stent to the muscular wall of the ureter.

Adson forceps are used to grasp a small section of the ileal serosa to which the left ureter will reach. This site is ideally approximately 2 cm from the butt end of the conduit on the anterior side of the antimesenteric surface. Metzenbaum scissors remove a small, full-thickness section of bowel wall (Fig. 46-7.3). The ileal mucosa should be easily visible.

A long tonsil clamp is inserted into the open end of the conduit, and the ureteral stent is grasped and pulled through. The prepared ureteral end is then sewn to the ileum. For this, the first suture is placed at the apex of the spatulation with a full-thickness bite through the ureteral wall and bowel mucosa

(Fig. 46-7.4). Two or three adjoining mucosa-to-mucosa sutures are placed. The left ureteral anastomosis is completed with additional circumferential sutures to achieve a watertight closure.

The anastomotic site for the right ureter is selected at least 2 to 3 cm distal to that of the left along the length of the conduit. The entire procedure is then repeated. Saline with methylene blue dye is used to fill the conduit and observe for watertight integrity. Any anastomotic leaks must be reinforced with additional sutures and retested. If

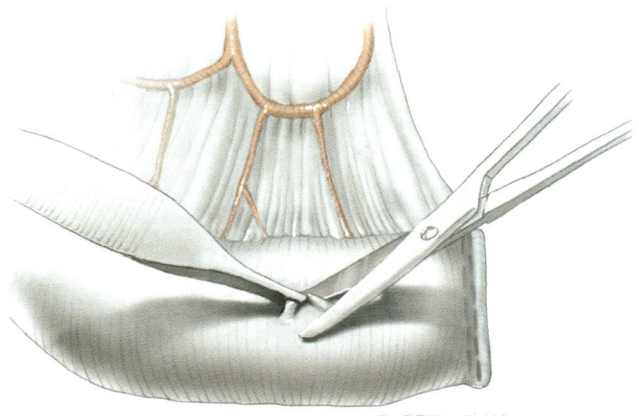

FIGURE 46-7.3 Ileal conduit: ileal incision.

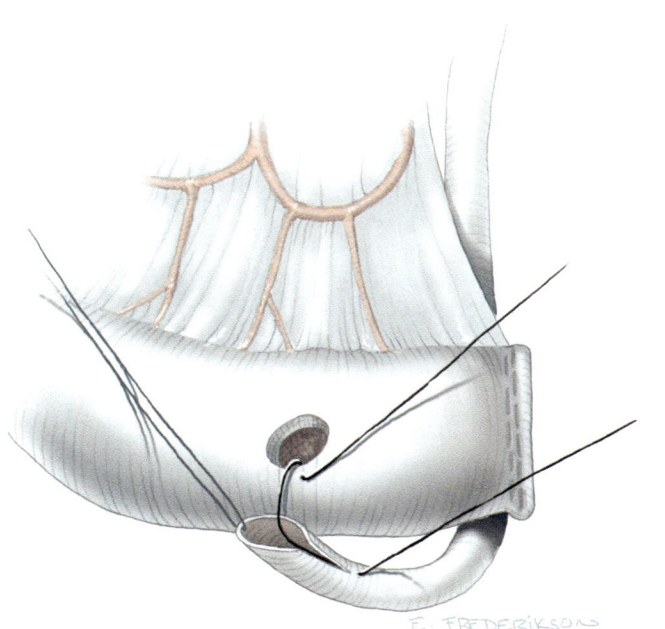

FIGURE 46-7.4 Ileal conduit: suturing ureter and ileal segment.

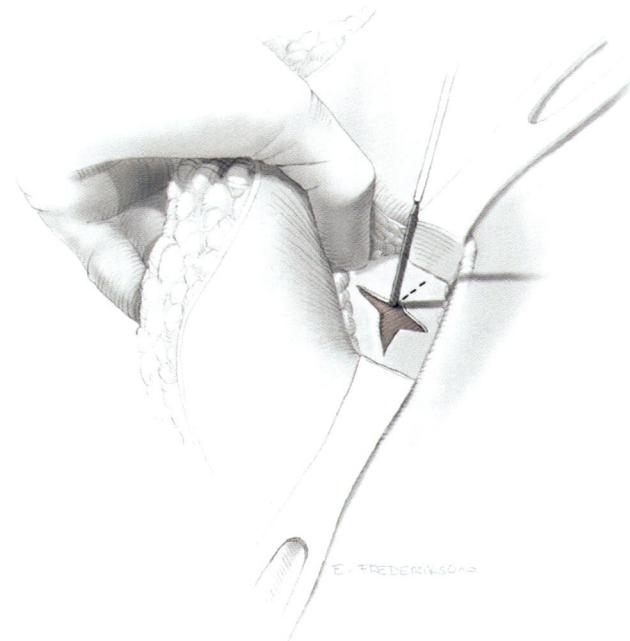

FIGURE 46-7.5 Ileal conduit: making the stoma.

leakage persists or if there is concern about the mucosa-to-mucosa apposition, the entire anastomosis should be redone.

This butt end of the conduit is next secured to the sacral promontory, iliopsoas muscle, or posterior peritoneum with two or three delayed-absorbable sutures through the seromuscular layer of the conduit. Stabilizing the conduit in this way will prevent undue tension on the ureteral anastomoses when the patient is upright and gravity allows the intestines to slide into the pelvis.

❻ Ileal Conduit: Stoma Creation. The skin at the proposed stoma site is elevated with a Kocher clamp. An electrosurgical blade, set on cutting mode, is used to excise a small circle of skin. The subcutaneous fat is separated by blunt dissection until the fascia is visible. A cruciate incision is made with an electrosurgical blade (Fig. 46-7.5). The rectus abdominis muscle is split longitudinally and another cruciate incision is created in the peritoneum. The opening is bluntly expanded until it easily accommodates two fingers.

The stoma and stents are carefully pulled through the incision until at least 2 cm of ileum protrudes through the skin (Fig. 46-7.6). The mesentery may need to

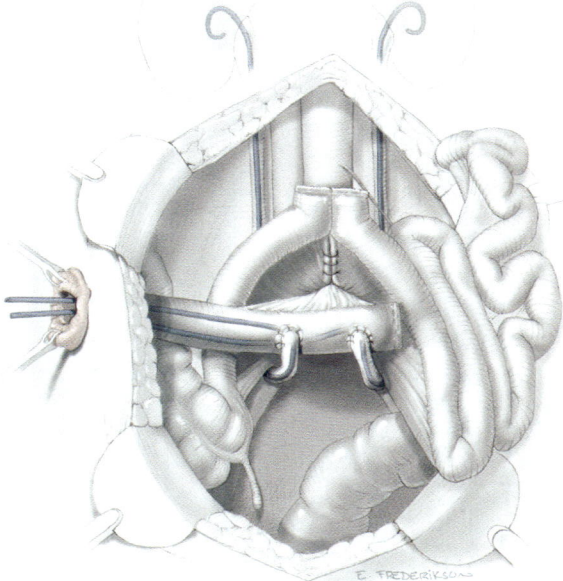

FIGURE 46-7.6 Ileal conduit: stoma with stents carefully pulled through abdominal incision.

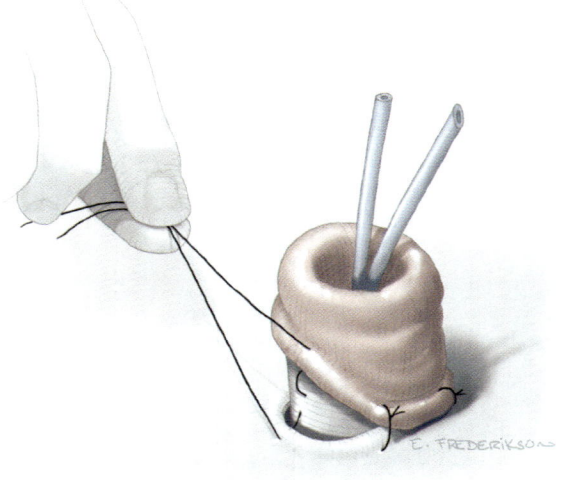

FIGURE 46-7.7 Ileal conduit: suturing the stoma.

be trimmed or the abdominal wall opening further dissected to accommodate the conduit. The mucosal edge of the bowel is everted. The stoma is completed with 3-0 gauge delayed-absorbable "rosebud" stitches that include the ileal mucosa, intervening bowel serosa, and skin dermis (Fig. 46-7.7). Circumferential sutures are placed.

Both stents are trimmed to fit in the stoma bag. To enable correct identification postoperatively, the right ureteral stent is cut at a "right" angle. Individual silk sutures placed through each stent may be secured at the skin to prevent stent dislodgment over the first few postoperative days.

❼ **Transverse Colon Conduit.** For this type of conduit, the hepatic and splenic flexures of the transverse colon are fully mobilized. In addition, the omentum is detached. Division points are marked with Penrose drains and transected (Fig. 46-7.8). The transverse mesocolon is then divided, as shown by the dotted lines, to provide sufficient mobility while preserving the middle colic artery. When performed in the usual setting of an exenteration with left lower quadrant colostomy, the bowel segment must measure approximately 20 cm to reach the right lower quadrant. Often, this requires incorporation of the hepatic flexure into the conduit and yields an antiperistaltic orientation, that is, urine ultimately flows through the conduit in the opposite direction that fecal waste would normally be propelled. Thus, the proximal bowel segment (nearest the cecum) will be the end of the conduit that eventually is brought through the abdominal wall.

Ureters are sufficiently mobilized in the retroperitoneal space, and both are brought out through a commodious peritoneal opening to reach the conduit. The left ureter will need to be brought across the aorta *proximal* to the IMA (unlike the ileal conduit). The ureteral anastomoses are then completed, ideally at the teniae coli, over stents. To prevent postoperative sliding and tension on the anastomoses, the conduit's butt end is secured to the sacrum, iliopsoas muscle, or posterior peritoneum with interrupted delayed-absorbable suture. Intestinal continuity is reestablished anterior to the conduit by a functional end-to-end anastomosis using EEA and TA staplers, as described in Section 46-18 (p. 1220). The stoma can be made at the preselected site, but it can be repositioned almost anywhere that the conduit will comfortably reach. The stomal end of the conduit is brought through the anterior abdominal wall and secured (Fig. 46-7.9).

❽ **Final Steps.** Mesenteric defects are closed to prevent internal hernias but not so tightly as to compromise blood supply. A suction drain may be placed if integrity of

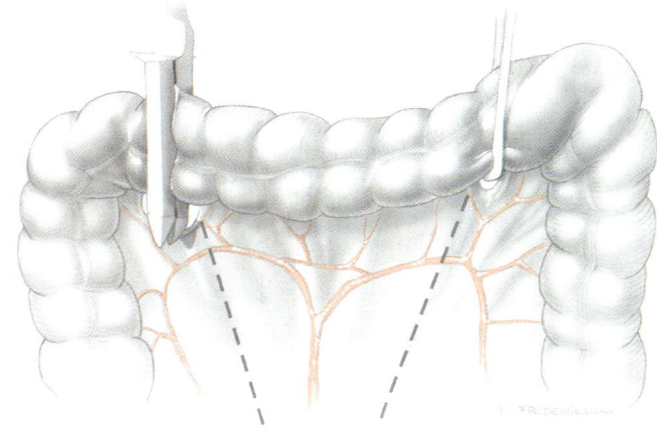

FIGURE 46-7.8 Transverse colon conduit: preparing the bowel segment.

the anastomoses and leakage is a concern. If the stoma appears dusky, the abdominal wall tunnel may be too tight, the mesentery may be twisted or placed on too much tension, or the blood supply may not be sufficient. The last circumstance is the worst, and it generally requires trimming of the distal end of the bowel or occasionally redoing the entire conduit. Either is preferable to avoid problematic retraction, stricture, or necrosis.

POSTOPERATIVE

The stoma is regularly checked for viability during the immediate postoperative recovery period and should show a pink, moist mucosa. Both stents should be functioning. A dry stent that does not respond to irrigation should prompt an IVP or CT urography to exclude ureteral obstruction. Urinary fistula or ureteral obstruction is uncommon but can lead to potentially life-threatening sepsis or

renal failure if not addressed with percutaneous drainage or reoperation. Prolonged bowel dysfunction may indicate an anastomotic urine leak or obstruction of the small bowel.

Patients often are readmitted within a few weeks of surgery due to partial small bowel obstruction, urinary infection, wound separation, or other relatively minor complications of exenteration. These typically resolve with targeted supportive care. Long-term complications include ureteral stenosis and renal loss. Renal function may deteriorate due to chronic infection and reflux. When patients cannot be otherwise managed, they may require long-term percutaneous nephrostomy tubes, indwelling stents, or reoperation and conduit or stoma revision.

Predictably, the overall morbidity of creating an incontinent conduit is much higher in previously irradiated patients (Houvenaeghel, 2004). Tissue quality and mobility are especially important in these patients.

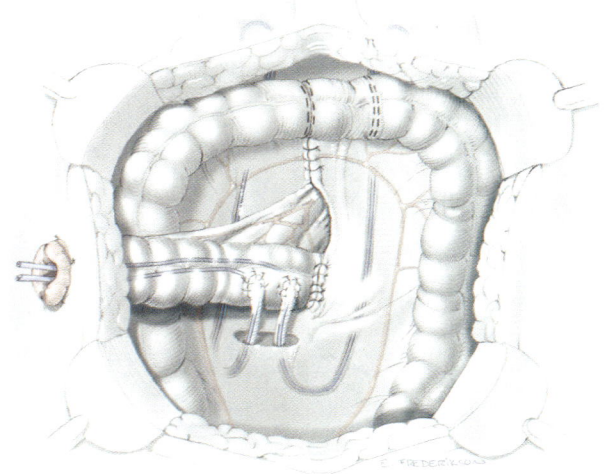

FIGURE 46-7.9 Transverse colon conduit: final appearance.

46-8

Continent Urinary Conduit

Removal of the bladder during total or anterior exenteration is the main indication for a continent urinary conduit. Vesicovaginal fistulas and disabling incontinence following radiation therapy are other less common reasons. Following cystectomy, urine is diverted into a reservoir created from a resected bowel segment. Depending on their construction, these diversions may render a woman continent or incontinent. An incontinent conduit reservoir chronically drains into an ostomy bag, whereas that of a continent conduit does not leak urine. Patients empty the reservoir by intermittent self-catheterization.

Continent conduits, however, may not be appropriate for all patients. The operation is more complex than an incontinent diversion procedure and may lead to more postoperative complications (Karsenty, 2005). It also requires a highly motivated patient who is capable of long-term self-catheterization. An ideal candidate for a continent conduit is a young, otherwise healthy woman without a colostomy.

There are several continent diversion methods. In gynecologic oncology, the continent ileocolonic urinary reservoir (Miami pouch) has become the most popular choice (Salom, 2004). This pouch is technically straightforward to construct and uses tissues that characteristically lie in nonirradiated areas (Penalver, 1998).

A Miami pouch includes a distal ileum segment, the ascending colon, and a portion of transverse colon. The basic steps involve opening the colon segment along the length of the tenia and folding it onto itself. The walls of the ascending and transverse colon are then sewn together to achieve a reservoir with low intraluminal pressure. The ileal segment is tapered and purse-string sutures are placed at the level of the ileocecal valve to achieve continence. The free ileal segment end is then exteriorized as a stoma to allow catheterization (Penalver, 1989).

PREOPERATIVE

Patient Evaluation

Preoperative evaluation is usually dictated by the preceding exenterative procedure. The specific decision is whether to plan for an incontinent or continent urinary conduit. Patients are extensively counseled regarding the differences. The presence of a permanent colostomy removes the apparent advantage of a continent conduit and an abdominal wall without draining stomas. Catheterization may be more problematic in very obese women. In addition, some patients with prior high-dose radiation or chronic bowel disease also may not be good candidates due to poor tissue quality and increased associated risks of anastomotic leaks, ureteral stricture, or fistula.

Consent

Patients are advised that intraoperative findings such as poor bowel appearance and dense adhesions may dictate a change in surgical plans. In addition, complications are common and should be reviewed. Even in experienced centers, half of patients will have one or more early pouch-related complications: ureteral stricture with obstruction, anastomotic leak, fistula, difficulty in catheterization, pyelonephritis, or sepsis. One third will develop late complications beyond 6 weeks. Ten percent of patients will ultimately require reoperation to revise the Miami pouch (Penalver, 1998). As a result, many patients would not choose the continent urinary conduit again (Goldberg, 2006).

Patient Preparation

Oral bowel preparation is mandatory but generally other presurgical steps are dictated by the preceding exenterative surgery. Ideally, an enterostomal therapist is available to mark a conduit stoma site in the right lower abdomen that is unobstructed in the supine, sitting, and standing positions.

INTRAOPERATIVE

Surgical Steps

❶ Initial Steps. To avoid unnecessary traction on anastomoses, the continent urinary conduit is constructed as the last major intraabdominal procedure during exenterative surgery. Before beginning the conduit, hemostasis should be achieved. Anesthesia, patient positioning, and skin incisions are typically dictated by the preceding operation.

❷ Exploration. The conduit bowel segment is carefully inspected. It must appear healthy and lack severe radiation injury. At this point, the final decision to proceed with creation of a Miami pouch is made.

❸ Preparing the Bowel Segment. The right colon is freed along the white line of Toldt from the cecum, around the hepatic flexure, to the proximal transverse colon. The white line of Toldt marks the lateral attachment of ascending and descending colon's peritoneum to the posterior abdomen's parietal peritoneum. The conduit will

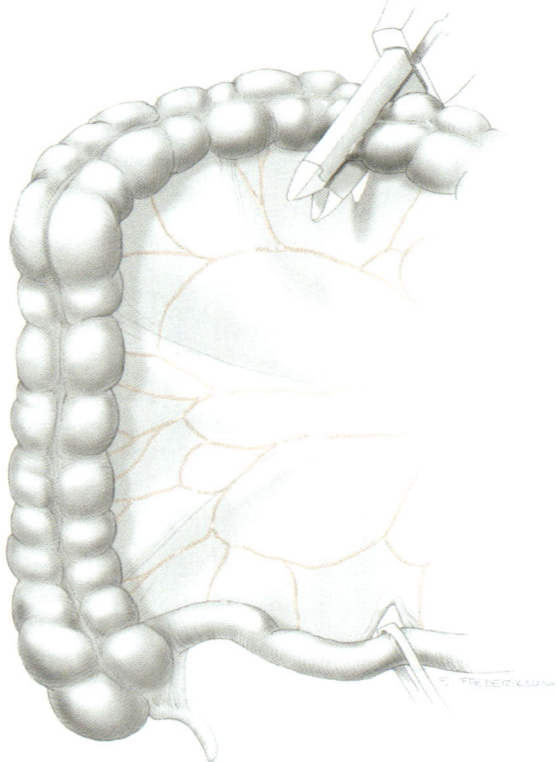

FIGURE 46-8.1 Preparing the bowel segment.

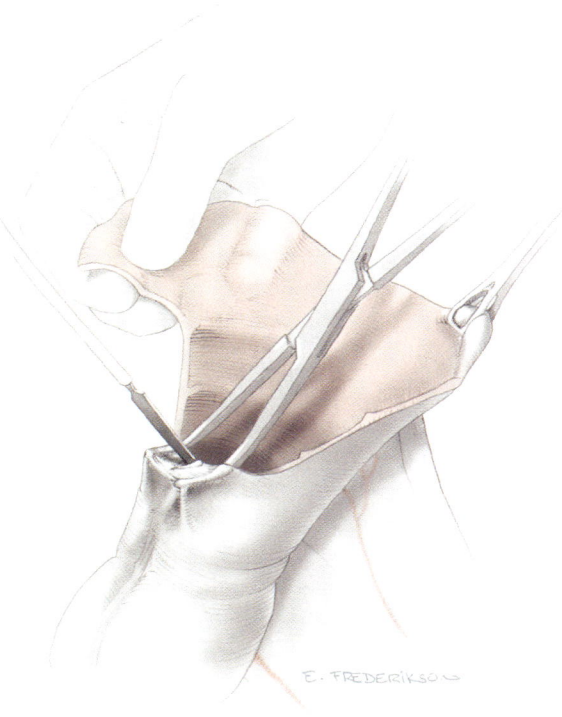

FIGURE 46-8.2 Detubularizing the bowel.

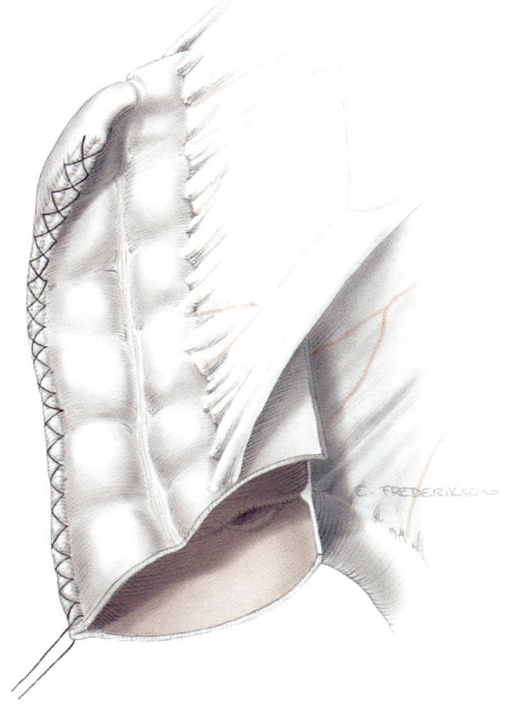

FIGURE 46-8.3 Creating the reservoir.

require approximately 25 to 30 cm of colon and at least 10 cm of ileum. With these measurements in mind, a surgeon selects sites to divide the bowel.

The mesentery is scored with an electrosurgical blade, and a Penrose drain is placed around the sections to be divided. Within the mesentery, the underlying vasculature is reviewed to ensure sufficient conduit blood supply. A gastrointestinal anastomosis (GIA) stapler is used to divide the bowel at both sites marked with the Penrose drains (Fig. 46-8.1).

The mesenteries are incised down through the avascular areas to the posterior peritoneum. At this point, intestinal continuity is reestablished by a functional end-to-end stapled ileotransverse enterocolostomy using the GIA and transverse anastomosis (TA) staplers. The mesenteric defect is closed with 0-gauge delayed-absorbable suture in a running fashion to prevent internal herniation.

❹ **Detubularizing the Bowel.** The conduit staple lines on both ends of the bowel segment are removed with Metzenbaum scissors, and the bowel is irrigated into a basin. Of this bowel segment, the entire colonic portion is opened with an electrosurgical blade along the tenia of the antimesenteric border to "detubularize" the bowel (Fig. 46-8.2). This is extended to remove the appendix.

❺ **Creating the Pouch.** The colon segment is folded in half and four delayed-absorbable stay sutures are placed at the corners to begin creation of the pouch. The lateral edge is closed in two layers with 2-0 and 3-0 gauge delayed-absorbable suture in a running fashion (Fig. 46-8.3).

❻ **Tapering the Ileum.** A 14F red rubber catheter is inserted through the terminal ileum segment into the pouch. Then,

two purse-string, 0-gauge delayed-absorbable sutures are placed 1 cm apart at the ileocecal junction. The ileum is elevated with Babcock clamps, and a GIA stapler is used to taper the terminal ileum on its antimesenteric border over the catheter (Fig. 46-8.4). Continence is attained by these two steps. An anterior abdominal wall opening is made in the right lower quadrant so that the ileal segment of the conduit can be pulled through to approximate its final position.

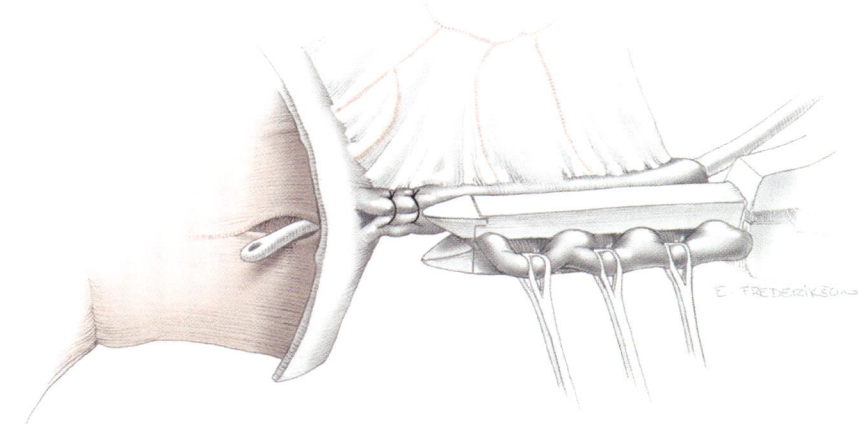

FIGURE 46-8.4 Tapering the ileum.

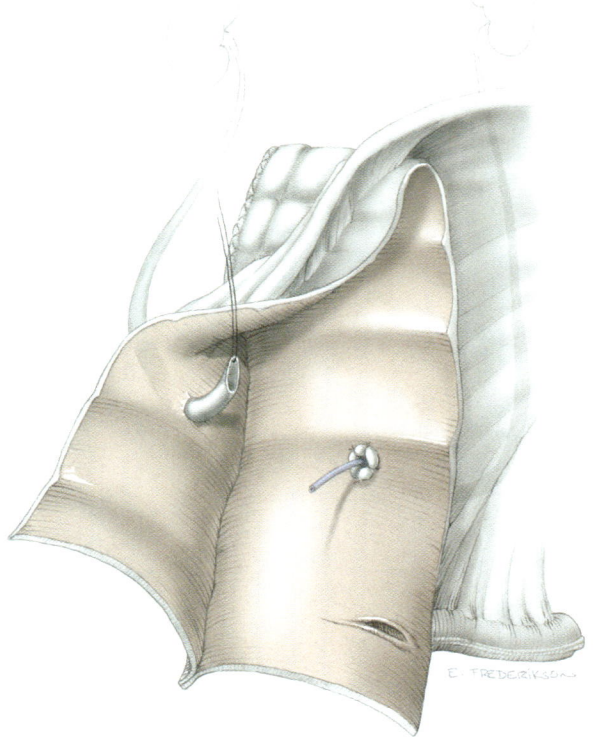

FIGURE 46-8.5 Ureteral anastomoses.

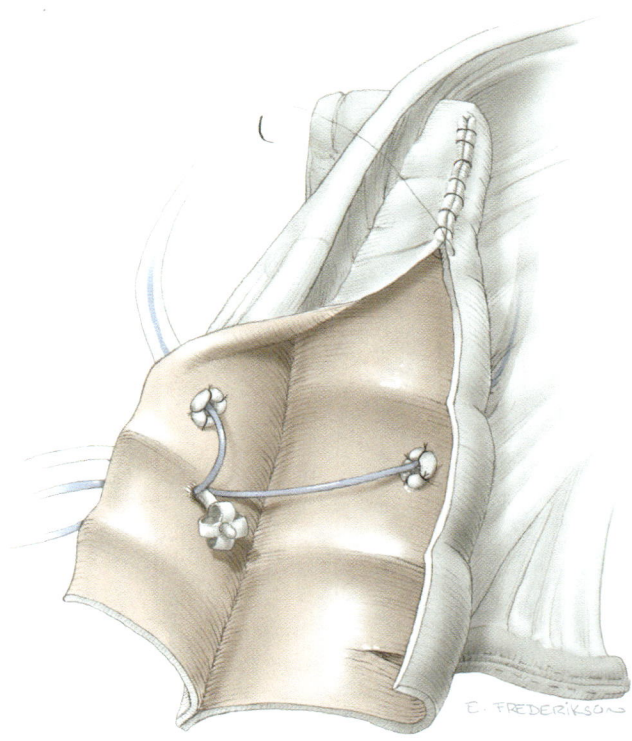

FIGURE 46-8.6 Closing the reservoir.

❼ **Ureteral Anastomoses.** Both ureters are further mobilized from their retroperitoneal attachments and brought into position under the ascending mesocolon using a 4-0 gauge delayed-absorbable stay suture at the tip. Manipulation with this suture avoids crush injury by forceps and subsequent necrosis. As in the transverse colon conduit, the left ureter is brought over the aorta and *above* the origin of the inferior mesenteric artery (IMA).

The ureteral anastomotic sites to the pouch are selected based on ureter length and their ability to have a straight course to the pouch. One ureter is usually brought through on either side of the pouch suture line. The ureters are trimmed and spatulated (see Fig. 46-7.2, p. 1183). In creating the openings for the ureters, the bowel mucosa is incised at sites away from the suture line. A hemostat is poked through the bowel wall, grasps the ureteral stay suture, and thereby pulls 2 cm of each ureter into the pouch.

Each ureter is secured to the bowel mucosa with interrupted stitches of 4-0 gauge delayed-absorbable suture (Fig. 46-8.5). Single-J ureteral stents (7F) are inserted and sutured to the bowel wall with 3-0 gauge chromic to stabilize their placement. To enable correct identification postoperatively, the distal end of the right ureteral stent is cut at a "right" angle.

❽ **Closing the Pouch.** A large Malecot catheter is brought into the pouch through an incision made away from the ileocecal valve. The ureteral stents are brought out through the pouch and next to the Malecot (Fig. 46-8.6). At the site where these tubes exit the pouch, a watertight purse string using 3-0 plain catgut suture is placed. Absorbable suture is used for this purse string, as the Malecot catheter will be removed only 2 to 3 weeks postoperatively.

The remaining edges of the pouch are closed with two layers of 2-0 and 3-0 gauge delayed-absorbable suture in a running fashion. Continence may be tested by inserting a red rubber catheter through the plicated ileum, filling the pouch with 250 to 300 mL of saline, removing the red rubber catheter, and gently squeezing the pouch. Additional purse-string sutures may be placed at the ileocecal valve if incontinence is demonstrated. The completed pouch (Fig. 46-8.7) is now ready to be brought to the abdominal wall.

❾ **Final Steps.** The two stents and the Malecot drain are brought out through a separate stab wound on the abdominal wall away from the stoma site. The Malecot drain is individually fixed to the skin with nylon sutures. The ileal segment is pulled through the abdominal wall and may require trimming to sit flush. The pouch is stabilized by

suturing it to the undersurface of the abdominal wall, and the stoma is created by placing interrupted stitches of 3-0 gauge delayed-absorbable suture between the dermis and ileal mucosa as described in Section 46-7, Step 6 (p. 1184). A red rubber catheter is inserted and withdrawn to make sure that the pouch can be easily accessed. A Jackson-Pratt (JP) drain is then placed near the pouch to monitor for urine leakage and is brought out through a separate stab wound away from the stoma.

POSTOPERATIVE

The Miami pouch initially requires more care than an incontinent urinary conduit. Mucus will be produced by the colonic bowel segment. Therefore, the Malecot catheter is irrigated every few hours to permit urine drainage. In contrast, the ureteral stents are irrigated only if one of the catheters becomes obstructed. Two to 3 weeks postoperatively, an intravenous pyelogram (IVP) and gravity pouchogram are performed. The IVP excludes anastomotic leaks, ureteral stricture, and fistulas. The pouchogram involves retrograde filling of the conduit to search for leaks. If these tests are normal, the ureteral stents, Malecot catheter, and JP suction drainage tube may all be removed. The hole

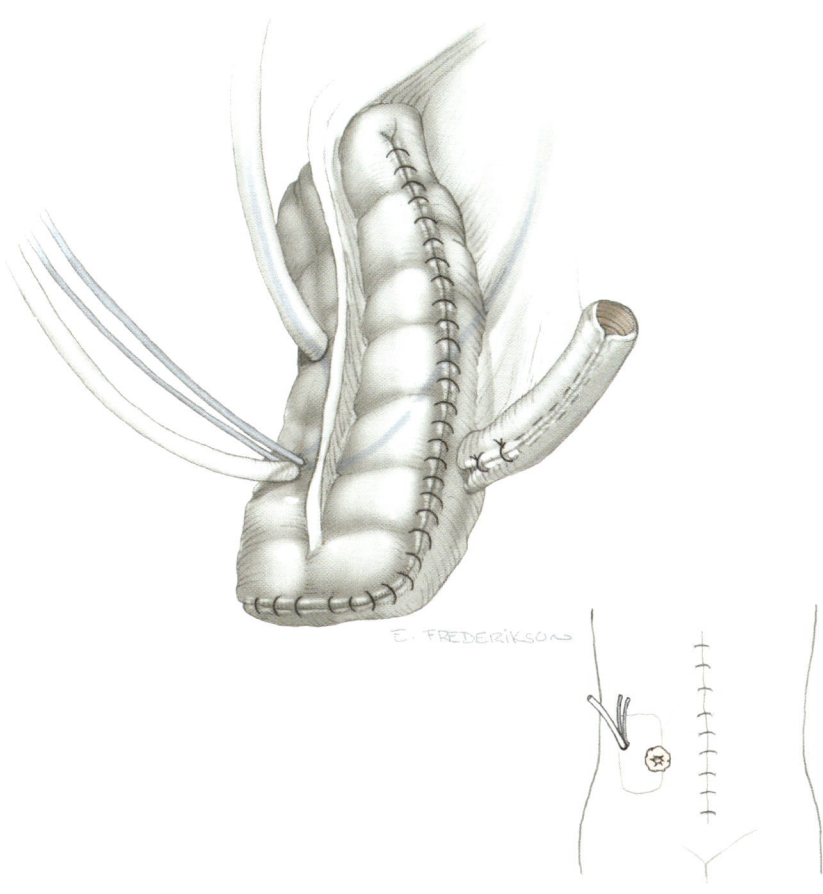

FIGURE 46-8.7 Final steps.

in the conduit that housed these tubes will heal secondarily.

A patient is taught self-catheterization using an 18F to 22F red rubber catheter and antiseptic technique. The interval between catheterizations is progressively increased over weeks to reach 6 hours during the day and span sleep hours at night. In addition, the pouch requires periodic irrigation to remove mucus. An IVP, pouchogram, and serum electrolyte and creatinine level measurement are performed at 3 months postoperatively and then every 6 months to evaluate the pouch, renal function, and upper urinary tracts.

More than half of patients will have a conduit-related complication postoperatively. Fortunately, most may be successfully managed conservatively without the need for reoperation (Ramirez, 2002). The most common urinary complications are ureteral stricture or obstruction, difficult catheterization, and pyelonephritis (Angioli, 1998; Goldberg, 2006). The gastrointestinal (GI) complication rate attributed to Miami pouch is less than 10 percent and includes fistulas (Mirhashemi, 2004).

46-9

Vaginal Reconstruction

Patients undergoing exenterative surgery are typical candidates for creation of a new vagina. Other less common indications include congenital absence of the vagina, postirradiation stenosis, and total vaginectomy. The procedure can be completed in innumerable ways, and the type of reconstruction is typically determined by both the surgeon's personal experience and the patient's clinical circumstances.

Vaginal reconstruction at the time of exenteration is a very personal choice. Not every woman will desire a new vagina, and others will be unhappy with the functional result (Gleeson, 1994a). Moreover, reconstruction may significantly prolong an already lengthy operation and lead to additional perioperative morbidity (Mirhashemi, 2002). However, proponents suggest that filling the large pelvic defect and bringing in a new source of blood supply may actually prevent postoperative fistula or abscess formation (Goldberg, 2006; Jurado, 2000). For perspective, in the United States from 2011 to 2015, vaginal reconstruction was completed in approximately one fourth of women undergoing pelvic exenteration (Matsuo, 2019).

To create a functional neovagina, one of the following is performed: (1) surrounding skin and subcutaneous tissue is mobilized and positioned into the defect (skin flap), (2) skin from another part of the body is harvested and transferred to replace the vaginal mucosa (split-thickness skin graft), or (3) skin and underlying tissue outside the radiated field are mobilized on an attached section of muscle with its dominant blood supply (myocutaneous flap). Of the three choices for vaginal reconstruction, skin flaps, such as *rhomboid flaps*, *pudendal thigh fasciocutaneous flaps*, and *advancement* or *rotational flaps*, are technically the easiest to perform (Burke, 1994; Gleeson, 1994b; Lee, 2006). *Split-thickness skin grafts (STSG)* provide the ability to cover large surfaces if primary closure is not possible. However, these require that most of the native subcutaneous tissue has been retained at the neovagina site and require months of stenting with a vaginal mold to prevent stricture (Kusiak, 1996). *Rectus abdominis myocutaneous (RAM) flaps* and *gracilis myocutaneous flaps* are technically more challenging and take longer to perform, but they provide the most satisfying functional results (Lacey, 1988; Smith, 1998). Importantly, RAM flaps may be inappropri-

ate in those with a prior Maylard incision or any other procedure that resulted in ligation of the inferior epigastric artery, which is the dominant blood supply to this type of flap.

Regardless of reconstruction technique, sexual function is often significantly impaired in women after pelvic exenteration (Hockel, 2008; Ratliff, 1996). Other techniques are used less commonly and are not covered in this section.

PREOPERATIVE

Patient Evaluation

The surgeon should have an open discussion with the patient regarding the risks and benefits of vaginal reconstruction. Some women may have unrealistic expectations that are important to address preoperatively. Others may not wish to incur additional morbidity. The patient should also be aware that intraoperative complications may dictate a change of plans and the need to abort reconstruction.

Consent

The potential morbidity of the neovagina depends on the type of reconstruction. Flap necrosis, prolapse, wound separation, or other complications may require reoperation and/or lead to an unsatisfying end result. Postoperative patient concerns are expected and include self-consciousness about being seen in the nude by their partner and vaginal dryness or discharge (Ratliff, 1996).

Patient Preparation

The preceding exenterative surgery typically dictates needed preoperative preparation.

Modifications may be required, depending on the type of neovaginal reconstruction. For example, the legs may need to be surgically prepped beyond the knees for a gracilis flap or a suitable donor site identified for STSG.

INTRAOPERATIVE

Surgical Steps

❶ Anesthesia and Patient Positioning. General anesthesia is required for vaginal reconstruction. The abdomen, perineum, and vagina are surgically prepared, and a Foley catheter inserted. Legs are positioned in standard lithotomy in booted support stirrups to permit adequate perineal access. For VTE prophylaxis, lower-extremity pneumatic compression devices are placed.

❷ Pudendal Thigh Fasciocutaneous Flap. Colloquially and formerly known as a "Singapore flap," this flap uses skin and subcutaneous tissue from the both labiocrural folds to create a tubular vagina. Blood supply derives from each posterior labial artery, which is a branch of the internal pudendal artery and then the perineal artery. Presurgical transperineal Doppler imaging can help to confirm patency (Ohmaru, 2017).

From a perineal approach, the planned incisions are marked along the skin from the non-hair-bearing areas just lateral to the labia majora. Flaps are roughly 15 × 6 cm. The most inferior skin margin should be level with the lower part of the gaping perineal defect. The skin incision is begun at the superior flap margin and dissected to include the underlying subcutaneous tissue and fascia lata (Fig. 46-9.1).

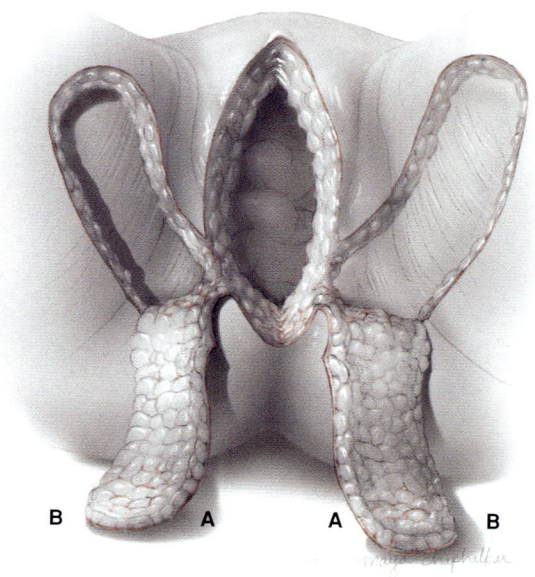

B   A   A   B

FIGURE 46-9.1 Raising the perineal flaps.

a cylinder for a new vagina. This is then lined by a STSG from the lateral thigh. Notably, in thin patients, a thin, poorly vascularized, attenuated omentum may be inadequate to form a substantial cylinder and cover the mold.

From an abdominal approach, the omentum is detached from the stomach with a ligate-divide-staple (LDS) device or electrosurgical bipolar coagulation device (LigaSure, ENSEAL). Resection is usually from right to left, until it will comfortably reach the pelvis as a J-flap (Section 46-14, p. 1211). Only three quarters of the omentum is divided, so as to preserve the left gastroepiploic artery for blood supply. The distal omentum is rolled into a cylinder and sutured together with interrupted stitches of 3-0 gauge delayed-absorbable suture (Fig. 46-9.3).

The proximal end can be closed abdominally with similar interrupted sutures or the transverse anastomosis (TA) stapler without dividing it entirely. From the perineal side, the omental cylinder is then sutured to the vaginal introitus.

Next, the STSG is harvested from the donor site and sutured over a vaginal mold with 4-0 gauge delayed-absorbable suture in a manner similar to the McIndoe procedure described in Section 43-26 (p. 996). The mold is placed into the neovaginal space and sutured into place at the introitus (Fig. 46-9.4). Each of the remaining smaller perineal

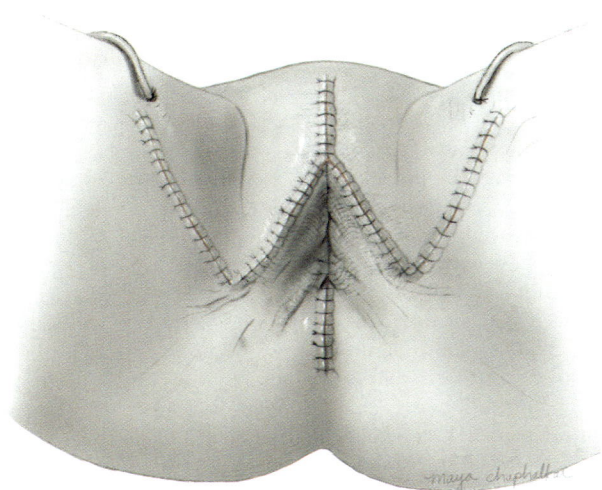

FIGURE 46-9.2 Perineal flap closure.

The flap's edges are approximated in a running, subcuticular suture line with 4-0 gauge delayed-absorbable suture. The edges both marked "A" in the figure are joined, as are both edges marked "B" (Fig. 46-9.2). The tubular neovagina is inserted into the perineal defect such that the end labeled with letters becomes the new vaginal apex. The perineal defect requires sculpting of tissue folds and suturing to form a functional end result.

The apex of the neovagina may then be abdominally sutured to the hollow of the sacrum as in a traditional sacrocolpopexy (Section 45-17, p. 1124). The neovagina is then covered with an omental J-flap to provide additional neovascularization.

The harvest site incisions are closed with interrupted stitches of 3-0 gauge delayed-absorbable suture. Bilateral JP drains are placed beneath these suture lines.

❸ Split-Thickness Skin Graft with Omental J-Flap. Modification of the omental flap, which is normally used to close off the pelvic inlet after exenteration, can create

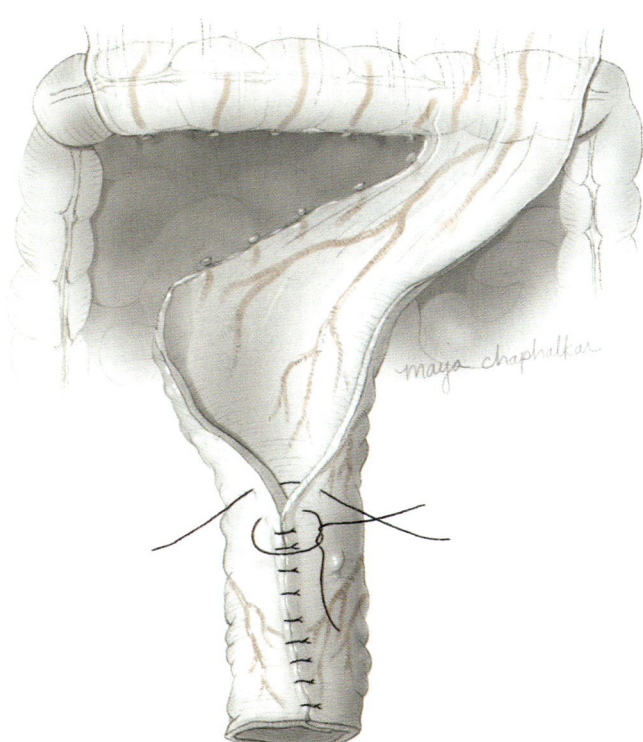

FIGURE 46-9.3 Raising the omental J-flap.

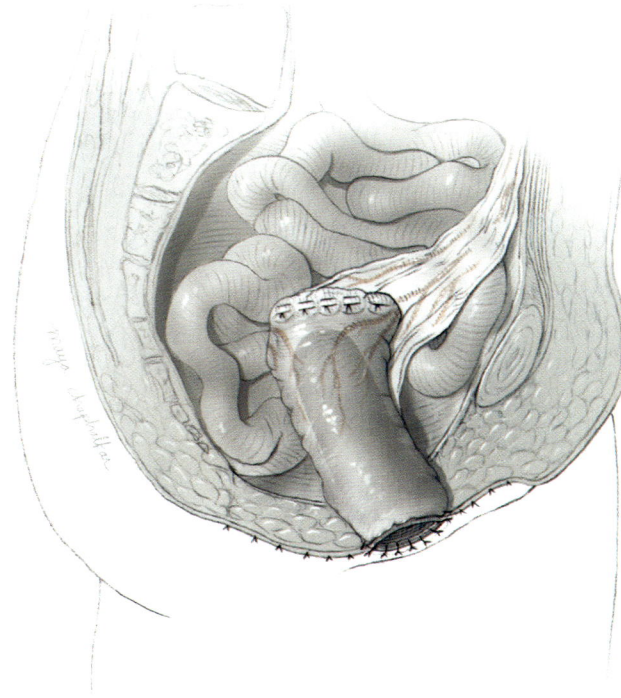

FIGURE 46-9.4 Insertion of the split-thickness skin graft.

defects, now above and below the neovagina, is closed in the midline with interrupted stitches of 3-0 gauge delayed-absorbable suture. The harvest sites are sprayed with a topical hemostatic agent and dressed with a clear occlusive dressing (Tegaderm).

❹ **Gracilis Myocutaneous Flap.** This flap uses the belly of both gracilis muscles and their overlying skin and subcutaneous tissue to fashion the vaginal tube. Blood supply derives from a branch of the medial femoral circumflex artery.

From a perineal approach, a reference line is drawn on the medial thigh from the pubic tubercle to the medial tibial plateau following the adductor longus muscle. Inferior to this line, an island of skin, its associated subcutaneous tissue, and the gracilis muscle will serve as the flap. The planned elliptic incision is marked, and a full-thickness skin incision through the reference line is continued through the subcutaneous fat and the fascia lata. The belly of the gracilis muscle is isolated at its distal margin and divided. The remainder of the incision is completed around the marked skin island margin (Fig. 46-9.5). The gracilis muscle is fully mobilized with blunt and sharp dissection from distal to proximal. This preserves its dominant vascular supply as it enters the deep anterior belly of the muscle 6 to 8 cm from the pubic tubercle.

Through the operative site on the thigh, a subfascial tunnel is bluntly developed medially to the open perineal defect. The left gracilis muscle flap is rotated *clockwise* against the thigh, that is, rotated first posteriorly and then medially (see Fig. 46-9.5). It is placed through the tunnels and allowed to hang freely between the patient's legs. The right flap is rotated *counterclockwise* and similarly positioned.

Beginning at the distal tip, the tubular gracilis neovagina is constructed by suturing the skin edges of the right and left skin islands together with interrupted stitches using 4-0 gauge delayed-absorbable suture. The proximal opening should accommodate two or three fingers.

The neovagina is then rotated cephalad into the pelvis. Through an abdominal approach, it is posteriorly anchored to the inner surface of the levator plate with interrupted stitches of 0-gauge delayed-absorbable suture to prevent vaginal prolapse.

At the perineum, redundant flap skin is trimmed, and the proximal skin is sutured to the introitus with interrupted stitches of 3-0 gauge delayed-absorbable suture. Each of the remaining smaller perineal defects, now above and below the neovagina, is closed in the midline with interrupted stitches of 3-0 gauge delayed-absorbable suture. Each thigh incision is similarly closed.

❺ **Rectus Abdominis Myocutaneous (RAM) Flap.** This flap uses the one belly of the rectus abdominis muscle and its overlying skin and subcutaneous tissue to fashion the vaginal tube. Blood supply derives from the inferior epigastric muscle (Fig. 38-3, p. 794). As such, this flap is avoided in those patients with significant peripheral vascular disease, who may rely on the inferior epigastric vessels for collateral blood supply to their lower extremities (Salom, 2007).

For this flap, a skin and muscle island can be harvested from any location on the abdominal wall as long as the base of its shape is at the umbilicus. Typically, a 10 × 15 cm skin island is marked. At the superior border of the island, which will ultimately form the vaginal opening, the skin, subcutaneous tissue, and anterior rectus sheath are incised. One belly of the rectus abdominis muscle is freed with blunt dissection from its posterior sheath. The belly is divided proximally,

and its anastomotic vessels connecting to the superior epigastric system are ligated.

The remaining borders of the skin island are incised deeply to the anterior rectus sheath and distally to the arcuate line. The subcutaneous fat is mobilized along the lateral and medial margins of the rectus muscle belly. The rectus muscle is then bluntly dissected from its posterior sheath until reaching the arcuate line, which is the caudal margin of this sheath. Next, the posterior peritoneum is cut inferiorly, well beyond the flap, along the full length of the midline incision.

The RAM flap is now fully detached but must be further mobilized on its vascular pedicle to be able to swing into the pelvis. At the distal portion of the skin island, the rectus muscle is then bluntly dissected inferiorly from the anterior sheath to its insertion onto the pubic bone.

The flap consists of skin, subcutaneous tissue, anterior sheath, rectus belly, and blood supply from the inferior epigastric vessels. The flap is coiled around a syringe to form a tube (Fig. 46-9.6). The skin edges are approximated with 4-0 gauge delayed-absorbable suture. The syringe is removed, and the tube is placed into the pelvis. The pelvic end is closed. The RAM flap must be put into the pelvis without tension to prevent occlusion of its dominant vascular supply from the inferior epigastric artery. An omental J-flap also may be prepared to provide additional blood supply.

The open end of the neovagina is brought out under the symphysis pubis to the perineum. Here, it is attached to the vulvar defect with interrupted vertical mattress stitches using 0-gauge delayed-absorbable suture. Each of the remaining smaller perineal defects, now above and below the neovagina, is closed in the midline with interrupted stitches of 3-0 gauge delayed-absorbable suture.

To close the midline abdominal incision, the abdominal wall's posterior rectus fascia on the harvested side is reapproximated to the opposing linea alba with no. 1 polydioxanone monofilament (PDS). Skin is closed with staples.

POSTOPERATIVE

The presence of a vagina significantly improves quality of life for many women and reduces sexual problems after exenteration (Hawighorst-Knapstein, 1997). Reconstruction may benefit a woman's self-image, and the knowledge that intercourse is possible may be reassuring even if she chooses not to be sexually active postoperatively. Morbidity from the procedure largely depends on the type of neovagina.

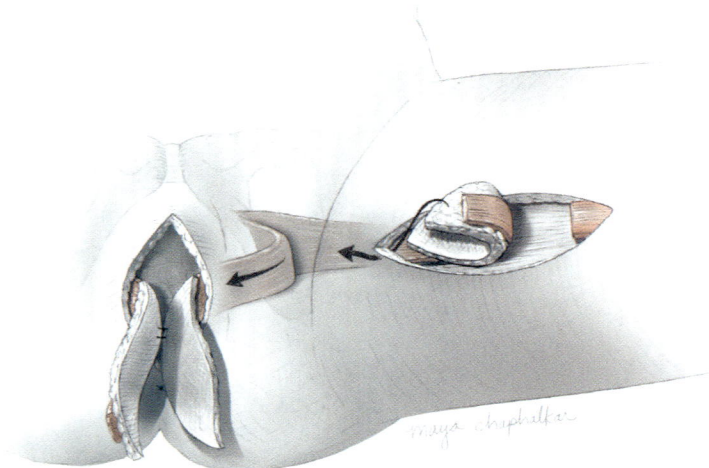

FIGURE 46-9.5 Gracilis myocutaneous flap.

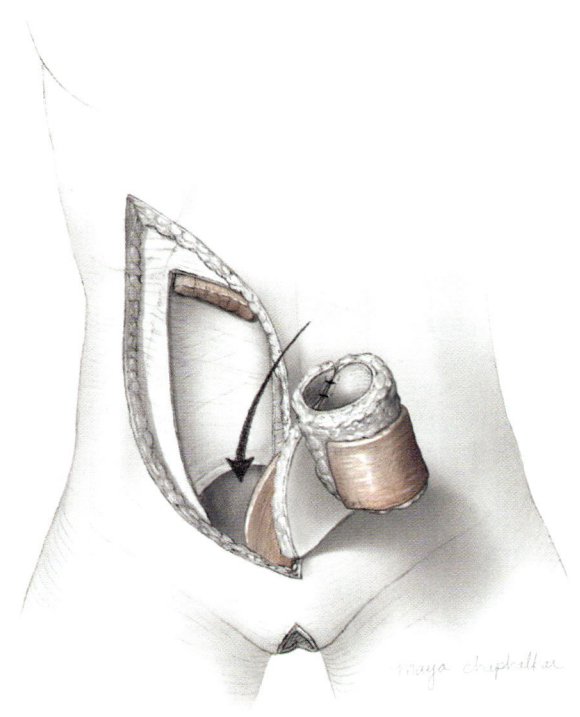

FIGURE 46-9.6 Rectus abdominis myocutaneous flap.

Pudendal thigh flaps are reliable and easy to harvest, but perhaps are the most likely to be nonfunctional. Long-term sequelae may include vulvar pain, chronic vaginal discharge, hair growth, and protrusion of the flaps. These symptoms may discourage patients and their partners from attempting sexual activity (Gleeson, 1994b).

STSG neovaginas may become infected at the donor or recipient site. Graft sloughing due to vascular compromise or development of a seroma is another common complication. Postoperatively, patients must initially be immobilized to aid healing, and stenting with a vaginal mold is required for months to prevent vaginal stenosis or contracture (Fowler, 2009).

Gracilis myocutaneous flaps may be difficult to pass into the pelvis during the procedure and have the potential for partial or complete tissue loss due to necrosis from an inherently tenuous blood supply (Cain, 1989). Flap loss is significantly more common if rectosigmoid anastomosis is performed concurrently during exenteration (Soper, 1995). Long-term prolapse is another relatively common problem. Residual scarring on the legs is a frequent, albeit relatively minor, complaint postoperatively.

Rectus abdominis muscle flaps are perhaps the best choice for vaginal reconstruction at the time of pelvic exenteration (Jurado, 2009). Ideally, they fill pelvic dead space, reduce the risk of fistulas, and provide satisfactory sexual activity (Goldberg, 2006). However, the donor site may be difficult to close primarily or may lead to a postoperative hernia or dehiscence. The operating time is also increased because, unlike a gracilis flap where the abdominal team can proceed with exenteration while the perineal team is beginning the reconstruction, two surgical teams are not possible when performing a RAM flap. Flap necrosis, enterocutaneous fistula, and vaginal stenosis are other frequent complications (Soper, 2005).

46-10

Pelvic Lymphadenectomy

Pelvic lymph node removal and evaluation is a fundamental tool in accurate cancer staging. As such, it is commonly indicated in women undergoing surgery for uterine, ovarian, or cervical cancer. Also, in those with grossly involved nodes, pelvic lymphadenectomy may serve to optimally debulk tumor burden.

The aim of lymphadenectomy is bilateral *complete* removal of all fatty lymphatic tissue from the areas predicted to carry nodal metastases (Cibula, 2010). These nodes lie within well-defined anatomic boundaries that include: the midportion of the common iliac artery (cephalad), deep circumflex iliac vein (caudad), psoas muscle (laterally), ureter (medially), and obturator nerve (dorsally) (Whitney, 2010). Ideally, the procedure yields numerous pelvic nodes from multiple sites within these boundaries (Huang, 2010). Groups specifically sampled are the external iliac artery, internal iliac artery, obturator, and common iliac artery nodal groups. Removal of at least four lymph nodes from each side (right and left) is a minimum requirement to validate that an "adequate" lymphadenectomy has been performed (Whitney, 2010). In general, the extent of pelvic lymphadenectomy will depend on the clinical circumstances, such as degree of associated scarring and patient habitus.

Additional definitions are commonly used in association with lymphadenectomy. For example, pelvic lymph node "sampling" is a more limited procedure within the same anatomic boundaries and is particularly intended to remove any enlarged or suspicious nodes (Whitney, 2010). Sampling is limited to easily accessible pelvic regions and does not address all nodal groups (Cibula, 2010). Pelvic lymph node "dissection" is a vague term that may range from sampling to lymphadenectomy.

Pelvic lymphadenectomy can be performed via laparotomy or a MIS abdominal approach (p. 1204). In contrast, although the pelvic lymph nodes lie retroperitoneally, a lateral abdominal wall approach to reach these without entering the peritoneal cavity, that is, *extraperitoneal pelvic lymphadenectomy*, is not commonly performed (Larciprete, 2006). Last, emerging advancements in lymphatic mapping and sentinel node techniques are designed to limit the short- and long-term complications associated with extensive lymphatic resection.

PREOPERATIVE

Patient Evaluation

Imaging studies such as CT, MR, or PET imaging may suggest pelvic lymphadenopathy and help guide a surgeon to suspicious areas. However, the ability to preoperatively detect microscopic metastases is limited.

Consent

With proper technique, pelvic lymphadenectomy is a straightforward procedure with relatively few complications. These include postoperative lymphocele, nerve and vascular injury, acute hemorrhage, infection, and chronic lymphedema.

Patient Preparation

Bleeding is a common problem with pelvic lymphadenectomy and may be exacerbated with obese patients, grossly enlarged or densely adhered lymph nodes, and pelvic vessel anatomic variants. Accordingly, units of packed red blood cells are typed and crossmatched. Topical hemostatic agents also may prove valuable (Table 40-6, p. 860).

Routine oral bowel preparation and antibiotic prophylaxis are not required for lymphadenectomy but may be indicated for other concurrent surgeries. Prevention of VTE is warranted, and options are listed in Table 39-10 (p. 834).

INTRAOPERATIVE

Surgical Steps

❶ **Anesthesia and Patient Positioning.** This surgery may be performed under general or regional anesthesia with a patient supine. For VTE prophylaxis, lower-extremity compression devices are placed. A Foley catheter is inserted, and the abdomen is surgically prepared.

❷ **Abdominal Entry.** A midline vertical or transverse abdominal incision that allows access to the previously noted anatomic boundaries is appropriate for this procedure. A Pfannenstiel incision offers limited exposure and is reserved for selected patients.

❸ **Abdominal Exploration.** Pelvic and paraaortic lymph nodes are routinely inspected during initial abdominal exploration. Unexpected grossly positive nodes may indicate that a proposed operative plan should be abandoned (for example, radical hysterectomy for cervical cancer) or revised (Whitney, 2000).

❹ **Retroperitoneal Exploration.** Typically, the retroperitoneal space has already been entered through the round ligament during preceding surgical procedures. However, to extend retroperitoneal access, a surgeon may further incise the anterior and posterior leaves of the broad ligament.

Palpation of the external iliac artery pulsation just medial to the psoas major muscle is the starting point. Its identification permits a surgeon to locate relevant anatomy, as vascular anomalies are regularly encountered. Blunt dissection is then performed cephalad to see the common iliac artery bifurcate into the external and internal iliac arteries. The ureter is isolated as previously described (p. 1162). The remaining pelvic sidewall structures are covered with fatty-lymphoid tissue and are not yet easily visible.

To summarize the planned en bloc specimen excision, dissection begins at a proximal site along the psoas major muscle and external iliac artery and proceeds distally to reach the inguinal ring. Here, the nodal specimen is reflected medially and off the external iliac vein. Next, dissection along the internal iliac artery begins cephalad and moves caudad. Last, dissection enters the obturator space for nodal dissection here. The entire nodal bundle is lifted and removed. Separately, nodes excised from along the distal common iliac artery can be included in the final specimen.

❺ **External Iliac Nodes.** For this nodal group, an index finger is placed atop the psoas major muscle and lateral to the external iliac artery at a point distal to the common iliac artery bifurcation. The finger bluntly dissects caudally and parallel to the external iliac artery to separate the lateral preperitoneal fat from the fatty-lymphoid tissue covering the external iliac vessels (Fig. 46-10.1). The general absence of lateral branches from these vessels enables more aggressive blunt separation to be performed unless there is significant fibrosis. The genitofemoral nerve, which is visible parallel to the external iliac artery, can often be spared with careful dissection. Injury to this nerve results in ipsilateral labium majus and proximal thigh numbness.

Next, beginning at the common iliac artery bifurcation, forceps traction is typically required to lift upward all adventitial tissue that overlies the external iliac artery. This countertraction helps maintain the correct dissection plane moving distally as bands between nodal tissue and the artery are divided using electrosurgical cutting (Fig. 46-10.2).

As dissection continues caudally, the distal self-retaining retractor blade may be temporarily removed to allow resection of all pelvic nodes heading toward the inguinal canal. For

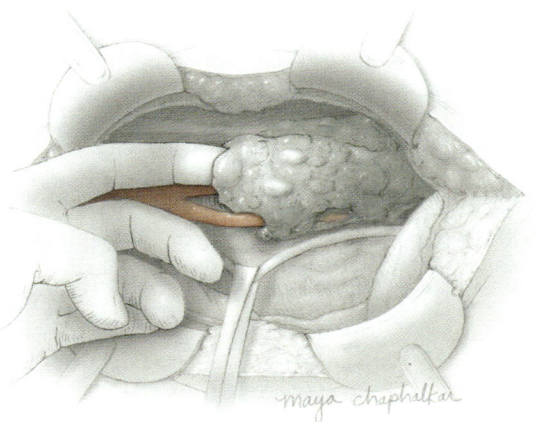

FIGURE 46-10.1 Mobilizing the lateral nodal tissue.

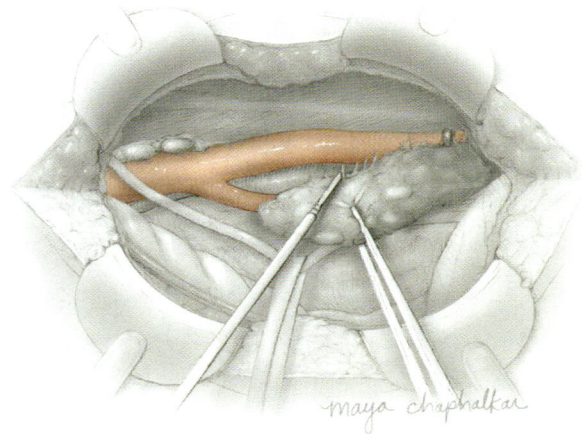

FIGURE 46-10.2 Medial dissection over the vein.

this, the fatty nodal tissue overlying the caudal portions of the psoas major muscle and external iliac artery is grasped with forceps. With an incision made parallel and superficial to the artery, distal nodal tissue is freed. Mobilization of this tissue exposes the deep circumflex iliac vein, which crosses laterally over the distal external iliac artery. The deep circumflex iliac vein originates from the distal part of the external iliac vein and serves as the caudal boundary for this nodal group.

The mobilized nodal tissue is next reflected medially to reveal the entire external iliac artery. Medial traction is applied with forceps, and fine adventitial bands that connect the nodes to the underlying external iliac vein are transected using electrocautery cutting or Metzenbaum scissors. Once completed, this external iliac nodal group dissection later permits safe entry into the obturator space, outlined in Step 7.

❻ Internal Iliac Nodes. Next, the ureter is moved and held medially by a Penrose drain or narrow retractor for protection and improved pelvic sidewall visualization. Spatially, nodes that have been dissected off the external iliac vessels and the fatty nodal tissue bridging the external iliac vein and the internal iliac artery lie in the same plane. Beginning at the common iliac artery bifurcation, the free nodal bundle is elevated and placed on tension. Initial sharp dissection of the internal iliac nodal group continues caudally along the internal iliac vessels and then along the superior vesical artery. As dissection approaches the distal aspect of the superior vesical artery, the nodal attachments are fine and enable electrosurgical dissection without the need for clips or ligatures. At this point, both the external iliac and internal iliac nodes are completely dissected and can be submitted as one specimen or combined

with obturator fossa lymph nodes, depending on surgeon preference.

❼ Obturator Fossa Node Group. To reach this nodal group, an index finger is gently inserted between the psoas major muscle and external iliac artery, and blunt dissection progresses downward to the obturator fossa. Lateral arterial or venous branches may need vascular clip application and transection. During this dissection, nodal tissue may be identified behind the external iliac vessels and added to the specimen.

As a result, the external iliac vein is mobile and can be retracted laterally by a vessel retractor to expose the obturator fossa (Fig. 46-10.3). If present, nodal tissue along the inferomedial wall of the external iliac vein is transected with blunt and electrosurgical blade dissection. Also, accessory venous branches may be identified and clipped.

With the vein retractor in place, the obturator nodal tissue is grasped with forceps.

This nodal bundle lies deep to the external iliac vein but superficial to the obturator nerve. With upward traction applied, blunt forceps or a suction tip moved gently side-to-side disrupts nodal tissue attachments to the obturator nerve. The blunt dissection is performed in the center of the fossa to minimize injury to surrounding deep pelvic vasculature. This also clears off tissue to permit obturator nerve identification.

Once this nerve is localized, dissection should purposefully remain superficial to it. Firm fibrotic attachments may be electrosurgically transected under direct visualization. As the caudal end of the bundle is reached, it is usually tethered to the sidewall. To free it, a vascular clip is placed distal to the bundle, and the tethered attachment is divided proximal to the clip. At the cephalad end of the bundle, nodes are carefully separated sharply from the inferior aspect of the external iliac vein while avoiding obturator nerve injury.

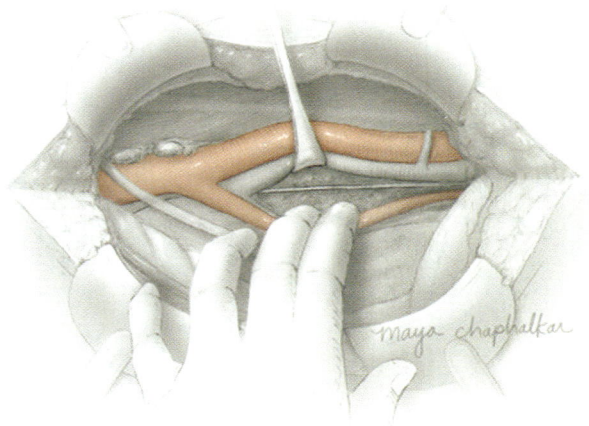

FIGURE 46-10.3 Obturator fossa dissection.

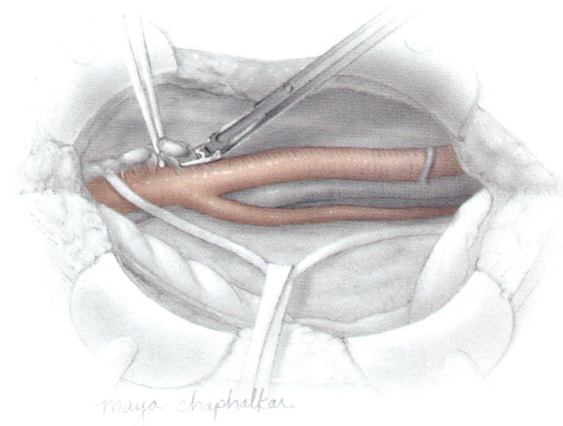

FIGURE 46-10.4 Distal common iliac dissection.

Nodal tissue deep to the obturator nerve is not routinely removed since the obturator artery and vein traverse this area. Laceration of either vessel can result in retraction and catastrophic hemorrhage that is difficult to control.

8 Distal Common Iliac Lymph Nodes. To remove this group, the upper retractor blade is readjusted to expose the distal half of the common iliac artery. The colon may require mobilization using electrosurgical dissection along the white line of Toldt. Once this line is incised, bowel can then be retracted sufficiently to allow access to the common iliac nodes. The ureter is further mobilized medially before beginning node dissection.

Lateral fatty-lymphoid tissue may be removed by first grasping and elevating with forceps and using electrosurgical dissection to establish a plane. Blunt dissection to further separate the nodal tissue from the artery is continued cephalad. Electrosurgical coagulation or clips plus sharp incision are used to detach these nodes (Fig. 46-10.4). Laterally, the nodes are dissected off the psoas major muscle. Importantly, on the patient's right side, the common iliac vein and inferior vena cava (IVC) lie beneath the lateral margin of the common iliac artery, and thus, careful dissection is warranted. Further dissection is performed atop the distal common iliac artery, which serves as the medial border of dissection for this nodal group.

9 Final Steps. Gauze sponges may be opened and tightly placed into the obturator fossa and medial to the external iliac vein to tamponade any surface oozing while additional procedures are performed. Topical hemostatic agents are employed as needed. Closing the retroperitoneal space and using suction drainage does not minimize hematoma or lymphocele development (Charoenkwan, 2017).

POSTOPERATIVE

Neurologic injuries involving the obturator, ilioinguinal, iliohypogastric, genitofemoral, or femoral nerves may result from direct surgical trauma, stretch injury, suture entrapment, or retractor placement (Cardosi, 2002). Their specific neurologic deficits and management are described in Chapter 40 (p. 842). Notably, transection of the obturator nerve is ideally immediately noted intraoperatively and an epineural repair performed (Vasilev, 1994).

Surgical blunt dissection techniques decrease the risk of inadvertent vessel or nerve injury, but these may increase the chance of postoperative lymphocele formation. Also known as lymphocyst, these usually asymptomatic and transient lymph collections may form a thick fibrotic wall. Postoperative pelvic hematomas also are not uncommon.

46-11

Paraaortic Lymphadenectomy

Removal of paraaortic lymph nodes typically follows pelvic lymphadenectomy to surgically stage women with uterine and ovarian cancer because of these cancers' unpredictable lymphatic dissemination patterns (Burke, 1996; Negishi, 2004). Moreover, removal of enlarged paraaortic nodes may provide optimal debulking of ovarian cancer and may also confer a survival benefit in selected endometrial and cervical cancer patients (Cosin, 1998; Havrilesky, 2005).

Paraaortic lymphadenectomy implies the bilateral complete removal of all nodal tissue from within an area with well-defined anatomic boundaries: inferior mesenteric artery (cephalad), midlength of common iliac artery (caudad), ureter (lateral), and aorta (medial). The completeness of the procedure will vary by clinical setting, but an adequate dissection requires that lymphatic tissue at least be demonstrated pathologically from both the right and left sides (Whitney, 2010).

Paraaortic lymphadenectomy can be performed via laparotomy or MIS approach (p. 1201). The proximal dissection is usually only extended to the inferior mesenteric artery (IMA), unless a "high" lymphadenectomy is indicated (Whitney, 2010). With this modification, a surgeon extends dissection to reach the renal veins. Most often, this is performed during ovarian cancer staging or in high-risk endometrial cancer cases to debulk tumor and more accurately stage these cancers (Mariani, 2008; Morice, 2003).

PREOPERATIVE

Patient Evaluation

As described earlier, imaging studies may help guide a surgeon to the most suspicious lymph nodes but are not entirely reliable in identifying small nodal metastases.

Consent

Paraaortic lymphadenectomy is not routinely performed worldwide due to the procedure's technical difficulty and potential for complications (Fujita, 2005). Of these, acute hemorrhage and postoperative ileus occur most often. Other complications should be infrequent. In obese women, operative visibility is hindered, and thus procedure complexity and operative times are considerably greater.

Patient Preparation

Bleeding is a common problem with this lymphadenectomy. Accordingly, units of packed red blood cells are typed and crossmatched. Topical hemostatic agents also may prove valuable (Table 40-6, p. 860). Routine bowel preparation and antibiotic prophylaxis are not typically required. However, other concurrent surgeries may dictate their use. Prevention of VTE is warranted, and options are listed in Table 39-10 (p. 834).

INTRAOPERATIVE

Surgical Steps

❶ Anesthesia and Patient Positioning. Lymphadenectomy may be performed under general or regional anesthesia with a patient supine. For VTE prophylaxis, lower-extremity compression devices are placed. A Foley catheter is inserted, and the abdomen is surgically prepared.

❷ Abdominal Entry. A midline vertical abdominal incision that allows access to the previously noted anatomic boundaries is appropriate for this procedure. Low transverse incisions offer limited exposure and are reserved for selected patients.

❸ Abdominal Exploration. The paraaortic lymph nodes are routinely palpated during initial abdominal exploration. A hand is placed beneath the small bowel mesentery to palpate the aorta. The index and middle fingers are then used to straddle the aorta and palpate for lymphadenopathy. Suspicious or grossly positive paraaortic nodes are typically removed as an initial step. Unexpected positive nodes may indicate that the proposed operative plan should be abandoned or revised (Whitney, 2000). For most instances, in which no adenopathy is present, the dissection is usually performed last due to the possibility of triggering catastrophic bleeding that might otherwise limit further surgery.

❹ Visualization. Exposure and proper retractor positioning is perhaps the most important part of this procedure. Thus, a self-retaining retractor is positioned to allow access to the aorta. The sigmoid colon and descending colon are gently retracted in a lower left direction, whereas small bowel and transverse colon are packed into the upper abdomen by laparotomy sponges. Modified Trendelenburg patient positioning also is helpful to shift bowel from the operative field. Additional sharp dissection along the right paracolic gutter peritoneum (white line of Toldt) may be necessary to sufficiently mobilize and move

the cecum from the dissection field. Once bowel has been cleared, the peritoneum overlying the aorta and right common iliac artery should be visible. Both vessels are palpated before proceeding. Also, as described on page 1162, the ureter is isolated and held laterally on a Penrose drain to avoid its injury.

❺ Opening the Retroperitoneal Space. Beginning atop the midportion of the right common iliac artery, a right-angle clamp is used to guide electrosurgical blade incision of the posterior parietal peritoneum. Following each vessel's course, the incision moves cephalad and medially over the right common iliac artery and then cephalad atop the aorta (Fig. 46-11.1). Staying directly above these arteries is recommended to avoid inadvertent laceration of the right common iliac vein or IVC. Continuing cephalad in the midline, sharp incision of the peritoneum is extended through the caudal and then left lateral aspect of the duodenal peritoneal reflection to mobilize the duodenum cephalad. An upper midline self-retaining retractor blade is repositioned to retract this bowel.

❻ Right Paraaortic Nodes. For the right-sided nodal group, dissection begins caudad and moves cephalad. With the ureter still held laterally, the surgeon first establishes the medial border of the right paraaortic nodal group. Atop the midportion of the right common iliac artery, the lymph node bundle is elevated with forceps to reveal fibrous bands connecting it to the artery. A right-angle clamp is placed beneath these bands, which are then sharply divided to free the distal bundle from the artery. Using electrosurgical cutting atop the right common iliac artery, cephalad and slightly medial dissection continues following the vessel course. Once the aortic bifurcation is reached, cephalad dissection progresses atop the right lateral border of the aorta to reach the level of the IMA. Small perforating vessels may be encountered and are coagulated.

To establish the lateral border of this nodal group, the ureter is again held laterally. Blunt cephalad dissection with a suction tip atop the iliopsoas muscle separates the retroperitoneal fat from the right border of the IVC. The upper right abdominal retractor blade may need to be repositioned to improve visibility.

At this point, the right paraaortic node bundle has been largely detached medially, distally, and laterally. Next, the bundle is again grasped distally with forceps and elevated as gentle sharp dissection beneath this bundle in the midline is directed cephalad. Delicate perforating veins along the IVC warrant meticulous dissection to reduce

caused by inadvertent avulsion of perforating venous tributaries. Hemorrhage may be copious and immediate. Initially, pressure is applied with a sponge-stick or finger, and anesthesia staff is informed of the potential for increased blood loss. Second, exposure is assessed. Blood is suctioned from the abdominal cavity, retractors are repositioned, and incisions are extended if necessary. Last, proper vascular instruments are obtained. Lacerated veins can usually be simply repaired with vascular clips (Fig. 46-11.3).

❽ Left Paraaortic Nodes. In contrast to the right-sided nodal group, dissection for this bundle begins cephalad and moves caudally. The medial border of this nodal group is developed using electrosurgical dissection that begins at the IMA. To advance, the medial side of the bundle is elevated with forceps to create tension across fibrous bands connecting it to the aorta. These fibers are sharply divided and free the proximal bundle. Moving caudally, continued similar dissection progresses atop the left border of the aorta toward its bifurcation. Upon reaching the bifurcation, dissection then advances caudally and slightly lateral to follow atop the left common iliac artery's course. This artery's midlength marks the caudad border.

Once this medial dissection is completed, fibrovascular attachments between the sigmoid colon mesentery and left side of the distal aorta are sharply transected. This aids access to laterally located paraaortic nodes.

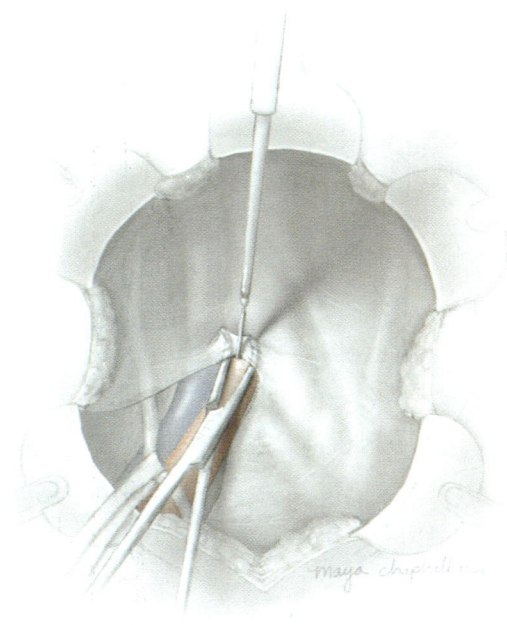

FIGURE 46-11.1 Opening the retroperitoneal spaces.

bleeding. One of these, the "fellow's vein," is routinely encountered near the level of the aortic bifurcation and is occluded with a vascular clip for hemostasis (Fig. 46-11.2). Upon reaching the level of the IMA, the nodal bundle can be removed by placing large vascular clips across the cephalad end

and transecting it before the clip. Once excised, this right nodal bundle is sent as a separate specimen.

❼ Repair of Venous Bleeding. A surgeon should prepare for small lacerations in the wall of the IVC or common iliac veins

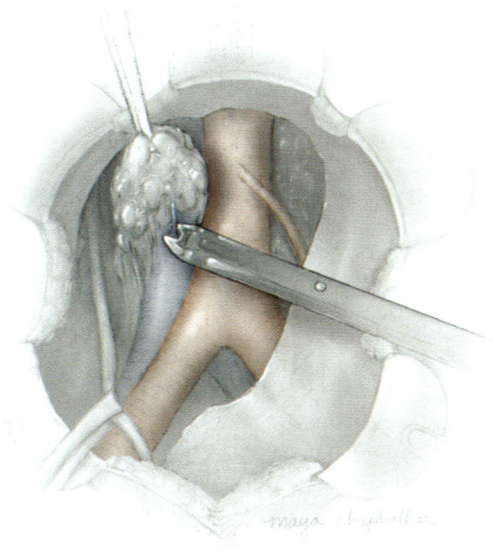

FIGURE 46-11.2 Removal of right paraaortic nodes.

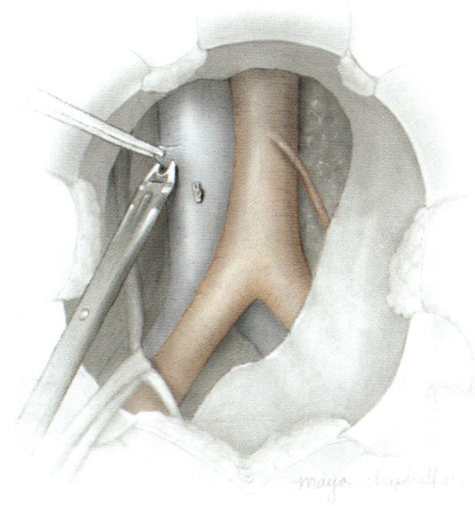

FIGURE 46-11.3 Repair of venous bleeding.

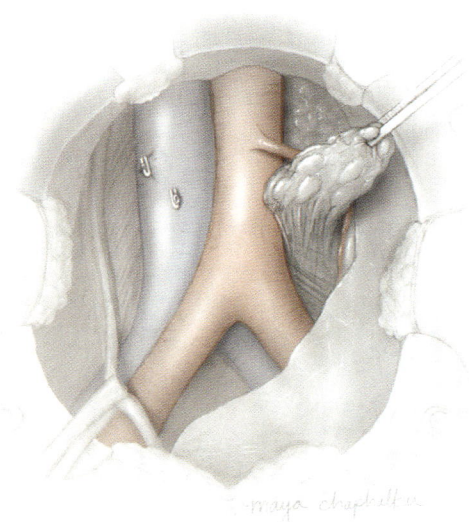

FIGURE 46-11.4 Removal of left paraaortic nodes.

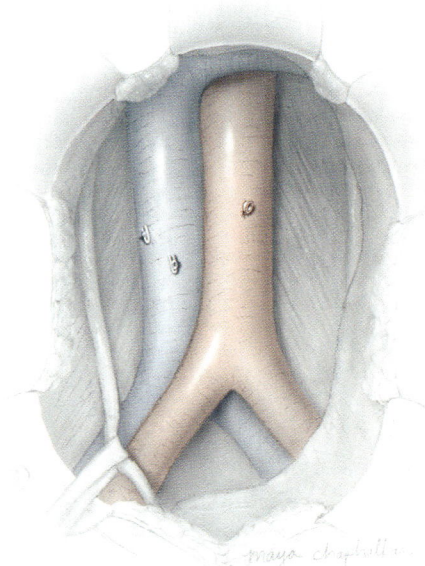

FIGURE 46-11.5 High paraaortic lymphadenectomy.

To develop the lateral border of this nodal group, fingers or suction tip carefully separate the lateral fatty lymphoid tissue from the overlying sigmoid colon mesentery and from the adjacent ovarian vessels and ureter. Opening this potential space allows clear identification of the ureter and the ovarian vessels, which lie medial to the ureter. A handheld vein retractor is positioned to gently lift up the sigmoid colon mesentery, its adjoining vessels, and ureter.

Establishing these medial and lateral borders delineates the left paraaortic lymph node bundle for removal. To free this bundle caudally, nodal tissue over the common iliac artery is elevated on traction with forceps. A vascular clip is placed across the bundle's caudal end, which is transected before the clip and freed. The distal nodal bundle is next elevated and lifted cephalad (Fig. 46-11.4). Fibrovascular attachments between the bundle and the medial aorta and lateral iliopsoas muscle are transected with electrosurgical blade or with vascular clips and Metzenbaum scissors as dissection moves progressively cephalad to the level of the IMA. Importantly, dissection into the lumbar vessels, which originate from the aorta's posteromedial aspect, is avoided. At the level of the IMA, the cephalad end of the left paraaortic lymph node bundle is clipped and transected. The entire nodal group is removed in toto and submitted as an individual specimen.

❾ Interiliac Nodes. Optionally, additional lymph nodes may be removed by excising the fatty tissue between the common iliac vessels. For this, the posterior peritoneum at the aortic bifurcation is grasped, and electrosurgical incision is extended caudally atop the inner side of both common iliac arteries. The crossing left common iliac vein is visible directly beneath.

The peritoneum is reflected caudally, and the fatty tissue beneath is grasped and placed on tension. Sharp dissection is performed along the surface of both common iliac veins, which have very few small perforating vessels. Once mobilized between the common iliac vessels, the triangle-shaped area of fatty-lymphoid tissue is freed by electrosurgical division of bands connecting it to the sacrum.

❿ High Paraaortic Lymphadenectomy. For this extended lymph node removal, anatomic boundaries begin caudally at the level of the IMA and reach cephalad to the entry level of the right ovarian vein and left renal vein (Whitney, 2010). To begin, the former midline peritoneal incision atop the aorta is incised further cephalad, and the duodenal loop is bluntly dissected off the aorta. Repositioning of the retractor blade to move this loop cephalad aids exposure.

On the aorta's right side, the caudal end of the high paraaortic nodal bundle is grasped with blunt forceps, and dissection atop the right lateral border of the aorta is continued cephalad until the right ovarian vein, before its insertion into the IVC. Here, the nodal bundle can be clipped, divided, and incorporated within the specimen.

On the left side, high paraaortic node dissection begins with identification, clipping, and cutting of the IMA between ties, which allows access to upper nodal tissue. The mesenteric circulation has an extensive collateral network that permits IMA ligation without subsequent bowel ischemia. Alternatively, the IMA may be preserved if adequate exposure is available. This avoids potential bowel ischemia in those with poorly developed collateral vessels.

Dissection continues cephalad atop the left border of the aorta and reaches the left renal vein, which was exposed by prior cephalad displacement of the duodenum.

The high paraaortic nodes may also be accessed from a lateral approach. The descending colon is mobilized medially by incising the line of Toldt on the left. The areolar tissue between the colon and the renal fascia that invests the kidney and adrenal gland (Gerota fascia) is bluntly dissected. This allows the colon to be retracted medially and superiorly to expose the left renal vein.

With either access, removal of the left paraaortic nodes includes elevation of the distal nodal bundle and sharp dissection to isolate and electrosurgically divide lymphatic attachments. At the left renal vein, the bundle is clipped and transected (Fig. 46-11.5).

⑪ Retroaortic Lymphadenectomy. This more extended dissection is optional and begins after left-sided paraaortic lymphadenectomy has been completed. The left-sided lumbar arteries can be seen branching directly from the aorta. These vessels may be clipped and cut to allow manual rolling of the aorta from left to right, which provides access to the retroaortic nodal chain. Typically, this procedure is performed when imaging studies have demonstrated suspicious nodes in the region.

⑫ Final Steps. Gauze sponges may be opened and gently placed in areas of nodal dissection to tamponade any surface oozing. Closing the retroperitoneal space or routinely using suction drainage does not minimize hematoma or lymphocele development (Morice, 2001).

POSTOPERATIVE

The postoperative course following paraaortic lymphadenectomy in general follows that after laparotomy. However, the incidence of postoperative ileus is increased due to longer operative time, increased bowel manipulation, incision extension, and additional blood loss. As with pelvic lymphadenectomy, lymphoceles and hematomas may develop.

Minimally Invasive Staging for Gynecologic Malignancies

Minimally invasive surgery can often be used for surgical staging that includes pelvic and paraaortic lymph node excision and sometimes omentectomy and peritoneal biopsy. Also, for those without comprehensive staging at their primary surgery, MIS may allow a less morbid completion of cancer staging. Specific MIS qualities that are suited to lymphadenectomy include expanded magnified views within deep or narrow spaces and the ability to achieve fine dissection. In terms of landmarks and fields of dissection, MIS lymphadenectomy procedural steps are the same as those with the open abdominal approach described in the prior two sections. However, with an MIS approach to cancer staging, paraaortic lymphadenectomy is typically completed first. The needed pneumoperitoneum gradually distends bowel, and thus surgery higher in the abdomen is performed early to permit adequate bowel manipulation and displacement.

PREOPERATIVE

Patient Evaluation

A thorough pelvic examination and history reveal factors that help determine the optimal surgical route for an individual patient. As described in Chapter 41 (p. 873), when considering MIS, patients with suspected extensive adhesive disease, morbid obesity, or significant cardiopulmonary disease may be poor candidates. Regardless of approach, preoperative imaging studies prior to lymphadenectomy may help guide the surgeon to suspicious lymph nodes.

Consent

General contraindications for MIS are discussed in Chapter 41 (p. 873). MIS-related complications include entry injury to major vessels, bladder, ureters, and bowel. More specific to MIS staging, acute hemorrhage is the most commonly associated complication. Additionally, ureteral damage, postoperative lymphocele, and nerve injuries can occur, particularly to the obturator and genitofemoral nerves. In addition, the risk of conversion to an open procedure is discussed. Conversion to laparotomy may be necessary if exposure and organ manipulation are limited or if acute hemorrhage cannot be controlled with MIS techniques. Finally, port-site metastasis is a rare but possible complication.

Patient Preparation

As mentioned, bleeding is a frequent problem with pelvic lymphadenectomy and may be exacerbated by retroperitoneal fibrosis. Accordingly, units of packed red blood cells are typed and crossmatched. Topical hemostatic agents also may prove valuable (Table 40-6, p. 860). Routine oral bowel preparation and antibiotic prophylaxis are not required for lymphadenectomy but may be indicated for other concurrent surgeries. Thromboembolism prophylaxis is warranted because of the VTE risk associated with cancer. Options are listed in Table 39-10 (p. 834).

INTRAOPERATIVE

Instruments

Important basic MIS tools for laparoscopy include blunt graspers and scissors, whereas the EndoWrist monopolar scissors and the EndoWrist bipolar Maryland grasper are used with the robot. Additional instruments needed for lymphadenectomy include a combined irrigation/suction device, which clears fluid and bluntly dissects; endoscopic bag for node removal; two to three 5-mm instrument trocars; 10-mm laparoscope trocar; 12-mm endoscopic-bag trocar; and energy devices for cutting and vessel sealing. For the last, several electrosurgical and ultrasonic energy-based devices are adapted for either laparoscopic or robotic cases. These include Harmonic scalpel, electrosurgical monopolar instruments, and electrosurgical bipolar coagulation devices (LigaSure, ENSEAL, PK Dissecting Forceps). For laparoscopy, the argon-beam coagulator is another option. Laparoscope selection varies by surgeon, and a 0-degree scope is frequently used. For others, a 30-degree scope permits greater visibility in tight or angulated spaces.

Surgical Steps

1 Anesthesia and Patient Positioning. Laparoscopic lymphadenectomy is performed under general anesthesia. For VTE prophylaxis, lower-extremity compression devices are placed, and legs are then positioned in adjustable booted support stirrups. Typically, low lithotomy position is selected due to concurrent hysterectomy, although supine may be appropriate for restaging procedures. As described in Chapter 41 (p. 877), appropriate positioning of legs within the stirrups and arms at the side is crucial to reduce nerve injury risks. Also, the patient is secured to the bed by means of a gel pad or bean bag with appropriate protective padding. This keeps the patient from sliding when placed in steep Trendelenburg position, which is needed to reflect bowel for retroperitoneal access.

To avoid stomach puncture by a trocar during primary abdominal entry, an orogastric or nasogastric tube is placed to decompress the stomach. To avert similar bladder injury, a Foley catheter is inserted. The abdomen is then surgically prepared. If hysterectomy is planned, then vaginal preparation also is done.

2 Placement of Ports. As described in Section 46-3 (p. 1168), a 10-mm primary trocar for the laparoscope is placed either at or approximately 1 to 2 cm above the umbilicus using an open abdominal entry method. For paraaortic dissection, this port is placed far enough cephalad to permit visualization of the lower aorta. Accessory ports include a right and left lateral abdominal site and one above one of the anterior superior iliac spines.

Additional trocars are inserted according to surgeon preference or clinical circumstances. All port sites ideally have a minimum of 8 cm between them to allow ample range of motion. For robotic procedures, this avoids robot arm collision.

3 Visual Inspection. Following insertion of the laparoscope, lymph nodes are grossly inspected during initial abdominal exploration. Unexpected positive nodes may alter a proposed operative plan in certain cases, particularly with cervical cancer. In addition, a decision is made to proceed with an MIS approach or convert to laparotomy.

4 Paraaortic Lymphadenectomy: Opening the Retroperitoneal Space. With the patient in steep Trendelenburg position, the small bowel is gently moved into the right and left upper quadrants. The first landmarks identified are the aortic bifurcation and right common iliac artery. The peritoneum over the midlength of the right common iliac artery is grasped, elevated, and sharply incised. This peritoneal incision is extended superiorly atop the right common iliac artery and then atop the aorta. Following each vessel's course, the incision progresses to the curve of duodenum overlying the aorta (Fig. 46-12.1).

Once the peritoneum is opened at this level, it is held anteriorly and cephalad by an assistant surgeon using graspers. Blunt and sharp dissection is performed by the surgeon to lift and displace the duodenum cephalad

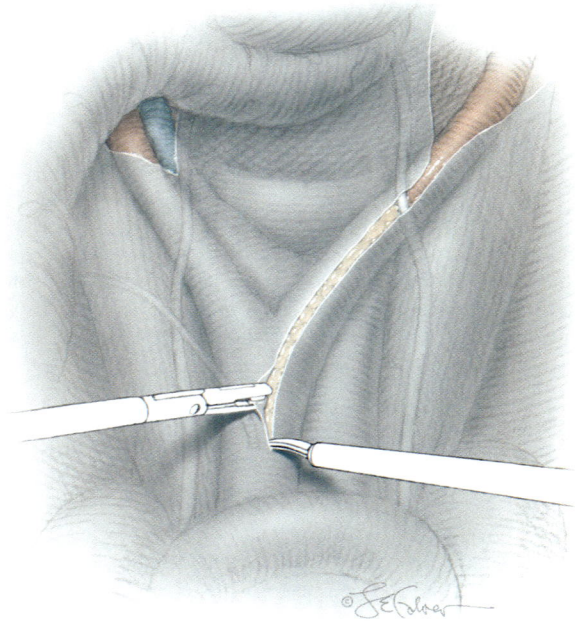

FIGURE 46-12.1 Opening peritoneum over common iliac artery and aorta.

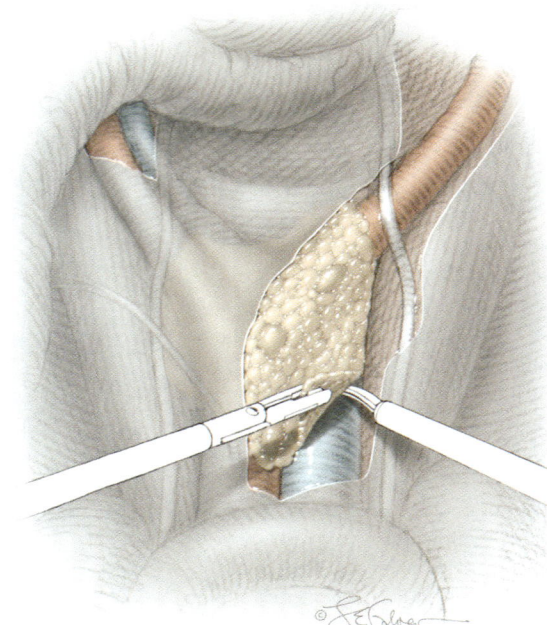

FIGURE 46-12.2 Dissection over the inferior vena cava.

to expose the inferior vena cava and aorta. The duodenum is progressively dissected off the aorta and lifted anteriorly until the level of the left renal vein is reached.

⑤ Ureter Identification. For this, the lateral peritoneal cut edge atop the right common iliac artery is grasped and elevated. Blunt dissection beneath this peritoneum progresses laterally until the right ureter is located as it crosses the common iliac artery. Once identified, the ureter is dissected laterally with gentle blunt traction until the lateral edge of the vena cava is exposed. This lowers ureteral injury risks during the remaining nodal dissection.

⑥ Right Paraaortic Lymph Nodes. To summarize lymphadenectomy within this anatomic area, the caudal end of the fatty, lymph node–containing tissue bundle is freed first. The surgeon then develops medial, lateral, and deep bundle margins and last frees the cephalad tip to permit bundle removal.

To begin, with the ureter held laterally and the inferolateral peritoneal edge elevated, the surgeon first develops the caudal border of this nodal group. Dissection begins at the midlength of the right common iliac artery and atop this artery's lateral border. Within the overlying fatty tissue, small spaces are bluntly developed to create fibrous pedicles that can be lysed or coagulated and divided. In doing so, the distal end of the nodal bundle is progressively freed from the artery and can be elevated and brought cephalad.

Dissection then follows the artery's course and moves medially atop its lateral border. During this dissection, small fibrous bands between the nodal bundle and the right common iliac artery are sequentially transected. Crossing the IVC and reaching the lower aorta, dissection continues atop the right lateral margin of the aorta until reaching the level of the IMA. Dissection may continue to the level of the right ovarian vein if an extended or "high" lymphadenectomy is planned.

To establish the lateral border of this nodal group, the surgeon revisits the dissection's starting point at the right common iliac artery's midlength. Here, a plane is bluntly developed between the lateral border of the IVC and psoas major muscle. Blunt dissection in this plane frees the retroperitoneal fat and is extended cephalad to the level of the IMA.

At this point, the right paraaortic node bundle has been largely detached medially, distally, and laterally, and division of the deep bundle attachments can be performed. The nodal tissue is elevated and separated from the underlying IVC with gentle blunt dissection (Fig. 46-12.2). This dissection moves cephalad atop the IVC to reach the level of the IMA. During this progression, small pedicles that often contain minor vessels are developed. These pedicles and their multiple perforating vessels are sequentially isolated, clipped or coagulated, and divided. Typically, this is the most difficult part of

the dissection because inadvertently avulsed vessels may bleed profusely. For control, hemostatic clips or coagulation can be used. Moreover, a small gauze sponge can be prophylactically placed into the abdomen early in the case to provide quick tamponade if required.

At the level of the IMA, the nodal bundle can be excised by placing vascular clips across the cephalad end and transecting it before the clip. Lymph nodes are extracted intact using an endoscopic bag through a 12-mm port. Once removed, this right nodal bundle is sent as an individual specimen.

⑦ Left Paraaortic Lymph Nodes. Acquisition of the left paraaortic lymph nodes begins atop the aorta at the level of the IMA. As on the right side, after the initial bundle tip is freed, the medial, lateral, and deep margins are developed. However, dissection moves caudally rather than cephalad and ends at the left common iliac artery's midlength.

To begin, the cephalad end of this nodal group is first developed using sharp or electrosurgical dissection that begins just below the IMA (Fig. 46-12.3). Small spaces within the fatty tissue are bluntly opened to create fibrous pedicles that can be lysed or coagulated and divided. This frees the proximal end of the nodal bundle.

To advance this medial border of the nodal group, the lateral peritoneal edge and colon mesentery are elevated to the left on

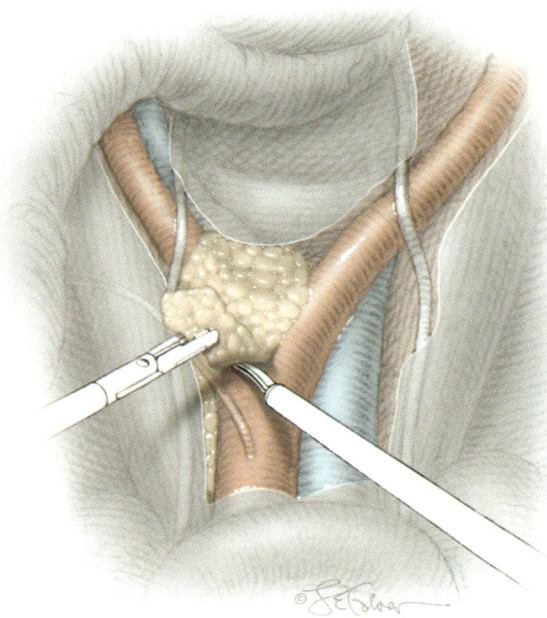

FIGURE 46-12.3 Dissection over the aorta.

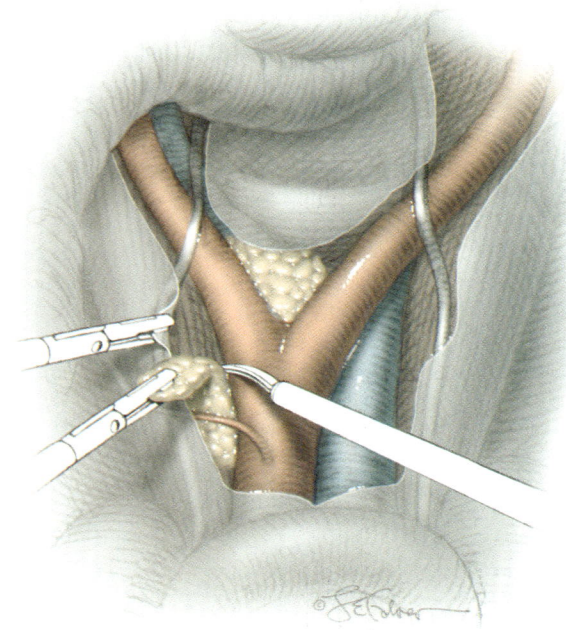

FIGURE 46-12.4 Dissection to the level of the inferior mesenteric artery.

tension, and fibrovascular attachments to the left side of the distal aorta are sharply transected. This permits lateral retraction of the colon mesentery for exposure. The medial side of the bundle is next elevated with forceps to create tension across fibrous bands connecting the nodal bundle and aorta. These fibers are sharply divided. Similar dissection continues caudally atop the left border of the aorta toward its bifurcation. Upon reaching the bifurcation, dissection moves caudally and slightly laterally atop the left common iliac artery's lateral border to finish at this artery's midlength.

To access the lateral border of this nodal group, a blunt tip carefully sweeps laterally to separate the lateral fatty lymphoid tissue from the overlying sigmoid colon mesentery and from the underlying ureter. The ureter serves as the lateral boundary of this nodal group. Opening this potential space allows the ureter and the ovarian vessels, which lie medial to the ureter, to be clearly identified. A blunt probe is then repositioned to gently lift the colon mesentery, its adjoining vessels, and ureter. With this lateral border now developed, dissection of nodal attachments continues caudad, staying medial to the ureter and reaching the midlength of the left common iliac artery.

After establishing the medial and lateral boundaries of the left paraaortic nodal group, the caudad tip of the nodal bundle is again grasped and elevated. From the midlength of the left common iliac artery, dissection beneath the bundle moves cephalad while

transecting deep attachments between it and the lateral aorta and between it and the psoas major muscle (Fig. 46-12.4). Upon reaching the level of the IMA, the cephalad end of the fatty tissue is clipped and transected. The entire nodal group bundle is removed in toto within an endoscopic bag through the 12-mm port. It is submitted as an individual specimen.

❽ High Paraaortic Lymphadenectomy. In some instances, a surgeon may elect an extended laparoscopic dissection. The anatomic boundaries of a high paraaortic lymphadenectomy begin distally at the IMA and reach proximally to the entry level of the right ovarian vein and left renal vein into the IVC, respectively (Whitney, 2010). Typically, this extension is possible only in selected patients with favorable anatomy, such as thin body habitus. Otherwise, upper abdominal exposure is problematic. Two other helpful maneuvers include having a second surgical assistant and placing additional right and left upper quadrant trocars.

To begin, the peritoneum overlying the aorta at the level of the IMA is grasped and elevated cephalad to displace small intestine into the upper abdomen and provide exposure to the aorta. The surgeon dissects retroperitoneally atop the aorta to further mobilize the duodenum and displace it cephalad. Often a laparoscopic fan retractor positioned in the retroperitoneal space aids exposure of the upper aorta.

To develop the medial border of the right high paraaortic nodal group, the nodal bundle overlying the IVC is regrasped and held on traction to dissect and divide the fibrous attachments from the aorta's anterior surface and right border. This begins caudally at the level of the IMA and ends cephalad at the right ovarian vein.

For the lateral border of this nodal group, the right ureter is identified and again retracted to the right. The lateral portion of the nodal bundle is then bluntly separated from the psoas muscle in a proximal direction. The ovarian vein will be encountered and may be individually sealed and divided depending on its proximity to lymph nodes slated for removal.

With both lateral and medial borders defined, the deep middle attachments of this nodal bundle are freed by gentle cephalad dissection over the IVC until the level of the right ovarian vein is reached. Last, the proximal border of the nodal bundle is detached and removed as described earlier.

Dissection of the high left paraaortic nodal group begins by placing laparoscopic clips on the IMA. It is divided between clips using a vessel-sealing device. Alternatively, the IMA may be preserved if adequate exposure is available. This avoids potential bowel ischemia in those with poorly developed collateral vessels. The left ureter is again identified as the lateral border of this high nodal group and is held laterally by an assistant.

The surgeon performs blunt dissection with intermittent coagulation and division of fibrous or vascular pedicles to detach the nodal bundle in a cephalad direction. Dissection continues until it reaches the left renal vein, where the bundle is detached and removed.

❾ Pelvic Lymphadenectomy: Retroperitoneal Entry. For this nodal resection, lymphoid tissue is removed within the area bounded by the psoas major muscle (lateral), the superior vesical artery (medial), the midlength of the common iliac artery (cephalad), and the deep circumflex iliac vein (caudad). To begin, the round ligament is transected, and the peritoneal leaf between the round and IP ligament is grasped, elevated, and incised parallel to the IP ligament. Gentle traction is again applied to the round ligament, and the broad ligament's anterior peritoneal leaf is opened to reach the vesicouterine fold in the midline. If radical hysterectomy is planned after pelvic lymphadenectomy, then pararectal and paravesical spaces are completely developed as described on page 1169 prior to pelvic lymph node removal.

❿ External Iliac Nodes. Bowel is first retracted sufficiently to allow access to the distal half of the common iliac artery. To remove this nodal group, the prior peritoneal incision atop the common iliac artery is extended from its midlength caudally to expose the artery. Ureterolysis, if not previously performed, is completed as described in Section 46-3, Step 4 (p. 1169). The ureter is then bluntly retracted medially before beginning node dissection.

Removal of the external iliac lymph node group starts by freeing its lateral border. Dissection then extends caudally along the lateral side of the external iliac artery until reaching the deep circumflex iliac vein. This vein crosses the distal external iliac artery and serves as the caudal boundary of this nodal group. Along this path, dissection bluntly develops a plane between medially located lymphoid tissue and lateral preperitoneal fat found above the psoas major muscle (Fig. 46-12.5). During dissection, the genitofemoral nerve running atop the psoas major muscle is ideally identified and protected.

Next, grasper traction is typically required to lift the nodal bundle above the external iliac artery beginning at the common iliac artery bifurcation. During caudal dissection, a blunt tool gently pushes into the fibrofatty tissue to create distinct pedicles that attach the nodal bundle to the artery. These pedicle attachments can then be coagulated and divided. Electrosurgery can also be used to obtain hemostasis as the lymph node bundle is progressively excised caudally.

The mobilized nodal bundle is next reflected medially to reveal the entire external iliac artery (Fig. 46-12.6). Medial traction is applied with forceps, and fine adventitial bands that connect nodes to the underlying external iliac vein are transected using electrosurgical cutting. In contrast to open surgery, the pneumoperitoneum and Trendelenburg position used during laparoscopy result in vein collapse. As a result, the external iliac vein is harder to distinguish and can be easily injured. Once completed, this external iliac nodal group dissection later permits safe entry into the obturator space, outlined in Step 12.

⓫ Internal Iliac Nodes. The ureter is moved and held medially by a blunt instrument for protection and improved pelvic sidewall visualization. Beginning at the distal aspect of the superior vesical artery, the free nodal bundle is again elevated and placed on tension. Initial sharp excision of the internal iliac nodal group continues cephalad along the superior vesical artery and then along the internal iliac vessels (Fig. 46-12.7). As dissection approaches the common iliac artery bifurcation, the nodal attachments are fine and allow blunt disruption. At this point, both the external iliac and internal iliac nodes are completely dissected and can be submitted as one specimen or combined with obturator fossa lymph nodes, depending on surgeon preference.

⓬ Obturator Fossa Nodes. With the assistant surgeon holding medial traction on the superior vesical artery, the obturator fossa

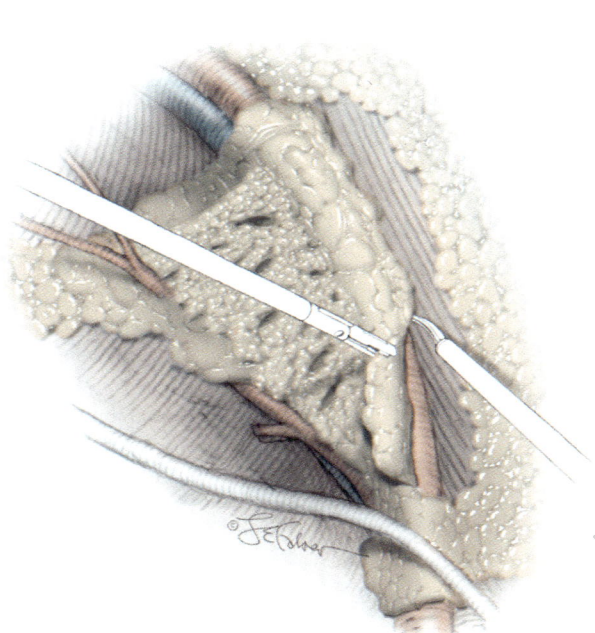

FIGURE 46-12.5 Dissection between the external iliac artery and psoas major muscle.

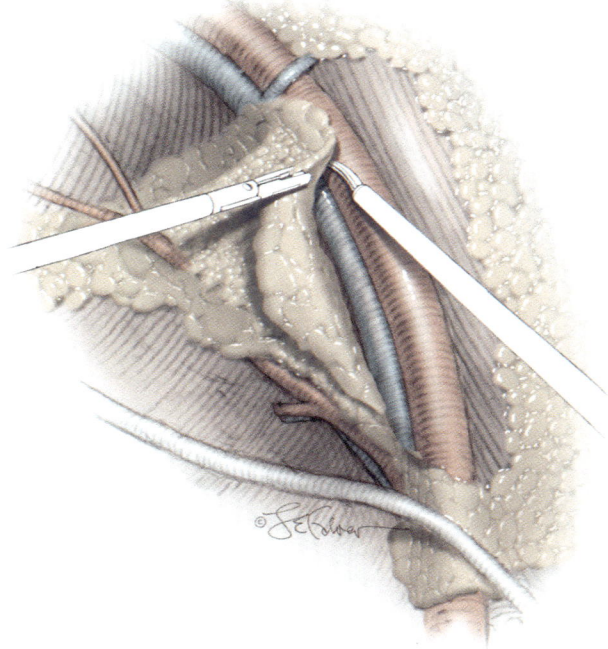

FIGURE 46-12.6 Dissection off the external iliac vessels.

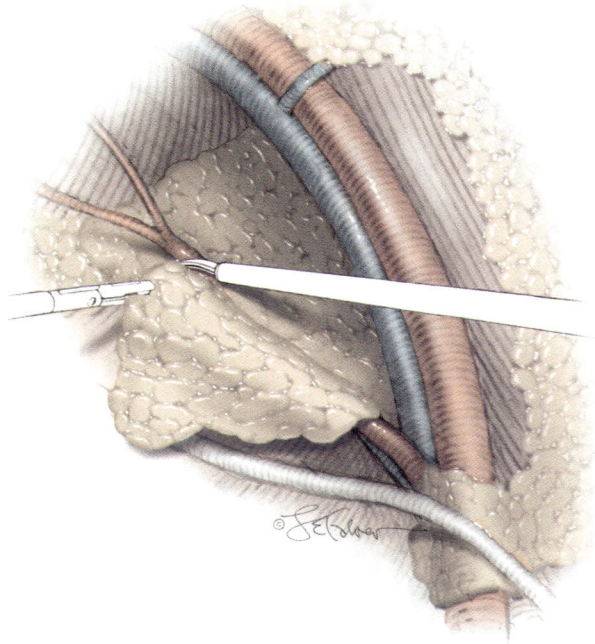

FIGURE 46-12.7 Dissection off the internal iliac artery.

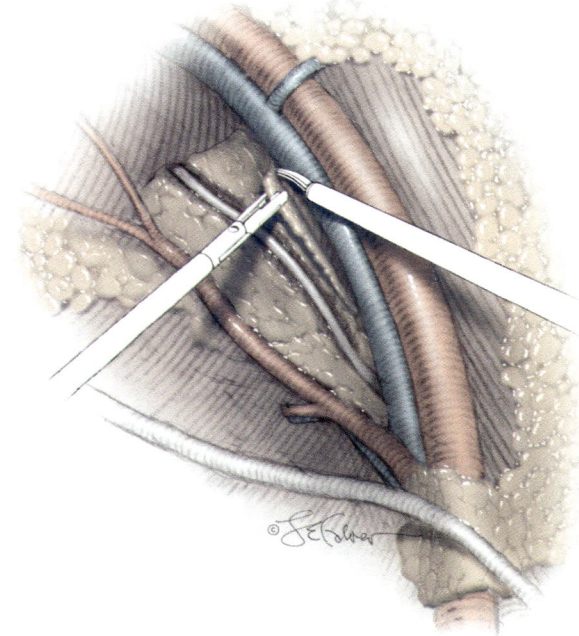

FIGURE 46-12.8 Dissection above the obturator artery.

can be exposed. This fossa may be entered medially, under the external iliac vein. If present, nodal tissue along the inferomedial wall of the external iliac vein is transected with blunt and electrosurgical dissection. Also, accessory venous branches may be identified and coagulated.

Within the exposed fossa, obturator nodal tissue is grasped with forceps. This nodal bundle lies deep to the external iliac vein but superficial to the obturator nerve. With upward traction applied, blunt forceps or a suction/irrigation device tip moved gently side-to-side disrupts nodal tissue attachments to the obturator nerve (Fig. 46-12.8). This blunt dissection is performed in the center of the fossa to minimize injury to surrounding deep pelvic vasculature. This also clears off tissue to permit obturator nerve identification.

Once this nerve is localized, dissection should purposely remain superficial to it. Firm fibrotic attachments may be electrosurgically transected under direct visualization. As the caudal end of the bundle is reached, it is usually tethered to the sidewall and freed sharply. At the cephalad end of the bundle, nodes are carefully separated sharply from the inferior aspect of the external iliac vein while avoiding obturator nerve injury. Nodal tissue deep to the obturator nerve is not routinely removed since the obturator artery and vein traverse this area. Laceration of either vessel can result in retraction and catastrophic hemorrhage that is difficult to control.

⑬ Pelvic Lymphadenectomy: Distal Common Iliac Nodes. Lateral fatty lymphoid tissue may be removed by first elevating it with a blunt grasper and using electrosurgical dissection atop the common iliac artery's lateral margin to establish a plane between the nodal bundle and artery. Blunt dissection to further separate the nodal tissue from the artery is continued caudad. Electrosurgical coagulation plus sharp incision is used to detach these nodes. Importantly, on the patient's right side, the common iliac vein and inferior vena cava lie beneath the common iliac artery's lateral margin, and thus careful node excision is prudent. Further dissection is performed atop the distal common iliac artery, which serves as the medial border for this nodal group. The common iliac artery bifurcation is the distal margin for this group.

Pelvic lymph nodes are then removed in toto via endoscopic bag. The identical procedure is performed on the contralateral side.

⑭ Completion of Laparoscopic Staging and Omentectomy. The staging procedure for ovarian cancer includes obtaining multiple peritoneal biopsies from the cul-de-sac, pelvic sidewalls, and pelvic gutters, and from the diaphragm bilaterally. This can be performed with a blunt grasper and laparoscopic scissors, with or without electrosurgical coagulation. The surgical staging for ovarian cancer and for certain histologic subtypes of endometrial cancer (papillary

serous and clear cell carcinoma) also includes omentum removal.

A laparoscopic omentectomy is performed by identifying and elevating the omentum away from the transverse colon. Avascular windows are created within the proximal omentum. The intervening vascular attachments are then ligated with a vessel-sealing energy tool or endoscopic stapler. Once completely dissected, the omentum is placed in an endoscopic bag and removed through a transabdominal 12-mm port. In many women, the omentum is large and therefore is brought through the vagina if a laparoscopic hysterectomy is performed. All specimens undergo minimal manipulation and are removed through an endoscopic bag to help decrease the risk of port-site or intraabdominal tumor implantation.

⑮ Cannula Removal and Fascial Closure. Once procedures are completed, areas are inspected for bleeding. Topical hemostatic agents may be used. If hemostasis is achieved, cannulas are removed and port sites closed. Fascial defects >10 mm are sutured to decrease the risk of herniation at those sites (Boone, 2013; Lambertz, 2017). Interrupted stitches of 0-gauge delayed-absorbable suture are used to reapproximate this fascia. Alternatively, a dedicated port-site closure device, described in Chapter 41 (p. 895), can be used. Regardless of technique, the defect is palpated to confirm adequate closure.

POSTOPERATIVE

The postoperative course following MIS staging lymphadenectomy generally follows that after other major laparoscopic surgery. Patients usually are quickly able to tolerate clear liquids, which are followed by a regular diet and discharge on postoperative day 1. With their pain typically controlled with oral pain medication, patients ambulate early.

Postoperative complications may include pelvic and paraaortic lymphocele formation, hematomas, ureteral injuries, bowel injuries, neurologic injuries, or port-site herniation. One long-term potential complication of pelvic lymphadenectomy is chronic lymphedema. The exact incidence is unknown, but estimates range from 1 to 27 percent after surgical staging for endometrial cancer (Todo, 2010). The risk increases if more lymph nodes are removed or if pelvic radiation is administered after surgery. Treatments, which may or may not be successful, often include compression stockings, lower-extremity wrapping, and massage therapy to manipulate lymph channels. Although generally not associated with an adverse outcome, this complication can significantly lower a patient's quality of life postoperatively.

46-13

En Bloc Pelvic Resection

Ovarian cancer with contiguous encasement of the reproductive organs, pelvic peritoneum, cul-de-sac, and sigmoid colon is the main indication for en bloc pelvic resection. Also known as radical oophorectomy, this effective technique aids a maximal cytoreductive surgical effort. Although neoadjuvant chemotherapy use continues to rise, the overall complexity of primary and interval debulking surgery also has increased (Horner, 2019). As a result, this procedure holds important value by removing all microscopic and infiltrative peritoneal tumor in the pelvis, with the expectation of improved survival rates in patients with advanced epithelial ovarian cancer (Aletti, 2006b). Moreover, pelvic recurrence rates are low and reflect the completeness of pelvic tumor eradication (Hertel, 2001). Many of the principles of en bloc pelvic resection mirror those of other procedures in gynecologic oncology.

PREOPERATIVE

Patient Evaluation

Pelvic examination may reveal a relatively immobile mass, and abdominopelvic CT images typically demonstrate a pelvic mass and ascites. With the presumed diagnosis of advanced ovarian cancer, patients are prepared for anticipated cytoreductive surgery. However, the need for en bloc resection is usually dictated by intraoperative findings rather than preoperative testing.

Consent

In general, women with advanced ovarian cancer undergoing cytoreductive surgery are at significant risk for complications. Minor postoperative problems such as incisional cellulitis, superficial wound dehiscence, urinary tract infection, or ileus are common. Major postoperative complications of en bloc resection include anastomotic leaks and various fistulas (Bristow, 2003; Park, 2006).

Patient Preparation

Primary anastomosis without colostomy is typical for most patients. Thus, bowel preparation is commonplace for any type of cytoreductive ovarian cancer surgery, but particularly if en bloc pelvic resection is a possibility. One or more bowel resections may be required to achieve optimal debulking, and often, preoperative determination of the exact location of tumor infiltration is not entirely accurate. The combination of pneumatic compression devices and subcutaneous heparin is particularly important due to the anticipated longer operation length, coagulability risk associated with malignancy, and possibility of extended postoperative recovery. Moreover, patients are routinely typed and crossmatched for packed red blood cell replacement, as transfusions are frequently indicated (Bristow, 2003).

INTRAOPERATIVE

Instruments

En bloc pelvic resection requires access to multiple sizes of bowel staplers, including gastrointestinal anastomosis (GIA), transverse anastomosis (TA), and end-to-end anastomosis (EEA) staplers. Additionally, a ligate-divide-staple (LDS) device or electrothermal bipolar coagulator (LigaSure) may be used to divide vascular tissue pedicles.

Surgical Steps

❶ **Anesthesia and Patient Positioning.** Bimanual examination under general anesthesia is especially important to confirm the need for low lithotomy leg positioning in booted support stirrups. For VTE prophylaxis, lower-extremity pneumatic compression devices are placed. Access to the perineum is crucial any time the EEA device may need to be placed in the rectum. Sterile preparation of the abdomen, perineum, and vagina is performed, and a Foley catheter is inserted.

❷ **Abdominal Entry.** Typically, a vertical incision is selected for ovarian cancer debulking surgery since the extent of disease cannot be precisely known beforehand and upper abdominal disease requires excision. At first, the incision extends up to the umbilicus. After exploration and determination of tumor resectability, it can be lengthened as needed.

❸ **Exploration.** The abdomen is thoroughly explored to first determine whether all gross disease can be safely removed. For example, unresectable upper abdominal tumor makes the prospect of a radical pelvic operation less attractive.

Frequently during exploration, it is difficult to distinguish uterus, adnexa, and adjacent tumor. As shown in Figure 46-13.1, both ovaries may be grossly enlarged with tumor and densely fixed into the posterior cul-de-sac with contiguous involvement of the uterus, rectosigmoid, and lateral sidewalls. Moreover, superficial implants often coat the fallopian tubes, the vesicouterine fold, and much of the surrounding pelvic peritoneum. En bloc pelvic resection will allow removal of all this gross disease.

❹ **Lateral Pelvic Dissection.** If the round ligaments cannot be located with certainty, the lateral peritoneum is grasped with an Allis

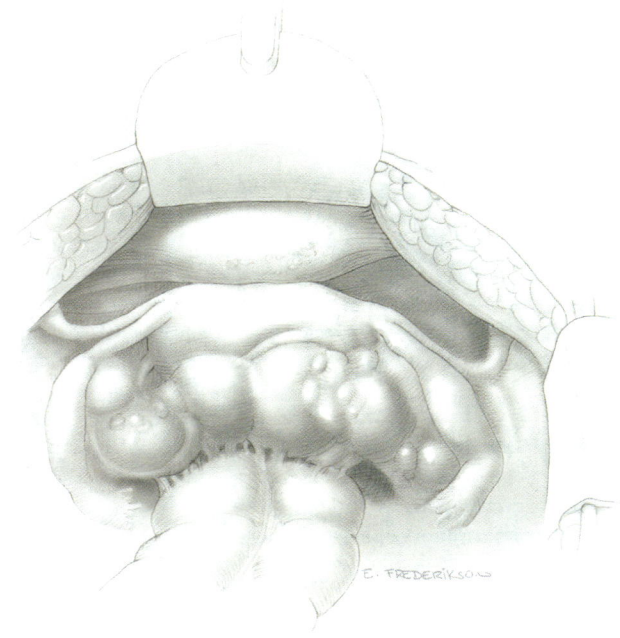

FIGURE 46-13.1 Extensive ovarian cancer.

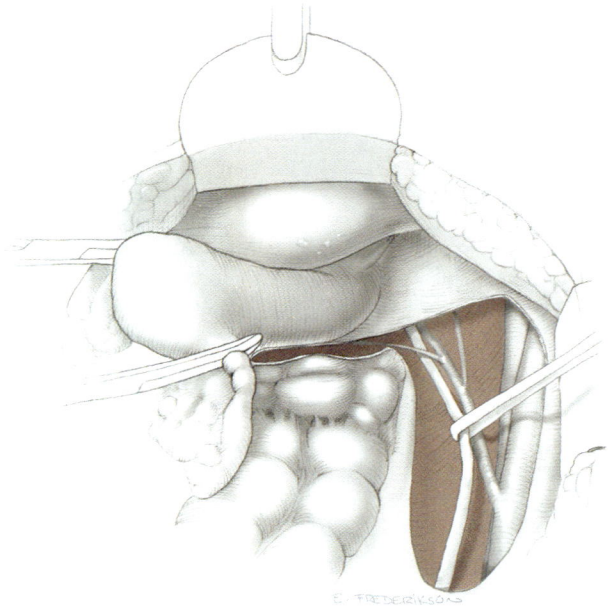

FIGURE 46-13.2 Lateral pelvic dissection.

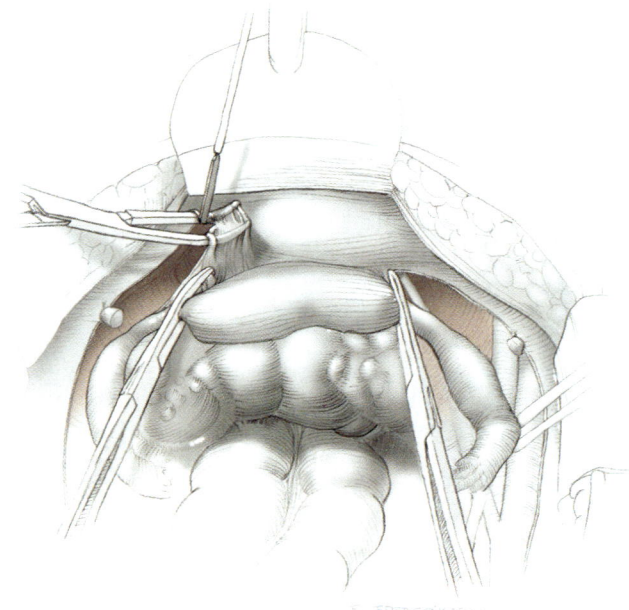

FIGURE 46-13.3 Vesicouterine dissection.

clamp, and an electrosurgical blade is used to enter the retroperitoneum (Fig. 46-13.2). The loose areolar connective tissue of this space is bluntly dissected, and the overlying peritoneum is sharply incised to create an opening in which the external iliac artery can be palpated. This artery is bluntly followed to the bifurcation with the internal iliac artery. The medial peritoneal leaf of the broad ligament is elevated to identify the ureter, around which a one-quarter inch Penrose drain is looped.

The IP ligament will typically not be entirely distinguishable due to induration and anatomic distortion by tumor. A window is bluntly opened just superior to the ureter as it crosses above the pelvic brim to isolate a tissue pedicle that will include the IP ligament. The ligament is isolated, clamped, cut, and tied with 0-gauge delayed-absorbable suture. The entire sequence is repeated on the contralateral side. The ureter may then be mobilized distally, and the anterior portion of the broad ligament is incised toward the vesicouterine fold using an electrosurgical blade. The round ligament will be identified during this dissection and separately divided.

5 Vesicouterine Dissection. The anterior broad ligament dissection is continued with a right-angle clamp guiding the electrosurgical blade (Fig. 46-13.3). The peritoneum is typically edematous and thick. En bloc removal of tumor implants within the vesicouterine fold will require a wide excision of gyne peritoneum over the bladder dome. Thus, the proximal end of the

vesicouterine fold may be held on traction, and an electrosurgical blade used to sharply dissect in a caudal direction toward the cervix while encompassing the tumor. The bladder mucosa is typically not entered, but it may be simply repaired if an inadvertent cystotomy occurs (Chap. 45, p. 1081). After removal of this peritoneum, the bladder may then be advanced distally in the usual manner as for simple hysterectomy. The whitish cervix will be visualized through the anterior vaginal wall. The ureters are held laterally while the uterine vessels are freed of surrounding connective tissue (skeletonized), clamped, cut, and ligated.

6 Dividing the Sigmoid Colon. This step mirrors those in Steps 5 and 6 of low anterior resection, shown on page 1226. First, the ureters are held laterally, while a right-angle clamp guides an electrosurgical blade during posterior peritoneum incision. This incision moves medially on each side to reach the midline sigmoid colon mesentery. The sigmoid colon segment that lies proximal to the tumor is selected, and the underlying mesentery is superficially incised on each side with the electrosurgical blade. A GIA stapler is then inserted to divide the bowel.

After colon division, the remaining mesentery is scored superficially with the electrosurgical blade and divided with the electrothermal bipolar coagulator. Larger pedicles, such as those including the inferior mesenteric vessels, will need to be clamped, cut, and ligated separately. As during total pelvic exenteration, the avascular retrorectal space between the rectum and the sacrum may then be bluntly dissected

to completely mobilize the rectosigmoid down to the cervix (Fig. 46-13.4).

7 Retrograde Hysterectomy. The bladder is separated from the upper vagina with sharp electrosurgical blade dissection. The anterior vaginal wall distal to the tumor margin is grasped with a Kocher clamp. The anterior vaginal wall is then incised at 12 o'clock with the electrosurgical blade, and the incision is extended laterally to the right and left. The cervix is grasped with a Kocher clamp and retracted to expose the posterior vaginal wall. An electrosurgical blade is used to incise this wall transversely and enter the rectovaginal space. Two Allis clamps grasp the upper vagina to apply caudad traction and aid further dissection. A retrorectal hand is placed to assess whether the tumor extends into the rectovaginal septum beyond the cervix. With large masses, distal dissection may be required into the rectovaginal septum to reach a point distal to the tumor's leading edge. If so, further distal vaginal wall excision may be needed to reach tumor-free margins. Alternatively, smaller tumors may allow proximal dissection in the rectovaginal septum. This gains additional rectal length distal to the tumor and allows for creation of a higher colon reanastomosis. Finally, the remaining uterosacral and cardinal ligaments are clamped, analogous to a radical hysterectomy (p. 1164), but in a retrograde fashion. With this, distal portions of the cardinal ligament are transected first, and then more cephalad portions are clamped, cut, and ligated. For protection, ureters are held laterally (Fig. 46-13.5).

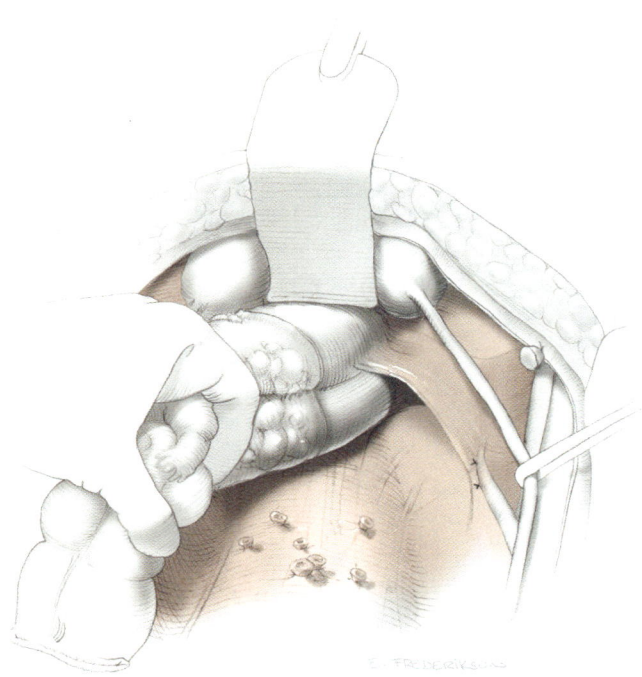

FIGURE 46-13.4 Dividing the rectosigmoid.

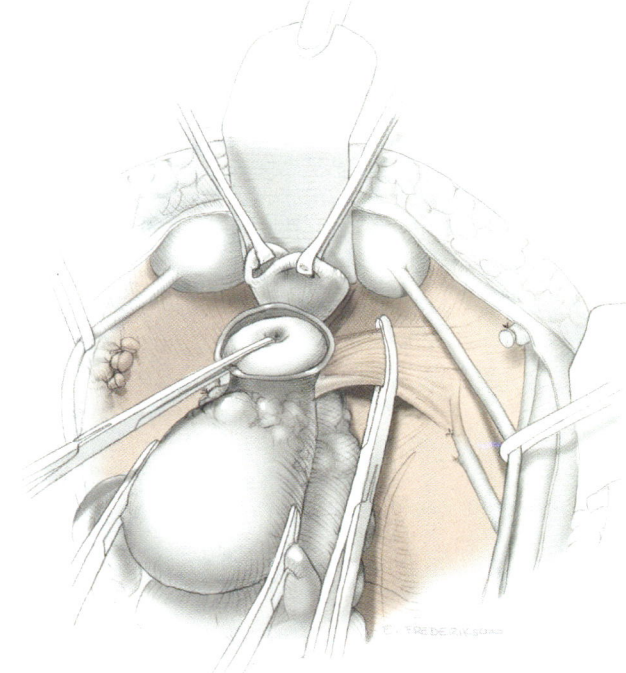

FIGURE 46-13.5 Retrograde hysterectomy.

❽ Distal Rectal Division. The mucosa of the rectal segment distal to the tumor is circumferentially dissected free of mesenteric attachments and rectal pillars by constant traction on the en bloc specimen. The TA or curved cutter (Contour) stapler is inserted into the pelvis and fired to transect the rectum (Fig. 46-13.6). The specimen, which contains the uterus, adnexa, rectosigmoid, and surrounding peritoneum, is then lifted out of the pelvis. The vaginal opening is closed in a running fashion with 0-gauge delayed-absorbable suture. The final appearance (Fig. 46-13.7) is shown with completed rectosigmoid anastomosis, which is described in Section 46-21 (p. 1227).

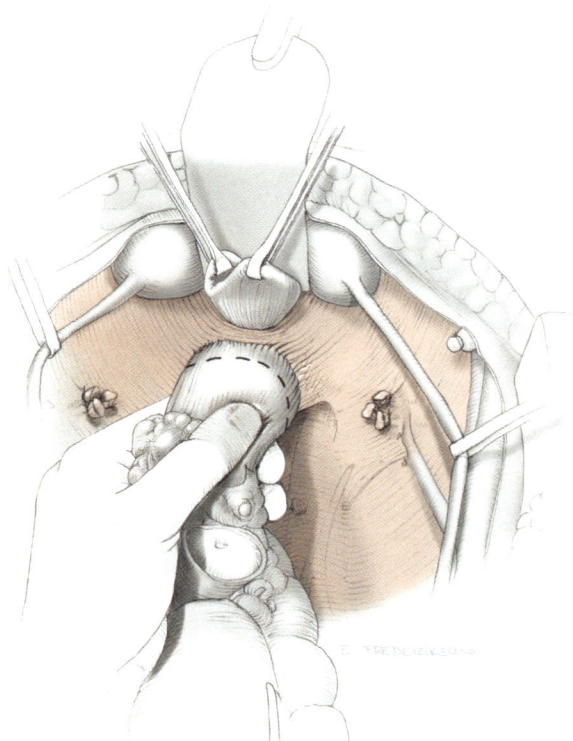

FIGURE 46-13.6 Rectosigmoid resection.

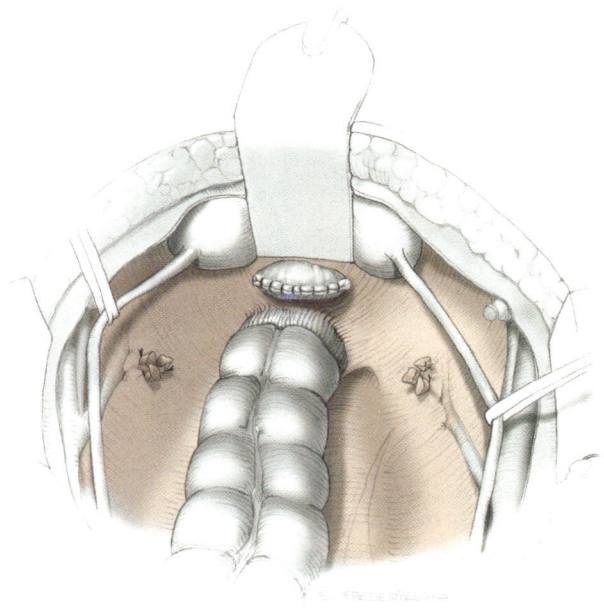

FIGURE 46-13.7 Final appearance.

❾ Final Steps. A surgeon then proceeds with additional procedures if necessary to complete the ovarian cancer debulking surgery. A colostomy or rectosigmoid anastomosis may require mobilization of the splenic flexure and is performed near the end of surgery. Postoperative drains may be placed at the surgeon's discretion. Occasionally, the bladder may also be retrograde filled to exclude cystotomy during vesicouterine dissection. All pedicles sites are reexamined for hemostasis.

POSTOPERATIVE

En bloc pelvic resection of primary and recurrent ovarian cancer permits a high rate of complete debulking with acceptable morbidity and mortality rates (Yildirim, 2014). Urinary tract infection, pneumonia, deep-vein thrombosis, wound cellulitis, and postoperative ileus are relatively common events following major abdominal surgery for ovarian cancer. Reoperation for anastomotic breakdown or postoperative hemorrhage specific to en bloc pelvic resection is uncommon (Tozzi, 2017).

Omentectomy

The omentum is typically removed for two reasons: tumor debulking or cancer staging. First, patients who present with advanced ovarian cancer almost invariably have metastases to the omentum. The extent of this "omental cake" may be massive and involve the upper gastrocolic ligament, anterior abdominal wall, splenic hilum, and transverse colon (Fig. 35-13, p. 746). Thus, a surgeon is prepared to encompass the entire tumor with an adequate resection. Second, omentectomy is routinely indicated for staging patients with ovarian cancer or with uterine papillary serous carcinoma who do not have obvious metastatic disease (Armstrong, 2019; Whitney, 2010).

As a reminder, the proximal omentum has two leaves. Its anterior leaf attaches to the greater curvature of the stomach via the gastrocolic ligament. Its posterior leaf attaches to the caudal margin of the transverse colon. The lesser omental sac lies between these two leaves. *Infracolic omentectomy* describes transection of the anterior leaf (gastrocolic ligament) at a level below the transverse colon. This is sufficient for most clinical circumstances. Supracolic (total) omentectomy describes transection of the anterior leaf (gastrocolic ligament) at a level above the transverse colon and close to the stomach's greater curvature. It may be indicated for a large omental cake.

Omentectomy may be completed by laparotomy, as described here. It is also amenable to a MIS approach, as described in Section 46-12, Step 14 (1205).

PREOPERATIVE

Patient Evaluation

Imaging studies may suggest an omental cake, but its extent is difficult to ascertain until exploration in the operating room.

Consent

Although bleeding may follow inadequate vessel ligation, complications from omentectomy are rare. Obesity and intraabdominal adhesive disease, however, may increase these risks. Obesity results in a much thicker omentum that has thicker vascular pedicles, which may slip from clamps or ligatures. Additionally, prior upper abdominal surgery—particularly gastric bypass—may cause adhesions and a more difficult resection. In addition to these risks, women with

an omental cake are informed of a possible need for bowel resection, splenectomy, or other radical debulking procedures to remove the entire tumor.

Patient Preparation

The risk of infection following omentectomy is low. However, this surgery is typically performed with other gynecologic procedures that warrant antibiotics and VTE prophylaxis, as listed in Tables 39-8 and 39-10 (p. 832). The decision to administer a bowel preparation regimen is individualized by surgeon preference and clinical setting. Suitable options are found in Chapter 39 (p. 833).

INTRAOPERATIVE

Surgical Steps

① **Anesthesia and Patient Positioning.** Omentectomy is typically performed as an inpatient procedure under general anesthesia. For VTE prophylaxis, lower-extremity pneumatic compression devices are placed. A patient is positioned supine, a Foley catheter is placed, and the abdomen is surgically prepared.

② **Abdominal Entry.** Infracolic omentectomy may be performed through any type of incision. However, because of the uncertain extent of disease that accompanies these cases, a midline vertical incision is most commonly selected. If only a portion of the omentum needs to be removed for staging purposes, the incision does not necessarily need to be extended above the umbilicus since the omentum is often accessible. In all other situations, the incision is extended cephalad to provide sufficient exposure.

③ **Exploration.** Palpation of the omentum is often the first step in exploring the abdomen. This organ is directly beneath a midline vertical incision and should be readily visible. Omentectomy is typically the first procedure performed in women with an omental cake and presumed ovarian cancer. The omentum can usually be quickly removed and sent for frozen-section analysis while a surgeon places a self-retaining retractor and proceeds with the remainder of a planned operation.

④ **Visualization.** A surgeon gently grasps the infracolic omentum and pulls it out of the abdomen through the incision. The borders of any omental cake can be seen directly or palpated. The extent of resection can then be determined, and the abdominal wall incision extended if necessary.

⑤ **Entrance into the Lesser Sac.** The posterior leaf of the omentum is best accessed by flipping the omental drape cephalad. Filmy adventitial tissue with some traversing small vessel tributaries joins this leaf and colon, and these attachments are electrosurgically cut and vessels divided by a ligate-divide-staple (LDS) device or an electrothermal bipolar coagulator (LigaSure). Dissection generally begins as far to the right as possible and continues as far to the left as possible. A right-angle clamp is opened beneath the omentum to guide the direction of the electrosurgical blade (Fig. 46-14.1). Once the posterior leaf is transected, the lesser sac is entered.

Entrance into the lesser sac mobilizes the colon and provides access to the tumor-free proximal gastrocolic ligament.

⑥ **Gastrocolic Ligament Division.** Next, attention turns to the anterior omental leaf, and the omental drape is now flipped caudad. For an infracolic omentectomy, dissection of the omentum is performed inferior to the level of the transverse colon. Dissection again generally begins on the far right and moves to the left. Numerous vertically coursing vessels can be seen, but others are covered by fatty tissue and difficult to appreciate. A right-angle clamp is used by the surgeon to "pop" through an avascular portion of the gastrocolic ligament that is near, but safely distal to, the colon. The clamp is then opened in a vertical direction (parallel to the vessels) and held in place to guide the LDS or electrothermal bipolar coagulator in safely and quickly dividing the tissue (Fig. 46-14.2).

This procedure is continued across the entire gastrocolic ligament, and the omental specimen is handed off. However, if a J-flap is planned instead of an omentectomy, then only three quarters of the omentum is divided from right to left. This preserves the left gastroepiploic artery for blood supply. The distal tip of the flap is brought into the pelvis and tacked to adjoining peritoneum with 2-0 or 3-0 gauge delayed-absorbable suture to provide additional blood supply wherever desired. Regardless of whether removing the infracolic omentum or fashioning a J-flap, the drape will need to be rotated back and forth intermittently to make certain that dissection remains away from the colon.

⑦ **Supracolic Omentectomy.** In cases in which an omental cake has extended proximally, a supracolic (total) omentectomy is indicated. This procedure requires a midline vertical incision to provide better exposure to the upper abdomen. Resection may simply involve transecting the omentum at a higher level in the gastrocolic ligament. Alternatively, anatomic boundaries of resection may need to be extended to the hepatic

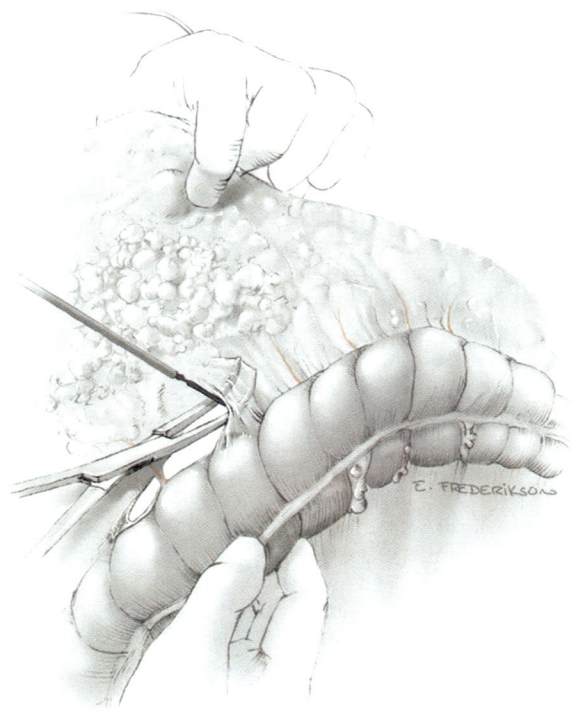

FIGURE 46-14.1 Posterior omental leaf transection to enter the lesser sac.

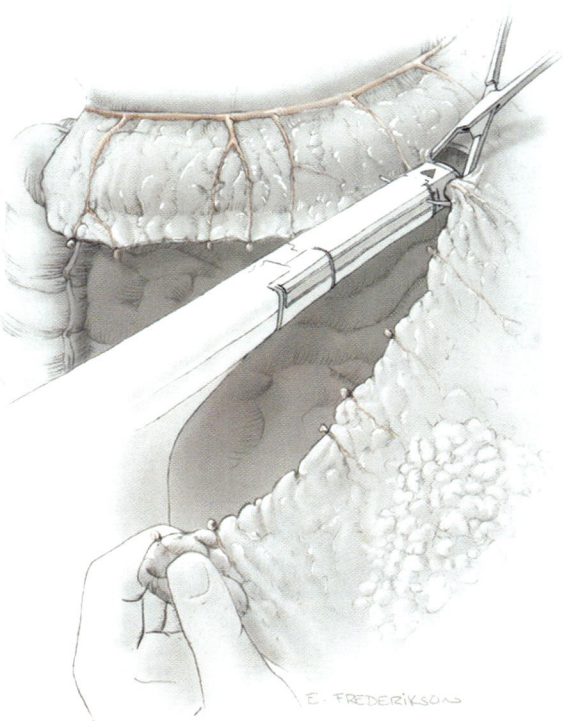

FIGURE 46-14.2 Anterior ligation of gastrocolic ligament.

flexure, the stomach, and the splenic flexure to encompass the entire tumor.

Dissection again proceeds from right to left, detaching the posterior leaf of the omentum from its attachment to the transverse colon. Mobilization of the ascending colon around the hepatic flexure may be necessary to perform a gastrocolic omentectomy. The right gastroepiploic artery is ligated, and the dissection is continued to the left by dividing the short gastric vessels until the lateral-most portion of the tumor is reached. Mobilization

of the descending colon and takedown of the splenic flexure may be required if tumor extends that far laterally.

❽ **Incision Closure.** The remaining omentum should be reexamined at the completion of surgery before closing the abdomen. Occasionally, small bleeding vessels or a hematoma will need to be addressed with additional ligation. The abdominal entry incision is then closed as described in Section 43-1 (p. 932).

POSTOPERATIVE

Nasogastric tube placement is required only if a total omentectomy has been performed. Decompression of the stomach for 48 hours protects the ligated gastric vessels from postoperative dislodgement due to gastric dilation. The remaining postoperative course follows that for laparotomy or for other specific concurrent surgeries performed.

46-15

Splenectomy

In gynecologic oncology, removal of the spleen is occasionally required to achieve optimal surgical cytoreduction of metastatic ovarian cancer. Most commonly, tumor is found directly extending from the omentum into the splenic hilum during primary debulking surgery. Splenectomy and other extensive upper abdominal resection techniques have been shown to improve survival with acceptable morbidity (Chi, 2010; Eisenhauer, 2006). However, the number of patients who will actually have their spleen removed during their initial operation ranges from 1 to 14 percent (Eisenkop, 2006; Goff, 2006). Splenectomy is also indicated for selected patients with isolated parenchymal recurrences to assist optimal secondary surgical cytoreduction of ovarian cancer. In some instances, a laparoscopic or robotic approach may be possible (Gallotta, 2016, 2018). Last, intraoperative splenic trauma is the least common indication and usually is unanticipated (Magtibay, 2006).

PREOPERATIVE

Patient Evaluation

Preoperative diagnosis of splenic involvement is often difficult to predict with certainty prior to primary cytoreduction. Typically, in such cases, an omental cake is seen on CT images, but its proximity to the spleen is difficult to ascertain. Splenic involvement is more commonly distinguishable at the time of secondary cytoreduction. Ideally, relapsed patients have isolated disease and have had an extended progression-free survival of at least 12 months before they are considered for splenectomy.

Consent

Patients with presumed advanced ovarian cancer are consented for possible splenectomy, but the decision to perform the procedure will only be finalized intraoperatively. Although removal of the spleen results in a longer operative time, greater blood loss, and longer hospital stay, it may ultimately determine whether tumor is optimally debulked (Zapardiel, 2012). Possible serious complications include hemorrhage, infection, and pancreatitis.

INTRAOPERATIVE

Surgical Steps

❶ Anesthesia and Patient Positioning. Splenectomy is performed under general anesthesia and with the patient supine. For VTE prophylaxis, lower-extremity pneumatic compression devices are placed. The abdomen is surgically prepared, and a Foley catheter is inserted.

❷ Abdominal Entry and Exploration. During laparotomy, splenectomy requires a vertical incision for adequate exposure. Following entry, a surgeon carefully assesses the entire abdomen and pelvis to confirm the ability to resect all gross disease. Ideally, splenectomy is performed only if optimal tumor debulking can thereby be achieved. The spleen is grasped to assess its mobility, degree of tumor involvement, and potential difficulty in removal. As a brief review, the spleen has ligamentous attachments to its surrounding organs. These include the gastrosplenic, splenocolic, and splenophrenic ligaments. All are transected during splenectomy.

❸ Entrance into the Lesser Sac. The gastrocolic ligament, which lies between the stomach's greater curvature and the transverse colon, is opened to the left of midline by dividing vascular pedicles as described in Section 46-14, Step 6 (p. 1211). Dissection is continued in two directions (Fig. 46-15.1). For one, dissection moves along the superior transverse colon with mobilization of the entire splenic flexure of the colon to reach the splenocolic ligament. For the other, dissection progresses upward to the greater curvature of the stomach toward the gastrosplenic ligament. The intervening portion of omentum is often involved with tumor and is removed.

❹ Mobilization of the Spleen. The spleen is grasped, elevated, and pulled medially to expose the splenophrenic ligament. A surgeon uses alternating electrosurgical blade and blunt finger dissection to further mobilize the spleen. Additional blunt and sharp dissection is then performed circumferentially to free the spleen from the gastrosplenic and splenocolic ligaments. Notably, the gastrosplenic is the most vascular and contains the short gastric arteries. These are carefully ligated and divided. To avoid pancreatic injury, it is important to continually review the anatomy.

❺ Ligating the Splenic Vessels. The spleen is elevated into the incision, and the peritoneum overlying the splenic hilum is carefully incised. To aid this approach, a left index finger is held against the spleen. Also, the pancreatic tail, which lies close to

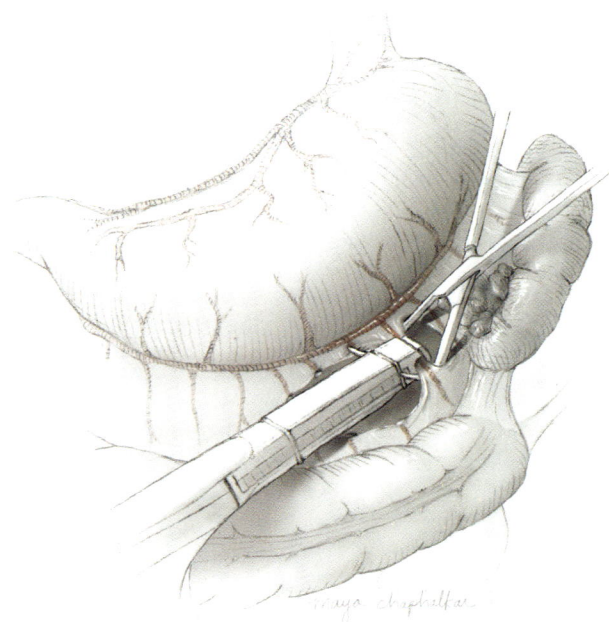

FIGURE 46-15.1 Mobilizing the spleen.

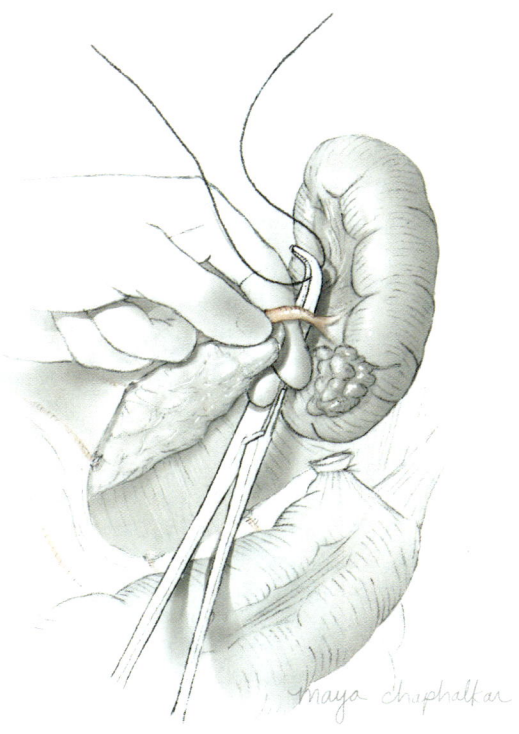

FIGURE 46-15.2 Vessel ligation.

the splenic hilum (often within 1 cm), is displaced medially with the left thumb.

Blunt dissection parallel to the expected course of the splenic artery and vein aids identification of these vessels. The artery, vein, and vascular tributaries are individually ligated. The artery is first isolated to prevent splenic engorgement (Fig. 46-15.2). A right-angle clamp is placed beneath the artery, and a 2-0 silk suture is pulled through and tied. A second silk tie is placed more distally, directly at the hilum. The proximal end of the artery is again tied or occluded with a vascular clip. The artery is then divided, and the procedure is repeated for the splenic vein. Vascular tributaries are similarly divided. The remaining peritoneal attachments are incised with an electrosurgical blade to remove the spleen.

6 Final Steps. The distal pancreas is carefully inspected to exclude injury. The splenic vessels also are reexamined prior to abdominal closure. Suspicion of pancreatic trauma or bleeding usually prompts placement of a suction drain in the splenic bed. Otherwise, drainage is not routinely required. A nasogastric tube is placed to decompress the stomach and prevent displacement of gastric vessel staples.

POSTOPERATIVE

Hemorrhage is the most serious immediate complication and, typically, originates from the short gastric or splenic vessels. Bleeding can be profuse, and thus the initial 12 to 24 postoperative hours require particular vigilance (Magtibay, 2006).

The most common postoperative "complication" is left lower lobe lung atelectasis. This will typically resolve with ambulation, pulmonary therapy, and time. Development of a postoperative intraabdominal abscess usually results from inadvertent injury to the stomach, splenic flexure, or distal pancreas.

Excessive pancreatic manipulation or laceration may lead to pancreatitis or leaking. When a distal pancreatectomy is required due to tumor adherence or injury, approximately one quarter of patients will develop a pancreatic leak. According to one set of criteria, this leak is defined by a left upper quadrant collection of fluid seen on imaging after postoperative day 3, and this fluid contains an amylase level >3 times that of serum amylase. If a drain has been placed, fluid may be sent to the laboratory if this complication is suspected. Pancreatic leak usually presents early in the postoperative period and can be managed conservatively with percutaneous drainage (Kehoe, 2009).

Patients undergoing splenectomy will be at lifelong risk for episodes of overwhelming sepsis. Accordingly, the pneumococcal and meningococcal vaccines are recommended and the *Haemophilus influenzae* type b is considered postoperatively (Kim, 2015a). Importantly, these vaccines may be given together but are not administered earlier than 14 days following splenectomy. In addition, patients are instructed to seek immediate medical attention for fevers, which may rapidly progress to serious illness.

46-16

Diaphragmatic Surgery

Patients with advanced ovarian cancer will often have tumor implants or confluent plaques involving the diaphragm. The right hemidiaphragm is most frequently affected. Implants are typically superficial, but invasive disease can extend through the peritoneum to the underlying muscle. Accordingly, gynecologic oncologists are prepared to perform diaphragmatic ablation, stripping (peritonectomy), or full-thickness resection. These surgical procedures increase the rate of optimal tumor debulking and correlate with improved survival (Aletti, 2006a; Tsolakidis, 2010). Although this procedure can be attempted using MIS, the open approach is described here (Magrina, 2019).

PREOPERATIVE

Patient Evaluation

Imaging studies may suggest diaphragmatic nodularity, but the extent is difficult to ascertain until exploration in the operating room.

Consent

Patients with presumed advanced ovarian cancer are informed of the possible need for extensive upper abdominal surgery to achieve optimal cytoreduction. Pulmonary complications after diaphragmatic surgical techniques most commonly include atelectasis and/or pleural effusion. However, pneumonia, empyema, and pneumothorax also are possible (Ye, 2017).

INTRAOPERATIVE

Instruments

It is generally advisable to have a cavitational ultrasonic surgical aspiration (CUSA) system and/or argon beam coagulator (ABC) available for ovarian cancer debulking procedures, since one or both can be useful in eradicating diaphragmatic disease. These tools are discussed further in Chapter 40 (p. 858).

Surgical Steps

❶ Anesthesia and Patient Positioning. As with other major intraabdominal surgeries, diaphragmatic surgery requires general anesthesia. For VTE prophylaxis, lower-extremity pneumatic compression devices are placed. The patient is positioned supine, the abdomen is surgically prepared to accommodate an incision to the sternum, and a Foley catheter is inserted.

❷ Abdominal Entry. Diaphragmatic surgery requires a vertical midline incision that has been extended to the sternum, passing to the right side of xiphoid process, for maximum exposure. Following abdominal entry, a surgeon carefully assesses the entire abdomen and pelvis to confirm the ability to resect all gross disease. Ideally, diaphragmatic surgery is performed only if optimal tumor debulking can thereby be achieved.

❸ Diaphragmatic Ablation. A few scattered, small tumor implants on the surface of the right or left hemidiaphragm can usually be easily ablated with the CUSA or ABC. This simple technique may be all that is required.

❹ Diaphragmatic Stripping. Confluent plaques of tumor or extensive implants indicate the need for resection of the peritoneum. For this, the right side of the anterior rib cage is retracted sharply upward. The liver is manually retracted downward and medially to aid division of the falciform ligament, right coronary ligament, and right triangular ligament of the liver with sharp dissection using an electrosurgical blade. This maneuver significantly mobilizes the liver and allows it to be held medially away from the diaphragm.

Dissection begins on the right side of the diaphragm, where the diaphragmatic peritoneum meets the anterior abdominal wall. Allis clamps are used to grasp the peritoneum above the tumor plaque and place it on tension. The peritoneal incision is created transversely above the tumor with an electrosurgical blade, and a plane is developed with blunt dissection to separate the peritoneum from the underlying muscle fibers of the diaphragm. The free peritoneal edge is placed on tension with Allis clamps to maintain traction. The incision is then extended medially and laterally to encompass the implants (Fig. 46-16.1). The specimen eventually becomes large enough to grasp with a left hand to aid in "stripping" the peritoneum off the diaphragm. Electrosurgical blade dissection proceeds dorsally until all implants are contained within the peritoneal specimen. At this point, it can be detached.

❺ Diaphragmatic Resection. Occasionally, tumor has penetrated through the peritoneum, and a plane cannot be developed to strip the diaphragm. In these circumstances, full-thickness diaphragmatic resection is required. A self-retaining retractor is placed, and the liver mobilized. A transverse peritoneal incision is made above the tumor plaque, and at this point, the inadequacy of stripping is determined.

The ventilator is temporarily turned off to avoid lung parenchymal injury, and an electrosurgical blade is used to cut through the diaphragmatic muscle into the pleural cavity above the tumor. Ventilation may then be resumed while Allis clamps are placed to retract the specimen into the peritoneal cavity. Both pleural and peritoneal surfaces should be visible to aid in complete resection of the disease. After resection, primary mass closure of the diaphragmatic defect is then performed with a running stitch using 0-gauge polydioxanone monofilament (PDS) suture or interrupted stitches of silk suture.

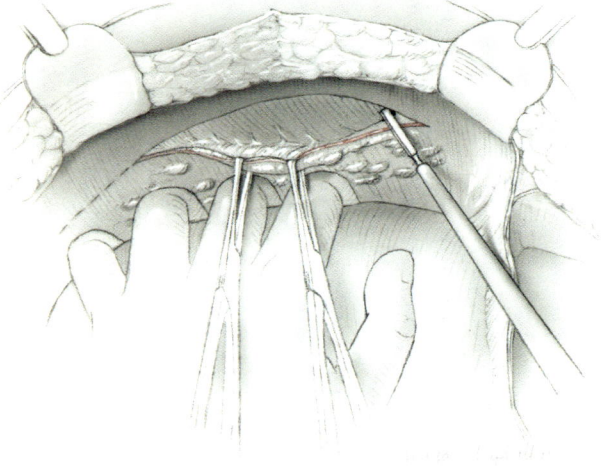

FIGURE 46-16.1 Diaphragm stripping.

To evacuate the pneumothorax, a red rubber catheter is placed through the defect into the pleural space prior to securing the final knot. The ventilator is turned off at the end of inspiration to maximally inflate the lungs while the catheter is placed on suction. The catheter is removed concomitantly with tying the knot, and mechanical ventilation is resumed (Bashir, 2010). Grafts are not typically needed, even for large defects (Silver, 2004).

❻ Final Steps. The patient is placed in Trendelenburg position at the completion of stripping or resection to check the integrity of the diaphragmatic closure. The upper abdomen is filled with saline and observed for air leaks as the patient is ventilated. The presence of air bubbles indicates the need to reintroduce the red rubber catheter through the hole, resuture the defect, and retest the closure. Chest tubes are not routinely required.

POSTOPERATIVE

Atelectasis is common with any diaphragmatic surgery, and routine postoperative respiratory expansion techniques are appropriate (Chap. 42, p. 911). Diaphragmatic stripping is associated with an increased incidence of pleural effusion, especially when the pleural space is entered. Fortunately, most will self-resolve, and only a few will require postoperative thoracentesis (Dowdy, 2008). Patients having full-thickness diaphragmatic resection are carefully monitored with chest radiographs for evidence of a pneumo- or hemothorax. Those few who do not resolve with supportive care measures may require chest tube drainage to aid lung reexpansion (Bashir, 2010).

46-17

Colostomy

A colostomy is a surgical anastomosis between created openings in the colon and anterior abdominal wall to divert bowel contents into an external collection bag. Colostomies serve several purposes and may be used: (1) to protect distal bowel repair from disruption or contamination by feces, (2) to decompress an obstructed colon, and (3) to evacuate feces if the distal colon or rectum is excised. In gynecologic oncology, specific indications for performing a colostomy are innumerable. Some of the more common ones include rectovaginal fistula, severe radiation proctosigmoiditis, bowel perforation, and rectosigmoid resection in which reanastomosis is not feasible.

A colostomy may be temporary or permanent, and its duration is dictated by clinical circumstances. For instance, recurrent end-stage cervical cancer with obstruction may warrant a permanent colostomy. In contrast, only temporary diversion is needed to allow healing of an intraoperative bowel injury that occurred during benign gynecologic surgery.

In addition, the location of the stoma and the decision to perform an end or loop colostomy are clinically based. A loop colostomy is constructed by creating an opening in a loop of colon and bringing both ends through the stoma. Alternatively, an end colostomy stoma contains only the proximal end of the transected colon. The distal end is stapled and left intraabdominally.

Regardless of the circumstances, the same surgical principles apply during colostomy: adequate bowel mobilization, sufficient blood supply, and a tension-free tunnel through the abdominal wall without bowel constriction. Strict attention to these seemingly straightforward steps ensures the best possible outcome. In some circumstances, a laparoscopic colostomy may be possible (Jandial, 2008).

PREOPERATIVE

Patient Evaluation

The colostomy site, typically on the patient's left, is ideally marked preoperatively by an enterostomal therapist to ensure that the postoperative stoma will be located in an easily accessible area when sitting and standing.

Consent

Concerns regarding postoperative quality of life changes are common with this procedure. Accordingly, a surgeon carefully describes a colostomy's medical purpose and its expected temporary or permanent duration. Much of the fear regarding "wearing a bag" can be assuaged with compassionate preoperative counseling and education. Many times, postoperative results are actually superior to a patient's current symptoms and quality of life.

Perioperative complications may include fecal leakage into the abdomen or retraction of the stoma. Long-term complications involve parastomal hernia, stricture, and the potential need for surgical revision.

Patient Preparation

To minimize fecal contamination during bowel incision, aggressive bowel preparation such as with a polyethylene glycol with electrolyte solution (GoLYTELY) may be considered the day prior to surgery unless contraindicated, such as with bowel obstruction or perforation. Additionally, broad-spectrum antibiotics are given preoperatively due to the possibility of stool contamination of the operative site. With stool spill, postoperative antibiotic doses for 24 to 48 hours and a drain near the anastomosis are reasonable.

INTRAOPERATIVE

Surgical Steps

1 Anesthesia and Patient Positioning. Colostomy is performed under general anesthesia with the patient positioned supine. For VTE prophylaxis, lower-extremity pneumatic compression devices are placed. Prior to surgery, the abdomen is surgically prepared, and a Foley catheter is inserted.

2 Abdominal Entry and Exploration. Although concurrent surgery may dictate the approach, a midline vertical incision, due to its superior exposure, is generally preferred when colostomy is a possibility. The bowel segment is selected as distally as possible to preserve normal bowel. Dissection and adhesiolysis are performed as necessary to mobilize the bowel to obtain sufficient length before creating the abdominal wall stoma opening. The colon is elevated to ensure that it will reach the selected stoma site without tension. If the bowel fails to reach the selected site without tension despite maximal mobilization, then the proposed stoma site is moved to accommodate the available bowel length.

3 End Colostomy. This type of diversion is commonly used for rectovaginal fistulas and severe proctosigmoiditis after radiation. Ideally, a more distal colon site is used since bowel content becomes progressively more solid and less voluminous as it moves from the cecum to the rectum. As a result, the ostomy bag does not need to be changed as often, and the risk of dehydration or electrolyte abnormalities is reduced. If performing an end sigmoid colostomy, the distal bowel may simply be stapled closed and left in the pelvis (Hartmann pouch). In contrast, a more proximal end colostomy performed for a distal colonic obstruction will require that the distal bowel also be brought to the abdominal wall and opened, either at the same site or as a second ostomy. This distal-bowel-loop ostomy serves as a "mucus fistula" to prevent a closed loop obstruction and subsequent colonic perforation from mucus or gas accumulation.

The stoma site for a sigmoid colostomy is selected based on an imaginary line drawn from the umbilicus to the left-sided anterior superior iliac spine. The site is sufficiently lateral from the midline to allow application of the ostomy appliance. But, it is located sufficiently medial because stoma support from the rectus muscle lowers stoma-site hernia risks.

To begin, a Kocher clamp is used to elevate the skin and an electrosurgical blade, set to a cutting mode, is used to remove a 3-cm circle of skin. The fascia is exposed by blunt dissection. In obese patients, a cone through the subcutaneous fat with its tip at the fascia may need to be removed to prevent bowel constriction. A cruciate incision is made on the anterior sheath. The fibers of the rectus abdominis muscle are bluntly separated, and another cruciate incision is cut on the posterior sheath. The opening is bluntly expanded to accommodate two or three fingers.

After the colon is divided as described in Section 46-21, Step 5 (p. 1226), the proximal bowel is mobilized by incising the peritoneum toward the splenic flexure along the white line of Toldt, which is the reflection of posterior abdominal parietal peritoneum over the mesentery of the descending colon. A Babcock clamp is then placed through the skin opening to grasp the stapled end of bowel and lift it through the abdominal opening (Fig. 46-17.1). The bowel should appear pink, and its mesentery must not be twisted. The primary vertical abdominal incision is then closed.

The stoma is not ordinarily "matured" until the abdominal wall and skin are closed, with a dressing in place. First, the table is tilted to the left to minimize bowel spillage and fecal contamination of the incision site, and then the intestinal staple line is excised. Circumferential interrupted 3-0 and 4-0 gauge delayed-absorbable sutures are placed through the bowel mucosa and skin dermis (Fig. 46-17.2). The ostomy bag appliance may then be attached.

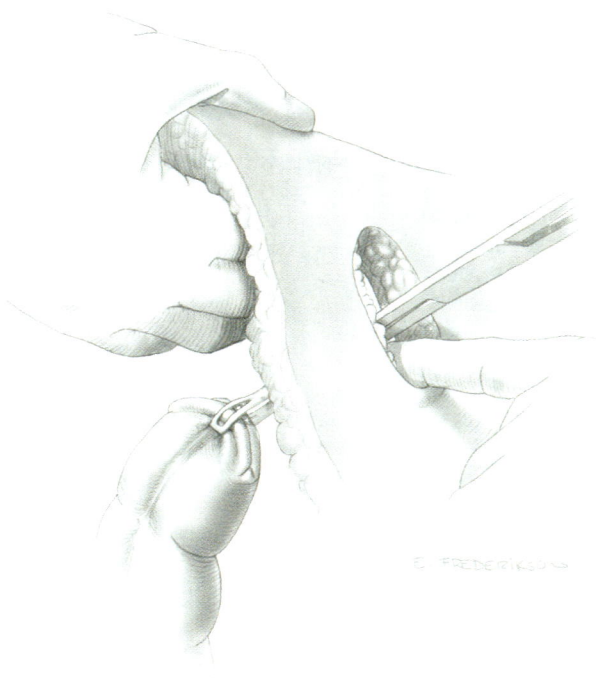

FIGURE 46-17.1 End-sigmoid colostomy: bowel pulled through abdominal wall incision.

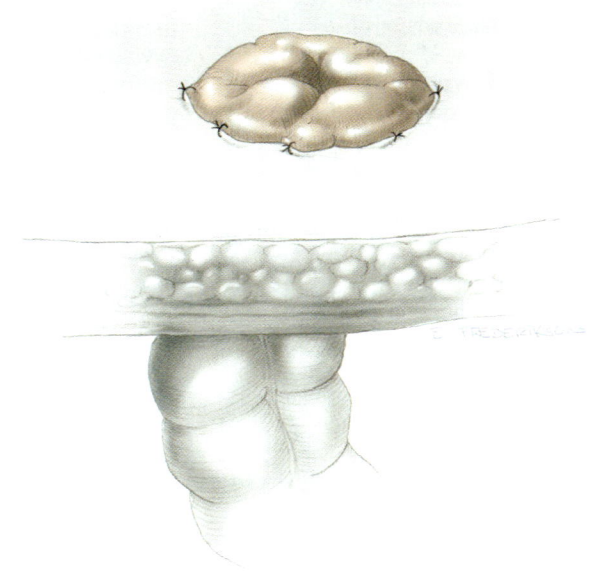

FIGURE 46-17.2 End-sigmoid colostomy: bowel mucosa sutured to skin.

❹ Loop Colostomy Principles. The usual indications for this type of procedure include protection of a distal anastomosis, relief of colonic obstruction, and colonic perforation. Accordingly, loop colostomy can be performed at any site along the colon where indicated. A loop colostomy in general is intended to be a temporary or palliative procedure. It is easier to take down, often simpler to perform, and does not necessarily require designation of loops as distal or proximal. However, fecal matter will eventually pass through to the distal segment. As a result, this type of colostomy is not a permanent solution to a fistula or proctosigmoiditis.

❺ Transverse Loop Colostomy. As a stand-alone procedure, a transverse loop colostomy is most often performed to relieve a distal obstruction and can be used in an emergent or palliative setting. This colostomy is performed in the left upper quadrant by creating a 5-cm transverse incision over the rectus abdominis muscle midway between the costal margin and the umbilicus. The anterior and posterior fascia, rectus abdominis muscle, and peritoneum are opened longitudinally by sharp and blunt dissection. The omentum is separated from the underlying transverse colon along enough length to allow the bowel segment to be pulled up through the incision without it. Next, a one-quarter inch Penrose drain may be placed through the

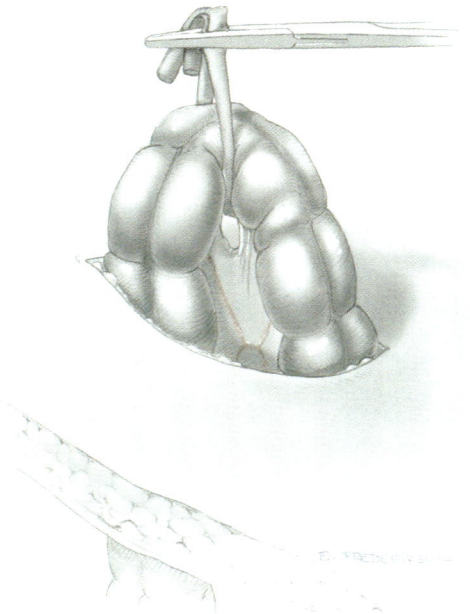

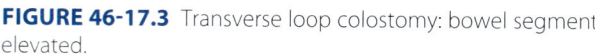

FIGURE 46-17.3 Transverse loop colostomy: bowel segment elevated.

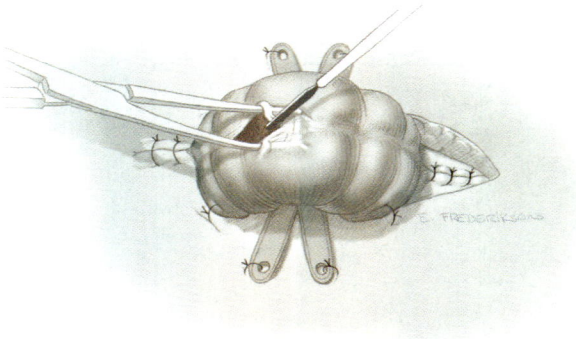

FIGURE 46-17.4 Transverse loop colostomy: bowel opened.

mesocolon for traction, and the bowel loop is brought through the incision (Fig. 46-17.3). A Hollister bridge or similar device may be passed through the mesenterotomy in place of the Penrose drain. However, this time-honored approach does not prevent retraction and results in more complications (Franklyn, 2017). The skin incision is then closed around the bowel loop without constricting it.

The bowel is then "matured" by opening the antimesenteric half of the bowel along the tenia with an electrosurgical blade and leaving a 1-cm margin on each end (Fig. 46-17.4). The colostomy edges are sutured to the skin with interrupted stitches of 3-0 gauge delayed-absorbable suture.

❻ Final Steps. The stoma is carefully inspected and ideally is pink and comfortably positioned. A dusky color may indicate bowel ischemia, which can lead to sloughing, necrosis, and retraction. Tension on the bowel may be improved with additional colon mobilization. Constriction of a loop colostomy within the abdominal wall opening can be improved by broadening the fascial incision or removing additional subcutaneous fat. With end colostomy, on occasion, the tip may need to be transected further distally to reach a viable bowel segment. All of these steps are cumbersome but are much easier to perform during the operation rather than postoperatively after complications become obvious.

POSTOPERATIVE

Morbidity is comparable for end and loop colostomies. Complications may be immediate or not evident for several months. Common complications specific to a colostomy may include wound infection, necrosis, bowel obstruction, hematoma, retraction, fistula, fecal leakage, sepsis, stricture, and parastomal herniation (Carlsson, 2016). Many of these complications are manageable with supportive care and local measures. Dramatic symptoms are infrequent but may require operative revision. Careful attention during initial surgery will prevent most of these morbidities.

46-18

Large Bowel Resection

Partial colectomy is most often performed as part of cytoreductive surgery for ovarian cancer, although other indications include radiation injury and colonic fistula. Surgical principles are similar, whether a bowel segment to be removed is from the ascending, transverse, or descending colon. Rectosigmoid (low anterior) resection is somewhat more complex and is reviewed in Section 46-21 (p. 1225).

Ideally during colectomy, a surgeon will achieve meticulous hemostasis, remove the smallest required length of colon, avoid fecal spill, and confirm bowel continuity by excluding possible sites of proximal or distal intestinal obstruction. In addition, bowel must be sufficiently mobilized to create a tension-free anastomosis that is watertight, large caliber, and supported by adequate blood supply. During surgery planning, insufficient bowel length for reanastomosis, a malnourished patient, questionable vascular supply, or undue anastomosis tension may instead require a permanent or temporary diverting colostomy.

A general familiarity with colonic blood supply is important for partial colectomy. The ascending and transverse colon are supplied by the superior mesenteric artery via the ileocolic, right colic, and middle colic branches. The descending and sigmoid colon are supplied by the left colic and sigmoid branches of the inferior mesenteric artery. As a result, these vessels form an effective anastomotic vascular network that allows large bowel resection at virtually any segment of the colon.

PREOPERATIVE

Patient Evaluation

The need for partial colectomy during ovarian cancer cytoreductive surgery is usually decided intraoperatively and is based on clinical circumstances. For example, although preoperative CT images may suggest tumor at multiple sites near the colon, these lesions are often superficial and may be removed without colectomy. Typically, the need for colectomy is more obvious preoperatively for those with radiation damage or fistula. However, the extent of resection will still generally be unclear until the operation is underway.

Consent

Patients are fully informed of the potential for colostomy, anastomotic leak, and abscess formation. A postoperative ileus also should be anticipated.

Patient Preparation

To minimize fecal contamination during bowel incision, with the intention of reducing surgical-site infection rates, most surgeons still recommend aggressive bowel preparation (McChesney, 2019). One choice, a polyethylene glycol with electrolyte solution (GoLYTELY), may be considered the day prior to surgery unless contraindicated, such as with bowel obstruction or perforation. However, there is no evidence that patients benefit from this practice, and bowel preparation may not lower the risk of postoperative complications (Koskenvuo, 2019; Suzuki, 2019). If a bowel obstruction is present, then cleansing only the distal colon with enemas is a secondary option. The patient is also marked for a colostomy if that is a possibility. Moreover, if a complicated resection or prolonged recovery is anticipated, postoperative TPN administration is considered. Preoperative antibiotics and perioperative VTE prophylaxis are warranted, and options are listed in Tables 39-8 and 39-10 (p. 832).

INTRAOPERATIVE

Instruments

To prepare for complicated resections, a surgeon should have access to all types and sizes of bowel staplers. These include end-to-end anastomosis (EEA), gastrointestinal anastomosis (GIA), and transverse anastomosis (TA) staplers. Additionally, a ligate-divide-staple (LDS) device or electrothermal bipolar coagulator (LigaSure) may aid in vessel ligation.

Surgical Steps

❶ **Anesthesia and Patient Positioning.** Rectovaginal examination under anesthesia is mandatory before positioning any patient for abdominal gynecologic cancer surgery. A palpable mass with compression of the rectum or rectovaginal septum indicates the need for low lithotomy with legs comfortably positioned in booted support stirrups to prepare for possible low anterior resection and anastomosis. Supine positioning is otherwise appropriate, and for VTE prophylaxis, lower-extremity pneumatic compression devices are placed. Sterile preparation of the abdomen, perineum, and vagina is completed, and a Foley catheter is inserted.

❷ **Abdominal Entry.** A midline vertical incision is preferable if partial colectomy is anticipated, as this incision provides access to the entire abdomen. Required dissection, adhesiolysis, or other unanticipated findings may render exposure from a transverse incision inadequate.

❸ **Exploration.** A surgeon first explores the entire abdomen to lyse adhesions, to "run" the bowel and evaluate its appearance from duodenum to rectum, to exclude other potential sites of obstruction proximally or distally, and to determine the extent of the bowel resection. Colonic blood supply at the splenic flexure, hepatic flexure, and ileocecal valve can be tenuous. As a result, resection boundaries ideally lie beyond these areas if possible. For example, in Figure 46-18.1, because of the known tenuous blood supply at the hepatic flexure, the proximal line of transection includes several centimeters of transverse colon. Similarly, the distal line of transection includes 8 to 10 cm of the terminal ileum because the ileocecal artery is sacrificed. Leaving this terminal ileum would render it vulnerable to necrosis from insufficient remaining vascular support.

Once the segment is selected, a window is made in the mesocolon proximal and distal

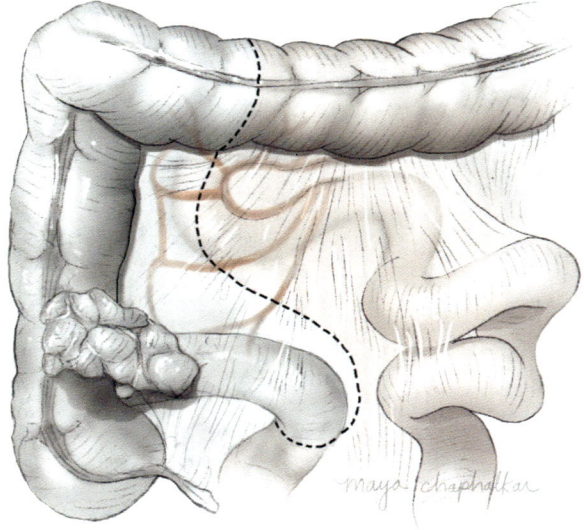

FIGURE 46-18.1 Area of resection encompasses tumor.

to the lesion. A one-quarter inch Penrose drain is pulled through each location's opening to provide traction.

❹ Mobilization of the Colon. The bowel is next mobilized by incising peritoneum along the white line of Toldt and/or along the hepatic or splenic flexures—depending on the resection site. For the case shown in Figure 46-18.1, the right retroperitoneal space is entered at the mid-ascending colon, continued along the white line of Toldt, and extended toward and around the cecum to a site beyond the distal Penrose drain. The entry opening is created with an electrosurgical blade just lateral to the colon. This space is bluntly expanded, and electrosurgical dissection is next guided cephalad past the proximal Penrose drain while providing countertraction on the colon. The bowel segment may be bluntly mobilized medially as necessary. Partial infracolic omentectomy may be required for resections involving the transverse colon.

❺ Resection. A GIA stapler is inserted to replace one Penrose drain, is positioned around the entire colon diameter, and is fired. This stapler lays two rows of staples and transects interposed bowel. A second stapling and transection is then repeated at the other Penrose drain site. Staying close to the bowel segment's wall, the bowel segment may then be detached from its underlying mesentery, using an LDS device, electrothermal bipolar coagulator, or individual clamps and 0-gauge delayed-absorbable suture ligation. During this process, as much of the mesentery as possible is preserved to provide adequate blood supply to the anastomosis. The specimen is then removed.

❻ Side-to-Side Anastomosis. The proximal and distal bowel ends are held parallel against each other to estimate their position following anastomosis. Typically, additional mobilization of the bowel by incising adhesions and peritoneum is required using a combination of electrosurgical blade and blunt dissection. The two segments must comfortably approximate antimesenteric borders without tension. For larger resections, the mesentery of each segment may also need to be dissected to achieve sufficient mobility. The proximal and distal stapled bowel ends are skeletonized of fatty tissue to create an anastomosis with maximal mucosa-to-mucosa contact. To accomplish this, the proximal staple line is elevated with two Allis clamps at its lateral edges. DeBakey forceps grasp surrounding fatty tissue and place it on traction, while an electrosurgical blade is used to dissect this tissue away from the bowel serosa. The dissection is then performed on the distal segment in similar fashion.

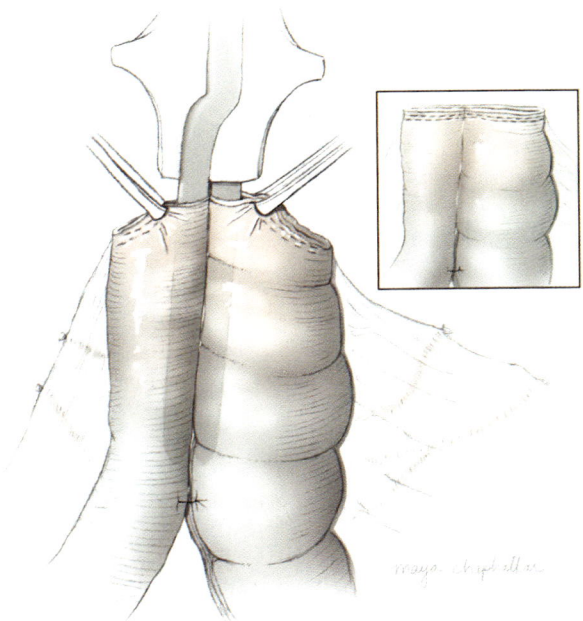

FIGURE 46-18.2 GIA stapler creates a side-to-side anastomosis of the ileum (*left*) and transverse colon (*right*). **Inset:** TA stapler line closes the distal end of the anastomosis.

The antimesenteric tip of each staple line is excised with scissors, and the bowel is held vertically by Allis clamps to prevent fecal spill. One or two seromuscular silk stay sutures may be placed distally on each bowel end to help align the correct position and prevent slippage. One fork of the GIA stapler is then inserted as deeply as possible into each of the bowel lumens (Fig. 46-18.2). The bowel segments are evenly positioned, and the device is then fired along the antimesenteric surfaces and removed. This stapler places two staggered rows of titanium staples and simultaneously transects tissue between these rows.

The bowel interior should be examined for bleeding sites, which may be electrosurgically coagulated. The remaining opening may then be stapled across with a TA stapler, and residual bowel tissue above the TA staple line is excised. The mesenteric defect is reapproximated with interrupted or running 0-gauge delayed-absorbable suture to prevent an internal hernia.

❼ Final Steps. The abdomen is irrigated with copious warmed saline at the conclusion of any bowel resection, especially if feces have spilled during the procedure. Drains are not routinely required and may impair healing.

POSTOPERATIVE

Morbidity after large bowel resection is significantly increased by various factors, but especially by preexisting obstruction, malignancy, obesity, radiation damage, or sepsis. Moreover, patients undergoing multiple bowel resections have greater blood loss and longer hospital stay (Salani, 2007). Anastomotic leaks are the most specific complication and typically present as an abscess or fistula, or as peritonitis within days or weeks of surgery. Some localized leaks can be managed with initiation of TPN, CT-guided drainage, antibiotic administration, and bowel rest for a couple of weeks. However, urgent reoperation is indicated for nonlocalized intraperitoneal perforation and its resulting peritonitis. This will usually require temporary colostomy (Lago, 2019).

Pelvic abscesses also may result from intraoperative fecal spillage or hematoma superinfection. Usually these will resolve with CT-guided drainage and antibiotics. Gastrointestinal hemorrhage should be rare with stapled procedures. In addition, symptomatic anastomotic strictures are infrequent and often present as colonic obstruction. Some strictures can be managed with endoscopic stents, but often they require reoperation. Small or large bowel may also become obstructed by postoperative adhesions or tumor progression. Last, a prolonged ileus can develop and be slow to resolve. Most of these complications will depend primarily on the patient's underlying nutrition and the clinical circumstances prompting the primary surgery.

46-19

Ileostomy

Relatively few patients will require ileostomy for management of a gynecologic malignancy. For those who do, loop ileostomy is usually a temporary procedure that is performed to protect a distal anastomosis (Koscielny, 2019). Palliation of a large-bowel obstruction or diversion of a colonic fistula may be other indications (Tsai, 2006). On occasion, ovarian cancer will involve the entire colon, requiring colectomy with a permanent end ileostomy and formation of a Hartmann pouch (Song, 2009). Occasionally, this procedure can be performed by an MIS approach, depending on the clinical circumstances (Schorge, 2019).

PREOPERATIVE

Patient Evaluation

Stoma placement is particularly important for an ileostomy since the effluent will be more corrosive than that of a colostomy. Ideally, the site is marked preoperatively by an enterostomal therapist.

Consent

In general, many of the complications from this procedure mirror those of colostomy: retraction, stricture, obstruction, and herniation. Patients are informed that temporary loop ileostomies can be taken down later without a laparotomy.

Patient Preparation

Bowel preparation is preferred whenever there is a potential for more extensive bowel resection. However, ileostomy can safely be performed in virtually all circumstances without cleansing. Antibiotics and VTE prophylaxis are warranted, and options are listed in Tables 39-8 and 39-10 (p. 832).

INTRAOPERATIVE

Surgical Steps

❶ **Anesthesia and Patient Positioning.** Ileostomy is performed under general anesthesia. Patients are generally supine, but low lithotomy is acceptable. For VTE prophylaxis, lower-extremity pneumatic compression devices are placed.

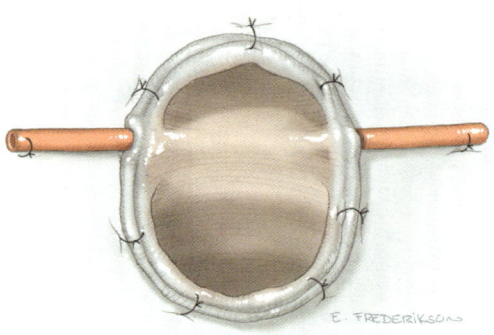

FIGURE 46-19.1 Ileal loop opened with cautery.

❷ **Abdominal Entry.** A midline vertical incision is preferable for most situations in which an ileostomy is considered.

❸ **Exploration.** After abdominal entry, a surgeon first explores the abdomen, lyses adhesions, "runs" the bowel length to identify obstructive sites, and determines the need for ileostomy. An ileum loop is selected that will reach several centimeters above the skin. Additionally, to reduce the effluent volume, the selected loop is located as distally along the bowel length as possible. On occasion, tethering of small bowel by carcinomatosis or radiation injury will significantly reduce mobility and will require a more proximal diversion.

❹ **Loop Ileostomy.** A one-quarter inch Penrose drain is placed through a mesenterotomy at the selected loop's apex. The loop can then be approximated to the stoma site, which is created to accommodate two fingers as described for an ileal conduit (Section 46-7, p. 1184). The loop is pulled through the abdominal wall opening so that several centimeters protrude above the skin surface. The Penrose drain is removed and replaced with either the cut end of a red rubber catheter or another device that can be sewn to the skin to elevate the loop. The loop should be tension-free and patent. The proximal end of the loop is placed in the lower position to reduce fecal flow into the distal bowel. The skin of the abdominal wall is then closed around the stoma.

The ileostomy is "matured" by longitudinally incising the bowel loop and everting its walls with Allis clamps. Circumferential interrupted stitches of 3-0 and 4-0 gauge delayed-absorbable sutures are placed through the dermis and bowel mucosa (Fig. 46-19.1). An ostomy bag may then be applied.

❺ **End Ileostomy.** If a total colectomy is performed or if the bowel is too tethered or the patient too obese for a loop to reach the abdominal wall, the distal ileum may need to be divided instead of brought out as a loop. The segment is selected, a mesenterotomy is made, and the GIA stapler is fired. An appropriate stoma site is identified, and with a few modifications, the end ileostomy is matured as in colostomy (Section 46-17, p. 1217). Typically, the abdominal wall opening will be smaller in diameter. Unless there is a distal colon obstruction necessitating creation of a mucus fistula, the distal bowel segment can be left in the peritoneal cavity or just under the fascia.

An attempt is made to evert the single stoma by turning the bowel wall over on itself using Allis clamps. In each quadrant of the stoma, stitches of 3-0 gauge delayed absorbable suture are placed through the dermis, the seromuscular layer of the bowel at the skin level, and a full-thickness bite at the cut edge of the everted bowel (p. 1184).

POSTOPERATIVE

The stoma is carefully examined postoperatively for its appearance and function. The loop supporting rod may be removed in 1 to 2 weeks, but potentially earlier if the stoma becomes dusky or the loops seem constricted or are obstructed.

Ileostomy may be associated with significant postoperative complications. High-output effluent may result in electrolyte abnormalities that are difficult to correct. Reversal is very successful, and overall survival rates are not compromised (Tseng, 2016). Long-term complications such as a peristomal hernia or retraction are possible.

Small Bowel Resection

Indications for small bowel resection in gynecologic oncology are numerous and include obstruction, tumor invasion, perforation, intraoperative injury, fistulas, or radiation damage. Unlike the large bowel, where greater attention is required to ensure an adequate blood supply to the anastomotic site, the small intestine has a consistent cascade of vessels that all arise from the superior mesenteric artery. However, unique situations such as radiation damage, obstructive dilatation, and edema can compromise this vasculature dramatically. In these situations, meticulous dissection is especially crucial to prevent inadvertent removal of the bowel serosa, enterotomy, and bowel damage that will impair anastomotic healing. In general, surgical principles with this procedure are much the same as those for large bowel resection (Section 46-18, p. 1220).

PREOPERATIVE

Patient Evaluation

Small bowel obstructions (SBOs) that do not resolve with nasogastric suction decompression and bowel rest may result from postoperative adhesions or tumor progression. Patients with recurrent gynecologic malignancy, particularly those with ovarian cancer, are preoperatively imaged by abdominopelvic CT with oral contrast. Numerous sites of obstruction may be suspected to indicate a woman with end-stage disease who might be better served by placement of a palliative percutaneous draining gastrostomy tube. Patients with an SBO following pelvic radiation often have stenosis at the terminal ileum. This vulnerability stems from its proximity to the radiation field of many gynecologic cancers and its limited mobility compared with other small-bowel segments.

Consent

Depending on circumstances, patients are counseled regarding the intraoperative decision-making process to decide on anastomosis, bypass, or ileostomy. Leaking, obstruction, and/or fistula formation are possible complications. Less common outcomes include short-bowel syndrome and vitamin B_{12} deficiency, both described later.

Patient Preparation

Aggressive bowel preparation is often contraindicated, particularly in patients with obstruction. Antibiotics and VTE prophylaxis are provided (Chap. 39, p. 832). If a complex fistula is present or an extensive resection for radiation damage is anticipated, then postoperative TPN may be advisable.

INTRAOPERATIVE

Instruments

The surgeon should have access to all types and sizes of bowel staplers, such as end-to-end anastomotic (EEA), gastrointestinal anastomotic (GIA), and transverse anastomotic (TA) staplers, to prepare for complicated resections.

Surgical Steps

❶ Anesthesia and Patient Positioning. Small bowel resection is performed under general anesthesia. Patients are generally supine, but low lithotomy or other positioning with access to the anterior abdominal wall is acceptable. For VTE prophylaxis, lower-extremity pneumatic compression devices are placed.

❷ Abdominal Entry. A midline vertical incision is preferable for most situations in which a small-bowel resection is considered.

❸ Exploration. The surgeon explores the entire abdomen first to identify the obstruction. Infrequently, an adhesion may be located and lysed to quickly relieve an obstruction, thereby avoiding small bowel resection. More often, an area is discovered that warrants removal. Importantly, the remainder of the bowel must be examined to exclude other obstructive sites.

Peritoneum and adhesions attached to the involved portion of small bowel are dissected to mobilize the bowel. The small intestine can be damaged easily by rough handling and by extensive blunt dissection—particularly if the bowel is edematous, densely adhered, or previously irradiated. Trauma is minimized to reduce spillage of intestinal contents by inadvertent enterotomy. Ideally, healthy-appearing serosa for anastomosis is identified at sites both proximal and distal to the lesion while preserving a maximum amount of intestine.

❹ Dividing Small Bowel. The involved bowel is brought through the abdominal incision. A one-quarter inch Penrose drain is pulled through a mesenterotomy at the proximal and distal sites to be approximated. A GIA stapler is inserted to replace the Penrose drain and is fired. This is repeated at the other bowel site (Fig. 46-20.1). These staple lines minimize contamination of the abdomen with bowel contents.

A wedge of mesentery then is "scored" by superficially creating a V shape with an electrosurgical blade. The mesentery is divided by a ligate-divide-staple (LDS) device, electrothermal bipolar coagulator (LigaSure), or clamps and 0-gauge delayed-absorbable suture ligatures. Achieving hemostasis will be more difficult with edematous or inflamed tissue, and thus smaller mesentery pedicles should be sequentially divided. The bowel specimen is then removed.

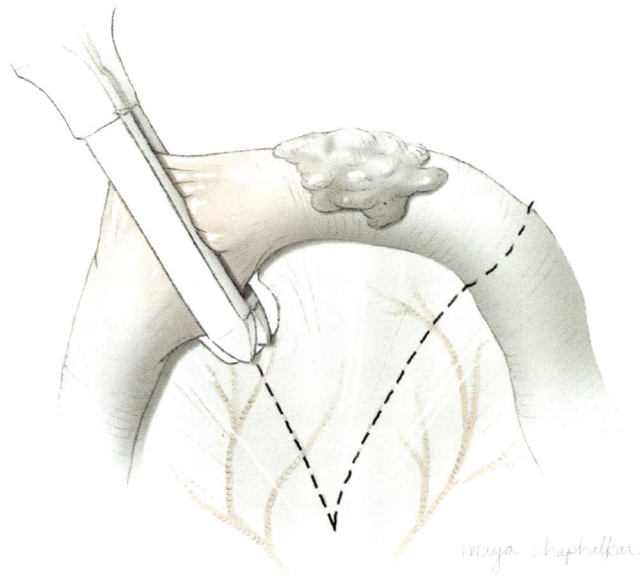

FIGURE 46-20.1 Identifying proximal and distal sites.

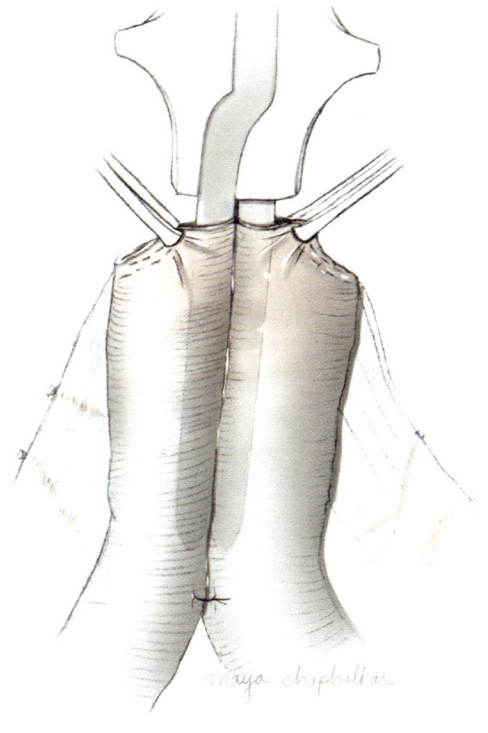

FIGURE 46-20.2 Side-to-side anastomosis.

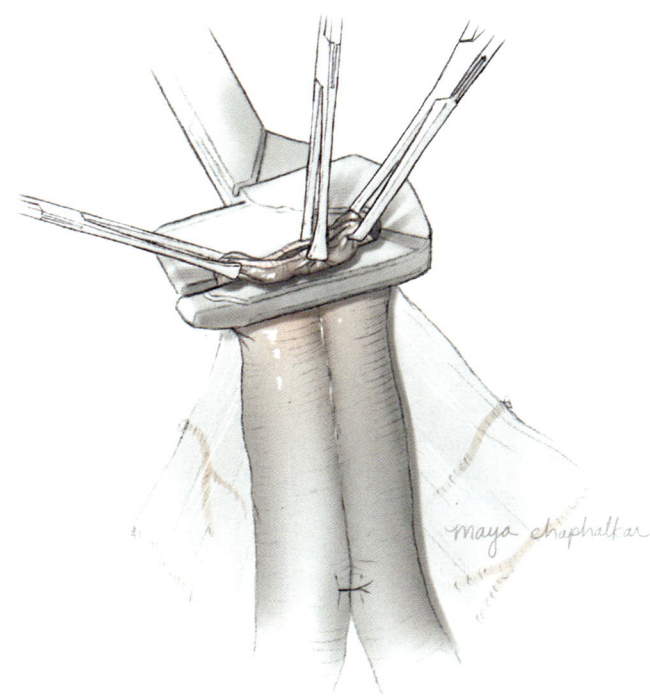

FIGURE 46-20.3 Closing the enterotomy.

❺ **Performing Side-to-Side Anastomosis.** The proximal and distal bowel segments are elevated with Allis clamps and matched parallel along their antimesenteric borders. To help alignment, one or two silk stay sutures are placed through the antimesenteric border of each segment beyond the tip of where the GIA stapler fork will reach. The antimesenteric corner of each segment is excised at the staple line just deeply enough to enter the lumen and sufficiently widely to permit passage of one GIA stapler fork. Massively distended bowel from an obstruction may be decompressed by inserting a pool suction tip into the proximal bowel end.

Allis clamps are replaced on the bowel at the edge of each opening. These clamps and silk stay sutures assist insertion of one fork of the GIA stapler into each segment and aid in bowel positioning (Fig. 46-20.2). The bowel is rotated to bring the antimesenteric borders together, Allis clamps are removed, and the GIA stapler is closed and fired.

The remaining enterotomy is regrasped with three Allis clamps to approximate for closure. The TA stapler is placed around the bowel beneath the Allis clamps and is closed (Fig. 46-20.3). The Allis clamps elevate the enterotomy and assist with correct positioning of the TA stapler. The stapler is fired, excess tissue above the stapler is trimmed sharply, and the stapler is opened

and removed. The mesenteric defect may be closed next with running 0-gauge delayed-absorbable suture to prevent internal herniation—that is, herniation of bowel or omentum through the mesenteric defect.

❻ **Final Steps.** The abdomen is copiously irrigated with warmed saline. This is performed at the conclusion of any bowel resection, but particularly if bowel contents spill during the procedure. Drains are not required routinely and may impair healing. In general, it is prudent to place a nasogastric tube to decompress the stomach postoperatively until bowel function has resumed. Palpation of the stomach will confirm correct placement, or else the anesthesiologist can be directed to advance or pull back the tube as needed. If this is overlooked, correct location can be reliably confirmed postoperatively only by chest radiography.

POSTOPERATIVE

The underlying health of the patient, diagnosis, and indications for small bowel resection will dictate much of the potential postoperative morbidity. Ileus is common. Fistula formation, anastomotic leakage, and obstruction are more serious problems that may require reoperation. Two specific complications are unique to extensive small bowel surgery.

First, short-bowel syndrome may develop. More than half the small intestine can be removed without impairing nutritional absorption as long as the remaining bowel is functional. Accordingly, this syndrome is more likely to develop from extensive radiation damage than from surgical resection. Symptoms include diarrhea and dehydration. Maldigestion, malabsorption, nutritional deficiencies, and electrolyte imbalance are often noted. As a result, home TPN may be required in some patients (Carroll, 2016).

A second complication, vitamin B_{12} deficiency, results from inadequate absorption and depletion of available stores. The ileum measures on average 300 cm in length, and vitamin B_{12} and bile salts are absorbed only in the ileum's distal 100 cm. Malabsorption in this segment may result from radiotherapy or extensive intestinal resection (Bandy, 1984). If vitamin B_{12} deficiency is suspected, a complete blood count (CBC), peripheral blood smear, and serum cobalamin (B_{12}) level are collected as part of an initial laboratory assessment. Accepted lower limits of serum vitamin B_{12} levels in adults range between 170 and 250 ng/L. One option for replacement is 1 mg intramuscularly weekly for 8 weeks, followed by long-term monthly injections (Centers for Disease Control and Prevention, 2019).

46-21

Low Anterior Resection

Rectosigmoid resection, also known as low anterior resection, is mainly used in gynecologic oncology to achieve optimal cytoreduction of primary or recurrent ovarian cancer (Fournier, 2018). This procedure is distinguished from other types of large bowel resection in that it requires mobilization and transection of the rectum distally, below the peritoneal reflection. Following resection of the involved rectosigmoid segment, proximal and distal bowel ends are usually anastomosed.

Low anterior resection is the most common bowel operation for primary tumor debulking (Hoffman, 2005). For example, en bloc pelvic resection combines low anterior resection with hysterectomy, bilateral salpingo-oophorectomy, and removal of surrounding peritoneum (Section 46-13, p. 1207) (Aletti, 2006b). In addition, total and posterior pelvic exenterations incorporate many of the same principles of tissue dissection to remove centrally recurrent cervical cancer and achieve widely negative soft tissue margins. Other less common indications for low anterior resection are radiation proctosigmoiditis and intestinal endometriosis (Urbach, 1998). Occasionally, additional large- or small-bowel resections will be performed concomitantly with low anterior resection. These do not raise the overall risk of anastomotic leak (Grimm, 2017).

PREOPERATIVE

Patient Evaluation

Bowel symptoms may or may not be present in women with rectosigmoid involvement of ovarian cancer. However, a surgeon should have greater suspicion if patients describe rectal bleeding or progressive constipation. A rectovaginal examination may help predict a need for low anterior resection. Additionally, CT images may suggest rectosigmoid invasion of tumor. However, prediction prior to surgery is difficult. Many ovarian cancers intraoperatively may be easily lifted away from the bowel, or surface tumors may be removed without resection.

Consent

Patients should be prepared for the possibility of low anterior resection any time ovarian cytoreductive surgery is discussed. The survival benefit of achieving minimal residual disease warrants the risks of this procedure. However, low anterior resection significantly extends operative time, and hemorrhage may contribute to a need for blood transfusion (Pereitti, 2012).

In general, progressively higher complication rates and poorer long-term bowel function follow anastomoses that are more distal and approach the anal verge. However, the operation is designed to encompass the tumor. Thus, an end sigmoid colostomy with Hartmann pouch is another, albeit less attractive, option for very low resections. In general, a protective loop colostomy or ileostomy is not required, but patients are counseled for that possibility in the event of poor nutrition, tenuous bowel blood supply, or anastomosis tension. With attention to risk factors that would instead indicate a need to divert, anastomotic leaks should develop in fewer than 5 percent of procedures (Kalogera, 2017).

Patient Preparation

To minimize fecal contamination during resection, bowel preparation such as with a polyethylene glycol with electrolyte solution (GoLYTELY) is generally considered prior to surgery. Antibiotics and VTE prophylaxis are warranted, and suitable options are found in Tables 39-8 and 39-10 (p. 832).

INTRAOPERATIVE

Instruments

All types and sizes of bowel staplers such as end-to-end anastomosis (EEA), gastrointestinal anastomosis (GIA), and transverse anastomosis (TA) staplers should be available. Additionally, a ligate-divide-staple (LDS) device or electrothermal bipolar coagulator (LigaSure) may be used for vessel ligation.

Surgical Steps

1 Anesthesia and Patient Positioning. Low anterior resection via laparotomy requires general anesthesia. Rectovaginal examination under anesthesia is performed before positioning any patient for abdominal gynecologic cancer surgery. A palpable mass with compression of the rectum or rectovaginal septum prompts patient positioning in low lithotomy with legs safely placed in boot support stirrups. This allows access to the rectum in cases requiring EEA stapler insertion for anastomosis. Alternatively, supine positioning may be appropriate if no mass is palpable by rectovaginal examination. In such cases, if a mass is more proximally located, low rectal anastomosis can be performed entirely within the pelvis. Lower-extremity pneumatic compression devices are placed for VTE prophylaxis.

2 Abdominal Entry. A midline vertical incision provides generous operating space and upper abdominal access. This is preferable if low rectal anastomosis is anticipated because the descending colon may need to be mobilized around and beyond the splenic flexure of the colon. Transverse incisions often fail to provide sufficient exposure.

3 Exploration. A surgeon first explores the entire abdomen to determine if disease is resectable. If not, then the procedure's benefit is reevaluated. On occasion, imminent bowel obstruction, infection, or other clinical circumstances may dictate resection regardless of residual tumor. The pelvis and rectosigmoid are palpated to mentally plan for the resection and determine whether en bloc pelvic resection or an exenterative procedure is indicated.

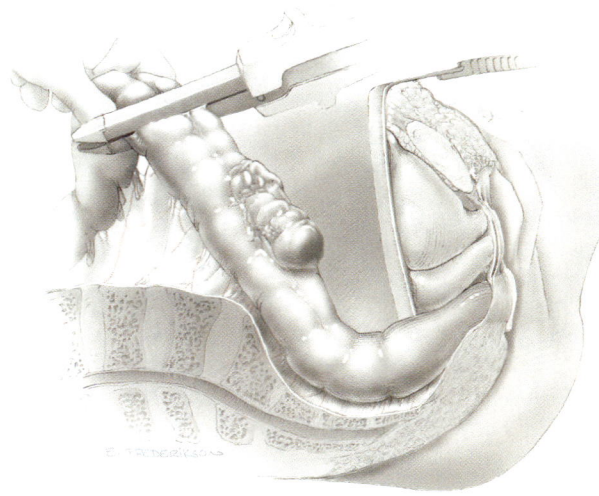

FIGURE 46-21.1 Dividing the proximal end.

④ Visualization. The bowel is packed into the upper abdomen, and retractor blades are positioned to allow access to the deep pelvis and the entire rectosigmoid colon. Ureters are identified at the pelvic brim and are held laterally on Penrose drains to expose the peritoneum and mesentery that can next be safely dissected.

⑤ Dividing the Proximal Sigmoid Colon. The sigmoid colon is held on traction proximal to the tumor and in the approximate area where it will be divided. The ureter is located, and a right-angle clamp is used to guide superficial electrosurgical blade dissection of the peritoneum and mesentery up to the bowel serosa. A similar dissection is repeated on the other side. Blunt dissection may then be performed to define the entire circumference of the sigmoid colon. Epiploica and adjacent fatty tissue are held with DeBakey forceps and dissected away with an electrosurgical blade from the proposed area of transection. The GIA stapler is placed across the sigmoid colon, fired, and removed (Fig. 46-21.1).

⑥ Dividing the Mesentery. Occasionally, the tumor is small and superficially located, requiring only a wedge resection of underlying mesentery to remove it with the bowel segment. More frequently, the entire mesentery needs to be divided to provide access to the avascular plane between the rectosigmoid and the sacrum (retrorectal space). For this, a right-angle clamp is placed through sections of the mesentery, and an LDS device or electrothermal bipolar coagulator divides this tissue. Dissection is continued caudally to divide the mesentery (Fig. 46-21.2). Typically, one or more pedicles will have a blood vessel that slips out and requires clamping with a right-angle clamp and ligation with 0-gauge delayed-absorbable suture.

Blunt dissection is performed in the pelvic midline to identify the large superior rectal vessels, which are branches of the inferior mesenteric artery. This artery and vein are large and are separately doubly clamped, cut, and ligated with 0-gauge delayed-absorbable suture. From this midline, dissection then progresses laterally on both sides until no tissue is visible between the ureters. The common iliac artery bifurcation and sacrum are entirely visible.

⑦ Dividing the Rectum. The proximal sigmoid colon and attached mesentery are repacked into the upper abdomen to improve pelvic exposure. The rectosigmoid is held superiorly, and blunt dissection is performed caudally in the retrorectal space to mobilize the distal bowel beyond the tumor

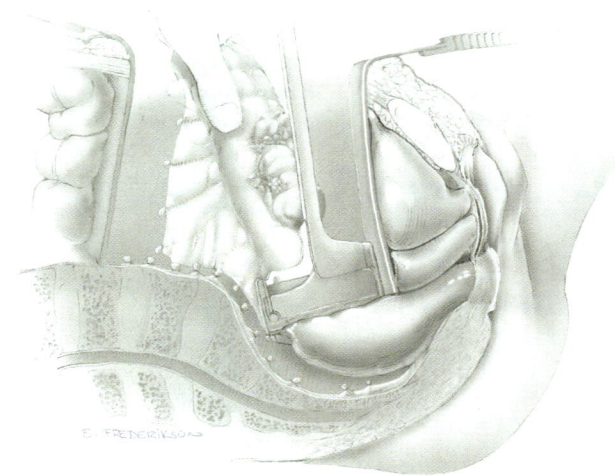

FIGURE 46-21.2 Dividing the distal end after mesentery freed.

to define the location of planned resection. The ureters are traced along the pelvic sidewall. Lateral blunt dissection is performed to further mobilize the rectosigmoid. Lateral mesenteric attachments are isolated and divided with an LDS device or electrothermal bipolar coagulator or are grasped between Pean clamps, cut, and ligated. Self-retaining retractor blades may require repositioning as dissection proceeds more distally.

The anterior bowel serosa is generally visible throughout its course beyond the peritoneal reflection and into the levator muscles. Lateral and posterior bowel margins are surrounded by fatty tissue, mesentery, and rectal pillars. The distal rectum beyond the tumor is grasped and rotated to aid exposure of these attachments. Attachments are divided using alternating electrosurgical blade dissection and vascular pedicle division and/or right-angle clamping and transection. Division continues circumferentially until the rectal serosa is entirely visible.

The curved cutter stapler (Contour) is a good choice for the limited space of the deep pelvis. The rectosigmoid is held on traction, while the stapler is gently inserted into the pelvis around the rectal segment. The ureters

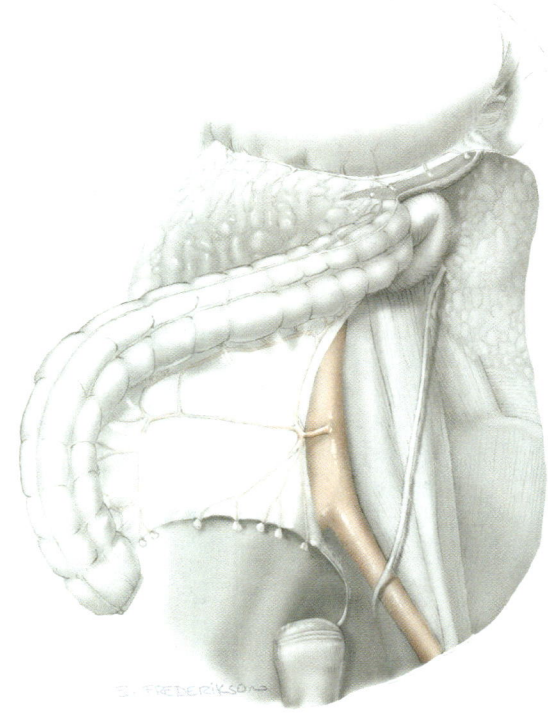

FIGURE 46-21.3 Mobilizing the descending colon.

and any lateral tissue are pushed safely away, the stapler is fired, and the low anterior resection specimen is removed (see Fig. 46-21.2). The pelvis is irrigated, and a laparotomy sponge is left in place to tamponade any surface oozing.

❽ Mobilization. The final decision is now made to perform an anastomosis instead of an end sigmoid colostomy. The upper abdominal retractors are removed, and the proximal sigmoid colon is mobilized by incising peritoneum along the white line of Toldt toward and/or around the splenic flexure. A combination of electrosurgical blade and blunt dissection is typically used. The proximal sigmoid colon is intermittently placed into the deep pelvis to assess the extent of further dissection needed to achieve a tension-free anastomosis. Ideally, the proximal sigmoid colon sits comfortably on top of the distal rectum. To achieve this, mobilization may encompass the entire splenic flexure of the colon (Fig. 46-21.3). Occasionally, the hepatic flexure also may need to be mobilized. Sufficient mobility is critical to ensure a tension-free anastomosis.

❾ Preparing the Anastomotic Sites. The proximal and distal stapled bowel ends now must be cleared of fatty tissue or epiploica to allow sufficient mucosa-to-mucosa contact during anastomosis. The staple line of the proximal sigmoid colon is grasped with two Allis clamps at the lateral edges and elevated. Adson forceps are used to delicately place any surrounding fatty tissue on traction, and an electrosurgical blade is used to dissect these away from the bowel serosa. This can be particularly difficult in patients

with prominent diverticulosis. A similar dissection also may be required on the distal rectal segment.

❿ Placing the Anvil. The largest possible EEA circular stapler that will fit the bowel segments, typically the 31-mm size, is used. This provides a commodious anastomosis that will lessen the chances of symptomatic rectal stenosis. The proximal sigmoid colon is again held with Allis clamps, and scissors are used to remove the entire staple line. The Allis clamps are replaced to grasp the mucosa/serosa and hold open the proximal sigmoid colon. Sizing instruments may be used if necessary to decide which EEA instrument is best. The EEA device contains an anvil that will be placed in the proximal bowel and a stapler that is placed in the distal bowel. Articulation of the anvil and stapler head allows firing of a staple ring at this articulation site to form the anastomosis.

First, the anvil is detached from the stapler, lubricated, and gently inserted by rotating it into the proximal sigmoid colon. Its concave surface faces proximally, away from the anticipated anastomotic site (Fig. 46-21.4 inset). Sequential stitches that pierce through bowel serosa, muscularis, and mucosa create a purse string around the anvil. These "through-and-through" stitches using 2-0 Prolene suture are placed 5 to 7 mm from the mucosal edge. The purse string begins and ends on the outside of the bowel serosa around the anvil spike and is then tied securely. Allis clamps are removed. A quicker alternative is to use a stapler purse-string suture device. Irrigation may be performed if bowel contents have spilled.

⓫ Placing the Stapler. The distal rectal stump is reexamined to ensure that all surrounding fatty tissue has been dissected free. The surgical team then reviews the details of using an EEA instrument. A phantom application is helpful. After this, the shaft of the stapler is extended and its spike is attached. The shaft and spike are then retracted into the instrument. The EEA is lubricated and gently inserted into the anus until the circular outline is visible and seen to be gently pressing on the rectal staple line. A wing nut located on the device handle is gently rotated, and this extends the shaft and its spike. This is guided by the abdominal surgeon so that the spike is brought out just posterior to the staple midline. In the abdomen, gentle countertraction against the rectum may be helpful as the sharp spike tip pops through the entire bowel wall thickness. The shaft subsequently becomes visible and the spike is removed.

⓬ Stapling. The abdominal surgeon lowers the proximal sigmoid colon to the distal rectum and connects the hollow tip of the anvil into the metal shaft of the EEA. An audible "click" should be heard to confirm articulation. The tip of the EEA is held perfectly still, while the wing nut is again rotated to retract the shaft back into the EEA until the handle indicator is in the correct position (Fig. 46-21.4). This draws the anvil into apposition with the stapler head. The safety is released, and the instrument is fired by squeezing and depressing the handles completely. Incomplete squeezing can result in partial stapling. The wing nut is then turned to the specified position to release the staple line. The EEA with its now attached anvil is gently rotated and slowly removed from the rectum.

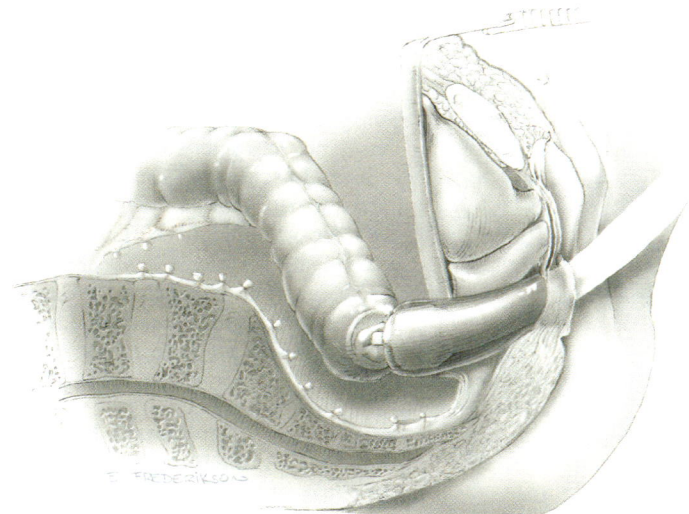

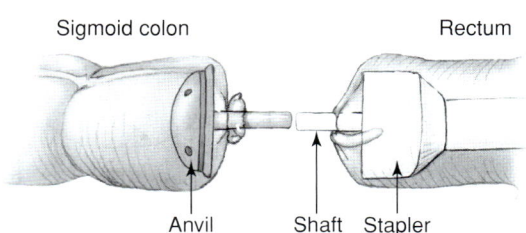

Sigmoid colon · Rectum

Anvil · Shaft · Stapler

FIGURE 46-21.4 Performing end-to-end anastomosis. **Inset:** The EEA stapler device head.

SECTION 6

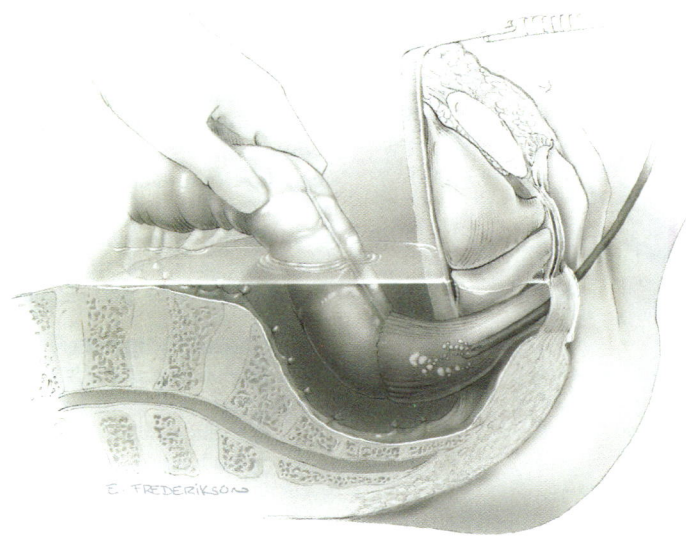

E. FREDERIKSON

FIGURE 46-21.5 Testing the anastomosis.

The anastomosis is visualized by the abdominal surgeon throughout the process. Distal retraction of the anastomosis or inability to remove the EEA suggests that the stapler was not completely fired. This situation may be salvaged by gently pulling the EEA through the anus and cutting inside the staple line to release the anastomosis. The anvil is removed from the EEA instrument and inspected to confirm that two completely intact circular "donuts" of rectal tissue are present.

⓭ Rectal Insufflation. Warmed saline is irrigated into the pelvis. The integrity of the anastomosis may now be checked by gently inserting a proctoscope or red rubber catheter into the anus, but distal to the anastomosis. Air is then insufflated into the bowel.

The abdominal surgeon gently palpates the sigmoid colon to make certain that air is entering the sigmoid colon proximal to the anastomotic site. No air bubbles are visible if the connection is watertight (Fig. 46-21.5). The appearance of bubbles suggests a leak, but this should be double-checked for authenticity. Occasionally, air is being erroneously pumped into the vagina rather than the rectum due to incorrect placement of the red rubber catheter. If there is any valid suspicion for a leak, the distal rectum should be divided again and the anastomosis redone. Reinforcing interrupted suture to close the air leak may be attempted in select situations, but this is riskier. Diverting colostomy may also be considered if the problem cannot otherwise be managed.

⓮ Final Steps. All pedicle sites are rechecked for hemostasis, and the pelvis is irrigated. Nasogastric suction is not routinely required. In addition, prophylactic suction drainage of the pelvis does not improve outcome or influence the severity of complications (Merad, 1999).

POSTOPERATIVE

The most common early postoperative complications are similar to those for other major abdominal operations and include fever, self-limiting ileus, wound separation, and anemia requiring transfusion. Serious events such as bowel obstruction and fistula develop infrequently (Gillette-Cloven, 2001). In the long term, some patients will have a poor functional result, including fecal incontinence or chronic constipation (Rasmussen, 2003).

Low rectal anastomoses have much higher intraperitoneal leakage rates than large bowel anastomoses. Leakage of stool leads to fever, leukocytosis, lower abdominal pain, and ileus. These should prompt abdominopelvic CT imaging with oral contrast. If a leak is present, it may appear as a pelvic abscess, or at times, contrast extravasation can be demonstrated into the fluid collection. Occasionally, this complication can be successfully managed with percutaneous drainage of the abscess, bowel rest, and broad-spectrum antibiotics. Otherwise, a temporary diverting loop ileostomy or colostomy may be required (Tseng, 2016). Risk factors for postoperative leakage include previous pelvic irradiation, diabetes mellitus, low preoperative serum albumin, a low anastomosis (≤6 cm from the anal verge), and lengthy surgical duration (Kalogera, 2017).

46-22

Intestinal Bypass

This bowel anastomotic procedure typically connects a section of the ileum to the ascending or transverse colon and thereby "bypasses" a portion of diseased bowel. Following anastomosis, the closed, bypassed small-bowel segment remains.

There are relatively few indications for intestinal bypass in gynecologic oncology, and this procedure accounts for less than 5 percent of all bowel operations performed for these cancers (Barnhill, 1991; Winter, 2003). In all circumstances, removal of diseased bowel and end-to-end anastomosis is preferable. However, some patients will have unresectable tumor, dense adhesions, extensive radiation injury, or other prohibitive factors. In these cases, a poor decision to proceed with an aggressive dissection can result in numerous enterotomies, hemorrhage, or other intraoperative catastrophes with major postoperative sequelae. Instead, an intestinal bypass can often quickly be performed with minimal morbidity. Many times a bypass is selected because it is the easiest palliative maneuver for a terminally ill patient. The main purpose is to relieve an obstruction, reestablish an adequate bowel communication, and restore the patient's ability to take oral nourishment.

PREOPERATIVE

Patient Evaluation

The intestinal tract is evaluated by CT scanning. Invariably, pelvic radiation injuries are located at the terminal ileum, but there may be complex fistulas or multiple sites of obstruction to be addressed. In most circumstances in which a bypass is considered, a surgeon should anticipate limitations in adequately exploring the abdomen intraoperatively. Careful analysis of preoperative findings will help ensure that bypass encompasses the entire lesion and does not leave a distal obstruction.

Consent

Patients usually have a miserable quality of life when bypass is considered, and the operation's goal is mainly to improve patient symptoms. The counseling process should emphasize that intraoperative judgment will dictate whether a small-bowel resection, ileostomy, large-bowel resection, colostomy, or bypass is indicated. Many risks are similar to those of other intestinal surgical procedures and include anastomotic leaks, obstruction,

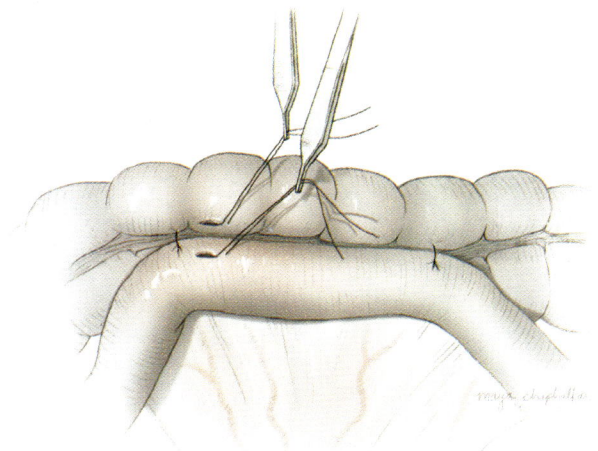

FIGURE 46-22.1 Aligning the bowel.

abscess formation, and fistula. Blind loop syndrome, discussed later, is one long-term complication that is specific to the bypass procedure.

Patient Preparation

Aggressive bowel preparation with oral agents is usually contraindicated due to bowel obstruction or other dire circumstances. Broad-spectrum antibiotics are given perioperatively due to the possibility of stool contamination, and VTE prophylaxis is provided. If a prolonged recovery is anticipated, postoperative TPN is considered.

INTRAOPERATIVE

Instruments

To prepare for complicated resections, bowel staplers such as an end-to-end anastomosis (EEA), gastrointestinal anastomosis (GIA), and transverse anastomosis (TA) staplers should be available.

Surgical Steps

1 Anesthesia and Patient Positioning. Bypass is performed under general anesthesia with the patient positioned supine. For VTE prophylaxis, lower-extremity pneumatic compression devices are placed. Prior to surgery, the abdomen is surgically prepared, and a Foley catheter is inserted.

2 Abdominal Entry and Exploration. Colostomy, if needed, usually requires a midline vertical incision for exposure. A surgeon first explores the entire abdomen to identify bowel lesions. In addition, the remaining bowel is examined to exclude other obstructive sites. Healthy-appearing bowel proximal

and distal to the lesion is selected with the intent of preserving the maximal amount of intestine. Typically, the bypass will entail connecting a section of the ileum to the ascending or transverse colon.

3 Aligning the Bowel. The two bowel segments selected for the anastomosis are aligned side-to-side without tension or twisting. The hepatic or splenic flexure of the transverse colon may require mobilization from its peritoneal attachments to achieve a tension-free connection. The antimesenteric borders of the bowel segments are held in position by 2-0 gauge silk stay sutures placed approximately 6 cm apart along the length of the aligned bowel segments. Two Adson forceps are used to hold up the small bowel serosa laterally and transversely on traction. An electrosurgical blade is used to enter the small bowel lumen on its antimesenteric surface (Fig. 46-22.1). The same maneuver is performed on the teniae coli to enter the colon.

4 Performing the Side-to-Side Anastomosis. One fork of the GIA stapler is inserted into each bowel segment lumen. The bowel is adjusted, if necessary, to position the antimesenteric surfaces between the stapler forks. The stapler is then closed and fired (Fig. 46-22.2). With stapling, the initial small bowel openings that were cut to admit the stapler forks are fused into one open defect. This opening can be closed with the TA stapler and the excess bowel trimmed. As a result of the other side of this TA staple line, the end of the diseased bowel loop also is simultaneously sealed.

5 Final Steps. Occasionally, small bleeding sites on the staple line will need spot electrosurgical coagulation. The anastomosis is also palpated to verify an adequate lumen. The bowel is reexamined to make certain

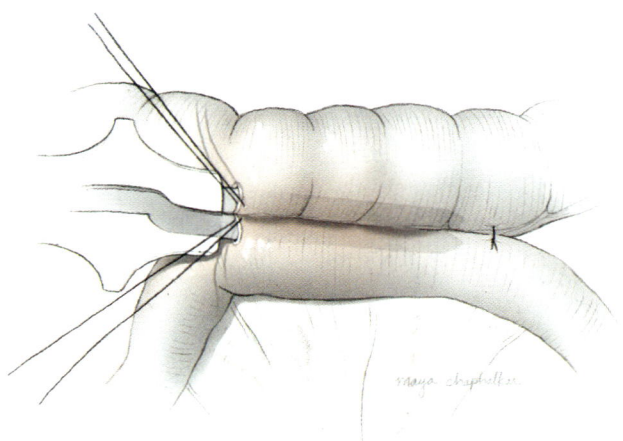

FIGURE 46-22.2 Performing side-to-side anastomosis.

that the connection is watertight and that there is no tension on the anastomosis.

POSTOPERATIVE

Recovery after bypass surgery should initially be rapid compared with that following a large resection with anastomosis. In general, postoperative ileus will resolve in several days, and patients may begin oral alimentation. Long-term, the underlying clinical situation prompting the need for bypass surgery will dictate most of the clinical course. Relatively minor complications such as febrile morbidity and wound infection or wound separation occur commonly. Fistulas, obstruction, anastomotic leaks, abscesses, peritonitis, and perforation are more difficult to manage and often lead to a prolonged postoperative course or death.

Blind loop syndrome is a condition of vitamin B_{12} malabsorption, steatorrhea, and bacterial overgrowth of the small intestine. The usual scenario is a bypass procedure that leaves a segment of nonfunctional, severely irradiated bowel behind. Stasis of the intestinal contents leads to dilatation and mucosal inflammation. Symptoms resemble a partial small bowel obstruction and include nausea, vomiting, diarrhea, abdominal distention, and pain. Bowel perforation is possible. Antibiotics will often alleviate the condition, but recolonization and resumption of the blind loop syndrome is common (Swan, 1974). The only definitive therapy for recurrent episodes is exploration with resection of the bypassed segment. To avoid this syndrome, a surgeon may still perform the side-to-side anastomosis. But, the closed loop can be relieved by creation of a mucus fistula at the abdominal wall.

46-23

Appendectomy

Removal of the appendix may be indicated during gynecologic surgery for various reasons. The need, however, is commonly not recognized until an operation is already underway, as signs and symptoms of benign gynecologic conditions can mimic appendicitis.

In addition, malignancies may involve the appendix. Ovarian cancer frequently metastasizes to the appendix, which thereby often warrants removal (Ayhan, 2005). Primary tumors of the appendix are rare but commonly metastasize to the ovaries. Thus, the initial surgical intervention is often performed by a gynecologic oncologist (Dietrich, 2007). Pseudomyxoma peritonei is the classic type of mucinous tumor of appendiceal origin that spreads to the ovaries and may implant throughout the abdomen (Mittal, 2017).

Elective coincidental appendectomy is defined as the removal of an appendix at the time of another surgical procedure unrelated to appreciable appendiceal pathology. Possible benefits include preventing a future emergency appendectomy and excluding appendicitis in patients with chronic pelvic pain or endometriosis. Other groups that may benefit include women in whom pelvic or abdominal radiation or chemotherapy is anticipated, women undergoing extensive pelvic or abdominal surgery in which major adhesions are anticipated postoperatively, and patients such as the developmentally disabled in whom making the diagnosis of appendicitis may be difficult because of diminished ability to perceive or communicate symptoms (American College of Obstetricians and Gynecologists, 2019).

PREOPERATIVE

Specific preoperative tests or preparations are not required prior to appendectomy. In general, the consenting process for gynecologic surgery includes a discussion of possible "other indicated procedures" such as appendectomy when anticipated intraoperative findings and the potential for performing an appendectomy are uncertain.

Most studies suggest that there is, at most, a small increased risk of nonfatal complications associated with elective coincidental appendectomy at the time of gynecologic surgery, whether performed during laparotomy or during laparoscopy (Salom, 2003). Hematoma formation at the mesoappendix may cause an ileus or partial small bowel obstruction. Perforation of the stump is rare and typically follows insecure suture placement.

INTRAOPERATIVE

Surgical Steps

❶ **Anesthesia and Patient Positioning.** Appendectomy is performed under general anesthesia in a supine position. For VTE prophylaxis, lower-extremity pneumatic compression devices are placed. Postoperative hospitalization is individualized and is dependent on concurrent surgeries and associated clinical symptoms.

❷ **Abdominal Entry.** Appendectomy can be performed through almost any incision. A laparoscopic approach or an oblique McBurney incision in the right lower quadrant of the abdomen is traditionally selected for appendectomy. However, in gynecologic cases, the needs of planned concurrent procedures will commonly dictate incision choice.

❸ **Locating the Appendix.** The appendix is located by first grasping the cecum and gently elevating it upward into the incision. Insertion of the terminal ileum should be visible, and the appendix is typically obvious at this point. Infrequently, an appendix is retrocecal or otherwise difficult to identify. In this situation, the convergence of the three teniae coli can be followed to locate the appendiceal base.

❹ **Mesoappendix Division.** The appendix tip is elevated with a Babcock clamp, and the cecum is held laterally to place the mesoappendix on gentle traction. The appendiceal artery is usually very difficult to distinguish reliably due to abundant surrounding fatty tissue. Thus, curved hemostats are used to successively clamp the mesoappendix and its vessels to reach the appendiceal base (Fig. 46-23.1).

The first hemostat is placed horizontally—aiming directly toward the base of the appendix. The second hemostat is placed at a 30-degree angle so that the tips meet but Metzenbaum scissors have room to cut between the two clamps. The mesoappendix pedicle is ligated with 3-0 gauge delayed-absorbable suture. This step is typically repeated once or twice to comfortably reach the base of the appendix. An alternative is to use an electrothermal bipolar coagulator (LigaSure) to divide the mesoappendix.

❺ **Appendix Ligation.** At this point, the appendix has been completely isolated from

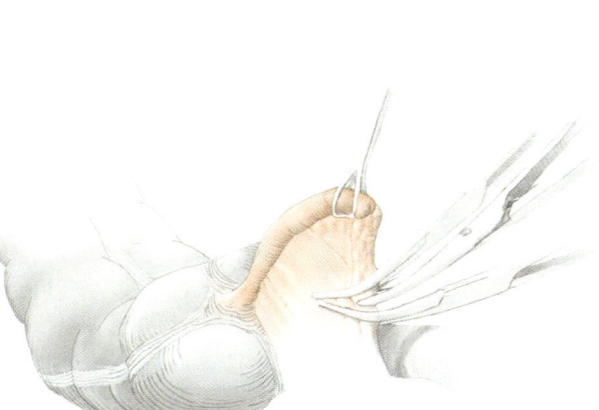

FIGURE 46-23.1 Clamping the mesoappendix.

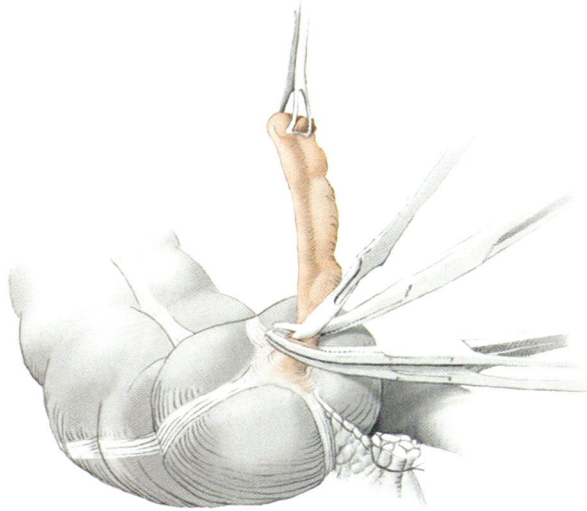

FIGURE 46-23.2 Ligation of the appendix.

the mesoappendix and is still held vertically by a Babcock clamp. A first hemostat is placed at the appendiceal base, and a second is positioned directly above (Fig. 46-23.2). A third hemostat is closed with a few millimeters of intervening tissue to allow for passage of a knife blade. The knife then cuts between the second and third clamps, and the appendix is removed. The contaminated knife and appendix are then handed off the field.

A 2-0 silk suture is tied beneath the first hemostat as that clamp is slowly removed. A separate suture is then tied underneath the second hemostat for added security of the appendiceal stump. Gentle electrosurgical coagulation at the stump surface also may be performed.

❻ **Final Steps.** There is no need to invert the stump or to place a purse-string suture around it. The cecum may be returned to the abdomen, and remaining concurrent surgeries completed.

POSTOPERATIVE

Patient care postoperatively is dictated by other surgeries performed. Delayed initiation of oral intake or administration of additional antibiotics is not required for appendectomy alone.

Skinning Vulvectomy

The term *skinning vulvectomy* implies a wide, superficial resection that encompasses both sides of the vulva, that is, a complete simple vulvectomy. It is distinguished from a *radical complete vulvectomy* in that skinning vulvectomy removes only the squamous epithelium and dermis and preserves the subcutaneous fat and deeper tissues. A less extensive, unilateral procedure is better referred to as *wide local excision* or *partial simple vulvectomy* (Section 43-29, p. 1006).

The usual indication for skinning vulvectomy is a woman with confluent, bilateral vulvar intraepithelial neoplasia (VIN) 2 to 3 who is not a candidate for directed ablation with carbon dioxide (CO_2) laser or cavitational ultrasonic surgical aspirator (CUSA) (Section 43-29, p. 1007). Fortunately, patients with such extensive VIN are infrequently encountered. Paget disease without underlying adenocarcinoma and vulvar dystrophies refractory to standard therapy are other rare indications (Ayhan, 1998; Curtin, 1990; Rettenmaier, 1985).

Despite its less radical resection, skinning vulvectomy can still be disfiguring and psychologically devastating. In addition, the defect is often large and cannot be closed primarily without a split-thickness skin graft (STSG) or other type of flap (Section 46-28, p. 1244) (Lavoué, 2013).

PREOPERATIVE

Patient Evaluation

Colposcopy with directed diagnostic biopsy is required to exclude a squamous lesion with invasion, which would warrant a more radical procedure. Familiarity with an array of possible STSGs or flaps is crucial to planning the operation in the event primary closure is not possible.

Consent

Patients are informed that other more limited treatment options either have been exhausted or are inappropriate. The surgery may result in significant sexual changes, which may be permanent. Accordingly, surgeons emphasize that all efforts will be made to restore a functional, normal-appearing vulva. Fortunately, most physical complications are minor and include cellulitis or partial wound dehiscence.

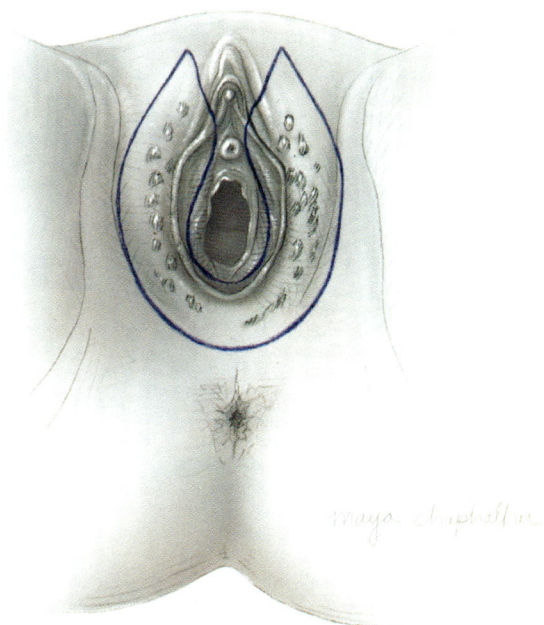

FIGURE 46-24.1 Marking the incisions.

Patient Preparation

VTE prophylaxis is individualized to patient risks, and prophylactic antibiotics similar to those for hysterectomy are provided. Grafts are typically taken from the upper thigh, and donor site selection for STSG is described in Section 43-26 (p. 997). Bowel preparation is not recommended to minimize fecal soiling and permit initial wound healing prior to the first stool.

INTRAOPERATIVE

Surgical Steps

❶ Anesthesia and Patient Positioning. Regional or general anesthesia is generally required. The patient is placed in standard lithotomy position, and adjustments are made to provide access to the entire lesion. For VTE prophylaxis, lower-extremity pneumatic compression devices are placed. Vulvar hair is clipped. Intraoperative colposcopy may be needed to better delineate VIN lesion margins. The vulva is surgically prepared, and a Foley catheter is inserted.

❷ Skin Incision. The inner and outer incision lines are drawn to encompass the disease with margins of at least a few millimeters (Fig. 46-24.1). As an overview, once final markings are placed, the skin is dissected off one side of the vulva. The skin

on the opposite side of the vulva is then removed, and the bridging skin overlying the perineal body is excised last. In performing this, the clitoris may be spared in many cases by making a horseshoe-shaped incision (as shown).

To begin, if preserving the clitoris, the outer incision is started on one side of the vulva at the anterolateral margin of the clitoris and is continued inferiorly along the length of the labium majus at least halfway to the perineal body. The inner incision on that same side of the vulva is then also taken through the full skin thickness to the same inferior halfway point. Incising the skin in stages reduces blood loss.

❸ Beginning the Dissection. After this initial incision, the specimen edge is reflected with an Allis clamp to provide traction as the avascular plane underneath the skin is dissected from the subcutaneous fatty tissue (Fig. 46-24.2). When the anterior skin edge is large enough, a hand is placed underneath to reflect the specimen more firmly and guide dissection inferiorly. The outer and inner skin incision is then extended on that same side downward toward the perineal body. Electrosurgical coagulation is used to achieve hemostasis before repeating the process on the contralateral side.

❹ Removal of the Specimen. The left and right outer skin incisions are joined in

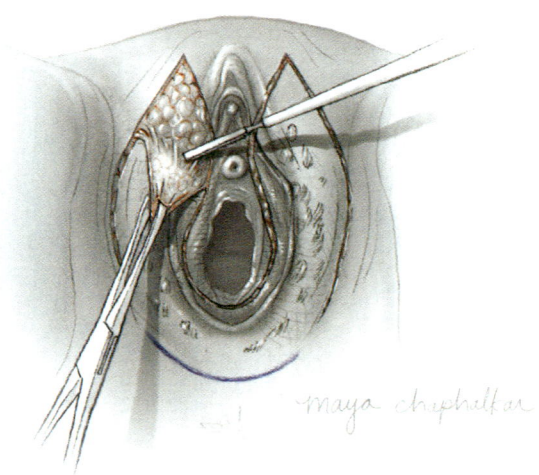

FIGURE 46-24.2 Performing the dissection.

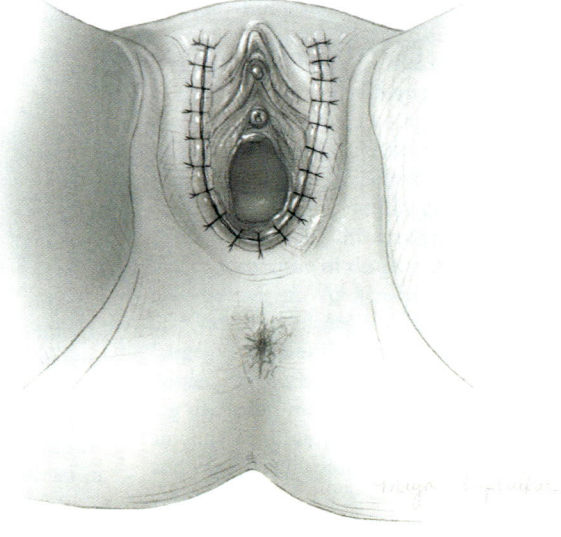

FIGURE 46-24.3 Primary closure.

the midline superficial to the perineal body. The inner incision is made sufficiently proximal to encompass disease. The posterior vulvar tissue margin is held with an Allis clamp to provide traction for upward dissection toward the inner incision. This portion of the skinning vulvectomy is typically performed last because an avascular tissue plane superficial to the subcutaneous tissue is absent, and bleeding can be brisk. The specimen can be removed following detachment from the inner incision.

The skinning vulvectomy specimen is carefully examined to grossly determine margins. A frozen section may be warranted if close VIN margins are suspected, to determine if more tissue requires excision. However, the margins of vulvar Paget disease cannot reliably be judged visually or by frozen-section

analysis (Fishman, 1995). A stitch is placed on the specimen and noted on the pathology requisition form to orient the pathologist.

❺ **Closure of the Defect.** A dry laparotomy pad is held against the vulvar defect and slowly rolled downward to halt surface bleeding and aid meticulous electrosurgical coagulation of vessels. The operative site is irrigated and assessed.

If the width of the defect is sufficiently narrow to permit primary closure, the surrounding tissue is mobilized. Lateral undermining may be particularly useful for a tension-free closure. Usually, 0- or 2-0 gauge delayed-absorbable vertical mattress sutures are then placed circumferentially around the introitus with the knots positioned laterally (Fig. 46-24.3). However, if a split-thickness

skin graft is required, the graft is now harvested and placed as described on page 1244.

❻ **Final Steps.** A CO_2 laser may be used to vaporize multifocal lesions outside the operative field. This is described in Section 43-29 (p. 1008).

POSTOPERATIVE

If a primary closure is performed, postoperative care is essentially the same as described for patients undergoing radical partial vulvectomy (p. 1237). Long-term surveillance is mandatory regardless of margin status to identify recurrent or de novo sites of preinvasive disease. The Foley catheter can be removed without regard to urine spill unless a graft is placed or the patient is otherwise immobile.

46-25

Radical Partial Vulvectomy

For vulvar cancer, to reduce the high morbidity associated with radical complete vulvectomy yet avoid sacrificing a cure, a less extensive resection may be used. Patients with well-localized, unifocal, clinical stage I invasive lesions are ideal candidates (Koh, 2018b; Stehman, 1992). *Radical partial vulvectomy* is a somewhat ambiguously defined operation that generally refers to complete removal of the tumor-containing portion of the vulva, wherever it is located, with 1- to 2-cm skin margins and excision to the perineal membrane (Whitney, 2010). *Radical hemivulvectomy* refers to a larger resection that may be anterior, posterior, right, or left. Vulvectomy is typically performed concurrently with inguinofemoral lymphadenectomy to add prognostic information. However, in those with microinvasive disease undergoing wide local excision or skinning vulvectomy, lymphadenectomy is not required.

The chief concern in performing a less extensive operation for vulvar cancer is the possible increased risk of local recurrence due to multifocal disease. However, survival after partial or complete radical vulvectomy is comparable if negative margins are obtained (Chan, 2007; Landrum, 2007; Tantipalakorn, 2009). Following radical partial vulvectomy, 10 percent of patients will develop a recurrence on the ipsilateral vulva, and this may be treated by reexcision (Desimone, 2007).

PREOPERATIVE

Patient Evaluation

Biopsy confirmation of invasive cancer is mandatory. An isolated squamous lesion with <1 mm of invasion, that is, microinvasion, may be adequately managed with only wide local excision (Section 43-29, p. 1006). Multiple microinvasive lesions may require skinning vulvectomy (p. 1233). In general, patients undergoing radical partial vulvectomy do not require reconstructive grafts or flaps to cover operative defects.

Consent

Morbidity after radical vulvar surgery is common. Wound separation or cellulitis develops frequently (Mert, 2019). Long-term changes may include displacement of the urine stream, dyspareunia, and vulvar pain. Similarly, sexual dysfunction is prevalent (Hazelwinkel, 2012). Surgeons should be sensitive to these possible sequelae and counsel patients appropriately, emphasizing the curative intent and limited scope of the operation.

Patient Preparation

Antibiotics similar to that for hysterectomy prophylaxis and VTE prophylaxis are typically given prior to incision (Tables 39-8 and 39-10, p. 832). Bowel preparation is not recommended to minimize fecal soiling and permit initial wound healing prior to the first stool.

INTRAOPERATIVE

Surgical Steps

❶ Anesthesia and Patient Positioning. Radical partial vulvectomy has been performed under local anesthesia combined with sedation in medically compromised patients (Manahan, 1997). However, regional or general anesthesia is typically required. For VTE prophylaxis, lower-extremity pneumatic compression devices are placed.

An inguinal lymphadenectomy (p. 1241) is typically performed before vulvar resection. Patients may then be repositioned to standard lithotomy position to provide full exposure to the vulva. Vulvar hair is clipped, this area is surgically prepared, and a Foley catheter is inserted.

❷ Radical Partial Vulvectomy: Variations. The area of tissue to be removed when radically excising a small cancer depends on the size and location of the tumor. In Figure 46-25.1, the dotted line indicates a planned skin incision for: (A) a 1-cm right labium majus tumor with 2-cm margins, (B) a 2.5-cm periclitoral tumor necessitating anterior hemivulvectomy, and (C) a 2.5-cm midline posterior fourchette tumor requiring posterior hemivulvectomy.

❸ Right Hemivulvectomy: Making the Lateral Incision. The planned excision is drawn on the vulva with a surgical marking pen to provide 2-cm margins (Fig. 46-25.2). Tapering the incision anteriorly and posteriorly will aid in a tension-free closure. The

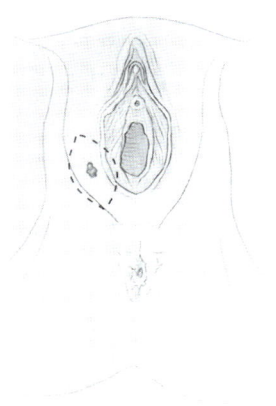

A

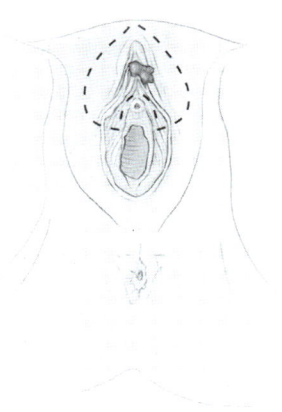

B

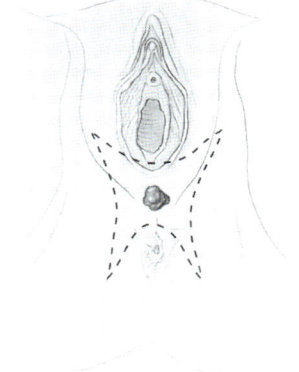

C

FIGURE 46-25.1 Partial radical vulvectomy: variations.

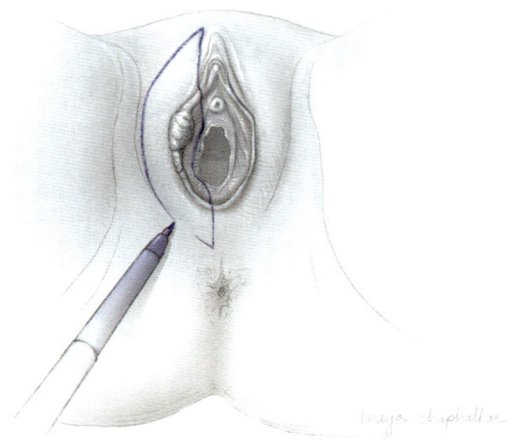

FIGURE 46-25.2 Right hemivulvectomy: outlining the skin incision.

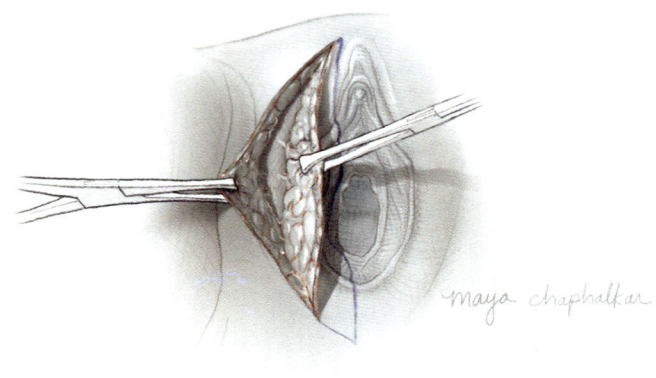

FIGURE 46-25.3 Right hemivulvectomy: lateral dissection to the fascia lata.

lateral skin incision is made with a knife (no. 15 blade) into the subcutaneous fat. Forceps are used to place the skin edges on traction and aid electrosurgical dissection to a depth that reaches the perineal membrane (Fig. 46-25.3). An index finger can then be used to develop the plane between the fat pad of the labium majus and the subcutaneous tissue of the lateral thigh.

❹ **Right Hemivulvectomy: Completing the Resection.** Tissue medial to this lateral resection border is next mobilized by blunt and electrosurgical dissection directed medially along the perineal membrane.

The skin edge of the specimen is then placed on lateral traction, and the medial (vaginal mucosa) incision is incised from anterior to posterior. The labial fat pad is transected anteriorly, and the entire radical right hemivulvectomy specimen is placed on downward traction to aid final dissection along the mucosal incision in an anterior-to-posterior direction (Fig. 46-25.4). Notably, the vascular vestibular bulb is typically encountered as the posterior resection is completed (Fig. 38-26, p. 815). Suture ligation of bleeding sites is often required.

After completed resection, the specimen is examined to ensure adequate margins. It is marked at 12 o'clock with an orienting stitch, and this is noted on the pathology requisition form.

❺ **Right Hemivulvectomy: Closing the Defect.** A gauze sponge may be held firmly in the cavity and gradually rolled downward to guide the electrosurgical blade in achieving hemostasis. The defect can then be irrigated and evaluated to determine requirement for a tension-free closure while minimizing anatomic distortion (Fig. 46-25.5). Several pedicles are visible, particularly at the vaginal margin, where vessels were clamped and tied.

In general, lateral undermining of the subcutaneous tissue will provide sufficient mobility to allow primary closure. Interrupted 0-gauge delayed-absorbable suture is used to create a layered reapproximation of deeper tissues. Interrupted vertical mattress sutures, often alternating 0- and 2-0 gauge suture, with knots placed laterally are used to close the skin (Fig. 46-25.6).

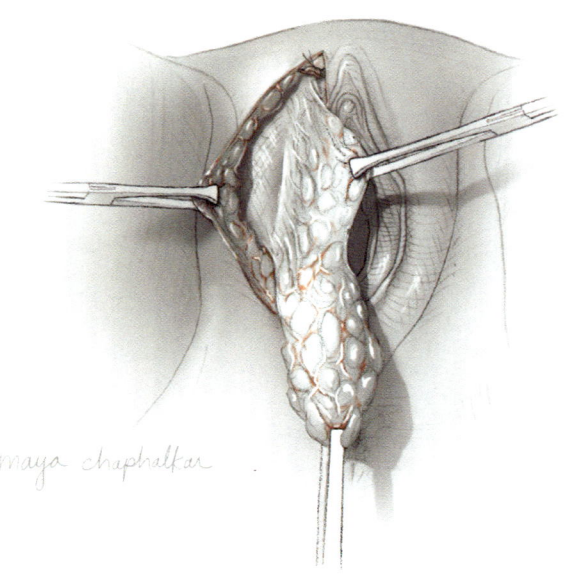

FIGURE 46-25.4 Right hemivulvectomy: removal of the specimen.

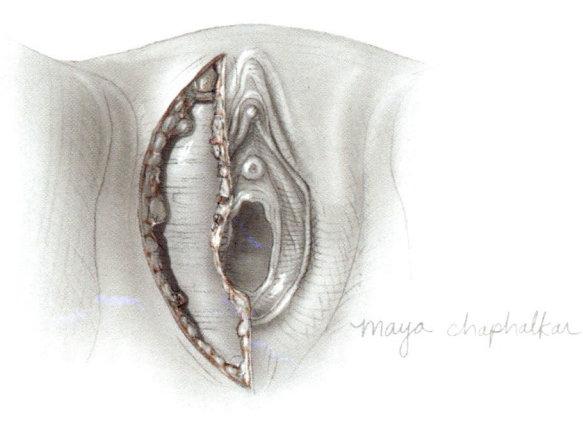

FIGURE 46-25.5 Right hemivulvectomy: evaluation of the surgical defect.

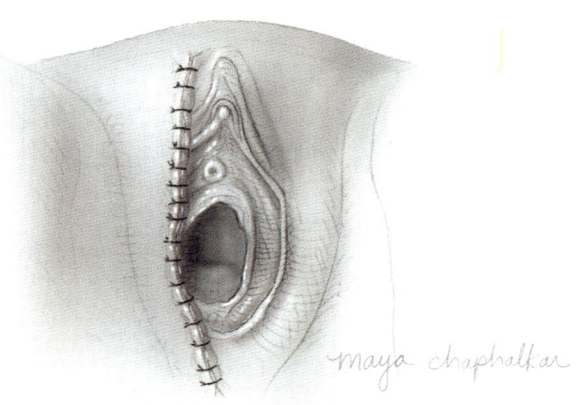

FIGURE 46-25.6 Right hemivulvectomy: closure of the surgical defect.

❻ Anterior Hemivulvectomy. This variation requires removal of the clitoris and partial resection of the labia minora, labia majora, and mons pubis (see Fig. 46-25.1B). The most anterior portion of the incision is first created on the mons and carried down to the symphysis pubis. The specimen is reflected posteriorly to guide dissection. In the midline, the dorsal artery and vein of the clitoris are separately clamped, divided, and ligated with 0-gauge delayed-absorbable suture (Fig. 38-28, p. 816).

The posterior incision is made superior to the urethral meatus. Careful attention to Foley catheter location helps avoid urethral injury.

After specimen excision, layers of interrupted 0-gauge delayed-absorbable sutures are used to reapproximate deep tissues. Next, 3-0 gauge absorbable suture is used to close the defect superficially. Suture lines are oriented either horizontally or vertically to create a suture line off tension. Usually, the area surrounding the urethral meatus is left to granulate in secondarily.

❼ Partial Urethral Resection (Optional). If an anterior lesion encroaches on the urethral meatus, a distal urethrectomy may be required to achieve a negative margin. Prior to this, the radical partial vulvectomy should otherwise be almost entirely completed.

The urethra may be transected anywhere distal to the pubic arch. For this, the meatus is held with an Allis clamp, and the specimen placed on traction. The posterior urethra is incised with a knife, and the underlying uroepithelium and mucosa are sewn jointly to the adjacent vestibule skin at the 6 o'clock position with 4-0 gauge delayed-absorbable

suture. The urethral incision is extended laterally, followed by additional sutures at 3 and 9 o'clock. The Foley balloon is deflated and removed from the bladder. Transection is completed, and a final stitch is placed at 12 o'clock. The Foley catheter is then replaced. Alternatively, the surgeon may forgo stitch placement altogether and allow the meatus to heal by secondary intent. Although urethral plication may be indicated in selected cases, resection of 1 to 1.5 cm of the distal urethra does not ordinarily result in a significant increase in the rates of urinary incontinence (de Mooij, 2007).

❽ Posterior Hemivulvectomy. This variation entails removal of a portion of both labia majora, the Bartholin glands, and upper perineal body (see Fig. 46-25.1C). It is generally necessary to compromise the deep margin in this resection because of proximity to the anal sphincter and rectum. The skin is first incised posteriorly, and a finger is placed into the rectum to guide proximal dissection. The specimen is gradually retracted upward off the sphincter. The perineal body, superficial to the level of the perineal membrane, is removed with the specimen. From the midline, dissection then proceeds laterally on each side until the anterior margin at the introitus can be incised to complete the resection.

Remaining perineal body is reinforced with interrupted 0-gauge delayed-absorbable sutures to provide bulk and allow reapproximation of skin edges for a tension-free closure. Rectal examination is done at the end of surgery to confirm the absence of palpable stitches or stenosis. Incontinence of flatus or stool may develop postoperatively despite efforts to preserve the sphincter.

❾ Final Steps. Suction drains are not typically required but are at least considered in some circumstances. Copious irrigation is indicated at various times during closure of the defect to minimize postoperative infection. No formal dressing is applied. However, fluffed-out gauze may be placed at the perineum and held in place with mesh underwear to tamponade any subcutaneous bleeding and to promote a clean and dry operative site in the immediate postoperative period.

POSTOPERATIVE

Meticulous care of the vulvar wound is mandatory to prevent morbidity. The vulva is kept dry by use of a blow dryer or fan. Within a few days, brief sitz baths or bedside irrigation followed by air drying will help keep the incision clean. Patients are instructed not to wear tight-fitting underwear upon discharge from the hospital. Moreover, instructions encourage loose-fitting gowns to aid healing and efforts to minimize wound tension. For posteriorly located defects near the anus, a low-residue diet and stool softeners will prevent straining and potential perineal incision disruption.

Typically, the Foley catheter is removed postprocedure or at least on postoperative day 1. If a distal urethrectomy was performed or extensive periurethral dissection was required, the catheter is removed within a few days. This permits tissue swelling and obstructive urinary retention concerns to abate. Early removal prevents ascending urinary infection. If immobility is encouraged to aid reconstructive graft or flap healing, the timing of catheter removal is individualized. Notably, urine that comes in contact with the vulvar incision during normal voiding is of little clinical concern. VTE prophylaxis is continued for 4 weeks postoperatively.

Incision separation is the most common postoperative complication and often will involve only a portion of the incision (Burke, 1995). Stitches are removed as needed, and affected portions of the wound are debrided. Efforts to keep the site clean and dry are continued. Granulation tissue will eventually allow healing by secondary intention, but recovery time will be significantly extended. Although negative-pressure wound therapy (wound vacuum-assisted closure) may be practical in rare instances, the location of most defects precludes effective device placement.

Sexual dysfunction may stem from a sense of disfigurement. Scarring may also result in discomfort or altered sensation that lowers a woman's sexual satisfaction. Clinician sensitivity to these concerns enables a dialogue to develop that can lead to possible management options (Janda, 2004).

Radical Complete Vulvectomy

If cancers are so extensive that no meaningful portion of the vulva can be preserved, radical complete vulvectomy is indicated rather than the more limited radical partial vulvectomy (p. 1235). The operation is typically performed concurrently with bilateral inguinofemoral lymphadenectomy (p. 1241). With the radical complete vulvectomy technique currently used, intact skin bridges remain between the three incisions (vulvectomy incision and two lymphadenectomy incisions) to aid wound healing. Traditionally, the en bloc incision, colloquially termed the *butterfly* or *longhorn incision*, removed these skin bridges and the underlying lymphatic channels that potentially harbored tumor emboli "in transit" between the vulvar tumor and nodes (Gleeson, 1994c). However, such recurrences are rare, and the en bloc technique has been largely abandoned (Rose, 1999). Thus, the three-incision procedure is preferred because survival rates are equivalent and major morbidity is dramatically reduced (Helm, 1992).

Removal of an extensive vulvar lesion with an adequate margin and with resection down to the perineal membrane usually creates a large surgical defect. In some cases, wound margins may be primarily closed without tension by undermining and mobilizing adjacent tissues. On other occasions, a split-thickness skin graft, lateral skin transposition, rhomboid flap, or other reconstructive procedure, described on page 1244, will be indicated to reduce the chances of wound separation.

PREOPERATIVE

Patient Evaluation

Biopsy confirmation of invasive cancer should precede surgery. Depending on the location of the tumor, the clitoris-sparing modification of radical complete vulvectomy is an option (Chan, 2004). Frequently, patients are elderly, are obese, or have significant coexisting medical problems that must be considered.

Consent

Major morbidity is common soon after radical complete vulvectomy, and partial wound separation or cellulitis occurs frequently. Complete wound breakdown is more problematic, and weeks of aggressive hospital care may be required to promote secondary healing.

Premature hospital discharge may result in poor home wound care, and subsequent tissue necrosis often requires readmission and surgical debridement. Thus, meticulous attention to the wound is critical during initial patient admission and during frequent office visits thereafter.

Long-term changes may include displacement of the urine stream, dyspareunia, vulvodynia, and sexual dysfunction. Accordingly, surgeons counsel on these possible sequelae yet emphasize the curative intent of the operation and the need for adequate tumor-free margins to lessen local recurrence risks.

Patient Preparation

Evaluation of potential graft donor sites is completed. Antibiotics and VTE prophylaxis are typically given prior to initial incision. Bowel preparation is not recommended to minimize fecal soiling and permit initial wound healing prior to the first stool.

INTRAOPERATIVE

Surgical Steps

❶ Anesthesia and Patient Positioning. Regional or general anesthesia is required, and inguinofemoral lymphadenectomy is performed first in low lithotomy position. The patient is then placed in standard lithotomy position. For VTE prophylaxis, lower-extremity pneumatic compression devices are placed. Exposure and surgical preparation of the operative field is planned to accommodate resection and reconstruction. Vulvar hair is clipped, this area is surgically prepared, and a Foley catheter is inserted. Sites of potential donor graft harvest are prepared as described on page 1244.

❷ Planning the Skin Incision. The medial and lateral incisions are drawn to encompass the tumor and provide a 1- to 2-cm margin around the tumor. The clitoris is included if necessary. Tapering the incision anteriorly and posteriorly will also aid in a tension-free closure (Fig. 46-26.1).

❸ Anterior Dissection. The skin incision begins anteriorly with the knife (no. 15 blade) cutting into the subcutaneous fat. The incision is extended downward approximately three quarters of its length. The remainder of the posterior skin incision is completed later to decrease blood loss. Much of the anterior dissection is described in the preceding section on radical partial vulvectomy (Section 46-25, Step 6, p. 1237). However, use of the Harmonic scalpel or bipolar electrocoagulation device (LigaSure, ENSEAL) in this more extensive resection may decrease operative time and blood loss compared with use of a conventional electrosurgical blade (Pellegrino, 2008).

Briefly, the incision is carried down to the symphysis pubis. The specimen is reflected downward on traction to guide dissection. The vascular base of the clitoris is clamped in the midline, transected, and suture ligated with 0-gauge delayed-absorbable suture (Fig. 46-26.2). Electrosurgical or Harmonic scalpel dissection then proceeds dorsally off the pubic bone until the inner incision line is reached anteriorly. This inner anterior incision is made above the urethral meatus to avoid injury to the urethra unless a distal urethrectomy is required (Section 46-25, Step 7, p. 1237).

❹ Lateral Dissection. Blunt finger dissection is performed to establish a plane lateral to the labial fat pads and at a depth to reach the perineal membrane. The vulvectomy specimen is placed on traction to guide dissection

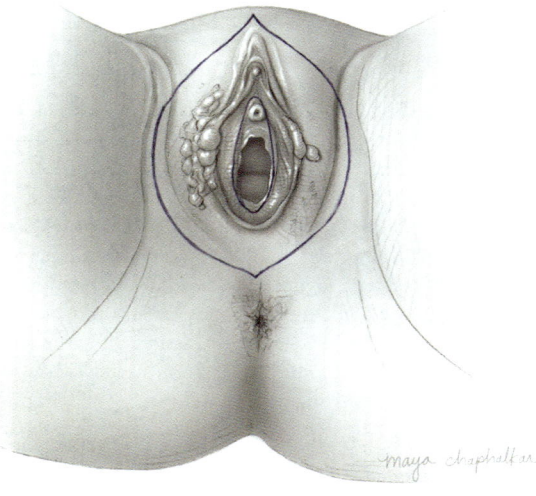

FIGURE 46-26.1 Incisions.

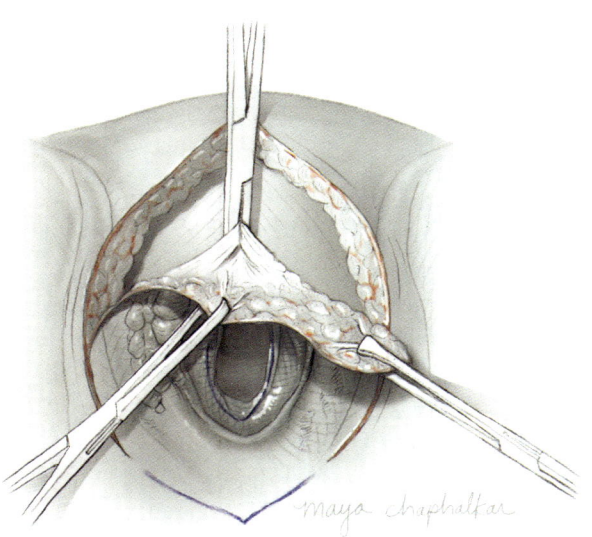

FIGURE 46-26.2 Anterior dissection.

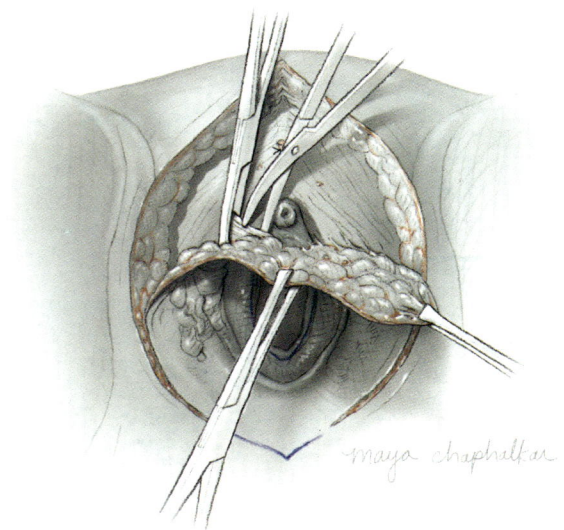

FIGURE 46-26.3 Medial dissection.

medially to reach the vaginal walls. Along the lower lateral sides of the vagina, each vascular vestibular bulb is encountered. Vessels are divided with the Harmonic scalpel or clamped, cut, and ligated with 0-gauge delayed-absorbable suture to reduce bleeding (Fig. 46-26.3).

❺ Posterior Dissection. The outer skin incision is completed inferiorly with a knife as the vulvectomy proceeds posteriorly toward the perineal body. A finger is then placed into the rectum to prevent inadvertent injury, and the specimen is now held upward

on traction (Fig. 46-26.4). Electrosurgical dissection along the deep fascia plane extends the outer incisions toward the midline. The dissection continues anteriorly away from the anus until the inner incision can be made. With this, the entire complete radical vulvectomy specimen is detached.

❻ Evaluating the Specimen. A stitch is placed at 12 o'clock on the specimen and noted on the laboratory requisition form to orient the pathologist. Skin retraction of the specimen will make it appear narrower

and smaller than the defect. However, it is carefully inspected to assess its margins. Additional lateral or medial tissue margins can be separately sent if necessary. Alternatively, a frozen-section analysis can be requested to evaluate an equivocal margin.

❼ Closing the Defect. The wound is copiously irrigated, and hemostasis is achieved with a combination of electrosurgical coagulation and clamping with suturing. The defect is then evaluated to determine the best method of closure (Fig. 46-26.5).

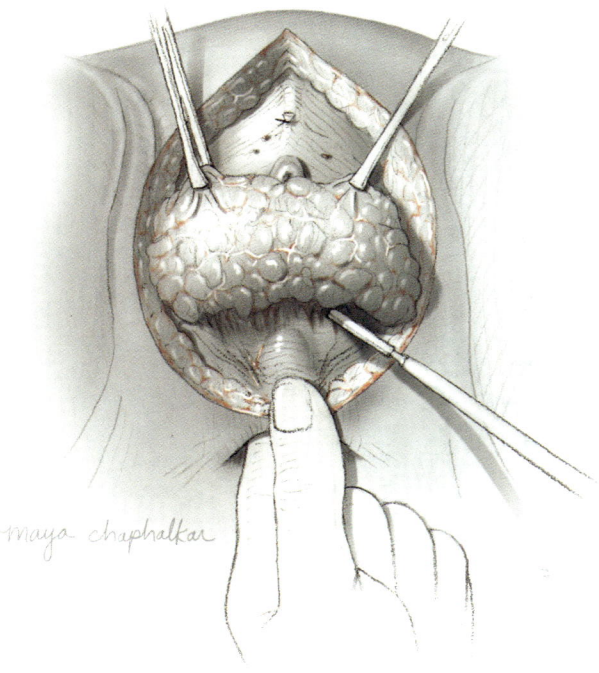

FIGURE 46-26.4 Posterior dissection.

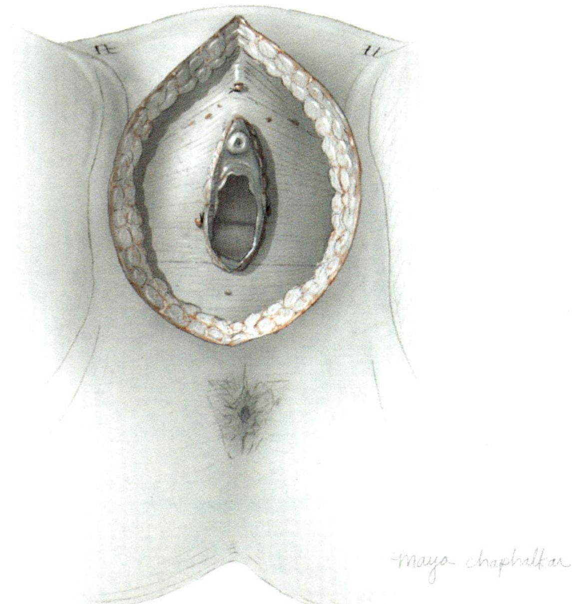

FIGURE 46-26.5 Surgical defect.

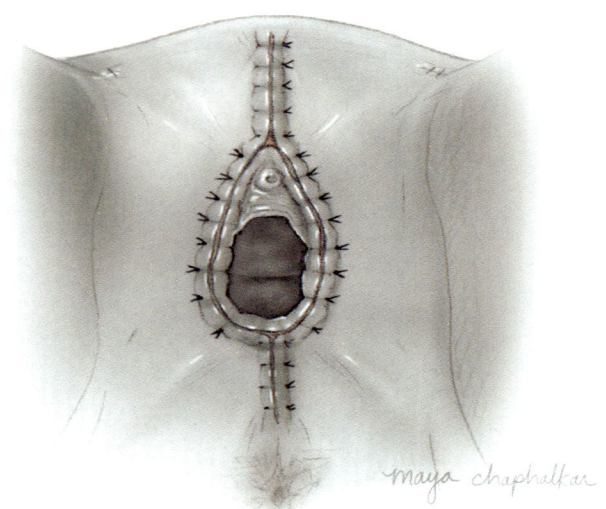

FIGURE 46-26.6 Simple closure.

Undermining lateral tissues will aid a tension-free primary closure. Deeper tissues are first reapproximated with 0-gauge delayed-absorbable suture and interrupted stitches. The vulvar skin is then closed solely with 0-gauge, or alternating with 2-0 gauge, delayed-absorbable vertical mattress sutures (Fig. 46-26.6). No stitches are placed between the skin and urethra if this displaces the urethra or creates tension on it. Instead, this area can be allowed to heal secondarily by granulation. If a split-thickness skin graft or flap is required to close the incision, the graft is now harvested and placed as described on page 1244.

❽ Final Steps. Suction drains do not prevent wound infection or breakdown but may be considered in some cases if the defect is large (Hopkins, 1993). If primary closure is performed, then fluffed-out gauze may be placed at the perineum and held in place with mesh underwear to keep the operative site clean and dry in the immediate postoperative period.

POSTOPERATIVE

If a primary closure is performed, postoperative care is essentially the same as described for patients undergoing radical partial vulvectomy (p. 1237). Because of a larger operative defect, the likelihood of morbidity is correspondingly increased. Management of reconstructive grafts and flaps is reviewed on page 1246.

46-27

Inguinofemoral Lymphadenectomy

Vulvar cancer staging is the primary indication for removal of groin nodes. Inguinal metastases are the most significant prognostic factor in vulvar squamous cancer, and their detection will necessitate additional therapy (Chap. 31, p. 679) (Homesley, 1991). Occasionally, in patients with ovarian or uterine cancer, suspicion of inguinal metastases will prompt removal.

In general, lymphatic drainage from the vulva rarely bypasses the superficial nodes. Thus, a superficial node dissection is integral. These lymph nodes lie within the fatty tissue along the saphenous, superficial external pudendal, superficial circumflex iliac, and superficial epigastric veins (Fig. 38-31, p. 819). After superficial nodes are addressed, deep nodes may be removed. These nodes are consistently located just medial and parallel to the femoral vein within the fossa ovalis. To reach these, cribriform fascia preservation is recommended to avoid major morbidity (Bell, 2000).

Generally, for patients with unilateral lesions distant from the midline, ipsilateral lymphadenectomy is usually sufficient (Gonzalez Bosquet, 2007). For bilateral lesions or those that encroach on the midline, bilateral lymphadenectomy is indicated.

Sentinel lymph node mapping is a promising modality that has demonstrated great potential in reducing the radicality of detecting inguinal metastases (Lawrie, 2014; Levenback, 2012; Te Grootenhuis, 2016). This minimally invasive strategy is emerging as the future standard for vulvar cancer staging and is described in Chapter 31 (p. 683).

PREOPERATIVE

Patient Evaluation

Clinical palpation is not an accurate means of evaluating the groin nodes (Homesley, 1993). MR imaging and PET scanning are also relatively insensitive (Bipat, 2006; Cohn, 2002; Kataoka, 2010). Fixed, large, clinically obvious groin metastases that appear unresectable are treated preoperatively with radiation before attempting removal.

Consent

Patients should understand the need for unilateral or bilateral groin dissection and its relationship to their cancer treatment.

They should be prepared for a potentially several-week recovery in which postoperative complications are common and may include cellulitis, wound breakdown, chronic lymphedema, and lymphocyst formation. These events may develop within a few days, several months, or even years later. In contrast, intraoperative complications are less common, and hemorrhage from the femoral vessels is rarely encountered.

Patient Preparation

When both groins are dissected, a two-team approach is ideal to reduce operative time. Prophylactic antibiotics may be administered, but they have not been shown to prevent complications (Gould, 2001). VTE prophylaxis is also provided (Table 39-10, p. 834).

INTRAOPERATIVE

Surgical Steps

❶ Anesthesia and Patient Positioning. General or regional anesthesia may be used. Inguinal lymphadenectomy is performed prior to partial or complete radical vulvectomy. Legs are placed in booted support stirrups in low lithotomy position, are abducted approximately 30 degrees, and are flexed minimally at the hip to flatten the groin. Rotation of the thigh a few degrees outward will open the femoral triangle. For VTE prophylaxis, lower-extremity pneumatic compression devices are placed. If concurrent vulvectomy is planned, vulvar hair is clipped, this area is surgically prepared, and a Foley catheter is inserted.

❷ Skin Incision. The groin is incised 2 cm below and parallel to the inguinal ligament starting 3 cm caudal and medial to the

anterior superior iliac spine—aiming toward the adductor longus tendon (Fig. 46-27.1). The incision is 8 to 10 cm long and is taken through full skin thickness and 3 to 4 mm into the fat.

❸ Developing the Upper Flap. Adson forceps elevate and provide traction to the upper skin edge while a hemostat is opened underneath to begin cephalad dissection down through the subcutaneous fat and Scarpa fascia—aiming for a position in the midline of the incision and 3 cm above the inguinal ligament. Dissection proceeds downward to a depth that reveals the glistening white aponeurosis of the external oblique muscle. Adson forceps are then replaced with skin hooks to provide better traction.

A semicircle of fatty tissue is rolled inferiorly and laterally along the aponeurosis using electrosurgical dissection and intermittent blunt dissection. During dissection, the superficial circumflex iliac vessels are divided with a Harmonic scalpel or clamped and ligated. Additionally, superficial epigastric and superficial external pudendal vessels are divided as they are encountered (Fig. 38-31, p. 819). Dissection proceeds until the lower margin of the inguinal ligament is exposed (Fig. 46-27.2).

❹ Developing the Lower Flap. The posterior skin flap is now raised in a similar manner to the upper flap. Dissection progresses through the subcutaneous fat to the deep fascia of the thigh—aiming approximately 6 cm from the inguinal ligament toward the apex of the femoral triangle. As shown in Figure 46-27.1, the femoral triangle is bordered by the inguinal ligament superiorly, by the sartorius muscle laterally, and by the adductor longus muscle medially. Blunt finger dissection along the inner portion of the sartorius and adductor longus muscles aids development of the lower

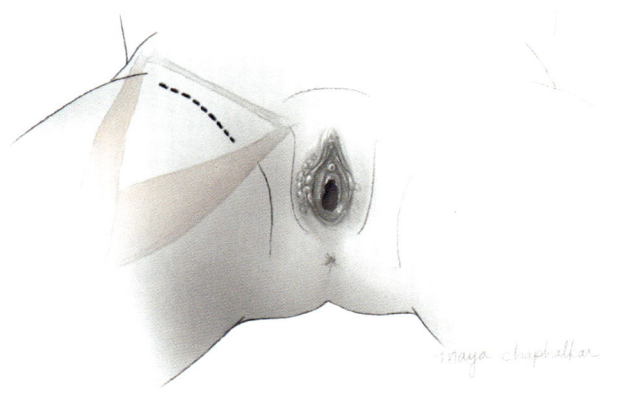

FIGURE 46-27.1 Incision.

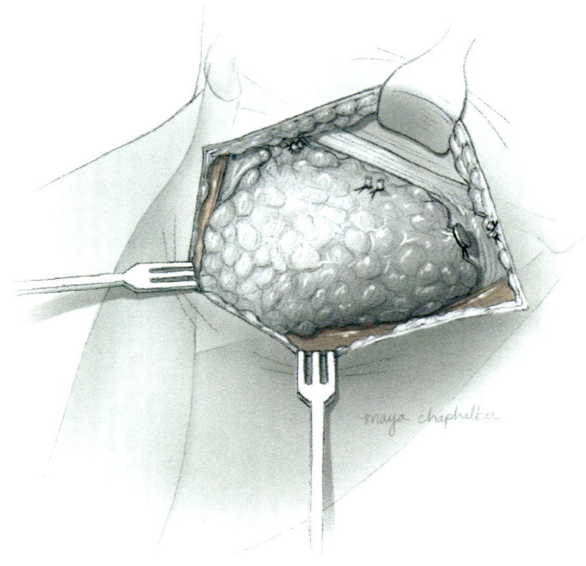

FIGURE 46-27.2 Dissection of the upper flap.

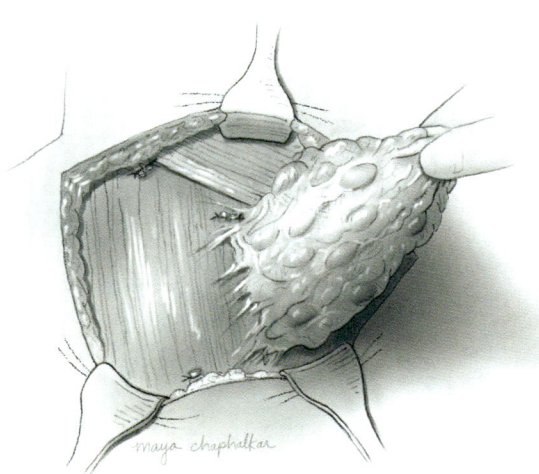

FIGURE 46-27.3 Dissection of the lower flap and removal of superficial nodes.

flap boundaries. The dissection progressively becomes deeper into the subcutaneous tissue of the thigh, but remains superficial to the fascia lata. The tissue exiting at the apex of the femoral triangle is similarly divided.

From these three boundaries, dissection moves in a circumferential path as it progresses toward the fossa ovalis. Node-bearing tissue is held on traction to aid its dissection. Venous tributaries are ligated as they are encountered.

❺ Removal of the Superficial Nodes. The superficial lymph nodes lie within the fatty tissue just mobilized. During the dissection of the medial side of the fat pad, the saphenous vein is encountered. The distal end of this vein is individually transected and ligated with permanent suture for identification. If desired, saphenous vein transection can be avoided, and the vein can be salvaged by dissecting it from the fat pad. Vein sparing may lower rates of postoperative cellulitis and chronic lymphedema in some patients without lowering survival rates (Dardarian, 2006; Zhang, 2000, 2007).

Circumferential dissection is next performed to isolate and remove the nodal bundle as it overlies the fossa ovalis (Fig. 46-27.3). The proximal end of the saphenous vein is separately ligated, unless the vessel has been preserved and can be dissected away from the nodal bundle. Remaining attachments are dissected from the cribriform fascia or clamped and cut to remove the specimen. The cribriform fascia is a multiperforated layer covering the fossa ovalis.

❻ Removal of the Deep Nodes. The femoral vein should be visible within the fossa ovalis. The deep groin nodes lie just medial and parallel to this vessel. Of these, Cloquet node is the uppermost. The residual deep femoral nodal tissue is excised by removing any fatty tissue along the anterior and medial surfaces of the femoral vein above the deep limit of the fossa ovalis. The femoral sheath and cribriform fascia remain intact if possible (Bell, 2000).

If a clinically positive deep node cannot otherwise be reached, the cribriform fascia may be unroofed by making a longitudinal incision distally along the overlying femoral sheath (Fig. 46-27.4). Seven or eight underlying deep inguinal nodes are revealed, and these deep nodes are typically located in a more orderly fashion than the superficial nodes. Fatty-lymphoid tissue is then dissected from the anterior and medial surfaces of the femoral vein. Following node removal, the femoral

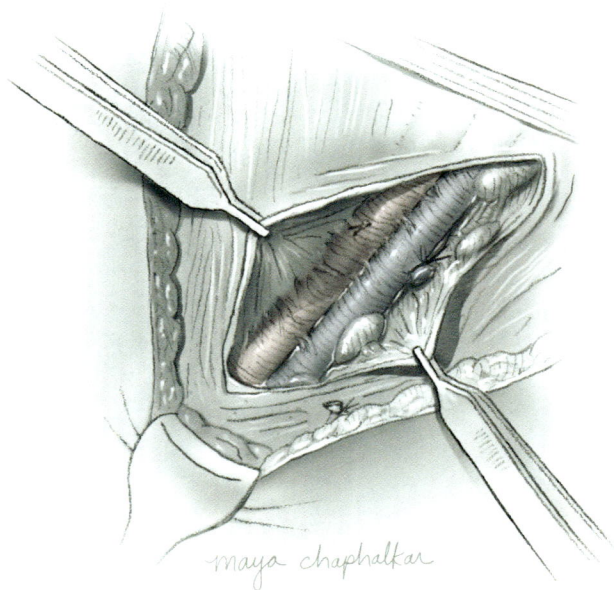

FIGURE 46-27.4 Unroofing the cribriform fascia to remove deep nodes.

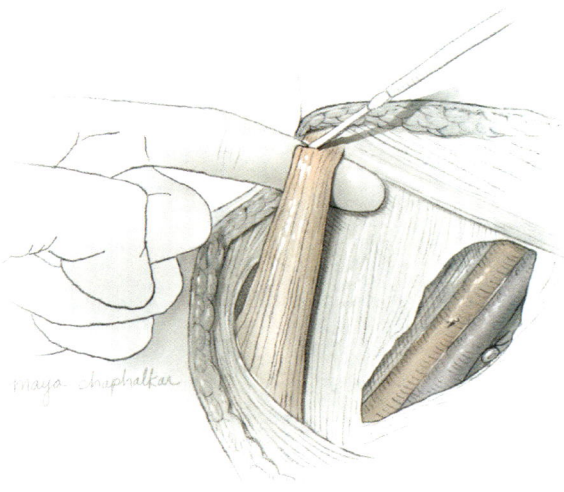

FIGURE 46-27.5 Sartorius muscle transposition.

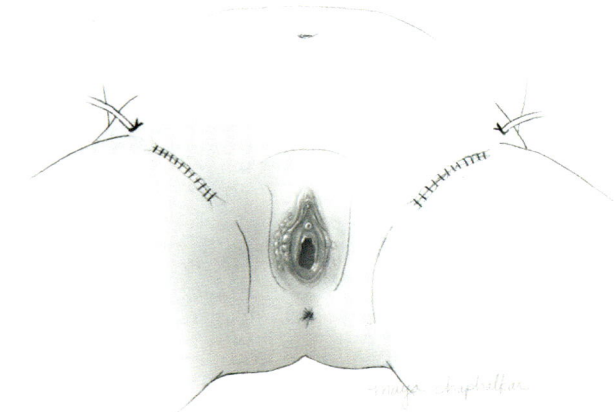

FIGURE 46-27.6 Wound closure.

sheath edges may then be reapproximated using 3-0 gauge delayed-absorbable suture and/or covered with the sartorius muscle.

❼ Sartorius Muscle Transposition (Optional). Unroofing the cribriform fascia can expose the femoral vessels to erosion or sudden hemorrhage. A protective sartorius muscle transposition may be indicated in these selected situations to prevent morbidity (Judson, 2004; Paley, 1997).

The fascia lata is incised to allow blunt dissection of the sartorius muscle (**Fig. 46-27.5**). The proximal sartorius muscle is then transected at its insertion to the anterior superior iliac spine. A finger is wrapped around the upper part of the muscle to aid electrosurgical blade transection directly off the spine. Transection is as high as possible, with care taken to avoid the lateral femoral cutaneous nerve. The muscle is then further mobilized

to cover the femoral vessels and is sutured to the inguinal ligament with 2-0 gauge delayed-absorbable suture.

❽ Wound Closure. The surgical defect is carefully examined, made hemostatic, and irrigated. The groin is closed with layers of delayed-absorbable suture, and a Blake or Jackson-Pratt drain is brought out superolaterally and tied in place at the skin with permanent suture (**Fig. 46-27.6**). Staples are placed to reapproximate skin edges.

POSTOPERATIVE

Suction drainage enables the incision to heal and the underlying space to be obliterated. Drain tubing is manually milked or stripped three times daily with index finger and thumb toward the suction device to prevent blockage. Drains may be removed when output

declines to 20 to 25 mL per day. Typically, this requires approximately 2 weeks (Gould, 2001). Premature removal may result in a symptomatic lymphocyst that requires drain reinsertion or outpatient needle aspiration (Pouwer, 2017).

The groin incision remains uncovered and is regularly examined. Postoperative complications are common, particularly wound cellulitis and breakdown. Preoperative radiation and removal of bulky, fixed nodes increase the risk of these.

Chronic lymphedema is another frequent complication of inguinal lymphadenectomy. As noted, saphenous vein preservation may reduce the incidence. Regardless, this condition is typically much more problematic with the addition of groin radiation. Supportive management is meant to minimize the edema and prevent symptomatic progression. Foot elevation, compression stockings, and, on occasion, diuretic therapy may be helpful.

Reconstructive Grafts and Flaps

Primary closure of a vulvar wound is typically not advised if closure of a large defect would create excessive incision tension or if other untoward factors are present. In these cases, a reconstructive skin graft or flap is preferable to a defect healing by secondary intent. In general, the simplest procedure that will achieve the best functional result should be selected.

The decision to perform a split-thickness skin graft (STSG), lateral skin transposition, or rhomboid skin flap depends on clinical circumstances and surgeon experience. Variations of these techniques are occasionally used in gynecologic oncology (Hand, 2018; Kim, 2015b). Typical candidates for a skin graft or flap have undergone a large wide local excision, skinning vulvectomy, or partial or complete radical vulvectomy. Myocutaneous flaps, most commonly using the rectus abdominis and gracilis muscles, are used primarily in patients with prior radiation, very large defects, or a need for vaginal reconstruction (Section 46-9, p. 1190). However, a full description of the innumerable types of local flaps is beyond the scope of this section.

PREOPERATIVE

Patient Evaluation

Fortunately, a broad range of operative procedures are available—each with their advantages and disadvantages (Weikel, 2005). The size of the lesion and the anticipated postsurgical defect will largely dictate reconstructive options. In some complicated cases, plastic surgery consultation may be indicated.

Consent

A woman's body image may be significantly altered following extensive vulvar surgery, and sexual dysfunction may be a problem (Green, 2000). When discussing these effects, patient responses vary widely. Some express minimal concern, whereas others are devastated by the thought of a disfiguring result. Accordingly, counseling is individualized, specifically addressing patient concerns.

In addition, wound separation, infection, and wound healing by secondary intention are common. Moreover, patients are advised that recurrences of their underlying disease may recur within the graft or flap (DiSaia, 1995).

Patient Preparation

Prophylactic antibiotics are typically given, and bowel preparation is generally influenced by surgeon preference. Early ambulation may be detrimental to graft or flap healing. Therefore, to prevent VTE, use of pneumatic compression devices or subcutaneous heparin is especially warranted (Tables 39-8 and 39-10, p. 832).

For patients undergoing STSG, the hip, buttock, and inner thigh are carefully examined. The selected donor sites should contain healthy skin, should be hidden by a patient's clothing postoperatively, and must be accessible in the operating room. Typically, a graft is taken from the upper thigh.

INTRAOPERATIVE

Surgical Steps

❶ Anesthesia and Patient Positioning. General or regional anesthesia is required. For VTE prophylaxis, lower-extremity pneumatic compression devices are placed. The patient will need to be positioned in low lithotomy with complete access to the vulva, upper thighs, and mons pubis. Sterile preparation of the lower abdomen, perineum, thighs, and vagina is performed, and a Foley catheter is placed. Infrequently, the buttock or hip will be selected as the STSG donor site—this will require additional repositioning.

❷ Evaluating the Surgical Defect. After the vulvar resection has been completed and hemostasis is achieved, the wound is examined to confirm that primary closure is impossible (Fig. 46-28.1). The best graft or flap that will adequately cover a defect is determined.

❸ Split-thickness Skin Graft (STSG). A dermatome device is required to harvest the graft from the donor site when performing a STSG. At a setting of 18/1000ths to 22/1000ths, normal epithelium is harvested from the donor site (Fig. 43-26.3, p. 997). The STSG is placed in a basin and moistened with saline. The donor site is then sprayed with thrombin, covered with a transparent film dressing (Tegaderm), and wrapped firmly with gauze.

The recipient site is irrigated with antibiotic solution, and hemostasis must be absolute. The graft is then held over the defect and cut to fit so that there is some overlap. Meticulous care is required to smooth graft

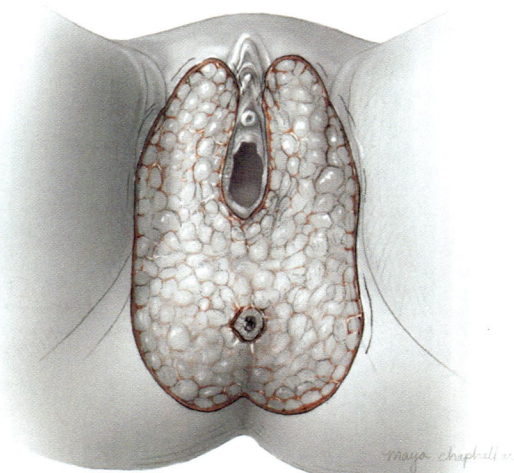

FIGURE 46-28.1 Large vulvar surgical defect.

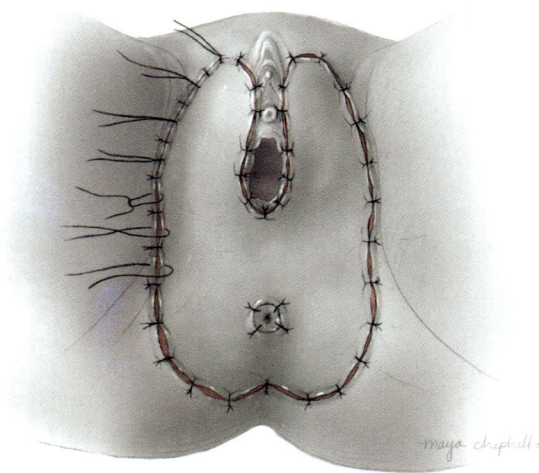

FIGURE 46-28.2 Split-thickness skin graft.

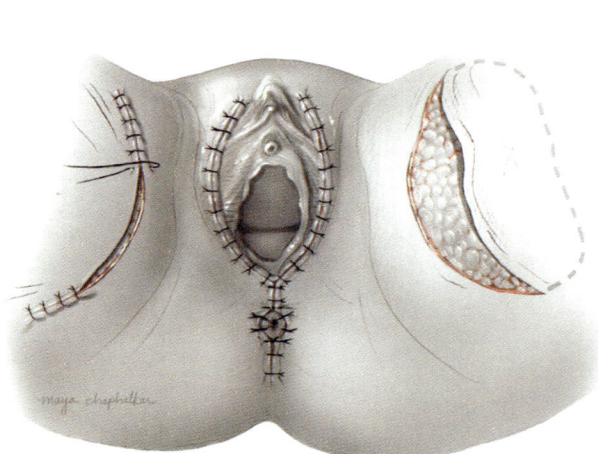

FIGURE 46-28.3 Lateral skin transposition.

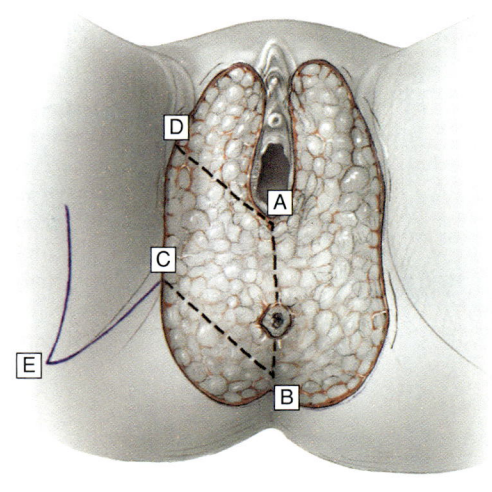

FIGURE 46-28.4 Rhomboid flap: incisions.

wrinkles and avoid graft tension. Edges are then sutured to the skin with interrupted 3-0 gauge nylon suture (Fig. 46-28.2). Moistened gauze or cotton balls are placed over the graft and covered with opened and fluffed gauze squares to provide light pressure. To create a stable dressing, a few ties are usually placed through the covering dressing and lateral to the graft site. Alternatively, fibrin tissue adhesives and/or vacuum-assisted closure devices may further augment graft adherence and viability (Dainty, 2005).

❹ Lateral Skin Transposition. In some cases, the skin lateral to the surgical defect is extensively undermined but still may not be able to cover a large defect and reach the medial skin margin. To perform a lateral skin

transposition, a surgeon makes separate curvilinear relaxing upper thigh skin incisions bilaterally. The relaxing incisions are each undermined laterally out to the dotted line as shown in Figure 46-28.3. The resulting mobility of the intervening vulvar skin bridge should allow for a tension-free primary closure using interrupted vertical mattress sutures. Last, the relaxing incisions are closed with interrupted 0-gauge delayed-absorbable suture.

❺ Rhomboid Flaps. A rhomboid is a four-sided parallelogram with unequal angles at its corners. When creating a rhomboid flap from adjacent tissue, a marking pen is used to draw all sides the same length as the short axis of the defect (A-C; Fig. 46-28.4).

This minimizes wound tension and prevents necrosis. The diagonal A-C is continued in a straight line onto the adjacent vulvar skin lateral to the defect, and marked so that the length of AC = CE. The remaining rhomboid sides are drawn in parallel.

Incisions are made through the skin and into the subcutaneous fat. A flap is developed to include underlying fatty tissue and is mobilized medially to cover the surgical defect (Fig. 46-28.5). In repositioning the flap, (as shown by the arrow), line CE swings medially to appose line AB and is secured with stay sutures at the corners CA and EB. Flap edges are reapproximated with vertical mattress stitches using 0-gauge delayed-absorbable suture (Fig. 46-28.6). Typically, excess tissue folding at the corners requires

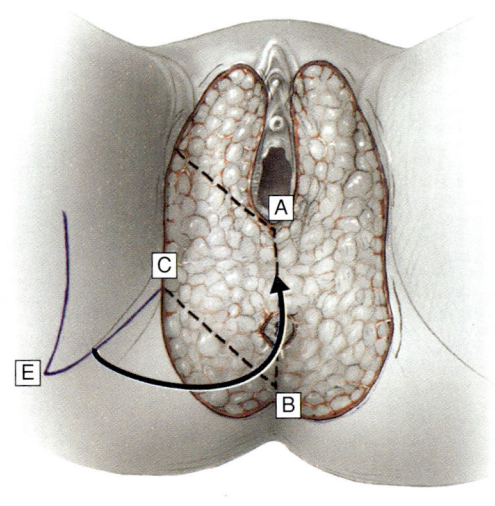

FIGURE 46-28.5 Rhomboid flap: flap positioning.

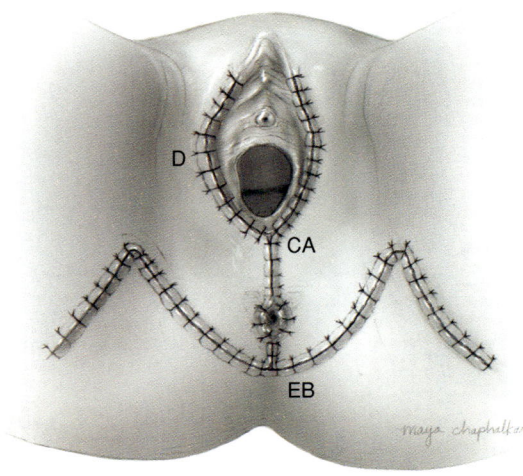

FIGURE 46-28.6 Rhomboid flap: closure.

significant trimming or undermining to provide a reasonably smooth contour and is needed to aid closure of the remaining defects above and below the flap. Finally, a suction drain is placed at the donor site to prevent seromas caused by extensive tissue dissection and that could otherwise result in wound dehiscence.

POSTOPERATIVE

Patients are kept relatively immobile for the first 5 to 7 postoperative days to prevent tension on the reconstruction. Foley catheter drainage is also continued during these initial postoperative days. A low-residue diet, diphenoxylate hydrochloride (Lomotil), or loperamide hydrochloride (Imodium) tablets will aid healing by delaying defecation and preventing straining (Table 25-5, p. 566). Thromboembolic prophylaxis is continued until the patient is ambulatory.

During the first few days postoperatively, the wound is examined frequently to identify signs of hematoma or infection. For STSGs, the transparent dressing may be removed from the donor site after approximately 7 days, and an antibiotic ointment applied. For skin flaps, positioning changes or release of some sutures may be helpful if ischemia is noted at the margins. Suction drains are discontinued when output is less than 30 mL per 24 hours.

Women experience significant sexual dysfunction after vulvectomy. However, the extent of the surgery and need for reconstruction is less important than preexisting depression and hypoactive sexual dysfunction. Accordingly, postoperative psychologic counseling and treatment of depression may be particularly helpful (Hellinga, 2018).

REFERENCES

Aletti GD, Dowdy SC, Podratz KC, et al: Surgical treatment of diaphragm disease correlates with improved survival in optimally debulked advanced stage ovarian cancer. Gynecol Oncol 100:283, 2006a

Aletti GD, Podratz KC, Jones MB, et al: Role of rectosigmoidectomy and stripping of pelvic peritoneum in outcomes of patients with advanced ovarian cancer. J Am Coll Surg 203:521, 2006b

American College of Obstetricians and Gynecologists: Elective coincidental appendectomy. Committee Opinion No. 323, November 2005, Reaffirmed 2019

Angioli R, Estape R, Cantuaria G, et al: Urinary complications of Miami pouch: trend of conservative management. Am J Obstet Gynecol 179:343, 1998

Angioli R, Estape R, Salom E, et al: Radical hysterectomy for cervical cancer: hysterectomy before pelvic lymphadenectomy or vice versa? Int J Gynecol Cancer 9:307, 1999

Armstrong DK, Alvarez RD, Bakkum-Gamez JN, et al: NCCN guidelines insights: ovarian cancer, version 1.2019. J Natl Compr Canc Netw 17(8):896, 2019

Ayhan A, Gultekin M, Taskiran C, et al: Routine appendectomy in epithelial ovarian carcinoma: is it necessary? Obstet Gynecol 105:719, 2005

Ayhan A, Tuncer ZS, Dogan L, et al: Skinning vulvectomy for the treatment of vulvar intraepithelial neoplasia 2–3: a study of 21 cases. Eur J Gynaecol Oncol 19:508, 1998

Backes FJ, Billingsley CC, Martin DD, et al: Does intra-operative radiation at the time of pelvic exenteration improve survival for patients with recurrent, previously irradiated cervical, vaginal, or vulvar cancer? Gynecol Oncol 135(1):95, 2014

Bandy LC, Clarke-Pearson DL, Creasman WT: Vitamin-B$_{12}$ deficiency following therapy in gynecologic oncology. Gynecol Oncol 17:370, 1984

Barnhill D, Doering D, Remmenga S, et al: Intestinal surgery performed on gynecologic cancer patients. Gynecol Oncol 40:38, 1991

Bashir S, Gerardi MA, Giuntoli RL 2nd, et al: Surgical technique of diaphragm full-thickness resection and trans-diaphragmatic decompression of pneumothorax during cytoreductive surgery for ovarian cancer. Gynecol Oncol 119:255, 2010

Bell JG, Lea JS, Reid GC: Complete groin lymphadenectomy with preservation of the fascia lata in the treatment of vulvar carcinoma. Gynecol Oncol 77:314, 2000

Benezra V, Lambrou NC, Salom EM, et al: Conversion of an incontinent urinary conduit to a continent urinary reservoir (Miami pouch). Gynecol Oncol 94:814, 2004

Benn T, Brooks RA, Zhang Q, et al: Pelvic exenteration in gynecologic oncology: a single institution study over 20 years. Gynecol Oncol 122(1):14, 2011

Berek JS, Howe C, Lagasse LD, et al: Pelvic exenteration for recurrent gynecologic malignancy: survival and morbidity analysis of the 45-year experience at UCLA. Gynecol Oncol 99:153, 2005

Bipat S, Fransen GA, Spijkerboer AM, et al: Is there a role for magnetic resonance imaging in the evaluation of inguinal lymph node metastases in patients with vulva carcinoma? Gynecol Oncol 103(3):1001, 2006

Bizzarri N, Chiantera V, Ercoli A, et al: Minimally invasive pelvic exenteration for gynecologic malignancies: a multi-institutional case series and review of the literature. J Minim Invasive Gynecol 26(7):1316, 2019

Boitano TK, Smith HJ, Rushton T, et al: Impact of enhanced recovery after surgery (ERAS) protocol on gastrointestinal function in gynecologic oncology patients undergoing laparotomy. Gynecol Oncol 151(2):282, 2018

Boone JD, Fauci JM, Barr ES, et al: Incidence of port site hernias and/or dehiscence in robotic-assisted procedures in gynecologic oncology patients. Gynecol Oncol 131(1):123, 2013

Bouma J, Dankert J: Infection after radical abdominal hysterectomy and pelvic lymphadenectomy: prevention of infection with a two-dose peri-operative antibiotic prophylaxis. Int J Gynaecol Cancer 3:94, 1993

Bristow RE, del Carmen MG, Kaufman HS, et al: Radical oophorectomy with primary stapled colorectal anastomosis for resection of locally advanced epithelial ovarian cancer. J Am Coll Surg 197:565, 2003

Buekers TE, Anderson B, Sorosky JI, et al: Ovarian function after surgical treatment for cervical cancer. Gynecol Oncol 80:85, 2001

Burke TW, Levenback C, Coleman RL, et al: Surgical therapy of T1 and T2 vulvar carcinoma: further experience with radical wide excision and selective inguinal lymphadenectomy. Gynecol Oncol 57:215, 1995

Burke TW, Levenback C, Tornos C, et al: Intraabdominal lymphatic mapping to direct selective pelvic and paraaortic lymphadenectomy in women with high-risk endometrial cancer: results of a pilot study. Gynecol Oncol 62:169, 1996

Burke TW, Morris M, Levenback C, et al: Closure of complex vulvar defects using local rhomboid flaps. Obstet Gynecol 84:1043, 1994

Butler-Manuel SA, Summerville K, Ford A, et al: Self-assessment of morbidity following radical hysterectomy for cervical cancer. J Obstet Gynaecol 19:180, 1999

Cai HB, Chen HZ, Zhou YF, et al: Class II radical hysterectomy in low-risk IB squamous cell carcinoma of cervix: a safe and effective option. Int J Gynecol Cancer 19:46, 2009

Cain JM, Diamond A, Tamimi HK, et al: The morbidity and benefits of concurrent gracilis myocutaneous graft with pelvic exenteration. Obstet Gynecol 74:185, 1989

Cardosi RJ, Cox CS, Hoffman MS: Postoperative neuropathies after major pelvic surgery. Obstet Gynecol 100:240, 2002

Carlsson E, Fingren J, Hallén AM, et al: The prevalence of ostomy-related complications 1 year after ostomy surgery: a prospective, descriptive, clinical study. Ostomy Wound Manage 62(10):34, 2016

Carroll RE, Benedetti E, Schowalter JP, et al: Management and complications of short bowel syndrome: an updated review. Curr Gastroenterol Rep 18(7):40, 2016

Centers for Disease Control and Prevention: Vitamin B$_{12}$: dietary supplement fact sheet. 2019. Available at: https://ods.od.nih.gov/factsheets/VitaminB12-HealthProfessional/. Accessed September 8, 2019

Chamberlain DH, Hopkins MP, Roberts JA, et al: The effects of early removal of indwelling urinary catheter after radical hysterectomy. Gynecol Oncol 43:98, 1991

Chan JK, Sugiyama V, Pham H, et al: Margin distance and other clinico-pathologic prognostic factors in vulvar carcinoma: a multivariate analysis. Gynecol Oncol 104:636, 2007

Chan JK, Sugiyama V, Tajalli TR, et al: Conservative clitoral preservation surgery in the treatment of vulvar squamous cell carcinoma. Gynecol Oncol 95:152, 2004

Charoenkwan K, Kietpeerakool C: Retroperitoneal drainage versus no drainage after pelvic lymphadenectomy for the prevention of lymphocyst formation in women with gynaecological malignancies. Cochrane Database Syst Rev 6:CD007387, 2017

Chen GD, Lin LY, Wang PH, et al: Urinary tract dysfunction after radical hysterectomy for cervical cancer. Gynecol Oncol 85:292, 2002

Chi DS, Abu-Rustum NR, Sonoda Y, et al: Ten-year experience with laparoscopy on a gynecologic oncology service: analysis of risk factors for complications and conversion to laparotomy. Am J Obstet Gynecol 191:1138, 2004

Chi DS, Zivanovic O, Levinson KL, et al: The incidence of major complications after the performance of extensive upper abdominal surgical procedures during primary cytoreduction of advanced ovarian, tubal, and peritoneal carcinomas. Gynecol Oncol 119:38, 2010

Chung HH, Kim SK, Kim TH, et al: Clinical impact of FDG-PET imaging in post-therapy surveillance of uterine cervical cancer: from diagnosis to prognosis. Gynecol Oncol 103(1):165, 2006

Cibula D, Abu-Rustum NR: Pelvic lymphadenectomy in cervical cancer—surgical anatomy and proposal for a new classification system. Gynecol Oncol 116:33, 2010

Cohn DE, Dehdashti F, Gibb RK, et al: Prospective evaluation of positron emission tomography for the detection of groin node metastases from vulvar cancer. Gynecol Oncol 85:179, 2002

Cohn DE, Swisher EM, Herzog TJ, et al: Radical hysterectomy for cervical cancer in obese women. Obstet Gynecol 96:727, 2000

Coleman RL, Keeney ED, Freedman RS, et al: Radical hysterectomy for recurrent carcinoma of the uterine cervix after radiotherapy. Gynecol Oncol 55:29, 1994

Cosin JA, Fowler JM, Chen MD, et al: Pretreatment surgical staging of patients with cervical carcinoma: the case for lymph node debulking. Cancer 82:2241, 1998

Curtin JP, Rubin SC, Jones WB, et al: Paget's disease of the vulva. Gynecol Oncol 39:374, 1990

Dainty LA, Bosco JJ, McBroom JW, et al: Novel techniques to improve split-thickness skin graft viability during vulvo-vaginal reconstruction. Gynecol Oncol 97:949, 2005

Dardarian TS, Gray HJ, Morgan MA, et al: Saphenous vein sparing during inguinal lymphadenectomy to reduce morbidity in patients with vulvar carcinoma. Gynecol Oncol 101(1):140, 2006

de Mooij Y, Burger MP, Schilthuis MS, et al: Partial urethral resection in the surgical treatment of vulvar cancer does not have a significant impact on urinary incontinence. A confirmation of an authority-based opinion. Int J Gynecol Cancer 17:294, 2007

Desimone CP, Van Ness JS, Cooper AL, et al: The treatment of lateral T1 and T2 squamous cell carcinomas of the vulva confined to the labium majus or minus. Gynecol Oncol 104(2):390, 2007

Dietrich CS III, Desimone CP, Modesitt SC, et al: Primary appendiceal cancer: gynecologic manifestations and treatment options. Gynecol Oncol 104:602, 2007

DiSaia PJ, Dorion GE, Cappuccini F, et al: A report of two cases of recurrent Paget's disease of the vulva in a split-thickness graft and its possible pathogenesis-labeled "retrodissemination." Gynecol Oncol 57:109, 1995

Dowdy SC, Loewen RT, Aletti G, et al: Assessment of outcomes and morbidity following diaphragmatic peritonectomy for women with ovarian carcinoma. Gynecol Oncol 109:303, 2008

Eisenhauer EL, Abu-Rustum NR, Sonoda Y, et al: The addition of extensive upper abdominal surgery to achieve optimal cytoreduction improves survival in patients with stages III-IV epithelial ovarian cancer. Gynecol Oncol 103(3):1083, 2006

Eisenkop SM, Spirtos NM, Lin WC: Splenectomy in the context of primary cytoreductive operations for advanced epithelial ovarian cancer. Gynecol Oncol 100:344, 2006

Eisenkop SM, Spirtos NM, Lin WM, et al: Laparoscopic modified radical hysterectomy: a strategy for a clinical dilemma. Gynecol Oncol 96:484, 2005

Eskandar N, Holley JL: Hyperkalaemia as a complication of ureteroileostomy: a case report and literature review. Nephrol Dial Transplant 23(6):2081, 2008

Estape R, Lambrou N, Diaz R, et al: A case matched analysis of robotic radical hysterectomy with lymphadenectomy compared with laparoscopy and laparotomy. Gynecol Oncol 113:357, 2009

Fagotti A, Fanfani F, Ercoli A, et al: Mini-laparotomy for type II and III radical hysterectomy: technique, feasibility, and complications. Int J Gynaecol Cancer 14:852, 2004

Fedele L, Bianchi S, Zanconato G, et al: Tailoring radicality in demolitive surgery for deeply infiltrating endometriosis. Am J Obstet Gynecol 193:114, 2005

Fishman DA, Chambers SK, Schwartz PE, et al: Extramammary Paget's disease of the vulva. Gynecol Oncol 56:266, 1995

Foley OW, Rauh-Hain JA, Clark RM, et al: Intraoperative radiation therapy in the management of gynecologic malignancies. Am J Clin Oncol 39(4):329, 2016

Fotopoulou C, Neumann U, Kraetschell R, et al: Long-term clinical outcome of pelvic exenteration in patients with advanced gynecological malignancies. J Surg Oncol 101:507, 2010

Fournier M, Huchon C, Ngo C, et al: Morbidity of rectosigmoid resection in cytoreductive surgery for ovarian cancer. Risk factor analysis. Eur J Surg Oncol 44(6):750, 2018

Fowler JM: Incorporating pelvic/vaginal reconstruction into radical pelvic surgery. Gynecol Oncol 115:154, 2009

Franchi M, Trimbos JB, Zanaboni F, et al: Randomised trial of drains versus no drains following radical hysterectomy and pelvic lymph node dissection: a European Organisation for Research and Treatment of Cancer–Gynaecological Cancer Group (EORTC-GCG) study of 234 patients. Eur J Cancer 43:1265, 2007

Franklyn J, Varghese G, Mittal R, et al: A prospective randomized controlled trial comparing early postoperative complications in patients undergoing loop colostomy with and without a stoma rod. Colorectal Dis 19(7):675, 2017

Frumovitz M, Sun CC, Schover LR, et al: Quality of life and sexual functioning in cervical cancer survivors. J Clin Oncol 23:7428, 2005

Fujii S, Takakura K, Matsumura N, et al: Precise anatomy of the vesico-uterine ligament for radical hysterectomy. Gynecol Oncol 104(1):186, 2007

Fujita K, Nagano T, Suzuki A, et al: Incidence of postoperative ileus after paraaortic lymph node dissection in patients with malignant gynecologic tumors. Int J Clin Oncol 10:187, 2005

Fujiwara K, Kigawa J, Hasegawa K, et al: Effect of simple omentoplasty and omentopexy in the prevention of complications after pelvic lymphadenectomy. Int J Gynaecol Cancer 13:61, 2003

Gallotta V, D'Indinosante M, Nero C, et al: Robotic splenectomy for isolated splenic recurrence of endometrial adenocarcinoma. J Minim Invasive Gynecol 25(5):774, 2018

Gallotta V, Nero C, Lodoli C, et al: Laparoscopic splenectomy for secondary cytoreduction in ovarian cancer patients with localized spleen recurrence: feasibility and technique. J Minim Invasive Gynecol 23(3):425, 2016

Gillette-Cloven N, Burger RA, Monk BJ, et al: Bowel resection at the time of primary cytoreduction for epithelial ovarian cancer. J Am Coll Surg 193:626, 2001

Gleeson N, Baile W, Roberts WS, et al: Surgical and psychosexual outcome following vaginal reconstruction with pelvic exenteration. Eur J Gynaecol Oncol 15:89, 1994a

Gleeson NC, Baile W, Roberts WS, et al: Pudendal thigh fasciocutaneous flaps for vaginal reconstruction in gynecologic oncology. Gynecol Oncol 54:269, 1994b

Gleeson NC, Hoffman MS, Cavanagh D: Isolated skin bridge metastasis following modified radical vulvectomy and bilateral inguinofemoral lymphadenectomy. Int J Gynaecol Cancer 4(5):356, 1994c

Goff BA, Matthews BJ, Wynn M, et al: Ovarian cancer: patterns of surgical care across the United States. Gynecol Oncol 103(2):383, 2006

Goldberg GL, Sukumvanich P, Einstein MH, et al: Total pelvic exenteration: the Albert Einstein College of Medicine/Montefiore Medical Center experience (1987–2003). Gynecol Oncol 101:261, 2006

Goldberg JM, Piver MS, Hempling RE, et al: Improvements in pelvic exenteration: factors responsible for reducing morbidity and mortality. Ann Surg Oncol 5:399, 1998

Gonzalez Bosquet J, Magrina JF, Magtibay PM, et al: Patterns of inguinal groin metastases in squamous cell carcinoma of the vulva. Gynecol Oncol 105(3):742, 2007

Gould MK, Garcia DA, Wren SM, et al: Prevention of VTE in nonorthopedic surgical patients: Antithrombotic Therapy and Prevention of Thrombosis, 9th ed: American College of Chest Physicians Evidence-Based Clinical Practice Guidelines. Chest 141(2 Suppl):e227S, 2012

Gould N, Kamelle S, Tillmanns T, et al: Predictors of complications after inguinal lymphadenectomy. Gynecol Oncol 82:329, 2001

Green MS, Naumann RW, Elliot M, et al: Sexual dysfunction following vulvectomy. Gynecol Oncol 77:73, 2000

Grimm C, Harter P, Alesina PF, et al: The impact of type and number of bowel resections on anastomotic leakage risk in advanced ovarian cancer surgery. Gynecol Oncol 146(3):498, 2017

Guimarães GC, Baiocchi G, Ferreira FO, et al: Palliative pelvic exenteration for patients with gynecological malignancies. Arch Gynecol Obstet 283(5):1107, 2011

Hand LC, Maas TM, Baka N, et al: Utilizing V-Y fasciocutaneous advancement flaps for vulvar reconstruction. Gynecol Oncol Rep 26:24, 2018

Havrilesky LJ, Cragun JM, Calingaert B, et al: Resection of lymph node metastases influ-

ences survival in stage IIIC endometrial cancer. Gynecol Oncol 99:689, 2005

Hawighorst-Knapstein S, Schonefusrs G, Hoffmann SO, et al: Pelvic exenteration: effects of surgery on quality of life and body image—a prospective longitudinal study. Gynecol Oncol 66:495, 1997

Hazewinkel MH, Laan ET, Sprangers MA, et al: Long-term sexual function in survivors of vulvar cancer: a cross-sectional study. Gynecol Oncol 126(1):87, 2012

Hazewinkel MH, Sprangers MA, van der Velden J, et al: Long-term cervical cancer survivors suffer from pelvic floor symptoms: a cross-sectional matched cohort study. Gynecol Oncol 117:281, 2010

Hellinga J, Te Grootenhuis NC, Werker PM, et al: Quality of life and sexual functioning after vulvar reconstruction with the lotus petal flap. Int J Gynecol Cancer 28(9):1728, 2018

Helm CW, Hatch K, Austin JM, et al: A matched comparison of single and triple incision techniques for the surgical treatment of carcinoma of the vulva. Gynecol Oncol 46:150, 1992

Hertel H, Diebolder H, Herrmann J, et al: Is the decision for colorectal resection justified by histopathologic findings: a prospective study of 100 patients with advanced ovarian cancer. Gynecol Oncol 83:481, 2001

Hockel M, Dornhofer N: Vulvovaginal reconstruction for neoplastic disease. Lancet Oncol 9:559, 2008

Hoffman MS, Griffin D, Tebes S, et al: Sites of bowel resected to achieve optimal ovarian cancer cytoreduction: implications regarding surgical management. Am J Obstet Gynecol 193:582, 2005

Homesley HD, Bundy BN, Sedlis A, et al: Assessment of current International Federation of Gynecology and Obstetrics staging of vulvar carcinoma relative to prognostic factors for survival (a Gynecologic Oncology Group study). Am J Obstet Gynecol 164:997, 1991

Homesley HD, Bundy BN, Sedlis A, et al: Prognostic factors for groin node metastasis in squamous cell carcinoma of the vulva (a Gynecologic Oncology Group study). Gynecol Oncol 49:279, 1993

Hopkins MP, Reid GC, Morley GW: Radical vulvectomy: the decision for the incision. Cancer 72:799, 1993

Horner W, Peng K, Pleasant V, et al: Trends in surgical complexity and treatment modalities utilized in the management of ovarian cancer in an era of neoadjuvant chemotherapy. Gynecol Oncol 154(2):283, 2019

Houvenaeghel G, Moutardier V, Karsenty G, et al: Major complications of urinary diversion after pelvic exenteration for gynecologic malignancies: a 23-year mono-institutional experience in 124 patients. Gynecol Oncol 92:680, 2004

Hu T, Wu L, Xing H, et al: Development of criteria for ovarian preservation in cervical cancer patients treated with radical surgery with or without neoadjuvant chemotherapy: a multicenter retrospective study and meta-analysis. Ann Surg Oncol 20(3):881, 2013

Huang M, Chadha M, Musa F, et al: Lymph nodes: is total number or station number a better predictor of lymph node metastasis in endometrial cancer? Gynecol Oncol 119:295, 2010

Husain A, Akhurst T, Larson S, et al: A prospective study of the accuracy of [18]Fluorodeoxyglucose positron emission tomography ([18]FDG PET) in identifying sites of metastasis prior to pelvic exenteration. Gynecol Oncol 106:177, 2007

Jackson LA, Ramirez DM, Carrick KS, et al: Gross and histologic anatomy of the pelvic ureter: clinical applications to pelvic surgery. Obstet Gynecol 133(5):896, 2019

Janda M, Obermair A, Cella D, et al: Vulvar cancer patients' quality of life: a qualitative assessment. Int J Gynecol Cancer 14:875, 2004

Jandial DD, Soliman PT, Slomovitz BM, et al: Laparoscopic colostomy in gynecologic cancer. J Minim Invasive Gynecol 15:723, 2008

Jensen PT, Groenvold M, Klee MC, et al: Early-stage cervical carcinoma, radical hysterectomy, and sexual function: a longitudinal study. Cancer 100:97, 2004

Judson PL, Jonson AL, Paley PJ, et al: A prospective, randomized study analyzing sartorius transposition following inguinal-femoral lymphadenectomy. Gynecol Oncol 95:226, 2004

Jurado M, Bazan A, Alcazar JL, et al: Primary vaginal reconstruction at the time of pelvic exenteration for gynecologic cancer: morbidity revisited. Ann Surg Oncol 16:121, 2009

Jurado M, Bazan A, Elejabeitia J, et al: Primary vaginal and pelvic floor reconstruction at the time of pelvic exenteration: a study of morbidity. Gynecol Oncol 77:293, 2000

Kalogera E, Nitschmann CC, Dowdy SC, et al: A prospective algorithm to reduce anastomotic leaks after rectosigmoid resection for gynecologic malignancies. Gynecol Oncol 144(2):343, 2017

Karsenty G, Moutardier V, Lelong B, et al: Long-term follow-up of continent urinary diversion after pelvic exenteration for gynecologic malignancies. Gynecol Oncol 97:524, 2005

Kataoka MY, Sala E, Baldwin P, et al: The accuracy of magnetic resonance imaging in staging of vulvar cancer: a retrospective multi-centre study. Gynecol Oncol 117(1):82, 2010

Kehoe SM, Eisenhauer EL, Abu-Rustum NR, et al: Incidence and management of pancreatic leaks after splenectomy with distal pancreatectomy performed during primary cytoreductive surgery for advanced ovarian, peritoneal and fallopian tube cancer. Gynecol Oncol 112:496, 2009

Key NS, Khorana AA, Kuderer NM, et al: Venous thromboembolism prophylaxis and treatment in patients with cancer: ASCO clinical practice guideline update. J Clin Oncol August 5, 2019 [Epub ahead of print]

Kim DK, Bridges CB, Harriman HK, et al: Advisory Committee on Immunization Practices recommended immunization schedule for adults aged 19 years or older: United States, 2015. Ann Intern Med 162:214, 2015a

Kim SR, Lee YY, Brar H, et al: Utility of 18F-FDG-PET/CT imaging in patients with recurrent gynecological malignancies prior to pelvic exenteration. Int J Gynecol Cancer March 28, 2019 [Epub ahead of print]

Kim SW, Lee WM, Kim JT, et al: Vulvar and vaginal reconstruction using the "angel wing" perforator-based island flap. Gynecol Oncol 137(3):380, 2015b

Koh WJ, Abu-Rustum NR, Bean S, et al: Cervical cancer, version 3.2019, NCCN clinical practice guidelines in oncology. J Natl Compr Canc Netw 17(1):64, 2019

Koh WJ, Abu-Rustum NR, Bean S, et al: Uterine neoplasms, version 1.2018, NCCN clinical practice guidelines in oncology. J Natl Compr Canc Netw 16(2):170, 2018a

Koh WJ, Abu-Rustum NR, Bean S, et al: Vulvar Cancer, Version 2.2019. Plymouth Meeting, National Comprehensive Cancer Network, 2018b

Kohler C, Tozzi R, Possover M, et al: Explorative laparoscopy prior to exenterative surgery. Gynecol Oncol 86:311, 2002

Kong TW, Kim J, Son JH, et al: Preoperative nomogram for prediction of microscopic parametrial infiltration in patients with FIGO stage IB cervical cancer treated with radical hysterectomy. Gynecol Oncol 142(1):109, 2016

Koscielny A, Ko A, Egger EK, et al: Prevention of anastomotic leakage in ovarian cancer debulking surgery and its impact on overall survival. Anticancer Res 39(9):5209, 2019

Koskenvuo L, Lehtonen T, Koskensalo S, et al: Mechanical and oral antibiotic bowel preparation versus no bowel preparation for elective colectomy (MOBILE): a multicentre, randomised, parallel, single-blinded trial. Lancet 394(10201):840, 2019

Kusiak JF, Rosenblum NG: Neovaginal reconstruction after exenteration using an omental flap and split-thickness skin graft. Plast Reconstr Surg 97:775, 1996

Lacey CG, Stern JL, Feigenbaum S, et al: Vaginal reconstruction after exenteration with use of gracilis myocutaneous flaps: the University of California, San Francisco, experience. Am J Obstet Gynecol 158:1278, 1988

Lago V, Fotopoulou C, Chiantera V, et al: Risk factors for anastomotic leakage after colorectal resection in ovarian cancer surgery: a multi-centre study. Gynecol Oncol 153(3):549, 2019

Lambert A, Stüben BO, Bock B, et al: Port-site incisional hernia—a case series of 54 patients. Ann Med Surg 14:8, 2017

Landoni F, Maneo A, Cormio G, et al: Class II versus class III radical hysterectomy in stage IBIIA cervical cancer: a prospective, randomized study. Gynecol Oncol 80:3, 2001

Landrum LM, Lanneau GS, Skaggs VJ, et al: Gynecologic Oncology Group risk groups for vulvar carcinoma: improvement in survival in the modern era. Gynecol Oncol 106:521, 2007

Larciprete G, Casalino B, Segatore MF, et al: Pelvic lymphadenectomy for cervical cancer: extraperitoneal versus laparoscopic approach. Eur J Obstet Gynaecol Reprod Biol 126:259, 2006

Lavoué V, Lemarrec A, Bertheuil N, et al: Quality of life and female sexual function after skinning vulvectomy with split-thickness skin graft in women with vulvar intraepithelial neoplasia or vulvar Paget disease. Eur J Surg Oncol 39(12):1444, 2013

Lawrie TA, Patel A, Martin-Hirsch PP, et al: Sentinel node assessment for diagnosis of groin lymph node involvement in vulval cancer. Cochrane Database Syst Rev 6:CD010409, 2014

Leath CA III, Straughn JM Jr, Estes JM, et al: The impact of aborted radical hysterectomy in patients with cervical carcinoma. Gynecol Oncol 95:204, 2004

Lee PK, Choi MS, Ahn ST, et al: Gluteal fold V-Y advancement flap for vulvar and vaginal reconstruction: a new flap. Plast Reconstr Surg 118:401, 2006

Leon-Casasola OA, Karabella D, Lema MJ: Bowel function recovery after radical hysterectomies: thoracic epidural bupivacaine-morphine versus intravenous patient-controlled analgesia with morphine: a pilot study. J Clin Anesth 8:87, 1996

Levenback CF, Ali S, Coleman RL, et al: Lymphatic mapping and sentinel lymph node biopsy in women with squamous cell carcinoma of the vulva: a gynecologic oncology group study. J Clin Oncol 30(31):3786, 2012

Likic IS, Kadija S, Ladjevic NG, et al: Analysis of urologic complications after radical hysterectomy. Am J Obstet Gynecol 199:644.e1, 2008

Maas CP, ter Kuile MM, Laan E, et al: Objective assessment of sexual arousal in women with a history of hysterectomy. BJOG 111:456, 2004

Maggioni A, Roviglione G, Landoni F, et al: Pelvic exenteration: ten-year experience at the European Institute of Oncology in Milan. Gynecol Oncol 114:64, 2009

Magrina JF, Guardiola TC, Magtibay PM 3rd, et al: Minimally invasive surgery for resection of diaphragm metastases in ovarian cancer. J Minim Invasive Gynecol 26(7):1268, 2019

Magrina JF, Stanhope CR, Weaver AL: Pelvic exenterations: supralevator, infralevator, and with vulvectomy. Gynecol Oncol 64:130, 1997

Magtibay PM, Adams PB, Silverman MB, et al: Splenectomy as part of cytoreductive surgery in ovarian cancer. Gynecol Oncol 102:369, 2006

Manahan KJ, Hudec J, Fanning J: Modified radical vulvectomy without lymphadenectomy under local anesthesia in medically compromised patients. Gynecol Oncol 67:166, 1997

Mariani A, Dowdy SC, Cliby WA, et al: Prospective assessment of lymphatic dissemination in endometrial cancer: a paradigm shift in surgical staging. Gynecol Oncol 109:11, 2008

Martinez A, Filleron T, Vitse L, et al: Laparoscopic pelvic exenteration for gynaecological malignancy: is there any advantage? Gynecol Oncol 120(3):374, 2011

Martino MA, Borges E, Williamson E, et al: Pulmonary embolism after major abdominal surgery in gynecologic oncology. Obstet Gynecol 107:666, 2006

Matsuo K, Mandelbaum RS, Adams CL, et al: Performance and outcome of pelvic exenteration for gynecologic malignancies: a population-based study. Gynecol Oncol 153(2):368, 2019

McChesney SL, Zelhart MD, Green RL, et al: Current U.S. pre-operative bowel preparation trends: a 2018 survey of the American Society of Colon and Rectal Surgeons members. Surg Infect (Larchmt) July 30 2019, [Epub ahead of print]

Melamed A, Margul DJ, Chen L, et al: Survival after minimally invasive radical hysterectomy for early-stage cervical cancer. N Engl J Med 379(20):1905, 2018

Merad F, Hay JM, Fingerhut A, et al: Is prophylactic pelvic drainage useful after elective rectal or anal anastomosis? A multicenter controlled randomized trial. Surgery 125:529, 1999

Mert I, Cliby WA, Bews KA, et al: Evidence-based wound classification for vulvar surgery: implications for risk adjustment. Gynecol Oncol 154(2):280, 2019

Miller B, Morris M, Rutledge F, et al: Aborted exenterative procedures in recurrent cervical cancer. Gynecol Oncol 50:94, 1993

Minig L, Biffi R, Zanagnolo V, et al: Reduction of postoperative complication rate with the use of early oral feeding in gynecologic oncologic patients undergoing a major surgery: a randomized controlled trial. Ann Surg Oncol 16(11):3101, 2009

Mirhashemi R, Averette HE, Lambrou N, et al: Vaginal reconstruction at the time of pelvic exenteration: a surgical and psychosexual analysis of techniques. Gynecol Oncol 87:39, 2002

Mirhashemi R, Lambrou N, Hus N, et al: The gastrointestinal complications of the Miami pouch: a review of 77 cases. Gynecol Oncol 92:220, 2004

Mittal R, Chandramohan A, Moran B: Pseudomyxoma peritonei: natural history and treatment. Int J Hyperthermia 33(5):511, 2017

Morice P, Joulie F, Camatte S, et al: Lymph node involvement in epithelial ovarian cancer: analysis of 276 pelvic and paraaortic lymphadenectomies and surgical implications. J Am Coll Surg 197:198, 2003

Morice P, Lassau N, Pautier P, et al: Retroperitoneal drainage after complete para-aortic lymphadenectomy for gynecologic cancer: a randomized trial. Obstet Gynecol 97:243, 2001

Naik R, Jackson KS, Lopes A, et al: Laparoscopic assisted radical vaginal hysterectomy versus radical abdominal hysterectomy—a randomized phase II trial: perioperative outcomes and surgicopathological measurements. BJOG 117:746, 2010

Naik R, Maughan K, Nordin A, et al: A prospective, randomised, controlled trial of intermittent self-catheterisation vs supra-pubic catheterisation for post-operative bladder care following radical hysterectomy. Gynecol Oncol 99:437, 2005

Negishi H, Takeda M, Fujimoto T, et al: Lymphatic mapping and sentinel node identification as related to the primary sites of lymph node metastasis in early stage ovarian cancer. Gynecol Oncol 94:161, 2004

Nelson G, Altman AD, Nick A, et al: Guidelines for postoperative care in gynecologic/oncology surgery: Enhanced Recovery After Surgery (ERAS®) Society recommendations—Part II. Gynecol Oncol 140(2):323, 2016a

Nelson G, Altman AD, Nick A, et al: Guidelines for pre- and intra-operative care in gynecologic/oncology surgery: Enhanced Recovery After Surgery (ERAS®) Society recommendations—Part I. Gynecol Oncol 140(2):313, 2016b

Nelson G, Bakkum-Gamez J, Kalogera E, et al: Guidelines for perioperative care in gynecologic/oncology: Enhanced Recovery After Surgery (ERAS) Society recommendations-2019 update. Int J Gynecol Cancer 29(4):651, 2019

Nick AM, Lange J, Frumovitz M, et al: Rate of vaginal cuff separation following laparoscopic or robotic hysterectomy. Gynecol Oncol 120(1):47, 2011

Ohmaru Y, Sakata K, Hashiguchi SI, et al: A new modified pudendal thigh flap of vaginoplasty including reconstruction of vaginal vestibule. Case Reports Plast Surg Hand Surg 4(1):21, 2017

Orr JW Jr, Orr PJ, Bolen DD, et al: Radical hysterectomy: does the type of incision matter? Am J Obstet Gynecol 173:399, 1995

Paley PJ, Johnson PR, Adcock LL, et al: The effect of sartorius transposition on wound morbidity following inguinal-femoral lymphadenectomy. Gynecol Oncol 64:237, 1997

Park JY, Kim DY, Kim JH, et al: Laparoscopic compared with open radical hysterectomy in obese women with early-stage cervical cancer. Obstet Gynecol 119(6):1201, 2012

Park JY, Seo SS, Kang S, et al: The benefits of low anterior en bloc resection as part of cytoreductive surgery for advanced primary and recurrent epithelial ovarian cancer patients outweigh morbidity concerns. Gynecol Oncol 103(3):977, 2006

Patsner B, Hackett TE: Use of the omental J-flap for prevention of postoperative complications following radical abdominal hysterectomy: report of 140 cases and literature review. Gynecol Oncol 65:405, 1997

Pellegrino A, Fruscio R, Maneo A, et al: Harmonic scalpel versus conventional electrosurgery in the treatment of vulvar cancer. Int J Gynaecol Obstet 103:185, 2008

Penalver MA, Angioli R, Mirhashemi R, et al: Management of early and late complications of ileocolonic continent urinary reservoir (Miami pouch). Gynecol Oncol 69:185, 1998

Penalver MA, Bejany DE, Averette HE, et al: Continent urinary diversion in gynecologic oncology. Gynecol Oncol 34:274, 1989

Peiretti M, Bristow RE, Zapardiel I, et al: Rectosigmoid resection at the time of primary cytoreduction for advanced ovarian cancer. A multi-center analysis of surgical and oncological outcomes. Gynecol Oncol 126(2):220, 2012

Plante M, Roy M: Operative laparoscopy prior to a pelvic exenteration in patients with recurrent cervical cancer. Gynecol Oncol 69:94, 1998

Pouwer AW, Hinten F, van der Velden J, et al: Volume-controlled versus short drainage after inguinofemoral lymphadenectomy in vulvar cancer patients: a Dutch nationwide prospective study. Gynecol Oncol 146(3):580, 2017

Puntambekar S, Kudchadkar RJ, Gurjar AM, et al: Laparoscopic pelvic exenteration for advanced pelvic cancers: a review of 16 cases. Gynecol Oncol 102(3):513, 2006

Pycha A, Comploj E, Martini T, et al: Comparison of complications in three incontinent urinary diversions. Eur Urol 54:825, 2008

Ramirez PT, Frumovitz M, Pareja R, et al: Minimally invasive versus abdominal radical hysterectomy for cervical cancer. N Engl J Med 379(20):1895, 2018

Ramirez PT, Modesitt SC, Morris M, et al: Functional outcomes and complications of continent urinary diversions in patients with gynecologic malignancies. Gynecol Oncol 85:285, 2002

Rasmussen OO, Petersen IK, Christiansen J: Anorectal function following low anterior resection. Colorectal Dis 5:258, 2003

Ratliff CR, Gershenson DM, Morris M, et al: Sexual adjustment of patients undergoing gracilis myocutaneous flap vaginal reconstruction in conjunction with pelvic exenteration. Cancer 78:2229, 1996

Rettenmaier MA, Braly PS, Roberts WS, et al: Treatment of cutaneous vulvar lesions with skinning vulvectomy. J Reprod Med 30:478, 1985

Rezk YA, Hurley KE, Carter J, et al: A prospective study of quality of life in patients undergoing pelvic exenteration: interim results. Gynecol Oncol 128(2):191, 2013

Ripperda CM, Jackson LA, Phelan JN, et al: Anatomic relationships of the pelvic autonomic nervous system in female cadavers: clinical applications to pelvic surgery. Am J Obstet Gynecol 216(4):388.e1, 2017

Rose PG: Skin bridge recurrences in vulvar cancer: frequency and management. Int J Gynaecol Cancer 9:508, 1999

Rose PG: Type II radical hysterectomy: evaluating its role in cervical cancer. Gynecol Oncol 80:1, 2001

Salani R, Zahurak ML, Santillan A, et al: Survival impact of multiple bowel resections in patients undergoing primary cytoreductive surgery for advanced ovarian cancer: a case-control study. Gynecol Oncol 107:495, 2007

Salom EM, Mendez LE, Schey D, et al: Continent ileocolonic urinary reservoir (Miami pouch): the University of Miami experience over 15 years. Am J Obstet Gynecol 190:994, 2004

Salom EM, Penalver M: Complications in gynecologic surgery. In Cohn SM, Barquist E, Byers PM, et al (eds): Complications in Surgery and Trauma. New York, Informa Healthcare USA, 2007, p 554

Salom EM, Schey D, Penalver M, et al: The safety of incidental appendectomy at the time of abdominal hysterectomy. Am J Obstet Gynecol 189:1563, 2003

Scambia G, Ferrandina G, Distefano M, et al: Is there a place for a less extensive radical surgery in locally advanced cervical cancer patients? Gynecol Oncol 83:319, 2001

Schorge JO: Laparoscopic diverting loop ileostomy for spontaneous colon perforation in advanced ovarian cancer. Gynecol Oncol Rep 28:84, 2019

Scribner DR Jr, Kamelle SA, Gould N, et al: A retrospective analysis of radical hysterectomies done for cervical cancer: is there a role for the Pfannenstiel incision? Gynecol Oncol 81(3):481, 2001

Segreti EM, Morris M, Levenback C, et al: Transverse colon urinary diversion in gynecologic oncology. Gynecol Oncol 63:66, 1996

Serati M, Salvatore S, Uccella S, et al: Sexual function after radical hysterectomy for early-stage cervical cancer: is there a difference between laparoscopy and laparotomy? J Sex Med 6:2516, 2009

Sevin BU, Ramos R, Gerhardt RT, et al: Comparative efficacy of short-term versus long-term cefoxitin prophylaxis against postoperative infection after radical hysterectomy: a prospective study. Obstet Gynecol 77:729, 1991

Sharma S, Odunsi K, Driscoll D, et al: Pelvic exenterations for gynecological malignancies: twenty-year experience at Roswell Park Cancer Institute. Int J Gynaecol Cancer 15:475, 2005

Shimada M, Kigawa J, Nishimura R, et al: Ovarian metastasis in carcinoma of the uterine cervix. Gynecol Oncol 101(6):234, 2006

Silver DF: Full-thickness diaphragmatic resection with simple and secure closure to accomplish complete cytoreductive surgery for patients with ovarian cancer. Gynecol Oncol 95:384, 2004

Slomovitz BM, Ramirez PT, Frumovitz M, et al: Electrothermal bipolar coagulation for pelvic exenterations. Gynecol Oncol 102:534, 2006

Smith HO, Genesen MC, Runowicz CD, et al: The rectus abdominis myocutaneous flap: modifications, complications, and sexual function. Cancer 83:510, 1998

Soliman PT, Frumovitz M, Sun CC, et al: Radical hysterectomy: a comparison of surgical approaches after adoption of robotic surgery in gynecologic oncology. Gynecol Oncol 123(2):333, 2011

Song YJ, Lim MC, Kang S, et al: Total colectomy as part of primary cytoreductive surgery in advanced Mullerian cancer. Gynecol Oncol 114:183, 2009

Sood AK, Nygaard I, Shahin MS, et al: Anorectal dysfunction after surgical treatment for cervical cancer. J Am Coll Surg 195:513, 2002

Soper JT, Berchuck A, Creasman WT, et al: Pelvic exenteration: factors associated with major surgical morbidity. Gynecol Oncol 35:93, 1989

Soper JT, Havrilesky LJ, Secord AA, et al: Rectus abdominis myocutaneous flaps for neovaginal reconstruction after radical pelvic surgery. Int J Gynaecol Cancer 15:542, 2005

Soper JT, Rodriguez G, Berchuck A, et al: Long and short gracilis myocutaneous flaps for vulvovaginal reconstruction after radical pelvic surgery: comparison of flap-specific complications. Gynecol Oncol 56:271, 1995

Stehman FB, Bundy BN, Dvoretsky PM, et al: Early stage I carcinoma of the vulva treated with ipsilateral superficial inguinal lymphadenectomy and modified radical hemivulvectomy: a prospective study of the Gynecologic Oncology Group. Obstet Gynecol 79:490, 1992

Stevens A, Parsa MA, Paka C, et al: Vaginal cuff dehiscence in a series of 12,398 hysterectomies: effect of different types of colpotomy and vaginal closure. Obstet Gynecol 121(1):189, 2013

Sutton GP, Bundy BN, Delgado G, et al: Ovarian metastases in stage IB carcinoma of the cervix: a Gynecologic Oncology Group study. Am J Obstet Gynecol 166(1 Pt 1):50, 1992

Suzuki T, Sadahiro S, Tanaka A, et al: Usefulness of preoperative mechanical bowel preparation in patients with colon cancer who undergo elective surgery: a prospective randomized trial using oral antibiotics. Dig Surg May 3, 2019 [Epub ahead of print]

Swan RW: Stagnant loop syndrome resulting from small-bowel irradiation injury and intestinal bypass. Gynecol Oncol 2:441, 1974

Tantipalakorn C, Robertson G, Marsden DE, et al: Outcome and patterns of recurrence for International Federation of Gynecology and Obstetrics (FIGO) stages I and II squamous cell vulvar cancer. Obstet Gynecol 113:895, 2009

Te Grootenhuis NC, van der Zee AG, van Doorn HC, et al: Sentinel nodes in vulvar cancer: long-term follow-up of the GROningen INternational Study on Sentinel nodes in Vulvar cancer (GROINSS-V) I. Gynecol Oncol 140(1):8, 2016

Todo Y, Yamamoto R, Minobe S, et al: Risk factors for postoperative lower-extremity lymphedema in endometrial cancer survivors who had treatment including lymphadenectomy. Gynecol Oncol 119:60, 2010

Tortorella L, Casarin J, Mara KC, et al: Prediction of short-term surgical complications in women undergoing pelvic exenteration for gynecological malignancies. Gynecol Oncol 152(1):151, 2019

Tozzi R, Hardern K, Gubbala K, et al: En-bloc resection of the pelvis (EnBRP) in patients with stage IIIC-IV ovarian cancer: a 10 steps standardised technique. Surgical and survival outcomes of primary vs. interval surgery. Gynecol Oncol 144(3):564, 2017

Tsai MS, Liang JT: Surgery is justified in patients with bowel obstruction due to radiation therapy. J Gastrointest Surg 10:575, 2006

Tseng JH, Suidan RS, Zivanovic O, et al: Diverting ileostomy during primary debulking surgery for ovarian cancer: Associated factors and postoperative outcomes. Gynecol Oncol 142(2):217, 2016

Tsolakidis D, Amant F, Van Gorp T, et al: Diaphragmatic surgery during primary debulking in 89 patients with stage IIIB-IV epithelial ovarian cancer. Gynecol Oncol 116:489, 2010

Uccella S, Ceccaroni M, Cromi A, et al: Vaginal cuff dehiscence in a series of 12,398 hysterectomies: effect of different types of colpotomy and vaginal closure. Obstet Gynecol 120(3):516, 2012

Uccella S, Malzoni M, Cromi A, et al: Laparoscopic vs transvaginal cuff closure after total laparoscopic hysterectomy: a randomized trial by the Italian Society of Gynecologic Endoscopy. Am J Obstet Gynecol 218(5):500.e1, 2018

Urbach DR, Reedijk M, Richard CS, et al: Bowel resection for intestinal endometriosis. Dis Colon Rectum 41:1158, 1998

Urh A, Soliman PT, Schmeler KM, et al: Postoperative outcomes after continent versus incontinent urinary diversion at the time of pelvic exenteration for gynecologic malignancies. Gynecol Oncol 129(3):580, 2013

Vasilev SA: Obturator nerve injury: a review of management options. Gynecol Oncol 53:152, 1994

Walker JL, Powell CB, Chen LM, et al: Society of Gynecologic Oncology recommendations for the prevention of ovarian cancer. Cancer 121(13):2108, 2015

Weikel W, Hofmann M, Steiner E, et al: Reconstructive surgery following resection of primary vulvar cancers. Gynecol Oncol 99:92, 2005

Westin SN, Rallapalli V, Fellman B, et al: Overall survival after pelvic exenteration for gynecologic malignancy. Gynecol Oncol 134(3):546, 2014

Whitney CW: GOG Surgical Procedures Manual. Gynecologic Oncology Group, 2010. Available at: https://gogmember.gog.org/manuals/pdf/surgman.pdf. Accessed October 4, 2019

Whitney CW, Stehman FB: The abandoned radical hysterectomy: a Gynecologic Oncology Group study. Gynecol Oncol 79:350, 2000

Winter WE, McBroom JW, Carlson JW, et al: The utility of gastrojejunostomy in secondary cytoreduction and palliation of proximal intestinal obstruction in recurrent ovarian cancer. Gynecol Oncol 91:261, 2003

Yang YC, Chang CL: Modified radical hysterectomy for early Ib cervical cancer. Gynecol Oncol 74:241, 1999

Ye S, He T, Liang S, et al: Diaphragmatic surgery and related complications in primary cytoreduction for advanced ovarian, tubal, and peritoneal carcinoma. BMC Cancer 17(1):317, 2017

Yildirim Y, Ertas IE, Nayki U, et al: En-bloc pelvic resection with concomitant rectosigmoid colectomy and immediate anastomosis as part of primary cytoreductive surgery for patients with advanced ovarian cancer. Eur J Gynaecol Oncol 35(4):400, 2014

Zapardiel I, Peiretti M, Zanagnolo V, et al: Splenectomy as part of primary cytoreductive surgery for advanced ovarian cancer: a retrospective cohort study. Int J Gynecol Cancer 22(6):968, 2012

Zhang SH, Sood AK, Sorosky JI, et al: Preservation of the saphenous vein during inguinal lymphadenectomy decreases morbidity in patients with carcinoma of the vulva. Cancer 89(7):1520, 2000

Zhang X, Sheng X, Niu J, et al: Sparing of saphenous vein during inguinal lymphadenectomy for vulval malignancies. Gynecol Oncol 105(3):722, 2007

INDEX

Note: Page numbers followed by f indicates figure and t for tables respectively.